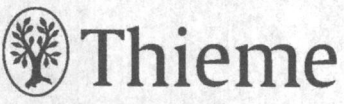

Greenberg's Handbook of Neurosurgery

Mark S. Greenberg, MD, FAANS
Associate Professor
Director, Residency Training Program
Department of Neurosurgery and Brain Repair
University of South Florida Morsani College of Medicine
Tampa, Florida

Tenth Edition

486 illustrations

Thieme
New York • Stuttgart • Delhi • Rio de Janeiro

Library of Congress Cataloging-in-Publication Data

Available upon request from the publisher.

First edition, 1990
Second edition, 1991
Third edition, 1994
Fourth edition, 1997
Fifth edition, 2001
Sixth edition, 2006
Seventh edition, 2010
Eighth edition, 2016
Ninth edition, 2020

Important note: Medicine is an ever-changing science undergoing continual development. Research and clinical experience are continually expanding our knowledge, in particular our knowledge of proper treatment and drug therapy. Insofar as this book mentions any dosage or application, readers may rest assured that the authors, editors, and publishers have made every effort to ensure that such references are in accordance with **the state of knowledge at the time of production of the book.**

Nevertheless, this does not involve, imply, or express any guarantee or responsibility on the part of the publishers in respect to any dosage instructions and forms of applications stated in the book. **Every user is requested to examine carefully** the manufacturers' leaflets accompanying each drug and to check, if necessary in consultation with a physician or specialist, whether the dosage schedules mentioned therein or the contraindications stated by the manufacturers differ from the statements made in the present book. Such examination is particularly important with drugs that are either rarely used or have been newly released on the market. Every dosage schedule or every form of application used is entirely at the user's own risk and responsibility. The authors and publishers request every user to report to the publishers any discrepancies or inaccuracies noticed. If errors in this work are found after publication, errata will be posted at www.thieme.com on the product description page.

Some of the product names, patents, and registered designs referred to in this book are in fact registered trademarks or proprietary names even though specific reference to this fact is not always made in the text. Therefore, the appearance of a name without designation as proprietary is not to be construed as a representation by the publisher that it is in the public domain.

Thieme addresses people of all gender identities equally. We encourage our authors to use gender neutral or gender-equal expressions wherever the context allows.

Thieme Medical Publishers, Inc.
333 Seventh Avenue, 18th Floor
New York, NY 10001, USA
www.thieme.com
+1 800 782 3488, customerservice@thieme.com

Cover design: Thieme Publishing Group,
illustration by Karl Wesker and Markus Voll

All illustrations in the text by the author.

Typesetting: DiTech Process Solutions

Printed in Germany by GGP Media   1 2 3 4 5 6

DOI: 10.1055/b000000751
ISBN: 978-1-68420-504-2

Also available as eBook:
eISBN (PDF) 978-1-68420-505-9
eISBN (epub) 978-1-68420-506-6

Dedication

In recognition of the immeasureable positive influence my late mother, Mary Ann Greenberg née Arkes, had on our entire extended family, my late uncle Benjamin Arkes, her brother, sagely suggested that I dedicate my next edition to her. As my uncle Ben passed away just shy of his 100th birthday before the publication of this 10th edition, I am dedicating this book to both my mother, Mary Ann Greenberg, and my uncle Benjamin Arkes. And at his suggestion, I am using the honorific name Mark Arkes Greenberg for this edition.

Contributors

Naomi A. Abel, MD
Assistant Professor
Department of Neurosurgery and Brain Repair
University of South Florida Morsani College of
  Medicine
Tampa, Florida
Failure of carpal tunnel and ulnar nerve surgery
Electrodiagnostics (EDX)
Pseudotumor cerebri syndrome

Puya Alikhani, MD
Associate Professor
Director of Spine Surgery
Department of Neurosurgery and Brain Repair
University of South Florida Morsani College of
  Medicine
Tampa, Florida
Spine infections

Siviero Agazzi, MD, MBA
Professor and Vice Chairman
Department of Neurosurgery and Brain Repair
University of South Florida Morsani College of
  Medicine
Tampa, Florida
Vestibular schwannomas

Norberto Andaluz, MD
Attending neurosurgeon
The Christ Hospital
Cincinnati, Ohio
Carotid stenosis and endarterectomy*
Emergency carotid endarterectomy*
Totally occluded carotid artery*

Ramsey Ashour, MD
Assistant Professor
The University of Texas at Austin
Dell Medical School
Austin, Texas
Dural arteriovenous fistulae*

Ali A. Baaj, MD
Assistant Professor
Department of Neurological Surgery
Weill Cornell Medical College
New York Presbyterian Hospital
New York, New York
Moyamoya disease*

Joshua M. Beckman, MD
Attending neurosurgeon
Fort Sam Houston
San Antonio, Texas
Concussion (mTBI)*

Davide M. Croci, MD
Assistant Professor
Department of Neurosurgery and Brain Repair
University of South Florida Morsani College of
  Medicine
Tampa, Florida
Vestibular schwannomas

Travis Dailey, MD
Attending physician
Advent Hospital, Tampa
Tampa, Florida
  Catheter tip granuloma (p.1389)*

Angela Downes, MD
Assistant Professor
School of Medicine
University of Colorado
Lone Tree, Colorado
Stereotactic radiosurgery*
Spontaneous subdural hematoma*

Zeegan George
Medical Student III
University of South Florida Morsani College of
  Medicine
Tampa, Florida
Dural substitutes (p.1719)

Melissa Giarratano, PharmD, BCPS
Clinical Pharmacist – Neurosciences
Tampa General Hospital
Tampa, Florida
Antibiotics*

Alexander Haas, MD
Attending physician
Department of Neurosurgery and Brain Repair
University of South Florida Morsani College of
  Medicine
Tampa, Florida
Colloid cysts*
Rhabdomyolysis (p.136)*

Ghaith Habboub, MD
Resident physician
Neurological Institute
Cleveland Clinic
Cleveland, Ohio
EVD-related infections*

Kevin Heinsimer, MD
Assistant Professor
Department of Urology
University of South Florida Morsani College of
  Medicine
Tampa, Florida
Bladder neurophysiology (p.92)*

Srinivasa Prasad Kanuparthi
Resident physician
Temple University Hospital
Philadelphia, Pennsylvania
Pneumorrhachis (p. 1387)*

Shah-Naz H. Khan, MD, FRCS(C), FAANS
Chair and Director
Institute of General and Endovascular
 Neurosurgery
Clinical Assistant Professor
Department of Surgery
Michigan State University
Flint, Michigan
Endovascular neurosurgery

Paul R. Krafft, MD
Attending physician
University of Florida, Halifax Health
Daytona Beach, Florida
Cerebellar mutism

Tsz Y. Lau, MD
Assistant Professor
Houston Methodist Department of
 Neurosurgery
Sugar Land, Texas
Subarachnoid hemorrhage
Cerebral bypass

Cheryl Reese Lawing, MD
Assistant Professor
Department of Orthopaedics and Sports
 Medicine
University of South Florida Morsani College of
 Medicine
Attending physician
Shriners Healthcare for Children - Florida
Tampa, Florida
Idiopathic adolescent scoliosis (p. 1319)

Shih-Sing Liu, MD
Assistant Professor
Department of Neurosurgery and Brain Repair
University of South Florida Morsani College of
 Medicine
Tampa, Florida
Jugular foramen
Anticoagulation & antiplatelet therapy

Jotham Manwaring, MD
Attending physician
Southern Utah Neurosciences Institute
St. George, Utah
Third ventriculostomy (ETV)
X-linked hydrocephalus

Carlos R. Martinez, MD, FACR
Courtesy Clinical Professor of Radiology
University of South Florida Morsani College of
 Medicine
Neuroradiologist
Bay Pines VA Hospital
St. Petersburg, Florida
Intracranial hypotension

Maxim Mokin, MD, PhD
Associate Professor of Neurology and
 Neurosurgery
Medical Director, Endovascular Neurosurgery at
 Tampa General Hospital
Director of Research, Department of Neurosur-
 gery and Brain Repair
University of South Florida Morsani College of
 Medicine
Tampa, Florida
Endovascular neurosurgery, update

Jose Montero, MD
Associate Professor
Department of Internal Medicine
University of South Florida Morsani College of
 Medicine
Tampa, Florida
Antibiotics

Brooks Osburn, MD
Attending physician
Florida Orthopedic Institute
Tampa, Florida
Neuromyelitis optica (NMO) (p. 1698)*

Glen A. Pollock, MD
Attending physician
Raleigh Neurosurgical Clinic
Raleigh, North Carolina
PRES

Edwin Ramos, MD
Associate Professor of Neurological Surgery
Program Director, Neurosurgery Residency
The University of Chicago Medicine
Chicago, Illinois
Hypothalamic hamartomas (p. 277)*

Stephen L. Reintjes Jr., MD
Attending physician
Meritas Health Neurosurgery
North Kansas City, Missouri
Anticoagulation & antiplatelet therapy
Spinal cord stimulator

Juan S. Uribe, MD
Professor and Vice Chairman
Department of Neurological Surgery
Chief, Spinal Disorders
Barrow Neurologic Institute
Phoenix, Arizona
*Transpsoas approach**
*Lhermitte-Duclos disease**
*Bone graft materials**
*New spine fusion techniques**

Fernando L. Vale, MD
Professor and Chairman
Department of Neurosurgery
Augusta University Medical Center
Augusta, Georgia
Seizure surgery (p. 1889)*

Jamie J. Van Gompel, MD
Professor
Departments of Neurosurgery and Otorhinolar-
  yngology/Head and Neck Surgery
Mayo Clinic
Rochester, Minnesota
*Olfactory neuroblastoma (esthesioneuroblas-
  toma)* (p. 935)*

Rohit Vasan, MD
Attending physician
James A. Haley Veterans Hospital
Tampa, Florida
*Syncope**

Andrew Vivas, MD
Health Sciences Assistant Clinical Professor
University of California
Los Angeles, California
Deep brain stimulation (DBS)
Sympathectomy
Scheuermann's kyphosis (p. 1374)*

Lucas Wiegand, MD
Assistant Professor
Department of Urology
University of South Florida Morsani College of
  Medicine
Tampa, Florida
Bladder neurophysiology (p. 92)*

Charles E. Wright, MD
Medical Director
LifeLink of Florida
Tampa, Florida
*Brain death & organ donation**

Chun-Po Yen, MD
Associate Professor
University of Virginia Health System
Charlottesville, Virginia
*Transpsoas approach**
*Stereotactic radiosurgery**

* Originally contributed to previous edition of the Handbook of Neurosurgery

Preface

During the preparation of this, the 10th edition of the *Handbook of Neurosurgery*, it dawned on me that the origins and the perpetuation of this book are probably antithetical to that of the majority of medical books. Instead of creating a book in an effort to help take care of patients, this book arose as a result of taking care of patients. It began as a collection of notes that I kept as my needs emerged, first as a resident, and later as a practicing neurosurgeon. I added to it during my residency as we presented weekly grand rounds on patients whom we were treating in the OR, the wards, and the ICU. Later, in my practice, when I encountered a condition or a treatment that I had to research, I included the results of that research in the book for future reference. The book grew organically, instead of arising from a preplanned blueprint. I feel that this has probably been part of the book's success, as well as a source of some of the unevenness of coverage, for which I gradually make amends. While it may not have occurred to me that this was likely a different genesis than most books, I have always said that my patients appear on all the pages of this book. And it is to them that I am eternally grateful.

Acknowledgments

I would like to take this opportunity to acknowledge the fantastic folks at Thieme Medical Publishers. Their support and willingness to take my opinions seriously has made it a pleasure to bring out this new edition. Special thanks go out to Thieme's amazing wizard of XML, Dr. Michael Wachinger, Senior Director International Business, Karen Edmonson, Senior Content Portfolio Manager, and Torsten Scheihagen, Senior Content Service Manager. Without their extraordinary help, this edition would not have been possible.

On the Neurosurgical side, I thank those who put up with me during my training (with special fondness for my chairman, Dr. John M. Tew, Jr.), and those who I am now happy to count among my friends and colleagues, especially my chairman and most trusted source for advice, Dr. Harry van Loveren.

Abbreviations and Symbols

Abbreviations used only locally are defined in that section using boldface type. Numbers following entries below indicate the page number for the relevant section.

Abbreviations	
a.	artery (aa. = arteries)
ABC	aneurysmal bone cyst (p. 979) *or* airway, breathing, circulation
Abx.	antibiotics
AC	arachnoid cyst (p. 260)
ACA	anterior cerebral artery
ACAS	asymptomatic carotid artery stenosis (p. 1548) *or* Asymptomatic Carotid Atherosclerosis Study (p. 1549)
ACDF	anterior cervical discectomy & fusion (p. 1284)
ACE	angiotensin-converting enzyme
ACEP	American College of Emergency Physicians
ACh	acetylcholine (neurotransmitter)
AChA	anterior choroidal artery
AComA	anterior communicating artery
AC-PC line	anterior commissure-posterior commissure line (p. 58)
ACTH	adrenocorticotropic hormone (corticotropin) (p. 151)
AD	autosomal dominant
ADH	antidiuretic hormone (p. 153)
ADI	atlantodental interval (p. 223)
ADPKD	autosomal dominant polycystic kidney disease (p. 1455)
ADQ	abductor digiti quinti (or minimi)
AED	antiepileptic drug (p. 485) (antiseizure medication (ASM))
AFO	ankle-foot-orthosis (p. 564)
AFP	alpha-fetoprotein (p. 635)
Ag	antigen
AHA	American Heart Association
AHCPR	Agency for Health Care Policy and Research (of the U. S. Public Health Service)
AICA	anterior inferior cerebellar artery (p. 81)
AIDP	acute inflammatory demyelinating polyradiculoneuropathy (p. 193)
AIDS	acquired immunodeficiency syndrome (p. 353)
AIM	astrocytoma, IDH-mutated (p. 658)
AIN	anterior interosseous neuropathy (p. 545)
AIS	acute ischemic stroke (p. 1536)
AKA	also known as
ALIF	anterior lumbar interbody fusion (p. 1795)
ALARA	As Low As Reasonably Achievable (p. 235) (radiation)
A-line	arterial line
ALL	anterior longitudinal ligament
ALS	amyotrophic lateral sclerosis (p. 1301)
AMS	acute mountain sickness (p. 1028)
AN	acoustic neuroma (p. 777)
ANA	antinuclear antibodies
AOD	atlantooccipital dislocation (p. 1153)
AOI	atlantooccipital interval (p. 1154)
AP	antero-posterior

APAG	antipseudomonal aminoglycoside
APAP	acetaminophen (p. 144)
APD	afferent pupillary defect (p. 592)
APTT	(or PTT) activated partial thromboplastin time
ARDS	adult respiratory distress syndrome
ASA	American Society of Anesthesiologists or aspirin (acetylsalicylic acid)
aSAH	aneurysmal subarachnoid hemorrhage (p. 1453)
ASAP	as soon as possible
ASM	antiseizure medication (p. 485)
ASD	antisiphon device
ASHD	atherosclerotic heart disease
ASPECTS	Alberta stroke program early CT score (p. 1559)
AT	anterior tibialis (tibialis anterior)
AT/RT	atypical teratoid/rhabdoid tumor (p. 754)
ATT	antitubercular therapy (p. 358)
AVM	arteriovenous malformation (p. 1504)
AVP	arginine vasopressin (p. 153)
β-hCG	beta-human chorionic gonadotropin (p. 634)
BA	basilar artery
BBB	blood-brain barrier (p. 90)
BC	basal cisterns (p. 1109)
BCP	birth control pills (oral contraceptives)
BCVI	blunt cerebrovascular injury (p. 1028)
BG	basal ganglia
BI	basilar impression/invagination (p. 228)
BMD	bone mineral density (p. 1209)
BMP	bone morphogenetic protein (p. 1723)
BOB	benign osteoblastoma (p. 990)
BP	blood pressure
BR	bed rest (activity restriction)
BSF	basal skull fracture (p. 1064)
BSG	brainstem glioma (p. 695)
Ca	cancer
CA	cavernous malformation (p. 1525)
CAA	cerebral amyloid angiopathy (p. 1612)
CABG	coronary artery bypass graft
CAD	coronary artery disease
CAT	(or CT) computerized (axial) tomography
CBF	cerebral blood flow (p. 1536)
CBV	cerebral blood volume
CBZ	carbamazepine (p. 490)
CCAA	cavernous carotid aneurysms (p. 1477)
CCB	calcium-channel blocker
CCF	carotid-cavernous (sinus) fistula (p. 1519)
CCHD	congenital cyanotic heart disease
CCTHR	Canadian CT Head Rule (p. 1007)
CCI	condyle-C1 interval (p. 1154) (atlantooccipital interval)
cCO	continuous cardiac output
CD	Cushing's disease (p. 867)
CEA	carotid endarterectomy (p. 1565) or carcinoembryonic antigen (p. 635)
CECT	contrast enhanced CT

cf	(Latin: confer) compare
cGy	centi-Gray (1 cGy = 1 rad)
CHF	congestive heart failure
CI	confidence interval (statistics)
CIDP	chronic inflammatory demyelinating polyneuropathy (p. 195)
CIP	critical illness polyneuropathy (p. 569)
CJD	Creutzfeldt-Jakob disease (p. 399)
CM	cavernous malformation (p. 1525)
CMAP	compound motor action potential (EMG)
$CMRO_2$	cerebral metabolic rate of oxygen consumption (p. 1537)
CMT	Charcot-Marie-Tooth (p. 568)
CMV	cytomegalovirus
CNL	chemonucleolysis
CNS	central nervous system
CO	cardiac output *or* carbon monoxide (p. 216)
CPA	cerebellopontine angle
CPM	central pontine myelinolysis (p. 119)
CPN	common peroneal nerve (p. 563)
CPP	cerebral perfusion pressure (p. 1036)
Cr. N.	cranial nerve(s)
CRH	corticotropin-releasing hormone (p. 151)
CRP	C-reactive protein
CRPS	complex regional pain syndrome (p. 525)
CSCS (CS^2)	chronic subthreshold cortical stimulation (p. 1892)
CSF	cerebrospinal fluid (p. 414)
CSM	cervical spondylotic myelopathy (p. 1297)
CSO	craniosynostosis (p. 264)
CSVL	central sacral vertical line (p. 1314)
CSW	cerebral salt wasting (p. 122)
CTA	CT angiogram (p. 238)
CTP	CT perfusion (p. 239)
CTS	carpal tunnel syndrome (p. 546)
CTV	CT venogram
CVA	coronal vertical axis (p. 1314)
CVP	central venous pressure
CVR	cerebrovascular resistance (p. 1536)
CVS	cerebral vasospasm (p. 1439)
CVT	cerebral venous thrombosis (p. 1594)
CXR	chest X-ray
DACA	distal anterior cerebral artery (p. 1475)
DAI	diffuse axonal injury (p. 1026)
DBM	demineralized bone matrix (p. 1723)
DC	decompressive craniectomy
D/C	discontinue
DCI	delayed cerebral ischemia (p. 1432)
DDAVP	1-deamino-8-D-arginine vasopressin (desmopressin) (p. 129)
DDx	differential diagnosis (p. 1683)
DBS	deep brain stimulation (p. 1839)
DESH	disproportionately enlarged subarachnoid space hydrocephalus (p. 441)
DI	diabetes insipidus (p. 124)
DIG	desmoplastic infantile astrocytoma and ganglioglioma (p. 708)

DIND	delayed ischemic neurologic deficit (p. 1440)
DIPG	diffuse infiltrating pontine glioma (see diffuse midline glioma (p. 683))
DISH	diffuse idiopathic skeletal hyperostosis (p. 1373)
DJK	distal junctional kyphosis
DKA	diabetic keto-acidosis
DLC	disco-ligamentous complex (p. 1181)
DLIF	direct lateral lumbar interbody fusion (p. 1802)
DOC	drug of choice
DM	diabetes mellitus
DMZ	dexamethasone
DNT or DNET	dysembryoplastic neuroepithelial tumors (p. 709)
DOE	dyspnea on exertion
DOMS	delayed onset muscle soreness (p. 1333)
DPL	diagnostic peritoneal lavage
DREZ	dorsal root entry zone lesion (p. 1886)
DSA	digital subtraction angiogram
DSD	degenerative spine disease (p. 1327)
DST	dural sinus thrombosis (p. 1594)
DTN	"door to needle"
DTs	delirium tremens (p. 214)
DTT	diffusion tensor tractography MRI (p. 245)
DVT	deep-vein thrombosis (p. 176)
DWI	diffusion-weighted imaging (p. 243) (MRI sequence)
EAC	external auditory canal
EAM	external auditory meatus
EAST	Eastern Association for the Surgery of Trauma
EBRT	external beam radiation therapy
EBV	Epstein-Barr Virus
ECM	erythema chronicum migrans (p. 364)
EDC	electrolytically detachable coils
EDH	epidural hematoma (p. 1072)
EHL	extensor hallucis longus
ELISA	enzyme-linked immunosorbent assay
ELST	endolymphatic sac tumors (p. 648)
EM	electron microscope (microscopy)
ENG	electronystagmography (p. 782)
ENT	ear, nose and throat (otolaryngology)
EOM	extra-ocular muscles (p. 596)
EOO	external oculomotor ophthalmoplegia
E/R	emergency room or department
ESR	erythrocyte sedimentation rate
EST	endodermal sinus tumor (p. 832)
EtOH	ethyl alcohol (ethanol)
ET tube	endotracheal tube
ETV	endoscopic third ventriculostomy (p. 453)
EVD	external ventricular drain (ventriculostomy)
EVT	endovascular therapy (p. 1913)
FCU	flexor carpi ulnaris
FDI	flexion-distraction injury (p. 1202)
FDP	flexor digitorum profundus
FIESTA	Fast Imaging Employing Steady-state Acquisition (p. 241) (MRI sequence)

FIM	Functional Independence Measure (p. 1643)
FLAIR	fluid-attenuated inversion recovery (p. 240) (MRI sequence)
FM	face mask
FMD	fibromuscular dysplasia (p. 209)
FSH	follicle stimulating hormone (p. 153)
F/U	follow-up
FUO	fever of unknown origin
GABA	gamma-aminobutyric acid
GBM	glioblastoma (p. 664) (obsolete: glioblastoma multiforme)
GBS	Guillain-Barré syndrome (p. 193)
GCA	giant cell arteritis (p. 203)
GCS	Glasgow coma scale (p. 318)
GCT	granular cell tumor (p. 853) or germ cell tumor (p. 831)
GD	Graves' disease
GFAP	glial fibrillary acidic protein (p. 631)
GGE	genetic generalized epilepsy (p. 481)
GGT	gamma glutamyl transpeptidase
GH	growth hormone (p. 153)
GH-RH	growth hormone releasing hormone (p. 153)
GMH	germinal matrix hemorrhage (p. 1630)
GNR	gram-negative rods
GnRH	gonadotropin-releasing hormone (p. 153)
GSW	gunshot wound
GTC	generalized tonic-clonic (seizure)
GTR	gross total resection
H/A	headache (p. 182)
H&H	Hunt and Hess (SAH grade) (p. 1424)
H&P	history and physical exam
HBsAg	hepatitis B surface antigen
HCD	herniated cervical disc (p. 1280)
hCG	human chorionic gonadotropin (p. 634)
HCP	hydrocephalus (p. 426)
HDT	hyperdynamic therapy (p. 1447)
HGB	hemangioblastoma (p. 822)
Hgb-A1C	hemoglobin A1C
hGH	human growth hormone
HH	hypothalamic hamartomas (p. 277) or homonymous hemianopsia
HHT	hereditary hemorrhagic telangiectasia (p. 1524)
HIV	human immunodeficiency virus
HLD	herniated lumbar disc (p. 1250)
HLA	human leukocyte antigen
H.O.	house officer
HNP	herniated nucleus pulposus (herniated disc) (p. 1250)
HNPP	hereditary neuropathy with liability to pressure palsies (p. 568)
HOB	head of bed
HPA	hypothalamic-pituitary-adrenal axis
HPF	high power field (used in histology, corresponds to 0.23 mm^2)
HRQOL	health related quality of life
HSE	herpes simplex encephalitis (p. 397)
HTN	hypertension
IAC	internal auditory canal

IASDH	infantile acute subdural hematoma (p. 1081)
ICA	internal carotid artery
ICG	indocyanine green (p. 1466)
ICH	intracerebral hemorrhage (p. 1608)
IC-HTN	intracranial hypertension (increased ICP)
ICP	intracranial pressure (p. 1036)
ICU	intensive care unit
IDDM	insulin-dependent diabetes mellitus
IDET	intradiscal endothermal therapy (p. 1258)
IDH	isocitrate dehydrogenase ▶ Table 37.2
IEP	immune electrophoresis
IG	image guidance (intraoperative)
IGF-1	insulin-like growth factor-1 (AKA somatomedin-C) (p. 153)
IIH	idiopathic intracranial hypertension (pseudotumor cerebri) (p. 955)
IJV	internal jugular vein
IMRT	intensity modulated radiation therapy
INO	internuclear ophthalmoplegia (p. 596)
iNPH	(idiopathic) normal pressure hydrocephalus (p. 438)
INR	international normalized ratio (p. 172)
IPS	inferior petrosal sinus
IPA	idiopathic paralysis agitans (Parkinson's disease) (p. 184)
ISAT	International Subarachnoid Hemorrhage Aneurysm Trial (p. 1458)
IT	intrathecal
ITB	intrathecal baclofen (p. 1847)
IVC	intraventricular catheter or inferior vena cava
IVH	intraventricular hemorrhage (p. 1671)
IVP	intravenous push (medication route) or intravenous pyelogram (X-ray study)
JPS	joint position sense
LBP	low back pain (p. 1226)
LDD	Lhermitte-Duclos disease (p. 716)
LE	lower extremity
LFTs	liver function tests
LGB	lateral geniculate body
LGG	low-grade glioma
LH	luteinizing hormone (p. 153)
LH-RH	luteinizing hormone releasing hormone (p. 153)
LMD	low-molecular-weight dextran
LMN	lower motor neuron (p. 531)
LMWH	low-molecular-weight heparin
LOC	loss of consciousness
LOH	loss of heterozygosity
LP	lumbar puncture (p. 1811)
LSO	lumbo-sacral orthosis
LOVA	lonstanding overt ventriculomegaly in an adult (p. 437)
MAOI	monoamine oxidase inhibitor
MAP	mean arterial pressure
MAST®	military anti-shock trousers
MB	medulloblastoma (p. 750)
MBEN	medulloblastoma with extensive nodularity (p. 746)
MBI	modified Barthel index ▶ Table 98.6
MCA	middle cerebral artery

mcg	(or µg) microgram
MCP	mean carotid pressure *or* metacarpal phalangeal
MDCTA	multidetector CT angiography
MDB	medulloblastoma (p. 750)
MDMA	methylenedioxymethamphetamine (p. 185)
mg	milligram
MGMT	O^6-methylguanine-DNA methyltransferase (p. 673)
MGUS	monoclonal gammopathy of undetermined significance (p. 575)
MHT	meningohypophyseal trunk (p. 77)
MI	myocardial infarction
MIB-1	monoclonal anti-Ki-67 antibody (p. 632)
MIC	minimum inhibitory concentration (for antibiotics)
MID	multi-infarct dementia
MISS	minimally invasive spine surgery
mJOA scale	modified Japanese Orthopedic Association (p. 1299) scale
MLF	medial longitudinal fasciculus
MLS	midline shift (p. 1110)
MM	myelomeningocele (p. 281) *or* multiple myeloma (p. 928)
MMD	moyamoya disease (p. 1581)
MMN	multifocal motor neuropathy (p. 1700)
MMPI	Minnesota Multiphasic Personality Inventory
mos	months
MPTP	1-methyl-4-phenyl-1,2,3,6-tetrahydropyridine (p. 185)
MRA	MRI angiogram (p. 243)
mRS	modified Rankin Scale ▶ Table 98.5
MRS	MRI spectroscopy (p. 244)
MRSA	methicillin resistant *Staphylococcus aureus*
MS	microsurgery *or* multiple sclerosis (p. 187)
MSO$_4$	morphine sulfate
mTICI	modified treatment in cerebral ischemia (scale) ▶ Table 116.2
MTP	metatarsal phalangeal
MTS	mesial temporal sclerosis (p. 482)
MTT	mean transit time (p. 239) (on CT perfusion)
MUAP	motor unit action potential (p. 256)
MVA	motor vehicle accident
MVD	microvascular decompression (p. 1867)
MW	molecular weight
n.	nerve (nn. = nerves)
Na	(or Na⁺) sodium
N$_2$O	nitrous oxide (p. 109)
NAA	N-acetyl aspartate (p. 244)
NAP	nerve action potential (p. 535)
NASCET	North American Symptomatic Carotid Endarterectomy Trial (p. 1565)
NB	(Latin: *nota bene*) note well
NC	nasal cannula
NCCN	National Comprehensive Cancer Network
NCD	neurocutaneous disorders (p. 637)
NCV	nerve conduction velocity
NEC	neurenteric cyst (p. 313) *or* necrotizing enterocolitis
NEXUS	National Emergency X-Radiography Utilization Study (p. 1142)
NF	(or NFT) neurofibromatosis (p. 637)

NF1	neurofibromatosis type 1 (p.638)
NF2	neurofibromatosis type 2 (p.640)
NG tube	nasogastric tube
NGGCT	non-germinomatous germ cell tumors (p.832)
NFPA	nonfunctioning pituitary adenoma (p.866)
NIHSS	NIH (National Institute of Health) Stroke Scale (p.1554)
NMBA	neuromuscular blocking agent (p.141)
NMO	neuromyelitis optica (Devic syndrome) (p.1698)
NOS	not otherwise specified (as used in WHO CNS5 (p.616))
NPH	normal pressure hydrocephalus (p.438)
NPS	neuropathic pain syndrome (p.518)
NS	normal saline
NSAID	non-steroidal anti-inflammatory drug (p.144)
NSCLC	non-small-cell cancer of the lung (p.911)
NSF	nephrogenic systemic fibrosis (p.243)
NSM	neurogenic stunned myocardium (p.1438)
N/V	nausea and vomiting
NVB	neurovascular bundle
OAD	occipital atlantal dislocation, see atlantooccipital dislocation (p.1153)
OALL	ossification of the anterior longitudinal ligament (p.1372)
OC	occipital condyle
OCB	oligoclonal bands (in CSF) (p.190)
OCF	occipital condyle fracture (p.1156)
ODG	oligodendroglioma (p.662)
OEF	oxygen extraction fraction
OFC	occipital-frontal (head) circumference (p.427)
OGST	oral glucose suppression test (for growth hormone) (p.882)
OMO	open-mouth odontoid (C-spine X-ray view)
OMP	oculomotor (third nerve) palsy
ONSF	optic nerve sheath fenestration (p.966)
OP	opening pressure (on LP) (p.1812)
OPG	optic pathway glioma (p.694)
OPLL	ossification of the posterior longitudinal ligament (p.1370)
OR or O.R.	operating room
ORIF	open reduction/internal fixation
OS	overall survival
OTC	over the counter (i.e., without prescription)
PACU	post-anesthesia care unit (AKA recovery room, PAR)
PADI	posterior atlantodental interval (p.223)
PAID	paroxysmal autonomic instability with dystonia (p.1048)
PAN	poly- (or peri-) arteritis nodosa (p.208)
PBPP	perinatal brachial plexus palsy (p.579)
PbtO$_2$	brain tissue oxygen tension (p.1045)
PC	pineal cyst (p.948)
PCA	pilocytic astrocytoma (p.689) *or* posterior cerebral artery
PCB	pneumatic compression boot
PCC	prothrombin complex concentrate (p.174)
PCI	prophylactic cranial irradiation
PCN	penicillin
PCNSL	primary CNS lymphoma (p.840)
PComA	posterior communicating artery

PCV	procarbazine, CCNU, & vincristine (p. 628) (chemotherapy)
PCR	polymerase chain reaction
PCWP	pulmonary capillary wedge pressure
PDA	patent ductus arteriosus
PDN	painful diabetic neuropathy (p. 518)
PDR	Physicians Desk Reference®
peds	pediatrics (infants & children)
PEEK	poly-ether-ether-ketone (graft material)
PET	positron emission tomography (scan)
p-fossa	posterior fossa
PFS	progression-free survival
PFT	pulmonary function test
PHN	postherpetic neuralgia (p. 522)
PHT	phenytoin (Dilantin®) (p. 488)
PICA	posterior inferior cerebellar artery (p. 81)
PIF	prolactin release inhibitory factor (p. 153)
PIN	posterior interosseous neuropathy (p. 559)
PION	posterior ischemic optic neuropathy (p. 1261)
PitNET	pituitary neuroendocrine tumor (p. 854) (formerly pituitary adenoma)
PIVH	periventricular-intraventricular hemorrhage (p. 1630)
PJK	proximal junctional kyphosis
PLAP	placental alkaline phosphatase (p. 832)
PLEDs	periodic lateralizing epileptiform discharges
PLIF	posterior lumbar interbody fusion
PM	pars marginalis (p. 57)
PMA	progressive muscular atrophy (p. 191) *or* pilomyxoid astrocytoma (p. 689)
PMD	perimetric mean deviation (p. 589) (visual fields)
PMH	pure motor hemiparesis
PML	progressive multifocal leukoencephalopathy (p. 353)
PMMA	polymethylmethacrylate (methylmethacrylate)
PMR	polymyalgia rheumatica (p. 206)
PMV	pontomesencephalic vein
PNEA	psychogenic non-epileptic attack (p. 507)
POD	postoperative day
POVL	postoperative visual loss (p. 1261)
PPV	positive predictive value: in unselected patients who test positive, PPV is the probability that the patient has the disease
PR	per rectum
PRES	posterior reversible encephalopathy syndrome (p. 202)
PRF	prolactin releasing factor (p. 153)
PIF	prolactin (releasing) inhibitory factor (p. 153)
PRN	as needed
PRSP	penicillinase resistant synthetic penicillin
PSNP	progressive supra-nuclear palsy (p. 186)
PSR	percutaneous stereotactic rhizotomy (for trigeminal neuralgia) (p. 1861)
PSVL	posterior sacral vertical line (p. 1355)
PSW	positive sharp waves (on EMG) (p. 255)
pt	patient
PT	physical therapy *or* prothrombin time
PTC	pituicytoma (p. 853)
PTCS	pseudotumor cerebri syndrome (p. 955)

PTR	percutaneous trigeminal rhizotomy (p. 1861)
PTT	(or APTT) partial thromboplastin time
PUD	peptic ulcer disease
PVP	percutaneous vertebroplasty (p. 1212)
PWI	perfusion-weighted imaging (p. 244) (MRI sequence)
PXA	pleomorphic xanthoastrocytoma (p. 698)
q	(Latin: *quaque*) every (medication dosing)
RA	rheumatoid arthritis
RAH	recurrent artery of Heubner (p. 74)
RAPD	relative afferent pupillary defect (p. 592)
RASS	Richmond agitation-sedation scale (p. 139)
RCVS	reversible cerebral vasoconstrictive syndrome (p. 1418)
rem	roentgen-equivalent man
REZ	root entry zone
RFR	radiofrequency rhizotomy (p. 1861)
rFVIIa	recombinant (activated) factor VII
rhBMP	recombinant human bone morphogenetic protein (p. 1723)
R/O	rule out
RNS®	responsive neurostimulation (p. 1892)
ROM	range of motion
ROP	retro-odontoid pseudotumor (p. 1678)
RPA	recursive partitioning analysis
RPDB	randomized prospective double-blind
RPLS	reversible posterior leukoencephalopathy syndrome; see posterior reversible encephalopathy syndrome (p. 202) (PRES)
RPNB	randomized prospective non-blinded
RTOG	Radiation Therapy Oncology Group
RTP	return to play (sports)
rt-PA or tPA	recombinant tissue-type plasminogen activator (AKA tissue plasminogen activator) e.g., alteplase
RT-QuIC	Real-Time Quaking-Induced Conversion assay (p. 403) (for CJD)
RTX	(or XRT) radiation therapy (p. 1898)
S/S	signs and symptoms
S2AI screws	S2-alar-iliac screws (p. 1807)
SAH	subarachnoid hemorrhage (p. 1453) *or* Selective amygdalo-hippocampectomy (p. 1893)
SBE	subacute bacterial endocarditis
SBO	spina bifida occulta (p. 280)
SBP	systolic blood pressure
SCA	superior cerebellar artery
SCD	sequential compression device
SCLC	small-cell lung cancer (p. 910)
SCI	spinal cord injury (p. 1132)
SCIWORA	spinal cord injury without radiographic abnormality (p. 1196)
SCM	sternocleidomastoid (muscle)
SD	standard deviation
SDE	subdural empyema (p. 350)
SDH	subdural hematoma (p. 1076)
SE	status epilepticus (for seizures) (p. 510)
SEA	spinal epidural abscess (p. 381)
SEGA	subependymal giant cell astrocytoma (p. 645)
SEP	(or SSEP) somatosensory evoked potential (p. 250)

SG	specific gravity
SHH	sonic hedgehog
SIAD	syndrome of inappropriate antidiuresis (p. 117)
SIADH	syndrome of inappropriate antidiuretic hormone (ADH) secretion (p. 118)
SIDS	sudden infant death syndrome
SIH	spontaneous intracranial hypotension (p. 421)
sICH	spontaneous intracerebral hemorrhage (p. 1608)
SIRS	septic inflammatory response syndrome
SjVO$_2$	jugular venous oxygen saturation (p. 1045)
SLE	systemic lupus erythematosus
SLIC	subaxial injury classification (p. 1181)
SMC	spinal meningeal cyst (p. 1400)
SMT	spinal manipulation therapy (p. 1238)
SNAP	sensory nerve action potential (EMG) (p. 255)
SNUC	sinonasal undifferentiated carcinoma (p. 1674)
SOMI	sternal-occipital-mandibular immobilizer (p. 1124)
SON	supraorbital neuralgia (p. 521)
S/P	status-post
SPAM	subacute progressive ascending myelopathy (p. 1221)
SPECT	single positron emission computed tomography (scan)
SPEP	serum protein electrophoresis
SQ	subcutaneous injection
SRS	stereotactic radiosurgery (p. 1903)
SRT	stereotactic radiotherapy (p. 1903)
SSEP	(or SEP) somatosensory evoked potential (p. 250)
SSPE	subacute sclerosing panencephalitis (p. 249)
SSRI	selective serotonin reuptake inhibitors
SSS	superior sagittal sinus
SSV	sagittal stable vertebra (p. 1355)
STA	superficial temporal artery
STAT	immediately (abbreviation of Latin *statim*)
STICH	Surgical Trial in Intracerebral Haemorrhage (p. 1624)
STIR	short tau inversion recovery (p. 241) (MRI sequence)
STN	subthalamic nucleus
STSG	Spine Trauma Study Group
SUDEP	sudden unexplained death in epilepsy (p. 480)
SUNCT	short-lasting unilateral neuralgiform H/A with conjunctival injection and tearing (p. 520)
SVC	superior vena cava
SVM	spinal vascular malformations (p. 1395)
SVR	systemic venous resistance
SVT	supraventricular tachycardia
SWN	schwannomatosis (p. 642)
SWS	Sturge–Weber syndrome (p. 652)
SXR	skull X-ray
Sz.	seizure (p. 480)
T1WI	T1 weighted image (p. 239) (MRI sequence)
T2WI	T2 weighted image (p. 240) (MRI sequence)
TAL	transverse atlantal ligament (p. 69)
TBA	total bilateral adrenalectomy (p. 891)
TBI	traumatic brain injury (p. 999)
TBM	tuberculous meningitis (p. 360)

TCA	tricyclic antidepressants
TCD	transcranial Doppler (p. 1443)
TDL	tumefactive demyelinating lesions (p. 190)
TE	time to echo (p. 239) (on MRI)
TEE	transesophageal echocardiogram
TEN	toxic epidermal necrolysis
TENS	transcutaneous electrical nerve stimulation
TGN	trigeminal neuralgia (p. 1857)
T-H lines	Taylor-Haughton lines (p. 61)
TIA	transient ischemic attack (p. 1536)
TICH	traumatic intracerebral hemorrhage (hemorrhagic contusion) (p. 1071)
TICI (mTICI)	treatment in cerebral ischemia (scale) (modified) ▶ Table 116.2
TIVA	total intravenous anesthesia
TLIF	transforaminal lumbar interbody fusion (p. 1801)
TLISS	thoracolumbar injury severity score (p. 1206)
TLJ	thoracolumbar junction
TLSO	thoracolumbar-sacral orthosis
TM	tympanic membrane
TP53	tumor protein 53
t-PA or tPA	tissue plasminogen activator
TR	time to repetition (p. 239) (on MRI)
TRH	thyrotropin releasing hormone; AKA TSH-RH (p. 153)
TS	transverse sinus
tSAH	traumatic subarachnoid hemorrhage (p. 1453)
TSC	tuberous sclerosis complex (p. 644)
TSE	transmissible spongiform encephalopathy (p. 399) (prion disease)
TSH	thyroid-stimulating hormone (thyrotropin) (p. 153)
TSV	thalamostriate vein
TTP	thrombotic thrombocytopenic purpura
TVO	transient visual obscurations (p. 961)
Tx.	treatment
UBOs	unidentified bright objects (on MRI)
UE	upper extremity
UMN	upper motor neuron (p. 531)
UTI	urinary tract infection
URI	upper respiratory tract infection
U/S	ultrasound
VA	vertebral artery or ventriculoatrial
VB	vertebral body
VBI	vertebrobasilar insufficiency (p. 1591)
VEMP	vestibular evoked myogenic potential (p. 782)
VHL	von Hippel-Lindau (disease) (p. 646)
VKA	vitamin K antagonist (e.g., warfarin)
VMA	vanillylmandelic acid
VP	ventriculoperitoneal
VS	vestibular schwannoma (p. 777)
VTE	venous thromboembolism
VZV	(herpes) varicella zoster virus
WBC	white blood cell (count)
WBXRT	whole brain radiation therapy (p. 919)
WFNS	World Federation of Neurosurgical Societies (grading SAH) (p. 1424)

WHO	World Health Organization
WHO CNS5	WHO Classification of Tumors of the Central Nervous System, 5th edition (p. 616)
wks	weeks
WNL	within normal limits
WNT	wingless/integrated (signal transduction pathway)
w/o	without
WRS	word recognition score (p. 780)
W/U	work-up (evaluation)
XLIF™	extreme lateral lumbar interbody fusion (p. 1802)
XRT	(or RTX) radiation therapy (p. 1898)
Symbols	
℞	prescribing information
→	causes or leads to
Δ	change
✓	check (e.g., lab or exam item to check)
↑	increased
↓	decreased
≈	approximately
↳	innervates (nerve distribution)
⇒	vascular supply
↳	a branch of the preceding nerve
★	crucial point
✘	caution; possible danger; negative factor...
Σ	summary
∴	therefore
Instrumentation: the following shorthand allows rapid identification of metrics for spinal instrumentation:	
ENTRY	screw entry site
TRAJ	screw trajectory
TARGET	object to aim for
SCREWS	typical screw specifications

Conventions

▶ **Box types.** The *Handbook of Neurosurgery* uses the following seven box types:

Drug info

Drug description & dosage.

Key concepts

Foundational knowledge in brief.

Practice guideline

Evidence-based guidelines. See below (in this section) for definitions. For a listing of evidence-based guidelines contained in this book, see the index under "Practice guideline."

Booking the case

These sections appear under certain specific operations to help when scheduling that surgery. Default information appears below (in this section); for example, a specific type of anesthesia will only be mentioned if something other than general anesthesia is typically used. A list of operations addressed by this means can be found in the index under "Booking the case."

Σ

Summarizing or synthesizing information from the associated text.

Side information

E.g., Greenberg IMHO.

Signs / symptoms

A description of signs and symptoms.

▶ **Grading scales.** Many grading scales are presented in table format, and to assist the reader in using them, a table cell has been included where an entry is to be made that shows the possible values for that cell. In many cases, those values are summed with those in other similar cells to arrive at the "grade."

▶ **Cross references.** The terms "see below" and "see above" are normally used when the referenced item is on the same page, or at most on the following (or preceding) page. When further excursions are needed, the page number will usually be included.

▶ **Default values.** These details are not repeated in each section or "Booking the case" box.
1. position: (depends on the operation)
2. pre-op:
   a) NPO after midnight the night before except meds with sips of water
   b) antithrombotics: discontinue Coumadin® ≥ 3 days prior to surgery, Plavix® 5–7 d pre-op, aspirin 7–10 d pre-op, other NSAIDs 5 d pre-op
3. cardiology/medical clearance as needed
4. anesthesia: default = general anesthesia, unless otherwise specified
5. equipment: special devices such as ultrasonic aspirator, image guidance…
6. instrumentation: standard surgical instrument trays for a specific operation are assumed. Special instrumentation resident in the hospital will be listed
7. implants: this usually requires scheduling with a vendor (manufacturers representative/distributor) to provide
8. neuromonitoring will be listed if typically used
9. post-op: default care is on the ward (ICU is typically needed after craniotomy)
10. blood availability: specified if recommended
11. consent (these items use lay terms for the patient—not all-inclusive):
    ★ **Disclaimers**: *informed consent* for surgery requires disclosure of risks and benefits that would substantively affect a normal person's decision to have the operation. It cannot and should not attempt to include every possibility. The items listed in this section are included as memory joggers for some items for various procedures, but are not meant to be all-inclusive. The omission of information from this memory aid is not to be construed as implying that the omitted item is not important or should not be mentioned.
    a) procedure: the typical operation and some possible common contingencies
    b) alternatives: non-surgical (AKA "conservative") treatment is almost always an option
    c) complications:
       • risks of general anesthesia include: heart attack, stroke, pneumonia
       • infection: a risk with any invasive procedure
       • usual **craniotomy** complications include: bleeding intra-op and postop, seizure, stroke, coma, death, hydrocephalus, meningitis, and neurologic deficit related to the area of surgery including (for applicable locations): paralysis, language or sensory disturbances, coordination impairment…
       • usual **spine surgery** complications include: injury to nerve or spinal cord with possible numbness, weakness or paralysis, failure of the operation to achieve the desired result, dural opening which may cause a CSF leak, which occasionally needs surgical repair. Hardware complications (when used) include: breakage, pull-out, malposition. Although a rare complication, it is serious enough that it bears mentioning in cases positioned prone with possible significant blood loss (> 2 L): blindness (due to PION (p. 1261))

► **Evidence-Based Medicine: Definitions.** These definitions are referred to in the "Practice guide-line" boxes.

Strength of recommendation		Description
Level I, II, III[a]	Level A, B, C, D[b]	
Level I High degree of clinical certainty	**Level A**	Based on consistent Class I evidence (well-designed, prospective randomized controlled studies)
	Level B	Single Class I study or consistent Class II evidence or strong Class II evidence especially when circumstances preclude randomized clinical trials
Level II Moderate degree of clinical certainty	**Level C**	Usually derived from Class II evidence (one or more well-designed comparative clinical studies or less well-designed randomized studies) or a preponderance of Class III evidence
Level III Unclear clinical certainty	**Level D**	Generally based on Class III evidence (case series, historical controls, case reports and expert opinion). Useful for educational purposes and to guide future research
	Level U[c]	Lack of studies meeting Level A, B or C criteria

[a] as used in the Guidelines for the Management of Severe Traumatic Brain Injury, 3rd edition (Brain Trauma Foundation, et al.: Guidelines for the management of severe traumatic brain injury. IX. Cerebral perfusion thresholds. J Neurotrauma 2007;24 (Suppl 1): S59-64).
[b] as used in the Guidelines for the Surgical Management of Cervical Degenerative Disease (Matz PG, et al.: Introduction and methodology: guidelines for the surgical management of cervical degenerative disease. J Neurosurg Spine 2009;11 (2): 101–3).
[c] as used in the 2016 American Epilepsy Guidelines for treatment of Convulsive Status Epilepticus (Glauser T, et al.: Evidence-Based Guideline: Treatment of Convulsive Status Epilepticus in Children and Adults: Report of the Guideline Committee of the American Epilepsy Society. Epilepsy Curr 2016;16 (1): 48-61).

Contents

Anatomy and Physiology

Imaging and Diagnostics

Developmental Anomalies

Peripheral Nerves

Neurophthalmology and Neurotology

Tumors of the Nervous and Related Systems

Head Trauma

Subarachnoid Hemorrhage and Aneurysms

Vascular Malformations

Stroke and Occlusive Cerebrovascular Disease

Procedures, Interventions, Operations

Part I

Anatomy and Physiology

I

1 Gross Anatomy, Cranial and Spine

1.1 Cortical surface anatomy

1.1.1 Lateral cortical surface

▶ Fig. 1.1. For abbreviations, see ▶ Table 1.1 and ▶ Table 1.2. The middle frontal gyrus (MFG) is usually more sinuous than the IFG or SFG, and it often connects to the pre-central gyrus via a thin isthmus.[1] The central sulcus joins the Sylvian fissure in only 2% of cases (i.e., in 98% of cases there is a "subcentral" gyrus). The intraparietal sulcus (ips) separates the superior and inferior parietal lobules. The IPL is composed primarily of the AG and SMG. The Sylvian fissure terminates in the SMG (Brodmann's area 40). The superior temporal sulcus terminates in the AG.

1.1.2 Brodmann's areas

▶ Fig. 1.1 also identifies the clinically significant areas of Brodmann's (Br.) map of the cytoarchitectonic fields of the human brain. Functional significance of these areas is as follows:
1. Br. areas 3, 1, 2: primary somatosensory cortex
2. Br. areas 41 & 42: primary auditory areas (transverse gyri of Heschl)
3. Br. area 4: precentral gyrus, primary motor cortex (AKA "motor strip"). Large concentration of giant pyramidal cells of Betz
4. Br. area 6: premotor area or supplemental motor area. Immediately anterior to motor strip, it plays a role in contralateral motor programming
5. Br. area 44: (dominant hemisphere) Broca's area (classically "motor speech area" see speech & language (p. 90))

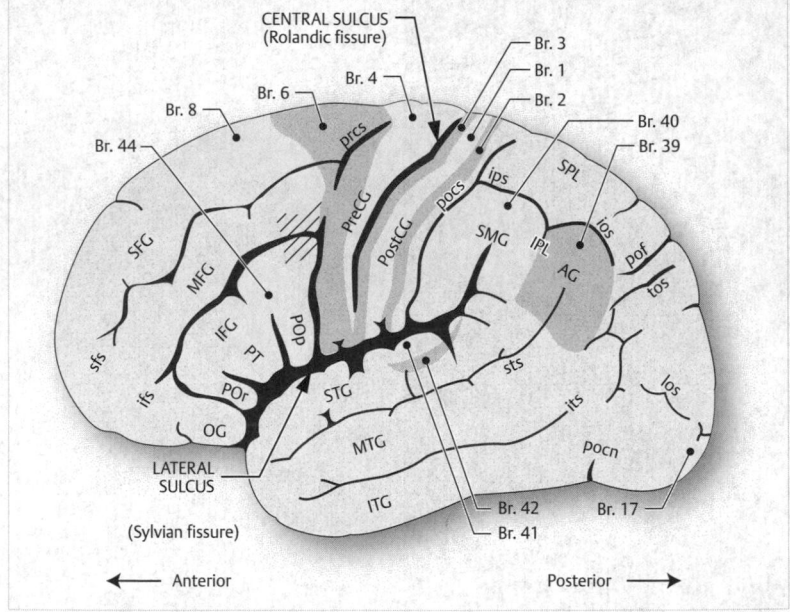

Fig. 1.1 Left lateral cerebral cortical surface anatomy.
Br. = Brodmann's area (shaded). See ▶ Table 1.1 and ▶ Table 1.2 for abbreviations (lowercase = sulci, UPPERCASE = gyri).

Table 1.1 Cerebral sulci (abbreviations)

Abbreviation	Sulcus
cins	cingulate sulcus
cs	central sulcus
ips-ios	intraparietal-intraoccipital sulcus
los	lateral occipital sulcus
pM	pars marginalis
pocn	pre-occipital notch
pocs	post-central sulcus
pof	parieto-occipital fissure
pos	parieto-occipital sulcus
prcs	pre-central sulcus
sfs, ifs	superior, inferior frontal sulcus
sps	superior parietal sulcus
sts, its	superior, inferior temporal sulcus
tos	trans occipital sulcus

Table 1.2 Cerebral gyri and lobules (abbreviations)

Abbreviation	Gyrus / lobule
AG	angular gyrus
CinG	cingulate gyrus
Cu	cuneus
LG	lingual gyrus
MFG, SFG	middle & superior frontal gyrus
OG	orbital gyrus
PCu	precuneus
PreCG, PostCG	pre- and post-central gyrus
PL	paracentral lobule (upper SFG and PreCG and PostCG)
IFG • POp • PT • POr	inferior frontal gyrus • pars opercularis • pars triangularis • pars orbitalis
STG, MTG, ITG	superior, middle & inferior temporal gyrus
SPL, IPL	superior & inferior parietal lobule
SMG	supramarginal gyrus

6. Br. area 17: primary visual cortex
7. Wernicke's area: (dominant hemisphere) most of Br. area 40 and a portion of Br. area 39 (may also include ≈ posterior third of STG). Significant in speech & language (p.90)
8. the striped portion of Br. area 8 in ▶ Fig. 1.1 (frontal eye field) initiates voluntary eye movements to the opposite direction

1.1.3 Medial surface

Pars marginalis

▶ Fig. 1.2. The cingulate sulcus terminates posteriorly in the pars marginalis (pM) (plural: partes marginales). On axial imaging, the pMs are visible on 95% of CTs and 91% of MRIs,[2] they are usually the most prominent of the paired grooves straddling the midline, and they extend a greater distance into the hemispheres.[2] On axial CT or MRI, the pM is posterior to the widest biparietal diameter.[2] The pMs curve posteriorly in lower slices and anteriorly in higher slices (here, the paired pMs form the "pars bracket"—a characteristic "handlebar" configuration straddling the midline).

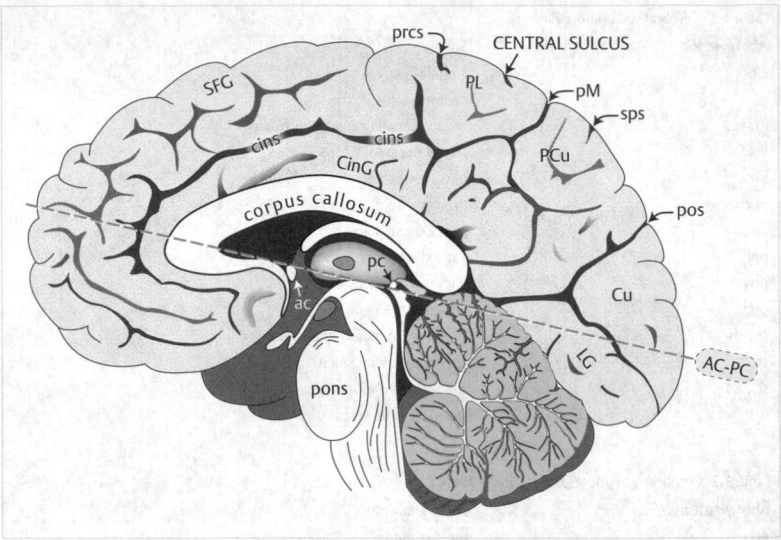

Fig. 1.2 Medial aspect of the right hemisphere.
Abbreviations: see ► Table 1.1 for sulci and ► Table 1.2 for gyri; ac = anterior commissure, pc = posterior commissure, AC-PC = AC-PC line (see text) which is illustrated here according to the Talairach definition.

AC-PC line

The "AC-PC line" connects the anterior commissure (AC) and the posterior commissure (PC) on a midline sagittal image (► Fig. 1.2). The AC is the horizontally oriented white matter tract connecting the left and right cerebral hemispheres that crosses in front of the fornix. The PC is the white-matter band at the level of the pineal that crosses at the posterior third ventricle. The AC-PC line is used in functional neurosurgery and is also used as the baseline for axial MRI scans (and for recent CT scanners). In the more entrenched Talairach definition,[3] it passes through the superior edge of the AC and the inferior edge of the PC (as illustrated in ► Fig. 1.2). Alternative Schaltenbrand definition[4]: the line passing through the midpoint of the AC & PC, allowing both AC & PC to be imaged on a single thin axial MRI slice. These definitions differ by 5.81° ± 1.07°.[5] The orbitomeatal line (p. 238) (used in older CT scanners) is ≈ 9° steeper than the Talairach AC-PC line.[5]

1.1.4 Somatotopic organization of primary sensory and motor cortex

The primary motor cortex (AKA "motor strip") and primary (somato)sensory cortex are organized somatotopically so that specific regions of the brain map correspond to specific areas of the body as shown in ► Fig. 1.3.

The regions are often drawn with a caricature of a human figure (the homunculus—Latin for "little man") along with the labels shown here.

Some key points: the representation of the arm and face are draped over the convexity of the brain, while the foot and leg areas are located along the upper aspect of the medial surface. Areas with fine motor or sensory function (e.g., fingers, tongue) have a larger area of representation.

1.2 Central sulcus on axial imaging

See ► Fig. 1.4. Identification of the central sulcus is important to localize the motor strip (contained in the PreCG). The central sulcus (CS) is visible on 93% of CTs and 100% of MRIs.[2] It curves posteriorly as it approaches the interhemispheric fissure (IHF), and often terminates in the paracentral lobule, just anterior to the pars marginalis (pM) within the pars bracket (see above)[2] (i.e., the CS often does not reach the midline).

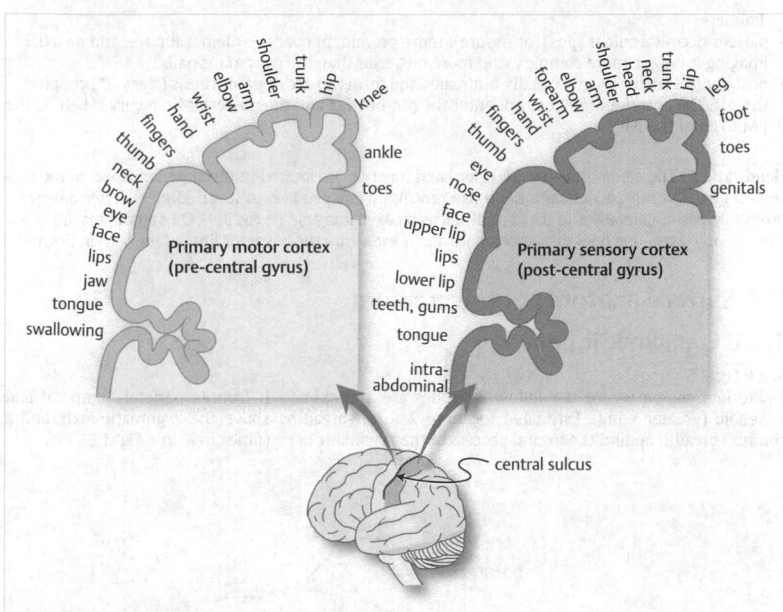

Fig. 1.3 Somatotopic organization of primary sensory and motor cortex.
The labels are placed along a cross section of the brain taken through the motor (blue) and the sensory (pink) cortex indicated on the drawing of the brain shown below the slices.

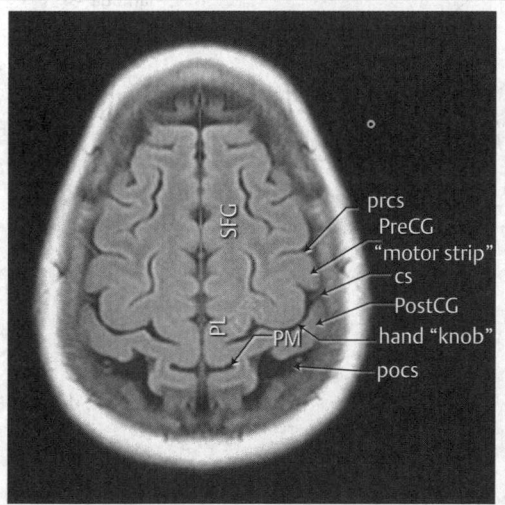

Fig. 1.4 Motor strip and hand knob.
Retouched axial FLAIR MRI with labels for gyri/sulci shown in the left hemisphere, and an unlabeled mirror image shown as the right hemisphere for reference. The inverted blue Ω (omega) illustrates the hand "knob" (see text).
See ► Table 1.1 and ► Table 1.2 for abbreviations.

1

Pointers:
- parieto-occipital sulcus (pos) (or fissure): more prominent over the medial surface, and on axial imaging is longer, more complex, and more posterior than the pars marginalis[6]
- post-central sulcus (pocs): usually bifurcates and forms an arc or parenthesis ("lazy-Y") cupping the pM. The anterior limb does not enter the pM-bracket and the posterior limb curves behind the pM to enter the IHF

Hand "knob": The alpha motor neurons for hand function are located in the superior aspect of the pre-central gyrus[7] which appears as a knob-like protrusion (shaped like an inverted greek letter omega Ω) projecting posterolaterally into the central sulcus on axial imaging[8] (▶ Fig. 1.4). On sagittal imaging it has a posteriorly projecting hook-like appearance and is even with the posterior limit of the Sylvian fissure.[8]

1.3 Surface anatomy of the cranium

1.3.1 Craniometric points

See ▶ Fig. 1.5.
Pterion: region where the following bones are approximated: frontal, parietal, temporal and sphenoid (greater wing). Estimated location: 2 finger-breadths above the zygomatic arch, and a thumb's breadth behind the frontal process of the zygomatic bone (blue circle in ▶ Fig. 1.5).

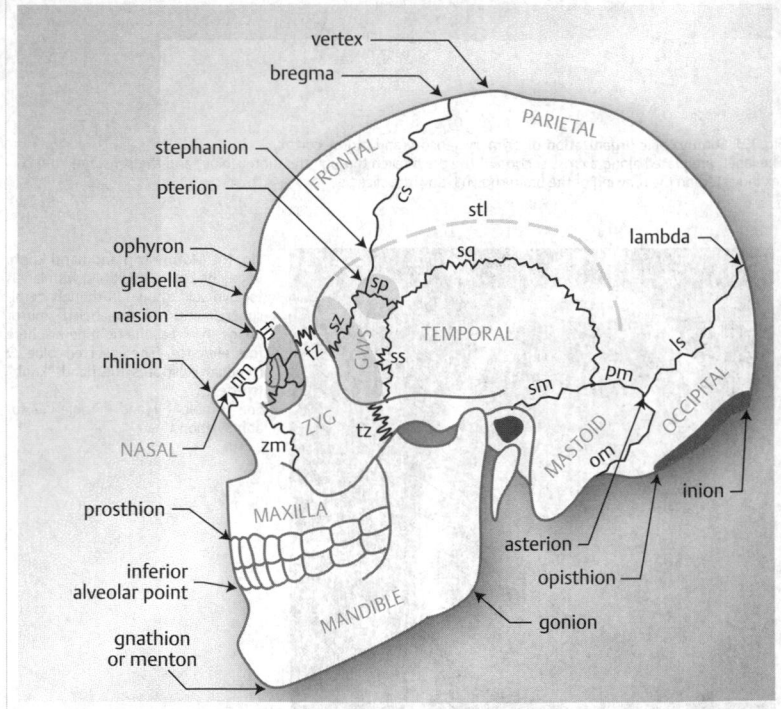

Fig. 1.5 Craniometric points & cranial sutures.
Named bones appear in all upper case letters. The blue circle is the pterion.
Abbreviations: GWS = greater wing of sphenoid bone; stl = superior temporal line; ZYG = zygomatic.
For basion, see ▶ Fig. 12.1.
Sutures: cs = coronal, fn = frontonasal, fz = frontozygomatic, ls = lambdoid, nm = nasomaxillary, om = occipitomastoid, pm = parietomastoid, sm = squamomastoid, sp = sphenoparietal, sq = squamosal, ss = sphenosquamous, sz = sphenozygomatic, tz = temporozygomatic, zm = zygomaticomaxillary.

Asterion: junction of lambdoid, occipitomastoid and parietomastoid sutures. Usually lies within a few millimeters of the posterior-inferior edge of the junction of the transverse and sigmoid sinuses (not always reliable[9]—may overlie either sinus).

Vertex: the topmost point of the skull.

Lambda: junction of the lambdoid and sagittal sutures.

Stephanion: junction of coronal suture and superior temporal line.

Glabella: the most forward projecting point of the forehead at the level of the supraorbital ridge in the midline.

Opisthion: the posterior margin of the foramen magnum in the midline.

Bregma: the junction of the coronal and sagittal sutures.

Sagittal suture: midline suture from coronal suture to lambdoid suture. Although often assumed to overlie the superior sagittal sinus (SSS), the SSS lies to the right of the sagittal suture in the majority of specimens[10] (but never by > 11 mm).

The most anterior mastoid point lies just in front of the sigmoid sinus.[11]

1.3.2 Relation of skull markings to cerebral anatomy

Taylor-Haughton lines

Taylor-Haughton (T-H) lines can be constructed on an angiogram, CT/MRI scout film, or skull X-ray. They can be constructed on the patient in the O.R. based on visible external landmarks.[12] T-H lines are shown as dashed lines in ▶ Fig. 1.6.

1. Frankfurt plane, AKA baseline: line from inferior margin of orbit through the *upper* margin of the external auditory meatus (EAM) (as distinguished from Reid's base line: from inferior orbital margin through the center of the EAM)[13(p 313)]
2. the distance from the nasion to the inion is measured across the top of the calvaria and is divided into quarters (can be done simply with a piece of tape which is then folded in half twice)
3. posterior ear line: perpendicular to the baseline through the mastoid process
4. condylar line: perpendicular to the baseline through the mandibular condyle
5. T-H lines (p. 61) can then be used to approximate the Sylvian fissure (see below) and the motor cortex

Motor cortex

Numerous methods utilize external landmarks to locate the motor strip (precentral gyrus) or the *central sulcus* (Rolandic fissure) which separates motor strip anteriorly from primary sensory cortex posteriorly. These are just approximations since individual variability causes the motor strip to lie anywhere from 4 to 5.4 cm behind the coronal suture.[14] The central sulcus cannot even be reliably identified visually at surgery.[15]

1. method 1: the superior aspect of the motor cortex is almost straight up from the EAM near the midline
2. method 2[16]: the central sulcus is approximated by connecting:
   a) the point 2 cm posterior to the midposition of the arc extending from nasion to inion (illustrated in ▶ Fig. 1.6), to
   b) the point 5 cm straight up from the EAM
3. method 3: using T-H lines, the central sulcus is approximated by connecting
   a) the point where the "posterior ear line" intersects the circumference of the skull (▶ Fig. 1.6; usually about 1 cm behind the vertex, and 3–4 cm behind the coronal suture), to
   b) the point where the "condylar line" intersects the line representing the Sylvian fissure
4. method 4: a line drawn 45° to Reid's base line starting at the pterion points in the *direction* of the motor strip[17(p 584–5)]

Sylvian fissure AKA lateral fissure

On the skin surface: approximated by a line connecting the lateral canthus to the point 3/4 of the way posterior along the arc running over convexity from nasion to inion (T-H lines).

On the skull (once it is exposed in surgery): the anterior portion of the Sylvian fissure follows the squamosal suture (▶ Fig. 1.7)[18] and then deviates superiorly to terminate at **Chater's point**, which is located 6 cm above the EAM on a line perpendicular to the orbitomeatal line; it is also ≈ 1.5 cm above the squamosal suture along the same perpendicular line. A 4 cm craniotomy centered at Chater's point provides access to potential recipient vessels in the angular gyrus for EC/IC bypass surgery.[19,20]

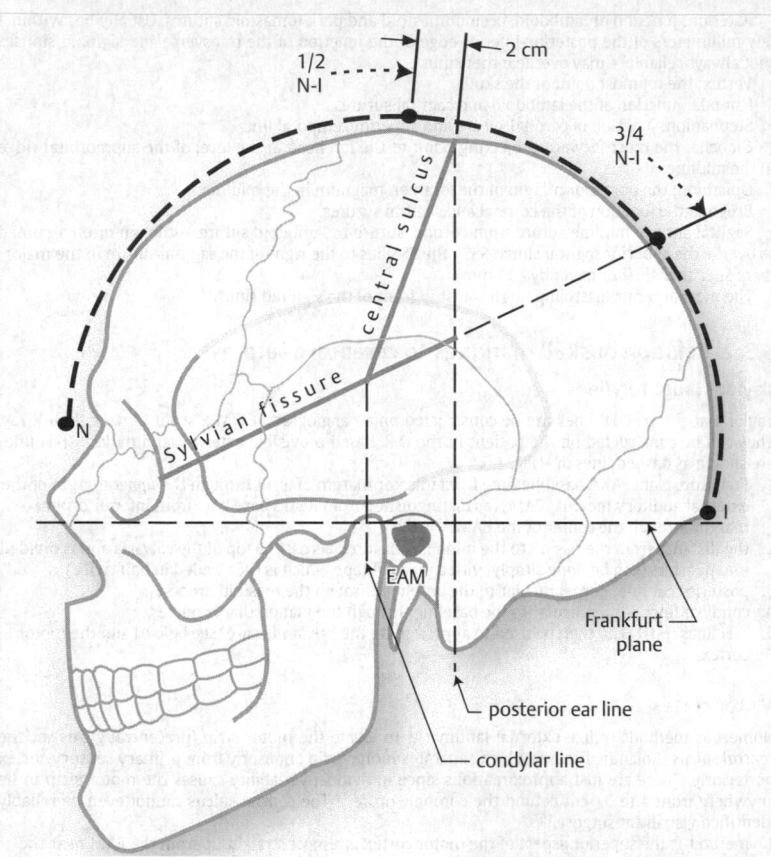

Fig. 1.6 Taylor-Haughton lines and other localizing methods.
N = nasion. I = inion.

Angular gyrus

Located just above the pinna, important on the dominant hemisphere as part of Wernicke's area (p. 90). Note: there is significant individual variability in the location.[21]

1.3.3 Relationship of ventricles to skull

▶ Fig. 1.8 shows the relationship of non-hydrocephalic ventricles to the skull in the lateral view. Some dimensions of interest are shown in ▶ Table 1.3.[22]

In the non-hydrocephalic adult, the lateral ventricles lie 4–5 cm below the outer skull surface. The center of the body of the lateral ventricle sits in the midpupillary line, and the frontal horn is intersected by a line passing perpendicular to the calvaria along this line.[23] The anterior horns extend 1–2 cm anterior to the coronal suture.

Average length of third ventricle ≈ 2.8 cm.

The midpoint of Twining's line (• in ▶ Fig. 1.8) should lie within the 4th ventricle.

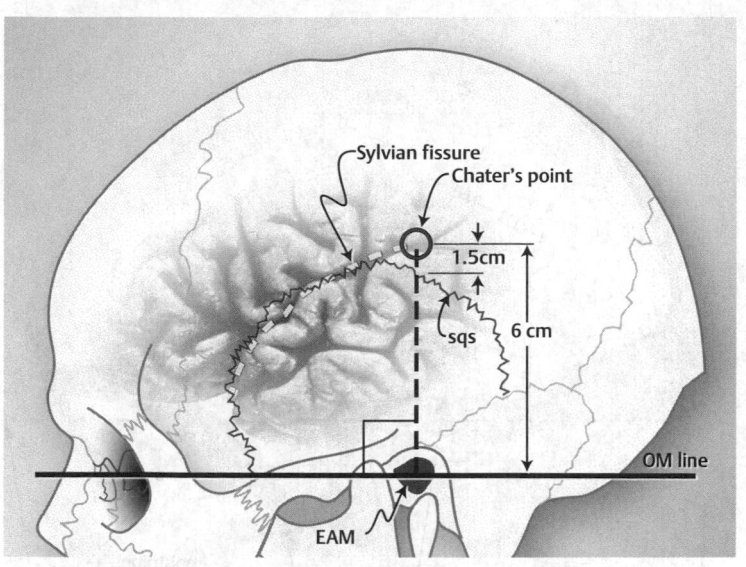

Fig. 1.7 Chater's point. Note the relationship of the Sylvian fissure to the squamosal suture.
Abbreviations: EAM = external auditory meatus; sqs = squamosal suture; OM line = orbitomeatal line (p. 238) (a line sometimes used in CT scanning that connects the lateral canthus to the midpoint of the EAM).
The dashed black line is perpendicular to the OM line. The red circle indicates Chater's point. The Sylvian fissure is highlighted by the broken yellow line and is situated under the anterior portion of the sqs.

1.4 Surface landmarks of spine levels

Estimates of cervical levels for anterior cervical spine surgery may be made using the landmarks shown in ▶ Table 1.4. Intraoperative C-spine X-rays are essential to verify these estimates.

The scapular spine is located at about T2–3.

The inferior scapular pole is ≈ T6 posteriorly.

Intercristal line: a line drawn between the highest point of the iliac crests across the back will cross the midline either at the interspace between the L4 and L5 spinous processes, or at the L4 spinous process itself.

1.5 Cranial foramina and their contents

1.5.1 Summary

See ▶ Table 1.5.

1.5.2 Porus acusticus

AKA internal auditory canal (▶ Fig. 1.9).

The filaments of the acoustic portion of VIII penetrate tiny openings of the lamina cribrosa of the cochlear area.[25]

Transverse crest: separates superior vestibular area and facial canal (above) from the inferior vestibular area and cochlear area (see below).[25]

Vertical crest (AKA Bill's bar—named after Dr. William House): separates the meatus to the facial canal anteriorly (containing VII and nervus intermedius) from the vestibular area posteriorly (containing the superior division of vestibular nerve). Bill's bar is deeper in the IAC than the transverse crest.

1

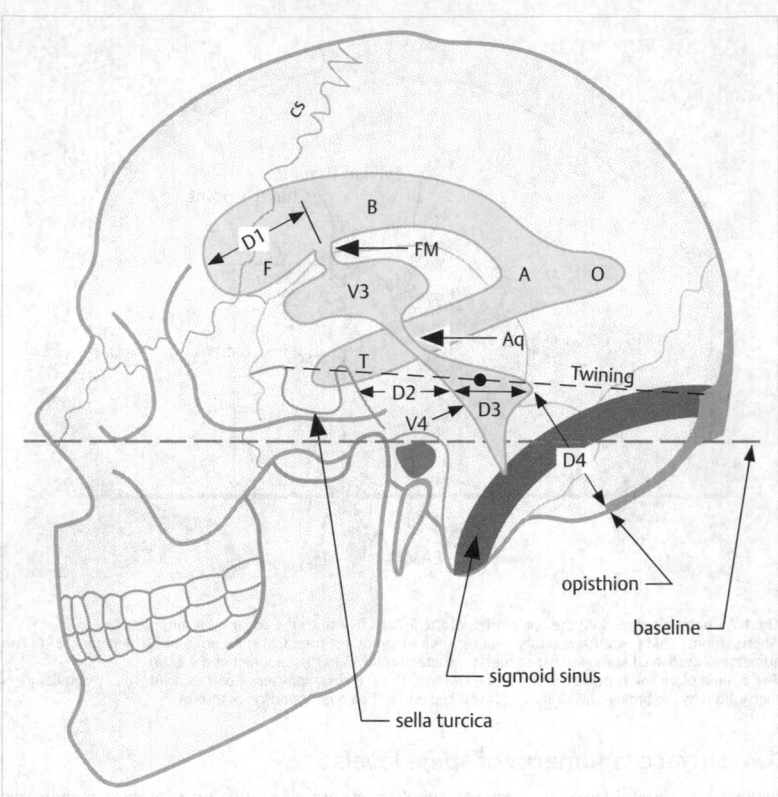

Fig. 1.8 Relationship of ventricles to skull landmarks.
Abbreviations: (F = frontal horn, B = body, A = atrium, O = occipital horn, T = temporal horn) of lateral ventricle. FM = foramen of Monro. Aq = Sylvian aqueduct. V3 = third ventricle. V4 = fourth ventricle. cs = coronal suture. Dimensions D1–4 see ▶ Table 1.3.

Table 1.3 Dimensions from ▶ Fig. 1.8

Dimension (▶ Fig. 1.8)	Description	Lower limit (mm)	Average (mm)	Upper limit (mm)
D1	length of frontal horn anterior to FM		25	
D2	distance from clivus to floor of 4th ventricle at level of fastigium[a]	33.3	36.1	40.0
D3	length of 4th ventricle at level of fastigium[a]	10.0	14.6	19.0
D4	distance from fastigium[a] to opisthion	30.0	32.6	40.0

[a] fastigium: the apex of the 4th ventricle within the cerebellum

Table 1.4 Cervical levels[24]

Level	Landmark
C1–2	angle of mandible
C3–4	1 cm above thyroid cartilage (≈ hyoid bone)
C4–5	level of thyroid cartilage
C5–6	crico-thyroid membrane
C6	carotid tubercle
C6–7	cricoid cartilage

Table 1.5 Cranial foramina and their contents[a]

Foramen	Contents
nasal slits	anterior ethmoidal nn., a. & v.
superior orbital fissure	Cr. Nn. III, IV, VI, all 3 branches of V1 (ophthalmic division divides into nasociliary, frontal, and lacrimal nerves); superior ophthalmic vv.; recurrent meningeal br. from lacrimal a.; orbital branch of middle meningeal a.; sympathetic filaments from ICA plexus
inferior orbital fissure	Cr. N. V-2 (maxillary div.), zygomatic n.; filaments from pterygopalatine branch of maxillary n.; infraorbital a. & v.; v. between inferior ophthalmic v. & pterygoid venous plexus
foramen lacerum	usually nothing (ICA *traverses* the upper portion but doesn't enter, 30% have vidian a.)
carotid canal	internal carotid a., ascending sympathetic nerves
incisive foramen	descending septal a.; nasopalatine nn.
greater palatine foramen	greater palatine n., a., & v.
lesser palatine foramen	lesser palatine nn.
internal acoustic meatus	Cr. N. VII (facial); Cr. N. VIII (stato-acoustic)—see text & ▶ Fig. 1.9
hypoglossal canal	Cr. N. XII (hypoglossal); a meningeal branch of the ascending pharyngeal a.
foramen magnum	spinal cord (medulla oblongata); Cr. N. XI (spinal accessory nn.) *entering* the skull; vertebral aa.; anterior & posterior spinal arteries
foramen cecum	occasional small vein
cribriform plate	olfactory nn.
optic canal	Cr. N. II (optic); ophthalmic a.
foramen rotundum	Cr. N. V2 (maxillary div.), a. of foramen rotundum
foramen ovale	Cr. N. V3 (mandibular div.) + portio minor (motor for Cr. N. V)
foramen spinosum	middle meningeal a. & v.
jugular foramen	internal jugular v. (beginning); Cr. Nn. IX, X, XI
stylomastoid foramen	Cr. N. VII (facial); stylomastoid a.
condyloid foramen	v. from transverse sinus
mastoid foramen	v. to mastoid sinus; branch of occipital a. to dura mater

[a]Abbreviations: a. = artery, aa. = arteries, v. = vein, vv. = veins, n. = nerve, nn. = nerves, br. = branch, Cr. N. = cranial nerve, fmn. = foramen, div. = division

The "5 nerves" of the IAC:
1. facial nerve (VII) (mnemonic: "7-up" as VII is in superior portion)
2. nervus intermedius: the somatic sensory branch of the facial nerve primarily innervating mechanoreceptors of the hair follicles on the inner surface of the pinna and deep mechanoreceptors of nasal and buccal cavities and chemoreceptors in the taste buds on the anterior 2/3 of the tongue
3. acoustic portion of the VIII nerve (mnemonic: "Coke down" for cochlear portion)
4. superior branch of vestibular nerve: passes through the superior vestibular area to terminate in the utricle and in the ampullæ of the superior and lateral semicircular canals (mnemonic superior = LSU (Lateral & Superior semicircular canals and the Utricule))
5. inferior branch of vestibular nerve: passes through inferior vestibular area to terminate in the saccule

1

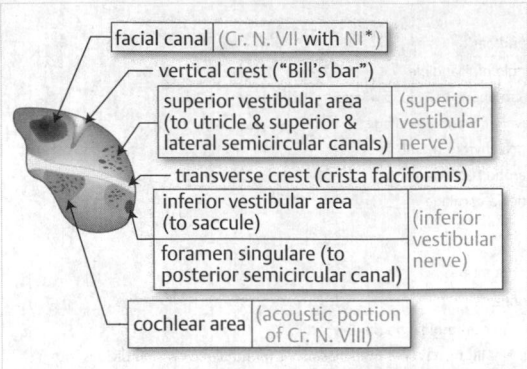

Fig. 1.9 Right internal auditory canal (porus acusticus) & nerves. Abbreviations: Cr. N. = cranial nerve; NI = nervus intermedius.

1.6 Internal capsule

1.6.1 Architectural anatomy

For a schematic diagram, see ▶ Fig. 1.10; ▶ Table 1.6 delineates the thalamic subradiations.
Most IC lesions are caused by vascular accidents (thrombosis or hemorrhage).

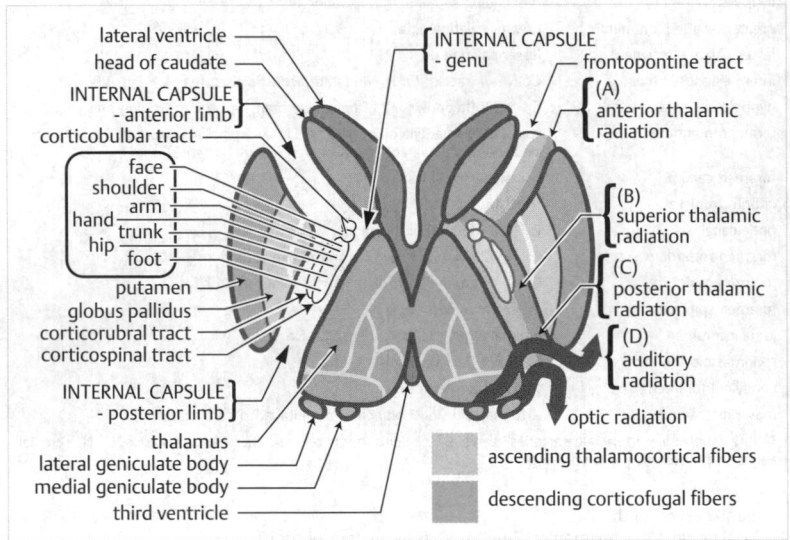

Fig. 1.10 Internal capsule schematic diagram.
Axial cut. The left side of the diagram shows tracts; the right side shows radiations.

1.6.2 Vascular supply of the internal capsule (IC)

1. anterior choroidal: ⇒ all of retrolenticular part (includes optic radiation) and ventral part of posterior limb of IC
2. lateral striate branches (AKA capsular branches) of middle cerebral artery: ⇒ most of anterior AND posterior limbs of IC
3. genu usually receives some direct branches of the internal carotid artery

Table 1.6 Four thalamic "subradiations" (AKA thalamic peduncles), labeled A-D in ▶ Fig. 1.10

Radiation		Connection		Comments
anterior (A)	medial & anterior thalamic nucleus	↔	frontal lobe	
superior (B)	rolandic areas	↔	ventral thalamic nuclei	general sensory fibers from body & head to terminate in postcentral gyrus (areas 3,1,2)
posterior (C)	occipital & posterior parietal	↔	caudal thalamus	
inferior (D)	transverse temporal gyrus of Heschl	↔	MGB	(small) includes auditory radiation

1.7 Cerebellopontine angle anatomy

For normal anatomy of right cerebellopontine angle, see ▶ Fig. 1.11.

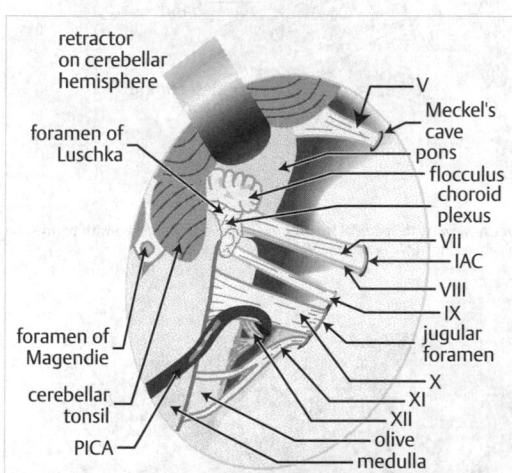

Fig. 1.11 Right cerebellopontine angle. Normal anatomy viewed from behind (as in a suboccipital approach).[25]

1.8 Occipitoatlantoaxial-complex anatomy

▶ **Ligaments of the occipitoatlantoaxial complex.** Stability of the occipitoatlantal joint is primarily due to ligaments, with little contribution from bony articulations and joint capsules (see ▶ Fig. 1.12, ▶ Fig. 1.13, ▶ Fig. 1.14):

1. ligaments that connect the atlas to the occiput:
   a) anterior atlantooccipital membrane: cephalad extension of the anterior longitudinal ligament. Extends from anterior margin of foramen magnum (FM) to anterior arch of C1
   b) posterior atlantooccipital membrane: connects the posterior margin of the FM to posterior arch of C1
   c) the ascending band of the cruciate ligament
2. ligaments that connect the axis (viz. the odontoid) to the occiput:
   a) tectorial membrane: some authors distinguish 2 components
      • superficial component: cephalad continuation of the posterior longitudinal ligament. A strong band connecting the dorsal surface of the dens to the ventral surface of the FM above, and dorsal surface of C2 & C3 bodies below
      • accessory (deep) portion: located laterally, connects C2 to occipital condyles
   b) alar ligaments (AKA check ligaments of the odontoid) [26]
      • occipito-alar portion: connects side of the dens to occipital condyle
      • atlanto-alar portion: connects side of the dens to the lateral mass of C1

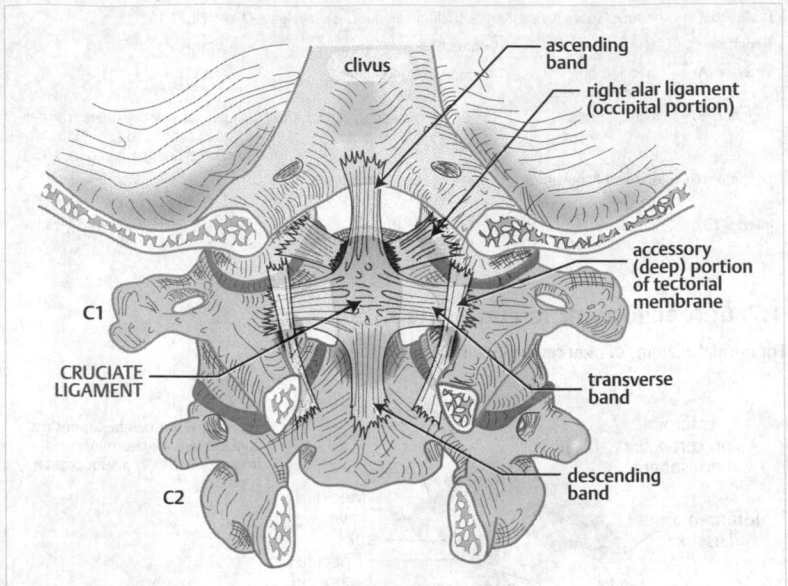

Fig. 1.12 Cruciate and alar ligaments. Dorsal view (with tectorial membrane removed). (Modified with permission from "In Vitro Cervical Spine Biomechanical Testing" BNI Quarterly, Vol. 9, No. 4, 1993.)

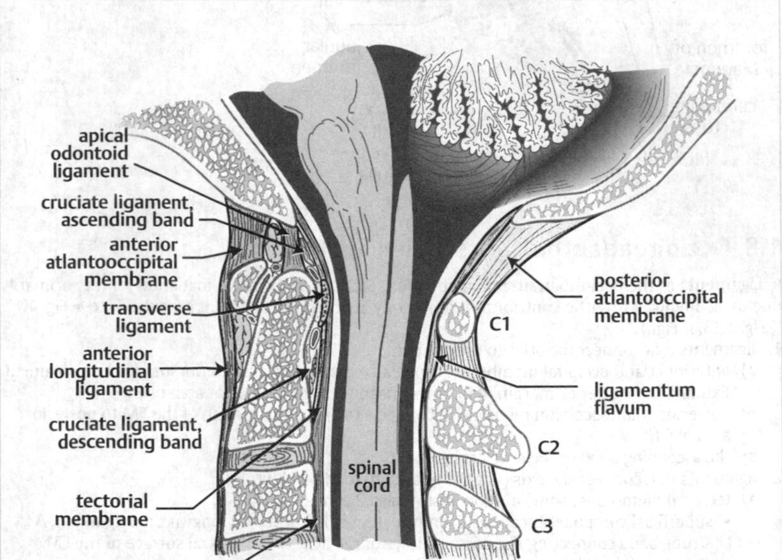

Fig. 1.13 Ligaments of the craniovertebral junction. Sagittal view. (Modified with permission from "In Vitro Cervical Spine Biomechanical Testing" BNI Quarterly, Vol. 9, No. 4, 1993.)

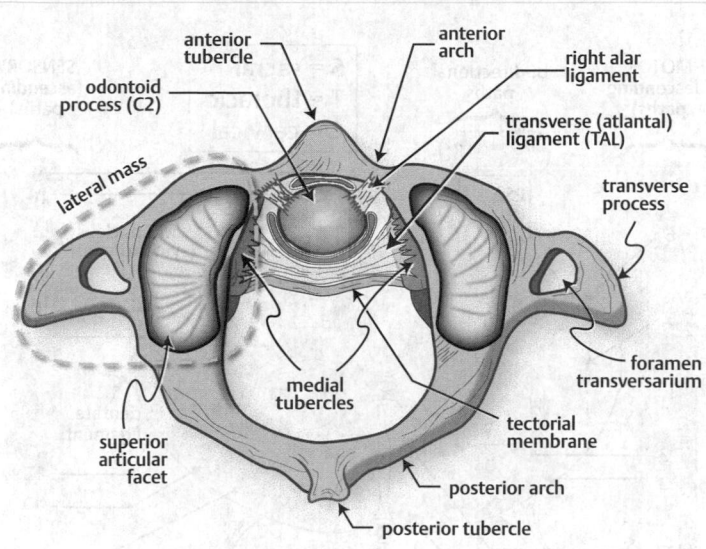

Fig. 1.14 C1 vertebral body. Viewed from above, showing the transverse and alar ligaments, and the critially important transverse atlantal ligament (TAL) AKA transverse ligament. (Modified with permission from "In Vitro Cervical Spine Biomechanical Testing" BNI Quarterly, Vol. 9, No. 4, 1993.)

   c) apical odontoid ligament: connects tip of dens to the FM. Little mechanical strength
3. ligaments that connect the axis to the atlas:
   a) transverse atlantal ligament (TAL) or (usually) just transverse ligament: the horizontal component of the cruciate ligament. Attaches at the medial tubercles of C1. Traps the dens against the anterior atlas via a strap-like mechanism (▶ Fig. 1.14). Provides the majority of the strength ("the strongest ligament of the spine"[27])
   b) atlanto-alar portion of the alar ligaments (see above)
   c) descending band of the cruciate ligament

The most important structures in maintaining atlantooccipital stability are the tectorial membrane and the alar ligaments. Without these, the remaining cruciate ligament and apical dentate ligament are insufficient.

1.9 Spinal cord anatomy

1.9.1 Dentate ligament

The dentate ligament separates dorsal from ventral nerve roots in the spinal nerves. The spinal accessory nerve (Cr. N. XI) is dorsal to the dentate ligament.

1.9.2 Spinal cord tracts

Anatomy

▶ Fig. 1.15 depicts a cross-section of a typical spinal cord segment, combining some elements from different levels (e.g., the intermediolateral gray nucleus is only present from T1 to ≈ L1 or L2 where there are sympathetic [thoracolumbar outflow] nuclei). It is schematically divided into ascending and descending halves; however, in actuality, ascending and descending paths coexist on both sides.
▶ Fig. 1.15 also depicts some of the laminae according to the scheme of Rexed. Lamina II is equivalent to the substantia gelatinosa. Laminae III and IV are the nucleus proprius. Lamina VI is located in the base of the posterior horn.

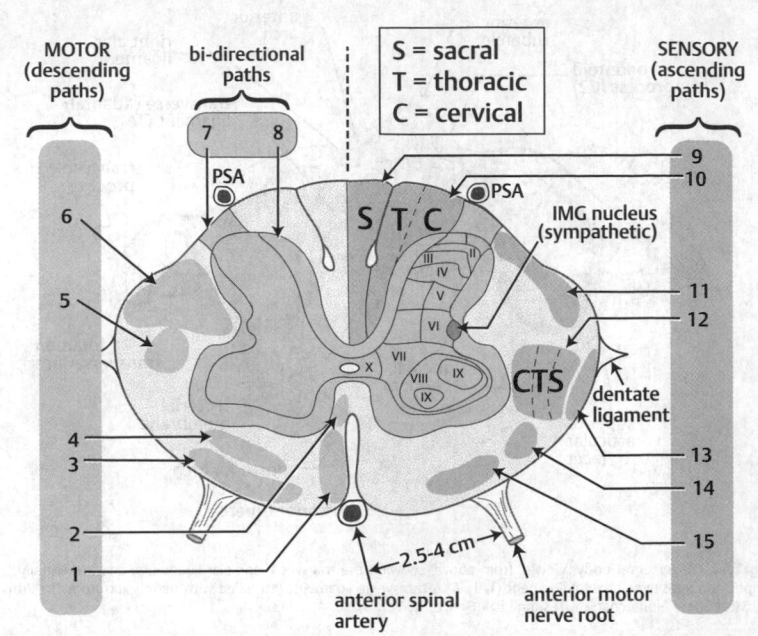

Fig. 1.15 Schematic cross-section of spinal cord. See ▶ Table 1.7, ▶ Table 1.8 and ▶ Table 1.9 for path names. Abbreviations: IMG = intermediolateral gray nucleus, PSA = posterior spinal artery. Roman numerals refer to laminae of Rexed.

Table 1.7 Descending (motor) tracts (↓) in ▶ Fig. 1.15

Number (▶ Fig. 1.15)	Path	Function	Side of *body*
1	anterior corticospinal tract	skilled movement	opposite[a]
2	medial longitudinal fasciculus	?	same
3	vestibulospinal tract	facilitates extensor muscle tone	same
4	medullary (ventrolateral) reticulospinal tract	automatic respirations?	same
5	rubrospinal tract	flexor muscle tone	same
6	lateral corticospinal (pyramidal) tract	skilled movement	same

[a]The terminal fibers of this uncrossed tract usually cross in the anterior white commissure to synapse on alpha motor neurons or on internuncial neurons. A minority of the fibers do remain ipsilateral. Also, an anterior corticospinal tract is easily identified only in the cervical and upper thoracic regions.

Motor

The lateral **corticospinal tract** (AKA pyramidal tract) is the largest and most significant motor tract of the spinal cord (often referred to simply as the corticospinal tract (CST) even though there is also an anterior CST). It consists of large axons of upper motor neuron (Betz cells) that originate in the motor cortex (precentral gyrus) in a somatotopic organization (p. 58). The nerve fibers pass through the corona radiata and then the posterior limb of the internal capsule (IC), still somatotopically organized (▶ Fig. 1.10). The CST progressively loses its somatotopic organization as it passes through the cerebral peduncles and basis pontis.[28] About 10% of the fibers enter the ipsilateral anterior CST,

Table 1.8 Bi-directional tracts in ▶ Fig. 1.15

Number (▶ Fig. 1.15)	Path	Function
7	dorsolateral fasciculus (of Lissauer)	?
8	fasciculus proprius	short spinospinal connections

Table 1.9 Ascending (sensory) tracts (↑) in ▶ Fig. 1.15

Number (▶ Fig. 1.15)	Path	Function	Side of *body*
9	fasciculus gracilis	joint position, fine touch, vibration	same
10	fasciculus cuneatus		
11	posterior spinocerebellar tract	stretch receptors	same
12	lateral spinothalamic tract	pain & temperature	opposite
13	anterior spinocerebellar tract	whole limb position	opposite
14	spinotectal tract	unknown, ? nociceptive	opposite
15	anterior spinothalamic tract	light touch	opposite

whereas the remaining fibers cross at the medullary decussation and continue as the lateral CST along with some fibers from the supplemental motor area (SMA) (Brodmann area 6, ▶ Fig. 1.1) and primary somatosensory cortex.

Contrary to classic teaching (which was that the CST is somatotopically organized with cervical fibers located medially, and thoracic and lumbar fibers situated progressively more laterally) evidence shows that the motor fibers of the CST In the spinal cord are diffusely distributed, unlike the situation with the sensory tracts (spinothalamic, and the gracilis and cuneatus fasciculi).[28] Axons of the CST terminate on alpha motor neurons (lower motor neurons) in the ventral gray horn of the spinal cord (Rexed lamina IX).

Sensation

Pain and temperature: body
Receptors: free nerve endings (probable).

1st order neuron: small, finely myelinated afferents; soma in dorsal root ganglion (no synapse). Enter cord at dorsolateral tract (zone of Lissauer). Synapse: substantia gelatinosa (Rexed II).

2nd order neuron: axons cross obliquely in the anterior white commissure ascending ≈ 1–3 segments while crossing to enter the lateral spinothalamic tract.

Synapse: VPL thalamus. 3rd order neurons pass through internal capsule to the postcentral gyrus (Brodmann's areas 3, 1, 2).

Fine touch, deep pressure and proprioception: body
Fine touch AKA discriminative touch. Receptors: Meissner's & pacinian corpuscles, Merkel's discs, free nerve endings.

1st order neuron: heavily myelinated afferents; soma in dorsal root ganglion (no synapse). Short branches synapse in nucleus proprius (Rexed III & IV) of posterior gray; long fibers enter the ipsilateral posterior columns without synapsing (below T6: fasciculus gracilis; above T6: fasciculus cuneatus).

Synapse: nucleus gracilis/cuneatus (respectively), just above pyramidal decussation. 2nd order neuron axons form internal arcuate fibers, decussate in lower medulla as medial lemniscus.

Synapse: VPL thalamus. 3rd order neurons pass through IC primarily to postcentral gyrus.

Light (crude) touch: body
Receptors: as fine touch (see above), also peritrichial arborizations.

1st order neuron: large, heavily myelinated afferents (Type II); soma in dorsal root ganglion (no synapse). Some ascend uncrossed in posterior columns (with fine touch); most synapse in Rexed VI & VII.

2nd order neuron: axons cross in anterior white commissure (a few don't cross); enter anterior spinothalamic tract.

Synapse: VPL thalamus. 3rd order neurons pass through IC primarily to postcentral gyrus.

1.9.3 Dermatomes and sensory nerves

Dermatomes are areas of the body where sensation is subserved by a single nerve root.

Peripheral nerves generally receive contributions from more than one dermatome.

Lesions in peripheral nerves and lesions in nerve roots may sometimes be distinguished in part by the pattern of sensory loss. A classic example is splitting of the ring finger in median nerve or ulnar nerve lesions, which does not occur in C8 nerve root injuries.

▶ Fig. 1.16 shows anterior and posterior view, each schematically separated into sensory dermatomes (segmental) and peripheral sensory nerve distribution.

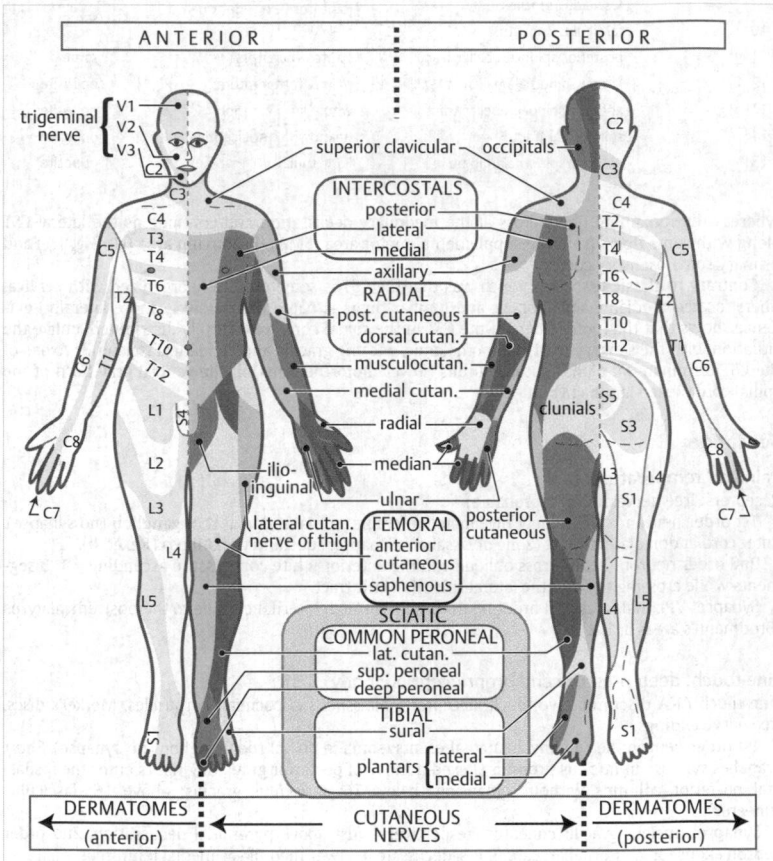

Fig. 1.16 Dermatomal and sensory nerve distribution. (Redrawn from "Introduction to Basic Neurology," by Harry D. Patton, John W. Sundsten, Wayne E. Crill and Phillip D. Swanson, © 1976, pp 173, W. B. Saunders Co., Philadelphia, PA, with permission.)

References

[1] Naidich TP. MR Imaging of Brain Surface Anatomy. Neuroradiology. 1991; 33:S95–S99

[2] Naidich TP, Brightbill TC. The pars marginalis, I: A "bracket" sign for the central sulcus in axial plane CT and MRI. International Journal of Neuroradiology. 1996; 2:3–19

[3] Talairach J, Tournoux P, Talairach J, et al. Practical examples for the use of the atlas in neuroradiogic examinations. In: Co-planar stereotactic atlas of the human brain. New Tork: Thieme Medical Publishers, Inc.; 1988:19–36

[4] Schaltenbrand G, Bailey P. Introduction to Stereotaxis with an Atlas of Human Brain. Stuttgart 1959

[5] Weiss KL, Pan H, Storrs J, et al. Clinical brain MR imaging prescriptions in Talairach space: technologist- and computer-driven methods. AJNR Am J Neuroradiol. 2003; 24:922–929

[6] Valente M, Naidich TP, Abrams KJ, et al. Differentiating the pars marginalis from the parieto-occipital sulcus in axial computed tomography sections. International Journal of Neuroradiology. 1998; 4:105–111

[7] Penfield W, Boldrey E. Somatic motor and sensory representation in the cerebral cortex of man as studied by electrical stimulation. Brain. 1937; 60:389–443

[8] Yousry TA, Schmid UD, Alkadhi H, et al. Localization of the motor hand area to a knob on the precentral gyrus. A new landmark. Brain. 1997; 120 (Pt 1):141–157

[9] Day JD, Tschabitscher M. Anatomic position of the asterion. Neurosurgery. 1998; 42:198–199

[10] Tubbs RS, Salter G, Elton S, et al. Sagittal suture as an external landmark for the superior sagittal sinus. J Neurosurg. 2001; 94:985–987

[11] Barnett SL, D'Ambrosio AL, Agazzi S, et al. Petroclival and Upper Clival Meningiomas III: Combined Anterior and Posterior Approach. In: Meningiomas. London: Springer-Verlag; 2009:425–432

[12] Willis WD, Grossman RG. The Brain and Its Environment. In: Medical Neurobiology. 3rd ed. St. Louis: C V Mosby; 1981:192–193

[13] Warwick R, Williams PL. Gray's Anatomy. Philadelphia 1973

[14] Kido DK, LeMay M, Levinson AW, et al. Computed tomographic localization of the precentral gyrus. Radiology. 1980; 135:373–377

[15] Martin N, Grafton S, Viñuela F, et al. Imaging Techniques for Cortical Functional Localization. Clin Neurosurg. 1990; 38:132–165

[16] Anderson JE. Grant's Atlas of Anatomy. Baltimore: Williams and Wilkins; 1978; 7

[17] Wilkins RH, Rengachary SS. Neurosurgery. New York 1985

[18] Rahmah NN, Murata T, Yako T, et al. Correlation between squamous suture and sylvian fissure: OSIRIX DICOM viewer study. PLoS One. 2011; 6. DOI: 10.1371/journal.pone.0018199

[19] Chater N, Spetzler R, Tonnemacher K, et al. Microvascular bypass surgery. Part 1: anatomical studies. J Neurosurg. 1976; 44:712–714

[20] Spetzler R, Chater N. Microvascular bypass surgery. Part 2: physiological studies. J Neurosurg. 1976; 45:508–513

[21] Ojemann G, Ojemann J, Lettich E, et al. Cortical Language Localization in Left, Dominant Hemisphere. An Electrical Stimulation Mapping Investigation in 117 Patients. J Neurosurg. 1989; 71:316–326

[22] Lusted LB, Keats TE. Atlas of Roentgenographic Measurement. 3rd ed. Chicago: Year Book Medical Publishers; 1972

[23] Ghajar JBG. A Guide for Ventricular Catheter Placement: Technical Note. J Neurosurg. 1985; 63:985–986

[24] Watkins RG. Anterior Cervical Approaches to the Spine. In: Surgical Approaches to the Spine. New York: Springer-Verlag; 1983:1–6

[25] Rhoton AL,Jr. The cerebellopontine angle and posterior fossa cranial nerves by the retrosigmoid approach. Neurosurgery. 2000; 47:S93–129

[26] Dvorak J, Panjabi MM. Functional anatomy of the alar ligaments. Spine (Phila Pa 1976). 1987; 12:183–189

[27] Dickman CA, Crawford NR, Brantley AGU, et al. In vitro cervical spine biomechanical testing. BNI Quarterly. 1993; 9:17–26

[28] Levi AD, Schwab JM. A critical reappraisal of corticospinal tract somatotopy and its role in traumatic cervical spinal cord syndromes. J Neurosurg Spine. 2021:1–7

2 Vascular Anatomy

2.1 Cerebral vascular territories

▶ Fig. 2.1 depicts approximate vascular distributions of the major cerebral arteries. There is considerable variability of the major arteries[1] as well as the central distribution.

Lenticulostriates may originate from different segments of the middle or anterior cerebral artery. **Recurrent artery of Heubner** (RAH) (AKA medial striate artery) origin: junction of the ACA and AComA in 62.3%, proximal A2 in 23.3%, A1 in 14.3%.[2]

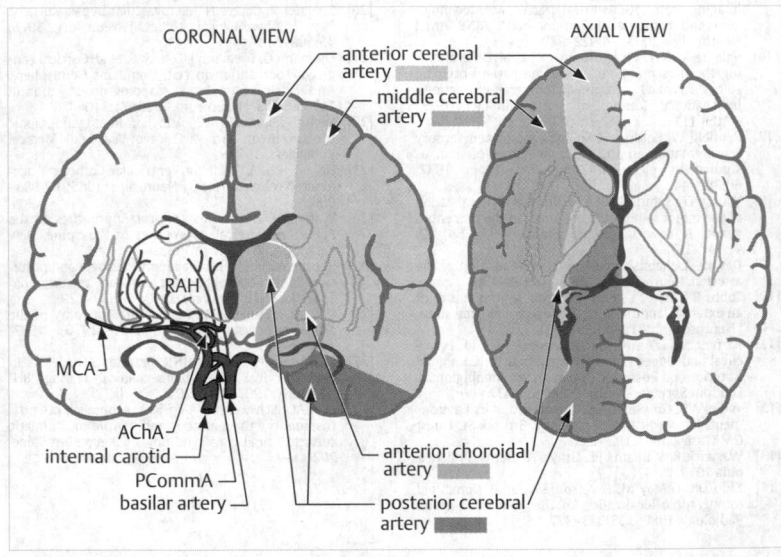

Fig. 2.1 **Vascular territories of the cerebral hemispheres**. RAH = recurrent artery of Heubner.

2.2 Cerebral arterial anatomy

2.2.1 General information

The symbol "⇒" is used to denote a region supplied by the indicated artery. See Angiography (cerebral) (p. 247) for angiographic diagrams of the following anatomy.

2.2.2 Circle of Willis

See ▶ Fig. 2.2. A balanced configuration of the Circle of Willis is present in only 18% of the population. Hypoplasia of 1 or both PComAs occurs in 22–32%; absent or hypoplastic A1 segments occur in 25%.

Key point: the anterior cerebral arteries pass over the superior surface of the optic chiasm.

2.2.3 Anatomical segments of intracranial cerebral arteries

1. carotid artery: see below for segments
2. anterior cerebral[3]:
   a) A1 (precommunicating): ACA from origin to AComA
   b) A2 (postcommunicating): ACA from AComA to branch-point of callosomarginal artery
   c) A3 (precallosal): from branch-point of callosomarginal curving around the genu of the corpus callosum to superior surface of corpus callosum 3 cm posterior to the genu

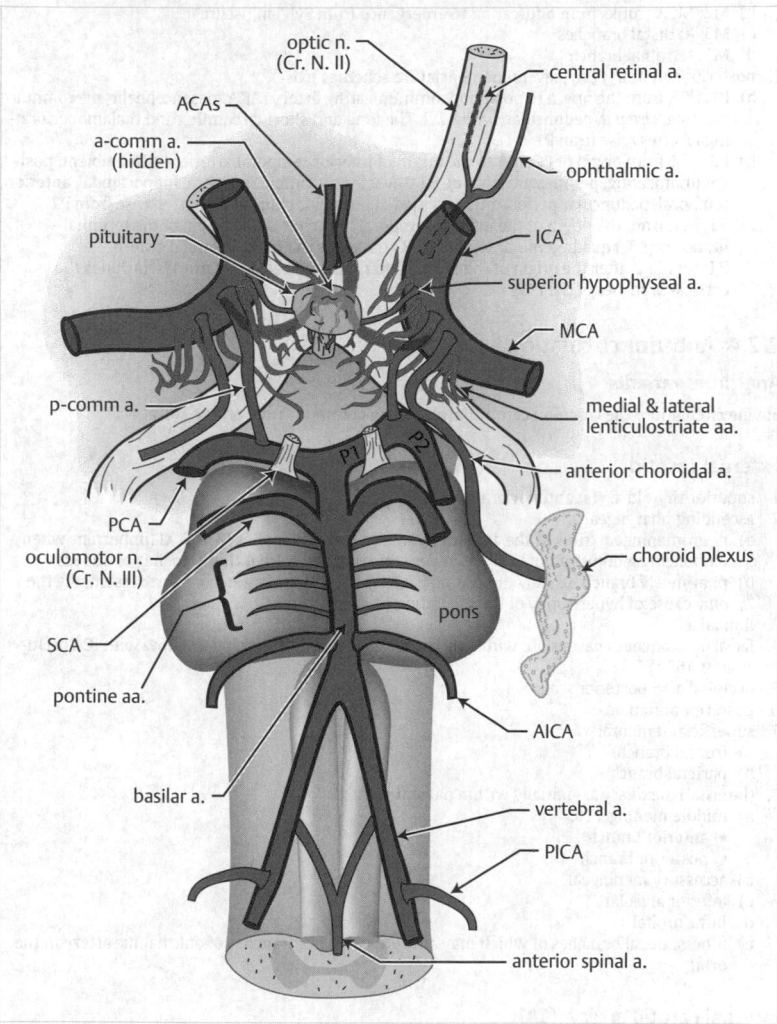

optic n.
(Cr. N. II)
ACAs
a-comm a.
(hidden)
pituitary
p-comm a.
PCA
oculomotor n.
(Cr. N. III)
SCA
pontine aa.
basilar a.

central retinal a.
ophthalmic a.
ICA
superior hypophyseal a.
MCA
medial & lateral
lenticulostriate aa.
anterior choroidal a.
choroid plexus
pons
AICA
vertebral a.
PICA
anterior spinal a.

P1 P2

Fig. 2.2 Circle of Willis. Viewed from anterior and inferior to the brain.

d) A4: (supracallosal)
e) A5: terminal branch (postcallosal)
3. middle cerebral[4]:
   a) M1: MCA from origin to bifurcation (horizontal segment on AP angiogram). A classical bifurcation into relatively symmetrical superior and inferior trunks is seen in 50%, no bifurcation occurs in 2%, 25% have a very proximal branch (middle trunk) arising from the superior (15%) or the inferior (10%) trunk creating a "pseudo-trifurcation," a pseudo-tetrafurcation occurs in 5%
      • lateral fronto-orbital and prefrontal branches arise from M1 or superior M2 trunk
      • precentral, central, anterior and posterior parietal arteries arise from a superior (60%), middle (25%), or inferior (15%) trunk
      • the superior M2 trunk does not give any branches to the temporal lobe

b) M2: MCA trunks from bifurcation to emergence from Sylvian fissure
c) M3–4: distal branches
d) M5: terminal branch
4. posterior cerebral (PCA) (several nomenclature schemes exist[3,5]):
   a) P1: PCA from the origin to posterior communicating artery (AKA mesencephalic, precommunicating, circular, peduncular, basilar…). The long and short circumflex and thalamoperforating arteries arise from P1
   b) P2: PCA from origin of PComA to the origin of inferior temporal arteries (AKA ambient, postcommunicating, perimesencephalic), P2 traverses the ambient cistern, hippocampal, anterior temporal, peduncular perforating, and medial posterior choroidal arteries arise from P2
   c) P3: PCA from the origin of the inferior temporal branches to the origin of the terminal branches (AKA quadrigeminal segment). P3 traverses the quadrigeminal cistern
   d) P4: segment after the origin of the parieto-occipital and calcarine arteries, includes the cortical branches of the PCA

2.2.4 Anterior circulation

Anatomic variants

Bovine circulation: the common carotids arise from a common trunk off the aorta.

External carotid

1. superior thyroid a.: 1st anterior branch
2. ascending pharyngeal a.
   a) neuromeningeal trunk of the ascending pharyngeal a.: supplies IX, X & XI (important when embolizing glomus tumors, 20% of lower cranial nerve palsy if this branch is occluded)
   b) pharyngeal branch: usually the primary feeder for jugular foramen tumors (essentially the *only* cause of hypertrophy of the ascending pharyngeal a.)
3. lingual a.
4. facial a.: branches anastamose with ophthalmic a.; important in collateral flow with ICA occlusion (p. 1537)
5. occipital a. ⇒ posterior scalp
6. posterior auricular
7. superficial temporal
   a) frontal branch
   b) parietal branch
8. (internal) maxillary a.—initially within parotid gland
   a) middle meningeal a.
      • anterior branch
      • posterior branch
   b) accessory meningeal
   c) inferior alveolar
   d) infra-orbital
   e) others: distal branches of which may anastomose with branches of ophthalmic artery in the orbit

Internal carotid artery (ICA)

Lies posterior & medial to the external carotid (ECA).

Segments of the ICA and its branches

See ▶ Fig. 2.3 for angiographic appearance, and ▶ Fig. 2.4 [6] for anatomic illustration.
1. **C1 (cervical):** begins in the neck at the carotid bifurcation where the common carotid artery divides into internal and external carotid arteries. Encircled with postganglionic sympathetic nerves (PGSN), the ICA travels in the carotid sheath with the IJV and vagal nerve. C1 ends where the ICA enters the carotid canal of the petrous bone. *No branches*
2. **C2 (petrous):** still surrounded by PGSNs. Ends at the posterior edge of the foramen lacerum (f-Lac) (inferomedial to the edge of the Gasserian ganglion in Meckel's cave). Three subdivisions:
   a) vertical segment: ICA ascends then bends as the…
   b) posterior loop: anterior to the cochlea, bends antero-medially becoming the…

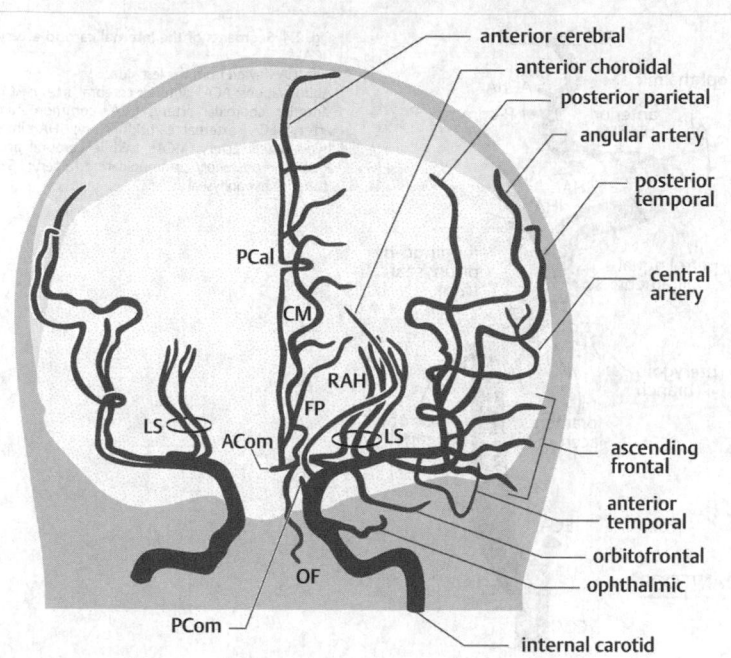

Fig. 2.3 Internal carotid arteriogram (AP view).
ACom: anterior communicating artery
CM: callosomarginal artery
FP: frontopolar artery
LS: lenticulostriate arteries
OF: orbitofrontal artery
PCal: pericallosal artery
PCom: posterior communicating artery
RAH: recurrent artery of Heubner (Reprinted courtesy of Eastman Kodak Company)

   c) horizontal segment: deep and medial to the greater and lesser superficial petrosal nerves, anterior to the tympanic membrane (TM)
3. **C3 (lacerum)**: the ICA passes over (but not through) the foramen lacerum (f-Lac) forming the lateral loop. Ascends in the canalicular portion of the f-Lac to the juxtasellar position, piercing the dura as it passes the petrolingual ligament to become the cavernous segment. Branches (usually not visible angiographically):
   a) caroticotympanic (inconsistent) ⇒ tympanic cavity
   b) pterygoid (vidian) branch: passes through the f-Lac, present in only 30%, may continue as the artery of the pterygoid canal
4. **C4 (cavernous)**: covered by a vascular membrane lining the sinus, still surrounded by PGSNs. Passes anteriorly then supero-medially, bends posteriorly (medial loop of ICA), travels horizontally, and bends anteriorly (part of anterior loop of ICA) to the anterior clinoid process. Ends at the proximal dural ring (incompletely encircles ICA). Many branches, main ones include
   a) meningohypophyseal trunk (MHT) (largest & most proximal). 2 causes of a prominent MHT: (1) tumor (usually petroclival meningioma—see below), (2) dural AVM (p.1514). 3 branches:
      1. a. of tentorium (AKA artery of Bernasconi & Cassinari): the blood supply of petroclival meningiomas
      2. dorsal meningeal a. (AKA dorsal clival a.)
      3. inferior hypophyseal a. (⇒ posterior lobe of pituitary): post-partum occlusion causes pituitary infarcts (Sheehan's necrosis); however, DI is rare because the stalk is spared
   b) anterior meningeal a.

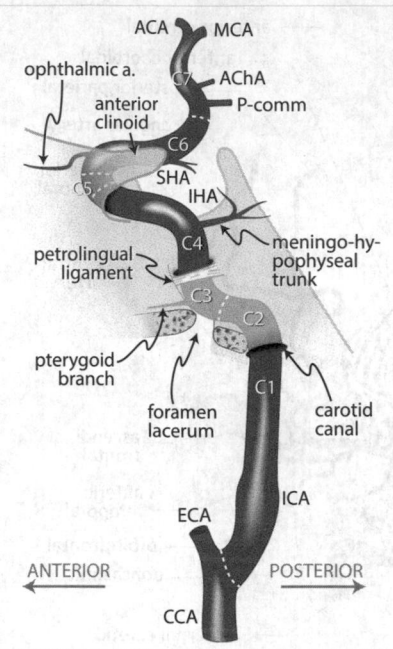

Fig. 2.4 Segments of the internal carotid artery (ICA).[6]
Left ICA viewed from the left side.
Abbreviations: ACA = anterior cerebral artery; AChA = anterior choroidal artery; CCA = common carotid artery; ECA = external carotid artery; IHA = inferior hypophyseal artery; MCA = middle cerebral artery; P-comm = posterior communicating artery; SHA = superior hypophyseal artery.

   c) a. to inferior portion of cavernous sinus (present in 80%)
   d) capsular aa. of McConnell (in 30%): supply the capsule of the pituitary[7]
5. **C5 (clinoid):** begins at the proximal dural ring, ends at the distal dural ring (which completely encircles ICA) where the ICA becomes intradural
6. **C6 (ophthalmic):** begins at distal dural ring, ends just proximal to the PComA. Branches:
   a) ophthalmic a.: the origin from the ICA is distal to the cavernous sinus in 89% (intracavernous in 8%, the ophthalmic artery is absent in 3%[8]) and can vary from 5 mm anterior to 7 mm posterior to the anterior clinoid.[7] Passes through the optic canal into the orbit (the intracranial course is very short, usually 1–2 mm[7]). Has a characteristic bayonet-like "kink" or "L" shape (depending on whether it passes above or below the optic nerve) on lateral angiogram
   b) superior hypophyseal a. branches ⇒ anterior lobe of pituitary & stalk (1st branch of supraclinoid ICA)
7. **C7 (communicating):** begins just proximal to the PComA origin, travels between Cr. N. II & III, terminates just below anterior perforated substance where it bifurcates into the ACA & MCA
   a) posterior communicating a. (PComA)
     • few anterior thalamoperforators (⇒ optic tract, chiasm & posterior hypothalamus): below
     • plexal segment: enters supracornual recess of temporal horn, ⇒ only this portion of choroid plexus
     • cisternal segment: passes through crural cistern
   b) anterior choroidal artery[9]: takeoff 2–4 mm distal to PComA ⇒ (variable) portion of optic tract, medial globus pallidus, genu of internal capsule (IC) (in 50%), inferior half of posterior limb of IC, uncus, retrolenticular fibers (optic radiation), lateral geniculate body; for occlusion syndromes (p. 1539)
8. "Carotid siphon": not a segment, but a region incorporating the cavernous, ophthalmic and communicating segments. Begins at the posterior bend of the cavernous ICA, and ends at the ICA bifurcation

Differentiating PComA from ACh on arteriogram

1. PComA origin is proximal to that of the anterior choroidal artery (ACh)
2. PComA is usually larger than ACh
3. PComA usually goes up or down a little, then straight back & usually bifurcates
4. ACh usually has a superior "hump" (plexal point) where it pass through the choroidal fissure to enter the ventricle

Anterior cerebral artery (ACA)

Passes between Cr. N. II and anterior perforated substance. See ▶ Fig. 2.5. Branches:
1. recurrent artery (of Heubner): typically arises from the area of the A1/A2 junction. Various statistics can be found in the literature regarding the percentage that arise from distal A1 vs. proximal A2.[2] It is most important to be mindful that the takeoff is variable, e.g., when treating aneurysms (one of the larger medial lenticulostriates, remainder of lenticulostriates may arise from this artery) ⇒ head of caudate, putamen, and anterior internal capsule
2. medial orbitofrontal artery
3. frontopolar artery
4. callosomarginal
   a) internal frontal branches:
      • anterior
      • middle
      • posterior
   b) paracentral artery
5. pericallosal artery (continuation of ACA)
   a) superior internal parietal (precuneate) artery
   b) inferior internal parietal artery

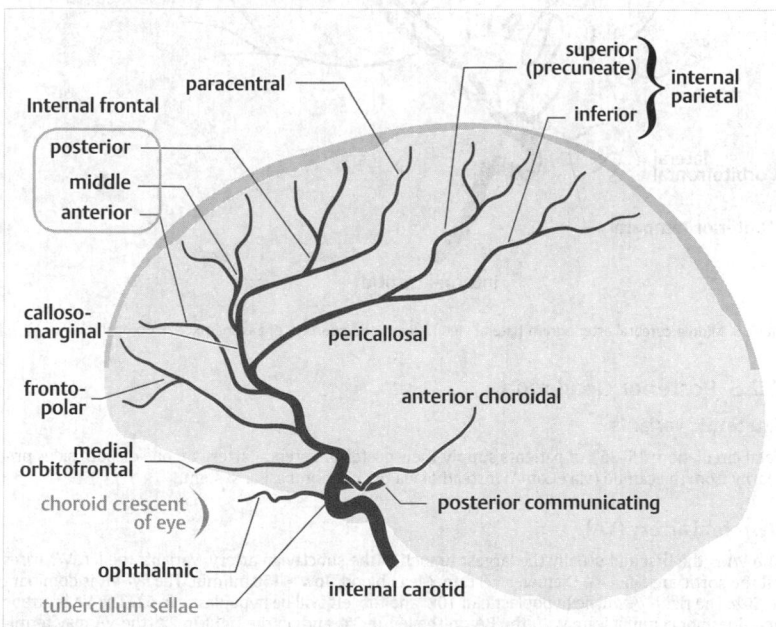

Fig. 2.5 Anterior cerebral arteriogram (lateral view). (Reprinted courtesy of Eastman Kodak Company.)

2

Anatomic variants
Hypoid: having only one anterior cerebral artery (as in a horse).

Middle cerebral artery (MCA)

See ▶ Fig. 2.6 and anatomy (p.75). Branches vary widely, 10 common ones:
1. medial (3–6 per side) and lateral lenticulostriate arteries
2. anterior temporal
3. posterior temporal
4. lateral orbitofrontal
5. ascending frontal (candelabra)
6. precentral (prerolandic)
7. central (rolandic)
8. anterior parietal (postrolandic)
9. posterior parietal
10. angular

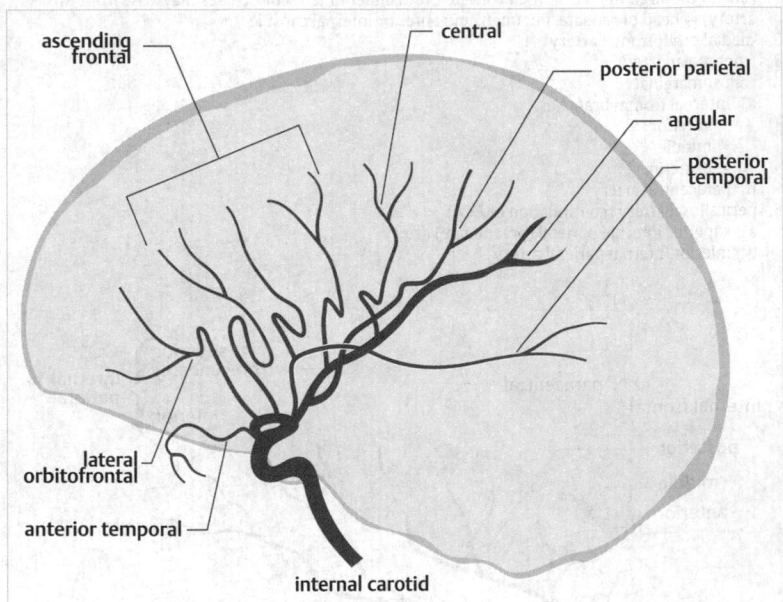

Fig. 2.6 **Middle cerebral arteriogram** (lateral view). (Reprinted courtesy of Eastman Kodak Company.)

2.2.5 Posterior circulation

Anatomic variants

Fetal circulation: 15–35% of patients supply their posterior cerebral artery on one or both sides primarily from the carotid (via PComA) instead of via the vertebrobasilar system.

Vertebral artery (VA)

The VA is the first and usually the largest branch of the subclavian artery. Variant: the left VA arises off the aortic arch in ≈ 4%. Diameter ≈ 3 mm. Mean blood flow ≈ 150 ml/min. The *left* VA is dominant in 60%. The right VA will be hypoplastic in 10%, and the left will be hypoplastic in 5%. The VA is atretic and does not communicate with the BA on the left in 3%, and on the right in 2% (the VA may terminate in PICA).

Four segments:
- **V1 prevertebral**: from subclavian artery, courses superiorly and posteriorly and enters the foramen transversarium, usually of the 6th vertebral body
- **V2** ascends vertically within the transverse foramina of the cervical vertebrae surrounded by sympathetic fibers (from the stellate ganglion) and a venous plexus. It is situated *anterior* to the cervical roots. It turns laterally to enter the foramen within the transverse process of the axis
- **V3** exits the foramen of the axis and curves posteriorly and medially in a groove on the upper surface of the atlas and enters the foramen magnum
- **V4** pierces the dura (location somewhat variable) and immediately enters the subarachnoid space. Joins the contralateral VA at the vertebral confluens located at the lower pontine border to form the basilar artery (BA)

Branches

▶ **Anterior meningeal.** Arises at body of C2 (axis), may feed chordomas or foramen magnum meningiomas, may also act as collateral in vascular occlusion

▶ **Posterior meningeal.** May be a source of blood for some dural AVMs (p.1514)

▶ **Medullary (bulbar) aa.**
▶ **Posterior spinal**
▶ **Posterior inferior cerebellar artery (PICA) (largest branch).** Usually arises ≈ 10 mm distal to point where VA becomes intradural, ≈ 15 mm proximal to the vertebrobasilar junction (▶ Fig. 2.7)
1. anatomic variants:
    a) in 5–8% the PICA has an extradural origin
    b) "AICA-PICA": origin is off basilar trunk (where AICA would usually originate)
2. 5 segments[10] (some systems describe only 4). During surgery, the first three must be preserved, but the last 2 may usually be sacrificed with minimal deficit[11]:
    a) anterior medullary: from PICA origin to inferior olivary prominence. 1 or 2 short medullary circumflex branches ⇒ ventral medulla
    b) lateral medullary: to origin of nerves IX, X & XI. Up to 5 branches that supply brainstem
    c) tonsillomedullary: to tonsillar midportion (contains *caudal loop* on angio)
    d) telovelotonsillar (supratonsillar): ascends in tonsillomedullary fissure (contains *cranial loop* on angio)
    e) cortical segments
3. 3 branches
    a) choroidal a. (BRANCH 1) arises from cranial loop (*choroidal point*), ⇒ choroid plexus of 4th ventricle
    b) terminal branches:
        - tonsillohemispheric (BRANCH 2)
        - inferior vermian (BRANCH 3) inferior inflection = *copular point* on angio

▶ **Anterior spinal**

Basilar artery (BA)

Formed by the junction of the 2 vertebral arteries. Branches:
1. anterior inferior cerebellar artery (AICA): from lower part of BA, runs posterolaterally anterior to VI, VII & VIII. Often gives off a loop that runs into the IAC and gives off the labyrinthine artery and then emerges to supply the anterolateral inferior cerebellum and then anastomoses with PICA
2. internal auditory (labyrinthine)
3. pontine branches
4. superior cerebellar a. (SCA)
    a) sup. vermian
5. posterior cerebral: joined by PComAs ≈ 1 cm from origin (the PComA is the major origin of the PCA in 15% and is termed "fetal" circulation, bilateral in 2%).
    3 segments (named for surrounding cistern) and their branches:
    a) peduncular segment (P1)
        - mesencephalic perforating aa. (⇒ tectum, cerebral peduncles, and these nuclei: Edinger-Westphal, oculomotor and trochlear)
        - interpeduncular thalamoperforators (1st of 2 groups of posterior thalamoperforating aa.)
        - medial post. choroidal (most from P1 or P2)

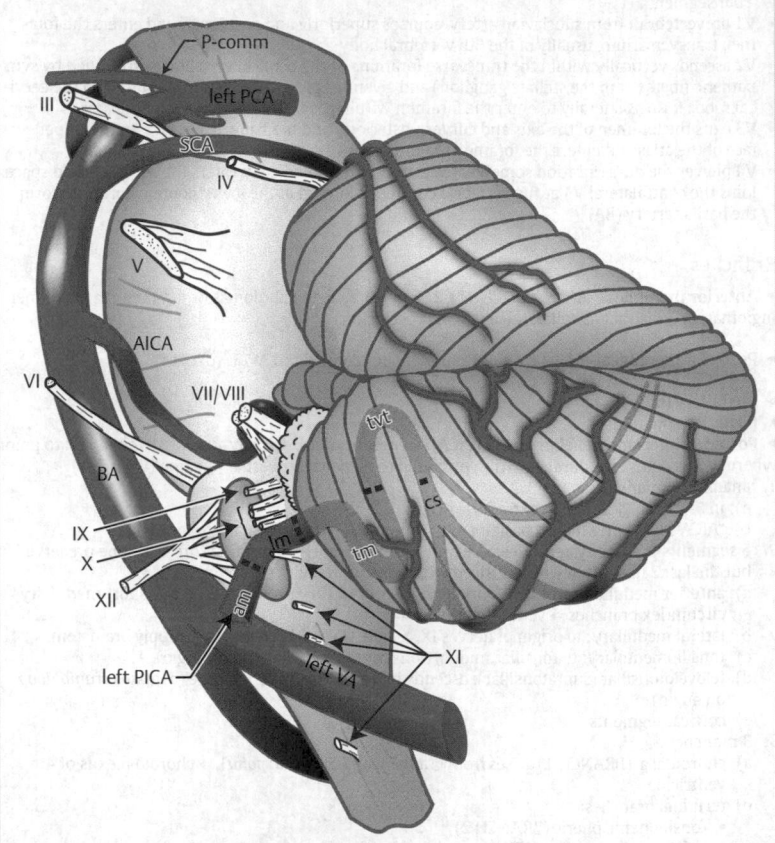

Fig. 2.7 Intradural VA and PICA segments. Lateral view. (Modified with permission from Lewis SB, Chang DJ, Peace DA, Lafrentz PJ, Day AL. Distal posterior inferior cerebellar artery aneurysms: clinical features and management. J Neurosurg 2002;97(4):756-66.)

- "artery of Percheron": a rare anatomic variant[12] in which a solitary arterial trunk arising from the proximal segment of one PCA supplies the paramedian thalami and rostral mid-brain bilaterally
  b) ambient segment (P2)
    - lateral post. choroidal (most from P2)
    - thalamogeniculate thalamoperforators (2nd of 2 groups of posterior thalamoperforating aa.) ⇒ geniculate bodies + pulvinar
    - anterior temporal (anastomoses with anterior temporal br. of MCA)
    - posterior temporal
    - parieto-occipital
    - calcarine
  c) quadrigeminal segment (P3)
    - quadrigeminal & geniculate branches ⇒ quadrigeminal plate
    - post. pericallosal (splenial) (anastomoses with pericallosal of ACA)

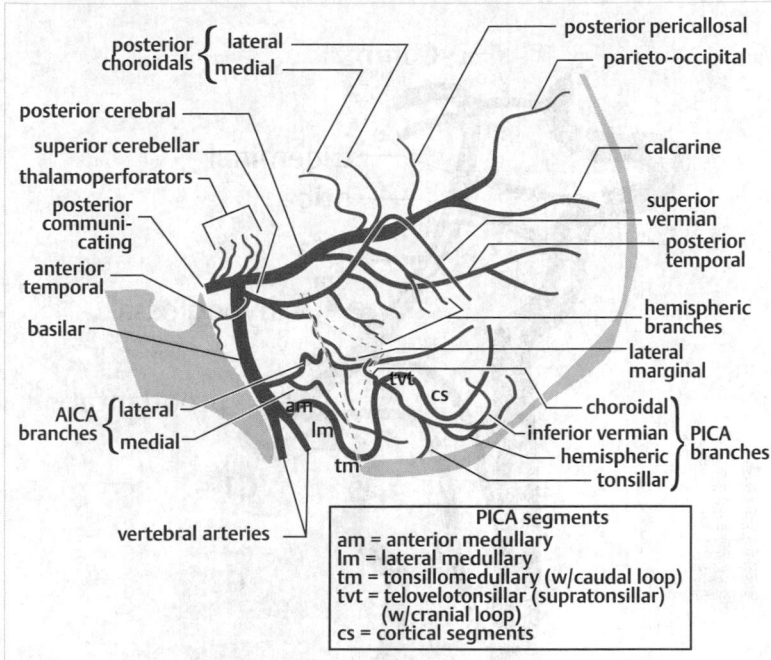

Fig. 2.8 Vertebrobasilar arteriogram. Lateral view. (Reprinted courtesy of Eastman Kodak Company.)

Posterior cerebral artery (PCA)

See ▶ Fig. 2.8.

2.2.6 Fetal carotid-vertebrobasilar anastomoses

PComA artery: the "normal" (most common) anastomosis.

Persistent fetal anastamoses[13] (▶ Fig. 2.9) result from failure to involute as the VAs and PComAs develop (order of involution: otic, hypoglossal, primitive trigeminal, proatlantal). Most are asymptomatic. However, some may be associated with vascular anomalies such as aneurysms or AVMs, and occasionally cranial nerve symptoms (e.g., trigeminal neuralgia with PPTA) can occur.

Four types (from cranial to caudal—the 1st 3 are named for the associated cranial nerve):
1. persistent primitive trigeminal artery (PPTA): seen in ≈ 0.6% of cerebral angiograms. The most common of the persistent fetal anastamoses (83%). May be associated with trigeminal neuralgia (p. 1857). Connects the cavernous carotid to the basilar artery. Arises from the ICA proximal to the origin of the meningohypophyseal trunk (50% go through sella, 50% exit the cavernous sinus & course with the trigeminal nerve) and connects to the upper basilar artery between AICA & SCA. The VAs may be small. Saltzman type 1 variant: the PComAs are hypoplastic and the PPTA provides significant blood supply to the distributions of the distal BA, PCA and the SCAs (the basilar artery is often hypoplastic). Saltzman type 2: PComA supplies PCA. Saltzman type 3: PPTA joins the SCA (instead of the BA). It is critical to recognize a PPTA before doing a Wada test (p. 1890) because of the risk of anesthetizing the brainstem, and in doing transsphenoidal surgery because of risk of arterial injury. May rarely be an explanation of posterior fossa symptoms in a patient with carotid disease
2. otic: the first to involute, and the rarest to persist (8 cases reported). Passes through IAC to connect petrous carotid to basilar artery

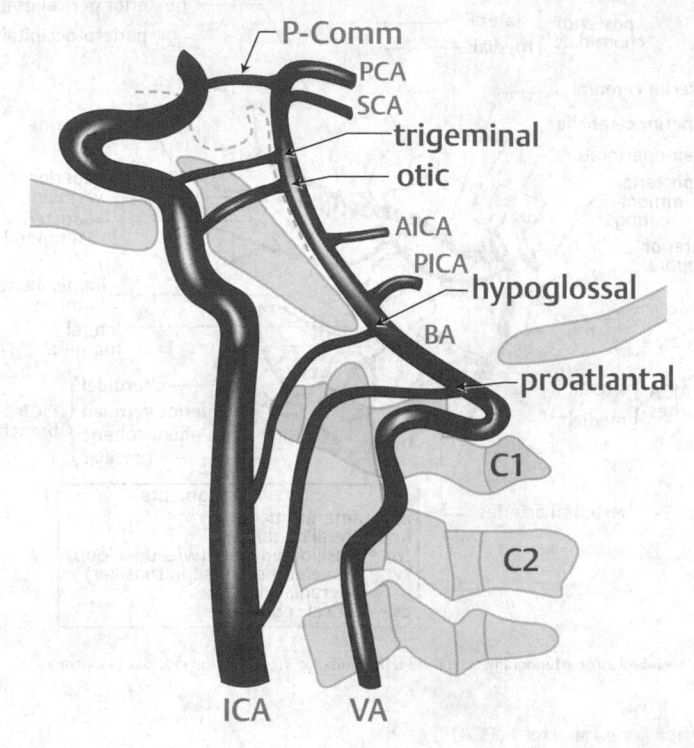

Fig. 2.9 Fetal carotid-vertebrobasilar anastomoses.
Normal adult arteries: P-Comm = posterior communicating, PCA = posterior cerebral, SCA = superior cerebellar, AICA = anterior inferior cerebellar, PICA = posterior inferior cerebellar, BA = basilar, ICA = internal carotid, VA = vertebral artery.

3. hypoglossal: connects petrous or distal cervical ICA (origin usually between C1–3) to VA. Traverses the hypoglossal canal. Does not cross foramen magnum
4. proatlantal intersegmental: connects cervical ICA to VA. May arise from: bifurcation of common carotid, ECA, or ICA from C2–4. Anastomosis with VA in suboccipital region. 50% have hypoplastic proximal VA. 40 cases reported

2.3 Cerebral venous anatomy

2.3.1 Supratentorial venous system

Major veins and tributaries

See ► Fig. 2.10 for angiogram and branches.

The left and right internal jugular veins (IJVs) are the major source of outflow of blood from the intracranial compartment. The *right* IJV is usually dominant. Other sources of outflow include orbital veins and the venous plexuses around the vertebral arteries. Diploic and scalp veins may act as collateral pathways, e.g., with superior sagittal sinus obstruction.[14] The following outline traces the venous drainage back from the IJVs.

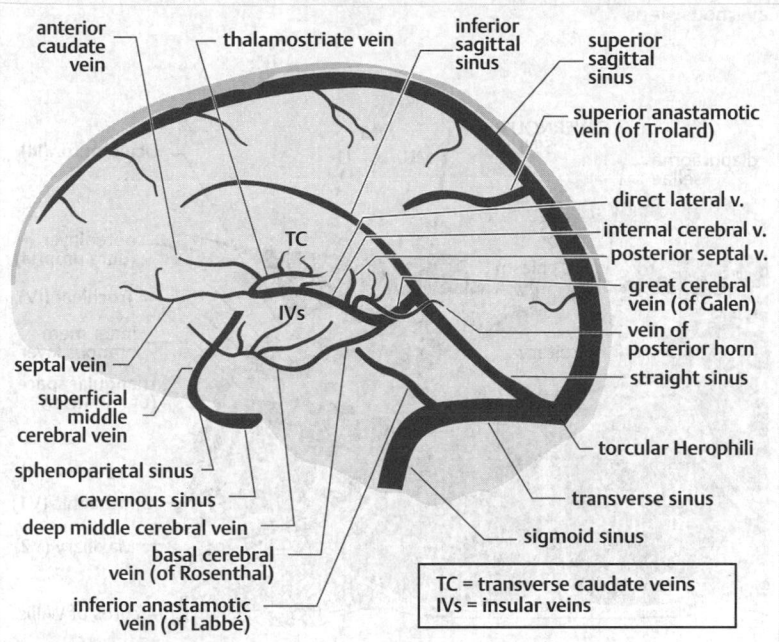

Fig. 2.10 Internal carotid venogram (lateral view). (Reprinted courtesy of Eastman Kodak Company.)

Inferior petrosal sinus
Drains to IJV near junction with sigmoid sinus.

Sigmoid sinus
Superior petrosal sinus
Terminates at sigmoid sinus within 1 cm of the junction of the sigmoid and transverse sinuses.

Transverse sinus
The right transverse sinus is dominant (i.e., R > L) in 65%.

▶ **V. of Labbe.** (Inferior anastomotic v.)

▶ **Confluence of sinuses.** (AKA torcular Herophili AKA torcula AKA confluens sinuum [TA]). Located at the internal occipital protuberance, a coming together of:
1. occipital sinus
2. superior sagittal sinus, fed by
    a) v. of Trolard (superior anastomotic v.): the prominent superficial vein on the *non-dominant* side (Labbé is more prominent on the dominant side)
    b) cortical veins
3. straight sinus, fed by
    a) inferior sagittal sinus
    b) great cerebral v. (of Galen)
        • pre-central cerebellar v.
        • basal vein of Rosenthal
        • internal cerebral v.: joined at the foramen of Monro (venous angle) by:
            anterior septal v.
            thalamostriate v.

2

Cavernous sinus

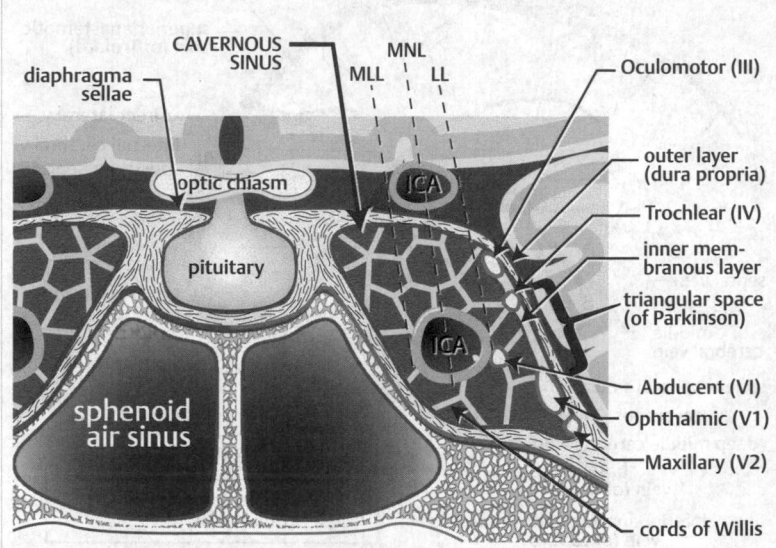

Fig. 2.11 Right cavernous sinus (colored in blue).
Stylized diagram of coronal cut through the cavernous sinuses.
3 lines passing through the intracavernous and supracavernous portion of the ICA may be used to classify the degree of tumor invasion: MLL (medial line) tangent to the medial borders of ICA cuts, MNL (median line) through middle of ICA cuts, & LL (lateral line) tangent to the lateral edges of ICA cuts (p. 884).

Originally named for its superficial resemblance to the corpora cavernosa. Although classical teaching depicts the cavernous sinus as a large venous space with multiple trabeculations, injection studies[15] and surgical experience[16] instead support the concept of the cavernous sinus as a plexus of veins. It is highly variable between individuals and from side-to-side. ▶ Fig. 2.11 is an oversimplified schematic of one section through the right cavernous sinus.

1. inflowing veins:
   a) superior & inferior ophthalmic veins
   b) superficial middle cerebral veins
   c) sphenoparietal sinus
   d) superior & inferior petrosal sinus
2. outflow:
   a) sphenoparietal sinus
   b) superior petrosal sinus
   c) basilar plexus (which drains to the inferior petrosal sinus)
   d) pterygoid plexus
   e) the right and left cavernous sinuses communicate anteriorly and posteriorly via the circular sinus
3. contents[17]
   a) oculomotor n. (cranial nerve III)
   b) trochlear n. (IV)
   c) ophthalmic division of trigeminal n. (V1)
   d) maxillary division of trigeminal n. (V2): the only nerve of the cavernous sinus that doesn't exit the skull through the superior orbital fissure (it exits through foramen rotundum)
   e) internal carotid artery (ICA). 3 segments within the cavernous sinus
      • posterior ascending segment: immediately after ICA enters the sinus

- horizontal segment: after ICA turns anteriorly (the longest segment of the intracavernous ICA)
- anterior ascending segment: ICA turns superiorly
  f) abducens n. (VI): the only nerve NOT attached to lateral dural wall, therefore sometimes considered as the only cranial nerve *inside* the cavernous sinus
4. triangular space (of Parkinson): superior border formed by Cr. N. III & IV, and the lower margin formed by V1 & VI (a landmark for surgical entrance to the cavernous sinus)[18,19(p 3007)]

2.3.2 Posterior fossa venous anatomy

See ▶ Fig. 2.12.

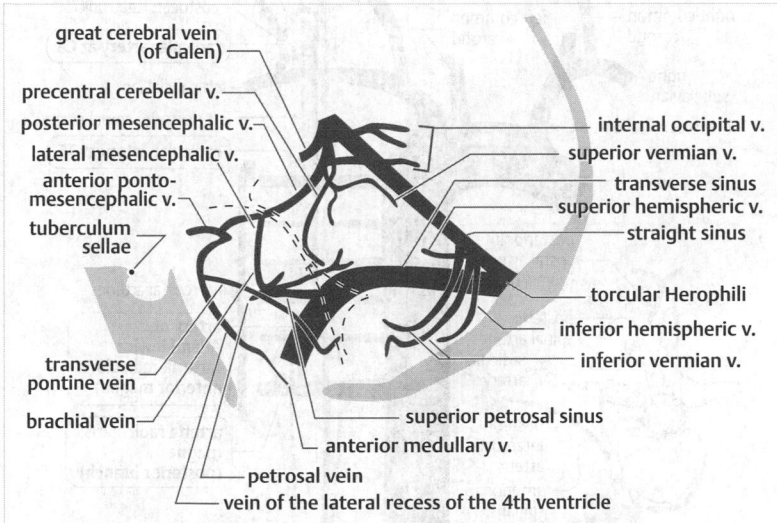

great cerebral vein (of Galen)
precentral cerebellar v.
posterior mesencephalic v.
lateral mesencephalic v.
anterior ponto-mesencephalic v.
tuberculum sellae
transverse pontine vein
brachial vein

internal occipital v.
superior vermian v.
transverse sinus
superior hemispheric v.
straight sinus
torcular Herophili
inferior hemispheric v.
inferior vermian v.
superior petrosal sinus
anterior medullary v.
petrosal vein
vein of the lateral recess of the 4th ventricle

Fig. 2.12 Vertebrobasilar venogram. Lateral view. (Reprinted courtesy of Eastman Kodak Company.)

2.4 Spinal cord vasculature

See ▶ Fig. 2.13. Although a radicular artery from the aorta accompanies the nerve root at many levels, most of these contribute little flow to the spinal cord itself. The anterior spinal artery is formed from the junction of two branches, each from one of the vertebral arteries. It supplies blood to the anterior 2/3 of the spinal cord (▶ Fig. 2.14). Branches include sulcal arteries which also supply the anterior horns of the gray matter. Major contributions to the anterior spinal cord are from 6–9 radicular arteries in variable locations, which may include the following ("radiculomedullary arteries," the levels listed are fairly consistent, but the side varies[20(p 1180–1)]):

1. C3—arises from vertebral artery
2. C6 and C8 (≈ 10% of population lack an anterior radicular artery in lower cervical spine[21])
   a) C6—usually arises from deep cervical artery
   b) C8—usually from costocervical trunk
3. T4 or T5
4. artery of Adamkiewicz AKA arteria radicularis anterior magna
   a) the main arterial supply for the spinal cord from ≈ T8 to the conus
   b) located on the left in 80%[22]
   c) situated between T9 & L2 in 85% (between T9 & T12 in 75%); in remaining 15% between T5 & T8 (in these latter cases, there may be a supplemental radicular artery further down)

2

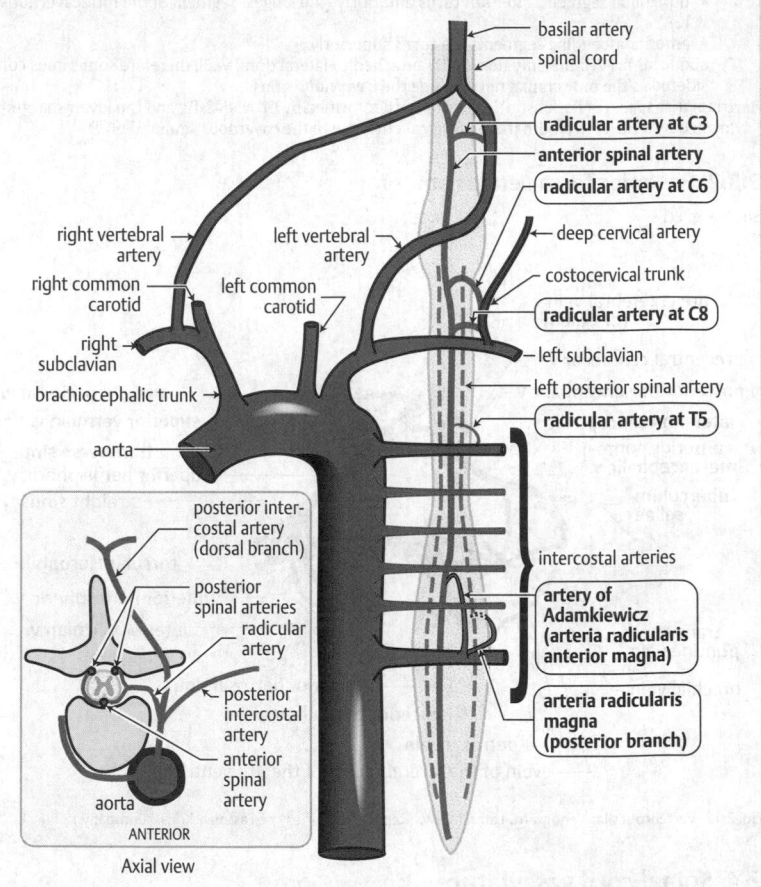

Fig. 2.13 Spinal cord arterial supply. Schematic diagram. (Modified from Diagnostic Neuroradiology, 2nd ed., Volume II, pp. 1181, Taveras J M, Woods EH, editors, © 1976, the Williams and Wilkins Co., Baltimore, with permission.)

    d) usually fairly large, gives off cephalic and caudal branch (latter is usually larger) giving a characteristic hair-pin appearance on angiography

The paired posterior spinal arteries are less well-defined than the anterior spinal artery, and are fed by 10–23 radicular branches. Anastamotic vessels between the anterior and posterior spinal arteries are called vasocorona.

The midthoracic region has a tenuous vascular supply ("watershed zone"), possessing only the above noted artery at T4 or T5. It is thus more susceptible to vascular insults.

▶ **Anatomic variants.** Arcade of Lazorthes: normal variant where the anterior spinal artery joins with the paired posterior spinal arteries at the conus medullaris.

2

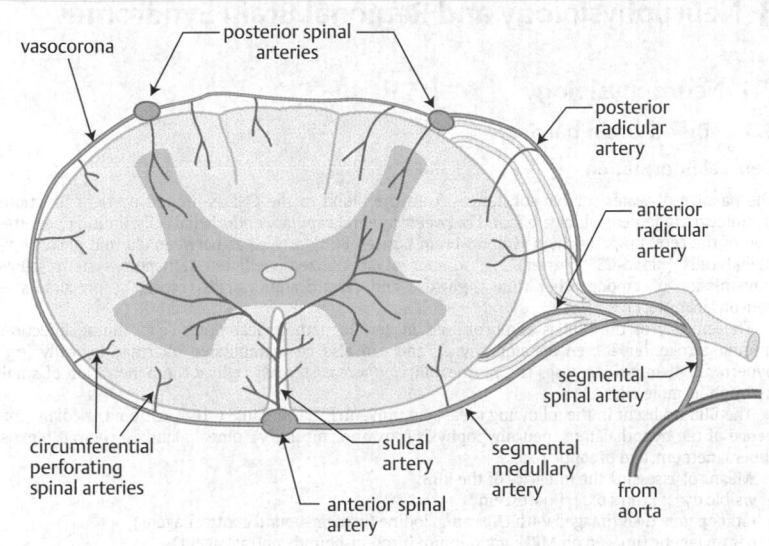

Fig. 2.14 Segmental blood supply to the spinal cord.

References

[1] van der Zwan A, Hillen B, Tulleken CAF, et al. Variability of the Territories of the Major Cerebral Arteries. Journal of Neurosurgery. 1992; 77:927–940

[2] Loukas M, Louis RG,Jr, Childs RS. Anatomical examination of the recurrent artery of Heubner. Clin Anat. 2006; 19:25–31

[3] Krayenbühl HA, Yasargil MG. Cerebral Angiography. 2nd ed. London: Butterworths; 1968:80–81

[4] Krayenbühl H, Yasargil MG, Huber P. Rontgenanatomie und Topographie der Hirngefasse. In: Zerebrale Angiographie fur Klinik und Praxis. Stuttgart: Georg Thieme Verlag; 1979:38–246

[5] Ecker A, Riemenschneider PA. Angiographic Localization of Intracranial Masses. Springfield, Illinois: Charles C. Thomas; 1955

[6] Bouthillier A, van Loveren HR, Keller JT. Segments of the internal carotid artery: A new classification. Neurosurgery. 1996; 38:425–433

[7] Gibo H, Lenkey C, Rhoton AL. Microsurgical Anatomy of the Supraclinoid Portion of the Internal Carotid Artery. Journal of Neurosurgery. 1981; 55:560–574

[8] Renn WH, Rhoton AL. Microsurgical Anatomy of the Sellar Region. Journal of Neurosurgery. 1975; 43:288–298

[9] Rhoton AL,Jr. The supratentorial arteries. Neurosurgery. 2002; 51:S53–120

[10] Lister JR, Rhoton AL, Matsushima T, et al. Microsurgical Anatomy of the Posterior Inferior Cerebellar Artery. Neurosurgery. 1982; 10:170–199

[11] Getch CC, O'Shaughnessy B A, Bendok BR, et al. Surgical management of intracranial aneurysms involving the posterior inferior cerebellar artery. Contemporary Neurosurgery. 2004; 26:1–7

[12] Percheron G. The anatomy of the arterial supply of the human thalamus and its use for the interpretation of the thalamic vascular pathology. Z Neurol. 1973; 205:1–13

[13] Luh GY, Dean BL, Tomsick TA, et al. The persistent fetal carotid-vertebrobasilar anastomoses. AJR Am J Roentgenol. 1999; 172:1427–1432

[14] Schmidek HH, Auer LM, Kapp JP. The Cerebral Venous System. Neurosurgery. 1985; 17:663–678

[15] Taptas JN. The So-Called Cavernous Sinus: A Review of the Controversy and Its Implications for Neurosurgeons. Neurosurgery. 1982; 11:712–717

[16] Sekhar LN, Sekhar LN, Schramm VL. Operative Management of Tumors Involving the Cavernous Sinus. In: Tumors of the Cranial Base: Diagnosis and Treatment. Mount Krisco: Futura Publishing; 1987:393–419

[17] Umansky F, Nathan H. The Lateral Wall of the Cavernous Sinus: With Special Reference to the Nerves Related to It. J Neurosurg. 1982; 56:228–234

[18] van Loveren HR, Keller JT, El-Kalliny M, et al. The Dolenc Technique for Cavernous Sinus Exploration (Cadaveric Prosection). Journal of Neurosurgery. 1991; 74:837–844

[19] Youmans JR. Neurological Surgery. Philadelphia 1982

[20] Taveras JM, Wood EH. Diagnostic Neuroradiology. 2nd ed. Baltimore: Williams and Wilkins; 1976

[21] Turnbull IM, Breig A, Hassler O. Blood Supply of the Cervical Spinal Cord in Man. A Microangiographic Cadaver Study. Journal of Neurosurgery. 1966; 24:951–965

[22] El-Kalliny M, Tew JM, van Loveren H, et al. Surgical approaches to thoracic disk herniations. Acta Neurochirurgica. 1991; 111:22–32

3 Neurophysiology and Regional Brain Syndromes

3.1 Neurophysiology

3.1.1 Blood-brain barrier

General information

The passage of water-soluble substances from the blood to the CNS is limited by tight junctions (zonulae occludentes) which are found between cerebral capillary endothelial cells, limiting penetration of the cerebral parenchyma (blood-brain barrier, BBB), as well as between choroid plexus epithelial cells (blood-CSF barrier).[1] A number of specialized mediated transport systems allow transmission of, among other things, glucose and certain amino acids (especially precursors to neurotransmitters).

The efficacy of the BBB is compromised in certain pathological states (e.g., tumor, infection, trauma, stroke, hepatic encephalopathy...), and can also be manipulated pharmacologically (e.g., hypertonic mannitol increases the permeability, whereas steroids reduce the penetration of small hydrophilic molecules).

The BBB is absent in the following areas: circumventricular organs[2] (area postrema, median eminence of the hypothalamus, neurohypophysis (posterior pituitary), pineal gland...) choroid plexus, tuber cinereum, and preoptic recess.

Means of assessing the integrity of the BBB:
* visible dyes: Evan's blue, fluorescein
* radioopaque dyes (imaged with CT scan[3]): iodine (protein-bound contrast agent)
* paramagnetic (imaged on MRI): gadolinium (protein-bound contrast agent)
* microscopic: horseradish peroxidase
* radiolabeled: albumin, sucrose

Cerebral edema and the blood-brain barrier

Two basic types of cerebral edema; diffusion-weighted MRI (p.243) may be able to differentiate:
1. cytotoxic: BBB is closed, therefore no protein extravasation, therefore no enhancement on CT or MRI. Cells swell then shrink. Classic examples: cell death due to head trauma or stroke
2. vasogenic: BBB is disrupted. Protein (serum) leaks out of vascular system, and therefore may enhance on imaging. Extracellular space (ECS) expands. Cells are stable. Responds to corticosteroids (e.g., dexamethasone). Seen, e.g., surrounding metastatic brain tumor

Cerebral edema related to ischemia may be a combination of the above. BBB is closed initially, but then may open. ECS shrinks then expands. Fluid extravasates late. May cause delayed deterioration following intracerebral hemorrhage (p.1615)

3.1.2 Language and speech function

Localizing language function

Caveat: Language function cannot be reliably localized on anatomic grounds alone due to individual variability. In order to perform maximal brain resections (e.g., for tumor) while minimizing the risk of aphasia, techniques such as awake intraoperative brain mapping (p.1735)[4] need to be employed.

Classic model

The model of speech and language function that was accepted for years was that of 2 primary areas, Wernicke's area (Brodmann area 40 and part of 39), which subserved language, and Broca's area (Brodmann area 44), which was considered the "motor speech" area, both located in the dominant hemisphere (▶ Fig. 1.1). These two areas were thought to communicate via the arcuate fasciculus (p.246).

Lesions in Wernicke's area were classically thought to produce "receptive aphasias," wherein the patient could not understand language. Some of these patients demonstrated "fluent aphasia," in which they generated speech without content. Conversely, patients with lesions in Broca's area would exhibit "expressive aphasia," wherein they could comprehend language, but lacked the motor ability to generate speech. "Conduction aphasia" was considered to be the result of damage to the arcuate fasciculus.

Dual stream model of language

A model that incorporates current understanding of speech and language[5] (▶ Fig. 3.1).

Region 1: (primary auditory areas) initial processing of language.

The ventral stream flows from Region 1 to Region 2 (anterior and middle temporal lobe) and is involved in speech recognition and lexical concepts.

The dorsal stream maps phonological information onto motor areas (Regions 4 (premotor cortex) & 5 (≈ Broca's area)).

Regions 3 (≈ Wernicke's area), 4 & 5 are all involved in dorsal stream processing.

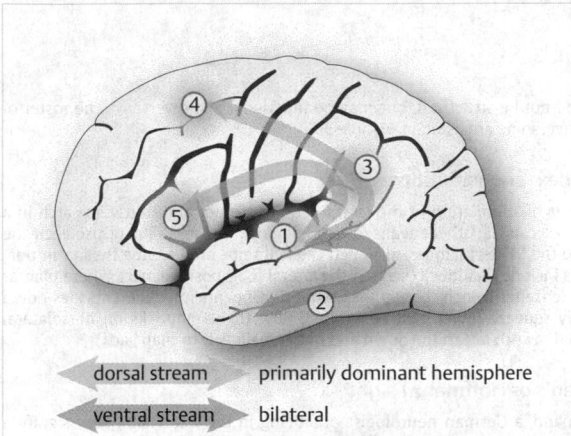

Fig. 3.1 Dual stream model of language function.
See text for descriptions of numbered green shaded Regions 1–5.

dorsal stream — primarily dominant hemisphere

ventral stream — bilateral

3.1.3 Babinski sign and Hoffmann sign

Introduction

Although the Babinski sign is regarded as the most famous sign in neurology, there is still disagreement over what constitutes a normal response and when abnormal responses should occur.[6] The following represents one interpretation.

The plantar reflex (PR) (AKA Babinski sign after Joseph François Félix Babinski [1857–1932], a French neurologist of Polish descent) is a primitive reflex, present in infancy, consisting of extension of the great toe in response to a noxious stimulus applied to the foot. The small toes may fan, but this is not a consistent nor clinically important component. The PR disappears usually at ≈ 10 months of age (range: 6 mos to 12 yrs), presumably under inhibitory control as myelination of the CNS occurs, and the normal response then converts to plantarflexion of the great toe. An upper motor neuron (UMN) lesion anywhere along the pyramidal (corticospinal) tract from the motor strip down to ≈ L4 will result in a loss of inhibition, and the PR will be "unmasked" producing extension of the great toe. With such an UMN lesion, there may also be associated flexor synergy resulting in concurrent dorsiflexion of the ankle, and flexion of the knee and hip (AKA triple flexor response) in addition to extension of the great toe.

Neuroanatomy

The afferent limb of the reflex originates in cutaneous receptors restricted to the first sacral dermatome (*S1*) and travels proximally via the tibial nerve. The spinal cord segments involved in the reflex-arc lie within *L4–2*. The efferent limb to the toe extensors travels via the *peroneal nerve*.

Table 3.1 Differential diagnosis of the plantar reflex (PR)

Etiologies
• spinal cord injuries[a]
• cervical spinal myelopathy
• lesions in motor strip or internal capsule (stroke, tumor, contusion…)
• subdural or epidural hematoma
• hydranencephaly
• toxic-metabolic coma
• seizures
• trauma
• TIAs
• hemiplegic migraine
• motor neuron disease (ALS)

[a]In spinal cord injuries, the PR may initially be absent during the period of spinal "shock" (p. 1119)

Differential diagnosis

Etiologies

Lesions producing a PR need not be structural, but may be functional and reversible. The roster of possible etiologies is extensive, some are listed in ▶ Table 3.1.

Eliciting the plantar reflex, and variations

The optimal stimulus consists of stimulation of the lateral plantar surface and transverse arch in a single movement lasting 5–6 seconds.[7] Other means for applying noxious stimuli may also elicit the plantar reflex (even outside the S1 dermatome, although these do not produce toe flexion in normals). Described maneuvers include Chaddock (scratch the lateral foot; positive in 3% where plantar stimulation was negative), Schaeffer (pinch the Achilles tendon), Oppenheim (slide knuckles down shin), Gordon (momentarily squeeze lower gastrocnemius), Bing (light pinpricks on dorsolateral foot), Gonda or Stronsky (pull the 4th or 5th toe down and out and allow it to snap back).

Hoffmann's (or Hoffman's or Hoffmann) sign

Attributed to Johann Hoffmann, a German neurologist practicing in the late 1800s. May signify a similar UMN interruption to the upper extremities. Elicited by flicking downward on the nail of the middle or ring finger: a positive (pathologic) response consists of involuntary flexion of the adjacent fingers and/or thumb (may be weakly present in normals).[8] Differs from the plantar reflex since it is monosynaptic (synapse in Rexed lamina IX).

Can sometimes be seen as normal in a young individual with diffusely brisk reflexes & positive jaw jerk, usually symmetric. When present pathologically, represents disinhibition of a C8 reflex, ∴ indicates lesion above C8.

Hoffmann sign was observed in 68% of patients operated on for cervical spondylotic myelopathy.[8] In 11 patients presenting with lumbar symptoms but no myelopathy, a bilateral Hoffman sign was associated with occult cervical spinal cord compression in 10 (91%).[8] The Hoffmann test has a sensitivity of 33–68%, a specificity of 59–78%, a positive predictive value of 26–62% and a negative predictive value of 67–75%.[9]

Conclusion: Hoffmann sign has too low a predictive value for it to be relied upon by itself as a screening tool for, or as an indication of the presence of, myelopathy.[9,10]

3.1.4 Bladder neurophysiology

Central pathways

The primary coordinating center for bladder function resides within the nucleus locus coeruleus of the pons. This center synchronizes bladder contraction with relaxation of the urethral sphincter during voiding.[11]

Voluntary cortical control primarily involves inhibition of the pontine reflex, and originates in the anteromedial portion of the frontal lobes and in the genu of the corpus callosum. In an uninhibited bladder (e.g., infancy), the pontine voiding center functions without cortical inhibition and the detrusor muscle contracts when the bladder reaches a critical capacity. Voluntary suppression from the cortex via the pyramidal tract may contract the external sphincter and may also inhibit detrusor contraction. Cortical lesions in this location → urgency incontinence with inability to suppress the micturition reflex.[12 (p 1031)]

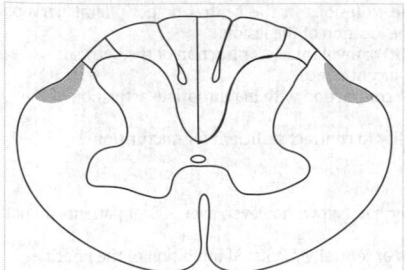

Fig. 3.2 Location of spinal cord bladder efferents in the spinal cord (shaded).

Efferents to the bladder travel in the dorsal portion of the lateral columns of the spinal cord (shaded areas in ▶ Fig. 3.2).

Motor

There are two sphincters that prevent the flow of urine from the bladder: internal (autonomic, involuntary control), and external (striated muscle, voluntary control).

Parasympathetics (PSN)

The detrusor muscle of the bladder contracts and the internal sphincter relaxes under PSN stimulation. PSN preganglionic cell bodies reside in the intermediolateral gray of spinal cord segments S2–4. Fibers exit as ventral nerve roots and travel via pelvic splanchnic nerves (nervi erigentes) to terminate on ganglia within the wall of the detrusor muscle in the body and dome of the bladder. These are the target receptors of anticholinergic medications and onabotulinumtoxinA (Botox™).[13]

Sympathetics

Sympathetic cell bodies lie within the intermediolateral gray column of lumbar spinal cord from segments T12–L2. Preganglionic axons pass through the sympathetic chain (without synapsing) to the inferior mesenteric ganglion. Postganglionic fibers pass through the inferior hypogastric plexus to the bladder wall and internal sphincter. Sympathetics heavily innervate the bladder neck and trigone. Stimulation of alpha-1 adrenergic receptors results in bladder neck closure allowing bladder filling and urine storage. Beta-3 adrenergic receptor stimulation results in detrusor smooth muscle relaxation during bladder filling and storage.[14]

Pelvic nerve stimulation → increased sympathetic tone → detrusor relaxation & increased bladder neck tone (allowing a larger volume to be accommodated).

Somatic nerves

Somatic voluntary control descends in the pyramidal tract to synapse on motor nerves in S2–4, and then travels via the pudendal nerve to the external sphincter. This sphincter may be voluntarily contracted, but relaxes reflexly with opening of the internal sphincter at the initiation of micturition. Primarily maintains continence during ↑ vesical pressure (e.g., Valsalva).

Sensory

Bladder wall stretch receptors sense bladder filling and send afferent signals via myelinated A-delta fibers (aid sensation during filling and emptying) and unmyelinated C fibers (sense noxious stimuli, thought to be involved in involuntary detrusor overactivity in neurogenic bladder[15]). These fibers run through the pelvic, pudendal, and hypogastric nerves to spinal cord segments T10–2 & S2–4. Fibers ascend primarily in the spinothalamic tract.

Urinary bladder dysfunction

General information

Bladder management is vital to protect the kidneys from obstruction and subsequent loss of renal function.

3

Neurogenic bladder: bladder dysfunction due to lesions in the central or peripheral nervous systems. Clinical manifestations differ based on the location of the lesion.
* detrusor hyperreflexia (detrusor overactivity (DO)): involuntary contraction of the detrusor muscle → sensation of urgency & possible urge incontinence
* detrusor-sphincter dyssynergia (DSD): detrusor contraction with inappropriate activation of the external urethral sphincters
* detrusor areflexia: loss of bladder tone → inability to contract sufficient for micturition[16]

Specific injuries affecting the bladder

Classic descriptions of location of lesions are described below; however, over 50% of patients do not have classic presentation or symptoms.

1. supraspinal (lesions above the brainstem): loss of centrally mediated inhibition of the pontine voiding reflex. Voluntary inhibition of micturition is lost. Coordination of detrusor filling and contraction with smooth and striated urinary sphincters is intact, allowing maintenance of normal bladder pressures with low risk of high pressure renal damage. Patients have DO without DSD. Detrusor hypertrophy is less pronounced. Symptoms: urinary frequency or urgency, urgency incontinence, and nocturia.[11] If sensory pathways are interrupted, unconscious incontinence occurs (insensate incontinence AKA incontinence of the unawares type). Voluntary bladder emptying may be maintained and timed voiding together with anticholinergic medications (see below) are used in management. Areflexia may sometimes occur

2. complete (or near complete) spinal cord lesions:
    a) suprasacral (lesion *above* the S2 spinal *cord* level, which is ≈ T12/L1 vertebral body level in an adult): loss of innervation to the pontine micturition center results in reflexive voiding modulated by the sacral voiding center (located in the conus medullaris).[17]
    Etiologies: spinal cord injuries, tumors, transverse myelitis.
       * initially following spinal cord injury, there may be spinal shock. During spinal shock (p. 1119), the bladder is acontractile and areflexic (detrusor areflexia); sphincter tone usually persists and urinary retention is the rule (urinary incontinence generally does not occur except with overdistention). This requires catheter drainage (intermittent or indwelling) due to retention until the spinal shock resolves typically within 6 months[17]
       * after spinal shock subsides, most develop *detrusor hyperreflexia* → involuntary bladder contractions without sensation (automatic bladder), smooth sphincter synergy, but striated dyssynergy (involuntary contraction of the external sphincter during voiding which produces a functional outlet obstruction with poor emptying and high vesical pressures which is transmitted to the kidneys and may result in loss of renal function). Bladder fills and empties spontaneously due to reflexive voiding.[17] Bladder hypertrophy occurs due to contraction against a closed sphincter and bladder storage pressure increases. Patients have DO with DSD. Management goals: decrease bladder pressures and preserve renal function, usually with pharmaceuticals and intermittent catheterizations. The frequency of bladder drainage is determined by urodynamic pressures to ensure urine volumes consistent with safe storage pressures (see below).
    b) infrasacral lesions (lesion below the S2 spinal cord level): includes injury to conus medullaris, cauda equina or peripheral nerves (formerly referred to as lower motor neuron lesions). Etiologies: large HLD, trauma with compromise of spinal canal or peripheral nerve injuries (traumatic or iatrogenic with pelvic surgery). Detrusor areflexia usually ensues, and do not have voluntary or involuntary bladder contractions. Reduced urinary flow rate or retention results, and voluntary voiding may be lost. Overflow incontinence develops. Usually associated with loss of bulbocavernosus (BCR) and anal wink reflexes (preserved in suprasacral lesions, except when spinal shock is present (p. 1119)) and perineal sensory loss. NB: up to 20% of neurologically normal patients do not exhibit a BCR[18]

3. specific disease processes
    a) herniated lumbar disc (p. 1250): most consist initially of difficulty voiding, straining, or urinary retention. Later, irritative symptoms may develop
    b) spinal stenosis (lumbar or cervical): urologic symptoms vary, and depend on the spinal level (s) involved and the type of involvement (e.g., in cervical spinal stenosis, detrusor hyperactivity or underactivity may occur depending on whether the involvement of the micturition neural axis is compression of the inhibitory reticulospinal tracts or myelopathy involving the posterior funiculus)
    c) cauda equina syndrome (p. 1254): usually produces urinary retention, although sometimes incontinence may occur (some cases are overflow incontinence)

  d) peripheral neuropathies: such as with diabetes, usually produce impaired detrusor activity
  e) neurospinal dysraphism: most myelodysplastic patients have an areflexic bladder with an open bladder neck. The bladder usually fills until the resting residual fixed external sphincter pressure is exceeded and the leakage occurs
  f) multiple sclerosis: 50–90% of patients develop voiding symptoms at some point. The demyelination primarily involves the posterior and lateral columns of the cervical spinal cord. Detrusor hyperreflexia is the most common urodynamic abnormality (in 50–99% of cases), with bladder areflexia being less common (5–20%). Patients have DO with DSD without upper tract injury or loss of compliance
  g) tethered cord: urologic complaints are present on initial presentation 30–70% of the time. Most common urologic symptoms are urgency and incontinence. Urodynamic findings show DO with DSD.[19] Urinary dysfunction improves in more than half, but not all patients, after surgical correction[20]

Urinary retention

Etiologies of urinary retention:
1. bladder outlet obstruction (a brief differential diagnosis list is presented here)
   a) urethral stricture: retention tends to be progressive over time
   b) prostatic enlargement in males:
      • benign prostatic hypertrophy (BPH) & prostate cancer: retention tends to be progressive over time
      • acute prostatitis: onset of retention may be *sudden*
   c) women: bladder or vaginal prolapse which can produce a urethral kink
   d) obstructing thrombus from hematuria (clot retention)
   e) bladder calculi
   f) bladder or urethral foreign bodies
   g) urethral cancer: rare
2. detrusor areflexia or hypotonia
   a) spinal cord lesion
      • trauma
      • tumor
      • myelomeningocele
   b) cauda equina syndrome (p. 1254)
   c) medications: anticholinergics, narcotics
   d) diabetes mellitus (autonomic neuropathy)
   e) herpes zoster at the level of the sacral dorsal root ganglia[21] (p 967)
3. postoperative urinary retention (POUR): occurs in ~ 4% of all surgeries, and 20–40% in neurosurgical patients after general anesthesia.[22,23] Felt to be secondary to combination of patient predisposition (eg BPH) along with anesthetic. Propofol, narcotics, benzodiazepines, inhaled anesthetics, and local intrathecal and epidural have all been shown to impact bladder contraction and coordination of micturition. POUR should be managed with CIC or indwelling catherization along with alpha blockers (see below) in men. Voiding trial may be done as soon as postoperative day 1 to avoid prolonged catheterization but keeping the Foley for 3–4 days has been shown to decrease need for replacement of the catheter.[23] POUR may persist > 1 week. Preoperative use of alpha blockers in at risk patients has shown protective against POUR in some studies, but not significant difference in other studies.[24] Urgent intervention is recommended to avoid long term sequela of bladder distention

Evaluation of bladder function

Urodynamics (UDS)

Usually combined with X-ray (cystometrogram [CMG]) or fluoro (videourodynamics). Measures intravesicular pressures during retrograde bladder filling through a urethral catheter, usually combined with sphincter electromyography. Assesses intravesical pressures during filling and voiding. Objectively assesses detrusor muscle at time of sensation to void. Most importantly, assesses bladder compliance, bladder storage pressures and risk for long term upper tract deterioration. Bladder pressures: < 40 cm H_2O is the cut off for safe storage pressures.[25] If bladder pressure > 40 cm H_2O during storage of urine, there is a high risk of progressive CKD. Routine UDS can help ensure safe management of a neurogenic bladder. UDS can also be used in the neurologically intact patient to determine if urinary retention is secondary to obstruction versus bladder areflexia.[26]

Voiding cystourethrogram and intravenous pyelography (IVP)

Voiding cystourethrogram (VCUG) detects urethral pathology (diverticula, strictures…), abnormalities of bladder (diverticula, detrusor trabeculations associated with long-standing contractions against high resistance…), and vesical-ureteral reflux. VCUG can be performed at the time of UDS (video urodynamics).

Urologic follow-up

Routine follow-up is needed to ensure bladder pressures < 40 cm H_2O, and subsequently for periodic renal imaging and monitoring of serum creatinine.

Changes in voiding symptoms should trigger prompt reevaluation.

NB: patient with indwelling catheters (Foley, suprapubic tube…) or intermittent catheterization will have colonization of their urine. Treatment for positive urine cultures is only indicated when related symptoms develop or when undergoing instrumentation.

Pharmacologic treatment for bladder dysfunction

Muscarinic anticholinergics

Bladder contraction is produced by ACh-mediated stimulation of postganglionic parasympathetic muscarinic cholinergic receptors on bladder smooth muscle. Anticholinergics bind M2 and M3 choline receptors and prevent stimulation. This increases bladder capacity by 50 ml and decreases bladder storage pressures by 15 cm H_2O.[27] They are a pillar in treating neurogenic bladders.

All are contraindicated in glaucoma as anticholinergics induce mydriasis. Overdosage results in the classic anticholinergic symptoms ("red as a beet, hot as a stove, dry as a rock, mad as a hatter"). Use is often limited by side effects including dry mouth, constipation, dry eyes, blurry vision, urinary retention & indigestion.

Anticholinergics may negatively impact cognition and memory.[28,29] Newer agents (tolterodine, darifenacin) have less impact on memory. Trospium, a quaternary amine, crosses the blood-brain barrier less readily than other anticholinergics and may have less negative impact.[29]

Drug info: Oxybutynin (Ditropan®)

Widely prescribed agent. Combines anticholinergic activity with independent musculotropic relaxant effect and local anesthetic activity. Immediate release (IR) produces the most side effects (including cognitive) in the class, which are better with extended release (ER).

℞ Adult IR: 5–30 mg divided TID. ER: 10–30 mg/d. Patch (Oxytrol) 3.7 mg q 3 d. ℞ Peds: not recommended for age < 5 years; usual dose is 5 mg BID (maximum 5 mg TID). **Supplied:** 5 mg tablets, 5 mg/5 ml syrup.

Drug info: Tolterodine (Detrol®)

Milder side effects than oxybutynin, but may also be less effective.[30] Side effects with IR > ER.

℞ IR: 2–8 mg PO divided BID. Can be lowered to 1 mg PO BID in some patients. ER: 2–8 mg qd. **Supplied:** 1 & 2 mg tablets. Detrol® LA 2 & 4 mg capsule

Drug info: Solifenacin (Vesicare®)

Most constipation in class.

℞ 5–10 mg qd. **Supplied:** ER & 10 mg tablets.

Drug info: Darifenacin (Enablex®)

℞ 5–10 mg po qd. **Supplied:** ER 7.5 & 15 mg tablets.

Drug info: Fesoterodine (Toviaz®)

R:4 mg PO qd, may increase up to 8 mg po qd PRN. **Supplied:** ER 4 & 8 mg tablets.

Drug info: Trospium (Sanctura®, Sanctura® XR)

R:IR: 20–60 mg po divided BID, ER: capsule 60 mg po qd. **Supplied:** IR: 20 mg tablets, ER: 60 mg capsule.

Alpha blockers

Alpha-adrenoreceptor antagonists block alpha-1 receptors on the bladder neck which results in smooth muscles relaxation and decreased bladder outlet resistance. This increases bladder compliance and decreases storage pressures with neurogenic bladders. Terazosin also decreases the frequency and severity of symptoms of autonomic dysreflexia.[27] Side effects include postural hypotension, rhinitis and retrograde ejaculation. Hypotension is more common in less selective alpha blockers and therefore dose escalation is required with terazosin and doxazosin.

Drug info: Tamsulosin (Flomax®)

A prostate alpha$_{1A}$ adrenoreceptor antagonist. Used to treat voiding difficulties resulting from outlet obstruction due to benign prostatic hypertrophy (BPH). Has some effectiveness in women via other mechanisms. Similar to terazosin (Hytrin®) and doxazosin (Cardura®), but has an advantage for acute relief because the dose of tamsulosin does not need to be gradually ramped up (it can be started at the therapeutic dose). It takes at least 5–7 days to work.

Side effects : very few. Rhinitis, retrograde or diminished ejaculation, or postural hypotension may occur.[31]

R: 0.4 mg PO qd (usually given 30 minutes after the same meal each day). If there is no response by 2–4 weeks, a dose of 0.8 mg PO qd can be tried.[31]

Botulinum toxin (Botox™)

Botulinum toxin A (BTX-A) inhibits acetylcholine exocytosis from parasympathetic postganglionic nerves to the M2 and M3 receptors of the detrusor, inhibiting detrusor contraction. BTX-A (100–200u) is injected into the detrusor muscle during cystoscopy. It decreases overactivity, urgency, and storage pressures.[32] Efficacy lasts 3–12 months and repeat injections are required. Maximum Botox dose is 360 u per 90 day from all sources. Side effects include urinary tract infection and urinary retention. In patient not already managed with catherization, must be aware of the risk of urinary retention and need for temporary catheterization in 2–20% of patients.[32] This is usually self-limited to weeks or months as the BTX-A wears off.

Neuromodulation for bladder dysfunction

Permanent implantable neuromodulation (e.g., InterStim™ by Medtronic) is indicated for refractory urinary urgency, frequency, urge incontinence, non-obstructive urinary retention, and fecal incontinence. If a trial with a temporary lead placed adjacent to the sacral nerve via the S3 foramen produces > 50% reduction in symptoms, it is connected to an implantable pulse generator. Mechanism of action is poorly understood but may modulate the afferent signals of the micturition reflex.[33] Improvement in symptoms is seen in up to 70% of patients with complete resolution in incontinence around 39%.[34] Contraindications to implantation include failure to improve with trial and the likely need for repeated MRIs in the future (the device is MRI conditional for head only with ≤ 1.5 tesla MRI).

3

Bladder management after acute urinary retention

In situations where there is urinary retention (e.g., following cauda equina compression) with some prospect of return of function (e.g., following surgery for acute cauda equina compression) the following bladder management regimen may be employed:

- early bladder management is key to avoid bladder overdistention & permanent injury to the detrusor
- use of intermittent catheterization (if able to be performed), or indwelling catheter (Foley or suprapubic) to drain bladder with a goal of < 400 ml each time (or volumes lower than patient's safe bladder capacity if known)
- initiate alpha blockers (e.g., tamsulosin (Flomax®) (p. 97) 0.4 mg PO q d (see above)
- urology consultation for assistance with long-term follow-up & bladder management

3.2 Regional brain syndromes

This section serves to briefly describe typical syndromes associated with lesions in various areas of the brain. Unless otherwise noted, the described syndromes occur with *destructive* lesions.

3.2.1 Overview

1. frontal lobe
   a) unilateral injury:
      - may produce few clinical findings except with very large lesions
      - bilateral or large unilateral lesions: apathy, abulia
      - the frontal eye field (for contralateral gaze) is located in the posterior frontal lobe (Br. area 8, shown as the striped area in ▶ Fig. 1.1). Destructive lesions impair gaze to the contralateral side (patient looks *toward* the side of the lesion), whereas irritative lesions (i.e., seizures) cause the center to activate, producing contralateral gaze (patient looks *away* from the side of the lesion). See also **Extraocular muscle (EOM) system** (p. 596) for more details.
   b) bilateral injury: may produce apathy, abulia
   c) olfactory groove region: may produce Foster Kennedy syndrome (p. 100)
   d) prefrontal lobes control "executive function": planning, prioritizing, organizing thoughts, suppressing impulses, understanding the consequences of decisions
2. parietal lobe: major features (see below for details)
   a) either side: cortical sensory syndrome, sensory extinction, contralateral homonymous hemianopia, contralateral neglect
   b) dominant parietal lobe lesion (left in most): language disorders (aphasias), Gerstmann syndrome (p. 99), bilateral astereognosis
   c) non-dominant parietal lobe lesions: topographic memory loss, anosognosia and dressing apraxia
3. occipital lobe: homonymous hemianopsia
4. cerebellum
   a) lesions of the cerebellar hemisphere cause ataxia in the *ipsilateral* limbs
   b) lesions of the cerebellar vermis cause truncal ataxia
5. brainstem: usually produces a mixture of cranial nerve deficits and long tract findings (see below for some specific brainstem syndromes)
6. pineal region
   a) Parinaud's syndrome (p. 101)

3.2.2 Parietal lobe syndromes

See reference.[35](p 308–12)

Parietal lobe anatomy

The parietal lobe is located behind the central sulcus, above the Sylvian fissure, merging posteriorly into the occipital lobe (the border on the medial surface of the brain is defined by a line connecting the parieto-occipital sulcus to the pre-occipital notch).

3

Parietal lobe neurophysiology

- either side: anterior parietal cortex organizes tactile precepts (probably contralateral) and integrates with visual and auditory sensation to build awareness of body and its spatial relations
- dominant side (on left in 97% of adults): understanding language, includes "cross-modal matching" (auditory-visual, visual-tactile, etc.). Dysphasia present with dominant lobe lesions often impedes assessment
- non-dominant side (right in most): integrates visual and proprioceptive sensation to allow manipulation of body and objects, and for certain constructional activities

Clinical syndromes of parietal lobe disease

Overview

1. *unilateral* parietal lobe disease (dominant or non-dominant):
   a) cortical sensory syndrome (see below) and sensory extinction (neglecting 1 of 2 simultaneously presented stimuli). Large lesion → hemianesthesia
   b) congenital injury → mild hemiparesis & contralateral muscle atrophy
   c) homonymous hemianopia or visual inattentiveness
   d) occasionally: anosognosia
   e) neglect of contralateral half of body and visual space (more common with right side lesions)
   f) abolition of *optokinetic nystagmus* to one side
2. additional effects of dominant parietal lobe lesion (left in most people):
   a) language disorders (aphasias)
   b) speech-related or verbally mediated functions, e.g., cross-modal matching (e.g., patient understands spoken words and can read, but cannot understand sentences with elements of relationships)
   c) Gerstmann syndrome, named for Josef Gerstmann (1887-1969). Localizes to the angular and supramarginal gyrus (Brodmann area 39 & 40 respectively) of the dominant hemispehre. Classically:
      - agraphia without alexia (patients cannot write but can still read)
      - left-right confusion
      - digit agnosia: inability to identify finger by name
      - acalculia (or dyscalculia): difficulty with math
   d) tactile agnosia (bilateral astereognosis)
   e) bilateral ideomotor apraxia (inability to carry out verbal commands for activities that can otherwise be performed spontaneously with ease)
3. additional effects of non-dominant parietal lobe lesions (usually right):
   a) topographic memory loss
   b) anosognosia and dressing apraxia

Cortical sensory syndrome

Lesion of postcentral gyrus, especially area that maps to hand.
- sensory deficits:
  a) loss of position sense and of passive movement sense
  b) inability to localize tactile, thermal, and noxious stimuli
  c) astereognosis (inability to judge object size, shape, and identity by feel)
  d) agraphesthesia (cannot interpret numbers written on hand)
  e) loss of two point discrimination
- preserved sensations: pain, touch, pressure, vibration, temperature
- other features
  a) easy fatigability of sensory perceptions
  b) difficulty distinguishing simultaneous stimulations
  c) prolongation of superficial pain with hyperpathia
  d) touch hallucinations

Anton-Babinski syndrome

A unilateral asomatognosia. May seem more common with non-dominant (usually right) parietal lesions because it may be obscured by the aphasia that occurs with dominant (left) sided lesions.

1. anosognosia (indifference or unawareness of deficits, patient may deny that paralyzed extremity is theirs)
2. apathy (indifference to failure)
3. allocheiria (one-sided stimuli perceived contralaterally)
4. dressing apraxia: neglect of one side of body in dressing and grooming
5. extinction: patient is unaware of contralateral stimulus when presented with double-sided simultaneous stimulation
6. inattention to an entire visual field (with or without homonymous hemianopia), with deviation of head, eyes, and torsion of body to unaffected side

3.2.3 Foster Kennedy syndrome

Named after neurologist Robert Foster Kennedy. Usually from olfactory groove or medial third sphenoid wing tumor (usually meningioma). Now less common due to earlier detection by CT or MRI. Classic triad:
1. ipsilateral anosmia
2. *ipsilateral* central scotoma (with optic *atrophy* due to pressure on optic nerve)
3. *contralateral* papilledema (from elevated ICP)

Occasionally ipsilateral proptosis will also occur due to orbital invasion by tumor.

3.2.4 Cerebellar mutism & syndromes of the posterior fossa

General information

▸ **Cerebellar mutism (CM).** AKA mutism with subsequent dysarthria.
   Definition: speechlessness that develops following various cerebellar injuries[36] including cerebellar trauma,[37,38] stroke,[39] hemorrhage,[40] and viral cerebellitis.[41] However, it is most frequently encountered in children subsequent to resection of posterior fossa brain tumors.
   Essentially always improves, but almost never back to normal. The anatomical substrate has not been definitively identified
   Cerebellar mutism (CM) may occur in isolation, or may be encountered as part of other more global syndromes that involve the posterior fossa:
1. cerebellar mutism syndrome: CM, ataxia, hypotonia & irritability, which may be encountered as part of #2 (the following item)[42]
2. posterior fossa syndrome: cerebellar mutism syndrome + cranial nerve deficits, neurobehavioral changes & urinary incontinence or retention

▸ **Cerebellar syndrome.** Ataxia, dysmetria & nystagmus.[42] CM is *not* part of the cerebellar syndrome.

Epidemiology

Incidence of CM: 11–29% of children following surgery for cerebellar tumors[36] including medulloblastoma (53%), ependymoma (33%) & pilocytic astrocytoma (11%).[43] Risk factors for post-op CM following surgery for medulloblastoma in children: brainstem involvement & midline location.[44]
   Post-op CM has been observed in ≈ 1% of adults following p-fossa surgery.[45]

Clinical characteristics

CM is characterized by delayed onset (mean: 1.7 days post-op, range: 1–6 days),[46] limited duration (mean: 6.8 weeks, range: 4 d–4 months),[46] and long-term linguistic sequelae (in 98.8% of patients).[47]

Pathophysiological correlate

The underlying disease mechanism remains elusive. Theories include: postoperative vasospasm, cerebellar ischemia, and edema, as well as transient dysregulation of neurotransmitter release. However, the most widely accepted explanation is cerebellar diaschisis[47] (from the Greek: διάσχισις meaning "shocked throughout"): metabolic hypofunction in a brain region distant but connected to an area of brain injury. Specifically: CM has been linked to the disruption of cerebello-cerebral circuits, such as the dentate thalamocortical tract, which originates in the dentate nucleus, extends through the superior cerebellar peduncle, and decussates to the contralateral cerebral hemisphere, where it connects the ventrolateral nucleus of the thalamus to diverse cortical areas.[48] SPECT scans demonstrated transient reduction of cerebral perfusion in frontal, parietal, and temporal cortices of patients with post-op CM.[49,50] In this manner, a supratentorial condition is provoked by disruption of connections to the cerebellum as a result of cerebellar injury.

Treatment & prevention

Treatment is limited to supportive measures: speech & rehabilitation therapy.

Post-op CM may be prevented by avoiding midline splitting of the cerebellar vermis (e.g., by using the telovelar approach to the 4th ventricle). However, results are conflicting and general recommendation for surgical strategies to avoid CM cannot be made at this time.

3.2.5 Brainstem and related syndromes

Weber's syndrome

Cr. N. III palsy with contralateral hemiparesis; also see Lacunar strokes (p. 1540). Third nerve palsies from parenchymal lesions may be relatively pupil sparing.

Benedikt's syndrome

Similar to Weber's, plus red nucleus lesion. Cr. N. III palsy with contralateral hemiparesis except arm which has hyperkinesia, ataxia, and a coarse intention tremor. Lesion: midbrain tegmentum involving red nucleus, brachium conjunctivum, and fascicles of III.

Millard-Gubler syndrome

Facial (VII) & abducens (VI) palsy + contralateral hemiplegia (corticospinal tract) from lesion in base of pons (usually ischemic infarct, occasionally tumor).

3.2.6 Parinaud's syndrome

Definition

AKA dorsal midbrain syndrome, AKA pretectal syndrome. As originally described, a supranuclear paralysis of vertical gaze resulting from damage to the mesencephalon.[51]

There are a number of somewhat varying descriptions; however, most include:

- supranuclear upward gaze palsy (i.e., upgaze palsy affecting both voluntary saccadic and pursuit movements, with preservation of vestibulo-ocular or oculocephalic [doll's eyes] reflexes in most cases). Horizontal eye movements are spared
- lid retraction (Collier's sign): NB: upgaze palsy + lid retraction produces the "setting sun sign"
- convergence palsy
- accommodation palsy
- less common associations: pseudoabducens palsy (AKA thalamic esotropia), see-saw nystagmus, fixed pupils, dissociated light-near response (pseudo-Argyll Robertson), convergence spasm, nystagmus retractorius, internuclear ophthalmoplegia (INO)

Skew deviation may be a unilateral variant of Parinaud's syndrome.

Syndrome of the Sylvian aqueduct: Parinaud's syndrome (PS) combined with downgaze palsy.

Differential diagnosis

Etiologies
1. masses pressing directly on quadrigeminal plate (e.g., pineal region tumors)
2. elevated ICP: secondary to compression of mesencephalic tectum by dilated suprapineal recess, e.g., in hydrocephalus
3. stroke or hemorrhage in upper brainstem
4. multiple sclerosis (MS)
5. occasionally seen with toxoplasmosis

Conditions affecting ocular motility that could mimic the upgaze palsy of PS:
1. Guillain-Barré syndrome
2. myasthenia gravis

3. botulism
4. hypothyroidism
5. there may be a gradual benign loss of upgaze with senescence

3.3 Jugular foramen syndromes

3.3.1 Applied anatomy

The jugular foramen (JF) is one of a pair of openings between the lateral part of the occipital bone and the petrous part of the temporal bone. The foramen is usually divided in 2 by a bony spine from the petrous temporal bone that attaches via a fibrous bridge (which is bony in 26%) to the jugular process of the occipital bone.[52] The right JF is usually larger than the left.[52,53] The carotid ridge separates the JF from the nearby carotid canal. Contents of jugular foramen (JF): Cr. N. IX, X, XI, petrosal sinus, sigmoid sinus, some meningeal branches from the ascending pharyngeal and occipital arteries.[54]

Nearby: Cr. N. XII passes through the hypoglossal canal just above the occipital condyle. The carotid artery with the sympathetic plexus enters the carotid canal.

Compartmentalization of the jugular foramen remains controversial. As many as 4 foramina have been described over the years. Although it had been recognized previously, an early 2-compartment description was published in 1967 by Hovelacque.[55] In this, the bony spine (± its fibrous septum) divides the foramen into:

- pars vascularis: the larger posterolateral compartment containing the vagal nerve (and branching Arnold's nerve), spinal accessory nerve and the internal jugular vein
- pars nervosa: the smaller anteromedial compartment containing the glossopharyngeal nerve (and branching Jacobson's nerve), inferior petrosal sinus and meningeal branch of the ascending pharyngeal artery

A publication in 1997 described these 3 compartments[56]:

- sigmoid: large posterolateral compartment containing sigmoid sinus
- petrosal: smaller anteromedial compartment containing petrosal sinus
- intrajugular or neural: CN IX, X, and XI

3.3.2 Clinical syndromes

General information

A number of eponymous syndromes with some conflicting findings in the literature have been described. See ▶ Table 3.2 for a summary and ▶ Fig. 3.3 for a schematic diagram of deficits in various jugular foramen syndromes.

Table 3.2 Cranial nerve dysfunction in jugular foramen syndromes

Nerve	Result of lesion	Syndrome					
		Vernet	Collet Sicard	Villaret	Tapia	Jackson	Schmidt
IX	loss of taste and sensation in posterior third of tongue	X	X	X			
X	paralysis of vocal cords & palate, anesthesia of pharynx & larynx	X	X	X	X	X	X
XI	weak trapezius & SCM	X	X	X	±	X	X
XII	tongue paralysis & atrophy		X	X	X	X	
sympathetics	Horner syndrome			X	±		

Key: X indicates dysfunction / deficit (lesion) of that nerve; ± indicates involvement may or may not occur

Vernet's syndrome: CN IX, X & XI palsy

AKA syndrome of the jugular foramen. Usually due to intracranial lesion.

Etiologies include: jugular foramen tumors, ICA dissections, mycotic aneurysms of the external carotid, thrombosis of the jugular vein, following carotid endarterectomy.

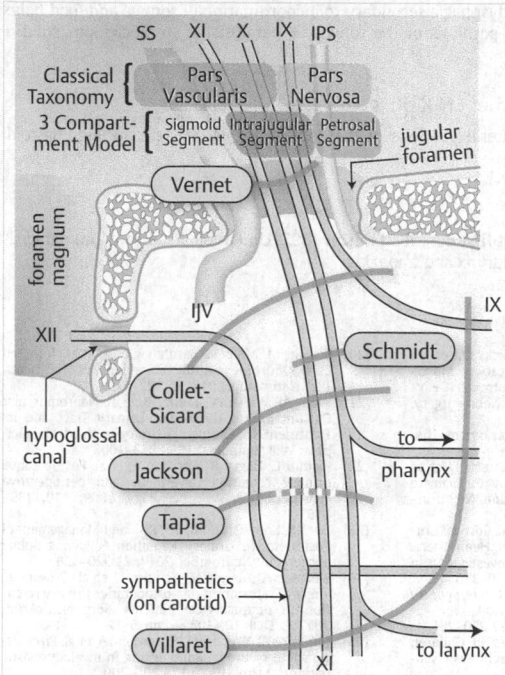

Fig. 3.3 Jugular foramen. Schematic diagram (coronal section through left jugular foramen viewed from the front). Includes the classic 2 compartment model and the 3 compartment classification of Katsuta et al.[56]

Jugular foramen syndromes are illustrated: a solid line through a nerve indicates a deficit, dashed line indicates ± involvement.

Abbreviations: SS = sigmoid sinus; IJV = inferior jugular vein; IPS = inferior petrosal sinus; Roman numerals denote cranial nerve numbers.

Symptoms: unilateral paralysis of the palate, vocal cords, sternocleidomastoid, trapezius, with loss of taste in the posterior 1/3 tongue, anesthesia of the soft palate, larynx and pharynx.

Collet-Sicard syndrome

Palsies of CN IX, X, XI & XII without sympathetic involvement. More likely with lesion outside skull. If caused by an intracranial lesion, it would have to be of such a large size that it would usually produce brainstem compression → long tract findings.

Etiologies include condylar and Jefferson's fractures, internal carotid dissection, primary and metastatic tumors, Lyme disease, and fibromuscular dysplasia.

Symptoms: unilateral paralysis of the palate, vocal cords, sternocleidomastoid, trapezius, tongue, loss of taste in posterior 1/3 tongue, anesthesia of soft palate, larynx and pharynx.

Villaret's syndrome: CN IX, X, XI & XII palsy + sympathetic dysfunction

AKA posterior retropharyngeal syndrome, AKA the nervous syndrome of the posterior retroparotid space). Collet-Sicard syndrome with sympathetic involvement. Usually due to retropharyngeal leasions.

Etiologies include: parotid tumors, metastases, external carotid aneurysm and osteomyelitis of the skull base.

Symptoms: as with Collet-Sicard + Horner syndrome.

Tapia syndrome: CN X & XII palsy (± XI)

AKA Matador's disease (first described in a bullfighter by Antonio Garcia Tapia). Some authors describe an intracranial and extracranial form.[57]

Etiologies include: oral intubation (majority of cases prior to 2013), metastases, rarely associated with carotid or vertebral artery dissections.

Symptoms: hoarseness of voice, dysphagia secondary to incoordination of tongue and food bolus propulsion, unilateral atrophy and paralysis of the tongue, ± paralysis of sternocleidomastoid & trapezius, sparing the soft palate.

(Hughlings) Jackson's syndrome: CN X, XI & XII palsy

First described in 1864 with unilateral paralysis of the soft palate, larynx, sternocleidomastoid, trapezius and tongue.

Schmidt syndrome: CN X & XI

AKA vago-spinal syndrome. Schmidt first described this in 1892. Unilateral vocal cord and paralysis of sternocleidomastoid, soft palate, larynx and trapezius.

References

[1] Neuwelt EA, Barnett PA, McCormick CI, et al. Osmotic Blood-Brain Barrier Modification: Monoclonal Antibody, Albumin, and Methotrexate Delivery to Cerebrospinal Fluid and Brain. Neurosurgery. 1985; 17:419–423

[2] Kaur C, Ling EA. The circumventricular organs. Histol Histopathol. 2017; 32:879–892

[3] Neuwelt EA, Maravilla KR, Frenkel EP, et al. Use of Enhanced Computerized Tomography to Evaluate Osmotic Blood-Brain Barrier Disruption. Neurosurgery. 1980; 6:49–56

[4] Ojemann G, Ojemann J, Lettich E, et al. Cortical Language Localization in Left, Dominant Hemisphere. An Electrical Stimulation Mapping Investigation in 117 Patients. J Neurosurg. 1989; 71:316–326

[5] Chang EF, Raygor KP, Berger MS. Contemporary model of language organization: an overview for neurosurgeons. J Neurosurg. 2015; 122:250–261

[6] Marcus JC. Flexor Plantar Responses in Children With Upper Motor Neuron Lesions. Archives of Neurology. 1992; 49:1198–1199

[7] Dohrmann GJ, Nowack WJ. The Upgoing Great Toe: Optimal Method of Elicitation. Lancet. 1973; 1:339–341

[8] Houten JK, Noce LA. Clinical correlations of cervical myelopathy and the Hoffmann sign. Journal of Neurosurgery (Spine). 2008; 9:237–242

[9] Glaser JA, Cure JK, Bailey KL, et al. Cervical spinal cord compression and the Hoffmann sign. Iowa Orthopaedic Journal. 2001; 21:49–52

[10] Grijalva RA, Hsu FP, Wycliffe ND, et al. Hoffmann sign: clinical correlation of neurological imaging findings in the cervical spine and brain. Spine (Phila Pa 1976). 2015; 40:475–479

[11] MacDiarmid SA. The ABCs of Neurogenic Bladder for the Neurosurgeon. Contemporary Neurosurgery. 1999; 21:1–8

[12] Youmans JR. Neurological Surgery. Philadelphia 1982

[13] Hegde SS. Muscarinic receptors in the bladder: from basic research to therapeutics. Br J Pharmacol. 2006; 147 Suppl 2:S80–S87

[14] Bragg R, Hebel D, Vouri SM, et al. Mirabegron: a Beta-3 agonist for overactive bladder. Consult Pharm. 2014; 29:823–837

[15] Consortium for Spinal Cord Medicine. Bladder management for adults with spinal cord injury: a clinical practice guideline for health-care providers. J Spinal Cord Med. 2006; 29:527–573

[16] Gajewski JB, Schurch B, Hamid R, et al. An International Continence Society (ICS) report on the terminology for adult neurogenic lower urinary tract dysfunction (ANLUTD). Neurourol Urodyn. 2018; 37:1152–1161

[17] Taweel WA, Seyam R. Neurogenic bladder in spinal cord injury patients. Res Rep Urol. 2015; 7:85–99

[18] Blaivas JG, Zayed AA, Labib KB. The bulbocavernosus reflex in urology: a prospective study of 299 patients. J Urol. 1981; 126:197–199

[19] Giddens JL, Radomski SB, Hirshberg ED, et al. Urodynamic findings in adults with the tethered cord syndrome. J Urol. 1999; 161:1249–1254

[20] Selcuki M, Mete M, Barutcuoglu M, et al. Tethered Cord Syndrome in Adults: Experience of 56 Patients. Turk Neurosurg. 2015; 25:922–929

[21] Wein AJ, Walsh PC, Retik AB, et al. Neuromuscular Dysfunction of the Lower Urinary Tract and Its Treatment. In: Campbell's Urology. 7th ed. Philadelphia: W.B. Saunders; 1998:953–1006

[22] Baldini G, Bagry H, Aprikian A, et al. Postoperative urinary retention: anesthetic and perioperative considerations. Anesthesiology. 2009; 110:1139–1157

[23] Lee KS, Koo KC, Chung BH. Risk and Management of Postoperative Urinary Retention Following Spinal Surgery. Int Neurourol J. 2017; 21:320–328

[24] Basheer A, Alsaidi M, Schultz L, et al. Preventive effect of tamsulosin on postoperative urinary retention in neurosurgical patients. Surg Neurol Int. 2017; 8. DOI: 10.4103/sni.sni_5_17

[25] McGuire EJ, Woodside JR, Borden TA, et al. Prognostic value of urodynamic testing in myelodysplastic patients. J Urol. 1981; 126:205–209

[26] Nitti VW. Pressure flow urodynamic studies: the gold standard for diagnosing bladder outlet obstruction. Rev Urol. 2005; 7 Suppl 6:S14–S21

[27] Cameron AP. Medical management of neurogenic bladder with oral therapy. Transl Androl Urol. 2016; 5:51–62

[28] Moga DC, Carnahan RM, Lund BC, et al. Risks and benefits of bladder antimuscarinics among elderly residents of Veterans Affairs Community Living Centers. J Am Med Dir Assoc. 2013; 14:749–760

[29] Kay GG, Ebinger U. Preserving cognitive function for patients with overactive bladder: evidence for a differential effect with darifenacin. Int J Clin Pract. 2008; 62:1792–1800

[30] Tolterodine for Overactive Bladder. Medical Letter. 1998; 40:101–102

[31] Tamsulosin for Benign Prostatic Hyperplasia. Medical Letter. 1997; 39

[32] Weckx F, Tutolo M, De Ridder D, et al. The role of botulinum toxin A in treating neurogenic bladder. Transl Androl Urol. 2016; 5:63–71

[33] Sukhu T, Kennelly MJ, Kurpad R. Sacral neuromodulation in overactive bladder: a review and current perspectives. Res Rep Urol. 2016; 8:193–199

[34] Herbison GP, Arnold EP. Sacral neuromodulation with implanted devices for urinary storage and voiding dysfunction in adults. Cochrane Database Syst Rev. 2009. DOI: 10.1002/14651858.CD004202.pub2

[35] Adams RD, Victor M. Principles of Neurology. 2nd ed. New York: McGraw-Hill; 1981

[36] Gudrunardottir T, Sehested A, Juhler M, et al. Cerebellar mutism: review of the literature. Childs Nerv Syst. 2011; 27:355–363

[37] Ersahin Y, Mutluer S, Saydam S, et al. Cerebellar mutism: report of two unusual cases and review of the literature. Clin Neurol Neurosurg. 1997; 99:130–134

[38] Turgut M. Transient "cerebellar" mutism. Childs Nerv Syst. 1998; 14:161–166

[39] Nishikawa M, Komiyama M, Sakamoto H, et al. Cerebellar mutism after basilar artery occlusion–case report. Neurol Med Chir (Tokyo). 1998; 38:569–573

[40] De Smet HJ, Marien P. Posterior fossa syndrome in an adult patient following surgical evacuation of an intracerebellar haematoma. Cerebellum. 2012; 11:587–592

[41] Kubota T, Suzuki T, Kitase Y, et al. Chronological diffusion-weighted imaging changes and mutism in the course of rotavirus-associated acute cerebellitis/cerebellopathy concurrent with encephalitis/encephalopathy. Brain Dev. 2011; 33:21–27

[42] Gudrunardottir T, Sehested A, Juhler M, et al. Cerebellar mutism: definitions, classification and grading of symptoms. Childs Nerv Syst. 2011; 27:1361–1363

[43] Catsman-Berrevoets C E, Van Dongen HR, Mulder PG, et al. Tumour type and size are high risk factors for the syndrome of "cerebellar" mutism and subsequent dysarthria. J Neurol Neurosurg Psychiatry. 1999; 67:755–757

[44] Pitsika M, Tsitouras V. Cerebellar mutism. J Neurosurg Pediatr. 2013; 12:604–614

[45] Dubey A, Sung WS, Shaya M, et al. Complications of posterior cranial fossa surgery–an institutional experience of 500 patients. Surg Neurol. 2009; 72:369–375

[46] Ersahin Y, Mutluer S, Cagli S, et al. Cerebellar mutism: report of seven cases and review of the literature. Neurosurgery. 1996; 38:60–5;discussion 66

[47] De Smet HJ, Baillieux H, Catsman-Berrevoets C, et al. Postoperative motor speech production in children with the syndrome of 'cerebellar' mutism and subsequent dysarthria: a critical review of the literature. Eur J Paediatr Neurol. 2007; 11:193–207

[48] van Baarsen KM, Grotenhuis JA. The anatomical substrate of cerebellar mutism. Med Hypotheses. 2014; 82:774–780

[49] Germano A, Baldari S, Caruso G, et al. Reversible cerebral perfusion alterations in children with transient mutism after posterior fossa surgery. Childs Nerv Syst. 1998; 14:114–119

[50] Catsman-Berrevoets C E, Aarsen FK. The spectrum of neurobehavioural deficits in the Posterior Fossa Syndrome in children after cerebellar tumour surgery. Cortex. 2010; 46:933–946

[51] Pearce JM. Parinaud's syndrome. J Neurol Neurosurg Psychiatry. 2005; 76

[52] Rhoton AL,Jr, Buza R. Microsurgical anatomy of the jugular foramen. J Neurosurg. 1975; 42:541–550

[53] Osunwoke EA, Oladipo GS, Gwuinereama IU, et al. Morphometric analysis of the foramen magnum and jugular foramen in adult skulls in southern Nigerian population. American Journal of Scientific and Industrial Research. 2012; 3:446–448

[54] Svien HJ, Baker HL, Rivers MH. Jugular Foramen Syndrome and Allied Syndromes. Neurology. 1963; 13:797–809

[55] Hovelacque A. Osteologie. Paris, France: G. Doin and Cie; 1967; 2

[56] Katsuta T, Rhoton AL,Jr, Matsushima T. The jugular foramen: microsurgical anatomy and operative approaches. Neurosurgery. 1997; 41:149–201; discussion 201-2

[57] Krasnianski M, Neudecker S, Schluter A, et al. Central Tapia's syndrome ("matador's disease") caused by metastatic hemangiosarcoma. Neurology. 2003; 61:868–869

Part II

General and Neurology

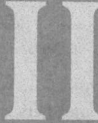

4 Neuroanesthesia

4.1 ASA classification

▶ Table 4.1 shows the American Society of Anesthesiologists (ASA) grading system to estimate anesthetic risk for various conditions.

Table 4.1 ASA classification (modified[1a])

ASA class	Description	% mortality <48 hrs[2]	% mortality <7 days[3]
I	normally healthy patient	0.08	0.06
II	mild systemic disease; no functional limitation	0.27	0.4
III	severe systemic disease (SSD); definite functional limitation	1.8	4.3
IV	SSD that is a constant threat to life	7.8	23.4
V	moribund, expected to die in 24 hrs with or without surgery	9.4	50.7
VI	organ donor		
"e"	appended for emergency operation	triple that for elective	

[a]NB: in this study, no reference is made to type of operation (intracranial and abdominal vascular surgery have higher mortality)

4.2 Neuroanesthesia parameters

For issues related to intracranial pressure (ICP), cerebral perfusion pressure (CPP), intracranial constituents, etc., see ICP principles (p. 1036). For cerebral blood flow (CBF) and cerebral metabolic rate of oxygen consumption ($CMRO_2$), see CBF and oxygen utilization (p. 1536).

Parameters of primary relevance to neurological surgery that can be modulated by the anesthesiologist:
1. blood pressure: one of the factors that determines CPP as well as spinal cord perfusion. May need to be manipulated (e.g., reduced when working on an aneurysm, or increased to enhance collateral circulation during cross clamping). Measurement by arterial line is most accurate and depending on the patient's presentation and the planned procedure, often should be placed prior to induction of anesthesia. For intracranial procedures, the arterial line should be calibrated at the external auditory meatus to most closely reflect intracranial blood pressure
2. jugular venous pressure: one of the factors that influences ICP
3. arterial CO_2 tension ($PaCO_2$): CO_2 is the most potent cerebral vasodilator. Hyperventilation reduces $PaCO_2$ (hypocapnea), which decreases CBV but also CBF. Goal is generally end tidal CO_2 ($ETCO_2$) of 25–30 mm Hg with a correlating $PaCO_2$ of 30–35. Use with care for stereotactic procedures to minimize shift of intracranial contents when using this method to control ICP[4]
4. arterial O_2 tension
5. hematocrit: in neurosurgery it is critical to balance oxygen carrying capacity (decreased by anemia) against improved blood rheology (impaired by elevated Hct)
6. patient temperature: mild hypothermia provides some protection against ischemia by reducing the cerebral metabolic rate of oxygen ($CMRO_2$) by ≈ 7% for each 1 °C drop
7. blood glucose level: hyperglycemia exacerbates ischemic deficits[5]
8. $CMRO_2$: reduced with certain neuro-protective agents and by hypothermia which helps protect against ischemic injury
9. in cases where a lumbar drain or a ventricular drain has been placed: CSF output
10. elevation of the head of the patient: lowering the head increases arterial blood flow, but also increases ICP by impairing venous outflow
11. intravascular volume: hypovolemia can impair blood flow in neurovascular cases. In surgery in the prone position, excessive fluids may contribute to facial edema which is one of the risk factors for PION (p. 1261)
12. positioning injuries: during the procedure, the patient's position may change and be unnoticed due to draping. Careful and frequent examination of the patient's position may prevent injuries associated with prolonged malpositioning
13. postoperative nausea and vomiting (PONV): may adversely affect ICP and may negatively impact recent cervical surgical procedures. Avoidance of anesthetic agents known to cause PONV or pretreatment to prevent PONV may be prudent

4.3 Drugs used in neuroanesthesia

4.3.1 Inhalational agents

General information

Most reduce cerebral metabolism (except nitrous oxide) by suppressing neuronal activity. These agents disturb cerebral autoregulation and cause cerebral vasodilatation, which increases cerebral blood volume (CBV) and can increase ICP. With administration > 2 hrs they increase CSF volume, which can also potentially contribute to increased ICP. Most agents increase the CO_2 reactivity of cerebral blood vessels. These agents affect intraoperative EP monitoring (p. 112).

4

Drug info: Nitrous oxide

A potent vasodilator that markedly increases CBF and minimally increases cerebral metabolism. Contributes to post-op N/V (PONV).

Nitrous oxide, pneumocephalus and air embolism: The solubility of nitrous oxide (N_2O) is ≈ 34 times that of nitrogen.[6] When N_2O comes out of solution in an airtight space it can increase the pressure which may convert pneumocephalus to "tension pneumocephalus." It may also aggravate air embolism. Thus caution must be used especially in the sitting position where significant post-op pneumocephalus and air embolism are common. The risk of tension pneumocephalus may be reduced by filling the cavity with fluid in conjunction with turning off N_2O about 10 minutes prior to completion of dural closure. See Pneumocephalus (p. 1067).

Halogenated agents

Agents in primary usage today are shown below. All suppress EEG activity and may provide some degree of cerebral protection.

Drug info: Isoflurane (Forane®)

Can produce isoelectric EEG without metabolic toxicity. Improves neurologic outcome in cases of incomplete global ischemia (although in experimental studies on rats, the amount of tissue injury was greater than with thiopental[7]).

Drug info: Desflurane (Suprane®)

A cerebral vasodilator, increases CBF and ICP. Decreases $CMRO_2$ which tends to cause a compensatory vasoconstriction.

Drug info: Sevoflurane (Ultane®)

Mildly increases CBP and ICP, and reduces $CMRO_2$. Mild negative inotrope, cardiac output not as well maintained as with isoflurane or desflurane.

4.3.2 Intravenous anesthetic agents

Agents generally used for induction

1. propofol: exact mechanism of action unknown. Short half–life with no active metabolites. May be used for induction and as a continuous infusion during total intravenous anesthesia (TIVA). Causes dose dependent decrease in mean arterial blood pressure (MAP) and ICP. See also information other than use in induction (p. 110). Is more rapidly cleared than, and has largely replaced, thiopental

2. barbiturates: produce significant reduction in $CMRO_2$ and scavenge free radicals among other effects (p. 1464). Produce dose-dependent EEG suppression which can be taken all the way to iso-electric. Minimally affect EPs. Most are anticonvulsant, but methohexital (Brevital®) (p. 139) can lower the seizure threshold. Myocardial suppression and peripheral vasodilatation from barbiturates may cause hypotension and compromise CPP, especially in hypovolemic patients
   ★ sodium thiopental (Pentothal®): the most common agent. Rapid onset, short acting. Minimal effect on ICP, CBF and $CMRO_2$
3. etomidate (Amidate®): a carboxylated imidazole derivative. Anesthetic and amnestic, but no analgesic properties. Sometimes produces myoclonic activity which may be confused with seizures. Impairs renal function and should be avoided in patients with known renal disease. May produce adrenal insufficiency. See Miscellaneous drugs in neuroanesthesia (p. 110) for information other than use in induction.
4. ketamine: NMDA receptor antagonist. Produces a dissociative anesthesia. Maintains cardiac output. May slightly increase both heart rate and blood pressure. ICP increases in parallel with increased cardiac output.

Narcotics in anesthesia

Nonsynthetic narcotics
Narcotics increase CSF absorption and minimally reduce cerebral metabolism. They slow the EEG but will *not* produce an isoelectric tracing. ✖ All narcotics cause dose-dependent respiratory depression which can result in hypercarbia and concomitant increased ICP in non-ventilated patients. Often also contribute to post-op N/V (PONV).
   Morphine: does not significantly cross the BBB.
   ✖ Disadvantages in neuro patients:
1. causes histamine release which
   a) may produce hypotension
   b) may cause cerebrovascular vasodilation → increased ICP[8 (p 1593)]
   c) the above together may compromise CPP
2. in renal or hepatic insufficiency, the metabolite morphine-6-glucuronide can accumulate which may cause confusion

Synthetic narcotics
These do *not* cause histamine release, unlike morphine and meperidine.
   ★ Remifentanil (Ultiva®); see also detailed information (p. 140): reduces $CMRO_2$, CBV and ICP. Large doses may be neurotoxic to limbic system and associated areas. May be used for awake craniotomy (p. 1732).
   Fentanyl: crosses the BBB. Reduces $CMRO_2$, CBV and ICP. May be given as bolus and/or as a continuous infusion.
   Sufentanil: more potent than fentanyl. Does not increase CBF. ✖ Raises ICP (may be due to hypoventilation, which can occur with any narcotic) and is thus often not appropriate for neurosurgical cases. Expensive.

4.3.3 Miscellaneous drugs in neuroanesthesia

▶ **Benzodiazepines.** These drugs are GABA agonists and decrease $CMRO_2$. They also provide antiseizure action and produce amnesia. See also agents and reversal (p. 213).

▶ **Etomidate** (p. 110). Used primarily for induction.
- a cerebrovasoconstrictor which therefore: reduces CBF and ICP; reduces $CMRO_2$ but no longer promoted as a cerebral protectant based on experimental studies[9] and a drop in $pBtO_2$ with temporary MCA clipping[10]
- does not suppress brainstem activity
- suppresses adrenocortical function cortisol production. This usually occurs with prolonged administration, but can occur even after single dose for induction and may persist up to 8 hrs (no adverse outcomes from short-term suppression have been reported)
- increases activity of seizure foci which may be used for mapping foci during seizure surgery but may also induce seizures

▶ **Propofol.** A sedative hypnotic. Useful for induction (p. 109). Reduces cerebral metabolism, CBF and ICP. Has been described for cerebral protection (p. 1466) and for sedation (p. 140). Short half–life permits rapid awakening which may be useful for awake craniotomy (p. 1733). Not analgesic.

▶ **Lidocaine.** Given IV, suppresses laryngeal reflexes which may help blunt ICP elevations that normally follow endotracheal intubation or suctioning. Anticonvulsant at low doses; may provoke seizures at high concentrations.

▶ **Esmolol.** Selective beta-1 adrenergic antagonist, blunts the sympathetic response to laryngoscopy and intubation. Less sedating than equipotent doses of lidocaine or fentanyl used for the same purpose. Half life: 9 minutes. See also dosing, etc. (p. 132).

▶ **Dexmedetomidine (Precedex®).** Alpha 2 adrenergic receptor agonist, used for control of hypertension post operatively, as well as for its sedating qualities during awake craniotomy either alone or in conjunction with propofol (p. 109). Also used to help patients tolerate endotracheal tube without sedatives/narcotics to facilitate extubation.

4.3.4 Paralytics for intubation

Paralytics (neuromuscular blocking agents [NMBA]): administered to facilitate tracheal intubation and to improve surgical conditions when indicated. Administration of paralytics ideally should always be guided by neuromuscular twitch monitoring. Also see Sedatives & paralytics (p. 139). In addition to paralytics, all conscious patients should also receive a sedative to blunt awareness.

Paralytics should not be given until it has been determined that patient can be ventilated manually, unless treating laryngospasm (may be tested with thiopental). Use with caution in non-fixated patients with unstable C-spine.

Due to long action, pancuronium (Pavulon®) is not indicated as the primary paralytic for intubation, but may be useful once patient is intubated or in *low* dose as an adjunct to succinylcholine.

Drug info: Succinylcholine (Anectine®)

The only depolarizing agent. May be used to secure airway for emergency intubation, but due to possible side effects (p. 141), should not be used acutely following injury or in adolescents or children (a short acting nondepolarizing blocker is preferred). May transiently increase ICP. Prior dosing with 10% of the ED95 dose of a non-depolarizing muscle relaxant reduces muscle fasciculations.

℞ Intubating dose: 1–1.5 mg/kg (supplied as 20 mg/ml → 3.5–5 cc for a 70 kg patient), onset 60–90 sec, duration 3–10 min, may repeat same dose × 1.

Drug info: Rocuronium (Zemuron®)

Intermediate acting, aminosteroid, non-depolarizing muscle relaxant. The only nondepolarizing neuromuscular blocking agent approved for rapid sequence intubation (RSI). Duration of action and onset are dose dependent. ℞ (p. 142).

Drug info: Vecuronium (Norcuron®)

See details (p. 142).
Aminosteroid with activity similar to that of rocuronium, however, does not cause histamine release and is not approved for rapid sequence intubation. ℞.

Drug info: Cisatracurium (Nimbex®)

See details (p. 143).
Metabolized by Hoffman degradation (temperature dependent), intermediate acting, no significant increases in histamine. ℞

4.4 Anesthetic requirements for intraoperative evoked potential monitoring

For details of intraoperative evoked potential (EP) monitoring itself, see **Intraoperative evoked potentials** (p.251).

All volatile anesthetics produce dose-dependent reduction in SSEP peak amplitude and an increase in peak latency. Adding nitrous oxide increases this sensitivity to anesthetic agents.

Anesthesia issues related to intraoperative evoked potential (EPs) monitoring:

1. induction: minimize pentothal dose (produces ≈ 30 minutes of suppression of EPs), or use eto-midate (which increases both SSEP amplitude and latency[11])
2. total intravenous anesthesia (TIVA) is ideal (i.e., no inhalational agents)
3. nitrous/narcotic technique is a distant second choice
4. if inhalational anesthetic agents are required:
   a) use < 1 MAC (maximal alveolar concentration), ideally < 0.5 MAC
   b) avoid older agents such as Halothane
5. nondepolarizing muscle relaxants have little effect on EP (in monkeys[12])
6. propofol has a mild effect on EP: total anesthesia with propofol causes less EP depression than inhalational agents at the same depth of anesthesia[13]
7. benzodiazepines have a mild-to-moderate depressant effect on EPs
8. continuous infusion of anesthetic drugs is preferred over intermittent boluses
9. SSEPs can be affected by hyper- or hypothermia, and changes in BP
10. hypocapnia (down to end tidal CO_2 = 21) causes minimal reduction in peak latencies[14]
11. antiseizure medications: phenytoin, carbamazipine and phenobarbital do not affect SSEP[15]

4.5 Malignant hyperthermia

4.5.1 General information

Malignant hyperthermia (MH) is a hypermetabolic state of skeletal muscle due to idiopathic block of Ca^{++} re-entry into sarcoplasmic reticulum. Transmitted by a multifactorial genetic predisposition. Total body O_2 consumption increases × 2–3.

Incidence: 1 in 15,000 anesthetic administrations in peds, 1 in 40,000 adults. 50% had previous anesthesia without MH. Frequently associated with administration of halogenated inhalational agents and the use of succinylcholine (fulminant form: muscle rigidity almost immediately after suc-cinylcholine, may involve masseters → difficulty intubating). Initial attack and recrudescence may also occur post-op. 30% mortality.[16]

4.5.2 Presentation

1. earliest possible sign: *increase* in end-tidal pCO_2
2. tachycardia (early) and other arrhythmias
3. with progression:
   a) coagulation disorder (DIC) (bleeding from surgical wound and body orifices)
   b) ABG: increasing metabolic acidosis & decreasing pO_2
   c) pulmonary edema
   d) elevated body temperature (may reach ≥ 44 °C (113 °F) at rate of 1 °C/5-min) (normal patients become hypothermic with general anesthesia)
   e) limb muscle rigidity (common, but late)
   f) rhabdomyolysis → elevated CPK & myoglobin (late)
4. terminal:
   a) hypotension
   b) bradycardia
   c) cardiac arrest

4.5.3 Treatment

1. eliminate offending agents (stop the operation, D/C inhalation anesthesia and change tubing on anesthesia machine)
2. dantrolene sodium (Dantrium®) 2.5 mg/kg IV usually effective, infuse until symptoms subside, up to 10 mg/kg

3. hyperventilation with 100% O_2
4. surface and cavity cooling: IV, in wound, per NG, PR
5. bicarbonate 1–2 mEq/kg for acidosis
6. IV insulin and glucose (lowers K^+, glucose acts as energy substrate)
7. procainamide for arrhythmias
8. diuresis: volume loading + osmotic diuretics

4.5.4 Prevention

1. identification of patients at risk:
   a) only reliable test: 4 cm viable muscle biopsy for in-vitro tests at a few regional test centers (abnormal contracture to caffeine or halothane)
   b) family history: any relative with syndrome puts patient at risk
   c) related traits: 50% of MH patients have heavy musculature, Duchenne type muscular dystrophy, or scoliosis
   d) patients who exhibit masseter spasm in response to succinylcholine
2. in patients at risk: avoid succinylcholine (nondepolarizing blockers preferred if paralysis essential), may safely have non-halogenated anesthetics (narcotics, barbiturates, benzodiazepines, droperidol, nitrous...)
3. prophylactic oral dantrolene: 4–8 mg/kg/day for 1–2 days (last dose given 2 hrs before anesthesia) is usually effective

References

[1] Schneider AJ. Assessment of Risk Factors and Surgical Outcome. Surg Clin N Am. 1983; 63:1113–1126
[2] Vacanti CJ, VanHouten RJ, Hill RC. A Statistical Analysis of the Relationship of Physical Status to Postoperative Mortality in 68,388 Cases. Anesth Analg Curr Res. 1970; 49:564–566
[3] Marx GF, Mateo CV, Orkin LR. Computer Analysis of Postanesthetic Deaths. Anesthesiology. 1973; 39:54–58
[4] Benveniste R, Germano IM. Evaluation of factors predicting accurate resection of high-grade gliomas by using frameless image-guided stereotactic guidance. Neurosurgical Focus. 2003; 14
[5] Martin A, Rojas S, Chamorro A, et al. Why does acute hyperglycemia worsen the outcome of transient focal cerebral ischemia? Role of corticosteroids, inflammation, and protein O-glycosylation. Stroke. 2006; 37:1288–1295
[6] Raggio JF, Fleischer AS, Sung YF, et al. Expanding Pneumocephalus due to Nitrous Oxide Anesthesia: Case Report. Neurosurgery. 1979; 4:261–263
[7] Drummond JC, Cole DJ, Patel PM, et al. Focal Cerebral Ischemia during Anesthesia with Etomidate, Isofluorane, or Thiopental: A Comparison of the Extent of Cerebral Injury. Neurosurgery. 1995; 37:742–749
[8] Shapiro HM, Miller RD. Neurosurgical Anesthesia and Intracranial Hypertension. In: Anesthesia. 2nd ed. New York: Churchill Livingstone; 1986:1563–1620
[9] Drummond JC, McKay LD, Cole DJ, et al. The role of nitric oxide synthase inhibition in the adverse effects of etomidate in the setting of focal cerebral ischemia in rats. Anesthesia and Analgesia. 2005; 100:841–6, table of contents
[10] Hoffman WE, Charbel FT, Edelman G, et al. Comparison of the effect of etomidate and desflurane on brain tissue gases and pH during prolonged middle cerebral artery occlusion. Anesthesiology. 1998; 88:1188–1194
[11] Koht A, Schutz W, Schmidt G, et al. Effects of etomidate, midazolam, and thiopental on median nerve somatosensory evoked potentials and the additive effects of fentanyl and nitrous oxide. Anesthesia and Analgesia. 1988; 67:435–441
[12] Sloan TB. Nondepolarizing neuromuscular blockade does not alter sensory evoked potentials. Journal of Clinical Monitoring. 1994; 10:4–10
[13] Liu EH, Wong HK, Chia CP, et al. Effects of isoflurane and propofol on cortical somatosensory evoked potentials during comparable depth of anaesthesia as guided by bispectral index. British Journal of Anaesthesia. 2005; 94:193–197
[14] Schubert A, Drummond JC. The effect of acute hypocapnia on human median nerve somatosensory evoked responses. Anesthesia and Analgesia. 1986; 65:240–244
[15] Borah NC, Matheshwari MC. Effect of antiepileptic drugs on short-latency somatosensory evoked potentials. Acta Neurologica Scandinavica. 1985; 71:331–333
[16] Nelson TE, Flewellen EH. The Malignant Hyperthermia Syndrome. N Engl J Med. 1983; 309:416–418

5 Sodium Homeostasis and Osmolality

5.1 Serum osmolality and sodium concentration

Clinical significance of various serum osmolality values is shown in ▶ Table 5.1.

▶ **Serum osmolality.** May be estimated using Eq (5.1).

$$\text{Osmolality (mOsm/kg)} = 2 \times \{ [Na^+] + [K^+] \} + \frac{[BUN]}{2.8} + \frac{[glucose]}{18} \tag{5.1}$$

(with [Na^+] in mEq/L or mmol/L, and glucose and BUN in mg/dl).
   NB: terms in square brackets [] represent the serum concentrations (in mEq/L for electrolytes).

▶ **Sodium content.** In the diet: usually expressed in grams Na^+ (not NaCl), a low sodium diet is considered 2 g of Na^+ per day or less.
   1 teaspoon of table salt (NaCl) has 2.3 gm of Na^+.
   1 mg NaCl has 17 mEq Na^+. 1 mg Na^+ has 43 mEq Na^+.
   Normal saline has 0.9 gm of NaCl/100 ml. 3% NaCl has 3 gm NaCl/100 ml.

Table 5.1 Clinical correlates of serum osmolality

Value (mOsm/kg)	Comment
282–295	normal
< 240 or > 321	panic values
> 320	risk of renal failure
> 384	produces stupor
> 400	risk of generalized seizures
> 420	usually fatal

5.2 Hyponatremia

5.2.1 General information

Key concepts

- definition: serum [Na^+] < 135 mEq/L. Common etiologies:
  - SIADH: hypotonic hyponatremia (effective serum osmolality < 275 mOsm/kg) with inappropriately high urinary concentration (urine osmolality > 100 mOsm/kg) and euvolemia or hypervolemia
  - cerebral salt wasting **(CSW)**: similar to SIADH but with extracellular fluid volume *depletion* due to renal sodium loss (urinary [Na] > 20 mEq/L)
- minimum W/U: ✓ serum [Na^+], ✓ serum osmolality, ✓ urine osmolality, ✓ clinical assessment of volume status. If volume status is high or low: ✓ urinary [Na^+] ✓ TSH (to R/O hypothyroidism)
- treatment: based on acuity, severity, symptoms & etiology; see SIADH (p. 119) or CSW (p. 122) as appropriate
- risk of overly rapid correction: osmotic demyelination (including central pontine myelinolysis)

▶ **Classification.** Severity of hyponatremia: [Na^+] < 135 mEq/L = mild, < 130 = moderate, < 125 = severe hyponatremia.
   See ▶ Fig. 5.1 for flow chart.

▶ **Hyponatremia in neurosurgical patients.** Chiefly seen in:
- syndrome of inappropriate antidiuretic hormone secretion (SIADH) (p. 118): dilutional hyponatremia with normal or *elevated intravascular volume*. The most common type of hyponatremia.[1]

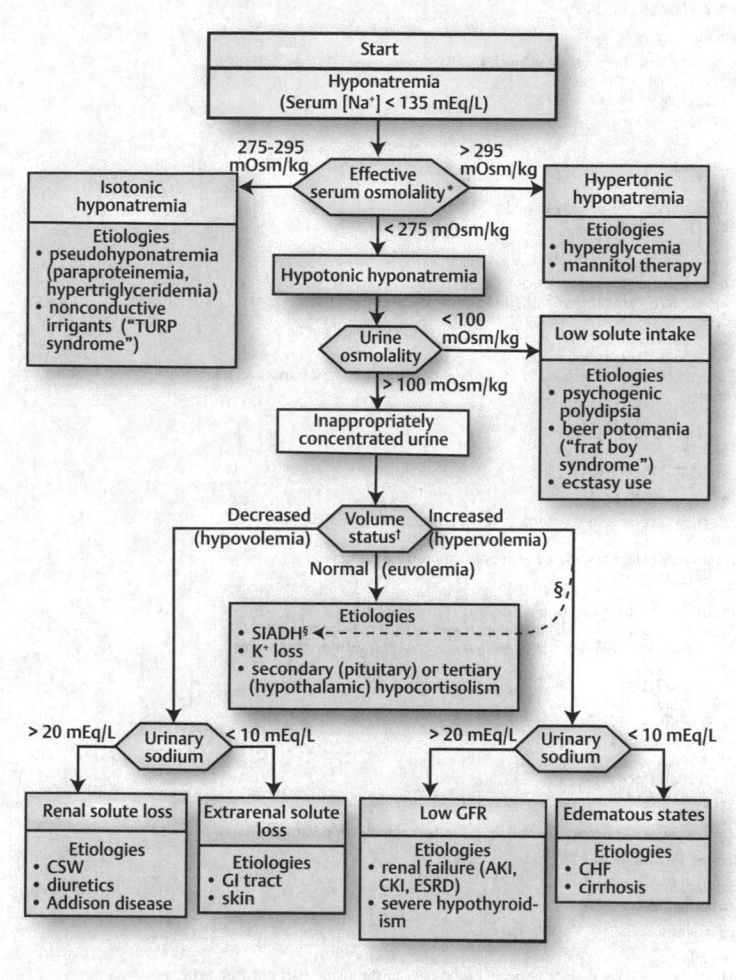

Fig. 5.1 Etiologies of hyponatremia (adapted[5,9]).
* effective serum osmolality = measured osmolality − [BUN]/2.8 (see formula in text (p. 117)).
† volume status is usually assessed clinically, but this may be insensitive to volume depletion.
§ SIADH may be associated with euvolemia or hypervolemia.
Abbreviations: AKI = acute kidney injury; CHF = congestive heart failure; CKI = chronic kidney injury; CSW = cerebral salt wasting; [Na+]$_{urine}$ = urinary concentration of sodium; SIADH = syndrome of inappropriate antidiuretic hormone secretion.

Usually treated with *fluid restriction*. May be associated with numerous intracranial abnormalities (▶ Table 5.2) and following transsphenoidal surgery
- cerebral salt wasting (CSW): inappropriate natriuresis with *volume depletion*. Treated with *volume replacement* (opposite to SIADH) and *sodium*; symptoms from derangements due to CSW may be exacerbated by fluid restriction (p. 122).[2] It is the etiology of 6–23% of cases of moderate-to-severe hyponatremia following aneurysmal SAH[3,4] (compared to 35% for SIADH)

5

Table 5.2 Etiologies of SIAD[a]

Malignant tumors

1. especially bronchogenic small-cell Ca
2. tumors of GI or GU tract
3. lymphomas
4. Ewing's sarcoma

CNS disorders

1. infection:
   a) encephalitis
   b) meningitis: especially in peds
   c) TB meningitis
   d) AIDS
   e) brain abscess
2. head trauma: 4.6% prevalence
3. increased ICP: hydrocephalus, SDH...
4. SAH
5. brain tumors
6. cavernous sinus thrombosis
7. ★ post craniotomy, especially following surgery for pituitary tumors, craniopharyngiomas, hypothalamic tumors
8. MS
9. Guillain-Barré
10. Shy-Drager
11. delirium tremens (DTs)

Pulmonary disorders

1. infection: pneumonia (bacterial & viral), abscess, TB, aspergillosis
2. asthma
3. respiratory failure associated with positive pressure respiration

Drugs

1. drugs that release ADH or potentiate it
   a) chlorpropamide (Diabinese®): increases renal sensitivity to ADH
   b) carbamazepine (Tegretol®), even more common with oxcarbazepine
   c) HCTZ
   d) SSRIs, TCAs
   e) clofibrate
   f) vincristine
   g) antipsychotics
   h) NSAIDs
   i) MDMA ("ecstasy")
2. ADH analogues
   a) DDAVP
   b) oxytocin: ADH cross activity, may also be contaminated with ADH

Endocrine disturbances

1. adrenal insufficiency
2. hypothyroidism

Miscellaneous

1. anemia
2. stress, severe pain, nausea or hypotension (all can stimulate ADH release), postoperative state
3. acute intermittent porphyria (AIP)

[a]excerpted and modified[1,11]

▶ **Other forms of hyponatremia:**
1. isotonic hyponatremia (effective serum osmolality: 275–295 mOsm/kg):
   a) pseudohyponatremia: an artifact of *indirect* lab techniques.[5] Unusually high levels of lipids (e.g., hypertriglyceridemia) or proteins (e.g., immunoglobulins as can occur in multiple myeloma[6]) reduce the aqueous fraction of plasma and produce artifactually low sodium lab values. This error does not occur with direct measurement methods
   b) nonconductive irrigants, e.g., as used in cystoscopy to allow coagulation, when large volumes are inadvertently absorbed through a severed vein ("TURP syndrome")

2. hypertonic hyponatremia (effective serum osmolality: > 295 mOsm/kg): excess of osmotically active solutes. Hyperglycemia is the most common example. For every 100 mg/dl increase of glucose, serum [Na^+] decreases by 1.6–2.4 mEq/L. Can also occur with mannitol
3. hypotonic hyponatremia (effective serum osmolality: typically < 275 mOsm/kg. Exceptions: in the presence of solutes with total body water distribution: e.g., EtOH, urea). Examples:
   a) renal failure: associated with hypervolemia and [Na^+]$_{urine}$ > 20 mEq/L
   b) CHF, cirrhosis: associated with hypervolemia and [Na^+]$_{urine}$ < 10 mEq/L
4. postoperative hyponatremia: a rare condition usually described in young, otherwise healthy women undergoing elective surgery[7] and may be related to administration of even only mildly hypotonic fluids (sometimes in modest amounts)[8] and the actions of ADH (which may be increased due to stress, pain, or medications)

5.2.2 Evaluation of hyponatremia

5

▶ Fig. 5.1 shows an algorithm for evaluating the etiology of hyponatremia[9] which drives treatment decisions. Work-up requires assessment of:
1. serum sodium: must be < 135 mEq/L to qualify as hyponatremia
2. the *effective* serum osmolality (AKA tonicity) is shown in this equation:

$$\text{effective serum osmolality} = \text{measured osmolality} - \frac{[BUN](mg/dl)}{2.8}$$

and should be used when the blood urea nitrogen (BUN) level is elevated (for a normal [BUN] of 7–18 mg/dl, just subtract 5 from the measured osmolality). Values < 275 mOsm/kg indicate hypotonic hyponatremia
3. urine osmolality: values > 100 mOsm/kg are inappropriately high if serum tonicity is < 275 mOsm/kg
4. volume status: differentiates SIADH from CSW
   a) clinical assessment: better for hypervolemia (edema, upward trend in patient weights) but is insensitive in identifying extracellular fluid depletion as an etiology of hyponatremia[10] (look for dry mucous membranes, loss of skin turgor, orthostatic hypotension)
   b) normal saline infusion test used in uncertain cases. If baseline urine osmolality is < 500 mOsm/kg, it is usually safe to infuse 2 L of 0.9% saline over 24–48 hours. Correction of the hyponatremia suggests extracellular fluid volume depletion was the cause
   c) central venous pressure (CVP) may be used: CVP < 5–6 cm H_2O suggests hypovolemia in patients with normal cardiac function[3,9]
5. check urinary [Na^+] if volume status is high or low
6. determine duration of hyponatremia:
   a) duration documented as < 48 hours is considered acute
   b) hyponatremia of > 48 hours duration or of unknown duration is chronic
   c) hyponatremia that occurs outside the hospital is usually chronic and asymptomatic except in marathoners and MDMA ("ecstasy") drug users

5.2.3 Symptoms

Due to slow compensatory mechanisms in the brain, a gradual decline in serum sodium is better tolerated than a rapid drop. Symptoms of mild ([Na] < 130 mEq/L) or gradual hyponatremia include: anorexia, headache, difficulty concentrating, irritability, dysgeusia, and muscle weakness. Severe hyponatremia (< 125 mEq/L) or a rapid drop (> 0.5 mEq/hr) can cause neuromuscular excitability, cerebral edema, muscle twitching and cramps, nausea/vomiting, confusion, seizures, respiratory arrest and possibly permanent neurologic injury, coma or death.

5.2.4 Syndrome of inappropriate antidiuresis (SIAD)

This term covers excess water retention in the face of hyponatremia, including cases due to inappropriate ADH secretion (SIADH) as well as others without increased circulating levels of ADH (e.g., heightened response to ADH, certain drugs…). A partial list of etiologies is shown in ▶ Table 5.2 (see references[1,11] for details).

The diagnostic criteria of SIAD is shown in ▶ Table 5.3. It is critical to *measure serum osmolality* to rule out pseudohyponatremia (p. 116), an artifact of indirect lab techniques.

Table 5.3 Diagnostic criteria for SIAD[1]

Essential features

- decreased effective serum osmolality[a] (< 275 mOsm/kg of water)
- simultaneous urine osmolality > 100 mOsm/kg of water
- clinical euvolemia
  a) no clinical signs of extracellular (EC) volume orthostatic hypotension (orthostasis, tachycardia, decreased skin turgor, dry mucous membranes...)
  b) no clinical signs of excess EC volume (edema, ascites...)
- urinary [Na] > 40 mEq/L with normal dietary Na intake
- normal thyroid and adrenal function
- no recent diuretic use

Supplemental features

- plasma [uric acid] < 4 mg/dl
- [BUN] < 10 mg/dl
- fractional Na excretion > 1%; fractional urea excretion > 55%
- NS infusion test: failure to correct hyponatremia with IV infusion of 2 L 0.9% saline over 24–48 hrs
- correction of hyponatremia with fluid restriction[b]
- abnormal result on water load test[c]:
  a) < 80% excretion of 20 ml of water/kg body weight over 5 hours, or
  b) inadequate urinary dilution (< 100 mOsm/kg of water)
- elevated plasma [ADH] with hyponatremia and euvolemia

[a]effective osmolality (AKA tonicity) = (measured osmolality) − [BUN]/2.8 with [BUN] measured in mg/dl
[b]this test is used in uncertain cases (corrects volume depletion), and is usually safe when baseline urine osmolality is < 500 mOsm/L
[c]water load test & [ADH] levels are rarely recommended; see text for details (p.119)

5.2.5 Syndrome of inappropriate antidiuretic hormone secretion (SIADH)

General information

Key concepts

- definition: release of ADH in the absence of physiologic (osmotic) stimuli
- results in hyponatremia with hypervolemia (occasionally with euvolemia) with inappropriately high urine osmolality (> 100 mOsm/kg)
- may be seen with certain malignancies and many intracranial abnormalities
- critical to distinguish from cerebral salt wasting which produces hypovolemia
- treatment: initial guidelines in brief, see details (p.119)
  ○ avoid rapid correction or overcorrection to reduce risk of osmotic demyelination (p.119). Check serum [Na$^+$] q 2–4 hours and do not exceed 1 mEq/L per hour, or 8 mEq/L in 24 hrs or 18 mEq/L in 48 hrs
  ○ severe ([Na$^+$] < 125 mEq/L of < 48 hrs duration or with severe symptoms (coma, Sz): start 3% saline at 1–2 ml/kg body weight/hr + furosemide 20 mg IV qd
  ○ severe ([Na$^+$] < 125 mEq/L of duration > 48 hours or unknown without severe symptoms: normal saline infusion @ 100 ml/hr + furosemide 20 mg IV qd
  ○ chronic or unknown duration and asymptomatic: fluid restriction (▶ Table 5.4) with dietary salt and protein, and, if necessary, adjuvant drugs (demeclocycline, conivaptan...)

SIADH, AKA Schwartz-Bartter syndrome, was first described with bronchogenic cancer which is one cause of SIAD. SIADH is the release of antidiuretic hormone (ADH), AKA arginine vasopressin (AVP) (p.153), in the absence of physiologic (osmotic) stimuli. Result: elevated urine osmolality, and expansion of the extracellular fluid volume leading to a dilutional hyponatremia which can produce fluid overload (hypervolemia), but SIADH may also occur with euvolemia. For unclear reasons, edema does not occur.

The hyponatremia of SIADH must be differentiated from that due to cerebral salt wasting (CSW) (p.122) because of differences in treatment recommendations.

Etiologies: ▶ Table 5.2.

Table 5.4 Fluid restriction recommendations[1]

Solute ratio[a]	Recommended fluid intake
>1	<500 ml/d
1	500–700 ml/d
<1	<1 L/d

[a]solute ratio defined as: $\frac{\text{urinary [Na]} + \text{urinary [K]}}{\text{plasma [Na]}}$

Diagnosis of SIADH

In general, 3 diagnostic criteria are: hyponatremia, inappropriately concentrated urine, and no evidence of renal or adrenal dysfunction. In more detail:
1. low serum sodium (hyponatremia): usually <134 mEq/L
2. low effective serum osmolality: <275 mOsm/kg
3. high urinary sodium (salt wasting): at least >18 mEq/L, often 50–150. Note: there has not been an adequate explanation of the high urinary sodium in SIADH
4. high ratio of urine:serum osmolality: often 1.5–2.5:1, but may be 1:1
5. normal renal function (check BUN & creatinine): BUN commonly <10
6. normal adrenal function (no hypotension, no hyperkalemia)
7. no hypothyroidism
8. no signs of dehydration or overhydration (in many patients with acute brain disease, there is significant hypovolemia often due to CSW (p.122) and as this is a stimulus for ADH secretion, the ADH release may be "appropriate"[12]). In uncertain cases, the normal saline infusion test (p.117) may be used.

If further testing is required, the following are options, but are rarely recommended:
1. measure serum or urinary levels of ADH. Rarely indicated since urine osmolality >100 mOsm/kg is usually sufficient to indicate excessive ADH.[1] ADH is normally undetectable in etiologies of hyponatremia other than SIADH
2. water-load test: considered to be the definitive test.[13] The patient is asked to consume a water load of 20 ml/kg up to 1500 ml. In the absence of adrenal or renal insufficiency, the failure to excrete 65% of the water load in 4 hrs or 80% in 5 hrs indicates SIAD.
   ✖ CONTRAINDICATIONS: this test is dangerous if the starting serum [Na⁺] is ≤124 mEq/L or if the patient has symptoms of hyponatremia

Symptoms of SIADH

Symptoms of SIADH are those of hyponatremia (p.117) and possibly fluid overload. If mild, or if descent of [Na⁺] is gradual, it may be tolerated. [Na⁺] <120–125 mEq/L is almost always symptomatic. These patients often have a paradoxical (inappropriate) thirst.

Treatment of hyponatremia with SIADH

Management is based on the severity and duration of hyponatremia, and the presence of symptoms. Two caveats:
1. ✖ be sure that hyponatremia is not due to CSW (p.122) before restricting fluids
2. avoid too rapid correction and avoid correcting to normal or supranormal (overcorrection) sodium to reduce the risk of osmotic demyelination syndrome

Osmotic demyelination syndrome

A complication associated with some cases of treatment for hyponatremia. While excessively slow correction of acute hyponatremia is associated with increased morbidity and mortality,[14] some cases of inordinately rapid treatment have been associated with osmotic demyelination syndrome (which includes central pontine myelinolysis (CPM) a rare disorder of pontine white matter[15] (▶ Fig. 5.2) and extrapontine myelinolysis (▶ Fig. 5.3), as well as other areas of cerebral white matter). First described in alcoholics,[16] producing insidious flaccid quadriplegia, mental status changes, and cranial nerve abnormalities with a pseudobulbar palsy appearance. In one review,[17] no patient developed CPM when treated slowly as outlined below. And yet, the rate of correction correlates poorly with CPM; it may be that the magnitude is another critical variable.[18] Features common to patients who develop CPM are[17]:

5

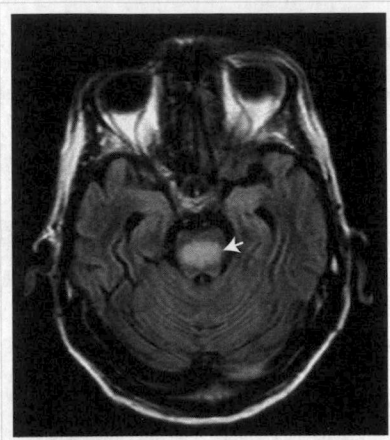

Fig. 5.2 Central pontine myelinolysis (*arrowhead*). Image: axial FLAIR MRI.

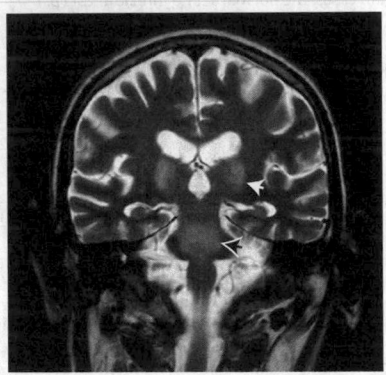

Fig. 5.3 Osmotic demyelination. Seen in pons (*black arrowhead*) & thalamus (*white arrowhead*). Image: coronal T2WI MRI.

- delay in the diagnosis of hyponatremia with resultant respiratory arrest or seizure with probable hypoxemic event
- rapid correction to normo- or hypernatremia (> 135 mEq/L) within 48 hours of initiating therapy
- increase of serum sodium by > 25 mEq/L within 48 hours of initiation of therapy
- over-correcting serum sodium in patients with hepatic encephalopathy
- NB: many patients developing CPM were victims of chronic debilitating disease, malnourishment, or alcoholism and never had hyponatremia. Many had an episode of hypoxia/anoxia[19]
- presence of hyponatremia > 24 hrs prior to treatment[18]

The only definitive treatment is treatment of the underlying cause.
- if caused by anemia: usually responds to transfusion
- if caused by malignancy, may respond to antineoplastic therapy
- most drug-related cases respond rapidly to discontinuation of the offending drug

Treatment algorithms
▶ Fig. 5.4 is an algorithm for selecting the correct SIADH treatment protocol (detailed below).

▶ **Aggressive treatment protocol.** Indications (also refer to ▶ Fig. 5.4):
1. severe hyponatremia (serum [Na⁺] < 125 mEq/L)

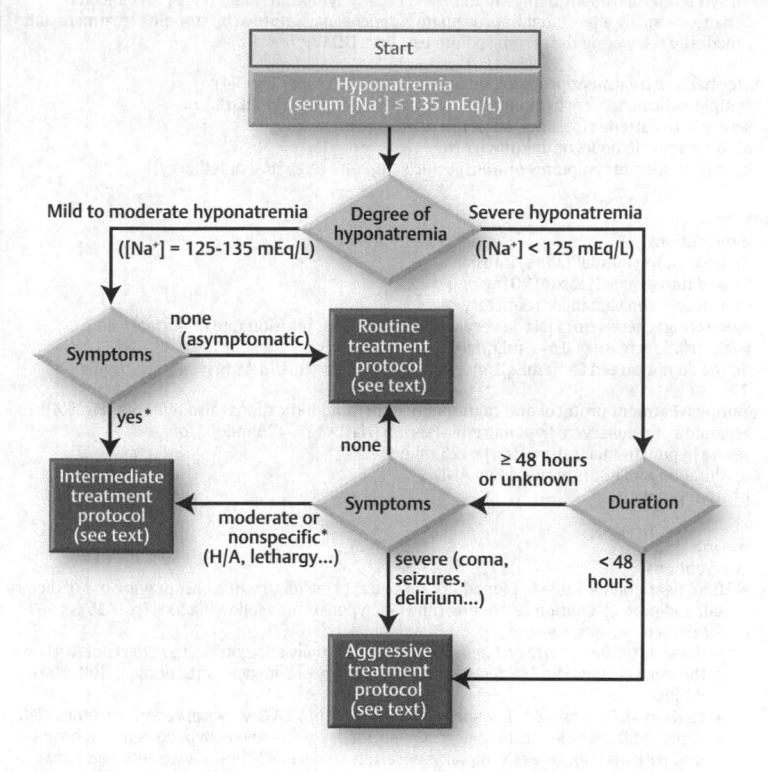

Fig. 5.4 Treatment protocol selection for hyponatremia in SIADH (see text for protocol details).
* mild to moderate symptoms include: anorexia, headache, difficulty concentrating, irritability, dysgeusia, muscle weakness...

2. AND either
   a) duration known to be < 48 hours
   b) or severe symptoms (coma, seizures)

Treatment
- transfer patient to ICU
- interventions
  - 3% saline: start infusion 1–2 ml/kg body weight per hour (infusion rate may be doubled to 2–4 ml/kg/hr for limited periods in patients with coma or seizures[1])
  - and furosemide (Lasix®) 20 mg IV q d (furosemide accelerates the increase in [Na$^+$] and prevents volume overload with subsequent increase in atrial natriuretic factor and resultant urinary dumping of the extra Na$^+$ being administered)
- monitoring and adjustments
  - check serum [Na$^+$] every 2–3 hours and adjust infusion rate of 3% saline
    - goal: raise serum sodium by 1–2 mEq/L/hr[20] (use lower end of range for hyponatremia > 48 hours duration or unknown duration)
    - limits: do not exceed 8–10 mEq/L in 24 hrs and 18–25 mEq/L in 48 hrs[1] (use lower end of these ranges for hyponatremia > 48 hours duration or unknown duration) to reduce risk of CPM
  - measure K$^+$ lost in urine and replace accordingly

○ if symptoms of osmotic demyelination occur (early symptoms are lethargy and affective changes, usually after initial improvement): deficits may improve by stopping treatment and modestly relowering the serum sodium e.g., with DDAVP[21,22]

▶ **Intermediate treatment protocol.** Indications (also refer to ▶ Fig. 5.4):
1. symptomatic nonsevere hyponatremia (serum [Na⁺] = 125–135 mEq/L), or
2. severe hyponatremia (serum [Na⁺] < 125 mEq/L), AND
   a) duration > 48 hours or unknown AND
   b) only moderate symptoms or nonspecific symptoms (e.g., H/A, or lethargy)

Treatment
1. interventions
   a) 0.9% saline (normal saline) infusion
   b) and furosemide (Lasix®) 20 mg IV q d
   c) consider conivaptan for refractory cases
2. monitoring: check serum [Na⁺] every 4 hours and adjust infusion rate of normal saline
3. goals: [Na⁺] increase of 0.5–2 mEq/L/hr
4. limits: do not exceed 8–10 mEq/L in 24 hrs and 18–25 mEq/L in 48 hrs[1]

▶ **Routine treatment protocol and maintenance therapy.** Indications (also refer to ▶ Fig. 5.4):
1. asymptomatic nonsevere hyponatremia (serum [Na⁺] = 125–135 mEq/L), or
2. severe hyponatremia (serum [Na⁺] < 125 mEq/L) AND
   a) duration > 48 hours or unknown AND
   b) asymptomatic

Treatment
1. interventions
   a) fluid restriction ▶ Table 5.4 for adults, for peds: 1 L/m²/day) while encouraging use of dietary salt and protein. Caution restricting fluids in hyponatremia following SAH (p. 1435).
   b) for refractory cases, consider
      • demeclocycline: a tetracycline antibiotic that partially antagonizes the effects of ADH on the renal tubules.[23,24,25] Effects are variable, and nephrotoxicity may occur. ℞ 300–600 mg PO BID
      • conivaptan (Vaprisol®): a nonpeptide antagonist of V1A & V2 vasopressin receptors. FDA approved for euvolemic and hypervolemic moderate-to-severe hyponatremia in hospitalized patients (NB: severe symptoms of seizures, coma, delirium… warrants aggressive treatment with hypertonic saline[1]). Use in the neuro-ICU has been described for treating elevated ICP when serum [Na] is not responding to traditional methods[26] (off-label use— use with caution). ℞ loading dose 20 mg IV over 30 minutes, followed by infusions of 20 mg over 24 hours × 3 days. If serum [Na⁺] are not rising as desired, the infusion may be increased to the maximal dose of 40 mg over 24 hours. Use is approved for up to 4 days total. Caution re drug interactions
      • lithium: not very effective and many side effects. Not recommended

5.2.6 Cerebral salt wasting

Cerebral salt wasting (CSW): renal loss of sodium as a result of intracranial disease, producing hyponatremia and a decrease in extracellular fluid volume.[13] CAUTION: CSW after aneurysmal SAH may mimic SIADH; however, there is usually also hypovolemia in CSW. In this setting, fluid restriction may exacerbate vasospasm induced ischemia.[13,27,28,29]

The mechanism whereby the kidneys fail to conserve sodium in CSW is not known, and may be either a result of a natriuretic factor or direct neural control mechanisms.

Laboratory tests (serum and urinary electrolytes and osmolalities) may be identical with SIADH and CSW.[30] Furthermore, hypovolemia in CSW may stimulate ADH release. To differentiate: CVP, PCWP, and plasma volume (a nuclear medicine study) are low in hypovolemia (i.e., CSW). ▶ Table 5.5 compares some features of CSW and SIADH, the two most important differences being extracellular volume and salt balance. An elevated serum [K⁺] with hyponatremia is incompatible with the diagnosis of SIADH.

Table 5.5 Comparison of CSW and SIADH[13]

Parameter	CSW	SIADH
★ Plasma volume	↓ (<35 ml/kg)	↑ or WNL
★ Salt balance	negative	variable
Signs & symptoms of dehydration	present	absent
Weight	↓	↑ or no Δ
PCWP	↓ (<8 mm Hg)	↑ or WNL
CVP	↓ (<6 mm Hg)	↑ or WNL
Orthostatic hypotension	+	±
Hematocrit	↑	↓ or no Δ
Serum osmolality	↑ or WNL[a]	↓
Ratio of serum [BUN]:[creatinine]	↑	WNL
Serum [protein]	↑	WNL
Urinary [Na⁺]	↑↑	↑
Serum [K⁺]	↑ or no Δ	↓ or no Δ
Serum [uric acid]	WNL	↓

Abbreviations: ↓ = decreased, ↑ = increased, ↑↑ = significantly increased, WNL = within normal limits, no Δ = no change, [ ] = concentration, + = present, ± = may or may not be present
[a]In reality, serum osmolality is usually ↓ in CSW

Treatment of cerebral salt wasting (CSW)

✖ Caution! Restricting fluids (which is the treatment for SIADH) may be hazardous in the case of CSW (SIADH or CSW may occur after SAH) since dehydration increases blood viscosity, which exacerbates ischemia from vasospasm.[28] See Treatment of hyponatremia with SIADH (p. 119).
Treatment goals:
1. volume replacement to achieve *euvolemia* (avoid hypovolemia & induced hypervolemia)
2. positive salt balance
3. avoid excessively rapid correction of hyponatremia or overcorrection which may be associated with osmotic demyelination (p. 119) (as discussed under SIADH (p. 119))
4. ✖ avoid hyperchloremic acidosis due to overuse of NS or 3% sodium (see below)

Interventions:
1. treat hypovolemia aggressively
   a) start with infusions of crystalloid, usually 0.9% NS at 100–125 ml/hr
   b) for severe cases, 3% saline at 25–50 cc/hr is occasionally needed. It is effective in correcting hyponatremia[31] and appears to increase regional cerebral blood flow, brain tissue oxygen, and pH in patients with high-grade aSAH[32]
   c) if fluid requirements remain large, switch to balanced crystalloid (e.g., Plasma-Lyte) to avoid hyperchloremic acidosis (see below)
   d) PRBCs as needed (see discussion of optimal Hgb)
   e) colloids may be used to supplement. Expensive as a replacement for crystalloids
2. ✖ do not give furosemide for CSW
3. salt may also be simultaneously replaced orally. Table salt is ≈ 99% NaCl: 1 tsp salt = 6 g salt ≈ 2300 mg Na⁺ = 100 mEq Na⁺. Salt tablets typically contain 1 g salt/tablet (other concentrations may be available) = 16.7 mEq Na⁺
4. blood products may be administered if anemia is present
5. medications
   a) fludrocortisone acetate acts directly on the renal tubule to increase sodium absorption and helps correct hyponatremia, with a reduced need for fluids,[33,34] but significant complications of pulmonary edema, hypokalemia and HTN may occur. Dose: 0.2 mg IV or PO q d for CSW[33]
   b) hydrocortisone administration has been associated with reduced natriuresis and a lower rate of hyponatremia[35]
   c) urea: an alternative treatment using urea, may be applicable to the hyponatremia of either SIADH or CSW, and therefore may be used before the cause has been ascertained: urea

(Ureaphil®) 0.5 grams/kg (dissolve 40 gm in 100–150 ml NS) IV over 30–60 mins q 8 hrs.[36] Use NS + 20 mEq KCl/L at 2 ml/kg/hr as the main IV until the hyponatremia is corrected (unlike mannitol, urea does not increase ADH secretion). They supplemented with colloids (viz. 250 ml of 5% albumin IV q 8–12 hrs x 72 hrs)

▶ **Hyperchloremic acidosis.** The sodium burden accompanying NS and even hypertonic saline is usually better tolerated by post-aSAH patients than other critically ill patients because hyponatremia after aSAH is usually due to CSW, which is sodium losing. However, the chloride load associated with NS or 3% saline can produce hyperchloremic acidosis (HCA), a metabolic acidosis that augments the inflammatory response, decreases renal cortical blood flow,[37,38] reduces gastric mucosal perfusion, and → tachypnea → hypocapnia → ↑ risk of cerebral vasoconstriction. Rationale: normally serum Na^+ is 140 and Cl^- is 100, but NS contains 154 mEq/L of Na^+ and Cl^- (representing excess Cl^-). Treating HCA is harder than prevention. To prevent HCA, avoid overuse of NS and reserve hypertonic saline for severe hyponatremia or acute increases in ICP. Consider using isotonic balanced crystalloid solutions, such as Plasma-Lyte A (pH = 7.4, osmolality = 294 mOsm/L, electrolytes (in mEq/L): Na^+ = 140, K^+ = 5, Cl^- = 98, Mg^+ = 1.5, acetate = 27, gluconate = 23) or Isolyte® for the main IV.

Treatment of hyperchloremic acidosis: substitute chlorine-free fluid for maintenance IV
- sodium bicarbonate ($NaHCO_3$): 3 amps (150 mEq) in 1 L sterile water: produces a slightly hypertonic solution for sodium (1.26%), or
- sodium acetate: 140 mEq/L of sodium acetate is isotonic

5.3 Hypernatremia

5.3.1 General information

Definition: serum sodium > 150 mEq/L. In neurosurgical patients, this is most often seen in the setting of diabetes insipidus (DI).

Since normal total body water (TBW) is ≈ 60% of the patient's normal body weight, the patient's current TBW may be estimated by Eq (5.2).

$$TBW_{current} = \frac{[Na^+]_{normal} \times TBW_{normal}}{[Na^+]_{current}} = \frac{140 mEq/L \times 0.6 \times usual\ body\ wt(kg)}{[Na^+]_{current}} \tag{5.2}$$

The free water deficit to be replaced is given by Eq (5.3). Correction must be made slowly to avoid exacerbating cerebral edema. *One half* the water deficit is replaced over 24 hours, and the remainder is given over 1–2 additional days. Judicious replacement of deficient ADH in cases of true DI must also be made.

$$free\ water\ deficit = 0.6 \times usual\ body\ wt\ (kg) - TBW_{current}$$
$$= \frac{[Na^+]_{current} - 140 mEq/L}{[Na^+]_{current}} \times 0.6 \times usual\ body\ wt\ (kg) \tag{5.3}$$

5.3.2 Diabetes insipidus

General information

Key concepts

- due to low levels of ADH (or, rarely, renal insensitivity to ADH)
- high output of dilute urine (< 300 mOsmol/kg or SG < 1.003) with normal or high serum osmolality and high serum sodium
- often accompanied by craving for water, especially ice-water
- if not managed carefully, there is a danger of severe dehydration, hypernatremia and, if severe, brain shrinkage with intracranial hemorrhage[39]

Diabetes insipidus (DI) is due to insufficient ADH activity at the kidneys, and results in the excessive renal loss of water (polyuria) and electrolytes. The name comes from the fact that the excessive urine is *insipid* (no taste) compared to the excessive urine of diabetes mellitus (mellitus meaning sweet, due to the spilling of sugar into the urine).

DI may be produced by two different etiologies:
* central or neurogenic DI: subnormal levels of ADH caused by hypothalamic-pituitary axis dysfunction. This is the type most often seen by neurosurgeons
* "nephrogenic DI": due to relative resistance of the kidney to normal or supra-normal levels of ADH. Seen with some drugs (drugs: I)

Etiologies of DI[40]:
1. neurogenic (AKA central) diabetes insipidus: dysfunction of hypothalamus or pituitary
   a) familial (autosomal dominant)
   b) idiopathic
   c) posttraumatic (brain injury, including surgery affecting the pituitary gland)
   d) tumor: craniopharyngioma, metastasis, lymphoma…
   e) granuloma: neurosarcoidosis, histiocytosis
   f) infectious: hypophysitis, meningitis, encephalitis
   g) autoimmune
   h) vascular: aneurysm, Sheehan's syndrome (rarely causes DI)
   i) dipsogenic DI: hypothalamic disorder that causes inappropriate thirst. Other causes include: psychogenic polydipsia (a mental health problem)
2. nephrogenic diabetes insipidus
   a) familial (X-linked recessive)
   b) hypokalemia
   c) hypercalcemia
   d) Sjögren's syndrome
   e) drugs: lithium, demeclocycline, colchicine…
   f) chronic renal disease: pyelonephritis, amyloidosis, sickle cell disease, polycystic kidney disease, sarcoidosis

Central DI

85% of ADH secretory capacity must be lost before clinical DI ensues. Characteristic features: high urine output (polyuria) with low urine osmolality, and (in the conscious patient) craving for water (polydipsia), especially ice-water.

Differential diagnosis of DI:
1. (neurogenic) diabetes insipidus (true DI)
2. nephrogenic diabetes insipidus (see above)
3. psychogenic
   a) idiopathic: from resetting of the osmostat (dipsogenic)
   b) psychogenic polydipsia (excess free water intake)
4. osmotic diuresis: e.g., following mannitol, or with renal glucose spilling
5. diuretic use: furosemide, hydrochlorothiazide…

Central DI may be seen in the following situations:
1. following transsphenoidal surgery or removal of craniopharyngioma: (usually transient, therefore avoid long-acting agents until it can be determined if long-term replacement is required). Injury to the posterior pituitary or stalk usually causes one of three patterns of DI[41]:
   a) transient DI: supra-normal urine output (UO) and polydipsia which typically normalizes ≈ 12–36 hrs post-op
   b) "prolonged" DI: UO stays supra-normal either for a prolonged period (may be months - about two–thirds of these patients will return to near-normal at one year post-op due to release of ADH directly from the hypothalamus) or permanently
   c) "triphasic response": least common
      * phase 1: injury to pituitary reduces ADH levels for 4–5 days → DI (polyuria/polydipsia producing **hypernatremia**)
      * phase 2: cell death liberates ADH for the next 4–5 days → transient normalization or even SIADH-like water retention producing **normonatremia or hyponatremia**
      (✖ *NB*: there is a danger of inadvertently continuing vasopressin therapy beyond the initial phase 1 DI into this phase which can produce iatrogenic SIADH)

- phase 3: reduced or absent ADH secretion → DI (transient DI as in "a" above, or "prolonged" DI as in "b" above) producing **hypernatremia**
2. central herniation (p.325): shearing of pituitary stalk may occur
3. brain death: hypothalamic production of ADH ceases
4. with certain tumors:
   a) PitNET/adenomas: DI is rare even with very large macroadenomas. DI may occur with pituitary apoplexy (p.865)
   b) craniopharyngioma: DI usually only occurs postoperatively since damage to pituitary or lower stalk does not prevent production and release of ADH by hypothalamic nuclei
   c) suprasellar germ cell tumors
   d) rarely with a colloid cyst
   e) hypothalamic tumors: Langerhans cell histiocytosis
5. mass lesions pressing on hypothalamus: e.g., AComA aneurysm
6. following head injury: primarily with basal (clival) skull fractures (p.1065)
7. with encephalitis or meningitis
8. drug induced:
   a) ethanol and phenytoin can inhibit ADH release
   b) exogenous steroids may seem to "bring out" DI because they may correct adrenal insufficiency (see below) and they inhibit ADH release
9. granulomatous diseases
   a) Wegener's granulomatosis (p.207): a vasculitis
   b) neurosarcoidosis involving the hypothalamus (p.198)
10. inflammatory: autoimmune hypophysitis (p.1656)[42] or lymphocytic infundibuloneurohypophysitis[43] (distinct conditions)

Diagnosis
The following are usually adequate to make the diagnosis of DI, especially in the appropriate clinical setting:
1. dilute urine:
   a) urine osmolality < 300 mOsm/kg (usually 50–150). (NB: normally, urine osmolality averages between 500–800 mOsm/kg; extreme range: 50–1400). Urine osmolality > 800 mOsm/kg rules out DI and polydipsia
   b) urine specific gravity (USG) in DI is usually **< 1.003** (range: 1.001 to 1.005).
   USG is often used as a quick bedside test, but is not as accurate as urine osmolality since it can be affected by the *size* of the solute particles.
   NB: moieties that produce osmotic diuresis can falsely elevate USG and therefore mask DI by making the urine look more concentrated than it really is. Agents include: large doses of mannitol as may be used in head trauma, glucose (as in poorly controlled diabetes mellitus)
2. or the inability to concentrate urine to > 300 mOsm/kg in the presence of clinical dehydration
3. **polyuria**: urine output (UO) > 50 ml/kg/24 hours in adults and children ≥ 2 years (which is 3.5 L/day for a 70 kg patient).
   Pediatrics: > 150 ml/kg/24 hours at birth (gestational DI); > 100-110 ml/kg/24 hours up to age 2 years.
4. serum sodium: > 135 mmol/L (normal or above-normal)
5. normal adrenal function: DI cannot occur in primary adrenal insufficiency because a minimum of mineralocorticoid activity is needed for the kidney to make free water, thus steroids may "bring out" or "unmask" underlying DI by correcting adrenal insufficiency

▶ **Interpretation**
- absence of polyuria rules out DI and psychogenic polydipsia (pathological water drinking)
- polyuria with urine osmolality > 800 mOsm/kg also rules out DI and polydipsia
- polyuria with serum sodium < 135 mmol/L (normal or low normal) and plasma osmolality ≤ 280 mOsm/kg is diagnostic of primary polydipsia

Plotting simultaneous urine and serum osmolality on the graph in ▶ Fig. 5.5 may help.
1. low serum osmolality (≤ 280 mOsm/kg) usually indicates psychogenic polydipsia
2. if the point falls in the "normal" range, a *supervised* water deprivation test is needed to determine if the patient can concentrate their urine with dehydration (caution: see below)
3. high serum osmolality:
   - diagnosis of DI is established and no further testing to establish the diagnosis is required

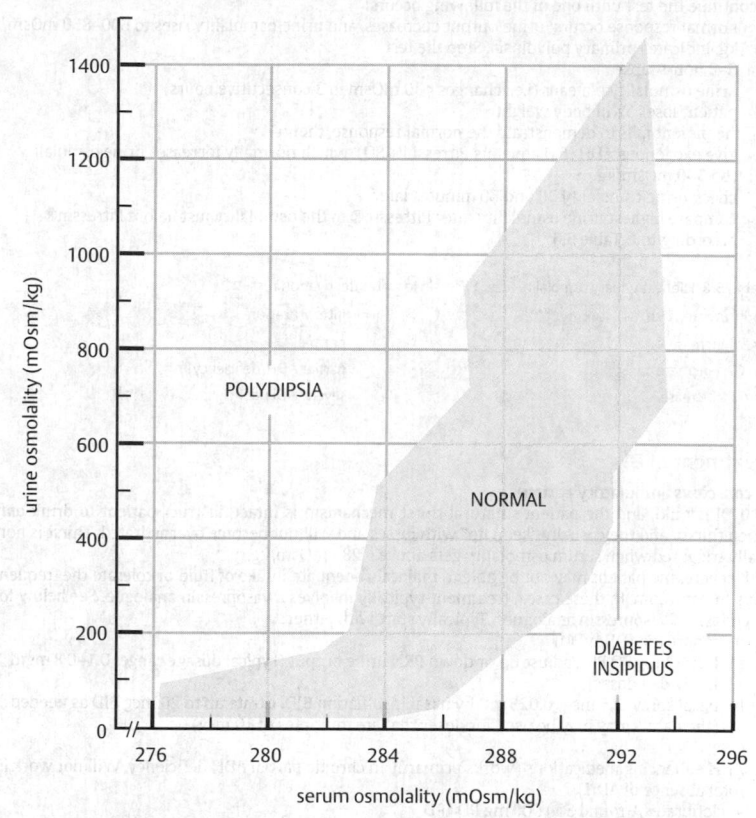

Fig. 5.5 Interpretation of simultaneous serum vs. urine osmolality in patients with polyuria. (Provided by Arnold M. Moses, MD, used with permission.)

- further testing is only needed to differentiate central from nephrogenic DI.
  If desired to differentiate central from nephrogenic DI, give aqueous Pitressin® 5 U SQ: in central DI the urine osmolality should double within 1–2 hours
4. plotting more than one data point may help as some patients tend to "vacillate" around the border zones

Water deprivation test
For indeterminate cases, polyuria due to DI can be differentiated from psychogenic polydipsia by the water deprivation test (✖ CAUTION: perform only under close supervision as rapid and potentially fatal dehydration may ensue in DI). (Note: in compensated DI, serum osmolality is more likely to be lower and to overlap with normal.[44]) There is also a hypertonic saline infusion test (not covered here).

Water deprivation test protocol:
- stop IVs and make the patient NPO
- monitoring:
  ○ check urine osmolality q hr
  ○ check patient weight q 1 hr

- continue the test until one of the following occurs:
  - normal response occurs: urine output decreases, and urine osmolality rises to 600–850 mOsm/kg. Indicates primary polydipsia. Stop the test
  - 6–8 hours lapse
  - urine osmolality plateaus (i.e., changes < 30 mOsm in 3 consecutive hours)
  - patient loses 3% of body weight
- if the patient fails to demonstrate the normal response, then:
  - give exogenous ADH (5 U aqueous Pitressin® SQ), which normally increases urine osmolality to > 300 mOsm/kg
  - check urine osmolality 30 and 60 minutes later
  - compare highest urine osmolality after Pitressin® to the osmolality just before Pitressin® according to ▶ Table 5.6

Table 5.6 Highest urinary osmolality after Pitressin in water deprivation test

Δ in urinary Osm	Interpretation
<5% increase	normal
6–67% increase	partial ADH deficiency
>67% increase	severe ADH deficiency

Treatment of DI

In *conscious* ambulatory patient

If DI is mild, and the patient's natural thirst mechanism is intact, instruct patient to drink *only* when thirsty and they usually "keep up" with losses and will not become overhydrated. Thirst is normally triggered when serum osmolality gets above ≈ 285 mOsm/kg.

If severe, the patient may not be able to maintain adequate intake of fluid or tolerate the frequent trips to bathroom. In these cases, treatment typically involves a vasopressin analogue. See below for a synopsis of vasopressin analogues. Typically start with either:
1. desmopressin (DDAVP®)
   a) PO: 0.1 mg PO BID, adjust up or down PRN urine output (typical dosage range: 0.1–0.8 mg/d in divided doses)
   b) nasal spray: 2.5 mcg (0.025 ml) by nasal insufflation BID, titrate up to 20 mcg BID as needed (the nasal spray may be used for doses that are multiples of 10 mcg)
   OR
2. ADH enhancing medications (works primarily in chronic partial ADH deficiency. Will not work in total absence of ADH)
   - clofibrate (Atromid S®) 500 mg PO QID
   - chlorpropamide: increases renal sensitivity to ADH
   - hydrochlorothiazide: thiazide diuretics may act by depleting Na^+ which increases reabsorption in proximal tubules and shifting fluid away from distal tubules which is where ADH works. ℞: e.g., Dyazide® 1 PO q d (may increase up to 2 per day PRN)

In *conscious* ambulatory patient with impaired thirst mechanisms

Conscious ambulatory patients whose thirst mechanism is *not* intact run the risk of dehydration (adipsic DI) or fluid overload. For these patients:
1. have patient follow UO and daily weights, balance fluid intake and output using antidiuretic medication as needed to keep UO reasonable
2. check serial labs (approximately q weekly) including serum sodium, BUN

In non-ambulatory, comatose/stuporous, or brain-dead patient; see also Medical Management of the Potential Organ Donor (p. 336)
1. follow I's & O's q 1 hr, with urine specific gravity (**SG**) q 4 hrs and whenever urine output (**UO**) > 250 ml/hr
2. labs: serum electrolytes with osmolality q 6 hrs
3. IV fluid management:
   BASE IV: D5 1/2 NS + 20 mEq KCl/L at appropriate rate (75–100 ml/hr)
   PLUS: replace UO above base IV rate ml for ml with 1/2 NS
   NB: for post-op patients, if the patient received significant intraoperative fluids, then they may have an *appropriate* post-op diuresis, in this case use 1/2 NS to replace only ≈ 2/3 of UO that exceeds the basal IV rate

4. if unable to keep up with fluid loss with IV (or NG) replacement (usually with UO > 300 ml/hr), then EITHER
   - 5 U arginine vasopressin (aqueous Pitressin®) IVP/IM/SQ q 4–6 hrs (avoid tannate oil suspension due to erratic absorption and variable duration)
     OR
   - vasopressin IV drip: start at 0.2 U/min & titrate (max: 0.9 U/min)
     OR
   - desmopressin injection SQ/IV titrated to UO, usual adult dose: 0.5–1 ml (2–4 mcg) daily in 2 divided doses

Vasopressin analogues
► Table 5.7 and ► Table 5.8 show dosing forms and duration of action of vasopressin analogues.

Pitressin® is aqueous solution of 8-arginine vasopressin and should be used with caution in patients with vascular disease (especially coronary arteries). ✖ Caution – soundalikes: sometimes pitocin is confused with pitressin because of similarities of the names.

DDAVP (1-deamino-8-D-arginine vasopressin) AKA desmopressin. More potent and longer acting than vasopressin.

Table 5.7 Available preparations of vasopressin analogues

Generic name	Trade name	Route	Concentration	Availability	Manufacturer
desmopressin	DDAVP®	SQ, IM, IV	4 mcg/ml	1 & 10 ml	Aventis
desmopressin	DDAVP® Nasal Spray	nasal spray	100 mcg/ml, each spray delivers 10 mcg	50 doses per bottle	Aventis
desmopressin	DDAVP® Tablets	PO		0.1 & 0.2 mg	Aventis
arginine vasopressin	aqueous Pitressin®	SQ, IM	20 U/ml (50 mcg/ml)	0.5 and 1 ml	Parke-Davis

Table 5.8 Mean time of hypertonic urine[a] (relative to plasma)[b]

Generic name	Route	Dose	Mean duration of action[c]
desmopressin	SQ, IM, IV	0.5 mcg	8 hrs
desmopressin[d]	SQ, IM, IV	1.0 mcg	12 hrs
desmopressin	SQ, IM, IV	2.0 mcg	16 hrs
desmopressin	SQ, IM, IV	4.0 mcg	20 hrs
desmopressin	intranasal	10 mcg (0.1 ml)	12 hrs
desmopressin	intranasal	15 mcg (0.15 ml)	16 hrs
desmopressin	intranasal	20 mcg (0.2 ml)	20 hrs
arginine vasopressin	SQ, IM	5 U (12.5 mcg)	4 hrs (range: 4–8)

[a]provided by Arnold M. Moses, M.D., used with permission
[b]onset of antidiuretic action of these preparations is 30–45 minutes following administration (except pituitary powder in oil which takes 2–4 hrs to start working)
[c]times may vary from patient to patient, but are usually consistent in any individual
[d]Note: 1 mcg BID of desmopressin is as effective as 4 mcg q d, but would obviously be less expensive

References

[1] Ellison DH, Berl T. Clinical practice. The syndrome of inappropriate antidiuresis. N Engl J Med. 2007; 356:2064–2072

[2] Diringer M, Ladenson PW, Borel C, et al. Sodium and Water Regulation in a Patient With Cerebral Salt Wasting. Arch Neurol. 1989; 46:928–930

[3] Sherlock M, O'Sullivan E, Agha A, et al. The incidence and pathophysiology of hyponatraemia after subarachnoid haemorrhage. Clinical Endocrinology. 2006; 64:250–254

[4] Kao L, Al-Lawati Z, Vavao J, et al. Prevalence and clinical demographics of cerebral salt wasting in patients with aneurysmal subarachnoid hemorrhage. Pituitary. 2009; 12:347–351

[5] Rondon-Berrios H, Agaba EI, Tzamaloukas AH. Hyponatremia: pathophysiology, classification,

manifestations and management. Int Urol Nephrol. 2014; 46:2153–2165

[6] Weisberg LS. Pseudohyponatremia: a reappraisal. American Journal of Medicine. 1989; 86:315–318

[7] Arieff AI. Hyponatremia, Convulsions, Respiratory Arrest and Permanent Brain Damage After Elective Surgery in Healthy Women. New England Journal of Medicine. 1986; 314:1529–1535

[8] Steele A, Gowrishankar M, Abrahamson S, et al. Postoperative Hyponatremia despite Near-Isotonic Saline Infusion: A Phenomenon of Desalination. Annals of Internal Medicine. 1997; 126:20–25

[9] Powers CJ, Friedman AH. Diagnosis and management of hyponatremia in neurosurgical patients. Contemporary Neurosurgery. 2007; 29:1–5

[10] Chung HM, Kluge R, Schrier RW, et al. Clinical assessment of extracellular fluid volume in hyponatremia. American Journal of Medicine. 1987; 83:905–908

[11] Lester MC, Nelson PB. Neurological Aspects of Vasopressin Release and the Syndrome of Inappropriate Secretion of Antidiuretic Hormone. Neurosurgery. 1981; 8:725–740

[12] Kröll M, Juhler M, Lindholm J. Hyponatremia in Acute Brain Disease. J Int Med. 1992; 232:291–297

[13] Harrigan MR. Cerebral salt wasting syndrome: A Review. Neurosurgery. 1996; 38:152–160

[14] Ayus JC, Krothapalli RK, Arieff AI. Changing Concepts on Treatment of Severe Symptomatic Hyponatremia: Rapid Correction and Possible Relation to Central Pontine Myelinolysis. Am J Med. 1985; 78:879–902

[15] Fraser CL, Arieff AI. Symptomatic Hyponatremia: Management and Relation to Central Pontine Myelinolysis. Sem Neurol. 1984; 4:445–452

[16] Adams RD, Victor M, Mancall EL. Central Pontine Myelinolysis: A Hitherto Undescribed Disease Occurring in Alcoholic and Malnourished Patients. Arch Neurol Psychiatr. 1959; 81:154–172

[17] Ayus JC, Krothapalli RK, Arieff AI. Treatment of Symptomatic Hyponatremia and Its Relation to Brain Damage. N Engl J Med. 1987; 317:1190–1195

[18] Berl T. Treating Hyponatremia: What is All the Controversy About? Ann Intern Med. 1990; 113:417–419

[19] Arieff AI. Hyponatremia Associated with Permanent Brain Damage. Adv Intern Med. 1987; 32:325–344

[20] Adrogue HJ, Madias NE. Hyponatremia. N Engl J Med. 2000; 342:1581–1589

[21] Soupart A, Ngassa M, Decaux G. Therapeutic relowering of the serum sodium in a patient after excessive correction of hyponatremia. Clin Nephrol. 1999; 51:383–386

[22] Oya S, Tsutsumi K, Ueki K, et al. Reinduction of hyponatremia to treat central pontine myelinolysis. Neurology. 2001; 57:1931–1932

[23] De Troyer A, Demanet JC. Correction of Antidiuresis by Demeclocycline. N Engl J Med. 1975; 293:915–918

[24] Perks WH, Mohr P, Liversedge LA. Demeclocycline in Inappropriate ADH Syndrome. Lancet. 1976; 2

[25] Forrest JN, Cox M, Hong C, et al. Superiority of Demeclocycline over Lithium in the Treatment of Chronic Syndrome of Inappropriate Secretion of Antidiuretic Hormone. N Engl J Med. 1978; 298:173–177

[26] Wright WL, Asbury WH, Gilmore JL, et al. Conivaptan for hyponatremia in the neurocritical care unit. Neurocrit Care. 2009; 11:6–13

[27] Maroon JC, Nelson PB. Hypovolemia in Patients with Subarachnoid Hemorrhage: Therapeutic Implications. Neurosurgery. 1979; 4:223–226

[28] Wijdicks EFM, Vermeulen M, Hijdra A, et al. Hyponatremia and Cerebral Infarction in Patients with Ruptured Intracranial Aneurysms: Is Fluid Restriction Harmful? Ann Neurol. 1985; 17:137–140

[29] Wijdicks EFM, Vermeulen M, ten Haaf JA, et al. Volume Depletion and Natriuresis in Patients with a Ruptured Intracranial Aneurysm. Ann Neurol. 1985; 18:211–216

[30] Nelson PB, Seif SM, Maroon JC, et al. Hyponatremia in Intracranial Disease. Perhaps Not the Syndrome of Inappropriate Secretion of Antidiuretic Hormone (SIADH). Journal of Neurosurgery. 1981; 55:938–941

[31] Suarez JI, Qureshi AI, Parekh PD, et al. Administration of hypertonic (3%) sodium chloride/acetate in hyponatremic patients with symptomatic vasospasm following subarachnoid hemorrhage. J Neurosurg Anesthesiol. 1999; 11:178–184

[32] Al-Rawi PG, Tseng MY, Richards HK, et al. Hypertonic saline in patients with poor-grade subarachnoid hemorrhage improves cerebral blood flow, brain tissue oxygen, and pH. Stroke. 2010; 41:122–128

[33] Hasan D, Lindsay KW, Wijdicks EFM, et al. Effect of Fludrocortisone Acetate in Patients with Subarachnoid Hemorrhage. Stroke. 1989; 20:1156–1161

[34] Mori T, Katayama Y, Kawamata T, et al. Improved efficiency of hypervolemic therapy with inhibition of natriuresis by fludrocortisone in patients with aneurysmal subarachnoid hemorrhage. J Neurosurg. 1999; 91:947–952

[35] Katayama Y, Haraoka J, Hirabayashi H, et al. A randomized controlled trial of hydrocortisone against hyponatremia in patients with aneurysmal subarachnoid hemorrhage. Stroke. 2007; 38:2373–2375

[36] Reeder RF, Harbaugh RE. Administration of Intravenous Urea and Normal Saline for the Treatment of Hyponatremia in Neurosurgical Patients. Journal of Neurosurgery. 1989; 70:201–206

[37] Chowdhury AH, Cox EF, Francis ST, et al. A randomized, controlled, double-blind crossover study on the effects of 2-L infusions of 0.9% saline and plasma-lyte(R) 148 on renal blood flow velocity and renal cortical tissue perfusion in healthy volunteers. Ann Surg. 2012; 256:18–24

[38] Yunos NM, Bellomo R, Hegarty C, et al. Association between a chloride-liberal vs chloride-restrictive intravenous fluid administration strategy and kidney injury in critically ill adults. Jama. 2012; 308:1566–1572

[39] Adrogue HJ, Madias NE. Hypernatremia. N Engl J Med. 2000; 342:1493–1499

[40] Thibonnier M, Barrow DL, Selman W. Antidiuretic Hormone: Regulation, Disorders, and Clinical Evaluation. In: Neuroendocrinology. Baltimore: Williams and Wilkins; 1992:19–30

[41] Verbalis JG, Robinson AG, Moses AM. Postoperative and Post-Traumatic Diabetes Insipidus. Front Horm Res. 1985; 13:247–265

[42] Abe T, Matsumoto K, Sanno N, et al. Lymphocytic Hypophysitis: Case Report. Neurosurgery. 1995; 36:1016–1019

[43] Imura H, Nakao K, Shimatsu A, et al. Lymphocytic Infundibuloneurohypophysitis as a Cause of Central Diabetes Insipidus. New England Journal of Medicine. 1993; 329:683–689

[44] Miller M, Dalakos T, Moses AM, et al. Recognition of partial defects in antidiuretic hormone secretion. Annals of Internal Medicine. 1970; 73:721–729

6 General Neurocritical Care

6.1 Parenteral agents for hypertension

Drug info: ★ Nicardipine (Cardene®)

Calcium channel blocker (CCB) that may be given IV. Does not require arterial line, *does not raise ICP.* Does not reduce heart rate, but may be used in conjunction with, e.g., labetalol or esmolol if that is desired. **Side effects:** H/A 15%, nausea 5%, hypotension 5%, reflex tachycardia 3.5%.

℞ start at 5 mg/hr IV (off label: 10 mg/hr may be used in situations where urgent reduction is needed). Increase by 2.5 mg/hr every 5–15 minutes up to a maximum of 15 mg/hr. Decrease to 3 mg/hr once control is achieved. ✖ Ampules contain 25 mg and *must be diluted* before administration.

Drug info: ★ Clevidipine (Cleviprex®)

IV calcium channel blocker (CCB) that is selective for vascular smooth muscle, with minimal effect on myocardial contractility or cardiac conduction. Reduces MAP by decreasing systemic vascular resistance. Is rapidly degraded by esterases in blood and extravascular tissues ∴ dosing does not need to be adjusted for liver or renal insufficiency. It is even metabolized rapidly in pseudocholinesterase deficient patients. Onset and end time are rapid which is an advantage for finely titrating blood pressure. Does not require arterial line, *does not raise ICP.* Does not reduce heart rate, but may be used in conjunction with, e.g., labetalol or esmolol if that is desired. **Side effects:** H/A 15%, nausea 5%, hypotension 5%, reflex tachycardia 3.5%. It is a lipid emulsion, with milky white appearance similar to propofol (possible confusion) and may induce hypertriglyceridemia when used simultaneously.[1]

In perioperative setting there is a 4–5% reduction in SBP within 4–5 minutes after infusion is started, and BP fully recovers in 5–15 minutes in most patients.

℞ start at 1–2 mg/hr IV. Titrate up by doubling the dose every 90 seconds until nearing the desired BP then smaller increments are made less frequently up to a maximum of 32 mg/hr (control is usually achieved at ≤ 16 mg/hr). The drug is *not diluted* before administration. ✖ Because of lipid loading, it is recommended to limit infusion to ≤ 1000 ml per 24 hours (an average of 21 mg/hr). There is little information regarding infusions > 72 hours.

Drug info: Nitroglycerin (NTG)

Raises ICP (less than with nitroprusside due to preferential venous action[2]). Vasodilator, venous > arterial (large coronaries > small). Result: decreases LV filling pressure (pre-load). Does not cause "coronary steal" (cf nitroprusside).

℞ 10–20 mcg/min IV drip (increase by 5–10 mcg/min q 5–10 min). For angina pectoris: 0.4 mg SL q 5 min × 3 doses, check BP before each dose.

Drug info: Labetalol (Normodyne®, Trandate®)

Blocks α_1 selective, β non-selective (potency < propranolol). ICP reduces or no change.[3] Pulse rate: decreases or no change. Cardiac output does not change. Does not exacerbate coronary ischemia. May be used in controlled CHF, but not in overt CHF. Contraindicated in asthma. Renal failure: same dose. **Side effects:** fatigue, dizziness, orthostatic hypotension.

Intravenous (IV)
Onset 5 mins, peak 10 mins, duration 3–6 hrs.

℞ IV: patient supine; check BP q 5 min; give each dose slow IVP (over 2 min) q 10 minutes until desired BP achieved; dose sequence: 20, 40, 80, 80, then 80 mg (300 mg total). Once controlled, use ≈ same total dose IVP q 8 hrs.

6

℞ *IV drip* (alternative): add 40 ml (200 mg) to 160 ml of IVF (result: 1 mg/ml); run at 2 ml/min (2 mg/min) until desired BP (usual effective dose = 50–200 mg) or until 300 mg given; then titrate rate (bradycardia limits dose, increase slowly since effect takes 10–20 minutes).

Oral (PO)

Undergoes first pass liver degradation, therefore requires higher doses PO. PO onset: 2 hrs, peak: 4 hrs.
℞ *PO*: to convert IV → PO, start with 200 mg PO BID. To start with PO, give 100 mg BID, and increase 100 mg/dose q 2 day; max. = 2400 mg/day.

Drug info: Enalaprilat (Vasotec®)

An angiotensin-converting enzyme (ACE) inhibitor. The active metabolite of the orally administered drug enalapril (see below). Acts within ≈ 15 mins of administration.
Side effects: hyperkalemia occurs in ≈ 1%. Do not use during pregnancy.
℞ IV: start with 1.25 mg slow IV over 5 mins, may increase up to 5 mg q 6 hrs PRN.

Drug info: Esmolol (Brevibloc®)

Cardioselective short-acting beta blocker.[4] Being investigated for hypertensive emergencies. Metabolized by RBC esterase. Elimination half-life: 9 mins. Therapeutic response (> 20% decrease in heart rate, HR < 100, or conversion to sinus rhythm) in 72%. **Side effects:** dose related hypotension (in 20–50%), generally resolves within 30 mins of D/C. Bronchospasm less likely than other beta blockers. Avoid in CHF.
℞ 500 mcg/kg loading dose over 1 min, follow with 4 min infusion starting with 50 mcg/kg/min. Repeat loading dose and increment infusion rate by 50 mcg/kg/min q 5 mins. Rarely > 100 mcg/kg/min required. Doses > 200 mcg/kg/min add little.

Drug info: Fenoldopam (Corlopam®)

Vasodilator. Onset of action < 5 minutes, duration 30 mins.
℞ IV infusion (no bolus doses): start with 0.1–0.3 mcg/kg/min, titrate by 0.1 mcg/kg/min q 15 min up to a maximum of 1.6 mcg/kg/min.

Drug info: Propranolol (Inderal®)

Main use IV is to counteract tachycardia with vasodilators (usually doesn't lower BP acutely when used alone), but esmolol and labetalol are more commonly used for this.
℞ IV: load with 1–10 mg slow IVP, follow with 3 mg/hr. PO: 80–640 mg q d in divided doses.

6.2 Hypotension (shock)

6.2.1 Classification

1. hypovolemic: first sign usually tachycardia. > 20–40% of blood volume loss must occur before perfusion of vital organs is impaired. Includes:
   a) hemorrhage (external or internal)
   b) bowel obstruction (with third spacing)

2. septic: most often due to gram-negative sepsis
3. cardiogenic: includes MI, cardiomyopathy, dysrhythmias (including A-fib)
4. neurogenic: e.g., paralysis due to spinal cord injury. Blood pools in venous capacitance vessels
5. miscellaneous
   a) anaphylaxis
   b) insulin reaction

6.2.2 Cardiovascular agents for shock

Plasma expanders. Includes:
1. crystalloids: normal saline has less tendency to promote cerebral edema than others; see IV fluids (p.1050), under control of elevated ICP
2. colloids: e.g., hetastarch (Hespan®). ✖ CAUTION: repeated administration over a period of days may prolong PT/PTT and clotting times and may increase the risk of rebleeding in aneurysmal SAH (p.1437).[5]
3. blood products: expensive. Risk of transmissible diseases or transfusion reaction

Drug info: Dopamine

See ▶ Table 6.1 for a summary of the effects of dopamine (DA) at various dosages. DA is primarily a vasoconstrictor (β_1 effects usually overridden by α-activity). 25% of dopamine given is rapidly converted to norepinephrine (NE). At doses > 10 mcg/kg/min one is essentially giving NE. May cause significant hyperglycemia at high doses.

   ℞ Start with 2–5 mcg/kg/min and titrate.

Table 6.1 Dopamine dosage

Dose (mcg/kg/min)	Effect	Result
0.5–2.0 (sometimes up to 5)	dopaminergic	renal, mesenteric, coronary, & cerebral vasodilatation, (+) inotrope
2–10	β_1	positive inotrope
>10	α, β & dopaminergic	releases nor-epi (vasoconstrictor)

Drug info: Dobutamine (Dobutrex®)

Vasodilates by β_1 (primary) and by increased CO from (+) inotropy (β_2); result: little or no fall in BP, less tachycardia than DA. No alpha release nor vasoconstriction. May be used synergistically with nitroprusside. Tachyphylaxis after ≈ 72 hrs. Pulse increases > 10% may exacerbate myocardial ischemia, more common at doses > 20 mcg/kg/min. Optimal use requires hemodynamic monitoring. Possible platelet function inhibition.

   ℞ usual range 2.5–10 mcg/kg/min; rarely doses up to 40 used (to prepare: put 50 mg in 250 ml D5 W to yield 200 mcg/ml).

Drug info: Amrinone (Inocor®)

Nonadrenergic cardiotonic. Phosphodiesterase inhibitor, effects similar to dobutamine (including exacerbation of myocardial ischemia). 2% incidence of thrombocytopenia.

   ℞ 0.75 mg/kg initially over 2–3 min, then drip 5–10 mcg/kg/min.

Drug info: Phenylephrine (Neo-Synephrine®)

Pure alpha sympathomimetic. Useful in hypotension associated with tachycardia (atrial tachyarrhythmias). Elevates BP by increasing SVR via vasoconstriction, causes reflex increase in parasympathetic tone (with resultant slowing of pulse). Lack of β action means non-inotropic, no cardiac acceleration, and no relaxation of bronchial smooth muscle. Cardiac output and renal blood flow may decrease. Avoid in spinal cord injuries (p. 1139).

℞ pressor range: 100–180 mcg/min; maintenance: 40–60 mcg/min. To prepare: put 40 mg (4 amps) in 500 ml D5 W to yield 80 mcg/ml; a rate of 8 ml/hr = 10 mcg/min.

Drug info: Norepinephrine

Primarily vasoconstrictor (? counterproductive in cerebral vasospasm, ? decreases CBF). β-agonist at low doses. Increases pulmonary vascular resistance.

Drug info: Epinephrine (adrenalin globally)

℞ 0.5–1.0 mg of 1:10,000 solution IVP; may repeat q 5 minutes (may bolus per ET tube). Drip: start at 1.0 mcg/min, titrate up to 8 mcg/min (to prepare: put 1 mg in 100 ml NS or D5W).

Drug info: Isoproterenol (Isuprel®)

Positive chronotropic and inotropic, → increased cardiac O_2 consumption, arrhythmias, vasodilatation (by $β_1$ action) skeletal muscle > cerebral vessels.

Drug info: Levophed

Direct β stimulation (positive inotropic and chronotropic).
℞ start drip at 8–12 mcg/min; maintenance 2–4 mcg/min (0.5–1.0 ml/min) (to prepare: put 2 mg in 500 ml NS or D5 W to yield 4 mcg/cc).

6.3 Acid inhibitors

6.3.1 Stress ulcers in neurosurgery

See reference.[6]

The risk of developing stress ulcers (SU) AKA Cushing's ulcers is high in critically ill patients with CNS pathology. These lesions are AKA Cushing's ulcers due to Cushing's classic treatise.[7] 17% of SUs produce clinically significant hemorrhage. CNS risk factors include intracranial pathology: brain injury (especially Glasgow Coma scale score < 9), brain tumors, intracerebral hemorrhage, SIADH, CNS infection, ischemic stroke, as well as spinal cord injury. The odds are increased with the coexistence of extra-CNS risk factors including long-term use of steroids (usually > 3 weeks), burns > 25% of body surface area, hypotension, respiratory failure, coagulopathies, renal or hepatic failure and sepsis.

The pathogenesis of SUs is incompletely understood, but probably results from an imbalance of destructive factors (acid, pepsin & bile) relative to protective factors (mucosal blood flow, mucus-bicarbonate layer, endothelial cell replenishment & protaglandins).[6] CNS pathology, especially that involving the diencephalon or brainstem, can lead to reduction of vagal output which leads to hypersecretion of gastric acid and pepsin. There is a peak in acid and pepsin production 3–5 days after CNS injury.

6.3.2 Prophylaxis for stress ulcers

There is strong evidence that reduction of gastric acid (whether by antacids or agents that inhibit acid secretion) reduces the incidence of GI bleeding from stress ulcers in critically ill patients. Elevating gastric pH > 4.5 also inactivates pepsin.

Other therapies that don't involve alterations of pH that may be effective include sucralfate (see below) and enteral nutrition (controversial).[6] Titrated antacids or sucralfate appear to be superior to H2 antagonists in reducing the incidence of SUs.

Routine prophylaxis when steroids are used is not warranted unless one of the following risk factors are present: prior PUD, concurrent use of NSAIDs, hepatic or renal failure, malnourishment, or prolonged steroid therapy > 3 weeks.

6.3.3 Possible increased pneumonia and mortality from altering gastric pH

Whereas bringing gastric pH to a more neutral level reduces the risk of SUs, pH > 4 permits bacterial colonization of the normally sterile stomach. This may increase the risk of pneumonia from aspiration, and there is a suggestion that mortality may also be increased.[8] Sucralfate may be as effective in reducing bleeding, but may be associated with lower rates of pneumonia and mortality. There is insufficient data to determine the net result of sucralfate compared to no treatment.[8]

6.3.4 Histamine2 (H2) antagonists

Drug info: Ranitidine (Zantac®)

℞ Adult age ≤ 65 yrs: 150 mg PO BID, or 50 mg IVPB q 8 hrs. For age > 65 with normal renal function: 50 mg IV q 12 hrs.

IV drip (provides a more consistently higher pH without peaks and troughs; some controversy that this may increase gastric bacterial concentration with increased risk of aspiration pneumonia has not been borne out): 6.25 mg/hr (e.g., inject 150 mg into 42 ml of IVF yielding 3.125 mg/ml, run at 2 ml/hr).

Drug info: Famotidine (Pepcid®)

℞ Adult: 20 mg PO q hs for maintenance; 40 mg PO q hs for active ulcer therapy; IV: 20 mg q 12 hrs (for hypersecretory conditions, 20 mg IVPB q 6 hrs).[9] **Supplied:** 20 & 40 mg tablets, 40 mg/5 ml suspension, and 20 & 40 mg orally disintegrating tablets as Pepcid RPD. Available OTC in 10 mg tablets as Pepcid AC. Available IV.

Drug info: Nizatidine (Axid®)

℞ 300 mg PO q d or 150 mg PO BID. **Supplied:** 150 & 300 mg pulvules. Available OTC in 75 mg tablets as Axid AR.

6.3.5 Gastric acid secretion inhibitors (proton pump inhibitors)

These agents reduce gastric acid by specific inhibition of the final step in acid secretion by gastric parietal cells (by inhibiting the (H^+, K^+)-ATPase enzyme system on the cell surface, the so-called "acid pump"). They block acid secretion regardless of the stimulus (Zollinger-Ellison syndrome, hypergastrinemia...). Full recovery of acid secretion upon discontinuation may not occur for weeks. ✖ Not indicated for long-term treatment as the trophic effects of the resultant elevated levels of gastrin may lead to gastric carcinoid tumors.

Drug info: Omeprazole (Prilosec®)

Inhibition of some hepatic P-450 enzymes results in reduced clearance of warfarin and phenytoin. Decreases the effectiveness of prednisone.

℞ *Adult*: for peptic ulcers and gastro-esophageal reflux disease (GERD) 20–40 mg PO daily. For Zollinger-Ellison syndrome: 20 mg PO q d to 120 mg PO TID (dose adjusted to keep basal acid output < 60 mEq/hr). **Side effects:** N/V, H/A, diarrhea, abdominal pain, or rash in 1–5% of patients. **Supplied:** 10, 20 & 40 mg delayed-release capsules. Available OTC in 20.6 mg tablets as Prilosec OTC.

Drug info: ★ Lansoprazole (Prevacid®)

Found *not* to have an affect on a number of other drugs metabolized by cytochrome P-450 including phenytoin, warfarin, and prednisone.

℞ *Adult*: 15 mg (for duodenal ulcer, GERD, or maintenance therapy) or 30 mg (for gastric ulcer or erosive esophagitis) PO q d, short-term treatment × 4 wks. **Supplied:** 15 & 30 mg delayed-release capsules.

Drug info: Pantoprazole (Protonix®)

℞ PO: 40 mg PO q d for up to 8 wks. IV: 40 mg IV q d × 7–10 d. **Supplied:** PO: 40 mg delayed-release capsules.

6.3.6 Miscellaneous

Drug info: Sucralfate (Carafate®)

Minimally absorbed from GI tract. Acts by coating ulcerated areas of mucosa, does not inhibit acid secretion. This may actually result in a lower incidence of pneumonia and mortality than agents that affect gastric pH (see above).

℞ 1 gm PO QID on an empty stomach. Do not give antacids within one half-hour of sucralfate.

6.4 Rhabdomyolysis

6.4.1 Background and pathophysiology

1. rhabdomyolysis (RM): a syndrome caused by injury to skeletal muscle → leakage of intracellular contents (potassium, phosphate, CPK, urate, and myoglobin) into plasma that may be toxic to kidneys
2. clinical triad: muscle weakness, myalgias, and dark urine
3. **myoglobin (Mgb)** is an oxygen binding protein in muscle that accepts oxygen from circulating hemoglobin. After muscle injury, plasma Mgb levels may exceed the capacity of the normal clearing mechanisms (which includes haptoglobin binding) and Mgb can precipitate in glomerular filtrate causing renal tubular obstruction, direct nephrotoxicity, intrarenal vasoconstriction, and acute kidney injury. Mgb appears quickly in the blood and is rapidly cleared within 24 hours. If Mgb spills into the urine (myoglobinuria) it can cause urine to test positive for "blood." Reference blood levels: 0–85 ng/mL
4. **creatine phosphokinase (CPK)** AKA creatine kinase (CK) is found mainly in the brain (CK-BB), skeletal muscle (CK-MM) and cardiac muscle (CK-MB & CK-MM). In muscle, CPK replenishes ATP by catalyzing a reaction between creatine phosphate and ADP. The appearance of CPK in the blood lags behind Mgb by a few hours, peaks in 24–36 hours, decreases at 30–40% per day, and

remains elevated for several days. It is used as a marker for the diagnosis and assessment of the severity of muscular injury. Reference range: 60–174 IU/L
5. acute kidney injury (AKI) is due to:
    a) decreased extracellular volume + vasoactive substances → renal vasoconstriction and
    b) ferrihemate, which is formed from myoglobin at a pH < 5.6
6. vasoconstriction/ischemia deplete renal tubular ATP formation, enhancing tubular cell damage and myoglobin precipitation causes formation of obstructive casts
7. risk of renal injury is low when initial CPK levels are < 15,000–20,000 IU/L (though may occur at lower levels in patients with sepsis, dehydration, or acidosis)

6.4.2 Etiology and epidemiology

1. trauma & muscle compression/crush → direct injury to sarcolemma & occlusion of muscular vessels
2. excluding trauma, neurosurgeons are most likely to encounter RM in the setting of prolonged operations, especially spine surgery in the prone position, but also possibly even with minimally invasive lateral approach[10]
3. other nontraumatic etiologies: infection, metabolic derangement, neuroleptic malignant syndrome, malignant hyperthermia, drugs, EtOH, environmental toxins, extreme muscular activity, sickle cell trait
4. incidence of myoglobin-induced AKI in adult rhabdomyolysis (all causes) ranges from 17–35%
5. ≈ 28–37% of adult patients require short-term hemodialysis
6. rhabdomyolysis accounts for 5–20% of all adult cases of AKI

6.4.3 Management and treatment

Proactive intervention: for patients at risk for rhabdomyolysis (e.g., spine surgery lasting > 5 hours), it may be helpful to proactively check CPK & myoglobin (Mgb) levels post-op, and, when elevated, to aggressively hydrate before the full-blown syndrome develops
    Predictors of potential AKI include[11]:
1. peak CPK level > 6000 IU/L, and especially if > 15,000 IU/L
2. dehydration: hematocrit > 50, serum sodium level > 150 mEq/L, orthostatic hypotension, pulmonary capillary wedge pressure < 5 mm Hg, urinary fractional excretion of sodium < 1%
3. sepsis
4. hyperkalemia or hyperphosphatemia on admission
5. hypoalbuminemia

Treatment: there is no Level 1 evidence for the treatment of rhabdomyolysis (RM).[12] Traditionally, RM has been treated with IV fluids with bicarbonate (in an effort to alkalinize the urine) along with PRN diuretics. These adjuncts to IV hydration have been called into question,[13] and it appears that prompt recognition and appropriate volume replacement may be all that is needed to avoid AKI in most patients.
    The following is one possible protocol for adults (modified[12] available online).
    In an adult with RM and CPK ≥ 5000 IU/L AND acute renal failure (Cr ≥ 2.9 mg/dl):
1. general measures:
    a) ABCs, I/O monitoring (foley catheter), correction of electrolyte abnormalities, correction of underlying cause if possible to prevent end organ complications, invasive hemodynamic monitoring may be needed to ensure adequate volume resuscitation
    b) minimize other potential renal stressors: nephrotoxic antibiotics, iodinated IV contrast, ACE inhibitors, NSAIDs… (Level III[12])
    c) EKG if hyperkalemia present
2. the mainstay of treatment is expansion of extracellular volume → increased glomerular filtration rate (GFR), oxygen delivery and dilution of myoglobin and other renal tubular toxins
3. start with IV fluid (IVF): lactated ringers (LR) is preferred over NS (Level II[12]) to maintain urine output (UO) ≥ 1 ml/kg/hr
4. if this not possible with IVF alone, add sodium bicarbonate ($NaHCO_3$) and mannitol as follows until CPK shows a steady downtrend or falls below 5000 IU/L or UO averages > 100 ml/hr for 12 consecutive hours
    a) if serum sodium ≤ 147 mEq/L: use 1/2 NS + 100 mEq $NaHCO_3$/L @ 125 ml/hr
    b) if serum sodium > 147 mEq/L: use D5W + 100 mEq $NaHCO_3$/L @ 125 ml/hr
    c) mannitol: 12.5 g IV q 6 hours

5. in patients receiving NaHCO₃, check daily ABG & electrolytes
   a) if serum pH < 7.15 or serum $NaHCO_3 \leq 15$ mg/dL: bolus with 100 mEq NaHCO₃ and recheck ABG in 3 hours, repeat until pH is > 7.5 AND serum NaHCO₃ is > 15
   b) discontinue bicarbonate if pH ≥ 7.5
   c) hold NaHCO₃ for hypernatremia
6. serial CPK measurements are not required after the peak is passed (Level III[12])
7. dialysis may be required in patients with oliguric renal failure, persistent hyperkalemia, pulmonary edema, congestive heart failure, or persistent metabolic acidosis

References

[1] Kaur H, Nattanamai P, Qualls KE. Propofol and Clevidipine-induced Hypertriglyceridemia. Cureus. 2018; 10. DOI: 10.7759/cureus.3165

[2] Cottrell JE, Patel K, Turndorf H, et al. ICP Changes Induced by Sodium Nitroprusside in Patients with Intracranial Mass Lesions. J Neurosurg. 1978; 48:329–331

[3] Orlowski JP, Shiesley D, Vidt DG, et al. Labetalol to Control Blood Pressure After Cerebrovascular Surgery. Crit Care Med. 1988; 16:765–768

[4] Esmolol - A Short-Acting IV Beta Blocker. Medical Letter. 1987; 29:57–58

[5] Trumble ER, Muizelaar JP, Myseros JS. Coagulopathy with the Use of Hetastarch in the Treatment of Vasospasm. Journal of Neurosurgery. 1995; 82:44–47

[6] Lu WY, Rhoney DH, Boling WB, et al. A Review of Stress Ulcer Prophylaxis in the Neurosurgical Intensive Care Unit. Neurosurgery. 1997; 41:416–426

[7] Cushing H. Peptic Ulcers and the Interbrain. Surgery Gynecology and Obstetrics. 1932; 55:1–34

[8] Cook DJ, Reeve BK, Guyatt GH, et al. Stress Ulcer Prophylaxis in Critically Ill Patients: Resolving Discordant Meta-Analyses. JAMA. 1996; 275:308–314

[9] Famotidine (Pepcid). Medical Letter. 1987; 29:17–18

[10] Dakwar E, Rifkin SI, Volcan IJ, et al. Rhabdomyolysis and acute renal failure following minimally invasive spine surgery: report of 5 cases. J Neurosurg Spine. 2011; 14:785–788

[11] Ward MM. Factors predictive of acute renal failure in rhabdomyolysis. Arch Intern Med. 1988; 148:1553–1557

[12] Bada Alvaro, Smith Nathan. Rhabdomyolysis: Prevention and Treatment. 2018. http://www.surgicalcriticalcare.net/Guidelines/Rhabdomyolysis%202018.pdf

[13] Brown CV, Rhee P, Chan L, et al. Preventing renal failure in patients with rhabdomyolysis: do bicarbonate and mannitol make a difference? J Trauma. 2004; 56:1191–1196

7 Sedatives, Paralytics, Analgesics

7.1 Sedatives and paralytics

7.1.1 Richmond agitation-sedation scale (RASS)

A validated scale[1,2] for quantitating the level of sedation, e.g., when titrating sedatives for agitated patients (▶ Table 7.1). Positive numbers = agitation, negative numbers = sedation

Procedure for performing RASS assessment:
1. on observation, patient is alert, restless or agitated: score 0 to +4
2. if patient is not alert, state patient's name and verbally instruct to open eyes and look at speaker: score –1 to –3
3. if no response to verbal stimulus, physically stimulate by shaking shoulder and/or sternal rub: score –4 or –5

Table 7.1 Richmond agitation-sedation scale

	Score	Term	Description	
Agitation	+4	combative	overly combative, violent, immediate danger to staff	
	+3	very agitated	pulls or removes tubes or catheters; aggressive	
	+2	agitated	frequent non-purposeful movements, fights ventilator	
	+1	restless	anxious, but movements not aggressive/vigorous	
	0	alert & calm		
Sedation	–1	drowsy	not fully alert, but has sustained awakening (eye-opening/contact) to voice (≥ 10 seconds)	verbal stimulation
	–2	light sedation	briefly awakens with eye contact to voice (< 10 seconds)	
	–3	moderate sedation	movement or eye opening to voice (no eye contact)	
	–4	deep sedation	no response to voice, but movement or eye-opening to physical stimulation	physical stimulation
	–5	unarousable	no response to voice or physical stimulation	

7.1.2 Conscious sedation

Use of these agents requires ability to provide immediate emergency ventilatory support (including intubation). Agents include:
1. midazolam (Versed®) (p.1050) with fentanyl
2. fentanyl
3. pentobarbital (Nembutal®): a barbiturate. ℞ for 70 kg adult: 100 mg slow IVP

Drug info: Methohexital (Brevital®)

More potent and shorter acting than thiopental (useful e.g., for percutaneous rhizotomy where patient needs to be sedated and awakened repeatedly). Lasts 5–7 min. Similar cautions with the added problem that methohexital may *induce* seizures. May no longer be available in the U.S.

℞ Adult: 1 gm% solution (add 50 ml diluent to 500 mg to yield 10 mg/ml), 2 ml test dose, then 5–12 ml IVP at rate of 1 ml/5 secs, then 2 to 4 ml q 4–7 min PRN.

7.1.3 Sedation

Generally requires intubation and mechanical ventilatory support in the ICU. Doses are generally lower than those used by anesthesiologists for general anesthesia.

Drug info: Thiopental (Pentothal®)

A short acting barbiturate. 1st dose causes unconsciousness in 20–30 secs (circulation time), depth increases up to 40 secs, duration = 5 mins (terminated by redistribution), consciousness returns over 20–30 mins.

Side effects: dose-related respiratory depression, irritation if extravasated, intra-arterial injection → necrosis, agitation if injected slowly, an *antianalgesic*, myocardial depressant, hypotension in hypovolemic patients.

℞ Adult: initial concentration should not exceed 2.5%, give 50 mg test dose moderately rapid IVP, then if tolerated give 100–200 mg IVP over 20–30 secs (500 mg may be required in large patient).

Drug info: ★ Remifentanil (Ultiva®)

Ultrashort acting micro-opioid receptor agonist. Potency similar to fentanyl. Rapidly crosses BBB. Onset: < 1 min. Offset: 3–10 mins. *Lowers ICP.* Metabolism: non-hepatic hydrolysis by nonspecific blood and tissue esterases, ∴ no accumulation. Synergy with thiopental, propofol, isoflurane, midazolam requires reducing doses of these agents by up to 75%. **Side effects:** bradycardia, hypotension (these side effects may be blunted by pretreatment with anticholinergics), N/V, muscle rigidity, pruritus (especially facial) dose-dependent respiratory depression at doses > 0.05 mcg/kg/min.

℞ Adult: avoid bolus doses. Start with drip of 0.05 mcg/kg/min. Titrate in 0.025 mcg/kg/min increments to a maximum of 0.1–0.2 mcg/kg/min. Add a sedative if adequate sedation not achieved at maximum dose. Wean infusion in 25% decrements over 10 minutes after extubation. **Supplied:** vials of 1, 2 or 5 mg powder to be reconstituted to 1 mg/ml solution.

Drug info: Fentanyl (Sublimaze®)

Narcotic, potency ≈ 100 × morphine. High lipid solubility → rapid onset. Offset (small doses): 20–30 mins. Unlike morphine and meperidine, does not cause histamine release. *Lowers ICP.* **Side effects:** dose dependent respiratory depression, large doses given rapidly may cause chest wall rigidity. Repeated dosing may cause accumulation. Diminished sensitivity to CO_2 stimulation, may persist longer than the depression of respiratory rate (up to 4 hours).

℞ Adult: 25–100 mcg (0.5–2 ml) IVP, repeat PRN. **Supplied:** 50 mcg/ml; requires refrigeration.

Drug info: ★ Propofol (Diprivan®)

A sedative hypnotic. Also useful in high doses during aneurysm surgery as a neuroprotectant (p. 1466). Protection seems to be less than with barbiturates. Offset time increases after ≈ 12 hours of use.

℞ for sedation: start at 5–10 mcg/kg/min. Increase by 5–10 mcg/kg/min q 5–10 minutes PRN desired sedation (up to a max of 50 mcg/kg/min).

Side effects: include Propofol infusion syndrome: hyperkalemia, hepatomegaly, lipemia, metabolic acidosis, myocardial failure, rhabdomyolysis, renal failure and sometimes death.[3] First identified in children, but may occur at any age. NB: *metabolic acidosis* of unknown etiology in a patient on propofol is propofol infusion syndrome until proven otherwise. Use with caution at doses > 50 mcg/kg/min or at any dose for > 48 hrs. Also note that the lipid carrier provides 1.1 kCal/ml and hypertriglyceridemia may occur.

Supplied: 500 mg suspended in a 50 ml bottle of fat emulsion. The bottle and tubing must be changed every 12 hours since it contains no bacteriostatic agent.

Drug info: ★ Precedex® (Dexmedetomidine)

An alpha-2 adrenoceptor agonist. Acts in locus ceruleus and dorsal root ganglia. Has both sedative and analgesic properties and dramatically reduces the risk of respiratory depression and the amount of narcotic analgesics required. Reduces shivering.

℞: usual loading dose is 1 mcg/kg IV over 10 minutes (loading dose not needed if patient already sedated with other agents), followed by continuous IV infusion of 0.2–1.0 mcg/kg/hr titrated to desired effect, not to exceed 24 hours (for short sedation or use as a "transition" drug). **Side effects:** clinically significant bradycardia and sinus arrest have occurred in young, healthy volunteers with increased vagal tone (anticholinergics such as atropine 0.2 mg IV or glycopyrrolate 0.2 mg IV may help). Use with caution in patients with advanced heart block, baseline bradycardia, using other drugs that lower heart rate, and hypovolemia. **Supplied:** 2 ml vials of 100 mcg/ml to be diluted in 48 ml NS for a final concentration of 4 mcg/ml for IV use.

7.2 Paralytics (neuromuscular blocking agents)

7.2.1 General information

CAUTION: requires ventilation (intubation or Ambu-bag/mask). Reminder: paralyzed patients may still be conscious and therefore able to feel pain, thus the simultaneous use of sedation is required for conscious patients.

Early routine use in head-injured patients lowers ICP (e.g., from suctioning[4]) and mortality, but does not improve overall outcome.[5]

Neuromuscular blocking agents (NMBAs) are classified clinically by time to onset and duration of paralysis as shown in ▶ Table 7.2. Additional information for some agents follows the table along with some considerations for neurosurgical patients.

Table 7.2 Onset and duration of muscle relaxants

Clinical class	Agent	Trade name (®)	Onset (min)	Duration (min)	Spontaneous recovery (min)	Comment
Ultra-short	succinylcholine	Anectine	1	5–10	20	shortest onset and duration; plasma cholinesterase dependent; many side effects
Short	rocuronium	Zemuron	1–1.5	20–35	40–60	close to succinylcholine in onset in large doses; some vagolytic action in children
Intermediate	vecuronium	Norcuron	3–5	20–35	40–60	minimal cardiovascular side effects (bradycardia reported); no histamine release
	cisatracurium	Nimbex	1.5–2	40–60	60–80	no histamine release at recommended doses

7.2.2 Ultra-short acting paralytics

Drug info: Succinylcholine (Anectine®)

The only depolarizing ganglionic blocker (the rest are competitive blockers). Rapidly inactivated by plasma pseudocholinesterases. A single dose produces fasciculations then paralysis. Onset: 1 min. Duration of action: 5–10 min.

7

Indications

Due to significant side effects (see below), use is now limited primarily to the following indications. Adults: generally recommended only for emergency intubations where the airway is not controlled. In children: only when intubation is needed with a full stomach, or if laryngospasm occurs during attempted intubation using other agents.

Side effects

✖ CAUTIONS: usually increases serum K^+ by 0.5 mEq/L (on rare occasion causes severe *hyperkalemia* ($[K^+]$ up to 12 mEq/L) in patients with neuronal or muscular pathology, causing cardiac complications which cannot be blocked), therefore contraindicated in acute phase of injury following major burns, multiple trauma or extensive denervation of skeletal muscle or upper motor neuron injury. Do not use for routine intubations in adolescents and children (may cause cardiac arrest even in apparently healthy youngsters, many of whom have undiagnosed myopathies). Linked to malignant hyperthermia (p. 112).

May cause dysrhythmias, especially sinus bradycardia (treat with atropine). May get autonomic stimulation from ACh-like action → HTN, and brady- or tachycardia (especially in peds with repeated doses). The fasciculations may increase ICP, intragastric pressure, and intraocular pressure (contraindicated in penetrating eye injury, especially to anterior chamber; OK in glaucoma).

Precurarization with a "priming dose" of a nondepolarizing blocker (usually ≈ 10% of the intubating dose, e.g., *pancuronium* 0.5–1 mg IV 3–5 minutes prior to succinylcholine) in patients with elevated ICP or increased intraocular pressure (to ameliorate further pressure increases during fasciculation phase) and in patients who have eaten recently (controversial[6]). Phase II block (similar to nondepolarizing blocker) may develop with excessive doses or in patients with abnormal pseudocholinesterase.

Dosing

℞ Adult: 0.6–1.1 mg/kg (2–3 ml/70 kg) IVP (err on high side to allow time for procedure & to avoid multi-dosing complications), may repeat this dose × 1.

℞ Peds (CAUTION: *Not* recommended for routine use, see above) *Children*: 1.1 mg/kg. *Infants* (< 1 month): 2 mg/kg.

Supplied: 20 mg/ml concentration.

7.2.3 Short acting paralytics

Drug info: Rocuronium (Zemuron®)

In large doses, has speed of onset that approaches succinylcholine. However, in these doses, paralysis usually lasts ≈ 1–2 hrs. Expensive.

℞ Adult: initial dose 0.6–1 mg/kg. May be used as infusion of 10–12 mcg/kg/min.

7.2.4 Intermediate acting paralytics

Drug info: ★ Vecuronium (Norcuron®)

Nondepolarizing (competitive) NMBA. Adequate paralysis for intubation within 2.5–3 minutes of administration. About one–third more potent than pancuronium, shorter duration of action (lasts ≈ 30 minutes after initial dose). Unlike pancuronium, very little vagal (i.e., cardiovascular) effects. No CNS active metabolites. Does not affect ICP or CPP. Hepatically metabolized. Due to active metabolites, paralysis has been reported to take 6 hrs to 7 days to recede following discontinuation of the drug after ≥ 2 days use in patients with renal failure.[7] Must be mixed to use.

Dosing

Supplied: 10 mg freeze-dried cakes requiring reconstitution. Use within 24 hrs of mixing.

℞ Adult and children > 10 years of age: 0.1 mg/kg (for most adults use 8–10 mg as initial dose). May repeat q 1 hr PRN. Infusion: 1–2 mcg/kg/min.

℞ Pediatric: *children* (1–10 yrs) require slightly higher dose and more frequent dosing than adult. *Infants* (7 weeks–1 yr): slightly more sensitive on a mg/kg basis than adults, takes ≈ 1.5 × longer to recover. Use in neonates and continuous infusion in children is insufficiently studied.

Drug info: ★ Cisatracurium (Nimbex®)

Nondepolarizing (competitive) blocker. This isomer of atracurium does not release histamine unlike its parent compound (see below). Provides about 1 hour of paralysis. Also undergoes Hofmann degradation, with laudanosine as one of its metabolites.

℞ Adult and children > 12 years of age: 0.15 or 0.2 mg/kg as part of propofol/nitrous oxide/oxygen induction-intubation technique produces muscle paralysis adequate for intubation within 2 or 1.5 minutes, respectively. Infusion: 1–3 mcg/kg/min.

℞ Pediatric: *children* (2–12 yrs): 0.1 mg/kg given over 5–10 seconds during inhalational or opioid anesthesia.

7.2.5 Reversal of competitive muscle blockade

Reversal is usually not attempted until patient has at least 1 twitch to a train of 4 stimuli, otherwise reversal may be incomplete if patient is profoundly blocked and blockade may reoccur as the reversal wears off (a response of 1/4 indicates 90% muscle blockade).

- neostigmine (Prostigmin®): ℞ 2.5 mg (minimum) to 5 mg (maximum) IV
  (start low, no efficacy from > 5 mg and can produce severe weakness especially if the maximum dose is exceeded in the absence of neuromuscular blockade)
- *PLUS* (to prevent bradycardia…),
  ◦ EITHER
    atropine ℞ 0.5 mg for each mg of neostigmine
  ◦ OR
    glycopyrrolate (Robinul®) ℞ 0.2 mg for each mg of neostigmine

▶ **Reversal of rocuronium or vecuronium.** Sugammadex (Bridion©) is the first selective relaxant binding agent and is specific for aminosteroid non-depolarizing NMBAs (e.g., rocuronium or vecuronium). In the European Union, in children & adolescents, sugammadex should be only used to reverse rocuronium. Sugammadex encapsulates the NMBA molecule so that it is unable to bind to the acetylcholine receptor at the neuromuscular junction. Unlike neostigmine, sugammadex does not inhibit acetylcholinesterase which would produce cholinergic side effects, so co-administration of antimuscarinic agents (e.g., atropine or glycopyrrolate) is not required except for the rare occasion when clinically significant bradycardia follows administration.

Dosing: sugammadex is given as an IV bolus over 10 secs
- for moderate block (reappearance of the second twitch in TOF): ℞ 2 mg/kg IV bolus over 10 secs
- for deep block (1-2 posttetanic count (PTC) but no twitch response to TOF): ℞ 4 mg/kg IV bolus

7.3 Analgesics

7.3.1 General information

For a discussion of types of pain and pain procedures (p.518).

Three types of pain medication
1. non-opioid pain medication (see below)
   a) nonsteroidal anti-inflammatory drugs: aspirin, ibuprofen…
   b) acetaminophen
2. opioids (p.146)
   a) agonists
   b) partial agonists
   c) mixed agonist/antagonists
3. drugs that are not strictly analgesics, but which act as adjuvants (p.149) when added to any of the above: tricyclic antidepressants, antiseizure medications, caffeine, hydroxyzine, corticosteroids (p.149)

7.3.2 Guiding principles

The key to good pain control is the early use of adequate levels of effective analgesics. For cancer pain, scheduled dosing is superior to PRN dosing, and "rescue" medication should be available.[8]

Nonopioid analgesics should be continued as more potent medications and invasive techniques are utilized.

7.3.3 Analgesics for some specific types of pain

Visceral or deafferentation pain

May sometimes be effectively treated with tricyclic antidepressants (p.519).
Tryptophan may be effective (p.149).
Carbamazepine (Tegretol®) may be useful for paroxysmal, lancinating pain.

Pain from metastatic bone disease

Steroids, aspirin, or NSAIDs are especially helpful, probably by reducing prostaglandin mediated sensitization of A-delta and C fibers, and therefore may be preferred to APAP.

7.3.4 Nonopioid analgesics

Acetaminophen

For dosing information, see ▶ Table 7.3.

Table 7.3 Acetaminophen dosing

Medication	Dosage

acetaminophen (APAP) (Tylenol®)	• adult dose: 650 or 1000 mg PO/PR q 4–6 hrs, not to exceed 4000 mg/day[a]
	• pediatric dose:
	  ○ infants: 10–15 mg/kg PO/PR q 4–6 hrs
	  ○ children: 1 grain/yr of age (= 65 mg/yr up to 650 mg) PO/PR q 4–6 hrs not to exceed 15 mg/kg q 4 hrs

[a]hepatic toxicity from APAP: usually with doses ≥ 10 gm/day, rare at doses < 4000 mg. However, may occur at lower doses (even at high therapeutic doses) in alcoholics, fasting patients, and those taking cytochrome P-450 enzyme-inducing drugs

Nonsteroidal anti-inflammatory drugs (NSAIDs)

The anti-inflammatory properties of NSAIDs is primarily due to inhibition of the enzyme cyclooxygenase (COX) which participates in the synthesis of prostaglandins and thromboxanes.[9] For dosage information, see ▶ Table 7.4.

Characteristics of nonselective nonsteroidal anti-inflammatory drugs:

1. all are given orally except ketorolac tromethamine (Toradol®) (see below)
2. no dependence develops
3. additive effect improves the pain relief with opioid analgesics
4. NSAIDs (and APAP) demonstrate a ceiling effect: a maximum dose above which no further analgesia is obtained. For aspirin and APAP, this is usually between 650–1300 mg, and is often higher for other NSAIDs which may also have a longer duration of action
5. risk of GI upset is common, more serious risks of hepatotoxicity,[10] or GI ulceration, hemorrhage, or perforation are less common
6. taking medication with meals or antacids has not been proven effective in reducing GI side effects. Misoprostol (Cytotec®), a prostaglandin, may be effective in mitigating NSAID-induced gastric erosion or peptic ulcer. Contraindicated in pregnancy. ℞ 200 mcg PO QID with food as long as patient is on NSAIDs. If not tolerated, use 100 mcg. ✖ CAUTION: an abortifacient. Should not be given to pregnant women or women of childbearing potential
7. most reversibly inhibit platelet function and prolong bleeding time (nonacetlyated salicylates have less antiplatelet action, e.g., salsalate, trisalicylate, nabumetome). Aspirin, unlike all other NSAIDS, *irreversibly* binds to cyclooxygenase and thus inhibits platelet function for the 8–10 day life of the platelet
8. all cause sodium and water retention and carry the risk of NSAID-induced nephrotoxicity[11] (by reducing synthesis of renal vasodilator prostaglandins → reduced renal blood flow which can → renal insufficiency, interstitial nephritis, nephrotic syndrome, hyperkalemia)
9. non-aspirin NSAIDs increase the risk of heart attack or stroke[12]

Table 7.4 Nonsteroidal anti-inflammatory drugs (NSAIDs)[a]

Generic name (proprietary name [®])	Typical adult oral dose[b]	Tabs/caps availability (mg)[c]	Daily maximum dose (mg)
aspirin[d] (many)	500–1000 mg PO q 4–6 hrs (ceiling dose ≈ 1 gm)	325, 500	4000
diclofenac (Voltaren, Cataflam)	start at 25 mg QID; additional dose q hs PRN; increase up to 50 mg TID or QID, or 75 mg BID	25, 50, 75	200
etodolac	for acute pain: 200–400 mg q 6–8 hrs	200, 300 caps, 400 tabs	1200
fenoprofen (Nalfon)	200 mg q 4–6 hrs; for rheumatoid arthritis 300–600 mg TID-QID	200, 300, 600	3200
flurbiprofen (Ansaid)	50 mg TID-QID or 100 mg TID	50, 100	300
ketoprofen	immediate release: start at 75 mg TID or 50 mg QID, ↑ to 150–300 mg daily DIV TID-QID	25, 50, 75	300
	extended release: 150 mg q d	ER[c] 150	
ketorolac	see below	see below	
ibuprofen[e] (Motrin)	400–800 mg QID (ceiling dose: 800 mg)	300, 400, 600, 800	3200
indomethacin	25 mg TID, ↑ by 25 mg total per day PRN	25, 50, SR 75	150–200
meclofenamate	50 mg q 4–6 hrs; ↑ to 100 mg QID if needed	50, 100	400
mefenamic (Ponstel)	500 mg initial; then 250 mg q 6 hrs	250	
nabumetome[f] (Relafen)	1000–2000 mg/d given in 1 or 2 doses	500, 750	2000
naproxen (Naprosyn)	500 mg, then 250 mg q 6–8 hrs	250, 375, 500	<1250
naproxen sodium (Anaprox)	550 mg, followed by 275 mg q 6–8 hrs	275, DS = 550	1375
oxaprozin (Daypro)	1200 mg q d (1st day may take 1800)	600	1800
piroxicam (Feldene)	10–20 mg q d (steady state takes 7–12 d)	10, 20	
sulindac	200 mg BID; ↓ to 150 BID when pain controlled	150, 200	400
salsalate	3000 mg divided BID-TID (e.g., 500 mg 2-tabs TID)	500, 750	
tolmetin	400 mg TID (bioavailability is reduced by food)	200, DS = 400, 600	1800

[a]NSAIDs increase the risk of cardiovascular thrombotic events (heart attack or stroke)[12]
[b]when dosage ranges are given, use the smallest effective dose
[c]abbreviations: DS = double strength; SR = slow release; ER = extended release; DOC = drug of choice
[d]aspirin: has unique effectiveness in pain from bone metastases
[e]ibuprofen: is available as a suspension (PediaProfen®) 100 mg/ml; dose for children 6 mos to 12 yrs of age is 5–10 mg/kg with a maximum of 40 mg/kg/day (not FDA approved for children because of possible Reye's syndrome)
[f]unlike most NSAIDs, nabumetome does not interfere with platelet function

Drug info: Ketorolac tromethamine (Toradol®)

The only parenteral NSAID approved for use in pain control in the U.S. Analgesic effect is more potent than anti-inflammatory effect. Half-life ≈ 6 hrs. May be useful to control pain in the following situations:
1. where the avoidance of sedation or respiratory depression is critical
2. when constipation cannot be tolerated
3. for patients who are nauseated by narcotics
4. where narcotic dependency is a serious concern
5. when epidural morphine has been used and further analgesia is needed without risk of respiratory depression (agonist type narcotics are contraindicated)
6. cautions:
   a) not indicated for use > 72 hrs (complications have been reported primarily with prolonged use of the oral form)

b) use with caution in postoperative patients since (as with most NSAIDs) bleeding time is pro-longed by platelet function inhibition (risk of GI or op-site hemorrhage is small, but is increased in patients > 75 yrs old, when used > 5 days, and when used in higher doses[13])

c) even though IM dosing circumvents the GI system, gastric mucosal irritation and erosions may occur as with all NSAIDs (avoid use with PUD)

d) as with all NSAIDs, use with caution in patients at risk for renal side effects

℞ Parenteral: For single dose administration: 30 mg IV or 60 mg IM in healthy adult. For multiple dos-ing: 30 mg IV or IM q 6 hrs PRN. Maximum dosage: 120 mg/day. Parenteral use should not exceed 5 days (3 days may be a better guideline).

For patient weight < 50 kg, age > 65 yrs, or reduced renal function (creatinine clearance < 50 ml/min), all of the above dosages are halved (max daily dose: 60 mg). Creatinine clearance can be esti-mated using the Cockcroft-Gault equation[14] shown in Eq (7.1), with normal values ≥ 60 ml/min.

$$\text{Creatinine clearance(ml/min)} = \frac{[140 - \text{age(years)}] \times \text{ideal wt(kg)}}{72 \times \text{serum creatinine (mg/dl)}} \times (0.85 \text{ for females}) \qquad (7.1)$$

℞ PO: Indicated only as a continuation of IV or IM therapy, not for routine use as an NSAID. Switching from IM to PO: start with 10 mg PO q 4–6 hrs (combined PO and IM dose should be ≤ 120 mg on the day of transition). **Supplied:** 10 mg tablets.

7.3.5 Opioid analgesics

General information

Narcotics are most commonly used for moderate to severe acute pain or cancer pain (some experts characterize cancer pain as recurrent acute pain and not chronic pain).

Characteristics of narcotics:

1. no ceiling effect (p. 144): i.e., increasing dosage increases the effectiveness (although with weak opioids for moderate pain, side effects may limit dosages to relatively low levels[8])
2. with chronic use, tolerance develops (physical and psychological)
3. overdose possible (p. 215), with the potential for respiratory depression with all, and seizures with some

Mild to moderate pain

Some useful medications are shown in ▶ Table 7.5.

Codeine and congener pentazocine, are usually no more effective that ASA or APAP and are usu-ally combined with these drugs.

Table 7.5 Weak opioids for mild to moderate pain

Medication	Dosage	
codeine	usual adult dose: 30–60 mg IM/PO q 3 hrs PRN; use with caution in nursing mothers[a] and children (30 mg PO is equivalent to 300 mg aspirin) pediatric dose: 0.5–1 mg/kg/dose q 4–6 hrs PO or IV PRN	
pentazocine	pentazocine is a mixed agonist-antagonist	
	Talwin®	→ 12.5 mg pentazocine, 325 mg ASA. ℞: 2 PO TID-QID PRN
	with naloxone	→ 50 mg pentazocine, 0.5 mg naloxone. ℞: 1–2 PO q 3–4 hrs PRN up to 12 tabs/day
tramadol (Ultram®)	(see below)	

[a]1–28% of women are ultrafast metabolizers of codeine and the resultant morphine may be passed on to the infant via the breast milk

Drug info: Tramadol (Ultram®)

An oral opioid agonist that binds to μ-opioid receptors, and is also a centrally acting analgesic that inhibits reuptake of norepinephrine and serotonin. For acute pain, 100 mg is comparable to codeine 60 mg with ASA or APAP.[15,16] There has been no report of respiratory depression when oral dosing recommendations are followed. Seizures and opioid-like dependence have been reported.[16]

℞ 50 to 100 mg PO q 4–6 hrs PRN pain up to a maximum of 400 mg/day (or 300 mg/d for older patients). For moderately severe acute pain, an initial dose of 100 mg followed by 50 mg doses may suffice. **Supplied:** 50 mg tabs.

Moderate to severe pain

See ▶ Table 7.6.

Table 7.6 Opioids for moderate to severe pain

Medication	Dosage
hydrocodone	(Vicodin®, Lorcet®, Lortab®...): 5 mg hydrocodone + 500 mg acetaminophen; (Vicodin ES®, Lortab 7.5/500®): 7.5 mg hydrocodone + 500 mg APAP; ℞ 1 tab PO q 6 hrs PRN (may increase up to 2 tabs PO q 3–4 hrs not to exceed 8 pills/24 hrs).
	(Lorcet® Plus, Lorcet® 10/650): 7.5 or 10 mg hydrocodone (respectively) + 650 mg APAP; ℞ 1 tab PO q 6 hrs PRN (not to exceed 6 tabs in 24 hrs).
	(Lortab® 10/500: 10 mg. hydrocodone + 500 mg APAP); ℞: 1–2 PO q 4 hrs PRN up to 6 tabs/day.
	(Norco®): 10 mg hydrocodone + 325 mg APAP scored tabs; ℞: 1 PO q 4 hrs PRN up to 6 tabs/day.
oxycodone	**Supplied:** usually available in combination as: aspirin 325 mg with oxycodone 5 mg (Percodan®) or acetaminophen (APAP) (Tylox® = APAP 500 mg + oxycodone 5 mg) (Percocet® = oxycodone/APAP in 2.5/325, 5/325, 7.5/500, 10/650) dose: 1 PO q 3–4 hrs PRN (may increase up to 2 PO q 3 hrs[a]) **Supplied:** also available alone as OxyIR® 5 mg, OxyFast® oral solution of 20 mg/ml, or in controlled-release tablets as OxyContin® 10, 20, 40, 80[b] & 160[b] mg (which last 12 hours, achieving steady state in 24–36 hours). ℞ Adult: OxyContin® tablets are taken whole and are not to be divided, chewed or crushed. It is intended for management of moderate to severe pain when continuous around-the-clock analgesic is needed for an extended period of time and is not intended for use as a PRN analgesic. For opiate naive patients, start with 10 mg PO q 12 hrs. For patients on narcotic medications, a conversion table is provided below for some medications. Titrate dose every 1–2 days, increasing dose by 25–50% q 12 hrs.

Conversion table for starting OxyContin®

Preparation currently being used	Dose	Suggested starting dose of OxyContin®
oxycodone combination pills (Tylox, Percodan...) or Lortab, Vicodin or Tylenol #3	1–5 pills/day	10–20 mg PO q 12 hrs
	6–9 pills/day	20–30 mg PO q 12 hrs
	10–12 pills/day	30–40 mg PO q 12 hrs
IV PCA morphine	determine total MSO_4 dose used per 24 hrs	multiply total MSO_4 dose in 24 hrs × 1.3 for total OxyContin dose in 24 hrs

hydromorphone	Dilaudid®: (see ▶ Table 7.7)
morphine	used in low doses (see ▶ Table 7.7)

[a]not to exceed 4000 mg of acetaminophen/24 hrs (see footnote to ▶ Table 7.3)
[b]for use only in opioid-tolerant patients

Severe pain

See ▶ Table 7.7 and ▶ Table 7.8.

7

Table 7.7 *Equianalgesic* doses for SEVERE pain, AGONIST opioids (parenteral route is referenced to 10 mg IM morphine)

Drug name: generic (proprietary®)	Route	Dose (mg)	Peak (hrs)	Duration (hrs)	Comments
morphine	IM	10	0.5–1	4–6	respiratory depression
	PO	20–60[a]	1.5–2	4–7	long acting PO forms: MS Contin®, Avinza® (see below)
codeine (not recommended at these doses)	IM	130		3–5	these high doses cause unaccept-able side effects
	PO	200			
methadone[b] (Dolophine®)	IM	10	0.5–1	4–6	long half-life[b]
	PO	20	1.5–2	4–7	
oxycodone (e.g., Tylox®[c]) (OxyContin®)	IM	15			
	PO	30	1	3–4	combination (Tylox®) or liquid
	PO	30–40		12	*OxyContin*, see ▶ Table 7.6
oxymorphone	IM	1		3–5	available as suppository
	PR	10			
hydromorphone (Dilaudid®)	IM	1.5	0.5–1	3–4	
	PO	7.5	1.5–2	3–4	supplied: 1, 2, 3, & 4 mg tabs
fentanyl (Sublimaze®)	IV	0.1		1–2	not recommended for acute pain control, esp. in narcotic naive pts.
transdermal fentanyl patch (Duragesic®)[d]	transdermal	[e]	12–24	72	patches of 25, 50, 75, 100 or 125 mcg/hr (use lowest effective)

[a]IM:PO potency ratio for morphine is 1:6 for single doses, but changes to 1:2–3 with chronic dosing
[b]due to long half-life, repeated dosing can lead to accumulation and CNS depression (must reduce dose after ≈ 3 days, even though the analgesic half-life does not change), especially in the elderly or debilitated patient. Use should be limited to physicians with experience using these drugs
[c]may not be practical for use in severe pain since 1 Tylox® contains only 5 mg oxycodone (the acetaminophen limits the dosage), may use OxyContin® for higher doses of oxycodone
[d] ✖ should not be used as routine post-op analgesic (risk of respiratory depression). Apply 1 patch to upper torso, replace q 72 hrs PRN.
[e]conversion from total daily parenteral morphine as follows:
8–27 mg MSO$_4$/day → Duragesic 25 mcg/hr
28–37 mg MSO$_4$/day → Duragesic 50 mcg/hr
38–52 mg MSO$_4$/day → Duragesic 75 mcg/hr
53–67 mg MSO$_4$/day → Duragesic 100 mcg/hr
68–82 mg MSO$_4$/day → Duragesic 125 mcg/hr

Table 7.8 *Equianalgesic* doses for SEVERE pain, AGONIST/ANTAGONIST opioids (referenced to 10 mg IM morphine)

Drug name: generic (proprietary®)	Route	Dose (mg)	Peak (hrs)	Duration (hrs)	Comments
buprenorphine (Buprenex®)	IM	0.4			partial agonist
	SL	0.3			
Mixed agonist/antagonist[a]					
butorphanol	IM	2	0.5–1	4–6	
nalbuphine	IM	10	1	3–6	no sigma receptor occupation[b]
	IV	140 mcg/kg	0.5	2–5	
pentazocine (Talwin®[c])	IM[b]	20–40	0.5–1	4–6	
	PO[b]	180 (start @ 50)	1.5–2	4–7	

[a]all can precipitate withdrawal symptoms in patients physically dependent on agonists
[b]most agonist/antagonist drugs occupy sigma receptors (Stadol > Nubain), which may cause hallucinations
[c]Talwin injectable (for IM use) contains only pentazocine. Talwin® Compound tablets contain ASA; therefore for high PO doses, use Talwin Nx, which contains no ASA (▶ Table 7.5)

Drug info: Avinza® (extended release morphine)

Once daily oral morphine formulation using a spherical oral drug absorption system (SODAS) (numerous ammonio-methacrylate copolymer beads, ≈ 1 mm dia.). Potential for overdosage and/or abuse.

℞: Dosage is titrated based on patient's opioid tolerance and degree of pain. Taken as 1 capsule PO q d. Not to be taken "PRN." Not for post-op pain. ✖ CAUTION: To prevent potentially fatal doses of morphine, capsules are to be swallowed whole, and are not to be chewed, crushed or dissolved. However, the contents of the capsule (the beads) may be sprinkled on apple-sauce for those unable to swallow the capsules, but the beads are not to be chewed or crushed. **Side effects**: Due to the potentially nephrotoxic effect of fumaric acid used in SODAS, the maximum dose of Avinza is 1600 mg/d. Doses ≥ 60 mg are for opioid tolerant patients only. **Supplied**: 30, 60, 90 & 120 mg capsules.

7.3.6 Adjuvant pain medications

The following may enhance the effectiveness of opioid analgesics (and thereby may reduce the required dose).

Tricyclic antidepressants:

Tryptophan: an amino acid and a precursor of serotonin, may work by increasing serotonin levels. Requires high doses and has hypnotic effects; therefore 1.5–2 g given usually q hs. Must give daily MVI as chronic tryptophan therapy depletes vitamin B6.

Antihistamines: histamines play a role in nociception. Antihistamines, which are also anxiolytic, antiemetic, and mildly hypnotic, are effective as analgesics or as adjuvants. Hydroxyzine (Atarax®, Vistaril®): ℞ start with 50 mg PO q AM and 100 mg PO q hs. May increase up to ≈ 200 mg daily.

Antiseizure medication-class drugs: carbamazepine, clonazepam, phenytoin, gabapentin or pregabalin tend to be more effective in neuropathic pain, e.g., from diabetic neuropathy, trigeminal neuralgia, post-herpetic neuralgia, glossopharyngeal neuralgia, and neuralgias due to nerve injury or infiltration with cancer.[16] See index for entries.

Phenothiazines: some cause mild reduction in nociception. Most are tranquilizing and antiemetic. Best known for this use is fluphenazine (Prolixin®), usually given with a tricyclic antidepressant for neuropathic pain, **Diabetic neuropathy, Treatment** (p. 572). Phenothiazines may reduce the seizure threshold.

Corticosteroids: in addition to the reduction of toxic effects of radiation or chemotherapy, they may potentiate narcotic analgesics. There are also a number of nonspecific beneficial effects: increased appetite, sense of well being, antiemetic. Steroid side effects (p. 156) may limit usefulness.

Caffeine: although it possesses no intrinsic analgesic properties, doses of 65–200 mg enhance the analgesic effect of APAP, ASA, or ibuprofen for pain including H/A, oral surgery pain, and postpartum pain.

References

[1] Sessler CN, Gosnell MS, Grap MJ, et al. The Richmond Agitation-Sedation Scale: validity and reliability in adult intensive care unit patients. American Journal of Respiratory and Critical Care Medicine. 2002; 166:1338–1344

[2] Ely EW, Truman B, Shintani A, et al. Monitoring sedation status over time in ICU patients: reliability and validity of the Richmond Agitation-Sedation Scale (RASS). JAMA. 2003; 289:2983–2991

[3] Kang TM. Propofol infusion syndrome in critically ill patients. Ann Pharmacother. 2002; 36:1453–1456

[4] Werba A, Weinstabi C, Petricek W, et al. Vecuronium Prevents Increases in Intracranial Pressure During Routine Tracheobronchial Suctioning in Neurosurgical Patients. Anaesthetist. 1991; 40:328–331

[5] Hsiang JK, Chesnut RM, Crisp CD, et al. Early, Routine Paralysis for Intracranial Pressure Control in Severe Head Injury: Is It Necessary? Critical Care Medicine. 1994; 22:1471–1476

[6] Ohlinger MJ, Rhoney DH. Neuromuscular Blocking Agents in the Neurosurgical Intensive Care Unit. Surgical Neurology. 1998; 49:217–221

[7] Segredo V, Caldwell JE, Matthay MA, et al. Persistent Paralysis in Critically Ill Patients After Long-Term Administration of Vecuronium. New England Journal of Medicine. 1992; 327:524–528

[8] Marshall KA. Managing Cancer Pain: Basic Principles and Invasive Treatment. Mayo Clinic Proceedings. 1996; 71:472–477

[9] Celecoxib for Arthritis. Medical Letter. 1999; 41:11–12

[10] Helfgott SM, Sandberg-Cook J, Zakim D, et al. Diclofenac-Associated Hepatotoxicity. JAMA. 1990; 264:2660–2662

[11] Henrich WL. Analgesic Nephropathy. Am J Med Sci. 1988; 295:561–568

[12] U.S. Food and Drug Administration (FDA). FDA Drug Safety Communication: FDA strengthens warning that non-aspirin nonsteroidal anti-inflammatory drugs (NSAIDs) can cause heart attacks or strokes. 2015

[13] Strom BL, Berlin JA, Kinman JL, et al. Parenteral Ketorolac and Risk of Gastrointestinal and Operative Site Bleeding. Journal of the American Medical Association. 1996; 275:376–382

[14] Cockcroft DW, Gault MH. Prediction of creatinine clearance from serum creatinine. Nephron. 1976; 16:31–41

[15] Tramadol - A new oral analgesic. Medical Letter. 1995; 37:59–60

[16] Drugs for Pain. Medical Letter. 1998; 40:79–84

7

8 Endocrinology

8.1 Pituitary embryology and neuroendocrinology

8.1.1 Embryology and derivation of the pituitary gland

The posterior pituitary (neurohypophysis AKA pars nervosa) derives from downward evagination of neural crest cells (brain neuroectoderm) from the floor of the third ventricle. The residual recess in the floor of the third ventricle is called the median eminence. The anterior pituitary gland (adenohypophysis) develops from an upward evagination of epithelial ectoderm of the oropharynx, the evagination is known as Rathke's pouch and is eventually separated from the oropharynx by the sphenoid bone. Failure of this separation results in a craniopharyngeal duct which can be a source of recurrent meningitis. The posterior surface of Rathke's pouch forms the pars intermedius, while the anterior portion forms the pars distalis. Remnants of Rathke's pouch may persist (Rathke's cleft [▶ Fig. 8.1]) in the pars intermedius. The adenohypophysis is comprised of the pars distalis (anterior lobe), the pars intermedia (intermediate lobe) and the pars tuberalis (extension of adenohypophyseal cells surrounding the base of the pituitary stalk[1]). The pituitary gland is functionally *outside* the blood-brain barrier.

8.1.2 Pituitary hormones, their targets and their controls

General information

The pituitary gland releases 8 hormones, 6 from the anterior pituitary and 2 from the posterior pituitary (▶ Fig. 8.1).

The anterior pituitary is one of only two sites in the body having a portal circulation (the other being the liver). Six hypothalamic hormones are released in a pulsatile fashion from neurons of the tuber cinereum (a hypothalamic nucleus) that are conveyed via the tubero-hypophyseal tract (a parvocellular system) to their terminus in the median eminence of the pituitary stalk. These hypophyseal hormones are released into capillaries of the hypophyseal portal circulation, which carries them via the pituitary stalk to a second capillary bed in the anterior pituitary where they control release of hormones by adenohypophyseal gland cells.[1]

Posterior pituitary hormones (ADH & oxytocin) are synthesized in magnocellular neuroendocrine *neurons* (*not* gland cells) in the supraoptic and paraventricular nuclei of the hypothalamus and are conveyed along their *axons* in the supraoptic-hypophyseal tract, also via the pituitary stalk, to the posterior pituitary gland where they are released into the circulation.

The complete homeostatic loops (including negative feedback involving hypothalamic hormones) will not be covered here, and the reader is referred to physiology texts.

Propiomelanocortin (POMC), AKA proopiomelanocortin

241 amino acid polypeptide hormone precursor synthesized primarily in corticotroph cell of the anterior pituitary (but also found in the hypothalamus). Contains amino acid sequences for ACTH, alpha-melanocyte-stimulating hormone (α-MSH), β-lipotropin, γ-lipotropin, β-endorphin and metenkephalin.

Corticotropin AKA adrenocorticotrophic hormone (ACTH)

A 39 amino acid trophic hormone synthesized from POMC. The first 13 amino acids at the amino terminal of ACTH are identical to α-MSH. Active half-life is ≈ 10 minutes. Produces a diurnal peak in cortisol (the highest peak occurs in the early morning, with a second, lesser peak in the late afternoon) and also increases in response to stress.

Control: CRH from the hypothalamus stimulates the release of ACTH.

Prolactin

AKA somatomammotropin. 199 amino-acid protein weighing 23,000 daltons. Levels are higher in females than males, and are higher still in pregnancy (see ▶ Table 52.3). Secreted in pulsatile fashion with a frequency and amplitude that varies during menstrual cycle (range: 5–27 ng/ml) (≈ 9 pulses/24 hours in the late luteal phase, ≈ 14 pulses/24 hours in the late follicular phase, the pulse amplitude increases from early to late follicular and luteal phases). There is also diurnal variation: levels begin to

8

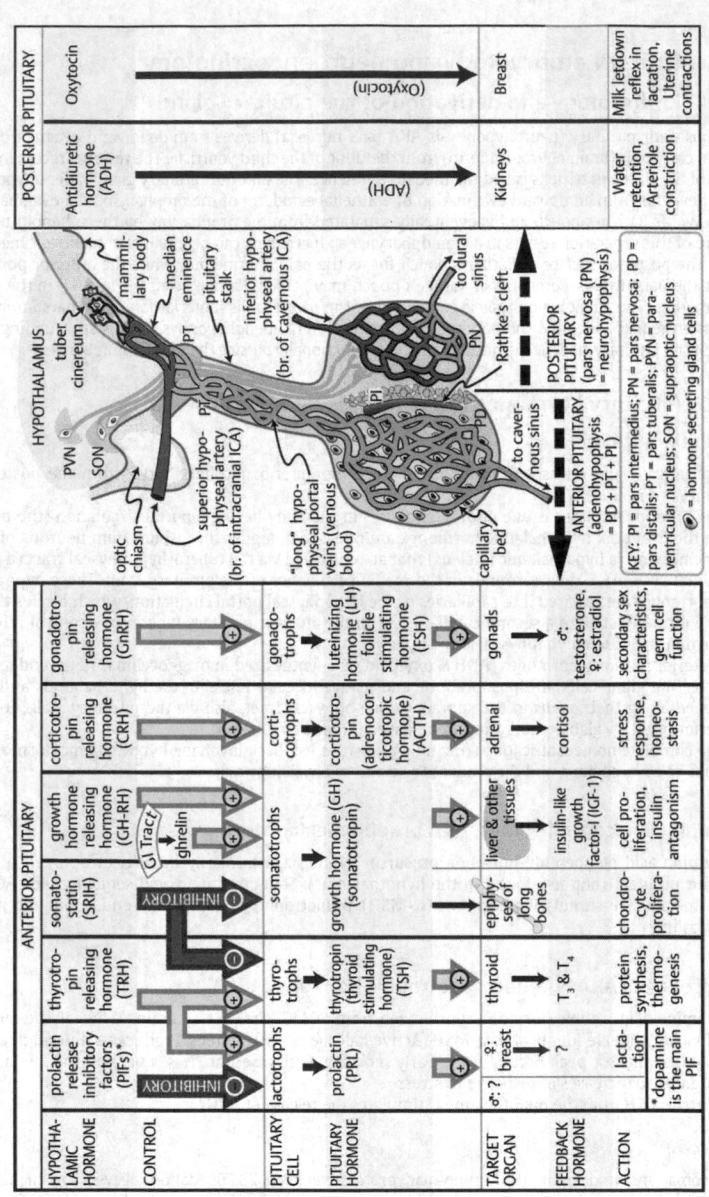

Fig. 8.1 Pituitary neuroendocrinology.

rise 1 hour after the onset of sleep, peak ≈ 5:00–7:00 AM, and nadir in midmorning after awakening. Heterogeneity of the molecule may produce different results between bioassays and immunoassays.

Control: prolactin is the only pituitary hormone predominantly under *inhibitory* control from the hypothalamus by prolactin releasing inhibitory factors (PIFs), with dopamine being the primary PIF. Prolactin releasing factors (PRFs) include thyrotropin-releasing hormone (TRH) and vasoactive intestinal peptide (VIP). The physiologic role of PRFs is not established. For DDx of hyperprolactinemia see ▶ Table 52.4.

Growth hormone (GH)

A 191 amino-acid polypeptide trophic hormone. GH normally has pulsatile secretion (≈ 5–10 pulses/24 hours, primarily at night, up to 30 mcg/L), levels may be undetectable (< 0.2 mcg/L) by standard assays between pulses.[2] Insulin-like growth factor-1 (IGF-1) (formerly known as somatomedin-C) is the protein secreted primarily by the liver in response to GH that is responsible for most of GH's systemic effects (see levels (p.881)). GH also acts directly on epiphyseal endplates of long bone to stimulate chondrocyte proliferation.

Control: GH is under dual hypothalamic control via the hypophysial portal system. GH-releasing hormone (GHRH) from the arcuate nucleus stimulates pituitary *secretion* and *synthesis* of GH and induces GH gene transcription. Somatostatin from the periventricular nucleus suppresses GH *release* only, and has no effect on synthesis. GH *release* is also stimulated by ghrelin,[3] a peptide synthesized primarily in the GI tract in response to certain nutrients (may act partially or totally via hypothalamic GHRH).

Thyrotropin AKA thyroid stimulating hormone (TSH)

Glycoprotein trophic hormone secreted by thyrotroph cells of the anterior pituitary.

Control: TSH is also under dual hypothalamic control. TRH stimulates production and release of TSH. Somatostatin inhibits the release of TSH.

Gonadotropins

Follicle stimulating hormone (FSH) and luteinizing hormone (LH) (AKA lutropin) are released from the pituitary in response to gonadotropin releasing hormone 1 (GnRH, formerly luteinizing hormone releasing hormone LH-RH) synthesized primarily in the preoptic area of the hypothalamus.

Antidiuretic hormone (ADH)

AKA arginine vasopressin (AVP). The major source of this nanopeptide hormone is the magnocellular portion of the supraoptic nucleus of the hypothalamus. It is conveyed along *axons* in the supraoptic-hypophyseal tract to the posterior pituitary gland where it is released into the systemic circulation. All actions of ADH result from binding of the hormone to specific membrane-bound receptors on the surface of target cells.[4] One of the major effects of ADH is to increase the permeability of the distal renal tubules resulting in increased reabsorption of water, diluting the circulating blood and producing a concentrated urine. The most powerful physiologic stimulus for ADH release is an increase in serum osmolality; a less potent stimulus is a reduction of intravascular volume. ADH is also released in glucocorticoid deficiency, and is inhibited by exogenous glucocorticoids and adrenergic drugs. ADH is also a potent vasoconstrictor.

Oxytocin

A nonapeptide. Oxytocin is a neurotransmitter as well as a hormone. The hypothalamus is the main source of pituitary oxytocin which is stored in nerve endings in the neurohypophysis and is involved in the milk letdown reflex for breastfeeding as well as in uterine contraction during labor.

8.2 Corticosteroids

8.2.1 General information

Under normal, basal conditions, the zona fasciculata of the adrenal cortex secretes 15–25 mg/day of cortisol (hydrocortisone is the name for the identical pharmaceutical compound for administration), and 1.5–4 mg/day of corticosterone. Cortisol has a half-life of ≈ 90 minutes. The release of cortisol by the adrenal glands is stimulated by adrenocorticotrophic hormone (ACTH) from the pituitary which in turn is stimulated by corticotropin releasing hormone (CRH) from the hypothalamus.

8.2.2 Replacement therapy

In primary adrenocortical insufficiency (Addison's disease), both glucocorticoids and mineralocorticoids must be replaced. In secondary adrenal insufficiency caused by deficient corticotropin (ACTH) release by the pituitary, mineralocorticoid secretion is usually normal and only glucocorticoids need to be replaced.
▶ Table 8.1 shows equivalent daily corticosteroid doses for replacement therapy.

Table 8.1 Equivalent corticosteroid doses[a]

Steroid: generic (proprietary)	Equiv dose (mg)	Route	Dosing	Mineralocorticoid potency	Oral dosing forms
cortisone acetate	25	PO, IM	2/3 in AM, 1/3 in PM	2+	tabs: 5, 10 & 25 mg
hydrocortisone AKA **cortisol (Cortef®)** (Solu-Cortef®)	20	PO IV, IM[b]	2/3 in AM, 1/3 in PM	2+	tabs: 5, 10 & 20 mg
prednisone	5	PO only	divided BID-TID	1+	tabs: 1, 2.5, 5, 10, 20, 50 mg[c]
methylprednisolone	4	PO, IV, IM		0	tabs[d]: 2, 4, 8, 16, 24, 32 mg
dexamethasone	0.75	PO, IV	divided BID-QID	0	scored tabs: 0.25, 0.5, 0.75, 1.5, 4, 6 mg

[a]doses given are daily doses. Steroids listed are used primarily as glucocorticoids: equivalent glucocorticoid PO or IV dose is given; IM may differ
[b]IM route recommended only for emergencies where IV access cannot be rapidly obtained
[c]Sterapred Uni-Pak® contains 21 tabs of 5 mg prednisone and tapers dosage from 30 to 5 mg over 6 days; "DS" contains 10 mg tabs and tapers from 60 mg to 10 mg over 6 days; "DS 12-Day" contains 48 10 mg tabs and tapers from 60 mg to 20 mg over 12 days
[d]Medrol Dosepak® contains 21 tabs of 4 mgs methylprednisolone and tapers dosage from 24 mg/d to 4 mg/d over 6 days

Physiologic replacement (in the absence of stress) can be accomplished with either:
1. hydrocortisone: 20 mg PO q AM and 10 mg PO q PM
2. or prednisone: 5 mg PO q AM and 2.5 mg PO q PM

Cortisol and cortisone are useful for chronic primary adrenocortical insufficiency or for Addisonian crisis. Because of mineralocorticoid activity, use for chronic therapy of other conditions (e.g., hypopituitarism) may result in salt and fluid retention, hypertension, and hypokalemia.

8.2.3 Hypothalamic-pituitary-adrenal axis suppression

General information

Chronic steroid administration suppresses the hypothalamic-pituitary-adrenal (HPA) axis, and eventually causes adrenal atrophy. When the HPA is suppressed, if exogenous steroids are abruptly stopped or if acute illness develops (which increases the steroid requirements), symptoms of adrenocortical insufficiency (AI) may ensue (▶ Table 8.2). Severe cases of AI may progress to Addisonian crisis (p.157). Recovery of adrenal cortex lags behind the pituitary, so basal ACTH levels increase before cortisol levels do.

Table 8.2 Symptoms of adrenal insufficiency (AI)

- fatigue
- weakness
- arthralgia
- anorexia
- nausea
- hypotension
- orthostatic dizziness
- hypoglycemia
- dyspnea
- Addisonian crisis (p. 157) (if severe; with risk of death)

HPA suppression depends on the specific glucocorticoid used, the route, frequency, time, and duration of treatment. Suppression is unlikely with < 40 mg prednisone (or equivalent) given in the morning for less than ≈ 7 days, or with every-other-day therapy of < 40 mg for ≈ 5 weeks.[5] Some adrenal atrophy may occur after 3–4 days of high dose steroids, and some axis suppression will almost certainly occur after 2 weeks of 40–60 mg hydrocortisone (or equivalent) daily. After a month or more of steroids, the HPA axis may be depressed for as long as one year.

Measuring morning plasma hydrocortisone can evaluate the degree of recovery of basal adrenocortical function, but does *not* assess adequacy of stress response.

Steroid withdrawal

See reference.[5]

In addition to the above dangers of hypocortisolism in the presence of HPA suppression, too rapid a taper may cause a flare-up of the underlying condition for which steroids were prescribed.

When the risk of HPA suppression is low (as is the case with short courses of steroids for less than ≈ 5–7 days[6] generally prescribed for most neurosurgical indications) abrupt discontinuation usually carries a low risk of AI. For up to ≈ 2 weeks of use, steroids are usually safely withdrawn by tapering over 1–2 weeks. For longer treatment, or when withdrawal problems develop, use the following *conservative taper*:

1. make small decrements (equivalent to 2.5–5 mg prednisone) every 3–7 d. Patient may experience mild withdrawal symptoms of[7]:
   a) fatigue
   b) anorexia
   c) nausea
   d) orthostatic dizziness
2. "backtrack" (i.e., increase the dose and resume a more gradual taper) if any of the following occur:
   a) exacerbation of the underlying condition for which steroids were used
   b) evidence of steroid withdrawal symptoms (► Table 8.2)
   c) intercurrent infection or need for surgery; see Stress doses (p. 155)
3. once "physiologic" doses of glucocorticoid have been reached (about 20 mg hydrocortisone/day or equivalent (► Table 8.1):
   a) the patient is switched to 20 mg hydrocortisone PO q AM (do not use long acting preparations)
   b) after ≈ 2–4 weeks, a morning cortisol level is checked (prior to the AM hydrocortisone dose), and the hydrocortisone is tapered by 2.5 mg weekly until 10 mg/d is reached (lower limits of physiologic)
   c) then, every 2–4 weeks, the AM cortisol level is drawn (prior to AM dose) until the 8 AM cortisol is > 10 mcg/100 ml, indicating return of baseline adrenal function
   d) when this return of baseline adrenal function occurs:
      • daily steroids are stopped, but stress doses must still be given when needed (see below)
      • monthly cosyntropin stimulation (p. 880) tests are performed until normal. The need for stress doses of steroids ceases when a positive test is obtained. The risk for adrenal insufficiency persist ≈ 2 years after cessation of chronic steroids (especially the first year)

Steroid stress doses

During physiologic "stress" the normal adrenal gland produces ≈ 250–300 mg hydrocortisone/day. With chronic glucocorticoid therapy (either at present, or within last 1–2 yrs), suppression of the normal "stress-response" necessitates supplemental doses.

In patients with a suppressed HPA axis:
• for mild illness (e.g., UTI, common cold), single dental extraction: double the daily dose (if off steroids, give 40 mg hydrocortisone BID)
• for moderate stress (e.g., flu), minor surgery under local anesthesia (endoscopy, multiple dental extractions…): give 50 mg hydrocortisone BID
• for major illness (pneumonia, systemic infections, high fever), severe trauma, or emergency surgery under general anesthesia: give 100 mg hydrocortisone IV q 6–8 hrs for 3–4 days until the stress is resolved
• for elective surgery, see ► Table 8.3 for guidelines

8

Table 8.3 Steroid stress doses for elective surgery

On day of surgery, 50 mg cortisone acetate IM, followed by 200 mg hydrocortisone IV infused over 24 hrs			
Post-op day	Hydrocortisone (mg)		
	8 AM	4 PM	10 PM
1	50	50	50
2	50	25	25
3	40	20	20
4	30	20	10
5	25	20	5
6	25	15	–
7	20	10	–

8.2.4 Steroid side effects

Although deleterious side effects of steroids are more common with prolonged administration,[8] some can occur even with short treatment courses. Some evidence suggests that low-dose glucocorticoids (≤ 10 mg/d of prednisolone or prednisone equivalent) for rheumatoid arthritis does not increase osteoporotic fractures, blood pressure, cardiovascular disease, or peptic ulcers,[9] but weight gain and skin changes are common. Possible side effects include[7,10]:

- cardiovascular and renal
  - hypertension
  - sodium and water retention
  - hypokalemic alkalosis
- CNS
  - progressive multifocal leukoencephalopathy (PML) (p. 354)
  - mental agitation or "steroid psychosis"
  - spinal cord compression from spinal epidural lipomatosis (p. 1381): rare
  - pseudotumor cerebri (p. 955)
- endocrine
  - caution: because of growth suppressant effect in children, daily glucocorticoid dosing over prolonged periods should be reserved for the most urgent indications
  - secondary amenorrhea
  - suppression of hypothalamic-pituitary-adrenal axis: reduces endogenous steroid production → risk of adrenal insufficiency with steroid withdrawal (see above)
  - Cushingoid features with prolonged usage (iatrogenic Cushing's syndrome): obesity, hypertension, hirsutism…
- GI: risk increased only with steroid therapy > 3 weeks duration and regimens of prednisone > 400–1000 mg/d or dexamethasone > 40 mg/d[11]
  - gastritis and steroid ulcers: incidence lowered with the use of antacids and/or H2 antagonists (e.g., cimetidine, ranitidine…)
  - pancreatitis
  - intestinal or sigmoid diverticular perforation[12]: incidence ≈ 0.7%. Since steroids may mask signs of peritonitis, this should be considered in patients on steroids with abdominal discomfort, especially in the elderly and those with a history of diverticular disease. Abdominal X-ray usually shows free intraperitoneal air
- inhibition of fibroblasts
  - impaired wound healing or wound breakdown
  - subcutaneous tissue atrophy
- metabolic
  - glucose intolerance (diabetes) and disturbance of nitrogen metabolism
  - hyperosmolar nonketotic coma
  - hyperlipidemia
  - tend to increase BUN as a result of protein catabolism
- ophthalmologic
  - posterior subcapsular cataracts
  - glaucoma
- musculoskeletal

- ○ avascular necrosis (AVN) of the hip or other bones: usually with prolonged administration →cushingoid habitus and increased marrow fat within the bone[13] (prednisone 60 mg/d for several months is probably the minimum necessary dose, whereas 20 mg/d for several months will probably *not* produce AVN[14]). Many cases blamed on steroids may instead be due to alcohol use, cigarette smoking,[15] liver disease, underlying vascular inflammation...
  - ○ osteoporosis: may predispose to vertebral compression fractures which occur in 30–50% of patients on prolonged glucocorticoids. Steroid induced bone loss may be reversed with cyclical administration of etidronate[16] in 4 cycles of 400 mg/d ✖ 14 days followed by 76 days of oral calcium supplements of 500 mg/d (not proven to reduced rate of VB fractures)
  - ○ muscle weakness (steroid myopathy): often worse in proximal muscles
- infectious
  - ○ immunosuppression: with possible superinfection, especially fungal, parasitic
  - ○ possible reactivation of TB, chickenpox
- hematologic
  - ○ hypercoagulopathy from inhibition of tissue plasminogen activator
  - ○ steroids cause demargination of white blood cells, which may artifactually elevate the WBC count even in the absence of infection
- miscellaneous
  - ○ hiccups: may respond to chlorpromazine (Thorazine®) 25–50 mg PO TID-QID ✖ 2–3 days (if symptoms persist, give 25–50 mg IM)
  - ○ steroids readily cross the placenta, and fetal adrenal hypoplasia may occur with the administration of large doses during pregnancy

8

8.2.5 Hypocortisolism

General information

AKA adrenal insufficiency.

Assessment: 8 A.M. serum cortisol level is the best way to test for hypocortisolism. Each lab should provide a lower limit of normal for their lab, which may be broken down further by age and gender.

Addisonian crisis

General information

AKA adrenal crisis. An adrenal insufficiency emergency.

Symptoms: mental status changes (confusion, lethargy, or agitation), muscle weakness.

Signs: postural hypotension or shock, hyperthermia (as high as 105 °F, 45.6 C)

Labs

Hyponatremia, hyperkalemia, hypoglycemia.

Treatment of Addisonian crisis

If possible, draw serum for cortisol determination (do not wait for these results to institute therapy). Give fluids sufficient for dehydration and shock.

For "glucocorticoid emergency"

- hydrocortisone sodium succinate (Solu-Cortef®): 100 mg IV STAT and then 50 mg IV q 6 hrs AND
- cortisone acetate 75–100 mg IM STAT, and then 50–75 mg IM q 6 hrs

For "mineralocorticoid emergency"

Usually not necessary in secondary adrenal insufficiency (e.g., panhypopituitarism)

- desoxycorticosterone acetate (Doca®): 5 mg IM BID OR
- fludrocortisone (Florinef®): 0.05- 0.2 mg PO q d

✖ methylprednisolone is NOT recommended for emergency treatment.

8.3 Hypothyroidism

8.3.1 General information

Chronic primary hypothyroidism may result in (non-pathologic) enlargement of the pituitary gland. Plasma TSH determination will distinguish primary hypothyroidism (high TSH) from secondary hypothyroidism (low TSH). Wound healing and cardiac function may be compromised, and surgery under general anesthesia should be postponed if possible until thyroid levels are normalized. Effects of anesthesia may be markedly prolonged, and dosages should be adjusted accordingly.

8.3.2 Thyroid replacement

Caution in patients with adrenal insufficiency

Primary hypothyroidism may be associated with immunologic destruction of adrenal cortex (Schmidt syndrome). Secondary hypothyroidism may be associated with and may mask reduced adrenal function. ✖ Thyroid replacement without adrenal replacement in patients with adrenal insufficiency (as may occur in panhypopituitarism) may precipitate adrenal crisis (thus give ≈ 300–400 mg hydrocortisone IV over 24 hrs in addition to thyroid replacement).

8.3.3 Routine thyroid replacement dosing

8

Drug info: Levothyroxine (Synthroid®)

Almost pure T4 (contains no T3 as most T3 is produced peripherally from T4).
  Dose required to prevent myxedema coma (not to achieve euthyroidism):
- Maintenance: ℞ 0.05 mg po q d
- when patient has been hypothyroid: ℞ start at 0.05 mg po q d and increase by 0.025 mg every 2–3 weeks

For euthyroidism (approximate dose, follow levels and clinical evaluation):
- for most adults < 60 years of age: ℞ 0.18 mg/day
- for elderly patients: ℞ 0.12 mg/day

Drug info: Desiccated thyroid (e.g., Armour thyroid®)

Typical dose: ℞ 60 mg (1 grain) to 300 mg daily.

Thyroid replacement in myxedema coma

Myxedema coma is an emergency of hypothyroidism and carries 50% mortality.
  Symptoms: altered mental status or unresponsiveness.
  Signs: hypotension, bradycardia, hyponatremia, hypoglycemia, hypothermia, hypoventilation, occasionally seizures.

Treatment

Drugs may need to be given IV due to reduced gastric motility.
1. general supportive care:
    a) hypotension: treat with IV fluids (responds poorly to pressors until thyroid replacement accomplished)
    b) hyponatremia: will correct with thyroid replacement; avoid hypertonic saline
    c) hypoglycemia: IV glucose
    d) symptoms of hypocortisolism: thyroid replacement may precipitate adrenal crisis (*see caution above*); give 300–400 mg hydrocortisone IV over 24 hrs
    e) hypothermia: avoid active warming since this increases metabolic demand, use blankets to warm gradually
    f) hypoventilation: check ABG, intubate if necessary

2. thyroid replacement (for average-sized adult):
   a) IV replacement: ℞ 0.5 mg of levothyroxine IV, followed by 0.05–0.2 mg/d IV until patient is able to tolerate PO or NG meds
   b) nasogastric replacement: liothyronine (Cytomel®) is primarily T_3, has a rapid onset of action, much shorter half-life than T4, and should be reserved for emergencies.
      ℞: liothyronine 0.05–0.1 mg per NG initially, followed by 0.025 mg BID per NG

References

[1] Prieto R, Castro-Dufourny I, Carrasco R, et al. Craniopharyngioma recurrence: the impact of tumor topography. J Neurosurg. 2016; 125:1043–1049

[2] Peacey SR, Toogood AA, Veldhuis JD, et al. The relationship between 24-hour growth hormone secretion and insulin-like growth factor I in patients with successfully treated acromegaly: impact of surgery or radiotherapy. Journal of Clinical Endocrinology and Metabolism. 2001; 86:259–266

[3] Tannenbaum GS, Epelbaum J, Bowers CY. Interrelationship between the novel peptide ghrelin and somatostatin/growth hormone-releasing hormone in regulation of pulsatile growth hormone secretion. Endocrinology. 2003; 144:967–974

[4] Thibonnier M, Barrow DL, Selman W. Antidiuretic Hormone: Regulation, Disorders, and Clinical Evaluation. In: Neuroendocrinology. Baltimore: Williams and Wilkins; 1992:19–30

[5] Byyny RL. Withdrawal from Glucocorticoid Therapy. N Engl J Med. 1976; 295:30–32

[6] Szabo GC, Winkler SR. Withdrawal of Glucocorticoid Therapy in Neurosurgical Patients. Surgical Neurology. 1995; 44

[7] Kountz DS. An Algorithm for Corticosteroid Withdrawal. Am Fam Physician. 1989; 39:250–254

[8] Marshall LF, King J, Langfitt TW. The Complication of High-Dose Corticosteroid Therapy in Neurosurgical Patients: A Prospective Study. Ann Neurol. 1977; 1:201–203

[9] Da Silva JA, Jacobs JW, Kirwan JR, et al. Safety of low dose glucocorticoid treatment in rheumatoid arthritis: published evidence and prospective trial data. Ann Rheum Dis. 2006; 65:285–293

[10] Braughler JM, Hall ED. Current Application of "High-Dose" Steroid Therapy for CNS Injury: A Pharmacological Perspective. J Neurosurg. 1985; 62:806–810

[11] Lu WY, Rhoney DH, Boling WB, et al. A Review of Stress Ulcer Prophylaxis in the Neurosurgical Intensive Care Unit. Neurosurgery. 1997; 41:416–426

[12] Weiner HL, Rezai AR, Cooper PR. Sigmoid Diverticular Perforation in Neurosurgical Patients Receiving High-Dose Corticosteroids. Neurosurgery. 1993; 33:40–43

[13] Zizic TM, Marcoux C, Hungerfold DS, et al. Corticosteroid Therapy Associated with Ischemic Necrosis of Bone in Systemic Lupus Erythematosus. Am J Med. 1985; 79:597–603

[14] Zizic TM. Avascular Necrosis of Bone. Current Opinions in Rheumatology. 1990; 2:26–37

[15] Matsuo K, Hirohata T, Sugioka T, et al. Influence of Alcohol Intake, Cigarette Smoking and Occupational Status on Idiopathic Necrosis of the Femoral Head. Clin Orthop. 1988; 234:115–123

[16] Struys A, Snelder AA, Mulder H. Cyclical Etidronate Reverses Bone Loss of the Spine and Proximal Femur in Patients With Established Corticosteroid-Induced Osteoporosis. American Journal of Medicine. 1995; 99:235–242

8

9 Hematology

9.1 Circulating blood volume

Circulating blood volumes for adults and peds are shown in ▶ Table 9.1.

Table 9.1 Circulating blood volume

Age	Vol (cc/kg[a])
premature infant	85–100
term infant < 1 month	85
age > 1 mo (including adult)	75

[a]cc per kg of body weight

9.2 Blood component therapy

9.2.1 Massive transfusions

Definition: replacement of > 1 blood volume (in average adult ≈ 20 U) in < 24 hrs for adult, or > 2 × circulating blood volume in peds, may cause dilution of effective platelets and coagulation factors, which requires platelet transfusion and fresh frozen plasma (FFP). When operating on a pediatric patient, you can usually safely replace up to 1.5 × the circulating blood volume before problems with coagulopathy ensue.

Blood component therapy required for massive transfusions:

9.2.2 Cellular component

Red blood cell therapy

General information

Major histocompatibilities of blood are shown in ▶ Table 9.2.

Table 9.2 Blood compatibility (AB0)

Blood type	Antibody present	Compatible blood (PRBC)	Compatible plasma	Compatible platelets or cryo-precipitate
A	B	A, O	A, AB	The same ABO type as the patient is preferred, but any ABO type may be used
B	A	B, O	B, AB	
AB	none	AB, A, B, O	AB	
O	A, B	O	AB, A, B, O	

Whole blood

1 U (≈ 510 cc) = 450 cc blood + 63 cc preservative.

Recommended transfusion criteria:

- exchange transfusions in neonates
- acute burn debridement and grafting in children

Packed red blood cells (PRBCs)

Recommended transfusion criteria:

1. acute blood loss ≥ 15% of patient's blood volume
2. in asymptomatic patient: hemoglobin (Hb) ≤ 8 gm or Hct ≤ 24%
3. symptoms of anemia at rest
4. preoperative Hb ≤ 15 gm or Hct < 45% in the neonate

Amount to transfuse:

Adult: 1 U (250–300 cc) raises Hct by 3–4%.

For peds, use Eq (9.1).

$$\text{ml of PRBC to transfuse} = \frac{(\text{estimated blood volume [ml]}) \times (\text{Hct increment desired [\%]})}{70\%} \quad (9.1)$$

(where the Hct of PRBCs ranges 70–80%)

Give no faster than 2–3 cc/kg/hr.

Autologous blood transfusion

Predonated whole blood may be stored 35 days. PRBCs may be stored 42 days.

Patients may donate every 3 days to 1 week as long as they maintain Hct ≥ 34% (supplement with ferrous sulfate). The following patients require physician release before donating: patients with coronary artery disease, angina, cerebrovascular disease, seizure disorder, pregnancy (because of possible vasovagal episode) or patients with malignancy.

Try to time last donation > 72 hrs prior to surgery to allow patient to replenish some of the depleted RBCs before surgery.

9.2.3 Platelets

General information

Normal platelet count (PC) is 150K–400K (abbreviation used here: 150K = 150,000/mm^3 = 150 × 10^9/l). Thrombocytopenia is defined as PC < 150K. Bleeding (spontaneously or with invasive procedures) is rarely a problem with PC > 50K. Spontaneous hemorrhage is very likely with PC < 5K. Spontaneous intracranial hemorrhage is uncommon with PC > 30K, and is more common in adults than children. Based on patients with ITP, the risk of fatal hemorrhage in patients with PC < 30K is 0.0162–0.0389 cases per patient-year[1] (risk of death from infection is higher). Intracranial bleeding is usually subarachnoid or intraparenchymal, with petechial hemorrhages common.

1 unit of platelets contains 5.5 × 10^{10} (minimum) to 10 × 10^{10} platelets. The volume of 6 units is 250–300 ml. Platelets may be stored up to 5 days.

Recommended platelet transfusion criteria

Indications for platelet transfusion[2]:
1. thrombocytopenia due to ↓ production (with or without increased destruction) (the most common causes are aplastic anemia and leukemia)
   a) PC < 10K even if no bleeding (prophylactic transfusion to prevent bleeding)
   b) PC < 20K and bleeding
   c) PC < 30K and patient at risk for bleeding: complaints of H/A, presence of confluent (c.f. scattered) petechiae, continuous bleeding from a wound, increasing retinal hemorrhage
   d) PC < 50K AND
      • major surgery planned within 12 hours
      • PC rapidly falling
      • patient < 48 hours post-op
      • patient requires lumbar puncture
      • acute blood loss of > 1 blood volume in < 24 hours
2. platelet transfusions have limited usefulness when thrombocytopenia is due to platelet destruction (e.g., by antibodies as in ITTP) or consumption (if production is adequate or increased, platelet transfusion usually will not be useful)
3. documented platelet dysfunction in a patient scheduled for surgery or in a patient with advanced hepatic and/or renal insufficiency (consider pharmacologic enhancement of platelet function, e.g., desmopressin[3])

Other indications for platelet transfusion:
1. patients who have been on Plavix® or aspirin who need urgent surgery that cannot be postponed for ≈ 5 days to allow new platelets to be synthesized

Dosage

Approximately 25% of platelets are lost just with transfusion.

Peds: 1 U/m^2 raises PC by ≈ 10K, usually give 4 U/m^2.

Adult: 1 U raises platelet count by ≈ 5–10K. Typical dose for thrombocytopenic bleeding adult: 6–10 U (usual order: "8-pack"). Alternatively, 1 U of pheresed platelets may be given (obtained from a single donor by apheresis, equivalent to 8–10 U of pooled donor platelets).

Check PC 1–2 hrs after transfusion. The increase in PC will be less in DIC, sepsis, splenomegaly, with platelet antibodies, or if the patient is on chemotherapy. In the absence of increased consumption, platelets will be needed q 3–5 days.

9.2.4 Plasma proteins

FFP (fresh frozen plasma)

General information
1 bag = 200–250 ml (usually referred to as a "unit," not to be confused with 1 unit of factor activity which is defined as 1 ml). FFP is plasma separated from RBCs and platelets, and contains all coagulation factors and natural inhibitors. FFP has an out-date period of 12 months. The risk of AIDS and hepatitis for each unit of FFP is equal to that of a whole unit of blood.

Recommended transfusion criteria
Recommendations (modified[2]):
1. history or clinical course suggestive of coagulopathy due to congenital or acquired coagulation factor deficiency with active bleeding or pre-op, with PT > 18 sec or APTT > 1.5 × upper limit of normal (usually > 55 sec), fibrinogen functioning normally and level > 1 g/l, and coagulation factor assay < 25% activity
2. proven coagulation factor deficiency with active bleeding or scheduled for surgery or other invasive procedure
   a) congenital deficiency of factor II, V, VII, X, XI or XII
   b) deficiency of factor VIII or IX if safe replacement factors unavailable
   c) von Willebrand's disease unresponsive to DDAVP
   d) multiple coagulation factor deficiency as in hepatic dysfunction, vitamin K depletion or DIC
3. reversal of warfarin (Coumadin®) (p. 174) effect (PT > 18 sec, or INR > 1.6) in patient actively bleeding or requiring emergency surgery or procedure with insufficient time for vitamin K to correct (which usually requires > 6–12 hrs)
4. deficiency of antithrombin III, heparin cofactor II, or protein C or S
5. massive blood transfusion: replacement of > 1 blood volume (≈ 5 L in 70 kg adult) within several hours with evidence of coagulation deficiency as in (1) and with continued bleeding
6. treatment of thrombotic thrombocytopenic purpura, hemolytic uremic syndrome
7. ✖ because of associated hazards and suitable alternatives, the use of FFP as a volume expander is relatively contraindicated

Dosage
Usual starting dose is 2 bags of FFP (400–600 ml). If PT is 18–22 secs or APTT is 55–70 secs, 1 bag may suffice. Doses as high as 10–15 ml/kg may be needed for some patients. Monitor PT/PTT (or specific factor assay) and clinical bleeding. Since factor VII has a shorter half-life (≈ 6 hrs) than the other factors, PT may become prolonged before APTT.

Remember: if patient is also receiving platelets, that for every 5–6 units of platelets the patient is also receiving coagulation factors equivalent to ≈ 1 bag of FFP.

Albumin and plasma protein fraction (PPF, AKA Plasmanate®)
Usually from outdated blood, treated to inactivate hepatitis B virus. Ratio of albumin:globulin percentage in "albumin" is 96%:4%, in PPF it is 83%:17%. Available in 5% (oncotically and osmotically equivalent to plasma) and 25% (contraindicated in dehydrated patients). 25% albumin may be diluted to 5% by mixing 1 volume of 25% albumin to 4 volumes of D5 W or 0.9% NS (✖ caution: mixing with sterile water will result in a hypotonic solution that can cause hemolysis and possible renal failure).

Expensive for use simply as a volume expander (≈ $60–80 per unit). Indicated only when total protein < 5.2 gm% (otherwise, use crystalloid which is equally effective). Rapid infusion (> 10 cc/min) has been reported to cause hypotension (due to Na-acetate and Hageman factor fragments). Use in ARDS is controversial. In neurosurgical patients, may be considered as an adjunct for volume expansion (along with crystalloids) for hyperdynamic therapy (p. 1447) when the hematocrit is < 40% following SAH where there is concern about increasing the risk of rebleeding e.g., with the use of hetastarch (p. 1434).

Cryoprecipitate

Recommended transfusion criteria:

1. hemophilia A
2. von Willebrand disease
3. documented fibrinogen/factor VIII deficiency
4. documented disseminated intravascular coagulation (DIC): along with other modes of therapy

Prothrombin complex concentrate (PCC) (Kcentra® and others)

Derived from fresh-frozen human plasma, contains clotting factors II, VII, IX and X, with protein C & S to prevent thrombosis. Primary indication is to be given IV to reverse warfarin in emergency situations. However it is also used in other settings. Requires much lower volume than FFP to work. Also, when the INR gets down to about 1.4, PCC will continue to reduce the INR whereas FFP will have little or no benefit (the INR of FFP itself is ≈ 1.3–1.4).

Optimal dosing is not known. Doses of 15–50 IU/kg have been given to hemophiliacs, but the clotting deficit differs in vitamin-K depletion than in clotting factor absence. A reasonable dose that is often used is 25 IU/kg.

9.3 Anticoagulation considerations in neurosurgery

9.3.1 General information

Most of these issues have not been studied in a rigorous, prospective fashion. Yet, these questions frequently arise. The following is to be considered a framework of guidelines, and is not to be construed as a standard of care. ▶ Table 9.3 acts as an index to the topics discussed below.

Choice of oral anticoagulant: compared to vitamin K antagonists (VKAs) (e.g., warfarin), the novel oral anticoagulants (NOACs) dabigatran, rivaroxaban & edoxaban are at least as effective in preventing ischemic stroke and systemic embolization in patient with atrial fibrillation. And compared to warfarin, NOACs reduce ICH by about 50%,[4] have a more rapid onset of action, a shorter half-life, more predictable pharmacokinetics, fewer drug-drug interactions, and do not require routine monitoring.[5]

Table 9.3 Anticoagulation issues in neurosurgery

General neurosurgical contraindications to full anticoagulation with heparin (p. 163)
Starting/continuing anticoagulation in the presence of the following neurosurgical conditions

• incidental aneurysm (p. 164)
• subarachnoid hemorrhage (p. 164)
• brain tumor (p. 164)
• following craniotomy (p. 164)
• acute epidural/subdural hematoma
• chronic subdural hematoma
• ischemic stroke
  ○ after tPA (p. 1564)
  ○ for prevention of (p. 1543)
• intracerebral hemorrhage (p. 1622)

Managing patients who are already anticoagulated who need a neurosurgical procedure
• warfarin (Coumadin®) (p. 164) • heparin (p. 168) • LMW-heparin (p. 168) • antiplatelet drugs (aspirin, Plavix, NSAIDs) (p. 168)
Recommendations for DVT prophylaxis in neurosurgical patients (p. 177)

9.3.2 Contraindications to heparin

Contraindications to heparin therapy are constantly being reevaluated. Massive PE producing hemodynamic compromise should be treated with anticoagulation in most cases despite intracranial risks. Contraindications to full anticoagulation with heparin include:

- recent severe head injury
- recent craniotomy: see below
- patients with coagulopathies
- hemorrhagic infarction
- bleeding ulcer or other inaccessible bleeding site
- uncontrollable hypertension

- severe hepatic or renal disease
- < 4–6 hours before an invasive procedure (see below)
- brain tumor: see below

9.3.3 Patients with unruptured (incidental) cerebral aneurysms

Anticoagulation may not increase the risk of hemorrhage (i.e., rupture); however, should rupture occur, anticoagulation would most likely increase volume of hemorrhage and thus increase morbidity and mortality.

The decision to start/continue anticoagulant depends on the indication for the drugs, the size of the aneurysm (a small aneurysm < 4 mm is not as worrisome). Patients needing antiplatelet therapy (e.g., Plavix®) for drug-eluting cardiac stents should probably be left on their drugs.

9.3.4 Patients on anticoagulation/antiplatelet drugs who develop SAH

Coumadin and antiplatelet drugs are usually reversed.

9.3.5 In patients with brain tumor

Some authors are reluctant to administer full-dose heparin to a patient with a brain tumor,[6] although a number of studies found no higher risk in these patients when treated with heparin or oral anticoagulation[7,8,9] (PT should be followed very closely, one study recommended maintaining PT ≈ 1.25 × control[9]).

9.3.6 Postoperatively following craniotomy

Requires individualization based on the reason for the craniotomy. Surgery for parenchymal lesions where the surgery disrupts small vessels (e.g., brain tumor) is probably higher risk for hemorrhage than, e.g., aneurysm surgery (expert opinion). Options:

Full anticoagulation: most neurosurgeons would probably not fully anticoagulate patients < 3–5 days following craniotomy,[10] and some recommend at least 2 weeks. However, one study found no increased incidence of bleeding when anticoagulation was resumed 3 days post craniotomy.[11]

Low-dose (prophylactic) anticoagulation: either with mini-dose heparin (5000 U SQ 2 hrs prior to craniotomy and continuing q 12 hrs post-op × 7 d) or enoxaparin (Lovenox) (30 mg SQ BID or as a single dose of 40 MG SQ q d). RPDB study[12]: assessed *safety* (not efficacy), 55 patients undergoing craniotomy for tumor received mini-dose heparin as indicated had no increased bleeding tendency by any of the parameters measured. RPNB study[13]: incidence of post-op hemorrhage increased to 11% with enoxaparin.

9.3.7 Management of anticoagulants prior to neurosurgical procedures

Preoperative laboratory assessment of the coagulation pathway and platelet function is routinely used even though these studies rarely contribute critical information in the patient with a negative history for bleeding tendencies. There are no randomized studies to assess the value of coagulation laboratory measurements to patient care. This section encompasses the use of antiplatelet and anticoagulation medicines, their monitoring, and their reversal.

▶ Table 9.4 summarizes this information.

Warfarin

Management guidelines

Patients on warfarin who must be anticoagulated as long as possible (e.g., mechanical heart valves) may be "bridged" to LMW heparin injections (e.g., Lovenox (p. 173)), as follows: stop warfarin at least 3 days prior to the procedure, and begin self-administered LMW heparin injections which are discontinued, as outlined in ▶ Table 9.4.

Patients with less critical anticoagulation needs (e.g., chronic a-fib) can usually stop the warfarin at least 4–5 days before the procedure, and a PT/INR is then checked on admission to the hospital. Patients must be advised that during the time that they are not anticoagulated, they are at risk of possible complications from the condition for which they are receiving the agents (*annual risk for mechanical valve*: ≈ 6%; for a-fib: depends on several factors including age and history of prior stroke, an average for patients > 65 years of age is ≈ 5–6%; see details (p. 1590)).

Table 9.4 Anticoagulants

Drug Name (Brand)	Administration	Mechanism	Monitoring	Metabolism	Reversal strategy	Hold time[a]	Comments
Unfractionated heparin	IV for therapeutic anticoagulation; SQ for prophylaxis	Binds antithrombin III. Inhibits conversion of prothrombin → thrombin and fibrinogen → fibrin	aPTT, ACT, or antifactor Xa	Liver; excreted in urine; $T_{1/2}$ 60–90 min	1 mg protamine sulfate/100 u heparin administered	Full anticoagulation 4–6 hrs, consider repeat aPTT; SQ "minidose" 12 hrs	Heparin produced since 2009 is 10% less potent; incidence of HIT is variable and reportedly 1–2%; "heparin rebound" may occur 8–9 hrs after protamine infusion[33,34]
Enoxaparin (Lovenox, Sanofi Aventis) (an LMWH)	SQ for DVT prophylaxis and therapeutic anticoagulation	Binds antithrombin III and accelerates activity; inhibits thrombin and factor Xa	Antifactor Xa (therapeutic level 0.4–0.8 units/l)	Liver; renal clearance, caution in patients with CrCl < 30 ml/min	protamine sulfate (1 mg/1 mg enoxaparin given in last 8 hrs); will only partially reverse effects (60%)	12 hrs after prophylactic dose; 24 hrs after therapeutic dose	more selective inhibitor of factor Xa than thrombin[33,34,35]
Fondaparinux (Arixtra, GlaskoSmithKline)	SQ for DVT prophylaxis and therapeutic anticoagulation	Inhibits factor Xa	Antifactor Xa; Prophylactic dose (0.4–0.5 mg/l); Therapeutic dose (1.2–1.26 mg/l)	Unknown; Excreted in urine; $T_{1/2}$ 17–21 hrs	No approved antidote; consider rVIIa; no studies examining the role of rVIIa in reversing fondaparinaux in the setting of bleeding; hemodialysis reduces ≈ 20%	2–4 days in patients with normal renal function	Does not cause HIT, useful in patients with HIT; recommend 50% dose reduction if CrCl 30–50, contraindicated if CrCl < 30[33,34,35]
Warfarin (Coumadin, Bristol-Myers Squibb)	PO	Vitamin K antagonist. (Vitamin K dependent factors are II, VII, IX, X, protein C & S)	PT; INR (goal varies with indication)	Liver; excreted in urine ≈ 92%, bile; $T_{1/2}$ 20–60 hrs (highly variable)	Vitamin K 10mg IV × 3 days and/or PCC (25–100 UI/kg) or FFP (15 ml/kg)[b,33]	5 days	Consider decreasing dose with hepatic impairment
Argatroban (GlaskoSmithKline)	IV for prophylaxis and treatment of thrombosis in patients with HIT	Direct thrombin inhibitor	aPTT (goal 1.5–3x normal); ACT	Liver; excreted in feces ≈ 65% and urine ≈ 22%; $T_{1/2}$ 39–51 min	No reversal agent; supportive care; Hemodialysis can remove some drug from bloodstream, but unknown effect on bleeding, consider FFP or cryoprecipitate	2–4 hrs	Liver disease, consider decreasing start dose and titrate slowly[30,34]
Dabigatran (Pradaxa®, Boehringer Ingelheim)	PO, BID dosing	Direct thrombin inhibitor, reversible	No routine monitoring; normal aPTT implies no effect	Liver; renal clearance in urine; $T_{1/2}$ 12–17 hrs	idarucizumab (Praxbind®) (see text below)	1–2 days, longer if renal CrCl<50 ml/min (see ▶ Table 9.5)	For prevention of stroke with atrial fibrillation (afib); PCC shown to be most effective but unproven in human studies[33,34,36]

9

(continued)

9

Table 9.4 continued

Drug Name (Brand)	Administration	Mechanism	Monitoring	Metabolism	Reversal strategy	Hold time[a]	Comments
Rivaroxaban (Xarelto®, Bayer HealthCare)	PO daily dosing	Factor Xa inhibitor	No routine monitoring; normal antifactor Xa indicates no effect	Liver; renal clearance ≈ 66%, feces ≈ 28%; $T_{1/2}$ 5–9h	AndexXa® (p. 175). If not available, consider rVIIa (partial reversal in animals	24 hrs (see ▲ Table 9.5)	For prevention of stroke in afib and DVT treatment; Caution: use with CrCl 15–50; CrCl <30 avoid use.[36,37] Not dialyzable[33]
Apixaban (Eliquis®, Bristol-Myers Squibb)	PO, BID dosing	Factor Xa inhibitor	No routine monitoring; normal antifactor Xa indicates no effect	Liver ≈ 75% renal clearance ≈ 25%; $T_{1/2}$ 12h	AndexXa® (p. 175). If not available, consider PCC, or rVIIa. rVIIa decreases bleeding time in animal model but does not reverse anticoagulant effect.	48 hrs (see ▲ Table 9.5)	For prevention of stroke in afib and DVT prophylaxis after orthopedic surgery. Decrease dose if Cr >1.5; do not use with severe hepatic impairment.[33,36] Not dialyzable[33]
Edoxaban (Savaysa™, Daiichi Sankyo Co.)	PO, daily dosing. Do not use if CrCl >95 mL/min	Factor Xa inhibitor	No routine monitoring. Changes in PT & INR are small and not useful. Normal antifactor Xa indicates no effect	renal ≈ 50% (unchanged drug). Remainder: biliary/ intestinal excretion & minimal metabolism. $T_{1/2}$ 10–14h	No specific antagonist	48 hrs	For DVT & PE after 5–10 d of parenteral anticoagulant; to reduce risk of stroke and embolism in nonvalvulat a-fib
Antithrombin, recombinant (ATryn, Lundbeck)	IV	Inhibits thrombin and factor Xa	AT levels	$T_{1/2}$ 11.6–17.7h			For thromboembolism prophylaxis in hereditary antithrombin deficiency
Antithrombin III (Thrombate III, Grifols)	IV	Forms bond with thrombin	AT levels	$T_{1/2}$ 2–3 days			For thromboembolism prophylaxis in hereditary antithrombin deficiency
Dalteparin (Fragmin, Eisai)	SQ for DVT prophylaxis and therapeutic anticoagulation	Accelerates activity of antithrombin III (inhibits thrombin and factor Xa)		Liver, urine; $T_{1/2}$ 3–5h (longer with renal impairment)			Caution when use with CrCl <30; caution with hepatic impairment
Bivalirudin (Angiomax®, The Medicines Company)	IV	Direct thrombin inhibitor (reversible)	ACT	Plasma; excreted in urine; $T_{1/2}$ 25 min (longer with renal impairment)	None		Caution when use with CrCl <30

Table 9.4 continued

Drug Name (Brand)	Administration	Mechanism	Monitoring	Metabolism	Reversal strategy	Hold time[a]	Comments
Desirudin (Ipri-vask®, Canyon)	SC	Direct thrombin inhibitor (selectively inhibits free and clot-bound thrombin	aPTT	Kidney; excreted in urine; $T_{1/2}$ 2h (longer with renal impairment)	None		CrCl < 60 use caution, decrease initial dose[33]

Abbreviations: PCC = prothrombin complex concentrate; IV = intravenous; SQ = subcutaneous; aPTT = partial thromboplastin time; DVT = deep venous thrombosis; HIT = heparin induced thrombocytopenia; ACT = activated clotting time; AT = anti-thrombin; CrCl = creatinine clearance.

[a]Hold time is the recommended time to wait after discontinuing the drug before doing an elective operation in order to eliminate the effects of the drug

[b]Intravenous vitamin K has a more rapid onset than subcutaneous vitamin K and current formulations, made with micelles of lecithin and glycol, seem to have a lower complication profile than older formulations containing polyethylated castor oil.[38]

9

Table 9.5 Recommendations for holding oral anticoagulants prior to invasive procedures related to renal function.[33]

	dabigatran (Pradaxa®)	apixaban (Eliquis®)	rivaroxaban (Xarelto®)
CrCl > 80 ml/min	≥ 72 hr	≥ 48 hr	≥ 48 hr
CrCl 50–80 ml/min	≥ 72 hr	≥ 48 hr	≥ 48 hr
CrCl 30–49 ml/min	≥ 96 hr	≥ 72 hr	≥ 72 hr
CrCl < 30 ml/min	≥ 120 hr	≥ 96 hr	≥ 96 hr

The recommended minimum interval between last dose and procedure is based on renal function and procedure risk. Generally, neurosurgical procedures including minor procedures such as LPs are considered interventions with a high bleeding risk

For non-emergent neurosurgical procedures

For procedures where post-op mass effect from bleeding would pose serious risk (which includes most neurosurgical operations), it is recommended that the PT should be ≈ ≤13.5 sec (i.e., ≤ upper limits of normal) or the INR should be ≈ ≤ 1.4 (e.g., for reference, this INR is considered safe for performing a percutaneous needle liver biopsy). See also reversal of anticoagulation (p. 174).

For emergent neurosurgical procedures

Give FFP (start with 2 units) and vitamin K (10–20 mg IV at ≤ 1 mg/min) as soon as possible; see also reversal of anticoagulation (p. 174). The timing of surgery is then based on the urgency of the situation and the nature of the procedure (e.g., the decision might be to evacuate a spinal epidural hematoma in an acutely paralyzed patient before anticoagulation is fully reversed).

Heparin

For emergencies: if it would be deleterious to wait 4–6 hours after discontinuing heparin and then repeating the PTT to verify that anticoagulation has been corrected, then heparin can be reversed with protamine (p. 174).

For non-emergencies

IV heparin: stop the drip ≈ 4–6 hours prior to the planned procedure. Option: recheck PTT just prior to starting the procedure.

"Mini-dose" SQ heparin: not mandatory to stop for craniotomy, but if desired to discontinue, then give last dose ≥ 12 hours prior to surgery.

Low-molecular weight heparins (LMWH)

For emergencies: can be reversed with protamine (p. 174).

Non-emergencies: See ▶ Table 9.4. Longer times are needed in renal failure. A factor Xa level can be used to check anticoagulation status, but this usually must be sent out, making it unsuitable for acute management.

Antiplatelet drugs and neurosurgical procedures

Platelet mechanistics and platelet function tests

Platelets are important for maintaining vascular endothelial integrity and are involved with hemostasis in conjunction with coagulation factors. Severe thrombocytopenia can result in petechial hemorrhages or spontaneous intracerebral hemorrhage (ICH). Vascular wall disturbance is the initial stimulus for platelet deposition and activation. Platelets adhere to collagen via surface receptors GPIb-V-IX and von Willebrand factor. This adhesion sets off a cascade of reactions, which result in platelet aggregation forming a hemostatic plug. Historically, bleeding time (BT) was used as the screening test for abnormalities of platelet function. Due to unreliability, many institutions have replaced the BT with the platelet function assay (PFA) using the PFA-100 (platelet function analyzer). There are limited studies confirming its use according to the International Society of Thrombosis and Hemostasis.[14,15]

In the PFA-100, primary hemostasis is simulated under "high-shear" flow by movement of citrated blood through a membrane-impregnated capillary in two collagen-coated cartridges; one stimulates platelets with adenosine diphosphate (ADP) and the other with epinephrine.[16] This interaction with the collagen induces a platelet plug, which closes an aperture. Results are reported as closure time in seconds. This method is eligible as a screening test for primary hemostatic disease such as von Willebrand disease as well as for monitoring the effect of antiplatelet therapy. The PFA-100 works for testing with aspirin but not with thienopyridine drug class (e.g., clopidogrel). Newly available PFA cartridges detect P2Y12 receptor blockade in patients on theinopyridine drugs.[17] VerifyNow® measures agonist-induced aggregation as an increase in light transmittance. The system contains a preparation of human fibrinogen-coated beads, which cause a change in light transmittance by ADP-induced platelet aggregation.[17] There is little correlation between the PFA-100 results and VerifyNow Assay.

Agents

▶ **Plavix® (clopidogrel)** (p.1548) **and aspirin.** Cause permanent inhibition of platelet function that persists ≈ 5 days after discontinuation of the drug and can increase the risk of bleeding. For elective cases, 5–7 days off these drugs is recommended (surveys of German neurosurgeons[18,19]: an average of 7 days was used for low-dose ASA, with a few who do *spine* surgery even while the patient is on ASA).

Cardiac stents: dual antiplatelet therapy (e.g., ASA + Plavix®) are mandatory for 4 weeks (90 days is preferable[20]) after placement of a bare metal cardiac stent, and for at least 1 year with drug-eluting stents (DES) (the risk declines from ≈ 6% to ≈ 3%).[21] Even short gaps in drug therapy (e.g., to perform neurosurgical procedures) is associated with significant risk of acute stent occlusion (and therefore elective surgery during this time is discouraged[22]). DES are so effective in suppressing endothelialization that lifetime dual antiplatelet therapy may be required. Bridging DES patients with antithrombin, anticoagulants, or glycoprotein IIb/IIIa agents has not been proven effective.[22]

Reversal of antiplatelet drugs: While heparin and warfarin can be reliably and measurably reversed, the situation is less clear with antiplatelet agents.[23] Agents used pre-op to reverse these drugs include Desmopressin (p.175) (DDAVP®)[18,19] and FFP.[18]

Reversal of Plavix for emergency surgery (p.161): platelets may be given; however, the Plavix effect persists for up to a couple of days after the last dose, and can actually inhibit platelets given after the drug is discontinued (the half-life of aspirin is lower and should not be an issue after 1 day). In cases with continued oozing in the first day or so after discontinuing Plavix, the following regimen is an option:

1. recombinant activated coagulation factor VII (rFVIIa): even though the defect is in the platelets, rFVIIa works, via a mechanism not mediated by protein clotting factors. Very expensive (≈ $10,000 per dose), but this must be balanced against the cost of repeat craniotomy, increased ICU stay and additional morbidity
    a) initial dose[24]: 90–120 mcg/kg
    b) same dose 2 hrs later
    c) 3rd dose 6 hrs after initial dose
2. platelets every 8 hours for 24 hours, *either*
    a) 6 U of regular platelets
    b) if patient is on fluid or volume restriction: 1 unit of pheresed platelets

▶ **Herbal products and supplements.** Herbal products and supplements often affect platelet aggregation and the coagulation cascade by means that cannot be detected by laboratory tests. The increasing popularity of these unregulated products requires screening patients for their use. There are limited studies regarding the use of herbal supplements in neurosurgery and, as a precaution for an elective operation, waiting 7–14 days after cessation of their use is suggested.

Fish Oil (Omega-3 Fatty Acids) is used for treatment of dyslipidemia and hypertriglyceridemia. Fish oil may affect platelet aggregation by a reduction in arachidonic acid and thromboxane and adenosine diphosphate receptor blockade. Fish oil may also potentially lengthen bleeding times.[25,26,27]

Garlic (Allium sativum): purported benefits include lowering blood pressure, preventing infection and myocardial infarction, and treating hypercholesterolemia. Garlic has an antiplatelet effect through ADP receptor blockade, and reducing calcium and thromboxane.[28] Garlic may potentiate the antiplatelet or anticoagulant effect of aspirin or warfarin.[29]

Ginkgo (Ginkgo biloba) is found in many formulations from capsules to energy drinks. It has been used to treat memory loss, depression, anxiety, dizziness, claudication, erectile dysfunction, tinnitus and headache. Ginkgo affects bleeding via an antiplatelet effect and antagonism of platelet-activating factor.[30,31] See Ginkgo biloba under Spontaneous subdural hematoma (p.1085).

Ginseng (Panax ginseng) also has antiplatelet activity through thromboxane inhibition and platelet-activating factor.[32]

Some authors also advocate cautious use of **ginger** and **vitamin E** when planning surgery, but the exact antiplatelet mechanism is unclear.[27]

9.3.8 Anticoagulants

See also ▶ Table 9.6 for platelet function inhibitors.

9

Table 9.6 Platelet function inhibitors

Drug Name (Brand)	Class/Target	Mechanism	Administration	Monitoring	Metabolism	Reversal strategy	Hold time[a]	Comments
Aspirin (Acetylsalicylic acid)	COX-1	Direct action, irreversible	PO	PFA, Arachidonic acid-based tests (VerifyNow)	Gut, plasma, and liver; renal clearance; $T_{1/2}$ 15–20 min	Platelet transfusion; Desmopressin[b]	7–10 days	Prevalence of aspirin resistance is 5–60%; therapeutic effect for lifetime of platelets (9 days), 10% of circulating platelets are replaced in 24-hr period[33,34,39]
Clopidogrel (Plavix®, Sanofi Aventis)	Thienopyridines/P2Y$_{12}$	Prodrug, irreversible	PO	PFA, VerifyNow P2Y12 (PRU Test)	Liver; renal clearance $T_{1/2}$ 8 hrs	Platelet transfusion (10 concentrate units every 12 hrs for 48 hrs); Desmopressin[b]	7–10 day	Prevalence of clopidogrel resistance is 8–35%[33,34,39]
Ticlodipine (Ticlid®, Roche)	Thienopyridines/P2Y$_{12}$	Prodrug, irreversible	PO	Bleeding time	Liver; renal clearance; $T_{1/2}$ 4–5 days	NA		Effective in ≈ 96% of patients with clopidogrel resistance
Prasugrel (Effient®, Eli Lilly)	Thienopyridines/P2Y$_{12}$	Prodrug, irreversible	PO	PFA, VerifyNow P2Y12 (PRU Test)	Liver; renal clearance ≈ 68%, feces ≈ 27%; $T_{1/2}$ 3.7 hrs	Platelet transfusion; active metabolite removed by dialysis		Used for coronary artery disease[33]
Ticagrelor (Brilinta®, AstraZeneca)	Cyclopentyltriazolopyrimidine/P2Y$_{12}$	Direct-acting, reversible	PO	NA	Liver; excreted in bile primarily; $T_{1/2}$ 9 hrs (active metabolite)	NA, not removed by dialysis		5 days[40]
Dipyridamole (Persantine®, Boehringer Ingelheim)	cGMP V	Prodrug, reversible	PO	NA	Liver; excretion in bile; $T_{1/2}$ 10–12 hrs	Dialysis is no benefit		
Abciximab (ReoPro®, Eli Lilly)	GPIIb/IIIa	Reversible	IV	aPTT, ACT, VerifyNow IIb/IIIa test	Proteolytic cleavage; $T_{1/2}$ 30 min	Platelet transfusion, no antagonist		Platelet function returns to ≈ 50% of baseline 24hrs after infusion; low-level inhibition may continue for up to 7 weeks[34]

Table 9.6 continued

Drug Name (Brand)	Class/Target	Mechanism	Administration	Monitoring	Metabolism	Reversal strategy	Hold time[a]	Comments
Eptifibatide (Integrilin, Millennium/ Merck)	GPIIb/IIIa	Reversible	IV	aPTT, ACT, VerifyNow IIb/IIIa test	Renal clearance 75%; $T_{1/2}$ 2.5 hrs	May be removed by dialysis		CrCl < 50 adjust infusion rate; platelet function returns to ≈ 50% 4hrs after infusion D/C'd[34]
Tirofiban (Aggrastat, Medicure)	GPIIb/IIIa	Reversible	IV		Renal clearance 65%; feces 25%; $T_{1/2}$ 2–3 hrs	May be removed by dialysis		CrCl < 30 adjust infusion rate; platelet coagulation is inhibited within 5 min, and remains inhibited for 3–8h[34]

Abbreviations: PCC = prothrombin complex concentrate; IV = intravenous; SQ = subcutaneous; aPTT = partial thromboplastin time; ACT = activated clotting time; CrCl = creatinine clearance; D/C = discontinue.

[a]Hold time is the recommended time to wait after discontinuing the drug before doing an elective operation in order to eliminate the effects of the drug

[b]Desmopressin enhances platelet adhesion to vessel wall by increased concentrations of factor VIII and von Willebrand factor. Desmopressin increased platelet adhesion in randomized trial in both aspirin group and control group.[41]

9

Warfarin

Drug info: Warfarin (Coumadin®)

An oral vitamin K antagonist. To anticoagulate average-weight patient, give 10 mg PO q d × 2–4 days, then ≈ 5 mg q d. Follow coagulation studies, titrate to PT = 1.2–1.5 × control (or INR ≈ 2–3) for most conditions (e.g., DVT, single TIA). Higher PT ratios of 1.5–2 × control (INR ≈ 3–4) may be needed for recurrent systemic embolism, mechanical heart valves... (the recommended ranges for the International Normalized Ratio (INR) are shown in ▶ Table 9.7).

✖ Contraindicated in pregnancy: in addition to risk of bleeding, warfarin is associated with spontaneous abortion and stillbirth. Warfarin also crosses the placenta and is teratogenic, causing birth defects in 5–30%, including fetal warfarin syndrome during 1st trimester (including scoliosis, brachydactyly, vertebral column calcifications, ventriculomegaly, agenesis of the corpus callosum) and spasticity/seizures and eye defects after the 1st trimester.

Starting warfarin: During the first ≈ 3 days of warfarin therapy, patients may actually be hypercoagulable (secondary to reduction of vitamin-K dependent anticoagulation factors protein C and protein S), putting them at risk of "Coumadin necrosis." Therefore patients should be "bridged" by starting either Lovenox (p. 173) which can be self-administered as an outpatient, or heparin (with a therapeutic PTT).

Supplied: scored tabs of 1, 2, 2.5, 5, 7.5 and 10 mg. IV form: 5 mg/vial.

9

Table 9.7 Recommended INRs[42]

Indication	INR
• mechanical prosthetic heart valve • prevention of recurrent MI	2.5–3.5
antiphospholipid antibody syndrome (p. 1542) [43]	≥ 3
all other indications (*DVT prophylaxis* and treatment, PE, atrial fibrillation, recurrent systemic embolism, tissue heart valves)	2–3

Heparin

Drug info: Heparin

℞ Full anticoagulation in an average-weight patient, give 5000 U bolus IV, follow with 1000 U/hr IV drip. Titrate to therapeutic anticoagulation of APTT = 2–2.5 × control (for DVT, some recommend 1.5–2 × control[44]).

℞ prophylactic AKA low-dose ("mini-dose") heparin: 5000 IU SQ q 8 or 12 hrs. Routine monitoring of APTT is usually not done, although occasionally patients may become fully anticoagulated on this regimen.

Side effects: (see Anticoagulant considerations in neurosurgery above): hemorrhage, thrombosis[45] (heparin activates anti-thrombin III and can cause platelet aggregation) which can result in MIs, DVTs, PEs, strokes, etc. Heparin induced thrombocytopenia (HIT): transient mild thrombocytopenia is fairly common in the first few days after initiating heparin therapy; however, severe thrombocytopenia occurs in 1–2% of patients receiving heparin > 4 days (usually has a delayed onset of 6–12 days, and is due to consumption in heparin-induced thrombosis or to antibodies formed against a heparin-platelet protein complex). The incidence of HIT in SAH is 5–6% and was similar with enoxaparin.[46] Consider use of fondaparinux in thrombocytopenic patients. Chronic therapy may cause osteoporosis.

Low molecular weight heparins

See references.[47,48]

Low molecular weight heparins (LMWH) (average molecular weight = 3000–8000 daltons) are derived from unfractionated heparin (average MW = 12,000–15,000 daltons). LMWHs differ from unfractionated heparin because they have a higher ratio of anti-factor Xa to anti-factor IIa (antithrombin) activity which theoretically should produce antithrombic effects with fewer hemorrhagic complications. Realization of this benefit has been very minor in clinical trials. LMWH have greater bioavailability after sub-Q injection leading to more predictable plasma levels which eliminates the need to monitor biologic activity (such as APTT). LMWH have a longer half-life and therefore require fewer doses per day. LMWH have a lower incidence of thrombocytopenia. More effective in DVT prophylaxis than warfarin in orthopedic surgery.[49]

Spinal epidural hematomas: There have been a number of case reports of spinal epidural hematomas occurring in patients on LMWH (primarily enoxaparin) who also underwent spinal/epidural anesthesia or lumbar puncture, primarily in elderly women undergoing orthopedic surgery. Some have had significant neurologic sequelae, including permanent paralysis.[50] The risk is further increased by the use of NSAIDs, platelet inhibitors, or other anticoagulants, and with traumatic or repeated epidural or spinal puncture.

▶ **Available low molecular weight heparins.** Drugs include:
- enoxaparin (Lovenox®): see below
- dalteparin (Fragmin®): R 2500 anti-Xa U SQ q d
- ardeparin (Normiflo®): half-life = 3.3 hrs. R 50 anti-Xa U/kg SQ q 12 hrs
- danaparoid (Orgaran®): a heparinoid. Even higher anti-Xa:anti-IIa ratio than LMWHs. Does not require laboratory monitoring. R 750 anti-Xa U SQ BID
- tinzaparin (Logiparin®, Innohep®): not available in U.S. R 175 anti-Xa U per kg SQ once daily

Drug info: Enoxaparin (Lovenox®)

R dosage established following hip replacement is 30 mg SQ BID × 7–14 days (alternative: 40 mg SQ q d). **Pharmacokinetics:** After SQ injection, peak serum concentration occurs in 3–5 hrs. Half-life: 4.5 hrs.

9

Direct thrombin inhibitors

Drug info: Dabigatran (Pradaxa®, Rendix®)

An oral anticoagulant in the class of direct thrombin inhibitors. Administered as the prodrug dabigatran etexilate. Must be stopped 24 hrs prior to surgery.

Reversal of anticoagulation: Praxbind® (idarucizumab) IV for emergencies. Pradaxa reversal begins within 12 minutes, maximum reversal within 4 hrs, lasts 24 hrs.[51]

Drug info: Bivalirudin (Angiomax® or Angiox®)

A reversible direct thrombin inhibitor (DTI) that increases the rapidity of plasminogen activator-mediated recanalization. No effective reversal.
R: IV loading dose of 0.5 mg/kg IV, followed by continuous infusion of 1.75 mg/kg/hr. Intra-arterial: inject 15 mg in 10 ml of heparinized saline via a microcatheter.

Factor Xa inhibitors

Drug info: Fondaparinux (Arixtra®)

A synthetic analog of the pentasaccharide binding sequence of heparin. Increases factor Xa inhibition without affecting factor IIa (thrombin).[52] Unlike heparin, fondaparinux does not bind to other plasma proteins or platelet factor-4 and does not cause heparin-induced thrombocytopenia (HIT) and can therefore be used in patients with HIT. May be more effective than enoxaparin (Lovenox®) for preventing post-op DVTs. **Side effects:** Bleeding is the most common side effect (may be increased by concurrent NSAID use). ✖ Contraindicated with severe renal impairment (CrCl < 30 ml/min).[53]

R: 2.5 mg SQ injection q d. **Supplied:** 2.5 mg single-dose syringes. **Pharmacokinetics:** Peak activity occurs in 2–3 hrs. Half-life: 17–21 hrs. Anticoagulation effect lasts 3–5 half-lives. Elimination: in urine (in renal insufficiency reduce dose by 50% for CrCl 30–50 ml/min). STOP: 2–4 days pre-op (longer with kidney dysfunction)

9.3.9 Coagulopathies

Correction of coagulopathies or reversal of anticoagulants

Also refer to recommended normal values for coagulation studies in neurosurgery (p. 164).

Platelets

See indications and administration guidelines (p. 161).

Fresh frozen plasma

To reverse warfarin anticoagulation, use the following as a starting point and recheck PT/PTT afterward:
- when patient is "therapeutically anticoagulated" start with 2–3 units FFP (approximately 15 ml/kg is usually needed)
- for severely prolonged PT/PTT, start with 6 units FFP

Prothrombin complex concentrate (PCC)

Warfarin induced anticoagulation may be reversed up to 4 or 5 times more quickly with PCC (Kcentra®) (contains coag factors II, IX, and X) compared to FFP.[54] Patient may become hyperthrombotic with PCC.

Drug info: Vitamin K (Mephyton®)

To reverse elevated PT from *warfarin* , give aqueous colloidal solution of vitamin K1 (phytonadione, Mephyton®). Doses > 10 mg may produce warfarin resistance for up to 1 week. FFP may be administered concurrently for more rapid correction (see above). See recommended levels of PT (p. 164).

R adult: start with 10–15 mg IM; the effect takes 6–12 hrs (in absence of liver disease). Repeat dose if needed. The average total dose needed to reverse therapeutic anticoagulation is 25–35 mg.

IV administration has been associated with severe reactions (possibly anaphylactic), including hypotension and even fatalities (even with proper precautions to dilute and administer slowly), therefore IV route is reserved only for situations where other routes are not feasible and the serious risk is justified. R IV (when IM route not feasible): 10–20 mg IV at a rate of injection not to exceed 1 mg/min (e.g., put 10 mg in 50 ml of D5 W and give over 30 minutes).

Drug info: Protamine sulfate

For heparin: 1 mg protamine reverses ≈ 100 U *heparin* (give slowly, not to exceed 50 mg in any 10 min period). Therapy should be guided by coagulation studies.

Reversal of low molecular weight heparins (LMWH): slow IV injection of a 1% solution of protamine can also be used to reverse LMWHs as follows:

Enoxaparin (Lovenox®): ≈ 60% of Lovenox can be reversed with 1 mg of protamine for every mg of Lovenox given (maximum dose = 50 mg) within the last 8 hrs, and 0.5 mg of protamine for every mg of Lovenox given from 8–12 hrs prior. Protamine is probably not needed for Lovenox given > 12 hrs earlier.

Dalteparin (Fragmin®) or ardeparin (Normiflo®): 1 mg of protamine for every 100 anti-Xa IU of the LMWH (maximum dose = 50 mg) with a second infusion of 0.5 mg protamine for every 100 anti-Xa IU of LMWH if the APTT remains elevated 2–4 hours after the first dose is completed.

Danaparoid and Hirudin: no known reversing agent.

Drug info: Andexanet alfa (AndexXa®)

A recombinant DNA manufactured derivative of clotting factor Xa (fXa) that binds to certain fXa-inhibitors inhibiting their action. FDA-approved for reversal of rivaroxaban (Xarelto®) or apixaban (Eliquis®) for life-threatening or uncontrolled bleeding.[55]

Reduces anti-fXa activity in healthy volunteers, but improvement in hemostasis has not been established (studies ongoing). ✖ Has not been shown effective for, and is not indicated for, reversal of other fXa inhibitors (e.g., fondaparinux).
* Use low dose regimen described below for:
  * rivaroxaban dose ≤ 10 mg (any timing from last dose)
  * apixaban dose ≤ 5 mg (any timing from last dose)
  * rivaroxaban dose > 10 mg or dose unknown (≥ 8 hrs from last dose)
  * apixaban dose > 5 mg or dose unknown (≥ 8 hrs from last dose)
* Use high dose regimen described below for:
  * rivaroxaban dose > 10 mg or dose unknown (< 8 hrs from last dose or unknown)
  * apixaban dose > 5 mg or dose unknown (< 8 hrs from last dose or unknown)

Dosing regimens
* ℞ Low dose regimen
  * Initial IV bolus: 400 mg IV. Target infusion rate: 10 mg/min.
  * Follow with 4 mg/min IV infusion for up to 120 min
* ℞ High dose regimen
  * Initial IV bolus: 800 mg IV. Target infusion rate: 10 mg/min.
  * Follow with 8 mg/min IV infusion for up to 120 min

Drug info: Desmopressin (DDAVP®)

Causes an increase in factor III coagulant activity and von Willebrand factor which helps coagulation and platelet activity in mild hemophilia A and in von Willebrand's disease Type I (where the factors are normal in makeup but low in concentration, ✖ but may cause thrombocytopenia in von Willebrand's disease Type IIB where factors may be abnormal or missing). May prevent abnormal bleeding in minor procedures. Not all patients with mild hemophilia A or von Willebrand disease respond to DDAVP.

℞ 0.3 mcg/kg (use 50 ml of diluent for doses ≤ 3 mcg, use 10 ml for doses > 3 mcg) given over 15–30 minutes, 30 minutes prior to a surgical procedure.

Elevated pre-op PTT

In a patient with no history of coagulopathy, a significantly elevated pre-op PTT is commonly due to either a factor deficiency or to lupus anticoagulant. Work-up:
1. mixing study
2. check serum lupus coagulant

If the mixing study corrects the elevated PTT, then there is probably a factor deficiency. Consult a hematologist.

Lupus anticoagulant: If the test for lupus anticoagulant is positive, then the major risk to the patient with surgery is *not* bleeding, rather it is thromboembolism. Management recommendations:
1. as soon as feasible post-op, start patient on heparin (p. 172) or LMW heparin (p. 172), e.g., Lovenox
2. at the same time start warfarin, and maintain therapeutic anticoagulation for 3–4 weeks (the risk of DVT/PE is actually highest in the first few weeks post-op)
3. mobilize as soon as possible post-op
4. consider vena-cava interruption filter in patients for whom anticoagulation is contraindicated

Disseminated intravascular coagulation (DIC)

General information
Abnormal intravascular coagulation which consumes clotting factors and platelets, coupled with abnormal activation of fibrinolytic system. Head trauma is an independent risk factor for DIC,

possibly because the brain is rich in thromboplastin which may be released into systemic circulation with trauma.[56] Other risk factors: shock, sepsis.

Presentation
Diffuse bleeding, cutaneous petechia, shock.

Labs
1. fibrinogen degradation products (FDP) > 16 mcg/ml (1–8 = normal; 8–16 = borderline; 32 = definitely abnormal; some labs require > 40 for diagnosis of DIC) (the most common abnormality)
2. fibrinogen < 100 mcg/dl (some use 130)
3. PT > 16; PTT > 50
4. platelets < 50,000 (relatively uncommon)

Chronic DIC
PT & PTT may be normal; platelet & fibrinogen low, fibrin split products elevated.
  Treatment
1. remove inciting stimulus if possible (treat infections, debride injured tissue, stop transfusions if suspected)
2. vigorous fluid resuscitation
3. anticoagulants, if not contraindicated (p. 163)
4. FFP if PT or PTT elevated, or fibrinogen < 130
5. platelet transfusion if platelet count < 100 K

Pseudo-DIC
Increased fibrin split products, normal fibrinogen.
  Seen in conditions such as liver failure.

9.3.10 Thromboembolism in neurosurgery

Deep-vein thrombosis (DVT)

DVT is of concern primarily because of the potential for material (clot, platelet clumps…) to dislodge and form emboli (including pulmonary emboli [PE]) which may cause pulmonary infarction, sudden death (from cardiac arrest), or cerebral infarction (from a paradoxical embolus, which may occur in the presence of a patent foramen ovale, see Cardiogenic brain embolism (p. 1590)). The reported mortality from DVT in the LEs ranges from 9–50%.[57] DVT limited to the calf has a low threat (< 1%) of embolization; however, these clots later extend into the proximal deep veins in 30–50% of cases,[57] from where embolization may occur (in 40–50%), or they may produce postphlebitic syndrome.
  Neurosurgical patients are particularly prone to developing DVTs (estimated risk: 19–50%), due at least in part to the relatively high frequency of the following:
1. long operating times of some procedures
2. prolonged bed rest pre- and/or post-op
3. alterations in coagulation status
   a) in patients with brain tumors (see below) or head injury[58]
      • related to the condition itself
      • due to release of brain thromboplastins during brain surgery
   b) increased blood viscosity with concomitant "sludging"
      • from dehydration therapy sometimes used to reduce cerebral edema
      • from volume loss following SAH (cerebral salt wasting)
   c) use of high-dose glucocorticoids

Specific "neurological" risk factors for DVT and PE include[57]:
1. spinal cord injury (p. 1141)
2. brain tumor: autopsy prevalence of DVT = 28%, of PE = 8.4%. Incidence using 125I-fibrinogen[59]: meningioma 72%, malignant glioma 60%, metastasis 20%. Risk may be reduced by pre-op use of aspirin[60]
3. subarachnoid hemorrhage
4. head trauma: especially severe TBI (p. 1106)
5. stroke: incidence of PE = 1–19.8%, with mortality of 25–100%
6. neurosurgical operation: risk is higher following craniotomy for supratentorial tumors (7% of 492 patients) than p-fossa tumors (0 out of 141)[61]

Prophylaxis against DVT

Options include:
1. general measures
   a) passive range of motion
   b) ambulate appropriate patients as early as possible
2. mechanical techniques (minimal risk of complications):
   a) pneumatic compression boots[62] (PCBs) or sequential compression devices (SCDs): reduces the incidence of DVTs and probably PEs. Do not use if DVTs already present. Continue use until patient is able to walk 3–4 hrs per day
   b) TED Stockings®: (TEDS) applies graduated pressure, higher distally. As effective as PCB. No evidence that the benefit is additive.[57] Care should be taken to avoid a tourniquet effect at the proximal end (note: TEDS® is a registered trademark. "TED" stands for thromboembolic disease)
   c) electrical stimulation of calf muscles
   d) rotating beds
3. anticoagulation; see also contraindications and considerations of anticoagulation in neurosurgery (p. 163)
   a) full anticoagulation is associated with perioperative complications[63]
   b) "low-dose" anticoagulation[64] (low-dose heparin): 5000 IU SQ q 8 or 12 hrs, starting 2 hrs pre-op or on admission to hospital. Potential for hazardous hemorrhage within brain or spinal canal has limited its use
   c) low molecular weight heparins and heparinoids (p. 172): not a homogeneous group. Efficacy in neurosurgical prophylaxis has not been determined
   d) aspirin: role in DVT prophylaxis is limited because ASA inhibits platelet aggregation, and platelets play only a minor role in DVT
4. combination of PCBs and "mini-dose" heparin starting on the morning of post-op day 1 (with no evidence of significant complications)[65]

Recommendations

Recommended prophylaxis varies with the risk of developing DVT, as illustrated in ▶ Table 9.8.[57] See also details of prophylaxis in cervical spinal cord injuries (p. 1141).

Table 9.8 Risk & prophylaxis of DVT in neurosurgical patients[a]

Risk group	Estimated risk of calf DVT	Typical neurosurgical patients	Treatment recommendation
low risk	< 10%	age < 40 yrs, minimal general risk factors, surgery with < 30 minutes general anesthesia	no prophylaxis, or PCB/TEDS
moderate risk	10–40%	age ≥ 40 yrs, malignancy, prolonged bed rest, extensive surgery, varicose veins, obesity, surgery > 30 minutes duration (except simple lumbar discectomy), SAH, head injury	PCB/TEDs; or for patients without ICH or SAH, mini-dose heparin
high risk	40–80%	history of DVT or PE, paralysis[b] (para- or quadriplegia or hemiparesis), brain tumor (especially meningioma or malignant glioma)	PCB/TEDS + (in patients without ICH or SAH) mini-dose heparin

[a]abbreviations: DVT = deep venous thrombosis, PCB = pneumatic compression device, TEDS = TED (thromboembolic disease) Stockings®, ICH = intracerebral hemorrhage, SAH = subarachnoid hemorrhage
[b]see specifics regarding DVT prophylaxis in cervical SCI (p. 1141)

Diagnosis of DVT

(For PE, see below). The clinical diagnosis of DVT is very unreliable. A patient with the "classic signs" of a hot, swollen, and tender calf, or a positive Homans' sign (calf pain on dorsiflexion of the ankle) will have a DVT only 20–50% of the time.[57] 50–60% of patients with DVT will not have these findings.

Laboratory tests
- contrast venography: the "gold standard," however it is invasive and carries risk of iodine reaction, occasionally produces phlebitis, not readily repeated
- Doppler ultrasound with high-resolution real-time B-mode imaging: 95% sensitive and 99% specific for proximal DVT. Less effective for calf DVT.[66] As a result, it is recommended that patients with initially negative studies undergo repeat studies over the next 7–10 days to R/O proximal

extension. Requires more skill on the part of the tester than IPG. May be used in immobilized or casted LE (unlike IPG). Widely accepted as the non-invasive test of choice for DVT[67]
* impedance plethysmography (IPG): looks for reduced electrical impedance produced by blood flow from the calf following relaxation of a pneumatic tourniquet. Good in detecting proximal DVT, not sensitive for calf DVT. A positive study indicates DVT that should be treated, a negative study can occur with non-occlusive DVT or with good collaterals, and should be repeated over a 2 week period
* 125I-fibrinogen: radiolabeled fibrinogen is incorporated into the developing thrombus. Better for calf DVT than proximal DVT. Expensive, and many false positives. Risk of HIV transmission has resulted in withdrawal of use
* D-dimer (a specific fibrin degradation product): high levels are associated with DVT and PE[68]

Treatment of DVT

1. bed rest, with elevation of involved leg(s)
2. unless anticoagulation is contraindicated (p.163): start heparin as outlined in Anticoagulation (p.163), aim for APTT = 1.5–2 × control; or fixed dose of LMW heparinoids, e.g., tinzaparin (Logiparin®,[69] or in the U.S. enoxaparin (Lovenox®) (p.173). *Simultaneously* initiate warfarin therapy. Heparin can be stopped after ≈ 5 days[70]
3. in patients where anticoagulation is contraindicated, consider inferior vena cava interruption or placement of a filter (e.g., Greenfield filter)
4. in non-paralyzed patients, cautiously begin to ambulate after ≈ 7–10 days
5. wear anti-embolic stocking on affected LE indefinitely (limb is always at risk of recurrent DVT)

Pulmonary embolism (PE)

See reference.[71]

Prevention of PE
Prevention of PE is best accomplished by prevention of DVT (p.177).[72]

Presentation of PE
Post-op PE generally occurs 10–14 days following surgery.[72] The reported incidence[72] ranges from 0.4–5%. A series (on a service with routine use of elastic stockings and, in high risk patients, "minidose" heparin) found a post-op incidence of ≈ 0.4%, with a doubling of this number if only patients with major pathology (brain tumor, head trauma, or cerebrovascular or spinal pathology) were considered[72] (another series dealing only with brain tumors found a 4% incidence[61]).

Clinical diagnosis is nonspecific (differential diagnosis of symptoms is large, and ranges from atelectasis to MI or cardiac tamponade).

Common findings: sudden dyspnea (the most frequent finding), tachypnea, tachycardia, fever, hypotension, 3rd or 4th heart sound. *Triad* (rare): hemoptysis, pleuritic chest pain, dyspnea. Auscultation: pleuritic friction rub or rales (rare). Shock and CHF (mimics MI) indicates massive life-threatening PE. Mortality reported ranges from 9–60%,[72] with a significant number of deaths within the first hour.

Diagnosis of PE
A negative D-dimer test (see above) reliably excludes PE in patients with a low clinical probability of PE[73] or in those with nondiagnostic VQ scan.[68]

Alternatively, one can check for DVT utilizing IPG, Doppler, or venography (see above). If positive, this indicates a possible source of PE, and since the treatment is similar for both, no further search for PE need be made and treatment is started. If negative, further testing may be needed (e.g.VQ scan, see below).

Laboratory tests
D-dimer: see above.

General diagnostic tests
None are very sensitive or specific.
* EKG: "classic" S1Q3T3 is rare. Usually just nonspecific-ST & T changes occur. Tachycardia may be the only finding

- CXR: normal in 25–30%. When abnormal, usually shows infiltrate and elevated hemidiaphragm
- ABG: not very sensitive. $pO_2 > 90$ on room air virtually excludes *massive* PE

Specific radiographic evaluation
- **test of choice**: contrast enhanced chest CT. Occasionally chest CTA may be employed. Can provide insight into alternate diagnoses
- pulmonary angiogram: historically, the "gold standard." Invasive, expensive, and labor intensive. 3–4% risk of significant complications. Not indicated in most cases
- ventilation-perfusion scan (VQ scan): CXR is also needed. A perfusion defect with no ventilation defect in a patient with no previous history of PE strongly suggests acute PE. Equivocal studies occur when an area of malperfusion corresponds to an area of reduced ventilation (on ventilation scan) or infiltrate (on CXR). Probabilities of PE based on VQ scan are shown in ▸ Table 9.9.[74] A technically adequate normal VQ scan virtually rules out PE. Patients with low or intermediate probability scans should have a test for DVT or quantitative D-dimer (see above). If test for DVT is positive, treat; if it is negative, the choice is to follow serial IPG or Doppler studies for 2 weeks, or (rarely) to do a pulmonary angiogram
- thin-section contrast-enhanced chest CT: more accurate in patients with COPD who often have an indeterminate VQ scan

Table 9.9 Probability of PE based on VQ scan

Scan results	Incidence of PE
high probability	90–95%
intermediate probability or indeterminate	30–40%
low probability	10–15%
normal	0–5%

Treatment

If diagnosis is seriously entertained, start *heparin* —unless contraindicated (p. 163)—without waiting for results of diagnostic studies. For an average 70 kg patient, begin with 5000–7500 unit IV bolus, followed by 1000 U/hr drip (less for smaller patient). Follow PTT and titrate drip rate for PTT 1.5 to 2 × control.

The use of heparin shortly after surgery and in patients with brain tumors is controversial, and vena caval interruption may be an alternate consideration (e.g., Greenfield filter).

Patients with massive PEs may be hemodynamically unstable. They usually require ICU care, often with PA catheter and pressors.

9.4 Extramedullary hematopoiesis

9.4.1 General information

In chronic anemias (especially thalassemia major, AKA Cooley's anemia), low hematocrit results in chronic overstimulation of bone marrow to produce RBCs. This results in systemic bony abnormalities, cardiomyopathy (due to hemochromatosis caused by increased breakdown of defective RBCs).

Pertinent to the CNS, there are three sites where extramedullary hematopoiesis (EMH) can cause findings:
- skull: produces "hair-on-end" appearance on skull X-ray
- vertebral bodies: may result in epidural cord compression[75] (see below)
- choroid plexus

9.4.2 Epidural cord compression from EMH

The exuberant tissue is very radiosensitive; however, the patient may be somewhat dependent on the hematopoietic capacity of the tissue.

9.4.3 Treatment

Surgical excision followed by radiation therapy has been the recommended treatment. Repeated blood transfusions may help reduce EMH and may be useful post-op instead of RTX except for refractory cases.[75]

Surgery on these patients is difficult because of:

1. low platelet count
2. poor condition of bone
3. cardiomyopathy: increased anesthetic risk
4. anemia, coupled with the fact that most of these patients are "iron-toxic" from multiple previous transfusions
5. total removal of the mass is not always possible

References

[1] Cohen YC, Djulbegovic B, Shamai-Lubovitz O, et al. The bleeding risk and natural history of idiopathic thrombocytopenic purpura in patients with persistent low platelet counts. Archives of Internal Medicine. 2000; 160:1630–1638

[2] Fresh-Frozen Plasma Cryoprecipitate and Platelets Administration Practice Guidelines Development Task Force of the College of American Pathologists. Practice Parameter for the Use of Fresh-Frozen Plasma, Cryoprecipitate, and Platelets. Journal of the American Medical Association. 1994; 271:777–781

[3] Mannucci PM. Desmopressin: A nontransfusion form of treatment for congenital and acquired bleeding disorders. Blood. 1988; 72:1449–1455

[4] Ruff CT, Giugliano RP, Braunwald E, et al. Comparison of the efficacy and safety of new oral anticoagulants with warfarin in patients with atrial fibrillation: a meta-analysis of randomised trials. Lancet. 2014; 383:955–962

[5] Bernhardt J, Zorowitz RD, Becker KJ, et al. Advances in Stroke 2017. Stroke. 2018; 49:e174–e199

[6] So W, Hugenholtz H, Richard MT. Complications of Anticoagulant Therapy in Patients with Known Central Nervous System Lesions. Can J Surg. 1983; 26:181–183

[7] Ruff R, Posner J. Incidence and Treatment of Peripheral Thrombosis in Patients with Glioma. Ann Neurol. 1983; 13:334–336

[8] Olin JW, Young JR, Graor RA, et al. Treatment of Deep Vein Thrombosis and Pulmonary Emboli in Patients with Primary and Metastatic Brain Tumors: Anticoagulants or Inferior Vena Cava Filter? Archives of Internal Medicine. 1987; 147:2177–2179

[9] Altschuler E, Moosa H, Selker RG, et al. The Risk and Efficacy of Anticoagulant Therapy in the Treatment of Thromboembolic Complications in Patients with Primary Malignant Brain Tumors. Neurosurgery. 1990; 27:74–77

[10] Stern WE, Youmans J. Preoperative Evaluation: Complications, Their Prevention and Treatment. In: Neurological Surgery. 2nd ed. Philadelphia: W. B. Saunders; 1982:1051–1116

[11] Kawamata T, Takeshita M, Kubo O, et al. Management of Intracranial Hemorrhage Associated with Anticoagulant Therapy. Surgical Neurology. 1995; 44:438–443

[12] Constantini S, Kanner A, Friedman A, et al. Safety of perioperative minidose heparin in patients undergoing brain tumor surgery: a prospective, randomized, double-blind study. J Neurosurg. 2001; 94:918–921

[13] Dickinson LD, Miller LD, Patel CP, et al. Enoxaparin increases the incidence of postoperative intracranial hemorrhage when initiated preoperatively for deep venous thrombosis prophylaxis in patients with brain tumors. Neurosurgery. 1998; 43:1074–1081

[14] Posan E, McBane RD, Grill DE, et al. Comparison of PFA-100 testing and bleeding time for detecting platelet hypofunction and von Willebrand disease in clinical practice. Thromb Haemost. 2003; 90:483–490

[15] Hayward CP, Harrison P, Cattaneo M, et al. Platelet function analyzer (PFA)-100 closure time in the evaluation of platelet disorders and platelet function. J Thromb Haemost. 2006; 4:312–319

[16] Beshay JE, Morgan H, Madden C, et al. Emergency reversal of anticoagulation and antiplatelet therapies in neurosurgical patients. J Neurosurg. 2010; 112:307–318

[17] Seidel H, Rahman MM, Scharf RE. Monitoring of antiplatelet therapy. Current limitations, challenges, and perspectives. Hamostaseologie. 2011; 31:41–51

[18] Korinth MC. Low-dose aspirin before intracranial surgery–results of a survey among neurosurgeons in Germany. Acta Neurochirurgica (Wien). 2006; 148:1189–96; discussion 1196

[19] Korinth MC, Gilsbach JM, Weinzierl MR. Low-dose aspirin before spinal surgery: results of a survey among neurosurgeons in Germany. European Spine Journal. 2007; 16:365–372

[20] Nuttall GA, Brown MJ, Stombaugh JW, et al. Time and cardiac risk of surgery after bare-metal stent percutaneous coronary intervention. Anesthesiology. 2008; 109:588–595

[21] Rabbitts JA, Nuttall GA, Brown MJ, et al. Cardiac risk of noncardiac surgery after percutaneous coronary intervention with drug-eluting stents. Anesthesiology. 2008; 109:596–604

[22] Landesberg G, Beattie WS, Mosseri M, et al. Perioperative myocardial infarction. Circulation. 2009; 119:2936–2944

[23] Ross IB, Dhillon GS. Ventriculostomy-related cerebral hemorrhages after endovascular aneurysm treatment. AJNR. American Journal of Neuroradiology. 2003; 24:1528–1531

[24] NovoSeven for non-hemophilia hemostasis. Medical Letter. 2004; 46:33–34

[25] Goodnight SH, Jr, Harris WS, Connor WE. The effects of dietary omega 3 fatty acids on platelet composition and function in man: a prospective, controlled study. Blood. 1981; 58:880–885

[26] Ang-Lee MK, Moss J, Yuan CS. Herbal medicines and perioperative care. JAMA. 2001; 286:208–216

[27] Stanger MJ, Thompson LA, Young AJ, et al. Anticoagulant activity of select dietary supplements. Nutr Rev. 2012; 70:107–117

[28] Allison GL, Lowe GM, Rahman K. Aged garlic extract and its constituents inhibit platelet aggregation through multiple mechanisms. J Nutr. 2006; 136:782S–788S

[29] Saw JT, Bahari MB, Ang HH, et al. Potential drug-herb interaction with antiplatelet/anticoagulant drugs. Complement Ther Clin Pract. 2006; 12:236–241

[30] Lee CJ, Ansell JE. Direct thrombin inhibitors. Br J Clin Pharmacol. 2011; 72:581–592

[31] Birks J, Grimley Evans J. Ginkgo biloba for cognitive impairment and dementia. Cochrane Database Syst Rev. 2009. DOI: 10.1002/14651858.CD003120.pub3

[32] Teng CM, Kuo SC, Ko FN, et al. Antiplatelet actions of panaxynol and ginsenosides isolated from ginseng. Biochim Biophys Acta. 1989; 990:315–320

[33] Baron TH, Kamath PS, McBane RD. Management of antithrombotic therapy in patients undergoing invasive procedures. N Engl J Med. 2013; 368:2113–2124

[34] Ryan J, Bolster F, Crosbie I, et al. Antiplatelet medications and evolving antithrombotic medication. Skeletal Radiology. 2013; 42:753–764

[35] Hirsh J, Bauer KA, Donati MB, et al. Parenteral anticoagulants: American College of Chest Physicians Evidence-Based Clinical Practice Guidelines (8th Edition). Chest. 2008; 133:141S–159S

[36] Kaatz S, Kouides PA, Garcia DA, et al. Guidance on the emergent reversal of oral thrombin and factor Xa inhibitors. Am J Hematol. 2012; 87 Suppl 1: S141–S145

[37] Rivaroxaban-once daily, oral, direct factor Xa inhibition compared with vitamin K antagonism for

prevention of stroke and Embolism Trial in Atrial Fibrillation: rationale and design of the ROCKET AF study. Am Heart J. 2010; 159:340–347 e1

[38] Tran HA, Chunilal SD, Harper PL, et al. An update of consensus guidelines for warfarin reversal. Med J Aust. 2013; 198:198–199

[39] James RF, Palys V, Lomboy JR, et al. The role of anti-coagulants, antiplatelet agents, and their reversal strategies in the management of intracerebral hemorrhage. Neurosurg Focus. 2013; 34. DOI: 10.3171/2 013.2.FOCUS1328

[40] Dimitrova G, Tulman DB, Bergese SD. Perioperative management of antiplatelet therapy in patients with drug-eluting stents. HSR Proc Intensive Care Cardiovasc Anesth. 2012; 4:153–167

[41] Lethagen S, Olofsson L, Frick K, et al. Effect kinetics of desmopressin-induced platelet retention in healthy volunteers treated with aspirin or placebo. Haemophilia. 2000; 6:15–20

[42] Hirsh J, Dalen JE, Deykin D, et al. Oral Anticoagulants: Mechanism of Action, Clinical Effectiveness, and Optimal Therapeutic Range. Chest. 1992; 102:312–326

[43] Khamashta MA, Cuadrado MJ, Mujic F, et al. The Management of Thrombosis in the Antiphospholipid-Antibody Syndrome. New England Journal of Medicine. 1995; 332:993–997

[44] Hyers TM, Hull RD, Weg JG. Antithrombotic Therapy for Venous Thromboembolic Disease. Chest. 1989; 95:37S–51S

[45] Atkinson JLD, Sundt TM, Kazmier FJ, et al. Heparin-induced thrombocytopenia and thrombosis in ischemic stroke. Mayo Clinic Proceedings. 1988; 63:353–361

[46] Kim GH, Hahn DK, Kellner CP, et al. The incidence of heparin-induced thrombocytopenia Type II in patients with subarachnoid hemorrhage treated with heparin versus enoxaparin. Journal of Neurosurgery. 2009; 110:50–57

[47] Dalteparin - Another Low-Molecular-Weight Heparin. Medical Letter. 1995; 37:115–116

[48] Ardeparin and Danaparoid for Prevention of Deep Vein Thrombosis. Medical Letter. 1997; 39:94–95

[49] Geerts WH, Bergqvist D, Pineo GF, et al. Prevention of venous thromboembolism: American College of Chest Physicians Evidence-Based Clinical Practice Guidelines (8th Edition). Chest. 2008; 133:381S–453S

[50] Reports of Epidural or Spinal Hematomas with the Concurrent Use of Low Molecular Weight Heparin and Spinal/Epidural Anesthesia or Spinal Puncture. Rockville, MD 1997

[51] U.S. Food and Drug Administration (FDA), . FDA approves Praxbind, the first reversal agent for the anticoagulant Pradaxa. 2015. https://wayback. archive-it.org/7993/20170111160812/http://www. fda.gov/NewsEvents/Newsroom/PressAnnounce-ments/ucm467300.htm

[52] Fondaparinux (Arixtra), a new anticoagulant. Medical Letter. 2002; 44:43–44

[53] Garcia DA, Baglin TP, Weitz JI, et al. Parenteral anti-coagulants: Antithrombotic Therapy and Prevention of Thrombosis, 9th ed: American College of Chest Physicians Evidence-Based Clinical Practice Guidelines. Chest. 2012; 141:e24S–e43S

[54] Fredriksson K, Norrving B, Stromblad LG. Emergency Reversal of Anticoagulation After Intracerebral Hemorrhage. Stroke. 1992; 23:972–977

[55] Siegal DM, Curnutte JT, Connolly SJ, et al. Andexanet Alfa for the Reversal of Factor Xa Inhibitor Activity. N Engl J Med. 2015; 373:2413–2424

[56] Kaufman HH, Hui K-S, Mattson JC, et al. Clinicopathological Correlations of Disseminated Intravascular Coagulation in Patients with Head Injury. Neurosurgery. 1984; 15:34–42

[57] Hamilton MG, Hull RD, Pineo GF. Venous Thromboembolism in Neurosurgery and Neurology Patients: A Review. Neurosurgery. 1994; 34:280–296

[58] Olson JD, Kaufman HH, Moake J, et al. The Incidence and Significance of Hemostatic Abnormalities in Patients with Head Injuries. Neurosurgery. 1989; 24:825–832

[59] Sawaya R, Zuccarello M, El-Kalliny M. Brain Tumors and Thromboembolism: Clinical, Hemostatic, and Biochemical Correlations. Journal of Neurosurgery. 1989; 70

[60] Quevedo JF, Buckner JC, Schmidt JL, et al. Thromboembolism in Patients With High-Grade Glioma. Mayo Clinic Proceedings. 1994; 69:329–332

[61] Constantini S, Karnowski R, Pomeranz S, et al. Thromboembolic Phenomena in Neurosurgical Patients Operated Upon for Primary and Metastatic Brain Tumors. Acta Neurochirurgica. 1991; 109:93–97

[62] Black PM, Baker MF, Snook CP. Experience with External Pneumatic Calf Compression in Neurology and Neurosurgery. Neurosurgery. 1986; 18:440–444

[63] Snyder M, Renaudin J. Intracranial Hemorrhage Associated with Anticoagulation Therapy. Surg Neurol. 1977; 7:31–34

[64] Cerrato D, Ariano C, Fiacchino F. Deep Vein Thrombosis and Low-Dose Heparin Prophylaxis in Neurosurgical Patients. J Neurosurg. 1978; 49:378–381

[65] Frim DM, Barker FG, Poletti CE, et al. Postoperative Low-Dose Heparin Decreases Thromboembolic Complications in Neurosurgical Patients. Neurosurgery. 1992; 30:830–833

[66] Rose SC, Zwiebel WJ, Murdock LE, et al. Insensitivity of Color Doppler Flow Imaging for Detection of Acute Calf Deep Venous Thrombosis in Asymptomatic Postoperative Patients. J Vasc Interv Radiol. 1993; 4:111–117

[67] Wells PS, Anderson DR, Bormanis J, et al. Value of Assessment of Pretest Probability of Deep-Vein Thrombosis in Clinical Management. Lancet. 1997; 350:1795–1798

[68] Ginsberg JS, Wells PS, Kearon C, et al. Sensitivity and Specificity of a Rapid Whole-Blood Assay for D-dimer in the Diagnosis of Pulmonary Embolism. Annals of Internal Medicine. 1998; 129:1006–1011

[69] Hull RD, Raskob GE, Pineo GF, et al. Subcutaneous Low-Molecular-Weight Heparin Compared with Continuous Intravenous Heparin in the Treatment of Proximal-Vein Thrombosis. New England Journal of Medicine. 1992; 326:975–982

[70] Hull RD, Raskob GE, Rosenbloom D, et al. Heparin for Five Days as Compared with Ten Days in the Initial Treatment of Proximal Venous Thrombosis. N Engl J Med. 1990; 322:1260–1264

[71] Wenger NK, Schwartz GR. Principles and Practice of Emergency Medicine. In: Philadelphia: W.B. Saunders; 1978:949–952

[72] Inci S, Erbengi A, Berker M. Pulmonary Embolism in Neurosurgical Patients. Surgical Neurology. 1995; 43:123–129

[73] Wells PS, Ginsberg JS, Anderson DR, et al. Use of a Clinical Model for Safe Management of Patients with Suspected Pulmonary Embolism. Annals of Internal Medicine. 1998; 129:997–1005

[74] The PIOPED Investigators. Value of the Ventilation/Perfusion Scan in Acute Pulmonary Embolism. Results of the Prospective Investigation of Pulmonary Embolism Diagnosis (PIOPED). Journal of the American Medical Association. 1990; 263:2753–2759

[75] Mann KS, Yue CP, Chan KH, et al. Paraplegia due to Extramedullary Hematopoiesis in Thalassemia: Case Report. Journal of Neurosurgery. 1987; 66:938–940

9

10 Neurology for Neurosurgeons

10.1 Dementia

▶ **Definition.** Loss of intellectual abilities previously attained (memory, judgment, abstract thought, and other higher cortical functions) severe enough to interfere with social and/or occupational functioning.[1] Memory deficit is the cardinal feature; however, the DSM-IV definition requires impairment in at least one other domain (language, perception, visuospatial function, calculation, judgment, abstraction, problem-solving skills). Affects 3–11% of community-dwelling adults > 65 yrs of age, with a greater presence among institutionalized residents.[2]

Risk factors: advanced age, family history of dementia, and apolipoprotein E-4 allele.

▶ **Delirium vs. dementia (critical distinction).** Delirium AKA acute confusional state. Distinct from dementia; however, patients with dementia are at increased risk of developing delirium.[3,4] A primary disorder of attention that subsequently affects all other aspects of cognition.[5] Often represents life-threatening illness, e.g., hypoxia, sepsis, uremic encephalopathy, electrolyte abnormality, drug intoxication, MI. 50% of patients die within 2 yrs of this diagnosis.

Unlike dementia, delirium has acute onset, motor signs (tremor, myoclonus, asterixis), slurred speech, altered consciousness (hyperalert/agitated or lethargic, or fluctuations), hallucinations may be florid. EEG shows pronounced diffuse slowing.

▶ **Brain biopsy for dementia.** Clinical criteria are usually sufficient for the diagnosis of most dementias. Biopsy should be reserved for cases of a chronic progressive cerebral disorder with an unusual clinical course where all other possible diagnostic methods have been exhausted and have failed to provide adequate diagnostic certainty.[6] Biopsy may disclose CJD, low grade astrocytoma, and AD among others. The high incidence of CJD among patients selected for biopsy under these criteria necessitates appropriate precautions; see Creutzfeldt-Jakob disease (p. 399). In a report of 50 brain biopsies performed to assess progressive neurodegenerative disease of unclear etiology,[7] the diagnostic yield was only 20% (6% were only suggestive of a diagnosis, 66% were abnormal but nonspecific, 8% were normal). The yield was highest in those with focal MRI abnormalities. Among the 10 patients with diagnostic biopsies, the biopsy result led to a meaningful therapeutic intervention in only 4.

▶ **Recommendations.** Based on the above, the following recommendations are made for patients with an otherwise unexplained neurodegenerative disease:
1. those with a focal abnormality on MRI: stereotactic biopsy
2. those without focal abnormality (possibly including SPECT or PET scan): brain biopsy should only be performed within an investigative protocol

▶ **Recommendations for specimen.** Ideally the biopsy specimen should[8]:
1. be large enough (usually 1 cm^3)
2. be taken from an affected area
3. include gray and white matter, pia and dura
4. be handled carefully to minimize artifact (electrocautery should not be used on the specimen side of the incision)

10.2 Headache

10.2.1 General information

Headache (H/A) may be broadly categorized as follows:
1. chronic recurring headaches
   a) vascular type (migraine): see below
   b) muscle contraction (tension) headaches
2. headache due to pathology
   a) systemic pathology
   b) intracranial pathology: a wide variety of etiologies including:
      • subarachnoid hemorrhage: *sudden* onset, severe, usually with vomiting, apoplexy, focal deficits possible; see differential diagnosis of paroxysmal H/A (p. 1418)
      • increased intracranial pressure from any cause (tumor, communicating hydrocephalus, inflammation, pseudotumor cerebri...)

- • irritation or inflammation of meninges: meningitis
- • tumor (p.623): with or without elevated ICP
- c) local pathology of the eye, nasopharynx, or extracranial tissues (including giant cell arteritis (p.203)
- d) following head trauma: postconcussive syndrome (p.1111)
- e) following craniotomy: "syndrome of the trephined" (p.1763)

A severe new H/A, or a change in the pattern of a long-standing or recurrent H/A (including developing associated N/V, or an abnormal neurologic exam) warrants further investigation with CT or MRI.[9]

Unilateral H/A that never changes side over a period ≥ 1 year warrants an MRI; this would be atypical in migraine and may be a presentation of an occipital AVM.

10.2.2 Migraine

General information

Migraine attacks usually occur in individuals predisposed to the condition, and may be activated by factors such as bright light, stress, diet changes, trauma, administration of radiologic contrast media (especially angiography) and vasodilators.

Classification

Based on the 1962 ad hoc committee on headache (H/A). See also index under Headache, e.g., for crash migraine (thunderclap headache) (p.1418), post-myelogram headache (p.1816).

Common migraine

Episodic H/A with N/V and photophobia, without aura or neurologic deficit.

Classic migraine

Common migraine + aura. May have H/A with occasional focal neurologic deficit(s) that resolve completely in ≤ 24 hrs.

Over half of the transient neurologic disturbances are visual, and usually consist of positive phenomena (spark photopsia, stars, complex geometric patterns, fortification spectra) which may leave negative phenomena (scotoma, hemianopia, monocular or binocular visual loss…) in their wake. The second most common symptoms are somatosensory involving the hand and lower face. Less frequently, deficits may consist of aphasia, hemiparesis, or unilateral clumsiness. A *slow march-like progression* of deficit is characteristic. The risk of stroke is probably increased in patients with migraine.[10]

Complicated migraine

Occasional attacks of classic migraine with minimal or no associated H/A, and complete resolution of neurologic deficit in ≤ 30 days.

Migraine equivalent

Neurologic symptoms (N/V, visual aura, etc.) without H/A (acephalgic migraine). Seen mostly in children. Usually develops into typical migraine with age. Aura may be shortened by opening and swallowing contents of a 10 mg nifedipine capsule.[11]

Hemiplegic migraine

H/A typically precedes hemiplegia which may persist even after H/A resolves.

Cluster headache

AKA histaminic migraine. Actually a neurovascular event, distinct from true migraine. Recurrent unilateral attacks of severe pain. Usually oculofrontal or oculotemporal with occasional radiation into the jaw, usually recurring on the same side of the head. Ipsilateral autonomic symptoms (conjunctival injection, nasal congestion, rhinorrhea, lacrimation, facial flushing) are common. Partial Horner syndrome (ptosis and miosis) sometimes occurs. Male:female ratio is ≈ 5:1. 25% of patients have a personal or family history of migraine.

10

Headaches characteristically have no prodrome, last 30–90 minutes, and recur one or more times daily, usually for 4–12 weeks, often at a similar time of day, following which there is typically a remission for an average of 12 months.[12]

Prophylaxis for cluster H/A is only minimally effective:
1. β-adrenergic blockers are less effective
2. lithium: becoming drug of choice (response rate 60–80%). 300 mg PO TID and follow levels (desired: 0.7–1.2 mEq/L)
3. occasionally ergotamines are used
4. naproxen (Naprosyn®)
5. methysergide (Sansert®) 2–4 mg PO TID is effective in 20–40% of cases, must cycle patient off the drug to prevent retroperitoneal fibrosis, etc. (also see below)

Treatment for cluster H/A (prophylaxis is only minimally effective):

Treatment is difficult because there is no prodrome and the H/A often stops after 1–2 hrs. Treatment of acute attacks includes:
- 100% O_2 by face mask with patient sitting for ≤ 15 min or until attack aborted
- ergotamine: see below
- SQ sumatriptan: usually aborts attack within 15 minutes (see below)
- steroids: see below
- refractory cases may be considered for:
  o percutaneous radiofrequency sphenopalatine ganglion blockade[13]
  o occipital nerve stimulation[14]
  o hypothalamic deep brain stimulation

Basilar artery migraine

Essentially restricted to adolescence. Recurrent episodes lasting minutes to hours of transient neurologic deficits in distribution of vertebrobasilar system. Deficits include vertigo (most common), gait ataxia, visual disturbance (scotomata, bilateral blindness), dysarthria, followed by severe H/A and occasionally nausea and vomiting.[15] Family history of migraine is present in 86%.

10.3 Parkinsonism

10.3.1 General information

Parkinsonism may be primary or secondary to other conditions. All result from a relative loss of dopamine mediated inhibition of the effects of acetylcholine in the basal ganglia.

10.3.2 Idiopathic paralysis agitans (IPA)

Clinical

Classical Parkinson's disease AKA shaking palsy. Affects ≈ 1% of Americans > age 50 yrs,[16] it is frequently underdiagnosed.[17] Male:female ratio is 3:2. Not clearly environmentally or genetically induced, but may be influenced by these factors.

The classic triad is shown in ▶ Table 10.1. Other signs may include: postural instability, micrographia, mask-like facies. Gait consists of small, shuffling steps (marche á petits pas) or festinating gait.

Table 10.1 Classic triad of Parkinson's disease

- tremor (resting, 4–7/second)
- rigidity (cogwheel)
- bradykinesia

Clinically distinguishing IPA from secondary parkinsonism (see below)

May be difficult early. IPA generally exhibits gradual onset of bradykinesia with tremor that is often asymmetrical, and initially responds well to levodopa. Other disorders are suggested with rapid progression of symptoms, when the initial response to levodopa is equivocal, or when there are early midline symptoms (ataxia or impairment of gait and balance, sphincter disturbance…), or with the presence of other features such as early dementia, sensory findings, profound orthostatic hypotension, or abnormalities of extraocular movements.[18,19]

Pathophysiology

Degeneration primarily of pigmented (neuromelanin-laden) dopaminergic neurons of the pars compacta of the substantia nigra, resulting in reduced levels of dopamine in the neostriatum (caudate nucleus, putamen, globus pallidus). This decreases the activity of inhibitory neurons with predominantly D2 class of dopamine receptors, which project directly to the internal segment of the globus pallidus (GPi), and also increases (by loss of inhibition) activity of neurons with predominantly D1 receptors which project indirectly to the globus pallidus externa (GPe) and subthalamic nucleus.[20] The net result is increased activity in GPi which has inhibitory projections to the thalamus which then suppresses activity in the supplemental motor cortex among other locations.

Histologically: Lewy bodies (eosinophilic intraneuronal hyaline inclusions) are the hallmark of IPA.

10.3.3 Secondary parkinsonism

General information

The differential diagnosis of Parkinson's disease includes the following etiologies of secondary parkinsonism or Parkinson-like conditions (these are sometimes referred to as "Parkinson plus" syndromes or parkinsonian disorders) (see above for distinguishing features):

1. olivopontocerebellar degeneration (OPC)
2. striato-nigral degeneration (SND): more aggressive than parkinsonism
3. postencephalitic parkinsonism: followed an epidemic of encephalitis lethargica (von Economo disease) in the 1920s, victims are no longer living. Distinguishing features: oculogyric crisis, tremor involves not only extremities but also trunk and head, asymmetrical, no Lewy bodies
4. progressive supranuclear palsy (PSNP): impaired vertical gaze (see below)
5. multiple system atrophy (Shy-Drager syndrome): see below
6. drug induced: includes:
   a) prescription drugs (elderly females seem more susceptible)
      - antipsychotics (AKA neuroleptics): haloperidol (Haldol®) which works by blocking post-synaptic dopamine receptors
      - phenothiazine antiemetics: prochlorperazine (Compazine®)
      - metoclopramide (Reglan®)
      - reserpine
   b) MPTP (1-methyl-4-phenyl-1,2,3,6-tetrahydropyridine): a commercially available chemical intermediate which is also a by-product of the synthesis of MPPP (a meperidine analog) that was synthesized and self-injected by a graduate student,[21] and later produced by illicit drug manufacturers to be sold as "synthetic heroin" and unwittingly injected by some IV drug abusers in northern California in 1983[22] (there is also a case report of a chemist who worked with MPTP who developed parkinsonism).[23] MPTP was subsequently discovered to be a potent neurotoxin for dopaminergic neurons (with continued toxic effects that persisted for years[24]). As a rule, the response to levodopa is dramatic, but short-lived with frequent side effects. In contrast to classic IPA, the locus coeruleus and dorsal motor vagus nucleus were essentially normal, and the symptoms differ slightly
   c) there is an as yet unproven assertion that methylenedioxymethamphetamine (MDMA) AKA "ecstasy" (on the street), may hasten the onset of Parkinsonism (a study demonstrating a link had to be withdrawn because of a mislabeling of drugs)
7. toxic: poisoning with
   a) carbon monoxide: symmetric low densities in the globus pallidus on CT
   b) manganese: may be seen in miners, welders, and pyrotechnics workers. Manganese is excreted by the liver, ∴ people with hepatic insufficiency are more susceptible. Imaging: symmetrical high signal abnormalities on T1WI primarily in the globus pallidus with essentially no findings on T2WI or T2* GRE (almost pathognomonic)
8. ischemic (lacunes in basal ganglia): produces so-called arteriosclerotic parkinsonism AKA vascular parkinsonism: "lower-half" parkinsonism (gait disturbance predominates[17]). Also causes pseudobulbar deficits, emotional lability. Tremor is rare
9. posttraumatic: parkinsonian symptoms may occur in chronic traumatic encephalopathy, see dementia pugilistica (p. 1112). There are usually other features not normally present in IPA (e.g., cerebellar findings)
10. normal pressure hydrocephalus (NPH) (p. 439): urinary incontinence…
11. neoplasm in the region of the substantia nigra
12. Riley-Day (familial dysautonomia)

13. parkinson-dementia complex of Guam: classic IPA + amyotrophic lateral sclerosis (ALS). Patho-logically has features of parkinsonism and Alzheimer's disease but no Lewy bodies nor senile plaques
14. Huntington's disease (HD): whereas adults typically show chorea, when HD manifests in a young person it may resemble IPA
15. (spontaneous) intracranial hypotension (p. 421) may present with findings mimicking IPA

Multiple system atrophy (MSA)

AKA Shy-Drager syndrome. Parkinsonism (indistinguishable from IPA), PLUS idiopathic orthostatic hypotension, PLUS other signs of autonomic nervous system (ANS) dysfunction (ANS findings may precede parkinsonism and may include urinary sphincter disturbance and hypersensitivity to nora-drenaline or tyramine infusions). Degeneration of preganglionic lateral horn neurons of thoracic spi-nal cord. Unlike IPA, most do not respond to dopa therapy. NB: classic IPA may eventually produce orthostatic hypotension from inactivity or as a result of progressive autonomic failure.

Progressive supranuclear palsy (PSNP)

AKA Steele-Richardson-Olszewski syndrome.[25]
   Triad:
1. progressive supranuclear ophthalmoplegia (chiefly vertical gaze): paresis of voluntary vertical eye movement, but still moves to vertical doll's eyes maneuver
2. pseudobulbar palsy (mask-like facies with marked dysarthria and dysphagia, hyperactive jaw jerk, emotional incontinence usually mild)
3. axial dystonia (especially of neck and upper trunk)

Associated findings: subcortical dementia (inconstant), motor findings of pyramidal, extrapyramidal and cerebellar systems. Average age of onset: 60 yrs. Males comprise 60%. Response to anti-parkinson drugs is usually very short-lived. Average survival after diagnosis: 5.7 yrs.

▶ **Differentiating from Parkinson's disease (IPA).** Patients with PSNP have a pseudo-parkinsonism. They have mask facies, but do not walk bent forward (they walk erect), and they do not have a tremor. They tend to fall backwards.

Course
1. early:
   a) many falls: due to dysequilibrium + downgaze palsy (can't see floor)
   b) eye findings may be normal initially, subsequently may develop difficulty looking down (especially to command, less to following), calorics have normal tonic component but absent nystagmus (cortical component)
   c) slurred speech
   d) personality changes
   e) difficulty eating: due to pseudobulbar palsy + inability to look down at food on plate
2. late:
   a) eyes fixed centrally (no response to oculocephalics or oculovestibulars): ocular immotility is due to frontal lobe lesions
   b) neck stiffens in extension (retrocollis)

Treatment for Parkinson's disease

Medical treatment for Parkinson's disease is beyond the scope of this book.

Surgical treatment
Before the introduction of L-dopa in the late 1960s, stereotactic thalamotomy was widely used for Parkinson's disease. The location ultimately targeted for lesioning was the ventrolateral nucleus. The procedure worked better for relieving the tremor than for the bradykinesia; however, it was the lat-ter symptom that was most disabling. This procedure cannot be done bilaterally without significant risk to speech function. The procedure fell out of favor when more effective drugs became available.[26]
   See Surgical treatment of Parkinson's disease (p. 1840) for further information.

10.4 Multiple sclerosis

Key concepts

- an idiopathic demyelinating disease of the CNS producing exacerbating and remitting symptoms disseminated in space and time
- classic clinical findings: optic neuritis, paresthesias, INO and bladder symptoms
- diagnostic criteria (McDonald criteria) use clinical and/or lab results (MRI, CSF...) to stratify patients as: MS, probable MS, or not MS
- MRI: multiple usually enhancing lesions involving optic nerves & white matter of brain (especially periventricular white matter), cerebellum and spinal cord

10.4.1 General information

An idiopathic demyelinating disease (thus affecting only white matter) of the cerebrum, optic nerves, and spinal cord (especially the corticospinal tracts and the posterior columns). Does *not* affect peripheral myelin. Pathologically produces multiple plaques of various age in diffuse locations in the CNS, especially in the periventricular white matter. Lesions initially evoke an inflammatory response with monocytes and lymphocytic perivascular cuffing, but with age settle down to glial scars.

10.4.2 Epidemiology

Usual age of onset: 10–59 years, with the greatest peak between ages 20–40 years. The female:male incidence is approximately 2:1.[27]

Prevalence varies with latitude, and is < 1 per 100,000 near the equator, and is ≈ 30–80 per 100,000 in the northern U.S. and Canada.

10.4.3 Classification

Typically causes exacerbations and remissions in various locations in the CNS (*dissemination in space and time*). Common symptoms: visual disturbances (diplopia, blurring, field cuts or scotoma), spastic paraparesis, and bladder disturbances. Nomenclature for the time course of MS is shown in ▶ Table 10.2.[28] Relapsing-remitting MS is the most common pattern (≥ 70%) at onset, and has the best response to therapy, but > 50% of cases eventually become secondary progressive MS. Only 10% have primary progressive MS, and these patients tend to be older at onset (40–60 years) and frequently develop progressive myelopathy.[29] Progressive relapsing MS is very uncommon. Deficits present > 6 months usually persist.

Table 10.2 Clinical categories of MS

Category	Definition
relapsing-remitting	episodes of acute worsening with recovery and a stable course between relapses
secondary progressive	gradual neurologic deterioration ± superimposed acute relapses in a patient who previously had relapsing-remitting MS
primary progressive	gradual, nearly continuous neurologic deterioration from the onset of symptoms
progressive relapsing	gradual neurologic deterioration from the onset of symptoms, but with subsequent superimposed relapses

10.4.4 Clinical signs and symptoms

Visual disturbances

Disturbances of visual acuity may be caused by optic or retrobulbar neuritis which is the presenting symptom of MS in 15% of cases, and which occurs at some time in 50% of MS patients. The percentage of patients with an attack of optic neuritis and no prior attack that will go on to develop MS ranges from 17–87%, depending on the series.[30] Symptoms: acute visual loss in one or both eyes with mild pain (often on eye movement).

Diplopia may be due to internuclear ophthalmoplegia (INO) (p.596) from a plaque in the MLF. INO is an important sign because it rarely occurs in other conditions besides MS or brainstem stroke.

Motor findings

Extremity weakness (mono, para, or quadriparesis) and gait ataxia are among the most common symptoms of MS. Spasticity of the LEs is often due to pyramidal tract involvement. Scanning speech results from cerebellar lesions.

Sensory findings

1. involvement of the posterior column of the spinal cord often causes loss of proprioception
2. paresthesias of extremities, trunk, or face
3. Lhermitte's sign (p.1712) (electric shock-like pain radiating down the spine on neck flexion) is common, but is not pathognomonic as it can occur in other conditions
4. trigeminal neuralgia occurs in ≈ 2%. It is more often bilateral and occurs at a younger age than in patients without MS[31]

Mental disturbances

Euphoria (la belle indifference) and depression occur in ≈ 50% of patients.

Reflex changes

Hyperreflexia and Babinski signs are common. *Abdominal cutaneous reflexes* disappear in 70–80%.

GU symptoms

Urinary frequency, urgency, and incontinence are common. Impotence in males and reduced libido in either sex is often seen.

10.4.5 Differential diagnosis

The plethora of possible signs and symptoms in MS causes the differential diagnosis to extend to almost all conditions causing focal or diffuse dysfunction of the CNS. Conditions that may closely mimic MS clinically and on diagnostic testing include:
1. acute disseminated encephalomyelitis (ADEM) (p.190): generally monophasic. May also have CSF-OCB (p.190). Corpus callosum involvement is uncommon
2. CNS lymphoma (p.840)
3. other closely related demyelinating diseases: e.g., Devic syndrome (p.1698)
4. vasculitis
5. encephalitis: patients are usually very ill
6. chronic white matter changes: seen in older patients

10.4.6 Diagnostic criteria

No single clinical feature or diagnostic test is adequate for the accurate diagnosis of MS. Therefore, clinical information is integrated with paraclinical studies. Diagnosing MS after a single, acute remitting clinically isolated syndrome (CIS) is very risky. 50–70% of patients with a CIS suggestive of MS will have multifocal MRI abnormalities characteristic of MS. The presence of these MRI abnormalities increases the risk of developing MS in 1–3 years (with greater prognostic significance than CSF-OCB). The more MRI lesions, the higher the risk.[32] Criteria for the diagnosis of MS[33] follows.

Definitions

See references.[33,34]

The following definitions are used in the classification system that follows:
1. attack (exacerbation, relapse): neurologic disturbance lasting > 24 hrs[35] typical of MS when clinicopathological studies determine that the cause is demyelinating or inflammatory lesions
2. remission: ≥ 30 days should separate the onset of the first attack from the onset of a second

3. historical information: reporting of symptoms by the patient (confirmation by observer desirable), adequate to locate a lesion of MS, and has no other explanation (i.e., manifestations must not be attributable to another condition)
4. clinical evidence (signs): neuro dysfunction recorded by competent examiner
5. paraclinical evidence: tests or procedures demonstrating CNS lesion which has not produced signs; e.g., Uthoff phenomenon or sign (worsening of symptoms with hot bath or shower), BAER, imaging procedures (CT, MRI), expert urological assessment
6. typical of MS: signs & symptoms (S/S) known to occur frequently in MS. Thus excludes gray matter lesions, peripheral nervous system lesions, and non-specific complaints such as H/A, depression, convulsive seizures, etc.
7. separate lesions: S/S cannot be explained on basis of single lesion (optic neuritis of both eyes simultaneously or within 15 days represents single lesion)
8. laboratory support: in this study, the only considerations were CSF oligoclonal bands (CSF-OCB) (see below) (OCB must not be present in serum) or increased CSF IgG production (CSF-IgG) (serum IgG must be normal). This assumes that syphilis, SSPE, sarcoidosis, etc. have been ruled out

Diagnosis of MS

The 2010 "McDonald MS Diagnostic criteria"[36] are shown in ▶ Table 10.3.

Table 10.3 2010 McDonald MS Diagnostic Criteria[36]

The diagnosis of MS requires elimination of more likely diagnoses and demonstration of lesions disseminated in space (DIS) and time (DIT)		
Clinical (attacks)	Lesions	Additional criteria to make the diagnosis
≥2	Objective clinical evidence of ≥2 lesions or objective clinical evidence of 1 lesion with reasonable historical evidence of a prior attack	None. If additional tests are done, results must still be consistent with MS
≥2	Objective clinical evidence of 1 lesion	DIS; or wait for further clinical attack implicating a different CNS location
1	Objective clinical evidence of ≥2 lesions	DIT; or wait for a second clinical attack
1	Objective clinical evidence of 1 lesion	DIS or wait for further clinical attack implicating a different CNS location and DIT; or wait for a second clinical attack
0 (progression from onset)		One year of disease progression (retrospective or prospective) and at least 2 of: • DIS in the brain based on ≥1 T2 MRI lesion in periventricular, juxtacortical or infratentorial regions • DIS in the spinal cord based on ≥2 T2 MRI lesions • or positive CSF
Paraclinical evidence in diagnosis of MS		
Evidence for DIS[37]	≥1 T2 MRI lesion in at least 2 out of 4 areas of the CNS: periventricular, juxtacortical, infratentorial or spinal cord • Gadolinium enhancement of lesions is not required • If the patient has a brainstem or spinal cord syndrome, the symptomatic lesions are excluded and do not contribute to lesion count	
Evidence for DIT[38]	• New T2 and/or gadolinium-enhancing MRI lesion(s) on follow-up MRI, with reference to a baseline study, irrespective of the timing of the baseline MRI or • Simultaneous presence of asymptomatic gadolinium-enhancing and non-enhancing lesions at any time	
Evidence for positive CSF	Oligoclonal bands in CSF (and not serum) or elevated IgG index	

MRI

MRI is the preferred imaging study in evaluating MS[39] and can demonstrate dissemination of lesions in time and space. Recommended[33] brain MRI criteria for diagnosing MS are shown in ▶ Table 10.3.[40,41] Lesions are normally > 3 mm diameter.[33] MRI shows multiple white matter abnormalities in 80% of patients with MS (compared to 29% for CT).[42,43] Lesions are high signal on T2, and acute lesions tend to enhance with gadolinium more than old lesions do. Periventricular lesions may blend in with the signal from CSF in the ventricles on T2; these lesions are shown to better advantage on FLAIR (fluid attenuation) MRI (p.240). These lesions are ovoid, are oriented perpendicular to the ependymal surface (▶ Fig. 10.1), and are sometimes called Dawson's fingers (after neuropathologist James Dawson).

Spinal cord lesions normally show little or no swelling, should be ≥ 3 mm but < 2 vertebral segments, occupy only a portion of the cross-section of the cord, and must be hyperintense on T2.[44]

Specificity of MRI is ≈ 94%[45]; however, encephalitis as well as UBOs seen in aging may mimic MS lesions. DWI should be normal; however, plaques can sometimes exhibit "shine through" (p.243), so the ADC map must be checked to rule out infarct.

Focal tumefactive demyelinating lesions (TDL) may occur in isolation or, more commonly, in patients with established MS (often blotchy in appearance, but may appear as bull's-eye targets in Balo's disease AKA concentric sclerosis of Balo). TDL may represent an intermediate position between MS and ADEM (p.190).[46] TDLs tend to be symmetric. TDLs may enhance, and show perilesional edema (but less than MS) and thus be mistaken for neoplasms. Biopsy results may be confusing. MRS may not be able to differentiate from neoplasm.[47]

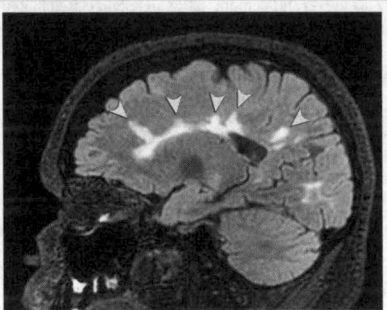

Fig. 10.1 Dawson's fingers (*yellow arrowheads*) in patient with multiple sclerosis (MS). Sagittal FLAIR MRI.

CSF

CSF analysis can support the diagnosis in some cases, but cannot document dissemination of lesions in time or space. The CSF in MS is clear and colorless. The OP is normal. Total CSF protein is < 55 mg/dl in ≈ 75% of patients, and < 108 mg/dl in 99.7% (values near 100 should prompt a search for an alternative diagnosis). The WBC count is ≤ 5 cells/mcl in 70% of patients, and only 1% have a count > 20 cells/mcl (high values may be seen in the acute myelitis).

In ≈ 90% of patients with MS, CSF-IgG is increased relative to other CSF proteins, and a characteristic pattern occurs. Agarose gel electrophoresis shows a few IgG bands in the gamma region (oligoclonal bands) that are not present in the serum (higher resolution isoelectric focusing can demonstrate 10–15 bands). CSF-OCB are not specific for MS, and can occur in CNS infections and less commonly with strokes or tumors. The predictive value of the absence of IgG in a patient with suspected MS has not been satisfactorily elucidated.

Recommended criteria have been published,[48] most of which pertain to specifics of laboratory analysis, pertinent clinical excerpts are shown in ▶ Table 10.4.

10.5 Acute disseminated encephalomyelitis

AKA ADEM. Acute demyelinating condition, has been associated with relatively recent history of vaccination. Like MS, may also demonstrate oligoclonal bands in CSF. ADEM is generally monophasic, and lesions occur within a couple of weeks. There is usuallly a good response to high-dose IV corticosteroids.

Table 10.4 CSF criteria for MS

1. qualitative assessment of IgG is the most informative analysis and is best performed using IEF with some form of immunodetection (blotting or fixation)
2. analysis should be performed on unconcentrated CSF and must be compared to simultaneously run serum sample in the same assay
3. runs should use the same amount of IgG from serum and CSF
4. each run should contain positive and negative controls
5. quantitative analysis should be made in terms of one of the 5 recognized staining patterns for OCB
6. an individual experienced in the techniques should report the results
7. all other tests performed on the CSF (including WBC, protein & glucose, lactate) should be taken into consideration
8. evaluation using light chains for immunodetection may be helpful in certain cases to resolve equivocal oligoclonal IgG patterns
9. if clinical suspicion is high but CSF results are equivocal, negative or show only a single band, consider repeating the LP
10. to measure IgG levels, nonlinear formulas that consider integrity of the blood-CSF barrier should be used (e.g., the ratio of CSF to serum albumin [AKA Qalb] is a measure of leakiness)
11. labs analyzing CSF should have internal as well as external quality assessment controls
12. quantitative IgG is a complementary test, but is not a substitute for qualitative IgG testing, which has the highest sensitivity and specificity

10.6 Motor neuron diseases

10.6.1 General information

Degenerative diseases of motor neurons. See also comparison of upper motor neurons (UMN) with lower motor neurons (LMN) (p. 531) and the paralysis they produce. There are five subtypes of degenerative motor neuron diseases, of which ALS is the most common (see below).

Three patterns of involvement:
1. mixed UMN & LMN degeneration: amyotrophic lateral sclerosis (ALS) (see below). The most common of the motor neuron diseases
2. UMN degeneration: primary lateral sclerosis. Rare, onset after age 50. No LMN signs. Slower progression than ALS (yrs to decades). Pseudobulbar palsy is common.[49] Usually does not shorten longevity. May present with falling due to balance problems or low back and neck pain due to axial muscle weakness
3. LMN degeneration: progressive muscular atrophy (PMA) and spinal muscular atrophy (SMA)

10.6.2 Amyotrophic lateral sclerosis

Key concepts

- degeneration of anterior horn cells and corticospinal tracts in the cervical spine and medulla (bulb) of unknown etiology
- a mixed upper and lower motor neuron disease (UMN → mild spasticity in LEs; LMN → atrophy and fasciculations in UEs)
- clinically: progressive muscle wasting, weakness, and fasciculations
- no cognitive, sensory, nor autonomic dysfunction

In the U.S. amyotrophic lateral sclerosis (ALS) is AKA Lou Gehrig's disease, named after the New York Yankees first baseman who announced that he had the disease in 1939. AKA motor neuron disease (singular).

Epidemiology

See reference.[30]

Prevalence: 4–6/100,000. Incidence: 0.8–1.2/100,000.

Familial in 8–10% of cases. Familial cases usually follow autosomal dominant inheritance, but occasionally demonstrate a recessive pattern.

Onset usually after 40 years of age.

10

Pathology

Etiology is not known with certainty. Histology: degeneration of anterior horn alpha-motoneurons (in the spinal cord *and* in brainstem motor nuclei) (LMNs) and corticospinal tracts (UMNs). Produces mixed UMN & LMN findings, with a great deal of variability depending on which predominates at any given time.

Clinical

Characterized by progressive muscle wasting, weakness, and fasciculations.

Involvement is of voluntary muscles, sparing the voluntary eye muscles and urinary sphincter.

Classically, presents initially with weakness and atrophy of the hands (lower motor neuron) with spasticity and hyperreflexia of the lower extremities (upper motor neuron). However, LEs may be hyporeflexic if the lower motor neuron deficits predominate.

Dysarthria and dysphagia are caused by a combination of upper and lower motor neuron pathology. Tongue atrophy and fasciculations may also occur.

Although cognitive deficits are generally considered to be absent in ALS, in actuality 1–2% of cases are associated with dementia, and cognitive changes may occasionally predate the usual features of ALS.[50]

Differential diagnosis

At times, it may be very difficult to distinguish ALS from cervical spondylotic myelopathy; see discussion of differentiating features (p. 1301).

Diagnostic studies

EMG

Not absolutely necessary to make diagnosis in most cases. Fibrillations and positive sharp waves are found in advanced cases (may be absent early, especially if upper motor neuron pathology predominates). LMN findings in the LE in the absence of lumbar spine disease, or fibrillation potentials in the tongue are suggestive of ALS.

LP (CSF)

May have slightly elevated protein.

Treatment

Much of care is directed toward minimizing disability:
1. risk of aspiration may be reduced with
   a) tracheostomy
   b) gastrostomy tube to allow continued feeding
   c) vocal cord injection with Teflon
2. noninvasive ventilation: e.g., BiPAP spasticity that occurs when upper motor neuron deficits predominate may be treated (usually with short-lived response) with:
   a) baclofen (p. 1846): also may relieve the commonly occurring cramps
   b) diazepam
3. riluzole (Rilutek®): inhibits presynaptic release of glutamate. Doses of 50–200 mg/d increases tracheostomy-free survival at 9 & 12 months, but the improvement is more modest or may be non-existent by ≈ 18 months[51,52]

Prognosis

Most patients die within 5 years of onset (median survival: 3–4 yrs). Those with prominent oropharyngeal symptoms may have a shorter life-span usually due to complications of aspiration.

10

10.7 Guillain-Barré syndrome

10.7.1 General

Key concepts

- acute onset of peripheral neuropathy with progressive muscle weakness (more severe *proximally*) with areflexia, reaches maximum over 3 days to 3 weeks
- cranial neuropathy: also common, may include facial diplegia, ophthalmoplegia
- little or no sensory involvement (paresthesias are not uncommon)
- onset often 3 days-5 weeks following viral URI, immunization, *Campylobacter jejuni enteritis*, or surgery
- pathology: focal segmental demyelination with endoneurial monocytic infiltrate
- elevated CSF protein without pleocytosis (albuminocytologic dissociation)

Guillain-Barré syndrome (GBS) AKA acute polyradiculoneuritis, among others, is actually a collection of syndromes having inflammatory polyradiculoneuropathy in common. Its most frequent form is acute inflammatory demyelinating polyradiculoneuropathy (AIDP). First described as an ascending paralysis, most forms are characterized by *symmetric* weakness and areflexia. Mild cases may present only with ataxia, whereas fulminant cases may ascend to complete tetraplegia with paralysis of respiratory muscles and cranial nerves. There are also a number of variants (p. 194).

GBS is the most common acquired demyelinating neuropathy. Incidence is ≈ 1–3/100,000. The lifetime risk for any one individual getting GBS is ≈ 1/1,000.

GBS is triggered by both humoral and cell mediated autoimmune response to an immune sensitizing event. Frequent (but not essential) antecedents: viral infection, surgery, immunization, mycoplasma infection, enteral infection with Campylobacter jejuni (≈ 4 days of intense diarrhea). Higher frequency in the following conditions than in general population: Hodgkin's disease, lymphoma, lupus.

Most cases involve antibodies to gangliosides and glycolipids in peripheral myelin (axon antibodies occur in some forms). For unknown reasons serum creatine kinase can be mildly elevated, and may correlate with muscle type pain.[53]

10.7.2 Diagnostic criteria

See reference.[54]

Features required for diagnosis:
- progressive motor weakness of more than 1 limb (from minimal weakness ± ataxia to paralysis, may include bulbar or facial or EOM palsy). Unlike most neuropathies, proximal muscles are affected more than distal
- areflexia (usually universal, but distal areflexia with definite hyporeflexia of biceps and knee jerks suffices if other features are consistent)

Features strongly supportive of diagnosis:
- clinical features (in order of importance)
  - progression: motor weakness peaks at 2 wks in 50%, by 3 wks in 80%, and by 4 wks in > 90%
  - relative symmetry
  - mild sensory symptoms/signs (e.g., mild paresthesias in hands or feet)
  - *cranial nerve* involvement: *facial weakness* in 50%, usually *bilateral*. GBS presents initially in EOMs or other Cr. N. in < 5% of cases. Oropharyngeal muscles may be affected
  - recovery usually by 2–4 wks after progression stops, may be delayed by months (most patients recover functionally)
  - autonomic dysfunction (may fluctuate): tachycardia and other arrhythmias, postural hypotension, HTN, vasomotor symptoms
  - afebrile at onset of neuritic symptoms
  - variants (not ranked):
    - fever at onset of neuritic symptoms
    - severe sensory loss with pain
    - progression > 4 wks
    - cessation of progression without recovery

– sphincter dysfunction (usually spared): e.g., bladder paralysis
– CNS involvement (controversial): e.g., ataxia, dysarthria, Babinski signs
- CSF: albuminocytologic dissociation (↑ protein without pleocytosis)
  - protein: elevated after 1 wk of symptoms, > 55 mg/dl
  - cells: 10 or fewer mononuclear leukocytes/ml
  - variants
    – no CSF protein rise 1–10 wks after onset (rare)
    – 11–50 monocytes/ml
    – electrodiagnostics: 80% have NCV slowing or block at some time (may take several weeks in some). NCV usually < 60% of normal, but not in all nerves

Features casting doubt on diagnosis:
- marked, persistent asymmetry of weakness
- persistent bowel or bladder dysfunction
- > 50 monocytes/ml CSF
- PMNs in CSF
- sharp sensory level
- features of conditions in the differential diagnosis (see below)

10.7.3 Guillain-Barré variants

General information

A number of variants have been described (some may simply be incomplete forms of typical Guillain-Barré). Autonomic dysfunction may occur in some.

Miller-Fisher variant of GBS

Ataxia, areflexia and ophthalmoplegia. May also have ptosis. 5% of cases of GBS. Serum marker: anti-GQ1b antibodies.

Acute motor axonal neuropathy (AMAN)

This variant and AIDP are the most common to follow Campylobacter jejuni enteritis.

Pharyngeal-cervical-brachial variant

Facial, oropharyngeal, cervical, and UE weakness, sparing the LEs.

Pure sensory variant

Sensory loss accompanied by areflexia.

Atypical GBS

May be accompanied by rhabdomyolysis.[55]

10.7.4 Differential diagnosis

Also see conditions in the differential diagnosis under Myelopathy (p. 1696)
1. Guillain-Barré syndrome (including one of its variants)
2. critical illness polyneuropathy (p. 569): EMG: ↓ CMAP & SNAP
3. current hexacarbon abuse: volatile solvents (n-hexane, methyl n-butyl ketone), glue sniffing
4. acute intermittent porphyria (AIP): a disorder of porphyrin metabolism. CSF protein is not elevated in AIP. Recurrent painful abdominal crises are common. Check urine delta-aminolevulinic acid or porphobilinogen
5. recent diphtheritic infection: diphtheritic polyneuropathy has a longer latency and a slower crescendo of symptoms
6. lead neuropathy: UE weakness with wrist drop. May be asymmetrical
7. poliomyelitis: usually *asymmetric*, has meningeal irritation
8. hypophosphatemia (may occur in chronic IV hyperalimentation)
9. botulism: difficult to distinguish clinically from GBS. Normal NCV and a facilitating response to repetitive nerve stimulation on electrodiagnostics

10. toxic neuropathy (e.g., from nitrofurantoin, dapsone, thallium or arsenic)
11. tick paralysis: may cause an ascending motor neuropathy without sensory impairment. Careful examination of the scalp for tick(s)
12. chronic immune demyelinating poly(radiculo)neuropathy (CIDP) AKA chronic relapsing GBS, chronic relapsing polyneuritis[56] AKA chronic immune demyelinating polyradiculoneuropathy. Similar to GBS, but longer time course (symptoms must be present > 2 mos). CIDP produces progressive, symmetrical, proximal & distal weakness, depression of muscle stretch reflexes, and variable sensory loss. Cranial nerves are usually spared (facial muscles may be involved). Balance difficulties are common. Need for respiratory support is rare. Peak incidence: age 40–60 yrs. Electrodiagnostics and nerve biopsy findings are indicative of demyelination. CSF findings are similar to GBS (see above). Most respond to immunosuppressive therapy (especially prednisolone & plasmapheresis) but relapses are common. Refractory cases may be treated with IV gamma-globulin, cyclosporin-A,[57] total body lymphoid irradiation or interferon-α[58]
13. critical illness myopathy: chronic illness myopathy. Muscles not excitable with direct stimulation. EMG: low or normal CMAP with normal SNAP. Muscle biopsy: abnormalities may range from Type II fiber atrophy to necrosis (severe necrosis may not recover)
14. motor neuron disease (p. 191): AKA ALS. Hyperreflexia in LEs
15. myasthenia gravis: weakness worsens towards the end of the day and with repeat efforts. Positive assay for circulating anti-acetylcholine receptor antibodies
16. spinal cord injury

10.7.5 Imaging

No characteristic finding; however, diffuse enhancement of cauda equina and nerve roots occurs in up to 95% of cases.[59] Thought to be due to disruption of the blood-nerve barrier from inflammation. Conspicuous nerve root enhancement correlates with pain, GBS disability grade, and duration of recovery.[59]

10.7.6 Treatment

Immunoglobulins may be helpful. In *severe* cases, early plasmapheresis hastens the recovery and reduces the residual deficit. Its role in mild cases is uncertain. Steroids are not helpful.[60] Mechanical ventilation and measures to prevent aspiration are used as appropriate. In cases of facial diplegia, the eyes must be protected from exposure (neuroparalytic) keratitis.

10.7.7 Outcome

Recovery may not be complete for several months. 35% of untreated patients have residual weakness and atrophy. Recurrence of GBS after achieving maximal recovery occurs in ≈ 2%.

10.8 Myelitis

10.8.1 General information

AKA acute transverse myelitis (ATM). The terminology is confusing: myelitis overlaps with "myelopathy." Both are pathologic conditions of the spinal cord. Myelitis indicates inflammation, and etiologies include infectious/post-infectious, autoimmune, and idiopathic. Myelopathy is generally reserved for compressive, toxic, or metabolic etiologies[61]; see also differential diagnosis (p. 1696).

10.8.2 Etiology

Many so-called "causes" remain unproven. Immunologic response against the CNS (most likely via cell mediated component) is the probable common mechanism. Animal model: experimental allergic encephalomyelitis (requires myelin basic protein of CNS, not peripheral).

Generally accepted etiologies include (items with an asterisk * may be more properly associated with myelopathy rather than myelitis):
1. infectious and post-infectious
   a) primary infectious myelitis
      • viral: poliomyelitis, myelitis with viral encephalomyelitis, herpes zoster, rabies
      • bacterial: including tuberculoma of spinal cord
      • spirochetal: AKA syphilitic myelitis. Causes syphilitic endarteritis

- fungal (aspergillosis, blastomycosis, cryptococcosis)
- parasitic (Echinococcus, cysticercosis, paragonimiasis, schistosomiasis)
  b) post-infectious: including post-exanthematous, influenza
2. posttraumatic
3. physical agents
   a) decompression sickness (dysbarism)
   b) electrical injury*
   c) post-irradiation
4. paraneoplastic syndrome (remote effect of cancer): most common primary is lung, but prostate, ovary and rectum have also been described[62]
5. metabolic
   a) diabetes mellitus*
   b) pernicious anemia*
   c) chronic liver disease*
6. toxins
   a) cresyl phosphates*
   b) intra-arterial contrast agents*
   c) spinal anesthetics
   d) myelographic contrast agents
   e) following chemonucleolysis[63]
7. arachnoiditis
8. autoimmune
   a) multiple sclerosis (MS), especially neuromyelitis optica (NMO) (p. 1698)
   b) following vaccination (smallpox, rabies)
9. collagen vascular disease
   a) systemic lupus erythematosus
   b) mixed connective tissue disease

10.8.3 Clinical

Presentation

34 patients with ATM[64]: age of onset ranged 15–55 yrs, with 66% occurring in 3rd and 4th decade. 12 patients (35%) had a viral-like prodrome. Presenting symptoms are shown in ▶ Table 10.5, with other presenting symptoms of unspecified frequency including[65]: fever and rash.

Table 10.5 Presenting symptoms in myelitis

Symptom	Series A[a]	Series B[b]
pain (back or radicular)	35%	35%
muscle weakness	32%	13%
sensory deficit or paresthesias	26%	46%
sphincter disturbance	12%	6%

[a]series A: 34 patients with ATM[64]
[b]series B: 52 patients with acute or subacute transverse myelitis[66]

Presenting level

The levels at presentation in 62 patients with ATM are shown in ▶ Table 10.6.[65] The thoracic level is the most common sensory level. Infrequently, ATM is the presenting symptom of MS (≈ 3–6% of patients with ATM develop MS).

Table 10.6 Level of sensory deficit

Level	%
cervical	8
high thoracic	36
low thoracic	32
lumbar	8
unknown	16

Progression

Progression is usually rapid, with 66% reaching maximal deficit by 24 hrs; however, the interval between first symptom and maximal deficit varies from 2 hrs-14 days.[65] Findings at the time of maximal deficit are shown in ▶ Table 10.7.

Table 10.7 Symptoms at time of *maximal* deficit (62 patients with ATM[65])

Symptom	%
sensory deficit or paresthesias	100
muscle weakness	97
sphincter disturbance (hesitancy, retention, overflow incontinence)	94
pain in back, abdomen, or limbs	34
fever	27
nuchal rigidity	13

10.8.4 Evaluation

Imaging should be done to rule out a compressive lesion. MRI or CT/myelogram: no characteristic finding. One paper reports 2 patients with fusiform cord enlargement.[67] MRI may be able to demonstrate the area of involvement within the cord. MRI may show the "central dot sign,"[68] an area of high signal on axial T2WI usually centrally located with a small dot of isointense signal in the core of the hyperintensity.

CSF: normal during acute phase in 38% of LPs. Remainder (62%) had elevated protein (usually > 40 mg%) or pleocytosis (lymphocytes, PMNs, or both) or both.

Evaluation scheme

In a patient developing acute myelopathy/paraplegia, especially when ATM is considered likely, the first test of choice is an emergency MRI. If not readily available, a myelogram (with CT to follow) directed at the region of the sensory level is performed (CSF may be sent in this circumstance once block is ruled out).

10.8.5 Treatment

No treatment has been studied in a randomized controlled trial.
1. steroids: not beneficial for some types of myelitis,[69] especially with ASIA A (complete paralysis); see ▶ 68.8.7 "ASIA impairment scale."[70] Rx: high-dose IV methylprednisolone 3–5 days (doses quoted include 500 mg/d, and 1000 mg/d[71]). The decision to introduce additional treatment measures is based on the response to steroids and the MRI appearance after ≈ 5 days of steroids
2. plasma exchange (PLEX) for patients that do not respond to steroids within 3–5 days
3. other forms of immune suppression may be attempted for failure of above therapies, including: cyclophosphamide (usually under the direction of an oncologist)
4. in cases of focal spinal cord enlargement, surgical decompression may be considered in cases that fail to respond to the above

10.8.6 Prognosis

In a series of 34 ATM patients with ≥ 5 yrs follow-up (F/U)[64]: 9 patients (26%) had good recovery (ambulate well, mild urinary symptoms, minimal sensory and UMN signs); 9 (26%) had fair recovery (functional gait with some degree of spasticity, urinary urgency, obvious sensory signs, paraparesis); 11 (32%) had poor recovery (paraplegic, absent sphincter control); 5 (15%) died within 4 mos of illness. 18 patients (62% of survivors) became ambulatory (in these cases, all could walk with support by 3–6 mos).

In a series of 59 patients[65] (F/U period unspecified): 22 (37%) had good recovery; 14 (24%) had poor recovery; 3 died in acute stage (respiratory insufficiency in 2, sepsis in 1). Recovery occurred between 4 weeks and 3 mos after onset (no improvement occurred after 3 mos).

10

10.9 Neurosarcoidosis

10.9.1 General information

> **Key concepts**
>
> - neurologic involvement of sarcoidosis (a systemic granulomatous disease)
> - may produce multiple cranial nerve palsies
> - the most common neurologic manifestation is diabetes insipidus
> - immunosuppressants (including corticosteroids) can improve systemic as well as neurologic symptoms

Sarcoidosis is a granulomatous disease that is usually systemic, and may include the CNS (so-called neurosarcoidosis AKA neurosarcoid). Only 1–3% of cases have CNS findings without systemic manifestations.[72] The cause of the disease is unknown. An exaggerated cellular immune response for unknown reasons is the currently favored hypothesis. Organs commonly involved include lungs, skin, lymph nodes, bones, eyes, muscles, and parotid glands.[30]

10.9.2 Pathology

Gross involvement

CNS sarcoidosis primarily involves the leptomeninges; however, parenchymal invasion often occurs. Adhesive arachnoiditis with nodule formation may also occur (nodules have a predilection for the posterior fossa). Diffuse meningitis or meningoencephalitis may occur, and may be most pronounced at the base of the brain (basal meningitis) and in the subependymal region of the third ventricle (including the hypothalamus).

Spinal involvement may include arachnoiditis, and lesions that may be intramedullary, extramedullary intradural and extramedullary extradural.

Microscopic features

Constant microscopic features of neurosarcoidosis include noncaseating granulomas with lymphocytic infiltrates. Langhans giant cells may or may not be present.

10.9.3 Epidemiology

Incidence of sarcoidosis is ≈ 3–50 cases/100,000 population; neurosarcoidosis occurs in ≈ 5% of cases (reported range: 1–27%). In one series, the median age of onset of neurologic symptoms was 44 years.

The spinal cord is involved in < 1% of patients with sarcoidosis,[73] and in 16% of these, the spinal cord was the only identifiable site of involvement.

10.9.4 Clinical findings

Clinical findings include multiple cranial nerve palsies in 50–70% (particularly facial n., including diplegia), peripheral neuropathy, and myopathy.[74] Occasionally the lesions may produce mass effect,[75] and hydrocephalus may result from adhesive basal arachnoiditis. Patients may have low grade fever. Intracranial hypertension is common and may be dangerous. Hypothalamic involvement may produce disorders of ADH (diabetes insipidus, disordered thirst...). Rare involvement of the pituitary may produce pituitary insufficiency. Seizures occur in 15%.

Spinal cord involvement may produce myelopathy.

10.9.5 Laboratory

CBC: mild leukocytosis and eosinophilia may occur.

Serum angiotensin-converting enzyme (ACE): abnormally elevated in 83% of patients with active pulmonary sarcoidosis, but in only 11% with inactive disease.[76] False positive rate: 2–3%; may also be elevated in primary biliary cirrhosis.

CSF: similar to any subacute meningitis: elevated pressure, mild pleocytosis (10–200 cells/mm^3) mostly lymphocytes, elevated protein (up to 2,000 mg/dl), mild hypoglycorrhachia (CSF glucose 15–40 mg/dl), CSF ACE is elevated in ≈ 55% of cases with neurosarcoidosis (normal in patients with sarcoidosis not involving the CNS).[77] No organisms are recovered on culture or gram stain.

10.9.6 Imaging

CXR

Usually demonstrates characteristic findings of sarcoidosis (hilar adenopathy, mediastinal lymph nodes…).

MRI

Gadolinium enhancement of the leptomeninges and/or optic nerve may be the only abnormal finding(s). Meningeal enhancement was seen in 38% of neurosarcoidosis patients.[78] Lesions may be solitary or multiple, and may be located intra- or extraparenchymal, periventricular, in basal cisterns, and/or intraspinal (intra- or extra medullary). Lesions may be seen on FLAIR that would otherwise have been missed. Hydrocephalus may occur.

Spinal involvement may involve intradural intramedullary spinal cord lesions.

Gallium scan

Nuclear medicine scan with 67Ga citrate (p. 248). Described findings include:
1. Panda sign[79]: uptake in lacrimal glands, parotid glands & nasopharynx (normal). Not specific for sarcoidosis
2. lambda distribution[80]: uptake in hilar lymph nodes
3. leopard man sign[81]: diffuse dappled pattern due to uptake in soft tissues, skin, muscles, mediastinum, and lacrimal glands

10.9.7 Differential diagnosis

1. Hodgkin's disease
2. chronic granulomatous meningitis:
   a) Hansen's disease (leprosy)
   b) syphilis
   c) cryptococcosis
   d) tuberculosis
3. multiple sclerosis
4. CNS lymphoma
5. pseudotumor cerebri
6. granulomatous angiitis

Differentiating granulomatous angiitis (**GA**) from neurosarcoidosis that involves only the CNS can be done on histologic criteria: the inflammatory reaction in sarcoidosis is not limited to the region immediately surrounding blood vessels as it is in GA, where extensive disruption of the vessel wall may occur.

10.9.8 Diagnosis

Making the diagnosis is relatively easy when systemic involvement occurs: characteristic findings on CXR, biopsy of skin or liver nodules, muscle biopsy, serum ACE assay.

Isolated neurosarcoidosis may be more difficult to diagnose, and may require biopsy (see below).

10.9.9 Biopsy

In uncertain cases, biopsy may be indicated. If a mass lesion cannot be biopsied, a meningeal biopsy may be done and should include all layers of meninges and cerebral cortex. Cultures and stains for fungus and acid-fast bacteria (TB) should be performed in addition to microscopic examination.

10

10.9.10 Treatment

Antibiotics have not been proven to be of benefit. Immunosuppression primarily with corticosteroids is beneficial for systemic as well as neurologic involvement. Therapy may be initiated with prednisone 60 mg PO qd in adults, and tapered based on response. Therapy with cyclosporine may allow a reduction in steroid dosage in refractory cases.[82] Treatment options for unresponsive cases include methotrexate, cytoxan, cyclophosphamide, azathioprine, Hydroxychloroquine (Plaquenil®) & low dose XRT. CSF shunting is indicated if hydrocephalus develops.

10.9.11 Prognosis

Usually a benign disease. Peripheral and cranial nerve palsies recover slowly.

References

[1] Consensus Conference. Differential Diagnosis of Dementing Diseases. JAMA. 1987; 258:3411–3416
[2] Fleming KC, Adams AC, Petersen RC. Dementia: Diagnosis and Evaluation. Mayo Clinic Proceedings. 1995; 70:1093–1107
[3] Lipowski ZJ. Delirium (Acute Confusional States). Journal of the American Medical Association. 1987; 258:1789–1792
[4] Pompei P, Foreman M, Rudberg MA, et al. Delirium in Hospitalized Older Persons: Outcomes and Predictors. J Am Geriatr Soc. 1994; 42:809–815
[5] Petersen RC. Acute Confusional State: Don't Mistake it for Dementia. Postgrad Med. 1992; 92:141–148
[6] Hulette CM, Earl NL, Crain BJ. Evaluation of Cerebral Biopsies for the Diagnosis of Dementia. Arch Neurol. 1992; 49:28–31
[7] Javedan SP, Tamargo RJ. Diagnostic Yield of Brain Biopsy in Neurodegenerative Disorders. Neurosurgery. 1997; 41:823–830
[8] Groves R, Moller J. The Value of the Cerebral Cortical Biopsy. Acta Neurol Scand. 1966; 42:477–482
[9] Forsyth PA, Posner JB. Headaches in Patients with Brain Tumors: A Study of 111 Patients. Neurology. 1993; 43:1678–1683
[10] Welch KMA, Levine SR. Migraine-related stroke in the context of the International Headache Society Classification of head pain. Arch Neurol. 1990; 47:458–462
[11] Lance JW. Treatment of Migraine. Lancet. 1992; 339:1207–1209
[12] Kittrelle JP, Grouse DS, Seybold ME. Cluster Headache: Local Anesthetic Abortive Agents. Arch Neurol. 1985; 42:496–498
[13] Sanders M, Zuurmond WWA. Efficacy of Sphenopalatine Ganglion Blockade in 66 Patients Suffering from Cluster Headache: A 12- to 70-Month Follow-Up Evaluation. Journal of Neurosurgery. 1997; 87:876–880
[14] Burns B, Watkins L, Goadsby PJ. Treatment of medically intractable cluster headache by occipital nerve stimulation: long-term follow-up of 8 patients. Lancet. 2007; 369:1099–1106
[15] Lapkin ML, Golden GS. Basilar Artery Migraine: A Review of 30 Cases. Am J Dis Child. 1978; 132:278–281
[16] Mitchell SL, Kiely DK, Kiel DP, et al. The Epidemiology, Clinical Characteristics, and Natural History of Older Nursing Home Residents with a Diagnosis of Parkinson's Disease. J Am Geriatr Soc. 1996; 44:394–399
[17] Lang AE, Lozano AM. Parkinson's Disease. First of Two Parts. New England Journal of Medicine. 1998; 339:1044–1053
[18] Koller WC, Silver DE, Lieberman A. An Algorithm for the Management of Parkinson's Disease. Neurology. 1994; 44:S5–52
[19] Young R. Update on Parkinson's Disease. American Family Physician. 1999; 59:2155–2167
[20] Kondziolka D, Bonaroti EA, Lunsford LD. Pallidotomy for Parkinson's Disease. Contemporary Neurosurgery. 1996; 18:1–6

[21] Davis GC, Williams AC, Markey SP, et al. Chronic Parkinsonism Secondary to Intravenous Injection of Meperidine Analogues. Psychiatry Res. 1979; 1:249–254
[22] Langston JW, Ballard P, Tetrud JW, et al. Chronic Parkinsonism in Humans Due to a Product of Meperidine-Analog Synthesis. Science. 1983; 219:979–980
[23] Langston JW, Ballard PA,Jr. Parkinson's Disease in a Chemist Working with 1-Methyl-4-phenyl-1,2,5,6-tetrahydropyridine. N Engl J Med. 1983; 309
[24] Langston JW, Forno LS, Tetrud J, et al. Evidence of Active Nerve Cell Degeneration in the Substantia Nigra of Humans Years After 1-Methyl-4-phenyl-1,2,3,6-tetrahydropyridine Exposure. Ann Neurol. 1999; 46:598–605
[25] Kristensen MO. Progressive Supranuclear Palsy - 10 Years Later. Acta Neurol Scand. 1985; 71:177–189
[26] Gildenberg PL. Whatever Happened to Stereotactic Surgery? Neurosurgery. 1987; 20:983–987
[27] Pugliatti M, Rosati G, Raine CS, et al. Epidemiology of multiple sclerosis. In: Multiple sclerosis: a comprehensive text. Philadelphia: Saunders Elsevier; 2008
[28] Lublin FD, Reingold SC. Defining the Clinical Course of Multiple Sclerosis: Results of an International Survey. Neurology. 1996; 46:907–911
[29] Rudick RA, Cohen JA, Weinstock-Guttman B, et al. Management of Multiple Sclerosis. New England Journal of Medicine. 1997; 22:1604–1611
[30] Rowland LP. Merritt's Textbook of Neurology. Philadelphia 1989
[31] Jensen TS, Rasmussen P, Reske-Nielsen E. Association of Trigeminal Neuralgia with Multiple Sclerosis. Archives of Neurology. 1982; 65:182–189
[32] Filippi M, Horsfield MA, Morrisey SP, et al. Quantitative Brain MRI Lesion Load Predicts the Course of Clinically Isolated Syndromes Suggestive of Multiple Sclerosis. Neurology. 1994; 44:635–641
[33] McDonald WI, Compston A, Edan G, et al. Recommended diagnostic criteria for multiple sclerosis: Guidelines from the international panel on the diagnosis of multiple sclerosis. Ann Neurol. 2001; 50:121–127
[34] Polman CH, Reingold SC, Edan G, et al. Diagnostic criteria for multiple sclerosis: 2005 revisions to the "McDonald Criteria". Ann Neurol. 2005; 58:840–846
[35] Poser CM, Paty DW, Scheinberg L, et al. New Diagnostic Criteria for Multiple Sclerosis: Guidelines for Research Protocols. Ann Neurol. 1983; 13:227–231
[36] Polman CH, Reingold SC, Banwell B, et al. Diagnostic criteria for multiple sclerosis: 2010 revisions to the McDonald criteria. Ann Neurol. 2011; 69:292–302
[37] Swanton JK, Rovira A, Tintore M, et al. MRI criteria for multiple sclerosis in patients presenting with clinically isolated syndromes: a multicentre retrospective study. Lancet Neurol. 2007; 6:677–686
[38] Montalban X, Tintore M, Swanton J, et al. MRI criteria for MS in patients with clinically isolated syndromes. Neurology. 2010; 74:427–434

10

[39] Swanson JW. Multiple Sclerosis: Update in Diagnosis and Review of Prognostic Factors. Mayo Clin Proc. 1989; 64:577–586

[40] Barkhof F, Filippi M, Miller DH, et al. Comparison of MR imaging criteria at first presentation to predict conversion to clinically definite multiple sclerosis. Brain. 1997; 120:2059–2069

[41] Tintore M, Rovira A, Martinez M, et al. Isolated demyelinating syndromes: comparison of different MR imaging criteria to predict conversion to clinically definite multiple sclerosis. American Journal of Neuroradiology. 2000; 21:702–706

[42] Stewart JM, Houser OW, Baker HL, et al. Magnetic Resonance Imaging and Clinical Relationships in Multiple Sclerosis. Mayo Clin Proc. 1987; 62:174–184

[43] Mushlin AI, Detsky AS, Phelps CE, et al. The Accuracy of Magnetic Resonance Imaging in Patients With Suspected Multiple Sclerosis. Journal of the American Medical Association. 1993; 269:3146–3151

[44] Kidd C, Thorpe JW, Thompson AJ, et al. Spinal cord imaging MRI using multi-array coils and fast spin echo. II. Findings in multiple sclerosis. Neurology. 1993; 43:2632–2637

[45] Kent DL, Larson EB. Magnetic Resonance Imaging of the Brain and Spine. Annals of Internal Medicine. 1988; 108:402–424

[46] Kepes JJ. Large focal tumor-like demyelinating lesions of the brain: intermediate entity between multiple sclerosis and acute disseminated encephalomyelitis? A study of 31 patients. Ann Neurol. 1993; 33:18–27

[47] Law M, Meltzer DE, Cha S. Spectroscopic magnetic resonance imaging of a tumefactive demyelinating lesion. Neuroradiology. 2002; 44:986–989

[48] Freedman MS, Thompson EJ, Deisenhammer D, et al. Recommended standard of cerebrospinal fluid analysis in the diagnosis of multiple sclerosis: A consensus statement. Archives of Neurology. 2005; 62:865–870

[49] Rowland LP. Diagnosis of amyotrophic lateral sclerosis. Journal of Neurological Science. 1998; 160: S6–24

[50] Peavy GM, Herzog AG, Rubin NP, et al. Neuropsychological Aspects of Dementia of Motor Neuron Disease: A Report of Two Cases. Neurology. 1992; 42:1004–1008

[51] Bensimon G, Lacomblez L, Meininger V, et al. A Controlled Trial of Riluzole in Amyotrophic Lateral Sclerosis. New England Journal of Medicine. 1994; 24:585–591

[52] Lacomblez L, Bensimon G, Guillet P, et al. Riluzole: A Double-Blind Randomized Placebo-Controlled Dose-Range Study in Amyotrophic Lateral Sclerosis (ALS). Electroenceph Clin Neurophysiol. 1995; 97

[53] Ropper AH, Shahani BT. Pain in Guillain-Barré syndrome. Arch Neurol. 1984; 41:511–514

[54] Asbury AK, Arnaso BGW, Karp HR, et al. Criteria for Diagnosis of Guillain-Barré Syndrome. Ann Neurol. 1978; 3:565–566

[55] Scott AJ, Duncan R, Henderson L, et al. Acute rhabdomyolysis associated with atypical Guillain-Barré syndrome. Postgrad Med J. 1991; 67:73–74

[56] Mendell JR. Chronic Inflammatory Demyelinating Polyradiculoneuropathy. Annual Review of Medicine. 1993; 44:211–219

[57] Mahattanakul W, Crawford TO, Griffin JW, et al. Treatment of Chronic Inflammatory Demyelinating Polyneuropathy with Cyclosporin-A. Journal of Neurology, Neurosurgery, and Psychiatry. 1996; 60:185–187

[58] Gorson KC, Ropper AH, Clark BD, et al. Treatment of Chronic Inflammatory Demyelinating Polyneuropathy with Interferon-a 2a. Neurology. 1998; 50:84–87

[59] Gorson KC, Ropper AH, Muriello MA, et al. Prospective evaluation of MRI lumbosacral nerve root enhancement in acute Guillain-Barré syndrome. Neurology. 1996; 47:813–817

[60] Guillain-Barré Syndrome Steroid Trial Group. Double-Blind Trial of Intravenous Methylprednisolone in Guillain-Barré Syndrome. Lancet. 1993; 341:586–590

[61] Kincaid JC, Dyken ML, Baker AB, et al. Myelitis and Myelopathy. In: Clinical Neurology. Hagerstown: Harper and Row; 1984:1–32

[62] Altrocchi PH. Acute Transverse Myelopathy. Arch Neurol. 1963; 9:111–119

[63] Eguro H. Transverse Myelitis following Chemonucleolysis: Report of a Case. J Bone Joint Surg. 1983; 65A:1328–1329

[64] Lipton HL, Teasdall RD. Acute Transverse Myelopathy in Adults: A Follow-Up Study. Arch Neurol. 1973; 28:252–257

[65] Berman M, Feldman S, Alter M, et al. Acute Transverse Myelitis: Incidence and Etiologic Considerations. Neurology. 1981; 31:966–971

[66] Ropper AH, Poskanzer DC. The Prognosis of Acute and Subacute Transverse Myelopathy Based on Early Signs and Symptoms. Ann Neurol. 1978; 4:51–59

[67] Merine D, Wang H, Kumar AJ, et al. CT Myelography and MRI of Acute Transverse Myelitis. J Comput Assist Tomogr. 1987; 11:606–608

[68] Berg B, Franklin G, Cuneo R, et al. Nonsurgical Cure of Brain Abscesses. Ann Neurol. 1978; 3:474–478

[69] Kalita J, Misra UK. Is methyl prednisolone useful in acute transverse myelitis? Spinal Cord. 2001; 39:471–476

[70] Greenberg BM, Thomas KP, Krishnan C, et al. Idiopathic transverse myelitis: corticosteroids, plasma exchange, or cyclophosphamide. Neurology. 2007; 68:1614–1617

[71] Britt RH, Enzmann DR, Yeager AS. Neuropathological and CT Findings in Experimental Brain Abscess. J Neurosurg. 1981; 55:590–603

[72] Stern BJ, Krumholz A, Johns C, et al. Sarcoidosis and its Neurological Manifestations. Arch Neurol. 1985; 42:909–917

[73] Saleh S, Saw C, Marzouk K, et al. Sarcoidosis of the spinal cord: literature review and report of eight cases. Journal of the National Medical Association. 2006; 98:965–976

[74] Oksanen V. Neurosarcoidosis: Clinical Presentation and Course in 50 Patients. Acta Neurol Scand. 1986; 73:283–290

[75] de Tribolet N, Zander E. Intracranial Sarcoidosis Presenting Angiographically as a Subdural Hematoma. Surg Neurol. 1978; 9:169–171

[76] Rohrbach MS, DeRemee RA. Pulmonary Sarcoidosis and Serum Angiotensin-Converting Enzyme. Mayo Clin Proc. 1982; 57:64–66

[77] Oksanen V. New Cerebrospinal Fluid, Neurophysiological and Neuroradiological Examinations in the Diagnosis and Follow-Up of Neurosarcoidosis. Sarcoidosis. 1987; 4:105–110

[78] Zajicek JP, Scolding NJ, Foster O, et al. Central nervous system sarcoidosis–diagnosis and management. QJM. 1999; 92:103–117

[79] Kurdziel KA. The Panda Sign. Radiology. 2000; 215:884–885

[80] Sulavik SB, Spencer RP, Weed DA, et al. Recognition of distinctive patterns of gallium-67 distribution in sarcoidosis. J Nucl Med. 1990; 31:1909–1914

[81] Fayad F, Duet M, Orcel P, et al. Systemic sarcoidosis: the "leopard-man" sign. Joint Bone Spine. 2006; 73:109–112

[82] Stern BJ, Schonfeld SA, Sewell C, et al. The Treatment of Neurosarcoidosis With Cyclosporine. Archives of Neurology. 1992; 49:1065–1072

10

11 Neurovascular Disorders and Neurotoxicology

11.1 Posterior reversible encephalopathy syndrome (PRES)

11.1.1 General information

AKA reversible posterior leukoencephalopathy syndrome (RPLS). A group of encephalopathies with characteristic pattern of widespread vasogenic brain edema seen on CT or MRI with some predominance in the parietal and occipital regions.[1] The most common PRES pattern involves watershed zones with involvement of the cortex, subcortical and deep white matter to a variable extent.[1] A small number of patients with PRES will go on to infarction.

Patients may present with headache, seizures, mental status changes and focal neurologic deficit. Intracerebral hemorrhage (ICH) and SAH may occur in up to 15%.[1]

11.1.2 Associated findings and conditions

Includes:
1. hypertensive encephalopathy: commonly seen in the setting of subacute blood pressure elevations (as may occur with malignant hypertension). Imaging studies show symmetric confluent lesions with mild mass effect and patchy enhancement primarily in the subcortical white matter of the *occipital lobes*[2] which may produce cortical blindness
   a) moderate to severe hypertension is seen in ≈ 75% of patients with PRES[1] although the upper limits of autoregulation are often not reached
   b) in addition to hemispheric patterns of edema, isolated brainstem and cerebellar edema have been described. Posterior fossa edema has been reported to cause obstructive hydrocephalus in a severe case[3]
2. preeclampsia/eclampsia associated with cerebral edema.[4] The condition is often temporary, but (permanent) infarctions also occur. Restricted diffusion on MR imaging is seen in 11–26% of cases. Abnormal DWI areas on MRI may be associated with a worse prognosis[5]
   a) may present (e.g., with blindness) during pregnancy complicated by preeclampsia or eclampsia[6]
   b) may develop 4–9 days post-partum and may be associated with vasospasm[7] even in patients not meeting clinical criteria for the diagnosis of eclampsia
   c) toxemia is attributed to the placenta. Delivery and removal of the placenta is felt to be curative[8]
3. infection, sepsis and shock: blood pressure was normal in 40% (edema was greater in the normotensive patients). Gram positive organisms predominate[9]
4. autoimmune disease: PRES has been described in patients with lupus, scleroderma, Wegener's granulomatosis and polyarteritis nodosa.[1] These patients often receive regimens of immunosuppressive medications (tacrolimus, cyclosporine), which have also been linked to cases of PRES
5. cancer chemotherapy: PRES occurs in patients receiving multi-drug high dose chemotherapy most commonly for hematopoietic malignancies
6. transplantation: PRES has been reported both with bone marrow and solid organ transplantation
   a) incidence: 3–16% with bone marrow transplantation depending on the preconditioning regimen and whether or not it is myeloablative[1]
   b) highest incidence in the first month following allogeneic bone marrow transplant[1]
   c) lower incidence following solid organ transplants. Occurs earlier following liver transplantation, usually within 2 months. Occurs later in renal transplants[1]
7. cyclosporine post-transplant neurotoxicity[9]

11.1.3 Treatment

Disordered autoregulation mandates tight control of blood pressure to reduce the risk of ICH. The underlying cause needs to be addressed (i.e., control HTN, hold immunosuppressives or chemotherapeutics, delivery of the placenta, etc.).

11.2 Crossed cerebellar diaschisis

Hypometabolism of cerebellar cortex contralateral to a cerebral hemispheric lesion (lesions include stroke, brain tumor...). Lesions in the motor cortex, anterior corona radiata, and thalamus produce the most marked suppression of metabolism. Theory: hypometabolism is due to disconnection of cerebro-ponto-cerebellar pathways → decreased oxygen and glucose consumption → decreased CO_2 production → local arterial constriction (down-regulation of cerebellar blood flow).

11.3 Vasculitis and vasculopathy

11.3.1 General information

The vasculitides are a group of disorders characterized by inflammation and necrosis of blood vessels. Vasculitis may be primary or secondary. Those that may affect the CNS are listed in ▶ Table 11.1; all of these cause tissue ischemia (even after the inflammation is quiescent) that may range in effect from neuropraxia to infarction.

Table 11.1 Vasculitides that may affect the CNS[10]

Vasculitis	Frequency of neuro involvement	Type of CNS involvement[a]				
		Acute encephalopathy	Seizure	Cranial nerve	Spinal cord	ICH or SAH
periarteritis nodosa[b] (PAN)[c]	20–40%	+ +	+ +	+	+	+
hypersensitivity vasculitis[b]	10%	+	+	0	0	+
giant cell (temporal) arteritis[b]	10%	+	0	+ +	0	0
Takayasu's arteritis	10–36%	+	+ +	+ +	+	+
Wegener's granulomatosis[b]	23–50%	+	+ +	+ +	+	+
lymphomatoid granulomatosis[b]	20–30%	+ +	+	+ +	+	0
isolated angiitis of the CNS[b]	100%	+ +	+	+ +	+ +	+
Behçet's disease[b]	10–29%	+ +	+	+ +	+	+

[a]KEY: 0 = uncommon or unreported; + = not uncommon; + + = common; ICH = intracerebral hemorrhage; SAH = subarachnoid hemorrhage; [b]see section that follows for these topics; [c]PAN: a group of disorders, frequencies may vary by subgroup

11.3.2 Giant cell arteritis (GCA)

Key concepts

- formerly often referred to as temporal arteritis
- a chronic vasculitis of large- and medium-caliber vessels, primarily involving cranial branches of the arteries arising from the aortic arch
- age > 50 years; affects women twice as often as men
- important possible late complications: blindness, stroke, thoracic aortic aneurysms, and aortic dissections
- temporal artery biopsy is recommended for all patients suspected of GCA
- corticosteroids are the drug of choice for treatment

AKA temporal arteritis (TA), AKA cranial arteritis. A chronic granulomatous arteritis of unknown etiology involving primarily the cranial branches of the aortic arch (especially the external carotid artery (ECA)),[11] which if untreated, may lead to blindness. Takayasu's arteritis is similar to GCA, but tends to affect large arteries in young women; it has 2 phases: inflammatory (treated with corticosteroids) and stenotic (treated with arterial bypasses).

11

Epidemiology

Seen almost exclusively in Caucasians > 50 yrs of age (mean age of onset is 70). Incidence: 17.8 per 100,000 people ≥ 50 years old[12] (range: 0.49–23). Prevalence: ≈ 223 (autopsy incidence may be much higher).[13] More common in northern latitudes and among individuals of Scandinavian descent, suggesting genetic and environmental causes.[11] Female:male ratio is ≈ 2:1 (reported range: 1.05–7.4:1). 50% of GCA patients also have polymyalgia rheumatica (PMR) (p. 206).

Pathology

Discontinuous (so-called "skip lesions") inflammatory reaction of lymphocytes, plasma cells, macrophages, ± giant cells (if absent, intimal proliferation may be prominent); predominantly in media of involved arteries. Arteries preferentially involved include the ophthalmic and posterior ciliary branches and the entire distribution of the external carotid system (of which the STA is a terminal branch). Other arteries in the body may be involved (reported involvement of abdominal aorta, femoral, brachial and mesenteric arteries are rarely symptomatic). Unlike PAN, GCA generally spares the renal arteries.

Clinical

Various combinations of symptoms of giant cell arteritis are listed in ▶ Table 11.2. Onset is usually insidious, although occasionally it may be abrupt.[14]
  Details of some findings:
1. H/A: the most common presenting symptom. May be nonspecific or located in one or both temporal areas, forehead, or occiput. May be superficial or burning with paroxysmal lancinating pain
2. symptoms relating to ECA blood supply (strongly suggestive of GCA, but not pathognomonic[16]): jaw claudication, tongue, or pharyngeal muscles
3. ophthalmologic symptoms: due to arteritis and occlusion of branches of ophthalmic artery or posterior ciliary arteries
   a) symptoms include amaurosis fugax (precedes permanent visual loss in 44%), blindness, visual field cuts, diplopia, ptosis, ocular pain, corneal edema, chemosis
   b) blindness: incidence is ≈ 7%, and once it occurs, recovery of sight is unlikely
4. systemic symptoms
   a) nonspecific constitutional symptoms: fever (may present as FUO in 15% of cases), anorexia, weight loss, fatigue, malaise
   b) 30% have neurologic manifestations. 14% are neuropathies including mononeuropathies and peripheral polyneuropathies of the arms or legs[17]
   c) musculoskeletal symptoms
      • PMR (p. 206) is the most common (occurs in 40% of patients)
      • peripheral arthritis, swelling & pitting edema of hands & feet in 25%
      • arm claudication from stenosis of subclavian and axillary arteries
   d) thoracic aortic aneurysms: 17 times as likely in GCA. Annual CXRs are adequate for screening
5. temporal arteries on physical examination may exhibit tenderness, swelling, erythema, reduced pulsations, or nodularity. Normal in 33%
6. the presence of systemic symptoms correlates with a *lower* incidence of blindness or stroke

Table 11.2 Signs and symptoms of GCA[11,15]

Frequent (> 50% of cases)	Occasional (10–50% of cases)	Rare (< 10% of cases)
H/A: 66% temporal artery tenderness	visual symptoms weight loss fever (low grade) proximal myalgias jaw claudication facial pain scalp tenderness	blindness extremity claudication tongue claudication ear pain synovitis stroke angina

Differential diagnosis

1. periarteritis nodosa (PAN) (p. 208)
2. hypersensitivity vasculitis

3. atherosclerotic occlusive disease
4. malignancy: shares common symptoms of low grade fever, malaise, and weight loss
5. infection
6. trigeminal neuralgia (p. 1857)
7. ophthalmoplegic migraine
8. dental problems

Evaluation

Laboratory studies

1. ESR > 40 mm/hr (usually > 50) by Westergren method (if > 80 mm/hr with above clinical syndromes, highly suggestive of GCA). ESR is normal in up to 22.5%[18]
2. C-reactive protein: another acute phase reactant that is more sensitive than ESR. Has the advantage that it can be performed on frozen sera
3. CBC: may show mild normochromic anemia[19]
4. rheumatoid factor, ANA, and serum complement usually normal
5. LFTs abnormal in 30% (usually elevated alkaline phosphatase)
6. tests for rheumatoid factor and ANA are usually negative
7. temporal artery angiography not helpful (angiography elsewhere indicated if suspicion of large artery involvement exists)
8. CT: usually not helpful, one report described calcified areas corresponding to the temporal arteries[20]
9. temporal artery biopsy: see below

Temporal artery biopsy

Sensitivity and specificity are shown in ▶ Table 11.3.

Table 11.3 Temporal artery biopsy	
sensitivity	≈ 90% (reported range[15,21] is 9–97%)
specificity	near 100%
predictive value	≈ 94%

Indications and timing

Recommendations: temporal artery biopsy in all patients suspected of having GCA.[11] May be controversial. Arguments for: toxicity of a long course of steroids in an elderly patient, and a high rate of false initial responses of other illnesses to steroids. Arguments against: since a negative biopsy cannot exclude the diagnosis, cases with a negative biopsy but a strong clinical suspicion are often treated as though they have GCA.[22] In general, however, biopsy is considered prudent before embarking on a long course of high-dose steroid therapy.[16] Complications of biopsy are rare and include bleeding, infection, and only in the setting of active vasculitis has scalp necrosis been reported (not linked to biopsy).

In general, perform biopsy before starting steroids if biopsy can be done immediately.[11] Otherwise, start steroids to preserve vision and perform biopsy usually within 1 week (pathologic changes can be seen after more than 2 weeks of therapy,[23] therefore do not withhold steroids to await biopsy).

Technique of temporal artery biopsy

Biopsy side of involvement if laterality exists. The yield is increased by removing a portion of the artery that is involved clinically (a tender or inflamed segment).[24] Mark the frontal branch of the STA with a skin marker (spare the main trunk and parietal branch if possible). Infiltrate local anesthetic. The incision is made parallel to the artery and if possible behind the hairline. The incision is taken down to the fascia of the temporalis muscle, to which the STA is superficial.[25] Optimal length of STA biopsy: 4–6 cm (if an abnormal segment of STA can be palpated, some say that a smaller biopsy to include this area may be sufficient, but this is probably unreliable as the muscle may be tender, etc.). Step-sectioning by pathologist through the entire length of the biopsy specimen also increases the yield.

Frozen sections can be performed. Biopsy of the contralateral side if the first side is negative (in cases where clinical suspicion is high) increases the yield only by 5–10%.

11

Treatment

No known cure. Steroids can produce symptomatic relief and usually prevent blindness (progression of ocular problems 24–48 hrs after institution of adequate steroids is rare). Totally blind patients or those with long-standing partial visual loss are unlikely to respond to any treatment.

1. for most cases:
   a) start with *prednisone*, 40–60 mg/d PO divided BID-QID (qod dosing is usually not effective in initial management)
   b) if no response after 72 hrs, and diagnosis certain, ↑ to 10–25 mg QID
   c) once response occurs (usually within 3–7 days), give entire dose as q AM dose for 3–6 weeks until symptoms resolved and ESR normalizes (occurs in 87% of patients within ≈ 4 weeks) or stabilizes at < 40–50 mm/hr
   d) once quiescent, a gradual taper is performed to prevent exacerbations: reduce by 10 mg/d q 2–4 weeks to 40 mg/d, then by 5 mg/d q 2–4 wks to 20 mg/d, then by 2.5 mg/d q 2–4 wks to 5–7.5 mg/d which is maintained for several months, followed by 1 mg/d decrements q 1–3 mos (usual length of treatment is 6–24 mos; do *not* D/C steroids when ESR normalizes)
   e) if symptoms recur during treatment, prednisone dose is temporarily increased until symptoms resolve (isolated rise in ESR is not sufficient reason to increase steroids[11])
   f) patients should be followed closely for ≈ 2 years
2. in severely ill patients: methylprednisolone, 15–20 mg IV QID
3. anticoagulant therapy: controversial
4. acute blindness (onset within 24–36 hrs) in a patient with giant cell arteritis:
   a) consider up to 500 mg methylprednisolone IV over 30–60 mins (no controlled studies show reversal of blindness)
   b) some have used intermittent inhalation of 5% carbon dioxide and oxygen

Outcome

Complications of steroid therapy occur in ≈ 50% of patients. Most are not life threatening, and include vertebral compression fractures in ≈ 36%, peptic ulcer disease in ≈ 12%, proximal myopathy, cataracts, exacerbation of diabetes; also see Possible deleterious side effects of steroids (p. 156).

30–50% of patients will have spontaneous exacerbations of GCA (especially during the first 2 years) regardless of the corticosteroid regimen.[11]

Survival parallels that of the general population. Onset of blindness after initiation of steroid therapy is rare.

11.3.3 Polymyalgia rheumatica (PMR)

General information

PMR and giant cell arteritis (GCA) (p. 203) may be different points on a continuum of the same disease. Both have an increased frequency of HLA-DR4 and systemic monocyte activation. 15% of patients with PMR eventually develop GCA.

Epidemiology

See reference.[11]

Both GCA & PMR occur in people ≥ 50 years old. The incidence increases with age and peaks between 70 and 80 years and is higher at higher latitudes.[11]

PMR is more common than GCA. Prevalence: 500/100,000).[26] Incidence: 52.5 per 100,000 people ≥ age 50, higher in females (61.7) than males (39.9).[27]

Features

See reference.[11]
- an inflammatory condition of unknown etiology
- clinical characteristics
   a) aching and morning stiffness in the cervical region and shoulder & pelvic girdles lasting > 1 month. The pain usually increases with movement
      ○ shoulder pain: present in 70–95% of patients. Radiates toward elbow
      ○ hip & neck pain: 50–70%. Hip pain radiates toward knees
   b) age ≥ 50 years
   c) ESR ≥ 40 mm/hr (7–20% have normal ESR[28])

d) usually responds rapidly to low dose corticosteroids (≤ 20 mg prednisone/day) see below
e) systemic symptoms (present in ≈ 33%): fever, malaise or fatigue, anorexia and weight loss
• favorable prognosis: usually remits in 1–3 years

Treatment

PMR responds either to low doses of steroids[26] (10–20 mg prednisone/day) or sometimes to NSAIDs (response to steroids is much more rapid). The initial dose of steroids is maintained for 2–4 weeks, and then by ≤ 10% of the daily dose every 1–2 weeks[11] while observing for signs of GCA.

11.3.4 ANCA-associated vasculitis

General information

Systemic autoimmune small vessel vasculitides associated with antineutrophil cytoplasmic autoantibodies (ANCAs). Composed of:
1. microscopic polyangiitis (MPA)
2. granulomatosis with polyangiitis (GPA) (p. 207): typically involves neutrophils
3. eosinophilis granulomatosis with polyangiitis (EGPA) (p. 208): typically involves eosinophils

The respiratory system is typically involved, with possible life-threatening alveolar hemorrhage.

Granulomatosis with polyangiitis (GPA)

General information
Formerly known as Wegener's granulomatosis. A systemic necrotizing granulomatous vasculitis involving the respiratory tract (lung → cough/hemoptysis, and/or nasal airways → serosanguinous nasal drainage ± septal perforation→ characteristic "saddle nose deformity") and frequently the kidneys (no reported cases of kidney involvement without respiratory).[29]

Nasal obstruction and crusting are the usual initial findings. Arthralgia (not true arthritis) is present in > 50%.

Neurologic involvement usually consists of cranial nerve dysfunction (usually II, III, IV, & VI; less often V, VII, & VIII; and least commonly IX, X, XI, & XII) and peripheral neuropathies, with diabetes insipidus (occasionally preceding other symptoms by up to 9 months). Focal lesions of the brain and spinal cord occur less frequently.

11

Differential diagnosis
Differential diagnosis includes:
• "lethal midline granuloma" (may be similar or identical to polymorphic reticulosis) may evolve into lymphoma. May cause fulminant local destruction of the nasal tissue. Differentiation is crucial as this condition is treated by radiation; one should avoid immune suppression (e.g., cyclophosphamide). Probably does not involve true granulomas. Renal and tracheal involvement do not occur
• fungal disease: Sporothrix schenckii & Coccidioides may cause identical syndrome
• other vasculitides: especially eosinophilic granulomatosis with polyangiitis (EGPA) (p. 208) (asthma and peripheral eosinophilia usually seen), and PAN (granulomas usually lacking)

Evaluation
Biopsy of upper airways consists of removing all crusts, and obtaining as much friable mucosa as possible. This tissue should be fixed in formaldehyde and examined pathologically within 24 hrs (do not freeze). A sample should also be cultured (including fungal and acid-fast cultures). Renal biopsy should not be done when more specific tissue is available from the upper airway.

Serum ANCA (Antineutrophil Cytoplasmic Antibodies): confusingly also known as cANCA, pANCA, 3-ANCA, Serine Protease 3 (PR3), Myeloperoxidase Antibodies (MPO), Proteinase 3 Antibodies (PR3-ANCA), MPO-ANCA. Elevated serum levels of autoantibodies to proteinase 3 (PR3) antigen are characteristic for GPA, and are detected in 95% of histologically proven cases.

Treatment
Untreated, GPA is rapidly fatal, with a median survival of 5 months, and more than 90% of patients are dead within 2 years of diagnosis.[30]

Therapy usually involves
1. steroids
2. immune modulators: includes cyclophosphamide (Cytoxan®), methotrexate,[30] mofetil (CellCept®)
3. antibodies: rituximab (Rituxan®) especially for disease relapse. Belimumab (Benlysta®) is under investigation
4. under investigation: plasma exchange, anti B- & T-cell biologics, and interleuken-5

Eosinophilic granulomatosis with polyangiitis (EGPA)

Formerly known as (Churg-Strauss syndrome).

11.3.5 Other vasculitides

Periarteritis nodosa

AKA polyarteritis nodosa. Actually a group of necrotizing vasculitides, including:
• classic periarteritis nodosa (PAN): a multisystem disease with inflammatory necrosis, thrombosis (occlusion), and hemorrhage of arteries and arterioles in every organ except lung & spleen. Nodules may be palpated along medium sized muscular arteries. Commonly produces mononeuritis multiplex, weight loss, fever, and tachycardia. Peripheral nerve manifestations are attributed to arteritic occlusion of vasa nervorum. CNS manifestations are uncommon and include H/A, seizures, SAH, retinal hemorrhages, and stroke in ≈ 13%
• systemic necrotizing vasculitis

These patients do better when treated with cyclophosphamide rather than steroids.

11.3.6 Lymphomatoid granulomatosis

Rare; affects mainly the lungs, skin (erythematous macules or indurated plaques in 40%) and nervous system (CNS in 20%, peripheral neuropathies in 15%). Sinuses, lymph nodes, and spleen are usually spared.

11.3.7 Behçet's syndrome

Relapsing ocular lesions and recurrent oral and genital ulcers, with occasional skin lesions, thrombophlebitis, and arthritis.[10] H/A occur in > 50%. Neurologic involvement includes pseudotumor, cerebellar ataxia, paraplegia, seizures, and dural sinus thrombosis. Only 5% have neurologic symptoms as the presenting complaint.

86% have CSF pleocytosis and protein elevation. Cerebral angiography is usually normal. CT may show focal areas of enhancing low density.

Steroids usually ameliorate ocular and cerebral symptoms, but usually have no effect on skin and genital lesions. Uncontrolled trials of cytotoxic agents → some benefit. Thalidomide may be effective (uncontrolled studies), but carries risk of serious adverse effects (teratogenicity, peripheral neuropathy…).[31]

Although painful, the disease is usually benign. Neurologic involvement portends a worse prognosis.

11.3.8 Isolated CNS vasculitis

General information

AKA isolated angiitis of the CNS. Rare (≈ 20 cases reported[32] as of 1983); limited to vessels of CNS. Small vessel vasculitis is ≈ always present → segmental inflammation and necrosis of small leptomeningeal and parenchymal blood vessels with surrounding tissue ischemia or hemorrhage.[10]

Presentation

Combinations of H/A, confusion, dementia, and lethargy. Occasionally seizures. Focal and multifocal brain disturbance occurs in > 80%. Visual symptoms are frequent (secondary either to involvement of choroidal and retinal arteries, or to involvement of visual cortex → visual hallucinations).

Evaluation

ESR & WBC count are usually normal. CSF may be normal or have pleocytosis and/or elevated protein. CT may show enhancing areas of low density.

Angiography (required for diagnosis): characteristically shows multiple areas of symmetrical narrowing ("string of pearls" configuration). If normal, it does not exclude diagnosis.

Histological diagnosis (recommended): all biopsy material should be cultured. Brain parenchyma biopsy infrequently shows vasculitis. Leptomeningeal biopsy invariably shows involvement.

Treatment and outcome

Reportedly fatal if untreated, but may smolder for years.

Rarity of this condition makes treatment uncertain. Recommended: cyclophosphamide (Cytoxan®) 2 mg/kg/d and prednisone 1 mg/kg/d qod therapy.

NB: this condition is thought to be T-cell mediated, but prednisone causes more B-cell suppression, therefore breakthrough during prednisone therapy is not uncommon.

11.3.9 Hypersensitivity vasculitis

Neurologic involvement is not a prominent feature of this group of vasculitides, which include:
- drug induced allergic vasculitis: A number of drugs are associated with the development of cerebral vasculitis. These include methamphetamines ("speed"), cocaine (frank vasculitis occurs[33] but is rare), heroin, and ephedrine
- cutaneous vasculitis
- serum sickness: may → encephalopathy, seizures, coma, peripheral neuropathy and brachial plexopathy
- Henoch-Schönlein purpura

11.3.10 Fibromuscular dysplasia

General information

A vasculopathy (angiopathy) affecting primarily branches of the aorta, with renal artery involvement in 85% of cases (the most common site) and commonly associated with hypertension. The disease has an incidence of ≈ 1%, and results in multifocal arterial constrictions and intervening regions of aneurysmal dilatation.

The second most commonly involved site is the cervical internal carotid (primarily near C1–2), with fibromuscular dysplasia (FMD) appearing on 1% of carotid angiograms, making FMD the second most common cause of extracranial carotid stenosis.[34] Bilateral cervical ICA involvement occurs in ≈ 80% of cases. 50% of patients with carotid FMD have renal FMD. Patients with FMD have an increased risk of intracranial aneurysms and neoplasms, and are probably at higher risk of carotid dissection.

Aneurysms and fibromuscular dysplasia: The reported incidence of aneurysms with FMD[35] ranges from 20–50%.

Etiology

The actual etiology remains unknown, although congenital defects of the media (muscular layer) and internal elastic layer of the arteries have been identified, which may predispose the arteries to injury from otherwise well-tolerated trauma. A high familial rate of strokes, HTN, and migraine have supported the suggestion that FMD is an autosomal dominant trait with reduced penetrance in males.[36]

Presentation

Most patients have recurrent, multiple symptoms as shown in ▶ Table 11.4.

Up to 50% of patients present with episodes of transient cerebral ischemia or infarction. However, FMD may also be an incidental finding and some cases have been followed for 5 years without recurrence of ischemic symptoms, suggesting that FMD may be a relatively benign condition.

Headaches are commonly unilateral and may be mistaken for typical migraine. Syncope may be caused by involvement of the carotid sinus.

Horner syndrome occurs in ≈ 8% of cases. T-wave changes on EKG may be seen in up to one-third of cases, and may be due to involvement of the coronary arteries.

11

Table 11.4 Previous symptoms in 37 cases of aortocranial FMD[36]

Symptom	%
H/A	78
mental distress	48
tinnitus	38
vertigo	34
cardiac arrhythmia	31
TIA	31
syncope	31
carotidynia	21
epilepsy	15
hearing impairment	12
abdominal angina	8
angina/MI	8

Diagnosis

The "gold-standard" for the diagnosis of FMD is the angiogram. The three angiographic types of FMD[37] are shown in ▶ Table 11.5.

Table 11.5 Angiographic classification of FMD

Type	Findings
1	most common (80–100% of reported cases). Multiple, irregularly spaced, concentric narrowings with normal or dilated intervening segments giving rise to the so-called "string of pearls" appearance. Corresponds with arterial medial fibroplasia
2	focal tubular stenosis, seen in ≈ 7% of cases. Less characteristic for FMD than Type 1, and may also be seen in Takayasu's arteritis and other conditions
3	"atypical FMD." Rare. May take on various appearances, most commonly consisting of diverticular outpouchings of one wall of the artery

Treatment

Medical therapy, including antiplatelet medication (e.g., aspirin), has been recommended.

Direct surgical treatment is problem-ridden due to the difficult location (high carotid artery, near the base of the skull) and to the friable nature of the vessels, which makes anastamosis or arteriotomy closure difficult.

Transluminal angioplasty has achieved some degree of success. Carotid-cavernous fistulas and arterial rupture have been reported as complications.

11.3.11 Miscellaneous vasculopathies

CADASIL

Key concepts

- clinical: migraines, dementia, TIAs, psychiatric disturbances
- MRI: white matter abnormalities
- autosomal dominant inheritance
- anticoagulants controversial, generally discouraged

An acronym for Cerebral Autosomal Dominant Arteriopathy with Subcortical Infarcts and Leukoencephalopathy.[38] A familial disease with onset in early adulthood (mean age at onset: 45 ± 11 yrs), mapped to chromosome 19. Clinical and neuroradiologic features are similar to those seen with multiple subcortical infarcts from HTN, except there is no evidence of HTN. The vasculopathy is distinct from that seen in lipohyalinosis, arteriosclerosis and amyloid angiopathy, and causes thickening of the media (by eosinophilic, granular material) of leptomeningeal and perforating arteries measuring 100–400 mcm in diameter.

Clinical involvement
Recurrent subcortical infarcts (84%), progressive or stepwise dementia (31%), migraine with aura (22%), and depression (20%). All symptomatic and 18% of asymptomatic patients had prominent subcortical white-matter and basal ganglia hyperintensities on T2WI MRI.

Treatment
Warfarin (Coumadin®) is used by some.

11.3.12 Paraneoplastic syndromes affecting the nervous system

General information

Paraneoplastic syndromes (PNS), AKA "remote effects of cancer." Develop acutely or subacutely. May mimic or be mimicked by metastatic disease. The neurologic disability is usually severe, and may precede other manifestations of the cancer by 6–12 mos. Often one particular neural cell type is predominantly affected. The presence of a PNS may portend a more benign course of the cancer.

16% of patients with lung Ca, and 4% with breast Ca will develop a PNS.

Pathogenesis unknown. Theories: ? toxin; ? competition for essential substrate; ? opportunistic infection; ? auto-immune process.

Types of syndromes

1. affecting cerebrum or cerebellum
   a) encephalitis
      - diffuse
      - limbic and brainstem: usually due to small-cell lung Ca or testicular Ca[39] as a result of serum antineuronal antibodies
   b) "limbic encephalitis" (mesial): dementia (decreased memory, psychiatric symptoms, hallucinations)
   c) pan-cerebellar degeneration (PCD) AKA subacute cerebellar degeneration*: (see below)
   d) opsoclonus-myoclonus syndrome*: in peds, usually indicates neuroblastoma
2. affecting spinal cord
   a) poliomyelitis (anterior horn syndrome): mimics ALS (weakness, hyporeflexia, fasciculations)
   b) subacute necrotizing (transverse) myelitis: rapid necrosis of spinal cord
   c) ganglionitis* (dorsal root ganglion): chronic or subacute. Pure sensory neuronopathy (not neuropathy)
3. affecting peripheral nervous system
   a) chronic sensory-motor: typical neuropathy (as in DM or EtOH abuse)
   b) pure sensory (p. 1541) [40]
   c) pure motor: rare. Almost always due to lymphoma (mostly Hodgkin's)
   d) acute inflammatory demyelinating polyradiculopathy, AKA Guillain-Barré (p. 193)
   e) Eaton-Lambert (EL) myasthenic syndrome*: rare. 66% of patients with this syndrome will have cancer, most common primary is oat cell Ca of lung. Pre-synaptic neuromuscular junction (PSNMJ) blockade due to antibodies against the PSNMJ; NB: true myasthenia gravis (MG) is a post-synaptic block. Worse in AM, improves during day with recruitment (opposite of MG, which is worse at night or with exercise due to depletion). Mostly motor, but often accompanied by paresthesias. MG affects mostly nicotinic receptors, but EL also affects muscarinic receptors, and therefore autonomic symptoms may occur: dry mouth, males may have impotence. Repetitive nerve stimulation on EMG: for MG use 2–5 Hz stimulation, for EL use > 10 Hz, MG: decremental response with low frequency, with EL there is incremental response (more response with repeat stimulation).
   f) myasthenia gravis: due to antibodies against the postsynaptic acetylcholine receptors of the neuromuscular junction
   g) polymyositis: in age > 60 yrs, 25% of patients with this have a malignancy*, most often linked to bronchogenic Ca
   h) type IIb muscle fiber atrophy: the most common paraneoplastic syndrome; mainly proximal muscle weakness (same as in other endocrine myopathies, e.g., hypothyroid, steroid)

11

* "classic" neurologic PNS. In a patient without previous cancer history presenting with one of these syndromes with an asterisk, work-up for occult malignancy has high yield.

Pan-cerebellar degeneration

Severe Purkinje cell loss (due to anti-Purkinje cell antibody) → severe pan-cerebellar dysfunction. Presents with vertigo, gait and upper and lower extremity ataxia, dysarthria, N/V, diplopia, oscillopsia, nystagmus, oculomotor dysmetria. Usually not treatable nor remitting even with immune suppression. 20% of patients improve with treatment of the primary cancer. CT is WNL early, late → cerebellar atrophy. In 70% of cases, cerebellar findings precede diagnosis of cancer.

The most common primary malignancies in pan-cerebellar degeneration are shown in ▶ Table 11.6.

Table 11.6 Common primaries with pan-cerebellar degeneration

Women	Men
ovarian Ca breast uterus Hodgkin's lymphoma	lung Ca Hodgkin's lymphoma

Evaluation

- LP: CSF for cell count, cytology and IgG. Typically WBCs and IgG are elevated
- Evaluation for primary
  - CT of chest/abdomen/pelvis
  - lymph node exam
  - pelvic exam and mammogram in women

11.4 Neurotoxicology

11.4.1 Ethanol

General information

The acute and chronic effects of ethyl alcohol (ethanol, EtOH) abuse on the nervous system (not to mention the effects of EtOH on other organ systems) are protean,[41] and are beyond the scope of this text). Neuromuscular effects include:

1. acute intoxication: see below
2. effects of chronic alcohol abuse
   a) **Wernicke's encephalopathy** (p.214)
   b) cerebellar degeneration: due to degeneration of Purkinje cells in the cerebellar cortex, predominantly in the anterior superior vermis
   c) central pontine myelinolysis (p.119)
   d) stroke: increased risk of
      - intracerebral hemorrhage (p.1608)
      - ischemic stroke[42]
      - possibly aneurysmal SAH
   e) peripheral neuropathy (p.568)
   f) skeletal myopathy
3. effects of alcohol withdrawal: usually seen in habituated drinkers with cessation or reduction of ethanol intake
   a) alcohol withdrawal syndromes: see below
   b) seizures: up to 33% of patients have a generalized tonic-clonic seizure 7–30 hrs after cessation of drinking—see Alcohol withdrawal seizures (p.506)
   c) delirium tremens (**DTs**): see below

Acute intoxication

The primary effect of EtOH on the CNS is depression of neuronal excitability, impulse conduction, and neurotransmitter release due to direct effects on the cell membranes. ▶ Table 11.7 shows the clinical effects associated with specific EtOH concentrations. Mellanby effect: the severity of intoxication is greater at any given level when blood alcohol levels are rising than when falling.

In most jurisdictions, individuals with blood ethanol levels ≥ 21.7 mmol/l (100 mg/dl) are defined as legally intoxicated, and a number of states have changed this to 80 mg/dl. However, even levels of 10.2 mmol/l (47 mg/dl) are associated with increased risk of involvement in motor vehicle accidents.

Table 11.7 Blood ethanol concentrations

Blood alcohol concentration		Clinical effect
mmol/liter	mg/dl	
5.4	25	mild intoxication: altered mood, impaired cognition, incoordination
>21.7	100	vestibular and cerebellar dysfunction: increased nystagmus, diplopia, dysarthria, ataxia
>108.5	500	usually fatal from respiratory depression

Chronic alcoholism leads to increased tolerance; in habituated individuals survival with levels exceeding 1000 mg/dl has been reported.

Alcohol withdrawal syndrome

General information
Compensation for the CNS depressant effects of EtOH occurs in chronic alcoholism. Consequently, rebound CNS hyperactivity may result from falling EtOH levels. Clinical signs of EtOH withdrawal are classified as major or minor (the degree of autonomic hyperactivity and the presence/absence of DTs differentiates these), as well as early (24–48 hrs) or late (> 48 hrs).

Signs/symptoms include tremulousness, hyperreflexia, insomnia, N/V, agitation, myalgias, mild confusion, autonomic hyperactivity (tachycardia, systolic HTN), agitation, myalgias, mild confusion. If EtOH withdrawal seizures (p. 506) occur, they tend to be early. Perceptual disturbances or frank hallucinosis may also occur early. Hallucinosis consists of visual and/or auditory hallucinations with an otherwise clear sensorium (which distinguishes this from the hallucinations of DTs). DTs can occur 3–4 days after cessation of drinking (see below).

Suppressed by benzodiazepines, resumption of drinking, β-adrenergic antagonists, or α2-agonists.

Prevention of and treatment for alcohol withdrawal syndrome
See reference.[43]

Mild EtOH withdrawal is managed with a quiet, supportive environment, reorientation and one-to-one contact. If symptoms progress, institute pharmacologic treatment.

Benzodiazepines
Benzodiazepines (BDZs) are the mainstay of treatment. They reduce autonomic hyperactivity, and may prevent seizures and/or DTs. All BDZs are effective. Initial doses are shown in ▶ Table 11.8 and are higher than those used for treating anxiety. Symptom triggered dosing with repeated evaluation utilizing a standardized protocol (e.g., CIWA-Ar[44]) may be more efficacious than fixed-dose schedules.[45] Avoid IM administration (erratic absorption).

Table 11.8 Guidelines for BDZ doses for EtOH withdrawal[a]

Drug	Dose	
	Oral	IV
chlordiazepoxide (Librium®)	100 mg initially, then 25–50 mg PO TID-QID, gradually taper over ≈ 4 days). Additional doses may be needed for continuing agitation, up to 50 mg PO hourly[46]	–
lorazepam (Ativan®)	4 mg initially, then 1–2 mg PO q 4 hrs	1–2 mg q 1–2 hrs
diazepam (Valium®)	20 mg PO initially, then 10 mg PO BID-QID	5–10 mg initially
midazolam (Versed®)		titrate drip to desired effect

[a]modify as appropriate based on patient response

Adjunctive medications
Associated conditions commonly seen in patients experiencing alcohol withdrawal syndrome include dehydration, fluid and electrolyte disturbances, infection, pancreatitis, and alcoholic ketoacidosis, and should be treated accordingly.

Other medications used for EtOH withdrawal itself include:
1. drugs useful for controlling HTN (caution: these agents should not be used alone because they do not prevent progression to more severe levels of withdrawal, and they may mask symptoms of withdrawal)

a) β-blockers: also treat most associated *tachyarrhythmias*
  - *atenolol* (Tenormin®): reduces length of withdrawal and BDZ requirement
  - ✖ avoid propranolol (psychotoxic reactions)
b) α-agonists: do not use together with β-blockers

2. phenobarbital: an alternative to BDZs. Long acting, and helps prophylax against seizures
3. baclofen: a small study[47] found 10 mg PO q d X 30 days resulted in rapid reduction of symptoms after the initial dose and continued abstinence
4. "supportive" medications
   a) *thiamine*: 100 mg IM q d × 3 d (can be given IV if needed, but there is risk of adverse reaction). Rationale: high-concentration glucose may precipitate acute Wernicke's encephalopathy in patients with thiamine deficiency
   b) folate 1 mg IM, IV or PO q d × 3 d
   c) MgSO4 1 gm × 1 on admission: helpful only if magnesium levels are low, reduces seizure risk. Be sure renal function is normal before administering
   d) vitamin B12 for macrocytic anemia: 100 mcg IM (do not give before folate)
   e) multivitamins: of benefit only if patient is malnourished
5. seizures: see indications for treatment (p. 506)
   a) **phenytoin** (Dilantin®) (p. 488): load with 18 mg/kg = 1200 mg/70 kg
   b) continued seizures may sometimes be effectively treated with *paraldehyde* if available
6. ethanol drip: not widely used. 5% EtOH in D5 W, start at 20 cc/hr, and titrate to a blood level of 100–150 mg/dl

Delirium tremens (DTs)

When DTs occur, they usually begin within 4 days of the onset of EtOH withdrawal, and typically persist for 1–3 days.

Signs and symptoms include: profound disorientation, agitation, tremor, insomnia, hallucinations, severe autonomic instability (tachycardia, HTN, diaphoresis, hyperthermia).[48] Mortality is 5–10% (higher in elderly), but can be reduced with treatment (including treating associated medical problems and treatment for seizures).

Haloperidol and phenothiazines may control hallucinations, but can lower the seizure threshold. HTN and tachyarrhythmias should be treated as outlined above under Alcohol withdrawal syndrome (p. 213).

Wernicke's encephalopathy (WE)

General information
AKA Wernicke-Korsakoff encephalopathy (not to be confused with Korsakoff's syndrome or Korsakoff's psychosis). Classic triad: encephalopathy (consisting of global confusion), ophthalmoplegia, and ataxia (NB: all 3 are present in only 10–33% of cases).

Due to thiamine deficiency. Body stores of thiamine are adequate only for up to ≈ 18 days. May be seen in:
1. a certain susceptible subset of thiamine deficient alcoholics. Thiamine deficiency here is due to a combination of inadequate intake, reduced absorption, decreased hepatic storage, and impaired utilization
2. hyperemesis (as in some pregnancies)
3. starvation: including anorexia nervosa, rapid weight loss
4. gastroplication (bariatric surgery)
5. hemodialysis
6. cancers
7. AIDS
8. prolonged IV hyperalimentation

Clinical
Oculomotor abnormalities occur in 96% and include nystagmus (horizontal > vertical), lateral rectus palsy, conjugate-gaze palsies.

Gait ataxia is seen in 87%, and results from a combination of polyneuropathy, cerebellar dysfunction, and vestibular impairment.

Systemic symptoms may include vomiting, fever.

Diagnostic testing
MRI: May show high signal in T2WI and FLAIR images in the paraventricular (medial) thalamus, the floor of the 4th ventricle, and periaqueductal gray of the midbrain. These changes may resolve with treatment.[49] Atrophy of the mammillary bodies may also be seen. Normal MRI does not R/O the diagnosis.

Treatment
Wernicke's encephalopathy (WE) is a medical emergency. When WE is suspected, 100 mg thiamine should be given IM or IV (oral route is unreliable, see above) daily for 5 days. ✖ IV glucose can precipitate acute WE in thiamine deficient patients, ∴ give thiamine before glucose.

Thiamine administration improves eye findings within hours to days; ataxia and confusion improve in days to weeks. Many patients that survive are left with horizontal nystagmus, ataxia, and 80% have Korsakoff's syndrome (AKA Korsakoff's psychosis), a disabling memory disturbance involving retrograde and anterograde amnesia.

11.4.2 Opioids

Includes heroin (which is usually injected IV, but the powder can be snorted or smoked) as well as prescription drugs. Opioids produce small pupils (miosis).

Overdose may produce:
1. respiratory depression
2. pulmonary edema
3. coma
4. hypotension and bradycardia
5. seizures
6. fatal overdose may occur with any agent, but is more likely with synthetic opioids such as fentanyl (Sublimaze®) among users unfamiliar with their high potency

Reversal of intoxication[50]

A test dose of naloxone (Narcan®) 0.2 mg IV avoids sudden complete reversal of all opioid effects. If no significant reaction occurs, an additional 1.8 mg (for a total dose of 2 mg) will reverse the toxicity of most opioids. If needed, the dose may be repeated q 2–3 minutes up to a total of 10 mg, although even larger doses may be needed with pentazocine or buprenorphine (Buprenex®). Naloxone may precipitate narcotic withdrawal symptoms in opioid-dependent patients, with anxiety or agitation, piloerection, yawning, sneezing, rhinorrhea, nausea, vomiting, diarrhea, abdominal cramps, muscle spasms… which are uncomfortable but not life threatening. Clonidine (Catapres®) may be helpful for some narcotic withdrawal symptoms.

With longer acting opioids, especially methadone (Dolophine®), repeat doses of naloxone may be obviated by the use of nalmefene (Revex®), a long-acting narcotic antagonist which is not appropriate for the initial treatment of opioid overdosage.

11.4.3 Cocaine

Cocaine is extracted from Erythroxylon coca leaves (and other Erythroxylon species) and is thus unrelated to opioids. It blocks the re-uptake of norepinephrine by presynaptic adrenergic nerve terminals. It is available in 2 forms: cocaine hydrochloride (heat labile and water soluble, it is usually taken PO, IV or by nasal insufflation) and as the highly purified cocaine alkaloid (free base or crack cocaine, which is heat stable but insoluble in water and is usually smoked).

Peak toxicity occurs 60–90 minutes after ingestion (except for "body packers"), 30–60 minutes after snorting, and minutes after IV injection or smoking (freebase or crack).[50]

Acute pharmacologic effects of cocaine

Effects on body systems outside the nervous system include tachycardia, acute myocardial infarction, arrhythmias, rupture of ascending aorta (aortic dissection), abruptio placenta, hyperthermia, intestinal ischemia, and sudden death.

Acute pharmacologic effects pertinent to the nervous system include:
1. mental status: initial CNS stimulation that first manifests as a sense of well-being and euphoria. Sometimes dysphoric agitation results, occasionally with delirium. Stimulation is followed by

11

depression. Paranoia and toxic psychosis may occur with overdosage or chronic use. Addiction may occur
2. pupillary dilatation (mydriasis)
3. hypertension: from adrenergic stimulation

Non-pharmacologic effects related to the nervous system
1. pituitary degeneration: from chronic intranasal use
2. cerebral vasculitis: less common than with amphetamines
3. seizures: possibly related to the local anesthetic properties of cocaine
4. stroke[51]
   a) intracerebral hemorrhage: see Intracerebral hemorrhage, Etiologies (p. 1610)
   b) subarachnoid hemorrhage[52,53]: possibly as a result of HTN in the presence of aneurysms or AVMs, however, sometimes no lesion is demonstrated on angiography.[54] May possibly be due to cerebral vasculitis
   c) ischemic stroke[55]: may result from vasoconstriction
   d) thrombotic stroke[50]
   e) TIA[56]
5. anterior spinal artery syndrome[56]
6. effects of maternal cocaine use on the fetal nervous system include[57] microcephaly (p. 312), disorders of neuronal migration, neuronal differentiation and myelination, cerebral infarction, subarachnoid and intracerebral hemorrhage, and sudden infant death syndrome (SIDS) in the postnatal period

Treatment of toxicity
Most cocaine toxicity is too short-lived to be treated. Anxiety, agitation or seizures may be treated with IV benzodiazepines, e.g., lorazepam (p. 513). Refractory HTN may be treated with clevidipine (p. 131) or phentolamine (Regitine®) (p. 131). IV lidocaine used to treat cardiac arrhythmias may cause seizures.[50]

11.4.4 Amphetamines

Toxicity is similar to that of cocaine (see above), but longer in duration (may last up to several hours). Cerebral vasculitis may occur with prolonged abuse which may lead to cerebral infarction.

Elimination of amphetamines requires adequate urine output. Antipsychotic drugs such as haloperidol (Haldol®) should not be used because of risk of seizures.

11.4.5 Carbon monoxide

General information

Carbon monoxide (CO) is the largest source of death from poisoning in the U.S.A.

Normal cellular function requires $\approx$ 5 ml O_2/100 ml blood. Blood normally contains $\approx$ 20 ml O_2/100 ml.

CO binds to hemoglobin (Hb) with an affinity $\approx$ 250 times that of O_2, and it causes a left shift of the Hb/O_2 dissociation curve. It also binds to intracellular myoglobin.

Only $\approx$ 6% of patients show the classic "cherry-red" color of blood.

Clinical findings

Clinical findings related to CO-Hb levels are shown in ▶ Table 11.9.

Diagnostic studies

EKG changes are common, usually non-specific ST-T wave changes.

In cases of severe intoxication, CT may show symmetrical low attenuation in the globus pallidus; see differential diagnosis (p. 1673).

Outcome

Prognosticators
1. outcome is more closely correlated with hypotension than with actual CO-Hb level
2. coma

Table 11.9 Levels of CO-Hb

CO-Hb level (%)	Signs/symptoms[a]
0–10	none
10–20	mild H/A, mild DOE
20–30	throbbing H/A
30–40	severe H/A, dizziness, dimming of vision, impaired judgment
40–50	confusion, tachypnea, tachycardia, possible syncope
50–60	syncope, seizures, coma
60–70	coma, hypotension, respiratory failure, death
>70	rapidly fatal

[a]NB: cigarette smokers may have CO-Hb levels of 15% without signs or symptoms

3. metabolic acidosis
4. EEG
5. CT/MRI changes: in one study, the presence of MRI lesions after 1 month did not accurately predict subsequent outcome
6. CO-Hb level
7. other factors probably have an effect, including: age, severity of exposure

Approximately 40% of patients exposed to significant levels of CO die. 30–40% have transient symptoms but make a full recovery. 10–30% have persistent neurological sequelae including CO-encephalopathy (may be delayed in onset) – impaired memory, irritability, parietal lobe symptoms including various agnosias.
   Brain lesions:
1. white matter lesions:
   a) multifocal small necrotic lesions in deep hemispheres
   b) extensive necrotic zones along lateral ventricles
   c) Grinker's myelinopathy (not necrosis)
2. gray matter lesions:
   a) bilateral necrosis of globus pallidus
   b) lesions of hippocampal formation and focal cortical necrosis

11.4.6 Heavy metal toxicity

General information

Heavy metals causing clinical toxicities include lead, mercury, cadmium, and arsenic. Effects depend on the metal, the route, the dose, and whether the exposure is acute or chronic.

Lead poisoning

1. possible sources of exposure
   a) ingesting lead-based paint: usually occurs in infants and small children
   b) consuming water conveyed by lead pipes in plumbing
   c) fumes from gasoline containing lead
   d) workplace exposure: e.g., workers involved in manufacturing lead-acid batteries
2. systemic symptoms and effects
   a) GI: abdominal colic, nausea/vomiting, GI hemorrhage
   b) renal: lead is excreted by the kidneys and is toxic to them, producing proteinuria and renal failure
   c) bone marrow: suppression leads to anemia (see below) and leukopenia
3. neurologic involvement
   a) in children: hyperactivity, low IQ, encephalopathy (the adult brain is relatively resistant[58])
   b) peripheral neuropathy: essentially only occurs in industrial exposure. Findings: purely motor (unusual in toxic neuropathies which are usually length-dependent, sensory, and involve the feet first), primarily weakness of ankle dorsiflexors (producing wrist drop) and finger extensors. Lower extremity involvement is less common and is usually confined to weakness of foot dorsiflexion (foot drop) and toe extension

11

4. labs
   a) CBC: microcytic microchromic anemia with basophilic stippling of erythrocytes
   b) elevated blood lead levels: > 10 micrograms/dl
5. radiographs: lead lines e.g., on knee X-rays

References

[1] Bartynski WS. Posterior reversible encephalopathy syndrome, part 1: fundamental imaging and clinical features. AJNR Am J Neuroradiol. 2008; 29:1036–1042

[2] Port JD, Beauchamp NJ. Reversible Intracerebral Pathologic Entities Mediated by Vascular Autoregulatory Dysfunction. Radiographics. 1998; 18:353–367

[3] Lin KL, Hsu WC, Wang HS, et al. Hypertension-induced cerebellar encephalopathy and hydrocephalus in a male. Pediatric Neurology. 2006; 34:72–75

[4] Schaefer PW, Buonanno FS, Gonzalez RG, et al. Diffusion-Weighted Imaging Discriminates Between Cytotoxic and Vasogenic Edema in a Patient with Eclampsia. Stroke. 1997; 28:1082–1085

[5] Covarrubias DJ, Luetmer PH, Campeau NG. Posterior reversible encephalopathy syndrome: prognostic utility of quantitative diffusion-weighted MR images. AJNR. American Journal of Neuroradiology. 2002; 23:1038–1048

[6] Beeson JH, Duda EE. Computed Axial Tomography Scan Demonstration of Cerebral Edema in Eclampsia Preceded by Blindness. Obstetrics and Gynecology. 1982; 60:529–532

[7] Raps EC, Galetta SL, Broderick M, et al. Delayed Peripartum Vasculopathy: Cerebral Eclampsia Revisited. Annals of Neurology. 1993; 33:222–225

[8] Dekker GA, Sibai BM. Etiology and pathogenesis of preeclampsia: current concepts. American Journal of Obstetrics and Gynecology. 1998; 179:1359–1375

[9] Bartynski WS, Boardman JF, Zeigler ZR, et al. Posterior reversible encephalopathy syndrome in infection, sepsis, and shock. AJNR. American Journal of Neuroradiology. 2006; 27:2179–2190

[10] Moore PM, Cupps TR. Neurologic Complications of Vasculitis. Ann Neurol. 1983; 14:155–167

[11] Salvarani C, Cantini F, Boiardi L, et al. Polymyalgia rheumatica and giant-cell arteritis. New England Journal of Medicine. 2002; 347:261–271

[12] Salvarani C, Gabriel SE, O'Fallon WM, et al. The incidence of giant cell arteritis in Olmstead County, Minnesota: apparent fluctuations in a cyclic pattern. Annals of Internal Medicine. 1995; 123:192–194

[13] Machado EB, Michet CJ, Ballard DJ, et al. Trends in Incidence and Clinical Presentation of Temporal Arteritis in Olmstead County, Minnesota, 1950–1985. Arthritis Rheum. 1988; 31:745–749

[14] Hunder GG. Giant Cell (Temporal) Arteritis. Rheum Dis Clin N Amer. 1990; 16:399–409

[15] Allen NB, Studenski SA. Polymyalgia Rheumatica and Temporal Arteritis. Med Clin N Amer. 1986; 70:369–384

[16] Hall S, Hunder GG. Is Temporal Artery Biopsy Prudent? Mayo Clin Proc. 1984; 59:793–796

[17] Caselli RJ, Danube JR, Hunder GG, et al. Peripheral neuropathic syndromes in giant cell (temporal) arteritis. Neurology. 1988; 38:685–689

[18] Salvarani C, Hunder GG. Giant cell arteritis with low erythrocyte sedimentation rate: frequency of occurrence in a population-based study. Arthritis and Rheumatism. 2001; 45:140–145

[19] Baumel B, Eisner LS. Diagnosis and Treatment of Headache in the Elderly. Med Clin N Amer. 1991; 75:661–675

[20] Karacostas D, Taskos N, Nikolaides T. CT Findings in Temporal Arteritis: A Report of Two Cases. Neurorad. 1986; 28

[21] McDonnell PJ, Moore GW, Miller NR, et al. Temporal Arteritis: A Clinicopathologic Study. Ophthalmology. 1986; 93:518–530

[22] Hall S, Lie JT, Kurland LT, et al. The Therapeutic Impact of Temporal Artery Biopsy. Lancet. 1983; 2:1217–1220

[23] Achkar AA, Lie JT, Hunder GG, et al. How does previous corticosteroid treatment affect the biopsy findings in giant cell (temporal) arteritis? Annals of Internal Medicine. 1994; 120:987–992

[24] Hunder GG, Kelley WN, Harris ED, et al. Giant Cell Arteritis and Polymyalgia Rheumatica. In: Textbook of Rheumatology. 4th ed. Philadelphia: W. B. Saunders; 1993:1103–1112

[25] Kent RB, Thomas L. Temporal Artery Biopsy. Am Surg. 1989; 56:16–21

[26] Chuang TY, Hunder GG, Ilstrup DM, et al. Polymyalgia Rheumatica: A 10-Year Epidemiologic and Clinical Study. Ann Intern Med. 1982; 97:672–680

[27] Salvarani C, Gabriel SE, O'Fallon WM, et al. Epidemiology of polymyalgia rheumatica in Olmstead County, Minnesota, 1970-1991. Arthritis and Rheumatism. 1995; 38:369–373

[28] Cantini F, Salvarani C, Olivieri I, et al. Erythrocyte sedimentation rate and C-reactive protein in the evaluation of disease activity and severity in polymyalgia rheumatica: a prospective follow-up study. Seminars in Arthritis and Rheumatism. 2000; 30:17–24

[29] McDonald TJ, DeRemee RA. Wegener's Granulomatosis. Laryngoscope. 1983; 93:220–231

[30] Sneller MC. Wegener's Granulomatosis. Journal of the American Medical Association. 1995; 273:1288–1291

[31] New Uses of Thalidomide. Medical Letter. 1996; 38:15–16

[32] Cupps TR, Moore PM, Fauci AS. Isolated angiitis of the central nervous system: prospective diagnostic and therapeutic experience. Am J Med. 1983; 74:97–105

[33] Kaye BR, Fainstat M. Cerebral Vasculitis Associated with Cocaine Abuse. JAMA. 1987; 258:2104–2106

[34] Hasso AN, Bird CR, Zinke DE, et al. Fibromuscular Dysplasia of the Internal Carotid Artery: Percutaneous Transluminal Angioplasty. AJR. 1981; 136:955–960

[35] Mettinger KL. Fibromuscular Dysplasia and the Brain II: Current Concept of the Disease. Stroke. 1982; 13:53–58

[36] Mettinger KL, Ericson K. Fibromuscular Dysplasia and the Brain: Observations on Angiographic, Clinical, and Genetic Characteristics. Stroke. 1982; 13:46–52

[37] Osborn AG, Anderson RE. Angiographic Spectrum of Cervical and Intracranial Fibromuscular Dysplasia. Stroke. 1977; 8:617–626

[38] Chabriat H, Vahedi K, Iba-Zizen MT, et al. Clinical Spectrum of CADASIL: A Study of Seven Families. Lancet. 1995; 346:934–939

[39] Voltz R, Gultekin SH, Rosenfeld MR, et al. A Serologic Marker of Paraneoplastic Limbic and Brain-Stem Encepahlitis in Patients with Testicular Cancer. New England Journal of Medicine. 1999; 340:1788–1795

[40] Denny-Brown D. Primary Sensory Neuropathy with Muscular Changes Associated with Carcinoma. Journal of Neurology, Neurosurgery, and Psychiatry. 1948; 11:73–87

[41] Charness ME, Simon RP, Greenberg DA. Ethanol and the Nervous System. N Engl J Med. 1989; 321:442–454

[42] Gorelick PB. Alcohol and stroke. Stroke. 1987; 18:268–271

[43] Lohr RH. Treatment of Alcohol Withdrawal in Hospitalized Patients. Mayo Clinic Proceedings. 1995; 70:777–782

[44] Sullivan JT, Sykora K, Schneiderman J, et al. Assessment of Alcohol Withdrawal: The Revised Clinical Institute Withdrawal Assessment for Alcohol Scale (CIWA-Ar). Br J Addict. 1989; 84:1353–1357

[45] Saitz R, Mayo-Smith MF, Roberts MS, et al. Individualized Treatment for Alcohol Withdrawal: A Randomized Double-Blind Controlled Trial. Journal of the American Medical Association. 1994; 272: 519–523

[46] Lechtenberg R, Worner TM. Seizure Risk With Recurrent Alcohol Detoxification. Arch Neurol. 1990; 47:535–538

[47] Addolorato G, Caputo F, Capristo E, et al. Rapid suppression of alcohol withdrawal syndrome by baclofen. Am J Med. 2002; 112:226–229

[48] Treatment of Alcohol Withdrawal. Medical Letter. 1986; 28:75–76

[49] Watson WD, Verma A, Lenart MJ, et al. MRI in acute Wernicke's encephalopathy. Neurology. 2003; 61

[50] Acute Reactions to Drugs of Abuse. Medical Letter. 1996; 38:43–46

[51] Fessler RD, Esshaki CM, Stankewitz RC, et al. The Neurovascular Complications of Cocaine. Surgical Neurology. 1997; 47:339–345

[52] Lichtenfeld PJ, Rubin DB, Feldman RS. Subarachnoid Hemorrhage Precipitated by Cocaine Snorting. Archives of Neurology. 1984; 41:223–224

[53] Oyesiku NM, Collohan ART, Barrow DL, et al. Cocaine-Induced Aneurysmal Rupture: An Emergent Negative Factor in the Natural History of Intracranial Aneurysms? Neurosurgery. 1993; 32:518–526

[54] Schwartz KA, Cohen JA. Subarachnoid Hemorrhage Precipitated by Cocaine Snorting. Arch Neurol. 1984; 41

[55] Levine SR, Brust JCM, Futrell N, et al. Cerebrovascular Complications of the Use of the 'Crack' Form of Alkaloidal Cocaine. N Engl J Med. 1990; 323:699–704

[56] Mody CK, Miller BL, McIntyre HB, et al. Neurologic Complications of Cocaine Abuse. Neurology. 1988; 38:1189–1193

[57] Volpe JJ. Effect of Cocaine Use on the Fetus. New England Journal of Medicine. 1992; 327:399–407

[58] Thomson RM, Parry GJ. Neuropathies associated with excessive exposure to lead. Muscle Nerve. 2006; 33:732–741

11

Part III

Imaging and Diagnostics

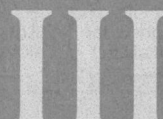

12 Plain Radiology and Contrast Agents

12.1 C-Spine X-rays

12.1.1 Normal findings

For radiographic signs of cervical spine trauma, see ▶ Table 69.2, and for guidelines for diagnosing clinical instability, see ▶ Table 71.4.

Contour lines

On a lateral C-spine X-ray, there are 4 contour lines (AKA arcuate lines). Normally each should form a smooth, gentle curve (▶ Fig. 12.1):
1. posterior marginal line (PML): along the posterior cortical surfaces of the vertebral bodies (VB). Marks the anterior margin of spinal canal

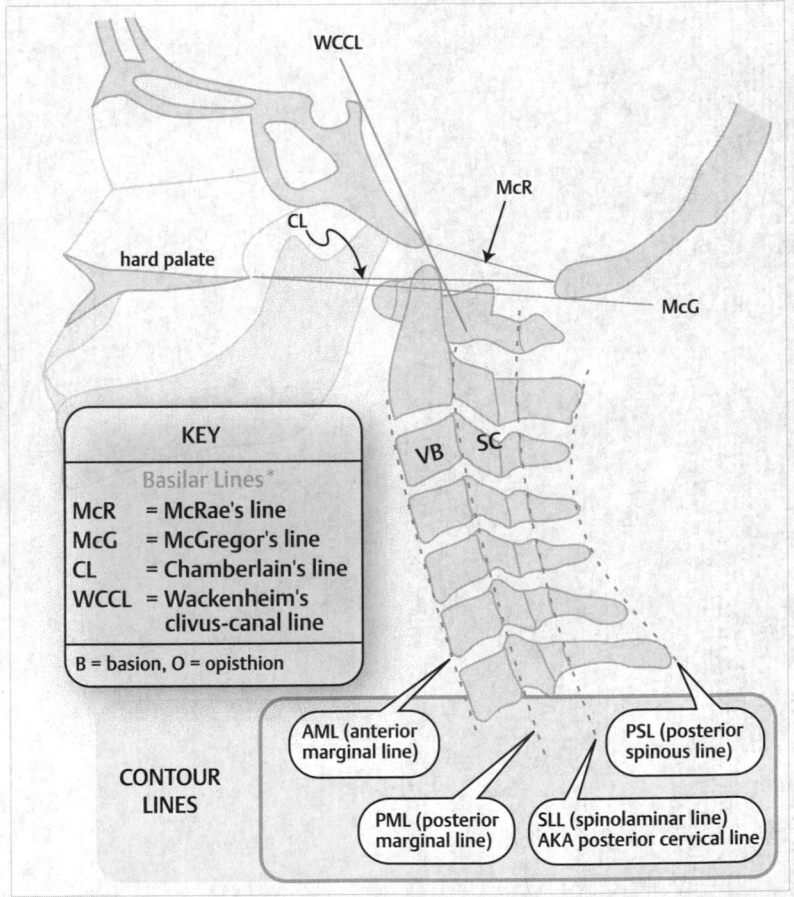

Fig. 12.1 Spinal contour lines and lines used to diagnose **basilar invagination.**
Image: lateral schematic of cervical spine and craniocervical junction.
* See discussion of the basilar lines (p. 228).

2. anterior marginal line (AML): along the anterior cortical surfaces of VBs
3. spinolaminar line (SLL) AKA posterior cervical line of Swischuk[1]. Along the base of the spinous processes. The posterior margin of the spinal canal
4. posterior spinous line (PSL): along tips of spinous processes

Relation of atlas to occiput

See also criteria for atlantooccipital dislocation (AOD) (p. 1153).

Relation of atlas to axis

These measurements are useful for atlantoaxial subluxation/dislocation (p. 1158) e.g., in trauma, rheumatoid arthritis (p. 1377) or Down syndrome (p. 1381).

12.1.2 Rule of Spence*

On AP or open-mouth odontoid X-ray, if the sum total overhang of both C1 lateral masses (so-called lateral mass displacement [LMD]) on C2 is ≥ 7 mm ($x + y$ in ► Fig. 12.8), the transverse atlantal ligament (TAL) is probably disrupted[2,3] (when corrected for an 18% magnification factor, it has been suggested that the criteria be increased to ≥ 8.2 mm[4]).

* NB: This rule is a surrogate marker for disruption of the TAL, and is insufficiently accurate (low sensitivity and low specificity) for clinical decisions.[5,6] Modern imaging methods are more accurate when they can be applied. It is therefore recommended that the use of this rule be discontinued. It is presented here for completeness as it appears in a number of management protocols.

12.1.3 (Anterior) atlantodental interval (ADI)

Note: ADI usually refers to the *anterior* atlantodental interval (there is also a posterior ADI (p. 223) as well as a lateral ADI which can be seen on AP radiographs).

AKA predental space or interval. The distance between the anterior margin of the dens and the closest point of the anterior arch of C1 ("C1 button") on a lateral C-spine X-ray (► Fig. 12.2). The normal maximal ADI is variously given in the range of 2 to 4 mm.[7,8] Commonly accepted upper limits are shown in ► Table 12.1. An abnormally increased ADI is a surrogate marker for TAL disruption.[9]

12

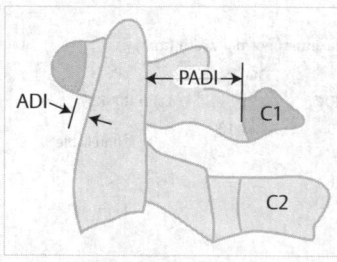

Fig. 12.2 **The atlantodental interval (ADI)** (p. 223) (AKA predental space or interval) and **posterior atlantodental interval (PADI)** (p. 223) on a lateral C-spine X-ray.

Table 12.1 Normal ADI		
Patient		**ADI**
adults	males	≤ 3 mm
	females	≤ 2.5 mm
pediatrics[10] (≤ 15 yrs)		≤ 4 mm

12.1.4 Posterior atlantodental interval (PADI)

AKA the neural canal width (NCW).[11] The PADI is the AP diameter of the *bony* canal at C1 and is measured from the back of the odontoid to the anterior aspect of the posterior C1 ring (► Fig. 12.2). It is more useful than the ADI for some conditions, e.g., AAS in rheumatoid arthritis (p. 1377) or Down syndrome (p. 1381).

12.1.5 Canal diameter

Definition: the spinal canal diameter (SCD in ▶ Fig. 12.1) as measured on an AP lateral spine X-ray (or sagittal CT/MRI) is defined as the distance from the posterior vertebral body to the spinolaminar line (SLL).

When a bony osteophyte is present on the posterior VB, the residual canal diameter (RCD in ▶ Fig. 12.1) can be measured from the posterior aspect of the osteophyte to the SLL.

X-ray technique: standard technique for lateral c-spine X-rays: patient positioned with the left shoulder resting against the film cassette or image detector and an X-ray source to image detector distance (SID) of 150-180 cm (roughly 5-6 feet) with the X-ray beam centered on C4.[12]

Values: the normal SCD measurement from C3 to T1 on a plain X-ray is 15 mm ± 5 mm.[13] Various cutoffs have been used,[14] but most agree that congenital bony stenosis of the spinal canal is present when the AP canal diameter on a plain lateral X-ray is **< 12 mm** in an adult.

Limitations: The X-ray technique described above allows for variablity in magnification that introduces measurement inaccuracies (noise). To compensate, a rule of thumb is that the SCD should be the same or greater than the AP diameter of the VB (VBD in ▶ Fig. 12.1). However, narrowing of the bony canal is a surrogate marker for spinal cord compression, which also depends on soft tissues not demonstrated on an X-ray (herniated discs, hypertrophied ligaments...), ligamentous ossification as well as the diameter of the spinal cord itself, all of which can be visualized directly on MRI or myelography.

12.1.6 Prevertebral soft tissue

Abnormally increased prevertebral soft tissue (PVST) may indicate the presence of a vertebral fracture, dislocation, or ligamentous disruption.[16] Normal values for lateral C-spine X-ray and CT scan are presented in ▶ Table 12.2 and illustrated for CT in ▶ Fig. 12.3. Plain films are subject to errors due to magnification and rotation. Multi-detector CT (MDCT) eliminates these shortcomings.[15]

Increased PVST is more likely with anterior than posterior injuries.[17] NB: the sensitivity of these measurements is only ≈ 60% at C3 and 5% at C6.[16] False positives may occur with basal skull/facial fractures, especially with fracture of the pterygoid plates. An ET-tube may allow fluid to accumulate in the posterior oropharynx which can obscure this measurement. In this setting, one can look for a thin fat layer between the prevertebral muscles and the posterior pharynx on cervical CT (▶ Fig. 12.3); the prevertebral tissue (posterior to this line) will be thickened (no measurements available at this time). MRI can also demonstrate abnormal signal within the prevertebral tissue.

Table 12.2 Normal prevertebral soft tissue

Space	Level	Maximum normal width (mm)		
		Adults		Peds
		MDCT		Lateral X-Ray
retropharyngeal	C1	8.5	10	unreliable
	C2–4	6–7[a]	5–7	
retrotracheal	C5–7	18	22	14

[a]CT data was deemed unreliable at C4[15]

12.1.7 Interspinous distances

C-spine AP: a fracture-dislocation or ligament disruption may be diagnosed if the interspinous distance is 1.5 times that at both adjacent levels (measured from center of spinous processes).[18] Also look for a malalignment of spinous processes below a certain level which may be evidence of rotation due to a unilaterally locked facet (p. 1187).

C-spine lateral: look for **"fanning"** or **"flaring"** which is an abnormal spread of one pair of spinous processes that may also indicate ligament disruption.

12.1.8 Pediatric C-spine

C1 (atlas)

Ossification centers[19]: usually 3 (▶ Fig. 12.4)
- 1 (sometimes 2) for body (not ossified at birth; appears on X-ray during 1st yr)
- 1 for each neural arch (appear bilaterally ≈ 7th fetal week)

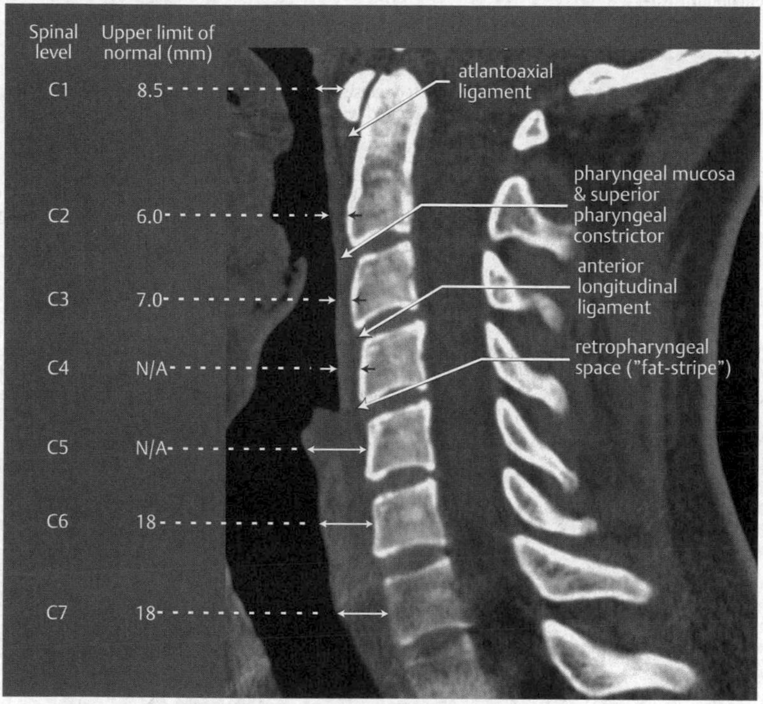

Spinal level	Upper limit of normal (mm)	
C1	8.5	atlantoaxial ligament
C2	6.0	pharyngeal mucosa & superior pharyngeal constrictor
C3	7.0	anterior longitudinal ligament
C4	N/A	retropharyngeal space ("fat-stripe")
C5	N/A	
C6	18	
C7	18	

Fig. 12.3 Sagittal CT scan through cervical spine showing normal prevertebral soft tissue dimensions.

12

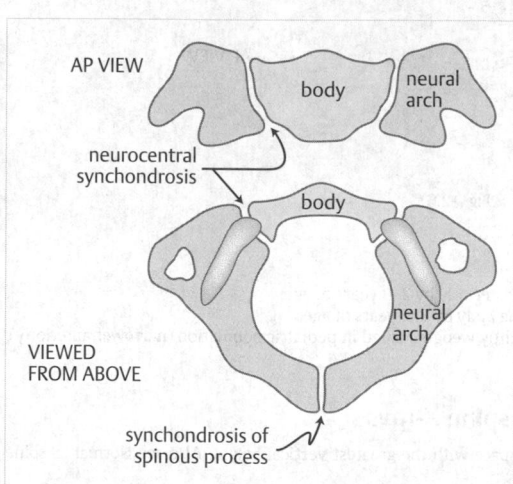

Fig. 12.4 Pediatric C1 (atlas).

AP VIEW

body

neural arch

neurocentral synchondrosis

body

neural arch

VIEWED FROM ABOVE

synchondrosis of spinous process

Synchondroses[19]:
- synchondrosis of the spinous process: fuses by ≈ 3 yrs of age
- 2 neurocentral synchondroses: fuse by ≈ 7 yrs of age

The ossification centers of C1 fail to completely close in 5% of adults (usually posteriorly). When present, the rare anterior defect is usually associated with a posterior defect.

C2 (axis)

Developmentally there are 5 ossification centers. The two halves of the odontoid fuse together in the midline (dashed line in ► Fig. 12.5) at 7 months development, so that at birth there are 4 primary ossification centers (► Fig. 12.5):
- odontoid process
- vertebral body
- 2 neural arches

The posterior arches fuse together by 2–3 years of age. The anterior synchondroses normally fuse between 3 and 6 years of age. However, the dentocentral synchondrosis (AKA subdental synchondrosis) may be visible on X-ray until ≈ 11 years of age. A secondary ossification center (os terminale) appears at the summit of the dens between 3 and 6 years of age, and fuses with the dens by age 12 years.[19]

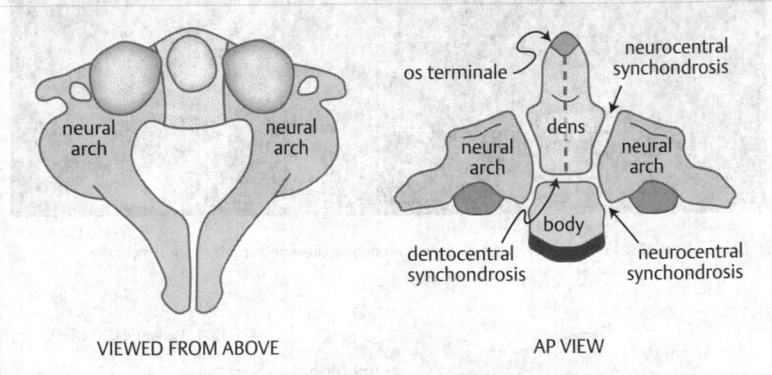

neurocentral synchondrosis

os terminale

dens

neural arch   neural arch

neural arch   neural arch

dentocentral synchondrosis   neurocentral synchondrosis

body

VIEWED FROM ABOVE   AP VIEW

Fig. 12.5 Pediatric C2 (axis).

C3–7

3 ossification centers at birth[20] (see ► Fig. 12.6).
- vertebral body
- 2 neural arches

The 2 neural arches fuse together posteriorly by 2–3 years of age.
   The neural arches each fuse to the body by 3–6 years of age.
   Cervical bodies are normally slightly wedge-shaped in pediatric population (narrower anteriorly). Wedging decreases with age.

12.2 Lumbosacral (LS) spine X-rays

L4–5 is normally the lumbar disc space with the greatest vertical height. Also see Normal LS spine measurements (p. 1333).
   AP view: look for defect or non visualization of the "owl's eyes" which is due to pedicle erosion, which may occur with lytic tumors (common with metastatic disease).
   Oblique views: look for discontinuity in neck of "Scotty dog" for defect in pars interarticularis.

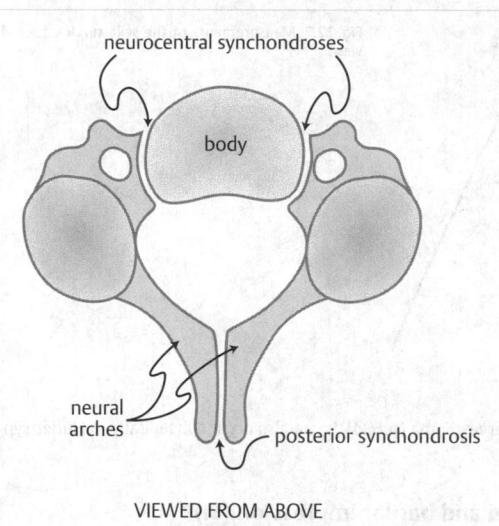

Fig. 12.6 Pediatric C3–7.

neurocentral synchondroses

body

neural arches

posterior synchondrosis

VIEWED FROM ABOVE

Butterfly vertebra: An uncommon congenital anomaly thought to arise from failure of fusion of the lateral halves of the VB due to persistent notochord tissue, producing a "butterfly" appearance on AP X-rays or coronal CT scan reconstructions. The involved VB is widened, and adjacent vertebrae may show a compensatory deformity as if to fill in some of the gap. May be associated with other spinal and rib malformations.[21] On lateral views may simulate compression fracture. In severe cases, there may be significant kyphosis and/or scoliosis. Often asymptomatic, requiring no treatment. May be associated with lipomyelomeningocele (p.284).

12.3 Skull X-rays

Water's view: AKA submental vertex view. X-ray tube angled up 45° (perpendicular to clivus). Towne's view: X-ray tube angled down 45°, to view occiput.

12.3.1 Sella turcica

Normal adult dimensions on skull X-ray

Technique: true lateral, 91 cm target to film distance, central ray 2.5 cm anterior and 1.9 cm superior to EAM. ▶ Table 12.3 shows normal values (▶ Fig. 12.7 shows how measurements are made).
  Depth (D): defined as the greatest measurement from floor to diaphragma sellae.
  Length (L): defined as the greatest AP diameter.

Table 12.3 Normal sella turcica dimensions (▶ Fig. 12.7)			
Dimension	Max	Min	Avg
D (depth) (mm)	12	4	8.1
L (length) (mm)	16	5	10.6

Abnormal findings

PitNet/adenomas tend to enlarge the sella, in contrast to craniopharyngiomas which erode the posterior clinoids. Empty sella syndrome tends to balloon the sella symmetrically, and also does not erode the clinoids. Tuberculum meningiomas usually do not enlarge the sella, and may be associated with enlargement of the sphenoid sinus; see sphenoid pneumosinus dilatans (p.1654).

12

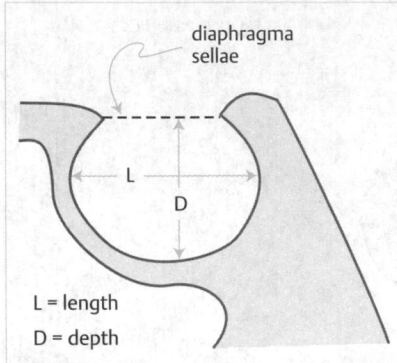

diaphragma
sellae

L = length
D = depth

Fig. 12.7 **Measurements of the sella turcica.** Lateral view.

"J" shaped sella suggests optic nerve glioma (p.694). It can also occur congenitally in Hurler syndrome (a mucopolysaccharidosis).

12.3.2 Basilar invagination and basilar impression (BI)

Terminology

The terms basilar impression and basilar invagination are often used interchangeably in the literature: historically, basilar invagination (AKA cranial settling) denoted upward indentation of the skull base, usually due to acquired softening of bone (see below); often associated with atlantooccipital fusion, while basilar impression implied normal bone. Making a distinction seems pointless (the abbreviation (BI) will be used for either). Common feature: upward displacement of the upper cervical spine (including odontoid process, AKA cranial migration of the odontoid) through the foramen magnum into the p-fossa.

Platybasia: flattening of the skull base. Originally assessed on plain X-rays (which are subject to error due to skull rotation or difficulty identifying landmarks), now more commonly evaluated on CT or MRI. May or may not be associated with BI, and may occur in association with craniofacial abnormalities, Chiari 1.5 malformation, Paget's disease…

Quantitated by measuring the basal angle, which on plain X-rays, measured the angle between lines drawn from the nasion to center of sella and then to the anterior foramen magnum,[22] but on MRI was felt to be better represented by the angle between a line drawn along the floor of the anterior fossa to the dorsum sellae and a second line drawn along the posterior clivus.[23] Normal mean basal angle: 130°. Platybasia: > 145° (abnormally obtuse basal angle).

Two subtypes of BI

See reference.[24]

Type I: BI without Chiari malformation. Tip of odontoid tends to be above CL, McR, and WCCL in ▶ Fig. 12.8. Brainstem compression is due to odontoid process invagination. 85% can be reduced with traction. Treatment: transoral surgery is recommended, usually accompanied by posterior fusion

Type II: BI + Chiari malformation. Odontoid tip tends to be above CL, but not McR or WCCL. Brainstem compression is due to reduced p-fossa volume. Only 15% can be reduced with traction. Foramen magnum decompression is appropriate

Measurements used in BI

(▶ Fig. 12.1 and ▶ Fig. 12.8):
1. McRae's line ("McR" in ▶ Fig. 12.1): drawn across foramen magnum (tip of clivus (basion) to opisthion).[25] The mean position of the odontoid tip below the line is 5 mm (± 1.8 mm SD) on CT and 4.6 mm (± 2.6 mm SD) on MRI.[26] No part of odontoid should be above this line (the most accurate measure for BI)

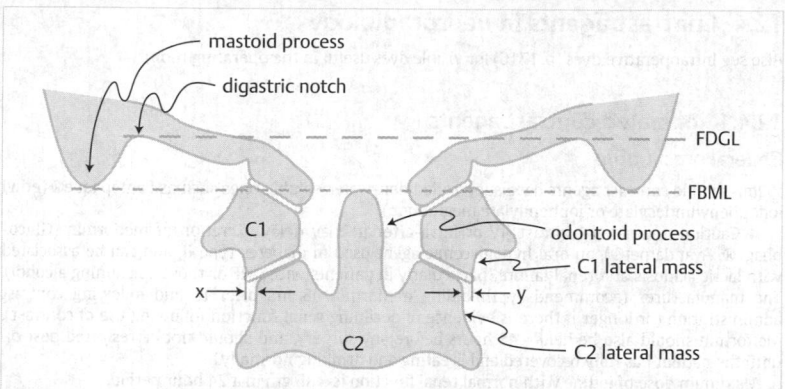

Fig. 12.8 Craniocervical junction. Image: diagram, AP view.
FDGL = Fischgold's digastric line; FBML = Fischgold's bimastoid line; x + y = total overhang of C1 on C2 (AKA lateral mass displacement); see Rule of Spence (p. 1161).

2. Chamberlain's line ("CL" in ▶ Fig. 12.1)[27]: posterior hard palate to posterior margin of foramen magnum (opisthion). Less than 3 mm or half of dens should be above this line, with 6 mm being definitely pathologic. Seldom used because the opisthion is often hard to see on plain film and may also be invaginated. On CT[28] and MRI[26] the normal odontoid tip is 1.4 mm (± 2.4) below the line

3. McGregor's baseline ("McG" in ▶ Fig. 12.1)[29]: posterior margin of hard palate to most caudal point of occiput. No more than 4.5 mm of dens should be above this. On CT[28] and MRI[26] the normal odontoid tip is 0.8 mm (± 2.4) above the line

4. Wackenheim's clivus-canal line ("WCCL" in ▶ Fig. 12.1): the odontoid should be tangential to or below the line that extends the course of the clivus (the clivus baseline). If the clivus is concave or convex, this baseline is drawn to connect the basion to the base of the posterior clinoids on the clivus[30]

5. (Fischgold's) digastric line ("FDGL" in ▶ Fig. 12.8): joins the digastric notches. The normal distance from this line to the middle of the atlantooccipital joint is 10 mm (decreased in BI).[31] No part of the odontoid should be above this line. More accurate than the bimastoid line (FBML)

6. Fischgold's bimastoid line ("FBML" in ▶ Fig. 12.8): joins tips of mastoid processes. The odontoid tip averages 2 mm above this line (range: 3 mm below to 10 mm above) and this line should cross the atlantooccipital joint

Conditions associated with BI

1. congenital conditions (BI is the most common congenital anomaly of the craniocervical junction; it is often accompanied by other anomalies[32(p 148–9)])
   a) Down syndrome
   b) Klippel-Feil syndrome (p. 289)
   c) Chiari malformation (p. 295): in a series of 100 patients, 92 had BI[33]
   d) syringomyelia
2. acquired conditions
   a) rheumatoid arthritis (in part due to incompetence of transverse ligament, see Basilar impression in rheumatoid arthritis (p. 1379)
   b) posttraumatic
3. conditions with BI associated with softening of bone include[34]:
   a) Paget's disease
   b) osteogenesis imperfecta: patients have blue discolored sclera and early hearing loss due to a genetic defect that causes defective Type 1 collagen. Bones are weak ("brittle-bone disease"). Autosomal dominant inheritance. There are 4 common types of OI and some uncommon ones
   c) osteomalacia
   d) rickets
   e) hyperparathyroidism

12

12.4 Contrast agents in neuroradiology

Also see Intraoperative dyes (p. 1716) for visible dyes useful in the operating room.

12.4.1 Iodinated contrast agents

General precautions

Water-soluble contrast agents have superseded non-water-soluble ones such as Pantopaque® (ethyl iodophenylundecylate or iophendylate meglumine).

✖ Caution: iodinated contrast (IV or intra-arterial) may delay excretion of metformin (Glucophage®, Avandamet®), an oral hypoglycemic agent used in diabetes type II, and can be associated with lactic acidosis and renal failure (particularly in patients with CHF or those consuming alcohol). The manufacturer recommends withholding metformin 48 hrs prior to and following contrast administration (or longer if there is evidence of declining renal function following use of contrast). Metformin should also be held ≈ 48 hours before any surgery, and should not be restarted post-op until the patient has fully recovered and is eating and drinking normally.

Maximum dose of iodine with normal renal function is ≈ 86 gm in a 24 hour period.

Intrathecal contrast agents

Inadvertent intrathecal injection of unapproved contrast agents

✖ Caution: serious reactions can occur with inadvertent intrathecal injection (e.g., for myelography, cisternography, ventriculography…) of iodinated contrast media that are not specifically indicated for intrathecal use (including ionic contrast agents as well as some non-ionic agents [e.g., Optiray®, Reno-60…]). This can cause uncontrollable seizures, intracerebral hemorrhage, cerebral edema, coma, paralysis, arachnoiditis, myoclonus (tonic-clonic muscle spasms), rhabdomyolysis with subsequent renal failure, hyperthermia, and respiratory compromise, with a significant fatality rate.[35]

Management suggestions for inadvertent intrathecal injection include:

1. immediately remove CSF + contrast if the error is recognized when the opportunity is available (e.g., withdraw fluid through myelography needle)
2. elevate head of bed ≈ 45° (to keep contrast out of head)
3. if there is a question about what may have occurred (i.e., it is not certain if an inappropriate contrast agent was used), send blood and CSF with contrast for high-performance liquid chromatography for identification of agent[36]
4. antihistamines: e.g., diphenhydramine (Benadryl®) 50 mg deep IM
5. respiration: supplemental oxygen, and if needed, intubation
6. control HTN
7. IV hydration
8. IV steroids
9. sedation if patient is agitated
10. treat fever with acetaminophen and if needed with a cooling blanket
11. pharmacologic paralysis if necessary to manage muscle activity
12. antiseizure medication: more than one agent may be required (e.g., phenytoin + phenobarbital + a benzodiazepine)
13. consider unenhanced brain CT scan: may help assess if contrast has diffused intracranially, but this requires placing patient flat and may not be advisable
14. insert lumbar subarachnoid drain with CSF drainage (e.g., 10 cc q hr)
15. monitor: electrolytes, antiseizure medication levels, creatine phosphokinase (CPK)
16. repeat EEGs to assess seizure activity while sedated/paralyzed

Iohexol (Omnipaque®)

The primary approved agent employed for intrathecal use today is iohexol (Omnipaque®).

A non-ionic triiodinated compound. Concentration is expressed as follows: e.g., Omnipaque 300 contains the equivalent of 300 mg of organic iodine per ml of media (300 mgI/ml).

Used for myelography, cisternography as well as IV contrasted CT. Uses and concentrations are shown in ▶ Table 12.4.

Table 12.4 Iohexol concentrations for adults

Procedure	Concentration (mgI/ml)	Volume (ml)
lumbar myelography via LP	180 240	10–17 7–12.5
thoracic myelography via LP or cervical injection	240 300	6–12.5 6–10
cervical myelography via LP	240 300	6–12.5 6–10
cervical myelography via C1–2 puncture	180 240 300	7–10 6–12.5 4–10
complete myelography via LP	240 300	6–12.5 6–10
cerebral arteriography[a]	300	≈ 6–12 ml/vessel
IV contrast-enhanced CT scan of the brain	240 350	120–250 ml IV drip 70–150 ml bolus[b]
CT cisternography via LP or C1–2 puncture	300 350	12 12
CT ventriculography via ventricular catheter	180[c]	2–3
plain film ventriculography via ventricular catheter	180	2–3
plain film "shunt-o-gram" injected via shunt into ventricles	180	2–3
plain film "shunt-o-gram" injected via shunt distal to valve so as not to enter into ventricles (to check distal shunt function)	300 350	10–12 10–12

[a]most centers use Optiray®, see text
[b]follow with 250 ml bolus of 0.45% NS to rehydrate patient
[c]180 will be very dense on CT, and some use 1–3 ml of 140 or diluted 180% (dilute approximately 2 parts contrast to 1 part preservative-free normal saline)

Intrathecal use

NB: only Omnipaque 180, 210, 240 and 300 are labeled for intrathecal use. 140 and 350 are *not* FDA approved for intrathecal use, however, some neuroradiologists will use Omnipaque 140 or diluted 180 e.g., for CT ventriculography (off-label usage).

Consider discontinuing neuroleptic drugs (including phenothiazines, e.g., chlorpromazine, prochlorperazine, and promethazine) at least 48 hours prior to procedure. Elevate HOB ≥ 30° for the first few hours after the procedure. Hydrate orally or IV.

Use with caution in patients with seizure history, severe cardiovascular disease, chronic alcoholism, or multiple sclerosis.

Iohexol undergoes slow diffusion from the intrathecal space to the systemic circulation and is eliminated by renal excretion with no significant metabolism or deiodination.

Maximum dosage: a total dose of 3060 mg iodine should not be exceeded in an adult during a single myelogram (some say up to 4500 mg is OK) (e.g., 15 cc of Omnipaque 300 = 15 ml × 300 mgI/ml = 4500 mg of iodine).

Iopamidol (e.g., Isovue 300, Isovue 370®)

Triiodinated, non-ionic, water-soluble. Used for intravascular and intrathecal radiographic contrast. Isovue 300 and 370 contains 300 and 270 mg iodine/ml, respectively.

Non-intrathecal contrast agents

For inadvertent intrathecal injection of contrast agents *not* intended for intrathecal use, see above.

Ioversol (Optiray®)

✖ Not for intrathecal use (see above).
  Uses and concentrations include:
• arteriography: Optiray 300 (ioversol 64%) or Optiray 320 (ioversol 68%). Total procedural dose should not usually exceed 200 ml

- IV contrast enhanced CT scan of brain:
  - a) adult: 50–150 ml of Optiray 300, 320, or 100–250 ml of Optiray 240.
    Typically: 100 ml of Optiray 320
  - b) pediatrics: 1–3 ml/kg of Optiray 320

Iopromide (Ultravist®)

✖ Not for intrathecal use (see above). Available in 150, 240, 300 & 370 mg iodine/ml. Osmolality of Ultravist 300 is 607.

Cerebral angiography (300 mg/ml): maximum dose is 150 ml per procedure.

Contrast enhanced CT (CECT) (300 mg/ml). ℞ *Pediatrics* (> 2 years of age): typical dose is 1–2 ml/kg IV, maximum dose is 3 ml/kg per procedure. *Adult*: typical dose is 50–200 ml, maximum dose is 200 ml.

Iodixanol (Visipaque®)

✖ Not for intrathecal use (see above). Triiodinated, non-ionic, *isosmolar* to blood. For intravascular use. FDA approved for CECT, some angiographers use Visipaque 270 for cerebral angiography (slightly lower opacification, but also slightly lower iodine dose). Available in 270 and 320 mg iodine/ml.

Iodinated contrast with allergies or renal insufficiency

Allergy prep

Indicated for patients with previous history of reaction to IV iodinated contrast material. Minor previous reactions such as hives and itching merit preparation with this regimen whenever possible. Patients with anaphylactic shock or severe edema causing compromise of the airway should probably not receive IV iodine even with this prep, unless absolutely necessary. ✖ Caution: in spite of this regimen, the patient may still have a serious reaction (modified[37]). This prep has also been used for the rare gadolinium allergy.

1. utilize non-ionic contrast medium (e.g., iohexol) whenever possible
2. have emergency equipment available during study
3. medications:
   - a) steroid (▶ Table 8.1 for further details of steroid dosing)
     - prednisone 50 mg PO: 20–24 hrs, 8–12 hrs & 2 hrs before study
     - equivalent dose of IV Solumedrol® (methylprednisolone): ≈ 25 mg
   - b) diphenhydramine (Benadryl®) 50 mg, *EITHER* IM 1 hr before,
     OR IV 5 min before study
   - c) optional: H2 antagonist, e.g., cimetidine 300 mg PO or IV 1 hr before study

Medications for an *emergency* scan when 24 hour prep is not possible:
- hydrocortisone 100 mg IV then scan within 2 hours

Prep for renal insufficiency or patients with DM

For patients with DM or mild renal insufficiency (e.g., slight serum creatinine elevation, > 1.2 mg/dl (U.S.) which is > 100 mcmol/L) 1 mg/dl of creatinine (used in the U.S.) = 88.4 mcmol/L, to mitigate against iodine contrast-induced nephropathy:
- N-acetyl cysteine (Mucomyst; the actual efficacy of NAC has not been proven, and may be no better than hydration alone): regimens all accompany hydration and include:
  - a) 800 mg PO q 8 hrs for 24 hours before the study,[38] followed by 600 mg PO BID for 24 hours after the study
  - b) 600 mg PO BID X 2 days before the study, 600 mg PO BID for 24 hours after
  - c) 600-mg IV bolus before the study, and 600 mg PO BID for 48 hours after[39]
- hydration: 1 L of sterile water with 3 amps of sodium bicarbonate IV at 100 ml/hr, start 1 hour prior to the study, and continue until entire L given

12.4.2 Reactions to intravascular contrast media

General information

See also treatment of inadvertent intrathecal injection of ionic contrast agents (p. 230).

✖ Beta blockers

Beta blockers can increase the risk of contrast media reactions, and may mask some manifestations of an anaphylactoid reaction. They also make use of epinephrine inadvisable since the alpha effects of epinephrine will predominate (bronchospasm, vasoconstriction, increased vagal tone). If treatment is required for hypotension after beta-blocker administration, may try glucagon 2–3 mg IV bolus, followed by 5 mg IV drip over 1 hour (glucagon has positive inotropic and chronotropic effect that is not mediated through adrenergic pathways).

Idiosyncratic reactions and treatment

Hypotension with tachycardia (anaphylactoid reaction)

1. mild: Trendelenburg position. IV fluids
2. if no response but remains mild:
   epinephrine (use with caution in patients with coronary artery disease, limited cardiac reserve, hypertension, or unclipped cerebral aneurysm)
   a) 0.3–0.5 ml of 1:1000 SQ (0.3–0.5 mg) q 15–20 mins (peds: 0.01 mg/kg)
   b) or ASEP recommendations (especially for elderly or patients in shock): 10 ml of 1:100,000 IV over 5 to 10 min (put 0.1 ml of 1:1000 in 10 ml of NS, or dilute 1 amp of 1:10,000 to 10 ml with NS)
3. moderate to severe or worsening (anaphylaxis): add:
   a) IV colloidal fluids, e.g., hetastarch (Hespan®) 6% (colloids are required since there is extravascular shift of fluids; these agents also carry a small risk of allergic reaction)
   b) epinephrine (see above). May repeat × 1
   c) O$_2$ 2–6 L/min per NC. Intubate if necessary
   d) EKG to R/O ischemic changes
4. if shock develops: add dopamine (p. 133), start at 5 mcg/kg/min

Hypotension with bradycardia (vasovagal reaction)

1. mild:
   a) Trendelenburg position
   b) IV fluids
2. if no response, add:
   a) atropine 0.75 mg IV, may repeat up to 2–3 mg over 15 mins PRN. Use with caution in patients with underlying heart disease
   b) EKG and/or cardiac monitor: especially if atropine or dopamine are used
3. if no response: add dopamine (p. 133), start at 5 mcg/kg/min

Urticaria

1. mild: self limited. No treatment necessary
2. moderate:
   a) diphenhydramine (Benadryl®) 50 mg PO or deep IM (avoid IV, can cause anaphylaxis itself)
   b) cimetidine (Tagamet®) 300 mg PO or IV diluted to 20 ml and given over 20 mins. H2 receptors contribute to wheal and flare of reaction
3. severe: treat as above for moderate reaction, and add:
   a) epinephrine (see above)
   b) maintain IV line

Facial or laryngeal angioedema

1. epinephrine: see above. May repeat up to 1 mg
2. if respiratory distress: O$_2$ 2–6 L/min. Intubate if necessary (orotracheal may be very difficult due to swelling of tongue, nasotracheal intubation or emergency cricothyrotomy may be required)
3. diphenhydramine: see above
4. cimetidine: see above
5. if angioedema is accessible, add ice pack
6. maintain IV line
7. steroids are usually effective only for *chronic* angioedema

Bronchospasm

1. mild to moderate:
   a) epinephrine: see above. May repeat up to 1 ml

12

b) if respiratory distress: O_2 2–6 L/min. Intubate if necessary
c) maintain IV line
d) inhalational therapy with a β-adrenergic agonist, e.g., albuterol (Proventil®) if respiratory therapy is available, otherwise, metered dose inhaler e.g., pirbuterol (Maxair®) or metaproterenol (Metaprel®), 2 puffs
2. severe: treat as above for moderate reaction, and add:
a) aminophylline 250–500 mg in 10–20 cc NS slow IV over 15–30 mins. Monitor for hypotension and arrhythmias
b) intubate
3. prolonged: add the following (will not have immediate effect):
a) hydrocortisone 250 mg IV
b) diphenhydramine: see above
c) cimetidine: see above

Pulmonary edema
1. O_2 2–6 L/min per NC. Intubate if necessary
2. raise head and body
3. furosemide (Lasix®) 40 mg IV
4. EKG
5. if hypoxia develops (may manifest as agitation or combativeness), add:
a) morphine 8–15 mg IV. May cause respiratory depression, be prepared to intubate
b) epinephrine: see above. ✖ CAUTION: use only if MI can be R/O as cause of the pulmonary edema. Patients with acute intracranial pathology may be at risk of neurogenic pulmonary edema (p. 1439)

Seizures
If seizure is not self limited, start with lorazepam (Ativan®) 2–4 mg IV for an adult. Take initial steps for status epilepticus (p. 512) and proceed with additional medications for generalized convulsive status epilepticus as indicated.

12.5 Radiation safety for neurosurgeons

12.5.1 General information
Radiation exposure has both a deterministic component (exposure over a certain threshold will cause a specific injury, e.g., cataracts) as well as a stochastic component (any dose increases the *chances* of an adverse event such as leukemia, and the higher the cumulative dose, the higher the chances).

12.5.2 Units
See reference.[40]

Absorbed dose: the amount of energy absorbed per unit mass. Expressed in Gray or rads.
Gray (Gy): the SI unit. 1 Gy = 100 cGy = 100 rads = an absorbed dose of 1 Joule/kg.
Rad: 1 rad = an absorbed dose of 100 ergs/gram = 0.01 joule/kg = 0.01 Gy = 1 cGy.
The biological effect (dose equivalent) of radiation: can be expressed in rem or Sieverts.
Sievert (Sv): the SI unit. The dose equivalent in sieverts is equal to the absorbed dose in grays multiplied by a "quality factor" (Q) which differs for different sources of radiation, e.g., high-energy protons have a Q of 10, X-rays have a Q of 1. 1 Sv=100 rems.
Roentgen-equivalent man (rem): the absorbed dose in rads multiplied by Q. 1 rem is estimated to cause ≈ 300 additional cases of cancer per million persons (one third of which are fatal). 1 rem = 0.01 sievert.

12.5.3 Typical radiation exposure
The average annual exposure to radiation is 360 mrem (about 30 mrem are due to background cosmic radiation, ≈ 20% of the total dose is due to radioactive potassium-40 which is in every cell). Exposure from a transcontinental airline flight is ≈ 5 mrem.
CXR: causes about 0.01–0.04 rem of exposure to the chest.
Spine X-ray with obliques: 5 rem.

CAT scan (brain, noncontrast): median effective dose to the head = 0.2 rem, but the range varied 13 fold within and across institutions.[41]

Spine CT: 5 rem.

Cerebral arteriogram: ≈ 10–20 rem (including fluoroscopy).[42]

Cerebral embolization: 34 rem.

Bone scan: 4 rem.

C-arm fluoroscopy[43]: exposure is shown in ► Table 12.5.

Doses during a minimally invasive TLIF[44]:

Patient exposure: mean 60 mGy to the skin in the AP plane (range: 8–250 mGy), 79 mGy in the lateral plane.

Surgeon exposure: 76 mrem to dominant hand, 27 mrem at the waist under a lead apron, and 32 mrem to an unprotected thyroid level detector.

Table 12.5 Radiation exposure with fluoroscopy[43a]

Distance from beam		Typical team member	Deep exposure	Superficial exposure
feet	meters		(mrem/min)	
Direct beam		patient	4000	—
1	0.3	surgeon	20	29
2	0.6	assistant	6	10
3	0.9	scrub tech	0	≤ 2
5	1.5	anesthesiologist	0[b]	0[b]

[a]in a mock OR set up for maximal scatter
[b]after 10 minutes of exposure

12.5.4 Occupational exposure

The U.S. Nuclear Regulatory Commission (NRC) maximal recommended annual occupational dose limits for radiation are shown in ► Table 12.6.[45] The 1990 recommendation of the International Commission on Radiological Protection (ICRP) was to keep exposure ≤ 2 rem/year averaged over 5 years.[46]

ALARA: an acronym for "As Low As Reasonably Achievable" by which the NRC means making every reasonable effort to keep radiation dose as far below the limits as possible, consistent with the purpose for which the licensed activity is undertaken.[47]

Steps to reduce occupational radiation dose (to staff) during surgery:

1. increase the distance from the radiation source: radiation exposure is proportional to the inverse *square* of the distance. Conventional wisdom is to stay 6 feet away from medical X-ray sources. An AANS publication recommends 3 m (10 ft)[48]
   Lead aprons/shields may or may not work, but distance ALWAYS works[49] (inverse square law—double the distance and get 1/4 the radiation).
2. shielding: shielding is less effective at higher keV (used with larger patients). Portable lead "doors" are more effective than aprons. Wrap-around 2-piece aprons are better than front/side aprons. With front aprons the wearer must always face the X-ray source, otherwise the posterior gap in the apron is not protective and the inside front of the apron can actually reflect some radiation back onto the wearer. Non-lead aprons may not provide the rated protection at levels > 100 keV.[50] Leaded surgical gloves reduce radiation exposure of the hands by only ≈ 33%.[51]
3. don't overuse magnification: fluoro systems increase the radiation emitted as much as 4 times to compensate for the associated reduction in image brightness
4. "boost" mode can double the radiation output. Use should be kept to a minimum
5. use live fluoro only when absolutely necessary

Table 12.6 Annual occupational radiation dose limits

Target organ	Recommended MAXIMAL dose (rem/yr)
whole body	5
lens of eye	15
skin, hands, feet	50
other organs (including thyroid)	15

6. for lateral imaging: scatter is the most significant cause of exposure here and is higher on the *source side*[52] (this asymmetry is not as significant for C-spine[53]). Therefore, whenever possible, stand on the "downstream" (image intensifier [Iml]) side of the C-arm
7. keep the Iml as close to the patient as possible (reduces patient & staff exposure and improves image quality)
8. on AP images (with the patient prone or supine): position the X-ray tube *under* the table with the Iml over the patient (reduces scatter exposure to staff)[54]
9. *collimate* the beam as much as possible: reduces radiation to patient and to staff, and results in less image degradation
10. keep hands, arms, etc. out of the primary beam at all times. Consider leaded surgical gloves if hands need to be close to the beam (see above)
11. minimize the number of images: plan your shot, avoid frequent "checks" or peeks
12. use image guided navigation when possible and practical
13. leaded glasses are recommended primarily for personnel with very high fluoro times: cataracts can be induced by single doses of 200 rads (very high); cumulative doses of 750 rads have not been associated with cataracts

References

[1] Swischuk LE. Anterior displacement of C2 in children: physiologic or pathologic? Radiology. 1977; 122:759–763

[2] Spence KF, Decker S, Sell KW. Bursting atlantal fracture associated with rupture of the transverse ligament. J Bone Joint Surg. 1970; 52A:543–549

[3] Fielding JW, Cochran GB, Lawsing JF,3rd, et al. Tears of the transverse ligament of the atlas. A clinical and biomechanical study. J Bone Joint Surg Am. 1974; 56:1683–1691

[4] Heller JG, Viroslav S, Hudson T. Jefferson fractures: the role of magnification artifact in assessing transverse ligament integrity. J Spinal Disord. 1993; 6:392–396

[5] Dickman CA, Greene KA, Sonntag VK. Injuries involving the transverse atlantal ligament: classification and treatment guidelines based upon experience with 39 injuries. Neurosurgery. 1996; 38:44–50

[6] Kopparapu S, Mao G, Judy BF, et al. Fifty years later: the "rule of Spence" is finally ready for retirement. J Neurosurg Spine. 2022:1–8

[7] Hinck VC, Hopkins CE. Measurement of the Atlanto-Dental Interval in the Adult. Am J Roentgenol Radium Ther Nucl Med. 1960; 84:945–951

[8] Meijers KAE, van Beusekom GT, Luyendijk W, et al. Dislocation of the Cervical Spine with Cord Compression in Rheumatoid Arthritis. J Bone Joint Surg. 1974; 56B:668–680

[9] Panjabi MM, Oda T, Crisco JJ,3rd, et al. Experimental study of atlas injuries. I. Biomechanical analysis of their mechanisms and fracture patterns. Spine. 1991; 16:S460–S465

[10] Powers B, Miller MD, Kramer RS, et al. Traumatic Anterior Atlanto-Occipital Dislocation. Neurosurgery. 1979; 4:12–17

[11] Brockmeyer D. Down syndrome and craniovertebral instability. Topic review and treatment recommendations. Pediatr Neurosurg. 1999; 31:71–77

[12] Murphy A. Cervical spine (lateral view). 2021. DOI: 10.53347/rID-58731

[13] Wolf BS, Khilnani M, Malis L. The Sagittal Diameter of the Bony Cervical Spinal Canal and its Significance in Cervical Spondylosis. J of Mount Sinai Hospital. 1956; 23:283–292

[14] Epstein N, Epstein JA, Benjamin V, et al. Traumatic Myelopathy in Patients With Cervical Spinal Stenosis Without Fracture or Dislocation: Methods of Diagnosis, Management, and Prognosis. Spine. 1980; 5:489–496

[15] Rojas CA, Vermess D, Bertozzi JC, et al. Normal thickness and appearance of the prevertebral soft tissues on multidetector CT. AJNR. American Journal of Neuroradiology. 2009; 30:136–141

[16] DeBenhe K, Havel C. Utility of Prevertebral Soft Tissue Measurements in Identifying Patients with Cervical Spine Injury. Ann Emerg Med. 1994; 24:1119–1124

[17] Miles KA, Finlay D. Is Prevertebral Soft Tissue Swelling a Useful Sign in Injury of the Cervical Spine? Injury. 1988; 19:177–179

[18] Naidich JB, Naidich TP, Garfein C, et al. The Widened Interspinous Distance: A Useful Sign of Anterior Cervical Dislocation. Radiology. 1977; 123:113–116

[19] Bailey DK. The Normal Cervical Spine in Infants and Children. Radiology. 1952; 59:712–719

[20] Yoganandan Narayan, Pintar FrankA, Lew SeanM, et al. Quantitative Analyses of Pediatric Cervical Spine Ossification Patterns Using Computed Tomography. Annals of Advances in Automotive Medicine / Annual Scientific Conference. 2011; 55:159–168

[21] Fischer FJ, Vandemark RE. Sagittal cleft (butterfly) vertebra. Journal of Bone and Joint Surgery. 1945; 27:695–698

[22] Poppel MH, Jacobson HG, Duff BK, et al. Basilar impression and platybasia in Paget's disease. British Journal of Radiology. 1953; 21:171–181

[23] Koenigsberg RA, Vakil N, Hong TA, et al. Evaluation of platybasia with MR imaging. AJNR. American Journal of Neuroradiology. 2005; 26:89–92

[24] Goel A, Bhatjiwale M, Desai K. Basilar invagination: a study based on 190 surgically treated patients. J Neurosurg. 1998; 88:962–968

[25] McRae DL. The Significance of Abnormalities of the Cervical Spine. AJR. 1960; 70:23–46

[26] Cronin CG, Lohan DG, Mhuircheartigh J N, et al. MRI evaluation and measurement of the normal odontoid peg position. Clinical Radiology. 2007; 62:897–903

[27] Chamberlain WE. Basilar Impression (Platybasia): Bizarre Developmental Anomaly of Occipital Bone and Upper Cervical Spine with Striking and Misleading Neurologic Manifestations. Yale J Biol Med. 1939; 11:487–496

[28] Cronin CG, Lohan DG, Mhuircheartigh J N, et al. CT evaluation of Chamberlain's, McGregor's, and McRae's skull-base lines. Clinical Radiology. 2009; 64:64–69

[29] McGregor J. The Significance of Certain Measurements of the Skull in the Diagnosis of Basilar Impression. Br J Radiol. 1948; 21:171–181

[30] VanGilder JC, Menezes AH, Dolan KD. Radiology of the Normal Craniovertebral Junction. In: The Craniovertebral Junction and Its Abnormalities. NY: Futura Publishing; 1987:29–58

[31] Hinck VC, Hopkins CE, Savara BS. Diagnostic Criteria of Basilar Impression. Radiology. 1961; 76

[32] The Cervical Spine Research Society. The Cervical Spine. Philadelphia 1983

[33] Menezes AH. Primary craniovertebral anomalies and the hindbrain herniation syndrome (Chiari I): data base analysis. Pediatr Neurosurg. 1995; 23:260–269

[34] Jacobson G, Bleeker HH. Pseudosubluxation of the Axis in Children. Am J Roentgenol. 1959; 82:472–481

[35] Rivera E, Hardjasudarma M, Willis BK, et al. Inadvertent Use of Ionic Contrast Material in Myelography: Case Report and Management Guidelines. Neurosurgery. 1995; 36:413–415

[36] Bohn HP, Reich L, Suljaga-Petchel K. Inadvertent Intrathecal Use of Ionic Contrast Media for Myelography. AJNR. 1992; 13:1515–1519

[37] Lasser EC, Berry CC, Talner LB, et al. Pretreatment with Corticosteroids to Alleviate Reactions to Intravenous Contrast Material. N Engl J Med. 1987; 317:825–829

[38] Allaqaband S, Tumuluri R, Malik AM, et al. Prospective randomized study of N-acetylcysteine, fenoldopam, and saline for prevention of radiocontrast-induced nephropathy. Catheterization and Cardiovascular Interventions. 2002; 57:279–283

[39] Marenzi G, Assanelli E, Marana I, et al. N-acetylcysteine and contrast-induced nephropathy in primary angioplasty. New England Journal of Medicine. 2006; 354:2773–2782

[40] Units of radiation dose. 1991. http://www.nrc.gov/reading-rm/doc-collections/cfr/part020/

[41] Smith-Bindman R, Lipson J, Marcus R, et al. Radiation dose associated with common computed tomography examinations and the associated lifetime attributable risk of cancer. Archives of Internal Medicine. 2009; 169:2078–2086

[42] Thompson TP, Maitz AH, Kondziolka D, et al. Radiation, Radiobiology, and Neurosurgery. Contemporary Neurosurgery. 1999; 21:1–5

[43] Mehlman CT, DiPasquale TG. Radiation exposure to the orthopaedic surgical team during fluoroscopy: "how far away is far enough?". Journal of Orthopaedic Trauma. 1997; 11:392–398

[44] Bindal RK, Glaze S, Ognoskie M, et al. Surgeon and patient radiation exposure in minimally invasive transforaminal lumbar interbody fusion. J Neurosurg Spine. 2008; 9:570–573

[45] Occupational dose limits for adults. 1991. http://www.nrc.gov/reading-rm/doc-collections/cfr/part020/

[46] 1990 Recommendations of the International Commission on Radiological Protection. Annals of the ICRP. 1991; 21

[47] Definitions. 1991. http://www.nrc.gov/reading-rm/doc-collections/cfr/part020/

[48] McCormick PW. Fluoroscopy: Reducing radiation exposure in the OR. Rolling Meadows, IL 2008

[49] Rechtine GR. Radiation satety for the orthopaedic surgeon: Or, C-arm friend or foe. Tampa, FL 2009

[50] Scuderi GJ, Brusovanik GV, Campbell DR, et al. Evaluation of non-lead-based protective radiological material in spinal surgery. Spine J. 2006; 6:577–582

[51] Rampersaud YR, Foley KT, Shen AC, et al. Radiation exposure to the spine surgeon during fluoroscopically assisted pedicle screw insertion. Spine (Phila Pa 1976). 2000; 25:2637–2645

[52] Boone JM, Pfeiffer DE, Strauss KJ, et al. A survey of fluoroscopic exposure rates: AAPM Task Group No. 11 Report. Medical Physics. 1993; 20:789–794

[53] Giordano BD, Baumhauer JF, Morgan TL, et al. Cervical spine imaging using standard C-arm fluoroscopy: patient and surgeon exposure to ionizing radiation. Spine. 2008; 33:1970–1976

[54] Faulkner K, Moores BM. An assessment of the radiation dose received by staff using fluoroscopic equipment. British Journal of Radiology. 1982; 55:272–276

12

13 Imaging and Angiography

13.1 CAT scan (AKA CT scan)

13.1.1 General information

CAT (computer assisted tomography) or just "CT" scans employ ionizing radiation (X-rays) with the attendant risks; see Radiation safety for neurosurgeons (p. 234). Computer algorithms are applied to multiple X-ray beams directed from different angles to create a virtual cross-sectional slice through an object being studied.

Attenuation of the X-ray beam on a CT scan is quantified in Hounsfield units. These units are not absolute, and vary between CT scanner models. Some sample values are shown in ▶ Table 13.1. Most imaging systems allow measurement of Hounsfield units for a user-defined region.

Originally, axial CT scan slices were taken parallel to the orbitomeatal line (OM line) AKA canthomeatal line, which connects the lateral canthus of the eye to the midpoint of the external auditory meatus. This practice was abandoned in favor of slices parallel to the roof of the orbit in order to reduce radiation to the radiosensitive lens of the eye. Current volumetric CT scanners tend to create axial slices parallel to the AC-PC line (p. 58) (as with MRI scanners, which is ironically within ≈ 9° of the original OM line).

Table 13.1 Hounsfield units for a sample CT scanner

Definitions	Hounsfield units	Comment
no attenuation (air)	−1000	definition
water	0	definition
dense bone	+1000	definition
Cranial CT		
brain (gray matter)	30 to 40	
brain (white matter)	20 to 35	
cerebral edema	10 to 14	
CSF	+5	
bone	+600	
blood clot[a]	75 to 80	acute SDH or EDH, fresh SAH
fat	−35 to −40	
calcium	100 to 300	
enhanced vessels	90–100	
Spine CT		
disc material	55–70	disc density is ≈ 2 × thecal sac
thecal sac	20–30	
[a]Hct < 23% will cause an acute SDH to be isodense with brain		

13.1.2 Noncontrast vs. IV contrast enhanced CT scan (CECT)

Noncontrast CT scans are often employed in emergency situations (to quickly rule out most acute abnormalities), to evaluate bone in great detail, or as a screening test. It excels in demonstrating acute blood (EDH, SDH, IPH, SAH), fractures, foreign bodies, pneumocephalus, and hydrocephalus. It is weak in demonstrating acute stroke (DWI MRI is preferred), and often has poor signal quality in the posterior fossa (due to bone artifact).

IV enhanced CT scans are used primarily for imaging neoplasms or vascular malformations, especially in patients with contraindications to MRI. All CT contrast agents contain iodine.

Typical IV dose of contrast: 60–65 ml of e.g., Isovue 300® (p. 231) which delivers 18–19.5 grams of iodine.

13.1.3 CT angiography (CTA)

Employs rapid injection of iodinated contrast at 3–4 cc/sec, typically 65–75 ml of e.g., Isovue 300®. Optimal results in patients who can hold their breath for 30–40 seconds (for spiral CT).

Various methods may be used to determine timing of CT after injection: may be based on time to peak in aorta after a small test injection, or can be based empirically on time, or give injection and look for peak in the region of interest.

Accuracy is diminished for vessels that are perpendicular to the axial CT plane. Also in the vicinity of dense clot, CTA has trouble resolving the adjacent vessels.

13.1.4 CT perfusion (CTP)

Requires use of iodinated contrast. Areas of interest are selected from an unenhanced CT scan in the 3 supratentorial vascular territories. Contrast is given at a standard rate (e.g., 40 ml IV at 5 ml/sec). Scans through the regions of interest are repeated at intervals, e.g., every 2 seconds for 1 minute.

Acetazolamide (ACZ) (Diamox®) challenge: after the above, a bolus of 1000 mg of IV ACZ is given, and scans are repeated at intervals for approximately 10 minutes, with a final scan usually at 15 minutes.

Parameters then calculated from the images: cerebral blood volume (CBV), CBF, mean transit times (MTT), and time to peak (TTP). In ischemic stroke, MTT is almost always increased and CBF is decreased.

Abnormalities that can be demonstrated:
1. flow significant stenosis: decreased CBV & CBF, increased MTT and TTP
2. steal: after ACZ challenge (see above), CBV & CBF decrease, often with increases in the corresponding contralateral territory; MTT increases

In comparison to perfusion weighted MRI (PWI) (p. 243):
1. PWI acquires multiple slices of the whole brain over and over. CTP is limited to a given slice or several slices (usually 10–20 mm thick), and one has to choose where to place that slice
2. PWI has more artifact than CTP

13.2 Pregnancy and CT scans

In general, unless there is a strong indication for a CT scan, they are usually avoided during pregnancy. The radiation dose to a fetus from a head or cervical spine CT is small, and can be reduced by lead shielding. However, abdominal CT scans expose the fetus directly to X-rays and should be considered with extreme care. The risk from fetal exposure to X-rays is highest during the first 2 weeks after conception (risk of miscarriage) and between 8-16 weeks of gestation (risk of cognitive disabilities).

13.3 Magnetic resonance imaging (MRI)

13

13.3.1 General information

Definitions.[1]
Abbreviations in ▶ Table 13.2:
- TR: time to repetition
- TE: time to echo
- T_I: time to inversion
- T_1: spin-lattice relaxation time ("time to magnetize") (regrowth)
- T_2: spin-spin relaxation time ("time to demagnetize") (decay)

Table 13.2 Range of acquisition data

	short TE (te < 50)	long TE (te > 80)
short TR (TR < 1000)	T1WI	
long TR (TR > 2000)	proton density or spin density	T2WI

13.3.2 Specific imaging sequences

T_1 weighted image (T1WI)

Short T_1 → high signal (bright). "Anatomic image," somewhat resembles CT. Shorter acquisition time than T2WI. Proton rich tissue (e.g., H_2O) has long T1.

Table 13.3 T1WI, MRI intensity change				
fat (including bone marrow), blood > 48 hrs old, melanin	white matter	gray matter	calcium	CSF, bone

(note: gray bar illustrates direction of intensity change and does not show actual gray on MRI)

Clues to recognizing T1WI: CSF is black, subcutaneous fat is white, TR and TE are short (hundreds and double digits, respectively); see ▶ Table 13.3.

★ The only objects that appear white on T1WI are: fat, melanin, Onyx® (p. 1927), and subacute blood (> 48 hrs old). White matter is higher signal than gray matter (myelin has a high fat content). Most pathology is low signal on T1WI.

T₂ weighted image (T2WI)

Long T_2 → high signal (bright). "Pathological image." Most pathology shows up as high signal, including surrounding edema.

Clues to recognizing T2WI: CSF is white, TR & TE are long (thousands and hundreds, respectively); see ▶ Table 13.4.

Table 13.4 T2WI, MRI intensity change				
brain edema/water, fat	CSF	gray matter	white matter	bone

(note: gray bar illustrates direction of intensity change and does not show actual gray level on MRI)

Spin density image

AKA balanced image, AKA proton density image. Partway between T1WI and T2WI. CSF = gray, approximately isodense with brain. Becoming less commonly used.

FLAIR

Acronym: FLuid-Attenuated Inversion Recovery. Long TR and TE. Resembles a T2WI except the CSF is nulled out (appears dark). The gray/white intensity pattern is reversed from T1WI and is more prominent. Most abnormalities including MS plaques, other white matter lesions, tumors, edema, encephalomalacia, gliosis, and acute infarcts appear bright. Periventricular lesions such as MS plaques become more conspicuous. Also good for demonstrating abnormalities in CSF.

Differential diagnosis of increased signal in subarachnoid spaces on FLAIR:

1. subarachnoid hemorrhage (SAH): ★ FLAIR is the best sequence for detecting acute SAH on MRI
2. meningitis: occurs in some cases
3. meningeal carcinomatosis
4. superior sagittal sinus thrombosis
5. stroke
6. adjacent tumor: ? if related to higher protein
7. previous administration of gadolinium
8. high levels of FIO_2 especially at levels nearing 100% as may be used in patients getting MRI under general anesthesia.[2] Shows up in basal cisterns and in sulci over the convexity, but not in ventricles

Echo train (AKA fast spin echo [FSE])

TR is held constant, TE is progressively increased utilizing multiple echoes (8–16) rather than one. Image approaches T2WI but with substantially reduced acquisition time (fat is brighter on FSE, which may be rectified by fat suppression techniques).

Gradient echo

AKA T2* GRE (called T2-star). Some manufacturers have trademarked names for this, e.g., "GRASS" (a GE trademarked acronym for Gradient Recalled Acquisition in a Steady State) or FISP (a Siemens trade name). A "fast" T2WI utilizing a partial flip angle. CSF and flowing vessels appear white. Bone, calcium, and heavy metals are *dark*. Typical acquisition data: TR = 22, TE = 11, angle 8°. Used e.g., in cervical spine to produce a "myelographic" image, improves MRI's ability to delineate bony spurs. Also shows small old cerebral hemorrhages (seen in 60% of patients presenting with hemorrhagic infarction, and in 18% with ischemic infarcts[3]); these patients may be at increased risk of hemorrhage from anticoagulation.

★ T2* GRE MRI is 3–4 times more sensitive test than FLAIR for demonstrating intraparenchymal blood (which appears as a *hypointense* bloom) due to high sensitivity to paramagnetic artifact. It is not as sensitive as SWI (susceptibility weighted imaging).

"STIR" image

Acronym for "Short Tau Inversion Recovery." Summates T1 & T2 signals. Causes fat to drop out— sometimes also called fat suppression or "fat sat" (for fat saturation). Allows gadolinium enhancement to show up better in areas of fat. Very good for showing bone edema (can help in dating spine fractures), periventricular lesions (subtracts out CSF), and orbit intra-orbital pathology. The dorsal spinal nerve root ganglion may enhance on fat suppression images.

FIESTA imaging

An acronym for Fast Imaging Employing Steady-state Acquisition (a GE trademarked name). Uses CSF as the contrast medium, (∴ does *not* use gadolinium). Useful in the cerebellopontine angle (CPA) e.g., to visualize vestibular schwannomas or neurovascular compression in trigeminal neuralgia.

3D CISS

An acronym for constructive interference in steady state. Accentuates the visualization between pathologic structures and CSF.[4] May be useful for imaging cranial nerves, CSF leaks, aqueductal stenosis…

13.3.3 MRI protocols

Many facilities have developed imaging "protocols" for specific diagnoses or situations. While these are not standardized, some are presented here to aid in understanding & ordering individual sequences.

▶ **Pituitary protocol.** Detailed imaging through the pituitary gland and its environs, with sequences to improve visualization of PitNet/adenomas.
  Sequences:
- brain MRI and pituitary MRI without and with contrast, including navigation compliant images (thin cuts for navigation systems such as BrainLab™ or Stealth™…)
- pituitary images: thin coronal cuts through the sella, cavernous sinuses and optic chiasm with "dynamic imaging" (images taken at intervals following contrast administration to try and differentiate an adenoma from the normal pituitary gland since the pituitary [which is outside the blood-brain barrier] usually enhances *before* the adenoma (differential enhancement). Especially helpful when looking for an microadenoma [see ▶ Fig. 52.2 for an example])

▶ **IAC protocol.** Detailed imaging through the internal auditory canals (IACs), with sequences to improve visualization of cranial nerves and vessels in the cerebellopontine angle (CPA) as well as the IACs themselves.
  Sequences:
1. thin cut images through each IAC individually without & thin cut with contrast, with vertically oriented images perpendicular to the long axis of the IACs
2. FIESTA or (3D)-CISS imaging sequences that enhance the differentiation of the CPA contents from CSF

13.3.4 Contraindications to MRI

General information

Safety issues are detailed in reference.[5] Web sites for MRI safety include: *www.MRIsafety.com* and *www.IMRSER.org* . Some issues that come up frequently in neurosurgical patients follows.

Pregnancy and MRI

During the first trimester, MRI can cause reabsorption of products of conception (miscarriage). There are no studies to determine the long term effects of MRI on a fetus after the first trimester (the low risk of MRI in this situation is probably preferable to the known dangers of ionizing radiation of X-rays (including CT).[6]) Gadolinium contrast is contraindicated during all of pregnancy, and is not approved for use in age < 2 years. Breast-feeding must be interrupted for 2 days after administration of gadolinium to the mother.

Common contraindications to MRI

1. cardiac pacemakers/defibrillator, implanted neurostimulators, cochlear implants, infusion pumps: may cause temporary or permanent malfunction
2. ferromagnetic aneurysm clips (see below): some centers exclude all patients with any type of aneurysm clip
3. metallic implants or foreign bodies with large component of iron or cobalt (may move in field, or may heat up)
4. Swann-Ganz catheter (pulmonary artery catheter)
5. metallic fragments within the eye
6. placement of a vascular stent, coil or filter within the past 6 weeks
7. shrapnel: BBs (some bullets are OK)
8. *relative* contraindications:
   a) claustrophobic patients: may be able to sedate adequately to perform study
   b) critically ill patients: ability to monitor and access to patient are impaired. Specially designed non-magnetic ventilator may be required. Cannot use most brands of electronic IV pumps/regulators
   c) obese patients: may not physically fit into many closed bore MRI scanners. Open bore scanners may circumvent this but many utilize lower field strength magnets and generally produce inferior quality images in large patients
   d) non-MRI compatible metal implants in the region of interest (or previous surgery with high speed drills which may leave metal filings): may produce susceptibility artifact which can distort the image in that area
   e) programmable shunt valve (p. 456): most will tolerate up to a 3 T MRI without permanent damage; however, the pressure setting may be altered and therefore should be rechecked after having an MRI for any reason

Aneurysm clips and MRI

Potential MRI concerns in patients with a cerebral aneurysm clip:
1. the danger of the MRI magnetic field causing the aneurysm clip to be pulled or torqued off the aneurysm or to tear the neck. This is a risk in older ferromagnetic aneurysm clips. Aneurysm clips *manufactured* since 1990 are non-ferromagnetic and are therefore MRI compatible. MRI is contraindicated if it is not known with certainty that an aneurysm clip is MRI compatible
2. the artifact produced by the metal of the clip in the magnetic field
3. heat generated in the region of the clip: not clinically significant

13.3.5 MRI contrast

Current agents are mostly based on gadolinium (a rare earth metal which is paramagnetic in solutions). Gadolinium based contrast agents (GBCAs) include gadopentetate dimeglumine (Magnevist®), gadodiamide (Omniscan®), gadoversetamide (OptiMARK®), gadobenate dimeglumine (MultiHance®) and gadoteridol (ProHance®).
  Adverse reactions:
1. anaphylactic reactions: rare (prevalence: 0.03–0.1%)
2. nephrotoxicity: incidence is lower than with iodinated agents used with angiograms or CT and X-ray contrast

3. nephrogenic systemic fibrosis (NSF): a rare, but serious illness characterized by fibrosis of skin, joints and other organs, which is associated with certain GBCAs in patients with severe renal failure (most were on dialysis). ✖ Gadolinium is relatively contraindicated with a GFR of 30–60 ml/min, and is contraindicated with GFR < 30.[7] In patients with end-stage renal disease, the risk is ≈ 2.4% per GBCA MRI[8]

   Safest agents have a macrocyclic structure and include Dotarem, Gadovist and ProHance.[9] (although it can still occur with these agents.[10] GBCAs with a linear structure appear to be associated with a higher risk of NSF and include: Omniscan, MultiHance, Magnevist, Evovist & OptiMARK

4. gadolinium allergy: use the same allergy prep for iodine allergy (p. 232)

5. trace amounts of gadolinium are retained in the body (including in brain tissue) after an MRI scan using a GBCAs.[11] This may accumulate after repeated use. Linear GBCAs (see entry above) exhibit more retention than macrocyclic GBCAs. As of this FDA update,[11] no adverse effects have been directly linked to GBCA use in individuals with normal kidney function. The FDA is recommending retention characteristics be considered in patients at higher risk, including: those requiring multiple lifetime GBCA doses, pregnant women, children and patients with inflammatory conditions. Also, repeated use of GBCAs should be limited, especially soon after a previous dose. However, a necessary GBCA MRI should not be deferred

6. see also issues related to pregnancy (p. 242)

13.3.6 Magnetic resonance angiography (MRA)

There are 2 ways to obtain an MRA

• gadolinium enhanced: usually for extracranial vessels (e.g., carotids)

• noncontrast images using flow-related enhancement techniques (most common: 2D time of flight [2D TOF]). Usually for intracranial vessels. Anything that appears bright on T1WI will also show up on MRA, but doesn't necessarily represent blood flow. This includes fat and fat-laden macrophages in an area of old stroke. Using fat-sat T1WI can mitigate this. Has some utility in screening for aneurysms (p. 1422), and for angiographically occult vascular malformations (p. 1524). High-flow AVMs are hard to resolve because arterialized veins can appear similar to arteries.

13.3.7 Diffusion-weighted imaging (DWI) and perfusion-imaging (PWI)

Diffusion-weighted imaging

Primary uses: early detection of ischemia (stroke) and differentiating active MS plaques from old ones. DWI is sensitive to random Brownian motion of water molecules.

13

Two images are generated, an apparent diffusion coefficient (ADC) map (based on a number of variables [time, slice orientation…]), and a trace image (the actual DWI).[12] Freely diffusing water (e.g., in CSF) appears dark on DWI.

The DWI is based on a T2WI, and anything that is bright on T2WI can also be bright on DWI (so-called "shine-through"). Since bright areas on DWI can represent either restricted diffusion or T2 "shine-through" ∴ check the ADC map: if the area is black on the ADC map, then this likely represents true restricted diffusion (recent infarct is the most common etiology).

★ Intraparenchymal areas of bright signal on DWI that are not bright on the ADC map are abnormal and represent regions of restricted diffusion such as acute stroke.

Differential diagnosis of areas of increased signal (bright) on DWI:

1. ischemic brain: *acute* stroke and areas with hypoperfusion (penumbra). While restricted diffusion usually indicates irreversible cell injury (death), it can sometimes indicate tissue that is just near cell death (penumbra). Acute brain ischemia can light up within minutes.[12,13] The DWI abnormality will persist for ≈ 1 month. The ADC map usually normalizes after ≈ 1 week

2. cerebral abscess (p. 346): DWI = bright, ADC = dark

3. *active* MS plaque (old plaques will not be bright)

4. some tumors: most tumors are dark on DWI, but highly cellular tumors may have decreased diffusion (bright on DWI) (e.g., epidermoids, lymphoma, some meningiomas, small cell lung cancer…). Restricted diffusion with tumors is usually not as bright as with stroke or abscess

Other possible uses of DWI:

TIAs: some, but not all,[14] are associated with DWI abnormalities. However, factors other than focal ischemia (e.g., global ischemia, hypoglycemia, status epilepticus…) can produce ADC decline and the DWI images must therefore be interpreted in relation to the clinical setting.[12]

DWI may also be able to distinguish cytotoxic from vasogenic edema (p. 90).[15,16]

Perfusion-weighted MRI

Provides information related to the perfusion status of the microcirculation. PWI is the most sensitive study for ischemia of the brain (more sensitive than DWI and FLAIR which primarily show *infarcted* tissue). There are several methods currently in use; the bolus-contrast approach is the most widely employed.[12] Ultrafast gradient imaging is used to monitor the gradual reduction to normal following administration of contrast (usually gadolinium). A signal wash-out curve is derived and is compared to contrast in an artery. In practical terms, PWI is not widely used because of technical challenges. Time to peak and mean transit time are 2 common parameters that are displayed (higher signal = longer times beyond normal).

DWI and PWI mismatch

DWI and PWI may be combined to locate areas of diffusion-perfusion mismatch (deficit on PWI that exceeds the zone of diffusion deficit on DWI), thus identifying salvageable brain tissue at risk of infarction—"penumbra" (p. 1464)—e.g., to screen for potential candidates for thrombolytic therapy.[17]

13.3.8 Magnetic resonance spectroscopy (MRS)

General information

This section specifically covers proton (H+) MRS which can be performed on almost any MRI scanner (especially units ≥ 1.5 T) with the appropriate software. Spectroscopy of other nuclei (e.g., phosphorous) can be evaluated only with specialized equipment.

Single voxel MRS

General information

A small area is selected on the "scout" MRI and the spectroscopic peaks for that region are displayed in resonance as a function of parts-per-million (ppm). Since only small regions are selected, may be subject to "sampling" error.

Clinically important characteristic peaks are delineated in ▶ Table 13.5.

Table 13.5 Important peaks on proton MRS

Moiety	Resonance (ppm)	Description
lipid	0.5–1.5	slightly overlaps lactate peak at TE ≈ 35
lactate	1.3	a couplet peak. Not present in normal brain. End product of anaerobic glycolysis, ∴ a marker of hypoxia. Present in ischemia, infection, demyelinating disease, inborn errors of metabolism... At higher TE (e.g., TE = 144), the peak inverts which can help distinguish it from the lipid peak
N-acetyl aspartate (NAA)	2	a neuronal marker. Normally the tallest peak (higher than Cr or Cho). ↓ in ≈ all focal and regional brain abnormalities (tumor, MS, epilepsy, Alzheimer's disease, abscess, brain injury...)
creatine (Cr)	3[a]	useful primarily as a reference for choline. Higher in gray matter than white matter
choline (Cho)	3.2	marker of membrane synthesis. ↑ in neoplasms and some rare conditions of increased cell growth & in the developing brain. ★ Stroke is low in choline

[a]Cr has another less important peak

Illustrative patterns

Normal brain: See ▶ Fig. 13.1.

Tumor: See ▶ Fig. 13.1. ↓ NAA, ↑ lactate, ↑ lipid, ↑ choline (rule of thumb: with gliomas, the higher the choline, the higher the grade up to WHO grade 3, thereafter necrosis reduces relative choline levels and the lipid peak may be utilized).

Stroke: ↑ lactate peak predominates. Choline is characteristically low.

Abscess[18]: Reduced NAA, Cr & choline peaks, and "atypical peaks" (succinate, acetate...) from bacterial synthesis is pathognomonic for abscess (not always present). Lactate may be elevated.

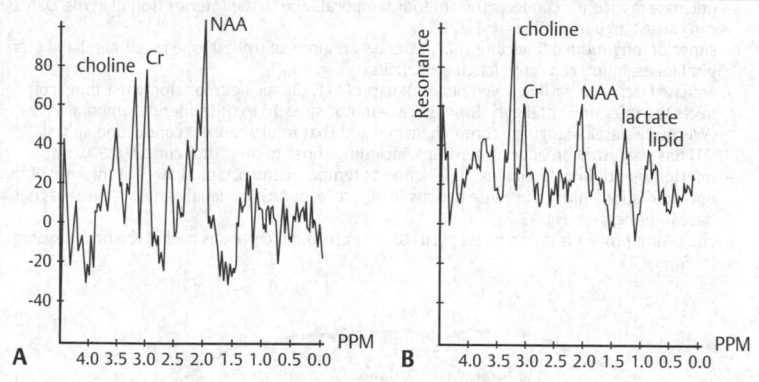

Fig. 13.1 Proton MRS. Image: A: normal brain, B: high grade glioma.

Multiple sclerosis: Bland pattern. NAA slightly reduced. Lactate and lipid slightly elevated. Choline not elevated.

Possible uses of MRS
1. differentiating abscess from neoplasm
2. post-op enhancement vs. recurrence of tumor
3. distinguishing tumor from MS plaques: occasionally cannot be differentiated
4. in AIDS: may be able to help differentiate toxo from lymphoma from PML (PML: ↓ NAA, no significant increase in choline, lactate or lipid)
5. the promise of differentiating tumor infiltration from edema has not materialized
6. some utility in distinguishing tumor from radiation necrosis (p. 1899)
7. large inositol peak may distinguish hemangiopericytoma from meningioma[19]

Multi-voxel MRS

Color coded scan with selected overlay for NAA, choline... one at a time. May reduce risk of sampling error.

13.3.9 Diffusion tensor imaging (DTI) MRI and white matter tracts

AKA diffusion tensor tractography (DTT) MRI. An MRI technique that demonstrates *white matter tracts* by exploiting the difference in diffusion parallel to the nerve axons that comprise white matter tracts from diffusion perpendicular to their course.

Available only with specialized software for specific MRI scanners.

Contraindications are same as for MRI in general (p. 242).

Probably most useful to permit planning surgical approaches that minimize disruption of critical white matter tracts during intraparenchymal brain surgery for deep lesions, especially when a lesion (e.g., tumor, AVM, cerebral hemorrhage...) may displace these tracts from their expected position.

The major divisions of white matter tracts demonstrable by DTT MRI are (▶ Fig. 13.2):
* projection fibers: tend to be oriented rostro-caudally
  ○ corticospinal tract coalesces as corona radiata funnels into internal capsule and forms pyramidal tract
* commisural fibers: mediolaterally oriented, connecting the cerebral hemispheres (▶ Fig. 13.2)
  ○ corpus callosum
  ○ anterior commissure
  ○ posterior commissure
* association fibers: connect regions within the same hemisphere
  ○ U-fibers: connect adjacent gyri (▶ Fig. 13.2)
  ○ long association fibers: connect more distant areas
    – optic radiations: connect lateral geniculate bodies to visual cortex. Pass lateral to the body of the lateral ventricles.

13

- uncinate fasciculus: connects the anterior temporal lobe to the inferior frontal gyrus. Damage can cause language deficits (▶ Fig. 13.2)
- superior longitudinal fasciculus (SLF): connects regions of frontal lobe to temporal and occipital lobes. Injury can cause language deficits (▶ Fig. 13.2)
- arcuate fasciculus (latin: curved bundle): part of SLF. Classic neuroanatomy teaching: connects the inferior frontal gyri (Broca's area = motor speech) to the superior temporal gyrus (Wernicke's area = language comprehension) and that injury causes "conduction aphasia." DTI has suggested broader connections, including those to premotor cortex (p. 90).
- inferior longitudinal fasciculus (ILF): connects temporal and occipital lobes at the level of the optic radiation. Injury can cause deficits in object recognition, visual agnosias, prosopagnosia (face blindness) (▶ Fig. 13.2)
- cingulum: project from cingulate gyrus to the entorhinal cortex as part of the limbic system (▶ Fig. 13.2)

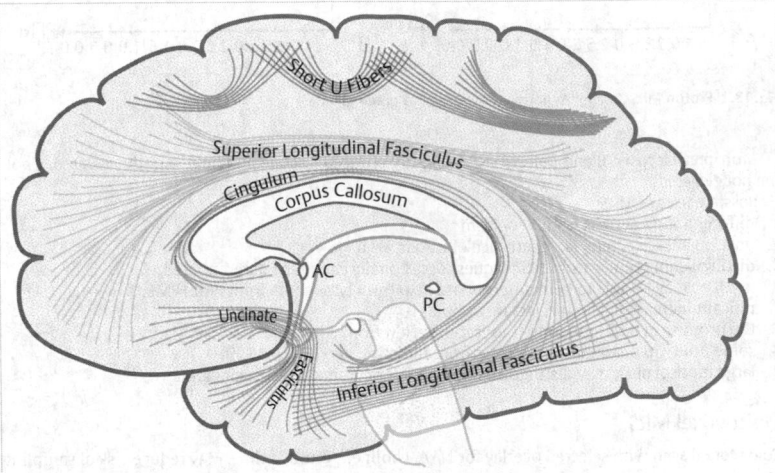

Fig. 13.2 White matter tracts (color conventions for DTI are not used in this anatomic diagram). Short U-fibers are located throughout the brain, but are illustrated here for only a few gyri. Abbreviations: AC = anterior commissure; PC = posterior commissure.

Convention for color coding tracts on DTI[20]:
- blue: superior-inferior tracts
- red: mediolateral (horizontal) tracts
- green: anterior-posterior tracts

Owing to a number of technical considerations, DTI is somewhat more operator-dependent than conventional MRI.

For surgical planning, the goal is to keep the surgical trajectory roughly parallel (at < 30° angle) to the long axis of the white matter tract that one is trying to preserve (unproven hypothesis[21]).

Surgical "corridors" have been described taking into consideration preservation of white matter tracts:
- anterior corridor: parallel to association fibers, between the SLF and the cingulum (e.g., can be through eyebrow or forehead incision)
- posterior corridor: enters at the parieto-occipital sulcus, passes adjacent to the optic radiations
- lateral corridor

13

13.4 Angiography

See Endovascular Neurosurgery section (p. 1913).

13.5 Myelography

Contraindications:
1. anticoagulation
2. allergy to iodinated contrast: requires iodine allergy prep (p. 232). NB: risk of adverse reaction still persists
3. infection at the desired puncture site
4. extensive midline lumbar spinal fusion may preclude needle access to the subarachnoid space

Lumbar myelogram
   Using iohexol (Omnipaque® 140 or 180) as shown in ▶ Table 12.4.
   Cervical myelogram with water soluble contrast via LP
   Use iohexol (Omnipaque® 300 or 240) as shown in ▶ Table 12.4. Insert spinal needle into lumbar subarachnoid space, tilt the head of the myelogram table down with the patient's neck extended and then inject dye. If a complete cervical block is seen, have patient flex neck. If the block cannot be traversed, patient may need C1–2 puncture or MRI (first obtain a CT which may show dye above the block that cannot be appreciated on myelography alone).
   Post myelographic CT
   Increases sensitivity and specificity of myelography (p. 1234). In cases of complete block on myelogram, CT will often show dye distal to the apparent site of the block.

13.6 Radionuclide scanning

13.6.1 Three phase bone scan

Technetium-99 (99mTc) pertechnetate is a radioisotope that may be attached to various substrates for use in bone scanning. It may be used to label polyphosphate (rarely used today), diphosphonate[22] (MDP), or phosphorous (HDP) (the most widely used agent currently). Accumulates in areas of osteoblastic activity.

Three-phase bone scan: uses technetium 99m-HDP. Images are obtained immediately after injection (flow phase), at 15 min (blood pooling) and in 4 hours (bone imaging). Cellulitis shows up as increased activity in the first 2 phases, and there is little or diffuse increased activity in the 3rd. Osteomyelitis causes increased uptake in all 3 phases.

Used in evaluation of acute osteomyelitis with sensitivity and specificity of ≈ 95% each, and is usually positive within 2–3 days. False positives can occur in conditions involving increased bone turnover, e.g., fracture, septic arthritis, tumors. False negative can occur in cases with associated bone infarction.

Applications for bone scans include:
1. infection
   a) osteomyelitis of the spine—vertebral osteomyelitis (p. 389)—or skull
   b) discitis (p. 390)
2. tumor
   a) spine metastases (p. 925)
   b) primary bone tumors of the spine (p. 989)
   c) skull tumors (p. 972)
3. diseases involving abnormal bone metabolism
   a) Paget's disease: of the skull or spine (p. 1362)
   b) hyperostosis frontalis interna (p. 975)
4. craniosynostosis (p. 265)
5. fractures: spine or skull
6. "low back problems" (p. 1235): to help identify some of the above conditions

13

13.6.2 Gallium scan

Nuclear medicine scan with 67Ga citrate which accumulates in areas of inflammation and some malignancies. Utility in neurosurgery for sarcoidosis (p. 198), chronic vertebral osteomyelitis; see also comparison to bone scan (p. 389).

References

[1] Jackson EF, Ginsberg LE, Schomer DF, et al. A Review of MRI Pulse Sequences and Techniques in Neuroimaging. Surgical Neurology. 1997; 47:185–199

[2] Anzai Y, Ishikawa M, Shaw DW, et al. Paramagnetic effect of supplemental oxygen on CSF hyperintensity on fluid-attenuated inversion recovery MR images. AJNR. American Journal of Neuroradiology. 2004; 25:274–279

[3] Alemany M, Stenborg A, Terent A, et al. Coexistence of microhemorrhages and acute spontaneous brain hemorrhage: Correlation with signs of microangiopathy and clinical data. Radiology. 2006; 238:240–247

[4] Yang D, Korogi Y, Ushio Y, et al. Increased conspicuity of intraventricular lesions revealed by three-dimensional constructive interference in steady state sequences. AJNR Am J Neuroradiol. 2000; 21:1070–1072

[5] Shellock FG. Reference Manual for Magnetic Resonance Safety. Salt Lake City, Utah: Amirsys, Inc.; 2003

[6] Edelman RR, Warach S. Magnetic Resonance Imaging (First of Two Parts). New England Journal of Medicine. 1993; 328:708–716

[7] Kanal E, Barkovich AJ, Bell C, et al. ACR guidance document for safe MR practices: 2007. American Journal of Roentgenology. 2007; 188:1447–1474

[8] Deo A, Fogel M, Cowper SE. Nephrogenic systemic fibrosis: a population study examining the relationship of disease development to gadolinium exposure. Clinical Journal of the American Society of Nephrology. 2007; 2:264–267

[9] Penfield JG, Reilly RF. Nephrogenic systemic fibrosis risk: is there a difference between gadolinium-based contrast agents? Semin Dial. 2008; 21:129–134

[10] Elmholdt TR, Jorgensen B, Ramsing M, et al. Two cases of nephrogenic systemic fibrosis after exposure to the macrocyclic compound gadobutrol. NDT Plus. 2010; 3:285–287

[11] U.S. Food and Drug Administration (FDA). FDA Drug Safety Communication: FDA warns that gadolinium-based contrast agents (GBCAs) are retained in the body; requires new class warnings. 2017. https://www.fda.gov/Drugs/DrugSafety/ucm589213.htm

[12] Fisher M, Albers GW. Applications of diffusion-perfusion magnetic resonance imaging in acute ischemic stroke. Neurology. 1999; 52:1750–1756

[13] Prichard JW, Grossman RI. New reasons for early use of MRI in stroke. Neurology. 1999; 52:1733–1736

[14] Ay H, Buonanno FS, Rordorf G, et al. Normal diffusion-weighted MRI during stroke-like deficits. Neurology. 1999; 52:1784–1792

[15] Ay H, Buonanno FS, Schaefer PW, et al. Posterior Leukoencephalopathy Without Severe Hypertension: Utility of Diffusion-Weighted MRI. Neurology. 1998; 51:1369–1376

[16] Schaefer PW, Buonanno FS, Gonzalez RG, et al. Diffusion-Weighted Imaging Discriminates Between Cytotoxic and Vasogenic Edema in a Patient with Eclampsia. Stroke. 1997; 28:1082–1085

[17] Marks MP, Tong DC, Beaulieu C, et al. Evaluation of Early Reperfusion and IV tPA Therapy Using Diffusion- and Perfusion-Weighted MRI. Neurology. 1999; 52:1792–1798

[18] Martinez-Perez I, Moreno A, Alonso J, et al. Diagnosis of brain abscess by magnetic resonance spectroscopy. Report of two cases. Journal of Neurosurgery. 1997; 86:708–713

[19] Barba I, Moreno A, Martinez-Perez I, et al. Magnetic resonance spectroscopy of brain hemangiopericytomas: high myoinositol concentrations and discrimination from meningiomas. Journal of Neurosurgery. 2001; 94:55–60

[20] Douek P, Turner R, Pekar J, et al. MR color mapping of myelin fiber orientation. J Comput Assist Tomogr. 1991; 15:923–929

[21] Kassam AB, Labib MA, Bafaquh M, et al. Part I: The challenge of functional preservation: an integrated systems approach using diffusion-weighted, image guided, exoscopic-assisted, transsulcal radial corridors. Innovative Neurosurgery. 2015

[22] Handa J, Yamamoto I, Morita R, et al. 99mTc-Polyphosphate and 99mTc-Diphosphonate Bone Scintigraphy in Neurosurgical Practice. Surgical Neurology. 1974; 2:307–310

14 Electrodiagnostics

14.1 Electroencephalogram (EEG)

14.1.1 General information

The primary use of EEG is in the diagnosis and management of seizure disorders. Non-convulsive use of EEG is essentially limited to monitoring for burst suppression (see below) (e.g., induced barbiturate coma) or for differential diagnosis of diffuse encephalopathy, including:

1. differentiating psychogenic unresponsiveness from organic: a normal EEG indicates either psychiatric unresponsiveness or locked-in syndrome
2. non-convulsive status epilepticus (seizures): absence or complex partial status
3. subclinical focal abnormalities: e.g., PLEDs (see below), focal slowing...
4. specific patterns diagnostic for certain pathologies: e.g.:
   a) periodic lateralizing epileptiform discharges (PLEDs): may occur with any acute focal cerebral insult (e.g., herpes simplex encephalitis (HSE), abscess, tumor, embolic infarct): seen in 85% of cases of HSE (onset 2–5 d after presentation), if bilateral is ≈ diagnostic of HSE
   b) subacute sclerosing panencephalitis (SSPE) (pathognomonic pattern): periodic high voltage with 4–15 secs separation with accompanying body jerks, no change with painful stimulation (differential diagnosis includes PCP overdose)
   c) Creutzfeldt-Jakob disease (p. 399): myoclonic jerks. EEG → bilateral sharp wave 1.5–2 per second (early → slowing; later → triphasic). May resemble PLEDs, but are reactive to painful stimulation (most PLEDs are not)
   d) triphasic waves: not really specific. May be seen in hepatic encephalopathy, post-anoxia, and hyponatremia
5. objective measure of severity of encephalopathy: usually used for anoxic encephalopathy (e.g., periodic spikes with seizures indicates < 5% chance of normal neurologic outcome, with high mortality). Alpha coma, burst suppression, and electrocerebral silence are all poor prognosticators
6. differentiating hydranencephaly (p. 309) from severe hydrocephalus
7. as a clinical confirmatory test in the determination of brain death (p. 333)

14.1.2 Common EEG rhythms

Common EEG rhythms are shown in ▶ Table 14.1.

Table 14.1 Common EEG rhythms

Rhythm	Symbol	Frequency
delta	Δ	0–3 Hz
theta	θ	4–7 Hz
alpha	α	8–13 Hz
beta	β	> 13 Hz

14.1.3 Burst suppression

Bursts of 8–12 Hz electrical activity (lasting 1–10 s)[1] that diminish to 1–4 Hz prior to intervals of electrical silence (no excursions ≥ 5 microvolts, lasting > 10 s)[2] (▶ Fig. 14.1).

Often used as an endpoint for titrating neuroprotective drugs such as barbiturates, propofol... e.g., for temporary clipping (p. 1465) during cerebrovascular surgery, traumatic or intracranial hypertension (p. 1056) refractory to lower tier interventions.

14.2 Evoked potentials

14.2.1 General information

Evoked potentials are averaged EEG waveforms recorded following repetitive stimulation. The process of averaging nulls out EEG activity that is not time-locked to the stimulus. Resultant waveforms

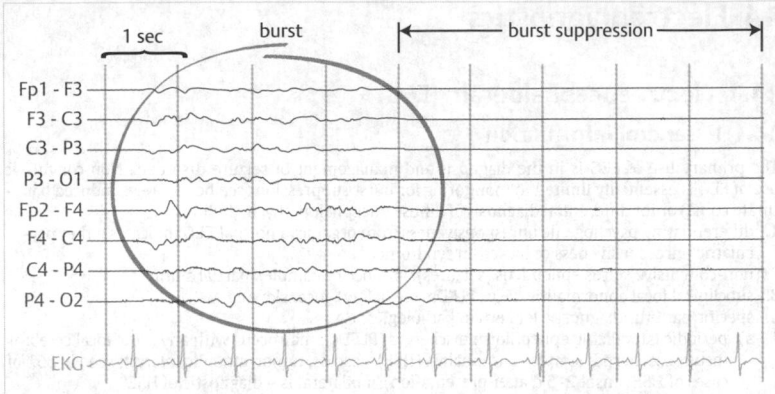

Fig. 14.1 Burst suppression. Image: EEG illustrating burst suppression.

contain peaks that are named N (negative—upward deflection) or P (positive—downward deflection) followed by the latency in milliseconds to the onset of the peak.

14.2.2 (Somato) sensory evoked potentials (SSEP or SEP)

General information

May use electrical stimulation of peripheral nerves (somatosensory or [SSEP]), auditory clicks through earphones (auditory or AEP, AKA BAER [brainstem auditory evoked response]) or flashing lights through goggles (visual EP or VEP).

Evoked potentials are most commonly used by neurosurgeons for intraoperative monitoring purposes. SSEP (especially from median nerve stimulation) also has prognostic significance in cervical spondylotic myelopathy,[3] although use for this purpose is limited.

Typical waveforms

Abbreviations

Abbreviations used in ► Table 14.2, ► Table 14.3, ► Table 14.4, and ► Table 14.5: BAER = brainstem auditory evoked response; UE/LE SSEP = upper/lower extremity somatosensory evoked potential; PR VER = pattern reversal visual evoked response which requires patient cooperation and visual attention as opposed to flash VER which may even be done through closed eyelids. See also references.[4,5]

Table 14.2 Typical stimulus values for intra-op evoked potentials

Test	Stimulus			Comment
	Freq (Hz)	Duration (mcS)	Magnitude	
BAER	23.5	150	85–100 dB	rarefaction usually better than compression
UE SSEP (median nerve at wrist)	4.7	300–700	up to 50 mA	supramaximal stimulus (sensory threshold + motor threshold)
LE SSEP (posterior tibial at ankle)	4.7	300–700	up to 100 mA	supramaximal stimulus
PR VER	1.97			16 × 16 checks, 1.6 cm each, at 1 meter (subtends 55° arc visual angle)

Table 14.3 Input characteristics for acquiring evoked potentials

Test	Analysis				Electrode derivations
	Input filter (Hz)	Sensitive (mcV)	Duration (mS)	Reps	
BAER	150–3000	25	15	1500	$M_1{}^a$-C_ZZ, $M_2{}^*$-C_Z, ground = FZ
UE SSEP	30–3000	50	55–60	600	F_Z-Erb's point, C_{V7}-F_{PZ}, C_3-F_{PZ}, C_3'-NC (non-cephalic, e.g., shoulder)
LE SSEP	30–3000	50	60	600	popliteal fossa (front to back), C_Z-F_{PZ}, back (L_5-T_{12}) (difficult in obese or elderly), C_I-C_C (optional: somato-sensory ipsilateral to contralateral)
PR VER	5–100	50	500	100	O_1-A_1, O_Z-A_1, O_2-A_1, O_Z-C_Z

^{a}M= mastoid ("i" is ipsilateral to stimulus, and "c" is contralateral)

Table 14.4 Evoked potential waveforms (note: values may differ from lab to lab)

Test	Figure	Possible generators	
BAER		CM	cochlear microphonic
		P_1	distal VIII nerve,
		P_2	proximal VIII or cochlear nucleus,
		P_3	lower pons (? superior olivary complex),
		P_4	mid-upper pons,
		P_5	upper pons or inferior colliculus
UE SSEP		N_9	(on F_Z-E_P where E_P is Erb's point) AKA EP: entry of volley into distal brachial plexus,
		N_{11}	(on C_{V7}-F_{PZ}): root entry zone (cervical region),
		N_{13}	cervicomedullary junction (recorded from C2),
		N_{19}	primary sensory cortex,
		P_{22}	(early) motor cortex,
		P_{22}	(late) IPSP "reaction" to N_{18}
LE SSEP		P_{22}	(on L_5-T_{12}): lumbo-sacral plexus,
		P_{40}	(on C_Z-F_{PZ}): sensory cortex (analogous to N18 in UE SSEP, reversed in polarity for ? reason),
		N_{27}	(on C_{V7}-F_{PZ}): ? dorsal column nucleus
		N_{30}	
PR VER		P_{100}	(striate & pre-striate occipital cortex, with contributions from thalamocortical volleys

14.2.3 Intraoperative evoked potentials

General information

EPs may be used for intraoperative monitoring (e.g., monitoring hearing during resection of vestibular schwannomas, or monitoring SSEPs during some spine surgery); however, the need to average a

Table 14.5 Normal values for evoked potentials[a] (note: values may differ from lab to lab)

Test	Parameters measured	Normal values		Comment
		Mean	+2.5 std dev	
BAER	I-V peak latency	4.01 mS	4.63 mS	
	I-III peak latency	2.15 mS	2.66 mS	prolongation suggests lesion between pons & colliculus, often **vestibular schwannoma**
	V absolute latency	5.7 mS	6.27 mS	
	III-V peak latency			prolongation suggests lesion between lower pons & midbrain, may be seen in M.S.
UE SSEP	N_9-N_{18} peak latency	9.38 mS	11.35 mS	
LE SSEP	P_{22}-P_{40} peak latency	15.62 mS	20.82 mS	
	P_{40} absolute latency	37.20 mS	44.16 mS	
PR VER	P_{100} absolute latency		+3 S.D.	
	P_{100} inter-eye difference	8–10 mS		Inter-eye difference is more sensitive with full field stimulation. Monocular defect suggests conduction defect in that optic nerve anterior to chiasm (e.g., M.S., glaucoma, compression retinal degeneration). Bilateral defect does not localize.

[a] normal values in boldface are critical values used as cutoff for abnormal results

number of waveforms results in a short delay which limits their usefulness in avoiding acute intra-operative injury. A 10% increased latency of a major EP peak, or a drop in amplitude of ≥ 50% is significant and should cause the surgeon to assess all variables (retractors, instruments, blood pressure…). Intraoperative SSEPs may also be used to localize primary sensory cortex in anesthetized patients (as opposed to using brain mapping techniques in awake patients) by looking for phase reversal potentials across the central sulcus.[6,7]

Brainstem auditory evoked responses (BAER)

14

AKA auditory brainstem response (ABR), AKA auditory evoked potential (AEP). Auditory clicks are delivered to the patient by earphones. Peaks (▶ Table 14.4). Once used for assistance in diagnosing vestibular schwannomas, their use for intraoperative monitoring is limited and has been largely replaced by direct eighth cranial nerve monitoring which provides more rapid information for the surgeon.

SSEP monitoring during spine surgery

Paralytics actually improve SSEP recordings by reducing muscle artifact, but will abolish the visible twitch that confirms that the stimulus is being received.

Typical stimulus sites: median, ulnar, and tibial nerves. Impulses ascend in the *ipsilateral* posterior column. UE SSEPs travel primarily in the dorsal columns, but LE SSEPs are carried mostly in the dorsolateral fasciculus (p. 71) which is supplied by the *anterior* spinal artery. Thus, UE and LE SSEPs are more sensitive to direct mechanical effects primarily on the *posterior* spinal cord (sensory) and may remain unchanged with some injuries to the anterior cord (motor); however, LE SSEPs can detect ischemic effects on the anterior cord by virtue of involvement of the anterior spinal artery.

In a personal series of 809 patients,[8] 17 had SSEP degradation, 14 of these (82%) responded to intra-op interventions (see below), and in 13 of these 14 (93%) there were no new deficits. In the 3 that did not respond, 2 had significant new neurologic deficits.

Transcranial motor evoked potentials (TCMEPs)

Anesthetic requirements: in addition to EP anesthetic requirements, neuromuscular blockade must be minimized to permit ≥ 2 out of 4 twitches.

AKA motor evoked potentials (MEP): transcranial electrical or magnetic stimulation of motor cortex and descending motor axons with EMG recording of motor potentials from representative muscle groups. Using direct electrical stimulation is limited in awake patients by local pain. Due to the large potentials, the acquisition time is shorter and feedback to the surgeon is almost immediate. However, due to patient movement from the muscle contractions, continuous recording is usually not possible (a variation allows monitoring the response over the spinal cord). Useful for surgery involving the spinal cord (cervical or thoracic), no utility for lumbar spine surgery. Seizures occur rarely, usually in patients with increased seizure risk and with high-rate stimulation frequency.

Contraindications to MEP:
1. history of epilepsy/seizures
2. past surgical skull defects
3. metal in head or neck
4. use special care with implanted electronic devices

Descending evoked potentials (DEP)

(Formerly referred to by the misleading term "neurogenic motor evoked potentials"). Rostral stimulation of the spinal cord with recording of a caudal neurogenic response from the spinal cord or peripheral nerve, or a myogenic response from a distal muscle. DEPs can be mediated primarily by sensory nerves and therefore do not represent true motor potentials. However, shown to be sensitive to spinal cord changes and may be useful when TCMEPs cannot be obtained.

Direct waves (D-waves)

See entry under intramedullary spinal cord tumors (p. 989).

14.2.4 Intraoperative electrophysiologic monitoring changes

EP change criteria to trigger notification of surgeon

Any of the following:
1. SSEP:
   a) 50% decrease in peak signal amplitude from baseline
   b) increase in peak latency > 10%
   c) complete loss of a waveform
2. TCMEP: sustained 50% decrease in signal amplitude. As a convention, if the same response can be obtained by an increase in stimulating voltage of no more than 100 V above the baseline voltage used, then this is considered stable from baseline
3. DEP: decrease in signal of > 60%

Interventions for SSEP/TCMEP changes during spine surgery

When loss or degradation of SSEP/TCMEP during spine surgery is due to compression, the prognosis may be good. Vascular injuries generally do not fare as well.

Options/suggestions include (adapted/excerpted from the "**Vitale checklist**"[9]) (this is a list, not a step-by-step protocol - items are not necessarily performed in order listed):
1. verify that the change is real. Technical considerations include:
   a) rule out 60 Hz interference from other equipment (OR table, C-arm, microscope… anything with a plug)
   b) check connections
   c) verify that stimulating electrodes & recording leads are making good contact
2. place OR on alert status
   a) announce intraoperative pause and stop the case
   b) eliminate possible distractions (music, unnecessary conversations…)
   c) "muster the troops": the attending anesthesiologist, senior neurologist or neurophysiologist and experienced nurse are called to the room. Consult a surgical colleague if necessary (even if by phone)
   d) if special imaging (CT, MRI, angiogram…) may be required, alert appropriate personnel
3. anesthetic/metabolic considerations
   a) optimize mean arterial pressure (MAP usually > 85 mm Hg preferred). Raising the MAP alone restores monitoring loss in 20% of cases[10]
   b) check hematocrit for anemia (could contribute to cord ischemia)
   c) optimize blood pH (rule out acidemia) and pCO_2

14

d) normalize patient body temperature
e) check anesthetic technical factors: assess extent of paralytics, inhalational agents…
f) discuss possibility of "Stagnara wake up test (p. 254)" with attending anesthesiologist and scrub nurse
4. surgical considerations (maneuvers are restricted to those that do not destabilize the spine):
   a) visually check patient position on table: arms, legs, shift in torso, malfunction of positioning frame; reverse step that immediately preceded change in potentials (if feasible).
   b) remove traction if used
   c) decrease distraction or other corrective forces
   d) remove rods
   e) remove screw that could correlate with the change, and re-probe for breach
   f) perform intra-op X-ray to rule out shift in patient position
   g) rule out spinal cord and/or nerve root compression
      1. as a result of instrumentation
      2. in scoliosis, consider resecting the apical pedicle or reducing the scoliosis
      3. in patients with spinal stenosis, consider emergently decompressing the spinal cord (for cervical stenosis) or cauda equina (for lumbar stenosis) if not already done
   h) check for nerve root compression at osteotomy sites
   i) obtain intraoperative axial imaging (e.g., CT or O-arm) if available
   j) consider staging operation if practical
5. perform Stagnara wake-up test if feasible (see below)
6. consider IV steroids

Other considerations that may be helpful that are not part of the Vitale checklist:
1. knowledge of neuroanatomy and comparison to the deficit pattern can be helpful in narrowing down the source of the problem. Examples: loss of MEPs from the vastus lateralis (innervation: L2, 3 & 4) during an L4-5 TLIF cannot be caused by a surgical site complication (hematoma, screw malposition…) and other etiologies should be sought. Loss of motor potentials in the hands during surgery on thoracic or lumbar spine: consider repositioning the arms to avoid traction on the brachial plexus or compression of ulnar nerves at the elbows
2. **dynamic spinal cord mapping** can also be used to localize the problem area when MEPs decrease or are completely lost.[11] Ideally, prior to beginning the procedure, a baseline is obtained by sequentially inserting a percutaneous monopolar electrode between lamina above and below the level of the surgery, and responses are recorded in distal musculature (they used sciatic nerves and popliteal fossa). During the operation, electrodes are placed on 2 adjacent spinous processes and the monitoring is performed continuously. If a change in monitoring occurs, an epidural stimulus is applied at individual levels until the level of the conduction loss is localized
3. for unexplained global loss of spinal cord function with a level caudal to the level of surgery, check for abdominal compression by bolsters on the OR table (increased intraabdominal pressure may increase venous pressure transmitted to the spinal cord, impairing blood flow to the cord)
4. loss of function in 1 limb: reposition the limb or padding if distal pulses are diminished

▶ **(Stagnara) wake-up test**[12]. An intraoperative test of voluntary motor function. The patient is allowed to wake up enough from anesthesia to be able to wiggle the toes on command (the patient is kept intubated and the wound is not closed). Less commonly used in the current era of electrophysiologic monitoring (EPM), but may be employed in cases where EPM is felt to be possibly unreliable. And since no specialized equipment is required, it can be used in times or places where access to EPM is limited. Is more efficacious if planned in advance, in which case short-acting anesthetic agents are employed and the patient can be briefed ahead of time.

Cons: can only be performed sparingly during surgery (time consuming and often challenging), so it may delay detection of any other change that might be identified earlier by EPM. Patients often will try to get up or move. Tests only motor function, and may miss subtle deficits.

14.3 NCS/EMG

14.3.1 General information

Electrodiagnostic studies are clinical tests usually performed by a neurologist or a physical medicine and rehabilitation physician. Electrodiagnostic studies of peripheral nerves consist of two parts:
1. conduction measurements: typically referred to as "NCV" (nerve conduction velocity) study but technically should be called NCS (nerve conduction studies) since amplitude, latency, and

duration of motor and sensory nerves are also evaluated. An electrical stimulation is applied through surface electrodes at specified locations and electrical responses are recorded in receiving electrodes. Since needles are almost never used, NCS can be done in patients on anticoagulants or antiplatelet drugs

2. electromyogram (EMG) AKA "needle exam" (see below). This part of the exam consists of inserting needle electrodes into muscles and analyzing muscle electrical activity at rest and under condiitons outlined below. Some electromyographers will not do an EMG in patients on anticoagulants or antiplatelet drugs due to risk of hematoma which could produce a compartment syndrome

14.3.2 Electromyography (EMG)

Definitions

SNAP: sensory nerve action potential. Key concept: since the ganglion of the sensory nerves lies within the neural foramen, preganglionic lesions (injury to the nerve root *proximal* to the neural foramen, e.g., root compression by herniated disc or root avulsion) does not affect the cell body, and therefore the distal SNAP is unaffected.[13] Postganglionic lesions (distal to the neural foramen, e.g., peripheral nerve injury) reduces SNAP amplitudes and/or slows the sensory conduction velocity.

F-wave: stimulation of a nerve causes orthodromic (normal conduction along the axon away from the cell body) and antidromic conduction. Some anterior horn cells that are stimulated antidromically will fire orthodromically, producing the F-wave. F-wave latency may be prolonged in multilevel radiculopathy (not sensitive). Most helpful in evaluating proximal root slowing, e.g., GBS (p. 193).

H-reflex: practical ≈ only in S1 nerve root. Provides information equivalent to the ankle jerk. Stimulation of Ia afferent fibers passes through a monosynaptic connection causing an orthodromic alpha-motor action potential that can be measured in the triceps surae (the two heads of the gastrocnemius and the soleus).

Volitional activity: the motor unit action potential (MUAP) can be assessed only with voluntary muscle contraction by the patient. Components of the MUAP measured include amplitude, rise time, duration, and number of phases (crossings of the baseline).

Polyphasic potentials: MUAPs with > 4 phases. Normally comprise < 15% of MUAPs. Following a nerve injury, reinnervation produces abnormally increased polyphasic potentials after 3-6 months (can be seen 6–8 weeks) which gradually increase over several months, and then begin to wane (as firing becomes more synchronous).

Myotonia: there are a number of myotonic conditions, including myotonic dystrophy in which there is sustained contraction of the muscle. Classic EMG finding: "dive bomber" sound due to myotonic discharges.

Exam overview

There are 3 phases of an EMG exam:

▶ **Phase 1 - insertional activity.** The electric response of the muscle to mechanical irritation caused by small movements of the needle.

▶ **Phase 2 - spontaneous activity.** In muscle at rest.
1. normal: silent with stationary needle once insertional activity has subsided
2. spontaneous activity: independently produced electrical activity. Usually abnormal (although sometimes seen in normal volunteers)
   a) after denervation (secondary to a nerve injury) or muscle injury:
      • positive sharp waves (PSW)
      • fibrillation potentials (AKA fibrillations or fibs): action potentials arising from *single* muscle fibers. Detectable on EMG (not visible to the naked eye, c.f. fasciculations (p. 531)). Typically develop ≈ 21 days after the death of the lower motor neuron (earliest onset 7–10 days after denervation, sometimes not for 3–4 weeks). If the nerve recovers, it may reinnervate the muscle, but with larger motor units (greater amplitude) resulting in longer duration and decreased numbers
      • increased insertional activity: due to the increase in acetycholine receptors in response to denervation
   b) myotonic discharges ("dive bomber" sound on speaker monitor)
   c) complex repetitive discharge (CRD): ephaptic conduction of groups of adjacent muscle fibers. Occurs in neuropathic or myopathic disorders

14

d) fasciculation potentials: nonspecific, but typically associated with motor neuron disease (ALS) (p.191)
e) other less common spontaneous activity includes: myokymic, neuromytonic and cramp discharges

▶ **Phase 3 - volitional activity.** Evaluated with patient exert minimal volitional effort and again with maximal effort.

1. motor unit action potential (MUAP) analysis: stimulation of a motor neuron produces contraction of the motor fibers supplied by its axon (the motor unit). Analysis includes evaluation of motor unit amplitude, duration, polyphasia and stability. In general, increased amplitude and duration suggest a disorder of the LMN, and reduced amplitude and duration suggest a primary myopathic disorder
2. recruitment with minimal volitional effort: normally with increasing effort motor units fire at an increasing rate and additional motor units begin to fire in an orderly manner. Two possible *abnormal* findings:
   a) reduced recruitment (or fast firing): overly fast firing of a reduced number of MUAPs. Always indicative of a neuropathic process
   b) early or increased recruitment: indicative of a myopathic process
3. with maximal effort

EMG for radiculopathy

EMG pearls for the neurosurgeon
General principles:
- if a reliable motor exam can be done, the EMG will not likely add any information. A normal motor exam will usually be associated with a normal EMG
- EMG is *not* extremely sensitive for radiculopathy (e.g., especially with sensory-only radiculopathy, which is more common in the cervical region than lumbar). However, when abnormal, EMG is very specific
- EMG is best reserved for cases with documented weakness where additional localizing or prognostic information is needed, or when the patient's strength cannot be reliably assessed (inability to cooperate, functional overlay...)
- timing
  ○ "acute changes" (see spontaneous activity, above) begin at about 3 weeks and can last up to about 6 months
  ○ chronic changes can be seen starting at about 6 months, and may persist indefinitely

Cervical EMG:
- EMG is most helpful for nerve roots C5–T1. There are no good muscles to reliably test C3–4, and compression here may cause findings in lower nerve roots

Lumbar EMG:
- if the lumbar MRI is normal in a patient with evidence of motor weakness (e.g., foot drop), get an EMG to look for peripheral neuropathy (again, a good motor exam can give the same info). If the EMG is negative for peripheral neuropathy (e.g., peroneal nerve palsy) then do an MRI (or CT) of abdomen and pelvis to look for pelvic floor tumor

Findings
Include spontaneous activity: fibs, PSWs and increased insertional activity (see above).

The earliest possible finding (within 2–3 d) is reduced recruitment with volitional activity, but this occurs only with significant compression of motor fibers.

EMG is useful if there is a concern about possible overlapping peripheral neuropathy (e.g., carpal tunnel syndrome vs. C6 radiculopathy).

EMG criteria for radiculopathy
1. fibrillations and/or positive sharp waves in at least 2 muscles innervated by a single nerve root in question, but by 2 different *peripheral* nerves
2. abnormal paraspinals: this supports the diagnosis, but is not required since paraspinals will be normal in ≈ 50%

Lumbar radiculopathy from herniated disc

With radiculopathy, SNAP is usually normal (see above). Paraspinal muscle fibrillations may occur. Accuracy in predicting level of involvement[14] is ≈ 84%.

Foot drop: the short head of the biceps femoris in the LE is the first muscle innervated by the peroneal division of the sciatic nerve at or just above the popliteal fossa just after the nerve splits off from the sciatic nerve. In cases e.g., of foot drop it is a good muscle to test to determine if there is a peroneal neuropathy vs. a more proximal lesion (i.e., above the popliteal fossa).

Findings with healing radiculopathy (e.g., following discectomy or spontaneous healing):
• motor potentials return first (if nerve injury were "complete," it would take a month to return)
• if lost, sensory potentials return last or may not return
• following laminectomy, paraspinal muscle potentials may no longer be useful for EMG because cutting the muscles during surgery alters their electrical signals resulting in effective denervation due to *muscle* injury. Fibs and PSWs decrease in amplitude over time but may remain present indefinitely

Interpreting the report

What the report says: e.g., "Chronic cervical radiculopathy"

What this usually means: there are large amplitude fast firing motor units (sometimes termed "decreased recruitment").

Neurosurgical implications: this does not imply anything about ongoing compression.

If report further qualifies it e.g., as "without evidence of ongoing denervation" this usually means no sharp waves (PSWs) or fibrillation potentials (fibs) were seen. This implies that there was some nerve injury at some point, but that there has been healing and unlikely that there is ongoing compression.

EMG in plexopathy

Reduction of SNAP with *no paraspinal* muscle fibrillations (the dorsal rami exit proximally to innervate the paraspinals, and are involved ≈ *only* with root lesions).

EMG in nerve root avulsion

Produces muscles weakness and sensory loss with normal SNAP since the lesion is proximal to the dorsal root ganglion (where the cell bodies for the sensory nerves are located).

References

[1] Bhattacharyya S, Biswas A, Mukherjee J, et al. Detection of artifacts from high energy bursts in neonatal EEG. Comput Biol Med. 2013; 43:1804–1814
[2] Donnegan JH, Blitt CD. The Electroencephalogram. In: Monitoring in Anesthesia and Critical Care Medicine. New York: Churchill Livingstone; 1985:323–343
[3] Holly LangstonT, Matz PaulG, Anderson PaulA, et al. Clinical prognostic indicators of surgical outcome in cervical spondylotic myelopathy. Journal of Neurosurgery: Spine. 2009; 11:112–118
[4] Chiappa KH. Evoked Potentials in Clinical Medicine (First of Two Parts). N Engl J Med. 1982; 306:1140–1150
[5] Chiappa KH. Evoked Potentials in Clinical Medicine (Second of Two Parts). N Engl J Med. 1982; 306:1205–1211
[6] Gregori EM, Goldring S. Localization of Function in the Excision of Lesions from the Sensorimotor Region. Journal of Neurosurgery. 1984; 61:1047–1054
[7] Woolsey CN, Erickson TC, Gibson WE. Localization in Somatic Sensory and Motor Areas of Human Cerebral Cortex as Determined by Direct Recording of Evoked Potentials and Electrical Stimulation. Journal of Neurosurgery. 1979; 51:476–506
[8] Roh MS, Wilson-Holden TJ, Padberg AM, et al. The utility of somatosensory evoked potential monitoring during cervical spine surgery: how often does it prompt intervention and affect outcome? Asian Spine J. 2007; 1:43–47
[9] Vitale MichaelG, Skaggs DavidL, Pace GregoryI, et al. Best Practices in Intraoperative Neuromonitoring in Spine Deformity Surgery: Development of an Intraoperative Checklist to Optimize Response. Spine Deformity. 2014; 2:333–339
[10] Yang J, Skaggs DL, Chan P, et al. Raising Mean Arterial Pressure Alone Restores 20% of Intraoperative Neuromonitoring Losses. Spine (Phila Pa 1976). 2018; 43:890–894
[11] Silva FE, Lenke L. Importance of intraoperative dynamic spinal cord mapping (DSCM) during complex spinal deformity surgery. Spine Deform. 2020; 8:1131–1134
[12] Vauzelle C, Stagnara P, Jouvinroux P. Functional monitoring of spinal cord activity during spinal surgery. Clin Orthop Relat Res. 1973:173–178
[13] Benecke R, Conrad B. The distal sensory nerve action potential as a diagnostic tool for the differentiation of lesions in dorsal roots and peripheral nerves. J Neurol. 1980; 223:231–239
[14] Young A, Getty J, Jackson A, et al. Variations in the Pattern of Muscle Innervation by the L5 and S1 Nerve Roots. Spine. 1983; 8:616–624

14

Part IV

Developmental Anomalies

IV

15 Primary Intracranial Anomalies

15.1 Arachnoid cysts, intracranial

15.1.1 General information

> ### Key concepts
>
> - a congenital fluid-containing abnormality of the arachnoid membrane that displaces brain and typically remodels bone
> - most common in middle fossa, cerebellopontine angle (CPA), suprasellar region, and posterior fossa. May also occur in the spine
> - most are asymptomatic (i.e., an incidental finding) except in the suprasellar region
> - imaging often shows remodeling of bone; imaging characteristics exactly mimic CSF on CT or MRI in most cases
> - recommendation for incidentally discovered arachnoid cyst in adults: a single follow-up imaging study in 6–8 months is usually adequate to rule out any increase in size. Subsequent studies only if concerning symptoms develop

AKA leptomeningeal cysts, distinct from posttraumatic leptomeningeal cysts (p. 1100) (AKA growing skull fractures), and unrelated to infection. Arachnoid cysts (AC) are congenital lesions that arise during development from splitting of arachnoid membrane (thus they are technically intra-arachnoid cysts) and contain fluid that is usually identical to CSF. They do not communicate with the ventricles or subarachnoid space. May be unloculated or may have septations. Typically lined with meningothelial cells positive for epithelial membrane antigen (EMA) and negative for carcinoembryonic antigen (CEA). AC may also occur in the spinal canal.

"Temporal lobe agenesis syndrome" is an obsolete label used with middle cranial fossa ACs (brain volumes on each side are actually the same,[1] bone expansion and shift of brain matter account for the parenchyma that appears to be replaced by the AC).

Two types of histological findings[2]:
1. "simple arachnoid cysts": arachnoid lining with cells that appear to be capable of active CSF secretion. Middle fossa cysts seem to be exclusively of this type
2. cysts with more complex lining which may also contain neuroglia, ependyma, and other tissue types

15.1.2 Epidemiology of intracranial arachnoid cysts

Incidence: 5 per 1000 in autopsy series. Comprise ≈ 1% of intracranial masses.
  Male:female ratio is 4:1. More common on the left side.
  Bilateral arachnoid cysts may occur in Hurler syndrome (a mucopolysaccharidosis).

15.1.3 Distribution

Almost all occur in relation to an arachnoid cistern (exception: intrasellar, the only one that is extra-dural, ▶ Table 15.1).

▶ **Intraventricular arachnoid cysts.** Intraventricular arachnoid cysts occur uncommonly.
  Evaluation: MRI preferred, CT if MRI not an option. Fluid should be nearly identical to CSF in MRI signal characteristics (or density on CT). Obtain contrast study to rule out a mural nodule. Before performing surgery, consider a CT cisternogram which can rule out communication with the ventricles (contrast may eventually seep into the cyst through the cyst walls).
  Arachnoid cysts of the 4th ventricle are even rarer. These often present with hydrocephalus. Other symptoms may be related to cerebellar or brainstem compression. May be mistaken for a dilated 4th ventricle. Shunting can ameliorate symptoms related to hydrocephalus, however, definitive treatment of the cyst may offer long-term relief from other symptoms as well.[4] A midline suboccipital approach may be used.[5] Ventriculoscopic treatment is an option.[4,6]

▶ **Sylvian fissure arachnoid cysts.** See ▶ Fig. 15.1 for the classification scheme of Galassi et al for middle fossa cysts

15

Table 15.1 Distribution of arachnoid cysts[3]

Location	%
Sylvian fissure ▶ Fig. 15.1	49
CPA*	11
supracollicular	10
vermian	9
sellar & suprasellar	9
interhemispheric	5
cerebral convexity	4
clival	3

* Epidermoid cysts in the cerebellopontine angle (CPA) may mimic an arachnoid cyst, but are high signal on DWI MRI

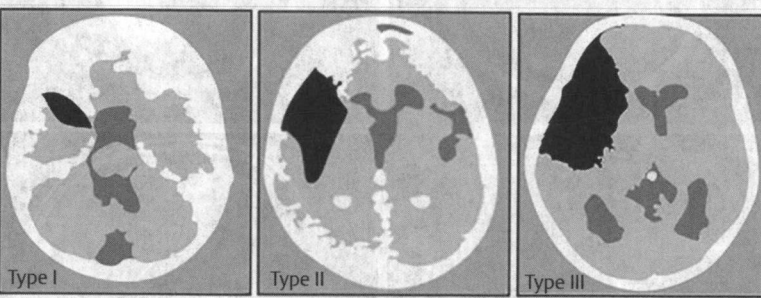

Fig. 15.1 Classification of Sylvian fissure arachnoid cysts.[7]
Type I: small, biconvex, located in anterior temporal tip. No mass effect. Communicates with subarachnoid space on water-soluble contrast CT cisternogram (WS-CTC).
Type II: involves proximal and intermediate segments of Sylvian fissure. Completely open insula gives rectangular shape. Partial communication on WS-CTC.
Type III: involves entire Sylvian fissure. Marked midline shift. Bony expansion of middle fossa (elevation of lesser wing of sphenoid, outward expansion of squamous temporal bone). Minimal communication on WS-CTC. Surgical treatment usually does not result in total reexpansion of brain (may approach type II lesion).

▶ **Pineal region arachnoid cyst.** Arachnoid cysts may occur in the pineal region (AKA quadrigeminal plate arachnoid cysts) (▶ Fig. 15.2). Hydrocephalus may be present and is usually due to compression of the Sylvian aqueduct.

See also differential diagnosis of midline posterior fossa arachnoid cysts (p.271).

15.1.4 Presentation

Most ACs are asymptomatic. Those that become symptomatic usually do so in early childhood.[8] The presentation varies with location and size of the cyst, and oftentimes appear mild considering the large size of some cysts. Obstructive hydrocephalus may occur e.g., with a suprasellar or with a quadrigeminal plate arachnoid cyst (▶ Fig. 15.2).

Typical presentations are shown in ▶ Table 15.2 [8] and include:
1. intracranial hypertension (elevated ICP): symptoms include H/A, N/V, lethargy
2. seizures
3. sudden deterioration:
    a) due to hemorrhage (into cyst or subdural compartment): middle fossa cysts are the most common ones to hemorrhage due to tearing of bridging veins, usually on the surface of the cyst. Some sports organizations do not allow participation in contact sports for these patients
    b) due to rupture of the cyst
4. as a focal protrusion of the skull
5. with focal signs/symptoms of a space occupying lesion
6. incidental finding discovered during evaluation for unrelated condition
7. suprasellar cysts may additionally present with[9]:
    a) hydrocephalus: probably due to compression of the third ventricle

15

15

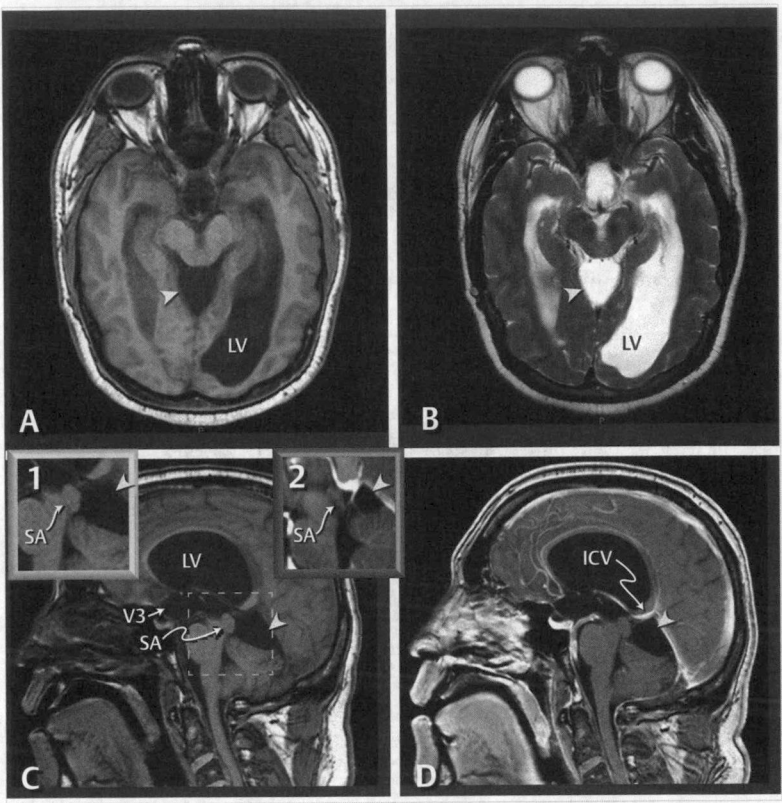

Fig. 15.2 Arachnoid cyst of the pineal region (*yellow arrowheads*).
The cyst abuts the quadrigeminal plate anteriorly, and is inferior to the internal cerebral vein (ICV). The cerebellum is displaced inferiorly. Hydrocephalus, demonstrated by the dilated third ventricle (V3) and the lateral ventricles (LV), is due to compression of the Sylvian aqueduct (SA) (which is occluded as seen in inset 1, compared to inset 2 which shows a patent SA in a different patient with a pineal region arachnoid cyst who did not have hydrocephalus).
Image: A: axial T1WI, B: axial T2WI, C: sagittal T1WI: D: sagittal T1WI + contrast.

Table 15.2 Typical presentations of arachnoid cysts

Middle fossa cysts	Suprasellar cysts with hydrocephalus	Diffuse supra- or infratentorial cysts with hydrocephalus
seizures	intracranial hypertension (see text)	intracranial hypertension
headache	craniomegaly	craniomegaly
hemiparesis	developmental delay	developmental delay
	visual loss	
	precocious puberty	
	bobble-head doll syndrome	

b) endocrine symptoms: occurs in up to 60%. Includes precocious puberty
c) "bobble-head doll syndrome"[10]): rare. Repetitive antero-posterior head movements (head bobbing) usually associated with expansile lesions in the region of the third ventricle.[11] Occurs in < 10% of suprasellar arachnoid cysts. Neuroendoscopic ventriculocystocisternostomy is the recommended treatment[11]
d) visual impairment

15.1.5 Evaluation

General information

Routine evaluation with CT or MRI is usually satisfactory. Further evaluation with CSF contrast or flow studies (cisternograms, ventriculograms…) are only occasionally necessary for the diagnosis of midline suprasellar and posterior fossa lesions[8]; for differential diagnosis, see Intracranial cysts (p. 1656).

CT scan

Smooth bordered non-calcified extraparenchymal cystic mass with density similar to CSF and no enhancement with IV contrast. Expansion of nearby bone by remodelling is usually seen, confirming their chronic nature. Often associated with ventriculomegaly (in 64% of supratentorial and 80% of infratentorial cysts).

Convexity or middle fossa cysts exert mass effect on adjacent brain and may compress ipsilateral lateral ventricle and cause midline shift. Suprasellar, quadrigeminal plate, and midline posterior-fossa cysts may compress the third and fourth ventricle and cause hydrocephalus by obstructing the foramina of Monro or the Sylvian aqueduct.

MRI

Better than CT in differentiating the CSF contained in arachnoid cysts from the fluid of neoplastic cysts. May also show cyst walls.

Cisternograms and/or ventriculograms

Using either iodinated contrast or radionuclide tracers. Variable rate of opacification has resulted in difficulty correlating results with operative findings. Some cysts are actually diverticula, and may fill with radiotracer or contrast.

15.1.6 Treatment

General information

Many (but not all) authors recommend not treating arachnoid cysts that do not cause symptoms, regardless of their size and location. For incidentally discovered arachnoid cyst in an adult not considered for surgery, a single follow-up imaging study in 6–8 months is usually adequate to rule out any changes (since they occasionally grow in size). Subsequent studies may be done if concerning symptoms develop. Pediatric patients may need to be followed until adulthood.

Treatment considerations for cysts (excluding suprasellar cysts)

Surgical treatment options are summarized in ▶ Table 15.3.

Cyst shunting

Probably the best overall treatment. For shunting into peritoneum, use a *low pressure* valve. If there is concurrent ventriculomegaly, one may simultaneously place a ventricular shunt (e.g., through a "Y" connector). Ultrasound, ventriculoscope, or image guidance may assist in locating suprasellar cysts. Shunting of middle fossa ACs may also be accomplished through the lateral ventricle, thus shunting both compartments.[13]

✖ NB: in running the distal shunt tubing from the middle fossa, it should be routed behind the ear (do not tunnel in front of ear to avoid injury to facial nerve—if this anterior route is unavoidable, it may help to solicit the services of a plastic surgeon to help avoid the facial nerve).

Treatment of suprasellar cysts

These cysts present with some unique treatment options, which include:
- transcallosal cystectomy[14]
- percutaneous ventriculo-cystostomy: procedure of choice of Pierre-Kahn et al.[9] Performed via a paramedian coronal burr hole through the lateral ventricle and foramen of Monro (may be facilitated by using a ventriculoscope[12])
- subfrontal approach (for fenestration or removal): dangerous and ineffective[9]

15

Table 15.3 Surgical treatment options for arachnoid cysts

Procedure	Advantages	Disadvantages
drainage by needle aspiration or burr hole evacuation	• simple • quick	• high rate of recurrence of cyst and neurologic deficit
craniotomy, excising cyst wall and fenestrating it into basal cisterns	• permits direct inspection of cyst (may help with diagnosis) • loculated cysts (rare) treated more effectively • avoids permanent shunt (in some cases) • allows visualization of bridging vessels (small advantage)	• subsequent scarring may block fenestration, allowing reaccumulation of cyst • flow through subarachnoid space may be deficient; many patients develop shunt dependency post-op • significant morbidity and mortality (may be due to abrupt decompression)
endoscopic cyst fenestration through a burr hole[12]	• as above	• as above
shunting of cyst into peritoneum or into vascular system	• definitive treatment • low morbidity/mortality • low rate of recurrence	• patient becomes "shunt dependent" • risk of infection of foreign body (shunt)

✖ ventricular drainage is ineffective (actually promotes cyst enlargement) and should not be routinely considered.

15.1.7 Outcome

Even following successful treatment a portion of the cyst may remain due to the remodeling of the bone and chronic shift of brain contents. Hydrocephalus may develop following treatment. Endocrinopathies tend to persist even after successful treatment of suprasellar cysts.

15.2 Craniofacial development

15.2.1 Normal development

Fontanelles

Anterior fontanelle: the largest fontanelle. Diamond shaped, 4 cm (AP) × 2.5 cm (transverse) at birth. Normally closes by age 2.5 yrs.

Posterior fontanelle: triangular. Normally closes by age 2–3 mos.

Sphenoid and *mastoid fontanelles*: small, irregular. Normally, former closes by age 2–3 mos, latter by age 1 yr.

Cranial vault

Growth: largely determined by growth of brain. 90% of adult head size is achieved by age 1 yr; 95% by age 6 yrs. Growth essentially ceases at age 7 yrs. By end of 2nd yr, bones have interlocked at sutures and further growth occurs by accretion and absorption.

Skull is unilaminar at birth. Diplöe appear by 4th yr and reach a maximum by age 35 yrs (when diploic veins form).

Mastoid process: formation commences by age 2 yrs, air cell formation occurs during 6th yr.

15.2.2 Craniosynostosis

General

Craniosynostosis (CSO) was originally called craniostenosis, and is the premature ossification of a cranial suture. Incidence: ≈ 0.6/1000 live births. It may occur in isolation, but may also be syndromic or secondary. Once the suture ossifies, normal growth of the skull perpendicular to the suture terminates and tends to proceed parallel to the suture.

Primary CSO is usually a prenatal deformity. Etiologies of secondary CSO include: metabolic (rickets, hyperthyroidism...), toxic (drugs such as phenytoin, valproate, methotrexate...), hematologic

15

(sickle cell, thalassemia…), and structural (lack of brain growth due to e.g., microcephaly, lissence-phaly, micropolygyria…). CSO is rarely associated with hydrocephalus (HCP).[15] The assertion that CSO may follow CSF shunting for HCP is unproven.

Treatment is usually surgical. In most instances, the indication for surgery is for cosmesis and to prevent the severe psychological effects of having a disfiguring deformity. However, with multisu-tural CSO, brain growth may be impeded by the unyielding skull. Also, ICP may be pathologically elevated, and although this is more common in multiple CSO,[16] elevated ICP occurs in ≈ 11% of cases with a single stenotic suture. Coronal synostosis can cause amblyopia. Most cases of single suture involvement can be treated with linear excision of the suture. Involvement of multiple sutures of the skull base usually requires the combined efforts of a neurosurgeon and craniofacial surgeon, and may need to be staged in some cases. Risks of surgery include blood loss, seizures, and stroke.

Diagnosis

Some cases of "synostosis" are really deformities caused by positional flattening (e.g., "lazy lamb-doid," see below). If this is suspected, instruct parents to keep head off of flattened area and recheck patient in 6–8 weeks: if it was positional, it should be improved, if it was CSO then it usually declares itself. The diagnosis of CSO may be aided by:

1. palpation of a bony prominence over the suspected synostotic suture (exception: lambdoidal synostosis may produce a trough, see below)
2. gentle firm pressure with the thumbs fails to cause relative movement of the bones on either side of the suture
3. plain skull X-rays:
   a) lack of normal lucency in center of suture. Some cases with normal X-ray appearance of the suture (even on CT) may be due to focal bony spicule formation[17]
   b) beaten copper calvaria (p. 267), sutural diastasis and erosion of the sella may be seen in cases of increased ICP[18]
4. CT scan:
   a) helps demonstrate cranial contour
   b) may show thickening and/or ridging at the site of synostosis
   c) will demonstrate hydrocephalus if present
   d) may show expansion of the frontal subarachnoid space[19]
   e) three-dimensional CT may help better visualize abnormalities
5. in questionable cases, a technetium bone scan can be performed[20]:
   a) there is little isotope uptake by any of the cranial sutures in the first weeks of life
   b) in prematurely closing sutures, increased activity compared to the other (normal) sutures will be demonstrated
   c) in completely closed sutures, no uptake will be demonstrated
6. MRI: usually reserved for cases with associated intracranial abnormalities. Often not as helpful as CT
7. measurements, such as occipito-frontal-circumference may not be abnormal even in the face of a deformed skull shape

Increased ICP

Evidence of increased ICP in the newborn with craniosynostosis include:
1. radiographic signs (on plain skull X-ray or CT, see above)
2. failure of calvarial growth (unlike the non-synostotic skull where increased ICP causes macrocra-nia in the newborn, here it is the synostosis that causes the increased ICP and lack of skull growth)
3. papilledema
4. developmental delay

Types of craniosynostosis

General information

▶ Fig. 15.3 illustrates 4 basic single-suture craniosynostoses.

Sagittal synostosis
General information
See ▶ Fig. 15.3. The most common CSO affecting a single suture. 80% male. Produces a palpable keel-like sagittal ridge and dolichocephaly (elongated skull with high forehead/frontal bossing) or

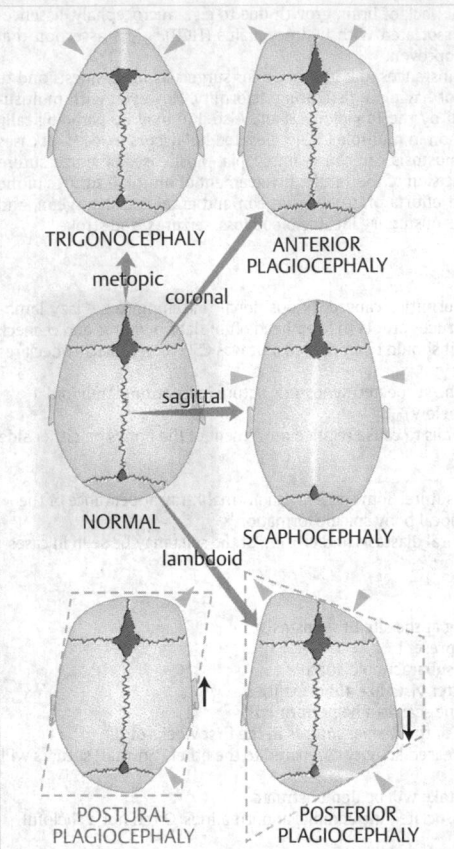

Fig. 15.3 Craniosynostosis.
Image: diagram of 4 types of single suture craniosynostosis and 1 type of positional deformity.
Red arrows identify the involved suture which is depicted as a white line. Blue arrowheads depict the direction of the deformities.
Postural plagiocephaly is a positional deformity and is *not* a craniosynostosis.
Broken lines illustrate the concept that posterior plagiocephaly produces a trapezoidal-shaped deformity (note the ipsilateral ear is displaced *posteriorly* with *contralateral* frontal bossing), whereas postural plagiocephaly bears more resemblance to a parallelogram (with the ipsilateral ear shifted *anteriorly* and *ipsilateral* frontal bossing).[21]

scaphocephaly ("boat shaped skull" with prominent occiput). OFC remains close to normal, but the biparietal diameter is markedly reduced. As many as 44% of patients with nonsyndromic sagittal synostosis have elevated ICP.[22]

Surgical treatment
Skin incision may be longitudinal or transverse. A linear "strip" craniectomy is performed, excising the sagittal suture from the coronal to the lambdoid suture, preferably within the first 3–6 months of life. The width of the strip should be at least 3 cm; no proof exists that interposing artificial substances (e.g., silastic sheeting over the exposed edges of the parietal bone) retards the recurrence of synostosis. Great care is taken to avoid dural laceration with potential injury to the underlying superior sagittal sinus. The child is followed and reoperated if fusion recurs before 6 months of age. After ≈ 1 yr of age, more extensive cranial remodelling is usually required.

Coronal synostosis
General information
Accounts for 18% of CSO, more common in females. In Crouzon's syndrome this is accompanied by abnormalities of sphenoid, orbital, and facial bones (hypoplasia of midface), and in Apert's syndrome is accompanied by syndactyly.[23] Unilateral coronal CSO → anterior plagiocephaly (▸ Fig. 15.3) with

the forehead on the affected side flattened or concave above the eye and compensatory prominence of the contralateral forehead. The supra-orbital margin is higher than the normal side, producing the harlequin eye sign. The orbit rotates out on the abnormal side, and can produce amblyopia. Without treatment, flattened cheeks develop and the nose deviates to the normal side (the root of the nose tends to rotate towards the deformity).

Bilateral coronal CSO (usually in craniofacial dysmorphism with multiple suture CSO, e.g., Apert's) → brachycephaly with broad, flattened forehead (acrocephaly), is more common than unilateral. When combined with premature closure of frontosphenoidal and frontoethmoidal sutures, it results in a foreshortened anterior fossa with maxillary hypoplasia, shallow orbits, and progressive proptosis.

Surgical treatment
Simple strip craniectomy of the involved suture has been used, often with excellent cosmetic result. However, some argument that this may not be adequate has been presented. Therefore, a more current recommendation is to do frontal craniotomy (uni- or bilateral) with lateral canthal advancement by taking off orbital bar.

Metopic synostosis
At birth, the frontal bone consists of two halves separated by the frontal or metopic suture. Abnormal closure produces trigonocephaly (pointed or triangular shaped) forehead with a midline ridge (▶ Fig. 15.3) and hypotelorism. Incidence: 1/15,000 live births. 75% are male. Many of these have a 19p chromosome abnormality and are mentally retarded.

Lambdoid synostosis
Epidemiology
Rare, with a reported incidence of 1–9% of CSO.[24] More common in males (male:female = 4:1). Involves the right side in 70% of cases. Usually presents between 3–18 months of age, but may be seen as early as 1–2 months of age.

Clinical findings
Flattening of the occiput. May be unilateral or bilateral. If unilateral, it produces posterior plagiocephaly. Bilateral lambdoid synostosis produces brachycephaly with both ears displaced anteriorly and inferiorly.[24] Unlike the palpable ridge of sagittal or coronal synostosis, an *indentation* may be palpated along the synostotic lambdoid suture (although a perisutural ridge may be found in some).

▶ **Mimic: "lazy lamboid" (positional flattening).** Lambdoid synostosis must be distinguished from positional flattening, the so-called "lazy lambdoid." Flattening of the occiput here is associated with anterior displacement of the ipsilateral ear (▶ Fig. 15.3). There is bulging of the ipsilateral cheek and forehead.

Positional flattening (or molding) may be produced by:
1. decreased mobility: patients who constantly lie supine with the head to the same side, e.g., cerebral palsy, mental retardation, prematurity, chronic illness
2. abnormal postures: *congenital torticollis*,[25] congenital disorders of the cervical spine
3. intentional positioning: due to the recommendation in 1992 to place newborns in a supine sleeping position to reduce the risk of sudden infant death syndrome (SIDS),[26] sometimes with a foam wedge to tilt the child to one side to reduce the risk of aspiration
4. intrauterine etiologies[27]: intrauterine crowding (e.g., from multiparous births or large fetal size), uterine anomalies

Diagnostic evaluation
The physical exam is the most important aspect of diagnosis. Skull X-ray may help differentiate (see below). If the skull X-ray is equivocal, prevent the infant from laying on the affected side for several weeks. A bone scan should be obtained if no improvement occurs (see below). In definite cases of synostosis, and for some cases of refractory positional flattening (which usually corrects with time, but may take up to 2 years), surgical treatment may be indicated.

Skull X-ray: Shows a sclerotic margin along one edge of the lambdoid suture in 70% of cases. Local "beaten copper cranium" (BCC) occasionally may be seen due to indentations in the bone from underlying gyri, which may be due to locally increased ICP. BCC produces a characteristic mottled appearance of the bone with lucencies of varying depth having round and poorly marginated edges. BCC correlates with generalized ↑ ICP only when it is seen with sellar erosion and sutural diastasis.[18]

CT scan: Bone windows may show eroded or thinned inner table in the occipital region in 15–20% of cases,[28] > 95% are on the side of the involvement. The suture may appear closed. Brain windows show parenchymal brain abnormalities in < 2%: heterotopias, hydrocephalus, agenesis of the corpus callosum; but ≈ 70% will have significant expansion of the frontal subarachnoid space (may be seen in synostosis of other sutures, see above).

Bone scan: Isotope uptake in the lambdoid suture increases during the first year, with a peak at 3 months of age[29] (following the usual inactivity of the first weeks of life). The findings with synostosis are those typical for CSO (p. 265).

Treatment

Early surgical treatment is indicated in cases with severe craniofacial disfigurement or those with evidence of increased ICP. Otherwise, children may be managed nonsurgically for 3–6 months. The majority of cases will remain static or will improve with time and simple nonsurgical intervention. Approximately 15% will continue to develop a significant cosmetic deformity.

Nonsurgical management[30]:

Although improvement can usually be attained, some degree of permanent disfigurement is frequent.

Repositioning will be effective in ≈ 85% of cases. Patients are placed on the unaffected side or on the abdomen. Infants with occipital flattening from torticollis should have aggressive physical therapy and resolution should be observed within 3–6 months.

More severe involvement may be treated with a trial of molding helmets[31] (however, no controlled study has proven the efficacy).

Surgical treatment:

Required in only ≈ 20% of cases. The ideal age for surgery is between 6 and 18 months. The patient is positioned prone on a well-padded cerebellar headrest (the face should be lifted and gently massaged every ≈ 30 minutes by the anesthesiologist to prevent pressure injuries).

Surgical options range from simple unilateral craniectomy of the suture to elaborate reconstruction by a craniofacial team.

Linear craniectomy extending from the sagittal suture to the asterion is often adequate for patients ≤ 12 weeks of age without severe disfigurement. Great care is taken to avoid dural laceration near the asterion, which is in the region of the transverse sinus. The excised suture demonstrates an *internal* ridge. Better results are obtained with earlier surgery, more radical surgery may be necessary after the age of 6 months.

Average blood loss for uncomplicated cases is 100–200 ml, and therefore transfusion is often required.

Multiple synostoses

Fusion of many or all cranial sutures → oxycephaly (tower skull with undeveloped sinuses and shallow orbits). These patients have elevated ICP.

Craniofacial dysmorphic syndromes

Over 50 syndromes have been described; ▶ Table 15.4 shows a few selected ones.

Table 15.4 Selected craniofacial dysmorphic syndromes (modified[32 (p 123–4)])

Syndrome	Genetics		Craniofacial findings	Associated findings
	Sporadic	Inherited		
Crouzon (craniofacial dysostosis)	yes (25%)	FGFR AD	CSO of coronal & basal skull sutures, maxillary hypoplasia, shallow orbits, proptosis	HCP rare
Apert (acrocephalosyndactyly)	yes (95%)	FGFR AD	same as Crouzon	syndactyly of digits 2,3,4; shortened UE, HCP common
Kleeblattschädel	yes	AD	CSO with trilobular skull	isolated, or with Apert's or thanatophoric dwarfism

Abbreviations: AD = autosomal dominant; CSO = craniosynostosis; FGFR = fibroblast growth factor receptor gene-related; HCP = hydrocephalus; UE = upper extremities

A number of craniosynostosis syndromes are due to mutations in the FGFR (fibroblast growth factor receptor) genes. FGFR gene-related craniosynostosis syndromes include some classic syndromes (Apert, Crouzon, Pfeiffer...) as well as several newer entities (Beare-Stevenson, Muenke, Jackson-Weiss syndromes). All exhibit autosomal dominant inheritance.

15.2.3 Encephalocele

General information

Cranium bifidum is a defect in the fusion of the cranial bone, it occurs in the midline, and is most common in the occipital region. If meninges and CSF herniate through the defect, it is called a meningocele. If meninges and cerebral tissue protrude, it is called an encephalocele.

Encephalocele AKA cephalocele is an extension of intracranial structures outside the normal confines of the skull. One case was seen for every five cases of spinal myelomeningoceles.[33] A nasal polypoid mass in a *newborn* should be considered an encephalocele until proven otherwise. See also Differential diagnosis (p. 1674).

Classification

System based on Suwanwela and Suwanwela[34]:
1. occipital: often involves vascular structures
2. cranial vault: comprises ≈ 80% of encephaloceles in Western hemisphere
   a) interfrontal
   b) anterior fontanelle
   c) interparietal: often involves vascular structures
   d) temporal
   e) posterior fontanelle
3. fronto-ethmoidal: AKA sincipital; 15% of encephaloceles; external opening into face in one of the following 3 regions:
   a) nasofrontal: external defect in the nasion
   b) naso-ethmoidal: defect between nasal bone and nasal cartilage
   c) naso-orbital: defect in the antero-inferior portion of medial orbital wall
4. basal: 1.5% of encephaloceles; (see below)
   a) transethmoidal: protrudes into nasal cavity through defect in cribriform plate
   b) spheno-ethmoidal: protrudes into posterior nasal cavity
   c) transsphenoidal: protrudes into sphenoid sinus or nasopharynx through patent craniopharyngeal canal (foramen cecum)
   d) fronto-sphenoidal or spheno-orbital: protrudes into orbit through superior orbital fissure
5. posterior fossa: usually contains cerebellar tissue and ventricular component

Basal encephalocele

The only group that does not produce a visible soft tissue mass. May present as CSF leak or recurrent meningitis. May be associated with other craniofacial deformities, including cleft lip, bifid nose, optic-nerve dysplasia, coloboma and microphthalmia, hypothalamic-pituitary dysfunction.

Iniencephaly is characterized by defects around the foramen magnum, rachischisis and retrocollis. Most are stillborn, some survive up to age 17.

Etiology

Two main theories:
1. arrested closure of normal confining tissue allows herniation through persistent defect
2. early outgrowth of neural tissue prevents normal closure of cranial coverings

Treatment

Occipital encephalocele

Surgical excision of the sac and its contents with water-tight dural closure. It must be kept in mind that vascular structures are often included in the sac. Hydrocephalus is often present and may need to be treated separately.

15

Basal encephalocele

Caution: a transnasal approach to a basal encephalocele (even for biopsy alone) may be fraught with intracranial hemorrhage, meningitis, or persistent CSF leak. Usually a combined intracranial approach (with amputation of the extracranial mass) and transnasal approach is used.

Outcome

Occipital encephalocele

The prognosis is better in occipital meningocele than in encephalocele. The prognosis is worse if a significant amount cerebral tissue is present in the sac, if the ventricles extend into the sac, or if there is hydrocephalus. Less than ≈ 5% of infants with encephalocele develop normally.

15.3 Dandy Walker malformation

15.3.1 General information

Key concepts

- a congenital condition with an incidence of 1 per 25,000–35,000 live births
- classic triad
  - complete or near complete absence of the cerebellar vermis
  - cystic dilation of the 4th ventricle projecting posteriorly
  - hydrocephalus: present in 75-95%
- posterior fossa is often enlarged → elevated tentorium & torcula-lambdoid inversion
- other CNS and systemic abnormalities are frequent. Be aware of the possibility of cardiovascular anomalies when considering surgery
- treatment: antiepileptic meds for seizures. Surgery is indicated for symptoms of brainstem compression by the cyst or hydrocephalus
- surgical options: shunting (the cyst and/or the ventricles, usually both), cyst fenestration (open or endoscopic), ETV is occasionally used (aqueduct must be open)
- outcome: 50% are cognitively impaired. Ataxia, spasticity, and poor fine motor control are common. Seizures occur in 15%

Definition: complete agenesis or hypoplasia of the cerebellar vermis and cystic dilatation of the fourth ventricle (▶ Fig. 15.4) which is distorted and encased in a neuroglial vascular membrane. The posterior fossa is usually enlarged and hydrocephalus is common.

First described by Dandy & Blackfan in 1914, dubbed Dandy Walker malformation (DWM) forty years later by Benda to acknowledge Taggart and Walker's contributions in 1942.[35]

DWM is likely on a continuum with variable presence of the definitional components. The term Dandy Walker variant (DWV) or Dandy Walker Complex (DWC) may be used when not all of the Dandy Walker criteria are present (e.g., vermian hypoplasia with cystic dilatation of the 4th ventricle, without enlargement of the posterior fossa), but a standardized nomenclature for this is lacking.

▶ **Associated CNS abnormalities.** Include:
1. hydrocephalus is frequent (75-95%). Argument is made whether hydrocephalus is[36] or is not[37] a component of DWM by definition
2. enlargement of the posterior fossa with accompanying elevation of the tentorium cerebelli producing torcula-lambdoid inversion (the torcular Herophili is situated above the lambdoid suture, oppostie of normal)
3. callosal dysgenesis 17-33%[37,38]
4. occipital encephalocele in 7%
5. other findings: heterotopias, polymicrogyria, agyria, schizencephaly, aqueductal stenosis, microcephaly, lipomas, cephaloceles & lumbosacral meningoceles, dermoid cysts, porencephaly, spina bifida, syringomyelia, and Klippel-Feil deformity
6. atresia of the foramina of Magendie and Luschka[39]

▶ **Systemic abnormalities.** Include[37]: facial abnormalities (e.g., angiomas, cleft palates, macroglossia, facial dysmorphia), ocular abnormalities (e.g., coloboma, retinal dysgenesis, microphthalmia),

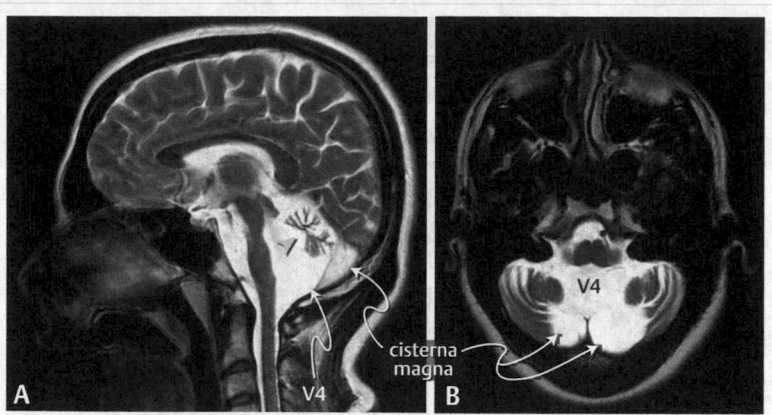

Fig. 15.4 Dandy Walker malformation.
Dandy Walker malformation in a 29 year old woman.
Hypoplastic cerebellar vermis (*blue arrowhead*).
Image: T2 MRI, A: sagittal, B: axial.
V4 = 4th ventricle. Note the membrane between the cystic 4th ventricle and the cisterna magna (better appreciated on the sagittal image).

and cardiovascular anomalies (e.g., septal defects, patent ductus arteriosus, aortic coarctation, dextrocardia). Note: be aware of the possibility of a cardiovascular abnormality when considering surgery on these patients.

15.3.2 Differential diagnosis

Disorders with posterior fossa CSF (or CSF-like) collections include[40]:
1. Dandy Walker malformation (DWM)
2. Dandy Walker variant (DWV): see above
3. persistent Blake's pouch cyst (BPC): tetraventricular hydrocephalus, communicating 4th ventricle and posterior fossa cyst. The vermis and medial aspects of the cerebellar hemispheres may *appear* hyoplastic, but they usually reexpand after shunting (although some atrophy from the pressure may occur)
4. retrocerebellar arachnoid cyst: anteriorly displaces the 4th ventricle and cerebellum, which can produce significant mass effect. Vermis is intact (▶ Fig. 15.5)
5. epidermoid cyst (p. 937) of the posterior fossa: restrict on DWI imaging (p. 938)
6. cerebellar atrophy
7. Joubert's syndrome: absence or underdevelopment of the cerebellar vermis
8. enlarged cisterna magna (AKA mega cisterna magna): a normal variant, present in about 1% of brains imaged. May have a secondarily enlarged posterior fossa. There is a normal vermis and fourth ventricle and no mass effet on the cerebellum
9. cystic posterior fossa tumor: e.g., pilocytic astrocytoma (p. 689). Usually have an enhancing mural nodule (▶ Fig. 39.3)

Differentiating features: DWM and DWV are difficult to distinguish, and may represent a continuum of developmental anomalies which may be grouped together as Dandy Walker complex (DWC).[41]

Retrocerebellar arachnoid cysts and BPCs may mimic DWM, but these do *not* have vermian agenesis. The position of the choroid plexus in the 4th ventricle is normal in arachnoid cysts, absent in Dandy Walker malformations, and displaced into the superior cyst wall in BPC. An intrathecal enhanced CT scan (performed after instilling iodinated contrast into a ventricular catheter) would identify a mega cisterna magna which communicates with the ventricles, while DWM and most but not all arachnoid cysts do not.

15

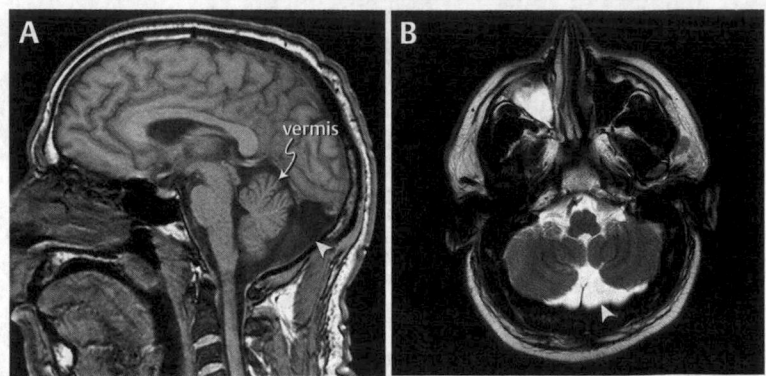

Fig. 15.5 Mega cisterna magna/posterior fossa arachnoid cyst (*yellow arrowheads*).
It was not determined which of these 2 entities this represents. Compare to Dandy Walker cyst (▶ Fig. 15.4).
Image: MRI, A: T1 sagittal, B: T2 axial.
Note in Panel A that the cerebellar vermis still forms a posterior border to the 4th ventricle.

15.3.3 Pathophysiology

The etiology of DWM is unknown. DWM is likely due to dysembryogenesis of the roof of the rhombencephalon, and not due to failure of formation of the fourth ventricle outlets as previously believed.[41] This results in agenesis of the cerebellar vermis with a large posterior fossa cyst communicating with an enlarged 4th ventricle.[35,41]

Hydrocephalus occurs in 75–95% of cases, and Dandy Walker malformation is present in 2–4% of all cases of hydrocephalus.

15.3.4 Risk factors and epidemiology

Gestational exposure to rubella, CMV, toxoplasmosis, warfarin, alcohol, and isotretinoin are thought to be predisposing factors. Autosomal recessive inheritance has been identified in a few cases, but a genetic basis is lacking in most. Incidence: 1 per 25,000–35,000 live births.[35] Male:female=1:3. May be associated with PHACES syndrome (p.1647).

15.3.5 Treatment

Antiseizure medication therapy for seizures. PT and speech therapy may aid development.

Early treatment for ventriculomegaly is recommended to achieve maximum cognitive development. In the absence of hydrocephalus or symptoms of brainstem compression, DWM may be followed during the first year of life to rule out hydrocephalus since this is the period during which most patients will develop symptoms (expectant management).

▶ **Surgical management.** Indications for surgery: symptoms of brainstem compression by the cyst or hydrocephalus.

Optimal surgical intervention is controversial, and has to be individualized. Options include:
1. posterior fossa craniectomy with excision of the membrane: currently less favored due to high complication rate and the fact that many patients still require shunting. May be considered for patients with frequent shunt malfunctions
2. lateral ventricular shunting alone: patients often develop aqueductal stenosis afterwards[42] and the cyst frequently persists, requiring additional treatment. Risk of upward cerebellar herniation (p.325) [43]
3. shunting of the cyst alone: requires patency of the sylvian aqueduct, otherwise the supratentorial ventricles will enlarge
4. concurrent ventricular and cyst shunting
5. shunting the lateral ventricles alone:

15

6. endoscopic third ventriculostomy: only viable in cases where the aqueduct is patent[44,45]
7. cyst fenestration: may be considered for older patients[42]

15.3.6 Prognosis

Prognosis ranges widely as there are various levels of severity of the malformation. Some pediatric neurosurgical literature quotes 12–50% mortality rates, although this is improving with modern shunting techniques. Only 50% have normal IQ. Ataxia, spasticity, and poor fine motor control are common. Seizures occur in 15%.

15.4 Aqueductal stenosis

15.4.1 General information

Aqueductal stenosis (AqS) is narrowing or complete blockage of the sylvian aqueduct which connects the third to the fourth ventricle. Blockage produces **triventricular hydrocephalus**, characterized by enlarged third and lateral ventricles and a normal sized 4th ventricle on MRI or CT. Most cases occur in children; however some present for the first time in adulthood.

15.4.2 Etiologies

1. a congenital malformation: may be associated with Chiari malformation or neurofibromatosis
2. acquired
   a) due to inflammation (following hemorrhage or infection, e.g., syphilis, T.B.)
   b) neoplasm: especially brainstem astrocytomas—including tectal gliomas (p. 697), lipomas
   c) quadrigeminal plate arachnoid cysts

15.4.3 Aqueductal stenosis in infancy

AqS is a frequent cause of congenital hydrocephalus (HCP) (up to 70% of cases[32]), but occasionally may be the *result* of HCP. Patients with congenital AqS usually have HCP at birth or develop it within ≈ 2–3 mos. Congenital AqS may be due to an X-linked recessive gene.[33] Four types of congenital AqS described by Russell (summarized[46]):
1. forking: multiple channels (often narrowed) with normal epithelial lining that do not meet, separated by normal nervous tissue. Usually associated with other congenital abnormalities (spina bifida, myelomeningocele)
2. periaqueductal gliosis: luminal narrowing due to subependymal astrocytic proliferation
3. true stenosis: aqueduct histologically normal
4. septum blocking the aqueduct

15.4.4 Aqueductal stenosis in adulthood

General information

AqS may be an overlooked cause of what may be mistaken as "normal pressure hydrocephalus" in the adult.[47] Some cases of AqS would remain occult, and manifest only in adulthood. In one series of 55 cases,[48] 35% had duration of symptoms < 1 year, 47% for 1–5 years; the longest was 40 yrs. Although most follow this long-standing benign course, there are reports of elevated ICP and sudden death.

Symptoms

See ▶ Table 15.5. Headache was the most common symptom, and had characteristics of H/A associated with elevated ICP. Visual changes were next, and usually consisted of blurring or loss of acuity. Endocrine changes included menstrual irregularities, hypothyroidism, and hirsutism.

Signs

Papilledema was the most common finding (53%). Visual fields were normal in 78%, the remainder having reduced peripheral vision, increased blind spots, quadrantic or hemianopic field cuts, or scotomata. Intellectual impairment was present in at least 36%. Other signs included: ataxia (29%), "pyramidal tract signs" in 44% (mild hemi- or para-paresis [22%], spasticity [22%], or Babinski's [20%]), and anosmia (9%).

15

Table 15.5 Symptoms of aqueductal stenosis presenting in adulthood (55 patients > 16 years of age[48])

Symptom	No.	%
H/A	32	58
visual disturbances	22	40
mental deterioration	17	31
gait disturbance	16	29
frequent falling	13	24
endocrine disturbance	10	18
nausea/vomiting	9	16
seizures	8	15
incontinence	7	13
vertigo	6	11
LE weakness	4	7
hemiparesis or hemianesthesia	4	7
diplopia	3	5
dysarthria	1	
deafness	1	

Evaluation

MRI is the test of choice. Contrast should be given to rule out tumor. Demonstrates the absence of the normal flow void in the Sylvian aqueduct. Sometimes an obstruction within the aqueduct can be identified (▶ Fig. 15.6). May produce "funneling" (widening that tapers to the obstruction) of the aqueduct.

Treatment (of non-tumoral AqS)

Although treatments of the primary lesion have been attempted (e.g., lysis of aqueductal septum), this has fallen into disfavor with the improved efficacy of CSF shunting and endoscopic third ventriculostomy (ETV).
1. shunting: CSF is usually shunted to the peritoneum or the vascular system, however shunting to subarachnoid space is also feasible (once obstruction at the level of the arachnoid granulations has been ruled out)
2. a Torkildsen shunt (shunting a lateral ventricle to the cisterna magna[49]) may work in adult cases[46]; however, pediatric patients with obstructive hydrocephalus may not have an adequately developed subarachnoid space for this to function properly
3. endoscopic third ventriculostomy (p. 453)

Follow-up of at least two years to rule out tumor is recommended.

15.5 Agenesis of the corpus callosum

15.5.1 General information

A failure of commissuration occurring ≈ 2 weeks after conception. Results in expansion of the third ventricle and separation of the lateral ventricles (which develop dilated occipital horns and atria, and concave medial borders).

The corpus callosum (CC) forms from rostrum (genu) to splenium,[50] ∴ in agenesis there may be an anterior portion with absence of the posterior segment (the converse occurs infrequently). Absence of the anterior CC with presence of some posterior CC is indicative of some form of holoprosencephaly.

15.5.2 Incidence

1 in 2,000–3,000 neuroradiological examinations.

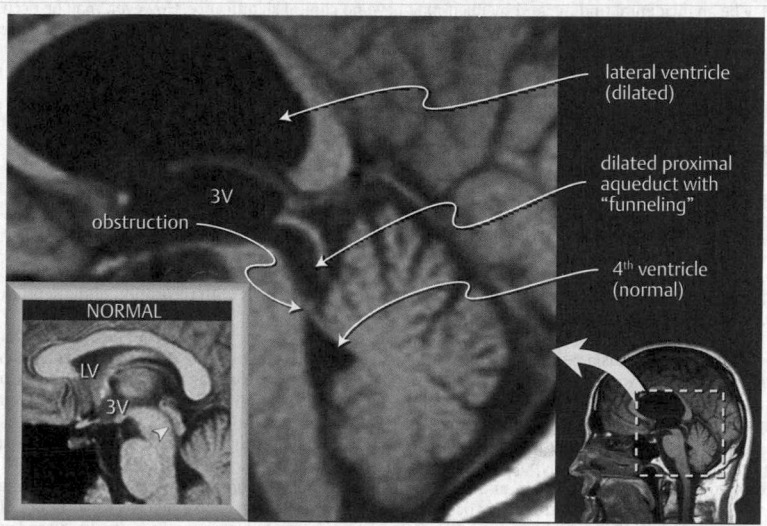

Fig. 15.6 Aqueductal stenosis in an adult.
Image: sagittal T2 MRI showing a weblike obstruction of the Sylvian aqueduct in a patient with dilated third ventricle (V3) and lateral ventricles with normal-sized 4th ventricle. The aqueduct proximal to the obstruction is dilated (and demonstrates "funneling").
Lower right inset depicts the location in the sagittal T2 brain MRI from where the detail is obtained.
Lower left inset in blue rectangle shows a patient with a normal aqueduct (*yellow arrowhead*) and normal third ventricle ("3V") for comparison.

15.5.3 Associated neuropathologic findings

See reference.[51]
- porencephaly
- microgyria
- interhemispheric *lipomas* and lipomas of the corpus callosum (p.276)
- arhinencephaly
- optic atrophy
- colobomas
- hypoplasia of the limbic system
- bundles of Probst: aborted beginnings of corpus callosum, bulge into lateral ventricles
- loss of horizontal orientation of cingulate gyrus
- schizencephaly (p.309)
- anterior and hippocampal commissures may be totally or partially absent[52]
- hydrocephalus
- cysts in the region of the corpus callosum
- spina bifida with or without myelomeningocele
- absence of the septum pellucidum (p.276)

15.5.4 Possible presentation

- hydrocephalus
- microcephaly
- seizures (rare)
- precocious puberty
- disconnection syndrome: more likely with *acquired* CC defect than with congenital

15

May be an incidental finding, and by itself may have no clinical significance. However, may be occur as part of a more complex clinical syndrome or chromosomal abnormality (e.g., Aicardi syndrome: agenesis of CC, seizures, retardation, patches of retinal pigmentation).

15.6 Absence of the septum pellucidum

Etiologies[53 (p 178)]
1. holoprosencephaly (p. 311)
2. schizencephaly (p. 309)
3. agenesis of the corpus callosum (p. 274)
4. Chiari type 2 malformation (p. 303)
5. basal encephalocele
6. porencephaly/hydranencephaly
7. may occur in severe hydrocephalus: thought to be due to necrosis with resorption of the septum
8. septo-optic dysplasia: see below

▶ **Septo-optic dysplasia**[54,53 (p 175–8)]. AKA de Morsier syndrome. Incomplete early morphogenesis of anterior midline structures produces hypoplasia of the optic nerves and possibly optic chiasm (affected patients are blind) and pituitary infundibulum. The septum pellucidum (p. 1657) is absent in about half the cases. About half the cases also have schizencephaly (p. 309).

Presentation may be due to secondary hypopituitarism manifesting as dwarfism, isolated growth hormone deficiency, or panhypopituitarism. Occasionally hypersecretion of growth hormone, corticotropin or prolactin may occur, and precocious puberty may occur. Most patients are of normal intelligence although retardation may occur. Septo-optic dysplasia may be a less severe form of holoprosencephaly (p. 311), and occasionally may occur as part of this anomaly (with its attendant poorer prognosis for function or survival). The ventricles may be normal or dilated. May be seen by the neurosurgeon because of concerns of possible hydrocephalus.

15.7 Intracranial lipomas

15.7.1 General information

Intracranial and intraspinal lipomas are felt to be of maldevelopmental origin[55 (p 706)] and may arise from failure of involution of the primitive meninges.[56]

15.7.2 Epidemiology of intracranial lipomas

Incidence: 8 in 10,000 autopsies. Usually found in or near the midsagittal plane, particularly over the corpus callosum; lipomas in this region are frequently associated with agenesis of the corpus callosum (p. 274). The tuber cinereum and quadrigeminal plate are less frequently affected.[51] Rarely, the CP angle or cerebellar vermis may be involved. May occur in isolation, but also has been described in association with a number of congenital anomalies, including trisomy 21, Pai's syndrome, frontal encephalocele, facial anomalies…. Other midline abnormalities may also be found: agenesis of the corpus callosum, myelomeningocele, and spina bifida.[56]

15.7.3 Evaluation

May be diagnosed by CT, MRI (study of choice), and by ultrasound in infants.

CT: Low density, may have peripheral calcification (difficult to appreciate on MRI).[56] Differential diagnosis on CT: primarily between dermoid cyst, teratoma[57] and germinoma.[56]

MRI: characteristic finding is a midline lesion with signal characteristics of fat (high intensity on T1WI, low intensity on T2WI).

15.7.4 Presentation

Often discovered incidentally. Large lipomas may be associated with seizures, hypothalamic dysfunction, or hydrocephalus (possibly from compression of the aqueduct). Associated findings that may or may not be directly related: mental retardation, behavioral disorders and headache.

15.7.5 Treatment

Direct surgical approach is seldom necessary for intracranial lipomas.[57] Shunting may be required for cases where hydrocephalus results from obstruction of CSF circulation.[57]

15.8 Hypothalamic hamartomas

15.8.1 General information

Key concepts

- rare, non-neoplastic congenital malformation, usually occurs in tuber cinereum
- may be parahypothalamic (pedunculated) or intrahypothalamic (sessile)
- presentation: precocious puberty due to gonadotropin-releasing hormone (GnRH), seizures (usually starting with gelastic seizures [brief unprovoked laughter]), developmental delay
- treatment: GnRH analogs for precocious puberty. Latero-basal craniotomy for pedunculated lesions, transcallosal interforniceal approach for intrahypothalamic lesions, option of endoscopic approach for lesions ≤ 1.5 cm dia, stereotactic radiosurgery may be an alternative

A hamartoma is an abnormal conglomeration of cells normally found in the same area. Hypothalamic hamartomas (HH) AKA diencephalic hamartomas or hamartomas of the (tuber cinereum [▶ Fig. 8.1]) are, non-neoplastic congenital malformations arising from inferior hypothalamus or tuber cinereum (floor of the third ventricle between the infundibular stalk and the mammillary bodies). May occur as part of Pallister-Hall syndrome (genetics: AD inherited defect in GL13 gene, resulting in abnormally short GL13 protein, which participates in normal shaping of many organs).

15.8.2 Clinical findings

1. specific types of seizures:
   a) **gelastic seizures** (brief episodes of unprovoked laughter[58]) are the most characteristic type and are the earliest seizure manifestation. Present in up to 92% of patients.[59] They are resistant to medical management and can lead to cognitive and behavioral deficits.[60] Not pathognomonic. A neocortical origin has been described[61]
   b) epileptic encephalopathy: gelastic fits gradually increase in frequency and other seizure types accrue: complex partial seizures, drop attacks, tonic seizures, tonic-clonic seizures, and secondarily generalized seizures. This phase is associated with marked deterioration of cognitive and behavioral abilities. Develops in 52% by a mean age of 7 years[59]
2. precocious puberty: believed to be due to release of gonadotropin-releasing hormone (GnRH) found within hamartoma cells.[62] HH are the most common CNS tumor to cause precocious puberty, other causes include other CNS tumors (astrocytoma, ependymoma, pineal tumors (p. 758), optic/hypothalamic gliomas [especially in NFT patients]), CNS XRT, hydrocephalus, CNS inflammation, septo-optic dysplasia (p. 276), and chronic hypothyroidism
3. developmental delay: primarily in patients with seizure disorder (severity correlates with duration of seizures). 46% of patients have borderline intellectual function (mental retardation)
4. behavioral disturbances[63]: aggressive behavior, rage attacks...

15.8.3 Imaging

MRI: nonenhancing, isointense on T1WI, slightly hyperintense or isointense on T2WI.[64]

15.8.4 Pathology

Two subtypes of hypothalamic hamartomas[59,64]:
1. pedunculated or parahypothalamic: narrower base attached to the floor of the hypothalamus (not arising within hypothalamus). No distortion of 3rd ventricle. Generally associated with precocious puberty more than seizures

2. intrathalamic or sessile: within hypothalamus (distorting the 3rd ventricle) or broad attachment to hypothalamus. More often associated with seizures. 66% have developmental delay, 50% have precocious puberty

Microscopic pathology: Clusters of disorganized small neurons surrounded by large pyramidal-like neurons in an astrocyte-rich neuropil[65] (in contrast to the usual ganglion cells surrounded by oligodendrocytes found in the hypothalamus).

15.8.5 Treatment

Precocious puberty usually responds well to GnRH analogs (they constantly stimulate the pituitary which reduces secretion of gonadotropins (LH & FSH)).[66]

▶ **Indications for surgery:**
1. precocious puberty that fails to respond to medical therapy (GnRH analogs)
2. seizures that cannot be adequately controlled medically. Post-op seizure control is related to completeness of resection
3. neurologic deficit from mass effect of the tumor

▶ **Options:**
1. surgical resection
   a) pedunculated lesions: approaches include[67] subtemporal, subfrontal, pterional, orbitozygomatic (most commonly recommended). Risks: cranial neuropathy, stroke[67]
   b) sessile lesions with intraventricular component: transcallosal anterior interforniceal approach.[68,69,70] Risks: memory impairment (forniceal injury), endocrine disturbances, weight gain[68,70]
   c) neuroendoscopic approach: considered for HH ≤ 1.5 cm diameter.[71] Risks: 25% incidence of thalamic cerebrovascular injury
2. stereotactic radiosurgery: especially for small sessile lesions, subtotal resection, or patients refusing or not candidates for surgery. In small series, 3-year outcome showed improvement similar to surgical resection with less neurologic and endocrinologic morbidity[72,73]

References

[1] Van Der Meche F, Braakman R. Arachnoid Cysts in the Middle Cranial Fossa: Cause and Treatment of Progressive and Non-Progressive Symptoms. J Neurol Neurosurg Psychiatry. 1983; 46:1102–1107

[2] Mayr U, Aichner F, Bauer G, et al. Supratentorial Extracerebral Cysts of the Middle Cranial Fossa: A Report of 23 Consecutive Cases of the So-called Temporal Lobe Agenesis Syndrome. Neurochirugia. 1982; 25:51–56

[3] Rengachary SS, Watanabe I. Ultrastructure and Pathogenesis of Intracranial Arachnoid Cysts. J Neuropathol Exp Neurol. 1981; 40:61–83

[4] Westermaier T, Vince GH, Meinhardt M, et al. Arachnoid cysts of the fourth ventricle - short illustrated review. Acta Neurochir (Wien). 2010; 152:119–124

[5] Bonde V, Muzumdar D, Goel A. Fourth ventricle arachnoid cyst. J Clin Neurosci. 2008; 15:26–28

[6] Aljohani H, Romano A, Iaccarino C, et al. Pure Endoscopic Management of Fourth Ventricle Arachnoid Cyst: Case Report and Literature Review. Asian J Neurosurg. 2018; 13:184–187

[7] Galassi E, Tognetti F, Gaist G, et al. CT scan and Metrizamide CT Cisternography of the Arachnoid Cysts of the Middle Cranial Fossa. Surg Neurol. 1982; 17:363–369

[8] Harsh GR, Edwards MSB, Wilson CB. Intracranial Arachnoid Cysts in Children. J Neurosurg. 1986; 64:835–842

[9] Pierre-Kahn A, Capelle L, Brauner R, et al. Presentation and Management of Suprasellar Arachnoid Cysts: Review of 20 Cases. J Neurosurg. 1990; 73:355–359

[10] Altschuler EM, Jungreis CA, Sekhar LN, et al. Operative Treatment of Intracranial Epidermoid Cysts and Cholesterol Granulomas: Report of 21 Cases. Neurosurgery. 1990; 26:606–614

[11] Reddy OJ, Gafoor JA, Suresh B, et al. Bobble head doll syndrome: A rare case report. J Pediatr Neurosci. 2014; 9:175–177

[12] Hopf NJ, Perneczky A. Endoscopic Neurosurgery and Endoscope-Assisted Microneurosurgery for the Treatment of Intracranial Cysts. Neurosurgery. 1998; 43:1330–1337

[13] Page LK. Comment on Albright L: Treatment of Bobble-Head Doll Syndrome by Transcallosal Cystectomy. Neurosurgery. 1981; 8

[14] Albright L. Treatment of Bobble-Head Doll Syndrome by Transcallosal Cystectomy. Neurosurgery. 1981; 8:593–595

[15] Golabi M, Edwards MSB, Ousterhout DK. Craniosynostosis and Hydrocephalus. Neurosurgery. 1987; 21:63–67

[16] Renier D, Sainte-Rose C, Marchac D, et al. Intracranial Pressure in Craniostenosis. J Neurosurg. 1982; 57:370–377

[17] Burke MJ, Winston KR, Williams S. Normal Sutural Fusion and the Etiology of Single Suture Craniosynostosis: The Microspicule Hypothesis. Pediatr Neurosurg. 1995; 22:241–246

[18] Tuite GF, Evanson J, Chong WK, et al. The Beaten Copper Cranium: A Correlation between Intracranial Pressure, Cranial Radiographs, and Computed Tomographic Scans in Children with Craniosynostosis. Neurosurgery. 1996; 39:691–699

[19] Chadduck WM, Chadduck JB, Boop FA. The Subarachnoid Spaces in Craniosynostosis. Neurosurgery. 1992; 30:867–871

[20] Gates GF, Dore EK. Detection of Craniosynostosis by Bone Scanning. Radiology. 1975; 115:665–671

[21] Huang MH, Gruss JS, Clarren SK, et al. The differential diagnosis of posterior plagiocephaly: true lambdoid synostosis versus positional molding. Plast Reconstr Surg. 1996; 98:765–74; discussion 775-6

[22] Wall SA, Thomas GP, Johnson D, et al. The preoperative incidence of raised intracranial pressure in nonsyndromic sagittal craniosynostosis is

underestimated in the literature. J Neurosurg Pediatr. 2014; 14:674–681

[23] Renier D, Arnaud E, Cinalli G, et al. Prognosis for Mental Function in Apert's Sydrome. Journal of Neurosurgery. 1996; 85:66–72

[24] Muakkassa KF, Hoffman HJ, Hinton DR, et al. Lambdoid Synostosis: Part 2: Review of Cases Managed at The Hospital for Sick Children, 1972-1982. J Neurosurg. 1984; 61:340–347

[25] Morrison DL, MacEwen GD. Congenital Muscular Torticollis: Observations Regarding Clinical Findings, Associated Conditions, and Results of Treatment. J Pediatr Orthop. 1982; 2:500–505

[26] American Academy of Pediatrics Task Force on Infant Positioning and SIDS. Positioning and SIDS. Pediatrics. 1992; 89:1120–1126

[27] Higginbottom MC, Jones KL, James HE. Intrauterine Constraint and Craniosynostosis. Neurosurgery. 1980; 6

[28] Keating RF, Goodrich JT. Lambdoid Plagiocephaly. Contemporary Neurosurgery. 1996; 18:1–7

[29] Hinton DR, Becker LE, Muakkassa KF, et al. Lambdoid Synostosis: Part 1: The Lambdoid Suture: Normal Development and Pathology of 'Synostosis'. J Neurosurg. 1984; 61:333–339

[30] McComb JG. Treatment of Functional Lambdoid Synostosis. Neurosurg Clin North Am. 1991; 2

[31] Clarren SK. Plagiocephaly and Torticollis: Etiology, Natural History, and Helmet Treatment. J Pediatr. 1981; 98

[32] Section of Pediatric Neurosurgery of the American Association of Neurological Surgeons. Pediatric Neurosurgery. New York 1982

[33] Matson DD. Neurosurgery of Infancy and Childhood. 2nd ed. Springfield: Charles C Thomas; 1969

[34] Suwanwela C, Suwanwela N. A Morphological Classification of Sincipital Encephalomeningoceles. J Neurosurg. 1972; 36:201–211

[35] Incesu L, Khosia A. Dandy-Walker malformation. 2008. http://emedicine.medscape.com/article/408059-overview

[36] Hart MN, Malamud N, Ellis WG. The Dandy-Walker syndrome. A clinicopathological study based on 28 cases. Neurology. 1972; 22:771–780

[37] Hirsch JF, Pierre-Kahn A, Renier D, et al. The Dandy-Walker Malformation: A Review of 40 Cases. J Neurosurg. 1984; 61:515–522

[38] Abdel Razek AA, Castillo M. Magnetic Resonance Imaging of Malformations of Midbrain-Hindbrain. J Comput Assist Tomogr. 2016; 40:14–25

[39] Raimondi AJ, Samuelson G, Yarzagaray L, et al. Atresia of the Foramina of Luschka and Magendie: The Dandy-Walker Cyst. J Neurosurg. 1969; 31:202–216

[40] Calabro F, Arcuri T, Jinkins JR. Blake's pouch cyst: an entity within the Dandy-Walker continuum. Neuroradiology. 2000; 42:290–295

[41] Forzano F, Mansour S, Ierullo A, et al. Posterior fossa malformation in fetuses: a report of 56 further cases and a review of the literature. Prenatal Diagnosis. 2007; 27:495–501

[42] Kumar R, Jain MK, Chhabra DK. Dandy-Walker syndrome: different modalities of treatment and outcome in 42 cases. Childs Nerv Syst. 2001; 17:348–352

[43] Mohanty A, Biswas A, Satish S, et al. Treatment options for Dandy-Walker malformation. Journal of Neurosurgery. 2006; 105:348–356

[44] Garg A, Suri A, Chandra PS, et al. Endoscopic third ventriculostomy: 5 years' experience at the All India Institute of Medical Sciences. Pediatr Neurosurg. 2009; 45:1–5

[45] Sikorski CW, Curry DJ. Endoscopic, single-catheter treatment of Dandy-Walker syndrome hydrocephalus: technical case report and review of treatment options. Pediatr Neurosurg. 2005; 41:264–268

[46] Nag TK, Falconer MA. Non-Tumoral Stenosis of the Aqueduct in Adults. Brit Med J. 1966; 2:1168–1170

[47] Vanneste J, Hyman R. Non-Tumoral Aqueduct Stenosis and Normal Pressure Hydrocephalus in the Elderly. J Neurol Neurosurg Psychiatry. 1986; 49:529–535

[48] Harrison MJG, Robert CM, Uttley D. Benign Aqueduct Stenosis in Adults. J Neurol Neurosurg Psychiatry. 1974; 37:1322–1328

[49] Alp MS. What is a Torkildsen shunt? Surg Neurol. 1995; 43:405–406

[50] Davidson HD, Abraham R, Steiner RE. Agenesis of the Corpus Callosum: Magnetic Resonance Imaging. Radiology. 1985; 155:371–373

[51] Atlas SW, Zimmerman RA, Bilaniuk LT, et al. Corpus Callosum and Limbic System: Neuroanatomic MR Evaluation of Developmental Anomalies. Radiology. 1986; 160:355–362

[52] Loeser JD, Alvord EC. Agenesis of the Corpus Callosum. Brain. 1968; 91:553–570

[53] Taveras JM, Pile-Spellman J. Neuroradiology. 3rd ed. Baltimore: Williams and Wilkins; 1996

[54] Jones KL. Smith's Recognizable Patterns of Human Malformation. 4th ed. Philadelphia: W.B. Saunders; 1988

[55] Russell DS, Rubenstein LJ. Pathology of Tumours of the Nervous System. 5th ed. Baltimore: Williams and Wilkins; 1989

[56] Rubio G, Garcci Guijo C, Mallada JJ. MR and CT Diagnosis of Intracranial Lipoma. American Journal of Radiology. 1991; 157:887–888

[57] Kazner E, Stochdorph O, Wende S, et al. Intracranial Lipoma. Diagnostic and Therapeutic Considerations. Journal of neurosurgery. 1980; 52:234–245

[58] Daly D, Mulder D. Gelastic epilepsy. Neurology. 1957; 7:189–192

[59] Nguyen D, Singh S, Zaatreh M, et al. Hypothalamic hamartomas: seven cases and review of the literature. Epilepsy Behav. 2003; 4:246–258

[60] Striano S, Meo R, Bilo L, et al. Gelastic epilepsy: symptomatic and cryptogenic cases. Epilepsia. 1999; 40:294–302

[61] Kurle PJ, Sheth RD. Gelastic seizures of neocortical origin confirmed by resective surgery. J Child Neurol. 2000; 15:835–838

[62] Culler FL, James HE, Simon ML, et al. Identification of gonadotropin-releasing hormone in neurons of a hypothalamic hamartoma in a boy with precocious puberty. Neurosurgery. 1985; 17:408–412

[63] Prigatano GP. Cognitive and behavioral dysfunction in children with hypothalamic hamartoma and epilepsy. Semin Pediatr Neurol. 2007; 14:65–72

[64] Arita K, Ikawa F, Kurisu K, et al. The relationship between magnetic resonance imaging findings and clinical manifestations of hypothalamic hamartoma. J Neurosurg. 1999; 91:212–220

[65] Coons SW, Rekate HL, Prenger EC, et al. The histopathology of hypothalamic hamartomas: study of 57 cases. J Neuropathol Exp Neurol. 2007; 66:131–141

[66] Chamouilli JM, Razafimahefa B, Pierron H. [Precocious puberty and hypothalamic hamartoma: treatment with triptorelin during eight years]. Arch Pediatr. 1995; 2:438–441

[67] Feiz-Erfan I, Horn EM, Rekate HL, et al. Surgical strategies for approaching hypothalamic hamartomas causing gelastic seizures in the pediatric population: transventricular compared with skull base approaches. J Neurosurg. 2005; 103:325–332

[68] Rosenfeld JV, Harvey AS, Wrennall J, et al. Transcallosal resection of hypothalamic hamartomas, with control of seizures, in children with gelastic epilepsy. Neurosurgery. 2001; 48:108–118

[69] Ng Y, Rekate HL, Kerrigan JF, et al. Transcallosal resection of a hypothalamic hamartoma: Case report. BNI Quarterly. 2004; 20:13–17

[70] Ng YT, Rekate HL, Prenger EC, et al. Transcallosal resection of hypothalamic hamartoma for intractable epilepsy. Epilepsia. 2006; 47:1192–1202

[71] Rekate HL, Feiz-Erfan I, Ng YT, et al. Endoscopic surgery for hypothalamic hamartomas causing medically refractory gelastic epilepsy. Childs Nerv Syst. 2006; 22:874–880

[72] Regis J, Scavarda D, Tamura M, et al. Gamma knife surgery for epilepsy related to hypothalamic hamartomas. Semin Pediatr Neurol. 2007; 14:73–79

[73] Mathieu D, Kondziolka D, Niranjan A, et al. Gamma knife radiosurgery for refractory epilepsy caused by hypothalamic hamartomas. Stereotact Funct Neurosurg. 2006; 84:82–87

15

16 Primary Spinal Developmental Anomalies

16.1 Spinal arachnoid cysts

16.1.1 General information

Almost always dorsal, most common in thoracic spine. With a ventral cyst, consider a neurenteric cyst (see below). Most are actually extradural and these are sometimes referred to as arachnoid diverticula—these may be associated with kyphoscoliosis in juveniles or with spinal dysraphism.

Usually asymptomatic, even if large.

Etiologies

1. congenital
2. posttraumatic
3. post-infectious

16.1.2 Treatment

Indications for surgery

Symptomatic lesions causing myelopathy are usually strong indications for surgery.

Pain is a soft indication as it may be difficult to determine if the pain is due to the lesion.

Surgical options

When surgery is indicated, treatment options include:
1. percutaneous procedures: may be done under MRI[1] or CT guidance. CT guidance usually requires use of intrathecal contrast to delineate the cyst
   a) needle aspiration
   b) needle fenestration[1]
2. open procedures:
   a) surgical resection
   b) fenestration
   c) cyst shunting: e.g., cyst peritoneal shunt

16.2 Spinal dysraphism (spina bifida)

16.2.1 Definitions

See reference.[2]

▶ **Spina bifida occulta.** Congenital absence of a spinous process and variable amounts of lamina. No visible exposure of meninges or neural tissue.

The following two entities are grouped together under the term spina bifida aperta (aperta from the Latin for "open") or spina bifida cystica.

▶ **Meningocele.** Congenital defect in vertebral arches with cystic distension of meninges, but no abnormality of neural tissue. One third have some neurologic deficit.

▶ **Myelomeningocele.** Congenital defect in vertebral arches with cystic dilatation of meninges and structural or functional abnormality of spinal cord or cauda equina.

16.2.2 Spina bifida occulta (SBO)

Reported prevalence range of SBO: 5–30% of North Americans (5–10% is probably more realistic). The defect may be palpable, and there may be overlying cutaneous manifestations (in ▶ Table 16.4).

Often an incidental finding, usually of no clinical importance *when it occurs alone*. Numerous reviews have shown no statistical association of SBO with nonspecific LBP.[3,4] An increased incidence of disc herniation was shown in one study.[5]

SBO may occasionally be associated with diastematomyelia, tethered cord, lipoma, or dermoid tumor. When symptomatic from one of these associated conditions, the presentation is usually that of tethered cord; gait disturbance, leg weakness and atrophy, urinary disturbance, foot deformities…, see Tethered cord syndrome (p. 290).

16.2.3 Myelomeningocele

Embryology

The anterior neuropore closes at gestation day 25. The caudal neuropore closes at day 28.

Epidemiology/genetics

Incidence of spina bifida with meningocele or myelomeningocele (MM) is 1–2/1000 live births (0.1–0.2%). Risk increases to 2–3% if there is one previous birth with MM, and 6–8% after two affected children. The risk is also increased in families where close relatives (e.g., siblings) have given birth to MM children, especially when on the mother's side of the family. Incidence may increase in times of war, famine or economic disasters, but it may be gradually declining overall.[6] Transmission follows non-Mendelian genetics, and is probably multifactorial. Prenatal folate (in the form of folic acid) lowers the incidence of MM (p. 313).

Hydrocephalus in myelomeningocele

Hydrocephalus (HCP) develops in 65–85% of patients with MM, and 5–10% of MM patients have clinically overt HCP at birth.[7] Over 80% of MM patients who will develop HCP do so before age 6 mos. Most MM patients will have an associated Chiari type 2 malformation (p. 303). Closure of the MM defect may convert a latent HCP to active HCP by eliminating a route of egress of CSF.

Latex allergy in myelomeningocele

Up to 73% of MM patients are allergic to proteins present in latex (the milky sap from the rubber tree Hevea brasiliensis), found only in naturally occurring rubber products (and which are not present in synthetics, such as silicone, vinyl, plastic, neoprene, nitrile…). The allergy is thought to arise from early and frequent exposure to latex products during medical care for these patients, and there is a suggestion that latex-free surgery on these infants may reduce the risk of the development of latex allergy.[8]

Prenatal diagnosis

See Prenatal detection of neural tube defects (p. 313).

Intrauterine closure of MM defect

Controversial. Does reduce incidence of Chiari II defect, but it has not been determined if this is clinically significant. Argued whether this reduces incidence of hydrocephalus. Does not improve distal neurologic function.

General management

Assessment and management of lesion
- measure size of defect
- assess whether lesion is ruptured or unruptured
  - ruptured: start antibiotics (e.g., nafcillin and gentamicin; D/C 6 hrs after MM closure, or continue if shunt anticipated in next 5 or 6 days)
  - unruptured: no antibiotics necessary
- cover lesion with telfa, then sponges soaked in lactated ringers or normal saline (form a sterile gauze ring around the lesion if it is cystic and protruding) to prevent desiccation
- Trendelenburg position, patient on stomach (keeps pressure off lesion)
- perform surgical closure within 36 hrs unless there is a contraindication to surgery (simultaneous shunt is not usually done except if overt hydrocephalus [HCP] at birth): see below

Neurological assessment and management
- items related to spinal lesion

16

- ○ watch for spontaneous movement of the LEs (good spontaneous movement correlates with better later functional outcome[9])
- ○ assess lowest level of neurologic function (▶ Table 16.1) by checking response of LEs to painful stimulus: although some infants will have a clear demarcation between normal and abnormal levels, at least 50% show some mixture of normal, reflex, and autonomous activity (arising from uninhibited anterior horn motor neurons)[9]
  - – differentiating reflex movement from voluntary may be difficult. In general, voluntary movement is not stereotyped with repetitive stimulus and reflex movement usually only persists as long as the noxious stimulus is applied
- • items related to the commonly associated Chiari type 2 malformation:
  - ○ measure OFC: risk of developing hydrocephalus (see above). Use OFC graphs (p. 427), and also look for abnormal rate of growth (e.g., > 1 cm/day)
  - ○ head U/S within ≈ 24 hrs
  - ○ check for inspiratory stridor, apneic episodes

Table 16.1 Findings in various levels of MM lesion[10]

Paralysis below	Findings
T12	complete paralysis of all muscles in LEs
L1	weak to moderate hip flexion, palpable contraction in sartorius
L2	strong hip flexion and moderate hip adduction
L3	normal hip adduction & almost normal knee extension
L4	normal hip adduction, knee extension & dorsiflexion/inversion of foot; some hip abduction in flexion
L5	normal adduction, flexion & lateral rotation of hip; moderate abduction; normal knee extension, moderate flexion; normal foot dorsiflexion; hip extension absent; • produces dorsiflexed foot and flexed thigh
S1	normal hip flexion & abduction/adduction, moderate extension and lateral rotation; strong knee flexion & inversion/eversion of foot; moderate plantarflexion of foot; extension of all toes, but flexion only of terminal phalanx of great toe; normal medial & lateral hip rotation; complete paralysis of foot intrinsic (except abductor and flexor hallucis brevis); • produces clawing of toes and flattening of sole of foot
S2	difficult to detect abnormality clinically; • with growth this produces clawing of the toes due to weakness of intrinsic muscles of sole of foot (innervated by S3)

Ancillary assessment and management

- • evaluation by neonatologist to assess for other abnormalities, especially those that may preclude surgery (e.g., pulmonary immaturity). There is an average incidence of 2–2.5 additional anomalies in MM patients
- • bladder: start patient on regular urinary catheterizations, obtain urological consultation (nonemergent)
- • AP & lat spine films: assess scoliosis (baseline)
- • orthopedic consultation for severe kyphotic or scoliotic spine deformities and for hip or knee deformities

Surgical management

Timing of MM closure

Early closure of MM defect is *not* associated with improvement of neurologic function, but evidence supports lower infection rate with early closure. MM should be closed within 24 hrs whether or not membrane is intact (after ≈ 36 hrs the back lesion is colonized and there is increased risk of postoperative infection).

Simultaneous MM defect closure and VP shunting

In patients without hydrocephalus, most surgeons wait at least ≈ 3 days after MM repair before shunting. In MM patients with clinically overt HCP at birth (ventriculomegaly with enlarged OFC and/or symptoms), MM repair and shunting may be performed in the same sitting without increased incidence of infection, and with shorter hospitalization.[11,12] It may also reduce the risk of MM repair breakdown previously seen during the interval before shunting. Patient is positioned prone, head turned to *right* (to expose the right occiput), right knee and thigh flexed to expose right flank (consider using left flank to prevent confusion with appendectomy scar later in life).

Surgical technique of myelomeningocele repair

Key concepts

- critical goals: 1) free placode from dura (to avoid tethering), 2) water-tight dural closure, 3) skin closure (can be accomplished in essentially all cases). Closure does not restore any neurologic function
- timing goal: surgical closure with latex-free setup ideally ≤ 36 hours after birth
- helpful tips: start at normal dura, open as wide as the defect, trim placode if necessary to close dura, undermine skin to achieve closure (avoid trapping skin → dermoid tumor)
- post-op CSF leak usually means a shunt is required

General principles[13]: prevent desiccation—keep the exposed neural tissue moist. Use latex-free environment (reduces development of latex allergy, as well as attack by maternal antibodies that may have crossed through the placenta). Do not allow scrub solutions or chemical antimicrobials to contact neural placode. Do not use monopolar cautery. At every point during the closure, avoid placing tension on the neural placode.

Multiple layer closure is advocated, 5 layers should be attempted, although occasionally only 2 or so layers may be closed. There is no evidence that multiple layer closure either improves neurologic function or prevents later tethering, but there is a suggestion that when tethering does occur, it may be easier to release when a previous multilayered closure was performed. Silastic does not prevent adherence in series with long follow-up (> 6 yrs), and may even render untethering procedures more difficult.

Begin by dividing the abnormal epithelial covering from the normal skin. The pia-arachnoid may be separated from the neural tissue. The placode is folded into a tube and the pia-arachnoid is then approximated around it with 7–0 suture (absorbable suture, e.g., PDS, may make future reoperation easier). It often helps to start with normal dura above, and then work down. The dura can then be isolated around the periphery and followed deep to the spinal canal superiorly. The dura is then also formed into a tube and approximated in a water-tight closure. If the dura cannot be closed, the placode may be judiciously trimmed. The filum terminale should be divided if it can be located. The skin is then mobilized and closed. Dermoid tumors may result from retained skin during the closure, but alternatively dermoids may also be present congenitally.[14]

If there is a kyphotic deformity, it is repaired at the same sitting as the MM defect closure. The kyphotic bone is rongeured, and 2–0 Vicryl is used to suture the adjacent bones. Some surgeons use a brace post-op, some do not.

Post-op management of MM repair
1. keep patient off all incisions
2. bladder catheterization regimen
3. daily OFC measurements
4. *avoid narcotics* (midbrain malformation renders these patients more sensitive to respiratory depression from narcotics)
5. if not shunted
   a) regular head U/S (twice weekly to weekly)
   b) keep patient flat to ↓ CSF pressure on incision
6. if a kyphectomy was done, use of a brace is optional (surgeon preference)

Late problems/issues

Include:
1. hydrocephalus: may mimic ≈ anything listed below. *ALWAYS RULE OUT SHUNT MALFUNCTION* when an MM patient deteriorates
2. syringomyelia (p. 1405) (and/or syringobulbia):
3. Tethered cord syndrome (p. 290) as many as 70% of MM patients have a tethered cord radiographically (some quote 10–20%), but only a minority are symptomatic. Unfortunately there is no good test to check for symptomatic retethering (SSEPs may deteriorate,[15] myelography may help)

16

a) scoliosis: early untethering of cord may improve scoliosis; see Scoliosis in tethered cord (p. 291)

b) symptomatic tethering may manifest as delayed neurological deterioration[16]

4. dermoid tumor (p. 980) at the MM site[17]: incidence ≈ 16%
5. medullary compression at foramen magnum, see symptomatic Chiari II malformation (p. 303)
6. short stature: use of growth hormone to increase stature is controversial

Outcome

Without any treatment, only 14–30% of MM infants survive infancy; these usually represent the least severely involved; 70% will have a normal IQ, 50% are ambulatory.

With modern treatment, ≈ 85% of MM infants survive. The most common cause of early mortality are complications from the Chiari malformation (respiratory arrest, aspiration…), where late mortality is usually due to shunt malfunction. 80% will have normal IQ. Mental retardation is most closely linked to shunt infection. 40–85% are ambulatory with bracing; however, most choose to use wheelchairs for ease. 3–10% have normal urinary continence, but most may be able to remain dry with intermittent catheterization.

16.2.4 Lipomyeloschisis

General information

Dorsal spinal dysraphism with lipoma. Six forms are described,[18] the following three are clinically important as possible causes of progressive neurologic dysfunction via tethering (p. 290) and/or compression:

1. (intra)dural lipoma
2. lipomyelomeningocele (see below)
3. fibrolipoma of the filum terminale (p. 286) ("fatty filum")

Lipomyelomeningocele

General information

A subcutaneous lipoma that passes through a midline defect in the lumbodorsal fascia, vertebral neural arch, and dura, and merges with an abnormally low tethered cord (▶ Fig. 16.1).[18] These may be terminal, dorsal, or transitional (between the two).

The intradural fatty tumor may also be known as lipoma of the cauda equina. In addition to being abnormally low, the conus medullaris is split in the midline dorsally usually at the same level as the bifid spine, and this dorsal myeloschisis may extend superiorly under intact spinal arches.[19] There is a thick fibrovascular band that joins the lamina of the most cephalic vertebrae with the bifid lamina. This band constricts the meningocele sac and neural tissue, causing a kink in the superior surface of the meningocele. Asymptomatic lipomas of the filum terminale occur in 0.2–4%[20,21] of MRIs.

The dura is dehiscent at the level of the dorsal myeloschisis, and reflects onto the placode. The lipoma passes through this dehiscence to become attached to the dorsal surface of the placode, and may continue cephalad under intact arches with the possibility of extension into the central canal superiorly to levels without dorsal myeloschisis. The lipoma is distinct from the normal epidural fat which is looser and more areolar. The subarachnoid space typically bulges to the side contralateral to the lipoma. These lipomas account for 20% of covered lumbosacral masses.

Presentation

In a pediatric series, 56% presented with a back mass, 32% with bladder problems, and 10% because of foot deformities, paralysis or leg pain.[22]

Physical examination

Almost all patients have cutaneous stigmata of the associated spina bifida: fatty subcutaneous pads (located over the midline and usually extends asymmetrically to one side) with or without dimples, port-wine stains, abnormal hair, dermal sinus opening, or skin appendages.[23] Clubbing of the feet (talipes equinovarus) may occur.

The neurologic exam may be normal in up to 50% of patients (most presenting with skin lesion only). The most common neurologic abnormality was sensory loss in the sacral dermatomes.

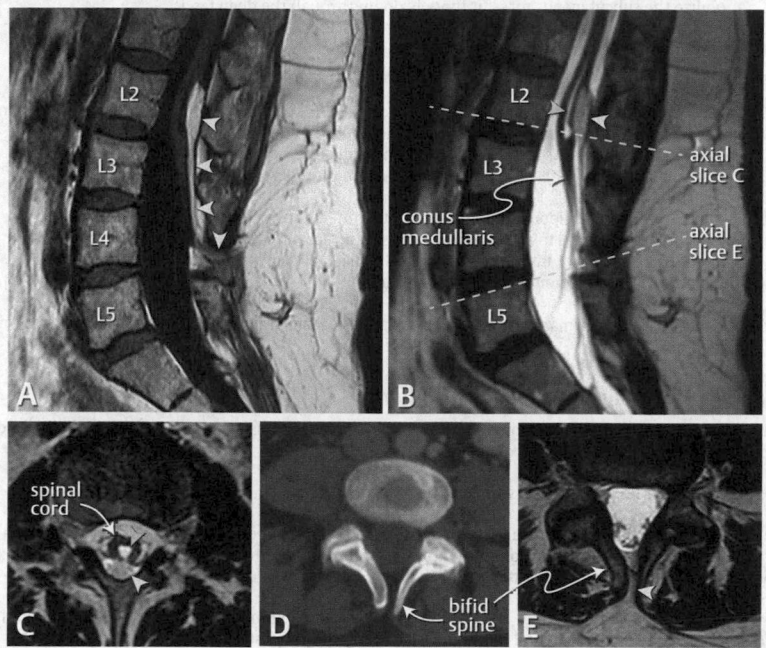

Fig. 16.1 Lipomyelomeningocele in a 53 year old female.
Image: A: T1 sagittal MRI, B: T2 sagittal MRI, C: T2 axial MRI (slice location shown in panel B), D: axial CT bone window, E: T2 axial MRI (slice location shown in panel B).
The lipoma (*yellow arrowheads*) extends up to L2, and extends down to exit the spinal canal through the bifid L4. Note the low lying conus at L3, the small syrinx (*blue arrowheads*), the splitting of the dorsal spinal cord by the lipoma (panel C). The lipoma did not enhance with contrast (not shown).

Evaluation

Plain LS spine X-rays will show spina bifida in most cases. Present in almost all by definition, but some may have segmentation anomalies instead, such as butterfly vertebra (p.227). Abnormalities of fusion and sacral defects may also be seen.

The abnormally low conus can be demonstrated on myelogram/CT or on MRI. MRI also demonstrates the lipomatous mass (high signal on T1WI, low signal on T2WI).

All patients should have pre-op urological evaluation to document any deficit.

Treatment

Since symptoms are due to (1) tethering of the spinal cord, especially during growth spurts, and (2) compression due to progressive deposition of fat, especially during periods of rapid weight gain; the goals of surgery are to release the tethering and reduce the bulk of fatty tumor. Simple cosmetic treatment of the subcutaneous fat pad does not prevent neurologic deficit, and may make later definitive repair more difficult or impossible.

Surgical treatment is indicated when the patient reaches 2 months of age, or at the time of diagnosis if the patient presents later in life. Adjuncts to surgical treatment include evoked potential monitoring and laser. Overall, with surgery, 19% will improve, 75% will be unchanged, and 6% will worsen. Foot deformities often progress regardless.

Surgical technique (modified)

See reference.[19]

16

1. mobilize the subcutaneous mass; it funnels down through the deep fascia
2. open last intact vertebral arch (work from normal dura)
3. identify the fibrovascular band that crosses the most cephalic widely bifid lamina
4. sectioning the fibrovascular band frees the dural tube and releases the sharp kink in the superior surface of the meningocele
5. taking care to preserve dorsal nerve roots, the dura is incised anterior to the dura-lipoma junction
6. a similar procedure is carried out with arachnoid membrane
7. dural/arachnoid incisions are continued around entire extent of tethered conus
8. cord and placode are untethered; monitoring techniques described in Tethered cord syndrome (p. 290) are an option
9. ★ subtotal removal of lipoma: lipoma is then trimmed as completely as possible, intentionally leaving some fat behind to avoid injury to dorsal surface of placode. Superior extension along dorsal surface of cord or into central canal is debulked as much as is safely possible
10. the placode is reformed into a closed neural tube
11. close the pial margins
12. the dura is closed (primarily if possible, or using fascia lata graft if too much tension is placed on folded placode)

Filum terminale lipoma (FTL) ("fatty filum")

AKA fibrolipoma of the filum terminale, AKA fatty filum. A lumbosacral lipoma with the fat limited to the filum terminale and not involving the conus medullaris.

▶ **Prevalence.** 4-6% on cadaveric studies,[18] 0.24-4% on MRI.[24]

▶ **Associated findings.** Additional vertebral anomalies may be seen including hemivertebrae, congenital fusion and abnormalities of segmentation. Other findings include low lying conus and syrinx which are more common in children with FTL than adults (▶ Table 16.2).

▶ **Symptoms.** As many as 95% of cases seen on MRI are asymptomatic, with most FTLs identified in adults considered to be incidental findings. Occasionaly may be associated with symptomatic tethering of the spinal cord, and this occurs more commonly in children and young adults.[24] Findings include: urological abnormalities (59%), back pain (32%) and leg pain (32%), and were more common the lower the conus was located.[24]

▶ **Evaluation.** In addition to MRI, urodynamics should be routinely performed.

▶ **Natural history.** Asymptomatic patients rarely develop symptoms over mean follow-up of 3.47 years (range: 0.5-16.4).[24]

▶ **Indications for surgery.** Prophylactic division of a fatty filum has been advocated in the older literature by some[25] to prevent symptomatic tethering—this is controversial. Fatty filum sectioning for asymptomatic lesions seems reasonable if lumbar spine surgery is being done for another reason (e.g., scoliosis correction). Surgical intervention is generally considered for cases with symptoms compatible with tethered cord (usually urologic symptoms).

Table 16.2 Additional conditions found when fatty filum was identified on MRI[24]

Condition	Prevalence	
	In pediatrics (N = 154)	In adults (N = 282)
low lying conus	30%	8%
syrinx	12%	1%

16.2.5 Dermal sinus

General information

A tract beginning at the skin surface, lined with epithelium. Usually located at either end of neural tube: cephalic or caudal. Most common location is lumbosacral. Probably results from failure of the cutaneous ectoderm to separate from the neuro-ectoderm at the time of closure of the neural groove.[2]

16

Spinal dermal sinus

General information

May appear as a dimple or as a sinus, with or without hairs, usually very close to midline, with an opening of only 1–2 mm. Surrounding skin may be normal, pigmented ("port wine" discoloration), or distorted by an underlying mass.

The sinus may terminate superficially, may connect with the coccyx, or may traverse between normal vertebrae or through bifid spines to the dural tube. It may widen at any point along its path to form a cyst; called an epidermoid cyst if lined with stratified squamous epithelium and containing only keratin from desquamated epithelium, or called a dermoid cyst if also lined with dermis (containing skin appendages, such as hair follicles and sebaceous glands) and also containing sebum and hair.

Although innocuous in appearance, they are a potential pathway for intradural infection which may result in meningitis (sometimes recurrent) and/or intrathecal abscess. Less serious, a local infection may occur. The lining dermis contains normal skin appendages which may result in hair, sebum, desquamated epithelium and cholesterol, within the tract. As a result, the contents of the sinus tract are irritating and can cause a sterile (chemical) meningitis with possible delayed *arachnoiditis* if it enters the dural space.

Incidence of a presumed sacral sinus (a dimple whose bottom could not be seen on skin retraction): 1.2% of neonates.[26]

Dermal sinuses are similar but distinct from **pilonidal cysts**, which may also be congenital (although some authors say they are acquired), contain hair, are located superficial to the postsacral fascia, and may become infected.

If the tract expands intrathecally to form a cyst, the mass may present as a tethered cord or as an intradural tumor. Bladder dysfunction is usually the first manifestation.

The tract from a spinal dermal sinus always courses cephalad as it dives inward from the surface. An occipital sinus may penetrate the skull and can communicate with dermoid cysts as deep as the cerebellum or fourth ventricle.

Evaluation

These tracts are NOT to be probed or injected with contrast as this can precipitate infection or sterile meningitis.

Exam is directed towards detecting abnormalities in sphincter function (anal and urinary), lumbosacral reflexes, and lower extremity sensation and function.

Radiologic evaluation

When seen at birth, *ultrasound* is the best means to evaluate for spina bifida and a possible mass inside the canal.

If seen initially following birth, an MRI should be obtained. Sagittal images may demonstrate the tract and its point of attachment. MRI also optimally demonstrates masses (lipomas, epidermoids...) within the canal.

Plain X-rays and CT are unable to demonstrate the fine tract which may exist between the skin and the dura.

Plain X-rays must be done when embarking on surgery as part of operative planning, as preparation for the possibility of a complete laminectomy.

16

Treatment

Sinuses above the lumbosacral region should be surgically removed. More caudally located sinuses are slightly controversial. Although ≈ 25% of presumed sacral sinuses seen at birth will regress to a deep dimple on follow-up (time not specified), it is recommended that all dermal sinuses should be surgically explored and fully excised *prior* to the development of neurologic deficit or signs of infection. The results following intradural infection are never as good as when undertaken prior to infection. Surgery within the week of diagnosis is appropriate. Sinuses that terminate on the tip of the coccyx rarely penetrate the dura, and may not need to be treated unless local infection occurs.

Surgical technique

An ellipse is cut around the opening, and the sinus is followed deep until the termination of the tract is encountered. Careful insertion of a lacrimal duct probe under direct vision may facilitate excision without violating the tract. If the tract penetrates the spine, laminectomy must be performed and the tract followed to its full extent (even if necessary to extend the laminectomy to T12). An extradural cyst may be present. If the tract enters the dura, it usually does so in the midline, and in these cases the dura should be opened and inspected. Extreme care is taken to prevent spilling cyst contents into the subdural space.

Cranial dermal sinus

General information
Stalk begins with a dimple in the occipital or nasal region. Cutaneous stigmata of hemangioma, subcutaneous dermoid cyst, or abnormal hair formation may occur. Occipital sinuses extend caudally, and if they enter the skull, they do so caudal to the torcular Herophili. Presentation may include recurrent bacterial (usually S. aureus) or aseptic meningitis. Evaluation should include MRI to look for intracranial extension and associated anomalies, including an intracranial dermoid cyst.

Treatment
When operating on a cranial dermal sinus, use a sagittally based incision to permit deep exploration. The tract must be followed completely. Be prepared to enter the posterior fossa.

16.3 Failure of vertebral segmentation and formation

16.3.1 General information

Classification

Multiple classification systems that have been proposed over the years.[27] No system that can cover every possible configuration. Some major concepts are illustrated in ▶ Fig. 16.2. They may be multiple, and formation/segmentation failures may be mixed. Often associated with other congenital abnormalities including cardiac, renal & other skeletal anomalies. May be detected on prenatal ultrasound.

1. failure of formation: hemivertebra (see below)
    a) fully segmented: fully formed disc space above and below with no attachment to adjacent vertebrae. This form has the highest risk for scoliosis progression (100% in one series[28])
    b) semi-segmented: the incomplete VB is fused without a disc to either the VB above or the VB below
    c) non segmented: connected to the VBs above and below. No disc. No potential for progression
    d) incarcerated: VB above and below compensate for the abnormal level, neutralizing the scoliosis ("balanced hemivertebra"[28])
2. failure of segmentation:
    a) unilateral: bar. Osseous bridging of the of one side between adjacent VBs and or posterior elements (a so-called "bar") which produces scoliosis, concave on the side of the bar
    b) bilateral: block vertebra (as in Klippel-Feil (p. 289))

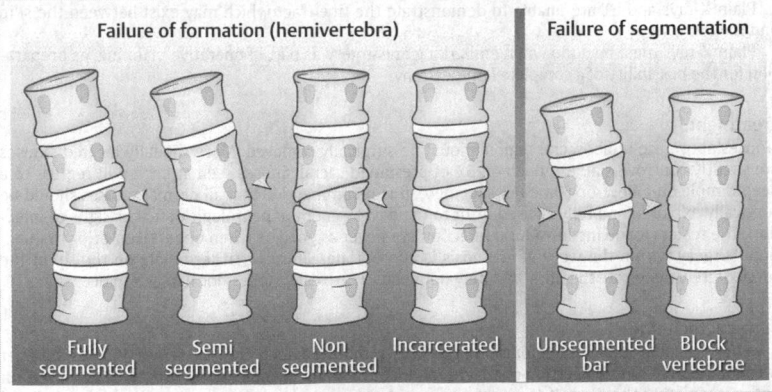

Fig. 16.2 Failure of spinal segmentation and formation.
Image: schematic AP view of involved vertebra (*yellow arrowheads*). Gray ovals represent pedicles on the posterior aspect of the vertebral bodies (VBs).

Evaluation

CT scan: demonstrates the bony anatomy and allows classification according to the above.
   MRI: important to rule out tethered cord, spina bifida, diastematomyelia.

16.3.2 Hemivertebra

Hemivertebra (HVB) (▶ Fig. 16.3) result from unilateral failure of vertebral formation, most commonly producing a lateral wedge of bone having a single pedicle and hemilamina. HVB are one of the leading causes of congenital scoliosis (p. 1319). Incidence is 1-10 per 10,000 live births.[29]
   Variations:
* HVB may be multiple
* associated segmentation failure is seen in > 40% of multiple HVBs[28]
* associated extra rib
* rare forms exist, such as anterior hemivertebrae

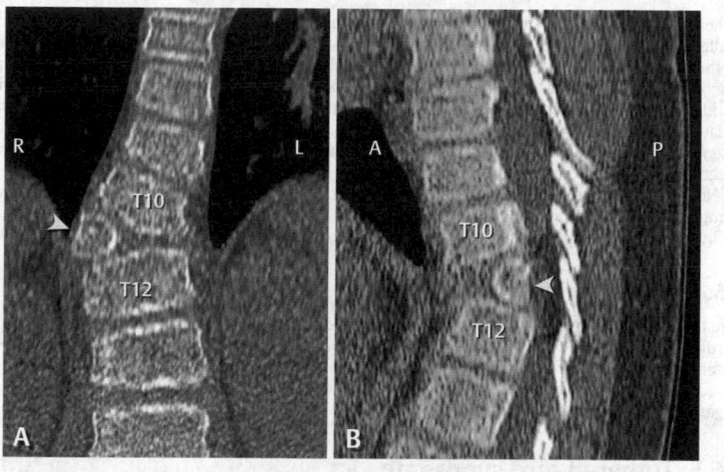

Fig. 16.3 Hemivertebra right T11 (*yellow arrowheads*) in an 8-year-old boy with back pain.
Image: curvilinear multiplanar reformatted CT scans, bone windows. A: coronal showing 38° segmental dextroscoliosis, B: sagittal through the right side of the canal showing 24° of focal kyphosis.

▶ **Treatment.** Indications for surgery: when 5° of progression occurs.
   Treatment consists of complete resection of the hemivertebra usually accompanied by a short-segment fusion.
   Points of controversy:
Optimal age for surgery: most recommend early surgery after 1 year age.
Posterior approach alone vs. an anterior-posterior approach.
Fuse 1 level above and below, or 2 levels.[30]
   Complications:
Crankshafting may occur with a posterior fusion, thought to be due to continued growth of the anterior spine producing VB rotation.

16.4 Klippel-Feil syndrome

16.4.1 General information

Congenital fusion of two or more cervical vertebrae. Ranges from fusion of only the bodies (congenital block vertebrae, ▶ Fig. 16.2) to fusion of the entire vertebrae (including posterior elements). Results from failure of normal segmentation of cervical somites between 3 and 8 weeks' gestation.

16

Involved VBs are often flattened, and associated disc spaces are absent or hypoplastic. Hemivertebrae may also occur. Neural foramina are smaller than normal and oval. Central canal stenosis is rare. Complete absence of the posterior elements with an enlarged foramen magnum and fixed hyperextension posture is called iniencephaly and is rare. Incidence of Klippel-Feil is unknown due to its rarity and the fact that it is frequently asymptomatic.

May occur in conjunction with other congenital cervical spine anomalies such as basilar impression and atlantooccipital fusion.

16.4.2 Presentation

Classic clinical triad (all 3 are present in < 50%):
1. low posterior hairline
2. shortened neck (brevicollis)
3. limitation of neck motion (may not be evident if < 3 vertebrae are fused, if fusion is limited only to the lower cervical levels,[31] or if hypermobility of nonfused segments compensates). Limitation of movement is more common in rotation than flexion–extension or lateral bending

Other clinical associations include scoliosis in 60%, facial asymmetry, torticollis, webbing of the neck (called pterygium colli when severe), Sprengel's deformity in 25–35% (raised scapula due to failure of the scapula to properly descend from its region of formation high in the neck to its normal position about the same time as the Klippel-Feil lesion occurs), synkinesis (mirror motions, primarily of hands but occasionally arms also), and less commonly facial nerve palsy, ptosis, cleft or high arched palate. Systemic congenital abnormalities may also occur, including: genitourinary (the most frequent being unilateral absence of a kidney), cardiopulmonary, CNS, and deafness in ≈ 30%[32] (due to defective development of the osseous inner ear).

No neurologic symptoms have ever been directly attributed to the fused vertebrae, however symptoms may occur from nonfused segments (less common in short-segment fusions) which may be hypermobile, possibly leading to instability or degenerative arthritic changes.

16.4.3 Treatment

Usually directed at detecting and managing the associated systemic anomalies. Patients should have cardiac evaluation (EKG), CXR, and a renal ultrasound. Serial examinations with lateral flexion–extension C-spine X-rays to monitor for instability. Occasionally, judicious fusion of an unstable nonfused segment may be needed at the risk of further loss of mobility. See also recommendations regarding athletic competition (p. 1126).

16.5 Tethered cord syndrome

16.5.1 General information

Abnormally low conus medullaris. Usually associated with a short, thickened filum terminale, or with an intradural lipoma (other lesions, e.g., lipoma extending through dura, or diastematomyelia, are considered as separate entities). Most common in myelomeningocele (MM). Diagnosis must be made clinically in MM, as almost all of these patients will have tethering radiographically.

16.5.2 Presentation

Presenting signs and symptoms in patients with tethered cord are shown in ▶ Table 16.3.

16.5.3 Myelomeningocele patients

If an MM patient has increasing scoliosis, increasing spasticity, worsening gait (in those previously ambulatory), or deteriorating urodynamics[34]:
- always make sure that there is a working shunt with normal ICP
- if painful, should be considered tethered cord until proven otherwise
- if painless, should be considered syringomyelia until proven otherwise
- may be due to brainstem compression—see symptomatic Chiari II malformation (p. 303)—requiring posterior fossa decompression

Table 16.3 Presenting signs and symptoms of tethered cord[33 (p 1331–2)]

Finding	%
cutaneous findings	54
• hypertrichosis	• 22
• sub-Q lipoma (no intraspinal extension)	• 15
• miscellaneous (hemangiomatous discoloration, dermal sinus, multiple manifestations)	• 17
gait difficulty with LE weakness	93
visible muscle atrophy, short limb, or ankle deformity	63
sensory deficit	70
bladder dysfunction	40
bladder dysfunction as only deficit	4
pain in back, leg, or foot arches	37
scoliosis or kyphosis[a]	29
posterior spina bifida (lumbar or sacral)	98
[a]high incidence of scoliosis and kyphosis due to inclusion of series by Hoffman	

16.5.4 Scoliosis in tethered cord

Progressive scoliosis may be seen in conjunction with tethered cord. Early untethering of the cord may result in improvement of scoliosis; however, untethering must be done when the scoliosis is mild. When cases of ≤ 10° scoliosis were untethered, 68% had neurologic improvement and the remaining 32% were stabilized, whereas when scoliosis is severe (≥ 50°) ≈ 16% deteriorated.

16.5.5 Tethered cord in adults

General information

Although most cases of tethered cord present in childhood, cases of adult tethered cord also occur. For comparison of adult and childhood forms, see ▶ Table 16.4.

Table 16.4 Comparison of childhood and adult tethered cord syndrome[35]

Finding	Childhood tethered cord	Adult tethered cord
pain	uncommon. Usually in back and legs, not perianal nor perineal	present in 86%, often perianal & perineal. Diffuse & bilateral. Occasionally shock-like
foot deformities	Common early. Usually progressive cavovarus deformity (club foot)	not seen
progressive spinal deformity	common. Usually progressive scoliosis	uncommon (< 5%)
motor deficits	common. Usually gait abnormalities & regression of gait training	usually presents as leg weakness
urological symptoms	common. Usually continuous urinary dribbling, delayed toilet training, recurrent UTIs, enuresis	common. Usually urinary frequency, urgency, sensation of incomplete emptying, stress incontinence, overflow incontinence
trophic ulcerations	relatively common in LEs	rare
cutaneous stigmata of dysraphism	present in 80–100% (tuft of hair, dimple, capillary angioma [naevus flammeus])	present in < 50%
aggravating factors	growth spurts	trauma, maneuvers associated with stretching conus, lumbar spondylosis, disc herniation, spinal stenosis
From J Neurosurg, D. Pang and J.E. Wilberger, Vol. 57, pp. 40, 1982, with permission.		

16

Evaluation

Radiographically: low conus medullaris (below L2) and thickened filum terminale (definition of thickened filum: normal diameter < 1 mm; diameters > 2 mm are pathological). NB: apparent filum diameter on CT-myelogram may vary with concentration of contrast material. Tethered cord syndrome can also occur in patients without a low-lying conus, here symptoms may be explained by taughtness of the cord.[36]

It is difficult to differentiate a tethered cord from a congenitally low lying conus (filum diameter is generally normal in the latter and the conus should not be below L3[37]).

16.5.6 Pre-op evaluation

Preoperative *cystometrogram* is strongly recommended, especially if the patient seems continent (postoperative changes in bladder function are not uncommon, possibly due to stretching of the lower fibers of the cauda equina).

Surgical treatment

If the only abnormality is a thickened, shortened filum, then a limited lumbosacral laminectomy may suffice, with division of the filum once identified.

If a lipoma is found, it may be removed with the filum if it separates easily from neural tissues.

For patients suffering from multiple recurrences, an alternative procedure is a spine shortening vertebral osteotomy via a posterior[38] or lateral approach.[39]

Distinguishing features of the filum terminale intraoperatively

The filum is differentiated from nerve roots by presence of characteristic squiggly vessel on the surface of the filum. Also, under the microscope, the filum has a distinctively whiter appearance than the nerve roots, and ligamentous-like strands can be seen running through it. NB: intra-op electrical stimulation and recording of anal sphincter EMG are more definitive.

Outcome

In MM: it is usually impossible to permanently untether a cord; however, in a growing MM child, it may be that after 2–4 untetherings, the child will be finished growing and tethering may cease to be a problem. Cases that are untethered early in childhood may recur later, especially during the adolescent growth spurt. Incidence of post-op CSF leak: 15%.

Adult form: surgical release is usually good for pain relief. However, it is poor for return of bladder function. Improvement after first-time release have been reported in 50% of patients.[39]

16.6 Split cord malformation

16.6.1 General information

There is no uniformly accepted nomenclature for malformations characterized by duplicate or split spinal cords. Pang et al[40] have proposed the following.

The term split cord malformation (SCM) should be used for all double spinal cords, all of which appear to have a common embryologic etiology.

16.6.2 Type I SCM

Defined as two hemicords, each with its own central canal and surrounding pia, each within a separate dural tube separated by a dural-sheathed rigid osseocartilaginous (bony) median septum. This has often (but not consistently) been referred to as diastematomyelia. There are abnormalities of the spine at the level of the split (absent disc, dorsal hypertrophic bone where the median "spike" attaches).[41] Two-thirds have overlying skin abnormalities including: nevi, hypertrichosis (tuft of hair), lipomas, dimples, or hemangiomas. These patients often have an orthopedic foot deformity (neurogenic high arches).

Treatment: symptoms are most commonly due to tethering of the cord; and are usually improved by untethering. In addition to untethering, the bony septum must be removed and the dura reconstituted as a single tube (these spines are often very distorted and rotated, and therefore start at normal anatomy and work toward defect). ✖ DO NOT cut the tethered filum until *after* the median septum is removed to avoid having the cord retract up against the septum.

16.6.3 Type II SCM

Consists of two hemicords within a single dural tube, separated by a nonrigid fibrous median septum. This has sometimes been referred to as diplomyelia. Each hemicord has nerve roots arising from it. There is usually no spine abnormality at the level of the split, but there is usually spina bifida occulta in the lumbosacral region.

Treatment: consists of untethering the cord at the level of the spina bifida occulta, and occasionally at the level of the split.[41]

16.7 Lumbosacral nerve root anomalies

Congenital anomalies of nerve roots are rare. This possibility should be considered in cases of failed back surgery for herniated disc.

Classification system of Cannon et al[42]:

- Type 1 anomalies: include conjoined nerve root (2 nerve roots arise from a common dural sheath). They separate at various distances from the thecal sac, and exit through the same or separate neural foramina. Neurosurgeons need to be aware of this anomaly to avoid inadvertent injury, e.g., during surgery for herniated disc
- Type 2 anomalies: 2 nerve roots exit through one foramen. Variants[43]:
  a) leaves an unoccupied neural foramen
  b) all foramina occupied, but one foramen has 2 nerve roots
- Type 3 anomalies: adjacent nerve roots are connected by an anastomosis

References

[1] Takahashi S, Morikawa S, Egawa M, et al. Magnetic resonance imaging-guided percutaneous fenestration of a cervical intradural cyst. Case report. J Neurosurg. 2003; 99:313–315

[2] Matson DD. Neurosurgery of Infancy and Childhood. 2nd ed. Springfield: Charles C Thomas; 1969

[3] van Tulder MW, Assendelft WJ, Koes BW, et al. Spinal radiographic findings and nonspecific low back pain. A systematic review of observational studies. Spine. 1997; 22:427–434

[4] Steinberg EL, Luger E, Arbel R, et al. A comparative roentgenographic analysis of the lumbar spine in male army recruits with and without lower back pain. Clin Radiol. 2003; 58:985–989

[5] Avrahami E, Frishman E, Fridman Z, et al. Spina bifida occulta of S1 is not an innocent finding. Spine. 1994; 19:12–15

[6] Lorber J, Ward AM. Spina Bifida - A Vanishing Nightmare? Arch Dis Child. 1985; 60:1086–1091

[7] Stein SC, Schut L. Hydrocephalus in Myelomeningocele. Childs Brain. 1979; 5:413–419

[8] Cremer R, Kleine-Diepenbruck U, Hoppe A, et al. Latex allergy in spina bifida patients–prevention by primary prophylaxis. Allergy. 1998; 53:709–711

[9] Sharrard WJW, McLaurin RL. Assessment of the Myelomeningocele Child. In: Myelomeningocele. New York: Grune and Stratton; 1977:389–410

[10] Sharrard WJW. The Segmental Innervation of the Lower Limb Muscles in Man. Ann R Coll Surgeons (Engl). 1964; 34:106–122

[11] Epstein NE, Rosenthal RD, Zito J, et al. Shunt Placement and Myelomeningocele Repair: Simultaneous versus Sequential Shunting. Childs Nerv Syst. 1985; 1:145–147

[12] Hubballah MY, Hoffman HJ. Early Repair of Myelomeningocele and Simultaneous Insertion of VP Shunt: Technique and Results. Neurosurgery. 1987; 20:21–23

[13] McLone DG. Technique for Closure of Myelomeningocele. Childs Brain. 1980; 6:65–73

[14] Ramos E, Marlin AE, Gaskill SJ. Congenital dermoid tumor in a child at initial myelomeningocele closure: an etiological discussion. J Neurosurg Pediatrics. 2008; 2:414–415

[15] Larson SJ, Sances A, Christenson PC. Evoked Somatosensory Potentials in Man. Arch Neurol. 1966; 15:88–93

[16] Heinz ER, Rosenbaum AE, Scarff TB, et al. Tethered Spinal Cord Following Meningomyelocele Repair. Radiology. 1979; 131:153–160

[17] Scott RM, Wolpert SM, Bartoshesky LE, et al. Dermoid tumors occurring at the site of previous myelomeningocele repair. Journal of Neurosurgery. 1986; 65:779–783

[18] Emery JL, Lendon RG. Lipomas of the Cauda Equina and Other Fatty Tumors Related to Neurospinal Dysraphism. Developmental Medicine and Child Neurology. 1969; 11:62–70

[19] Naidich TP, McLone DG, Mutluer S. A new understanding of dorsal dysraphism with lipoma (lipomyeloschisis): radiologic evaluation and surgical correction. AJNR. 1983; 4:103–116

[20] Uchino A, Mori T, Ohno M. Thickened fatty filum terminale: MR imaging. Neuroradiology. 1991; 33:331–333

[21] Brown E, Matthes JC, Bazan C,3rd, et al. Prevalence of incidental intraspinal lipoma of the lumbosacral spine as determined by MRI. Spine. 1994; 19:833–836

[22] Bruce DA, Schut L. Spinal Lipomas in Infancy and Childhood. Childs Brain. 1979; 5:192–203

[23] Sato K, Shimoji T, Sumie H, et al. Surgically Confirmed Myelographic Classification of Congenital Intraspinal Lipoma in the Lumbosacral Region. Childs Nerv Syst. 1985; 1:2–11

[24] Cools MJ, Al-Holou WN, Stetler WR,Jr, et al. Filum terminale lipomas: imaging prevalence, natural history, and conus position. J Neurosurg Pediatr. 2014; 13:559–567

[25] La Marca F, Grant JA, Tomita T, et al. Spinal lipomas in children: outcome of 270 procedures. Pediatr Neurosurg. 1997; 26:8–16

[26] Powell KR, Cherry JD, Horigan TJ, et al. A Prospective Search for Congenital Dermal Abnormalities of Craniospinal Axis. J Pediatr. 1975; 87:744–750

[27] Ghita RA, Georgescu I, Muntean ML, et al. Burnei-Gavriliu classification of congenital scoliosis. J Med Life. 2015; 8:239–244

[28] Nasca RJ, Stilling FH,3rd, Stell HH. Progression of congenital scoliosis due to hemivertebrae and hemivertebrae with bars. J Bone Joint Surg Am. 1975; 57:456–466

[29] Johal J, Loukas M, Fisahn C, et al. Hemivertebrae: a comprehensive review of embryology, imaging,

16

[30] Wang C, Meng Z, You DP, et al. Individualized Study of Posterior Hemivertebra Excision and Short-Segment Pedicle Screw Fixation for the Treatment of Congenital Scoliosis. Orthop Surg. 2021; 13:98–108

[31] Gray SW, Romaine CB, Skandalakis JE. Congenital Fusion of the Cervical Vertebrae. Surg Gynecol Obstet. 1964; 118

[32] Hensinger RN, Lang JR, MacEwen GD. Klippel-Feil Syndrome: A Constellation of Associated Anomalies. J Bone Joint Surg. 1974; 56A

[33] Youmans JR. Neurological Surgery. Philadelphia 1982

[34] Park TS, Cail WS, Maggio WM, et al. Progressive Spasticity and Scoliosis in Children with Myelomeningocele: Radiological Investigation and Surgical Treatment. Journal of Neurosurgery. 1985; 62:367–375

[35] Pang D, Wilberger JE. Tethered Cord Syndrome in Adults. J Neurosurg. 1982; 57:32–47

[36] Bui CJ, Tubbs RS, Oakes WJ. Tethered cord syndrome in children: a review. Neurosurg Focus. 2007; 23. DOI: 10.3171/foc.2007.23.2.2

[37] Wilson DA, Prince JR. John Caffey award. MR imaging determination of the location of the normal conus medullaris throughout childhood. AJR Am J Roentgenol. 1989; 152:1029–1032

[38] Hsieh PC, Stapleton CJ, Moldavskiy P, et al. Posterior vertebral column subtraction osteotomy for the treatment of tethered cord syndrome: review of the literature and clinical outcomes of all cases reported to date. Neurosurg Focus. 2010; 29. DOI: 10.3171/2010.4.FOCUS1070

[39] Steinberg JA, Wali AR, Martin J, et al. Spinal Shortening for Recurrent Tethered Cord Syndrome via a Lateral Retropleural Approach: A Novel Operative Technique. Cureus. 2017; 9. DOI: 10.7759/cureus.1632

[40] Pang D, Dias MS, Ahab-Barmada M. Split Cord Malformation: Part I: A Unified Theory of Embryogenesis for Double Spinal Cord Malformations. Neurosurgery. 1992; 31:451–480

[41] Hoffman HJ. Comment on Pang D, et al.: Split Cord Malformation: Part I: A Unified Theory of Embryogenesis for Double Spinal Cord Malformations. Neurosurgery. 1992; 31

[42] Cannon BW, Hunter SE, Picaza JA. Nerve-root anomalies in lumbar-disc surgery. J Neurosurg. 1962; 19:208–214

[43] Neidre A, MacNab I. Anomalies of the lumbosacral nerve roots. Review of 16 cases and classification. Spine. 1983; 8:294–299

16

17 Primary Craniospinal Anomalies

17.1 Chiari malformations

17.1.1 General information

The term "Chiari malformation" is preferred for type 1 malformations (due to the more significant contribution of pathologist, Hans Chiari), with the term "Arnold–Chiari malformation" reserved for type 2 malformation.

The Chiari malformations consists of four types of hindbrain abnormalities, probably unrelated to each other. The majority of Chiari malformations are types 1 or 2 (▶ Table 17.1); a very limited number of cases comprise the remaining types. Chiari zero is a novel condition (p.305).

17.1.2 Type 1 Chiari malformation

General information

Key concepts

- a heterogeneous entity with the common feature of impaired CSF circulation through the foramen magnum
- may be congenital or acquired
- most common symptom: occipital H/A, exacerbated by coughing (tussive H/A)
- evaluation: MRI of brain and cervical spine (to assess compression at the foramen magnum and to R/O syringomyelia). Cine MRI to evaluate CSF flow through foramen magnum in uncertain cases
- cerebellar tonsillar herniation on MRI: criteria vary, > 5 mm below the foramen magnum is often cited, but is neither essential nor diagnostic of the condition
- treatment, when indicated, is surgical, but aspects of what that surgery should entail are controversial (enlargement of foramen magnum is usually involved)
- associated with syringomyelia in 30–70%, which almost always improves with treatment of the Chiari malformation

AKA primary cerebellar ectopia,[2] AKA adult Chiari malformation (since it tends to be diagnosed in the 2nd or 3rd decade of life). A heterogeneous group of conditions, with the underlying commonality of disruption of normal CSF flow through the foramen magnum (FM). Some cases are congenital, but others are acquired (this topic is positioned here in the developmental section for historical and organizational reasons).

Classically described as a rare abnormality restricted to caudal displacement of cerebellum with tonsillar herniation below the foramen magnum (see below for criteria) and "peg-like elongation of tonsils." Unlike Chiari type 2, the medulla is *not* caudally displaced (some authors disagree on this

Table 17.1 Comparisons of Chiari type 1 and 2 anomalies (adapted[1])

Finding	Chiari type 1 (see below)	Chiari type 2 (p.303)
caudal dislocation of medulla	unusual	yes
caudal dislocation into cervical canal	tonsils	inferior vermis, medulla, 4th ventricle
spina bifida (myelomeningocele)	may be present	rarely absent
hydrocephalus	may be absent	rarely absent
medullary "kink"	absent	present in 55%
course of upper cervical nerves	usually normal	usually cephalad
usual age of presentation	young adult	infancy
usual presentation	cervical pain, suboccipital H/A	progressive hydrocephalus, respiratory distress

17

point[3]), the brainstem is not involved, lower cranial nerves are not elongated, and upper cervical nerves do not course cephalad. Syringomyelia of the spinal cord is present in 30–70% of cases.[4] True hydromyelia probably doesn't occur; CSF flow has not been documented in humans, and it is generally not possible to find communication between the syrinx and the central canal in Chiari 1 patients. Hydrocephalus occurs in 7–9% of patients with Chiari type 1 malformation and syringomyelia.[4]

Cerebellar tonsil descent below FM with impaction, while common, is no longer a sine qua non of diagnosis.

Associations

May be associated with
1. a small posterior fossa
    a) underdevelopment of the occipital bone due to a defect in the occipital somites originating from the para-axial mesoderm
    b) low lying tentorium (the roof of the p-fossa)
    c) thickened or elevated occipital bone (the floor of the p-fossa)
    d) space occupying lesion in p-fossa: arachnoid cyst (retrocerebellar or supracerebellar[5]), tumor (e.g., FM meningioma or cerebellar astrocytoma), hypervascular dura
2. has been described with just about anything that takes up intracranial space
    a) chronic subdural hematomas
    b) hydrocephalus
3. following lumboperitoneal shunt (p. 456) or multiple (traumatic) LPs[6]: this is considered **acquired Chiari 1 malformation** and the causal relationship has been established. May be asymptomatic
4. arachnoid web or scar or fibrosis around brainstem and tonsils near FM
5. abnormalities of the upper cervical spine
    a) hypermobility of the craniovertebral junction
    b) Klippel-Feil syndrome (p. 289)
    c) occipitalization of the atlas
    d) anterior indentation at foramen magnum: e.g., basilar invagination or retroversion of the odontoid process
6. Ehlers-Danlos syndrome
7. pseudotumor cerebri (Chiari-pseudotumor cerebri syndrome (p. 301)): may explain some treatment failures of suboccipital craniectomy
8. craniosynostosis: especially cases involving all sutures
9. retained rhomboid roof: rare

Epidemiology

Prevalence of Chiari I malformation (CIM) (radiographically): ≈ 0.5%.[7,8]

Average age at presentation is 41 years (range: 12–73 yrs). Slight female preponderance (female:male = 1.3:1). Average duration of symptoms clearly related to Chiari malformation is 3.1 yrs (range: 1 month-20 yrs); if nonspecific complaints, e.g., H/A, are included, this becomes 7.3 years.[9] This latency is probably lower in the MRI era.

Clinical correlates

Patients with Chiari type 1 malformation may present due to any or all of the following:
1. compression of brainstem at the level of the foramen magnum
2. hydrocephalus
3. syringomyelia
4. isolation of the intracranial pressure compartment from the spinal compartment causing transient elevations of ICP intracranial pressure
5. 15–30% of patients with adult Chiari malformation are asymptomatic[10]

Symptoms

Presenting symptoms are shown in ▶ Table 17.2. The most common symptom is pain (69%), especially headache, which is usually felt in the suboccipital region. H/A are often brought on or exacerbated by neck extension or Valsalva maneuver including cough (tussive headache). Weakness is also prominent, especially unilateral grasp. Lhermitte's sign (p. 1712) may also occur. Lower extremity

Table 17.2 Presenting *symptoms* in Chiari 1 malformation (71 cases[3])

Symptom	%
pain • H/A: 34% • neck (suboccipital, cervical): 13% • girdle: 11% • arm: 8% • leg: 3%	69
weakness (1 or more limbs)	56
numbness (1 or more limbs)	52
loss of temperature sensation	40
painless burns	15
unsteadiness	40
diplopia	13
dysphasia	8
tinnitus	7
vomiting	5
dysarthria	4
miscellaneous	
• dizziness	3
• deafness	3
• fainting	3
• facial numbness	3
• hiccough	1
• facial hyperhidrosis	1

involvement usually consists of bilateral spasticity. Some patients may develop acute neurologic deficit after craniocervical trauma.[11]

Signs

Downbeat nystagmus (p. 586) is considered a characteristic of this condition. 10% will have a normal neurologic exam with occipital H/A as their only complaint. Some patients may present primarily with spasticity.

See ▶ Table 17.3. Three main patterns of clustering of signs[3]:
1. *foramen magnum compression syndrome* (22%): ataxia, corticospinal and sensory deficits, cerebellar signs, lower cranial nerve palsies. 37% have severe H/A
2. *central cord syndrome* (p. 1132) (65%): dissociated sensory loss (loss of pain & temperature sensation with preserved touch & JPS), occasional segmental weakness, and long tract signs (syringomyelic syndrome[12]). 11% have lower cranial nerve palsies
3. *cerebellar syndrome* (11%): truncal and limb ataxia, nystagmus, dysarthria

Natural history

The natural history is not known with certainty (only 2 reports on "natural history" exist). A patient may remain stable for years, with intermittent periods of deterioration. Rarely, spontaneous improvement may occur (debated).

Evaluation

General information

A Chiari malformation is often times first identified or suspected based on a cervical MRI. It is important to follow-up with an MRI of the brain to rule out an intracranial process that might be driving the malformation (e.g. a posterior fossa mass), to fully assess the degree of occlusion at the foramen magnum (axial images on cervical MRIs rarely go as high as the foramen magnum) and to look for signs of elevated ICP (empty sella, optic nerve sheath dilation…) that could e.g., be part of an associated pseudotumor cerebri syndrome (PTCS) (p. 955) (6-21% of PTCS patients have tonsillar descent ≥ 5 mm below the FM[14,15,16]).

17

Table 17.3 Presenting *signs* in Chiari I malformation (127 patients[9])

Sign	%
hyperactive lower extremity reflexes	52
nystagmus[a]	47
gait disturbance	43
hand atrophy	35
upper extremity weakness	33
"cape" sensory loss	31
cerebellar signs	27
hyperactive upper extremity reflexes	26
lower cranial nerve dysfunction	26
Babinski sign	24
lower extremity weakness	17
dysesthesia	17
fasciculation	11
Horner sign	6

[a]classically: downbeat nystagmus on vertical movement, and rotatory nystagmus on horizontal movement; also includes oscillopsia[13]

Plain X-rays
Usually not extremely helpful. Of 70 skull X-rays, only 36% were abnormal (26% showed basilar impression, 7% platybasia, and 1 patient each with Paget's and concave clivus). In 60 C-spine X-rays, 35% were abnormal (including assimilation of atlas, widened canal, cervical fusions (i.e., Klippel–Feil deformity (p.289)), and agenesis of posterior arch of atlas).

MRI
MRI of brain and C-spine are the diagnostic tests of choice (▶ Fig. 17.1). Readily shows many of the classic abnormalities described earlier, including tonsillar herniation, as well as hydrosyringomyelia which occurs in 20–30% of cases. Also demonstrates ventral brainstem compression when present. Other findings may include hydrocephalus, empty sella.

Tonsillar herniation: Criteria for the descent of the tonsillar tips below the foramen magnum (FM) to diagnose Chiari type 1 malformation have gone through a number of reconsiderations.

Σ: Significance of tonsillar descent in Chiari I malformation

Tonsillar herniation identified radiographically is of limited prognostic value in diagnosing Chiari I malformation, and requires clinical correlation.

Initially, > 5 mm was defined as clearly pathologic[17] (with 3–5 mm being borderline). Barkovich[18] found tonsillar positions as shown in ▶ Table 17.4, and ▶ Table 17.5 shows the effect of utilizing 2 vs. 3 mm as the lowest normal position.

The tonsils normally ascend with age,[19] as shown in ▶ Table 17.6.

Patients with syringohydromyelia without hindbrain herniation that responded to p-fossa decompression have been described[20] (so-called "Chiari zero malformation"). Conversely, 14% of patients with tonsillar herniation > 5 mm are asymptomatic[8] (average extent of ectopia in this group was 11.4 ± 4.86 mm).

Potentially more significant than the absolute tonsillar descent is the amount of compression of the brainstem at the FM, best appreciated on axial T2WI MRI through the FM. Complete obliteration of CSF signal and brainstem deformity due to compression at the FM by impacted tonsils is a common significant finding.

Cine MRI
AKA CSF flow study. May demonstrate blockage of CSF flow at FM. Not widely available. Accuracy is not high, and therefore usually does not alter management.

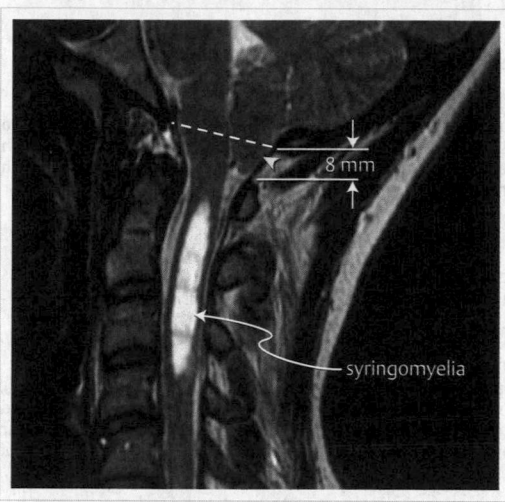

Fig. 17.1 Chiari 1 malformation.
Cerebellar tonsils (*yellow arrowhead*) descend 8 mm below the foramen magnum (*broken line*). Syringomyelia appears as high signal within the spinal cord.
Image: T2 sagittal MRI.

Table 17.4 Location of cerebellar tonsils below foramen magnum[18]

Group	Mean[a]	Range
normal	1 mm above	8 mm above to 5 mm below
Chiari I	13 mm below	3–29 mm below

[a]based on measurements in 200 normals and 25 Chiari I patients taken in relation to the lower part of the foramen magnum

Table 17.5 Criteria for Chiari I[18]

Criteria for lowest extent of tonsils accepted as normal	Sensitivity for Chiari I	Specificity for Chiari I
2 mm below FM	100%	98.5%
3 mm below FM	96%	99.5%

Table 17.6 Tonsillar position relative to FM at various ages[19]

Age (years)	Normal (mm)[a]	2 S.D.[b] (mm)
0–9	–1.5	–6
10–19	–0.4	–5
20–29	–1.1	
30–39	0.0	–4
40–49	0.1	
50–59	0.2	
60–69	0.2	
70–79	0.6	
80–89	1.3	–3

[a]negative number indicates distance below FM
[b]S.D. = standard deviation. Descent > 2 S.D. beyond normal is suggested as a criteria for tonsillar ectopia

17

Myelography
Generally used only when MRI cannot be obtained. Only 6% false negative. It is critical to run the intrathecal contrast (dye) all the way up to the foramen magnum. Usually combined with CT scan.

CT
Unenhanced CT is poor for evaluating the neural structures in the foramen magnum region due to bony artifact. It is very good at demonstrating hydrocephalus (as is MRI). When combined with intrathecal iodinated contrast (myelogram), reliability improves. Findings: tonsillar descent with possible complete blockage of dye at foramen magnum.

Treatment

Patients with Chiari malformation and hydrocephalus
Treatment of the hydrocephalus with CSF shunting may also resolve the tonsillar descent and syringomyelia, when present.[21]

Indications for surgical decompression
Since patients respond best when operated on within 2 years of the onset of symptoms (see below), early surgery is recommended for symptomatic patients. Asymptomatic patients may be followed and operated upon if and when they become symptomatic. Patients who have been symptomatic and stable for years may be considered for observation, with surgery indicated for signs of deterioration.

Surgical techniques
Surgical technique for suboccipital decompression (p. 306).

Operative findings
See ► Table 17.7.

Tonsillar herniation is present in all cases (by definition), the most common position being at C1 (62%). Fibrous adhesions between dura, arachnoid and tonsils with occlusion of foramina of Luschka and Magendie in 41%. The tonsils separated easily in 40%.

Table 17.7 Operative findings in Chiari I (71 patients[3])

Finding	%
tonsillar descent • below foramen magnum: 4% • C1: 62% • C2: 25% • C3: 3% • unspecified level: 6%	100
adhesions	41
syringomyelia	32
dural band (at foramen magnum or C1 arch)	30
vascular abnormalities[a]	20
skeletal abnormalities	
inverted foramen magnum	10
keel of bone	3
C1 arch atresia	3
occipitalization of C1 arch	1
cervicomedullary "hump"	12

[a]vascular abnormalities: PICA dilated or abnormal course in 8 patients (PICA often descends to lower margin of tonsils[12]); large dural venous lakes in 3

Surgical complications

After suboccipital craniectomy plus C1–3 laminectomy in 71 patients, with dural patch grafting in 69, one death due to sleep apnea occurred 36 hrs post-op. Respiratory depression was the most common post-op complication (in 10 patients), usually within 5 days, mostly at night. Close respiratory monitoring is therefore recommended.[3] Other risks of the procedure include CSF leak, herniation of cerebellar hemispheres, vascular injuries (to PICA…).

Operative results

See ▶ Table 17.8.

Patients with pre-op complaints of pain generally respond well to surgery. Weakness is less responsive to surgery, especially when muscle atrophy is present.[22] Sensation may improve when the posterior columns are unaffected and the deficit is due to spinothalamic involvement alone.

Rhoton feels that the main benefit of operation is to arrest progression.

The most favorable results occurred in patients with cerebellar syndrome (87% showing improvement, no late deterioration). Factors that correlate with a worse outcome are the presence of atrophy, ataxia, scoliosis, and symptoms lasting longer than 2 years.[22]

In patients who fail to improve despite adequate decompression, the diagnosis of pseudotumor cerebri syndrome should be ruled out (see below).

Table 17.8 Long-term follow-up after surgery for Chiari I malformation (69 patients, 4 years mean F/U[3])

early improvement of pre-op symptoms	82%
• percent of above that relapsed[a]	21%
early improvement of pre-op signs	70%
no change from pre-op status	16%
worse than pre-op	0

[a]these patients deteriorated to pre-op status (none deteriorated further) within 2–3 years of surgery; relapse occurred in 30% with foramen magnum compression syndrome, and in 21% with central cord syndrome

Chiari-pseudotumor cerebri syndrome (CPCS)

Chiari malformation and pseudotumor cerebri syndrome (PTCS) (p. 955) may coexist in the same patient. The cause and effect in this situation is uncertain (CSF obstruction at the foramen magnum can cause elevated ICP sometimes without hydrocephalus, conversely, elevated ICP with PTCS can cause tonsillar herniation).

Diagnosing PTCS pre-operatively may be difficult in a patient with Chiari malformation, as LP is relatively contraindicated (LP is considered safe in patients with mild tonsillar descent that is not causing a block at the foramen magnum). Papilledema is uncommon in CIM,[23,24] its presence may be suggestive of PTCS, but is not considered to be a reliable indicator[25] (due to inadequate specificity and sensitivity).

PTCS should be considered in a patient with Chiari I who has failed to respond to adequate posterior fossa decompression (PFD)[26] (verified radiographically) or in those who deteriorate after PFD.[27] In one series of mostly pediatric patients who failed PFD, PTCS was found in 42%[26]).

▶ **Treatment.** Optimal treatment for CPCS is controversial. Issues include:
- it is possible that CSF shunting as an initial therapy in patients suspected of having CPCS may avoid the need for PFD[21]
- some authors advocate PFD for patients with Chiari and papilledema[24]
- rarely, a patient with Chiari malformation will deteriorate following PFD due to underlying PTCS
- tonsillar ectopia is not uncommon in PTCS and may be asymptomatic
- papilledema occurs infrequently in CIM without PTCS
- there are reports of resolution of tonsillar herniation in patients with PTCS following treatment of elevated ICP (by CSF shunt placement or acetazolamide[25])

One possible approach in a Chiari patient with papilledema:
1. for patients with fulminant PTCS (p. 967) (rapid vision loss), urgent treatment for PTCS (CSF shunt or ONSF) is indicated
2. for patients with typical PTCS profile (obese females with papilledema ± visual field constriction, no neurologic deficit except possible abducens palsy)
   a) if it is safe to do LP (no block at foramen magnum), and OP is ≥ 25 cm CSF: consider treating the PTCS first (as outlined elsewhere (p. 967))
   b) if LP is not safe, consider placing an external ventricular drain (EVD) to measure the ICP and to assess the response to CSF drainage
      - if PTCS is diagnosed, treat the PTCS as outlined elsewhere (p. 967)
      - if the findings are not suggestive of PTCS or if EVD is not desired, perform PFD

17

3. for patients who do not have typical PTCS profile (women of childbearing age who are either obese (BMI ≥ 30 kg/m²) or who have recently gained weight), or whose symptoms are more suggestive of CIM, perform PFD and reserve treatment for PTCS for those who fail to respond who have documented ICP ≥ 25 cm CSF on LP (which can be more safely performed after PFD)

Chiari malformation and pregnancy

Optimal management of CIM in pregnancy is unclear.[28]

Issues during pregnancy:

1. increased ICP during vaginal labor & delivery elevates the risk of acute tonsillar herniation (p. 325). Etiologies of increased ICP may include any of: Valsalva maneuver as part of maternal pushing during active labor, uterine contractions, associated pain, or other factors
2. Cesarian section carries associated risks such as neonatal respiratory distress, increased blood loss, longer hospital stays and possible complications during subsequent deliveries, and it requires anesthesia, either spinal/epidural or, rarely, general anesthesia
3. anesthetic risks
   a) spinal or epidural anesthesia: commonly used during labor to relieve pain or for C-section. Risks spinal fluid leak with spinal anesthesia or with a "wet tap" (inadvertent entry into subarachnoid space during attempted epidural anesthesia) which may precipitate tonsillar herniation (p. 1815)
   b) general anesthesia for C-section: associated risks including those related to endotracheal intubation

▶ **Literature.** A literature review,[28] found no report of fatal intrapartum herniation of a patient with CIM (NB: absence of proof is not proof of absence). 79% of the patients were symptomatic from the CIM during the pregnancy. 51% of the 36 deliveries were performed by C-section—the criteria for deciding whether or not to perform C-section was not systematically investigated. Most patients had unremarkable vaginal or C-section deliveries without reported neurologic complications. Notable cases among the 4 adverse neurologic events:

- two cases were likely post-anesthetic spinal H/A—unrelated to the CIM— which were successfully treated with epidural blood patch
- a patient who likely had pre-conception symptoms from CIM but was not diagnosed before delivery had an inadvertent dural puncture during attempted epidural anesthesia, had no reported intrapartum issues but became more symptomatic from CIM during the year after delivery and then underwent suboccipital decompression with relief of symptoms[29]

In an institutional series[30] of 95 pregnancies in patients with CIM, 51 delivered vaginally, 44 via C-section. There were no complications attributable to CIM in the 62 patients who had neuraxial anesthesia (38 epidural, 24 spinal). There was no neurologic deterioration in the 51 vaginal deliveries. C-section was performed in 10 patients (23%) just because they had CIM, but the remainder were performed for obstetrical indications.

NB: CIM is present in ≈ 0.5% of the population. Undoubtedly many women with undiagnosed CIM undergo routine labor and delivery or C-section with various forms of anesthesia and there is not widespread reporting of complications related to CIM. Patients with known CIM may be referred more often for C-section which theoretically could avoid some complications and bias the statistics.

▶ **Recommendations (proposed guidelines)**
1. before pregnancy in a patient with known CIM
   - MRI of brain and cervical spine to assess degree of obstruction at the foramen magnum and to look for cervical syrinx
   - lumbar MRI to evaluate for occult spinal dysraphism that could complicate spinal or epidural anesthesia
   - if the patient has symptoms from CIM (other than H/A) or has hydrocephalus: suboccipital decompression is recommended before pregnancy[28]
2. patients with CIM considering pregnancy or already pregnant
   - consultation from a multidisciplinary team composed of maternal–fetal medicine, anesthesia, and neurosurgery is recommended
   - management at a specialized center may be considered since there is *limited* (biased) data that women with CIM have increased risk of medical and obstetrical complications including ARDS, stroke, seizures, sepsis, pre-eclampsia and eclampsia*.[31]
   *NB: based on data mining the Nationwide Inpatient Sample[32] which would not account for patients who delivered and had CIM that was not known. The prevalence of CIM patients in

the analysis sample was 0.08% compared to the known prevalence of CIM of 0.5% in the general population, meaning there might be as many as 79,000 women in the reference cohort who had undetected CIM and delivered without any of the indexed complications

3. pregnant patients with CIM who are asymptomatic or only have H/A
   • mode of delivery should be based on obstetrical considerations[30]
   • epidural or spinal anesthesia are low risk and should be made available[30]
4. pregnant CIM patients with more symptoms than just headache during pregnancy[28]
   • for vaginal delivery, minimizing Valsalva maneuvers seems reasonable. Some obstetricians utilize forceps or vacuum assistance to achieve this
   • C-section under regional anesthesia or general anesthesia is another option
5. pregnant CIM patients with unshunted hydrocephalus or findings of increased ICP (e.g., papilledema) may be considered high-risk for vaginal delivery and neuraxial anesthesia[30]:
   • C-section under general anesthesia should be considered[30]
   • suboccipital decompression may be considered if the fetus has not reached viability

17.1.3 Type 2 (Arnold)–Chiari malformation

General information

Key concepts

• almost always associated with myelomeningocele, often accompanied by hydrocephalus
• pathology, includes: caudally displaced cervicomedullary junction, small posterior fossa, tectal beaking
• is probably not just due to tethering
• major clinical findings: swallowing difficulties, apnea, stridor, opisthotonos, downbeat nystagmus
• when symptomatic: always check the shunt first! Then, consider surgical decompression (which cannot correct intrinsic brainstem abnormalities)
• cranial and cervical MRI is the diagnostic test of choice

Almost always associated with myelomeningocele (MM), or, rarely, spina bifida occulta.

Pathophysiology

Probably does *not* result from tethering of the cord by the associated MM. More likely due to primary dysgenesis of the brainstem with multiple other developmental anomalies.[33]

Major findings

Caudally dislocated cervicomedullary junction, pons, 4th ventricle and medulla. Cerebellar tonsils located at or below the foramen magnum. Replacement of normal cervicomedullary junction flexure with a "kink-like deformity."
   Other possible associated findings:

1. beaking of tectum
2. absence of the septum pellucidum with enlarged interthalamic adhesion: absence of the septum pellucidum is thought to be due to necrosis with resorption secondary to hydrocephalus, and not a congenital absence[34(p 178)]
3. poorly myelinated cerebellar folia
4. hydrocephalus: present in most
5. heterotopias
6. hypoplasia of falx
7. microgyria
8. degeneration of lower cranial nerve nuclei
9. bony abnormalities:
   a) of cervicomedullary junction
   b) assimilation of atlas
   c) platybasia
   d) basilar impression
   e) Klippel–Feil deformity (p. 289)
10. syringomyelia
11. craniolacunia of the skull (see below)

17

Presentation

Findings are due to brainstem and lower cranial nerve dysfunction. Onset is rare in adulthood. The presentation of neonates differs substantially from older children, and neonates were more likely to develop rapid neurological deterioration with profound brainstem dysfunction over a period of several days than were older children in whom symptoms were more insidious and rarely as severe.[35]
Findings include[35,36]:

1. swallowing difficulties (neurogenic dysphagia) (69%).[37] Manifests as poor feeding, cyanosis during feeding, nasal regurgitation, prolonged feeding time, or pooling of oral secretions. Gag reflex often decreased. More severe in neonates
2. apneic spells (58%): due to impaired ventilatory drive. More common in neonates
3. stridor (56%): more common in neonates, usually worse on inspiration (abductor and occasionally adductor vocal cord paralysis seen on laryngoscopy) due to 10th nerve paresis; usually transient, but may progress to respiratory arrest
4. aspiration (40%)
5. arm weakness (27%) that may progress to quadriparesis[38]
6. opisthotonos (18%)
7. nystagmus: especially downbeat nystagmus
8. weak or absent cry
9. facial weakness

Diagnostic evaluation

Skull films

May demonstrate cephalofacial disproportion from congenital HCP. Craniolacunia (AKA Lückenschädel) in 85% (round defects in the skull with sharp borders, separated by irregularly branching bands of bone; *not* due to increased ICP). Low lying internal occipital protuberance (foreshortened posterior fossa). Enlarged foramen magnum in 70%; elongation of upper cervical lamina.[1]

CT and/or MRI findings

Cranial and cervical MRI is the diagnostic test of choice.
- primary findings
  a) "Z" bend deformity of medulla*
  b) cerebellar peg
  c) tectal fusion ("tectal beaking"): the quadrigeminal plate fuses into a posterior point
  d) enlarged massa intermedia (interthalamic adhesion)*
  e) elongation/cervicallization of medulla
  f) low attachment of tentorium
- associated findings
  a) hydrocephalus
  b) syringomyelia in the area of the cervicomedullary junction (reported incidence in pre-MRI era[22] ranges from 48–88%)
  c) trapped fourth ventricle
  d) cerebellomedullary compression
  e) agenesis/dysgenesis of corpus callosum*

17

* items with an asterisk are best appreciated on MRI

Laryngoscopy

Performed in patients with stridor to rule out croup or other upper respiratory tract infections.

Treatment

General information

- insert CSF shunt for hydrocephalus (or check function of existing shunt)
- if neurogenic dysphagia, stridor, or apneic spells occur, expeditious posterior fossa decompression is recommended (see below) (required in 18.7% of MM patients[36]); before recommending decompression, always make sure the patient has a functioning shunt!
- tracheostomy (usually temporary) is recommended if stridor and abductor laryngeal palsy are present pre-op. Close post-op respiratory monitoring is needed for obstruction *and* reduced ventilatory drive (mechanical ventilation is indicated for hypoxia or hypercarbia).

Surgical decompression

NB: it has been argued that part of the explanation for the poor operative results in infants is that many of the neurological findings may be due in part to intrinsic (uncorrectable) abnormalities which surgical decompression cannot improve.[39,40] A dissenting view is that the histologic lesions are due to chronic brainstem compression and concomitant ischemia, and that expeditious brainstem decompression should be carried out when any of the following critical warning signs develop: *neurogenic dysphagia, stridor, apneic spells*.[35]

Surgical technique

Surgical technique for suboccipital decompression (p. 306).

Outcome

68% had complete or near-complete resolution of symptoms, 12% had mild to moderate residual deficits, and 20% had no improvement (in general, neonates fared worse than older children).[35]

Respiratory arrest is the most common cause of mortality (8 of 17 patients who died), with the rest due to meningitis/ventriculitis (6 patients), aspiration (2 patients), and biliary atresia (1 patient).[36]

In follow-up ranging 7 mos-6 yrs, 37.8% mortality in operated patients.

Pre-op status and the rapidity of neurologic deterioration were the most important prognosticators. Mortality rate is 71% in infants having cardiopulmonary arrest, vocal cord paralysis or arm weakness within 2 weeks of presentation, compared to 23% mortality in patients with a more gradual deterioration. Bilateral vocal cord paralysis was a particularly poor prognosticator for response to surgery.[35]

17.1.4 Other Chiari malformations

Chiari type 0

Patients with syringohydromyelia without hindbrain herniation that respond to p-fossa decompression have been described[20] (so-called "Chiari zero malformation"). Some cases may be due to outlet obstruction of the 4th ventricle or crowded foramen magnum with arachnoid webs.

Chiari type 0.5

Cerebellar tonsils descend less than 5 mm below the foramen magnum, but exhibit ventral herniation defined as unilateral or bilateral crossing of the cerebellar tonsils anterior to the horizontal anatomic line bisecting the caudal medulla at the level of the foramen magnum.

Symptoms include: dysphagia & sleep apnea in very young children, and exertion induced H/A and paresthesias in older children. Other possible symptoms: ataxia, behavioral changes.

Chiari type 1.5

Severe form of Chiari 1. Entire cervicomedullary junction (and obex) is situated below the foramen magnum (▶ Fig. 17.2). Many of these cases have platybasia (p. 228). Clinical manifestations and response to suboccipital decompression are similar to Chiari I with the exception that syringomyelia persisted in almost twice as many Chiari 1.5 cases (13.6%) as Chiari I (6.9%).[41,42]

Chiari type 3

Rare. Both the definition and even the existence are controversial. Most descriptions are based on 1 or 2 cases. Original description cited dislocation of the cerebellum below the foramen magnum into an occipital encephalocele.[43] Some have added herniation of the medulla, fourth ventricle and all of the cerebellum into an occipital and high cervical encephalocele. Some have sided with Raimondi who included occipital encephaloceles associated with caudal displacement of the cerebellum and medulla.[44,45]

Prognosis is poor for most, as it is usually incompatible with life.

Chiari type 4

Originally described as cerebellar hypoplasia without cerebellar herniation.[46] Associated with a small posterior fossa. Existence as a distinct clinical entity is debated.[43]

17

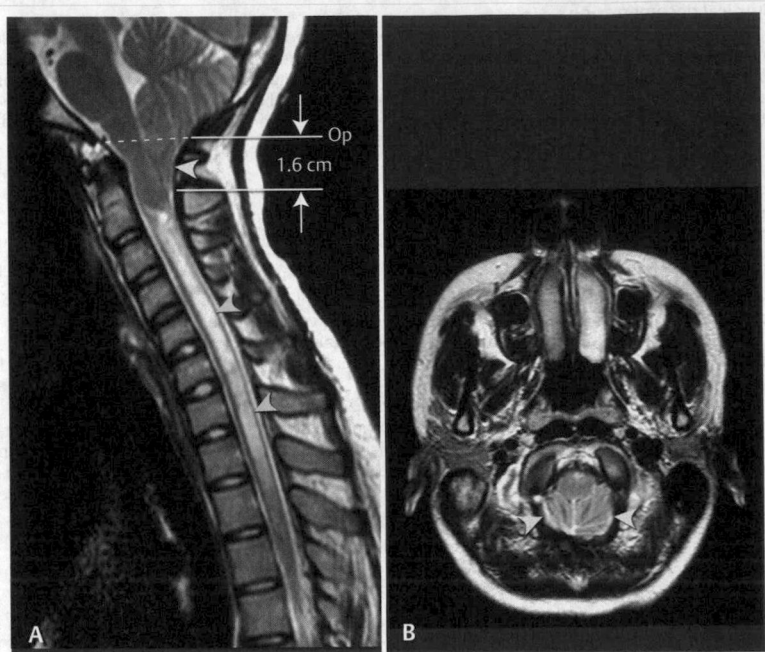

Fig. 17.2 Chiari 1.5 malformation in 18-year-old female.
Image: T2 MRI, A: sagittal, B: axial through the foramen magnum.
Tonsils (*yellow arrowheads*) descend 1.6 cm below the foramen magnum (broken line in A), and compress the cervico-medullary junction with complete obliteration of CSF signal (B).
Syringomyelia (*blue arrowheads*) appears as high signal with the spinal cord.
Op = opisthion (posterior lip of foramen magnum).

17.1.5 Surgical technique for suboccipital decompression

Booking the case: Chiari malformation

Also see defaults & disclaimers (p. 25).
1. position: prone
2. equipment:
   a) optional microscope
   b) intra-op Doppler, if used (primarily in pediatrics)
3. consent:
   a) procedure: surgery through the back of the neck to open the bone at the base of the skull and to insert a "patch" to make more room for the brainstem
   b) alternatives: non-surgical management is usually not effective
   c) complications: CSF leak, brainstem injury/stroke, apnea, failure to improve syrinx (if present)

General information

The most frequently performed operation is posterior fossa decompression of the cerebellar tonsils using a suboccipital craniectomy, with or without other procedures (usually combined with dural patch grafting and cervical laminectomy, which must be carried down to the bottom of the tonsillar tip,[38] which usually includes C1, and sometimes C2 or C3). Options for grafts: same incision (pericranium), separate incision (e.g., fascia lata), and allograft (avoided by many authors because of dissatisfaction with ability to provide water-tight closure and because of infectious risks).

Goals of surgery: decompress the brainstem and reestablish normal flow of CSF at the craniocervical junction.

Positioning

Prone on chest rolls with the head in a Mayfield head-holder or in a horseshoe headrest. Flex the neck to open the interspace between the occiput and posterior arch of C1 (be sure to leave room to insert two fingers between the chin and the chest). The shoulders are retracted inferiorly with adhesive tape. If a fascia lata graft is planned, elevate one thigh on a sandbag.

Approach

▶ **Skin incision.** Midline incision from inion to ≈ C2 spinous process. The fascia is "T'd" at the top to leave a cuff of tissue attached to the occiput to assist in a watertight closure.

▶ **Bone removal.** The posterior rim of the foramen magnum (FM) is the inferior part of the occipital bone. The FM is enlarged no higher than ≈ 3 cm above the FM and approximately as wide as the FM (also ≈ 3 cm).

NB: the compression is at the foramen magnum, *not* in the p-fossa, so keep the posterior-fossa exposure *small*; the emphasis is to decompress the tonsils by opening the FM and the upper cervical spine as far inferiorly as the tonsils extend. Excessive removal of occipital bone may allow the cerebellar hemispheres to herniate through the FM ("cerebellar ptosis" AKA "cerebellar sag," ▶ Fig. 17.3), which may re-create the compression at the foramen magnum.

If a pericranial graft is planned, it should be harvested at this time to reduce the amount of blood entering the subsequent dural opening.[47] Pericranial graft can be procured without extending the incision above the inion, using the technique of Dr. Robert Ojemann[47] with subgaleal dissection and using a monopolar cautery with a bent tip to incise the periosteum and then a Penfield #1 dissector to free it from the bone surface.

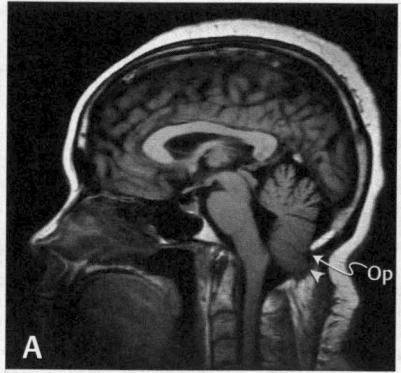 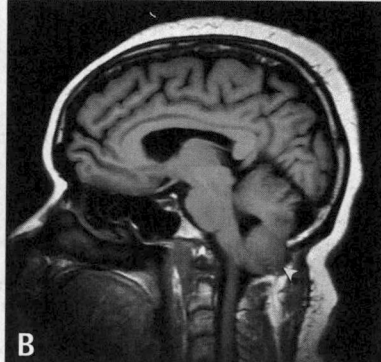

Fig. 17.3 Cerebellar ptosis with cerebellar tissue (*yellow arrowheads*) herniating into the foramen magnum on this MRI done when symptoms recurred 2 years following suboccipital craniectomy for Chiari malformation which initially relieved the symptoms (no ptosis was present on MRI 1 year post-op).
Abbreviations: Op = opisthion (posterior lip of foramen magnum).
Image: T1 sagittal MRI. A: midline cut. B: cut slightly lateral to midline.

17

Decompression

A thick constricting dural band is usually found between the C1 arch and foramen magnum and may be lysed separately. Open the dura in a "Y" shaped incision, and excise the triangular top flap. CAUTION: the transverse sinuses are usually abnormally *low* in Chiari malformations. Also, infants may have a well-developed occipital sinus with associated large dural lakes.[36] Suture the patch graft to provide more room for the contents (tonsils + medulla).

An option that is sometimes used in pediatrics is to not initially open the dura but to lyse constricting bands over the dura at the foramen magnum and then use intraoperative ultrasound to determine if there is adequate room for CSF flow; the dura is then opened only if there is not.

Supplementay options

The following or other additional procedures beyond dural patch grafting are probably not routinely warranted, but may be appropriate in special circumstances.

Shrinking the tonsils with bipolar cautery may be employed if it seems like the bony decompression and dural patch alone will not provide enough room for CSF circulation.

Some authors recommend cautiously dividing adhesions to separate the tonsils from each other as well as from the underlying medulla. Others repeatedly admonish *not* to do this because of the risk of injuring vital structures, including PICAs and medulla.

Historical adjuncts (no longer widely used): plugging the obex (with muscle or teflon), drainage of syrinx if present (fenestration, usually through dorsal root entry zone, with or without stent or shunt[35]), 4th ventricular shunting, terminal ventriculostomy, and opening the foramen of Magendie if obstructed (see reference for illustrations[12]).

17.1.6 Closure

Dura is closed in a watertight fashion. Supplemental dural sealants are optional. A Valsalva maneuver is used to check for CSF leak. Tight fascial closure is critical. Skin is usually closed with running or interrupted suture which is usually more watertight than staples.

17.1.7 Managing ventral compression

In cases with ventral brainstem compression, some authors advocate performing a transoral clivus-odontoid resection as they feel these patients may potentially deteriorate with posterior fossa decompression alone.[22] Since this deterioration was reversible with odontoidectomy, it may be reasonable to perform this procedure on patients who show signs of deterioration or progression of basilar impression on serial MRIs after posterior fossa decompression.

17.2 Neural tube defects

17.2.1 Classification

General information

There is no universally accepted classification system. Two are presented below.

Lemire classification

A system adapted from Lemire.[48]
1. neurulation defects: non-closure of the neural tube results in open lesions
   a) craniorachischisis: total dysraphism. Many die as spontaneous abortion
   b) anencephaly: AKA exencephaly. Due to failure of fusion of the anterior neuropore. Neither cranial vault nor scalp covers the partially destroyed brain. Uniformly fatal. Risk of recurrence in future pregnancies: 3%
   c) meningomyelocele: most common in lumbar region
      • myelomeningocele (MM) (p. 281)
      • myelocele
2. postneurulation defects: produces skin-covered (AKA closed) lesions (some may also be considered "migration abnormalities"; see below)
   a) cranial
      • microcephaly (p. 312)
      • hydranencephaly (p. 309): loss of most of cerebral hemispheres, replaced by CSF. Must distinguish from severe hydrocephalus (p. 310)
      • holoprosencephaly: see below
      • lissencephaly: see below
      • porencephaly: see below to distinguish from schizencephaly
      • agenesis of corpus callosum (p. 274)
      • cerebellar hypoplasia/Dandy Walker syndrome (p. 270)
      • macroencephaly AKA megalencephaly: see below

b) spinal
- diastematomyelia, diplomyelia: see Split cord malformation (p. 292)
- hydromyelia/syringomyelia (p. 1405)

Migration abnormalities

A slightly different classification scheme defines the following as abnormalities of neuronal migration (some are considered postneurulation defects; see above):

1. **lissencephaly**: The most severe neuronal migration abnormality. Maldevelopment of cerebral convolutions (probably an arrest of cortical development at an early fetal age). Infants are severely retarded and usually don't survive > 2 yrs
   a) agyria: completely smooth surface
   b) pachygyria: few broad & flat gyri with shallow sulci
   c) polymicrogyria: small gyri with shallow sulci. May be difficult to diagnose by CT/MRI, and may be confused with pachygyria
2. **heterotopia**: abnormal foci of (nonenhancing) gray matter which may be located anywhere from the subcortical white matter to (most commonly) the subependymal lining of the ventricles. May manifest as nodules or as a band of cortex. An early migration defect that results from arrest of radial migration. Almost always presents with seizures
3. **cortical dysplasia**: a cleft that does not communicate with the ventricle. Heterotopias are common. A migration abnormality not quite as severe as schizencephaly
4. **schizencephaly**:
   a) sine qua non: cleft that communicates with the ventricle (communication may be confirmed with CT cisternogram if necessary)
   b) cleft lined with cortical gray matter (often abnormal, may have polymicrogyria). In comparison, porencephaly is a cystic lesion lined with glial tissue (white matter) or connective tissue (see below)
   c) two forms:
      - open lipped: large cleft to ventricle (▶ Fig. 17.4). Very severe forms may mimic hydranencephaly (see below)
      - close lipped (walls fused): ★ look for a dimple in the lateral wall of the lateral ventricle immediately under the cortical cleft (the appearance of which may mimic an enlarged sulcus)
   d) may be unilateral or bilateral
   e) pia and arachnoid fuse
   f) there may be an "abnormal" vein that represents a cortical vein that now looks medullary because it follows the cortex into the cleft)
   g) absence of septum pellucidum in 80–90%
   h) presentation may range from seizures to hemiparesis, depending on size and location

Porencephaly

Not a migration nor neurulation defect—included here to contrast with schizencephaly. Usually arises from in-utero insult (usually infection, hemorrhage, infarct or penetrating trauma including repeated ventricular punctures). Some authors require communication with the ventricle to distinguish it from encephalomalacia, but this distinction is not universally accepted.

Imaging: MRI signal follows CSF exactly (▶ Fig. 17.5). Lined by white matter (c.f. schizencephaly which is lined with gray matter, or arachnoid cysts which displace gray matter) that may or may not be gliotic.

Symptoms: depend on the location, the amount of brain involved and the timing of the injury. Spasticity and seizures are common manifestations. May be associated with macrocephaly. May also be an incidental finding with no associated signs or symptoms.

17.2.2 Examples of neural tube defects

Hydranencephaly

General information

A post-neurulation defect. Total or near-total absence of the cerebrum (small bands of cerebrum may be consistent with the diagnosis[49]), with intact cranial vault and meninges, the intracranial cavity being filled with CSF. There is usually progressive macrocrania, but head size may be normal (especially at birth), and, occasionally, microcephaly may occur. Facial dysmorphism is rare.

17

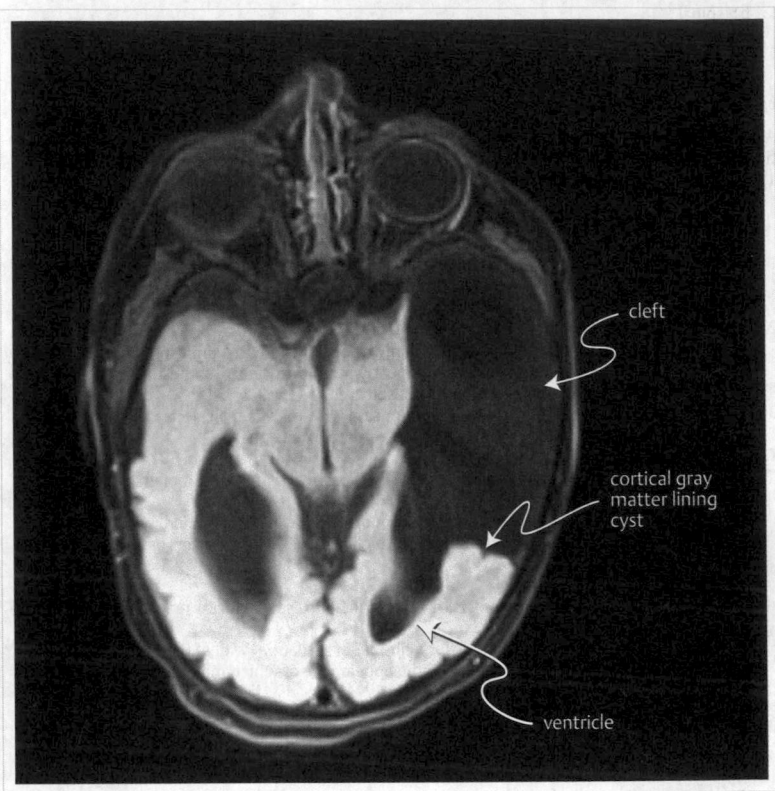

cleft

cortical gray matter lining cyst

ventricle

Fig. 17.4 Schizencephaly. Open lipped form.
Image: axial T2 FLAIR MRI.

May be due to a variety of causes; the most commonly cited is bilateral ICA infarcts (which results in absence of brain tissue supplied by the anterior and middle cerebral arteries with preservation in the distribution of the PCA). May also be due to infection (congenital or neonatal herpes, toxoplasmosis, equine virus).

Less affected infants may appear normal at birth, but are often hyperirritable and retain primitive reflexes (Moro, grasp, and stepping reflex) beyond 6 mo. They rarely progress beyond spontaneous vowel production and social smiling. Seizures are common.

Differentiation from severe ("maximal") hydrocephalus

Progressive enlargement of CSF spaces may occur, which can mimic severe ("maximal") hydrocephalus (HCP). It is critical to differentiate the two, since true HCP may be treated by shunting, which may produce some re-expansion of the cortical mantle. Many means to distinguish hydranencephaly and HCP have been described, including:

1. EEG: shows no cortical activity in hydranencephaly (maximal HCP typically produces an abnormal EEG, but background activity will be present throughout the brain[49]) and is one of the best ways to differentiate the two

2. CT,[49,50] MRI, or ultrasound: majority of intracranial space is occupied by CSF. Usually do not see frontal lobes or frontal horns of lateral ventricles (there may be remnants of temporal, occipital or subfrontal cortex). A structure consisting of brainstem nodule (rounded thalamic masses, hypothalamus) and medial occipital lobes sitting on the tentorium occupies a midline position surrounded by CSF. Posterior fossa structures are grossly intact. The falx is usually intact (unlike

17

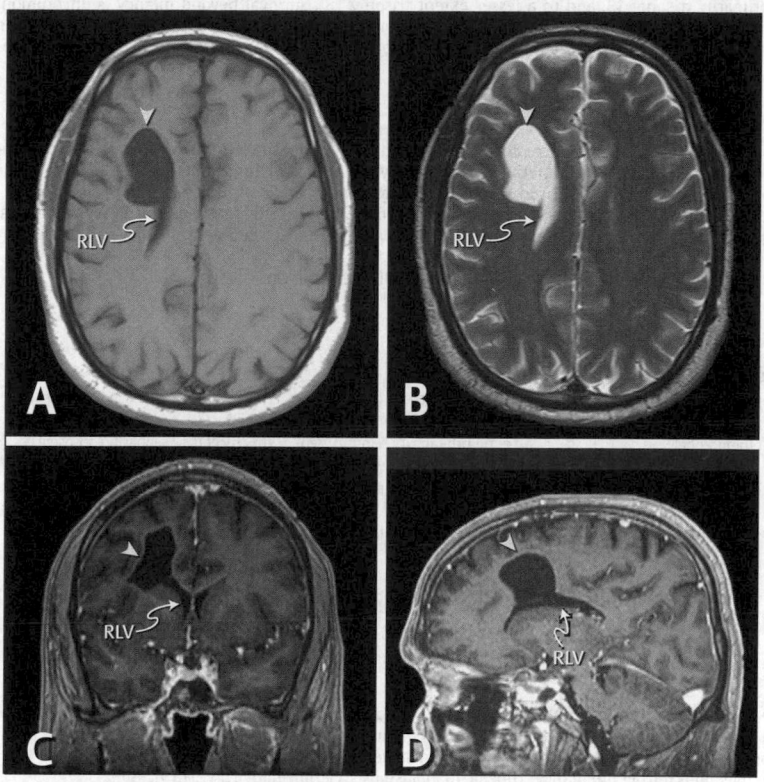

Fig. 17.5 Porencephalic cyst (*yellow arrowheads*).
Image: MRI, A: axial T1. B: axial T2. C: coronal T1 post-contrast. D: sagittal T1-post contrast.
Abbreviations: RLV = right lateral ventricle.

alobar holoprosencephaly) and is not thickened, but it may be displaced laterally. In HCP, some cortical mantle is usually identifiable

3. transillumination of the skull: in a darkened room, a bright light is placed against the surface of the skull. To transilluminate, the patient must be < 9 mos old and the cortical mantle under the light source must be < 1 cm thick,[51(p215)] but it can also occur if fluid displaces the cortex inward (e.g., subdural effusions). Too insensitive to be very helpful

4. angiography: in "classic" cases resulting from bilateral ICA occlusion, no flow through supraclinoid carotids and a normal posterior circulation is expected

Treatment
Shunting may be performed to control head size, but unlike the case with maximal hydrocephalus, there is no restitution of the cerebral mantle.

Holoprosencephaly

AKA arhinencephaly. Failure of the telencephalic vesicle to cleave into two cerebral hemispheres. The degree of cleavage failure ranges from the severe alobar (single ventricle, no interhemispheric fissure) to semilobar and lobar (less severe malformations). The olfactory bulbs are usually small and the cingulate gyrus remains fused. Median faciocerebral dysplasia is common, and the degree of severity parallels the extent of the cleavage failure (▶ Table 17.9). 80% are associated with trisomy

17

(primarily trisomy 13, and to a lesser extent trisomy 18). Survival beyond infancy is uncommon; most survivors are severely retarded, and a minority are able to function in society. Some develop shunt-dependent hydrocephalus. The risk of holoprosencephaly is increased in subsequent pregnancies of the same couple.

Microcephaly

Definition: head circumference more than 2 standard deviations below the mean for sex and gestational age. Terms that are sometimes used synonymously: microcrania, microcephalus. Not a single entity. Many of the conditions in ▶ Table 17.9 may be associated with microcephaly. It is important to differentiate the small skull of microcephaly from that due to craniosynostosis in which surgical treatment may provide the opportunity for improved cerebral development.

Epidemiology
Estimated incidence is 2–12 babies per 10,000 live births in the U.S.[53]

Table 17.9 The five facies of severe holoprosencephaly[52]

Type of face	Facial features	Cranium and brain findings
cyclopia	single eye or partially divided eye in single orbit; arhinia with proboscis	microcephaly; alobar holoprosencephaly
ethmocephaly	extreme orbital hypotelorism; separate orbits; arhinia with proboscis	microcephaly; alobar holoprosencephaly
cebocephaly	orbital hypotelorism; proboscis-like nose; no median cleft lip	microcephaly; usually has alobar holoprosencephaly
with median cleft lip	orbital hypotelorism; flat nose	microcephaly; sometimes has trigonocephaly; usually has alobar holoprosencephaly
with median philtrum-premaxilla anlage	orbital hypotelorism; bilateral lateral cleft lip with median process representing philtrum-premaxillary anlage; flat nose	microcephaly; sometimes has trigonocephaly; semilobar or lobar holoprosencephaly

▶ **Risk factors for microcephaly.** In most cases no definitivce cause can be identified. There may be a genetic component in some cases. Since the main stimulus for growth of the skull is growth of the brain, risk factors for microcephaly include maladies that impede brain growth which include:
• infections during pregnancy: rubella, toxoplasmosis, cytomegalovirus, Zika virus
• severe malnutrition
• maternal exposure to certain drugs during pregnancy: cocaine,[54] alcohol
• interruption of the blood supply to the brain during pregnancy

The effects depend on the severity of the microcephaly. Associated conditions:
• seizures
• developmental delay
• intellectual disability
• hearing problems
• vision problems
• feeding problems: including difficulty swallowing

Macroencephaly

Adapted.[55 (p 109)] AKA macrencephaly, AKA megalencephaly. Not to be confused with macrocephaly (p.1691), which is enlargement of the skull. Not a single pathologic entity. An enlarged brain may be due to hypertrophy of gray matter alone, gray and white matter, presence of additional structures (glial overgrowth, diffuse gliomas, heterotopias, metabolic storage diseases...).

Conditions in which macrocephaly may be seen include:
• neurocutaneous disorders (p.637) (especially neurofibromatosis)
• megalencephaly-capillary malformation syndrome (MCAP): an overgrowth syndrome with megalencephaly (often with hydrocephalus, Chiari malformation, polymicrogyria and seizures) and capillary malformations in the skin (usually on the face)

17

Brains may weigh up to 1600–2850 grams. IQ may be normal, but developmental delay, retardation, spasticity and hypotonia may occur. Head circumference is 4–7 cm above mean. The usual signs of hydrocephalus (frontal bossing, bulging fontanelle, "setting sun" sign, scalp vein engorgement) are absent. Imaging studies (CT or MRI) show normal-sized ventricles and can be used to rule out extra-axial fluid collections.

17.2.3 Risk factors

1. lack of prenatal folic acid: early administration of folic acid[56,57,58] (0.4 mg/d if no history of neural tube defects; 4 mg/d in a carrier or with previous child with NTD was associated with a 71% reduction in recurrence of NTD[59]) (confirm that vitamin B12 levels are normal)
2. folate antagonists (e.g., carbamazepine) doubles the incidence of MM
3. mothers with 5, 10-methylenetetrahydrofolate reductase (MTHFR) gene polymorphism. The common variant, C677 T, substitutes an alanine residue for valine at position 222 in the folate dependent MTHFR enzyme → decreased enzyme activity → reduced levels of tissue folate, and increased levels of homocysteine in the plasma. This polymorphism may be homozygous (TT genotype) or heterozygous (CT genotype); present in ≈ 10% and 38% of the population, respectively. The effects with the TT genotype are more pronounced than with the heterozygous CT form, and there is an increased risk of neural tube defects, as well as a lesser increased risk of cardiovascular disease[60]
4. use of valproic acid (Depakene®) during pregnancy is associated with a 1–2% risk of NTD[61]
5. maternal heat exposure in the form of hot-tubs, saunas or fever (but not electric blankets) in the first trimester was associated with an increased risk of NTDs[62]
6. obesity (before and during pregnancy) increases the risk of NTD[63,64]
7. maternal cocaine abuse may increase the risk of microcephaly, disorders of neuronal migration, neuronal differentiation, and myelination[54]

17.2.4 Prenatal detection of neural tube defects

Serum alpha-fetoprotein (AFP)

See Alpha-fetoprotein (p. 635) for background. A high maternal serum AFP (≥ 2 multiples of the median for the appropriate week of gestation) between 15 and 20 weeks gestation carries a relative risk of 224 for neural tube defects, and an abnormal value (high or low) was associated with 34% of all major congenital defects.[65] The sensitivity of maternal serum AFP for spina bifida was 91% (10 of 11 cases), it was 100% for 9 cases of anencephaly. However, other series show a lower sensitivity. Closed lumbosacral spine defects, accounting for ≈ 20% of spina bifida patients,[66] will probably be missed by serum AFP screening, and may also be missed on ultrasound. Since maternal serum AFP rises during normal pregnancy, an overestimate of gestational age may cause an elevated AFP to be interpreted as normal, and an underestimate may cause a normal level to be interpreted as elevated.[67]

Ultrasound

Prenatal ultrasound will detect 90–95% of cases of spina bifida, and thus in cases of elevated AFP, it can help differentiate NTDs from non-neurologic causes of elevated AFP (e.g., omphalocele), and can help to more accurately estimate gestational age.

Amniocentesis

For pregnancies subsequent to an MM, if prenatal ultrasound does not show spinal dysraphism, then amniocentesis is recommended (even if abortion is not considered, it may allow for optimal postpartum care if MM is diagnosed). *Amniotic* fluid AFP levels are elevated with open neural tube defects, with a peak between weeks ≈ 13 and 15 of pregnancy. Amniocentesis also carries a ≈ 6% risk of fetal loss in this population.

17.3 Neurenteric cysts

17.3.1 General information

No uniformly accepted nomenclature. Working definition: CNS cyst lined by epithelium primarily resembling that of the GI tract, or less often, the respiratory tract. Congenital. Not true neoplasms.

17

Most common alternate term: enterogenous cyst. Less common terms include: teratomatous cyst, intestinoma, archenteric cyst,[68] enterogene cyst, and endodermal cyst. Usually affect the upper thoracic and lower cervical spine.[69] Associated developmental vertebral anomalies (e.g., diastematomyelia) are common.[70] Rarely intracranial (see below). Spinal neurenteric cysts (NEC) may have a fistulous or fibrous connection to the GI tract (through a spinal dysraphism) and some call these endodermal sinus cysts. Occurs as a result of persistence of the neurenteric canal (temporary duct between the notochord and the primitive gut (amniotic and yolk sacs) formed during week 3 of embryogenesis by breakdown of the floor of the notochordal canal).

17.3.2 Intracranial neurenteric cysts

General information

Rare, most common in p-fossa. Initially, may be difficult to rule out metastasis from an extremely well-differentiated primary adenocarcinoma of unknown origin (absence of progressive disease suggests NEC). Locations:
1. posterior fossa
   a) cerebellopontine angle (CPA)[68]: usually intradural, extraaxial (case report of extradural lesion with bone destruction[71])
   b) in midline anterior to brainstem[69]
   c) cisterna magna[72]
2. supratentorial: only 15 case reports as of 2004.[73] Locations: suprasellar[74] (possible confusion with Rathke's cleft cyst), frontal lobe intraparenchymal,[73] quadrigeminal plate region, dural-based extra-axial. Source of endoderm is controversial since the primitive foregut extends cranially only to the midbrain.[75] Theory: colloid cysts, Rathke cleft cysts, and supratentorial NECs may all arise from remnants of Seesel's pouch, a transient endodermally derived diverticulum of the cranial end of the embryonic foregut[76]

Clinical

Most commonly present during the first decade of life.[70] Pain or myelopathy from the intraspinal mass are the most common presentations in older children and adults. Neonates and young children may present with cardiorespiratory compromise from an intrathoracic mass, or with cervical spinal cord compression.[70] Meningitis may occur from the fistulous tract, especially in newborns and infants.

Imaging

Intracranial NEC:
- CT: usually low density, nonenhancing[77]
- T1WI MRI: isointense or slightly hyperintense to CSF (may be hyperintense if there are blood products). T2WI isointense to CSF.[77] Nonenhancing

Histology

Most are simple cysts lined by cuboidal-columnar epithelium and mucin-secreting goblet cells. Less common types of epithelium described include stratified squamous and pseudostratified columnar, and ciliated epithelial cells. Mesodermal components may be present, including smooth muscle and adipose tissue, and some have called these teratomatous cysts,[78,79] not to be confused with teratomas, which are true germinal cell neoplasms. May be histologically identical to colloid cysts.

Treatment

Spinal NEC
Surgical removal usually reverses the symptoms. Recurrence is uncommon with complete removal of cyst wall.

Intracranial NEC
Capsule adherent to brainstem may prevent complete resection, which predisposes to delayed recurrence. Apparently successful treatment by evacuation of contents and marsupialization has been reported (5 cases, mean follow-up: 5 yrs[80]). Incomplete removal requires long-term follow-up. Hydrocephalus is shunted if indicated.

References

[1] Carmel PW. Management of the Chiari Malformations in Childhood. Clinical Neurosurg. 1983; 30:385–406

[2] Spillane JD, Pallis C, Jones AM. Developmental Abnormalities in the Region of the Foramen Magnum. Brain. 1957; 80:11–52

[3] Paul KS, Lye RH, Strang FA, et al. Arnold-Chiari Malformation: Review of 71 Cases. J Neurosurg. 1983; 58:183–187

[4] Guinto G, Zamorano C, Dominguez F, et al. Chiari I malformation: Part I. Contemporary Neurosurgery. 2004; 26:1–7

[5] Bahuleyan B, Rao A, Chacko AG, et al. Supracerebellar arachnoid cyst - a rare cause of acquired Chiari I malformation. Journal of Clinical Neuroscience. 2006; 14:895–898

[6] Sathi S, Stieg PE. "Acquired" Chiari I Malformation After Multiple Lumbar Punctures: Case Report. Neurosurgery. 1993; 32:306–309

[7] Milhorat TH, Chou MW, Trinidad EM, et al. Chiari I malformation redefined: clinical and radiographic findings for 364 symptomatic patients. Neurosurgery. 1999; 44:1005–1017

[8] Meadows J, Kraut M, Guarnieri M, et al. Asymptomatic Chiari Type I malformations identified on magnetic resonance imaging. J Neurosurg. 2000; 92:920–926

[9] Levy WJ, Mason L, Hahn JF. Chiari Malformation Presenting in Adults: A Surgical Experience in 127 Cases. Neurosurgery. 1983; 12:377–390

[10] Bejjani GK, Cockerham KP. Adult Chiari malformation. Contemporary Neurosurgery. 2001; 23:1–7

[11] Woodward JA, Adler DE. Chiari I malformation with acute neurological deficit after craniocervical trauma: Case report, imaging, and anatomic considerations. Surg Neurol Int. 2018; 9. DOI: 10.4103/sni.sni_304_16

[12] Rhoton AL. Microsurgery of Arnold-Chiari Malformation in Adults with and without Hydromyelia. J Neurosurg. 1976; 45:473–483

[13] Gingold SI, Winfield JA. Oscillopsia and Primary Cerebellar Ectopic: Case Report and Review of the Literature. Neurosurgery. 1991; 29:932–936

[14] Banik R, Lin D, Miller NR. Prevalence of Chiari I malformation and cerebellar ectopia in patients with pseudotumor cerebri. J Neurol Sci. 2006; 247:71–75

[15] Johnston I, Hawke S, Halmagyi M, et al. The Pseudotumor Syndrome: Disorders of Cerebrospinal Fluid Circulation Causing Intracranial Hypertension Without Ventriculomegaly. Archives of Neurology. 1991; 48:740–747

[16] Aiken AH, Hoots JA, Saindane AM, et al. Incidence of cerebellar tonsillar ectopia in idiopathic intracranial hypertension: a mimic of the Chiari I malformation. AJNR Am J Neuroradiol. 2012; 33:1901–1906. http://www.ajnr.org/content/33/10/1901.full.pdf

[17] Aboulezz AO, Sartor K, Geyer CA, et al. Position of cerebellar tonsils in the normal population and in patients with Chiari malformation: a quantitative approach with MR imaging. Journal of Computer Assisted Tomography. 1985; 9:1033–1036

[18] Barkovich AJ, Wippold FJ, Sherman JL, et al. Significance of cerebellar tonsillar position on MR. AJNR Am J Neuroradiol. 1986; 7:795–799

[19] Mikulis DJ, Diaz O, Egglin TK, et al. Variance of the position of the cerebellar tonsils with age: preliminary report. Radiology. 1992; 183:725–728

[20] Iskandar BJ, Hedlund GL, Grabb PA, et al. The resolution of syringohydromyelia without hindbrain herniation after posterior fossa decompression. J Neurosurg. 1998; 89:212–216

[21] Mathkour M, Keen JR, Huang B, et al. "Two-Birds-One-Stone" Approach for Treating an Infant with Chiari I Malformation and Hydrocephalus: Is Cerebrospinal Fluid Diversion as Sole Treatment Enough? World Neurosurg. 2020; 137:174–177

[22] Dyste GN, Menezes AH, VanGilder JC. Symptomatic Chiari Malformations: An Analysis of Presentation, Management, and Long-Term Outcome. J Neurosurg. 1989; 71:159–168

[23] Vaphiades MS, Eggenberger ER, Miller NR, et al. Resolution of papilledema after neurosurgical decompression for primary Chiari I malformation. Am J Ophthalmol. 2002; 133:673–678

[24] Zhang JC, Bakir B, Lee A, et al. Papilloedema due to Chiari I malformation. BMJ Case Rep. 2011; 2011. DOI: 10.1136/bcr.08.2011.4721

[25] Smith V, MacMahon P, Avellino A, et al. Commentary: The Dilemma of Papilledema in Chiari I Malformation. Neurosurgery. 2018; 82:E73–E74

[26] Fagan LH, Ferguson S, Yassari R, et al. The Chiari pseudotumor cerebri syndrome: symptom recurrence after decompressive surgery for Chiari malformation type I. Pediatr Neurosurg. 2006; 42:14–19

[27] Furtado SV, Visvanathan K, Reddy K, et al. Pseudotumor cerebri: as a cause for early deterioration after Chiari I malformation surgery. Childs Nerv Syst. 2009; 25:1007–1012

[28] Sastry R, Sufianov R, Laviv Y, et al. Chiari I malformation and pregnancy: a comprehensive review of the literature to address common questions and to guide management. Acta Neurochir (Wien). 2020; 162:1565–1573

[29] Barton JJ, Sharpe JA. Oscillopsia and horizontal nystagmus with accelerating slow phases following lumbar puncture in the Arnold-Chiari malformation. Ann Neurol. 1993; 33:418–421

[30] Waters JFR, O'Neal MA, Pilato M, et al. Management of Anesthesia and Delivery in Women With Chiari I Malformations. Obstet Gynecol. 2018; 132:1180–1184

[31] Orth T, Gerkovich M, Babbar S, et al. Maternal and pregnancy complications among women with Arnold Chiari malformation: A national database review. Am J Ob Gyn. 2015; 212

[32] Agency for Healthcare Research and Quality. Overview of the National (Nationwide) Inpatient Sample (NIS). 2021. https://www.hcup-us.ahrq.gov/nisoverview.jsp

[33] Peach B. The Arnold-Chiari Malformation. Morphogenesis. Arch Neurol. 1965; 12:527–535

[34] Taveras JM, Pile-Spellman J. Neuroradiology. 3rd ed. Baltimore: Williams and Wilkins; 1996

[35] Pollack IF, Pang D, Albright AL, et al. Outcome Following Hindbrain Decompression of Symptomatic Chiari Malformations in Children Previously Treated with Myelomeningocele Closure and Shunts. Journal of Neurosurgery. 1992; 77:881–888

[36] Park TS, Hoffman HJ, Hendrick EB, et al. Experience with Surgical Decompression of the Arnold-Chiari Malformation in Young Infants with Myelomeningocele. Neurosurgery. 1983; 13:147–152

[37] Pollack IF, Pang D, Kocoshis S, et al. Neurogenic Dysphagia Resulting from Chiari Malformations. Neurosurgery. 1992; 30:709–719

[38] Hoffman HJ, Hendrick EB, Humphreys RP. Manifestations and Management of Arnold-Chiari Malformation in Patients with Myelomeningocele. Childs Brain. 1975; 1:255–259

[39] Gilbert JN, Jones KL, Rorke LB, et al. Central Nervous System Anomalies Associated with Myelomeningocele, Hydrocephalus, and the Arnold-Chiari Malformation: Reappraisal of Theories Regarding the Pathogenesis of Posterior Neural Tube Closure Defects. Neurosurgery. 1986; 18:559–564

[40] Bell WO, Charney EB, Bruce DA, et al. Symptomatic Arnold-Chiari Malformation: Review of Experience with 22 Cases. Journal of Neurosurgery. 1987; 66:812–816

[41] Tubbs RS, McGirt MJ, Oakes WJ. Surgical experience in 130 pediatric patients with Chiari I malformations. J Neurosurg. 2003; 99:291–296

[42] Tubbs RS, Iskandar BJ, Bartolucci AA, et al. A critical analysis of the Chiari 1.5 malformation. J Neurosurg. 2004; 101:179–183

[43] Brownlee R, Myles T, Hamilton MG, et al. The Chiari III and IV malformations. In: Syringomyelia and the Chiari Malformations. Park Ridge, IL: American Association of Neurological Surgeons; 1997:83–90

[44] Raimondi AJ. Pediatric neuroradiology. Philadelphia: W. B. Saunders; 1972

[45] Castillo M, Quencer RM, Dominguez R. Chiari III malformation: imaging features. AJNR. American Journal of Neuroradiology. 1992; 13:107–113

[46] Chiari H. Über Veränderungen des Kleinhirns infolge von Hydrocephalie des Grosshirns. Deutsche medicinische Wochenschrif, Berlin. 1891; 17:1172–1175

[47] Stevens EA, Powers AK, Sweasey TA, et al. Simplified harvest of autologous pericranium for duraplasty in Chiari malformation Type I. Technical note. J Neurosurg Spine. 2009; 11:80–83

[48] Lemire RJ. Neural Tube Defects. JAMA. 1988; 259:558–562

[49] Sutton LN, Bruce DA, Schut L. Hydranencephaly versus Maximal Hydrocephalus: An Important Clinical Distinction. Neurosurgery. 1980; 6:35–38

[50] Dublin AB, French BN. Diagnostic Image Evaluation of Hydranencephaly and Pictorially Similar Entities with Emphasis on Computed Tomography. Radiology. 1980; 137:81–91

[51] Matson DD. Neurosurgery of Infancy and Childhood. 2nd ed. Springfield: Charles C Thomas; 1969

[52] DeMyer W, Zeman W, Palmer CG. The Face Predicts the Brain: Diagnostic Significance of Median Facial Anomalies for Holoprosencephaly (Arhinencephaly). Pediatrics. 1964; 34:256–263

[53] State birth defects surveillance program data. Birth Defects Research Part A: Clinical and Molecular Teratology. 2013; 97:S1–122

[54] Volpe JJ. Effect of Cocaine Use on the Fetus. New England Journal of Medicine. 1992; 327:399–407

[55] Section of Pediatric Neurosurgery of the American Association of Neurological Surgeons. Pediatric Neurosurgery. New York 1982

[56] Werler MM, Shapiro S, Mitchell AA. Periconceptual Folic Acid Exposure and Risk of Occurent Neural Tube Defects. Journal of the American Medical Association. 1993; 269:1257–1261

[57] Centers for Disease Control. Recommendations for Use of Folic Acid to Reduce Number of Spina Bifida Cases and Other Neural Tube Defects. Morbidity and Mortality Weekly Report. 1992; 41:RR–14

[58] Daly LE, Kirke PN, Molloy A, et al. Folate Levels and Neural Tube Defects. Journal of the American Medical Association. 1995; 274:1698–1702

[59] Wald N, Sneddon J. Prevention of neural tube defects: Results of the Medical Research Council Vitamin Study. Lancet. 1991; 338:131–137

[60] Kirke PN, Mills JL, Molloy AM, et al. Impact of the MTHFR C677 T polymorphism on risk of neural tube defects: case-control study. Bmj. 2004; 328:1535–1536

[61] Oakeshott P, Hunt GM. Valproate and Spina Bifida. Br Med J. 1989; 298:1300–1301

[62] Milunsky A, Ulcickas M, Rothman J, et al. Maternal Heat Exposure and Neural Tube Defects. Journal of the American Medical Association. 1992; 268:882–885

[63] Werler MM, Louik C, Shapiro S, et al. Prepregnant Weight in Relation to Risk of Neural Tube Defects. Journal of the American Medical Association. 1996; 275:1089–1092

[64] Shaw GM, Velie EM, Schaffer D. Risk of Neural Tube Defect-Affected Pregnancies Among Obese Women. Journal of the American Medical Association. 1996; 275:1093–1096

[65] Milunsky A, Jick SS, Bruell CL, et al. Predictive Values, Relative Risks, and Overall Benefits of High and Low Maternal Serum Alpha-Fetoprotein Screening in Singleton Pregnancies: New epidemiologic data. American Journal of Obstetrics and Gynecology. 1989; 161:291–297

[66] Burton BK. Alpha-Fetoprotein Screening. Adv Pediatr. 1986; 33:181–196

[67] Bennett MJ, Blau K, Johnson RD, et al. Some Problems of Alpha-Fetoprotein Screening. Lancet. 1978; 2:1296–1297

[68] Enyon-Lewis NJ, Kitchen N, Scaravilli F, et al. Neurenteric Cyst of the Cerebellopontine Angle. Neurosurgery. 1998; 42:655–658

[69] Lin J, Feng H, Li F, et al. Ventral brainstem enterogenous cyst: an unusual location. Acta Neurochir (Wien). 2004; 146:419–20; discussion 420

[70] LeDoux MS, Faye-Petersen OM, Aronin PA. Lumbosacral Neurenteric Cyst in an Infant. Journal of Neurosurgery. 1993; 78:821–825

[71] Inoue T, Kawahara N, Shibahara J, et al. Extradural neurenteric cyst of the cerebellopontine angle. Case report. J Neurosurg. 2004; 100:1091–1093

[72] Boto GR, Lobato RD, Ramos A, et al. Enterogenous cyst of the cisterna magna. Acta Neurochir (Wien). 2000; 142:715–716

[73] Christov C, Chretien F, Brugieres P, et al. Giant supratentorial enterogenous cyst: report of a case, literature review, and discussion of pathogenesis. Neurosurgery. 2004; 54:759–63; discussion 763

[74] Fandino J, Garcia-Abeledo M. [Giant intraventricular arachnoid cyst: report of 2 cases]. Rev Neurol. 1998; 26:763–765

[75] Harris CP, Dias MS, Brockmeyer DL, et al. Neurenteric cysts of the posterior fossa: recognition, management, and embryogenesis. Neurosurgery. 1991; 29:893–7; discussion 897–8

[76] Graziani N, Dufour H, Figarella-Branger D, et al. Do the suprasellar neurenteric cyst, the Rathke cleft cyst and the colloid cyst constitute a same entity? Acta Neurochir (Wien). 1995; 133:174–180

[77] Shin JH, Byun BJ, Kim DW, et al. Neurenteric cyst in the cerebellopontine angle with xanthogranulomatous changes: serial MR findings with pathologic correlation. AJNR Am J Neuroradiol. 2002; 23:663–665

[78] Morita Y. Neurenteric Cyst or Teratomatous Cyst. Journal of Neurosurgery. 1994; 80

[79] Hes R. Neurenteric Cyst or Teratomatous Cyst. Journal of Neurosurgery. 1994; 80:179–180

[80] Goel A. Comment on Lin J, et al.: Ventral brainstem enterogenous cyst: an unusual location. Acta Neurochir (Wien). 2004; 146

17

Part V

Coma and Brain Death

V

18 Coma

18.1 Coma and coma scales

Consciousness has two components: arousal and content. Impairment of arousal can vary from mild (drowsiness or somnolence), to obtundation, to stupor to coma. Coma is the severest impairment of arousal, and is defined as the inability to obey commands, speak, or open the eyes to pain.

Coma results from one or more of the following:
- dysfunction of high brainstem (central upper pons) or midbrain
- bilateral diencephalic dysfunction
- diffuse lesions in both cerebral hemispheres (cortical or subcortical white matter)

▶ **Glasgow coma scale (GCS).** The Glasgow coma scale (▶ Table 18.1) is a widely used grading system for assessing level of consciousness (is not designed for following neurologic deficits). It has good repeatability. For intubated patients (in whom the verbal axis cannot be evaluated), general practice is to award 1 point for the verbal score and to affix a "T" notation to the total (e.g., "GCS = 6T").[1] No single GCS score defines a cutoff for coma, however, 90% of patients with GCS ≤ 8 and none with GCS ≥ 9 meet the above definition of coma. Thus, GCS ≤ 8 is a generally accepted operational definition of coma.

A number of scales for use in children have been proposed. One is shown in ▶ Table 18.2.[3]

Table 18.1 Glasgow coma scale[2] (recommended for age ≥ 4 yrs)

Points	1	2	3	4	5	6	Score[a]
Best eye opening	none	to pain[b]	to speech	spontaneous	- -	- -	(1 - 4)
Best verbal	none	incomprehensible	inappropriate	confused	oriented	- -	(1 - 5)
Best motor[c]	none[d]	extensor (decerebrate (p. 319))	flexion (decorticate (p. 319))	withdraws to pain	localizes pain	obeys	(1 - 6)
Glasgow coma scale score; range: 3 (worst) to 15 (normal) → TOTAL							(3 - 15)

[a]the number at the head of the column fitting the description is entered here, e.g., if the Best eye opening is to pain, a 2 would be entered for the Best eye opening row
[b]when testing eye opening to pain, use peripheral stimulus (the grimace associated with central pain may cause eye closure)
[c]motor response is tested using central pain
[d]if no motor response, it is important to exclude complete spinal cord injury with spinal shock

Table 18.2 Children's coma scale[a] (for age < 4 yrs)

Points		1	2	3	4	5	6	Score[b]
Best eye opening		none	to pain	to speech	spontaneous	- -	- -	(1 - 4)
Best "verbal"	Crying	none	inconsolable	inconsistently consolable	consolable	smiles, oriented to sound, follows objects, interacts	- -	(1 - 5)
	Interaction	none	restless	moaning	inappropriate			
Best motor		none	extensor (decerebrate)	flexion (decorticate)	withdraws to pain	localizes pain	obeys	(1 - 6)
Children's coma scale score; range: 3 (worst) to 15 (normal) → TOTAL								(3 - 15)

[a]identical to the adult Glasgow coma scale except for verbal score[3]
[b]the total of the 3 scores for Best Eye, Verbal & Motor is the Children's coma scale score

18

18.2 Posturing

18.2.1 General information

The following terms do not accurately localize the site of the lesion. Decorticate posturing implies a more rostral lesion than extensor posturing, and prognosis may be slightly better.

18.2.2 Decorticate posturing

Classically attributed to disinhibition by removal of corticospinal pathways above the midbrain.
  Overview: abnormal flexion in UE and extension in LE.
  Detail:
• UE: slow flexion of arm, wrist and fingers with adduction
• LE: extension, internal rotation, plantarflexion

18.2.3 Decerebrate posturing

Classically attributed to disinhibition of vestibulospinal tract (more caudal) and pontine reticular formation (RF) by removing inhibition of medullary RF (transection at intercollicular level, between vestibular and red nuclei).
  Overview: abnormal extension in UE and LE.
  Detail:
• Head & trunk: opisthotonos (head and trunk extended), teeth clenched
• UE: arms extended, adducted and hyperpronated (internally rotated), wrists flexed, fingers flexed
• LE: extended and internally rotated, feet plantarflexed and inverted, toes plantarflexed.

18.3 Etiologies of coma

18.3.1 Toxic/metabolic causes of coma

1. electrolyte imbalance: especially hypo- or hypernatremia, hypercalcemia, renal failure with elevated BUN & creatinine, liver failure with elevated ammonia
2. endocrine: hypoglycemia, nonketotic hyperosmolar state, DKA (diabetic ketoacidosis, AKA diabetic coma), myxedema coma, Addisonian crisis (hypoadrenalism)
3. vascular: vasculitis, DIC, hypertensive encephalopathy (p. 202)
4. toxic: EtOH, drug overdose (including narcotics, iatrogenic polypharmacy, barbiturates), lead intoxication, carbon monoxide (CO) poisoning, cyclosporine (causes an encephalopathy that shows white-matter changes on MRI that is often reversible with discontinuation of the drug)
5. infectious/inflammatory: meningitis, encephalitis, sepsis, lupus cerebritis, neurosarcoidosis (p. 198), toxic-shock syndrome
6. neoplastic: leptomeningeal carcinomatosis, rupture of neoplastic cyst
7. nutritional: Wernicke's encephalopathy, vitamin B_{12} deficiency
8. inherited metabolic disorders: porphyria, lactic acidosis
9. organ failure: uremia, hypoxemia, hepatic encephalopathy, Reye's syndrome, anoxic encephalopathy (e.g., post-resuscitation from cardiac arrest), CO_2 narcosis
10. epileptic: status epilepticus (including non-convulsive status), post-ictal state (especially with unobserved seizure)

18.3.2 Structural causes of coma

1. vascular:
   a) bilateral cortical or subcortical infarcts (e.g., with cardioembolism due to SBE, mitral stenosis, A-fib, mural thrombus...)
   b) occlusion of vessel supplying both cerebral hemispheres (e.g., severe bilateral carotid stenosis)
   c) bilateral diencephalic infarcts: well described syndrome. May be due to occlusion of a thalamo-perforator supplying both medial thalamic areas or with "top-of-the-basilar" occlusion. Initially resembles metabolic coma (including diffuse slowing on EEG), patient eventually arouses with apathy, memory loss, vertical gaze paresis

18

2. infectious: abscess with significant mass effect, subdural empyema, herpes simplex encephalitis
3. trauma: hemorrhagic contusions, edema, hematoma (see below)
4. neoplastic: primary or metastatic
5. herniation from mass effect: presumably brainstem compression causes dysfunction of reticular activating system or mass in one hemisphere, causing compression of the other, and resulting in bilateral hemisphere dysfunction
6. increased intracranial pressure: reduces CBF
7. acute lateral shift (midline shift) of the brain: e.g., due to hematoma (subdural or epidural) (▶ Table 18.3)

Table 18.3 Effect of lateral shift on level of consciousness[4]

Amount of midline shift	Level of consciousness
0–3 mm	alert
3–4 mm	drowsy
6–8.5 mm	stuporous
8–13 mm	comatose

18.3.3 Pseudocoma

Differential diagnosis:
1. locked-in syndrome: ventral pontine infarction
2. psychiatric: catatonia, conversion reaction
3. neuromuscular weakness: myasthenia gravis, Guillain-Barré

18.3.4 Approach to the comatose patient

General information

This section addresses nontraumatic coma. See Head trauma (p. 1000) for that topic.

Initial evaluation: includes measures to protect brain (by providing CBF, O_2, and glucose), assesses upper brainstem (Cr. N. VIII), and rapidly identifies surgical emergencies. Keep "pseudocoma" as a possible etiology in back of mind.

Outline of approach to comatose patient

1. cardiovascular stabilization: establish airway, check circulation (heartbeat, BP, carotid pulse), CPR if necessary
2. obtain blood for tests
   a) STAT: electrolytes (especially Na, glucose, BUN), CBC + diff, ABG
   b) others as appropriate: toxicology screen (serum and urine), calcium, ammonia, antiseizure medication (ASM) levels (if patient is taking ASMs)
3. administer emergency supportive medications
   a) glucose: at least 25 ml of D50 IVP. Due to potentially harmful effect of glucose in global ischemia, if possible check fingerstick glucose first, otherwise glucose is given without exception, unless it is known with certainty that serum glucose is normal
   b) naloxone (Narcan®): in case of narcotic overdose. 1 amp (0.4 mg) IVP
   c) flumazenil (Romazicon®): in case of benzodiazepine overdose. Start with 0.2 mg IV over 30 seconds, wait 30 secs, then give 0.3 mg over 30 secs at 1 minute intervals up to 3 mg or until patient arouses
   d) thiamine: 50–100 mg IVP (3% of Wernicke's present with coma)
4. core neuro exam (assesses midbrain/upper pons, allows emergency measures to be instituted rapidly, more thorough evaluation possible once stabilized): see Core neuro exam for coma below
5. if herniation syndrome or signs of expanding p-fossa lesion with brainstem compression (▶ Table 18.4): initiate measures to lower ICP—see Treatment measures for elevated ICP (p. 1046)—then get a CT scan if patient begins improving, otherwise emergency surgery. ✱ Do NOT do LP
6. if meningitis is suspected (altered mental status + fever, meningeal signs…)
   a) if no indication of herniation, p-fossa mass (▶ Table 18.4), focal deficit indicating mass effect or papilledema: perform LP, start antibiotics immediately (do not wait for CSF results); see Meningitis (p. 340)

18

b) if evidence of possible mass effect, coagulopathy or herniation, CT to R/O mass. If significant delay anticipated, consider empiric antibiotics or careful LP with small gauge needle (≤22 Ga), measure opening pressure (OP), remove only a small amount of CSF if OP high, replace CSF if patient deteriorates; LP in this setting may be risky, see Lumbar puncture (p. 1811).

7. treat generalized seizures if present. If status epilepticus is suspected, treat as indicated (p. 512); obtain emergency EEG if available

8. treat metabolic abnormalities
   a) restore acid-base balance
   b) restore electrolyte imbalance
   c) maintain body temperature

9. obtain as complete history as possible once stabilized

10. administer specific therapies

Table 18.4 Signs of herniation syndrome or posterior fossa lesion

Herniation syndromes	Signs of p-fossa lesion
also see Herniation syndromes (p. 324)	also see Posterior fossa (infratentorial) tumors (p. 624)
• unilateral sensory or motor deficit • progressive obtundation → coma • unilateral 3rd nerve palsy • decorticate or decerebrate posturing (especially if unilateral)	• initial symptoms of diplopia, vertigo, bilateral limb weakness, ataxia, occipital H/A • rapid onset of deterioration/coma • bilateral motor signs at onset • miosis • absent "doll's eyes" to horizontal movement, possibly with preserved vertical movements • ocular bobbing • ophthalmoplegia • multiple cranial nerve abnormalities with long tract signs • apneustic, cluster or ataxic respirations

Core neuro exam for coma

Pupil

Record size (in mm) in ambient light, and in reaction to direct/consensual light

1. ★ equal and reactive pupils indicates toxic/metabolic cause with few exceptions (see below) (may have hippus). The light reflex is the most useful sign in distinguishing metabolic from structural coma
   a) the *only* metabolic causes of fixed/dilated pupil: glutethimide toxicity, anoxic encephalopathy, anticholinergics (including topically applied atropine), occasionally with botulism toxin poisoning
   b) narcotics cause small pupils (*miosis*) with a small range of constriction and sluggish reaction to light (in severe overdose, the pupils may be so small that a magnifying glass may be needed to see reaction)

2. unequal; note: an afferent pupillary defect does *not* produce anisocoria, see Alterations in pupillary diameter (p. 591)
   a) fixed and dilated pupil: usually due to oculomotor palsy. Possible herniation, especially if larger pupil associated with ipsilateral 3rd nerve EOM palsy (eye deviated "down and out")
   b) possible Horner syndrome: consider carotid occlusion/dissection (NB: in Horner syndrome, the miotic (smaller) pupil is the abnormal one)

3. bilateral pupil abnormalities
   a) pinpoint with minute reaction that can be detected with magnifying glass[5]: pontine lesion (sympathetic input is lost; parasympathetics emerge at Edinger-Westphal nucleus and are unopposed)
   b) bilateral fixed and dilated (7–10 mm): subtotal damage to medulla or immediate post-anoxia or hypothermia (core temperature < 90 °F [32.2 °C])
   c) midposition (4–6 mm) and fixed: more extensive midbrain lesion, presumably due to interruption of sympathetics and parasympathetics

Respiratory rate and pattern

The most common disorder in impaired consciousness (this information is often lacking in patients that are intubated early in their course):

• Cheyne-Stokes (► Fig. 18.1 A): breathing gradually crescendos in amplitude and then trails off, followed by an expiratory pause, and then the pattern repeats. Hyperpneic phase is usually longer

18

than apneic. Usually seen with diencephalic lesions or bilateral cerebral hemisphere dysfunction (non-specific), e.g., early increased ICP or metabolic abnormality. Results from an increased ventilatory response to CO_2

- hyperventilation: usually in response to hypoxemia, metabolic acidosis, aspiration, or pulmonary edema. True central neurogenic hyperventilation is rare, and usually results from dysfunction within the pons. If no other brainstem signs are present, may suggest psychiatric disorder
- cluster breathing (▶ Fig. 18.1 **B**): periods of rapid irregular breathing separated by apneic spells, may appear similar to Cheyne-Stokes, may merge with various patterns of gasping respirations. High medulla or lower pons lesion. Often an ominous sign
- apneustic (rare; ▶ Fig. 18.1 **C**): a pause at full inspiration. Indicates pontine lesion, e.g., with basilar artery occlusion
- ataxic (Biot's breathing; ▶ Fig. 18.1 **D**): no pattern in rate or depth of respirations. Seen with medullary lesion. Usually preterminal

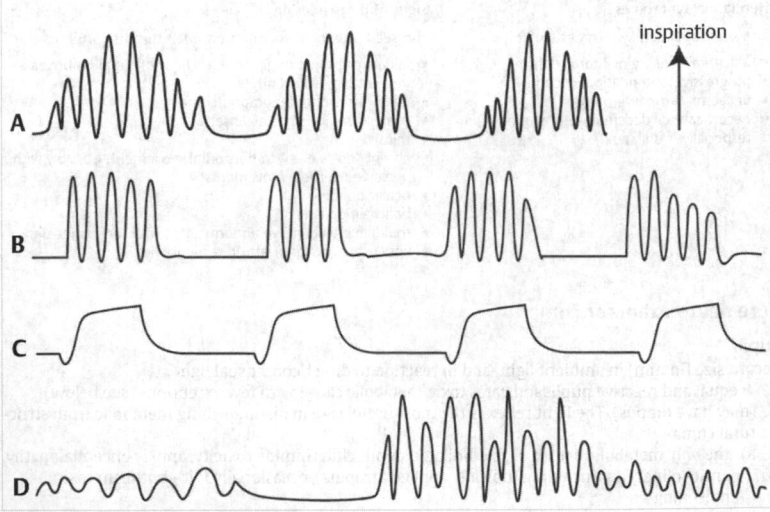

Fig. 18.1 Respiratory rate and pattern.
(A) Cheyne-Stokes respiratory pattern.
(B) Cluster breathing.
(C) Apneustic respiratory pattern.
(D) Ataxic respirations.

Extraocular muscle function

1. deviations of ocular axes at rest
   a) bilateral conjugate deviation:
      - frontal lobe lesion (frontal center for contralateral gaze): looks toward side of destructive lesion (away from hemiparesis). Looks away from side of seizure focus (looks at jerking side), may be status epilepticus. Reflex eye movements (see below) are normal
      - pontine lesion: eyes look *away* from lesion and toward hemiparesis; calorics impaired on side of lesion
      - "wrong way gaze": medial thalamic hemorrhage. Eyes look away from lesion and toward hemiparesis (an exception to the axiom that the eyes look *toward* a destructive supratentorial lesion)[5]
      - downward deviation: may be associated with unreactive pupils, Parinaud's syndrome (p. 101). Etiologies: thalamic or midbrain pretectal lesions, metabolic coma (especially barbiturates), may follow a seizure
   b) unilateral outward deviation on side of larger pupil (III palsy): uncal herniation
   c) unilateral inward deviation: VI (abducens) nerve

d) skew deviation
- III or IV nerve/nucleus lesion
- infratentorial lesion (frequently dorsal midbrain)

2. spontaneous eye movements
   a) "windshield wiper eyes": random roving conjugate eye movements. Non-localizing. Indicates an intact III nucleus and medial longitudinal fasciculus
   b) periodic alternating gaze, AKA "ping-pong gaze": eyes deviate side to side with frequency of ≈ 3–5 per second (pausing 2–3 secs in each direction). Usually indicates bilateral cerebral dysfunction
   c) **ocular bobbing** (p. 601): repetitive rapid vertical deviation downward with slow return to neutral position.

3. internuclear ophthalmoplegia (INO) (p. 596): due to lesion in medial longitudinal fasciculus (MLF) (fibers crossing to contralateral III nucleus are interrupted). Eye ipsilateral to MLF lesion does not adduct on spontaneous eye movement or in response to reflex maneuvers (e.g., calorics)

4. reflex eye movements (maneuvers to test brainstem)
   a) oculovestibular reflex[a], AKA ice water calorics: first rule out TM perforation and occlusion of the EAC by cerumen. Elevate the HOB 30°, irrigate one ear with 60–100 ml of ice water[b]. NB: response is inhibited by neuromuscular blocking agents (NMBA)
   - a comatose patient with an *intact* brainstem will have tonic conjugate eye deviation to side of cold stimulus which may be delayed up to one minute or more. There will be no fast component (nystagmus) (the cortical component) even if the brainstem is intact. (NB: ocu-locephalic reflex[c] (doll's eyes) provides similar information as oculovestibular reflex[d], but poses a greater risk to the spinal cord if C-spine not cleared)
   - no response: symmetrical, could be specific toxin (e.g., neuromuscular block or barbitu-rates), metabolic cause, brain death or possibly massive infratentorial lesion
   - asymmetric: infratentorial lesion, especially if response is inconsistent with 3rd nerve palsy (herniation). Usually maintained in toxic/metabolic coma
   - nystagmus without tonic deviation (i.e., eyes remain in primary position), virtually diagnos-tic of psychogenic coma
   - contralateral eye fails to adduct: INO (MLF lesion)
   b) optokinetic nystagmus presence strongly suggests psychogenic coma

Notes:
[a] **Oculovestibular reflexes** (calorics): the anticipated response is commonly misunderstood. In a normal **awake** patient **there is slow deviation toward the side of the cold stimulus with nystag-mus** (which is named for the rapid, cortical phase) in the opposite direction (hence the mnemonic "COWS" [cold-opposite, warm-same]). Nystagmus will be **absent** in the comatose patient.
[b] HOB at 30° places the horizontal semicircular canal (SCC) vertically for maximal response.[6(p 56)] Cold water → downward endolymphatic currents, **away** from the ampulla of the horizontal SCC.[6(p 57)]
[c] **Oculocephalic reflex** ("doll's eyes" or "doll's head"): do not perform if there is any uncertainty about cervical-spine stability. In an **awake** patient, the eyes will either move with the head, or, if the movement is slow enough and the patient is fixating on an object, there will be contraversive conju-gate eye movement[7] (c.f. oculovestibular reflex which does not depend on patient's level of coopera-tion). In a comatose patient with an intact brainstem and cranial nerves, there will also be contraversive conjugate eye movement (a positive doll's eyes response).
[d] Oculovestibular reflexes are absent but oculocephalic are maintained only when vestibular inputs are interrupted, e.g., streptomycin toxicity of labyrinths or bilateral vestibular schwannomas.

Motor

Record muscle tone and reflexes, response to pain, plantar reflex (Babinski). Note asymmetries
1. appropriate: implies corticospinal tracts and cortex intact
2. asymmetric: supratentorial lesion (tone usually increased), unlikely in metabolic
3. inconsistent/variable: seizures, psychiatric
4. symmetric: metabolic (usually decreased). Asterixis, tremor, myoclonus may be present in meta-bolic coma
5. hyporeflexia: consider myxedema coma, especially in patient presenting weeks after transsphe-noidal surgery
6. patterns
   a) decorticate posturing: arms flex, legs extend: large cortical or subcortical lesion
   b) decerebrate posturing: arms and legs extend: brainstem injury at or below lower midbrain

18

c) arms flexed, legs flaccid: pontine tegmentum
d) arms flaccid, legs appropriate ("man-in-the-barrel syndrome"): anoxic injury (poor prognosis)

Ciliospinal reflex
Pupillary dilatation to noxious cutaneous stimuli: tests integrity of sympathetic pathways
1. bilaterally present: metabolic
2. unilaterally present: possible 3rd nerve lesion (herniation) if on side of larger pupil. Possible pre-existing Horner syndrome if on side of smaller pupil
3. bilaterally absent: usually not helpful

18.4 Herniation syndromes

18.4.1 General information

Classic teaching has been that shifts in brain tissue (e.g., caused by masses or increased intracranial pressure) through rigid openings in the skull (herniation) compress other structures of the CNS producing the observed symptoms. In actuality it may be that herniation is an epiphenomenon that occurs late in the process and is not actually the cause of the observations.[8] However, herniation models still serve as useful models.

The five most common herniation syndromes are:
- supratentorial herniation
  - central (transtentorial) herniation (p. 325)
  - uncal herniation (p. 327)
- cingulate herniation: cingulate gyrus herniates under falx (AKA subfalcine herniation). Usually asymptomatic unless ACA kinks and occludes causing bifrontal infarction. Usually warns of impending transtentorial herniation
- infratentorial herniation
  - upward cerebellar (see below)
  - tonsillar herniation (see below)

18.4.2 Coma from supratentorial mass

See reference.[6]

General information

Central and uncal herniation each causes a different form of rostral-caudal deterioration. Central herniation results in sequential failure of diencephalon, midbrain, pons, medulla (p. 326). See also uncal herniation (p. 327). "Classic" signs of increased ICP (HTN, bradycardia, altered respiratory pattern) usually seen with p-fossa lesions may be absent in slowly developing supratentorial masses.

Distinction between central and uncal herniation is difficult when dysfunction reaches the midbrain level or below. Predicting the location of the lesion based on the herniation syndrome is unreliable.

Clinical characteristics differentiating uncal from central herniation

- decreased consciousness occurs early in central herniation, late in uncal
- uncal herniation syndrome *rarely* gives rise to decorticate posturing

Differential diagnosis of supratentorial etiologies

1. vascular: stroke, intracerebral hemorrhage, SAH
2. inflammatory: cerebral abscess, subdural empyema, herpes simplex encephalitis
3. neoplastic: primary or metastatic
4. traumatic: epidural or subdural hematoma, depressed skull fracture

18.4.3 Coma from infratentorial mass

General information

NB: it is essential to identify patients with primary posterior fossa lesions (▶ Table 18.4) as they may require emergent surgical intervention.

Etiologies of infratentorial masses:

1. vascular: brainstem infarction (including basilar artery occlusion), cerebellar infarction or hematoma
2. inflammatory: cerebellar abscess, central pontine myelinolysis, brainstem encephalitis
3. neoplasms: primary or metastatic
4. traumatic: epidural or subdural hematoma

Hydrocephalus

Infratentorial masses can produce obstructive hydrocephalus by compressing the Sylvian aqueduct and/or 4th ventricle (▶ Fig. 18.2).

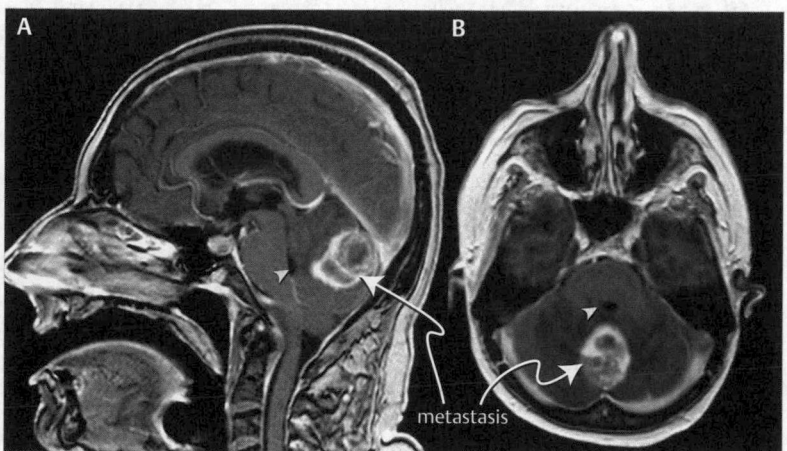

Fig. 18.2 Posterior fossa metastasis causing compression of the 4th ventricle (*yellow arrowheads*) resulting in obstructive hydrocephalus.
Image: enhanced T1 MRI. A: sagittal, B: axial image.

Upward cerebellar herniation

Occasionally seen with p-fossa masses, may be exacerbated by ventriculostomy. Cerebellar vermis ascends above tentorium, compressing the midbrain, and possibly occluding SCAs → cerebellar infarction. May compress Sylvian aqueduct → hydrocephalus.

Tonsillar herniation

Cerebellar tonsils "cone" through the foramen magnum, compressing the medulla → respiratory arrest. Usually rapidly fatal.

Can occur with any of: supra- or infratentorial masses (tumor, abscess, hematoma…), elevated ICP from cerebral edema, obstruction to CSF flow at the foramen magnum (e.g., as in Chiari malformation (p.295)), obstructive hydrocephalus. May be precipitated by LP in these situations. In many cases, there may simply be pressure on the brainstem without actual herniation.[9] There are also cases with significant cerebellar herniation through the foramen magnum with the patient remaining alert.[8]

18.4.4 Central herniation

General information

AKA transtentorial herniation AKA tentorial herniation. Usually more chronic than uncal herniation, e.g., due to tumor, especially of frontal, parietal or occipital lobes.

The diencephalon is gradually forced through the tentorial incisura. The pituitary stalk may be sheared, resulting in diabetes insipidus. PCAs may be trapped along the open edge of the incisura,

18

and may occlude producing cortical blindness; see Blindness from hydrocephalus (p. 429). The brainstem suffers ischemia from compression and shearing of perforating arteries from the basilar artery → hemorrhages within the brainstem (Duret hemorrhages).

Imaging

MRI or CT: the perimesencephalic cisterns may be compressed.

Skull X-rays: downward displacement of the pineal gland may be identified.[10]

Stages of central herniation

Diencephalic stage

Early. May be due to diffuse bilateral hemisphere dysfunction (e.g., from decreased blood flow from increased ICP) or (more likely) from bilateral diencephalic dysfunction due to downward displacement. This stage warns of impending (irreversible) midbrain damage but is frequently reversible if the cause is treated.

Consciousness: Altered alertness is first sign; usually lethargy, agitation in some. Later: stupor → coma.

Respiration: Sighs, yawns, occasional pauses. Later: Cheyne-Stokes.

Pupils: Small (1–3 mm), small range of contraction.

Oculomotor: Conjugate or slightly divergent roving eyes; if conjugate then brainstem intact. Usually positive DOLL'S EYES and conjugate ipsilateral response to cold water calorics (CWC). Impaired upgaze due to compression of superior colliculi and diencephalic pretectum: Parinaud's syndrome (p. 101)

Motor: Early: appropriate response to noxious stimuli, bilateral Babinski, gegenhalten (paratonic resistance). If previously hemiparetic contralateral to lesion: may worsen. Later: motionlessness & grasp reflexes, then DECORTICATE (initially contralateral to lesion in most cases).

Midbrain—upper pons stage

When midbrain signs fully developed (in adults), prognosis is very poor (extreme ischemia of midbrain). Fewer than 5% of cases will have a good recovery if treatment is successfully undertaken at this stage.

Respiration: Cheyne-Stokes → sustained tachypnea.

Pupils: Moderately dilated midposition (3–5 mm), fixed. Note: in pontine hemorrhage pinpoint pupils appear because the loss of sympathetics leaves the parasympathetics unopposed, whereas in herniation, the parasympathetics are usually lost, too (3rd nerve injury).

Oculomotor: Doll's eyes & CWC impaired, may be dysconjugate. MLF lesion → internuclear ophthalmoplegia (when doll's or CWC elicited and dysconjugate, medially moving eye moves less than laterally moving eye).

Motor: Decorticate → bilaterally DECEREBRATE (occasionally spontaneously).

Lower pons—upper medullary stage

Respiration: Regular, shallow and rapid (20–40/min).

Pupils: Midposition (3–5 mm), fixed.

Oculomotor: Doll's eyes and CWC unelicitable.

Motor: Flaccid. Bilateral Babinski. Occasionally LE flexion to pain.

Medullary stage (terminal stage)

Respiration: Slow, irregular rate and depth, sighs/gasps. Occasionally hyperpnea alternating with apnea.

Pupils: Dilate widely with hypoxia.

Outcome after central herniation

In a series of 153 patients with signs of central herniation (altered level of consciousness, anisocoria or fixed pupils, abnormal motor findings) 9% had good recovery, 18% had functional outcome, 10% were severely disabled, and 60% died.[11]

Factors associated with a better result were young age (especially age ≤ 17 yrs), anisocoria with deteriorating Glasgow Coma Score and nonflaccid motor function. Factors associated with poor outcome were bilaterally fixed pupils, with only 3.5% of these patients having a functional recovery.

18

18.4.5 Uncal herniation

General information

Usually occurs in rapidly expanding traumatic hematomas, frequently in the lateral middle-fossa or temporal lobe pushing medial uncus and hippocampal gyrus over edge of tentorium, entrapping third nerve and directly compressing midbrain. PCA may be occluded (as with central herniation). For CT criteria see below.

Impaired consciousness is NOT a reliable early sign. Earliest consistent sign: unilaterally dilating pupil. However, it is unlikely that a patient undergoing early uncal herniation would be completely neurologically intact except for anisocoria (do not dismiss confusion, agitation, etc.). Once brainstem findings appear, deterioration may be rapid (deep coma may occur within hours).

CT and/or MRI criteria

See reference.[12]

The tentorial incisura surrounds the interpeduncular and pre-pontine cisterns and brainstem. There is great interpersonal variability in the amount of space in the incisura.

Impending uncal or hippocampal herniation may be indicated by encroachment on lateral aspect of suprasellar cistern → flattening of normal pentagonal shape. Once herniation occurs CT may show: brainstem displacement and flattening, compression of contralateral cerebral peduncle, midbrain rotation with slight increase of ipsilateral subarachnoid space. Also, contralateral hydrocephalus may occur.[13]

Obliteration of parasellar and interpeduncular cisterns occurs as uncus and/or hippocampus are forced through hiatus. Brainstem is elongated in AP direction due to lateral compression. Since dural structures enhance with IV contrast, this may be used to help delineate tentorial margins when necessary.

Stages of uncal herniation

Early third nerve stage

This is *not* a brainstem finding, it is due to 3rd nerve compression.

Pupils: Approach to the comatose patient

Oculomotor: Doll's eyes (oculocephalic reflex) = normal or dysconjugate. CWC (oculovestibular reflex) = slow ipsilateral deviation, impaired nystagmus, may be dysconjugate if external oculomotor ophthalmoplegia (**EOO**).

Respirations: Normal.

Motor: Appropriate response to nociceptive stimulus. Contralateral Babinski.

Late third nerve stage

Midbrain dysfunction occurs almost immediately after symptoms extend beyond those due to focal cerebral lesion (i.e., may skip diencephalic stage, due to lateral pressure on midbrain). Treatment delays may result in irreversible damage.

Pupils: Pupil fully dilates.

Oculomotor: Once pupil blown, then external oculomotor ophthalmoplegia (EOO).

Consciousness: Once EOO occurs: stupor→coma.

Respirations: Sustained hyperventilation, rarely Cheyne-Stokes.

Motor: Usually produces contralateral weakness. However, the contralateral cerebral peduncle may be compressed against the tentorial edge, causing ipsilateral hemiplegia (*Kernohan's phenomenon*, a false localizing sign). Then bilateral decerebration (decortication unusual).

Midbrain—upper pons stage

Contralateral pupil fixes in midposition or full dilation. Eventually, both midposition (5–6 mm) and fixed.

Oculomotor: Impaired or absent.

Respirations: Sustained hyperpnea.

Motor: Bilateral decerebrate rigidity.

Following the midbrain—upper pons stage

From this point onward, the uncal syndrome is indistinguishable from central herniation (see above).

18

18.5 Hypoxic coma

Anoxic encephalopathy may be due to anoxemic anoxia (drop in pO_2) or anemic anoxia (following exsanguination or cardiac arrest). Myoclonus is common.

Vulnerable cells:

1. cerebral gray matter: lesions predominate in 3rd cortical layer (white matter is usually better preserved due to lower O_2 requirements)
2. Ammon's horn is also vulnerable, especially the Sommer section
3. in the basal ganglia (BG):
   a) anoxemic anoxia severely affects globus pallidus
   b) anemic anoxia affects the caudate nucleus and putamen
4. in the cerebellum: Purkinje cells, dentate nuclei, and inferior olives are affected

Multivariate analysis yields outcome prognosticators shown in ▶ Table 18.5 and ▶ Table 18.6. NB: this analysis applies *only* to hypoxic-ischemic coma; and is based retrospectively on 210 patients, most S/P cardiac arrest with many medical complications.[14] More recent studies confirm the poor prognosis of unreactive pupils and lack of motor response to pain[15]; if either of these findings are seen within a few hours after cardiac arrest there is an 80% risk of death or permanent vegetative state, and if present at 3 days, this rate rose to 100%.

Glucocorticoids (steroids) have been shown to have no beneficial effect on survival rate or neurological recovery rate after cardiac arrest.[16]

Table 18.5 Patients with BEST chance of regaining independence

Time of exam	Finding
<6 hrs from onset	(pupillary light reflex present) *AND* (GCS-motor > 1) *AND* (spontaneous EOM WNL, i.e., orienting or conjugate roving)
1 day	(GCS-motor > 3) *AND* (GCS-eye improved ≥ 2 from initial)
3 days	(GCS-motor > 3) *AND* (spontaneous EOM WNL)
1 week	GCS-motor = 6
2 weeks	oculocephalic WNL

Abbreviations: EOM = extraocular muscle; GCS = Glasgow Coma Scale ("GCS-motor" refers to the motor score...); WNL = within normal limits.

Table 18.6 Patients with virtually NO chance of regaining independence

Time of exam	Finding
<6 hrs	no pupillary light reflex
1 day	(GCS-motor < 4) *AND* (spontaneous eye movements not orienting nor conjugate roving)
3 days	GCS-motor < 4
1 week	(GCS-motor < 6) *AND* (at < 6 hrs spontaneous EOM not orienting nor conjugate roving) *AND* (at 3 d GCS-eye < 4)
2 week	(oculocephalic not WNL) *AND* (at 3 d GCS-motor < 6) *AND* (at 3 d GCS-eye < 4) *AND* (at 2 wk GCS-eye not improved at least 2 points from initial)

Abbreviations: EOM = extraocular muscle; GCS = Glasgow Coma Scale ("GCS-motor" refers to the motor score...); WNL = within normal limits.

18

References

[1] Valadka AB, Narayan RK, Narayan RK, et al. Emergency Room Management of the Head-Injured Patient. In: Neurotrauma. New York: McGraw-Hill; 1996:119–135

[2] Teasdale G, Jennett B. Assessment of Coma and Impaired Consciousness: a Practical Scale. Lancet. 1974; 2:81–84

[3] Hahn YS, Chyung C, Barthel MJ, et al. Head Injuries in Children Under 36 Months of Age: Demography and Outcome. Child's Nervous System. 1988; 4:34–40

[4] Ropper AH. Lateral Displacement of the Brain and Level of Consciousness in Patients with an Acute Hemispheral Mass. New England Journal of Medicine. 1986; 314:953–958

[5] Fisher CM. Some Neuro-Ophthalmological Observations. Journal of Neurology, Neurosurgery, and Psychiatry. 1967; 30:383–392

[6] Plum F, Posner JB. The Diagnosis of Stupor and Coma. 3rd ed. Philadelphia: F A Davis; 1980:87–130

[7] Buettner UW, Zee DS. Vestibular Testing in Comatose Patients. Arch Neurol. 1989; 46:561–563

[8] Fisher CM. Acute Brain Herniation: A Revised Concept. Sem Neurology. 1984; 4:417–421

[9] Fisher CM, Picard EH, Polak A, et al. Acute Hypertensive Cerebellar Hemorrhage: Diagnosis and Surgical Treatment. J Nerv Ment Dis. 1965; 140:38–57

[10] Hahn F, Gurney J. CT Signs of Central Descending Transtentorial Herniation. Am J Neuroradiol. 1985; 6:844–845

[11] Andrews BT, Pitts LH. Functional Recovery After Traumatic Transtentorial Herniation. Neurosurgery. 1991; 29:227–231

[12] Osborn AG. Diagnosis of Descending Transtentorial Herniation by Cranial CT. Radiology. 1977; 123:93–96

[13] Stovring J. Descending Tentorial Herniation: Findings on Computerized Tomography. Neuroradiology. 1977; 14:101–105

[14] Levy DE, Caronna JJ, Singer BH, et al. Predicting Outcome from Hypoxic-Ischemic Coma. JAMA. 1985; 253:1420–1426

[15] Zandbergen EGJ, de Haan RJ, Stoutenbeek CP, et al. Systematic Review of Early Prediction of Poor Outcome in Anoxic-Ischemic Coma. Lancet. 1998; 352:1808–1812

[16] Jastremski M, Sutton-Tyrell K, Vaagenes P, et al. Glucocorticoid Treatment Does Not Improve Neurological Recovery Following Cardiac Arrest. JAMA. 1989; 262:3427–3430

18

19 Brain Death and Organ Donation

19.1 Brain death in adults

The President's Commission for the Study of Ethical Problems in Medicine first published guidelines for the determination of death in 1981[1] which contributed to the approval of the Uniform Determination of Death Act (UDDA; policy statement, see box).[2]

Uniform determination of death act, 1980 (verbatim quote)

"An individual who has sustained either
1. irreversible cessation of circulatory and respiratory functions, or
2. irreversible cessation of all functions of the entire brain, including the brainstem,
is dead.
   A determination of death must be made with accepted medical standards."

Most states have adopted the UDDA, although some have enacted amendments stipulating qualifications of the determining clinician(s). Individual hospitals may also mandate that certain protocols be followed.

As was reaffirmed in 2010,[3] when the clinical determination of brain death is made in accordance with the original published guidelines,[4] there has been no report of recovery of neurologic function in adults.

19.2 Brain death criteria

19.2.1 General information

This section deals with brain death in adults. For individuals < 5 years of age, see Brain death in children (p. 335).

When the cause of death is other than natural causes the Medical Examiner or Coroner (depending on the authority in your jurisdiction) will be contacted per hospital policy.

Key point: Criteria shown below may be used to determine the clinical absence of brain and brainstem function. Then to ensure that the total cessation of brain function is *irreversible*, the clinician must take into consideration the cause of the absence, and exclude conditions that can mimic the clinical appearance of brain death. This may require ancillary confirmatory tests and observation for a period of time.

Waiting periods: There is insufficient evidence to support a specific observation period to ensure that the cessation of neurologic function is irreversible.[3] This requires that the determination of brain death take into consideration all of the available information and circumstances.

19.2.2 Establishing the cause of cessation of brain activity

The cause of the cessation of brain activity (CBA) can usually be determined by a combination of history, physical examination, laboratory tests and imaging studies.

19.2.3 Clinical criteria

See ▸ Table 19.1 for a summary of basic requirements and clinical findings that may be used in determining brain death. Details follow below.

Recommendations[1,3,5]:
1. absence of **brainstem reflexes**:
   a) ocular examination:
   - *fixed* pupils: no response to bright light (caution after resuscitation: see below). The size of the pupils is unimportant, they are usually midposition (4–6 mm) but may vary to dilated (≈ 9 mm). Dilated pupils can be compatible with brain death because cervical sympathetic pathways may remain intact
   - absent corneal reflexes (corneal reflex: eye closing to corneal, not scleral, stimulation)

Table 19.1 Summary of findings in brain death (see text for details)[3]

Vital signs & general criteria	
• Core temp > 36 °C (96.8 °F)	
• SBP ≥ 100 mm Hg (with or without pressors)	
• Absence of drugs that could simulate brain death (e.g., NMBAs, drug intoxication, blood alcohol content (BAC) should be < 0.08%...)	
Absence of brainstem reflexes	
• Fixed pupils	No pupillary reaction to light
• Absent corneal reflexes	Touching cornea with a gauze does not cause eye closure
• Absent oculovestibular reflex (calorics)	No eye movement of any sort to ice water in ear with HOB elevated to 30°
• Absent oculocephalic reflex: "Doll's eyes" (p. 323)	Turning the head does not cause contralateral eye deviation (clear C-spine first)
• Absent gag reflex	No gagging reaction to movement of ET tube
• Absent cough reflex	No coughing in response to bronchial suctioning
Absence of any cerebrally mediated response to auditory and tactile noxious stimulation peripherally and in the cranium	**Stimulate areas like supraorbital ridge. No limb movement, no eye movement, no facial movement**
Apnea confirmed with apnea challenge	**No respirations with $pCO_2 > 60$ mm Hg**

- absent oculocephalic "doll's eyes" reflex (p. 323), contraindicated if C-spine not cleared
- absent oculovestibular reflex (cold water calorics): instill 60–100 ml ice water into one ear (✖ do not do if tympanic membrane perforated) with HOB at 30°. Brain death is excluded if *any* eye movement. Wait at least 1 minute for response, and ≥ 5 min before testing the opposite side (to avoid canceling out of opposing response)
  b) absent oropharyngeal reflex (gag) to stimulation of posterior pharynx
  c) no cough response to bronchial suctioning
2. apnea test AKA apnea challenge (assesses function of medulla). Disconnection from ventilator causes an increase in $PaCO_2$ (the most potent stimulus for respirations, except in patients with severe COPD whose respiratory drive is simultaed by low PaO_2). Apnea is confirmed if there are no spontaneous respirations after disconnection from ventilator as detailed below. Respirations are defined as abdominal or chest excursions that produce adequate tidal volumes; if there is any question, a spirometer may be connected to the patient.[4] Since elevating $PaCO_2$ increases ICP which could precipitate herniation and vasomotor instability, this test should be reserved for last and only used when the diagnosis of brain death is reasonably certain. Guidelines[6,7]:
   a) to prevent hypoxemia during the test (with the danger of cardiac arrhythmia or myocardial infarction):
      - preoxygenate for ≥ 10 minutes before the test with 100% FIO_2 to $PaO_2 > 200$ mm Hg
      - monitor oxygen saturation continuously with pulse oximeter during test
      - prior to the test, reduce the ventilator rate to bring the $PaCO_2$ to normocarbia (35–40 mm Hg) (to shorten the test time and thus reduce the risk of hypoxemia)
      - during the test, administer passive O_2 flow at 6 L/min through either a pediatric oxygen cannula or a No. 14 French tracheal suction catheter (with the side port covered with adhesive tape) passed to the estimated level of the carina
   b) starting from normocapnea, the average time to reach $PaCO_2 = 60$ mm Hg is **6 minutes** (classic teaching is that $PaCO_2$ rises 3 mm Hg/min, but in actuality the rate at which $PaCO_2$ rises varies widely, with an average of 3.7 ± 2.3,[6] or 5.1 mm Hg/min if starting at normocarbia[7]). Sometimes as long as 12 minutes may be necessary
   c) apnea is confirmed if no respirations for > 2 minutes with $PaCO_2 > 60$ mm Hg or $PaCO_2 > 20$ mm Hg over baseline or pH < 7.3 (if patient does not breathe by this point, they won't breathe at a higher $PaCO_2$)
   d) the test is aborted if:
      - the patient breathes (chest or abdominal movement, gasps): incompatible with brain death
      - SBP < 90 mm Hg (hypotension)
      - if O_2 saturation drops < 80% for > 30 seconds (on pulse oximeter)
      - significant cardiac arrhythmias occur
   e) if patient does not breathe, send ABG at regular intervals and at the completion of test, regardless of reason for termination. If the patient does not breathe for at least 2 minutes *after*

19

a $PaCO_2 > 60$ mm Hg is documented, then the test is valid and is compatible with brain death (if the patient is stable and ABG results are available within a few minutes, the apnea challenge may be continued while waiting for results, in case the $PaCO_2$ is < 60)

f) if $PaCO_2$ stabilizes below 60 mm Hg and the pO_2 remains adequate, try reducing the passive O_2 flow rate slightly (O_2 flow may be washing out CO_2 from lungs)

g) the test is positive (i.e., compatible with brain death) if there are no respirations and $PaCO_2$ is ≥ 60 mm Hg (or there is a 20 mm Hg rise in $PaCO_2$ above baseline)

3. no motor function
   a) no cerebrally mediated response to auditory and tactile noxious stimulation peripherally or centrally: there should be no movement of limbs (stereotypical spinal cord mediated movements in response to peripheral pain are excluded and may be confusing), no eye opening or eye movement, no facial movement
   b) true decerebrate or decorticate posturing or seizures are incompatible with the diagnosis of brain death
   c) spinal cord mediated reflex movements (including flexor plantar reflexes, flexor withdrawal, muscle stretch reflexes,[8] and even abdominal and cremasteric reflexes) can be compatible with brain death, and may occasionally consist of complex movements,[9] including bringing one or both arms up to the face,[10] or sitting up (the "Lazarus" sign[11]), especially with hypoxemia (thought to be due to spinal cord ischemia stimulating surviving motor neurons in the upper cervical cord). If complex integrated motor movements occur, it is recommended that confirmatory testing be performed prior to pronouncement of brain death[12]

4. absence of *complicating conditions* (that could simulate brain death on exam):
   a) hypothermia: core temp should be > 36 °C (96.8 °F). Below this temp, pupils may be fixed and dilated,[13] respirations may be difficult to detect, and recovery is possible.[14] It may be necessary to wait 48–72 hours after rewarming to declare brain death due to a case report of transient return of brainstem reflexes after therapeutic hypothermia[15]
   b) no evidence of remediable exogenous or endogenous intoxication, including drug or metabolic (blood alcohol level should be < 0.08%, barbiturates, benzodiazepines, meprobamate, methaqualone, trichloroethylene, paralytics, hepatic encephalopathy, hyperosmolar coma...). If there is doubt, depending on circumstances, lab tests including drug levels (serum and urine) may be sent. Pseudocholinesterase deficiency is present in 1/3000 patients, which can cause succinylcholine to last up to 8 hours (instead of 5 mins). A twitch monitor can rule out NMB (place the electrodes immediately behind the eye or across the zygomatic arch)
   c) shock (neuro exam should be reliable if SBP ≥ 100 mm Hg) and anoxia. Loss of > 45% of circulating blood volume can produce lethargy
   d) immediately post-resuscitation: shock or anoxia may cause fixed and dilated pupils. Atropine (p. 335) may cause slight dilatation but *not* unreactivity. Neuromuscular blockage (e.g., for intubation) does not affect pupils because the iris lacks nicotinic receptors
   e) patients coming out of pentobarbital coma (wait until level ≈ ≤ 10 mcg/ml)

5. confirmation of brain death by use of ancillary confirmatory tests (preferred tests[3]: angiography, EEG, or CRAG, see below) is not required. May be used at the discretion of the physician, generally if there is uncertainty about the reliability of other parts of the exam

6. recommended observation periods: there is insufficient evidence to determine a minimal observation period to ensure that neurologic function has irreversibly ceased[3]:
   a) in a situation where overwhelming brain damage from an irreversible condition is well-established (e.g., massive intracerebral hemorrhage, gunshot wound traversing the brain...), and there is no uncertainty in the clinical exam, ancillary confirmatory tests would usually not be necessary
   b) in clear-cut situations as outlined above, if several hours have passed since the onset of the brain insult, a single neurologic examination consistent with brain death should suffice, although many states require two examinations by statute[3] (see state and local laws below)
   c) in less clear-cut situations (e.g., anoxic brain injury, hypothermia...) longer observation periods are appropriate and ancillary confirmatory tests may be considered (see below)

19.2.4 State and local laws

Most states have adopted the Uniform Determination of Death Act (UDDA) regarding brain death. State amendments and local regulations or hospital policies may dictate that more than one practitioner must concur on the diagnosis. It is incumbent that the practitioner know the applicable regulations before making the diagnosis.

19.2.5 Ancillary confirmatory tests

General information

There is insufficient evidence that any ancillary test can accurately determine brain death.[3] Preferred tests[3]: angiography, EEG, or CRAG.

Cerebral angiography

Requires absence of cerebral blood flow, which is incompatible with brain survival. Pros: highly sensitive for determining death of cerebral hemispheres. Cons: costly, time-consuming, requires transport of the patient to X-ray department, invasive, potentially damaging to organs that may be used for donation, and is not optimal for detecting small amount of blood flow to brainstem. Requires a radiologist and technician. Criteria: absence of intracranial flow at the level of the carotid bifurcation or circle of Willis.[5] Filling of the superior sagittal sinus may occur in a delayed fashion and is not incompatible with brain death. Interobserver validity has not been studied. Not routinely used in the diagnosis of brain death, but may be employed in difficult situations.

EEG

Can be done at bedside. Requires experienced interpreter. Does not detect brainstem activity, and electrocerebral silence (ECS) (i.e., isoelectric EEG) does not exclude the possibility of reversible coma. ∴ Use ECS as a clinical confirmatory test only in patients without drug intoxication, hypothermia, or shock, and not in patients where brainstem activity might be preserved (i.e., situations where the clinical brainstem exam cannot be performed). Note: a practical problem with EEG for brain-death determination is that it is often difficult to get a tracing that is totally free of electrical signal, even in patients who are brain dead by other criteria.

Definition of electrocerebral silence on EEG: no electrical activity > 2 mcV with the following requirements:
1. recording from scalp or referential electrode pairs ≥ 10 cm apart
2. 8 scalp electrodes and ear lobe reference electrodes
3. inter-electrode resistance < 10,000 Ω (or impedance < 6,000 Ω) but over 100 Ω
4. sensitivity of 2 mcV/mm
5. time constants 0.3–0.4 sec for part of recording
6. no response to stimuli (pain, noise, light)
7. record > 30 mins
8. repeat EEG in doubtful cases
9. qualified technologist and electroencephalographer with ICU EEG experience
10. telephone transmission not permissible

Cerebral radionuclide angiogram (CRAG)

General information

Can be done using a gamma camera, or more contemporary HMPAO SPECT (for 99mTechnetium hexamethylpropyleneamine oxime single-photon emission CT). May not detect minimal blood flow to the brain, especially brainstem. Necessitates transport to the radiology/nuclear medicine department and requires an experienced interpreter.

May be useful to confirm clinical brain death in the following settings:
1. where complicating conditions are present, e.g., hypothermia, hypotension (shock), drug intoxication… (e.g., patients emerging from barbiturate coma), metabolic abnormalities
2. in patients with severe facial trauma where evaluation of ocular findings may be difficult or confusing
3. in patients with severe COPD or CHF where apnea testing may not be valid
4. to shorten the observation period

Technique
Using gallium camera
1. scintillation camera is positioned for an AP head and neck view
2. inject 20–30 mCi of 99mTc-labeled serum albumin or pertechnetate in a volume of 0.5–1.5 ml into a proximal IV port, or a central line, followed by a 30 ml NS flush

19

3. perform serial dynamic images at 2 second intervals for ≈ 60 seconds
4. then, obtain static images with 400,000 counts in AP and then lateral views at 5, 15, and 30 minutes after injection
5. if a study needs to be repeated because of a previous non-diagnostic study or a previous exam incompatible with brain death, a period of 12 hours should lapse to allow the isotope to clear from the circulation

Findings

No uptake in brain parenchyma = "hollow skull phenomenon" (▶ Fig. 19.1). Termination of carotid circulation at the skull base, and lack of uptake in the ACA and MCA distributions (absent "candelabra effect"). There may be delayed or faint visualization of dural venous sinuses even with brain death,[16] due to connections between the extracranial circulation and the venous system.

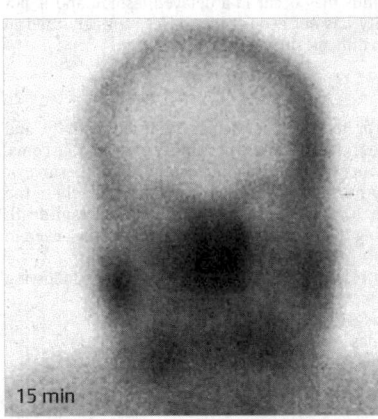

Fig. 19.1 "Hollow-skull" sign on CRAG radionuclide CBF study (static AP view taken 15 minutes after injection).

MRI and MR angiography (MRA)

MRA is very sensitive for detecting loss of blood flow in cavernous ICA; however, the specificity has not been accurately evaluated[3] (i.e., might give false positives for brain death in comatose patients) and is not considered a valid confirmatory test.

CT angiography (CTA)

Blood flow on CTA (i.e., not consistent with brain death) was seen in patients with isoelectric EEG. False positive rate had not been determined in comatose non-brain dead patients. CTA is not considered to be a valid confirmatory test for brain death.[3]

Transcranial Doppler

Not widely used. See reference.[4]
1. small peaks in early systole without diastolic flow or reverberating flow (indicative of significantly increased ICP)
2. initial absence of Doppler signals cannot be used as criteria for brain death since 10% of patients do not have temporal insonation windows

SSEPs

One protocol requires bilateral absence of N20-P22 response with median nerve stimulation. An alternative criteria is disappearance of the P14 peak[17] (substrate: medial lemniscus and nucleus cuneatus) on nasopharyngeal electrode recordings. Studies were judged as Class III data, and that while P14 recordings could be a valuable confirmatory test, interobserver variability needed to be studied.[3]

19

Atropine

In brain death, 1 amp of atropine (1 mg) IV should not affect the heart rate due to the absence of vagal tone (the normal response to atropine of increased heart rate rules out brain death, but absence of the response is not helpful since some conditions such as Guillain-Barré may blunt the response).

Systemic atropine in usual doses causes slight pupillary dilatation,[18,19] but does not eliminate reaction to light (therefore, to eliminate uncertainty, it is prudent to examine the pupils before giving the atropine).

19.2.6 Pitfalls in brain death determination

The following pitfalls may complicate the determination of brain death:
- Movement of body parts after brain death. Movements are sometimes complex in nature, and may occur as long as 32 hours after brain death. Many are mediated by spinal cord discharges as it undergoes cell death. Documented observations include facial movements, finger tremor, repetitive leg movements, and even sitting up. These movements are often repetitive, usually stereotypical, and do not change with changing stimuli.
- The appearance of breathing. This typically occurs with a ventilator that is set to trigger on detecting respiratory effort. Ventilators may be sensing air movement created by transmission of arterial pulses of the great vessels to the lung or actions of a chest tube.

19.3 Brain death in children

19.3.1 General information

The following is based on 2011 guidelines[20] that are endorsed by the Society of Critical Care Medicine, The Section for Critical Care and Section of Neurology of the American Academy of Pediatrics and the American College of Critical Care Medicine.

Key points[20]:
- The diagnosis of brain death in term newborns, infants and children is a clinical diagnosis requiring absence of neurologic function and a known irreversible cause of loss of function.
- These guidelines are not supported for infants < 37 weeks gestational age because of insufficient data
- Ancillary tests are not required and are not a substitute for a correctly performed neurologic exam
- Two examinations that include apnea testing separated by an observation period is recommended
- Treat and correct conditions that can interfere with the neurologic exam, including hypothermia, hypotension, interfering drugs (high levels of sedatives, analgesics, paralytics, high doses of anti-seizure medication), and metabolic disturbances

19.3.2 Clinical examination

Two examinations, each including apnea testing, each consistent with brain death, and each performed by different attending physicians separated by an observation period are required. Apnea testing may be performed by the same physician.

Apnea testing requires documentation of arterial $PaCO_2$ that is 20 mm Hg above the baseline and ≥ 60 mm Hg with no respiratory effort. If apnea testing cannot be safely completed, an ancillary study should be done.

Recommended observation periods between exams:
- For term newborns (37 weeks gestational age) through 30 days of age: 24 hours
- For infants and children (> 30 days to 18 years): 12 hours
- Following cardiopulmonary resuscitation, the diagnosis of brain death should be deferred ≥ 24 hrs if there are concerns or inconsistencies in the examination

19

19.3.3 Ancillary studies

These tests are not required to make the determination of brain death. Use may be considered:
- When apnea testing cannot be safely completed, e.g., due to underlying medical conditions or desaturation to < 85% or inability to achieve $paCO_2$ ≥ 60 mm Hg
- If there is uncertainty about results of the neurologic examination

- If drugs that interfere with the neurologic exam may be present
- To reduce the inter-examination observation period

When ancillary tests are employed, a second neurologic examination and apnea test should be performed to the extent possible, and there should not be any finding inconsistent with brain death.

19.4 Organ and tissue donation

19.4.1 General considerations

The Center for Medicare Services' (CMS) conditions of participation require all hospitals that receive Medicare funds to refer all imminent deaths to the local Organ Procurement Organization (OPO).[21] The OPO is responsible for the determination of suitability and for discussion of donation with the legal next of kin. The discussion must be by trained personnel. The OPO is also responsible for organ donor management, allocation and facilitating recovery of organs in the OR.[21]

19.4.2 Referral of the potential organ donor

Most OPOs have developed a process for referral of the potential organ donor by educating the critical care nurses to referral by a set of "triggers." The triggers usually include patients with a neurologic injury (anoxia, hemorrhage, trauma, etc.), on a ventilator and either losing brainstem reflexes, GCS < 5, or discussion of withdrawal of support. This set of triggers results in the referral of many patients not suitable for donation but allows for the early notification of the OPO and reduces the risk of missed referrals.

19.4.3 Medical management of the potential organ donor

Brain death results in several predictable physiologic aberrations. Many hospitals have developed "Catastrophic Brain Injury" order sets to address these predictable consequences.

Hypotension

With hypovolemia due to diabetes insipidus and destruction of the pontine and medullary vasomotor centers most brain dead patients are hypotensive. Treatment requires restoration of a euvolemic state and support with vasopressors. Usually norepinephrine to supply inotropic support and neosynephrine to increase peripheral vascular resistance is sufficient to support the blood pressure.

Diabetes insipidus

With loss of hypothalamic function brain dead individuals frequently have posterior pituitary dysfunction and diabetes insipidus. This is manifest by large volume dilute urinary output, hypernatremia and hyperosmolar serum. Management options include DDAVP injection (1–2 mcg SC/IV q 12 hours) or a vasopressin drip (0.01–0.04 units/min IV). The vasopressin drip may be preferable because the shorter duration of action can help avoid oliguria due to overdosing.

Hypothermia

Loss of temperature regulation frequently causes hypothermia which can worsen coagulopathy and invalidate brain death testing. Application of a warming blanket to support temperature will help restore normal physiology.

19.4.4 Organ Procurement Organization (OPO) process

Authorization

OPO staff will respond to referrals and after discussion with medical staff and nursing staff engage the family in a discussion involving authorization for organ donation. The term "authorization" is preferred to "consent" because the donor is dead and there is no potential benefit to them. United Network for Organ Sharing (UNOS) data has demonstrated that OPO trained staff have higher authorization rates than medical staff. This may be due to the fact that only having the OPO staff advocating for donation reduces the sense of abandonment by the treatment team.

19

Donor evaluation

The OPO staff will evaluate donor suitability. Donors will be ruled out if there is thought to be a high potential for transmission of malignancy. The OPO will screen for blood-borne pathogens (HIV, HCV, HBV). Each organ will be evaluated for suitability.
- Heart: EF > 50%, no LVH, no CAD
- Lungs: P/F Ratio > 300, normal bronchoscopy
- Liver: ALT, AST, GGTP and bilirubin WNL or returning to normal and no known liver disease
- Kidneys: BUN and Creatinine WNL
- Pancreas: normal lipase, amylase and HgbA1c

Allocation and recovery

Once brain death occurs in a patient authorized for organ donation, the OPO will allocate organs according to UNOS allocation policy and UNOS-generated allocation lists. When the transplant centers have accepted organs, an OR time will be set and the teams will come to the donor hospital for organ recovery. The time frame from authorization until organ recovery frequently takes 24 to 36 hours or longer.

19.4.5 Organ donation after cardiac death

General information

Key concepts

- candidates: ventilator-dependent patients (typically with brain or spinal cord injury) where the family has decided to withdraw support and the medical team expects the patient would progress to asystole less than 60 minutes after withdrawal
- consent from legal next of kin for: organ donation, heparin, and femoral lines
- clearance from medical examiner when applicable (usually, cases of unnatural death)
- counsel the family that the procedure cannot be done in ≈ 20% of cases. They are to be notified immediately if this happens and end-of-life care continues
- the transplant team cannot participate in end-of-life care or declaration of death, and should not be in O.R. until after cardiac death is declared

Candidates for organ donation after cardiac death are typically ventilator-dependent patients with brain or spinal cord injuries who are so near death that further treatment is futile, but who do not meet brain death criteria. Organs typically recovered in this manner: kidneys, liver, pancreas, lungs, and, rarely, the heart.[22]

Ethical concerns related to DCD organ recovery have been raised.[23] The Institute of Medicine has reviewed DCD twice (1997 and 2000) and determined DCD to be ethically sound and OPOs have been encouraged to pursue DCD donation.[24]

Consent

Prior to any discussion of donation, the family should have made their decision to withdraw support and allow the patient to progress to death. After the family has had this discussion with the treating physician, the OPO can discuss DCD with the legal next of kin. Consent must also be obtained for any donation-related procedures prior to death (which typically includes heparin infusion to prolong organ viability[25] and the possibility of femoral catheters). The discussion should also include the process to return to ICU if the patient does not progress to asystole.

Clearance from the medical examiner must be obtained in applicable cases (including deaths due to accident, homicide, suicide...).

19

Procedure

Life sustaining measures are discontinued (typically consisting of extubation) usually in the operating room. Death is pronounced typically ≈ 2 to 5 minutes after cardiac activity becomes insufficient to generate a pulse, because limited data indicates that circulation will not spontaneously return[26] (NB: EKG activity does not need to cease). After declaration of death, cold perfusion of organs is performed and they are procured.

To avoid potential conflicts of interest, no member of the transplant team can participate in end-of-life care nor the declaration of death.[22] About 20% of the time, the progression to cardiac death does not occur in a timeframe that permits organ retrieval. In these cases, organ donation is cancelled, the family must be immediately notified, and end-of-life care continues.

References

[1] Guidelines for the determination of death. Report of the medical consultants on the diagnosis of death to the President's Commission for the Study of Ethical Problems in Medicine and Biomedical and Behavioral Research. JAMA. 1981; 246:2184–2186

[2] National Conference of Commissioners on Uniform State Laws. Uniform Determination of Death Act. 645 N. Michigan Ave., Suite 510, Chicago, IL 60611 1980. https://www.uniformlaws.org/HigherLogic/System/DownloadDocumentFile.ashx?DocumentFileKey=341343fa-1efe-706c-043a-9290fdcfd9009&forceDialog=0

[3] Wijdicks EF, Varelas PN, Gronseth GS, et al. Evidence-based guideline update: determining brain death in adults: report of the Quality Standards Subcommittee of the American Academy of Neurology. Neurology. 2010; 74:1911–1918

[4] Wijdicks EF. Determining Brain Death in Adults. Neurology. 1995; 45:1003–1011

[5] Quality Standards Subcommittee of the American Academy of Neurology. Practice Parameters for Determining Brain Death in Adults (Summary Statement). Neurology. 1995; 45:1012–1014

[6] Benzel EC, Gross CD, Hadden TA, et al. The apnea test for the determination of brain death. J Neurosurg. 1989; 71:191–194

[7] Benzel EC, Mashburn JP, Conrad S, et al. Apnea Testing for the Determination of Brain Death: A Modified Protocol. Journal of Neurosurgery. 1992; 76:1029–1031

[8] Ivan LP. Spinal Reflexes in Cerebral Death. Neurology. 1973; 23:650–652

[9] Turmel A, Roux A, Bojanowski MW. Spinal Man After Declaration of Brain Death. Neurosurgery. 1991; 28:298–302

[10] Heytens L, Verlooy J, Gheuens J, et al. Lazarus Sign and Extensor Posturing in a Brain-Dead Patient. J Neurosurg. 1989; 71:449–451

[11] Ropper AH. Unusual Spontaneous Movements in Brain-Dead Patients. Neurology. 1984; 34:1089–1092

[12] Jastremski MS, Powner D, Snyder J, et al. Spontaneous Decerebrate Movement After Declaration of Brain Death. Neurosurgery. 1991; 29:479–480

[13] Treatment of Hypothermia. Medical Letter. 1994; 36:116–117

[14] Antretter H, Dapunt OE, Mueller LC. Survival After Prolonged Hypothermia. New England Journal of Medicine. 1994; 330

[15] Webb AC, Samuels OB. Reversible brain death after cardiopulmonary arrest and induced hypothermia. Crit Care Med. 2011; 39:1538–1542

[16] Goodman JM, Heck LL, Moore BD. Confirmation of Brain Death with Portable Isotope Angiography: A Review of 204 Consecutive Cases. Neurosurgery. 1985; 16:492–497

[17] Wagner W. Scalp, earlobe and nasopharyngeal recordings of the median nerve somatosensory evoked P14 potential in coma and brain death. Detailed latency and amplitude analysis in 181 patients. Brain. 1996; 119 (Pt 5):1507–1521

[18] Greenan J, Prasad J. Comparison of the Ocular Effects of Atropine and Glycopyrrolate with Two IV Induction Agents. Br J Anaesth. 1985; 57:180–183

[19] Goetting MG, Contreras E. Systemic Atropine Administration During Cardiac Arrest Does Not Cause Fixed and Dilated Pupils. Ann Emerg Med. 1991; 20:55–57

[20] Nakagawa TA, Ashwal S, Mathur M, et al. Guidelines for the determination of brain death in infants and children: an update of the 1987 Task Force recommendations. Crit Care Med. 2011; 39:2139–2155

[21] U.S. Electronic Code of Federal Regulations. Condition of Participation for Hospitals. 1998

[22] Steinbrook R. Organ donation after cardiac death. New England Journal of Medicine. 2007; 357:209–213

[23] DuBois JM, DeVita M. Donation after cardiac death in the United States: how to move forward. Critical Care Medicine. 2006; 34:3045–3047

[24] Committee on Non-Heart-Beating Transplantation II, Division of Health Care Services - Institute of Medicine. Non-Heart-Beating Organ Transplantation: Practice and Protocols. Washington, D.C.: National Academy Press; 2000

[25] Bernat JL, D'Alessandro A M, Port FK, et al. Report of a National Conference on Donation after cardiac death. Am J Transplant. 2006; 6:281–291

[26] DeVita MA. The death watch: certifying death using cardiac criteria. Prog Transplant. 2001; 11:58–66

Part VI

Infection

VI

20 Bacterial Infections of the Parenchyma and Meninges and Complex Infections

20.1 Meningitis

20.1.1 Community acquired meningitis

General information

Community acquired meningitis (CAM) is generally more fulminant than meningitis following neurosurgical procedures or trauma. CAM tends to involve certain specific organisms in patients with an intact immune system (viz. in adults: Neisseria meningitidis, Streptococcus pneumoniae, Hamophilus influenza type B…), but can be caused by less virulent organisms in individuals with impaired host defenses.

Waterhouse-Friderichsen syndrome: occurs in 10–20% of children with meningococcal infection (usually disseminated infection in age < 10 yrs), produces large petechial hemorrhages in the skin and mucous membranes, fever, septic shock, adrenal failure (due to hemorrhage into adrenal glands) and DIC. Focal neurologic signs are rare in acute purulent meningitis; however, increased ICP may occur.

Community acquired meningitis is a medical emergency, and should be treated immediately with corticosteroids, e.g., IV betamethasone 0.12 mg/kg[1] or dexamethasone before or at least with the first dose of antibiotics.[2] See Lumbar puncture (p.345) for a discussion about when to perform an LP.

External ventricular drain (EVD) for community acquired meningitis

External ventricular drainage for community acquired meningitis or ventriculitis to measure and treat ICP may be indicated for comatose patients who are not localizing pain.[1] EVD is sometimes employed for administering intrathecal antibiotics. Decompressive craniectomy may be considered for ICP refractory to medical management and CSF drainage. EVD may also be needed for acute hydrocephalus, which is not uncommon with cryptococcal meningitis (p.409).

20.1.2 Post-neurosurgical procedure meningitis

1. usual organisms: coagulase-negative staphylococci, S. aureus, Enterobacteriaceae, Pseudomonas sp., pneumococci (usually with basilar skull fractures and otorhinologic surgery)
2. empiric antibiotics: vancomycin (to cover MRSA), adult ℞ 15 mg/kg q 8–12 hrs to achieve trough 15–20 mg/dl + cefipime 2 g IV q 8 hrs
3. if severe PCN allergy, use aztreonam 2 g IV q 6–8 hrs or ciprofloxacin 400 mg IV q 8 hrs
4. if severe infection, consider intrathecal therapy delivered daily (use only preservative-free drug)
   • vancomycin
   • tobramycin/gentamicin
   • amikacin
   • colistin
5. streamline ABX based on sensitivities, e.g., if organism turns out to be MSSA, change vancomycin, oxacillin, or nafcillin
6. also, consider the possibility of chemical meningitis (see below)

For suspected CSF fistula
1. usual organisms: streptococci; see CSF fistula (cranial) (p.415)
2. treatment/work-up; see CSF fistula (cranial) (p.415)
3. immunocompromised host (e.g., AIDS)
   a) usual organisms: as above PLUS Cryptococcus neoformans, M. tuberculosis, HIV aseptic meningitis, L. monocytogenes
   b) empiric antifungal agents for cryptococcal meningitis: Induction therapy: Liposomal amphotericin B 3–4 mg/kg IV daily + flucytosine 25 mg/kg PO QID for at least 2 weeks followed by
   c) consolidation therapy: fluconazole 400 mg PO daily for at least 8 weeks followed by
   d) chronic maintenance therapy: fluconazole 200 mg PO daily

20

20.1.3 Post craniospinal trauma meningitis (posttraumatic meningitis)

Epidemiology

Occurs in 1–20% of patients with moderate to severe head injuries.[3] Most cases occur within 2 weeks of trauma, although delayed cases have been described.[4] 75% of cases have demonstrable basal skull fracture (p.1064), and 58% have obvious CSF rhinorrhea.

Pathogens

As expected from above, there is a high rate of infection with organisms indigenous to the nasal cavity. The most common organisms in a series from Greece were Gram-positive cocci (Staph. hemoliticus, S. warneri, S. cohnii, S. epidermidis, and Strep. pneumonia) and Gram-negative bacilli (E. coli, Klebsiella pneumonia, Acinetobacter anitratus).[3]

Treatment

1. see also CSF Fistula, Treatment (p.420)
2. antibiotics: appropriate antibiotics are selected based on CSF penetration and organism sensitivities (adapted to the pathogens common in the patient's locale). For empiric antibiotics: Vancomycin 15 mg/kg IV q 8–12 hours to achieve trough 15–20 mg/dl + meropenem 2 g IV q 8 hrs
3. **pneumococcal vaccine**: (Note: these recommendations are specific for patients with CSF leaks and differ from vaccination recommendations in other situations)
   a) pediatrics (age 2-18 years)
      - in the U.S. children are routinely vaccinated with pneumococcal conjugate vaccine (PCV13, Prevnar 13, Pfizer) at ages 2, 4, & 6 months with a booster at age 12-15 months
      - children 6-18 years age with a CSF leak who have not received PCV13 before: give a single dose of PCV13[5]
      - children age 2-18 with a CSF leak should receive a dose of pneumococcal polysaccharide vaccine (PPSV23) (e.g., Pneumovax, Merck) **at least 8 weeks** after any dose of PCV13[5]
   b) adults (age ≥ 19 years) with CSF leak who have not received any pneumococcal vaccines, or for those with unknown vaccination history, the CDC recommends[6]
      - 1 dose of pneumococcal conjugate vaccine (PCV13) (e.g., Prevnar 13, Pfizer)
      - 1 dose of pneumococcal polysaccharide vaccine (PPSV23) PPSV23 (pneumococcal vaccine) (e.g., Pneumovax, Merck) **at least 8 weeks** later
      - one final dose of PPSV23 at age ≥ 65 years, given ≥ 5 years after the most recent dose of PPSV23
4. surgical treatment vs. "conservative treatment": controversial. Some feel that any case of posttraumatic CSF rhinorrhea should be explored,[7,8] and that cases of spontaneous cessation often represent obscuration by incarcerated brain, so-called "sham healing" with the potential for later CSF leak and/or meningitis.[4] Others support the notion that cessation (possibly with the assistance of lumbar spinal drainage) is acceptable
5. continue antibiotics for 1 week after CSF is sterilized. If rhinorrhea persists at this time, surgical repair is recommended

20.1.4 Recurrent meningitis

Patients with recurrent meningitis must be evaluated for the presence of abnormal communication with the intraspinal/intracranial compartment. Etiologies include dermal sinus (p.286) (either spinal or cranial), CSF fistula (p.415), or neurenteric cyst (p.313).

20.1.5 Chronic meningitis

Usually due to one of the following etiologies:
1. tuberculosis
2. fungal infections
3. cysticercosis, neurocysticercosis (p.404)

Differential diagnosis includes:
1. sarcoidosis
2. meningeal carcinomatosis

20

20.1.6 Chemical meningitis

Aseptic meningitis refers to meningitis that is not caused by bacteria. The most common etiology is viral meningitis (e.g., Mollaret's meningitis, a lymphocytic meningitis that is now believed to be due to Herpes Simplex type 2 virus). Carcinomatous meningitis (p.920) should also be in the differential.

Chemical meningitis is a subset of aseptic meningitis with meningeal inflammation that is non-infectious in nature. It may be related to use of certain drugs, including those administered intrathe-cally, especially with intraventricular delivery (it was reported in 3% of patients given IT methotrexate[9]) including contrast agents.

Some cases of chemical meningitis occur following intracranial operations, particularly posterior fossa surgery[10] or in the presence of intraventricular hemorrhage or debris from certain tumors or cyst contents (classically epidermoid cysts[11] or craniopharyngiomas). It may also occur spontaneously, e.g., from a leaking craniopharyngioma[12] or epidermoid.

Post-operative chemical meningitis: symptom onset is usually 3-7 days following surgery,[13] but can be delayed for weeks.[14] Clinically, there may be fever and meningeal signs (p.1419). However, classic signs of meningitis may be lacking.

▶ **Evaluation.** CSF for analysis is crucial. While CSF leucocyte and CSF glucose values may be similar to infectious meningitis, the WBC:RBC ratio is usually not as high and glucose is not as low.[10] In one series, no patient with chemical meningitis had CSF WBC > 7.5K/microliter *and* CSF glucose < 10 mg/dl.[15] Cultures are critical (routine, plus fungal, TB and viral cultures). Also send CSF for cytology to look for malignant cells.

▶ **Treatment.** Removal of the offending tumor when possible is indicated for spontaneous tumor-related cases.

The condition is usually self-limited, but use of systemic steroids and CSF removal by serial lumbar punctures or lumbar drain[13] has been described for patients with a protracted course. There is no consensus on appropriate steroid doasge, however, since the condition is generally benign, it would be appropriate to find the lowest dose that controls symptoms. Persistent H/A may respond to closure of pseudomeningocele if present.[14]

20.1.7 Antibiotics for specific organisms in meningitis

Specific antibiotics

See reference.[16]

Route is IV unless specified otherwise.

1. S. pneumoniae: PCN G
   a) if MIC ≤ 0.06: PCN G or ampicillin, alternative: third generation cephalosporin (ceftriaxone)
   b) if MIC ≥ 0.12: third generation cephalosporin (ceftriaxone)
   c) if cephalosporin resistance: vancomycin
   d) alternative: moxifloxacin
2. N. meningitidis: PCN G
   a) if MIC ≤ 0.1 PCN G or ampicillin
   b) if MIC ≥ 0.1: third generation cephalosporin (ceftriaxone)
   c) alternative: moxifloxacin, meropenem
3. H. influenza:
   a) beta lactamase negative: ampicillin
   b) beta lactamase positive
      • third generation cephalosporin (ceftriaxone)
      • alternative: aztreonam, ciprofloxacin
4. Group B strep
   a) ampicillin
   b) alternative: vancomycin
5. L. monocytogenes
   a) ampicillin ± IV gentamicin
   b) alternative: IV sulfamethoxazole/trimethoprim
6. S. aureus
   a) if methicillin susceptible
      • oxacillin or nafcillin
      • PCN allergy: vancomycin

b) if methicillin resistant
- • vancomycin ± rifampin
- • alternative: linezolid ± rifampin

7. aerobic Gram-negative bacilli (GNB)
- a) ceftriaxone, or cefotaxime, or moxifloxacin (in order of preference, make alterations based on sensitivities)
- b) if aminoglycoside required, intraventricular therapy may be indicated after the newborn period

8. P. aeruginosa
- a) ceftazidime or cefepime
- b) alternative meropenem or aztreonam
- c) if ventriculitis: consider IT gentamicin or tobramycin

9. Candida spp: Liposomal amphotericin B 3–4 mg/kg IV daily + flucytosine 25 mg/kg PO QID

Length of treatment for meningitis

Generally continue antibiotics for 10–14 days total. Duration is dependent on organism and clinical response. Treatment should be 21 days for listeria, group B strep and some GN bacilli.

20.2 Cerebral abscess

20.2.1 General information

Key concepts

- • may arise from hematogenous spread, contiguous spread, or direct trauma
- • risk factors: pulmonary abscess or AV fistulas, congenital cyanotic heart disease, immune compromise, chronic sinusitis/otitis, dental procedures
- • symptoms are similar to any other mass lesions but tend to progress rapidly
- • peripheral WBC may be normal or slightly ↑, CRP usually ↑
- • organisms: Streptococcus is most common, up to 60% are polymicrobial
- • imaging: usually round with thin enhancing ring on CT or MRI. T2WI → high signal lesion with thin rim of low intensity surrounded by hi signal (edema). Unlike with tumor, DWI often shows core of restricted diffusion (not reliable)
- • treatment: IV antibiotics, needle drainage for some, excision infrequently (for fungal or resistant abscess)

20.2.2 Epidemiology

Approximately 1500–2500 cases per year in the U.S. Incidence is higher in developing countries. Male:female ratio is 1.5–3:1.

20.2.3 Risk factors

Risk factors include pulmonary abnormalities (infection, AV-fistulas…, see below), congenital cyanotic heart disease (see below), bacterial endocarditis, penetrating head trauma (see below), chronic sinusitis or otitis media, and immunocompromised host (transplant recipients on immunosuppressants, HIV/AIDS).

20.2.4 Vectors

General information

Prior to 1980, the most common source of cerebral abscess was from contiguous spread. Now, hematogenous dissemination is the most common vector. In 10–60% no source can be identified.[17]

20

Hematogenous spread

Abscesses arising by this means are multiple in 10–50% of cases.[18] No source can be found in up to 25% of cases. The chest is the most common origin:

1. in adults: lung abscess (the most common), bronchiectasis and empyema
2. in children: congenital cyanotic heart disease (CCHD) (estimated risk of abscess is 4–7%, which is ≈ 10-fold increase over general population), especially tetralogy of Fallot (which accounts for ≈ 50% of cases). The increased Hct and low PO_2 in these patients provides an hypoxic environment suitable for abscess proliferation. Those with right-to-left (veno-atrial) shunts additionally lose the filtering effects of the lungs (the brain seems to be a preferential target for these infections over other organs). Streptococcal oral flora is frequent, and may follow dental procedures. Coexisting coagulation defects often further complicate management[19]
3. pulmonary arteriovenous fistulas: ≈ 50% of these patients have Osler-Weber-Rendu syndrome (AKA hereditary hemorrhagic telangectasia), and in up to 5% of these patients a cerebral abscess will eventually develop
4. bacterial endocarditis: only rarely gives rise to brain abscess.[20] More likely to be associated with acute endocarditis than with subacute form
5. dental abscess
6. GI infections: pelvic infections may gain access to the brain via Batson's plexus

In patients with septic embolization, the risk of cerebral abscess formation is elevated in areas of previous infarction or ischemia.[21]

Contiguous spread

1. from purulent sinusitis: spreads by local osteomyelitis or by phlebitis of emissary veins. Virtually always singular. Rare in infants because they lack aerated paranasal and mastoid air cells. This route has become a less common source of cerebral abscess due to improved treatment of sinus disease (with antibiotics and, especially with surgery for chronic otitis media and mastoiditis)
   a) middle-ear and mastoid air sinus infections → temporal lobe and cerebellar abscess. The risk of developing a cerebral abscess in an adult with active chronic otitis media is ≈ 1/10,000 per year[22] (this risk appears low, but in a 30-year-old with active chronic otitis media the lifetime risk becomes ≈ 1 in 200)
   b) ethmoidal and frontal sinusitis → frontal lobe abscess
   c) sphenoid sinusitis: the least common location for sinusitis, but with a high incidence of intracranial complications due to venous extension to the adjacent cavernous sinus → temporal lobe
2. odontogenic → frontal lobe. Rare. Associated with a dental procedure in the past 4 weeks in most cases.[23] May also spread hematogenously

Following penetrating cranial trauma or neurosurgical procedure

Following penetrating trauma: The risk of abscess formation following civilian gunshot wounds to the brain is probably very low with the use of prophylactic antibiotics, except in cases with CSF leak not repaired surgically following traversal of an air sinus. An abscess following penetrating trauma cannot be treated by simple aspiration as with other abscesses; open surgical debridement to remove foreign matter and devitalized tissue is required.

Post-neurosurgical: especially with traversal of an air sinus. Abscess has been reported following use of intracranial pressure monitors and halo traction.[24]

20.2.5 Pathogens

1. cultures from cerebral abscesses are sterile in up to 25% of cases
2. organisms recovered varies with the primary source of infection
3. in general: Streptococcus is the most frequent organism; 33–50% are anaerobic or microaerophilic. Multiple organisms may be cultured to varying degrees (depends on care of technique), usually in only 10–30% of cases, but can approach 60%,[17] and usually includes anaerobes (Bacteroides sp. common)
4. when secondary to fronto-ethmoidal sinusitis: Strep. milleri and Strep. anginosus may be seen
5. from otitis media, mastoiditis, or lung abscess: usually multiple organisms, including anaerobic strep., Bacteroides, Enterobacteriaceae (Proteus)
6. posttraumatic: usually due to S. aureus or Enterobacteriaceae
7. odontogenic (dental) source: may be associated with Actinomyces

8. following neurosurgical procedures: Staph. epidermidis and aureus may be seen
9. immunocompromised hosts, including transplant patients (both bone marrow and solid organ) and AIDS: fungal infections are more common than otherwise would be seen. Organisms include:
    a) Toxoplasma gondii (p. 357); see also treatment (p. 356)
    b) Nocardia asteroides (p. 366)
    c) Candida albicans
    d) Listeria monocytogenes
    e) mycobacterium
    f) Aspergillus fumigatus often from a primary pulmonary infection
10. infants: Gram-negatives are common because IgM fraction of antibodies don't cross the placenta

20.2.6 Presentation

Adults: no findings are specific for abscess, and many are due to edema surrounding the lesion. Most symptoms are due to increased ICP (H/A, N/V, lethargy). Hemiparesis and seizures develop in 30–50% of cases. Symptoms tend to progress more rapidly than with neoplasms.

Newborns: patent sutures and poor ability of infant brain to ward off infection → cranial enlargement. Papilledema is rare before 2 yrs of age. Common findings: seizures, meningitis, irritability, increasing OFC, and failure to thrive. Most newborns with abscess are afebrile. Prognosis is poor.

20.2.7 Stages of cerebral abscess

▶ Table 20.1 shows the four well-recognized histologic stages of cerebral abscess, and correlates this with the resistance to insertion of an aspirating needle at the time of surgery. It takes at least 2 weeks to progress through this maturation process, and steroids tend to prolong it.

Table 20.1 Histologic staging of cerebral abscess

Stage	Histologic characteristics (days shown are general estimates)	Resistance to aspirating needle
1	early cerebritis: (days 1–3) early infection & inflammation, poorly demarcated from surrounding brain, toxic changes in neurons, perivascular infiltrates	intermediate resistance
2	late cerebritis: (days 4–9) reticular matrix (collagen precursor) & developing necrotic center	no resistance
3	early capsule: (days 10–13) neovascularity, necrotic center, reticular network surrounds (less well-developed along side-facing ventricles)	no resistance
4	late capsule: (> day 14) collagen capsule[a], necrotic center, gliosis around capsule	firm resistance, "pop" on entering

[a] abscess is ≈ the only process in the brain that leaves a collagen scar; all other scars are glial scars

20.2.8 Evaluation

Bloodwork

Peripheral WBC: may be normal or only mildly elevated in 60–70% of cases (usually > 10,000).

Blood cultures: should be obtained when abscess is suspected, usually negative.

ESR: may be normal (especially in congenital cyanotic heart disease CCHD where polycythemia lowers the ESR).

C-reactive protein (CRP): hepatic synthesis increases with inflammatory conditions; however, infection anywhere in body (including brain abscess and dental abscess) can raise the CRP level. May also be elevated in noninfectious inflammatory conditions and brain tumor. Sensitivity for abscess is ≈ 90%, specificity is ≈ 77%.[25] See also normal values (p. 378).

Lumbar puncture (LP)

The role of LP is *very* dubious in abscess. Although LP is abnormal in > 90%, there is no characteristic finding diagnostic of abscess. The OP is usually increased, and the WBC count and protein may be elevated. The offending organism can rarely be identified from CSF obtained by LP (unless abscess ruptures into ventricles) with positive cultures in ≈ 6–22%.[26] There is a risk of transtentorial herniation, especially with large lesions.

Σ: Lumbar puncture with suspected cerebral abscess

✖ Due to the risk involved and the low yield of useful information, avoid the use of LP in evaluating patients with suspected cerebral abscess if not already done.

Brain imaging

CT
Ring enhancing. Sensitivity ≈ 100%. For CT staging of abscess; see below.

MRI
See ► Table 20.2 for findings. Enhanced T1WI → thin-walled ring enhancement surrounding low intensity central region (► Fig. 99.1). Fluid-fluid levels may be seen. Occasionally gas-producing organisms may cause pneumocephalus.

Diffusion MRI: DWI → bright, ADC → dark (restricted diffusion suggesting viscous fluid)[27] (► Fig. 99.1). Unlike most tumors which are *dark* on DWI (► Fig. 99.2). More reliable with pyogenic abscess, less reliable e.g., with fungal[28] or TB abscess).

MR-spectroscopy: presence of amino acids and either acetate or lactate are diagnostic for abscess.

Table 20.2 MRI findings with cerebral abscess

Stage	T$_1$WI	T$_2$WI
cerebritis	hypointense	hi signal
capsular	lesion center → low signal, capsule → mildly hyperintense, perilesional edema → low signal	center → iso- or hyperintense, capsule → dark (collagen), perilesional edema → hi signal

Infrequently used imaging
Leukocyte scan with 99mTc-HMPAO: patient's own WBCs are tagged and reinjected. Close to 100% sensitivity and specificity (sensitivity will be reduced if patient is treated with steroids within 48 hrs prior to the scan).[25]

Staging cerebral abscess on imaging
CT staging
Late cerebritis (stage 2) has similar features to early capsule (stage 3) on routine contrast and non-contrast CT. There is some therapeutic importance in differentiating these two stages; the following aids in distinguishing[29]:
1. cerebritis: tends to be more ill-defined
   a) ring-enhancement: usually appears by late cerebritis stage, usually *thick*
   b) further diffusion of contrast into central lumen, and/or lack of decay of enhancement on delayed scan 30–60 min after contrast infusion
2. capsule:
   a) faint rim present on pre-contrast CT (necrotic center with edematous surrounding brain cause collagen capsule to be seen)
   b) *thin* ring enhancement AND (more importantly) delayed scans → decay of enhancement

NB: Thin ring enhancement but lack of delayed decay correlates better with cerebritis
NB: Steroids reduce degree of contrast enhancement (especially in cerebritis)

MRI staging

▶ Table 20.2 shows MRI findings in cerebral abscess. In the cerebritis stage, the margins are ill defined.

Additional evaluation

CXR and chest CT (if indicated) to look for pulmonary source.

Cardiac echo (including TEE, Doppler and/or echo with agitated saline injection (bubble study)): for suspected hematogenous spread, to look for patent foramen ovale or cardiac vegetations.

20.2.9 Treatment

General information

There is no single best method for treating a brain abscess. Treatment usually involves:
- Surgical treatment: needle drainage or excision
- correction of the primary source
- long-term use of antibiotics: often IV x 6–8 weeks and possibly followed by oral route x 4–8 weeks. Duration should be guided by clinical and radiographic response

Surgical vs. pure medical management

General information

In a patient with suspected cerebral abscess, tissue should be obtained in almost every case to confirm diagnosis and to isolate pathogens (preferably before initiation of antibiotics).

Medical treatment

In general, surgical drainage or excision is employed in the treatment. Purely medical treatment of *early* abscess (cerebritis stage)[30] is controversial. NB: pathogens were cultured from well-encapsulated abscesses despite adequate levels of appropriate antibiotics in 6 patients who failed medical therapy.[31] Failure may be due to poor blood supply and acidic conditions within the abscess (which may inactivate antibiotics in spite of concentrations exceeding the MIC).

Medical therapy alone is more successful if:
1. treatment is begun in cerebritis stage (before complete encapsulation), even though many of these lesions subsequently go on to become encapsulated
2. small lesions: diameter of abscesses successfully treated with antibiotics alone were 0.8–2.5 cm (1.7 mean). Those that failed were 2–6 cm (4.2 mean).
   ★ 3 cm is suggested as a cutoff,[32] above this diameter surgery should be included
3. duration of symptoms ≤ 2 wks (correlates with higher incidence of cerebritis stage)
4. patients show definite clinical improvement within the first week

Medical management alone considered if:
1. poor surgical candidate (NB: with local anesthesia, stereotactic biopsy can be done in almost any patient with normal blood clotting)
2. multiple abscesses, especially if small
3. abscess in poorly accessible location: e.g., brainstem[33]
4. concomitant meningitis/ependymitis

Indications for surgical treatment

Indications for initial *surgical* treatment include:
1. significant mass effect exerted by lesion (on CT or MRI)
2. difficulty in diagnosis (especially in adults)
3. proximity to ventricle: indicates likelihood of intraventricular rupture which is associated with poor outcome[19,34]
4. evidence of significantly increased intracranial pressure
5. poor neurologic condition (patient responds only to pain, or does not even respond to pain)
6. traumatic abscess associated with foreign material

20

7. fungal abscess
8. multiloculated abscess
9. follow-up CT/MRI scans cannot be obtained every 1–2 weeks
10. failure of medical management: neurological deterioration, progression of abscess towards ventricles, or after 2 wks if the abscess is enlarged. Also considered if no decrease in size by 4 wks.

Management

General outline
- obtain blood cultures
- initiate antibiotic therapy (preferably after biopsy specimen is obtained), regardless of which mode of treatment (medical vs. surgical) is chosen (see below)
- LP (p. 345): avoid in most cases of cerebral abscess
- antiseizure medications: indicated for seizures, prophylactic use is optional
- steroids: controversial. Reduces edema, but may impede therapy (see below)

Antibiotic selection
1. initial antibiotics of choice when pathogen is unknown, and especially if S. aureus is suspected (if there is no history of trauma or neurosurgical procedure, then the risk of MRSA is low):
   - **vancomycin**: covers MRSA. 15 mg/kg IV q 8–12 hours to achieve trough 15–20 mg/dl
     PLUS
   - a 3rd generation cephalosporin (ceftriaxone); utilize cefepime if post surgical
     PLUS
   - **metronidazole** (Flagyl®). Adult: 500 mg q 6–8 hours
   - alternative to cefepime + metronidazole: meropenem 2 g IV q 8 hours
   - make appropriate changes as sensitivities become available
2. if culture shows only strep, may use PCN G (high dose) alone or with ceftriaxone
3. if cultures show methicillin-sensitive staph aureus and the patient does not have a beta lactam allergy, can change vancomycin to nafcillin (adult: 2 g IV q 4 hrs. peds: 25 mg/kg IV q 6 hrs)
4. Cryptococcus neoformans, Aspergillus sp., Candida sp.: Liposomal amphotericin B 3–4 mg/kg IV daily + flucytosine 25 mg/kg PO QID.
5. in AIDS patients: Toxoplasma gondii is a common pathogen, and initial empiric treatment with sulfadiazine + pyrimethamine + leucovorin is often used (p. 355)
6. for suspected or confirmed nocardia asteroides, see details (p. 366)

Antibiotic duration
IV antibiotics for 6–8 wks (most commonly 6), may then D/C *even if the CT abnormalities persist* (neovascularity remains). NB: CT improvement may lag behind clinical improvement. Duration of treatment may be reduced if abscess and capsule entirely are excised surgically. Oral antibiotics may be used following IV course.

Glucocorticoids (steroids)
Reduces edema and decreases likelihood of fibrous encapsulation of abscess. May reduce penetration of antibiotics into abscess.[32] Immune suppression may also be deleterious.

★ Reserved for patients with clinical and imaging evidence of deterioration from marked mass effect, and duration of therapy should be minimized.

Follow-up imaging
If therapy is successful, imaging should show decrease in:
1. degree of ring enhancement
2. edema
3. mass effect
4. size of lesion: takes 1 to 4 wks (2.5 mean). 95% of lesions that will resolve with antibiotics alone decrease in size by 1 month

Surgical treatment
Options
See reference.[35]

1. needle aspiration: the mainstay of surgical treatment. Especially well-suited for multiple or deep lesions (see below); may also be used with thin-walled or immature lesions
2. surgical excision: Shortens length of time on antibiotics and reduces risk of recrudescence. Recommended in traumatic abscess to debride foreign material (especially bone), and in fungal abscess because of relative antibiotic resistance (see below)
3. external drainage: controversial. Not frequently used
4. instillation of antibiotics directly into the abscess: has not been extremely efficacious, although it may be used for refractory Aspergillus abscesses

Needle aspiration
Most often implemented with stereotactic localization especially for deep lesions.[36] May be performed under local anesthesia if necessary (e.g., in patients who are poor surgical candidates for general anesthesia). May be combined with antibiotic or normal saline irrigation. Repeated aspirations are required in up to 70% of cases. May be the only surgical intervention required (in addition to antibiotics), but sometimes must be followed with excision (especially with multiloculated abscess).

Performed through a trajectory chosen to:
1. minimize the path length through the brain
2. avoid traversing the ventricles or vital neural or vascular structures
3. avoid traversing infected structures outside the intracranial compartment (infected bone, paranasal sinuses, and scalp wounds)
4. in cases of multiple abscesses, target[18]:
   a) when the diagnosis is unknown: the largest lesion or the one causing the most symptoms
   b) once the diagnosis of abscess is confirmed
      - any lesion ≥ 2.5 cm diameter
      - lesions causing significant mass effect
      - enlarging lesions

Cultures
Send aspirated material for the following:
1. stains
   a) Gram stain
   b) acid-fast stain for Mycobacterium (AFB stain, acid-fast resist decolorization with an acid-alcohol mixture and retain the initial dye carbolfuchsin and appear red. The genus Mycobacterium and the genus Nocardia are acid-fast, all other bacteria will be decolorized and stain blue, the color of the counterstain methylene blue)
   c) modified acid-fast stain (for Nocardia, see below) looking for branching acid-fast bacillus
   d) special fungal stains (e.g., methenamine silver, mucicarmine)
2. culture
   a) routine cultures: aerobic and anaerobic
   b) fungal culture: this is not only helpful for identifying fungal infections, but since these cultures are kept for longer periods and any growth that occurs will be further characterized, fastidious or indolent bacterial organisms may sometimes be identified
   c) TB culture
   d) molecular testing: PCR (mycobacteria, EBV, JC virus)

Excision
Can only be performed during the "chronic" phase (late capsule stage). Abscess is removed as any well-encapsulated tumor. The length of time on antibiotics can be shortened to ≈ 3 days in some cases, following total excision of an accessible, mature abscess (e.g., located in pole of brain). Recommended for abscesses associated with foreign body and most Nocardia abscesses (see below). May also be necessary for fungal abscess, multiloculated or resistant lesions.

20.2.10 Outcome

In the pre-CT era, mortality ranged from 40–60%. With advances in antibiotics, surgery, and the improved ability to diagnose and follow response with CT and/or MRI, mortality rate has been reduced to ≈ 10%, but morbidity remains high with permanent neurologic deficit or seizures in up to 50% of cases. Current outcomes are shown in ▶ Table 20.3. A worse prognosis is associated with poor neurologic function, intraventricular rupture of abscess, and almost 100% mortality with fungal abscesses in transplant recipients.

20

Table 20.3 Outcomes with cerebral abscess

mortality (CT era data)[18,37]	0–10%
neurologic disability	45%
late focal or generalized seizures	27%
hemiparesis	29%

20.3 Subdural empyema

20.3.1 General information

Referred to as subdural abscess prior to 1943.[38] Subdural empyema (**SDE**) is a suppurative infection that forms in the space between the dura and the arachnoid membranes, which has no anatomic barrier to spread over the convexity and into the interhemispheric fissure[39] (and occasionally to the opposite hemisphere and posterior fossa). Antibiotic penetration into this space is poor. Distinguished from abscess which forms within brain substance, surrounded by tissue reaction with fibrin and collagen capsule formation. Hence, SDE tends to be more emergent.

SDE may be complicated by cerebral abscess (seen in 20–25% of imaging studies in patients with SDE), cortical venous thrombosis with risk of venous infarction, or localized cerebritis. Spinal subdural empyema (p. 385) may also develop as an extension of intracranial SDE.

20.3.2 Epidemiology

Less common than cerebral abscess (ratio of abscess:empyema is ≈ 5:1). Found in 32 cases in 10,000 autopsies. Male:female ratio is 3:1.

Location: 70–80% are over the convexity, 10–20% are parafalcine.

20.3.3 Etiologies

See ▶ Table 20.4 for etiologies. Most often occurs as a result of direct extension of local infection (rarely following septicemia). Spread of the infection to the intracranial compartment may occur through the valveless diploic veins, often with associated thrombophlebitis.[40]

Chronic otitis media was the leading cause of SDE in the preantibiotic era, but in the U.S. this has now been surpassed by paranasal sinus disease, especially with frontal sinus involvement[41] (may also follow mastoid sinusitis). SDE is a rare but sometimes fatal complication of cranial traction devices.[41,42] Infection of preexisting subdural hematomas (both treated and untreated, in infants and adults) has been reported[41] (bacteremic seeding of an unoperated SDH is very rare).

Trauma includes compound skull fractures and penetrating injuries. Other etiologies include: osteomyelitis, pneumonia, unrelated infection (e.g., foot cellulitis) in diabetics.

Table 20.4 Etiologies of SDE

Location	%
paranasal sinusitis (especially frontal)[a]	67–75
otitis (usually chronic otitis media)[b]	14
post surgical (neuro or ENT)	4
trauma	3
meningitis (more common in peds[43])	2
congenital heart disease	2
misc. (including pulmonary suppuration)	4
undetermined	3

[a]more common in adults
[b]no cases from otitis in a recent series[41]

20

20.3.4 Organisms

The causative organism varies with the specific source of the infection. SDE associated with sinusitis is often caused by aerobic and anaerobic streptococci (▶ Table 20.5). Following trauma or

Table 20.5 Organisms in SDE associated with sinusitis

Organisms	%
Adult cases	
aerobic streptococcus	30–50
staphylococci	15–20
microaerophilic and anaerobic strep	15–25
aerobic Gram-negative rods	5–10
other anaerobes	5–10
Childhood	
Organisms are similar to meningitis for the same age group. Antibiotics choice is the same as for meningitis	

neurosurgical procedures, staphylococci and Gram-negative species predominate (whereas S. aureus was not a common pathogen in sinusitis-related SDE). Sterile cultures occur in up to 40% (some of which may be due to fastidious anaerobes and/or previous exposure to antibiotics).

20.3.5 Presentation

Neurologic findings are shown in ▶ Table 20.6. Symptoms are due to mass effect, inflammatory involvement of the brain and meninges, and thrombophlebitis of cerebral veins and/or venous sinuses. SDE should be suspected in the presence of meningismus + unilateral hemisphere dysfunction. Marked tenderness to percussion or pressure over affected air sinuses is common.[39] Forehead or eye swelling (from emissary vein thrombosis) may occur.

Focal neurologic deficit and/or seizures usually occur late.

Table 20.6 Findings on presentation with SDE[a]

Finding	%
fever	95
H/A	86
meningismus (nuchal rigidity…)	83
hemiparesis	80
altered mental status	76
seizures	44
sinus tenderness, swelling or inflammation	42
nausea and/or vomiting	27
homonymous hemianopsia	18
speech difficulty	17
papilledema	9

[a]from a review of multiple articles[41]

20.3.6 Evaluation

- imaging: IV contrast is usually helpful. Crescentic or lenticular extracerebral lesion with dense enhancement of medial membrane (▶ Fig. 20.1). As with any subdural collection, there is inward displacement of the gray-white interface, ventricular compression and possible effacement of basal cisterns[44]
  - CT: unenhanced CT may miss small lesions. Lesion is hypodense (but denser than CSF)
  - MRI: low signal on T1WI, high signal on T2WI
- LP: ✘ potentially hazardous (risk of herniation). Organisms are usually present only in cases originating from meningitis. If no meningitis, usually see findings consistent with a parameningeal inflammatory process: moderate sterile pleocytosis (150–600 WBC/mm³) with PMNs predominating; glucose normal; opening pressure is usually high[39]; protein is usually elevated (range: 75–150 mg/dl)

20

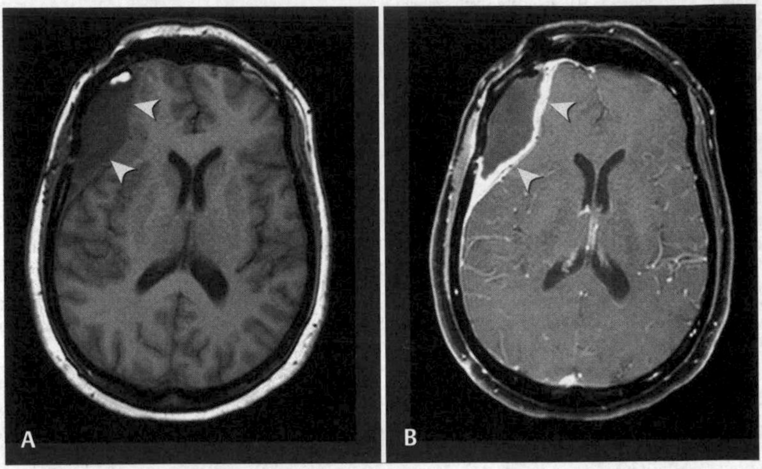

Fig. 20.1 Subdural empyema (*yellow arrowheads*).
Axial T1 MRI, A: without contrast. B: with contrast.

20.3.7 Treatment

1. surgical drainage: indicated in most cases (nonsurgical management has been reported,[45] but should only be considered with minimal neurologic involvement, limited extension and mass effect of SDE, and early favorable response to antibiotics), usually done relatively emergently
2. early in the course, the pus tends to be more fluid and may be more amenable to burr hole drainage; later, loculations develop which may necessitate craniotomy
3. there has been controversy over the optimal surgical treatment. Early studies indicated a better outcome with craniotomy than with burr holes. Recent studies show less difference
   a) critically ill patients with localized SDE may be candidates for burr hole drainage (usually inadequate if loculations are present). Repeat procedures may be needed, and up to 20% will later require a craniotomy
   b) craniotomy: to debride and, if possible, drain. A wide craniotomy is often required because of septations. The dura appears white because of pus underneath. Open and wash out subdural space. Do not try to remove material adherent to cortex (may cause infarction)
4. antibiotics: similar to treatment for cerebral abscess
5. antiseizure medications: usually used prophylactically, mandatory if seizures occur

20.3.8 Outcome

See ▶ Table 20.7. Mortality has dropped from near 100% in the pre-antibiotic era to ≈ 10%. Neurologic deficits tend to improve following treatment, but were present in 55% of patients at the time of discharge from the hospital.[41] Age ≥ 60 years, obtundation or coma at presentation, and SDE related to surgery or trauma (rather than sinusitis) carry a worse prognosis.[41] Burr-hole drainage may be associated with a worse outcome than with craniotomy, but this may have been influenced by the poorer condition of these patients. Fatal cases may have associated venous infarction of the brain.

Table 20.7 Outcome with SDE

Outcome	%
persistent seizures	34
residual hemiparesis	17
mortality	10–20

20.4 Neurologic involvement in HIV/AIDS

20.4.1 Types of neurologic involvement

General information

40–60% of all patients with acquired immunodeficiency syndrome (AIDS) will develop neurologic symptoms, with one–third of these presenting initially with their neurologic complaint.[46,47] Only ≈ 5% of patients that die with AIDS have a normal brain on autopsy. One study found the CNS complications of AIDS shown in ▶ Table 20.8.

The most common conditions producing *focal* CNS lesions in AIDS[49]:
1. toxoplasmosis
2. primary CNS lymphoma
3. progressive multifocal leukoencephalopathy (PML)
4. cryptococcal abscess
5. TB (tuberculoma)

Table 20.8 CNS complications of AIDS (320 patients[46])

Complication	%
Viral syndromes	
subacute encephalitis[a]	17
atypical aseptic meningitis	6.5
herpes simplex encephalitis	2.8
★ progressive multifocal leukoencephalopathy (PML)	1.9[b]
viral myelitis	0.93
varicella zoster encephalitis	0.31
Non-viral infections	
★ Toxoplasma gondii	> 32
Cryptococcus neoformans	13
Candida albicans	1.9
coccidiomycosis	0.31
Treponema pallidum (neurosyphilis)	0.62
atypical Mycobacteria	1.9
Mycobacterium tuberculosis	0.31
Aspergillus fumigatus	0.31
bacteria (E. coli)	0.31
Neoplasms	
★ primary CNS lymphoma	4.7
systemic lymphoma with CNS involvement	3.8
Kaposi's sarcoma (including brain mets)	0.93
Stroke	
infarct	1.6
intracerebral hemorrhage	1.2
miscellaneous/unknown	7.8

[a]CMV encephalitis occasionally occurs
[b]more recent estimate[48] of the incidence of PML in AIDS: 4%

Primary effects of HIV infection

Aside from opportunistic infection and tumors caused by the immunodeficient state, infection with the Human Immunodeficiency Virus (HIV) itself can cause direct neurologic involvement including:
1. AIDS encephalopathy: the most common neurologic involvement, occurs in ≈ 66% of patients with AIDS involving the CNS
2. AIDS dementia AKA HIV dementia complex
3. aseptic meningitis
4. cranial neuropathies: including "Bell's palsy" (occasionally bilateral)

20

5. AIDS-related myelopathy: vacuolization of spinal cord; see Myelopathy (p. 1696)
6. peripheral neuropathies

CNS toxoplasmosis in AIDS

May present as:
1. mass lesion (toxoplasmosis abscess): the most common lesion-causing mass effect in AIDS patients (70–80% of cerebral mass lesions in AIDS[50]) (see below for CT/MRI findings)
2. meningoencephalitis
3. encephalopathy

CNS toxoplasmosis occurs late in the course of HIV infection, usually when CD4 counts are < 200 cells/mm^3.

PML in HIV/AIDS

Progressive multifocal leukoencephalopathy (PML):
1. is caused by a ubiquitous polyomavirus (a subgroup of papova virus, small nonenveloped viruses with a closed circular double DNA-stranded genome) called "JC virus" (JCV, named after the initials of the patient in whom it was first discovered, not to be confused with Jakob-Creutzfeldt—a prion disease—nor with Jamestown Canyon virus, also confusingly called JC virus, a single-stranded RNA virus that occasionally causes encephalitis in humans). 60–80% of adults have antibodies to JCV[51]
2. frequently manifests in patients with suppressed immune systems, including
   a) AIDS: currently the most common underlying disease associated with PML
   b) prior to AIDS, the most common associated diseases were chronic lymphocytic leukemia & lymphoma
   c) allograft recipients: due to immunosuppression[52]
   d) chronic steroid therapy
   e) PML also occurs with other malignancies, and with autoimmune disorders (e.g., SLE)
3. pathologic findings: focal myelin loss (demyelination, ∴ affects white matter) with sparing of axon cylinders, surrounded by enlarged astrocytes and bizarre oligodendroglial cells with eosinophilic intranuclear inclusion bodies. EM can detect the virus. Sometimes occurs in brainstem and cerebellum
4. clinical findings: mental status changes, blindness, aphasia, progressive cranial nerve, motor, or sensory deficits and ultimately coma. Seizures are rare
5. imaging findings: see below
6. clinical course: usually rapidly progressive to death within a few months, occasionally longer survival occurs inexplicably.[53] There is no effective treatment. Some promise initially with anti-retroviral therapy[54]
7. definitive diagnosis requires brain biopsy (sensitivity: 40–96%), although it is infrequently employed. JCV has been isolated from brain and urine. Polymerase chain reaction (PCR) of JCV DNA from CSF has been reported, and is specific but not sensitive for PML

Primary CNS lymphoma (PCNSL) in AIDS

Occurs in ≈ 10% of patients with AIDS.[55] PCNSL is associated with the Epstein-Barr virus (p. 842).

Neurosyphilis

1. AIDS patients can develop neurosyphilis in as little as 4 mos from infection[56] (unlike the 15–20 yrs usually required in non-immunocompromised patients)
2. neurosyphilis can develop in spite of what would otherwise be adequate treatment for early syphilis with benzathine PCN[56,57]
3. CDC recommendations[58]: treat patients having symptomatic or asymptomatic neurosyphilis with:
   • penicillin G 3–4-million units IV q 4 hrs (total of 24-million units/d) for 10–14 days or
   • penicillin G procaine 2.4 million units IM daily + probenecid 500 mg QID orally, both for 10–14 days
   • alternative: Rocephin 2 g IV once daily for 10–14 days for patients with a mild beta-lactam allergy
   • for severe beta-lactam allergy: PCN desensitization

20.4.2 Neuroradiologic findings in AIDS

Overview

MR with gadolinium is recommended as the initial screening procedure of choice for AIDS patients with CNS symptoms (lower false negative rate than CT[49]).

See ▶ Table 20.9 for a comparison of neuroradiologic findings in toxoplasmosis, PCNSL, and PML.

Table 20.9 Comparison of neuroradiologic lesions in AIDS[a]

Feature	Toxo	PCNSL	PML
Multiplicity	usually > 5 lesions	multiple but < 5 lesions	may be multiple
Enhancement	ring	homogeneous	none
Location	basal ganglia and gray-white junction	subependymal	usually limited to white matter
Mass effect	mild-moderate	mild	none-minimal
Miscellaneous	lesions surrounded by edema	may extend across corpus callosum	high signal on T2WI, low on T1WI

[a]abbreviations: Toxo = toxoplasmosis, PCNSL = primary CNS lymphoma, PML = progressive multifocal leukoencephalopathy

CT/MRI findings in toxoplasma abscess

See ▶ Table 20.9.
1. most common findings: large area (low density on CT) with mild to moderate edema, ring enhancement with IV contrast in 68% compatible with abscess (of those that did not ring-enhance, many showed hypodense areas with less mass effect, with slight enhancement adjacent to lesion), well-circumscribed margins[59]
2. most commonly located in *basal ganglia*, are also often subcortical
3. often multiple (typically > 5 lesions[60]) and bilateral
4. usually with little to moderate mass effect[49] (in BG, may compress third ventricle and Sylvian aqueduct, causing obstructive hydrocephalus)
5. most patients with toxoplasmosis had evidence of cerebral atrophy

CT/MRI findings in PML

See ▶ Table 20.9. Note: the appearance of PML may differ in AIDS patients from its appearance in non-AIDS patients.
1. CT: diffuse areas of low density. MRI: high intensity on T2WI
2. normally involves only white matter (spares cortex); however, in AIDS patients gray matter involvement has been reported
3. no enhancement (on either CT or MRI), unlike most toxoplasmosis lesions
4. no mass effect
5. no edema
6. lesions may be solitary on 36% of CTs and on 13% of MRIs
7. borders are usually more ill-defined than in toxoplasmosis[59]

CT/MRI findings in primary CNS lymphoma (PCNSL)

See ▶ Table 20.9. NB: the appearance of PCNSL may differ in AIDS patients from non-AIDS patients.
1. multiple lesions with mild mass effect and edema that tend to ring-enhance on CT, or appear as areas of hypointensity surrounding central area of high intensity (target lesions) on T2WI MRI (unlike non-AIDS cases which tend to enhance homogeneously[61])
2. there is a greater tendency to multicentricity in AIDS patients than in the nonimmunosuppressed population[62]

20.4.3 Management of intracerebral lesions

Neurosurgical consultation is often requested for biopsy in an AIDS patient with questionable lesion (s). The diagnostic dilemma is usually for low-density lesions on CT, and in the United States is primarily between the following:
• toxoplasmosis: treated with pyrimethamine and sulfadiazine + leucovorin (see below)

20

- PML: no proven effective treatment (initiating or optimizing antiretroviral therapy may help[54])
- CNS lymphoma: usually treated with RTX; see CNS lymphoma (p. 840)
- note: cryptococcus is more common than PML or lymphoma, but usually manifests as cryptococcal meningitis (p. 409), and *not* as a *ring-enhancing* lesion

Recommendations

PML can usually be identified radiographically. However, radiographic imaging alone cannot reliably differentiate toxoplasmosis from lymphoma or from some other concurrent conditions (patients with toxoplasmosis may have other simultaneous diseases). Therefore, the following recommendations are made:

1. obtain baseline toxoplasmosis serology (IgG) on all known AIDS patients (NB: 50% of the general population have been infected by toxo and have positive titer by age 6 years, 80–90% will be positive by middle adulthood).

2. multiple enhancing lesions with basal ganglion involvement in a patient whose toxo titer is positive have a high probability of being toxo

3. primary CNS lymphoma (PCNSL): with a *single* lesion, lymphoma is more likely than toxo. If the possibility of PCNSL is strong
   a) consider LP (contraindicated in presence of mass effect)
      - high volume LP for cytology: PCNSL can be diagnosed in ≈ 10–25% of cases using ≈ 10 ml of CSF
      - or send CSF for polymerase chain reaction (PCR) amplification of viral DNA of Epstein-Barr virus or JC-virus[63] (the agents responsible for AIDS-related PCNSL and PML, respectively)
   b) some centers recommend early biopsy to identify PCNSL cases to avoid delaying RTX for 3 weeks while assessing response to antibiotics[49]; instead of biopsy, a few centers advocate empiric radiation treatment (for possible lymphoma)

4. in patient with possible toxoplasmosis (i.e., positive toxo serology (tests may include: dye test (DT), indirect fluorescent antibody test (IFA) enzyme immunoassays, agglutination test, and avidity test) even if other conditions have not been excluded (Note: serologic tests may be unreliable in immunocompromised patients)[64,65]:
   a) initial therapy: sulfadiazine 1000 mg four times daily for patients < 60 kg or 1500 mg four times daily for patients ≥ 60 kg + pyrimethamine 200 mg loading dose, then 50 mg daily for patients < 60 kg or 75 mg daily for patients ≥ 60 kg + folinic acid (leucovorin) 10–25 mg daily to prevent pyrimethamine induced hematologic toxicity
   b) for patients who cannot take sulfadiazine (including those who develop sulfa allergy), change sulfadiazine to clindamicin 600 mg IV or PO q 6 hrs
   c) alternative regimens:
      - atovaquone 1500 mg PO BID + pyrimethamine 200 mg loading dose, then 50 mg daily for patients < 60 kg or 75 mg daily for patients ≥ 60 kg + folinic acid 10–25 mg daily
      - atovaquone 1500 mg PO BID + sulfadiazine 1000 mg four times daily for patients < 60 kg or 1500 mg four times daily for patients ≥ 60 kg
   d) there should be a clinical and radiographic response within 2–3 weeks[66]
   e) if no response to therapy after 3 weeks (some recommend 7–10 days[67]), then consider alternative diagnosis (brain biopsy should be considered)
   f) if response is good, reduce dosage of sulfadiazine after 6 weeks to 50% of the above dose for chronic maintenance therapy: sulfadiazine 1000 mg twice daily for patients < 60 kg or 1500 mg twice daily for patients ≥ 60 kg + pyrimethamine 25–50 mg daily + folinic acid 10–25 mg daily
   g) chronic maintenance therapy can be discontinued in asymptomatic patients who have completed initial therapy if they are receiving antiretroviral therapy (ART), have a suppressed HIV viral load, and have maintained a CD4 count > 200 cells/mcl for at least six months

5. perform biopsy in the following settings:
   a) in patient with a negative toxo titer (note: patients occasionally have negative titer because of anergy)
   b) accessible lesion(s) atypical for toxo (i.e., non-enhancing, sparing basal ganglia, periventricular location)
   c) in the presence of extraneural infections or malignancies that may involve the CNS
   d) lesion that could be either lymphoma or toxo (e.g., single lesion, see 3. a.)
   e) in patients who have lesions not inconsistent with toxo but fail to respond to appropriate anti-toxo medications in the recommended time (see above)
   f) the role of biopsy for *non-enhancing* lesions is less well-defined as the diagnosis does not influence therapy (most are PML or biopsies are non-diagnostic); it may be useful only for prognostic purposes[67]

g) note: the risk of open biopsy in AIDS patients may be higher than in nonimmunocompromised patients. Stereotactic biopsy may be especially well-suited, with up to 96% efficacy, fairly low morbidity (major risk: significant hemorrhage, ≈ 8% incidence), and low mortality[68,69]

6. stereotactic biopsy guidelines:
   a) if multiple lesions are present, choose the most accessible lesion in the least eloquent brain area, or the lesion not responding to treatment
   b) biopsy the center of non-enhancing lesions, or the enhancing portion of ring-enhancing lesions
   c) recommended studies on biopsy: histology; immunoperoxidase stain for Toxoplasma gondii; stains for TB and fungus; culture for TB, fungi, pyogens

20.4.4 Prognosis

Patients with CNS toxo have a median survival of 446 days, which is similar to that with PML but longer than AIDS-related PCNSL.[60]

Patients with CNS lymphoma in AIDS survive on average a shorter time than similarly treated CNS lymphoma in nonimmunosuppressed patients (3 months vs. 13.5 mos). Median survival is < 1 month with no treatment. CNS lymphoma in AIDS tends to occur late in the disease, and patients often die of unrelated causes (e.g., *Pneumocystis carinii* pneumonia).[67]

20.5 Tuberculosis of the CNS (neurotuberculosis)

20.5.1 General information

Tuberculosis (TB) is a multi-system disease caused by the airborne bacterial pathogen, *Mycobacterium tuberculosis*. Forms of central nervous system (CNS) involvement includes[70,71]:
1. intracranial
   a) tuberculous meningitis (p. 360) (TBM)
   b) CNS tuberculoma (see below)
   c) tuberculous brain abscess (p. 363)
   d) tuberculous encephalopathy (p. 364)
   e) tuberculous vasculopathy (p. 363)
2. spinal
   a) spinal meningitis
   b) spinal arachnoiditis
   c) spinal tuberculoma
   d) tuberculous spondylitis (p. 387) (Pott's disease)

Despite being a preventable and treatable disease, it is a leading cause of morbidity and mortality with 10 million new cases and 1.5 million TB-related deaths annually.[72] TB in its most severe form involves the CNS in 5-10% of extrapulmonary TB cases, and accounts for approximately 1% of all TB cases.[73]

20.5.2 Epidemiology & risk factors

Globally, an estimated 1.7 billion people are infected with *M. tuberculosis* and most of them reside in the WHO South-East Asia, Western-Pacific, and Africa regions.[74]

Risk factors for contracting TB[73]:
1. young age
2. coinfection with HIV
3. malnutrition
4. malignancies
5. immunosuppression
6. alcoholism
7. endemic TB in the community

20.5.3 Pathogenesis

M. tuberculosis is an aerobic, non-spore-forming, nonmotile, acid-fast bacillus (AFB) with a unique waxy coating. It is highly aerobic and primarily infects humans. Once an aerosolized droplet

20

containing bacilli is inhaled and reaches the lung alveoli, it interacts with alveolar macrophages through several receptors. Innate immune cells are triggered, and release chemokines and cytokines. T-helper cell-mediated immune response occurs and a granuloma forms. During this process, some bacilli are filtered into draining lymph nodes and some hematogenous dissemination occurs to the highly oxygenated parts of the body (such as the brain) before actual containment of the infection.[75,76] Once the bacilli enters the body, they are suppressed by the immune system and re-activation of infection only occurs if the immune system is compromised.

20.5.4 Medical treatment for TB

Antitubercular therapy (ATT) for neuro-TB

Most recommendations come from TBM. The consensus among several societies[77,78,79] is to use oral antitubercular drugs as:

- **Intensive Phase**: "HRZE" = Isoniazid (H), Rifampin (AKA Rifampicin) (R), Pyrazinamide (Z), and Ethambutol (E) for initial 2 months followed by
- **Continuation Phase**: after 2 months of IP therapy, for TBM known or presumed to be caused by susceptible strains of TB:
  HR for the next 7-10 months

Multidrug resistant TB

Approximately 4.8% of new TB cases worldwide are due to multi-drug resistant (MDR) *Mycobacterium tuberculosis* strains.[75] The strain has to be resistant to isoniazid and rifampin to be labeled as MDR TB. The WHO recommends the use of at least five effective drugs initially including a fluoroquinolone and an injectable second-line agent and that the treatment should last for 18–24 months.[80]

BCG vaccine

BCG vaccine (bacille or bacillus Calmette-Guérin) is a live-attenuated *Mycobacterium bovis* strain vaccine against TB. Though not routinely given to infants in the United States, it is included in the immunization programs of highly endemic regions of the world. It provides limited and variable protection against adult pulmonary TB[81] but its protection against CNS TB is uncertain. There is evidence that it reduces the likelihood of CNS tuberculoma.[82] Several studies have shown that BCG vaccine provided effective protection against TBM, as well against the death of newborns caused by tuberculosis.[83,84,85] Children with TBM who have been vaccinated with BCG appear to have fewer symptoms and fared better than those who did not receive it.[86] Trunz et al. showed an efficacy of 73% in TBM and 77% in miliary TB.[87]

20.5.5 Intracranial tuberculoma

General information

A tuberculoma is a well-defined intraparenchymal granulomatous lesion that is firm, avascular and ranges in size from 2-8 cm with surrounding edema and gliosis.[70] They favor the frontoparietal region and basal ganglia, and occur rarely in the cerebellar hemispheres, brainstem, corpus callosum, cerebellopontine angle, retro-orbital and quadrigeminal cistern.[88] Infratentorial lesions are more common among the pediatric age group.[89] They are usually solitary, but multiple lesions are also seen. Tuberculomas account for 5-30% of all intracranial space-occupying lesions among children and half of all non-neoplastic lesions in patients in endemic regions.[90] Lesions may be noncaseous, or may be caseating with either solid or liquid centers comprised of clear, straw-colored fluid secondary to liquefactive necrosis.

Clinical features

Tuberculomas generally present as a slow-growing mass with signs and symptoms of raised intracranial pressure (headache, seizures, nausea, vomiting, and focal neurological deficits).[90] Focal seizures are frequently the initial symptom. Fever may be present in ≈ 25% of patients. Tuberculoma should be suspected in patients with active TB or TBM in an endemic area with constitutional symptoms of weight loss, malaise and low-grade nocturnal fever.

20

Diagnostics

Laboratory

ESR may be normal or may peak as high as 40.[91]

Mantoux Tuberculin Skin test is positive in most cases. A negative test, however does not eliminate the diagnosis and a positive test does not necessarily establish the diagnosis.

Lumbar puncture is contraindicated in the presence of intracranial mass due to the risk of herniation. When it is done, CSF analysis is usually nonspecific.[92]

Imaging

▶ **Plain X-rays.** Skull X-rays: provide limited information. Calcifications may be seen.

Chest X-ray: may disclose a pulmonary TB lesion. Chest CT is more sensitive.

▶ **Brain CT.** Tuberculomas appear as a hypo to iso dense, irregular lesions with perilesional edema out of proportion to the size of the mass.[70,93] Contrast produces ring enhancement with solid or noncaseating lesions. A central nidus of calcification with surrounding ring-like enhancement (post-contrast) is sometimes seen ("target sign"[93]) which suggests tuberculoma but is not pathognomonic (neurocysticercosis (p. 404) NCC may produce similar appearing lesions but they are < 20 mm diameter and may have a mural nodule (scolex) whereas, tuberculomas are > 20 mm and irregular with significant edema[70] and never a mural nodule).[79] Occasionally, healed tuberculomas may appear as calcified foci on nonenhanced CT.[93]

▶ **Brain MRI.** The imaging study of choice. The appearance varies depending upon the type of granuloma (solid, noncaseating, caseating with a solid center, or caseating with a liquified center). Like CT, a pattern of ring-like enhancement is seen with perilesional edema in caseating tuberculomas with solid and liquid centers. DWI typically shows low central signal (no restricted diffusion). In the presence of liquefactive necrosis, the signal may be high centrally.

▶ **MRS (MR spectroscopy).** Commonly shows lipid peaks (due to large lipid fractions in TB bacilli), as well as increased choline levels and decreased N-acetyl aspartate and creatine levels. The choline:creatine ratio is usually > 1, however, higher Cho:Cr ratios favor malignancy over granuloma.

Biopsy

In case of doubt, image-guided stereotactic biopsy can confirm the diagnosis and simultaneously be used in management as well.

Treatment of tuberculomas

Medical treatment of tuberculomas

▶ **Antitubercular therapy (p. 358) (ATT).** Institute ATT as soon as there is a strong suspicion of tuberculoma (do not wait for confirmation).

ATT duration ranges from 9-12 months, extending beyond the radiographic resolution of lesions and cessation of symptoms which may go well up to 18 months and beyond.[90]

Treatment of multidrug resistant TB (p. 358) (MDR-TB) and extensive drug resistant TB (XDR-TB) is difficult, and requires prolonged drug therapy in special combination with first- and second-line drugs. Follow-up CT or MR studies are useful in monitoring the response to medical treatment.

▶ **Steroids.** Systemic corticosteroids as adjuvant therapy are indicated when there is peri-lesional edema, meningeal involvement or paradoxical progression during treatment.[94,95]

▶ **Antiseizure medication (ASM).** Due to the high incidence of seizures, ASMs should be routinely used. Commonly used drugs are phenytoin, levetiracetam, carbamazepine, oxcarbazepine, and sodium valproate.[96] NB: phenytoin and isoniazid can induce toxicity due to drug-drug interaction.

▶ **Treatment monitoring. Paradoxical enlargement** of a preexisting tuberculoma or development of a new intracranial or spinal tuberculoma may occur during ATT in ≈ 1% of all patients with active TB and in 4.5-28% of those with tuberculous meningitis.[97] This does not necessarily represent treatment failure or a second process. Most patients remain asymptomatic and clinical deterioration occurs in only ≈ 6-29%.[98] With continuation of ATT and steroids, resolution of the tuberculomas usually eventually occurs.[93]

20

Surgical treatment of tuberculomas

Surgical resection may be required to resolve the mass effect, in cases of drug resistance or paradoxical worsening or whenever there is a dilemma in diagnosis, brainstem compression or impending herniation.[99] A well-developed plane exists between the firm, avascular tuberculoma and the surrounding edematous brain. While gross total resection is preferred, sub-total resection with post-op ATT is equally efficacious if the proximity to eloquent brain or the nature of the lesion does not allow complete removal.[90] ATT is usually started before or during surgery to reduce the risk of port-op tuberculous meningitis (TBM).

VP-shunt or ETV is used for significant or symptomatic hydrocephalus.

20.5.6 Tuberculous meningitis (TBM)

General information

Tuberculous meningitis is the most common form of CNS TB and represents 1% of all extra-pulmonary cases and 5% of all cases of meningitis.[100] It is common in developing countries, and is rare in developed countries with about 100 to 150 cases occurring annually in the US.[101] It carries high morbidity and mortality, particularly in patients with HIV coinfection.[102] It is more common in pediatrics (6 months to 4 years of age) in the developing world.[103] In contrast, in the developed world, the adult population is frequently affected due the to re-activation of TB seen among the immunocompromised because of alcoholism, DM, chronic steroid use or in those with HIV. Hydrocephalus is a common complication of TBM, and may be responsible for some of the clinical findings (p. 361).

Clinical manifestations of TBM

Illness begins with a prodrome of non-specific signs and symptoms, e.g., low-grade fever (most common), anorexia, malaise and fatigue. A previous history of TB is present in ≈ 50% of children and in 10% of adults.[70] The prodrome typically lasts 2-3 weeks after which a meningitic phase commences with severe headache, meningismus, vomiting and sometimes with altered state of consciousness, focal neurological deficits, CN palsy and long-tract signs.[71] Seizure, though not common in adult patients, was seen in up to 50% of pediatric patients.[104] CN VI is the most common cranial nerve palsy observed followed by CN III and CN IV.[105]

Without prompt treatment, morbidity and mortality are high. Even with timely initiation of appropriate antitubercular therapy (p. 358) (ATT), the mortality rate ranges from 20–67.2%. Among survivors, it causes serious disability in 5–40% of patients.[100]

Diagnostics for TBM

General measures

Search should be made for evidence of TB elsewhere in the body by means of sputum for AFB, Gene Xpert PCR test (see below), chest X-ray or preferably high-resolution chest CT and U/S of the abdomen.

CSF through lumbar puncture

CSF analysis through LP is one of the most important tests for the diagnosis of TBM. Classically, the CSF is described as yellow and opalescent, with fibrin clot on standing.

▶ **CSF cytology.** Characteristic CSF findings are lymphocytic pleocytosis with high WBC count (100-500), elevated protein (100-500), low glucose (less than 45 mg/dL)[101] and elevated opening pressure.[76] Neutrophilic predominance can occasionally occur later in cases with ongoing ATT. This paradoxical immunological response is due to a hypersensitivity reaction to tubercular protein during treatment.[76]

▶ **Microbiology.** The gold standard diagnostic is isolation of the organism through culture or detection of its presence by acid-fast staining.[106]

When TBM is suspected, CSF should be examined by Ziehl-Neelsen (ZN) staining for acid-fast bacilli (AFB). However, the sensitivity of conventional ZN staining is rarely > 60% and thus unreliable to identify AFB in the smear.[107]

Similarly, identification of AFB by conventional Lowenstein Jensen (LJ) culture is quite low, especially in cerebrospinal fluid (CSF) which contains a small number of organisms.[106]

CSF mycobacterium cultures have variable yield and are only positive 40-83% of the time and can take from 6 to 8 weeks to grow.

PCR: nucleic acid amplification (NAA) assays for the diagnosis of TBM is 56% sensitive and 98-100% specific and the diagnostic yield increases with larger volumes of CSF.[73]

Xpert MTB/RIF assay: recommended in 2013 by the WHO[108] as the initial test for CSF of patients with suspicion of TBM for rapid (within 2 hours) and simultaneous detection of MTB and rifampin resistance in preference to conventional microscopy and culture. With centrifugation of CSF it has sensitivity of 72% and specificity of 100%.

Imaging for TBM

▶ **Chest imaging.** Chest X-ray is suggestive of active or previous pulmonary TB in ≈ 50% of cases.[102] Chest CT scan is more sensitive in detecting cavitary lung lesions in TB.[109]

▶ **Brain imaging.** TBM is characterized radiologically by the triad of basal meningeal enhancement, hydrocephalus and cerebral infarction, though a range of other features are common.[110] MRI is superior to CT in assessing cerebral infarcts (thalamus, basal ganglia, internal capsule regions),[70] cerebral edema, and meningeal enhancement while CT imaging is best used to rule out hydrocephalus in emergency situations which requires immediate neurosurgical intervention. CT imaging can also show thick basilar exudates in basal cisterns and Sylvian fissures.[70]

Treatment

▶ **Antimicrobial therapy.** Start empiric treatment with ATT once there is high index of suspicion clinically and through CSF analysis even before microbiological confirmation. Standard treatment consists of Intensive Phase (p. 358) with HRZE for 2 months followed by Continuation Phase with HR for 7-10 months.[101]

▶ **Adjunctive corticosteroid therapy.** Corticosteroids are given along with ATT to dampen the host immunological response.[101] WHO recommends dexamethasone or prednisolone tapered over 6-8 weeks. Dexamethasone reduces mortality in HIV-uninfected individuals but probably does not prevent disability.[80,103] There were lower rates of mortality, death or severe disability, and disease relapse when given with ATT. A concern that corticosteroids may decrease the CSF penetration of ATT was debunked by Kaojarern et al.[111]

Prognosis with TBM

▶ **Mortality.** Reported mortality rate with TBM is 20–67% even with the administration of appropriate ATT. Mortality is higher in patients with HIV. Disability and impairment is observed in 5–40% of patients treated with ATT.[100]

▶ **Morbidity.** Even those who are cured are often left with significant neurological deficits and complete neurological recovery occurs in only 21.5%.[112]

Complications include: hydrocephalus (see below), meningeal adhesions, ventriculitis, vasculitis, ischemic stroke, tuberculoma, hyponatremia, cranial neuropathies, optico-chiasmatic arachnoiditis leading to vision impairment.[112,113]

TBM and hydrocephalus

Hydrocephalus is one of the most common complications of TBM and may occur during, before or after treatment. It develops in most (87-95%) pediatric patients[114,115] who have had TBM for 4-6 weeks, and in ≈ 12% of adults.[115] Late onset is also reported.[115] The hydrocephalus may be purely communicating type (the most common, especially late[116,117]), or purely non-communicating type (more common early in the course[116,117]) or a complex-mixed type, depending on where the CSF pathway has been blocked by the thick gelatinous inflammatory exudates (subarachnoid cisterns or ventricular pathways).[115,116,118] The fact that not all patients respond to treatment of the hydrocephalus indicates that the clinical findings are multifactorial and not attributable solely to the hydrocephalus.[116,119]

▶ **Treatment of hydrocephalus in TBM.** Treatment decisions may be guided by the severity of the illness. The validated modified Vellore grading (mVG) system is shown in ▶ Table 20.10.

Medical management includes antitubercular therapy (p. 358) (ATT), steroids and diuretics.

Surgical options primarily involves CSF diversion: shunt, external ventricular drainage (EVD) or endoscopic third ventriculostomy (ETV).

20

Table 20.10 Vellore grading system[116] (modified[117]) (mVG) for hydrocephalus in tuberculous meningitis

Grade	Sensorium[a]	Clinical/Neurologic Deficit	Outcome[b]
I	GCS 15 (normal sensorium)	H/A, vomiting, fever and or neck stiffness,no neurologic deficit	(5 patients) 3 good, 1 moderate disability, 1 death
II	GCS 15 (normal sensorium)	neurologic deficit present	(75 patients) 31 good, 15 moderate disability, 3 severe disability, 26 deaths
III	GCS 9-14 (altered sensorium but easily arousable)	± dense neurologic deficit	(27 patients) 7 good, 6 moderate disability, 14 deaths
IV	GCS 3-8 (deeply comatose)	decerebrate or decorticate posturing	(7 patients) 7 deaths

[a] The GCS (Glasgow Coma Scale (p. 318) score) is used in the modified grading system, the original Vellore grading is described below that in parentheses).
[b] Outcome among 114 patients with ≥ 6 months follow-up[116]

The following statements are pertinent to shunting in TBM hydrocephalus.
- mVG grade at presentation is the most consistent predictor of outcome from shunting (better outcome with lower mVG)[119]
- mVG III patients: the response to EVD was not highly correlated with outcome, so shunting is recommended in all[117]
- mVG IV patients: patients who did not improve with EVD within 48 hours did not improve with shunting, ∴ EVD placement for up to 48 hours is recommended, and then shunting only if there is a positive response[117]
- **EVD** (external ventricular drainage):
  a) **emergency EVD**: when urgent CSF diversion is indicated (e.g., for deterioration in an mVG III patient) and a shunt cannot be done immediately, EVD may be used as a temporizing measure until the shunt can be performed[117]
  b) EVD may also help with mVG IV patients to determine appropriateness of shunting (see ▶ Fig. 20.2)
- **ETV** can be an effective treatment for TBM with HCP[120] and is regarded as the preferred long-term intervention by some.[121] However, these points need to be considered:
  a) ETV requires a surgeon experienced in the technique
  b) with TBM, the floor of the third ventricle may be thickened and the subarachnoid space may be obliterated.[119] ETV can be unsafe in patients with these findings due to increased risk of injury to the basilar artery
  c) overall success rates of ETV in TBM hydrocephalus is 41-81%. The following factors influence the success rate
  d) the median duration of TBM was 4 days in patients with successful ETV, and 1.5 days in the unsuccessful group (statistically significant difference)[121]
  e) the median duration of pre-op ATT was 30 days in patients with successful ETV, and 1 day in the unsuccessful group (a trend, not statistically significant)[121]
  f) the role of ETV is controversial in communicating hydrocephalus and in the acute phase of disease[118]
- **VP vs. VA shunt**: because of concerns of hematogenous dissemination of infection,[122] ventriculo-peritoneal shunting is generally preferred over ventriculoatrial shunting (despite studies showing the safety of VA shunting[123])
- **timing**: shunting 2 days after the decision to shunt was associated with a better outcome compared to waiting 3 weeks[124]
- **type of hydrocephalus**: obstructive hydrocephalus is a strong indication for shunting.[125] The case been made for initially attempting medical management in communicating hydrocephalus,[125] however this necessitates close continuous monitoring (some advocate with ICP monitoring[124]) and risks some patients having irreversible damage from deterioration[119]

Based on the above, a management algorithm is shown in ▶ Fig. 20.2 (NB: this algorithm has not been validated).

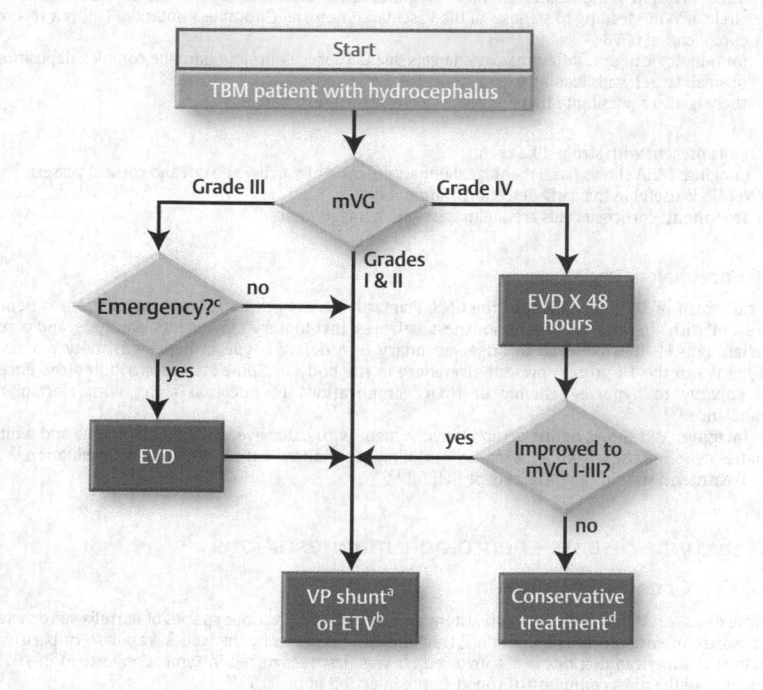

Fig. 20.2 Algorithm for shunting hydrocephalus in TB meningitis.
[a] VP shunting is ideally performed early, e.g. within 2 days of the decision to shunt (timing is less urgent if an EVD is in place)
[b] ETV is recommended by some, but VP shunt may be preferred early in the course of MTB and early in the course of ATT and for other reasons (see text)
[c] emergency EVD is used for patients who deteriorate and cannot be shunted immediately
[d] remove the EVD and provide ATT and other supportive measures as indicated
Abbreviations: ATT = antitubercular therapy (p. 358), ETV = endoscopic third ventriculostomy, EVD = external ventricular drain, mVG = modified Vellore grade (▶ Table 20.10), TBM = TB meningitis.

20.5.7 Other forms of TB involvement

TB brain abscess

Rare, compared to tuberculoma. Abscesses tend to be larger (> 3 cm) and present with fever, H/A and focal neurologic deficit.[126] They are more common in immunocompromised patients (20%) who do not form granulomas, compared to immunocompetent patients (4-7.5%).[127]

Imaging: CT and MRI appearance are similar to pyogenic abscesses. DWI MRI demonstrates restricted diffusion, unlike a tuberculoma.[110]

Management: antitubercular therapy (p. 358) (ATT) is the cornerstone of treatment. Surgical intervention is indicated for failure to respond, and options include stereotactic one-time drainage, continuous drainage, repeat aspiration and total excision.[128]

TB vasculopathy

Generally occurs as a sequelae of TBM, but may rarely occur without neuro-TB.[129]

Infections in general can cause vasculitis by a number of mechanisms. However, in neuro-TB, the primary mechanisms appear to be[129]:

20

1. direct invasion of the vessel wall: basal exudates cause inflammatory changes in vessels of the circle of Willis leading to stenosis of the vascular lumen and thrombus formation. This is a severe complication of TB
2. immunologic injury: inflammatory changes due to tuberculoprotein immune complex deposition in small vessel walls leading to
3. there is also a possibility that antibodies form against host antigens

Patients present with stroke-like events.

Imaging: MRA shows basal meningeal enhancement and narrowed basal and cortical vessels.[129]
DWI MRI is useful in the early detection of infarction.[130]

Treatment: corticosteroids are the mainstay in management.[129]

TB encephalopathy

A rare form of TB involvement of the CNS. Primarily occurs in the pediatric population. Patients present with altered level of consciousness, seizures, involuntary movements, paralysis, and cerebellar signs.[131] It is believed to arise secondary to a delayed-type of hypersensitivity reaction (Type IV) to the TB protein present elsewhere in the body.[132] Some studies attributed the encephalopathy to hypoxic–ischemic or toxic complications of infection along with electrolyte imbalance.[133]

Imaging: MRI shows diffuse cerebral involvement with extensive white matter edema and white matter hyperintense lesions with marked gadolinium enhancement representing demyelination.[73]

Treatment: steroids and ATT may be helpful.[134]

20.6 Lyme disease—neurologic manifestations

20.6.1 General information

Lyme disease (LD) is a complex multisystem disease caused by various species of Borrelia spirochetes (in North America: Borrelia burgdorferi) transmitted to humans by the Ixodes scapularis or pacificus ticks (the American dog tick is not involved). It was first recognized in Lyme, Connecticut in 1975, and is now the most common arthropod-borne infection in the U.S.[135]

20.6.2 Clinical findings

There are 3 clinical stages which can overlap or occur separately.

▶ **Stage 1 (early localized disease, erythema migrans and flu-like illness).** Systemic signs of infection usually begin with a flu-like illness within days to weeks of infection, symptoms include: fever, chills, malaise, fatigue or lethargy, backache, headache, arthralgia, and myalgia. Regional or generalized lymphadenopathy may occur.

The hallmark of LD is erythema chronicum migrans (ECM) (classically a "bulls-eye rash") which begins 3–30 days after the tick bite, and occurs in 60–75% of patients. ECM usually begins in the thigh, inguinal region, or axilla, and consists of an expanding macular rash with bright red borders and central clearing and induration that usually fades without scarring in 3–4 weeks. In addition to ECM, other dermatologic findings include: malar rash (13%), diffuse erythema, and urticaria. Within 30 days of the tick bite, spirochetes may be demonstrated in acellular spinal fluid.

▶ **Stage 2 (early disseminated disease).** Several weeks to months after infection, untreated patients develop signs of more serious organ involvement. Cardiac and neurologic involvement may occur. Manifestations include:
1. cardiac: occurs in 8%. Conduction defects (usually A-V block, generally brief and mild) and myopericarditis
2. ocular: panophthalmitis, ischemic optic atrophy, and interstitial keratitis occur rarely
3. neurologic: occurs in 10–15% of patients with stage 2 disease
   a) the clinical triad of neurologic manifestations of Lyme disease is[136]:
      • cranial neuritis (especially that mimicking Bell's palsy: Lyme disease is the most common cause of bilateral "Bell's palsy" [facial diplegia] in endemic areas)
      • meningitis
      • radiculopathy
   b) other possible neurologic involvement includes: encephalitis, myelitis, peripheral neuritis

Neurologic findings are frequently migratory, and ≈ 60% of patients have multiple neurologic findings simultaneously. In Europe, Bannwarth's syndrome (chronic lymphocytic meningitis, peripheral neuropathy, and radiculopathy) is the most common manifestation, and primarily affects the peripheral nervous system.[137] Neurologic symptoms usually resolve gradually.

▶ **Stage 3 (late disease)**. Arthritis and chronic neurologic syndromes may occur in this stage. Arthralgias are common in stage 1, but true arthritis usually does not begin for months to years after infection, and is seen in ≈ 60% of cases.[138] When arthritis occurs, it may affect the knee (89%), hip (9%), shoulder (9%), ankle (7%), and/or elbow (2%).[139] Neurologic involvement includes[140]:
1. encephalopathy (chronic, manifestation may be subtle)
2. encephalomyelitis (chronic, manifestation may be subtle)
3. peripheral neuropathy (chronic, manifestation may be subtle)
4. ataxia
5. dementia
6. sleep disorder
7. neuropsychiatric disease and fatigue syndromes

20.6.3 Diagnosis

Diagnostic criteria

There is no test indicative of active infection. The spirochete is difficult to culture from infected humans. Diagnosis is easy if a history of travel to endemic areas, tick bite, and ECM are identified.
▶ Table 20.11 shows the CDC criteria for diagnosis.

Table 20.11 CDC criteria for diagnosis of Lyme disease[141]

Area	Criteria
In endemic area	• erythema chronicum migrans (ECM) • antibody titer ≥ 1:256 by IFA[a] and involvement of ≥ 1 organ system[b]
In non-endemic area	• ECM with antibody titer ≥ 1:256 • ECM with involvement of ≥ 2 organ systems[b] • antibody titer ≥ 1:256 by IFA[a] and involvement of ≥ 1 organ system[b]

[a]IFA = immunofluorescence antibody
[b]either musculoskeletal, neurologic, or cardiac

Serology

It takes 7–10 days from initial infection to develop antibodies to B. burgdorferi, but it takes ≈ 2–3 wks before antibodies can be reliably detected in untreated patients (antibiotics can reduce the immune response).[142] If the first serum test is negative, it should be repeated in 4–6 weeks if the clinical suspicion of LD is strong (seroconversion from negative to positive is supportive of B. burgdorferi infection). False positives can occur with other borrelial and treponemal infections (e.g., syphilis); however, VDRL test will differentiate the two.

Enzyme-linked immunosorbent assay (ELISA) detects IgM or IgG. Antibodies to B. burgdorferi is the usual test method. IgM is elevated acutely, and IgG gradually rises and is elevated in almost all patients at 4–6 weeks and is usually highest in patients with arthritis.[135] Western blot may help identify false-positive ELISA results (more sensitive and specific than ELISA; however, results may vary between labs). Amplification of B. burgdorferi DNA by polymerase chain reaction (PCR) yields a more sensitive test that may have significant false positives, and can be positive even if the DNA is from dead organisms.

CSF

Elevated CSF IgG antibody titer to B. burgdorferi may occur with neurologic involvement.[143] CSF findings in late disease are usually compatible with aseptic meningitis. Oligoclonal bands and increased ratio of IgG to albumin may occur.[144]

20.6.4 Treatment

See references.[140,145,146]
Antibiotic therapy is more effective early in the illness.

20

20.7 Nocardia brain abscess

20.7.1 General information

Nocardia infections may involve the CNS in multiple ways.

Nocardiosis is caused primarily by *Nocardia asteroides* (other Nocardia species such as *N. brasiliensis* are less common), a gram-positive beaded branching bacillus that is a soil-born obligate aerobic actinomycete (a bacteria, not a fungus). Usually inoculated through the respiratory tract and produces a localized or disseminated infection. Hematogenous spread frequently results in cutaneous lesions and CNS involvement. Nocardia is responsible for 2% of all brain abscesses, the majority of these are *N. asteroides*.

Nocardiosis occurs primarily in patients with chronic debilitating illnesses including:
1. neoplasms: leukemia, lymphoma…
2. conditions requiring long-term corticosteroid treatment
3. Cushing's disease
4. Paget's disease of bone
5. AIDS
6. renal or cardiac organ transplant recipients

The diagnosis is suspected in high-risk patients presenting with soft-tissue abscesses and CNS lesions. CNS involvement occurs in about one-third and includes:
1. cerebral abscess: often multiloculated. Restricted diffusion on MRI
2. meningitis
3. ventriculitis in patients with CSF shunt[147]
4. epidural spinal cord compression from vertebral osteomyelitis[148]

20.7.2 Diagnosis

Serologic tests are unreliable.

Gram stain of specimens is the most sensitive test for diagnosis. Characteristic finding: gram-positive beaded branching filaments. Weakly stain in acid-fast preparations.

Brain biopsy may not be needed in high-risk patients with confirmed nocardia infection in other sites,[147] except possibly in AIDS patients where the risk of multiple organism infections or infection plus tumor (particularly lymphoma) is considerable.

20.7.3 Treatment

General information

Surgical indications (p. 347) are the same as for other abscesses.

Antibiotics

See references.[149,150]
- primary choice: trimethoprim-sulfamethoxazole (TMP-SMZ 15 mg/kg IV of trimethoprim component per day in two to four divided doses PLUS imipenem 500 mg IV q 6h ± amikacin 7.5 mg/kg IV q 12h (if CNS disease with multiorgan involvement)
- alternative if sulfa allergy: imipenem 500 mg IV q 6h PLUS amikacin 7.5 mg/kg IV q 12h

Antimicrobial susceptibility testing should be conducted on all isolates.

Duration: because of risks of relapse or hematogenous spread, treatment is recommended for at least one year with CNS involvement, possibly indefinitely for immunocompromised hosts.

References

[1] Edberg M, Furebring M, Sjolin J, et al. Neurointensive care of patients with severe community-acquired meningitis. Acta Anaesthesiol Scand. 2011; 55:732–739

[2] Tunkel AR, Hartman BJ, Kaplan SL, et al. Practice guidelines for the management of bacterial meningitis. Clin Infect Dis. 2004; 39:1267–1284

[3] Baltas I, Tsoulfa S, Sakellariou P, et al. Posttraumatic Meningitis: Bacteriology, Hydrocephalus, and Outcome. Neurosurgery. 1994; 35:422–427

[4] Eljamel MSM, Foy PM. Post-Traumatic CSF Fistulae, the Case for Surgical Repair. Br J Neurosurg. 1990; 4:479–483

[5] Immunization Action Coalition. Pneumococcal Vaccines (PCV13 and PPSV23). 2020. http://www.immunize.org/askexperts/experts_pneumococcal_vaccines.asp

[6] Centers for Disease Control (CDC). Pneumococcal vaccine timing for adults. 2020. https://www.cdc.gov/vaccines/vpd/pneumo/downloads/pneumo-vaccine-timing.pdf

[7] Lewin W. Cerebrospinal Fluid Rhinorrhea in Closed Head Injuries. Clinical Neurosurgery. 1966; 12:237–252

[8] Horwitz NH, Levy CS. Comment on Baltas I, et al.: Posttraumatic Meningitis: Bacteriology, Hydrocephalus, and Outcome. Neurosurgery. 1994; 35

[9] Glantz MJ, Jaeckle KA, Chamberlain MC, et al. A randomized controlled trial comparing intrathecal sustained-release cytarabine (DepoCyt) to intrathecal methotrexate in patients with neoplastic meningitis from solid tumors. Clin Cancer Res. 1999; 5:3394–3402

[10] Sanchez GB, Kaylie DM, O'Malley MR, et al. Chemical meningitis following cerebellopontine angle tumor surgery. Otolaryngol Head Neck Surg. 2008; 138:368–373

[11] Abramson RC, Morawetz RB, Schlitt M. Multiple Complications from an Intracranial Epidermoid Cyst: Case Report and Literature Review. Neurosurgery. 1989; 24:574–578

[12] Hakizimana D, Poulsgaard L, Fugleholm K. Chemical meningitis from a leaking craniopharyngioma: a case report. Acta Neurochir (Wien). 2018; 160:1203–1206

[13] He Xuzhi, Wang ZXuhui, Xu Minhui, et al. Diagnosis and treatment of postoperative aseptic meningitis. Scientific Research and Essays. 2011; 6:2221–2224

[14] Hillier CE, Stevens AP, Thomas F, et al. Aseptic meningitis after posterior fossa surgery treated by pseudomeningocele closure. J Neurol Neurosurg Psychiatry. 2000; 68:218–219

[15] Forgacs P, Geyer CA, Freidberg SR. Characterization of chemical meningitis after neurological surgery. Clin Infect Dis. 2001; 32:179–185

[16] van de Beek D, Brouwer MC, Thwaites GE, et al. Advances in treatment of bacterial meningitis. Lancet. 2012; 380:1693–1702

[17] Calfee DP, Wispelwey B. Brain abscess. Semin Neurol. 2000; 20:353–360

[18] Mamelak AN, Mampalam TJ, Obana WG, et al. Improved Management of Multiple Brain Abscesses: A Combined Surgical and Medical Approach. Neurosurgery. 1995; 36:76–86

[19] Takeshita M, Kagawa M, Yato S, et al. Current treatment of brain abscess in patients with congenital cyanotic heart disease. Neurosurgery. 1997; 41:1270–1279

[20] Kanter MC, Hart RG. Neurologic Complications of Infective Endocarditis. Neurology. 1991; 41:1015–1020

[21] Garvey G. Current Concepts of Bacterial Infections of the Central Nervous System: Bacterial Meningitis and Bacterial Brain Abscess. J Neurosurg. 1983; 59:735–744

[22] Nunez DA, Browning GG. Risks of Developing an Otogenic Intracranial Abscess. J Laryngol Otol. 1990; 104:468–472

[23] Hollin SA, Hayashi H, Gross SW. Intracranial Abscesses of Odontogenic Origin. Oral Surg. 1967; 23:277–293

[24] Williams FH, Nelms DK, McGaharan KM. Brain Abscess: A Rare Complication of Halo Usage. Arch Phys Med Rehabil. 1992; 73:490–492

[25] Grimstad IA, Hirschberg H, Rootwelt K. 99mTc-hexamethylpropyleneamine oxime leukocyte scintigraphy and C-reactive protein levels in the differential diagnosis of brain abscesses. Journal of Neurosurgery. 1992; 77:732–736

[26] Fritz DP, Nelson PB, Roos KL. Brain Abscess. In: Central Nervous System Infectious Diseases and Therapy. New York: Marcel Dekker; 1997:481–498

[27] Desprechins B, Stadnik T, Koerts G, et al. Use of diffusion-weighted MR imaging in differential diagnosis between intracerebral necrotic tumors and cerebral abscesses. AJNR Am J Neuroradiol. 1999; 20:1252–1257

[28] Mueller-Mang C, Castillo M, Mang TG, et al. Fungal versus bacterial brain abscesses: is diffusion-weighted MR imaging a useful tool in the differential diagnosis? Neuroradiology. 2007; 49:651–657

[29] Britt RH, Enzmann DR. Clinical Stages of Human Brain Abscesses on Serial CT Scans After Contrast Infusion. J Neurosurg. 1983; 59:972–989

[30] Heineman HS, Braude AI, Osterholm JL. Intracranial Suppurative Disease. JAMA. 1971; 218:1542–1547

[31] Black P, Graybill JR, Charache P. Penetration of Brain Abscess by Systemically Administered Antibiotics. J Neurosurg. 1973; 38:705–709

[32] Rosenblum ML, Hoff JT, Norman D, et al. Nonoperative Treatment of Brain Abscesses in Selected High-risk Patients. J Neurosurg. 1980; 52:217–225

[33] Ruelle A, Zerbi D, Zuccarello M, et al. Brain Stem Abscess Treated Successfully by Medical Therapy. Neurosurgery. 1978; 49:658–668

[34] Zeidman SM, Geisler FH, Olivi A. Intraventricular Rupture of a Purulent Brain Abscess: Case Report. Neurosurgery. 1995; 36:189–193

[35] Stephanov S. Surgical Treatment of Brain Abscess. Neurosurgery. 1988; 22:724–730

[36] Hollander D, Villemure J-G, Leblanc R. Thalamic Abscess: A Stereotactically Treatable Lesion. Appl Neurophysiol. 1987; 50:168–171

[37] Rosenblum ML, Hoff JT, Norman D, et al. Decreased Mortality from Brain Abscesses Since Advent of CT. J Neurosurg. 1978; 49:658–668

[38] Stephanov S, Sidani AH. Intracranial subdural empyema and its management. A review of the literature with comment. Swiss Surg. 2002; 8:159–163

[39] Kubik CS, Adams RD. Subdural Empyema. Brain. 1943; 66:18–42

[40] Maniglia AJ, Goodwin WJ, Arnold JE, et al. Intracranial Abscess Secondary to Nasal, Sinus, and Orbital Infections in Adults and Children. Arch Otolaryngol Head Neck Surg. 1989; 115:1424–1429

[41] Dill SR, Cobbs CG, McDonald CK. Subdural Empyema: Analysis of 32 Cases and Review. Clin Inf Dis. 1995; 20:372–386

[42] Garfin SR, Botte MJ, Triggs KJ, et al. Subdural Abscess Associated with Halo-Pin Traction. Journal of Bone and Joint Surgery. 1988; 70A:1338–1340

[43] Jacobson PL, Farmer TW. Subdural Empyema Complicating Meningitis in Infants: Improved Prognosis. Neurology. 1981; 31:190–193

[44] Weisberg L. Subdural Empyema: Clinical and Computed Tomographic Correlations. Archives of Neurology. 1986; 43:497–500

[45] Mauser HW, Ravijst RAP, Elderson A, et al. Nonsurgical Treatment of Subdural Empyema: Case Report. Journal of Neurosurgery. 1985; 63:128–130

[46] Levy RM, Bredesen DE, Rosenblum ML. Neurological manifestations of the acquired immunodeficiency syndrome (AIDS): Experience at UCSF and review of the literature. J Neurosurg. 1985; 62:475–495

[47] Simpson DM, Tagliati M. Neurologic Manifestations of HIV Infection. Annals of Internal Medicine. 1994; 121:769–785

[48] Berger JR, Kaszovitz B, Post JD, et al. Progressive Multifocal Leukoencephalopathy Associated with Human Immunodeficiency Virus Infection: A Review of the Literature with a Report of Sixteen Cases. Ann Intern Med. 1987; 107:78–87

[49] Ciricillo SF, Rosenblum ML. Use of CT and MR Imaging to Distinguish Intracranial Lesions and to Define the Need for Biopsy in AIDS Patients. J Neurosurg. 1990; 73:720–724

[50] Chaisson RE, Griffin DE. Progressive Multifocal Leukoencephalopathy in AIDS. JAMA. 1990; 364:79–82

[51] Demeter LM, Mandell GL, Bennett JE. JC, BK, and other polyomaviruses; progressive multifocal leukoencephalopathy. In: Mandell, Douglas and Bennett Principles and Practice of Infectious Diseases. 4th ed. New York: Churchill Livingstone; 1995:1400–1406

[52] Krupp LB, Lipton RB, Swerdlow ML, et al. Progressive Multifocal Leukoencephalopathy: Clinical and Radiographic Features. Annals of Neurology. 1985; 17:344–349

20

[53] Berger JR, Mucke L. Prolonged Survival and Partial Recovery in AIDS-Associated Progressive Multifocal Leukoencephalopathy. Neurology. 1988; 38:1060–1065

[54] Elliot B, Aromin I, Gold R, et al. 2.5 year remission of AIDS-associated progressive multifocal leukoencephalopathy with combined antiretroviral therapy. Lancet. 1997; 349

[55] Jean WC, Hall WA. Management of Cranial and Spinal Infections. Contemporary Neurosurgery. 1998; 20:1–10

[56] Johns DR, Tierney M, Felenstein D. Alterations in the Natural History of Neurosyphilis by Concurrent Infection with the Human Immunodeficiency Virus. N Engl J Med. 1987; 316:1569–1592

[57] Lukehart SA, Hook EW, Baker-Zander SA, et al. Invasion of the Central Nervous System by Treponema pallidum: Implications for Diagnosis and Treatment. Ann Int Med. 1988; 109:855–862

[58] Workowski KA, Bolan GA. Sexually transmitted diseases treatment guidelines, 2015. MMWR Recomm Rep. 2015; 64:1–137

[59] Jarvik JG, Hesselink JR, Kennedy C, et al. Acquired Immunodeficiency Syndrome: Magnetic Resonance Patterns of Brain Involvement with Pathologic Correlation. Archives of Neurology. 1988; 45:731–736

[60] Sadler M, Brink NS, Gazzard BG. Management of Intracerebral Lesions in Patients with HIV: A Retrospective Study with Discussion of Diagnostic Problems. Q J Med. 1998; 91:205–217

[61] Schwaighofer BW, Hesselink JR, Press GA, et al. Primary Intracranial CNS Lymphoma: MR Manifestations. AJNR. 1989; 10:725–729

[62] So YT, Beckstead JH, Davis RL. Primary central nervous system lymphoma in acquired immune deficiency syndrome: A clinical and pathological study. Ann Neurol. 1986; 20:566–572

[63] Cinque P, Brytting M, Vago L, et al. Epstein-Barr Virus DNA in Cerebrospinal Fluid from Patients with AIDS-Related Primary Lymphoma of the Central Nervous System. Lancet. 1991; 342:398–401

[64] Montoya JG, Liesenfeld O. Toxoplasmosis. Lancet. 2004; 363:1965–1976

[65] CDC (Centers for Disease Control and Prevention). Parasites - Toxoplasmosis (Toxoplasma infection). Resources for health professionals. 2018. https://www.cdc.gov/parasites/toxoplasmosis/health_professionals/index.html

[66] Cohn JA, Meeking MC, Cohen W, et al. Evaluation of the policy of empiric treatment of suspected toxoplasma encephalitis in patients with the acquired immunodeficiency syndrome. Am J Med. 1989; 86:521–527

[67] Chappell ET, Guthrie BL, Orenstein J. The Role of Stereotactic Biopsy in the Management of HIV-Related Focal Brain Lesions. Neurosurgery. 1992; 30:825–829

[68] Levy RM, Russell E, Yungbluth M, et al. The efficacy of image-guided stereotactic brain biopsy in neurologically symptomatic acquired immunodeficiency syndrome patients. Neurosurgery. 1992; 30:186–190

[69] Nicolato A, Gerosa M, Piovan E, et al. Computerized Tomography and Magnetic Resonance Guided Stereotactic Brain Biopsy in Nonimmunocompromised and AIDS Patients. Surgical Neurology. 1997; 48:267–277

[70] Garg RK. Tuberculosis of the central nervous system. Postgrad Med J. 1999; 75:133–140

[71] Leonard JM. Central Nervous System Tuberculosis. Microbiol Spectr. 2017; 5. DOI: 10.1128/microbiolspec.TNMI7-0044-2017

[72] MacNeil A, Glaziou P, Sismanidis C, et al. Global Epidemiology of Tuberculosis and Progress Toward Meeting Global Targets - Worldwide, 2018. MMWR Morb Mortal Wkly Rep. 2020; 69:281–285

[73] Cherian A, Thomas SV. Central nervous system tuberculosis. Afr Health Sci. 2011; 11:116–127

[74] Houben RM, Dodd PJ. The Global Burden of Latent Tuberculosis Infection: A Re-estimation Using Mathematical Modelling. PLoS Med. 2016; 13. DOI: 10.1371/journal.pmed.1002152

[75] Be NA, Kim KS, Bishai WR, et al. Pathogenesis of central nervous system tuberculosis. Curr Mol Med. 2009; 9:94–99

[76] Rock RB, Olin M, Baker CA, et al. Central nervous system tuberculosis: pathogenesis and clinical aspects. Clin Microbiol Rev. 2008; 21:243–61, table of contents

[77] Sharma SK, Ryan H, Khaparde S, et al. Index-TB guidelines: Guidelines on extrapulmonary tuberculosis for India. Indian J Med Res. 2017; 145:448–463

[78] Thwaites G, Fisher M, Hemingway C, et al. British Infection Society guidelines for the diagnosis and treatment of tuberculosis of the central nervous system in adults and children. J Infect. 2009; 59:167–187

[79] Ramachandran R, Muniyandi M, Iyer V, et al. Dilemmas in the diagnosis and treatment of intracranial tuberculomas. J Neurol Sci. 2017; 381:256–264

[80] Davis A, Meintjes G, Wilkinson RJ. Treatment of Tuberculous Meningitis and Its Complications in Adults. Curr Treat Options Neurol. 2018; 20. DOI: 1 0.1007/s11940-018-0490-9

[81] Pokkali S, Jain S. Novel vaccine strategies against tuberculosis: a road less travelled. Expert Rev Vaccines. 2013; 12:1373–1375

[82] Wasay M, Ajmal S, Taqui AM, et al. Impact of bacille Calmette-Guerin vaccination on neuroradiological manifestations of pediatric tuberculous meningitis. J Child Neurol. 2010; 25:581–586

[83] Awasthi S, Moin S. Effectiveness of BCG vaccination against tuberculous meningitis. Indian Pediatr. 1999; 36:455–460

[84] Kumar P, Kumar R, Srivastava KL, et al. Protective role of BCG vaccination against tuberculous meningitis in Indian children: a reappraisal. Natl Med J India. 2005; 18:7–11

[85] Puvacic S, Dizdarevic J, Santic Z, et al. Protective effect of neonatal BCG vaccines against tuberculous meningitis. Bosn J Basic Med Sci. 2004; 4:46–49

[86] Kumar R, Dwivedi A, Kumar P, et al. Tuberculous meningitis in BCG vaccinated and unvaccinated children. J Neurol Neurosurg Psychiatry. 2005; 76:1550–1554

[87] Trunz BB, Fine P, Dye C. Effect of BCG vaccination on childhood tuberculous meningitis and miliary tuberculosis worldwide: a meta-analysis and assessment of cost-effectiveness. Lancet. 2006; 367:1173–1180

[88] Sonmez G, Ozturk E, Sildiroglu HO, et al. MRI findings of intracranial tuberculomas. Clin Imaging. 2008; 32:88–92

[89] Trivedi R, Saksena S, Gupta RK. Magnetic resonance imaging in central nervous system tuberculosis. Indian J Radiol Imaging. 2009; 19:256–265

[90] DeLance AR, Safaee M, Oh MC, et al. Tuberculoma of the central nervous system. J Clin Neurosci. 2013; 20:1333–1341

[91] Bhagwati SN, Parulekar GD. Management of intracranial tuberculoma in children. Childs Nerv Syst. 1986; 2:32–34

[92] Mohammadian M, Butt S. Symptomatic central nervous system tuberculoma, a case report in the United States and literature review. IDCases. 2019; 17. DOI: 10.1016/j.idcr.2019.e00582

[93] Sanei Taheri M, Karimi MA, Haghighatkhah H, et al. Central nervous system tuberculosis: an imaging-focused review of a reemerging disease. Radiol Res Pract. 2015; 2015. DOI: 10.1155/2015/202806

[94] Monteiro R, Carneiro JC, Costa C, et al. Cerebral tuberculomas - A clinical challenge. Respir Med Case Rep. 2013; 9:34–37

[95] Zahrou F, Elallouchi Y, Ghannane H, et al. Diagnosis and management of intracranial tuberculomas: about 2 cases and a review of the literature. Pan Afr Med J. 2019; 34. DOI: 10.11604/pamj.2019.34.23.17587

[96]   Patwari AK, Aneja S, Chandra D, et al. Long-term anticonvulsant therapy in tuberculous meningitis–a four-year follow-up. J Trop Pediatr. 1996; 42:98–103

[97]   Das A, Das SK, Mandal A, et al. Cerebral tuberculoma as a manifestation of paradoxical reaction in patients with pulmonary and extrapulmonary tuberculosis. J Neurosci Rural Pract. 2012; 3:350–354

[98]   Marais S, Van Toorn R, Chow FC, et al. Management of intracranial tuberculous mass lesions: how long should we treat for? Wellcome Open Res. 2019; 4. DOI: 10.12688/wellcomeopenres.15501.2

[99]   Salway RJ, Sangani S, Parekh S, et al. Tuberculoma-Induced Seizures. West J Emerg Med. 2015; 16:625–628

[100] Lee SA, Kim SW, Chang HH, et al. A New Scoring System for the Differential Diagnosis between Tuberculous Meningitis and Viral Meningitis. J Korean Med Sci. 2018; 33. DOI: 10.3346/jkms.2018.33.e201

[101] Marx GE, Chan ED. Tuberculous meningitis: diagnosis and treatment overview. Tuberc Res Treat. 2011; 2011. DOI: 10.1155/2011/798764

[102] Chin JH. Tuberculous meningitis: Diagnostic and therapeutic challenges. Neurol Clin Pract. 2014; 4:199–205

[103] Buonsenso D, Serranti D, Valentini P. Management of central nervous system tuberculosis in children: light and shade. Eur Rev Med Pharmacol Sci. 2010; 14:845–853

[104] Farinha NJ, Razali KA, Holzel H, et al. Tuberculosis of the central nervous system in children: a 20-year survey. J Infect. 2000; 41:61–68

[105] Pehlivanoglu F, Yasar KK, Sengoz G. Tuberculous meningitis in adults: a review of 160 cases. ScientificWorldJournal. 2012; 2012. DOI: 10.1100/2012/169028

[106] Pasco PM. Diagnostic features of tuberculous meningitis: a cross-sectional study. BMC Res Notes. 2012; 5. DOI: 10.1186/1756-0500-5-49

[107] Zou Y, Bu H, Guo L, et al. Staining with two observational methods for the diagnosis of tuberculous meningitis. Exp Ther Med. 2016; 12:3934–3940

[108] World Health Organization. Automated Real-Time Nucleic Acid Amplification Technology for Rapid and Simultaneous Detection of Tuberculosis and Rifampicin Resistance: Xpert MTB/RIF Assay for the Diagnosis of Pulmonary and Extrapulmonary TB in Adults and Children: Policy Update. Geneva 2013. https://www.ncbi.nlm.nih.gov/books/NBK258608/

[109] Alkabab YM, Enani MA, Indarkiri NY, et al. Performance of computed tomography versus chest radiography in patients with pulmonary tuberculosis with and without diabetes at a tertiary hospital in Riyadh, Saudi Arabia. Infect Drug Resist. 2018; 11:37–43

[110] Helmy A, Antoun N, Hutchinson P. Cerebral tuberculoma and magnetic resonance imaging. J R Soc Med. 2011; 104:299–301

[111] Kaojarern S, Supmonchai K, Phuapradit P, et al. Effect of steroids on cerebrospinal fluid penetration of antituberculous drugs in tuberculous meningitis. Clin Pharmacol Ther. 1991; 49:6–12

[112] Raberahona M, Rakotoarivelo RA, Razafinambinintsoa T, et al. Clinical Features and Outcome in Adult Cases of Tuberculous Meningitis in Tertiary Care Hospital in Antananarivo, Madagascar. Biomed Res Int. 2017; 2017. DOI: 10.1155/2017/9316589

[113] Luo M, Wang W, Zeng Q, et al. Tuberculous meningitis diagnosis and treatment in adults: A series of 189 suspected cases. Exp Ther Med. 2018; 16:2770–2776

[114] Bhargava S, Gupta AK, Tandon PN. Tuberculous meningitis–a CT study. Br J Radiol. 1982; 55:189–196

[115] Sharma D, Shah I, Patel S. Late onset hydrocephalus in children with tuberculous meningitis. J Family Med Prim Care. 2016; 5:873–874

[116] Palur R, Rajshekhar V, Chandy MJ, et al. Shunt surgery for hydrocephalus in tuberculous meningitis: a long-term follow-up study. J Neurosurg. 1991; 74:64–69

[117] Mathew JM, Rajshekhar V, Chandy MJ. Shunt surgery in poor grade patients with tuberculous meningitis and hydrocephalus: effects of response to external ventricular drainage and other variables on long term outcome. J Neurol Neurosurg Psychiatry. 1998; 65:115–118

[118] Yadav YR, Parihar VS, Todorov M, et al. Role of endoscopic third ventriculostomy in tuberculous meningitis with hydrocephalus. Asian J Neurosurg. 2016; 11:325–329

[119] Rajshekhar V. Management of hydrocephalus in patients with tuberculous meningitis. Neurol India. 2009; 57:368–374

[120] Aranha A, Choudhary A, Bhaskar S, et al. A Randomized Study Comparing Endoscopic Third Ventriculostomy versus Ventriculoperitoneal Shunt in the Management of Hydrocephalus Due to Tuberculous Meningitis. Asian J Neurosurg. 2018; 13:1140–1147

[121] Chugh A, Husain M, Gupta RK, et al. Surgical outcome of tuberculous meningitis hydrocephalus treated by endoscopic third ventriculostomy: prognostic factors and postoperative neuroimaging for functional assessment of ventriculostomy. J Neurosurg Pediatr. 2009; 3:371–377

[122] Murray HW, Brandstetter RD, Lavyne MH. Ventriculoatrial shunting for hydrocephalus complicating tuberculous meningitis. Am J Med. 1981; 70:895–898

[123] Bhagwati SN. Ventriculoatrial shunt in tuberculous meningitis with hydrocephalus. J Neurosurg. 1971; 35:309–313

[124] Kemaloglu S, Ozkan U, Bukte Y, et al. Timing of shunt surgery in childhood tuberculous meningitis with hydrocephalus. Pediatr Neurosurg. 2002; 37:194–198

[125] Lamprecht D, Schoeman J, Donald P, et al. Ventriculoperitoneal shunting in childhood tuberculous meningitis. Br J Neurosurg. 2001; 15:119–125

[126] Nelson CA, Zunt JR. Tuberculosis of the central nervous system in immunocompromised patients: HIV infection and solid organ transplant recipients. Clin Infect Dis. 2011; 53:915–926

[127] Ansari MK, Jha S. Tuberculous brain abscess in an immunocompetent adolescent. J Nat Sci Biol Med. 2014; 5:170–172

[128] Kumar R, Pandey CK, Bose N, et al. Tuberculous brain abscess: clinical presentation, pathophysiology and treatment (in children). Childs Nerv Syst. 2002; 18:118–123

[129] Wang Y, Li Q, Zhen X, et al. Immunologic Cerebral Vasculitis and Extrapulmonary Tuberculosis: An Uncommon Association. J Clin Diagn Res. 2015; 9: OD03–OD05

[130] Shukla R, Abbas A, Kumar P, et al. Evaluation of cerebral infarction in tuberculous meningitis by diffusion weighted imaging. J Infect. 2008; 57:298–306

[131] Li J, Afroz S, French E, et al. A Patient Presenting with Tuberculous Encephalopathy and Human Immunodeficiency Virus Infection. Am J Case Rep. 2016; 17:406–411

[132] Dev N, Bhowmick M, Chaudhary S, et al. Tuberculous encephalopathy without meningitis: A rare manifestation of disseminated tuberculosis. Int J Mycobacteriol. 2019; 8:406–408

[133] Lammie GA, Hewlett RH, Schoeman JF, et al. Tuberculous encephalopathy: a reappraisal. Acta Neuropathol. 2007; 113:227–234

[134] Kim HJ, Shim KW, Lee MK, et al. Tuberculous encephalopathy without meningitis: pathology and brain MRI findings. Eur Neurol. 2011; 65:156–159

[135] Nocton JJ, Steere AC. Lyme Disease. Advances in Internal Medicine. 1995; 40:69–117

[136] Pachner AR, Steere AC. The Triad of Neurologic Manifestations of Lyme Disease: Meningitis, Cranial Neuritis, and Radiculoneuritis. Neurology. 1985; 35:47–53

[137] Pachner AR, Duray P, Steere. Central Nervous System Manifestations of Lyme Disease. Arch Neurol. 1990; 46:790–795

[138] Steere AC, Schoen RT, Taylor E. The Clinical Evolution of Lyme Arthritis. Ann Intern Med. 1987; 107:735–731

[139] Centers for Disease Control. Lyme Disease – Connecticut. Morbidity and Mortality Weekly Report. 1988; 37:1–3

[140] Sigal LH. Lyme Disease Overdiagnosis: Cause and Cure. Hospital Practice. 1996; 31:13–15

[141] Weinstein A, Bujak Dl. Lyme Disease: A Review of its Clinical Features. NY State J Med. 1989; 89:566–571

[142] Magnarelli LA. Current Status of Laboratory Diagnosis for Lyme Disease. American Journal of Medicine. 1995; 98 (S4A):10–2S

[143] Wilkse B, Scheirz G, Preac-Mursic V, et al. Intrathecal Production of Specific Antibodies Against Borrelia burgdorferi in Patients with Lymphocytic Meningoradiculitis (Bannwarth's Syndrome). J Infect Dis. 1986; 153:304–314

[144] Henriksson A, Link H, Cruz M, et al. Immunoglobulin Abnormalities in Cerebrospinal Fluid and Blood Over the Course of Lymphocytic Meningoradiculitis (Bannwarth's Syndrome). Ann Neurol. 1986; 20:337–345

[145] Treatment of Lyme Disease. Medical Letter. 1988; 30:65–66

[146] Steere AC. Lyme Disease. New England Journal of Medicine. 1989; 321:586–596

[147] Byrne E, Brophy BP, Pettett LV. Nocardia Cerebral Abscess: New Concepts in Diagnosis, Management, and Prognosis. Journal of Neurology, Neurosurgery, and Psychiatry. 1979; 42:1038–1045

[148] Awad I, Bay JW, Petersen JM. Nocardial Osteomyelitis of the Spine with Epidural Spinal Cord Compression - A Case Report. Neurosurgery. 1984; 15:254–256

[149] Sorrell TC, Iredell JR, Mandell GL, et al. Principles and Practice of Infectious Diseases. 6th ed. Philadelphia: Elsevier; 2005

[150] Lerner PI. Nocardiosis. Clin Infect Dis. 1996; 22:891–903; quiz 904-5

21 Skull, Spine, and Post-Surgical Infections

21.1 Shunt infection

21.1.1 Epidemiology

Acceptable shunt infection rate[1]: < 5–7% (although many published series have a rate near 20%,[2] possibly due to different patient population).

Risk of early infection after shunt surgery: reported range is 3–20% per procedure (typically ≈ 7%).

Over 50% of staph infections occur within 2 weeks post-shunt, 70% within 2 mos. Source is often the patient's own skin.[1] It is estimated that in ≈ 3% of operations for shunt insertion the CSF is already infected (therefore CSF during shunt insertion is recommended).

21.1.2 Morbidity of shunt infections in children

Children with shunt infections have an increased mortality rate and risk of seizure than those without shunt infection. Those with myelomeningocele who develop ventriculitis after shunting have a lower IQ compared to those without infection.[3] Mortality ranges from 10–15%.

21.1.3 Risk factors for shunt infection

Many factors have been blamed. Some that seem to be better documented include:
- young age of patient[2]: in myelomeningocele (MM) patients, waiting until the child is 2 weeks old may significantly lower the infection rate
- length of procedure
- open neural tube defect

21.1.4 Pathogens

Early infection

Most commonly:
- Staph. epidermidis (coagulase-negative staph): 60–75% of infections (most common)
- S. aureus
- Gram-negative bacilli (GNB): 6–20% (may come from intestinal perforation)

In neonates E. coli and Strep. hemolyticus dominate.

Late infection (> 6 months after procedure)

Risk: 2.7–31% per patient (typically 6%). Almost all are S. epidermidis. 3.5% of patients account for 27% of infections.[4]

"Late" shunt infections may be due to:
- an indolent infection due to Staph. epidermidis
- seeding of a vascular shunt during episode of septicemia (probably very rare)
- colonization from an episode of meningitis

Fungal infections

Candida spp. infections

Candida spp. are responsible for the majority of fungal ventricular shunt infections. Usually occurs in children < 1 year of age. Incidence: 1–7%.[5] The 4th leading pathogen causing meningitis in neurosurgical patients in 1 study,[6] possibly related to the use of prophylactic antibiotics used for ICP monitoring and CSF drainage. Higher incidence in VP shunt patients with abdominal infections and shunts placed in patients with previous bacterial meningitis.[7] CSF typically shows: elevated WBCs and protein, normal glucose. Management recommendations:
1. completely remove the contaminated shunt (may be more important than with bacterial infections)

2. place a fresh external ventricular drain (if patient is shunt-dependent)
3. treat with antifungal therapy
4. place a fresh shunt after ≥ 5–7 days of therapy and clinical response is apparent
5. continue antifungal agents for 6–8 weeks

21.1.5 Presentation

Signs and symptoms

Non-specific syndrome: fever, N/V, H/A, lethargy, anorexia, irritability. May also present as shunt malfunction; 29% of patients presenting with shunt malfunction had positive cultures.

Erythema and tenderness along shunt tubing may occur.

Distal infection of ventriculoperitoneal shunts may mimic acute abdomen.

In neonates may manifest as apneic episodes, anemia, hepatosplenomegaly, and stiff neck.[8] S. epidermidis infections tend to be indolent (smoldering). GNB infections usually cause more severe illness; abdominal findings are more common; main clinical manifestation is fever, usually intermittent and low grade.

Shunt nephritis[9]: may occur with chronic low level infection of a ventriculovascular shunt, causing immune complex deposition in renal glomeruli, characterized by proteinuria and hematuria.

Blood tests

WBC: < 10K in one fourth of shunt infections. It is > 20K in one–third.

ESR: rarely normal in shunt infections.

Blood cultures: positive in less than one–third of cases.

CSF: WBC is usually not > 100 cells/mm^3. Gram stains may be positive ≈ 50% (yield with S. epidermidis is much lower). Protein is often elevated, glucose may be low or normal. Rapid antigen tests used for community acquired meningitis are usually not helpful for the organisms that tend to cause shunt infections. CSF cultures are negative in 40% of cases (higher culture yield if CSF WBC count is > 20K).

Evaluation of shunt for infection

1. history and physical directed at determining presence of above signs and symptoms with emphasis on
   a) history suggestive of infection at another site
      • exposure to others with viral syndromes, including sick siblings
      • GI source (e.g., acute gastroenteritis). Often associated with diarrhea.
      • otitis media (check tympanic membranes)
      • tonsillitis/pharyngitis
      • appendicitis (peritoneal inflammation may impede VP shunt outflow)
      • URI
      • UTI
      • pneumonia
   b) physical exam to R/O meningismus (stiff neck, photophobia…)
2. bloodwork
   a) serum WBC count with differential
   b) acute phase reactants: ESR & CRP
   c) blood cultures
3. shunt tap: should be done in cases of suspected shunt infection. Clip hair (do not shave) and prep carefully to avoid introducing infection. GNB requires different therapy and has higher morbidity than staph; thus it is desirable to identify these rare patients: > 90% of these had positive Gram-stained CSF smear (only a few Gram-positive infections have positive results). GNB have higher protein and lower glucose, and neutrophils predominate in differential (unpublished data[1])
4. imaging
   a) CT: usually not helpful for diagnosing infection. Ependymal enhancement when it occurs is diagnostic of ventriculitis. CT may demonstrate shunt malfunction
   b) abdominal U/S or CT: the presence of an abdominal pseudocyst is suggestive of infection
5. LP: usually NOT recommended. ✖ May be hazardous in obstructive hydrocephalus (HCP) with a nonfunctioning shunt. Often does not yield the pathogen even in communicating HCP, especially if the infection is limited to a ventriculitis. If positive, may obviate a shunt tap

21.1.6 Treatment

Antibiotics alone (without removal of shunt hardware)

Although eradication of shunt infections without removal of hardware has been reported,[10(p 595-7),11] this has a lower success rate than with shunt removal,[12] and may require protracted treatment (up to 45 days in some); risks problems associated with draining infected CSF into the peritoneum (reduced CSF absorption, abdominal signs/symptoms including tenderness to full-blown peritonitis[10(p 235)]) or vascular system—shunt nephritis (p. 372), sepsis…—and often requires at least partial shunt revision at some point in most cases. Treatment with antibiotics without shunt removal is therefore recommended only in cases where the patient is terminally ill, is a poor anesthetic risk, or has slit ventricles that might be difficult to catheterize.

Removal of shunt hardware

In most instances, during the initial treatment with antibiotics the shunt is either externalized (i.e., tubing is diverted at some point distal to the ventricular catheter and connected to a closed drainage system), or sometimes the entire shunt may be removed. In the latter case, some means of CSF drainage must be provided in shunt-dependent cases, either by insertion of an external ventricular drain (EVD), or by intermittent ventricular taps (rarely employed) or LPs (with communicating HCP). EVD allows easy monitoring of CSF flow, control of ICP, and repeated sampling for signs of resolution of infection (normalization of WBC count and surveillance cultures). In addition, EVD allows for possible administration of intrathecal antibiotics. In symptomatic patients or those with a positive CSF culture,[13] any hardware removed should be cultured, as only ≈ 8% are sterile in shunt infections. Skin organisms are fastidious and may take several days to grow.

If there is an abdominal pseudocyst, the fluid should be drained through the peritoneal catheter before removing it.

Antibiotics

Empiric antibiotics
See reference.[14]
1. vancomycin (adult) 15 mg/kg IV q 8–12 hours to achieve trough 15–20 mg/dl for MRSA coverage + cefepime 2 g IV q 8h or meropenem 2 g q 8h to cover gram-negative pathogens. Streamline therapy based on culture and sensitivity results
2. intraventricular injection of preservative-free antibiotics may be used in addition to IV therapy. Clamp EVD for one hour after injection

Treatment for specific organisms
Positive cultures from shunt hardware removed at the time of shunt revision in the absence of clinical symptoms or a positive CSF culture may be due to contamination and do not always require treatment.[13]
1. S. aureus and S. epidermidis
   a) if methicillin sensitive: nafcillin or oxacillin ± IT vancomycin
   b) if methicillin resistant: continue IV vancomycin + PO rifampin ± IT vancomycin
2. Enterococcus: IV ampicillin ± IT gent
3. other streptococci: either antistreptococcal or above enterococcal regimen
4. aerobic GNR: base on susceptibilities. Both IV beta-lactam & IT aminoglycoside indicated
5. Serratia marcescens: a rare cause of VP shunt infection[15] but the high morbidity may warrant aggressive antibiotic therapy (IV ceftriaxone + IT aminoglycoside) and surgical therapy
6. Corynebacterium spp. & Proprionibacterium spp. (diphtheroids)
   a) if PCN sensitive: use enterococcal regimen above
   b) if PCN resistant: IV + IT vancomycin
7. Candida spp.: see protocol and drugs (p. 343). Systemic antifungal therapy and removal of shunt is warranted. Avoid echinocandins (antifungal drugs that inhibit synthesis of glucan in the fungal cell wall) as they have poor CNS penetration

Subsequent management

Once the CSF is sterile × 3 days, convert the EVD to a shunt (if an EVD was not used, it is still recommended that the shunt be replaced with new hardware). Continue antibiotics an additional 10–14 days.

21

Managing ventriculoperitoneal shunts in patients with peritonitis

Peritonitis may occur as a result of:
1. perforation of a viscus (sometimes as a result of penetration by the peritoneal catheter tip,[16] more common with obsolete Raimondi wire-reinforced tubing)
2. spontaneous bacterial peritonitis (SBP): absence of an identifiable intra-abdominal source. Most commonly diagnosed in patients with cirrhotic ascites[17]
3. seeding through a VP shunt in a patient with a shunt infection: predominantly gram-positive, cutaneous organisms[18]

Concerns following an episode of peritonitis in a patient with VP shunt:
1. ascending infection into the CNS: uncommon, especially in the acute setting while on appropriate antibiotics with shunts containing a 1-way valve (as most do). CSF grows predominantly mixed, gram-negative intestinal flora[18]
2. contamination of the distal shunt: prevents permanent eradication of infection (appendicitis in the absence of peritonitis does not produce shunt infection[18])
3. shunt malfunction due to distal shunt obstruction: often as a result of walling off of the catheter tip, usually by omentum in reaction to the infection

Management recommendations following an episode of peritonitis (many viable options):
1. immediate appropriate treatment of peritonitis, usually managed by general surgeon (e.g., for ruptured appendix: appendectomy and appropriate antibiotics), with initial attempt to address shunt not being mandatory
2. anecdotally, cases have been managed successfully by cleaning off the peritoneal catheter with bacitracin solution, and then wrapping the catheter in a bacitracin-soaked lap sponge until the time comes to close the abdomen
3. if the peritonitis was diffuse or if the shunt catheter is believed to have been contaminated, an option is to externalize the distal catheter, preferably once the patient has stabilized from the peritonitis (afebrile, stable vital signs, normal WBC)
   a) externalization is done in a manner to avoid pulling the contaminated catheter up towards hopefully sterile portions of the shunt. This can be accomplished by reopening the skin incision used for inserting the peritoneal catheter, and making a second incision over the shunt tubing, well above this entry point. The catheter is then divided at the upper incision. The catheter is grasped at the lower incision and is pulled, extracting both ends (the peritoneal end and the end just cut). The remaining catheter coming from above is connected to an external drainage system
   b) CSF cultures are monitored daily
   c) if 3 consecutive cultures are negative, a new distal catheter may be implanted
   d) if cultures continuously grow organisms, then the shunt may be contaminated and should then be replaced with an entirely new shunt system
   e) when it is time to replace the shunt, some authors[19,20] recommend using an alternative site other than the peritoneum, but this is not mandatory[18]

21.2 External ventricular drain (EVD)-related infection

21.2.1 General information

Key concepts

- Common organisms: S. epidermidis and S. aureus followed by gram-negative bacilli and proprionibacterium acne.
- Diagnosis: Hypoglycorrhea (CSF glucose/Blood glucose < 0.2), rising cell index, and CSF pleocytosis > 1000 in the presence of positive CSF culture suggests EVD-related infection
- In CSF drain-related ventriculitis the diagnostic utility of CSF leucocyte count, glucose, and protein is limited, as noninfectious entities like intracranial hemorrhage and neurosurgical procedures can also cause abnormalities in these parameters.
- Management: remove EVD when clinically acceptable. Empiric coverage with IV vancomycin (for gram-positives) + IV ceftazidime or cefepime (for gram-negatives). Consider intraventricular/intrathecal antimicrobial for resistant organisms or non-responsiveness to IV antimicrobials.
- Prevention: antibiotic-coated catheters and catheter tunneling decrease infection rate.

21.2.2 Definitions

Suggested classification system and approach to a patient with suspected external ventricular drain (EVD) AKA ventriculostomy infection (modification of Lozier's definitions).[21]
- **cell index**, see Eq (21.1) [22,23]
- **contamination:** isolated positive CSF culture and/or Gram stain, with expected CSF cell count and glucose with NO attributable symptoms or signs.
- **ventriculostomy colonization:** Multiple positive CSF cultures and/or Gram stain, with expected CSF cell count and glucose levels with NO attributable symptoms or signs.
- **possible ventriculostomy-related infection:** Progressive rise in cell index or progressive decrease in CSF: blood glucose ratio or an extreme value for CSF WBC count (> 1000/micro L) or CSF:blood glucose ratio (< 0.2), with attributable symptoms and signs, but NEGATIVE Gram stain & cultures
- **probable ventriculostomy-related infection:** CSF WBC count or CSF:blood glucose ratio MORE abnormal than expected, but NOT an extreme value (CSF WBC count 1000/micro L or CSF:blood glucose ratio < 0.2) and stable (not progressively worsening) attributable symptoms and signs and POSITVE Gram stain & cultures
- **definitive meningitis:** Progressive rise in cell index or progressive decrease in CSF:blood glucose ratio or an extreme value for CSF WBC count (> 1000/micro L) or CSF:blood glucose ratio (< 0.2), with attributable symptoms or signs and a POSITIVE Gram stain & cultures

$$\text{Cell index} = \frac{Leucocytes\ (CSF)\ /\ Erythroctyes\ (CSF)}{Leucocytes\ (Blood)\ /\ Erythrocytes\ (Blood)} \tag{21.1}$$

21.2.3 Epidemiology

▶ **Incidence.** The incidence of EVD infection is approximately 9.5%.[24]

▶ **Risk factors.** Factors associated with EVD infections[21]:
- duration of EVD[21,25,26]
- site leakage
- blood in CSF (IVH and SAH)[27]
- irrigation and flushing[25,26]

21.2.4 Microbiology

- unlike organisms that cause acute community-acquired meningitis, those causing neurosurgical procedure-related meningitis are slow to grow on cultures and may require anaerobic media.
- the usual organisms that cause EVD-related infections are either:
  - organisms that usually colonize the skin, especially the scalp (coagulase negative Staphylococcus, Staphylococcus aureus, and Propionibacterium acnes).
  - organisms that can be present in the healthcare environment: S. aureus, both methicillin-sensitive and -resistant, gram-negative bacteria like E. coli, Klebsiella, pseudomonas, and Acinitobacter species, some of which can be multi-drug resistant.
- infectious organisms can form a polysaccharide layer (biofilm) on the surface of catheters, which increases the resistance to antimicrobials.

21.2.5 Clinical presentation

Clinical signs and symptoms may include the following; however, these symptoms are nonspecific as they are commonplace in the neuro-ICU as a result of the underlying pathology (e.g., intracranial hemorrhage or hydrocephalus)[28]
- change in mental status
- fever: alternative sources of fever may include intracranial hemorrhage, central fever, thrombotic episodes, and drug fevers, in addition to non-CNS infection like blood-borne infections, hospital-acquired pneumonias, and urinary tract infections
- meningismus: stiff neck, Brudzinski or Kernig sign.

21.2.6 Diagnosis

▶ **Blood parameters.** These parameters can suggest the diagnosis but should not be relied upon exclusively.
- a prospective study showed likely EVD infections in the presence of these parameters[29]: peripheral WBC count > 15 in EVD infections (vs. < 11 in non-infected)
- serum inflammatory markers: there is very limited literature on the diagnostic utility of ESR and CRP. Procalcitonin alone was found not to be helpful.[30]

▶ **CSF parameters.** There are limited studies on the diagnostic accuracy of CSF parameters in post-craniotomy meningitis and ventriculitis. Sometimes the surgery itself may produce "chemical meningitis (p. 342)." The following could help in confirming underlying EVD infection.
- hypoglycorrhachia (low CSF glucose): ratio of [CSF glucose]/[blood glucose] < 0.2
- CSF pleocytosis > 1000 or rising cell index (p. 375)
- CSF protein was not a reliable predictor for incipient ventricular catheter infection[31]

Routine CSF sampling: CSF sampling should be performed only when symptoms appear. There is no evidence of benefit to obtaining CSF cultures or cell count at the time of EVD insertion (false positive cultures may occur from contamination).[32]

21.2.7 Principles of management

- it is difficult to achieve high CSF antimicrobial levels due to blood-CSF barrier
- some hospital-acquired organisms have higher MICs (minimal inhibitory concentration) for antimicrobials than community-acquired organisms
- organisms often form biofilms on the catheters which resist antimicrobial penetration. For this reason, catheter should be removed if it is safe to do so
- empiric antibiotics: initiate if ventriculitis is suspected once the appropriate sampling has been obtained
  - if no penicillin allergy:
    - vancomycin as a continuous infusion or divided doses (2–3) of 60 mg per kg of body weight per day after a loading dose of 15 mg per kg of body weight, aiming for trough (15–25 mcg/ml) PLUS
    - ceftazidime 2 g IV q 8 hrs or cefepime 2 g IV q 8 hrs
  - for penicillin allergy:
    - vancomycin as a continuous infusion or divided doses (2–3) of 60 mg per kg of body weight per day after a loading dose of 15 mg per kg of body weight PLUS
    - meropenem 2 g IV q 8 hrs or aztreonam 2 g IV q 6 hrs
- switch to more selective agents as appropriate, based on culture and susceptibility when they become available (see ▶ Table 21.1)
- duration of treatment should be individualized to the patient, but as a rule of thumb: treat for 2 weeks if the infection was with S. aureus and S. epidermidis, and 3 weeks if it was gram-negative[33]

Table 21.1 Selective antibacterial agents (based on culture and susceptibility)

Bacteria	Specific antimicrobial regimen
MRSA and MRSE (with an MIC ≤ 1 mcg/ml)	Vancomycin continuous infusion or divided doses (2–3/d) of 60 mg per kg of body weight per day after a loading dose of 15 mg per kg of body weight. If the catheter is retained, can add rifampin 300 mg IV q 12 hrs
MRSA and MRSE (with MIC > 1 mcg/ml) or patient with vancomycin allergy	Linezolid 600 mg IV or PO q 12 hrs
MSSA and MSSE	Nafcillin 2 g IV q 4 hrs
Propionobacter acne	Penicillin G 2 MU IV q 4 hrs
Pseudomonas	Ceftazidime 2 g IV q 8 hrs, Cefepime 2 g IV q 8 hrs, or Meropenem 2 g q 8 hrs
E. coli or other enterobacteriaceae	Ceftriaxone 2 g IV q 12 hrs or meropenem 2 g IV q 8 hrs
Enterobacter or Citrobacter	Cefepime 2 g IV q 8 hrs or meropenem 2 g IV q 8 hrs

- failing to respond to systemic treatment or infection with a resistant organism might require intrathecal/intraventricular antibiotic administration. Choose the antimicrobial based on susceptibility. Dosages for intraventricular antibiotics:
  - vancomycin: 5 mg for slit ventricles, 10 mg with normal-sized ventricles, 15–20 mg for patients with enlarged ventricles
  - aminoglycoside: Dosing can also be tailored to ventricular size. Frequency can be adjusted based on drain output as well: once daily for drain output > 100 ml/day, every other day if drain output = 50–100 ml/day, every third day if drainage < 50 ml/day
    - gentamicin: 4–8 mg
    - tobramycin: 5–20 mg
    - amikacin: 5–30 mg
  - colistimethate sodium: 10 mg CMS, which is 125,000 IU or 3.75 mg CBA (Colistin Base units)
  - daptomycin: 2–5 mg
- after IT administration of an antimicrobial, clamp the drain for 15–60 minutes to allow the antimicrobial concentration to equilibrate in the CSF before opening the drain[34]
- expert opinion: wait at least 7–10 days after the CSF cultures become sterile to implant a shunt if needed

21.2.8 Prevention

- tunneling > 5 cm away from the burr hole[35]
- antibiotic coated catheters (e.g., Rifampin + minocycline) significantly reduce the risk of EVD infection[36,37,38,39,40]
- routine catheter exchange at day 5 *did not* show reduction in the rate of infection[41,42,43] Therefore a single catheter may be employed as long as clinically required.[44]
- prolonged antibiotic prophylaxis while the EVD is in place does not decrease the risk of infection and may select for resistant organisms. *However one dose pre-procedure antimicrobial may be administered*

21.3 Wound infections

21.3.1 Laminectomy wound infection

General information

Occurs in 0.9–5% of cases.[45] May range from superficial to severe dehiscent wound infection to deeper infection (discitis/osteomyelitis ± epidural abscess). The risk is increased with age, long term steroid use, obesity, and possibly DM. Intraoperative mild hypothermia (as commonly occurs in the operating room) may also increase the risk of wound infection (as demonstrated with colorectal resection[46]). Most are caused by *S. aureus*.

Superficial wound infection

Management
1. culture the wound and/or any purulent drainage
2. start the patient empirically on vancomycin plus cefepime or meropenem
3. modify antibiotics appropriately when culture and sensitivity results available
4. debride wound of all necrotic and devascularized tissue and any visible suture material (foreign bodies). Superficial wound infections may be debrided in the office or treatment room, deep infections must be done in OR
5. shallow defects may be allowed to heal by secondary intention, and the following is one possible regimen
   a) pack the wound defect with 1/4" Iodophor® gauze
   b) dressing changes at least BID (for hospitalized patients, change q 8 hrs), remove and trim ≈ 0.5–1" of packing with each dressing change
      - while wound is purulent, utilize 1/2 strength Betadine® wet to dry dressings
      - when purulence subsides, switch to normal saline wet to dry
   c) antibiotics, may be useful as an adjunct to wound treatment initially, switch to oral antibiotics as early as possible, a duration of 10–14 days total is probably adequate if local wound care is being done
6. some prefer to close wound by primary intention,[47] it is critical that there be no tension on the wound for healing to occur. Some close over an irrigation system or antibiotic beads. Retention sutures may be helpful[48]

7. with large defects or when bone and/or dura becomes exposed, the use of a muscle flap (often performed by a plastic surgeon) is probably required[45]
8. CSF leakage requires exploration in the OR with watertight dural closure to prevent meningitis

Postoperative discitis

Epidemiology
Incidence after lumbar discectomy[49]: 0.2–4% (realistic estimate is probably at the lower end of this range). May also occur after LP, myelogram, cervical laminectomy, lumbar sympathectomy, discography, fusions (with or without instrumentation) and other procedures. Very rare after ACDF. Risk factors include advanced age, obesity, immunosuppression, systemic infection at the time of surgery.

Pathophysiology
There is some controversy as to whether some cases of post-op discitis are not infectious,[50] an autoimmune process has been implicated in some of these so-called "avascular" or "chemical" or "aseptic" discitis cases. These cases are less common than infectious ones. ESR and CRP abnormalities may be less pronounced in these patients, and biopsy of the disc space fails to grow organisms or show signs of infection (infiltrates of lymphocytes or PMNS) on microscopy.[50]

In septic cases, various mechanisms for infection have been proposed: direct inoculation at the time of surgery, infection following aseptic necrosis of disc material…

Pathogens
See ▶ Table 21.2. Most studies report *S. aureus* as the most commonly identified organism, accounting for ≈ 60% of positive cultures,[49] followed by other staph species. Also reported: Gram-negative organisms (including E. coli), Strep viridans, Streptococcus species anaerobes, TB and fungi. Enteric flora in post-op discitis may be due to unrecognized breach of the anterior longitudinal ligament with bowel perforation.

Blood cultures were positive in 2 of 6 patients (both *S. aureus*) in one series.[51]

For culture techniques, see surgical management section below.

Table 21.2 Culture results (14 patients, Craig needle biopsy)

Organism	No. of patients
Staphylococcus epidermidis	4
S. aureus	3
No growth	7

Clinical
1. interval from operation to onset of symptoms: 3 days to 8 mos (most commonly 1–4 wks post-op, usually after an initial period of pain relief and recovery from surgery). 80% present by 3 wks
2. symptoms:
   a) moderate to (usually) severe back pain at the site of operation was the most common symptom, exacerbated by virtually any motion of the spine, often accompanied by paraspinal muscle spasms. Back pain is usually out of proportion to the findings
   b) fever (> 38 °C in 9 patients; literature reports only 30–50% are febrile) and chills
   c) pain radiating to hip, leg, scrotum, groin, abdomen or perineum (true sciatica is uncommon)
3. signs: in 27 patients,[51] all had paravertebral muscle spasm and limited range of motion of the spine. 13 (48%) were virtually immobilized by pain. Point tenderness over the infected level occurred in 9, expressible pus in 2 (literature reports 0–8%). No new neurologic deficits were noted. Only 10–12% have associated wound infection[52]
4. lab findings:
   a) ESR: in a series of 27 patients,[51] 96% had ESR > 20 mm/hr (60 = ave.; > 40 in 17 patients; > 100 in 5 patients; the single patient < 20 was on steroids). ESR increases after uncomplicated discectomy, peaking at 2–5 days, and can fluctuate for 3–6 weeks before normalizing.[53] An elevated ESR that never decreases after surgery is a strong indicator of discitis. NB: ESR in anemic patients is unreliable and no reference range can be established (use CRP in these cases)
   b) *C-reactive protein* (CRP)[53]: an acute phase protein synthesized by hepatocytes that because of rapid decomposition may be a more specific indicator of post-op infection than ESR. Values vary from lab to lab, but CRP is normally not detectable in the blood (i.e., < 0.6 mg/dl = 6 mg/L).

After uncomplicated discectomy (i.e., in the absence of discitis), CRP peaks ≈ 2–3 days post-op (to 4.6 ± 2.1 mg/dl after lumbar microdiscectomy, 9.2 ± 4.7 after conventional lumbar discectomy, 7.0 ± 2.3 after anterior lumbar fusion, and 17.3 ± 3.9 after PLIF), and returns to normal between 5 and 14 days post-op

c) *WBC*: > 10,000 in only 8/27 patients[51] (prevalence in literature: 18–30%)

Radiographic evaluation

In postoperative discitis (POD), the average time from surgery to changes on plain X-ray is 3 mos (range: 1–8 mos). Average time from first change to spontaneous spinal fusion: 2 yrs.

MRI: The triad of gadolinium enhancement shown in ▶ Table 21.3 is strongly suggestive of discitis (some asymptomatic patients may have some of these findings, but they rarely have all).[54]

MRI also rules out other causes of post-op pain (epidural abscess, recurrent/residual disc herniation…).

Table 21.3 Gadolinium enhancement in discitis

Location of gadolinium enhancement	Number (out of 15 post-op patients without discitis)	Number (out of 7 patients with discitis)
1. vertebral bone marrow	1	7
2. disc space	3	5
3. posterior annulus fibrosus	13	7

Management

1. initial labs (in addition to routine): ESR, C-reactive protein, CBC, blood cultures
2. analgesics + muscle relaxants (e.g., diazepam (Valium®) 10 mg PO TID)
3. antibiotics:
   a) IV antibiotics for 1–6 wks then PO for 1–6 mos
   b) most start with anti-staphylococcal antibiotics (initial empiric therapy: vancomycin ± PO rifampin) and cefepime or meropenem. Modify based on sensitivities if positive cultures are obtained
   c) duration of therapy depends on depth of infection and presence of hardware
      • superficial infection: 1–2 weeks
      • deep infection 4–8 weeks, possibly up to 12 weeks in complex cases
      • consider chronic PO therapy if hardware not removed
4. activity restriction (one of the following used, usually until significant pain relief):
   a) spinal immobilization with brace
   b) strict bed rest
   c) advance activity with brace as tolerated
5. some authors recommend steroid therapy initially to assist pain relief
6. cultures: performed if radiographs suspicious, usually performed utilizing percutaneous CT-guided technique
   a) sites
      • disc aspiration if evidence of disc space involvement
      • needling of paraspinal mass if present
   b) send culture for the following
      • Stains: (a) Gram stain (b) fungal stain (c) AFB stain
      • Cultures: (a) routine cultures: aerobic and anaerobic; (b) fungal culture: this is not only helpful for fungus, but since these cultures are kept for longer period and any growth that occurs will be further characterized, fastidious or indolent bacterial organisms may sometimes be identified; (c) AFB (TB) culture
7. 3 out of 27 patients underwent anterior discectomy and fusion after unsuccessful medical therapy[51]

Outcome

9 patients developed bony bridging in 12–18 mos; 10 developed bony fusion in 18–24 mos.[51]

All patients eventually become pain free (or significantly improve). This is not the case in all series, where some report 60% were pain free at F/U, others found slight back pain in most patients, and yet others report severe chronic LBP in 75%.[49] 67–88% returned to their previous work, and 12–25% received disability pension; these numbers are similar to the outcome from disc surgery in general.

No difference in outcome was found for the various activity restrictions specified, except for earlier pain relief with first two types listed above.

21.3.2 Craniotomy wound infection

Also, see under meningitis, post-neurosurgical procedure (p. 340).

C-reactive protein

Following uncomplicated craniotomy for microsurgery for brain tumors, C-reactive protein (CRP) peaked on post-op day (POD) 2 with a mean value of 32 ± 38 mg/l.[55] Values declined from POD 3 through 5, reaching a mean of 6.7 ± 11 on POD 5. These values may be lower than with most post-op infections.

21.4 Osteomyelitis of the skull

21.4.1 General information

The skull is normally very resistant to osteomyelitis, and hematogenous infection is rare. Most infections are due to contiguous spread (usually from an infected air sinus, occasionally from scalp abscess) or to penetrating trauma (including surgery and fetal scalp monitors[56]). With long-standing infection, edema and swelling in the area may become visible (usually over the forehead, but also may occur over the mastoids), and is called "Pott puffy tumor" (after Percival Pott).

21.4.2 Pathogens

Staphylococcus is the most common organism, with S. aureus predominating, followed by S. epidermidis. In neonates, E. coli may be the infecting organism.

21.4.3 Imaging

Imaging findings may include: bony resorption, periosteal reaction, contrast enhancement.

21.4.4 Treatment

Antibiotics alone are rarely curative. Treatment usually involves surgical debridement of infected skull, biting off infected bone with rongeurs until a normal snapping sound replaces the more muted sound made by rongeuring infected bone. In the case of an infected craniotomy bone flap, the flap usually must be removed and discarded, and the edges of the skull rongeured back to healthy bone. Bone suspected of infection should be sent for cultures.

Closure of the scalp is then performed either leaving a bone defect (for later cranioplasty) or cranioplasty can be performed using titanium mesh.

Debridement surgery is followed by at least 6–12 weeks of antibiotics.[57] Until MRSA is ruled out: vancomycin + cefepime or meropenem. Culture results guide choice of antibiotic. Once MRSA is ruled out, vancomycin may be changed to a penicillinase-resistant synthetic penicillin (e.g., nafcillin). Most treatment failures occurred in patients treated with < 4 weeks of antibiotics following surgery.

Cranioplasty may be performed ≈ 6 months post-op if there are no signs of residual infection.

21.5 Spine infections

21.5.1 General information

Spine infections may be divided into the following major categories:
1. vertebral osteomyelitis (p. 386) (spondylitis):
   a) pyogenic
   b) nonpyogenic, granulomatous
      - tuberculous spondylitis (p. 387) (Pott's disease)
      - brucellosis
      - aspergillosis
      - blastomycosis
      - coccidiomycosis
      - infection with Candida tropicalis

2. discitis (p. 390): usually associated with vertebral osteomyelitis (spondylodiscitis) (p. 386)
   a) spontaneous
   b) postoperative/post-procedure
3. spinal epidural abscess (p. 381)
4. spinal subdural empyema
5. meningitis
6. spinal cord abscess

MRI experience suggests that patients with infectious spondylitis will develop an associated epidural abscess if untreated, and that epidural empyema is unusual in the absence of vertebral osteomyelitis.[58] Thus, the discovery of one of these conditions should prompt a search for the other.

21.5.2 Spinal epidural abscess

General information

Key concepts

- should be considered in a patient with back pain, fever, and spine tenderness
- major risk factors: diabetes, IV drug abuse, chronic renal failure, alcoholism, previous spine surgery
- may produce progressive myelopathy, sometimes with precipitous deterioration, therefore early surgery has been advocated by some even if no neuro deficit
- fever, sweats, or rigors are common, but normal WBC and temperature can occur
- classical presentation of a skin boil (furuncle) occurs in only ≈ 15% somewhere on the body
- treatment: controversial. Many patients improve with antibiotics alone, but some may deteriorate precipitously

Epidemiology

Incidence: 0.2–1.2 per 10,000 hospital admissions annually,[59] possibly on the rise.[60] Average age: 57.5 ± 16.6 years.[61]

Thoracic level is the most common site (≈ 50%), followed by lumbar (35%) then cervical (15%).[61] 82% were posterior to the cord, and 18% anterior in one series.[59] SEA may span from 1 to 13 levels.[62]

Spinal epidural abscess (SEA) is often associated with vertebral osteomyelitis (in one series of 40 cases, osteomyelitis occurred in all cases of anterior SEA, in 85% of circumferential SEA, and no cases of posterior SEA) and intervertebral discitis.

Co-morbid conditions

Chronic diseases associated with compromised immunity were identified in 65% of 40 cases.[63] Associated conditions included diabetes mellitus (32%), IV drug abuse (18%), chronic renal failure (12%), alcoholism (10%), and the following in only 1 or 2 patients: cancer, recurrent UTI, Pott's disease, and positivity for HIV. Chronic steroid use and recent spinal procedure or trauma (e.g., GSW) are also risk factors.[62] Skin infection (e.g., furuncle).

Clinical features

Usually presents with excruciating pain localized over spine with tenderness to percussion. Radicular symptoms follow with subsequent distal cord findings, often beginning with bowel/bladder disturbance, abdominal distension, weakness progressing to para- and quadriplegia. Average time is 3 days from back pain to root symptoms; 4.5 days from root pain to weakness; 24 hrs from weakness to paraplegia.

Fever, sweats or rigors are common, but are not always present.[62]

A furuncle (skin boil) somewhere on the body may be identified in 15%.

Patients may be encephalopathic. This may range from mild to severe and may further delay diagnosis. Meningismus (p. 1419) with a positive Kernig sign may occur.

Patients with postoperative SEA may demonstrate surprisingly few signs or symptoms (including lack of leukocytosis, lack of fever) aside from local pain.[64]

Pathophysiology of spinal cord dysfunction

Although some cord symptoms may be due to mechanical compression (including that due to vertebral body collapse), this is not always found.[65] A vascular mechanism has also been postulated, and various combinations of arterial and venous pathology have been described[59] (one autopsy series showed little arterial compromise, but did show venous compression and thrombosis, thrombophlebitis of epidural veins, and venous infarction and edema of the spinal cord[66]). Occasionally, there may be infection of the spinal cord itself, possibly by extension through the meninges.

Differential diagnosis

SEA should be considered in any patient with backache, fever, and spine tenderness,[67] especially diabetics, IV drug abusers or immunocompromised patients. Also see Differential diagnosis, Myelopathy (p. 1696).

Differential diagnosis:
1. meningitis
2. acute transverse myelitis (paralysis is usually more rapid, radiographic studies are normal)
3. intervertebral disc herniation
4. spinal cord tumors
5. post-op SEA may appear similar to pseudomeningocele[64]

Source site of infection

1. hematogenous spread is the most common source (26–50% of cases) either to the epidural space or to the vertebra with extension to epidural space. Reported foci include:
   a) skin infections (most common): furuncle may be found in 15% of cases
   b) parenteral injections, especially with *IV drug abuse*[68]
   c) bacterial endocarditis
   d) UTI
   e) respiratory infection (including otitis media, sinusitis, or pneumonia)
   f) pharyngeal or dental abscess
2. direct extension from:
   a) decubitus ulcer
   b) psoas abscess (p. 393)
   c) penetrating trauma, including abdominal wounds, neck wounds, GSW
   d) pharyngeal infections
   e) mediastinitis
   f) pyelonephritis with perinephric abscess
   g) dermal sinus
3. following spinal procedures (3 of 8 of these patients had readily identified perioperative infections of periodonta, UTI, or AV-fistula[63])
   a) open procedures: especially lumbar discectomy (incidence[64] ≈ 0.67%)
   b) closed procedures: e.g., epidural catheter insertion for spinal epidural anesthesia,[69,70,71] lumbar puncture[72]…
4. a history of recent back trauma is common (in up to 30%)
5. no source can be identified in up to 50% of patients in some series[73]

Organisms

Operative cultures are most useful in identifying the responsible organism, these cultures may be negative (possibly more common in patients previously on antibiotics) and in these cases blood cultures may be positive. No organism may be identified in 29–50% of cases.
1. *Staph. aureus*: the most common organism (cultured in > 50%) possibly due to its propensity to form abscesses, its ubiquity, and its ability to infect normal and immunocompromised hosts (these facts help explain why many SEA arise from skin foci)
2. aerobic and anaerobic streptococcus: second most common
3. E.coli
4. Pseudomonas aeruginosa
5. Diplococcus pneumoniae
6. Serratia marcescens
7. Enterobacter
8. chronic infections:

a) TB is the most common of these, and although it has become less widespread in the U.S. it is still responsible for 25% of cases of SEA,[74] it is usually associated with vertebral osteomyelitis, see Pott's disease (p. 387)
b) brucellosis
c) fungal: cryptococcosis, aspergillosis
d) parasitic: Echinococcus
9. multiple organisms in ≈ 10%
10. anaerobes cultured in ≈ 8%

Laboratory tests

CBC: leukocytosis common in acute group (average WBC = 16,700/mm³), but usually normal in chronic (ave. WBC = 9,800/mm³).[59]

ESR elevated in most,[75] usually > 30,[63] CRP.

LP: performed cautiously in suspected cases at a level distant to the clinically suspected site (C1–2 puncture may be needed to do myelogram) with constant aspiration while approaching thecal sac to detect pus (danger of transmitting infection to subarachnoid space); if pus is encountered, stop advancing, send the fluid for culture, and abort the procedure. CSF protein & WBC usually elevated; glucose normal (indicative of parameningeal infection). 5 of 19 cases grew organisms identical to abscess.

Blood cultures: may be helpful in identifying organism in some cases.

Anergy battery: (e.g., mumps and Candida) to assess immune system.

Radiographic studies

Plain films

Usually normal unless there is osteomyelitis of adjacent vertebral bodies (more common in infections anterior to dura). Look for lytic lesions, demineralization, and scalloping of endplates (may take 4–6 weeks after onset of infection).

MRI

Imaging study of choice. Differentiates other conditions (especially transverse myelitis or spinal cord infarction) better than myelo/CT, and doesn't require LP.

Typical findings: T1WI → hypo- or isointense epidural mass, vertebral osteomyelitis shows up as reduced signal in bone. T2WI → high intensity epidural mass that often enhances with gadolinium (3 patterns of enhancement: 1) dense homogeneous, 2) inhomogeneous with scattered areas of sparse or no uptake, and 3) thin peripheral enhancement[76]) but may show minimal enhancement in the acute stage when comprised primarily of pus with little granulation tissue. Vertebral osteomyelitis shows up as increased signal in bone, associated discitis produces increased signal in disc and loss of intranuclear cleft. Unenhanced MRI may miss some SEA,[77] gadopentetate dimeglumine enhancement may slightly increase sensitivity.[78]

Myelogram-CT

Usually shows findings of extradural compression (e.g., "paintbrush appearance" when complete block is present). In the event of complete block, C1–2 puncture may be needed to delineate upper extent (unless post-myelographic CT shows dye above the lesion). See cautions above regarding LP.

CT scan

Intraspinal gas has been described on plain CT.[79] Post-myelographic CT is more sensitive.

Biopsy

Image guided needle aspiration to identify infecting organism(s). Usually done percutaneously with local anesthesia. May be performed by interventional radiologist or spine surgeon.

Treatment

General information

Controversial, including surgical vs. nonsurgical management. In most cases, treatment consists of early surgical evacuation combined with antibiotics as the treatment of choice. Argument: although there are reports of management with antibiotics alone[80,81,82] ± immobilization,[58] rapid and irreversible deterioration has occurred even in patients treated with appropriate antibiotics who were initially neurologically intact.[61,63] 86% of those who deteriorated were initially treated with antibiotics alone.[62] Therefore it has been recommended that nonsurgical management be reserved for the following patients (reference[80] modified[62]):

1. those with prohibitive operative risk factors
2. involvement of an extensive length of the spinal canal
3. complete paralysis for > 3 days

To add to the complexity, in many cases, at the time of surgery, instead of a true abscess, inflammatory tissue that is not easily or effectively debrided is encountered.

Surgery

▶ **Surgical indications**

1. open biopsy
2. progression of infection or failure of infectious markers (CRP, ESR...) to trend towards normal, despite antibiotic therapy (failure of conservative management)
3. neurologic deficit
4. epidural abscess with neural element compression
5. instability: due to tumor or iatrogenic
6. deformity correction or prevention

▶ **Surgical goals.** Goals are establishing diagnosis and causative organism, drainage of pus and debridement of granulation tissue, and bony stabilization if necessary.

▶ **Surgical considerations.** Most SEA are posterior to the dura and are approached with extensive laminectomy. Alternatively, skip laminectomies may be used (leaving one or several intact levels between laminectomies and irrigating between open levels using e.g., a red rubber catheter). For posteriorly located SEA with no evidence of vertebral osteomyelitis, instability will usually not follow simple laminectomy and appropriate postoperative antibiotics.[73] Thorough antibiotic irrigation is employed intraoperatively. Primary closure is often employed. Post-op drainage is not necessary in cases with only granulation tissue and no pus. For recurrent infections, reoperation and post-op suction-irrigation may be needed.[83]

Patients with associated osteomyelitis of the vertebral body may develop instability after laminectomy alone,[84] especially if significant bony destruction is present. Thus for anterior SEA, usually with osteomyelitis (especially Pott's disease), a posterolateral extracavitary approach is utilized whenever possible (to avoid transabdominal or transthoracic approach in these debilitated patients) with removal of devitalized bone usually followed by posterior instrumentation and fusion. Strut grafting with autologous bone (rib or fibula) can be done acutely in Pott's disease with little risk of graft infection.

Surgical instrumentation: With purulent osteomyelitis, metal hardware is not contraindicated (titanium is more resistant to harboring bacteria than stainless steel for several reasons, including the fact that titanium does not permit bacteria to form a glycocalyx on its surface), but bone grafting may run the risk of perpetuating the infection. In this situation, some surgeons use beads of calcium sulfate bone void filler impregnated with antibiotic (e.g., Stimulan® Rapid Cure™ antibiotic beads). Instrumentation has been shown to be effective and safe when used in conjunction with a prolonged course of antibiotics.[85]

Specific antibiotics

If organism and source unknown, S. aureus most likely. Empiric antibiotics:

- Ceftriaxone or cefepime (use when pseudomonas is a concern)
  PLUS
- metronidazole
  PLUS
- vancomycin:
  ○ until methicillin resistant S. aureus (MRSA) can be ruled out
  ○ once MRSA is ruled out switch to synthetic penicillin (e.g., nafcillin or oxacillin)
- ± rifampin PO

Modify antibiotics based on culture results or knowledge of source (e.g., IV drug abusers have a higher incidence of Gram-negative organisms).

Duration of treatment

For spinal epidural abscess (SEA), treatment should continue for a minimum of 6 weeks. Longer therapy may be warranted in complicated infections and for patients who have spinal implants or hardware. Immobilization for at least 6 weeks during antibiotic therapy is recommended.

Outcome

Fatal in 4–31%[86] (the higher end of the range tends to be in older patients and in those paralyzed before surgery[63]). Patients with severe neurologic deficit rarely improve, even with surgical intervention within 6–12 hrs of onset of paralysis, although a few series have shown a chance for some recovery with treatment within 36 hrs of paralysis.[67,87] Reversal of paralysis of caudal spinal cord segments if present for more than a few hours is rare (exception: Pott's disease has 50% return). Mortality is usually due to original focus of infection or as a complication of residual paraplegia (e.g., pulmonary embolism).

21.5.3 Spinal subdural empyema (AKA spinal subdural abscess)

General information

A rare infection of the space between the dura and arachnoid membranes of the spine. May be primary, or may be an exension of intracranial subdural empyema (p. 350). It is so uncommon that no large case series have been reported.[88]

Based on a literature review of 70 cases,[89] spinal levels involved in decreasing frequency are: lumbar (53%), thoracic (43%), cervical (37%) and sacral (11%). Multiple spinal areas may be involved as there is essentially no barrier to spread in the subarachnoid space. Adjacent structures such as vertebral bodies and psoas muscles may become involved.

Clinical

Patients often present with fever, back pain and radiculopathy. In contrast to spinal epidural abscess, spinal tenderness is less common, being described in only 23%.[89]

Neurologic deficit (motor and/or sensory) is reported in 74%.

Etiologies

The source of infection is hematogenous (43%), contiguous spread (28%).

Infectious routes mechanisms: IV drug abuse, 25% of cases were iatrogenic, most commonly following lumbar puncture including blood patch for CSF leak.

Comorbidities that may increase the risk of developing SSDE: DM, HIV, dermal sinus tracts, Crohn's disease, pneumonia.

Staphylococcus aureus is the most common bacterial species. Streptococcus is second most common. Polymicrobial infections are also common.

Diagnostics

Labs: 57% had leukocytosis.[89]

MRI without and with contrast is the optimal imaging modality.

Treatment

For symptomatic collections, urgent surgical intervention with laminectomy and durotomy with washout is recommended, followed by appropriate IV antibiotics. Antibiotic treatment alone may be considered for small asymptomatic collections that are too small to drain:[88] these may be monitored closely with serial imaging and neuro exams (infection progresses at a faster rate than most neoplasms).

Antibiotics are essential. Levels within the emypema are not well studied. Penetration into CSF is also important due to the high incidence of associated meningitis.

Outcome

Reported mortality of surgically treated SSDE is 13%, vs. 43% in patients treated only medically[89] (not statistically significant because data is retrospective observational).

21

21.5.4 Vertebral osteomyelitis

General information

Key concepts

- presentation and risk factors similar to spinal epidural abscess (p. 381)
- percutaneous needle biopsy (typically CT-guided) for C&S and to rule out tumor; can usually be done by neurosurgeon or interventional radiologist
- treatment: most cases can be managed nonsurgically with long-term antibiotics
- surgery is considered for instability, and infrequently for severe resistance to Abx

For differential diagnosis, see Destructive lesions of the spine (p. 1679). Often associated with discitis, which may be grouped together under the term spondylodiscitis. VO has features similar to spinal epidural abscess (SEA) (p. 381).

Vertebral body collapse and kyphotic deformity may occur with possible retropulsion of necrotic bone and disc fragments, compressing the spinal cord or cauda equina.

Complications that may accrue:

1. spinal epidural abscess (SEA) (p. 381)
2. subdural abscess
3. meningitis
4. bony instability
5. progressive neurologic impairment
6. unique to cervical spine involvement: pharyngeal abscess
7. unique to thoracic spine involvement: mediastinitis

Epidemiology

Vertebral osteomyelitis (VO) comprises 2–4% of all cases of osteomyelitis.[90] Incidence is 1:250,000 in general population. Incidence appears to be rising. Male:female ratio is 2:1. Incidence increases with age; most patients are > 50 years old. The lumbar spine is the most common site, followed by thoracic, cervical and sacrum.[91] Thoracic VO may → empyema.

Risk factors

1. IV drug abuse[92]
2. diabetes mellitus: susceptible to unusual bacterial infections and even fungal osteomyelitis
3. hemodialysis: a diagnostic challenge since radiographic changes of osteomyelitis can occur even in the absence of infection; see Destructive lesions of the spine (p. 1679)
4. immunosuppression
   a) AIDS
   b) chronic corticosteroid use
   c) ethanol abuse
5. infectious endocarditis
6. following spinal surgery or invasive diagnostic or therapeutic procedures
7. may occur in elderly patients with no other identifiable risk factors[93]

Clinical

Signs/symptoms: localized pain (90%), fever (52%, with fever spikes and chills being rare), weight loss, paraspinal muscle spasm, radicular symptoms (50–93%) or myelopathy. VO sometimes produces few systemic effects (e.g., WBC and/or ESR may be normal). ≈ 17% of patients with VO have neurologic symptoms. The risk of paralysis may be higher in the older patient, in cervical VO (vs. thoracic or lumbar), in those with DM or rheumatoid arthritis, and in those with VO due to S. aureus.[84] Neurologic findings are uncommon initially, which may delay the diagnosis.[94] Sensory involvement is less common than motor and long-tract signs because compression is primarily anterior.

Pathogenesis

Source of infection

21

Sources of spontaneous VO: UTI (the most common), respiratory tract, soft-tissues (e.g., skin boils, IV drug abuse…), dental flora. In 37% of cases a source is never identified.[95]

Potential routes of spread

Three main routes: arterial, venous, and direct extension:
1. hematogenous: hematogenously disseminated spondylodiscitis in adults usually involves bone initially, and once infection is established in the subchondral space, spread is to the adjacent disc and thence to the next VB[96]
   a) arterial
   b) venous: via spinal epidural venous plexus (Batson's plexus[97])
2. direct extension (e.g., following surgery/LP, trauma, or local infection)

Organisms

1. *Staphylococcus aureus* is the most common pathogen (> 50%) as in SEA
2. E. coli is a distant second
3. organisms associated with some primary infection sites[98]:
   a) IV drug abusers: Pseudomonas aeruginosa and *S. aureus* are common
   b) urinary tract infections: E. coli & Proteus spp. are common
   c) respiratory tract infections: Streptococcus pneumoniae
   d) alcohol abuse: Klebsiella pneumoniae
   e) endocarditis:
      • acute endocarditis: Staph. aureus
      • subacute endocarditis: Streptococcus spp.
4. tuberculous VO: Mycobacterium tuberculosis (see below)
5. unusual organisms include: nocardia (p. 366)
6. *Mycobacterium avium* complex (*M. avium* and *M. intracellulare*) (MAC) can cause pulmonary disease in nonimmunocompromised patients (usually elderly or on chronic steroids), but can also cause VO similar to TB[99] as part of disseminated disease which usually occurs in HIV patients
7. polymicrobial infections: *rare* (< 2.5% of pyogenic VO infections)

Tuberculous vertebral osteomyelitis: AKA tuberculous spondylitis, AKA Pott's disease. More common in third world countries. Typically symptomatic for many months. Usually affects more than one level. The most common levels involved are the lower thoracic and upper lumbar levels. Has a predilection for the vertebral body, sparing the posterior elements, and characteristically, sparing the intervertebral disc (▶ Fig. 21.1) unlike most pyogenic infections. Psoas abscess is common (the psoas major muscle attaches to the bodies and intervertebral discs from T12–5). Sclerosis of the involved vertebral body may occur. Definitive diagnosis requires the identification of acid-fast bacilli on culture or Gram stain of biopsy material (may be done percutaneously).

Neurologic deficit develops in 10–47% of patients,[100] and may be due to medullary and radicular artery inflammation in most cases. The infection itself rarely extends into the spinal canal[101]; however, epidural granulation tissue or fibrosis or a kyphotic bony deformity may cause cord compression.[100]

The role of surgical debridement and fusion with TB is controversial, and good results may be obtained with either medical treatment or surgery. Surgery may be more appropriate when definite cord compression is documented or for complications such as abscess or sinus formation[102] or spinal instability.

Diagnostic tests

Laboratories

WBC: elevated in only ≈ 35% (rarely > 12,000), associated with poor prognosis.

ESR: elevated in almost all. Usually > 40 mm/hr. Mean: 85.

CRP: may be more sensitive than ESR, and may tend to normalize more quickly with appropriate treatment.[103] See also normal values (p. 378).

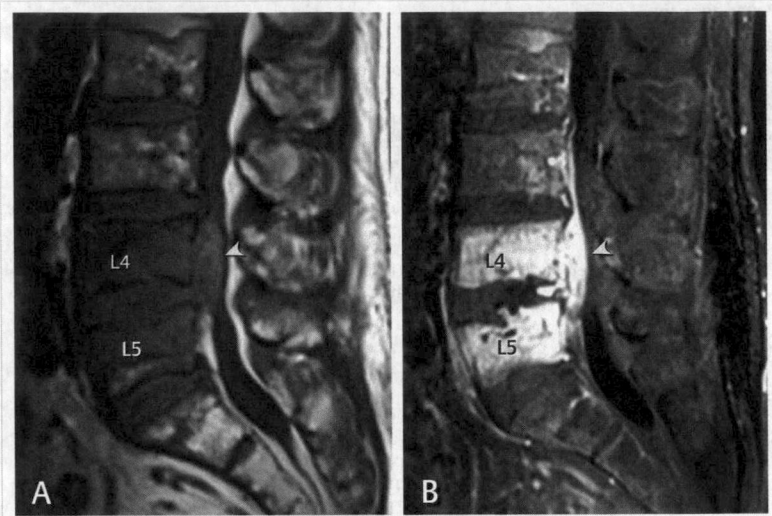

Fig. 21.1 **Tuberculous vertebral osteomyelitis** (Pott's disease) of L4 & L5 with spinal epidural abscess (*yellow arrowheads*).
Image: sagittal MRI, A: T1 without contrast, B: T1 FLAIR + contrast.
Note the sparing of the intervertebral disc, which is characteristic for Pott's disease.

Cultures/biopsy

Culture: blood (positive in ≈ 50%), urine and any focal suppurative process.

Needle biopsy with cultures: can usually be done percutaneously via transpedicular approach with CT or fluoroscopic guidance. May be helpful even if blood cultures are positive (different organisms retrieved in 15%[104]) ∴ an attempt at direct culture from the involved site should be made. Ideally, cultures should be done before antibiotics are started. The yield of needle biopsy cultures ranges from 60–90%. Open biopsy is more sensitive, but morbidity is higher.

Imaging

A comparison of sensitivities and specificities of various imaging modalities is shown in ▶ Table 21.4.
NB: CT may be negative if done too early in the course.

MRI: T1WI → confluent low signal in vertebral bodies and intervertebral disc space. T2WI → increased intensity of involved VBs and disc space.[105] Contrast: enhancement of VB and disc, also look for paraspinal and epidural mass.

CT scan: helpful for demonstrating bony involvement as well as detailed bony anatomy in case instrumentation is required during treatment.

Plain X-ray: changes take from 2–8 weeks from the onset of infection to develop. Earliest changes are loss of cortical endplate margins and loss of disc space height.

Table 21.4 Accuracy of various imaging modalities for vertebral osteomyelitis[105]

Modality	Sensitivity	Specificity	Accuracy
plain X-rays	82%	57%	73%
bone scan	90%	78%	86%
gallium scan	92%	100%	93%
bone scan + gallium scan	90%	100%	94%
MRI	96%	92%	94%

Bone scan: three phase bone scan (p. 247) has reasonably good sensitivity and specificity. Gallium scan (p. 248) has better accuracy, findings include increased uptake in the 2 adjacent VBs with loss of intervening disc.[106] Indium-111 labeled WBC scan: low sensitivity for vertebral osteomyelitis.

Work-up

In patients with suspected vertebral osteomyelitis (VO) (see text above for details):
1. clinical: history of IV drug abuse, DM, immunocompromise, skin boil
2. physical exam: R/O radiculopathy & myelopathy, point tenderness over spine
3. diagnostic tests:
   a) bloodwork: WBC, ESR & CRP (a normal ESR is almost incompatible with VO), blood cultures
   b) imaging:
      • MRI without and with contrast
      • If MRI is contraindicated: CT-myelogram assesses bony anatomy and can demonstrate spinal canal compromise. Bone scan may occasionally be helpful if the diagnosis is still uncertain when suspicion is high
   c) percutaneous needle biopsy with cultures: usually by radiologist. Cultures should include: fungal, aerobic and anaerobic bacterial, and TB

Treatment

Also see more details (p. 383). 90% of cases can be managed non-surgically with antibiotics and immobilization. Characteristics of potential candidates for non-surgical treatment are listed in ▶ Table 21.5. Must also take into account level(s) involved and patient's condition.

Table 21.5 Candidates for non-surgical treatment in pyogenic spontaneous spondylodiscitis[98]

- organism identified
- antibiotic sensitivity
- single disc space involvement with little VB involvement
- minimal or no neurologic deficit
- minimal or no spinal instability

In cases with high suspicion for VO, antibiotics may be started as soon as biopsy has been performed (some treat even earlier). For details of antimicrobials, see Treatment (p. 383) under spinal epidural abscess.

Improvement on imaging can lag behind clinical response and ESR/CRP.

Indications for neurosurgical intervention (note: intervention by a general surgeon may be indicated for empyema, psoas abscess...):
1. progression of disease despite adequate best-case antibiotic therapy
2. spinal instability
3. spinal epidural abscess (p. 381)
4. chronic infection refractory to medical management

For patients not being treated surgically:
1. percutaneous biopsy to obtain ID & sensitivity of organism
2. antibiotics:
   a) IV antibiotics for at least 6 weeks (the rate of treatment failure is increased when IV antibiotics are given for < 4 weeks[98]; longer, e.g., 12 weeks, if ESR not normalizing or if extensive bone involvement and paravertebral infection)
   b) followed by 6–8 weeks of oral agents[98]
3. pain medication as appropriate for pain
4. TLSO brace: to reduce pain (due to movement at involved site) and to reduce stress on weakened bone until healing
5. check upright films in the TLSO to verify stability in the brace
6. follow-up at approximately 8 and 12 weeks with X-rays in brace, then consider discontinuing brace if infection and pain are under control

Surgical treatment

Decompression of neural elements, removal of inflammatory tissue and infected bone to decrease bioburden. Use of instrumented fusion is not contraindicated even for pyogenic infections. Although not routinely used, bone morphogenetic protein (rhBMP-2) in 14 patients undergoing circumferential fusion for refractory infections did not produce complications.[107]

21.5.5 Discitis

General information

Infection of the nucleus pulposus. May start in the cartilaginous endplate and spread to the disc and vertebral body (VB). Similar to vertebral osteomyelitis, except osteomyelitis primarily involves the VB and spreads secondarily to the disc space.

Setting: may be "post-op" or "spontaneous."
- Spontaneous discitis: Occurs in the absence of any procedure. Discussed below.
- Post-op discitis: Can occur following a number of procedures; see Postoperative discitis (p. 378). This is covered under post-op infections.

Many radiographic features of spondylodiscitis and tumor (metastatic and primary) are similar, but tumors rarely involve the disc space, whereas most infections begin in, or before too long, involve the disc space; for more details, see Differentiating factors (p. 1680).

Two distinct types:
1. juvenile: age usually < 20 yrs (see below)
2. adult: usually occurs in susceptible patients (diabetics, IV drug abusers)

Juvenile discitis

Age usually < 20 yrs, with a peak between 2 and 3 years. Probably due to the presence of primordial feeding arteries that nourish the nucleus pulposus and which involute at ≈ 20–30 yrs of age. Lumbar spine is more commonly involved than thoracic or cervical.

Common presentation in young children: refusal to walk or stand progressing to refusal to sit. Back pain is most common in children > 9 yrs of age. Low-grade fever may be present. ESR is usually 2–3 × normal. WBC is sometimes elevated. *H. flu* is a more commonly seen pathogen in this group.

In most cases, there is complete resolution in 9–22 weeks without recurrence in long-term follow-up studies.[100(p 365–71)] Surgery is reserved for the rare case that progresses in spite of antibiotics, for spinal instability, or for recurrent cases.

Most authors reserve antibiotics for patients with[100(p 365–71)]:
1. positive cultures (blood cultures or biopsy cultures)
2. elevated WBC count, constitutional symptoms, or high fever
3. poor response to rest or immobilization
4. neurologic sequelae (very rare)

Antibiotics should be given for a total of 4–6 weeks. Start with IV antibiotics, and when clinical symptoms improve convert to PO for the remainder of therapy.

Clinical

1. symptoms:
   a) pain (the primary symptom)
      - local pain, moderate to severe, exacerbated by virtually any motion of the spine, usually well-localized to the level of involvement
      - radiating to abdomen,[108] hip, leg, scrotum, groin, or perineum
      - radicular symptoms: occurs in 50%[52] to 93%[109] depending on the series
   b) fever and chills: up to 70% are afebrile
2. signs:
   a) localized tenderness
   b) paravertebral muscle spasm
   c) limitation of movement

Work-up

Overview
See following sections for details.

- blood tests
  - WBC
  - ESR & CRP
  - blood cultures
- imaging
  - MRI of the region of concern without and with contrast: the diagnostic test of choice.
  - If MRI is contraindicated: CT-myelogram, bone scan
- percutaneous needle biopsy: usually performed by interventional radiologist
- a source of the infection should be sought
  - thorough history for possible risk factors: skin lesions, IV drug abuse, immunocompromise
  - echocardiogram TEE: rule out endocarditis or valvular vegetations

Radiographic evaluation
General information
A characteristic radiographic finding that helps distinguish infection from metastatic disease is that destruction of the disc space is highly suggestive of infection, whereas in general, *tumor* does *not* cross the disc space; see Differentiating factors (p. 1680).

Plain X-rays
Usually not helpful for early diagnosis. Sequence of changes on plain films:
- earliest changes: interspace narrowing with some demineralization of the VB. Not seen < 2–4 wks following onset of clinical symptoms, nor later than 8 wks
- sclerosis (eburnation) of adjacent cortical margins with increased density of adjacent areas of VB representing new bone formation, starting 4–12 weeks following onset of clinical symptoms
- irregularity of the adjacent vertebral endplates, with sparing of the pedicles (except for tuberculosis, which may involve the pedicles)
- in 50% of cases, the infection remains confined to the disc space, in the other 50% it spreads to adjacent VB
- a late finding is widening (ballooning) of the disc space with erosion of the VB
- circumferential bone formation may lead to exuberant spur formation between VBs 6–8 months into course of illness
- spontaneous fusion of the VB may occur

MRI
Without and with gadolinium contrast. Demonstrates involvement of disc space and of VBs. MRI can R/O paravertebral or epidural spinal abscess but is poor in assessing bony fusion and bone integrity. As sensitive as radionuclide bone scan. Characteristic finding: decreased signal from the disc and adjacent portion of VBs on T1WI, and increased signal from these structures on T2WI. Enhancement is common. Characteristic findings may occur 3–5 days after onset of *symptoms.*

CT and myelo-CT
Like MRI, may also R/O paravertebral or epidural spinal abscess, and while it is better for assessing bony fusion and integrity, by itself it is poor for demonstrating canal compromise. With the addition of water soluble intrathecal contrast (myelo-CT), also assesses the spinal canal for compromise.

Diagnostic criteria
Three basic changes on CT[110] (if all 3 are present, pathognomonic for discitis; if only the 1st 2 are present, then only 87% specific for discitis):
1. endplate fragmentation
2. paravertebral soft-tissue swelling with obliteration of fat planes
3. paravertebral abscess

Nuclear medicine
Very sensitive for discitis and vertebral osteomyelitis (85% sensitivity), but may be negative in up to 85% of patients with Pott's disease. Uses either technetium-99 (abnormal as early as 7 days following onset of clinical symptoms) or gallium-67 (abnormal within 14 days). A positive scan shows focal increased uptake in adjacent endplates, and may be differentiated from osteomyelitis which will involve only one endplate. A positive scan is not specific for infection, and may also occur with neoplasms, fractures, and degenerative changes.

Laboratory studies

ESR: In non-immunocompromised patients, ESR will be elevated in almost all cases with an average value of 60 mm/hr (although discitis with a normal ESR occurs rarely, it should call the diagnosis into question. ESR may be useful to follow as an indicator of response to treatment.

C-reactive protein (CRP): Often used in conjunction with ESR.

WBC: Peripheral WBC is often normal, and rarely is elevated above 12,000.

PPD (Purified Protein Derivative, AKA Mantoux screening test): May be helpful to R/O Pott's disease in cases of spontaneous discitis (p. 387). May be negative in 14% of cases.[111]

Cultures: An attempt should be made to obtain direct cultures from the involved disc space. These may be obtained percutaneously (e.g., Craig needle biopsy) with CT or other radiographic guidance (reported up to 60% positive culture rate), or from intraoperative specimen (NB: open surgery solely to obtain a biopsy is usually not indicated). Staining for acid-fast bacilli (AFB) to identify *Mycobacterium tuberculosis* (TB) should be done in all cases.

Blood cultures may be positive in ≈ 50% of cases, and can be helpful in guiding choice of antimicrobial agent when positive.

Pathogens

Staphylococcus aureus is the most common organism when direct cultures are obtained, followed by S. albus and S. epidermidis. Gram-negative organisms may also be found, including E. coli and Proteus species.

Pseudomonas aeruginosa may be more common in IV drug abusers.

H. flu is common in juvenile discitis (p. 390).

Mycobacterium tuberculosis: Tuberculous spondylitis (Pott's disease) may also occur.

Treatment

General information

Outcome is generally good, and antibiotics together with spinal bracing (immobilization) are adequate treatment in ≈ 75% of cases. Occasionally surgery is required. See also under postoperative discitis for other aspects of management (p. 379).

Most patients are started on strict bed rest, and are then mobilized with or without a brace as tolerated.

Spinal bracing

Probably does not affect final outcome. Affords earlier pain relief for some, and may allow return to activity at an earlier time. For thoracic or upper lumbar discitis, the patient is fitted with a clamshell-type body jacket which is used for 6–8 weeks on the average. As a practical matter, most patients find that the discomfort from the brace is worse than that without the brace. Alternative forms of immobilization include spica cast (provides better immobilization for lower lumbar discitis) or a corset-type brace (less immobilization but better tolerated).

Antibiotics

Choice of antibiotics is guided by the results of direct cultures when positive. In the 40–50% of cases where no organism is isolated, broad spectrum antibiotics should be used. Positive blood culture results may also help guide choice of antibiotics.

Two alternative treatment plans suggested:

1. treat with IV antibiotics for an arbitrary period of time, usually ≈ 4–6 weeks, followed with oral antibiotics for an additional 4–6 weeks
2. treat with IV antibiotics until the ESR normalizes, then change to PO

Surgery

Required in only ≈ 25% of cases.

Indications for surgery:

1. situations where the diagnosis is uncertain, especially when neoplasm is a strong consideration (CT-guided needle biopsy usually helps here)
2. decompression of neural structures, especially with associated spinal epidural abscess or compression by reactive granulation tissue. Ascending numbness, weakness, or onset of neurogenic bladder herald cauda equina syndrome
3. drainage of associated abscess, especially septated abscesses that might be recalcitrant to CT-guided percutaneous needling
4. rarely, to fuse an unstable spine. Most cases go on to spontaneous fusion

Approaches
- anterior approaches: generally used in the cervical or thoracic regions. Removes some or most of the offending infected tissue
  - cervical spine: anterior discectomy and fusion for limited involvement; corpectomy with strut graft and plating with posterior instrumentation (360° fusion) for more extensive involvement
  - thoracic spine: a posterolateral approach (e.g., transpedicular or costotransversectomy approach) or lateral approach (e.g., trans-thoracic or retro-coelomic) may be used
- posterior laminectomy
  - may be used in the lumbar region (below the conus medullaris)
  - ✖ laminectomy alone is not appropriate in the thoracic or cervical spine when there is anterior compression of the spinal cord

21.5.6 Psoas abscess

General information

1. applied anatomy of psoas muscle:
   a) one of 2 heads of the iliopsoas muscle (the other head is iliacus)
   b) origin: inner surface of ilium, base of sacrum, and transverse processes, vertebral bodies (VB) and intervertebral discs of spinal column starting from the inferior margin of T12 VB, extending to the upper part of L5 VB. Insertion: lesser trochanter of the femur. Psoas is the primary hip flexor
   c) 30% of people also have a psoas minor which lies anterior to the psoas major
   d) innervation: branches of L2–4 nerve roots proximal to the formation of the femoral nerve
   e) susceptibility to infection
      - rich vascular supply makes it vulnerable to hematogenous spread
      - proximity to structures that may be a source of infection: sigmoid colon, jejunum, vermiform appendix, ureters, aorta, renal pelvis, pancreas, iliac lymph nodes and spine
2. may be primary (no identifiable underlying disease) or secondary, in which case it may be associated with one of the conditions shown in ▶ Table 21.6
3. risk factors: IV drug abuse, HIV/AIDS, age > 65 years, DM, immunosuppression, renal failure

Table 21.6 Conditions associated with secondary psoas abscess[114]

Organ system	Condition
gastrointestinal	diverticulitis, appendicitis, Crohn's disease, colorectal cancer
genitourinary	UTI, cancer
musculoskeletal infections	vertebral osteomyelitis, infectious sacroiliitis, septic arthritis
other	endocarditis, femoral artery catheterization, infected abdominal aortic aneurysm graft, hepatocellular Ca, intrauterine contraceptive device, trauma, sepsis, dialysis (peritoneal or long-term hemodialysis)

Clinical findings
Physical findings: signs of iliopsoas inflammation include:
1. active: pain on flexing the hip against resistance
2. passive: with the patient lying on the unaffected side, hyperextension of the affected hip stretches the psoas muscle and produces pain

Diagnostic tests
1. routine infection work-up: WBC (often elevated), blood cultures, U/A + C&S (pyuria may be seen)
2. AP abdominal X-ray: psoas shadow may be obliterated
3. CT: sensitivity is 80–100% (MRI is not better).[112] Enlargement of psoas muscle on affected side best seen inside iliac wing

Treatment often includes drainage of the psoas abscess either surgically or percutaneously with CT guidance.

Mortality rates associated with psoas abscess: 2.4% with primary, 19% with secondary, with sepsis being the usual cause of death.[113]

21

References

[1] Yogev R. Cerebrospinal Fluid Shunt Infections: A Personal View. Pediatr Infect Dis. 1985; 4:113–118

[2] Ammirati M, Raimondi A. Cerebrospinal Fluid Shunt Infections in Children: A Study of the Relationship between the Etiology of the Hydrocephalus, Age at the Time of Shunt Placement, and Infection. Child's Nervous System. 1987; 3:106–109

[3] McLone D, Czyzewski D, Raimondi A, et al. Central Nervous System Infection as a Limiting Factor in the Intelligence of Children with Myelomeningocele. Pediatrics. 1982; 70:338–342

[4] Amacher AL, Wellington J. Infantile Hydrocephalus: Long-Term Results of Surgical Therapy. Childs Brain. 1984; 11:217–229

[5] Sanchez-Portocarrero J, Martin-Rabadan P, Saldana CJ,. et al. Candida cerebrospinal fluid shunt infection. Report of two new cases and review of the literature. Diagnostic Microbiology and Infectious Disease. 1994; 20:33–40

[6] Nguyen MH, Yu VL. Meningitis caused by Candida species: an emerging problem in neurosurgical patients. Clinical Infectious Diseases. 1995; 21:323–327

[7] Geers TA, Gordon SM. Clinical significance of Candida species isolated from cerebrospinal fluid following neurosurgery. Clinical Infectious Diseases. 1999; 28:1139–1147

[8] O'Brien M, Parent A, Davis B. Management of Ventricular Shunt Infections. Childs Brain. 1979; 5:304–309

[9] Wald SL, McLaurin RL. Shunt-Associated Glomerulonephritis. Neurosurgery. 1978; 3:146–150

[10] Section of Pediatric Neurosurgery of the American Association of Neurological Surgeons. Pediatric Neurosurgery. New York 1982

[11] Frame PT, McLaurin RL. Treatment of CSF Shunt Infections with Intrashunt Plus Oral Antibiotic Therapy. Journal of Neurosurgery. 1984; 60:354–360

[12] James HE, Walsh JW, Wilson HD, et al. Prospective Randomized Study of Therapy in Cerebrospinal Fluid Shunt Infection. Neurosurgery. 1980; 7:459–463

[13] Steinbok P, Cochrane DD, Kestle JRW. The Significance of Bacteriologically Positive Ventriculoperitoneal Shunt Components in the Absence of Other Signs of Shunt Infection. Journal of Neurosurgery. 1996; 84:617–623

[14] van de Beek D, Drake JM, Tunkel AR. Nosocomial bacterial meningitis. N Engl J Med. 2010; 362:146–154

[15] Tumialan LM, Lin F, Gupta SK. Spontaneous bacterial peritonitis causing Serratia marcescens and Proteus mirabilis ventriculoperitoneal shunt infection. Case report. J Neurosurg. 2006; 105:320–324

[16] Vinchon M, Baroncini M, Laurent T, et al. Bowel perforation caused by peritoneal shunt catheters: diagnosis and treatment. Neurosurgery. 2006; 58: ONS76–82; discussion ONS76-82

[17] Gaskill SJ, Marlin AE. Spontaneous bacterial peritonitis in patients with ventriculoperitoneal shunts. Pediatr Neurosurg. 1997; 26:115–119

[18] Rush DS, Walsh JW, Belin RP, et al. Ventricular Sepsis and Abdominally Related Complications in Children with Cerebrospinal Fluid Shunts. Surgery. 1985; 97:420–427

[19] Bayston R. Epidemiology, diagnosis, treatment, and prevention of cerebrospinal fluid shunt infections. Neurosurg Clin N Am. 2001; 12:703–8, viii

[20] Salomao JF, Leibinger RD. Abdominal pseudocysts complicating CSF shunting in infants and children. Report of 18 cases. Pediatr Neurosurg. 1999; 31:274–278

[21] Lozier AP, Sciacca RR, Romanoli M, et al. Ventriculostomy-related infection: a critical review of the literature. Neurosurgery. 2002; 51:170–182

[22] Pfausler B, Beer R, Engelhardt K, et al. Cell index–a new parameter for the early diagnosis of ventriculostomy (external ventricular drainage)-related ventriculitis in patients with intraventricular

hemorrhage? Acta Neurochir (Wien). 2004; 146:477–481

[23] Beer R, Lackner P, Pfausler B, et al. Nosocomial ventriculitis and meningitis in neurocritical care patients. J Neurol. 2008; 255:1617–1624

[24] Kim JH, Desai NS, Ricci J, et al. Factors contributing to ventriculostomy infection. World Neurosurg. 2012; 77:135–140

[25] Aucoin PJ, Kotilainen HR, Gantz NM, et al. Intracranial pressure monitors. Epidemiologic study of risk factors and infections. Am J Med. 1986; 80:369–376

[26] Mayhall CG, Archer NH, Lamb VA, et al. Ventriculostomy-related infections. A prospective epidemiologic study. New England Journal of Medicine. 1984; 310:553–559

[27] Mayhall CG, Archer NH, Lamb VA, et al. Ventriculostomy-related infections. A prospective epidemiologic study. New England Journal of Medicine. 1984; 310:553–559

[28] Schade RP, Schinkel J, Roelandse FW, et al. Lack of value of routine analysis of cerebrospinal fluid for prediction and diagnosis of external drainage-related bacterial meningitis. J Neurosurg. 2006; 104:101–108

[29] Schuhmann MU, Ostrowski KR, Draper EJ, et al. The value of C-reactive protein in the management of shunt infections. J Neurosurg. 2005; 103:223–230

[30] Martinez R, Gaul C, Buchfelder M, et al. Serum procalcitonin monitoring for differential diagnosis of ventriculitis in adult intensive care patients. Intensive Care Med. 2002; 28:208–210

[31] Pfisterer W, Muhlbauer M, Czech T, et al. Early diagnosis of external ventricular drainage infection: results of a prospective study. J Neurol Neurosurg Psychiatry. 2003; 74:929–932

[32] Hader WJ, Steinbok P. The value of routine cultures of the cerebrospinal fluid in patients with external ventricular drains. Neurosurgery. 2000; 46:1149–53; discussion 1153-5

[33] The management of neurosurgical patients with postoperative bacterial or aseptic meningitis or external ventricular drain-associated ventriculitis. Infection in Neurosurgery Working Party of the British Society for Antimicrobial Chemotherapy. Br J Neurosurg. 2000; 14:7–12

[34] Cook AM, Mieure KD, Owen RD, et al. Intracerebroventricular administration of drugs. Pharmacotherapy. 2009; 29:832–845

[35] Friedman WA, Vries JK. Percutaneous tunnel ventriculostomy. Summary of 100 procedures. J Neurosurg. 1980; 53:662–665

[36] Harrop JS, Sharan AD, Ratliff J, et al. Impact of a standardized protocol and antibiotic-impregnated catheters on ventriculostomy infection rates in cerebrovascular patients. Neurosurgery. 2010; 67:187–91; discussion 191

[37] Zabramski JM, Spetzler RF, Sonntag VK. Impact of a standardized protocol and antibiotic-impregnated catheters on ventriculostomy infection rates in cerebrovascular patients. Neurosurgery. 2011; 69. DOI: 10.1227/NEU.0b013e31821756ca

[38] Sonabend AM, Korenfeld Y, Crisman C, et al. Prevention of ventriculostomy-related infections with prophylactic antibiotics and antibiotic-coated external ventricular drains: a systematic review. Neurosurgery. 2011; 68:996–1005

[39] Zabramski JM, Whiting D, Darouiche RO, et al. Efficacy of antimicrobial-impregnated external ventricular drain catheters: a prospective, randomized, controlled trial. J Neurosurg. 2003; 98:725–730

[40] Poon WS, Ng S, Wai S. CSF antibiotic prophylaxis for neurosurgical patients with ventriculostomy: a randomised study. Acta Neurochir Suppl. 1998; 71:146–148

[41] Holloway KL, Barnes T, Choi S, et al. Ventriculostomy Infections: The Effect of Monitoring Duration and Catheter Exchange in 584 Patients. Journal of Neurosurgery. 1996; 85:419–424

[42] Wong GK, Poon WS, Wai S, et al. Failure of regular external ventricular drain exchange to reduce cerebrospinal fluid infection: result of a randomised controlled trial. J Neurol Neurosurg Psychiatry. 2002; 73:759–761

[43] Lo CH, Spelman D, Bailey M, et al. External ventricular drain infections are independent of drain duration: an argument against elective revision. J Neurosurg. 2007; 106:378–383

[44] Khalil BA, Sarsam Z, Buxton N. External ventricular drains: is there a time limit in children? Childs Nerv Syst. 2005; 21:355–357

[45] Shektman A, Granick MS, Solomon MP, et al. Management of Infected Laminectomy Wounds. Neurosurgery. 1994; 35:307–309

[46] Kurz A, Sessler DI, Lenhardt R. Perioperative Normothermia to Reduce the Incidence of Surgical-Wound Infection and Shorten Hospitalization. New England Journal of Medicine. 1996; 334:1209–1215

[47] Dernbach PD, Gomez H, Hahn J. Primary Closure of Infected Spinal Wounds. Neurosurgery. 1990; 26:707–709

[48] Ebersold MJ. Comment on Shektman A, et al.: Primary Closure of Infected Spinal Wounds. Neurosurgery. 1994; 35

[49] Iversen E, Nielsen VAH, Hansen LG. Prognosis in Postoperative Discitis. A Retrospective Study of 111 Cases. Acta Orthop Scand. 1992; 63:305–309

[50] Fouquet B, Goupille P, Jattiot F, et al. Discitis After Lumbar Disc Surgery. Features of "Aseptic" and "Septic" Forms. Spine. 1992; 17:356–358

[51] Rawlings CE, Wilkins RH, Gallis HA, et al. Postoperative Intervertebral Disc Space Infection. Neurosurgery. 1983; 13:371–376

[52] Malik GM, McCormick P. Management of Spine and Intervertebral Disc Space Infection. Contemp Neurosurg. 1988; 10:1–6

[53] Thelander U, Larsson S. Quantitation of C-Reactive Protein Levels and Erythrocyte Sedimentation Rate After Spinal Surgery. Spine. 1992; 17:400–404

[54] Boden SD, Davis DO, Dina TS, et al. Postoperative Diskitis: Distinguishing Early MR Imaging Findings from Normal Postoperative Disk Space Changes. Radiology. 1992; 184:765–771

[55] Mirzayan MJ, Gharabaghi A, Samii M, et al. Response of C-reactive protein after craniotomy for microsurgery of intracranial tumors. Neurosurgery. 2007; 60:621–5; discussion 625

[56] Listinsky JL, Wood BP, Ekholm SE. Parietal Osteomyelitis and Epidural Abscess: A Delayed Complication of Fetal Monitoring. Pediatr Radiol. 1986; 16:150–151

[57] Bernard L, Dinh A, Ghout I, et al. Antibiotic treatment for 6 weeks versus 12 weeks in patients with pyogenic vertebral osteomyelitis: an open-label, non-inferiority, randomised, controlled trial. Lancet. 2015; 385:875–882

[58] Cahill DW. Infections of the Spine. Contemporary Neurosurgery. 1993; 15:1–8

[59] Baker AS, Ojemann RG, Swartz MN, et al. Spinal Epidural Abscess. New England Journal of Medicine. 1975; 293:463–468

[60] Nussbaum ES, Rigamonti D, Standiford H, et al. Spinal Epidural Abscess: A Report of 40 Cases and Review. Surgical Neurology. 1992; 38:225–231

[61] Danner RL, Hartman BJ. Update of Spinal Epidural Abscess: 35 Cases and Review of the Literature. Rev Infect Dis. 1987; 9:265–274

[62] Curry WT,Jr, Hoh BL, Amin-Hanjani S, et al. Spinal epidural abscess: clinical presentation, management, and outcome. Surgical Neurology. 2005; 63:364–71; discussion 371

[63] Hlavin ML, Kaminski HJ, Ross JS, et al. Spinal epidural abscess: a ten-year perspective. Neurosurgery. 1990; 27:177–184

[64] Spiegelmann R, Findler G, Faibel M, et al. Postoperative Spinal Epidural Empyema: Clinical and Computed Tomography Features. Spine. 1991; 16:1146–1149

[65] Browder J, Meyers R. Pyogenic Infections of the Spinal Epidural Space. Surgery. 1941; 10:296–308

[66] Russell NA, Vaughan R, Morley TP. Spinal Epidural Infection. Can J Neurol Sci. 1979; 6:325–328

[67] Heusner AP. Nontuberculous Spinal Epidural Infections. New England Journal of Medicine. 1948; 239:845–854

[68] Koppel BS, Tuchman AJ, Mangiardi JR, et al. Epidural spinal infection in intravenous drug abusers. Arch Neurol. 1988; 45:1331–1337

[69] Abdel-Magid RA, Kotb HIM. Spinal Epidural Abscess After Spinal Anesthesia: A Favorable Outcome. Neurosurgery. 1990; 27:310–311

[70] Loarie DJ, Fairley HB. Epidural Abscess Following Spinal Anesthesia. Anesth Analg. 1978; 57:351–353

[71] Strong WE. Epidural Abscess Associated with Epidural Catheterization: A Rare Event? Report of Two Cases with Markedly Delayed Presentation. Anesthesiology. 1991; 74:943–946

[72] Bergman I, Wald ER, Meyer JD, et al. Epidural Abscess and Vertebral Osteomyelitis following Serial Lumbar Punctures. Pediatrics. 1983; 72:476–480

[73] Rea GL, McGregor JM, Miller CA, et al. Surgical Treatment of the Spontaneous Spinal Epidural Abscess. Surgical Neurology. 1992; 37:274–279

[74] Kaufman DM, Kaplan JG, Litman N. Infectious agents in spinal epidural abscesses. Neurology. 1980; 30:844–850

[75] Wilkins RH, Rengachary SS. Neurosurgery. New York 1985

[76] Post MJD, Sze G, Quencer RM, et al. Gadolinium-Enhanced MR in Spinal Infection. Journal of Computer Assisted Tomography. 1990; 14:721–729

[77] Post MJD, Quencer RM, Montalvo BM, et al. Spinal infection: evaluation with MR imaging and intraoperative ultrasound. Radiology. 1988; 169:765–771

[78] Sandhu FS, Dillon WP. Spinal Epidural Abscess: Evaluation with Contrast-Enhanced MR Imaging. AJNR. 1991; 158:1087–1093

[79] Kirzner H, Oh YK, Lee SH. Intraspinal Air: A CT Finding of Epidural Abscess. AJR. 1988; 151:1217–1218

[80] Leys D, Lesoin F, Viaud C, et al. Decreased Morbidity from Acute Bacterial Spinal Epidural Abscess using Computed Tomography and Nonsurgical Treatment in Selected Patients. Ann Neurol. 1985; 17:350–355

[81] Mampalam TJ, Rosegay H, Andrews BT, et al. Nonoperative Treatment of Spinal Epidural Infections. J Neurosurg. 1989; 71:208–210

[82] Hanigan WC, Asner NG, Elwood PW. Magnetic Resonance Imaging and the Nonoperative Treatment of Spinal Epidural Abscess. Surgical Neurology. 1990; 34:408–413

[83] Garrido E, Rosenwasser RH. Experience with the Suction-Irrigation Technique in the Management of Spinal Epidural Infection. Neurosurgery. 1983; 12:678–679

[84] Eismont FJ, Bohlman HH, Soni PL, et al. Pyogenic and Fungal Vertebral Osteomyelitis with Paralysis. Journal of Bone and Joint Surgery. 1983; 65A:19–29

[85] Rayes M, Colen CB, Bahgat DA, et al. Safety of instrumentation in patients with spinal infection. J Neurosurg Spine. 2010; 12:647–659

[86] Pereira CE, Lynch JC. Spinal epidural abscess: an analysis of 24 cases. Surg Neurol. 2005; 63:S26–S29

[87] Curling OD, Gower DJ, McWhorter JM. Changing Concepts in Spinal Epidural Abscess: A Report of 29 Cases. Neurosurgery. 1990; 27:185–192

[88] Greenlee JE. Subdural empyema. Curr Treat Options Neurol. 2003; 5:13–22

[89] Marciano RD, Buster W, Karas C, et al. Isolated spinal subdural empyema: A case report & review of the literature. Open Journal of Modern Neurosurgery. 2017; 7:112–119

[90] Schmorl G, Junghanns H. The Human Spine in Health and Disease. New York: Grune & Stratton; 1971

[91] Waldvogel FA, Vasey H. Osteomyelitis: The Past Decade. New England Journal of Medicine. 1980; 303:360–370

[92] Holzman RS, Bishko R. Osteomyelitis in heroin addicts. Annals of Internal Medicine. 1971; 75:693–696

[93] Cahill DW, Love LC, Rechtine GR. Pyogenic Osteomyelitis of the Spine in the Elderly. Journal of Neurosurgery. 1991; 74:878–886

[94] Burke DR, Brant-Zawadzki MB. CT of Pyogenic Spine Infection. Neuroradiology. 1985; 27:131–137

[95] Sapico FL, Montgomerie JZ. Pyogenic Vertebral Osteomyelitis: Report of Nine Cases and Review of the Literature. Rev Infect Dis. 1979; 1:754–776

[96] Skaf GS, Fehlings MG, Bouclaous CH. Medical and surgical management of pyogenic and nonpyogenic spondylodiscitis: Part I. Contemporary Neurosurgery. 2004; 26:1–5

[97] Batson OV. The Function of the Vertebral Veins and Their Role in the Spread of Metastases. Ann Surg. 1940; 112

[98] Skaf GS, Fehlings MG, Bouclaous CH. Medical and surgical management of pyogenic and nonpyogenic spondylodiscitis: Part II. Contemporary Neurosurgery. 2004; 26:1–5

[99] Weiner BK, Love TW, Fraser RD. Mycobacterium avium intracellulare: vertebral osteomyelitis. Journal of Spinal Disorders. 1998; 11:89–91

[100] Rothman RH, Simeone FA. The Spine. Philadelphia 1992

[101] Kinnier WSA. Tuberculosis of the Skull and Spine. In: Neurology. London: Edward Arnold; 1940:575–583

[102] Medical Research Council Working Party on Tuberculosis of the Spine. Controlled Trial of Short-Course Regimens of Chemotherapy in the Ambulatory Treatment of Spinal Tuberculosis: Results at Three Years of a Study in Korea. Journal of Bone and Joint Surgery. 1993; 75B:240–248

[103] Rath SA, Nelf U, Schneider O, et al. Neurosurgical management of thoracic and lumbar vertebral osteomyelitis and discitis in adults: a review of 43 consecutive surgically treated patients. Neurosurgery. 1996; 38:926–933

[104] Patzakis MJ, Rao S, Wilkins J, et al. Analysis of 61 cases of vertebral osteomyelitis. Clinical Orthopaedics and Related Research. 1991; 264:178–183

[105] Modic MT, Feiglin DH, Piraino DW, et al. Vertebral Osteomyelitis: Assessment Using MR. Radiology. 1985; 157:157–166

[106] Hadjipavlou AG, Cesani-Vazquez F, Villaneuva-Meyer J, et al. The effectiveness of gallium citrate Ga 67 radionuclide imaging in vertebral osteomyelitis revisited. American Journal of Orthopedics. 1998; 27:179–183

[107] Allen RT, Lee YP, Stimson E, et al. Bone morphogenetic protein-2 (BMP-2) in the treatment of pyogenic vertebral osteomyelitis. Spine. 2007; 32:2996–3006

[108] Sullivan CR, Symmonds RE. Disk Infections and Abdominal Pain. JAMA. 1964; 188:655–658

[109] Kemp HBS, Jackson JW, Jeremiah JD, et al. Pyogenic Infections Occurring Primarily in Intervertebral Discs. J Bone Joint Surg. 1973; 55B:698–714

[110] Kopecky KK, Gilmor RL, Scott JA, et al. Pitfalls of CT in Diagnosis of Discitis. Neuroradiology. 1985; 27:57–66

[111] Lifeso RM, Weaver P, Harder EH. Tuberculous Spondylitis in Adults. J Bone Joint Surg. 1985; 67A:1405–1413

[112] Taiwo B. Psoas abscess: a primer for the internist. South Med J. 2001; 94:2–5

[113] Gruenwald I, Abrahamson J, Cohen O. Psoas abscess: case report and review of the literature. J Urol. 1992; 147:1624–1626

[114] Riyad NYM, Sallam A, Nur A. Pyogenic psoas abscess: Discussion of its Epidemiology, Etiology, Bacteriology, Diagnosis, Treatment and Prognosis - Case Report. Kuwait Medical Journal. 2003; 35:44–47

22 Other Nonbacterial Infections

22.1 Viral encephalitis

Encephalitides that come to the attention of the neurosurgeon usually cause imaging findings that may mimic mass lesions, for cases where biopsy may be helpful, and shunting for hydrocephalus is needed. Those covered in this book:
1. herpes simplex encephalitis: see below
2. multifocal herpes varicella-zoster virus leukoencephalitis (p. 399)
3. progressive multifocal leukoencephalopathy (PML) (p. 354)

22.1.1 Herpes simplex encephalitis
General information

> ### Key concepts
>
> - a hemorrhagic viral encephalitis with a predilection for the temporal lobes
> - definitive diagnosis requires brain biopsy
> - optimal treatment: early administration of IV acyclovir

Herpes simplex encephalitis (HSE) AKA multifocal necrotizing encephalomyelitis, is caused by the herpes simplex virus (HSV) type I. It produces an acute, often (but not always) hemorrhagic, necrotizing encephalitis with edema. There is a predilection for the temporal and orbitofrontal lobes and limbic system.

Epidemiology

Estimated incidence of HSE: 1 in 750,000 to 1 million persons/yr. Equally distributed between male and females, in all races, in all ages (over 33% of cases occur in children 6 mos to 18 yrs), throughout the year.[1]

Presentation

Patients are often confused and disoriented at onset, and progress to coma within days. Adult presentations are shown in ► Table 22.1, and for pediatrics in ► Table 22.2. Other symptoms include headache.

Diagnostic studies

Diagnosis can often be made on the basis of history, CSF, and MRI. Treatment should be instituted rapidly without waiting for biopsy, before the onset of coma.
1. CSF: leukocytosis (mostly monocytes), RBCs 500–1000/mm³, (NB: 3% have no pleocytosis), protein rises markedly as disease progresses. HSV antibodies may appear in the CSF but takes at least ≈ 14 days and is thus not useful for early diagnosis

Table 22.1 Herpes simplex encephalitis—adult presentation

Symptom	%
altered consciousness	97
fever	90
seizures (usually focal onset)	67
personality changes	71
hemiparesis	33

22

Table 22.2 Herpes simplex encephalitis—presentation in age < 10 yrs

irritability
altered mentation
malaise
seizure
disorientation
dysphasia
hemiparesis
fever
papilledema (except in age ≤ 2 yrs)

2. EEG: periodic lateralizing epileptiform discharges (PLEDs) (triphasic high-voltage discharges every few seconds) usually from the temporal lobe. EEG may vary rapidly over a few days (unusual in conditions mimicking HSE)
3. CT: edema predominantly localized in temporal lobes (poorer prognosis once hemorrhagic lesions are visible). In one review, 38% of initial CTs were normal[2] (many were on early generation CT scanners or were done within 3 days of onset). Hemorrhages were apparent in only 12% of the initially abnormal CTs
4. MRI: more sensitive than CT,[3] demonstrates edema as high signal on T2WI, primarily within the temporal lobe, with some extension across Sylvian fissure ("transsylvian sign"),[2] especially suggestive of HSE if bilateral. Differentiate from MCA infarct (which may also span Sylvian fissure) by typical arterial distribution of the latter. Enhancement doesn't occur until the 2nd week
5. technetium brain scan: process localized to temporal lobes
6. brain biopsy: false negatives may occur[4]; see details below

Brain biopsy

Indications: reserved for questionable cases. May not be necessary in patients with fever, encephalopathy, compatible CSF findings, focal neuro findings (focal seizure, hemiparesis, or cranial nerve palsy), and supporting evidence of at least one of the following: focal EEG, CT, MRI or technetium brain scan abnormality.

Should be performed within ≤ 48 hrs of starting acyclovir (otherwise false negatives may occur).

Biopsy results: of 432 brain biopsies performed using the technique below, 45% had HSE, 22% had identifiable but non-HSE pathology (e.g., vascular disease, other viral infection, adrenal leukodystrophy, bacterial infection…), and 33% remained without a diagnosis.[5]

Technique
1. anterior inferior temporal lobe is preferred site
   a) the side chosen for biopsy is the one showing maximal involvement based on clinical information (e.g., localizing seizures), EEG and/or imaging studies[6]
   b) 10 × 10 × 5 mm deep specimen obtained from anterior portion of the inferior temporal gyrus with NO COAGULATION on specimen side (cut surface with #11 blade, then cauterize pial surface on *non*-specimen side)
   c) 2nd specimen obtained from beneath surface specimen with fenestrated pituitary biopsy forceps
2. virus isolation is the most specific (100%) and sensitive (96–97%) test for HSE. Other findings (less accurate): perivascular cuffing, lymphocytic infiltration, hemorrhagic necrosis, neuronophagia, intranuclear inclusions (present in 50%)
3. if electron microscopy (EM) or immunohistofluorescence is available, 70% may be diagnosed within ≈ 3 hrs of biopsy
4. biopsy tissue handling
   a) avoid macerating specimens for histology
   b) tissue for EM: placed in glutaraldehyde
   c) tissue for permanent histology: placed in formalin
   d) tissue for culture:
      • handling: specimen is placed in sterile specimen container and sent directly to virology lab. If lab is closed, tissue may be placed in regular refrigerator for up to 24 hrs or placed in –70 °C freezer for indefinite time (virus remains viable for up to 5 yrs). ✖ DO NOT place specimen in regular *freezer* (destroys virus)
      • cultures generally take at least 1 week to become positive
      • cultures checked for 3 weeks before being declared negative

Treatment

General treatment measures
General supportive measures: to control elevated ICP from edema, includes elevate HOB, mannitol, hyperventilation (dexamethasone unproven efficacy); also see Treatment measures for elevated ICP (p. 1046). Antiseizure medications are used for seizure prophylaxis.

Antiviral medications
Acyclovir is the drug of choice for HSE.

Drug info: Acyclovir (Zovirax®)

℞ Adult: 30 mg/kg/day, in divided q 8 hr doses in minimum volume of 100 ml IV fluid over 1 hr (caution: this fluid load may be hazardous, especially since cerebral edema is already usually problematic) for 14–21 days (some relapses have been reported after only 10 days of treatment).
℞ Children > 6 mos age: 500 mg/m^2 IV q 8 hrs × 10 days.
℞ Neonatal: 10 mg/kg IV q 8 hrs for 10 days.

Drug info: Vidarabine (Vira-A®)

Six month mortality following treatment with acyclovir was influenced by:
- age (6% under age 30, 36% over age 30)
- Glasgow coma score (GCS) at time of treatment initiation (25% for GCS ≤ 10, 0% for GCS > 10)
- duration of disease before therapy (0% for initiating therapy within 4 days of onset of symptoms, 35% if after 4 days)

22.1.2 Multifocal varicella-zoster leukoencephalitis

Caused by the herpes varicella-zoster virus (VZV) which is responsible for varicella (chickenpox), herpes zoster (HZ) (shingles), and post-herpetic neuralgia (p. 522). VZV is a herpes virus that is distinct from the herpes simplex virus.

Symptomatic zoster-related encephalitis occurs in < 5% of immunocompromised patients (including AIDS patients) with cutaneous zoster.[7] It typically follows cutaneous HZ by a short time (average time: 9 days), although cases have been reported where many months have lapsed.[8]

Manifestations include: altered level of consciousness, headache, photophobia, meningismus. Although focal neurologic deficits may occur, these are uncommon.

Recently, vasculopathy following VZV reactivation has been increasingly recognized.[9]

MRI may show multiple, discrete, round and oval lesions with minimal edema (best seen on T2WI) and minimal enhancement.

Unlike herpes simplex virus, VZV is difficult to isolate in culture. On brain biopsy, look for multiple discrete lesions within gray and white matter, with Cowdry type A intranuclear inclusion bodies in oligodendrocytes, astrocytes, and neurons, and a positive direct fluorescent antibody test directed against VZV.

There is a case report of VZV encephalitis treated with IV acyclovir.[7]

22.2 Creutzfeldt-Jakob disease

22.2.1 General information

Key concepts

- an invariably fatal encephalopathy characterized by rapidly progressive dementia, ataxia and myoclonus
- death usually occurs within 1 yr of onset of symptoms

- 3 forms: 1) transmissible (likely via prions [proteinaceous particles]), 2) autosomal dominant inherited, 3) sporadic
- pathologic process: abnormal protease resistant protein (PrP^{Sc}) induces abnormal folding in the normal PrP^{C} protein, forming large beta-sheets which accumulate in neurons producing vacuolization and cell death
- histology: status spongiosus without inflammatory response
- EEG: characteristic finding is bilateral sharp waves (0.5–2 per second)
- MRI: hyperintensity (on DWI or FLAIR) in the striatum or in at least two cortical regions is characteristic but nonspecific
- labs: a positive RT-QuIC (p. 403) in CSF is a higly accurate indicator of prion disease

Creutzfeldt-Jakob disease (CJD) is one of 4 known rare human diseases associated with transmissible spongiform encephalopathy (TSE) agents, also called prions (proteinaceous infectious particles). The other 3 human prion diseases are Gerstmann-Sträussler-Scheinker disease, fatal familial insomnia,[10, 11,12] and variably protease-sensitive prionopathy (VPSPr). Although sometimes also referred to as a "slow virus," these agents contain no nucleic acids and are also resistant to processes that inactivate conventional viruses (▶ Table 22.4). Prions do not provoke an immune response. The famed choreographer George Balanchine died of CJD in 1983.

The protease-resistant protein associated with disease is designated PrPres or PrP^{Sc}, and is an isoform of a naturally occurring protease-sensitive protein designated PrPsen or PrP^{C}. In pathologic cases, PrP^{C}, which is a predominantly alpha-helical structure, undergoes a post-translational conformational change to PrP^{Sc}, which has large abnormally folded beta-sheets which propagates the the misfolding of PrP^{C} and accumulates in neural cells, disrupting function and leading to cell death and vacuolization.[13]

CJD occurs in 3 forms: transmissible (possibly via prions), inherited (autosomal dominant) and sporadic, which will be discussed below.

22.2.2 Epidemiology

Annual incidence of CJD: 0.5–1.5 per million population[13] with little change over time and no geographic clustering (except in locations with large numbers of familial cases). Over 200 people die of CJD in the U.S. each year.

22.2.3 Acquired prion diseases

The natural route of infection is unknown and virulence appears low, with lack of significant dissemination by respiratory, enteric, or sexual contact. There is no increased incidence in spouses (only a single conjugal pair of cases has been verified), physicians, or laboratory workers. There is no evidence of transplacental transmission. Horizontal transmission of CJD has occurred iatrogenically (see below). Transmission also occurred primarily in the 1950-60 s via handling and ingestion of infected brains in ritualistic funereal cannibalism practiced among the Fore (pronounced: "fore-ay") linguistic group in the eastern highlands of Papua, New Guinea,[14] a practice which has been gradually abandoned. The affliction (called "kuru" which means "to tremble" in the local language[15 (p 6)]) is a subacute, uniformly fatal disease involving cerebellar degeneration.

Most noniatrogenically transmitted cases of CJD occur in patients > 50 yrs old, and is rare in age < 30. The incubation period can range from months to decades. The onset of symptoms following direct inoculation is usually faster (common range: 16–28 mos), but still may be much longer (up to 30 years with corneal transplant,[16] and 4–21 yrs with hGH transmission). In experimental models of CJD, higher inoculation doses produce shorter incubation periods.[17]

22.2.4 Inherited CJD

5–15% of cases of CJD occur in an autosomal dominant inheritance pattern with abnormalities in the amyloid gene[18] on chromosome 20 with a penetrance of 0.56.[19] Since familial CJD is dominantly inherited, analysis for the PrP gene is not indicated unless there is a history of dementia in a first-degree relative.

22.2.5 Sporadic CJD (sCJD)

In ≈ 90% of cases of CJD, no infectious or familial source can be identified,[18] and these cases are considered sporadic. 80% occur in persons 50–70 yrs old.[13] Sporadic cases show no abnormality in the PrP gene. Molecular biology and phenotyping have resulted in identification of at least 6 subtypes of sCJD.

There appears to be a genetic susceptibility in the sporadic and iatrogenically transmitted CJD cases, with the majority of these showing specific changes in the human prion protein.

22.2.6 New variant CJD

Cases of atypical CJD are well-recognized. A variant of CJD (vCJD) was identified in 10 cases of unusually young individuals (median age at death: 29 yrs) during 1994–95 in the United Kingdom,[20] and has been strongly linked to the 1980s epidemic of bovine spongiform encephalopathy (BSE), dubbed "mad cow" disease by the lay press. The BSE epidemic may have been exacerbated by the practice of feeding discarded sheep organs (called offals) to the cows (a practice banned since 1989). This raises the question of possible transmission and mutation of the sheep slow-virus disease, scrapie (which resembles kuru in man) to cows. None of the vCJD patients had periodic spikes on EEG characteristic of classic CJD, the clinical course was atypical (having prominent psychiatric symptoms and early cerebellar ataxia, somewhat similar to kuru), and brain plaques showed unusual features also reminiscent of amyloid plaques seen in kuru. A comparison of vCJD to sporadic CJD is shown in ▶ Table 22.3.

Table 22.3 Comparison of vCJD to sporadic CJD[13]

Characteristic	vCJD	sporadic
mean age at onset (yr)	29	60
mean duration of disease (mo)	14	5
most consistent and prominent early signs	psychiatric abnormalities, sensory symptoms	dementia, myoclonus
cerebellar signs (%)	100	40
periodic complexes on EEG (%)	0	94
pathological changes	diffuse amyloid plaques	sparse plaques in 5–10%

22.2.7 Iatrogenic transmission of CJD

Described only in cases of direct contact with infected organs, tissues, or surgical instruments. Has been reported with: corneal transplants,[16,21] intracerebral EEG electrodes sterilized with 70% alcohol and formaldehyde vapor after use on a CJD patient,[22] operations in neurosurgical ORs after procedures on CJD patients, in recipients of pituitary-derived human growth hormone (hGH)[23] (most cases have occurred in France[17]; there is no longer a risk of CJD with growth hormone in the U.S. since distribution of pituitary derived hGH was halted in 1985 and current hGH is obtained from recombinant DNA technology), and dural graft with cadaveric dura mater (Lyodura®) (most cases have occurred in Japan[17]). Ethylene oxide, autoclaving, formalin, and ionizing radiation do not inactivate the CJD agent[24,25,26] (see ▶ Table 22.4 for other ineffective procedures). Recommended sterilization procedures for suspected CJD tissues and contaminated materials also appear in ▶ Table 22.4.

22.2.8 Pathology

The typical form of CJD produces the classic histologic triad of neuronal loss, astrocytic proliferation, and cytoplasmic vacuoles in neurons and astrocytes (status spongiosus), all in the absence of an inflammatory response. There is a predilection for cerebral cortex and basal ganglia, but all parts of the CNS may be involved. In 5–10% of cases, these changes are accompanied by the deposition of amyloid plaques (plaques are common in kuru, vCJD and some familial spongiform encephalopathies). Immunostaining for PrPres is definitive.

22

Table 22.4 Operating room sterilization procedures for CJD[27]

Fully effective (recommended) procedures
- steam autoclaving for 1 hr at 132 °C, or
- immersion in 1N sodium hydroxide (NaOH) for 1 hr at room temperature

Partially effective procedures
- steam autoclaving at either 121 °C or 132 °C for 15–30 mins, or
- immersion in 1N NaOH for 15 mins, or lower concentrations (<0.5N) for 1 hr at room temp, or
- immersion in sodium hypochlorite (household bleach) undiluted or up to 1:10 dilution (0.5%) for 1 hr[28]

✖ *Ineffective* procedures:
- boiling, UV or ionizing radiation, ethylene oxide, ethanol, formalin, beta-propiolactone, detergents, quaternary ammonium compounds, Lysol®, alcoholic iodine, acetone, potassium permanganate, routine autoclaving

22.2.9 Presentation

One-third initially express vague feelings of fatigue, sleep disorders, or reduced appetite. Another third have neurologic symptoms including memory loss, confusion, or uncharacteristic behavior. The last third have focal signs including cerebellar ataxia, aphasia, visual deficits (including cortical blindness), or hemiparesis.

The typical course is inexorable, progression of dementia, often noticeably worse week by week, with subsequent rapid development of pyramidal tract findings (limb weakness and stiffness, pathologic reflexes), late extrapyramidal findings (tremor, rigidity, dysarthria, bradykinesia), and myoclonus (often stimulus-triggered). Clinical signs of sporadic CJD are shown in ▶ Table 22.5.

Supranuclear gaze palsy is an occasional finding, also usually late.[19] In early stages, CJD may resemble Alzheimer's disease (SDAT). 10% of cases present as ataxia without dementia or myoclonus. Cases with predominant spinal cord findings may be initially mistaken for ALS.

Myoclonus subsides in the terminal phases, and akinetic mutism ensues.

Table 22.5 Major clinical signs in sporadic CJD[13]

Sign	Freq (%)
cognitive deficits[a]	100
myoclonus	>80
pyramidal tract signs	>50
cerebellar signs	>50
extrapyramidal signs	>50
cortical visual deficits	>20
abnormal extraocular movements	>20
lower motor-neuron signs	<20
vestibular dysfunction	<20
seizures	<20
sensory deficits	<20
autonomic abnormalities	<20

[a]dementia, psychiatric and behavioral abnormalities

22.2.10 Diagnosis

Diagnostic criteria

The complete "diagnostic triad" (dementia, myoclonus, and periodic EEG activity) may be absent in up to 25% of cases. Diagnostic criteria have been published[29] as shown in ▶ Table 22.6. No patients in their series with a diagnosis other than CJD fulfilled the criteria for clinically definite CJD. The most common condition other than CJD fulfilling the criteria for clinically probable CJD was SDAT (especially difficult to distinguish in the early stages). There is a CSF immunoassay for the 14–3–3 brain protein (see below).

Table 22.6 Diagnostic criteria[a] of CJD[29]

Pathologically confirmed (with unequivocal spongiform changes)					
• clinically: requires brain biopsy (see text)					
• found at autopsy					
Clinical criteria	Mental deterioration	Myoclonus	1–2 Hz periodic EEG complexes	Any movement disorder or periodic EEG activity	Duration of illness (months)
clinically definite	+	+	+		<12
clinically probable	+	+ OR +			<18
clinically possible	+			+	<24

[a]in patients with normal metabolic status and spinal fluid. If there are early cerebellar or visual symptoms and then muscular rigidity, or if another family member has died of pathologically verified CJD, then upgrade the degree of certainty to the next higher category

Differential diagnosis

CSF examination to exclude SSPE or infections such as tertiary syphilis or is recommended. Toxicity from bismuth, bromides, and lithium must be ruled out. Myoclonus is usually more prominent early in toxic/metabolic disorders than in CJD, and seizures in CJD are usually late.[13]

Diagnostic tests

1. imaging: no pathognomonic CT or MR finding. These studies may be normal, but are essential to rule out other conditions, (e.g., herpes-simplex encephalitis, recent stroke…). Diffuse atrophy may be present, especially late. Characteristic MRI findings: hyperintensity (on DWI or FLAIR sequences) in the striatum or in at least two cortical regions, which are present in up to 79% of cases (retrospectively).[30] This is nonspecific but may help differentiate CJD from SDAT[31]
2. blood tests: serum assays for S-100 protein are so insensitive and nonspecific[32] that it can only be used as a diagnostic adjunct
3. CSF
   a) routine labs: usually normal, although protein may occasionally be elevated
   b) abnormal proteins:
      • surrogate markers of CJD in CSF include proteins 130 & 131 and t-tau proteins. However, assays for these proteins are not practical for routine use, and confirmatory tests such as post-mortem identification of PrP^{Sc} in brain tissue are still required for diagnosis
      • protein amplification: using the self-replicating property of PrP^{SC}, the first specific test for TSE diseases appeared in 2011[33] and refinement produced the second generation (IQ-CSF) Real-Time Quaking-Induced Conversion (RT-QuIC) assay[34] which appears to have high accuracy[35]
4. EEG: characteristic finding of bilateral, symmetrical, periodic bi- or triphasic synchronous sharp-wave complexes, AKA periodic spikes, AKA pseudoperiodic sharp-wave complexes (0.5–2 per second) have ≈ 70% sensitivity and 86% specificity.[36] They resemble PLEDs (p. 249), but are responsive to noxious stimulus (may be absent in familial CJD[19] and in the recent UK variant [see above])
5. SPECT scan: may be abnormal in vCJD even when EEG is normal[37]; however, the findings are not specific for vCJD
6. brain biopsy: see below
7. tonsillar biopsy: patients with variant CJD (vCJD) may have detectable levels of variant type 4 of the abnormal prion protein (PrPSc) in their lymphoreticular system, which may be accessed by a 1 cm wedge-biopsy of one palatine tonsil (using careful aseptic precautions)[38]

Brain biopsy

Due to lack of an effective treatment and the potential for iatrogenic infection in surgery, biopsy is reserved for cases where establishing the diagnosis is deemed important, or as part of a research study,[6] or when diagnostic tests are equivocal and other potentially treatable etiologies are suspected.

22

Technique: to prevent aerosolization of the infectious agent, a manual saw is recommended over a power craniotome, and every effort should be made to avoid cutting the dura with the saw. Recommended decontamination procedures should be followed (▶ Table 22.4 and references). Specimens should be clearly labeled as being from suspected CJD patients to alert laboratory personnel to the hazard. Tissue should be fixed in a saturated 15% phenolized formalin (15 g of phenol per dl of 10% neutral buffered formalin with the undissolved phenol layering at the bottom of the solution).[39]

Analysis for classic histologic findings (see above) and/or immunostaining for PrPres are the gold standards of diagnosis.

22.2.11 Treatment and prognosis

Given the lack of demonstrated infectivity (with tissues other than brain or CSF), isolation precautions such as gowns or masks are felt to be unnecessary.[13]

There is no known treatment. The disease is rapidly progressive. Median survival is 5 months, and 80% of patients with sporadic CJD die within 1 year of diagnosis.[13]

22.3 Parasitic infections of the CNS

22.3.1 General information

A number of parasitic infections may involve the central nervous system. Immunosuppression (including HIV) increases the susceptibility.[40] CNS parasitic infections include:
1. cysticercosis†: see Neurocysticercosis below
2. toxoplasmosis†: may occur as a congenital TORCH infection, or in the adult usually with AIDS; see Neurologic manifestations of AIDS (p. 353). Toxoplasma gondii is an obligate intracellular protozoan that is ubiquitous but does not cause clinical infection except in immunocompromised hosts. Histologic features: necrosis containing 2–3 nm tachyzoites (cysts)
3. echinococcus† (p. 408)
4. amebiasis†: ≈ exclusively Naegleria fowleri (p. 410)
5. schistosomiasis
6. malaria
7. African trypanosomiasis

† parasitic infections with a dagger are those that are more likely to come to neurosurgical attention

22.3.2 Neurocysticercosis

General information

Key concepts

- intracranial encystment of larva of Taenia solium (pork tapeworm)
- the most common parasitic infection of the CNS
- neurological symptoms: seizures or progressive intracranial hypertension
- occurs from ingesting the parasite's eggs, not from eating infested meat
- characteristic imaging finding: low density cysts with eccentric punctate high density (the scolex = tapeworm head). Hydrocephalus is common
- medical treatment: all patients get steroids. Start anthelmintic drugs (praziquantel or albendazole) when no signs of intracranial hypertension are present
- biopsy sometimes needed for diagnosis. Surgery: may be required for spinal, intraventricular or subarachnoid cysts (more refractory to medical therapy) or for giant cysts (> 50 mm) when intracranial hypertension persists despite steroids

Cysticercosis is the most common parasitic infection involving the CNS[41] and in some low-income countries it is the most common cause of acquired epilepsy.[42] It is caused by Cysticercus cellulosae, the larval stage of the pork tapeworm Taenia solium, which has a marked predilection for neural tissue. Cysticercosis is endemic in areas of Mexico, Eastern Europe, Asia, Central and South America, and Africa. The incidence of neurocysticercosis (encystment of larva in the brain) may reach 4% in some areas.[43] The incubation period varies from months to decades, but 83% of cases show symptoms within 7 years of exposure.

Life cycle of T. Solium

Stages

There are 3 stages to the life cycle: larva, embryo (or oncosphere), and adult. T. solium can infect a person in two different ways: as the adult worm or as the larva.

Infection with the adult worm (taeniasis—a parasitic infection)

Human intestinal tapeworm infection (taeniasis) results from eating undercooked infested (measly) pork. The encysted larvae are released in the small bowel and can then mature within the intestine into an adult over about 2 months. The scolex (head) of the segmented adult worm attaches by means of four suckers and two rows of hooklets to the wall of the small intestine where the worm absorbs food directly through its cuticle. Humans are the only known definitive hosts for the adult tapeworm, for which the GI tract is the sole habitat. Proglottids (mature segments, each containing reproductive organs) produce eggs which are liberally excreted along with gravid proglottid segments in the feces.

Infection with the larva

The disease *cysticercosis* occurs when animals or humans become an intermediate host for the larval stage by ingesting viable *eggs* produced by the proglottid. The most common routes of ingestion of viable eggs are:

1. food (usually vegetables) or water contaminated with human feces containing eggs or gravid proglottids (this is the means whereby pigs acquire the disease)
2. fecal-oral autoinoculation in an individual harboring the adult form of the tapeworm due to lack of good sanitary habits or facilities
3. autoinfection by reverse peristalsis of gravid proglottids from the intestine into the stomach (unproven theoretical possibility)

In the duodenum of man and pig, the shell of the ova dissolves and the thusly hatched embryos (oncospheres) burrow through the small bowel wall to enter the lymphatics or systemic circulation and gain access to the following commonly involved sites:

- brain: involved in 60–92% of cases of cysticercosis. Latency from ingestion of eggs to symptomatic neurocysticercosis: 2–5 years[44]
- skeletal muscle
- eye: immunologically privileged, like brain
- subcutaneous tissue
- heart

Once in the tissue of the intermediary host, embryos develop a cyst wall in ≈ 2 months (immature cyst) which matures in ≈ 4 months to a larva. Larval cysts are usually rapidly eliminated by the immune system. Many larvae die naturally within 5–7 yrs or with cysticidal therapy producing an inflammatory reaction with collapse of the cyst (granular nodular stage); these sometimes calcify (nodular calcified stage). In pigs, the larva lie dormant in the muscle, "waiting" to be eaten, after which the cycle repeats.

Types of neurologic involvement

Spinal cord and peripheral nerve involvement is rare.
Giant cysts: definition: cyst with diameter > 50 mm.[45]
Two types of cysts tend to develop in the brain[46]:
1. cysticercus cellulosae: regular, round or oval thin-walled cyst, ranging in size from ≈ 3 to 20 mm tending to form in the *parenchyma* or narrow *subarachnoid* spaces. This cyst contains a scolex (head), is usually static, and produces only mild inflammation during the active phase
2. cysticercus racemosus: larger (4–12 cm), grows actively producing grape-like clusters in the basal subarachnoid spaces and produces intense inflammation. There are *no larvae* in these cysts. These cysts usually degenerate in 2–5 years, during which the capsule thickens and the clear cyst contents are replaced by a whitish gel which undergoes calcium deposition with concomitant shrinkage of the cyst

22

Location of the cysts tends to fall into 1 of 4 groups:
1. meningeal: found in 27–56% of cases with neural involvement. Cysts are adherent or free-floating and are located either in:
   a) dorsolateral subarachnoid space: usually *C. cellulosae* type, causing minimal symptoms
   b) basal subarachnoid space: usually the expanding *C. racemosus* form producing arachnoiditis and fibrosis comprising a chronic meningitis with hypoglycorrhachia. Can obstruct foramina of Luschka and Magendie producing hydrocephalus, or can cause entrapment of basal cisterns → cranial neuropathies (including visual disturbance). Extremely high mortality with this form
2. parenchymal: found in 30–63%; focal or generalized seizures occurs in ≈ 50% of cases (up to 92% in some series)
3. ventricular: found in 12–18%, possibly gaining access via the choroid plexus. Pedunculated or free floating cysts occur, can block CSF flow and cause hydrocephalus with intermittent intracranial hypertension (Brun syndrome). There may be adjacent ependymal enhancement (ependymitis)
4. mixed lesions: found in ≈ 23%

Clinical

Presentation: seizures, signs of elevated ICP (36% of patients with CNS cysticercosis present with increased ICP[47]), focal deficits related to the location of the cyst, and altered mental status are the most common findings. Increased ICP may be due to hydrocephalus or to giant cysts. Symptoms may also be produced by the immunologic reaction to the infestation (cysticercotic encephalitis). Cranial nerve palsies can occur with basal arachnoiditis. Subcutaneous nodules may sometimes be felt.

Diagnosis

General information
Diagnosis is usually made by imaging studies and confirmatory serologic tests.

Laboratory evaluation
Mild peripheral eosinophilia can occur, but is inconsistent and thus unreliable.

CSF may be normal. Eosinophils are seen in 12–60% of cases and suggests parasitic infection. Protein may be elevated.

Stool: less than 33% of cases have T. solium ova in the stool.

Serology
Most centers use enzyme-linked immunoelectrotransfer blot (EITB) against glycoprotein antigens (western blot), which is ≈ 100% specific and 98% sensitive,[48] although sensitivity is less (70%) in cases with a solitary cyst.[49] May be used on serum or CSF. EIBT has effectively superseded ELISA where titer is considered significant at 1:64 in serum, and 1:8 in the CSF; checking for titer exceeding these thresholds in the serum produces a test that is more sensitive and in the CSF is more specific for cysticercosis. False negative rates are higher in cases without meningitis.

Radiographic evaluation
Soft-tissue X-rays may show calcifications in subcutaneous nodules, and in thigh and shoulder muscles.

Skull X-rays show calcifications in 13–15% of cases with neurocysticercosis. May be single or multiple. Usually circular or oval in shape.

CT
The following findings on brain CT have been described (modified[46,50]):
1. ring-enhancing cysts of various sizes representing living cysticerci. Little inflammatory response (edema) occurs as long as the larva is alive. Characteristic finding: small (< 2.5 cm) low density cysts with eccentric punctate high density that may represent the scolex
2. low density with ring enhancement seen as an intermediate stage between living cyst and calcified remnant representing intermediate stage in granuloma formation. Resultant inflammatory reaction can cause edema, and basal arachnoiditis in cysts located in basal subarachnoid space. Often ring-enhancing
3. intraparenchymal punctate calcifications (granuloma) sometimes with, but usually without surrounding enhancement; seen with dead parasites

4. hydrocephalus. Sometimes with intraventricular cysts, which may be isointense with CSF on plain CT[51] and may require contrast CT ventriculography[52] or MRI to be demonstrated

MRI

Early findings: nonenhancing cystic structure(s) with eccentric T1WI hyperintensity (scolex) with no inflammatory response. Lesions may be seen in parenchyma, ventricle, and subarachnoid space. The cyst collapses in later stages of parasitic evolution, with initial edema that gradually resolves with time.

Treatment

Overview

Combination of:
1. anthelmintic medication: antiparasitic and/or cysticidal regimens
2. antiepileptics: to treat seizures, which may sometimes be medically refractory
3. steroids (see below)
4. surgery:
   a) surgical resection of lesions when appropriate
   b) ventricular CSF diversionary procedures

Steroids

Corticosteroids should be used in all patients. May temporarily relieve symptoms, and may help decrease edema that tends to occur initially during treatment with anthelmintic drugs. If possible, start 2–3 d before anthelmintics (e.g., dexamethasone 8 mg q 8 hours[45]), on day 3 decrease to 4 mg q 8 hours, and on day 6 change to prednisone 0.4 mg/kg per day divided TID. Taper steroids after anthelmintics are discontinued. In patients with symptoms of intracranial hypertension: anthelmintic treatment is started after symptoms subside (usually after 3 doses). ✖ Any cysticercocidal drug may cause irreversible damage when used to treat ocular or spinal cysts, even with corticosteroid use.

Antiepileptics

Seizures usually respond to a single ASM. However, the risk of seizures may be lifelong. Risk factors for recurrent seizures: calcified brain lesions, multiple seizures, multiple brain cysts.[53]

Anthelmintic drugs

Since many lesions resolve on their own, and there are significant side effects to these drugs, their use is controversial.[54]

Praziquantel (Biltricide®) is an anthelmintic with activity against all known species of schistosomas. Several regimens have been published:
- 50 mg/kg/d divided in 3 doses (same dose for pediatrics) for 15 days (doses of 100 mg/kg/d have been recommended[45] because steroids reduce serum concentration by 50%[55]). Produces a significant reduction in symptoms and in number of cysts seen on CT[41]
- 10–100 mg/kg/d × 3–21 days
- high dose single day regimen: 25–30 mg/kg q 2 hrs × 3 doses
- for intestinal infestation: single oral dose of 5–10 mg/kg

Albendazole (Zentel®) 15 mg/kg per day divided in 2–3 doses, taken with a fatty meal to enhance absorption (same dose for pediatrics), may be given for 3 months,[56,57] can be stopped sooner if imaging shows resolution.[45] More parasiticidal than praziquantel and may have fewer side effects.

Niclosamide (Niclocide® and others) may be given orally to treat adult tapeworms in the *GI tract*. ℞ 1 gm (2 tablets) chewed PO, repeated in 1 hour (total = 2 g).

Intraventricular disease: There is no consensus on the efficacy of medical treatment for intraventricular cysts.[45,47,58]

Surgery

Surgery may sometimes be necessary to establish the diagnosis. Stereotactic biopsy may be well suited for some cases, especially with deep lesions.

CSF diversion is necessary for patients with symptomatic hydrocephalus, although tubing may become obstructed by granulomatous inflammatory debris.[59]

22

Surgery may be indicated for spinal cysts[43] and for intraventricular cysts, which may be less responsive to medical therapy. The latter may sometimes be dealt with using stereotactic techniques and/or endoscopic instrumentation[52]; however, shunting and anthelmintics may suffice.[58] Surgery may also be needed for giant cysts when intracranial hypertension does not respond to steroids.[45] Anthelmintics may be required even after complete surgical removal because of possibility of relapse.[45]

Follow-up

CT or MRI scan every 6 months until lesions disappear or calcify.[45]

Contacts

Both patients with cysticercosis and their personal contacts should be screened for tapeworm infection since a single dose of niclosamide or praziquantel will eliminate the tapeworm.[60] Close contacts of persons with tapeworms should have screening by medical history and serologic testing for cysticercosis; if suggestive of cysticercosis a neurologic exam and CT or MRI should be done.

22.3.3 Echinococcosis

General information

AKA hydatid (cyst) disease. Caused by encysted larvae of the dog tapeworm Echinococcus granulosa in endemic areas (Uruguay, Australia, New Zealand...). The dog is the primary definitive host of the adult worm. Intermediate hosts for the larval stage include sheep and man. Ova are excreted in dog feces and contaminate herbage eaten by sheep. After ingestion, the embryos hatch and the parasite burrows through the duodenal wall to gain hematogenous access to multiple organs (liver, lungs, heart, bone, brain). Dogs eat these infested organs and the parasite enters the intestine where it remains.

Man is infected either by eating food contaminated with ova, or by direct contact with infected dogs. CNS involvement occurs in only ≈ 3%. Produces cerebral cysts that are confined to the white matter. Primary cysts are usually solitary, secondary cysts (e.g., from embolization from cardiac cysts that rupture or from iatrogenic rupture of cerebral cysts) are usually multiple. The CT density of the cyst is similar to CSF, it does not enhance (although rim enhancement may occur if there is an inflammatory reaction), and there is little surrounding edema. It contains germinating parasitic particles called "hydatid sand" containing ≈ 400,000 scoleces/ml. The cyst enlarges slowly (rates of ≈ 1 cm per year are quoted, but this is variable and may be higher in children), and usually does not present until quite large with findings of increased ICP, seizures, or focal deficit. Patients often have eosinophilia and may have positive serologic tests for hydatid disease.

Treatment

Treatment is surgical removal of the intact cyst. Every effort must be made to avoid rupturing these cysts during removal, or else the scoleces may contaminate the adjacent tissues with possible recurrence of multiple cysts or allergic reaction. May use adjunctive medical treatment with albendazole (Zentel®) 400 mg PO BID (pediatric dose: 15 mg/kg/d) × 28 days, taken with a fatty meal, repeated as necessary.[57]

The Dowling technique is recommended[61]:
1. the head is positioned so that the cyst points straight up towards the ceiling when the OR table is 30° head up
2. drilling burr holes and performing craniotomy must be done very carefully to avoid rupturing the cyst or tearing the dura, which is thin and under tension
3. do not coagulate with anything but low-power bipolar (to avoid cyst rupture)
4. open the dura circumferentially away from the dome of the cyst as it may be adherent to the dura
5. keep the surface of the cyst moist to prevent desiccation and rupture
6. open the thinned overlying cortex gently, separating it from the cyst with irrigation and cottonoids. The cortical opening need only be ≈ 3/4 the cyst diameter but no less
7. insert a soft rubber catheter between the cyst and the brain, and gently irrigate with saline as the head of the OR table is slowly lowered 45° while the surgeon supports the adjacent cortex with his/her fingers
8. continue irrigating more saline and float the cyst out and into a saline filled receptacle

9. if the cyst is ruptured during the procedure, immediately place a sucker in the cyst to aspirate the contents, remove the capsule, and wash the cavity with saline for 5 minutes. Change instruments and gloves. Placing 10% formalin soaked cottonoids on the cavity for a few minutes is controversial[62(p 3750)]

22.4 Fungal infections of the CNS

22.4.1 General information

Most are medically treated conditions that do not require neurosurgical intervention. They tend to present either with chronic meningitis or brain abscess. Some of the more common ones or those of particular relevance to neurosurgery include:

1. cryptococcosis: see below
   a) cryptococcal meningitis
   b) cryptococcoma (mucinous pseudocyst): rare
2. candidiasis: the most common fungal infection of the CNS, but rarely diagnosed before autopsy. Very rare in healthy individuals. Most are C. albicans
   a) candidal meningitis (p. 343): the most common CNS infection; see R (p. 343)
   b) parenchymal infection: candida brain abscesses are rare
   c) following ventricular shunt placement: almost all fungal VP shunt infections are due to Candida spp. (p. 371) [63]
3. aspergillosis (p. 345): may be associated with cerebral abscess in organ transplant patients
4. coccidiomycosis: caused by the dimorphic fungus Coccidioides immitis. Endemic in southwestern U.S. (including San Joaquin Valley in southern California), Mexico, and Central America. Usually presents as meningitis, with rare reports of parenchymal lesions[64]
5. mucormycosis (phycomycosis) (p. 599): usually occurs in diabetics

22.4.2 Cryptococcal involvement of the CNS

General information

Cryptococcal CNS involvement with cryptococcus is diagnosed more frequently in living patients than any other fungal disease. Occurs in healthy or immunocompromised patients. In HIV, Cryptococcus neoformans is the typical agent.

1. cryptococcoma (mucinous pseudocyst): a parenchymal collection which occurs almost exclusively in AIDS patients. Much less common than cryptococcal meningitis. No enhancement of the lesion or the meninges. Usually 3–10 mm in diameter and are frequently located in the basal ganglia (due to spread by small perforating vessels)
2. cryptococcal meningitis (p. 409)
   a) occurs in 4–6% of patients with AIDS.[65] Typical symptoms: fever, malaise and H/A.[66] Meningeal signs (nuchal rigidity, photophobia…) occur in only ≈ 25%. Encephalopathic symptoms (lethargy, altered mentation…), usually from increased ICP, occur in a minority
   b) can also occur without AIDS: gatti variety can infect the brain of immunocompetent hosts[67]
   c) may be associated with increased ICP (with or without hydrocephalus on CT/MRI), decreased visual acuity, and/or cranial nerve deficits. Dilation of Virchow-Robbins spaces may be seen on imaging; on MRI the signal is similar to CSF on T1WI & T2WI, but will be higher on FLAIR
   d) late deterioration in the absence of documented infection may respond to decadron 4 mg q 6 hrs transitioned to prednisone 25 mg PO q d[68]

Diagnosis

LP

Opening pressure (OP) should be measured in the lateral decubitus position.[69] OP is usually elevated, and is > 20 cm H_2O in up to 75%.

CSF: cryptococcal antigen titer is invariably high with cryptococcal meningitis or meningoencephalitis.

Serum cryptococcal antigen: almost always elevated with CNS involvement.[69]

Management

2009 CDC guidelines for CNS cryptoccal infection in *HIV*-infected adolescents/adults[69]:

22

1. antifungal agents: the recommended initial standard treatment[69] is amphotericin B deoxycholate (Amphocin®) 0.7 mg/kg IV q d, plus fluconazole (an oral triazole) 100 mg/kg PO q d in 4 divided doses
2. patients with clinical signs of increased ICP (confusion, blurred vision, papilledema, LE clonus…) should have LP to measure ICP
3. management of intracranial hypertension (ICHT) (OP ≥ 25 cm H$_2$O) with or without hydrocephalus; corticosteroids, acetazolamide, and mannitol have not been shown to be effective[70]:
   a) daily LPs: drain enough CSF to reduce ICP by 50% (typically 20–30 ml)[71]
   b) daily LPs may be suspended when pressures are normal for several consecutive days
   c) lumbar drain: occasionally needed for extremely high OPs (> 40 cm H$_2$O) when frequent LPs are required to or fail to control symptoms[70]
   d) CSF shunt: considered when daily LPs are no longer tolerated or when signs and symptoms of ICHT are not being relieved (neither dissemination of infection through the distal shunt nor creation of a nidus of infection refractory to medical therapy has been described[72]). Options:
      • lumboperitoneal shunt
      • VP or VA shunt[73,74]
4. antifungal treatment is continued for ≥ 2 weeks if renal function is normal (most immunocompetent patients will be successfully treated with 6 weeks of therapy[70])
5. after 2 weeks of treatment, repeat the LP to look for clearance of the organism from the CSF. Positive CSF cultures after 2 weeks of treatment are predictive of future relapse and are associated with worse outcome
6. treatment failures: defined as lack of clinical improvement after 2 weeks of appropriate therapy, including management of ICHT, or relapse after an initial response (defined as either a positive CSF culture and/or rising CSF cryptococcal Ag titer with a compatible clinical picture). Management:
   a) optimal management has not been defined
   b) trials with alternative antifungals (e.g., flucytosine) or higher doses of fluconazole
7. maintenance therapy (secondary prophylaxis): HIV patients who have completed 10 weeks of treatment should be maintained on fluconazole 200 mg q d until immune reconstitution occurs, otherwise lifetime treatment is indicated[69]
8. the risk of recurrence is low for patients who remain asymptomatic after a complete course of therapy and have sustained increase (> 6 months) of CD4 + counts to ≥ 200 cells/mcl. Some experts perform an LP to document negative CSF culture and antigen before stopping maintenance therapy

22.5 Amebic infections of the CNS

22.5.1 General information

Naegleria fowleri: the only ameba (alternative spelling: amoeba) known to cause CNS infection in humans → primary amebic meningoencephalitis (PAM): diffuse encephalitis with hemorrhagic necrosis and purulent meningitis involving brain and spinal cord. Rare (only 95 cases in the U.S. as of 2002, and ≈ 200 cases worldwide as of 2004). The ameba lives in fresh water and soil and typically gains entry to the CNS by invading nasal olfactory mucosa. PAM typically occurs within 5 days of exposure, usually from diving in warm freshwater.

Associated cerebral edema may cause increased ICP and, ultimately, herniation. Fatal in ≈ 95% of cases, usually within 1 week.

CSF: cloudy and often hemorrhagic, ↑ leukocytes, ↑ protein, normal or ↓ glucose, Gram stain negative (no bacteria or fungi), wet prep → motile trophozoites (may be confused with WBCs).

22.5.2 Treatment

Drug of choice: amphotericin B (lipid preparations (Abelcet®) achieve higher MICs (minimal inhibitory concentrations) than other amphotericin preparations. Miconazole may be synergistic with amphotericin B.

Surgical intervention: ventriculostomy with CSF drainage may be indicated when findings are suggestive of increased ICP. In one survivor, surgical drainage of a brain abscess was performed in addition to treatment with a 6-week course of amphotericin B, rifampicin, and chloramphenicol (withdrawn from U.S. market).

References

[1] Wilkins RH, Rengachary SS. Neurosurgery. New York 1985

[2] Neils EW, Lukin R, Tomsick TA, et al. Magnetic Resonance Imaging and Computerized Tomography Scanning of Herpes Simplex Encephalitis. Journal of Neurosurgery. 1987; 67:592–594

[3] Schroth G, Gawehn J, Thron A, et al. The Early Diagnosis of Herpes Simplex Encephalitis by MRI. Neurology. 1987; 37:179–183

[4] Whitley RJ, Soong S-J, Dolin R, et al. Adenosine Arabinoside Therapy of Biopsy-Proved Herpes Simplex Encephalitis: National Institute of Allergy and Infectious Diseases Collaborative Antiviral Study. New England Journal of Medicine. 1977; 297:289–294

[5] Whitley RJ, Cobbs CG, Alford CA, et al. Diseases that Mimic Herpes Simplex Encephalitis: Diagnosis, Presentation, and Outcome. JAMA. 1989; 262:234–239

[6] Schlitt MJ, Morawetz RB, Bonnin JM, et al. Brain Biopsy for Encephalitis. Clinical Neurosurgery. 1986; 33:591–602

[7] Carmack MA, Twiss J, Enzmann DR, et al. Multifocal Leukoencephalitis Caused by Varicella-Zoster Virus in a Child with Leukemia: Successful Treatment with Acyclovir. Pediatr Infect Dis J. 1993; 12:402–406

[8] Horten B, Price RW, Jiminez D. Multifocal Varicella-Zoster Virus Leukoencephalitis Temporally Remote from Herpes Zoster. Annals of Neurology. 1981; 9:251–266

[9] Gilden Don, Cohrs RandallJ, Mahalingam Ravi, et al. Varicella zoster virus vasculopathies: diverse clinical manifestations, laboratory features, pathogenesis, and treatment. Lancet neurology. 2009; 8. DOI: 10.1016/s1474-4422(09)70134-6

[10] Medori R, Montagna P, Tritschler HJ, et al. Fatal Familial Insomnia: A Second Kindred with Mutation of Prion Protein Gene at Codon 178. Neurology. 1992; 42:669–670

[11] Medori R, Tritschler HJ, LeBlanc A, et al. Fatal Familial Insomnia, a Prion Disease with a Mutation at Codon 178 of the Prion Protein Gene. New England Journal of Medicine. 1992; 326:444–449

[12] Manetto V, Medori R, Cortelli P, et al. Fatal familial insomnia: Clinical and pathologic study of five new cases. Neurology. 1992; 42:312–319

[13] Johnson RT, Gibbs CJ. Creutzfeldt-Jakob Disease and Related Transmissible Spongiform Encephalopathies. New England Journal of Medicine. 1998; 339:1994–2004

[14] Gajdusek DC. Unconventional Viruses and the Origin and Disappearance of Kuru. Science. 1977; 197:943–960

[15] Klitzman R. The Trembling Mountain. A Personal Account of Kuru, Cannibals, and Mad Cow Disease. New York: Plenum Trade; 1998

[16] Heckmann JG, Lang CJG, Petruch F, et al. Transmission of Creutzfeldt-Jakob Disease via a Corneal Transplant. Journal of Neurology, Neurosurgery and Psychiatry. 1997; 63:388–390

[17] Brown P, Preece M, Brandel J-P, et al. Iatrogenic Creutzfeldt-Jakob Disease at the Millennium. Neurology. 2000; 55:1075–1081

[18] Hsiao K, Prusiner SB. Inherited Human Prion Diseases. Neurology. 1990; 40:1820–1827

[19] Bertoni JM, Brown P, Goldfarb LG, et al. Familial Creutzfeldt-Jakob Disease (Codon 200 Mutation) With Supranuclear Palsy. Journal of the American Medical Association. 1992; 268:2413–2415

[20] Will RG, Zeidler JW, Cousens SN, et al. A new variant of Creutzfeldt-Jakob disease in the UK. Lancet. 1996; 347:921–925

[21] Duffy P, Wolf J, Collins G, et al. Possible Person to Person Transmission of Creutzfeldt-Jakob Disease. New England Journal of Medicine. 1974; 290:692–693

[22] Bernoulli C, Siegfried J, Baumgartner G, et al. Danger of Accidental Person-To-Person Transmission of Creutzfeldt-Jakob Disease by Surgery. Lancet. 1977; 1:478–479

[23] Fradkin JE, Schonberger LB, Mills JL, et al. Creutzfeldt-Jakob Disease in Pituitary Growth Hormone Recipients in the United States. Journal of the American Medical Association. 1991; 265:880–884

[24] Centers for Disease Control (Morbidity and Mortality Weekly Report). Rapidly Progressive Dementia in a Patient Who Received a Cadaveric Dura Mater Graft. JAMA. 1987; 257:1036–1037

[25] Thadani V, Penar PL, Partington J, et al. Creutzfeldt-Jakob disease probably acquired from a cadaveric dura mater graft. J Neurosurg. 1988; 69:766–769

[26] Centers for Disease Control. Creutzfeldt-Jakob Disease in a Second Patient Who Received a Cadaveric Dura Mater Graft. Morbidity and Mortality Weekly Report. 1989; 39:37–43

[27] Rosenberg RN, White CL, Brown P, et al. Precautions in Handling Tissues, Fluids and Other Contaminated Materials from Patients with Documented or Suspected Creutzfeldt-Jakob Disease. Ann Neurol. 1986; 12:75–77

[28] Brown P, Gibbs CJ, Amyx JL, et al. Chemical disinfection of Creutzfeldt-Jakob virus. New England Journal of Medicine. 1982; 306:1279–1282

[29] Brown P, Cathala F, Castaigne P, et al. Creutzfeldt-Jakob Disease: Clinical Analysis of a Consecutive Series of 230 Neuropathologically Verified Cases. Annals of Neurology. 1986; 20:597–602

[30] Finkenstaedt M, Szudra A, Zerr I, et al. MR Imaging of Creutzfeldt-Jakob Disease. Radiology. 1996; 199:793–798

[31] Gertz H-J, Henkes H, Cervos-Navarro J. Creutzfeldt-Jakob disease: Correlation of MRI and neuropathologic findings. Neurology. 1988; 38:1481–1482

[32] Otto M, Wiltfang J, Schutz E, et al. Diagnosis of Creutzfeldt-Jakob Disease by Measurement of S100 Protein in Serum: Prospective Case-Control Study. British Medical Journal. 1998; 316:577–582

[33] Atarashi R, Satoh K, Sano K, et al. Ultrasensitive human prion detection in cerebrospinal fluid by real-time quaking-induced conversion. Nat Med. 2011; 17:175–178

[34] Orru CD, Groveman BR, Hughson AG, et al. Rapid and sensitive RT-QuIC detection of human Creutzfeldt-Jakob disease using cerebrospinal fluid. mBio. 2015; 6. DOI: 10.1128/mBio.02451-14

[35] Franceschini A, Baiardi S, Hughson AG, et al. High diagnostic value of second generation CSF RT-QuIC across the wide spectrum of CJD prions. Sci Rep. 2017; 7. DOI: 10.1038/s41598-017-10922-w

[36] Steinhoff BJ, Räcker S, Herrendorf G, et al. Accuracy and Reliability of Periodic Sharp Wave Complexes in Creutzfeldt-Jakob Disease. Archives of Neurology. 1996; 53:162–166

[37] de Silva R, Patterson J, Hadley D, et al. Single photon emission computed tomography in the identification of new variant Creutzfeldt-Jakob disease: Case reports. British Medical Journal. 1998; 316:593–594

[38] Hill AF, Butterworth RJ, Joiner S, et al. Investigation of Variant Creutzfeldt-Jakob Disease and Other Human Prion Diseases with Tonsil Biopsy Samples. Lancet. 1999; 353:183–189

[39] Brumbach RA. Routine Use of Phenolized Formalin in Fixation of Autopsy Brain Tissue to Reduce Risk of Inadvertent Transmission of Creutzfeldt-Jakob Disease. N Engl J Med. 1988; 319

[40] Walker M, Kublin JG, Zunt JR. Parasitic central nervous system infections in immunocompromised hosts: malaria, microsporidiosis, leishmaniasis, and African trypanosomiasis. Clin Infect Dis. 2006; 42:115–125

[41] Sotelo J, Escobedo F, Rodriguez-Carbajal J, et al. Therapy of parenchymal brain cysticercosis with praziquantel. N Engl J Med. 1984; 310:1001–1007

[42] Garcia HH, Gonzales AE, Evans CAW, et al. Taenia solium cysticersosis. Lancet. 2003; 362:547–556

[43] Sotelo J, Guerrero V, Rubio F. Neurocysticercosis: A new classification based on active and inactive forms. Arch Intern Med. 1985; 145:442–445

[44] Garcia HH, Del Brutto OH, for The Cysticercosis Working Group in Peru. Neurocysticercosis: updated concepts about an old disease. Lancet Neurology. 2005; 4:653–661

[45] Proano JV, Madrazo I, Avelar F, et al. Medical treatment for neurocysticercosis characterized by giant subarachnoid cysts. N Engl J Med. 2001; 345:879–885

[46] Leblanc R, Knowles KF, Melanson D, et al. Neurocysticercosis: Surgical and Medical Management with Praziquantel. Neurosurgery. 1986; 18:419–427

[47] Colli BO, Carlotti CG, Machado HR, et al. Treatment of Patients with Intraventricular Cysticercosis. Contemporary Neurosurgery. 1999; 21:1–7

[48] Wilson M, Bryan RT, Fried JA, et al. Clinical Evaluation of the Cysticercosis Enzyme-Linked Immunoelectrotransfer Blot in Patients with Neurocysticercosis. J Infect Dis. 1991; 164:1007–1009

[49] Prabhakaran V, Rajshekhar V, Murrell KD, et al. Taenia solium metacestode glycoproteins as diagnostic antigens for solitary cysticercus granuloma in Indian patients. Transactions of the Royal Society of Tropical Medicine and Hygiene. 2004; 98:478–484

[50] Enzman DR. Cysticercosis. In: Imaging of Infections and Inflammations of the Central Nervous System: Computed Tomography, Ultrasound, and Nuclear Magnetic Resonance. New York: Raven Press; 1984:103–122

[51] Madrazo I, Renteria JAG, Paredes G, et al. Diagnosis of Intraventricular and Cisternal Cysticercosis by Computerized Tomography with Positive Intraventricular Contract Medium. J Neurosurg. 1981; 55:947–951

[52] Apuzzo MLJ, Dobkin WR, Zee C-S, et al. Surgical Considerations in Treatment of Intraventricular Cysticercosis: An Analysis of 45 Cases. Journal of Neurosurgery. 1984; 60:400–407

[53] Del Brutto OH. Prognostic factors for seizure recurrence after withdrawal of entiepileptic drugs in patients with neurocysticercosis. Neurology. 1994; 44:1706–1709

[54] Abba K, Ramaratnam S, Ranganathan LN. Anthelmintics for people with neurocysticercosis. Cochrane Database Syst Rev. 2010. DOI: 10.1002/1 4651858.CD000215.pub3

[55] Jung H, Hurtado M, Sanchez M, et al. Plasma and CSF levels of albendazole and praziquantel in patients with neurocysticercosis. Clin Neuropharmacol. 1990; 13:559–564

[56] Sotelo J, Penagos P, Escobedo F, et al. Short Course of Albendazole Therapy for Neurocysticercosis. Arch Neurol. 1988; 45:1130–1133

[57] Drugs for Parasitic Infections. Medical Letter. 1995; 37:99–108

[58] Bandres JC, White AC,Jr, Samo T, et al. Extraparenchymal neurocysticercosis: report of five cases and review of management. Clin Infect Dis. 1992; 15:799–811

[59] McCormick GF, Zee C-S, Heiden J. Cysticercosis Cerebri. Arch Neurol. 1982; 39:534–539

[60] Centers for Disease Control. Locally acquired neurocysticercosis. Morbidity and Mortality Weekly Report. 1992; 41:1–4

[61] Carrea R, Dowling E, Guevara JA. Surgical Treatment of Hydatid Cysts of the Central Nervous System in the Pediatric Age (Dowling's Technique). Childs Brain. 1975; 1:4–21

[62] Youmans JR. Neurological Surgery. Philadelphia 1990

[63] Sanchez-Portocarrero J, Martin-Rabadan P, Saldana CJ,. et al. Candida cerebrospinal fluid shunt infection. Report of two new cases and review of the literature. Diagnostic Microbiology and Infectious Disease. 1994; 20:33–40

[64] Mendel E, Milefchik EN, Ahmadi J, et al. Coccidioidomycotic Brain Abscess: Case Report. Journal of Neurosurgery. 1994; 80:140–142

[65] Chuck SL, Sande MA. Infections with cryptococcus neoformans in the acquired immunodeficiency syndrome. New England Journal of Medicine. 1989; 321:794–799

[66] Aberg JA, Powderly WG, Dolin R, et al. Cryptococcosis. In: AIDS Therapy. New York: Churcill Livingstone; 2002:498–510

[67] Lan S, Chang W, Lu C, et al. Cerebral infarction in chronic meningitis: a comparison of tuberculous meningitis and cryptococcal meningitis. Quarterly Journal of Medicine. 2001; 94:247–253

[68] Lane M, McBride J, Archer J. Steroid responsive late deterioration in Cryptococcus neoformans variety gattii meningitis. Neurology. 2004; 63:713–714

[69] Kaplan JE, Benson C, Holmes KH, et al. Guidelines for prevention and treatment of opportunistic infections in HIV-infected adults and adolescents. MMWR Recomm Rep. 2009; 58:1–207; quiz CE1-4

[70] Saag MS, Graybill RJ, Larsen RA, et al. Practice guidelines for the management of crytpococcal disease. Clinical Infectious Diseases. 2000; 30:710–718

[71] Fessler RD, Sobel J, Guyot L, et al. Management of elevated intracranial pressure in patients with Cryptococcal meningitis. Journal of Acquired Immune Deficiency Syndromes and Human Retrovirology. 1998; 17:137–142

[72] Park MK, Hospenthal DR, Bennett JE. Treatment of hydrocephalus secondary to cryptococcal meningitis by use of shunting. Clin Infect Dis. 1999; 28:629–633

[73] Bach MC, Tally PW, Godofsky EW. Use of cerebrospinal fluid shunts in patients having acquired immunodeficiency syndrome with cryptococcal meningitis and uncontrollable intracranial hypertension. Journal of Neurosurgery. 1997; 41:1280–1283

[74] Liliang PC, Liang CL, Chang WN, et al. Use of ventriculoperitoneal shunts to treat uncontrollable intracranial hypertension in patients who have cryptococcal meningitis without hydrocephalus. Clin Infect Dis. 2002; 34:E64–E68

Part VII

Hydrocephalus and Cerebrospinal Fluid (CSF)

VII

23

23 Cerebrospinal Fluid

23.1 General CSF characteristics

Cerebrospinal fluid (CSF) surrounds the brain and spinal cord, and may function as a shock absorber for the CNS. It may also serve an immunological function analogous to the lymphatic system (so-called "glymphatics" a portmanteau word from glia and lymphatic).[1,2] It circulates within the subarachnoid space, between the arachnoid and the pial membranes.

CSF is normally a clear colorless fluid with a specific gravity of 1.007 and a pH of ≈ 7.33–7.35.

23.2 Bulk flow model

23.2.1 General information

The classic bulk flow model of CSF ascribes discrete sites of CSF production, absorption, as well as circulation routes. While this model may be useful for understanding and treating some aspects of CSF physiology, it is becoming clear that it is inadequate to explain many of the details. Pulsatile flow, lymphatic channels (glymphatics) and distributed sites of production and absorption all appear to participate in CSF dynamics. For the time being, the bulk flow model with its shortcomings will be presented here.

23.2.2 Production

Location

80% of CSF is produced by the choroid plexuses, located in both lateral ventricles (accounts for ≈ 95% of CSF produced in the choroid plexuses) and in the 4th ventricle. Most of the rest of intracranial production occurs in the interstitial space.[3] CSF is also produced by the ependymal lining of the ventricles, and in the spine within the dura of the nerve root sleeves. ▶ Table 23.1 shows properties of CSF production, volumes and pressures.

Production rate

In the adult, CSF is produced at a rate of about 0.3 ml/min (▶ Table 23.1). In terms that are clinically relevant, this approximates 450 ml/24hrs, which means that in an adult (where the average total CSF volume in the body is 150 ml), the CSF is "turned over" ≈ 3 times every day. The rate of formation is independent of the intracranial pressure[4] (except in the limiting case when ICP becomes so high that cerebral blood flow is reduced[5]).

Table 23.1 Normal CSF production, volumes, and pressure (bulk flow model)

Property	Peds		Adult
	Newborn	1–10 yrs	
total volume (ml)	5		150 (50% intracranial, 50% spinal)
formation rate	25 ml/d		≈ 0.3–0.35 ml/min (≈ 450–750 ml/d)
pressure[a] (cm of fluid)	9–12	mean: 10 normal: < 15	adult: 7–15 (> 18 usually abnormal) young adult: < 18–20

[a]as measured in the lumbar subarachnoid space, with the patient relaxed in the lateral decubitus position

23.2.3 Absorption

CSF is absorbed primarily by arachnoid villi (granulations) that extend into the dural venous sinuses. Other sites of absorption include the choroid plexuses and glymphatics. The rate of absorption is pressure-dependent.[6]

23.3 CSF constituents

23.3.1 Cellular components of CSF

In normal adult CSF, there are 0–5 lymphocytes or mononuclear cells per mm³, and no polys (PMNs) or RBCs. In the absence of RBCs, 5–10 WBCs per mm³ is suspicious, and > 10 WBCs per mm³ is definitely abnormal.

23.3.2 Noncellular components of CSF

See ▶ Table 23.2.

Table 23.2 CSF solutes.[7 (p 169),8] For CEA, AFP, & hCG, see Tumor markers (p.631)

Constituent	Units	CSF	Plasma	CSF:plasma ratio
osmolarity	mOsm/L	295	295	1.0
H_2O content		99%	93%	
sodium	mEq/L	138	138	1.0
potassium	mEq/L	2.8	4.5	0.6
chloride	mEq/L	119	102	1.2
calcium	mEq/L	2.1	4.8	0.4
pCO_2	mm Hg	47	41[a]	1.1
pH		7.33	7.41	
pO_2	mm Hg	43	104[a]	0.4
glucose	mg/dl	60	90	0.67
lactate	mEq/L	1.6	1.0[a]	1.6
pyruvate	mEq/L	0.08	0.11[a]	0.73
lactate:pyruvate		26	17.6[a]	
total protein[b]	mg/dl	35	7000	0.005
albumin	mg/L	155	36600	0.004
IgG	mg/L	12.3	9870	0.001

[a]arterial plasma
[b]Note: CSF protein is lower in ventricular fluid than in lumbar subarachnoid space
Data from Table 6–1 of "Cerebrospinal Fluid in Diseases of the Nervous System" by Robert A. Fishman, M.D., © 1980, W. B. Saunders Co., Philadelphia, PA, used with permission

23.3.3 Variation with site

The composition of CSF differs slightly in the ventricles where the majority of it is produced compared to the lumbar subarachnoid space.

23.3.4 CSF variations with age

See ▶ Table 23.3. For further variations in CSF findings specifically in adults, see ▶ Table 23.4.

23.4 Cranial CSF fistula

Key concepts

- suspect in posttraumatic otorrhea/rhinorrhea or recurrent meningitis
- management strategy: 1) confirm the fluid is CSF, 2) identify the site of origin of the leak, 3) determine etiology/mechanism
- most bedside tests are unreliable and include "reservoir sign," target/halo sign, qualitative glucose
- most accurate confirmatory test is β2-transferrin
- CT cisternography is the test of choice for localizing site of fistula

23

Table 23.3 Variations with age

Age group	WBC/mm³	RBC/mm³	Protein (mg/dl)	Glucose (mg/dl)	Glucose ratio (CSF:plasma)
newborn					
preemie	10	many	150	20–65	0.5–1.6
term	7–8	mod	80	30–120	0.4–2.5
infants					
1–12 mos	5–6	0	15–80		
1–2 yrs	2–3	0	15		
young child	2–3	0	20		
child 5–15 yrs	2–3	0	25		
adolescent & adult	3	0	30	40–80	0.5
senile	5	0	40[a]		

[a]normal CSF protein rises ≈ 1 mg/dl per year of age in the adult

23.4.1 General information

AKA CSF leak. CSF fistula should be suspected in patients with otorrhea or rhinorrhea after head trauma, or in patients with recurrent meningitis.

23.4.2 Possible routes of egress of CSF

1. mastoid air cells (especially after p-fossa surgery, e.g., for vestibular schwannoma [VS])
2. sphenoid air cells (especially post-transsphenoidal surgery)
3. cribriform plate/ethmoidal roof (floor of frontal fossa)
4. frontal sinus air cells
5. herniation into empty sella and then into sphenoid air sinus
6. along path of internal carotid artery
7. Rosenmüller's fossa: located just inferior to cavernous sinus, may be exposed by drilling off anterior clinoids to allow access to ophthalmic artery aneurysms
8. site of the opening of the transient lateral craniopharyngeal canal
9. percutaneously through a surgical or traumatic wound
10. petrous ridge or internal auditory canal: following temporal bone fracture or vestibular schwannoma surgery. Then either:
    a) rhinorrhea: through middle ear → eustachian tube → nasopharynx
    b) otorrhea: via perforated tympanic membrane → external auditory canal

23.4.3 Traumatic vs. nontraumatic etiology

Description

Two major subgroups of CSF fistula (omitting the ambiguous category of "spontaneous")[9]:
1. traumatic (or posttraumatic): may occur acutely or may be delayed
    a) post-procedure (iatrogenic). Including: post-transsphenoidal surgery and post skull base surgery
    b) posttraumatic (more common): 67–77% of cases
2. nontraumatic
    a) high pressure
       • hydrocephalus
       • tumor
    b) normal pressure
       • congenital defects
       • bony erosion from infection or necrosis
       • focal atrophy (olfactory or sellar)

Traumatic fistula

Occur in 2–3% of all patients with head injury, 60% occur within days of trauma, 95% within 3 months.[10] 70% of cases of CSF rhinorrhea stop within 1 wk, and usually within 6 mos in the rest.

Table 23.4 CSF findings in various pathologic conditions (adult values)[a]

Condition	OP (cm H₂O)	Appearance	Cells (per mm³)	Protein (mg%)	Glucose (% serum)	Miscellaneous
normal	7–18	clear colorless	0 PMN, 0 RBC 0–5 monos	15–45	50	
acute purulent meningitis	Freq ↑	turbid	few–20K WBCs (mostly PMNs)	100–1000	<20	few cells early or if treated
viral meningitis & encephalitis	nl	nl	few–350 WBCs (mostly monos)	40–100	nl	PMNs early
Guillain-Barré	nl	nl	nl	50–1000	nl	protein↑ freq IgG
polio	nl	nl	50–250 (monos)	40–100	nl	
TB meningitis[b]	freq ↑	opalescent, yellow, fibrin clot on standing	50–500 (lymphocytes and monocytes)	60–700	20–40	PMN early, (+) AFB culture, (+) Ziel-Neelson stain
fungal meningitis	Freq ↑	opalescent	30–300 (monos)	100–700	<30	(+) India ink prep with cryptococcus
amebic meningoencephalitis (Naegleria)	freq ↑	cloudy, may be hemorrhagic	↑ WBCs (400–26K), ↑ RBCs	↑	nl or ↓	negative Gram stain; wet mount → motile trophozoites (p. 410)
parameningeal infection	↑ if block	nl	WBCs nl or ↑ (0–800)	↑	nl	e.g., spinal epidural abscess
traumatic[c] (bloody) tap	nl	bloody; supernatant colorless	RBC:WBC ratio ≈ as in peripheral	slight ↑	nl	RBCs ↓ in successive tubes; no xanthochromia
SAH[c]	↑	bloody; supernatant xanthochromic	early: ↑RBCs	50–400	nl or ↓	RBCs disappear in 2 wks, xanthochromia may persist for weeks
			late: ↑WBCs	100–800		
multiple sclerosis (MS)[d]	nl	nl	5–50 monos	nl–800	nl	usually ↑ gamma globulins (oligoclonal)

[a]abbreviations: OP = opening pressure; nl = normal; ↑ = increased; ↓ = decreased; freq = frequently
[b]the CSF findings in TB meningitis are almost pathognomonic when they occur in combination; 20–30% have acid-fast bacilli in their CSF sediment smears
[c]to differentiate traumatic tap from SAH, see Differentiating SAH from traumatic tap (p. 1814)
[d]see more information on the CSF in MS (p. 190)

Non-traumatic cases cease spontaneously in only 33%. Adult:child ratio is 10:1, rare before age 2 yrs. In children the incidence of CSF leaks is less than 1% of closed head injuries.[11] Anosmia is common in traumatic leaks (78%), and is rare in spontaneous.[12] Most (80–85%) CSF otorrhea ceases in 5–10 days.

CSF fistula occurred in 8.9% of 101 cases of penetrating trauma, and increases the infection rate over those penetrating injuries without fistula (50% vs. 4.6%).[13] It is reported to occur post-op in up to 30% of cases of skull-base surgery.[14]

23

Nontraumatic CSF fistula

General information

Nontraumatic leaks primarily occur in adults > 30 yrs. Often insidious. May be mistaken for allergic rhinitis. Unlike traumatic leaks, these tend to be intermittent, the sense of smell is usually preserved, and pneumocephalus is uncommon.[15]

Sometimes associated with the following[16]:

1. agenesis of the floor of the anterior fossa (cribriform plate) or middle fossa
2. empty sella syndrome (p.952): primary or post-transsphenoidal surgery
3. increased ICP and/or hydrocephalus
4. infection of the paranasal sinuses
5. tumor: including PitNET/adenomas (p.854), meningiomas
6. a persistent remnant of the craniopharyngeal canal[17]
7. AVM[15]
8. congenital anomalies: most involve dehiscence of bone
   a) dehiscence of the footplate of the stapes (a congenital abnormality) which can produce CSF rhinorrhea via the eustachian tube[15]
   b) dehiscence below foramen rotundum

Spontaneous posterior fossa CSF fistula

1. pediatric: usually presents with either meningitis or hearing loss
   a) preserved labyrinthine function (hearing and balance): these usually present with meningitis. 3 usual routes of fistula:
      • facial canal: can fistulize into middle ear
      • petromastoid canal: along path of arterial supply to mucosa of mastoid air sinuses
      • Hyrtl's fissure (AKA tympanomeningeal fissure): links p-fossa to hypotympanum
   b) anomalies of labyrinth (hearing lost): one of several types of Mundini dysplasias, usually presenting with rounded labyrinth/cochlea that permits CSF to erode through oval or round window into auditory canal
2. adult: usually presents with conductive hearing loss with serous effusion, meningitis (often following an episode of otitis media), or cerebral abscess. Occurs most commonly through middle fossa. May be due to arachnoid granulations eroding into air sinus compartment

23.5 Spinal CSF fistula

Often presents with postural headache associated with neck stiffness and tenderness.[18]

23.6 Meningitis in CSF fistula

Incidence with posttraumatic CSF leak: 5–10%, increases as leak persists > 7 days. Meningitis is more common with spontaneous fistula. Risk may be higher in fistula following a neurosurgical procedure than in posttraumatic fistula possibly due to elevated ICP common in latter (forces CSF outward).

Meningitis may promote inflammatory changes at the site of the leak, with a resultant cessation of the leak. However, this often proves to be a temporary resolution, providing a false sense of security.

Pneumococcal meningitis is the most common pathogen (83% of cases[19]), mortality is lower than in pneumococcal meningitis without underlying fistula (< 10% vs. 50%), possibly because the latter is frequently seen in elderly debilitated patients. Prognosis in children is worse.[10]

23.7 Evaluation of the patient with CSF fistula

23.7.1 Determining if rhinorrhea or otorrhea is due to a CSF fistula

1. characteristics of the fluid suggesting the presence of CSF
   a) fluid is as clear as water (unless infected or admixed with blood)
   b) fluid does not cause excoriation within or outside the nose
   c) patients with CSF rhinorrhea describe the taste as salty
2. confirmatory tests
   a) β_2-transferrin: present in CSF, but absent in tears, saliva, nasal exudates and serum (except for newborns and patients with liver disease).[20,21] The only other source is the vitreous fluid of the eye. It may be detected by protein electrophoresis. A minimum of ≈ 0.5 ml needs to be

collected, placed in a sterile urine container, packed in dry ice, and shipped to a lab that can perform this study. Very sensitive and specific

b) collect fluid and obtain *quantitative* glucose (urine glucose detection strips are too sensitive, and may be positive even with excess mucus). Test the fluid shortly after collection to mini-mize fermentation. Normal CSF glucose is > 30 mg% (usually lower with meningitis), whereas lacrimal secretions and mucus are usually < 5 mg%. A negative test is more helpful since it rules out CSF (except in hypoglycorrhachia [low glucose in the CSF]), but there is a 45–75% chance of false positive[22 (p 1638)]

c) "ring sign": when a CSF leak is suspected but the fluid is blood tinged, allow the fluid to drip onto linen (sheet or pillowcase). A ring of blood with a larger concentric ring of clear fluid (so-called "double ring" or halo sign) suggests the presence of CSF. An old, but unreliable, sign

d) reservoir sign: a gush of fluid that occurs with a certain head position. Most common when first sitting up after a period of recumbency. Thought to indicate drainage of CSF pooled in the sphenoid sinus. Not reliable[23]

3. radiographic signs: pneumocephalus on CT or skull X-ray. Pneumocephalus occurs in ≈ 20% of patients with CSF leaks[24 (p 280)]

4. cisternogram: intrathecal injection of radionuclide tracer followed by scintigram or injection of radiopaque contrast followed by CT scan (see below)

5. anosmia is present in ≈ 5% of CSF leaks

6. following skull-base surgery (especially involving greater superficial petrosal nerve), there may be a pseudo-CSF rhinorrhea, possibly due to nasal hypersecretion from imbalanced autonomic regulation of the nasal mucosa[14] ipsilateral to the surgery. Often accompanied by nasal stuffiness and absent ipsilateral lacrimation, and occasionally by facial flushing

23.7.2 Localizing the site of CSF fistula

90% of the time, localization does not require water-soluble contrast CT cisternography (WS-CTC) (see below).

1. CT: to detect pneumocephalus, fractures, skull base defects, hydrocephalus and obstructive neo-plasms. Include thin *coronal* cuts or reconstructions through anterior fossa all the way back to the sella turcica
   a) non-contrast (optional): to demonstrate bony anatomy
   b) with IV contrast: leak site is usually associated with abnormal enhancement of adjacent brain parenchyma (possibly from inflammation)

2. water-soluble contrast CT cisternography (procedure of choice): see below

3. plain skull X-ray (helpful in only 21%)

4. MRI: may provide additional information for localization and can R/O p-fossa mass, tumor, and empty sella better than CT. Both CT and MRI can R/O hydrocephalus. T2WI fast spin-echo sequen-ces with fat suppression and video image reversal have been used to visualize CSF flow (sensitiv-ity and specificity are 0.87 and 0.57, respectively)[25]

5. older tests (abandoned in favor of above):
   a) radionuclide cisternography (RNC): not a contemporary test. Poor localization. Some of the studied radiopharmaceuticals are no longer available
   b) intrathecal (visible) dye studies: some success with indigo carmine or fluorescein (p. 1716) with little or no complications.
      ✖ methylene blue (p. 1716) is neurotoxic and should not be used

Water-soluble contrast CT cisternography

Procedure of choice. This test is performed if:

1. no site identified on plain CT (with coronals)

2. when patient is leaking clinically (the site is only sometimes identified in the absence of an active leak)

3. when multiple bony defects are identified, and it is essential to determine which site is actively leaking

4. if a bony defect seen on plain CT does not have associated changes of abnormal enhancement of adjacent brain parenchyma

Technique[26]: Use iohexol (p. 230) 6–7 ml of 190–220 mg/ml injected into lumbar subarachnoid space via 22 gauge spinal needle (or 5 ml via C1–2 puncture). Patient positioned in -70° Trendelen-burg × 3 min prone with neck gently flexed, in CT they are kept prone with head hyperextended with 5 mm coronal cuts with 3 mm overlap (use 1.5 mm cuts if necessary). May need provocative maneuvers (coronal scans prone (brow up) or in position of leak, intrathecal saline infusion (requires Harvard pump)[27]...).

Look for accumulation of contrast in air sinuses. Apparent discontinuity of bone on CT without extravasation of contrast is probably not the site of leakage (bone discontinuities may be mimicked by partial volume averaging on CT).

23.8 Treatment for CSF fistula

23.8.1 Initial treatment

Acutely after trauma, observation is justified as most cases cease spontaneously.

Prophylactic antibiotics: Controversial. There was no difference in the incidence or morbidity of meningitis between treated and untreated patients.[28] Furthermore, the risk of selecting resistant strains appears real[10] and is therefore usually avoided.

Pneumococcal vaccine: recommended for most patients ≥ 2 years age, see details (p. 341)

23.8.2 For persistent posttraumatic or post-op leaks

Non-surgical treatment

1. measures to lower ICP:
   a) bed rest: although recumbency may ameliorate symptoms, there is no other benefit from bed rest[29]
   b) avoid straining (stool softeners) and avoid blowing nose
   c) acetazolamide (250 mg PO QID) to reduce CSF production
   d) modest fluid restriction. Use with caution following transsphenoidal adenoma resection because of possible DI (p. 124): 1500 ml/day in adults, 75% of maintenance/day in peds
2. if leak persists (caution: first R/O obstructive hydrocephalus with CT or MRI)
   NB: see box below regarding lumbar drainage of CSF
   a) LP: q d to BID (lower pressure to near atmospheric or until H/A)
      OR
   b) continuous lumbar drainage (CLD): via percutaneous catheter. Two (of many) management options:
      • keep HOB elevated 10–15° and place drip chamber at shoulder level (lower the chamber if leak persists) and leave open to drain (uses pressure to regulate drainage—may be dangerous e.g., if drainage bag falls to floor)
      • allow 15–20 cc to drain, then clamp tubing. Repeat q 1 hour
   c) CLD may require ICU monitoring. If patient deteriorates with drain in place: immediately stop drainage, place patient flat in bed (or slight Trendelenburg), start 100% O_2, get CT or bedside cross-table skull X-ray (to R/O tension pneumocephalus due to drawing in of air)
3. surgical treatment in persistent cases (see below)

Greenberg IMHO

A CSF leak following transsphenoidal surgery is rarely definitely treated with lumbar drainage of CSF alone (via LP or lumbar drain). If the leak is identified at the time of surgery, a septal mucosal flap is more frequently successful. If the leak manifests post-op, the best course of action is usually to take the patient back to the OR for reclosure. These procedures may then be *augmented* with lumbar drainage of CSF.

Surgical treatment

General information

If the site of leakage is not identified prior to attempted surgical treatment, 30% develop a recurrent leak post-op, with 5–15% of these developing meningitis before leak is stopped.[27]

Indications for surgical intervention

1. **traumatic** CSF leak that persists > 2 weeks in spite of non-surgical measures

2. **spontaneous** leaks and those of **delayed onset following trauma** or surgery: usually require surgery because of a high incidence of recurrence
3. leaks complicated by recurrent **meningitis**

Leaks through cribriform plate/ethmoidal roof

Extradural approach: Generally preferred by ENT surgeons.[30] If a frontal craniotomy is being performed, an intradural approach should be used since problems may arise in dissecting the dura off of the floor of the frontal fossa, wherein the dura almost always tears and then it is difficult to know if an identified tear is the cause of the leak or if it is iatrogenic. Fluorescein dye mixed with CSF injected intrathecally may help demonstrate the leak intraoperatively. *CAUTION*: must be diluted with CSF to reduce risk of seizures (p. 1716).

Intradural approach

Generally the procedure of choice.[31] If the fistula site is unidentified preoperatively, use a bifrontal bone flap.

General techniques of *intradural* approach:

Close bone defects with fat, muscle, cartilage, or bone.

Close dural defect with fascia lata, temporalis muscle fascia, or pericranium. Fibrin glue may be used to help hold tissue in place.

If the leak is unidentified pre-op and intra-op, then pack both cribriform plates and sphenoid sinus (incise dura over tuberculum sellae, drill through bone to reach sphenoid sinus, remove mucosa or pack it inferiorly, pack with fat).

Post op: lumbar drain after craniotomy is controversial. Some feel CSF pressure may help enhance the seal.[32] If used, place the drip chamber at the level of shoulder for 3–5 days (for precautions, see above).

Consider shunt (LP or VP) if elevated ICP or hydrocephalus is demonstrated.

Leaks into sphenoid sinus (including post-transsphenoidal surgery leak)

1. LP BID or CLD: as long as pressure > 150 mm H_2O or CSF xanthochromic
   a) if leak persists > 3 days: repack sphenoid sinus and pterygoid recesses with fat, muscle, cartilage and/or fascia lata (must reconstruct floor of sella, packing alone is inadequate). Some recommend against muscle since it putrefies and shrinks. Continue LP or CLD as above for 3–5 days post-op
   b) if leak persists > 5 days: lumboperitoneal shunt (first R/O obstructive hydrocephalus)
2. more difficult surgical approach: intracranial (intradural) approach to medial aspect of middle cranial fossa
3. consider transnasal sellar injection of fibrin glue under local anesthesia[33]

Petrous bone

May present as otorrhea or as rhinorrhea (via the eustachian tube).

1. following posterior fossa surgery: see also treatment following vestibular schwannoma surgery (p. 797)
2. following mastoid bone fractures: may be approached via extensive mastoidectomy[15]
3. due to dehiscence of the footplate of the stapes: may require obliteration of the middle ear and eustachian tube through a tympanomeatal flap[15]

23.9 Spontaneous intracranial hypotension (SIH)

23.9.1 General information

Intracranial hypotension may be spontaneous or posttraumatic. This section deals with spontaneous intracranial hypotension. Posttraumatic intracranial hypotension includes iatrogenic etiologies and may follow head trauma or cranial surgery with CSF leak, lumbar puncture (LP), or CSF shunting with lumbar or ventricular shunts (see "overshunting" (p. 462)).

Key concepts

- low CSF pressure (generally < 6 cm H_2O)
- typically associated with orthostatic headache (H/A that is improved in recumbency)

23

- characteristic findings on imaging (not required for dx): mnemonic: "SEEPS" (sagging brain, pachy-meningeal enhancement, engorged veins, pituitary hyperemia, subdural fluid)
- *spontaneous* intracranial hypotension (SIH)
  - excludes patients with history of dural puncture, penetrating spinal trauma, spinal surgery or procedures
  - epidural blood patch provides relief in the majority of patients

23.9.2 Epidemiology of spontaneous intracranial hypotension (SIH)

Incidence 5:100,000, prevalence 1:50,000.[34,35] More common in females[34,35,36,37] with mean age of presentation in the 40 s.[35,36]

23.9.3 Clinical

The syndrome of spontaneous intracranial hypotension is characterized by the following in the absence of antecedent trauma or dural puncture:
1. low CSF pressure (generally < 6 cm H_2O)
2. typically associated with orthostatic headache: dramatically worse when upright, improved in recumbency
3. diffuse pachymeningeal enhancement (cerebral and/or spinal) on MRI

For SIH, most patients have orthostatic headache with sudden onset, but other headaches have been described such as thunderclap, non-positional, exertional headaches, headaches at the end of the day, and even paradoxical headaches with worsening upon lying.[37,38] Atypical patients have been described without headache, without pachymeningeal enhancement on MRI,[39] with clinical signs of encephalopathy, cervical myelopathy or parkinsonism.[40] Since some patients may have normal intracranial pressure, the term "CSF hypovolemia" has been suggested.[41]

23.9.4 Diagnosis

Diagnostic criteria of headache attributed to low CSF pressure (per IHS Classification (ICHD-III)[42]):
1. any headache that developed in temporal relation to low CSF pressure or CSF leakage or has led to its discovery
2. low CSF pressure (< 6 cm of water) and/or evidence of CSF leakage on imaging
3. not better accounted for by another ICHD-III

Radiographic criteria are not required for diagnosis since no characteristic findings are seen in 20–25% of patients.[34,37,38,43]

Median delay from presentation to diagnosis of SIH is 4 months.[35,36] This delay may be detrimental to patient outcomes. Therefore, brain MRI without and with contrast is recommended in patients with new onset orthostatic headaches.[36]

23.9.5 Pathophysiology

The underlying cause of SIH is usually a spontaneous CSF leak,[35] however some cases may be due to low CSF volume. Evidence supports an underlying weakness of the meninges as a contributing factor; for instance, connective tissue disorders like Marfan syndrome, and Ehlers-Danlos syndrome.[18,34,35,44] Spinal diverticula, at the cervicothoracic junction or thoracic spine (thoracic being more common[35,37,38]), and excluding lumbosacral perineural cysts, are thought to be the source of CSF leak in most patients. Some cases of SIH may be due to pseudotumor cerebri syndrome (p. 955).[45] No relationship has been found between cranial leaks and SIH.[34,46] Other causes of dural injury are degenerative disc disease, osteophytes and bony spurs.[35] The orthostatic headache is believed to be caused by the descent of the brain, causing strain on intracranial structures sensitive to pain.[34,38,47]

23.9.6 Evaluation

1. radiographic studies
   a) MRI (brain): findings (mnemonic **SEEPS**)

- Sagging of the brain caused by the loss of buoyancy from low CSF volume.[34,38] Associated with low-lying cerebellar tonsils (seen in 36% of patients[40]) effacement of perichiasmatic and prepontine cisterns, bowing of the optic chiasm, flattening of pons, and ventricular collapse[34,37,38,48]
- Enhancement of the pachymeninges, sparing the leptomeninges, is common from dilation of subdural blood vessels[34,46,48]
- Engorgement of veins. Can also see venous distension sign as transverse sinus becomes dilated and convex[49]
- Pituitary hyperemia
- Subdural fluid collections seen in 50% of patients.[35,50] Can be hygromas versus hematomas, with hygromas being twice as frequent as hematomas. Occasionally may require intervention

b) CT (brain): not as conclusive but can help identify these changes. 11% of SIH patients also have pseudo-SAH finding on CT caused by effacement of basal cisterns due to sagging of the brain[51,52]

c) CT myelogram with iodinated contrast: study of choice for diagnosis and localization of a CSF leak. Timed images immediately after contrast injection or at delayed intervals after injections can help localize intermittent leaks[35,38]

d) MRI with intrathecal gadolinium: alternative to CT myelogram. Injection of 0.5 ml of gadolinium followed by full spine T1 with fat suppression imaging an hour after injection. Contrast remains for 24 hours, hence it can aide in detection of intermittent leaks. Prospective cohort study localized leak in 67% of patients with SIH. In another study, MRI 15 minutes after gadolinium injection identified CSF leak in 21% of SIH patients with a negative CT myelogram. No side effects were reported, but intrathecal gadolinium is not FDA approved (off-label use)[53,54,55]

e) spinal MRI: may show evidence of CSF leak, but is more likely to help localize extrathecal fluid collections for patients with local symptoms.[34] If there is focal spine pain, the leak will often be near this location. Other findings include dural enhancement, dilated veins, deformed dural sac, meningeal diverticula, syringomyelia, and retrospinal fluid collections at C1–2.[35,56,57,58,59,60,61,62,63]

f) radioisotope cisternography: poor resolution, may leave as many as one third of leaks unidentified.[35,38] Can be used especially if CT myelogram fails

2. lumbar puncture: CSF pressure < 6 cm of water is part of the diagnostic criteria. Patients have been identified with normal CSF pressure.[35,43,64] Associated CSF findings that have been identified include lymphocytic pleocytosis, high protein level, and xanthochromia[35,38,51]

3. positive response to EBP also supports the diagnosis

23.9.7 Treatment

None of these treatments have been evaluated by randomized clinical trials.

- conservative medical management: bed rest, hydration, analgesics, caffeine, and abdominal binder. Limited effect has been reported with intravenous caffeine, steroids and theophylline[34,35,37,38]
- epidural blood patch (EBP): see technique (p. 1817). Injection of autologous blood (10–20 ml) into epidural space. Evidence shows patients respond well and usually immediately.[35,52] However, some patients require more than one EBP and relief in headache may not be permanent.[65] If unsuccessful, can repeat blood patch with same or larger amount of blood. Positioning the patient in Trendelenberg position after injection aides in movement of blood to cover more segments for increased effectiveness.[35,38] May not be effective in up to 25–33%[34,35,37,53,66]
- directed epidural blood patch to site of leak if the above fails
- percutaneous placement of fibrin sealant at site of leak: can provide relief in patients that fail to improve with conservative measures and epidural blood patch[35,38,66,67]
- surgical intervention: last resource for patients without relief with conservative measures, EBP or fibrin sealant in which the exact site of the leak has been identified. Meningeal diverticula can be ligated with suture, aneurysm clips or muscle pledget with gel foam and fibrin sealant, a technique that may also be effective if a dural defect is identified[35,38]

23.9.8 Outcome

After appropriate treatment, clinical improvement is seen and precedes radiographic improvement. MRI usually takes days to weeks to normalize. Complete resolution of HA was achieved in 70% of patients (usually in days to weeks). Resolution was more likely if receiving EBP and less likely if they had multiple sites of CSF leak.[40] Patients with MRI changes characteristic of SIH and an identifiable focal CSF leak have better outcomes when compared to patients with multilevel CSF leaks.[35,38,68] CSF leak can recur in approximately 10% of patients. An association between longer interval from symptom onset to diagnosis and poorer outcome has been reported.[36]

Pseudotumor cerebri syndrome (p.955) (PTCS) has been implicated as a potential cause of SIH, and patients may not manifest symptoms of PTCS until several weeks after the repair of CSF leak.[45]

23

References

[1] Iliff JJ, Lee H, Yu M, et al. Brain-wide pathway for waste clearance captured by contrast-enhanced MRI. J Clin Invest. 2013; 123:1299–1309

[2] Iliff JJ, Goldman SA, Nedergaard M. Implications of the discovery of brain lymphatic pathways. Lancet Neurol. 2015; 14:977–979

[3] Sato O, Bering EA. Extraventricular Formation of Cerebrospinal Fluid. Brain Nerv. 1967; 19:883–885

[4] Lorenzo AV, Page LK, Walters GV. Relationship Between Cerebrospinal Fluid Formation, Absorption, and Pressure in Human Hydrocephalus. Brain. 1970; 93:679–692

[5] Bering EA, Sato O. Hydrocephalus: Changes in Formation and Absorption of Cerebrospinal Fluid within the Cerebral Ventricles. J Neurosurg. 1963; 20:1050–1063

[6] Griffith HB, Jamjoom AB. The Treatment of Childhood Hydrocephalus by Choroid Plexus Coagulation and Artificial Cerebrospinal Fluid Perfusion. Br J Neurosurg. 1990; 4:95–100

[7] Fishman RA. Cerebrospinal Fluid in Diseases of the Nervous System. Philadelphia: W. B. Saunders; 1980

[8] Felgenhauer K. Protein Size and Cerebrospinal Fluid Composition. Klin Wochenschr. 1974; 52:1158–1164

[9] Ommaya AK. Spinal fluid fistulae. Clinical Neurosurgery. 1975; 23:363–392

[10] Spetzler RF, Zabramski JM. Cerebrospinal Fluid Fistula. Contemp Neurosurg. 1986; 8:1–7

[11] Shulman K. Later complications of head injuries in children. Clinical Neurosurgery. 1971; 19:371–380

[12] Manelfe C, Cellerier P, Sobel D, et al. CSF Rhinorrhea: Evaluation with Metrizamide Cisternography. AJNR. 1982; 3:25–30

[13] Meirowsky AM, Ceveness WF, Dillon JD, et al. CSF Fistulas Complicating Missile Wounds of the Brain. J Neurosurg. 1981; 54:44–48

[14] Cusimano MD, Sekhar LN. Pseudo-Cerebrospinal Fluid Rhinorrhea. Journal of Neurosurgery. 1994; 80:26–30

[15] Calcaterra TC, English GM. Cerebrospinal Rhinorrhea. In: Otolaryngology. Philadelphia: Lippincott-Raven; 1992:1–7

[16] Nutkiewicz A, DeFeo DR, Kohout RI, et al. Cerebrospinal Fluid Rhinorrhea as a Presentation of Pituitary Adenoma. Neurosurgery. 1980; 6:195–197

[17] Jonhston WH. Cerebrospinal Rhinorrhea: The Study of One Case and Reports of Twenty Others Collected from the Literature Published Since Nineteen Hundred. Ann Otolaryngol. 1926; 35

[18] Schievink WI, Meyer FB, Atkinson JLD, et al. Spontaneous Spinal Cerebrospinal Fluid Leaks and Intracranial Hypotension. Journal of Neurosurgery. 1996; 84:598–605

[19] Hand WL, Sanford JP. Posttraumatic Bacterial Meningitis. Ann Int Medicine. 1970; 72:869–874

[20] Ryall RG, Peacock MK, Simpson DA. Usefulness of ß2-Transferrin Assay in the Detection of Cerebrospinal Fluid Leaks Following Head Injury. Journal of Neurosurgery. 1992; 77:737–739

[21] Fransen P, Sindic CJM, Thauvoy C, et al. Highly Sensitive Detection of Beta-2 Transferrin in Rhinorrhea and Otorrhea as a Marker for Cerebrospinal Fluid (CSF) Leakage. Acta Neurochirurgica. 1991; 109:98–101

[22] Wilkins RH, Rengachary SS. Neurosurgery. New York 1985

[23] Kaufman B, Nulsen FE, Weiss MH, et al. Acquired spontaneous, nontraumatic normal-pressure cerebrospinal fluid fistulas originating from the middle fossa. Radiology. 1977; 122:379–387

[24] Bakay L. Head Injury. Boston: Little Brown; 1980

[25] El Gammal T, Sobol W, Wadlington VR, et al. Cerebrospinal fluid fistula: detection with MR cisternography. AJNR. American Journal of Neuroradiology. 1998; 19:627–631

[26] Ahmadi J, Weiss MH, Segall HD, et al. Evaluation of CSF Rhinorrhea by Metrizamide CT Cisternography. Neurosurgery. 1985; 16:54–60

[27] Naidich TP, Moran CJ. Precise Anatomic Localization of Atraumatic Sphenoethmoidal CSF Rhinorrhea by Metrizamide CT Cisternography. J Neurosurg. 1980; 53:222–228

[28] Klastersky J, Sadeghi M, Brihaye J. Antimicrobial Prophylaxis in Patients with Rhinorrhea or Otorrhea: A Double Blind Study. Surgical Neurology. 1976; 6:111–114

[29] Allen C, Glasziou P, Del Mar C. Bed Rest: A Potentially Harmful Treatment Needing More Careful Evaluation. Lancet. 1999; 354:1229–1233

[30] Calcaterra TC. Extracranial Repair of Cerebrospinal Rhinorrhea. Ann Otol Rhinol Laryngol. 1980; 89:108–116

[31] Lewin W. Cerebrospinal Fluid Rhinorrhea in Closed Head Injuries. Br J Surgery. 1954; 17:1–18

[32] Dagi TF, George ED, Schmidek HH, et al. Surgical Management of Cranial Cerebrospinal Fluid Fistulas. In: Operative Neurosurgical Techniques. 3rd ed. Philadelphia: W.B. Saunders; 1995:117–131

[33] Fujii T, Misumi S, Onoda K, et al. Simple Management of CSF Rhinorrhea After Pituitary Surgery. Surg Neurol. 1986; 26:345–348

[34] Hoffmann J, Goadsby PJ. Update on intracranial hypertension and hypotension. Curr Opin Neurol. 2013; 26:240–247

[35] Schievink WI. Spontaneous spinal cerebrospinal fluid leaks. Cephalalgia. 2008; 28:1345–1356

[36] Mea E, Chiapparini L, Savoiardo M, et al. Clinical features and outcomes in spontaneous intracranial hypotension: a survey of 90 consecutive patients. Neurol Sci. 2009; 30 Suppl 1:S11–S13

[37] Schievink WI, Maya MM, Louy C, et al. Diagnostic criteria for spontaneous spinal CSF leaks and intracranial hypotension. AJNR. American Journal of Neuroradiology. 2008; 29:853–856

[38] Schievink WI. Spontaneous spinal cerebrospinal fluid leaks and intracranial hypotension. JAMA. 2006; 295:2286–2296

[39] Schievink WI, Tourje J. Intracranial hypotension without meningeal enhancement on magnetic resonance imaging. Journal of Neurosurgery. 2000; 92:475–477

[40] Chung SJ, Kim JS, Lee MC. Syndrome of cerebral spinal fluid hypovolemia: clinical and imaging features and outcome. Neurology. 2000; 55:1321–1327

[41] Mokri B. Spontaneous cerebrospinal fluid leaks, from intracranial hypotension to cerebrospinal fluid hypovolemia: evolution of a concept. Mayo Clinic Proceedings. 1999; 74:1113–1123

[42] Headache Classification Committee of the International Headache Society (IHS). The International Classification of Headache Disorders, 3rd edition. Cephalalgia. 2018; 38:1–211

[43] Schoffer KL, Benstead TJ, Grant I. Spontaneous intracranial hypotension in the absence of magnetic resonance imaging abnormalities. Can J Neurol Sci. 2002; 29:253–257

[44] Schievink WI, Gordon OK, Tourje J. Connective tissue disorders with spontaneous spinal cerebrospinal fluid leaks and intracranial hypotension: a prospective study. Neurosurgery. 2004; 54:65–70; discussion 70-1

[45] Perez MA, Bialer OY, Bruce BB, et al. Primary spontaneous cerebrospinal fluid leaks and idiopathic intracranial hypertension. J Neuroophthalmol. 2013; 33:330–337

[46] Schievink WI, Schwartz MS, Maya MM, et al. Lack of causal association between spontaneous intracranial hypotension and cranial cerebrospinal fluid leaks. J Neurosurg. 2012; 116:749–754

[47] Mea E, Franzini A, D'Amico D, et al. Treatment of alterations in CSF dynamics. Neurol Sci. 2011; 32 Suppl 1:S117–S120

[48] Fishman RA, Dillon WP. Dural enhancement and cerebral displacement secondary to intracranial hypotension. Neurology. 1993; 43:609–611

[49] Farb RI, Forghani R, Lee SK, et al. The venous distension sign: a diagnostic sign of intracranial hypotension at MR imaging of the brain. AJNR. American Journal of Neuroradiology. 2007; 28:1489–1493

[50] Schievink WI, Maya MM, Moser FG, et al. Spectrum of subdural fluid collections in spontaneous intracranial hypotension. J Neurosurg. 2005; 103:608–613

[51] Ferrante E, Regna-Gladin C, Arpino I, et al. Pseudosubarachnoid hemorrhage: a potential imaging pitfall associated with spontaneous intracranial hypotension. Clin Neurol Neurosurg. 2013; 115:2324–2328

[52] Zada G, Pezeshkian P, Giannotta S. Spontaneous intracranial hypotension and immediate improvement following epidural blood patch placement demonstrated by intracranial pressure monitoring. Case report. J Neurosurg. 2007; 106:1089–1090

[53] Vanopdenbosch LJ, Dedeken P, Casselman JW, et al. MRI with intrathecal gadolinium to detect a CSF leak: a prospective open-label cohort study. Journal of Neurology, Neurosurgery, and Psychiatry. 2011; 82:456–458

[54] Akbar JJ, Luetmer PH, Schwartz KM, et al. The role of MR myelography with intrathecal gadolinium in localization of spinal CSF leaks in patients with spontaneous intracranial hypotension. AJNR Am J Neuroradiol. 2012; 33:535–540

[55] Albayram S, Kilic F, Ozer H, et al. Gadolinium-enhanced MR cisternography to evaluate dural leaks in intracranial hypotension syndrome. AJNR. American Journal of Neuroradiology. 2008; 29:116–121

[56] Moayeri NN, Henson JW, Schaefer PW, et al. Spinal dural enhancement on magnetic resonance imaging associated with spontaneous intracranial hypotension. Report of three cases and review of the literature. J Neurosurg. 1998; 88:912–918

[57] Rabin BM, Roychowdhury S, Meyer JR, et al. Spontaneous intracranial hypotension: spinal MR findings. AJNR Am J Neuroradiol. 1998; 19:1034–1039

[58] Dillon WP. Spinal manifestations of intracranial hypotension. AJNR Am J Neuroradiol. 2001; 22:1233–1234

[59] Yousry I, Forderreuther S, Moriggl B, et al. Cervical MR imaging in postural headache: MR signs and pathophysiological implications. AJNR Am J Neuroradiol. 2001; 22:1239–1250

[60] Sharma P, Sharma A, Chacko AG. Syringomyelia in spontaneous intracranial hypotension. Case report. J Neurosurg. 2001; 95:905–908

[61] Chiapparini L, Farina L, D'Incerti L, et al. Spinal radiological findings in nine patients with spontaneous intracranial hypotension. Neuroradiology. 2002; 44:143–50; discussion 151-2

[62] Burtis MT, Ulmer JL, Miller GA, et al. Intradural spinal vein enlargement in craniospinal hypotension. AJNR Am J Neuroradiol. 2005; 26:34–38

[63] Watanabe A, Horikoshi T, Uchida M, et al. Diagnostic value of spinal MR imaging in spontaneous intracranial hypotension syndrome. AJNR Am J Neuroradiol. 2009; 30:147–151

[64] Mokri B, Piepgras DG, Miller GM. Syndrome of orthostatic headaches and diffuse pachymeningeal gadolinium enhancement. Mayo Clin Proc. 1997; 72:400–413

[65] The International Classification of Headache Disorders, 3rd edition (beta version). Cephalalgia. 2013; 33:629–808

[66] Schievink WI, Maya MM, Moser FM. Treatment of spontaneous intracranial hypotension with percutaneous placement of a fibrin sealant. Report of four cases. J Neurosurg. 2004; 100:1098–1100

[67] Gladstone JP, Nelson K, Patel N, et al. Spontaneous CSF leak treated with percutaneous CT-guided fibrin glue. Neurology. 2005; 64:1818–1819

[68] Schievink WI, Maya MM, Louy C. Cranial MRI predicts outcome of spontaneous intracranial hypotension. Neurology. 2005; 64:1282–1284

24 Hydrocephalus – General Aspects

24.1 Basic definition

An abnormal accumulation of cerebrospinal fluid within the ventricles of the brain.

24.2 Epidemiology

Estimated prevalence: 1–1.5%.

Incidence of congenital hydrocephalus is ≈ 0.9–1.8/1000 births (reported range from 0.2 to 3.5/1000 births[1]).

24.3 Etiologies of hydrocephalus

24.3.1 General information

Hydrocephalus (HCP) is either due to subnormal CSF reabsorption or, rarely, CSF overproduction.
- subnormal CSF reabsorption. Two main functional subdivisions:
  1. obstructive hydrocephalus (AKA non-communicating): block proximal to the arachnoid granulations (AG). On CT or MRI: enlargement of ventricles proximal to block (e.g., obstruction of aqueduct of Sylvius → lateral and 3rd ventricular enlargement out of proportion to the 4th ventricle, so-called triventricular hydrocephalus)
  2. communicating hydrocephalus (AKA non-obstructive): defect in CSF reabsorption by the AG
- CSF overproduction: rare. As with some choroid plexus papillomas; even here, reabsorption is probably defective in some as normal individuals could probably tolerate the slightly elevated CSF production rate of these tumors.

24.3.2 Specific etiologies of hydrocephalus

The etiologies in one series of pediatric patients is shown in ► Table 24.1.
1. congenital
   a) Chiari Type 2 malformation and/or myelomeningocele (MM) (usually occur together)
   b) Chiari Type 1 malformation: HCP may occur with 4th ventricle outlet obstruction
   c) primary aqueductal stenosis (usually presents in infancy, rarely in adulthood)
   d) secondary aqueductal gliosis: due to intrauterine infection or germinal matrix hemorrhage[3]
   e) Dandy Walker malformation (p. 270): atresia of foramina of Luschka & Magendie. The incidence of this in patients with HCP is 2.4%
   f) X-linked inherited disorder (p. 434): rare
2. acquired
   a) infectious (the most common cause of communicating HCP)
      • post-meningitis; especially purulent and basal, including TB, cryptococcus (p. 409)
      • cysticercosis
   b) post-hemorrhagic (2nd most common cause of communicating HCP)
      • post-SAH
      • post-intraventricular hemorrhage (IVH): many will develop *transient* HCP. 20–50% of patients with large IVH develop permanent HCP, requiring a shunt
   c) secondary to masses
      • non neoplastic: e.g., vascular malformation

Table 24.1 Etiologies of HCP in 170 pediatric patients with HCP[2]	
congenital (without myelomeningocele)	38%
congenital (with MM)	29%
perinatal hemorrhage	11%
trauma/subarachnoid hemorrhage	4.7%
tumor	11%
previous infection	7.6%

- neoplastic: most produce obstructive HCP by blocking CSF pathways, especially tumors around aqueduct (e.g., medulloblastoma). A colloid cyst can block CSF flow at the foramen of Monro. Pituitary tumor: suprasellar extension of tumor or expansion from pituitary apoplexy

d) post-op: 20% of pediatric patients develop permanent hydrocephalus (requiring shunt) following p-fossa tumor removal. May be delayed up to 1 yr

e) neurosarcoidosis (p.198)

f) "constitutional ventriculomegaly": asymptomatic. Needs no treatment

g) associated with spinal tumors[4]: ? due to ↑ protein?, ↑ venous pressure?, previous hemorrhage in some?

24.3.3 Special forms of hydrocephalus

These are covered in other sections
- normal pressure hydrocephalus (NPH) (p.438)
- entrapped fourth ventricle (p.436)
- arrested hydrocephalus (p.435)
- "triventricular hydrocephalus" (p.273)

24.4 Signs and symptoms of HCP

24.4.1 In older children (with rigid cranial vault) and adults

Findings are those of increased ICP, including papilledema, H/A, N/V, gait changes, upgaze and/or abducens palsy. Slowly enlarging ventricles may initially be asymptomatic.

24.4.2 In young children

Symptoms

- irritability
- poor head control
- N/V
- failure to thrive or developmental delay

Signs

- abnormalities in head circumference (OFC) (see below)
- cranium enlarges at a rate > facial growth
- fontanelle full and bulging
- frontal bossing (protuberance of the frontal bone manifesting as a prominent forehead)
- enlargement and engorgement of scalp veins: due to reversal of flow from intracerebral sinuses, due to increased intracranial pressure[5]
- Macewen's sign: cracked pot sound on percussing over-dilated ventricles
- 6th nerve (abducens) palsy: the long intracranial course is postulated to render this nerve very sensitive to pressure
- "setting sun sign" (p.101) (upward gaze palsy): Parinaud's syndrome (p.101) from pressure on region of suprapineal recess
- hyperactive reflexes
- irregular respirations with apneic spells

Occipital-frontal circumference

The occipital-frontal circumference (OFC) should be followed in every growing child (as part of a "well-baby" check-up, and especially in infants with documented or suspected hydrocephalus [HCP]). As a rule of thumb, the OFC of a normal infant should equal the distance from crown to rump.[6 (rule No. 335)] Also see differential diagnosis of macrocephaly (p.1691).

▶ **Measurement technique[7].** Using a non-stretchable tape, measure the circumference of the head just above the supraorbital ridge anteriorly and around the most prominent part of the occiput posteriorly (staying above the ears). Pull the tape snug to compress hair (exclude any braids or hairclips). Take 2 separate measurements (reposition the tape each time); if the measurements are within

24

2 mm, record the largest value. If the measurements disagree by > 2 mm, take a third measurement and record the average of the 2 closest measures.

Normal head growth: parallels normal curves as seen on the graphs in ▶ Fig. 24.1, or in ▶ Fig. 24.2 and ▶ Fig. 24.3 for preemies. Any of the following may signify treatable conditions such as active HCP, subdural hematoma, or subdural effusions, and should prompt an evaluation of the intracranial contents (e.g., CT, head U/S …):

1. progressive upward deviations from the normal curve (crossing curves)
2. continued head growth of more than 1.25 cm/wk
3. OFC approaching 2 standard deviations (SD) above normal

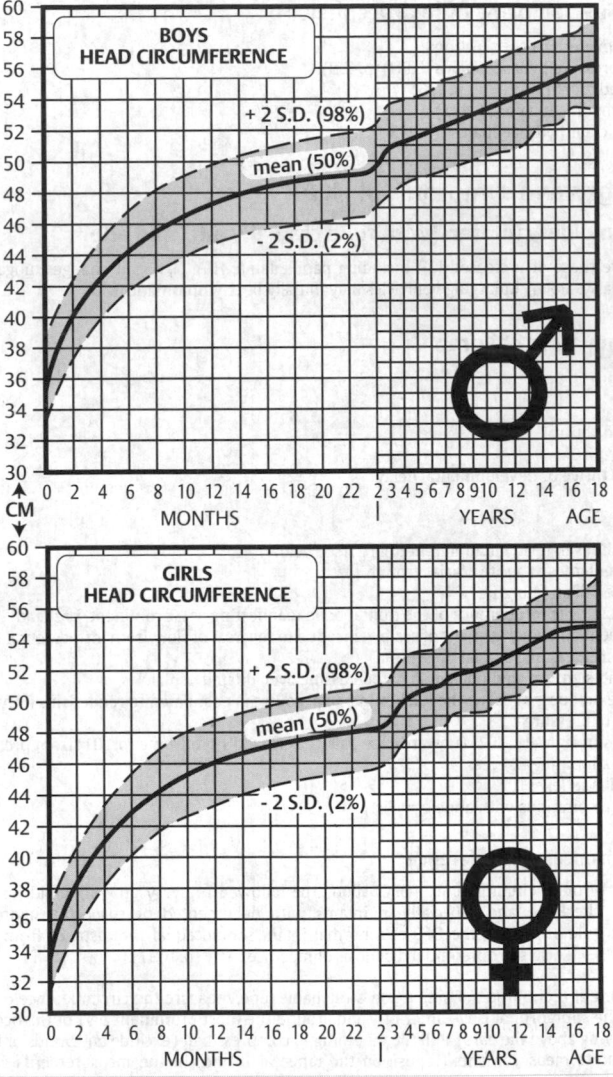

Fig. 24.1 Boys' & girls' head circumference. (Reproduced by permission of Pediatrics 1968, Vol 41, page 107-108.)

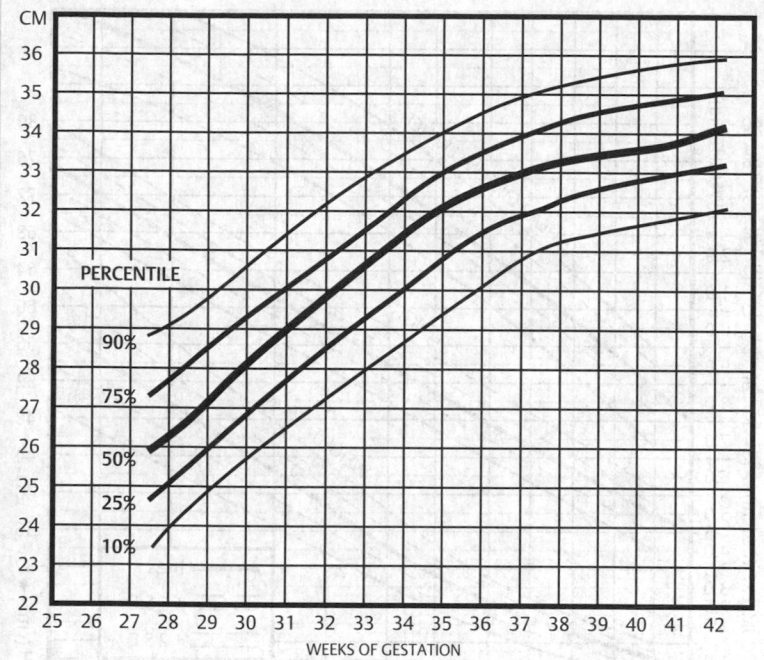

Fig. 24.2 OFC for premature infants as a function of gestational age.

4. head circumference out of proportion to body length or weight, even if within normal limits for age (▶ Fig. 24.3)[8]

These conditions may also be seen in the "catch-up phase" of brain growth in premature infants after they recover from their acute medical illnesses; see **Catch-up phase of brain growth** (p. 1636). Deviations below the curves or head growth in the premature infant in the neonatal period of less than 0.5 cm/wk (excluding the first few weeks of life) may indicate microcephaly (p. 312).

The graph in ▶ Fig. 24.3 shows the relationship of head circumference, weight and length for various gestational ages.

24.4.3 Blindness from hydrocephalus

General information

Blindness is a rare complication of hydrocephalus and/or shunt malfunction. Possible causes include:

1. occlusion of posterior cerebral arteries (**PCA** caused by downward transtentorial herniation)
2. chronic papilledema causing injury to optic nerve at the optic disc
3. dilatation of the 3rd ventricle with compression of optic chiasm

Ocular motility or visual field defects are more common with shunt malfunction than is blindness.[9,10,11,12] One series found 34 reported cases of permanent blindness in children attributed to shunt malfunction with concomitant increased ICP[13] (these authors were based in a referral center for visually impaired children, thus incidence was not estimated). Another series of 100 patients with tentorial herniation (most from acute EDH and/or SDH) proven by CT; 48 patients operated; only 19 of 100 survived > 1 month (all were in operated group); 9 of 100 developed occipital lobe infarct (2 died, 3 vegetative state, remaining 4 moderate to severe disability).[14]

24

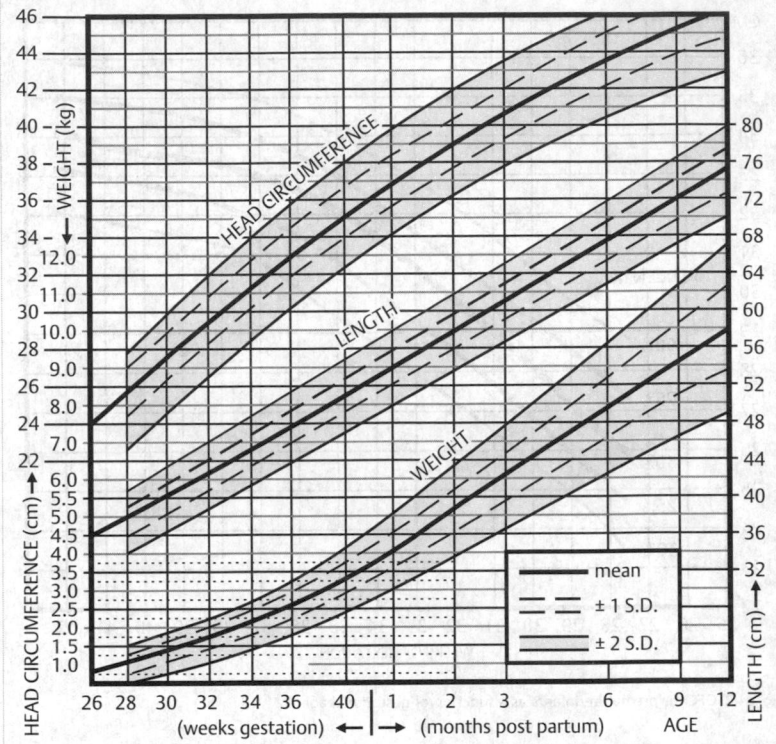

Fig. 24.3 **Head circumference, weight and length.** (Redrawn from Journal of Pediatrics, "Growth Graphs for the Clinical Assessment of Infants of Varying Gestational Age," Babson S G, Benda G I, vol 89, pp 815, with permission.)

Types of visual disturbance

9 of 14 had pregeniculate (anterior visual pathway) blindness with marked optic nerve atrophy (early), and reduced pupillary light reflexes. 5 of 14 had postgeniculate (cortical) blindness with normal light responses and minimal or no optic nerve atrophy (or atrophy late). A few patients had evidence of damage in both sites.

Cortical blindness: due to lesions posterior to lateral geniculate bodies (LGB), may also be seen with hypoxic injuries or trauma.[15] Occasionally associated with Anton's syndrome (denial of visual deficit) and with Ridoch's phenomenon (appreciation of moving objects without perception of stationary stimuli).

Pathophysiology

In patients with occipital lobe infarction

Occipital lobe infarctions (OLI) in PCA distribution are seen either bilaterally, or if unilateral are associated with other injuries to optic pathways posterior to LGB. The most often cited mechanism is compression of PCA resulting from brain herniating downward through the tentorial notch, where the PCA or its branches lie on the surface of the hippocampal gyrus and tend to cross the free edge of the tentorium[16] (some authors implicate parahippocampal gyral compression in tentorial notch directly injuring LGBs; this may never produce permanent blindness). Alternatively, upward cerebellar herniation (e.g., from ventricular puncture in face of a p-fossa mass) may impinge on PCA or branches with the same results.[17]

OLIs are more likely with a rapid rise in ICP (doesn't allow compensatory shifts and collateral circulation to develop).[18] Macular sparing is common, possibly due to potential dual blood supply of occipital poles (sometimes filled both by PCA and MCA collaterals[19]); alternatively the calcarine cortex may be supplied by a distinct branch of the PCA that fortuitously escapes compression.[20]

Reported causes of OLI include posttraumatic edema, tumor, abscess, SDH, unshunted hydrocephalus, and shunt malfunction.[16,21,22]

The occipital poles are also particularly vulnerable to diffuse hypoxia[23]; attested to by cases of cortical blindness after cardiac arrest.[24] Hypotension superimposed on compromised PCA circulation (from herniation or elevated ICP) may thus increase the risk of postgeniculate blindness.[13,18]

Both coup and contrecoup trauma may produce OLI. Unlike a PCA occlusion infarct, macular sparing is not expected in traumatic occipital lobe injury.[16]

24

In patients with pregeniculate blindness

Elevated ICP transmits pressure to retina → bloodflow stasis, as well as mechanical trauma to optic chiasm from enlarging third ventricle (latter more commonly thought to be responsible for bitemporal hemianopia,[9] but could, if unchecked, progress to complete visual loss). Also, if hypotension and anemia were present, consider the possibility of ischemic optic neuropathy,[25,26,27] which may be anterior, or posterior (the latter of which carries a poorer prognosis).

Presentation

These deficits are frequently unsuspected (altered mental state and the youth of many of these patients[13] makes detection difficult); an examiner must persevere to detect homonymous hemianopsias in an obtunded patient.[16]

Pregeniculate blindness is less often associated with depressed sensorium than is postgeniculate (where direct compression and vascular compromise of midbrain are more likely[13]).

Prognosis

Cortical blindness after diffuse anoxia frequently improves (occasionally to normal); usually slowly (weeks to years quoted; several mos usually adequate).[24] Many reports of blindness after shunt malfunction are pre-CT era; thus, the presence or extent of occipital lobe infarction cannot be ascertained. Some optimistic outcomes are reported[28]; however, permanent blindness or severe visual handicap are also described[16,22]; no reliable predictor has been identified. As with infarcts elsewhere, younger patients fare better,[23] but extensive calcarine infarcts are probably incompatible with significant visual recovery.

24.5 Imaging diagnosis of hydrocephalus

24.5.1 General information

Currently, hydrocephalus (HCP) is most often diagnosed on CT or MRI. Ultrasound may be used in infants with open fontanelles. There are angiographic correlates of HCP, but this is infrequently the means for detecting HCP.

Most experienced clinicians can recognize the ventriculomegaly associated with HCP by its radiographic appearance. Quantitative criteria for hydrocephalus (HCP) have also been defined, typically for use e.g., to create guidelines or for research purposes. See also radiologic features of chronic HCP (p. 432). NB: ventricular size normally increases with age.[29]

24.5.2 Specific imaging criteria for hydrocephalus

Attempts have been made to define hydrocephalus using linear measurements, often for use in research studies or for guidelines (e.g., for diagnosing NPH). None have proven completely satisfactory. Alternative measurements (including total ventricular volume) have been proposed for more accurate assessment, but have yet to be embraced in stardardized guidelines.

▶ **Evans ratio (AKA Evans index).** The Evans ratio or index was originally described for ventriculography (pneumoencephalogram)[30] and was later adapted to axial imaging.[31] To calculate the Evans index on axial CT or MRI images, find the slice with the largest internal biparietal diameter (BPD) of the skull (▶ Fig. 24.4-A). The frontal horns (FH) are then measured on that same slice. The Evans ratio is given by FH/BPD, and the interpretation is shown in ▶ Table 24.2.

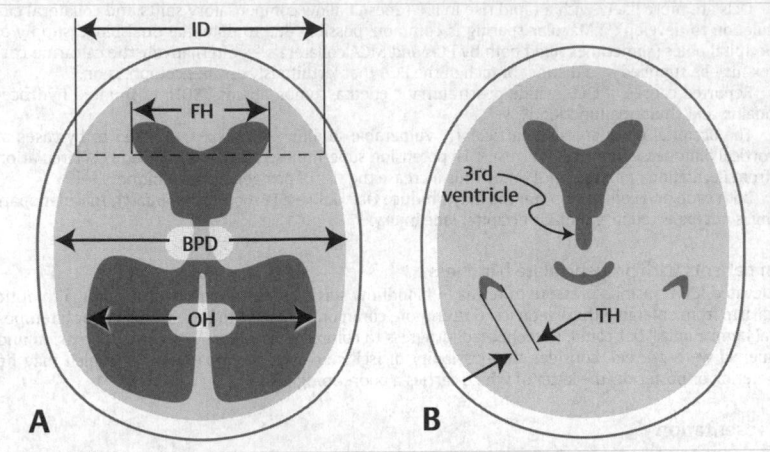

Fig. 24.4 Linear ventricular measurements for CT, MRI or U/S.
Image: A: Axial slice having the largest BPD. B: Axial slice at the level of the temporal horns of the lateral ventricles (typically best seen at the level of the petrous apex).
Abbreviations: BPD = biparietal diameter of the skull from inner-table to inner-table; FH = width of the frontal horns on the same slice; ID = internal diameter of the skull at the level of the maximal FH; OH = occipital horns; TH = temporal horns.

Table 24.2 Evans ratio[30] adapted to axial imaging

Evans ratio	Value	Interpretation
$\frac{FH}{ID} > 0.5$	0.2–0.25	normal
	0.25–0.3	borderline
	> 0.3	ventricular enlargement

Problems with the Evans ratio as adapted to axial imaging:
1. it varies with the angle of the slice[32]
2. the maximal BPD may not be on the same slice as the maximal FH[32] (the original ventriculo-graphic description divides the width of the frontal horns by the maximal BPD)
3. measurements that rely on the frontal horn diameter tend to underestimate hydrocephalus in pediatrics possibly because of disproportionate dilatation of the occipital horns[33]
4. in reality, the variability of the ratio may be greater than the value of FH[34]

▶ **Temporal horns.** On axial CT, the TH are often best visualized on the highest cut through the petrous temporal bone. In the absence of HCP, the TH should be barely visible. HCP is suggested when either[35]:
1. the size of both TH is ≥ 2 mm in width (▶ Fig. 24.4), and the Sylvian & interhemispheric fissures and cerebral sulci are not visible
   OR
2. both TH are ≥ 2 mm, *and* the ratio $\frac{FH}{ID} > 0.5$ (where FH is the largest width of the frontal horns, and ID is the internal diameter from inner-table to inner-table at this level - this is *not* the Evans ratio) (▶ Fig. 24.4-B)

24.5.3 Other findings suggestive of hydrocephalus

- ballooning of frontal horns of lateral ventricles (sometimes called "Mickey Mouse" ventricles)
- widening of the 3rd ventricle (the 3rd ventricle should normally be slit-like)
- periventricular low density on CT, or periventricular high intensity signal on T2WI MRI suggesting transependymal flow of CSF (note: this is likely a misnomer. CSF does not actually penetrate the ependymal lining, proven with CSF labeling studies. This finding probably represents stasis of fluid in the brain adjacent to ventricles)

24.5.4 Chronic hydrocephalus

Features indicative of chronic hydrocephalus (as opposed to acute hydrocephalus):
1. beaten copper cranium (some refer to beaten silver appearance) on plain skull X-ray.[36] By itself, does not correlate with increased ICP, however when associated with #3 and #4 below, does suggest ↑ ICP. May be seen in craniosynostosis (p. 264)
2. 3rd ventricle herniating into the sella (seen on CT or MRI)
3. erosion of sella turcica (may be due to #2 above) which sometimes produces an empty sella, and erosion of the dorsum sella
4. the temporal horns may be less prominent on imaging than in acute HCP
5. **macrocrania**: by convention, OFC greater than 98th percentile[37 (p 203)] (2 standard deviations above the mean)
6. corpus callosum: changes are best appreciated on sagittal MRI or CT. Findings include:
    a) atrophy (or thinning)
    b) upward bowing of the corpus callosum
7. in infants
    a) sutural diastasis (splaying of cranial sutures) may be seen on plain skull X-ray or CT
    b) delayed closure of fontanelles

24.6 Differential diagnosis of hydrocephalus

Etiologies: see etiologies of hydrocephalus (p. 426).

Mimics: conditions that may mimic HCP but are not due to inadequate CSF absorption are occasionally referred to as "pseudohydrocephalus" and include:
- "hydrocephalus ex vacuo": enlargement of the ventricles due to loss of cerebral tissue (cerebral atrophy), usually as a function of normal aging, but accelerated or accentuated by certain disease processes (e.g., Alzheimer's disease, Creutzfeldt-Jakob disease (p. 399), traumatic brain injury). Does not represent altered CSF hydrodynamics, but rather the loss of brain tissue (p. 433). See means of differentiating from true hydrocephalus (p. 1108)
- developmental anomalies where the ventricles or portions of the ventricles appear enlarged:
    ○ agenesis of the corpus callosum (p. 274): may occasionally be associated with HCP, but more often merely represents expansion of the third ventricle and separation of the lateral ventricles
    ○ septo-optic dysplasia (p. 276)
    ○ hydranencephaly (p. 309): a post-neurulation defect. Total or near-total absence of the cerebrum, most commonly due to bilateral ICA infarcts. It is critical to differentiate this from severe ("maximal") hydrocephalus (HCP) since shunting for true HCP may produce some re-expansion of the cortical mantle; see means to differentiate (p. 310)

Conditions that have been dubbed "hydrocephalus" but do not actually mimic the appearance of HCP:
- otitic hydrocephalus: obsolete term used to describe the increased intracranial pressure seen in patients with otitis media. This was also an early term for pseudotumor cerebri (p. 955)
- external hydrocephalus (p. 433): seen in infancy, enlarged subarachnoid space with increasing OFCs and normal or mildly dilated ventricles

24.7 External hydrocephalus (AKA benign external hydrocephalus)

24.7.1 General information

Key concepts

- enlarged subarachnoid spaces primarily over the frontal poles in the first year of life
- ventricles are normal or minimally enlarged
- the "cortical vein sign" (p. 434) (when present) helps distinguish from subdural hematoma
- usually resolves spontaneously by 2 years of age

24

A dissarray of terminology

Unfortunately, there are numerous terms that are used inconsistently in the context of extraaxial intracranial fluid collections. They include:
- external hydrocephalus or benign external hydrocephalus
- extraventricular hydrocephalus
- subdural effusion or benign subdural effusion of infancy
- benign subdural collection of infancy
- benign extra-axial collections
- benign enlargement of subarachnoid space (BESS) in infancy
- subdural hygroma

External hydrocephalus (EH) is enlarged subarachnoid space (usually over the cortical sulci of the frontal poles) seen in infancy (primarily in the first year of life), usually accompanied by abnormally increasing head circumference with normal or mildly dilated ventricles.[38] There are often enlarged basal cisterns and widening of the anterior interhemispheric fissure. No other symptoms or signs should be present (although there may be slight delay only in motor milestones due to the large head). Etiology is unclear, but a defect in CSF resorption is postulated. EH may be a variant of communicating hydrocephalus.[39] No predisposing factor may be found in some cases, although EH may be associated with some craniosynostoses[40] (especially plagiocephaly), or it may follow intraventricular hemorrhage or superior vena cava obstruction.

24.7.2 Differential diagnosis

EH may be distinct from **benign subdural collections (or extra-axial fluid) of infancy** (p. 1087).

★ EH must be distinguished from **symptomatic chronic extra-axial fluid collections** (p. 1088) (or chronic subdural hematoma), which may be accompanied by seizures, vomiting, headache… and may be the result of nonaccidental trauma (p. 1103). With EH, MRI or CT may demonstrate cortical veins extending from the surface of the brain to the inner table of the skull coursing through the fluid collection ("**cortical vein sign**" [▶ Fig. 64.7]), whereas the collections in subdural hematomas compress the subarachnoid space, which apposes the veins to the surface to the brain.[41,42]

24.7.3 Treatment

EH usually compensates by 12–18 mos age without shunting.[43] Recommended: follow serial ultrasound and/or CT to rule out abnormal ventricular enlargement. Emphasize to parents that this does not represent cortical atrophy. Due to increased risk for positional molding, parents may need to periodically reposition the head while the child is sleeping.[44]

A shunt may rarely be indicated when the collections are bloody (consider the possibility of child abuse) or for cosmetic reasons for severe macrocrania or frontal bossing.

24.8 X-linked hydrocephalus

24.8.1 General information

Inherited hydrocephalus (HCP) with phenotypic expression in males, passed on through carrier mothers who are phenotypically normal. Classical phenotypic expression will skip single generations.

Incidence: 1/25,000 to 1/60,000. Prevalence: ≈ 2 cases per 100 cases of hydrocephalus.

Gene located on Xq28.[45,46,47]

24.8.2 Pathophysiology

L1CAM membrane-bound receptor plays a significant role in CNS development for axonal migration to appropriate target locations through Integrin cell adhesion molecules and MAP Kinase signal cascade.[45,46,47]

Abnormal gene expression results in poor differentiation and maturation of cortical neurons, macroscopic anatomical abnormalities (bilateral absence of pyramidal tracts, see below).

Cytoplasmic domain loss of function mutations result in severe L1 syndrome, whereas mutations retaining expression of some functional protein (component imbedded in cell membrane) leads to mild L1 syndrome.

24.8.3 L1 syndromes

Classical syndromes include CRASH (corpus callosum hypoplasia, retardation, adducted thumbs (clasp thumbs), spastic paralysis, HCP), MASA (mental handicap, aphasia, shuffling gait, adducted thumbs), and HSAS (HCP with stenosis of the aqueduct of sylvius). Spectrum of disease also includes x-linked agenesis of the corpus callosum (ACC), and spastic paraparesis type 1.[45,46]
   Recent deliniations[47]:
- mild L1 syndrome: adducted thumbs, spastic paralysis, hypoplasia of CC
- severe L1 syndrome: as in mild L1 syndrome plus anterior cerebellar vermis hypoplasia, large massa intermedia, enlarged quadrigeminal plate, rippled ventricular wall following VP shunt placement (pathognomonic for X-linked HCP). Profound mental retardation in virtually all cases

Radiographic findings likely present if severe L1[48]:
1. severe symmetric HCP with predominant posterior horn dilation
2. hypoplastic CC/ACC
3. hypoplastic anterior cerebellar vermis
4. large massa intermedia
5. large quadrigeminal plate
6. rippled ventricular wall following VP shunt placement (pathognomonic)

Treatment: no intervention demonstrates improvement in retardation status in observational papers.
1. VP shunt: main purpose is management of head size for improved care by caregiver. Does not improve neurologic outcome
2. there are no current genetic therapies for L1CAM protein abnormalities
3. prenatal U/S: early (≈ 20–24 weeks gestational age) with frequent repeat scan in known carrier mothers. May allow for medically indicated termination early on
4. male infants with HCP and ≥ 2 clinical/radiographic signs should undergo genetic testing for L1CAM mutation detection for future pregnancy counseling[45]

24.9 "Arrested hydrocephalus" in pediatrics

24.9.1 General information

The exact definition of this term is not generally agreed upon, and some use the term "compensated hydrocephalus" interchangeably. Most clinicians use these terms to refer to a situation where there is no progression or deleterious sequelae due to hydrocephalus that would require the presence of a CSF shunt. Patients and families should be advised to seek medical attention if they develop symptoms of intracranial hypertension (decompensation), which may include headaches, vomiting, ataxia, or visual symptoms.[44]
   Arrested hydrocephalus satisfies the following criteria in the absence of a CSF shunt:
1. near normal ventricular size
2. normal head growth curve
3. continued psychomotor development

24.9.2 Shunt independence

The concept of becoming independent of a shunt is not universally accepted.[49] Some feel that shunt independence occurs more commonly when the HCP is due to a block at the level of the arachnoid granulations (communicating hydrocephalus),[50] but others have shown that it can occur regardless of the etiology.[51] These patients must be followed closely, as there are reports of death as late as 5 years after apparent shunt independence, sometimes without warning.[50]

24.9.3 When to remove a disconnected or non-functioning shunt?

Note: a disconnected shunt may continue to function by CSF flow through an endothelialized subcutaneous tract. Recommendations on whether or not to repair vs. remove a disconnected or non-functioning shunt:
1. when in doubt, shunt
2. indications for shunt repair (vs. removal)
   a) marginally functioning shunts

b) the presence of any signs or symptoms of increased ICP (vomiting, upgaze palsy, sometimes H/A alone[52]...)

c) changes in cognitive function, ↓ attention span, or emotional changes

d) patients with aqueductal stenosis or spina bifida: most are shunt-dependent

3. because of risks associated with shunt removal, surgery for this purpose alone should be performed only in the situation of a shunt infection[53] (and then, and EVD is usually placed)

4. patients with a nonfunctioning shunt should be followed closely with serial CTs, and possibly with serial neuropsychological evaluations

24.10 Entrapped fourth ventricle

24.10.1 General information

AKA isolated fourth ventricle: 4th ventricle that neither communicates with the 3rd ventricle (through Sylvian aqueduct) nor with the basal cisterns (through foramina of Luschka or Magendie). Usually seen with chronic shunting of the lateral ventricles, especially with post-infectious hydrocephalus (fungal, in particular) or in those with repeated shunt infections. Possibly as a result of adhesions forming from prolonged apposition of the ependymal lining of the aqueduct due to the diversion of CSF through the shunt. Occurs in 2–3% of shunted patients.[54] May also occur in Dandy Walker malformation (p.270) if the aqueduct is also obstructed. The choroid plexus of the 4th ventricle continues to produce CSF, which enlarges the ventricle when there is 4th ventricular outlet obstruction or obstruction at the level of the arachnoid granulations.

24.10.2 Presentation

Presentation may include:
1. headache
2. lower cranial nerve palsies: swallowing difficulties
3. pressure on the floor of the 4th ventricle may compress the facial colliculus (p.607) → facial diplegia and bilateral abducens palsy
4. ataxia
5. reduced level of consciousness
6. nausea/vomiting
7. may also be an incidental finding (NB: some "atypical" findings, such as reduced attention span, may be related)

24.10.3 Treatment

Treatment of the entrapped 4th ventricle may alleviate associated slit ventricles.[55] Most surgeons advocate shunting the ventricle either with a separate VP shunt, or by linking into an existing shunt. Options:
1. usual first choice: insertion from below the tonsils under direct vision. The catheter may be brought out at the dural suture line, and may be anchored here by use of an angle adapter sutured to the dura
2. passage through a cerebellar hemisphere: potential complications include delayed injury to the brainstem by the catheter tip as the brainstem moves into its normal position with drainage of the 4th ventricle. This may be avoided by bringing the catheter into the 4th ventricle at a slight angle through the cerebellar hemisphere
3. Torkildsen shunt (ventriculocisternal shunt) is an option for obstructive hydrocephalus if it is certain that the arachnoid granulations are functional (usually not the case with hydrocephalus of infantile onset)
4. an LP shunt may be considered when the 4th ventricle outlets are patent

Cranial nerve palsies may occur with shunting of the 4th ventricle, usually as a result of penetration of the brainstem by the catheter, either at the time of catheter insertion or in a delayed fashion as the 4th ventricle decreases in size,[56] but also possibly as a result of overshunting causing traction on the lower cranial nerves as the brainstem shifts posteriorly.[54]

24.11 Ventriculomegaly in adults

24.11.1 General information

Semantically, ventriculomegaly (VM) means ventricular enlargement. VM may be due to increased pressure of CSF within the ventricles (hydrocephalus) or it may be due to loss of brain parenchyma (sometime called "hydrocephalus ex vacuo") or brain maldevelopment (as in benign macrocrania of infancy). In some cases, determining if ventriculomegaly is due to hydrocephalus versus other causes can be difficult or impossible. Some authors use VM in a sense that is intended to differentiate it from hydrocephalus, but this is ambiguous.

Ventricular size increases with age.[29] The rate of increase is higher in patients with Alzheimer disease compared to controls.[29]

24.11.2 Long-standing overt ventriculomegaly in an adult (LOVA)

LOVA is a heterogeneous group of conditions. Terms that have been used for some of these conditions include arrested hydrocephalus, compensated hydrocephalus, aqueductal stenosis.

Adult head circumference (OFC) (p.427) > 59 cm in males, or > 57.5 cm in females, suggests the possibility of congenital hydrocephalus[29,57] that was undetected or untreated.

▶ **Definition of LOVA[58].** An adult with
1. ventriculomegaly involving the lateral and third ventricles (but excluding the fourth) with obliterated sulci
2. clinical flindings including: macrocephaly with or without sub-normal IQ, H/A, dementia, gait disturbance, urinary incontinence, vegetative state, akinetic mutism, apathetic consciousness, parkinsonism
3. expanded or destroyed sella turcica on imaging studies (evidence of long-standing ventriculomegaly)

Most cases cluster into 1 of 4 categories (with a fifth category used for patients with panventriculomegaly (i.e., including the fourth ventricle) as follows[59]

▶ **Cluster 1—incidental ventriculomegaly (normal ICP).** The fewest symptoms, including asymptomatic ventriculomegaly discovered incidentally on workup of unrelated issues (e.g., post-trauma) or headache. Mean age ≈ 40 years. ICP is normal. Some patients demonstrate spontaneous third ventriculostomy which might explain the paucity of symptoms in those cases. NB: arrested hydrocephalus does not always remain asymptomatic.

Management recommendation: annual surveillance. H/A may be controlled with analgesics or sometimes with acetazolamide (p.496).

▶ **Cluster 2—decompensated ventriculomegaly (high ICP).** Highly symptomatic, often present acutely with gait disturbance, visual changes, H/A, urinary incontinence, and in 25% cognitive deficit. Some extreme cases have rapidly deteriorating GCS. Typically don't present until middle-aged. 33% had *severe* aqueductal stenosis. Elevated ICP (mean: 14 mm Hg).

Management recommendation: CSF diversion (VP shunt or ETV). Following treatment, ventricles tend to remain enlarged.

▶ **Cluster 3—early presenting ventriculomegaly (normal ICP, abnormal pulsatility).** Patients tend to be younger (mean age: 29 ± 11 years standard deviation), have the largest ventricles, and all have H/A. 30% have nausea. ICP is normal, but **pulsatility** (high peak-to-low peak of CSF pressure wave) was abnormal (mean: 5.2 mm Hg). 25% of patients had a history of prematurity with germinal matrix hemorrhage (p.1630).

Management recommendations: the majority of these patients were treated with a shunt.

▶ **Cluster 4—late ventriculomegaly.** Older age (mean 59 ± 17 years). Much more common in women. Main complaint: headache. Symptomatically may mimic NPH (p.438) (with cognitive deficits, gait disturbance and urinary incontinence, but magnetic gait was not seen). ICP was not measured in most due to contraindications.

Management recommendations: CSF diversion usually produces improvement, but overdrainage is common with a high incidence of associated subdural hematoma; therefore a programmable valve should be considered.

▶ **Cluster 5—panventriculomegaly.** Patients with panventriculomegaly. 50% had a history of prenatal injury. Symptoms: gait disturbance (50%), cognitive deficits (50%) and epilepsy (88%). Dysphagia may occur with a dilated 4th ventricle.

Management recommendations: ventricular shunt.

24.12 Normal pressure hydrocephalus (NPH)

24.12.1 General information

Key concepts

- triad (not pathognomonic): dementia, gait disturbance, urinary incontinence
- communicating hydrocephalus on CT or MRI
- normal pressure on random LP (so called "secondary NPH" patients may have higher pressures around 20 cm CSF)
- symptoms may be remediable with CSF shunting

Normal pressure hydrocephalus (NPH), AKA Hakim-Adams syndrome, first described in 1965,[60] may cause treatable symptoms, including one of the few forms of remediable dementia.

As originally described, the hydrocephalus of NPH was considered to be *idiopathic* (iNPH). However, in some cases of hydrocephalus with normal pressure, a predisposing condition may be identified, suggesting that the ICP may have been elevated at some point in time. These "secondary NPH" patients tend to have a higher pressure on LP (e.g., around 20 cm CSF, compared to < 10-12 cm for "primary NPH") may also respond to shunting.

Etiologies of "secondary NPH" include risk factors for communicating hydrocephalus:

1. post-SAH
2. posttraumatic (including concussion)
3. post-infectious: meningitis or cerebral abscess
4. following posterior fossa surgery
5. following radiation therapy to the brain
6. tumors, including carcinomatous meningitis
7. also seen in ≈ 15% of patients with Alzheimer's disease (AD)
8. enlarged head circumference[61]
9. deficiency of the arachnoid granulations
10. aqueductal stenosis may be an overlooked cause

To further complicate things, some patients considered to have NPH may actually have episodic elevations in ICP.

Throughout this text, discussion focuses on *idiopathic* NPH (iNPH) unless stated otherwise.

It is becoming increasingly clear that the ventricular enlargement is likely not the primary underlying pathologic entity. Furthermore, the simplistic model of bulk flow of CSF (production by choroid plexus and absorption by arachnoid granulations and nerve root sheaths) is proving to be inadequate for an in-depth understanding of iNPH. Concepts of CNS lymphatics ("glymphatics"[62]) are gaining acceptance but are currently beyond the scope of this text. Research continues in an effort to improve the understanding of this complicated condition.

24.12.2 Epidemiology

Incidence for idiopathic NPH (iNPH) may be as high as 5.5 per 100,000 per year.[63]

The mean age for iNPH is older than that for secondary NPH.

24.12.3 Clinical

Clinical triad

See reference.[64]

The triad is not pathognomonic, and similar features may also be seen e.g., in vascular dementia,[65] Alzheimer's dementia, and Parkinson's disease.

1. gait disturbance: usually precedes other symptoms. Almost all iNPH patients have gait disturbance. Gait is wide-based with short, shuffling steps and unsteadiness on turning. Patients often feel like they are "glued to the floor" (so-called "magnetic gait") and may have difficulty initiating steps or turns. Other features: multistep turns, retropulsion, and frequent falls. Appendicular ataxia is characteristially absent

2. dementia: primarily memory impairment with bradyphrenia (slowness of thought) and bradykinesia. Other features that are shared with various frontal subcortical disorders: apathy or lack of motivation, daytime sleepiness. Findings that are not characteristic: expressive or receptive dyphasias, dysnomia (impaired naming), difficulty recognizing familiar people, or hallucinations.
   ▶ Table 24.3 shows some differentiating features with Alzheimer's disease

3. urinary incontinence: typically urinary urgency with impaired ability to inhibit bladder emptying. Incontinence without awareness is not characteristic and may suggest other dementing processes.

Table 24.3 Comparison of cognitive deficits in Alzheimer's disease (AD) and NPH[a,b]

Feature	AD	NPH
memory	↓	± auditory memory
executive function[c]	↓	±
attention concentration	↓	±
orientation	↓	
writing	↓	
learning	↓	
fine motor speed and accuracy	±	↓
psychomotor skills	±	slowed
language and reading	±	
behavioral or personality changes		±

[a]modified[66]
[b]Key: ↓ = impaired; ± = borderline impaired
[c]see ▶ Table 24.7 for definition of executive function

Other clinical features

Age usually > 60 yrs. Slight male preponderance. Also see below for other clinical information.

True aphasia is unusual, but speech output may be disturbed by impaired motivation or executive dysfunction.[66] As NPH progresses, cognitive impairment may become more generalized and less responsive to treatment.[66] Symptoms identical to those of idiopathic parkinsonism may occur in 11%.[67]

Case reports of a variety of psychiatric disturbances associated with NPH include depression,[68] bipolar disorder,[69] aggressiveness,[70] paranoia.[71]

Symptoms not expected with NPH

Although a variety of clinical features have been demonstrated to occur infrequently (e.g., SIADH,[72] syncope…), clinical features *not* expected solely as a result of NPH include papilledema, seizures (prior to shunting), headaches, spasticity, hyperreflexia and lateralizing findings.[66,73] See also unanticipated findings listed under iNPH triad (p. 439).

24

24.12.4 Other conditions that may be present

Differential diagnosis of NPH

▶ Table 24.4 shows conditions with presentations similar to findings in NPH in the differential diagnosis.[66,74] ▶ Table 24.5 compares some features of NPH, Alzheimer's disease, and Parkinson's disease.

Tests used to rule out common NPH mimics:
1. "dementia blood testing"
   1. CBC
   2. electrolytes
   3. B_{12}
   4. folate
   5. thyroid-stimulating hormone
   6. additional blood tests when indicated:
      1. rapid plasma reagin (RPR): screening for syphilis antibodies (in neurosyphilis)
      2. ELISA screening test for Lyme disease; then if positive, Western blot to confirm
      3. vitamin D level
2. neuropsychological testing
3. MRI
   1. cervical and/or thoracic as appropriate if concern about myelopathy
   2. lumbar if there is pain with ambulating
4. electrodiagnostic studies (EMG/NVC) if peripheral neuropathy is possible
5. urology consultation

Table 24.4 Conditions with similar presentation to NPH

Neurodegenerative disorders	• Alzheimer's disease • Parkinson's disease • Lewy body disease • Huntington's disease • frontotemporal dementia • corticobasal degeneration • progressive supranuclear palsy • amyotrophic lateral sclerosis • multisystem atrophy • spongiform encephalopathy
Vascular dementia	• cerebrovascular disease • multi-infarct dementia • Binswanger's disease • CADASIL • vertebrobasilar insufficiency (VBI)
Other hydrocephalic disorders	• aqueductal stenosis • arrested hydrocephalus • other forms of ventriculomegaly in adults: long-standing overt ventriculomegaly in adult (LOVA) syndrome (p.437) • noncommunicating hydrocephalus
Infectious disease	• Lyme disease • HIV • syphilis
Urological disorders	• urinary tract infection • bladder or prostate cancer • benign prostatic hypertrophy (BPH)
Miscellaneous	• vitamin B12 deficiency • collagen vascular diseases • epilepsy • depression • traumatic brain injury • spinal stenosis • Chiari malformation • Wernicke's encephalopathy • carcinomatous meningitis • spinal cord tumor

Table 24.5 Comparison of NPH, Alzheimer's & Parkinson's disease[a]

Feature	NPH	AD	IPA
gait disturbance[b]	+	±	±
postural instability	±		+
urinary disturbance	±	±	±
memory or cognitive impairment	±	+	±
difficulty performing familiar tasks	±	+	±
behavioral changes	±	+	±
limb rigidity			+
limb tremor			+
bradykinesia			+

[a]abbreviations: AD + Alzheimer's disease; IPA = idiopathic paralysis agitans (Parkinson's disease); + = feature present; ± = feature partial or late
[b]in NPH, the gait is often wide based, in IPA often narrow stance

24

Treatment of other conditions

Current recommendations are to treat other disorders (e.g., cervical spinal myelopathy) and to reach stable dosages when adding or withdrawing medications (e.g., thyroid replacement, trials of carbidopa/levodopa…) before embarking on NPH testing.[73] This avoids confusion about what condition is causing which symptoms, and can cloud interpretation of response e.g., to CSF removal. This is not, however, a hard and fast rule.

24.12.5 Imaging in iNPH

CT and MRI

MRI is preferred over CT because it provides more information and does not involve ionizing radiation (X-rays).

Features on CT[75] and MRI[76]:

1. prerequisite: ventricular enlargement without block (i.e., communicating hydrocephalus). MRI excels at ruling out obstructive hydrocephalus due to aqueductal stenosis (p. 273)
2. features that correlate with favorable response to shunt. These features suggest that the hydrocephalus is *not* due to atrophy alone. Note: atrophy / hydrocephalus ex vacuo, as in conditions such as Alzheimer's disease, lessens the chance of, but does not preclude responding to a shunt (cortical atrophy is a common finding in healthy individuals of advanced age[77])
   a) periventricular low density on CT or high intensity on T2WI MRI: may represent transependymal absorption of CSF. May resolve with shunting
   b) compression of convexity sulci (as distinct from dilatation in atrophy). Note: focal sulcal dilation may sometimes be seen and may represent atypical reservoirs of CSF, which may diminish after shunting and should not be considered as atrophy[78]
   c) rounding of the frontal horns

Other helpful findings in iNPH that require MRI
1. Japanese guidelines[79] for iNPH also identify the following features:
   a) **DESH** (disproportionately enlarged subarachnoid space hydrocephalus) (▶ Fig. 24.5): hydrocephalus with enlarged subarachnoid spaces primarily in the Sylvian fissure and basal cisterns and effacement of the subarachnoid space over the convexity (so-called "tight high convexity").[79,80,81] In comparison, dilated subarachnoid space in the high convexity is suggestive of atrophy
   b) ventricular enlargement in iNPH deforms the corpus callosum, including:
      • upward bowing and thinning (best appreciated on sagittal MRI)[82]
      • impingement on the falx, producing an **acute callosal angle** ($\leq 90°$, ▶ Fig. 24.6), demonstrated on a coronal MRI perpedicular to the AC-PC line (p. 58), passing through the posterior commissure (PC)
2. phase-contrast MRI may demonstrate hyperdynamic flow of CSF through the aqueduct

24

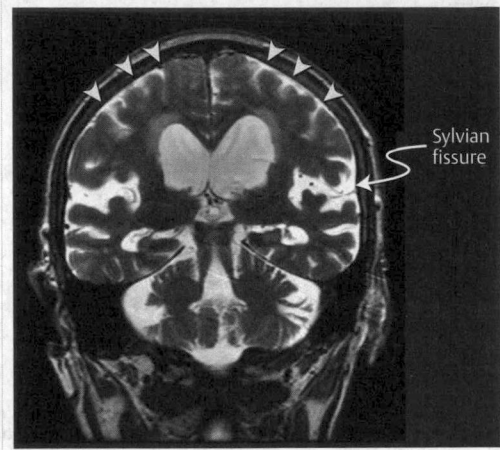

Fig. 24.5 Disproportionately enlarged subarachnoid space hydrocephalus (DESH).
Image: coronal T2 MRI showing enlarged Sylvian fissures with narrow sulci over the convexity (*yellow arrowheads*) with ventriculomegaly.

Sylvian fissure

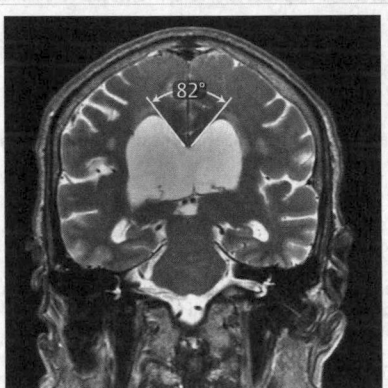

Fig. 24.6 Callosal angle.
Image: coronal MRI passing through the posterior commissure (PC) perpendicular to the AC-PC line.
The callosal angle is demonstrated, and in this patient measures 82° (since it is <90°, it is consistent with iNPH).

Although some patients improve with no change in ventricles,[83] clinical improvement most often accompanies reduction of ventricular size.

Radionuclide cisternography

✖ High false-positive rate. One study found that the cisternogram does not increase the diagnostic accuracy of clinical and CT criteria.[84] Use has been abandoned by most researchers[85] and it is not recommended in the International[73] and Japanese[79] guidelines.

iNPH Radscale

Numerous grading scales attempt to identify patients who are likely to respond to shunting. The iNPH Radscale (▶ Table 24.6)[86] assigns point values to currently favored radiologic findings to form a summative iNPH Radscale score that is used in conjunction with clinical findings. The higher the score, the more it supports the diagnosis of iNPH.

Table 24.6 iNPH Radscale[86]

Feature	Finding	Points	Score
Evans index (p. 431): ratio of the maximum width of the frontal horns of the lateral ventricles to the maximum BPD on the same CT or MRI slice	≤0.25	0	(0 - 2)
	0.25–0.3	1	
	>0.3	2	
tight high convexity (► Fig. 24.5): narrow CSF spaces in high convexity & high parafalcine sulci on coronal and upper axial MRI slices*[87]	none	0	(0 - 2)
	parafalcine	1	
	vertex	2	
Sylvian fissure enlargement in the coronal plane compared to surrounding sulci*[82]	normal	0	(0 - 1)
	enlarged	1	
focally enlarged sulci in coronal or transverse planes compared to surrounding sulci[78]	absent	0	(0 - 1)
	present	1	
temporal horns, TH (► Fig. 24.4: the mean width of the left & right TH measured on axial images[82]	<4 mm	0	(0 - 2)
	≥4 and <6 mm	1	
	≥6	2	
callosal angle (p. 441): angle between the frontal horns of the lateral ventricles under the falx (on a coronal MRI slice perpendicular to the AC-PC line passing through the PC)	>90°	0	(0 - 2)
	>60° and ≤90°	1	
	≤60°	2	
periventricular hypodensities in the vicinity of the lateral ventricles: anterior to the frontal horns ("caps") or diffusely surrounding the ventricle[88]	absent	0	(0 - 2)
	frontal horn caps	1	
	diffusely surrounding	2	
iNPH Radscale score → TOTAL			(0 - 12)

* these two items are components of DESH (p. 441)

24.12.6 Ancillary tests for NPH

Lumbar puncture (LP)

Opening pressure

Normal LP opening pressure (OP) in the left lateral decubitus position averages 12.2 ± 3.4 cm H_2O (8.8 ± 0.9 mm Hg)[89] and should be < 180 mm H_2O (OP > 24 cm H_2O suggests noncommunicating hydrocephalus rather than NPH[66,90]). In NPH the average OP is 15 ± 4.5 cm H_2O (11 ± 3.3 mm Hg), slightly higher than, but overlapping with, normal. Based on expert opinion, an upper limit of 24 cm H_2O (17.6 mm Hg) is suggested for the definition of NPH. Patients with an initial OP > 10 cm H_2O have a higher response rate to shunting.

CSF labs

Send CSF for routine labs (p. 1813) to R/O infection, elevated protein (e.g., with tumor), SAH.
If there is a concern for Alzheimer's disease (AD), CSF can be sent for amyloid β_{1-42} which is low in AD, and t-tau and p-tau which are high in AD, all 3 are low in iNPH.[91]

"Tap Test" (AKA Miller Fisher test)

Consists of lumbar puncture with removal of a specific quantity of CSF and assessment of response.

The tap test has not undergone rigorous prospective evaluation. A *positive* response to withdrawal of 40–50 ml of CSF has a PPV in the range of 73–100%,[92,93,94] but sensitivity is low (26–61%). (Note: what constitutes a *significant* "response" has not been standardized; most experts prefer demonstrating objective improvement in gait, taking into account the fact that NPH patients can have day-to-day fluctuations in symptoms).

Some measurements that are commonly compared before and after CSF removal:
1. TUG (Timed Up & Go) test[95]
   1. patient wearing their usual footwear and walking aid (if needed) sits back in a standard armchair. A line 3 meters (10 feet) in front is identified
   2. the patient is instructed that when the examiner says "Go" to stand up from the chair, walk to the line at their normal pace, turn, walk back to the chair and sit down again
   3. the activity is timed from the word "Go" until the patient sits back down

   4. in addition to recording the time, notate: slow tentative pace, loss of balance, short stride, little or no arm swing, steadying self on walls or furniture, shuffling, en bloc turning, improper use of assistive device
   5. additional notes: stay by the patient for safety. An older adult who takes ≥ 12 seconds to complete the TUG test is at increased risk for falls
2. 10 meter walk
3. 6 minute walk
4. sit to stand
5. TUG cognitive
6. Tennetti balance and gait test

Resistance testing

CSF Ro is considered to be the impedance of CSF absorptive mechanisms. 1/Ro is the conductance. Techniques and thresholds are center-specific. No clinical study has adequately addressed the fact that Ro normally increases with age.[96]

Determination of CSF Ro *may* have a higher sensitivity (57–100%) but a similar PPV (75–92%) to the tap test.

Methodology
Numerous methods have been devised to measure Ro. Two illustrative methods:
1. bolus method[97]: a known volume (usually ≈ 4 ml) is injected via LP at a rate of 1 ml/sec
2. Katzman test[98]: infuse saline through LP at a known rate, Ro is given by Eq (24.1) (up to 19% of patients experience H/A after infusion studies[99])

$$Ro = \frac{(\text{final steady state pressure}) - (\text{initial pressure})}{\text{infusion rate}} \tag{24.1}$$

Ambulatory lumbar drainage (ALD)

See reference.[92]

A lumbar subarachnoid drain is placed with Tuohy needle and connected through a drip chamber to a closed drainage system. The drip chamber is placed at the level of the patient's ear when they are recumbent, or at the level of the shoulder when sitting or ambulating. A properly functioning drain should put out ≈ 300 ml of CSF per day. Alternatively, instead of leaving the tubing open to drain against pressure, 10 cc of CSF may be withdrawn every hour

If symptoms of nerve root irritation develop during the drainage, the catheter should be withdrawn several millimeters. Daily surveillance CSF cell counts and cultures should be performed (NB: a pleocytosis of ≈ 100 cells/mm³ can be seen normally just as a result of the presence of a drain).

A 5-day trial is recommended (mean time to improvement: 3 days).

Continuous CSF pressure monitoring

Some patients with a normal OP on LP demonstrate pressure peaks > 270 mm H_2O or recurrent B-waves.[100] These patients may also have a higher response to shunting than those without these findings.

Miscellaneous

Cerebral blood flow (CBF) measurements: Although some studies indicate otherwise, CBF measurements show no specific findings in NPH, and are not helpful in predicting who will respond to shunting. However, increased CBF after shunting correlates with clinical improvement.[101]

EEG: There are no specific EEG findings in NPH.

24.12.7 Diagnostic criteria

Practice guideline: Diagnosis of NPH

Level II[66]: Since strict diagnostic criteria cannot be formulated for NPH because of a lack of knowledge of the underlying pathophysiology at this time, it is recommended that the diagnosis be made in terms of Probable, Possible, and Unlikely NPH as described in ▶ Table 24.7.

Table 24.7 Diagnostic guidelines[a] for NPH[66]

Probable NPH

History[b]: must include:

1. insidious onset (vs. acute)
2. onset age ≥ 40 years
3. duration ≥ 3–6 months
4. no antecedent head trauma, ICH, meningitis, or other known cause of secondary hydrocephalus
5. progression over time
6. no other neurological, psychiatric, or general medical conditions that are sufficient to explain the presenting symptoms

Brain imaging: CT or MRI _after_ onset of symptoms must show:

1. ventricular enlargement not attributable to cerebral atrophy or congenital enlargement (Evans index[c] > 0.3 or comparable measure)
2. no macroscopic obstruction to CSF flow
3. ≥ 1 of the following supportive features
   a) enlarged temporal horns not entirely attributable to hippocampal atrophy
   b) callosal angle[d] ≥ 40°
   c) evidence of altered brain water content, including periventricular changes not attributable to microvascular ischemic changes or demyelination
   d) aqueductal or 4th ventricle flow void on MRI

Other imaging findings that may support _Probable_ designation but are not required:
1. pre-morbid study showing smaller or nonhydrocephalic ventricles
2. radionuclide cisternogram showing delayed clearance of radiotracer over the convexities after 48–72 hours[e]
3. cine-MRI or other technique showing increased ventricular flow rate[f]
4. SPECT showing decreased periventricular perfusion that is not altered by acetazolamide challenge

Physiological

CSF opening pressure (OP) on lateral decubitus LP: 5–18 mm Hg (70–245 mm H_2O)

Clinical: must show gait/balance disturbance, plus impairment in cognition and/or urinary function

1. **gait/imbalance:** ≥ 2 of the following (not entirely attributable to other conditions
   a) decreased step height
   b) decreased step length
   c) decreased cadence (speed of walking)
   d) increased trunk sway while walking
   e) widened standing base
   f) toes turn outward while walking
   g) retropulsion (spontaneous or provoked)
   h) en bloc turning (≥ 3 steps to turn 180°)
   i) impaired walking balance: ≥ 2 corrections out of 8 tandem steps
2. **cognition:** documented impairment (adjusted for age & education) and/or decrease in performance on cognitive screening instrument (e.g., Mini-Mental State Examination[102]), or evidence of ≥ 2 of the following not fully attributable to other conditions:
   a) psychomotor slowing (increased response latency)
   b) decreased fine motor speed
   c) decreased fine motor accuracy
   d) difficulty dividing or maintaining attention
   e) impaired recall, especially for recent events
   f) executive dysfunction: e.g., impairment in multistep procedures, working memory, formulation of abstractions/similarities, insight
   g) behavioral or personality changes
3. **urinary dysfunction:**
   a) any one of the following
      • episodic or persistent incontinence not attributable to primary urological disorder
      • persistent urinary incontinence
      • urinary and fecal incontinence
   b) or any 2 of the following:
      • urinary urgency: frequent perception of a pressing need to void
      • urinary frequency (pollakiuria): voiding > 6 times in 12 hours with normal fluid intake
      • nocturia: needing to void > 2 times in an average night

Possible NPH

History: reported symptoms may:

1. have subacute or indeterminate mode of onset
2. onset at any age after childhood
3. duration: < 3 months or indeterminate
4. may follow events such as mild head trauma, remote history of ICH, or childhood or adult meningitis or other conditions judged not likely to be causally related

(continued)

Table 24.7 continued

Probable NPH
5. coexist with other neurological, psychiatric, or general medical disorders but judged not to be entirely attributable to these conditions
6. be nonprogressive or not clearly progressive

Clinical: symptoms of either:

1. incontinence and/or cognitive impairment in the absence of observable gait/balance disturbance
2. gait disturbance or dementia alone

Brain imaging: ventricular enlargement consistent with hydrocephalus but associated with any of the following:

1. cerebral atrophy of sufficient severity to potentially explain ventricular enlargement
2. structural lesions that may influence ventricular size

Physiological

OP not available or outside of the range delineated for *Probable NPH*

Unlikely NPH
1. no ventriculomegaly
2. signs of increased ICP (e.g., papilledema)
3. no component of the clinical triad of NPH
4. symptoms explained by other causes (e.g., spinal stenosis)

[a]these guidelines are often referred to as "The International Guidelines" as opposed to "The Japanese Guidelines"[79]
[b]history should be verified by an individual familiar with premorbid and current condition
[c]see definition and illustration of Evans index (p. 431). A threshold of 0.3 is used for the guidelines, but a criteria of ≥ 0.33 is probably more specific in elderly subjects[73]
[d]this callosal angle is different than the one discussed by Ishii[103]
[e]radionuclide cisternography has a high false positive rate and ∴ its use is currently not recommended[73]
[f]only 1 Class II and 3 Class III studies available. Conclusion: high aqueductal flow velocity on MRI coupled with an abnormal CSF infusion test are possibly more likely to respond to shunting[104]

24.12.8 Treatment

Management algorithm

1. based on history, physical exam, and imaging, classify the patient as probable, possible, or unlikely NPH (see ► Table 24.7). For probable and possible NPH, without further testing, the degree of certainty of the diagnosis of NPH is ≈ 50–61%.[84,105,106] In an otherwise healthy patient in whom the diagnosis of NPH seems highly probable, it is not unreasonable to proceed to shunting[90]
2. to increase the certainty of response to shunting, one or more of the following is recommended[90]
   a) "tap test" (AKA Miller Fisher test): withdrawal of 40–50 ml of CSF via LP
      • positive response (p. 443) increases likelihood of responding to a shunt (PPV) to the range of 73–100%
      • due to low sensitivity (26–61%), a negative response does not rule out the possibility of responding, and a subsequent supplemental test should be performed[90]
      • if OP > 17.6 mm Hg (24 cm H_2O), consider further search for cause of secondary hydrocephalus (does not rule out shunting as a treatment)
   b) resistance testing: sensitivity (57–100%) > tap test, similar PPV (75–92%)
   c) external lumbar drainage

CSF diversionary procedures

VP shunt is the procedure of choice. Lumbar-peritoneal shunts have been used, but disadvantages include: tendency to overshunt, difficult to tap, tendency to migrate. For most, use a *medium pressure* valve[107] (closing pressure 65–90 mm H_2O) to minimize the risk of subdural hematomas (see below), although response rate may be higher with a low-pressure valve.[108] Gradually sit patient up over a period of several days; proceed more slowly in patients who develop low-pressure headaches. Alternatively, the risk of developing SDH may be decreased with use of a programmable shunt valve, set initially at a high pressure (to reduce risk of subdural hematoma) and gradually decreasing the pressure setting over a number of weeks.

Follow patients clinically and with CT for ≈ 6–12 months.

Patients who do not improve and whose ventricles do not change on imaging should be evaluated for shunt malfunction. If not obstructed, and if no subdural fluid collections have developed, a lower pressure valve may be tried (or a lower pressure selected on a programmable shunt).

Potential complications of shunting for NPH

Complication rates may be as high as ≈ 35% (due in part to the frailty of the elderly brain).[109,110]
Potential complications include[111]:

1. subdural hematomas or hygroma (p.464): higher risk with low pressure valve and older patients who tend to have cerebral atrophy. Usually accompanied by headache, most resolve spontaneously or remain stable. Approximately one–third require evacuation and tying off of shunt (temporarily or permanently). Risk may be reduced by gradual mobilization post-op
2. shunt infection
3. intracerebral hemorrhage
4. seizures (p.455)
5. delayed complications include above, plus shunt obstruction or disconnection

Endoscopic third ventriculostomy (ETV)

Initially reported for NPH in 1999.[112] Mechanistically, it is difficult to explain why ETV would work for NPH, but it has been advocated by some[113] in highly selected patients, using nonvalidated outcome measures, quoting post-op improvement in 69% of patients. At this time, ETV should not be considered a first line treatment for most cases of NPH.

24.12.9 Outcome

The most likely symptom to improve with shunting is *incontinence*, then gait disturbance, and lastly dementia. Black et al[107] give the following markers for good candidates for improvement with shunting:

- clinical: presence of the classic triad (p.439).[109] Also 77% of patients with gait disturbance as the primary symptom improved with shunting. Patients with dementia and *no* gait disturbance rarely respond to shunting
- LP: OP > 100 mm H_2O
- continuous CSF pressure recording: pressure > 180 mm H_2O or frequent Lundberg B waves (p.1045)
- CT or MRI: large ventricles with flattened sulci (little atrophy)

Response is better when symptoms have been present for a shorter time.

NB: NPH patients with co-existing Alzheimer's disease (AD) may still improve with VP shunts; thus AD should not exclude these patients from shunting.[114] However, patients with AD *alone* (without NPH) did not respond to shunting in an RPDB placebo-controlled trial.[115]

In general, most responders eventually relapse, often after ≈ 5–7 years of good response. Shunt malfunction and subdural collections must be ruled out before ascribing this to the natural course of the underlying condition.

24.13 Hydrocephalus and pregnancy

24.13.1 General information

Patients with CSF shunts may become pregnant, and there are case reports of patients developing hydrocephalus during pregnancy requiring shunting.[116]

Any of the shunt problems discussed in the following sections may occur in a pregnant patient with a shunt. With VP shunts, distal shunt problems may be higher in pregnancy. The following are management suggestions modified from Wisoff et al.[116]

24.13.2 Preconception management of patients with shunts

1. evaluation, including:
   a) evaluation of shunt function: preconception baseline MRI or CT. Further evaluation of shunt patency if any suspicion of malfunction. Patients with slit ventricles may have reduced compliance and may become symptomatic with very small changes in volume
   b) assessment of medications, especially antiseizure medications
2. counselling, including:
   a) genetic counselling: if the HCP is due to a neural tube defect (NTD), then there is a 2–3% chance that the baby will have an NTD
   b) other recommendations include early administration of prenatal vitamins and avoiding teratogenic drugs and excessive heat (e.g., hot-tubs). Neural tube defects, Risk factors (p.313)

24.13.3 Gravid management

1. close observation for signs of increased ICP: headache, N/V, lethargy, ataxia, seizures... Caution: these signs may mimic preeclampsia (which must also be ruled out). 58% of patients exhibit signs of increased ICP, which may be due to:
   a) decompensation of partial shunt malfunction
   b) shunt malfunction
   c) some show signs of increased ICP in spite of adequate shunt function, may be due to increased cerebral hydration and venous engorgement
   d) enlargement of tumor during pregnancy
   e) cerebral venous thrombosis: including dural sinus thrombosis & cortical venous thrombosis
   f) encephalopathy related to disordered autoregulation
2. patients developing symptoms of increased ICP should have CT or MRI to compare ventricle size to preconception baseline study
   a) if no change from preconception study, puncture shunt to measure ICP and culture CSF. Consider radioisotope shunt-o-gram
   b) if all studies are negative, then physiologic changes may be responsible. Treatment is bed rest, fluid restriction, and, in severe cases, steroids and/or diuretics. If symptoms do not abate, then early delivery is recommended as soon as fetal lung maturity can be documented (give prophylactic antibiotics for 48 hrs before delivery)
   c) if ventricles have enlarged and/or shunt malfunction is demonstrated on testing, shunt revision is performed
      • in first two trimesters: VP shunt is preferred (do not use peritoneal trocar method after first trimester) and is tolerated well
      • in third trimester: VA or ventriculopleural shunt is used to avoid uterine trauma or induction of labor

24.13.4 Intrapartum management

1. prophylactic antibiotics are recommended during labor and delivery to reduce the incidence of shunt infection. Since coliforms are the most common pathogen in L&D, Wisoff et al recommend ampicillin 2 g IV q 6 hrs, and gentamicin 1.5 mg/kg IV q 8 hrs in labor and × 48 hrs post partum[116]
2. in patients without symptoms: a vaginal delivery is performed if obstetrically feasible (lower risk of forming adhesions or infection of distal shunt). A shortened second stage is preferred since the increase in CSF pressure in this stage is probably greater than during other Valsalva maneuvers[117]
3. in the patient who becomes symptomatic near term or during labor, after stabilizing the patient a C-section under general anesthesia (epidurals are contraindicated with elevated ICP) is performed with careful fluid monitoring and, in severe cases, steroids and diuretics

References

[1] Lemire RJ. Neural Tube Defects. JAMA. 1988; 259:558–562

[2] Amacher AL, Wellington J. Infantile Hydrocephalus: Long-Term Results of Surgical Therapy. Childs Brain. 1984; 11:217–229

[3] Hill A, Rozdilsky B. Congenital Hydrocephalus Secondary to Intra-Uterine Germinal Matrix/Intraventricular Hemorrhage. Dev Med Child Neurol. 1984; 26:509–527

[4] Kudo H, Tamaki N, Kim S, et al. Intraspinal Tumors Associated with Hydrocephalus. Neurosurgery. 1987; 21:726–731

[5] Schmidek HH, Auer LM, Kapp JP. The Cerebral Venous System. Neurosurgery. 1985; 17:663–678

[6] Parker T. Never Trust a Calm Dog: And Other Rules of Thumb. New York: Harper Perennial; 1990

[7] U.S. Department of Health and Human Services - Health Resources and Services Administration. Accurately Weighing and Measuring: Technique. . https://depts.washington.edu/growth/module5/text/page5a.htm

[8] Babson SG, Benda GI. Growth Graphs for the Clinical Assessment of Infants of Varying Gestational Age. J Pediatr. 1976; 89:814–820

[9] Humphrey PRD, Moseley IF, Russell RWR. Visual Field Defects in Obstructive Hydrocephalus. J Neurol Neurosurg Psychiatry. 1982; 45:591–597

[10] Calogero JA, Alexander E. Unilateral Amaurosis in a Hydrocephalic Child with an Obstructed Shunt. J Neurosurg. 1971; 34:236–240

[11] Kojima N, Kuwamura K, Tamaki N, et al. Reversible Congruous Homonymous Hemianopia as a Symptom of Shunt Malfunction. Surg Neurol. 1984; 22:253–256

[12] Black PM, Chapman PH. Transient Abducens Paresis After Shunting for Hydrocephalus. J Neurosurg. 1981; 55:467–469

[13] Arroyo HA, Jan JE, McCormick AQ, et al. Permanent Visual Loss After Shunt Malfunction. Neurology. 1985; 35:25–29

[14] Sato M, Tanaka S, Kohama A, et al. Occipital Lobe Infarction Caused by Tentorial Herniation. Neurosurgery. 1986; 18:300–305

[15] Joynt RJ, Honch GW, Rubin AJ, et al. Occipital Lobe Syndromes. In: Handbook of Clinical Neurology. Holland: Elsevier Science Publishers; 1985:49–62

[16] Hoyt WF. Vascular Lesions of the Visual Cortex with Brain Herniation Through the Tentorial Incisura. Arch Ophthalm. 1960; 64:44–57

[17] Rinaldi I, Botton JE, Troland CE. Cortical Visual Disturbances Following Ventriculography and/or Ventricular Decompression. J Neurosurg. 1962; 19:568–576

24

[18] Lindenberg R, Walsh FB. Vascular Compressions Involving Intracranial Visual Pathways. Tr Am Acad Ophth Otol. 1964; 68:677–694

[19] Glaser JS, Duane TD, Jaeger EA. Topical Diagnosis: Retrochiasmal Visual Pathways and Higher Cortical Function. In: Clinical Ophthalmology. 2nd ed. Philadelphia: Harper and Row; 1983:4–10

[20] Lindenberg R. Compression of Brain Arteries as Pathogenetic Factor for Tissue Necrosis and their Areas of Predilection. J Neuropath Exp Neurol. 1955; 14:223–243

[21] Barnet AB, Manson JI, Wilner E. Acute Cerebral Blindness in Childhood. Neurology. 1970; 20:1147–1156

[22] Keane JR. Blindness Following Tentorial Herniation. Ann Neurol. 1980; 8:186–190

[23] Hoyt WF, Walsh FB. Cortical Blindness with Partial Recovery Following Cerebral Anoxia from Cardiac Arrest. Arch Ophthalm. 1958; 60:1061–1069

[24] Weinberger HA, van der Woude R, Maier HC. Prognosis of Cortical Blindness Following Cardiac Arrest in Children. JAMA. 1962; 179:126–129

[25] Slavin ML. Ischemic Optic Neuropathy After Cardiac Arrest. Am J Ophthalmol. 1987; 104:435–436

[26] Sweeney PJ, Breuer AC, Selhorst JB, et al. Ischemic Optic Neuropathy: A Complication of Cardiopulmonary Bypass Surgery. Neurology. 1982; 32:560–562

[27] Drance SM, Morgan RW, Sweeney VP. Shock-Induced Optic Neuropathy. A Cause of Nonprogressive Glaucoma. N Engl J Med. 1973; 288:392–395

[28] Lorber J. Recovery of Vision Following Prolonged Blindness in Children with Hydrocephalus or Following Pyogenic Meningitis. Clin Pediatr. 1967; 6:699–703

[29] Jack CR,Jr, Shiung MM, Gunter JL, et al. Comparison of different MRI brain atrophy rate measures with clinical disease progression in AD. Neurology. 2004; 62:591–600

[30] Evans WA. An encephalographic ratio for estimating ventricular and cerebral atrophy. Archives of Neurology and Psychiatry. 1942; 47:931–937

[31] Meese W, Kluge W, Grumme T, et al. CT evaluation of the CSF spaces of healthy persons. Neuroradiology. 1980; 19:131–136

[32] Toma AK, Holl E, Kitchen ND, et al. Evans' index revisited: the need for an alternative in normal pressure hydrocephalus. Neurosurgery. 2011; 68:939–944

[33] O'Hayon BB, Drake JM, Ossip MG, et al. Frontal and Occipital Horn Ratio: A Linear Estimate of Ventricular Size for Multiple Imaging Modalities in Pediatric Hydrocephalus. Pediatric Neurosurgery. 1998; 29:245–249

[34] Zatz LM. The Evans ratio for ventricular size: a calculation error. Neuroradiology. 1979; 18. DOI: 10.1007/BF00344827

[35] LeMay M, Hochberg FH. Ventricular Differences Between Hydrostatic Hydrocephalus and Hydrocephalus Ex Vacuo by CT. Neuroradiology. 1979; 17:191–195

[36] Tuite GF, Evanson J, Chong WK, et al. The Beaten Copper Cranium: A Correlation between Intracranial Pressure, Cranial Radiographs, and Computed Tomographic Scans in Children with Craniosynostosis. Neurosurgery. 1996; 39:691–699

[37] Section of Pediatric Neurosurgery of the American Association of Neurological Surgeons. Pediatric Neurosurgery. New York 1982

[38] Alvarez LA, Maytal J, Shinnar S. Idiopathic External Hydrocephalus: Natural History and Relationship to Benign Familial Macrocephaly. Pediatrics. 1986; 77:901–907

[39] Barlow CF. CSF Dynamics in Hydrocephalus - With Special Attention to External Hydrocephalus. Brain Dev. 1984; 6:119–127

[40] Chadduck WM, Chadduck JB, Boop FA. The Subarachnoid Spaces in Craniosynostosis. Neurosurgery. 1992; 30:867–871

[41] McCluney KW, Yeakley JW, Fenstermacher JW. Subdural Hygroma Versus Atrophy on MR Brain Scans: "The Cortical Vein Sign". American Journal of Neuroradiology. 1992; 13:1335–1339

[42] Kuzma BB, Goodman JM. Differentiating External Hydrocephalus from Chronic Subdural Hematoma. Surgical Neurology. 1998; 50:86–88

[43] Ment LR, Duncan CC, Geehr R. Benign Enlargement of the Subarachnoid Spaces in the Infant. J Neurosurg. 1981; 54:504–508

[44] Sutton LN. Current Management of Hydrocephalus in Children. Contemporary Neurosurgery. 1997; 19:1–7

[45] Weller S, Gartner J. Genetic and clinical aspects of X-linked hydrocephalus (L1 disease): Mutations in the L1CAM gene. Human Mutation. 2001; 18:1–12

[46] Grupe A, Hultgren B, Ryan A, et al. Transgenic knockouts reveal a critical requirement for pancreatic beta cell glucokinase in maintaining glucose homeostasis. Cell. 1995; 83:69–78

[47] Yamasaki M, Arita N, Hiraga S, et al. A clinical and neuroradiological study of X-linked hydrocephalus in Japan. Journal of Neurosurgery. 1995; 83:50–55

[48] Kanemura Y, Okamoto N, Sakamoto H, et al. Molecular mechanisms and neuroimaging criteria for severe L1 syndrome with X-linked hydrocephalus. Journal of Neurosurgery. 2006; 105:403–412

[49] Foltz EL, Shurtleff DB. Five-Year Comparative Study of Hydrocephalus in Children with and without Operation (113 Cases). J Neurosurg. 1963; 20:1064–1079

[50] Rekate HL, Nulsen FE, Mack HL, et al. Establishing the Diagnosis of Shunt Independence. Monogr Neural Sci. 1982; 8:223–226

[51] Holtzer GJ, De Lange SA. Shunt-Independent Arrest of Hydrocephalus. J Neurosurg. 1973; 39:698–701

[52] Hemmer R. Can a Shunt Be Removed? Monogr Neural Sci. 1982; 8:227–228

[53] Epstein F. Diagnosis and Management of Arrested Hydrocephalus. Monogr Neural Sci. 1982; 8:105–107

[54] Pang D, Zwienenberg-Lee M, Smith M, et al. Progressive cranial nerve palsy following shunt placement in an isolated fourth ventricle: case report. J Neurosurg. 2005; 102:326–331

[55] Oi S, Matsumoto S. Slit ventricles as a cause of isolated ventricles after shunting. Childs Nerv Syst. 1985; 1:189–193

[56] Eder HG, Leber KA, Gruber W. Complications after shunting isolated IV ventricles. Childs Nerv Syst. 1997; 13:13–16

[57] Krefft TA, Graff-Radford NR, Lucas JA, et al. Normal pressure hydrocephalus and large head size. Alzheimer Dis Assoc Disord. 2004; 18:35–37

[58] Oi S, Shimoda M, Shibata M, et al. Pathophysiology of long-standing overt ventriculomegaly in adults. J Neurosurg. 2000; 92:933–940

[59] Craven CL, Ramkumar R, D'Antona L, et al. Natural history of ventriculomegaly in adults: a cluster analysis. J Neurosurg. 2019; 132:741–748

[60] Hakim S, Adams RD. The Special Clinical Problem of Symptomatic Hydrocephalus with Normal CSF Pressure. J Neurol Sci. 1965; 2:307–327

[61] Wilson RK, Williams MA. Evidence that congenital hydrocephalus is a precursor to idiopathic normal pressure hydrocephalus in only a subset of patients. J Neurol Neurosurg Psychiatry. 2007; 78:508–511

[62] Iliff JJ, Lee H, Yu M, et al. Brain-wide pathway for waste clearance captured by contrast-enhanced MRI. J Clin Invest. 2013; 123:1299–1309

[63] Brean A, Eide PK. Prevalence of probable idiopathic normal pressure hydrocephalus in a Norwegian population. Acta Neurol Scand. 2008; 118:48–53

[64] Adams RD, Fisher CM, Hakim S, et al. Symptomatic Occult Hydrocephalus with 'Normal' Cerebrospinal Fluid Pressure. N Engl J Med. 1965; 273:117–126

[65] Thal LJ, Grundman M, Klauber MR. Dementia: Characteristics of a Referral Population and Factors Associated with Progression. Neurology. 1988; 38:1083–1090

[66] Relkin N, Marmarou A, Klinge P, et al. INPH Guidelines, Part II: Diagnosing idiopathic normal-pressure hydrocephalus. Neurosurgery. 2005; 57: S2–4 to 16

[67] Knutsson E, Lying-Tunell U. Gait apraxia in normal-pressure hydrocephalus. Neurology. 1985; 35:155–160

[68] Rosen H, Swigar ME. Depression and normal pressure hydrocephalus. A dilemma in neuropsychiatric differential diagnosis. J Nerv Ment Dis. 1976; 163:35–40

[69] Schneider U, Malmadier A, Dengler R, et al. Mood cycles associated with normal pressure hydrocephalus. Am J Psychiatry. 1996; 153:1366–1367

[70] Crowell RM, Tew JM,Jr, Mark VH. Aggressive dementia associated with normal pressure hydrocephalus. Report of two unusual cases. Neurology. 1973; 23:461–464

[71] Bloom KK, Kraft WA. Paranoia–an unusual presentation of hydrocephalus. Am J Phys Med Rehabil. 1998; 77:157–159

[72] Yoshino M, Yoshino Y, Taniguchi M, et al. Syndrome of inappropriate secretion of antidiuretic hormone associated with idiopathic normal pressure hydrocephalus. Internal Medicine. 1999; 38:290–292

[73] Williams MA, Relkin NR. Diagnosis and management of idiopathic normal-pressure hydrocephalus. Neurol Clin Pract. 2013; 3:375–385

[74] Bech-Azeddine R, Waldemar G, Knudsen GM, et al. Idiopathic normal pressure hydrocephalus: Evaluation and findings in a multidisciplinary memory clinic. European Journal of Neurology. 2001; 8:601–611

[75] Vassilouthis J. The Syndrome of Normal-Pressure Hydrocephalus. J Neurosurg. 1984; 61:501–509

[76] Jack CR, Mokri B, Laws ER, et al. MR Findings in Normal Pressure Hydrocephalus: Significance and Comparison with Other Forms of Dementia. J Comput Assist Tomogr. 1987; 11:923–931

[77] Schwartz M, Creasey H, Grady CL, et al. Computed Tomographic Analysis of Brain Morphometrics in 30 Healthy Men, Aged 21 to 81 Years. Ann Neurol. 1985; 17:146–157

[78] Holodny AI, George AE, de Leon MJ, et al. Focal Dilation and Paradoxical Collapse of Cortical Fissures and Sulci in Patients with Normal-Pressure Hydrocephalus. Journal of Neurosurgery. 1998; 89:742–747

[79] Mori E, Ishikawa M, Kato T, et al. Guidelines for management of idiopathic normal pressure hydrocephalus: second edition. Neurol Med Chir (Tokyo). 2012; 52:775–809

[80] Hashimoto M, Ishikawa M, Mori E, et al. Diagnosis of idiopathic normal pressure hydrocephalus is supported by MRI-based scheme: a prospective cohort study. Cerebrospinal Fluid Res. 2010; 7. DOI: 10.1186/1743-8454-7-18

[81] Kiefer M, Unterberg A. The differential diagnosis and treatment of normal-pressure hydrocephalus. Dtsch Arztebl Int. 2012; 109:15–25; quiz 26

[82] Virhammar J, Laurell K, Cesarini KG, et al. Preoperative prognostic value of MRI findings in 108 patients with idiopathic normal pressure hydrocephalus. AJNR Am J Neuroradiol. 2014; 35:2311–2318

[83] Shenkin HA, Greenberg JO, Grossman CB. Ventricular Size After Shunting For Idiopathic Normal Pressure Hydrocephalus. J Neurol Neurosurg Psychiatry. 1975; 38:833–837

[84] Vanneste J, Augustijn P, Davies GAG, et al. Normal-Pressure Hydrocephalus: Is Cisternography Still Useful in Selecting Patients for a Shunt? Arch Neurol. 1992; 49:366–370

[85] Relkin N. Neuroradiology Assessment of iNPH. Banff, Alberta, Canada 2015

[86] Kockum K, Lilja-Lund O, Larsson EM, et al. The idiopathic normal-pressure hydrocephalus Radscale: a radiological scale for structured evaluation. Eur J Neurol. 2018; 25:569–576

[87] Sasaki M, Honda S, Yuasa T, et al. Narrow CSF space at high convexity and high midline areas in idiopathic normal pressure hydrocephalus detected by axial and coronal MRI. Neuroradiology. 2008; 50:117–122

[88] Fazekas F, Chawluk JB, Alavi A, et al. MR signal abnormalities at 1.5 T in Alzheimer's dementia and normal aging. AJR Am J Roentgenol. 1987; 149:351–356

[89] Bono F, Lupo MR, Serra P, et al. Obesity does not induce abnormal CSF pressure in subjects with normal cerebral MR venography. Neurology. 2002; 59:1641–1643

[90] Marmarou A, Bergsneider M, Klinge P, et al. INPH Guidelines, Part III: The value of supplemental prognostic tests for the preoperative assessment of idiopathic normal-pressure hydrocephalus. Neurosurgery. 2005; 57:S2–17 to 28

[91] Graff-Radford NR, Jones DT. Normal Pressure Hydrocephalus. Continuum (Minneap Minn). 2019; 25:165–186

[92] Haan J, Thomeer RTWM. Predictive Value of Temporary External Lumbar Drainage in Normal Pressure Hydrocephalus. Neurosurgery. 1988; 22:388–391

[93] Malm J, Kristensen B, Karlsson T, et al. The predictive value of cerebrospinal fluid dynamic tests in patients with the idiopathic adult hydrocephalus syndrome. Arch Neurol. 1995; 52:783–789

[94] Walchenbach R, Geiger E, Thomeer RT, et al. The value of temporary external lumbar CSF drainage in predicting the outcome of shunting on normal pressure hydrocephalus. J Neurol Neurosurg Psychiatry. 2002; 72:503–506

[95] Centers for Disease Control. Timed Up & Go (TUG). 2017. https://www.cdc.gov/steadi/pdf/TUG_test-print.pdf

[96] Czosnyka M, Czosnyka ZH, Whitfield PC, et al. Age dependence of cerebrospinal pressure-volume compensation in patients with hydrocephalus. J Neurosurg. 2001; 94:482–486

[97] Marmarou A, Shulman K, Rosende RM. A nonlinear analysis of the cerebrospinal fluid system and intracranial pressure dynamics. J Neurosurg. 1978; 48:332–344

[98] Katzman R, Hussey F. A simple constant-infusion manometric test for measurement of CSF absorption. I. Rationale and method. Neurology. 1970; 20:534–544

[99] Meier U, Bartels P. The importance of the intrathecal infusion test in the diagnostic of normal-pressure hydrocephalus. Eur Neurol. 2001; 46:178–186

[100] Symon L, Dorsch NWC, Stephens RJ. Pressure Waves in So-Called Low-Pressure Hydrocephalus. Lancet. 1972; 2:1291–1292

[101] Tamaki N, Kusunoki T, Wakabayashi T, et al. Cerebral Hemodynamics in Normal-Pressure Hydrocephalus: Evaluation by 133Xe Inhalation Method and Dynamic CT Study. J Neurosurg. 1984; 61:510–514

[102] Folstein MF, Folstein SE, McHugh PR. "Mini-Mental State": A Practical Method for Grading the Cognitive State of Patiets for the Clinician. J Psychiatr Res. 1975; 12:189–198

[103] Ishii K, Kanda T, Harada A, et al. Clinical impact of the callosal angle in the diagnosis of idiopathic normal pressure hydrocephalus. Eur Radiol. 2008; 18:2678–2683

[104] Halperin JJ, Kurlan R, Schwalb JM, et al. Practice guideline: Idiopathic normal pressure hydrocephalus: Response to shunting and predictors of response: Report of the Guideline Development, Dissemination, and Implementation Subcommittee of the American Academy of Neurology. Neurology. 2015; 85:2063–2071

[105] Vanneste J, Augustijn P, Tan WF, et al. Shunting normal pressure hydrocephalus: The predictive value of combined clinical and CT data. Journal of Neurology, Neurosurgery and Psychiatry. 1993; 56:251–256

[106] Takeuchi T, Kasahara E, Iwasaki M, et al. Indications for shunting in patients with idiopathic normal pressure hydrocephalus presenting with dementia and brain atrophy (atypical idiopathic normal pressure hydrocephalus). Neurol Med Chir (Tokyo). 2000; 40:38–47

[107] Black PM, Ojemann RG, Tzouras A. CSF Shunts for Dementia, Incontinence and Gait Disturbance. Clin Neurosurg. 1985; 32:632–651

[108] McQuarrie IG, Saint-Louis L, Scherer PB. Treatment of Normal-Pressure Hydrocephalus with Low versus Medium Pressure Cerebrospinal Fluid Shunts. Neurosurgery. 1984; 15:484–488

[109] Black PM. Idiopathic Normal-Pressure Hydrocephalus: Results of Shunting in 62 Patients. J Neurosurg. 1980; 52:371–377

[110] Peterson RC, Mokri B, Laws ER. Surgical Treatment of Idiopathic Hydrocephalus in Elderly Patients. Neurology. 1985; 35:307–311

[111] Udvarhelyi GB, Wood JH, James AE. Results and Complications in 55 Shunted Patients with Normal Pressure Hydrocephalus. Surg Neurol. 1975; 3:271–275

[112] Mitchell P, Mathew B. Third ventriculostomy in normal pressure hydrocephalus. British Journal of Neurosurgery. 1999; 13:382–385

[113] Gangemi M, Maiuri F, Naddeo M, et al. Endoscopic third ventriculostomy in idiopathic normal pressure hydrocephalus: an Italian multicenter study. Neurosurgery. 2008; 63:62–7; discussion 67-9

[114] Golomb J, et al. Alzheimer's Disease Comorbidity in Normal Pressure Hydrocephalus: Prevalence and Shunt Response. Journal of Neurology, Neurosurgery and Psychiatry. 2000; 68:778–781

[115] Silverberg GD, Mayo M, Saul T, et al. Continuous CSF drainage in AD: results of a double-blind, randomized, placebo-controlled study. Neurology. 2008; 71:202–209

[116] Wisoff JH, Kratzert KJ, Handwerker SM, et al. Pregnancy in Patients with Cerebrospinal Fluid Shunts: Report of a Series and Review of the Literature. Neurosurgery. 1991; 29:827–831

[117] Marx GF, Zemaitis MT, Orkin LR. CSF Pressures During Labor and Obstetrical Anesthesia. Anesthesiology. 1981; 22:348–354

24

25 Treatment of Hydrocephalus

25.1 Medical treatment of hydrocephalus

HCP remains a surgically treated condition. Acetazolamide may be helpful for temporizing (see below).

25.1.1 Diuretic therapy

May be tried in premature infants with bloody CSF (as long as there is no evidence of active hydrocephalus) while waiting to see if there will be resumption of normal CSF absorption. However, at best this should only be considered as an adjunct to definitive treatment or as a temporizing measure.

Satisfactory control of HCP was reported in ≈ 50% of patients of age < 1 year who had stable vital signs, normal renal function and no symptoms of elevated ICP (apnea, lethargy, vomiting) using the following[1]:

1. acetazolamide (a carbonic anhydrase inhibitor): 25 mg/kg/day PO divided TID × 1 day, increase 25 mg/kg/day each day until 100 mg/kg/day is reached
2. simultaneously start furosemide: 1 mg/kg/day PO divided TID
3. to counteract acidosis, use tricitrate (Polycitra®):
   a) start 4 ml/kg/day divided QID (each ml is equivalent to 2 mEq of bicarbonate, and contains 1 mEq K^+ and 1 mEq Na^+)
   b) measure serial electrolytes, and adjust dosage to maintain serum HCO_3 > 18 mEq/L
   c) change to Polycitra-K® (2 mEq K^+ per ml, no Na^+) if serum potassium becomes low, or to sodium bicarbonate if serum sodium becomes low
4. watch for electrolyte imbalance and acetazolamide side effects: lethargy, tachypnea, diarrhea, paresthesias (e.g., tingling in the fingertips)
5. perform weekly U/S or CT scan and insert ventricular shunt if progressive ventriculomegaly occurs. Otherwise, maintain therapy for a 6 month trial, then taper dosage over 2–4 weeks. Resume 3–4 mos of treatment if progressive HCP occurs

25.2 Spinal taps

HCP after intraventricular hemorrhage may be only transient. Serial taps (ventricular or LP[2]) may temporize until resorption resumes but LPs can only be performed for *communicating* HCP. If reabsorption does not resume when the protein content of the CSF is < 100 mg/dl, then it is unlikely that spontaneous resorption will occur in the near future (i.e., a shunt will usually be necessary).

25.3 Surgical

25.3.1 Goals of therapy

Normal sized ventricles is not the goal of therapy (some children have a paucity of brain tissue). Goals are optimum neurologic function (which usually requires normal intracranial pressure) and a good cosmetic result.

25.3.2 Surgical options

Options include
- third ventriculostomy: currently, endoscopic method is preferred (see below)
- shunting (p. 1825): various shunts are described below. The techniques of shunt placement are covered for VP shunts (p. 1826), for VA shunt (p. 1827), for ventriculopleural shunts (p. 1827), and for LP shunt (p. 1829)
- eliminating the obstruction: e.g., opening a stenosed Sylvian aqueduct. Often higher morbidity and lower success rate than simple CSF diversion with shunts, except perhaps in the case of tumor
- choroid plexectomy: described by Dandy in 1918 for communicating hydrocephalus.[3] May reduce the rate of, but does not totally halt, CSF production (only a portion of CSF is secreted by the choroid plexus, other sources include the ependymal lining of the ventricles and the dural sleeves of spinal nerve roots). Open surgery was associated with a high mortality rate (possibly due to

replacement of CSF by air). Endoscopic choroid plexus coagulation was originally described in 1910 and was recently resurrected[4]

25.4 Endoscopic third ventriculostomy

25.4.1 Indications

Endoscopic third ventriculostomy (ETV) may be used in patients with obstructive HCP. May also be an option in managing shunt infection (as a means to remove all hardware without subjecting the patient to increased ICP). ETV has also been proposed as an option for patients who developed subdural hematomas after shunting (the shunt is removed before the ETV is performed). ETV may also be indicated for slit ventricle syndrome (p. 463).

25.4.2 Contraindications

Communicating hydrocephalus has traditionally been considered a contraindication to ETV. However, it has been occasionally used for NPH.[5] Relative contraindications to ETV would be the presence of any of the conditions associated with a low success rate (see below).

25.4.3 Complications

- hypothalamic injury: may result in hyperphagia
- injury to pituitary stalk or gland: may result in hormonal abnormalities, including diabetes insipidus, amenorrhea
- transient 3rd and 6th nerve palsies
- injury to basilar artery, PComA, or PCA: a fixed endoscope sheath seated just distal to the foramen of Monro within the third ventricle may allow for safe egress of blood extacranially
- uncontrollable bleeding
- cardiac arrest[6]
- traumatic basilar artery aneurysm[7]: possibly related to thermal injury from use of laser in performing ETV

25.4.4 Technique

See dedicated section on technique (p. 1829).

25.4.5 Success rate

Overall success rate is ≈ 56% (range of 60–94% for nontumoral aqueductal stenosis[7] [AqS]). Highest maintained patency rate is with previously untreated acquired AqS. Success rate in infants may be poor because they may not have a normally developed subarachnoid space. There is a low success rate (only ≈ 20% of TVs will remain patent) if there is pre-existing pathology including:

1. tumor
2. previous shunt
3. previous SAH
4. previous whole brain radiation (success with focal stereotactic radiosurgery is not known)
5. significant adhesions visible when perforating through the floor of the third ventricle at the time of performance of ETV

▶ **ETV Success Score**[8,9]. A validated[10,11] tool for predicting the likelihood of success of ETV, which therefore may assist in selecting appropriate patients for the procedure. Shown in ▶ Table 25.1.

The total of the 3 scores (1 from each category: age, etiology, and shunt history) expressed as a percent is the approximate chance of an ETV lasting 6 months without failure. Scores < 40% correlated with a very low chance of success. Scores > 80% correlated with a better chance of success compared to shunting from the outset.

Intermediate scores (50–70%): ETV had a higher initial failure rate compared to shunting, but after 3–6 months the balance shifted in favor of ETV.[9]

In one series, clinical improvement after ETV was achieved in 76% (72 of 95 patients), including 6 patients requiring second ETVs (three of which had partially functioning shunts that were left in place at the time of ETV).

Table 25.1 ETV Success Score

Category	Finding	Value	Score
Age	< 1 month	0%	
	1 to < 6 months	10%	
	6 months to < 1 year	30%	(0 - 50%)
	1 to < 10 years	40%	
	≥ 10 years	50%	
Etiology	• post-infectious	0%	
	• myelomeningocele • post IVH • non-tectal brain tumor	20%	(0 - 30%)
	• aqueductal stenosis • tectal tumor • other	30%	
Previous Shunt?	yes	0%	(0 - 10%)
	no	10%	
ETV Success Score → TOTAL			(0 - 90%)

25.5 Shunts

25.5.1 Types of shunts

1. ventriculoperitoneal (VP) shunt:
   a) most commonly used shunt in modern era
   b) lateral ventricle is the usual proximal location
   c) intraperitoneal pressure: normal is near atmospheric
2. ventriculo-atrial (VA) shunt ("vascular shunt"):
   a) shunts ventricles through jugular vein to superior vena cava; so-called "ventriculo-atrial" shunt because it shunts the cerebral ventricles to the vascular system with the catheter tip in the region of the right cardiac atrium
   b) treatment of choice when abdominal abnormalities are present (extensive abdominal surgery, peritonitis, morbid obesity, in preemies who have had NEC and may not tolerate VP shunt...)
   c) shorter length of tubing results in lower distal pressure and less siphon effect than VP shunt; however, pulsatile pressures may alter CSF hydrodynamics
3. Torkildsen shunt:
   a) shunts ventricle to cisternal space
   b) rarely used
   c) effective only in acquired obstructive HCP, as patients with congenital HCP frequently do not develop normal subarachnoid CSF pathways
4. miscellaneous: various distal projections used historically or in patients who have had significant problems with traditional shunt locations (e.g., peritonitis with VP shunt, SBE with vascular shunts):
   a) pleural space (ventriculopleural shunt): not a first choice, but a viable alternative if the peritoneum is not available.[12] To avoid symptomatic hydrothorax necessitating relocating distal end, it is recommended only for patients > 7 yrs of age (although some feel that these may be placed as young as 2 yrs of age, and that hydrothorax is primarily a sign of infection regardless of age). Pressure in pleural space is less than atmospheric
   b) gallbladder (p. 1828)
   c) ureter or bladder: can cause electrolyte imbalances due to losses through urine
5. lumboperitoneal (LP) shunt; see insertion technique (p. 1830)
   a) only for communicating HCP: useful in situations with small ventricles (e.g., pseudotumor cerebri) or CSF fistula[13]
   b) over age 2 yrs, percutaneous insertion with Tuohy needle is preferred
6. cyst or subdural shunt: from arachnoid cyst or subdural hygroma cavity, usually to peritoneum

25.5.2 Disadvantages/complications of various shunts

Complications that may occur with any shunt

1. obstruction: the most common cause of shunt malfunction
   a) proximal: ventricular catheter (the most common site)
   b) valve mechanism
   c) distal: reported incidence of 12–34%.[14] Occurs in peritoneal catheter in VP shunt (see below), in atrial catheter in VA shunt
2. disconnection at a junction, or break at any point
3. infection: may produce obstruction
4. hardware erosion through skin, usually only in debilitated patients (especially preemies with enlarged heads and thin scalp from chronic HCP, who lay on one side of head due to elongated cranium). May also indicate silicone allergy (see below)
5. *seizures* (ventricular shunts only): there is ≈ 5.5% risk of seizures in the first year after placement of a shunt which drops to ≈ 1.1% after the 3rd year[15] (NB: this does not mean that the shunt was the cause of all of these seizures). Seizure risk is questionably higher with frontal catheters than with parieto-occipital
6. act as a conduit for extraneural metastases of certain tumors (e.g., medulloblastoma). This is probably a relatively low risk[16]
7. silicone allergy[17]: rare (if it occurs at all). May resemble shunt infection with skin breakdown and fungating granulomas. CSF is initially sterile but later infections may occur. May require fabrication of a custom silicone-free device (e.g., polyurethane)

Disadvantages/complications with VP shunt

1. inguinal hernia: incidence = 17% (many shunts are inserted while processus vaginalis is patent)[18]
2. need to lengthen catheter with growth: may be obviated by using long peritoneal catheter (p. 1826)
3. obstruction of peritoneal catheter:
   a) may be more likely with distal slit openings ("slit valves") due to occlusion by omentum or by trapping debris from the shunt system[14]
   b) by peritoneal cyst (or pseudocyst)[19]: usually associated with infection, may also be due to reaction to talc from surgical gloves (the omentum tends to "wall off" a nidus of irritation). It may rarely be necessary to differentiate a CSF collection from a urine collection in patients with overdistended bladders that have ruptured (e.g., secondary to neurogenic bladder). Fluid can be aspirated percutaneously and analyzed for BUN and creatinine (which should be absent in CSF)
   c) severe peritoneal adhesions: reduce surface area for CSF resorption
   d) malposition of catheter tip:
      • at time of surgery: e.g., in preperitoneal fat
      • tubing may pull out of peritoneal cavity with growth
4. peritonitis from shunt infection
5. hydrocele
6. CSF ascites
7. tip migration
   a) into scrotum[20]
   b) perforation of a viscus[21]: stomach,[22] bladder… More common with older spring-reinforced (Raimondi) shunt tubing
   c) through the diaphragm[23]
8. intestinal obstruction (as opposed to perforation): rare
9. volvulus[24]
10. intestinal strangulation: occurred only in patients in whom attempt was made to remove peritoneal tubing using traction on the catheter applied at the cephalad incision with subsequent breakage of the tubing leaving a residual intraabdominal segment (immediate peritoneal exploration is recommended under these circumstances)[25]
11. overshunting (p. 461): more likely than with VA shunt. Some recommend LP shunt for communicating hydrocephalus

25

Disadvantages/complications with VA shunt

1. requires repeated lengthening in growing child
2. higher risk of infection, septicemia
3. possible retrograde flow of blood into ventricles if valve malfunctions (rare)
4. shunt embolus
5. vascular complications: perforation, thrombophlebitis, pulmonary micro-emboli may cause pulmonary hypertension[26] (incidence ≈ 0.3%)

Disadvantages/complications with LP shunt

1. if at all possible, should not be used in growing child unless ventricular access is unavailable (e.g., due to slit ventricles):
   a) because of laminectomy in children causes scoliosis in 14%[27]
   b) due to risk of progressive cerebellar tonsillar herniation (acquired Chiari I malformation)[28] in up to 70% of cases[29,30]
2. overshunting: may be more common than with ventricular shunts. Treatment options include:
   a) horizontal-vertical (H-V) valve: increases resistance when upright (see below)
   b) flow reducing valves: e.g., inline miter valves (p. 1829) or specialized programmable Strata® NSC valve (p. 1829)
3. difficult access to proximal end for revision or assessment of patency; see Lumboperitoneal (LP) shunt evaluation (p. 1830).
4. lumbar nerve root irritation (radiculopathy)
5. leakage of CSF around catheter
6. pressure regulation can be difficult
7. bilateral 6th and even 7th cranial nerve dysfunction from overshunting
8. risk of arachnoiditis and adhesions
9. in severely obese, the peritoneal catheter may gradually spontaneously withdraw from the peritoneal compartment and coil up in the subcutaneous tissue

25.5.3 Shunt valves

X-ray appearance of some shunt valves

► Fig. 25.1 depicts *idealized* X-ray appearances of some common shunt valvess (to differentiate shunt systems on X-ray, not to scale). Appearance may vary with orientation relative to the X-ray beam. Manufacturer's diagrams of these shunts appear in section 25.7.

Abbreviations: P/L = performance level.

Programmable shunt valves

A number of externally programmable shunts available in the U.S., including:
- Strata by Medtronic (p. 469) (as Strata II or Strata NSC)
- Polaris by Sophysa (p. 469)
- Codman Hakim (p. 469)
- Certas Plus (p. 469) by Codman
- ProGav (p. 470) by Aesculap

All are programmed externally with a magnet, and can potentially be inadvertently reprogrammed by external magnetic fields including those encountered during an MRI (the Polaris valve and the Certas Plus valve are promoted as being less susceptible to inadvertent reprogramming. ★ Therefore, valve settings should be rechecked after an MRI scan performed for any reason, or if there is ever a concern about shunt function. The pressure setting on all of these valves can be checked on a plain X-ray taken perpendicular to the shunt valve (see ► Fig. 25.1 to identify the programmable valve type, then see the corresponding section for that valve to determine the shunt pressure setting). Some can also be checked using a special hand-held compass-like device provided by the manufacturer to most hospitals and clinics that deal with their valves.

In all systems on the market, increasing the programmed number results in higher valve opening pressures and therefore *less* CSF drainage at any given CSF pressure.

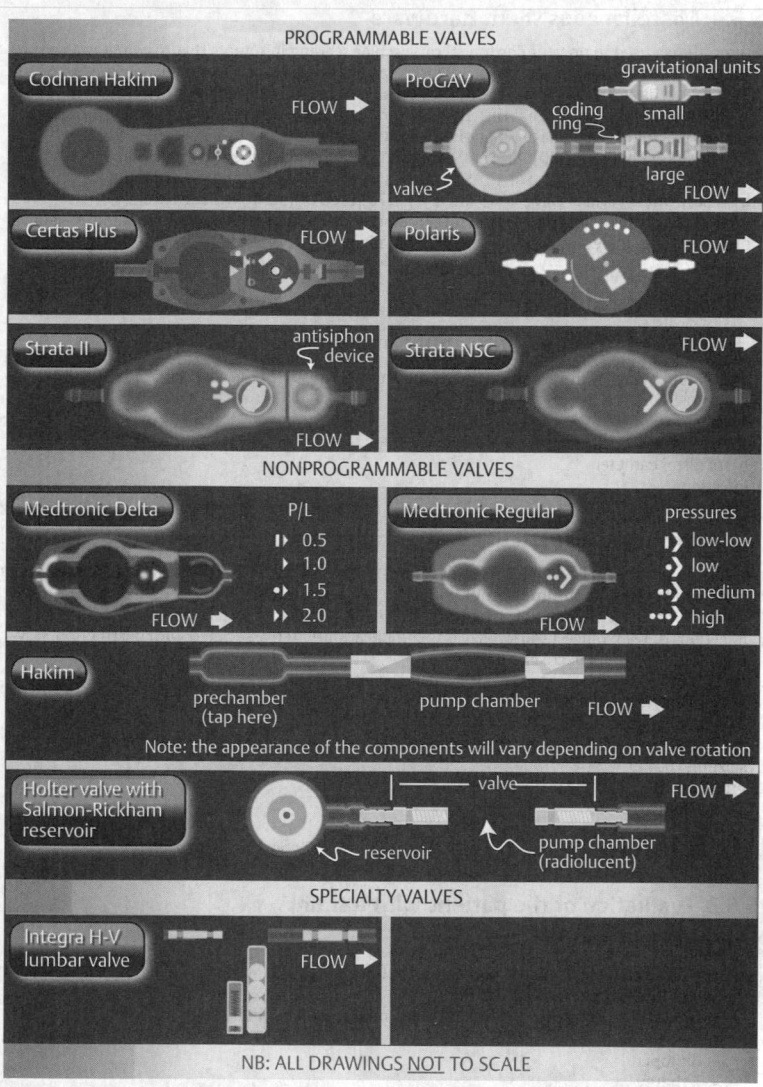

Fig. 25.1 Common shunt valves. X-ray appearance of some common shunt valves.
For X-ray appearance of different pressure settings for programmable valves, see the entry for that individual valve: Codman Hakim (p.469), ► Fig. 25.9; ProGAV (p.470), ► Fig. 25.12; Certas Plus (p.469), ► Fig. 25.10; Polaris (p.469), ► Fig. 25.11; Strata (II and NSC) (p.469), ► Fig. 25.8; nonprogrammable valves, ► Fig. 25.4; Integra H-V lumbar valve (p.470), ► Fig. 25.15.

25

25.5.4 Miscellaneous shunt hardware

1. tumor filter: used to prevent peritoneal or vascular seeding in tumors that may metastasize through CSF (e.g., medulloblastoma,[31] PNETs, ependymoma); may eventually become occluded by tumor cells and need replacement; may be able to radiate tumor filter to "sterilize" it. Not often used despite the fact that the risk of "shunt mets" appears to be low[16]
2. devices to avoid overdrainage when the patient is upright
   a) antisiphon devices (ASD): prevents siphoning effect when patient is erect. Some valves have ASDs integrated into the valve. ASDs always increase the resistance of the shunt
   b) "horizontal-vertical valve" (H-V valve) (p. 470) used primarily with LP shunts
3. with a standard 90-cm long 1.2 mm inner diameter distal catheter, the hydrodynamic resistance of most shunts increases by 2–2.5 mm Hg/(ml/min)[32]

25.6 Shunt problems

25.6.1 Risks associated with shunt insertion

1. intraparenchymal or intraventricular hemorrhage: risk ≈ 4% (in the absence of coagulopathy[33])
2. seizures
3. malposition
   a) of ventricular catheter
   b) of distal catheter
4. infection

25.6.2 Problems in patients with established CSF shunt

Shunt "problems" usually involve one or more of the following (**undershunting and infection account for most common shunt problems**):
1. undershunting (see below): obstruction (rate: ≈ 10% per year), breakage, migration...
2. infection (p. 371): range 1–40%. A serious complication. Often associated with obstruction. Having a shunt infection decreases IQ
3. overshunting:
   a) slit ventricle syndrome
   b) subdural hematomas… (p. 461)
   c) "spinal headache" (postural H/A, worse when upright, relieved by recumbency)
4. seizures (p. 455)
5. problems related to the distal catheter
   a) peritoneal (p. 455)
   b) atrial (p. 456)
6. skin breakdown over hardware (p. 455): may indicate infection or silicone allergy

25.6.3 Evaluation of the patient with a shunt

History and physical

1. history directed at determining presence of shunt-related symptoms
   a) acute symptoms of increased ICP
      - H/A: effect of posture, position, activity, migraine-like symptoms (visual aura...)
      - N/V
      - diplopia
      - lethargy
      - ataxia
      - infants: apnea and/or bradycardia; irritability; poor feeding
      - seizures: either new onset, or if pre-existing, an increase in frequency, or difficulty in control
   b) symptoms of infection: fever, chills, night-sweats, erythema and/or tenderness over shunt tubing. Diarrhea may indicate infection unrelated to shunt. Exposure to other sick individuals
2. physical exam: the following includes signs of increased intracranial pressure
   a) for children: OFC (p. 427). Plot on graph of normal curves (use existing chart for that patient if available) look for OFC crossing curves
   b) fontanelle tension (if open): a soft pulsating fontanelle varying with respirations is normal, a tense bulging fontanelle suggests obstruction, a sunken fontanelle may be normal or may represent overshunting

    c) upward gaze palsy: "setting sun sign," Parinaud's syndrome (p. 101)
    d) abducens palsy (p. 598): false localizing sign
    e) field cut, or blindness; see Blindness from hydrocephalus (p. 429)
    f) swelling around shunt tubing: caused by CSF dissecting along tract of an obstructed shunt
3. shunt history
    a) type of shunt: VP, VA, pleural, LP
    b) initial insertion of shunt: reason (MM, post-meningitis, etc.) and patient age
    c) date of last revision and reason for revision
    d) presence of accessory hardware in system (e.g., antisiphon device, etc.)
4. ability of shunt to pump and refill
    a) ✖ caution: may exacerbate obstruction, especially if shunt is occluded by ependyma due to overshunting: controversial
    b) difficult to depress: suggests distal occlusion
    c) slow to refill (generally, any valve should refill in 15–30 secs): suggests proximal (ventricular) occlusion or slit ventricles
5. evidence of CSF dissecting along tract outside of shunt tubing
6. in children presenting only with vomiting, especially those with cerebral palsy and feeding gastrostomy tubes, rule out gastroesophageal reflux

Radiographic evaluation

1. "shunt series" (plain X-rays to visualize entire shunt)
    a) purpose: R/O disconnection/breakage or migration of tip (NB: a disconnected shunt may continue to function by CSF flow through a subcutaneous fibrous tract)
    b) for a VP shunt: AP & lateral skull, CXR and abdominal X-ray
    c) the following hardware may be radiolucent and can mimic disconnection:
       • the central silastic part of older Holter style valves
       • connectors ("Y" & "T" as well as straight)
       • antisiphon devices
       • tumor filters
    d) obtain most recent X-rays available to compare for breaks (essential for "complicated" shunts involving multiple ventricular or cyst ends or accessory hardware)
2. in infants with open fontanelles, ultrasound is optimal method of evaluation (especially if previous U/S available)
3. *brain CT* required if fontanelles closed, may be desirable in complicated shunt systems (e.g., cyst shunts). Minimize the number of CTs in pediatric patients
4. *brain MRI*: best for assessing specific issues related to hydrocephalus (aqueductal stenosis, transependymal absorption of CSF, loculations… Shunt hardware is difficult to see on MRI. Programmable valves must be evaluated and reprogrammed after an MRI
5. "shunt-o-gram" if it is still unclear if shunt is functioning
    a) radionuclide: see below
    b) X-ray: using iodinated contrast: see below
6. abdominal CT or abdominal ultrasound: when undershunting is unexplained or if there is an index of suspicion of abdominal obstruction (e.g., abdominal symptoms such as pain or bloating)

"Shunt-o-gram"

General information
Two types: radionuclide shunt-o-gram (a nuclear medicine study) and iodinated contrast shunt-o-gram (an X-ray study)

Indications
When shunt function cannot be reliably ascertained using other methods.

Procedure
Clip hair over reservoir & prep (e.g., with Betadine). With patient supine, tap the shunt by inserting a 25 gauge butterfly needle into the reservoir. Measure the pressure with a manometer. Patients with multiple ventricular catheters need to have each injected to verify its patency.

▶ **Radionuclide "shunt-o-gram".** AKA radionuclide shuntography[34]: after tapping the shunt, drain 2–3 ml of CSF and send 1 ml of CSF for C&S. Inject radio-isotope (e.g., for VP shunt in an adult, use

1 mCi of 99m-Tc (technetium) pertechnetate (usable range: 0.5 to 3 mCi) in 1 cc of fluid) while occluding distal flow (by compressing valve or occluding ports). Flush in isotope with remaining CSF.

Immediately image the abdomen with the gamma camera to rule out direct injection into distal tubing. Image the cranium to verify flow into ventricles (proximal patency) for diffusion of the isotope within the abdomen to rule out pseudocyst formation around catheter.

Interpretation: If spontaneous flow into abdomen occurs within 20 minutes, the shunt is patent. If there is no flow on delayed imaging, it is occluded. The valve can be pumped to look for diffusion of isotope within the abdomen to rule out pseudocyst formation around the catheter tip. If it takes > 20 minutes, or if the patient has to be stood up to get flow, this is indeterminate and you should use other information to decide whether or not to revise the shunt.

▶ **X-ray "shunt-o-gram".** after tapping the shunt, drain ≈ 1 ml of CSF and send for C&S. Inject e.g., iohexol (Omnipaque 180) (p. 230) while occluding distal flow (by compressing valve or occluding ports).

Tapping a shunt

Indications
Indications to tap a shunt or ventricular access device (e.g., Ommaya reservoir) include:
1. to obtain CSF specimen
   a) to evaluate for shunt infection
   b) for cytology: e.g., in PNET to look for malignant cells in CSF
   c) to remove blood: e.g., in intraventricular hemorrhage
2. to evaluate shunt function
   a) measuring pressures
   b) contrast studies:
      • proximal injection of contrast (iodinated or radio-labeled)
      • distal injection of contrast
3. as a temporizing measure to allow function of a distally occluded shunt[35,36]
4. to inject medication
   a) antibiotics: for shunt infection or ventriculitis
   b) chemotherapeutic (antineoplastic) agents
5. for catheters placed within tumor cyst (not a true shunt):
   a) periodic withdrawal of accumulated fluid
   b) for injection of radioactive liquid (usually phosphorous) for ablation

Technique
For LP shunt, see Lumboperitoneal (LP) shunt evaluation (p. 1830).

There is a risk of introducing infection with every entry into the shunt system. With care, this may be kept to a minimum.
1. shave area
2. prep: e.g., povidone iodine solution × 5 minutes
3. use 25 gauge butterfly needle or smaller (ideally a noncoring needle should be used): for routine taps, the needle should only be introduced into shunt components specifically designed to be tapped

To measure pressures
A 25 Ga butterfly needle and an LP tray (with manometer, specimen tubes, 3-way stopcock valve...) are helpful. Steps are outlined in ▶ Table 25.2.

25.6.4 Undershunting

General information
The shunt malfunction rate is ≈ 17% during the first year of placement in the pediatric population.

Etiologies
May be due to one or a number of the following:
1. blockage (occlusion)
   a) possible causes of occlusion:
      • proximal obstruction by choroid plexus

Table 25.2 Steps in tapping a shunt

Step	Information provided
• After shave and prep, insert 25 Ga butterfly needle into the reservoir and look for spontaneous flow into butterfly tubing • measure pressure in manometer	• spontaneous flow indicates that the proximal end is not completely occluded • pressure is that of ventricular system (normal is < 15 cm of CSF in relaxed recumbent patient)
• measure the pressure with distal occluder compressed (if present)	• rise in pressure indicates some function of valve and distal shunt
• if no spontaneous flow, try to aspirate CSF with syringe	• if CSF is easily aspirated, it may be that pressure seen by ventricular system is very low. There should be spontaneous flow after that when the end of the tubing is lowered • if no CSF obtained or if difficult to aspirate, indicates proximal occlusion
• if still no flow, carefully inject 1–2 ml of preservative-free saline into ventricular catheter and see if spontaneous flow of more than the amount injected occurs	• may dislodge clot or debris from catheter • if only the 1–2 ml that were injected or less returns, indicates there is not a patent catheter in an open CSF space (possibilities include: occluded catheter, tip lodged in brain, slit ventricles)
• send any CSF for C&S, protein/glucose, cell count	• checks for infection
• fill manometer with sterile saline with the valve turned off to the shunt • compress *proximal* (inlet) occluder if present • open valve to shunt and measure runoff pressure after ≈ 60 seconds	• measures forward transmission pressure (through valve and peritoneal catheter in valves with a proximal occluder); forward pressure should be less than ventricular pressure (and absolute pressure should be < 8 cm H_2O)
• if no distal flow, keep inlet occluder compressed and inject 3–5 ml of saline into distal shunt and recheck distal runoff pressure • ✖ do not inject more than ≈ 1–2 ml into ventricles to avoid increasing ICP	• if the peritoneal catheter is in a loculated compartment the pressure will be considerably higher after injection

    • buildup of proteinaceous accretions
    • blood
    • cells (inflammatory or tumor)
    • secondary to infection
  b) site of blockage
    • blockage of ventricular end (most common): usually by choroid plexus, may also be due to glial adhesions, intraventricular blood
    • blockage of intermediate hardware (valves, connectors, etc.; tumor filters may become obstructed by tumor cells, antisiphon devices may close due to variable overlying subcutaneous tissue pressures[37])
    • blocked distal end, also see VP shunt (p.455)
2. disconnection, kinking or breakage of system at any point: with age, silicone elastomers used in catheters calcify and break down, and become more rigid and fragile and more likely to adhere to subcutaneous tissue.[38] Barium impregnation may accelerate this process. Tube fractures often occur near the clavicle, presumably due to the increased motion there

Signs and symptoms of undershunting

Signs and symptoms are those of active hydrocephalus. See "Evaluation of patient with shunt" (p.458).

25.6.5 Shunt infection

See Shunt infection (p.371) for evaluation and treatment.

25.6.6 "Overshunting"

General information

Possible complications of overshunting include[39]:
1. slit ventricles: including slit ventricle syndrome (see below)

2. intracranial hypotension: see below
3. subdural hematomas (p.464)
4. craniosynostosis and microcephaly (p.466): controversial
5. stenosis or occlusion of Sylvian aqueduct

10–12% of long-term ventricular shunt patients will develop one of the above problems within 6.5 yrs of initial shunting.[39] Some experts feel that problems related to overshunting could be reduced by utilizing LP shunts for communicating hydrocephalus, and reserving ventricular shunts for obstructive HCP.[39] VP shunts may also be more likely to overdrain than VA shunts because of the longer tubing → greater siphoning effect.

Intracranial hypotension following CSF shunting

AKA low ICP syndrome. Symptoms include "spinal H/A" (postural H/A that are worse when the patient is upright, *relieved by recumbency*). The following symptoms uncommonly occur[39,40]: N/V, lethargy, or neurologic signs (e.g., diplopia, upgaze palsy). Symptoms sometimes resemble those of high ICP, except that they are relieved when prostrate. Acute effects that may occur include[39]: tachycardia, loss of consciousness, or other brainstem deficits due to a rostral shift of the intracranial contents or to low ICP.

Etiology may be as simple as a shunt valve pressure that is too low, allowing excessive CSF to be drained, alternatively a siphoning effect may occur due to the column of CSF in the shunt tube when the patient is erect.[41]

Ventricles may be slit-like (▶ Fig. 25.2) (as in slit ventricle syndrome (SVS)) or may be normal in appearance. Other possible findings include thickening of the meninges best appreciated on MRI (▶ Fig. 25.2). Sometimes it is necessary to document a drop in ICP when going from supine to erect to diagnose this condition. These patients may also develop shunt occlusion and then the distinction from SVS blurs (see below).

With short-term symptoms, an increase in the valve pressure (requires re-operation if a non-programmable valve is present) or insertion of an antisiphon device (ASD) is the treatment of choice. However, patients with long-standing overshunting may not tolerate efforts to return intraventricular pressures to normal levels.[39,42]

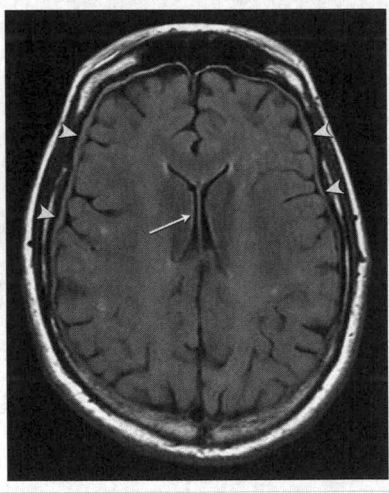

Fig. 25.2 Intracranial hypotension following VP shunting for hydrocephalus.
Image: axial FLAIR MRI. Findings include slit-ventricles (*white arrow*) and thickening of the meninges (*yellow arrowheads*).

Slit ventricles

"Slit ventricles" refers to complete collapse of the ventricles. In a survey, a frontal-occipital horn ratio[43] < 0.2 was most often interpreted as representing SVS. May be demonstrated in:
1. a significant number of shunted patients (especially younger ones) as a normal occurrence

2. overshunting
3. with entrapped (isolated) fourth ventricle (p. 436)
4. some patients with pseudotumor cerebri (p. 955) have slit-like ventricles with consistently elevated ICP

Slit ventricles may be:
1. asymptomatic:
   a) slit ventricles (totally collapsed lateral ventricles) may be seen on CT in 3–80% of patients after shunting,[40,44] most are asymptomatic
   b) these patients may occasionally present with symptoms unrelated to the shunt, e.g., true migraine
2. slit ventricle syndrome (SVS): seen in < 12% of all shunted patients. Subtypes:
   a) intermittent shunt occlusion: overshunting leads to ventricular collapse (slit ventricles) which causes the ependymal lining to occlude the inlet ports of the ventricular catheter (by coaptation), producing shunt obstruction. With time, many of these patients develop low ventricular compliance,[45] where even minimal dilatation results in high pressure which produces symptoms. Expansion then eventually reopens the inlet ports, allowing resumption of drainage (hence the intermittent symptoms). Symptoms may resemble shunt malfunction: intermittent headaches unrelated to posture, often with N/V, drowsiness, irritability, and impaired mentation. Signs may include 6th cranial nerve palsy. Incidence in shunted patients: 2–5%.[40,46] CT or MRI scans may also show evidence of transependymal absorption of CSF
   b) total shunt malfunction (AKA normal volume hydrocephalus[45]): may occur and yet ventricles remain slit-like if the ventricles cannot expand because of subependymal gliosis, or due to the law of Laplace (which states that the pressure required to expand a large container is lower than the pressure required to expand a small container)
   c) venous hypertension with normal shunt function: may result from partial venous occlusion that occurs in some conditions (e.g., at the level of the jugular foramen in Crouzon's syndrome). Usually subsides by adulthood
3. intracranial hypotension: symptoms often relieved by recumbency (see above)

Evaluation of slit ventricles

1. slit ventricles may be demonstrated on brain CT or MRI without contrast as total collapse of the ventricles (▶ Fig. 25.3)
2. physical exam: the shunt valve often fills slowly. If it is already known that the patient has slit ventricles, pumping the valve should be undertaken with caution since pumping may aggravate the situation, and slow filling of the valve in SVS is not unusual and so adds little useful information

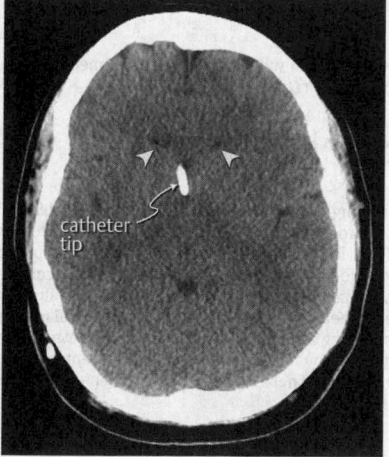

Fig. 25.3 Slit ventricles.
Image: noncontrast axial head CT scan. The frontal horns of the lateral ventricles are barely visible (*yellow arrowheads*). The tip of the ventricular catheter is seen in the collapsed third ventricle.

25

3. radionuclide "shunt-o-gram" (see above): can confirm distal patency
4. CSF pressure monitoring: either via lumbar drain, or with a butterfly needle inserted into the shunt reservoir ("sump" drain). Follow the pressure during postural changes to look for negative pressure when upright. Also monitor for pressure spikes, especially during sleep

Treatment

In treating a patient with slit ventricles on imaging studies, it is important to ascertain into which of the categories (see above) the patient falls. If the patient can be categorized, then the specific treatment listed below should be employed. Otherwise, it is probably most common to initially treat the patient empirically as intracranial hypotension, and then to move on to other methods for treatment failures.

Treatment of asymptomatic slit ventricles

Prophylactic upgrading to a higher pressure valve or insertion of an antisiphon device as initially advocated has largely been abandoned. However, this may be appropriate at the time of shunt revision when done for other reasons.[44]

Treatment of intracranial hypotension

Postural H/A due to intracranial hypotension (true overshunting) is usually self limited; however, if symptoms persist after ≈ 3 days of bed-rest and analgesics and a trial with a tight abdominal binder, the valve should be checked for proper closing pressure. If it is low, replace with a higher pressure valve. If it is not low, an ASD (which, by itself, also increases the resistance of the system) alone or together with a higher pressure valve may be needed.[47]

Treatment of slit ventricle syndrome

Patients with symptoms of SVS are actually suffering from intermittent high pressure. If total shunt malfunction is the cause, then shunt revision is indicated. For intermittent occlusion, treatment options include:

1. if symptoms occur early after shunt insertion or revision, initial expectant management may be indicated, because symptoms will spontaneously resolve in many patients as they equilibrate to the new intracranial pressure
2. revision of the proximal shunt. This may be difficult due to the small size of the ventricles. One can attempt to follow the existing tract and insert a longer or shorter length of tubing based on the pre-op imaging studies. Some advocate the placement of a second ventricular catheter, leaving the first one in place
3. patients may "respond" (fortuitously) to either of the following interventions because the slight ventricular enlargement elevates the ependyma off of the inlet ports (this may *not* always be the therapy of choice):
   a) valve upgrade[48] or
   b) ASD insertion[40,47]: the procedure of choice in some opinions.[39] First described in 1973[49]
4. subtemporal decompression[50,51,52] sometimes with dural incision.[50] This results in dilatation of the temporal horns (evidence for elevated pressure) in most, but not all[52] cases
5. third ventriculostomy (p. 453)[53]

25.6.7 Problems unrelated to shunting

For H/A consistent with migraine that are not postural, a trial with migraine-specific medications is warranted (Fiorinal®). See treatment of pseudotumor cerebri (p. 964).

25.6.8 Subdural hematomas in patients with CSF shunts

General information

May be due to collapse of brain with tearing of bridging veins. Incidence: 4–23% in adults, 2.8–5.4% in children, and is higher with normal pressure hydrocephalus (20–46%) than with "hypertensive hydrocephalus" (0.4–5%).[54,55] The risk of SDH is higher in the setting of long-standing hydrocephalus with a large head and little brain parenchyma (craniocerebral disproportion) with a thin cerebral mantle, as usually occurs in children with macrocephaly and large ventricles on initial evaluation. These patients have an "extremely delicate balance between subdural and intraventricular pressure."[54] By the same token, SDH can also follow shunting in elderly patients who have severe brain atrophy. The development of SDH may also be facilitated by negative pressures in the ventricles as a result of a siphoning effect when the patient is upright.[55,56] There is also a low risk of epidural hematoma following CSF shunting.[55]

Characteristics of the fluid

The collections may be on the same side as the shunt in 32%, on the opposite side in 21%, and bilateral in 47%.[55]

At the time of discovery, the SDHs are usually subacute to chronic, and the previously large ventricles are usually collapsed. Only 1 of 19 cases showed colorless fluid.[55] In all cases tested (even the 1 with clear fluid), the protein was elevated compared to CSF.

Treatment

Indications for treatment

Small (< 1–2 cm thick) asymptomatic collections in patients with closed cranial sutures may be followed with serial imaging studies. SDH were symptomatic in ≈ 40% of cases (symptoms often resemble those of shunt malfunction), and these require treatment. Treatment of SDH in children with open sutures has been advocated[55] to prevent later symptoms and/or development of macrocrania. The controversy arises with large asymptomatic SDH in older children or adults. Many authors recommend not treating asymptomatic lesions regardless of appearance,[54,57] whereas others vary their recommendations based on diverse criteria including size, appearance (chronic, acute, mixed…), etc.

Treatment techniques

A number of techniques have been described. Most involve evacuation of the SDHs by any of the usual methods (e.g., burr holes for chronic collections, craniotomy for acute collections) together with:

1. reducing the degree of shunting (i.e., to establish a lower pressure in the subdural space than in the intraventricular space, to cause the ventricles to re-expand and to prevent reaccumulation of the SDH)
   a) in shunt-dependent cases
      - replacing the valve with a higher pressure unit (upgrading the valve)
      - increasing the pressure on a programmable pressure valve[58,59]
      - using a Portnoy device that can be turned off and on externally. Be sure that care providers can reliably open the device in an emergency
   b) in non–shunt-dependent cases
      - any of the methods outlined above for shunt-dependent cases, or
      - temporarily tying off the shunt[60]
   c) insertion of an anti-siphon device[49]
2. drainage of the subdural space to
   a) the cisterna magna[61]
   b) to the peritoneum (subdural peritoneal shunt) with a low pressure valve (or no valve[55]). Some authors have the care-giver frequently pump the subdural valve

The goal is to achieve a delicate balance between undershunting (producing symptoms of active hydrocephalus) and overshunting (promoting the return of the SDH). Following surgery the patient should be mobilized slowly to prevent recurrence of the SDH.

25.6.9 Abdominal (peritoneal) pseudocyst with VP shunt

An abdominal pseudocyst is usually an indication of infection.

The following treatment algorithm is one of many valid protocols to deal with this:
1. open abdominal incision over tubing, and divide tubing at this site
2. verify which cut end is the peritoneal end and which is the distal shunt (with a working shunt, pumping the valve should cause CSF to come out the distal shunt)
3. attempt to drain the cyst through the remaining peritoneal end
   a) when you can't draw any more fluid, or if you don't get any to begin with, withdraw the catheter a little at a time and aspirate at each step
   b) send any fluid obtained for culture
   c) if tubing does not pull out smoothly, the abdomen may need to be opened (consider consulting general surgeon)
4. verify function of remaining shunt
   a) if the remaining shunt is functioning
      - connect it to sterile collection system

25

- monitor output volumes & send surveillance cultures of CSF qod
- after 3 consecutive cultures are negative, internalize distal end of shunt (using fresh distal catheter). The choice of target for distal end (peritoneum, pleura, vein) depends on whether abdominal cyst fluid is infected and if the peritoneal cavity still seems suitable)
  b) if the shunt is not functioning, a new external ventricular catheter should be inserted and connected to a collection system
    - monitor output volumes & send surveillance cultures of CSF qd
    - after 3 consecutive cultures are negative, remove the old shunt and place a totally new shunt. The choice of target for distal end (peritoneum, pleura, vein…) depends on whether abdominal cyst fluid is infected and if the peritoneal cavity still seems suitable)
5. shunt tap: indications vary, generally performed if occlusion is suspected or if surgical exploration is considered or if infection is strongly suspected; see Tapping a shunt (p. 460)
6. shunt exploration: sometimes even after thorough evaluation, the only means to definitively prove or disprove the functioning of various shunt components is to operate and isolate and test each part of the system independently. Even when infection is not suspected, CSF and any removed hardware should be cultured.

25.6.10 Miscellaneous shunt issues

Craniosynostosis, microcephaly and skull deformities

See also Craniosynostosis (p. 264). A number of skull changes have been described in infants after shunting, including[62]: thickening and inward growth of the bone of the skull base and cranial vault, decrease in size of the sella turcica, reduction in size of the cranial foramina, and craniosynostosis. The most common skull deformity was dolichocephaly from sagittal synostosis.[63] Microcephaly accounted for ≈ 6% of skull deformities after shunting (about half of these had sagittal synostosis). Some of these changes were reversible (except when complete synostosis was present) if intracranial hypertension recurred.

Laparoscopic surgery in patients with VP shunts

Issues regarding safety of laparoscopic surgery in patients with VP shunts:
1. laparoscopic surgery: abdominal insufflation with CO_2 is used to create a pneumoperitoneum, permitting the general surgeon to work. Typical insufflation pressure: 15 mm Hg (see conversion factors between mm Hg and cm of water (p. 1041)). In thin patients, 10 mm Hg may suffice. Transient additional increases in pressure may occur, e.g., when the surgeon leans on the patient's abdomen
2. concerns for patients with VP shunts:
   a) in some cases insufflation → ↑ ICP[64] which may be due to:
     - compression of vena cava → reduced venous return from head, as in Valsalva maneuver (independent of presence of a shunt)
     - absorption of CO_2 from the peritoneum → ↑ in arterial CO_2, causing cerebral arterial dilatation, thereby increasing ICP
     - ↓ CSF drainage due to ↑ pressure against which CSF must flow
     - retrograde passage of air/debris into intracranial compartment through an incompetent shunt valve (this also has potential for infection in the presence of peritonitis). This risk is minimal even with in vitro back-pressures up to 80 mm Hg.[65] Retrograde flow may also occur with a valveless shunt (rarely used)
     - in one case report monitoring TCDs,[66] there was no change during laparoscopic surgery in a patient with a VP shunt (except during periods of very high pressure)
   b) occlusion of the distal catheter by air, debris[67] or soft tissue
   c) extremely high intraabdominal pressures (> 80 mm Hg in vitro) may damage the valve,[65] which could cause malfunction after the laparoscopy

Prophylactic management options:
1. very controversial, special precautions may not be necessary[68]
2. one can temporarily occlude the peritoneal catheter (e.g., by a hemoclip applied by the general surgeon through the laparoscope under minimal initial insufflation pressure; the clip is removed at the end of the procedure), or temporary externalization of the shunt may be performed by the neurosurgeon, with internalization at the end of the procedure (this engenders an increased risk of infection)
3. ICP monitoring during laparoscopy
4. using low insufflation pressures (e.g., < 10 mm Hg)

25.7 Specific shunt systems

The following describes the salient features of some commonly used shunt systems. Diagrams are for general information only, and are not to scale.

25.7.1 Comparison of nonprogrammable shunt valves

▶ Fig. 25.4 compares opening pressures for some common nonprogrammable shunt valves.

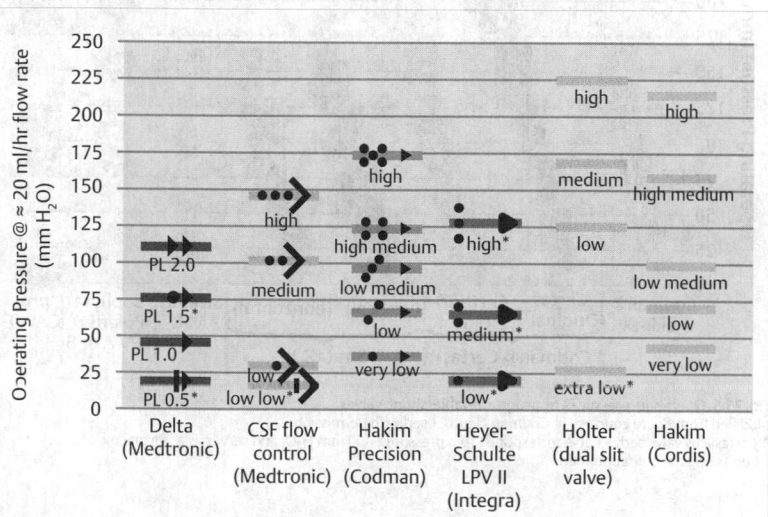

Fig. 25.4 **Opening pressures of nonprogrammable shunt valves.**
Symbols superimposed on the colored pressure bars depict the X-ray markings on the valves.
* Data provided by manufacturer, all others from Czosnyka Z, Czosnyka M, Richards HK, et al.[32]

25.7.2 Comparison of programmable shunt valves

▶ Fig. 25.5 shows a comparison of operating pressures of some common programmable shunt valves.

25.7.3 PS Medical/Medtronic CSF flow controlled valve

Manufactured by Medtronic Inc.

A single one-way membrane valve design. The radio-opaque arrowhead points in the direction of flow (▶ Fig. 25.6).

Pumping the valve

To pump the shunt in the "forward" direction, first occlude the inlet port (▶ Fig. 25.7) with pressure from one finger on the "inlet occluder" (prevents back-flow into the ventricle during the next step). Then while maintaining this pressure, depress the reservoir dome with a second finger. Release both fingers, and repeat. The one-way valve regulates shunt pressure and prevents reflux of CSF during normal use and during the release phase of shunt pumping.

X-ray characteristics

The three available valve pressures are indicated by radio-opaque dots on the valve (allows X-ray identification of valve pressure): one dot = low pressure, two dots = medium, three dots = high.

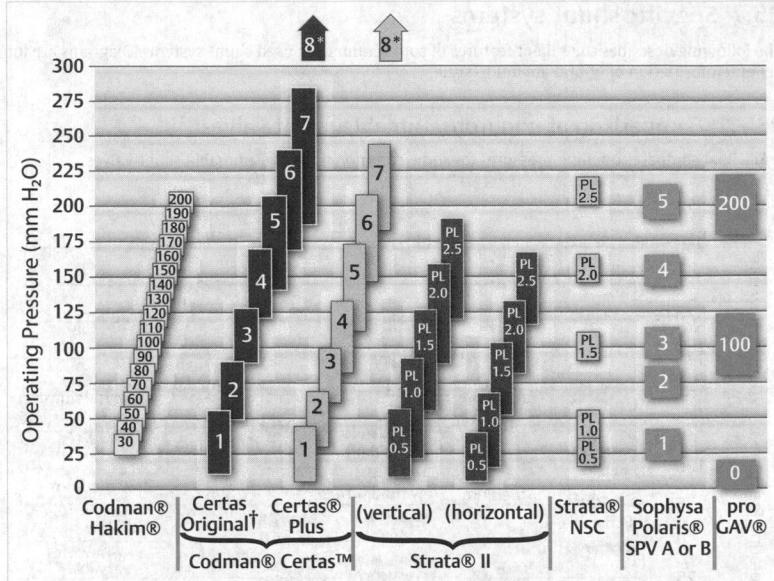

Fig. 25.5 Operating pressures of programmable shunt valves.
Modified from figure courtesy of Codman Neuro, used with permission.
* Certas Plus valve setting of 8 corresponds to a pressure > 400 mm H₂O, and serves as a "virtual off".
† Certas original is discontinued.

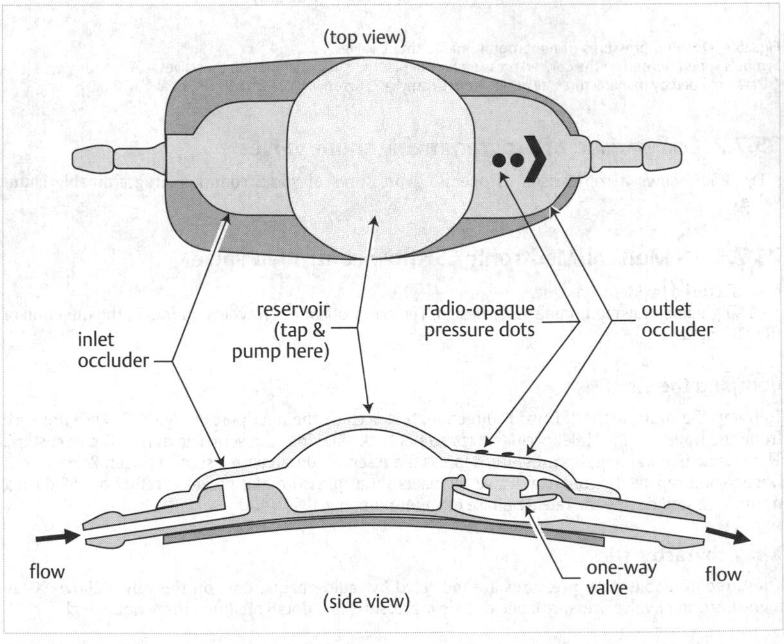

(top view)

reservoir
(tap &
pump here)

radio-opaque
pressure dots

inlet
occluder

outlet
occluder

flow

one-way
valve

flow

(side view)

Fig. 25.6 PS Medical standard contoured valve.

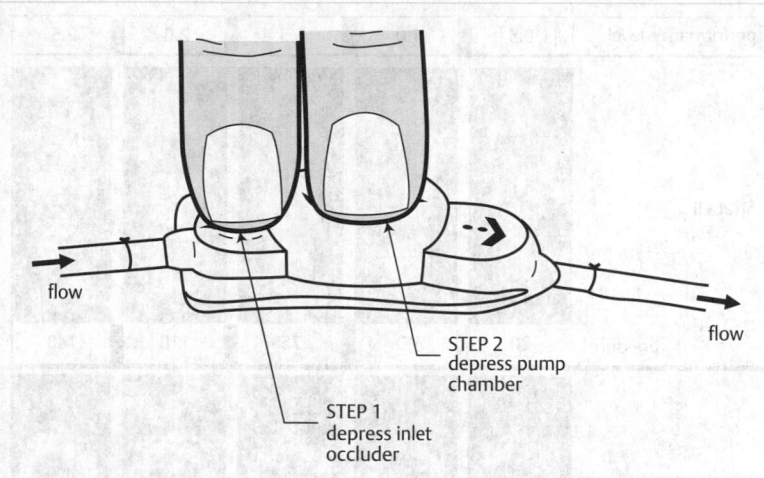

Fig. 25.7 Pumping the PS Medical valve.

flow

STEP 2
depress pump
chamber

STEP 1
depress inlet
occluder

flow

25.7.4 Strata® programmable valve

The Medtronic Strata valve is an externally adjustable valve that is programmed (using a magnet) to one of five performance level settings ("P/L" 0.5 to 2.5 in 0.5 increments) (► Fig. 25.8). It is available as Strata II (with an integrated antisiphon device) or as Strata NSC ("no siphon control"). A specialized Strata NSC valve for lumboperitoneal shunts (p. 1829) is also available as part of a kit.

Also, see general information regarding programmable valves (p. 456).

25.7.5 Codman Hakim programmable valve

Manufactured by Codman Inc.

18 pressure settings. Programmed by an AC-powered programming unit that requires confirmatory X-ray after re-programming. Newer programming units with acoustic monitoring may obviate the need for X-ray. The manufacturer advises not to increase the pressure by > 40 mm H_2O in a 24-hour period.

X-ray appearance for various settings are shown in ► Fig. 25.9. (Note: settings of 70, 120 & 170 mm H_2O align with an arm of the central cross of the valve). NB: when X-rayed correctly, the X-ray beam passes first through the valve and then the patient, which causes the radio-opaque marker to appear as a solid circle to the right of center as shown in ► Fig. 25.9. If the marker is on the left side, the beam is passing from the bottom of the valve, and the actual pressure reading should be based on a mirror image of the X-ray.

25.7.6 Certas Plus programmable valve

Manufactured by Codman Inc.

The X-ray appearance is shown in ► Fig. 25.10, and the pressure settings appear in ► Table 25.3.

25.7.7 Polaris programmable valve

Manufactured by Sophysa.

The Polaris valve is an externally programmable valve that uses two attracting Samarium-Cobalt magnets to lock the pressure setting and to resist inadvertent reprogramming by environmentally encountered magnets such as MRI scanners, cell phones, headphones...

Available in 4 models (different pressure ranges, each identified by a unique number of radio-opaque dots), each with 5 externally adjustable positions. The X-ray appearance and corresponding pressures are shown in ► Fig. 25.11.

25

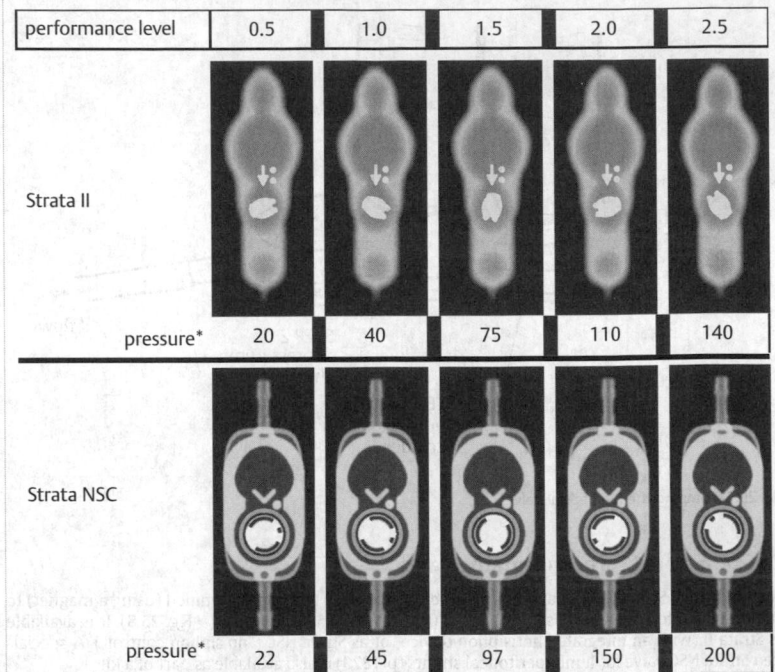

performance level	0.5	1.0	1.5	2.0	2.5
Strata II					
pressure*	20	40	75	110	140
Strata NSC					
pressure*	22	45	97	150	200

Fig. 25.8 Performance level (P/L) settings for the regular size Strata II valve and Strata NSC along with X-ray appearance.
* pressures in mm H_2O at flow rate of 20 ml/hr with patient recumbent and 0 mm H_2O distal pressure.

25.7.8 ProGAV programmable valve

See ▶ Fig. 25.12.

25.7.9 Heyer-Schulte

Distributed by Integra Neurosciences.

The LPV® II valve is shown in ▶ Fig. 25.13. To pump the shunt, occlude inlet port with one finger, then depress reservoir with another finger (as for the PS Medical valve, see above). This valve may be injected in either direction by depressing the appropriate occluder while injecting into the reservoir.

25.7.10 Hakim (Cordis) shunt

Distributed by Integra Neurosciences.

A dual ball-valve mechanism (▶ Fig. 25.14). To pump shunt, depress the indicated portion of the valve. NB: *do not* tap here, as the silicone elastomer housing is not self-sealing. The antechamber is provided for this type of access.

25.7.11 Integra (Cordis) horizontal-vertical lumbar valve

▶ Fig. 25.15. May be used in lumboperitoneal shunt to increase the transmission pressure when the patient is upright to prevent overshunting. Markings used to orient the device during implantation:

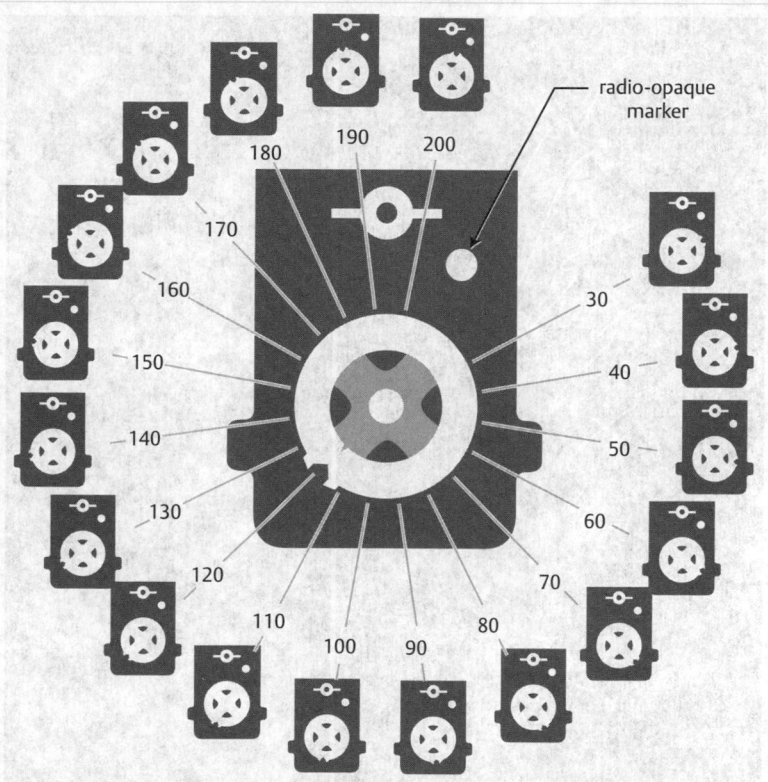

radio-opaque
marker

25

Fig. 25.9 Rotor of the Codman Hakim programmable valve. Detailed appearance at the various settings in mm Hg (e.g., the large central image shows a setting of 120 mm H$_2$O).

1. an arrow on the inlet side of the unit indicates direction of flow
2. inlet tubing is clear
3. inlet tubing has smaller diameter than outlet tubing
4. outlet tubing is white
5. before positioning the valve and fastening it to the fascia with permanent suture, the valve should be connected to both the subarachnoid catheter (inlet) and the peritoneal catheter (outlet). The arrow on the inlet valve should point towards the patient's feet

25.7.12 Holter valve

A dual slit valve mechanism (▶ Fig. 25.16). Usually used in combination with a reservoir (e.g., Rickham or Salmon-Rickham reservoir) (▶ Fig. 25.17). Letter markings on the valves (H, M, L, EL for "high," "medium," "low," and "extra low") visible at surgery indicates the pressure range of that valve.

To pump the shunt, simply depress the indicated portion of the valve.

X-ray characteristics

The silastic tube between the two one-way valves is radiolucent (▶ Fig. 25.1). There are no radiographic markings that allows differentiation between the various available pressure valves.

25

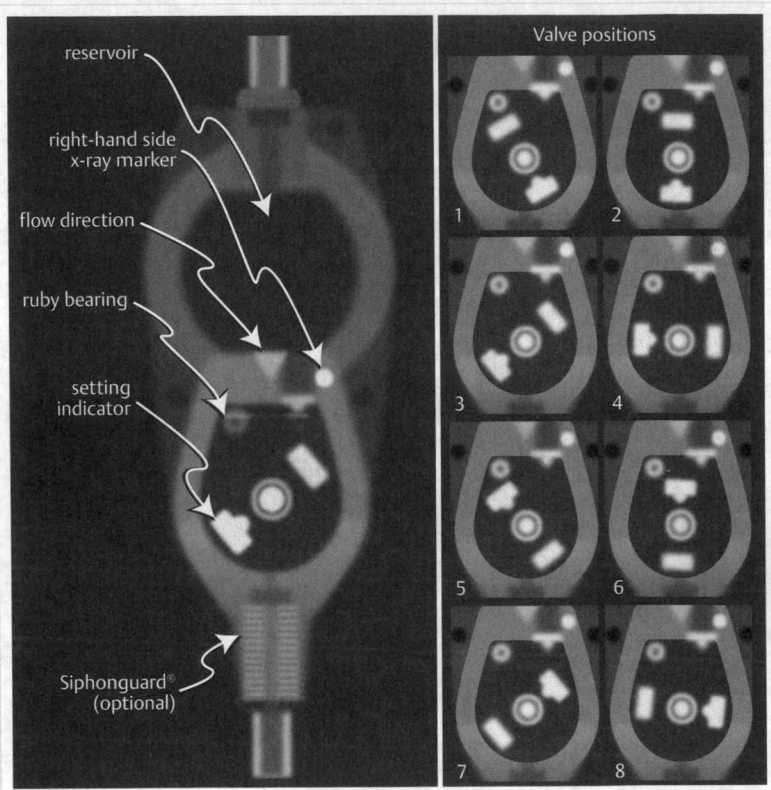

Fig. 25.10 Certas Plus valve. X-ray appearance.

Table 25.3 Certas pressure settings

Setting number	Mean pressure (mm H$_2$O) measured at 20 ml/hr flow rate	
	Certas (discontinued)	Certas Plus
1	36	25
2	71	50
3	109	80
4	146	110
5	178	145
6	206	180
7	238	215
8 (virtual off)	>400	>400

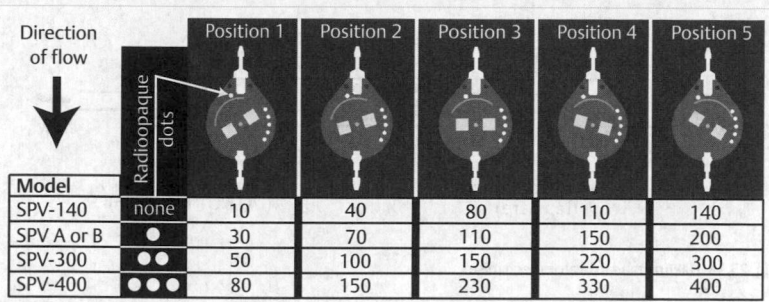

Fig. 25.11 Polaris valve. Programmable settings for models as seen on X-ray (pressures in mm H₂O).

Model	Radioopaque dots	Position 1	Position 2	Position 3	Position 4	Position 5
SPV-140	none	10	40	80	110	140
SPV A or B	●	30	70	110	150	200
SPV-300	●●	50	100	150	220	300
SPV-400	●●●	80	150	230	330	400

25

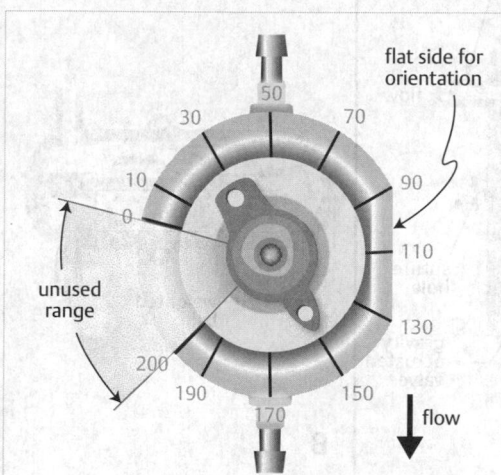

Fig. 25.12 ProGAV programmable valve, schematic diagram. Numbers represent opening pressure (in mm H₂O). In this illustration the valve is set at 150 (at the 5:00 position).

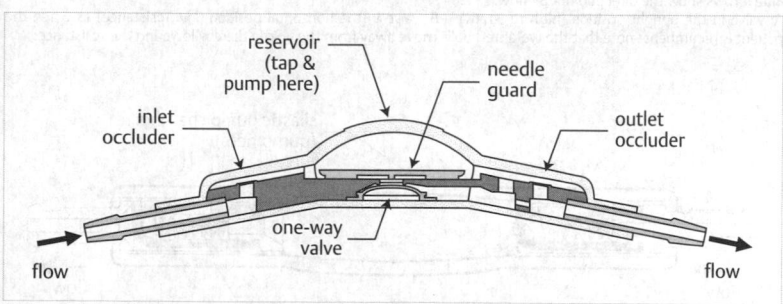

Fig. 25.13 Heyer-Schulte LPV® II valve (low-profile, side view).

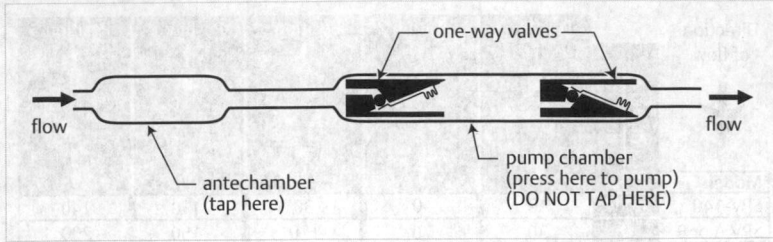

Fig. 25.14 Hakim standard valve mechanism.

25

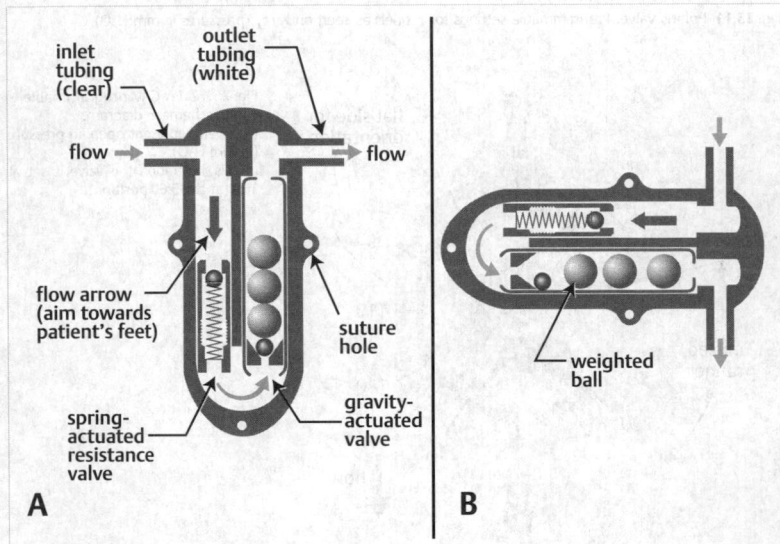

Fig. 25.15 Cordis H-V valve.
Blue arrows show the direction of CSF flow.
A: valve in the upright position (high resistance). B: valve in the horizontal position (low resistance) as when the patient is recumbent—note that the weighted balls move away from the nozzle thereby lowering the resistance.

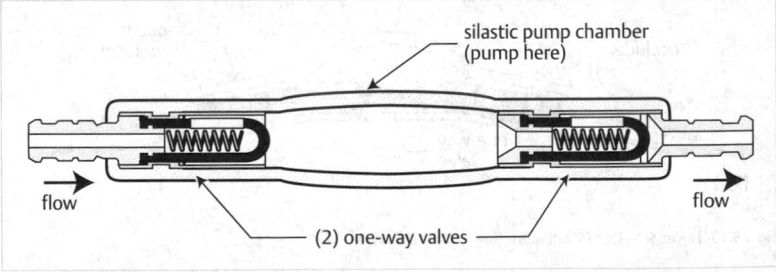

Fig. 25.16 Holter valve.

25.7.13 Salmon-Rickham reservoir

Similar to standard Rickham reservoir except for lower profile (▶ Fig. 25.17). A metal base provides a positive stop for needles. The smaller dome size may make needle access more challenging than with a dedicated ventricular access device.

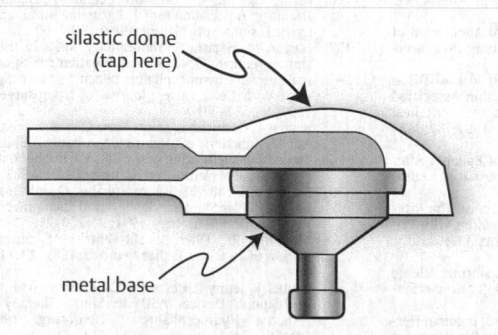

silastic dome
(tap here)

metal base

Fig. 25.17 Salmon-Rickham reservoir.

25.8 Surgical insertion techniques

For surgical techniques, refer to the section on insertion of Ventricular shunts (p. 1825).

25.9 Instructions to patients

All patients and families of patients with hydrocephalus should be instructed regarding the following:

1. signs and symptoms of shunt malfunction or infection
2. not to pump the shunt unless instructed to do so for a specific purpose
3. prophylactic antibiotics: for the following situations (mandatory in vascular shunts, sometimes recommended in other shunts)
   a) dental procedures other than routine cleaning
   b) instrumentation of the bladder: not practical for patients who catheterize to void. Important for cystoscopy, CMG, etc., where septicemia may occur
4. in a growing child: the need for periodic evaluation, including assessment of distal shunt length
5. parents and/or patients should take photos with their smart phone showing what a CT or MRI scan looks like when their shunt is functioning for reference when they are evaluated for shunt issues when prior images are not otherwise readily available

References

[1] Shinnar S, Gammon K, Bergman EW, et al. Management of Hydrocephalus in Infancy: Use of Acetazolamide and Furosemide to Avoid Cerebrospinal Fluid Shunts. J Pediatr. 1985; 107:31–37

[2] Kreusser KL, Tarby TJ, Kovnar E, et al. Serial LPs for at Least Temporary Amelioration of Neonatal Posthemorrhagic Hydrocephalus. Pediatrics. 1985; 75:719–724

[3] Dandy WE. Extirpation of the Choroid Plexus of the Lateral Ventricle in Communicating Hydrocephalus. Annals of Surgery. 1918; 68:569–579

[4] Griffith HB, Jamjoom AB. The Treatment of Childhood Hydrocephalus by Choroid Plexus Coagulation and Artificial Cerebrospinal Fluid Perfusion. Br J Neurosurg. 1990; 4:95–100

[5] Gangemi M, Maiuri F, Naddeo M, et al. Endoscopic third ventriculostomy in idiopathic normal pressure hydrocephalus: an Italian multicenter study. Neurosurgery. 2008; 63:62–7; discussion 67-9

[6] Handler MH, Abbott R, Lee M. A Near-Fatal Complication of Endoscopic Third Ventriculostomy: Case Report. Neurosurgery. 1994; 35:525–528

[7] McLaughlin MR, Wahlig JB, Kaufmann AM, et al. Traumatic Basilar Aneurysm After Endoscopic Third Ventriculostomy: Case Report. Neurosurgery. 1997; 41:1400–1404

[8] Kulkarni AV, Drake JM, Mallucci CL, et al. Endoscopic third ventriculostomy in the treatment of childhood hydrocephalus. J Pediatr. 2009; 155:254–9 e1

[9] Kulkarni AV, Drake JM, Kestle JR, et al. Predicting who will benefit from endoscopic third ventriculostomy compared with shunt insertion in childhood hydrocephalus using the ETV Success Score. J Neurosurg Pediatr. 2010; 6:310–315

[10] Naftel RP, Reed GT, Kulkarni AV, et al. Evaluating the Children's Hospital of Alabama endoscopic third ventriculostomy experience using the Endoscopic Third Ventriculostomy Success Score: an external

validation study. J Neurosurg Pediatr. 2011; 8:494–501

[11] Durnford AJ, Kirkham FJ, Mathad N, et al. Endoscopic third ventriculostomy in the treatment of childhood hydrocephalus: validation of a success score that predicts long-term outcome. J Neurosurg Pediatr. 2011; 8:489–493

[12] Jones RFC, Currie BG, Kwok BCT. Ventriculopleural Shunts for Hydrocephalus: A Useful Alternative. Neurosurgery. 1988; 23:753–755

[13] James HE, Tibbs PA. Diverse Clinical Application of Percutaneous Lumboperitoneal Shunts. Neurosurgery. 1981; 8:39–42

[14] Cozzens JW, Chandler JP. Increased Risk of Distal Ventriculoperitoneal Shunt Obstruction Associated With Slit Valves or Distal Slits in the Peritoneal Catheter. Journal of Neurosurgery. 1997; 87:682–686

[15] Dan NG, Wade MJ. The Incidence of Epilepsy After Ventricular Shunting Procedures. Journal of Neurosurgery. 1986; 65:19–21

[16] Berger MS, Baumeister B, Geyer JR, et al. The Risks of Metastases from Shunting in Children with Primary Central Nervous System Tumors. J Neurosurg. 1991; 74:872–877

[17] Jimenez DF, Keating R, Goodrich JT. Silicone Allergy in Ventriculoperitoneal Shunts. Child's Nervous System. 1994; 10:59–63

[18] Moazam F, Glenn JD, Kaplan BJ, et al. Inguinal Hernias After Ventriculoperitoneal Shunt Procedures in Pediatric Patients. Surg Gynecol Obstet. 1984; 159:570–572

[19] Bryant MS, Bremer AM, Tepas JJ, et al. Abdominal Complications of Ventriculoperitoneal Shunts. Am Surg. 1988; 54:50–55

[20] Ram Z, Findler G, Guttman I, et al. Ventriculoperitoneal Shunt Malfunction due to Migration of the Abdominal Catheter into the Scrotum. J Pediatr Surg. 1987; 22:1045–1046

[21] Rush DS, Walsh JW. Abdominal Complications of CSF-Peritoneal Shunts. Monogr Neural Sci. 1982; 8:52–54

[22] Alonso-Vanegas M, Alvarez JL, Delgado L, et al. Gastric Perforation due to Ventriculo-Peritoneal Shunt. Pediatr Neurosurg. 1994; 21:192–194

[23] Lourie H, Bajwa S. Transdiaphragmatic Migration of a Ventriculoperitoneal Catheter. Neurosurgery. 1985; 17:324–326

[24] Sakoda TH, Maxwell JA, Brackett CE. Intestinal Volvulus Secondary to a Ventriculoperitoneal Shunt. Case Report. Journal of Neurosurgery. 1971; 35:95–96

[25] Couldwell WT, LeMay DR, McComb JG. Experience with Use of Extended Length Peritoneal Shunt Catheters. Journal of Neurosurgery. 1996; 85:425–427

[26] Pascual JMS, Prakash UBS. Development of Pulmonary Hypertension After Placement of a Ventriculoatrial Shunt. Mayo Clinic Proceedings. 1993; 68:1177–1182

[27] Chumas PD, Kulkarni AV, Drake JM, et al. Lumboperitoneal Shunting: A Retrospective Study in the Pediatric Population. Neurosurgery. 1993; 32:376–383

[28] Welch K, Shillito J, Strand R, et al. Chiari I "malformation": An acquired disorder? Journal of Neurosurgery. 1982; 55:604–609

[29] Chumas PD, Armstrong DC, Drake JM, et al. Tonsillar Herniation: The Rule Rather than the Exception After Lumboperitoneal Shunting in the Pediatric Population. Journal of Neurosurgery. 1993; 78:568–573

[30] Payner TD, Prenger E, Berger TS, et al. Acquired Chiari Malformations: Incidence, Diagnosis, and Management. Neurosurgery. 1994; 34:429–434

[31] Kessler LA, Dugan P, Concannon JP. Systemic Metastases of Medulloblastoma Promoted by Shunting. Surg Neurol. 1975; 3:147–152

[32] Czosnyka Z, Czosnyka M, Richards HK, et al. Laboratory testing of hydrocephalus shunts – conclusion of the U.K. Shunt evaluation programme. Acta Neurochir (Wien). 2002; 144:525–38; discussion 538

[33] Savitz MH, Bobroff LM. Low incidence of delayed intracerebral hemorrhage secondary to

[34] French BN, Swanson M. Radionuclide Imaging Shuntography for the Evaluation of Shunt Patency. Monogr Neural Sci. 1982; 8:39–42

[35] Chan KH, Mann KS. Prolonged Therapeutic External Ventricular Drainage: A Prospective Study. Neurosurgery. 1988; 23:436–438

[36] Mann KS, Yue CP, Ong GB. Percutaneous Sump Drainage: A Palliation for Oft-Recurring Intracranial Cystic Lesions. Surg Neurol. 1983; 19:86–90

[37] Hassan M, Higashi S, Yamashita J. Risks in using siphon-reducing devices in adult patients with normal-pressure hydrocephalus: bench test investigations with Delta valves. Journal of Neurosurgery. 1996; 84:634–641

[38] Boch A-L, Hermelin É, Sainte-Rose C, et al. Mechanical Dysfunction of Ventriculoperitoneal Shunts Caused by Calcification of the Silicone Rubber Catheter. Journal of Neurosurgery. 1998; 88:975–982

[39] Pudenz RH, Foltz EL. Hydrocephalus: Overdrainage by Ventricular Shunts. A Review and Recommendations. Surgical Neurology. 1991; 35:200–212

[40] McLaurin RL, Olivi A. Slit-Ventricle Syndrome: Review of 15 Cases. Pediat Neurosci. 1987; 13:118–124

[41] Gruber R, Jenny P, Herzog B. Experiences with the Anti-Siphon Device (ASD) in Shunt Therapy of Pediatric Hydrocephalus. J Neurosurg. 1984; 61:156–162

[42] Foltz EL, Blanks JP. Symptomatic Low Intraventricular Pressure in Shunted Hydrocephalus. Journal of Neurosurgery. 1988; 68:401–408

[43] O'Hayon BB, Drake JM, Ossip MG, et al. Frontal and Occipital Horn Ratio: A Linear Estimate of Ventricular Size for Multiple Imaging Modalities in Pediatric Hydrocephalus. Pediatric Neurosurgery. 1998; 29:245–249

[44] Teo C, Morris W. Slit Ventricle Syndrome. Contemporary Neurosurgery. 1999; 21:1–4

[45] Engel M, Carmel PW, Chutorian AM. Increased Intraventricular Pressure Without Ventriculomegaly in Children with Shunts: "Normal Volume" Hydrocephalus. Neurosurgery. 1979; 5:549–552

[46] Kiekens R, Mortier W, Pothmann R. The Slit-Ventricle Syndrome After Shunting in Hydrocephalic Children. Neuropediatrics. 1982; 13:190–194

[47] Hyde-Rowan MD, Rekate HL, Nulsen FE. Reexpansion of Previously Collapsed Ventricles: The Slit Ventricle Syndrome. J Neurosurg. 1982; 56:536–539

[48] Salmon JH. The Collapsed Ventricle: Management and Prevention. Surgical Neurology. 1978; 9:349–352

[49] Portnoy HD, Schult RR, Fox JL, et al. Anti-Siphon and Reversible Occlusion Valves for Shunting in Hydrocephalus and Preventing Postshunt Subdural Hematoma. Journal of Neurosurgery. 1973; 38:729–738

[50] Epstein FJ, Fleischer AS, Hochwald GM, et al. Subtemporal Craniectomy for Recurrent Shunt Obstruction Secondary to Small Ventricles. J Neurosurg. 1974; 41:29–31

[51] Holness RO, Hoffman HJ, Hendrick EB. Subtemporal Decompression for the Slit-Ventricle Syndrome After Shunting in Hydrocephalic Children. Childs Brain. 1979; 5:137–144

[52] Linder M, Diehl J, Sklar FH. Subtemporal Decompressions for Shunt-Dependent Ventricles: Mechanism of Action. Surgical Neurology. 1983; 19:520–523

[53] Reddy K, Fewer HD, West M, et al. Slit Ventricle Syndrome with Aqueduct Stenosis: Third Ventriculostomy as Definitive Treatment. Neurosurgery. 1988; 23:756–759

[54] Puca A, Fernandez E, Colosimo C, et al. Hydrocephalus and Macrocrania: Surgical or Non-Surgical Treatment of Postshunting Subdural Hematoma. Surgical Neurology. 1996; 45:76–82

[55] Hoppe-Hirsch E, Sainte Rose C, Renier D, et al. Pericerebral Collections After Shunting. Child's Nervous System. 1987; 3:97–102

[56] McCullogh DC, Fox JL. Negative Intracranial Pressure Hydrocephalus in Adults with Shunts and its

Relationship to the Production of Subdural Hematoma. Journal of Neurosurgery. 1974; 40:372–375

[57] Schut L. Comment on Puca A, et al.: Hydrocephalus and Macrocrania: Surgical or Non-Surgical Treatment of Postshunting Subdural Hematoma. Surgical Neurology. 1996; 45

[58] Dietrich U, Lumenta C, Sprick C, et al. Subdural Hematoma in a Case of Hydrocephalus and Macrocrania: Experience with a Pressure-Adjustable Valve. Child's Nervous System. 1987; 3:242–244

[59] Kamano S, Nakano Y, Imanishi T, et al. Management with a Programmable Pressure Valve of Subdural Hematomas Caused by a Ventriculoperitoneal Shunt: Case Report. Surgical Neurology. 1991; 35:381–383

[60] Illingworth RD. Subdural Hematoma After the Treatment of Chronic Hydrocephalus by Ventriculocaval Shunts. Journal of Neurology, Neurosurgery, and Psychiatry. 1970; 33:95–99

[61] Davidoff LM, Feiring EH. Subdural Hematoma Occurring in Surgically Treated Hydrocephalic Children with a Note on a Method of Handling Persistent Accumulations. Journal of Neurosurgery. 1963; 10:557–563

[62] Kaufman B, Weiss MH, Young HF, et al. Effects of Prolonged Cerebrospinal Fluid Shunting on the Skull and Brain. Journal of Neurosurgery. 1973; 38:288–297

[63] Faulhauer K, Schmitz P. Overdrainage Phenomena in Shunt Treated Hydrocephalus. Acta Neurochirurgica. 1978; 45:89–101

[64] Al-Mufarrej F, Nolan C, Sookhai S, et al. Laparoscopic procedures in adults with ventriculoperitoneal shunts. Surg Laparosc Endosc Percutan Tech. 2005; 15:28–29

[65] Neale ML, Falk GL. In vitro assessment of back pressure on ventriculoperitoneal shunt valves. Is laparoscopy safe? Surg Endosc. 1999; 13:512–515

[66] Ravaoherisoa J, Meyer P, Afriat R, et al. Laparoscopic surgery in a patient with ventriculoperitoneal shunt: monitoring of shunt function with transcranial Doppler. Br J Anaesth. 2004; 92:434–437

[67] Baskin JJ, Vishteh AG, Wesche DE, et al. Ventriculoperitoneal shunt failure as a complication of laparoscopic surgery. Journal of the Society of Laparoendoscopic Surgeons. 1998; 2:177–180

[68] Collure DW, Bumpers HL, Luchette FA, et al. Laparoscopic cholecystectomy in patients with ventriculoperitoneal (VP) shunts. Surg Endosc. 1995; 9:409–410

25

Part VIII

Seizures

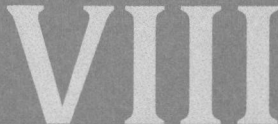

26 Seizure Classification and Syndromes

26.1 Seizure definitions and classification

26.1.1 Definitions

Epileptic seizure: "a transient occurrence of signs and/or symptoms due to abnormal excessive or synchronous neuronal activity in the brain."[1]

Epilepsy: "a disorder of the brain characterized by an enduring predisposition to generate epileptic seizures and by the neurobiologic cognitive, psychological, and social consequences of this condition. The definition of epilepsy requires the occurrence of at least one epileptic seizure."[1] However, one single seizure does not usually qualify as epilepsy.

Provoked seizure: AKA "acute symptomatic seizure," occurs within 2 weeks of an acute disturbance of brain structure or metabolism known to increase risk of seizures (e.g., metabolic insult, toxic insult, CNS infection, stroke, brain trauma, cerebral hemorrhage, medication toxicity, alcohol or other drug intoxication or withdrawal, or a patient with a known seizure disorder with subtherapeutic levels of seizure medication).

Unprovoked seizure: AKA cryptogenic seizure, due to unknown cause but presumed to be primarily structural. Not associated with prior CNS insult known to increase the risk of epilepsy.

26.1.2 Miscellaneous seizure information

Factors that lower the seizure threshold

Factors that lower the seizure threshold (i.e., make it easier to provoke a seizure) in individuals with or without a prior seizure history include many items listed under etiologies of New onset seizures (p.503), as well as:
1. sleep deprivation
2. hyperventilation
3. photic stimulation (in some)
4. infection: systemic (febrile seizures (p.509)), CNS (meningitis…)
5. metabolic disturbances: electrolyte imbalance (especially profound hypoglycemia), pH disturbance (especially alkalosis), drugs… (see below)
6. head trauma: closed head injury, penetrating trauma (p.505)
7. cerebral ischemia: stroke (see below)
8. "kindling": a concept that repeated seizures may facilitate the development of later seizures

Todd's paralysis

A post-ictal phenomena in which there is partial or total paralysis usually in areas involved in a partial seizure. More common in patients with structural lesions as the source of the seizure. The paralysis usually resolves slowly over a period of an hour or so. Thought to be due to depletion of neurons in the wake of the extensive electrical discharges of a seizure. Other similar phenomena include post-ictal aphasia and hemianopsia.

Mortality in epilepsy

Mortality in patients with epilepsy is 2-4 times that of the general population.
1. 10% are directly due to seizures, including status epilepticus
2. 5% are due to accidents that occur during a seizure
3. 7-22% are suicides
4. 10% are **sudden unexplained death in epilepsy** (SUDEP). Sudden death in a person with epilepsy with no other identifiable cause of death. Incidence is 1-2 per 1000 people with epilepsy annually. In one third there is no evidence of a seizure having occurred. Most have generalized tonic-clonic seizure disorder

26.1.3 Classification of seizure types

Seizure grouping based on etiology

See reference.[2]
1. **symptomatic seizure** (AKA "secondary"): seizures resulting from a structural abnormality (e.g., …).[3]
   a) cavernous malformation

b) stroke

c) brain tumor

d) mesial temporal sclerosis (p.482) producing mesial temporal lobe epilepsy

e) hypothalamic hamartoma (p.277) producing gelastic seizures

2. **genetic generalized epilepsies** (GGE): formerly called idiopathic generalized epilepsies (IDEs) AKA "primary" or **idiopathic seizure**. No identifiable underlying cause. Some are due primarily to inherited abnormalities of neurotransmission.[3] Some of the gene alterations are known, others are presumed. Includes:

a) GGE with tonic-clonic seizures alone (GGE with GTC)

b) childhood absence epilepsy

c) juvenile absence epilepsy

d) juvenile myoclonic epilepsy (p.484)

e) genetic epilepsy with febrile seizures plus (GEFS+)[2]

3. **cryptogenic seizures**: unknown underlying etiology.[3] Includes:

a) West syndrome (p.484) (infantile spasms, Blitz-Nick-Salaam Krämpfe)

b) Lennox-Gastaut (p.484) syndrome

4. **provoked seizures**: situation-related seizures

a) febrile seizures (p.509)

b) seizures occurring only with acute metabolic or toxic event: e.g., alcohol withdrawal

2017 ILAE classification of seizures

An overview of the major seizure types delineated in the 2017 International League Against Epilepsy (ILAE) classification[2,4] is presented below.

▶ **Onset.** Classification starts with a determination of whether a seizure is of focal *onset*, generalized *onset*, unknown onset or unclassified. A seizure that is referred to as a "focal seizure" is understood to mean "focal *onset* seizure," and a "generalized seizure" is shorthand for "generalized *onset* seizure."[4]

Focal onset seizures (focal seizures)

Comprise ≈ 57% of all seizures. They originate within networks restricted to one cerebral hemisphere.[5] Focal seizures are classified based on level of awareness and by motor vs. nonmotor onset.

Rule of thumb: the first occurrence of a focal seizure represents a structural lesion until proven otherwise.

▶ **Level of awareness**

• **retained awareness**: the patient is aware of self and environment during the seizure (even if they are immobile). Formerly called "simple partial seizure"

• **impaired awareness**: awareness is impaired during any part of the seizure. Formerly called "complex partial seizure"

• this descriptor may be omitted if not applicable (see items with an asterisk below) or if unknown

▶ **Motor vs. nonmotor.** Focal seizures are also categorized as motor vs. nonmotor signs and symptoms based on the *first* prominent feature at onset (if both are present at onset, motor signs usually dominate). The earliest feature may not be the most significant behavioral feature. This classification has an anatomic basis.

1. motor onset

a) automatisms

b) atonic*

c) clonic

d) epileptic spasms*

e) hyperkinetic: agitated thrashing or leg pedaling movements

f) myoclonic

g) tonic

2. nonmotor onset

a) autonomic

b) behavior arrest

c) cognitive: e.g., aphasia, apraxia, neglect, déjà vu, jamais vu, illusions, or hallucinations

d) emotional: e.g., fear, joy and affective manifestations with the appearance of emotions without subjective emotionality, e.g., as with some gelastic seizures (p.277) or dacrystic seizures

e) sensory

* level of awareness descriptor is usually omitted for these seizure types

▶ **Focal to bilateral tonic-clonic seizure.** A propagation pattern of a seizure, rather than a specific seizure type. Formerly called "partial onset with secondary generalization."

Generalized onset seizures

Represents ≈ 40% of all seizures. Originate within and rapidly engage bilaterally distributed networks.[5] Manifestations of generalized onset seizures can be asymmetrical, mimicking focal-onset seizures.
1. motor seizure
    a) tonic-clonic (formerly called grand-mal seizure): generalized seizure that evolves from tonic to clonic motor activity. This is a specific type and does *not* include focal seizures that generalize secondarily
    b) clonic: fairly symmetric, bilateral synchronous semirhythmic jerking of the UE and LE, usually with elbow flexion and knee extension
    c) tonic: sudden sustained increased tone with a characteristic guttural cry or grunt as air is forced through adducted vocal cords
    d) myoclonic: shocklike body jerks (1 or more in succession) with generalized EEG discharges
    e) myoclonic-tonic-clonic: common in juvenile myoclonic epilepsy
    f) myotonic-atonic: e.g., as part of Doose syndrome
    g) atonic: (AKA astatic seizures or "drop attacks"): sudden brief loss of tone that may cause falls
    h) epileptic spasms*
2. nonmotor (absence) seizure (formerly: petit-mal seizure): impaired consciousness with mild or no motor involvement (automatisms occur more commonly with bursts lasting > 7 secs). *No postictal confusion.* Aura rare. May be induced by hyperventilation × 2–3 mins. EEG shows spike and wave at exactly 3 per second
    a) typical absence seizure
    b) atypical: more heterogeneous with more variable EEG pattern then typical absence. Seizures may last longer
    c) myoclonic
    d) eyelid myoclonia: most significant as a feature of absence seizure

Unknown onset seizures

A placeholder until the seizure can be better characterized. May be referred to as "unclassified" alone or with one of a limited number of qualifiers as follows. This may allow further description for activity observed during the seizure when the type of onset is not known to be focal or generalized with ≈ 80% confidence.
1. motor seizure
    a) tonic-clonic
    b) epileptic spasms: can be of focal, generalized or unknown onset
2. nonmotor (absence) seizure
    a) behavior arrest

Unclassified seizures

Used when there is inadequate information of inability to place in other categories.

26.2 Epilepsy syndromes

26.2.1 General information

Epilepsy syndromes are conditions sharing similar seizure types, EEG findings and imaging features. They do not necessarily have a distinct etiology.

26.2.2 Mesial temporal lobe epilepsy/ mesial temporal sclerosis

Mesial temporal sclerosis (MTS) is the most common cause of intractable temporal lobe epilepsy. Pathologic basis: hippocampal sclerosis[6,7] (cell loss in hippocampus on one side) (▶ Fig. 26.1). See also differential diagnosis (p. 1672).

▶ **Applied anatomy.** The hippocampus is located in the medial temporal lobe, and is composed of Ammon's horn (the "hippocampus proper" in some texts) and the dentate gyrus (▶ Fig. 26.1). The dorsal hippocampus subserves aspects of spatial memory, verbal memory, and learning conceptual information.

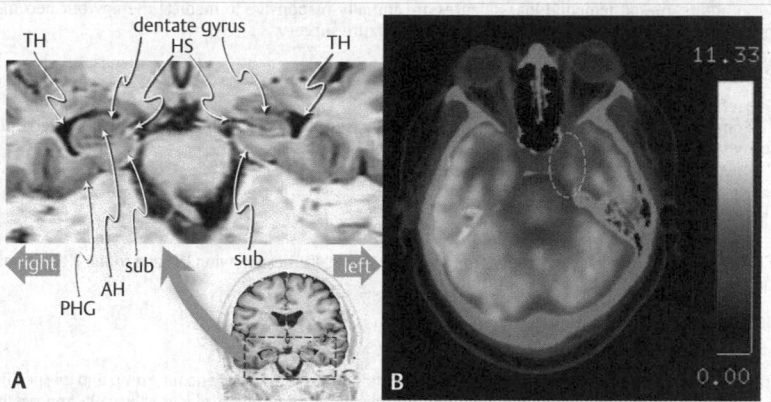

Fig. 26.1 Mesial temporal sclerosis (left side).
Image: A: Inversion recovery coronal MRI (black/white inverted to enhance visualization). Dashed lines in inset shows from where the detail in (A) is taken. Note atrophy of the left hippocampus (hippocampus = Ammon's horn + dentate gyrus) compared to the right.
B: PET scan (taken 45 minutes after injecting 10.65 millicurie Fluorodeoxyglucose IV) fused with a CT scan. Shows subtle decrease in activity in the medial left temporal lobe (less of the higher activity yellow pixels in the green oval) compared to the right. In a patient with epilepsy, this is suggestive of a seizure focus in this region.
Abbreviations: AH = Ammon's horn; HS = hippocampal sulcus; PHG = parahippocampal gyrus; sub = subiculum; TH = temporal horn of the lateral ventricle.

Characteristics of seizures originating in the inferior medial temporal lobe are shown in ▶ Table 26.1.

Some of these seizures have been called uncinate seizures (obsolete term: "uncal fits"). Well known symptoms include olfactory hallucinations (kakosmia (alternative spelling: cacosmia): the perception of bad odors where none exist).

Table 26.1 Syndrome of mesial temporal lobe epilepsy[8]

History

- higher incidence of complicated febrile seizures than in other types of epilepsy
- common family history of epilepsy
- onset in latter half of first decade of life
- auras in isolation are common
- infrequent secondarily generalized seizures
- seizures often remit for several years until adolescence or early adulthood
- seizures often become medically refractory
- common interictal behavioral disturbances (especially depression)

Clinical features of seizures

- most have aura (especially epigastric, emotional, olfactory or gustatory) × several secs
- complex partial seizures (CPS) often begin with arrest & stare. Oroalimentary & complex automatisms are common. Posturing of contralateral arm may occur. Seizure usually lasts 1–2 mins
- postictal disorientation, recent-memory deficit, amnesia of ictus and (in dominant hemisphere) aphasia usually lasts several mins

Neurologic and laboratory features

- neuro exam: normal except memory deficit
- MRI: hippocampal atrophy (▶ Fig. 26.1 A) and signal alteration with ipsilateral dilatation of temporal horn of lateral ventricle
- unilateral or bilateral independent anterior temporal EEG spikes with maximal amplitude in basal electrodes
- external ictal EEG activity only with CPS, usually initial or delayed focal rhythmic onset pattern of 5–7 Hz, maximal in 1 basal temporal derivation
- interictal fluorodeoxyglucose PET scan: hypometabolism in temporal lobe (▶ Fig. 26.1 B) and possibly ipsilateral thalamus and basal ganglia
- neuropsychological testing: memory dysfunction specific to involved temporal lobe
- Wada test (p. 1890): amnesia with contralateral amobarbital injection

In adults, mesial temporal lobe seizures are initially responsive to medical therapy but become more varied and refractory, and may respond to seizure surgery.

26.2.3 Juvenile myoclonic epilepsy

See reference.[9]

Sometimes called bilateral myoclonus. 5–10% of cases of epilepsy. An idiopathic generalized epilepsy syndrome with age-related onset consisting of 3 seizure types:
1. myoclonic jerks: predominantly after waking
2. generalized tonic-clonic seizures
3. absence

EEG → polyspike discharges. Strong family history (some studies showing linkage to the HLA region on the short arm of chromosome 6).

Most are responsive to depakene.

26.2.4 West syndrome

This term is being used less frequently as it appears not to be a homogeneous group and as specific etiologies for infantile spasms are identified. Classically a seizure disorder that usually appears in first year of life, and consists of recurrent, gross flexion and occasionally extension of the trunk and limbs (massive myoclonus, AKA infantile spasms, AKA salaam seizures, AKA jackknife spasms). Seizures tend to diminish with age, often abating by 5 yrs. Usually associated with mental retardation. 50% may develop complex-partial seizures, some of the rest may develop Lennox-Gastaut syndrome (see below). An associated brain lesion may be found in some.

EEG → the majority show either interictal hypsarrhythmia (huge spike/wave plus slow wave resembling muscle artifact) or modified hypsarrhythmia at some point.

Usually dramatic response of seizures and EEG findings to ACTH or corticosteroids.

26.2.5 Lennox-Gastaut syndrome

Rare condition that begins in childhood as atonic seizures ("drop attacks"). Often develops into tonic seizures with mental retardation. Seizures are often polymorphic, difficult to treat medically, and may occur as often as 50 per day. May also present with status epilepticus. Approximately 50% of patients have reduced seizures with valproic acid. Corpus callosotomy may reduce the number of atonic seizures.

References

[1] Fisher RS, van Emde Boas W, Blume W, et al. Epileptic seizures and epilepsy: definitions proposed by the International League Against Epilepsy (ILAE) and the International Bureau for Epilepsy (IBE). Epilepsia. 2005; 46:470–472

[2] Scheffer IE, Berkovic S, Capovilla G, et al. ILAE classification of the epilepsies: Position paper of the ILAE Commission for Classification and Terminology. Epilepsia. 2017; 58:512–521

[3] Kwan P, Brodie MJ. Early identification of refractory epilepsy. N Engl J Med. 2000; 342:314–319

[4] Fisher RS, Cross JH, French JA, et al. Operational classification of seizure types by the International League Against Epilepsy: Position Paper of the ILAE Commission for Classification and Terminology. Epilepsia. 2017; 58:522–530

[5] Berg AT, Berkovic SF, Brodie MJ, et al. Revised terminology and concepts for organization of seizures and epilepsies: report of the ILAE Commission on Classification and Terminology, 2005-2009. Epilepsia. 2010; 51:676–685

[6] French JA, Williamson PD, Thadani VM, et al. Characteristics of Medial Temporal Lobe Epilepsy. I. Results of History and Physical Examination. Annals of Neurology. 1993; 34:774–780

[7] Williamson PD, French JA, Thadani VM, et al. Characteristics of Medial Temporal Lobe Epilepsy. II. Interictal and Ictal Scalp Electroencephalography, Neuropsychological Testing, Neuroimaging, Surgical Results, and Pathology. Annals of Neurology. 1993; 34:781–787

[8] Engel JJ. Surgery for Seizures. New England Journal of Medicine. 1996; 334:647–652

[9] Grunewald RA, Panayiotopoulos CP. Juvenile Myoclonic Epilepsy: A Review. Archives of Neurology. 1993; 50:594–598

27 Antiseizure Medication (ASM)

27.1 General information

Formerly sometimes called antiepileptic drugs (AEDs) or anticonvulsants, the goal of treatment with ASM is seizure control (a contentious term, usually taken as reduction of seizure frequency and severity to the point of permitting the patient to live a normal lifestyle without epilepsy-related limitations) with minimal or no drug toxicity. ≈ 75% of epileptics can achieve satisfactory seizure control with medical therapy.[1]

27.2 Antiseizure medications (ASM) for various seizure types

27.2.1 General information

Aside from some specific agents for a few select seizure types, there is generally no significant difference in efficacy of ASMs. There is also little difference in Type I side effects. Choices then tend to be made based on tolerability, adverse effects, effects on comorbidities, drug-drug interactions, and availability of dosing forms (IV, oral, rectal…).

Newer drugs (some of which are shown in ▶ Table 27.1) often have differing mechanisms of action than older ones, and they obtain approval based on RCTs as add-ons compared to placebos, and so it make sense use in combination with older drugs for dual agent therapy.[2] They also often have a tolerability advantage.[3]

Table 27.1 Antiseizure medications introduced since 2010 (U.S.)

Agent	Year
clobazam	2011
ezogabine	2011
perampanel	2012
eslicarbazepine	2014
brivaracetam	2016
stiripentol	2018
cannabidiol	2018
cenobamate	2020
fenfluramine	2020

27.2.2 Indications

General considerations

The following agents are considered "broad spectrum" (treat a variety of seizure types):
1. valproic acid
2. lamotrigine (Lamictal®)
3. levetiracetam (Keppra®)
4. zonisamide (Zonegran®)

These agents are not considered broad spectrum:
1. phenytoin (Dilantin® and others)
2. carbamazepine (Tegretol®)

Agents that interfere with platelet function and may increase the risk of bleeding complications:
1. valproic acid
2. phenytoin (Dilantin® and others)

Specific indications

Indications for some ASMs are shown in ▶ Table 27.2.
Boldface drugs are drug of choice (DOC).
1. primary generalized onset (GOS)
   a) GTC (generalized tonic-clonic):
      • **valproic acid (VA)** (p. 492): if no evidence of focality some studies show fewer side effects and better control than PHT

Table 27.2 Antiseizure medication (ASM) indications (used with permission from Abou-Khalil BW. Update on Antiseizure Medications 2022. Continuum (Minneap Minn). 2022; 28: 500–535. https://journals.lww.com/continuum/Abstract/2022/04000/Update_on_Antiseizure_Medications_2022.13.aspx)[3]

Drug	Indications[a]					
	FOS	GTC	ABS	MYO	STAT	MISC
brivaracetam	+			+ [b]		
cannabidiol	+					LG, DRA, TS
carbamazepine (Tegretol®, Carbatrol®)	+	+ [b]	–			
cenobamate	+					
clobazam	+ [b]			–	–	adj-LG
eslicarbazepine	+	+ [b]	+ [b]	+ [b]		LG
ethosuximide (Zarontin®)	–	–	+	–		
felbamate (Felbatol®)	+	+ [b]				LG
fenfluramine						DRA
gabapentin (Neurontin®)	+	–	–	–		
lacosamide	+		–	–		
lamotrigine (Lamictal®)	+	+	+ [b]	±		LG
levetiracetam (Keppra®)	+	+	+ [b]	+		
oxcarbazepine (Trileptal®)	+		–	–		
perampanel	+	+		+ [c]		
phenobarbital	+	+ [b]		+ [c]	IV	
phenytoin (Dilantin®)	+	+ [b]	–	–	+	
pregabalin (Lyrica®)	+	–	–	–		
primidone (Mysoline®)	+	+				
rufinamide (Banzel®)	+	+ [b]				LG
stiripentol (Diacomit®)						DRA
tiagabine (Gabitril®)	+	–	–	–		
topiramate (Topamax®)	+	+	± [d]			LG
valproate (Depakene®...)	+	+ [b]	+	+ [b]		
vigabatrin (Sabril®...)	+	–	–	–		INF
zonisamide (Zonegran®)	+	+ [b]	+ [b]	+ [b]		

[a] indications for seizure types (does not include other uses, e.g., for chronic pain).
[b] suggested but not proven in Class I trials
[c] class IV evidence
[d] not effective in 1 Class I trial
Abbreviations: + = effective, – = not effective; ± = variable; blank cells = no information/unknown; adj = use as adjunctive therapy; ABS = absence; DRA = Dravet syndrome; FOS = focal onset seizure; GTC = generalized tonic-clonic; INF = infantile spasms; IV = intravenous form; LG= Lennox-Gastaut syndrome; MYO = generalized myoclonic seizures; STAT = status epilepticus; TS = tuberous sclerosis

- carbamazepine (p. 490)
- **phenytoin (PHT)** (p. 488)
- phenobarbital (PB) (p. 493)
- primidone (PRM) (p. 493)

b) absence:
- **ethosuximide**
- **valproic acid (VA)**
- clonazepam
- methsuximide (p. 494)

c) myoclonic →

d) tonic or atonic:
- benzodiazepines
- felbamate (p. 494)
- vigabatrin (p. 498)

2. focal onset (FOS) with or without retained awareness, with or without secondary generalization

   a) the well controlled Veterans Administration Cooperative Study[4] ranked the following 4 drugs (based on seizure control and side effects) in this order (VA may compare favorably with CBZ for secondarily GTC, but is less effective for complex partial seizures[5])
      1. **carbamazepine (CBZ)**: most effective, least side effects
      2. **phenytoin (PHT)**
      3. phenobarbital (PB)
      4. **primidone (PRM)** slightly less effective, more side effects
   b) cenobamate (p.499): a newer drug with exceptional efficacy for FOS.[6] May become DOC as usage data accrues
3. second line drugs for any of the above seizure types:
   a) valproate
   b) lamotrigine (p.497): effective for many types of generalized seizures, but is not FDA approved for this yet
   c) topiramate (p.498): effective for many types of generalized seizures, but is not FDA approved for this yet
4. agents for specific syndromes
   a) genetic generalized epilepsy (p.481) (GGE) with GTC: valproate is the most effective medication, and should be the fist drug of choice for men with this condition[7]

27.3 Antiseizure medication pharmacology

27.3.1 General guidelines

See reference.[8]

Monotherapy versus polytherapy

1. increase a given medication until seizures are controlled or side effects become intolerable (do not rely solely on therapeutic levels, which is only the range in which *most* patients have seizure control without side effects)
2. try monotherapy with different drugs before resorting to two drugs together. 80% of epileptics can be controlled on monotherapy; however, failure of monotherapy indicates an 80% chance that the seizures will not be controllable pharmacologically. Only ≈ 10% benefit significantly from the addition of a second drug.[5] When > 2 ASMs are required, consider nonepileptic seizures (p.507)
3. when first evaluating patients on multiple drugs, withdraw the most sedating ones first (usually barbiturates and clonazepam)

Generally, dosing intervals should be less than one half-life. Without loading dose, it takes about 5 *half-lives* to reach steady state.

Many ASMs affect liver function tests (LFTs); however, only rarely do the drugs cause enough hepatic dysfunction to warrant discontinuation. Guideline: discontinue an ASM if the GGT exceeds twice normal.

27.3.2 Specific antiseizure medications

For abbreviations, see ► Table 27.3.

Table 27.3 Antiseizure medication: abbreviations

ASM	antiseizure medication
ABS	absence seizure
EC	enteric coated
DIV	divided
DOC	drug of choice
FOS	focal onset seizures (p.481)
GGE	genetic generalized epilepsies (p.481)
GOS	generalized onset seizures (p.482)
GTC	generalized tonic-clonic seizure
Pharmacokinetics: Unless otherwise specified, numbers are given for *oral* dosing form.	
$t_{1/2}$	half-life
t_{PEAK}	time to peak serum level
t_{SS}	time to steady state (approximately $5 \times t_{1/2}$)
$t_{D/C}$	time to discontinue (recommended withdrawal period over which drug should be tapered)
MDF	minimum dosing frequency. "Therapeutic level" is the average therapeutic range.

27

Drug info: Phenytoin (PHT) (Dilantin®)

Uses

Infrequently used due to complicated pharmacokinetics, cytochrome P450 enzyme induction, narrow therapeutic window, drug-drug interactions (see side effects below).

May be used for FOS and GTC. Not effective against: generalized myoclonic or ABS (∴ avoid in GGE).[3]

Pharmacokinetics (▶ Table 27.4)

PHT has saturable nonlinear kinetics: at low concentrations, kinetics are 1st order (elimination proportional to concentration), metabolism saturates near the therapeutic level resulting in zero-order kinetics (elimination at a constant rate). ≈ 90% of total drug is protein bound. Oral bioavailability is ≈ 90% whereas IV bioavailability is ≈ 95%; this small difference may be significant when patients are near limits of therapeutic range (due to zero-order kinetics).

Table 27.4 Pharmacokinetics of phenytoin

$t_{1/2}$ (half-life)	t_{PEAK} (peak serum levels)	t_{SS} (steady state)	$t_{D/C}$ (discontinue)	Therapeutic level[a]
≈ 24 hrs (range: 9–140 hrs)[b]	oral suspension: 1.5–3 hrs regular capsules: 1.5–3 hrs extended release capsules: 4–12 hrs	7–21 days	4 wks	10–20 mcg/ml

[a]therapeutic level as measured in most labs: 10–20 mcg/ml (NB: it is the free PHT that is the important moiety; this is usually ≈ 1% of total PHT, thus therapeutic free PHT levels are 1–2 mcg/ml; some labs are able to measure free PHT directly)
[b]$t_{1/2}$ for phenytoin

Renal failure: dosage adjustment not needed. However, serum protein binding may be altered in uremia, which can obfuscate interpretation of serum phenytoin levels. Eq (27.1) may be used to convert serum PHT concentration in a uremic patient C (observed), to the expected PHT level in nonuremic patients C (nonuremic).

$$C(nonuremic) = \frac{C(observed)}{0.1 \times albumin + 0.1} \tag{27.1}$$

Oral dose

℞ Adult: usual maintenance dose = 300–600 mg/d divided BID or TID (MDF = q d, for single daily dosing, either the phenytoin-sodium capsules or the extended release form should be used). Oral *loading* dose: 300 mg PO q 4 hrs until 17 mg/kg are given. Peds: oral maintenance: 4–7 mg/kg/d (MDF = BID). **Supplied:** (oral forms): 100 mg tablets of phenytoin-sodium (sodium-salt); 30 & 100 mg Kapseals® (extended release); 50 mg chewable Infatabs® (phenytoin-acid); oral suspension 125 mg/5-ml in 8 oz. (240 ml) bottles or individual 5 ml unit dose packs; pediatric suspension 30 mg/5-ml. Phenytek® 200 & 300 mg capsules.

Dosage changes (▶ Table 27.5)

Table 27.5 Guidelines for changing phenytoin dosage

Present level (mg/dl)	Change to make
<6	100 mg/day
6–8	50 mg/day
>8	25–30 mg/day

Because of zero-order kinetics, at near-therapeutic levels a small dosage change can cause large level changes. Although computer models are necessary for a high degree of accuracy, the dosing change guidelines in ▶ Table 27.5 or the nomogram in ▶ Fig. 27.1 [9] may be used as a quick approximation.

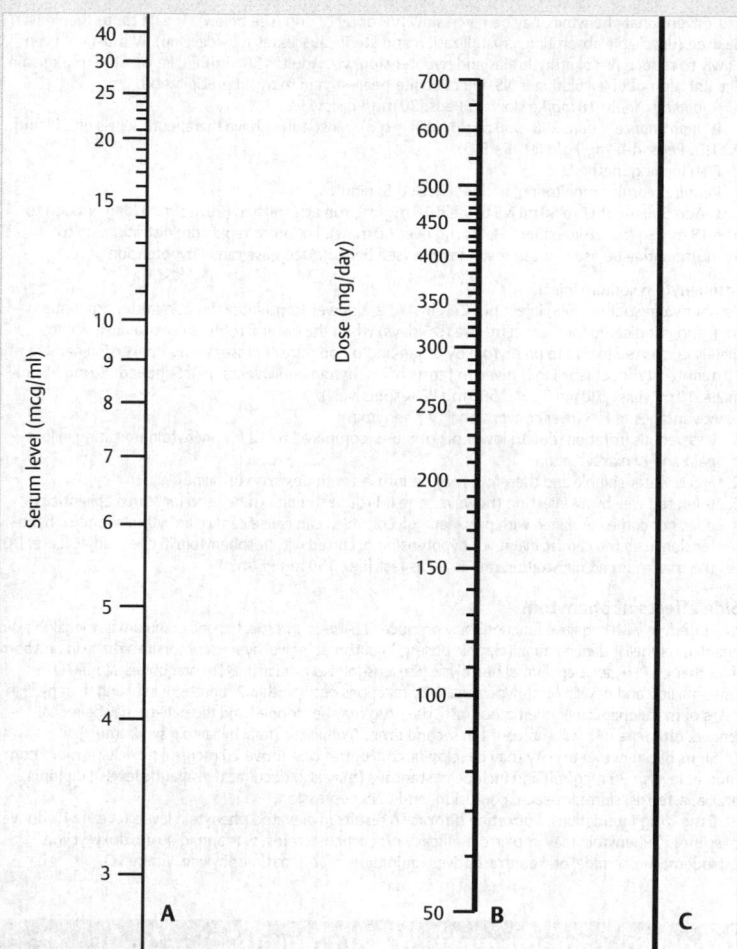

Fig. 27.1 Nomogram for adjusting phenytoin dose.
Directions for using nomogram (assumes steady state).
(a) draw line connecting serum level on line A with current dose on line B.
(b) mark point where this line intersects line C.
(c) connect point on C to the desired serum level on A.
(d) read new dosage on line B.
Reproduced from Therapeutic Drug Monitoring, "Predicting Phenytoin Dose - A Revised Nomogram," Rambeck B, et al, Vol. 1, pp. 325–33, 1979, with permission.

GI absorption of phenytoin suspension or capsules may be decreased by up to 70% when given with nasogastric feedings of Osmolyte® or Isocal®,[10,11] and the suspension has been reported to have erratic absorption. Hold NG feeding for 2 hrs before and 1 hour after phenytoin dose.

Parenteral dose
Phenytoin is a negative inotrope and can cause hypotension.

Conventional phenytoin may be given slow IVP or by IV drip (see below). The IM route should NOT be used (unreliable absorption, crystallization and sterile abscesses may develop). IV must be given slowly to reduce risk of arrhythmias and hypotension, viz. Adult: < 50 mg/min, Peds: < 1–3 mg/kg/min. The only compatible solution is NS, inject at site nearest vein to avoid precipitation.

R *loading*. Adult: 18 mg/kg slow IV. Peds: 20 mg/kg slow IV.

R *maintenance*. Adult: 200–500 mg/d (MDF = q d). Most adults have therapeutic levels on 100 mg PO TID. Peds: 4–7 mg/kg/d (MDF = BID).

Drip loading method:

Requires cardiac monitoring, and BP check q 5 minutes.

R Add 500 mg PHT to 50 ml NS to yield 10 mg/ml, run at 2 ml/min (20 mg/min) long enough to give 18 mg/kg (for 70 kg patient: 1200 mg over 60 mins). For more rapid administration, up to 40 mg/min may be used, or use fosphenytoin (see below). Decrease rate if hypotension occurs.

Fosphenytoin sodium injection

Fosphenytoin sodium (FPS) injection (Cerebyx®) is a newer formulation for administering IV phenytoin, and is indicated for short term use (≤ 5 days) when the enteral route is not usable. It is completely converted in vivo to phenytoin by organ and blood phosphatases with a conversion half-life of 10 minutes. Product labeling is given in terms of phenytoin equivalents (PE). **Supplied:** 50 mg PE/ml in 2 & 10 ml vials (100 mg PE and 500 mg PE respectively).

Advantages of FPS (over conventional IV phenytoin):

1. less venous irritation (due to lower pH of 8.6–9 compared to 12 for phenytoin) resulting in less pain and IV extravasation
2. FPS is water soluble and therefore may be infused with dextrose or saline
3. tolerated well by IM injection (however, the IM route should not be used for status epilepticus)
4. does not come combined with propylene glycol which can cause cardiac arrhythmias and/or hypotension itself (no cardiac events or hypotension occurred with fosphenytoin in one study[12] [Level B])
5. the maximum administration rate is 3 × as fast (i.e., 150 mg PE/min)

Side effects of phenytoin

May interfere with cognitive function. May produce SLE-like syndrome, hepatic granulomas, megaloblastic anemia, cerebellar degeneration (chronic doses), hirsutism, gingival hypertrophy, hemorrhage in newborn if mother on PHT, toxic epidermal necrolysis (Stevens-Johnson variant). PHT antagonizes vitamin D → osteomalacia and rickets. Most hypersensitivity reactions occur within 2 months of initiating therapy.[10] In cases of maculopapular erythematous rash, the drug may be stopped and the patient may be rechallenged; often the rash will not recur the second time. *Teratogenic* (fetal hydantoin syndrome[13]).

Signs of phenytoin toxicity may develop at concentrations above 20 mcg/ml (toxicity is more common at levels > 30 mcg/ml) and include nystagmus (may also occur at therapeutic levels), diplopia, ataxia, asterixis, slurred speech, confusion, and CNS depression.

Drug-drug interactions: fluoxetine (Prozac®) results in elevated phenytoin levels (ave: 161% above baseline).[14] Phenytoin may impair the efficacy of: corticosteroids, warfarin, digoxin, doxycycline, estrogens, furosemide, oral contraceptives, quinidine, rifampin, theophylline, vitamin D.

Drug info: Carbamazepine (CBZ) (Tegretol®)

Indications

FOS, GTC. with or without secondary generalization. Trigeminal neuralgia. An IV form for use in e.g., status epilepticus was approved in 2016.

May exacerbate ABS, myotonic and atonic seizures (∴ avoid in GGE).[3] Newer medications have more favorable pharmacokinetics.

Dose

R oral route. Adult range: 600–2000 mg/d. Peds: 20–30 mg/kg/d. MDF = BID.

Before starting, check: CBC & platelet count (consider reticulocyte count) & serum Fe. Package insert says "recheck at frequent intervals, perhaps q week × 3 mos, then q month × 3 yrs."

Do not start CBZ (or discontinue it if patient already on CBZ) if: WBC < 4K, RBC < 3 × 106, Hct < 32%, platelets < 100K, reticulocytes < 0.3%, Fe > 150 mcg%.

Start low and increment slowly: 200 mg PO q d × 1 wk, BID × 1 wk, TID × 1 wk. As an inpatient, dosage changes may be made every 3 days, monitoring for signs of side effects. As an outpatient, changes should be made only ≈ weekly, with levels after each change. Carbatrol® (extended release CBZ) is usually dosed BID.

Supplied: oral form. Scored tabs 200 mg. Chewable scored tabs 100 mg. Suspension 100 mg/5-ml. IV form:. Carbatrol® (extended release CBZ): 200 & 300 mg tablets.

Caveats with oral forms: oral absorption is erratic, and smaller, more frequent doses are preferred.[15] Oral suspension is absorbed more readily, and also ✖ should *not* be administered simultaneously with other liquid medicines, as it may result in the precipitation of a rubbery, orange mass. ✖ May aggravate hyponatremia by SIADH-like effect.

Pharmacokinetics (▶ Table 27.6)

Table 27.6 Pharmacokinetics of carbamazepine

$t_{1/2}$ (half-life)	t_{PEAK} (peak levels)	t_{SS} (steady state)	$t_{D/C}$ (discontinue)	Therapeutic level (mcg/ml)[a]
single dose: 20–55 hrs after chronic therapy: 10–30 hrs (adults), 8–20 hrs (peds)	4–24 hrs	up to 10 days[b]	4 wks	6–12

[a]may be misleading since the active metabolite carbamazepine-10,11-epoxide may cause toxicity and must be assayed separately
[b] t_{SS} may subsequently fall due to autoinduction, which plateaus at 4–6 wks

CBZ induces hepatic enzymes that result in increased metabolism of itself (autoinduction) therefore as well as other drugs over a period of ≈ 3–4 weeks.

Side effects

✖ Drug-drug interaction: caution, cimetidine, erythromycin, and isoniazid may cause dramatic elevation of CBZ levels due to inhibition of hepatic cytochrome oxidase that degrades CBZ.[16] Side effects include:
1. drowsiness and GI upset: minimized by slow dose escalation
2. relative leukopenia in many: usually does not require discontinuing drug
3. transient diplopia
4. ataxia
5. less effect on cognitive function than PHT
6. hematological toxicity: rare. May be serious → agranulocytosis & aplastic anemia
7. Stevens-Johnson syndrome
8. SIADH
9. hepatitis (occasionally fatal) reported
10. severe rash especially in patients of Asian descent with HLA-B1502 allele

Drug info: Oxcarbazepine (OCZ) (Trileptal®)

Very similar efficacy profile to carbamazepine (and also may exacerbate ABS, myotonic and atonic seizures (∴ avoid in GGE)[3]) with the following differences:
1. there is no autoinduction (C-P450 is not involved in metabolism) and therefore minimal drug-drug interactions
2. no blood testing is required since:
    a) there is no liver toxicity
    b) there is no hematologic toxicity
    c) there is no need to check drug levels
3. dosing is BID
4. kinetics are linear
5. more expensive

OCZ is more likely to cause hyponatremia than CBZ.[3]

Dose

℞: starting dose for pain control is 150 mg PO BID, for seizures 300 mg PO BID. Maximum dose 2400 mg/day total. **Supplied:** 150, 300 & 600 mg scored tablets. 300 mg/5 ml oral suspension. When transitioning a patient from CBZ overnight, administer 200 mg OCZ for every 200 mg of CBZ when the dose of CBZ is < 800 mg (a slower conversion and lower ratio should be used at higher doses).[3]

Drug info: Eslicarbazepine (Aptiom®)

A prodrug that is converted to S-licarbezepine. Similar adverse effects to OCZ, but less frequent.

Uses
First approved for FOS. Like OCZ, avoid in GGE.[3]

Pharmacokinetics
$t_{1/2}$ is 13 to 20 hours in plasma, & 20-24 hours in CSF, justifying once-daily dosing.

Dose
Avoid combining with a classic sodium channel drug (including the phenytoins, CBZ...).

℞: start at 400 mg PO once daily. Increase to 800 mg/d after 1 week. Most patients do not need more than 800 mg/d, but If needed, increase to 1200 mg/d after 1 week. **Supplied:** 200, 400, 600 & 800 mg tablets.

27 | Drug info: Valproate

Available as valproic acid (Depakene®) and divalproex sodium (Depakote®).

Indications
The most effective ASM for GGE with GTC. Also effective for all FOS and GOS including ABS and myoclonic seizures, but ethosuximide is as effective as for ABS in children but has fewer adverse cognitive effects.[3] The divalproex sodium formulation is also FDA approved for migraine prophylaxis and bipolar disorder. Note: severe GI upset and short half-life make valproic acid much less useful than Depakote® (divalproex sodium).

Dose
Adult range: 600–3000 mg/d. Peds range: 15–60 mg/kg/d. MDF = q d.

℞ Start at 15 mg/kg/d, increment at 1 wk intervals by 5–10 mg/kg/d. Max recommended adult dose: 60 mg/kg/d. If daily dose > 250 mg is required, it should be divided. **Supplied:** Oral: capsules 250 mg. Syrup 250 mg/5-ml. Depakote® (enteric coated) tabs: 125, 250, & 500 mg; sprinkle capsules 125 mg. IV: Depacon® for IV injection 500 mg/5 ml vial.

Pharmacokinetics (▶ Table 27.7)

Table 27.7 Pharmacokinetics of valproate

$t_{1/2}$ (half-life)	t_{PEAK} (peak serum levels)	t_{SS} (steady state)	$t_{D/C}$ (discontinue)	Therapeutic level (mcg/ml)
8–20 hrs	(uncoated) 1–4 hrs	2–4 days	4 wks	50–100

Valproic acid (VA) is 90% protein bound. ASA displaces VA from serum proteins.

Side effects
Serious side effects are rare. *Pancreatitis* has been reported, sometimes life-threatening. Fatal liver failure has occurred especially if age < 2 yrs and in combination with other ASMs. *Teratogenic* (below). Drowsiness (temporary), minimal cognitive deficits, N/V (minimized with Depakote), liver dysfunction, hyperammonemia (even without liver dysfunction), weight gain, mild hair loss, tremor (dose related; similar to benign familial tremor; if severe and valproic acid is absolutely necessary, the tremor may be treated with beta blockers). May interfere with platelet function, caution with surgery on these patients.

Contraindications
✘ Pregnancy: causes neural tube defects (NTD) in ≈ 1–2% of patients.[17] Since a correlation between peak VA levels and the risk of NTDs has been found, if VA must be used, some experts recommend changing from BID to TID dosing. There was a correlation with autism spectrum disorder (ASD) (hazard ratio = 2.3) and attention-deficit/hyperactivity disorder (ADHD) (HR = 1.18) in mothers taking VA during the first trimester.[18]

✘ Patients ≤ 2 yrs of age (risk of hepatotoxicity).

Drug info: Phenobarbital

Indications
Used as alternative in GTC and partial (not DOC). Had been DOC for febrile seizures, dubious bene-fit.[19] About as effective as PHT, but very sedating. Also used for status epilepticus (p. 513).

Dose
Same dose PO, IV, or IM. MDF = q d.[20,21] Start slowly to minimize sedation.
℞ Adult *loading*: 20 mg/kg *slow* IV (administer at rate < 100 mg/min). *Maintenance*: 30–250 mg/d (usually divided BID-TID). Peds *loading:* 15–20 mg/kg. *Maintenance:* 2–6 mg/kg/d (usually divided BID). **Supplied:** tabs 15 mg, 30 mg, 60 mg, 100 mg; elixir 20 mg/5-ml.

Pharmacokinetics (▶ Table 27.8)

Table 27.8 Pharmacokinetics of phenobarbital

$t_{1/2}$ (half-life)	t_{PEAK} (peak levels)	t_{SS} (steady state)	$t_{D/C}$ (discontinue)	Therapeutic level
adult: 5 d (range: 50–160 hrs) peds: 30–70 hrs	PO & IM: 1–6 hrs	16–21 days (may take up to 30 days)	≈ 6–8 wks (reduce ≈ 25% per week)	15–30 mcg/ml

Phenobarbital is a potent inducer of hepatic enzymes that metabolize other ASMs.

Side effects
Cognitive impairment (may be subtle and may outlast administration of the drug by at least several months[19]), thus avoid in peds; sedation; paradoxical hyperactivity (especially in peds); may cause hemorrhage in newborn if mother is on phenobarbital.

Drug info: Primidone (Mysoline®)

Indications
Same as phenobarbital (not DOC). NB: when used in combination therapy, low doses (50–125 mg/day) may add significant seizure control to the primary ASM with few side effects.

Dose
℞ Adult: 250–1500 mg/d. Peds: 15–30 mg/kg/d; MDF = BID.
Start at 125 mg/d × 1 wk, and inc. slowly to avoid sedation. **Supplied:** (oral only): scored tabs 50 mg, 250 mg; suspension 250 mg/5-ml.

Pharmacokinetics (▶ Table 27.9)
Metabolites include phenylethylmalonamide (PEMA) and phenobarbital. Therefore always check phenobarbital level at same time as primidone level.

Table 27.9 Pharmacokinetics of primidone

$t_{1/2}$ (half-life)	t_{PEAK} (peak levels)	t_{SS} (steady state)	$t_{D/C}$ (discontinue)	Therapeutic level (mcg/ml)
primidone: 4–12 hrs derived phenobarbital: 50–160 hrs	2–5 hrs	up to 30 days	same as phenobarbital	primidone: 1–15 derived phenobarbital: 10–30

Side effects
Same as phenobarbital, plus: loss of libido, rare macrocytic anemia.

27

27

Drug info: Ethosuximide (Zarontin®)

Indications
DOC in ABS.

Dose
℞ Adult: 500–1500 mg/d. Peds: 10–40 mg/kg/d; MDF = q d. **Supplied:** oral only; capsules 250 mg; syrup 250 mg/5-ml.

Pharmacokinetics (▶ Table 27.10)

Table 27.10 Pharmacokinetics of ethosuximide

$t_{1/2}$ (half-life)	t_{PEAK} (peak levels)	t_{SS} (steady state)	Therapeutic level (mcg/ml)
adult: 40–70 hrs peds: 20–40 hrs	1–4 hrs	adult: up to 14 days peds: up to 7 days	40–100

Side effects
N/V; lethargy; hiccups; H/A; rarely: eosinophilia, leukopenia, erythema multiforme, Stevens-Johnson syndrome, SLE-like syndrome. Toxic levels→ psychotic behavior.

Drug info: Methsuximide (Celontin®)

Indications
Indicated for absence seizures refractory to other drugs.

Dose
℞ optimum dose must be determined by trial. Start with 300 mg PO q d, increase by 300 mg at weekly intervals PRN to a maximum of 1200 mg/d. **Supplied:** 150 & 300 mg capsules.

Drug info: Felbamate (Felbatol®)

✖ CAUTION: Due to an unacceptably high rate of aplastic anemia and hepatic failure, felbamate (FBM) should not be used except in those circumstances where the benefit clearly outweighs the risk; then, hematologic consultation is recommended by the manufacturer. See Side effects below (also for drug-drug interactions).

FBM is efficacious for monotherapy and adjunctive therapy for partial seizures (complex and secondary generalization), and reduces the frequency of atonic and GTC seizures in Lennox-Gastaut syndrome.

Pharmacokinetics (▶ Table 27.11)

Table 27.11 Pharmacokinetics of felbamate

$t_{1/2}$ (half-life)	t_{PEAK} (peak levels)	t_{SS} (steady state)	Therapeutic level (mcg/ml)
20–23 hrs	1–3 hrs	5–7 days	not established

Dose

Table 27.12 Effect of felbamate on other ASM levels

ASM	Change in level	Recommended dosing change
phenytoin	↑ 30–50%	↓ 20–33%
carbamazepine	↓ 30% total ↑ 50–60% epoxide	↓ 20–33%
valproic acid	↑ 25–100%	↓ 33%

℞: CAUTION see above. Felbamate is *not* to be used as a first-line drug. Patient or guardian should sign informed consent release. Start with 1200 mg/d divided BID, TID, or QID, and decrease other ASMS by one-third. Increase felbamate biweekly in 600 mg increments to usual dose of 1600–3600 mg/d (max: 45 mg/kg/d). Slow down increments and/or reduce other ASMs further if side effects become severe. Administer at upper end of range when used as monotherapy. **Supplied:** (oral only) 400 & 600 mg scored tablets; suspension 600 mg/5-ml.

Side effects
Felbamate has been associated with aplastic anemia (usually discovered after 5–30 wks of therapy) in ≈ 2–5 cases per million persons per yr, and hepatic failure (some fatal, necessitating baseline and serial LFTs every 1–2 wks). Other side effects: insomnia, anorexia, N/V, H/A. Felbamate is a potent metabolic inhibitor; thus it is necessary to reduce the dose of phenytoin, valproate or carbamazepine when used with felbamate[22] (▶ Table 27.12, general rule: drop dose by one third).

Drug info: Levetiracetam (Keppra®)

No identified drug-drug interactions. Less than 10% protein bound. Linear pharmacokinetics, no level monitoring needed.

Indications
Adjunctive therapy for partial onset Sz with secondary generalization in patients 4 years of age and older. Myoclonic seizures (juvenile myoclonic epilepsy). Generalized tonic-clonic.

Dose
℞ start with 500 mg PO BID. Increment by 1000 mg/d q 2 weeks PRN to a maximum of 3000 mg/d. Keppra XR: the same dose of levetiracetam can be converted to Keppra XR for q d dosing.
   IV: 500–1500 mg diluted in 100 ml of diluent (LR, D5 W, normal saline) infused over 15 minutes BID.
   Supplied: 250, 500, 750 & 1000 mg scored film-coated tabs; 100 mg/ml oral solution. Keppra XR (extended release) 500 mg.
   IV: 1 vial (5 ml) contains 500 mg.

Side effects
PO or IV: somnolence and fatigue in 15%. Dizziness in 9%. Asthenia 15% and infection 13% (nasopharyngitis and influenza may or may not have been related).
   Keppra XR: somnolence 8%, irritability 6%.

Drug info: Clonazepam (Klonopin®)

A benzodiazepine derivative.

Indications
✖ *Not* a recommended drug for seizures (see below).
   Used for myoclonic, atonic, and absence seizures (in absence, less effective than valproate or ethosuximide, and tolerance may develop).
   NB: clonazepam usually works very well for several months, and then tends to become less effective, leaving only the sedating effects. Also, many cases have been reported of patients having seizures during withdrawal, including status epilepticus (even in patients with no history of status). Thus, may need to taper this drug over 3–6 months.

Dose
℞ Adult: start at 1.5 mg/d DIV TID, increase by 0.5–1 mg q 3 d, usual dosage range is 1–12 mg/d (max 20 mg/d); MDF = q d. Peds: start at 0.01–0.03 mg/kg/d DIV BID or TID, increase by 0.25–0.5 mg/kg/d q 3 d; usual dosage range is 0.01–0.02 mg/kg/d; MDF = q d. **Supplied:** oral only; scored tabs: 0.5 mg, 1 mg, 2 mg.

27

Pharmacokinetics (▶ Table 27.13)

Table 27.13 Pharmacokinetics of clonazepam

t$_{1/2}$ (half-life)	t$_{PEAK}$ (peak levels)	t$_{SS}$ (steady state)	t$_{D/C}$ (discontinue)	Therapeutic level (mcg/ml)
20–60 hrs	1–3 hrs	up to 14 days	≈ 3–6 months[a]	0.013–0.072

[a]CAUTION: withdrawal seizures are common, see text above

Side effects
Ataxia; drowsiness; behavior changes.

Drug info: Zonisamide (Zonegran®)

Indications
A broad spectrum ASM, FDA approved as adjunctive therapy for FOS in adults.

Side effects
Cognitive slowing, especially at higher doses (but less severe than tipiramate).

Dose
℞ Initiate therapy with 100 mg PO q PM × 2 wks, then increase dose by 100 mg/d q 2 wks up to 400 mg/d. Bioavailability is not affected by food. Steady state is achieved within 14 days of dosage changes. **Supplied :** 25, 50 & 100 mg capsules. 100 mg/5 ml strawberry flavored liquid.

Drug info: Acetazolamide (Diamox®)

The anti-epileptic effect may be either due to direct inhibition of CNS carbonic anhydrase (which also reduces CSF production rate) or due to the slight CNS acidosis that results.

Indications
Centricephalic epilepsies (absence, nonfocal seizures). Best results are in absence seizures; however benefit has also been observed in GTC, myoclonic jerk.

Side effects
✖ Do not use in first trimester of pregnancy (may be teratogenic, although this is disputed). The diuretic effect causes renal loss of HCO3 (bicarbonate), which may lead to an acidotic state with long-term therapy. A sulfonamide, therefore any typical reaction to this class may occur (anaphylaxis, fever, rash, Stevens-Johnson syndrome, toxic epidermal necrolysis...). Paresthesias: medication should be discontinued.

Dose
℞ Adult: 8–30 mg/kg/d in divided doses (max 1 gm/d, higher doses do not improve control). When given with another ASM, the suggested starting dose is 250 mg once daily, and this is gradually increased. **Supplied:** tablets 125, 250 mg. Diamox sequels® are sustained release 500 mg capsules. Sterile cryodessicated powder is also available in 500 mg vials for parenteral (IV) use.

Drug info: Gabapentin (Neurontin®)

Although developed to be a GABA agonist, it does not interact at any known GABA receptor. Efficacious for primary generalized seizures and FOS (with or without secondary generalization). Ineffective for absence seizures. Very low incidence of known side effects. No known drug interactions (probably because it is renally excreted). Also used for central pain

Dose

℞ Adult: 300 mg PO × 1 day 1; 300 mg BID day 2; 300 mg TID day 3; then increase rapidly up to usual doses of ≈ 800–1800 mg per day. Doses of 1800–3600 mg may be needed in intractable patients.
✖ Dosage must be reduced in patients with renal insufficiency or on dialysis, see Eq (7.1) to estimate.
Supplied: 100, 300, 400, 600, 800 mg capsules. 50 mg/ml suspension.

Pharmacokinetics (▶ Table 27.14)

Gabapentin is not metabolized, and 93% is excreted unchanged renally with plasma clearance directly proportional to creatinine clearance.[23] Does not affect hepatic microsomal enzymes, and does not affect metabolism of other ASMs. Antacids decrease bioavailablilty by ≈ 20%, therefore give gabapentin > 2 hrs after the antacid.[24]

Table 27.14 Pharmacokinetics of gabapentin

$t_{1/2}$ (half-life)	t_{PEAK} (peak levels)	t_{SS} (steady state)	Therapeutic level (mcg/ml)
5–7 hrs[a]	2–3 hrs	1–2 days	not established

[a]with normal renal function

Side effects

Somnolence, dizziness, ataxia, fatigue, nystagmus; all reduce after 2–3 weeks of drug therapy. Increased appetite. Not known to be teratogenic.

Drug info: Lamotrigine (Lamictal®)

Anticonvulsant effect may be due to presynaptic inhibition of glutamate release.[23]

Efficacious as *adjunctive* therapy for partial seizures (with or without secondary generalization) and Lennox-Gastaut syndrome. Preliminary data suggest it may also be useful as an adjunct for refractory generalized seizures, or as monotherapy for newly diagnosed partial or generalized seizures.[25] Also FDA approved for bipolar disorder.

Side effects

Somnolence, dizziness, diplopia. ✖ Serious rashes requiring hospitalization and discontinuation of therapy have been reported (rash usually begins 2 weeks after initiating therapy and may be severe and potentially life-threatening, including Stevens-Johnson syndrome (more of a concern with simultaneous use of valproate), and rarely, toxic epidermal necrolysis (TEN)). Incidence of significant epidermal reaction may be decreased by a slow ramping-up of dosage. May increase seizure frequency in some patients with severe myoclonic epilepsy of infancy.[26] Metabolism of lamotrigine is affected by concurrent use of other ASMs.

Dose

℞ Adult: In adults receiving enzyme-inducing ASMs (PHT, CBZ, or phenobarbital), start with 50 mg PO q d x 2 wks, then 50 mg BID × 2 wks, then ↑ by 100 mg/d q week until the usual maintenance dose of 200–700 mg/d (divided into 2 doses) is reached. For patients on valproic acid (VA) alone, the maintenance dose was 100–200 mg/d (divided into 2 doses), and VA levels drop by ≈ 25% within a few weeks of starting lamotrigine. For patients on both enzyme-inducing ASMs *and* VA, the starting dose is 25 mg PO qod × 2 wks, then 25 mg qd × 2 wks, then ↑ by 25–50 mg/d q 1–2 wks up to a maintenance of 100–150 mg/d (divided into 2 doses). Instruct patients that rash, fever or lymphadenopathy may herald a serious reaction and that a physician should be contacted immediately. Peds: not indicated for use in patients < 16 yrs old due to higher incidence of potentially life-threatening rash in the pediatric population.[23] **Supplied:** 25, 100, 150 & 200 mg tablets. 2, 5 & 25 mg chewable dispersible tablets.

Pharmacokinetics[25] (▶ Table 27.15)

Table 27.15 Pharmacokinetics of lamotrigine

$t_{1/2}$ (half-life)	t_{PEAK} (peak levels)	t_{SS} (steady state)	Therapeutic level (mcg/ml)
24 hrs[a]	1.5–5 hrs	4–7 days	controversial[27]

[a]half-life is shortened to ≈ 15 hrs by PHT and CBZ, whereas valproic acid increases it to 59 hrs

27

Drug info: Vigabatrin (Sabril®, Vigadrone®)

Irreversible GABA transaminase inhibitor, causing an increase in synaptic GABA.

Indications
A narrow spectrum drug used for FOS. Also effective against infantile spasms especially as part of tuberous sclerosis.

✖ May worsen absence and myoclonic seizures in GGE.

Side effects
✖ Causes a progressive and permanent concentric visual field constriction in 30-40% of patients, the higher the risk with the higher the dose and the duration of treatment.

Less severe adverse effects include sedation, fatigue, irritability, behavior changes, psychosis, depression and weight gain.

Dose
Because of visual toxicity, visual fields should be monitored every 3 months.

℞ Adult: 1500–3000 mg/d. Start at 500 mg BID, titrating upwards by 500 mg/d every week up to a maximum of 1.5 gm BID. Discontinue the drug if significant benefit does not occur in the 1st 3 months.

Drug info: Topiramate (Topamax®)

May block voltage-sensitive sodium channels and enhance GABA activity at GABA-A receptors and attenuate some glutamate receptors.[23]

Indications[28]
A broad spectrum ASM. FDA approved for initial monotherapy for FOS and GTC, but is not a drug of first choice due to cognitive side effects.

Dose
NB: titrate slowly to deal with adverse cognitive efects.

℞ Adult: start with 50 mg/d and increase slowly up to 200–400 mg/d,[29] with no significant benefit noted at dosages > 600 mg/d.[30] **Supplied:** 25, 100, & 200 mg tabs.

Pharmacokinetics (▶ Table 27.16)
30% is metabolized in the liver, the rest is excreted unchanged in the urine.

Table 27.16 Pharmacokinetics of topiramate

$t_{1/2}$ (half-life)	t_{ss} (steady state)	Therapeutic level
19–25 hrs	5–7 days	not established

Side effects
May increase phenytoin concentration by up to 25%. Levels of topiramate are reduced by other ASMs (phenytoin, carbamazepine, valproic acid, and possibly others).

Cognitive impairment (word-finding difficulty, problems with concentration, more pronounced than with lamotrigine...), weight loss, dizziness, ataxia, diplopia, paresthesias, nervousness, and confusion have been troublesome. ≈ 1.5% incidence of renal stones which usually pass spontaneously.[23]

Oligohidrosis (reduced sweating) and hyperthermia, primarily in children in association with elevated environmental temperatures and/or vigorous physical activity.

Drug info: Tiagabine (Gabitril®)

A GABA uptake inhibitor, with cognitive problems of a similar frequency to that with topiramate.[31]

℞ Adult: start with 4 mg/d, increase weekly by 4–8 mg to a maximum of 32–56 mg (divided BID to QID). **Supplied:** 4, 12, 16 & 20 mg tablets.

Drug info: Cenobamate (XCOPRI®)

2 mechanisms of action: 1) blocking the sodium channel (predominantly attenuating the persistent sodium current rather than the transient voltage-gated sodium current), and 2) enhancing GABA activity.

Indications
FDA approved for FOS (it showed exceptional efficacy as adjunctive therapy in this regard[6]).

Dose
℞ Adult: taken once daily, start at 12.5 mg/d for 2 weeks, then 25 mg/d for 2 weeks, then 50 mg/d for 2 weeks, and then 100 mg/d. Thereafter, increase by 50 mg every 2 weeks to a maximum of 400 mg/d. (NB: slow titration appears to be important to reduce the occurrence of DRESS (drug rash with eosinophilia and systemic symptoms).[32] **Supplied:** 12.5, 25, 50, 150 & 200 mg tabs.

Drug info: Lacosamide (Vimpat®)

Enhances slow inactivation of voltage gated sodium channels, affecting only neurons that are depolarized or active over a prolonged period (as in a seizure).

Indications
FOS & GTC. Painful diabetic neuropathy.

Dose
℞ Adult: start at 100 mg/d, either once at bedtime or divided into 2 daily doses. Increase by 100 mg/d every 1-2 weeks to the range of 200-400 mg/d (maximum: 600 mg/d). **Supplied:** 50, 100, 150 & 200 mg tablets. 200 mg/20 ml single use vial for IV use.

27.4 Withdrawal of antiseizure medications

27.4.1 General information

Most seizure recurrences develop during the first 6 months after ASM withdrawal.[33]

27.4.2 Indications for ASM withdrawal

There is no agreement on how long a patient should be seizure-free before withdrawal of antiseizure medications, nor is there agreement on the prognostic value of EEGs and on the best time period over which to withdraw ASMs.

The following is based on a study of 92 patients with *idiopathic* epilepsy, who had been free of seizures for two years.[34] Generalization, e.g., to posttraumatic seizures, may not be appropriate. Taper was by 1 "unit" q 2 weeks (where a unit is defined as 200 mg for CBZ or valproic acid, or 100 mg for PHT). Follow-up: mean = 26 mos (range: 6–62).

31 patients (34%) relapsed, with the average time to relapse being 8 mos (range: 1–36). Using actuarial methods, the risk for recurrence is 5.9%/month for 3 months, then 2.7%/month for 3 months, then 0.5%/month for 3 months. Factors found to affect the likelihood of relapse include:
1. seizure type: 37% relapse rate for generalized seizures; 16% for complex or simple partial; 54% for complex partial with secondary generalization
2. number of seizures before control attained: those with ≥ 100 seizures before control had statistically significant higher relapse rate than those with < 100
3. the number of drugs that had to be tried before single drug therapy successfully controlled seizures: 29% if 1st drug worked, 40% if a change to a 2nd drug was needed, and 80% if a change to a 3rd drug was required
4. EEG class (▶ Table 27.17): class 4 had worst prognosis for relapse. Epileptiform discharges on EEG serves to discourage ASM withdrawal[35]

In a larger randomized study,[36] the most important factors identified to predict freedom from recurrent seizures were:
1. longer seizure-free period

Table 27.17 EEG class and seizure relapse rate

Class	EEG description		Relapse rate	No. of relapses/ patients at risk
	Before treatment	Before withdrawal		
1	normal	normal	34%	11/31
2	abnormal	normal	11%	4/35
3	abnormal	improved	50%	2/4
4	abnormal	unchanged	74%	14/19

2. use of only one ASM (vs. multiple ASMs)
3. seizures other than tonic-clonic seizures

27.4.3 Withdrawal times

The recommended withdrawal times in ▶ Table 27.18 should be used only as guidelines.

Table 27.18 Recommended ASM withdrawal times

ASM	Recommended withdrawal period
phenytoin, valproic acid, carbamazepine	2–4 weeks
phenobarbital	6–8 weeks (25% per week)
clonazepam	3–6 months; see CAUTION (p. 496)

27.5 Pregnancy and antiseizure medications

27.5.1 General information

Women of childbearing potential with epilepsy should undergo counseling regarding pregnancy.[37]

27.5.2 Birth control

ASMs that induce liver microsomal cytochrome P450 enzymes (▶ Table 27.19) increase the failure rate of oral contraceptives up to fourfold.[38] Patients desiring to use BCPs should employ barrier contraceptive measures until ovulation is consistently suppressed, and they should watch for breakthrough bleeding which may indicate a need for a change in the hormone dosage.[33] Non-oral hormonal contraceptives (e.g., levonorgestrel implant [Norplant®]) circumvent first pass liver degradation but should be combined with a barrier method because of declining effectiveness with time.

Table 27.19 Effect of ASMs on liver cytochrome P_{450}[a]

Inducers	Noninducers
carbamazepine phenobarbital phenytoin felbamate primidone	valproic acid benzodiazepines gabapentin lamotrigine

[a]references[33,39]

27.5.3 Complications during pregnancy

Women with epilepsy have more complications with pregnancy than mothers without epilepsy, but > 90% of pregnancies have a favorable outcome.[33]

There is an increase in the number of gravid seizures in ≈ 17% (reported range: 17–30%) of epileptic women, which may be due to noncompliance or to changes of free drug levels of ASMs during pregnancy (▶ Table 27.20). Isolated seizures can occasionally be deleterious, but usually cause no problem. Status epilepticus poses serious risk to mother and fetus during pregnancy and should be treated aggressively.

There is also a slightly increased risk of toxemia (HTN of pregnancy) and fetal loss.

Table 27.20 Changes in free ASM levels during pregnancy[40]

Drug	Change
carbamazepine	↓ 11%
phenobarbital	↓ 50%
phenytoin	↓ 31%
valproic acid	↑ 25%

27.5.4 Birth defects

The incidence of fetal malformations in offspring of patients with a known seizure disorder is ≈ 4–5%, or approximately double that of the general population.[41] The degree to which this is due to the use of ASMs vs. genetic and environmental factors is unknown. All ASMs have the potential to cause deleterious effects on the infant. Polytherapy is associated with an increased risk over monotherapy in a more than additive manner.

Generally, the risk of seizures (with possible concomitant maternal and fetal hypoxia and acidosis) is felt to outweigh the teratogenic risk of most ASMs, but this must be evaluated on a case-by-case basis. Occasionally patients may be weaned off ASMs.

Specific drugs

Carbamazepine (CBZ) produced an increased incidence of "minor" malformations (but not of "major" malformations) in one study[42] (this study may have had methodologic problems), and may increase the incidence of neural tube defects (NTD).[43] In utero exposure to phenytoin may lead to the fetal hydantoin syndrome[13,44] and a child with an IQ lower by ≈ 10 points.[45] Phenobarbital produced the highest incidence of major malformations (9.1%) in one prospective study[46] and was also associated with most of the increase in fetal death or anomalies in another study.[47] Valproate (VA) causes the highest incidence of NTD (1–2%[17]), which can be detected with amniocentesis and allow an abortion if desired. TID dosing may reduce the risk of NTD (p.492). Benzodiazepines given shortly before delivery can produce the "floppy infant syndrome."[48] Similar effects may occur with other sedating ASMs such as phenobarbital.

Drug recommendations

A general consensus is that for most women of childbearing potential who require ASMs, that monotherapy with the lowest dose of CBZ that is effective is the method of choice if the seizure disorder is responsive to it.[49] If ineffective, then monotherapy with valproic acid (with TID dosing) is currently the recommended second choice. Folate supplementation (after confirming normal B12 levels) should be used in all.

References

[1] Brodie MJ, Dichter MA. Antiepileptic Drugs. New England Journal of Medicine. 1996; 334:168–175

[2] Park KM, Kim SE, Lee BI. Antiepileptic Drug Therapy in Patients with Drug-Resistant Epilepsy. J Epilepsy Res. 2019; 9:14–26

[3] Abou-Khalil BW. Update on Antiseizure Medications 2022. Continuum (Minneap Minn). 2022; 28:500–535

[4] Mattson RH, Cramer JA, Collins JF, et al. Comparison of Carbamazepine, Phenobarbital, Phenytoin, and Primidone in Partial and Secondarily Generalized Tonic-Clonic Seizures. N Engl J Med. 1985; 313:145–151

[5] Mattson RH, Cramer JA, Collins JF, et al. A Comparison of Valproate with Carbamazepine for the Treatment of Complex Partial Seizures and Secondarily Generalized Tonic-Clonic Seizures in Adults. New England Journal of Medicine. 1992; 327:765–771

[6] Chung SS, French JA, Kowalski J, et al. Randomized phase 2 study of adjunctive cenobamate in patients with uncontrolled focal seizures. Neurology. 2020; 94:e2311–e2322

[7] Marson AG, Al-Kharusi AM, Alwaidh M, et al. The SANAD study of effectiveness of valproate, lamotrigine, or topiramate for generalised and unclassifiable epilepsy: an unblinded randomised controlled trial. Lancet. 2007; 369:1016–1026

[8] Drugs for Epilepsy. Medical Letter. 1986; 28:91–93

[9] Rambeck B, Boenigk HE, Dunlop A, et al. Predicting Phenytoin Dose - A Revised Nomogram. Ther Drug Monit. 1979; 1:325–333

[10] Saklad JJ, Graves RH, Sharp WP. Interaction of Oral Phenytoin with Enteral Feedings. J Parent Ent Nutr. 1986; 10:322–323

[11] Worden JP, Wood CA, Workman CH. Phenytoin and Nasogastric Feedings. Neurology. 1984; 34

[12] DeToledo JC, Ramsay RE. Fosphenytoin and phenytoin in patients with status epilepticus: improved tolerability versus increased costs. Drug Saf. 2000; 22:459–466

[13] Buehler BA, Delimont D, van Waes M, et al. Prenatal Prediction of Risk of the Fetal Hydantoin Syndrome. N Engl J Med. 1990; 322:1567–1572

[14] Public Health Service. Fluoxetine-Phenytoin Interaction. FDA Medical Bulletin. 1994; 24:3–4

[15] Winkler SR, Luer MS. Antiepileptic Drug Review: Part 1. Surgical Neurology. 1998; 49:449–452

[16] Oles KS, Waqar M, Penry JK. Catastrophic Neurologic Signs due to Drug Interaction: Tegretol and Darvon. Surgical Neurology. 1989; 32:144–151

[17] Oakeshott P, Hunt GM. Valproate and Spina Bifida. Br Med J. 1989; 298:1300–1301

[18] Wiggs KK, Rickert ME, Sujan AC, et al. Anti-seizure medication use during pregnancy and risk of ASD and ADHD in children. Neurology. 2020. DOI: 10.1212/WNL.0000000000010993

[19] Farwell JR, Lee YJ, Hirtz DG, et al. Phenobarbital for Febrile Seizures - Effects on Intelligence and on Seizure Recurrence. N Engl J Med. 1990; 322:364–369

[20] Wroblewski BA, Garvin WH. Once-Daily Administration of Phenobarbital in Adults: Clinical Efficacy and Benefit. Arch Neurol. 1985; 42:699–700

[21] Davis AG, Mutchie KD, Thompson JA, et al. Once-Daily Dosing with Phenobarbital in Children with Seizure Disorders. Pediatrics. 1981; 68:824–827

[22] Felbamate. Medical Letter. 1993; 35:107–109

[23] Winkler SR, Luer MS. Antiepileptic Drug Review: Part 2. Surgical Neurology. 1998; 49:566–568

[24] Gabapentin - A new anticonvulsant. Medical Letter. 1994; 36:39–40

[25] Lamotrigine for Epilepsy. Medical Letter. 1995; 37:21–23

[26] Guerrini R, Dravet ,C, Genton P, et al. Lamotrigine and Seizure Aggravation in Severe Myoclonic Epilepsy. Epilepsia. 1998; 39:508–512

[27] Sondergaard Khinchi M, Nielsen KA, Dahl M, et al. Lamotrigine therapeutic thresholds. Seizure. 2008; 17:391–395

[28] Topiramate for Epilepsy. Medical Letter. 1997; 39:51–52

[29] Faught E, Wilder BJ, Ramsay RE, et al. Topiramate Placebo-Controlled Dose-Ranging Trial in Refractory Partial Epilepsy using 200-, 400-, and 600-mg Daily Dosages. Neurology. 1996; 46:1684–1690

[30] Privitera M, Fincham R, Penry J, et al. Topiramate Placebo-Controlled Dose-Ranging Trial in Refractory Partial Epilepsy using 600-, 800-, and 1,000-mg Daily Dosages. Neurology. 1996; 46:1678–1683

[31] Tiagabine for Epilepsy. Medical Letter. 1998; 40:45–46

[32] Sperling MR, Klein P, Aboumatar S, et al. Cenobamate (YKP3089) as adjunctive treatment for uncontrolled focal seizures in a large, phase 3, multicenter, open-label safety study. Epilepsia. 2020; 61:1099–1108

[33] Shuster EA. Epilepsy in Women. Mayo Clinic Proceedings. 1996; 71:991–999

[34] Callaghan N, Garrett A, Goggin T. Withdrawal of Anticonvulsant Drugs in Patients Free of Seizures for Two Years. N Engl J Med. 1988; 318:942–946

[35] Anderson T, Braathen G, Persson A, et al. A Comparison Between One and Three Years of Treatment in Uncomplicated Childhood Epilepsy: A Prospective Study. II. The EEG as Predictor of Outcome After Withdrawal of Treatment. Epilepsia. 1997; 38:225–232

[36] Medical Research Council Antiepileptic Drug Withdrawal Study Group. Randomized study of antiepileptic drug withdrawal in patients in remission. Lancet. 1991; 337:1175–1180

[37] Delgado-Escueta A, Janz D. Consensus Guidelines: Preconception Counseling, Management, and Care of the Pregnant Woman with Epilepsy. Neurology. 1992; 42:149–160

[38] Mattson RH, Cramer JA, Darney PD, et al. Use of Oral Contraceptives by Women with Epilepsy. Journal of the American Medical Association. 1986; 256:238–240

[39] Perucca E, Hedges A, Makki KA, et al. A Comparative Study of the Relative Enzyme Inducing Properties of Anticonvulsant Drugs in Epileptic Patients. Br J Clin Pharmacol. 1984; 18:401–410

[40] Yerby MS, Freil PN, McCormick K. Antiepileptic Drug Disposition During Pregnancy. Neurology. 1992; 42:12–16

[41] Dias MS, Sekhar LN. Intracranial Hemorrhage from Aneurysms and Arteriovenous Malformations during Pregnancy and the Puerperium. Neurosurgery. 1990; 27:855–866

[42] Jones KL, Lacro RV, Johnson KA, et al. Patterns of Malformations in the Children of Women Treated With Carbamazepine During Pregnancy. N Engl J Med. 1989; 310:1661–1666

[43] Rosa FW. Spina Bifida in Infants of Women Treated with Carbamazepine During Pregnancy. New England Journal of Medicine. 1991; 324:674–677

[44] Hanson JW, Smith DW. The Fetal Hydantoin Syndrome. J Pediatr. 1975; 87:285–290

[45] Scolnik D, Nulman I, Rovet J, et al. Neurodevelopment of Children Exposed In Utero to Phenytoin and Carbamazepine Monotherapy. Journal of the American Medical Association. 1994; 271:767–770

[46] Nakane Y, Okuma T, Takahashi R, et al. Multi-Institutional Study of the Teratogenicity and Fetal Toxicity of Antiepileptic Drugs: A Report of a Collaberative Study Group in Japan. Epilepsia. 1980; 21:663–680

[47] Waters CH, Belai Y, Gott PS, et al. Outcomes of Pregnancy Associated with Antiepileptic Drugs. Archives of Neurology. 1994; 51:250–253

[48] Kanto JH. Use of Benzodiazepines During Pregnancy, Labor, and Lactation, with Particular Reference to Pharmacokinetic Considerations. Drugs. 1982; 23:354–380

[49] Saunders M. Epilepsy in Women of Childbearing Age: If Anticonvulsants Cannot be Avoided, Use Carbamazepine. Br Med J. 1989; 199

28 Special Seizure Considerations

28.1 New onset seizures

28.1.1 General information

The age adjusted *incidence* of new onset seizures in Rochester, Minnesota was 44 per 100,000 person-years.[1]

28.1.2 Etiologies

In patients presenting with a first-time seizure, etiologies include (modified[2]) (the first 3 items would be considered provoked):
1. following neurologic insult*: either acutely (i.e., < 1 week) or remotely (> 1 week, and usually < 3 mos from insult)
   a) stroke: 4.2% had a seizure within 14 days of a stroke. Risk increased with severity of stroke[3]
   b) head trauma: closed head injury, penetrating trauma (p. 505)
   c) CNS infection: meningitis, cerebral abscess, subdural empyema
   d) febrile seizures (p. 509)
   e) birth asphyxia
2. underlying CNS abnormality*
   a) congenital CNS abnormalities
   b) degenerative CNS disease
   c) CNS tumor: metastatic or primary
   d) hydrocephalus
   e) AVM
3. acute systemic metabolic disturbance*
   a) electrolyte disorders: uremia, hyponatremia, hypoglycemia (especially profound hypoglycemia), hypercalcemia
   b) drug related, including:
      • alcohol-withdrawal (p. 506)
      • cocaine toxicity (p. 216)
      • opioids (narcotics)
      • phenothiazine antiemetics (p. 149)
      • with administration of flumazenil (Romazicon®) to treat benzodiazepine (BDZ) overdose (especially when BDZs are taken with other seizure lowering drugs such as tricyclic antidepressants or cocaine)
      • phencyclidine (PCP): originally used as an animal tranquilizer
      • cyclosporine: can affect Mg^{++} levels
   c) eclampsia
4. idiopathic

* Items with an asterisk would be considered provoked seizures.

In 166 *pediatric* patients presenting to an emergency department with either a chief complaint of, or a discharge diagnosis of a first-time seizure[4]:
1. 110 were found to actually have either a recurrent seizure or a non-ictal event
2. of the 56 patients actually thought to have had a first-time seizure
   a) 71% were febrile seizures
   b) 21% were idiopathic
   c) 7% were "symptomatic" (hyponatremia, meningitis, drug intoxication…)

In a prospective study of 244 patients with a new-onset unprovoked seizure, only 27% had further seizures during follow-up.[2,5] Recurrent seizures were more common in patients with a family seizure history, spike-and-waves on EEG, or a history of a CNS insult (stroke, head injury…). No patient seizure-free for 3 years had a recurrence. Following a second seizure, the risk of further seizures was high.

28

28.1.3 Evaluation

Adults

A new-onset seizure in an *adult* in the absence of obvious cause (e.g., alcohol withdrawal) should prompt a search for an underlying basis (the onset of idiopathic seizures, i.e., epilepsy, is most common before or during adolescence). An MRI (without and with enhancement) should be performed (CT without and with contrast if MRI cannot be done). A systemic work-up should be done to identify the presence of any provoking factors listed above. If all this is negative, a repeat MRI (or CT if MRI cannot be done) should be done in ≈ 6 months and at 1 and possibly 2 years to rule out a tumor which might not be evident on the initial study.

Pediatrics

Among pediatric patients with first-time seizures, laboratory and radiologic evaluations were often costly and not helpful.[4] A detailed history and physical exam were more helpful.

Management

Management of an adult with the new onset of idiopathic seizures (i.e., no abnormality found on CT or MRI, no evidence of a provoking etiology) is controversial.

▶ **Electroencephalogram (EEG).** An EEG is a brief (20 minute) sample of electrical activity of the brain, and is normal in > 50% of patients later proven to have epilepsy (poor sensitivity). However, it is highly specific when abnormal.

In one study, an EEG was performed, which, if normal, was followed by a sleep deprived EEG with the following observations[6]:
1. there is substantial interobserver variation in interpreting such EEGs
2. if both EEGs were normal, the 2-yr recurrence rate of seizures was 12%
3. if one or both EEGs showed epileptic discharges, the 2-yr recurrence rate was 83%
4. the presence of nonepileptic abnormalities in one or both EEGs had a 41% 2-yr recurrence rate
5. the recurrence rate with focal epileptic discharges (87%) was slightly higher than for generalized epileptic discharges (78%)

Conclusion: EEGs thus obtained have moderate predictive value, and may be factored into the decision of whether or not to treat such seizures with ASMs.

▶ **Ambulatory EEG.** Permits home recording typically for 1-3 days (similar to a Holter monitor used for cardiac arrhythmias).

▶ **Video-EEG.** The patient is monitored with continuous EEG and video recording, usually in a specialized video-EEG monitoring unit (some home video-EEGs have been trialed) to correlate symptoms with electrical activity of the brain. The most accurate means of diagnosing seizures (including ruling out non-epileptic seizures (p. 507)). However, with only scalp (surface) electrodes, even video-EEG may miss some seizures.

▶ **Additional evaluation.** Further evaluation may be needed for uncharacterized disabling episodes. See details (p. 1890).

28.2 Posttraumatic seizures

28.2.1 General information

Key concepts

- 2 categories: early (≤ 7 days) and late (> 7 days) after head trauma
- antiseizure medications (ASMs) may be used to prevent early posttraumatic seizures (PTS) in patients at high risk for seizures
- prophylactic ASMs do NOT reduce the frequency of late PTS
- discontinue ASMs after 1 week except for cases meeting specific criteria (see text)

Posttraumatic seizures (PTS) are often divided (arbitrarily) into early (occurring within 1 week of injury) and late (thereafter).[7] There may be justification for a third category: "immediate," i.e., within minutes to an hour or so.

28.2.2 Early PTS (≤ 7 days after head trauma)

30% incidence in severe head injury ("severe" defined as: LOC > 24 hrs, amnesia > 24 hrs, focal neuro deficit, documented contusion, or intracranial hematoma) and ≈ 1% in mild to moderate injuries. Occurs in 2.6% of children < 15 yrs of age with head injury causing at least brief LOC or amnesia.[8]

Early PTS may precipitate adverse events as a result of elevation of ICP, alterations in BP, changes in oxygenation, and excess neurotransmitter release.[9]

28.2.3 Late onset PTS (< 7 days after head trauma)

Estimated incidence 10–13% within 2 yrs after "significant" head trauma (includes LOC > 2 mins, GCS < 8 on admission, epidural hematoma…) for all age groups.[10,11] Relative risk: 3.6 times control population. Incidence in severe head injury > moderate > mild.[8]

The incidence of early PTS is higher in children than adults, but late seizures are much less frequent in children (in children who have PTS, 94.5% develop them within 24 hrs of the injury[12]). Most patients who have not had a seizure within 3 yrs of penetrating head injury will not develop seizures.[13] Risk of late PTS in children does not appear related to the occurrence of early PTS (in adults: only true for mild injuries). Risk of developing late PTS may be higher after repeated head injuries.

28.2.4 Penetrating trauma

The incidence of PTS is higher with penetrating head injuries than with closed head injuries (occurs in 50% of penetrating trauma cases followed 15 yrs[14]).

28.2.5 Treatment

General information

Some early retrospective studies suggested that early administration of PHT prevents early PTS, and reduces the risk of late PTS even after discontinuation of the drug. Later prospective studies disputed this but were criticized for not maintaining satisfactory levels and for lacking statistical power.[7,11] A prospective double blind study of patients at high risk of PTS (excluding penetrating trauma) showed a 73% reduction of risk of *early* PTS by administering 20 mg/kg loading dose of PHT within 24 hrs of injury and maintaining high therapeutic levels; but after 1 week there was no benefit in continuing the drug (based on intention to treat).[15] Carbamazepine (Tegretol®) has also been shown to be effective in reducing the risk of early PTS.

Phenytoin has adverse cognitive effects when given long-term as prophylaxis against PTS.[16]

Treatment guidelines

Based on available information (see above) it appears that:
1. no treatment studied effectively impedes epileptogenesis (i.e., neuronal changes that ultimately lead to late PTS)
2. in high-risk patients (▶ Table 28.1), ASMS reduce the incidence of *early* PTS
3. however, no study has shown that reducing early PTS improves outcome[17]
4. once epilepsy has developed, continued ASMs reduce the recurrence of further seizures

The following are therefore offered as guidelines.

Table 28.1 High risk criteria for PTS

1. acute subdural, epidural, or intracerebral hematoma (SDH, EDH or ICH)
2. open-depressed skull fracture with parenchymal injury
3. seizure within the first 24 hrs after injury
4. Glasgow Coma Scale score < 10
5. penetrating brain injury
6. history of significant alcohol abuse
7. ± cortical (hemorrhagic) contusion on CT

28

Initiation of ASMs

ASMs may be considered for short term use, especially if a seizure could be detrimental. Early post-traumatic seizures were effectively reduced when phenytoin was used for 2 weeks following head injury with no significant increased risk of adverse effects.[18]

Acutely, seizures may elevate ICP, and may adversely affect blood pressure and oxygen delivery, and may worsen other injuries (e.g., spinal cord injury in the setting of an unstable cervical spine). There may also be negative psychological effects on the family, loss of driving privileges, and possibly deleterious effects of excess neurotransmitters.[9]

Option: begin ASMs (usually levetiracetam, phenytoin or carbamazepine) within 24 hrs of injury in the presence of any of the high risk criteria shown in ▶ Table 28.1 (modified[9,12,15,19]). When using PHT, load with 20 mg/kg and maintain high therapeutic levels. Switch to phenobarbital if PHT is not tolerated.

Discontinuation of ASMs

1. taper ASMs after 1 week of therapy except in the following cases:
   a) penetrating brain injury
   b) development of late PTS (i.e., a seizure > 7 days following head trauma)
   c) prior seizure history
   d) patients undergoing craniotomy[20]
2. for patients *not* meeting the criteria to discontinue ASMs after 1 week (see above):
   a) maintain ≈ 6–12 mos of therapeutic ASM levels
   b) recommend EEG to rule out presence of a seizure focus before discontinuing ASMs (shown to have poor predictive value, but probably advisable for legal purposes) for the following:
      • repeated seizures
      • presence of high risk criteria shown in ▶ Table 28.1.

28.3 Alcohol withdrawal seizures

28.3.1 General information

Also, see Alcohol withdrawal syndrome (p. 213). The withdrawal syndrome may begin hours after the EtOH peak; see also prevention and treatment (p. 213). Ethanol withdrawal seizures are classically seen in up to 33% (some say 75%) of habituated drinkers within 7–30 hours of cessation or reduction of ethanol intake. They typically consist of 1–6 tonic-clonic generalized seizures without focality within a 6-hour period.[21] Seizures usually occur before delirium develops. They may also occur during intoxication (without withdrawal).

The seizure risk persists for 48 hrs (risk of delirium tremens [DTs] continues beyond that); thus a single loading dose of PHT is frequently adequate for prophylaxis. However, since most EtOH withdrawal seizures are single, brief, and self-limited, PHT has *not* been shown to be of benefit in uncomplicated cases and is thus *usually not indicated*. Chlordiazepoxide (Librium®) or other benzodiazepines (p. 213) administered during detoxification reduces the risk withdrawal seizures.[22]

28.3.2 Evaluation

The following patients should have a CT scan of the brain, and should be admitted for further evaluation as well as for observation for additional seizures or for DTs:
1. those with their first EtOH withdrawal seizure
2. those with focal findings
3. those having more than 6 seizures in 6 hrs
4. those with evidence of trauma

Other causes of seizure should also be considered, e.g., a febrile patient may require an LP to rule out meningitis.

28.3.3 Treatment

A brief single seizure may not warrant treatment, except as outlined below. A seizure that continues beyond 3–4 minutes may be treated with diazepam or lorazepam, with further measures used as in status epilepticus (p. 510) if seizures persist. Loading with phenytoin (18 mg/kg = 1200 mg/70 kg) and long-term treatment is indicated for:
1. a history of previous alcohol withdrawal seizures

2. recurrent seizures after admission
3. history of a prior seizure disorder unrelated to alcohol
4. presence of other risk factors for seizure (e.g., subdural hematoma)

28.4 Nonepileptic seizures

28.4.1 General information

AKA pseudoseizures (this term has fallen out of favor since it may connote voluntary feigning of seizures), with the term psychogenic non-epileptic attacks (PNEA) being preferred for nonepileptic seizures (NES) with a psychologic etiology (PNEAs are real events and may not be under voluntary control).[23]

One of the hazards of NES is that patients may end up needlessly taking ASMs, which in some cases may worsen NES. Possible etiologies of NES are given in ▶ Table 28.2. Most NES are psychogenic.

NES comprise 20-30% of medically refractory presentations resembling seizures. The incidence is ≈ 4 per 1000,000. They may mimic any seizure type.

DDx for seizures:
1. psychogenic: comprise 20–90% of patients with intractable seizures referred to epilepsy centers. These patients carry the diagnosis of seizures from 5–7 years. Up to 50% of these may have bona fide seizures at some time as well.[24]
2. tic: can be suppressed, is not repetitive (if repetitive, may be hemifacial spasm)
3. movement disorder: myoclonus (can be epileptic or non-epileptic)
   a) cataplexy: e.g., with narcolepsy often provoked by laughter or other emotional stimulus (can rarely be caught on EEG, and when it is, it shows REM intrusion into wakefulness)
   b) parasomnia: a sleep movement disorder (occurs during sleep). Includes: night terrors (occurs in slow wave sleep, vs. nightmare which occurs in REM), sleep walking, REM behavior disorders (usually occurs in older men), and there is a high probability they will go on to have degenerative brain disease (used to be called paroxysmal nocturnal PNT). Head banging is a benign parasomnia
4. syncope: 90% of the time people who faint have myoclonic jerks or shaking[25]
5. TIA

Table 28.2 Differential diagnosis of nonepileptic seizures[23]

psychologic disorders (PNEAs)	a) somatoform disorders: especially conversion disorder b) anxiety disorders: especially panic attack and posttraumatic stress disorder c) dissociative disorders d) psychotic disorders e) impulse control disorders f) attention-deficit disorders[a] g) factitious disorders: including Munchausen's syndrome
cardiovascular disorders	a) syncope b) cardiac arrhythmias c) transient ischemic attacks (TIAs) d) breath-holding spells[a]
migraine syndromes	a) complicated migraines[a] b) basilar migraines
movement disorders	a) tremors b) dyskinesias c) tics[a], spasms d) other (including shivering)
parasomnias & sleep-related disorders	a) night terrors[a], nightmares[a], somnambulism[a] b) narcolepsy, cataplexy c) rapid eye movement behavior disorder d) nocturnal paroxysmal dystonia
gastrointestinal disorders	a) episodic nausea or colic[a] b) cyclic vomiting syndrome[a]
other	a) malingering b) cognitive disorders with episodic behavioral or speech symptoms c) medication effects or toxicity d) daydreams[a]

[a]usually encountered in children

28.4.2 Differentiating NES from epileptic seizures

General information

Distinguishing between epileptic seizures (ES) and NES is a common clinical dilemma. There are unusual seizures that may fool experts.[26] Some frontal lobe and temporal lobe complex partial seizures may produce bizarre behaviors that do not correspond to classic ES findings and may not produce discernible abnormalities with scalp-electrode EEG (and therefore may be misdiagnosed even with video-EEG monitoring, although this is more likely with partial seizures than with generalized). A multidisciplinary team approach may be required.

▶ Table 28.3 contrasts some features of true seizures vs. NES, and ▶ Table 28.4 lists some features often associated with NES. However, no characteristics are definitively diagnostic of NES since a number of them may also occur with ES.

Table 28.3 Features of ES vs. NES[24]

Feature	Epileptic seizure	NES
% males	72%	20%
Clonic UE movement		
in-phase	96%	20%
out-of-phase	0	56%
Clonic LE movement		
in-phase	88%	16%
out-of-phase	0	56%
Vocalizations		
none	16%	56%
start of seizure	24%	44%
middle	60% "epileptic cry"	0
types	only sounds of tonic or clonic respiratory muscle contraction	moans, screams, grunts, snorts, gagging, retching, understandable statements, gasps
Head turning		
unilateral	64%	16%
side-to-side	8% (slow, low amplitude)	36% (violent, high amplitude)

Table 28.4 Features often associated with NES[23]

- frequent seizures despite therapeutic ASMs
- multiple different-physician visits
- lingering prodrome or gradual ictal onset (over minutes)
- prolonged duration (>5 mins)
- manifestations altered by distraction
- suggestible or inducible seizures
- intermittent arrhythmic and out-of-phase convulsive activity
- fluctuating intensity and severity during Sz
- side-to-side rolling, pelvic thrusting, wild movements
- bilateral motor activity with preserved consciousness
- nonphysiologic spread of neurologic signs
- absence of labored breathing or drooling after generalized convulsion
- expression of relief or indifference
- crying or whimpering
- no postictal confusion or lethargy
- disproportionate postictal mental status changes
- absence of stereotypy

Features common to both true seizures and NES: verbal unresponsiveness, rarity of automatisms and whole-body flaccidity, rarity of urinary incontinence. Reminder: some seizures can be bizarre and can resemble NES (sometimes called pseudo-pseudoseizures). 10% of patients with psychogenic seizures actually have epilepsy.

Features suggestive of non-epileptic seizures:

1. arching of the back: 90% specific for NES

2. asynchronous movement
3. stop & go: seizures usually build and then gradually subside
4. forced eye closing during entire seizure
5. provoked with stimuli that would not cause a seizure (e.g., tuning fork to the head, alcohol pad to the neck, IV saline…)
6. bilateral shaking with preserved awareness. Exception: supplementary motor area seizures (mesial frontal area)—these seizures are usually tonic (not clonic)
7. weeping (whining): highly specific
8. multiple or variable seizure types (ES is usually stereotypical), fluctuating level of consciousness, denial of correlation of Sz with stress

If any two of the following are demonstrated, 96% of time this will be NES:
1. out-of-phase clonic UE movement
2. out-of-phase clonic LE movement
3. no vocalization or vocalization at start of event

Clinical features in favor of seizures:
1. injuries: especially lateral tongue laceration which is very specific for seizures[27]
2. very stereotyped
3. duration < 2 minutes
4. eyes open
5. incontinence

History

Attempt to document: prodromal symptoms, precipitating factors, time and environment of Sz, mode and duration of progression, ictal and postictal events, frequency and stereotypy of manifestations. Determine if patient has history of psychiatric conditions, and if they are acquainted with individuals who have ES.

Psychological testing

May help. Differences occur in ES and NES on the Minnesota Multiphasic Personality Inventory (MMPI) scales in hypochondriasis, depression hysteria, and schizophrenia.[28]

28.5 Febrile seizures

28.5.1 Definitions

▶ **Febrile seizure.** See reference.[29]
   A seizure in infants or children associated with fever with no defined cause and unaccompanied by acute neurologic illness (includes seizures during post- vaccination fevers). Some may be inerited as in Genetic Epilepsy with Febrile Seizures Plus (GEFS +).

▶ **Complex febrile seizure.** A convulsion that lasts longer than 15 minutes, is focal, or multiple (more than one convulsion per episode of fever).

▶ **Simple febrile seizure.** Not complex.

▶ **Recurrent febrile seizure.** More than one episode of fever associated with seizures.

28.5.2 Epidemiology

See reference.[29]
   Febrile convulsions are the most common type of seizure. Excluding children with pre-existing neurologic or developmental abnormalities, the prevalence of febrile seizures is ≈ 2.7% (range: 2–5% in U.S. children aged 6 mos-6 yrs). The risk for developing epilepsy after a simple febrile seizure is ≈ 1%, and for a complex febrile seizure is 6% (9% for prolonged seizure, 29% for focal seizure). An underlying neurological or developmental abnormality or a family history of epilepsy increases the risk of developing epilepsy. The notion that the younger the child with a febrile seizure the greater the risk of epilepsy is unproven.

28.5.3 Treatment

In one study, the IQ in the group treated with phenobarbital was 8.4 points lower (95% confidence interval) than the placebo group, and there remained a significant difference several months after discontinuing the drug.[30] Furthermore, there was no significant reduction in seizures in the phenobarbital group. And yet, no other drug really appears well suited to treating this entity: carbamazepine and phenytoin appear ineffective, valproate may be effective but has serious risks in the < 2 yrs of age group. Given the low incidence (1%) of having afebrile seizures (i.e., epilepsy) after a *simple* febrile seizure and the fact that ASMs probably do not prevent this development, there is little support for prescribing antiseizure medications in these cases. The recurrence rate of febrile seizures in children with a history of one or more febrile seizure can be reduced by administering diazepam 0.33 mg/kg PO q 8 hrs during a febrile episode (temp > 38.1 °C) and continuing until 24 hrs after the fever subsides.[31]

28.6 Status epilepticus

28.6.1 General information

Key concepts

- definition: > 30 mins of either 1) continuous seizure activity or 2) ≥ 2 sequential seizures without full recovery of consciousness between seizures
- morbidity and mortality are high in untreated status epilepticus (SE)
- most common etiology: patient with known seizure disorder with low ASM levels
- de novo SE in acute illness is considered a manifestation of the illness which should be treated at the same time as the SE
- begin treatment as soon as a seizure persists > 5 minutes
- see treatment measures (p. 512)
- treatment goal: rapid termination of all clinical and electrical seizure activity

▶ **Definitions. Brief seizure:** seizure lasting < 5 minutes.
  Prolonged seizure: seizure lasting 5-30 minutes
  Status epilepticus: more than 30 minutes of either 1) continuous seizure activity or 2) ≥ 2 sequential seizures without full recovery of consciousness between seizures.[32] Status epilepticus lasting > 30 minutes may lead to permanent neurologic damage[33]

▶ **Important things to know about management**
- since 61% of seizures that persist > 5 mins will continue > 1 hour,[34] and permanent neurologic damage can occur after 30 minutes, treatment should be initiated once a seizure has persisted > 5 minutes (even though technically this is not long enough to be considered SE yet)
- in patients with no prior seizure history, status epilepticus (SE) is usually a manifestation of illness-related cortical irritation or injury[35] and treatment of the underlying disorder (in addition to treating the SE) is critical
- a relapse of seizure in a patient with a known seizure disorder and subtherapeutic ASM levels usually responds to a bolus of the maintenance ASMs. However, true SE should be treated by the standard protocol[35]
- most cases of convulsive status in adults start as partial seizures that generalize secondarily
- treatment goal: rapid termination (not just reduction) of clinical *and* electrical seizure activity
- prognosis is related to seizure etiology, duration of SE, and patient age
- the choice of 1st and 2nd-line ASMs is arbitrary, *dose*[35] and starting treatment in < 30 minutes[36] are more important determinants of success in aborting SE

28.6.2 Types of status epilepticus

See reference.[37]
- generalized status
  1. convulsive status epilepticus (SE): repeated generalized (tonic-clonic, tonic-clonic-tonic, or clonic) seizues with persistent postictal neurologic dysfunction between seizures. This is the most common type of SE.[38] A medical emergency

2. absence (note: in status, this may present in "epileptic twilight" state)
3. secondarily generalized: accounts for ≈ 75% of generalized SE
4. myoclonic
5. atonic (drop attack): especially in Lennox-Gastaut syndrome (p. 484)
- partial status (usually related to an anatomic abnormality)
  1. simple (AKA epilepsy partialis continua): not associated with altered mental status
  2. complex (note: in status, this may present in "epileptic twilight" state) most often from frontal lobe focus. Urgent treatment is required (several case reports of permanent deficits following this)
  3. secondarily generalized
- nonconvulsive SE
  1. benign variants (typical absence SE, complex partial SE)
  2. electrical SE during sleep
  3. atypical absence SE
  4. tonic SE (associated with learning disability in children), SE in coma

Alternatively, SE can be broken down as follows:
- with prominent motor effects
- without prominent motor effects
- boundary syndromes (syndromes which combine encephalopathy, behavioral disturbances, delirium, or psychosis with SE-like EEG findings)

28.6.3 Epidemiology

Incidence: 50,000 to 150,000 new cases/year in the U.S. in the outpatient setting.[35] Most cases occur in young children (among children, 73% were < 5 yrs old[39]); the next most affected group is patients > 60 yrs of age. In > 50% of cases, SE is the patient's first seizure.[38] One out of six patients presenting with a first time seizure will present in SE.

Mortality in children is estimated at < 3%, but is up to 30% in adults.[40]

28.6.4 Etiologies

The most common causes (the short list):
- low level of prescribed ASM in a patient with a seizure disorder (34%)
- remote symptomatic cause (24%)
- stroke (22%)
- metabolic disturbances (15%)
- hypoxia (13%)

The long list:
1. a patient with a known seizure disorder having low ASM levels for any reason (non-compliance, intercurrent infection preventing PO intake of meds, drug-drug interactions → lowering effectiveness of ASMs…)
2. febrile seizures: a common precipitator in young patients. 5–6% of patients presenting with SE have a history of prior febrile seizures
3. stroke: the most commonly identified cause in the elderly
4. CNS infection: in children, most are bacterial, the most common organisms were H. influenza and S. pneumoniae
5. idiopathic: accounts for ≈ one-third (in children, usually associated with fever)
6. epilepsy: is present or is subsequently diagnosed in ≈ 50% of patients presenting with SE. About 10% of adults ultimately diagnosed as having epilepsy will present in SE
7. electrolyte imbalance: hyponatremia (most common in children, usually due to water intoxication[39]), hypoglycemia, hypocalcemia, uremia, hypomagnesemia…
8. illicit drug intoxication: especially cocaine, amphetamines
9. precipitous drug withdrawal: barbiturates, benzodiazepines, alcohol, or narcotics
10. proconvulsant drugs, including: β-lactam antibiotics (penicillins, cephalosporins), certain antidepressants (bupropion), clonazapine, bronchodilators, immunosuppressants
11. traumatic brain injury: acute as well as old
12. hypoxia/ischemia
13. tumor

28

In children < 1 yr of age, 75% had an acute cause: 28% were secondary to CNS infection, 30% due to electrolyte disorders, 19% associated with fever.[39] In adults, a structural lesion is more likely. In an adult, the most common cause of SE is subtherapeutic ASM levels in a patient with a known seizure disorder.

28.6.5 Morbidity and mortality from SE

Outcomes are related to underlying cause and duration of SE. Mean duration of SE in patients without neurologic sequelae is 1.5 hrs (therefore, proceed to pentobarbital anesthesia before ≈ 1 hour of SE). Recent mortality: < 10–12% (only ≈ 2% of deaths are directly attributable to SE or its complications; the rest are due to the underlying process producing the SE). Mortality is lowest among children (≈ 6%[39]), patients with SE related to subtherapeutic ASMs, and patients with unprovoked SE.[41] The highest mortality occurs in elderly patients and those with SE resulting from anoxia or stroke.[41] 1% of patients die during the episode itself.

Morbidity and mortality is due to[42]:

1. CNS injury from repetitive electric discharges: irreversible changes begin to appear in neurons after as little as 20 minutes of convulsive activity. Cell death is very common after 60 mins
2. systemic stress from the seizure (cardiac, respiratory, renal, metabolic)
3. CNS damage by the acute insult that provoked the SE

28.6.6 Treatment

Prehospital phase

1. impending SE: may be heralded by a crescendo in seizures. A 1–3 d course of lorazepam may preempt the development of SE
2. SE treatment may be initiated in the home setting with buccal midazolam or rectal diazepam. For children with SE, midazolam (IM or intranasal or buccal) is probably more effective than diazepam (IV or rectal)[40] (Level B)

General treatment measures for status epilepticus

Treatment success, like morbidity/mortality, may be time-dependent. First-line ASM therapy aborts SE in 60% of patients if initiated within the first 30 minutes, and efficacy decreases as seizure duration increases.[43] As such, treatment should be initiated as soon as possible and should be directed at stabilizing the patient, rapid termination (not just reduction) of clinical and electrical seizure activity, identifying the cause (determining if there is an acute insult to the brain), and, if possible, also treating any underlying process identified. Treatment often must be initiated prior to the availability of test results to confirm the diagnosis and may even be initiated in the pre-hospital setting. The following is modified from the American Epilepsy Society guidelines[40]

0-5 Minutes

Stabilization phase

1. "ABCs"
   a) Airway: oral airway if feasible. Turn patient on their side to avoid aspiration
   b) Breathing: O_2 by nasal cannula or bag-valve-mask. Consider intubation if respirations compromised or if seizure persists > 30 min.
      NB: if paralytics are used to intubate, use short acting agents and be aware that muscle paralysis alone may stop visible seizure manifestations, but does not stop the electrical seizure activity in the brain, which can lead to permanent neurologic damage if prolonged
   c) Circulation: CPR if needed. Large bore proximal IV access (2 if possible: 1 for phenytoin (PHT) (Dilantin®), not necessary if fosphenytoin is available): start with NS KVO
2. begin tracking time from onset of seizure
3. baseline vital signs. Frequent blood pressure checks

4. assess oxygenation: O_2 saturation (via pulse oximeter) or ABG. Administer oxygen via nasal cannula or mask as needed. Intubate if hypoxia or respiratory distress
5. monitor EKG
6. blood glucose: if fingerstick glucose can be obtained immediately and it shows hypoglycemia (glucose < 60 mg/dl), or if no fingerstick glucose can be done, give glucose as below. If it won't delay giving glucose, draw blood for definitive serum glucose first (don't wait for results to give glucose)
    • adult: 100 mg thiamine IV then 50 ml of D50 W IV push.
      NB: thiamine is given first because giving glucose in thiamine deficiency (e.g., patients with poor nutrition such as alcoholics) can precipitate Wernicke's encephalopathy (p.214)
    • children ≥ 2 years: 2 ml/kg of D25 W IV push
    • children < 2 years: 4 ml/kg of D12.5 W IV push
7. secure IV access: large bore proximal IV access (2 if possible, 1 for possible phenytoin)
    • use this opportunity to obtain blood for labs: electrolytes, CBC, LFTs, Mg^{++}, Ca^{++}, ASM levels, toxicology, ABG
    • start maintenance IV fluid with NS @ KVO
8. neurologic exam

As acuity permits

Additional initial measures

28

• EEG monitor if possible (EEG electrodes typically take 45-60 minutes just to apply)
• head CT (usually without contrast)
• correct any electrolyte imbalance (SE due to electrolyte imbalance responds more readily to correction than to ASMs[39])
• if CNS infection is a major consideration, perform LP for CSF analysis (especially in febrile children) unless contraindicated (p.1811). WBC pleocytosis up to 80×10^6/L can occur following SE (benign postictal pleocytosis), and these patients should be treated with antibiotics until infection can be ruled out by negative cultures
• *general* meds for unknown patient:
    a) naloxone (Narcan®) 0.4 mg IVP (in case of narcotics)
    b) ± bicarbonate to counter acidosis (1–2 amps depending on length of seizure)
    c) for neonate < 2 years: consider pyridoxine 100 mg IV push (pyridoxine-dependent seizures constitute a rare autosomal recessive condition that generally presents in the early neonatal period[34])

If seizures continue:

5-20 minutes

Initial therapy phase

• **A benzodiazepine is the drug therapy of choice** (Level A)
  Choose one of the following (they are equivalent in level of recommendation)
    ○ IM midazolam: (for weight > 40 kg give 10 mg; wt 13-40 kg give 5 mg) X 1 dose, OR
    ○ IV lorazepam: 0.1 mg/kg/dose up to max 4 mg/dose, may repeat X 1, OR
    ○ IV diazepam: 0.15-0.2 mg/kg/dose up to max 10 mg/dose, may repeat X 1
• If none of the 3 above options are available or if all are contraindicated, choose one of:
    ○ IV phenobarbital: 15 mg/kg/dose, single dose (Level A), OR
    ○ rectal diazepam (Diastat® gel): 0.2-0.5 mg/kg up to max 20 mg/dose X 1 (Level B), OR
    ○ intranasal midazolam (Level B) or buccal midazolam (Level B)

If seizures continue:

20-40 minutes

Second therapy phase

* **There is no evidence to guide choice of second therapy** (Level U = lack of studies meeting criteria for levels A, B or C).
  Choose one of the following (give as single dose)
  ○ IV fosphenytoin: 20 mg PE/ up to max 1500 mg PE/dose X 1, OR
  ○ IV valproic acid: 40 mg/kg/dose up to max 3000 mg/dose X 1, OR
  ○ IV levitiracetam: 60 mg/kg/dose up to max 4500 mg/dose X 1
* If none of the 3 above options are available or if all are contraindicated:
  ○ IV phenobarbital (if not already given): 15 mg/kg/dose, single dose (Level B)

If seizures continue:

40-60 minutes

Third therapy phase

* **There is no evidence to guide therapy in the 3rd phase** (Level U).
  Options include
  ○ repeat 2nd line therapy, OR
  ○ anesthetic doses of one of thiopental, midazolam, pentobarbital or propofol, together with continuous EEG monitoring

28.6.7 Medications for non-convulsive status epilepticus

In non-convulsive status epilepticus, the first and second line ASMs listed in section 28.6.6 should be utilized. However, many practitioners avoid escalating to the anesthetic options, instead opting for trials of additional ASMs first (carbamazepine, oxcarbazepine, topiramate, lamotrigine, etc).
  Absence status epilepticus almost always responds to diazepam.

28.6.8 Myoclonic status epilepticus

Treatment: valproic acid (drug of choice). Place NG, give 20 mg/kg per NG loading dose. Maintenance: 40 mg/kg/d divided.
  Can add lorazepam (Ativan®) or clonazepam (Klonopin®) to help with acute control.

References

[1] Hauser WA, Annegers JF, Kurland LT. Incidence of Epilepsy and Unprovoked Seizures in Rochester, Minnesota, 1935-1984. Epilepsia. 1993; 34:453–468

[2] Hauser WA, Anderson VE, Loewenson RB, et al. Seizure Recurrence After a First Unprovoked Seizure. New Engl J Med. 1982; 307:522–528

[3] Reith J, Jorgensen HS, Nakayama H, et al. Seizures in acute stroke: Predictors and prognostic significance. The Copenhagen stroke study. Stroke. 1997; 28:1585–1589

[4] Landfish N, Gieron-Korthals M, Weibley RE, et al. New Onset Childhood Seizures: Emergency Department Experience. Journal of the Florida Medical Association. 1992; 79:697–700

[5] Hauser WA, Rich SS, Jacobs MP, et al. Patterns of Seizure Occurrence and Recurrence Risks in Patients with Newly Diagnosed Epilepsy. Epilepsia. 1983; 24:516–517

[6] van Donselaar C, Schimsheimer R-J, Geerts AT, et al. Value of the Electroencephalogram in Adult Patients With Untreated Idiopathic First Seizures. Arch Neurol. 1992; 49:231–237

[7] Young B, Rapp RP, Norton JA, et al. Failure of Prophylactically Administered Phenytoin to Prevent Late Posttraumatic Seizures. J Neurosurg. 1983; 58:236–241

[8] Annegers JF, Grabow JD, Groover RV, et al. Seizures After Head Trauma: A Population Study. Neurology. 1980; 30:683–689

[9] Bullock R, Chesnut RM, Clifton G, et al. Guidelines for the Management of Severe Head Injury. 1995

[10] McQueen JK, Blackwood DHR, Harris P, et al. Low Risk of Late Posttraumatic Seizures Following Severe Head Injury. J Neurol Neurosurg Psychiatry. 1983; 46:899–904

[11] Young B, Rapp RP, Norton JA, et al. Failure of Prophylactically Administered Phenytoin to Prevent

Early Posttraumatic Seizures. J Neurosurg. 1983; 58:231–235

[12] Hahn YS, Fuchs S, Flannery AM, et al. Factors Influencing Posttraumatic Seizures in Children. Neurosurgery. 1988; 22:864–867

[13] Weiss GH, Salazar AM, Vance SC, et al. Predicting Posttraumatic Epilepsy in Penetrating Head Injury. Archives of Neurology. 1986; 43:771–773

[14] Temkin NR, Dikmen SS, Winn HR. Posttraumatic Seizures. Neurosurgery Clinics of North America. 1991; 2:425–435

[15] Temkin NR, Dikmen SS, Wilensky AJ, et al. A Randomized, Double-Blind Study of Phenytoin for the Prevention of Post-Traumatic Seizures. N Engl J Med. 1990; 323:497–502

[16] Dikmen SS, Temkin NR, Miller B, et al. Neurobehavioral Effects of Phenytoin Prophylaxis of Posttraumatic Seizures. JAMA. 1991; 265:1271–1277

[17] Brain Trauma Foundation, Povlishock JT, Bullock MR. Antiseizure prophylaxis. J Neurotrauma. 2007; 24:S83–S86

[18] Haltiner AM, Newell DW, Temkin NR, et al. Side Effects and Mortality Associated with Use of Phenytoin for Early Posttraumatic Seizure Prophylaxis. Journal of Neurosurgery. 1999; 91:588–592

[19] Yablon SA. Posttraumatic seizures. Arch Phys Med Rehabil. 1993; 74:983–1001

[20] North JB, Penhall RK, Hanieh A, et al. Phenytoin and Postoperative Epilepsy: A Double-Blind Study. J Neurosurg. 1983; 58:672–677

[21] Charness ME, Simon RP, Greenberg DA. Ethanol and the Nervous System. N Engl J Med. 1989; 321:442–454

[22] Lechtenberg R, Worner TM. Seizure Risk With Recurrent Alcohol Detoxification. Arch Neurol. 1990; 47:535–538

[23] Chabolla DR, Krahn LE, So EL, et al. Psychogenic Nonepileptic Seizures. Mayo Clinic Proceedings. 1996; 71:493–500

[24] Gates JR, Ramani V, Whalen S, et al. Ictal Characteristics of Pseudoseizures. Arch Neurol. 1985; 42:1183–1187

[25] Lempert T, Bauer M, Schmidt D. Syncope: a videometric analysis of 56 episodes of transient cerebral hypoxia. Ann Neurol. 1994; 36:233–237

[26] King DW, Gallagher BB, Marvin AJ, et al. Pseudoseizures: Diagnostic Evaluation. Neurology. 1982; 32:18–23

[27] Benbadis SR, Wolgamuth BR, Goren H, et al. Value of tongue biting in the diagnosis of seizures. Arch Intern Med. 1995; 155:2346–2349

[28] Henrichs TF, Tucker DM, Farha J, et al. MMPI Indices in the Identification of Patients Evidencing Pseudoseizures. Epilepsia. 1988; 29:184–187

[29] Verity CM, Golding J. Risk of Epilepsy After Febrile Convulsions: A National Cohort Study. BMJ. 1991; 303:1373–1376

[30] Farwell JR, Lee YJ, Hirtz DG, et al. Phenobarbital for Febrile Seizures - Effects on Intelligence and on Seizure Recurrence. N Engl J Med. 1990; 322:364–369

[31] Rosman NP, Colton T, Labazzo J, et al. A Controlled Trial of Diazepam Administered During Febrile Illnesses to Prevent Recurrence of Febrile Seizures. New England Journal of Medicine. 1993; 329:79–84

[32] Glauser TA. Designing practical evidence-based treatment plans for children with prolonged seizures and status epilepticus. J Child Neurol. 2007; 22:38S–46S

[33] Treatment of convulsive status epilepticus. Recommendations of the Epilepsy Foundation of America's Working Group on Status Epilepticus. Journal of the American Medical Association. 1993; 270:854–859

[34] Abend NS, Dlugos DJ. Treatment of refractory status epilepticus: literature review and a proposed protocol. Pediatric Neurology. 2008; 38:377–390

[35] Costello DJ, Cole AJ. Treatment of acute seizures and status epilepticus. Journal of Intensive Care Medicine. 2007; 22:319–347

[36] Eriksson K, Metsaranta P, Huhtala H, et al. Treatment delay and the risk of prolonged status epilepticus. Neurology. 2005; 65:1316–1318

[37] Varelas PN, Spanaki MV, Mirski MA. Status epilepticus: an update. Curr Neurol Neurosci Rep. 2013; 13. DOI: 10.1007/s11910-013-0357-0

[38] Hauser WA. Status Epilepticus: Epidemiologic Considerations. Neurology. 1990; 40:9–13

[39] Phillips SA, Shanahan RJ. Etiology and Mortality of Status Epilepticus in Children. Archives of Neurology. 1989; 46:74–76

[40] Glauser T, Shinnar S, Gloss D, et al. Evidence-Based Guideline: Treatment of Convulsive Status Epilepticus in Children and Adults: Report of the Guideline Committee of the American Epilepsy Society. Epilepsy Curr. 2016; 16:48–61

[41] Delorenzo RJ, Pellock JM, Towne AR, et al. Epidemiology of Status Epilepticus. J Clin Neurophysiol. 1995; 12:312–325

[42] Fountain NB, Lothman EW. Pathophysiology of Status Epilepticus. J Clin Neurophysiol. 1995; 12:326–342

[43] Lowenstein DH. The management of refractory status epilepticus: an update. Epilepsia. 2006; 47 Suppl 1:35–40

28

Part IX

Pain

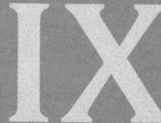

29 Pain

29.1 Major types of pain

Major types of pain:
1. nociceptive pain
   a) somatic: well localized. Described as sharp, stabbing, aching or cramping. Results from tissue injury or inflammation, or from nerve or plexus compression. Responds to treating the underlying pathology or by interrupting the nociceptive pathway
   b) visceral: poorly localized. Poor response to primary pain medications
2. deafferentation pain: poorly localized. Described as crushing, tearing, tingling or numbness. Also causes burning dysesthesia numbness often with lancinating pain, and hyperpathia. Unaffected by ablative procedures
3. "sympathetically maintained" pain and the likes, e.g., causalgia (p.525)

29.2 Neuropathic pain syndromes

29.2.1 General information

Definition: Neuropathic pain: pain caused by a lesion of the peripheral and/or central nervous system manifesting with sensory symptoms and signs (Backonja[1] modified from the International Association for the Study of Pain[2]).

Neuropathic pain syndromes (NPS) are typified by painful diabetic neuropathy (PDN) and postherpetic neuralgia (PHN). Common chronic NPSs are shown in ▶ Table 29.1,[3] divided into central or peripheral nervous system origin of the pain. The pain of PDN and PHN is typically burning and aching, is continuous, and is characteristically refractory to medical and surgical treatment.

29

Table 29.1 Common neuropathic pain syndromes

Peripheral neuropathic pain
acute & chronic inflammatory demyelinating polyneuropathy (CIDP)
alcoholic polyneuropathy
chemotherapy-induced polyneuropathy
complex regional pain syndrome (CRPS)
entrapment neuropathies
HIV sensory neuropathy
iatrogenic neuralgias (e.g., postthoracotomy pain)
idiopathic sensory neuropathy
neoplastic nerve compression or infiltration
nutritional-deficiency neuropathies
painful diabetic neuropathy (PDN)
phantom limb pain
postherpetic neuralgia (PHN)
postradiation plexopathy
radiculopathy
toxic exposure-related neuropathies
trigeminal neuralgia
posttraumatic neuralgias

Central neuropathic pain
cervical spondylotic myelopathy
HIV myelopathy
multiple sclerosis-related pain
Parkinson's disease-related pain
postischemic myelopathy
postradiation myelopathy
poststroke pain
posttraumatic spinal cord injury pain
syringomyelia

29.2.2 Medical treatment of neuropathic pain

General information

Treatment traditionally includes narcotic analgesics,[4] and tricyclic antidepressants (see below). For further details and other treatment measures, see PHN (p. 523).

Tricyclic antidepressants

Use is often limited by anticholinergic and central effects and by limited pain relief.[5,6] Possibly because serotonin potentiates the analgesic effect of endorphins and elevates pain thresholds, serotonin re-uptake blockers are more effective than norepinephrine re-uptake blockers, e.g., trazodone (Desyrel®) blocks only serotonin. Also useful: amitriptyline (Elavil®) 75 mg daily; desipramine (Norpramin®) 10–25 mg/d; doxepin (Sinequan®) 75–150 mg/d. Some benefit may also derive from the fact that many patients with chronic pain are depressed. **Side effects:** anticholinergic effects and orthostatic hypotension, especially in the elderly. ✖ Not recommended for use in patients with ischemic heart disease.

Gabapentin

Effective in postherpetic neuralgia (PHN) (p. 524) and painful diabetic neuropathy. Benefit also reported in pain associated with trigeminal neuralgia, cancer,[7] multiple sclerosis, HIV-related sensory neuropathy, CRPS, spinal cord injury, postoperative state,[8] migraine[9] (a number of these studies may have been sponsored by the manufacturer[10]). See also side effects, dosing & availability... (p. 496)

Lidocaine patch (Lidoderm®)

May be effective.[3] ℞: apply patch for up to 12 hrs/day up to a maximum of 3 patches at a time to the intact skin over the most painful area (may trim patch to appropriate size). **Supplied:** 5% lidocaine (p. 525).

Tramadol (Ultram®)

A centrally acting analgesic (p. 147).[3]

29.3 Craniofacial pain syndromes

29.3.1 General information

Possible pathways for *facial* pain include trigeminal nerve (portio major as well as portio minor [motor root]), facial nerve (usually deep facial pain), and eighth nerve.[11] Etiologies (adapted[12(p 2328),13]):
1. cephalic neuralgias
   a) trigeminal neuralgia (p. 1857)
      • vascular compression of Cr. N. V by the SCA at root entry zone: the most common cause
      • MS: plaque within Cr. N. V nucleus
   b) glossopharyngeal neuralgia (p. 1873): pain usually in base of tongue and adjacent pharynx
   c) geniculate neuralgia (p. 1873): otalgia and deep prosopalgia
   d) tic convulsif (p. 1873): geniculate neuralgia with hemifacial spasm
   e) occipital neuralgia (p. 541)
   f) superior laryngeal neuralgia: a branch of the vagus, results primarily in laryngeal pain and occasionally pain on the auricle
   g) sphenopalatine neuralgia
   h) herpes zoster: pain is continuous (not paroxysmal). Characteristic vesicles and crusting usually follow pain, most often in distribution of V1 (isolated V1 TGN is rare). In rare cases without vesicles, diagnosis may be difficult
   i) postherpetic neuralgia (p. 1873)
   j) Ramsay-Hunt syndrome: reactivation of herpes zoster in the geniculate ganglion (AKA herpes zoster oticus). Triad: ispilateral facial paralysis, ear pain and veiscles on the face, ear, or in the ear
   k) supraorbital neuralgia (SON) (p. 521)
   l) trigeminal neuropathic pain (AKA trigeminal deafferentation pain)[13]: may follow injuries from sinus or dental surgery, head trauma

29

m) trigeminal deafferentation pain: follows trigeminal denervation, including therapeutic measures to treat trigeminal neuralgia[13]

n) short-lasting unilateral neuralgiform headache with conjunctival injection and tearing (SUNCT)[14]: rare. Usually affects males 23–77 years old. Brief (< 2 minutes) pain (burning, stabbing or shock-like) usually near the eye, occurring multiple times per day. Associated autonomic findings (the "hallmark of SUNCT"): ptosis, conjunctival injection, lacrimation, rhinorrhea, hyperemia. May be due to CPA AVM. Microvascular decompression or trigeminal rhizotomy may be effective in some cases refractory to medical treatment with ASMs or corticosteroids. Note: lacrimation (the most common) or other autonomic signs may occur in V1 trigeminal neuralgia but are usually mild, and appear only in the later stages of the condition and with long lasting attacks.[15] Dramatic lacrimation and conjunctival injection from the onset of symptoms with SUNCT are the best characteristics to distinguish this from trigeminal neuralgia.[16] May also occur in cluster headache (p. 183).

2. ophthalmic pain
   a) Tolosa-Hunt syndrome (p. 600): painful ophthalmoplegia
   b) (Raeder's) paratrigeminal neuralgia (p. 601): unilateral Horner syndrome + trigeminal neuralgia
   c) orbital pseudotumor (p. 600): proptosis, pain, and EOM dysfunction
   d) diabetic (oculomotor) neuritis
   e) optic neuritis
   f) iritis
   g) glaucoma
   h) anterior uveitis

3. otalgia (see below)

4. masticatory disorders
   a) dental or periodontal disease
   b) nerve injury (inferior and/or superior alveolar nerves)
   c) temporo-mandibular joint (TMJ) dysfunction
   d) elongated styloid process
   e) temporal & masseter myositis

5. vascular pain syndromes
   a) migraine headaches: see Migraine (p. 183)
      • simple migraine: includes classic migraine, common migraine
      • complicated migraine: includes hemiplegic migraine, ophthalmoplegic migraine
   b) cluster H/A (p. 183); subtypes: episodic, chronic, chronic paroxysmal hemicrania
   c) giant cell arteritis (p. 203) (temporal arteritis). Tenderness over STA
   d) toxic or metabolic vascular H/A (fever, hypercapnia, EtOH, nitrites, hypoxia, hypoglycemia, caffeine withdrawal)
   e) hypertensive H/A
   f) aneurysm or AVM (due either to mass effect or hemorrhage)
   g) carotidynia: e.g., with carotid dissection (p. 1578)
   h) basilar dolichoectasia with fifth n. compression or indentation of the pons

6. sinusitis (maxillary, frontal, ethmoidal, sphenoidal)

7. dental disease

8. neoplasm: may cause referred pain or fifth nerve compression
   a) extracranial
   b) intracranial tumor: primarily posterior fossa lesions, neoplastic compression of trigeminal nerve usually causes sensory deficit (p. 1859)

9. atypical facial pain (AFP) (prosopalgia): traditionally a "wastebasket" category used for many things. It has been proposed[13] to reserve this term for a psychogenic disorder

10. primary (nonvascular) H/A: including
    a) tension (muscle contraction) H/A
    b) posttraumatic H/A

29.3.2 Otalgia

General information

Because of redundant innervation of the region of the ear, *primary* otalgia may have its source in the 5th, 7th, 9th, or 10th cranial nerves or the occipital nerves.[17] As a result, sectioning of the 5th, 9th or 10th nerve or a component of the 7th (nervus intermedius, chorda tympani, geniculate ganglion) has been performed with varying results.[18] Also, microvascular decompression (MVD) of the corresponding nerve may also be done.[19]

Work-up includes neurotologic evaluation to rule out causes of secondary otalgia (otitis media or externa, temporal bone neoplasms…). CT or MRI should be done in any case where no cause is found.

Primary otalgia

Primary otalgia is unilateral in most (≈ 80%). Trigger mechanisms are identified in slightly more than half, with cold air or water being the most common.[18] About 75% have associated aural symptoms: hearing loss, tinnitus, vertigo. Pain relief upon cocainization or nerve block of the pharyngeal tonsils suggests glossopharyngeal neuralgia (p.1873); however, the overlap of innervation limits the certainty.

An initial trial with medications used in trigeminal neuralgia (carbamazepine, phenytoin, baclofen…) (p.1860) is the first line of defense. In intractable cases not responding to pharyngeal anesthesia, suboccipital exploration of the 7th (nervus intermedius) and lower cranial nerves may be indicated. If significant vascular compression is found, one may consider MVD alone. If MVD fails, or if no significant vessels are found, Rupa et al recommend sectioning the nervus intermedius, the 9th and upper 2 fibers of 10th nerve, and a geniculate ganglionectomy (or, if glossopharyngeal neuralgia is strongly suspected, just 9th and upper 2 fibers of 10th).[18]

29.3.3 Supraorbital and supratrochlear neuralgia

Anatomy

The supraorbital and supratrochlear nerves arise from the frontal nerve and are 2 of the 5 branches of V1 (ophthalmic division of the trigeminal nerve). The supraorbital nerve is the largest branch. It exits the orbit through the supraorbital notch or foramen, usually within the medial third of the orbital roof (mean distance from exit to medial angle of orbit: 20 mm (range: 5–47)[20]). The supratrochlear nerve exits the orbit without a foramen or notch 3–38 mm medial to the supraorbital nerve (mean: 15.3 mm[20]); the most medial branch varies from 8–30 mm lateral to the patient's midline.[20]

Supraorbital neuralgia characteristics

Trigeminal neuralgia (TGN) may present with pain in the distribution of the supraorbital nerve; however, the supraorbital nerve may be involved in supraorbital neuralgia (SON), a distinct syndrome with different clinical characteristics. SON is a rare condition slightly more common in women, with onset typically 40–50 years of age.[21] Characteristics[22]: 1) unilateral pain in the distribution of the supraorbital nerve (▶ Fig. 104.2), 2) tenderness in the region of the supraorbital notch or along the distribution of the nerve, and 3) temporary relief with nerve block.

The pain is usually chronic-continuous or remitting-intermittent.[21]

SON may be:
1. primary (no identifiable etiology): these cases lack any sensory loss
2. secondary (e.g., due to trauma to the area, or resulting from chronic pressure such as with wearing swim goggles): more common than primary SON. Most cases remit within one year[21] with elimination of the offending pressure

Supratrochlear neuralgia

Cases of pain isolated to the supratrochlear nerve appear to exist. Supratrochlear neuralgia (STN) may be differentiated from SON by restriction of pain in the more medial forehead, and with relief on blockade of the supratrochlear nerve alone.

Differential diagnosis

1. migraine: suggested by nausea, vomiting, and photophobia
2. associated autonomic activity is rare with SON, and should prompt consideration of cluster H/A (p.183) or SUNCT (p.520)
3. TGN: typical TGN features *lacking* in SON include characteristic triggers and pain consisting exclusively of paroxysmal/ultra-brief electric-shock–like pain
4. hemicrania continua: continuous unilateral pain that tends to be located more posteriorly and is absolutely responsive to indomethacin[22]
5. trochleitis: inflammation of the trochlea/superior-oblique muscle complex, may mimic supratrochlear neuralgia with pain of the medial upper orbit extending a short distance to the forehead.[23]

The pain is typically exacerbated by supraduction of the eye and to palpation of the trochlea, and is relieved with injection of local anesthetic or by the usually definitive treatment of infiltration of corticosteroids close to the trochlea. Diplopia is rare and minimal

6. nummular (coin-like) H/A[24]: round or oval 2–6 cm diameter area of pressure-like continuous head pain without underlying structural abnormality. In 13 patients, 9 (70%) the area was located at the parieto-occipital junction. 9 (70%) demonstrated hypoesthesia and touch provoked paresthesias in the affected area

Treatment

Gabapentin (800–2400 mg/d) or pregabalin (150 mg/d) is helpful for some.[25]

Topical capsaicin (p. 1861) applied to the symptomatic area may help.

Refractory cases may respond to rhizotomy with alcohol (providing an average of 8.5 months relief[26]) or with radiofrequency ablation.

Persistent cases may require exploration and decompression of the nerve by lysing bands overlying the supraorbital notch,[27] or, ultimately, to neurectomy (p. 1862) which provides an average of 33.2 months relief.[28]

29.4 Postherpetic neuralgia

29.4.1 General information

Herpes zoster (HZ) (Greek: zoster – girdle) (shingles in lay terms): painful vesicular cutaneous eruptions caused by the herpes varicella zoster virus (VZV) (the etiologic agent of chickenpox, a herpes virus that is distinct from herpes simplex virus). It occurs in a dermatomal distribution over one side of the thorax in ≈ 65% of cases (rarely, infections occur without vesicles, called zoster sine herpete). In 20% of cases it involves the trigeminal nerve (with a predilection for the ophthalmic division, called herpes zoster ophthalmicus). Pain usually resolves after 2–4 weeks. When the pain persists > 1 month after the vesicular eruption has healed, this pain syndrome is known as postherpetic neuralgia (PHN). PHN can follow a herpes varicella infection in any site and is difficult to treat by any means (medical or surgical). It can occasionally be seen in a limb, and follows a dermatomal distribution (*not* a peripheral nerve distribution). PHN may remit spontaneously, but if it hasn't done so by 6 mos this is unlikely.

29.4.2 Epidemiology

Incidence of herpes zoster is ≈ 125/100,000/year in the general population, or about 850,000 cases per year in the U.S.[29] Both sexes are equally affected. There is no seasonal variance. HZ is also more common in those with reduced immunity and in those with a coexistent malignancy (especially lympho-proliferative).[30,31] PHN occurs in ≈ 10% of cases of HZ.[29] Both HZ and PHN are more common in older patients (PHN is rare in age < 40 yrs, and usually occurs in age > 60) and in those with diabetes mellitus. PHN is more likely after ophthalmic HZ than after spinal segmental involvement.

29.4.3 Etiology

It is postulated that the VZV lies dormant in the sensory ganglia (dorsal root ganglia of the spine, trigeminal (semilunar) ganglion for facial involvement) until such time that the patient's immune system is weakened and then the virus erupts. Inflammatory changes within the nerve are present early and are later replaced by fibrosis.

29.4.4 Clinical

PHN is usually described as a constant burning and aching. There may be superimposed shocks or jabs. It rarely produces throbbing or cramping pain. Pain may be spontaneous, or may be triggered by light cutaneous stimulation (allodynia) (e.g., by clothing), and may be relieved by constant pressure. The pain is present to some degree at all times with no pain-free intervals. Scars and pigmentary changes from the acute vesicular eruption are usually visible. It is not known if PHN can follow zoster sine herpete. The involved area may demonstrate hypesthesia, hypalgesia, paresthesias and dysesthesias.

29.4.5 Medical treatment

For herpes zoster

Varicella vaccination of older individuals can increase immunity to herpes zoster, but it will be several years before it can be determined if this will reduce PHN.[29]

Treatment for the pain of the *acute* attack of herpes zoster may be accomplished with epidural or paravertebral somatic (intercostal) nerve block.[32(p 4018)]

Oral antiherpetic drugs: Also effective (they shorten the duration of pain), and also reduce the incidence of PHN. They may cause thrombotic thrombocytopenic purpura/hemolytic uremic syndrome (TTP/HUS) when used in severely immunocompromised patients at high doses. These drugs include:

Acyclovir (Zovirax®): poorly absorbed from the GI tract (15–30% bioavailability). ℞ 800 mg PO q 4 hrs 5 times/d × 7 d.

Valacyclovir (Valtrex®)[33] is a prodrug of acyclovir and is more completely absorbed and should be equally as effective with fewer daily doses. ℞ 1,000 mg PO TID starting within 72 hrs of onset of the rash × 7 days.

Famciclovir (Famvir®): ℞ 500 mg PO TID × 7 d.

For post-herpetic neuralgia

General information

Most drugs useful for trigeminal neuralgia (p. 1860) are less effective for PHN. Some treatment alternatives for PHN are summarized in ▶ Table 29.2. Details of some drugs follows. It is suggested to initiate therapy with lidocaine skin patches (p. 525) since this modality has the lowest potential for serious side effects.[29]

29

Table 29.2 Medical treatments for PHN[a]

Treatment	Efficacy
PHN treatments that appear effective	
tricyclic antidepressants	widely used for PHN (see text)
lidocaine patch (Lidoderm®)[34]	effective, few side effects (p. 525)
intrathecal steroids + lidocaine (see text)	appears very effective, larger studies & long-term follow-up needed
Gabapentin	proven efficacy (see text)
oxycodone CR 10 mg PO BID[4]	proven efficacy
Treatments of questionable efficacy	
SSRIs[b]	may be effective
SNRIs	may be effective
Tramadol	may be effective
topical capsaicin	controversial (see text)
Iontophoresis	insufficient evidence
nonsteroidal creams	questionable
aspirin suspended in acetone, ether or chloroform	questionable
EMLA cream	questionable
Treatments that are not useful	
dextromethorphan, benzodiazepines, acyclovir, acupuncture	no benefit[35]
ketamine (NMDA receptor antagonist)	may be beneficial, but hepatotoxic
Preventative treatment	
oral antiherpetic drugs given during HZ infection	shortens length of HZ, may reduce incidence of PHN
varicella vaccination of older patients	trials of this strategy are in progress[29]

[a]modified with permission from Rubin M, Relief for postherpetic neuralgia, **Neurology Alert**, 6: 33–4, 2001
[b]abbreviations: oxycodone CR = controlled release (Oxycontin®); HZ = herpes zoster; PHN = postherpetic neuralgia; SNRIs = serotonin-norepinephrine reuptake inhibitor; SSRIs = selective serotonin reuptake inhibitors (e.g., Prosac®),

Antiseizure medications for post-herpetic neuralgia

Drug info: Gabapentin (Neurontin®)

FDA approved only for partial seizures and postherpetic neuralgia (PHN).
Side effects: dizziness and somnolence (usually during titration, often diminish with time). Ataxia, fatigue, peripheral edema, confusion and depression may occur.

℞ For PHN, start with 300 mg on Day 1, 300 mg BID on Day 2, and 300 mg TID on Day 3. Dose may be titrated up to 1800 mg/d divided TID. To limit daytime drowsiness, patients may need to start with 100 mg at hs and increase slowly over 3–8. Although doses up to 3600 mg/day (the antiseizure dose) were studied[36] there was no significant benefit for PHN over 1800 mg/d. Lower doses are required for renal insufficiency. **Supplied:** 100, 300 & 400 mg capsules; 600 & 800 mg scored tabs. 50 mg/ml suspension.

Drug info: Oxcarbazepine (Trileptal®)

℞ 150 mg PO BID.

Drug info: Zonisamide (Zonegran®)

℞ Initiate therapy with 100 mg PO q PM × 2 wks, then increase dose by 100 mg/d q 2 wks up to 400 mg/d. Bioavailability is not affected by food. Steady state is achieved within 14 days of dosage changes. **Supplied :** 100 mg capsules.

Tricyclic antidepressants (TCA)

Drug info: Amitriptyline (Elavil®)

Helpful in ≈ 66% of patients at a mean dose of 75 mg/d even without antidepressant effect.[5] **Side effects:** see Amitriptyline, side effects (p. 572), minimized by starting low and slowly incrementing dose.

℞ Start with 12.5–25 mg PO q hs, and increase by the same amount q 2–5 days to a maximum of 150 mg/d.

Drug info: Nortriptyline (Pamelor®)

Fewer side effects than amitriptyline.
℞ Start with 10–20 mg PO q hs, and increase gradually.

Topical treatment

Drug info: Capsaicin (Zostrix®)

A vanillyl alkaloid derived from hot peppers, available without prescription for topical treatment of the pain of herpes zoster and diabetic neuropathy. Beneficial in some patients with either of these conditions (response rate at 8 weeks was 90% for PHN, 71% for diabetic neuropathy, vs. 50% with placebo in either group), although the high placebo response rate is disturbing and many authorities are skeptical.[37] Expensive. **Side effects:** include burning and erythema at the application site (usually subsides by 2–4 weeks).

R Manufacturer recommends massaging the medication into the affected area of the skin TID-QID (apply a very thin coat). Some authorities recommend q 2 hr application. Avoid contact with eyes or damaged skin. Supplied as Zostrix® (0.25% capsaicin) or Zostrix-HP® (0.75%).

Drug info: Lidocaine patch 5% (Lidoderm®)

Often better tolerated by elderly patients than TCAs (due to pre-existing cognitive impairments, cardiac disease, or systemic illness).

R Apply up to 3 patches of 5% lidocaine (to cover a maximum of 420 cm^2) to intact skin q 12 hrs to cover as much of the area of greatest pain as possible.[34]

Intrathecal steroids

Over 90% of patients receiving intrathecal methylprednisolone (60 mg) + 3% lidocaine (3 ml) given once per week for up to 4 weeks, reported good to excellent pain relief for up to 2 years.[38] This technique was not studied for use in PHN involving the trigeminal nerve. Further clinical trials are needed to verify the efficacy and safety[29] (potential long-term side effects include adhesive arachnoiditis).

Surgical treatment

There is no operation that is uniformly successful in treating PHN. Numerous operations have been shown to work occasionally. Procedures that have been tried include:

1. nerve blocks: once PHN is established, nerve blocks provide only temporary relief[39]
2. cordotomy: although percutaneous cordotomy (p. 1878) may work when the level of PHN is at least 3–4 segments below the cordotomy, this procedure is not recommended for pain of benign etiology because of possible complications and the high likelihood of pain recurrence
3. rhizotomy: including retrogasserian for facial involvement
4. neurectomies
5. sympathectomy
6. DREZ (p. 1886)[40]: often offers good early relief, but recurrence rate is high
7. acupuncture[41]
8. TENS
9. spinal cord stimulation (p. 1883)
10. undermining the skin
11. motor cortex stimulation: for *facial* PHN

29.5 Complex regional pain syndrome (CRPS)

29.5.1 General information

The terminology is confusing. Formerly also called causalgia (reflex sympathetic dystrophy). The term causalgia (Greek: kausis – burning, algos – pain) was introduced by Weir Mitchell in 1864. It was used to describe a rare syndrome that followed a minority of *partial* peripheral nerve injuries in the American civil war. *Triad*: burning pain, autonomic dysfunction, and trophic changes.

CRPS Type II (AKA major causalgia) follows nerve injury (originally described after high velocity missile injuries). CRPS Type I (AKA reflex sympathetic dystrophy or causalgia minor) denoted less severe forms, and has been described after non-penetrating trauma.[42] Shoulder-hand syndrome and Sudeck's atrophy are other variant designations. In 1916, the autonomic nervous system was implicated by René Leriche, and the term reflex sympathetic dystrophy (RSD) later came into use[43] (but RSD may be distinct from causalgia[44]).

Post-op CRPS has been described following carpal tunnel surgery as well as surgery on the lumbar[45] and cervical spine.

A contemporary definition might be: a disproportionate pain syndrome caused by nerve damage and resultant sympathetic dysfunction.[46] It may arise from direct injury to a nerve (type 1), or indirectly due to damage to surrounding tissue (type 2).[47]

At best, CRPS must be regarded as a symptom complex, and not as a discrete syndrome nor medical entity (for a cogent editorial on the subject, see the essay by Ochoa[48]). Patients exhibiting CRPS phenomenology are not a homogeneous group, and include[49]:

1. actual CRPS (for these, Mailis proposes the term "physiogenic RSD"): a complex set of neuropathic phenomena that may occur with or without nerve injury
2. medical conditions distinct from CRPS but with signs and symptoms that mimic CRPS: vascular, inflammatory, neurologic...
3. the product of mere immobilization: as in severe pain avoidance behavior, or at times psychiatric disorders
4. part of a factitious disorder with either a psychological basis (e.g., Munchausen's syndrome) or for secondary gain (financial, drug seeking...) i.e., malingering

29.5.2 Pathogenesis

Early theories invoked ephaptic transmission between sympathetics and afferent pain fibers. This theory is rarely cited currently. Another more recent postulate involves norepinephrine released at sympathetic terminals together with hypersensitivity secondary to denervation or sprouting. Many modern hypotheses do not even embrace involvement of the autonomic nervous system in all cases.[43,44,49]

Thus, many of the alterations seen in CRPS may simply be epiphenomena rather than part of the etiopathogenetic mechanism.

29.5.3 Clinical

CRPS may be described as a phenomenology, i.e., a variable complex of signs and symptoms due to multiple etiologies included in this nonhomogeneous group.[49] No diagnostic criteria for the condition have been established, and various investigators select different factors to include or exclude patients from their studies.

29.5.4 Symptoms

Pain: affecting a limb, usually burning, and prominent in the hand or foot. Onset in the majority is within 24 hrs of injury (unless injury causes anesthesia, then hrs or days may intervene); however, CRPS may take days to weeks to develop. Median, ulnar and sciatic nerves are the most commonly cited involved nerves. However, it is not always possible to identify a specific nerve that has been injured. Almost any sensory stimulus worsens the pain (allodynia is pain induced by a nonnoxious stimulus).

29.5.5 Signs

The physical exam is often difficult due to pain.

Vascular changes: either vasodilator (warm and pink) or vasoconstrictor (cold, mottled blue). Trophic changes (may be partly or wholly due to immobility): dry/scaly skin, stiff joints, tapering fingers, ridged uncut nails, either long/coarse hair or loss of hair, sweating alterations (varies from anhidrosis to hyperhidrosis).

29.5.6 Diagnostic aids

In the absence of an agreed upon etiology or pathophysiology, there can be no basis for specific tests, and the lack of a "gold-standard" diagnostic criteria makes it impossible to verify the authenticity of any diagnostic marker. Numerous tests have been presented as aids to the diagnosis of CRPS, and essentially all have eventually been refuted. Candidates have included:

1. thermography: discredited in clinical practice
2. three-phase bone scan: typical CRPS changes also occur after sympathectomy,[50] which has traditionally been considered curative of CRPS
3. osteoporosis on X-ray,[51] particularly periarticular demineralization: nonspecific
4. response to sympathetic block (once thought to be the sine qua non for causalgia major and minor, the response sought was relief (complete or significant) with sympathetic block of appropriate trunk (stellate for UE, lumbar for LE)): has failed to hold up once stringent placebo-controlled trials were executed

5. various autonomic tests[52]: resting sweat output, resting skin temperature, quantitative sudomotor axon reflex test

29.5.7 Treatment

In the absence of a delineated pathophysiology, treatment is judged purely by subjective impression of improvement. CRPS treatment studies have had an unusually high placebo response rate.[53] Medical therapy is usually ineffective. Proposed treatments include:
1. tricyclic antidepressants
2. 18–25% have satisfactory long-lasting relief after a series of sympathetic blocks, see Stellate ganglion block (p. 1834) and Lumbar sympathetic block (p. 1835), although one report found no long-lasting benefit in any of 30 patients[54]
3. intravenous regional sympathetic block, particularly for UE CRPS: agents used include *guanethedine*[55] 20 mg, reserpine, bretylium…, injected IV with arterial tourniquet (sphygmomanometer cuff) inflated for 10 min. If no relief, repeat in 3–4 wks. No better than placebo in several trials[56, 57]
4. surgical sympathectomy (p. 1853): some purport that this relieves pain in > 90% of patients (with a few retaining some tenderness or hyperpathia). Others opine that there is no rational reason to consider sympathectomy since sympathetic blocks have been shown to be no more effective than placebo[43]
5. spinal cord stimulation: some success has been reported

References

29

[1] Backonja MM. Defining neuropathic pain. Anesth Analg. 2003; 97:785–790
[2] Merskey H, Bogduk N. Classification of Chronic Pain: Descriptions of Chronic Pain Syndromes and Definitions of Pain Terms. 2nd ed. Seattle, WA: IASP Press; 1994
[3] Dworkin RH, Backonja M, Rowbotham MC, et al. Advances in neuropathic pain: diagnosis, mechanisms, and treatment recommendations. Arch Neurol. 2003; 60:1524–1534
[4] Watson CPN, Babul N. Efficacy of oxycodone in neuropathic pain: a randomized trial in postherpetic neuralgia. Neurology. 1998; 50:1837–1841
[5] Watson CP, Evans RJ, Reed K, et al. Amitriptyline versus Placebo in Postherpetic Neuralgia. Neurology. 1982; 32:671–673
[6] Max MB, Lynch SA, Muir J, et al. Effects of Desipramine, Amitriptyline, and Fluoxetine on Pain in Diabetic Neuropathy. N Engl J Med. 1992; 326:1250–1256
[7] Bennett MI, Simpson KH. Gabapentin in the treatment of neuropathic pain. Palliat Med. 2004; 18:5–11
[8] Dierking G, Duedahl TH, Rasmussen ML, et al. Effects of gabapentin on postoperative morphine consumption and pain after abdominal hysterectomy: a randomized, double-blind trial. Acta Anaesthesiol Scand. 2004; 48:322–327
[9] Mathew NT, Rapoport A, Saper J, et al. Efficacy of gabapentin in migraine prophylaxis. Headache. 2001; 41:119–128
[10] Gabapentin (Neurontin®) for chronic pain. Medical Letter. 2004; 46:29–31
[11] Keller JT, van Loveren H. Pathophysiology of the Pain of Trigeminal Neuralgia and Atypical Facial Pain: A Neuroanatomical Perspective. Clin Neurosurg. 1985; 1985
[12] Wilkins RH, Rengachary SS. Neurosurgery. New York 1985
[13] Burchiel KJ. A new classification for facial pain. Neurosurgery. 2003; 53:1164–1167
[14] Pareja JA, Sjaastad O. SUNCT syndrome. A clinical review. Headache. 1997; 37:195–195
[15] Sjaastad O, Pareja JA, Zukerman E, et al. Trigeminal neuralgia. Clinical manifestations of first division involvement. Headache. 1997; 37:346–357
[16] Pareja JA, Baron M, Gili P, et al. Objective assessment of autonomic signs during triggered first division trigeminal neuralgia. Cephalalgia. 2002; 22:251–255

[17] Yeh HS, Tew JM. Tic Convulsif, the Combination of Geniculate Neuralgia and Hemifacial Spasm Relieved by Vascular Decompression. Neurology. 1984; 34:682–683
[18] Rupa V, Saunders RL, Weider DJ. Geniculate Neuralgia: The Surgical Management of Primary Otalgia. Journal of Neurosurgery. 1991; 75:505–511
[19] Young RF. Geniculate Neuralgia. Journal of Neurosurgery. 1992; 76
[20] Andersen NB, Bovim G, Sjaastad O. The frontotemporal peripheral nerves. Topographic variations of the supraorbital, supratrochlear and auriculotemporal nerves and their possible clinical significance. Surgical and Radiologic Anatomy. 2001; 23:97–104
[21] Pareja JA, Caminero AB. Supraorbital neuralgia. Curr Pain Headache Rep. 2006; 10:302–305
[22] Headache Classification Committee of the International Headache Society. Classification and diagnostic criteria for headache disorders, cranial neuralgias, and facial pain, 2nd edition. Cephalalgia. 2004; 24:9–160
[23] Pareja JA, Pareja J, Yanguela J. Nummular headache, trochleitis, supraorbital neuralgia, and other epicranial headaches and neuralgias: the epicranias. Journal of Headache and Pain. 2003; 4:125–131
[24] Pareja JA, Caminero AB, Serra J, et al. Numular headache: a coin-shaped cephalgia. Neurology. 2002; 58:1678–1679
[25] Caminero AB, Pareja JA. Supraorbital neuralgia: a clinical study. Cephalalgia. 2001; 21:216–223
[26] Stookey B, Ransohoff J. Trigeminal Neuralgia: Its History and Treatment. Springfield, IL: Charles C Thomas; 1959
[27] Sjaastad O, Stolt-Nielsen A, Pareja JA, et al. Supraorbital neuralgia: on the clinical manifestations and a possible therapeutic approach. Headache. 1999; 39:204–212
[28] Grantham EG, Segerberg LH. An evaluation of palliative surgical procedures in trigeminal neuralgia. Journal of Neurosurgery. 1952; 9:390–394
[29] Watson CPN. A new treatment for postherpetic neuralgia. New England Journal of Medicine. 2000; 343:1563–1565
[30] Loeser JD. Herpes Zoster and Postherpetic Neuralgia. Pain. 1986; 25:149–164
[31] Schimpff S, Serpick A, Stoler B, et al. Varicella-Zoster Infection in Patients with Cancer. Annals of Internal Medicine. 1972; 76:241–254
[32] Youmans JR. Neurological Surgery. Philadelphia 1990

[33] Valacyclovir. Medical Letter. 1996; 38:3–4

[34] Rowbotham MC, Davies PS, Verkempinck C, et al. Lidocaine patch: double-blind controlled trial of a new treatment method for postherpetic neuralgia. Pain. 1996; 65:39–44

[35] Alper BS, Lewis PR. Treatment of postherpetic neuralgia: a systematic review of the literature. J Fam Pract. 2002; 51:121–128

[36] Rowbotham MC, Harden N, Stacey B, et al. Gabapentin for the treatment of postherpetic neuralgia: A randomized controlled trial. Journal of the American Medical Association. 1998; 280:1837–1842

[37] Capsaicin - A Topical Analgesic. Medical Letter. 1992; 34:62–63

[38] Kotani N, Kushikata T, Hashimoto H, et al. Intrathecal methylprednisolone for intractable postherpetic neuralgia. New England Journal of Medicine. 2000; 343:1514–1519

[39] Dan K, Higa K, Noda B, et al. Nerve block for herpetic pain. In: Advances in Pain Research and Therapy. New York: Raven Press; 1985:831–838

[40] Friedman AH, Nashold BS. Dorsal Root Entry Zone Lesions for the Treatment of Postherpetic Neuralgia. Neurosurgery. 1984; 15:969–970

[41] Lewith GT, Field J, Machin D. Acupuncture Compared with Placebo in Post-Herpetic Pain. Pain. 1983; 17:361–368

[42] Sternschein MJ, Myers SJ, Frewin DB, et al. Causalgia. Arch Phys Med Rehabil. 1975; 56:58–63

[43] Schott GD. An Unsympathetic View of Pain. Lancet. 1995; 345:634–636

[44] Ochoa JL, Verdugo RJ. Reflex Sympathetic Dystrophy: A Common Clinical Avenue for Somatoform Expression. Neurol Clin. 1995; 13:351–363

[45] Sachs BL, Zindrick MR, Beasley RD. Reflex Sympathetic Dystrophy After Operative Procedures on the Lumbar Spine. Journal of Bone and Joint Surgery. 1993; 75A:721–725

[46] Hsu ES. Practical management of complex regional pain syndrome. Am J Ther. 2009; 16:147–154

[47] Groeneweg G, Huygen FJ, Coderre TJ, et al. Regulation of peripheral blood flow in complex regional pain syndrome: clinical implication for symptomatic relief and pain management. BMC Musculoskelet Disord. 2009; 10. DOI: 10.1186/1471-2474-10-116

[48] Ochoa JL. Reflex? Sympathetic? Dystrophy? Triple Questioned Again. Mayo Clinic Proceedings. 1995; 70:1124–1125

[49] Mailis A. Is Diabetic Autonomic Neuropathy Protective Against Reflex Sympathetic Dystrophy? Clin J Pain. 1995; 11:77–81

[50] Mailis A, Meindok H, Papagapiou M, et al. Alterations of the Three-Phase Bone Scan After Sympathectomy. Clin J Pain. 1994; 10:146–155

[51] Kozin F, Genant HK, Bekerman C, et al. The Reflex Sympathetic Dystrophy Syndrome. Am J Med. 1976; 60:332–338

[52] Chelimsky TC, Low PA, Naessens JM, et al. Value of Autonomic Testing in Reflex Sympathetic Dystrophy. Mayo Clinic Proceedings. 1995; 70:1029–1040

[53] Ochoa JL. Pain Mechanisms in Neuropathy. Curr Opin Neurol. 1994; 7:407–414

[54] Dotson R, Ochoa JL, Cline M, et al. A Reassessment of Sympathetic Blocks as Long Term Therapeutic Modality for "RSD". Pain. 1990; 5

[55] Hannington-Kiff JG. Relief of Sudek's Atrophy by Regional Intravenous Guanethidine. Lancet. 1977; 1:1132–1133

[56] Blanchard J, Ramamurthy W, Walsh N, et al. Intravenous Regional Sympatholysis: A Double-Blind Comparison of Guanethedine, Reserpine, and Normal Saline. J Pain Symptom Manage. 1990; 5:357–361

[57] Jadad AR, Carroll D, Glynn CJ, et al. Intravenous Regional Sympathetic Blockade for Pain Relief in Reflex Sympathetic Dystrophy: A Systematic Review and a Randomized, Double-Blind Crossover Study. J Pain Symptom Manage. 1995; 10:13–20

29

Part X

Peripheral Nerves

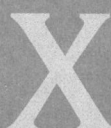

30 Peripheral Nerves

30.1 Peripheral nerves – definitions and grading scales

30.1.1 Peripheral nervous system definition

The peripheral nervous system (PNS) consists of those structures (including cranial nerves III-XII, spinal nerves, nerves of the extremities, and the cervical, brachial and lumbosacral plexi) containing nerve fibers or axons that connect the central nervous system (CNS) with motor and sensory, somatic and visceral, end organs.[1] ▶ Table 30.1 shows classification of motor and sensory nerves.

Table 30.1 Motor & sensory classification of nerves

Sensory	Sensory & motor	Greatest fiber diameter (mcm)	Greatest conduction velocity (m/sec)	Motor/ sensory	Comments
Ia	A-alpha	22	120	motor	large alpha motor neurons of lamina IX (extrafusal) sensory-primary afferents (anulospiral of muscle spindles for proprioception)
Ib	A-alpha	22	120	sensory	Golgi tendon organs, touch & pressure receptors
II	A-beta	13	70	sensory	secondary afferents (flower spray) of muscle spindles, crude touch, pressure receptors, Pacinian corpuscles (vibratory) (to posterior columns[a])
	A-gamma	8	40	motor	small γ motor neurons of lamina IX (intrafusal)
III	A-delta	5	15	sensory	small, lightly myelinated, fine touch, pressure, pain & temperature
	B	3	14	motor	small, lightly myelinated preganglionic autonomic fibers
IV	C	1	2	motor	all post-ganglionic autonomic
				sensory	unmyelinated pain & temp (to spinothalamic tract)

[a]these fibers to the posterior columns are more medial in the root entry zone than the C-fibers (important in DREZ lesions where the goal is to lesion C-fibers and spare A-beta)

30.1.2 Grading strength and reflexes

Muscle strength grading most commonly employs the Royal Medical Research Council of Great Britain (MRC) scale,[2] a common modification of which is shown in ▶ Table 30.2. Muscle stretch reflexes may be graded as shown in ▶ Table 30.3.[2]

Table 30.2 Muscle grading (modified Medical Research Council (MRC) system)

Grade	Strength	
0	no contraction (total paralysis)	
1	flicker or trace contraction (palpable or visible)	
2	active movement with gravity eliminated	
3	active movement through full ROM against gravity	
4	active movement against resistance; subdivisions →	4 – Slight resistance 4 Moderate resistance 4 + Slight resistance
5	normal strength (against full resistance)	
NT	not testable	

Table 30.3 A sample muscle stretch reflex (deep tendon reflex) grading scale. Various scales are in use. Typically go from 0 to 4 + where 4 + is sustained clonus.

Grade	Definition
0	no contraction (total paralysis)
0.5 +	elicitable only with reinforcement[a]
1 +	low normal
2 +	normal
3 +	more brisk than normal (hyperreflexic)
4 +	hyperreflexic with clonus
5 +	sustained clonus

[a]In the LEs, reinforcement consists of having the patient hook the tips of the fingers of the left hand into the tips of the hooked fingers of the right hand and pulling (Jendrassik maneuver). Reinforcement in the UEs consists of having the patient clench their teeth

30.1.3 Upper motor neuron vs. lower motor neuron

Upper motor neurons (UMN) (first-order motor neurons): some soma reside in the primary motor cortex (precentral gyrus) of the brain. Axons project to LMNs.

Lower motor neurons (LMN) (second-order motor neuron): cell bodies (soma) reside in spinal cord (in anterior gray matter) or in brainstem (for cranial nerve motor nuclei). Axons connect directly to neuromuscular junction of muscles.

See ▶ Table 30.4 for comparison of weakness due to UMN vs. LMN.

Table 30.4 Upper vs. lower motor neuron paralysis

	Upper motor neuron paralysis	Lower motor neuron paralysis
possible etiologies	stroke (motor strip (p. 56), internal capsule...), spinal cord injury, cervical spondylotic myelopathy	herniated intervertebral disc, nerve entrapment syndrome, polio, progressive muscular atrophy (PMA)
muscle tone	initially flaccid; later spastic with clasp-knife resistance	flaccid
tendon reflexes	hyperactive; clonus may be present	absent
pathologic reflexes (e.g., Babinski, Hoffman)	present (after days to weeks)	absent
muscle manifestations	spontaneous spasms may occur; some *atrophy of disuse* may occur	fibrillations, fasciculations. *Atrophy* after days to weeks due to trophic influence

30.1.4 Fasciculations vs. fibrillations

Fasciculations are coarse muscle contractions that are visible to the naked eye, whereas fibrillations are *not* visible and require EMG to detect; AKA fibrillation potentials (p. 255).

Fasciculations represent discharge of a group of muscle fibers (all or part of an entire motor unit), and occur most often in diseases involving anterior horn cells, including:

1. amyotrophic lateral sclerosis (ALS) (p. 191)
2. spinal muscular atrophy (p. 1702)
3. polio
4. syringomyelia

30.2 Muscle innervation

30.2.1 Muscles, roots, trunks, cords and nerves of the upper extremities

See ▶ Table 30.5.

Table 30.5 Muscle innervation—shoulder & upper extremity[a]

	Muscle	Action to test	Roots[b]	Trunk[c]	Cord[d]	Nerve
	deep neck	flex, ext, rotation of neck	C1–4	–	–	cervical
	trapezius	elevates shoulder, abducts arm > 90°	XI, C3, 4			(spinal acc + roots)
	diaphragm	inspiration	C3–5			phrenic
•	serratus anterior	forward shoulder thrust	C5–7	–	–	long thoracic
	levator scapulae	elevate scapula	C3, 4, **5**			dorsal scapular
	rhomboids	adduct & elevate scapula	C4, 5			
	supraspinatus	abduct arm (15–30°)	C4, **5**, 6	S		suprascapular
•	infraspinatus	exorotation of humerus	**C5**, 6	S	–	
	latissimus dorsi	adduct arm	C5, 6, **7**, 8			thoracodorsal
	teres major, subscapularis		C5–7			subscapular
•	deltoid	abduct arm (30–90°)	**C5**, 6	S	P	axillary
	teres minor	exorotate & adduct humerus	C4,5			
•	biceps brachii	flex forearm (with hand supinated), & supinate forearm	**C5**, C6	S	L	musculocutaneous
	coracobrachialis	flex humerus at shoulder	C5–7			
	brachialis	flex forearm	C5, 6			
•	flexor carpi ulnaris	ulnar flexion of wrist	C7, **8**, T1	M, I	M	ulnar
•	flexor digitorum profundus III & IV (ulnar part)	flex distal phalanx of Dig 4–5	C7, **8**, T1	M, I	M	
	adductor pollicis	thumb adduction	C8, **T1**		M	
	abductor digiti minimi	abduction Dig 5	C8, T1		M	
	opponens digiti minimi	opposition Dig 5	C7, 8, T1			
	flexor digiti minimi brevis	flexion Dig 5	C7, **8**, **T1**		M	
•	interossei	flex proximal phalanx, extend 2 distal phalanges, abduct or adduct fingers	C8, **T1**	I	M	
	lumbricals 3 & 4	flex proximal phalanges & extend 2 distal phalanges of Dig 4–5	C7, **8**			
•	pronator teres	forearm pronation	C6, 7	S,M	L	median
•	flexor carpi radialis	radial flexion of wrist	C6, 7	S,M	L	
	palmaris longus	wrist flexion	C7, 8, T1			
•	flexor digitorum superficialis	flexion middle phalanx Dig 2–5, flex wrist	C7, **8**, T1	M, I	M	
•	abductor pollicis brevis	abduct thumb metacarpal	C8, **T1**	I	M	
	flexor pollicis brevis	flex prox phalanx thumb	C8, **T1**			

(continued)

Table 30.5 continued

	Muscle	Action to test	Roots[b]	Trunk[c]	Cord[d]	Nerve
•	opponens pollicis	opposes thumb metacarp	C8, **T1**	I	M	
	lumbricals 1 & 2	flex proximal phalanx & extend 2 distal phalanges Dig 2–3	C8, **T1**			
•	flexor digitorum profundus I & II (radial part)	flex distal phalanx of Dig 2–3; flex wrist	C7, **8**, T1	M, I	M	anterior interosseous
•	flexor pollicis longus	flex distal phalanx thumb	C7, **8**, T1			
•	triceps brachii	forearm extension	C6, **7**, 8	all	P	radial
•	brachioradialis	forearm flexion (with thumb pointed up)	C5, **6**	S	P	
•	extensor carpi radialis	radial wrist extension	C5, **6**	S,M	P	
•	supinator	forearm supination	**C6**, 7	S	P	
•	extensor digitorum	extension of wrist & phalanges of Dig 2–5	**C7**, C8	M, I	P	posterior interosseous (PIN)
	extensor carpi ulnaris	ulnar wrist extension	**C7**, C8			
•	abductor pollicis longus	abduction thumb metacarpal & radial wrist extension	**C7**, C8	M, I	P	
	extensor pollicis brevis & longus	thumb extension & radial wrist extension	**C7**, C8			
	extensor indicis proprius	extension Dig 2 & wrist extension	**C7**, C8			
	pectoralis major: clavicular head	push arm forward against resistance	**C5**, 6			lateral pectoral
	pectoralis major: sternocostal head	adduct arm	C6, **7**, 8			lateral & medial pectoral

[a]NB: items marked with a bullet (•) are clinically important muscle/nerves.
NB: Dig ® U.S. digit numbering convention: 1=thumb, 2=index finger, 3=middle, 4=ring, 5=little.
[b]Major innervation is indicated in boldface. Differing opinions exist, most shown are based on reference.[3]
[c] Trunk (trunks of brachial plexus): S = superior, M = middle, I = inferior, all = all three.
[d] Cord (cords of brachial plexus): P = posterior, L = lateral, M = medial.

30.2.2 Thumb innervation/movement

See ▶ Table 30.6.
Flexion/extension: occurs in the plane of the palm.
Abduction/adduction: occur in a plane at right angles to palm.
Opposition: bringing the thumb across the hand.

Table 30.6 The 3 innervations of the thumb

Action	Nerve	Muscle(s)
abduction, flexion, opposition[a]	median	abductor pollicis brevis, flexor pollicis brevis, opponens pollicis
adduction	ulnar	adductor pollicis
extension	radial[b]	extensor pollicis brevis & longus

[a]occasional anomalous innervation by ulnar nerve
[b]via the posterior interosseous nerve

30.2.3 Muscles, roots, trunks, cords and nerves of the lower extremities

See ▶ Table 30.7.

Table 30.7 Muscle innervation—hip & lower extremity[a]

	Muscle	Action	Roots[b]	Plexus[c]	Nerves
•	iliopsoas[d]	hip flexion	**L1, 2,** 3	L	femoral & L1, 2, 3
	sartorius	hip flex & thigh evert	L2, 3		femoral
•	quadriceps femoris	leg (knee) extension	L2, 3, **4**	L	
	pectineus	thigh adduction	L2, 3		obturator
•	adductor longus		**L2,** 3, 4	L	
	adductor brevis		L2–4		
	adductor magnus		L3, 4		
	gracilis		L2–4		
	obturator externus	thigh adduction & lateral rotation	L3, 4		
•	gluteus medius/minimus	thigh abduction & medial rotation	**L4, 5,** S1	S	superior gluteal
	tensor fasciae lata	thigh flexion	L4, 5		
	piriformis	lateral thigh rotation	L5, S1		
•	gluteus maximus	thigh abduction (patient prone)	**L5, S1,** 2	S	inferior gluteal
	obturator internus	lateral thigh rotation	L5, S1	S	muscular branches
	gemelli		L4, 5, S1	S	
	quadratus femoris		L4, 5, S1	S	
•	biceps femoris[e]	leg flexion (& assist thigh extension)	L5, **S1,** 2		sciatic (trunk)
•	semitendinosus[e]		L5, **S1,** 2		
•	semimembranosus[e]		L5, **S1,** 2		
•	tibialis anterior	foot dorsiflexion & supination	L4, 5[f]	S	deep peroneal
•	extensor digitorum longus	extension toes 2–5 & foot dorsiflexion	**L5,** S1		
•	extensor hallucis longus (EHL)[g]	great toe extension & foot dorsiflexion	L5[f], S1	S	
•	extensor digitorum brevis	extension great toe & toes 2–5	**L5,** S1	S	
•	peroneus longus & brevis	P-flex pronated foot & eversion	L5, S1	L/S	superficial peroneal
•	posterior tibialis	P-flex supinated foot & inversion	L4, 5	S	tibial
	flexor digitorum longus	P-flex sup foot, flex terminal phalanx toes 2–5	L5, **S1,** 2		
	flexor hallucis longus	P-flex sup foot, flex terminal phalanx great toe	L5, **S1,** 2		
	flexor digitorum brevis	flex mid phalanx toes 2–5	S2, 3		
	flexor hallucis brevis	flex proximal phalanx great toe	L5, **S1,** 2		
•	gastrocnemius	knee flexion, ankle P-flex	**S1,** 2	S	
	plantaris		**S1,** 2		
•	soleus	ankle P-flex	**S1,** 2	S	

(continued)

Table 30.7 continued

	Muscle	Action	Roots[b]	Plexus[c]	Nerves
•	abductor hallucis[h]	(cannot test[h])	**S1**, 2	S	
	perineal & sphincters	voluntary contract pelvic floor	S2–4		pudendal

NB: items marked with a bullet (•) are clinically important muscle/nerves.
[a]Abbreviations: P-flex = plantarflexion, D-flex = dorsiflexion.
[b]Major innervation is indicated in boldface type. e.g., when roots are shown as L4, **5**, this indicates L5 is the main innervation, but both L4 & L5 contribute.
[c]Plexus: L = lumbar, S = sacral
[d]iliopsoas is the term for the combined iliacus and psoas major muscles
[e]"**hamstrings**": familiar term for the grouped: semitendinosus and semimembranosus (together, the medial hamstrings) and the biceps femoris (lateral hamstrings)
[f]although many references, including some venerable ones, cite AT as being primarily L4, many clinicians agree that L5 innervation is probably more significant
[g]EHL is the best L5 muscle to test clinically (although S1 radiculopathy can also weaken this muscle)
[h]abductor hallucis cannot be tested clinically, but is important for EMG

30.3 Peripheral nerve injury/surgery

30.3.1 Nerve action potentials

Stimulating a healthy nerve fiber with an electrical stimulus of an amplitude and duration that exceeds its threshold will produce a conducted impulse, or nerve action potential (NAP).[4(p 103)] Medium-sized axons (fibers) have a lower threshold than large ones, which have a lower threshold than small or fine axons.[4(p 103)]

30.3.2 Use of NAP with lesion in continuity

There is some degree of continuity in ≥ 60% of nerve injuries.[4(p 104)]

For a lesion in continuity (LIC), if surgical repair is needed, it may be too late if one waits until there is failure of anticipated clinical improvement. Presence of a NAP (regardless of amplitude or latency) distal to an LIC in the first few months after an injury usually indicates that operative intervention will not be needed. For recommended timing to obtain NAP recording, see ▶ Table 30.8.[4(p 106)]

Table 30.8 Recommended timing to obtain NAP recording

Injury	Timing
relatively focal contusions	2–4 months
stretch injuries (esp. brachial plexus)	4–5 months
partial injuries & entrapments, compressive lesions and tumors	any time
to identify an area of conduction block (regardless if lesion is from neuropraxia, axonotmesis, or neurotmesis)	acutely

30.3.3 Timing of surgical repair

The longer the distance from the injury site to the functional unit to be reinnervated, the earlier surgical intervention should be considered.[4(p 74)]

24 month rule[4(p 74)]: after 24 months of denervation, most muscles cannot recover useful function even with reinnervation. Exceptions: facial muscles, large bulky muscles such as biceps, brachialis, gastrocs, and some lesions in continuity with some preserved innervation.

30.3.4 Brachial plexus

General information

Formed by *ventral* rami (the dorsal rami innervate the paraspinal muscles), most commonly of nerve roots C5–1 (schematically depicted in ▶ Fig. 30.1).

▶ Table 30.5 shows action, etc. of specific muscles. Also see ▶ Fig. 30.1. ↳ indicates that the nerve supplies the muscles listed; ↳ denotes a branch of the preceding nerve.

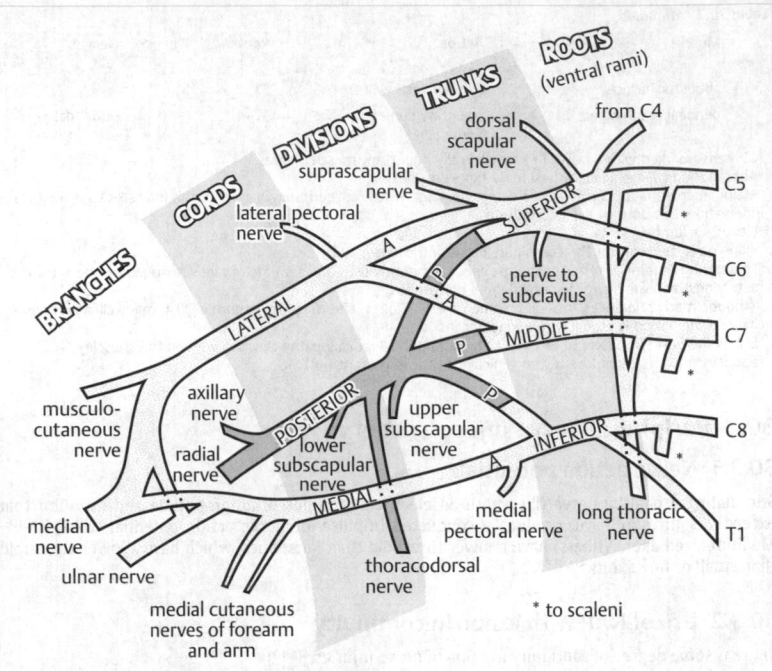

Fig. 30.1 Schematic diagram of the brachial plexus. (By permission: Churchill Livingstone, Edinburgh, 1973, R. Warwick & P. Williams: Gray's Anatomy 35th Edition © Longman Group UK Limited.)

Nerves arising from the brachial plexus

Radial nerve (C5–8)

See ▶ Fig. 30.2. The radial nerve (and its branches) innervate the extensors of arm and forearm:

- ↓ triceps (all 3 heads)
- ↓ anconeus
- ↓ brachioradialis
- ↓ extensor carpi radialis longus & brevis (latter originates ≈ at terminal branch)
- ↓ supinator (originates near the terminal branch)
- ↳ continues into forearm as **posterior interosseous nerve** (C7, C8)
  - ○ ↓ extensor carpi ulnaris
  - ○ ↓ extensor digitorum
  - ○ ↓ extensor digiti minimi
  - ○ ↓ extensor pollicis brevis & longus
  - ○ ↓ abductor pollicis longus
  - ○ ↓ extensor indicis

Axillary nerve (C5, C6)

See ▶ Fig. 30.2.
- ↓ teres minor
- ↓ deltoid

Median nerve (C5–1)

See ▶ Fig. 30.3, also see Martin-Gruber anastomosis (p. 540).
- nothing in arm
- all forearm pronators and flexors except the two supplied by ulnar nerve

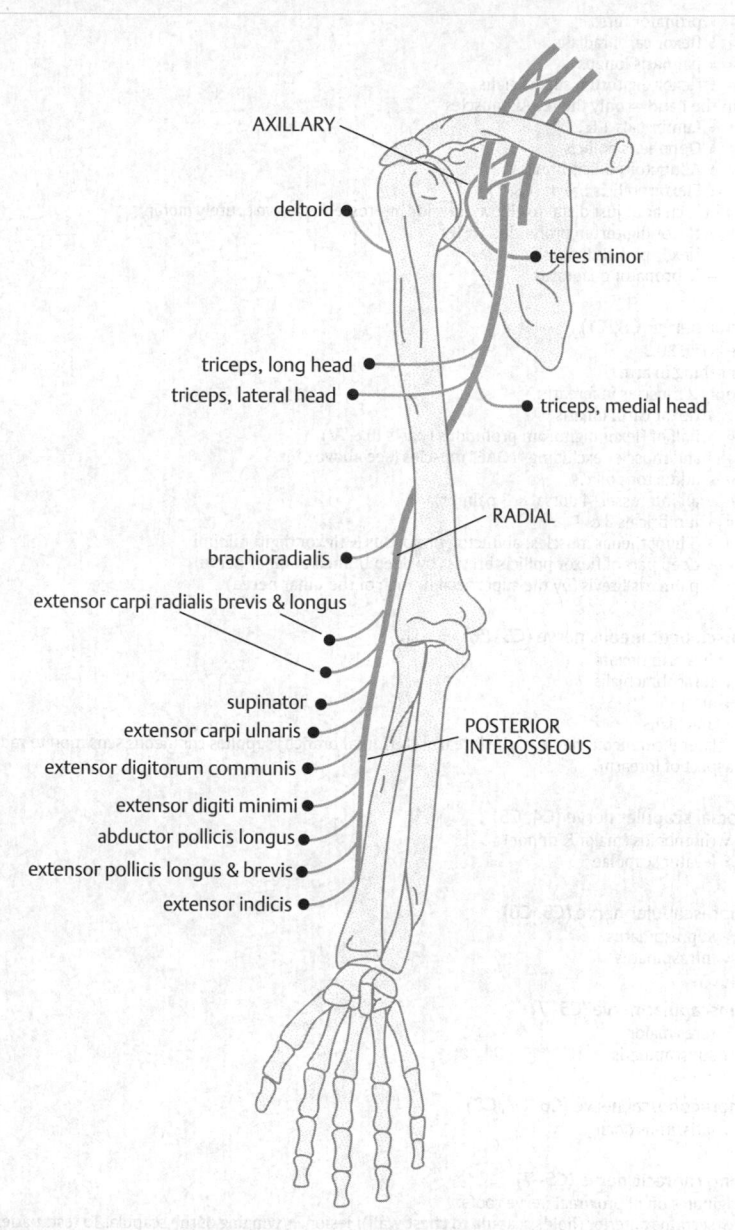

AXILLARY

deltoid

teres minor

triceps, long head
triceps, lateral head

triceps, medial head

RADIAL

brachioradialis

extensor carpi radialis brevis & longus

supinator
extensor carpi ulnaris
extensor digitorum communis
extensor digiti minimi
abductor pollicis longus
extensor pollicis longus & brevis
extensor indicis

POSTERIOR
INTEROSSEOUS

30

Fig. 30.2 Muscles of the radial and axillary nerves.

- ○ ↕ pronator teres
- ○ ↕ flexor carpi radialis
- ○ ↕ palmaris longus
- ○ ↕ flexor digitorum superficialis
- in the hand ⇒ only the "LOAF muscles"
  - ○ ↕ **L**umbricals 1 & 2
  - ○ ↕ **O**pponens pollicis
  - ○ ↕ **A**bductor pollicis brevis
  - ○ ↕ **F**lexor pollicis brevis (C8, T1)
- ↳ branch at or just distal to elbow anterior interosseous nerve (purely *motor*)
  - ○ ↕ flexor digitorum profundus I & II
  - ○ ↕ flexor pollicis longus
    - – ↕ pronator quadratus

Ulnar nerve (C8, T1)
See ► Fig. 30.3.
- nothing in arm
- only 2 muscles in forearm:
  - ○ ↕ flexor carpi ulnaris
  - ○ ↕ half of flexor digitorum profundus (parts III & IV)
- all hand muscles excluding "LOAF" muscles (see above), viz.:
  - ○ ↕ adductor pollicis
  - ○ ↕ all interossei (4 dorsal & 3 palmar)
  - ○ ↕ lumbricals 3 & 4
  - ○ ↕ 3 hypothenar muscles: abductor, opponens & flexor digiti minimi
  - ○ ↕ deep part of flexor pollicis brevis (by deep branch of ulnar nerve)
  - ○ ↕ palmaris brevis (by the superficial branch of the ulnar nerve)

Musculocutaneous nerve (C5, C6)
Supplies arm flexors
- ↕ coracobrachialis
- ↕ biceps
- ↕ brachialis
- ↳ lateral cutaneous nerve of the forearm (terminal branch) supplies cutaneous sensation to radial aspect of forearm

Dorsal scapular nerve (C4, C5)
- ↕ rhomboids (major & minor)
- ↕ levator scapulae

Suprascapular nerve (C5, C6)
- ↕ Supraspinatus
- ↕ Infraspinatus

Subscapular nerve (C5–7)
- ↕ teres major
- ↕ subscapularis

Thoracodorsal nerve (C6, C7, C8)
- ↕ latissimus dorsi

Long thoracic nerve (C5–7)
Originates off of proximal nerve roots.
- ↕ serratus anterior (holds scapula to chest wall): lesion → winging of the scapula. To test: patient leans forward against wall with arms outstretched, scapula separates from posterior chest wall if the serratus anterior is not contracting. (note: this describes classic winging of the scapula. A variant of winging can occur with loss of trapezius muscle, e.g., with accessory nerve injury, and typically manifests when the patient pushes forward with the elbow held at the side of the thorax.)

30

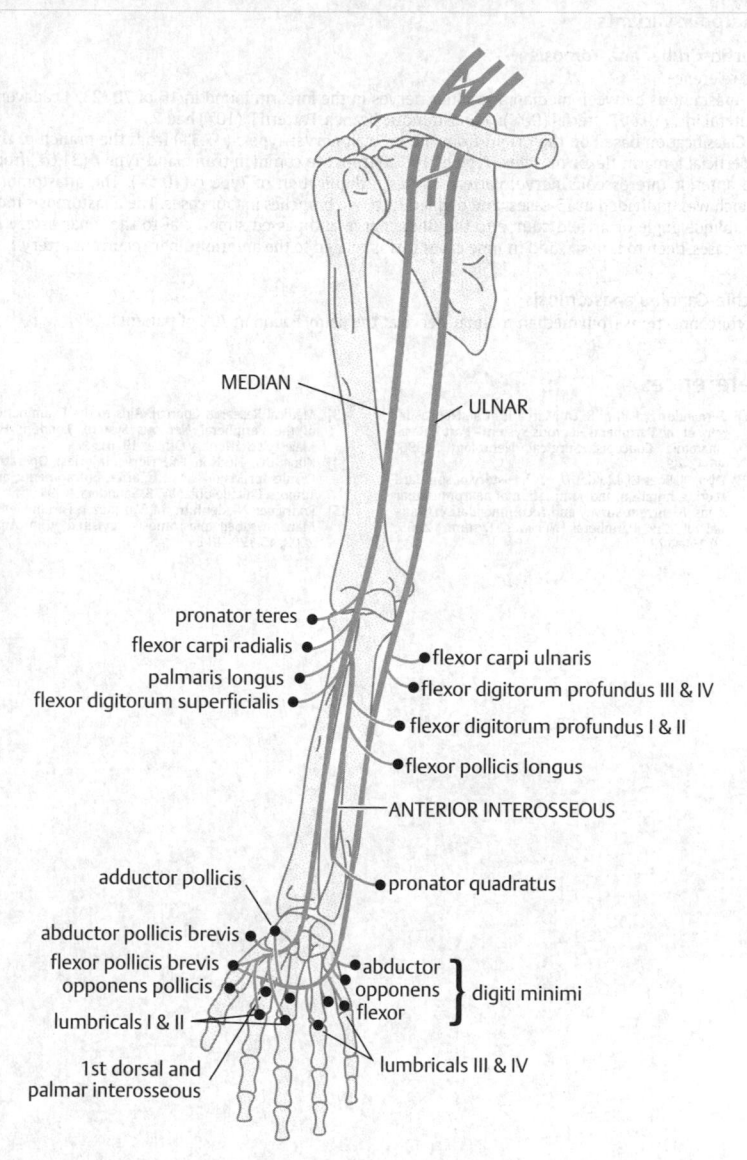

MEDIAN

ULNAR

pronator teres
flexor carpi radialis
palmaris longus
flexor digitorum superficialis

flexor carpi ulnaris
flexor digitorum profundus III & IV
flexor digitorum profundus I & II
flexor pollicis longus
ANTERIOR INTEROSSEOUS

adductor pollicis
abductor pollicis brevis
flexor pollicis brevis
opponens pollicis
lumbricals I & II
1st dorsal and
palmar interosseous

pronator quadratus

abductor
opponens } digiti minimi
flexor

lumbricals III & IV

30

Fig. 30.3 Muscles of the median and ulnar nerves.

Anatomic variants

Martin-Gruber anastomosis
See reference.[5]

Anastamosis between median and ulnar nerves in the forearm found in 16 of 70 (23%) cadavers, bilateral in 3 (19%). Pattern I (90%): 1 anastomotic branch, Pattern II (10%) had 2.

Classification based on the origin from the median nerve: Type a (47.3%) from the branch to the superficial forearm flexor muscles, Type b (10.6%) from the common trunk, and Type c (31.6%) from the anterior interosseous nerve. Pattern II was a duplication of Type c (10.5%). The anastomotic branch was undivided in 15 cases, and divided into two branches in four cases. The anastomosis took an oblique angle or arched course to the ulnar nerve and passed superficial to the ulnar artery in four cases, deep to it in six, and in nine cases it was related to the anterior ulnar recurrent artery.[5]

Richie-Cannieu anastomosis
Motor connections from median to ulnar nerve at the palm. Found in 70% of patients.

References

[1] Fernandez E, Pallini R, La Marca F, et al. Neurosurgery of the Peripheral Nervous System - Part I: Basic Anatomic Concepts. Surgical Neurology. 1996; 46:47–48

[2] Dyck PJ, Boes CJ, Mulder D, et al. History of standard scoring, notation, and summation of neuromuscular signs. A current survey and recommendation. Journal of the Peripheral Nervous System. 2005; 10:158–173

[3] Medical Research Council. Aids to the Examination of the Peripheral Nervous System. London: Her Majesty's Stationery Office; 1976

[4] Kline DG, Hudson AR. Nerve Injuries: Operative Results for Major Nerve Injuries, Entrapments, and Tumors. Philadelphia: W. B. Saunders; 1995

[5] Rodriguez-Niedenfuhr M, Vazquez T, Parkin I, et al. Martin-Gruber anastomosis revisited. Clin Anat. 2002; 15:129–134

30

31 Entrapment Neuropathies

31.1 Entrapment neuropathy – definitions and associations

Entrapment neuropathy is a peripheral nerve injury resulting from compression either by external forces or from nearby anatomic structures. Mechanism can vary from one or two significant compressive insults to many localized, repetitive mild compressions of a nerve. Certain nerves are particularly vulnerable at specific locations by virtue of being superficial, fixed in position, traversing a confined space, or in proximity to a joint. The most common symptom is pain (frequently at rest, more severe at night, often with retrograde radiation causing more proximal lesion to be suspected) with tenderness at the point of entrapment. Referred pain is so common that Frank Mayfield once said that patients with nerve entrapment don't know where the problem is located. Always consider the possibility of a systemic cause. Entrapment neuropathies may be associated with:

1. diabetes mellitus
2. hypothyroidism: due to glycogen deposition in Schwann cells
3. acromegaly
4. amyloidosis: primary or secondary (as in multiple myeloma)
5. carcinomatosis
6. polymyalgia rheumatica (p. 206)
7. rheumatoid arthritis: 45% incidence of 1 or more entrapment neuropathies
8. gout

31.2 Mechanism of injury

Brief compression primarily affects myelinated fibers, and classically spares unmyelinated fibers (except in cases of severe acute compression). Acute compression compromises axoplasmic flow which can reduce membrane excitability. Chronic compression affects both myelinated and unmyelinated fibers and can produce segmental demyelination in the former, and if the insult persists, axolysis and wallerian degeneration will occur in both types. The issue of ischemia is more controversial.[1] Some contend that simultaneous venous stasis at the site of compression can produce ischemia, which can lead to edema outside the axonal sheath, which may further exacerbate the ischemia. Eventually, fibrosis, neuroma formation, and progressive neuropathy can occur.

31

31.3 Occipital nerve entrapment

31.3.1 General information

Greater occipital nerve (nerve of Arnold) is a sensory branch of C2 (▶ Fig. 112.1 for dermatome). Entrapment presents as occipital neuralgia: pain in occiput usually with a trigger point near the superior nuchal line. Pressure here reproduces pain radiating up along back of head towards vertex.

More common in women.

31.3.2 Differential diagnosis

1. headache
   a) may be mimicked by migraine headache
   b) may be part of muscle contraction (tension) headache
2. myofascial pain[2]: the pain may be widely separated from the trigger point
3. vertebrobasilar disease including aneurysm and SAH
4. cervical spondylosis
5. pain from Chiari I malformation (p. 295)

31.3.3 Possible causes of entrapment

1. trauma
   a) direct trauma (including iatrogenic placement of suture through the nerve during surgical procedures, e.g., in closing a posterior fossa craniectomy)

b) following traumatic cervical extension[3] which may crush the C2 root and ganglion between the C1 arch and C2 lamina

c) fractures of the upper cervical spine

2. atlanto-axial subluxation (AAS) (e.g., in rheumatoid arthritis) or arthrosis
3. entrapment by hypertrophic C1–2 (epistrophic) ligament[4]
4. neuromas
5. arthritis of the C2–3 zygapophyseal joint

31.3.4 Treatment

General information

> ## Σ: Optimal treatment for idiopathic occipital neuralgia
>
> For idiopathic occipital neuralgia: available evidence is from small, retrospective, case series studies and is insufficient to conclude that either local injection or surgery are effective. Nerve blocks with steroids and local anesthetics provide only temporary relief. Surgical procedures such as nerve root decompression or neurectomy may provide effective pain relief for some patients; however, patient-selection criteria for these procedures have not been defined, and recurrence is common.

In idiopathic cases with no neurologic deficit, the condition is usually self limited.

Non surgical treatment

1. greater occipital nerve block with local anesthetic and steroids (see below)
   a) may provide relief typically lasting ≈ 1 month[5]
   b) is no longer considered diagnostic because it is not sufficiently specific
2. physical therapy: massage and daily stretching exercises
3. TENS unit: provided ≥ 50% relief in 13 patients for up to 5 yrs[6]
4. oral antiinflammatory agents
5. centrally acting pain medications: Neurontin, Paxil, Elavil…
6. botulinum toxin injection[7]: although this study had quite a few placebo responders

If these measures do not provide permanent relief in *disabling* cases, surgical treatment may be considered, although caution is advised by many due to poor results.[2,8] Alcohol neurolysis may be tried. A collar is *not* indicated as it may irritate the condition.

Occipital nerve block

Inject trigger point(s) if one or more can be identified (there is usually a trigger point near the superior nuchal line). The nerve may also be blocked at the point where it emerges from the dorsal neck muscles.

If the pathology is more proximal (e.g., at C2 spinal ganglion), then block of the ganglion may be required. Technique[9] (done under fluoroscopy): shave hair below the mastoid process; prep with iodine; infiltrate with local; insert a 20 gauge spinal needle midway between C1 and C2, halfway between the midline and the lateral margin of the dorsal neck muscles. Aim rostrally, the final target is the midpoint of the C1–2 joint on AP fluoro, and almost but not touching the inferior articular process of C1. Infiltrate 1–3 ml of anesthetic and check for analgesia in the C2 distribution.

Surgical treatment

1. decompression of C2 nerve root if compressed between C1 and C2[4]
2. in cases of AAS, decompression and atlanto-axial fusion (p.1778) may work

Surgical treatment options for *idiopathic* occipital neuralgia:
1. peripheral occipital nerve procedures: these may not be effective for proximal compression of the C2 root or ganglion:
   a) occipital neurectomy (see below)
      • peripheral avulsion of the nerve

31

- avulsion of the greater occipital nerve as it exits between the transverse process of C2 and the inferior oblique muscle
b) alcohol injection of greater occipital nerve
2. occipital nerve stimulators
3. release of the nerve within the trapezius muscle. Immediate results: relief in 46%, improvement in 36%. Only 56% reported improvement at 14.5 mos[10]
4. intradural division of the C2 dorsal route via a posterior intradural approach
5. ganglionectomy

Occipital neurectomy: The occipital nerve usually pierces the cervical muscles ≈ 2.5 cm lateral to the midline, just below the inion. Palpation or Doppler localization of the pulse of the accompanying greater occipital artery sometimes helps to locate the nerve. However, relief only occurs in ≈ 50%, and recurrence, usually within a year, is common.

31.4 Median nerve entrapment

31.4.1 General information

The two most common sites of entrapment of the median nerve:
1. at the wrist by the transverse carpal ligament: carpal tunnel syndrome (p. 546)
2. in upper forearm by pronator teres muscle: pronator teres syndrome (p. 548)

31.4.2 Anatomy

Contributing nerve roots: C5 through T1. The median nerve arises from the medial and lateral cords of the brachial plexus (▶ Fig. 30.1), and descends the upper arm adjacent to the lateral side of the brachial artery. It crosses to the medial side of the artery at the level of the coracobrachialis. In the cubital fossa, the median nerve passes behind the lacertus fibrosus (bicipital aponeurosis) and enters the upper forearm between the two heads of the pronator teres and supplies this muscle.

Just beyond this point, it branches to form the purely motor anterior interosseous nerve, which supplies all but 2 muscles of finger and wrist flexion. It descends adherent to deep surface of flexor digitorum superficialis (FDS), lying on the flexor digitorum profundus. Near the wrist, it emerges from the lateral edge of FDS becoming more superficial, lying medial to the tendon of flexor carpi radialis, just lateral to and partially under the cover of the palmaris longus tendon. It passes under the transverse carpal ligament (TCL) through the carpal tunnel, which also contains the tendons of the flexor digitorum profundus and superficialis deep to the nerve (9 tendons total, 2 to each finger, 1 to the thumb[11]). The motor branch arises deep to the TCL, but may anomalously pierce the TCL. It supplies the "LOAF muscles" (Lumbricals 1 & 2, Opponens pollicis, and Abductor and Flexor pollicis brevis).

The TCL attaches medially to pisiform and hook of hamate, laterally to trapezium and tubercles of scaphoid. TCL is continuous proximally with fascia over FDS and antebrachial fascia, distally with the flexor retinaculum of the hand. The TCL extends distally into the palm to ≈ 3 cm beyond the distal wrist crease. The palmaris longus tendon, which is absent in 10% of population, partially attaches to the TCL.

Palmar cutaneous branch (PCB) of median nerve: arises from the radial aspect of the median nerve approximately 5.5 cm proximal to styloid process of the radius, underneath the cover of FDS of the middle finger. It crosses the wrist *above* the TCL to provide sensory innervation to the base of the thenar eminence (and is thus spared in carpal tunnel syndrome).

The sensory distribution of the *average* median nerve is shown in ▶ Fig. 31.1.

31.4.3 Injuries to the main trunk of the median nerve

General information

Above the elbow, the median nerve may rarely be compressed by Struther's ligament (see below). At the elbow and forearm, the median nerve may rarely be trapped at any of three sites: 1) lacertus fibrosus (bicipital aponeurosis),[12] 2) pronator teres, 3) sublimis bridge. Neuropathy may also result from direct or indirect trauma or external pressure ("honeymoon paralysis").[12] Longstanding

31

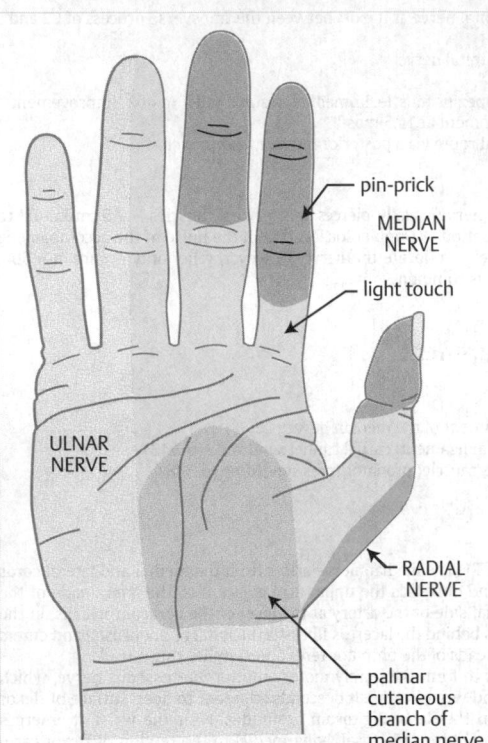

Fig. 31.1 **Cutaneous sensory innervation of the hand** illustrating the distribution of the median, ulnar & radial nerves in the hand, palmar surface.
Blue areas = median nerve (dark blue = pin-prick, light blue = light touch), green area = radial nerve, remainder = ulnar nerve.

pin-prick
MEDIAN NERVE

light touch

ULNAR NERVE

RADIAL NERVE

palmar cutaneous branch of median nerve

compression of the main trunk of the median nerve produces a "benediction hand" when trying to make a fist (index finger extended, middle finger partially flexed; due to weakness of flexor digitorum profundus I & II).

Struther's ligament

Distinct from struthers arcade (p. 554) which is a normal finding. The supracondylar process (SCP) is an anatomical variant located 5–7 cm above medial epicondyle, present in 0.7–2.7% of population. Struther's ligament bridges the SCP to the medial epicondyle. The median nerve and brachial artery pass underneath, the ulnar nerve may also. Usually asymptomatic, but occasionally may cause typical median nerve syndrome.

Pronator (teres) syndrome

From direct trauma or repeated pronation with tight hand-grip. Trapped where nerve dives between 2 heads of pronator teres. Causes vague aching and easy fatiguing of forearm muscles with weak grip and poorly localized paresthesias in index finger and thumb. Nocturnal exacerbation is *absent*. Pain in palm distinguishes this from carpal tunnel syndrome (CTS) since the median palmar cutaneous branch (PCB) exits before the TCL and is spared in CTS.

Treat with resting forearm. Surgical decompression indicated for cases that progress while on rest or when continued trauma is unavoidable.

Anterior interosseous neuropathy

General information

Key concepts

- weakness of 3 muscles: FDP I & II, FPL, & pronator quadratus. No sensory loss
- loss of flexion of the distal phalanges of the thumb and index finger (pinch sign)

The anterior interosseous nerve is a purely motor branch of the median nerve that arises in the upper forearm. Anterior interosseous neuropathy (AIN) produces no sensory loss and weakness of the 3 muscles supplied by the nerve:

1. flexor digitorum profundus (FDP) I & II: flexion of distal phalanx of digits 2 & 3
2. flexor pollicis longus (FPL): flexion of distal phalanx of thumb
3. pronator quadratus (in the distal forearm): difficult to isolate clinically

Etiologies of AIN

Include: idiopathic, amyotrophy, ulna/radius fractures, penetrating injuries, forearm lacerations.

Clinical

Symptoms: Patients complain of difficulty grasping small objects between the thumb and the index finger. Idiopathic cases may be preceded with forearm aching.

    Physical exam: Sensory: *no* sensory loss.

    Strength: digits 1, 2 & 3 are examined individually. The proximal interphalangeal joints are stabilized by the examiner and the patient is asked to flex the DIP. With AIN, there is no significant flexion of the DIP.

    Pinch sign: the patient attempts to forcefully pinch the *tips* of the index finger and thumb as in making an "OK" sign (▶ Fig. 31.2, left); with AIN the terminal phalanges extend and the pulps touch instead of the tips[13] (▶ Fig. 31.2, right).

31

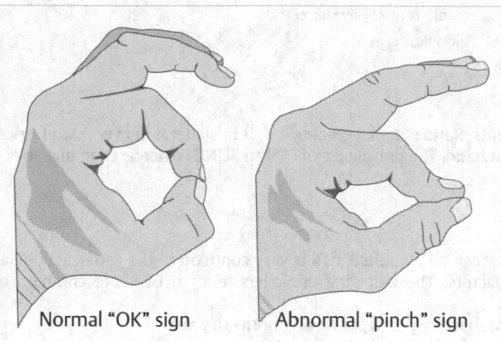

Normal "OK" sign   Abnormal "pinch" sign

Fig. 31.2 "Pinch sign" seen with anterior interosseous neuropathy (AIN).

Diagnosis

In addition to the physical exam, EMG may be helpful.

    EMG: primarily assesses pronator quadratus & flexor pollicis longus (FDP I & II is difficult on EMG because it has dual innervation with the ulnar nerve innervated portion being more superficial than the median nerve innervated portion). Important to evaluate pronator teres (abnormalities suggest involvement more proximal than forearm).

Management

In the absence of an identifiable cause of nerve injury, expectant management is recommended for 8–12 weeks, following which exploration is indicated, which may reveal a constricting band near the origin.

31.4.4 Carpal tunnel syndrome

General information

Key concepts

- the most common compression neuropathy. Involves median nerve in the wrist
- symptoms: tingling in the hand, worse at night and with elevation of hands
- physical exam is not very sensitive:
  ○ sensory: decreased pinprick in digits 1–3 and the radial half of 4
  ○ sensitivity: Tinels (tapping on wrist) 60%, Phalens (flexion of wrist) 80%
- electrodiagnostics: sensory latency @ wrist > 3.7 ms is the most sensitive test
- treatment:
  ○ mild cases: nonsurgical treatment (NSAIDs, neutral position splint...)
  ○ unresponsive or severe cases (neurologic deficits, duration > 1 year): surgical neurolysis (decompression) of the median nerve at the wrist has 70% satisfaction rate

Carpal tunnel syndrome (CTS) is the most common entrapment neuropathy in the upper extremity.[14,15,16] Carpal tunnel release (CTR) is one of the most frequently performed hand procedures.[17,18] The majority of patients have a satisfactory outcome from surgical treatment; see Outcome of surgical treatment (carpal tunnel release) (p.553). The median nerve is compressed within its course through the carpal tunnel just distal to the wrist crease. ► Table 31.1 shows the effect of pressure within the carpal tunnel.

Table 31.1 Pressure within carpal tunnel

Pressure (mm Hg)	Description
< 20	normal
20–30	venular flow retarded
30	axonal transport impaired
40	sensory & motor dysfunction
60–80	blood flow ceases

Epidemiology

Usually occurs in middle aged patients. Ratio of female:male = 4:1. It is bilateral in over 50% of cases, but is usually worse in the dominant hand. The prevalence of CTS and UNE is increased in diabetics.

Common etiologies

See reference.[19]

In most cases, no specific etiology can be identified. CTS is very common in the geriatric population without any additional risk factors. The following etiologies tend to be more common in younger patients:

1. "classic" CTS: chronic time course, usually over a period of months to years
   a) trauma: often job-related (may also be associated with avocations)
      - repetitive movements of hand and/or wrist: e.g., carpenter's
      - repeated forceful grasping or pinching of tools or other objects
      - awkward positions of hand and/or wrist, including wrist extension, ulnar deviation, or especially forced wrist flexion
      - direct pressure over carpal tunnel
      - use of vibrating hand tools
   b) systemic conditions: in addition to the listed systemic causes of entrapment neuropathies (p.541)—especially rheumatoid arthritis, diabetes—also consider:
      - obesity
      - local trauma
      - pregnancy: 54% remained symptomatic 1 year post-partum, and patients with onset early in pregnancy were less likely to improve[20]

- mucopolysaccharidosis V
- tuberculous tenosynovitis
- multiple myeloma (p. 928) (amyloid deposition in flexor retinaculum)
- the incidence of CTS may be increased in sarcoidosis (especially those with extrapulmonary involvement)[21]

c) local etiologies
  - patients with A-V dialysis shunts in the forearm have an increased incidence of CTS, possibly on an ischemic basis (steal and/or venous stasis) or possibly from the underlying renal disorder
  - carpal-metacarpal (CMC) osteoarthritis involving the thumb is common after age 40 (and is more prevalent in women), and in addition to the pain (with grasping) & tenderness at the base of the thumb, patients may develop secondary CTS

2. "acute" CTS: an uncommon condition where the symptoms of CTS appear suddenly and severely, usually following some type of exertion or trauma. Etiologies:
   a) median artery thrombosis: < 10% of individuals have a persistent median artery
   b) hemorrhage or hematoma in the transverse carpal ligament

Signs and symptoms

The physical exam for CTS is fairly insensitive. Signs and symptoms may include:

1. dysesthesias:
   a) characteristically patients are awakened at night by a painful numbness in the hand (often described as the "hand falling asleep") that often subjectively feels like a loss of circulation of blood. They often seek relief by: shaking the hand (flick sign[22]) or dangling or swinging the hand, opening and closing or rubbing the fingers, running hot or cold water over the hand, slapping the hand on the thigh, or pacing the floor. It may radiate up the forearm, and occasionally as far as the shoulder
   b) daytime activities that characteristically elicit symptoms usually involve prolonged hand elevation: holding a book or newspaper or cell phone to read, driving a car, holding a telephone to the ear, brushing hair, shaving the face
   c) distribution of symptoms:
      - on palmar side in radial 3.5 fingers (palmar side of thumb, index finger, middle finger, and radial half of ring finger)
      - dorsal side of these same fingers distal to the PIP joint
      - radial half of palm
      - subjective involvement of little finger occurs not infrequently for reasons that are not clear

2. hand weakness, especially grip. Characteristically manifests as difficulty opening jars. May be associated with thenar atrophy (late change, severe atrophy is seldom seen with current awareness of CTS by most physicians). An occasional patient may present with severe atrophy and no history of pain

3. clumsiness of the hand and/or difficulty with fine motor skills: probably due more to numbness than to a motor deficit. Often presents as difficulty buttoning buttons or zipping zippers, putting on earrings, fastening bra straps, handwriting changes…

4. hypesthesia in median nerve sensory distribution: usually best appreciated in finger *tips*, loss of 2-point discrimination may be more sensitive test

5. Phalen's test: 30–60 secs wrist flexion to a 90° angle exaggerates or reproduces pain or tingling. Positive in 80% of cases (80% sensitive)[23]

6. Tinel's sign at the wrist: paresthesias or pain in median nerve distribution produced by gently percussing over the carpal tunnel. Positive in 60% of cases. May also be present in other conditions. Reverse Tinel's sign: produces symptoms radiating up the forearm for variable distance

7. ischemic testing: place blood pressure cuff proximal to wrist, inflation x 30–60 seconds may reproduce CTS pain

Differential diagnosis

Differential diagnosis includes (modified[24]):

1. cervical radiculopathy: coexists in 70% of patients with either median or ulnar neuropathy (C6 radiculopathy may mimic CTS). Usually relieved by rest, and exacerbated by neck movement. Sensory impairment has dermatomal distribution. It has been postulated that cervical nerve root compression may interrupt axoplasmic flow and predispose the nerve to compressive injury distally (the term double-crush syndrome was coined to describe this[25]), and although this has been challenged,[26] it has not been disproven

2. thoracic outlet syndrome (p. 581): loss of bulk in hand muscles other than thenar. Sensory impairment in ulnar side of hand and forearm

31

3. pronator teres syndrome (p. 544): more prominent palmar pain than with CTS (median palmar cutaneous branch does not pass through carpal tunnel)
4. de Quervain's syndrome: tenosynovitis of the abductor pollicis longus and extensor pollicis brevis tendons often caused by repetitive hand movements. Results in *pain and tenderness* in the wrist near the thumb. Onset in 25% of cases is during pregnancy, and many in 1st postpartum year. Usually responds to wrist splints and/or steroid injections. NCVs should be normal. Finkelstein's test: the thumb is passively abducted while thumb abductors are palpated, positive if this aggravates the pain[27]
5. reflex sympathetic dystrophy: may respond to sympathetic block (p. 1835)
6. tenosynovitis of any of the flexor ligaments: may occasionally be due to TB or fungus. Usually a long, indolent course. Fluid accumulation may be present

Diagnostic tests

Electrodiagnostics (EDX)

Electromyogram (EMG) and nerve conduction study (NCS) which includes measurement of nerve conduction velocities (NCV): may help confirm the diagnosis of CTS and distinguish it from cervical root abnormalities and from tendonitis.

CTS is predominantly a demyelinating injury, although it can progress to axonal loss.[28] Two sensory comparison techniques that clearly agree (either normal or abnormal) are adequate to confirm or refute the diagnosis. For borderline abnormalities, additional sensory comparison testing or the combined sensory index (CSI) can clarify the diagnosis. If sensory responses are absent, the median motor latency in comparison to the ulnar latency can help localize a focal abnormality.[29]

Practice guideline: Electrodiagnostic criteria for CTS

The practice guideline for CTS recommends diagnostic examination strategies[30,31,32]:

1. Standard: perform a median sensory nerve conduction study (NCS) across the wrist with conduction distance of 13 to 14 cm. If abnormal, compare to an adjacent sensory nerve in the symptomatic limb
2. Standard: if the initial median sensory NCS across the wrist is normal then additional comparison studies are recommended
3. Guideline: record motor NCS of the median nerve from the thenar muscle and of 1 other nerve in the symptomatic limb
4. Option: supplementary NCS
5. Option: needle electromyography (EMG) of cervical root screen muscles including a thenar muscle

NCV: Electrophysiologic studies support a diagnosis of carpal tunnel syndrome (CTS) using median nerve conduction studies across the transverse carpal ligament. Characteristic abnormalities: prolongation of sensory and motor distal latencies, slowing of the conduction velocity and decreased amplitudes of sensory and motor responses. Guidelines regarding recommended studies are published by the American Association of Neuromuscular and Electrodiagnostic Medicine (AANEM), AAPM&R, and AAN. Adhering to the guidelines, sensitivity is greater than 85% and specificity is greater than 95%.[30] Sensory latencies are more sensitive than motor. (Note: although up to 15% of cases may have normal electrodiagnostic studies, great reservation should be exercised in considering operating on CTS with normal sensory NCV and amplitude.)

Normal findings are shown in ▶ Table 31.2. Abnormal values also listed are a rough guide, but the correlation between severity of EDX findings and symptoms in CTS is not well-established.[29] Nevertheless, classification as follows can in part predict the outcome of carpal tunnel release (surgery), with normal and very severe NCS abnormalities having a worse prognosis than patients with moderate NCS abnormalities.[29,33]

EDX interpretation (reports may also include the degree of slowing in the summary of findings or interpretation[29,34,35]):

* mild: prolonged (relative or absolute) median nerve sensory latencies with normal motor studies. No evidence of axonal loss.
* moderate: prolonged (relative or absolute) median nerve sensory latencies with prolongation of motor distal latency. No evidence of axonal loss.
* severe: any of the aforementioned NCS abnormalities with evidence of axonal loss on EMG.

Table 31.2 Distal conduction latencies through *carpal tunnel*[a]

Degree of involvement[b]	Sensory		Motor	
	latency[c] (mSec)	amplitude (mcV)	latency[d] (mSec)	amplitude (mV)
normal	<3.7	>25	<4.5	>4
mild[b]	3.7–4.0		4.4–6.9	
moderate[b]	4.1–5.0		7.0–9.9	
severe[b]	>5 or unobtainable		>10	

[a]assumes normal proximal NCV
[b]severity does not reliably correlate with latency (see text)
[c]to index finger. Sensory latency is measured to the peak of the waveform
[d]to abductor pollicis brevis

Additional comparison studies for uncertain cases compare median nerve sensory conduction velocity to that of the ulnar nerve (or radial nerve): normal median nerve should be at least 4 m/sec faster than the ulnar; reversal of this pattern suggests median nerve injury. Alternatively, the sensory latencies for the palmar median and ulnar nerves can be compared; the median nerve latency should not be ≥ 0.3 mS longer than the ulnar.

EMG: normal in up to 31% of cases of CTS. In relatively advanced CTS, it may show increased polyphasicity, positive waves, fibrillation potentials, and decreased motor unit numbers on maximal voluntary thenar muscle contraction. EMG may detect cervical radiculopathy if motor involvement is present.

With severe "end stage" CTS, sensory and motor potentials may not be recordable, and EMG is not helpful in localizing (i.e., differentiating CTS from other etiologies).

Laboratory tests

Recommended in cases where an underlying peripheral neuropathy is suspected (e.g., a young individual with no risk factors such as repetitive hand use). This same protocol is a useful initial workup for any case of peripheral neuropathy:
1. thyroid hormone levels (T4 (total or free) & TSH): to R/O myxedema
2. CBC: anemia is common in multiple myeloma
3. electrolytes:
   a) standard panel (Na, K, Cl, BUN, creatinine, glucose): to R/O chronic renal failure that could cause uremic neuropathy
   b) HgA1c and blood glucose: R/O diabetes
4. vitamin B12, folate & MMA (methylmalonic acid) levels to R/O clinically significant vitamin B12 deficiency[36]
5. in cases suspicious for multiple myeloma: (summary, see for details) (p.928)
   a) 24 hour urine for kappa Bence-Jones protein (p.930)
   b) bloodwork: SPEP with reflex IFE and FLC (p.930)
   c) skeletal radiologic survey
6. light-chain assay: in patients with associated kidney failure to R/O light-chain deposition disease (LCDD) which differs from amyloid because light chain immunoglobulins are deposited in the absence of amyloid granules[37]
7. hTTR: genetic testing for TTR gene mutations in suspected cases (peripheral neuropathy with cardiac and GI symptoms) to rule out hereditary TTR (hTTR) amyloidosis, an autosomal dominant hereditary form of amyloidosis where one of many possible mutations of the TTR (transthyretin) gene causes deposition of abnormal TTR (amyloid) which may produce CTS, often also associated with cardiac and GI symptoms beginning between ages 40-65 years[38]

Imaging studies

Not routinely done unless a mass lesion is suspected.

Wrist MRI: very sensitive. Findings with CTS include flattening or swelling of the nerve, palmar bowing of the flexor retinaculum. May also demonstrate ganglion cysts, lipomas… Enhancement may occur with hypervascular edema.

Diagnostic ultrasound: faster and less expensive than MRI, and can assess blood flow and changes with different wrist positions. 18 MHz probes may improve images.

31

Management of CTS

Practice guideline: Management of CTS

American Association of Orthopedic Surgeons (AAOS) Clinical Practice Guideline endorsed by American Association of Neurological Surgeons, Congress of Neurological Surgeons, American Society of Plastic Surgeons, American Academy of PM&R and AANEM[39]

1. a course of non-operative treatment is an option in patients diagnosed with CTS. Early surgery is an option when there is clinical evidence of median nerve denervation or the patient elects to proceed directly to surgical treatment (Grade C, Level V)
2. another non-operative treatment or surgery is suggested when the current treatment fails to resolve the symptoms within 2–7 weeks (Grade B, Level I and II)
3. there is not sufficient evidence to provide specific treatment recommendations for CTS when found in association with diabetes*, coexisting cervical radiculopathy, hypothyroidism, polyneuropathy, pregnancy, rheumatoid arthritis, and CTS in the workplace (inconclusive)
4. management specifics
   • local steroid injection or splinting is suggested when treating patients with CTS before considering surgery (Grade B, Level I and II)
   • oral steroids or ultrasound are options for treatment of CTS (Grade C, Level II)
   • carpal tunnel release is recommended for treatment of CTS (Grade A, level I)

* Notwithstanding the AAOS recommendations, multiple studies report that the results of carpal tunnel release in diabetics are good even when polyneuropathy is present.[40,41]

Non-surgical management

Options include:
1. rest
2. medications: non-steroidal anti-inflammatory drugs (NSAIDs), diuretics, and pyridoxine (vitamin B6) have been studied with no evidence of efficacy[11]
3. treatment of associated conditions (e.g., hypothyroidism or DM) is appropriate, but there is no data as to whether this relieves CTS[11]
4. **neutral position splints**: alleviates symptoms in > 80% of patients[42] (usually within a few days) and reduces prolonged sensory latencies.[43] Relapse is common (works best when patient does not return to heavy manual labor). A trial of at least 2–4 weeks is recommended
5. *steroid injection*: symptoms improve in > 75% of patients.[11] 33% relapse within 15 mos. Repeat injections are possible, but most clinicians limit to 3/year
   a) use 10–25 mg hydrocortisone. *Avoid local anesthetics* (may mask symptoms of intra-neural injection)
   b) inject into carpal tunnel (deep to transverse carpal ligament) to *ulnar side* of palmaris longus to avoid median nerve (in patients without palmaris longus, inject in line with fourth digit)
   c) median nerve injuries have been reported with this technique,[44] primarily due to intra-neural injection (all steroids are neurotoxic upon intrafascicular injection, and so are some of the carrier agents)
   d) risk factors for recurrence: severe electrodiagnostic abnormalities, constant numbness, impaired sensation, & weakness or atrophy of thenar muscles[11]

Surgical treatment

General information
The operation is commonly called a carpal tunnel release (CTR), AKA neurolysis or neuroplasty of the median nerve at the wrist.

Indications
Surgical intervention is recommended for constant numbness, symptoms > 1 year duration, sensory loss, or thenar weakness/atrophy.[11] Surgical treatment of cases due to amyloidosis from multiple myeloma is also effective.

With bilateral CTS, in general one operates on the more *painful* hand first. However if the condition is severe in both hands (on EMG) and if it has progressed beyond the painful stage and is only causing weakness and/or numbness, it may be best to operate on the "better" hand first in order to try and maximize recovery of the median nerve, at least on that side. Simultaneous bilateral procedures may also be done.[45] In severe cases, nerve recovery may not occur; it may be necessary to wait up to a year to determine extent of recovery.

Applied anatomy

The carpal tunnel is a space in the wrist bounded by the transverse carpal ligament (TCL) as the "roof," and the "floor" composed of 4 carpal bones: trapezium, trapezoid, capitate and hamate. Through the carpal tunnel passes:
• 4 tendons of the flexor digitorum profundus
• 4 tendons of the flexor digitorum superficialis
• tendon of the flexor pollicus longus
• median nerve

The TCL is contiguous proximally with the deep investing fascia of the forearm, and distally with the flexor retinaculum of the palm of the hand. The fibers of the TCL are oriented transversely, compared to the longitudinal fibers of the flexor retinaculum. 4 points of attachment of the TCL to the carpal bones:
• 2 radial (lateral) points of attachment: scaphoid and trapezium
• 2 ulnar (medial) points of attachment: pisiform and hook of the hamate

Median nerve (MN): positioned slightly to the radial side of midline in the carpal tunnel. 2 branches (KEY: both usually run on the radial side of the MN):
• palmar cutaneous branch (PCB): sensory to skin of base of the thenar eminence (see ▸ Fig. 31.1) (roots: C6&7). Arises from the radial aspect of the MN proximal to the carpal tunnel and travels along the ulnar aspect of the flexor carpi radialis tendon superficial to the flexor retinaculum/TCL (i.e., passes over, not through, the carpal tunnnel), ∴ *spared* in carpal tunnel syndrome
• recurrent motor branch: innervates the muscles of the thenar eminence. AKA thenar motor branch, AKA the "million dollar nerve" because injury to the nerve during carpal tunnel surgery will lead to loss of function of the thumb and a possible malpractice lawsuit. Arises from MN usually distal to the TCL (reports that it arises proximal to the TCL in 20% of cases seem exaggerated)

The radial artery and ulnar artery anastomose via a superficial and a deep palmar arch in the palm.

Kaplan's cardinal line: there are multiple variations of the definition of this line. For discussion here, it runs from the base of the thumb web space to the hook of the hamate (see ▸ Fig. 31.3). The superfical palmar arch, which is vulnerable during carpal tunnel syurgery, is distal to this line.

Surgical techniques

A number of techniques are popular, including incision through palm of hand, transverse incision through wrist crease (with or without a retinaculatome (e.g., Paine retinaculatome)[46]), and endoscopic techniques (using single or dual incisions). The efficacies of the various approaches have not been compared in an adequately powered randomized study[11] and there is no consensus on the superiority of any one technique,[14,47,48,49] including endoscopic vs. open CTR.

Transpalmar approach (▸ Fig. 31.3): Magnification (e.g., operating loupes) is helpful.

Incision along an imaginary line extending proximally from the space between digits 3 and 4 (usually stay just to the ulnar side of the interthenar crease to avoid the PCB). The location of the median nerve may also be estimated by the palmaris longus tendon (stay slightly to ulnar side of tendon). Incision starts at distal wrist flexion crease, and the length depends on thickness of hand (it may extend as far distally as Kaplan's cardinal line (p.551)). Optionally: curve ulnarward at proximal wrist flexion crease (to facilitate retraction).

The flexor retinaculum flexor (longitudinally oriented fibers) is incised after the skin, and then the median nerve is carefully approached through the transversely oriented fibers of the TCL with progressively deepening incisions made e.g., with a 15 blade. All approaches to CTS surgery require complete division of the TCL at and distal to the wrist. If tendons of the flexor digitorum superficialis are encountered, you are too deep and need to back out and look more radially (toward the thumb) to find the nerve. In selected cases, the epineurium may be opened; however, internal neurolysis probably does more harm than good and in general should be avoided.

Close with absorbable 4–0 inverted sutures. Approximate skin edges with 4–0 nylon running or interrupted vertical mattress. Pad palm with several fluffs (opened dressing sponge). Cover with Kerlix®.

31

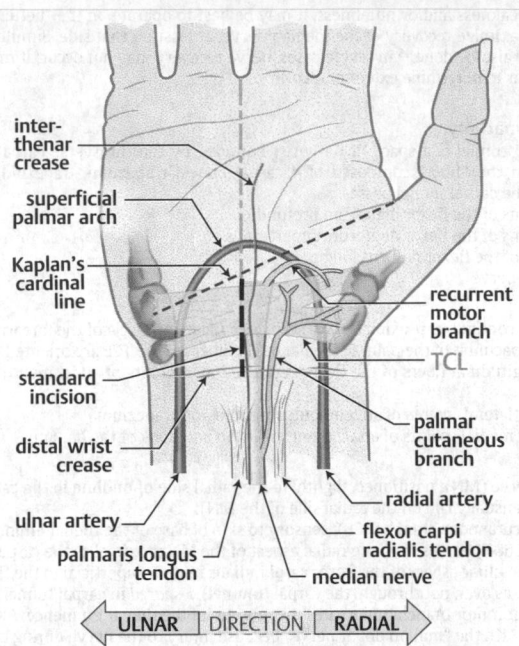

31

Fig. 31.3 Transpalmar incision for carpal tunnel syndrome surgery (right hand)—broken black line.
Broken green line = trajectory of incision (parallel to interspace between digits #3 & 4).
Broken red line = Kaplan's cardinal line. TCL = transverse carpal ligament (in blue).
NB: the superficial palmar arch (artery) is illustrated, the deep palm arch is generally not at risk and is not shown.

Post-op: wrap hand with thumb exposed. Wrist elevation and rest is recommended for several days. Analgesics for mild-to-moderate pain (e.g., acetaminophen with codeine) for 3–4 days. Sutures are removed at 7–10 days. No heavy work with hand for 2–3 weeks.

Complications of carpal tunnel surgery
See reference.[50]
1. pain due to neuroma formation following transection of **palmar cutaneous branch** (PCB) of the median nerve
    a) branches of PCB may cross interthenar crease
    b) avoid by using magnification and making incision slightly to ulnar side of interthenar crease
    c) treated by ligating this branch where it originates from median nerve in forearm (results in small area of numbness at base of thenar eminence)
2. neuroma of dorsal sensory branch of radial nerve
    a) caused by extending incision proximally and radially
    b) may be treated by neurolysis of neuroma
3. injury to recurrent thenar (motor) branch of median nerve
    a) anomaly may cause nerve to lie above or to pierce TCL
    b) avoided by: staying to *ulnar side* of midline
4. direct injury to median nerve
5. volar displacement and entrapment of median nerve in healing edges of TCL
6. hypertrophic scar causing compression of median nerve
    a) usually caused by incision crossing wrist perpendicular to flexion crease
    b) avoid by not crossing flexion crease, or in cases where necessary (e.g., in releasing Guyon's canal entrapment of ulnar nerve, in tenosynovectomy for rheumatoid arthritis, or in dealing with an anomalous superficialis or palmaris muscle) by crossing wrist obliquely at 45° angle directed toward ulnar side[50] (see optional extension line in ▶ Fig. 31.3)

7. failure to improve symptoms
    a) incorrect diagnosis: if EMG or NCV not done pre-op, they should be done after surgical failure (to R/O e.g., cervical root involvement [look for posterior myotome involvement], or generalized peripheral neuropathy)
    b) incomplete transection of TCL: the most common cause for failure if diagnosis is correct (also possibility of accessory ligament or fascial band proximal to TCL in cases where division was complete). When this is identified on re-exploration, 75% of patients will be cured or improved after division is completed
8. joint stiffness: caused by excessively long immobilization of wrist and fingers
9. injury to superficial palmar arch (arterial): usually results from "blind" distal division of TCL
10. bowstringing of flexor tendons
11. complex regional pain syndrome AKA reflex sympathetic dystrophy: exact incidence is unknown, reported in 4 of 132 patients in one series (probably too high, most surgeons will see only one or two cases in their career). Treatment with IV phentolamine has been suggested, but most cases are self limited after ≈ 2 weeks
12. infection: usually causes exquisite tenderness
13. hematoma: also usually quite painful and tender

Outcome of surgical treatment (carpal tunnel release)

75–90% of patients have symptom resolution or are improved to a satisfactory state following carpal tunnel release.[17,47,51] Clinical improvement peaks at 6 months post-op,[52,53,54] although paresthesias may take ≥ 9 months to resolve.[47,55,56,57] 70–90% are free of nocturnal pain.[58,59]

Diabetic patients: the results of decompression are good in diabetics with CTS even when a generalized peripheral neuropathy is present.[60] In contrast, ulnar neuropathy at the elbow is often poorly responsive in diabetics (p. 557).[40]

Managing surgical treatment failures

Less than satisfactory outcomes following CTR should be categorized as:
1. new symptoms: may include neuropathic pain out of proportion to the surgery, new areas of numbness/paresthesias or marked weakness of the thenar muscles.[61] When present immediately post-op, this suggests iatrogenic injury to branches of the median nerve
2. persistent symptoms (primary failure or failure to improve) defined as symptoms that remain unchanged compared to preop. Etiologies include incorrect initial diagnosis, incomplete release of the transverse carpal ligament, and severe (i.e., irreversible) CTS at initial diagnosis.[14]
3. or recurrent symptoms: requires symptom-free interval before return of symptoms (there is no standardization of either the level of recurrent symptoms or length of interval,[47] although 6 months has been used in some studies[61]). Etiologies include circumferential fibrosis around the median nerve, soft tissue adhesions, synovial proliferation, tenosynovitis, ganglions, amyloid deposits, and subtle palmar subluxation.[14,61]

▶ **Electrodiagnostic (EDX) studies.** Following CTR, distal motor latency improves after 3 months and 6 months and may continue to improve for up to 2 years.[53,62,63] Electrophysiologic abnormalities may improve but may not return to normal range after CTR even with clinical improvement.[47,54] Electrophysiologic studies are most helpful when it is possible to compare to pre-op studies.[14,17,61,64,65] There are no guidelines or standard recommendations for when to obtain postoperative studies for surgical failures. It is reasonable to obtain repeat studies at 3 to 6 months following carpal tunnel release for persistent symptoms and at onset for new or recurrent symptoms. If the repeat nerve conduction studies are worse or if the EMG needle exam has findings of denervation (fibrillation potentials and positive sharp waves) not previously present, then repeat surgery is indicated.[17,61] If the preoperative study is not available, repeating the EDX study with comparison at 2 points in time to evaluate for improvement or worsening is advised. Prolonged latencies alone are not an indication for reoperation.[66]

31.5 Ulnar nerve entrapment

31.5.1 General information

Ulnar nerve has components of C7, C8, and T1 nerve roots. Even though this is the second most prevalent entrapment neuropathy after CTS, it is still relatively uncommon. Potential sites of compression:
1. above elbow: possibly by the arcade of Struthers

31

2. at the elbow: retroepicondylar groove ("ulnar groove"): between the medial epicondyle and the olecranon process. Compression by fascia or by dynamic compression or repetitive trauma. This is also the location of the "funny bone" where the nerve can be acutely impacted to produce transient numbness and tingling in the 2 little fingers
3. cubital tunnel: just distal to the ulnar groove, under the aponeurosis spanning the heads of the flexor carpi ulnaris (FCU) known as Osborne's ligament[67] or cubital tunnel retinaculum
4. at the point of exit from the FCU
5. wrist: Guyon's canal

Etiologies: structural, mechanical or idiopathic.

Motor findings include:
1. wasting of the interossei may occur, and is most evident in the first dorsal interosseous (in the thumb web space)
2. Wartenberg's sign: one of the earliest findings of ulnar nerve entrapment (abducted little finger due to weakness of the third palmar interosseous muscle—patient may complain that the little finger doesn't make it in when they reach into their pocket)
3. Froment's prehensile thumb sign: grasping a sheet of paper between thumb and the extended index finger results in extension of the proximal phalanx of the thumb and flexion of the distal phalanx as a result of substituting flexor pollicis longus (which is spared since it is innervated by anterior interosseous nerve) for the weak adductor pollicis[68 (p 18)]
4. claw deformity of the hand (main en griffe): in severe ulnar nerve injuries on attempted finger *extension* (some have called this "benediction hand," which differs from that with the same name in median nerve injury where the named sign occurs on trying to make a fist. Fingers 4 and 5 and to a lesser extent 3 are hyperextended at the MCP joints (extensor digitorum is unopposed by interossei and "ulnar" lumbricals III & IV) and flexed at the interphalangeal joints (due to pull of long flexor muscles). NB: C8 radiculopathy can also cause benediction sign[69])

Sensory findings. Disturbance of sensation involving:
1. the little finger and ulnar half of the ring finger (▶ Fig. 31.1)
2. sensory loss over the ulnar side of the dorsum of the hand. This will be spared in ulnar nerve entrapment at the wrist (dorsal ulnar cutaneous nerve branches proximal to the wrist)

31.5.2 Injury above elbow

May occur with injury to the medial cord of the brachial plexus.

In the upper arm, the ulnar nerve descends anterior to the medial head of triceps; in 70% of people it passes under arcade of Struthers—distinct from Struther's ligament (p. 544)—a flat, thin, aponeurotic band. This is not normally a point of entrapment, but may cause kinking after ulnar nerve transposition if not adequately divided.[70 (p 1781)]

31.5.3 Ulnar nerve entrapment at elbow (UNE)

General information

Entrapment at or just distal to the elbow produces the cubital tunnel syndrome. (Technically, the cubital tunnel is formed by the fibrous arch between the two heads of the FCU,[71 (p 877)] the proximal entrance to which is just distal to the retrocondylar groove. However, common vernacular usually includes entrapment within the groove itself as being "cubital tunnel syndrome.")

Can also present as so-called tardy ulnar palsy because of delayed onset following bony injury at the elbow, initial case reports occurred ≥ 12 years later, with the majority commencing > 10 years following the original injury. The elbow is the most vulnerable point of the ulnar nerve: here the nerve is superficial, fixed, and crosses a joint. Most cases are idiopathic, although there may be a history of elbow fracture (especially lateral condyle of the humerus, with associated cubitus valgus deformity), dislocation, arthritis, or repeated minor trauma. The aponeurotic arch extending over the ulnar groove and attaching on the medial epicondyle may become thickened and can compress the nerve, especially with elbow flexion.[71 (p 884)] The ulnar nerve may also be injured during anesthesia (p. 575).[72] In contrast to CTS, which is predominantly demyelinating, UNE has more axonal loss even when chronic.[33]

Presentation

Typically presents with discomfort (pain, numbness and/or tingling) in little finger and ulnar half of ring finger, elbow pain, and hand weakness. Early symptoms may be purely motor (see Froment's sign and claw deformity above), unlike the median nerve where sensory involvement is almost always present. Symptoms may be exacerbated by the cold, and are often somewhat vague and may be described as a loss of finger coordination or clumsiness. Cramping and easy fatiguing of the ulnar innervated muscles in the hand may occur. Pain may *not* be a significant feature, but if present tends to be aching in nature along the ulnar aspect of the elbow or forearm. Atrophy of interossei is common by the time of presentation.

The ulnar nerve is usually tender and may be palpably enlarged in the ulnar groove. Tinel's sign may be positive over the elbow, but this is not very specific.

Grading: the classification system proposed by Stewart[73] is shown in ▶ Table 31.3.

Table 31.3 Stewart classification system for severity of ulnar nerve injury (Stewart[73] after Bartels[74])

Grade	Description
1 (mild)	sensory symptoms ± motor symptoms; ± sensory loss; no muscle atrophy or weakness
2 (moderate)	sensory symptoms with detectable sensory loss. Mild atrophy; 4 or 4 + muscle strength
3 (severe)	usually constant sensory symptoms with detectable sensory loss. Moderate to marked atrophy; 4 - or less muscle strength.

Evaluation

Electrodiagnostic studies

The literature review from AANEM Practice Parameters for EDX studies in ulnar neuropathy at the elbow (UNE) reports sensitivities to range from 37% to 86% with specificities of 95%.[30,31,32]

EDX interpretation: Reports should include localization and may comment on whether the lesion is predominantly demyelinating or axonal. Reports may use grading classification.[75]

The following suggest a focal lesion involving the ulnar nerve at the elbow. Multiple internally consistent abnormalities are more convincing than isolated abnormalities. These are listed in order of strength of evidence.

Sensory abnormalities of the distal sensory or mixed nerve action potential (NAP), especially loss of amplitude, are not localizing for ulnar neuropathy (in contradistinction to median nerve/carpal tunnel), the motor component of the exam for the ulnar nerve is more useful for localization of the site of entrapment.

31

Practice guideline: Electrodiagnostic criteria for ulnar neuropathy at the elbow

Not all criteria need to be present and an EMG needle exam is not required[31,76]:
1. absolute motor nerve conduction velocity (NCV) < 50 m/sec from below elbow (BE) to above elbow (AE)
2. drop of NCV > 10 m/sec, comparing BE to wrist segment to the AE to BE segment
3. amplitude of compound motor action potential (CMAP) normally decreases with distance, but a drop > 20% from BE to AE is abnormal (in the absence of anomalous innervation, e.g., Martin-Gruber anastomosis (p. 540))
4. if ulnar motor studies are inconclusive (with stimulation at the wrist, above the elbow and below the elbow, while recording from ADQ) the following may be of benefit:
   • NCS recorded from the FDI (first dorsal interosseus muscle, innervated by ulnar nerve)
   • inching study recording latencies and amplitudes at cm increments.
   • with severe UNE and wallerian degeneration, comparison of AE to BE with axilla to AE
   • needle EMG should always include FDI and ulnar innervated forearm muscles (flexor digitorum profundus (FDP) to ring or little finger and/or abductor digiti quinti/minimi [ADQ]). If abnormal then extend to include non-ulnar innervated C8, medial cord, lower trunk muscles and cervical paraspinals to exclude brachial plexopathy/cervical radiculopathy.

The 2 most important parameters that predict a good outcome are preserved compound muscle action potential (CMAP) amplitudes in ulnar hand muscles and conduction block (CB) with slowed conduction velocity across the elbow, which is consistent with demyelination and has a better prognosis.[28,77] Poor prognosis correlates with small or absent CMAP and no CB consistent with axonal loss.[28]

Diagnostic ultrasound

Localizing ulnar nerve lesions with electrodiagnostic studies can be difficult. There has been a recent renewed interest in diagnostic ultrasound using high frequency (18 MHz) probes to help with localization, and also for identification of pathology, including nerve swelling, transection,[78] and neuroma, that exceeds MRI in some aspects and at a lower cost and with faster acquisition time.

Management of ulnar neuropathy at the elbow

There are no Clinical Practice Guidelines for treatment of UNE endorsed by AANEM, AAOS, CNS, AANS, AAPM&R, or Am Society of Plastic Surgeons. A fundamental difficulty in treating UNE are the multiple etiologies and locations so that the natural history and responses to treatment vary widely. The primary management decision is conservative versus surgical treatment.

A Cochrane Database Review concluded the available evidence is not sufficient to identify the best treatment for UNE on the basis of clinical, neurophysiologic and imaging characteristics.[79,80]

Nonsurgical treatment (see below) may be considered for the patient with intermittent symptoms, no atrophy and mild EDX findings. Surgical intervention has been advised for patients who fail conservative management, although the best nonsurgical management and duration of treatment are not well defined.[80]

Suggested protocol:

- mild or moderate UNE (grade 1 and 2, ▶ Table 31.3): treat conservatively as studies report improvement or complete recovery in 30–90%.[33,73] Follow clinically every 2 months to detect deterioration. If worsening occurs, image with CT or MRI. Surgical exploration is indicated regardless of imaging results
- severe (grade 3) UNE: initiate conservative treatment, obtain imaging and f/u in 1 month. If there is worsening or if a structural abnormality is found, or both, then proceed with surgical intervention. If stable or improving and imaging is normal, then follow clinically at monthly intervals. Surgical intervention for worsening.[73]

There is a probable increased prevalence of UNE in diabetics. The UNE is often more severe with predominant axonal injury, and these patients do not respond well to surgery.[40]

Non-surgical treatment

Patient education on positions to avoid (prolonged elbow bending to ≥ 90° flexion). Avoid trauma to the elbow, including resting it on firm surfaces (tables, rigid armrests in motor vehicles…); a soft elbow gel-pad may help. Results are often better when definite traumatic etiology can be identified and eliminated.

Surgical treatment

General approach

Most operations utilize a "lazy omega" skin incision centered over the medial epicondyle, extending at least ≈ 6 cm proximal and distal to the elbow with the central "hump" directed anteriorly. The ulnar nerve is most constant and therefore most easily found immediately at the entrance to the ulnar groove. It may then be followed proximally and distally. Nerve branches that should be preserved include: posterior branches of the medial antebrachial cutaneous nerve (or else numbness or dysesthesias along medial forearm may occur) and branches to the flexor carpi ulnaris (which may branch early). Small articular branches at or proximal to the elbow joint can be preserved with simple decompression but may need to be sacrificed in transposition if they cannot be dissected far enough along the ulnar nerve. Internal neurolysis should be avoided as it may promote intraneural fibrosis.

The choice of one of the options below will determine subsequent steps.

Surgical options primarily consist of:

1. simple nerve decompression without transposition[81] (see below). Includes all of the following:
   a) at the elbow: division of the cubital tunnel retinaculum
   b) distal to the elbow: dividing the aponeurosis connecting the two heads of the flexor carpi ulnaris, some advocate resuturing the aponeurosis underneath the nerve
   c) proximal to the elbow: dividing the medial intermuscular septum (between distal biceps and triceps muscles) and the arcade of Struthers (if present)
   d) preservation of the branch to the flexor carpi ulnaris and the dorsal cutaneous branch to the hand (arises 5 cm proximal to wrist)

31

2. nerve decompression and transposition (extent of surgery differs because degree of entrapment varies; all forms of transposition require fashioning a sling to retain the nerve in its new location). Transposition may be to:
   a) subcutaneous tissue: this leaves the nerve fairly superficial and vulnerable to further trauma
   b) within the flexor carpi ulnaris muscle (intramuscular transposition): some contend this actually worsens the condition due to intramuscular fibrosis
   c) a submuscular position: see below
3. medial epicondylectomy. Usually combined with decompression. Normally reserved for patients with a bony deformity
4. sometimes excision of neuroma and possibly jump graft may be required

Submuscular transposition

Placement under pronator teres, within a groove fashioned in the flexor carpi ulnaris (FCU). Usually requires general anesthesia (endotracheal or laryngeal mask airway).
Some key concepts[82 (p 247,260–5),83]:
1. the skin incision must extend at least ≈ 8 cm distal and proximal to the medial epicondyle to mobilize the nerve (spare the medial antecubital cutaneous nerve in the subcutaneous fatty tissue just distal to the elbow)
2. the nerve is mobilized, sparing branches to flexor carpi ulnaris (FCU) and the ulnar flexor profundi branch(es) (usually arise 2–4 cm distal to olecranon)
3. the medial intermuscular septum (between distal biceps and triceps muscles) must be cut in the distal arm to prevent the nerve from being kinked over it
4. the pronator teres muscle must be sectioned completely through just distal to the medial epicondyle
   a) start by undermining the muscle just distal to the medial epicondyle
   b) a mosquito hemostat may be passed under the muscle to assist
   c) the muscle is cut sharply, leaving a cuff to reattach it
5. a trough is cut in the volar aspect of the FCU to accommodate the nerve
6. after the pronator teres is reattached over the nerve, make sure that the nerve can slide back and forth easily under the muscle
7. test the elbow through a range of motion after the transposition to look for snapping of the medial portion of the triceps over the medial epicondyle[84]

31

Transposition vs. decompression

Σ: Ulnar transposition vs. simple decompression

For most cases, simple decompression is recommended over transposition. Possible exceptions include: bony deformity, nerve subluxation

Randomized studies have shown similar success but lower complication rate with simple decompression vs. transposition.[79,85,86] Advantages of simple decompression include[74,87] shorter operation that can be done more easily under local anesthesia, avoidance of nerve kinking and muscular fibrosis around the transposed nerve, reduced risk of wound infection[79] and scar formation,[73] and preservation of cutaneous branches, ulnar branches, and nourishing blood vessels (vasa nervorum[73]) that are sometimes sacrificed with transposition, rendering portions of the nerve ischemic.

Arguments against simple decompression: continued dynamic compression with elbow flexion, possible nerve subluxation (if present pre-op, simple decompression may make this worse; to avoid nerve subluxation and loss of vascular supply with simple decompression, avoid a 360° freeing of the nerve), and incomplete release of pressure points.

Results with surgery

Not as good as with CTS, possibly due in part to the fact that patients tend to present much later. Overall, a good to excellent result is obtained in 60%, a fair result in 25%, and a poor result (no improvement or worsening) in 15%.[88 (p 2530)] These results may be worse in patients with symptoms present > 1 year, with only 30% of these symptomatically improved in one series.[81] Pain and sensory changes respond better than muscle weakness and atrophy.

Patients with comorbidities: lower success rate is seen in older patients and those with certain medical conditions (diabetes, alcoholism…). Ulnar neuropathy at the elbow is often severe in diabetics and predominantly motor with axonal injury and usually does not respond well to surgery.[40]

31.5.4 Entrapment in the forearm

Very rare. Just distal to the elbow, the ulnar nerve exits the retroepicondylar groove to pass under the fascial band (Osborne's ligament) connecting the two heads of the flexor carpi ulnaris (FCU), superficial to the flexor superficialis and pronator teres. Findings with entrapment in the forearm are similar to tardy ulnar nerve palsy (see above).

Surgical treatment consists of steps outlined for nerve distal to the elbow in ulnar nerve decompression (see above). A technique for locating the course of the ulnar nerve distal to the elbow: the surgeon takes the little finger of his/her own hand (using the hand contralateral to the patient's side that is being decompressed) and places the proximal phalanx in the ulnar groove aiming it toward the ulnar side of the wrist.[82 (p 262)]

31.5.5 Entrapment in the wrist or hand

At the wrist, the terminal ulnar nerve enters Guyon's canal, the roof of which is the palmar fascia and palmaris brevis, and the floor of which is the flexor retinaculum of the palm and the pisohamate ligament.

▶ **Guyon's canal.** Is *superficial* to the transverse carpal ligament (which overlies the carpal tunnel and compresses the median nerve in carpal tunnel syndrome).

The canal contains no tendons, only the ulnar nerve and artery. At the middle of the canal the nerve divides into a deep and superficial branch. The superficial branch is mostly sensory (except for the branch to palmaris brevis), and supplies hypothenar eminence and ulnar half of ring finger. The deep (muscular) branch innervates hypothenar muscles, lumbricals 3 & 4, and all interossei. Occasionally the abductor digiti minimi branch arises from the main trunk or superficial branch.

Shea and McClain[89] divided lesions of the ulnar nerve in Guyon's canal into 3 types shown in ▶ Table 31.4. Injury to the distal motor branch can also occur in the palm and produces findings similar to a Type II injury.

Table 31.4 Types of ulnar nerve lesions in Guyon's canal

Type	Location of compression	Weakness	Sensory deficit
Type I	just proximal to or within Guyon's canal	all intrinsic hand muscles innervated by ulnar n.	palmar ulnar distribution[a]
Type II	along deep branch	muscles innervated by deep branch[b]	none
Type III	distal end of Guyon's canal	none	palmar ulnar distribution[a]

[a]palmar ulnar distribution: the hypothenar eminence and ulnar half of ring finger, both on the palmar surface only (the dorsum is innervated by the dorsal cutaneous nerve)
[b]depending on the location, may spare hypothenar muscles

Injury is most often due to a ganglion of the wrist,[90] but also may be due to trauma (use of pneumatic drill, pliers, repetitively slamming a stapler, leaning on palm while riding bicycle). Symptoms are similar to those of ulnar nerve involvement at the elbow, except there will never be sensory loss in the *dorsum* of the hand in the ulnar nerve territory because the dorsal cutaneous branch leaves the nerve in the forearm 5–8 cm proximal to the wrist (sparing of flexor carpi ulnaris and flexor digitorum profundus III & IV is not helpful in localizing because these are so rarely involved even in proximal lesions). Electrodiagnostics are usually helpful in localizing the site of the lesion. Pain, when present, may be exacerbated by tapping over pisiform (Tinel's sign). It may also radiate up the forearm.

Surgical decompression may be indicated in refractory cases. To locate: find the ulnar artery, and the nerve is on the ulnar side of the artery. Controversial whether simple decompression vs. subcutaneous transposition is best; the outcome is similar but there may be more complications in the transposition group,[85,86] but studies are small.

31.6 Radial nerve injuries

See reference.[91 (p 1443–45)]

31.6.1 Applied anatomy

The radial nerve arises from the posterior divisions of the 3 trunks of the brachial plexus (▶ Fig. 30.1). It receives contributions from C5 to C8. The nerve winds laterally along the spiral groove of the humerus where it is vulnerable to compression or injury from fracture.

Distinguish radial nerve injury from injury of posterior cord of brachial plexus by sparing of deltoid (axillary nerve) and latissimus dorsi (thoracodorsal nerve).

31.6.2 Axillary compression

Etiologies: crutch misuse; poor arm position during (drunken) sleep.

31.6.3 Mid-upper arm compression

Etiologies

1. "Saturday night palsy": improper positioning of arm in sleep (especially when drunk and therefore less likely to self-reposition in response to the accompanying discomfort, e.g., due to a bedmate's head resting on the arm)
2. from positioning under general anesthesia
3. from callus due to old humeral fracture

Clinical

Weakness of wrist extensors (wrist drop) and finger extensors. ★ Key: *triceps is normal* because takeoff of nerve to triceps is proximal to spiral groove. Involvement of distal nerve is variable, may include thumb extensor palsy and paresthesias in radial nerve distribution.

Differential diagnosis

1. isolated wrist and finger extensor weakness can also occur in lead poisoning (usually bilateral, more common in adults)
2. C7 radiculopathy: triceps will be weak

31.6.4 Forearm compression

General information

The radial nerve enters the anterior compartment of the arm just above the elbow. It gives off branches to brachialis, brachioradialis, and extensor carpi radialis (ECR) longus before dividing into the posterior interosseous nerve and the superficial radial nerve. The posterior interosseous nerve dives into the supinator muscle through a fibrous band known as the arcade of Fröhse.

Posterior interosseous neuropathy

Posterior interosseous neuropathy (often referred to by its acronym "PIN") may result from lipomas, ganglia, fibromas, rheumatoid arthritis changes at elbow, entrapment at the arcade of Fröhse (rare), and occasionally from strenuous use of the arm.

Treatment: cases that do not respond to 4–8 weeks of expectant management should be explored, and any constrictions lysed (including arcade of Fröhse).

Radial tunnel syndrome

AKA supinator syndrome. Controversial. The "radial tunnel" extends from just above the elbow to just distal to it, and is composed of different structures (muscles, fibrous bands…) depending on the level.[92] It contains the radial nerve and its two main branches (posterior interosseous and superficial radial nerves). Repeated forceful supination or pronation or inflammation of supinator muscle attachments (as in tennis elbow) may traumatize the nerve (sometimes by ECR brevis). Characteristic finding: pain in the region of the common extensor origin at the lateral epicondyle on resisted extension of the middle finger which tightens the ECR brevis. May be mistakenly diagnosed as resistant "tennis elbow" (lateral epicondylitis must be excluded). There may also be peristhesias in the distribution of the superficial radial nerve and local tenderness along the radial nerve anterior to the

31

radial head. Even though the site of entrapment is similar to PIN, unlike PIN, there is usually no muscle weakness. Surgery: rarely required, consists of nerve decompression.[92]

31.7 Injury in the hand

The distal cutaneous branches of the superficial radial nerve cross the extensor pollicis longus tendon, and can often be palpated at this point with the thumb in extension. Injury to the medial branch of this nerve occurs commonly e.g., with handcuff injuries, and causes a small area of sensory loss in the dorsal web-space of the thumb.

31.8 Axillary nerve injuries

Isolated neuropathy of the axillary nerve may occur in the following situations[93]:
1. shoulder dislocation: the nerve is tethered to the joint capsule[94]
2. sleeping in the prone position with the arms abducted above the head
3. compression from a thoracic harness
4. injection injury in the high posterior aspect of the shoulder
5. entrapment of the nerve in the quadrilateral space (bounded by the teres major and minor muscles, long head of triceps, and neck of humerus) which contains the axillary nerve and the posterior humeral circumflex artery. Arteriogram may show loss of filling of the artery with the arm abducted and externally rotated

31.9 Suprascapular nerve

31.9.1 General information

The suprascapular nerve is a mixed peripheral nerve arising from the superior trunk of the brachial plexus, with contributions from C5 & C6. There is often a history of shoulder trauma or frozen shoulder. Entrapment results in weakness & atrophy of infra- and supra-spinatus (IS & SS) and deep, poorly localized (referred) shoulder pain (the sensory part of the nerve innervates the posterior joint capsule but has no cutaneous representation).

31.9.2 Etiologies

1. nerve entrapment within the suprascapular notch beneath the transverse scapular (suprascapular) ligament (TSL)[95]
2. repetitive shoulder trauma: may be bilateral when the injury is from activities such as weight-lifting
3. ganglion or tumor[96] (MRI is the test of choice for imaging these)
4. paralabral cyst from labral tear (the tendon of the long head of the biceps attaches to the superior glenoid labrum; test of choice for labral tears is MR arthrography)

31.9.3 Differential diagnosis

1. pathology in or around shoulder joint[95]
   a) rotator cuff injuries (distinction may be very difficult)
   b) adhesive capsulitis
   c) bicipital tenosynovitis
   d) arthritis
2. Parsonage-Turner syndrome limited to the suprascapular nerve; see Neuralgic amyotrophy (p.570)
3. the following two etiologies will also produce rhomboid and deltoid weakness and, usually, cutaneous sensory loss:
   a) cervical radiculopathy (≈ C5)
   b) upper brachial plexus lesion

31.9.4 Diagnosis

Diagnosis requires temporary relief with nerve block, and EMG abnormalities of SS & IS (in rotator cuff tears, fibrillation potentials will be absent). Transient pain relief with a suprascapular nerve block helps verify the diagnosis.[97]

31.9.5 Treatment

In cases where a mass is not the underlying cause, initial treatment consists of resting the affected UE, PT (including gentle conditioning), NSAIDs, topical capsaicin cream, and sometimes corticosteroid injection.

Surgical treatment is indicated for documented cases that fail to improve with conservative treatment (PT, NSAIDs, steroid/local anesthetic injection…). Position: lateral decubitus. Incision: 2 cm above and parallel to the scapular spine (atrophy of SS facilitates this). Only the trapezius needs to be split along its fibers (caution re spinal accessory nerve). To locate suprascapular notch, follow omohyoid to where it attaches to scapula and palpate just lateral to this. The suprascapular artery and vein pass over the TSL and should be preserved. Elevate the TSL with a dull nerve hook and divide it (exposure of the nerve and/or resection of the bony notch are not necessary).

31.10 Meralgia paresthetica

31.10.1 General information

AKA Originally known as the Bernhardt-Roth syndrome, and sometimes called "swashbuckler's disease," meralgia paresthetica (MP) (Greek: meros – thigh, algos – pain) is a condition often caused by entrapment of the lateral femoral cutaneous nerve (LFCN) of the thigh (a purely sensory branch with contributions from L2 and L3 nerve roots, see ▶ Fig. 1.16 for distribution), where it enters the thigh through the opening between the inguinal ligament and its attachment to the anterior superior iliac spine (ASIS). Anatomic variation is common, and the nerve may actually pass through the ligament, and as many as four branches may be found. May also be an initial manifestation of diabetes (diabetic neuropathy).

31.10.2 Signs and symptoms

Burning dysesthesias in the lateral aspect of the upper thigh, occasionally just above the knee, usually with increased sensitivity to clothing (hyperpathia). There may be decreased sensation in this distribution. Spontaneous rubbing or massaging the area in order to obtain relief is very characteristic.[98] MP may be bilateral in up to 20% of cases. Sitting or lying prone usually ameliorates the symptoms.

There may be point tenderness at the site of entrapment (where pressure may reproduce the pain), which is often located where the nerve exits the pelvis medial to the ASIS. Hip extension may also cause pain.

31.10.3 Occurrence

Usually seen in obese patients, may be exacerbated by wearing tight belts or girdles, and by prolonged standing or walking. Recently found in long distance runners. Higher incidence in diabetics. May also occur post-op in slender patients positioned prone, tends to be *bilateral* (p. 576).

Possible etiologies are too numerous to list; more common ones include tight clothing or belts, surgical scars post-abdominal surgery, cardiac catheterization (p. 577), pregnancy, iliac crest bone graft harvesting, ascites, obesity, metabolic neuropathies, and abdominal or pelvic mass.

31.10.4 Differential diagnosis

1. femoral neuropathy: sensory changes tend to be more anteromedial than MP
2. L2 or L3 radiculopathy: look for motor weakness (thigh flexion or knee extension)
3. nerve compression by abdominal or pelvic tumor (suspected if concomitant GI or GU symptoms)

The condition can usually be diagnosed on clinical grounds. When it is felt to be necessary, confirmatory tests may help (but frequently are disappointing), including:
1. EMG: may be difficult (the electromyographer cannot always find the nerve)
2. MRI or CT/myelography: when disc disease is suspected
3. pelvic imaging (MRI or CT)
4. somatosensory evoked potentials
5. response to local anesthetic injections
6. recent promise of diagnostic ultrasound using high frequency (18 MHz) probes

31.10.5 Treatment

Nonsurgical management

Tends to regress spontaneously, but recurrence is common. Nonsurgical measures achieve relief in ≈ 91% of cases and should be tried prior to considering surgery[99]:
1. remove offending articles (constricting belts, braces, casts, tight garments…)
2. in obese patients: weight loss and exercises to strengthen the abdominal muscles is usually effective, but is rarely achieved by the patient
3. elimination of activities involving hip extension
4. application of ice to the area of presumed constriction × 30 minutes TID
5. NSAID of choice × 7–10 days
6. capsaicin ointment applied TID (p. 524)
7. lidoderm patches (p. 519) in areas of hyperesthesia may help[100]
8. centrally acting pain medications (e.g., gabapentin, carbamazepine…) are rarely effective
9. if the above measures fail, injection of 5–10 ml of local anesthetic (with or without steroids) at the point of tenderness, or medial to the ASIS may provide temporary or sometimes long-lasting relief, and confirms the diagnosis

Surgical treatment

Options include:
1. surgical decompression (neurolysis) of the nerve: higher failure and recurrence rate than neurectomy
2. decompression and transposition
3. selective L2 nerve stimulation
4. division of the nerve (neurectomy) may be more effective, but risks denervation pain, and leaves an anesthetic area (usually a minor nuisance). May be best reserved for treatment failures

Technique

See references.[99,101]

The operation is best performed under general anesthesia. A 4–6 cm oblique incision is centered 2 cm distal to the point of tenderness. Since the course of the nerve is variable, the operation is exploratory in nature, and generous exposure is required. If the nerve can't be located, it is usually because the exposure is too superficial. If the nerve still cannot be found, a small abdominal muscle incision can be made and the nerve may be located in the retroperitoneal area. CAUTION: cases have occurred where the femoral nerve has erroneously been divided.

If neurectomy instead of neurolysis is elected, electrical stimulation should be performed prior to sectioning to rule out a motor component (which would disqualify the nerve as the LFCN). If the nerve is to be divided, it should be placed on stretch and then cut to allow the proximal end to retract back into the pelvis. Any segment of apparent pathology should be resected for microscopic analysis. Neurectomy results in anesthesia in the distribution of the LFCN that is rarely distressing and gradually reduces in size.

A supra-inguinal ligament approach has also been described.[101]

31.11 Obturator nerve entrapment

Controversial if this exists. The obturator nerve is composed of L2–4 roots. It courses along the pelvic wall to provide sensation to the inner thigh, and motor to the thigh adductors (gracilis and adductors longus, brevis, and magnus). It may be compressed by pelvic tumors, also from the pressure of the fetal head or forceps during parturition.

The result is numbness of the medial thigh and weak thigh adduction.

31.12 Femoral nerve entrapment

Composed of roots L2–4. Entrapment is a rare cause of femoral neuropathy. More commonly due to fracture or surgery. See Femoral neuropathy (p. 573).

31.13 Common peroneal nerve palsy

31.13.1 General information and applied anatomy

The peroneal nerve is the most common nerve to develop acute compression palsy.

Functional anatomy: the sciatic nerve (L4–S3) consists of 2 separate nerves within a common sheath that separate at a variable location in the thigh (the peroneal division of the sciatic nerve is more vulnerable to injury than the tibial division). See ▶ Fig. 102.2.

1. posterior tibial nerve, or just tibial nerve (AKA medial popliteal nerve), which provides for foot inversion among other motor functions
2. common peroneal nerve (CPN), or just peroneal nerve (AKA lateral popliteal nerve): high injuries may involve the lateral hamstring (short head of the biceps femoris) in addition to the following. The CPN passes behind the fibular head where it is superficial and fixed, making it vulnerable to pressure or trauma (e.g., from crossing the legs at the knee). Just distal to this, the CPN divides into:
   a) deep peroneal nerve (AKA anterior tibial nerve): primarily motor
      - motor: foot and toe extension (extensor hallucis longus [EHL], anterior tibialis [AT], extensor digitorum longus [EDL])
      - sensory: very small area between great toe and second toe
   b) superficial peroneal nerve (AKA musculocutaneous nerve)
      - motor: foot eversion (peroneus longus and brevis)
      - sensory: lateral distal leg and dorsum of foot

31.13.2 Causes of common peroneal nerve injury

The most frequent cause of serious peroneal nerve injury is knee injury ± fracture; see also causes of foot drop other than peroneal nerve palsy (p. 1708).

1. entrapment as it crosses the fibular neck or as it penetrates the peroneus longus
2. diabetes mellitus and other metabolic peripheral neuropathies
3. inflammatory neuropathy: including Hansen's disease (leprosy)
4. traumatic: e.g., clipping injury in football players, stretch injury due to dislocating force applied to the knee, fibular fracture, injury during hip or knee replacement surgery
5. penetrating injury
6. masses in the area of the fibular head/proximal lower leg: popliteal fossa cysts (Baker cyst), anterior tibial artery aneurysm[102] (rare)
7. pressure at fibular head: e.g., from crossing the legs at the knee, casts, obstetrical stirrups…
8. traction injuries: severe inversion sprains of the ankle
9. intraneural tumors: neurofibroma, schwannoma, neurogenic sarcoma, ganglion cysts
10. vascular: venous thrombosis
11. weight loss

31.13.3 Findings in peroneal nerve palsy

General information

1. sensory changes (uncommon): involves lateral aspect of lower half of leg
2. muscle involvement: See ▶ Table 31.5

Table 31.5 Muscle involvement in peroneal nerve palsy

Nerve	Muscle	Action	Involvement
deep peroneal	EHL	great toe dorsiflexion	Most commonly involved
	anterior tibialis	ankle dorsiflexion	↓
	EDL	toe extension	↓
superficial peroneal	peroneus longus & brevis	foot eversion	Least commonly involved (often spared)

Common peroneal nerve palsy (most common) produces weak ankle dorsiflexion (foot drop) due to anterior tibialis palsy, weak foot eversion, and sensory impairment in areas innervated by deep and superficial peroneal nerve (lateral calf and dorsum of foot). There may be a Tinel's sign with percussion over the nerve near the fibular neck. Occasionally, only the deep peroneal nerve is involved, resulting in foot drop with minimal sensory loss. Must differentiate from other causes of foot drop (p. 1706).

Examination/clinical correlation

See reference.[82 (p 293)]
- buttock level injury: unless the injury is one that permits spontaneous regeneration, prognosis is poor for return of peroneal nerve function even with surgery
- thigh level injury: also difficult to get improvement with surgical repair. Some peroneus function may occur at ≥ 6 mos, early contraction of AT may take ≥ 1 yr
- knee level injury: with successful regeneration, peroneus contraction may begin by 3–5 months. First signs: quivering of muscle lateral to the proximal fibula on attempted foot eversion, or tightening of tendon posterior and behind the lateral malleolus on attempted ankle dorsiflexion

31.13.4 Evaluation

EMG

EMG takes 2–4 weeks from the onset of symptoms to become positive. Stimulate above and below fibular head for prognostic information: if absent in both sites, the prognosis is poor (indicates retrograde degeneration has occurred). Wallerian degeneration takes ≈ 5 days to cause deterioration.

In addition to the expected findings of denervation—PSWs & fibs (p. 255)—in the anterior tibialis, evaluate:
1. L5 innervated muscles outside the distribution of the common peroneal nerve:
   a) posterior tibialis
   b) flexor digitorum longus
2. L5 muscles whose nerve originates above the knee (these muscles are *spared* in cases of compression of the peroneal nerve at the fibular head due to the fact that the nerve takeoff is proximal to the popliteal fossa):
   a) biceps femoris (short or long head)
   b) tensor fascia lata
3. paraspinal muscles: signs of denervation solidifies the location of the lesion as nerve root; not helpful if negative

MRI

May demonstrate causes such as tumor or a ganglion cyst arising from the superior tibiofibular articulation.

31.13.5 Treatment

General information

When treatment can eliminate a reversible cause, the outcome is usually good. Surgical exploration and decompression may be considered when there is no reversible cause or when improvement does not occur.

Nonsurgical management

Bracing: ankle-foot-orthosis (AFO) compensates for loss of ankle dorsiflexion which inserts unobtrusively into a shoe. If this is inadequate, or to stabilize the ankle, a spring-loaded kick-up foot brace built into a shoe may be used. The patient should be instructed in techniques to avoid contracture of the Achilles tendon (heel cord), which would impair ankle dorsiflexion if nerve function returns.

Surgical management

At the level of the popliteal fossa, the skin incision is made just medial to the tendon of the short head of the biceps femoris (lateral hamstring) as the peroneal nerve is best located deep to or slightly medial to this tendon. The incision is carried distally slightly laterally along the surgical neck of the fibula. The biceps femoris is retracted laterally and the nerve is isolated and tagged with a Penrose drain. The sensory sural nerve branches off the peroneal nerve at variable sites ranging from the sciatic portion of the nerve (proximal to the flexor crease) or distal to this.

In cases of compression, the fascia from the lateral gastrocnemius and soleus overlying the nerve distal to the fibular head is lysed and the nerve is exposed in 360°. As the nerve crosses the fibular neck it divides into superficial and deep branches. The superficial branch travels directly distally to supply the peroneus longus and brevis (foot evertors). The deep branches curve anteriorly to the anterior tibialis, EHL, and toe extensors.

If a graft is needed, the contralateral sural nerve is usually used, which may be supplemented with the ipsilateral sural nerve if needed.

31.14 Tarsal tunnel

31.14.1 General information

Entrapment of (posterior) tibial nerve may occur in the tarsal tunnel, posterior and inferior to *medial* malleolus. The tunnel is covered by the flexor retinaculum (laciniate ligament) which extends downward from the medial malleolus to the tubercle of the calcaneus. There is often (but not necessarily) a history of old ankle dislocation or fracture. The nerve may be trapped at the retinacular ligament. This results in pain and paresthesias in the toes and sole of foot (often sparing the heel because the sensory branches often originate proximal to the tunnel), typically worse at night. May cause clawing of toes secondary to weakness of intrinsic foot muscles. Often caused by fracture or dislocation, also rheumatoid arthritis, rarely tumors.

31.14.2 Exam

Percussion of nerve at medial malleolus produces paresthesias that radiate distally (Tinel's sign). Maximal inversion and eversion of the foot tend to exacerbate. Dorsiflexion-eversion test: examiner maximally everts and dorsiflexes the ankle while dorsiflexing the toes at the MTP joints for 5–10 seconds. Positive test reproduces the pain.

31.14.3 Diagnosis

EMG and NCV studies may help.

31.14.4 Nonsurgical management

External ankle support to improve foot mechanics.

31.14.5 Surgical management

Surgical decompression is indicated for confirmed cases that fail to improve. A curvilinear incision is used, ≈ 1.5 cm posterior and inferior to the medial malleolus. The flexor retinaculum is divided, as are any septa underneath, and the distal branches should be followed until they dive into the muscle.

References

[1] Neary D, Ochoa JL, Gilliatt RW. Subclinical Entrapment Neuropathy in Man. J Neurol Sci. 1975; 24:283–298

[2] Graff-Radford SB, Jaeger B, Reeves JL. Myofascial Pain May Present Clinically as Occipital Neuralgia. Neurosurgery. 1986; 19:610–613

[3] Hunter CR, Mayfield FH. Role of the Upper Cervical Roots in the Production of Pain in the Head. Am J Surg. 1949; 48:743–751

[4] Poletti CE, Sweet WH. Entrapment of the C2 Root and Ganglion by the Atlanto-Epistrophic Ligament: Clinical Syndrome and Surgical Anatomy. Neurosurgery. 1990; 27:288–291

[5] Anthony M. Headache and the greater occipital nerve. Clin Neurol Neurosurg. 1992; 94:297–301

[6] Weiner RL, Reed KL. Peripheral neurostimulation for control of intractable occipital neuralgia. Neuromodulation. 1999; 2:217–221

[7] Freund BJ, Schwartz M. Treatment of chronic cervical-associated headache with botulinum toxin A: a pilot study. Headache. 2000; 40:231–236

[8] Weinberger LM. Cervico-Occipital Pain and Its Surgical Treatment. Am J Surg. 1978; 135:243–247

[9] Bogduk N. Local Anesthetic Blocks of the Second Cervical Ganglion. A Technique with Application in Occipital Headache. Cephalalgia. 1981; 1:41–50

[10] Bovim G, Fredriksen TA, Stolt-Nielsen A, et al. Neurolysis of the greater occipital nerve in cervicogenic headache. A follow up study. Headache. 1992; 32:175–179

[11] Katz JN, Simmons BP. Clinical practice. Carpal tunnel syndrome. New England Journal of Medicine. 2002; 346:1807–1812

[12] Laha RK, Lunsford LD, Dujovny M. Lacertus Fibrosus Compression of the Median Nerve. Journal of Neurosurgery. 1978; 48:838–841

31

[13] Nakano KK, Lundergan C, Okihiro M. Anterior Interosseous Nerve Syndromes: Diagnostic Methods and Alternative Treatments. Archives of Neurology. 1977; 34:477–480

[14] Stewart JD. Median Nerve. In: Focal Peripheral Neuropathies. 4th ed. West Vancouver, Canada: JBJ Publishing; 2010:214–239

[15] Yasargil MG, Antic J, Laciga R, et al. Microsurgical Pterional Approach to Aneurysms of the Basilar Bifurcation. Surg Neurol. 1976; 6

[16] Atroshi I, Gummesson C, Johnsson R, et al. Prevalence of carpal tunnel syndrome in a general population. JAMA. 1999; 282:153–158

[17] Mosier BA, Hughes TB. Recurrent carpal tunnel syndrome. Hand Clin. 2013; 29:427–434

[18] Jain NB, Higgins LD, Losina E, et al. Epidemiology of musculoskeletal upper extremity ambulatory surgery in the United States. BMC Musculoskelet Disord. 2014; 15. DOI: 10.1186/1471-2474-15-4

[19] Feldman RG, Goldman R, Keyserling WM. Classical Syndromes in Occupational Medicine: Peripheral Nerve Entrapment Syndromes and Ergonomic Factors. Am J Ind Med. 1983; 4:661–681

[20] Padua L, Aprile I, Caliandro P, et al. Carpal tunnel syndrome in pregnancy: multiperspective follow-up of untreated cases. Neurology. 2002; 59:1643–1646

[21] Yanardag H, Pamuk ON, Kiziltan M, et al. An increased frequency of carpal tunnel syndrome in sarcoidosis. Results of a study based on nerve conduction study. Acta Medica (Hradec Kralove). 2003; 46:201–204

[22] Pryse-Phillips W E. Validation of a diagnostic sign in carpal tunnel syndrome. J Neurol Neurosurg Psychiatry. 1984; 47:870–872

[23] Phalen GS. The Carpal Tunnel Syndrome. Clinical Evaluation of 598 Hands. Clin Ortho Rel Res. 1972; 83

[24] Sandzen SC. Carpal Tunnel Syndrome. Am Fam Physician. 1981; 24:190–204

[25] Upton RM, McComas AJ. The Double Crush in Nerve Entrapment Syndromes. Lancet. 1973; 11:359–362

[26] Wilbourn AJ, Gilliatt RW. Double-Crush Syndrome: A Critical Analysis. Neurology. 1997; 49:21–29

[27] Rempel DM, Harrison RJ, Barnhart S. Work-Related Cumulative Trauma Disorders of the Upper Extremity. JAMA. 1992; 267:838–842

[28] Robinson LR. How electrodiagnosis predicts clinical outcome of focal peripheral nerve lesions. Muscle Nerve. 2015; 52:321–333

[29] Werner RA, Andary M. Electrodiagnostic evaluation of carpal tunnel syndrome. Muscle Nerve. 2011; 44:597–607

[30] Jablecki CK, Andary MT, Floeter MK, et al. Practice parameter: Electrodiagnostic studies in carpal tunnel syndrome. Report of the American Association of Electrodiagnostic Medicine, American Academy of Neurology, and the American Academy of Physical Medicine and Rehabilitation. Neurology. 2002; 58:1589–1592

[31] Campbell WW. Guidelines in electrodiagnostic medicine. Practice parameter for electrodiagnostic studies in ulnar neuropathy at the elbow. Muscle Nerve Suppl. 1999; 8:S171–S205

[32] American Association of Electrodiagnostic Medicine. Chapter 9: Practice parameter for needle electromyographic evaluation of patients with suspected cervical radiculopathy: Summary statement. Muscle and Nerve. 1999; 22:S209–S211

[33] Bland JD. A neurophysiological grading scale for carpal tunnel syndrome. Muscle Nerve. 2000; 23:1280–1283

[34] Robinson L, Kliot M. Stop using arbitrary grading schemes in carpal tunnel syndrome. Muscle Nerve. 2008; 37. DOI: 10.1002/mus.21012

[35] Bland JD. Stop using arbitrary grading schemes in carpal tunnel syndrome. Muscle Nerve. 2008; 38:1527; author reply 1527–1527; author reply 1528

[36] Leishear K, Boudreau RM, Studenski SA, et al. Relationship between vitamin B12 and sensory and motor peripheral nerve function in older adults. J Am Geriatr Soc. 2012; 60:1057–1063

[37] Ronco PM, Alyanakian MA, Mougenot B, et al. Light chain deposition disease: a model of glomerulosclerosis defined at the molecular level. J Am Soc Nephrol. 2001; 12:1558–1565

[38] Gertz MA, Benson MD, Dyck PJ, et al. Diagnosis, prognosis, and therapy of transthyretin amyloidosis. J Am Coll Cardiol. 2015; 66:2451–2466

[39] Keith MW, Masear V, Chung KC, et al. American Academy of Orthopaedic Surgeons clinical practice guideline on the treatment of carpal tunnel syndrome. J Bone Joint Surg Am. 2010; 92:218–219

[40] Stewart JD. Mononeuropathies in Diabetics. 2012

[41] Thomsen NO, Cederlund R, Rosen I, et al. Clinical outcomes of surgical release among diabetic patients with carpal tunnel syndrome: prospective follow-up with matched controls. J Hand Surg Am. 2009; 34:1177–1187

[42] Burke DT, Burke MM, Stewart GW, et al. Splinting for carpal tunnel syndrome: in search of the optimal angle. Archives of Physical Medicine and Rehabilitation. 1994; 75:1241–1244

[43] Walker WC, Metzler M, Cifu DX, et al. Neutral wrist splinting in carpal tunnel syndrome: a comparison of night-only versus full-time wear instructions. Archives of Physical Medicine and Rehabilitation. 2000; 81:424–429

[44] Linskey ME, Segal R. Median Nerve Injury from Local Steroid Injection in Carpal Tunnel Syndrome. Neurosurgery. 1990; 26:512–515

[45] Pagnanelli DM, Barrer SJ. Bilateral Carpal Tunnel Release at One Operation: Report of 228 Patients. Neurosurgery. 1992; 31:1030–1034

[46] Pagnanelli DM, Barrer SJ. Carpal Tunnel Syndrome: Surgical Treatment Using the Paine Retinaculatome. Journal of Neurosurgery. 1991; 75:77–81

[47] Louie D, Earp B, Blazar P. Long-term outcomes of carpal tunnel release: a critical review of the literature. Hand (N Y). 2012; 7:242–246

[48] Atroshi I, Larsson GU, Ornstein E, et al. Outcomes of endoscopic surgery compared with open surgery for carpal tunnel syndrome among employed patients: randomised controlled trial. BMJ. 2006; 332. DOI: 10.1136/bmj.38863.632789.1F

[49] Atroshi I, Hofer M, Larsson GU, et al. Open compared with 2-portal endoscopic carpal tunnel release: a 5-year follow-up of a randomized controlled trial. J Hand Surg Am. 2009; 34:266–272

[50] Louis DS, Greene TL, Noellert RC. Complications of Carpal Tunnel Surgery. J Neurosurg. 1985; 62:352–356

[51] Louie DL, Earp BE, Collins JE, et al. Outcomes of open carpal tunnel release at a minimum of ten years. J Bone Joint Surg Am. 2013; 95:1067–1073

[52] Guyette TM, Wilgis EF. Timing of improvement after carpal tunnel release. J Surg Orthop Adv. 2004; 13:206–209

[53] Zyluk A, Puchalski P. A comparison of the results of carpal tunnel release in patients in different age groups. Neurol Neurochir Pol. 2013; 47:241–246

[54] Padua L, Lo Monaco M, Padua R, et al. Carpal tunnel syndrome: neurophysiological results of surgery based on preoperative electrodiagnostic testing. J Hand Surg Br. 1997; 22:599–601

[55] Nancollas MP, Peimer CA, Wheeler DR, et al. Long-term results of carpal tunnel release. J Hand Surg Br. 1995; 20:470–474

[56] Katz JN, Fossel KK, Simmons BP, et al. Symptoms, functional status, and neuromuscular impairment following carpal tunnel release. J Hand Surg Am. 1995; 20:549–555

[57] Pensy RA, Burke FD, Bradley MJ, et al. A 6-year outcome of patients who cancelled carpal tunnel surgery. J Hand Surg Eur Vol. 2011; 36:642–647

[58] Katz JN, Keller RB, Simmons BP, et al. Maine Carpal Tunnel Study: outcomes of operative and nonoperative therapy for carpal tunnel syndrome in a

community-based cohort. J Hand Surg Am. 1998; 23:697–710

[59] Brown RA, Gelberman RH, Seiler JG,3rd, et al. Carpal tunnel release. A prospective, randomized assessment of open and endoscopic methods. Journal of Bone and Joint Surgery. 1993; 75:1265–1275

[60] Thomsen NO, Rosen I, Dahlin LB. Neurophysiologic recovery after carpal tunnel release in diabetic patients. Clin Neurophysiol. 2010; 121:1569–1573

[61] Jones NF, Ahn HC, Eo S. Revision surgery for persistent and recurrent carpal tunnel syndrome and for failed carpal tunnel release. Plast Reconstr Surg. 2012; 129:683–692

[62] Ginanneschi F, Milani P, Reale F, et al. Short-term electrophysiological conduction change in median nerve fibres after carpal tunnel release. Clin Neurol Neurosurg. 2008; 110:1025–1030

[63] Shurr DG, Blair WF, Bassett G. Electromyographic changes after carpal tunnel release. J Hand Surg Am. 1986; 11:876–880

[64] Schrijver HM, Gerritsen AA, Strijers RL, et al. Correlating nerve conduction studies and clinical outcome measures on carpal tunnel syndrome: lessons from a randomized controlled trial. J Clin Neurophysiol. 2005; 22:216–221

[65] Rotman MB, Enkvetchakul BV, Megerian JT, et al. Time course and predictors of median nerve conduction after carpal tunnel release. J Hand Surg Am. 2004; 29:367–372

[66] Stolp KA. Upper extremity Focal Neuropathies. 2013

[67] Granger A, Sardi JP, Iwanaga J, et al. Osborne's Ligament: A Review of its History, Anatomy, and Surgical Importance. Cureus. 2017; 9. DOI: 10.7759/cureus.1080

[68] Brazis PW, Masdeu JC, Biller J. Localization in Clinical Neurology. 2nd ed. Boston: Little Brown and Company; 1990

[69] Harrop JS, Hanna A, Silva MT, et al. Neurological manifestations of cervical spondylosis: an overview of signs, symptoms, and pathophysiology. Neurosurgery. 2007; 60:S1–14–20

[70] Wilkins RH, Rengachary SS. Neurosurgery. New York 1985

[71] Dumitru D. Electrodiagnostic Medicine. Philadelphia: Hanley and Belfus; 1995

[72] Bonney G. Iatrogenic Injuries of Nerves. Journal of Bone and Joint Surgery. 1986; 68B:9–13

[73] Stewart JD. Ulnar Nerve. In: Focal Peripheral Neuropathies. 4th ed. West Vancouver, Canada: JBJ Publishing; 2010:258–313

[74] Bartels RHMA, Menovsky T, Van Overbeeke JJ, et al. Surgical Management of Ulnar Nerve Compression at the Elbow: An Analysis of the Literature. Journal of Neurosurgery. 1988; 89:722–727

[75] Padua L, Aprile I, Mazza O, et al. Neurophysiological classification of ulnar entrapment across the elbow. Neurol Sci. 2001; 22:11–16

[76] Practice parameter: electrodiagnostic studies in ulnar neuropathy at the elbow. American Association of Electrodiagnostic Medicine, American Academy of Neurology, and American Academy of Physical Medicine and Rehabilitation. Neurology. 1999; 52:688–690

[77] Beekman R, Wokke JH, Schoemaker MC, et al. Ulnar neuropathy at the elbow: follow-up and prognostic factors determining outcome. Neurology. 2004; 63:1675–1680

[78] Cartwright MS, Chloros GD, Walker FO, et al. Diagnostic ultrasound for nerve transection. Muscle and Nerve. 2007; 35:796–799

[79] Caliandro P, La Torre G, Padua R, et al. Treatment for ulnar neuropathy at the elbow. Cochrane Database Syst Rev. 2012; 7. DOI: 10.1002/14651858.CD006839.pub3

[80] Elhassan B, Steinmann SP. Entrapment neuropathy of the ulnar nerve. J Am Acad Orthop Surg. 2007; 15:672–681

[81] Le Roux PD, Ensign TD, Burchiel KJ. Surgical Decompression Without Transposition for Ulnar Neuropathy: Factors Determining Outcome. Neurosurgery. 1990; 27:709–714

[82] Kline DG, Hudson AR. Nerve Injuries: Operative Results for Major Nerve Injuries, Entrapments, and Tumors. Philadelphia: W. B. Saunders; 1995

[83] Janjua RM, Fernandez J, Tender G, et al. Submuscular transposition of the ulnar nerve for the treatment of cubital tunnel syndrome. Neurosurgery. 2008; 63:321–4; discussion 324-5

[84] Spinner RJ, O'Driscoll S W, Jupiter JB, et al. Unrecognized dislocation of the medial portion of the triceps: another cause of ulnar nerve transposition. Journal of Neurosurgery. 2000; 92:52–57

[85] Bartels RH, Verhagen WI, van der Wilt GJ, et al. Prospective randomized controlled study comparing simple decompression versus anterior subcutaneous transposition of the ulnar nerve at the elbow for idiopathic neuropathy of the ulnar nerve at the elbow: Part 1. Neurosurgery. 2005; 56:522–30; discussion 522-30

[86] Biggs M, Curtis JA. Randomized, prospective study comparing ulnar neurolysis in situ with submuscular transposition. Neurosurgery. 2006; 58:296–304; discussion 296-304

[87] Tindall SC. Comment on LeRoux P D, et al.: Surgical Decompression without Transposition for Ulnar Neuropathy: Factors Determining Outcome. Neurosurgery. 1990; 27

[88] Youmans JR. Neurological Surgery. Philadelphia 1990

[89] Shea JD, McClain EJ. Ulnar-Nerve Compression Syndromes at and Below the Wrist. Journal of Bone and Joint Surgery. 1969; 51A:1095–1103

[90] Cavallo M, Poppi M, Martinelli P, et al. Distal Ulnar Neuropathy from Carpal Ganglia: A Clinical and Electrophysiological Study. Neurosurgery. 1988; 22:902–905

[91] Dyck PJ, Thomas PK. Peripheral Neuropathy. 2nd ed. Philadelphia: W. B. Saunders; 1984

[92] Roles NC, Maudsley RH. Radial Tunnel Syndrome: Resistant Tennis Elbow as a Nerve Entrapment. Journal of Bone and Joint Surgery. 1972; 54B:499–508

[93] McKowen HC, Voorhies RM. Axillary Nerve Entrapment in the Quadrilateral Space: Case Report. Journal of Neurosurgery. 1987; 66:932–934

[94] de Laat EAT, Visser CPJ, Coene LNJEM, et al. Nerve Lesions in Primary Shoulder Dislocations and Humeral Neck Fractures. Journal of Bone and Joint Surgery. 1994; 76B:381–383

[95] Hadley MN, Sonntag VKH, Pittman HW. Suprascapular Nerve Entrapment: A Summary of Seven Cases. J Neurosurg. 1986; 64:843–848

[96] Fritz RC, Helms CA, Steinbach LS, et al. Suprascapular nerve entrapment: Evaluation with MR imaging. Radiology. 1992; 182:437–444

[97] Callahan JD, Scully TB, Shapiro SA, et al. Suprascapular Nerve Entrapment: A Series of 27 Cases. Journal of Neurosurgery. 1991; 74:893–896

[98] Stevens HI. Meralgia Paresthetica. Arch Neurol Psychiatry. 1957; 77:557–574

[99] Williams PH, Trzil KP. Management of Meralgia Paresthetica. J Neurosurg. 1991; 74:76–80

[100] Devers A, Galer BS. Topical lidocaine patch relieves a variety of neuropathic pain conditions: an open-label study. Clinical Journal of Pain. 2000; 16:205–208

[101] Aldrich EF, Van den Heever C. Suprainguinal Ligament Approach for Surgical Treatment of Meralgia Paresthetica. Technical Note. J Neurosurg. 1989; 70:492–494

[102] Kars HZ, Topaktas S, Dogan K. Aneurysmal Peroneal Nerve Compression. Neurosurgery. 1992; 30:930–931

31

32 Non-Entrapment Peripheral Neuropathies

32.1 General information

Lesions of peripheral nerves which may produce somatic findings (combinations of weakness, sensory disturbance, and/or reflex changes) and/or autonomic disturbances.

▶ **Mononeuropathy.** A disorder of a single nerve, often due to trauma or entrapment.

▶ **Mononeuropathy multiplex.** Involvement of 2 or more nerves, usually due to a systemic abnormality (e.g., vasculitis, rheumatoid arthritis, DM…). Treatment is directed at the underlying disorder.

32.2 Etiologies of peripheral neuropathy

A mnemonic for etiologies of peripheral neuropathies is "GRAND THERAPIST" (see ▶ Table 32.1). Diabetes, alcoholism, and Guillain-Barré (italicized in table) account for 90% of cases. Other etiologies include: arteritis/vasculitis, monoclonal gammopathy (p. 574), hepatitis C virus-associated cryoglobulinemia, acute idiopathic polyneuritis, Sjögren's syndrome (disease), amyloidosis, HIV/AIDS.

Table 32.1 Mnemonic for etiologies of peripheral neuropathy

G-R-A-N-D	T-H-E-R-A-P-I-S-T
Guillain-Barré (p. 193) Renal; uremic neuropathy (p. 576) Alcoholism (see below) Nutritional (B12 deficiency…) *Diabetes*; see below or Drugs (p. 573)	Traumatic Hereditary and HIV Endocrine or Entrapment Radiation Amyloid (p. 576) or AIDS (p. 574) Porphyria (should be under hereditary) or Psychiatric or Paraneoplastic (see below) or Pseudoneuropathy (see below) or PMR (p. 206) or Polycythema vera[1] Infectious/post-infectious (e.g., Hansen's disease) Sarcoidosis, see neurosarcoidosis (p. 198), or "Systemic" Toxins, including heavy metals, e.g., lead toxicity (plumbism) (p. 1219)

32.3 Classification

1. inherited neuropathies. Examples include:
   a) Charcot-Marie-Tooth (CMT) (AKA peroneal muscular atrophy, AKA Hereditary Motor and Sensory Neuropathy [HMSN]): Up to 7 types (the most common form is autosomal dominant, but X-linked recessive forms also exist). CMT Types 1 & 2 together make up the most common inherited disorder of peripheral nerves (up to 40/100,000). The most common forms involve demyelination. Progressive loss of motor (primarily *distal* LE) and, to a lesser degree, sensory function (predominantly proprioception and vibration), with atrophy in UEs & LEs. Earliest findings: pes cavus with hammer toes, foot drop and frequent ankle sprains. Patients are more susceptible to entrapment neuropathies due to underlying compromise of peripheral nerves. Patients with Type 1 usually maintain ability to ambulate, whereas Type 2 usually lose ambulation by their teenage years
   b) hereditary neuropathy with liability to pressure palsies (HNPP): similar to CMT but due to focal areas of irregular thickening of myelin sheaths ("tomaculous" changes), mild trauma or pressure can produce nerve palsies that may last for months
2. acquired neuropathies: see sections below for details
   a) acquired pure *sensory* neuropathies (in the absence of autonomic dysfunction) are rare. May be seen with pyridoxine therapy or paraneoplastic syndromes (see below)
   b) entrapment neuropathies (p. 541)
3. pseudoneuropathy
   a) definition: psychogenic somatoform disorders or malingering, reproducing the pains, paresthesias, hyperalgesia, weakness, and even objective findings such as changes in color and temperature which may mimic neuropathic symptoms[2]

32.4 Clinical

32.4.1 Presentation

Peripheral neuropathies can present as loss of sensation, pain, weakness, incoordination and difficulty ambulating as well as with autonomic symptoms.

32.4.2 Evaluation

Initial (screening) work-up for peripheral neuropathies of unknown etiology:
1. bloodwork:
   a) fasting electrolytes
   b) Hgb-A1C
   c) CBC: anemia is common in multiple myeloma
   d) TSH
   e) ESR & CRP
   f) vitamin B_{12} & methylmalonic acid (p. 1699)
   g) SPEP with reflex to IFE (serum protein electrophoresis (SPEP), with additional test of serum immunofixation (IFE) if M-spike is present) (see multiple myeloma (p. 930) for details)
   h) optional (if multifocal motor neuropathy (MMN) (p. 1700) is suspected): Anti GM-1 antibodies
2. electrodiagnostics (EMG/NCV) (p. 254)

32.5 Syndromes of peripheral neuropathy

32.5.1 Length-dependent peripheral neuropathy

The most common clinical pattern related to neuropathy is that of length-dependent peripheral neuropathy. Symptoms are symmetric and begin in the feet (the longest nerves in the body) and gradually progress proximally. Upper limb involvement may occur late or not at all.

32.5.2 Critical illness polyneuropathy (CIP)

AKA neuropathy of critical illness, ICU neuropathy... See DDx under Guillain-Barré syndrome (p. 194).

May occur in up to 70% of septic patients (not all are significantly symptomatic). Affects primarily distal muscles.

Diagnostic criteria:
1. presence of sepsis, multi-organ failure, respiratory failure, or septic inflammatory response syndrome (SIRS)
2. difficulty weaning from ventilator or extremity weakness
3. EMG: ↓ amplitudes of compound muscle action potentials (CMAP) & SNAP
4. widespread muscle denervation potentials
5. normal or only mild increase in serum CPK levels

Recovery occurs in weeks to months (faster than Guillain-Barré).
Treatment is supportive. Complete recovery occurs in 50%.

32.5.3 Paraneoplastic syndromes affecting the nervous system

Occurs in < 1% of cancer patients. Peripheral *sensory* neuropathy of unknown etiology has been associated with cancer since its earliest description.[3] Therefore, in patients with sensory neuropathy of unknown etiology, occult neoplasms should be ruled out. If the work-up is negative, the patient should be followed since up to 35% of patients will be found to have cancer after a mean interval of 28 months after the onset of neuropathy (range: 3–72 months)[4] (no one particular cancer type predominated, in spite of the fact that historically lung cancer is the most frequent neoplasm associated with sensory neuropathy[5]).

32.5.4 Alcohol neuropathy

Characteristically produces a diffuse sensory neuropathy, with absent Achilles reflexes.

32

32.5.5 Brachial plexus neuropathy

Evaluation

When the etiology is unclear, check CXR (with apical lordotic view), glucose, ESR, and ANA.

If no improvement by ≈ 4 weeks, obtain MRI of the plexus (idiopathic brachial plexitis will usually start to show some improvement by this time; therefore tumor should be ruled out if no improvement).

Differential diagnosis of etiologies of brachial plexopathy

1. Pancoast syndrome or Pancoast tumor AKA superior sulcus tumor. Clinical: various combinations of pain in the shoulder radiating into the upper extremity in the ulnar nerve distribution from involvement of the lower brachial plexus, atrophy of hand muscles, Horner syndrome (p. 594), UE edema. Etiologies:
   a) neoplasms:
      - most common: bronchogenic cancer, usually non-small cell (NSCLC) (squamous cell or adenocarcinoma) arising in the pulmonary apex
      - metastases
   b) infections
   c) inflammatory: granulomas, amyloid
2. (idiopathic) brachial plexitis AKA neuralgic amyotrophy: most commonly upper plexus or diffuse (see below)
3. cervical rib
4. viral
5. following radiation treatment: often diffuse (see below)
6. diabetes
7. vasculitis
8. inherited: dominant genetics
9. trauma (p. 579)

Neuralgic amyotrophy of the upper extremity

General information

AKA idiopathic brachial plexus neuropathy, AKA (paralytic) brachial neuritis, AKA brachial plexitis, AKA Parsonage-Turner syndrome,[6] AKA immune-mediated brachial plexus neuropathy, among others. Idiopathic. Not clearly infectious or inflammatory; allergic mechanism possible. Prognosis is generally good. Common patterns: single or multiple mononeuropathy, plexopathy, or some combination. Demographics are shown in ▶ Table 32.2.

Table 32.2 Neuralgic amyotrophy of the upper extremity

incidence	1.64 per 100,000 population
male:female	2.4:1
age range at onset	3 mos–75 years
prodrome	• ≈ 45% had viral prodrome (URI in 25%) • may follow vaccination
onset	rapid onset of pain or paralysis/paresis
initial symptom	pain in 95%
weakness	• 50% confined to shoulder girdle • 10% confined to a single peripheral nerve
sensory deficit	67%, usually axillary and antebrachial cutaneous
laterality	• 66% unilateral (right side 54%) • 34% bilateral
lab tests	normal

In a review of 99 cases[7]: predominant symptom is acute onset of intense *pain*, with weakness developing simultaneously or after a variable period (70% occur within 2 weeks of pain), usually as the pain lessened.[6,8] Weakness never preceded pain, onset of weakness was sudden in 80%. Pain was usually constant, and described as "sharp", "stabbing", "throbbing," or "aching." Arm movement exacerbated the pain, and muscle soreness was noted in 15%. Pain lasted hours to several weeks. Paresthesias occurred in 35%. Pain usually lacked radicular features. When bilateral, weakness is usually asymmetric.

Exam

Weakness or paralysis in 96%, confined to shoulder girdle in 50%. In descending order of involvement: deltoid, spinati, serratus anterior, biceps brachii, and triceps. Winging of the scapula occurred in 20%. Sensory loss occurred in 60% of plexus lesions, of mixed variety (superficial cutaneous and proprioceptive). Sensory loss most common in outer surface of upper arm (circumflex nerve distribution) and radial aspect of forearm. Reflexes were variable.

Overall distribution judged to predominantly involve *upper* plexus in 56%, diffuse plexus in 38%, and lower in 6%.

EMG/NCV

May help localize the portion of the plexus involved, and may detect subclinical involvement of the contralateral extremity. Must wait ≥ 3 weeks from onset for findings. Differentiating from cervical radiculopathy: SNAP (p.255) should be normal in radiculopathy whereas some involvement usually occurs in plexitis. Cervical paraspinals will usually be normal in plexitis (except for very severe cases where there can be some retrograde involvement), and will be abnormal (fibrillations) in radiculopathy (except in cases where there has been enough time that significant recovery has occurred).

Outcome

Functional recovery is better in patients with primarily upper plexus involvement. After 1 year, 60% of upper plexus lesions were functioning normally, whereas none with lower involvement were (latter took 1.5–3 years). Rate of recovery estimated to be 36% within 1 year, 75% within 2, and 89% by 3 years. Recurrence was seen in only 5%. No evidence that steroids altered the course of the disease although it is still often prescribed in the acute phase.

Radiation induced brachial plexus neuropathy

Often follows external beam irradiation in the region of the axilla for breast carcinoma. Produces sensory loss with or without weakness. CT or MRI or biopsy may be needed to rule out tumor invasion of the brachial plexus.

32.5.6 Lumbosacral plexus neuropathy

32

General information

Analogous to idiopathic brachial plexitis (see above).[9] It is controversial whether this actually exists in isolation without diabetes. Often starts with LE pain of abrupt onset, followed in days or a few weeks by weakness with or without muscle atrophy. Sensory symptoms are less prominent, and usually involve paresthesias. Objective sensory loss is only occasionally seen. There may be tenderness over the femoral nerve.

Differential diagnosis

May be confused with femoral neuropathy or L4 radiculopathy when quadriceps weakness and wasting occurs. Similarly, L5 radiculopathy or peroneal neuropathy may be erroneously suspected when foot drop is seen. Straight leg raising may occasionally be positive. Conspicuously absent are back pain, exacerbation of pain by Valsalva maneuver or back motion, and significant sensory involvement. See differential diagnosis of foot drop (p.1708) and other causes of sciatica (p.1700).

Etiologies

Other etiologies are similar to that for brachial plexus neuropathy (see above) except that under tumor, a pelvic mass should also be included (check prostate on rectal exam).

Evaluation

Evaluation is as for brachial plexus neuropathy (see above), except that instead of a brachial plexus MRI, a lumbar MRI and pelvic CT should be done to rule out masses.

EMG is key to diagnosis: evidence of patchy denervation (fibrillation potentials, and motor unit potentials that are either decreased in number or increased in amplitude or duration and polyphasic) involving at least 2 segmental levels with *sparing* of the paraspinal muscles is highly diagnostic (once diabetes, etc. have been ruled out).

Outcome

Recovery from pain precedes return of strength. Improvement is generally monophasic, slow (years), and incomplete.

32.5.7 Diabetic neuropathy

General information

≈ 50% of patients with DM develop neuropathic symptoms or show slowing of nerve conduction velocities on electrodiagnostic testing. Neuropathy may sometimes be the initial manifestation of diabetes. Diabetic neuropathy is reduced by tight control of blood glucose.[10]

Syndromes

Disagreement exists over the number of distinct clinical syndromes; there is probably a continuum[11] and they likely occur in various combinations. Some of the more readily identified syndromes include:

1. primary sensory polyneuropathy: symmetric, affecting feet and legs more than hands. Chronic, slowly-progressive. Often with accelerated loss of distal vibratory sense (normal loss with aging is ≈ 1% per year after age 40). Presents as pain, paresthesias, and dysesthesias. Soles of feet may be tender to pressure. Meralgia paresthetica (p. 561) may be first manifestation
2. autonomic neuropathy: involving bladder, bowel, and circulatory reflexes (resulting in ortho-static hypotension). May produce impotence, impaired micturition, diarrhea, constipation, impaired pupillary light response
3. diabetic plexus neuropathy[12] or proximal neuropathy: possibly secondary to vascular injury to nerves (similar to a diabetic mononeuritis):
   a) one that occurs in patients > 50 years old with mild diabetes type II that is often confused with femoral neuropathy. Causes severe pain in the hip, anterior thigh, knee, and sometimes medial calf. Weakness of the quadriceps, iliopsoas, and occasionally thigh adductors. Loss of patellar reflex (knee jerk). Possible sensory loss over medial thigh and lower leg. Pain usually improves in weeks, the weakness in months
   b) ★ diabetic amyotrophy: occurs in similar patient population, often with recently diagnosed DM. Alternative names include[13]: Bruns-Garland syndrome, ischemic mononeuropathy mul-tiplex….[14] Abrupt onset of asymmetric pain (usually deep aching/burning with superimposed lancinating paroxysms, most severe at night) in back, hip, buttocks, thigh, or leg. Progressive weakness in proximal or proximal and distal muscles, often preceded by weight loss. Patellar reflexes are absent or reduced. Sensory loss is minimal. Proximal muscles (especially thigh) may atrophy. EMG findings consistent with demyelination invariably accompanied by axonal degeneration, with involvement of paraspinals and no evidence of myopathy. Symptoms may progress steadily or stepwise for weeks or even up to 18 months, and then gradually resolve. Opposite extremity may become involved during the course or may occur months or years later. Sural nerve biopsy (p. 1832) may suggest demyelination
   c) diabetic proximal neuropathy (DPN): fairly similar findings to diabetic amyotrophy, except for subacute onset of symmetric LE involvement that usually start with weakness, may be a var-iant.[15] ▶ Table 32.3 (adapted[15]) compares DPN to diabetic amyotrophy and chronic inflamma-tory demyelinating polyneuropathy (CIDP)

Treatment

Treatment of Bruns-Garland syndrome is primarily expectant, although immunotherapy (steroids, immune globulin, or plasma exchange) may be considered in severe or progressive cases (efficacy is unproven).[15]

For sensory polyneuropathy, good control of blood sugar contributes to reduction of symptoms. Adjunctive agents that have been used include:

1. mexiletine (Mexitil®): start at 150 mg q 8 hrs, and titrate to symptoms to a maximum of 10 mg/kg/d
2. amitriptyline (Elavil®) and fluphenazine (Prolixin®): ℞: start with 25 mg amitriptyline PO q hs and 1 mg fluphenazine PO TID; and work up to 75 mg amitriptyline PO q hs[16] (≈ 100 mg qd ami-triptyline alone may also be effective[17]). Usefulness has been challenged,[18] but many studies do show benefit.[17,19] **Side effects:** that may limit use include sedation, confusion, fatigue, malaise, hypomania, rash, urinary retention, and orthostatic hypotension

Table 32.3 Comparison of diabetic amyotrophy, diabetic proximal neuropathy (DPN), & CIDP

Description	Diabetic amyotrophy	DPN	CIDP
Onset	acute	subacute	gradual
Initial symptoms	asymmetric pain→ weakness	symmetric weakness	symmetric weakness
UE weakness	no	uncommon	yes
Sensory loss	minimal	minimal	moderate
Areflexia	LE	LE	generalized
CSF protein	variable	increased	increased
Axonal pathologic changes	common	typical	uncommon
Conduction slowing	patchy	patchy	diffuse
Prognosis	good	good	poor without treatment
Response to immuno-therapy	unknown	possible	yes
Course	monophasic	monophasic	progressive

3. desipramine (Norpramin®): more selective blocker of norepinephrine reuptake (which seems more effective for this condition than serotonin reuptake blockers). Effectiveness at mean doses of 110 mg/day ≈ same as amitriptyline and therefore may be useful for patients unable to tolerate amitriptyline.[17] **Side effects:** include insomnia (may be minimized by AM dosing), orthostatic hypotension, rash, bundle branch block, tremor, pyrexia. **Supplied:** 10, 25, 50, 75, 100 & 150 mg tablets

4. capsaicin (Zostrix®) (p. 524): effective in some

5. paroxetine (Paxil®): a selective serotonin reuptake inhibitor (SSRI) antidepressant. ℞: 20 mg PO q AM. If necessary, increase by 10 mg/d q week up to a maximum of 50 mg/day (except in elderly, debilitated, or renal or hepatic failure where maximum is 40 mg/day). **Supplied:** 20 mg (scored) & 30 mg tablets

6. gabapentin (Neurontin®) doses of 1800–3600 mg/d produces at least moderate pain relief in painful diabetic neuropathy in 60% of patients[20] and was ≈ as efficacious as amitriptyline.[21] Dosage must be reduced with renal insufficiency. See details (p. 496)

7. pregabalin (Lyrica®) ℞: start with 50 mg TID and increase up to a maximum of 100 mg PO TID within 1 week in patients with creatinine clearance ≥ 60 ml/min, see Eq (7.1) to estimate. Dosage must be reduced with renal insufficiency. **Supplied:** 25, 50, 75, 100, 150, 200, 225, 300 mg capsules

32

32.5.8 Drug-induced neuropathy

Many drugs have been implicated as possible causes of peripheral neuropathy. Those that are better established or more notorious include:

1. thalidomide: neuropathy may occur with chronic use, and may be irreversible[22]
2. metronidazole (Flagyl®)
3. phenytoin (Dilantin®)
4. amitriptyline (Elavil®)
5. dapsone: a rare complication reported with use in nonleprosy patients is a reversible peripheral neuropathy that may be due to axonal degeneration, producing a Guillain-Barré-like syndrome (p. 193).
6. nitrofurantoin (Macrodantin®): may additionally cause optic neuritis
7. cholesterol-lowering drugs: e.g., lovastatin (Mevacor®), indapamide (Lozol®), gemfibrozil (Lopid®)
8. thallium: may produce tremors, leg pains, paresthesias in the hands and feet, polyneuritis in the LE, psychosis, delirium, seizures, encephalopathy
9. arsenic: may produce numbness, burning and tingling of the extremities
10. chemotherapy: cisplatin, vincristine...

32.5.9 Femoral neuropathy

Clinical findings

1. motor deficits:
   a) wasting and weakness of the quadriceps femoris (knee extension)

b) ± weakness of iliopsoas (hip flexion): if present, indicates very proximal pathology (lumbar root or plexus lesion) as the branches to the iliopsoas arise just distal to the neural foramina
2. diminution of the patellar (knee jerk) reflex
3. sensory findings:
   a) sensory loss over the anterior thigh and medial calf
   b) pain in same distribution may occur
4. mechanical signs: positive femoral stretch test (p. 1252)

Etiologies

1. diabetes: the most frequent cause
2. femoral nerve entrapment: rare
   a) may occur secondary to inguinal hernia or may be injured by deep sutures placed during herniorrhaphy
   b) secondary to prolonged pelvic surgery from retractor compression (usually bilateral)
3. intraabdominal tumor
4. femoral arterial catheterization: see below
5. retroperitoneal hematoma (e.g., in hemophiliac or on anticoagulants)
6. during surgery (p. 576)

Differential diagnosis

1. L4 radiculopathy: L4 radiculopathy should not cause iliopsoas weakness; see L4 involvement (p. 1702)
2. diabetic plexus neuropathy (see above)
3. (idiopathic) lumbosacral plexus neuropathy (see above)

32.5.10 AIDS neuropathy

General information

3.3% of patients with AIDS will develop peripheral nerve disorders[23] (whereas none who were just HIV positive developed neuropathy). The most common disorder is distal symmetric polyneuropathy (DSP), usually consisting of vague numbness and tingling, and sometimes painful feet (although it may also be painless). There may be subtle reduction of light touch and vibratory sense. Other neuropathies include mononeuropathies—usually meralgia paresthetica (p. 561)—mononeuropathy multiplex, or lumbar polyradiculopathy. Drugs used to treat HIV can also cause neuropathies (see below).

The DSP in AIDS patients is often associated with CMV infection, Mycobacterium avium intracellulare infection, or may be due to lymphomatous invasion of the nerve or lymphomatous meningitis. May demonstrate a mixed axonal demyelinating type of neuropathy on electrodiagnostic testing.

Neuropathies associated with drugs used to treat HIV

1. nucleoside reverse transcriptase inhibitors
   a) zidovudine (Retrovir®) (formerly AZT)
   b) didanosine (ddI; Videx®): (formerly dideoxyinosine) can cause a painful dose-related neuropathy[24]
   c) stavudine (d4T; Zerit®): can cause sensory neuropathy which usually improves when d4 T is discontinued, and may not recur if restarted at lower dose[24]
   d) zalcitabine (ddC; Hivid®): the least potent of the nucleoside analogs, therefore rarely used; dose-related neuropathy can be severe and persistent. More common in patients with DM or didanosine treatment[24]
2. protease inhibitors
   a) ritonavir (Norvir®): can cause peripheral paresthesias
   b) amprenavir (Agenerase®): can cause perioral paresthesias

32.5.11 Neuropathy associated with monoclonal gammopathy

General information

Abnormal immunoglobulin protein (paraproteins) are found in the blood.

Monoclonal gammopathies include:
1. (multiple) myeloma (p. 928)
2. Waldenstrom's macroglobulinemia
3. non-malignant entities such as monoclonal gammopathy of undetermined significance (MGUS). MGUS patients will develop multiple myeloma (MM) at a rate of 1.5%/year, but the risk of developing a lymphoproliferative disorder before they die is only 11%. Most cases of MM are preceded by MGUS. MGUS can also progress to Waldenstroms macroglobulinemia, amyloidosis, B-cell lymphoma, or lymphocytic leukemia. Criteria for MGUS:
   a) monoclonal paraprotein band < 30 g/l (which is less than with MM)
   b) plasma cells < 10% on bone marrow biopsy
   c) no evidence of bone lesions of MM, hypercalcemia, or renal insufficiency related to the paraprotein, and
   d) no evidence of another β-cell proliferative disorder

Much effort has gone into determining which benign gammopathies are or are not likely to progress, and will not be addressed here.

≈ 10% of patients with neuropathy with no apparent etiology will be determined to have a monoclonal gammopathy (malignant or otherwise).

Etiologies

1. antibodies directed primarily against oligosaccharides of peripheral nerves, e.g., myelin associated glycoprotein (MAG), producing demyelinating neuropathy
2. cryoglobulins may damage vaso-nervorum (small blood vessels nourishing peripheral nerves)
3. in malignant gammopathies, tumor cells can invade the peripheral nerves (lymphomatosis)
4. amyloidosis (p. 576): deposition of amyloid in peripheral nerves
5. thalidomide (p. 573) used to treat some myelomas, may cause neuropathy

Treatment

1. IgM monoclonal gammopathies: reduce the IgM antibody concentration
2. IgG or IgA monoclonal gammopathies:
   a) treatment for myeloma-related neuropathy is directed at treating the myeloma
   b) solitary plasmacytoma: excision or XRT can improve the neuropathy

32.5.12 Perioperative neuropathies

General information

Also, below. Represent ≈ 1/3 of all anesthesia-associated malpractice claims in the U.S.[25] Most often involves ulnar nerve or brachial plexus. In many cases, a nerve that is abnormal but asymptomatic may become symptomatic as a result of any of the following factors: stretch or compression of the nerve, generalized ischemia or metabolic derangement. The injury may be permanent or temporary. Occurs almost exclusively in adults.[26]

Types of perioperative neuropathies

Examples include:
1. ulnar neuropathy: controversial. Often blamed on external nerve compression or stretch as a result of malpositioning. Although this may be true in some cases, in one series this was felt to be a factor in only ≈ 17% of cases.[27] Patient-related characteristics associated with these neuropathies are shown in ▶ Table 32.4.[28] Many of these patients have abnormal contralateral nerve conduction, suggesting a possible predisposing condition.[29] Many patients do not complain of symptoms until > 48 hours post-op[28,29,30] (if it were due to compression, deficit would be

Table 32.4 Patient-related characteristics in anesthesia-related ulnar neuropathy

male gender
obesity (body mass index ≥ 38)
prolonged post-op bed rest

maximal immediately post-op). Risk may be reduced by padding the arm at, and especially distal to, the elbow, and avoiding flexion of the elbow (especially avoiding > 110° flexion which tightens the cubital tunnel retinaculum), and by reducing the amount of time spent convalescing in the recumbent position with leaning on the elbows[30]

2. brachial plexus neuropathy: may be mistaken for ulnar neuropathy. May be associated with:
   a) median sternotomy (most common with internal mammary dissection). Posterior sternal retraction displaces the upper ribs and may stretch or compress the C6 through T1 roots (which are major contributors to the ulnar nerve)
   b) head-down (Trendelenburg) positions where the patient is stabilized with a shoulder brace. The brace should be placed over the acromioclavicular joint(s), and non-slip mattresses and flexion of the knees may be used as adjuncts[26]
   c) prone position (rare): especially with shoulder abduction and elbow flexion with contralateral head rotation[26]

3. median neuropathy: perioperative median nerve injury may result from stretch of the nerve. Rare. Seems to occur primarily in middle-aged muscular males with reduced extension of the elbows due to muscle mass. This may result in stretching of the nerve after muscle relaxants are given. Padding should be placed under the forearms and hands of these patients to maintain mild elbow flexion[26]

4. lower extremity neuropathies: most occur in patients undergoing procedures in the lithotomy position.[26] Frequency of involvement in a large series of patients undergoing procedures in the lithotomy position[31]: common peroneal 81%, sciatic 15%, and femoral 4%. Risk factors other than position: prolonged duration of procedure, extremely thin body habitus, and cigarette smoking in the preoperative period
   a) common peroneal neuropathy: susceptible to injury in the posterior popliteal fossa where it wraps around the fibular head. May be compressed by leg holders, which should be padded in this area
   b) femoral neuropathy: compression of the nerve by self-retaining abdominal wall retractor or rendering the nerve ischemic by occlusion of the external iliac artery.[26] Hemorrhage into the iliopsoas muscle may also compress the nerve. Cutaneous branches of the femoral nerve may be injured during labor and/or delivery[32] (most are transient)
   c) sciatic neuropathy: stretch injuries may occur with hyperflexion of the hip and extension of the knee as may occur in some variants of the lithotomy position
   d) meralgia paresthetica[33]: tends to occur bilaterally in young, slender males positioned prone, with operations lasting 6–10 + hours. Onset: 1–8 days post-op. Spontaneous recovery typically occurs over an average of 5.8 months

Management

Once a neuropathy is detected, determine if it is sensory, motor, or both. Pure sensory neuropathies are more often temporary than motor,[28] and expectant management for ≈ 5 days is suggested (have the patient avoid postures or activities that may further injure the nerve). Neurologic consultation should be requested for all motor neuropathies and for sensory neuropathies persisting > 5 days[26] (EMG evaluation will not usually be helpful earlier than ≈ 3 weeks after onset).

32.5.13 Other neuropathies

Amyloid neuropathy

Amyloid is an insoluble extracellular protein aggregate that can be deposited in peripheral nerves. Amyloidosis occurs in a number of conditions, e.g., in ≈ 15% of patients with **multiple myeloma** (p. 928). The neuropathy predominantly produces a progressive autonomic neuropathy and symmetric dissociated sensory loss (reduced pain and temperature, preserved vibratory sense). There is usually less prominent motor involvement. May predispose to pressure injury of nerves—especially carpal tunnel syndrome, see laboratory tests (p. 549).

Uremic neuropathy

Occurs in chronic renal failure. Early symptoms include calf cramps ("Charlie horses"), dysesthetic pain in feet (similar to painful diabetic neuropathy) and "restless legs." Achilles reflexes are lost. A stocking sensory loss is followed later by LE weakness that starts distally and ascends. The offending toxin is not known. Dialysis or renal transplantation relieves the symptoms.

Neuropathy after cardiac catheterization

In a series of ≈ 10,000 patients followed after femoral artery catheterization[34] (e.g., for coronary angiography or angioplasty), neuropathy occurred in 0.2% (with an estimated range in the literature up to ≈ 3%). Risk factors identified include patients developing retroperitoneal hematomas or pseudo-aneurysms after the procedure, procedures requiring larger introducer sheaths (e.g., angioplasty & stent placement > diagnostic catheterization), excessive anticoagulation (PTT > 90 for at least 12 hours).

Two groups of patients were identified and are shown in ▶ Table 32.5.

Table 32.5 Neuropathy after cardiac catheterization (N = 9585)[34]

Catheterization complication	Neurologic complication
Group I (4 patients)	
groin hematoma or pseudoaneurysm	sensory neuropathy in all 4 cases • in distribution of medial & intermediate femoral cutaneous nerves → isolated sensory neuropathy (dysesthesia & sensory loss) of the anterior and medial thigh • no motor deficit
Group II (16 patients)	
large retroperitoneal hematoma	femoral neuropathy • sensory in all 16 cases: dysesthesia of the anterior/medial thigh & medial calf • motor in 13 cases: iliopsoas & quadriceps weakness
	obturator neuropathy in 4 cases • sensory: upper medial thigh • motor: obturator weakness
	lateral femoral cutaneous nerve → meralgia paresthetica

Excruciating pain after the catheterization procedure often preceded the development or recognition of neuropathy.

Treatment

After considering available information, the recommendation is to repair pseudoaneurysms surgically, but to treat the neuropathy conservatively. A case could *not* be made that surgical drainage of hematoma reduced the risk of neuropathy. Weakness from femoral or obturator neuropathy was treated with inpatient rehabilitation.

Outcome

Group I patients all had resolution in < 5 mos. In group II, 50% had complete resolution in 2 mos. 6 patients had persistent symptoms, 5 had mild femoral *sensory* neuropathy (1 of whom felt it was at least somewhat disabling), 1 had mild persistent quadriceps weakness and occasionally walks with a cane.

32.6 Peripheral nerve injuries

32.6.1 General information

Anatomy of peripheral nerves

See ▶ Fig. 32.1. Endoneurium surrounds myelinated and unmyelinated axons. These bundles are gathered into fascicles surrounded by perineurium. The epineurium encases the nerve trunk, containing fascicles separated by interfascicular epineurium or mesoneurium.

Nerve regeneration

Peripheral nerves regenerate ≈ 1 mm/day (about 1 inch/month). Divide this figure into the distance that the nerve has to traverse (from knowledge of anatomy) for guide as to how long to wait before considering failure of therapy (either operative or non-operative). However, this rule may not be

32

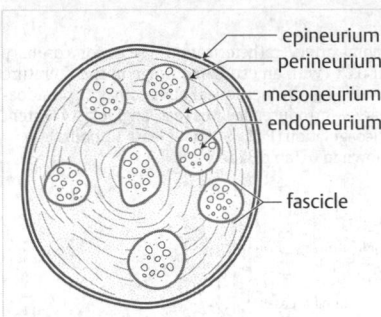

epineurium
perineurium
mesoneurium
endoneurium

fascicle

Fig. 32.1 Cross-sectional anatomy of a peripheral nerve.

applicable to long distances (> ≈ 12 inches), and it may take longer to traverse regions of entrapment, scar or nerve injury. There may also be fibrosis of the muscle beyond salvage.

Peripheral nerve injury classification

See ▶ Table 32.6.

There are numerous classification systems. The Seddon classification is an older 3-tiered system, The Sunderland system has 5 tiers, essentially dividing axonotmesis into 3 subgroups. Others have added a 6th category as shown in ▶ Table 32.6.

Table 32.6 Classification of peripheral nerve injury[a]

Seddon system	Sunderland system
Neuropraxia	**First-degree**
Features common to both systems: Physiologic transection (nerve in continuity). Basement membrane intact. Compression or ischemia → local conduction block (impaired axonal transport). ★ No wallerian degeneration[b]. Motor involvement is typically > sensory. Autonomic function is preserved	
Recovers in hours to months; average is 6–8 weeks	Focal demyelination may occur. Recovery is usually complete in 2–3 weeks (not the "1 mm/day rule")
Axonotmesis	**Second-degree**
Features common to both systems: Complete interruption of axons and myelin sheaths. Supporting structures (including endoneurium) intact. ★ Wallerian degeneration occurs	
	Recovers at 1 mm/day as axon follows "tubule." Sometimes may only be diagnosed retrospectively. Recovery is poor in lesions requiring > 18 months to reach target muscle
	Third-degree
	Endoneurium disrupted, epineurium & perineurium intact. Nerve may not appear seriously damaged on gross inspection. Recovery may range from poor to complete and depends on degree of intrafascicular fibrosis
	Fourth-degree
	Interruption of all neural & supporting elements. Epineurium intact. Grossly: nerve is usually indurated & enlarged
Neurotmesis	**Fifth-degree**
Nerve completely severed or disorganized by scar tissue. Spontaneous regeneration impossible	Complete transection with loss of continuity
	Sixth-degree[c]
	Mixed lesion. Combination of elements of first through fourth degree. There may be some preserved sensory fascicles (may produce a positive Tinel's sign)

[a]comparing and showing approximate equivalence of Seddon and Sunderland systems
[b]wallerian degeneration after British physiologist Augustus Volney Waller (1816–1870), AKA orthograde degeneration, AKA secondary degeneration: degeneration of the axon distal to a focal lesion
[c]not part of original Sunderland system

32

32.6.2 Brachial plexus injuries

Etiologies

Etiologies include:
1. penetrating trauma
2. traction (stretch injuries): more likely to affect the posterior and lateral cords than the medial cord and median nerve
3. first rib fractures
4. compression by hematoma

Differentiating preganglionic from postganglionic injuries

Initial exam seeks to differentiate preganglionic injuries (proximal to dorsal root ganglion) which cannot be repaired surgically, from postganglionic injuries. Clues to a preganglionic injury include:
1. Horner syndrome: pre-ganglionic injury interrupts white rami communicantes
2. paralysis of serratus anterior (long thoracic nerve): produces winging of scapula
3. paralysis of rhomboids (dorsal scapular nerve)
4. early neuropathic pain suggests nerve root avulsion. MRI or myelogram will show pseudomeningoceles at the avulsed levels
5. EMG: requires ≥ 3 weeks from injury for some findings. Look for:
   a) denervation potentials in paraspinal muscles due to loss of neural input. The posterior ramus of the spinal nerve originates just distal to the dorsal root ganglion. Due to overlap, cannot localize to a specific segment
   b) normal sensory nerve action potential (SNAP): preganglionic injuries leave the dorsal ganglion sensory cell body and the distal axon intact, so that normal SNAP can be recorded proximally even in an anesthetic region
6. pseudomeningocele on myelography or MRI: suggests nerve root avulsion (very proximal); however, 15% of pseudomeningoceles are not associated with avulsions, and 20% of avulsions do not have pseudomeningoceles[35,36]

Types of brachial plexus injuries

(Duchene)-Erb's palsy

Upper brachial plexus injury (C5 & 6, some authors include C7) e.g., from forceful separation of humeral head from shoulder, commonly due to difficult parturition (see below) or motorcycle accident (downward force on shoulder can cause traumatic nerve root avulsion from the spinal cord). Paralysis of deltoid, biceps, rhomboids, brachioradialis, supra- & infraspinatus, and occasionally supinator. C7 involvement produces weak wrist extension.

Motor: arm hangs at side internally rotated & extended at elbow and flexed at the wrist ("Bellhop's tip position"). Hand motion is unaffected.

Klumpke's palsy

Injury to lower brachial plexus (C8 & T1, some authors include C7), from traction of abducted arm e.g., in catching oneself during a fall from a height, or by Pancoast tumor (lung apex tumor—check CXR with apical lordotic view). Characteristic claw deformity (also seen with ulnar nerve injury) with weakness and wasting of small hand muscles. Possible Horner syndrome if T1 involved.

Birth brachial plexus injury (BBPI)

Incidence is 0.3–2.0 per 1000 live births (0.1% in infants with birthweight < 4000 gm[37]). Rarely, a congenital case may be mistaken for BBPI.[38] Some contend that the plexus injury may occur when uterine contractions push the shoulder against the mother's pubic bone or with lowering of the shoulder with opposite inclination of the cervical spine.[38]

Classification of BBPI injuries: Upper plexus injuries are most common, with about half having C5 & C6 injuries, and 25% involving C7 also.[39] Combined upper and lower lesions occur in ≈ 20%. Pure lower lesions (C7–1) are rare, constituting only ≈ 2% and seen most commonly in breech deliveries. Lesions are bilateral in ≈ 4%. A 4-level scale of intensity is shown ► Table 32.7.[40]

Risk factors:
1. shoulder dystocia
2. high birth weight
3. primiparous mother
4. forceps[41] or vacuum assisted delivery

32

Table 32.7 Birth brachial plexus injury

Group	Lesion	Manifestation	Spontaneous recovery rate
1	C5 or C6 roots or superior trunk	paralysis of shoulder abduction, elbow flexion & forearm supination. Finger flexion is normal	90%
2	above + involvement of C7 or medial trunk	above + paralysis of finger extensors (but not flexors)	65%
3	above + finger flexors	essentially no hand movement. No Horner syndrome	≈ < 50%
4	complete brachial plexus	flail arm + Horner syndrome	0%
	"dominant C7" paralysis variant	selective loss of shoulder abduction & elbow extension	

5. breech presentation[42]
6. prolonged labor
7. previous birth complicated by BBPI

Management of BBPI: Most surgeons observe all patients until age 3 months. Conservative surgeons may wait up to 9 months. More aggressive surgeons will explore the plexus at age 3 months if not antigravity in deltoid, biceps or triceps. In cases of proven avulsion (pseudomeningocele and EMG indicative of a preganglionic injury), nerve transfers are a valid option at 3 months.[43] EMG may show signs of reinnervation, but the recovery may not be robust enough.

Management of brachial plexus injuries

1. most injuries show maximal deficit at onset. Progressive deficit is usually due to vascular injuries (pseudoaneurysm, A-V fistula, or expansile clot); these should be explored immediately
2. clean, sharp, relatively fresh lacerating injuries (usually iatrogenic, scalpel-induced) should be explored acutely and repaired with tension-free end-to-end anastamoses within 24–48 hours (after that, ends will be more edematous and therefore more difficult to suture)
3. penetrating non-missile injuries with severe or complete deficit should be explored as soon as the primary wound heals
4. gunshot wounds (GSW) to the brachial plexus: deficit is usually due to axonotmesis or neurotmesis (see below). Sometimes nerves may be divided. Nerves showing partial function usually recover spontaneously; those with complete dysfunction rarely do so. Surgery is of little benefit for discrete injuries to the lower trunk, medial cord, or C8/T1 roots. Most are managed conservatively for 2–5 months. Indications for surgery are shown in ▶ Table 32.8

Table 32.8 Indications for neurosurgical intervention in GSW to the brachial plexus[44]

1. complete loss in the distribution of at least one element
   a) no improvement clinically or on EMG in 2–5 months
   b) deficit in distribution that is responsive to surgery (e.g., C5, C6, C7, upper or middle trunk, lateral or posterior cords or their outflows)
   c) injuries with loss only in lower elements are *not* operated
2. incomplete loss with failure to control pain medically
3. pseudoaneurysm, clot, or fistula involving plexus
4. true causalgia requiring sympathectomy

5. traction injuries: incomplete postganglionic injuries tend to improve spontaneously. If recovery is not satisfactory, perform EMG at 4–5 months and explore at 6 months
6. neuromas in continuity: those that do not conduct a SNAP (p. 255) have complete internal disruption and require resection and grafting. Methods of repair:
   a) neurolysis:
      • external neurolysis: most commonly performed in exploration. Value is questionable
      • internal neurolysis: splitting the nerve into fascicles. Not recommended unless a clear neuroma in continuity is found eccentric in the nerve that conducts SNAP
   b) nerve grafting. Sural nerve is the most commonly used interposition graft following resection of neuroma in continuity

c) nerve transfers. Donor nerve options:
- spinal accessory nerve
- intercostal nerves to musculocutaneous nerve
- fascicles of the ulnar nerve for the median nerve (Oberlin procedure)
- anterior interosseus nerve to median nerve

32.7 Missile injuries of peripheral nerves

This section deals primarily with gunshot wounds (GSW). Most injuries from a single bullet are due to shock and cavitation from the missile causing axonotmesis or neurotmesis, and are not from direct nerve transection. Approximately 70% will recover with expectant management.

However, if there is a lack of improvement on serial examinations, including electrodiagnostic studies, intervention should be undertaken by about 5–6 months to avoid further difficulties due to nerve fibrosis and muscle atrophy.

See ▶ Table 32.8 for indications for surgery for missile injuries of the brachial plexus.

32.8 Thoracic outlet syndrome

32.8.1 General information

The thoracic outlet is a confined area at the apex of the lung bordered by the 1st rib below and the clavicle above through which passes the subclavian artery, vein, and brachial plexus.

Thoracic outlet syndrome (TOS) is a term implying compression of one or more of the enclosed structures producing a heterogeneous group of disorders. TOS tends to be diagnosed more often by general and vascular surgeons than by neurologists and neurosurgeons. Four unrelated conditions with different structures involved:
1. "noncontroversial," with characteristic symptom complex, reproducible clinical findings, confirmatory laboratory tests. Low incidence[45]
   - arterial vascular: producing arm, hand, and finger pallor and ischemia
   - venous vascular: producing arm swelling and edema
   - true neurologic: compressing the lower trunk or median cord of the brachial plexus (see below)
2. disputed neurologic: includes scalenus anticus syndrome (see below)

32.8.2 Differential diagnosis

1. herniated cervical disc
2. cervical arthrosis
3. lung cancer (pancoast tumor)
4. tardy ulnar nerve palsy
5. carpal tunnel syndrome
6. orthopedic shoulder problems
7. complex regional pain syndrome (reflex sympathetic dystrophy)

32.8.3 True neurologic TOS

General information

A rare condition primarily affecting adult women, usually unilateral.
  Neurologic structures involved
1. most common: compression of the C8/T1 roots
2. or proximal lower trunk of the brachial plexus (BP)
3. less common: compression of the median cord of the BP

Etiologies

1. constricting band extending from the first rib to a rudimentary "cervical rib" or to an elongated C7 transverse process
2. scalenus (anticus) syndrome: controversial (see below)
3. compression beneath the pectoralis minor tendon under the coracoid process: may result from repetitive movements of the arms above the head (shoulder elevation and hyperabduction)

32

Signs and symptoms

1. ★ sensory changes in distribution of median cord (mainly along medial forearm), *sparing* median nerve sensory fibers (pass through upper and middle trunks)
2. hand clumsiness or weakness and wasting, especially abductor pollicis brevis and ulnar hand intrinsics (C8/T1 denervation/atrophy)
3. there may be tenderness over Erb's point (2 to 3 cm above the clavicle in front of the C6 transverse process)
4. may be painless
5. usually unilateral

Confirmatory tests

1. EMG: unreliable (may be negative). Most common abnormality in neurogenic TOS is loss of medial antebrachial cutaneous SNAP (p. 255)
2. MRI does not show bony abnormalities well, but may occasionally demonstrate a kink in the lower BP. Can also rule out conditions that may mimic TOS, such as herniated cervical disc
3. cervical spine X-rays with obliques and apical lordotic CXR may demonstrate bony abnormalities. However, not every cervical rib produces symptoms (some patients with bilateral cervical ribs may have unilateral TOS).

Treatment

Controversial. Conservative treatment (usually including stretching and physical therapy) is about equally as effective as surgery and avoids attendant risks.

Decompression can be achieved by removing the muscles that surround the nerves (scalenectomy), by transaxillary first rib resection, or both.

32.8.4 Scalenus (anticus) syndrome (disputed neurologic TOS)

Controversial. More commonly diagnosed in the 1940s and 1950s. There is a lack of consensus regarding the pathophysiology (including structures involved), clinical presentation, helpful tests, and optimal treatment. Removal of first thoracic rib is often advocated for treatment, frequently via a transaxillary approach. Unfortunately, injuries, especially to the lower trunk of the brachial plexus, may result from the surgery.

Other variations include an "upper plexus" type for which total anterior scalenectomy is advocated. Again, very controversial.

References

[1] Poza JJ, Cobo AM, Marti-Masso JF. Peripheral neuropathy associated with polycythemia vera. Neurologia. 1996; 11:276–279
[2] Ochoa JL, Verdugo RJ. Reflex Sympathetic Dystrophy: A Common Clinical Avenue for Somatoform Expression. Neurol Clin. 1995; 13:351–363
[3] Denny-Brown D. Primary Sensory Neuropathy with Muscular Changes Associated with Carcinoma. Journal of Neurology, Neurosurgery, and Psychiatry. 1948; 11:73–87
[4] Camerlingo M, Nemni R, Ferraro B, et al. Malignancy and Sensory Neuropathy of Unexplained Cause: A Prospective Study of 51 Patients. Archives of Neurology. 1998; 55:981–984
[5] McLeod JG, Dyck PJ, Thomas PK. Paraneoplastic Neuropathies. In: Peripheral Neuropathy. Philadelphia: W.B. Saunders; 1993:1583–1590
[6] Turner JW, Parsonage MJ. Neuralgic amyotrophy (paralytic brachial neuritis); with special reference to prognosis. Lancet. 1957; 273
[7] Tsairis P, Dyck PJ, Mulder DW. Natural History of Brachial Plexus Neuropathy: Report on 99 Patients. Arch Neurol. 1972; 27:109–117
[8] Misamore GW, Lehman DE. Parsonage-Turner syndrome (acute brachial neuritis). Journal of Bone and Joint Surgery. 1996; 78:1405–1408
[9] Evans BA, Stevens JC, Dyck PJ. Lumbosacral Plexus Neuropathy. Neurology. 1981; 31:1327–1330
[10] The Diabetes Control and Complications Trial Research Group. The Effect of Intensive Treatment of Diabetes on the Development and Progression of Long-Term Complications in Insulin-Dependent Diabetes Mellitus. New England Journal of Medicine. 1993; 329:977–986
[11] Asbury AK. Proximal Diabetic Neuropathy. Ann Neurol. 1977; 2:179–180
[12] Dyck PJ, Thomas PK. Peripheral Neuropathy. 2nd ed. Philadelphia: W. B. Saunders; 1984
[13] Garland H. Diabetic Amyotrophy. BMJ. 1955; 2:1287–1290
[14] Barohn RJ, Sahenk Z, Warmolts JR, et al. The Bruns-Garland Syndrome (Diabetic Amyotrophy): Revisited 100 Years Later. Arch Neurol. 1991; 48:1130–1135
[15] Pascoe MK, Low PA, Windebank AJ. Subacute Diabetic Proximal Neuropathy. Mayo Clinic Proceedings. 1997; 72:1123–1132
[16] Davis JL, Lewis SB, Gerich JE, et al. Peripheral Diabetic Neuropathy Treated with Amitriptyline and Fluphenazine. JAMA. 1977; 21:2291–2292
[17] Max MB, Lynch SA, Muir J, et al. Effects of Desipramine, Amitriptyline, and Fluoxetine on Pain in Diabetic Neuropathy. N Engl J Med. 1992; 326:1250–1256
[18] Mendel CM, Klein RF, Chappell DA, et al. A Trial of Amitriptyline and Fluphenazine in the Treatment of Painful Diabetic Neuropathy. JAMA. 1986; 255:637–639
[19] Mendel CM, Grunfeld C. Amitriptyline and Fluphenazine for Painful Diabetic Neuropathy. JAMA. 1986; 256:712–714

[20] Backonja M, Beydoun A, Edwards KR, et al. Gabapentin for the symptomatic treatment of painful neuropathy in patients with diabetes mellitus: a randomized controlled trial. JAMA. 1998; 280:1831–1836

[21] Morello CM, Leckband SG, Stoner CP, et al. Randomized double-blind study comparing the efficacy of gabapentin with amitriptyline on diabetic peripheral neuropathy pain. Arch Intern Med. 1999; 159:1931–1937

[22] New Uses of Thalidomide. Medical Letter. 1996; 38:15–16

[23] Fuller GN, Jacobs JM, Guiloff RJ. Nature and Incidence of Peripheral Nerve Syndromes in HIV Infection. Journal of Neurology, Neurosurgery, and Psychiatry. 1993; 56:372–381

[24] Drugs for HIV Infection. Medical Letter. 2000; 42:1–6

[25] Kroll DA, Caplan RA, Posner K, et al. Nerve Injury Associated with Anesthesia. Anesthesiology. 1990; 73:202–207

[26] Warner MA. Perioperative Neuropathies. Mayo Clinic Proceedings. 1998; 73:567–574

[27] Wadsworth TG, Williams JR. Cubital Tunnel External Compression Syndrome. British Medical Journal. 1973; 1:662–666

[28] Warner MA, Marner ME, Martin JT. Ulnar Neuropathy: Incidence, Outcome, and Risk Factors in Sedated or Anesthetized Patients. Anesthesiology. 1994; 81:1332–1340

[29] Alvine FG, Schurrer ME. Postoperative Ulnar-Nerve Palsy: Are There Predisposing Factors? Journal of Bone and Joint Surgery. 1987; 69A:255–259

[30] Stewart JD, Shantz SH. Perioperative ulnar neuropathies: A medicolegal review. Canadian Journal of Neurological Sciences. 1994; 81

[31] Warner MA, Martin JT, Schroeder DR, et al. Lower-Extremity Motor Neuropathy Associated with Surgery Performed on Patients in a Lithotomy Position. Anesthesiology. 1994; 81:6–12

[32] O'Donnell D, Rottman R, Kotelko D, et al. Incidence of Maternal Postpartum Neurologic Dysfunction. Anesthesiology. 1994; 81

[33] Sanabria EAM, Nagashima T, Yamashita H, et al. Postoperative bilateral meralgia paresthetica after spine surgery: An overlooked entity? Spinal Surgery. 2003; 17:195–202

[34] Kent CK, Moscucci M, Gallagher SG, et al. Neuropathies After Cardiac Catheterization: Incidence, Clinical Patterns, and Long-Term Outcome. J Vasc Surg. 1994; 19:1008–1014

[35] Carvalho GA, Nikkhah G, Matthies C, et al. Diagnosis of root avulsions in traumatic brachial plexus injuries: value of computerized tomography myelography and magnetic resonance imaging. Journal of Neurosurgery. 1997; 86:69–76

[36] Hashimoto T, Mitomo M, Hirabuki N, et al. Nerve root avulsion of birth palsy: comparison of myelography with CT myelography and somatosensory evoked potential. Radiology. 1991; 178:841–845

[37] Rouse DJ, Owen J, Goldenberg RL, et al. The effectiveness and costs of elective cesarean delivery for fetal macrosomia diagnosed by ultrasound. Jama. 1996; 276:1480–1486

[38] Gilbert A, Brockman R, Carlioz H. Surgical Treatment of Brachial Plexus Birth Palsy. Clinical Orthopedics. 1991; 264:39–47

[39] Boome RS, Kaye JC. Obstetric Traction Injuries of the Brachial Plexus: Natural History, Indications for Surgical Repair and Results. Journal of Bone and Joint Surgery. 1988; 70B:571–576

[40] van Ouwerkerk WJ, van der Sluijs J A, Nollet F, et al. Management of obstetric brachial plexus lesions: state of the art and future developments. Childs Nerv Syst. 2000; 16:638–644

[41] Piatt JH, Hudson AR, Hoffman HJ. Preliminary Experiences with Brachial Plexus Explorations in Children: Birth Injury and Vehicular Trauma. Neurosurgery. 1988; 22:715–723

[42] Hunt D. Surgical Management of Brachial Plexus Birth Injuries. Developmental Medicine and Child Neurology. 1988; 30:821–828

[43] Anand P, Birch R. Restoration of sensory function and lack of long-term chronic pain syndromes after brachial plexus injury in human neonates. Brain. 2002; 125:113–122

[44] Kline DG, Hudson AR. Nerve Injuries: Operative Results for Major Nerve Injuries, Entrapments, and Tumors. Philadelphia: W. B. Saunders; 1995

[45] Wilbourn AJ. The Thoracic Outlet Syndrome is Overdiagnosed. Arch Neurol. 1990; 47:328–330

32

Part XI

Neurophthalmology and Neurotology

XI

33 Neurophthalmology

33.1 Nystagmus

33.1.1 Definition

Involuntary rhythmic oscillation of the eyes, usually conjugate. Most common form is jerk nystagmus, in which the direction of the nystagmus is defined for the direction of the fast (cortical) component (which is *not* the abnormal component). Horizontal or upward gaze-provoked nystagmus may be due to sedatives or ASMs; otherwise vertical nystagmus is indicative of posterior fossa pathology.

33.1.2 Localizing lesion for various forms of nystagmus

1. seesaw nystagmus: intorting eye moves up, extorting eye moves down, pattern then reverses. Lesion in diencephalon. Also reported with chiasmal compression (occasionally accompanied with bitemporal hemianopia in parasellar masses)
2. convergence nystagmus: slow abduction of eyes followed by adducting (converging) jerks, usually associated with features of Parinaud's syndrome. May be associated with nystagmus retractorius (see below) with similar location of lesion
3. nystagmus retractorius: resulting from co-contraction of all EOM's. May accompany convergence nystagmus. Lesion in upper midbrain tegmentum (usually vascular disease or tumor, especially pinealoma)
4. downbeat nystagmus: nystagmus with the fast phase downward while in primary position. Most patients have a structural lesion in the posterior fossa, especially at the *cervicomedullary junction* (foramen magnum (FM)),[1] including *Chiari I malformation*, basilar impression, p-fossa tumors, syringobulbia.[2] Uncommonly occurs in multiple sclerosis (MS), spinocerebellar degeneration, and in some metabolic conditions (hypomagnesemia, thiamine deficiency, alcohol intoxication or withdrawal, or treatment with phenytoin, carbamazepine or lithium[3])
5. upbeat nystagmus: lesion in medulla
6. abducting nystagmus occurs in INO. Lesion in pons (MLF)
7. Brun's nystagmus: lesion in pontomedullary junction (PMJ)
8. vestibular nystagmus: lesion in PMJ
9. ocular myoclonus: lesion in myoclonic triangle
10. periodic alternating nystagmus (PAN): lesion in FM and cerebellum
11. square wave jerks, macro square wave jerks, macro saccadic oscillations. Lesion in cerebellar pathways
12. "nystagmoid" eye movements (not true nystagmus)
    a) ocular bobbing (p.601): lesion in pontine tegmentum
    b) ocular dysmetria: overshoot of eye on attempted fixation followed by diminishing oscillations until eye "hones in" on target. Lesion in cerebellum or pathways (may be seen in Friedreich's ataxia)
    c) ping-pong gaze (p.323)
    d) "windshield wiper eyes" (p.323)

33.2 Papilledema

33.2.1 General information

AKA choked (optic) disc. The term papilledema is reserved for optic disc swelling caused by increased intracranial pressure, as distinguished from papillitis.

Pathomechnics: elevated ICP is transmitted through the subarachnoid space of the optic nerve sheath to the region of the optic disc → axoplasmic stasis. Elevated ICP will usually obliterate retinal venous pulsation if the pressure is transmitted to the point where the central retinal vein passes through the subarachnoid space (≈ 1 cm posterior to the globe). Papilledema (PPD) may also be dependent on the ratio of retinal arterial to retinal venous pressure, with ratios < 1.5:1 more commonly associated with papilledema than higher ratios.

Elevated ICP usually causes *bilateral* papilledema (see below for unilateral papilledema).

Papilledema typically takes 24–48 hours to develop following a sustained rise in ICP. It is rarely seen as early as ≈ 6 hours after onset, but not earlier. Papilledema does not cause visual blurring or reduction of visual fields unless very severe and prolonged.

33.2.2 Findings on funduscopy (ophthalmoscopy)

Funduscopic exam is best performed with pharmacologically dilated pupils, usually by an ophthalmologist. Findings include:
- venous engorgement: usually the earliest sign
- loss of venous pulsations
- blurring of optic margins
- elevation of optic disc
- although not part of papilledema, associated findings may include retinal hemorrhages (subretinal, pre-retinal, intraretinal), retinal and choroidal folds, Paton's folds, venous tortuosity, retino-choroidal collateral veins, partial macular star

Papilledema is often graded using the Frisén scale (0–5)[4] (▶ Table 33.1).

Table 33.1 Modified Frisén grading scale[5] for papilledema

Frisén grade	Description
0	Normal optic disc • minimal swelling of nasal margin of optic disc • nerve fiber layer (NFL) clear • vessels not obscurred • cup, if present, not obscured
1	Minimal papilledema • 230° "C-shaped" swelling of nasal, superior & inferior borders • normal (sharp) temporal margin (temporal gap) • cup, if present, is maintained
2	Low degree of papilledema • elevation of nasal margin • 360° disc swelling (circumferential halo) • no obscuration of major vessels
3	Moderate degree of papilledema • elevation of entire disc • 360° disc swelling • obscuration of ≥ 1 segment of major blood vessel at disc margin • cup may be obscured
4	Marked degree of papilledema • NFL opaque, 360° disc swelling • vessels obscured at disc margin, not completely obscured on disc surface
5	Severe papilledema • NFL opaque, 360° disc swelling • all vessels obscured on disc surface & leaving disc

33.2.3 Imaging findings in papilledema

Papilledema is primarily an ophthalmologic diagnosis. Some imaging correlates that may be associated:
- MRI or CT: flattening of the posterior globe (▶ Fig. 33.1) or elevation of the optic nerve head are specific findings. An empty sella may be seen with increased intracranial pressure, independent of papilledema
- MRI, CT or ultrasound: dilation of the optic nerve sheath (▶ Fig. 33.1) (optic nerve sheath hydrops) may be demonstrated (with current improved imaging techniques this is also now being seen more frequently in normal patients), enlargement of Meckel's cave (▶ Fig. 57.1)

33.2.4 Differential diagnosis

▶ **Mimics of papilledema on on funduscopy**
1. optic neuritis. Usually associated with more severe visual loss and tenderness to eye pressure over the eye. Etiologies:
   a) infection: Lyme disease, syphilis, measles, mumps, herpes. Cat-scratch fever (infection with Bartonella henselae) can rarely cause optic neuritis (AKA Bartonella papillitis)
   b) inflammatory/granulomatous: sarcoidosis, lupus, Behçet's disease

33

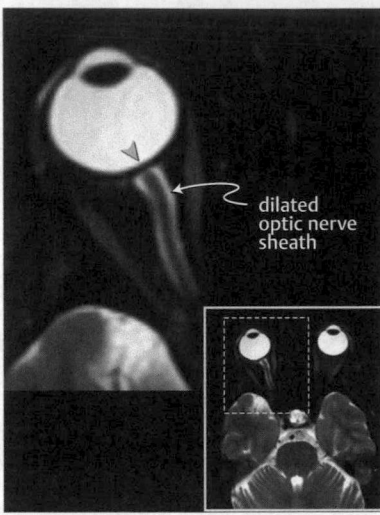

Fig. 33.1 Dilated optic nerve sheath and flattened posterior globe (*green arrowhead*).
Image: T2 axial MRI. Yellow broken line in inset shows from where the detail is taken.

dilated
optic nerve
sheath

2. pseudopapilledema: anomalous elevation of the optic nerve head. The optic disc may appear swollen, but, unlike true papilledema, the peripapillary vessels are not obscured and retinal venous pulsations are usually present. It may be unilateral or bilateral. Benign conditions that can cause pseudopapilledema include: hyperopia (farsightedness), a small optic cup, buried disc drusen (p. 1659)… Extensive workup is generally not indicated

3. non-arteritic anterior ischemic optic neuropathy (NAAION) can cause optic nerve head swelling

4. optic nerve edema. Can occur e.g., in malignant hypertension

▶ **Etiologies of unilateral papilledema**
1. compressive lesions
    a) orbital tumors: meningiomas…
    b) tumors of optic nerve sheath: schwannoma
    c) optic nerve tumors (optic pathway gliomas)
2. local inflammatory disorder
3. Foster Kennedy syndrome (p. 100)
4. demyelinating disease (e.g., multiple sclerosis)
5. elevated ICP in the setting of something that prevents manifestation in the other eye, including:
    a) blockage that prevents transmission of elevated CSF pressure to that optic disc[6]
    b) prosthetic eye (artificial eye)

33.3 Visual fields

33.3.1 General information

From a point of fixation, the normal eye can detect stimuli as far as 60° superiorly, 70° inferiorly, 60° nasally, and 100° temporally[7] (this varies with size, color and brightness of the stimuli). The normal physiological blind spot (caused by absence of light receptors in the optic disc due to penetration of the retina by the optic nerve and vessels) is located on the temporal side of the macular visual area in each eye.

The fibers from the temporal retina pass directly to the ipsilateral lateral geniculate body (LGB), whereas the nasal fibers cross in the optic chiasm (▶ Fig. 33.2).

33.3.2 Visual field testing

Visual fields may be evaluated by:
1. bedside confrontational testing: detects only gross peripheral field deficits. Using "finger wiggle" with the patient's gaze fixated on the examiner's nose while covering one of their eyes is the least

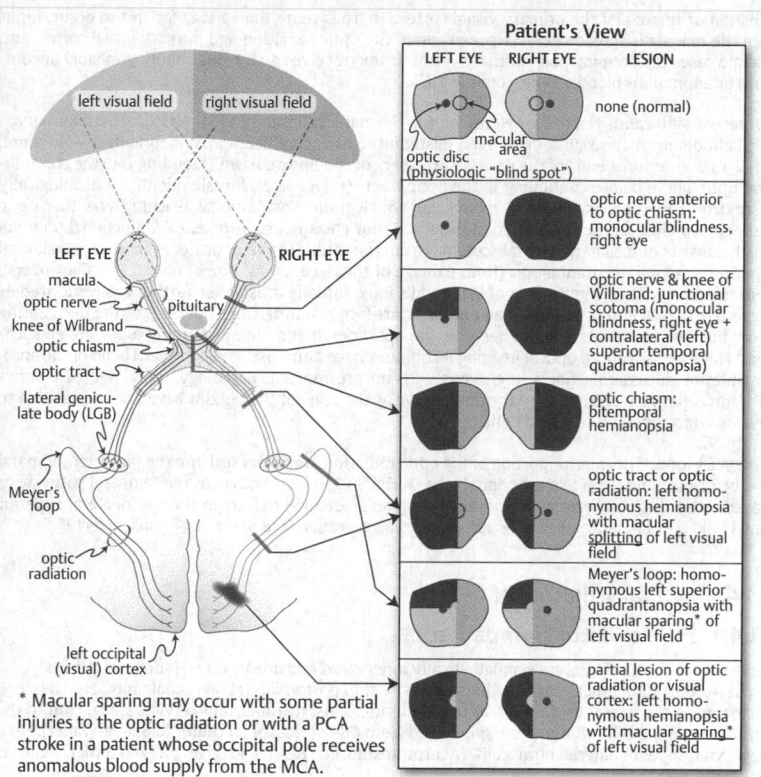

Patient's View

LEFT EYE	RIGHT EYE	LESION
		none (normal)
		optic nerve anterior to optic chiasm: monocular blindness, right eye
		optic nerve & knee of Wilbrand: junctional scotoma (monocular blindness, right eye + contralateral (left) superior temporal quadrantanopsia)
		optic chiasm: bitemporal hemianopsia
		optic tract or optic radiation: left homonymous hemianopsia with macular splitting of left visual field
		Meyer's loop: homonymous left superior quadrantanopsia with macular sparing* of left visual field
		partial lesion of optic radiation or visual cortex: left homonymous hemianopsia with macular sparing* of left visual field

* Macular sparing may occur with some partial injuries to the optic radiation or with a PCA stroke in a patient whose occipital pole receives anomalous blood supply from the MCA.

Fig. 33.2 Visual field deficits.

accurate. Presenting simultaneous fingers extended in the temporal fields and asking the patient to add the total number of fingers seen is somewhat better, and assesses homonymous hemianopsia

2. formal perimetry
   a) using a tangent screen (typically using Goldmann perimetry). Stimulus is brought in from non-seeing to seeing field (towards macular vision area) along 8 meridians
   b) automated perimetry exam: Humphrey visual field (HVF) (Zeiss) or Octopus (Haag-Streit) perimeters. Requires good patient cooperation to be valid

▶ **Perimetric mean deviation.** With automated perimetry, a "perimetric mean deviation" (PMD) is calculated as an average deviation from age and race matched normal sighted individuals at multiple locations in the visual field. A positive score means the subject sees dimmer stimuli than controls, a negative score means they require brighter stimuli. A PMD of -2 to -7 would be consistent with a mild visual loss.

33.3.3 Visual field deficits

▶ **Visual field deficits patterns.** Visual field deficit patterns are shown in ▶ Fig. 33.2.

▶ **Macular sparing/splitting.** Macular splitting can occur both in lesions anterior or posterior to the lateral geniculate body (LGB). However, macular sparing tends to occur with lesions posterior to the LGB. Homonymous hemiaonpsia with macular sparing usually occurs with lesions of the optic radiation or infarcts of the primary visual cortex. There is more than 1 way for this to occur: input from the macula is spread over a large portion of the optic radiation and primary visual cortex, and in some cases the occipital pole (primary visual cortex) receives dual blood supply (probably uncommon) or anomalous blood supply from the MCA.

▶ **Knee of Wilbrand.** Named for Hermann (or Herman) Wilbrand (1851–1935), a German neuroophthalmologist, whose surname is often misreported as von Willebrand, Willebrand, or Wildbrand. A 1–2-mm anterior "bend" of the decussating fibers of the optic chiasm extending into the contralateral optic nerve before continuing to the optic tract[8] (▶ Fig. 33.2). Initially identified histologically postmortem in subjects who had monocular enucleation. Conventional teaching was that optic nerve injury close to the chiasm produces an anterior chiasmal syndrome, AKA junctional scotoma which consists of ipsilateral central scotoma (from the injury to the optic nerve) and a contralateral superior temporal quadrantanopia (from damage of the decussating "knee" fibers).[8,9,10] Controversy as to the existence or significance of Wilbrand's knee initially arose after further cadaveric studies suggested that Wilbrand's knee is an anatomic artifact resulting from buckling of the decussating fibers into the contralateral optic nerve as the optic nerve and chiasm atrophy following enucleation.[8] However, advanced optical imaging techniques have demonstrated a forward bend of the anterior inferior decussating fibers in chiasms with no pre-mortem pathology.[11] And yet, case series with intraoperative sectioning of the optic nerve at the level of the chiasm have not been shown to develop contralateral visual field deficits.[12,13]

▶ **Meyer's loop.** The inferior portion of the optic radiation loops forward into the posterior temporal lobe before coninuing on to the occipital lobe (▶ Fig. 33.2) and is known as the temporal pathway or Meyer's loop. Lesions here cause homonymous wedge-shaped defects in the contralateral superior visual field (i.e., bilateral superior quadrantanopsia), so-called "pie in the sky" visual defect.[14]

33.4 Pupillary diameter

33.4.1 Pupilodilator (sympathetic)

Pupilodilator muscle fibers are sympathetically innervated and are arranged radially in the iris.

First-order sympathetic nerve fibers arise in the posterolateral hypothalamus, and descend uncrossed in the lateral tegmentum of the midbrain, pons, medulla, and cervical spinal cord to the intermediolateral cell column of the spinal cord from C8–2 (ciliospinal center of Budge-Waller). Here they synapse with lateral horn cells (neurotransmitter: ACh) and give off 2nd order neurons (preganglionics).

Second-order neurons exit the spinal cord at T1 and enter the sympathetic chain and ascend but do not synapse until they reach the superior cervical ganglion, where they give rise to 3rd order neurons.

Third-order neurons (postganglionics) course upward with the common carotid artery. Those that mediate sweat in the face split off with the ECA (exception: fibers to the medial forehead do not branch off[15]). The rest travel with the ICA passing over the carotid sinus, entering the skull through the carotid canal, traversing the cavernous sinus where they follow the VI nerve for a short distance before they accompany V1 (ophthalmic division of trigeminal nerve), entering the orbit through the superior orbital fissure with the nasociliary nerve, passing through (without synapsing) the ciliary ganglion. Upon exiting the ciliary ganglion the sympathetic fibers divide, some reach the pupilodilator muscle of the eye as 2 long ciliary nerves (neurotransmitter: NE). Other fibers travel with the ophthalmic artery to innervate the lacrimal gland and Müller's muscle (the accessory levator muscle of the upper eyelid).

33.4.2 Pupilloconstrictor (parasympathetic)

Pupilloconstrictor muscle fibers are parasympathetically innervated and are arranged as a sphincter (i.e., circular) in the iris.

Parasympathetic preganglionic fibers arise in the Edinger-Westphal nucleus (in high midbrain, superior colliculus level) and are situated peripherally on the intracranial portion of the oculomotor nerve (p. 596).

33.4.3 Pupillary light reflex

Involves cranial nerves II & III, and neurons in 2 brainstem nucleii (Edinger-Westphal and pretectal nuclear complex).

Mediated by rods and cones of the retina which are stimulated by light, and transmit via their axons in the optic nerve. As with the visual path, temporal retinal fibers remain ipsilateral, whereas nasal retinal fibers decussate in the optic chiasm. Fibers subserving the light reflex bypass the lateral geniculate body (LGB) (unlike fibers for vision which enter the LGB) to synapse in the pretectal nuclear complex at the level of the superior colliculus. Intercalating neurons connect to both Edinger-Westphal parasympathetic motor nuclei. The preganglionic fibers travel within the third nerve to the ciliary ganglion as described above under Pupilloconstrictor (parasympathetic).

Monocular light normally stimulates bilaterally symmetric (i.e., equal) pupillary constriction (ipsilateral response is called the direct response, contralateral response is the consensual response).

33.4.4 Pupillary exam

To perform a complete bedside pupillary exam (see following sections for rationale for various aspects of the pupillary exam):

1. measure pupil size in a dimly lit room: anisocoria augmented in the dark indicates the smaller pupil is abnormal and suggests a sympathetic lesion
2. measure pupil size in a lighted room: anisocoria intensified in the light suggests the larger pupil is abnormal and that the defect is in the parasympathetics
3. note the reaction to bright light (direct and consensual)
4. near response (it is necessary to check this only if the light reaction is not good): the pupil normally constricts on convergence, and this response should be greater than the light reflex (accommodation is not necessary, and a visually handicapped patient can be instructed to follow their own finger as it is brought in)
   a) light-near dissociation: pupillary constriction on convergence but absent light response (Argyll Robertson pupil). Etiologies:
      • classically described in syphilis
      • Parinaud's syndrome (p. 100): dorsal midbrain lesion
      • oculomotor neuropathy (usually causes a tonic pupil as in oculomotor compression, see below): DM, EtOH
      • Adie's pupil: see below
5. swinging flashlight test: alternate the flashlight from one eye to the other with as little delay as possible; watch ≥ 5 seconds for the pupil to redilate (dilation after initial constriction is called pupillary escape and is normal due to retinal adaptation). Normal: direct and consensual light reflexes are equal. Afferent pupillary defect (see below): consensual reflex is stronger than the direct (i.e., pupil is larger on direct illumination than contralateral illumination)

33.4.5 Alterations in pupillary diameter

Anisocoria

General information

▶ **Definition.** Unequal pupil sizes (usually ≥ 1 mm difference).

▶ **Note.** An afferent pupillary defect (APD) (even with total blindness in one eye) alone does *not* produce anisocoria (i.e., an APD together with anisocoria indicates two separate lesions).

Evaluation

1. history is critically important. Check for exposure to drugs that affect pupillary size, trauma. Look at old photos (e.g., driver's license) for physiologic anisocoria
2. exam: see Pupillary exam above
3. a non-contrast CT is usually not helpful and can provide a false sense of security

Differential diagnosis

1. physiologic anisocoria: occurs in ≈ 20% of population (more common in people with a light iris). Familial and nonfamilial varieties exist. The difference in pupils is usually < 0.4 mm. The inequality is the same in a light and dark room (or slightly worse in the dark)
2. pharmacologic pupil (see below): the most common cause of *sudden onset* of anisocoria. Drugs include:
   a) mydriatics (pupillary dilators):
      • sympathomimetics (stimulate the dilator pupillae): usually cause only 1–2 mm of dilation, may react slightly to light. Includes phenylephrine, clonidine, naphazoline (an ingredient in OTC eye drops for allergies), eye contact with cocaine, certain plants (e.g., jimsonweed)

33

- parasympatholytics (inhibit the sphincter pupillae): cause maximal dilation (up to 8 mm) that does *not* react to light. Includes tropicamide, atropine, scopolamine (including patches for motion sickness), certain plants (e.g., deadly nightshade)

   b) miotics (pupillary constrictors): pilocarpine, organophosphates (pesticides), flea powders containing anticholinesterase

3. Horner syndrome: interruption of sympathetics to pupilodilator. The abnormal pupil is the *smaller* (miotic) pupil. If there is ptosis it will be on the side of the *small* pupil. See etiologies, etc. (p. 594)
4. third nerve palsy (p. 596). If there is ptosis, it will be on the side of the *large* pupil
   a) oculomotor neuropathy ("peripheral" neuropathy of the third nerve): usually spares the pupil. Etiologies: DM (usually resolves in ≈ 8 weeks), EtOH…
   b) third nerve compression: tends *not* to spare pupil (i.e., pupil is dilated). Produces loss of para-sympathetic tone. Etiologies include:
      - aneurysm:
        PComA (the most common aneurysm to cause this)
        basilar bifurcation (occasionally compresses the posterior III nerve)
      - uncal herniation: below
      - tumor
      - cavernous sinus lesions: including cavernous internal carotid aneurysm, carotid-caver-nous fistula, cavernous sinus tumors
5. Adie's pupil (AKA tonic pupil): see below
6. local trauma to the eye: traumatic iridoplegia. Injury to the pupillary sphincter muscle may pro-duce mydriasis or, less often, miosis, shape may be irregular
7. pontine lesions
8. eye prosthesis (artificial eye) AKA pseudoanisocoria
9. occasionally some patients have anisocoria that occurs only during migraine[16]
10. iritis
11. keratitis or corneal abrasion

Marcus Gunn pupil ([relative] afferent pupillay defect [RAPD])

AKA (relative) afferent pupillary defect (APD or RAPD), AKA amaurotic pupil. Finding: consensual pupillary reflex to light is stronger than the direct (normal responses are equal). Contrary to some textbooks, the amaurotic pupil is *not* larger than the other.[17] The presence of the consensual reflex is evidence of a preserved third nerve (with parasympathetics) on the side of the impaired direct reflex. Almost always associated with some visual loss in the affected eye. There are other causes of visual loss that do *not* produce an RAPD, such as a vitreous hemorrhage.

Testing: best detected with the swinging flashlight test (see above).

NB: Pupils should remain equal to each other throughout the test. In a dimly lit room, when you shine a light into a normal eye, both pupils constrict equally. If you move the light from a normal eye to an eye with RAPD, both pupils will dilate slightly because less signal is being transmitted through the pre-chiasmal optic nerve.

Etiologies

Lesion *anterior to the chiasm* ipsilateral to the side of the impaired direct reflex:
1. either in the retina (e.g., retinal detachment, retinal infarct e.g., from embolus)
2. or optic nerve, as may occur in:
   a) optic or retrobulbar neuritis: commonly seen in MS, but may also occur after vaccinations or viral infections, and usually improves gradually
   b) trauma to the optic nerve: indirect (p. 1014) or direct
   c) compression by tumor anterior to the chiasm

Adie's pupil (tonic pupil)

An iris palsy resulting in a dilated pupil, due to impaired postganglionic parasympathetics. Thought to be due to a viral infection of the ciliary ganglion. When associated with loss of all muscle tendon reflexes it is called Holmes-Adie's (is not limited to knee jerks, as some texts indicate). Typically seen in a woman in her twenties.

Slit-lamp exam shows some parts of iris contract and others don't.

These patients exhibit light-near dissociation (see above): in checking near response it is neces-sary to wait a few seconds.

33

Denervation supersensitivity: usually occurs after several weeks (not in acute phase). Administer two drops of dilute pilocarpine (0.1–0.125%), a parasympathomimetic, in each eye. Miosis (constriction) will occur in Adie's pupil within 30 minutes (normal pupils will react only to ≈ 1% pilocarpine).

Pharmacologic pupil

General information
Follows administration of a mydriatic agent. The mydriatic agent may be "occult" when other care providers have not been alerted that this has been used on a patient (this should always be noted in the chart), or when health care personnel unwittingly inoculate agents, e.g., scopolamine, atropine[18]... into a patient's eye or into their own eye. May present with accompanying H/A, and if it is unknown that a mydriatic is involved, this may be misinterpreted e.g., as a warning of an expanding PComA aneurysm.

A pharmacologically dilated pupil is very large (7–8 mm), and is larger than typical mydriasis due to third nerve compression (5–6 mm).

To differentiate pharmacologic pupil from a third nerve lesion: instill 1% pilocarpine (a parasympathomimetic) in both eyes (for comparison). A pharmacologic pupil does *not* constrict, whereas the normal side and a dilated pupil from a third nerve palsy will.

Agents
Drugs intentionally used by physicians to dilate the pupils (e.g., Mydriacyl, see below). For other mydriatics, see above.

Management
Option: admit and observe overnight, pupil should normalize.

Using mydriatic agents to produce pupillary dilatation
Indications: to improve the ability to examine the retina. NB: ability to follow bedside examination of pupils will be lost for duration of drug effect. This could mask pupillary dilatation from third nerve compression due to herniation. Always alert other caregivers and place a note in the chart to document that the pupil has been pharmacologically dilated (see above), including the agent(s) used and the time administered.

℞: 2 gtt of 0.5% or 1% tropicamide (Mydriacyl®) blocks the parasympathetic supply to pupil, and produces a mydriasis that lasts a couple hrs to half a day. This can be augmented with 1 gtt 2.5% phenylephrine ophthalmic (Mydfrin®, Neofrin®, Phenoptic® and others) which stimulates the sympathetics.

33

Oculomotor nerve compression

Third nerve compression may manifest initially with a mildly dilated pupil (5–6 mm). Possible etiologies include uncal herniation or expansion of a PComA or basilar bifurcation aneurysm. However, within 24 hours, most of these cases will also develop an oculomotor palsy (with down and out deviation of the eye and ptosis). These pupils respond to mydriatics and to miotic agents (the latter helps differentiate this from a pharmacologic pupil, see above).

Although it is possible for a unilaterally dilated pupil alone to be the initial presentation in uncal herniation, in actuality almost all of these patients will have some other finding, e.g., alteration in mental status (confusion, agitation, etc.) before midbrain compression occurs (i.e., it would be rare for a person undergoing early uncal herniation with a dilating pupil to be awake, talking, appropriate and neurologically intact).

Neuromuscular blocking agents (NMBAs)

Due to the absence of nicotinic receptors on the iris, non-depolarizing muscle blocking agents, such as pancuronium (Pavulon®) normally do not alter pupillary reaction to light[19] except in large doses where some of the first and second order neurons may be blocked.

Paradoxical pupillary reaction

Pupils constrict when light is removed.
1. congenital stationary night blindness
2. Best disease: autosomal dominant hereditary progressive macular dystrophy
3. optic nerve hypoplasia
4. retinitis pigmentosa

33.4.6 Horner syndrome

General information

Horner syndrome (**HS**) is caused by interruption of sympathetics to the eye and face anywhere along their path; see Pupilodilator (sympathetic) (p. 590). Unilateral findings on the involved side in a fully developed Horner syndrome are shown in ▶ Table 33.2.

Table 33.2 Findings in (complete) Horner syndrome

- miosis (constricted pupil)
- ptosis
- enophthalmos
- hyperemia of eye
- anhidrosis of half of face

Miosis in HS

The miosis (pupillary constriction) in Horner syndrome is only ≈ 2–3 mm. This will be accentuated by darkening the room, which causes the normal pupil to dilate.

Ptosis and enophthalmos

Ptosis is due primarily to paralysis of the superior and inferior tarsal muscles (weakness of the inferior tarsal muscle is technically called "inverse ptosis"). Enophthalmos is due to Müller's muscle paralysis, which also contributes a maximum of ≈ 2 mm to the ptosis. Ptosis in HS is partial, c.f. complete ptosis, which is due to weakness of levator palpebra superioris, which is not involved in Horner syndrome.

Possible sites of disruption of sympathetics

General information

See also anatomy of 1st, 2nd, and 3rd order sympathetic neurons (p. 590).

1st order neuron (central neuron)

Interruption is often accompanied by other brainstem abnormalities. Etiologies of dysfunction: infarction from vascular occlusion (usually PICA), syringobulbia, intraparenchymal neoplasm.

2nd order neuron (preganglionic)

Etiologies of dysfunction: lateral sympathectomies, significant chest trauma, apical pulmonary neoplasms[20] (Pancoast tumor), high thoracic or cervical neuroblastoma.

3rd order neuron (postganglionic)

The most common type. Etiologies of dysfunction: neck trauma, carotid vascular disease/studies (e.g., carotid dissections (p. 1578)), cervical bony abnormalities, migraine, skull base neoplasms, cavernous sinus lesions (e.g., meningioma). With involvement only of fibers on ICA, anhidrosis does not occur (i.e., sweating is preserved) on ipsilateral face since fibers to facial sweat glands travel with ECA.

Pharmacologic testing in Horner syndrome

Establishing the diagnosis

The following may be used if the diagnosis of Horner syndrome is in doubt. It is not necessary when a pupil lag upon darkening the room can be demonstrated in the affected eye. This test does *not* localize the lesion, e.g., as 1st order, 2nd order or 3rd order, and prevents localizing testing the same day.

Cocaine. R: 1 gtt 4% *cocaine* OU (not the 10% solution that is commonly used in ENT procedures which will also anesthetize the sphincter pupillae, thus preventing miosis), repeat in 10 min. Observe pupils over 30 min. Cocaine blocks the NE re-uptake of postganglionics at the neuroeffector junction. In HS, no NE is released and cocaine will not dilate the pupil (▶ Fig. 33.3). HS is not present if the pupil dilates normally. Delayed dilatation occurs in partial HS.

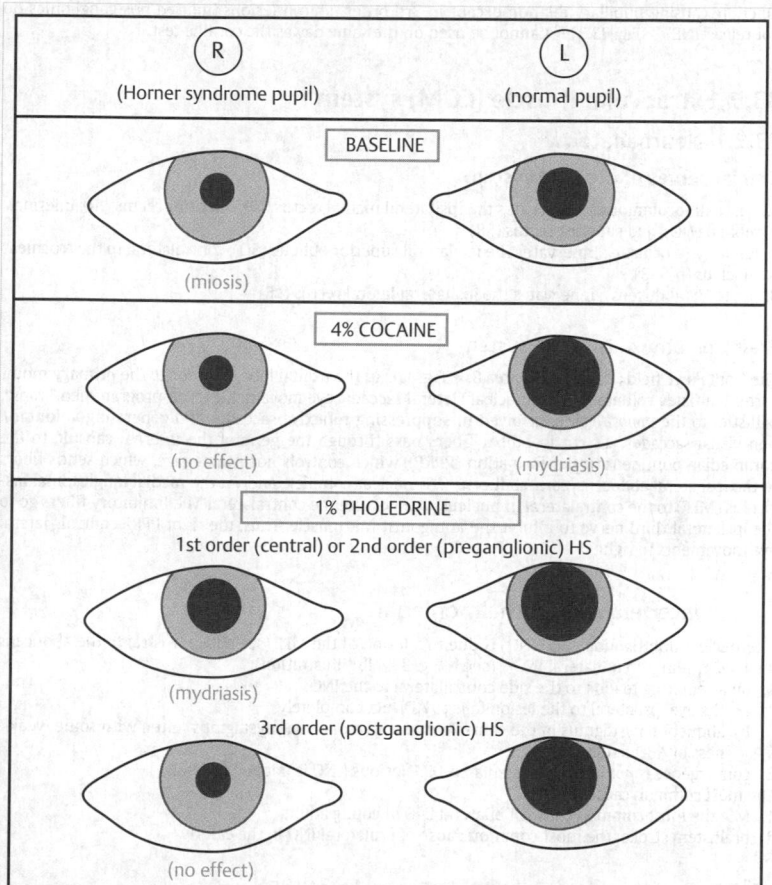

Fig. 33.3 Pharmacologic testing in Horner syndrome (HS).
This figure illustrates the findings in a right-sided HS.
Baseline: the abnormal right pupil will be smaller (miosis). This is accentuated in a darkened room where the unaffected left pupil dilates normally.
Cocaine is used when the diagnosis is uncertain. Only the normal pupil dilates (mydriasis).
Pholedrine is used to distinguish a 3rd order HS (where the affected pupil does not dilate) from a 1st or 2nd order HS (where it dilates some).
See text for details.

1% apraclonidine ophthalmic (Iopidine®): an alpha-agonist, can replace cocaine for establishing the diagnosis. It produces mydriasis in the affected eye due to denervation hypersensitivity in the pupilodilator muscle fibers, while the unaffected eye dilates 0–0.5 mm.[21]

Localizing the site of the lesion
First order (central) HS: is generally easy to diagnosis as it is usually accompanied by other hypothalamic, brainstem, or medullary findings.

To differentiate a first or second-order from a third-order HS: *1% pholedrine* (a substitute for the no longer available hydroxyamphetamine) releases NE from nerve endings at the neuroeffector

33

junction, causing pupillary dilation except in 3rd order neuron lesions (injured postganglionics do not release NE) (▶ Fig. 33.3).[22] Cannot be used on the same day as the cocaine test.

33.5 Extraocular muscle (EOM) system

33.5.1 Neuroanatomy

Cranial nerves of the EOM system

1. Cr. N. III (oculomotor): innervates the ipsilateral medial rectus (MR), inferior rectus (IR), inferior oblique (IO), and superior rectus (SR)
2. Cr. N. IV (trochlear): innervates the ipsilateral superior oblique (SO), contralateral to the trochlear nucleus (p. 598)
3. Cr. N. VI (abducens): innervates the ipsilateral lateral rectus (LR)

Brain anatomy of the EOM system

The frontal eye field (Brodmann's area 8, ▶ Fig. 1.1) in the frontal lobe, anterior to the primary motor cortex) initiates voluntary (supranuclear) lateral saccadic eye movements ("pre-programmed," rapid, ballistic) to the *opposite* side, involved in suppressing reflexive saccades and generating voluntary, non-visual saccades. It's corticobulbar fibers pass through the genu of the internal capsule to the paramedian pontine reticular formation (PPRF), which controls horizontal gaze, which sends fibers to the ipsilateral abducens/para-abducens (VI) nuclear complex, and via the medial longitudinal fasciculus (MLF) to the contralateral III nucleus to innervate the contralateral MR. Inhibitory fibers go to the ipsilateral third nerve to inhibit the antagonist MR muscle. Thus, the right PPRF controls lateral eye movements to right.

33.5.2 Internuclear ophthalmoplegia

Internuclear ophthalmoplegia (INO) is due to a lesion of the MLF (see above) rostral to the abducens nucleus. Findings in unilateral INO[23] (see ▶ Fig. 33.4 for illustration):
1. on attempting to look to the side contralateral to the INO:
   a) the eye ipsilateral to the lesion fails to ADDuct completely
   b) abduction nystagmus in the contralateral eye (monocular nystagmus) often with some weakness of ABDuction
2. convergence is *not* impaired in isolated MLF lesions (INO is not an EOM palsy)

The most common causes of INO:
1. MS: the most common cause of bilateral INO in young adults
2. brainstem stroke: the most common cause of unilateral INO in the elderly

33.5.3 Oculomotor (Cr. N. III) nerve palsy (OMP)

General information

The oculomotor nerve exits the brainstem ventrally and has two components: motor neurons which originate in the oculomotor nucleus, and more *peripherally situated* parasympathetic fibers which arise from the Edinger-Westphal nucleus. The nerve passes through the cavernous sinus and enters the superior orbital fissure where it divides into a superior division (innervating the superior rectus and the levator palpebrae superioris) and an inferior division (supplying the medial rectus, inferior rectus and inferior oblique). The parasympathetic fibers travel with the inferior division and branch off to the ciliary ganglion where they synapse. Postganglionic fibers enter the posterior globe to innervate the ciliary muscle (relaxes the lens which "thickens" and accommodates for near vision) and the constrictor pupillae muscle.

Oculomotor nerve *motor* palsy causes ptosis with eye deviated "down & out." Nuclear involvement of 3rd nerve is rare. NB: 3rd nerve palsy alone can cause up to 3 mm exophthalmos (proptosis) from relaxation of the rectus muscles.

Also see Painful ophthalmoplegia (p. 599) and Painless ophthalmoplegia (p. 600). For brainstem syndromes, see Benedikt's syndrome (p. 101) and Weber's syndrome (p. 101). Also, see Anisocoria (p. 591).

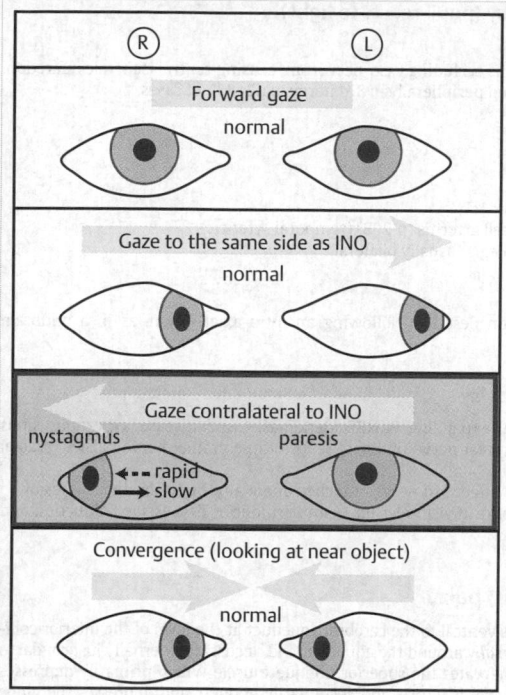

Fig. 33.4 Internuclear ophthalmo-plegia (INO). Illustration of gaze findings with a left medial longitudinal fasciculus (MLF) lesion producing a left INO.
(Red box illustrates the abnormal findings.)

Non pupil-sparing oculomotor palsy

33

The rule of the pupil in third nerve palsy

Elucidated in 1958 by Rucker. In effect, the rule states, "Third nerve palsy due to *extrinsic* compression of the nerve will be associated with impaired pupillary constriction." However, it is often overlooked that in 3% the pupil is spared.[24]

Etiologies

Most cases are due to extrinsic compression of 3rd nerve. Etiologies include:

1. tumor: the most common tumors affecting 3rd nerve:
   a) chordomas
   b) clival meningiomas
2. vascular: the most common vascular lesions:
   a) aneurysms of PComA artery (pupil sparing with aneurysmal oculomotor palsy occurs in < 1%).
      ★ Development of a new 3rd nerve palsy ipsilateral to a PComA aneurysm may be a sign of expansion with the possibility of imminent rupture, and is traditionally considered an indication for urgent treatment
   b) aneurysms of the distal basilar artery or bifurcation (basilar tip)
   c) carotid-cavernous fistula (p. 1519): look for pulsatile proptosis and chemosis
3. uncal herniation
4. cavernous sinus lesions: usually cause additional cranial nerve findings (V1, V2, IV, VI); see Cavernous sinus syndrome (p. 1689). Classically the third nerve palsy, e.g., from enlarging cavernous aneurysm, will *not* produce a dilated pupil because the sympathetics which dilate the pupil are also paralyzed[1 (p 1492)]

Pupil sparing oculomotor palsy (pupil reacts to light)

General information

Usually from intrinsic vascular lesions occluding vaso-nervorum, causing central ischemic infarction. Spares parasympathetic fibers located peripherally in 3rd nerve in 62–83% of cases.[24]

Etiologies

Etiologies include:
1. diabetic neuropathy
2. atherosclerosis (as seen in chronic HTN)
3. vasculopathies: including giant cell arteritis (p.203) (temporal arteritis)
4. chronic progressive ophthalmoplegia: usually bilateral
5. myasthenia gravis

Rarely, pupil-sparing OMP has been described following an intra-axial lesion, as in a midbrain infarction.[25]

Other causes of oculomotor palsy

Trauma, uncal herniation, laterally expanding PitNET/adenomas, Lyme disease, cavernous sinus lesions: usually cause additional cranial nerve findings; see Multiple cranial nerve palsies (cranial neuropathies) (p.1687).

Lesions within the orbit tend to affect 3rd nerve branches unequally. Superior division lesion → ptosis and impaired elevation; inferior division lesion → impairment of depression, adduction and pupillary reaction.

33.5.4 Trochlear nerve (IV) palsy

Anatomy: the trochlear nucleus lies ventral to the cerebral aqueduct at the level of the inferior colliculi. Trochlear nerve axons pass *dorsally* around the aqueduct and decussate internally just caudal to the inferior colliculi. The nerve innervates the superior oblique muscle which primarily depresses the adducted eye, but in primary gaze it intorts and secondarily abducts and depresses the globe (i.e., it moves the eye down & out).

Some unique features of the trochlear nerve:
1. the only cranial nerve to decussate internally (i.e., the trochlear nucleus is on the contralateral side to the nerve that exits and to the superior oblique it goes to)
2. the only cranial nerve to exit posteriorly on the brainstem
3. the only cranial nerve passing through the superior orbital fissure that does not pass through the annulus of Zinn (AKA annulus tendineus or annular tendon)

Trochlear palsy results in eye deviation "up and in." Patients tend to spontaneously tilt the head to the side *opposite* the IV palsy to "intort" the paretic eye and eliminate the diplopia. Diplopia is exacerbated when looking down (e.g., on descending stairs) especially when also looking inward, or when the examiner tilts the head *toward* the paretic side.

Isolated fourth nerve palsy is uncommon. It may occasionally occur with lesions of the cerebral peduncle or injury to the floor of the fourth ventricle near the aqueduct.

33.5.5 Abducens (VI) palsy

Anatomy: the abducens n. (Cr. N VI) leaves the abducens nucleus in the pons just beneath the floor of the 4th ventricle, exiting at the pontomedullary junction. It has a long intracranial course, and passes between the pons and clivus to enter the cavernous sinus via Dorello's canal.

Abducens palsy produces a lateral rectus palsy (inability to abduct the eye). Clinically produces diplopia that is exaggerated with lateral gaze to the side of the palsy. Etiologies of isolated 6th nerve palsy include[26]:
1. vasculopathy: including diabetes and giant cell arteritis. Most cases resolve within 3 months (alternative cause should be sought in cases lasting longer)
2. increased intracranial pressure: palsy may occur with increased ICP even in the absence of direct compression of the nerve (a "false localizing" sign in this setting). Postulated to occur due to the fact that the VI nerve has a long intracranial course, which may render it more sensitive to increased pressure. May be bilateral. Etiologies include:

a) traumatically increased ICP
b) increased ICP due to hydrocephalus (p.624), e.g., from p-fossa tumor
c) pseudotumor cerebri syndrome (p.955)
3. cavernous sinus lesions: cavernous carotid aneurysm (p.1489), neoplasm (meningioma...), carotid-cavernous fistula (p.1519)
4. inflammatory:
a) Gradenigo's syndrome (p.601), involvement at Dorello's canal
b) sphenoid sinusitis
5. intracranial neoplasm: e.g., clivus chordoma, chondrosarcoma
6. pseudoabducens palsy: may be due to
a) thyroid eye disease: the most common cause of chronic VI palsy. Will have positive forced duction test (eye cannot be moved by examiner)
b) myasthenia gravis: responds to edrophonium (Tensilon®) test
c) long-standing strabismus
d) Duane's syndrome (p.601)
e) fracture of the medial wall of the orbit with medial rectus entrapment
7. following lumbar puncture (p.1815): almost invariably unilateral
8. fracture through clivus (p.1065)
9. idiopathic

33.5.6 Multiple extraocular motor nerve involvement

Lesions in cavernous sinus (see below) involve cranial nerves III, IV, VI and V1 & V2 (ophthalmic and maxillary divisions of trigeminal nerve), and spare II and V3.
Superior orbital fissure syndrome: dysfunction of nerves III, IV, VI and V1.
Orbital apex syndrome: involves II, III, IV, VI and partial V1.
4th nerve palsy may result from a contrecoup injury in frontal head trauma.

33.5.7 Painful ophthalmoplegia

Definition

Pain and dysfunction of ocular motility (may be due to involvement of one or more of cranial nerves III, IV, V & VI).

Etiologies

33

1. intraorbital
a) inflammatory pseudotumor (idiopathic orbital inflammation): see below
b) contiguous sinusitis
c) invasive fungal sinus infection producing orbital apex syndrome. Rhinocerebral *mucormycosis* (AKA zygomycosis): sinusitis with painless black palatal or nasal septal ulcer or eschar with hyphal invasion of blood vessels by fungi of the order Mucorales, especially rhizopus.[27] Usually seen in diabetic or immunocompromised patients, occasionally in otherwise healthy patients.[28] Often involves dural sinuses and may cause cavernous sinus thrombosis
d) mets
e) lymphoma
2. superior orbital fissure/anterior cavernous sinus
a) Tolosa-Hunt syndrome: see below
b) mets
c) nasopharyngeal Ca
d) lymphoma
e) herpes zoster
f) carotid-cavernous fistula
g) cavernous sinus thrombosis
h) intracavernous aneurysm
3. parasellar region
a) PitNet/adenoma
b) mets
c) nasopharyngeal Ca
d) sphenoid sinus mucocele
e) meningioma/chordoma
f) apical petrositis (Gradenigo's syndrome): see below

4. posterior fossa
   a) PComA aneurysm
   b) basilar artery aneurysm (rare)
5. miscellaneous
   a) diabetic ophthalmoplegia
   b) migrainous ophthalmoplegia
   c) cranial arteritis
   d) tuberculous meningitis: may cause ophthalmoplegia, usually incomplete, most often primarily oculomotor nerve

33.5.8 Painless ophthalmoplegia

Differential diagnosis:
1. chronic progressive ophthalmoplegia: pupil sparing, usually bilateral, slowly progressive
2. myasthenia gravis: pupil sparing, responds to edrophonium (Tensilon®) test
3. myositis: usually also produces symptoms in other organ systems (heart, gonads...)

33.6 Neurophthalmologic syndromes

33.6.1 Pseudotumor (of the orbit)

General information

AKA "chronic granuloma" (a misnomer, since true epithelioid granulomas are rarely found). An idiopathic inflammatory disease confined to the orbit that may mimic a true neoplasm. Lymphocytic infiltration of extraocular muscles. Usually unilateral.

Typically presents with rapid onset of proptosis, pain, and EOM dysfunction (painful ophthalmoplegia with diplopia). Often follows URI, may be associated with scleral inflammation. Most commonly involves the superior orbital tissues.

Differential diagnosis

See Orbital lesions (p. 1658) for list.

Key points for Graves' disease (GD): the histologic appearance of GD (hyperthyroidism) may be indistinguishable from pseudotumor. Involvement with GD is usually bilateral.

Treatment

Surgery tends to cause a flare up, and is thus usually best avoided.

Steroids are the treatment of choice. ℞: 50–80 mg prednisone q d. Severe cases may necessitate treatment with 30–40 mg/d for several months.

Radiation treatment with 1000–2000 rads may be needed for cases of reactive lymphocytic hyperplasia.

33.6.2 Tolosa-Hunt syndrome

Nonspecific inflammation in the region of the superior orbital fissure, often with extension into the cavernous sinus, sometimes with granulomatous features. A diagnosis of exclusion. May be a topographical variant of orbital pseudotumor (see above). Clinical diagnostic criteria:
1. painful ophthalmoplegia
2. involvement of any nerve traversing the cavernous sinus. The pupil is usually spared (frequently not the case with aneurysms, specific inflammation, etc.)
3. symptoms last days to weeks
4. spontaneous remission, sometimes with residual deficit
5. recurrent attacks with remissions of months or years
6. no systemic involvement (occasional N/V, due to pain?)
7. dramatic improvement with systemic steroids: 60–80 mg prednisone PO q day (slow taper), relief within about 1 day
8. occasional inflammation of rectus muscle from contiguous inflammation

33

33.6.3 Raeder's paratrigeminal neuralgia

Two essential components[29]:
1. unilateral oculosympathetic paresis (AKA partial Horner syndrome [HS]; this usually lacks anhidrosis, and in this syndrome, possibly ptosis also)
2. homolateral trigeminal nerve involvement (usually tic-like pain, but may be analgesia or masseter weakness; pain, if present, must be tic-like and does not include e.g., unilateral head, face or vascular pain)

Localizing value of syndrome: region adjacent to trigeminal nerve in middle fossa. The cause is often not determined, but may rarely be due to aneurysm[30] compressing V1 with sympathetics.

33.6.4 Gradenigo's syndrome

AKA apical petrositis. Mastoiditis with involvement of petrous apex (if pneumatized). Usually seen by ENT physicians. Classic triad:
1. abducens palsy: from inflammation of 6th nerve at Dorello's canal, which is where it enters the cavernous sinus just medial to the petrous apex
2. retro-orbital pain: due to inflammation of V1
3. draining ear

33.7 Miscellaneous neurophthalmologic signs

▶ **Corneal mandibular reflex.** Eliciting the corneal reflex produces a jaw jerk or contralateral jaw movement (ipsilateral pterygoid contraction). A primitive pontine reflex, may be seen in a variety of insults to the brain (trauma, intracerebral hemorrhage…).

▶ **Duane syndrome.** AKA retraction syndrome: paradoxical innervation causing co-contraction of the lateral and medial rectus muscles on attempted adduction with relaxation on abduction, produces mild enophthalmos with pseudoptosis. May be congenital (e.g., part of one of the following syndromes: acrorenal-ocular syndrome, Okihiro syndrome…).

▶ **Hippus.** Rhythmic, irregular pupillary oscillations, changing by ≥ 2 mm. May confuse examination when checking pupillary responses; record the *initial* response. May be normal. No localizing value.

▶ **Marcus Gunn phenomenon.** Not to be confused with Marcus Gunn pupil (p. 592). Opening the mouth causes opening of a ptotic eye (abnormal reflex between proprioception of pterygoid muscles and third nerve). Reverse Marcus Gunn phenomenon: normal eye that closes with opening the mouth. Seen only in patients with peripheral facial nerve injuries, and probably results from aberrant regeneration.

▶ **Ocular bobbing**[31]. Abrupt, spontaneous, conjugate downward eye deviation with slow return to midposition, 2 to 12 times per min. It is associated with bilateral paralysis of horizontal gaze, including doll's-eyes and calorics. Most commonly seen with destructive lesions of the pontine tegmentum (usually hemorrhage, but also infarction, glioma, trauma), but has also been described with compressive lesions.[32] Atypical bobbing is similar except that horizontal gaze is preserved, and can be seen with cerebellar hemorrhage, hydrocephalus, trauma, metabolic encephalopathy…

▶ **Opsoclonus**[33]. (Rare.) Rapid, conjugate, irregular, non-rhythmic (differentiates this from nystagmus) eye movements vertically or horizontally, persist (attenuated) during sleep (opsochoria if dysconjugate). Usually associated with diffuse myoclonus (fingers, chin, lips, eyelid, forehead, trunk and LEs); also, malaise, fatigability, vomiting and some cerebellar findings. Often resolves spontaneously within 4 mos.

▶ **Oscillopsia.** Visual sensation that stationary objects are swaying side-to-side or vibrating.[34] Rarely the sole manifestation of Chiari I malformation[35] (often associated with downbeat nystagmus). Other causes include MS, or injury to both vestibular nerves; e.g., aminoglycoside ototoxicity,[36] bilateral vestibular neurectomies, see Dandy's syndrome (p. 603).

33

► **Pseudo von Grafe sign.** Lid retraction on downward gaze (true von Grafe sign is lid lag in hyperthyroidism) seen in aberrant nerve regeneration (inferior rectus innervation → activation of levator palpebrae).

► **Optic atrophy.** Chronic, progressive optic atrophy is due to a compressive lesion (aneurysm, meningioma, osteopetrosis…) until proven otherwise.

References

[1] Wilkins RH, Rengachary SS. Neurosurgery. New York 1985

[2] Pinel JF, Larmande P, Guegan Y, et al. Down-Beat Nystagmus: Case Report with Magnetic Resonance Imaging and Surgical Treatment. Neurosurgery. 1987; 21:736–739

[3] Williams DP, Troost BT, Rogers J. Lithium-Induced Downbeat Nystagmus. Archives of Neurology. 1988; 45:1022–1023

[4] Frisen L. Swelling of the optic nerve head: a staging scheme. J Neurol Neurosurg Psychiatry. 1982; 45:13–18

[5] Scott CJ, Kardon RH, Lee AG, et al. Diagnosis and grading of papilledema in patients with raised intracranial pressure using optical coherence tomography vs clinical expert assessment using a clinical staging scale. Arch Ophthalmol. 2010; 128:705–711

[6] Sher NA, Wirtschafter J, Shapiro SK, et al. Unilateral Papilledema in 'Benign' Intracranial Hypertension (Pseudotumor Cerebri). JAMA. 1983; 250:2346–2347

[7] Anderson DR, Patella VM. Automated Static Perimetry. 2nd ed. C V Mosby; 1998

[8] Horton JC. Wilbrand's knee of the primate optic chiasm is an artefact of monocular enucleation. Trans Am Ophthalmol Soc. 1997; 95:579–609

[9] Grzybowski A. Harry Moss Traquair (1875-1954), Scottish ophthalmologist and perimetrist. Acta Ophthalmol. 2009; 87:455–459

[10] Donaldson LC, Eshtiaghi A, Sacco S, et al. Junctional Scotoma and Patterns of Visual Field Defects Produced by Lesions Involving the Optic Chiasm. J Neuroophthalmol. 2022; 42:e203–e208

[11] Shin RK, Li TP. Visualization of Wilbrand's knee. Snowbird, UT 2013

[12] Lee JH, Tobias S, Kwon JT, et al. Wilbrand's knee: does it exist? Surg Neurol. 2006; 66:11–7; discussion 17

[13] Zweckberger K, Unterberg AW, Schick U. Prechiasmatic transection of the optic nerve can save contralateral vision in patients with optic nerve sheath meningiomas. Clin Neurol Neurosurg. 2013; 115:2426–2431

[14] Cho J, Liao E, Trobe JD. Visual Field Defect Patterns Associated With Lesions of the Retrochiasmal Visual Pathway. J Neuroophthalmol. 2022; 42:353–359

[15] Walton KA, Buono LM. Horner syndrome. Curr Opin Ophthalmol. 2003; 14:357–363

[16] Kawasaki A. Physiology, assessment, and disorders of the pupil. Current Opinion in Ophthalmology. 1999; 10:394–400

[17] Walsh FB, Hoyt WF. Clinical Neuro-Ophthalmology. Baltimore 1969

[18] Nakagawa TA, Guerra L, Storgion SA. Aerosolized atropine as an unusual cause of anisocoria in a child with asthma. Pediatr Emerg Care. 1993; 9:153–154

[19] Wijdicks EF. Determining Brain Death in Adults. Neurology. 1995; 45:1003–1011

[20] Lepore FE. Diagnostic Pharmacology of the Pupil. Clin Neuropharmacol. 1985; 8:27–37

[21] Morales J, Brown SM, Abdul-Rahim AS, et al. Ocular effects of apraclonidine in Horner syndrome. Arch Ophthalmol. 2000; 118:951–954

[22] Bates AT, Chamberlain S, Champion M, et al. Pholedrine: a substitute for hydroxyamphetamine as a diagnostic eyedrop test in Horner's syndrome. J Neurol Neurosurg Psychiatry. 1995; 58:215–217

[23] Zee DS. Internuclear ophthalmoplegia: pathophysiology and diagnosis. Baillieres Clin Neurol. 1992; 1:455–470

[24] Trobe JD. Third nerve palsy and the pupil. Footnotes to the rule. Arch Ophthalmol. 1988; 106:601–602

[25] Breen LA, Hopf HC, Farris BK, et al. Pupil-Sparing Oculomotor Nerve Palsy due to Midbrain Infarction. Arch Neurol. 1991; 48:105–106

[26] Galetta SL, Smith JL. Chronic Isolated Sixth Nerve Palsies. Archives of Neurology. 1989; 46:79–82

[27] DeShazo RD, Chapin K, Swain RE. Fungal Sinusitis. New England Journal of Medicine. 1997; 337:254–259

[28] Radner AB, Witt MD, Edwards JE. Acute Invasive Rhinocerebral Zygomycosis in an Otherwise Healthy Patient: Case Report and Review. Clin Infect Dis. 1995; 20:163–166

[29] Mokri B. Raeder's Paratrigeminal Syndrome. Arch Neurol. 1982; 39:395–399

[30] Kashihara K, Ito H, Yamamoto S, et al. Raeder's Syndrome Associated with Intracranial Internal Carotid Artery Aneurysm. Neurosurgery. 1987; 20:49–51

[31] Fisher CM. Ocular Bobbing. Arch Neurol. 1964; 11:543–546

[32] Sherman DG, Salmon JH. Ocular Bobbing with Superior Cerebellar Artery Aneurysm: Case Report. J Neurosurg. 1977; 47:596–598

[33] Smith JL, Walsh FB. Opsoclonus - Ataxic Conjugate Movements of the Eyes. Arch Ophthalm. 1960; 64:244–250

[34] Brickner R. Oscillopsia: A new symptom commonly occurring in multiple sclerosis. Arch Neurol Psychiatry. 1936; 36:586–589

[35] Gingold SI, Winfield JA. Oscillopsia and Primary Cerebellar Ectopie: Case Report and Review of the Literature. Neurosurgery. 1991; 29:932–936

[36] Marra TR, Reynolds NC, Stoddard JJ. Subjective Oscillopsia ("Jiggling Vision") Presumably Due to Aminoglycoside Ototoxicity: A Report of Two Cases. J Clin Neuro Ophthalmol. 1988; 8:35–38

33

34 Neurotology

34.1 Dizziness and vertigo

34.1.1 Differential diagnosis of dizziness

▶ **Near syncope.** Some overlap with syncope; see Syncope and apoplexy (p. 1684)
1. orthostatic hypotension
2. cardiogenic hypotension
   a) arrhythmia
   b) valvular disease
3. vasovagal episode
4. hypersensitive carotid sinus; see Syncope and apoplexy (p. 1684)

▶ **Dysequilibrium**
1. multiple sensory deficits: e.g., peripheral neuropathy, visual impairment
2. cerebellar degeneration

▶ *Vertigo.* Sensation of movement (usually spinning)
1. inner ear dysfunction
   a) labyrinthitis
   b) Meniere disease (see below)
   c) trauma: endolymphatic leak
   d) *drugs*: especially aminoglycosides
   e) **benign (paroxysmal) positional vertigo**[1]: AKA *cupulolithiasis.* Attacks of severe vertigo when the head is turned to certain positions (usually in bed). Due to calcium concretions in the semicircular canals. Self limited (most cases do not last > 1 year). No hearing loss
   f) syphilis
   g) vertebrobasilar insufficiency (p. 1591)
2. vestibular nerve dysfunction
   a) vestibular neuronitis: sudden onset of vertigo, gradual improvement
   b) compression:
      - meningioma
      - vestibular schwannoma: usually slowly progressive ataxia instead of severe vertigo. BAER latencies usually abnormal. CT or MRI usually abnormal
3. **disabling positional vertigo:** as described by Jannetta et al,[2] *constant* disabling positional vertigo or dysequilibrium, causing ≈ constant nausea, no vestibular dysfunction nor hearing loss (tinnitus may be present). One possible cause is vascular compression of the vestibular nerve which may respond to microvascular decompression
4. brainstem dysfunction
   a) vascular disease; see Vertebrobasilar insufficiency (p. 1591): less distinct vestibular symptoms, prominent nonvestibular symptoms
   b) migraine: especially basilar artery migraine
   c) demyelinating disease: e.g., multiple sclerosis
   d) *drugs*: antiseizure medications, alcohol, sedatives/hypnotics, salicylates
5. dysfunction of cervical proprioceptors: as in cervical osteoarthritis

▶ **Poorly defined lightheadedness.** Mostly psychiatric. May also include:
1. hyperventilation
2. hypoglycemia
3. anxiety neurosis
4. hysterical

34

34.1.2 Vestibular neurectomy

General information

Complete loss of vestibular function from one side is thought to produce transient vertigo due to the mismatch of vestibular input from the two ears. Theoretically, a central compensatory mechanism (the "cerebellar clamp") results in the amelioration of symptoms. In cases of unilateral *fluctuating* vestibular dysfunction, this compensatory mechanism may be impaired. Unilateral selective vestibular neurectomy

(SVN) may convert the fluctuating or partial loss to a complete cessation of input and facilitate compensation. Bilateral SVN is often complicated by oscillopsia (p.601)—AKA Dandy's syndrome, with difficulty in maintaining balance in the dark due to loss of the vestibulo-ocular reflex—and is to be avoided.

Indications

The two conditions for which SVN is most commonly employed are Meniere disease (see below) and partial vestibular injury (viral or traumatic). SVN may be indicated in disabling cases refractory to medical or non-destructive surgical treatment when vestibular studies demonstrate continued or progressive uncompensated vestibular dysfunction.[3]

SVN preserves hearing and in Meniere disease is > 90% effective in eliminating episodic vertiginous spells (≈ 80% success rate in non-Meniere cases), but is unlikely to improve stability with rapid head movement.

Surgical approaches for SVN

1. retrolabyrinthine, AKA postauricular approach: anterior to sigmoid sinus. Primary choice in patients with Meniere disease who have not had previous endolymphatic sac (ELS) procedures since it permits simultaneous SVN and decompression of the endolymphatic sac. Requires mastoidectomy with skeletonization of the semicircular canals and ELS. The dural opening is bounded anteriorly by the posterior semicircular canal, posteriorly by the sigmoid sinus. Water-tight dural closure is difficult
2. retrosigmoid, AKA posterior fossa, AKA suboccipital approach: posterior to sigmoid sinus. The original approach applied by Dandy in pre-microsurgical era, usually sacrificed hearing, and occasionally facial nerve function. Better results are achieved today with microscopic techniques. Indicated for cases other than Meniere disease where there is no need for identification of the ELS. Also the best approach for positive identification of eighth nerve
3. middle fossa (extradural) approach: the fibers of the vestibular division may be more segregated from the cochlear fibers in the IAC than in the CPA, thus permitting more complete section of the vestibular nerve. May be appropriate for failed response to SVN by the above approaches. Disadvantages: requires temporal lobe retraction, does not allow exposure of ELS, and higher morbidity and risk of damage to facial nerve[4] than retrolabyrinthine approach

Surgical considerations for selective vestibular neurectomy

(Also, see ▶ Fig. 1.9)
1. the vestibular nerve is in the superior half of the eighth nerve complex, and is slightly more *gray* in color than the cochlear division (due to less myelin[5]). They may be separated by a small vessel or by an indentation in the bundle
2. facial (VII) nerve:
   a) whiter than the VIII nerve complex
   b) lies anterior and superiorly to the VIII nerve
   c) EMG monitoring of the facial nerve is recommended
   d) direct stimulation confirms the identification
3. any vessels present on eighth nerve bundle must be preserved to save hearing (primarily, the artery of the auditory canal must be preserved)
4. if no plane of cleavage can be defined between vestibular & cochlear divisions, the superior half of the nerve bundle is divided
5. the endolymphatic sac lies ≈ midway between the posterior edge of the internal auditory meatus and the sigmoid sinus

34.2 Meniere disease

34.2.1 General information

Key concepts

- increased endolymphatic pressure
- clinical triad: vertigo, tinnitus & fluctuating hearing loss
- surgical options for failure of medical management include endolymphatic shunt or selective vestibular neurectomy

Probably due to a derangement of endolymphatic fluid regulation (a consistent finding is endolymphatic hydrops: increased endolymphatic volume and pressure with dilatation of endolymph spaces), with resultant fistulization into the perilymphatic spaces.

34.2.2 Epidemiology

Incidence: ≈ 8–46 per 100,000 population per year.[6] Most cases have onset between 30 and 60 years of age, rarely in youth or in the elderly.

Prevalence range: 3.5–513 per 100,000 population.[6] Health claims data found prvalence 190 per 100,000 with a female:male ratio of1.89 to 1.[6] May become bilateral in 20%.

34.2.3 Clinical

Clinical triad

1. attacks of violent vertigo (due to vestibular nerve dysfunction): usually the earliest and the most disabling symptom. Nausea, vomiting, and diaphoresis are frequent concomitants. Severe attacks may cause prostration. Vertigo may persist even after complete deafness. Balance is normal between attacks
2. tinnitus: often described as resembling the sound of escaping steam, not a true "ringing"
3. fluctuating low frequency hearing loss: may fluctuate for a periods of weeks to years, and may progress to permanent deafness if untreated (a sensation of fullness in the ear is commonly described[7]; however, this is nonspecific and may occur with hearing loss for any reason)

Other clinical features

Drop attacks ("otolithic crises of Tumarkin") occasionally occur.

Attack duration: ≈ 5–30 minutes (some say 2–6 hours), with a "post-ictal" period of fatigue lasting several hrs.

Frequency: varies from one or two attacks a year to several times per week.

Two subtypes differ from classical form: vestibular Meniere (episodic vertigo with normal hearing) and cochlear Meniere (few vestibular symptoms).

Natural course of syndrome is characterized by periods of remission. Eventually the vertiginous attacks either progress in severity, or "burn out" (being replaced by constant unsteadiness[7]).

Differential diagnosis

Also see Differential diagnosis: Dizziness and vertigo (p. 603) for more details.

1. benign (paroxysmal) positional vertigo: AKA *cupulolithiasis*. Self limited (most cases last < 1 year). No hearing loss
2. disabling positional vertigo: *constant* disabling positional vertigo or dysequilibrium, ≈ constant nausea, no vestibular dysfunction nor hearing loss (tinnitus may be present)
3. vestibular schwannoma: usually slowly progressive ataxia instead of episodic severe vertigo. BAER latencies usually abnormal. CT or MRI usually positive
4. vestibular neuronitis: sudden onset of vertigo with gradual improvement
5. vertebrobasilar insufficiency (VBI) (p. 1591): less distinct vestibular symptoms, and prominence of nonvestibular symptoms

Diagnostic studies

1. electronystagmography (ENG) with bithermal caloric stimulation usually abnormal, may show blunted thermal responses
2. audiogram: low frequency hearing loss, fairly good preservation of discrimination and loudness recruitment, negative tone decay on impedance testing
3. BAER usually shows normal latencies
4. radiographic imaging (CT, MRI, etc.): no findings in Meniere disease
5. in bilateral cases, a VDRL should be checked to R/O luetic disease

Treatment

Medical treatment

1. reduced intake of salt (strict salt restriction is as effective as any medication) and caffeine

34

2. diuretics: taken daily until ear fullness abates, then PRN ear pressure (usually once or twice weekly suffices)
   a) acetazolamide: ℞ Diamox® sequels 500 mg PO q d × 1 week, increase to BID if symptoms persist. D/C if paresthesias develop. Do not use during 1st trimester of pregnancy
3. vestibular suppressants
   a) diazepam (Valium®): probably the most effective
   b) meclizine HCl (Antivert®): ℞ Adult dose for vertigo associated with the vestibular system (during attacks): 25–100 mg/day PO divided. Dose for motion sickness: 25–50 mg PO one hr prior to stimulus. Supplied: 12.5, 25 & 50 mg tabs. **Side effects:** drowsiness
4. vasodilators: postulated to be mediated by increased cochlear blood flow: inhalation of 5–10% CO_2 works well, but relief is short lived

Surgical treatment

Reserved for *incapacitating* cases *refractory* to medical management. When functional hearing exists, procedures that spare hearing are preferred because of high incidence of bilateral involvement. Procedures include:

1. endolymphatic shunting procedures: to mastoid cavity (Arenberg shunt) or to subarachnoid space. Reserved for cases with serviceable hearing. ≈ 65% success rate (see below). If symptoms are relieved ≥ 1 year, then a recurrence would be treated by shunt revision, if < 1 year then vestibular neurectomy
2. direct application of corticosteroids to the inner ear
3. nonselective vestibular ablation (in cases with nonserviceable hearing on the side of involvement)
   a) surgical labyrinthectomy
   b) middle ear perfusion with gentamicin
   c) translabyrinthine section of the 8th nerve
4. selective vestibular neurectomy (p. 603), in cases with serviceable hearing

Outcome

Endolymph shunting procedures

Outcomes from 112 endolymphatic shunting procedures are shown in ▶ Table 34.1.

Table 34.1 Outcome in 112 endolymphatic-subarachnoid shunts[7]

	Vertigo	Tinnitus	Hearing[a]	Ear pressure
improved	79 (70%)[b]	53 (47%)	19 (17%)	57 (51%)
stable	33 (29%)	49 (43%)	50 (45%)	24 (21%)
worse	(none)	10 (10%)	39 (35%)	31 (28%)

[a]improved hearing considered serviceable (50 dB pure tone, 70% speech discrimination); additional 4 patients had improved but non-serviceable hearing
[b]5 patients had recurrence of vertigo after 1–3 years

Neurectomy procedures

Vestibulocochlear nerve section (based on early posterior fossa surgery by Dandy; entire eighth nerve bundle was sectioned in 587 patients; all were deaf post-op): 90% relieved of vertigo, 5% unchanged and 5% worse; 9% incidence of facial paralysis (3% incidence of permanent paralysis).

Selective vestibular nerve section (sparing cochlear portion, 95 patients from Dandy): 10% had improved hearing, 28% unchanged, 48% worse, 14% deaf.

Retrolabyrinthine approach: in 32 patients with Meniere syndrome (25 failed endolymph shunt) responding to survey, 85% had complete relief of vertigo, 6% improved, 9% no relief (one of whom responded to middle fossa neurectomy).[5]

Complications and untoward effects

Patients with little vestibular nerve function pre-op (determined by ENG) usually have little difficulty immediately following vestibular neurectomy; patients with more function may have a transient worsening post-op until they accommodate.

Among 42 patients undergoing retrolabyrinthine approach: none lost hearing as a result of surgery, no facial weakness, one CSF rhinorrhea requiring reoperation, and one meningitis with good outcome.[5]

In post-op failures, check ENG. If any vestibular nerve function is demonstrated on operated side, then the nerve section was incomplete; consider re-operating.

34.3 Facial nerve palsy

34.3.1 Severity grading

Severity of facial palsy is often graded with the House and Brackmann scale (see ▶ Table 45.3).

34.3.2 Localizing site of lesion

Central facial palsy (AKA supranuclear facial palsy)

The cortical representation for facial movement occurs in the motor strip along the lateral aspect (just above the most inferior opercular portion of the precentral gyrus (▶ Fig. 1.3)). The keys to differentiating central paralysis (due to *supranuclear* lesions) from peripheral facial palsy are that *central* palsies:
1. are confined primarily to the lower face due to some bilateral cortical representation of upper facial movement
2. may spare emotional facial expression[8] (e.g., smiling at a joke)

Nuclear facial palsy

The motor nucleus of the seventh nerve is located at the pontomedullary junction. Nuclear VII palsy results in paralysis of all VII nerve motor function. In nuclear facial palsies, other neurologic findings also often occur from involvement of adjacent neural structures by the underlying process (stroke, tumor…); e.g., in Millard-Gubler syndrome (p.101), there is ipsilateral abducens palsy + contralateral limb weakness. Tumors invading the floor of the 4th ventricle (e.g., medulloblastoma) may also cause nuclear facial palsy (from involvement of facial colliculus in the floor of 4th ventricle).

Facial nerve lesion

Motor fibers ascend within the pons and form a sharp bend ("internal genu") around the sixth nerve (abducens) nucleus, forming a visible bump in the floor of the 4th ventricle (facial colliculus). The seventh nerve exits from the brainstem at the ponto-medullary junction (▶ Fig. 2.7) where it may be involved in CPA tumors. It enters the supero-anterior portion of the internal auditory canal (▶ Fig. 1.9). The geniculate ganglion ("external genu") is located within the temporal bone. The first branch from the ganglion is the greater superficial petrosal nerve (GSPN), which passes to the pterygopalatine ganglion and innervates the nasal and palatine mucosa and the lacrimal gland of the eye; lesions proximal to this point produce a dry eye. The next branch is the branch to the stapedius muscle; lesions proximal to this point produce hyperacusis. Next, the chorda tympani joins the facial nerve bringing taste sensation from the anterior two–thirds of the tongue. Basal skull fractures may injure the nerve just proximal to this point. Travelling with the chorda tympani are fibers to the submandibular and sublingual glands. The facial nerve exits the skull at the stylomastoid foramen. It then enters the parotid gland, where it splits into the following branches to the facial muscles (cranial to caudal): temporal, zygomatic, buccal, mandibular, and cervical. Lesions within the parotid gland (e.g., parotid tumors) may involve some branches but spare others.

34.3.3 Etiologies

These etiologies produce primarily facial nerve palsy, also see Multiple cranial nerve palsies (cranial neuropathies) (p.1687). **Note:** 90–95% of all cases of facial palsy are accounted for by the first 3 items: Bell's palsy, herpes zoster oticus, and trauma (basal skull fractures).[9]
1. Bell's palsy (p.608)
2. herpes zoster oticus (auris) (p.609)
3. trauma: basal skull fracture
4. birth:
   a) congenital
      - *bilateral facial palsy (facial diplegia) of Möbius syndrome (p.1687) : unique in that it affects upper face more than lower face
      - *congenital facial diplegia may be part of facioscapulohumeral or myotonic muscular dystrophy
   b) traumatic

34

5. otitis media: with acute otitis media, facial palsy usually improves with antibiotics. With chronic suppurative otitis surgical intervention is required
6. central facial paralysis and nuclear facial paralysis: see Localizing site of lesion above
7. neoplasm: usually causes hearing loss, and (unlike Bell's palsy) *slowly progressive* facial paralysis
   a) most are either benign schwannomas of the facial or auditory nerve, or malignancies metastatic to the temporal bone. Facial neuromas account for ≈ 5% of peripheral facial nerve palsies[10]; the paralysis tends to be slowly progressive
   b) parotid tumors may involve some branches but spare others
   c) Masson's vegetant intravascular hemangioendothelioma (p. 961)
8. *neurosarcoidosis (p. 198): VII is the most commonly affected cranial nerve
9. diabetes: 17% of patients > 40 yrs old with peripheral facial palsy (PFP) have abnormal glucose tolerance tests. Diabetics have 4.5 times the relative risk of developing PFP than nondiabetics[11]
10. *stage II Lyme disease (p. 364)[12]: facial diplegia is a hallmark
11. *Guillain-Barré syndrome: facial diplegia occurs in ≈ 50% of fatal cases
12. occasionally seen in Klippel-Feil syndrome
13. *isolated 4th ventricle (p. 436): compression at the facial colliculus

* Items with an asterisk are often associated with facial *diplegia* (i.e., bilateral facial palsy), see also multiple cranial neuropathies (p. 1687).

34.3.4 Bell's palsy

General information

Bell's palsy (BP), AKA idiopathic peripheral facial palsy (PFP), is the most common cause of facial paralysis (50–80% of PFPs). Incidence: 150–200/1-million/yr.

Etiology: by definition, PFP is called Bell's palsy when it is not due to known causes of PFP (e.g., infection, tumor, or trauma) and there are no other neurological (e.g., involvement of other cranial nerves) or systemic manifestations (e.g., fever, diabetes, possibly hypertension[13]).[14] Thus, true BP is idiopathic, and is a diagnosis of exclusion. Most cases probably represent a viral inflammatory demyelinating polyneuritis[15] usually due to the herpes simplex virus.[16] Facial palsy due to Lyme disease can usually be recognized on clinical grounds.[17] Severity may be graded on the House & Brackmann grading scale (see ▶ Table 45.3).

Presentation

A viral prodrome is frequent: URI, myalgia, hypesthesia or dysesthesia of the trigeminal nerve, N/V, diarrhea... Paralysis may be incomplete and remain so (Type I); it is complete at onset in 50% (Type II), the remainder progress to completion in 1 week. Usually exhibits distal to proximal progression: motor branches, then chorda tympani (loss of taste and decreased salivation), then stapedial branch (hyperacusis), then geniculate ganglion (decreased tearing). Associated symptoms are shown in ▶ Table 34.2, and are usually, but not always, ipsilateral. Herpes zoster vesicles develop in 4% of patients 2–4 days after onset of paralysis; and in 30% of patients 4–8 days after onset. During the recovery phase excessive lacrimation may occur (aberrant nerve regeneration).

Table 34.2 Associated symptoms with Bell's palsy

Symptom	%
facial & retroauricular pain	60
dysgeusia	57
hyperacusis	30
reduced tearing	17

Evaluation

Patients with PFP should be examined at an early stage to optimize outcome.

Electrodiagnostics: EMG may detect re-innervation potentials, aids prognostication. Nerve conduction study: electrical stimulation of the facial nerve near the stylomastoid foramen while recording EMG in facial muscles (a facial nerve may continue to conduct for up to ≈ 1 week even after complete transection).

Management

General measures

Eye protection: protection of the eye is critical. Artificial tears during the day, eye ointment at night, avoid bright light (using dark glasses during the day).

Medical management

Steroids: prednisolone 25 mg p.o. BID × 10 days, started within 72 hours of onset of symptoms, improves the chances of complete recovery at 3 & 9 months.

Acyclovir: does *not* help (alone or in combination with prednisolone).[18]

Surgical management

Surgical decompression: controversial. The definitive study has not been done. Rarely utilized. Indications may include:

1. complete facial nerve degeneration without response to nerve stimulation (although this absence is also used as an argument against surgery[9])
2. progressively deteriorating response to nerve stimulation
3. no clinical nor objective (nerve testing) improvement after 8 wks (however, in cases where the diagnosis of Bell's palsy is felt to be certain, the active disease will have abated by ≈ 14 days after onset[9])

Prognosis

Essentially all cases show some recovery (if none by 6 mos, other etiologies should be sought). Extent of recovery: 75–80% of cases recover completely, 10% partial, remainder poor. If recovery begins by 10–21 d, tends to be complete; if not until 3–8 wks → fair, if not until 2–4 mos → poor recovery. If paralysis is complete at onset, 50% will have incomplete recovery. Cases of incomplete paralysis at onset that do not progress to complete paralysis → complete recovery; incomplete paralysis at onset that progresses to complete → incomplete recovery in 75%. A worse prognosis is associated with: more proximal involvement, hyperacusis, decreased tearing, age > 60 yrs, diabetes, HTN, psychoneuroses, and aural, facial, or radicular pain.

34.3.5 Herpes zoster oticus facial paralysis

Symptoms are more severe than Bell's palsy, herpetic vesicles are usually present, and antibody titers to varicella-zoster virus rise. These patients have a higher risk of facial nerve degeneration.

34.3.6 Surgical treatment of facial palsy

General information

For cases with focal injury to the facial nerve (e.g., trauma, injury during surgery for CPA tumor...), dynamic reconstruction by nerve anastamoses are usually considered superior to static methods.[19] For nonfocal causes, e.g., Bell's palsy, only "static" methods may be applicable. A functional neural repair is not possible if the facial muscles have atrophied or fibrosed.

Surgical options

Surgical treatment options include:

1. for intracranial injury to facial nerve (e.g., during CPA tumor surgery): intracranial reapproximation (with or without graft) offers the best hope for the most normal facial reanimation
   a) timing
      - at time of tumor removal (for a divided facial nerve during removal of vestibular schwannoma[20,21,22]): the best result that can be achieved with this is House-Brackmann Grade III (▶ Table 45.3). The operation fails to produce good results in ≈ 33% of cases[22]
      - in delayed fashion, especially if the nerve was left in anatomic continuity
   b) techniques
      - direct reanastamosis: difficult due to the frail nature of the VII nerve (especially when it has been stretched by a tumor)
      - cable graft: e.g., using greater auricular nerve[23] or sural nerve

34

2. extracranial facial nerve anastomosis
    a) hypoglossal nerve (Cr. N. XII)-facial nerve anastomosis (see below)
    b) spinal accessory nerve (Cr. N. XI)-facial nerve anastomosis (see below)
    c) phrenic nerve-facial nerve anastamosis
    d) glossopharyngeal (Cr. N. IX)-facial nerve anastamosis
    e) crossface grafting (VII-VII): results have not been very good
3. "mechanical" or "static" means
    a) facial suspension: e.g., with polypropylene (Marlex®) mesh[24]
    b) eye closure techniques (protects the eye from exposure and reduced tearing)
        - tarsorrhaphy: partial or complete
        - gold weights in eyelid
        - stainless-steel spring in eyelid

Timing of surgery

If the facial nerve is known to be interrupted (e.g., transected during removal of vestibular schwannoma) then early surgical treatment is indicated. When the status of the nerve is unknown or if in continuity but not functioning, then several months of observation and electrical testing should be allowed for spontaneous recovery. Very late attempts at anastomosis have less chance for recovery due to facial muscle atrophy.

Hypoglossal nerve-facial nerve (XII-VII) anastomosis

General information

Cannot be used bilaterally in patients with facial diplegia or in those with other lower cranial nerve deficits (or potential for same). In spite of some suggestions to the contrary, sacrificing the XII nerve does create some morbidity (tongue atrophy with difficulty speaking, mastication and swallowing in ≈ 25% of cases, exacerbated when the facial muscles do not function on that side; aspiration may occur if vagus (Cr. N. X) dysfunction coexists with loss of XII).

Not as effective as would theoretically seem possible. The resultant facial reanimation is often less than ideal (may permit mass movement). To avoid severe disappointment, the patient should thoroughly understand the likely side effects and that the facial movement will probably be much less than normal, often with poor voluntary control.

Usually performed in conjunction with anastamosis of the descendens hypoglossi to the distal hypoglossal nerve to try and reduce hemiatrophy of the tongue. Atrophy may also be reduced by using a "jump graft" without completely interrupting XII.[25]

Technique

Position: supine, head turned slightly to the opposite side. Skin incision: 6–8 cm incision from just above the mastoid process obliquely downward across the neck to 2 cm below the angle of the jaw. The platysma is opened, and the tip of the mastoid is exposed by incising the insertion of the SCM and using a periosteal elevator. Incise the deep fascia; avoid the parotid gland, which is retracted superiorly. Rongeur the anterior third of the mastoid process (wax any exposed air cells) and identify the facial nerve as it exits the stylomastoid foramen between the mastoid process and the styloid process. Retract the posterior belly of the digastric inferiorly to aid the exposure.

The SCM is retracted laterally until the carotid sheath is identified, revealing the hypoglossal nerve. It loops around the occipital artery at this level (where it gives off the descendens hypoglossi) to pass between the carotid artery and jugular vein. The nerve is freed proximally to the point where it enters the carotid sheath and distally to the submandibular triangle where it is sharply divided.

The facial nerve is divided at the stylomastoid foramen and is approximated to the proximal hypoglossal nerve. The descendens hypoglossi is divided as far distally as possible and is then anastomosed to the distal stump of the hypoglossal nerve.

Variations

1. interposition jump grafts: spares function in the XII nerve (to minimize glottic denervation, the incision of XII should be distal to the descendens hypoglossi[25])
    a) using cutaneous nerve jump graft[25]
    b) using muscle interposition jump graft[26]
2. mobilizing the intratemporal portion of VII out of the fallopian canal (as previously described[27]) and then anastamosing it using bevelled cuts to a partially incised XII[28]

Outcome

Results are better if performed early, although good results can occur up to 18 mos after injury. In 22 cases, 64% had good results, 14% fair, 18% poor, and 1 patient had no evidence of reinnervation. In 59% of cases, evidence of reinnervation was seen by 3–6 mos; in the remaining patients with reinnervation improvement was noted by 8 mos.[29] Recovery of forehead movement occurs in only ≈ 30%. Return of tone precedes movement by ≈ 3 months.

Spinal accessory nerve-facial nerve (XI-VII) anastamosis

General information

First described in 1895 by Sir Charles Ballance.[30] Sacrifices some shoulder movement rather than use of tongue. Initial concerns about significant shoulder disability and pain resulted in the technique of using only the SCM branch of XI[31]; however these problems have not occurred in the majority of patients even with use of the major division.[32]

Technique

See reference.[32]

Skin incision: curves across the mastoid tip along the anterior margin of the SCM. Strip and remove the anterior third of the mastoid process (wax any exposed air cells), identify the facial nerve and divide it as close to its exit from the stylomastoid foramen as possible. Locate the XI nerve 3–4 cm below the mastoid tip, and divide it distal to the SCM division. Mobilize the free end and anastamose it to the distal stump of VII. Results in loss of trapezius function, which may not cause deficit even if done bilaterally. Alternatively, the SCM branch of XI may be used, sparing the trapezius function; however, the shorter length may be difficult to work with and in some individuals there may only be multiple small branches to the SCM.

34.4 Hearing loss

Two anatomic types: conductive and sensorineural.

34.4.1 Conductive hearing loss

1. patients tend to speak with normal or low volume voice
2. etiologies: anything that interferes with ossicular movement. Included:
   a) otitis media with middle ear effusion
   b) otosclerosis
3. clinical findings with unilateral hearing loss (see ▶ Table 34.3):
   a) *Weber test* will lateralize to side of hearing loss (Weber test: place a vibrating 256 or 512 Hz tuning fork on the center of the forehead; the sound will lateralize (i.e.sound louder) on the side of conductive hearing loss, or opposite to the side of SNHL)
      The "hum test" can provide the same information as the Weber test by having the patient hum, anddoes not require special equipment and can be done remotely (e.g., over the phone).[33]
   b) *Rinne test* will be abnormal (BC > AC) on the side of hearing loss, called a *negative* Rinne (Rinne test: place a vibrating 256 or 512 Hz tuning fork on the mastoid process; when sound is no longer heard, move the fork to just outside the ear to see if air conduction [AC] is > bone conduction [BC])
4. middle ear impedance measurements are abnormal

34

Table 34.3 Interpretation of Weber and Rinne test results

Weber	Rinne	Interpretation
nonlateralizing	AC > BC bilat	normal[a]
lateralizes to side A	normal bilaterally (AC > BC)	sensorineural hearing loss (SNHL) side B
lateralizes to side A	abnormal in side A (BC > AC)	conductive hearing loss side A
lateralizes to side A	abnormal in side B (BC > AC)	combined conductive + SNHL side B

[a]normal, or symmetric hearing loss

34.4.2 Sensorineural hearing loss (SNHL)

1. patients tend to speak with loud voice
2. clinical findings with unilateral hearing loss (▶ Table 34.3):
   a) *Weber test* will lateralize to side of better hearing (Weber test: place a vibrating 256 or 512 Hz tuning fork on the center of the forehead; the sound will lateralize—sound louder—on the side of conductive hearing loss, or opposite to the side of SNHL)
   b) *Rinne test* will be normal (AC > BC), called a *positive* Rinne (Rinne test: place a vibrating 256 or 512 Hz tuning fork on the mastoid process; when sound is no longer heard, move the fork to just outside the ear to see if air conduction [AC] is > bone conduction [BC])
3. further divided into sensory or neural. Distinguished by otoacoustic emissions (only produced by a cochlea with functioning hair cells) or BSAERs
   a) sensory: loss of outer hair cells in the cochlea. Etiologies: cochlear damage (usually causes high-frequency hearing loss) from noise exposure, ototoxic drugs (e.g., aminoglycosides), senile cochlear degeneration, viral labyrinthitis. Speech discrimination may be relatively preserved
   b) neural: due to compression of the 8th cranial nerve. Etiologies: CP angle tumor (e.g., vestibular schwannoma). Typically much greater loss of word discrimination out of proportion to pure tone audiogram abnormalities

Sensory hearing loss may be distinguished from neural hearing loss by
1. otoacoustic emissions which are only produced by a cochlea with functioning hair cells
2. or BSAERs
3. an elevated stapedial reflex threshold out of proportion to PTA abnormalities is also highly diagnostic of a retrocochlear (neural) lesion

References

[1] Brandt T, Daroff RB. The Multisensory Physiological and Pathological Vertigo Syndromes. Ann Neurol. 1980; 7:195–203

[2] Jannetta PJ, Moller MB, Moller AR. Disabling Positional Vertigo. N Engl J Med. 1984; 310:1700–1705

[3] Arriaga MA, Chen DA. Vestibular Nerve Section in the Treatment of Vertigo. Contemporary Neurosurgery. 1997; 19:1–6

[4] McElveen JT, House JW, Hitselberger WE, et al. Retrolabyrinthine Vestibular Nerve Section: A Viable Alternative to the Middle Fossa Approach. Otolaryngol Head Neck Surg. 1984; 92:136–140

[5] House JW, Hitelsberger WE, McElveen J, et al. Retrolabyrinthine Section of the Vestibular Nerve. Otolaryngol Head Neck Surg. 1984; 92:212–215

[6] Alexander TH, Harris JP. Current epidemiology of Meniere's syndrome. Otolaryngol Clin North Am. 2010; 43:965–970

[7] Glassock ME, Miller GW, Drake FD, et al. Surgical Management of Meniere's Disease with the Endolymphatic Subarachnoid Shunt. Laryngoscope. 1977; 87:1668–1675

[8] Shambaugh GE. Facial Nerve Decompression and Repair. In: Surgery of the Ear. Philadelphia: W. B. Saunders; 1959:543–571

[9] Adour KK. Diagnosis and Management of Facial Paralysis. N Engl J Med. 1982; 307:348–351

[10] Shambaugh GE, Clemis JD, Paparella MM, et al. Facial Nerve Paralysis. In: Otolaryngology. Philadelphia: W. B. Saunders; 1973

[11] Adour KK, Wingerd J, Doty HE. Prevalence of Concurrent Diabetes Mellitus and Idiopathic Facial Paralysis (Bell's Palsy). Diabetes. 1975; 24:449–451

[12] Treatment of Lyme Disease. Medical Letter. 1988; 30:65–66

[13] Abraham-Inpijn L, Devriese PP, Hart AAM. Predisposing Factors in Bell's Palsy: A Clinical Study with Reference to Diabetes Mellitus, Hypertension, Clotting Mechanism and Lipid Disturbance. Clin Otolaryngol. 1982; 7:99–105

[14] Devriese PP, Schumacher T, Scheide A, et al. Incidence, Prognosis and Recovery of Bell's Palsy: A Survey of About 1000 Patients (1974-1983). Clin Otolaryngol. 1990; 15:15–27

[15] Adour KK, Byl FM, Hilsinger RL, et al. The True Nature of Bell's Palsy: Analysis of 1000 Consecutive Patients. Laryngoscope. 1978; 88:787–801

[16] Adour KK, Bell DN, Hilsinger RL. Herpes simplex virus in idiopathic facial paralysis (Bell palsy). JAMA. 1975; 233:523–530

[17] Kuiper H, Devriese PP, de Jongh BM, et al. Absence of Lyme Borreliosis Among Patients With Presumed Bell's Palsy. Archives of Neurology. 1992; 49:940–943

[18] Sullivan FM, Swan IR, Donnan PT, et al. Early treatment with prednisolone or acyclovir in Bell's palsy. N Engl J Med. 2007; 357:1598–1607

[19] Conley J, Baker DC. Hypoglossal-Facial Nerve Anastomosis for Reinnervation of the Paralyzed Face. Plast Reconstr Surg. 1979; 63:63–72

[20] Pluchino F, Fornari M, Luccarelli G. Intracranial Repair of Interrupted Facial Nerve in Course of Operation for Acoustic Neuroma by Microsurgical Technique. Acta Neurochirurgica. 1986; 79:87–93

[21] Stephanian E, Sekhar LN, Janecka IP, et al. Facial Nerve Repair by Interposition Nerve Graft: Results in 22 Patients. Neurosurgery. 1992; 31:73–77

[22] King TT, Sparrow OC, Arias JM, et al. Repair of Facial Nerve After Removal of Cerebellopontine Angle Tumors: A Comparative Study. Journal of Neurosurgery. 1993; 78:720–725

[23] Alberti PWRM. The Greater Auricular Nerve. Donor for Facial Nerve Grafts: A Note on its Topographical Anatomy. Arch Otolaryngol. 1962; 76:422–424

[24] Strelzow VV, Friedman WH, Katsantonis GP. Reconstruction of the Paralyzed Face With the Polypropylene Mesh Template. Arch Otolaryngol. 1983; 109:140–144

[25] May M, Sobol SM, Mester SJ. Hypoglossal-Facial Nerve Interpositional-Jump Graft for Facial Reanimation without Tongue Atrophy. Otolaryngology - Head and Neck Surgery. 1991; 104:818–825

[26] Drew SJ, Fullarton AC, Glasby MA, et al. Reinnervation of Facial Nerve Territory Using a Composite Hypoglossal Nerve-Muscle Autograft-Facial Nerve Bridge. An Experimental Model in Sheep. Clin Otolaryngol. 1995; 20:109–117

[27] Hitselberger WE, House WF, Luetje CM. Hypoglossal-Facial Anastomosis. In: Acoustic Tumors:

Management. Baltimore: University Park Press; 1979:97–103

[28] Atlas MD, Lowinger DSG. A new technique for hypoglossal-facial nerve repair. Laryngoscope. 1997; 107:984–991

[29] Pitty LF, Tator CH. Hypoglossal-Facial Nerve Anastomosis for Facial Nerve Palsy Following Surgery for Cerebellopontine Angle Tumors. Journal of Neurosurgery. 1992; 77:724–731

[30] Duel AB. Advanced Methods in the Surgical Treatment of Facial Paralysis. Ann Otol Rhinol Laryngol. 1934; 43:76–88

[31] Poe DS, Scher N, Panje WR. Facial Reanimation by XI-VII Anastomosis Without Shoulder Paralysis. Laryngoscope. 1989; 99:1040–1047

[32] Ebersold MJ, Quast LM. Long-Term Results of Spinal Accessory Nerve-Facial Nerve Anastomosis. J Neurosurg. 1992; 77:51–54

[33] Ahmed OH, Gallant SC, Ruiz R, et al. Validity of the Hum Test, a Simple and Reliable Alternative to the Weber Test. Ann Otol Rhinol Laryngol. 2018; 127:402–405

34

Part XII

Tumors of the Nervous and Related Systems

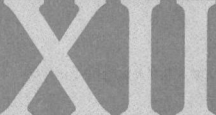

XII

35 Tumor Classification and General Information

35.1 WHO classification of tumors of the nervous system

The fifth edition of the WHO Classification of Tumors of the Central Nervous System (**WHO CNS5**)[1] published in 2021 is shown in ► Table 35.1 and incorporates recommendations of the cIMPACT-NOW (the Consortium to Inform Molecular and Practical Approaches to CNS Tumor Taxonomy–Not Official WHO).[2] Some noteworthy general features:

1. tumors are classified by types, some of which are divided into subtypes. Some subtypes are actual variations of the parent tumor, while others are just differing grades of the tumor
2. the suffixes NOS & NEC are used as follows[3]:
   - NOS (not otherwise specified): indicates that molecular testing was either not done or that the results were uncertain
   - NEC (not elsewhere classified): is used when there is nonconcordance between histologic features and molecular testing, or when results show noncanonical results e.g., as might occur with a new or emerging tumor type
3. molecular alterations are integral to the accurate diagnosis of CNS neoplasms. The most common diagnostic findings are listed in ► Table 35.7
4. in the following sections, descriptions such as histology and molecular biology do not cover the gamut of each tumor—for that the reader is referred to the definitive WHO Classification publication[1]—but excerpts are included to show where the tumors fit into the overall scheme and to highlight some features that might be of relevance or interest to the clinician treating patients with these conditions

35

Table 35.1 WHO classification of tumors of the central nervous system (5th edition)[1] (modified, used with permission from WHO Classification of Tumours Editorial Board. Central Nervous System Tumours. Lyon (France): International Agency for Research on Cancer; 2021. (WHO classification of tumours series, 5th ed.; vol. 6). Available from: https://tumourclassification.iarc.who.int/.)

Tumor[a]	WHO grade[b]	ICD-O[c]
Gliomas, glioneuronal tumors, and neuronal tumors (p. 657)		
Adult-type diffuse gliomas (p. 658)		
astrocytoma, IDH mutant (p. 658)		
• astrocytoma, IDH-mutant, grade 2	2	9400/3
• astrocytoma, IDH-mutant, grade 3	3	9401/3
• astrocytoma, IDH-mutant, grade 4	4	9405/3
oligodendroglioma, IDH-mutant & 1p/19q codeleted (p. 662)		
• oligodendroglioma, IDH-mutant & 1p/19q codeleted, grade 2	2	9450/3
• oligodendroglioma, IDH-mutant & 1p/19q codeleted, grade 3	3	9451/3
glioblastoma, IDH-wildtype (p. 664)	4	9400/3
• giant cell glioblastoma (p. 665)	4	
• gliosarcoma (p. 665)	4	
• epithelioid glioblastoma (p. 666)	4	
Pediatric-type diffuse low-grade gliomas (p. 679)		
diffuse astrocytoma, MYB- or MYBL1-altered (p. 679)	1	9421/1
angiocentric glioma (p. 679)	1	9431/1
polymorphous low-grade neuroepithelial tumor of the young (p. 680)	1	9413/0
diffuse low-grade glioma, MAPK pathway-altered (p. 682)	1	9421/1
Pediatric-type diffuse high-grade gliomas (p. 683)		
diffuse midline glioma, H3 K27-altered (p. 683)	4	9385/3
diffuse hemispheric glioma, H3 G34-mutant (p. 685)	4	
diffuse pediatric-type high-grade glioma, H3-wildtype & IDH-wildtype (p. 686)	4	
infant-type hemispheric glioma (p. 687)	N/A	

Table 35.1 continued

Tumor[a]	WHO grade[b]	ICD-O[c]
Circumscribed astrocytic gliomas (p. 689)		
pilocytic astrocytoma (p. 689)	1	9421/1
high-grade astrocytoma with piloid features (p. 698)	N/A	9421/3
pleomorphic xanthoastrocytoma (p. 698) (PXA)	2 or 3	9424/3
subependymal giant cell astrocytoma (p. 700) (SEGA)	1	
chordoid glioma (p. 702)	2	9444/1
astroblastoma, MN1-altered (p. 703)	1	9430/3
Glioneuronal and neuronal tumors		
ganglioglioma (p. 706)	1	9505/1
gangliocytoma (p. 707)	1	9492/0
desmoplastic infantile ganglioglioma (DIG)/ desmoplastic infantile astrocytoma (DIA) (p. 708)	1	9412/1
dysembryoplastic neuroepithelial tumor (p. 709) (DNT)	1	9413/0
diffuse glioneuronal tumor with oligodendroglioma-like features and nuclear clusters (p. 711) *(provisional entity)*	N/A	N/A
papillary glioneuronal tumor (p. 712) (PGNT)	1	9509/1
rosette-forming glioneuronal tumor (p. 713) (RGNT)	1	
myxoid glioneuronal tumor (p. 714)	1	
diffuse leptomeningeal glioneuronal tumor (p. 715) (DLGNT)	2 or 3	9509/3
multinodular and vacuolating neuronal tumor (p. 717) (MVNT)	1	9509/0
dysplastic cerebellar gangliocytoma (p. 716) (DCG) (Lhermitte-Duclos disease)	1	9493/0
central neurocytoma (p. 719)	2	9506/1
extraventricular neurocytoma (p. 720)	2	
cerebellar liponeurocytoma (p. 721)	2	
Ependymal tumors		
supratentorial ependymoma (p. 724)	2 or 3	9391/3
supratentorial ependymoma, ZFTA fusion-positive (p. 725)	2 or 3	9396/3
supratentorial ependymoma, YAP1 fusion-positive (p. 726)	N/A	
posterior fossa ependymoma (p. 727)	2 or 3	9391/3
posterior fossa group A (PFA) ependymoma (p. 730) (PFA)	2 or 3	9396/3
posterior fossa group B (PFB) ependymoma (p. 731) (PFB)	2 or 3	
spinal ependymoma (p. 732)	2 or 3	9391/3
spinal ependymoma, MYCN-amplified (p. 733)	N/A	9396/3
myxopapilary ependymoma (p. 734)	2	9394/1
subependymoma (p. 735)	1	9383/1
Choroid plexus tumors		
choroid plexus papilloma (p. 739) (CPP)	1	9390/0
atypical choroid plexus papilloma (p. 740)	2	9390/1
choroid plexus carcinoma (p. 741)	3	9390/3
Embryonal tumors (p. 744)		
Medulloblastomas, molecularly defined (p. 750)		
medulloblastoma, WNT-activated (p. 750)	4	9475/3
medulloblastoma, SHH-activated & *TP53-wildtype* (p. 751)	4	9471/3
medulloblastoma, SHH-activated & *TP53-mutant* (p. 752)	4	9476/3
medulloblastoma, non-WNT/non-SHH (p. 753)	4	9477/3
Medulloblastomas, histologically defined		
medulloblastoma, histologically defined (p. 748)		9470/3
• classic medulloblastoma (p. 749)	4	N/A

35

Table 35.1 continued

Tumor[a]	WHO grade[b]	ICD-O[c]
• medulloblastoma, desmoplastic/nodular (p. 749)	4	9471/3
• medulloblastoma, with extensive nodularity (p. 749) (MBEN)	4	
• large cell/anaplastic medulloblastoma (p. 749)	4	9474/3
Other CNS embryonal tumors		
atypical teratoid/rhabdoid tumor (p. 754) (AT/RT)	4	9508/3
cribriform neuroepithelial tumor (p. 755)	N/A	N/A
embryonal tumor with multilayered rosettes (p. 756) (ETMR)	4	9478/3
CNS neuroblastoma, FOXR2-activated	4	9500/3
CNS tumor with BCOR internal tandem duplication	N/A	
CNS embryonal tumor NEC/NOS	3 or 4	9473/3
Tumors of the pineal region (p. 758)		
Pineal tumors		
pineocytoma (p. 762)	1	9361/1
pineal parenchymal tumor of intermediate differentiation (p. 763) (PPTID)	2 or 3	9362/3
pineoblastoma (p. 764)	4	9362/3
papillary tumor of the pineal region (p. 765)	2 or 3	9395/3
Pineal region tumors of uncertain cell of origin		
desmoplastic myxoid tumor of the pineal region, SMARCB1-mutant	1	N/A
Pineal region tumors of non-pineal cell origin		
germ cell tumors (see Germ cell tumors section below)		
other non-pineal tumors (▶ Table 44.1). Includes: ependymomas, epidermoid or dermoid cysts, astrocytomas, paragangliomas...		
Cranial and paraspinal nerve tumors (p. 768)		
schwannoma (p. 768)		9560/0
• ancient schwannoma	1	
• cellular schwannoma	1	
• plexiform schwannoma	1	
• epitheliod schwannoma	1	
• microcystic/reticular schwannoma	1	
neurofibroma (p. 769)		9540/0
• cellular neurofibroma	1	
• atypical neurofibroma / atypical neurofibromatous neoplasm of uncertain biological potential (AN/ANNUBP)	N/A	
• plexiform neurofibroma	1	
• diffuse neurofibroma	1	
• nodular neurofibroma	1	
• plexiform neurofibroma	1	
• massive soft tissue neurofibroma	1	
perineurioma (p. 771)	1	9571/0
hybrid nerve sheath tumor (p. 772)		9563/0
malignant melanocytic nerve sheath tumor (p. 773)		9540/3
malignant peripheral nerve sheath tumor (MPNST) (p. 774)	2, 3 or 4	
cauda equina neuroendocrine tumor (p. 774)		8693/3
Meningiomas		
meningioma (p. 803)		9530/X
• meningothelial meningioma	1	9531/X
• fibrous meningioma	1	9532/X
• transitional meningioma	1	9537/X

35

Table 35.1 continued

Tumor[a]	WHO grade[b]	ICD-O[c]
• psammomatous meningioma	1	9533/X
• angiomatous meningioma	1	9534/X
• microcystic meningioma	1	9531/X
• secretory meningioma	1	9530/X
• lymphoplasmacyte-rich meningioma	1	9530/X
• metaplastic meningioma	1	9530/X
• chordoid meningioma	2	9538/2
• clear cell meningioma	2	9538/2
• rhabdoid meningioma	3	9538/X
• papillary meningioma	2 or 3	9538/X
• atypical meningioma	2	9539/X
• anaplastic (malignant) meningioma	3	9538/X
Mesenchymal, non-meningothelial tumors involving the CNS		
Soft tissue tumors		
Fibroblastic and myofibroblastic tumors		
solitary fibrous tumor (p. 820)	1 - 3	8815/X
Vascular tumors		
hemangioma (p. 821)	1	X
hemangioblastoma (p. 822)	1	9161/1
Skeletal muscle tumors		
rhabdomyosarcoma		8900/3
Tumors of uncertain differentiation		
intracranial mesenchymal tumor, FET::CREB fusion-positive		N/A
CIC-rearranged sarcoma		9367/3
primary intracranial sarcoma, DICER1-mutant		9480/3
Ewing sarcoma		9364/3
Chondro-osseous tumors		
Chondrogenic tumors		
mesenchymal chondrosarcoma		9240/3
chondrosarcoma		9920/3
Notochordal tumors		
chordoma (p. 825)		9370/3
Melanocytic tumors (p. 829)		
Diffuse meningeal melanocytic neoplasms		
meningeal melanocytosis (p. 829)		8728/0
meningeal melanomatosis (p. 829)		8728/3
Circumscribed meningeal melanocytic neoplasms		
meningeal melanocytoma (p. 830)		8728/1
meningeal melanoma (p. 830)		8720/3
Hematolymphoid tumors involving the CNS		
Lymphomas		
CNS lymphomas		
primary diffuse large B-cell lymphoma of the CNS (p. 840)		9680/3
immunodeficiency-associated CNS lymphomas (p. 845)		N/A
lymphomatoid granulomatosis		9766/1
• lymphomatoid granulomatosis, grade 1		9766/1
• lymphomatoid granulomatosis, grade 2		9766/1
• lymphomatoid granulomatosis, grade 3		9766/3

35

Table 35.1 continued

Tumor[a]	WHO grade[b]	ICD-O[c]
intravascular large B-cell lymphoma		9712/3
Miscellaneous rare lymphomas in the CNS		
MALT lymphoma of the dura		9699/3
other low-grade B-cell lymphomas of the CNS		
anaplastic large cell lymphoma (ALK+/ALK−)		9714/3
T-cell lymphomas		9702/3
NK/T-cell lymphomas		9719/3
Histiocytic tumors		
Erdheim-Chester disease		9749/3
Rosai-Dorfman disease		9749/3
juvenile xanthogranuloma		9749/1
Langerhans cell histiocytosis (p. 846)		9751/1
histiocytic sarcoma		9755/3
Germ cell tumors (p. 831)		
mature teratoma		9080/3
immature teratoma		9080/3
teratoma with somatic-type malignancy		9084/3
germinoma		9064/3
embryonal carcinoma		9070/3
yolk sac tumor		9071/3
choriocarcinoma		9100/3
mixed germ cell tumor		9085/3
Tumors of the sellar region (p. 849)[4]		
Tumors of non pituitary origin		
adamantinomatous craniopharyngioma (p. 849)		9351/1
papillary craniopharyngioma (p. 850)		9352/1
Tumors of the posterior pituitary gland & infundibulum		
pituicytoma (p. 853)		9432/1
granular cell tumor of the sellar region (p. 853)		9582/0
spindle cell oncocytoma/oncocytic pituicytoma (p. 854)		8290/0
ependymal pituicytoma		9391/1
Tumors of the anterior pituitary gland (p. 861) *(adenohypophyseal tumors)* *(Pituitary adenoma / pituitary neuroendocrine tumors (PitNET))*		
Pituitary neuroendocrine tumors of PIT1-lineage		
somatotroph PitNET/adenoma (p. 870) (GH & α-subunit secreting)		8272/3
lactotroph PitNET/adenoma (p. 867) (PRL secreting)		8271/3
mammosomatotroph PitNET/adenoma (p. 870) (GH > PRL & α-subunit secreting)		8272/3
thyrotroph PitNET/adenoma (p. 871) (TSH-β & α-subunit secreting)		8272/3
mature plurihormonal PIT1 lineage PitNET/adenoma (GH > PRL, α-subunit, TSH-β secreting)		8272/3
immature PIT1-lineage PitNET/adenoma (GH, PRL, α-subunit, TSH-β secreting)		8272/3
acidophil stem cell PitNET/adenoma (PRL > GH secreting)		8272/3
mixed somatotroph-lactotroph PitNET/adenoma (GH, PRL secreting)		8281/3
Pituitary neuroendocrine tumors of TPIT lineage		
corticotroph PitNET/adenoma (p. 867) (ACTH & other POMC secreting)		8272/3
Pituitary neuroendocrine tumors of SF1 lineage		
gonadotroph PitNET/adenoma (p. 870) (α-subunit, FSH-β, LH-β secreting)		8272/3

35

Table 35.1 continued

Tumor[a]	WHO grade[b]	ICD-O[c]
Pituitary neuroendocrine tumors without distinct lineage differentiation		
null cell PitNET (p. 861)/adenoma (non-secretory)		8272/3
Other sellar region tumors		
pituitary blastoma		8273/3
Metastasis to the CNS (p. 908)		
metastases to the brain parenchyma (p. 867)		
metastases to the spinal cord parenchyma		
metastases to the meninges		

[a]Tumor type based on the fifth edition of the WHO Classification of Tumors of the Central Nervous System (WHO CNS5)[1]
• bulleted tumors are subtypes (in some cases they arediffering grades of the parent tumo
[b]graded according to the 2013 WHO Classification of Tumors of Soft Tissues & Bone.
[c]ICD-O = morphology code of the International Classification of Diseases for Oncology (ICD-O), third edition, second revision (ICD-O-3.2) International Association of Cancer Registries (IACR) [Internet]. Lyon (France): International Agency for Research on Cancer; updated 2021 Jan 25. Available from (http://codes.iarc.fr).
The extension after the slash is the "behavior code": /0 = benign; /1 = unspecified, borderline, or uncertain behavior; /2 = carcinoma in situ and grade 3 intraepithelial neoplasia; /3 = malignant tumors, primary site; /6 = malignant tumors, metastatic site; X = designation and/or grade assigned by characteristics described in that section.
* indicates new codes for 2021 approved by the IARC/WHO Committee for ICD-O in May 2021.
N/A indicates that the WHO has "not assigned" a grade as of the 2021 publication.

35.2 Pediatric brain tumors

35.2.1 General information

Among all childhood cancers, brain tumors are the second only to leukemias in incidence (20%), and are the most common solid pediatric tumor,[5] comprising 40–50% of all tumors.[6] Annual incidence of CNS tumors by age is shown in ▶ Table 35.2.

Table 35.2 Incidence of CNS tumors by age in the U.S. (for the years 2014-2018)[7]

Age (years)	Incidence per 100,000
0-4	6.30
5-9	5.59
10-14	5.94
15-19	7.32

35

35.2.2 Types of tumors

The common pediatric brain tumors (age < 20 years) are gliomas and glioneural tumors (cerebellum, brainstem, and optic nerve) (which account for 45% of primary CNS tumors in this age group), embryonal tumors (12.3%) (67% of which are medulloblastoma), pituitary tumors (6.2%), nerve sheath tumors (4.2%), and craniopharyngiomas (3.8%).[7]

Among patients < 20 years of age, the incidence of the following tumors decrease with age: pilocytic astrocytoma, malignant glioma, ependymal tumors, choroid plexus tumors, and embryonal tumors.[7]

35.2.3 Infratentorial vs. supratentorial tumor location

It has traditionally been taught that most pediatric brain tumors (≈ 60%) are infratentorial, and that these are ≈ equally divided among brainstem gliomas, cerebellar astrocytomas, and medulloblastomas. In reality, the ratio of supratentorial to infratentorial tumors is dependent on the specific age group studied, as illustrated in ▶ Table 35.3.

▶ Table 35.4 shows the histological breakdown for infratentorial vs. supratentorial tumors. Astrocytomas are the most common supratentorial tumors in pediatrics as in adulthood.

Table 35.3 Percentage of infratentorial tumors by age

Age	% Infratentorial
0–6 mos	27%
6–12 mos	53%
12–24 mos	74%
2–16 yrs	42%

Table 35.4 Incidence of pediatric brain tumors[a]

Tumor type	% of total
infratentorial tumors	**54%**
cerebellar astrocytomas (p. 693)	15%
medulloblastomas (p. 750)	14%
brainstem gliomas (p. 695)	12%
ependymomas (p. 724) [8]	9%
supratentorial benign astrocytomas	**13%**

[a]data pooled from 1350 pediatric brain tumors[9 (p 368)]

35.2.4 Intracranial neoplasms during the first year of life

Brain tumors presenting during the first year of life are a different subset of tumors than those presenting later in childhood. In a busy neurosurgical unit in a children's hospital, they represented ≈ 8% of children admitted with brain tumors, an average of only ≈ 3 admissions per year.[10]

90% of brain tumors in *neonates* are of neuroectodermal origin, teratoma being the most common. Some of these tumors may be congenital.[11] Other supratentorial tumors include: astrocytoma, choroid plexus tumors, ependymomas, and craniopharyngiomas. Posterior fossa tumors include medulloblastoma and cerebellar astrocytoma.

Many of these tumors escape diagnosis until they are very large in size due to the elasticity of the infant skull, the adaptability of the developing nervous system to compensate for deficits, and the difficulty in examining a patient with limited neurologic repertoire and inability to verbalize or cooperate. The most common presenting manifestations are vomiting, arrest or regression of psychomotor development, macrocrania, poor feeding/failure to thrive. They may also present with seizures.

35.3 Brain tumors—general clinical aspects

35.3.1 Epidemiology

The average annual age-adjusted incidence rate (AAAIR) of all CNS tumors from 2014–2018 in the U.S. was 24.25 per 100,000[7] The AAAIR was 7.06 for malignant brain tumors, and 17.18 for non-malignant. Approximately 29% of all CNS tumors (including brain tumors) were malignant and 71% were non-malignant.

The 6 histological groups that have a younger median age of diagnosis than other types are: pilocytic astrocytoma (median age = 11 years), choroid plexus tumors (20 years), neuronal and mixed neuronal-glial tumors (26 years), pineal region tumors (32 years), embryonal tumors (8 years), and germ cell tumors (15 years).[7]

35.3.2 Presenting signs and symptoms

For details of presentation, see sections below for supratentorial and infratentorial tumors. Most brain tumors present with:
- progressive neurologic deficit (68%): usually motor weakness (45%). This is in distinction to the more rapid presentation e.g., of stroke or seizure
- headache: a presenting symptom in 54% (see below)
- seizures in 26%. Often focal in onset (due to cortical irritation in the area of the tumor), may generalize secondarily. Uncommon with p-fossa tumors

35

35.3.3 Focal neurologic deficits associated with brain tumors

In addition to nonfocal signs and symptoms (e.g., seizures, increased ICP...), as with any destructive brain lesion, tumors may produce progressive deficits related to the function of the involved brain. Some characteristic "syndromes":

1. frontal lobe: abulia, dementia, personality changes. Often nonlateralizing, but apraxia, hemiparesis or dysphasia (with dominant hemisphere involvement) may occur
2. temporal lobe: auditory or olfactory hallucinations, déja vu, memory impairment. Contralateral superior quadrantanopsia may be detected on visual field testing
3. parietal lobe: contralateral motor or sensory impairment, homonymous hemianopsia. Agnosias (with dominant hemisphere involvement) and apraxias may occur; see Clinical syndromes of parietal lobe disease (p.99)
4. occipital lobe: contralateral visual field deficits, alexia (especially with corpus callosum involvement with infiltrating tumors)
5. posterior fossa: (see above) cranial nerve deficits, ataxia (truncal or appendicular). Seizures generally do not occur with isolated posterior fossa lesions

35.3.4 Headaches with brain tumors

General information

Headache (H/A) may occur with or without elevated ICP. H/A are present equally in patients with primary or metastatic tumor (≈ 50% of patients[12]). Classically described as being worse in the morning (possibly due to hypoventilation during sleep)—this may actually be uncommon.[12] Often exacerbated by coughing, straining, or (in 30%) bending forward (placing head in dependent position). Associated with nausea and vomiting in 40%, may be temporarily relieved by vomiting (possibly due to hyperventilation during vomiting). These features along with the presence of a focal neurologic deficit or seizure were thought to differentiate tumor H/A from others. However, H/A in 77% of brain tumor patients were similar to tension H/A, and in 9% were migraine-like.[12] Only 8% showed the "classic" brain tumor H/A, two–thirds of these patients had increased ICP.

Etiologies of tumor headache

The brain itself is not pain sensitive. H/A in the presence of a brain tumor may be due to any combination of the following:

1. increased intracranial pressure (ICP): which may be due to
   a) tumor mass effect
   b) hydrocephalus (obstructive or communicating)
   c) mass effect from associated edema
   d) mass effect from associated hemorrhage
2. invasion or compression of pain sensitive structures:
   a) dura
   b) blood vessels
   c) periosteum
   d) cranial nerves with sensory function
3. difficulty with vision can cause headache
   a) diplopia due to dysfunction of nerves controlling extra-ocular muscles
      • direct compression of III, IV, or VI
      • abducens palsy from increased ICP, see diplopia (p.624)
      • internuclear ophthalmoplegia due to brainstem invasion/compression
   b) difficulty focusing: due to optic nerve dysfunction from invasion/compression
4. extreme hypertension resulting from increased ICP (part of Cushing's triad)
5. psychogenic: due to stress from loss of functional capacity (e.g., deteriorating job performance)

35.3.5 Supratentorial tumors

Signs and symptoms include[13]:

1. those due to increased ICP (see "increased ICP" under posterior fossa tumors below):
   a) from mass effect of tumor and/or edema
   b) from blockage of CSF drainage (hydrocephalus): less common in supratentorial tumors (classically occurs with colloid cyst, may also occur with entrapped lateral ventricle)

35

2. progressive focal deficits: includes weakness, dysphasia (which occurs in 37–58% of patients with left-sided brain tumors[14]): see below
   a) due to destruction of brain parenchyma by tumor invasion
   b) due to compression of brain parenchyma by mass and/or peritumoral edema and/or hemorrhage
   c) due to compression of cranial nerve(s)
3. headache: see above
4. seizures: not infrequently the first symptom of a brain tumor. Tumor should be aggressively sought in an idiopathic first time seizure in a patient > 20 years (if negative, the patient should be followed with repeat studies at later dates). Rare with posterior fossa tumors or pituitary tumors
5. mental status changes: depression, lethargy, apathy, confusion
6. symptoms suggestive of a TIA (dubbed "tumor TIA") or stroke, may be due to:
   a) occlusion of a vessel by tumor cells
   b) hemorrhage into the tumor: any tumor may hemorrhage, see Hemorrhagic brain tumors (p.1612)
   c) focal seizure
7. in the special case of pituitary tumors (p.861):
   a) symptoms due to endocrine disturbances
   b) pituitary apoplexy (p.865)
   c) CSF leak

Booking the case: Craniotomy for supratentorial tumor

Also see defaults & disclaimers (p.25). If awake craniotomy is required, see Booking the case: Awake craniotomy (p.1732).
1. position: (depends on location of tumor)
2. pre-op embolization (by neuroendovascular interventionalist) for some vascular tumors including some meningiomas
3. equipment:
   a) microscope
   b) ultrasonic aspirator
   c) image guidance system
4. blood availability: type and cross 2 U PRBC
5. post-op: ICU
6. consent (in lay terms for the patient—not all-inclusive):
   a) procedure: surgery through the skull to remove as much of the tumor as is safely possible
   b) alternatives: nonsurgical management, radiation therapy for some tumors
   c) complications: usual craniotomy complications (p.25) plus inability to remove all of the tumor

35

35.3.6 Infratentorial tumors

Signs and symptoms

Seizures are rare (unlike the situation with supratentorial tumors) since seizures arise from irritation of cerebral cortex.
1. increased intracranial pressure (ICP): most posterior fossa tumors present with signs and symptoms of increased ICP due to hydrocephalus (HCP). These include:
   a) headache: (see above)
   b) nausea/vomiting: due either to increased ICP from HCP, or from direct pressure on the vagal nucleus or the area postrema (so-called "vomiting center")
   c) papilledema: estimated incidence is ≈ 50–90% (more common when the tumor impairs CSF circulation). Chronic increased pressure can cause irreversible blindness from optic nerve atrophy
   d) gait disturbance/ataxia
   e) vertigo
   f) diplopia: may be due to VI nerve (abducens) palsy, which may occur with increased ICP in the absence of direct compression of the nerve

2. S/S indicative of mass effect in various locations within the p-fossa
   a) lesions in cerebellar *hemisphere* may cause: ataxia of the extremities, dysmetria, intention tremor
   b) lesions of cerebellar *vermis* may cause: broad based gait, truncal ataxia, titubation
   c) brainstem involvement usually results in multiple cranial nerve and long tract abnormalities, and should be suspected when nystagmus is present (especially rotatory or vertical)

Evaluation of the patient with a posterior fossa (infratentorial) tumor

See Posterior fossa lesions (p.1089) for differential diagnosis (includes non-neoplastic lesions as well.)

In pediatric patients with a posterior fossa tumor, an MRI of the lumbar spine should be done pre-op to rule out drop mets (post-op there may be artifact from blood).

In adults, most intraparenchymal p-fossa tumors will be metastatic, and work-up for a primary should be undertaken in most cases.

Treatment of associated hydrocephalus

In cases with hydrocephalus at the time of presentation, some authors advocate initial placement of VP shunt or EVD prior to definitive surgery (waiting ≈ 2 wks before surgery) because of possibly lower operative mortality.[15] Theoretical risks of using this approach include the following:
1. placing a shunt is generally a lifelong commitment, whereas not all patients with hydrocephalus from a p-fossa tumor will require a shunt
2. possible seeding of the peritoneum with malignant tumor cells e.g., with medulloblastoma. Consider placement of tumor filter (may not be justified given the high rate of filter occlusion and the low rate of "shunt metastases"[16])
3. some shunts may become infected prior to the definitive surgery
4. definitive treatment is delayed, and the total number of hospital days may be increased
5. upward transtentorial herniation (p.325) may occur if there is excessively rapid CSF drainage

Either approach (shunting followed by elective p-fossa surgery, or semi-emergent definitive p-fossa surgery) is accepted. At Children's Hospital of Philadelphia, dexamethasone is started and the surgery is performed on the next elective operating day, unless neurologic deterioration occurs, necessitating emergency surgery.[17]

Some surgeons place a ventriculostomy at the time of surgery. CSF is drained only after the dura is opened (to avoid upwards herniation) to help equilibrate the pressures between the infra- and supratentorial compartments. Post-op, the external ventricular drain (EVD) is usually set at a low height (≈ 10 cm above the EAM) for 24 hours, and is progressively raised over the next 48 hrs and should be D/C'd by ≈ 72 hrs post-op.

Booking the case: Craniotomy for infratentorial tumor   35

Also see defaults & disclaimers (p.25) and retromastoid surgery for vestibular schwannomas (p.793).
1. position: (typically either prone or park bench, depending on tumor type/location and surgeon preference)
2. pre-op embolization (by neuroendovascular interventionalist) for some vascular tumors such as hemangioblastoma
3. equipment:
   a) microscope
   b) ultrasonic aspirator
   c) image guidance system (optional)
4. blood availability: type and cross 2 U PRBC
5. post-op: ICU
6. consent (in lay terms for the patient—not all-inclusive):
   a) procedure: surgery through the skull, remove as much of the tumor as is safely possible
   b) alternatives: nonsurgical management, radiation therapy for some tumors
   c) complications: usual craniotomy complications (p.25) plus inability to remove all of the tumor, hydrocephalus, CSF leak

35.4 Management of the patient with a brain tumor

35.4.1 Initial evaluation and management

Approach to the patient with a newly demonstrated or suspected brain tumor

1. imaging:
   a) obtain an MRI of the brain without and with contrast. A CT without and with contrast is an alternative if the MRI is not available or is contraindicated. In the current era, ensure that a navigation compatible sequence is included for possible surgery
   b) if the lesion is likely a pituitary tumor, a brain MRI with pituitary protocol without and with contrast should be obtained
   c) a metastatic workup (p.914) is obtained if there is a possibility that the lesion could represent a metastasis. Indications for this include multiple brain lesions, a solitary round ring-enhancing lesion at the interface between the gray and white matter or in the posterior fossa of an adult, suspicion based on history (patient with known cancer, or symptoms suggestive of cancer such as unexplained weight loss…). If the suspicion of metastases is low, or if the craniotomy needs to be done urgently, the metastatic workup can be deferred until after the craniotomy and then undertaken if the pathology from the surgery is consistent with metastases
   d) obtain imaging of the entire neuraxis (cervical, thoracic and lumbar spinal MRI without and with contrast in addition to the brain) to rule out drop mets for pediatric patients with a posterior fossa tumor or if the tumor is suspicious for tumors that tend to seed in the CSF (e.g., ependymoma…)
   e) specialized imaging studies, such as diffusion tensor imaging (DTI) MRI, functional MRI, cerebral angiography… are usually obtained subsequently, based on a number of factors obtained during this initial evaluation phase
   f) cerebellopontine angle (CPA) tumors: FIESTA MRI and audiology screening should be obtained
   g) if cerebral abscess is suspected, an infectious workup should be performed
2. medication
   a) steroids: for lesions with significant or symptomatic edema or mass effect. If not acutely indicated, defer steroids until after biopsy in case the tumor could be a lymphoma (steroids can transiently suppress lymphoma). Typically decadron (see steroid use in brain tumors (p.626))
   b) antiseizure medications (ASMs): if patient is not on ASMs and has not had a seizure, prophylactic ASMs should not be administered before sugery (see prophylactic antiseizure medications with brain tumors (p.626))
3. labs (in addition to routine labs):
   a) for tumors that may involve the pituitary, obtain pituitary screening labs (p.874)
   b) for pineal region tumors: markers are of limited usefulness (p.758). If still desired, one can obtain serum markers for β-hCG & alpha-fetoprotein (AFP), and/or CSF markers (p.832) (usually via LP when not contraindicated by mass effect or hydrocephalus) for β-hCG, AFP, PLAP

Steroid use in brain tumors

The beneficial effect of steroids in metastatic tumors is often much more dramatic than with primary infiltrating gliomas.

Dexamethasone (Decadron®) dose for brain tumors:
* for patients not previously on steroids:
   ○ adult: 10 mg IVP loading, then 6 mg PO/IVP q 6 hrs.[18,19] In cases with severe vasogenic edema, doses up to 10 mg q 4 hrs may be used for a short time (< 48-72 hours)
   ○ peds: 0.5–1 mg/kg IVP loading, then 0.25–0.5 mg/kg/d PO/IVP divided q 6 hrs. NB: avoid prolonged treatment because of growth suppressant effect in children
* for patients already on steroids:
   ○ for acute deterioration, a dose of approximately double the usual dose should be tried
   ○ see also "stress doses" (p.155)
* patients on steroids should receive prophylaxis against Cushing ulcers (see stress ulcers in neurosurgery (p.134))

Prophylactic antiseizure medications with brain tumors

20–40% of patients with a brain tumor will have had a seizure by the time their tumor is diagnosed.[20] Antiseizure medications (ASMs) are indicated in these patients who have had a seizure.

20–45% more will ultimately develop a seizure.[20] Prophylactic ASMs do not provide substantial benefit (reduction of risk > 25% for seizure-free survival), and there are significant risks involved. Practice guidelines for ASM use with brain tumors are shown below. Prophylactic ASMs are not indicated for isolated posterior fossa tumors due to the fact that p-fossa tumors by themselves have a low risk of provoking seizures.

Practice guideline: Prophylactic antiseizure medications with brain tumors

Level I[20]: prophylactic ASMs should not be used routinely in patients with newly diagnosed brain tumors

Level II[20]: in patients with brain tumors undergoing craniotomy, prophylactic ASMs may be used, and if there has been no seizure, it is appropriate to taper off ASMs starting 1 week post-op

35.4.2 Surgical intervention

Almost all tumors require surgical intervention. Exceptions include situations with an extremely high confidence diagnosis of a slow growing benign lesion based on imaging (e.g., many meningiomas, asymptomatic central neurocytomas…) in which case surveillance mode with serial imaging and monitoring of symptoms is employed (see below).

Goals of surgery are usually cytoreduction (maximal safe resection) with the goal of gross total excision when feasible, but at a minimum for a biopsy for diagnostic, prognostic, and treatment planning purposes.

35.4.3 Surveillance mode

For appropriate tumors with low suspicion of malignancy (e.g., many asymptomatic meningiomas, asymptomatic hormonally inactive pituitary tumors…). Use with caution with suspected low-grade glioma as some of these may be high-grade glioma or encephalitis.[21]
1. an initial follow-up imaging study is usually performed ≈ 3 months after the initial study (so-called "stability scan") to rule-out rapid growth
2. if stability is demonstrated, studies are performed annually thereafter unless a change in symptoms prompts an earlier repeat study

35.5 Chemotherapy agents for brain tumors

35.5.1 General information

General information is presented here. Chemotherapy for some specific tumors is also included in the respective sections devoted to those tumors where appropriate. Some agents used for CNS tumors: see ▶ Table 35.5.[22,23]

35.5.2 Alkylating agents

Temozolomide (Temodar®), an oral alkylating agent, is a derivative of Dacarbazine (DTIC®). It is a prodrug which undergoes rapid non-enzymatic conversion at physiologic pH to the active metabolite monomethyl triazenoimidazole carboxamide (MTIC). The mutagenic/cytotoxic effect of MTIC is associated with alkylation (adding an alkyl group, the smallest of which is a methyl group) to DNA at various sites primarily at the O6 and N7 positions on guanine. Cells can repair this damage via O[6]-methylguanine-DNA methyltransferase (p.673) (MGMT), a protein which may be deficient to some degree in various tumors (especially astrocytomas, IDH-mutant (p.658)) which renders them more susceptible to temozolomide.

35.5.3 Nitrosoureas

Excellent BBB penetration (see below). Significant hematopoietic, pulmonary, and renal toxicity.

35

Table 35.5 Some chemotherapeutic agents used for CNS tumors

Agent	Mechanism
nitrosoureas: BCNU (carmustine), CCNU (lomustine), ACNU (nimustine)	DNA crosslinks, carbamoylation of amino groups
alkylating (methylating) agents: procarbazine, temozolomide (Temodar®) (p. 627)	DNA alkylation, interferes with protein synthesis
carboplatin, cisplatin	chelation via intrastrand crosslinks
nitrogen mustards: cyclophosphamide, isofamide, cytoxan	DNA alkylation, carbonium ion formation
vinca alkaloids: vincristine, vinblastine, paclitaxel	microtubule function inhibitors
epidophyllotoxins (ETOP-oside, VP16, teniposide, VM26)	topoisomerase II inhibitors
topotecan, irinotecan (CPT-11)	topoisomerase I inhibitors
tamoxifen	protein kinase C inhibitor at high doses
bevacizumab (Avastin®)	anti-VEGF antibody may be useful in vestibular neuromas or recurrent GBM

hydroxyurea
bleomycin
taxol (paxlitaxol)
methotrexate
cytosine, arabinoside
corticosteroids: dexamethasone, prednisone
fluorouracil (FU)

35.5.4 Combination chemotherapy

PCV: procarbazine, CCNU (lomustine), and vincristine combination therapy is used as either an adjunct (following XRT) or concomitant (simultaneously with XRT) therapy in a number of tumors. Sometimes carmustine (BCNU) is substituted for lomustine.

35.5.5 Blood-brain barrier (BBB) and chemotherapy agents

Traditionally, the BBB has been considered to be a major hindrance to the use of chemotherapy for brain tumors. In theory, the BBB effectively excludes many chemotherapeutic agents from the CNS, thereby creating a "safe haven" for some tumors, e.g., metastases. This concept has been challenged.[24] Regardless of the etiology, the response of most brain tumors to systemic chemotherapy is usually very modest, with a notable exception being a favorable response of tumors with deficient MGMT (p. 673) activity. Considerations regarding chemotherapeutic agents in relation to the BBB include:

1. some CNS tumors may partially disrupt the BBB, especially malignant gliomas[25]
2. lipophilic agents (e.g., nitrosoureas) may cross the BBB more readily
3. selective intra-arterial (e.g., intracarotid or intervertebral) injection[26]: produces higher local concentration of agents which increases penetration of the BBB, with lower associated systemic toxicities than would otherwise occur
4. the BBB may be iatrogenically disrupted (e.g., with mannitol) prior to administration of the agent
5. the BBB may be bypassed by intrathecal administration of agents via LP or ventricular access device, e.g., methotrexate for CNS lymphoma (p. 844)
6. biodegradable polymer wafers containing a chemotherapeutic agent may be directly implanted. At present, the only such prepartion is Gliadel wafers (p. 673) (BCNU and prolifeprosan)

35.5.6 Imaging studies following surgical removal of tumor

At many academic centers, it is common to get a noncontrast CT scan within 6–12 hours of surgery to assess for acute complications (primarily hematoma—intraparenchymal, epidural or subdural, amount of pneumocephalus, hydrocephalus...).

Then to assess the extent of tumor removal, a post-op brain MRI (or CT if MRI cannot be done) without and with contrast should either be obtained within 2–3 days,[27] or should be delayed at least ≈ 30 days. The *non*-contrast scan is important to help differentiate blood from enhancement. The contrast images demonstrates areas of enhancement, which may represent residual tumor.

As a result of inflammatory changes due to surgery, enhancement increases in the wall of the resection bed within 24–48 hrs of surgery (so-called "post-operative changes"). ∴ After ≈ 48 hours, one cannot reliably differentiate contrast enhancement due to postoperative changes from residual. This usually subsides by ≈ 30 days,[28] but may persist for 6–8 weeks.[29] The effect of steroids on contrast enhancement is controversial,[30,31] and may depend on many factors (including tumor type).

35.6 Intraoperative pathology consultations ("frozen section")

35.6.1 Accuracy of intraoperative pathology consultations

Accuracy of intraoperative pathologic diagnosis (IPD) can be increased by:
- providing the pathologist with information regarding: patient demographics, clinical history, imaging results, relevant previous pathologic diagnoses, and clinical impression
- larger specimen sizes when possible
- avoiding artifact created by excessive crushing or coagulation

Intraoperative pathology diagnoses (IPD) should be considered preliminary. The final diagnosis differs from the IPD in approximately 3–10% of cases.[32,33,34] If the IPD does not correlate with the clinical impression, direct discussion with the pathologist may be advisable.

35.6.2 Techniques for intraoperative tissue preparation

▶ **Touch preparation.** The specimen is gently "touched" with a glass slide which is then rapidly fixed, stained and dehydrated for examination. This technique is particularly useful for tumors with discohesive cells (e.g., lymphoma, PitNET/adenoma).

▶ **Smear or squash preparation.** A small portion of specimen is smeared or compressed with moderate pressure between two glass slides, rapidly fixed, stained, and dehydrated for examination. This technique can be particularly useful for: multiple sclerosis (identifying histiocytes), visualizing long cell processes in gliomas, and identifying cytoplasmic inclusions or intranuclear pseudoinclusions).[35 (p 5–6)] The cohesive nature often seen in tumors such as metastases and meningiomas is apparent, as are areas of necrosis.

Σ: Smears are good for cytology, but do not show architecture. Preserve more tissue for permanent pathology than frozen section.

▶ **Frozen section.** A portion of tissue is rapidly frozen in liquid nitrogen and cut into 4–6 micron sections, mounted on a slide, rapidly fixed, stained, and dehydrated for examination. Unlike touch and smear preparations, this allows more accurate assessment of lesion architecture, cellularity, and interface with adjacent brain tissue. Disadvantages include use of greater tissue with less available for permanent histology (important with small biopsies), as well as artifacts such as freezing ice crystal artifact (which, when present, suggests lesional tissue has been biopsied but limits interpretation of cellularity).[35 (p 6)] When possible, some tissue should be preserved for processing without freezing to avoid artifacts.

Σ: Frozen section is better for tumor achitecture, but creates artifact and uses more tissue.

At the time of frozen section interpretation, consideration for additional studies such as tissue cultures or flow cytometry should be entertained. With minute specimens, a discussion is warranted whether frozen section is required to preserve tissue for permanent studies.

35.6.3 Selected frozen section pitfalls or potential critical diagnoses

- **differentiating low grade gliomas** from **normal or reactive brain** tissue can be challenging.[32,33] Increased cellularity (best evaluated at low power), nuclear atypia when present, and increased perineuronal satellitosis can be helpful, though not always readily observed.[35 (p 72–3,174–7)]
  Pearl: Secondary structures of Scherer may be useful in identifying gliomas in challenging cases, and include increased perineuronal and perivascular satellitosis (limited perineuronal satellitosis is normal) and accumulation of neoplastic cells in the subpial molecular layer with subpial tumor spread[36]
- **metastasis vs. glioma:** usually not problematic on frozen section, except occasionally with markedly atypical gliomas with limited sampling.[32,33,34] In such rare cases immunohistochemistry is helpful

35

- **astrocytoma vs. oligodendroglioma**: usually not a critical distinction at the time of frozen section diagnosis. However, in part due to frozen section artifact imparted to the nuclei, oligodendrogliomas can be interpreted as astrocytomas on frozen section.[32] Smear preparations can at times be helpful due to decreased "freezing" artifact. Also, perineuronal satellitosis may in some cases be more pronounced in oligodendrogliomas. In WHO CNS5, the distinction is dependent on molecular genetics.
  Pearl: The "fried egg" appearance in oligodendrogliomas is an artifact of formalin fixation for permanent sections and is NOT present on frozen sections, also hindering intraoperative interpretation
- **glioma grading**: sampling bias, particularly in small biopsy specimens, can lead to undergrading (i.e., underrepresentation of mitotic figures, vascular proliferation or necrosis in the biopsy specimen). Conversely, overgrading of gliomas at the time of intraoperative consultation can occur, including with low-grade childhood gliomas such as pilocytic astrocytomas[32]
- **radionecrosis vs. recurrent tumor (higher grade astroctymoa or glioblastoma)**: despite the fact that a history of prior radiation therapy is usually known at the time of intraoperative consultation, differentiation of the two entities can at times be difficult.[32] Both lesions are often present simultaneously. Identifying obvious tumor cells and palisading necrosis suggests recurrent/residual glioblastoma. Radiation necrosis, which affects primarily white matter, is supported by large geographic areas of necrosis, sclerosis/hyalinization of vessels or fibrinoid necrosis of vessel walls, perivascular lymphocytes, calcifications, and the presence of macrophages
- **ischemic infarct**: may see ischemic red neuron change (if the biopsy includes gray matter), as well as histiocytes (similar to demyelinating lesions). Necrosis may mimic the center of ring enhancing lesions (such as glioblastoma or metastasis), though tumor necrosis will typically involve vessels and lack a macrophage response[35 (p 663-6)]
- **demyelinating lesions** (e.g., tumefactive MS): primarily affects white matter with discrete borders. Identifying histiocytes at the time of frozen section is critical for the diagnosis. The histiocytes can mimic astrocytes of gliomas on frozen section preparation; smear preparations are particularly helpful in the distinction
- **small cell carcinoma & lymphoma** (PCNSL): accurate frozen section diagnosis may be critical as both conditions typically require only biopsy without debulking unless there is significant mass effect (definitive treatment is chemo-radiation). The two entities may resemble each other on frozen section as well as resembling astrocytomas, oligodendrogliomas, and other types of metastatic carcinomas.[32,33,34,35 (p 395-7)] Touch preparations can be particularly useful in identifying PCNSL
- **meningioma vs. tumors with spindle cells** (e.g., schwannoma): distinguishing between these two can be difficult at times on intraoperative consultation.[32] Classic features of meningiomas (whorls, psammoma bodies, intranuclear pseudoinclusions) may be absent, and freeze artifact can create areas that resemble Antoni B fibers.[32] In addition, underdiagnosis of malignant meningiomas and sarcomas at the time of frozen section has been noted[32,33]
- **spinal cord astrocytoma vs. ependymoma**: On occasion these entities can be difficult to distinguish during intraoperative consultation, especially as most spinal cord biopsies for frozen interpretation are minute. Due to the critical surgical implications of the accuracy of the frozen section diagnosis for intramedullary spinal gliomas, a careful discussion should be had between the surgeon and pathologist at the time of intraoperative consultation (refer to section on tumors of the spine and spinal cord)

35.6.4 Tissue preparation for permanent sections

Tissue is processed overnight through a variety of alcohol/xylene steps to remove water. This allows for embedding into paraffin so that thin sections can be cut for slide mounting. The specimens are then rehydrated by essentially reversing the alcohol/xylene steps in preparation for staining, and then dehydrated again for permanent slide coverslipping. This produces better histology with fewer artifacts, allows for processing of larger specimen volumes for evaluation, and allows for application of special stains as needed.

▶ **Fresh specimens.** Tissue should be sent "fresh" (i.e., without preservatives such as formalin) when the following techniques are needed:
- electron microscopy
- flow cytometry: e.g., when lymphoma is suspected
- muscle
- cultures (typically: aerobic, anaerobic, acid-fast, and fungal) should be sent in situations where infection is a consideration

35.7 Select commonly utilized stains in neuropathology

35.7.1 Organism and special stains

1. organism stains:
   - tissue Gram stains (Brown & Brenn, Brown & Hopps)
   - fungi: Periodic acid–Schiff (PAS), Gomori methenamine silver (GMS)
   - acid-fast bacilli (tuberculosis is the most common): Ziehl-Neelsen, Kinyoun, FITE
2. special stains:
   - luxol fast blue: stains myelin. Absence of staining highlights demyelinating lesions. Presence within histiocytes demonstrates ingestion of myelin as seen in MS
   - trichrome and reticulin stain: both delineate the sarcomatous component of gliosarcomas. A reticulin stain demonstrates the connective tissue around acini of the normal pituitary gland, a feature that is lost with PitNET/adenomas

35.7.2 Immunohistochemical stains

General information

Staining patterns: An individual tumor may lack a marker that is typically representative of its type. ★ Therefore, a positive stain is typically more significant than a negative stain.[37] General staining patterns[37] are shown in ▶ Table 35.6.

Table 35.6 Immunohistochemical staining patterns for nervous system tumor masses of epithelioid cells[a]

Neoplasm	Immunohistochemical stain response[b,c]					
	GFAP	CAM5.2	EMA	S-100	CgA	Syn
oligodendroglioma	+		−			0
ependymoma	0	−		−	−	−
choroid plexus papilloma			0	+	0	+
chordoma						
craniopharyngioma		+				
carcinoma			+	−	0	0
PitNET	−					
paraganglioma			−	0	+	+
meningioma		0	+			
melanoma			−	+	−	−
hemangioblastoma	0	−	−	0	0	0

[a]modified from McKeever PE. Immunohistochemistry of the Nervous System. In: Dobbs DJ, ed. Diagnostic Immunohistochemistry. Churchill Livingstone, NY, © 2002
[b]abbreviations: GFAP = glial fibrillary acidic protein, EMA = epithelial membrane antigen, CAM5.2 = cytokeratin CAM5.2, CgA = chromogranin A, syn = synaptophysin
[c]a "+" or a "−" sign indicates presence or absence of the stain respectively; "0" entries indicate that the stain is not decisive for that particular tumor

Glial fibrillary acidic protein (GFAP)

Polypeptide, MW = 49,000 Daltons. Stains intermediate filaments classically identified in astrocytes/astrocytic tumors. However, it is also typically expressed in ependymomas, oligodendrogliomas (especially in minigemistocytes and gliofibrillary oligodendrocytes), and some choroid plexus papillomas.[38 (p 30–1),39 (p 56,76,83)] GFAP is only rarely found outside the CNS in such tissues as Schwann cells, epithelium of the lens, certain liver cells, chondrocytes, etc). ★ It would be unusual for a metastatic lesion to demonstrate staining for GFAP. However, GFAP expression may be limited in certain subsets of GBM (e.g., small cell GBM).[39 (p 37)]

S-100 protein

A low molecular weight (21,000 Daltons) calcium-binding protein that stains a variety of tissues including glia, neurons, chondrocytes, stellate cells of the adenohypophysis, myoepithelial cells, etc.[37 (p 75)] Stains a variety of CNS neoplasms such as gliomas (though less specific than GFAP),

35

ependymomas, chordomas, and craniopharyngiomas.[37,39] Primary uses in neuropathology include to support the diagnosis of metastatic melanoma, and, in the peripheral nervous system, to confirm the diagnosis of schwannoma or neurofibroma (less intense staining in the latter).[39(p 156)]

Clinically has been measured in serum (see below).

Cytokeratins (high and low molecular weight)

A variety of stains (low [e.g., CAM 5.2] and high molecular weight keratin, CK7, CK20, etc.) which stain epithelial cells. Useful to distinguish metastatic carcinoma (positive staining) from primary CNS tumors (note: cytokeratins can be expressed in choroid plexus papillomas, and GBM can express cytokeratins in rare cases).[39(p 39–40)] Different keratin staining combinations can be used to suggest possible sites of origin for metastatic tumors.

Epithelial membrane antigen (EMA)

Stains cell membranes in many carcinomas; useful to distinguish hemangioblastoma (negative) from metastatic renal cell carcinoma (positive). Also, meningiomas typically demonstrate positive staining, as do ependymomas.[39(p 169)]

MIB-1 (AKA monoclonal mouse anti-human Ki-67 antibody)

The Ki-67 antigen is expressed in all phases of the cell cycle except G0. Available since the early 1990s, it is a valuable marker of cell proliferation but can only be used with fresh-frozen specimens. MIB-1 is a monoclonal antibody developed using recombinant parts of the Ki-67 protein as an immunogen, and can be used on paraffin-embedded sections of fixed tissue. Cells leaving the G0/G1-phase and entering the S-phase (performing DNA synthesis) stain positive with MIB-1 immunohistochemical stain. This stain can be used to compute a semi-quantitative score. A high MIB-1 labeling index denotes high mitotic activity, which often correlates with degree of malignancy. Often used in lymphomas, endocrine tumors, carcinoids, etc. See also use in astrocytomas (p. 660) and in meningiomas (p. 805).

Neuroendocrine stains

In neuropathology, utilized in central neurocytoma, medulloblastoma, pineocytoma, ganglion cell tumors, paragangliomas, and choroid plexus tumors.[37] Metastases that are positive for neuroendocrine stains include small-cell carcinoma of the lung (most common), malignant pheochromocytoma, and Merkel cell tumor.

Includes:
1. chromogranin: stains synaptic vesicles. Perhaps less commonly utilized than synaptophysin in primary CNS tumor
2. synaptophysin: stains synaptic vesicles; has higher sensitivity but lower specificity than chromogranin.[37(p 200)] Often positive for central neurocytoma, which typically lacks chromogranin staining.[39(p 107)]
3. CD56 (Neural cell adhesion molecule): a family of glycoproteins present in nervous tissue as well as other tissues such as thyroid, liver, etc.[37(p 142–3,264)] Frequently used to confirm neuroendocrine differentiation.
4. neuron specific enolase (NSE): sensitive but not specific for neuronal or neuroendocrine differentiation despite its name (often referred to as "neuron non-specific enolase").[37(p 338)] Due to this, it is less often utilized as a neuroendocrine marker.

Cluster of differentiation (CD) markers

A number of immunohistochemical stains that detect antigens on the surface of leukocytes, though many stain other cell types as well. Examples include:
- CD45: General leukocyte marker
- CD3 and CD5: T-cells
- CD20: B-cells
- CD38 and CD138: Plasma cells
- CD68: Histiocytes
- CD56 (Neural cell adhesion molecule): Classically stains natural killer cells, but also a neuroendocrine marker (see above)
- organism-specific immunohistochemical stains are available to detect certain organisms that infect the nervous system including HSV, CMV, and *Toxoplasma gondii*

Metastases that are positive for neuroendocrine stains include: small-cell carcinoma of the lung, malignant pheochromocytoma, Merkel cell tumor. Metastatic small-cell tumors to the brain staining positive for neuroendocrine stains are almost all due to lung primaries (all other primaries are a distant possibility).

35.7.3 Molecular alterations in major CNS tumors

In the WHO CNS5,[1] molecular genetics plays a central role in the classification of CNS tumors. ▶ Table 35.7 shows key molecular alterations that are involved in the diagnostic classification of major CNS tumors. See reference for more details.

Table 35.7 Key diagnostic genes, mutations, molecules, pathways, and/or combinations in major primary CNS tumors[1,40] (used with permission from WHO Classification of Tumours Editorial Board. Central Nervous System Tumours. Lyon (France): International Agency for Research on Cancer; 2021. (WHO classification of tumours series, 5th ed.; vol. 6). Available from: https://tumourclassification.iarc.who.int/.)

Tumor type	Genes/molecular profiles characteristically altered[a]
Adult-type diffuse gliomas	
astrocytoma, IDH mutant (p.658)	*IDH1, IDH2, ATRX, TP53, CDKN2A/B*
oligodendroglioma, IDH-mutant & 1p/19q codeleted (p.662)	*IDH1, IDH2, 1p/19q, TERT* promoter, *CIC, FUBP1, NOTCH1*
glioblastoma, IDH-wildtype (p.664)	IDH-wildtype, *TERT* promoter, chromosomes 7/10, *EGFR*
Pediatric-type diffuse low-grade gliomas	
diffuse astrocytoma, MYB- or MYBL1-altered (p.679)	*MYB, MYBL1*
angiocentric glioma (p.679)	*MYB*
polymorphous low-grade neuroepithelial tumor of the young (p.680)	*BRAF, FGFR* family
diffuse low-grade glioma, MAPK pathway-altered (p.682)	*FGFR1, BRAF*
Pediatric-type diffuse high-grade gliomas	
diffuse midline glioma, H3 K27-altered (p.683)	H3 K27, *TP53, ACVR1, PDGFRA, EGFR, EZHIP*
diffuse hemispheric glioma, H3 G34-mutant (p.685)	H3 G34, *TP53, ATRX*
diffuse pediatric-type high-grade glioma, H3-wildtype & IDH-wildtype (p.686)	IDH-wildtype, H3-wildtype, *PDGFRA, MYCN, EGFR* (methylome)
infant-type hemispheric glioma (p.687)	NTRK family, *ALK, ROS, MET*
Circumscribed astrocytic gliomas	
pilocytic astrocytoma (p.689)	*KIAA1549-BRAF, BRAF, NF1*
high-grade astrocytoma with piloid features (p.698)	*BRAF, NF1, ATRX, CDKN2A/B* (methylome)
pleomorphic xanthoastrocytoma (p.698)	*BRAF, CDKN2A/B*
subependymal giant cell astrocytoma (p.700)	*TSC1, TSC2*
chordoid glioma (p.702)	*PRKCA*
astroblastoma, MN1-altered (p.703)	*MN1*
Glioneural and neuronal tumors	
ganglion cell tumors	*BRAF*
dysembryoplastic neuroepithelial tumor (p.709)	*FGFR1*
diffuse glioneuronal tumor with oligodendroglioma-like features and nuclear clusters (p.711)	chromosome 14, (methylome)
papillary glioneuronal tumor (p.712)	*PRKCA*
rosette-forming glioneuronal tumor (p.713)	*FGFR1, PIK3CA, NF1*
myxoid glioneuronal tumor (p.714)	*PDFGRA*
diffuse leptomeningeal glioneuronal tumor (p.715)	*KIAA1549-BRAF* fusion, 1p (methylome)

35

Table 35.7 continued

Tumor type	Genes/molecular profiles characteristically altered[a]
multinodular and vacuolating neuronal tumor (p. 717)	MAPK pathway
dysplastic cerebellar gangliocytoma (Lhermitte-Duclos disease) (p. 716)	*PTEN*
extraventricular neurocytoma (p. 720)	*FGFR* (*FGFR1-TACC1* fusion), IDH-wildtype
Ependymal tumors	
supratentorial ependymoma (p. 724)	*ZFTA, RELA, YAP1, MAML2*
posterior fossa ependymomas (p. 727)	H3 K27me3, *EZHIP* (methylome)
spinal ependymomas (p. 732)	*NF2, MYCN*
Embryonal tumors	
medulloblastoma, WNT-activated (p. 750)	*CTNNB1, APC*
medulloblastoma, SHH-activated (p. 751)	*TP53, PTCH1, SUFU, SMO, MYCN, GLI2* (methylome)
medulloblastoma, non-WNT/non-SHH (p. 753)	*MYC, MYCN, PRDM6, KDM6A* (methylome)
atypical teratoid/rhabdoid tumor (p. 754)	biallelic inactivation of *SMARCB1* (or rarely *SMARCA4*)
embryonal tumor with multilayered rosettes	*C19MC, DICER1*
CNS neuroblastoma, FOXR2-activated	*FOXR2*
CNS tumor with BCOR internal tandem duplication	*BCOR*
desmoplastic myxoid tumor of the pineal region, SMARCB1-mutant	*SMARCB1*
meningioma	*NF2, AKT1, TRAF7, SMO, PIK3CA; KLF4, SMARCE1, BAP1* in subtypes; H3K27me3; *TERT* promoter, *CDKN2A/B* in CNS WHO grade 3
solitary fibrous tumor	*NAB2-STAT6*
meningeal melanocytic tumors	*NRAS* (diffuse); *GNAQ, GNA11, PLCB4, CYSLTR2* (circumscribed)
Tumors of the sellar region	
adamantinomatous craniopharyngioma	*CTNNB1*
papillary craniopharyngioma	*BRAF*

Abbreviations: CNS, central nervous system; C19MC, chromosome 19 microRNA cluster; IDH, isocitrate dehydrogenase; SHH, sonic hedgehog. Some of these are definitional for specific diagnoses, while others are not definitional but are characteristically altered or not altered. For each tumor type, these distinctions are specified in the WHO CNS5[1] as well as the Essential and Desirable Criteria sections of the individual chapters.

[a] In this column, molecules that are definitional (including for those that are wildtype) are listed before others; for those tumor types without specific definitional changes, more commonly altered genes and molecules are listed before others. Most types have characteristic methylome patterns, but "(methylome)" is only listed for those types for which methylome testing offers particular diagnostic guidance, including for designating subtypes (as for Medulloblastoma, SHH-activated; Medulloblastoma, non-WNT/non-SHH; and Diffuse leptomeningeal glioneuronal tumor). H3 is a gene family (eg, H3F3A, HIST1H3B).

35.7.4 Tumor markers used clinically

Human chorionic gonadotropin (hCG)

A glycoprotein, MW = 45,000. Secreted by placental trophoblastic epithelium. Beta chain (β-hCG) is normally present only in the fetus or in gravid or postpartum females; otherwise it indicates disease. Classically associated with choriocarcinoma (uterine or testicular), it is also found in patients with embryonal cell tumors, teratocarcinoma of testis, and others.

CSF β-hCG is 0.5–2% of serum β-hCG in non-CNS tumors. Higher levels are diagnostic of cerebral mets from uterine or testicular choriocarcinoma, or primary choriocarcinoma or embryonal cell carcinoma of pineal (p. 758) or suprasellar region.

Alpha-fetoprotein

Alpha-fetoprotein (AFP) is a normal fetal glycoprotein (MW = 70,000) initially produced by the yolk sac, and later by the fetal liver. It is found in the fetal circulation throughout gestation, and drops rapidly during the first few weeks of life, reaching normal adult levels by age 1 yr. It is detectable only in trace amounts in normal adult males or nonpregnant females. It is present in amniotic fluid in normal pregnancies, and is detectable in maternal serum starting at ≈ 12–14 weeks gestation, increasing steadily throughout pregnancy until ≈ 32 weeks.[41]

Abnormally elevated serum AFP may occur in Ca of ovary, stomach, lung, colon, pancreas, as well as in cirrhosis or hepatitis and in the majority of gravid women carrying a fetus with an open neural tube defect; see Prenatal detection of neural tube defects (p.313). Serum AFP > 500 ng/ml usually means primary hepatic tumor.

CSF-AFP is elevated in some pineal region germ cell tumors (p.759). 16–25% of patients with testicular tumors develop cerebral mets, and elevated CSF AFP levels are reported in some.

Carcinoembryonic antigen (CEA)

A glycoprotein, MW = 200,000. Normally present in fetal endodermal cells. Originally described in the early 1960s in the serum in patients with colorectal adeno-Ca, it is now known to be elevated in many malignant and nonmalignant conditions (including cholecystitis, colitis, diverticulitis, hepatic involvement from any tumor, with 50–90% of terminal patients having elevation).

CSF CEA: levels > 1 ng/ml are reported with leptomeningeal spread of lung Ca (89%), breast Ca (60–67%), malignant melanoma (25–33%), and bladder Ca. May be normal even in CEA-secreting cerebral mets if they don't communicate with the subarachnoid space. Only carcinomatous meningitis from lung or breast Ca consistently elevates CSF CEA in the majority of patients.

S-100 protein

Serum S-100 protein levels rise after head trauma, and possibly after other insults to the brain. Levels may also be elevated in Creutzfeldt-Jakob disease.

References

[1] Bosman FT, Jaffe ES, Lakhani SR, et al. World Health Organization Classification of Tumors series, vol. 6. In: WHO Classification of Tumors Editorial Board (ed.) World Health Organization classification of tumors of the central nervous system. 5th ed. Lyon, France: International Agency for Research on Cancer; 2021

[2] Louis DN, Aldape K, Brat DJ, et al. Announcing cIM-PACT-NOW: the Consortium to Inform Molecular and Practical Approaches to CNS Tumor Taxonomy. Acta Neuropathol. 2017; 133:1–3

[3] Louis DN, Wesseling P, Paulus W, et al. cIMPACT-NOW update 1: Not Otherwise Specified (NOS) and Not Elsewhere Classified (NEC). Acta Neuropathol. 2018; 135:481–484

[4] Mete O, WHO Classification of Tumors Editorial Board. Pituitary gland. Lyon, France 2022. https://publications.iarc.fr/Book-And-Report-Series/Who-Classification-Of-Tumours

[5] Allen JC. Childhood Brain Tumors: Current Status of Clinical Trials in Newly Diagnosed and Recurrent Disease. Ped Clin N Am. 1985; 32:633–651

[6] Laurent JP, Cheek WR. Brain Tumors in Children. J Pediatr Neurosci. 1985; 1:15–32

[7] Ostrom QT, Cioffi G, Waite K, et al. CBTRUS Statistical Report: Primary Brain and Other Central Nervous System Tumors Diagnosed in the United States in 2014-2018. Neuro Oncol. 2021; 23:iii1–iii105

[8] Duffner PK, Cohen ME, Freeman AI. Pediatric Brain Tumors: An Overview. Ca. 1985; 35:287–301

[9] Section of Pediatric Neurosurgery of the American Association of Neurological Surgeons. Pediatric Neurosurgery. New York 1982

[10] Jooma R, Hayward RD, Grant DN. Intracranial Neoplasms During the First Year of Life: Analysis of One Hundred Consecutive Cases. Neurosurgery. 1984; 14:31–41

[11] Wakai S, Arai T, Nagai M. Congenital Brain Tumors. Surgical Neurology. 1984; 21:597–609

[12] Forsyth PA, Posner JB. Headaches in Patients with Brain Tumors: A Study of 111 Patients. Neurology. 1993; 43:1678–1683

[13] Mahaley MS, Mettlin C, Natarajan N, et al. National Survey of Patterns of Care for Brain-Tumor Patients. J Neurosurg. 1989; 71:826–836

[14] Whittle IR, Pringle A-M, Taylor R. Effects of Resective Surgery for Left-Sided Intracranial Tumors on Language Function: A Prospective Study. Lancet. 1998; 351:1014–1018

[15] Albright L, Reigel DH. Management of Hydrocephalus Secondary to Posterior Fossa Tumors. Preliminary Report. J Neurosurg. 1977; 46:52–55

[16] Berger MS, Baumeister B, Geyer JR, et al. The Risks of Metastases from Shunting in Children with Primary Central Nervous System Tumors. J Neurosurg. 1991; 74:872–877

[17] McLaurin RL, Venes JL. Pediatric Neurosurgery. Philadelphia 1989

[18] Galicich JH, French LA. Use of Dexamethasone in the Treatment of Cerebral Edema Resulting from Brain Tumors and Brain Surgery. Am Pract Dig Treat. 1961; 12:169–174

[19] French LA, Galicich JH. The Use of Steroids for Control of Cerebral Edema. Clinical Neurosurgery. 1964; 10:212–223

[20] Glantz MJ, Cole BF, Forsyth PA, et al. Practice Parameter: Anticonvulsant Prophylaxis in Patients with Newly Diagnosed Brain Tumors. Report of the Quality Standards Subcommittee of the American

35

Academy of Neurology. Neurology. 2000; 54:1886–1893

[21] Kondziolka D, Lunsford LD, Martinez AJ. Unreliability of contemporary neurodiagnostic imaging in evaluating suspected adult supratentorial (low-grade) astrocytoma. Journal of Neurosurgery. 1993; 79:533–536

[22] Chicoine MR, Silbergeld DL. Pharmacology for Neurosurgeons. Part I: Anticonvulsants, Chemotherapy, Antibiotics. Contemporary Neurosurgery. 1996; 18:1–6

[23] Prados MD, Berger MS, Wilson CB. Primary Central Nervous System Tumors: Advances in Knowledge and Treatment. Ca Cancer J Clin. 1998; 48:331–360

[24] Stewart DJ. A Critique of the Role of the Blood-Brain Barrier in the Chemotherapy of Human Brain Tumors. Journal of Neuro-Oncology. 1994;121–139

[25] Salcman M, Broadwell RD, Salcman M. The Blood Brain Barrier. In: Neurobiology of Brain Tumors. Baltimore: Williams and Wilkins; 1991:229–250

[26] Madajewicz S, Chowhan N, Tfayli A, et al. Therapy for Patients with High Grade Astrocytoma Using Intraarterial Chemotherapy and Radiation Therapy. Cancer. 2000; 88:2350–2356

[27] Barker FG, Prados MD, Chang SM, et al. Radiation Response and Survival Time in Patients with Glioblastoma Multiforme. Journal of Neurosurgery. 1996; 84:442–448

[28] Laohaprasit V, Silbergeld DL, Ojemann GA, et al. Postoperative CT Contrast Enhancement Following Lobectomy for Epilepsy. Journal of Neurosurgery. 1990; 73:392–395

[29] Jeffries BF, Kishore PR, Singh KS, et al. Contrast Enhancement in the Postoperative Brain. Radiology. 1981; 139:409–413

[30] Gerber AM, Savolaine ER. Modification of Tumor Enhancement and Brain Edema in Computerized Tomography by Corticosteroids: Case Report. Neurosurgery. 1980; 6:282–284

[31] Hatam A, Bergström M, Yu ZY, et al. Effect of Dexamethasone Treatment in Volume and Contrast Enhancement of Intracranial Neoplasms. Journal of Computer Assisted Tomography. 1983; 7:295–300

[32] Plesec TP, Prayson RA. Frozen section discrepancy in the evaluation of central nervous system tumors. Arch Pathol Lab Med. 2007; 131:1532–1540

[33] Shah AB, Muzumdar GA, Chitale AR, et al. Squash preparation and frozen section in intraoperative diagnosis of central nervous system tumors. Acta Cytol. 1998; 42:1149–1154

[34] Uematsu Y, Owai Y, Okita R, et al. The usefulness and problem of intraoperative rapid diagnosis in surgical neuropathology. Brain Tumor Pathol. 2007; 24:47–52

[35] Burger PC. Smears and Frozen Sections in Surgical Neuropathology: A manual. PB Medical Publishing; 2009

[36] Scherer HB. Structural Developments in Gliomas. American Journal of Cancer. 1938; 34:333–351

[37] McKeever PE, Dabbs DJ. Immunohistochemistry of the Nervous System. In: Diagnostic Immunohistochemistry. New York: Churchill Livingstone; 2002:559–624

[38] Russell DS, Rubenstein LJ. Pathology of Tumours of the Nervous System. 5th ed. Baltimore: Williams and Wilkins; 1989

[39] Louis DN, Ohgaki H, Wiestler OD, et al. WHO classification of tumors of the central nervous system. Lyon 2007

[40] Louis DN, Perry A, Wesseling P, et al. The 2021 WHO Classification of Tumors of the Central Nervous System: a summary. Neuro Oncol. 2021. DOI: 10.1093/neuonc/noab106

[41] Burton BK. Alpha-Fetoprotein Screening. Adv Pediatr. 1986; 33:181–196

36 Genetic Tumor Syndromes Involving the CNS

36.1 General information

At least 20 genetic syndromes with predisposition for central and peripheral nervous system tumors have been identified (see ▶ Table 36.1 for some). Several of them used to be grouped under the heading "neurocutaneous disorders" (or phakomatoses), viz., neurofibromatosis types I & II, tuberous sclerosis, and Sturge Weber syndrome (p. 652). This section covers some of these syndromes that are more likely to come to the attention of the neurosurgeon.

Table 36.1 Examples of genetic syndromes associated with CNS tumors

Syndrome	Associated CNS tumor(s)
neurofibromatosis type 1 (p. 638)	optic glioma, astrocytoma, neurofibroma
neurofibromatosis type 2 (p. 640)	bilateral vestibular schwannoma, meningioma, ependymoma, astrocytoma
schwannomatosis (p. 642)	multiple schwannomas, infrequently meningiomas
tuberous sclerosis (p. 644)	subependymal giant cell astrocytoma (SEGA)
von Hippel-Lindau syndrome (p. 646)	hemangioblastoma
Li-Fraumeni syndrome (p. 650)	children: medulloblastoma adult: astrocytoma, PNET
Cowden syndrome (p. 651)	dysplastic cerbellar gangliocytoma
constitutional mismatch repair deficiency syndrome (p. 651)	ultrahypermutated malignant gliomas, CNS embryonal tumors
familial adenomatous polyposis 1 (p. 651) (FAP1) + brain tumors (BTP2)	medulloblastoma WNT-activated
nevoid basal cell carcinoma syndrome (Gorlin syndrome)	desmoplastic/nodular subtype of medulloblastoma
rhabdoid tumor predisposition syndrome (RPTS)	atypical teratoid/rhabdoid tumors (AT/RTs)
Carney complex (p. 652)	malignant melanotic nerve sheath tumor, schwannoma, PitNET/adenoma
DICER1 syndrome	metastatic pleuropulmonary blastoma; pineoblastoma; embryonal tumor with multilayered rosettes; pituitary blastoma; primary intracranial sarcoma, DICER1-mutant
familial paraganglioma syndromes	paraganglioma (including pheochromocytoma)
melanoma-astrocytoma syndrome	astrocytoma, nerve sheath tumors
familial retinoblastoma	pineoblastoma
BAP1 tumor predisposition syndrome	meningioma
Fanconi anemia	medulloblastoma
ELP1-medulloblastoma syndrome	medulloblastoma SHH-activated

36

36.2 Neurofibromatosis

36.2.1 General information

Neurofibromatosis is a group of neurogenetic disorders with a predisposition to developing multiple nerve sheath tumors. There are as many as 6 distinct types of neurofibromatosis, the two most common of which (NF1 & NF2) are compared in ▶ Table 36.2. A third, less common type is schwannomatosis (p. 642).

▶ **Schwannoma vs. neurofibroma.** While similar in many ways, these tumors differ histologically. Schwannomas (formerly: neurilemmomas) arise from schwann cells, which produce myelin. Neurofibromas consist of neurites (axons or dendrites of immature or developing neurons), Schwann's cells, and fibroblasts within a collagenous or myxoid matrix. In contrast to schwannomas which displace axons (centrifugal), neurofibromas are unencapsulated and engulf the nerve of origin (centripetal). Neurofibromas may occur as solitary lesions, or may be multiple as part of NF1 in the setting of which there is potential for malignant transformation. Both tumors have Antoni A (compact) and Antoni B (loose) fibers, but neurofibromas tend to have more Antoni B fibers and the cells tend to be smaller than those of schwannomas. Markers of mature Schwann cells including S100, SOX10 and collagen IV, are present in both, but to a lesser extent in neurofibromas. A patient ≤ 30 years of age with a vestibular schwannoma is at increased risk of having NF2.

36.2.2 Neurofibromatosis type 1

General information

More common than NF2, representing > 90% of cases of neurofibromatosis.[2] For a comparison of NF1 and NF2, see ▶ Table 36.2.

Table 36.2 Comparison of neurofibromatosis 1 & 2[1]

current designation →	Neurofibromatosis 1 (NF1) (p. 638)	Neurofibromatosis 2 (NF2) (p. 640)
alternate term (not recommended)	von Recklinghausen's disease	bilateral acoustic NFT AKA MISME syndrome
obsolete term	peripheral NFT	central NFT
U.S. prevalence	100,000 people	≈ 3000 people
incidence	1/3000 births	1/40,000
inheritance	AD	AD
sporadic occurrence	30–50%	> 50%
gene locus	17 (17q11.2)	22 (22q12.2)
gene product	neurofibromin	schwannomin (merlin)
vestibular schwannomas (VS)	uncommon, ≈ never bilateral	bilateral VSs are the hallmark
cutaneous schwannomas	no	70%
Lisch nodules	very common	not associated
cataracts	not associated	60–80%
skeletal anomalies	common (scoliosis...)	not associated
pheochromocytoma	occasional	not associated
MPNST[a]	≈ 2%	not associated
intellectual impairment	in ≥ 50%	not associated
most common associated intramedullary spinal cord tumors	astrocytoma	ependymoma

[a]malignant peripheral nerve sheath tumor

Clinical

NF1 should be *suspected* in individuals who have any of the suggestive findings shown in ▶ Table 36.3 (1988 NIH criteria).

The NIH diagnostic criteria are met in an individual with 2 or more of the features listed in ▶ Table 36.3 (reference available online at https://www.ncbi.nlm.nih.gov/books/NBK1109/).[3] In *adults*, the diagnosis is usually made clinically using the NIH criteria which are highly specific and highly sensitive,[4] molecular genetic testing is rarely needed. In children, more care must be taken in assigning the diagnosis of NF1,[3] where molecular analysis may help differentiate NF1 from forms of Noonan syndrome that have multiple neurofibromas.

Associated conditions

1. Schwann-cell tumors on any nerve (but bilateral VSs are virtually nonexistent)
2. spinal and/or peripheral nerve neurofibromas
3. multiple skin neurofibromas
4. aqueductal stenosis (p. 273)
5. macrocephaly: secondary to aqueductal stenosis and hydrocephalus, increased cerebral white matter

Table 36.3 Suggestive findings of NF1[5]

Two or more of the following:

- ≥6 café au lait spots[a], each ≥5 mm in greatest diameter in prepubertal individuals, or ≥15 mm in greatest diameter in postpubertal patients
- ≥2 neurofibromas of any type, or one plexiform neurofibroma (neurofibromas are usually not evident until age 10–15 yrs). May be painful
- freckling (hyperpigmentation) in the axillary or intertriginous (inguinal) areas
- optic pathway glioma/pilocytic astrocytoma: see below
- ≥2 Lisch nodules: pigmented iris hamartomas that appear as translucent yellow/brown elevations that tend to become more numerous with age
- distinctive osseous abnormality, such as *sphenoid dysplasia* or thinning of long bone cortex with or without pseudarthrosis (e.g., of tibia or radius)
- a first degree relative (parent, sibling, or offspring) with NF1 by above criteria

[a]café au lait spots: hyperpigmented oval light brown skin macules (flat). May be present at birth, increase in number and size during 1st decade. Are present in >99% of NF1 cases. Rare on face.

6. intracranial tumors: hemispheric astrocytomas are the most common, solitary or multicentric meningiomas (usually in adults). Gliomas associated with NF1 are usually pilocytic astrocytomas. Brainstem astrocytomas include both contrast-enhancing pilocytic lesions and those that are non-enhancing and radiologically diffuse
7. unilateral defect in superior orbit → pulsatile exophthalmos
8. neurologic or cognitive impairment: 30–60% have mild learning disabilities
9. kyphoscoliosis (seen in 2–10%, often progressive, which then requires surgical stabilization)
10. visceral manifestations from involvement of autonomic nerves or ganglia within the organ. Up to 10% of patients have abnormal gastrointestinal motility/neuronal intestinal dysplasia related to neuronal hyperplasia within submucosal plexus
11. ≈ 20% develop plexiform neurofibromas: tumors from multiple nerve fascicles that grow along the length of the nerve. Almost pathognomonic for NF1[6]
12. syringomyelia
13. malignant tumors that have increased frequency in NFT: neuroblastoma, ganglioglioma, sarcoma, leukemia, Wilm's tumor, breast cancer[7]
14. pheochromocytoma: is occasionally present
15. "unidentified bright objects" (UBOs) on brain or spinal MRI in 53–79% of patients (bright on T2WI, isointense on T1WI) that may be hamartomas, heterotopias, foci of abnormal myelination or low grade tumors.[8] Tend to resolve with age

Epidemiology

An autosomal dominant disorder with an incidence of ≈ 1 case per every 3000 births.

Genetics

Simple autosomal dominant inheritance with variable expressivity but almost 100% penetrance after age 5 years. The NF1 gene is on chromosome 17q11.2, which codes for neurofibromin[9] (neurofibromin is a negative regulator of the RAS oncogene). Loss of neurofibromin results in elevation of growth-promoting signals. The spontaneous mutation rate is high, with 30–50% of cases representing new somatic mutations.[10]

Counselling: prenatal diagnosis is possible by linkage analysis only if there are 2 or more affected family members.[9] 70% of NF1 gene mutations can be detected using protein truncation analysis.

Neurofibromas

Dermal and plexiform neurofibromas are characteristic of NF1. Deep-seated intraneural variants are less common and may produce neurologic symptoms. The lifetime risk of malignant transformation of plexiform neurofibromas to MPNST (p. 774) is ≈ 10%.[11]

Management

1. optic gliomas
   a) unlike optic gliomas in the absence of NFT, these are rarely chiasmal (usually involving the nerve), are often multiple, and have a better prognosis
   b) most are non progressive, and should be followed ophthalmologically and with serial imaging (MRI or CT)

36

    c) surgical intervention probably does not alter visual impairment. Therefore, surgery is reserved for special situations (large disfiguring tumors, pressure on adjacent structures…)

2. other neural tumors in patients with NF1 should be managed in the same manner as in the general population
   a) focal, resectable, symptomatic lesions should be surgically removed
   b) MEK inhibitors are approved use in ages 2-18 years of age with for symptomatic, inoperable plexiform neurofibromas,[12] with surgery reserved for cases with increasing ICP
   c) when malignant degeneration is suspected (rare, but incidence of sarcomas and leukemias is increased), biopsy with or without internal decompression may be indicated

3. surveillance[3]
   a) annual exam by physician familiar with NF1
   b) annual ophthalmologic exam in children, less frequent in adults
   c) regular developmental assessment of children
   d) regular BP monitoring
   e) MRI for follow-up of clinically suspected intracranial and other internal tumors
   f) annual mammography in women starting at age 30 years and consider annual breast MRI in women age 30–50 years

36.2.3 Neurofibromatosis type 2 (NF2 AKA bilateral acoustic NFT)

General information

AKA MISME syndrome (acronym for **M**ultiple **I**nherited **S**chwannomas, **M**eningiomas, and **E**pendymomas).[13] An autosomal dominant disorder characterized by bilateral vestibular schwannomas (VS), with other neoplastic and dysplastic lesions that primarily affect the nervous system.[14] Multiple meningiomas are the second hallmark, occurring in about 50% of patients. For a comparison of NF1 and NF2, see ▶ Table 36.2.

There are 2 phenotypic subtypes[15]:
1. Wishart phenotype: severe. Early onset, myriad tumors and high tumor burden
2. Gardner phenotype: mild. Later presentation, VS are the only tumors, slower deterioration of hearing

Diagnostic criteria for neurofibromatosis type 2 (NF2)

Diagnostic criteria have been modified from the original NIH guidelines[16,17] (reference available online at https://www.ncbi.nlm.nih.gov/books/NBK1201/) with the revised Manchester criteria[18] shown in ▶ Fig. 36.1.

NF2 is diagnosed in a proband that meets the consensus diagnostic criteria, or if only 1 criteria is met in the presence of a heterozygous pathogenic variant of the NF2 gene.[19]

Clinical

Other clinical features:
1. seizures or other focal deficits
2. skin nodules, dermal neurofibromas, café au lait spots (less common than in NF1)
3. multiple intradural spinal tumors are common (less common in NF1)[20]: including intramedullary (especially ependymomas) and extramedullary (schwannomas, meningiomas…)
4. retinal hamartomas
5. antigenic nerve growth factor is increased (does not occur with NF1)
6. despite its name, is not associated with neurofibromas

Epidemiology

≈ 1 in 25,000 to 1 in 40,000 are affected. NF2 is considered an adult-onset disease, the average age of onset is 18–24 years.[17] By age 30 years, almost all affected patients will have bilateral VS.

Genetics

Autosomal dominant inheritance. There are a number of NF2 gene mutations that lead to the development of NF2. One is due to a mutation at chromosome 22q12.2, which results in the inactivation of schwannomin (AKA merlin, a semi-acronym for moesin-, ezrin-, and radixin-like proteins), a tumor suppression peptide. NF2 patients with nonsense and frameshift mutations are more likely to have intramedullary tumors (but not any other type of tumor) compared with other mutation types.

36

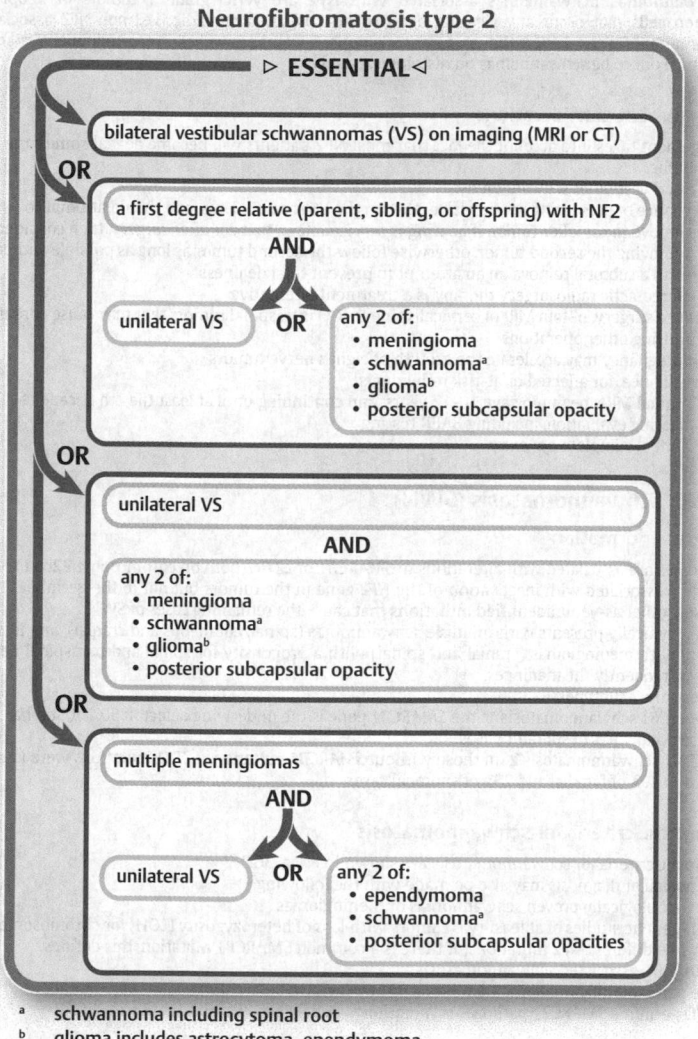

Neurofibromatosis type 2

▷ **ESSENTIAL** ◁

bilateral vestibular schwannomas (VS) on imaging (MRI or CT)

OR

a first degree relative (parent, sibling, or offspring) with NF2

AND

unilateral VS   **OR**   any 2 of:
- meningioma
- schwannoma[a]
- glioma[b]
- posterior subcapsular opacity

OR

unilateral VS

AND

any 2 of:
- meningioma
- schwannoma[a]
- glioma[b]
- posterior subcapsular opacity

OR

multiple meningiomas

AND

unilateral VS   **OR**   any 2 of:
- ependymoma
- schwannoma[a]
- posterior subcapsular opacities

[a] schwannoma including spinal root
[b] glioma includes astrocytoma, ependymoma

NB: with 1 of the clinical criteria, the diagnosis may be made if molecular gene testing shows a germline pathologic variant of the NF2 gene

Fig. 36.1 Diagnostic criteria for NF2. (Modified with permission from WHO Classification of Tumors Editorial Board, (ed.) World Health Organization classification of tumors of the central nervous system. 5th ed. Bosman F T, Jaffe E S, Lakhani S R, et al. (series eds.): World Health Organization Classification of Tumors series, vol. 6. International Agency for Research on Cancer, Lyon, France, 2021.)

36

► **Schwannomas.** Schwannomas associated with NF2 are WHO grade 1 tumors of neoplastic Schwann cells that occur at an earlier age (in the 20s) than sporadic (i.e., non-NF2 associated) schwannomas (in the 50s). Although cutaneous neurofibromas have been reported, in NF2 many of these turn out to be schwannomas on histological analysis.

Management considerations

Management takes into account the fact that most NF2 patients will become deaf at some time during their life.
1. bilateral vestibular schwannomas:
   a) chance of preserving hearing is best when the VS is small. Thus, one should attempt to remove the smaller tumor. If hearing is serviceable in that ear after surgery, then consider removing the second tumor, otherwise follow the second tumor as long as possible and perform a subtotal removal in an attempt to prevent total deafness
   b) stereotactic radiosurgery therapy is a treatment alternative
2. prior to surgery, obtain MRI of cervical spine to R/O intraspinal tumors that may cause cord injuries during other operations
3. NB: pregnancy may accelerate the growth of eighth nerve tumors
4. surveillance: for affected or at-risk individuals[17]
   a) annual MRIs beginning age 10-12 years, and continuing until at least the 4th decade of life
   b) hearing evaluation, including BAER testing
   c) annual complete eye exam

36.2.4 Schwannomatosis (SWN)

General information

Most cases are associated with alterations in *SMARCB1* or *LZTR1*(both on chromosome 22q11) which in turn is associated with inactivation of the *NF2* gene in the tumors but not in the germline. There are likely other as-yet unidentified mutations that cause the remaining cases of SWN.

SWN typically presents with multiple schwannomas (spinal, cutaneous and cranial), and less frequently with meningiomas (cranial and spinal) with a propensity for spinal and paraspinal nerves, and less frequently the meninges.

There are 2 subtypes:
1. *SMARCB1* schwannomatosis 1: the *SMARCB1* gene is the underlying defect in 50% of familial cases, and < 10% of sporadic cases.
2. *LZTR1* schwannomatosis 2: in those without *SMARCB1* mutation, *LZTR1* mutations were identified in 40% of familial and 25% of sporacid cases

Diagnostic criteria for schwannomatosis

Diagnostic criteria for schwannomatosis are shown in ► Fig. 36.2.[21]
    A molecular diagnosis may also be made with the following[22]:
* ≥ 2 pathologically proven schwannomas or meningiomas
  AND genetic studies of at least two tumors with loss of heterozygosity (LOH) for chromosome 22 and two different NF2 mutations; if there is a common SMARCB1 mutation, this defines SMARCB1-associated schwannomatosis
* one pathologically proven schwannoma or meningioma
  AND germline SMARCB1 pathogenic mutation

Patients with the following do not qualify for the diagnosis of schwannomatosis[22]:
1. germline pathogenic NF2 mutation
2. those fulfilling the diagnostic criteria for NF2 (especially bilateral vestibular schwannomas)
3. those with a first-degree relative with NF2
4. schwannomas only in previous field of radiation therapy

Epidemiology

Annual incidence is 0.58 cases per 1,000,000 persons.[23] There was a family history of SWN in 13% of 87 cases.[24]

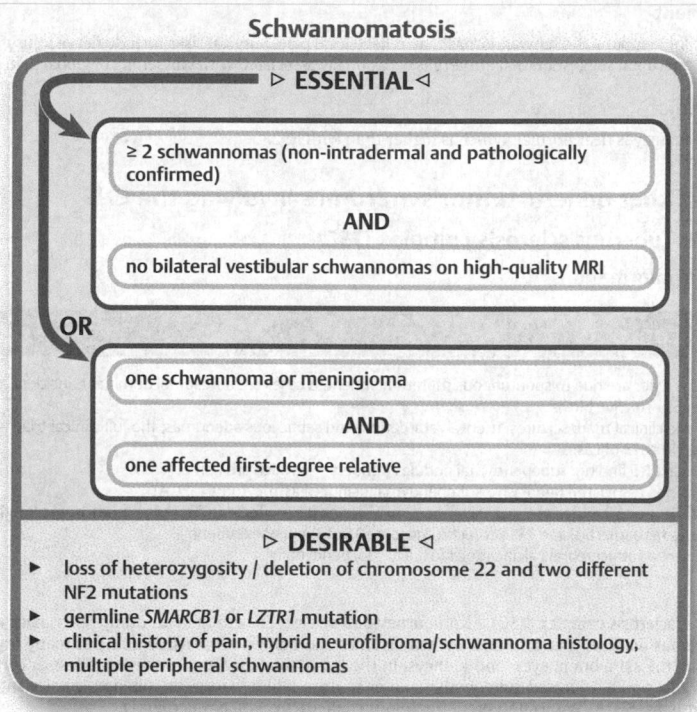

Fig. 36.2 Diagnostic criteria for schwannomatosis. (Modified with permission from WHO Classification of Tumors Editorial Board, (ed.) World Health Organization classification of tumors of the central nervous system. 5th ed. Bosman F T, Jaffe E S, Lakhani S R, et al. (series eds.): World Health Organization Classification of Tumors series, vol. 6. International Agency for Research on Cancer, Lyon, France, 2021.)

Presentation

There is considerable clinical (phenotypical) overlap with NF2, and molecular testing may be necessary to differentiate the two. In distinction to NF2, 68% of SWN patients have chronic pain, and 46% have pain unassociated with a mass.[24] It is debatable whether neurologic deficit is common[25] or not.[21] The pain has both neuropathic and nociceptive features and the relationship of the pain to the number, size and location of tumors is unclear.[22]

Evaluation

H&P: careful history to assess for 1st degree relatives with SWN or NF2 and physical exam for stigmata of NFT.

Imaging: MRI of the entire neuraxis, including high resolution brain MRI with attention to the internal auditory canals (IACs) with slices ≤ 3 mm thick. This can be accomplished with separate MRIs without and with contrast of the brain (with IACs), cervical, thoracic and lumbar spine, or, when available, with whole-body MRI without contrast using special commercially available software.[22,26]

Molecular genetic testing: including tumor biopsy for questionable cases (NB: patients with SWN-associated chronic pain should be made aware that risks include possibility of exacerbation of their pain; see below). Appropriate genetic counselling for confirmed cases.

36

Treatment

Surgery for symptomatic schwannomas may relieve local pain. Surgical risks include nerve injury, and there is anecdotal suggestion that surgery is occasionally associated with worsening of global pain.[22]

Prognosis

Life expectancy is near normal, which is higher than with NF2.

36.3 Other genetic tumor syndromes involving the CNS

36.3.1 Tuberous sclerosis complex (TSC)

General information

> ### Key concepts
>
> - most cases are due to spontaneous mutation. Inherited cases are autosomal dominant. Incidence: 1 in 6K–10K live births
> - classic clinical triad: seizures, mental retardation, and sebaceous adenomas; the full clinical triad is seen in < 1/3 of cases
> - typical CNS finding: subependymal nodules ("tubers") — which are hamartomas
> - common associated neoplasm: subependymal giant cell astrocytoma (SEGA)
> - TSC develops if either of these 2 tumor suppressor genes is affected: *TSC1* (on chromosome 9q34) codes for hamartin, and *TSC2* (on chromosome 16p13) encodes tuberin
> - CT shows intracerebral calcifications (usually subependymal)

Tuberous sclerosis complex (TSC), AKA Bourneville's disease, is a group of autosomal dominant neurocutaneous disorder characterized by hamartomas and benign neoplastic lesions of many organs including the skin, brain, eyes, and kidneys. In the brain, the hamartomas may manifest as cortical tubers, glial nodules located subependymally or in deep white matter, or subependymal giant cell astrocytomas (SEGA). Associated brain findings include pachygyria or microgyria.

Diagnostic criteria

General information

The diagnosis of TS is based primarily on clinical features, but the variability of phenotype and age at symptom onset can make this challenging. Molecular testing may help when the phenotype is strongly suspicious but a definitive diagnosis cannot be made clinically.

Clinical diagnostic criteria

Clinical diagnostic criteria are shown in ▶ Table 36.4.

In the infant, the earliest finding is of "ash leaf" macules (hypomelanotic, leaf shaped) that are best seen with a Wood's lamp. Infantile myoclonus may also occur.

In older children or adults, the myoclonus is often replaced by generalized tonic-clonic or partial complex seizures, which occur in 70–80%. Facial adenomas are not present at birth, but appear in > 90% by age 4 yrs (these are not really adenomas of the sebaceous glands, but are small hamartomas of cutaneous nerve elements that are yellowish-brown and glistening and tend to arise in a butterfly malar distribution, usually sparing the upper lip).

Retinal hamartomas occur in ≈ 50% (central calcified hamartoma near the optic disc or a more subtle peripheral flat salmon-colored lesion). A distinctive depigmented iris lesion may also occur.

Genetic diagnostic criteria

Identification of either a *TSC1* or a *TSC2* pathogenic mutation is sufficient to definitively diagnose TS (online resources: for *TSC1*, and for *TSC2*).

Subtypes

1. tuberous sclerosis 1
2. tuberous sclerosis 2

Table 36.4 Clinical diagnostic criteria of tuberous sclerosis complex[27]

- **Definitive diagnosis** 2 major criteria, or 1 major AND ≥ 2 minor
- **Possible diagnosis** 1 major or ≥ 2 minor

Major criteria

- ≥ 3 hypomelanotic macules ≥ 5 mm diameter
- ≥ 3 angiofibromas or fibrous cephalic plaque
- ≥ 2 ungual fibroma
- shagreen patch
- multiple retinal hamartomas
- cortical dysplasias (including tubers & cerebral white matter radial migration lines)
- subependymal nodules
- subependymal giant cell astrocytoma (SEGA)
- cardiac rhabdomyoma
- lymphangioleiomyomatosis
- ≥ 2 angiomyolipomas

Minor criteria

- "confetti" skin lesions
- ≥ 4 pits in dental enamel
- ≥ 2 intraoral fibromas
- achromic retinal patch
- multiple renal cysts
- nonrenal hamartomas

Epidemiology/genetics/epigenetics

Incidence: 1 in 6,000–10,000 live births.[28] Population prevalence: 1 in 20,000.[27]

Autosomal dominant inheritance; however, spontaneous mutation accounts for the majority of cases.[29] Two distinct tumor suppressor genes have been identified: the TSC1 gene (located on chromosome 9q34) codes for *TSC1* (AKA hamartin), and the *TSC2* gene (on chromosome 16p13.3) codes for TSC2 (tuberin). Only 1 gene needs to be affected to develop TSC. These proteins work together to inhibit activation of rapamycin (mTOR).

Genetic counseling for unaffected parents with one affected child: 1–2% chance of recurrence.

Histology

Subependymal nodules ("tubers") are benign hamartomas that are almost always calcified, and protrude into the ventricles.

▶ **Subependymal giant cell astrocytoma (SEGA).** A WHO grade 1 tumor—see Subependymal giant cell astrocytoma (SEGA) (WHO grade 1) (p. 700). Almost always located at the foramen of Monro. Occurs in 5–15% of patients with TSC.[30]

Evaluation

Plain skull X-rays

Not particularly helpful. May show calcified cerebral nodules.

CT scan

See reference.[31]

Intracerebral *calcifications* are the most common (97% of cases) and characteristic finding. Primarily located subependymally along the lateral walls of the lateral ventricles or near the foramina of Monro.

Low density lesions that do not enhance are seen in 61%. Probably represent heterotopic tissue or defective myelination. Most common in occipital lobe.

Hydrocephalus (HCP) may occur even without obstruction. In the absence of tumor, HCP is usually mild. Moderate HCP usually occurs only in the presence of tumor.

Subependymal nodules are usually calcified, and protrude into the ventricle ("**candle guttering**" described the appearance on pneumoencephalography).

Paraventricular tumors (mostly giant cell astrocytomas; see pathology (p. 645)) are essentially the *only* enhancing lesions in TSC.

36

MRI

Subependymal tubers are high on T2 and low on T1 and only ≈ 10% enhance.

Low signal in subependymal lesions may represent calcification. SEGA enhance intensely (enhancing subependymal lesions are almost always SEGAs).

Radial bands sign: abnormal signal intensity extending in a radial manner, representing cells of varying degrees of neuronal and astrocytic differentiation as well as difficult-to-classify cells.[32]

Treatment

Paraventricular tumors should be followed. Tubers grow minimally, but SEGA progress should be removed if they are symptomatic. A transcallosal approach or ventriculoscopic removal are options.

Infantile myoclonus may respond to steroids. Seizures are treated with ASMs.

Surgery for intractable seizures may be considered when a particular lesion is identified as a seizure focus. Better seizure control, not cure, is the goal in TSC.

Patients ≥ 3 years of age with increasing size of SEGA lesions have had sustained reduction of SEGA volume on everolimus.[33]

Prognosis

Lifespan is slightly shortened by TS.[34] When death occurs in the second decade of life, it is usually due to brain tumors and status epilepticus, followed by renal abnormalities. After age 40, mortality is usually associated with renal cysts or tumors or lymphangioleiomyomatosis.

36.3.2 Von Hippel-Lindau disease (VHL)

General information

> ### Key concepts
>
> - disorder with hemangioblastomas (HGB) primarily of cerebellum, retina, brainstem and spinal cord, endolymphatic sac tumors, as well as renal cysts/tumors, pheochromocytomas...
> - autosomal dominant, due to germline variants of the VHL tumor suppressor gene on 3p25.3
> - expression and age of onset are variable, but ≈ always manifests by age 60
> - mean age of developing HGBs is at least 10 years younger than sporadic HGBs

An autosomal dominant multisystem neoplastic disorder characterized by a tendency to develop hemangioblastomas (HGB) of the retina, brain and spinal cord (especially nerve roots), renal clear cell carcinoma (RCC), pheochromocytomas, endolymphatic sac tumors, and others[35,36] (retinal location is 2nd most common after cerebellar, ▶ Table 36.5). It is caused by germline variants of the VHL tumor tumor suppressor gene on chromosome 3p25.3. The variability of von Hippel-Lindau disease (VHL) has led some to suggest the use of the term hemangioblastomatosis.

Epidemiology

Incidence: 1 in 31,000 to 36,000 live births. ≈ 30% of patients with cerebellar HGB have VHL.[28]

Genetics

The VHL gene is a tumor suppressor gene on chromosome 3p25.3 that codes for VHL protein, which is part of protein complex VCB-CUL2. Biallelic inactivation (2-hit model) is required for tumor development.[28] Most patients inherit the autosomal dominant VHL gene (allele) with the germline mutation from the affected parent and a normal somatic (wild-type) VHL gene from the unaffected parent, with ≈ 95% penetrance by age 60 yrs.[35,39] However, about 20% of cases result from a spontaneous mutation that occurs in the egg or sperm, or very early in development.[40]

In either case, at some time during their life, the required second mutation occurs in susceptible organs, e.g., brain, kidney, retina... which causes the cell to not make functional VHL protein, which allows the cyst to develop.

4% of patients with the mutant VHL gene are asymptomatic carriers.

36

Table 36.5 Associations with von Hippel-Lindau disease[a]

Common lesions	Frequency in VHL
hemangioblastomas	
• cerebellum (solid or cystic)	80%
• retina	41–59%
• brainstem	10–25%
• spinal cord	10–50%
pancreatic tumors or cysts	22–80%
renal clear cell Ca & cysts	14–60%
polycythemia	9–20% of intracranial HGBs
Rare lesions (pertinent to nervous system)	**Frequency in VHL**
supratentorial hemangioblastoma	3–6%
cystadenomas of the broad ligament	10% of ♀
papillary cystadenomas of epididymis	25–60% ♂
endolymphatic sac tumors	10–15%
adrenal medullary *pheochromocytoma* (tends to be bilateral)	7–24%

[a]see references[35,37,38] for more

Subtypes of VHL

See reference.[41]

Type I: any manifestation of VHL (typically HGB and RCC) *except* pheochromocytoma.
Type 2A: pheochromocytoma is characteristic. RCC is rare.
Type 2B: high risk of HGB, RCC and pheochromocytoma.
Type 2C: risk of pheochromocytoma only (without risk of HGB or RCC).

Diagnostic criteria

Formal criteria for diagnosis of VHL have not been published; suggested diagnostic criteria appear here.[42]

▶ **Suspected VHL.** VHL should be suspected in an individual (with or without a family history of VHL) who has:
1. retinal angioma, especially at a young age
2. spinal or cerebellar hemangioblastoma
3. adrenal or extra-adrenal pheochromocytoma
4. renal cell carcinoma (RCC), if the individual is < 47 years old, or has a personal or family history of other tumors typical of VHL
5. multiple renal and pancreatic cysts
6. neuroendocrine tumors of the pancreas
7. endolymphatic sac tumors
8. less common: multiple papillary cystadenomas of the epididymis or broad ligament

▶ **Establishing the diagnosis of VHL.** The diagnosis of VHL is established in a proband with clinical features listed below and/or by identification of a heterozygous germline pathogenic variant in the VHL gene by molecular genetic testing. If the clinical features are absent, a patient with this variant is diagnosed with VHL and should be surveilled as such, even if clinical or radiographic findings are inconclusive.

Clinical diagnostic criteria
• an individual with no known family history of VHL with ≥ 2 charateristic lesions:
  ○ ≥ 2 HGB of the retina, spine or brain, or a single HGB in association with a visceral manifestation (e.g., multiple renal or pancreatic cysts)
  ○ renal cell carcinoma
  ○ adrenal or extra-adrenal pheochromocytoma
  ○ less common: endolymphatic sac tumors, papillary cystadenomas of the epididymis or broad ligament, or neuroendocrine tumors of the pancreas

36

- an individual with a family history of VHL with ≥ 1 of the following:
  - retinal angioma
  - spinal or cerebellar hemangioblastoma
  - adrenal or extra-adrenal pheochromocytoma retinal angioma
  - renal cell carcinoma
  - multiple renal and pancreatic cysts

Tumors associated with VHL

1. cerebellar hemangioblastomas (HGB):
   a) prevalence: 44–72% of VHL patients
   b) mean age of diagnosis in VHL patients with cerebellar hemangioblastomas is at least 10 years younger than sporadic cerebellar hemangioblastomas
   c) cysts are commonly associated with cerebellar, brainstem and spinal HGBs
   d) cysts grow at a faster rate than the HGBs, ∴ symptoms related to mass effect are frequently secondary to the cysts
   e) cerebellar HGBs were located in the superficial, posterior and superior half of the cerebellar hemispheres[43]
   f) 93% of the cerebellar HGBs were located in the cerebellar hemispheres and 7% in the vermis
   g) the HGBs are also more frequently found in the superficial posterior half of the brainstem and the spinal cord
   h) the HGBs have multiple sequential growth and quiescent phases
2. spinal cord hemangioblastomas
   a) occur in 13–44% of VHL patients
   b) 90% are located cranially within the cervical and thoracic cord. Almost all (96%) of the tumors are located in the posterior half of the spinal cord, 4% are located in the ventral half of the spinal cord. 1–3% are found in the lumbosacral nerve roots
   c) by way of comparison, 80% of spinal cord HGB are associated with VHL, whereas only 5–31% of cerebellar HGB are associated with VHL
   d) 95% of symptom-producing spinal HGBs are associated with syringomyelia
3. brainstem hemangioblastomas
   a) usually located in the posterior medulla oblongata usually around the obex and the region within the area postrema
4. pheochromocytomas (PCC): 20% of PCC are associated with VHL. PCC occur in 7–20% of families with VHL
5. endolymphatic sac tumors (ELST) (the endolymphatic sac is a cul-de sac in the petrous portion of the temporal bone in the middle fossa just deep to the dura that communicates with the saccule of the inner ear):
   a) locally invasive benign tumors that occur in 10–15% of VHL patients (30% of these will develop bilateral ELSTs—VHL is the only disease with bilateral ELSTs). Rarely metastasize
   b) presents with hearing loss in 95% (may be acute (86%) or insidious (14%), tinnitus (90%), vertigo or imbalance (66%), aural fullness (30%), and facial paresthesias (8%))
   c) mean age of onset of hearing loss: 22 years (range: 12–50)[44]
6. retinal hemangioblastomas[45]
   a) occur in > 50% of VHL patients. Mean age of presentation: 25 years
   b) frequently bilateral, multifocal, and recurrent
   c) often asymptomatic. Visual symptoms occur with progressive growth, edema, retinal detachments, and hard exudates
   d) typically located in the periphery and near or on the optic disc
   e) microangiomas measuring a few hundred microns without dilated feeding vessels may be located in the periphery
   f) retrobulbar HGB are rare (5.3% in NIH cohort)[46]
   g) severity of optic disease correlates with CNS and renal involvement
   h) early diagnosis and treatment with laser photocoagulation, and cryotherapy can prevent visual loss. Low dose external XRT may be an option for refractory cases
7. renal-cell carcinoma (RCC)[38,47,48,49,50,51,52,53]
   a) the most common malignant tumor in VHL. Usually a clear cell carcinoma
   b) lifetime risk for RCC in VHL: ≈ 70%.
   c) the growth rate of RCC is high variable
   d) RCC is the cause of death in 15–50% of patients

   e) metastases respond poorly to chemotherapy and radiation
   f) bilateral and multiple lesions are common
   g) partial nephrectomy or tumor enucleation is preferred to avoid/delay dialysis and transplantation
   h) nephron- or renal-sparing surgery recommended for tumors less < 3 cm
   i) promising techniques: cryo- and radiofrequency ablation of tumors < 3 cm
8. renal cysts[38,49,52,53,54]
   a) 50–70% of VHL patients have bilateral and multiple renal cysts
   b) rarely cause profound renal impairment
   c) chronic renal failure or renal hypertension not as common as with polycystic kidney disease
9. epididymal cystadenomas
   a) benign lesions that arise from the epididymal duct
   b) found in 10–60% of male VHL patients
   c) typically appear in the teenage years
   d) may cause infertility if bilateral
   e) may be multiple
10. broad ligament cystadenomas
   a) arise from the embryonic mesonephric duct
   b) true incidence unknown
   c) rarely reported and usually not recognized in women with VHL
11. pancreatic neuroendocrine tumors and cysts
   a) 35 to 70% of patients with VHL develop an endocrine tumor or cyst
   b) pancreatic cysts are generally asymptomatic and often multiple
   c) pancreatic neuroendocrine tumors are usually non-functional and 8% of them are malignant
   d) differential diagnosis: pancreatic islet cell tumors, MEN2

Treatment

Medical therapy with belzutifan (Welireg), an hypoxia-inducible factor inhibitor FDA approved for adults with VHL needing therapy for associated renal cell carcinoma (RCC), CNS hemangioblastomas, or pancreatic neuroendocrine tumors not requiring immediate surgery. More effective for the hemangioblastomas and pancreatic neuroendocrine tumors than RCC. Severe anemia and hypoxia can be significant side effects of belzutifan and are treated with transfusions (not erythropoietic agents). As always, follow full prescribing information.

   Surgical resection of individual CNS tumors is usually reserved until symptomatic to decrease the number of operations over a lifetime, since the tumors in VHL are usually multiple, tend to recur, and the growth pattern is saltatory. Surgery is the treatment of choice for accessible *cystic* HGBs. For details, see Treatment, under Hemangioblastoma (p. 825).

   Stereotactic radiosurgery (SRS)[55]: May provide local control rates of > 50% over 5 years. SRS has been recommended for asymptomatic HBG > 5 mm diameter if they are cystic or progressing in size during surveillance.[56] Cranial treatment plan: using a median dose of 22 Gy (range: 12–40 Gy) prescribed to the median 82% isodose line in 1–4 sessions. In cystic lesions, treatment is confined to the contrast enhancing mural nodule (the cyst wall is not treated). Spinal treatment plan: median dose of 21 Gy (range 20–25 Gy) prescribed to the median 77% isodose line in 1–3 sessions. Radiosurgery is usually contraindicated in hemangioblastomas with a cyst.

Surveillance

Because of the lifetime risk of developing tumors, regular surveillance is needed. Various protocols have been proposed,[58,59] including those by the NIH[38] and the Danish clinical recommendations.[60] The algorithm recommended by the VHL Family Alliance for patients with VHL and at-risk relatives is shown in ► Table 36.6. (Screening at-risk relatives can be stopped at age 60 years if no abnormalities have been detected.)

   Individuals who do not carry the altered gene on DNA testing do not require surveillance.

Prognosis

The lifespan of patients with VHL is decreased (median 49 years). 30–50% die of renal cell Ca (RCC). Metastases from RCC and neurologic complications from cerebellar HGB are the primary causes of death.
   Metastases respond poorly to chemotherapy and XRT.

36

Table 36.6 Health-care provider's surveillance guidelines for patients with or at risk for VHL[a]

Age	Surveillance
Any age	DNA testing for VHL marker is available to identify family members at risk
From conception	inform obstetrician of family history of VHL
From birth	check for neurologic disturbance: nystagmus, strabismus, white pupil... & refer to retinologist for abnormal findings. Newborn hearing screening
1–4 years	Annual: retina exam[b] (especially if positive for VHL mutation). Pediatrician to check for neurologic disturbance (nystagmus, strabismus, white pupil, hearing vision...) and abnormal BP
5–15 years	Annual: • PE[c] including orthostatic blood pressure measurement, exam for neurologic disturbance (as above) and other retinal problems, hearing disturbances, retina exam[b] • test for fractionated metanephrines (p. 940), especially normetanephrine in a "plasma-free metanephrine" blood test or in a 24-hour urine test. If abnormalities detected: abdominal MRI or MIBG scan (p. 940) • abdominal U/S starting at age 8 or earlier if indicated Every 2–3 years: complete audiology exam. Annually if hearing loss, tinnitus or vertigo. If repeated ear infections: thin cut MRI with contrast of the IACs to look for ELST
16 + years	Every 6 months: retina exam[b] Annual: • retina exam[b] • PE (including scrotal exam in males), neuro exam • 24° urine for catecholamines & metanephrines (p. 940). If elevated: abdominal MRI or MIBG scan (p. 940) • quality abdominal U/S (kidneys, pancreas & adrenals) (and at least every other year while not pregnant, abdominal MRI). If abnormal: abdominal MRI or CT (except in pregnancy) Every 2–3 years or if symptoms develop: • MRI without and with contrast on ≥ 1.5 T scanner to look for hemangioblastomas of brain with thin cuts of the posterior fossa with attention to the inner ear/petrous temporal bone to R/O ELST & spine (cervical, thoracic, lumbar). Annually at onset of puberty or before and after pregnancy (only for emergencies during pregnancy) • complete audiology exam. If abnormal, or if tinnitus or vertigo at any time: MRI of IAC to look for ELST
Prior to surgery or childbirth	• blood test or 24° urine for catecholamines & metanephrines (p. 940) to rule out pheochromocytoma

[a]adapted[57]
[b]dilated eye/retinal exam with indirect ophthalmoscope exam by retinologist familiar with VHL
[c]abbreviations: PE = physical exam by physician familiar with VHL, ELST = endolymphatic sac tumor

Resources

Genetic screening for VHL can be done at a few centers. Information for patients and families can be found at www.vhl.org.

36.3.3 Li-Fraumeni syndrome (LFS)

General information

A rare inherited autosomal dominant disorder of children and young adults with multiple tumors, 80% of which are of the following: soft-tissue sarcomas, osteosarcomas, breast cancer, brain tumors and adrenocortical carcinoma.[14] Usually caused by a germline mutation in the TP53 tumor suppressor gene on chromosome 17p13.1 which occurs in ≈ 1 of every 500 to 5000 live births.

Diagnostic criteria

Essential criterion is pathogenic germline alteration (mutation, rearrangement, or partial/complete deletion) in the *TP53* gene.[21]

There are 3 main sets of criteria for recommending *TP53* germline testing for diagnosing Li-Fraumeni-like syndrome: 1) classic criteria (shown below), 2) Birch or Eeles criteria for LFS-like syndromes, and 3) the Chompret criteria.[21]

Classic criteria[61]:
• sarcoma before age 45 years **AND**
• a first degree relative with any cancer before age 45 years **AND**
• a first or second degree relative with any cancer before age 45 years or a sarcoma at any age

Associated CNS tumors

3.5–14% of tumors are found in the CNS.

CNS tumors show a bimodal age distribution: 1) in children (primarily SHH-activated medullo-blastomas, IDH-wildtype high-grade gliomas and choroid plexus carcinomas), and 2) in age 20–40 (primarily IDH-mutant diffuse astrocytic neoplasms).[21]

Prognosis

Medulloblastomas in LFS have a very poor prognosis. Choroid plexus carcinoma in patients with *TP53* mutations fare worse than their sporadic counterparts; likewise for childhood IDH-wildtype astrocytomas occuring in childhood. IDH-mutant astrocytomas in young adults with LFS have similar OS to those without LSF. Close surveillance for tumors is associated with earlier detectection and improved outcomes.

36.3.4 Cowden syndrome

General information

AKA *PTEN* hamartoma tumor syndrome. An autosomal dominant syndrome resulting primarily from pathogenic germline mutations of *PTEN*, manifesting as multiple hamartomas derived from all three germ cell layers, accompanied by a high risk of cancers of the breast, thyroid, endometrium, kidneys and colon. Adult onset of dysplastic cerebellar gangliocytoma (p. 716) (Lhermitte-Duclos disease) is pathognomonic for Cowden syndrome. For diagnostic criteria, see reference.[21]

Subtypes

* Bannayan–Riley–Ruvalcaba syndrome
* Proteus syndrome: fewer than 200 confirmed cases worldwide (many undiagnosed cases are likely, especially when the manifestations are mild)

Prognosis

There is inadquate data as to whether tumors in patients with Cowden syndrome have a different prognosis than the same tumors in non-syndromic patients.

36.3.5 Constitutional mismatch repair deficiency syndrome

General information

Originally called brain tumor polyposis syndrome 1 (BTP1) as part of "Turcot syndrome" (both terms now obsolete).

An autosomal recessive syndrome caused by biallelic germline mutations in one of four mismatch repair genes, producing a predisposition to ultrahypermutated malignant gliomas, CNS embryonal tumors, in addition to other systemic cancers of childhood and early adulthood. A different condition (Lynch syndrome 1) is caused by heterozygous carriers.

> 90% present with café-au-lait macules and other dermatologic abnormalities.[14]

36.3.6 Familial adenomatous polyposis 1 (FAP1)

General information

FAP1 is an autosomal dominant syndrome resulting from an inactivating germline sequence variant in the tumor suppressor gene *APC* predisposing to gastrointestinal tumors (benign colonic polyposis and colorectal carcinomas). Patients with FAP1 who also develop a primary brain tumor are considered brain tumor polyposis syndrome 2 (BTP2) (see following).

Brain tumor polyposis syndrome 2 (BTP2)

Originally part of the now obsolete "Turcot syndrome." Extremely rare subset of FAP1 patients. The only primary brain tumor unequivocally associated with BPT2 is medulloblastoma WNT-activated). Other non-CNS cancers include osteomas, thyroid cancer, and hepatoblastoma. The OS and PFS of patients with BTP2 associated MDB WNT-activated appears similar to sporadic cases, which is excellent.

36

36.3.7 Carney complex (AKA Carney syndrome)

Obsolete terms include LAMB syndrome.

A rare (> 700 individuals worldwide[62]) autosomal dominant disorder which in > 70% is associated with a heterozygous inactivating variant in the *PRKAR1A* gene which codes for the type 1α regulatory (R1α) subunit of PKA (this variant has ≈ 100% penetrance). It is typified by cardiac myxomas, endocrine tumors or overactivity, schwannomas and pigmented skin lesions.[62] The most common endocrine tumor is primary pigmented nodular adrenocortical disease (PPNAD), which often produces ACTH-independent hypercortisolism (Cushing syndrome).

The primary nervous system association is the potentially lethal malignant melanotic nerve sheath tumor (p.773) (MMNST) which occurs in 8-10% of adults. A somatotroph pituitary adenoma (p.870) is found in 10-18%.[21]

Mean life expectancy is 50 years due to cardiac myxoma, MMNST, surgical complications, and other cancers.

36.3.8 Sturge–Weber syndrome

General information

Key concepts

- cardinal signs: 1) localized cerebral cortical atrophy and calcifications, 2) ipsilateral port-wine facial nevus in the distribution of the ophthalmic branch of the trigeminal nerve (V1)
- contralateral seizures usually present
- caused by somatic mosaicism, not a germline mutation
- skull x-rays classically show "tram-tracking" (double parallel lines) from cortical calcifications

AKA encephalotrigeminal angiomatosis AKA encephalofacial angiomatosis. Sturge-Weber syndrome (SWS) is a rare, congenital neurocutaneous disorder involving the brain, skin, and eye. It is not hereditary and is generally not associated with brain tumors. SWS consists of:
1. cardinal features:
   a) localized cerebral cortical atrophy and calcifications (especially cortical layers 2 and 3, with a predilection for the occipital and posterior parietal lobes):
      - calcifications appear as curvilinear double parallel lines ("tram-tracking") on plain X-rays
      - cortical atrophy usually causes contralateral hemiparesis, hemiatrophy, and homonymous hemianopia (with occipital lobe involvement)
   b) ipsilateral port-wine facial nevus (nevus flammeus) (a cutaneous capillary malformation) usually in the distribution of the 1st division of the trigeminal nerve (V1) typically involving the forehead and/or eyelid (rarely bilateral): not always present, alternatively sometimes in V2 or V3 regions[63]
2. other findings that may be present:
   a) ipsilateral exophthalmos and/or glaucoma, coloboma of the iris
   b) oculomeningeal capillary hemangioma
   c) cerebral venous malformation (leptomeningeal angiomatosis)[63]
   d) convulsive seizures: contralateral to the facial nevus and cortical atrophy. Present in most patients starting in infancy
   e) retinal angiomas
   f) endocrinopathies: growth hormone deficiency is more common in SWS patients. For suspected or confirmed SWS, screen for this in children ≥ age 2 years by measuring serum IGF-1 (p.881)

Diagnostic criteria

Diagnosis is made based on having 2 out of 3 of the following:
- facial port-wine birthmark
- increased intraocular pressure
- leptomeningeal angiomatosis

Patients with only leptomeningeal angiomatosis and no skin or eye involvement are considered to have the intracranial varient of SWS.[63]

▶ **Other clinical aspects.** Only 8–20% of patients with facial port-wine birthmarks (with or without ocular involvement) develop neurologic symptoms. Those with port-wine stain only in V2 and V3 have a lower risk of developing symptoms of SWS, and those with bilateral V1 birthmarks have a higher risk (≈ 35%).

Genetics

In contrast to other phakomatoses, SWS is not hereditary. It is caused by somatic mosaicism (two genetically distinct populations of cells brought about by a post-zygotic mutation). A single nucleotide substitution in the *GNAQ* gene on chromosome 9q21 that occurs early after conception in utero is found in affected tissues but not in unaffected tissues.[64]

Epidemiology

Incidence is ≈ 1 in 20,000 to 50,000 live births.[65]

Treatment

Treatment is supportive.
    Seizures: frequent and protracted seizures exacerbate the neurologic damage.
* antiseizure medications are the first-line treatment
    1. oxcarbazepine is a common initial drug. Side effects include central hypothyroidism, especially in girls
    2. levetiracetam and topiramate are alternatives
* refractory seizures may require lobectomy or hemispherectomy. Options include: functional hemispherectomy,[66] anatomic hemispherectomy, and hemispherotomy

Skin lesions: laser treatment (currently, flashlamp-pumped PDL is favored) can lighten the birthmark. It may also reduce hypertrophy of soft and bony tissue.
    Endocrinopathies: growth hormone deficiency can be replaced; however, there may be a risk of increasing seizures.[63]
    XRT: complications are common and benefits are lacking.

36.3.9 Neurocutaneous melanosis (NCM)

Background

1. a rare, congenital, nonheritable phakomatosis that usually presents before age 2 years in which large or numerous congenital melanocytic nevi are associated with benign and/or malignant melanocytic tumors of the leptomeninges[67]
2. pathogenesis: neuroectodermal defect during morphogenesis involving melanoblasts of skin and pia mater originating from neural crest cells[67]

Clinical features

1. two-thirds of patients with NCM have giant congenital melanocytic nevi[67]: pigmented nevi that are large, hairy, or both. (The chances that nevi represents NCM is higher when the nevi are located on head, posterior neck, or paravertebral area)
2. one-third have numerous lesions without a single giant lesion[67]
3. virtually all have large cutaneous melanocytic (pigmented) nevi located on the posterior torso[68]
4. neurologic manifestations: usually before age 2 years. Signs of intracranial hypertension (lethargy, vomiting…), focal seizures, motor deficits or aphasia[67]
5. hydrocephalus: in almost 66%. Usually due to obstruction of CSF flow or reduced absorption as a result of thickened leptomeninges[67]

Clinical diagnostic criteria

See reference.[69]
1. large or multiple congenital melanocytic nevi with meningeal melanosis or melanoma
2. absence of cutaneous melanoma, except in patients with benign meningeal lesions (i.e., must rule out meningeal metastases from cutaneous melanoma)
3. no evidence of meningeal melanoma, except in patients with benign cutaneous lesions

36

Associated conditions

NCM is sometimes associated with
1. neurocutaneous disorders[67]
   a) Sturge-Weber syndrome (p. 652)
   b) von Recklinghausen's neurofibromatosis (NF1) (p. 638)
2. posterior fossa cystic malformations: e.g., Dandy Walker malformation (p. 270); occurs in up to 10%. These cases have worse prognosis due to malignant transformation[67]
3. intraspinal lipoma and syringomyelia[67]

Diagnostic testing

1. MRI: T1 and T2 signal shortening produced by melanin. IV gadolinium may demonstrate enhancement of tumor-infiltrated meninges[67]
2. histological exam of CNS lesions shows leptomeningeal melanosis (benign) which develops from the melanocytes of the pia matter. Melanoma (malignant) occurs in 40–62% of cases but distinction has little prognostic significance because of the poor outcome of the symptomatic NCM patient even in the absence of melanoma[67]

Management

The benefit of resecting skin lesions is questionable in the presence of leptomeningeal lesions.[70] NCM appears refractory to radiation therapy and chemotherapy[70]
   Neurosurgical involvement is usually limited to[69]:
1. shunting for hydrocephalus
2. palliative operative decompression if early in the course
3. biopsy for tissue diagnosis in questionable cases

Prognosis

1. when neurological signs are present, prognosis is poor regardless of whether or not malignancy is present
2. > 50% of patients die within 3 years after the first neurologic manifestation[67]

References

[1] Burger PC, Scheithauer BW. AFIP Atlas of Tumor Pathology. Fourth series. Fascicle 7: Tumors of the Central Nervous System. Washington, D.C.: Armed Forces Institute of Pathology; 2007

[2] Riccardi VM. von Recklinghausen Neurofibromatosis. N Engl J Med. 1981; 305:1617–1627

[3] Friedman JM, Adam MP, Ardinger HH, et al. Neurofibromatosis 1. Seattle, WA 1998

[4] Ferner RE, Gutmann DH. Neurofibromatosis type 1 (NF1): diagnosis and management. Handb Clin Neurol. 2013; 115:939–955

[5] National Institutes of Health Consensus Development Conference. Neurofibromatosis: Conference Statement. Arch Neurol. 1988; 45:575–578

[6] Packer RJ, Gutmann DH, Rubenstein A, et al. Plexiform neurofibromas in NF1: toward biologic-based therapy. Neurology. 2002; 58:1461–1470

[7] Sharif S, Moran A, Huson SM, et al. Women with neurofibromatosis 1 are at a moderately increased risk of developing breast cancer and should be considered for early screening. Journal of Medical Genetics. 2007; 44:481–484

[8] Sevick RJ, Barkovich AJ, Edwards MS, et al. Evolution of white matter lesions in neurofibromatosis type 1: MR findings. AJR. American Journal of Roentgenology. 1992; 159:171–175

[9] Karnes PS. Neurofibromatosis: A Common Neurocutaneous Disorder. Mayo Clinic Proceedings. 1998; 73:1071–1076

[10] Walker L, Thompson D, Easton D, et al. A prospective study of neurofibromatosis type 1 cancer incidence in the UK. British Journal of Cancer. 2006; 95:233–238

[11] Hirbe AC, Gutmann DH. Neurofibromatosis type 1: a multidisciplinary approach to care. Lancet Neurol. 2014; 13:834–843

[12] Anderson MK, Johnson M, Thornburg L, et al. A Review of Selumetinib in the Treatment of Neurofibromatosis Type 1-Related Plexiform Neurofibromas. Ann Pharmacother. 2022; 56:716–726

[13] Martuza RL, Eldridge R. Neurofibromatosis 2: (Bilateral Acoustic Neurofibromatosis). N Engl J Med. 1988; 318:684–688

[14] Louis DN, Ohgaki H, Wiestler OD, et al. WHO classification of tumors of the central nervous system. Lyon, France 2016

[15] Parry DM, Eldridge R, Kaiser-Kupfer MI, et al. Neurofibromatosis 2 (NF2): clinical characteristics of 63 affected individuals and clinical evidence for heterogeneity. American Journal of Medical Genetics. 1994; 52:450–461

[16] Neurofibromatosis. Conference statement. National Institutes of Health Consensus Development Conference. Arch Neurol. 1988; 45:575–578

[17] Evans DG, Pagon RA, Adam MP, et al. Neurofibromatosis 2. Seattle, WA 1998

[18] Smith MJ, Bowers NL, Bulman M, et al. Revisiting neurofibromatosis type 2 diagnostic criteria to exclude LZTR1-related schwannomatosis. Neurology. 2017; 88:87–92

[19] Baser ME, Friedman JM, Joe H, et al. Empirical development of improved diagnostic criteria for neurofibromatosis 2. Genet Med. 2011; 13:576–581

[20] Egelhoff JC, Bates DJ, Ross JS, et al. Spinal MR Findings in Neurofibromatosis Types 1 and 2. American Journal of Neuroradiology. 1992; 13:1071–1077

[21] Bosman FT, Jaffe ES, Lakhani SR, et al. World Health Organization Classification of Tumors series, vol. 6. In: WHO Classification of Tumors Editorial Board (ed.) World Health Organization classification of tumors of the central nervous system. 5th ed. Lyon, France: International Agency for Research on Cancer; 2021

36

[22] Plotkin SR, Blakeley JO, Evans DG, et al. Update from the 2011 International Schwannomatosis Workshop: From genetics to diagnostic criteria. Am J Med Genet A. 2013; 161A:405–416

[23] Antinheimo J, Sankila R, Carpen O, et al. Population-based analysis of sporadic and type 2 neurofibromatosis-associated meningiomas and schwannomas. Neurology. 2000; 54:71–76

[24] Merker VL, Esparza S, Smith MJ, et al. Clinical features of schwannomatosis: a retrospective analysis of 87 patients. Oncologist. 2012; 17:1317–1322

[25] Li P, Zhao F, Zhang J, et al. Clinical features of spinal schwannomas in 65 patients with schwannomatosis compared with 831 with solitary schwannomas and 102 with neurofibromatosis Type 2: a retrospective study at a single institution. J Neurosurg Spine. 2016; 24:145–154

[26] Plotkin SR, Bredella MA, Cai W, et al. Quantitative assessment of whole-body tumor burden in adult patients with neurofibromatosis. PLoS One. 2012; 7. DOI: 10.1371/journal.pone.0035711

[27] Northrup H, Krueger DA, International Tuberous Sclerosis Complex Consensus Group. Tuberous sclerosis complex diagnostic criteria update: recommendations of the 2012 International Tuberous Sclerosis Complex Consensus Conference. Pediatr Neurol. 2013; 49:243–254

[28] Hottinger AF, Khakoo Y. Neurooncology of familial cancer syndromes. Journal of Child Neurology. 2009; 24:1526–1535

[29] Logue LG, Acker RE, Sienko AE. Best cases from the AFIP: angiomyolipomas in tuberous sclerosis. Radiographics. 2003; 23:241–246

[30] Thiele EA. Managing epilepsy in tuberous sclerosis complex. Journal of Child Neurology. 2004; 19:680–686

[31] McLaurin RL, Towbin RB. Tuberous Sclerosis: Diagnostic and Surgical Considerations. Pediat Neurosci. 1985; 12:43–48

[32] Bernauer TA. The radial bands sign. Radiology. 1999; 212:761–762

[33] Franz DN, Agricola K, Mays M, et al. Everolimus for subependymal giant cell astrocytoma: 5-year final analysis. Ann Neurol. 2015. DOI: 10.1002/ana.24523

[34] Shepherd CW, Gomez MR, Lie JT, et al. Causes of death in patients with tuberous sclerosis. Mayo Clin Proc. 1991; 66:792–796

[35] Catapano D, Muscarella LA, Guarnieri V, et al. Hemangioblastomas of central nervous system: molecular genetic analysis and clinical management. Neurosurgery. 2005; 56:1215–21; discussion 1221

[36] Glenn GM, Linehan WM, Hosoe S, et al. Screening for von Hippel-Lindau Disease by DNA Polymorphism Analysis. JAMA. 1992; 267:1226–1231

[37] Wanebo JE, Lonser RR, Glenn GM, et al. The natural history of hemangioblastomas of the central nervous system in patients with von Hippel-Lindau disease. Journal of Neurosurgery. 2003; 98:82–94

[38] Butman JA, Linehan WM, Lonser RR. Neurologic manifestations of von Hippel-Lindau disease. JAMA. 2008; 300:1334–1342

[39] Go RCP, Lamiell JM, Hsia YE, et al. Segregation and Linkage Analysis of von Hippel-Lindau Disease Among 220 Descendents from one Kindred. Am J Human Genet. 1984; 36:131–142

[40] Richards FM, Payne SJ, Zbar B, et al. Molecular analysis of de novo germline mutations in the von Hippel-Lindau disease gene. Hum Mol Genet. 1995; 4:2139–2143

[41] Friedrich CA. Genotype-phenotype correlation in von Hippel-Lindau syndrome. Hum Mol Genet. 2001; 10:763–767

[42] van Leeuwaarde RS, Ahmad S, Links TP, et al. Von Hippel-Lindau Disease. Seattle, WA 2000

[43] Jagannathan J, Lonser RR, Smith R, et al. Surgical management of cerebellar hemangioblastomas in patients with von Hippel-Lindau disease. Journal of Neurosurgery. 2008; 108:210–222

[44] Manski TJ, Heffner DK, Glenn GM, et al. Endolymphatic sac tumors. A source of morbid hearing loss in von Hippel-Lindau disease. JAMA. 1997; 277:1461–1466

[45] Chew EY. Ocular manifestations of von Hippel-Lindau disease: clinical and genetic investigations. Transactions of the American Ophthalmological Society. 2005; 103:495–511

[46] Meyerle CB, Dahr SS, Wetjen NM, et al. Clinical course of retrobulbar hemangioblastomas in von Hippel-Lindau disease. Ophthalmology. 2008; 115:1382–1389

[47] Niemela M, Lemeta S, Summanen P, et al. Long-term prognosis of haemangioblastoma of the CNS: impact of von Hippel-Lindau disease. Acta Neurochirurgica (Wien). 1999; 141:1147–1156

[48] Choyke PL, Glenn GM, Walther MM, et al. Hereditary renal cancers. Radiology. 2003; 226:33–46

[49] Meister M, Choyke P, Anderson C, et al. Radiological evaluation, management, and surveillance of renal masses in Von Hippel-Lindau disease. Clinical Radiology. 2009; 64:589–600

[50] Maher ER, Kaelin WG,Jr. von Hippel-Lindau disease. Medicine. 1997; 76:381–391

[51] Hes FJ, Feldberg MA. Von Hippel-Lindau disease: strategies in early detection (renal-, adrenal-, pancreatic masses). European Radiology. 1999; 9:598–610

[52] Bisceglia M, Galliani CA, Senger C, et al. Renal cystic diseases: a review. Advances in Anatomic Pathology. 2006; 13:26–56

[53] Truong LD, Choi YJ, Shen SS, et al. Renal cystic neoplasms and renal neoplasms associated with cystic renal diseases: pathogenetic and molecular links. Advances in Anatomic Pathology. 2003; 10:135–159

[54] Bradley S, Dumas N, Ludman M, et al. Hereditary renal cell carcinoma associated with von Hippel-Lindau disease: a description of a Nova Scotia cohort. Can Urol Assoc J. 2009; 3:32–36

[55] Moss JM, Choi CY, Adler JR,Jr, et al. Stereotactic radiosurgical treatment of cranial and spinal hemangioblastomas. Neurosurgery. 2009; 65:79–85; discussion 85

[56] Chang SD, Meisel JA, Hancock SL, et al. Treatment of hemangioblastomas in von Hippel-Lindau disease with linear accelerator-based radiosurgery. Neurosurgery. 1998; 43:28–34; discussion 34-5

[57] VHL Alliance. VHLA suggested active surveillance guidelines. 2016. https://www.vhl.org/wp-content/uploads/2017/07/Active-Surveillance-Guidelines.pdf

[58] Constans JP, Meder F, Maiuri F, et al. Posterior fossa hemangioblastomas. Surg Neurol. 1986; 25:269–275

[59] Hes FJ, van der Luijt RB. [Von Hippel-Lindau disease: protocols for diagnosis and periodical clinical monitoring. National Von Hippel-Lindau Disease Working Group]. Ned Tijdschr Geneeskd. 2000; 144:505–509

[60] Poulsen ML, Budtz-Jorgensen E, Bisgaard ML. Surveillance in von Hippel-Lindau disease (vHL). Clinical Genetics. 2009. DOI: 10.1111/j.1399-0004.2009.01281.x

[61] Li FP, Fraumeni JF,Jr, Mulvihill JJ, et al. A cancer family syndrome in twenty-four kindreds. Cancer Res. 1988; 48:5358–5362

[62] Stratakis CA, Raygada M, Adam MP, et al. Carney Complex. Seattle, WA 2003

[63] Bachur CD, Comi AM. Sturge-Weber syndrome. Curr Treat Options Neurol. 2013; 15:607–617

[64] Shirley MD, Tang H, Gallione CJ, et al. Sturge-Weber syndrome and port-wine stains caused by somatic mutation in GNAQ. N Engl J Med. 2013; 368:1971–1979

[65] Comi AM. Update on Sturge-Weber syndrome: diagnosis, treatment, quantitative measures, and controversies. Lymphat Res Biol. 2007; 5:257–264

[66] Schramm J, Kuczaty S, Sassen R, et al. Pediatric functional hemispherectomy: outcome in 92 patients. Acta Neurochir (Wien). 2012; 154:2017–2028

[67] Di Rocco F, Sabatino G, Koutzoglou M, et al. Neurocutaneous melanosis. Child's Nervous System. 2004; 20:23–28

36

[68] DeDavid M, Orlow SJ, Provost N, et al. Neurocutaneous melanosis: clinical features of large congenital melanocytic nevi in patients with manifest central nervous system melanosis. Journal of the American Academy of Dermatology. 1996; 35:529–538

[69] McClelland S,3rd, Charnas LR, SantaCruz KS, et al. Progressive brainstem compression in an infant with neurocutaneous melanosis and Dandy-Walker complex following ventriculoperitoneal shunt placement for hydrocephalus. Case report. Journal of Neurosurgery. 2007; 107:500–503

[70] Mena-Cedillos CA, Valencia-Herrera A M, Arroyo-Pineda AI, et al. Neurocutaneous melanosis in association with the Dandy-Walker complex, complicated by melanoma: report of a case and literature review. Pediatric Dermatology. 2002; 19:237–242

36

37 Adult Diffuse Gliomas

37.1 Incidence

These are the most common primary intra-axial brain tumors. For a list of tumors in this category, see ▶ Table 35.1. With the introduction of new diagnostic categories in the WHO CNS5 in 2021, statistics on incidence and prognosis for some of these tumors will have to wait until enough data is accumulated to reflect the fact that prior studies were unknowingly grouping disparate tumors together.

37.2 Risk factors for diffuse gliomas

The best-established causes for brain tumors are syndromic (p. 637) (familial diseases…) and radiation therapy used to treat other CNS tumors (most of these are IDH wildtype[1]).

▶ **Cell phones and cancer risk.** The following information is excerpted from the National Cancer Institute (NCI) web site.[2]

Concern over cell phones and cancer have arisen because cell phones emit radiofrequency electromagnetic radiation (RF-EMR) and the number of cell phones and duration of use has rapidly increased since their introduction. While ongoing studies continue to look into possible ramifications, a summary of findings to date is presented here.

- brain cancer incidence and mortality have remained stable over the past decade
- in May 2011, the WHO issued a warning of possible cancer risk related to the use of devices that emit nonionizing EMR, such as cellular phones[3]
- the American Cancer Society (ACS) states that the WHO classification means that while RF-EMR could pose some cancer risk, the evidence is not strong enough to be considered causal and further investigation is needed
- the National Institute of Environmental Health (NIEHS) indicates that the weight of current evidence has not conclusively linked cell phone use with any adverse health problems, but that more research is needed
- the US Food and Drug Administration (FDA) commented that the majority of human epidemiologic studies have failed to show a relationship between RF-EMR from cell phones and health problems
- the US Centers for Disease Control (CDC) states that no scientific information definitively answers the question of whether cell phones cause cancer
- the Federal Communications Commission (FCC) concludes that no scientific evidence establishes a causal link between cell phone use and cancer or other illnesses
- the European Commission Scientific Committee on Emerging and Newly Identified Health Risks concluded in 2015 that cell phone RF-EMR exposure did not show an increased risk of brain tumors or other head and neck cancers and that epidemiologic studies do not indicate increased risk for other malignant diseases, including childhood cancer

37.3 General features of gliomas

37.3.1 Neuroradiology

37

Astrocytomas typically arise in white matter (e.g., centrum semiovale) and traverse through white matter tracts (see Spread (p. 658)). See also MR-spectroscopy findings (p. 244).

▶ **CT scan & MRI grading.** Grading gliomas by CT or MRI is imprecise,[4] but may be used as a preliminary assessment (see ▶ Table 37.1). Neuroradiologic grading is *not* applicable to pediatric patients with astrocytomas that are not diffuse astrocytomas (e.g., pilocytic astrocytomas).

▶ **Positron emission tomography (PET) scan.** Astrocytoma, IDH-mutant, grade 2 tumors appear as hypometabolic "cold" spots with fluorodeoxyglucose PET scans. Hypermetabolic "hot" spots suggest grade 3 or 4, and may distinguish the uncommon grade 3 or 4 tumors that do not enhance on MRI from astrocytoma, IDH-mutant, grade 2.

Table 37.1 Grading gliomas by CT or MRI

WHO grade	Typical radiographic findings		Location
astrocytoma, IDH-mutant, grade 2	CT: low density MRI: abnormal signal on T2WI	no enhancement with little or no mass effect	temporal, posterior frontal & anterior parietal lobes
astrocytoma, IDH-mutant, grade 3	complex enhancement[a]		
astrocytoma, IDH-mutant, grade 4	solid enhancement[a]		frontal lobe predilection
glioblastoma, IDH-wildtype	central necrosis with ring enhancement[b]		temporal > parietal > frontal > occipital

[a]some may not enhance. Most glioblastomas enhance, but some rare ones do not.[4,5]
[b]the nonenhancing center may represent necrosis or associated cyst (see Tumor associated cysts (p.658)). The enhancing ring is cellular tumor; however, tumor cells also extend ≥ 15 mm beyond the ring[6]

37.3.2 Spread

Gliomas may spread by the following mechanisms[7] (note: < 10% of recurrent gliomas recur away from the original site[8]):
1. tracking through white matter
   a) corpus callosum (CC)
      • through genu or body of CC → bilateral frontal lobe involvement ("butterfly glioma")
      • through splenium of CC → bilateral parietal or occipital lobes
   b) cerebral peduncles → midbrain involvement
   c) internal capsule → encroachment of basal ganglion tumors into centrum semiovale
   d) uncinate fasciculus → simultaneous frontal and temporal lobe tumors
   e) interthalamic adhesion → bilateral thalamic gliomas
2. CSF pathways (subarachnoid seeding): 10–25% frequency of meningeal and ventricular seeding by high grade gliomas[9]
3. rarely, gliomas may spread systemically

37.3.3 Tumor-associated cysts

Gliomas may have cystic central necrosis, but may also have an associated cyst even without necrosis. When fluid from these cysts is aspirated it can be differentiated from CSF by the fact that it is usually xanthochromic and often clots once removed from the body (unlike e.g., fluid from a chronic subdural). Although they may occur with malignant gliomas, cysts are more commonly associated with pilocytic astrocytomas (p.693).

37.3.4 Molecular biomarker testing for diffuse gliomas

Recommendations for biomarker testing for diffuse gliomas is summarized in ▶ Table 37.2 [10]

37.4 Adult-type diffuse gliomas

37.4.1 Astrocytoma, IDH-mutant (WHO grade 2, 3 or 4) (AIM grades 2-4)

General information

A diffuse astrocytoma with mutation in either the *IDH1* or *IDH2* gene and absence of 1p/19q codeletion. *ATRX* and/or *TP53* mutations are common.

There is a predilection for the supratentorial compartment, usually near or within the frontal lobes (▶ Fig. 37.3).

Most present with seizures. The slower growth of grade 3 & 4 lesions compared to glioblastoma IDH-wildtype may provide more time for normal brain tissue to accommodate to the mass effect and may account for the longer clinical course (16.8 months).

Table 37.2 Biomarker testing recommendations for diffuse gliomas (DG)[10]

Recommendation	Strength of recommendation
• IDH mutational testing must be performed on all DGs	strong
• ATRX status should be assessed in all IDH-mutant DGs unless they show 1p/19q codeletion	strong
• TP53 status should be assessed in all IDH-mutant DGs unless they show 1p/19q codeletion	conditional
• 1p/19q codeletion must be assessed in IDH-mutant DGs unless they show ATRX loss or TP53 mutations	strong
• CDKN2A/B homozygous deletion testing should be performed on IDH-mutant astrocytomas	conditional
• MGMT promoter methylation (p.673) testing should be performed on all GBM, IDH-WT	strong
• for IDH-mutant DGs, MGMT promoter methylation testing may not be necessary	conditional
• TERT promoter mutation testing may be used to provide further support for the diagnosis of oligodendroglioma and IDH-WT GBM	conditional
• for histologic grade 2-3 DGs that are IDH-WT, testing should be performed for whole chromosome 7 gain/whole chromosome 10 loss, EGFR amplification, and TERT promoter mutation to establish the molecular diagnosis of GBM, IDH-WT, grade 4	strong
• H3 K27 M testing must be performed in DGs that involve the midline in the appropriate clinical and pathologic setting	strong
• H3 G34 testing may be performed in pediatric and young adult patients with IDH-WT DGs	conditional
• BRAF mutation testing (V600) may be performed in DGs that are IDH-WT and H3-WT	conditional
• MYB/MYBL1 and FGFR1 testing may be performed in children and young adults with DGs that are histologic grade 2-3 and are IDH-WT and H3-WT	conditional

Abbreviations: ATRX, ATRX chromatin remodeler; BRAF, B-Raf proto-oncogene; CDKN2A, cyclin-dependent kinase inhibitor 2A; CDKN2B, cyclindependent kinase inhibitor 2B; DGs, diffuse gliomas; EGFR, epidermal growth factor; FGFR1, fibroblast growth factor receptor 1; GBM, glioblastoma; H3, histone 3; IDH, isocitrate dehydrogenase; MGMT, O-6-methylguanine-DNA methltyransferase; MYB, MYB proto-oncogene; MYBL1, MYB-like; TERT, telomerase reverse transcriptase; TP53, tumor protein p53; WT, wild-type.

Reprinted from Brat DJ, Aldape K, Bridge JA et al "Molecular Biomarker Testing for the Diagnosis of Diffuse Gliomas: Guideline From the College of American Pathologists in Collaboration With the American Association of Neuropathologists, Association for Molecular Pathology, and Society for Neuro-Oncology" (Arch Pathol Lab Med. 2022;146(5):547-574) with permission from Archives of Pathology & Laboratory Medicine. Copyright 2022. College of American Pathologists.

Diagnostic criteria for astrocytoma, IDH-mutant (AIM)

Diagnostic criteria are shown in ▶ Fig. 37.1.[11]

Subtypes

See reference.[11]

- **astrocytoma, IDH-mutant, grade 2** (AIM grade 2)
  a) well differentiated
  b) lacking histologic features of anaplasia, with low or undetectable mitotic activity, and no microvascular proliferation, no necrosis
  c) no homozygous deletions of CDKN2A* or CDKN2B*
- **astrocytoma, IDH-mutant, grade 3** (AIM grade 3)
  a) focal or dispersed anaplasia
  b) significant mitotic activity
  c) no microvascular proliferation
  d) no necrosis
  e) no homozygous deletions of CDKN2A* or CDKN2B*

37

Astrocytoma, IDH-mutant (AIM)

▷ **ESSENTIAL** ◁

a diffusely infiltrating tumor

AND

IDH1 codon 132 or *IDH2* codon 172 missense mutation

AND

| loss of nuclear *ATRX* expression or *ATRX* mutation | **OR** | exclusion of combined whole-arm deletions of 1p &19q |

▷ **DESIRABLE** ◁

► *TP53* mutation or strong nuclear expression of p53 in > 10% of tumor cells
► methylation profile of astrocytoma, IDH-mutant
► astrocytic differentiation by morphology

Fig. 37.1 Diagnostic criteria for astrocytoma, IDH-mutant. (Modified with permission from WHO Classification of Tumors Editorial Board, (ed.) World Health Organization classification of tumors of the central nervous system. 5th ed. Bosman F T, Jaffe E S, Lakhani S R, et al. (series eds.): World Health Organization Classification of Tumors series, vol. 6. International Agency for Research on Cancer, Lyon, France, 2021.)

- **astrocytoma, IDH-mutant, grade 4**: (AIM grade 4) any combination of:
  a) microvascular proliferation
  b) necrosis
  c) homozygous deletions of *CDKN2A** and/or *CDKN2B**

* AIM with homozygous deletion of *CDKN2A* and/or *CDKN2B* are more aggressive, with shorter OS and are classified as AIM grade 4 regardless of histology.[12,13]

Lower grade AIMs can dedifferentiate to a higher grade (p.662).

► **Ki-67 (MIB-1) index.** It has been suggested that a MIB-1 index (p.632) ≥ 7–9% is indicative of a high-grade tumor. But this can overlap with grade 2 AIM at the low end or grade 4 AIM at the high end, and can vary within the tumor itself. This, together with the variability between observers and institutions precludes using the Ki-67 index as a sole discriminant between grade 2 & 3 or between grade 3 & 4 AIM.[14]

Imaging

AIM grade 2: usually hypodense on CT. Most are hypointense on T1WI MRI, and show high intensity changes on T2WI that extend beyond the tumor volume. See ► Fig. 37.2. Most do not enhance on CT or MRI. Calcifications and cysts may be seen.

AIM grades 2 & 3: may demonstrate **T2-FLAIR mismatch** where high signal areas on T2 may be hypointense on FLAIR.[15]

With higher grade AIM, there tends to be more edema, enhancement and necrosis (suggested by central hypodensity). Unlike their GBM, IDH-wildtype (► Fig. 37.6) counterpart, astrocytoma, IDH-mutant, grade 4 tumors (► Fig. 37.3) tend not to have large areas of central necrosis, are often larger at diagnosis, and have less perilesional edema.

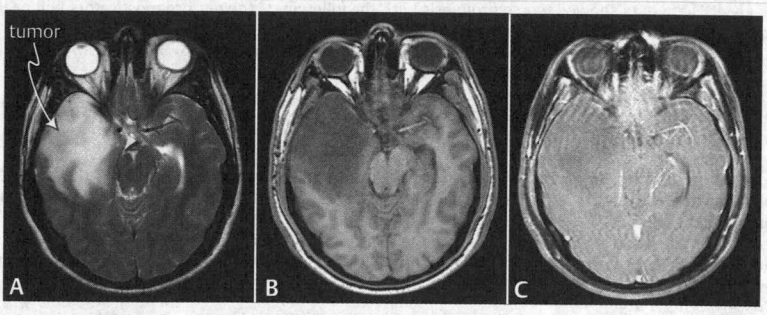

Fig. 37.2 Astrocytoma, IDH-mutant, grade 2 of the right temporal lobe.
Image: axial brain MRI, A: T2, B: T1, C: T1 with contrast.
White matter changes can be seen extending back from the temporal tip on the T2 image (A). Tumor is low intensity on the T1 image (B), and does not enhance with gadolinium contrast (C). The tumor is causing mass effect with compression of the right midbrain (*yellow arrowhead*), which could progress to uncal herniation.

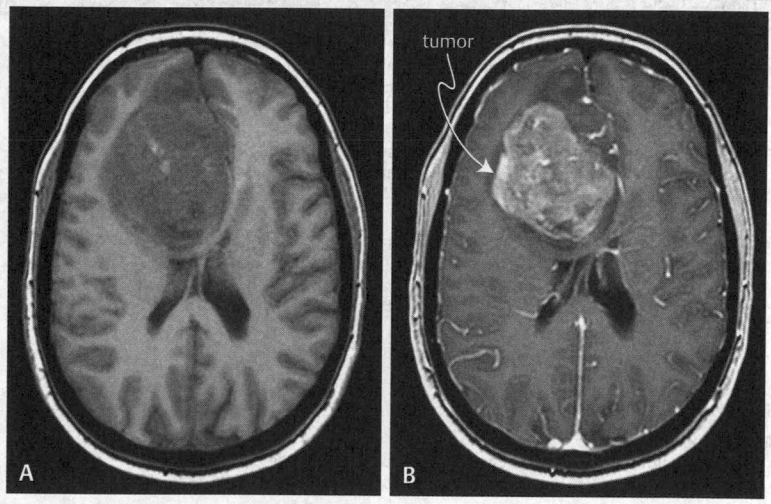

Fig. 37.3 Astrocytoma, IDH-mutant, grade 4 of the right frontal lobe.
Image: axial brain MRI, A: T1 non-contrast, B: T1 with contrast.
Note the location in the frontal lobe, and the lack of central necrosis, both of which are characteristic of astrocytoma, IDH-mutant (compare to GBM, IDH-wildtype, ▶ Fig. 37.6).

37

Treatment

See Treatment for adult-type diffuse infiltrating gliomas (p. 668) for grades 2-4.

Prognosis

One cohort demonstrated a median survival of 10.9 years.[16]

A recent study[13] demonstrated that there was no survival benefit of AIM grade 2 over AIM grade 3 as defined by the WHO CNS5 criteria.[13] They also found that post-operative residual tumor volume and preoperative tumor size were significant prognosticators, and that age was not.

Pre-IDH era data showed worse prognosis with the following[17] (newer prognosticators will need to be identified with known IDH status):

1. age > 40 years (perhaps the most important unfavorable prognosticator)
2. largest tumor diameter ≥ 6 cm
3. tumor crossing the midline
4. neurologic deficit prior to surgery
5. subtotal resection

▶ **Dedifferentiation.** Low-grade AIM are capable of malignant dedifferentiation, and the ultimate behavior of these tumors in adults is usually not benign, as 75% of adult tumors undergo anaplastic progression.

WHO grade 2 astrocytomas tend to undergo malignant transformation more quickly when diagnosed after age 45 years. Once dedifferentiation occurs, median survival is 2–3 years beyond that event (pre-IDH era data[18]).

37.4.2 Oligodendroglioma, IDH mutant and 1p/19q-codeleted (WHO grade 2 or 3) (ODG grade 2 or 3)

General information

Key concepts

- slow growing tumor that frequently presents with seizures
- occur primarily in adults, predilection for the frontal lobes > temporal lobe
- by definition: a diffusely infiltrating glioma with codeletion of *BOTH* chromosome arms 1p *AND* 19q, *AND* mutation of IDH1 *AND/OR* IDH2
- 2 grades: WHO 2 and 3
- histology: classic features of "fried egg" cytoplasm (on permanent pathology) and "chicken wire" vasculature are unreliable. Calcifications are common

Location: > 50% occur in the frontal lobes, followed by temporal, parietal, and occipital lobes.

Diagnostic criteria for oligodendroglioma, IDH mutant and 1p/19q-codeleted (ODG)

Diagnostic criteria are shown in ▶ Fig. 37.4.[11]

Subtypes

See reference.[11]
- **oligodendroglioma, IDH mutant and 1p/19q-codeleted, grade 2** (ODG grade 2)
- **oligodendroglioma, IDH mutant and 1p/19q-codeleted, grade 3** (ODG grade 3)

Grading oligodendroglioma

The criteria for distinguishing grade 2 from grade 3 ODG is not well characterized. WHO grade 2 has a more favorable prognosis.

Grade 3 ODGs usually have several of the following features:
- high cellularity
- marked cytological atypia
- brisk mitotic activity
- pathological microvascular proliferation
- necrosis with or without palisading

Other features that may be helpful in borderline cases are proliferation markers such as Ki-67 (MIB1) and clinical or radiologic evidence of rapid symptomatic growth and contrast enhancement.

The presence of several mitotic figures alone is not diagnostic of grade 3

Oligodendroglioma, IDH mutant and 1p/19q-codeleted

▷ **ESSENTIAL** ◁

a diffusely infiltrating tumor

AND

IDH1 codon 132 or *IDH2* codon 172 missense mutation[a]

AND

combined whole-arm deletions of 1p and 19q

▷ **DESIRABLE** ◁

► DNA methylation profile of oligodendroglioma, IDH-mutant and 1p/19q-codeleted
► retained nuclear expression of ATRX
► *TERT* promoter mutation

[a] IDH mutation analysis may not be required when DNA methylome profiling is performed and unequivocally assigns the tumor to the methylation class oligodendroglioma, IDH-mutant and 1p/19q-codeleted.

Fig. 37.4 Diagnostic criteria for oligodendroglioma, IDH mutant and 1p/19q-codeleted. (Modified with permission from WHO Classification of Tumors Editorial Board, (ed.) World Health Organization classification of tumors of the central nervous system. 5th ed. Bosman F T, Jaffe E S, Lakhani S R, et al. (series eds.): World Health Organization Classification of Tumors series, vol. 6. International Agency for Research on Cancer, Lyon, France, 2021.)

Clinical

Presenting symptoms are nonspecific for ODG. Seizures are the presenting symptoms in ≈ two thirds of cases.[19] Other symptoms are nonspecific for ODG, and are more often related to local mass effect and less commonly to ↑ ICP.

Imaging

Calcifications: seen in 28–60% of ODGs on plain radiographs,[20] and on 90% of CTs.

CT: hypodense to iso-dense.

MRI: poorly demarcated, hypointense on T1 and hyperintense on T2. Fewer than 20% of grade 2 ODG and over 70% of grade 3 ODG enhance with gadolinium.[21]

Histology

Oligodendroglial tumors cells are isomorphic with round nuclei and are slightly larger than normal oligodendrocytes. Tumors show moderate cellularity, often arranged in sheets.

73% of tumors have microscopic calcifications.[22] Isolated tumor cells consistently penetrate largely intact parenchyma; an associated solid tumor component may or may not be present.[23] When a solid portion is present, permanent (paraffin) pathology demonstrates lucent perinuclear halos, giving a "fried egg" or "honeycomb" appearance (which is actually an artifact of *formalin* fixation, and is not present on frozen section which may make diagnosis difficult on frozen). A "chicken-wire" vascular pattern has also been described.[24] These features are variable.

Nuclear atypia and an occasional mitotic figure is compatible with an ODG grade 2 tumor.[25] But extensive mitotic activity, prominent microvascular proliferation and spontaneous necrosis are indications of anaplasia corresponding to an oligodendroglioma, IDH-mutant 1p/19q codeleted (ODG) grade 3.

37

16% of hemispheric ODGs are *cystic*[22] (cysts generally form from coalescence of microcysts from microhemorrhages, unlike astrocytomas, which actively secrete fluid).

GFAP staining: Since most ODGs contain microtubules instead of glial filaments,[26] ODGs usually do not stain for GFAP (p. 631), although some do.[27]

CSF metastases

Metastases reportedly occur in 8–14%, mainly as a microscopic finding,[28] but 1% may be a more realistic estimate.[20] Symptomatic spinal metastases (drop mets) are even more uncommon.[28]

Treatment

See Treatment for adult-type diffuse infiltrating gliomas grades 2-4 (p. 668).

Prognosis

Median survival with ODG, IDH-mutant & 1p/19q codeletion is 8 years.[29]

Codeletion of 1p/19q by itself is also associated with longer median survival[30,31] compared to 6.4 years with astrocytoma, IDH mutant.

ODG grade 2 is an independent favorable prognosticator compared to ODG grade 3.

37.4.3 Glioblastoma, IDH-wildtype (WHO grade 4) (GBM)

General information

The term "glioblastoma *multiforme*" is obsolete,[32] although the abbreviation "GBM" persists. This tumor arises de novo, without any identifiable lower grade precursor and was formerly called "primary glioblastoma". All GBM are now, by definition, IDH-wildtype, and are WHO CNS5 grade 4.[11] The putative cell of origin of GBM is a neural precursor cell in the subventricular zone.[33]

Glioblastoma accounts for 14% of primary brain tumors, and is the most common adult *malignant* primary brain tumor (comprising 49% of them).[34] It is also the most lethal. It primarily affects older adults (mean age at diagnosis ≈ 62 years) with a peak incidence between 55-85 years of age. There is a male predominance of 1.6:1 in the U.S.[34]

GBM constitutes only 3% of pediatric brain tumors.

Infratentorial GBMs are rare, and often represent subarachnoid dissemination of a supratentorial GBM.[35]

Diagnostic criteria for glioblastoma, IDH-wildtype

Diagnostic criteria are shown in ▶ Fig. 37.5.[11]

Subtypes

See reference.[11]
- **giant cell glioblastoma** (p. 665)
- **gliosarcoma** (p. 665)
- **epithelioid glioblastoma** (p. 666)

Histopathology

▶ **Histology.** Glioblastomas are typicaly infiltrating, highly cellular tumors of poorly differentiated astrocytes with nuclear atypia, cellular pleomorphism, with marked mitotic activity. Characteristic findings include microvascular proliferation and/or necrosis with or without perinecrotic pseudopalisading. As the "multiforme" part of the obsolete term "gliobastoma mutiforme" implies, the histopathology of the tumor is highly variable. This feature may make it difficult to establish a reliable diagnosis with small specimens (e.g., needle biopsy).

Cell density is highest in the ring enhancing portion of the tumor, as viable cells may not be found in the necrtotic center.

▶ **Glial fibrillary acidic protein (GFAP).** Most astrocytomas stain positive for GFAP. Astrocytomas that may not stain GFAP positive: some poorly differentiated gliomas, tumors that have a paucity of fibrillary astrocytes (some of these tumors used to be called gemistocytic astrocytomas), since fibrillary astrocytes are required for a positive stain.

Glioblastoma

▷ ESSENTIAL ◁

a diffusely infiltrating astrocytic glioma

AND

IDH-wildtype and H3-wildtype

AND

one or more of the following:
- microvascular proliferation
- necrosis (with or without pseudopalisading)
- TERT promoter mutation (occurs in 72%)
- EGFR gene amplification (occurs in 35%)
- +7/−10 chromosome copy-number alterations

▷ DESIRABLE ◁

► DNA methylation profile of glioblastoma, IDH-wildtype

Fig. 37.5 Diagnostic criteria for glioblastoma, IDH-wildtype. (Modified with permission from WHO Classification of Tumors Editorial Board, (ed.) World Health Organization classification of tumors of the central nervous system. 5th ed. Bosman F T, Jaffe E S, Lakhani S R, et al. (series eds.): World Health Organization Classification of Tumors series, vol. 6. International Agency for Research on Cancer, Lyon, France, 2021.)

Tumor location

These tumors tend to favor the deep white matter of the temporal and parietal lobes (► Fig. 37.6) with frequency of locations shown in ► Table 37.3. Spinal cord or cerebellar involvement are rare.

Neuroradiology

IDH-wildtype GBMs tend to have a large area of central necrosis, which produces a ring-enhancement pattern on contrast CT or MRI (► Fig. 37.6) (unlike astrocytoma, IDH-mutant tumors which tend not to have central necrosis (► Fig. 37.3)).

Subtypes of glioblastoma, IDH-wildtype

Giant cell glioblastoma (WHO grade 4)

A rare variant of IDH-wildtype GBM comprising < 1% of glioblastomas. Histology features bizarre, multinucleated giant cells and, in some cases, abundant reticulin network.

Tends to develop in younger patients (mean age = 51 years) than classic GBM IDH-wildtype (62 years).

As with GBM IDH-wildtype, these tumors appear to arise de novo with no known precursor.

Mutations of TP53 (in 75–90%) and PTEN (in 33%) are characteristic.

Gliosarcoma (WHO grade 4)

A rare variant of IDH-wildtype GBM, comprising 2–8% of GBMs. Histology features a biphasic tissue pattern consisting of areas of glial differentiation alternating with areas of mesenchymal differentiation.

May arise de novo, or can develop following treatment of a GBM. May also appear in conjunction with ependymoma (ependymosarcoma) and oligodendroglioma (oligosarcoma).

37

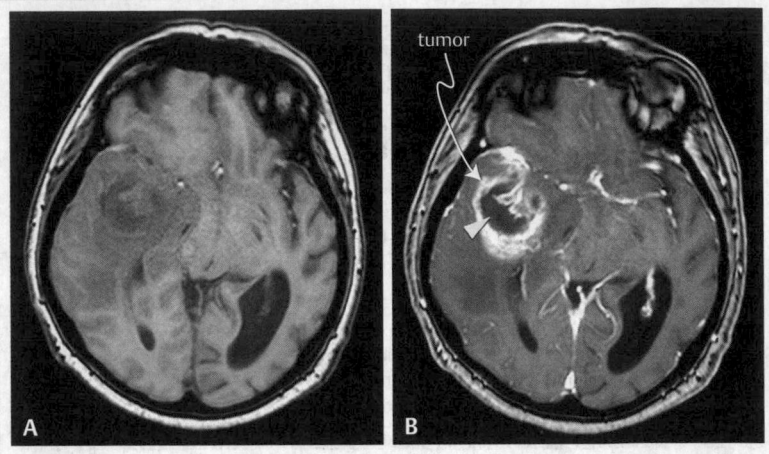

Fig. 37.6 Glioblastoma, IDH-wildtype of the right temporal lobe.
Image: axial brain MRI, A: T1 non-contrast, B: T1 with contrast.
Note the location in the temporal lobe, and the area of central necrosis (dark area indicated by *yellow arrowhead*) characteristic of GBM, IDH-wildtype.

Table 37.3 Location of glioblastoma IDH-wildtype tumors

Location	%
temporal	31
parietal	24
frontal	23
occipital	16

Gliosarcomas that are predominantly sarcomatous may enhance homogeneously and can mimic a meningioma.

Epithelioid glioblastoma (WHO grade 4)
A subtype of GBM IDH-wildtype featuring closely spaced epithelioid cells, as well as some rhabdoid cells, in addition to the characteristic GBM findings of mitoses, microvascular proliferation, and necrosis.

Affects young adults and children, with a predilection for the cerebellum and diencephalon.

Molecular genetics are notable for a higher incidence (50%) of BRAF V600E mutation.

Treatment
See Treatment for adult-type diffuse infiltrating gliomas (p.668) for grades 2–4.

Prognosis for high grade diffuse gliomas (WHO grades 3 & 4)
Univariate analysis[36] shows improved prognosis with the following:
1. preoperative performance status: e.g., Karnofsky score (KPS) (p.1640) ≥ 80
2. age: younger age is consistently found to be a very significant prognosticator (possibly in part because it is overrepresented with secondary GBM). Patients < 45 years in this study fared better
3. IDH1 mutation
4. methylation of MGMT promoter gene

Survival based on MGMT promotor gene methylation (p.673) (▶ Table 37.4)[37]

37

Table 37.4 Survival with GBM based on MGMT promotor gene status[37]

	MGMT promoter gene	
	Unmethylated	Methylated
Median OS (months)	12.2	18.2
2-year survival	7.8%	34.1%

Median overall survival among 206 patients: MGMT promoter gene methylation positive patients treated with temozolomide + RT was 21.7 months, RT only 15.3 months; no survival difference between treatments in patients with unmethylated MGMT.

Recursive partitioning analysis (RPA) with grade 4 diffuse glioma: RPA has been used to classify groups with distinct differences in survival. This is useful for refining stratification and phase III study design and can determine which patient subsets will likely benefit from specific treatments (and which may be spared unnecessary treatment).[38,39] RPA identified 3 classes shown in ▶ Table 37.5. To read this table, each RPA class can have more than one combination of characteristics to qualify, and each set of characteristics is a row in that class. Caveats for this particular analysis: only IDH1 mutations were assayed (IDH2 mutations are rare in GBM but were not included). There are some implications that appear contradictory (e.g., Class II patients with IDH-wildtype could have GTR or PR/biopsy and end up with the same prognosis).

The European Nomogram GBM Calculator[40]: http://www.eortc.be/tools/gbmcalculator. Data from randomized trials by EORTC and NCIC analyzed for the prediction of survival of GBM patients (based on factors such as WHO performance status, mini mental exam score...) which is updated periodically.

Table 37.5 recursive partitioning analysis (RPA) model of survival with AIM grade 4 or GBM[38,39]

RPA class	n	Median survival (months)	5-year survival	Characteristic				
				MGMT gene	IDH1 gene	Surgery	Age (years)	KPS
I	126	58.5 (range: 40.7–76.3)	13%	methyl	mut			
				methyl	wt	GTR		≥ 90
II	483	21 (range: 18.6–23.3)	3.8%	methyl	wt	GTR		< 90
				methyl	wt	PR/biopsy		
				unmeth		GTR	≥ 50	
				unmeth			< 50	
III	202	14.3 (range: 12.4-16.1)	0	unmeth		PR/biopsy	≥ 50	

Abbreviations: methyl = methylated MGMT promoter gene; unmeth = unmethylated; mut = IDH1 mutated; wt = wildtype; KPS = Karnofsky score (KPS) (p. 1640) at presentation; GTR = gross total resection; PR/biopsy = partial resection or biopsy.

37.4.4 Multiple gliomas

Discussion of multiple gliomatous masses has to acknowledge the concept that a diffuse glioma is an infiltrative disease. Some terms are probably artificial. The term gliomatosis cerebri has been abandoned. Widespread brain invasion involving ≥ 3 lobes, frequently with bilateral involvement and often with posterior fossa extension, is considered a special pattern of spread within several diffuse glioma subtypes.

0.5–35% of GBM are multiple

1. multifocal glioblastomas have contiguous pathways of spread by one of the mechanisms previously described (see above (p.658))
2. multiple primary gliomas: some of the following terms are inconsistently used interchangeably: "multicentric," "multifocal," and "multiple." Reported range of occurrence is 2–20% of gliomas[41,42] (lower end of range ≈ 2–4% is probably more accurate; the higher end of the range is probably accounted for by infiltrative extension[43 (p 3117)])
   a) commonly associated with neurofibromatosis and tuberous sclerosis
   b) rarely associated with multiple sclerosis and progressive multifocal leukoencephalopathy
3. meningeal gliomatosis: dissemination of glioma throughout the CSF, similar to carcinomatous meningitis (p.920). Occurs in up to 20% of autopsies on patients with high-grade gliomas. May

37

present with cranial neuropathies, radiculopathies, myelopathy, dementia, and/or communicating hydrocephalus

▶ **Treatment considerations for multiple gliomas.** There is little data available. In a nonrandomized study of 25 patients with multifocal glioma,[44] the 16 patients who underwent debulking did better than the 9 who did not. However, there was significant selection bias in choosing patients suitable for craniotomy.

Biopsy is generally required/recommended to confirm the diagnosis.

Σ: Treatment options with multiple gliomatous masses

Once the diagnosis of multiple gliomatous masses has been ascertained, local therapies (e.g., surgery, interstitial radiation...) are impractical. Whole brain radiation and possibly chemotherapy are indicated. An exception would be to consider debulking a tumor that threatens herniation in a patient deteriorating from mass effect (other conditions such as anticipated length of survival and quality of life would need to be factored in to the decision to operate).

37.5 Treatment for adult-type diffuse gliomas

37.5.1 General information

Tumors included in this section

- astrocytoma, IDH-mutant, grades 2–4 (AIM grades 2-4)
- oligodendroglioma, IDH mutant and 1p/19q-codeleted, grades 2 & 3 (ODG grades 2 & 3)
- glioblastoma, IDH-wildtype (GBM) (all are grade 4)

Initial management

When confronted with an adult with imaging studies suggestive of a diffuse (infiltrating) glioma, see evaluation and initial management (p.626) as outlined for brain tumors in general.

Clinical trials

Eligible patients should be considered for available clinical trials.

37.5.2 Surgical intervention for adult-type diffuse gliomas

General information

Surgical intervention (cytoreduction or biopsy) is indicated for almost all tumors suspected of being diffuse gliomas. Surgery alone is never curative for these infiltrating lesions where there is no margin between brain and tumor. Aside from biopsy, the objective for cytoreduction is maximal safe resection with the goal of gross total resection (see below for definition) when feasible. When maximal safe resection is anticipated to be severely limited or is not desirable at the time, at a minimum a biopsy (open or needle) for diagnostic, prognostic, and treatment planning purposes should be done since clinical and radiographic data are not definitive.[45] NB: the onset of new postoperative motor or speech deficits reduces OS.[46]

Relative contraindications to surgery

Careful consideration should be exercised in the decision to proceed with surgical debulking (cytoreduction surgery) with the following:

1. extensive dominant lobe high grade glioma
2. lesions with significant bilateral involvement. **Butterfly gliomas** refers to gliomas, typically IDH-wildtype glioblastoma (p.664) (grade 4), that cross into both cerebral hemispheres through the corpus callosum most commonly into frontal (68%) or parietal (8.9%) lobes.[47] Gliomas can also cross through the commissures. These tumors have a worse prognosis than their unilateral counterparts.[48] Debulking surgery for the purpose of reducing oncologic burden for these tumors is controversial, and is often not recommended due to the risk of neurologic deficit (in 32% in one

review, including supplementary motor area syndrome (in 5.1%), motor deficit (4.3%) and abulia (2.5%)[47]) with dubious survival benefit (improved survival at 6 months, but no difference at 12 and 18 months[49]). Limited surgery for large bulky portions of these tumors may be a consideration for reducing ICP and risk of herniation (which may occur if edema becomes a major issue during chemoradiation). Yet, there are advocates for maximal safe resection.[47,48,49] Shunting may be offered for hydrocephalus

3. elderly patients
4. Karnofsky score < 70 (in general, with infiltrating tumors, the neurologic condition on steroids is as good as it is going to get, and surgery rarely improves this)
5. multicentric gliomas
6. patients in poor medical condition

Maximal safe resection – considerations

Maximal safe resection (MSR) is an abstraction. In many cases, maximizing the resection increases the risk of surgery (decreasing the safety), and maximizing safety can mean compromising the extent of resection. It is not possible to know the exact correct stopping point for MSR in every case.

Gross total resection – definition

With diffuse (i.e., infiltrating) tumors, there is no line of demarcation (e.g., a tumor capsule) that separates brain from tumor. Tumor cells can be found beyond the enhancing margins demonstrated on MRI.
Definition of gross total resection (GTR) for diffuse gliomas:
1. lesions that enhance on pre-op imaging (most high-grade (grades 3 & 4) gliomas): complete removal of enhancing portions of the tumor and any nonenhacing portion contained within, as *verified by post-operative contrast imaging* within 48 hours of surgery
2. for nonenhancing lesions (most astrocytoma, IDH-mutant grade 2): removal of high intensity lesion on T2 MRI or very low intensity on T1 MRI, if safe, as *verified on post-operative imaging*[50]

Surgical goals

The objectives of surgery in diffuse astrocytomas are:
1. to obtain adequate tissue for histological and molecular study: can be accomplished with biopsy (open or needle [usually image-guided]) or cytoreductive surgery
2. cytoreduction—maximal safe resection, with a goal of GTR when feasible (see box)
   a) to reduce tumor burden, which facilitates adjuvant therapy (oncologic goal)
   b) to reduce mass effect which, when severe, can threaten herniation and can compress and inhibit adjacent brain tissue that is still capable of functioning
   c) to reduce intracranial pressure (with large lesions)
   d) may reduce peritumoral edema
   e) may reduce seizure frequency[51]
   f) for low grade gliomas, to prevent or delay malignant transformation[52]

NB: Partial resection of a high-grade glioma carries significant risk of postoperative hemorrhage and/or edema (wounded glioma syndrome) with risk of herniation. Furthermore, the benefit of subtotal resection is dubious. Retrospective evidence suggested survival benefits in gross total resection but not with incomplete resection.[53] Therefore, surgical excision should be considered carefully when the goal of gross total removal is not feasible.

37

Greenberg IMHO

A few words about gross total resection
The true effect of extent of resection (EOR) of diffuse gliomas on outcome is not known[54] and will likely never be known. To make the case for improved outcome with greater EOR, published series compare cases with varying degrees of resection. This begs the question: why would there be any patients with subtotal resections (STR) in a series of surgical cases published by experts in the field? A likely possibility that has not been excluded is that the surgery had to be stopped short of complete resection due to, e.g., concerns about neurologic injury to the patient or due to difficulty identifying tumor—and it may be that these tumors are associated with worse outcome by virtue of their location or possibly even differences in biology, and not solely because of extent of resection. It is

acknowledged that there is a strong *association* between EOR and outcome, but the causality has not been established. And it is unlikely that a trial will ever be conducted in which patients are randomized to intentionally leave portions of tumor behind. We have to be satisfied with the proposition that maximizing the extent of resection *likely* increases OS and PFS. But keep in mind the following:
   ★ **Caveat:** the onset of a new postoperative motor or speech deficit reduces OS.[46]

Resection – definitions and goals

▶ **Definitions.** **Extent of resection** (EOR) is reported as the percentage of the original tumor volume that was removed, and should be measured on imaging studies since the estimates made by surgeons based on intra-operative findings are grossly inaccurate. As a metric, EOR fails to communicate the residual tumor burden that requires monitoring and treatment.
   A credible case has been made that **residual tumor volume** (RTV) may be a more critical parameter to measure.[54,55]

▶ **Resection goals.** The extent of tumor removal and (in an inverse relationship) the residual tumor volume on post-op imaging studies[54] have a significant correlation with time to tumor progression and median survival.[56]
   Whenever feasible, gross total resection (p.669) of tumor with preservation of eloquent and critical structures should be the goal. NB: new onset post-operative deficit (motor or language) reduces OS.[46]
   Various threshholds have been quoted for minimal EOR to improve outcome. One study demonstrated that EOR ≥ 97% was *associated* with increased survival time.[57] Another study showed that the minimum required resection to improve OS and PFS in high grade glioma was 70% EOR, and $5 \, cm^3$ RTV.[55]

Technical enhancements at surgery

The extent of resection is limited by the infiltrative nature of diffuse gliomas and their frequent location at or near eloquent brain. The safely of resection may be enhanced using various techniques described below.
   Image-guidance (sometimes called stereotactic surgery) is extremely useful especially for deep tumors or in areas bordering on eloquent brain,[58] and for low-grade diffuse gliomas which may not be readily discernible at the time of surgery.
   Intraoperative MRI may also increase the extent of resection, although this is of questionable benefit depending on how it is used.
   Intraoperative (diagnostic) ultrasound may help identify tissue with altered echogenicity that differs from the normal brain.
   Preoperative mapping functional MRI (fMRI) can localize sensitive areas of brain. Diffusion tensor imaging (DTI) can help localize critical fiber tracts. Mapping can demonstrate when each of these are displaced, that may facilitate preservation. These techniques are even more helpful when merged with image guidance.
   Intraoperative mapping to localize critical structures. The motor strip and primary sensory cortex can be mapped with the patient awake or under anesthesia. Mapping the speech area requires awake craniotomy. A meta-analysis of 8091 patients showed that the use of intraoperative stimulation brain mapping achieved more gross total resection with less late severe neurological deficits, and is especially recommended if eloquent areas are involved.[59] For language function, the extent of resection may be safely increased using speech mapping.[60] Multicentric gliomas, previously considered unresectable, can also be debulked with the aid of awake intraoperative mapping.[61] Despite this advance, the role of surgery remains limited for widespread gliomas or very deep-seated lesions.
   Intraoperative dyes may help distinguish tumor from normal brain and are becoming more widely used primarily for high-grade gliomas. They include indocyanine green (ICG) and 5-aminolevulinic-acid (5-ALA) (Gleolan®).
   5-ALA is metabolized into fluorescent porphyrins, which accumulate in malignant glioma cells. This property permits use of ultraviolet illumination during surgery as an adjunct to visualize the tumor. This has been proven with RCT where use of 5-ALA leads to more complete resection (65% vs. 36%, p < 0.0001), which translates into a higher 6-month progression free survival (41% vs. 21.1%, p = 0.0003) but no effect on OS.[62]

37

37.5.3 Treatment of adult diffuse gliomas grade 2 (dLGG)

Tumors included in this section

These patients may be grouped together as "diffuse low grade gliomas" (dLGG)
- astrocytoma, IDH-mutant, grade 2 (AIM grade 2)
- oligodendroglioma, IDH-mutant, 1p/19q codeleted grade 2 (ODG grade 2)

Treatment options

✖ Caution: if any option is being considered that does not include surgical excision, a biopsy is essential to confirm the diagnosis as 43% of tumors that were thought to be dLGG on imaging turned out to have high grade gliomas.[4])
1. surveillance / "watchful waiting" (p. 627): no tumor specific treatment. Treat symptomatically (i.e., medical control of seizures and/or perilesional edema), and follow serial neurologic exams and imaging studies, with intervention reserved for progression of symptoms or radiographic progression. This has historically been very controversial and subject to biases. A Norwegian group has convincingly shown significantly lower median overall survival in a center favoring the watchful waiting approach (5.8 years) compared to 14.4 years at a center favoring early resection[63,64]
2. radiation: XRT is insufficient as monotherapy. As a post-op adjunct, late effects of radiation on cognition need to be considered in long-term survivors with dLGG
3. chemotherapy: the optimal agent and timing of chemotherapy is not well defined. Temozolamide (TMZ) or PCV improves PFS and OS when added to XRT. TMZ is less toxic than PCV, but is inadequate as monotherapy (at least for ODG[65]) and may induce hypermutation (resistant tumor cells)[66]
4. surgery: see "surgical intervention" above
5. combinations of radiation and chemotherapy, with or without surgery

Management recommendations

There is no Class I data. All studies are either retrospective surveys or prospective cohort series where patients were a selected subset of patients with dLGG. With that understanding,early maximal safe surgical resection is currently the recommended initial step for most grade 2 diffuse gliomas in adults[a,67,68]

Following maximal safe resection in patients with KPS ≥ 60:
- **low-risk patients**—characteristics: age < 40 years and gross total resection.
  Recommendation: routine imaging surveillance (e.g., every 3–6 months)
- **high-risk patients**—characteristics: age > 40 or subtotal resection. Tumor size and neurologic deficit are sometimes taken into consideration.
  Recommendation: options
  ○ XRT followed by PCV (p. 628)[b 69]
  ○ XRT + temozolamide (concurrent or after XRT)[70]
  ○ a period of close monitoring may be considered in select cases

Notes:
[a] more aggressive excision is associated with better outcome[71,72,73] and longer latency to malignant transformation (PFS—progression-free survival).[72] Even with recurrent diffuse astrocytomas, surgical resection is associated with a survival benefit.

[b] RTOG 9802 did not specify how long after XRT the PCV was to be administered.

Surgery for grade 2 diffuse gliomas

See section 37.5.2.

A case for supramaximal resection for dLGG has been made[74] in which intra-operative mapping is used to excise dLGG plus margins, and in carefully selected patients may result in increased tumor excision. The definition of supramaximal is not precise, and further study is needed to prove superior outcomes.[75]

Adjuvant therapy for grade 2 diffuse gliomas

See discussion of low risk vs. high risk patients following surgery (p. 671).

37

▶ **Radiation therapy (XRT).** Early post-op radiotherapy has been debated as an adjunct. It has been shown to prolong median progression-free survival from 3.4 to 5.3 years but does not affect overall survival.[76] Quality of life and cognition were not assessed. Typically given as 54 Gy in fractions of 1.8–2 Gy over 5–6 weeks. In patients with radical tumor resection, early RT did not prolong PFS and is recommended to be deferred until progression. Following incomplete resection, early RT significantly prolongs PFS and disease-specific survival.[77] Two prospective trials found no difference in OS or PFS between different XRT doses (EORTC trial[78]: 45 Gy in 5 weeks vs. 59.4 Gy in 6.6 weeks; Intergroup study[79]: 50.4 vs. 64.8 Gy). Side effects from whole brain XRT (WBXRT) include leukoencephalopathy and cognitive impairment (see Radiation injury and necrosis (p. 1899)). The frequency of side effects may[79] or may not[80] be higher at higher XRT doses.

▶ **Chemotherapy** . Usually reserved for high-risk patients or low-risk patients with tumor progression. RTOG 9802 showed benefit of PCV (p. 628) in PFS and OS in IDH-mutant, grade 2 astrocytomas,[69] but not for IDH-wildtype.

Temozolomide (Temodar®) initially appeared to be effective in progressive AIM grade 2 tumors (off label use).[81]

37.5.4 Treatment of diffuse gliomas, grades 3 & 4

Tumors included in this section

- astrocytoma, IDH mutant grades 3 & 4 (AIM grades 3 & 4)
- oligodendroglioma, IDH-mutant, 1p/19q codeleted grade 3 (ODG grade 3)
- glioblastoma, IDH-wildtype (GBM)

Surgery for newly diagnosed AIM grade 3 & 4 and glioblastoma, IDH-wildtype

See section 37.5.2.

Maximal safe cytoreductive surgery followed by external beam radiation and concurrent temozolomide has become the standard against which other treatments are compared.[82]

Adjuvant therapy for diffuse glioma grades 3 & 4

Stupp regimen
General information
The standard of care for newly diagnosed grade 3 & 4 gliomas is cytoreductive surgery followed by the "Stupp regimen"[82] which consists of concomitant and adjuvant radiotherapy and chemotherapy as detailed below. Chemoradiotherapy is started within six weeks after histological diagnosis. Alkylating agents (the current prototypical drug is temozolomide) are more effective in tumors that are deficient in the DNA repair enzyme, MGMT (see below for details).

Radiotherapy (XRT) in the Stupp regimen
XRT in the Stupp regimen consists of fractionated *focal* radiation at a dose of 2 Gy per fraction once daily five days per week over a period of six weeks, for a total dose of 60 Gy, with a 2–3 cm margin of clinical target volume. This is compared to the previous conventional XRT regiment for malignant gliomas of 50–60 Gy (usually 50 Gy to a margin 2–3 cm greater than the enhanced volume on MRI with a boost to the enhancing volume to bring the total to 60 Gy[83]).

Chemotherapy in the Stupp regimen
Concomitant chemotherapy employs temozolomide (TMZ), an oral alkylating agent that is a prodrug which undergoes rapid non-enzymatic conversion at physiologic pH to the active metabolite monomethyl triazenoimidazole carboxamide (MTIC). The cytotoxic effect of MTIC is associated with alkylation (primarily methylation) of DNA at various sites, including the O^6 and N^7 positions on guanine.

Temozolomide dosing
- initial treatment: 75 mg/m²/day, 7 days per week till the end of XRT
- 4 weeks later, start 6 cycles of *adjuvant* chemotherapy with each cycle consisting of 5 days of TMZ repeated every 28 days
  - first cycle dosing: 150 mg/m²/day
  - subsequent cycles dosing: 200 mg/m²/day

Side effects: Temozolomide may cause myelosuppression. It should not be given unless the neutrophil count is ≥ 1.5 x 10⁹/L and platelet count ≥ 100 x 10⁹/L. For all patients with newly diagnosed high-grade gliomas for concomitant TMZ and radiotherapy, prophylaxis against *Pneumocystis jirovecii* (formerly *P. carinii*) pneumonia is required for the initial 6-week regimen.

Adjuvant monotherapy with TMZ is also associated with malignant transformation in low grade diffuse gliomas on multivariate analysis.[84]

▶ **MGMT transcriptional silencing (epigenetics).** Alkylating chemotherapeutic agents (p. 627) (e.g., nitrosourea or temozolomide) damage DNA by attaching an alkyl group (the smallest of which is a methyl group) to guanine bases forming O^6-methylguanine which results in cell death. **MGMT** (O^6-methylguanine-DNA methyltransferase) is a DNA repair enzyme that specifically removes this cytotoxic alkyl group and restores guanine residues to their native state.[85,86] Compared to normal cells, ≈ 75% of grade 4 AIMs inherently have reduced MGMT activity (while only 36% of GBM, IDH-wildtype have reduced activity), most likely as a result of epigenetic transcriptional gene silencing through hypermethylation of the CpG islands (promoter areas) of the genome that codes for MGMT, located on chromosome 10q26.[87,88]

MGMT activity is an independent prognosticator for response to chemotherapy with alkylating agents. Longer survival is observed with higher grade AIMs that have reduced MGMT activity[37] (MGMT levels < 30 fmol/mg protein respond better to alkylating agents[89]).

The box below summarizes the implications of gene methylation and MGMT activity.

Notes: testing for promoter gene methylation is done by PCR (polymerase chain reaction) which is may need to be sent out to a lab which typically takes 1–2 weeks for results. Cost is in the range of $1000 U.S. Measuring MGMT is faster, but does not always produce reliable results, and requires frozen tumor specimens which may not always be available. Although methylation of > 10% of the promoter gene may be reported as "methylated," it is only when methylation is **> 30%** that the median OS with Temodar increases significantly to 25.2 months compared to 15.2 months for all others.[90] Promoter gene methylation may not be as accurate a predictor of outcome as the mRNA expression product.[89] Analysis of recurrent astrocytomas shows some tumors with methylated MGMT promoter genes may convert to unmethylated following treatment[91] (possibly as a result of Temodar toxicity giving selective advantage to resistant cells).

Σ: Transcriptional silencing of MGMT synthesis

Finding	Comment
Hypermethylation (sometimes reported simply as "methylation") of the MGMT promoter gene	This naturally occurs on chromosome 10q26 of the DNA in 75% of grade 4 AIMs. It usually leads to reduced levels of MGMT activity (see the next row in this table) which becomes very significant at > 30% methylation
Reduced (or undetectable) MGMT activity	MGMT is an enzyme that repairs the damage to DNA caused by alkylating chemotherapy drugs such as temozolomide (Temodar®). Tumors with reduced MGMT levels are more susceptible to cytotoxic effects of temozolomide than nontumor cells which have normal MGMT levels, and are better able to repair the DNA damage. This results in longer patient survival

37

Outcomes with the Stupp regimen

The median survival was 14.6 months with the Stupp regimen compared to 12.1 months with radiotherapy alone, with median survival benefit of 2.1 months. The five-year survival rate was 9.8% for the Stupp regimen in contrast to 1.9%.[92] Regardless of extent of resection and MGMT status, patients receiving the Stupp regimen had longer median survival. Patients with MGMT promoter gene methylation (75% of AIM grade 4 tumors, compare to 36% of GBM IDH-wildtype) had median survival time of 23.4 months compared to 12.6 months in the non-methylated group (see below). In the MGMT unmethylated group, the Stupp regimen only improved median survival from 11.8 months to 12.6 months. Some practitioners extend the adjuvant chemotherapy after the standard six-month regimen until tumor progression is observed; in one study this extended the median survival time from 16.5 months to 24.6 months.[93]

Other adjuvant treatment options for high-grade AIM and GBM

Gliadel® wafer: carmustine (BCNU) 7.7 mg in a 200 mg prolifeprosan 20 hydrophobic polymer carrier (wafer) that can be applied to resection cavity after tumor excision. The wafers are degraded by hydrolysis and the drug is released over 2–3 wks. This exposes the tumor to 113 times the concentration of BCNU compared to IV administration. Following tumor removal, up to 8 of the 1.4 cm × 1 mm (dime-sized) wafers are applied to the tumor resection bed at the time of surgery.

It increases median survival to 13.8 months compared with 11.6 months in placebo groups for newly diagnosed malignant gliomas.[94] It showed no survival benefit for recurrent disease.[95] Side effects: seizures, cerebral edema, healing complications, intracranial infection.

MRI-guided **laser interstitial thermal therapy** (LITT): This may be a consideration for patients needing treatment when surgery is not a consideration and when maximal XRT has already been given, oftentimes in the setting of radiation necrosis.[96]

Focused ultrasound (FUS) may become a non-invasive adjuvant therapy option for some deep situated tumors.[97] Transcranial FUS is not a viable option for tumors near the surface due to the inability to focus the ultrasound beams close to the convexity of the skull.

37.5.5 Response to treatment

Pseudoprogression

Since XRT + temozolomide became part of the standard of care for the treatment of many high grade difuse gliomas, there has been an increase in progressive contrast-enhancing areas on MRI that mimic tumor progression, typically seen ≤ 3 months after treatment. This phenomenon, called pseudoprogression, occurs in up to 28–60% of patients after XRT + temozolomide treatment. Histologically it resembles radiation necrosis and is believed to be associated with tumor kill by radiation. Increased tumor kill with chemotherapy results in more pseudoprogression; therefore it is more common with temozolomide treatment for tumors with methylated MGMT promoter genes (as in astrocytoma, IDH-mutant) (91%) vs. unmethylated (as in glioblastoma, IDH-wildtype) (41%).[98]

Diagnosis: There is no definitive diagnostic test to distinguish pseudoprogression from true progression or from radiation necrosis. Imaging methods that have been tried: MR perfusion, DWI with higher apparent diffusion co-efficient (ADC), MR spectroscopy, and PET have not achieved high sensitivity and specificity. Monitoring with serial MRIs and clinical exams seems to be an effective strategy. Rule of thumb: MRI changes suggestive of GBM recurrence within the first 6 months after treatment with XRT + temozolomide should be assumed to be pseudoprogression as long as it is within the radiation field.

Management: The MRI findings usually improve without treatment.[99] If significantly symptomatic, options to ameliorate symptoms include:

1. corticosteroids
2. bevacizumab (Avastin®): often used to treat radiation necrosis[100]
3. laser interstitial thermal therapy (LITT): as a salvage technique for *radiation necrosis*, LITT facilitated reduction of steroid dependency with stabilization of KPS, QOL and neurocognitive function[101]
4. ✖ hyperbaric oxygen: thus far, only case reports and small non-randomized studies support its use

Pseudoresponse

Gadolinium contrast agents used with MRI produce enhancement in areas where the blood-brain barrier (BBB) is disrupted. Just as pseudoprogression may represent increased enhancement without actual tumor regrowth (see above), agents that stabilize the BBB and thereby reduce enhancement may cause underestimation of tumor load or they may mask enhancement-free progression. This is called **"pseudoresponse"**.[102] It can occur while under treatment with angiogenesis inhibitors (including agents targeting VEGF and VEGF receptors such as bevacizumab). Enhancement may also be reduced by corticosteroids (however, the effect may be variable).

RANO (Response Assessment in Neuro-Oncology) criteria

The MacDonald criteria[103] were widely used to assess response to treatment in high-grade gliomas. However, it relied on contrast enhancment on CT. Enhancement may be affected by many factors (steroids, inflammation, angiogenesis inhibitors, chemotherapy wafers, gene and viral therapies, brachytherapy...), and can therfore produce pseudoprogression or pseudoresponse (see above). As a result, the MacDonald criteria have been superceded by the RANO (Response Assessment in Neuro-Oncology)[104] criteria (▶ Table 37.6).

Table 37.6 Response Assessment in Neuro-Oncology (RANO) criteria for high-grade gliomas[a]

Complete response

Requires all of the following:
1. complete disappearance of all disease (measurable and nonmeasurable) for ≥ 4 weeks
2. no new lesions
3. stable or improved nonenhancing lesions (on T2/FLAIR)
4. patient off corticosteroids (except for physiologic replacement)
5. clinically stable or improved

Patients with only nonmeasurable disease cannot have complete response (stable disease is best possible response)

Partial response

Requires all of the following:
1. (compared to baseline) ≥ 50% decrease of the sum of products of perpendicular diameters of all measurable enhancing lesions for ≥ 4 weeks
2. no progression of nonmeasurable disease
3. no new lesions
4. stable or improved nonenhancing lesions (on T2/FLAIR) on same or lower doses of corticosteroids compared to doses at baseline scan
5. corticosteroid dose at the time of the scan is no greater than dose at time of baseline scan
6. clinically stable or improved

Patients with only nonmeasurable disease cannot have partial response (stable disease is best possible response)

Stable disease

Requires all of the following:
1. does not qualify for complete response, partial response or progression
2. stable nonenhancing lesions (T2/FLAIR) on same or lower doses of corticosteroids compared to doses at baseline scan
3. if steroid dose was increased for new symptoms and signs without confirming progression on imaging, and subsequent imaging shows that the need for increased steroids was due to disease progression, the last scan considered to show stable disease will be the one obtained when the steroid dose was the same as at the baseline scan

Progression

Defined by any of the following:
1. ≥ 25% increase in sum of products of perpendicular diameters enhancing lesions compared with the smallest lesion measurement at either baseline (if no decrease) or best response, on stable or increasing doses of corticosteroids
2. significant increase in nonenhancing lesions (on T2/FLAIR) on equal or increased doses of steroids compared to dose at baseline or best response after initiation of therapy not caused by comorbid events (e.g., XRT, demyelination, ischemic injury, infection, seizures, post-op changes, or other treatment effects...)
3. any new lesion
4. clear clinical deterioration not attributable to causes other than tumor (e.g., seizures, adverse effects of medication, stroke, infection...) or changes in steroid dose
5. failure to return for evaluation due to death or deterioration
6. or clear progression of nonmeasurable disease

[a]see reference[104] for definitions (e.g., measurable and nonmeasurable disease...) and for measurement technique. All lesions (measurable and nonmeasurable) must be assessed using the same technique as baseline imaging.

References

[1] Lopez GY, Van Ziffle J, Onodera C, et al. The genetic landscape of gliomas arising after therapeutic radiation. Acta Neuropathol. 2019; 137:139–150

[2] National Cancer Institute. Cell Phones and Cancer Risk. 2018. https://www.cancer.gov/about-cancer/causes-prevention/risk/radiation/cell-phones-fact-sheet

[3] World Health Organization. Electromagnetic fields and public health: mobile phones. 2011. http://www.who.int/mediacentre/factsheets/fs193/en/

[4] Kondziolka D, Lunsford LD, Martinez AJ. Unreliability of contemporary neurodiagnostic imaging in evaluating suspected adult supratentorial (low-grade) astrocytoma. Journal of Neurosurgery. 1993; 79:533–536

[5] Chamberlain MC, Murovic J, Levin VA. Absence of Contrast Enhancement on CT Brain Scans of Patients with Supratentorial Malignant Gliomas. Neurology. 1988; 38:1371–1373

[6] Greene GM, Hitchon PW, Schelper RL, et al. Diagnostic Yield in CT-Guided Stereotactic Biopsy of Gliomas. Journal of Neurosurgery. 1989; 71:494–497

[7] Scherer HJ. The Forms of Growth in Gliomas and their Practical Significance. Brain. 1940; 63:1–35

[8] Choucair AK, Levin VA, Gutin PH, et al. Development of Multiple Lesions During Radiation Therapy and Chemotherapy. J Neurosurg. 1986; 65:654–658

[9] Erlich SS, Davis RL. Spinal Subarachnoid Metastasis from Primary Intracranial Glioblastoma Multiforme. Cancer. 1978; 42:2854–2864

[10] Brat DJ, Aldape K, Bridge JA, et al. Molecular Biomarker Testing for the Diagnosis of Diffuse Gliomas. Arch Pathol Lab Med. 2022; 146:547–574

[11] Bosman FT, Jaffe ES, Lakhani SR, et al. World Health Organization Classification of Tumors series, vol. 6. In: WHO Classification of Tumors Editorial Board (ed.) World Health Organization

37

classification of tumors of the central nervous system. 5th ed. Lyon, France: International Agency for Research on Cancer; 2021

[12] Brat DJ, Aldape K, Colman H, et al. cIMPACT-NOW update 5: recommended grading criteria and terminologies for IDH-mutant astrocytomas. Acta Neuropathol. 2020; 139:603–608

[13] Carstam L, Corell A, Smits A, et al. WHO Grade Loses Its Prognostic Value in Molecularly Defined Diffuse Lower-Grade Gliomas. Front Oncol. 2021; 11. DOI: 10.3389/fonc.2021.803975

[14] Kleihues P, Louis DN, Scheithauer BW, et al. The WHO classification of tumors of the nervous system. J Neuropathol Exp Neurol. 2002; 61:215–25; discussion 226-9

[15] Patel SH, Poisson LM, Brat DJ, et al. T2-FLAIR Mismatch, an Imaging Biomarker for IDH and 1p/19q Status in Lower-Grade Gliomas: A TCGA/TCIA Project. Clin Cancer Res. 2017; 23:6078–6085

[16] Reuss DE, Mamatjan Y, Schrimpf D, et al. IDH mutant diffuse and anaplastic astrocytomas have similar age at presentation and little difference in survival: a grading problem for WHO. Acta Neuropathol. 2015; 129:867–873

[17] Pignatti F, van den Bent M, Curran D, et al. Prognostic factors for survival in adult patients with cerebral low-grade glioma. Journal of Clinical Oncology. 2002; 20:2076–2084

[18] Shafqat S, Hedley-Whyte ET, Henson JW. Age-Dependent Rate of Anaplastic Transformation in Low-Grade Astrocytoma. Neurology. 1999; 52:867–869

[19] Zetterling M, Berhane L, Alafuzoff I, et al. Prognostic markers for survival in patients with oligodendroglial tumors; a single-institution review of 214 cases. PLoS One. 2017; 12. DOI: 10.1371/journal.pone.0188419

[20] Mork SJ, Lindegaard KF, Halvorsen TB, et al. Oligodendroglioma: Incidence and Biological Behavior in a Defined Population. J Neurosurg. 1985; 63:881–889

[21] Khalid L, Carone M, Dumrongpisutikul N, et al. Imaging characteristics of oligodendrogliomas that predict grade. AJNR Am J Neuroradiol. 2012; 33:852–857

[22] Roberts M, German W. A Long Term Study of Patients with Oligodendrogliomas. J Neurosurg. 1966; 24:697–700

[23] Daumas-Duport C, Varlet P, Tucker M-L, et al. Oligodendrogliomas: Part I - Patterns of Growth, Histological Diagnosis, Clinical and Imaging Correlations: A Study of 153 Cases. J Neurooncol. 1997; 34:37–59

[24] Coons SW, Johnson PC, Pearl DK, et al. The Prognostic Significance of Ki-67 Labeling Indices for Oligodendrogliomas. Neurosurgery. 1997; 41:878–885

[25] Louis DN, Ohgaki H, Wiestler OD, et al. WHO classification of tumors of the central nervous system. Lyon, France 2016

[26] Rutka JT, Murakami M, Dirks PB, et al. Role of Glial Filaments in Cells and Tumors of Glial Origin: A Review. Journal of Neurosurgery. 1997; 87:420–430

[27] Kros JM, Schouten WCD, Janssen PJA, et al. Proliferation of Gemistocytic Cells and Glial Fibrillary Acidic Protein (GFAP)-Positive Oligodendroglial Cells in Gliomas: A MIB-1/GFAP Double Labeling Study. Acta Neuropathol (Berl). 1996; 91:99–103

[28] Elefante A, Peca C, Del Basso De Caro M L, et al. Symptomatic spinal cord metastasis from cerebral oligodendroglioma. Neurol Sci. 2012; 33:609–613

[29] Cancer Genome Atlas Research Network, Brat DJ, Verhaak RG, et al. Comprehensive, Integrative Genomic Analysis of Diffuse Lower-Grade Gliomas. N Engl J Med. 2015; 372:2481–2498

[30] Cairncross JG, Ueki K, Zlatescu MC, et al. Specific Genetic Predictors of Chemotherapeutic Response and Survival in Patients with Anaplastic Oligodendrogliomas. J Natl Cancer Inst. 1998; 90:1473–1479

[31] Smith JS, Perry A, Borell TJ, et al. Alterations of chromosome arms 1p and 19q as predictors of survival in oligodendrogliomas, astrocytomas, and mixed oligoastrocytomas. J Clin Oncol. 2000; 18:636–645

[32] Louis DN, Ohgaki H, Wiestler OD, et al. WHO classification of tumors of the central nervous system. Lyon 2007

[33] Lee JH, Lee JE, Kahng JY, et al. Human glioblastoma arises from subventricular zone cells with low-level driver mutations. Nature. 2018; 560:243–247

[34] Ostrom QT, Cioffi G, Waite K, et al. CBTRUS Statistical Report: Primary Brain and Other Central Nervous System Tumors Diagnosed in the United States in 2014-2018. Neuro Oncol. 2021; 23:iii1–iii105

[35] Kopelson G, Linggood R. Infratentorial Glioblastoma: The Role of Neuraxis Irradiation. International Journal of Radiation Oncology and Biological Physics. 1982; 8:999–1003

[36] Yang P, Zhang W, Wang Y, et al. IDH mutation and MGMT promoter methylation in glioblastoma: results of a prospective registry. Oncotarget. 2015; 6:40896–40906

[37] Hegi ME, Diserens AC, Gorlia T, et al. MGMT gene silencing and benefit from temozolomide in glioblastoma. N Engl J Med. 2005; 352:997–1003

[38] Wee CW, Kim E, Kim N, et al. Novel recursive partitioning analysis classification for newly diagnosed glioblastoma: A multi-institutional study highlighting the MGMT promoter methylation and IDH1 gene mutation status. Radiother Oncol. 2017; 123:106–111

[39] Wee CW, Kim IH, Park CK, et al. Validation of a novel molecular RPA classification in glioblastoma (GBM-molRPA) treated with chemoradiation: A multi-institutional collaborative study. Radiother Oncol. 2018; 129:347–351

[40] Gorlia T, van den Bent MJ, Hegi ME, et al. Nomograms for predicting survival of patients with newly diagnosed glioblastoma: prognostic factor analysis of EORTC and NCIC trial 26981-22981/ CE.3. Lancet Oncol. 2008; 9:29–38

[41] Barnard RO, Geddes JF. The Incidence of Multifocal Cerebral Gliomas: A Histological Study of Large Hemisphere Sections. Cancer. 1987; 60:1519–1531

[42] van Tassel P, Lee Y-Y, Bruner JM. Synchronous and Metachronous Malignant Gliomas: CT Findings. AJNR. 1988; 9:725–732

[43] Harsh GR, Wilson CB, Youmans JR. Neuroepithelial Tumors of the Adult Brain. In: Neurological Surgery. 3rd ed. Philadelphia: W. B. Saunders; 1990:3040–3136

[44] Salvati M, Caroli E, Orlando ER, et al. Multicentric glioma: our experience in 25 patients and critical review of the literature. Neurosurgical Review. 2003; 26:275–279

[45] Berger MS, Apuzzo MLJ. Role of Surgery in Diagnosis and Management. In: Benign Cerebral Glioma. Park Ridge, Illinois: American Association of Neurological Surgeons; 1995:293–307

[46] McGirt MJ, Mukherjee D, Chaichana KL, et al. Association of surgically acquired motor and language deficits on overall survival after resection of glioblastoma multiforme. Neurosurgery. 2009; 65:463–9; discussion 469-70

[47] Palmisciano P, Ferini G, Watanabe G, et al. Gliomas Infiltrating the Corpus Callosum: A Systematic Review of the Literature. Cancers (Basel). 2022; 14. DOI: 10.3390/cancers14102507

[48] Chaichana KL, Jusue-Torres I, Lemos AM, et al. The butterfly effect on glioblastoma: is volumetric extent of resection more effective than biopsy for these tumors? J Neurooncol. 2014; 120:625–634

[49] Chojak R, Kozba-Gosztyla M, Slychan K, et al. Impact of surgical resection of butterfly glioblastoma on survival: a meta-analysis based on comparative studies. Sci Rep. 2021; 11. DOI: 10.1038/s41598-021-93441-z

[50] Kawaguchi T, Sonoda Y, Shibahara I, et al. Impact of gross total resection in patients with WHO

grade III glioma harboring the IDH 1/2 mutation without the 1p/19q co-deletion. J Neurooncol. 2016; 129:505–514

[51] Chang EF, Potts MB, Keles GE, et al. Seizure characteristics and control following resection in 332 patients with low-grade gliomas. J Neurosurg. 2008; 108:227–235

[52] van den Bent MJ, Snijders TJ, Bromberg JE. Current treatment of low grade gliomas. Magazine of European Medical Oncology. 2012; 5:223–227

[53] Kreth FW, Thon N, Simon M, et al. Gross total but not incomplete resection of glioblastoma prolongs survival in the era of radiochemotherapy. Ann Oncol. 2013; 24:3117–3123

[54] Grabowski MM, Recinos PF, Nowacki AS, et al. Residual tumor volume versus extent of resection: predictors of survival after surgery for glioblastoma. J Neurosurg. 2014; 121:1115–1123

[55] Chaichana KL, Jusue-Torres I, Navarro-Ramirez R, et al. Establishing percent resection and residual volume thresholds affecting survival and recurrence for patients with newly diagnosed intracranial glioblastoma. Neuro Oncol. 2014; 16:113–122

[56] Keles GE, Anderson B, Berger MS. The Effect of Extent of Resection on Time to Tumor Progression and Survival in Patients with Glioblastoma Multiforme of the Cerebral Hemisphere. Surgical Neurology. 1999; 52:371–379

[57] Lacroix M, Abi-Said D, Fourney DR, et al. A multivariate analysis of 416 patients with glioblastoma multiforme: prognosis, extent of resection, and survival. J Neurosurg. 2001; 95:190–198

[58] Kelly PJ, Apuzzo MLJ. Role of Stereotaxis in the Management of Low-Grade Intracranial Gliomas. In: Benign Cerebral Glioma. Park Ridge, Illinois: American Association of Neurological Surgeons; 1995:275–292

[59] De Witt Hamer PC, Robles SG, Zwinderman AH, et al. Impact of intraoperative stimulation brain mapping on glioma surgery outcome: a meta-analysis. J Clin Oncol. 2012; 30:2559–2565

[60] De Benedictis A, Moritz-Gasser S, Duffau H. Awake mapping optimizes the extent of resection for low-grade gliomas in eloquent areas. Neurosurgery. 2010; 66:1074–84; discussion 1084

[61] Terakawa Y, Yordanova YN, Tate MC, et al. Surgical management of multicentric diffuse low-grade gliomas: functional and oncological outcomes: clinical article. J Neurosurg. 2013; 118:1169–1175

[62] Stummer W, Pichlmeier U, Meinel T, et al. Fluorescence-guided surgery with 5-aminolevulinic acid for resection of malignant glioma: a randomised controlled multicentre phase III trial. Lancet Oncol. 2006; 7:392–401

[63] Jakola AS, Myrmel KS, Kloster R, et al. Comparison of a strategy favoring early surgical resection vs a strategy favoring watchful waiting in low-grade gliomas. JAMA. 2012; 308:1881–1888

[64] Jakola AS, Skjulsvik AJ, Myrmel KS, et al. Surgical resection versus watchful waiting in low-grade gliomas. Ann Oncol. 2017; 28:1942–1948

[65] Jaeckle KA, Ballman KV, van den Bent M, et al. CODEL: phase III study of RT, RT + TMZ, or TMZ for newly diagnosed 1p/19q codeleted oligodendroglioma. Analysis from the initial study design. Neuro Oncol. 2021; 23:457–467

[66] Yu Y, Villanueva-Meyer J, Grimmer MR, et al. Temozolomide-induced hypermutation is associated with distant recurrence and reduced survival after high-grade transformation of low-grade IDH-mutant gliomas. Neuro Oncol. 2021; 23:1872–1884

[67] Tandon A, Schiff D. Therapeutic decision making in patients with newly diagnosed low grade glioma. Curr Treat Options Oncol. 2014; 15:529–538

[68] Oberheim Bush NA, Chang S. Treatment Strategies for Low-Grade Glioma in Adults. J Oncol Pract. 2016; 12:1235–1241

[69] Bell EH, Zhang P, Shaw EG, et al. Comprehensive Genomic Analysis in NRG Oncology/RTOG 9802: A Phase III Trial of Radiation Versus Radiation Plus Procarbazine, Lomustine (CCNU), and Vincristine

in High-Risk Low-Grade Glioma. J Clin Oncol. 2020; 38:3407–3417

[70] Baumert BG, Hegi ME, van den Bent MJ, et al. Temozolomide chemotherapy versus radiotherapy in high-risk low-grade glioma (EORTC 22033-26033): a randomised, open-label, phase 3 intergroup study. Lancet Oncol. 2016; 17:1521–1532

[71] McGirt MJ, Goldstein IM, Chaichana KL, et al. Extent of surgical resection of malignant astrocytomas of the spinal cord: outcome analysis of 35 patients. Neurosurgery. 2008; 63:55–60; discussion 60-1

[72] Capelle L, Fontaine D, Mandonnet E, et al. Spontaneous and therapeutic prognostic factors in adult hemispheric World Health Organization Grade II gliomas: a series of 1097 cases: clinical article. J Neurosurg. 2013; 118:1157–1168

[73] Shaw EG, Berkey B, Coons SW, et al. Recurrence following neurosurgeon-determined gross-total resection of adult supratentorial low-grade glioma: results of a prospective clinical trial. J Neurosurg. 2008; 109:835–841

[74] Duffau H. A new philosophy in surgery for diffuse low-grade glioma (DLGG): oncological and functional outcomes. Neurochirurgie. 2013; 59:2–8

[75] de Leeuw CN, Vogelbaum MA. Supratotal resection in glioma: a systematic review. Neuro Oncol. 2019; 21:179–188

[76] van den Bent MJ, Afra D, de Witte O, et al. Long-term efficacy of early versus delayed radiotherapy for low-grade astrocytoma and oligodendroglioma in adults: the EORTC 22845 randomised trial. Lancet. 2005; 366:985–990

[77] Hanzely Z, Polgar C, Fodor J, et al. Role of early radiotherapy in the treatment of supratentorial WHO Grade II astrocytomas: long-term results of 97 patients. J Neurooncol. 2003; 63:305–312

[78] Karim ABMF, Maab B, Hatlevoll R, et al. A randomized trial on dose-response in radiation therapy of low-grade cerebral glioma: European Organization for Research and Treatment of Cancer (EORTC) Study 22844. International Journal of Radiation Oncology and Biological Physics. 1996; 36:549–556

[79] Shaw E, Arusell R, Scheithauer B, et al. Prospective randomized trial of low- versus high-dose radiation therapy in adults with supratentorial low-grade glioma: initial report of a North Central Cancer Treatment Group/Radiation Therapy Oncology Group/Eastern Cooperative Oncology Group study. Journal of Clinical Oncology. 2002; 20:2267–2276

[80] Laack NN, Brown PD, Ivnik RJ, et al. Cognitive function after radiotherapy for supratentorial low-grade glioma: a North Central Cancer Treatment Group prospective study. International Journal of Radiation Oncology, Biology, Physics. 2005; 63:1175–1183

[81] Quinn JA, Reardon DA, Friedman AH, et al. Phase II trial of temozolomide in patients with progressive low-grade glioma. J Clin Oncol. 2003; 21:646–651

[82] Stupp R, Mason WP, van den Bent MJ, et al. Radiotherapy plus concomitant and adjuvant temozolomide for glioblastoma. New England Journal of Medicine. 2005; 352:987–996

[83] Narayan P, Olson JJ. Management of anaplastic astrocytoma. Contemporary Neurosurgery. 2001; 23:1–6

[84] Johnson BE, Mazor T, Hong C, et al. Mutational analysis reveals the origin and therapy-driven evolution of recurrent glioma. Science. 2014; 343:189–193

[85] Margison GP, Kleihues P. Chemical carcinogenesis in the nervous system. Preferential accumulation of O6-methylguanine in rat brain deoxyribonucleic acid during repetitive administration of N-methyl-N-nitrosourea. Biochem J. 1975; 148:521–525

[86] Goth R, Rajewsky MF. Persistence of O6-ethylguanine in rat-brain DNA: correlation with nervous system-specific carcinogenesis by ethylnitrosourea. Proc Natl Acad Sci U S A. 1974; 71:639–643

[87] Qian XC, Brent TP. Methylation hot spots in the 5' flanking region denote silencing of the O6-

37

methylguanine-DNA methyltransferase gene. Cancer Res. 1997; 57:3672–3677

[88] Esteller M, Hamilton SR, Burger PC, et al. Inactivation of the DNA repair gene O6-methylguanine-DNA methyltransferase by promoter hypermethylation is a common event in primary human neoplasia. Cancer Res. 1999; 59:793–797

[89] Kreth S, Thon N, Eigenbrod S, et al. O-methylguanine-DNA methyltransferase (MGMT) mRNA expression predicts outcome in malignant glioma independent of MGMT promoter methylation. PLoS One. 2011; 6. DOI: 10.1371/journal.pone.0017156

[90] Brigliadori Giovanni, Foca Flavia, Dall'Agata Monia, et al. Defining the cutoff value of MGMT gene promoter methylation and its predictive capacity in glioblastoma. Journal of Neuro-Oncology. 2016; 128:333–339

[91] Wiewrodt D, Nagel G, Dreimüller N, et al. MGMT in primary and recurrent human glioblastomas after radiation and chemotherapy and comparison with p53 status and clinical outcome. Int J Cancer. 2008; 122:1391–1399

[92] Stupp R, Hegi ME, Mason WP, et al. Effects of radiotherapy with concomitant and adjuvant temozolomide versus radiotherapy alone on survival in glioblastoma in a randomised phase III study: 5-year analysis of the EORTC-NCIC trial. Lancet Oncol. 2009; 10:459–466

[93] Roldan Urgoiti G B, Singh AD, Easaw JC. Extended adjuvant temozolomide for treatment of newly diagnosed glioblastoma multiforme. J Neurooncol. 2012; 108:173–177

[94] Westphal M, Ram Z, Riddle V, et al. Gliadel wafer in initial surgery for malignant glioma: long-term follow-up of a multicenter controlled trial. Acta Neurochir (Wien). 2006; 148:269–75; discussion 275

[95] Hart MG, Grant R, Garside R, et al. Chemotherapy wafers for high grade glioma. Cochrane Database Syst Rev. 2011. DOI: 10.1002/14651858.CD007294. pub2

[96] de Franca SA, Tavares WM, Salinet ASM, et al. Laser interstitial thermal therapy as an adjunct therapy in brain tumors: A meta-analysis and comparison with stereotactic radiotherapy. Surg Neurol Int. 2020; 11. DOI: 10.25259/SNI_152_2020

[97] Bunevicius A, McDannold NJ, Golby AJ. Focused Ultrasound Strategies for Brain Tumor Therapy. Oper Neurosurg (Hagerstown). 2020; 19:9–18

[98] Brandes AA, Tosoni A, Spagnolli F, et al. Disease progression or pseudoprogression after concomitant radiochemotherapy treatment: pitfalls in neurooncology. Neuro Oncol. 2008; 10:361–367

[99] Brandsma D, Stalpers L, Taal W, et al. Clinical features, mechanisms, and management of pseudoprogression in malignant gliomas. Lancet Oncol. 2008; 9:453–461

[100] Liao G, Khan M, Zhao Z, et al. Bevacizumab Treatment of Radiation-Induced Brain Necrosis: A Systematic Review. Front Oncol. 2021; 11. DOI: 10.3389/fonc.2021.593449

[101] Ahluwalia M, Barnett GH, Deng D, et al. Laser ablation after stereotactic radiosurgery: a multicenter prospective study in patients with metastatic brain tumors and radiation necrosis. J Neurosurg. 2018; 130:804–811

[102] Clarke JL, Chang S. Pseudoprogression and pseudoresponse: challenges in brain tumor imaging. Curr Neurol Neurosci Rep. 2009; 9:241–246

[103] Macdonald DR, Cascino TL, Schold SCJr, et al. Response criteria for phase II studies of supratentorial malignant glioma. J Clin Oncol. 1990; 8:1277–1280

[104] Wen PY, Macdonald DR, Reardon DA, et al. Updated response assessment criteria for high-grade gliomas: response assessment in neuro-oncology working group. J Clin Oncol. 2010; 28:1963–1972

38 Pediatric-type Diffuse Tumors

38.1 Pediatric-type diffuse low-grade gliomas

38.1.1 Diffuse astrocytoma, MYB- or MYBL1-altered (CNS grade 1)

General information

See reference.[1]

A diffusely infiltrating astroglial tumor with *MYB* or *MYBL1* gene alterations.

Comprised of monomorphic cells with bland round, ovoid or spindled nuclei.

Typically presents with seizures that are refractory to medication.

Diagnostic criteria for diffuse astrocytoma, MYB- or MYBL1-altered

Diagnostic criteria are shown in ▶ Fig. 38.1.[1]

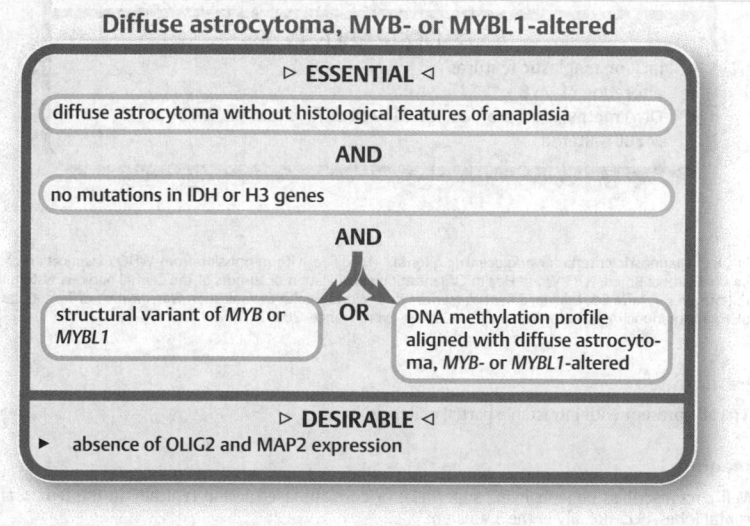

Fig. 38.1 Diagnostic criteria for diffuse astrocytoma, MYB- or MYBL1-altered. (Modified with permission from WHO Classification of Tumors Editorial Board, (ed.) World Health Organization classification of tumors of the central nervous system. 5th ed. Bosman F T, Jaffe E S, Lakhani S R, et al. (series eds.): World Health Organization Classification of Tumors series, vol. 6. International Agency for Research on Cancer, Lyon, France, 2021.)

Subtypes

See reference.[1]

* diffuse astrocytoma, MYB-altered
* diffuse astrocytoma, MYBL1-altered

38.1.2 Angiocentric glioma (WHO grade 1)

General information

A static or slow growing WHO grade 1 tumor primarily of children and young adults characterized by angiocentric pattern of growth, monomorphous bipolar cells and features of ependymal differentiation. Nearly all have *MYB::QKI* gene fusion, and the rest usually have another *MYB* alteration.

38

Behavior is usually indolent, with little change radiographically.

Diagnostic criteria for angiocentric glioma

Diagnostic criteria are shown in ▶ Fig. 38.2.[1]

Angiocentric glioma

▷ ESSENTIAL ◁

glioma with diffuse growth architecture & a focal angiocentric pattern

AND

monomorphic spindled cells with immunophenotypic and/or ultrastructural evidence of astrocytic and ependymal differentiation

▷ DESIRABLE ◁

► lack of anaplastic features
► alteration of MYB
► DNA methylation profile aligned with diffuse glioma, MYB- or MYBL1-altered

---

Fig. 38.2 Diagnostic criteria for angiocentric glioma. (Modified with permission from WHO Classification of Tumors Editorial Board, (ed.) World Health Organization classification of tumors of the central nervous system. 5th ed. Bosman F T, Jaffe E S, Lakhani S R, et al. (series eds.): World Health Organization Classification of Tumors series, vol. 6. International Agency for Research on Cancer, Lyon, France, 2021.)

Presentation

Typically present with intractable partial epilepsy.

Imaging

Well circumscribed nonenhancing superficial or cortical based lesion typically in the temporal or frontal lobes, occasionally in the brainstem.

Treatment

Gross total excision can be achieved in most cases and is usually curative.[2]

38.1.3 Polymorphous low-grade neuroepithelial tumor of the young (PLNTY) (WHO grade 1)

General information

An indolent tumor strongly with diffuse growth patterns, commonly with components resembling oligodendrogliomas, calcifications, CD34 immunoreactivity and MAPK pathway activating genetic abnormalities.

Behavior appears to be consistent with WHO grade 1.

Diagnostic criteria for polymorphous low-grade neuroepithelial tumor of the young

Diagnostic criteria are shown in ▶ Fig. 38.3.[1]

38

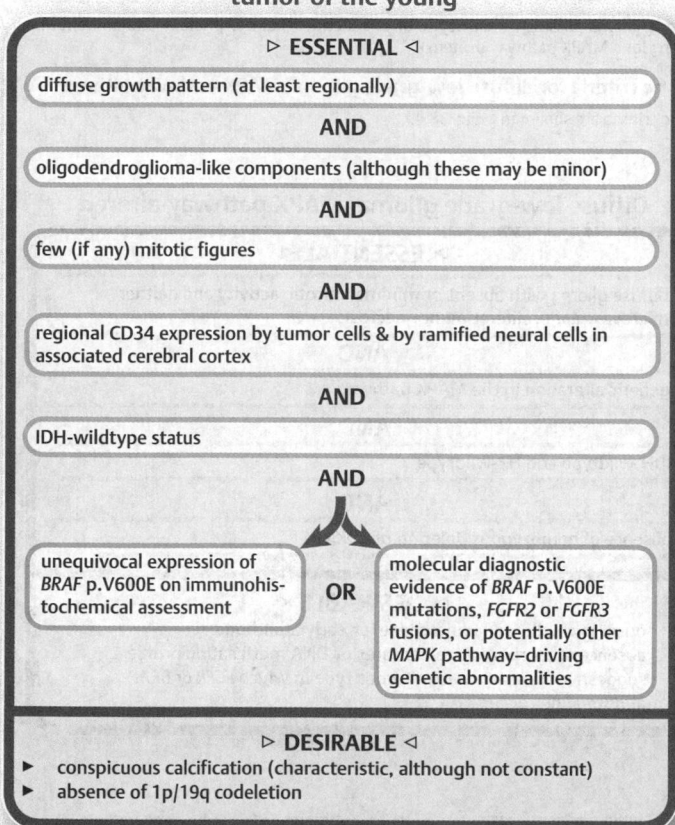

Fig. 38.3 Diagnostic criteria for polymorphous low-grade neuroepithelial tumor of the young. (Modified with permission from WHO Classification of Tumors Editorial Board, (ed.) World Health Organization classification of tumors of the central nervous system. 5th ed. Bosman F T, Jaffe E S, Lakhani S R, et al. (series eds.): World Health Organization Classification of Tumors series, vol. 6. International Agency for Research on Cancer, Lyon, France, 2021.)

38

Presentation

Typically presents with seizures in young patients.

Imaging

Cortical and subcortical components are typical. 80% involve the temporal lobes, usually on the right side.

Treatment

Tumor excision appears to be effective and improves seizures in most cases.[3]

38.1.4 Diffuse low-grade glioma, MAPK pathway-altered (WHO grade 1)

General information

A low-grade glioma possessing astrocytic or oligodendroglial morphology and an abnormality in a gene coding for a MAPK pathway protein.

Diagnostic criteria for diffuse low-grade glioma, MAPK pathway-altered

Diagnostic criteria are shown in ▶ Fig. 38.4.[1]

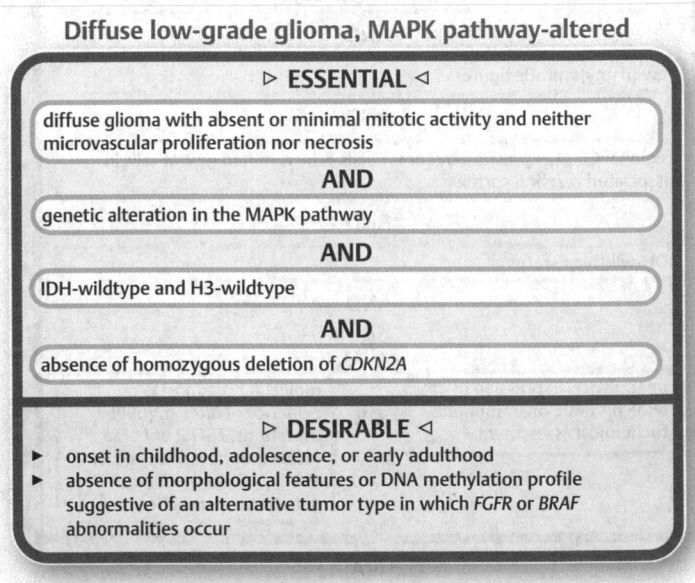

Diffuse low-grade glioma, MAPK pathway-altered

▷ **ESSENTIAL** ◁

diffuse glioma with absent or minimal mitotic activity and neither microvascular proliferation nor necrosis

AND

genetic alteration in the MAPK pathway

AND

IDH-wildtype and H3-wildtype

AND

absence of homozygous deletion of *CDKN2A*

▷ **DESIRABLE** ◁

► onset in childhood, adolescence, or early adulthood
► absence of morphological features or DNA methylation profile suggestive of an alternative tumor type in which *FGFR* or *BRAF* abnormalities occur

Fig. 38.4 Diagnostic criteria for diffuse low-grade glioma, MAPK pathway-altered. (Modified with permission from WHO Classification of Tumors Editorial Board, (ed.) World Health Organization classification of tumors of the central nervous system. 5th ed. Bosman F T, Jaffe E S, Lakhani S R, et al. (series eds.): World Health Organization Classification of Tumors series, vol. 6. International Agency for Research on Cancer, Lyon, France, 2021.)

Subtypes

See reference.[1]
- diffuse low-grade glioma, *FGFR1* tyrosine kinase domain–duplicated
- diffuse low-grade glioma, *FGFR1*-mutant
- diffuse low-grade glioma, *BRAF p.V600E*–mutant

Presentation

Seizures or symptoms related to mass effect, sometimes with increased intracranial pressure.

Imaging

Appearance may resemble that of pilocytic astrocytoma complete with cystic elements, but these tumors tend to be more extensive on T2-FLAIR images.

Treatment

Unresolved issues related to the behavior of this group, and possible subgroups.

38

38.2 Pediatric-type diffuse high-grade gliomas

38.2.1 Diffuse midline glioma, H3 K27M-altered (WHO grade 4)

General information

An infiltrating midline glioma with with loss of H3 p.K28me3 (K27me3) and usually either an H3 c.83A > T p.K28 M (K27M) substitution in one of the histone H3 isoforms, aberrant overexpression of EZHIP, or an *EGFR* mutation.

In children, involvement tends to be in brainstem (formerly called brainstem glioma), pons (formerly called diffuse infiltrating pontine glioma [DIPG]), or bithalamic. In adolescents or adults, they occur unilaterally in the thalamus or in the spinal cord.

Leptomeningeal involvement was found in 40% in autopsy series, and DIPG is the leading cause of brain tumor-related death in children.[4]

Diagnostic criteria for diffuse midline glioma, H3 K27M-altered

Diagnostic criteria are shown in ▶ Fig. 38.5.[1]

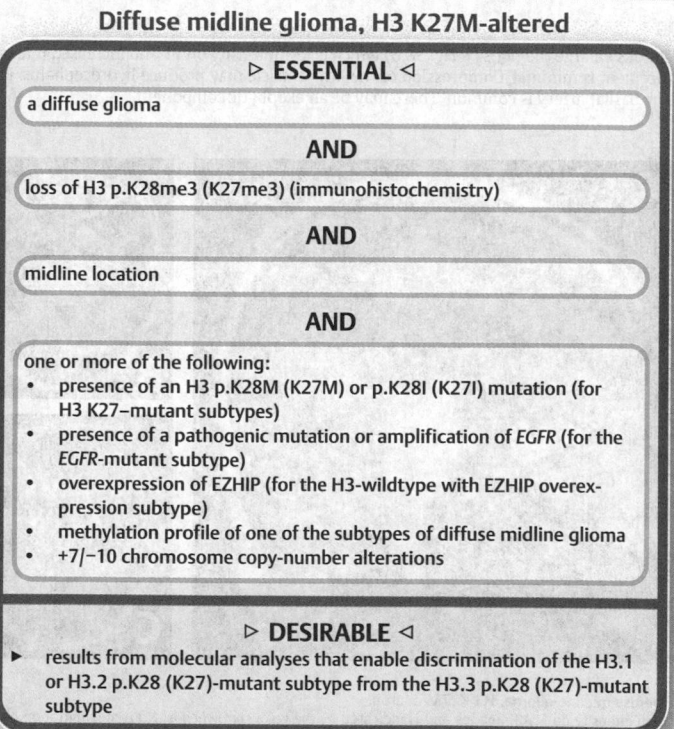

Diffuse midline glioma, H3 K27M-altered

▷ **ESSENTIAL** ◁

a diffuse glioma

AND

loss of H3 p.K28me3 (K27me3) (immunohistochemistry)

AND

midline location

AND

one or more of the following:
- presence of an H3 p.K28M (K27M) or p.K28I (K27I) mutation (for H3 K27–mutant subtypes)
- presence of a pathogenic mutation or amplification of *EGFR* (for the *EGFR*-mutant subtype)
- overexpression of EZHIP (for the H3-wildtype with EZHIP overexpression subtype)
- methylation profile of one of the subtypes of diffuse midline glioma
- +7/−10 chromosome copy-number alterations

▷ **DESIRABLE** ◁
▶ results from molecular analyses that enable discrimination of the H3.1 or H3.2 p.K28 (K27)-mutant subtype from the H3.3 p.K28 (K27)-mutant subtype

38

Fig. 38.5 Diagnostic criteria for diffuse midline glioma, H3 K27M-altered. (Modified with permission from WHO Classification of Tumors Editorial Board, (ed.) World Health Organization classification of tumors of the central nervous system. 5th ed. Bosman F T, Jaffe E S, Lakhani S R, et al. (series eds.): World Health Organization Classification of Tumors series, vol. 6. International Agency for Research on Cancer, Lyon, France, 2021.)

Subtypes

See reference.[1]
- **diffuse midline glioma, H3.3 K27–mutant**
- **diffuse midline glioma, H3.1 or H3.2 K27–mutant**
- **diffuse midline glioma, H3-wildtype with EZHIP overexpression**
- **diffuse midline glioma, *EGFR*-mutant**

Presentation

Patients with DMG typically present with a short course with brainstem findings[5] (triad: multiple cranial nerve palsies, long tract signs and ataxia) or obstructive hydrocephalus. Evidence of thalamic involvement includes signs of increased ICP, motor weakness (e.g., hemiparesis), and gait disturbance.

Evalutation

Given the high rate of leptomeningeal spread, imaging of the entire neuraxis is recommended.

Current trends favor obtaining a biopsy in most cases as ealy reports of high complications and lack of clinical utility have been debunked.[6] Biopsy confirms H3 K27M-mutation and can determine if there is MGMT promoter gene methylation.

Imaging

Pontine lesions enlarge the pons (▶ Fig. 38.6) which is low intensity on T1 and increased intensity on T2. Enhancement is minimal. Compression of the 4th ventricle may produce hydrocephalus. Encasement of the basilar artery is common. There may be an exophytic component.

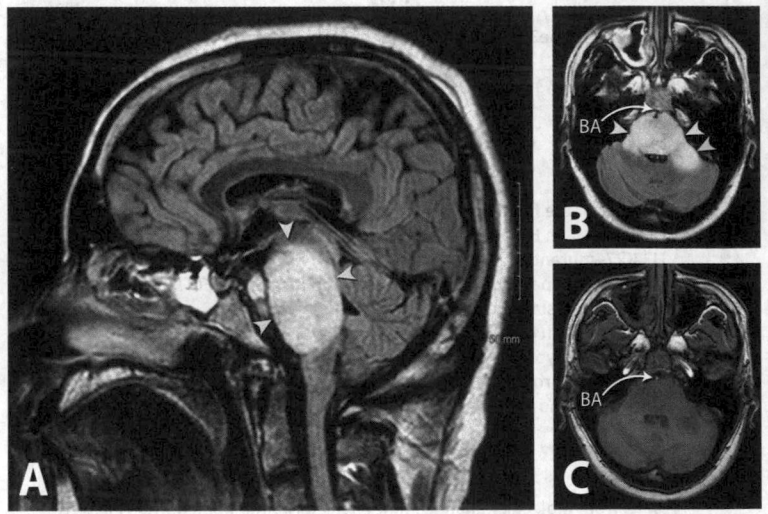

Fig. 38.6 Diffuse midline glioma, H3 K27M-altered.
Tumor is high intensity on FLAIR images and is indicated by the *yellow arrowheads*. Note the infiltration of the left cerebellar peduncle (*blue arrowhead*). Abbreviation: BA = the compressed basilar artery.
Image: MRI scans. A: sagittal FLAIR. B: Axial FLAIR. C: Axial T1 with contrast demonstrating lack of tumor enhancement.

Treatment and prognosis

Even with current therapies, 2-year survival is < 10%.[7]

The role for surgical intervention is limited due to the location of of these tumors.

Prognosis is better for subtypes involving H3.1 or H3.2 K27-mutation or EZHIP overexpression than the H3.3 K27 mutation.[1]

38.2.2 Diffuse hemispheric glioma, H3 G34-mutant (WHO grade 4)

General information

An infiltrative glioma located in the cerebral hemispheres having a missense mutation of the *H3-3A* gene resulting in one of the substitutions of the H3 protein shown in ▶ Fig. 38.7. The tumor occasionally extends to the midline.

Diagnostic criteria for diffuse hemispheric glioma, H3 G34-mutant

Diagnostic criteria are shown in ▶ Fig. 38.7.[1]

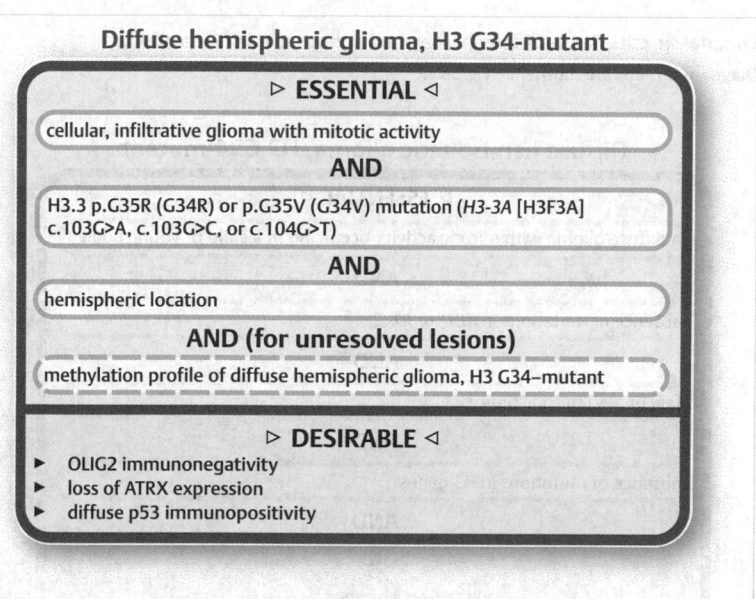

Fig. 38.7 Diagnostic criteria for diffuse hemispheric glioma, H3 G34-mutant. (Modified with permission from WHO Classification of Tumors Editorial Board, (ed.) World Health Organization classification of tumors of the central nervous system. 5th ed. Bosman F T, Jaffe E S, Lakhani S R, et al. (series eds.): World Health Organization Classification of Tumors series, vol. 6. International Agency for Research on Cancer, Lyon, France, 2021.)

Presentation

Non specific (seizures, mass effect from locally involved brain…).

Histology

Appearance similar to GBM (high cellularity, infiltrating margins, extensive mitoses…).

Evaluation

Spine imaging is recommended in addition to brain.

Imaging

Hemispheric lesion that typically contrast enhances. Occasionally multifocal.

38

Treatment and prognosis

Median PFS is 9 months, with median OS of 18-22 months.[8]

Recurrence after treatment is typically local, although leptomeningeal spread may occur.

MGMT promoter gene methylation (p.673) and absence of oncogene amplification (e.g., *PDGFRA, EGFR, CDK4, MDM2, CDK6, CCND2, MYC, MYCN*) may portend a better prognosis for OS.[8]

38.2.3 Diffuse pediatric-type high-grade glioma, H3-wildtype and IDH-wildtype (WHO grade 4)

General information

An infiltrative glioma located in the cerebral hemispheres having a missense mutation of the *H3-3A* gene resulting in one of the substitutions of the H3 protein shown in ▶ Fig. 38.7. The tumor occasionally extends to the midline.

Diagnostic criteria for diffuse hemispheric glioma, H3 G34-mutant

Diagnostic criteria are shown in ▶ Fig. 38.8.[1]

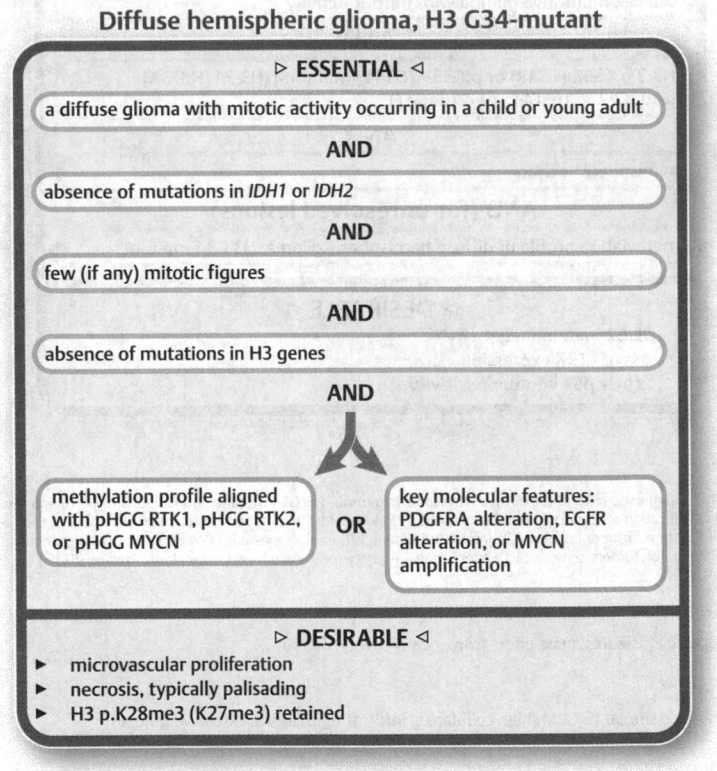

Fig. 38.8 Diagnostic criteria for diffuse pediatric-type high-grade glioma, H3-wildtype and IDH-wildtype. (Modified with permission from WHO Classification of Tumors Editorial Board, (ed.) World Health Organization classification of tumors of the central nervous system. 5th ed. Bosman F T, Jaffe E S, Lakhani S R, et al. (series eds.): World Health Organization Classification of Tumors series, vol. 6. International Agency for Research on Cancer, Lyon, France, 2021.)

Presentation

Nonspecific (seizures, mass effect from locally involved brain…).

Histology

Appearance similar to GBM (high cellularity, infiltrating margins, extensive mitoses…).

Evaluation

Spine imaging is recommended in addition to brain.

Imaging

Hemispheric lesion that typically contrast enhances. Occasionally multifocal.

Treatment and prognosis

Median PFS is 9 months, with median OS of 18–22 months.[8]

Recurrence after treatment is typically local, although leptomeningeal spread may occur.

MGMT promoter gene methylation (p.673) and absence of oncogene amplification (e.g., *PDGFRA, EGFR, CDK4, MDM2, CDK6, CCND2, MYC, MYCN*) may protend a better prognosis for OS.[8]

38.2.4 Infant-type hemispheric glioma (WHO grade N/A)

General information

A high-grade hemispheric glioma occurring in early childhood, having receptor tyrosine kinase (RTK) fusions including those in the NTRK family, or in *ROS1*, *ALK*, or *MET*.

Diagnostic criteria for infant-type hemispheric glioma

Diagnostic criteria are shown in ▶ Fig. 38.9.[1]

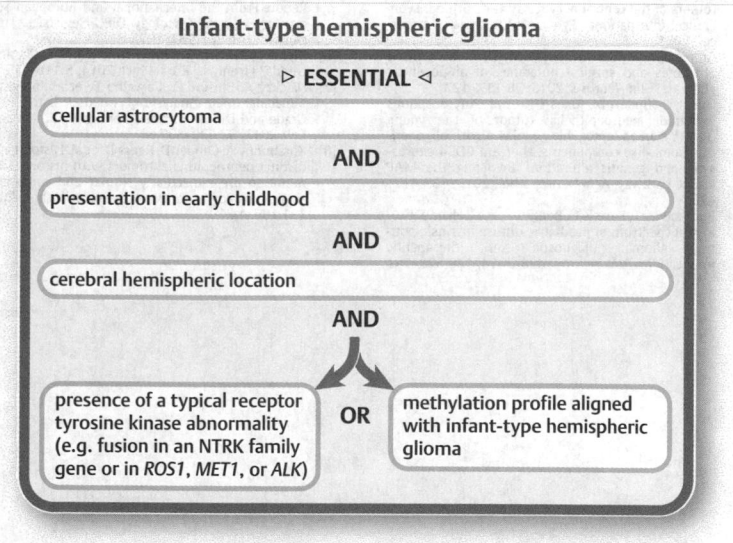

38

Fig. 38.9 Diagnostic criteria for infant-type hemispheric glioma. (Modified with permission from WHO Classification of Tumors Editorial Board, (ed.) World Health Organization classification of tumors of the central nervous system. 5th ed. Bosman F T, Jaffe E S, Lakhani S R, et al. (series eds.): World Health Organization Classification of Tumors series, vol. 6. International Agency for Research on Cancer, Lyon, France, 2021.)

Subtypes

See reference.[1]
- **infant-type hemispheric glioma, NTRK-altered**
- **infant-type hemispheric glioma, *ROS1*-altered**
- **infant-type hemispheric glioma, *ALK*-altered**
- **infant-type hemispheric glioma, *MET*-altered**

Presentation

All known cases occurred in early childhood, usually in the 1st year of life. Typically acute presentation. In infancy, may manifest as agitatin or lethargy, possibly with enlarged head circumference.

Histology

Typcially well-demarcated, cellular tumors involving brain parenchyma and leptomeninges.
   Initial diagnosis was a high-grade glioma or GBM in 84%.[1]

Evaluation

Owing to leptomeningeal involvement, spine imaging is recommended in addition to brain.

Treatment and prognosis

There is insufficient data on this recently designated entity. Stereotypically, infants with high-grade gliomas fare better than older children.

References

[1] Bosman FT, Jaffe ES, Lakhani SR, et al. World Health Organization Classification of Tumors series, vol. 6. In: WHO Classification of Tumors Editorial Board (ed.) World Health Organization classification of tumors of the central nervous system. 5th ed. Lyon, France: International Agency for Research on Cancer; 2021

[2] Ampie L, Choy W, DiDomenico JD, et al. Clinical attributes and surgical outcomes of angiocentric gliomas. J Clin Neurosci. 2016; 28:117–122

[3] Huse JT, Snuderl M, Jones DT, et al. Polymorphous low-grade neuroepithelial tumor of the young (PLNTY): an epileptogenic neoplasm with oligodendroglioma-like components, aberrant CD34 expression, and genetic alterations involving the MAP kinase pathway. Acta Neuropathol. 2017; 133:417–429

[4] Buczkowicz P, Bartels U, Bouffet E, et al. Histopathological spectrum of paediatric diffuse intrinsic pontine glioma: diagnostic and therapeutic implications. Acta Neuropathol. 2014; 128:573–581

[5] Hoffman LM, Veldhuijzen van Zanten S EM, Colditz N, et al. Clinical, Radiologic, Pathologic, and Molecular Characteristics of Long-Term Survivors of Diffuse Intrinsic Pontine Glioma (DIPG): A Collaborative Report From the International and European Society for Pediatric Oncology DIPG Registries. J Clin Oncol. 2018; 36:1963–1972

[6] Mohanty A. Biopsy of brain stem gliomas: Changing trends? J Neurosci Rural Pract. 2014; 5:116–117

[7] Mackay A, Burford A, Carvalho D, et al. Integrated Molecular Meta-Analysis of 1,000 Pediatric High-Grade and Diffuse Intrinsic Pontine Glioma. Cancer Cell. 2017; 32:520–537 e5

[8] Korshunov A, Capper D, Reuss D, et al. Histologically distinct neuroepithelial tumors with histone 3 G34 mutation are molecularly similar and comprise a single nosologic entity. Acta Neuropathol. 2016; 131:137–146

39 Circumscribed Astrocytic Gliomas

39.1 General meaning of "circumscribed"

Circumscribed astrocytic tumors have a more contained growth pattern which differs from the infiltrating gliomas. With diffuse gliomas, there is generally no tumor identifiable margin beyond which there there is tumor-free brain.

39.2 Specific tumor types

39.2.1 Pilocytic astrocytomas (PCAs) (WHO grade 1)

General information

Key concepts

- a subgroup of astrocytomas (WHO grade 1) with better prognosis (10-year survival: > 95%) than infiltrating fibrillary or diffuse astrocytomas
- the most common astrocytic tumor in children
- average age is lower than for typical astrocytomas (75% of patients are ≤ 20 yrs)
- common locations: cerebellar hemisphere, optic nerve/chiasm, hypothalamus
- CT/MRI appearance: discrete appearing, contrast enhancing lesion. Cerebellar PCAs are classically cystic with mural nodule
- the principal CNS tumor associated with NF1
- histology: biphasic. 1) compacted, 2) loose (myxoid) textured astrocytes with Rosenthal fibers and/or eosinophilic granular bodies
- associated with MAPK pathway gene alterations (typically *KIAA1549::BRAF* gene fusions)
- histology alone may be inadequate for diagnosis; knowledge of patient age & radiographic appearance is critical; there is a risk of overgrading and overtreating if decisions are made on histology alone
- complete surgical resection, when possible, is usually curative. ★ For cystic PCAs with enhancing mural nodule, only the nodule needs to be resected (the cyst wall is not neoplastic). XRT is used post-op only for nonresectable recurrence or malignant degeneration

Diagnostic criteria for pilocytic astrocytoma and pilomyxoid astrocytoma

Diagnostic criteria for pilocytic astrocytoma are shown in ▶ Fig. 39.1 and for pilomyxoid astrocytoma in ▶ Fig. 39.2.[1]

Subtypes

See reference.[1]

- **pilomyxoid astrocytoma** (PMA): a tumor of infancy that develops in the hypothalamic/chiasmatic region, and carries a higher rate of recurrence, worse outome, and tendency for CSF dissemination,[2] with a case report of extraneural peritoneal mets spread through a VP shunt.[3] Because not all PMAs behave differently than a WHO grade 1 PCA, a definite WHO grade was not recommended.[4] They are comprised of monomorphic piloid cells, have a diffusely myxoid background and increased cellularity compared with classic PCAs and angiocentric cell arrangement. By definition, does not contain Rosenthal fibers or eosinophilic granular bodies.[4] They may eventually morph into a classic PCA
  May also occur in spinal cord
- **pilocytic astrocytoma with histological features of anaplasia**: a proposed term for tumors morphologically similar to PCA but also possess mitotic features ± necrosis. These anaplastic features may be present on initial analysis, or may develop later

39

Background and terminology

Pilocytic astrocytoma (PCA) is the currently recommended nomenclature for these tumors previously referred to variously as cystic cerebellar astrocytomas and juvenile pilocytic astrocytomas

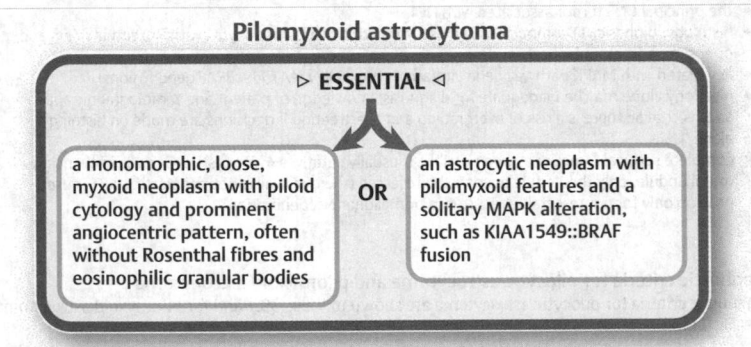

Pilocytic astrocytoma

▷ ESSENTIAL ◁

classic histological features of pilocytic astrocytoma, such as biphasic compact and loose growth patterns, piloid cytology, and low proliferative activity, with or without Rosenthal fibres and/or eosinophilic granular bodies

OR

a low-grade piloid astrocytic neoplasm with a solitary MAPK alteration, such as KIAA1549::BRAF fusion

Fig. 39.1 Diagnostic criteria for pilocytic astrocytoma. (Modified with permission from WHO Classification of Tumors Editorial Board, (ed.) World Health Organization classification of tumors of the central nervous system. 5th ed. Bosman F T, Jaffe E S, Lakhani S R, et al. (series eds.): World Health Organization Classification of Tumors series, vol. 6. International Agency for Research on Cancer, Lyon, France, 2021.)

Pilomyxoid astrocytoma

▷ ESSENTIAL ◁

a monomorphic, loose, myxoid neoplasm with piloid cytology and prominent angiocentric pattern, often without Rosenthal fibres and eosinophilic granular bodies

OR

an astrocytic neoplasm with pilomyxoid features and a solitary MAPK alteration, such as KIAA1549::BRAF fusion

Fig. 39.2 Diagnostic criteria for pilomyxoid astrocytoma. (Modified with permission from WHO Classification of Tumors Editorial Board, (ed.) World Health Organization classification of tumors of the central nervous system. 5th ed. Bosman F T, Jaffe E S, Lakhani S R, et al. (series eds.): World Health Organization Classification of Tumors series, vol. 6. International Agency for Research on Cancer, Lyon, France, 2021.)

39

(JPA), among others.[4] Based on location, these tumors may be called optic gliomas, hypothalamic gliomas, and cerebellar PCAs. Treatment decisions vary based on location and neural involvement.

PCAs differ markedly from the infiltrating diffuse astrocytomas in terms of their reduced tendency to invade tissue and their very low propensity for malignant degeneration.

Epidemiology

PCAs comprise 5% of primary brain tumors. They are the most common glioma in pediatrics (age 0–19 years) with an incidence of 0.82/100,000.[5] The incidence progressively declines after age 15. Slight male predilection.

Usually presents during second decade of life (ages 10–20).[5] 75% occur in age < 20 years.[6]

Most PCAs are sporadic, but they are the main tumor in neurodevelopmental diseases with germ-line mutations in the MAPK pathway genes including: NF1 (p.638), Noonan syndrome, and encephalocraniocutaneous lipomatosis.

Location

PCAs arise throughout the neuraxis (2003 study in adults and children[7]):
1. pilocytic astrocytoma of the cerebellum (p.693): 42%. Formerly referred to as cystic cerebellar astrocytoma
2. cerebral hemispheres: 35%. Rare in children, tends to occur more often in older patients (i.e., young adults) than optic nerve/hypothalamic lesions. These PCAs are potentially confused with infiltrating astrocytomas possessing more malignant potential. PCAs are often distinguished by a cystic component with an enhancing mural nodule (would be atypical for a diffuse astrocytoma), and some PCAs have dense calcifications[8]
3. optic gliomas & hypothalamic gliomas: 9%
   a) PCAs arising in the optic nerve are called optic gliomas (p.694). This is the most common site in neurofibromatosis type 1 (p.638) (NF1) patients (may be bilateral)[9]
   b) when they occur in the region of the chiasm they cannot always be distinguished clinically or radiographically from so-called hypothalamic gliomas (p.695) or gliomas of the third ventricular region
4. brainstem PCAs: 9%. Usually are fibrillary infiltrating type and only a small proportion are pilocytic. May comprise the majority of the prognostically favorable group described as "dorsally exophytic (p.696)" brainstem gliomas[9,10]
5. spinal cord: 2%. PCAs may also occur here, but little information is available on these. Again, patients tend to be younger than with infiltrating astrocytomas of the spinal cord

Molecular genetics

Detailed molecular genetics are available.[11] For most neurosurgeons, the salient aspects are:
• the most common genetic abnormality in PCAs is in the BRAF gene which activates the MAPK pathway which is involved in nearly all PCAs. This is common in all PCAs, but most prevalent (75%) in cerebellar PCAs
• 15–20% of patients with neurofibromatosis type 1 (NF1) develop PCAs,[12] which are the main CNS tumors associated with NF1. NF1 patients have only 1 NF1 wildtype gene copy. Loss of this copy by a "second hit" (by point mutation, LOH, or DNA hypermethylation[13]) results in overactivation of RAS and MAPK pathway[14]

Histology

PCAs are usually histologically WHO grade 1 (however, a rare anaplastic form in adults has been identified,[15] but a WHO grade 3 variant is not officially recognized).

▶ **Microscopy.** Low to moderate cellularity with two main cell populations (biphasic), best appreciated in cerebellar PCAs:
1. cells with long thin bipolar processes (resembling hairs—hence *pilo*cytic)[9] with Rosenthal fibers[8] (sausage or corkscrew shaped cytoplasmic eosinophilic inclusion bodies consisting of glial filament aggregates resembling hyaline; stain bright red on Masson trichrome smears)
2. loosely knit tissue comprising stellate astrocytes with microcysts and occasional eosinophilic granular bodies

PCAs easily break through the pia to fill the overlying subarachnoid space. PCAs may also infiltrate into the perivascular spaces. Vascular proliferation is common. Multinucleated giant cells with peripherally located nuclei are common, especially in PCAs of the cerebellum or cerebrum. Mitotic figures may be seen, but are clinically not as ominous as with fibrillary astrocytomas. Areas of necrosis may also be seen. In spite of well-demarcated margins grossly and on MRI, at least 64% of PCAs infiltrate the surrounding parenchyma, especially the white matter[16] (the clinical significance of this is uncertain; one study found no statistically significant decrease in survival[17]).

▶ **Differentiating from a diffuse or infiltrating astrocytoma.** Pathology alone may not be able to differentiate. This may be especially problematic with small specimens obtained e.g., with stereotactic biopsy. A young age may suggest the diagnosis, and knowledge of the radiographic appearance is often critical (see below).

39

▶ **Malignant degeneration.** Rare malignant degeneration has been reported, often after many years. Radiation therapy (XRT) had been administered in most cases[18] although this may occur without XRT.[19]

Radiographic evaluation

Preoperative MRI of the entire neuraxis (brain, cervical, thoracic, and lumbar spine) without and with contrast is recommended when possible to evaluate for dissemination through the CSF (rare) and in case it proves to be a different pathology.

On CT or MRI, PCAs are usually well circumscribed, 94% enhance with contrast[16] (unlike most low-grade diffuse astrocytomas), frequently have a cystic component with a mural nodule (especially cerebellar PCAs) (see ▶ Fig. 39.3), and have little or no surrounding edema. The cyst wall may or may not enhance. PCAs involving the optic apparatus are typically fusiform.

Although they may occur anywhere in the CNS, 82% are periventricular.[16] Calcifications are only occasionally present.[16] 4 main imaging patterns of cerebellar or cerebral PCAs are shown in ▶ Table 39.1.

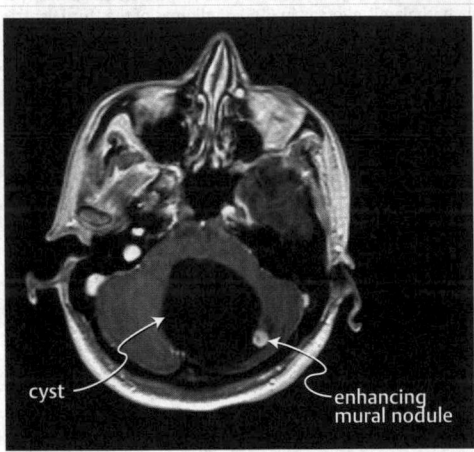

Fig. 39.3 Pilocytic astrocytoma of the posterior fossa.
Note characteristic nonenhancing cyst wall with enhancing mural nodule.
Image: axial T1 MRI with contrast.

cyst

enhancing mural nodule

Table 39.1 Common imaging characteristics of cerebellar or cerebral PCAs

%	Description	
21	nonenhancing cyst with enhancing mural nodule	over 66% are cystic with enhancing mural nodule
46	enhancing cyst with enhancing mural nodule	
16	mass with nonenhancing central area (necrosis)	
17	solid mass with minimal or no cyst	

Treatment

Treatment of choice is surgical excision of the maximal amount of the tumor that can be removed without producing deficit. In some, invasion of brainstem or involvement of cranial nerves or blood vessels may limit resection.

▶ **Cysts.** In tumors composed of a nodule with a true cyst, excision of the nodule is sufficient; the cyst wall need not be removed (the strength of this statement is based on the fact that the wall has been biopsy proven negative for neoplasm in 3 cases[20] and that patients do very well after excision of the nodule alone). In tumors with a so-called "false cyst" where the cyst wall is thick and enhances (on CT or MRI), this portion must also be removed.

▶ **XRT & chemotherapy.** Because of the high 5- and 10-year survival rates together with the high complication rate of radiation therapy over this time interval—see Radiation injury and necrosis (p. 1899)—and the fact that many incompletely resected tumors enlarge minimally if at all over periods of 5, 10, or even 20 years, it is recommended to *not* radiate these patients post-op. Rather, they should be followed with serial CT or MRI and be re-operated if there is recurrence.[21] Radiation therapy is indicated for nonresectable recurrence (i.e., reoperation is preferred if possible) or for recurrence with malignant histology. Chemotherapy is preferable to XRT in younger patients.[22]

Prognosis

The natural history of these tumors is slow growth. Survival rates at 5 and 10 years are 95% after surgical resection alone.

Tumor recurrence is relatively common, and although it has been said that they generally occur within ≈ 3 yrs of surgery,[23] this is controversial, and very late recurrences are documented,[21] violating Collins' law (which says that a tumor may be considered cured if it does not recur within a time period equal to the patient's age at diagnosis + 9 months). Also, some tumors excised partially fail to show further growth, representing a form of cure (long-term progression free survival).

About 20% of cerebellar PCAs develop hydrocephalus, requiring treatment following surgery.[24] So-called "drop metastases" occur rarely with PCAs.

Pilocytic astrocytoma (PCA) of the cerebellum

General information

Key concepts

- often cystic, half of these have mural nodule
- usually presents during the second decade of life (ages 10–20 yrs)
- also, see Key concepts for pilocytic astrocytomas in general (p. 689)

An informal subtype of pilocytic astrocytoma (PCA) (p. 689). Formerly referred to by the nonspecific and confusing term cystic cerebellar astrocytoma. One of the more common pediatric brain tumors (≈ 15% of primary brain tumors in patients < 19 years[7]), comprising 27–40% of pediatric p-fossa tumors.[25 (p 367–74),26 (p 3032)] They may also occur in adults, where the mean age is lower and the post-operative survival is longer than for diffuse astrocytomas.[27]

Presentation

Signs and symptoms of cerebellar PCAs are usually those of any p-fossa mass, i.e., those of hydrocephalus (headache, nausea/vomiting...) or cerebellar dysfunction (ataxia, cranial nerve deficits) (see Posterior fossa (infratentorial) tumors (p. 624)). Optic pathway gliomas typically present with loss of vision.

Imaging

"Classic" MRI finding: posterior fossa cyst with an enhancing mural nodule (see ▶ Fig. 39.3). The cyst wall sometimes enhances, usually as a thin rim (biopsy negative for neoplasm, enhancement may be reactive[20]).

Pathology

The classic "juvenile pilocytic astrocytoma" of the cerebellum is a distinctive entity with its macroscopic cystic architecture and microscopic spongy appearance.[8] For other microscopic findings, see PCAs in general, above.

These tumors may be solid, but are more often cystic (hence the older term "cystic cerebellar astrocytoma") with a mural nodule. They tend to be large at the time of diagnosis (cystic tumors: 4–5.6 cm diameter; solid tumors: 2–4.8 cm diameter). Cysts contain highly proteinaceous fluid (averaging ≈ 4 Hounsfield units higher density than CSF on CT[28]).

Treatment guidelines

For cystic cerebellar PCAs, excision of the nodule without removing the cyst wall is sufficient. See treatment of pilocytic astrocytomas in general (p. 692).

39

Also, see Posterior fossa (infratentorial) tumors (p. 624) for guidelines regarding hydrocephalus, etc.

Because of the high frequency of BRAF abnormalities, research is ongoing to evaluate the efficacy of BRAF and/or MEK inhibitors.[29]

Optic pathway glioma (OPG)

General information

Accounts for ≈ 2% of gliomas in adults, and 7% in children. The incidence is higher (≈ 25%) in neurofibromatosis type 1 (NF1) (p. 637). OPG may occur anywhere along the optic pathway from the optic disc to the occipital cortex.

OPG may arise in any of the following patterns:

1. one optic nerve (without chiasmal involvement): > 25% of OPGs are confined to the optic disc and nerve[30]
2. optic chiasm: 40-70% of OPGs.[30] Less commonly involved in patients with NF1 than in sporadic cases. Aggressive. 33-60% also invade the hypothalamus or third ventricle
3. multicentric in both optic nerves sparing the chiasm: seen almost exclusively in NF1
4. may occur in conjunction with, or be part of, a hypothalamic glioma (see below)

Pathology

Most OPGs are pilocytic astrocytomas (PCA) and are composed of low-grade (pilocytic) astrocytes. Rarely, a malignant chiasmal glioma occurs.

Presentation

Many OPGs remain asymptomatic.

Painless proptosis is an early sign in lesions involving one optic nerve. Chiasmal lesions produce variable and nonspecific visual defects (usually monocular) without proptosis. Large chiasmal tumors may cause hypothalamic and pituitary dysfunction (see diencephalic syndrome below), and may produce hydrocephalus by obstruction at the foramen of Monro. Gliosis of the optic nerve head may be seen on fundoscopy.

Evaluation

Plain X-rays: not usually helpful. The classic skull X-ray findings are enlargement of the optic canals and a "J"-shaped sella turcica.

CT/MRI: CT scan can readily demonstrate structures within the orbit. In addition to that, MRI also easily demonstrates chiasmal or hypothalamic involvement. On CT or MRI, involvement of the optic nerve produces fusiform enlargement of the nerve usually extending > 1 cm in length. Optic pathway gliomas in patients with NF1 are typically isolated to the optic nerve, whereas those not associated with NF1 usually involve the optic chiasm, may extend outside the optic apparatus, and are frequently cystic. Enhancement is usually only mild to moderate.

Biopsy is not needed in cases with characteristic findings.

Treatment

Tumor involving a single optic nerve, sparing the chiasm, producing proptosis and visual loss should be treated with a transcranial approach with excision of the nerve from the globe all the way back to the chiasm (a transorbital [Kronlein] approach is not appropriate since tumor may be left in the nerve stump). In addition to the anticipated blindness in the involved eye, this may produce a junctional scotoma (p. 875).

Chiasmal tumors are generally not treated surgically except for biopsy (especially when it is difficult to distinguish an optic nerve glioma from a hypothalamic glioma), CSF shunting, or to remove the rare exophytic component to try and improve vision.

▶ **Adjuvant therapy.** Chemotherapy[22] (preferred over XRT in younger patients) or XRT. Indications:

1. chiasmal tumors
2. multicentric tumors
3. post-op if tumor is found in the chiasmal stump end of the resected nerve
4. malignant tumor (rare)

Typical XRT treatment planning: 45 Gy in 25 fractions of 1.8 Gy.

Hypothalamic glioma

General information
Pilocytic astrocytomas of the hypothalamus and third ventricular region occur primarily in children. Radiographically, the lesion may have an intraventricular appearance. Many of these tumors have some chiasmal involvement and the distinction from optic nerve glioma cannot be made (see above).

Presentation
Possible presentations include:
- **"diencephalic syndrome"**: a rare syndrome seen in peds, usually caused by an infiltrating glioma of the anterior hypothalamus. Classically:
  a) cachexia (loss of subcutaneous fat)/failure to thrive, failure to gain weight
  b) hyperactivity/over-alertness
  c) an almost euphoric affect (in stark contrast to their gaunt appearance)
- endocrine disturbance
  a) hypoglycemia
  b) diabetes insipidus with attendant hypernatremia
  c) precocious puberty
- symptoms related to hydrocephalus
  a) macrocephaly
  b) headache
  c) nausea/vomiting

Treatment
When complete resection is not possible, adjuvant therapy may be needed as outlined under optic gliomas (above).

Brainstem glioma

General information

> ## Key concepts
>
> - not a homogeneous group. MRI can differentiate malignant from benign lesions
> - trend: lower grade tumors tend to occur in the upper brainstem, and higher grade tumors in the lower brainstem/medulla
> - usually presents with multiple cranial nerve palsies and long tract findings
> - most are malignant, have poor prognosis, and are not surgical candidates
> - role of surgery primarily limited to dorsally exophytic lesions and shunting

Brainstem gliomas (BSG) tend to occur during childhood and adolescence (77% are < 20 yrs old, they comprise 1% of adult tumors[31]). BSG are one of the 3 most common brain tumors in pediatrics—see Pediatric brain tumors (p.621)—comprising ≈ 10–20% of pediatric CNS tumors.[10]

Presentation
See reference.[32]

Upper brainstem tumors tend to present with cerebellar findings and hydrocephalus, whereas lower brainstem tumors tend to present with multiple lower cranial nerve deficits and long tract findings. Due to their invasive nature, signs and symptoms usually do not occur until the tumor is fairly extensive in size.

Signs and symptoms:
1. gait disturbance
2. headache (p.623)
3. nausea/vomiting
4. cranial nerve deficits: diplopia, facial asymmetry
5. distal motor weakness in 30%
6. papilledema in 50%

39

7. hydrocephalus in 60%, usually due to aqueductal obstruction (often late, except with periaqueductal tumors, e.g., below)
8. failure to thrive (especially in age ≤ 2 yrs)

Pathology

BSG is a heterogeneous group. There may be a tendency towards lower grade tumors in the upper brainstem (76% were low-grade) versus the lower brainstem (100% of the glioblastomas were in the medulla).[33] A cystic component is seen rarely. Calcifications are also rare. 4 growth patterns that can be identified by MRI[34] that may correlate with prognosis[35]:

1. diffuse: all are malignant (most are anaplastic astrocytomas, the rest are glioblastomas). On MRI these tumors extend into the adjacent region in vertical axis (e.g., medullary tumors extend into pons and/or cervical cord) with very little growth towards obex, remaining intra-axial. Diffuse midline glioma, H3 K27M-mutant (p. 683) is a specific tumor seen mostly in pediatrics (but also uncommonly in adults)
2. cervicomedullary: most (72%) are low-grade astrocytomas. The rostral extent of these tumors is limited to the spinomedullary junction. Most bulge into the obex of the 4th ventricle (some may have an actual exophytic component)
3. focal: extent limited to medulla (does not extend up into pons nor down into spinal cord). Most (66%) are low-grade astrocytomas
4. dorsally exophytic: may be an extension of "focal" tumors (see above). Many of these may actually be low grade gliomas including:
   a) pilocytic astrocytomas (p. 689)
   b) gangliogliomas (p. 706): very rare. Compared to other BSGs, these patients tend to be slightly older and the medulla is involved more frequently[36]

Evaluation

MRI

The diagnostic test of choice. MRI evaluates status of ventricles, gives optimal assessment of tumor (CT is poor in the posterior fossa) and detects exophytic component. See ▶ Fig. 38.6. T1WI: almost all are hypointense, homogeneous (excluding cysts). T2WI: increased signal, homogeneous (excluding cysts). Gadolinium enhancement is highly variable.[34]

CT

Most do not enhance on CT, except possibly an exophytic component. If there is marked enhancement, consider other diagnoses (e.g., high-grade vermian astrocytoma).

Treatment

Surgery

Biopsy: biopsy for diffuse non-exophytic infiltrating tumors was discouraged[37]; however, changing trends are leaning towards biopsy even when the MRI shows a diffuse infiltrating brainstem lesion (to look for H3 K27 M mutation (p. 683)).[38]

Treatment is usually non-surgical. Exceptions where surgery may be indicated:

1. tumors with a dorsally exophytic component[10]: see below; these may protrude into 4th ventricle or CP angle, tend to enhance with IV contrast, tend to be lower grade
2. some success has been achieved with non-exophytic tumors that are *not* malignant astrocytomas (surgery in malignant astrocytomas is without benefit)[35] (detailed follow-up is lacking)
3. shunting for hydrocephalus

Stereotactic biopsy can be transfrontal, of for lesions entering the cerebellar peduncle a transcerebellar approach with the patient positioned on their side mahy be used.

Dorsally exophytic tumors

These tumors are generally histologically benign (e.g., gangliogliomas) and are amenable to radical subtotal resection. Prolonged survival is possible, with a low incidence of disease progression at short-term follow-up.[10]

Surgical goals in exophytic tumors include:

1. enhanced survival by subtotal removal of exophytic component[39]: broad attachment to the floor of 4th ventricle is typical and usually precludes complete excision (although some "safe entry" zones have been described[40]). An ultrasonic aspirator facilitates debulking
2. establishing diagnosis: radiographic differentiation of exophytic brainstem glioma tumors from other lesions (e.g., medulloblastoma, ependymoma, and dermoids) may be difficult

3. tumors that demonstrate recurrent growth after resection remained histologically benign and were amenable to re-resection[10]

Complications of surgery generally consisted of exacerbation of preoperative symptoms (ataxia, cranial nerve palsies…) which usually resolved with time.

Medical

No proven chemotherapeutic regimen. Steroids are usually administered. In pediatrics, there is some indication of response to Temodar® (temozolomide) (p. 627).

Radiation

Traditionally given as 45–55 Gy over a six week period, five days per week. When combined with steroids, symptomatic improvement occurs in 80% of patients.

Possible improved survival with so called "hyperfractionation" where multiple smaller doses per day are used.

Prognosis

Most children with malignant BSG will die within 6–12 months of diagnosis. XRT may not prolong survival in patients with grade 3 or 4 tumors. A subgroup of children have a more slowly growing tumor and may have up to 50% five-year survival. Dorsally exophytic tumors composed of pilocytic astrocytomas may have a better prognosis.

Tectal gliomas

General information

A topically defined diagnosis generally consisting of low-grade astrocytomas. Considered a benign subgroup of brainstem glioma. Because of location, tends to present with hydrocephalus. Was dramatically referred to as "the smallest tumor in the body that can lead to the death of the patient."[41] Focal neurologic findings are rare—diplopia, visual field deficits, nystagmus, Parinaud's syndrome (p. 101), ataxia, seizures…—and are often reversible after the hydrocephalus is corrected.

Epidemiology

Comprises ≈ 6% of surgically treated pediatric brain tumors.[42] Presents primarily in childhood. Median age of patients becoming symptomatic = 6–14 years.[42]

Pathology

Since many of these are not biopsied, meaningful statistical analysis is not possible. Pathologies identified include: WHO grade 2 diffuse astrocytoma, pilocytic astrocytomas, WHO grade 2 ependymoma, anaplastic astrocytoma, oligodendroglioma, and oligoastrocytoma.

Radiographic evaluation

CT scan detects hydrocephalus, but may miss the tumor in ≈ 50%.[43] Calcification on CT has been described in 9–25%.[43,44]

MRI is the study of choice for diagnosis and follow-up. Typically appears as a mass projecting dorsally from the quadrigeminal plate. Isointense on T1WI, iso- or hyperintense on T2WI.[42,45] Enhancement with gadolinium occurs in 18% and is of uncertain prognostic significance.

Treatment
General information

Due to the indolent course, open surgery is not recommended. Options include:

1. VP shunt: the standard treatment for years. Long-term results are good with a functioning shunt
2. endoscopic third ventriculostomy: may avoid the need for a shunt. Endoscopic biopsy[46] may be done at the same time through the same burr hole if it is technically feasible (requires a dilated foramen of Monro, which is often present). Long-term results unknown
3. endoscopic aqueductoplasty (with or without stenting): an option for some. Long-term results unknown

Stereotactic radiosurgery: May be offered for tumor progression (criteria are not defined: radiographic progression may not be associated with clinical deterioration[45]). Dosing should be limited to ≤ 14 Gray at the 50–70% isodose line to avoid radiation-induced side effects.[47]

39

Prognosis

Tumor progression: described in 15–25%.

Follow-up: no accepted guidelines. Serial neurologic exams and MRIs every 6–12 months has been suggested.[42]

39.2.2 High-grade astrocytoma with piloid features (HGAP) (WHO grade N/A)

General information

A rare astrocytoma that often shows high-grade piloid and/or glioblastoma-like features, possessing a distinct DNA methylation profile. These tumors may arise de novo, but they can also develop from lower grade astrocytomas, including pilocytic astrocytoma. Prognostic information is limited, with a 5-year OS of 50%.[48]

Diagnostic criteria for high-grade astrocytoma with piloid features

Diagnostic criteria for high-grade astrocytoma with piloid features are shown in ▶ Fig. 39.4.[1]

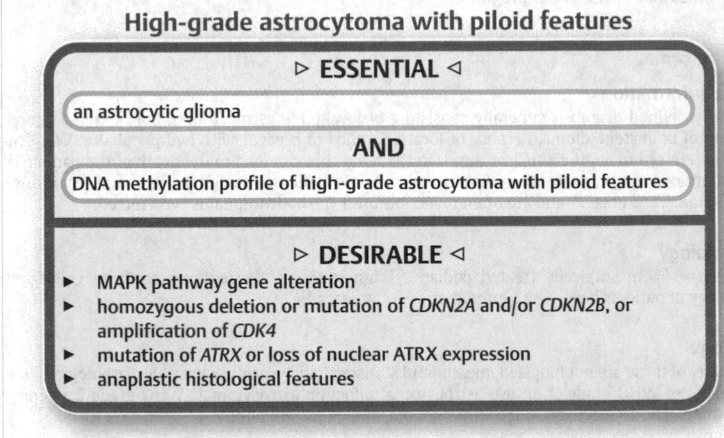

High-grade astrocytoma with piloid features

▷ **ESSENTIAL** ◁

an astrocytic glioma

AND

DNA methylation profile of high-grade astrocytoma with piloid features

▷ **DESIRABLE** ◁

► MAPK pathway gene alteration
► homozygous deletion or mutation of *CDKN2A* and/or *CDKN2B*, or amplification of *CDK4*
► mutation of *ATRX* or loss of nuclear ATRX expression
► anaplastic histological features

Fig. 39.4 **Diagnostic criteria for high-grade astrocytoma with piloid features.** (Modified with permission from WHO Classification of Tumors Editorial Board, (ed.) World Health Organization classification of tumors of the central nervous system. 5th ed. Bosman F T, Jaffe E S, Lakhani S R, et al. (series eds.): World Health Organization Classification of Tumors series, vol. 6. International Agency for Research on Cancer, Lyon, France, 2021.)

39.2.3 Pleomorphic xanthoastrocytoma (PXA) (WHO grade 2 or 3)

General information

39

Key concepts

- a glioma (usually WHO grade 2), possibly from subpial astrocytes → superficial location involving the leptomeninges in >67%
- 98% supratentorial, most common in children or young adults
- mural nodule with cystic component in 25%
- histology: large pleomorphic cells (xanthomatous [lipid-laden] cells, fibrillary and giant multi-nucleated astrocytes) often containing eosinophilic granular bodies and reticulin deposition
- characteristically with MAPK pathway gene alterations

- usually circumscribed, occasionally invasive
- WHO grade 2 (if ≥ 5 mitoses per HPF it qualifies as anaplastic, WHO grade 3)
- treatment: maximal safe resection

A low-grade glioma thought to arise from subpial astrocytes, which may explain their superficial location and abundance of reticulin fibers. Over 90% are supratentorial. Predilection for temporal lobes (50%), followed by parietal, occipital & frontal lobes. Most have a cystic component (may be multiloculated, but > 90% have a large, single cyst).

Diagnostic criteria for pleomorphic xanthoastrocytoma

Diagnostic criteria for pleomorphic xanthoastrocytoma are shown in ► Fig. 39.5.[1]

Pleomorphic xanthoastrocytoma

▷ ESSENTIAL ◁

an astrocytoma with pleomorphic tumor cells, including large multinucleated cells, spindle cells, xanthomatous (lipidized) cells, and eosinophilic granular bodies

▷ DESIRABLE ◁

► reticulin deposition
► *BRAF* mutation or other MAPK pathway gene alterations, combined with homozygous deletion of *CDKN2A* and/or *CDKN2B*
► DNA methylome profile of pleomorphic xanthoastrocytoma

Fig. 39.5 Diagnostic criteria for pleomorphic xanthoastrocytoma. (Modified with permission from WHO Classification of Tumors Editorial Board, (ed.) World Health Organization classification of tumors of the central nervous system. 5th ed. Bosman F T, Jaffe E S, Lakhani S R, et al. (series eds.): World Health Organization Classification of Tumors series, vol. 6. International Agency for Research on Cancer, Lyon, France, 2021.)

Epidemiology

≈ 1% of astrocytomas. Usually occurs in children or young adults (most are < 18 years of age). No gender difference. High prevalence of MAPK pathway alterations in PXA may explain the association with NF1.

Clinical

Usual presentation: seizures. May also produce focal deficit or increased ICP.

Differential diagnosis

1. imaging: meningioma is also superficial with dural tail. PXA may also resemble a low grade diffuse astrocytoma
2. pathology: may be confused with anaplastic astrocytoma

Histology

A compact, superficial tumor, usually circumscribed, occasionally infiltrates cortex. Marked cellular pleomorphism (fibrillary and giant multinucleated astrocytes, large xanthomatous (lipid laden) may cause these tumors to be mistaken for anaplastic astrocytoma. Cells stain for GFAP, bespeaking glial

39

origin. Abundant eosinophilic granular bodies, reticulin and frequent perivascular chronic inflammatory cells. The reticulin fibers surround two cell types:
1. spindle cells: fusiform cell shape with elongated nuclei
2. pleomorphic cells: round cells with heterochromic, pleomorphic nuclei that may be mononucleated or multinucleated. Variable intracellular lipid content

Grading

Most PXAs are WHO grade 2 with an MIB typically < 1%. A high mitotic index (≥ 5 mitoses per 10 HPF) qualifies as WHO grade 3.[49] Necrosis is common in grade 3 PXAs, but the significance of necrosis when encountered alone is not determined.

Dedifferentiation

PXAs have a tendency to recur and undergo anaplastic change.[50] There have also been several reported cases of malignant transformation to anaplastic astrocytoma or glioblastoma.[51]

Molecular genetics

Almost all PXAs demonstrate abnormal activation of MAPK pathway due to genetic alterations. The most common alteration is in *BRAF* V600E, and when seen in the absence of IDH mutation is strongly supportive of the diagnosis.

Other MAPK pathway gene alterations include homozygous *CDKN2A* and/or *CDKN2B* deletion.

Imaging

The cyst, when present, may partially enhance on CT or MRI. A mural nodule is present in 25%. May have "dural tail" (67% show leptomeningeal involvement, 13% show involvement of all 3 meningeal layers). Peritumoral edema may be mild to moderate, calcifications are rare.[52]

CT: solid portion of tumor is ill-defined and may be isodense to gray matter.

MRI: T1WI: hypointense cystic component with ill-defined isointense solid component that strongly enhances with gadolinium. T2WI: hyperintense cystic component with ill-defined isointense solid component.

Since PXAs tend to disseminate when they progress, spine MRI is recommended at the time of clinical progression.

Treatment

1. surgery: primary treatment
   a) gross total resection if it can be accomplished without unacceptable neurologic deficit, otherwise subtotal resection
   b) extent of resection: most strongly associated with recurrence free survival[53]
   c) incomplete resections should be followed since these tumors may grow very slowly over many years before retreatment is necessary, and repeat excision should be considered
2. radiation therapy: controversial
   a) literature suggests either no difference in overall survival or possibly a trend toward prolonged survival[54]
   b) considered with: residual disease, high mitotic index, or necrosis
3. chemotherapy: role not defined

Prognosis

PXAs frequently recur and malignant progression is more common than other WHO CNS5 grade 1 or 2 gliomas in young patients.

Grade 3 PXAs fare much worse than grade 2, with 5-year recurrence-free survival of 71% for grade 2 PXAs, and 49% for grade 3 (P = .0003).[55] OS is 54 months for grade 2 vs. 33 for grade 3.[56]

Extent of resection, mitotic index, and necrosis appear to be the best predictors of outcome.[52,53]

39.2.4 Subependymal giant cell astrocytoma (SEGA) (WHO grade 1)

General information

A circumscribed and often calcified WHO grade 1 tumor having a strong association with tuberous sclerosis (p. 644) (it is unclear if SEGAs develop in the absence of this condition).

39

Diagnostic criteria for subependymal giant cell astrocytoma

Diagnostic criteria for subependymal giant cell astrocytoma are shown in ▸ Fig. 39.6.[1]

Subependymal giant cell astrocytoma (SEGA)

▷ ESSENTIAL ◁

characteristic histological features, with multiple glial phenotypes including polygonal cells, gemistocyte-like cells, spindle cells, and ganglionic-like cells

AND

loss of H3 p.K28me3 (K27me3) (immunohistochemistry)

AND

immunoreactivity for glial markers (GFAP, S100)

AND

variable expression of neuronal markers (class III β-tubulin, neurofilament, synaptophysin, NeuN)

▷ DESIRABLE ◁

- ▸ nuclear immunoexpression of thyroid transcription factor 1 (TTF1)
- ▸ lost or reduced expression of tuberin and hamartin
- ▸ immunoexpression of phosphorylated S6
- ▸ DNA methylome profile of subependymal giant cell astrocytoma
- ▸ history of tuberous sclerosis
- ▸ TSC1 or TSC2 mutation

Fig. 39.6 Diagnostic criteria for subependymal giant cell astrocytoma. (Modified with permission from WHO Classification of Tumors Editorial Board, (ed.) World Health Organization classification of tumors of the central nervous system. 5th ed. Bosman F T, Jaffe E S, Lakhani S R, et al. (series eds.): World Health Organization Classification of Tumors series, vol. 6. International Agency for Research on Cancer, Lyon, France, 2021.)

Epidemiology & genetics

Incidence in patients with tuberous sclerosis is 5-15%. SEGAs rarely occur de novo after age ≈ 25 years.

SEGAs typically possess biallelic inactivation of TSC1 (15%) or TSC2 (56%) with the second hit being deletion or loss of heterozygosity. Deficient tuberin and hamartin epression are observed with these mutations.

Location

Arise from the lateral walls of the lateral ventricles next to the foramen of Monro. Rarely found in the third ventricle.

Histology

A wide variety of phenotypes occur. Large, plump cells resembling gemistocytic astrocytes are common, arrayed in fascicles, sheets and nests. Polygonal cells with ample cytoplasm may be seen. Areas

39

of necrosis and mitotic figures may be seen, but are not associated with the typical malignant aggressiveness that these features usually denote.[57] Mean Ki-67 (p. 632) is 3%.

Prognosis

Gross total resection is associated with a favorable prognosis. Larger lesions or symptomatic lesions have increased risk of surgical morbidity.[58]

Everolimus may reduce tumor size and progression.[59]

Because of the risk of late recurrence, long-tem follow-up is recommended.

39.2.5 Chordoid glioma (WHO grade 2)

General information

A glioma that occurs in the anterior third ventricle, possibly arising from tanycyte ependymal cells of the organum vasculosum of the lamina terminalis.

Diagnostic criteria for chordoid glioma

Diagnostic criteria for chordoid glioma are shown in ▶ Fig. 39.7.[1]

Chordoid glioma

▷ ESSENTIAL ◁

a glial neoplasm with chordoid features located in the anterior third ventricle

▷ DESIRABLE ◁

► nuclear thyroid transcription factor 1 (TTF1) immunopositivity
► *PRKCA* p.D463H mutation or DNA methylation profile aligning with chordoid glioma

Fig. 39.7 Diagnostic criteria for chordoid glioma. (Modified with permission from WHO Classification of Tumors Editorial Board, (ed.) World Health Organization classification of tumors of the central nervous system. 5th ed. Bosman F T, Jaffe E S, Lakhani S R, et al. (series eds.): World Health Organization Classification of Tumors series, vol. 6. International Agency for Research on Cancer, Lyon, France, 2021.)

Epidemiology & genetics

Comprise < 0.1% of primary brain tumors, typically occurring in adults. Female preponderance of 2:1.[60]

Presentation

- obstructive hydrocephalus: with typical symptoms of H/A, N/V, obtundation
- endocrine disturbance (hypothyroidism, amenorrhea, diabetes insipidus) from compression of the hypothalamus visual field deficit from compression of the chiasm
- psychiatric symptoms: personality changes, memory disturbance…

Imaging

MRI shows a well-circumscribed mass isotintense to brain on T1 images with avid enhancement, located in the anterior third ventricle (large tumors may occupy the entire third ventricle).

Histology

Typically comprised of clusters and cords of epitheliod cells embedded in a mucinous stroma. GFAP immunostaining is common. Mitotic activity is absent in most.

Treatment

Maximal safe resection is the primary treatment modality. Attachment to the wall of the 3rd ventricle (hypothalamus) may prevent total removal. Surgical risks include insufficiency of hypothalamic hormones, including diabetes insipidus. Post-op adjuvane therapy with XRT is of uncertain benefit.

39.2.6 Astroblastoma, MN1-altered (WHO grade 1)

General information

A circumscribed glial tumor with MN1 alteration.

Diagnostic criteria for astroblastoma, MN1-altered

Diagnostic criteria for astroblastoma, MN1-altered are shown in ► Fig. 39.8.[1]

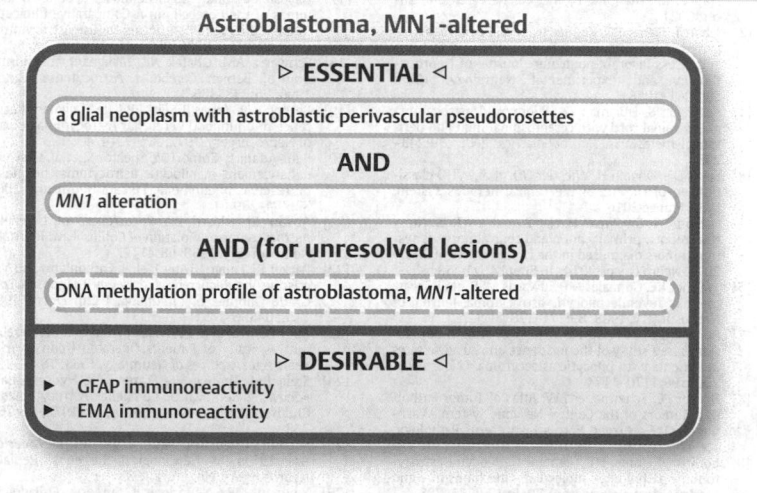

Fig. 39.8 Diagnostic criteria for astroblastoma, MN1-altered. (Modified with permission from WHO Classification of Tumors Editorial Board, (ed.) World Health Organization classification of tumors of the central nervous system. 5th ed. Bosman F T, Jaffe E S, Lakhani S R, et al. (series eds.): World Health Organization Classification of Tumors series, vol. 6. International Agency for Research on Cancer, Lyon, France, 2021.)

Epidemiology & genetics

Occurs almost exclusively in females.[61] Median age of presentation is 15 years (range: 3 months to 40 years).

Location

Primarily in the cerebral hemispheres, typically in the frontal or parietal lobes, but also may occur in the occipital or temporal lobes. Has also been described in the brainstem, intraventricular compartment and spinal cord.

39

Imaging

Solid or cystic mass that is iso- to hypo-intense to brain on T1 MRI, hyperintense on T2, and heterogeneous enhancement.

Histology

Hallmark is the astroblastic pseudorosette (tumor cells arranged in a radial pattern around blood vessels).

Treatment and prognosis

Maximal safe resection is associated with longer OS.[62] XRT and chemotherapy areoptions when surgery is not feasible.

5- and 10-year survival rates are 90% and 50% respectively.

References

[1] Bosman FT, Jaffe ES, Lakhani SR, et al. World Health Organization Classification of Tumors series, vol. 6. In: WHO Classification of Tumors Editorial Board (ed.) World Health Organization classification of tumors of the central nervous system. 5th ed. Lyon, France: International Agency for Research on Cancer; 2021

[2] Tihan T, Fisher PG, Kepner JL, et al. Pediatric astrocytomas with monomorphous pilomyxoid features and a less favorable outcome. Journal of Neuropathology and Experimental Neurology. 1999; 58:1061–1068

[3] Arulrajah S, Huisman TA. Pilomyxoid astrocytoma of the spinal cord with cerebrospinal fluid and peritoneal metastasis. Neuropediatrics. 2008; 39:243–245

[4] Louis DN, Ohgaki H, Wiestler OD, et al. WHO classification of tumors of the central nervous system. Lyon, France 2016

[5] Ostrom QT, Gittleman H, Liao P, et al. CBTRUS statistical report: primary brain and central nervous system tumors diagnosed in the United States in 2007-2011. Neuro Oncol. 2014; 16 Suppl 4:iv1–i63

[6] Wallner KE, Gonzales MF, Edwards MSB, et al. Treatment of juvenile pilocytic astrocytoma. Journal of Neurosurgery. 1988; 69:171–176

[7] Burkhard C, Di Patre PL, Schuler D, et al. A population-based study of the incidence and survival rates in patients with pilocytic astrocytoma. J Neurosurg. 2003; 98:1170–1174

[8] Burger PC, Scheithauer BW. Atlas of Tumor Pathology. Tumors of the Central Nervous System. Washington, D.C.: Armed Forces Institute of Pathology; 1994

[9] Collins VP, Jones DT, Giannini C. Pilocytic astrocytoma: pathology, molecular mechanisms and markers. Acta Neuropathol. 2015; 129:775–788

[10] Pollack IF, Hoffman HJ, Humphreys RP, et al. The Long-Term Outcome After Surgical Treatment of Dorsally Exophytic Brain-Stem Gliomas. Journal of Neurosurgery. 1993; 78:859–863

[11] Park SH, Won J, Kim SI, et al. Molecular Testing of Brain Tumor. J Pathol Transl Med. 2017; 51:205–223

[12] Listernick R, Charrow J, Greenwald M, et al. Natural history of optic pathway tumors in children with neurofibromatosis type 1: a longitudinal study. J Pediatr. 1994; 125:63–66

[13] Gutmann DH, McLellan MD, Hussain I, et al. Somatic neurofibromatosis type 1 (NF1) inactivation characterizes NF1-associated pilocytic astrocytoma. Genome Res. 2013; 23:431–439

[14] Gutmann DH, McLellan MD, Hussain I, et al. Somatic neurofibromatosis type 1 (NF1) inactivation characterizes NF1-associated pilocytic astrocytoma. Genome Res. 2013; 23:431–439

[15] Fiechter M, Hewer E, Knecht U, et al. Adult anaplastic pilocytic astrocytoma - a diagnostic challenge? A case series and literature review. Clin Neurol Neurosurg. 2016; 147:98–104

[16] Coakley KJ, Huston J, Scheithauer BW, et al. Pilocytic Astrocytomas: Well-Demarcated Magnetic Resonance Appearance Despite Frequent Infiltration Histologically. Mayo Clinic Proceedings. 1995; 70:747–751

[17] Hayostek CJ, Shaw EG, Scheithauer B, et al. Astrocytomas of the Cerebellum: A Comparative Clinicopathologic Study of Pilocytic and Diffuse Astrocytomas. Cancer. 1993; 72:856–869

[18] Schwartz AM, Ghatak NR. Malignant Transformation of Benign Cerebellar Astrocytoma. Cancer. 1990; 65:333–336

[19] Bernell WR, Kepes JJ, Seitz EP. Late Malignant Recurrence of Childhood Cerebellar Astrocytoma. Journal of Neurosurgery. 1972; 37:470–474

[20] Beni-Adani L, Gomori M, Spektor S, et al. Cyst wall enhancement in pilocytic astrocytoma: neoplastic or reactive phenomena. Pediatr Neurosurg. 2000; 32:234–239

[21] Austin EJ, Alvord EC. Recurrences of Cerebellar Astrocytomas: A Violation of Collins' Law. Journal of Neurosurgery. 1988; 68:41–47

[22] Packer RJ, Lange B, Ater J, et al. Carboplatin and Vincristine for Recurrent and Newly Diagnosed Low-Grade Gliomas of Childhood. J Clin Oncol. 1993; 11:850–856

[23] Bucy PC, Thieman PW. Astrocytomas of the Cerebellum. A Study of Patients Operated Upon Over 28 Years Ago. Archives of Neurology. 1968; 18:14–19

[24] Stein BM, Tenner MS, Fraser RAR. Hydrocephalus Following Removal of Cerebellar Astrocytomas in Children. Journal of Neurosurgery. 1972; 36:763–768

[25] Section of Pediatric Neurosurgery of the American Association of Neurological Surgeons. Pediatric Neurosurgery. New York 1982

[26] Youmans JR. Neurological Surgery. Philadelphia 1990

[27] Ringertz N, Nordenstam H. Cerebellar Astrocytoma. Journal of Neuropathology and Experimental Neurology. 1951; 10:343–367

[28] Zimmerman RA, Bilaniuk CT, Bruno LA, et al. CT of Cerebellar Astrocytoma. Am J Roentgenol. 1978; 130:929–933

[29] Schreck KC, Grossman SA, Pratilas CA. BRAF Mutations and the Utility of RAF and MEK Inhibitors in Primary Brain Tumors. Cancers (Basel). 2019; 11. DOI: 10.3390/cancers11091262

[30] Binning MJ, Liu JK, Kestle JR, et al. Optic pathway gliomas: a review. Neurosurg Focus. 2007; 23. DOI: 10.3171/FOC-07/11/E2

[31] Packer RJ, Nicholson HS, Vezina LG, et al. Brainstem gliomas. Neurosurg Clin N Am. 1992; 3:863–879

[32] Laurent JP, Cheek WR. Brain Tumors in Children. J Pediatr Neurosci. 1985; 1:15–32

[33] Reigel DH, Scarff TB, Woodford JE. Biopsy of Pediatric Brain Stem Tumors. Childs Brain. 1979; 5:329–340

[34] Epstein FJ, Farmaer J-P. Brain-Stem Glioma Growth Patterns. J Neurosurg. 1993; 78:408–412

[35] Epstein F, McCleary EL. Intrinsic Brain-Stem Tumors of Childhood: Surgical Indications. J Neurosurg. 1986; 64:11–15

[36] Garcia CA, McGarry PA, Collada M. Ganglioglioma of the Brain Stem. Case Report. Journal of Neurosurgery. 1984; 60:431–434

[37] Albright AL, Packer RJ, Zimmerman R, et al. Magnetic Resonance Scans Should Replace Biopsies for the Diagnosis of Diffuse Brain Stem Gliomas: A Report from the Children's Cancer Group. Neurosurgery. 1993; 33:1026–1030

[38] Mohanty A. Biopsy of brain stem gliomas: Changing trends? J Neurosci Rural Pract. 2014; 5:116–117

[39] Hoffman HJ, Becker L, Craven MA. A Clinically and Pathologically Distinct Group of Benign Brainstem Gliomas. Neurosurgery. 1980; 7:243–248

[40] Kyoshima K, Kobayashi S, Gibo H, et al. A Study of Safe Entry Zones via the Floor of the Fourth Ventricle for Brain-Stem Lesions. Journal of Neurosurgery. 1993; 78:987–993

[41] Kernohan WJ, Armed Forces Institute of Pathology. Tumors of the central nervous system. In: Atlas of Tumor Pathology. Washington, DC 1952:19–42

[42] Stark AM, Fritsch MJ, Claviez A, et al. Management of tectal glioma in childhood. Pediatr Neurol. 2005

[43] Bognar L, Turjman F, Villanyi E, et al. Tectal plate gliomas. Part II: CT scans and MR imaging of tectal gliomas. Acta Neurochir (Wien). 1994

[44] Pollack IF, Pang D, Albright AL. The long-term outcome in children with late-onset aqueductal stenosis resulting from benign intrinsic tectal tumors. J Neurosurg. 1994; 80:681–688

[45] Grant GA, Avellino AM, Loeser JD, et al. Management of intrinsic gliomas of the tectal plate in children. A ten-year review. Pediatr Neurosurg. 1999; 31:170–176

[46] Oka K, Kin Y, Go Y, et al. Neuroendoscopic approach to tectal tumors: a consecutive series. J Neurosurg. 1999; 91:964–970

[47] Kihlstrom L, Lindquist C, Lindquist M, et al. Stereotactic radiosurgery for tectal low-grade gliomas. Acta Neurochir Suppl. 1994; 62:55–57

[48] Reinhardt A, Stichel D, Schrimpf D, et al. Anaplastic astrocytoma with piloid features, a novel molecular class of IDH wildtype glioma with recurrent MAPK pathway, CDKN2A/B and ATRX alterations. Acta Neuropathol. 2018; 136:273–291

[49] Fouladi M, Jenkins J, Burger P, et al. Pleomorphic xanthoastrocytoma: favorable outcome after complete surgical resection. Neuro-oncol. 2001; 3:184–192

[50] Weldon-Linne CM, Victor TA, Groothuis DR, et al. Pleomorphic Xanthoastrocytoma: Ultrastructural and Immunohistochemical Study of a Case with a Rapidly Fatal Outcome Following Surgery. Cancer. 1983; 52:2055–2063

[51] Kumar S, Retnam TM, Menon G, et al. Cerebellar hemisphere, an uncommon location for pleomorphic xanthoastrocytoma and lipidized glioblastoma multiformis. Neurol India. 2003; 51:246–247

[52] Pahapill PA, Ramsay DA, Del Maestro RF. Pleomorphic xanthoastrocytoma: case report and analysis of the literature concerning the efficacy of resection and the significance of necrosis. Neurosurgery. 1996; 38:822–8; discussion 828-9

[53] Giannini C, Scheithauer BW, Burger PC, et al. Pleomorphic xanthoastrocytoma: what do we really know about it? Cancer. 1999; 85:2033–2045

[54] Kepes JJ, Rubinstein LJ, Eng LF. Pleomorphic Xanthoastrocytoma: A Distinctive Meningeal Glioma of Young Subjects with Relatively Favorable Prognosis. A Study of 12 Cases. Cancer. 1979; 44:1839–1852

[55] Ida CM, Rodriguez FJ, Burger PC, et al. Pleomorphic Xanthoastrocytoma: Natural History and Long-Term Follow-Up. Brain Pathol. 2015; 25:575–586

[56] Gandham EJ, Goyal-Honavar A, Beno D, et al. Impact of Grade on Survival in Pleomorphic Xanthoastrocytoma and Low Prevalence of BRAF V600E Mutation. World Neurosurg. 2022; 164:e922–e928

[57] Chow CW, Klug GL, Lewis EA. Subependymal Giant-Cell Astrocytoma in Children: An Unusual Discrepancy Between Histological and Clinical Features. J Neurosurg. 1988; 68:880–883

[58] de Ribaupierre S, Dorfmuller G, Bulteau C, et al. Subependymal giant-cell astrocytomas in pediatric tuberous sclerosis disease: when should we operate? Neurosurgery. 2007; 60:83–89; discussion 89-90

[59] Franz DN, Belousova E, Sparagana S, et al. Long-Term Use of Everolimus in Patients with Tuberous Sclerosis Complex: Final Results from the EXIST-1 Study. PLoS One. 2016; 11. DOI: 10.1371/journal.pone.0158476

[60] Ampie L, Choy W, Lamano JB, et al. Prognostic factors for recurrence and complications in the surgical management of primary chordoid gliomas: A systematic review of literature. Clin Neurol Neurosurg. 2015; 138:129–136

[61] Chen W, Soon YY, Pratiseyo PD, et al. Central nervous system neuroepithelial tumors with MN1-alteration: an individual patient data meta-analysis of 73 cases. Brain Tumor Pathol. 2020; 37:145–153

[62] Tauziede-Espariat A, Pages M, Roux A, et al. Pediatric methylation class HGNET-MN1: unresolved issues with terminology and grading. Acta Neuropathol Commun. 2019; 7. DOI: 10.1186/s40478-019-0834-z

39

40 Glioneuronal and Neuronal Tumors

40.1 Glioneuronal tumors

40.1.1 Ganglioglioma (WHO grade 1)

General information

Key concepts

- a well-circumscribed tumor composed of two cell types: ganglion cells (neurons) and glial cells
- extremely rare (<2% of intracranial neoplasms)
- seen primarily in the first 3 decades of life
- characterized by slow growth and a tendency to calcify

A very slow-growing well-differentiated (WHO grade 1) glioneuronal tumor that primarily affects children and young adults. Composed of two types of cells, dysplastic ganglion cells (neurons) in conjunction with neoplastic glial cells (usually astrocytic in any phase of differentiation).[1] The term "ganglioglioma" was introduced in 1930 by Courville.[2]

An anaplastic ganglioglioma may exist in which the glial component exhibits anaplasia in the form of pronounced mitotic activity with a high Ki-67 proliferation index, necrosis and microvascular proliferation, however, most studies have lacked molecular analysis to exclude other tumor types, and refined data is therefore needed.

Diagnostic criteria for ganglioglioma

Diagnostic criteria for ganglioglioma are shown in ▶ Fig. 40.1.[3]

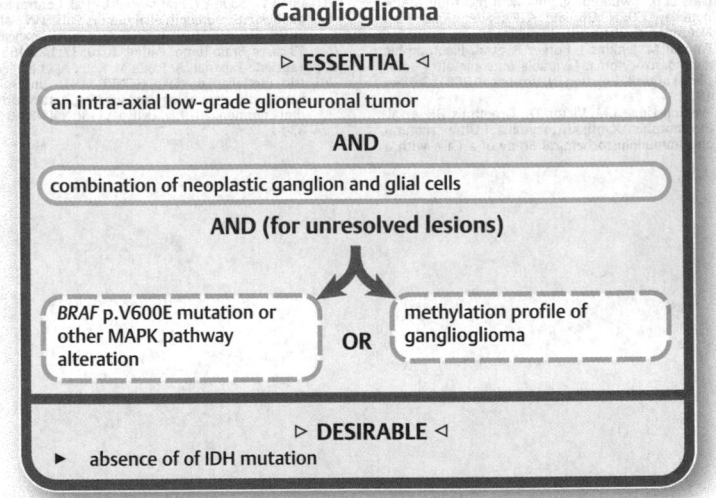

Fig. 40.1 **Diagnostic criteria for ganglioglioma.** (Modified with permission from WHO Classification of Tumors Editorial Board, (ed.) World Health Organization classification of tumors of the central nervous system. 5th ed. Bosman F T, Jaffe E S, Lakhani S R, et al. (series eds.): World Health Organization Classification of Tumors series, vol. 6. International Agency for Research on Cancer, Lyon, France, 2021.)

Epidemiology

Incidence: Typically quoted[4] as 0.3–0.6%. One series[5] found gangliogliomas in 1.3% of all brain tumors (including mets), or 3% of primary brain tumors.

Demographics: Occurs primarily in children and young adults (peak age of occurrence: 11 yrs). Considering only children and young adults, incidence ranges from 1.2–7.6% of brain tumors.[4]

Location

May occur in various parts of the nervous system (cerebral hemispheres, spinal cord, brainstem, cerebellum, pineal region, thalamus, intrasellar, optic nerve, and peripheral nerve have been reported[4]). Most occur above the tentorium, primarily in the temporal lobe (>70%) or near the 3rd ventricle, in the hypothalamus or in the frontal lobes.[6] Brainstem gangliogliomas (p.696) occur rarely.

Histology

Mixture of 2 types of neoplastic cells: neuronal (ganglion) and astrocytic (glial).

Grossly: white matter mass, well-circumscribed, firm, with occasional cystic areas and calcified regions. Most dissect easily from brain, but the solid portion may show an infiltrative tendency.[4]

Microscopically: ganglion cells demonstrate nerve cell differentiation, e.g., Nissl substance and axons or dendrites. Pitfall: differentiating neoplastic neurons from neurons entrapped by an invading astrocytoma may be difficult. Also, neoplastic astrocytes may resemble neurons on light microscopy. 2 of 10 patients had areas of oligodendroglioma. Also seen: necrotic areas, minimal calcification, and Rosenthal bodies.[7]

Radiologic evaluation

Neuroradiologic findings are not specific for this tumor.

CT: all of 10 patients had a low density lesion on non-contrast CT.[5] Tumor calcification are best appreciated on CT and are seen in 30%. Frequently appears cystic on CT, but still may be found to be solid at operation.

MRI: T1WI low to iso-intense with variable enhancement. T2WI hyperintense. Calcifications appear as low signal on both.

CT and MRI: the temporal lobe is favored. Mass effect rare (suggests slow growth). Enhancement varies from none to intense.

Plain skull X-ray: calcification may be noted.

Treatment

Recommendation is maximal safe resection. Close follow-up is recommended, and re-resection should be considered for recurrence. The role of XRT is unknown, and due to the deleterious effects together with the good long-term prognosis, it is not recommended initially but may be considered for recurrence.[8]

Prognosis

These benign tumors have a 97% 7.5-year recurrence-free survival rate.

Prognosis is better with temporal lobe location, gross total excision, and chronic epilepsy.

The correlation between histologic anaplasia and outcome is inconsistent.

The prognosis following subtotal resection of brainstem gangliogliomas is better than for brainstem gliomas as a group.[6]

40.1.2 Gangliocytoma (WHO grade 1)

General information

A rare, slow-growing well-differentiated (WHO grade 1) tumor that primarily affects children, characterized by clusters of neoplastic ganglion cells, frequently with dysplastic features.

Diagnostic criteria for gangliocytoma

Diagnostic criteria for gangliocytoma are shown in ▶ Fig. 40.2.[3]

40

Gangliocytoma

▷ ESSENTIAL ◁

a tumefactive lesion with presence of irregular groups of large, mature ganglion cells

AND

matrix resembling normal neuropil, sometimes more coarsely fibrillar or vacuolated

▷ DESIRABLE ◁

- **atypical and binucleated ganglion cells**
- **cytoplasmic ballooning or vacuolization**

Fig. 40.2 Diagnostic criteria for gangliocytoma. (Modified with permission from WHO Classification of Tumors Editorial Board, (ed.) World Health Organization classification of tumors of the central nervous system. 5th ed. Bosman F T, Jaffe E S, Lakhani S R, et al. (series eds.): World Health Organization Classification of Tumors series, vol. 6. International Agency for Research on Cancer, Lyon, France, 2021.)

Location

As with ganglioglioma, gangliocytomas can occur anywhere in the CNS. Most occur above the tentorium, primarily in the temporal lobe (> 70%) or near the 3rd ventricle, in the hypothalamus or in the frontal lobes.[6] They have been described in the pituitary.

Prognosis

Gangliocytomas are benign tumors with generallly good prognosis. No specific prognostic inidcators have been identified.

40.1.3 Desmoplastic infantile ganglioglioma (DIG) & desmoplastic infantile astrocytoma (DIA) (WHO grade 1)

General information

DIA & DIG are benign (WHO grade 1) glioneural tumor with a neuroepithelial population (restricted to either neoplastic astrocytes only (DIA) or to astrocytes with a variably mature neuronal component (DIG)) in a desmoplastic stroma.

DIA & DIG usually occur primarily in the cerebral hemispheres of infants, often as a large cystic lesion, frequently attached to dura. They are driven by MAPK pathway alteration.

These tumors rarely seed through the CSF.[9]

Diagnostic criteria for desmoplastic infantile ganglioglioma & desmoplastic infantile astrocytoma

Diagnostic criteria for desmoplastic infantile ganglioglioma & desmoplastic infantile astrocytoma are shown in ▶ Fig. 40.3.[3]

Prognosis

Prognosis is usually favorable with gross total resection, with no relapse in 5-15 years of follow-up. They can rarely recur with anaplastic transformation as long as 8-10 years after initial resection, and the reponse to re-resection is promising.[10]

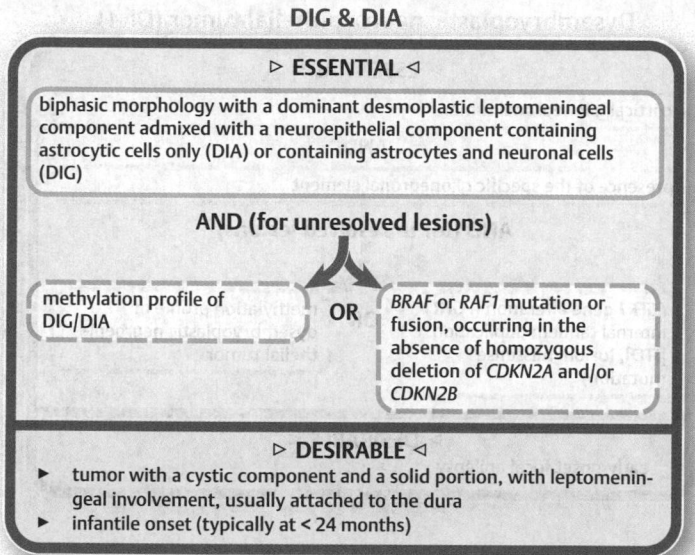

Fig. 40.3 Diagnostic criteria for desmoplastic infantile ganglioglioma & desmoplastic infantile astrocytoma.
(Modified with permission from WHO Classification of Tumors Editorial Board, (ed.) World Health Organization classification of tumors of the central nervous system. 5th ed. Bosman F T, Jaffe E S, Lakhani S R, et al. (series eds.): World Health Organization Classification of Tumors series, vol. 6. International Agency for Research on Cancer, Lyon, France, 2021.)

40.1.4 Dysembryoplastic neuroepithelial tumor (DNT) (WHO grade 1)

General information

A WHO grade 1 glioneuronal tumor usually cortically based in the temporal lobe of children and young adults, characterized by a multinodular architecture with neuroglial columns, with a pathognomonic glioneuronal element.

Thought to arise embryologically from the secondary germinal layer (which includes subependymal layer, cerebellar external granular layer, hippocampal dentate fascia, and subpial granular layer).

Most DNTs are sporadic, and result from *FGFR1* alterations present in 40-80% of DNTs which upregulate the MAPK and PI3K pathways. *BRAF* p.V600E mutations are found in up to 50% in some studies.

Diagnostic criteria for dysembryoplastic neuroepithelial tumor

Diagnostic criteria for dysembryoplastic neuroepithelial tumor are shown in ▶ Fig. 40.4.[3]

Epidemiology

Incidence: not accurately known because the diagnosis may be missed. Estimated range: 0.8–5% of all primary brain tumors. Typically occurs in children and young adults. Slight preponderance in males.

Location

DNTs have a predilection for the temporal lobes (67% of cases) and the frontal lobe (16%), with the remainder occurring in any other location within the cerebral cortex.

40

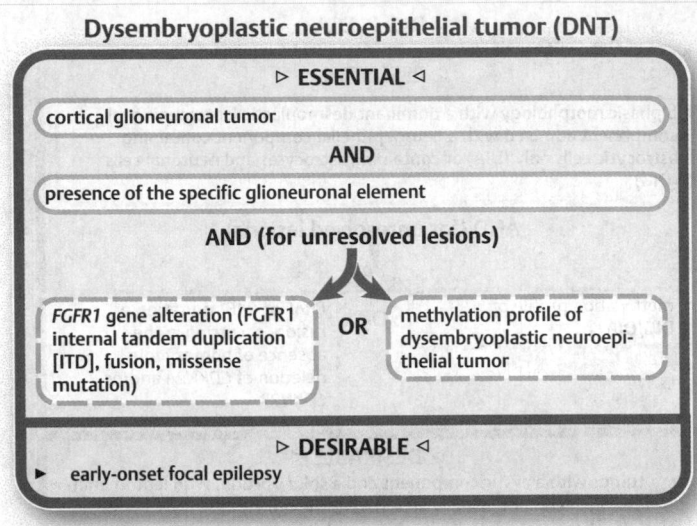

Fig. 40.4 Diagnostic criteria for dysembryoplastic neuroepithelial tumor. (Modified with permission from WHO Classification of Tumors Editorial Board, (ed.) World Health Organization classification of tumors of the central nervous system. 5th ed. Bosman F T, Jaffe E S, Lakhani S R, et al. (series eds.): World Health Organization Classification of Tumors series, vol. 6. International Agency for Research on Cancer, Lyon, France, 2021.)

Histology

Multinodularity at low-power is a key feature with neuroglial columns comprised of bundles of axons aligned perpendicular to the cortical surface. These columns are lined by oligodendriglial like cells incorporated within a mucoid matrix with interspersed neurons.[11] Occasionally difficult to differentiate from oligodendroglioma.

Two distinct forms[12] (do not appear to have different prognoses):
1. simple form: glioneural elements consisting of axon bundles perpendicular to the cortical surface, lined with oligodendroglial-like cells that are S-100 positive and GFAP negative. Normal appearing neurons floating in a pale eosinophilic matrix are scattered between these columns (no resemblance to ganglion cells, unlike gangliogliomas)
2. complex form: glioneural elements as described above in the simple form, with glial nodules scattered throughout. The glial component may mimic a low-grade fibrillary astrocytoma. Foci of cortical dysplasia occur

Clinical

Typically associated with longstanding medically intractable seizures, usually complex partial. Symptoms usually begin before age 20.

Imaging

Cortical lesions that traverse the entire cortical mantle with no surrounding edema and no midline mass effect.

CT: hypodense with distinct margins. Deformity of overlying calvaria is common.

MRI: T1WI: hypointense. T2WI: hyperintense, septations may be seen. If there is enhancement, it is usually nodular.

PET scan: hypometabolic with [18F]-fluorodeoxyglucose. Negative [11C]-methionine uptake (unlike all other gliomas).

40

Prognosis

Seizure control: usually improves after surgery. Degree of control seems to correlate with completeness of removal. Improvement in seizures correlates inversely with the duration of intractable seizures.

Recurrence/continued growth: recurrence after complete removal, or tumor growth after partial resection is rare. Adjuvant treatment (XRT, chemotherapy…) is of no benefit in these benign tumors. Mitoses or endothelial proliferation, seen on occasion, do not affect outcome. Malignant transformation is very rare.

40.1.5 Diffuse glioneuronal tumor with oligodendroglioma-like features and nuclear clusters (DGONC) (WHO grade N/A)

General information

DGONC is a provisional entity for a neuroepithelial tumor with variably differentiated cells, often possessing perinuclear haloes, scattered multinucleated cells and nuclear clusters, having a distinct DNA methylation profile and frequent chromosome 14 monosomy.

Diagnostic criteria for diffuse glioneuronal tumor with oligodendroglioma-like features and nuclear clusters (DGONC)

Diagnostic criteria for DGONC are shown in ► Fig. 40.5.[3]

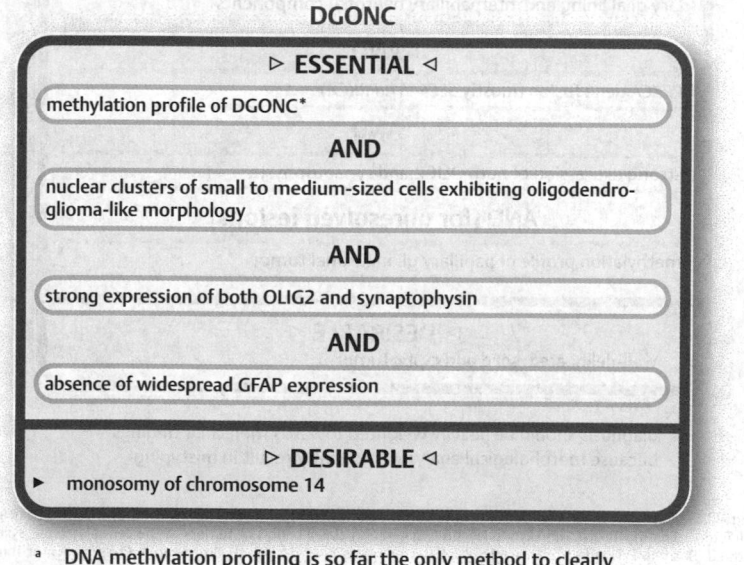

DGONC

▷ **ESSENTIAL** ◁

methylation profile of DGONC*

AND

nuclear clusters of small to medium-sized cells exhibiting oligodendroglioma-like morphology

AND

strong expression of both OLIG2 and synaptophysin

AND

absence of widespread GFAP expression

▷ **DESIRABLE** ◁

► monosomy of chromosome 14

a   DNA methylation profiling is so far the only method to clearly identify DGONC. If DNA methylation profiling is not available, morphological features may provide an approximation.

Fig. 40.5 Diagnostic criteria for DGONC. (Modified with permission from WHO Classification of Tumors Editorial Board, (ed.) World Health Organization classification of tumors of the central nervous system. 5th ed. Bosman F T, Jaffe E S, Lakhani S R, et al. (series eds.): World Health Organization Classification of Tumors series, vol. 6. International Agency for Research on Cancer, Lyon, France, 2021.)

40

Location

In the small number of cases reported, all were supratentorial.[13,14]

Prognosis

Outcome has been report only for 26 cases which showed 81% 5-year PFS, and 89% 5-year OS.[13,14] Treatment data are available only for 3 patients.

40.1.6 Papillary glioneuronal tumor (PGNT) (WHO grade 1)

General information

A rare glioneuronal tumor of young adults with a biphasic pattern and variable manifestation of pseudopapillary glial structures and interpapillary neuronal components, and possessing *PRKCA* gene fusion (primarily *SLC44A1::PRKCA* fusion).

Diagnostic criteria for papillary glioneuronal tumor

Diagnostic criteria for papillary glioneuronal tumor are shown in ▶ Fig. 40.6.[3]

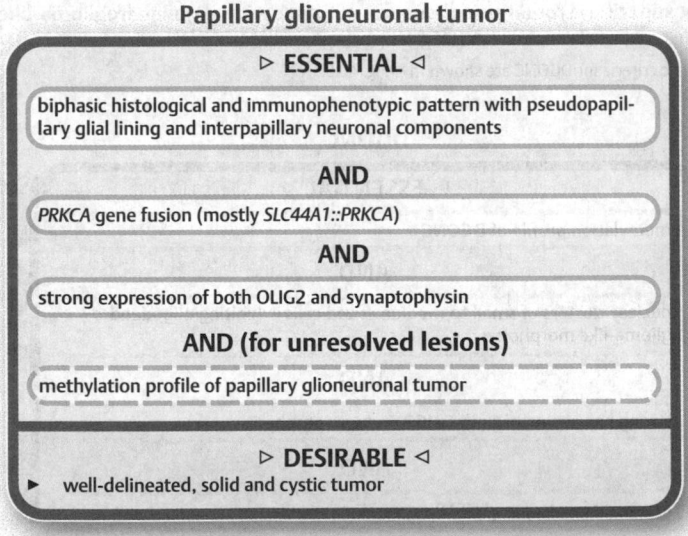

Fig. 40.6 Diagnostic criteria for papillary glioneuronal tumor. (Modified with permission from WHO Classification of Tumors Editorial Board, (ed.) World Health Organization classification of tumors of the central nervous system. 5th ed. Bosman F T, Jaffe E S, Lakhani S R, et al. (series eds.): World Health Organization Classification of Tumors series, vol. 6. International Agency for Research on Cancer, Lyon, France, 2021.)

Location

PGNT are supratentorial, most often in the temporal lobe (28%), frequently in proximity to the lateral ventricle (28%).[15]

Imaging

PGNT appear as well demarcated lesions with solid and cystic components and mild mass effect and edema. Portions may enhance with contrast.

Prognosis

The ability to achieve gross total excision is the primary prognostic factor.

40.1.7 Rosette-forming glioneuronal tumor (RGNT) (WHO grade 1)

General information

A rare, slow-growing WHO 1 glioneuronal tumor with two histological components: 1) uniform neurocytes forming rosettes and/or perivascular pseudorosettes, and 2) glial component with piloid and oligodendrogliocyte-like cells resembling a pilocytic astrocytoma.

Although WHO grade 1, they occasionally develop satellite lesions, leptomeningeal involvement or "drop mets" (dissemination of tumor through the CSF to dependent areas, e.g., spinal cord).

Diagnostic criteria for rosette-forming glioneuronal tumor (RGNT)

Diagnostic criteria for rosette-forming glioneuronal tumor are shown in ▶ Fig. 40.7.[3]

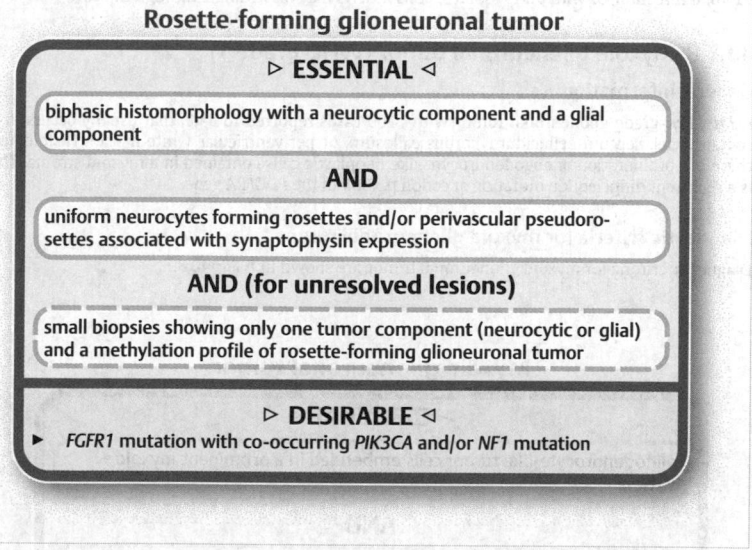

Fig. 40.7 Diagnostic criteria for rosette-forming glioneuronal tumor. (Modified with permission from WHO Classification of Tumors Editorial Board, (ed.) World Health Organization classification of tumors of the central nervous system. 5th ed. Bosman F T, Jaffe E S, Lakhani S R, et al. (series eds.): World Health Organization Classification of Tumors series, vol. 6. International Agency for Research on Cancer, Lyon, France, 2021.)

Epidemiology

The literature on RGNTs is limited to case reports and single center retrospective studies.[16] Slight female preponderance (male:female ratio of 1:1.36).[17] Mean age is 23.57 years (median 22.5, range 4-49).[16] There is no accepted theory for cytogenesis of these tumors.

Location

RGNTs are typically midline, arise from the 4th ventricle in 42%, and extend into adjacent structures.[16] However, they may also occur in the pineal region, third ventricle, optic chiasm, thalamus and temporal lobe. Spinal cord involvement has also been reported.

Histology

RGNTs demonstrate mixed glial and neuronal elements emblematic of tumors in the class of glioneural tumors.

Imaging

CT: RGNTs are hypodense.

MRI: appearance is variable. They are relatively well circumscribed. Most have solid and cystic components, but they can be either one alone. They tend to be hyperintense on T2WI, and iso- or hypo-intense on T1WI with variable enhancement.

Treatment

Treatment of choice is of choice is gross total resection (GTR) when possible.

Prognosis

Prognosis for OS is favorable. Recurrence is rare after GTR. However, neurologic deficit following surgery is common. Malignant progression has been reported in 2 cases[16]), and may be higher risk with subtotal resection, or with purely solid lesions. RGNTs may disseminate through the CSF.

40.1.8 Myxoid glioneuronal tumor (WHO grade 1)

General information

A rare, low-grade glioneuronal tumor with < 100 cases reported to date, that usually occurs in the septal nuclei, septum pellucidum, corpus callosum, or periventricular white matter. Histologically there is a proliferation of oligodendrocyte-like neoplastic cells contained in a myxoid stroma. There is a recurrent dinucleotide mutation at codon p.K385 in the *PDGFRA* gene.

Diagnostic criteria for myxoid glioneuronal tumor

Diagnostic criteria for myxoid glioneuronal tumor are shown in ▶ Fig. 40.8.[3]

Myxoid glioneuronal tumor

▷ **ESSENTIAL** ◁

oligodendrocyte-like tumor cells embedded in a prominent myxoid stroma

AND

location in septal nuclei, septum pellucidum, corpus callosum, or periventricular white matter

▷ **DESIRABLE**[a] ◁

► *PDGFRA* p.K385L/I dinucleotide mutation or (less commonly) other mutations in the extracellular domain of *PDGFRA*
► methylation profile of myxoid glioneuronal tumor

a   desirable diagnostic criteria can be essential for unresolved cases

Fig. 40.8 Diagnostic criteria for myxoid glioneuronal tumor. (Modified with permission from WHO Classification of Tumors Editorial Board, (ed.) World Health Organization classification of tumors of the central nervous system. 5th ed. Bosman F T, Jaffe E S, Lakhani S R, et al. (series eds.): World Health Organization Classification of Tumors series, vol. 6. International Agency for Research on Cancer, Lyon, France, 2021.)

Imaging

Well circumscribed tumor that is hypointense on T1 and hyperintense on T2 MRI. On SWI, susceptibility artifact may be seen, suggestive of previous hemorrhages. Septal lesions often produce obstructive hydrocephalus.

Prognosis

These slow growing tumors have a favorable prognosis for OS. A subset may recur locally or disseminate through the CSF, but their behavior remains indolent. Dedifferentiation has not been reported.

40.1.9 Diffuse leptomeningeal glioneuronal tumor (DLGNT) (WHO grade 2 or 3)

General information

A glioneuronal neoplasm comprised of oligodendrocyte-like cells that is characterized by chromosome arm 1p deletion and a MAPK pathway gene alteration, typically *KIAA1549::BRAF* fusion. Leptomeningeal involvement is common.

Diagnostic criteria for diffuse leptomeningeal glioneuronal tumor

Diagnostic criteria for diffuse leptomeningeal glioneuronal tumor are shown in ▶ Fig. 40.9.[3]

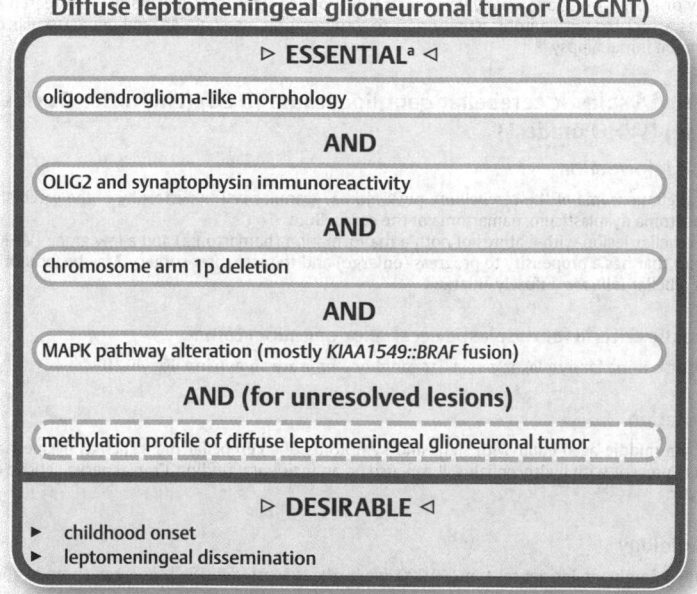

Fig. 40.9 Diagnostic criteria for diffuse leptomeningeal glioneuronal tumor. (Modified with permission from WHO Classification of Tumors Editorial Board, (ed.) World Health Organization classification of tumors of the central nervous system. 5th ed. Bosman F T, Jaffe E S, Lakhani S R, et al. (series eds.): World Health Organization Classification of Tumors series, vol. 6. International Agency for Research on Cancer, Lyon, France, 2021.)

40

Subtypes

See reference.[3]
- **diffuse leptomeningeal glioneuronal tumor with 1q gain**
- **diffuse leptomeningeal glioneuronal tumor, methylation class 1 (DLGNT-MC-1)**
- **diffuse leptomeningeal glioneuronal tumor, methylation class 2 (DLGNT-MC-2)**

Grading

Data for grading these tumors is limited. Most DLGNTs are well differentiated low-grade tumors. A subset may show anaplastic features on histology. For cases of conventional DLGNT and DLGNT-MC-1, the behavior has been consistent with WHO grade 2 entities. Whereas tumors with anaplastic features, 1 q gain and/or DLGNT-MC-2 profile have a clinical course more suggestive of a WHO grade 3 lesion.

Location

Predilection for the spinal and intracranial leptomeninges. Intracranially, leptomeningeal growth is tupically observed in the posterior fossa, around the brainstem and along the skull base.

Imaging

MRI usually shows diffuse leptomeningeal enhancement and thickening alongside the spinal cord with intracranial extension to the posterior fossa, brainstem and basal cisterns.

Prognosis

Stability or slow growth over many years may still produce significant morbidity.[18] Decreased survival was associated with mitotic activity, a Ki-67 proliferation index of ≥ 4%, and microvascular proliferation on initial biopsy.[18]

40.1.10 Dysplastic cerebellar gangliocytoma (DCG) (Lhermitte-Duclos disease) (WHO grade 1)

General information

AKA: ganglioneuroma of the cerebellum, purkinjoma, granular cell hypertrophy of the cerebellum, gangliocytoma dysplasticum, hamartoma of the cerebellum.

A cerebellar lesion with features of both a malformation (hamartoma) and a low grade (WHO 1) neoplasm that has a propensity to progress (enlarge) and to recur after surgery. May be focal or diffuse. Cerebellar folia are diffusely enlarged.

Diagnostic criteria for dysplastic cerebellar gangliocytoma

Diagnostic criteria for dysplastic cerebellar gangliocytoma are shown in ▸ Fig. 40.10.[3]

Presentation

Typically a middle-aged *adult* with signs and symptoms of a cerebellar mass such as dysmetria, or they may present with hydrocephalus. It can also be an incidental finding. Cranial nerve deficits may also occur.

Epidemiology

Autosomal dominant. Incidence: 1 in 250,000 live births.[19] Most identified cases have been in adults, but patients as young a 3 years have been reported. Strongly associated with Cowden syndrome (p. 651) (AKA PTEN hamartoma tumor syndrome) where the incidence is 1 in 200,000.[20] Associated with thyroid, breast, and uterine cancer, mucosal neuromas and meningiomas.

Histology

Derangement of normal laminar cellular architecture of the cerebellum with:
1. thickening of the outer molecular cell layer
2. loss of middle Purkinje cell layer
3. infiltration of inner granular cell layer with dysplastic ganglion cells

40

Dysplastic cerebellar gangliocytoma

▷ **ESSENTIAL** ◁

gangliocytic lesion enlarging cerebellar folia

AND

densely packed ganglionic cells of various sizes

AND

matrix resembling normal neuropil, sometimes more coarsely fibrillar or vacuolated

▷ **DESIRABLE** ◁

► *PTEN* mutation/deletion or loss of expression
► abnormal myelination and vacuolization in the outer molecular layer
► calcification and ectatic vessels

Fig. 40.10 Diagnostic criteria for dysplastic cerebellar gangliocytoma. (Modified with permission from WHO Classification of Tumors Editorial Board, (ed.) World Health Organization classification of tumors of the central nervous system. 5th ed. Bosman F T, Jaffe E S, Lakhani S R, et al. (series eds.): World Health Organization Classification of Tumors series, vol. 6. International Agency for Research on Cancer, Lyon, France, 2021.)

Imaging

CT: hypo- to isodense, nonenhancing lesion with mass effect.

MRI: T1WI: hypo- to isointense. T2WI: hyperintense, heterogeneous. Nonenhancing. Characteristic striated appearance[21] (tiger stripes) due to widened cerebellar folia. May contain calcifications. DWI: hyperintense. ADC map: hypointense.

NB: in a child with MRI findings of Lhermitte-Duclos disease (LDD) (even if classic), a medulloblastoma is statistically more likely[22,23] (especially medulloblastoma with extensive nodularity[24] (MBEN)).

Treatment

Controversial. A few cases with a benign course have been described.[25] Shunting is performed for hydrocephalus. Biopsy is recommended[23] particularly for pediatric cases to rule out medulloblastoma. Surgical excision may be considered when there is significant mass effect.[26] Efficacy of XRT is unknown.

Prognosis

Most patients are cured by surgery when indicated. Since DCG may be a harbinger of Cowden syndrome, patients should be monitored for other tumors, e.g., breast and thyroid cancer.

40.2 Neuronal tumors

40.2.1 Multinodular and vacuolating neuronal tumor (MVNT) (WHO grade 1)

40

General information

A rare tumor (17 case reports as of 2018[27]) comprised of uniform neuronal elements dispersed in discrete nodules with vacuolar changes. MVNTs favor the temporal lobes and characteristically involve the deep cortical ribbon and superficial white matter.

Diagnostic criteria for multinodular and vacuolating neuronal tumor

Diagnostic criteria for multinodular and vacuolating neuronal tumor are shown in ▶ Fig. 40.11.[3]

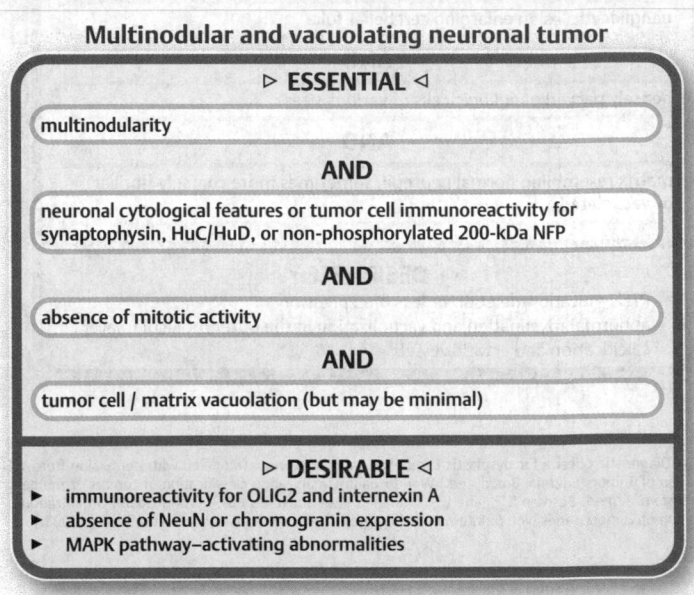

Multinodular and vacuolating neuronal tumor

▷ **ESSENTIAL** ◁

multinodularity

AND

neuronal cytological features or tumor cell immunoreactivity for synaptophysin, HuC/HuD, or non-phosphorylated 200-kDa NFP

AND

absence of mitotic activity

AND

tumor cell / matrix vacuolation (but may be minimal)

▷ **DESIRABLE** ◁

► immunoreactivity for OLIG2 and internexin A
► absence of NeuN or chromogranin expression
► MAPK pathway–activating abnormalities

Fig. 40.11 Diagnostic criteria for multinodular and vacuolating neuronal tumor. (Modified with permission from WHO Classification of Tumors Editorial Board, (ed.) World Health Organization classification of tumors of the central nervous system. 5th ed. Bosman F T, Jaffe E S, Lakhani S R, et al. (series eds.): World Health Organization Classification of Tumors series, vol. 6. International Agency for Research on Cancer, Lyon, France, 2021.)

Location

There is a predilection for the temporal lobes (75-80%) and frontal lobes (10-15%).[27]

Presentation

The most common presentation is seizures (60%) which may be complex partial ± secondary generalization, followed by headache (10-15%).

Prognosis

These are benign neoplasms. Following gross total excision there are no reports of recurrence, and subtotally resected tumors have not progressed.

40.2.2 Central neurocytoma (WHO grade 2)

General information

> ### Key concepts
>
> - rare, WHO grade 2 neuronal tumor primarily seen in young adults
> - typically intraventricular, attached to septum pellucidum
> - gross total resection can be curative (but some recur even after GTR)
> - if MIB-1 labeling index > 2–4%, there is an increased risk of recurrence after subtotal resection
> - if MIB-1 labeling is elevated, radiation therapy after subtotal resection can reduce the risk of recurrence

Central neurocytomas are rare WHO grade 2 neuronal tumors. They are generally attached to the septum pellucidum within the lateral ventricles, and less frequently occur within the third ventricle. The most common presentation is with increased intracranial pressure and ventriculomegaly.[28],[29] See also differential diagnosis for intraventricular lesions (p.1667).

Due to an uncertain relation of prognosis to Ki-67 index and anaplastic features, a distinction between a possible grade 1 vs. 2 was not made.[30]

Diagnostic criteria for central neurocytoma

Diagnostic criteria for central neurocytoma are shown in ► Fig. 40.12.[3]

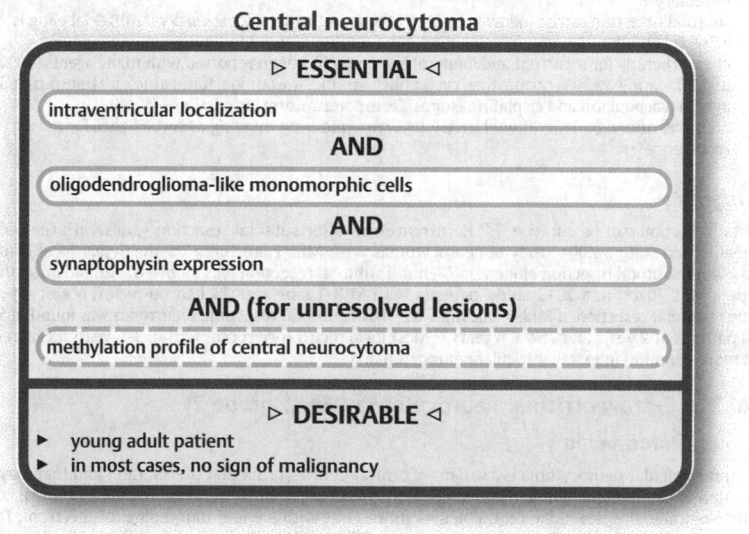

Central neurocytoma

▷ **ESSENTIAL** ◁

intraventricular localization

AND

oligodendroglioma-like monomorphic cells

AND

synaptophysin expression

AND (for unresolved lesions)

methylation profile of central neurocytoma

▷ **DESIRABLE** ◁

► young adult patient
► in most cases, no sign of malignancy

Fig. 40.12 Diagnostic criteria for central neurocytoma. (Modified with permission from WHO Classification of Tumors Editorial Board, (ed.) World Health Organization classification of tumors of the central nervous system. 5th ed. Bosman F T, Jaffe E S, Lakhani S R, et al. (series eds.): World Health Organization Classification of Tumors series, vol. 6. International Agency for Research on Cancer, Lyon, France, 2021.)

40

Epidemiology

Constitutes 0.1–0.5% of brain tumors. Incidence peaks in the 3rd decade, but they can also present in children and the elderly.[31] No gender predominates.

Histology

Central neurocytoma cells have small, round nuclei. Cells often have a "fried egg" appearance on H&E staining, which can mimic oligodendroglioma. There are two primary architectures: honeycomb (also mimicking oligodendroglioma) and fibrillary. Rosettes can also be seen. Immunohistochemistry is often positive for neuronal markers synaptophysin and Neu-N.

Electron microscopy: not necessary for diagnosis.[30] It has been used by some when the diagnosis is not clear, and demonstrates neuronal features, including: a prominent golgi apparatus, parallel microtubules, and dense core neurosecretory granules.[28,29]

Molecular genetics: 1p/19q deletion has not been reported in central neurocytoma, but it can be seen in extraventricular neurocytoma.[32]

Imaging

CT scan: 25–50% of these tumors show calcifications. Tumors are usually iso- to hyperdense, with hypodense areas that represent cystic degeneration.[28]

MRI: Tumors appear heterogeneously isointense on T1 and hyperintense on T2. MR spectroscopy often shows a high glycine peak.[33]

Moderate to strong contrast enhancement occurs on both CT and MR images.[29]

Treatment

1. total resection is often curative. After gross total resection, radiation therapy is generally not necessary[28]
2. subtotal resection can be followed by stereotactic radiosurgery, especially if MIB-1 labeling is > 2–4%[28,29,33,34]
3. chemotherapy for recurrent and inoperable tumors has been reported with many agents, including: alkylating agents (carmustine, cyclophosphamide, ifosfamide, lomustine), platinum-based agents (carboplatin and cisplatin), etoposide, topotecan, and vincristine[33,34]
4. after treatment, patients should have long-term follow-up imaging as surveillance for tumor recurrence[29]

Prognosis

Total resection can be curative.[28,33] Recurrence risk after subtotal resection varies with the MIB-1 labeling index. In a 2004 study of neurocytomas with MIB-1 labeling > 2%, the 5-year local control rate after subtotal resection alone was 7%, but if subtotal resection was followed with radiation therapy it was 70%.[34] In a 2013 study, patients with MIB-1 labeling < 4% had no recurrence at 4 years after subtotal resection. If MIB-1 labeling was > 4% at subtotal resection, recurrence was found in 50% of patients at 2 years and 75% at 4 years.[33] Most local recurrences occur within 3–6 years. Recurrence is more common in extraventricular neurocytoma.[34]

40.2.3 Extraventricular neurocytoma (WHO grade 2)

General information

Extraventricular neurocytoma is a variant of central neurocytoma that is even rarer and that may be located in the cerebral parenchyma, cerebellum, thalamus, brainstem, pineal region, and spinal cord. Histologically, they resemble central neurocytomas but with a wider morphological spectrum. They can be focally infiltrative into surrounding tissue. *FGFR1::TACC1* fusions are frequently identified.

Diagnostic criteria for extraventricular neurocytoma

Diagnostic criteria for extraventricular neurocytoma are shown in ▶ Fig. 40.13.[3]

Histology

Histology is similar to central neurocytoma.

Immunohistochemistry is positive for synaptophysin in the cytoplasm and neuropil. Neu-N staining is often positive.

40

Extraventricular neurocytoma

▷ **ESSENTIAL** ◁

extraventricular neurocytic neoplasm without IDH alteration

AND

synaptophysin expression

AND (for unresolved lesions)

methylation profile of extraventricular neurocytoma

▷ **DESIRABLE** ◁

► OLIG2 immunonegativity
► loss of ATRX expression
► diffuse p53 immunopositivity

ᵃ diagnosis should be heavily weighted towards molecular findings because morphological analyses frequently result in mistyping

Fig. 40.13 Diagnostic criteria for extraventricular neurocytoma. (Modified with permission from WHO Classification of Tumors Editorial Board, (ed.) World Health Organization classification of tumors of the central nervous system. 5th ed. Bosman F T, Jaffe E S, Lakhani S R, et al. (series eds.): World Health Organization Classification of Tumors series, vol. 6. International Agency for Research on Cancer, Lyon, France, 2021.)

Central neurocytoma can often be identified by its intraventricular location, however for extraventricular neurocytoma the reactivity for synaptophysin without either IDH mutation or 1p/19q codeletion can differentiate this tumor from oligodendroglioma.

Molecular genetics

The most common genetic alterations are *FGFR1::TACC1* fusions which were found in 60%, while other FGFR alterations were present in 13%.[35] Neither IDH1/2 mutation nor MGMT promoter gene methylation (p. 673) has been reported.[36]

Prognosis

The overall prognosis with this low-grade tumor is favorable. The rate of recurrence has been low and seizure control has been good following gross total resection.

40.2.4 Cerebellar liponeurocytoma (WHO grade 2)

General information

Formerly lipomatous medulloblastoma. A rare WHO grade 2 neoplasm with neuronal/neurocytic differentiation and clusters of neoplastic neurocytes with lipidization (resembling adipocytes) that occurs exclusively in cerebellum (typically in the cerebellar hemispheres, and less commonly the midline or CPA) of adults (mean age: 50 years). No gender preference.

Some authors suggest the more inclusive name "Liponeurocytoma" should replace the separate WHO classification of "Cerebellar liponeurocytoma." Others contend that the supratentorial exceptions are central neurocytomas which contain neurocytes that underwent lipidization, instead of having actual adipose metaplasia.[37]

Diagnostic criteria for cerebellar liponeurocytoma

Diagnostic criteria for cerebellar liponeurocytoma are shown in ► Fig. 40.14.[3]

40

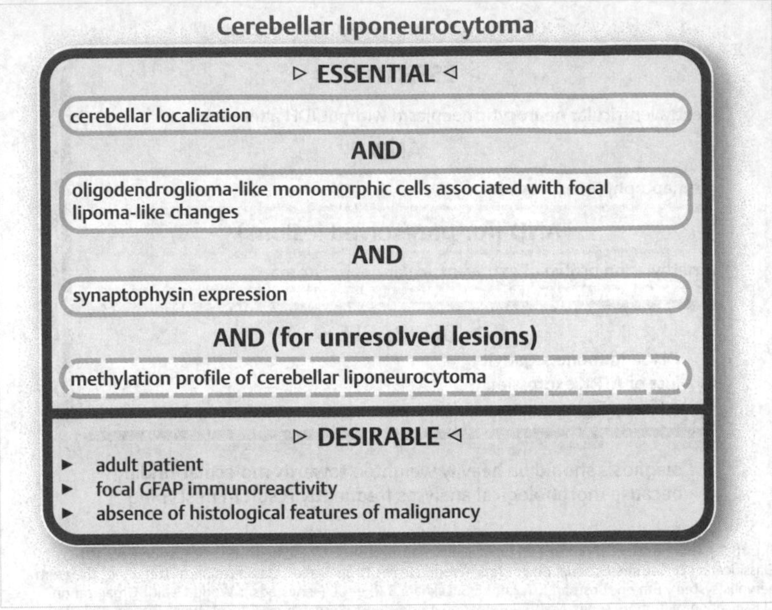

Fig. 40.14 **Diagnostic criteria for cerebellar liponeurocytoma.** (Modified with permission from WHO Classification of Tumors Editorial Board, (ed.) World Health Organization classification of tumors of the central nervous system. 5th ed. Bosman F T, Jaffe E S, Lakhani S R, et al. (series eds.): World Health Organization Classification of Tumors series, vol. 6. International Agency for Research on Cancer, Lyon, France, 2021.)

Imaging

CT: isodense in areas, with areas of very low density where the fat content is high.

MRI: lipid rich areas are hyperintense on T1 and T2. The suspicion about lipid content is supported when these areas drop out on fat suppression sequences.

Histology

Cells are uniform, neuocytic morphology with regular round to oval nuclei and clear cytoplasm with ill-defined cell mambranes arrayed in sheets and lobules. The distinctive feature are lipid containing cells resembling adipocytes.

Synaptophysin (p. 632) and MAP-2 immunostaining is consistent and diffuse, focal GFAP staining is common. Usually no mitotic figures. MIB-1 index is usually low (mean of 3.73% ± 4.01%).[38]

Prognosis

Cerebellar liponeurocytoma have a favorable prognosis. Following GTR, the 5-year survival rate was 71.3%, PFS rate 61%, mean OS was 16.3 years, and the mean PFS was 10 years.[38] Subtotal resection carried a 42% recurrence rate vs. 15% with GTR.[38] Post-op radiation improved the PFS from 55% (16/29 patients) to 92% (11 out of 12) with median follow-up of 52 months.[38] All recurrences were restricted to the posterior fossa.

40

References

[1] Rubinstein LJ. Tumors of the Central Nervous System. Atlas of Tumor Pathology, Second Series, Fascicle 6. Washington, DC: Armed Forces Institute of Pathology; 1972

[2] Courville CB. Ganglioglioma. Tumor of the Central Nervous System: Review of the Literature and Report of Two Cases. Archives of Neurology and Psychiatry. 1930; 24:439–491

[3] Bosman FT, Jaffe ES, Lakhani SR, et al. World Health Organization Classification of Tumors series, vol. 6. In: WHO Classification of Tumors Editorial Board (ed.) World Health Organization classification of tumors of the central nervous system. 5th ed. Lyon, France: International Agency for Research on Cancer; 2021

[4] Demierre B, Stichnoth FA, Hori A, et al. Intracerebral Ganglioglioma. J Neurosurg. 1986; 65:177–182

[5] Kalyan-Raman UP, Olivero WC. Ganglioglioma: A Correlative Clinicopathological and Radiological Study of Ten Surgically Treated Cases with Follow-Up. Neurosurgery. 1987; 20:428–433

[6] Garcia CA, McGarry PA, Collada M. Ganglioglioma of the Brain Stem. Case Report. Journal of Neurosurgery. 1984; 60:431–434

[7] Sutton LN, Packer RJ, Rorke LB, et al. Cerebral Gangliogliomas During Childhood. Neurosurgery. 1983; 13:124–128

[8] Lang FF, Epstein FJ, Ransohoff J, et al. Central Nervous System Gangliogliomas. Part 2: Clinical Outcome. Journal of Neurosurgery. 1993; 79:867–873

[9] Darwish B, Arbuckle S, Kellie S, et al. Desmoplastic infantile ganglioglioma/astrocytoma with cerebrospinal metastasis. J Clin Neurosci. 2007; 14:498–501

[10] Loh JK, Lieu AS, Chai CY, et al. Malignant transformation of a desmoplastic infantile ganglioglioma. Pediatr Neurol. 2011; 45:135–137

[11] Daumas-Duport C, Scheithauer BW, Chodkiewicz J-P, et al. Dysembryoplastic Neuroepithelial Tumor: A Surgically Curable Tumor of Young Patients with Intractable Seizures. Neurosurgery. 1988; 23:545–556

[12] Adada B, Sayed K. Dysembryoplastic neuroepithelial tumors. Contemporary Neurosurgery. 2004; 26:1–5

[13] Deng MY, Sill M, Sturm D, et al. Diffuse glioneuronal tumour with oligodendroglioma-like features and nuclear clusters (DGONC) - a molecularly defined glioneuronal CNS tumour class displaying recurrent monosomy 14. Neuropathol Appl Neurobiol. 2020; 46:422–430

[14] Pickles JC, Mankad K, Aizpurua M, et al. A case series of Diffuse Glioneuronal Tumours with Oligodendroglioma-like features and Nuclear Clusters (DGONC). Neuropathol Appl Neurobiol. 2021; 47:464–467

[15] Hou Y, Pinheiro J, Sahm F, et al. Papillary glioneuronal tumor (PGNT) exhibits a characteristic methylation profile and fusions involving PRKCA. Acta Neuropathol. 2019; 137:837–846

[16] Anyanwu CT, Robinson TM, Huang JH. Rosette-forming glioneuronal tumor: an update. Clin Transl Oncol. 2020; 22:623–630

[17] Schlamann A, von Bueren AO, Hagel C, et al. An individual patient data meta-analysis on characteristics and outcome of patients with papillary glioneuronal tumor, rosette glioneuronal tumor with neuropil-like islands and rosette forming glioneuronal tumor of the fourth ventricle. PLoS One. 2014; 9. DOI: 10.1371/journal.pone.0101211

[18] Rodriguez FJ, Perry A, Rosenblum MK, et al. Disseminated oligodendroglial-like leptomeningeal tumor of childhood: a distinctive clinicopathologic entity. Acta Neuropathol. 2012; 124:627–641

[19] Nelen MR, van Staveren WC, Peeters EA, et al. Germline mutations in the PTEN/MMAC1 gene in patients with Cowden disease. Human Molecular Genetics. 1997; 6:1383–1387

[20] Nelen MR, Kremer H, Konings IB, et al. Novel PTEN mutations in patients with Cowden disease: absence of clear genotype-phenotype correlations. Eur J Hum Genet. 1999; 7:267–273

[21] Meltzer CC, Smirniotopoulos J G, Jones RV. The striated cerebellum: an MR imaging sign in Lhermitte-Duclos disease (dysplastic gangliocytoma). Radiology. 1995; 194:699–703

[22] Chen KS, Hung PC, Wang HS, et al. Medulloblastoma or cerebellar dysplastic gangliocytoma (Lhermitte-Duclos disease)? Pediatr Neurol. 2002; 27:404–406

[23] Someshwar S, Hogg JP, Nield LS. Lhermitte-Duclos disease or neoplasm? Applied Neurology. 2007; 3:37–39

[24] Suresh TN, Santosh V, Yasha TC, et al. Medulloblastoma with extensive nodularity: a variant occurring in the very young-clinicopathological and immunohistochemical study of four cases. Childs Nerv Syst. 2004; 20:55–60

[25] Capone Mori A, Hoeltzenbein M, Poetsch M, et al. Lhermitte-Duclos disease in 3 children: a clinical long-term observation. Neuropediatrics. 2003; 34:30–35

[26] Carlson JJ, Milburn JM, Barre GM. Lhermitte-Duclos disease: case report. J Neuroimaging. 2006; 16:157–162

[27] Shitara S, Tokime T, Akiyama Y. Multinodular and vacuolating neuronal tumor: A case report and literature review. Surg Neurol Int. 2018; 9. DOI: 10.4103/sni.sni_348_17

[28] Patel DM, Schmidt RF, Liu JK. Update on the diagnosis, pathogenesis, and treatment strategies for central neurocytoma. J Clin Neurosci. 2013; 20:1193–1199

[29] Sharma MC, Deb P, Sharma S, et al. Neurocytoma: a comprehensive review. Neurosurg Rev. 2006; 29:270–85; discussion 285

[30] Louis DN, Ohgaki H, Wiestler OD, et al. WHO classification of tumors of the central nervous system. Lyon, France 2016

[31] Hassoun J, Soylemezoglu F, Gambarelli D, et al. Central neurocytoma: a synopsis of clinical and histological features. Brain Pathol. 1993; 3:297–306

[32] Agarwal S, Sharma MC, Sarkar C, et al. Extraventricular neurocytomas: a morphological and histogenetic consideration. A study of six cases. Pathology. 2011; 43:327–334

[33] Kaur G, Kane AJ, Sughrue ME, et al. MIB-1 labeling index predicts recurrence in intraventricular central neurocytomas. J Clin Neurosci. 2013; 20:89–93

[34] Rades D, Fehlauer F, Schild SE. Treatment of atypical neurocytomas. Cancer. 2004; 100:814–817

[35] Sievers P, Stichel D, Schrimpf D, et al. FGFR1:TACC1 fusion is a frequent event in molecularly defined extraventricular neurocytoma. Acta Neuropathol. 2018; 136:293–302

[36] Myung JK, Cho HJ, Park CK, et al. Clinicopathological and genetic characteristics of extraventricular neurocytomas. Neuropathology. 2013; 33:111–121

[37] Chakraborti S, Mahadevan A, Govindan A, et al. Supratentorial and cerebellar liponeurocytomas: report of four cases with review of literature. J Neurooncol. 2011; 103:121–127

[38] Gembruch O, Junker A, Monninghoff C, et al. Liponeurocytoma: Systematic Review of a Rare Entity. World Neurosurg. 2018; 120:214–233

40

41 Ependymal Tumors

41.1 Introduction to ependymal tumors

The WHO CNS5 classified ependymomas by site as well as by histology and molecular biology features.

41.2 Specific tumor types

41.2.1 Supratentorial ependymoma (WHO grade 2 or 3)

General information

A well-circumscribed supratentorial glioma with small uniform cells having round nuclei that form focal pseudorosettes or ependymal rosettes embedded in a fibrillary matrix. Cells are thought to derive from radial glial cells (bipolar progenitor cells that are thought to be a major source of neurons in the developing nervous system).

The following designations should be used:

- **supratentorial ependymoma, NEC** (not elsewhere classified): when genetic analysis has not identified a pathologic fusion gene involving *ZFTA* (*C11orf95*) or *YAP1*
- **supratentorial ependymoma, NOS** (not otherwise specified): when genetic analysis has not been successful or is not feasible

Diagnostic criteria for supratentorial ependymoma

Diagnostic criteria for supratentorial ependymoma are shown in ▸ Fig. 41.1.[1]

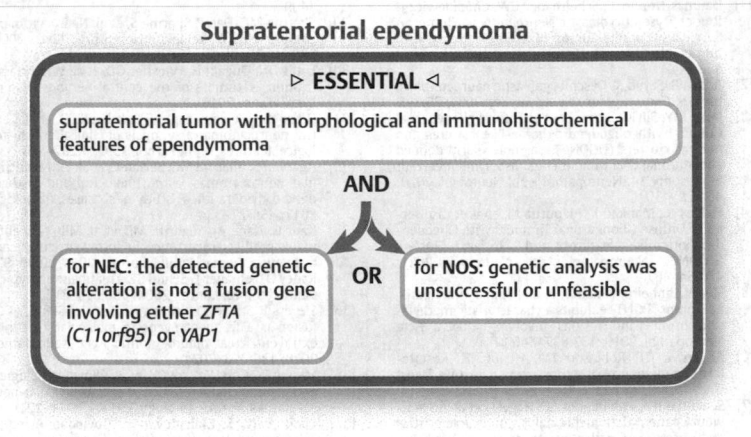

Fig. 41.1 Diagnostic criteria for supratentorial ependymoma. (Modified with permission from WHO Classification of Tumors Editorial Board, (ed.) World Health Organization classification of tumors of the central nervous system. 5th ed. Bosman F T, Jaffe E S, Lakhani S R, et al. (series eds.): World Health Organization Classification of Tumors series, vol. 6. International Agency for Research on Cancer, Lyon, France, 2021.)

Grading

The most important characteristics distinguishing grade 3 supratentorial ependymomas from grade 2 are abundant mitoses and the presence of microvascular proliferation. These are more influential than nuclear pleomorphism or necrosis.[2] NB: histopathological grading of ependymomas is not highly correlated with overall outome.

Location

These tumors are found in the cerebral hemispheres. A connection to the ventricular system may or may not be obvious. They favor the frontal or parietal lobes over the temporal or occipital lobes.

Epidemiology

These tumors affect all ages, but the proportion relative to the posterior fossa and spinal ependymomas decreases with age.[3] They comprise ≈ one third of intracranial ependymomas.

Prognosis

Most of the data comes from studies performed before molecular testing. The outcome is worse for supratentorial than infratentorial ependymomas in adults.

Gross total removal is the most important prognosticator of OS in adults and children. Post-op XRT lowers the risk of local recurrence.

41.2.2 Supratentorial ependymoma, ZFTA fusion-positive (WHO grade 2 or 3)

General information

A well-circumscribed supratentorial glioma with a *ZFTA* (formerly *C11orf95*) fusion gene (typically *ZFTA* is fused with *RELA*), with small uniform cells having round nuclei containing speckled chromatin and poorly delineated fibrillary cytoplasm. Pseudorosettes are usually not prominent, and true ependymal rosettes embedded are infrequent. There is often a network of branching capillary vasculature. Cells are thought to derive from radial glial cells.

Diagnostic criteria for supratentorial ependymoma, ZFTA fusion-positive

Diagnostic criteria for supratentorial ependymoma, ZFTA fusion-positive are shown in ► Fig. 41.2.[1]

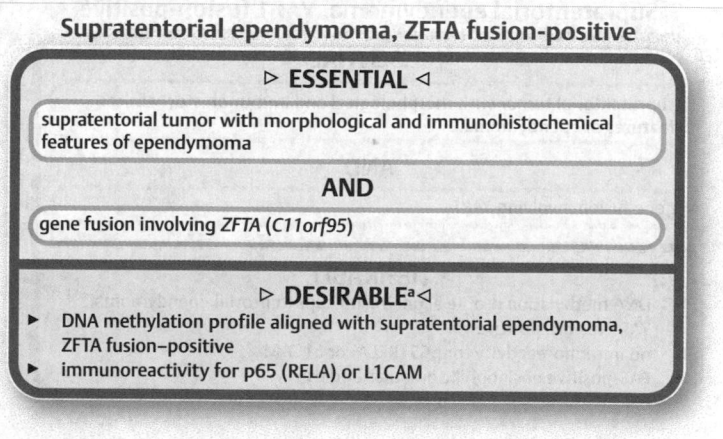

Fig. 41.2 **Diagnostic criteria for supratentorial ependymoma, ZFTA fusion-positive.** (Modified with permission from WHO Classification of Tumors Editorial Board, (ed.) World Health Organization classification of tumors of the central nervous system. 5th ed. Bosman F T, Jaffe E S, Lakhani S R, et al. (series eds.): World Health Organization Classification of Tumors series, vol. 6. International Agency for Research on Cancer, Lyon, France, 2021.)

Grading

These tumors are considered WHO grade 2 or 3 based on the degree of anaplasia observed.

Location

Most of these tumors are found in the frontal or parietal lobes. They occur infrequently in the thalamus, hypothalamic/thrid ventricular region, or extra-axially.

Epidemiology

Supratentorial ependymoma, ZFTA fusion-positive tumors comprise the majority of supratentorial ependymomas (20-58% in adults, 66-84% in pediatrics).[1]

Prognosis

Preliminary data suggest a worse outome than with other ependymomas, however, more experience with this recently molecularly defined group will be needed to make any definitive statements. Homozygous deletion of *CDKN2A* and/or *CDKN2B* are independent risk factors for worse OS in a series of supratentorial ependymomas with *ZFTA::RELA* fusions.[4]

41.2.3 Supratentorial ependymoma, YAP1 fusion-positive (WHO grade N/A)

General information

A well circumscribed supratentorial glioma with a *YAP1* fusion gene (typically YAP1 is fused with *MAMLD1*), with small uniform cells having round nuclei that form focal pseudorosettes or ependymal rosettes embedded in a fibrillary matrix. Cells are thought to derive from PAX6-positive radial glial neural stem cells.

Diagnostic criteria for supratentorial ependymoma, YAP1 fusion-positive

Diagnostic criteria for supratentorial ependymoma, YAP1 fusion-positive are shown in ▸ Fig. 41.3.[1]

Supratentorial ependymoma, YAP1 fusion-positive

▷ **ESSENTIAL** ◁

supratentorial tumor with morphological and immunohistochemical features of ependymoma

AND

gene fusion involving *YAP1*

▷ **DESIRABLE**[a] ◁
- ▸ DNA methylation profile aligned with supratentorial ependymoma, YAP1 fusion–positive
- ▸ no immunoreactivity for p65 (RELA) or L1CAM
- ▸ PAS-positive eosinophilic granular bodies

Fig. 41.3 Diagnostic criteria for supratentorial ependymoma, YAP1 fusion-positive. (Modified with permission from WHO Classification of Tumors Editorial Board, (ed.) World Health Organization classification of tumors of the central nervous system. 5th ed. Bosman F T, Jaffe E S, Lakhani S R, et al. (series eds.): World Health Organization Classification of Tumors series, vol. 6. International Agency for Research on Cancer, Lyon, France, 2021.)

Location

These tumors are usually found within or adjacent to the lateral ventricle.

Epidemiology

Supratentorial ependymoma, YAP1 fusion-positive tumors seem to be isolated to young children, and show a M:F ratio of 0.3:1.[1] They account for 6-7.4% of supratentorial ependymomas in pediatric cohorts.[1]

Prognosis

Prognosis appears favorable compared to other supratentorial ependymomas (retrospective analysis).[1]

41.2.4 Posterior fossa ependymoma (WHO grade 2 or 3)

General information

Key concepts

- usually benign tumors, often fibrillary with epithelial appearance. Perivascular pseudorosettes or ependymal rosettes may be seen
- most often occur in the floor of the 4th ventricle, presenting with hydrocephalus (increased ICP) and cranial nerve VI & VII palsies
- evaluation: includes imaging the entire neuraxis (MRI with and without enhancement: cervical, thoracic, lumbar & brain) because of potential for seeding through CSF
- worse prognosis the younger the patient (especially age < 24 months)
- treatment: the best outcomes are associated with gross total removal (no enhancing tumor on post-op MRI) followed by XRT. XRT may be withheld for age < 3 years due to side effects
- do LP ≈ 2 weeks post-op to send ≈ 10 cc of CSF for cytology for prognostication

---

A circumscribed posterior fossa glioma of monomorphic round cells with round nuclei that form focal pseudorosettes or ependymal rosettes embedded in a fibrillary matrix. This diagnosis should be employed when molecular analysis cannot assign a molecular group (NEC, not elsewhere classified) or is not feasible or the results were uncertain (NOS, not otherwise specified)

Diagnostic criteria for posterior fossa ependymoma

Diagnostic criteria for posterior fossa ependymoma are shown in ▶ Fig. 41.4.[1]

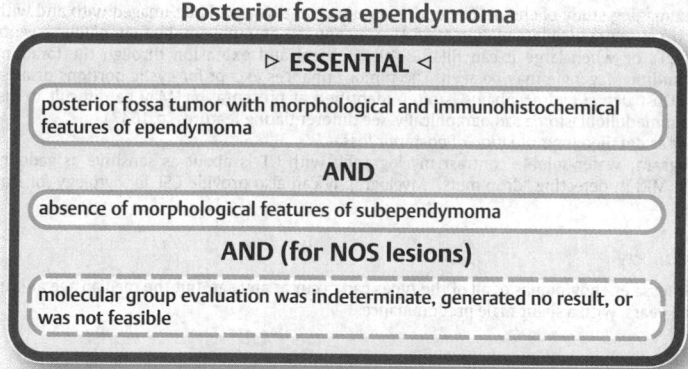

Fig. 41.4 Diagnostic criteria for posterior fossa ependymoma. (Modified with permission from WHO Classification of Tumors Editorial Board, (ed.) World Health Organization classification of tumors of the central nervous system. 5th ed. Bosman F T, Jaffe E S, Lakhani S R, et al. (series eds.): World Health Organization Classification of Tumors series, vol. 6. International Agency for Research on Cancer, Lyon, France, 2021.)

41

Grading

Should ideally be done in the context of an integrated diagnosis.[2] The most important characteristics distinguishing grade 3 posterior fossa ependymomas from grade 2 are abundant mitoses and the presence of microvascular proliferation. These are more influential than nuclear pleomorphism or necrosis.[2] NB: histopathological grading of ependymomas is not highly correlated with overall outome.

Location

These tumors generally occur in relation to the 4th ventricle (floor, lateral aspect, cerebellar peduncles, or roof).

Spread

Ependymomas have the potential to spread via the CSF through the neuraxis (including to the spinal cord), a process known as "seeding," resulting in so-called **"drop mets"** in the spinal cord in 11%. The incidence is higher with higher grade.[5] Systemic spread occurs on rare occasions.

Presentation

Mostly those of posterior fossa mass with increased ICP (from hydrocephalus) and cranial nerve involvement.

▶ **Symptoms.** Symptoms of increased ICP:
1. headache
2. N/V
3. ataxia or vertigo
4. obtundation/lethargy

Symptoms of cranial nerve involvement: diplopia, facial weakness...

▶ **Signs.** In infants: increasing head circumference crossing growth curves.
  Cranial nerve involvement: invasion of the floor of the 4th ventricle may impact the facial colliculus (a small bump in the floor of the 4th ventricle produced by the internal genu of the VII nerve as it deviates posteriorly around the VI nerve nucleus). This can produce peripheral facial nerve palsy (p. 607) (from VII nerve) and/or abducens palsy (p. 598) (from VI nucleus).

Imaging

MRI: the imaging study of choice. The entire craniospinal axis should be imaged with and without contrast because of possibility of drop mets. Usually appears as a mass in the floor of fourth ventricle (▶ Fig. 41.5), or when large it can fill the 4th ventrical and extension through the foramina of Luschka and/or Magengie may be seen. The tumor enhances except for cystic portions or areas of necrosis. Obstructive hydrocephalus is often identified at presentation. May be difficult to distinguish from medulloblastoma radiographically, see differentiating features (p. 1647).

  CT: not as detailed for evaluation of posterior fossa.

  Myelogram: water-soluble contrast myelography with CT is about as sensitive as gadolinium enhanced MRI in detecting "drop mets." Myelography can also provide CSF for cytology for staging purposes.

Epidemiology

Posterior fossa ependymomas of all of the types can occur at any age, but the median age at presentation is 6 years, with a slight male predominance.

Treatment

Surgical resection

Goal of surgery: maximal possible resection of intracranial portion without causing neurological deficits (since extent of resection is an important prognosticator). Gross total resection may not be possible when invasion of the floor is extensive, or when tumor extends through the foramen of Luschka (bradycardia may prevent GTR).

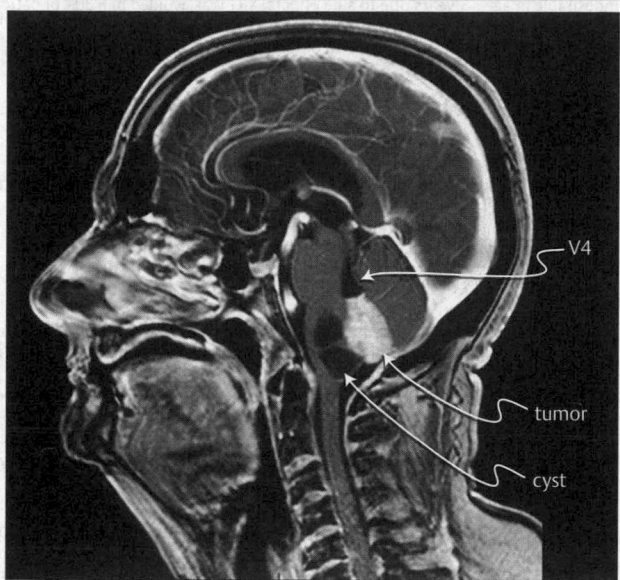

Fig. 41.5 Ependymoma (WHO grade 2) of the posterior fossa in a 71-year-old woman. Here, the tumor arises from the floor of the 4th ventricle and has a cystic component that invades the medulla. It displaces but does not invade the cerebellum. The 4th ventricle (V4) is obstructed and the patient had hydrocephalus.
Image: sagittal T1 contrast-enhanced MRI.

These tumors are usually circumscribed with a covering layer of ependyma, and are only rarely invasive to a significant degree.[6]

Operative morbidity: advise patients/families pre-op of the likelihood of need for post-op gastric feeding tube (G-tube) and tracheostomy (these may be temporary).

2 weeks postoperatively, perform LP to look for "drop mets": 10 cc of CSF is sent for cytology to quantitate (if any) number of malignant cells (may be used to follow treatment). If LP is positive, then by definition there are drop mets. If negative, it is not as helpful (sensitivity is not high). CSF from an EVD is not as sensitive as LP.

Lesions in fourth ventricle region are approached via midline suboccipital craniectomy.

Radiation therapy (XRT)

Ependymomas rank 2nd only to medulloblastomas in radiosensitivity. XRT is administered after surgical excision (survival is improved with post-op XRT[7,8]: 50% survival time was 2 yrs longer with XRT than without,[7] and 5-year survival increased from 20–40% without XRT to 40–80% with XRT[8]); however, for patients age < 3 years, see below.

1. cranial XRT
   a) traditional therapy: 45–48 Gy to tumor bed[8] (recurrence treated with additional 15–20 Gy)
   [9(p 2797)]
   b) recent recommendations: 3-D conformal XRT with higher doses (59.4 Gy delivered to tumor bed + 1 cm margins)[10]
   c) intensity modulated proton beam therapy appears equivalent in terms of local control, but may be better at sparing normal tissue[11]
2. spinal XRT: most radiate only if drop mets or if positive CSF cytology (however, prophylactic spinal is controversial[12])
   a) low dose XRT to entire spinal axis (median dose = 30 Gy in one series[8])
   b) boost to any regions showing drop mets

3. XRT is undesirable in age < 3 years due to side effects. XRT was avoided in ≈ 30% of patients < 3 years of age with comparable survival when XRT was reserved for treatment failures.[13,14] This concept of selective XRT may be applicable to older children as well[15]

Chemotherapy

Role is very limited.

1. has little impact on newly diagnosed cases. Adjuvant chemo after XRT in patients > 3 years showed no benefit
2. may reduce vascularity of ependymomas, which may facilitate GTR (sometimes in a second stage operation)
3. may be considered for infants < ≈ 3 years of age to delay use of XRT (see above)
4. chemo at the time of recurrence may arrest tumor progression for short periods

Prognosis

Extent of resection: the risk of recurrence is highest following subtotal resection. Gross total resection (GTR) (surgical) of primary intracranial tumor followed by craniospinal XRT as outlined above yields 41% 5-year survival.

Treatment failure: tumors tend to recur initially at the site of origin.[16] However, treatment failure in 9–25% of patients is due to drop mets.[17,18]

Age: peds vs. adults: 5-year survival (5YS) is 20–30% in the pediatric group,[5,19] compared with up to 80% in adults. Patients 24–35 months old did better (73% 5YS) than those younger than 24 months (26% 5YS) or those older than 36 months (36% 5YS).[17]

41.2.5 Posterior fossa group A (PFA) ependymoma (WHO grade 2 or 3)

General information

PFA ependymoma is a circumscribed posterior fossa glioma aligned with the PFA molecular groups of ependymomas (loss of nuclear H3 p.K28me3 (K27me3) expression in tumor cells or by DNA methylation profiling) having small uniform cells with round nuclei that form focal pseudorosettes or ependymal rosettes embedded in a fibrillary matrix. Cells are thought to derive from undifferentiated glial stem or progenitor cell in the developing hindbrain.

Diagnostic criteria for posterior fossa group A (PFA) ependymoma

Diagnostic criteria for posterior fossa group A (PFA) ependymoma are shown in ▶ Fig. 41.6.[1]

Grading

Grading of WHO grade 2 or 3 is based on the degree of anaplasia and reported in an integrated diagnosis.[2]

Location

These tumors arise more frequently from the roof or lateral aspect of the 4th ventricle.

Presentation

Similar to the presentation of posterior fossa ependymomas (p. 728) in general.

Epidemiology

PFA ependymomas predominantly occur in pre-adolescents with a median age of 3 years at presentation.[1]

Prognosis

Prognosis appears less favorable than with PFB ependymomas.[20] Extent of resection correlates with outcome.[21] Tiers of disease risk can be defined using chromosome 1q status and other variables.[21]

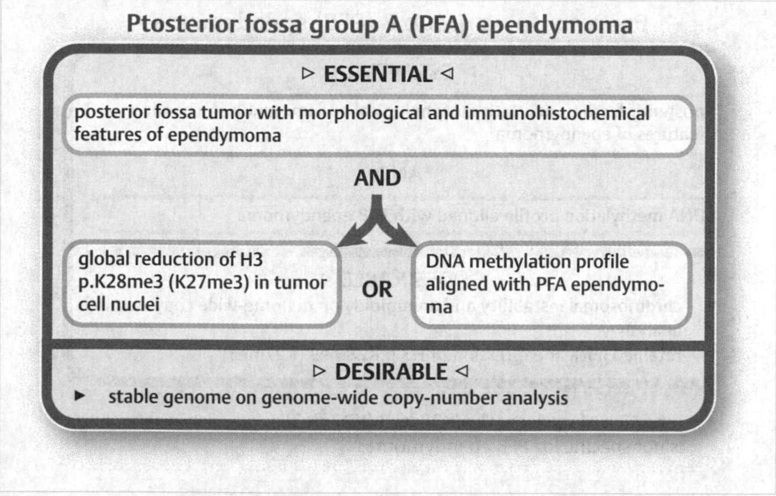

Fig. 41.6 **Diagnostic criteria for posterior fossa group A (PFA) ependymoma.** (Modified with permission from WHO Classification of Tumors Editorial Board, (ed.) World Health Organization classification of tumors of the central nervous system. 5th ed. Bosman F T, Jaffe E S, Lakhani S R, et al. (series eds.): World Health Organization Classification of Tumors series, vol. 6. International Agency for Research on Cancer, Lyon, France, 2021.)

41.2.6 Posterior fossa group B (PFB) ependymoma (WHO grade 2 or 3)

General information

PFB ependymoma is a circumscribed posterior fossa glioma aligned with the PFB molecular groups of ependymomas (by DNA methylation profiling) having small uniform cells with round nuclei that form focal pseudorosettes or ependymal rosettes embedded in a fibrillary matrix.[1]

Diagnostic criteria for posterior fossa group B (PFB) ependymoma

Diagnostic criteria for posterior fossa group B (PFB) ependymoma are shown in ▶ Fig. 41.7.[1]

Grading

Grading of WHO grade 2 or 3 is based on the degree of anaplasia and reported in an integrated diagnosis.[2] High-grade features, including brisk mitotic activity and microvascular proliferation, were observed in 41% of PFB ependymomas.[20]

Location

These tumors arise more frequently from the floor of the 4th ventricle.

Presentation

Similar to the presentation of posterior fossa ependymomas (p. 728) in general.

Epidemiology

PFB ependymomas are more common in adults and adolescents than in pre-adolescents, with a median age of 30 years (range: 1-72) at presentation.[1]

41

Posterior fossa group B (PFB) ependymoma

▷ **ESSENTIAL** ◁

posterior fossa tumor with morphological and immunohistochemical features of ependymoma

AND

DNA methylation profile aligned with PFB ependymoma

▷ **DESIRABLE** ◁

- ► chromosomal instability and aneuploidy on genome-wide copy-number analysis
- ► retained nuclear expression of H3 p.K28me3 (K27me3)[a]

a   retention of nuclear H3 p.K28me3 (K27me3) expression is seen, but is not specific for PFB ependymomas

Fig. 41.7 Diagnostic criteria for posterior fossa group B (PFB) ependymoma. (Modified with permission from WHO Classification of Tumors Editorial Board, (ed.) World Health Organization classification of tumors of the central nervous system. 5th ed. Bosman F T, Jaffe E S, Lakhani S R, et al. (series eds.): World Health Organization Classification of Tumors series, vol. 6. International Agency for Research on Cancer, Lyon, France, 2021.)

Prognosis

Subtotal resection and loss of 13q correlated with a poor prognosis, and gain of 1q did not appear to be correlated to OS.[22]

41.2.7 Spinal ependymoma (WHO grade 2 or 3)

General information

Spinal ependymomas are circumscribed intramedullary spinal gliomas having small uniform cells with round nuclei that form focal pseudorosettes or ependymal rosettes embedded in a fibrillary matrix. They typically have low levels of mitoses. Features of myxopapillary ependymoma or subependymoma are absent, by definition. *MYCN* amplification is absent when testing is possible.[1]

Diagnostic criteria for spinal ependymoma

Diagnostic criteria for spinal ependymoma are shown in ► Fig. 41.8.[1]

Grading

The vast majority of spinal ependymomas are WHO grade 2, with grade 3 tumors being rare. Grade 3 tumors have brisk mitotic activity, high cell density, and tend to invade adjacent spinal cord structures.

Location

These tumors arise anywhere along the spinal canal, but favor cervical or cervicothoracic levels.

Presentation

See presentation of intramedullary spinal cord tumors (p. 986).

Epidemiology

Spinal ependymomas comprise 17% of primary spinal tumors in the U.S.[23]

Spinal ependymoma

▷ ESSENTIAL ◁

spinal tumor with morphological and immunohistochemical features of ependymoma

AND

absence of morphological features of myxopapillary ependymoma or subependymoma

▷ DESIRABLE ◁
- ▶ DNA methylation profile aligned with spinal ependymoma
- ▶ loss of chromosome 22q
- ▶ no MYCN amplification

Fig. 41.8 Diagnostic criteria for spinal ependymoma. (Modified with permission from WHO Classification of Tumors Editorial Board, (ed.) World Health Organization classification of tumors of the central nervous system. 5th ed. Bosman F T, Jaffe E S, Lakhani S R, et al. (series eds.): World Health Organization Classification of Tumors series, vol. 6. International Agency for Research on Cancer, Lyon, France, 2021.)

Imaging

These are intramedullary tumors that are low intensity on T1 MRI, hyperintense on T2, and enhance readily. They tend to be more centrally located and more readily defined than spinal astrocytomas which are often eccentric and poorly demarcated.[24] 22% have a tumor cyst, and 62% are associated with a nontumoral cyst (e.g., syringomyelia).[24] Necrosis or calcifications may be seen.

Prognosis

Prognosis for grade 2 spinal ependymomas is favorable with PFS rates of 70% in children and 90% in adults over 5-10 years, and OS of 90% in children and 100% in adults over the same period.[25] Unfortunately, late recurrence is not uncommon.[26] The prognosis for grade 3 tumors is poor.[25]

41.2.8 Spinal ependymoma, MYCN-amplified (WHO grade N/A)

General information

MYCN-amplified spinal ependymomas are rare, circumscribed intramedullary spinal gliomas having small uniform cells with round nuclei that form focal pseudorosettes or ependymal rosettes embedded in a fibrillary matrix. Essentially all tumors demonstrate microvascular proliferation, necrosis and brisk mitotic activity. By definition, *MYCN* amplification is present.[1]

Diagnostic criteria for spinal ependymoma, MYCN-amplified

Diagnostic criteria for spinal ependymoma, MYCN-amplified are shown in ▶ Fig. 41.9.[1]

Grading

A WHO grade has not yet been assigned to these tumors.

Location

78% of cases involved the cervical or thoracic spinal cord, and 7% lumbar. They may be intramedullary, intramedullay with exophytic component, or mostly extramedullary. Leptomeningeal is frequent at diagnosis, or eventually occurs during the course.[1]

41

Spinal ependymoma, MYCN-amplified

> ▷ **ESSENTIAL** ◁

spinal tumor with morphological and immunohistochemical features of ependymoma

AND

MYCN amplification

> ▷ **DESIRABLE** ◁
> ► DNA methylation profile aligned with spinal ependymoma, *MYCN*-amplified
> ► high-grade histopathological features

Fig. 41.9 **Diagnostic criteria for spinal ependymoma, MYCN-amplified.** (Modified with permission from WHO Classification of Tumors Editorial Board, (ed.) World Health Organization classification of tumors of the central nervous system. 5th ed. Bosman F T, Jaffe E S, Lakhani S R, et al. (series eds.): World Health Organization Classification of Tumors series, vol. 6. International Agency for Research on Cancer, Lyon, France, 2021.)

Presentation

See presentation of intramedullary spinal cord tumors (p. 986).

Epidemiology

Only 27 cases were reported at the time the WHO CNS5 classification was published. 17 occurred in women, 10 in men. The median age at presentation was 31 years, with a range of 12-56 years.[1]

Imaging

These are intramedullary tumors that are low intensity on T1 MRI, hyperintense on T2, and enhance avidly. They tend to be more centrally located and more readily defined than spinal astrocytomas which are often eccentric and poorly demarcated.[24] 22% have a tumor cyst, and 62% are associated with a nontumoral cyst (e.g., syringomyelia).[24] Necrosis or calcifications may be seen.

Prognosis

Prognosis is poor for PFS and OS. Early spread throughout the neuraxis is frequent. Recurrence occurred in all patients with follow-up.[1]

41.2.9 Myxopapillary ependymoma (WHO grade 2)

General information

A distinctive variant of ependymoma. A WHO grade 2 glial neoplasm that essentially only occurs in the conus medullaris (the inferior terminus of the spinal cord) or the filum terminale (connective tissue band that extends inferiorly from the conus medullaris) characterized by tumor cells radially arranged around blood vessels with perivascular myxoid changes and microcyst formation.

Staining for GFAP can help differentiate this tumor from metastatic carcinoma, paragangliomas, schwannomas, chordomas, and myxoid chondrosarcomas.

Diagnostic criteria for myxopapillary ependymoma

Diagnostic criteria for smyxopapillary ependymoma are shown in ► Fig. 41.10.[1]

Myxopapillary ependymoma

▷ **ESSENTIAL** ◁

glioma with papillary structures and perivascular myxoid change or at least focal myxoid microcysts

AND

immunoreactivity for GFAP

AND (for unresolved lesions)

DNA methylation profile aligned with myxopapillary ependymoma

▷ **DESIRABLE** ◁

▶ papillary arrangements of tumor cells around vascularized fibromyxoid cores
▶ location in the filum terminale or conus medullaris

Fig. 41.10 Diagnostic criteria for myxopapillary ependymoma. (Modified with permission from WHO Classification of Tumors Editorial Board, (ed.) World Health Organization classification of tumors of the central nervous system. 5th ed. Bosman F T, Jaffe E S, Lakhani S R, et al. (series eds.): World Health Organization Classification of Tumors series, vol. 6. International Agency for Research on Cancer, Lyon, France, 2021.)

Treatment

Complete removal is often not possible due to invasion of the spinal cord parenchyma and/or CSF dissemination which is more common in pediatrics.

The high recurrence rate is an argument for early use of post-resection XRT, but proof of benefit in large series is lacking.[25]

Prognosis

Prognosis is relatively favorable with 10-year survival rates > 90% in adults and children.

41.2.10 Subependymoma (WHO grade 1)

General information

Key concepts

- slow growing, WHO grade 1 tumor
- arise from ependymal lining of, and protrude into, the ventricle. Noninvasive
- one of the only intraventricular tumors (excluding colloid cysts) that does not enhance
- almost always an incidental finding; hydrocephalus when symptomatic
- treatment: most are oberved with serial imaging. Gross total removal, when possible, is the goal if intervention is indicated

A slow growing (WHO grade 1) glioma arising from the ependymal lining of the ventricles characterized by clusters of bland to mildly pleomorphic cells in a fibrillary matrix, often with microcysts. Cells are mitotically inactive. 50-60% occur in the 4th ventricle, 30-40% in the lateral ventricles.

The tumors protrude into the ventricle and are noninvasive.

Diagnostic criteria for subependymoma

Diagnostic criteria for subependymoma are shown in ▸ Fig. 41.11.[1]

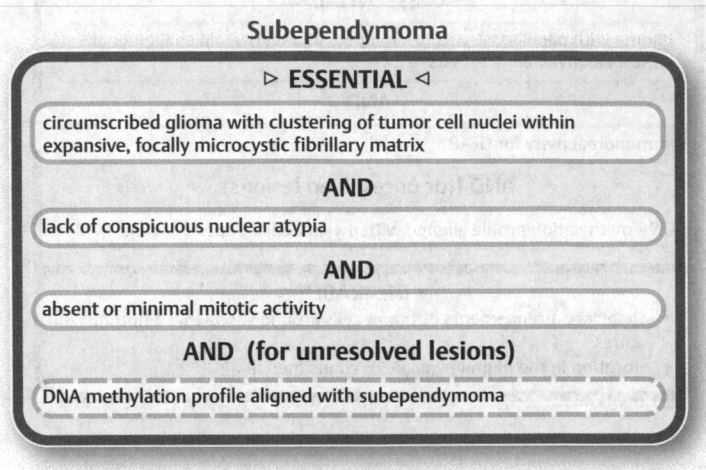

Fig. 41.11 **Diagnostic criteria for subependymoma.** (Modified with permission from WHO Classification of Tumors Editorial Board, (ed.) World Health Organization classification of tumors of the central nervous system. 5th ed. Bosman F T, Jaffe E S, Lakhani S R, et al. (series eds.): World Health Organization Classification of Tumors series, vol. 6. International Agency for Research on Cancer, Lyon, France, 2021.)

Epidemiology

Reliable data on incidence is difficult to come by since the majority are asymptomatic. A SEER registry database analysis found an incidence of 0.055 cases per 100,000 person years and a M:F ratio of about 2.5:1, and a peak incidence in adults 40-84 years old.[27]

Subependymomas make up ≈ 8% of ependymal tumors and < 1% of intracranial neoplasms.

Presentation

almost always an incidental finding on imaging performed for some other reason. The unusual exception to this is when a subependymoma causes obstructive hydrocephalus.

Neuroimaging

The typical appearance is a nonenhancing well-demarcated intraventricular mass (▸ Fig. 41.12). There are differences of opinion of the tendency for subependymomas to enhance; Jelinek et al[28] found that they did not. Also see differential diagnosis for intraventricular lesions (p. 1667).

Treatment

Almost always an incidental finding on imaging performed for some other reason. The unusual exception to this is when a subependymoma causes obstructive hydrocephalus.

Tumors meeting the typical imaging characterstics of subependymomas may be monitored with serial imaging. Usually the first follow-up image is obtained 3 months after initial discovery to rule out a mimic with rapid growth. Then, annual imaging should be done for a period of time (e.g., 5 years) and then at a less frequent basis.

Prognosis

Prognosis is excellent. When treatment is indicated, gross total resection (GTR) when possible is almost always curative. When GTR is not possible (e.g., tumors arising from the floor of the 4th ventricle) subtotal resection is usually satisfactory since the tumors are so slow growing.

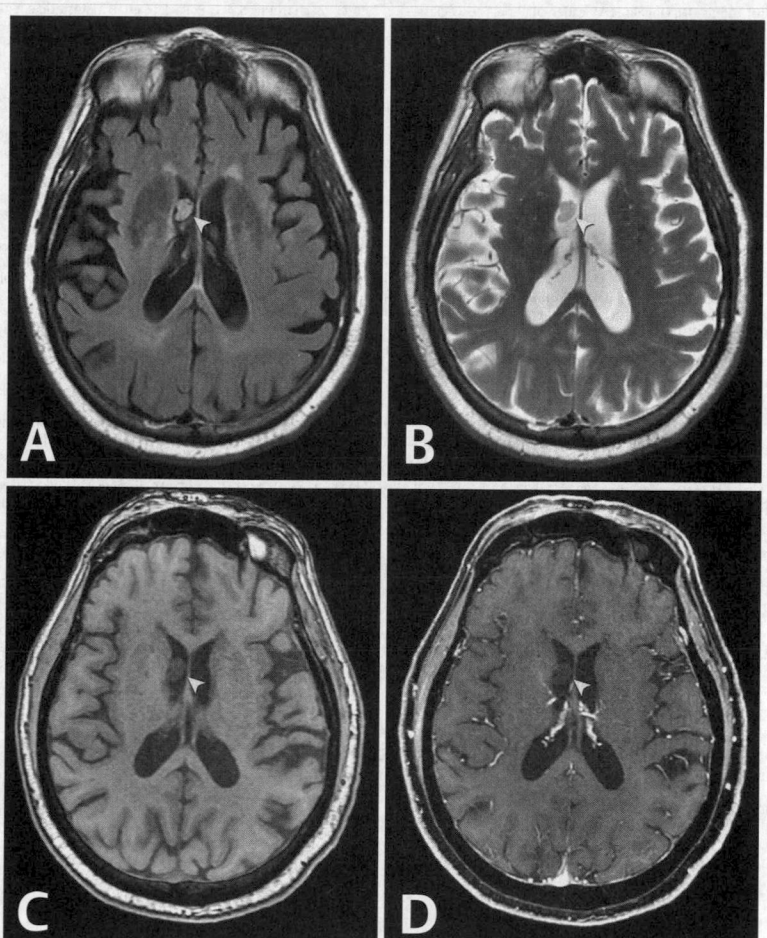

Fig. 41.12 Subependymoma (presumed, not biopsy proven). The lesion (*yellow arrowheads*) has remained unchanged over 10 years of observation.
Image: axial MRI A: FLAIR, B: T2, C: T1 non-contrast, D: T1 with contrast (note the lack of enhancement).

References

[1] Bosman FT, Jaffe ES, Lakhani SR, et al. World Health Organization Classification of Tumors series, vol. 6. In: WHO Classification of Tumors Editorial Board (ed.) World Health Organization classification of tumors of the central nervous system. 5th ed. Lyon, France: International Agency for Research on Cancer; 2021

[2] Louis DN, Perry A, Burger P, et al. International Society Of Neuropathology–Haarlem consensus guidelines for nervous system tumor classification and grading. Brain Pathol. 2014; 24:429–435

[3] Elsamadicy AA, Koo AB, David WB, et al. Comparison of epidemiology, treatments, and outcomes in pediatric versus adult ependymoma. Neurooncol Adv. 2020; 2. DOI: 10.1093/noajnl/vdaa019

[4] Junger ST, Andreiuolo F, Mynarek M, et al. CDKN2A deletion in supratentorial ependymoma with RELA alteration indicates a dismal prognosis: a retrospective analysis of the HIT ependymoma trial cohort. Acta Neuropathol. 2020; 140:405–407

[5] Duffner PK, Cohen ME, Freeman AI. Pediatric Brain Tumors: An Overview. Ca. 1985; 35:287–301

[6] Louis DN, Ohgaki H, Wiestler OD, et al. WHO classification of tumors of the central nervous system. Lyon, France 2016

[7] Mork SJ, Loken AC. Ependymoma: A Follow-Up Study of 101 Cases. Cancer. 1977; 40:907–915

[8] Shaw EG, Evans RG, Scheithauer BW, et al. Postoperative Radiotherapy of Intracranial Ependymoma in Pediatric and Adult Patients. International Journal of Radiation Oncology and Biological Physics. 1987; 13:1457–1462

[9] Youmans JR. Neurological Surgery. Philadelphia 1982

[10] Merchant TE, Mulhern RK, Krasin MJ, et al. Preliminary results from a phase II trial of conformal radiation therapy and evaluation of radiation-related CNS effects for pediatric patients with localized ependymoma. Journal of Clinical Oncology. 2004; 22:3156–3162

[11] MacDonald SM, Safai S, Trofimov A, et al. Proton radiotherapy for childhood ependymoma: initial clinical outcomes and dose comparisons. International Journal of Radiation Oncology, Biology, Physics. 2008; 71:979–986

[12] Vanuytsel L, Brada M. The Role of Prophylactic Apinal Irradiation in Localized Intracranial Ependymoma. International Journal of Radiation Oncology and Biological Physics. 1991; 21:825–830

[13] van Veelen-Vincent M L, Pierre-Kahn A, Kalifa C, et al. Ependymoma in childhood: prognostic factors, extent of surgery, and adjuvant therapy. Journal of Neurosurgery. 2002; 97:827–835

[14] Grundy RG, Wilne SA, Weston CL, et al. Primary postoperative chemotherapy without radiotherapy for intracranial ependymoma in children: the UKCCSG/SIOP prospective study. Lancet Oncol. 2007; 8:696–705

[15] Little AS, Sheean T, Manoharan R, et al. The management of completely resected childhood intracranial ependymoma: the argument for observation only. Child's Nervous System. 2009; 25:281–284

[16] Kawabata Y, Takahashi JA, Arakawa Y, et al. Long-term outcome in patients harboring intracranial ependymoma. Journal of Neurosurgery. 2005; 103:31–37

[17] Zacharoulis S, Ji L, Pollack IF, et al. Metastatic ependymoma: a multi-institutional retrospective analysis of prognostic factors. Pediatric Blood and Cancer. 2008; 50:231–235

[18] Foreman NK, Love S, Thorne R. Intracranial ependymomas: analysis of prognostic factors in a population-based series. Pediatr Neurosurg. 1996; 24:119–125

[19] Sutton LN, Goldwein J, Perilongo G, et al. Prognostic Factors in Childhood Ependymomas. Pediatr Neurosurg. 1990; 16:57–65

[20] Pajtler KW, Witt H, Sill M, et al. Molecular Classification of Ependymal Tumors across All CNS Compartments, Histopathological Grades, and Age Groups. Cancer Cell. 2015; 27:728–743

[21] Godfraind C, Kaczmarska JM, Kocak M, et al. Distinct disease-risk groups in pediatric supratentorial and posterior fossa ependymomas. Acta Neuropathol. 2012; 124:247–257

[22] Cavalli FMG, Hubner JM, Sharma T, et al. Heterogeneity within the PF-EPN-B ependymoma subgroup. Acta Neuropathol. 2018; 136:227–237

[23] Ostrom QT, Cioffi G, Waite K, et al. CBTRUS Statistical Report: Primary Brain and Other Central Nervous System Tumors Diagnosed in the United States in 2014-2018. Neuro Oncol. 2021; 23:iii1–iii105

[24] Koeller KK, Rosenblum RS, Morrison AL. Neoplasms of the spinal cord and filum terminale: radiologic-pathologic correlation. Radiographics. 2000; 20:1721–1749

[25] Benesch M, Frappaz D, Massimino M. Spinal cord ependymomas in children and adolescents. Childs Nerv Syst. 2012; 28:2017–2028

[26] Gomez DR, Missett BT, Wara WM, et al. High failure rate in spinal ependymomas with long-term follow-up. Neuro Oncol. 2005; 7:254–259

[27] Nguyen HS, Doan N, Gelsomino M, et al. Intracranial Subependymoma: A SEER Analysis 2004-2013. World Neurosurg. 2017; 101:599–605

[28] Jelinek J, Smirniotopoulos JG, Parisi JE, et al. Lateral ventricular neoplasms of the brain: Differential diagnosis based on clinical, CT, and MR findings. AJNR. 1990; 11:567–574

42 Choroid Plexus Tumors

42.1 General information

Choroid plexus tumors can occur anywhere there is choroid plexus. This is one of several groups of tumors with a younger median age at diagnosis than other histologies.[1]

Most are histologically benign.

All may produce drop mets in the CSF, but WHO grade 3 choroid plexus carcinomas do so more commonly.

Malignant degeneration from WHO grade 1 or 2 to grade 3 was seen in 2 out of 124 patients with 59 months mean follow-up.[2]

42.2 Choroid plexus tumor types

42.2.1 Choroid plexus papilloma (CPP) (WHO grade 1)

General information

A benign (WHO grade 1) intraventricular neoplasm resembling normal choroid plexus, with little or no mitotic activity.

Diagnostic criteria for choroid plexus papilloma

Diagnostic criteria for choroid plexus papilloma are shown in ▶ Fig. 42.1.[3]

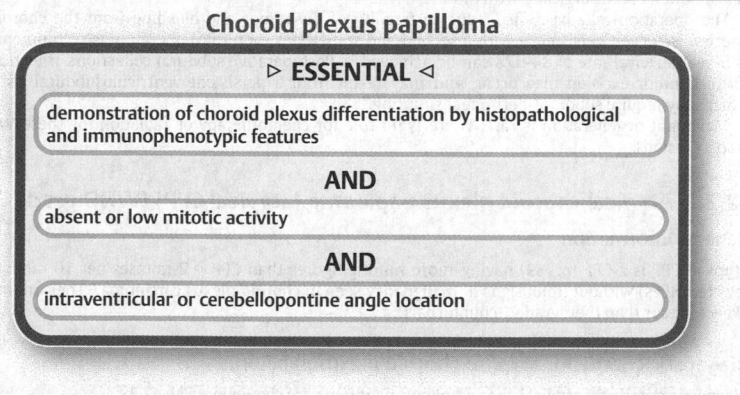

Fig. 42.1 Diagnostic criteria for choroid plexus papilloma. (Modified with permission from WHO Classification of Tumors Editorial Board, (ed.) World Health Organization classification of tumors of the central nervous system. 5th ed. Bosman F T, Jaffe E S, Lakhani S R, et al. (series eds.): World Health Organization Classification of Tumors series, vol. 6. International Agency for Research on Cancer, Lyon, France, 2021.)

Location

CPP are most frequently found in the lateral ventricles (with a predilection for the left side), followed by the fourth ventricles and then third ventricles. Rare ectopic cases have been reported. They may be found in the CPA from extension of choroid plexus through the foramen of Luschka. In adults these tumors are usually infratentorial, whereas in children they tend to occur supratentorially (a reverse from the situation for most other tumors) in the lateral ventricle.[4] See Intraventricular lesions (p. 1667) for differential diagnosis.

42

Epidemiology

Although they may occur at any age, 70% of patients are < 2 yrs old.[5] About 80% of lateral ventricle CPPs occur in patients < 20 years of age, unlike fourth ventricluar CPPs which are evenly distributed among all ages.[6]

CPP comprise 2.1% of all primary and CNS tumors in the U.S.,[1] and 2.1% of brain tumors in individuals < 15 years of age, and 10–20% of brain tumors in the first year of life. A portion of these tumors occur in neonates, supporting the hypothesis that some of these are congenital.[4]

Presentation

Most present with symptoms of increased ICP from hydrocephalus (H/A, N/V, craniomegaly), others may present with seizures, subarachnoid hemorrhage (with meningismus), or focal neurologic deficit (hemiparesis, sensory deficits, cerebellar signs, or cranial nerve palsies of III, IV, and VI).

Hydrocephalus, which may result from: overproduction of CSF (although total removal of these tumors does not always cure the hydrocephalus—especially in patients with high CSF protein, hemorrhage from tumor or surgery, or ependymitis), obstruction of CSF outflow, or communicating hydrocephalus from CSF-borne particulates.

Imaging

CT: iso- to hyper-dense.

MRI: T1 isointense, T2 hyperintense.

CT or MRI: intraventricular multilobulated mass, classically with projecting "fronds." Densely enhancing. Hydrocephalus is common.

Treatment & prognosis

CPP are often cured surgically with total removal.

The operation may be difficult due to fragility of the tumor and bleeding from the choroidal arteries. However, persistence with a second and sometimes even third operation is recommended as 5-year survival rate of 84-97% can be achieved.[4,7] Postoperative subdural collections after transcortical tumor excision may occur, and may result from a persistent ventriculosubdural fistula, which may require subdural-peritoneal shunting.[5]

Malignant degeneration is rare. There is no role for chemotherapy or radiation for these WHO grade 1 lesions.

42.2.2 Atypical choroid plexus papilloma (atypical CPP) (WHO grade 2)

General information

Atypical CPP is a CPP (p.739) having more mitotic figures than CPP (≥ 2 mitoses per 10 randomly selected HPFs) without frank signs of malignancy seen in choroid plexus carcinoma.[8] They are more likely to recur than their grade 1 counterpart.

Diagnostic criteria for atypical choroid plexus papilloma

Diagnostic criteria for atypical choroid plexus papilloma are shown in ► Fig. 42.2.[3]

Location

Unlike CPP which occur equally as ofter supratentorially as infratentorially, these grade 2 lesions are more common in the lateral ventricles. See Intraventricular lesions (p.1667) for differential diagnosis.

Epidemiology

Median age at diagnosis is younger than CPP (8-10 months vs. 26-35 months). All of the atypical CPP patients were < 10-11 years of age.

Atypical choroid plexus papilloma

▷ **ESSENTIAL** ◁

intraventricular or cerebellopontine angle location

AND

demonstration of choroid plexus differentiation by histopathological and immunophenotypic features

AND

demonstration of ≥ 1 mitosis/mm² in a minimum of 2.3 mm² (equating to ≥ 2 mitoses/10 HPF of 0.23 mm²)

AND

absence of criteria qualifying for the diagnosis of choroid plexus carcinoma

▷ **DESIRABLE** ◁

▶ *in select cases: demonstration of hyperploidy by genome-wide chromosomal copy-number analysis*

Fig. 42.2 Diagnostic criteria for atypical choroid plexus papilloma. (Modified with permission from WHO Classification of Tumors Editorial Board, (ed.) World Health Organization classification of tumors of the central nervous system. 5th ed. Bosman F T, Jaffe E S, Lakhani S R, et al. (series eds.): World Health Organization Classification of Tumors series, vol. 6. International Agency for Research on Cancer, Lyon, France, 2021.)

Imaging

Imaging appears the same as imaging with CPP (p. 740).

Prognosis

Prognosis is intermediate between CPP (grade 1) and choroid plexus carcinoma (grade 3). The definitional requirement of mitotic counts ≥ 2 per 10 HPF increased the 5-year recurrrence for atypical CPP by a factor of 5 over CPP.

42.2.3 Choroid plexus carcinoma (CPC) (WHO grade 3)

General information

A malignant (WHO grade 3) tumor of the choroid plexus that invades adjacent brain and is prone to metastasize through the CSF (present in 21% at diagnosis). Occurs primarily in the lateral ventricles of children.

Diagnostic criteria for choroid plexus carcinoma

Diagnostic criteria for choroid plexus carcinoma are shown in ▶ Fig. 42.3.[3]

Choroid plexus carcinoma

▷ **ESSENTIAL** ◁

demonstration of choroid plexus differentiation by histopathological and immunophenotypic features

AND

presence of at least four of the following five histological features:
- increased cellular density
- nuclear pleomorphism
- blurring of the papillary pattern with poorly structured sheets of tumor cells
- necrotic areas
- frequent mitoses, usually > 2.5 mitoses/mm^2 in a minimum of 2.3 mm^2 (equating to > 5 mitoses/10 HPF of 0.23 mm^2)

AND

intraventricular location

▷ **DESIRABLE** ◁

► *TP53* mutation analysis
► methylation profile of choroid plexus carcinoma
► in select cases: demonstration of hypoploidy by genome-wide chromosomal copy-number analysis

Fig. 42.3 **Diagnostic criteria for choroid plexus carcinoma.** (Modified with permission from WHO Classification of Tumors Editorial Board, (ed.) World Health Organization classification of tumors of the central nervous system. 5th ed. Bosman F T, Jaffe E S, Lakhani S R, et al. (series eds.): World Health Organization Classification of Tumors series, vol. 6. International Agency for Research on Cancer, Lyon, France, 2021.)

Epidemiology

80% of all CPCs are foud in children.

Most arise sporadically, but, since 40% occur as part of Li-Fraumeni syndrome (p. 650) with germline *TP53* pathogenic sequence variants, genetic counselling and TP53 testing is recommended for all patients and their family.[3]

Imaging

CPCs have heterogeneous signal on T1 & T2 MRI, irregular enhancing margins (suggesting subependymal invasion), edema in the adjacent brain, vascular flow voids in 55%, and often present with hydrocephalus and early CSF dissemination.[9] Imaging of the entire neuraxis is recommended due to the high incidence of drop mets.

Treatment

Even malignant choroid plexus tumors respond to surgery.

Chemotherapy benefits a subset of patients.[10]

XRT was not shown to improve survival in patients undergoing surgery.

Prognosis

3- and 5-year progression free survival rates are 58% and 38% respectively, and overall survival is 83% and 62% for the same time periods.[11]

Absence of TP53 mutation may be associated with a more favorable outcome.

References

[1] Ostrom QT, Cioffi G, Waite K, et al. CBTRUS Statistical Report: Primary Brain and Other Central Nervous System Tumors Diagnosed in the United States in 2014-2018. Neuro Oncol. 2021; 23:iii1–iii105

[2] Jeibmann A, Wrede B, Peters O, et al. Malignant progression in choroid plexus papillomas. Journal of Neurosurgery. 2007; 107:199–202

[3] Bosman FT, Jaffe ES, Lakhani SR, et al. World Health Organization Classification of Tumors series, vol. 6. In: WHO Classification of Tumors Editorial Board (ed.) World Health Organization classification of tumors of the central nervous system. 5th ed. Lyon, France: International Agency for Research on Cancer; 2021

[4] Ellenbogen RG, Winston KR, Kupsky WJ. Tumors of the Choroid Plexus in Children. Neurosurgery. 1989; 25:327–335

[5] Boyd MC, Steinbok P. Choroid Plexus Tumors: Problems in Diagnosis and Management. Journal of Neurosurgery. 1987; 66:800–805

[6] Wolff JE, Sajedi M, Brant R, et al. Choroid plexus tumours. Br J Cancer. 2002; 87:1086–1091

[7] Krishnan S, Brown PD, Scheithauer BW, et al. Choroid plexus papillomas: a single institutional experience. J Neurooncol. 2004; 68:49–55

[8] Jeibmann A, Hasselblatt M, Gerss J, et al. Prognostic implications of atypical histologic features in choroid plexus papilloma. Journal of Neuropathology and Experimental Neurology. 2006; 65:1069–1073

[9] Meyers SP, Khademian ZP, Chuang SH, et al. Choroid plexus carcinomas in children: MRI features and patient outcomes. Neuroradiology. 2004; 46:770–780

[10] Wrede B, Liu P, Wolff JE. Chemotherapy improves the survival of patients with choroid plexus carcinoma: a metaanalysis of individual cases with choroid plexus tumors. Journal of Neuro-Oncology. 2007; 85:345–351

[11] Zaky W, Dhall G, Khatua S, et al. Choroid plexus carcinoma in children: the Head Start experience. Pediatr Blood Cancer. 2015; 62:784–789

43 Embryonal Tumors

43.1 General information for embryonal tumors

Embryonal tumors are a diverse category of malignancies featuring immature tumor cells that resemble neural progenitors. It is divided into medulloblastomas (relatively common, occurring ≈ exclusively in the posterior fossa) and "other" rare non medulloblastoma CNS embryonal tumors (p. 754), many of which exhibit amplification of the C19MC region of chromosome 19.

Many of these tumors were formerly encompassed by the term primitive neuroectodermal tumor (PNET) which has been eliminated from the diagnostic lexicon.[1]

43.2 Medulloblastoma (a subset of embryonal tumors), general aspects

43.2.1 General information

Key concepts

- a small-cell embryonal WHO grade 4 neuroepithelial tumor that occurs predominantly in the posterior fossa of children (peak: 1st decade). The most common pediatric brain malignancy
- classified on 4 molecular and 4 histologic criteria
  - 4 molecularly defined types: 1) WNT-activated; 2) SHH-activated (TP53-mutant & -wildtype); 3) non-WNT/non-SHH, group 3; 4) non-WNT/non-SHH, group 4
  - 4 histologic types: 1) classic; 2) desmoplastic/nodular (D/N); 3) extensive nodularity (MBEN); 4) large cell/anaplastic (LC/A)
- brainstem invasion usually limits complete surgical excision
- staging: all patients must be evaluated for "drop mets" (imaging the entire neuraxis with contrast - brain + spine, pre-operatively if possible), and postoperatively with LP for CSF cytology

Medulloblastomas (MDB) are WHO grade 4 embryonal neuroepithelial tumors that typically occur in the posterior fossa (cerebellum or dorsal brainstem) of children. In the cerebellum, they typically arise in the vermis near the apex of the roof of the 4th ventricle (the fastigium [Latin for summit]). They acount for 68% of embryonal tumors.[2]

43.2.2 Seeding and metastases

≈ 10–35% have seeded the craniospinal axis at the time of diagnosis,[3] and extraneural mets occur in 5% of patients,[4] sometimes promoted by shunting[5] (although this is uncommon[6]).

43.2.3 Clinical

Clinical history is typically brief (6–12 weeks). Predilection for posterior fossa predisposes to early obstructive hydrocephalus. Usual presenting symptoms: H/A, N/V, and ataxia. Infants with hydrocephalus may present with irritability, lethargy, or progressive macrocrania.[7] Spinal drop mets may produce back pain, urinary retention, or leg weakness.

Common signs: papilledema, truncal and appendicular ataxia, nystagmus, EOM palsies. Macrocrania in infants and young children.

43.2.4 Classification

Classification of medulloblastomas based on a combination of molecular signatures combined with histopathological findings is recommended and provides optimal prognostic information. Molecularly defined MDBs are associated with specific morphological patterns to a high degree.

Molecular genetics: Transcriptome profiling (analysis of all RNA in a cell population), microRNA analysis and methylome profiling allows MDBs to be segregated into these 4 principal types[8] (which are covered individually in the following sections). NB: on a more granular level, additional subgroups have been identified and will continue to emerge.

1. WNT-activated (p. 750)
2. SHH-activated
   a) SHH-activated, TP53-wildtype (p. 751)
   b) SHH-activated, TP53-mutant (p. 752)
3. non-WNT/non-SHH (p. 753), group 3
4. non-WNT/non-SHH (p. 753), group 4

43

Histology: 4 histologic types are defined; see detailed descrition (p. 749)
1. classic (p. 749)
2. desmoplastic/nodular (p. 749) (D/N MDB)
3. extensive nodularity (p. 749) (MBEN)
4. large cell/anaplastic (p. 749) (LC/A MDB)

The distribution and prognosis of the histologic variants and prognostic information among the molecularly classified MDBs is depicted graphically in ▶ Fig. 43.1 (this is not the entire gamut, see reference[9] for more details).

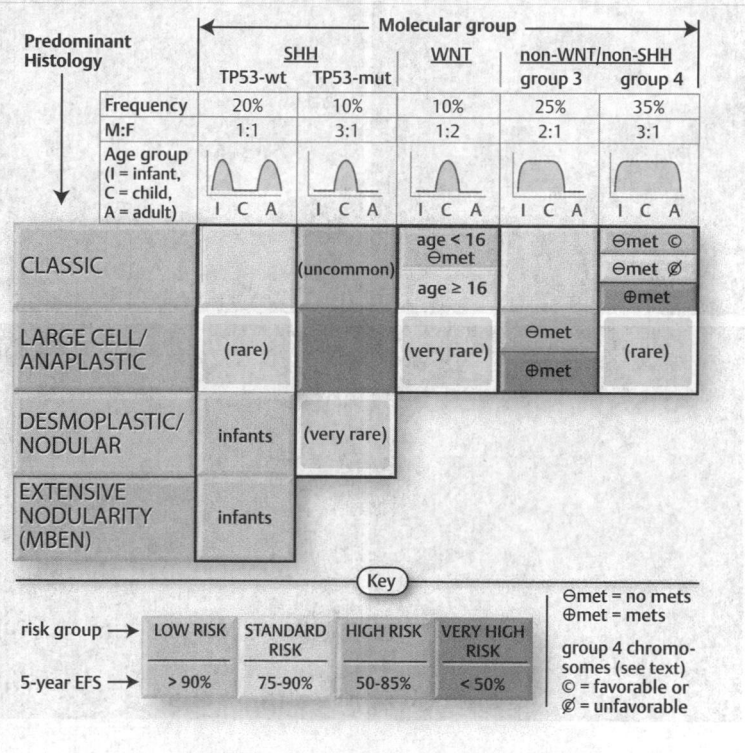

Fig. 43.1 Prognosis and distribution of histologic variants among molecular types of medulloblastoma. Box color indicates prognosis as follows:
5-year EFS rates: **low risk** >90%, **standard risk** 75-90%, **high risk** 50-75%, **very high risk** <50%
(see text for more details).[8,10,11] No risk is shown for tumors of uncertain clinicopathological significance.
Abbreviations: EFS = event-free survival; MDB = medulloblastoma; SHH = activated sonic hedgehog; TP53 = tumor protein 53; mut = mutant; wt = wildtype; WNT = activated wingless/integrated (signal transduction pathway).
© = favorable chromosomal findings for non-WNT/non-SHH group 4: chromosome 7 gain, chromosome 8 loss, chromosome 11 loss, chromosome 17 gain.

43.2.5 Evaluation

MDBs usually appear as a solid, IV-contrast-enhancing lesion on CT or MRI. Most are located in the midline in the region of the 4th ventricle (laterally situated tumors are more common in adults). Most have hydrocephalus at the time of presentation. Ependymoma (p. 1647) is the main entity from which to differentiate on imaging. MDBs tend to protrude into the 4th ventricle from the posterior aspect (the "roof") of the ventricle, whereas ependymomas more commonly arise from the floor.

CT: noncontrast → typically hyperdense (due to high cellularity). Contrast → most enhance. 20% have calcifications. CT has poor resolution in the posterior fossa due to bone interference

MRI: Can be variabled (▶ Fig. 43.2). T1WI → hypo- to isointense. T2WI → heterogeneous due to tumor cysts, vessels, and calcifications.[12] Most enhance. **MRS:** elevated choline and decreased NAA.

Spinal imaging: MRI with IV gadolinium or CT/myelography with water-soluble contrast should be done to rule out "drop mets." Staging is done either pre-op or within 2–3 weeks of surgery.

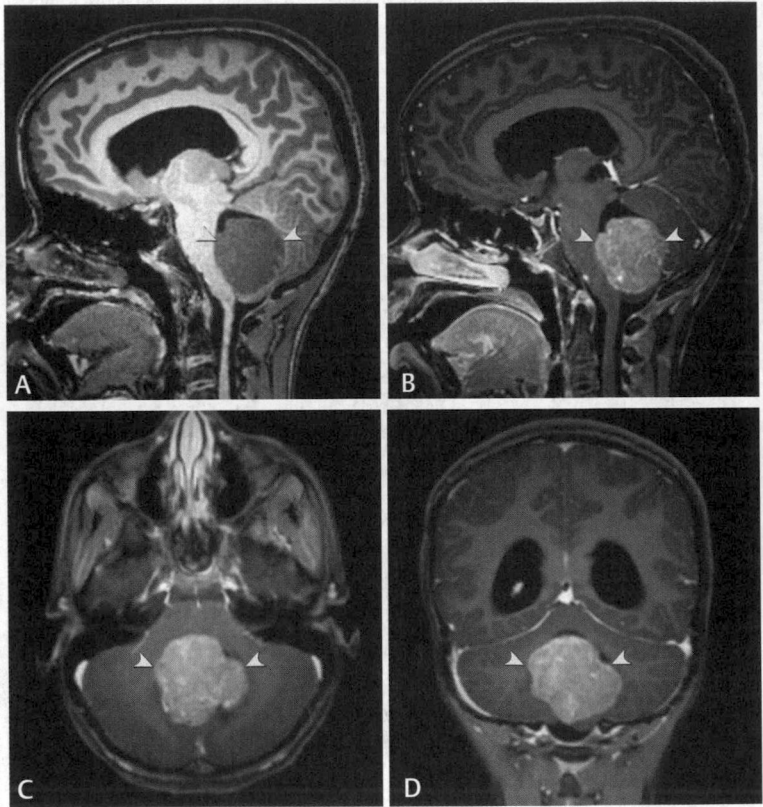

Fig. 43.2 Medulloblastoma. MRI of 10-year-old patient with medulloblastoma (*yellow arrowheads*) in the 4th ventricle producing obstructive hydrocephalus, presenting with progressive H/A, nausea and acute emesis. Image: A: sagittal T1 FLAIR without contrast, B: sagittal T1 FLAIR with contrast, C: axial T1 with contrast, D: coronal T1 with contrast.

▶ **Staging.** Staging employs MRI of the entire neuraxis without and with contrast and, postoperatively, CSF cytology obtained by LP. The grading system of Chang et al. (▶ Table 43.1) is still used.

Table 43.1 Post-operative staging system for medulloblastoma[13]

Stage	Description
M0	no metastasis
M1	microscopic tumor cells in the CSF
M2	gross nodular seeding in the cerebellar/cerebral subarachnoid space or in the third or lateral ventricles
M3	gross nodular seeding in the spinal subarachnoid space
M4	metastasis outside the CNS

43

43.2.6 Treatment

Surgical intervention

Surgical debulking of as much tumor as possible (without causing neurological injury) to obtain tissue for classification and to improve outcome is considered standard.

Invasion of or attachment to the floor of the fourth ventricle (brainstem in the region of the facial colliculus) often limits excision. It is better to leave a small residual on the brainstem (these patients do fairly well) than it is to chase every last remnant into the brainstem (neurologic deficit is more likely with this).

Surgical exposure of midline cerebellar medulloblastomas requires opening of the foramen magnum, usually removal of the posterior arch of C1, and occasionally the arch of C2. Tumor spread with arachnoidal thickening ("sugar coating") may occur.

Shunts: 30–40% of children require permanent VP shunts following p-fossa resection. The risk of shunt-related seeding has been quoted as high as 10–20%,[3] but this is probably overestimated.[6] In the past, tumor filters were sometimes used. They are less commonly used today because of the high incidence of obstruction.

Post-op adjuvant therapy

Following surgery, stratification of patients into risk groups guides subsequent therapy. One postoperative stratification scheme is shown in ▶ Table 43.2. Other systems have been published e.g., for pediatrics (age 3–17 years).[8]

In children: chemotherapy can be used to delay the need for XRT in 20–40% of children < 3–4 years of age with non-disseminated MBD.[15]

▶ **Low-risk and standard-risk patients**
- especially in pediatrics, may consider reduced dose XRT: 23.4 Gy with a boost to the primary site of 54–55.8 Gy with adjuvant chemotherapy
- or conventional fractionated XRT (see high-risk below)

▶ **High- and very high-risk patients**
- conventional fractionated XRT (once a day) for 54 Gy to the primary tumor and 18 Gy to the craniospinal axis
- chemotherapy[15]
  ○ agents that have been used include: cisplatin, lomustine, vincristine, cyclophosphamide, etoposide, simultaneous high-dose IV methotrexate and/or intrathecal methotrexate of mafosfamide, and/or intraventricular methotrexate
  ○ in adults: SHH-activated MDBs (which have higher prevalence of PTCH & SMO mutations) may be more responsive to SMO receptor inhibitors and SHH-inhibiting drugs such as vismodegib[15]

43.2.7 Prognosis

Prognostic details for specific tumor types will be found in the following sections. Poor prognosticators in general include[16]:
- in some cell types younger age (especially if < 3 yrs). For other cell types (e.g., desmoplastic/nodular or MBEN, the prognosis for infants is favorable)
- disseminated (metastatic) disease at the time of diagnosis except for MBEN
- inability to perform gross-total removal (especially if residual > 1.5 cm² with localized disease)
- poor Karnofsky performance scale score (p. 1640)

Most common site of recurrence is p-fossa.

43

Table 43.2 Postoperative risk stratification in medulloblastoma[14,15,11]

Standard-risk tumors

- total or near total surgical resection[a]
- no CNS metastases on MRI of brain and spine
- no tumor cells on cytospin of lumbar CSF
- no clinical evidence of extra-CNS metastases
- MDB classification
  - SHH-activated, TP53-wildtype with classic histology
  - or non-WNT/non-SHH, group 4, with classic histology and no metastases at diagnosis and no favorable chromosomal findings[b]
  - or non-WNT/non-SHH, group 3
  - or WNT with classic histology age ≥ 16 years

Low-risk tumors

- MDB classification
  - WNT-activated group
    - β-catenin mutation (mandatory testing)
    - β-catenin nuclear immunopositivity by immuno-histochemistry & monosomy 6 (optional testing)
  - or SHH-activated, TP53-wildtype in infants with
    - desmoplastic/nodular histology
    - or extensive nodularity histology
- total or near total surgical resection[a]

High-risk tumors

- large cell/anaplastic histology non-WNT/non-SHH, group 3 without metastases at diagnosis
- classic histology with
  - SHH-activated, TP53-mutant
  - or non-WNT/non-SHH, group 4 with metastases at diagnosis
- unresectable tumor or residual tumor > 1.5 cm² on axial-plane early post-op MRI
- extra-CNS metastases

Very high-risk tumors

- large cell/anaplastic histology with
  - SHH-activated, TP53-mutant
  - or non-WNT/non-SHH, group 3 with metastases at diagnosis

[a] near total resection: < 1.5 cm² on axial-plane early post-op MRI. This criteria is controversial as much of the data is from CT era[8]
[b] favorable chromosomal findings for non-WNT/non-SHH group 4: chromosome 7 gain, chromosome 8 loss, chromosome 11 loss, and chromosome 17 gain

Long-term survivors of MDB are at significant risk for permanent endocrinologic, cognitive, and psychological sequelae of treatments. Infants and very young children with MDB remain a difficult therapeutic challenge because they have the most virulent form of the disease and are at highest risk for treatment-related sequelae.

43.3 Medulloblastomas by definition criteria

43.3.1 Medulloblastoma, histologically defined

General information

An embryonal neuroepithelial tumor that occurs in the posterior fossa consisting of small, poorly differentiated cells with a high nuclear to cytoplasmic ratio with profuse mitotic activity and apoptosis. Divided into 4 histologic subtypes described below. On the rare occasion that any subtype shows myogenic and/or melanocytic differentiation, the terms "medullomyoblastoma" and "melanocytic medulloblastoma" respectively may be used in the description.

Diagnostic criteria for medulloblastoma, histologically defined

Diagnostic criteria for medulloblastoma, histologically defined are shown in ▶ Fig. 43.3.[9]

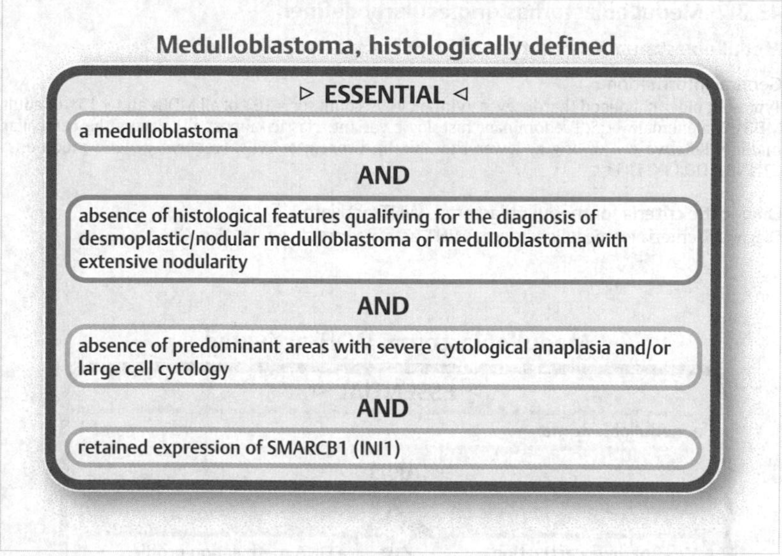

Medulloblastoma, histologically defined

▷ **ESSENTIAL** ◁

a medulloblastoma

AND

absence of histological features qualifying for the diagnosis of desmoplastic/nodular medulloblastoma or medulloblastoma with extensive nodularity

AND

absence of predominant areas with severe cytological anaplasia and/or large cell cytology

AND

retained expression of SMARCB1 (INI1)

Fig. 43.3 **Diagnostic criteria for medulloblastoma, histologically defined.** (Modified with permission from WHO Classification of Tumors Editorial Board, (ed.) World Health Organization classification of tumors of the central nervous system. 5th ed. Bosman F T, Jaffe E S, Lakhani S R, et al. (series eds.): World Health Organization Classification of Tumors series, vol. 6. International Agency for Research on Cancer, Lyon, France, 2021.)

Subtypes (histologic/morphologic variants)

- **MDB, classic:** densely packed undifferentiated small round cells with mild-to-moderate nuclear pleomorphism and high mitotic count. Comprise ≈ 72% of MDBs. Occur at any age, but predominate in childhood. Found in all 4 molecular MDB types.
- **desmoplastic/nodular MDB:** nodular, reticulin-free zones and intervening densely packed, poorly differentiated cells in an intercellular network of reticulin-positive collagen fibers. Account for ≈ 20% of all MDBs. Occurs in cerebellar hemispheres and midline. Bimodal age distribution: 1) young children and adolescents, 2) adults. Associated with Gorlin syndrome in early childhood. The prognosis in early childhood is excellent with surgery + chemotherapy alone, and is likely better than with any other histologic subtype.
- **MDB with extensive nodularity (MBEN):** numerous reticulin-free neurocytic nodules with a neuropil matrix and narrow internodular strands of poorly differentiated tumor cells in a desmoplastic matrix. Occurs primarily in infants. Accounts for < 5% of MDBs overall, but up to 50% of cases in age < 3 years. Outcome is favorable with near 100% 5-year OS in many (but not all) series. > 80% of these occur in the vermis. The presence of metastases at diagnosis in this group does not affect prognosis.
- **large cell/anaplastic MDB:** Undifferentiated cells with marked nuclear pleomorphism, prominent nucleoli, and hight mitotic and apoptotic counts. Accounts for 10% of MDBs. Found in all 4 molecular MDB types. The LC/A morphology is an independent prognosticator of poor outcome (5-year PFS is 30–40%) (very high-risk MDB) justifying aggressive adjuvant therapy. Molecular biology of MDB SHH-activated TP53-mut and non-WNT/non-SHH group 3 with MYC amplification can behave more aggressively.

Staging

See postoperative staging (p. 746).

Treatment

For treatment, see treatment for medulloblastomas (p. 747).

43.3.2 Medulloblastomas, molecularly defined

Medulloblastoma, WNT-activated (WHO grade 4)

General information
Typical in older childhood (hardly ever in infancy). Account for ≈ 10% of all MDBs and ≈ 15% of adult MDBs. Male:female = 1:2. Predominant histologic variant: classic (almost all). Favors the cerebellar midline. Putative cell of origin: lower rhombic lip progenitor cells. Frequent genetic mutations: CTNNB1, DDX3X, TP53.

Diagnostic criteria for medulloblastoma, WNT-activated
Diagnostic criteria for medulloblastoma, WNT-activated are shown in ▸ Fig. 43.4.[9]

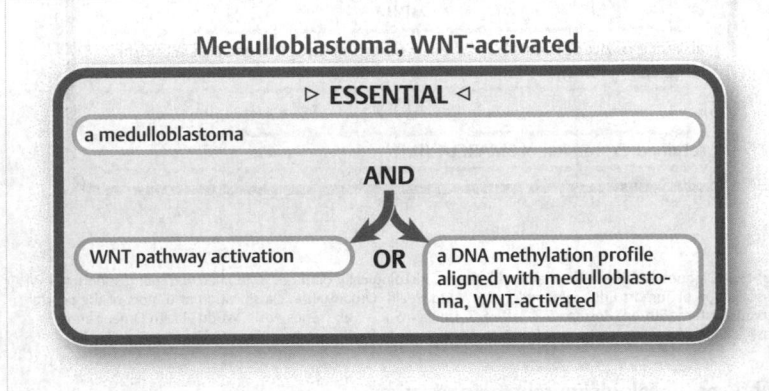

Fig. 43.4 Diagnostic criteria for medulloblastoma, WNT-activated. (Modified with permission from WHO Classification of Tumors Editorial Board, (ed.) World Health Organization classification of tumors of the central nervous system. 5th ed. Bosman F T, Jaffe E S, Lakhani S R, et al. (series eds.): World Health Organization Classification of Tumors series, vol. 6. International Agency for Research on Cancer, Lyon, France, 2021.)

Location
Generally either of the following:
- around the foramen of Luschka, arising from the brainstem or cerebellum
- or in the cerebellar midline, generally contiguous with the brainstem

Extension towards the CPA or cerebellar peduncle occurs in a significant number.

Histology
See section 43.3.1.

▸ **Classic morphology.** Almost all WNT-activated MDBs have classic morphology.

▸ **Large cell/anaplastic morphology.** Very rare. Uncertain clinical significance.

Staging
See postoperative staging (p. 746).

Treatment
For treatment, see treatment for medulloblastomas (p. 747).

Prognosis
In spite of being a grade 4 neoplasm, the prognosis for children is excellent with surgery and adjuvant therapy. In contrast, the prognosis is poor for adults.

Medulloblastoma, SHH-activated, TP53-wildtype (WHO grade 4)

Typical in infancy and adult. Male:female = 1:1. Predominant histologic variant: desmoplastic/nodular. Putative cell of origin: cerebellar granule neuron cell precursors of the external granule cell layer and cochlear nucleus; less likely neural stem cells of the subventricular zone. Frequent genetic mutations: PTCH1, SMO (adults), SUFU (infants), TERT promoter.

Diagnostic criteria for medulloblastoma, SHH-activated, TP53-wildtype

Diagnostic criteria for medulloblastoma, SHH-activated, TP53-wildtype are shown in ▶ Fig. 43.5.[9]

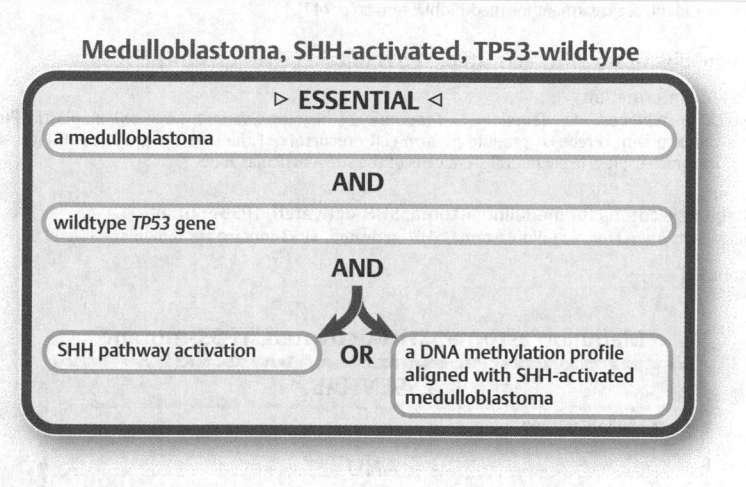

Fig. 43.5 Diagnostic criteria for medulloblastoma, SHH-activated, TP53-wildtype. (Modified with permission from WHO Classification of Tumors Editorial Board, (ed.) World Health Organization classification of tumors of the central nervous system. 5th ed. Bosman F T, Jaffe E S, Lakhani S R, et al. (series eds.): World Health Organization Classification of Tumors series, vol. 6. International Agency for Research on Cancer, Lyon, France, 2021.)

Subtypes

See reference.[9]

Four provisional molecular subgroups are determined by DNA methylation or transcriptome profiling
- **SHH-1**
- **SHH-2**
- **SHH-3**
- **SHH-4**

Location

Infants: the cerebellar vermis is much more frequently than the cerebellar hemispheres.
Older children and young adults: mainly involves the hemispheres.

Epidemiology

SHH activated meduloblastomas exhibit a bimodal age distribution with one peak in infants and the other in adults. M:F ratio is ≈ 1.5:1.

Histology

See section 43.3.1.
Most MDB, SHH activated TP53-wt tumors are desmoplastic/nodular or MBENS.

▶ **Classic morphology.** Prognosis: Standard risk tumor.

► **Large cell/anaplastic morphology.** Rare. Uncertain clinical significance.

► **Desmoplastic/nodular morphology.** Prognosis: low risk tumor. Prevalent in infants and adults.

► **Extensive nodularity morphology (MBEN).** Prognosis: low risk tumor. Prevalent in infants.

43

Staging
See postoperative staging (p. 746).

Treatment
For treatment, see treatment for medulloblastomas (p. 747).

Medulloblastoma, SHH-activated, TP53-mutant (WHO grade 4)

General information
Typical in childhood. Male:female = 1:1. Predominant histologic variant: large cell/anaplastic. Putative cell of origin: cerebellar granule neuron cell precursors of the external granule cell layer and cochlear nucleus; less likely neural stem cells of the subventricular zone.

Diagnostic criteria for medulloblastoma, SHH-activated, TP53-mutant
Diagnostic criteria for medulloblastoma, SHH-activated, TP53-mutant are shown in ► Fig. 43.6.[9]

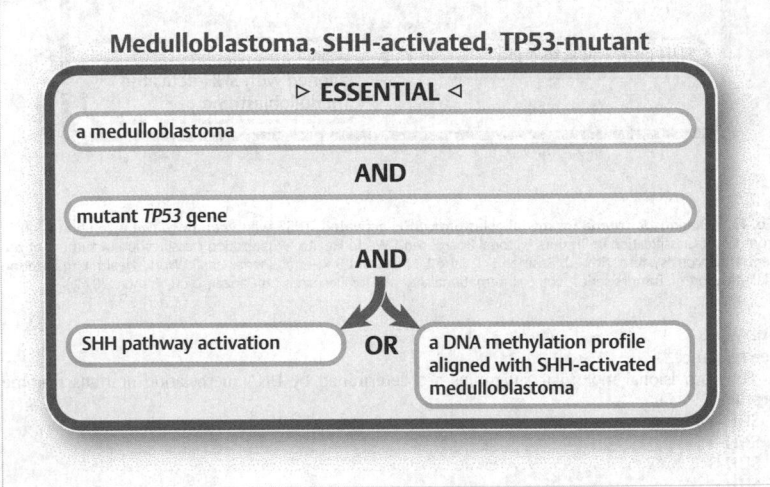

Fig. 43.6 **Diagnostic criteria for medulloblastoma, SHH-activated, TP53-mutant.** (Modified with permission from WHO Classification of Tumors Editorial Board, (ed.) World Health Organization classification of tumors of the central nervous system. 5th ed. Bosman F T, Jaffe E S, Lakhani S R, et al. (series eds.): World Health Organization Classification of Tumors series, vol. 6. International Agency for Research on Cancer, Lyon, France, 2021.)

Subtypes
The same four subtypes as MDB SHH-activated TP53-wildtype (viz. SHH 1-4).

Histology
See section 43.3.1.

Metastatic disease and MYCN amplification are independent poor prognosticators in children (not infants) and adolescents.

▶ **Classic morphology.** Prognosis: high-risk tumor. Uncommon.

▶ **Large cell/anaplastic morphology.** The predominant histologic type (70%). Prognosis: high-risk tumor. Prevalent in ages 7–17 years.

▶ **Desmoplastic/nodular morphology.** Very rare. Uncertain clinical significance.

Staging
See postoperative staging (p. 746).

Treatment
For treatment, see treatment for medulloblastomas (p. 747).

Medulloblastoma, non-WNT/non-SHH (WHO grade 4)

General information
An embryonal tumor of the cerebellum without a molecular signature. Classified as group 3 or group 4 tumors, with 8 molecular subgroups as determined by DNA methylation profiling. Typical in infancy and childhood. Male:female = 2:1. They occur exclusively in the inferior cerebellum, usually near the midline. Predominant histologic variants: classic; large cell/anaplastic. Putative cell of origin: cerebellar granule neuron cell precursors of the external granule cell layer. Frequent genetic mutations: PVT1-MYC, GFI1/GFI1B structural variants.

Diagnostic criteria for medulloblastoma, non-WNT/non-SHH
Diagnostic criteria for medulloblastoma, non-WNT/non-SHH are shown in ▶ Fig. 43.7.[9]

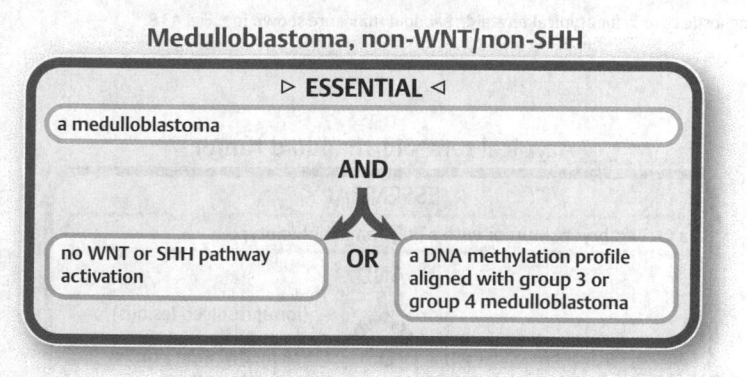

Fig. 43.7 Diagnostic criteria for medulloblastoma, non-WNT/non-SHH. (Modified with permission from WHO Classification of Tumors Editorial Board, (ed.) World Health Organization classification of tumors of the central nervous system. 5th ed. Bosman F T, Jaffe E S, Lakhani S R, et al. (series eds.): World Health Organization Classification of Tumors series, vol. 6. International Agency for Research on Cancer, Lyon, France, 2021.)

Subtypes
There are 8 subgroups of group 3/4 as differentiated by DNA methylation profiling.

Histology
See section 43.3.1.

▶ **Classic morphology.** The most common histology for this tumor. Prognosis: Standard risk tumor.

▶ **Large cell/anaplastic morphology.** This histology is more prevalent in group 3 than group 4. Prognosis: high risk tumor.

Staging
See postoperative staging (p. 746).

43

Treatment
For treatment, see treatment for medulloblastomas (p. 747).

Prognosis
In group 3 MDBs, MYC amplification is associated with poor outcome, but other markers also have prognostic impact.
Among group 4 MDBs, metastatic disease at the time of diagnosis is the strongest indicator of poor outcome. Favorable outcome in group 4 is associated with chromosome 7 gain, chromosome 8 loss, chromosome 11 loss, and chromosome 17 gain.

43.4 CNS embryonal tumors other than medulloblastoma

43.4.1 Atypical teratoid/rhabdoid tumor (AT/RT) (WHO grade 4)

General information

A high-grade malignant WHO grade 4 embryonal tumor of the CNS comprised of poorly differentiated elements and rhabdoid cells which exhibit biallelic inactivation of *SMARCB1* or rarely *SMARCA4* and which can differentiate along neuroepithelial, epithelial and mesenchymal cell lines. Many of these tumors were probably previously misdiagnosed as MDBs.

Diagnostic criteria for atypical teratoid/rhabdoid tumor

Diagnostic criteria for atypical teratoid/rhabdoid tumor are shown in ▶ Fig. 43.8.[9]

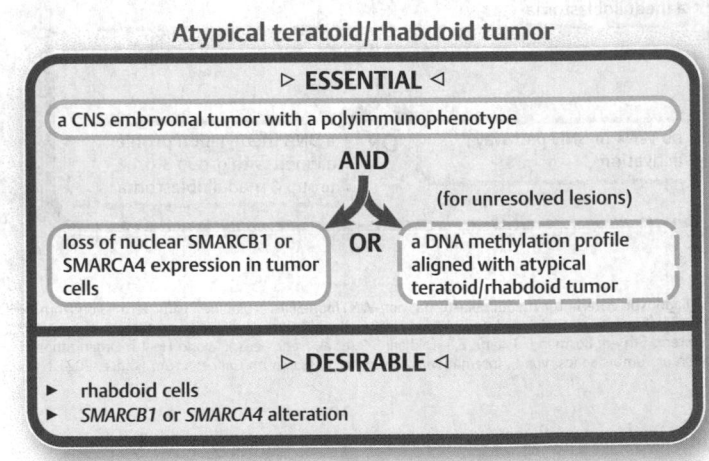

Fig. 43.8 **Diagnostic criteria for atypical teratoid/rhabdoid tumor.** (Modified with permission from WHO Classification of Tumors Editorial Board, (ed.) World Health Organization classification of tumors of the central nervous system. 5th ed. Bosman F T, Jaffe E S, Lakhani S R, et al. (series eds.): World Health Organization Classification of Tumors series, vol. 6. International Agency for Research on Cancer, Lyon, France, 2021.)

Subtypes

Three molecular subtypes are identifiable on DNA methylation profiling:
- AT/RT-SHH
- AT/RT-TYR
- AT/RT-MYC

Location

Anywhere along the neuraxis. Supratentorial location is more likely with advancing age, and includes the hemispheres, and less often the ventricles, or suprasellar or pineal region. Other locations include cerebellar hemispheres, cerebellopontine angle and brainstem. Spinal cord involvement is rare. 33% have CSF spread at presentation.

Epidemiology

Occurs primarily in infants and children (most are age < 2 years, 33% are ≤ 1 year old, and > 90% are < 5 years). Rare in adults. AT/RT account for 17% of embryonal tumors.[2]

Familial cases may occur in cohorts with rhabdoid tumor predisposition syndrome.

Staging

See postoperative staging (p. 746).

Prognosis

Althogh the prognosis is poor, not all AT/RTs have the same behavior. Pending validation studies, prognosis may be predicted based on molecular group, age, location and exent of resection.

43.4.2 Cribriform neuroepithelial tumor (CRINET) *(provisional)*

General information

A *provisional* non-rhabdoid neuroectodermal neoplasm identifiable by cribriform strands and ribbons with loss of SMARCB1 expression.

Diagnostic criteria for cribriform neuroepithelial tumor

Diagnostic criteria for cribriform neuroepithelial tumor are shown in ► Fig. 43.9.[9]

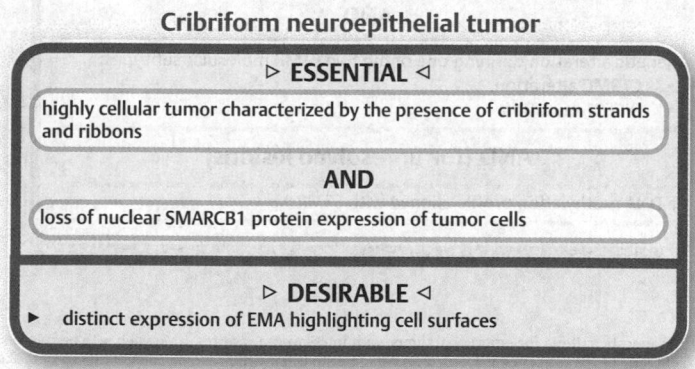

Fig. 43.9 Diagnostic criteria for cribriform neuroepithelial tumor. (Modified with permission from WHO Classification of Tumors Editorial Board, (ed.) World Health Organization classification of tumors of the central nervous system. 5th ed. Bosman F T, Jaffe E S, Lakhani S R, et al. (series eds.): World Health Organization Classification of Tumors series, vol. 6. International Agency for Research on Cancer, Lyon, France, 2021.)

43

Location
Near any of the ventricles (3rd, 4th, or lateral).

Epidemiology
Median age: 20 months (range: 10-129 months). M:F ratio 1.5:1.[17]

Prognosis
In 10 patients with CRINET, estimated mean OS was 125 months.[17]

43.4.3 Embryonal tumor with multilayered rosettes (ETMR) (WHO grade 4)

General information
A WHO grade 4 embryonal tumor with multilayered rosettes demonstrating one of three histological patterns (embryonal tumor with abundant neuropil and true rosettes, ependymoblastoma, or medulloepithelioma) typically exhibiting amplification in the C19MC region on chromosome 19 (19q13.42) or, rarely, a *DICER1* mutation. May develop in the cerebrum, brainstem, or cerebellum. Usually affect children < 4 years old (with the vast majority being < 2 years old).

Diagnostic criteria for embryonal tumor with multilayered rosettes

Diagnostic criteria for embryonal tumor with multilayered rosettes are shown in ▶ Fig. 43.10.[9]

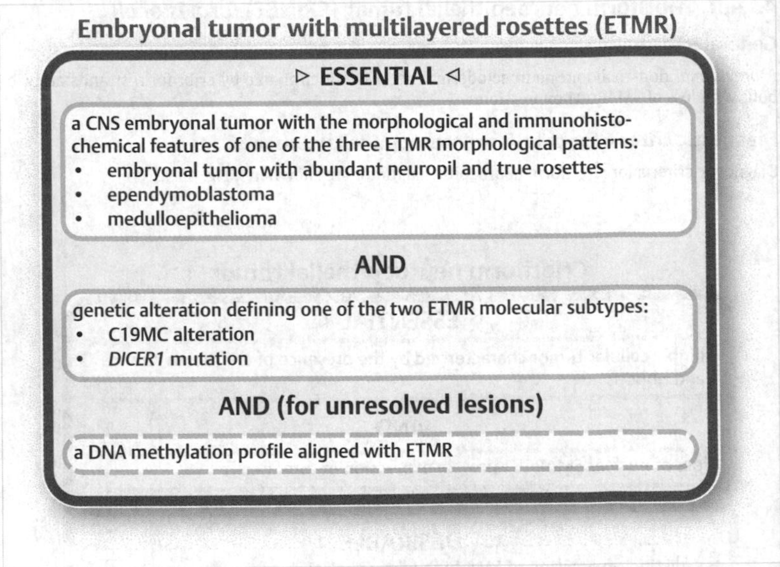

Embryonal tumor with multilayered rosettes (ETMR)

▷ **ESSENTIAL** ◁

a CNS embryonal tumor with the morphological and immunohisto-chemical features of one of the three ETMR morphological patterns:
- embryonal tumor with abundant neuropil and true rosettes
- ependymoblastoma
- medulloepithelioma

AND

genetic alteration defining one of the two ETMR molecular subtypes:
- C19MC alteration
- *DICER1* mutation

AND (for unresolved lesions)

a DNA methylation profile aligned with ETMR

Fig. 43.10 **Diagnostic criteria for embryonal tumor with multilayered rosettes.** (Modified with permission from WHO Classification of Tumors Editorial Board, (ed.) World Health Organization classification of tumors of the central nervous system. 5th ed. Bosman F T, Jaffe E S, Lakhani S R, et al. (series eds.): World Health Organization Classification of Tumors series, vol. 6. International Agency for Research on Cancer, Lyon, France, 2021.)

Subtypes

- embryonal tumor with multilayered rosettes, C19MC-altered
- embryonal tumor with multilayered rosettes, *DICER1*-mutated

Location

The cerebral hemispheres is the most common location, with 45% located elsewhere including the posterior fossa. Spinal cord involvement is rare.

43

Epidemiology

Data is sparse due to the rarity of the tumor. Primarily affects children < 4 years, with most younger than 2. M:F ratio is close to 1:1.

Staging

See postoperative staging (p. 746).

Prognosis

These aggressive tumors grow rapidly producing precipitous clinical deterioration. Mean OS is 12 months following intensive treatment.[9] Outcome is worse when metastases are present at diagnosis and with brainstem involvement. Gross total resection, XRT and aggressive chemotherapy are "probably helpful."

References

[1] Louis DN, Perry A, Reifenberger G, et al. The 2016 World Health Organization Classification of Tumors of the Central Nervous System: a summary. Acta Neuropathol. 2016; 131:803–820

[2] Ostrom QT, Cioffi G, Waite K, et al. CBTRUS Statistical Report: Primary Brain and Other Central Nervous System Tumors Diagnosed in the United States in 2014-2018. Neuro Oncol. 2021; 23:iii1–iii105

[3] Laurent JP, Cheek WR. Brain Tumors in Children. J Pediatr Neurosci. 1985; 1:15–32

[4] Allen JC. Childhood Brain Tumors: Current Status of Clinical Trials in Newly Diagnosed and Recurrent Disease. Ped Clin N Am. 1985; 32:633–651

[5] Kessler LA, Dugan P, Concannon JP. Systemic Metastases of Medulloblastoma Promoted by Shunting. Surg Neurol. 1975; 3:147–152

[6] Berger MS, Baumeister B, Geyer JR, et al. The Risks of Metastases from Shunting in Children with Primary Central Nervous System Tumors. J Neurosurg. 1991; 74:872–877

[7] Park TS, Hoffman HJ, Hendrick EB, et al. Medulloblastoma: Clinical Presentation and Management. J Neurosurg. 1983; 58:543–552

[8] Ramaswamy V, Remke M, Bouffet E, et al. Risk stratification of childhood medulloblastoma in the molecular era: the current consensus. Acta Neuropathol. 2016; 131:821–831

[9] Bosman FT, Jaffe ES, Lakhani SR, et al. World Health Organization Classification of Tumors series, vol. 6. In: WHO Classification of Tumors Editorial Board (ed.) World Health Organization classification of tumors of the central nervous system. 5th ed. Lyon, France: International Agency for Research on Cancer; 2021

[10] Juraschka K, Taylor MD. Medulloblastoma in the age of molecular subgroups: a review. J Neurosurg Pediatr. 2019; 24:353–363

[11] Goschzik T, Schwalbe EC, Hicks D, et al. Prognostic effect of whole chromosomal aberration signatures in standard-risk, non-WNT/non-SHH medulloblastoma: a retrospective, molecular analysis of the HIT-SIOP PNET 4 trial. Lancet Oncol. 2018; 19:1602–1616

[12] Blaser SI, Harwood-Nash DC. Neuroradiology of pediatric posterior fossa medulloblastoma. J Neurooncol. 1996; 29:23–34

[13] Chang CH, Housepian EM, Herbert C,Jr. An operative staging system and a megavoltage radiotherapeutic technic for cerebellar medulloblastomas. Radiology. 1969; 93:1351–1359

[14] Louis DN, Ohgaki H, Wiestler OD, et al. WHO classification of tumors of the central nervous system. Lyon, France 2016

[15] Cambruzzi E. Medulloblastoma, WNT-activated/SHH-activated: clinical impact of molecular analysis and histogenetic evaluation. Childs Nerv Syst. 2018; 34:809–815

[16] Gilbertson RJ. Medulloblastoma: signalling a change in treatment. Lancet Oncol. 2004; 5:209–218

[17] Johann PD, Hovestadt V, Thomas C, et al. Cribriform neuroepithelial tumor: molecular characterization of a SMARCB1-deficient non-rhabdoid tumor with favorable long-term outcome. Brain Pathol. 2017; 27:411–418

44 Pineal Tumors and Pineal Region Lesions

44.1 Pineal region lesions

44.1.1 General information

44

Key concepts

- wide variety of pathology: germ cell tumors (mostly germinomas, teratomas), astrocytomas, & pineal tumors (mostly pineoblastomas) account for most tumors. Non pineal neoplasms (meningiomas, metastases from other regions, ependymomas...) as well as non-neoplastic lesions (pineal cysts...) also occur in this region
- pineal region tumors are relatively rare and are more common in children than in adults
- in children, most tumors are germinomas or astrocytomas; in adults, meningiomas and gliomas predominate
- due to mixed tumors and many non-secretory tumors, tumor markers are no longer considered clinically useful for diagnosis or monitoring response to treatment → get a biopsy to avoid operating on a germinoma or just using XRT on a non-germinoma

Germ cell tumors (p.831) are covered in a separate section. Pineal cysts (p.948) are non-neoplastic and are covered elsewhere.

The pineal gland is a neuroendocrine gland that secretes melatonin in response to photic stimulation of the retina by bright light, and also regulates secretion of some pituitary hormones. It is outside the blood brain barrier and is supplied by choroidal branches of the posterior cerebral artery.

▶ **Pineal region.** The area of the brain bounded dorsally by the splenium of the corpus callosum and the tela choroidea, ventrally by the quadrigeminal plate and midbrain tectum, rostrally by the posterior aspect of the 3rd ventricle, and caudally by the cerebellar vermis.[1]

A striking feature of the pineal region is the diversity of lesions (neoplastic and nonneoplastic) that may occur in this location due to the variety of tissues and conditions normally present, as shown in ▶ Table 44.1.

Over 17 tumor types occur in this region.[2] Germinoma is the most common tumor (21–44% in American/European population, 43–70% in Japan), followed by astrocytoma, teratoma, and pineoblastoma.[3] Many tumors are of mixed cell type.

Table 44.1 Conditions giving rise to pineal region lesions

Substrate in pineal region	Tumor that may arise
pineal glandular tissue	pineocytomas, pineal parenchymal tumor of intermediate differentiation, pineoblastomas
glial cells	astrocytomas (including pilocytic astrocytomas & GBM), oligodendrogliomas, glial cysts (AKA pineal cyst)
arachnoid cells	meningiomas (characteristically displace the the internal cerebral vein inferiorly)
ependymal lining	ependymomas
sympathetic nerves	paragangliomas
rests of germ cells	germ cell tumors: choriocarcinoma, germinoma, embryonal carcinoma, endodermal sinus tumor (yolk sac tumor), and teratoma
absence of blood-brain barrier (BBB) in pineal gland	makes it a susceptible site for hematogenous metastases
remnants of ectoderm	epidermoid or dermoid cysts
non-neoplastic lesions that may mimic tumors	
• vascular	vein of Galen aneurysm (p.1518), AVM
• infectious	cysticercosis (p.404)
• arachnoid cyst (p.261)	fluid trapped between layers of arachnoid membrane

Germ cell tumors (GCT), ependymomas, and pineal cell tumors metastasize easily through the CSF ("drop metastases").

▶ **Pediatric.** Tumors in this region are rare and are more common in children (3–8% of pediatric brain tumors) than in adults (≤ 1%).[4]

A breakdown of pediatric pineal region tumors is shown in ▶ Table 44.2.

In 36 patients < 18 yrs of age, 17 distinct histological tumor types were identified: 11 germinomas (the most common tumor), 7 astrocytomas, and the remaining 18 had 15 different tumors.[5]

▶ **Adult.** GCTs and pineal cell tumors occur primarily in childhood and young adults. Thus, over the age of 40, a pineal region tumor is more likely to be a meningioma or a glioma. Series B in ▶ Table 44.2 includes both adult and pediatric patients.

44

Table 44.2 Pineal region tumors

Tumor	Series A (age ≤ 18 years)[a] (%)	Series B (ages 3-73)[b] (%)
germinoma	30	27
astrocytoma	19	26
pineocytoma	6	12
malignant teratoma	6	
unidentified germ cell tumor	6	
choriocarcinoma	3	1.1
malignant teratoma/embryonal cell tumor	3	1.6
glioblastoma	3	
teratoma	3	4.3
germinoma/yolk sac tumor	3	
dermoid	3	
embryonal cell tumor	3	
pineoblastoma	3	12
pineocytoma/pineoblastoma	3	
endodermal sinus tumor	3	
glial cyst (pineal cyst)[6]	3	2.7
arachnoid cyst	3	
metastases		2.7
meningioma		2.7
ependymoma		4.3
oligodendroglioma		0.54
ganglioglioneuroma		2.7
lymphoma		2.7

[a]36 children ≤ 18 yrs[5]
[b]370 tumors in patients 3–73 yrs old[4]

44.1.2 Clinical

Hydrocephalus: almost all patients have hydrocephalus by the time of presentation, producing typical signs and symptoms of headache, vomiting, lethargy, memory disturbance, abnormally increasing head circumference in infants, and seizures. Hydrocephalus is of the obstructive variety, and is usually due to compression of the sylvian aqueduct which occurs early in masses in the pineal region, and which produces triventricular enlagement (of the 2 lateral ventricles and the 3rd ventricle, but not the 4th ventricle which is distal to the obstruction).

Parinaud syndrome (p.101): AKA syndrome of the sylvian aqueduct, may be present. This can occur with hydrocephalus of any cause, but can also result from direct pressure on the dorsal midbrain.

Endocrinologic disturbances: precocious puberty may occur only in boys with choriocarcinomas or germinomas with syncytiotrophoblastic cells, due to luteinizing hormone-like effects of β-hCG secreted in the CSF. Suprasellar GCT: triad of diabetes insipidus, visual deficit, and panhypopituitarism.[7]

Spinal symptoms: Drop metastases from CSF seeding can produce radiculopathy and/or myelopathy.

44.1.3 Imaging of pineal region masses

Critical differentiating fact: intrinsic pineal tumors tend to cause upward displacement of the internal cerebral vein (▶ Fig. 44.5), whereas tentorial meningiomas tend to displace the vein inferiorly.

44.1.4 Management of pineal region masses

The optimal management strategy for pineal region tumors has yet to be determined.

✗ "Test dose" radiation: The practice of this is generally obsolete. The logic behind the test dose was that if a pineal region tumor enhanced uniformly and had the classic appearance of a germinoma on MRI, a test dose of 5 Gy was given, and if the tumor shrank then the diagnosis of germinoma was virtually certain and XRT was continued without surgery. This would needlessly expose a patient with benign or radioresistant tumors to the test dose of XRT.[4] "Test dose XRT" should especially be avoided in tumors suspected of being teratomas or epidermoid cyst on MRI, and the response may be misleading in the relatively common situation of tumors with mixed cell types. This practice is that giving way to the paradigm of surgery (p. 761) to ascertain histology in almost all cases (e.g., via endoscopic surgery) because of the harmful effects of XRT and because 36–50% of pineal tumors are benign or radioresistant.[8]

Management suggestions

The use of germ cell tumor markers are no longer considered to be useful for diagnosing tumors or for following response to therapy (p. 832)
1. MRI without and with contrast of: brain, as well as cervical, thoracic, and lumbar spine to assess for drop mets
2. pineal cysts do not require surgery unless they become large enough (usually > 2 cm) to cause obstructive hydroceephalus
3. biopsy, which should be generous (to avoid missing other histologies in mixed cell tumors)
   a) if hydrocephalus: transventricular biopsy
   b) if no hydrocephalus:
      • open biopsy or
      • stereotactic biopsy or
      • navigation-assisted endoscopic approach: see below
4. based on histology:
   a) germinoma: XRT + chemo
   b) all other tumors: one option is resection followed by adjuvant therapy (usually not very helpful)—see Indications (p. 761) for controversies

Hydrocephalus: Patients presenting acutely due to hydrocephalus may be best treated with external ventricular drainage (EVD). This permits control over the amount of CSF drained, prevents peritoneal seeding with tumor (a rare event[9]), and may avoid having a permanent shunt placed in the significant number of patients who will not need one after tumor removal (although ≈ 90% of patients with a pineal GCT require a shunt). In the event of acute post-operative hydrocephalus, ready ventricular access, via EVD or Frazier burr hole (p. 1742), is important.

Stereotactic surgical procedures: May be used to ascertain diagnosis (biopsy), or to treat symptomatic pineal region cysts.[10,11] Caution is advised since the pineal region has numerous vessels (vein of Galen, basal veins of Rosenthal, internal cerebral veins, posterior medial choroidal artery)[12] which may be displaced from their normal position. The complication rate of stereotactic biopsy is: ≈ 1.3% mortality, ≈ 7% morbidity, and 1 case of seeding in 370 patients, and the diagnostic rate is ≈ 94%.[4] A shortcoming of stereotactic biopsy is that it may fail to disclose the histologic heterogeneity of some tumors.

Two main stereotactic trajectories: 1) anterolateral (low frontal) approach below the internal cerebral veins, and 2) posterolateral trans-parieto-occipital.[2] One study found that the trajectory correlated with complications, and they recommended the anterolateral approach.[13] However, the correlation of trajectory and complications was not born out in another study,[4] and they found that the complication rate was higher in firm tumors (pineocytomas, teratomas, and astrocytomas) and they recommend an open approach when the tumor appears difficult to penetrate on the first attempt at biopsy.

Stereotactic radiosurgery may be appropriate for treatment of some lesions.

Navigation-assisted endoscopic approach: Various approaches including a supracerebellar infratentorial approach[2] that permits visualization and thus avoidance of neurovascular structures, or for patients with hydrocephalus a combined endoscopic third ventriculoscopy with pineal biopsy.[14]

Radiation treatment: See "Test dose" radiation (p. 760) for controversies related to that. Germinomas are very sensitive to radiation (and chemotherapy), and are probably best treated with these modalities and followed.

XRT is also utilized post-op for other malignant tumors. For highly malignant tumors or if there is evidence of CSF seeding, craniospinal XRT with a boost to the tumor bed is appropriate.

If possible, XRT is best avoided in the young child. Chemotherapy may be used for age < 3 yrs until the child is older, when XRT is better tolerated.[7]

44.1.5 Surgical treatment of the tumor

Indications

Controversial. Some authors feel that most tumors (except germinomas, which are best treated with XRT) are amenable to open resection.[15] Others feel that resection should be limited to ≈ 25% of tumors which are[4]:
1. radioresistant (e.g., malignant nongerminoma GCTs): 35–50% of pineal region tumors (larger numbers occur in series not limited to pediatric patients)
2. benign (e.g., meningioma, teratomas…)
3. well-encapsulated
4. NB: malignant germ cell tumors should be without evidence of metastases (those with metastases do not benefit from surgery on the primary tumor)
5. pineocytoma: recommendation is for surgical excision + SRS for any residual

Options

1. direct surgery: obtains generous tissue for biopsy. Curative for benign lesions. Not the optimum treatment for malignant tumors and germinomas without complications
2. biopsy followed by adjuvant therapy: the preferred management (p. 760) for malignancies and germinomatous germ cell tumors

Surgical approaches

Choice is aided by the pre-op MRI and includes:
1. most common approach: midline infratentorial-supracerebellar approach of Horsley and Krause as refined by Stein.[16] Cannot be used if the angle of the tentorium is too steep (best assessed on MRI). May be done in the sitting position (NB: risk of air embolism (p. 1738)) or in the Concorde position (p. 1737)
2. occipital transtentorial: wide view. Risk of injury to occipital visual cortex or splenium of corpus callosum. Recommended for lesions centered at or superior to the tentorial edge or located above the vein of Galen, or for rare cysts with superior extension. The occipital lobe is retracted laterally, and the tentorium is incised 1 cm lateral to the straight sinus
3. transventricular: indicated for large, eccentric lesions with ventricular dilatation. Usually via a cortical incision in the posterior portion of the superior temporal gyrus. Risks: visual defect, seizures, and on dominant side language dysfunction
4. lateral paramedian infratentorial
5. transcallosal: largely abandoned except for tumors extending into corpus callosum and third ventricle
6. paramedian infratentorial-supracerebellar approach may be used for cysts that do not extend superiorly or contralaterally[17]: avoids midline venous structures

Important surgical considerations: The base of the pineal gland is the posterior wall of the 3rd ventricle. The splenium of the corpus callosum lies above, and the thalamus surrounds both sides. The pineal projects posteriorly and inferiorly into the quadrigeminal cistern. The deep cerebral veins are a major obstacle to operations in this region. Venous drainage of the pineal region must be preserved.

44.1.6 Surgical outcome

Surgical mortality rate: 5–10%.[4] Postoperative complications include: new visual field deficits, epidural fluid collection, infection, and cerebellar ataxia.

44.2 Pineal tumors

44.2.1 Pineocytoma (WHO grade 1)

General information

A rare, well-differentiated WHO grade 1 tumor of the pineal parenchyma consisting of pineocytoma-tous rosettes of uniform cells and/or pleomorphic cells having gangliocytic differentiation. Thought to derive from pinealocytes which are photosensory neuroendocrine cells.

44

Diagnostic criteria for pineocytoma

Diagnostic criteria for pineocytoma are shown in ▶ Fig. 44.1.[18]

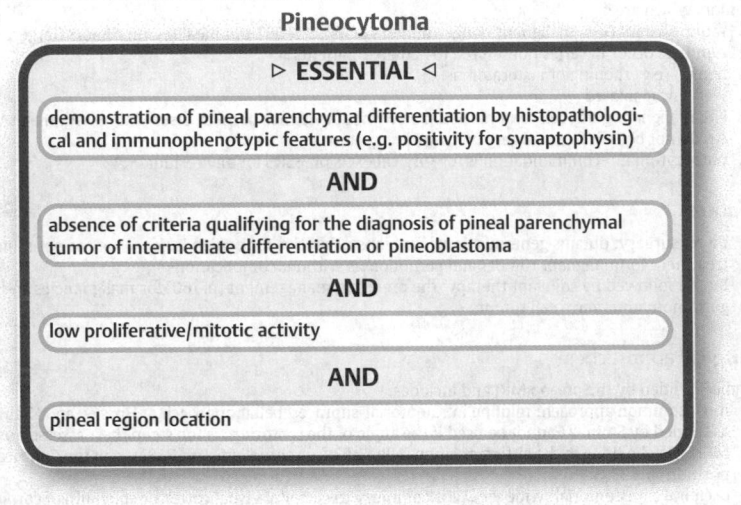

Fig. 44.1 Diagnostic criteria for pineocytoma. (Modified with permission from WHO Classification of Tumors Editorial Board, (ed.) World Health Organization classification of tumors of the central nervous system. 5th ed. Bosman F T, Jaffe E S, Lakhani S R, et al. (series eds.): World Health Organization Classification of Tumors series, vol. 6. International Agency for Research on Cancer, Lyon, France, 2021.)

Location

Found exclusively in the pineal gland. Not disseminating or infiltrating.[19]

Imaging

MRI: typically hypintense to isointense on T1WI, hyperintense on T2WI, with avid homogeneous enhancement.

Epidemiology

Typically affects adults (average age at diagnosis: 43 yrs). Comprises ≈ 25% of all pineal parenchymal neoplasms.

Prognosis

5-year survival rate is 86–91%.[20] Extent of surgical excision is a major predictor of prognosis.[21]

44.2.2 Pineal parenchymal tumor of intermediate differentiation (PPTID) (WHO grade 2 or 3)

General information

A pineal parenchymal tumor with clinical and biological behavior intermediate in malignancy between pineocytoma and pineoblastoma consisting of monomorphic round cells that appear more differentiated than those of pineoblastomas and are arrayed in sheets or lobules. Ki-67 index (p.632) is variable.

Biological behavior ranges from WHO grade 2 to 3, but qualifying histological criteria are not yet defined.[19]

Diagnostic criteria for pineal parenchymal tumor of intermediate differentiation (PPTID)

Diagnostic criteria for PPTID are shown in ▶ Fig. 44.2.[18]

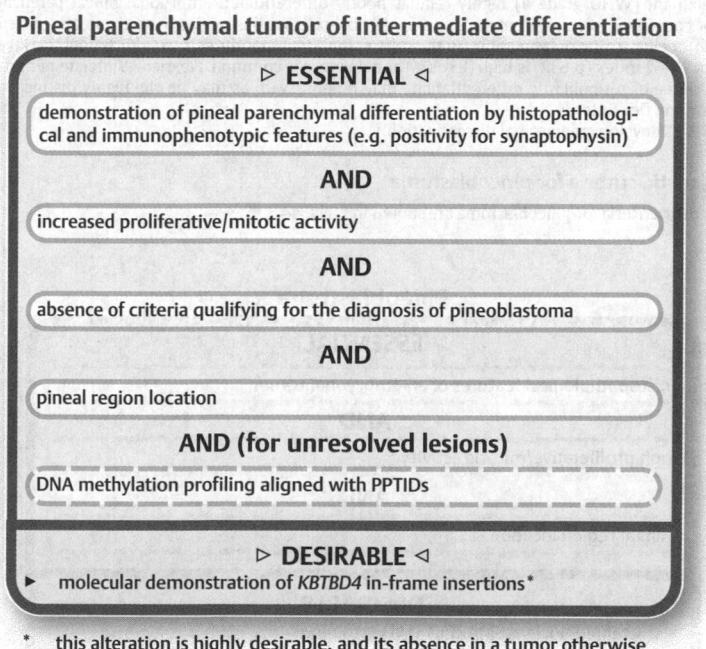

Pineal parenchymal tumor of intermediate differentiation

▷ **ESSENTIAL** ◁

demonstration of pineal parenchymal differentiation by histopathological and immunophenotypic features (e.g. positivity for synaptophysin)

AND

increased proliferative/mitotic activity

AND

absence of criteria qualifying for the diagnosis of pineoblastoma

AND

pineal region location

AND (for unresolved lesions)

DNA methylation profiling aligned with PPTIDs

▷ **DESIRABLE** ◁

▶ molecular demonstration of *KBTBD4* in-frame insertions*

* this alteration is highly desirable, and its absence in a tumor otherwise resembling PPTID, should prompt careful consideration as to whether an alternative diagnosis may be more suitable

Fig. 44.2 Diagnostic criteria for PPTID. (Modified with permission from WHO Classification of Tumors Editorial Board, (ed.) World Health Organization classification of tumors of the central nervous system. 5th ed. Bosman F T, Jaffe E S, Lakhani S R, et al. (series eds.): World Health Organization Classification of Tumors series, vol. 6. International Agency for Research on Cancer, Lyon, France, 2021.)

44

Although the behavior of the majority of PPTIDs are consistent with WHO grade 2, definitive criteria has not been defined for identifying more aggressive grade 3 lesions.

Imaging

MRI: typically larger and more heterogeneous than pineocytoma. Local invasion was seen in 9 out of 11 cases (82%).[22]

Epidemiology

44

Mean age at diagnosis is 41 years, median 33 years (range: 3.5-64). Slight female predominance (M:F ratio 1:1.25).[18]

Prognosis

Lower grade PPTIDs demonstrate frequent local and delayed recurrence, higher grade lesions may be more prone to produce craniospinal metastases. Median OS is 14 years, and 5-year OS is 84%.[23] Median PFS was 5.2 years, with a 52% 5-year PFS.

44.2.3 Pineoblastoma (WHO grade 4)

General information

A malignant (WHO grade 4) highly cellular poorly differentiated embryonal pineal parenchymal tumor comprised of small, immature neuroepithelial cells with irregular hyperchromatic nucleii and a high nuclear-to-cytoplasm ratio (with scant cytoplasm), poorly defined cell borders, arrayed in sheets. Ki-67 index (p. 632) is high (23-50%) and necrosis is common. Flexner–Wintersteiner rosettes —indicative of retinoblastic differentiation—may be observed, as may be the highly distinctive but uncommon fleurettes.[18]

25-33% develop craniospinal dissemination.[18]

Diagnostic criteria for pineoblastoma

Diagnostic criteria for pineoblastoma are shown in ► Fig. 44.3.[18]

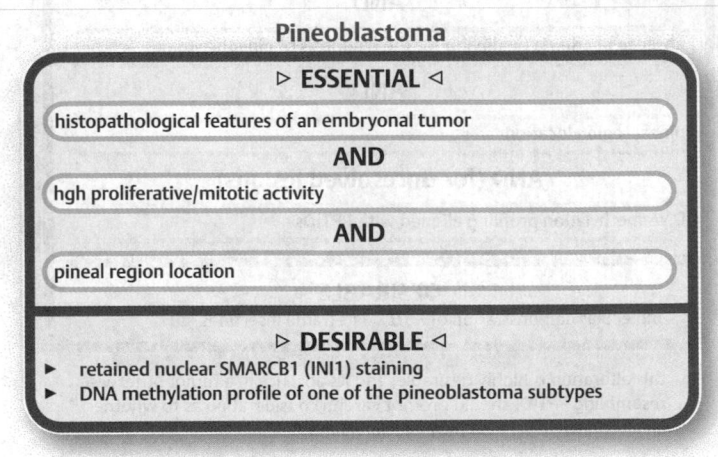

Fig. 44.3 Diagnostic criteria for pineoblastoma. (Modified with permission from WHO Classification of Tumors Editorial Board, (ed.) World Health Organization classification of tumors of the central nervous system. 5th ed. Bosman F T, Jaffe E S, Lakhani S R, et al. (series eds.): World Health Organization Classification of Tumors series, vol. 6. International Agency for Research on Cancer, Lyon, France, 2021.)

Subtypes

- pineoblastoma, miRNA processing-altered_1
- pineoblastoma, miRNA processing-altered_2
- pineoblastoma, *RB1*-altered (pineal retinoblastoma)
- pineoblastoma, MYC/FOXR2-activated

Imaging

MRI: at presentation, these tumors are usually large and invasion of surrounding structures is frequent. Typically hypintense to isointense on T1WI, isointense to mildly hyperintense on T2WI, with heterogeneous enhancement.

Epidemiology

Pineoblastomas constitute 35% of pineal parenchymal tumors.[18] Most occur in children (median age: 6 years) although they can occur at any age (range: 0–41.5 years).[24] Mean age at diagnosis is younger (17.8 years) than the less malignant counterparts.

Staging

The same principle for postoperative staging of medulloblastomas (p. 746) applies.

Prognosis

Clinical course is aggressive. CSF metastases are common. Median OS is 4.1–8.7 years[25,26]). Reported 5-year survival ranges 10–81%.[18]
   Poor prognosticators include:
- disseminated disease at time of diagnosis (evidenced by positive CSF cytology and/or spinal MRI)[25]
- young patient age
- partial surgical resection (extent of resection was more significant than M-staging in one study[26])

Molecular subgrouping holds promise for prognostication.[18]
   XRT appears to be a helpful adjuvant therapy to surgery.[25]

44.2.4 Papillary tumor of the pineal region (PTPR) (WHO grade 1 or 2)

General information

A neuroepithelial tumor of the pineal region with papillary and solid areas (▶ Fig. 44.5) comprised of epithelial-like cells and showing immunoreactivity for cytokeratins (especially CK18).
   Biological behavior ranges from WHO grade 2 to 3, but differentiating histological criteria are not yet defined.[19]

Diagnostic criteria for papillary tumor of the pineal region

Diagnostic criteria for papillary tumor of the pineal region are shown in ▶ Fig. 44.4.[18]

Epidemiology

Incidence data is lacking. Affects children and adults, with a median age of 35 years (range: 1-75).

Imaging

PTPRs are well-circumscribed lesions with cystic and solid components (▶ Fig. 44.5). Unlike other pineal parenchymal tumors, T1WI may show hyperintensity. Enhancement is heterogeneous.

Prognosis

Local recurrence is common. Spinal metastases can occur. Only gross total resection and younger age have been found to be better prognosticators for OS, whereas XRT and chemotherapy had no impact.[27]
   5-year and 10-year survival are both about 73%. Estimated 5-year PFS is 27%.[28]

Papillary tumor of the pineal region

▷ **ESSENTIAL** ◁

papillary growth pattern with epithelial-like cells

AND

characteristic immunohistochemical staining pattern (e.g. positivity for cytokeratins, SPDEF, CD56)

AND

pineal region location

AND (for unresolved lesions)

confirmatory DNA methylation profiling

Fig. 44.4 Diagnostic criteria for papillary tumor of the pineal region. (Modified with permission from WHO Classification of Tumors Editorial Board, (ed.) World Health Organization classification of tumors of the central nervous system. 5th ed. Bosman F T, Jaffe E S, Lakhani S R, et al. (series eds.): World Health Organization Classification of Tumors series, vol. 6. International Agency for Research on Cancer, Lyon, France, 2021.)

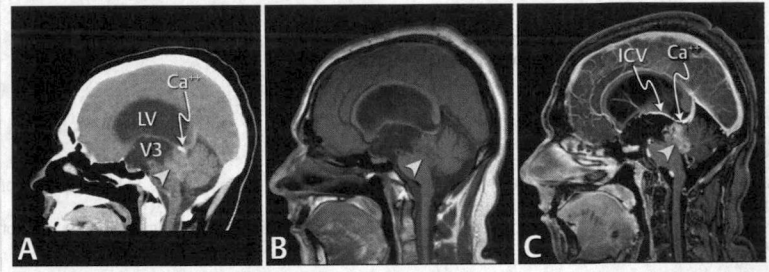

Fig. 44.5 Papillary tumor of the pineal region (*yellow arrowheads*) in a 27-year-old man. This patient experienced a local recurrence following surgery as well as spine metastases.
Image: A: sagittal noncontrast CT. V3 = enlarged third ventricle (V3) & lateral venticle (LV) due to hydrocephalus caused by tumor compressing the Sylvian aqueduct. Ca^{++} = physiologic calcificationis within the dorsally displaced pineal gland.
B: sagittal noncontrast T1 MRI. The tumor is ≈ isointense with brain.
C: sagittal contrasted T1 MRI. ICV = internal cerebral vein; Ca^{++} = calcifications within the pineal gland appear dark (which is difficult to see).

References

[1] Ringertz N, Nordenstam H, Flyger G. Tumors of the Pineal Region. Journal of Neuropathology and Experimental Neurology. 1954; 13:540–561

[2] Youssef AS, Keller JT, van Loveren HR. Novel application of computer-assisted cisternal endoscopy for the biopsy of pineal region tumors: cadaveric study. Acta Neurochir (Wien). 2007; 149:399–406

[3] Oi S, Matsumoto S. Controversy pertaining to therapeutic modalities for tumors of the pineal region: a

worldwide survey of different patient populations. Childs Nerv Syst. 1992; 8:332–336

[4] Regis J, Bouillot P, Rouby-Volot F, et al. Pineal Region Tumors and the Role of Stereotactic Biopsy: Review of the Mortality, Morbidity, and Diagnostic Rates in 370 Cases. Neurosurgery. 1996; 39:907–914

[5] Edwards MSB, Hudgins RJ, Wilson CB, et al. Pineal Region Tumors in Children. J Neurosurg. 1988; 68:689–697

[6] Todo T, Kondo T, Shinoura N, et al. Large Cysts of the Pineal Gland: Report of Two Cases. Neurosurgery. 1991; 29:101–106

[7] Hoffman HJ, Ostubo H, Hendrick EB, et al. Intracranial Germ-Cell Tumors in Children. Journal of Neurosurgery. 1991; 74:545–551

[8] Oi S, Matsuzawa K, Choi JU, et al. Identical characteristics of the patient populations with pineal region tumors in Japan and in Korea and therapeutic modalities. Childs Nerv Syst. 1998; 14:36–40

[9] Berger MS, Baumeister B, Geyer JR, et al. The Risks of Metastases from Shunting in Children with Primary Central Nervous System Tumors. J Neurosurg. 1991; 74:872–877

[10] Stern JD, Ross DA. Stereotactic Management of Benign Pineal Region Cysts: Report of Two Cases. Neurosurgery. 1993; 32:310–314

[11] Musolino A, Cambria S, Rizzo G, et al. Symptomatic Cysts of the Pineal Gland: Stereotactic Diagnosis and Treatment of Two Cases and Review of the Literature. Neurosurgery. 1993; 32:315–321

[12] Kelly PJ. Comment on Musolino A, et al.: Symptomatic Cysts of the Pineal Gland: Stereotactic Diagnosis and Treatment of Two Cases and Review of the Literature. Neurosurgery. 1993; 32:320–321

[13] Dempsey PK, Kondziolka D, Lunsford LD. Stereotactic Diagnosis and Treatment of Pineal Region Tumors and Vascular Malformations. Acta Neurochirurgica. 1992; 116:14–22

[14] Samadian M, Maloumeh EN, Shiravand S, et al. Pineal region tumors: Long-term results of endoscopic third ventriculostomy and concurrent tumor biopsy with a single approach in a series of 64 cases. Clin Neurol Neurosurg. 2019; 184. DOI: 10.1016/j.clineuro.2019.105418

[15] Kelly PJ. Comment on Regis J, et al.: Pineal Region Tumors and the Role of Stereotactic Biopsy: Review of the Mortality, Morbidity, and Diagnostic Rates in 370 Cases. Neurosurgery. 1996; 39:912–913

[16] Stein BM. The infratentorial supracerebellar approach to pineal lesions. J Neurosurg. 1971; 35:197–202

[17] Torres A, Krisht AF, Akouri S. Current Management of Pineal Cysts. Contemporary Neurosurgery. 2005; 27:1–5

[18] Bosman FT, Jaffe ES, Lakhani SR, et al. World Health Organization Classification of Tumors series, vol. 6. In: WHO Classification of Tumors Editorial Board (ed.) World Health Organization classification of tumors of the central nervous system. 5th ed. Lyon, France: International Agency for Research on Cancer; 2021

[19] Louis DN, Ohgaki H, Wiestler OD, et al. WHO classification of tumors of the central nervous system. Lyon, France 2016

[20] Fauchon F, Jouvet A, Paquis P, et al. Parenchymal pineal tumors: a clinicopathological study of 76 cases. Int J Radiat Oncol Biol Phys. 2000; 46:959–968

[21] Clark AJ, Sughrue ME, Ivan ME, et al. Factors influencing overall survival rates for patients with pineocytoma. J Neurooncol. 2010; 100:255–260

[22] Komakula S, Warmuth-Metz M, Hildenbrand P, et al. Pineal parenchymal tumor of intermediate differentiation: imaging spectrum of an unusual tumor in 11 cases. Neuroradiology. 2011; 53:577–584

[23] Mallick S, Benson R, Rath GK. Patterns of care and survival outcomes in patients with pineal parenchymal tumor of intermediate differentiation: An individual patient data analysis. Radiother Oncol. 2016; 121:204–208

[24] Liu APY, Li BK, Pfaff E, et al. Clinical and molecular heterogeneity of pineal parenchymal tumors: a consensus study. Acta Neuropathol. 2021; 141:771–785

[25] Farnia B, Allen PK, Brown PD, et al. Clinical outcomes and patterns of failure in pineoblastoma: a 30-year, single-institution retrospective review. World Neurosurg. 2014; 82:1232–1241

[26] Jakacki RI, Burger PC, Kocak M, et al. Outcome and prognostic factors for children with supratentorial primitive neuroectodermal tumors treated with carboplatin during radiotherapy: a report from the Children's Oncology Group. Pediatr Blood Cancer. 2015; 62:776–783

[27] Fauchon F, Hasselblatt M, Jouvet A, et al. Role of surgery, radiotherapy and chemotherapy in papillary tumors of the pineal region: a multicenter study. J Neurooncol. 2013; 112:223–231

[28] Fevre-Montange M, Hasselblatt M, Figarella-Branger D, et al. Prognosis and histopathologic features in papillary tumors of the pineal region: a retrospective multicenter study of 31 cases. J Neuropathol Exp Neurol. 2006; 65:1004–1011

45 Cranial and Paraspinal Nerve Tumors

45.1 General information

These slow-growing tumors may occur sporadiaclly or as part of a syndromic condition such as neurofibromatosis (type 1 or type 2), schwannomatosis, and Carney complex (p. 652). The WHO now considers paragangliomas which involve sympathetic and parasympathetic neuroendocrine cells to be grouped in this category in contrast to the historical classification as neuronal and mixed neuronal-glial tumors. Schwannomatosis may be associated with painful schwannomas.

45.2 Specific cranial and paraspinal nerve tumors

45.2.1 Schwannoma (WHO grade 1)

General information

A benign nerve sheath tumor exclusively or primarily comprised of differentiated neoplastic Schwann cells. May be sporadic or associated with syndromes. Over 90% are solitary and sporadic, and 50-75% of these show inactivating mutations of the NF2 suppressor gene located at 22q12.2 resulting in loss of expression of the growth inhibiting product, merlin (AKA schwannomin). Multiple schwannomas occur in NF2 (p. 640) (bilateral involvement of the vestibular division of Cr N VIII is diagnostic of NF2) and schwannomatosis (p. 642). Spinal schwannomas are typical in NF1 (p. 638).

Diagnostic criteria for schwannoma

Diagnostic criteria for schwannoma are shown in ▶ Fig. 45.1.[1]

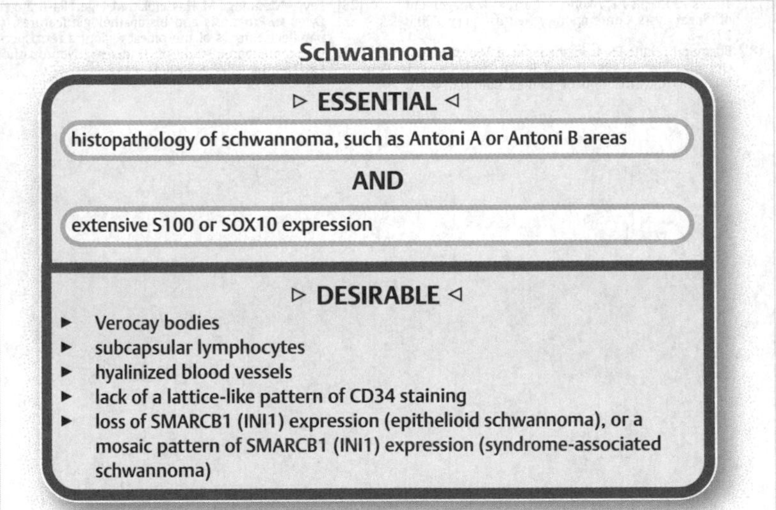

Schwannoma

▷ ESSENTIAL ◁

histopathology of schwannoma, such as Antoni A or Antoni B areas

AND

extensive S100 or SOX10 expression

▷ DESIRABLE ◁

▶ Verocay bodies
▶ subcapsular lymphocytes
▶ hyalinized blood vessels
▶ lack of a lattice-like pattern of CD34 staining
▶ loss of SMARCB1 (INI1) expression (epithelioid schwannoma), or a mosaic pattern of SMARCB1 (INI1) expression (syndrome-associated schwannoma)

Fig. 45.1 Diagnostic criteria for schwannoma. (Modified with permission from WHO Classification of Tumors Editorial Board, (ed.) World Health Organization classification of tumors of the central nervous system. 5th ed. Bosman F T, Jaffe E S, Lakhani S R, et al. (series eds.): World Health Organization Classification of Tumors series, vol. 6. International Agency for Research on Cancer, Lyon, France, 2021.)

Subtypes

See reference.[1]
- **ancient schwannoma**: contains dispersed cells with bizarre nuclei
- **cellular schwannoma**: Antoni A tissue predominates. Verocay bodies are absent. Small areas of necrosis may cause confusion with MPNST (p. 774). May contain foci of Ki-67 labeling (the index is usually < 20%, but not always)
- **plexiform schwannoma**: often arise in skin or sub-Q tissue. Most are sporadic, but may occur in HF2 or schwannomatosis. Histology may be classic (i.e., biphasic) or cellular subtype
- **epithelioid schwannoma**: demonstrate multilobulated single or nests of epithelioid cells in a myxoid or hyalinized matrix. Most are sporadic
- **microcystic/reticular schwannoma**: the least common subtype. Typically occur in viscera (usually the GI tract) where they are unencapsulated. Named for a rich microcystic network of spindle cells with eosiniphilic cytoplasm. Antoni A tissue is common, and they usualy lack features of hyalinized blood vessels and Verocay bodies

45

Location

Commonly arise from peripheral nerves in the skin and subcutaneous tissue of the head and neck, or on flexor surfaces of the limbs. Intracranially, they frequently involve the vestibular division of Cr. N. VIII (vestibular schwannoma (p. 777)), but can also arise from Cr. N. V or other cranial nerves. In the spine, they can form "dumbbell"-shaped tumors as they extend out through the neural foramen which constricts them.

Histology

Most are biphasic (composed of 2 cell types):
1. Antoni A tissue: compact. Occasional Verocay bodies (nuclear palisading)
2. Antoni B tissue: loosely arrayed with lipid-laden histiocytes and hyalinized vasculature.

Refer to the comparison of the histology to that of neurofibromas (p. 637).

Epidemiology

Peak incidence is the fourth to sixth decades.

Prognosis

The sporadic forms of these benign tumors usually do not recur following gross total resection. However, GTR is often difficult with the cellular and plexiform subtypes. Malignant transformation is exceedingly rare.

45.2.2 Neurofibroma (WHO grade 1)

General information

The most common peripheral nerve sheath tumor. A benign neoplasm composed of neoplastic Schwann cells interspersed with normal cells. They are WHO CNS5 grade 1 except for atypical neurofibromatous neoplasm of uncertain biological potential (ANNUBP), which is not assigned a grade. The finding of multiple or plexiform neurofibromas should prompt consideration of underlying NF1. Complete functional loss of neurofibromin (p. 639) is considered a prerequisite for tumor development. Refer to the comparison of the histology to that of schwannomas (p. 637).

Diagnostic criteria for neurofibroma

Diagnostic criteria for neurofibroma are shown in ▶ Fig. 45.2.[1]

Subtypes

See reference.[1]
- **cellular neurofibroma**
- **atypical neurofibroma / neurofibromatous neoplasm of uncertain biological potential (AN/ ANNUBP)** : characterized by 2 or more of the following concerning findings[2]

45

Neurofibroma

▷ **ESSENTIAL** ◁

infiltrative, low-cellularity spindle cell neoplasm associated with a variably myxoid to collagenous stroma and a mixed cell population

▷ **DESIRABLE** ◁

► S100 positivity in the Schwann cell population, with a lattice-like CD34 pattern, highlighting the stromal component
► intraneural localization
► patient has neurofibromatosis type 1
► atypical histological features (nuclear enlargement, hypercellularity, architectural loss, mitoses) for atypical neurofibroma / atypical neurofibromatous neoplasm of uncertain biological potential in the setting of neurofibromatosis type 1, often with loss of p16 expression

Fig. 45.2 **Diagnostic criteria for neurofibroma.** (Modified with permission from WHO Classification of Tumors Editorial Board, (ed.) World Health Organization classification of tumors of the central nervous system. 5th ed. Bosman F T, Jaffe E S, Lakhani S R, et al. (series eds.): World Health Organization Classification of Tumors series, vol. 6. International Agency for Research on Cancer, Lyon, France, 2021.)

- ○ cytological atypia
- ○ hypercellularity
- ○ loss of neurofibroma architecture (on H&E and/or CD34 staining)
- ○ mitotic count > 0.2 mitoses/mm^2 and < 1.5 mitoses/mm^2 (equating to > 1 mitosis/50 HPF and < 3 mitoses/10 HPF of 0.51 mm in diameter and 0.2 mm^2 in area)

AN/ANNUBP are considered premalignant or early malignant lesions that do not meet criteria for MPNST (p. 774) but have an increased risk of progression to MPNST.[3] They are not assigned a WHO grade

- **plexiform neurofibroma**
- **diffuse neurofibroma**
- **nodular neurofibroma**
- **massive soft tissue neurofibroma**: consistently benign lesions that may overlie an MPNST

Location

Usually located in the skin, typically in the dermal layer. Less commonly, may involve deeper nerves of medium-size, a nerve plexus or a major nerve trunk. They may also originate from spinal nerve roots.

Epidemiology

Most are sporadic and solitary. Multiple lesions usually occur in the context of NF1 and begin to appear around ages 5-10 years. Plexiform lesions are often congenital.[4] There is no age or gender bias.

Clinical

Cutaneous lesions are typically soft, mobile and asymptomatic. Deep tumors often produce sensory and/or motor symptoms related to the nerve of origin. The least common manifestation is a plaque-like cutaneous and subcutaneous mass of the head or neck, or as a massive enlargement of the shoulder or pelvis in a patient with NF1.

Prognosis

Isolated cutaneous neurofibromas are uniformly benign. Plexiform neurofibromas, ANNUBP and intraneural lesions originating in sizeable nerves may progress to MPNST (p. 774). Diffuse neurofibromas of the skin rarely progress.

45.2.3 Perineurioma (WHO grade 1)

General information

A benign tumor comprised exclusively of neoplastic perineural cells.

Diagnostic criteria for intraneural and soft tissue perineurioma

Diagnostic criteria for soft tissue perineurioma are shown in ▶ Fig. 45.3, and for intraneural perineurioma in ▶ Fig. 45.4.[1]

45

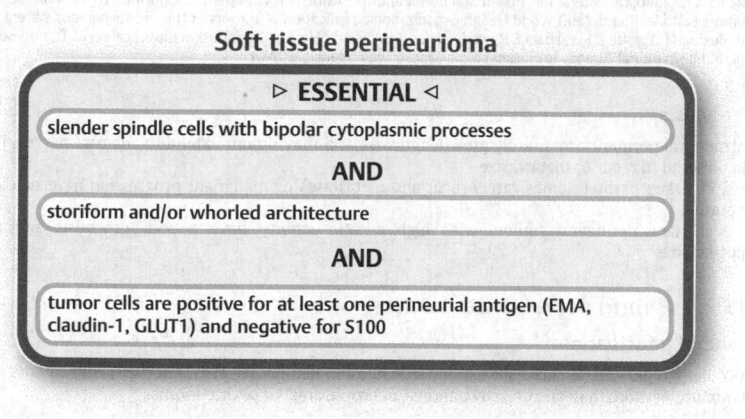

Soft tissue perineurioma

▷ **ESSENTIAL** ◁

slender spindle cells with bipolar cytoplasmic processes

AND

storiform and/or whorled architecture

AND

tumor cells are positive for at least one perineurial antigen (EMA, claudin-1, GLUT1) and negative for S100

Fig. 45.3 Diagnostic criteria for soft tissue perineurioma. (Modified with permission from WHO Classification of Tumors Editorial Board, (ed.) World Health Organization classification of tumors of the central nervous system. 5th ed. Bosman F T, Jaffe E S, Lakhani S R, et al. (series eds.): World Health Organization Classification of Tumors series, vol. 6. International Agency for Research on Cancer, Lyon, France, 2021.)

Subtypes

See reference.[1]

- **soft tissue perineurioma**: uncommon, only ≈ 1% of soft tissue neoplasms. Arise in deep soft tissues and present as a soft tissue mass with nonspecific symptoms. Only rarely can an associated nerve be identified. Almost exclusively benign, but malignant variety does occur. Female:male ratio = 2:1. In males, hands are often affected. Discrete, but not encapsulated, diameter = 1.5–20 cm. Treatment: gross total excision is curative
- **intraneural perineurioma**: rare, only ≈ 1% of nerve sheath tumors. Usually a solitary lesion of adolescence or young adulthood, affecting primarily peripheral nerves of the extremities (cranial nerve involvement is rare). Pseudo-onion bulb formation with cylindrical enlargement of the nerve over 2–10 cm. Mitotic activity is rare, MIB-1 labeling index is low. Chromosome 22 loss is characteristic,[5] no definite association with NF1 or NF2. No gender preference. Present primarily with weakness and atrophy more often than sensory symptoms of the related nerve. Treatment: conservative sampling of lesion, not resection
- **reticular perineurioma**
- **sclerosing perineurioma**

45

Intraneural perineurioma

> ▷ **ESSENTIAL** ◁

pseudo–onion bulb pattern on cross-section, with axons in the center

AND

tumor cells are positive for at least one perineurial antigen (EMA, claudin-1, GLUT1) and negative for S100

Fig. 45.4 Diagnostic criteria for intraneural perineurioma. (Modified with permission from WHO Classification of Tumors Editorial Board, (ed.) World Health Organization classification of tumors of the central nervous system. 5th ed. Bosman F T, Jaffe E S, Lakhani S R, et al. (series eds.): World Health Organization Classification of Tumors series, vol. 6. International Agency for Research on Cancer, Lyon, France, 2021.)

Prognosis

Intraneural perineuriomas rarely grow lengthwise and they do not extend to adjacent nerves. They do not tend to recur or metastasize.

Soft tissue perineuriomas rarely recur and metastases or malignant progression have not been reported.

Malignant perineural tumors with high mitotic activity have a poor prognosis and may metastasize.

45.2.4 Hybrid nerve sheath tumors

General information

AKA benign peripheral nerve sheath tumor NOS. Rare, benign peripheral nerve sheath tumors with a mixture of more than one of: schwannoma, neurofibroma, or perineurioma.

Diagnostic criteria for hybrid nerve sheath tumor

Diagnostic criteria for hybrid nerve sheath tumor are shown in ▶ Fig. 45.5.[1]

Hybrid nerve sheath tumor

> ▷ **ESSENTIAL** ◁

intermingled features of two types of benign nerve sheath tumors

AND

appropriate immunohistochemical staining for each component

Fig. 45.5 Diagnostic criteria for hybrid nerve sheath tumor. (Modified with permission from WHO Classification of Tumors Editorial Board, (ed.) World Health Organization classification of tumors of the central nervous system. 5th ed. Bosman F T, Jaffe E S, Lakhani S R, et al. (series eds.): World Health Organization Classification of Tumors series, vol. 6. International Agency for Research on Cancer, Lyon, France, 2021.)

Subtypes

See reference.[1]
- **schwannoma/perineurioma**: the most common subtype
- **neurofibroma/schwannoma**: the second most common subtype
- **neurofibroma/perineurioma**

Prognosis

Benign neoplasms which rarely recur following excision.

45.2.5 Malignant melanotic nerve sheath tumor (MMNST)

General information

AKA malignant melanotic Schwannian tumor. A peripheral nerve sheath tumor uniformly comprised of neoplastic cells with both Schwann cell and melanocytic features that frequently behaves aggressively. Usually arise from a spinal or autonomic nerve. There is variable association with Carney complex (p.652). Loss of PRKAR1A protein expression with *PRKAR1A* gene mutations are found in the vast majority.

Diagnostic criteria for malignant melanotic nerve sheath tumor

Diagnostic criteria for malignant melanotic nerve sheath tumor are shown in ▸ Fig. 45.6.[1]

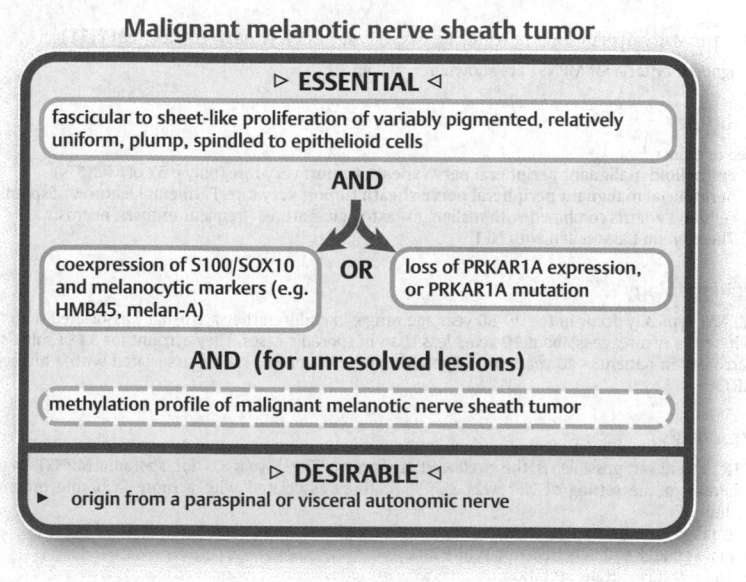

Fig. 45.6 Diagnostic criteria for malignant melanotic nerve sheath tumor. (Modified with permission from WHO Classification of Tumors Editorial Board, (ed.) World Health Organization classification of tumors of the central nervous system. 5th ed. Bosman F T, Jaffe E S, Lakhani S R, et al. (series eds.): World Health Organization Classification of Tumors series, vol. 6. International Agency for Research on Cancer, Lyon, France, 2021.)

Epidemiology

This rare tumor of adulthood tends occur at a later age with sporadic cases (mean age: 33.2 years) than in those associated with Carney complex (mean age: 22.5 years).[6] Tumors are multiple in 20%, and these patients have a greater chance of having Carney complex than those with solitary tumors.

Prognosis

Behavior is unpredictable, and 26-44% may recur locally or metastasize even without identifiable malignant features. Recurrence rate is 47% in patients followed for more than 5 years.[1]

45.2.6 Malignant peripheral nerve sheath tumor (MPNST) (no WHO grade)

General information

A malignant spindle-cell peripheral nerve sheath tumor typically originating from a peripheral nerve, a pre-existing benign nerve sheath tumor, or in a patient with NF1. Limited Schwann cell differentiation is often seen. Characteristic molecular findings are combined genetic inactivation of *NF1*, *CDKN2A* and/or *CDKN2B*, and *SUZ12* or *EED* genes, as well as complex genomic rearrangements.

Approximately 50% are associated with NF1 (p.638) (in NF1 they tend to occur in deep-seated plexiform neurofibromas or large intraneural neurofibromas). The lifetime risk of developing MPNST with NF1 is ≈ 9–13%.[7]

MPNSTs may spread along nerves, and 20% metastasize hematogenously, usually to lung.

Diagnostic criteria for malignant peripheral nerve sheath tumor (MPNST)

Diagnostic criteria for MPNST are shown in ▶ Fig. 45.7.[1]

Subtypes

See reference.[1]
- **epithelioid malignant peripheral nerve sheath tumor**: very rare (only ≈ 5% of MPNSTs)
- **perineurial malignant peripheral nerve sheath tumor**: very rare. Perineural features of spindle cells and whorls combined with malignant histologic features (frequent mitoses, necrosis…). These are not associated with NF1

Epidemiology

MPNST typically occur in the 20-50 year age range. In children they are usually associated with NF1 where the mean age is about 10 years less than in sporadic cases. They account for 5% of soft tissue sarcomas in patients <20 years old.[8] Approximately 10% of MPNST are associated with a history of XRT.[9]

Prognosis

GTR, whenever possible, is the preferred treatment. The 5-year OS for sporadic MPNST is 69%, whereas in the setting of NF1 was 35%.[10] Features associated with a more favorable prognosis include[1,8]:
- smaller tumor size
- male gender and non-Hispanic White race
- no metastases at presentation
- GTR
- no association with prior XRT
- epitheliod and perineural subtypes appear to be less aggressive than conventional MPNST

45.2.7 Cauda equina neuroendocrine tumor (WHO grade 1)

General information

AKA (and formerly) paraganglioma of the cauda equina, or cauda equina paraganglioma.

Malignant peripheral nerve sheath tumor (MPNST)

▷ **ESSENTIAL** ◁

histopathologically consistent malignant spindle cell tumor in a patient with NF1[a] or in a pre-existing neurofibroma

OR

malignant spindle cell tumor associated with a peripheral nerve
AND
no more than focal/patchy S100/SOX10 expression
AND
no SS18::SSX (SSX1, SSX2, or SSX4) fusion gene present

OR

malignant spindle cell tumor associated with a peripheral nerve
AND
evidence of PRC2 inactivation (molecularly or via loss of H3 p.K28me3 [K27me3] immunostaining)

OR

tumor with features of ANNUBP in a patient with NF1, but with a mitotic count of at least 1.5–4.5 mitoses/mm² (3–9 mitoses/10 HPF of 0.51 mm in diameter and 0.20 mm² in area)

OR

unresolved lesion with the methylation profile of MPNST

▷ **DESIRABLE** ◁

▶ loss of H3 p.K28me3 (K27me3)
▶ loss of neurofibromin expression

[a] this alteration is highly desirable, and its absence in a tumor otherwise resembling PPTID, should prompt careful consideration as to whether an alternative diagnosis may be more suitable

Fig. 45.7 Diagnostic criteria for MPNST. (Modified with permission from WHO Classification of Tumors Editorial Board, (ed.) World Health Organization classification of tumors of the central nervous system. 5th ed. Bosman F T, Jaffe E S, Lakhani S R, et al. (series eds.): World Health Organization Classification of Tumors series, vol. 6. International Agency for Research on Cancer, Lyon, France, 2021.)

A neuroendocrine tumor originating from specialized neural crest cells in the region of the cauda equina/filum terminale. CSF protein is usually increased.[11]

Diagnostic criteria for cauda equina neuroendocrine tumor

Diagnostic criteria for cauda equina neuroendocrine tumor are shown in ▶ Fig. 45.8.[1]

45

Cauda equina neuroendocrine tumor

▷ ESSENTIAL ◁

well-demarcated tumor with Zellballen architecture

AND

synaptophysin or chromogranin immunoreactivity in chief cells

AND

cauda equina location

AND (for unresolved lesions)

methylation profile of cauda equina neuroendocrine tumor*

▷ DESIRABLE ◁

- ► S100-positive sustentacular cells
- ► cytokeratin-positive chief cells
- ► reticulin silver stain showing typical architecture

* the DNA methylation profile and copy-number profiles of cauda equina neuroendocrine tumors are distinct from those of paragangliomas from other locations

Fig. 45.8 Diagnostic criteria for cauda equina neuroendocrine tumor. (Modified with permission from WHO Classification of Tumors Editorial Board, (ed.) World Health Organization classification of tumors of the central nervous system. 5th ed. Bosman F T, Jaffe E S, Lakhani S R, et al. (series eds.): World Health Organization Classification of Tumors series, vol. 6. International Agency for Research on Cancer, Lyon, France, 2021.)

Location

Most spinal paragangliomas occur in the region of the cauda equina, and most of these are intradural and are attached to the filum terminale.

Clinical

Typically present with low back bain and radiculopathy. Numbness, paraparesis and sphincter disturbance are less common. Even less common are cauda equina syndrome or symptoms of increased ICP (including papilledema). Acute paraparesis, spinal subarachnoid hemorrhage,[11] or neuroendocrine symptoms due to catecholamine secretion (paroxysmal or sustained hypertension, palpitations, diaphoresis and H/A) are extremely rare.

Imaging

On imaging, these tumors are usually indistinguishable from other common neoplasms of the area (schwannomas, myxopapillary ependymomas). The diagnosis may be suggested preoperatively in the infrequent case demonstrating serpiginous dilated and ectatic blood vessels, sometimes with a "cap sign" (low-intensity rim on T2WI or GRASS or SWI MRI due to hemosiderin from prior hemorrhages).[11]

Histology

The tumors are well differentiated. Uniform round or polygonal chief (type I) cells congregate in lobules (Zellballen) encompassed by a barely discernible single layer of susentacular (type II) cells.

Mature ganglion cells and a Schwann cell component (gangliocytic neuroendocrine tumors) are found in ≈ 25%. Scattered mitotic figures, areas of focal hemorrhagic necrosis and nuclear pleomorphism may be seen but are not prognostically significant.

Prognosis

The preponderance of these tumors are slow growing. The recurrence rate following GTR is very low.[12] Dissemination of tumor through the CSF may occur.

45.3 Vestibular schwannoma

45.3.1 General information

Key concepts

- histologically benign tumor of cranial nerve VIII located in the cerebellopontine angle (CPA)
- usually arises from inferior division (controversial) of the vestibular portion of the VIII nerve
- about 1 in 500 persons will develop this tumor during their lifetime
- 3 most common early symptoms (clinical triad): hearing loss (insidious and progressive), tinnitus (high pitched) and dysequilibrium (true vertigo is uncommon)
- W/U: All patients: ✔ MRI with IAC protocol (p. 241), ✔ audiometrics (pure tone audiogram and speech discrimination). In addition for small VSs (≤ 1.5 cm dia): ✔ ENG, ✔ cVEMP, ✔ ABR
- histology: comprised of Antoni A (narrow elongated bipolar cells) and Antoni B fibers (loose reticulated). Compared to most schwannomas, Antoni A fibers predominate
- choice of management option (observation, surgery, XRT or chemotherapy [Avastin®]) depends heavily on tumor size, growth, hearing status, VII function and presence of NF2 (see text)

Owing to the commonality and intricacies, this particular schwannoma receives a section devoted just to this tumor.

Vestibular schwannoma (VS) is a histologically benign Schwann-cell sheath tumor that usually arises from the inferior division of the *vestibular nerve* (not the cochlear portion). VSs arise as a result of the loss of a tumor-suppressor gene on the long arm of chromosome 22 (in sporadic cases this is a somatic mutation; in neurofibromatosis Type 2 (NF2) this is either inherited or represents a new mutation that may then be transmitted to offspring).

Obsolete terms, included for reference, should be avoided[13,14]: acoustic neuroma, acoustic neurinomas (neurinoma is an obsolete term for schwannoma), neurolemma or neurilemmoma.

45.3.2 Epidemiology

The most common non-malignant nerve sheath tumor, comprising 8–10% of tumors intracranial tumors.[15] Annual incidence quoted by CBTRUS is 1.51 cases per 100,000 population in the U.S.[16]— over the past couple decades the incidence has increased and the typical size at diagnosis has decreased, partially as a result of the proliferation of MRI scans.[17] Other estimates disclose a higher incidence of 3.0-5.2/100,000.[18,19] The highest incidence occurs in patients aged ≥ 70 years, peaking at 20.6 per 100,000 person-years.[19] There is no gender differential.[19] At least 95% are unilateral.

▶ **Neurofibromatosis Type 2.** The incidence of vestibular schwannomas (VS) is increased in in neurofibromatosis Type 2 (NFT2) (p. 640) (central NFT), with bilateral VS being a hallmark. Any patient < 40 yrs old with unilateral VS should be evaluated for NFT2. Cytologically, the VSs of NFT2 are identical to sporadic cases; however, in NFT2 the tumors form grape-like clusters that may infiltrate the nerve fibers (unlike most sporadic VSs which *displace* the eighth nerve).

45.3.3 Pathology

Tumors are composed of Antoni A fibers (narrow elongated bipolar cells) and Antoni B fibers (loose reticulated). Verocay bodies are also seen, and consist of acellular eosinophilic areas surrounded by parallel arrangement of spindle shaped schwann cells (they are not a cell type). Tumor-associated macrophages (TAMs) may be associated with increased risk of recurrence following STR.

45.3.4 Clinical

Symptoms

General information

VSs typically become symptomatic after age 30. Symptoms are shown in ▶ Table 45.1. The type of symptoms are closely correlated with tumor size. Most initially cause the triad of ipsilateral sensorineural hearing loss, tinnitus and balance difficulties. Larger tumors can cause facial numbness, weakness or twitching, and possibly brainstem symptoms. Rarely, a large tumor may produce hydrocephalus. With current imaging modalities (CT and especially MRI), increasing numbers of smaller lesions are being detected.

45

Table 45.1 Symptoms in vestibular schwannoma[15,20,21,22]

Symptom	%
hearing loss	95
tinnitus	55
dizziness/imbalance	61
H/A	32
facial numbness	18
facial weakness	17
diplopia	10
N/V	9
otalgia	9
change of taste	6
vertigo	8
continuous dizziness	3

Acoustic nerve (Cr N VIII) symptoms

Unilateral sensorineural hearing loss, tinnitus and dysequilibrium are the most frequent symptoms. For years it was taken for granted that hearing loss was due to compression and/or stretching of the VIII nerve by the tumor; however, recent evidence suggests possible toxic factors secreted by the tumor cause cochlear damage.[23,24]

Hearing loss is insidious and progressive in most (c.f. the hearing loss in Meniere disease which fluctuates); however, 10% report sudden hearing loss (see below). 70% have a high frequency loss pattern, and word discrimination is usually affected (especially noticeable in telephone conversation).

The tinnitus is usually high-pitched.

Unsteadiness manifests primarily as difficulty with balance; true vertigo occurs in < 20%.

Sudden hearing loss: The differential diagnosis for sudden hearing loss (SHL) is extensive.[25] *Idiopathic* SHL (i.e., no identified etiology: must rule out neoplasm, infection, autoimmune, vascular, and toxic causes) represents 90% of cases[26] and occurs in an estimated 5-20 per 100,000 population.[27] 1% of patients with SHL will be found to have a VS, and SHL may be the presenting symptom in 1–14% of patients with VS.[28] SHL with VS is presumably due to an infarction of the acoustic nerve, or acute occlusion of the cochlear artery. Treatment options for SHL include:

1. steroids: e.g., prednisone 60 mg PO q d × 10 d then tapered.[28] Ideally initiated within 2 weeks of onset of SHL[26]
2. there is no high-quality data supporting addition of antiviral therapy (e.g., famciclovir)[29,30]
3. ✖ not recommended
   • heparin has been shown *not* to be of help
   • there is also no high quality data to support: rest, restriction of salt, alcohol or tobacco, or use of thrombolytics

Trigeminal (Cr N V) and facial (Cr N VII) nerve symptoms

Otalgia, facial numbness and weakness, and taste changes occur as the tumor enlarges and compresses the fifth and seventh nerves. These symptoms usually do not occur until the tumor is > 2 cm. This highlights an interesting paradox: facial weakness is a rare or late occurrence, even though the 7th nerve is almost always distorted early; whereas facial numbness occurs sooner once trigeminal compression occurs (often in the presence of normal facial movement), despite the fact that the 5th nerve is farther away.[31] This may be due to the resiliency of motor nerves relative to sensory nerves.

Brainstem and other cranial nerve symptoms

Larger tumors cause brainstem compression (with ataxia, H/A, N/V, diplopia, cerebellar signs, and if unchecked, coma, respiratory depression and death) and lower cranial nerve (IX, X, XII) palsies (hoarseness, dysphagia…). Obstruction of CSF circulation by larger tumors (usually > 4 cm) may produce hydrocephalus with increased ICP.

Rarely, 6th nerve involvement may cause diplopia.

Signs

Hearing loss due to VIII involvement is the earliest cranial nerve finding. 66% of patients have no abnormal physical finding except for hearing loss (for other findings, see ▶ Table 45.2).

Since hearing loss is sensorineural, **Weber test** (p.611) will lateralize to the uninvolved side, and if there is enough preserved hearing, **Rinne test** (p.611) will be positive (i.e., normal; air conduction > bone conduction) on both sides.

Facial nerve (VII) dysfunction due to VS is uncommon before treatment. Facial nerve function is commonly graded on the House and Brackmann scale (▶ Table 45.3).

Vestibular involvement causes nystagmus (may be central or peripheral) and abnormal electronystagmography (ENG) with caloric stimulation.

Table 45.2 Signs in 131 vestibular schwannomas (excluding hearing loss)[15]

Sign	%
abnormal corneal reflex	33
nystagmus	26
facial hypoesthesia	26
facial weakness (palsy)	12
abnormal eye movement	11
papilledema	10
Babinski sign	5

Table 45.3 Clinical grading of facial nerve function (House and Brackmann[32])

Grade	Function	Description
1	normal	normal facial function in all areas

2	mild dysfunction	1. gross: slight weakness noticeable on close inspection; may have very slight synkinesis
		2. at rest: normal symmetry and tone
		3. motion:
		  a) forehead: slight to moderate movement
		  b) eye: complete closure with effort
		  c) mouth: slight asymmetry

3	moderate dysfunction	1. gross: obvious but not disfiguring asymmetry: noticeable but not severe synkinesis
		2. motion:
		  a) forehead: slight to moderate movement
		  b) eye: complete closure with effort
		  c) mouth: slightly weak with maximal effort

4	moderate to severe dysfunction	1. gross: obvious weakness and/or disfiguring asymmetry
		2. motion:
		  a) forehead: none
		  b) eye: incomplete closure
		  c) mouth: asymmetry with maximum effort

5	severe dysfunction	1. gross: only barely perceptible motion
		2. at rest: asymmetry
		3. motion:
		  a) forehead: none
		  b) eye: incomplete closure

6	total paralysis	no movement

45.3.5 Evaluation

Diagnostic studies – overview

1. brain MRI without and with contrast: include navigation and IAC protocol (p. 241) (if available). If MRI is contraindicated, then a CT scan without and with contrast. Tumor size is graded using the Koos system (▶ Table 45.7)[33]
2. temporal bone CT for detailed bony anatomy if surgery is contemplated
3. audiometric evaluation (see text below for explanation & indications):
   a) pure tone audiogram (see below)
   b) speech discrimination evaluation (see below)
   c) patients with small VSs (≤ 1.5 cm dia) also get:
      - ENG: (p. 782) assesses *superior* vestibular nerve
      - VEMP: (p. 782) assesses *inferior* vestibular nerve
      - ABR: (p. 782) prognosticates chance of hearing preservation

Audiometric and audiologic studies

General information
Baseline studies are helpful for management treatment decisions and for later comparison and to assess the contralateral ear.

Pure tone audiogram (PTA)
May be useful as first-step screening test. Air conduction assesses the entire system, bone conduction assesses from the cochlea and proximally. PTA assesses the functionality of hearing (to help in treatment decision making) and acts as a baseline for future comparison. The pure tone average (also abbreviated PTA) is a single numerical score that is an *average* of the thresholds for frequencies across the audio spectrum (at 500, 1000 & 2000 Hz). On a standard audiogram, X's denote the left ear (AS) and O's denote the right ear (AD).

Progressive unilateral or *asymmetric* sensorineural hearing loss of high tones occurs in > 95% of VSs.[34] High-frequency hearing loss also happens to be the most common type of hearing loss with age or with noise-induced sensorineural hearing loss, but is usually symmetrical. Only ≈ 1 in 1000 patients with asymmetric hearing have a VS.[13] Other causes of asymmetrical sensorineural hearing loss[35]: other CPA lesions (e.g., meningioma), inner ear lesions, intraaxial lesions (including brainstem infarctions), multiple sclerosis. On hearing screening tests, an unexplained PTA difference from one ear to the other > 10–15 dB is suspicious and should be investigated further.

Speech discrimination evaluation
Speech discrimination is maintained in conductive hearing loss, moderately impaired in cochlear hearing loss, and worst with retrocochlear lesions. No longer used for diagnostic purposes; a score of 4% suggests a retrocochlear lesion, as does a score that is worse than would be predicted based on PTA testing (the speech recognition threshold should be similar to PTA thresholds below 4 kHz). Useful in determining serviceability of hearing and prognosticating for hearing preservation surgery.

Table 45.4 Open-set word recognition score

Class	WRS (%)
I	70–100
II	50–69
III	1–49
IV	0

Open-set word recognition score (WRS ▶ Table 45.4) is a more sensitive measure of communication ability than PTA.

Definition of serviceable hearing

There are many definitions of what constitutes serviceable hearing. Also, even nonserviceable hearing can offer some benefit. If WRS is good (≥ 70%) but PTA is poor, a hearing aid may provide significant benefit.

Two commonly used scoring systems for hearing are shown here:
1. Modified **Gardener-Robertson** system for grading hearing: shown in ▶ Table 45.5. Class I patients may use a phone on that side, class II patients can localize sounds.
2. The American Academy of Otolaryngology – Head and Neck Surgery Foundation (AAO-HNS) hearing classification system[36]: shown in ▶ Table 45.6.

Some definitions of serviceable hearing (see text that follows for details):
1. AAO-HNS class A or B
2. Gardner-Robertson system
   • "50/50 rule": Gardner-Robertson class I or II (pure tone audiogram threshold ≤ 50 dB and speech discrimination score ≥ 50%)
   • some prefer a "70/30 rule" (70% WRS, 30 dB PTA)
3. in a patient with good hearing in the contralateral ear, a speech discrimination score (SDS) of < 70% in the affected ear is not considered good hearing; whereas if the contralateral ear is totally deaf, an SDS of ≥ 50% can be useful[39]

Table 45.5 Gardener and Robertson modified hearing classification[a]

Class	Pure tone audiogram[b](dB)	Speech discrimination[b]	Description	Clinical utility
I	**0–30**	**70–100%**	**good-excellent**	serviceable
II	**31–50**	**50–69%**	**serviceable**	serviceable
III	51–90	5–49%	non-serviceable	non-serviceable
IV	91-max	1–4%	poor	non-serviceable
V	not testable	0	none	

[a]modification[37] of the Silverstein and Norrell system[38]
[b]if PTA and speech discrimination score do not qualify in the same class, use the lower class
Boldface grades are generally considered serviceable hearing.

Table 45.6 American Academy of Otolaryngology–Head and Neck Surgery Foundation hearing classification system

Class	Pure tone threshold (dB)[a]		Speech discrimination score[b] (%)	Clinical utility
A	**≤ 30**	**AND**	**≥ 70**	"useful"
B	**> 30 AND ≤ 50**	**AND**	**≥ 50**	"useful"
C	> 50	AND	≥ 50	"aidable"
D	any level		< 50	"nonfunctional"

[a]average of pure tone hearing thresholds by air conduction at 0.5, 1, 2 & 3 kHz
[b]speech discrimination at 40 dB or maximum comfortable loudness
Boldface classes are generally considered serviceable hearing.

Additional audiometric tests that are helpful with small VSs (≤ 1.5 cm diameter)

The **ENG (caloric testing) and cVEMP** evaluate the superior and inferior division of the vestibular nerve (VN) respectively. The inferior VN is closer to the cochlear nerve than the superior VN (► Fig. 1.9), and small tumors (≤ 4 mm) of the inferior VN tend to be deeper and closer to the cochlear nerve than similarly sized tumors of the superior division which tend to be more superficial and more easily removed.

Electronystagmography (ENG): Only tests the horizontal semicircular canal ∴ assesses the *superior* vestibular nerve which innervates it. Normally, each ear contributes an equal portion of the response. The ENG is considered abnormal if there is > 20% difference between the two sides. Response may be normal with a small tumor arising from the *inferior* division of vestibular nerve. NB: the vestibular nerve may continue to function until almost all of the nerve fibers are affected. Mnemonic for the directionality of the nystagmus (direction is classified based on the fast phase of the nystagmus). COWS (Cold Opposite, Warm Same). NB: this differs from caloric testing for brain death (p. 323) and is a source of confusion.

Vestibular evoked myogenic potential (VEMP): Most commonly cVEMP ("c" for cervical to denote that the muscle recorded in the sternocleidomastoid, oVEMP (ocular) and tVEMP (triceps) are used much less frequently).

cVEMP assesses the *inferior* vestibular nerve by imparting acoustic energy to the saccule.[40] Independent of hearing (can be done even with deafness from profound sensorineural hearing loss). Electrodes are placed on sternocleidomastoid muscle (SCM).

Auditory brainstem responses (ABR): AKA BAER (p. 252). The most common findings are prolonged I-III and I-V interpeak latencies. No longer used for diagnostic purposes (sensitivity is only ≈ 88–90% (i.e., will miss 10–12% of VSs) and specificity is only 85%). ABR is useful for prognostication— poor wave morphology correlates with lower chance of preserving hearing (even with good hearing).

Radiographic evaluation

Imaging guidelines

Practice guideline: Imaging for vestibular schwannomas

For the full guideline, see reference.[41]

Initial pre-op evaluation to detect VS
- Level III[41]: high-resolution T2 and contrast-enhanced T1 MRI should be used
- Level III[41]: standard T1, T2 FLAIR & DWI MRI sequences in axial, coronal, and sagittal plane may be used

Pre-op surveillance for a known VS if an observation (an "watch-and-wait") approach is being used
- Level III[41]: pre-op surveillance for VS growth should be either contrast-enhanced 3-D T1 magnetization prepared rapid acquisition gradient echo (MPRAGE) or high-resolution T2 MRI (including FIESTA or CISS sequences[a])
- Level III[41]: MRIs should be obtained annually for 5 years, with lengthening of the interval after that if stable
- Level III[41]: because of more variable growth rates, NF2 patients with VS should be imaged more frequently at first and then annually once the growth rate is determined
- Level III[41]: in NF2 patients, consider non-contrast MRIs if high-resolution T2 (including CISS or FIESTA) MRI adequately visualizes the tumor

Pre-op evaluation in preparation for surgery
- Level III[41]: T2 MRI may be used to augment visualization of the course of the facial nerve
- Level III[41]: counsel adults with cystic VS that their tumors may more often exhibit rapid growth, lower rates of complete resection, and inferior outcome of facial nerve function immediately post-op but similar to noncystic VS over time
- Level III[41]: the degree of lateral IAC involvement adversely affects facial nerve and hearing outcomes

Postop evaluation
- Level II[41]: post-contrast 3-D T1 MPRAGE should be used for nodular enhancement suspicious for recurrence

- Level III[41]: post-op imaging
  - following GTR: an MRI may be considered as late as 1 yr post-op to confirm GTR
  - for < GTR: more frequent MRIs are suggested—annually for 5 years, with adjustments for changes in nodular enhancement. NB: tumor volume decreases by ≈ 35% in the 1st 3 months after STR, and 32% do not enhance in the immediate post-op period[42]
- Level III[41]: after resection of one VS in an NF2 patients with bilateral VS, the growth of the contralateral VS may accelerate and more frequent imaging should be considered until the growth pattern is established

Abbreviatons: GTR = gross total resection; STR = subtotal resection; IAC = internal auditory canal.
  [a] FIESTA (p. 241) or CISS (p. 241) may improve visualization of the tumor and nerves in CSF

45

Differential diagnosis

See Cerebellopontine angle (CPA) lesions (p. 1647). The major differentials on imaging are:
1. CPA meningioma; see differentiating features (p. 1648)
2. schwannoma of adjacent cranial nerve, including mainly:
   a) facial nerve (Cr. N. VII) schwannoma: can arise anywhere along the course of Cr. N. VII
      1. imaging: may be dumbbell shaped due to extension from the ICA fundus through the labyrinthine segment and into the geniculate fossa. When isolated to the CPA, they may be indistinguishable from VS[43]
      2. clinical: typically present with facial weakness (slowly progressive or sudden), often preceded by facial twitching, facial nerve pain, hemifacial spasm and decreased lacrimation.[44] In patients thought to have Bell's palsy, a facial nerve neuroma was found to be the cause in 5%, and 27% had normal facial nerve function[45]
   b) trigeminal (Cr. N. V) schwannoma

CT scan

CT with IV contrast is second choice for imaging modality. If MRI is contraindicated and clinical suspicion of VS is strong but the CT is negative, small lesions may be visualized by introducing 3–4 ml of subarachnoid air via lumbar puncture, and scanning the patient with the affected side up (to trap air in region of IAC), non-filling of the IAC is indicative of an intracanalicular mass. Even with air contrast, CT was normal in 6% in Mayo series.[15]

Many VSs enlarge the ostium of the IAC (called trumpeting). Normal diameter of the IAC: 5–8 mm. 3–5% of VSs do not enlarge the IAC on CT (percentage is likely higher in small VSs vs. large ones).

Thin-cut temporal bone CT should be obtained for operative planning. Important features to identify:
- for middle fossa approach: bony coverage of geniculate ganglion to identify dehiscence
- for translab approach:
  - extent of pneumatization of the mastoid and position of sigmoid sinus. An anterior sinus with poorly pneumatized mastoids can indicate a tight space for this approach
  - position of the jugular bulb. If high riding, can indicate a tight space in translab approach
- for retrosigmoid transmeatal approach: location and thickness of bone coverage over the posterior semicircular canal and vestibular aqueduct. The extent of peritubular air cells and retro facial air cells needs to be assessed in planning the approach and preventing CSF leaks

MRI

MRI (▶ Fig. 45.9) is the diagnostic procedure of choice (see Practice guideline (p. 782) for sequence recommendations) with sensitivity close to 98% and almost 0% false positive rate. Characteristic findings: round or oval enhancing tumor centered on IAC. Large VSs (> 3 cm dia) may show cystic appearing areas on CT or MRI; in actuality these areas are usually solid. Adjacent trapped CSF cisterns may also give cystic appearance. In a pilot study, hyperintensity on T2 has been associated with soft and suckable tumors at the time of surgery[46] and a trend towards better VII function preservation.

Tumor size is graded using the Koos system (▶ Table 45.7).[33]

45

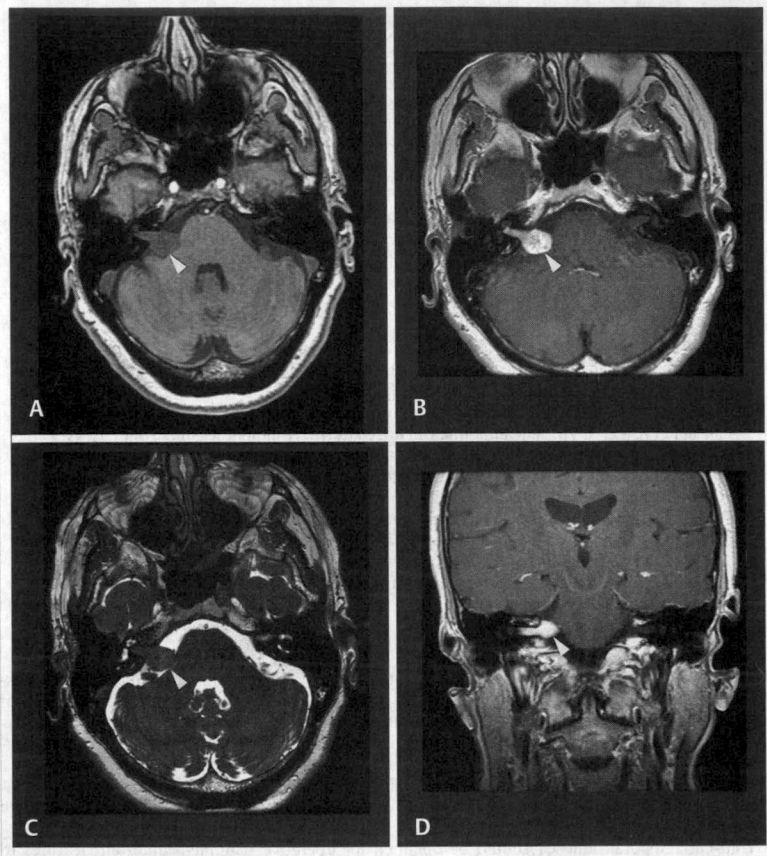

Fig. 45.9 Vestibular schwannoma, right-sided.
This Koos grade III tumor is identified by *yellow arrowheads*.
Image: MRI, A: axial T1 sequence, B: axial T1 + contrast, C: axial FIESTA scan, D: coronal T1 + contrast.

Table 45.7 Koos grading system for vestibular schwannomas & approximate corresponding volume[a]

Grade	Tumor extent[33]	Average tumor volume[b] [47] (cc)
I	intracanalicular tumor	0.3
II	protrusion into CPA, but not reaching the brainstem	0.6
III	extends to brainstem surface without displacing it	1.8
IV	displaces brainstem and cranial nerves	4.2[c]

[a]volume measurements are not part of the Koos grading system and are included for interest as it may impact stereotactic radiosurgery decisions
[b]volume measurements are from 235 patients undergoing gamma knife treatment and this may be a source of selection bias for volume measurement
[c]grade IV was a very heterogeneous group, and Minderman & Schlegel proposed adding a category V for tumors > 6 cc

45.3.6 Management

Management options

Management options include:

1. expectant management ("wait and scan" approach): follow symptoms, hearing (audiometrics) and tumor growth on serial imaging (MRI or CT) (see guidelines (p. 782) for imaging recommendations). Intervention is performed for progression. Growth patterns observed:
   a) little or no growth: applies to most (83%) VSs confined within the IAC (► Table 45.7, Koos grade I) and to 30% extending into CPA (► Table 45.7, Koos grade II) (see natural history of growth below)
   b) slow growth ≈ 2 mm/yr
   c) rapid growth: ≥ 10 mm/yr
   d) a few actually shrink[17]
2. radiation therapy (alone, or in conjunction with surgery)
   a) external beam radiation therapy (EBRT)
   b) stereotactic radiation
      • stereotactic radiosurgery (SRS) (p. 1903): single dose. As there is little difference in radiographic control at different doses, single dose SRS < 13 Gy is recommended for hearing preservation and to minimize new onset or worsening of cranial nerve deficits (Level III[48])
      • stereotactic radiotherapy (SRT) (p. 1903): fractionated
3. surgery: approaches include the following (see below for details)
   a) retrosigmoid (AKA suboccipital): may be able to spare hearing
   b) translabyrinthine (and its several variations): sacrifices hearing, may be slightly better for sparing VII
   c) middle fossa approach (extradural subtemporal): only for small lateral VSs
4. chemotherapy: some preliminary promise for progressive NF2-related vestibular schwannomas with bevacizumab (Avastin®), an anti-VEGF (vascular endothelial growth factor) monoclonal antibody (see below). Side effects: hemorrhage occurs in ≈ 7% due to vessel necrosis

Patient/tumor factors influencing management decisions

In addition to the usual factors involved in the decision process with brain tumors (e.g., the patient's general medical condition, age, natural history, etc.) elements unique to VSs include: chances of preserving VII & V nerve function and hearing (in those with serviceable hearing) (all of which are related to tumor size), and the presence of NF2.

Specifics:

1. natural history of growth
   a) usual quoted range: ≈ 1–10 mm/yr. However this can be quite variable
   b) strictly intracanalicular tumors: only 17% grew outside the meatus (in 552 VSs over 3.6 years mean follow-up (230 were intrameatal at time of diagnosis, 322 had extrameatal extension)[17])
   c) extrameatal tumors (with extension into CP angle): 30% grew > 2 mm (in 522 VSs over 3.6 years mean follow-up[17])
   d) VSs that did not grow in the 5 years after diagnosis did not grow after that
   e) 6% actually decrease in size[49]
2. natural history of hearing function in untreated intracanalicular VSs in AAO-HNS Group A (► Table 45.6) patients. Rule of thumb for patients presenting with serviceable hearing (SH): 75% retain SH at 3 years, 60% at 5 years, and 40% at 10 years.[50] Details[51]:
   a) 50% deteriorated to a lower class over 4.6 years (loss of ≥ 10 dB PTA or ≥ 10% SDS)
   b) after 4.6 years of observation, the proportion of patients eligible for hearing preservation treatment (as determined by a word recognition score class I [70–100% SDS]) was reduced to 28% (a 44% reduction) and by AAO-HNS class A to 9% (a 53% reduction)
   c) the risk of losing hearing was not related to: age, gender, VS size (all tumors were intracanalicular) or tumor sublocalization (fundus, central, porus)
   d) hearing loss was positively correlated to the absolute volumetric tumor growth rate (tumors that eventually expand out of the IAC have a faster rate and degree of hearing loss compared to tumors remaining in the IAC)
   e) the risk of losing hearing was significantly lower for patients with 100% word recognition score. Over 4.6 years observation, 89% remained in WRS class I (► Table 45.4) compared to only 43% for patients with only a small (1–10%) loss of WRS at diagnosis
3. size: as tumors exceed 15 mm diameter, treatment complications increase
   a) significantly lower chance for hearing preservation
   b) increased incidence of VII injury

45

4. presence of cysts: cystic tumors may display sudden and dramatic growth[17]
5. serviceable hearing: see Definition of serviceable hearing (p. 781)
6. hearing in contralateral ear

Surgical factors – hearing preservation following microsurgery (MS) in sporadic VS

The probability of maintaining serviceable hearing following GTR of an *intracanalicular* VS for retrosigmoid vs. middle fossa approach in experienced hands is shown in ▶ Table 45.8 and is so similar that the choice of approach with regard to hearing preservation should be made on the basis of the expertise of the surgical team.[52]

If class A hearing (≤ 30 dB PTA, ≥ 70% WRS) is initially preserved following gross total resection of a VS, the probability of maintaining serviceable hearing (≤ 50 dB PTA, ≥ 50% WRS) is 80–100% at 2 years, 80–100% at 5 years, and 70–90% at 10 years.[52]

Table 45.8 Probability of maintaining SH[a] after GTR microsurgery[b] [52]

Time post op	Probability of preserved SH[a]	
	Retrosigmoid approach	Middle fossa approach
immediate post-op	40-60%	50-70%
2 years	40-60%	40-60%
5 years	30-50%	40-60%
10 years	20-40%	20-40%

[a] SH (serviceable hearing): ≤ 50 dB PTA, ≥ 50% WRS
[b] following gross total resection (GTR) of a sporadic intracanalicular VS in experienced hands

Practice guidelines for management of sporadic VS

Practice guideline: Hearing preservation outcomes with vestibular schwannomas

For the full guideline, see reference.[53]
   Observation vs. intervention recommendation
- Level III[48]: for VS without tinnitus that are intracanalicular (▶ Table 45.7, Koos grade I) or < 2 cm, observation[a] is recommended since it does not have a negative impact on tumor growth or hearing preservation

Hearing preservation with observation[a] in sporadic VS
- Level III[53]: for VS < 2 cm with serviceable hearing, chances of hearing preservation are > 75–100% @ 2 years, > 50–75% @ 5 years, and > 25–50% @ 10 years
- Level III[53]: for VS < 2 cm with AAO-HNS class A or GR grade I (▶ Table 45.5) hearing, chances of hearing preservation are > 75%-100% @ 2 years, and > 50%-75% @ 5 years. Data was insufficient for chances @ 10 years

Hearing preservation following SRS[b] in sporadic VS
- Level III[53]: for serviceable hearing pre-SRS, chances of hearing preservation are > 50–75% @ 2 & 5 years, and > 25–50% @ 10 years
- Level III[53]: for AAO-HNS class A or GR grade I (▶ Table 45.5) hearing pre-SRS, chances of hearing preservation are > 75%-100% @ 2 years, > 50%-75% @ 5 years, and > 25–50% @ 10 years

Hearing preservation following middle fossa or retrosigmoid MS in sporadic VS
- Level III[53]: for sporadic VS < 2 cm with serviceable hearing pre-op, chances of hearing preservation are > 25%-50% immediately post-op, and @ 2, 5 & 10 years post-op
- Level III[53]: for sporadic VS < 2 cm with AAO-HNS class A or GR grade I (▶ Table 45.5) hearing pre-SRS, chances of hearing preservation are > 50%-75% immediately post-op and @ 2 & 5 years post op, and > 25%-50% @ 10 years

[a] observation consists of serial MRI evaluations as discussed in (p. 782)
   [b] single dose SRS using modern dose planning (generally ≤ 13 Gy to the tumor margin, or ≤ 12 Gy to the tumor margin and cochlear dose ≤ 4 Gy)
   Abbreviations: MS = microsurgery; SRS = stereotactic radiosurgery.

▶ **Modified Delphi Study Consensus for sporadic VS.** The Modified Delphi Study for sporadic VS published in 2020[52] issued 103 consensus statements related to this topic, and the reader is highly encouraged to review the results. Some FAQs derived from these statements are presented in ▶ Table 45.9, along with the strength of the opinion.

Table 45.9 Some FAQs based on the modified Delphi Study on VS[52]

FAQ & Answer	Statement numbers
Q: Is poorer baseline hearing associated with a greater probability of progression to non-serviceable hearing regardless of treatment[a]? A: Yes (strong consensus)	#10, 25, 44
Q: Does larger tumor size increase the probability of progression to non-serviceable hearing[a]? A: Yes (strong consensus)	#7, 24, 40
Q: What is the optimal form of radiation for treating VS? A: There is no clear clinical advantage of fractionated radiation vs. SF-SRS, or for LINAC vs. Gamma radiation. Proton beam and intensity modulated radiation are not established modalities for treating VS (strong consensus)	#4, 74
Q: Is GTR associated with a greater probability of losing SH compared to near-total & subtotal resection? A: Yes (strong consensus)	#31
Q: When should patients undergoing observation be treated? A: Treatment (MS, SF-SRS or fractionated-SRS) should be offered at the first sign of unequivocal tumor growth (strong consensus)	#72

[a] regardless of treatment: SF-SRS, MS or observation
Abbreviations: GTR = gross total resection; MS= microsurgery; SF-SRS = single fraction stereotactic radiosurgery; SH (serviceable hearing): ≤ 50 dB PTA, ≥ 50% WRS

Management algorithm

Note: there are no Level I recommendations for most aspects of VS management. Some recommendations here differ from the published guidelines quoted above. The reader is encouraged to review the available information and determine their preferred approach which may differ from either of these strategies.

- small tumors (< 15 mm diameter) with perfect hearing (WRS 100%):
  observe radiographically (CT or MRI scan) plus serial hearing tests (so-called "wait and scan"):
  ○ scan: recommend treatment for growth > 2 mm between studies. Scan schedule guide:
    – every 6 months × 2 years after diagnosis, then (if stable)
    – annually until 5 years after diagnosis, then (if stable)
    – at years 7, 9, and 14 after diagnosis[17]
  ○ annual audiology evaluations
    – hearing deterioration (WRS < 100%) but no growth: see below
    – rationale: in patients with small tumors and normal WRS, comparing the results of hearing preservation following surgery or SRS to the natural history, the conclusion is that *established tumor growth* should be the main determinant for treatment[39]
- small tumors with serviceable hearing: management is very controversial
  ○ in general, patients with serviceable hearing but WRS < 100% have a 50% chance of preserving their serviceable hearing (50/50 rule or AAO-HNS class A or B) with either observation, SRS or microsurgical resection. Observation is sstrongly recommended as the initial management[52]
  ○ hearing preservation rates better than 50% have been reported for both microsurgery and radiosurgery in very selected patients (smaller tumors, located medially in the IAC, intact pre-op ABR amplitudes and latencies)
  ○ decisions to try to beat the natural history (50% chance of hearing loss at 10 years) should be very individualized based on tumor factors (size, location) and patient factors (ABR, age, co-morbidities, preferences)

- final management decisions are often dictated by non medical reasons (patient's perception, social situation, financial considerations, support system, etc.)
- medium size tumors (15–25 mm diameter)
  - tumors > 15–20 mm should be treated.[17,39] This is mostly true for young patients
  - close observation to establish growth is a valid option in older patients or patients with medical co-morbidities
  - complication rate increases and facial outcome worsens with increasing tumor size
  - NF2 patients present a challenge and should be evaluated individually. In general the success rate in the management of their tumors is lower (higher cranial nerve deficit and higher recurrence rate).[54,55] Early management is considered more favorable for good outcome.[56] A retrospective study found significant hearing improvement and tumor shrinkage in > 50% of NF2 patients with progressive VS using bevacizumab (Avastin®) (see above)

45

- large tumors (> 25 mm diameter): treatment is recommended
  - microsurgical resection is favored to reduce mass effect and decompress the brainstem
  - SRS is also useful in larger tumors for older patients or those with significant co-morbidities
  - for tumors > 3 cm maximal p-fossa dimension with brainstem compression: intraoperative monitoring of trigeminal nerve (Cr. N. V), lower cranial nerves (Cr. N. IX, X) and use of SSEPs is not obligatory but should be considered[52]
  - for tumors > 3 cm diameter with symptomatic hydrocephalus: pre-op placement of EVD is optional. A VP shunt should be placed if the hydrocephalus does not resolve post-op[52]

Selection options for intervention

Once treatment is elected (see algorithm above), the type of treatment must be selected.
    Comparison of microsurgery vs. radiosurgery (SRS)

1. hearing preservation
   a) for patients with testable preoperative hearing
      - summary: radiosurgery or stereotactic radiation appears to be better at preserving hearing than microsurgery for VS < 2 cm up to 5 years post treatment. The chances of hearing preservation at 10 years is the same with SRS or MS. The difference is minor for tumors < 10 mm and very good preoperative hearing (70% SDS, and 30 dB PTA). The advantage of radiation is more pronounced for larger tumors and greater preoperative hearing loss. Details:
      - SRS: overall, at 2, 5, and 10 years, 50–75%, 50–75%, and 25–50% of the patients maintained their GR hearing class (▶ Table 45.5). Hearing preservation appears to be related to the radiation dose to the cochlea rather than to the tumor itself[57]
      - microsurgery: hearing preservation is significantly related to the tumor size and to the experience of the surgical team. Hearing preservation in Samii's series of 1000 VS[55] improved from 24% in the first 200 cases to 49% in later cases. Hearing preservation in microsurgery has improved with the use of direct cochlear nerve monitoring[58] compared to auditory brainstem responses monitoring only. Hearing preservation in patients with class A, small tumors and direct cochlear nerve monitoring (compound nerve action potential) was 91%.[59] With microsurgery, the durability of the hearing preservation is also excellent with only 15% of patients with class A hearing after surgery, and 33% of patients with class B hearing after surgery slipping one class at 5 years follow-up[60]
2. facial nerve preservation
   a) preservation has been excellent with both microsurgery and radiosurgery
   b) microsurgery: 98.5% overall[61] and 100% in tumors not touching the brainstem. Staged resection has been advocated by some to improve facial nerve preservation in giant VS (> 4–4.5 cm)[62]
   c) radiosurgery: 98% of patients.[63] The incidence of facial neuropathy has significantly decreased since the SRS dose was decreased to 12–13 Gy. Facial neuropathy in the recent series occurred in patients having received 18–20 Gy
3. trigeminal neuropathy (TGN)
   a) a complication classically feared in large tumors especially following SRS
   b) SRS: 7% incidence of TGN (mainly in patients receiving higher doses, i.e., 18 Gy). No patients who received a dose < 13 Gy developed TGN[63]
   c) microsurgery: post-op TGN is not reported in most series
4. tumor control (local control rate (LCR)):
   a) microsurgery: tumor recurrence has been poorly studied. Quoted rates in the literature vary between 0.5% at 6 years[61] and 9.2%[64]
   b) SRS: long term data are lacking with the currently favored dose of 12–14 Gy to the tumor margin. In 68 patients with sporadic VS with median follow-up of 43.5 months[65]:
      - intracanalicular VS: no growth after SRS (9 patients)

- extracanalicular VS: 97% LCR for VS that grew at a rate < 2.5 mm/year before SRS, vs. 69% LCR for VS that grew ≥ 2.5 mm/year before SRS
- 10-18% of patients show swelling ("pseudogrowth")[63,65] following SRS defined as enlargement ≥ 2 mm within 6-12 months that decreased or stabilized in size on follow-up

Vertigo and dizziness

Practice guideline: Balance problems with VS

Data is insufficient to support MS or SRS for balance problems due to VS[66]

For patients with episodic vertigo or balance difficulties as the predominant symptom; also, see points under Selection options for intervention (p.788):

1. remember: patients with VS are susceptible to other causes of vertigo as well, and patients should undergo ENG and functional balance assessment
2. vertigo that is due to the VS is often self-limited, and improves in 6–8 weeks to a reasonably tolerable level with no treatment (patients may do better with so-called "vestibular rehab")
3. residual dizziness and balance disturbances are common whether stereotactic radiosurgery (SRS) or microsurgery (MS) is used, but are typically less after MS
4. patients' reported vertigo intensity is improved by any treatment versus observation[67]
5. after SRS: a minimum of 5–6 mos, and sometimes up to 18 months may be required to produce beneficial effects. Symptoms are improved more rapidly after MS than with SRS
6. following MS: The severity of dizziness after MS depends on the preoperative vestibular function on the affected side. If the ipsilateral vestibular function is absent preoperatively, then patients will not suffer from dizziness or nausea post-op. If ipsilateral vestibular function is intact pre-op, then patients may be very dizzy and nauseated in particular for the first 24 hrs
7. conclusion:
   a) observation may be the best choice for ≈ 20% of patients ("wait and scan")
   b) when treatment is desired:
      - surgery is the best choice for most VSs producing vertigo
      - SRS may be the right choice for some, especially: elderly patients (> 70 yrs) with other health problems, for recurrence of VS, for intracanalicular tumors or tumors growing < 2 mm/year, and for individual preference

Hydrocephalus

When hydrocephalus is present, it may require separate treatment with a CSF shunt—see Surgical considerations (p.791)—and may possibly be done at the same time as surgery for the VS (if surgery for the VS is indicated).

45.3.7 Surgical treatment

Practice guidelines for surgical management of vestibular schwannomas

Practice guideline: Surgical management of vestibular schwannomas

For the full guideline, see reference.[66]

Choice of surgical approach or surgical team

- When serviceable hearing is present: data is insufficient to recommend either middle fossa (MF) or retrosigmoid (RS) approach over the other for complete resection and facial nerve (FN) preservation[66]
- When serviceable hearing is not present: data is insufficient to recommend either the RS or translabyrinthine (TL) approach over the other for GTR and FN preservation[66]
- Outcome data is insufficient to recommend a multispecialty team (neurosurgeon and neurotologist) over either specialty working alone[66]

45

Microsurgery (MS) for small VS
- Data is insufficient to support a firm recommendation that surgery should be the primary treatment for intracanalicular VS < 1.5 cm[66]
- Level III[66]: hearing preservation surgery may be attempted via the MF or RS approach for VS < 1.5 cm with good pre-op hearing

Microsurgery (MS) for VS in patients with neurofibromatosis type 2 (NF2)
- There is insufficient data that MS should be the initial treatment for VS in NF2[66]

Miscellaneous information regarding microsurgery (MS) for VS
- There is insufficient data that subtotal resection followed by SRS provides comparable hearing and FN preservation to patients having GTR[66]
- Level III[66]: trigeminal neuralgia with VS is better relieved with MS than with SRS
- Level III[66]: patients should be counseled that MS after SRS has an increased likelihood of STR and decreased FN function
- Level III[68]: FN monitoring is recommended during MS to improve long-term FN function (strong Delphi consensus[52])
- Level III[68]: favorable intraoperative FN response is a reliable predictor of good long-term FN outcome, but a poor response in the presence of an anatomically intact FN does not reliably predict long-term FN function & cannot be used to direct decisions for early reinnervation procedures
- Level III[68]: intraoperative VIII nerve monitoring should be used when hearing preservation surgery is a goal. Update: auditory brainstem reflexes (ABRs) should be utilized, and direct cochlear nerve action potential monitoring should be considered when feasible (strong Delphi consensus[52])

Abbreviations: FN = facial nerve; GTR = gross total resection; MF = middle fossa; MS = microsurgery; RS = retrosigmoid; STR = subtotal resection; TL = translabyrinthine approach.

Approaches

General information
Three basic surgical approaches:
1. those with possibility of hearing preservation
   a) middle fossa (MF): poor access to posterior fossa (see below)
   b) retrosigmoid (RS) (see below) AKA retrosigmoid-transmeatal approach
2. translabyrinthine (TL): non-hearing preserving (see below)

Excellent results have been reported with each of these approaches. These guidelines assume that the surgical team is comfortable with all three approaches.

Decision algorithm for approach
The choice of approach is dictated by hearing salvageability and tumor size as follows:
1. salvageable hearing (▶ Table 45.10 for definition and guidelines)
   a) if tumor is intracanalicular (no extension beyond a few mm into the posterior fossa (CPA); note: differences of opinion exist regarding how much tumor in the CPA can be removed via MF): use the middle fossa approach. Note: some authors exclusively use the retrosigmoid approach for hearing preservation even for these tumors with excellent results
   b) if tumor extends > few mm into the posterior fossa: use the retrosigmoid approach (it is generally accepted that the cisternal part of the tumor is not well exposed by the middle fossa approach, especially regarding the ability to dissect tumor off the nerves)
2. non salvageable hearing (see ▶ Table 45.10 for definition and guidelines)
   a) use translabyrinthine approach or retrosigmoid approach
   b) either can be used irrespective of tumor size. Surgical team preference is the main deciding factor. Some influencing aspects:
      - a young patient with no cerebellar atrophy might favor a translab approach
      - an anteriorly situated sigmoid sinus and/or a high riding jugular bulb restrict the working space in the translab approach, and might favor a retrosigmoid approach

Table 45.10 Hearing salvageability

Serviceable and unsalvageable hearing
Definition of serviceable hearing
A generous definition of serviceable hearing: PTA < 50 dB and SDS > 50%[a]
Unsalvageable hearing
Serviceable hearing is *unlikely* to be preserved post-op when 1. pre-op SDS < 75% 2. or pre-op PTA loss > 25 dB 3. or pre-op BAER has abnormal wave morphology 4. or tumor > 2–2.5 cm diameter

[a]see also other definitions of serviceable hearing (p. 781)

45

Surgical considerations

General information

The first surgical removal of a vestibular schwannoma was performed over a century ago in 1894.[69]

The facial nerve is pushed forward by the tumor in ≈ 75% of cases (range: 50–80%), but may occasionally be pushed rostrally, less often inferiorly, and rarely posteriorly. It may even continue to function while it is flattened to a mere ribbon on the tumor capsule surface.

Anesthesia with minimal muscle relaxants allows intra-op seventh nerve monitoring. In only ≈ 10% of large tumors is the cochlear nerve a separate band on the tumor capsule, in the remainder it is incorporated into the tumor.

Although total excision of tumor is usually the goal of surgery, facial nerve preservation must take precedence over degree of resection. Near total resection (very small sliver of tumor left on the facial nerve) or subtotal resection are all excellent options if the tumor is tightly adherent to the facial nerve or the brainstem. Both have excellent long term tumor control rate with either observation or post-op radiation.

If hydrocephalus is present, historically standard practice was to place a CSF shunt and wait ≈ 2 weeks before the definitive operation.[70] While still acceptable, this is less commonly done at present, and shunting or EVD is often performed under the same anesthesia.

Large tumors may be approached by a staged surgical approach to debulk tumor and preserve facial nerve, or a planned subtotal resection followed by radiation. For tumors > 3 cm, such an approach seems to lead to improved results of facial nerve function.[71]

The extra anesthesia time involved in translab approach may be detrimental in the elderly.

Middle fossa approach

- indications:
  a) hearing preservation
  b) laterally placed tumors
  c) small tumors (usually < 2.5 cm)
- pros:
  a) allows drilling and exposure of the IAC all the way to the geniculate ganglion (good for laterally placed tumors)
  b) basically an extradural subtemporal operation
- cons:
  a) potential damage to temporal lobe with risk of seizures
  b) facial nerve is the most superficial nerve in this exposure and therefore the surgeon works "around" the facial nerve (possibility of injury)
- technique summary
  a) lumbar drain
  b) usually straight incision, starting in front of the tragus, extending cephalad for 6 cm, held open with a self-retaining retractor
  c) the temporalis muscle is incised vertically (along the muscle fibers) along the most posterior aspect of the exposure and is reflected anteriorly
  d) craniotomy: 4 cm × 3 cm
  e) elevate the middle fossa dura, section the middle meningeal artery. Identify and preserve the greater superficial petrosal nerve (GSPN), arcuate eminence, V3, and true edge of the petrous bone (the false edge is the groove occupied by the superior petrosal sinus)

f) drill and expose the internal auditory canal all the way to Bill's bar (for tumors extending laterally)
g) localize the facial nerve with the nerve stimulator
h) open the IAC dura along the main axis of the IAC, avoiding VII
i) identify the vestibular, cochlear, and facial nerves
j) dissect the tumor off the nerves

Translabyrinthine approach

Often preferred by neurotologists.
1. pros & cons: See ▶ Table 45.11
2. technique summary
   a) position: supine head rotated to contralateral side, can be done either with pins or doughnut if it is anticipated that no retractors will be used
   b) prep the abdomen for fat graft (almost always used)
   c) skin incision should be tailored to the location of the sigmoid sinus (observe location of the sigmoid sinus and pinna of the ear on the pre-op MRI). Usually smaller opening than retrosigmoid approach
      • does not require a craniotomy. For large tumors requiring an "extended translab," 1–2 cm of retrosigmoid dura should be exposed during the mastoidectomy to allow for retraction of the sigmoid sinus
      • dural opening along the IAC after identification of VII with stimulator
      • for large tumor: section the superior petrosal sinus and section the tentorium to gain better intradural exposure
      • closure requires fat graft

Table 45.11 Pros & cons of translabyrinthine approach

Disadvantages	Advantages
• sacrifices hearing (acceptable when hearing is already non-functional or unlikely to be spared by other approach) • may take longer than retrosigmoid approach • possibly higher rate of post-op CSF leak	• early identification of VII may result in higher preservation rate • less risk to cerebellum and lower cranial nerves • patients do not get as "ill" from blood in cisterna magna, etc. (essentially an extracranial approach) • less trauma to musculature ∴ less H/A than retrosigmoid

Booking the case: Translabyrinthine approach for vestibular schwannoma

Also see defaults & disclaimers (p. 25).
1. position: supine with shoulder roll
2. equipment:
   a) microscope
   b) high speed drill
   c) ultrasonic aspirator
3. some surgeons work with neurotologist to assist with the IAC and for follow-up
4. neuromonitoring: facial EMG (does not require EEG tech), SSEPs for tumors involving the brainstem (requires EEG tech)
5. post-op: ICU
6. consent (in lay terms for the patient—not all-inclusive):
   a) procedure: surgery through an incision behind the ear to remove a tumor growing inside the skull on the nerve to the ear. Possible need for post-op lumbar drain. Fat graft (≈ always used)
   b) alternatives: nonsurgical management with follow-up MRIs, other surgical approaches, radiation (stereotactic radiosurgery)
   c) complications: CSF leak with possible meningitis, loss of hearing in ipsilateral ear (if not already lost), paralysis of facial muscles on the side of surgery with possible need for surgical procedures to help correct (correction is often far from perfect), facial numbness, post-op balance difficulties/vertigo, brainstem injury with stroke

Retrosigmoid approach

AKA posterior fossa, AKA suboccipital approach.[72,73]

- pros:
    - a) familiar to most neurosurgeons ∴ often preferred by neurosurgeons
    - b) quick access to the tumor
    - c) hearing preservation possible
    - d) NOTE: this approach is very versatile. Samii[55] resected all his acoustic tumors via a retrosigmoid approach; he achieved a significant amount of brain relaxation and improved exposure by using in the sitting position, which is generally not used in the U.S. because of associated complications (p. 1737)
- cons:
    - a) cerebellar retraction: not a problem for tumors < 4 cm, provided the craniotomy is sufficiently lateral and the cisterna magna and the CP angle cistern has been opened
    - b) headaches: it has been suggested that headaches are more common following retrosigmoid craniotomy than after translabyrinthine craniotomy. Postulated mechanisms: purely extra-dural drilling in translab with no bone dust in subarachnoid space. More anterior skin incision in translab and less disruption of the suboccipital musculature and greater occipital nerve

45

Booking the case: Retrosigmoid craniotomy for vestibular schwannoma

Also see defaults & disclaimers (p. 25).
1. position: lateral decubitus with tumor side up
2. equipment:
    - a) microscope
    - b) ultrasonic aspirator
    - c) image guided navigation system (if used) (may be helpful for placing skin incision and craniotomy more than for tumor localization)
3. some surgeons work with neurotologist to assist with the IAC and for follow-up
4. neuromonitoring: facial EMG (does not require EEG tech), BAERS, near field monitoring (CNAP: compound nerve action potential)
5. post-op: ICU
6. consent (in lay terms for the patient—not all-inclusive):
    - a) procedure: surgery through an incision behind the ear to remove a tumor growing inside the skull on the nerve to the ear. Possible need for post-op lumbar drain. Possible fat graft (optional)
    - b) alternatives: nonsurgical management with follow-up MRIs, other surgical approaches, radiation (stereotactic radiosurgery)
    - c) complications: CSF leak with possible meningitis, loss of hearing in ipsilateral ear (if not already lost), paralysis of facial muscles on the side of surgery with possible need for surgical procedures to help correct (correction is often far from perfect), facial numbness post-op balance difficulties/vertigo, brainstem injury with stroke. Facial numbness (infrequent)

Technique summary
1. position: lateral decubitus with tumor side up, head in pins rotated (might need shoulder roll), zygomatic arch horizontal. 30° elevation of the head is paramount; see Posterior fossa (suboccipital) craniectomy, Lateral oblique position (p. 1738)
2. percutaneous lumbar drain (optional)
3. incision is shaped like the pinna of the ear, 3 finger breaths behind the external auditory canal
4. the craniotomy has to be lateral enough to expose part of the sigmoid and part of the transverse sinuses and to allow a straight line of sight to the lateral end of the IAC
5. to prevent CSF leak, seal all bone edges with bone wax
6. dural opening along the lines of the craniotomy
7. exposure is enhanced by opening the cerebellopontine angle cistern and the cisterna magna under the microscope and draining CSF (20–40 ml of CSF can also be drained via a lumbar subarachnoid catheter)
8. the petrosal vein is often sacrificed at the beginning of the procedure to allow the cerebellum to relax and fall back and to avoid tearing off the transverse sinus. Be careful not to coagulate the SCA that often runs with the petrosal vein

9. using the facial nerve stimulator, the posterior aspect of the tumor is inspected to make sure the facial nerve has not been pushed posteriorly
10. the thin layer of arachnoid that covers most tumors is identified. Vessels within the arachnoid may contribute to cochlear function and may be preserved by keeping them with the arachnoid
11. the plane between tumor and cerebellum may be followed to the brainstem, and occasionally to the VII nerve (this plane is harder to follow once bleeding from tumor debulking occurs)
12. to help locate the origin of the VII nerve at the brainstem, see ▶ Table 45.12 and CPA anatomy in ▶ Fig. 1.11
13. the posterolateral tumor capsule is opened, and internal decompression is performed. The tumor is collapsed inward and the capsule is kept intact and is rolled laterally off of VII and is eventually removed. The most difficult area to separate VII from tumor is just proximal to the entrance to the porus acusticus. A general recommendation is to accept a subtotal or near total resection to preserve anatomic continuity of the facial nerve in cases where it is identified by stimulation but because it is so flattened it cannot be seen as a separate structure on the surface of the tumor.
14. after the extracanalicular portion of tumor is removed, the dura over the IAC is incised, and the IAC is drilled open and tumor is removed from this portion. To preserve hearing, the bony labyrinth must not be violated. The posterior semicircular canal (SCC) is the most vulnerable structure (▶ Fig. 45.10). The vestibule of the SCCs is also at risk but is less likely to be entered. The maximal amount of temporal bone drilling that can be accomplished without entering the posterior SCC can be determined from the pre-op CT. The operculum of the temporal bone is a small step-off palpable with a nerve hook posteriorly from the porus acusticus. It marks the location of the vestibular aqueduct and is a good landmark for the posterior extent of the drilling in the retrosigmoid exposure of the IAC. Measuring the distance from the IAC to the posterior semicircular canal on a pre-op CT and measuring the thickness of the bone overlying the posterior semicircular canal are recommended for safe exposure of the IAC, in particular for hearing preservation. However, opening the labyrinth cannot always be avoided; and any opening should be plugged with bone-wax or muscle.[74] If the facial nerve is not intact and is not going to be grafted, then the IAC should be plugged, e.g., by bone wax covered with a small piece of hammered muscle (hammering makes the muscle sticky by activating extrinsic clotting factors) and Gelfoam®.

Table 45.12 Aids in localizing VII nerve origin[76]

- VII nerve originates in the pontomedullary sulcus near the lateral end of the sulcus, 1–2 mm anterior to the VIII nerve
- the pontomedullary sulcus ends just medial to the foramen of Luschka (extending from the lateral recess of the IV ventricle, ▶ Fig. 1.11)
- a tuft of choroid plexus usually extends out of the foramen of Luschka on the posterior surface of IX and X nerve, just inferior to the origin of VII
- the flocculus of the cerebellum projects from the lateral recess into the CPA just posterior to the origin of VII and VIII
- VII origin is 4 mm cephalad and 2 mm anterior to that of the IX nerve

NB: *large tumors*: in some large tumors, the capsule may be adherent to the brainstem and so portions of tumor must be left; recurrence rate among these is ≈ 10–20%.[75] Large tumors may also involve V superiorly (sometimes VII is pushed up against V), and inferiorly may involve IX, X, and XI. The lower cranial nerves can usually be spared by dissecting them off of the tumor capsule, and protecting them with cottonoids.

Post-op care and care for complications

Practice guideline

Practice guideline: Perioperative nimodipine for VS surgery

Level III[77]: perioperative nimodipine (possibly with the addition of hydroxyethyl starch) should be considered to improve facial nerve functional outcome and may help with hearing outcome following microsurgery

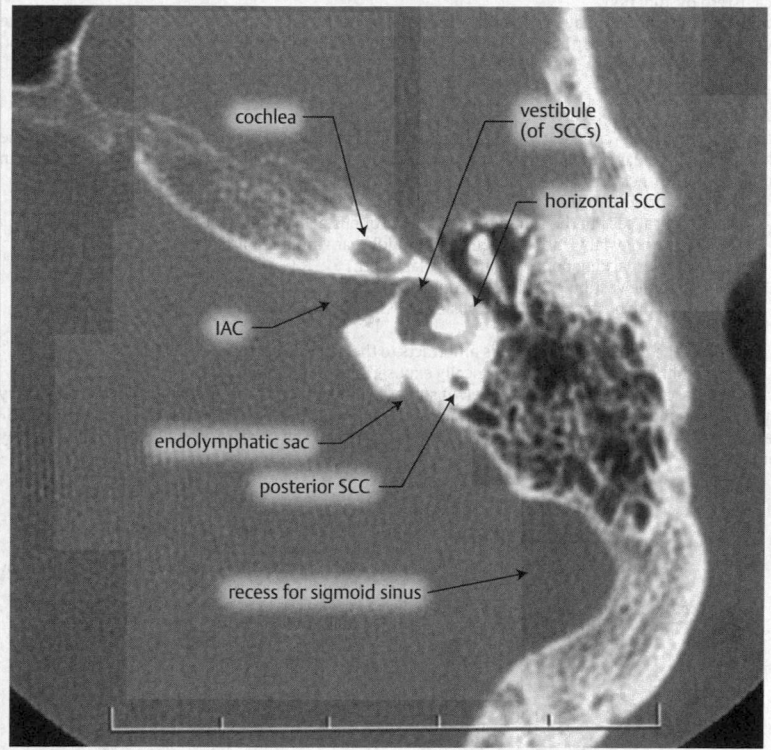

Fig. 45.10 Temporal bone structures. Image: CT scan, axial slice through left petrous bone with bone windows. Provided courtesy of Chris Danner, MD.

Cranial nerve and brainstem dysfunction

Facial nerve (VII)
If eye closure is impaired due to VII dysfunction: R natural tears 2 gtts to affected eye q 2 hrs and PRN. Apply Lacrilube® to affected eye and tape it shut q hs. If the eye is also insensate from Cr. N. V impairment, the eye is at risk of exposure and trophic keratitis and immediate consultation with ophthalmology for emergency tarsorrhaphy is indicated. Early tarsorrhaphy should also be considered If there is complete VII palsy with little chance of early recovery.

Facial re-animation (e.g., hypoglossal-facial anastamosis) is performed after 1–2 months if VII was divided, or if no function returns after 1 year with an anatomically intact nerve.

Vestibular nerve (VIII)
Vestibular dysfunction is common post-op, nausea and vomiting due to this (and also intracranial air) is common. Balance difficulties due to this clear rapidly; however, ataxia from brainstem dysfunction may have a permanent component.

Lower cranial nerves
The combination of IX, X, and XII dysfunction creates swallowing difficulties and creates a risk of aspiration.

Brainstem dysfunction

Brainstem dysfunction may occur from dissection of tumor off of the brainstem. This may produce ataxia, contralateral paresthesias in the body. Although there may be improvement, once present, there is often some permanent residual.

CSF fistula

Also, see CSF fistula (cranial) (p. 415) for general information. CSF fistula may develop through the skin incision, the ear (CSF otorrhea) through a ruptured tympanic membrane, or via the eustachian tube and then either through the nose (rhinorrhea) or down the back of the throat.

Rhinorrhea may occur through any of the following routes (circled numbers in ▶ Fig. 45.11):

* ① via the apical cells to the tympanic cavity (TC) or eustachian tube (the most common path)
* entry into the bony labyrinth—reaching the middle ear would require rupture (e.g., of the oval window by overpacking bone wax into the labyrinth)
  ○ ② through the vestibule of the horizontal semicircular canal (SCC)
  ○ ③ through the posterior SCC (the posterior SCC is the most common area that is entered by drilling)
* ④ follows the perilabyrinthine cells and tracts to the mastoid antrum
* ⑤ through the mastoid air cells surgically exposed at the craniotomy site

Most leaks are diagnosed within 1 week of surgery, although one presented 4 years post-op.[78] They appear to be more common with more lateral unroofing of the IAC.[78] Meningitis complicates a CSF leak in 5–25% of cases, and usually develops within days of the onset of leak.[78] Hydrocephalus may promote the development of a CSF fistula.

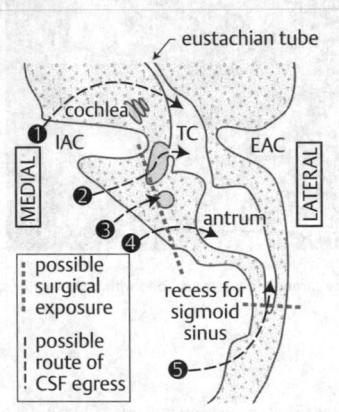

Fig. 45.11 **Possible routes for CSF rhinorrhea following vestibular schwannoma surgery** (see text). Image: schematic axial slice through right petrous bone. Adapted from Surgical Neurology, Vol. 43, Nutik S L, Korol H W, Cerebrospinal Fluid Leak After Acoustic Neuroma Surgery, 553–7, 1995, with permission from Elsevier Science.

Treatment: 25–35% of leaks stop spontaneously (one series reported 80%).[78] Treatment options include:

1. surgical treatment: in general, postoperative CSF leak (including rhinorrhea) is best addressed with immediate surgical re-exploration. Non-surgical measures (see following items) may be used to temporize
   a) in the case of a translabyrinthine approach with absent ipsilateral hearing: to treat rhinorrhea, pack and permanently close the Eustachian tube via a trans tympanic membrane approach. This is very effective and avoids re-opening the surgical incision and removing the previously placed fat graft.
   b) if hearing is preserved (which excludes translab), every effort should be made to preserve the Eustachian tube function to preserve middle ear function. Re-explore the surgical field, re-wax the aircells and place additional fat graft, fascia, pericranium, or other sealant over the exposed aircells. This aggressive management is the most definitive and rapid treatment, and avoids prolonged bed rest required by placing a lumbar drain and trying to control the leak in a conservative way
2. non-surgical: may be used to temporize, but early surgical treatment is recommended
   a) evaluate for infection, which is often associated with CSF leak
   b) elevate HOB

    c) for leaks through the incision, reinforcement with additional sutues may be attempted

    d) a percutaneous lumbar subarachnoid drain may be tried,[79,80] although some debate its effi-
cacy,[73] and there is a theoretical risk of drawing bacteria into the CNS

    e) placement of EVD

3. a CSF leak may be an indication of altered CSF hydrodynamics. Most of these patients demonstrate frank ventriculomegaly (hydrocephalus). In some patients the leak may function as a pressure relief valve and thereby ameliorate the ventriculomegaly (i.e., there would be hydrocephalus
if there wasn't a leak). Adjunctive CSF shunting is usually also necessary or the repair will be
more likely to fail

Outcome and follow-up

Complete surgical removal was reported in 97–99% of cases.[81]

45

Surgical morbidity and mortality

Also see Post-op considerations for p-fossa cranis (p. 1744). Estimated frequency of some complications[82]: the most common complication is CSF leakage in 4–27%[78] (see above), meningitis in 5.7%,
stroke in 0.7%, subsequent requirement for CSF shunt (for hydrocephalus or to treat leak) in 6.5%.

    The mortality rate is ≈ 1% at specialized centers.[55,81,83]

Cranial nerve dysfunction

▶ Table 45.13 shows statistics of VII and VIII cranial nerve preservation following suboccipital
removal of VSs in several combined groups of patients. For more details, see below.

    Post-radiation cranial neuropathies generally appear 6–18 months following stereotactic radio-
surgery (SRS),[85] and since more than half of these resolve within 3–6 months after the onset, the
recommendation is to treat these with a course of corticosteroids.

▶ **Facial nerve (VII).** See ▶ Table 45.3 for the House and Brackmann grading scale. Grades 1–3 are
associated with acceptable function. Facial nerve preservation is related to tumor size.

    Surgery: With the use of modern facial nerve monitoring techniques, anatomical integrity of the
facial nerve can be achieved in > 90% even for very large tumors and in close to 99% in medium-sized
tumors.[86] In cases where the nerve is so flattened that the tumor has to be left over the nerve to
preserve its anatomical integrity, functional outcome of the facial nerve is nevertheless lower, especially with larger tumors. Excellent outcome (HB grade I-III) was only achieved in 75% of the patients
with large tumors and 91% in medium-sized tumors.

    SRS for tumors ≤ 3 cm diameter: With modern SRS dosimetry (12–13 Gy for patients with service-
able hearing and 13–14 Gy for patients with non-serviceable hearing), the incidence of new facial
nerve weakness was 4%.[87]

Table 45.13 Cranial nerve preservation in retrosigmoid removal of VSs[a]

Size of tumor	Preserved function	
	VII nerve	VIII nerve
< 1 cm	95–100%	57%
1–2 cm	80–92%	33%
> 2 cm	50–76%	6%

[a]series of 135 VSs[84 (p 729)] and other sources[75 (p 3337),81]

▶ **Vestibulo-acoustic nerve (VIII).** Patients with unilateral VS and Class I or II hearing (▶ Table 45.5)
comprised ≈ 12% of cases in a large series.[88] Preservation of hearing is critically dependent on tumor
size, with little chance of preservation with tumors > 1–1.5 cm diameter. Chances of preserving hearing may possibly be improved by intraoperative brainstem auditory evoked potential monitoring.[89]
In centers treating large numbers of VSs, hearing *preservation* rates of 35–71% can be achieved with
tumors < 1.5 cm[88,90] (although a range of 14–48% may be more realistic[91]). Hearing may rarely be
improved post-op.[92]

    SRS: for tumors ≤ 3 cm diameter,[93] hearing was preserved in 26% of 65 cases with pre-op pure
tone threshold < 90 dB. Hearing loss has been correlated with increase in tumor size.[94] NB: there is a
high rate of hearing loss at 1 year. SRT: useful hearing was preserved in 93%.[95]

    Vestibular nerve function is rarely normal post-op. Attempts at "vestibular" sparing surgery have
shown no better results than surgery not specifically addressing this issue. Most patients with

unilateral loss of vestibular nerve function will learn to compensate to a significant degree with input from the contralateral side, if normal. Patients with ataxia as a result of brainstem injury from the tumor or the surgery will have more difficulties post-op. Some patients will seem to do well initially post-op with respect to vestibular nerve function, only to undergo a delayed deterioration several months post-op. These cases likely represent aberrant regeneration of the vestibular nerve fibers and may be extremely difficult to manage. Some experts advocate cutting the vestibular nerve, as for Meniere disease (p. 604).

▶ **Trigeminal nerve (V).** Postoperative trigeminal nerve symptoms occur transiently in 22% and permanently in 11% following microsurgery, similar to the results of SRS.[96] New facial numbness occurred in 2% with SRT.[95]

▶ **Lower cranial nerves.** Injuries to IX, X, and XI occur infrequently following surgery on large tumors that distort the nerves and displace them inferiorly against the occipital bone.

Recurrence
Following microsurgery (MS)
Recurrence is highly dependent on extent of removal. However, recurrence can develop in tumors that were apparently totally removed, or when subtotal resection was performed. This can occur many years after treatment. Tumor progression rate following subtotal resection is ≈ 20%.[91] All patients should be followed with imaging (CT or MRI). In older series with up to 15 yrs follow-up, local control rate (LCR) after "total resection" is ≈ 94%. More recent series with MRI follow-up indicate recurrence rates of 7–11% (3–16 yrs follow-up).[91]

Use of EBRT
EBRT may improve LCR in incompletely resected tumors as shown in ▶ Table 45.14 (note: with the long survival expected with benign tumors, post-XRT complications may occur).

Table 45.14 Local control rates of surgery vs. surgery + EBRT for VSs[97]

Extent of surgical removal	Local control rate (LCR)	
	Surgery	Surgery + EBRT[a]
gross total	60/62 (97%)	no data
near total (90–99%)	14/15 (93%)	2/2 (100%)
subtotal (< 90%)	7/13 (54%)	17/20 (85%)[a]
biopsy only	no data	3/3 (100%)

[a]with doses < 45 Gy, LCR was 33%; with > 45 Gy, LCR was 94%

Microsurgery vs. SRS
In a non-randomized retrospective study[96] of VSs < 3 cm dia, the *short-term* LCR (median 24 mos follow-up) was 97% for microsurgery vs. 94% for stereotactic radiosurgery (SRS). However, for benign tumors, long-term follow-up is critical (possibly 5–10 years[85]), and this study *suggests* that the long-term LCR will be better for MS than SRS. SRS studies with long-term follow-up[98] are not directly comparable because in the cases with longest follow-up, higher radiation doses were used with a resultant higher incidence of radiation complications, and an anticipated better LCR.

Initially there may be temporary enlargement of the tumor accompanied by loss of central contrast enhancement following SRS in ≈ 5% of patients[99] (with up to 2% of patients showing actual initial tumor growth), and so the need for further treatment after SRS should be postponed until there is evidence of sustained growth.[100] Surgery should therefore be avoided during the interval from 6 to 18 months after SRS because this is the time of maximum damage from the radiation.[100]

Although the numbers are small, the rate of VII nerve injury may be higher in patients undergoing MS following SRS failure to achieve LCR compared to cases where microsurgery was the initial procedure[101,102]; however, this has been disputed.[100] Lastly, there is a potential for malignant transformation of VSs following SRS, including triton tumors[103,104] (malignant neoplasms with rhabdoid features) or the induction of skull base tumors (which has been reported with external beam radiation[105]), as well as the risk of late arterial occlusion (the AICA lies near the surface of VSs), any of which may occur many years later. The observed malignant transformation rate is 0.3% and the annual incidence of malignant transformation is 0.02%.[106]

Level III[48]: patients should be informed that there is a minimal risk of malignant transformation of VS after SRS

Treatment for recurrence following microsurgery

Repeat surgery for recurrent VS is an option. One series of 23 patients[107] showed that 6 of 10 patients with moderate or normal VII function maintained at least moderate function after reoperation, 3 patients had increased ataxia, and 1 patient had a cerebellar hematoma. SRS offers a safe and effective long-term management strategy for residual or retained VS after MS.[108] Using SRS for recurrent VSs resulted in progression-free survival rate of 97% at 3 years, 95% at 5 years, and 90% at 10 years. Among patients with any facial dysfunction (▶ Table 45.3, HB II-VI) at the time of recurrence or progression, 19% had improvement after SRS, and 5.5% with some facial function (HB I-V) developed more facial weakness. Among patients with trigeminal neuropathy, 20% had improvement, 5.8% developed or had worsened trigeminal neuropathy after SRS.

45

Level III[48]: SRS is safe & effective to re-treat patients with VS progression after initial SRS

Hydrocephalus

May occur following treatment (MS or SRS) for VS, and may even occur years later. The increased CSF pressure may also predispose to development of a CSF fistula.

Quality of life

Being diagnosed with a VS creates anxiety and leads to a temporary reduction in quality of life (QoL). However, once a treatment modality is chosen, observational management for amenable tumors produced the highest QoL.[109]

Patients undergoing SRS or observation report a better total Penn Acoustic Neuroma Quality of Life (PANQOL) score and higher PANQOL facial, balance, and pain subdomain scores than those undergoing microsurgical resection. However, the differences in health related QOL outcomes following SRS, observation, and microsurgical resection are small.[110]

Long term QoL in patients with VS < than 3 cm in diameter was higher in those having gross total resection (GTR) than those with less than GTR despite having similar rates of facial nerve and hearing preservation. This may be due to psychological factors. Notwithstanding, functional preservation should be prioritized.

References

[1] Bosman FT, Jaffe ES, Lakhani SR, et al. World Health Organization Classification of Tumors series, vol. 6. In: WHO Classification of Tumors Editorial Board (ed.) World Health Organization classification of tumors of the central nervous system. 5th ed. Lyon, France: International Agency for Research on Cancer; 2021

[2] Miettinen MM, Antonescu CR, Fletcher CDM, et al. Histopathologic evaluation of atypical neurofibromatous tumors and their transformation into malignant peripheral nerve sheath tumor in patients with neurofibromatosis 1-a consensus overview. Hum Pathol. 2017; 67:1–10

[3] Higham CS, Dombi E, Rogiers A, et al. The characteristics of 76 atypical neurofibromas as precursors to neurofibromatosis 1 associated malignant peripheral nerve sheath tumors. Neuro Oncol. 2018; 20:818–825

[4] Pemov A, Li H, Patidar R, et al. The primacy of NF1 loss as the driver of tumorigenesis in neurofibromatosis type 1-associated plexiform neurofibromas. Oncogene. 2017; 36:3168–3177

[5] Emory TS, Scheithauer BW, Hirose T, et al. Intraneural perineurioma. A clonal neoplasm associated with abnormalities of chromosome 22. American Journal of Clinical Pathology. 1995; 103:696–704

[6] Torres-Mora J, Dry S, Li X, et al. Malignant melanotic schwannian tumor: a clinicopathologic, immunohistochemical, and gene expression profiling study of 40 cases, with a proposal for the reclassification of "melanotic schwannoma". Am J Surg Pathol. 2014; 38:94–105

[7] Evans DG, Huson SM, Birch JM. Malignant peripheral nerve sheath tumors in inherited disease. Clin Sarcoma Res. 2012; 2. DOI: 10.1186/2045-3329-2-17

[8] PDQ Pediatric Treatment Editorial Board. Childhood Soft Tissue Sarcoma Treatment (PDQ®): Health Professional Version. Bethesda, MD 2022

45

[9] Foley KM, Woodruff JM, Ellis FT, et al. Radiation-induced malignant and atypical peripheral nerve sheath tumors. Ann Neurol. 1980; 7:311–318

[10] Le Guellec S, Decouvelaere AV, Filleron T, et al. Malignant Peripheral Nerve Sheath Tumor Is a Challenging Diagnosis: A Systematic Pathology Review, Immunohistochemistry, and Molecular Analysis in 160 Patients From the French Sarcoma Group Database. Am J Surg Pathol. 2016; 40:896–908

[11] Nagarjun MN, Savardekar AR, Kishore K, et al. Apoplectic presentation of a cauda equina paraganglioma. Surg Neurol Int. 2016; 7. DOI: 10.4103/2152-7806.180093

[12] Rahimizadeh A, Ahmadi SA, Koshki AM, et al. Paraganglioma of the filum terminal: Case report and review of the literature. Int J Surg Case Rep. 2021; 78:103–109

[13] National Institutes of Health Consensus Development Conference. Acoustic Neuroma: Consensus Statement. Bethesda, MD 1991

[14] Eldridge R, Parry D. Summary: Vestibular Schwannoma (Acoustic Neuroma) Consensus Development Conference. Neurosurgery. 1992; 30:962–964

[15] Harner SG, Laws ER. Clinical Findings in Patients with Acoustic Neuromas. Mayo Clin Proc. 1983; 58:721–728

[16] Ostrom QT, Cioffi G, Waite K, et al. CBTRUS Statistical Report: Primary Brain and Other Central Nervous System Tumors Diagnosed in the United States in 2014-2018. Neuro Oncol. 2021; 23:iii1–iii105

[17] Stangerup SE, Caye-Thomasen P, Tos M, et al. The natural history of vestibular schwannoma. Otol Neurotol. 2006; 27:547–552

[18] Marinelli JP, Grossardt BR, Lohse CM, et al. Is Improved Detection of Vestibular Schwannoma Leading to Overtreatment of the Disease? Otol Neurotol. 2019; 40:847–850

[19] Marinelli JP, Beeler CJ, Carlson ML, et al. Global Incidence of Sporadic Vestibular Schwannoma: A Systematic Review. Otolaryngol Head Neck Surg. 2022; 167:209–214

[20] Matthies C, Samii M. Management of 1000 vestibular schwannomas (acoustic neuromas): clinical presentation. Neurosurgery. 1997; 40:1–9; discussion 9-10

[21] Carlson ML, Tveiten OV, Driscoll CL, et al. Long-term dizziness handicap in patients with vestibular schwannoma: a multicenter cross-sectional study. Otolaryngol Head Neck Surg. 2014; 151:1028–1037

[22] Sweeney AD, Carlson ML, Shepard NT, et al. Congress of Neurological Surgeons Systematic Review and Evidence-Based Guidelines for Patients With Vestibular Schwannomas. Neurosurgery. 2018; 82: E29–E31

[23] Edvardsson Rasmussen J, Laurell G, Rask-Andersen H, et al. The proteome of perilymph in patients with vestibular schwannoma. A possibility to identify biomarkers for tumor associated hearing loss? PLoS One. 2018; 13. DOI: 10.1371/journal.pone.0198442

[24] Dilwali S, Landegger LD, Soares VY, et al. Secreted Factors from Human Vestibular Schwannomas Can Cause Cochlear Damage. Sci Rep. 2015; 5. DOI: 10.1038/srep18599

[25] Jaffe B. Clinical Studies in Sudden Deafness. Adv Otorhinolaryngol. 1973; 20:221–228

[26] Rauch SD. Clinical practice. Idiopathic sudden sensorineural hearing loss. N Engl J Med. 2008; 359:833–840

[27] Byl FM,Jr. Sudden hearing loss: eight years' experience and suggested prognostic table. Laryngoscope. 1984; 94:647–661

[28] Berenholz LP, Eriksen C, Hirsh FA. Recovery From Repeated Sudden Hearing Loss With Corticosteroid Use in the Presence of an Acoustic Neuroma. Ann Otol Rhinol Laryngol. 1992; 101:827–831

[29] Awad Z, Huins C, Pothier DD. Antivirals for idiopathic sudden sensorineural hearing loss.

Cochrane Database Syst Rev. 2012. DOI: 10.1002/14651858.CD006987.pub2

[30] Chandrasekhar SS, Tsai Do BS, Schwartz SR, et al. Clinical Practice Guideline: Sudden Hearing Loss (Update) Executive Summary. Otolaryngol Head Neck Surg. 2019; 161:195–210

[31] Tarlov EC. Microsurgical Vestibular Nerve Section for Intractable Meniere's Disease. Clin Neurosurg. 1985; 33:667–684

[32] House WF, Brackmann DE. Facial Nerve Grading System. Otolaryngol Head Neck Surg. 1985; 93:184–193

[33] Koos WT, Day JD, Matula C, et al. Neurotopographic considerations in the microsurgical treatment of small acoustic neurinomas. J Neurosurg. 1998; 88:506–512

[34] Hardy DG, Macfarlane R, Baguley D, et al. Surgery for Acoustic Neurinoma: An Analysis of 100 Translabyrinthine Operations. J Neurosurg. 1989; 71:799–804

[35] Daniels RL, Swallow C, Shelton C, et al. Causes of unilateral sensorineural hearing loss screened by high-resolution fast spin echo magnetic resonance imaging: review of 1,070 consecutive cases. American Journal of Otology. 2000; 21:173–180

[36] Committee on Hearing and Equilibrium of the American Academy of Otolaryngology-Head and Neck Surgery Foundation. Guidelines for the evaluation of hearing preservation in acoustic neuroma (vestibular schwannoma). Otolaryngol Head Neck Surg. 1995; 113:179–180

[37] Gardner G, Robertson JH. Hearing Preservation in Unilateral Acoustic Neuroma Surgery. Ann Otol Rhinol Laryngol. 1988; 97:55–66

[38] Silverstein H, McDaniel A, Norrell H, et al. Hearing Preservation After Acoustic Neuroma Surgery with Intraoperative Direct Eighth Cranial Nerve Monitoring: Part II. A Classification of Results. Otolaryngol Head Neck Surg. 1986; 95

[39] Stangerup SE, Caye-Thomasen P, Tos M, et al. Change in hearing during 'wait and scan' management of patients with vestibular schwannoma. Journal of Laryngology and Otology. 2008; 122:673–681

[40] Murofushi T, Matsuzaki M, Mizuno M. Vestibular evoked myogenic potentials in patients with acoustic neuromas. Archives of Otolaryngology – Head and Neck Surgery. 1998; 124:509–512

[41] Dunn IF, Bi WL, Mukundan S, et al. Congress of Neurological Surgeons Systematic Review and Evidence-Based Guidelines on the Role of Imaging in the Diagnosis and Management of Patients With Vestibular Schwannomas. Neurosurgery. 2018; 82: E32–E34

[42] Heller RS, Joud H, Flores-Milan G, et al. Changing Enhancement Pattern and Tumor Volume of Vestibular Schwannomas After Subtotal Resection. World Neurosurg. 2021; 151:e466–e471

[43] Pathapati D, Barla K, Dayal M, et al. Facial Nerve Schwannoma: The Rare/Great Mimicker of Vestibular Schwannoma/Neuroma. Indian J Radiol Imaging. 2021; 31:510–513

[44] Latack JT, Gabrielsen TO, Knake JE, et al. Facial nerve neuromas: radiologic evaluation. Radiology. 1983; 149:731–739

[45] Sataloff RT, Frattali MA, Myers DL. Intracranial facial neuromas: total tumor removal with facial nerve preservation: a new surgical technique. Ear Nose Throat J. 1995; 74:244–6, 248-56

[46] Copeland WR, Hoover JM, Morris JM, et al. Use of preoperative MRI to predict vestibular schwannoma intraoperative consistency and facial nerve outcome. J Neurol Surg B Skull Base. 2013; 74:347–350

[47] Mindermann T, Schlegel I. Grading of vestibular schwannomas and corresponding tumor volumes: ramifications for radiosurgery. Acta Neurochir (Wien). 2013; 155:71–4; discussion 74

[48] Germano IM, Sheehan J, Parish J, et al. Congress of Neurological Surgeons Systematic Review and Evidence-Based Guidelines on the Role of Radiosurgery and Radiation Therapy in the Management of

Patients With Vestibular Schwannomas. Neurosurgery. 2018; 82:E49–E51

[49] Bederson JB, von Ammon K, Wichmann WW, et al. Conservative Treatment of Patients with Acoustic Tumors. Neurosurgery. 1991; 28:646–651

[50] Khandalavala KR, Saba ES, Kocharyan A, et al. Hearing Preservation in Observed Sporadic Vestibular Schwannoma: A Systematic Review. Otol Neurotol. 2022; 43:604–610

[51] Caye-Thomasen P, Dethloff T, Hansen S, et al. Hearing in patients with intracanalicular vestibular schwannomas. Audiology and Neuro-Otology. 2007; 12:1–12

[52] Carlson ML, Link MJ, Driscoll CLW, et al. Working Toward Consensus on Sporadic Vestibular Schwannoma Care: A Modified Delphi Study. Otol Neurotol. 2020; 41:e1360–e1371

[53] Carlson ML, Vivas EX, McCracken DJ, et al. Congress of Neurological Surgeons Systematic Review and Evidence-Based Guidelines on Hearing Preservation Outcomes in Patients With Sporadic Vestibular Schwannomas. Neurosurgery. 2018; 82:E35–E39

[54] Asthagiri AR, Parry DM, Butman JA, et al. Neurofibromatosis type 2. Lancet. 2009; 373:1974–1986

[55] Samii M, Matthies C. Management of 1000 Vestibular Schwannomas (Acoustic Neuromas): Surgical Management with an Emphasis on Complications and How to Avoid Them. Neurosurgery. 1997; 40:11–23

[56] Brackmann DE, Fayad JN, Slattery WH,3rd, et al. Early proactive management of vestibular schwannomas in neurofibromatosis type 2. Neurosurgery. 2001; 49:274–80; discussion 280-3

[57] Timmer FC, Hanssens PE, van Haren AE, et al. Gamma knife radiosurgery for vestibular schwannomas: results of hearing preservation in relation to the cochlear radiation dose. Laryngoscope. 2009; 119:1076–1081

[58] Danner C, Mastrodimos B, Cueva RA. A comparison of direct eighth nerve monitoring and auditory brainstem response in hearing preservation surgery for vestibular schwannoma. Otol Neurotol. 2004; 25:826–832

[59] Yamakami I, Yoshinori H, Saeki N, et al. Hearing preservation and intraoperative auditory brainstem response and cochlear nerve compound action potential monitoring in the removal of small acoustic neurinoma via the retrosigmoid approach. Journal of Neurology, Neurosurgery, and Psychiatry. 2009; 80:218–227

[60] Wang AC, Chinn SB, Than KD, et al. Durability of hearing preservation after microsurgical treatment of vestibular schwannoma using the middle cranial fossa approach. J Neurosurg. 2013; 119:131–138

[61] Samii M, Gerganov V, Samii A. Improved preservation of hearing and facial nerve function in vestibular schwannoma surgery via the retrosigmoid approach in a series of 200 patients. Journal of Neurosurgery. 2006; 105:527–535

[62] Patni AH, Kartush JM. Staged resection of large acoustic neuromas. Otolaryngology - Head and Neck Surgery. 2005; 132:11–19

[63] Lobato-Polo J, Kondziolka D, Zorro O, et al. Gamma knife radiosurgery in younger patients with vestibular schwannomas. Neurosurgery. 2009; 65:294–300; discussion 300-1

[64] Roche PH, Ribeiro T, Khalil M, et al. Recurrence of vestibular schwannomas after surgery. Prog Neurol Surg. 2008; 21:89–92

[65] Marston AP, Jacob JT, Carlson ML, et al. Pretreatment growth rate as a predictor of tumor control following Gamma Knife radiosurgery for sporadic vestibular schwannoma. J Neurosurg. 2017; 127:380–387

[66] Hadjipanayis CG, Carlson ML, Link MJ, et al. Congress of Neurological Surgeons Systematic Review and Evidence-Based Guidelines on Surgical Resection for the Treatment of Patients With Vestibular Schwannomas. Neurosurgery. 2018; 82:E40–E43

[67] Van Gompel JJ, Patel J, Danner C, et al. Acoustic neuroma observation associated with an increase in symptomatic tinnitus: results of the 2007-2008 Acoustic Neuroma Association survey. J Neurosurg. 2013; 119:864–868

[68] Vivas EX, Carlson ML, Neff BA, et al. Congress of Neurological Surgeons Systematic Review and Evidence-Based Guidelines on Intraoperative Cranial Nerve Monitoring in Vestibular Schwannoma Surgery. Neurosurgery. 2018; 82:E44–E46

[69] Pitts LH, Jackler RK. Treatment of Acoustic Neuromas. New England Journal of Medicine. 1998; 339:1471–1473

[70] Ojemann RG. Microsurgical Suboccipital Approach to Cerebellopontine Angle Tumors. Clin Neurosurg. 1978; 25:461–479

[71] Porter RG, LaRouere MJ, Kartush JM, et al. Improved facial nerve outcomes using an evolving treatment method for large acoustic neuromas. Otol Neurotol. 2013; 34:304–310

[72] Rhoton AL,Jr. The cerebellopontine angle and posterior fossa cranial nerves by the retrosigmoid approach. Neurosurgery. 2000; 47:S93–129

[73] Ebersold MJ, Harner SG, Beatty CW, et al. Current Results of the Retrosigmoid Approach to Acoustic Neurinoma. J Neurosurg. 1992; 76:901–909

[74] Tatagiba M, Samii M, Matthies C, et al. The Significance for Postoperative Hearing of Preserving the Labyrinth in Acoustic Neurinoma Surgery. Journal of Neurosurgery. 1992; 77:677–684

[75] Youmans JR. Neurological Surgery. Philadelphia 1990

[76] Rhoton AL. Microsurgical Anatomy of the Brainstem Surface Facing an Acoustic Neuroma. Surg Neurol. 1986; 25:326–339

[77] Van Gompel JJ, Agazzi S, Carlson ML, et al. Congress of Neurological Surgeons Systematic Review and Evidence-Based Guidelines on Emerging Therapies for the Treatment of Patients With Vestibular Schwannomas. Neurosurgery. 2018; 82:E52–E54

[78] Nutik SL, Korol HW. Cerebrospinal Fluid Leak After Acoustic Neuroma Surgery. Surgical Neurology. 1995; 43:553–557

[79] Symon L, Pell MF. Cerebrospinal Fluid Rhinorrhea Following Acoustic Neurinoma Surgery: Technical Note. J Neurosurg. 1991; 74:152–153

[80] Ojemann RG. Management of Acoustic Neuromas (Vestibular Schwannomas). Clinical Neurosurgery. 1993; 40:498–539

[81] Sekhar LN, Gormely WB, Wright DC. The Best Treatment for Vestibular Schwannoma (Acoustic Neuroma): Microsurgery or Radiosurgery? Am J Otol. 1996; 17:676–689

[82] Wiegand DA, Fickel V. Acoustic Neuromas. The Patient's Perspective. Subjective Assessment of Symptoms, Diagnosis, Therapy, and Outcome in 541 Patients. Laryngoscope. 1989; 99:179–187

[83] Gormley WB, Sekhar LN, Wright DC, et al. Acoustic Neuroma: Results of Current Surgical Management. Neurosurgery. 1997; 41:50–60

[84] Wilkins RH, Rengachary SS. Neurosurgery. New York 1985

[85] Flickinger JC, Kondziolka D, Pollock BE, et al. Evolution in Technique for Vestibular Schwannoma Radiosurgery and Effect on Outcome. International Journal of Radiation Oncology and Biological Physics. 1996; 36:275–280

[86] Samii M, Gerganov VM, Samii A. Functional outcome after complete surgical removal of giant vestibular schwannomas. J Neurosurg. 2010; 112:860–867

[87] Pollock BE, Driscoll CL, Foote RL, et al. Patient outcomes after vestibular schwannoma management: a prospective comparison of microsurgical resection and stereotactic radiosurgery. Neurosurgery. 2006; 59:77–85; discussion 77-85

[88] Glasscock ME, Hays JW, Minor LB, et al. Preservation of Hearing in Surgery for Acoustic Neuromas. Journal of Neurosurgery. 1993; 78:864–870

[89] Ojemann RG, Levine RA, Montgomery WM, et al. Use of Intraoperative Auditory Evoked Potentials to Preserve Hearing in Unilateral Acoustic Neuroma Removal. J Neurosurg. 1984; 61:938–948

[90] Brackmann DE, House JRIII, Hitselberger WE. Technical Modifications to the Middle Cranial Fossa

45

45

Approach in Removal of Acoustic Neuromas. Los Angeles, CA 1993

[91] Pollock BE, Lunsford LD, Flickinger JC, et al. Vestibular Schwannoma Management. Part I. Failed Microsurgery and the Role of Delayed Stereotactic Radiosurgery. Journal of Neurosurgery. 1998; 89:944–948

[92] Shelton C, House WF. Hearing Improvement After Acoustic Tumor Removal. Otolaryngol Head Neck Surg. 1990; 103:963–965

[93] Hirsch A, Norén G. Audiological Findings After Stereotactic Radiosurgery in Acoustic Neuromas. Acta Otolaryngol (Stockh). 1988; 106:244–251

[94] Flickinger JC, Lunsford LD, Coffey RJ, et al. Radiosurgery of Acoustic Neurinomas. Cancer. 1991; 67:345–353

[95] Selch MT, Pedroso A, Lee SP, et al. Stereotactic radiotherapy for the treatment of acoustic neuromas. J Neurosurg. 2004; 101:362–372

[96] Pollock BE, Lunsford LD, Kondziolka D, et al. Outcome Analysis of Acoustic Neuroma Management: A Comparison of Microsurgery and Stereotactic Radiosurgery. Neurosurgery. 1995; 36:215–229

[97] Wallner KE, Sheline GE, Pitts LH, et al. Efficacy of Irradiation for Incompletely Excised Acoustic Neurilemomas. Journal of Neurosurgery. 1987; 67:858–863

[98] Noren G, Hirsch A, Mosskin M. Long-Term Efficacy of Gamma Knife Radiosurgery in Vestibular Schwannomas. Acta Neurochirurgica. 1993; 122

[99] Linskey ME, Lunsford LD, Flickinger JC. Neuroimaging of Acoustic Nerve Sheath Tumors After Stereotactic Radiosurgery. American Journal of Neuroradiology. 1991; 12:1165–1175

[100] Pollock BE, Lunsford LD, Kondziolka D, et al. Vestibular Schwannoma Management. Part II. Failed Radiosurgery and the Role of Delayed Microsurgery. Journal of Neurosurgery. 1998; 89:949–955

[101] Slattery WH, Brackmann DE. Results of Surgery Following Stereotactic Irradiation for Acoustic Neuromas. Am J Otol. 1995; 16:315–321

[102] Wiet RJ, Micco AG, Bauer GP. Complications of the Gamma Knife. Arch Otolaryngol Head Neck Surg. 1996; 122:414–416

[103] Yakulis R, Manack L, Murphy AI. Postradiation Malignant Triton Tumor: A Case Report and Review of the Literature. Arch Pathol Lab Med. 1996; 120:541–548

[104] Comey CH, McLaughlin MR, Jho HD, et al. Death From a Malignant Cerebellopontine Angle Triton Tumor Despite Stereotactic Radiosurgery. Journal of Neurosurgery. 1998; 89:653–658

[105] Lustig LR, Jackler RK, Lanser MJ. Radiation-Induced Tumors of the Temporal Bone. Am J Otol. 1997; 18:230–235

[106] Hasegawa T, Kida Y, Kato T, et al. Long-term safety and efficacy of stereotactic radiosurgery for vestibular schwannomas: evaluation of 440 patients more than 10 years after treatment with Gamma Knife surgery. J Neurosurg. 2013; 118:557–565

[107] Beatty CW, Ebersold MJ, Harner SG. Residual and Recurrent Acoustic Neuromas. Laryngoscope. 1987; 97:1168–1171

[108] Huang MJ, Kano H, Mousavi SH, et al. Stereotactic radiosurgery for recurrent vestibular schwannoma after previous resection. J Neurosurg. 2017; 126:1506–1513

[109] Carlson ML, Tombers NM, Kerezoudis P, et al. Quality of Life Within the First 6 Months of Vestibular Schwannoma Diagnosis With Implications for Patient Counseling. Otol Neurotol. 2018. DOI: 10.1097/mao.0000000000001999

[110] Carlson ML, Tveiten OV, Driscoll CL, et al. Long-term quality of life in patients with vestibular schwannoma: an international multicenter cross-sectional study comparing microsurgery, stereotactic radiosurgery, observation, and nontumor controls. J Neurosurg. 2015; 122:833–842

46 Meningiomas (Intracranial)

46.1 General information

Meningiomas are a group of tumors that are believed to originate in meningothelial cells of the arachnoid membrane. They may be intracranial (the most common location), intraorbital, or intraspinal (p.981).

46.2 Meningioma tumor types

46.2.1 Meningioma (WHO grade 1, 2 or 3)

General information

46

Key concepts

- slow growing, extra-axial tumor, usually benign, arise from arachnoid (not dura)
- imaging (MRI or CT): classically broad-based attachment on dura often with dural tail, typically enhance densely, hyperostosis of adjacent bone is common
- MRI: isointense on T1WI, hypointense on T2WI
- 32% of incidentally discovered meningiomas do not grow over 3 years follow-up
- surgical indications: documented growth on serial imaging, symptoms referable to the lesion that are not satisfactorily controlled medically, edema (low density on CT, high signal on T2 MRI) changes in adjacent brain
- most (but not all) are cured if completely removed, which is not always possible
- most commonly located along falx, convexity, or sphenoid bone
- frequently calcified: classic histological finding with this are psammoma bodies

Meningiomas are the most common primary intracranial tumors in adults, representing 36.4% of CNS tumors.[1] They comprise 54.5% of non-malignant tumors.[2] They are usually slow growing, circumscribed (non-infiltrating), benign lesions. About 10% are histologically malignant and/or rapidly growing. Meningiomas arise from arachnoid cap cells (meningothelial cells) of the arachnoid layer (not dura). They can be multiple in up to 8% of cases,[3] which is more common in neurofibromatosis. Occasionally meningiomas form a diffuse sheet of tumor (**meningioma en plaque**).

They may occur anywhere that arachnoid cells are found (between brain and skull, within ventricles, intraorbital, and along the spinal cord). Ectopic meningiomas may arise within the bone of the skull (primary intraosseous meningiomas)[4] and others occur in the subcutaneous tissue with no attachment to the skull.

They are characteristically slow growing. Most are asymptomatic (see below).

Psammoma bodies (from the Greek word for sand) are common in some meningioma subtypes, as well as in other tumors, e.g., prolactinomas, schwannomas, papillary thyroid carcinoma... and some non-neoplastic conditions. They are round, microscopic calcified structures having a concentric laminated (onion-like) appearance. The calcification may be dystrophic, or possibly a tumoricidal defense mechanism.[5] They are eosinophilic, and stain positive for CEA and PAS.

Diagnostic criteria for meningioma

Diagnostic criteria for meningioma are shown in ► Fig. 46.1.[6]

Subtypes

See reference.[6]

There is a wide variety of histological morphology among meningiomas, leading to the 15 subtypes delineatd below. The most common ones are meningothelial, fibrous and transitional. Aggressiveness can vary within each subtype (p.805), but most are benign WHO CNS5 grade 1. However, the chordoid and clear cell subtypes have been assigned grade 2 because of a higher recurrence rate irrespective of the grading criteria discussed in the following section. Most, but not all, rhabdoid meningiomas are considered grade 3.

46

Meningioma

▷ **ESSENTIAL** * ◁

classic histopathological features matching at least one of the meningioma subtypes

OR

suggestive histopathological features combined with biallelic inactivation of *NF2* or other classic drivers of conventional meningioma (*TRAF7, AKT1, KLF4, SMO, PIK3CA*), clear cell meningioma (*SMARCE1*), or rhabdoid meningioma (*BAP1*)

OR

suggestive histopathological features combined with one of the defined DNA methylation classes of meningioma

▷ **DESIRABLE** ◁

► meningeal localization
► EMA immunoreactivity
► strong and diffuse SSTR2A immunoreactivity
► classic copy-number alterations of *NF2*-mutant meningioma, such as monosomy 22/22q in lower-grade meningiomas, with additional losses of 1p, 6, 10q, 14q, and/or 18 in higher-grade meningiomas

* diagnosis frequently requires matching of several criteria

Fig. 46.1 Diagnostic criteria for meningioma. (Modified with permission from WHO Classification of Tumors Editorial Board, (ed.) World Health Organization classification of tumors of the central nervous system. 5th ed. Bosman F T, Jaffe E S, Lakhani S R, et al. (series eds.): World Health Organization Classification of Tumors series, vol. 6. International Agency for Research on Cancer, Lyon, France, 2021.)

- **meningothelial meningioma:** syncytia-like lobules of epitheliod cells with some nuclei appearing to have holes and pseudoinclusions. May resemble arachnoid cap cells, which may mimic meningothelial hyperplasia which can be seen adjacent to other tumors, e.g., optic gliomas. Whorls and psammoma bodies are less frequent than in fibrous, transitional, and psammomatous subtypes. More common at the skull base than other subtypes
- **fibrous meningioma:** parallel, storiform, or interlacing fascicles of spindle cells in a collagen-rich matrix. Often found over the convexities. Consistency is more rubbery than meningothelial or transitional
- **transitional meningioma:** contains meningothelial and fibrous morphology as well as transitional features. Whorls and psammoma bodies are frequent. Often found over the convexities
- **psammomatous meningioma:** psammoma bodies predominate over meningioma cells (which may be hard to find), and can overlap to form large calcified masses. Often arises in the thoracic spine of middle-aged to elderly women
- **angiomatous meningioma:** small, often hyalinized blood vessels predominate over meningioma cells (which may be hard to find). Angiomatous areas may be scattered in regions consistent with microcystic or metaplastic subtypes, and can manifest nuclear atypia which meets one of the criteria for a higher grade (see next section). Hypervascular specimens may resemble hemangioblastoma. Often produce cerebral edema out of proportion to their size
- **microcystic meningioma:** cells with thin, elongated processes create microcysts with a cobweb-like background. These microcysts may form radiologically identifiable macrocysts. Most are

benign, but degenerative nuclear atypia meets one of the criteria for a higher grade (see next section). Often produce cerebral edema out of proportion to their size

* **secretory meningioma:** foci of cells with gland-like epithelial differentiation and psammoma bodies. Often produce cerebral edema out of proportion to their size
* **lymphoplasmacyte-rich meningioma:** rare. Mengothelial cells are often dominated by chronic inflammatory infiltrates, which may mimic inflammatory conditions having meningothelial hyperplasia
* **metaplastic meningioma:** focal or diffuse mesenchymal features (including one or more of osseous, cartilaginous, lipomatous, myxoid and xanthomatous tissue) which are of unknown clinical signficance. Features may overlap with angiomatous or microcystic subtypes. Ossification may mimic bone invasion or psammoma bodies of the psammomatous subtype
* **chordoid meningioma** (WHO grade 2): cords or trabeculae of small epitheliod cells in a mucin-rich matrix may resembles a chordoma. Chronic inflammatory infiltrates may be prominent. Typically large supratentorial tumors, with a younger average age of presentation (45 years). A high recurrence rate comparable to aytpical meningiomas has caused assignment of WHO grade 2 to these tumors independent of morphology
* **clear cell meningioma** (WHO grade 2): round to polygonal cells with clear, glycogen-rich cytoplasm and prominent PAS-positive staining embedded in perivascular and interstitial collagen arranged in a patternless or sheet architecture. The collagen may coalesce into large acellular structures. Whorls and psammoma bodies are infrequent. Predilection for the CPA and spine (especially the cauda equina) with a young average age (24 years). A high rate of recurrence and CSF seeding has caused assignment of WHO grade 2 to these tumors independent of morphology
* **rhabdoid meningioma:** defined by the identification of rhabdoid cells (plump cells with eccentric nuclei, open chromatin, macronuclei and conspicuous eosinophilis paranuclear inclusions or whorls or waxy spheres). Rhabdoid features alone may be seen in tumors behaving as WHO grade 1 or 2[7]; however, most are highly proliferative and have other malignant features, which together with a high recurrence and mortality rate supports the designation of WHO grade 3 for most, and justifies close follow-up for all. There may be overlap of histologic and genetic features with the papillary subtype
* **papillary meningioma:** defined by a predominant pattern of thin-walled vessels in a perivascular pseudorosette (pseudopapillary) pattern. These tumors have been reported in children and adults, and are commonly associated with peritumoral edema and bony hyperostosis or lysis. Invasion of brain parenchyma and metastases (primarily to lung) are associated with the papillary growth pattern, but in the absence of other higher grade features, focal papillary growth is insufficient for grade 2 or 3 designation
* **atypical meningioma** (WHO grade 2): a meningioma of intermediate grade with features delineated in ▶ Fig. 46.2, which includes elevated mitotic activity and parenchymal brain invasion (extension along Virchow-Robin spaces does not violate the pia and does not qualify as invasion). Nuclear atypia alone is inadequate to classify as grade 2 as it is often degenerative in nature and does not correlate with outcome. Associated with: male gender, non-skull base location and previous surgery. Recurrence rate is higher following GTR than with grade 1 meningiomas, with further elevation in the presence of bone invasion
* **anaplastic (malignant) meningioma** (WHO grade 3): a meningioma that meets grading criteria shown in ▶ Fig. 46.3, often exhibiting extensive necrosis and potential for brain parenchymal invasion. Comprise 1-3% of meningiomas. Loss of H3 p.K28me3 occurs in 10-20% of anaplastic meningiomas and corelates with shorter OS

Grading meningiomas

Grading criteria for Grade 2 meningiomas is shown in ▶ Fig. 46.2, and for Grade 3 meningiomas in ▶ Fig. 46.3.[6]

These criteria can be applied across all meningioma subtypes, but the CNS WHO grade 2 criteria must be met for a diagnosis of atypical meningioma, and the CNS WHO grade 3 criteria must be met for a diagnosis of anaplastic (malignant) meningioma.

▶ **Proliferation index.** Due to variation between institutions and observers, it is advised that proliferation indices (e.g., Ki-67 or MIB-1 (p. 632)) not be used as the sole discriminant for grading. However, these indices do correlate with prognosis (see ▶ Table 46.1).

Presentation

Symptoms from mass efect or peritumoral edema depend on the location of the tumor. Some specific locations are associated with well-described symptom complexes (see below).

46

> ▷ **Meningioma WHO Grade 2** ◁
>
> 4 to 19 mitotic figures in 10 consecutive HPF of each 0.16 mm^2 (at least 2.5/mm^2)
>
> **OR**
>
> unequivocal brain invasion (not only perivascular spread or indentation of brain without pial breach)
>
> **OR**
>
> specific morphological subtype (chordoid or clear cell; see text)
>
> **OR**
>
> at least 3 of the following:
> - increased cellularity
> - small cells with high N:C ratio
> - prominent nucleoli
> - sheeting (uninterrupted patternless or sheet-like growth)
> - foci of spontaneous (non-iatrogenic) necrosis

Fig. 46.2 Grading criteria for WHO Grade 2 meningioma.

> ▷ **Meningioma WHO Grade 3** ◁
>
> 20 or more mitotic figures in 10 consecutive HPF of each 0.16 mm^2 (at least 12.5/mm^2)
>
> **OR**
>
> frank anaplasia (sarcoma-, carcinoma-, or melanoma-like appearance)
>
> **OR**
>
> *TERT* promoter mutation
>
> **OR**
>
> homozygous deletion of *CDKN2A* and/or *CDKN2B*

Fig. 46.3 Grading criteria for WHO Grade 3 meningioma.

Table 46.1 Ki-67 proliferation index and recurrence rates in meningiomas[8a]

Description & WHO grade	Mean Ki-67 index[a]	Recurrence rate
common meningioma (WHO grade 1)	0.7%	9%
atypical meningioma (WHO grade 2)	2.1%	29%
anaplastic meningioma (WHO grade 3)	11%	50%

[a]not to be used as sole discriminant for grading (see text)

Seizures may occur with supratentorial meningiomas as a result of irritation of the cerebral cortex. Occasionally patients may feel a mass under their scalp with convexity tumors that invade the bone.

Asymptomatic meningiomas

Meningiomas are the most common primary intracranial tumors, and most remain asymptomatic throughout the patient's life.[9] The routine use of CT and MRI for numerous indications inevitably results in the discovery of incidental (asymptomatic) meningiomas. In a population-based study (the study population was middle class Caucasians and result, may not be generalizable to other demographic groups),[9] incidental meningiomas were seen in 0.9% of MRIs. In another series, 32% of primary brain tumors seen on imaging studies were meningiomas, and 39% of these were asymptomatic.[10] Of 63 cases followed for > 1 year with nonsurgical management, 68% showed no increase in size over an average follow-up of 36.6 mos, whereas 32% increased in size over 28 mos average follow-up.[10] Asymptomatic meningiomas with calcification seen on CT and/or hypointensity on T2WI MRI appeared to have a slower growth rate.[10]

Common locations

▶ Table 46.2 lists common locations. Other locations include: CP angle, clivus, planum sphenoidale and foramen magnum. ≈ 60–70% occur along the falx (including parasagittal), along sphenoid bone (including tuberculum sellae), or over the convexity. Childhood meningiomas are rare, 28% are intraventricular, and the posterior fossa is also a common site. Details on some of these appear in the sections that follow.

Table 46.2 Location of adult meningiomas (series of 336 cases[11])

Location	%
parasagittal	20.8
convexity	15.2
tuberculum sellae	12.8
sphenoidal ridge	11.9
olfactory groove	9.8
falx	8.0
lateral ventricle (intraventricular)	4.2
tentorial	3.6
middle fossa	3.0
orbital	1.2
spinal	1.2
intrasylvian	0.3
extracalvarial	0.3
multiple	0.9

Sphenoid wing (or ridge) meningiomas

Three basic categories[12]:

1. lateral sphenoid wing (or pterional): behavior and treatment are usually similar to convexity meningioma
2. middle third (or alar)
3. medial (clinoidal): tend to encase the ICA and the MCA as well as cranial nerves in the region of the superior orbital fissure and the optic nerve. May compress brainstem. Total removal is often not possible

46

Olfactory groove meningiomas

Presentation: usually asymptomatic until they are large. Findings may include:

1. Foster Kennedy syndrome (p. 100): can occur when the tumor is asymmetrically situated to one side. Anosmia (patient is usually unaware of this), ipsilateral optic atrophy, contralateral papilledema (from increased ICP)
2. mental status changes: often with frontal lobe findings (apathy, abulia...) mimicking dementia
3. urinary incontinence
4. posteriorly located lesions may compress the optic apparatus causing visual impairment
5. large lesions may compress the fornix and cause short-term memory loss
6. seizure

The morbidity, mortality, and difficulty in achieving total removal increase significantly for tumors > 3 cm in size.[13]

Pre-op MRA, CTA or angiogram may be helpful to assess location of anterior cerebral arteries relative to the tumor. 70–80% of these get the majority of their blood supply from the anterior ethmoidal artery, which is usually not embolized due to risk to ophthalmic artery (and blindness). If there are substantial middle meningeal feeders, these may be embolized, but the benefit tends to be small.

Paarasagittal and falx meningiomas

▶ Fig. 46.4 shows an example of a parafalcine meningioma (PFM).

PFM are grouped based on their location along the AP direction of the SSS as:

- anterior (ethmoidal plate to coronal suture): 44% (in a series of 75 parasagittal meningiomas[14]). Most often present with H/A and mental status changes
- middle (between noncoronal and lambdoidal sutures): 33%. Most often present as Jacksonian seizure and progressive monoplegia. At the level of the motor strip, a common initial is contralateral foot drop (see ▶ Fig. 1.3 for location of "ankle" area on motor strip)[15]

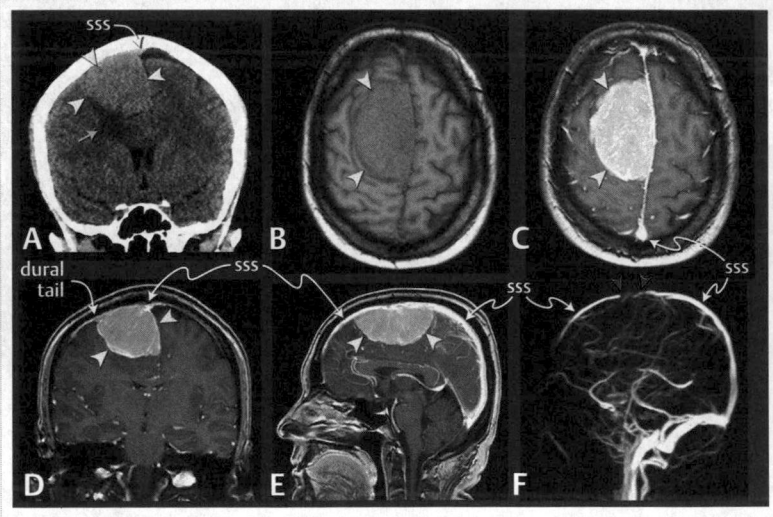

Fig. 46.4 Parafalcine meningioma (*yellow arrowheads*).
Sample images from a 49-year-old woman with a grade 2 (atypical) meningioma presenting with headache and left-sided weakness.
Image: A: coronal noncontrast brain window CT scan. *Blue arrow* denotes edema in the adjacent brain tissue.
B: axial T1 MRI without contrast, C: axial T1 MRI with contrast.
D: coronal T1 MRI with contrast. Note the dural tail which is characteristic of meningioma (but not pathognomonic, nor necessary to diagnose).
E: sagittal T1 MRI with contrast.
F: sagittal contrast MRV. Note the lack of opacification of the superior sagittal sinus between the two *red arrowheads* which is located within the borders of the tumor.
Abreviations: sss = superior sagittal sinus.

- posterior (lambdoidal suture to torcular Herophili): 23%. Most often present with H/A, visual symptoms, focal seizures, or mental status changes

Up to 50% of PFM invade the superior sagittal sinus (SSS). Classification systems for the extent of SSS invasion includes the one by Sindou et al[16] (▶ Fig. 46.5).

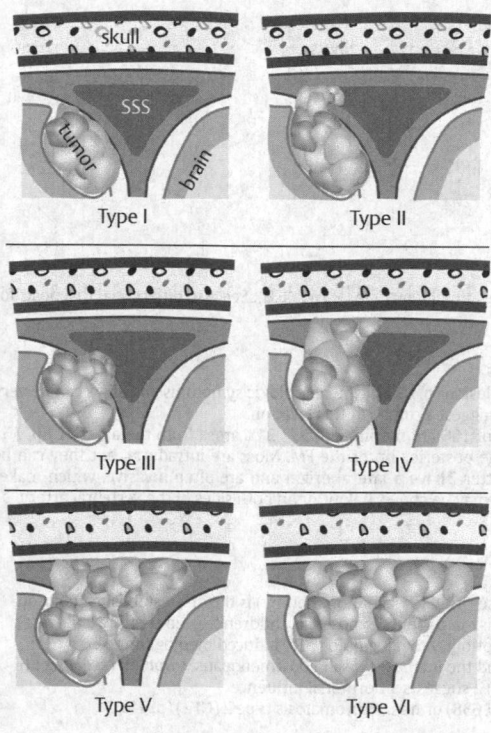

Type I

Type II

Type III

Type IV

Type V

Type VI

Fig. 46.5 Sindou grading system for meningioma invasion of the superior sagittal sinus.
(Modified from Sindou MP, et al. J Neurosurg. 2006;105:514–525.)
Image: schematic coronal sections through the superior sagittal sinus (SSS).
Type I = attachment to lateral wall of sinus.
Type II = invasion of lateral recess.
Type III = invasion of lateral wall.
Type IV = invasion of lateral wall and roof.
Type V = total sinus occlusion, contralateral wall spared.
Type VI = total sinus occlusion, invasion of all walls.

46

Planum sphenoidale meningiomas

These uncommon meningiomas arise from the flat horizontal portion of the sphenoid bone (▶ Fig. 46.6) anterior to the chiasmatic sulcus (the depression in the posterior part of the anterior cranial fossa where the optic chiasm perches). An example is shown in ▶ Fig. 46.7. With large meningiomas arising from the floor of the frontal fossa, it may not be possible to differentiate planum sphenoidale from olfactory groove meningiomas.

Tuberculum sellae meningiomas (TSM)

The site of origin of these tumors is only about 2 cm posterior to that of olfactory groove meningiomas.[13] The tuberculum sellae is the bony elevation between the chiasmatic sulcus and the sella turcica (see ▶ Fig. 46.6). By definition, the limbus sphenoidale (which is the anterior margin of the chiasmatic sulcus) is the demarcation between the anterior and middle cranial fossa. Therefore these tumors originate in the middle fossa (unlike planum sphenoidale meningiomas which are in the anterior fossa).

TSMs are notorious for producing visual loss (chiasmal syndrome = primary optic atrophy + bitemporal hemianopsia; see ▶ Fig. 33.2). When a TSM grows posteriorly into the sella turcica it may be mistaken for a pituitary macroadenoma (see ▶ Fig. 99.3 for MRI and differentiating features).

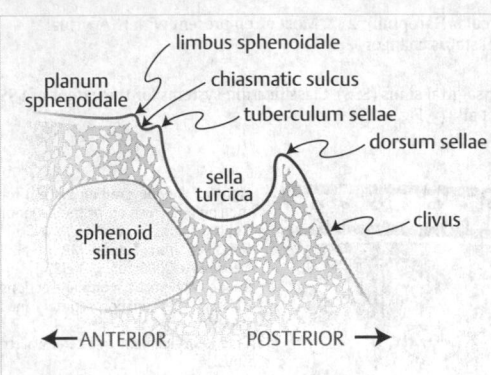

Fig. 46.6 Anatomic locations of planum sphenoidale and tuberculum sellae. The olfactory groove (not shown) is located in the floor of the frontal fossa immediately anterior to the planum sphenoidale.
Image: schematic sagittal section through the sella turcica.

Intraventricular meningiomas

Most are located in the atrium of the lateral ventricle (▶ Fig. 46.8). See also differential diagnosis for intraventricular lesions (p. 1667).

Foramen magnum meningiomas

As with any foramen magnum (FM) lesion (p. 1649); the neurologic symptoms and signs can be very confusing and often do not initially suggest a tumor in this location.

In the French Cooperative Study of 106 FM meningiomas,[17] 31% arose from the anterior lip, 56% were lateral, and 13% arose from the posterior lip of the FM. Most are intradural, but they can be extradural or a combination (the latter 2 have a lateral origin and are often invasive, which makes total removal more difficult).[18] They may be above, below, or on both sides of the vertebral artery.[18]

Epidemiology

▶ **Risk factors**
- ionizing radiation (typically in doses used for radiation therapy) is the only established environmental risk factor,[19] with higher risk in patients exposed as children (e.g., in treating leukemia). There appears to be genetic susceptibility to developing XRT induced meningiomas[20]
- the higher incidence in females and the increased risk in postmenopausal women receiving hormonal replacement therapy (HRT)[21] suggests a hormonal influence
- neurofibromatosis type 1 (NF1) (p. 638) or neurofibromatosis type 2 (NF2) (p. 640)

▶ **Genetics.** 50-60% of WHO grade 1 meningiomas have mutations of the NF2 tumor suppressor gene on chromosome 22q12.2 (which codes for merlin (p. 640)).[22]

Genetic mutations tend to be location dependent: convexity meningiomas and most spinal meningiomas harbor a 22q deletion and/or *NF2* mutation, skull base lesions carry *AKT1*, *TRAF7*, *SMO* and/or *PIK3CA* mutations.

▶ **General epidemiology.** As many as 3% of autopsies on patients > 60 yrs of age reveal a meningioma.[23] Meningiomas account for 39% of primary intracranial neoplasms and 54.5% of non-malignant tumors in the U.S.[2] Incidence peaks at 45 years of age. The median age at diagnosis is 65 years, and the risk increases with age (from an incidence of 1.49/100,000 for ages 20-34 years, to 57.29 for age > 85).[2] Female:male ratio is 2.3:1 in the U.S.[2]

Meningiomas comprise 1.7% of primary brain & CNS tumors in patients age 0-14 years, and 4.6% for ages 15-19 years.[2] 19-24% of adolescent meningiomas occur in patients with neurofibromatosis type I (von Recklinghausen's).

Evaluation

See "Imaging" below for specific findings.

Brain MRI, without and with contrast, is the diagnostic study of choice.

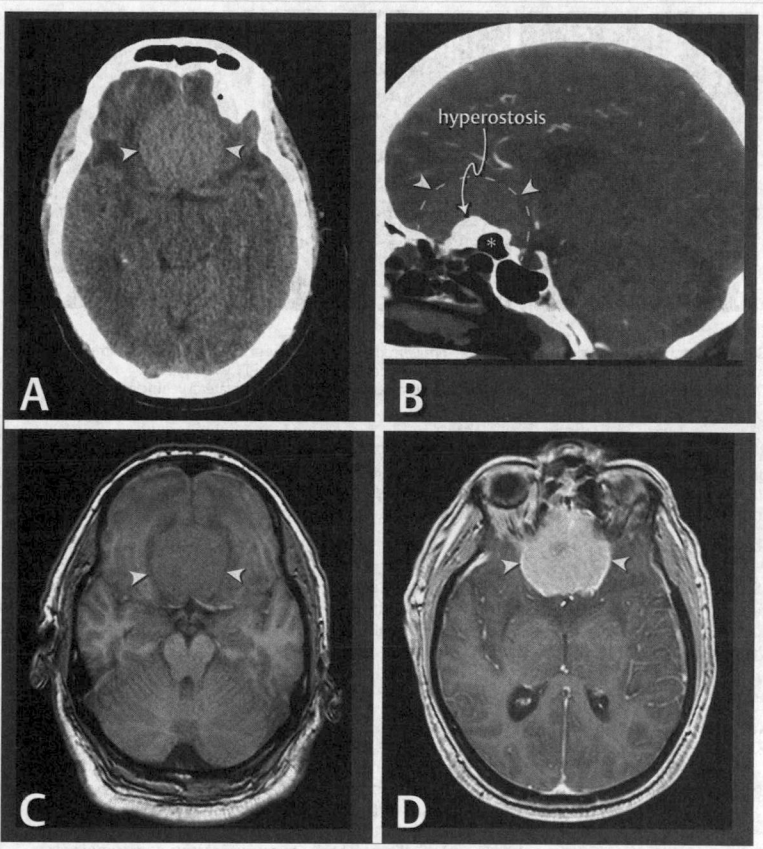

Fig. 46.7 Planum sphenoidal meningioma (*yellow arrowheads*).
Image: A: axial noncontrast CT scan. The tumor is visible although close to brain in density.
B: sagittal CTA. The tumor is barely visible, and has been outlined by a *broken blue line*. Note the hyperostosis of bone at the base of the tumor which is common with meningiomas. There is also enlargement of the underlying air sinus (*yellow asterisk* *), a condition that is termed pneumosinus dilitans.
C: axial noncontrast T1 MRI, and D: axial contrast T1 MRI.

CT without and with contrast scan is second choice when MRI cannot be done, and may also be considered when the identification of calcifications or reactive bone changes is considered crucial, or sometimes for surgical planning.

Angiography may be considered when more definitive assessment of dural sinus occlusion is desired, or to determine if pre-op embolization is a viable intervention.

In questionable cases, a metastatic workup (p.914) might be considered to rule out that possibility.

Imaging

CT

(See below for characteristic findings shared between CT and MRI). Without contrast, meningiomas are typically homogeneous, isodense or slightly hyperdense to brain on CT (▶ Fig. 46.4 panel A).

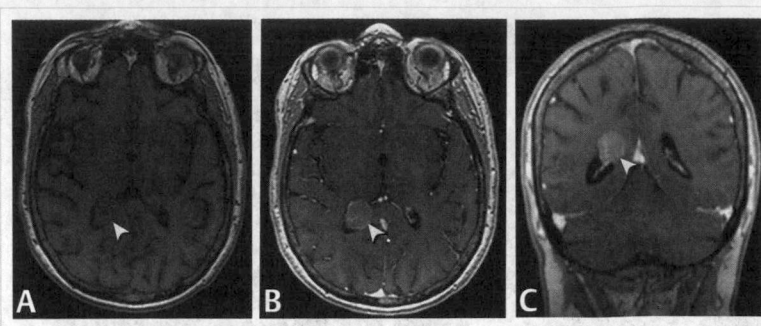

Fig. 46.8 Intraventricular meningioma (*yellow arrowheads*) in the atrium of the right lateral ventricle.
Image: MRI, A: axial T1 without contrast, B: axial T1 with contrast, C: coronal T1 with contrast.
The patient presented with entrapped occipital and temporal horns of the right lateral ventricle.

20-30% have areas of calcification (better appreciated on CT than MRI). Non-contrast Hounsfield numbers of 60–70 in a meningioma usually correlate with presence of psammomatous calcifications (p. 803). On CT, prostate cancer may mimic meningioma (prostate mets to brain are rare, but prostate frequently goes to bone, and may go to skull and can cause hyperostosis).

MRI
(See below for characteristic findings shared between CT and MRI). Meningiomas may be isointense to brain on T1 or T2 images (making them difficult to visualize) but most enhance with gadolinium. Calcifications appear as signal voids on MRI. MRI gives information regarding patency of dural venous sinuses (accuracy in predicting sinus involvement is ≈ 90%[24]).

Characteristic findings on CT or MRI
1. **broad base of attachment** to the meninges
2. **dural tail:** enhancing extension along the dura where the tumor attaches to the meninges
   (▶ Fig. 46.4 panel D) (this is not pathognomonic and can also occur with a lower incidence in many conditions such as pleomorphic xanthoastrocytoma (PXA), Rosai-Dorfman disease, plasmacytoma…). The dural tail may be comprised of tumor itself, reactive fibrovascular tissue, and to a limited extent and in only ≈ one third of cases, tumor infiltration of the dura[25]
3. **hyperostosis** (or sometimes blistering) of adjacent bone is very suggestive of meningioma
   (▶ Fig. 46.7 panel B). Usually better appreciated on CT than MRI
4. **edema** of the adjacent brain may be minimal or may be marked especially in certain meningioma subtypes (secretory, angiomatous/microcystic, lymphoplasmacyte-rich, and high-grade meningiomas).[26] Significant edema may be considered to be a criteria for surgical excision (p. 813). Intraventricular meningiomas: 50% produce extraventricular edema
5. **enhancement:** meningiomas usually enhance densely and uniformly, although there may be cystic areas and/or areas of calcification that do not enhance

Angiography
Classic pattern: appears early in arterial phase, blush persists beyond venous phase ("comes early, stays late"). The distinctive prolonged homogeneous tumor blush can also help confirm the diagnosis.
   Meningiomas characteristically have *external* carotid artery feeders. Some notable exceptions that feed from the ICA:
1. low frontal median meningiomas (e.g., olfactory groove): feed from ethmoidal branches of the ophthalmic artery
2. suprasellar meningiomas: may also be fed by large branches of the ophthalmic arteries
3. parasellar meningiomas: tend to feed from the ICA. Secondary vascular supply may be derived from pial branches of the anterior, middle, and posterior cerebral arteries
4. petroclival meningiomas: supplied via the artery of the tentorium (a branch of the meningohypophyseal trunk) AKA the **artery of Bernasconi & Cassinari** (the so-called "Italian" artery) which is enlarged in lesions involving tentorium (e.g., tentorial meningiomas)

Angiography also gives information about occlusion of dural venous sinuses, especially for parasagittal/falx meningiomas (may be more accurate than MRI for this). Oblique views are often best for evaluating patency of the superior sagittal sinus (SSS). Angiography also provides an opportunity for pre-op embolization (p.815) (see below).

Plain X-rays
May show: calcifications within the tumor (in ≈ 10%), hyperostosis or blistering of the skull (including floor of frontal fossa with olfactory groove meningiomas), enlargement of vascular grooves (especially middle meningeal artery). Most of these findings are better appreciated on bone window CT scan.

Differential diagnosis/diagnostic considerations of meningioma

1. pleomorphic xanthoastrocytoma (PXA) (p.698): may mimic meningiomas since they tend to be peripherally located and may have a dural tail
2. solitary fibrous tumor (▶ Fig. 47.2): (formerly hemangiopericytoma) a rapidly growing tumor
3. gliosarcomas (p.665), especially ones that are predominantly carcomatous
4. Rosai-Dorfman disease: especially if extracranial lesions are also identified. A connective tissue disorder with sinus histiocytosis and massive painless lymphadenopathy (most have cervical lymphadenopathy). Usually in young adults. Isolated intracranial involvement is rare. MRI: dural-based enhancing mass with signal characteristics similar to meningioma, may have dural tail. Most common intracranial locations: cerebral convexities, parasagittal, suprasellar, cavernous sinus. Pathology: dense fibrocollagenous connective tissue with spindle cells and lymphocytic infiltration, stains for CD68 & S-100. Histiocytic proliferation without malignancy. Foamy histiocytes are characteristic. Surgery and immunosuppressive therapy not effective. Low-dose XRT may be the best option
5. NB: multiple meningiomas suggests the possibility of neurofibromatosis 2 (p.640) (NF2)

Treatment in general

Indications for treatment
Treatment is indicated for meningiomas with any of the following:
1. symptoms that cannot be satisfactorily controlled medically (e.g., refractory seizures)
2. significant growth on serial imaging studies (see ▶ Table 46.3 for what may constitute "significant growth")
3. more than minimal edema on imaging

"**Significant growth**": the definition is controversial. Proposed criteria includes any of those shown in ▶ Table 46.3

Table 46.3 Various proposed criteria for "significant growth" of meningiomas

- 2-5 mm increase in diameter over 1 year[27]*
- 1 cc increase in volume in 1 year[28]
- or 15% increase in volume over 1 year[29]

* the concern with using a linear measurement such as diameter is that the volume of a sphere is proportional to the cube of the radius, so for a small tumor a small change in diameter results in a small increase in volume, but for a large tumor the increase in volume with even a small increase in diameter can be substantial

▶ **Asymptomatic meningiomas.** Data is lacking to make evidence-based management guidelines. Incidental meningiomas with no brain edema or those presenting only with seizures that are easily controlled medically may be managed expectantly with serial imaging as meningiomas tend to grow slowly, and some may "burn out" and cease growing.

A suggestion is to obtain a follow-up imaging study 3–4 months after the initial study to rule out rapid progression (often indicating a higher grade meningioma or other lesion), and then if growth is not significant (see ▶ Table 46.3), repeat annually for at least 2–3 years. If stable, follow-up studies could be spaced out further. Treatment would be recommended for significant growth. The development of symptoms should prompt performing a study at the time of the symptoms.

"**High-risk meningiomas**" (atypical meningiomas, rhabdoid meningiomas, malignant meningiomas, and any meningioma with a high proliferation index) tend to have higher growth rates.

Treatment options

Surgery is the treatment of choice for accessible meningiomas meeting indications for treatment (see above) in patients who are surgical candidates. The perioperative morbidity rate is statistically significantly higher in patients > 70 years old (23%) than in those < 70 (3.5%).[10] See below for details.

Radiation therapy is used most often as adjuvant therapy after surgery for some cases of tumor recurrence or incomplete resection (see post-op radiation (p. 814)). Use as a primary therapy might occasionally be considered for patients who are not surgical candidates or for some deep inaccessible tumors.

MRI-guided **laser interstitial thermal therapy** (LITT): early experience with recurrent meningiomas shows potential, demonstrating early (first few weeks) increase in tumor volume with a subsequent decrease at 3 months and subsequent re-growth in some,[30] requiring further study. This may be a consideration for patients needing treatment when surgery is not a consideration and when maximal XRT has already been given.

Focused ultrasound (FUS) may become a non-invasive adjuvant therapy option for some deep situated tumors. Superficially located meningiomas (especially convexity meningiomas) are generally not candidates for transcranial FUS due to the inability to focus the ultrasound beams near the convexity of the skull.

Radiation therapy (XRT)

▶ **As primary treatment.** Generally regarded as ineffective as primary modality of treatment. Also, due to long-term risks of XRT, it is usually avoided for "benign" lesions (WHO grade 1) if there are other effective options. Primary XRT may be considered for symptomatic or progressive tumors if the risks of surgical resection (including risks of patients who are poor surgical candidate) outweigh the benefits.

▶ **Post-op XRT.** Efficacy of XRT in preventing recurrence is controversial—see box for suggestions.

A retrospective series of 135 non-malignant meningiomas followed 5–15 years post-op at UCSF revealed a recurrence rate of 4% with total resection, 60% for partial resection without XRT, and 32% for partial resection with XRT.[31] Mean time to recurrence was longer in the XRT group (125 mos) than in the non-XRT group (66 mos). These results suggest that XRT may be beneficial in partially resected meningiomas. Alternatively, one can follow these patients with CT or MRI and use XRT for documented progression if repeat surgery is not desired.

Atypical meningioma (WHO grade 2): there are no large prospective studies. Retrospective and/ or small studies suggest a nonsignificant trend towards longer PFS with post op XRT, but no difference in OS.

Σ: Post-op XRT suggestions (these are not guidelines)

WHO grade 1 meningiomas: post-op XRT is not recommended even with subtotal resection unless there is progressive growth on follow-up imaging and repeat surgery is not viable (e.g., risky tumor location, poor medical condition...) or desired by patient and surgeon.

Post-op XRT is suggested for **high-risk meningiomas** defined as[32]:
1. anaplastic (WHO grade 3) regardless of extent of resection
2. new atypical meningiomas (WHO grade 2) with *subtotal* resection (Simpson grade ▶ Table 46.4 IV - V)
3. recurrent atypical meningiomas regardless of extent of resection

New atypical meningiomas (WHO grade 2) with gross total resection (Simpson grade ▶ Table 46.4 I - III): patient may be followed and then treated with XRT for recurrence.

Dosing for anaplastic or atypical meningioma: fractionated therapy to a dose of 55–60 Gy.

In addition to the usual side effects of XRT—see Radiation injury and necrosis (p. 1899)—there is a risk of radiation-induced tumors such as astrocytomas.[33]

Surgical treatment for meningiomas

General information

Surgical goals: complete resection when possible, with removal of involved meninges and bone when feasible. The Simpson grading system for extent of meningioma resection is shown in ▶ Table 46.4.

Table 46.4 Simpson grading system for removal of meningiomas[50]

Grade	Degree of removal	Recurrence rate (%)
I	macroscopically complete removal with excision of dural attachment and abnormal bone (including sinus resection when involved)	9
II	macroscopically complete with endothermy coagulation (electrocautery or laser) of dural attachment	19
III	macroscopically complete without resection or coagulation of dural attachment or of its extradural extensions (e.g., hyperostotic bone)	29
IV	partial removal leaving tumor in situ	44
V	simple decompression (± biopsy)	N/A

Meningiomas are often very bloody. Preoperative embolization may be helpful for specific tumors (see below). Pre-op autologous blood donation may also be a consideration.

General principles of meningioma surgery[34]:
1. early interruption of the arterial blood supply to the tumor: unfortunately, the blood supply is often on the deep aspect of the tumor and may be difficult to access early in the resection
2. to avoid excessive retraction on the brain, a common technique consists of
   a) internal decompression (debulking) of the tumor using ultrasonic aspirator, cautery loops…
   b) followed by collapsing the tumor capsule into the area of decompression and dissectiing the capsule from the brain by cutting and coagulating vascular and arachnoid attachments
3. removal of attached bone and dura when possible

Pre-op tumor embolization: Reduces the vascularity of these often bloody tumors, facilitating surgical removal. Timing of subsequent surgery is controversial. Some advocate waiting 7–10 days to permit tumor necrosis, which simplifies resection.[35,36] Complications include: hemorrhage (intratumoral and SAH), cranial nerve deficits (usually transient), stroke from embolization through ICA or VA anastomoses, scalp necrosis, retinal embolus, and potentially dangerous tumor swelling. Many meningiomas are not readily amenable to embolization (e.g., olfactory groove meningioma).

Position
As usual, the head should be elevated ≈ 30° above the right atrium.

For meningiomas involving the superior sagittal sinus (SSS)[37]:
- for tumors involving the anterior third of the SSS: supine semi-sitting position
- for tumors of the middle third of the SSS: lateral position with the side of the tumor *down*, the neck tilted 45° toward the upward shoulder
- for tumors of the posterior third of the SSS: prone position

Sinus involvement

Greenberg IMHO

Due to unappreciated venous drainage (see text), attempting to occlude or bypass the middle third of the superior sagittal sinus involved with meningioma is treacherous. Even in expert hands, there is significant risk of venous infarction/sinus occlusion with 8% morbidity and 3% mortality,[16] and complete removal is still not assured.[38] Rather than risking venous infarctions, it is almost always preferable to leave residual tumor and follow with serial imaging (especially for WHO grade 1 meningiomas, and with some grade 2 lesions (p. 814)) and consider treating with repeat surgery or radiation therapy as appropriate.

Alternatives for treatment of dural sinus involvement include:

▶ **Superior sagittal sinus (SSS).** If the tumor occludes the SSS, it has been suggested that the sinus can be resected carefully, preserving veins draining into the patent portions of the sinus. ✖ However, this should be undertaken under advisement since patients still not infrequently develop venous infarcts, probably as a result of loss of venous drainage of even minimal sinus flow, venous channels in the dura adjacent to the sinus, through the skin or bone of the skull, and even the tumor itself may participate. Before ligating the sinus, the lumen should be inspected for a tail of tumor within the sinus.

46

Partial occlusion of superior sagittal sinus:
1. anterior to the coronal suture, the sinus may usually be divided safely
2. posterior to the coronal suture (or, perhaps more accurately, posterior to the vein of Trolard), it must not be divided or else severe venous infarction will occur
   a) with superficial involvement (Type I, ▶ Fig. 46.5), tumor may be dissected off the sinus with care to preserve patency
   b) with extensive involvement:
      • sinus reconstruction: hazardous. Thrombosis rate using venous graft approaches 50%, and is close to 100% with artificial grafts (e.g., Gore-Tex) which should *not* be used
      • it may be best to leave residual tumor, and follow with CT or MRI. If the residual tumor grows, or if the Ki-67 score is high (p.805), SRS may be used; SRS (p.1903) may also be used as initial treatment for tumors that are < 2.3–3 cm diameter

▶ **Transverse sinus (TS).** A patent dominant TS must not be suddenly occluded.

Convexity meningiomas

NB: the tumor capsule of convexity meningiomas that straddle the Sylvian fissure may be adherent to branched of the middle meningeal artery and must be carefully dissected off of the tumor to avoid damage to them.

The craniotomy should be large enough (ideally 1-2 cm beyond the tumor attachment) to permit excising the invaded dura adjacent to the point of tumor attachment. Dura directly involved with the tumor must be resected, and an autograft (e.g., fascia lata or periosetum from an uninvolved location) or allograft will be required.

▶ **Dural tail.** The dural tail is infrequently comprised of dura invaded by tumor (p.812), and it is not always necessary to remove it all. Current practice is generally to excise as much of the dural tail as is reasonably possible without chasing it for long distances.

▶ **Bone involvement. Hyperostosis** of bone adjacent to a meningioma: occurs in 5-44%.[39] Various pathologic mechanisms have been invoked,[40] and only in some cases is frank tumor invasion present. MRI often shows increased T2 signal extending beyond the limits of hyperostosis. The hyperostotic bone can usually be drilled off the surface of the bone flap which may then be replaced.

Bone invasion: if extensive, the bone flap may have to be discarded and replaced with a cranioplasty (at the time of surgery, e.g., using titanium mesh, or at a later date). Alternatively, the invaded bone may be excised from the center of the flap and the resultant defect is often significantly smaller than the flap and is more easily patched, and the patched flap can then be reimplanted.

A study in which bone biopsies were taken 2 cm outside the hyperostotic margin were negative for tumor in all 12 cases of grade 1 & 2 meningiomas (even where there was increased signal on T2 MRI), whereas in the 2 cases of grade 3 meningioma all biopsies were positive.[41]

Sphenoid wing, parasagittal, or falx meningiomas (general principles)

Once tumor is exposed a partial internal debulking is performed. Then the point of attachment (to the falx or sphenoid bone) is peeled away using bipolar cautery to divide feeding vessels. Then the main portion of the tumor may be separated from the brain, with the tumor being avascular once the vascular pedicle has been transected.

Parasagittal and falx meningiomas

The inferior portion of the tumor may adhere to branches of the anterior cerebral artery. Middle or posterior third tumors are exposed using a horseshoe incision based in the direction of the major scalp feeding vessels. Alternatively, the patient may be placed in a lateral position, or the sitting position may be used with Doppler monitoring for air embolism (p.1738). Anterior third tumors are approached using a bicoronal skin incision with the patient supine. For tumors that cross the midline, burr holes are placed to straddle the SSS. For managing superior sagittal sinus involvement, see above.

Since these tumors are often debulked from the inside, removal tends to be bloodier than meningiomas that can be removed in 1 piece. The ability to embolize these tumors pre-op is somewhat limited, but may be an adjunct. For tumors involving the convexity dura, cut through tumor leaving a thin layer on dura. Then remove the now relatively avascular part that impresses the brain. Then make an incision through the dura near the tumor; it tends to be bloody, but once you have control of both sides of the dura you can begin to excise the dura around the tumor (you may need to leave a cuff on SSS if it is involved).

Sphenoid wing meningiomas

A pterional craniotomy (p. 1748) is utilized. The neck is extended to allow gravity to retract the brain off of the floor of the skull.

Lateral sphenoid wing meningiomas: The approach to these tumors is often similar to convexity meningiomas. The height of the skin incision and bone opening should be high enough to encompass the tumor.

Medial sphenoid wing meningiomas: A lumbar drain is used. The head is turned 30° off the vertical. Aggressive extradural removal of sphenoid wing is performed. An FTOZ approach may provide additional exposure. The Sylvian fissure is split widely. The ICA and MCA are often encased by tumor (look for the appearance of "grooves" on the surface of the tumor on MRI, which indicates vessels, e.g., MCA). To locate the ICA, identify MCA branches and follow them proximally into the tumor. The optic nerve is best identified at the optic canal. Avoid excessive retraction of the optic apparatus. The deep portion of the tumor often has numerous small parasitic vessels from the ICA (which makes this part very bloody), and may also invade the lateral wall of the cavernous sinus (which creates risk of cranial nerve deficits with attempted removal). Therefore, the recommendation is to leave some tumor behind and use radiosurgery to deal with it.

46

Olfactory groove meningiomas

Approached via a bifrontal craniotomy (preserving the periosteum to cover the frontal air sinus and floor of frontal fossa at the end of the case). Small tumors may be approached via unilateral craniotomy on the side with the most tumor.[42(p 3284)] For large tumors, a lumbar CSF drain will help with brain relaxation[13] and the head is rotated 20° to one side to facilitate dissection of the anterior cerebral arteries and optic nerve while preserving visualization of both sides of the tumor involvement.[43] The neck is slightly extended. The dura is opened low, and the superior sagittal sinus is ligated and divided at this location. Amputation of the frontal pole should be done if necessary to avoid excessive retraction. Vascular feeding arteries come through the floor of the frontal fossa in the midline. Initially, the anterior tumor capsule is opened and the tumor debulked from within, heading towards the floor of the frontal fossa to interrupt the blood supply. The posterior capsule of the tumor is dissected carefully as this portion of the tumor may encase branches of the anterior cerebral artery, and/or optic nerves and chiasm. A large tumor with suprasellar extension usually displaces the optic nerve and chiasm *inferiorly*.[13] If necessary, the frontopolar branch and other small branches may be sacrificed without problem.[44] Periosteum is laid over the floor of the frontal fossa. To hold it in place, one may attempt to suture it to the adjacent dura with a couple of retaining sutures, alternatively a small titanium plate (e.g., "dogbone") can be placed over the flap and screws are placed into the bone of the floor of the frontal fossa (both methods are challenging). Post-op risks include CSF leak through the ethmoid sinuses.

Tuberculum sellae meningiomas

These tumors typically displace both optic nerves posteriorly and laterally.[13] Occasionally, the nerves are completely engulfed by tumor.

Cerebellopontine angle meningiomas

Usually arise from the meninges covering the petrous bone. May be divided into those that occur anterior to, and those that occur posterior to the IAC.

Foramen magnum meningiomas

Tumors arising from the posterior or posterolateral lip of the foramen magnum (FM) are removed relatively easily. Anterior and lateral FM tumors may be operated by the posterolateral approach, and for anterior tumors,[18] a transcondylar approach may alternatively be used.[45]

With meningiomas below the vertebral artery (VA), the lower cranial nerves are displaced superiorly with the VA. However, when the tumor is above the VA, the position of the lower cranial nerves cannot be predicted.[18]

Large tumors may adhere to or encase neurovascular structures, and these should be internally debulked and then dissected free.

Posterior suboccipital approach: Used for meningiomas arising from the posterior lip of the FM or slightly posterolateral.

The patient is positioned prone or three-quarter prone. Neck flexion should be kept to a minimum to avoid brainstem compression by the tumor.[46] The surgeon must remain vigilant for the PICA and vertebral arteries, which may be encased.

Recurrence after surgery

The most powerful *histopathologic* predictor of recurrence is WHO grade, with grade 1 recurrence rate of 7-25%, grade 2 recur in 29-52%, and grade 3 in 50-94%. Some histologic subtypes are also more prone to recurrence (as noted under subtypes).

The extent of surgical tumor removal is the most important factor in the prevention of post-op recurrence. The Simpson grading system for the extent of meningioma removal is shown in ► Table 46.4. An often overlooked aspect of the Simpson grading system is that it refers exclusively to the removal of *intradural* tumor, and thus leaving the tumor e.g., in the sagittal sinus could still be considered "complete removal." Recurrence after gross total tumor removal occurred in 11–15% of cases, but was 29% when removal was incomplete (length of follow-up not specified)[11]; 5-year recurrence rates of 37%[47]-85%[48] after partial resection are also quoted. The overall recurrence rate at 20 years was 19% in one series,[49] and 50% in another.[48] Malignant meningiomas have a higher recurrence rate than benign ones.

Prognosis

5-year survival for patients with meningioma[51]: 91.3%. With anaplastic meningiomas, median survival ranges from < 2 years to > 5 years depending on completeness of removal and use of adjuvant XRT.[6]

References

[1] Achey RL, Gittleman H, Schroer J, et al. Non-malignant and malignant meningioma incidence and survival in the elderly from 2005-2015 using the Central Brain Tumor Registry of the United States. Neuro Oncol. 2018. DOI: 10.1093/neuonc/noy162

[2] Ostrom QT, Cioffi G, Waite K, et al. CBTRUS Statistical Report: Primary Brain and Other Central Nervous System Tumors Diagnosed in the United States in 2014-2018. Neuro Oncol. 2021; 23:iii1–iii105

[3] Sheehy JP, Crockard HA. Multiple Meningiomas: A Long-Term Review. J Neurosurg. 1983; 59:1–5

[4] Kulali A, Ilcayto R, Rahmanli O. Primary calvarial ectopic meningiomas. Neurochirurgia (Stuttg). 1991; 34:174–177

[5] Das DK. Psammoma body: a product of dystrophic calcification or of a biologically active process that aims at limiting the growth and spread of tumor? Diagn Cytopathol. 2009; 37:534–541

[6] Bosman FT, Jaffe ES, Lakhani SR, et al. World Health Organization Classification of Tumors series, vol. 6. In: WHO Classification of Tumors Editorial Board (ed.) World Health Organization classification of tumors of the central nervous system. 5th ed. Lyon, France: International Agency for Research on Cancer; 2021

[7] Vaubel RA, Chen SG, Raleigh DR, et al. Meningiomas With Rhabdoid Features Lacking Other Histologic Features of Malignancy: A Study of 44 Cases and Review of the Literature. J Neuropathol Exp Neurol. 2016; 75:44–52

[8] Kolles H, Niedermayer I, Schmitt C, et al. Triple approach for diagnosis and grading of meningiomas: histology, morphometry of Ki-67/Feulgen stainings, and cytogenetics. Acta Neurochir (Wien). 1995; 137:174–181

[9] Vernooij MW, Ikram A, Tanghe HL, et al. Incidental findings on brain MRI in the general population. New England Journal of Medicine. 2007; 357:1821–1828

[10] Kuratsu J-I, Kochi M, Ushio Y. Incidence and Clinical Features of Asymptomatic Meningiomas. Journal of Neurosurgery. 2000; 92:766–770

[11] Yamashita J, Handa H, Iwaki K, et al. Recurrence of Intracranial Meningiomas, with Special Reference to Radiotherapy. Surg Neurol. 1980; 14:33–40

[12] Cushing H, Eisenhardt L. Mengiomas of the Sphenoidal Ridge. A. Those of the Deep or Clinoidal Third. In: Meningiomas: Their Classification, Regional Behaviour, Life History, and Surgical End Results. Springfield, Illinois: Charles C Thomas; 1938:298–319

[13] Al-Mefty O, Sekhar LN, Janecka IP. Tuberculum Sella and Olfactory Groove Meningiomas. In: Surgery of Cranial Base Tumors. New York: Raven Press; 1993:507–519

[14] Ricci A, Di Vitantonio H, De Paulis D, et al. Parasagittal meningiomas: Our surgical experience and the reconstruction technique of the superior sagittal sinus. Surg Neurol Int. 2017; 8. DOI: 10.4103/2152-7806.198728

[15] Eskandary H, Hamzel A, Yasamy MT. Foot Drop Following Brain Lesion. Surgical Neurology. 1995; 43:89–90

[16] Sindou MP, Alvernia JE. Results of attempted radical tumor removal and venous repair in 100 consecutive meningiomas involving the major dural sinuses. J Neurosurg. 2006; 105:514–525

[17] George B, Lot G, Velut S. Tumors of the Foramen Magnum. Neuro-Chirurgie. 1993; 39:1–89

[18] George B, Lot G, Boissonnet H. Meningioma of the Foramen Magnum: A Series of 40 Cases. Surgical Neurology. 1997; 47:371–379

[19] Wiemels J, Wrensch M, Claus EB. Epidemiology and etiology of meningioma. J Neurooncol. 2010; 99:307–314

[20] Flint-Richter P, Sadetzki S. Genetic predisposition for the development of radiation-associated meningioma: an epidemiological study. Lancet Oncol. 2007; 8:403–410

[21] Andersen L, Friis S, Hallas J, et al. Hormone replacement therapy increases the risk of cranial meningioma. Eur J Cancer. 2013; 49:3303–3310

[22] Miller RJr, DeCandio ML, Dixon-Mah Y, et al. Molecular targets and treatment of meningioma. J Neurol Neurosurg. 2014; 1

[23] Nakasu S, Hirano A, Shimura T, et al. Incidental Meningiomas in Autopsy Studies. Surgical Neurology. 1987; 27:319–322

[24] Zimmerman RD, Fleming CA, Saint-Louis LA, et al. Magnetic Resonance of Meningiomas. American Journal of Neuroradiology. 1985; 6:149–157

[25] Sotoudeh H, Yazdi HR. A review on dural tail sign. World J Radiol. 2010; 2:188–192

[26] Osawa T, Tosaka M, Nagaishi M, et al. Factors affecting peritumoral brain edema in meningioma: special histological subtypes with prominently extensive edema. J Neurooncol. 2013; 111:49–57

[27] Yano S, Kuratsu JI, Demonte F, et al. Natural course of untreated meningiomas. In: Al-Mefty's Meningiomas. 2nd ed. New York: Thieme Medical Publishers, Inc.; 2011:63–67

[28] Yoneoka Y, Fujii Y, Tanaka R. Growth of incidental meningiomas. Acta Neurochir (Wien). 2000; 142:507–511

[29] Hashiba T, Hashimoto N, Izumoto S, et al. Serial volumetric assessment of the natural history and growth pattern of incidentally discovered meningiomas. J Neurosurg. 2009; 110:675–684

[30] Rammo R, Scarpace L, Nagaraja T, et al. MR-guided laser interstitial thermal therapy in the treatment of recurrent intracranial meningiomas. Lasers Surg Med. 2019; 51:245–250

[31] Barbaro NM, Gutin PH, Wilson CB, et al. Radiation Therapy in the Treatment of Partially Resected Meningiomas. Neurosurgery. 1987; 20:525–528

[32] Rogers CL, Won M, Vogelbaum MA, et al. High-risk meningioma: Initial outcomes from NRG Oncology/ RTOG 0539. Int J Radiat Oncol Biol Phys. 2020; 106:790–799

[33] Zuccarello M, Sawaya R, deCourten-Myers. Glioblastoma Occurring After Radiation Therapy for Meningioma: Case Report and Review of Literature. Neurosurgery. 1986; 19:114–119

[34] Ojemann RG. Management of Cranial and Spinal Meningiomas. Clinical Neurosurgery. 1992; 40:321–383

[35] Chun JY, McDermott MW, Lamborn KR, et al. Delayed surgical resection reduces intraoperative blood loss for embolized meningiomas. Neurosurgery. 2002; 50:1231–5; discussion 1235-7

[36] Kai Y, Hamada J, Morioka M, et al. Appropriate interval between embolization and surgery in patients with meningioma. AJNR Am J Neuroradiol. 2002; 23:139–142

[37] Colli BO, Carlotti CG. Parasagittal meningiomas. Contemporary Neurosurgery. 2007; 29:1–8

[38] Heros RC. Meningiomas involving the sinus. J Neurosurg. 2006; 105:511–513

[39] Dziuk TW, Woo S, Butler EB, et al. Malignant meningioma: an indication for initial aggressive surgery and adjuvant radiotherapy. J Neurooncol. 1998; 37:177–188

[40] Di Cristofori A, Del Bene M, Locatelli M, et al. Meningioma and Bone Hyperostosis: Expression of Bone Stimulating Factors and Review of the Literature. World Neurosurg. 2018; 115:e774–e781

[41] Fathalla H, Tawab MGA, El-Fiki A. Extent of Hyperostotic Bone Resection in Convexity Meningioma to Achieve Pathologically Free Margins. J Korean Neurosurg Soc. 2020; 63:821–826

[42] Youmans JR. Neurological Surgery. Philadelphia 1990

[43] Bogaev CA, Sekhar LN, Sekhar LN, et al. Olfactory groove and planum sphenoidale meningiomas. In: Atlas of Neurosurgical Techniques. New York: Thieme Medical Publishers, Inc.; 2006:608–617

[44] Ojemann RG, Schmidek HH, Sweet WH. Surgical Management of Olfactory Groove Meningiomas. In: Operative Neurosurgical Techniques. 3rd ed. Philadelphia: W.B. Saunders; 1995:393–401

[45] Hakuba A, Tsujimoto T, Sekhar LN, et al. Transcondyle Approach for Foramen Magnum Meningiomas. In: Surgery of Cranial Base Tumors. New York: Raven Press; 1993:671–678

[46] David CA, Spetzler R. Foramen Magnum Meningiomas. Clinical Neurosurgery. 1997; 44:467–489

[47] Mirimanoff RO, Dosoretz DE, Lingood RM, et al. Meningioma: Analysis of Recurrence and Progression Following Neurosurgical Resection. J Neurosurg. 1985; 62:18–24

[48] Adegbite AV, Khan MI, Paine KWE, et al. The Recurrence of Intracranial Meningiomas After Surgical Treatment. J Neurosurg. 1983; 58:51–56

[49] Jaaskelainen J. Seemingly complete removal of histologically benign intracranial meningioma: late recurrence rate and factors predicting recurrence in 657 patients. A multivariate analysis. Surgical Neurology. 1986; 26:461–469

[50] Simpson D. The recurrence of intracranial meningiomas after surgical treatment. J Neurol Neurosurg Psychiatry. 1957; 20:22–39

[51] Mahaley MS, Mettlin C, Natarajan N, et al. National Survey of Patterns of Care for Brain-Tumor Patients. J Neurosurg. 1989; 71:826–836

46

47 Mesenchymal, Non-meningothelial Tumors

47.1 General information

Benign and malignant mesenchymal tumors originating in the CNS are very rare and are organized using terminology and histologic features corresponding to their soft tissue and bone counterparts as outlined in the 2020 WHO Classification of Soft Tissue & Bone Tumors, 5th edition.[1]

Primary mesenchymal tumors relating to the brain and spine tend to arise in the meninges rather than in the parenchyma, and occur more often in the supratentorial compartment than in the p-fossa or spine.

47.2 Fibroblastic and myofibroblastic tumors

47.2.1 Solitary fibrous tumor (WHO grade 1, 2 or 3)

General information

A mesenchymal tumor of the fibroblastic type with genomic inversion at the 12q13 locus in most solitary lesions, producing *NAB2* and *STAT6* gene fusion and STAT6 nuclear expression, with a high chance of recurrence and metastases. Formerly included hemangiopericytomas—an obsolete term. Cells are spindle to ovoid, located amidst dilated thin-walled blood vessels. Calcifications including psammoma bodies have not been observed. There is a case report of a tumor releasing IGF-2 causing hypoglycemia.[2]

Diagnostic criteria for solitary fibrous tumor

Diagnostic criteria for solitary fibrous tumor are shown in ▶ Fig. 47.1.[3]

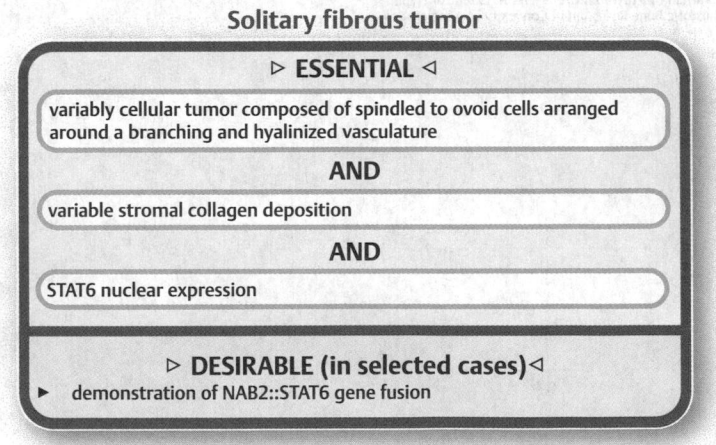

Fig. 47.1 Diagnostic criteria for solitary fibrous tumor. (Modified with permission from WHO Classification of Tumors Editorial Board, (ed.) World Health Organization classification of tumors of the central nervous system. 5th ed. Bosman F T, Jaffe E S, Lakhani S R, et al. (series eds.): World Health Organization Classification of Tumors series, vol. 6. International Agency for Research on Cancer, Lyon, France, 2021.)

Grading

The degree of mitotic activity and the presence of necrosis correlates with prognosis:
- WHO grade 1 (ICD-O 8815/0): hypocellular, collagenized tumor with a classic solitary fibrous tumor phenotype. < 2.5 mitoses/mm^2 (< 5 mitoses/10 high powered fields)

- WHO grade 2 (ICD-O 8815/1): more dense. ≥ 2.5 mitoses/mm² (≥ 5 mitoses/10 HPF)
- WHO grade 3 (ICD-O 8815/3): ≥ 2.5 mitoses/mm² (≥ 5 mitoses/10 HPF) with tumoral necrosis

Imaging

Radiographically may be mistaken for a meningioma (► Fig. 47.2).

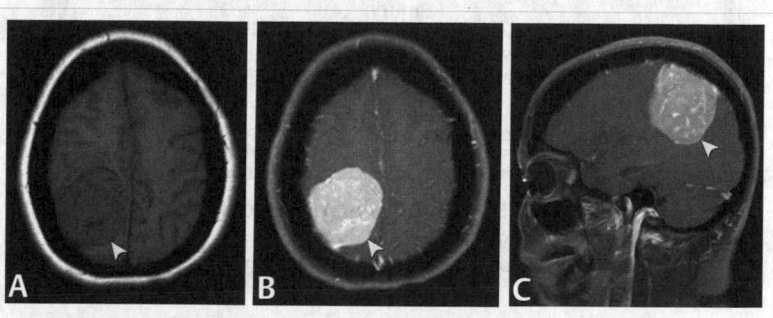

Fig. 47.2 Solitary fibrous tumor (*yellow arrowheads*), right parietal.
Image: MRI, A: T1 without contrast and B: with contrast; C: sagittal T1 with contrast. Note features that may be mistaken for meningioma: broad base of attachment, iso-intense with brain on T1 & T2 noncontrast sequences, dense enhancement with contrast.

Treatment

Surgery is the primary treatment. Grades 2 & 3 benefit from adjuvant XRT. Chemotherapy is used for metastases or for tumors failing local control measures.

Prognosis

SFTs tumors have a high rate of recurring and/or metastasizing, as late as decades after initial diagnosis. Therefore, long-term follow-up is advised. Unlike SFTs outside the CNS, advanced age does not correlate with worse outcome.

47.3 Vascular tumors

47.3.1 Hemangioma (WHO grade 1)

General information

Hemangiomas are benign neoplastic lesions with multiple closely approximated vessels lined by a single cell layer of bland endothelial cells with very rare mitoses. The vessels range in size from capillary-sized vessels (so-called **capillary hemangioma**, ICD-O 9131/0) to dilated vessels with flattened endothelial lining (so-called **cavernous hemangioma**, ICD-O 9131/0). They form lobules that are each supplied by a separate artery and separated by a fibrous septation. Hemangiomas may be solitary, multiple, or part of a *PIK3CA*-related overgrowth syndrome. Refer to details on vertebral hemangiomas (p. 992).

Diagnostic criteria for hemangioma

Diagnostic criteria for hemangioma are shown in ► Fig. 47.3.[3]

Location

Hemangiomas originate most frequently in the spine (p. 992), followed by the skull (p. 973), and uncommonly in the brain parenchyma, nerve roots and cauda equina. In the spine, there is a predilection for the thoracic and lumbar regions, and they are often multiple (p. 992).

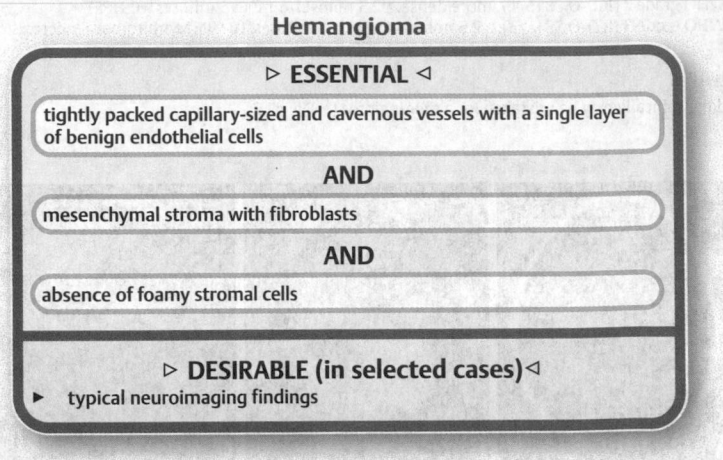

Fig. 47.3 **Diagnostic criteria for hemangioma.** (Modified with permission from WHO Classification of Tumors Editorial Board, (ed.) World Health Organization classification of tumors of the central nervous system. 5th ed. Bosman F T, Jaffe E S, Lakhani S R, et al. (series eds.): World Health Organization Classification of Tumors series, vol. 6. International Agency for Research on Cancer, Lyon, France, 2021.)

Imaging

In the spine, suggestive findings include polka-dot sign on axial images, or corduroy pattern on longitudinal images (p. 992). Calcifications are frequent, and are well demonstrated on CT.

T2-MRI shows mixed signal internally. The surrounding hemosiderin ring is low density on T2 with blooming artifact.

47.3.2 Hemangioblastoma (WHO grade 1)

General information

Key concepts

- highly vascular well-circumscribed benign solid or cystic neoplasm of CNS or retina
- the most common *primary intra-axial* tumor in the adult posterior fossa
- may occur sporadically (70%) or as part of von Hippel-Lindau disease (30%), and any patient with HGB should be screened for VHL
- on imaging, may be solid, or cystic with enhancing mural nodule (for cysts with mural nodule, surgically, the cyst wall does not need to be removed)
- ✓ CBC: may be associated with erythrocytosis (polycythemia)

Hemangioblastomas (HGB) are extremely vascular histologically benign slow growing tumors comprised of neoplastic stromal cells with clear to vacuolated cytoplasm and copious small vessels with characteristic immunohistochemical features (e.g., staining for inhibin) and molecular signatures (e.g., *VHL* laterations). They may occur sporadically or as part of von Hippel-Lindau disease (p. 646). HGBs are difficult to distinguish histologically from a renal cell carcinoma (which is common in VHL and adds to the difficulty of this differential).

Diagnostic criteria for hemangioblastoma (HGB)

Diagnostic criteria for hemangioblastoma are shown in ▶ Fig. 47.4.[3]

Hemangioblastoma

> ## ▷ ESSENTIAL ◁

a tumor composed of large, multivacuolated, and lipidized stromal cells with occasional hyperchromatic nuclei, as well as a rich capillary network

AND

stromal cells with immunohistochemical positivity for markers such as inhibin (at least focally)

OR

loss or inactivation of the VHL gene

OR

in a patient with von Hippel–Lindau syndrome

> ## ▷ DESIRABLE ◁

▶ in patients with von Hippel–Lindau syndrome, absence of immunohisto-chemical staining for markers of renal cell carcinoma

Fig. 47.4 Diagnostic criteria for hemangioblastoma. (Modified with permission from WHO Classification of Tumors Editorial Board, (ed.) World Health Organization classification of tumors of the central nervous system. 5th ed. Bosman F T, Jaffe E S, Lakhani S R, et al. (series eds.): World Health Organization Classification of Tumors series, vol. 6. International Agency for Research on Cancer, Lyon, France, 2021.)

Location

Intracranially, they occur almost exclusively in the p-fossa (hemangioblastomas are the most common *primary* intra-axial p-fossa tumor in adults). May occur in the cerebellar hemisphere, vermis, or brainstem. May also occur in the spinal cord (p.986) (1.5–2.5% of spinal cord tumors). Retinal HGB and/or angiomas occur in 6% of patients with cerebellar HGBs.

Epidemiology

HGB represent 1–2.5% of intracranial tumors. They comprise 7–12% of primary p-fossa tumors.[4]

70% of HGBs occur sporadically, but 30% occur as part of von Hippel-Lindau (VHL) disease (p.646).[5] 5–30% of cases of cerebellar HGB and 80% of spinal HGB are associated with VHL.

Sporadic cases tend to present in the 4th decade, whereas VHL cases present *earlier* (peak in 3rd decade). In sporadic cases, the HGB are solitary and originate in the cerebellum (83–95%), spinal cord (3–13%), medulla oblongata (2%)[6] or cerebrum (1.5%).[4] In 65% of patients with VHL the HGB are multiple.

Presentation

S/S of cerebellar HGB are usually those of any p-fossa mass—H/A, N/V, cerebellar findings...; see Posterior fossa (infratentorial) tumors (p.624)—and obstructive hydrocephalus may occur. HGB is rarely documented as a cause of apoplexy due to intracerebral hemorrhage (ICH) (lobar or cerebellar); however, some studies indicate that if cases of ICH are carefully examined, abnormal vessels consistent with HGB (and occasionally misidentified as AVM) may be found with surprising frequency (in spite of negative CT and/or angiography).[7]

Retinal HGBs tend to be located peripherally, and may hemorrhage and cause retinal detachment.

Erythrocytosis may be due to erythropoietin liberated by the tumor.

Histology

Invasion of adjacent neural tissue is rare. Mitotic figures are rare. No true capsule, but usually well circumscribed (narrow zone of infiltration). May be solid, or cystic with a mural nodule (70% of cerebellar lesions are cystic; nodules are very vascular, appear red, are often located near pial surface, and may be as small as 2 mm; cyst fluid is clear yellow with high protein). In cystic lesions, the cyst wall is lined with non-neoplastic compressed cerebellum. The cyst develops because the vessel walls are so thin that they leak water, and proteins don't cross as readily.

Cardinal feature: numerous capillary channels, lined by a single layer of endothelium, surrounded by reticulin fibers (stains positive with reticulin stain). Macrophages stain PAS positive.

Two main component cells:
1. stromal cells: polygonal. Characteristic and distinguishing finding: plentiful lipid laden vacuoles,
2. reactive vascular cells

Cyst patterns[8]:
1. no associated cysts: 28%
2. peritumoral cyst alone: 51%
3. intratumoral cyst: 17%
4. peritumoral AND intratumoral cysts: 4%

Evaluation

Patients with a p-fossa HGB (radiologically suspected or histologically proven) should undergo MRI of entire neuraxis because of possibility of spinal HGBs (may be distant from p-fossa lesion; may suggest possibility of VHL).

CT: solid lesions are usually isodense with intense contrast enhancement. Cystic HGBs remain low density with contrast, with the nodule enhancing.

MRI (▶ Fig. 47.5): preferable to CT due to the predilection of HGBs for the p-fossa. May show serpentine vascular signal voids, especially in the periphery of the lesion. Also, peripheral hemosiderin deposits may occur from previous hemorrhages.[4]

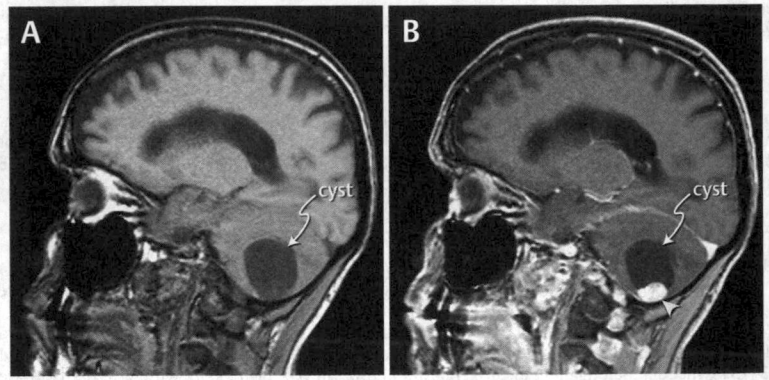

Fig. 47.5 Hemangioblastoma of the posterior fossa. Demonstrates cyst with enhancing mural nodule (*yellow arrowhead*). Image: Sagittal MRI, A: T1 noncontrast, B: T1 + contrast.

Vertebral angiography: usually demonstrates intense vascularity (most other tumors of the p-fossa are relatively avascular). May be required in HGBs where nodule is too small to be imaged on CT/MRI. 4 patterns: 1) vascular mural nodule on side of avascular cyst, 2) vascular lesion surrounding avascular cyst, 3) solid vascular mass, and 4) multiple, separate vascular nodules.

Labs: often discloses *polycythemia* (no hematopoietic foci within tumor). In cases with suggestive history, labwork to rule out catecholamine production from pheochromocytoma may be indicated; see Endocrine/laboratory studies (p. 942).

Treatment

Surgery

Surgical treatment may be curative in cases of sporadic HGB, not in VHL. GTR is considered the optimal treatment.[9]

Preoperative embolization may help reduce the vascularity.

Cystic HGBs require removal of mural nodule (otherwise, cyst will recur). The cyst wall is not removed unless there is evidence of tumor within the cyst wall on MRI (typically thick-walled cysts) or visually at the time of surgery.[8] 5-ALA fluorescence may aid in visual localization of small hemangioblastomas within the cyst wall.[10]

Solid HGBs tend to be more difficult to remove. They are treated like AVMs (avoid piecemeal removal), working along margin and devascularizing blood supply. A helpful technique is to shrink the tumor by laying a length of bipolar forceps along tumor surface and coagulating. HGBs with attachment to floor of 4th ventricle may be hazardous to remove (cardio-respiratory complications).

Multiple lesions: if ≥ 0.8–1 cm diameter: may treat as in solitary lesion. Smaller and deeper lesions may be difficult to locate at time of surgery.

Cystic brainstem HGB: the solid nodule of the tumor is removed under the microscope by bipolaring and cutting the gliotic adhesions to the parenchyma. ★ Removal of the cyst wall is not necessary. There is often a cleavage between the tumor and the floor of the fourth ventricle which facilitates tumor removal. To reduce bleeding, avoid piecemeal removal. Preserve large draining veins until the arterial feeders to the mural nodule have been isolated and resected.[11]

Radiation treatment

Effectiveness is dubious. May be useful to reduce tumor size or to retard growth, e.g., in patients who are not surgical candidates, for multiple small deep lesions, or for inoperable brainstem HGB. Does not prevent regrowth following subtotal excision.

Prognosis

Prognosis is excellent following GTR, and is better for sporadic HGB vs. those associated with VHL. No report of malignant change. May spread thru CSF after surgery, but remain benign.

Prognostic factors for *longer* OS in older patients (but not in younger patients) include: GTR vs. STR or biopsy (HR 0.62).

Prognostic factors for *shorter* OS include: age ≥ 40 years (HR 3.9), size, growth pattern, multifocality and brainstem location (vs. cerebellum) (HR 1.9).[9]

47.4 Notochordal tumors

47.4.1 Chordoma

General information

Key concepts

- primary malignant tumor, usually of clivus or sacrum, with high recurrence rate
- histology: characteristic physaliphorous cells (containing intracellular mucin)
- generally slow-growing and radioresistant
- treatment of choice: wide en bloc resection when possible (piecemeal removal carries risk of inducing metastases), proton-beam radiation may help

Rare tumors (incidence of ≈ 0.51 cases/million) of the remnant of the primitive notochord (which normally differentiates into the nucleus pulposus of the intervertebral discs). They represent less than 1% of intracranial tumors and 3% of primary spine tumors.[12]

They are slow growing, locally aggressive and osteodestructive.

47

Histologically, these tumors are considered low-grade malignancies. However, their behavior is more malignant because of the difficulty of total removal, a high recurrence rate (85% following surgery), and the fact that they metastasize (usually late) in 5–20%,[13] (often after multiple resections) typically to lung, liver, and bone. Therefore aggressive XRT is usually employed post-op. Malignant transformation into fibrosarcoma or malignant fibrous histiocytoma is rare. Four types have been identified:

1. conventional: median age: 55 years
2. chondroid: extracellular matrix resembles hyaline cartilage. Median age: 45 years
3. dedifferentiated: biphasic tumors comprised of conventional chordoma adjacent to high grade sarcoma. Nuclear and cytokeratin expression are retained in the conventional chordoma areas, but not in the sarcomatous component. Median age: 61 years
4. poorly differentiated: no physaliphorous cells. Median age: 7 years

Diagnostic criteria for chordoma

Diagnostic criteria for chordoma are shown in ▶ Fig. 47.6.[3]

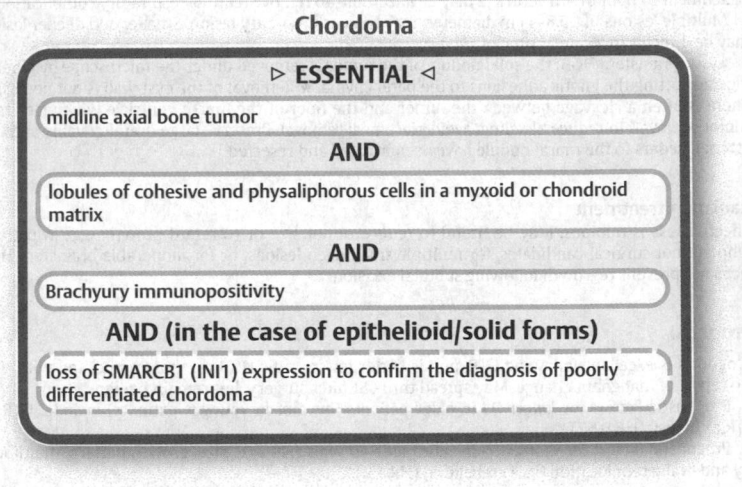

Fig. 47.6 Diagnostic criteria for chordoma. (Modified with permission from WHO Classification of Tumors Editorial Board, (ed.) World Health Organization classification of tumors of the central nervous system. 5th ed. Bosman F T, Jaffe E S, Lakhani S R, et al. (series eds.): World Health Organization Classification of Tumors series, vol. 6. International Agency for Research on Cancer, Lyon, France, 2021.)

Location

Chordomas can arise anywhere along the neuraxis where there is remnant of notochord; however, cases tend to cluster at the two ends of the primitive notochord: 35% cranially[14] in the spheno-occipital region (clivus), and 53%[14] in the spine at the sacrococcygeal region.[15] Less commonly, they may occur in the spine above the sacrum.[16]

Pathogenesis

The notochord is a flexible cartilage-like embryologic structure that requires the protein brachyury (coded for by the *TBXT* gene) to develop. In most individuals, the notochord regresses in utero and by birth has devolved into the nucleus pulposus (the center of spinal intervertebral discs). In a small number of people, remnants of the notochord persist, usually in the odontoid process or coccyx. The process of neoplastic transformation of these remnants is incompletely understood, but mutations have been identified including duplications of the *TBXT* gene in 27%.[17]

Histology

Physaliphorous cells are distinctive, vacuolated cells on histology that probably represent cytoplasmic mucus vacuoles seen ultrastructurally.

Radiographic appearance

Usually lytic, lobular midline lesions with frequent calcifications.[18]
  MRI: hypointense on T1WI, hyperintense on T2WI.
  Enhances on CT or MRI with contrast.[18] Rarely, they may appear as a sclerotic vertebra[19] ("ivory vertebra").

Cranial chordomas

Peak incidence of cranial chordomas is 50–60 years of age. These tumors are rare in patients < 30 years of age.[20] Male:female distribution is ≈ equal.
  Differential diagnosis: Primarily between other cartilaginous tumors of the skull base; see differential diagnosis of other foramen magnum region tumors (p. 1649):
1. chondrosarcomas
2. chondromas

47

Presentation: Usually produces cranial nerve palsies (usually oculomotor or abducens nerve).

Spinal chordomas

General information

Occur primarily in the sacrococcygeal region. Unlike cranial chordomas, sacrococcygeal chordomas show a male predominance,[14] and these patients tend to be older. May also arise in C2. Chordomas constitute over 50% of primary bone tumors of the sacrum. May produce pain, sphincter disturbance, or nerve root symptoms from local nerve root compression. They may occasionally extend cephalad into the lumbar spinal canal. They are usually confined anteriorly by the presacral fascia, and only rarely invades the wall of the rectum.[21] A firm fixed mass may be palpable between the rectum and the sacrum on a rectal exam.

Evaluation

Characteristic radiographic findings: centrally located destruction of several sacral segments, with an anterior soft-tissue mass that occasionally has small calcifications. CT and MRI show the bony destruction. This is usually difficult to see on plain X-rays. MRI also shows the soft-tissue mass.
  Open or CT guided percutaneous *posterior* biopsy can confirm the diagnosis. Transrectal biopsy should be avoided because of the potential of rectal spread of tumor.[22]
  Chest CT and bone scan: to R/O mets for staging purposes.

Treatment of spinal chordomas
Surgery

Wide en bloc excision with postoperative radiation is usually the best option, although this may also be only temporarily effective. Decompression is best avoided since entering the mass serves to spread tumor (surgically induced metastases) which will then regrow. Chordomas located in C2 are usually not amenable to en bloc resection.[23]
  Sacral chordomas: The particulars of the surgical procedure are highly dependent on the extent of the lesion. These tumors may spread through the gluteal musculature, and if significant muscular excision is required, then a pedicle-based rectus abdominis flap may be employed. A diverting colostomy may be required if it is necessary to resect the rectum or if a cephalic sacral resection is anticipated.[24]
  For chordomas caudal to the third sacral segment, most agree that a posterior approach is satisfactory. For more rostral lesions, some advocate a combined anterior-posterior approach. However, a posterior approach has also been used for these.[24]
  Adverse effects of sacrectomy: if S2 nerve roots are the most caudal nerve roots spared, there is ≈ 50% chance of normal bladder and bowel control.[24] If S1 or more cephalic roots are the most caudad nerve roots spared, most will have impaired bladder control and bowel problems.[24]

Radiation therapy (XRT)

Best results were obtained with en bloc excision (even if marginal), sometimes combined with high-dose XRT[16,25] (conventional XRT did not prevent recurrence when incorporated with palliative or debulking surgery,[16] but it did lengthen the interval to recurrence[25]). Early radiation was associated with longer survival.[26] Higher XRT doses can be used in the sacrococcygeal region (4500–8000 rads) than in the cervical spine (4500–5500 rads) because of concerns of radiation injury to the spinal cord. IMRT and stereotactic radiosurgery have also been used.[23]

Proton beam therapy, alone[13] or combined with high-energy X-ray (photon) therapy,[27,28] may be more effective than conventional XRT alone. However, proton beam therapy requires travel to one of a limited number of facilities with a cyclotron which may be difficult to arrange for what is typically ≈ 7 weeks of fractionated treatments.

Chemotherapy
Imatinib (Gleevec®) (a tyrosine kinase inhibitor) has some antitumor effect in chordoma.[29]

Prognosis
The prognosis is worse for dedifferentiated and poorly differentiated with median PFS of 6 months and 4 months respectively, and median OS of 15 months and 13 months. Conventional chordomas have a median PFS of 24 months, and median OS of 48 months.[3]

Median survival is 6.3 years.[23]

References

[1] WHO Classification of Tumors Editorial Board. Soft Tissue and Bone Tumors. 5th ed. Lyon, France: International Agency for Research on Cancer; 2020; 3. https://publications.iarc.fr/610

[2] Sohda T, Yun K. Insulin-like growth factor II expression in primary meningeal hemangiopericytoma and its metastasis to the liver accompanied by hypoglycemia. Hum Pathol. 1996; 27:858–861

[3] Bosman FT, Jaffe ES, Lakhani SR, et al. World Health Organization Classification of Tumors series, vol. 6. In: WHO Classification of Tumors Editorial Board (ed.) World Health Organization classification of tumors of the central nervous system. 5th ed. Lyon, France: International Agency for Research on Cancer; 2021

[4] Ho VB, Smirniotopoulos JG, Murphy FM, et al. Radiologic-Pathologic Correlation: Hemangioblastoma. American Journal of Neuroradiology. 1992; 13:1343–1352

[5] Hottinger AF, Khakoo Y. Neurooncology of familial cancer syndromes. Journal of Child Neurology. 2009; 24:1526–1535

[6] Catapano D, Muscarella LA, Guarnieri V, et al. Hemangioblastomas of central nervous system: molecular genetic analysis and clinical management. Neurosurgery. 2005; 56:1215–21; discussion 1221

[7] Wakai S, Inoh S, Ueda Y, et al. Hemangioblastoma Presenting with Intraparenchymatous Hemorrhage. J Neurosurg. 1984; 61:956–960

[8] Jagannathan J, Lonser RR, Smith R, et al. Surgical management of cerebellar hemangioblastomas in patients with von Hippel-Lindau disease. Journal of Neurosurgery. 2008; 108:210–222

[9] Huang Y, Chan L, Bai HX, et al. Assessment of care pattern and outcome in hemangioblastoma. Sci Rep. 2018; 8. DOI: 10.1038/s41598-018-29047-9

[10] Utsuki S, Oka H, Sato K, et al. Fluorescence diagnosis of tumor cells in hemangioblastoma cysts with 5-aminolevulinic acid. Journal of Neurosurgery. 2009. DOI: 10.3171/2009.5.JNS08442

[11] Agrawal A, Kakani A, Vagh SJ, et al. Cystic hemangioblastoma of the brainstem. J Neurosci Rural Pract. 2010; 1:20–22

[12] Wright D. Nasopharyngeal and Cervical Chordoma – Some Aspects of the Development and Treatment. J Laryngol Otol. 1967; 81:1335–1337

[13] Hug EB, Loredo LN, Slater JD, et al. Proton Radiation Therapy for Chordomas and Chondrosarcomas of the Skull Base. Journal of Neurosurgery. 1999; 91:432–439

[14] O'Neill P, Bell BA, Miller JD, et al. Fifty Years of Experience with Chordomas in Southeast Scotland. Neurosurgery. 1985; 16:166–170

[15] Heffelfinger MJ, Dahlin DC, MacCarty CS, et al. Chordomas and Cartilaginous Tumors at the Skull Base. Cancer. 1973; 32:410–420

[16] Boriani S, Chevalley F, Weinstein JN, et al. Chordoma of the Spine Above the Sacrum. Treatment and Outcome in 21 Cases. Spine. 1996; 21:1569–1577

[17] Tarpey PS, Behjati S, Young MD, et al. The driver landscape of sporadic chordoma. Nat Commun. 2017; 8. DOI: 10.1038/s41467-017-01026-0

[18] Meyer JE, Lepke RA, Lindfors KK, et al. Chordomas: Their CT Appearance in the Cervical, Thoracic and Lumbar Spine. Radiology. 1984; 153:693–696

[19] Schwarz SS, Fisher WS, Pulliam MW, et al. Thoracic Chordoma in a Patient with Paraparesis and Ivory Vertebral Body. Neurosurgery. 1985; 16:100–102

[20] Wold LE, Laws ER. Cranial Chordomas in Children and Young Adults. J Neurosurg. 1983; 59:1043–1047

[21] Azzarelli A, Quagliuolo V, Cerasoli S, et al. Chordoma: Natural History and Treatment Results in 33 Cases. J Surg Oncol. 1988; 37:185–191

[22] Mindell ER. Current Concepts Review. Chordoma. Journal of Bone and Joint Surgery. 1981; 63A:501–505

[23] Jiang L, Liu ZJ, Liu XG, et al. Upper cervical spine chordoma of C2-C3. European Spine Journal. 2009; 18:293–298; discussion 298-300

[24] Samson IR, Springfield DS, Suit HD, et al. Operative Treatment of Sacrococcygeal Chordoma. A Review of Twenty-One Cases. Journal of Bone and Joint Surgery. 1993; 75:1476–1484

[25] Klekamp J, Samii M. Spinal Chordomas - Results of Treatment Over a 17-Year Period. Acta Neurochir (Wien). 1996; 138:514–519

[26] Cheng EY, Özerdemoglu RA, Transfeldt EE, et al. Lumbosacral Chordoma. Prognostic Factors and Treatment. Spine. 1999; 24:1639–1645

[27] Suit HD, Goitein M, Munzenrider J, et al. Definitive Radiation Therapy for Chordoma and Chondrosarcoma of Base of Skull and Cervical Spine. Journal of Neurosurgery. 1982; 56:377–385

[28] Rich TA, Schiller A, Mankin HJ. Clinical and Pathologic Review of 48 Cases of Chordoma. Cancer. 1985; 56:182–187

[29] Magenau JM, Schuetze SM. New targets for therapy of sarcoma. Current Opinion in Oncology. 2008; 20:400–406

48 Melanocytic Tumors and CNS Germ Cell Tumors

48.1 Melanocytic tumors

48.1.1 General information

Rare. Diffuse or localized CNS tumors that presumably originate from leptomeningeal melanocytes.
Terminology:
1. **circumscribed** melanocytic tumors: rare
   a) meningeal melanocytoma: may be well differentiated. When increased mitotic activity or parenchymal invasion occurs, these qualify as intermediate grade tumors
   b) meningeal melanoma: the malignant counterpart to the above
2. **diffuse** melanocytic tumors are defined by involvement of large areas of the subarachnoid space, with or without focal nodularity
   a) meningeal melanocytosis: benign histology
   b) meningeal melanomatosis: malignant histology. Aggressive and resistant to XRT

These primary CNS lesions may be distinguished from other pigmented CNS neoplasms (e.g., malignant melanotic nerve sheath tumors) using molecular analysis (▶ Table 35.7) and methylation profiling.

48.1.2 Diffuse meningeal melanocytic neoplasms

General information

Rare, primary CNS neoplasms that involve the leptomeninges and spread diffusely throughout the subarachnoid space, sometimes with focal or multifocal nodularity, and frequentl invasion of the Virchow-Robin (perivascular) spaces. There is a predilection for the temporal lobes, cerebellum, pons, medulla, and spinal cord.

Distinguishing these primary tumors from metastases originating outside the CNS is critical for treatment decsions and prognostication, and often requires molecular testing in addition to microscopic histology.

These tumors frequently occur in the setting of neurocutaneous melanosis (p. 653) (a rare neurocutaneous disorder).

Symptoms may be due to hydrocephalus or from dysfunction of invaded brain. Other associations include arachnoid cysts, syringomyelia, other brain tumors (e.g., astrocytoma, ependymoma...), and other structural conditions (e.g., Chiari malformation). Symptoms progress rapidly when malignant transformation occurs.

MRI findings vary with the amount of melanin content, and these tumors may be isodense or hyperintense on T1WI, and hypodense on T2WI.[1]

There are case reports of tumor spreading to the peritoneal compartment when ventriculo-peritoneal shunting is used to treat hydrocephalus.[2]

Diagnostic criteria for diffuse meningeal melanocytic neoplasms

Diagnostic criteria for diffuse meningeal melanocytic neoplasms are shown in ▶ Fig. 48.1.[3]

Meningeal melanocytosis

A diffuse or multifocal proliferation of cytologically bland melanocytic cells. See ▶ Fig. 48.1 for diagnostic criteria. May spread into perivascular spaces without invasion of the brain. Symptoms related to meningeal melanocytosis will develop in 10-15% of patients with large congenital cutaneous melanocytic nevi. Meningeal melanocytosis may be asymptomatic.

Prognosis is poor once symptoms manifest.

Meningeal melanomatosis

Malignant histology distinguishes these tumors from meningeal melanocytosis. CNS invasion is a common finding. See ▶ Fig. 48.1 for diagnostic criteria. Usually aggressive with poor prognosis.

Diffuse meningeal melanocytic neoplasms

▷ **ESSENTIAL** ◁

diffuse or multifocal primary meningeal melanocytic neoplasm

AND

► for **meningeal melanocytosis**: absence of CNS parenchyma invasion, absence of marked cytological atypia, absence of mitotic activity, and absence of necrosis
► for **meningeal melanomatosis**: invasion of the CNS parenchyma and/or marked cytological atypia and/or mitotic activity and/or necrosis

▷ **DESIRABLE** ◁

► in children, meningeal melanocytosis/melanomatosis is often *NRAS*-mutant and rarely *BRAF*-mutant

Fig. 48.1 Diagnostic criteria for diffuse meningeal melanocytic neoplasms. (Modified with permission from WHO Classification of Tumors Editorial Board, (ed.) World Health Organization classification of tumors of the central nervous system. 5th ed. Bosman F T, Jaffe E S, Lakhani S R, et al. (series eds.): World Health Organization Classification of Tumors series, vol. 6. International Agency for Research on Cancer, Lyon, France, 2021.)

48.1.3 Circumscribed meningeal melanocytic neoplasms

General information

These tumors arise from leptomeningeal melanocytes and vary from well-differentiated neoplasms (meningeal melanocytoma) to aggressive, malignancies (meningeal melanoma). An intermediate grade between the two exhibits bland cytology but increased mitotic activity on invasion of parenchyma.

Diagnostic criteria for circumscribed meningeal melanocytic neoplasms

Diagnostic criteria for circumscribed meningeal melanocytic neoplasms are shown in ► Fig. 48.2.[3]

Meningeal melanocytoma

A well developed, solid, noninfiltrating melanocytic tumor that arises from the leptomeninges characterized by epithelioid fusiform, polyhedral or spindled melanocytes with no evidence of anaplasia, necrosis or increased mitoses. Rare reports of malignant transformation.[4] See ► Fig. 48.2 for diagnostic criteria.

Comprises 0.06–0.1% of brain tumors with an estimated incidence of 1 per 10 million.[5] Most commonly found in the cervical or thoracic spine. Less commonly, they originate in the leptomeninges of the posterior fossa or supratentorial intracranial compartment. A handful of patients with nevus of Ota (AKA oculodermal melanocytosis, which results from incomplete migration of melanocytes from the neural crest to the epidermis) have concurrent meningeal melanocytoma.[6]

Meningeal melanoma

A primary solitary malignant neoplasm that arises from leptomeningeal melanocytes characterized by aggressive growth. Histologically similar to melanomas occurring elsewhere.[5] See ► Fig. 48.2 for diagnostic criteria.

Circumscribed meningeal melanocytic neoplasms

▷ ESSENTIAL ◁

circumscribed/localized primary melanocytic neoplasm in the meninges

AND

- ▶ for **melanocytoma**: limited cytological atypia, (almost) no mitoses, no necrosis, and (in cases of evaluable CNS parenchyma) no CNS invasion
- ▶ for **intermediate-grade melanocytoma**: mitotic count[a] of 0.5–1.5 mitoses/mm^2 and/or CNS invasion, but limited cytological atypia and no necrosis
- ▶ for **melanoma**: mitotic count[a] > 1.5 mitoses/mm^2 and/or necrosis, often accompanied by marked cytological atypia

▷ DESIRABLE ◁

- ▶ demonstration of *GNAQ*, *GNA11*, *PLCB4*, or *CYSLTR2* mutation corroborates the CNS origin of the neoplasm, especially after exclusion of uveal or blue nevus–like melanoma
- ▶ additional molecular markers (*SF3B1*, *EIF1AX*, and *BAP1* mutations; chromosome 3 monosomy; complex copy-number variations) indicating aggressive behavior

[a] 1 mm^2 equates approximately to 5 HPF of 0.5 mm in diameter and 0.2 mm^2 in area.

Fig. 48.2 Diagnostic criteria for circumscribed meningeal melanocytic neoplasms. (Modified with permission from WHO Classification of Tumors Editorial Board, (ed.) World Health Organization classification of tumors of the central nervous system. 5th ed. Bosman F T, Jaffe E S, Lakhani S R, et al. (series eds.): World Health Organization Classification of Tumors series, vol. 6. International Agency for Research on Cancer, Lyon, France, 2021.)

Compared to melanocytoma, these are more pleomorphic, anaplastic, mitotically active and often invade CNS tissue and may demonstrate necrosis. May spread through CSF pathways. Occasional systemic metastases outside the CNS occur.[7]

Incidence of 0.5 per 10 million.[8] The peak age for this tumor is in the 4th decade (mean age: 43 years) compared to the 7th decade for primary cutaneous melanoma.[9]

They are aggressive and resistant to XRT. However, with GTR, the prognosis is better than with cutaneous melanoma metastatic to the CNS.

48.2 Germ cell tumors of the CNS

48.2.1 General information

Background

A family of morphological and immunophenotypic homologues of germ cell tumors of the gonads and other sites.

80–90% of GCTs occur in the midline, usually in the suprasellar and/or pineal region (simultaneous suprasellar and pineal region lesions is diagnostic of a GCT; so-called synchronous germ cell tumors, which comprise 13% of GCTs). GCTs are highly sensitive to XRT.[10] In the pineal region, these tumors occur predominantly in males. In females, GCTs are more common in the suprasellar region.[11] Aside from benign teratomas, all intracranial GCTs are malignant and may metastasize via CSF and systemically.

Epidemiology

GCTs primarily affect children and adolescents. They comprise 2–3% of primary intracranial tumors. Prevalence appears higher in eastern Asia.

Peak incidence: age 10–14 years. Affects males more than females, although in the suprasellar region girls are more prevalent.

CSF tumor markers

GCTs can (but not always) give rise to tumor markers in the CSF (see Tumor markers used clinically (p.634)). ▶ Table 48.1 summarizes these findings.
- beta-human chorionic gonadotropin (β-hCG): elevated CSF levels are classically associated with choriocarcinomas, but also occur in up to 50% of germinomas (which are more common)
- alpha-fetoprotein (AFP) is elevated with yolk sac tumors, embryonal carcinoma and occasionally with teratomas
- placental alkaline phosphatase (PLAP) may be elevated in serum or CSF with intracranial germinomas[12]

NB: tumor markers alone are no longer considered useful for making a definitive diagnosis or following response to treatment with a pineal region tumor since many of these tumors are mixed cell type and many pineal region tumors do not give rise to markers.

Table 48.1 Occurrence of CSF tumor markers with pineal germ cell tumors

Tumor	β-hCG[a]	AFP	PLAP[b]
choriocarcinoma	≈ 100%	–	–
germinoma	10–50%	–	+
embryonal carcinoma	–	+	–
yolk sac carcinoma	–	+	–
immature teratoma	–	+	–
mature teratoma	–	–	–

[a]abbreviations: β-hCG = beta human chorionic gonadotropin, AFP = alpha-fetoprotein, PLAP = placental alkaline phosphatase
[b]elevated PLAP may also occur in serum

▶ **General outline of GCTs.** This outline shows the hierarchy of germ cell tumors. Details are provided in following sections.
1. germinoma: malignant tumor of primitive germ cells that occurs in the gonads (called testicular seminomas in males, dysgerminomas in females) or in the CNS. Survival with these is much better than with nongerminomatous tumors
   - *variant*: syncytiotrophoblastic giant cell variant
2. nongerminomatous germ cell tumors (NGGCT) include:
   a) embryonal carcinoma:
   b) choriocarcinoma
   c) yolk sac tumor AKA endodermal sinus tumor (EST): usually malignant
   d) teratoma. A germ cell tumor composed of at least two of the three germ cell layers: ectoderm, endoderm, and mesoderm. Subclassifications:
      - mature teratoma: adult-type tissue elements. Minimal mitoses. All 3 skin layers
      - immature teratoma: contain immature embryonic or fetal tissue alone or in combination with mature tissues
      - teratoma with somatic-type malignancy: contain a component resulting from malignant transformation of a somatic tissue (usually a carcinoma or sarcoma)
3. mixed germ cell tumor

48.2.2 Mature teratoma

General information

Exclusively comprised of mature somatic tissue, consisting of 2 or more of the 3 skin layers:
1. endoderm: glands lined with respiratory or enteric epithelia (often as dilated cysts) are typical, and rarely GI and bronchial structures, and hepatic or pancreatic tissue

2. mesoderm: smooth and striated muscle, cartilage and bone
3. ectoderm: epidermis, skin appendage organs (sweat glands, hair follicles often with hair), CNS tissue, choroid plexus, salivary gland

Little or no mitotic activity. Ki-67 in the mature tissue may be unexpectedly high.

Diagnostic criteria for mature teratoma

Diagnostic criteria for mature teratoma are shown in ▶ Fig. 48.3.[3]

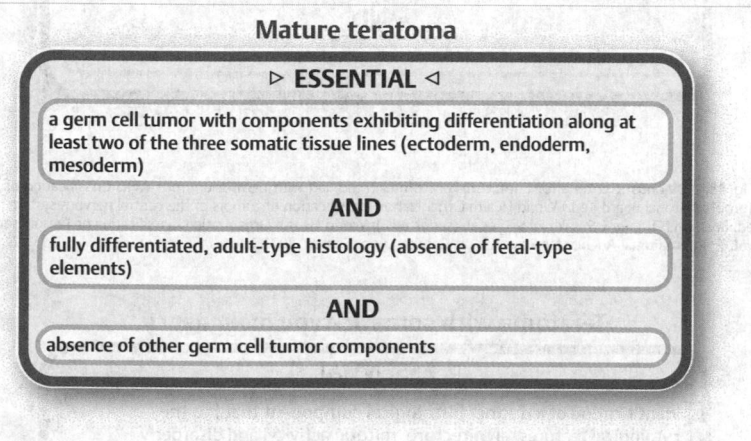

Fig. 48.3 **Diagnostic criteria for mature teratoma.** (Modified with permission from WHO Classification of Tumors Editorial Board, (ed.) World Health Organization classification of tumors of the central nervous system. 5th ed. Bosman F T, Jaffe E S, Lakhani S R, et al. (series eds.): World Health Organization Classification of Tumors series, vol. 6. International Agency for Research on Cancer, Lyon, France, 2021.)

48.2.3 Immature teratoma

General information

The presence of any incompletely differentiated or fetal-like tissue requires the tumor to be designated as immature teratoma. Hypercellular stromal elements resembling fetal gut and respiratory tissue with increased mitotic activity are common. Other unusual components may include primitive retinal tissue or neural tube elements.

Diagnostic criteria for immature teratoma

Diagnostic criteria for immature teratoma are shown in ▶ Fig. 48.4.[3]

48.2.4 Teratoma with somatic-type malignancy

General information

Somatic cancers that may occur include rhabdomyosarcomas and undifferentiated sarcomas, adenocarcinoma resembling GI tract lineage and squamous cell carcinoma. Other rare cancers may also be seen. The diagnosis of somatic-type malignancy should not be made based on cytologic atypia alone.

Diagnostic criteria for teratoma with somatic-type malignancy

Diagnostic criteria for teratoma with somatic-type malignancy are shown in ▶ Fig. 48.5.[3]

Immature teratoma

▷ **ESSENTIAL** ◁

identification of incompletely differentiated elements exhibiting differentiation along at least two of the three somatic tissue lines (ectoderm, endoderm, mesoderm) in a teratoma, or the identification of any such elements within a tumor otherwise qualifying as a mature teratoma

AND

absence of other germ cell tumor components

Fig. 48.4 Diagnostic criteria for immature teratoma. (Modified with permission from WHO Classification of Tumors Editorial Board, (ed.) World Health Organization classification of tumors of the central nervous system. 5th ed. Bosman F T, Jaffe E S, Lakhani S R, et al. (series eds.): World Health Organization Classification of Tumors series, vol. 6. International Agency for Research on Cancer, Lyon, France, 2021.)

48

Teratoma with somatic-type malignancy

▷ **ESSENTIAL** ◁

identification of a distinct histological component that has the cytological features, architecture, mitotic activity, and disorderly growth pattern expected of a sarcoma, carcinoma, or other defined type of somatic cancer in a mature or immature teratoma

Fig. 48.5 Diagnostic criteria for teratoma with somatic-type malignancy. (Modified with permission from WHO Classification of Tumors Editorial Board, (ed.) World Health Organization classification of tumors of the central nervous system. 5th ed. Bosman F T, Jaffe E S, Lakhani S R, et al. (series eds.): World Health Organization Classification of Tumors series, vol. 6. International Agency for Research on Cancer, Lyon, France, 2021.)

48.2.5 Germinoma

General information

Large, undifferentiated appearing cells resembling primordial germ cells with ample glycogen-rich clear cytoplasm containing round, vesicular and centrally place nuclei. The cells are arranged in sheets, lobules or cords with trabeculae. Necrosis is uncommon and mitotic activity is variable.

Some may have syncytiotrophoblastic giant cells seen on squash or smear preparations, but this alone does not qualify them as choriocarcinoma.

Diagnostic criteria for germinoma

Diagnostic criteria for germinoma are shown in ▶ Fig. 48.6.[3]

Germinoma

▷ ESSENTIAL ◁

a germ cell tumor containing large tumor cells with typical cytological characteristics

AND

nuclear OCT4 and widespread membranous KIT (or podoplanin [D2-40]) immunoreactivity, or absence of 5-methylcytosine expression

AND

absence of CD30 expression

AND

absence of AFP expression

AND

hCG immunoreactivity in syncytiotrophoblastic giant cells (for the specific diagnosis of germinoma with syncytiotrophoblastic elements)

AND

absence of other germ cell tumor components (except syncytiotrophoblastic giant cells for the specific diagnosis of germinoma with syncytiotrophoblastic giant cells)

Fig. 48.6 Diagnostic criteria for germinoma. (Modified with permission from WHO Classification of Tumors Editorial Board, (ed.) World Health Organization classification of tumors of the central nervous system. 5th ed. Bosman F T, Jaffe E S, Lakhani S R, et al. (series eds.): World Health Organization Classification of Tumors series, vol. 6. International Agency for Research on Cancer, Lyon, France, 2021.)

48.2.6 Embryonal carcinoma

General information

Large epithelioid cells resembling cells of the embryonic germ disc containing vesicular nuclei, macro-nuclei and clear to violet cytoplasm. Mitotic activity is often increased. Necrotic areas are common.

Diagnostic criteria for embryonal carcinoma

Diagnostic criteria for embryonal carcinoma are shown in ▶ Fig. 48.7.[3]

48.2.7 Yolk sac tumor

General information

Formerly called endodermal sinus tumor. Primitive appearing epithelial cells that may be associated with loose variably cellular stromal component. Bright eosinophil PAS-positive particles may appear in the cytoplasm of epithelial cells but are not a consistent feature.

48

Embryonal carcinoma

▷ ESSENTIAL ◁

a germ cell tumor with large epithelioid cells as described in the Histopathology subsection[a]

AND

CD30 and OCT4 expression

AND

absent or only focal, non-membranous KIT expression

AND

absence of hCG expression

AND

absence of AFP expression

AND

absence of other germ cell tumor components

▷ DESIRABLE ◁

► cytokeratin expression

Fig. 48.7 Diagnostic criteria for embryonal carcinoma.
[a] For histopathology details, refer to the WHO blue book[3] (Modified with permission from WHO Classification of Tumors Editorial Board, (ed.) World Health Organization classification of tumors of the central nervous system. 5th ed. Bosman F T, Jaffe E S, Lakhani S R, et al. (series eds.): World Health Organization Classification of Tumors series, vol. 6. International Agency for Research on Cancer, Lyon, France, 2021.)

Diagnostic criteria for yolk sac tumor

Diagnostic criteria for yolk sac tumor are shown in ► Fig. 48.8.[3] AFP (p.635) reactivity in the cytoplasm distinguishes these tumors from other germ cell tumors except for yolk sac tumors and possibly the glandular and hepatocellular components of some teratomas.

48.2.8 Choriocarcinoma

General information

Components of syncytiotrophoblast (the selective barrier between maternal and fetal blood in the placenta) are seen, characterized by giant cells that encompass cytotrophoblastic elements.

Diagnostic criteria for choriocarcinoma

Diagnostic criteria for choriocarcinoma are shown in ► Fig. 48.9.[3]

Yolk sac tumor

▷ ESSENTIAL ◁

a germ cell tumor with epithelioid cells arranged in any of the patterns described in the Histopathology subsection[a], with or without mesenchymal components

AND

absence of other germ cell tumor components

AND

AFP expression

AND

absent or only focal, non-membranous KIT expression

AND

absent or only focal CD30 expression

AND

absence of β-hCG expression

Fig. 48.8 Diagnostic criteria for yolk sac tumor.
[a] For histopathology details, refer to the WHO blue book[3] (Modified with permission from WHO Classification of Tumors Editorial Board, (ed.) World Health Organization classification of tumors of the central nervous system. 5th ed. Bosman F T, Jaffe E S, Lakhani S R, et al. (series eds.): World Health Organization Classification of Tumors series, vol. 6. International Agency for Research on Cancer, Lyon, France, 2021.)

48.2.9 Mixed germ cell tumor

General information

Combinations of germ cell subtypes which exhibit the same findings as the subtypes in pure form.

Diagnostic criteria for mixed germ cell tumor

Diagnostic criteria for mixed germ cell tumor are shown in ▶ Fig. 48.10.[3]

48

Choriocarcinoma

▷ ESSENTIAL ◁

a germ cell tumor with both syncytiotrophoblastic and cytotrophoblastic elements but no other germ cell tumor components

AND

β-hCG expression

AND

absence of KIT (or podoplanin [D2-40]) expression

AND

absence of AFP expression

AND

absent or only focal CD30 expression

AND

absence of OCT4 expression

Fig. 48.9 Diagnostic criteria for choriocarcinoma. (Modified with permission from WHO Classification of Tumors Editorial Board, (ed.) World Health Organization classification of tumors of the central nervous system. 5th ed. Bosman F T, Jaffe E S, Lakhani S R, et al. (series eds.): World Health Organization Classification of Tumors series, vol. 6. International Agency for Research on Cancer, Lyon, France, 2021.)

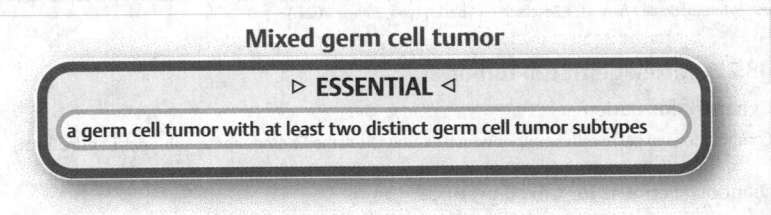

Mixed germ cell tumor

▷ ESSENTIAL ◁

a germ cell tumor with at least two distinct germ cell tumor subtypes

Fig. 48.10 Diagnostic criteria for mixed germ cell tumor. (Modified with permission from WHO Classification of Tumors Editorial Board, (ed.) World Health Organization classification of tumors of the central nervous system. 5th ed. Bosman F T, Jaffe E S, Lakhani S R, et al. (series eds.): World Health Organization Classification of Tumors series, vol. 6. International Agency for Research on Cancer, Lyon, France, 2021.)

References

[1] Smith AB, Rushing EJ, Smirniotopoulos J G. Pigmented lesions of the central nervous system: radiologic-pathologic correlation. Radiographics. 2009; 29:1503–1524

[2] Cajaiba MM, Benjamin D, Halaban R, et al. Metastatic peritoneal neurocutaneous melanocytosis. Am J Surg Pathol. 2008; 32:156–161

[3] Bosman FT, Jaffe ES, Lakhani SR, et al. World Health Organization Classification of Tumors series, vol. 6. In: WHO Classification of Tumors Editorial Board (ed.) World Health Organization classification of tumors of the central nervous system. 5th ed. Lyon, France: International Agency for Research on Cancer; 2021

[4] Roser F, Nakamura M, Brandis A, et al. Transition from meningeal melanocytoma to primary cerebral melanoma. Case report. J Neurosurg. 2004; 101:528–531

[5] Louis DN, Ohgaki H, Wiestler OD, et al. WHO classi-fication of tumors of the central nervous system. Lyon, France 2016

[6] Kuo KL, Lin CL, Wu CH, et al. Meningeal Melanocy-toma Associated with Nevus of Ota: Analysis of Twelve Reported Cases. World Neurosurg. 2019; 127:e311–e320

[7] Savitz MH, Anderson PJ. Primary Melanoma of the Leptomeninges: A Review. Mt Sinai J Med. 1974; 41:774–791

[8] Helseth A, Helseth E, Unsgaard G. Primary menin-geal melanoma. Acta Oncol. 1989; 28:103–104

[9] Gibson JB, Burrows D, Weir WP. Primary Melanoma of the Meninges. J Pathol Bacteriol. 1957; 74:419–438

[10] Sugiyama K, Uozumi T, Kiya K, et al. Intracranial germ-cell tumor with synchronous lesions in the pineal and suprasellar regions: report of six cases and review of the literature. Surg Neurol. 1992; 38:114–120

[11] Hoffman HJ, Ostubo H, Hendrick EB, et al. Intracra-nial Germ-Cell Tumors in Children. Journal of Neu-rosurgery. 1991; 74:545–551

[12] Shinoda J, Yamada H, Sakai N, et al. Placental alka-line phosphatase as a tumor marker for primary intracranial germinoma. J Neurosurg. 1988; 68:710–720

48

49 Hematolymphoid Tumors Involving the CNS

49.1 CNS lymphomas

49.1.1 Primary diffuse large B-cell lymphoma of the CNS (CNS-DLBCL)

General information

> ### Key concepts
>
> - may be histologically identical to secondary secondary CNS spread of systemic DLBCL
> - suspected with homogeneously enhancing lesion(s) in the central gray matter or corpus callosum (on MRI or CT) especially in AIDS patients
> - may present with multiple cranial-nerve palsies
> - diagnosis highly likely if tumor seen in conjunction with uveitis
> - very responsive initially to steroids → short-lived disappearance ("ghost tumors")
> - treatment: usually XRT ± chemotherapy. Role of neurosurgery usually limited to biopsy and/or placement of ventricular access reservoir for chemotherapy, and occasionally to debulking an extremely large tumor causing severe symptoms
> - risk factors: immunosuppression (AIDS, transplants), Epstein-Barr virus, collagen vascular diseases

49

AKA primary CNS lymphoma. CNS involvement with lymphoma may arise primarily, or may occur secondarily from a "systemic" lymphoma invading the CNS. CNS-DLBCL is a lymphoma confined to the CNS at presentation that has histological features and many molecular findings that replicate those of systemic lymphomas. 65% are solitary lesions, with the remainder being multifocal.

Diagnostic criteria for primary diffuse large B-cell lymphoma of the CNS (CNS-DLBCL)

Diagnostic criteria for CNS-DLBCL are shown in ▶ Fig. 49.1.[1]

Primary vs. secondary lymphoma

Secondary CNS lymphoma
Non CNS lymphoma is the fifth most common cause of cancer deaths in the U.S.; 63% of new cases are non-Hodgkin's. Secondary CNS involvement usually occurs late in the course. Metastatic spread of systemic lymphoma to the cerebral *parenchyma* occurs in 1–7% of cases at autopsy.[2]

Primary CNS lymphoma
Older names include: reticulum cell sarcoma and microglioma,[3] since they were thought to possibly arise from microglia which were considered part of the reticuloendothelial system.

A rare, malignant primary CNS form of non-Hodgkin lymphoma comprising 0.85–2% of all primary brain tumors and 0.2–2% of malignant lymphomas.[4] May occasionally metastasize outside the CNS.

Specific types of primary CNS lymphoma

1. diffuse large B-cell lymphoma of the CNS (CNS-DLBCL): excludes any of lymphomas listed below, as well as lymphomas with systemic involvement
2. immunodeficiency-associated CNS lymphoma: immunodeficiency (includes immunosuppression for organ transplantation, IgA deficiency, SLE…) inceases the risk for lymphoma. Lymphoma associated with HIV or post-transplant immunosuppression is usually EBV-related
   a) AIDS-related diffuse large B-cell lymphoma
   b) EBV + diffuse large B-cell lymphoma, NOS
   c) lymphomatoid granulomatosis
3. intravascular large B-cell lymphoma
4. miscellaneous rare lymphomas in the CNS
   a) low-grade B-cell lymphomas

Primary diffuse large B-cell lymphoma of the CNS

▷ ESSENTIAL ◁

biopsy-proven mature large B-cell lymphoma confined to the CNS at presentation

AND

expression of one or more B-cell markers (CD20, CD19, CD22, CD79a, PAX5)

▷ DESIRABLE ◁

► immunohistochemical phenotype of late germinal-center exit B cells (IRF4 [MUM1]+, BCL6+/−, CD10−); CD10 expression does not exclude the diagnosis, but it is uncommon and indicates possible systemic DLBCL
► immunohistochemical positivity for BCL2 and MYC
► absence of EBV-associated markers (in > 97% of cases)
► molecular detection of a clonal B-cell population in cases in which histology is not definitive, such as corticoid-mitigated CNS-DLBCL

49

Fig. 49.1 Diagnostic criteria for CNS-DLBCL. (Modified with permission from WHO Classification of Tumors Editorial Board, (ed.) World Health Organization classification of tumors of the central nervous system. 5th ed. Bosman F T, Jaffe E S, Lakhani S R, et al. (series eds.): World Health Organization Classification of Tumors series, vol. 6. International Agency for Research on Cancer, Lyon, France, 2021.)

    b) T-cell and NK/T-cell lymphomas
    c) anaplastic large cell lymphoma
5. extranodal marginal zone lymphoma of mucosa associated lymphoid tissue (MALT lymphoma) of the dura

Epidemiology

Incidence of primary CNS lymphoma (PCNSL) in the U.S.: 0.44 per 100,000,[5] making it the third most common of malignant primary brain tumors (behind GBM & diffuse astrocytoma). In the past 20 years, incidence has increased in patients > 60 years of age.[6]

    Male:female ratio = 1.22:1.[5]

    Median age at diagnosis: 52 yrs[7] (younger among immunocompromised patients: ≈ 34 yrs).

    Most common supratentorial locations: frontal lobes, then deep nuclei; periventricular also common. Infratentorially: cerebellum is the most common location.

Conditions with increased risk of primary CNS lymphomas (PCNSL)

1. collagen vascular disease
    a) systemic lupus erythematosus
    b) Sjögren's syndrome: an autoimmune connective tissue disorder
    c) rheumatoid arthritis
2. immunosuppression
    a) organ transplant recipients: related to chronic immunosuppression. Falls under category of post transplant lymphoproliferative disease (PTLD) (p. 845)[8]
    b) AIDS[9,10]: CNS lymphoma occurs in ≈ 10% of AIDS patients, and is the first presentation in 0.6%
    c) severe-congenital immunodeficiency syndrome ("SCIDS")
    d) possibly increased incidence in the elderly due to reduced competency of immune system

3. Epstein-Barr virus[11] is associated with a broad spectrum of lymphoproliferative disorders, and is detectable in ≈ 30–50% of systemic lymphomas; however, it has been associated with almost 100% of PCNSL,[12] especially AIDS-related cases[13(p 317)]

Presentation

General information
Presentation is similar with primary or secondary CNS lymphoma: the two most common neurologic manifestations are those due to epidural spinal cord compression and those of carcinomatous meningitis (multiple cranial nerve deficits) (p. 920). Seizures occur in up to 30% of patients.[14] Most lymphomas in patients first presenting with neurologic symptoms are PCNSL.[15]

Neurologic symptoms
1. presents with non-focal non-specific symptoms in over 50% of patients; at time of presentation most commonly includes:
   a) mental status changes in one–third
   b) symptoms of increased ICP (H/A, N/V)
   c) generalized seizures in 9%
2. focal symptoms in 30–42% of cases:
   a) hemimotor or hemisensory symptoms
   b) partial seizures
   c) multiple cranial-nerve palsies (due to carcinomatous meningitis)
3. combination of focal and non-focal symptoms

Signs
1. non-focal in 16%:
   a) papilledema
   b) encephalopathy
   c) dementia
2. focal findings in 45% of cases:
   a) hemimotor or hemisensory deficits
   b) aphasia
   c) visual field deficits
3. combination of focal and non-focal signs

Uncommon but characteristic syndromes
1. uveocyclitis, coincident with (in 6% of cases) or preceding the diagnosis of (in 11% of cases) lymphoma
2. subacute encephalitis with subependymal infiltration
3. MS-like illness with steroid-induced remission

Histology

Characteristic sites: corpus callosum, basal ganglia, periventricular.

The neoplastic cells are identical to those of systemic lymphomas. Most are bulky tumors that are contiguous with the ventricles or meninges.

Histologic distinguishing features: tumor cells form cuffs around blood vessels which demonstrate multiplication of basement membranes (best demonstrated with silver reticulum stain).

Frozen section distorts the cells and may lead to a misdiagnosis of malignant glioma.[13(p 320)]

Immunohistochemical stains differentiate B-cell lymphomas from T-cell lymphomas (B-cell types are more common, especially in PCNSL and in AIDS).

EM shows absence of junctional complexes (desmosomes) that are usually present in epithelial derived tumors.

Intravascular lymphomatosis[16]: Formerly: (malignant) angioendotheliomatosis. A rare lymphoma with no solid mass in which malignant lymphoid cells are found in the lumen of small blood vessels in affected organs. CNS involvement is reported in most cases. Presentation is non specific: patients are often febrile, and may present with progressive multifocal cerebrovascular events (including stroke or hemorrhage), spinal cord or nerve root symptoms including cauda equina syndrome (p. 1254), encephalopathy, or peripheral or cranial neuropathies.[17] Initial transient cerebral symptoms may mimic TIAs or seizures. The ESR is often elevated prior to initiation of steroids. Lymphoma cells may be seen in the CSF.

49

Painful skin nodules or plaques occur in ≈ 10% of cases, generally involving the abdomen or lower extremities, and these cases may be diagnosed with skin biopsy (differential diagnosis here includes angioendotheliomatosis, a benign capillary, and endothelial cell disorder). Otherwise, diagnosis often requires brain biopsy (open or stereotactic), in which involved areas on imaging studies are targeted. Pathology: malignant lymphoid cells distend and occlude small arteries, veins and capillaries with little or no parenchymal extension.[13 (p 324)] Treatment with combination chemotherapy can result in long-term remission in some patients, but early diagnosis before permanent damage occurs is critical (diagnosis is rarely made pre-mortem).

Evaluation

All patients should be assessed (history, physical and laboratory tests as appropriate) for any of the conditions associated with lymphoma (p.841). Since PCNSL is less common than secondary involvement, any patient with CNS lymphoma should have work-up for occult systemic lymphoma which may include:
1. careful physical exam of all lymph nodes (LN)
2. early detection of HIV and reflex CD4 + count nadir are important because HIV increases the risk of PCNSL and infection
3. contrast CT of chest, abdomen & pelvis or whole body PET/CT (evaluation of perihilar and pelvic LN)
4. routine blood (CBC, chemistries) and urine testing
5. LP for CSF (omit if not safe: anticoagulation, thrombocytopenia or intracranial mass effect): for routine tests (cell count, protein/glucose, culture) & cytology, flow cytometry
6. bone marrow biopsy
7. MRI of the entire spine
8. testicular ultrasound in males > 60 years of age (omit if PET scan is done and is negative)
9. ophthalmologic examination (including slit-lamp evaluation of both eyes) in all
    a) for possible uveitis
    b) ≈ 28% of patients with PCNSL will also have intraocular lymphoma. Often resistant to methotrexate, but responds to low dose ocular XRT (7–8 Gy)

Diagnostic tests

CT & MRI

▶ **Findings common to CT/MRI.** On imaging (CT or MRI) 50–60% occur in one or more cerebral lobes (in gray or white matter). 25% occur in deep midline structures (septum pellucidum, basal ganglion, corpus callosum). 25% are infratentorial. 10–30% of patients have multiple lesions at the time of presentation. In contrast, systemic lymphomas that spread to the CNS tend to present with leptomeningeal involvement instead of parenchymal tumors.[18]

Almost all PCNSLs enhance (except only 1.1% in immune intact, and 3.2% in immune compromised[5]).

Non–AIDS-related cases tend to enhance homogeneously, whereas AIDS-related cases are more likely to be ring-enhancing (necrotic center) and *multifocal*.[15,19]

Non–AIDS-related cases: CNS lymphomas should be suspected with homogeneously enhancing lesion(s) in the central gray or corpus callosum. 75% are in contact with ependymal or meningeal surfaces (this together with dense enhancement may produce a "pseudomeningioma pattern"; however, lymphomas lack calcifications and are more likely to be multiple).

▶ **CT (see also "Findings common to CT/MRI" above).** 60% are hyperdense to brain, only 10% are hypodense. Characteristically, > 90% of these tumors enhance; this is densely homogeneous in over 70%. As a result, when rare non-enhancing cases occur it often leads to a delay in diagnosis.[20] The appearance of enhanced PCNSL on CT has been likened to "fluffy cotton balls." There may be surrounding edema[21] and there is usually mass effect.

There is an almost diagnostic tendency of rapid partial to complete resolution on CT (and even at the time of surgery) following the administration of steroids, earning the nickname of "ghost-cell tumor"[15,22,23] or disappearing tumor.

▶ **MRI (see also "Findings common to CT/MRI" above).** No pathognomonic feature. Bright on DWI (restricted diffusion) in most cases, isointense to hypointense on ADC map. May be difficult to discern if tumor is located subependymally (signal characteristics similar to CSF); proton-weighted image may avoid this limitation.

Serologic tests

There are no blood tests that are diagnostic for PCNSL.

49

Serum lactate dehydrogenase (LDH) elevation indicates rapid cell turnover and is an independent poor prognosticator for non-Hodgkin, follicular and mantle cell lymphomas. In the absence of the diagnosis of lymphoma, this is nonspecific (occurs in liver failure, infection...).[15]

CSF studies

LP should only be performed if no mass effect. Some abnormality of routine CSF labs occurs in > 80%, but are non-specific. Most common abnormalities are elevated protein (in 45–67%), and increased cell count (in 40%). PCNSL can lower CSF glucose.[15]

Cytology is positive for lymphoma cells (preoperatively) in only 2–32%[15] (sensitivity may be higher with leptomeningeal involvement as in non-AIDS patients than with parenchymal involvement commonly seen in AIDS). Sensitivity is higher when ≥ 10.5 ml of CSF is analyzed.[15] Repeating up to 3 LPs may increase yield. The morphology of lymphoma cells can sometimes be difficult to distinguish from inflammatory lymphocytes, but sharp nuclear notches, cytoplasmic irregularity, and increased cell size (> 2.5 times the upper limit of normal) are suggestive of lymphoma. Although the diagnosis of lymphoma can be made from CSF, cells obtained in this manner are not adequate for detailed tissue typing which is possible with solid tissue from biopsy, ∴ LP alone rarely suffices.

Flow cytometry provides information about the immunophenotype of lymphocytes.

Immunoglobulin analysis can show a single elevated immunoglobulin heavy chain (IgH) band with lymphoma, compared to a wide band produced by lymphocytes involved in an inflammatory process.[15]

Proteomics have shown elevated levels of antithrombin III in the CSF. A cutoff of levels > 1.2 mcg/dl is 75% sensitive and 98.7% specific.[24]

Angiography

Rarely helpful. 60% of cases show only an avascular mass. 30–40% show diffuse homogeneous staining or blush.

Treatment

Surgery

Surgical decompression with partial or gross total removal does not alter patient's prognosis. The main indication for surgery:

* biopsy: obtain solid tissue to ascertain that the tumor is a lymphoma, and to determine the type of lymphoma. Stereotactic techniques are often well-suited for these often deep tumors[25]

Radiation therapy

The standard treatment after tissue biopsy is whole-brain radiation therapy. Doses used tend to be lower than for other primary brain tumors. ≈ 40–50 Gy total are usually given in 1.8–3 Gy daily fractions.

Chemotherapy

General information

In *non-AIDS* cases, chemotherapy combined with XRT prolongs survival compared to XRT alone.[26]

Methotrexate (MTX)

The addition of intraventricular MTX (rather than just intrathecal via LP) delivered through a ventricular access device (6 doses of 12 mg twice a week, with IV leucovorin rescue) may result in even better survival.[27] In the event of an intrathecal MTX overdose (OD), interventions recommended[28]: ODs of up to 85 mg can be well tolerated with little sequelae; immediate LP with drainage of CSF can remove a substantial portion of the drug (removing 15 ml of CSF can eliminate ≈ 20–30% of the MTX within 2 hrs of OD). This can be followed by ventriculolumbar perfusion over several hours using 240 ml of warmed isotonic preservative-free saline entering through the ventricular reservoir and exiting through a lumbar subarachnoid catheter. For major OD of > 500 mg, add intrathecal administration of 2,000 U of carboxypeptidase G2 (an enzyme that inactivates MTX). In cases of MTX OD, systemic toxicity should be prevented by treating with IV dexamethasone and IV (not IT) leucovorin.

Rituximab

Available since 1997 for treatment of refractory systemic B-cell non-Hodgkins lymphoma. Intrathecally, may be more effective for CD33 + lymphomas.

Prognosis

With no treatment, median survival is 1.8–3.3 months following diagnosis.

With radiation therapy,[14] median survival is 10 months, with 47% 1-year median survival, and 16% 2-year median survival. 3-year survival is 8%, and 5-year survival is 3–4%. With intraventricular MTX, median time to recurrence was 41 mos.[27] Occasionally, prolonged survival may be seen.[29]

About 78% of cases recur, usually ≈ 15 months after treatment (late recurrences also are seen). Of these recurrences, 93% are confined to the CNS (often at another site if the original site responded well), and 7% are elsewhere.

Although there are individual studies that show trends, there are no prognostic features that consistently correlate with survival.

49.1.2 Immunodeficiency-associated CNS lymphomas (IDA-CNSL)

General information

A family of CNS lymphomas occurring in patients with inherited or acquired immunodeficiency (HIV AIDS, immunosuppression…). The number of cases related to AIDS has declined due to the effectiveness of newer anti-retroviral therapy. Most immunodeficiency-associated lymphomas are Epstein-Barr virus (EBV) related. EBV-positive DLBCL of the elderly is coupled with immunosenescence and starts to ramp up after age 50 years.[30]

Imaging demonstrates multiplicity of lesions and necrotic areas more frequently than in immunocompetent patients.

Diagnostic criteria for immunodeficiency-associated CNS lymphomas (IDA-CNSL)

49

Diagnostic criteria for IDA-CNSL are shown in ► Fig. 49.2.[1]

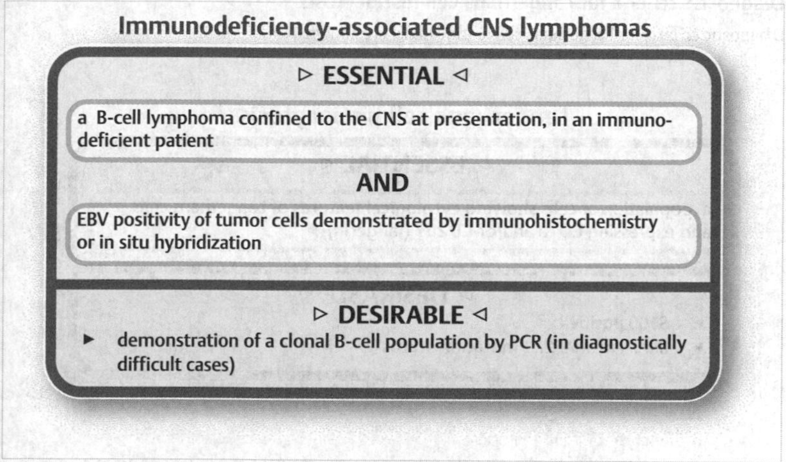

Immunodeficiency-associated CNS lymphomas

▷ **ESSENTIAL** ◁

a B-cell lymphoma confined to the CNS at presentation, in an immuno-deficient patient

AND

EBV positivity of tumor cells demonstrated by immunohistochemistry or in situ hybridization

▷ **DESIRABLE** ◁

► demonstration of a clonal B-cell population by PCR (in diagnostically difficult cases)

Fig. 49.2 **Diagnostic criteria for IDA-CNSL.** (Modified with permission from WHO Classification of Tumors Editorial Board, (ed.) World Health Organization classification of tumors of the central nervous system. 5th ed. Bosman F T, Jaffe E S, Lakhani S R, et al. (series eds.): World Health Organization Classification of Tumors series, vol. 6. International Agency for Research on Cancer, Lyon, France, 2021.)

Prognosis

The prognosis is worse than CNS-DLBCL. Although complete remission occurs in 20–50% following XRT, the median survival is only 3–5 months,[31,32] usually related to AIDS-related opportunistic infection. However, neurologic function and quality of life improve in ≈ 75%.[31]

49.2 Histiocytic tumors

49.2.1 General information

Histiocytic disorders may be classified as follows:
1. malignant (true histiocytic lymphoma)
2. reactive (benign histiocytosis)
3. Langerhans cell histiocytosis (LCH)
   a) **unifocal**: formerly eosinophilic granuloma and/or histiocytosis X. Rare (1/1200 new cases/yr in US). More common in children. Slowly progressing disease. May occur in bone, skin, lungs, or stomach (see below)
   b) **multifocal unisystem**: seen mostly in children. Fever, bone & skin lesions
   c) **multifocal multisystem**: formerly Letterer-Siwe disease (a fulminant, malignant lymphoma of infancy).[33] Hand-Schüller-Christian triad: DI (from invasion of pituitary stalk), exophthalmos (from intraorbital tumor), and lytic bone lesions (particularly of cranium).
4. Erdheim-Chester disease
5. Rosai-Dorfman disease
6. juvenile xanthogranuloma
7. histiocytic sarcoma

49.2.2 Langerhans cell histiocytosis of the CNS or meninges

General information

49

Formerly histiocytosis X (or eosinophilic granuloma, when solitary). A clonal proliferation of Langerhans-type cells involving the CNS, skull or meninges, with or without extra-CNS lesions. 36% of patients develop a leukoencephalopathy pattern, and 8% demonstrate cerebral atrophy.

Diagnostic criteria for Langerhans cell histiocytosis

Diagnostic criteria for Langerhans cell histiocytosis are shown in ▶ Fig. 49.3.[1]

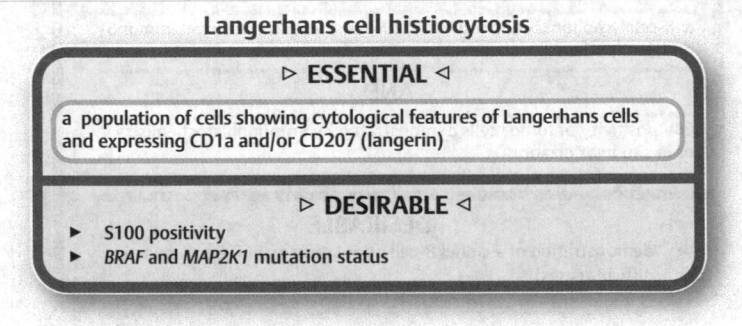

Fig. 49.3 Diagnostic criteria for Langerhans cell histiocytosis. (Modified with permission from WHO Classification of Tumors Editorial Board, (ed.) World Health Organization classification of tumors of the central nervous system. 5th ed. Bosman F T, Jaffe E S, Lakhani S R, et al. (series eds.): World Health Organization Classification of Tumors series, vol. 6. International Agency for Research on Cancer, Lyon, France, 2021.)

Location

There is a predilection for the craniofacial bones and skull base (56%) favoring the parietal and frontal bones.[33] Intracranial involvement may include the hypothalamic-pituitary region (25-50%), meninges (30%) and choroid plexus (6%).[1]

Epidemiology

Generally a condition of youth, 70% of patients are < 20 yrs of age. In a series of 26 patients,[33] age range was 18 mos–49 yrs (mean: 16 yrs). The incidence among patients < 15 years old is 0.5 per 100,000, with a M;F ratio of ≈ 1:2.[34]

Clinical

Most common presenting symptom: *tender*, enlarging skull mass (> 90%). May be asymptomatic and incidentally discovered on skull X-ray obtained for other reasons. Blood tests were normal in all except 1 who had eosinophilia of 23%.

Evaluation

Skull X-rays
Classic radiographic finding: round or oval non-sclerotic punched out skull lesion with sharply defined margins, involving both inner and outer tables (the disease begins in diploic space), often with bevelled edges. A central bone density is occasionally noted (rare, but diagnostic). No abnormal vascularity of adjacent bone. No periosteal reaction. Differentiate from hemangioma by absence of sunburst appearance.

CT scan
Characteristic appearance of a soft tissue mass within area of bony destruction having a central density.[35] Differentiate from epidermoid, which has dense surrounding sclerosis.

49

Pathology

Gross: pinkish gray to purple lesion extending out of bone and involving pericranium. Dural involvement occurs in only 1 of 26 patients, but with no dural penetration.

Microscopic: numerous histiocytes, eosinophils, and multinucleated cells in a reticulin fiber network. No evidence that this is a result of an infection.

▶ **Molecular biology.** The most frequent molecular correlate if BRAF p.V600E mutation, seen in ≈ 50%.[1]

Treatment

There is a tendency toward spontaneous regression; however, most single lesions are treated by curettage. Multiple lesions are usually associated with extracalvarial bony involvement and are often treated with chemotherapy and/or low dose radiation therapy. Very radiosensitive.

Outcome

After a mean 8 years follow-up, 8 patients (31%) developed additional lesions, 5 of these were ≤ 3 yrs of age (all of 5 patients < 3 yrs of age)[33] (may suggest a form of multifocal LCH, thus young patients should be followed closely). Recurrences were local in one case, and in others involved other bones (including the skull, femur, lumbar spine) or brain (including the hypothalamus, presenting with diabetes insipidus and growth delay).

References

[1] Bosman FT, Jaffe ES, Lakhani SR, et al. World Health Organization Classification of Tumors series, vol. 6. In: WHO Classification of Tumors Editorial Board (ed.) World Health Organization classification of tumors of the central nervous system. 5th ed. Lyon, France: International Agency for Research on Cancer; 2021

[2] Jellinger K, Radaszkiewicz T. Involvement of the Central Nervous System in Malignant Lymphomas. Virchows Arch (Pathol Anat). 1976; 370:345–362

[3] Helle TL, Britt RH, Colby TV. Primary Lymphoma of the Central Nervous System. J Neurosurg. 1984; 60:94–103

[4] Alic L, Haid M. Primary Lymphoma of the Brain: A Case Report and Review of the Literature. J Surg Oncol. 1984; 26:115–121

[5] Ostrom QT, Gittleman H, Liao P, et al. CBTRUS Statistical Report: Primary brain and other central nervous system tumors diagnosed in the United States in 2010-2014. Neuro Oncol. 2017; 19:v1–v88

[6] Villano JL, Koshy M, Shaikh H, et al. Age, gender, and racial differences in incidence and survival in primary CNS lymphoma. Br J Cancer. 2011; 105:1414–1418

[7] Murray K, Kun L, Cox J. Primary Malignant Lymphoma of the Central Nervous System: Results of Treatment of 11 Cases and Review of the Literature. J Neurosurg. 1986; 65:600–607

[8] Penn I. Development of Cancer as a Complication of Clinical Transplantation. Transplant Proc. 1977; 9:1121–1127

49

[9] Levy RM, Bredesen DE, Rosenblum ML. Neurological manifestations of the acquired immunodeficiency syndrome (AIDS): Experience at UCSF and review of the literature. J Neurosurg. 1985; 62:475–495

[10] Jean WC, Hall WA. Management of Cranial and Spinal Infections. Contemporary Neurosurgery. 1998; 20:1–10

[11] Hochberg FH, Miller G, Schooley RT, et al. Central-Nervous-System Lymphoma Related to Epstein-Barr Virus. N Engl J Med. 1983; 309:745–748

[12] MacMahon EME, Glass JD, Hayward SD, et al. Epstein-Barr Virus in AIDS-Related Primary Central Nervous System Lymphoma. Lancet. 1991; 338:969–973

[13] Burger PC, Scheithauer BW, Vogel FS. Surgical Pathology of the Nervous System and Its Coverings. 4th ed. New York: Churchill Livingstone; 2002

[14] O'Neill BP, Illig JJ. Primary Central Nervous System Lymphoma. Mayo Clinic Proceedings. 1989; 64:1005–1020

[15] Scott BrianJ, Douglas VanjaC, Tihan Tarik, et al. A Systematic Approach to the Diagnosis of Suspected Central Nervous System Lymphoma. JAMA neurology. 2013; 70:311–319

[16] Calamia KT, Miller A, Shuster EA, et al. Intravascular Lymphomatosis: A Report of Ten Patients with Central Nervous System Involvement and a Review of the Disease Process. Advances in Experimental Medicine and Biology. 1999; 455:249–265

[17] Glass J, Hochberg FH, Miller DC. Intravascular Lymphomatosis. A Systemic Disease with Neurologic Manifestations. Cancer. 1993; 71:3156–3164

[18] So YT, Beckstead JH, Davis RL Primary central nervous system lymphoma in acquired immune deficiency syndrome: A clinical and pathological study. Ann Neurol. 1986; 20:566–572

[19] Poon T, Matoso I, Tchertkoff V, et al. CT features of primary cerebral lymphoma in AIDS and non-AIDS patients. Journal of Computer Assisted Tomography. 1989; 13:6–9

[20] DeAngelis LM. Cerebral Lymphoma Presenting as a Nonenhancing Lesion of Computed Tomographic/Magnetic Resonance Scan. Annals of Neurology. 1993; 33:308–311

[21] Enzmann DR, Krikorian J, Norman D, et al. Computed Tomography in Primary Reticulum Cell Sarcoma of the Brain. Radiology. 1979; 130:165–170

[22] Vaquero J, Martinez R, Rossi E, et al. Primary Cerebral Lymphoma: the 'Ghost Tumor'. J Neurosurg. 1984; 60:174–176

[23] Gray RS, Abrahams JJ, Hufnagel TJ, et al. Ghost-cell tumor of the optic chiasm; primary CNS lymphoma. Journal of Clinical Neuro-Ophthalmology. 1989; 9:98–104

[24] Roy S, Josephson SA, Fridlyand J, et al. Protein biomarker identification in the CSF of patients with CNS lymphoma. J Clin Oncol. 2008; 26:96–105

[25] O'Neill BP, Kelly PJ, Earle JD, et al. Computer-Assisted Stereotactic Biopsy for the Diagnosis of Primary Central Nervous System Lymphoma. Neurology. 1987; 37:1160–1164

[26] DeAngelis LM, Yahalom J, Heinemann M-H, et al. Primary Central Nervous System Lymphomas: Combined Treatment with Chemotherapy and Radiotherapy. Neurology. 1990; 40:80–86

[27] DeAngelis LM, Yahalom J, Thaler HT, et al. Combined Modality Therapy for Primary CNS Lymphomas. J Clin Oncol. 1992; 10:635–643

[28] O'Marcaigh AS, Johnson CM, Smithson WA, et al. Successful Treatment of Intrathecal Methotrexate Overdose by Using Ventriculolumbar Perfusion and Intrathecal Instillation of Carboxypeptidase G2. Mayo Clinic Proceedings. 1996; 71:161–165

[29] Hochberg FH, Miller DC. Primary Central Nervous System Lymphoma. J Neurosurg. 1988; 68:835–853

[30] Oyama T, Yamamoto K, Asano N, et al. Age-related EBV-associated B-cell lymphoproliferative disorders constitute a distinct clinicopathologic group: a study of 96 patients. Clin Cancer Res. 2007; 13:5124–5132

[31] Baumgartner JE, Rachlin JR, Beckstead JH, et al. Primary Central Nervous System Lymphomas: Natural History and Response to Radiation Therapy in 55 Patients with Acquired Immunodeficiency Syndrome. Journal of Neurosurgery. 1990; 73:206–211

[32] Formenti SC, Gill PS, Lean E, et al. Primary Central Nervous System Lymphoma in AIDS: Results of Radiation Therapy. Cancer. 1989; 63:1101–1107

[33] Rawlings CE, Wilkins RH. Solitary Eosinophilic Granuloma of the Skull. Neurosurgery. 1984; 15:155–161

[34] Guyot-Goubin A, Donadieu J, Barkaoui M, et al. Descriptive epidemiology of childhood Langerhans cell histiocytosis in France, 2000-2004. Pediatr Blood Cancer. 2008; 51:71–75

[35] Mitnick JS, Pinto RS. CT in the Diagnosis of Eosinophilic Granuloma. J Comput Assist Tomogr. 1980; 4:791–793

50 Tumors of the Sellar Region

50.1 General information

The pituitary gland is composed of the adenohypophysis, a neuroendocrine structure with 6 hormone secreting cell types, and the neurohypophysis which is comprised of pituicytes. Tumors can arise from these structures, and other tumors can occur in this region including those from rests of oral ectoderm (craniopharyngiomas) as well as meningiomas, germ cell tumors, chordomas and metastases.

50.2 Sellar region tumors of non pituitary origin

50.2.1 Craniopharyngiomas

Key concepts

- epithelial tumors thought to arise from residual cells of Rathke's pouch (p. 151)
- histologically benign, but the location and propensity to invade critical neural structures makes them malignant in behavior
- initially regarded as 1 tumor with two subtypes, now considered to be two distinct tumors which may be differentiated by gene mutations:
  1. adamantinomatous craniopharyngioma: 95% show *CTNNB1* mutations and aberrant nuclear expression of beta-catenin. Bimodal distribution: 5–15 years & 45–60 years
  2. papillary craniopharyngioma: 1–95% of cases show BRAF V600E mutations. Mean age of 40–55 years.

50

Historically, craniopharyngioma was considered a tumor with 2 subtypes, adamantinomatous and papillary. It is now recognized that, although both of these tumors arise in the same region and display squamous lineage, that they are actually discinct tumors with differing epidemiology, radiology, histology, and molecular genetics.[1]

They are thought to develop from residual cells of Rathke's pouch (p. 151) (craniopharyngeal duct).

CP do not undergo malignant degeneration, but the fact that they may infiltrate neural tissue can make them difficult to cure (benign in histology, malignant in behavior). CP are distinct from Rathke's cleft cyst (p. 949), but share some similarities.

Epidemiology

0.8% of all brain tumors, with an incidence of 0.19 per 100,000 in the US.[2] They comprise 5–11% of pediatric brain tumors, making them the most common non-neuroepithelial intracerebral tumor in children.

50.2.2 Adamantinomatous craniopharyngioma (ACP) (WHO grade 1)

General information

A mixed solid and cystic squamous epithelial tumor with stellate reticulum, wet keratin and basal pallisades. Up to 95% of cases of this variant shows *CTNNB1* mutations and aberrant nuclear expression of beta-catenin.[3] Tend to arise from the anterior superior margin of the pituitary. Fluid in the cysts varies, but usually contains cholesterol crystals.

Diagnostic criteria for adamantinomatous craniopharyngioma

Diagnostic criteria for adamantinomatous craniopharyngioma are shown in ▶ Fig. 50.1.[4]

Epidemiology

Bimodal age distribution: childhood peak age 5–15 years, adult peak age 45–60 years.[3]

Adamantinomatous craniopharyngioma

▷ ESSENTIAL ◁

tumor in the sellar region

AND

squamous non-keratinizing epithelium, benign

AND

stellate reticulum and/or wet keratin

▷ DESIRABLE ◁

► nuclear immunoreactivity for β-catenin
► mutation in *CTNNB1*
► absence of *BRAF* p.V600E mutation

Fig. 50.1 Diagnostic criteria for adamantinomatous craniopharyngioma. (Modified with permission from WHO Classification of Tumors Editorial Board, (ed.) World Health Organization classification of tumors of the central nervous system. 5th ed. Bosman F T, Jaffe E S, Lakhani S R, et al. (series eds.): World Health Organization Classification of Tumors series, vol. 6. International Agency for Research on Cancer, Lyon, France, 2021.)

Location

Most occur in the region of the sella turcica and pituitary infundibulum. Purely sellar lesions are rare, with ≈ 95% extending into the suprasellar compartment. Pure involvement of the 3rd entricle is more common with papillary CP.

Imaging

Imaging mnemonic: "90% rule" 90% of adamantinomatous craniopharyngiomas exhibit at least 2 of the following "C" features: cyst formation, prominent calcifications, and contrast enhancement in the cyst walls.[5]

50.2.3 Papillary craniopharyngioma (RCP) (WHO grade 1)

General information

A craniopharyngioma with papillary features that occurs primarily in adults. 81–95% of cases show *BRAF* V600E mutations.[3] Usually solid, or partially cystic.

Diagnostic criteria for papillary craniopharyngioma

Diagnostic criteria for papillary craniopharyngioma are shown in ► Fig. 50.2.[4]

Location

Typically arises in the infundibular recess and tuber cinereum of the floor of the 3rd ventricle. Rarely occurs intrasellar.

Epidemiology

Comprise 1.2–4.6% of intracranial tumors, with an incidence of 0.5-1.5 cases per 1 million.[4] They are less common than adamantinomatous CP, constituting only ≈ 10% of all CP, but 12-33% in adults.[4]

Occurs almost exclusively in adults with a mean age of 40–55 years.

Papillary craniopharyngioma

▷ ESSENTIAL ◁

tumor in the sellar region

AND

non-keratinizing mature squamous epithelium covering fibrovascular cores or a cyst wall

▷ DESIRABLE ◁

- ▶ immunoreactivity for BRAF p.V600E
- ▶ presence of *BRAF* p.V600E mutation
- ▶ absence of nuclear β-catenin immunoreactivity
- ▶ absence of *CTNNB1* mutation

Fig. 50.2 Diagnostic criteria for papillary craniopharyngioma. (Modified with permission from WHO Classification of Tumors Editorial Board, (ed.) World Health Organization classification of tumors of the central nervous system. 5th ed. Bosman F T, Jaffe E S, Lakhani S R, et al. (series eds.): World Health Organization Classification of Tumors series, vol. 6. International Agency for Research on Cancer, Lyon, France, 2021.)

50

Imaging

Less frequently cystic than adamantinomatous CP. Usually spherical (c.f., lobulated) and infrequently contain calcifications. The pituitary stalk is often thickened.

50.2.4 Vascular anatomy

Arterial supply: usually small feeders from ACA and A-comm, or from ICA and P-comm (do not receive blood from PCA or BA-bifurcation unless blood supply of the floor of the third ventricle is parasitized).

50.2.5 Treatment options

GTR is associated with better PFS than STR alone, but the advantage of GTR over STR followed by adjuvant XRST is not as clear.[4]

BRAF and/or MEK inhibitors show promise in *BRAF* p.V600E–mutant papillary CP.[6]

50.2.6 Surgical treatment

Pre-op endocrinologic evaluation

As for pituitary tumor (p.876). Hypoadrenalism may be corrected rapidly, but hypothyroidism takes longer; either condition can increase surgical mortality.

Approach

Usually via large right frontotemporal flap as low as possible along base of frontal fossa (lateral sphenoid wing rongeured/drilled). Approach to tumor is extra-axial, whether subfrontal or frontotemporal. *All* tumors should be aspirated (even if they appear solid radiographically). Then, with microscope, possible approaches include:

1. subchiasmatic: through space between optic nerves and anterior to chiasm. It was thought that a "prefixed chiasm" (i.e., congenitally short optic nerves with chiasm unusually close to the planum sphenoidale) was more common in patients with CP, making this approach more difficult.

However, in reality the chiasm is probably bowed anteriorly by the tumor within the third ventricle, giving the illusion of a prefixed chiasm in most cases

2. opticocarotid (between right ICA and right optic nerve/tract)
3. lamina terminalis (tumor often needs to be brought down and removed subchiasmatically)[7,8]
4. lateral to carotid artery
5. transfrontal-transsphenoidal: drill off tuberculum sellae

Alternative approaches to frontotemporal
1. pure transsphenoidal: if dark fluid is aspirated with no CSF evident, it is possible to leave a stent from the tumor cavity to the sphenoid air-sinus to permit continued drainage
2. transcallosal: strictly for tumors limited to the third ventricle
3. a combined subfrontal/pterional approach capitalizes on the advantages of each (head is positioned with slight lateral rotation)
4. extended transnasal transsphenoidal endoscopic resection[9,10]

Spare the following structures: small arterial feeders to *undersurface* of the chiasm (major supply) and tract; at least a remnant of pituitary stalk (recognized by unique pattern of longitudinal striations which are the long portal veins). If the tumor easily pulls down from above then this is permissible; however, do not pull too hard, or else hypothalamic injury may result.
Post-op
1. steroids: these patients are all considered hypo-adrenal. Give hydrocortisone in physiologic doses (for mineralocorticoid activity) in addition to dexamethasone (glucocorticoid that treats edema) taper. Taper steroids slowly to avoid aseptic (chemical) meningitis
2. diabetes insipidus (DI) (p. 902): often shows up early. May be part of a "triphasic response." (p. 125) Best managed initially with fluid replacement. If necessary, use short acting vasopressin (prevents iatrogenic renal shutdown if an SIADH-like phase develops during vasopressin therapy)

50.2.7 Radiation

Controversial. **Side effects:** include endocrine dysfunction, optic neuritis, dementia. Post-op XRT probably helps prevent regrowth when residual tumor is left behind[11]; however, in pediatric cases it may be best to postpone XRT (to minimize deleterious effect on IQ), recognizing that reoperation may be necessary for recurrence.

50.2.8 Outcome

Most outcome data are derived from CP as a monolithic entity, and since papillary CP make up only a minority of CPs, their outcome data is sparse. It has been asserted that papillary CP have a better prognosis, but inconvertible proof of this is lacking.

5–10% mortality in most series, most from hypothalamic injury (unilateral hypothalamic lesions are rarely clinically evident; bilateral injuries may produce hyperthermia and somnolence; damage to anterior osmoreceptors may → loss of thirst sensation).

Five year survival is ≈ 55–85% (range from 30–93% has been reported).

50.2.9 Recurrence

Most recurrences are in < 1 year, few > 3 yrs (very delayed recurrence usually follow what was thought to be "total" removal). Morbidity/mortality is higher with reoperation.

50.3 Tumors of the neurohypophysis & infundibulum

50.3.1 General information

Description

This group of rare low-grade tumors that originate from pituicytes of the neurohypophysis (posterior pituitary) and infundibulum are probably a spectrum of a single entity, the members of the group being:
1. pituicytoma
2. granular cell tumor of the sellar region (GCT)

3. spindle cell oncocytoma (SCO)

These tumors all show nuclear expression of thyroid transcription factor 1 (TTF1). They are usually misidentified as PitNET/adenomas on imaging, and are rarely considered in the preoperative differential diagnosis.

Epidemiology

The rarity of these tumors has prevented robust epidemiologic analysis. A literature meta-analysis of 270 cases[12] found a mean age of 48 ± 22 years.

Location

These tumors originate in the posterior pituitary or infundibulum, and therefore their location is purely sellar (25%), sellar with suprasellar extension (48%), or suprasellar (23%).[12] Spindle cell oncocytoma can be more invasive (see below).

Presentation

Symptoms from mass effect are similar to other tumors of this location: visual field defects (in 58%) (classically bitemporal hemianopsia), hypopituitarism (34%), and H/A (40%).[12] Diabetes insipidus occurs infrequently (2.4%).

Associated endocrinologic overproduction syndromes include hypercortisolism (4.1%), and acromegaly (2.0%), some of which may be due to synchronous functional PitNET/adenomas.[13]

Imaging

These tumors may appear radiographically identical to adenomas. They are rarely considered in the differential diagnosis pre-op. Isodense on CT and isointense on T1WI MRI, with dense homogeneous enhancement on CT and MRI.

50

Treatment

GTR frequently cures these tumors, although SCO appears to have a higher recurrence rate. If the diagnosis is suspected pre-op, a transcranial approach is preferred over transsphenoidal because of the vascularity which has prevented total resection in 60–70% of reported cases.[14]

XRT may be considered for subtotal resection.[15]

50.3.2 Pituicytoma (WHO grade 1)

General information

Rare (mostly case reports). Circumscribed, with bipolar spindle cells arranged in a fascicular or storiform pattern (a cartwheel pattern).[3,16] Low mitotic activity. Cytoplasmic granules (found in granular cell tumors) are lacking. WHO grade 1. Reported only in adults.

Diagnostic criteria for pituicytoma

Diagnostic criteria for pituicytoma are shown in ▶ Fig. 50.3.[4]

50.3.3 Granular cell tumor of the sellar region (WHO grade 1)

General information

A circumscribed tumor with nests of large cells having granular, eosinophilic cytoplasm due to copious cytoplasmic lysosomes. Mitotic activity is rare.

While rare, GCTs are the most common primary tumor of the neurohypophysis and pituitary stalk/infundibulum[15] with a predilection for the stalk (causing suprasellar extension). GCTs have been identified in the gastrointestinal tract, genitourinary tract, orbital region as well as in other locations of the central nervous system with no connection to the pituitary gland or hypothalamus (e.g., spinal meninges[17]). Female:male ratio ≥ 2:1. Asymptomatic microscopic clusters of granular cells (tumorettes) are more common, with an incidence up to 17%.[18]

They usually follow a slow progression with benign behavior.

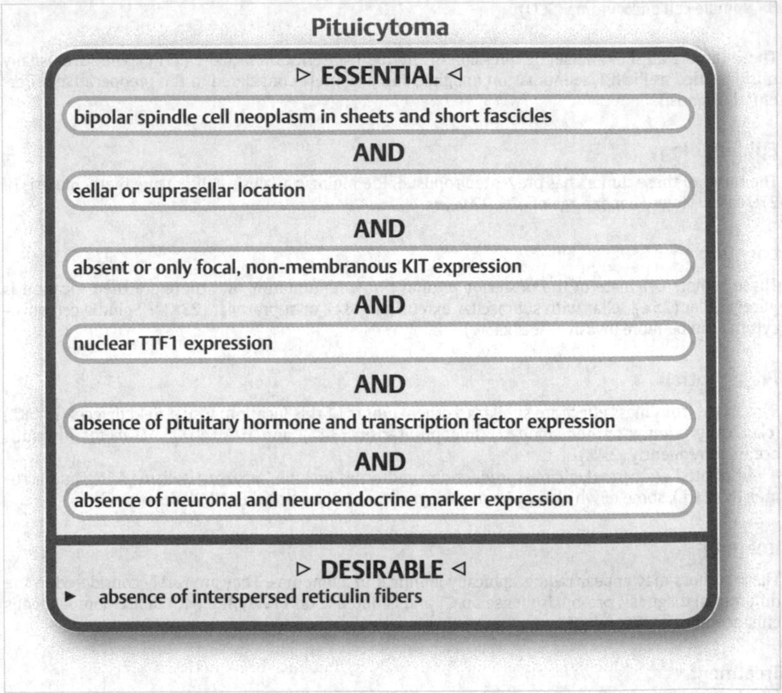

Fig. 50.3 Diagnostic criteria for pituicytoma. (Modified with permission from WHO Classification of Tumors Editorial Board, (ed.) World Health Organization classification of tumors of the central nervous system. 5th ed. Bosman F T, Jaffe E S, Lakhani S R, et al. (series eds.): World Health Organization Classification of Tumors series, vol. 6. International Agency for Research on Cancer, Lyon, France, 2021.)

Diagnostic criteria for granular cell tumor

Diagnostic criteria for granular cell tumor are shown in ▶ Fig. 50.4.[4]

50.3.4 Spindle cell oncocytoma (WHO grade 1)

General information

In addition to intrasellar and suprasellar involvement, there are reports of invasion of the cavernous sinus[19] and floor of the sella.[20] Their highly vascular nature makes them suscepitble to spontaneous hemorrhage and also to significant blood loss during surgery.

Diagnostic criteria for spindle cell oncocytoma

Diagnostic criteria for spindle cell oncocytoma are shown in ▶ Fig. 50.5.[4]

50.4 Tumors of the adenohypophysis

50.4.1 Pituitary neuroendocrine tumor (PitNET)/pituitary adenoma

General information

A clonal neoplasm of anterior pituitary hormone producing cells.

Granular cell tumor

▷ ESSENTIAL ◁

neoplasm composed of polygonal cells with granular cytoplasm

AND

sellar or suprasellar location

AND

absent or only focal, non-membranous KIT expression

AND

nuclear TTF1 expression

AND

absence of pituitary hormone and transcription factor expression

AND

absence of neuronal and neuroendocrine marker expression

▷ DESIRABLE ◁

► absence of interspersed reticulin fibers
► PAS-positive/diastase-resistant
► CD68 or α1-antitrypsin immunoreactivity

50

Fig. 50.4 Diagnostic criteria for granular cell tumor. (Modified with permission from WHO Classification of Tumors Editorial Board, (ed.) World Health Organization classification of tumors of the central nervous system. 5th ed. Bosman F T, Jaffe E S, Lakhani S R, et al. (series eds.): World Health Organization Classification of Tumors series, vol. 6. International Agency for Research on Cancer, Lyon, France, 2021.)

Terminology: traditionally, these tumors have been classified as adenomas, but they are actually neuroendocrine tumors since they contain neurosecretory granules. Thus the current nomenclature is pituitary neuroendocrine tumors (PitNETs). To transition the terminology, for the time being they may also be called **PitNET/adenomas** to denote that "pituitary adenoma" is still acceptable, but Pit-NET is preferred.[21]

Diagnostic criteria for PitNET/adenoma

Diagnostic criteria for PitNET/adenoma are shown in ► Fig. 50.6.[4]

Clinical considerations for PitNET/adenomas

Owing to the intricacies of PitNET/adenomas, a number of sections are devoted to their clinical aspects, starting with section 51.

50.4.2 Invasive pituitary tumors

General information

Tumors of the anterior pituitary can invade surrounding structures. Some of these are PitNETs (≈ 5% of PitNETs, and ≈ 30–40% of *surgically treated* PitNETs are invasive[22]). Non-functioning PitNETs have a

Spindle cell oncocytoma

▷ **ESSENTIAL** ◁

neoplasm composed of polygonal cells with granular cytoplasm

AND

sellar or suprasellar location

AND

absent or only focal, non-membranous KIT expression

AND

nuclear TTF1 expression

AND

absence of pituitary hormone and transcription factor expression

AND

absence of neuronal and neuroendocrine marker expression

▷ **DESIRABLE** ◁
► absence of interspersed reticulin fibers
► antimitochondrial antigen immunoreactivity

Fig. 50.5 Diagnostic criteria for spindle cell oncocytoma. (Modified with permission from WHO Classification of Tumors Editorial Board, (ed.) World Health Organization classification of tumors of the central nervous system. 5th ed. Bosman F T, Jaffe E S, Lakhani S R, et al. (series eds.): World Health Organization Classification of Tumors series, vol. 6. International Agency for Research on Cancer, Lyon, France, 2021.)

higher incidence of invasion.[23] However, more aggressive pituitary tumors can also be locally invasive, and are considered here.

Wilson's anatomic classification for invasive pituitary tumors[24] (modified from Hardy[25,26]) is shown in ► Table 50.1.

At times, a pituitary tumor may displace the medial wall of the cavernous sinus ahead of it without actually perforating this dural structure (i.e., not actually invading the sinus).[27] This is difficult to reliably identify on MRI, and the most definitive sign of cavernous sinus invasion is carotid artery encasement.[28]

The clinical course is variable, with some tumors being more aggressive than others. Occasionally, these tumors grow to sizes > 4 cm dia, and these are often very aggressive and follow a malignant course.[29]

Aggressive pituitary tumors

A subset of invasive pituitary tumors meet the European Society of Endocrinology (ESE) guidelines[30] definition of "aggressive pituitary tumors," viz., pituitary tumors that do not respond to standard therapies (surgery, conventional medical treatments and XRT) and present with multiple local recurrences. The WHO does not recognize this category in its current classification[4] (and the term "atypical adenoma" was dropped in the WHO 2017 classification).

Pituitary carcinoma

The definition of pituitary carcinoma is contentious. Both the ESE and WHO consider the presence of noncontiguous metastases as qualifying as pituitary carcinoma.[4,21] Only ≈ 0.16% of pituitary tumors

PitNET/adenoma

▷ ESSENTIAL ◁

sellar or suprasellar location

AND

histological features of a low-grade neuroendocrine tumor that displays destruction of the normal anterior gland acinar structure

AND

subclassification based on immunoreactivity for pituitary hormones and/or lineage-specific transcription factors

▷ DESIRABLE ◁

► reticulin fiber disruption
► low-molecular-weight cytokeratins, in particular for somatotroph and corticotroph tumors
► tumor proliferation as indicated by either mitotic count or Ki-67 (MIB1) expression

Fig. 50.6 Diagnostic criteria for PitNET/adenoma. (Modified with permission from WHO Classification of Tumors Editorial Board, (ed.) World Health Organization classification of tumors of the central nervous system. 5th ed. Bosman F T, Jaffe E S, Lakhani S R, et al. (series eds.): World Health Organization Classification of Tumors series, vol. 6. International Agency for Research on Cancer, Lyon, France, 2021.)

Table 50.1 Anatomic classification of invasive pituitary tumors (modified Hardy system)[24]

Extension

- **Suprasellar extension**
  0: none
  A: expanding into suprasellar cistern
  B: anterior recesses of 3rd ventricle obliterated
  C: floor of 3rd ventricle grossly displaced
- **Parasellar extension**
  D[a]: intracranial (intradural)
  E: into or beneath cavernous sinus (extradural)

Invasion/Spread

- **Floor of sella intact**
  I: sella normal or focally expanded; tumor < 10 mm
  II: sella enlarged; tumor ≥ 10 mm
- **Sphenoid extension**
  III: localized perforation of sellar floor
  IV: diffuse destruction of sellar floor
- **Distant spread[b]**
  V: spread via CSF or blood-borne

[a] specify: 1) anterior, 2) middle, or 3) posterior fossa
[b] this qualifies as pituitary carcinoma (see text)

give rise to noncontiguous metastases (spreading systemically or through the CSF).[31] Although the prognosis with metastases is worse, there are some aggressive tumors with similar behavior even in the absence of metastases.[22]

Nomenclature suggestion for pituitary tumor grades

Taking into account the areas of agreement and areas of uncertainty in classification, the suggestion shown in the box has been proposed[22,32]

Σ: Nomenclature suggestion for pituitary tumor grades[22,32]

- Noninvasive tumors on MRI (60-65%): **PitNET/adenomas**
- Invasive tumors on MRI (35-40%):
  - Persistent disease that is *controlled* (with or without XRT) after surgery and/or medical treatment: **Invasive PitNet**
  - Persistent disease that is *recurrent or progressive* (with or without XRT) after surgery and/or medical treatment[a]: **aggressive pituitary tumor** or **invasive PitNET with malignant potential**
  - Persistent disease with noncontiguous metastases[a]: **Pituitary carcinoma**

[a] many of these tumors will exhibit some combination of the following (only 2% exhibit all 3[33]): Ki67 ≥ 3%, positive P53 expression and/or mitotic rate > 2/10 HPF

Presentation of invasive pituitary tumors

1. visual system
   a) most present due to compression of the optic apparatus, usually producing gradual visual deficit (however, sudden blindness is not unheard of)
   b) extraocular muscle deficits may occur with cavernous sinus invasion, and usually develop after visual loss
   c) exophthalmos may occur with orbital invasion due to compromise of orbital venous drainage
2. hydrocephalus: suprasellar extension may obstruct one or both foramen of Monro
3. invasion of the skull base may lead to nasal obstruction. CSF rhinorrhea may occasionally be precipitated by tumor shrinkage in response to dopamine agonists (e.g., bromocriptine or cabergoline) as a result of uncovering areas of bone erosion. This carries the risk of ascending meningitis.[34]
4. invasive pituitary tumors that secrete prolactin (p. 863) often present with findings of hyperprolactinemia and with these, the prolactin levels are usually > 1000 ng/ml (caution: giant invasive adenomas with very high prolactin production may have a falsely low PRL due to "hook effect" (p. 877))

Management suggestions for invasive pituitary tumors

The European Society of Endocrinology (ESE) treatent guidelines include the following[30] (see reference for full details).
1. routine pituitary tumor screening ▶ Table 52.1 (pituitary hormone assessment and visual field testing)
2. the diagnosis of an aggressive pituitary tumor should be considered with invasive tumors exhibiting an unusually rapid growth rate, or clinically significant growth following optimal standard treatment (surgery, XRT and conventional medical treatment)
3. consider screening for metastatic disease for symptoms outside the sellar region or MRI findings suspicious for local noncontiguous spread
4. initial surgery by a surgeon with extensive experience in pituitary surgery
5. Ki67 proliferative index should be assessed in surgical specimens, and if the Ki67 is ≥ 3%, then p53 immunodetection and mitotic count should be evaluated as potential predictors of tumor aggressiveness
6. consideration of repeat surgery prior to proceeding to other treatment options
7. XRT
   a) recommended for progression after surgery for non-functioning tumors, or after surgery + standard medcial treatment in functioning tumors
   b) consideration of XRT recommended after surgery for clinically relevant tumor remnant with markers that suggest aggressive behavior (Ki67 ≥ 3% and/or positive P53 and/or mitotic rate > 2/10 HPF)

8. chemotherapy for tumors demonstrating continued growth*
   a) Stupp regimen (p.672): temozolamide (TMZ) monotherapy using the *adjuvant* dosing regimen (150–200 mg/m^2 for 5 consecurive days every 28 days) & XRT (if maximal XRT has not yet been given)
   b) assessment after 3 cycles of TMZ
      1. if there is clinical response, continue TMZ cycles for 5 days every 28 days for 6 months total, and consideration for longer duration if continued benefit is demonstrated
      2. if no response, then a trial with systemic toxic chemotherapy is suggested (no specific agent could be preferentially recommended)
9. for isolated metastases, local regional therapies in addition to systemic treatment as indicated
10. MRIs should be repeated every 3–12 months depending on tumor growth and risk to vital structures

* assessment of MGMT promoter gene methylation (p.673) expression is mentioned as a recommendation, but this may not alter the treatment paradigm.

References

[1] Muller HL, Merchant TE, Warmuth-Metz M, et al. Craniopharyngioma. Nat Rev Dis Primers. 2019; 5. DOI: 10.1038/s41572-019-0125-9

[2] Ostrom QT, Gittleman H, Liao P, et al. CBTRUS Statistical Report: Primary brain and other central nervous system tumors diagnosed in the United States in 2010-2014. Neuro Oncol. 2017; 19:v1–v88

[3] Louis DN, Ohgaki H, Wiestler OD, et al. WHO classification of tumors of the central nervous system. Lyon, France 2016

[4] Bosman FT, Jaffe ES, Lakhani SR, et al. World Health Organization Classification of Tumors series, vol. 6. In: WHO Classification of Tumors Editorial Board (ed.) World Health Organization classification of tumors of the central nervous system. 5th ed. Lyon, France: International Agency for Research on Cancer; 2021

[5] Johnson LN, Hepler RS, Yee RD, et al. Magnetic resonance imaging of craniopharyngioma. Am J Ophthalmol. 1986; 102:242–244

[6] Nussbaum PE, Nussbaum LA, Torok CM, et al. Case report and literature review of BRAF-V600 inhibitors for treatment of papillary craniopharyngiomas: A potential treatment paradigm shift. J Clin Pharm Ther. 2022; 47:826–831

[7] Klein HJ, Rath SA. Removal of Tumors of the III Ventricle Using Lamina Terminalis Approach: Three Cases of Isolated Growth of Craniopharyngiomas in the III Ventricle. Child's Nervous System. 1989; 5:144–147

[8] Patterson RH, Denylevich A. Surgical Removal of Craniopharyngiomas by a Transcranial Approach through the Lamina Terminalis and Sphenoid Sinus. Neurosurgery. 1980; 7:111–117

[9] Park HR, Kshettry VR, Farrell CJ, et al. Clinical Outcome After Extended Endoscopic Endonasal Resection of Craniopharyngiomas: Two-Institution Experience. World Neurosurg. 2017; 103:465–474

[10] Cao L, Wu W, Kang J, et al. Feasibility of endoscopic endonasal resection of intrinsic third ventricular craniopharyngioma in adults. Neurosurg Rev. 2022; 45:1–13

[11] Manaka S, Teramoto A, Takakura K. The Efficacy of Radiotherapy for Craniopharyngiomas. Journal of Neurosurgery. 1985; 62:648–656

[12] Guerrero-Perez F, Marengo AP, Vidal N, et al. Primary tumors of the posterior pituitary: A systematic review. Rev Endocr Metab Disord. 2019; 20:219–238

[13] Iglesias P, Guerrero-Perez F, Villabona C, et al. Adenohypophyseal hyperfunction syndromes and posterior pituitary tumors: prevalence, clinical characteristics, and pathophysiological mechanisms. Endocrine. 2020; 70:15–23

[14] Gueguen B, Merland JJ, Riche MC, et al. Vascular Malformations of the Spinal Cord: Intrathecal Perimedullary Arteriovenous Fistulas Fed by Medullary Arteries. Neurology. 1987; 37:969–979

[15] Schaller B, Kirsch E, Tolnay M, et al. Symptomatic granular cell tumor of the pituitary gland: case report and review of the literature. Neurosurgery. 1998; 42:166–70; discussion 170-1

[16] Wesseling P, Brat DJ, Fuller GN, et al. Pituicytoma. In: WHO classification of tumors of the central nervous system. 4th ed. Lyon: International Agency for Research on Cancer; 2007:243–244

[17] Markesbery WR, Duffy PE, Cowen D. Granular cell tumors of the central nervous system. J Neuropathol Exp Neurol. 1973; 32:92–109

[18] Fuller GN, Wesseling P, Louis DN, et al. Granular cell tumors of the neurohypophysis. In: WHO classification of tumors of the central nervous system. 4th ed. Lyon: International Agency for Research on Cancer; 2007:241–242

[19] Dahiya S, Sarkar C, Hedley-Whyte ET, et al. Spindle cell oncocytoma of the adenohypophysis: report of two cases. Acta Neuropathol. 2005; 110:97–99

[20] Kloub O, Perry A, Tu PH, et al. Spindle cell oncocytoma of the adenohypophysis: report of two recurrent cases. Am J Surg Pathol. 2005; 29:247–253

[21] Mete O, WHO Classification of Tumors Editorial Board. Pituitary gland. Lyon, France 2022. https://publications.iarc.fr/Book-And-Report-Series/Who-Classification-Of-Tumours

[22] Raverot G, Ilie MD, Lasolle H, et al. Aggressive pituitary tumours and pituitary carcinomas. Nat Rev Endocrinol. 2021; 17:671–684

[23] Lu L, Wan X, Xu Y, et al. Classifying Pituitary Adenoma Invasiveness Based on Radiological, Surgical and Histological Features: A Retrospective Assessment of 903 Cases. J Clin Med. 2022; 11. DOI: 10.3390/jcm11092464

[24] Wilson CB, Tindall GT, Collins WF. Neurosurgical Management of Large and Invasive Pituitary Tumors. In: Clinical Management of Pituitary Disorders. New York: Raven Press; 1979:335–342

[25] Hardy J, Kohler PO, Ross GT. Transsphenoidal Surgery of Hypersecreting Pituitary Tumors. In: Diagnosis and Treatment of Pituitary Tumors. New York: Excerpta Medica/American Elsevier; 1973:179–194

[26] Hardy J, Thompson RA, Green R. Transsphenoidal Surgery of Intracranial Neoplasm. In: Advances in Neurology. New York: Raven Press; 1976:261–274

[27] Laws ER. Comment on Knosp E, et al.: Pituitary Adenomas with Invasion of the Cavernous Sinus Space: A Magnetic Resonance Imaging Classification Compared with Surgical Findings. Neurosurgery. 1993; 33

[28] Scotti G, Yu CY, Dillon WP, et al. MR Imaging of Cavernous Sinus Involvement by Pituitary Adenomas. American Journal of Radiology. 1988; 151:799–806

[29] Krisht AF. Giant invasive pituitary adenomas. Contemporary Neurosurgery. 1999; 21:1–6

[30] Raverot G, Burman P, McCormack A, et al. European Society of Endocrinology Clinical Practice Guidelines for the management of aggressive pituitary

50

tumours and carcinomas. Eur J Endocrinol. 2018; 178:G1–G24

[31] Saeger W, Ludecke DK, Buchfelder M, et al. Pathohistological classification of pituitary tumors: 10 years of experience with the German Pituitary Tumor Registry. Eur J Endocrinol. 2007; 156:203–216

[32] Trouillas J, Burman P, McCormack A, et al. Aggressive pituitary tumours and carcinomas: two sides of the same coin? Eur J Endocrinol. 2018; 178:C7–C9

[33] Raverot G, Dantony E, Beauvy J, et al. Risk of Recurrence in Pituitary Neuroendocrine Tumors: A Prospective Study Using a Five-Tiered Classification. J Clin Endocrinol Metab. 2017; 102:3368–3374

[34] Barlas O, Bayindir C, Hepgul K, et al. Bromocriptine-induced cerebrospinal fluid fistula in patients with macroprolactinomas: report of three cases and a review of the literature. Surg Neurol. 1994; 41:486–489

51 PitNET/Adenomas – Clinical Considerations

51.1 General information

Key concepts

- most are benign, however some are locally aggressive and (rarely) metastasize
- presentation (p. 863): most common
  - symptoms from excess hormonal secretion: includes hyperprolactinemia, Cushing's syndrome (↑ cortisol), acromegaly (↑ growth hormone)...
  - mass effect. Most commonly: bitemporal hemianopsia from compression of optic chiasm, or infrequently hypopituitarism from compression of pituitary gland
  - H/A: some H/A are due to increased pressure within the sella
  - incidental finding
  - infrequent presentations: pituitary apoplexy (p. 865), spontaneous CSF rhinorrhea
- work-up for a newly diagnosed intrasellar lesion: endocrine screening, visual field evaluation, imaging to visualize the tumor, the parasellar carotid arteries and the sphenoid sinus (see ▶ Table 52.1)
- prolactinoma is the only type for which medical therapy (DA agonists) may be the primary treatment (p. 886). For other tumor types, options primarily consist of surgery (usually transsphenoidal, sometimes transcranial), or XRT
- post-op concerns include: diabetes insipidus, adrenal insufficiency, CSF leak, and rarely visual deterioration due to herniation of the optic chiasm into empty sella

See review of pituitary embryology and neuroendocrinology (p. 151), and, for a discussion of the change in classification to PitNET/adenomas as well as diagnostic criteria, see section 50.4.1.

Most primary pituitary tumors are benign and arise from the anterior pituitary gland (adenohypophysis) as a monoclonal proliferation. However, some can be locally aggressive and rarely may metastasize.

PitNETs have been classified by a number of schemes, including: by endocrine function (aided by immunostaining), by light microscopy (p. 871) with routine histological staining, by electron microscopic appearance, and by molecular biology.

Microadenoma: defined as a pituitary tumor ≤ 1 cm diameter. 50% of pituitary tumors are < 5 mm at time of diagnosis. These may be difficult to find at the time of surgery.

Macroadenomas: pituitary tumors > 1 cm diameter.

51.2 Diagnostic criteria and classification of PitNET/adenoma

Diagnostic criteria for PitNET/pituitary adenoma are shown in ▶ Fig. 50.6.[1]

PitNETs derive from the six adenohypophyseal cell types. Each tumor type may have multiple subtypes which are shown along with their secretion products and clinical syndromes in ▶ Table 51.1

▶ **Null cell tumor (adenoma).** A PitNET without cell-type-specific differentiation based on immunohistochemistry, transcription factors, negative PAS stain.[3] The term is not synonymous with nonfunctioning adenomas. No endocrine syndrome is associated with these tumors. They comprise 5-30% of surgically resected adenomas, and < 5% of non-functioning adenomas. They typically occur after age 60 years.

51.3 Epidemiology/pathology

Pituitary tumors represent ≈ 10% of intracranial tumors (incidence is higher in autopsy series). They are most common in the 3rd and 4th decades of life, and affect both sexes equally. Nonfunctioning PitNETs are the most common pituitary tumors.[4] Cushing's disease and prolactinomas are more common in females, and nonfunctioning, lactotroph and null tumors[3] are more common in males.

Table 51.1 Classification of PitNETs[1,2] (used with permission from WHO Classification of Tumours Editorial Board. Central Nervous System Tumours. Lyon (France): International Agency for Research on Cancer; 2021. (WHO classification of tumours series, 5th ed.; vol. 6). Available from: https://tumourclassification.iarc.who.int/.)

Tumor type[a]	Transcription factors	Hormones	Keratin (CAM5.2 or CK18)	Tumor subtypes (if applicable)	Hormone excess syndrome[b]
PIT1-lineage tumors					
Somatotroph tumors	PIT1	GH, α-subunit	perinuclear	densely granulated somatotroph tumor	florid acromegaly
		GH	fibrous bodies (> 70%)	sparsely granulated somatotroph tumor	subtle acromegaly
Lactotroph tumors	PIT1, ERα	PRL (paranuclear)	weak or negative	sparsley granulated lactotroph tumor	hyperprolactinemia[c]
		PRL (diffuse cytoplasmic)	weak or negative	densely granulated lactotroph tumor	hyperprolactinemia[c]
Mammosomatotroph tumor	PIT1, ERα	GH (often predominant), PRL, α-subunit	perinuclear		acromegaly and hyperprolactinemia[c]
Thyrotroph tumor	PIT1, GATA2/3[d]	α-subunit, TSH-β	weak or negative		hyperthyroidism
Mature PIT1-lineage tumor	PIT1, ERα, GATA2/3[d]	GH (often predominant), PRL, α-subunit, TSH-β	perinuclear		acromegaly, hyperprolactinemia[c] and hyperthyroidism
Acidophil stem cell tumor	PIT1, ERα	PRL (predominant), GH (focal/variable)	scattered fibrous bodies		hyperprolactinemia[c] and subclinical acromegaly
Immature PIT1-lineage tumor	PIT1, ERα, GATA2/3[d]	GH, PRL, α-subunit, TSH-β	focal/ variable		acromegaly, hyperprolactinemia[c] and hyperthyroidism
TPIT-lineage tumors					
Corticotroph tumors	TPIT (TBX19), NeuroD1 (β2)	ACTH and other POMC derivatives	strong	densely granulated corticotroph tumor	florid Cushing, often microtumor
			variable	sparsely granulated corticotroph tumor	subtle Cushing, often macrotumor
			intense ring-like perinuclear	Crooke cell tumor	variable, Cushing
SF1-lineage tumors					
Gonadotroph tumor	SF1, ERα, GATA2/3[d]	α-subunit, FSH-β, LH-β	variable		hypogonadism (virtually all) or hypergonadism (exceptional)
Tumors without distinct cell lineage					
Unclassified plurihormonal tumors	multiple combinations	multiple combinations	variable		variable
Null cell tumor[e]	none	none	variable		none

[a] mixed tumors also occur and can constitute any combination of tumors shown; the most common is mixed somatotroph–lactotroph tumor

[b] any tumor type can be clinically non-functioning

[c] moderate hyperprolactinaemia can occur with any sellar mass that has suprasellar extension, interrupting hypothalamic tonic dopaminergic inhibition; however, the PRL level rarely exceeds 150 ng/mL; lactotroph tumors usually show a characteristic correlation between tumor size and PRL levels, whereas other PRL-secreting tumors do not

[d] GATA2 and GATA3 are paralogues and show cross-reactivity with some available antisera

[e] null cell tumor: not synonymous with non-functioning tumor (see text for details)

Most PitNET/adenomas are sporadic,[5] and arise from a somatic mutation of single progenitor cells. However, PitNETs may also occur as part of syndromes, including:

1. multiple endocrine adenomatosis or neoplasia (MEA or MEN) (especially type I: autosomal dominant inheritance with high penetrance, also involves pancreatic islet cell tumors (which may produce gastrin and hence Zollinger-Ellison syndrome) and parathyroids (hyperparathyroidism), and in which the pituitary tumors are usually nonsecretory)
2. Carney complex (p.652). Autosomal dominant, cardiac and cutaneous myxomas and hyperpigmentation. Associated with PitNET/adenomas that secrete either GH or GH + prolactin
3. familial isolated pituitary adenoma (FIPA). Autosomal dominant. Criteria: ≥ 2 family members with PitNET/adenomas in the absence of MEN or Carney complex. The adenomas may be of the same type (homogeneous FIPA) or of different types (heterogeneous FIPA)
4. McCune-Albright syndrome: mammosomatotroph and somatotroph tumors or hyperplasia
5. tuberous sclerosis: corticotroph tumors

51.4 Differential diagnosis of pituitary tumors

See differential diagnosis (p.1653), which also includes non-neoplastic etiologies.

51.5 Clinical presentation of pituitary tumors

51.5.1 General information

Classically, pituitary tumors are divided into functional (or secreting), and non-functional (AKA endocrine-inactive, which are either nonsecretory or else secrete hormonally inactive products or ones that do not cause endocrinologic symptoms, e.g., gonadotropin.

Possible presentations:
1. endocrine syndromes
   a) due to hormonal excess (with *functional* tumors), (see below). Primarily, one of the following: prolactin, growth hormone, cortisol, thyroid hormone
   b) due to hormonal deficiency (p.864) as a result of compression of the normal pituitary
2. mass effect (p.864)
3. incidental finding on imaging done for unrelated reasons (primarily with macroadenomas) in up to 20% of the population[6]
4. pituitary apoplexy (p.865): paroxysmal H/A with nausea and meningismus, endocrinologic and/ or neurologic deficit (usually ophthalmoplegia or visual loss)
5. hydrocephalus e.g., when tumors with a large suprasellar component compresses the 3rd ventricle

Unless they are discovered on imaging performed for some other indication ("pituitary incidentaloma"[7]), functional tumors tend to present earlier as a result of symptoms caused by physiologic effects of excess hormones that they secrete[8] (this applies less to gonadotropins and to prolactinomas in males since the symptoms may be mild or unrecognized). Nonfunctional tumors usually do not present until they are large enough to cause neurologic deficits by mass effect.

51.5.2 Presentation due to hormone oversecretion (secretory tumor)

≈ 65% of adenomas secrete an active hormone (48% prolactin, 10% GH, 6% ACTH, 1% TSH)[9]:
1. prolactin (p.867): can cause amenorrhea-galactorrhea syndrome in females, impotence in males. Etiologies:
   a) prolactinoma (p.867): neoplasia of pituitary lactotrophs
   b) stalk effect (p.877): pressure on the pituitary stalk may reduce the inhibitory control over prolactin secretion causing a modest increase in serum prolactin levels (PRLs)
2. growth hormone (GH): elevated GH is due to a PitNET > 95% of the time
   a) in adults: causes acromegaly (p.870)
   b) in prepubertal children (before epiphyseal plate closure): produces pituitary gigantism (very rare)
3. corticotropin AKA adrenocorticotropic hormone (ACTH):
   a) Cushing's disease (endogenous hypercortisolism): see below
   b) Nelson syndrome (p.869): can develop only in patients who have had an adrenalectomy
4. thyrotropin (TSH) (p.871): secondary (central) hyperthyroidism

51

5. gonadotropins (follicle stimulating hormone (FSH) and less commonly luteinizing hormone (LH)): usually does not produce a clinical syndrome. Rarely produces ovarian hyperstimulation syndrome (p. 867) in women (menstrual disturbance, galacorrhea…) or testicular hypertrophy in men

51.5.3 Presentation due to mass effect

Presentation due to underproduction of pituitary hormones

May be caused by compression of the normal pituitary by large tumors. More common with non-secretory tumors than with secretory tumors. In order of sensitivity to compression (i.e., the order in which pituitary hormones become depressed from mass effect): GH (61–100%), gonadotropins (LH & FSH) (36–96%), TSH (8–81%), ACTH (17–62%),[10] prolactin (mnemonic: **Go Look For The Adenoma Please**). Chronic deficiency of all pituitary hormones (panhypopituitarism) may produce pituitary cachexia (AKA Simmonds' cachexia).

✗ NB: selective reduction of a single pituitary hormone is very atypical with PitNETs. May occur with autoimmune hypophysitis (p. 1656), which most commonly involves ACTH or ADH (causing diabetes insipidus[11]—see below)

Deficiency of specific hormones:
1. growth hormone deficiency (note: growth hormone stimulation test (p. 882) is more sensitive and specific for GH deficiency than measuring basal GH levels):
   a) in children: produces growth delay
   b) in adults: produces vague symptoms with metabolic syndrome (decreased lean body mass, centripetal obesity, reduced exercise tolerance, impaired sense of well-being)
   c) hypogonadism: amenorrhea (women), loss of libido, infertility
2. hypothyroidism: cold intolerance, myxedema, entrapment neuropathies (e.g., carpal tunnel syndrome), weight gain, memory disturbance, integumentary changes (dry skin, coarse hair, brittle nails), constipation, increased sleep demand
3. hypoadrenalism: orthostatic hypotension, easy fatigability
4. diabetes insipidus: almost never seen preoperatively with pituitary tumors (except possibly with pituitary apoplexy, see below). If DI is present, other etiologies should be sought, including:
   a) autoimmune hypophysitis (p. 1656)
   b) hypothalamic glioma
   c) suprasellar germ cell tumor
5. gonadotropin deficiency (hypogonadotrophic hypogonadism) with anosmia is part of Kallmann syndrome[12]

Presentation due to mass effect (other than compression of the pituitary gland)

Because they tend to get to a larger size before detection, this is more common with nonfunctioning tumors. Of functional tumors, prolactinoma is the most likely to become large enough to cause mass effect (especially in males or non-menstruating females); ACTH tumor is least likely. Nonspecific symptoms include headaches. ✗ Seizures are rarely attributable to a PitNET and other etiologies should be sought. Mass effect may occur suddenly as a result of expansion with pituitary apoplexy (see below).

Structures are commonly compressed and their manifestations include:
1. optic chiasm: from tumor growth superiorly through the diaphragma sella (▶ Fig. 52.1). Classically produces **bitemporal hemianopsia** (non-congruous) (▶ Fig. 33.2). May also cause decreasing visual acuity
2. involvement of third ventricle may produce obstructive hydrocephalus
3. cavernous sinus
   a) pressure on cranial nerves contained within (III, IV, V1, V2, VI): ptosis, facial pain, diplopia (see below)
   b) occlusion of the cavernous sinus: proptosis, chemosis
   c) encasement of the carotid artery by tumor: may cause slight narrowing, but complete occlusion is rare
4. invasive adenomas (p. 855) may present as nasal or paranasal masses
5. CSF rhinorrhea: usually with invasive adenomas often as a result of erosion of the skull base, sometimes precipitated by shrinkage of these large tumors resulting from medical treatment[13]
6. macroadenomas may produce H/A possibly via increased intrasellar pressure

51

51.5.4 Pituitary apoplexy

General information

Key concepts

- due to expansion of a PitNET from hemorrhage or necrosis
- typical presentation: paroxysmal H/A with nausea and meningismus, endocrinologic and/or neurologic deficit (usually ophthalmoplegia or visual field loss)
- a medical emergency due to potentially lethal adrenal insufficiency and threat of permanent visual loss
- management: immediate administration of fluids and empiric corticosteroids (hydrocortisone) for hemodynamic instability, altered mental status (GCS < 15), visual deficits (acuity or visual fields). Shunt or EVD for hydrocephalus and transsphenoidal decompression within 7 days for visual loss
- not an emergency if asymptomatic

Definition

Neurologic and/or endocrinologic deterioration due to sudden expansion of a mass within the sella turcica.

Etiology

Sudden intrasellar expansion may occur as a result of hemorrhage, necrosis,[14,15] and/or infarction within a pituitary tumor and adjacent pituitary gland. Occasionally, hemorrhage occurs into a normal pituitary gland or Rathke's cleft cyst.[16]

Epidemiology

Pituitary apoplexy (PA) occurs in an estimated 2-12% of patients with pituitary adenomas.[17] In some cases, PA may be the initial presentation of a pituitary tumor.[18] Furthermore, hemorrhage into a ptuitary tumor can be asymptomatic.

Clinical features of pituitary apoplexy

Patients often present with abrupt onset of H/A, visual disturbance, and loss of consciousness. The majority of patients present with potentially lethal adrenal insufficiency, and over 50% have visual loss and/or ophthalmoplegia.

Neurologic involvement includes:
1. visual disturbances: one of the most common findings. Includes:
   a) ophthalmoplegia (unilateral or bilateral): opposite the situation with a pituitary tumor, ophthalmoplegia occurs more often (78%) than visual pathway deficits (52–64%)[19]
   b) one of the typical field cuts (p. 875) seen in pituitary tumors
2. acute secondary adrenal insufficiency (hypocortisolism) occurs in 66% and is the major source of mortality
   a) fluid and electrolyte disturbances may be caused by vasopressin release from the posterior pituitary
   b) hemodynamic instability may result from reduced vascular response to catecholamines caused by hypocortisolism
3. reduced mental status (lethargy, stupor, or coma): due to ↑ ICP (from intracranial extension of blood or to hydrocephalus) or hypothalamic involvement
4. cavernous sinus compression can cause venous stasis and/or pressure on any of the structures within the cavernous sinus
   a) trigeminal nerve symptoms
   b) proptosis
   c) ophthalmoplegia (Cr. N. III palsy is more common than VI) in 70% of cases[20]
   d) ptosis may be an early symptom[21,22]

51

e) pressure on carotid artery
f) compression of sympathetics within the cavernous sinus may produce third order (incomplete) Horner syndrome with unilateral ptosis and miosis, but anhidrosis may be absent or limited to the central forehead[23]
g) carotid artery compression may cause stroke or vasospasm
5. when hemorrhage breaks through the tumor capsule and the arachnoid membrane into the chiasmatic cistern, signs and symptoms of SAH may be seen
a) N/V
b) meningismus
c) photophobia
6. hypothalamic involvement may produce
a) hypotension
b) thermal dysautoregulation
c) cardiac dysrhythmias
d) respiratory pattern disturbances
e) diabetes insipidus
f) altered mental status: lethargy, stupor, or coma
7. suprasellar expansion can produce acute hydrocephalus

Evaluation

In cases due to hemorrhage: CT or MRI shows hemorrhagic mass in sella turcica and/or suprasellar region, often distorting the anterior third ventricle.

Cerebral angiography or CTA should be considered in cases where differentiating pituitary apoplexy from aneurysmal SAH is difficult.

Management of pituitary apoplexy

Rapid empiric administration of corticosteroids is indicated for hemodynamic instabilty, altered mental status (GCS < 15), or visual deficits (acutiy or field cuts).[20] Typical dose: hydrocortisone 100-200 mg IV bolus followed by 2-4 mg/hr IV infusion.[20] ✖ Dexamethasone alone is not recommended as it is deficient in the necessary mineralocorticoid activity. Patients without the aforementioned emergency findings may be evaluated endocrinologically and have corticosteroid replacement if deficient.

In the absence of visual deficits, prolactinomas may be treated with dopamine agonists (bromocriptine, cabergoline…).

Rapid decompression is required for: sudden constriction of visual fields, severe and/or rapid deterioration of visual acuity, or neurologic deterioration due to hydrocephalus. Surgery in ≤ 7 days of pituitary apoplexy resulted in better improvement in ophthalmoplegia (100%), visual acuity (88%), and field cuts (95%) than surgery after 7 days, based on a retrospective study of 37 patients.[24] Decompression is usually via a transsphenoidal route (transcranial approach may be advantageous in some cases). Goals of surgery:
1. to decompress the following structures if under pressure: optic apparatus, pituitary gland, cavernous sinus, third ventricle (relieving hydrocephalus)
2. obtain tissue for pathology
3. complete removal of tumor is usually not necessary
4. for hydrocephalus: ventricular drainage is generally required

51.6 Specific types of pituitary tumors

51.6.1 Nonfunctioning PitNET/adenomas (NFPA)

Nonfunctioning PitNET/adenoma (NFPA) is a clinical definition, viz. a pituitary adenoma that does not produce signs or symptoms as a result of hormonal hypersecretion.[25] NFPAs are the most common pituitary tumors,[4] comprising 15–30% of PitNETs.[26] They are predominantly derived from gonadotroph cells[25] and most actually do secrete gonadotropins or gonadotropin subunits,[27] but this is rarely symptomatic (see below). Most are either found incidentally or present due to signs and/or symptoms due to mass effect (p.864). For management see section 53.1.3.

51.6.2 Gonadotropin (FSH, LH) secreting tumors

As indicated above, most of these tumors do not produce clinical symptoms and are therefore considered nonfunctioning adenomas (80–90% of "nonfunctioning adenomas" are gonadotroph adenomas[28]). Rarely, clinical findings may occur:

- FSH: may cause **ovarian hyperstimulation syndrome** in reproductive-age women causing menstrual irregularities (including amenhrrhea) and glactorrhea (as with prolactin) along with ovarian cysts,[25,29] and rarely testicular hypertrophy and sexual dysfunction in men
- LH: even more rare, reported as causing precocious puberty in 2 boys[25]

51.6.3 Prolactinomas (lactotroph tumor)

The most common secretory adenoma. Arise from neoplastic transformation of anterior pituitary lactotrophs. See ▶ Table 52.4 for the differential diagnosis of hyperprolactinemia.

Manifestations of prolonged hyperprolactinemia:

1. females: amenorrhea-galactorrhea syndrome (AKA Forbes-Albright syndrome, AKA Ahumadadel Castillo syndrome). Variants: oligomenorrhea, irregular menstrual cycles. 5% of women with primary amenorrhea will be found to have a prolactin-secreting pituitary tumor.[30] Remember: pregnancy is the most common cause of secondary amenorrhea in females of reproductive potential. The galactorrhea may be spontaneous or expressive (only on squeezing the nipples)
2. males: impotence, decreased libido. Galactorrhea is rare (estrogen is also usually required). Gynecomastia is rare. Prepubertal prolactinomas may result in small testicles and feminine body habitus
3. either sex:
   a) infertility is common
   b) bone loss (osteoporosis in women, and both cortical and trabecular osteopenia in men) due to a relative estrogen deficiency, not due to the elevated prolactin itself

At the time of diagnosis, 90% of prolactinomas in women are microadenomas, vs. 60% for males (probably due to gender-specific differences in symptoms resulting in earlier presentation in females). Some tumors secrete both prolactin and GH.

51.6.4 Cushing's disease

General information and Cushing's syndrome

Cushing's syndrome (CS) is a constellation of findings caused by hypercortisolism. Cushing's disease (p.867)—endogenous hypercortisolism due to hypersecretion of ACTH by an ACTH-secreting PitNET —is just one cause of CS. The most common cause of CS is iatrogenic (administration of exogenous steroids). Possible etiologies of *endogenous* hypercortisolism are shown in ▶ Table 51.2. To determine the etiology of CS, see Dexamethasone suppression test (p.879).

Table 51.2 Causes of endogenous hypercortisolism

Site of pathology	Secretion product	Percent of cases	ACTH levels
pituitary corticotroph adenoma: Cushing's disease (p.867)		60–80%	slightly elevated[a]
ectopic ACTH production (p.868); most are lung tumors, others: pancreas...	ACTH	1–10%	very elevated
adrenal (adenoma or carcinoma)	cortisol	10–20%	low
hypothalamic or ectopic secretion of corticotropin-releasing hormone (CRH) producing hyperplasia of pituitary corticotrophs; pseudo-Cushing's state (p.868)	CRH	rare	elevated

[a]ACTH may be normal or slightly elevated; normal ACTH levels in the presence of hypercortisolism are considered inappropriately elevated

51

Conversion factors[31] for ACTH and cortisol between U.S. units and SI units are shown in Eq (51.1) and (51.2).

$$\text{ACTH} : 1\text{pg/ml} = 1\text{ng/liter} \tag{51.1}$$

$$\text{Cortisol} : 1\mu\text{g/dl} = 27.59 \text{ nmol/liter} \tag{51.2}$$

Ectopic ACTH secretion

Hypercortisolism may also be due to ectopic secretion of ACTH usually by tumors, most commonly small-cell carcinoma of the lung, thymoma, carcinoid tumors, pheochromocytomas, and medullary thyroid carcinoma. In addition to findings of Cushing's syndrome, patients are typically cachectic due to the malignancy which is usually rapidly fatal.

Prevalence of Cushing's disease

40 cases/million population. ACTH-producing adenomas comprise 10–12% of pituitary adenomas.[32] Cushing's disease is 9 times more common in women, whereas *ectopic* ACTH production is 10 times more common in males. Non-iatrogenic CS is 25% as common as acromegaly.

At the time of presentation, over 50% of patients with Cushing's disease have pituitary tumors <5 mm in diameter, which are very difficult to image with CT or MRI. Most are basophilic, some (especially the larger ones) may be chromophobic. Only ≈ 10% are large enough to produce some mass effect, which may cause enlargement of the sella turcica, visual field deficit, cranial nerve involvement, and/or hypopituitarism.

Clinical findings in Cushing's disease

Findings are those of Cushing's syndrome (hypercortisolism from any cause) include:
1. weight gain
   a) generalized in 50% of cases
   b) centripetal fat deposition in 50%: trunk, upper thoracic spine ("buffalo hump"), supraclavicular fat pad, neck, "dewlap tumor" (episternal fat), with round plethoric face ("moon facies" AKA "Cushingoid facies") and slender extremities
2. hypertension
3. ecchymoses and purple striae, especially on flanks, breasts, and lower abdomen
4. amenorrhea in women, impotence in men, reduced libido in both
5. hyperpigmentation of skin and mucous membranes: due to MSH cross-reactivity of ACTH. Occurs only with elevated ACTH, i.e., Cushing's disease (not Cushing's syndrome) or ectopic ACTH production (also below)
6. atrophic, tissue-paper thin skin with easy bruising and poor wound healing
7. psychiatric: depression, emotional lability, dementia
8. osteoporosis
9. generalized muscle wasting with complaints of easy fatigability
10. elevation of other adrenal hormones: androgens may produce hirsutism and acne
11. sepsis: associated with advanced Cushing's syndrome

Laboratory findings in Cushing's disease

1. hyperglycemia: diabetes or glucose intolerance
2. hypokalemic alkalosis
3. loss of diurnal variation in cortisol levels
4. normal or elevated ACTH levels
5. failure to suppress cortisol with low-dose (1 mg) dexamethasone test (p.879)
6. elevated 24-hour urine-free cortisol

51

7. CRH levels will be low (not commonly measured)

Nelson's syndrome (or Nelson syndrome) (NS)

General information

Key concepts

- a rare condition that follows 10–30% of total bilateral adrenalectomies (TBA) performed for Cushing's disease; see indications for TBA (p. 892)
- classic triad: hyperpigmentation (skin & mucus membranes), abnormal ↑ ACTH, and progression of pituitary tumor (the last criteria is now controversial)
- treatment options: surgery (transsphenoidal or transcranial), XRT, medication

A rare condition that follows 10–30% of total bilateral adrenalectomies (TBA) performed for Cushing's disease; see indications for TBA (p. 891). NS is due to continued growth of corticotroph (ACTH-secreting) adenoma cells. Usually occurs 1–4 years after TBA (range: 2 mos-24 years).[32] Theoretical explanation (unproven)[33]: following TBA, hypercortisolism resolves, and CRH levels increase back to normal from the (reduced) suppressed state; corticotroph adenomas in patients with NS have an increased & prolonged response to CRH resulting in increased growth. Also, corticotrophs in NS and CD show reduced inhibition by glucocorticoids. It is controversial if some cases may be related to insufficient glucocorticoid replacement after TBA.[32]

Manifestations
See reference.[33]

1. hyperpigmentation (due to melanin stimulating hormone (MSH) cross reactivity of ACTH and actual increased levels of MSH due to increased proopiomelanocortin production). Often the earliest sign that Nelson's syndrome is developing. Look for linea nigra (midline pigmentation from pubis to umbilicus) and hyperpigmentation of scars, gingivae, and areolae. DDx of hyperpigmentation includes: primary adrenal insufficiency (high levels of ACTH), ectopic ACTH secretion, hemochromatosis (more bronze color), jaundice (yellowish)
2. tumor growth → increased mass effect (p. 864) or invasion: the most serious consequence. These corticotroph tumors are among the most aggressive of pituitary tumors.[34 (p 545)] May produce any of the problems associated with macroadenomas (optic nerve compression, cavernous sinus invasion, pituitary insufficiency, H/A, bony invasion...) as well as necrosis with precipitous intracranial hypertension[35]; see pituitary apoplexy (p. 865)
3. malignant transformation of the corticotroph tumor (very rare)
4. hypertrophy of adrenal tissue rests: may be located in the testes → painful testicular enlargement and oligospermia. Rarely the rests can secrete enough cortisol to normalize cortisol levels or even cause a recurrence of Cushing's disease despite the adrenalectomy

Evaluation

1. laboratories
    a) ACTH > 200 ng/L (usually thousands of ng/L) (normal: usually < 54 ng/L)
    b) exaggerated ACTH response to CRH (not required for diagnosis)
    c) other pituitary hormones may be affected as with any macroadenoma-causing mass effect (p. 864) and endocrine screening (► Table 52.1) should be done
2. formal visual field testing (p. 874): should be done in patients with suprasellar extension or in those being considered for surgery (as a baseline for comparison)

Treatment
See treatment (p. 888).

51

51.6.5 Acromegaly

General information

Key concepts

- abnormally high levels of growth hormone in an adult. > 95% of cases are due to a benign pituitary somatotroph adenoma, > 75% are > 10 mm at time of diagnosis
- effects include soft tissue and skeletal changes, cardiomyopathy, colon Ca
- work-up: endocrine tests (p. 874), cardiology consult, colonoscopy
- treatment (p. 889): surgery for most, and then if necessary, medical therapy (p. 889) and/or XRT (p. 893)
- suggested criteria for biochemical cure (p. 903): normal IGF-1, growth hormone level < 5 ng/ml, AND GH nadir of < 1 ng/ml after OGST (p. 882)

Incidence: 3 cases/1-million persons/year. > 95% of cases of excess GH result from a pituitary somato-troph adenoma. Ectopic GH secretion may occur uncommonly with: carcinoid tumor, lymphoma, pancreatic islet-cell tumor. By the time of diagnosis, > 75% of pituitary GH tumors are macroadeno-mas (> 10 mm dia) with cavernous sinus invasion and/or suprasellar extension.

25% of acromegalics have thyromegaly with normal thyroid studies. 25% of GH adenomas also secrete prolactin. Acromegaly occurs rarely as part of a genetic syndrome, including: multiple endo-crine neoplasia type 1 (MEN 1), McCune-Albright syndrome (p. 975), familial acromegaly, and Carney complex (p. 652).[36]

Clinical

Elevated levels of GH in children before closure of the epiphyseal plates in the long bones (shortly after puberty) produces gigantism. Usually presents in the teen years. Hypertension may also occur.

In adults, elevated GH levels produce acromegaly (age: usually > 50 yrs) with findings that may include[37,38] (also see ▶ Table 51.3):

1. skeletal overgrowth deformities
   a) increasing hand and foot size
   b) thickened heel pad
   c) frontal bossing
   d) prognathism
2. cardiovascular
   a) cardiac findings (structural and functional): arrhythmias, valvular disease, concentric myo-cardial hypertrophy
   b) hypertension (30%)
3. soft tissue swelling (includes macroglossia)
4. glucose intolerance
5. peripheral nerve entrapment syndromes (including carpal tunnel syndrome)
6. debilitating headache
7. excessive perspiration (especially palmar hyperhidrosis)
8. oily skin
9. joint pain
10. sleep apnea
11. fatigue
12. colon cancer: risk is ≈ 2 × risk of general population[39]

Patients with elevated levels of GH (including partially treated cases) have 2–3 times the expected mortality rate,[40] primarily due to hypertension, diabetes, pulmonary infections, cancer, and cardio-vascular disease (▶ Table 51.3). Soft-tissue swelling and nerve entrapment may be reversible with normalization of GH levels, but many disfiguring changes and health risks are permanent (see ▶ Table 51.3 for specifics).

Table 51.3 Risks of long-term exposure to excess growth hormone (GH)[40]

Arthropathy

1. unrelated to age of onset or GH levels
2. usually with longstanding acromegaly
3. reversibility[a]:
   a) rapid symptomatic improvement
   b) bone & cartilage lesions irreversible

Peripheral neuropathy

1. intermittent anesthesias, paresthesias
2. sensorimotor polyneuropathy
3. impaired sensation
4. reversibility[a]:
   a) symptoms may improve
   b) onion bulbs (whorls) do not regress

Cardiovascular disease

1. cardiomyopathy
   a) reduced LV diastolic function
   b) increased LV mass and arrhythmias
   c) fibrous hyperplasia of connective tissue
2. HTN: exacerbates cardiomyopathic changes
3. reversibility[a]: may progress even with normal GH

Respiratory disease

1. upper airway obstruction: caused by soft tissue overgrowth and decreased pharyngeal muscle tone with sleep apnea in ≈ 50%
2. reversibility[a]: generally improves

Neoplasia

1. increased risk of malignancies (especially colon-Ca) & soft-tissue polyps
2. reversibility[a]: unknown

Glucose intolerance

1. occurs in 25% of acromegalics (more common with family history of DM)
2. reversibility[a]: improves

[a]reversibility with normalization of GH levels

51

51.6.6 Thyrotropin (TSH)-secreting adenomas (thyrotroph adenoma)

General information

Rare: comprise ≈ 0.5–1% of pituitary tumors.[9,41] Produces central (secondary) hyperthyroidism (note: central hyperthyroidism may also occur with pituitary resistance to thyroid hormones[42]): elevated circulating T3 and T4 levels, with elevated or inappropriately normal TSH[42] (TSH should be undetectable in primary hyperthyroidism). Up to 33% of tumors positive for TSH immunostaining are nonsecretory.[42] Many of these tumors are plurihormonal, but the secondary hormone is usually clinically silent. Most of these tumors are aggressive and invasive and are large enough at presentation to also produce mass effect (especially if prior thyroid ablative procedures have been done, which occurs in up to 60% of cases due to lack of recognition of pituitary abnormality.[42,43])

Clinical

Symptoms of hyperthyroidism: anxiety, palpitations (due to a-fib), heat intolerance, hyperhidrosis, and weight loss despite normal or increased intake. Signs: hyperactivity, lid lag, tachycardia, irregular rhythm when a-fib is present, hyperreflexia, tremor. Exophthalmos and infiltrative dermopathy (e.g., pretibial myxedema) are present only in Graves' disease.

51.6.7 Pathological classification of pituitary tumors

Light microscopic appearance of adenomas

Obsolete classification system (presented for completeness). With newer techniques (EM, molecular biology, immunohistochemistry...), many tumors previously considered nonsecretory have been found to have all the components necessary to secrete hormones.

In order of decreasing frequency:
1. chromophobe: most common (ratio of chromophobe to acidophil is 4-20:1). Originally considered "non-secretory," in actuality may produce prolactin, GH, or TSH
2. acidophil (eosinophilic): produce prolactin, TSH, or usually *GH*
3. basophil→ gonadotropins, β-lipotropin, or usually *ACTH → Cushing's disease*

Classification of adenomas based on secretory products

1. endocrine-active tumors: ≈ 70% of pituitary tumors produce 1 or 2 hormones that are measurable in the serum and cause defined clinical syndromes; these are classified based on their secretory product(s)
2. endocrine-inactive (nonfunctional) tumors[44] (**note**: a and b constitute the bulk of endocrine-inactive adenomas):
   a) oncocytoma
   b) gonadotropin-secreting adenoma
   c) silent corticotropin-secreting adenoma
   d) glycoprotein-secreting adenoma

Tumors of the neurohypophysis and infundibulum

The most common tumors encountered in the posterior pituitary are metastases (owing to the rich blood supply and the rarity of posterior pituitary tumors).

See Tumors of the neurohypophysis and infundibulum (p.852) for details of specific tumor types (granular cell tumor, pituicytoma, and spindle cell oncocytoma).

References

[1] Bosman FT, Jaffe ES, Lakhani SR, et al. World Health Organization Classification of Tumors series, vol. 6. In: WHO Classification of Tumors Editorial Board (ed.) World Health Organization classification of tumors of the central nervous system. 5th ed. Lyon, France: International Agency for Research on Cancer; 2021

[2] Mete O, Pituitary gland: Chapter 8, Series 8. In: WHO Classification of Tumors Editorial Board (ed.) World Health Organization Classification of Tumors series, Vol. 8. Endocrine and Neuroendocrine tumors, 5th ed. Lyon, France: International Agency for Research on Cancer; 2022. https://publications.iarc.fr/Book-And-Report-Series/Who-Classification-Of-Tumours. Date accessed: October 12, 2022

[3] Moini Jahangir, Badolato C, Ahangari R. Pituitary Tumors. In: Epidemiology of Endocrine Tumors. Elsevier; 2020:151–200

[4] Cozzi R, Lasio G, Cardia A, et al. Perioperative cortisol can predict hypothalamus-pituitary-adrenal status in clinically non-functioning pituitary adenomas. J Endocrinol Invest. 2009; 32:460–464

[5] Herman V, Fagin J, Gonsky R, et al. Clonal origin of pituitary adenomas. J Clin Endocrinol Metab. 1990; 71:1427–1433

[6] Ezzat S, Asa SL, Couldwell WT, et al. The prevalence of pituitary adenomas: a systematic review. Cancer. 2004; 101:613–619

[7] Aghi MK, Chen CC, Fleseriu M, et al. Congress of Neurological Surgeons Systematic Review and Evidence-Based Guidelines on the Management of Patients With Nonfunctioning Pituitary Adenomas: Executive Summary. Neurosurgery. 2016; 79:521–523

[8] Ebersold MJ, Quast LM, Laws ER, et al. Long-Term Results in Transsphenoidal Removal of Nonfunctioning Pituitary Adenomas. J Neurosurg. 1986; 64:713–719

[9] Biller BM, Swearingen B, Zervas NT. A decade of the Massachusetts General Hospital Neuroendocrine Clinical Center. Journal of Clinical Endocrinology and Metabolism. 1997; 82:1668–1674

[10] Fleseriu M, Bodach ME, Tumialan LM, et al. Congress of Neurological Surgeons Systematic Review and Evidence-Based Guideline for Pretreatment Endocrine Evaluation of Patients With Nonfunctioning Pituitary Adenomas. Neurosurgery. 2016; 79:E527–E529

[11] Abe T, Matsumoto K, Sanno N, et al. Lymphocytic Hypophysitis: Case Report. Neurosurgery. 1995; 36:1016–1019

[12] Lieblich JM, Rogol AD, White BJ, et al. Syndrome of anosmia with hypogonadotropic hypogonadism (Kallmann syndrome): clinical and laboratory studies in 23 cases. American Journal of Medicine. 1982; 73:506–519

[13] Nutkiewicz A, DeFeo DR, Kohout RI, et al. Cerebrospinal Fluid Rhinorrhea as a Presentation of Pituitary Adenoma. Neurosurgery. 1980; 6:195–197

[14] Reid RL, Quigley ME, Yen SC. Pituitary Apoplexy: A Review. Arch Neurol. 1985; 42:712–719

[15] Cardoso ER, Peterson EW. Pituitary Apoplexy: A Review. Neurosurgery. 1984; 14:363–373

[16] Onesti ST, Wisniewski T, Post KD. Pituitary Hemorrhage into a Rathke's Cleft Cyst. Neurosurgery. 1990; 27:644–646

[17] Shepard MatthewJ, Snyder MHarrison, Soldozy Sauson, et al. Radiological and clinical outcomes of pituitary apoplexy: comparison of conservative management versus early surgical intervention. Journal of Neurosurgery. 2021; 135:1310–1318

[18] Rovit RL, Fein JM. Pituitary Apoplexy, A Review and Reappraisal. J Neurosurg. 1972; 37:280–288

[19] Liu JK, Couldwell W. Pituitary apoplexy: Diagnosis and management. Contemporary Neurosurgery. 2003; 25:1–5

[20] Rajasekaran S, Vanderpump M, Baldeweg S, et al. UK guidelines for the management of pituitary apoplexy. Clin Endocrinol (Oxf). 2011; 74:9–20

[21] Yen MY, Liu JH, Jaw SJ. Ptosis as the early manifestation of pituitary tumour. British Journal of Ophthalmology. 1990; 74:188–191

[22] Telesca M, Santini F, Mazzucco A. Adenoma related pituitary apoplexy disclosed by ptosis after routine cardiac surgery: occasional reappearance of a dismal complication. Intensive Care Medicine. 2009; 35:185–186

[23] Walton KA, Buono LM. Horner syndrome. Curr Opin Ophthalmol. 2003; 14:357–363

[24] Bills DC, Meyer FB, Laws ER,Jr, et al. A retrospective analysis of pituitary apoplexy. Neurosurgery. 1993; 33:602–8; discussion 608-9

[25] Greenman Y, Stern N. Non-functioning pituitary adenomas. Best Pract Res Clin Endocrinol Metab. 2009; 23:625–638

[26] Davis FG, Kupelian V, Freels S, et al. Prevalence estimates for primary brain tumors in the United States by behavior and major histology groups. Neuro Oncol. 2001; 3:152–158

[27] Kwekkeboom DJ, de Jong FH, Lambers SW. Gonadotropin release by clinically nonfunctioning and gonadotroph pituitary adenomas in vivo and in vitro: relation to sex and effects of thyrotropin-releasing hormone, gonadotropin-releasing hormone, and bromocriptine. J Clin Endocrinol Metab. 1989; 68:1128–1135

[28] Chaidarun SS, Klibanski A. Gonadotropinomas. Semin Reprod Med. 2002; 20:339–348

[29] Kawaguchi T, Ogawa Y, Ito K, et al. Follicle-stimulating hormone-secreting pituitary adenoma manifesting as recurrent ovarian cysts in a young woman–latent risk of unidentified ovarian hyperstimulation: a case report. BMC Res Notes. 2013; 6. DOI: 10.1186/1756-0500-6-408

[30] Amar AP, Couldwell WT, Weiss MH. Prolactinomas: Focus on Indications, Outcomes, and Management of Recurrences. Contemporary Neurosurgery. 1989; 21:1–6

[31] Esposito F, Dusick JR, Cohan P, et al. Early morning cortisol levels as a predictor of remission after transsphenoidal surgery for Cushing's disease. Journal of Clinical Endocrinology and Metabolism. 2006; 91:7–13

[32] Banasiak MJ, Malek AR. Nelson syndrome: comprehensive review of pathophysiology, diagnosis, and management. Neurosurgical Focus. 2007; 23

[33] Assie G, Bahurel H, Coste J, et al. Corticotroph tumor progression after adrenalectomy in Cushing's Disease: a reappraisal of Nelson's syndrome. Journal of Clinical Endocrinology and Metabolism. 2007; 49:381–386

[34] Bertagna X, Raux-Demay M-C, Guilhaume B, et al. Cushing's Disease. In: The Pituitary. 2nd ed. Malden, MA: Blackwell Scientific; 2002:496–560

[35] Kasperlik-Zaluska A A, Bonicki W, Jeske W, et al. Nelson's syndrome - 46 years later: clinical experience with 37 patients. Zentralblatt fur Neurochirurgie. 2006; 67:14–20

[36] Cook DM. AACE Medical Guidelines for Clinical Practice for the diagnosis and treatment of acromegaly. Endocr Pract. 2004; 10:213–225

[37] Melmed S. Acromegaly. N Engl J Med. 1990; 322:966–977

[38] Melmed S. Medical progress: Acromegaly. N Engl J Med. 2006; 355:2558–2573

[39] Renehan AG, Shalet SM. Acromegaly and colorectal cancer: risk assessment should be based on population-based studies. Journal of Clinical Endocrinology and Metabolism. 2002; 87:1909–1909

[40] Acromegaly Therapy Consensus Development Panel. Consensus Statement: Benefits Versus Risks of Medical Therapy for Acromegaly. American Journal of Medicine. 1994; 97:468–473

[41] Beck-Peccoz P, Brucker-Davis F, Persani L, et al. Thyrotropin-secreting pituitary tumors. Endocr Rev. 1996; 17:610–638

[42] Clarke MJ, Erickson D, Castro MR, et al. Thyroid-stimulating hormone pituitary adenomas. J Neurosurg. 2008; 109:17–22

[43] Beck-Peccoz P, Persani L. Medical management of thyrotropin-secreting pituitary adenomas. Pituitary. 2002; 5:83–88

[44] Wilson CB. Endocrine-Inactive Pituitary Adenomas. Clinical Neurosurgery. 1992; 38:10–31

51

52 Pituitary Tumors – Evaluation

52.1 History and physical

Directed to identify signs and symptoms of:
1. endocrine hyperfunction, including:
   a) prolactin: amenorrhea (women), nipple discharge (primarily in women since estrogen is also required), impotence (males)
   b) thyroid: heat intolerance, proptosis
   c) growth hormone. Adults: change in ring size or shoe size or coarsening of facial features (acromegaly). Children: gigantism
   d) cortisol: hyperpigmentation, Cushingoid features (moon facies, buffalo hump…)
2. endocrine deficits due to mass effect (p. 864) on pituitary: hypothyroidism, hypocortisolism, growth hormone deficit…
3. visual field deficit: classically bitemporal hemianopsia (▶ Fig. 33.2) due to compression of the optic chiasm. Use bedside confrontational testing (p. 588) as a screening test until formal visual fields can be obtained
4. deficits of cranial nerves within cavernous sinus
   a) III, IV, VI: disorder of pupil and extraocular muscles
   b) V1, V2: reduced sensation in forehead, nose, upper lip, and cheek

52.2 Diagnostic tests

52.2.1 Overview

Initial (screening) tests to work-up a patient presenting with a known or suspected pituitary mass are shown in ▶ Table 52.1. Further testing is indicated for abnormal results or for strong suspicion of specific syndromes.

52.2.2 Vision evaluation

General information

> ### Practice guideline: Visual evaluation with PitNET/adenomas[*]
>
> Level III[2]
> - evaluation by an ophthalmologist is recommended
> - automatic static perimetry is recommended to detect visual field defects
> - visual evoked potentials may be useful in certain situations (e.g., when acuity and visual fields cannot be assessed) but the usefulness for routine testing is limited by significant false negative and false positive results
> - older patients and those with visual loss > 4 months should be advised that the chances of return of vision post-op are reduced
> - optical coherence tomography (OCT): not a practice standard. May be used to document extent of damage to optic disc
>
> [*] these guidelines were developed for suspected *nonfunctioning* PitNET/adenomas, principles may not be generalizable

At a minimum, formal visual field testing should be done in all patients to detect visual field deficits and to serve as a baseline.

Visual fields

Formal visual field testing:
- by perimetry using a tangent screen (Goldmann perimetry). Use the small red stimulus since desaturation of color is an early sign of chiasmal compression
- or automated perimetry (p. 589) (recommended[2]). E.g., Humphrey perimeter

Table 52.1 Summary of initial (screening) work-up for pituitary tumors (see indicated page for details)

Evaluation	Rationale
Vision to detect visual field deficits and serve as a baseline	
✓ Formal visual fields (most commonly Humphrey automated visual fields (HVF))	• compression of optic chiasm → visual field deficit (classically bitemporal hemianopsia, ▶ Fig. 33.2)
Endocrine screening	
✓ 8 A.M. cortisol[a] and/or 24-hour urine free cortisol[a]	• cortisol ↓ in hypoadrenalism (primary or secondary) • cortisol ↑ in hypercortisolism (Cushing syndrome) (p.876)
✓ TSH & either free T4 or free T4 index (FTI)[b] (✗ total T4 is not recommended for this purpose[b])	**Hypothyroidism** • T4 ↓ & TSH ↑ in primary hypothyroidism (this may cause thyrotroph hyperplasia in the pituitary gland) • T4 ↓ & TSH nl or ↓ in secondary hypothyroidism (as in hypopituitarism) **Hyperthyroidism (thyrotoxicosis)** • T4 ↑ & TSH ↓ in primary hyperthyroidism • T4 ↑ & TSH ↑ in TSH-secreting PitNETs
✓ prolactin	• ↑ or ↑ ↑ with prolactinoma • slight ↑ with stalk effect (usually < 90 ng/ml)
✓ gonadotropins (FSH, LH) and sex steroids[c] (♀: estradiol, ♂: testosterone)	• ↓ in hypogonadotrophic hypogonadism (from mass effect causing compression of the pituitary gland) • ↑ with gonadotropin-secreting adenoma
✓ insulin-like growth factor-1 (IGF-1) AKA somatomedin-C[d]	• ↑ in acromegaly • ↓ in hypopituitarism (one of the most sensitive markers)
✓ fasting blood glucose	• ↓ in hypoadrenalism (primary or secondary) • ↑ with hyperadrenalism

Radiographic studies (p. 882) ✓ either:

• MRI without & with contrast brain & pituitary protocol (test of choice), include image navigation protocol if navigation is to be used. Some surgeons also get noncontrast brain CT to delineate bony anatomy (especially of sphenoid sinus)
• if MRI is contraindicated: CT without & with contrast (with coronal reconstruction) + cerebral angiogram

[a]8 A.M. cortisol is the best test for hypocortisolism (e.g., to look for pituitary insufficiency); 24-hour urine free-cortisol is the best test for hypercortisolism (p.876) [1] (e.g., to look for Cushing's syndrome)
[b]free T4 and TFI measure thyroid hormone available to tissues ("ignoring" protein bound hormone)
[c]elevated estrogen or testosterone from a pituitary tumor is extremely rare, and is usually related to exogenous hormone intake or dietary supplements (such as dehydroepiandrosterone (DHEA))
[d]IGF-1 is the primary test for excess growth hormone (GH); direct measurement of GH is unreliable due to pulsatile secretion

52

▶ **Visual field deficit patterns** (▶ Fig. 33.2). Depends in part on location of chiasm with respect to the sella turcica: the chiasm is located above the sella in most patients, but it is posterior to the sella turcica (postfixed chiasm) in 4% (on imaging); and anterior to the sella (pre-fixed chiasm) in 8%[3]
1. compression of the optic chiasm:
    a) bitemporal hemianopsia that obeys the vertical meridian (macular splitting): classic visual field deficit associated with a pituitary tumor. Due to impingement on crossing nasal fibers in the chiasm
    b) other reported patterns that occur rarely: monocular temporal hemianopsia
2. optic nerve compression: more likely in patients with a postfixed chiasm
    a) loss of vision in the ipsilateral eye. If carefully sought, there is usually a superior outer (temporal) quadrantanopsia in the contralateral eye[4(p 2135),5] ("pie in the sky" defect*) from compression of the anterior knee of Wilbrand (p. 1478); may also be an early finding even without a post-fixed chiasm (so-called junctional scotoma = monocular visual loss + superior temporal quadrantanopsia in the contralateral eye)
       * this "pie in the sky" defect is in the contralateral eye only, unlike the defect with Meyer's loop injuries which is bilateral
    b) may produce central scotoma or monocular reduction in visual acuity
3. compression of the optic tract: may occur with a pre-fixed chiasm. Produces homonymous hemianopsia

Ophthalmology consult

A recommended option, see Practice guideline: Visual evaluation with PitNET/adenomas (p.874). In addition to visual field testing, it provides evaluation of the optic disc and other visual deficits and may help provide prognostic information for any visual loss that may be present.

Ancillary visual testing

Visual evoked potentials: usefulness is limited, see Practice guideline: Visual evaluation with pituitary adenomas (p.874).

Optical coherence tomography (OCT): an option, see Practice guideline: Visual evaluation with PitNET/adenomas (p.874) Uses light waves to provide high-resolution information about the thickness of the retina (including the optic disc). Does not utilize ionizing radiation. May be able to provide prognostic information.[6]

52.2.3 Initial endocrinologic evaluation (screening)

Overview

Practice guideline: Endocrine evaluation of PitNET/adenomas *

- Level II[7]:
  - all anterior pituitary axes should be routinely evaluated
  - prolactin levels should be routinely tested
  - cutoff values to initiate thyroid and adrenal replacement may be different in patients with panhypopituitarism (as opposed to patients with isolated deficits)
  - adrenal insufficiency and significant hypothyroidism should be treated pre-op
- Level III[7]: IGF-1 should be routinely tested to rule out subclinical growth hormone hypersecretion

* these guidelines were developed for suspected *nonfunctioning* PitNET/adenomas, principles may not be generalizable

See ▶ Table 52.1. May give indication of tumor type, determines whether any hormones need to be replaced, and serves as a baseline for comparison following treatment. Includes clinical assessment for signs and symptoms, as well as laboratory tests. Screening tests for anterior pituitary hormones should be checked in all patients with pituitary tumors.[7] Note: selective loss of a *single* pituitary hormone together with thickening of the pituitary stalk is strongly suggestive of autoimmune hypophysitis (p.1656).

1. adrenal axis screening; see tests to assess **cortisol reserve** (p.880)
   a) cortisol levels generally peak between 7–8 AM. AM cortisol may normally be slightly elevated above the reference range. 8 AM cortisol level: better for detecting hypocortisolism.[1] Normal: 6–18 mcg/100 ml. Interpretation:
      - 8 AM cortisol < 6 mcg/100 ml: suggestive of adrenal insufficiency
      - 8 AM cortisol 6–14 mcg/100 ml: nondiagnostic
      - 8 AM cortisol > 14 mcg/100 ml: adrenal insufficiency is unlikely
   b) see distinguishing Cushing's disease from ectopic ACTH secretion (p.880) in questionable cases, including differentiating pseudo-Cushing states from Cushing's syndrome
   c) 24-hour urine free cortisol: more accurate for *hypercortisolism*[1] (almost 100% sensitive and specific, false negative rare except in stress or chronic alcoholism). If not elevated several times above normal, at least 2 additional determinations should be made[8]
2. thyroid axis: the basis for thyroid screening is shown in ▶ Table 52.2
   a) screening: T4 level (total or free), thyroid-stimulating hormone (TSH) (AKA thyrotropin). Normal values: free T4 index is 0.8–1.5, TSH 0.4–5.5 mcU/ml, total T4 4–12 mcg/100 ml (NB: be sure to check both T4 *AND* TSH)
   b) further testing: thyrotropin-releasing hormone *(TRH) stimulation test* (indicated if T4 is low or borderline): check baseline TSH, give 500 mcg TRH IV, check TSH at 30 & 60 mins. Normal response: peak TSH twice baseline value at 30 mins. Impaired response with a low T4 indicates pituitary deficiency. Exaggerated response suggests primary hypothyroidism

3. gonadal axis
   a) screening:
      - serum gonadotropins: FSH & LH
      - sex steroids: estradiol in women, testosterone in men (measure *total* testosterone)
   b) further testing: none dependable in differentiating pituitary from hypothalamic disorders
4. prolactin levels (PRLs): for prolactin neurophysiology (p. 151)
   a) interpretation is shown in ▶ Table 52.3. See ▶ Table 52.4 for differential diagnosis of hyperprolactinemia. With prolactinomas, PRL correlates with size of the tumor[9]: if PRL is < 200 ng/ml, ≈ 80% of tumors are microadenomas, and 76% of these will have normal PRL after surgery; if PRL > 200, only ≈ 20% are microadenomas
   b) blood samples should be obtained midmorning (i.e., not soon after awakening) and not after stress, breast stimulation, or physical examination, which may increase PRLs
   c) be aware of the following when interpreting PRLs:
      - because of variations in secretion (daily PRL fluctuations can be as high as 30%) and intrinsic inaccuracies of radioimmunoassay, PRLs should be rechecked if there is a reason to question a specific result
      - heterophilic antibodies (seen in individuals routinely exposed to animal serum products) can cause anomalous results
      - **stalk effect**: prolactin is the only pituitary hormone primarily under inhibitory regulation (p. 153). Injury to or compression of the hypothalamus or pituitary stalk from surgery or compression by any type of tumor can cause modest elevation of PRL due to decrease in prolactin inhibitory factors (PIFs). Rule of thumb: the percent chance of an elevated PRL being due to a prolactinoma is ≈ one half the PRL (details (p. 878))
      - lab report stating "prolactin level > X": if the lab reports the PRL as "> X" (where X is some high value, e.g., 500 ng/ml) instead of specifying an actual number, it usually indicates a PRL so high that it exceeds the upper limits of the assay. Determining the actual number usually requires performing serial dilutions on the specimen until the PRL is in a range that their assay can quantify. Some labs will do this reflexively. If not, contact the lab and ask them to do this (they may be able to be done with the specimen they have, or else the patient will need to have another blood draw). This is important for:
      treatment decisions: **PRL > 500** usually indicates that surgery alone will not be able to normalize the PRL (see management guidelines (p. 888));
      to assess response to treatment: it is essential to know what PRL you are starting with to determine response to medication, surgery, XRT…
      - hook effect: extremely high PRLs may overwhelm the assay (the large numbers of PRL molecules prevent the formation of the necessary PRL-antibody-signal complexes for radioimmunoassay) and produce falsely low results. Therefore, for large adenomas with a normal PRL and a high clinical suspicion of hyperprolactinemia, have the lab perform several dilutions of the serum sample and re-run the PRL
      - macroprolactinemia: occurs when prolactin molecules polymerize and bind to immunoglobulins. Prolactin in this form has reduced biological activity but produces lab values consistent with hyperprolactinemia. Clinical significance is controversial[10]; asymptomatic patients usually do not require treatment
5. growth hormone: due to pulsatile secretion of GH:
   a) IGF-1 (somatomedin-C) level (p. 881) is the recommended initial test (elevated IGF-1 is extremely sensitive for acromegaly)
   b) checking a single random GH level (p. 881) may not be a reliable indicator and is therefore *not* recommended
6. neurohypophysis (posterior pituitary): deficits are rare with pituitary tumors
   a) screening: check adequacy of ADH by demonstrating concentration of urine with water deprivation
   b) further testing: measurement of serum ADH in response to infusion of hypertonic saline

52

Thyroid screening

Table 52.2 Basis for thyroid screening (T4 snd TSH)

Rationale	T$_4$	TSH
Primary hypothyroidism[a] (problem with thyroid gland itself)	↓	↑
• chronic primary hypothyroidism may produce secondary pituitary hyperplasia (pituitary pseudotumor) indistinguishable from adenoma on CT or MRI. Must be considered in any patient with a pituitary mass[11,12] • pathophysiology: loss of negative feedback from thyroid hormones causes increased TRH release from the hypothalamus producing secondary hyperplasia of thyrotrophic cells in the adenohypophysis (thyrotroph hyperplasia). The patient may present due to pituitary enlargement (visual symptoms, elevated PRL from stalk effect, enlarged sella turcica on X-rays...) • chronic stimulation from elevated TRH may rarely produce thyrotroph adenomas • labs: T$_4$ low or normal, TSH elevated (> 90–100 in patients presenting with thyrotroph hyperplasia), prolonged and elevated TSH response to TRH stimulation test (see text)		
Secondary hypothyroidism[a] (insufficient TSH stimulation of thyroid)	↓	↓ or nl
• pituitary hypothyroidism accounts for only ≈ 2–4% of all hypothyroid cases[13] • secondary hypothyroidism was found in 8–81% of patients with nonfunctioning pituitary tumors[7] (pituitary compression reduces TSH) • labs: T$_4$ low, TSH low or normal, reduced response to TRH stimulation test (see text)		
Primary hyperthyroidism (problem with thyroid gland itself)	↑	↓
• etiologies: localized hyperactive thyroid nodule, circulating antibody that stimulates the thyroid, or diffuse thyroid hyperplasia (Graves' disease, AKA ophthalmic hyperthyroidism) • labs: T$_4$ elevated, TSH subnormal (usually *undetectable*)		
Secondary hyperthyroidism (central hyperthyroidism)	↑	↑ or nl

• etiologies
   ○ TSH-secreting PitNET/adenoma (rare)
   ○ pituitary resistance to thyroid hormones (disrupts negative feedback loop)
 • labs: T$_4$ elevated, TSH elevated or inappropriately normal		

[a] ✖ Caution: replacing thyroid hormone with inadequate cortisol reserves (as may occur in panhypopituitarism) can precipitate adrenal crisis; see management (p. 886)

Prolactin screening

Interpretation of prolactin levels (PRL) is shown in ► Table 52.3.

Table 52.3 Significance of prolactin levels[a]

PRL (ng/ml)	Interpretation	Situations observed in
3–30[b]	normal	non-pregnant female
10–400		pregnancy (► Table 52.4)
2–20		postmenopausal female
25[b]-150	moderate elevation	• prolactinoma • "stalk effect" (see text) • other causes[d]
> 150[c]	significant elevation	prolactinoma[d]

[a] note: ectopic sites of prolactin secretion have rarely been reported (e.g., in a teratoma[14])
[b] normal values vary, use your lab's reference range
[c] some authors recommend 200 ng/ml as the cutoff for probable prolactinomas[15]
[d] for DDx of hyperprolactinemia, see ► Table 52.4

For differential diagnosis of hyperprolactinemia, see ► Table 52.4.

► **Stalk effect.** Modest elevation of prolactin level (PRL) tue to loss of inhibitory effect of PRIF from hypothalamus. There is no Class I evidence to support a threshhold to distinguish between stalk effect and a prolactinoma.[7] Mean PRL in nonfunctioning PitNETs was 39 ng/ml, with a majority of patients with stalk effect having PRL < 200 ng/ml.[7] Rule of thumb: the percent chance of an elevated

52

Table 52.4 Differential diagnosis of elevated prolactin (PRL) level (hyperprolactinemia)[a]

1. pregnancy-related
   a) during pregnancy[b]: 10–400 ng/ml
   b) postpartum: PRL decreases ≈ 50% (to ≈ 100 ng/ml) in the first week postpartum, and is usually back to normal in 3 weeks
   c) in the lactating female: suckling increases prolactin, which is critical for lactogenesis (once initiated, nonpregnant PRLs can maintain lactation).
      First 2–3 months postpartum: basal PRL = 40–50 ng/ml, suckling → increases × 10–20. 3–6 months postpartum: basal PRLs become normal or slightly elevated, and double with suckling. PRL should normalize by 6 months after weaning
2. PitNET/adenoma
   a) prolactinoma: larger prolactin microadenomas and macroadenomas usually produce PRL > 100 ng/ml
   b) stalk effect (p. 877): rule of thumb, the percent chance of an elevated PRL being due to a prolactinoma is equal to one half the PRL
   c) some tumors secrete both PRL and GH
3. drugs: dopamine receptor antagonists (e.g., phenothiazines, metoclopramide), oral contraceptives (estrogens), tricyclic antidepressants, verapamil, H2 antagonists (e.g., ranitidine), some SSRIs, in particular paroxetine (Paxil®)[16], carbamazepine rarely produces clinically significant increases[17]...
4. primary hypothyroidism: TRH, a prolactin releasing factor (PRF) (p. 153), will be elevated
5. empty sella syndrome (p. 955)
6. transient elevations in human serum prolactin (HSP) levels occur following 80% of generalized motor, 45% of complex partial, and only 15% of simple partial seizures.[18] Peak levels are reached in 15–20 minutes, and gradually return to baseline over the subsequent hour.[19,20,21]
7. breast or chest-wall trauma/surgery: usually ≤ 50 ng/ml
8. excessive exercise: usually ≤ 50 ng/ml
9. stress: in some cases the stress of having the blood test is enough to elevate PRL, anorexia nervosa
10. ectopic secretion: reported in renal cell or hepatocellular tumors, uterine fibroids, lymphomas
11. infiltrating hypothalamic tumors
12. renal failure
13. cirrhosis
14. macroprolactinemia: see text

[a]hyperprolactinemia from causes other than prolactinomas rarely exceeds 200 ng/ml
[b]always R/O pregnancy as a cause of amenorrhea & hyerprolactinemia in a female with reproductive potential

PRL being due to a prolactinoma is equal to one half the PRL. Also, a very large tumor with a modest elevation of PRL suggests stalk effect and not a prolactinoma since large prolactinomas usually have a very high PRL. Persistent post-op PRL elevation may occur even with total tumor removal as a result of stalk injury (usually ≤ 90 ng/ml; stalk effect is doubtful if PRL > 150). For stalk effect, follow these patients, do not use bromocriptine.

52.2.4 Specialized endocrinologic tests

Cushing's syndrome

Table 52.5 Basis for biochemical tests in Cushing's syndrome (CS)

- normally, low dose DMZ suppress ACTH release through negative feedback on hypothalamic-pituitary axis, reducing urine and serum corticosteroids
- in ≥ 98% of cases of Cushing's syndrome, suppression occurs, but at a much higher threshold
- adrenal tumors and most (85–90%) cases of ectopic ACTH production (especially bronchial Ca) will not suppress even with high dose DMZ
- ACTH response to CRH is exaggerated in CS
- DMZ does not interfere with measurement of urinary and plasma cortisol and 17-hydroxycorticosteroids

Tests for hypercortisolism

These tests are used to determine if *hypercortisolism* (Cushing's syndrome, CS) is present or not, regardless of etiology. Usually only needed if the screening 24-hr urine free cortisol (p. 876) is equivocal (the basis of these tests is shown in ► Table 52.5).

1. overnight *low-dose* dexamethasone (DMZ) suppression tests[22]:
   a) overnight low dose test: give DMZ 1 mg PO @ 11 P.M. and draw serum cortisol the next day at 8 A.M. Results:

52

- cortisol < 1.8 mcg/dl (note: this is the currently accepted normal value; previously it was 5 mcg/dl): Cushing's syndrome is ruled out (except for a few patients with CS who suppress at low DMZ doses, possibly due to low DMZ clearance[23])
- cortisol 1.8–10 mcg/dl: indeterminate, retesting is necessary
- cortisol > 10 mcg/dl: CS is probably present. False positives can occur in the so-called pseudo-Cushing's state where ectopic CRH secretion produces hyperplasia of pituitary corticotrophs that is clinically indistinguishable from pituitary ACTH-producing tumors (requires further testing[23]). Seen in: 15% of obese patients, in 25% of hospitalized and chronically ill patients, in high estrogen states, in uremia, and in depression. The combined DMZ-CRH test can be used to identify this (see reference[23]). False positives also may occur in alcoholics or patients on phenobarbital or phenytoin due to increased metabolism of DMZ caused by induced hepatic microsomal degradation

b) 2 day low-dose test (used when overnight test is equivocal): give DMZ 0.5 mg PO q 6 hrs for 2 days starting at 6 A.M.; 24 hr urine collections are obtained prior to test and on the 2nd day of DMZ administration. Normal patients suppress urinary 17-hydroxycorticosteroids (OHCS) to less than 4 mg/24 hrs, whereas ≈ 95% of patients with CS have abnormal response (higher amounts in urine)[23]

2. 11 PM salivary cortisol: this is the time of the usual cortisol nadir. Test must be run at NIH-approved lab. Accuracy is as good as low-dose DMZ suppression test

Distinguishing Cushing's disease from ectopic ACTH secretion

These tests are used to distinguish primary Cushing's disease (CD) (pituitary ACTH hypersecretion) from ectopic ACTH production and adrenal tumors (may be required since 40% of CD patients have a normal MRI[1])

1. random serum ACTH: if < 5 ng/L indicates ACTH independent CS (e.g., adrenal tumor). Not sensitive or specific due to variability of ACTH levels
2. abdominal CT: usually shows unilateral adrenal mass with adrenal tumors, or normal or bilateral adrenal enlargement in ACTH-dependent cases
3. *high-dose* dexamethasone (DMZ) suppression test: (NB: up to 20% of patients with CD do not suppress with high-dose DMZ. Phenytoin may also interfere with high-dose DMZ suppression[24])
   a) overnight high-dose test: obtain a baseline 8 A.M. plasma cortisol level
   b) then give DMZ 8 mg PO @ 11 P.M. and measure plasma cortisol level the next morning at 8 A.M.
   c) in 95% of CD cases plasma cortisol levels are reduced to < 50% of baseline, whereas in ectopic ACTH or adrenal tumors it will usually be unchanged
4. **metyrapone** (Metopirone®) test: performed on an inpatient basis. Give 750 mg metyrapone (suppresses cortisol synthesis) PO q 4 hrs for 6 doses. Most patients with CD will have a rise in 17-OHCS in urine of 70% above baseline, or an increase in serum 11-deoxycortisol 400-fold above baseline
5. corticotropin-releasing hormone (CRH) stimulation test: CD responds to exogenous CRH 0.1 mcg/kg IV bolus with even further increased plasma ACTH and cortisol levels; ectopic ACTH and adrenal tumors do not[25]
6. inferior petrosal sinus (IPS) sampling (or cavernous sinus sampling is preferred by some): done by interventional neuroradiologist. Uses a microcatheter to measure ACTH levels on each side at baseline, and then at 2, 5, and 10 minutes after stimulation with IV CRH (with simultaneous peripheral ACTH levels at each interval). General information:
   a) IPS sampling is not needed when the following criteria of CD are met[26]:
      - ACTH-dependent Cushing's disease
      - suppression with high-dose dexamethasone test (see above)
      - visible PitNET/adenoma on MRI
   b) may also determine likely side of a microadenoma within the pituitary (thus may be able to avoid bilateral adrenalectomy, which requires lifelong gluco- and mineralo-corticoid replacement and risks Nelson's syndrome (p. 869) in 10–30%). 15–30%[1] of the time this test falsely lateralizes the tumor due to the communication through the circular sinus
   c) a baseline IPS ACTH to peripheral ACTH ratio > 1.4:1 is consistent with primary Cushing's disease
   d) a post CRH ratio > 3 is also consistent with primary Cushing's disease
   e) complication rate: 1–2%, includes puncture of the sinus wall

Assessing cortisol reserve

1. cosyntropin stimulation test[27]:

a) draw a baseline cortisol level (fasting is not required; test can be performed at any time of day)
b) give cosyntropin (Cortrosyn®) (a potent ACTH analogue) 1 ampoule (250 mcg) IM or IV
c) then check cortisol levels at 30 mins (optional) and at 60 mins
d) normal response: peak cortisol level > 18 mcg/dl AND an increment > 7 mcg/dl, or a peak > 20 mcg/dl regardless of the increment
e) subnormal response: indicates adrenal insufficiency. In primary adrenal insufficiency, pituitary ACTH secretion will be elevated. In secondary adrenal insufficiency, chronically reduced ACTH causes adrenal atrophy and unresponsiveness to acute stimulation with this exogenous ACTH analogue
f) normal response: rules out primary and overt secondary adrenal insufficiency, but may be normal in *mild* cases of reduced pituitary ACTH or *early* after pituitary surgery where adrenal atrophy has not occurred. In these cases further testing may be positive: see metyrapone test (p. 902) or ITT (see below)

2. insulin tolerance test (ITT): "gold standard" for assessing integrity of the hypothalamic-pituitary-adrenal axis. Cumbersome to do. Abnormal in 80% of CS. Assesses ACTH, cortisol & GH reserve
   a) rationale: an appropriate cortisol increment in response to insulin-induced hypoglycemia suggests patient will also be able to respond to other stresses (acute illness, surgery…)
   b) contraindications: seizure disorder, ischemic cardiac disease, untreated hypothyroidism
   c) pre-test preparation: D/C estrogen replacement for 6 weeks prior to test. Have 50 ml of D50 and 100 mg IV hydrocortisone available during test
   d) protocol: give regular insulin 0.1 U/kg IV push, and draw blood for glucose, cortisol and GH at 0, 10, 20, 30, 45, 60, 90 and 120 mins (monitor blood sugar by fingerstick during test, and give IV glucose if patient becomes symptomatic). If fingerstick blood sugar is not < 50 mg/dl by 30 minutes and patient is asymptomatic, give additional regular insulin 5 U IVP. There must be 2 specimens after adequate hypoglycemia
   e) results:
      • if adequate hypoglycemia (< 40 mg/dl) was not accomplished: cortisol or GH deficiency cannot be diagnosed
      • normal: cortisol increment > 6 mcg/dl to a peak > 20
      • peak cortisol = 16–20: steroids needed only for stress
      • peak cortisol < 16: glucocorticoid replacement needed
      • Cushing syndrome: increment < 6

52

Acromegaly

For suspected acromegaly, the most useful test is an IGF-1 level.

1. insulin-like growth factor-1 (IGF-1) (formerly somatomedin-C) level: an excellent integrative marker of average GH secretion. Normal levels depend on age (peaking during puberty), gender, pubertal stage and lab. Typical fasting levels by age are shown in ▶ Table 52.6. Estrogen may suppress IGF-1 levels

Table 52.6 Normal IGF-1 by age

Age (yrs)	Level (ng/ml)
1–5	49–327
6–8	52–345
9–11	74–551
12–15	143–996
16–20	141–903
21–39	109–358
40–54	87–267
> 54	55–225

2. growth hormone (GH): normal basal fasting level is < 5 ng/ml. In patients with acromegaly, GH is usually > 10 ng/ml but can be normal. Normal basal levels do not reliably distinguish normal patient from GH deficiency.[28] Furthermore, due to pulsatile secretion of GH, normal patients may have sporadic peaks up to 50 ng/ml.[29] Occasionally acromegaly may be present even with GH

levels as low as 37 pg/ml.[30] ∴ random GH levels are not generally useful for diagnosing acromegaly (see above for IGF-1)
3. other tests used uncommonly
   a) oral glucose suppression test (OGST): less precise and more expensive than measuring IGF-1; however, may be more useful than IGF-1 for monitoring initial response to therapy. GH levels are measured at 0, 30, 60, 90, and 120 minutes after a 75 gm oral glucose load. If the GH nadir is not < 1 ng/ml, the patient is acromegalic.[31,32] GH suppression may also be absent with liver disease, uncontrolled DM & renal failure. ✖ Relatively contraindicated in patients with DM and high glucose levels
   b) growth-hormone releasing hormone (GHRH) levels: may help diagnose ectopic GH secretion in a patient with proven acromegaly with no evidence of pituitary tumor on imaging. If an extrapituitary source is suspected, chest and abdominal CT and/or MRI should also be obtained[33]
   c) GHRH stimulation test: results may be discordant in up to 50% of patients with acromegaly[31] and is thus rarely used (as of this writing, pharmaceutical production of GHRF has been discontinued)
4. octreotide scan: SPECT imaging 4 and 24 hours after injection with 6.5 mCi of indium-111 OctreoScan, a somatostatin receptor imaging agent

52.2.5 Radiographic evaluation

General information

Practice guideline: Imaging of PitNET/adenomas*

- Level II[34]:
  - MRI without and with contrast with dedicated images through the pituitary spaced 1–2 mm apart is the imaging modality of choice
  - thin-cut CT through the sella/sphenoid region and/or CTA may be used to augment the MRI (or may be used in cases where MRI is contraindicated)
- Level III[34]: 3 T MRI scanners may provide finer anatomic resolution relative to 1.5 T scanners

* these guidelines were developed for suspected *nonfunctioning* PitNET/adenomas, principles may not be generalizable

≈ 50% of pituitary tumors causing Cushing's syndrome are too small to be imaged on CT or MRI at the time of initial presentation (therefore endocrinologic testing is required to prove the pituitary origin). See differential diagnosis of intrasellar lesions (p.1653); some are indistinguishable radiographically.

Normal AP diameter of pituitary gland: female of childbearing age (≈ 13–35 yrs): ≤ 11 mm, for all others normal is ≤ 9 mm. (Note: pituitary glands in adolescent girls may be physiologically enlarged (mean height: 8.2 ± 1.4 mm) as a result of hormonal stimulation of puberty.[35]

MRI

MRI is the imaging test of choice for pituitary tumors.
   Ordering the MRI:
1. a pituitary protocol (p.241) is especially helpful when searching for a microadenoma
2. for follow-up of macroadenomas: routine coronal and sagittal pituitary MRI without and with contrast with detailed coronal cuts through the pituitary often suffices (i.e., dynamic images are not required unless there is a specific need to visualize the pituitary gland as distinct from the tumor)

Findings: MRI provides information about invasion of cavernous sinus, and about location and/or involvement of parasellar carotids (▶ Fig. 52.1). MRI may fail to demonstrate microadenomas in 25–45% of cases of Cushing's disease.[36] 3 T vs. 1.5 T MRI: based on 5 cases of Cushing's disease, a 3 T MRI showed the adenoma more clearly in 2 cases, in 1 case it showed the tumor on the correct side opposite to where the 1.5 T MRI showed it, and in 2 cases neither 1.5 T nor 3 T MRI could show the microadenoma.[37]

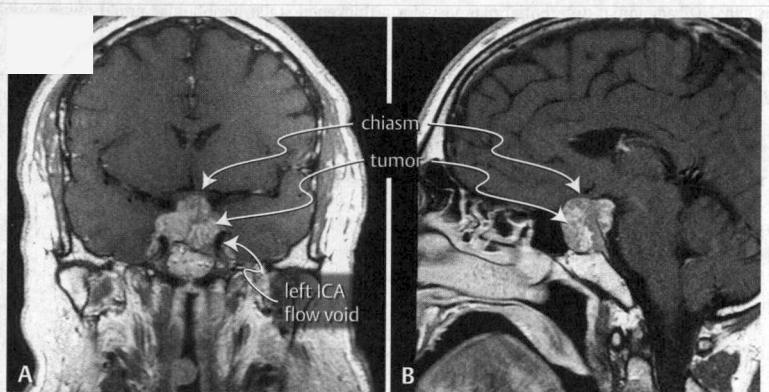

Fig. 52.1 Pituitary macroadenoma.
This 3 cm diameter tumor has grown superiorly through the diaphragma sella and is minimally elevating the optic chiasm. The tumor has invaded both cavernous sinuses, and flow voids within the cavernous segment of the internal carotid arteries (ICAs) are shown.
Image: T1 MRI with contrast. A: Coronal, B: Sagittal.

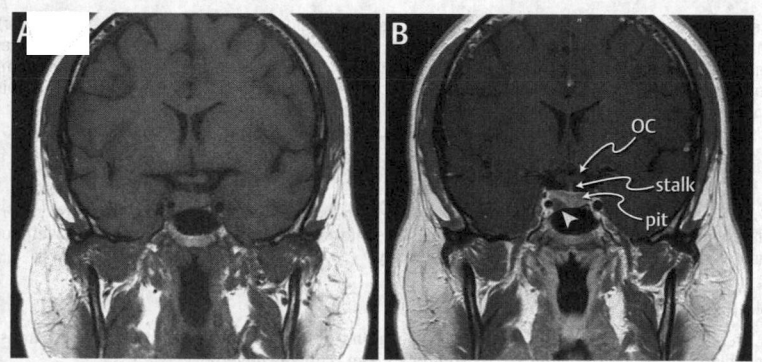

Fig. 52.2 Pituitary microadenoma in a 27-year-old woman with Cushing's disease.
Coronal MRI. A: T1WI noncontrast, B: T1WI with contrast.
The tumor is not visible on the noncontrast image (A), but shows up on the contrast image (B) as a hypointense area (*yellow arrowhead*) when scanned shortly after the administration of contrast.
Abbreviations: OC = optic chiasm, stalk = pituitary stalk, pit = pituitary gland.

Microadenoma: 75% are low signal on T1WI, and high signal on T2WI (but 25% can behave in any way, including completely opposite to above). Enhancement is very time-dependent. Imaging must be done with 5 minutes of contrast administration to see a discrete microadenoma. Initially, gadolinium enhances the normal pituitary (no blood-brain barrier) but *not* the pituitary tumor (▶ Fig. 52.2). After ≈ 30 minutes, the tumor enhances about the same. Dynamic MRI scans have been used to increase the sensitivity (contrast is injected while the MRI scanner is running).

Neurohypophysis: normally is high signal on T1WI[38] (possibly due to phospholipids). Absence of this "bright spot" often correlates with diabetes insipidus as may occur with autoimmune hypophysitis (p. 1656); however, failure to image the bright spot is not uniformly abnormal.

Deviation of the pituitary stalk may also indicate the presence of a microadenoma. Normal thickness of the pituitary stalk is approximately equal to basilar artery diameter. Thickening of stalk is usually NOT adenoma; differential diagnosis for a thickened stalk: lymphoma, autoimmune hypophysitis (p. 1656), granulomatous disease, hypothalamic glioma.

Cavernous sinus invasion: numerous criteria have been proposed to determine the degree of cavernous sinus invasion which correlates with degree of resectability. Knosp et al.[39] utilized 3 lines (MLL, MNL, and LL) as shown in ▶ Fig. 2.11, and the tumor invasion is graded as shown in ▶ Table 52.7.

Table 52.7 Knosp et al.[39] grading of cavernous sinus invasion as modified by Micko et al.[40] in 137 tumors grade ≥ 1

Grade	Feature	Percent invasive[a]	GTR	ER
0	tumor does not cross lateral to the MLL	0%		
1	tumor crosses the MLL but not the MNL (intercarotid line)	1.5%	83%	88%
2	tumor crosses MNL but not LL	10%	71%	60%
3A[b]	tumor extends lateral to LL superiorly (above ICA)	26%	85%	67%
3B[b]	tumor extends lateral to LL inferiorly (below ICA)	71%	64%	0%
4	tumor wraps completely around the intracavernous ICA	100%	0%	0%

[a]percentage of tumors in the grade that were invasive
[b]the original grade 3 was subdivided into 3A and 3B by Micko et al.[40]
Abbreviations: GTR = gross total resection, ER = endocrinologic remission in functioning tumors, MLL = medial line, MNL = median line (intercarotid line), LL lateral line (see ▶ Fig. 2.11 for illustration of the lines used)

CT

Generally superseded by MRI. May be appropriate when MRI is contraindicated (e.g., pacemaker). May also be considered as pre-op assessment in cases for transsphenoidal surgery (demonstrates shenoid septal anatomy with more detail[34]). If MRI cannot be done, consider also CTA to demonstrate parasellar carotid arteries and in questionable cases to R/O giant aneurysm which may mimic an adenoma (p. 1655).

Calcium in a pituitary tumor usually signifies previous hemorrhage or infarction within the tumor.

Angiography

Sometimes used pre-op for transsphenoidal surgery to localize the parasellar carotids (note: generally supplanted by CTA). NB: MRI also provides this information, and evaluates invasion of cavernous sinuses, usually obviating the need for angiography.

Skull X-ray

A lateral skull X-ray may help define the bony anatomy of the sphenoid sinus in cases where transsphenoidal surgery is contemplated (currently, CT scan is usually preferred).

References

[1] Chandler WF. Treatment of disorders of the pituitary gland: pearls and pitfalls from 30 years of experience. Clinical Neurosurgery. 2008; 56:18–22
[2] Newman SA, Turbin RE, Bodach ME, et al. Congress of Neurological Surgeons Systematic Review and Evidence-Based Guideline on Pretreatment Ophthalmology Evaluation in Patients With Suspected Nonfunctioning Pituitary Adenomas. Neurosurgery. 2016; 79:E530–E532
[3] Griessenauer CJ, Raborn J, Mortazavi MM, et al. Relationship between the pituitary stalk angle in prefixed, normal, and postfixed optic chiasmata: an anatomic study with microsurgical application. Acta Neurochir (Wien). 2014; 156:147–151
[4] Walsh FB, Hoyt WF. Clinical Neuro-Ophthalmology. Baltimore 1969
[5] Donaldson LC, Eshtiaghi A, Sacco S, et al. Junctional Scotoma and Patterns of Visual Field Defects Produced by Lesions Involving the Optic Chiasm. J Neuroophthalmol. 2022; 42:e203–e208

[6] Jacob M, Raverot G, Jouanneau E, et al. Predicting visual outcome after treatment of pituitary adenomas with optical coherence tomography. Am J Ophthalmol. 2009; 147:64–70 e2
[7] Fleseriu M, Bodach ME, Tumialan LM, et al. Congress of Neurological Surgeons Systematic Review and Evidence-Based Guideline for Pretreatment Endocrine Evaluation of Patients With Nonfunctioning Pituitary Adenomas. Neurosurgery. 2016; 79:E527–E529
[8] Watts NB. Cushing's Syndrome: An Update. Contemporary Neurosurgery. 1995; 17:1–7
[9] Gillam MP, Molitch ME, Lombardi G, et al. Advances in the treatment of prolactinomas. Endocrine Reviews. 2006; 27:485–534
[10] Olukoga AO. Macroprolactinemia is clinically important. Journal of Clinical Endocrinology and Metabolism. 2002; 87:4833–4834
[11] Bilaniuk LT, Moshang T, Cara J, et al. Pituitary Enlargement Mimicking Pituitary Tumor. Journal of Neurosurgery. 1985; 63:39–42

52

[12] Atchison JA, Lee PA, Albright L. Reversible Suprasellar Pituitary Mass Secondary to Hypothyroidism. JAMA. 1989; 262:3175–3177

[13] Watanakunakorn C, Hodges RE, Evans TC. Myxedema. A Study of 400 Cases. Arch Intern Med. 1965; 116:183–190

[14] Kallenberg GA, Pesce CM, Norman B, et al. Ectopic Hyperprolactinemia Resulting From an Ovarian Teratoma. JAMA. 1990; 263:2472–2474

[15] Randall RV, Scheithauer BW, Laws ER, et al. Pituitary Adenomas Associated with Hyperprolactinemia. Mayo Clin Proc. 1985; 60:753–762

[16] Cowen PJ, Sargent PA. Changes in plasma prolactin during SSRI treatment: evidence for a delayed increase in 5-HT neurotransmission. J Psychopharmacol. 1997; 11:345–348

[17] Torre DL, Falorni A. Pharmacological causes of hyperprolactinemia. Ther Clin Risk Manag. 2007; 3:929–951

[18] Wyllie E, Luders H, MacMillan JP, et al. Serum Prolactin Levels After Epileptic Seizures. Neurology. 1984; 34:1601–1604

[19] Dana-Haeri J, Trimble MR, Oxley J. Prolactin and Gonadotropin Changes Following Generalized and Partial Seizures. Journal of Neurology, Neurosurgery, and Psychiatry. 1983; 46:331–335

[20] Prichard PB, Wannamaker BB, Sagel J, et al. Serum Prolactin and Cortisol Levels in Evaluation of Pseudoepileptic Seizures. Ann Neurol. 1985; 18:87–89

[21] Laxer KD, Mullooly JP, Howell B. Prolactin Changes After Seizures Classified by EEG Monitoring. Neurology. 1985; 35:31–35

[22] Tyrell JB, Aron DC, Forsham PH, et al. Glucocorticoids and Adrenal Androgens. In: Basic and Clinical Endocrinology. 3rd ed. Norwalk: Appleton and Lange; 1991:323–362

[23] Yanovski JA, Cutler GB, Chrousos GP, et al. Corticotropin-releasing hormone stimulation following low-dose dexamethasone administration: A new test to distinguish Cushing's syndrome from pseudo-Cushing's states. Journal of the American Medical Association. 1993; 269:2232–2238

[24] McCutcheon IE, Oldfield EH, Barrow DL, et al. Cortisol: Regulation, Disorders, and Clinical Evaluation. In: Neuroendocrinology. Baltimore: Williams and Wilkins; 1992:117–173

[25] Chrousos GP, Schulte HM, Oldfield EH, et al. The Corticotropin-Releasing Factor Stimulation Test: An Aid in the Evaluation of Patients with Cushing's Syndrome. New England Journal of Medicine. 1984; 310:622–626

[26] Esposito F, Dusick JR, Cohan P, et al. Early morning cortisol levels as a predictor of remission after transsphenoidal surgery for Cushing's disease.

Journal of Clinical Endocrinology and Metabolism. 2006; 91:7–13

[27] Watts NB, Tindall GT. Rapid assessment of corticotropin reserve after pituitary surgery. JAMA. 1988; 259:708–711

[28] Abboud CF. Laboratory Diagnosis of Hypopituitarism. Mayo Clin Proc. 1986; 61:35–48

[29] Melmed S. Acromegaly. N Engl J Med. 1990; 322:966–977

[30] Dimaraki EV, Jaffe CA, DeMott-Friberg R, et al. Acromegaly with apparently normal GH secretion: implications for diagnosis and follow-up. J Clin Endocrinol Metab. 2002; 87:3537–3542

[31] Cook DM. AACE Medical Guidelines for Clinical Practice for the diagnosis and treatment of acromegaly. Endocr Pract. 2004; 10:213–225

[32] Melmed S. Medical progress: Acromegaly. N Engl J Med. 2006; 355:2558–2573

[33] Frohman LA. Ectopic hormone production by tumors: growth hormone-releasing factor. Neuroendocrine Perspect. 1984; 3:201–224

[34] Chen CC, Carter BS, Wang R, et al. Congress of Neurological Surgeons Systematic Review and Evidence-Based Guideline on Preoperative Imaging Assessment of Patients With Suspected Nonfunctioning Pituitary Adenomas. Neurosurgery. 2016; 79:E524–E526

[35] Peyster RG, Hoover ED, Viscarello RR, et al. CT Appearance of the Adolescent and Preadolescent Pituitary Gland. American Journal of Neuroradiology. 1983; 4:411–414

[36] Watson JC, Shawker TH, Nieman LK, et al. Localization of Pituitary Adenomas by Using Intraoperative Ultrasound in Patients with Cushing's Disease and No Demonstrable Pituitary Tumor on Magnetic Resonance Imaging. Journal of Neurosurgery. 1998; 89:927–932

[37] Kim LJ, Lekovic GP, White WL, et al. Preliminary Experience with 3-Tesla MRI and Cushing's Disease. Skull Base. 2007; 17:273–277

[38] Kucharczyk W, Davis DO, Kelly WM, et al. Pituitary adenomas: high-resolution MR imaging at 1.5 T. Radiology. 1986; 161:761–765

[39] Knosp E, Steiner E, Kitz K, et al. Pituitary Adenomas with Invasion of the Cavernous Sinus Space: A Magnetic Resonance Imaging Classification Compared with Surgical Findings. Neurosurgery. 1993; 33:610–618

[40] Micko AS, Wohrer A, Wolfsberger S, et al. Invasion of the cavernous sinus space in pituitary adenomas: endoscopic verification and its correlation with an MRI-based classification. J Neurosurg. 2015; 122:803–811

52

53 PitNET/Adenomas – General Management

53.1 Management/treatment recommendations

53.1.1 General information

For pituitary apoplexy (p. 865). For large invasive adenomas (p. 886).

Note: Prolactinoma is the only pituitary tumor for which medical therapy (dopamine agonist) is the primary treatment modality (in certain cases).

Hormone replacement therapy (HRT)

HRT may be required for patients with documented endocrine deficits pre-op or post-op in cases where pituitary function is not normal. Critical issues:

1. corticosteroids
   a) indications: inadequate cortisol reserve as demonstrated by failing a cosyntropin stimulation test (viz. failure to achieve a peak cortisol level > 18 mcg/dl in response to cosyntropin) (p. 880)
   b) may start cortisol immediately after bloodwork for cosyntropin test is drawn (do not need to wait for test results)—then, when test results are available, continue or stop therapy based on test results
   c) ℞ physiologic replacement dose: cortisol 20 mg PO q AM and 10 mg PO q 4 PM. Stress doses may be needed (p. 155) in some situations
2. thyroid hormone replacement
   a) ✖ thyroid replacement can precipitate adrenal crisis if started before cortisol in a patient with adrenal insufficiency (as may occur in panhypopituitarism)
      • ∴ do a cosyntropin stimulation test (p. 880) and start cortisol
      • thyroid replacement may be initiated after 1 full day of cortisol.
         ℞: start with synthroid 125 mcg/d
   b) although there are warnings not to do surgery on a hypothyroid patient, the reality is that it takes 3–4 weeks for adequate replacement, and hypothyroid patients frequently undergo surgery before then with no untoward effect
3. testosterone replacement: may increase intratumoral levels of estradiol, which may promote tumor growth. ∴ wait for stabilization of tumor before starting

53.1.2 Management of large, invasive adenomas

See reference.[1]

1. prolactinomas
   a) dopamine agonists (DA) (p. 888) unless there is unstable deficit
   b) for unstable deficit, or if the tumor does not respond to DAs: debulk the tumor transsphenoidally and then rechallenge with DA therapy
2. tumors secreting growth hormone or ACTH: an aggressive surgical approach is indicated with these tumors since the secretion product is harmful and effective medical adjuvants are lacking
   a) pre-treat invasive GH-secreting tumors with somatostatin analogue therapy before surgery to reduce surgical risks (general and cardiac)
   b) elderly patients or tumors > 4 cm diameter: debulk tumor transsphenoidally and/or adjuvant therapy (XRT and/or medications)
   c) young age and size < 4 cm: radical surgery (may utilize a cranio-orbito-zygomatic skull base approach; may be curative)
3. nonfunctional adenomas
   a) elderly patient: expectant management is an option, with intervention for signs of progression (radiographic or neurologic)
   b) central tumor or elderly patient with progression: transsphenoidal tumor debulking and/or XRT (residual tumor in the region of the cavernous sinus may show little or no change over several years, and with these nonfunctional tumors, there is less risk in following them than if there is a harmful secretion product)
   c) parasellar tumor and/or young age: radical surgery (often not curative)

53.1.3 Nonfunctioning PitNET/adenomas—management

Surgical indications

Surgical resection is recommended for *symptomatic* NFPAs (based on a large amount of class III data), as opposed to limited class III evidence that showed inconsistent benefits for: observation alone (2 studies), primary XRT (3 studies) or primary medical treatment (8 studies) for improving vision, H/A, hypopituitarism or tumor volume.[2]

Literature on nonsurgical treatment modalities for NFPAs

- medical management: reported tumor response rates using dopamine agonists (e.g., bromocriptine) in 0–60% of cases, somatostatin analogs (e.g., Octreotide) in 12–40%, and combination therapy in 60%.[2] These agents are therefore not recommended as primary treatment due to lack of a significant and consistent response[2]
- XRT: studies have not shown equivalence or superiority of XRT as primary management compared to surgical management. XRT has been demonstrated to be an effective adjuncdtive tharapy for post-op residual tumor or recurrence (p.893)
- natural history: NFPA *micro*adenomas have low growth propensity (estimated 3.2-12.5%), whereas ≈ 36% of NFPA *macro*adenomas enlarged (follow-up ranging 32-85 months).[3,4] Of the enlarging macroadenomas, 45% were asymptomatic. A minority of tumors actually shrink with time. Two studies showed tumor progression in 40–50%, and 21–28% required surgery.[5,6] Observation only is not recommended for *symptomatic* NFPAs[2]

Follow-up recommendations for NFPAs managed not meeting surgical criteria

Suggested management for incidental (asymptomatic) NFPAs that do not meet surgical criteria:
1. frequency of follow-up pituitary-MRI imaging[7]
   a) for microadenoma (≤1 cm maximal diameter): years 1, 2, 5 and ± 10 after the initial study, less frequently thereafter
   b) for macroadenoma (> 1 cm diameter): 6 months after initial study and then, if stable, annually for an additional 3 years, and then less frequently thereafter
2. duration of follow-up MRI: because growth may be very delayed, Dekkers recommended surveillance imaging for a total of 22 years[5]

Surgical indications for nonfunctioning pituitary macroadenomas

1. tumors causing symptoms by mass effect: visual field deficit (classically: bitemporal hemianopsia, panhypopituitarism)
2. some surgeons recommend surgery for macroadenomas that elevate the chiasm even in the absence of endocrine abnormalities or visual field deficit because of the possibility of injury to the optic apparatus
3. see invasive pituitary macroadenomas (p.855)
4. acute and rapid visual or other neurologic deterioration. May represent ischemia of the chiasm, or tumor hemorrhage/infarction causing expansion (pituitary apoplexy (p.865)). The immediate concern is irreversible blindness (hypopituitarism, while serious, can be treated with replacement therapy). Visual loss usually requires *emergent* decompression. Some surgeons feel that a transcranial approach is necessary, but transsphenoidal decompression is usually satisfactory[1,8]
5. to obtain tissue for pathological diagnosis in questionable cases

53

6. Nelson's syndrome (p. 869)
    a) surgery (transsphenoidal or transcranial): the primary treatment. The aggressiveness of the tumor sometimes requires total hypophysectomy
    b) XRT (possibly SRS) is used following subtotal excision
    c) medical therapy is usually ineffective. Agents that could be considered include[9]: dopamine agonists, valproic acid, somatostatin analogues, rosiglitazone, and serotonin agonists

53.1.4 Prolactinomas—management

Management guidelines

Prolactinomas are essentially the only PitNET/adenoma for which medical therapy is sometimes the primary treatment modality.

1. prolactin level (PRL) < 500 ng/ml in tumors that are not extensively invasive (see below for invasive tumors): PRL may be normalized with surgery
2. PRL > 500 ng/ml: the chances of normalizing PRL surgically are very low.[10] Algorithm:
    a) if no acute *progression* (worsening vision…), an initial attempt at purely medical control should be made as the chances of normalizing PRL surgically with pre-op levels > 500 ng/ml are very low[10] (these tumors may shrink dramatically with bromocriptine)
    b) response should be evident by 4–6 weeks (significant decrease in PRL, improvement of visual deficits, or shrinkage on MRI)
    c) if tumor *not* controlled medically (≈ 18% will not respond to bromocriptine, an attempt with cabergoline may also be considered): surgery followed by reinstitution of medical therapy may normalize PRL

Medical management with dopamine agonists

Dopamine agonists

Side effects[11]: (may vary with different preparations) nausea, H/A, fatigue, orthostatic hypotension with dizziness, cold induced peripheral vasodilatation, depression, nightmares and nasal congestion. Side effects are more troublesome during the first few weeks of treatment. Tolerance may be improved by bedtime dosing with food, slow dose escalation, sympathomimetics for nasal congestion, and acetaminophen 1–2 hrs before dosing to reduce H/A. Psychosis and vasospasm are rare side effects that usually necessitate discontinuation of the drug.

53

Drug info: Bromocriptine (Parlodel®)

A semi-synthetic ergot alkaloid that binds to dopamine receptors (dopamine agonist) on normal and tumor lactotrophs, inhibiting synthesis and secretion of PRL and other cell processes resulting in decreased cell division and growth. Bromocriptine lowers prolactin level, regardless of whether the source is an adenoma or normal pituitary (e.g., as a result of stalk effect), to < 10% of pretreatment values in most patients. It also frequently reduces the tumor size in 6–8 weeks in 75% of patients with macroadenomas, but only as long as therapy is maintained and only for tumors that actually produce prolactin. Only ≈ 1% of prolactinomas continue to grow while the patient is on bromocriptine. Prolactinomas may enlarge rapidly upon discontinuation of the drug. However, permanent normoprolactinemia can occur (see below).

Pregnancy issues: bromocriptine can restore fertility. Continued therapy during pregnancy is associated with a 3.3% incidence of congenital anomalies and 11% spontaneous abortion rate which is the same as for the general population. Estrogen elevation during pregnancy stimulates hyperplasia of lactotrophs and some prolactinomas, but the risk of symptomatic enlargement of microadenomas and totally intrasellar macroadenomas is < 3%, vs. 30% risk for macroadenomas.[12]

Prolonged treatment with bromocriptine may reduce the chances of surgical cure if this should be chosen at a later date. With a microadenoma, one year of bromocriptine may reduce the surgical cure rate by as much as 50%, possibly due to induced fibrosis.[13] Thus, it is suggested that if surgery is to be done that it be done in the first 6 months of bromocriptine therapy. Shrinkage of large tumors due to bromocriptine may cause CSF rhinorrhea.[14] **Side effects:** see above.

R: start with 1.25 mg (half of a 2.5 mg tablet) PO q hs (nighttime dosing reduces some side effects) (vaginal administration is an alternative). Add additional 2.5 mg per day as necessary (based on prolactin levels (PRLs)), making a dosage change every 2–4 weeks for microadenomas, or every 3–4 days for macroadenomas causing mass effect. Initial recheck of prolactin level after about 4 weeks at a reasonable dose to verify response. ★ To shrink large tumors or for extremely high PRLs, higher doses are usually needed initially (e.g., 7.5 mg TID for ≈ 6 mos), and then lower doses may be able to maintain normal levels (typical maintenance dosage: 5–7.5 mg daily (range: 2.5–15 mg) which may be given as a single dose or divided TID). **Supplied:** 2.5 mg scored tabs; 5 mg capsules.

Drug info: Cabergoline (Dostinex®)

An ergot alkaline derivative that is a selective D2 dopamine agonist (bromocriptine (see above) affects both D2 and D1 receptors).[15] The elimination half-life is 60–100 hrs which usually permits dosing 1–2 times weekly. Control of PRL and resumption of ovulatory cycles may be better than with bromocriptine.[16] **Side effects:** (see above) H/A and GI symptoms are reportedly less problematic than with bromocriptine. ✖ Cardiac valve disease[17] (incidence-rate ratio, 4.9; 95% CI) affecting the mitral, aortic, and tricuspid valves, possibly leading to regurgitation (the drug activates 5-HT2B receptors which induces prolonged mitogenic effects in fibromyoblasts, which may lead to valvular fibroplasia) which has not been observed at doses used for prolactinomas (it is associated with doses used for Parkinson's disease which are > 10 × pituitary doses): recommendation: do not discontinue cabergoline for this reason if dose is < 2 mg/wk. ✖Contraindications: eclampsia or preeclampsia, uncontrolled HTN. Dosage should be reduced with severe hepatic dysfunction.

R: Start with 0.25 mg PO twice weekly, and increase each dose by 0.25 mg every 4 weeks as needed to control PRL (up to a maximum of 3 mg per week). Typical dose is 0.5–1 mg twice weekly. Some combine the total dose and give it once weekly. Initial recheck of prolactin level after about 4 weeks to verify response. **Supplied:** 0.5 mg scored tablets.

Response to medical treatment

Treatment response to DA is assessed with serial prolactin levels as shown in ► Table 53.1. It is uncommon for a prolactinoma to enlarge without an increase in prolactin level.[18]

Discontinuation of dopamine agonists: Long-term therapy with DA agonists has some cytocidal effect on pituitary tissue. In an early report, discontinuation of treatment after 24 months was associated with > 95% recurrence rate.[19] There is a 20–30% chance of normoprolactinemia off medication in select patients.[20]

Recommendations[20]: if response to DA agonist is satisfactory, treat for 1–4 years (microadenomas: check prolactin yearly, macroadenomas are more likely to grow and should be checked more often). Microadenomas or macroadenomas that are no longer visible on MRI are candidates for DA agonist withdrawal. For microadenomas: discontinue the drug; for macroadenomas: slowly taper the drug then discontinue. Recurrence rate is highest during 1st year, ∴ check prolactin levels and clinical symptoms every 3 months during the 1st year. Long-term follow up is required, especially for macroadenomas.

53

Table 53.1 Prolactin level (PRL) with DA agonist treatment

PRL (ng/ml)	Recommendation
< 20	maintain
20–50	reassess dose
> 50	consider surgery

53.1.5 Acromegaly—management

See references.[21,22,23]

Surgery

Surgery is the primary treatment modality for acromegaly when treatment is indicated.
1. asymptomatic elderly patients do not require treatment since there is little evidence that intervention alters life expectancy in this group
2. if no contraindications, *surgery* (usually transsphenoidal) is currently the best initial therapy (worse prognosis with macroadenomas), providing more rapid reduction in GH levels and

decompression of neural structures (e.g., optic chiasm) and improving the efficacy of subsequent somatostatin analogues.[23] Surgery is not recommended for elderly patients

3. medical therapy (p. 889); reserved for:
   a) patients not cured by surgery (reoperation doesn't work very often for acromegaly). Note: the definition of "biochemical cure" with acromegaly is not standardized (p. 903). Surgery is still helpful for those "not cured" and improves efficacy of other therapies; IGF-1 may take months to normalize after surgery
   b) or for those who cannot tolerate surgery (e.g., due to cardiomyopathy, severe hypertension, airway obstruction…; these contraindications may improve with medical therapy and then surgery can be reconsidered)
   c) or for recurrence after surgery or XRT
4. XRT (p. 893): for failure of medical therapy. Not recommended as initial treatment. NB: some practitioners use XRT for surgical failure, and employ medical therapy while waiting for XRT to have an effect. GH levels decline very slowly after XRT, see details and side effects (p. 888)

Medical therapy

Overview

1. dopamine agonists (DAs): although not mentioned in the AACE guidelines,[24] it may be worth trying a DA to see if the tumor responds ($\approx$ 20% respond). If responsive, DAs are especially well suited for GH tumors that cosecrete PRL
   a) bromocriptine: (see below) although it benefits only a minority, a first line drug since it is cheaper than pegvisomant or octreotide and is given PO
   b) cabergoline (see above)
   c) others: lisuride, depo-bromocriptine (bromocriptine-LAR)
2. somatostatin analogues: indications: as initial medical therapy, or if no response to DAs, some also use this pre-op to improve surgical success rate
   a) octreotide and octreotide-LAR (see below)
   b) lanreotide, lanreotide SR and long-acting aqueous gel lanreotide (Autogel)
3. GH antagonists: pegvisomant (see below) considered for failures to above (not a primary therapy)
4. combination therapy: may be more effective than individual drugs. Pegvisomant or octreotide + dopamine agonist if no response to 1 drug alone

Specific agents

53

Drug info: Bromocriptine (Parlodel®)

Neoplastic somatotrophs may respond fortuitously to dopamine agonists and reduce growth hormone (GH) secretion. Bromocriptine lowers GH levels to < 10 ng/ml in 54% of cases, to < 5 ng/ml in only $\approx$ 12%. Tumor shrinkage occurs in only < 20%. Higher doses are usually required than for prolactinomas. If effective, the drug may be continued but should be periodically withdrawn to assess the GH level; see **Side effects** (p. 888). Estimated annual cost: $3,200 in the U.S.

℞ For growth hormone tumors that respond to bromocriptine, the usual dosage is 20–60 mg/d in divided doses (higher doses are unwarranted). The maximal daily dose is 100 mg.

Drug info: Octreotide (Sandostatin®)

A somatostatin analogue that is 45 times more potent than somatostatin in suppressing GH secretion but is only twice as potent in suppressing insulin secretion, has a longer half-life ($\approx$ 2 hrs after SQ injection, compared to $\approx$ minutes for somatostatin), and does not result in rebound GH hypersecretion. GH levels are reduced in 71%, IGF-1 levels are reduced in 93%. 50–66% have normal GH levels, 66% achieve normal IGF-1 levels. Tumor volume reduces significantly in about 30% of patients. Many symptoms including H/A usually improve within the first few weeks of treatment. Annual cost to the patient: at least $\approx$ $7,800 in the U.S. Usually given in combination with bromocriptine.

After 50 mcg SQ injection, GH secretion is suppressed within 1 hr, nadirs at 3 hrs, and remains reduced for 6–8 hrs (occasionally up to 12 hrs). **Side effects:** reduced GI motility and secretion, diarrhea, steatorrhea, flatulence, nausea, abdominal discomfort (all of these usually remit in 10 days), clinically insignificant bradycardia in 15%, cholesterol *cholelithiasis* (in 10–25%) or bile sludge.

Asymptomatic stones require no treatment and routine ultrasonography is not required. Mild hypo-thyroidism or worsening of glucose intolerance may occur.

℞: Start with 50–100 mcg SQ q 8 hrs. Increase up to a maximum of 1500 mcg/d (doses > 750 mcg/d are rarely needed). Average dose required is 100–200 mcg SQ q 8 hrs.

Sandostatin LAR Depot: long acting release (LAR) form given by IM injection. ℞: give a test dose of *short acting* octreotide SQ in the office, and if no reaction (e.g., N/V...) begin LAR injections with 20 mg IM q 4 weeks, increase to 30 mg if GH > 5 mU/L just before 4th dose. Control can be achieved in some patients with dosing q 8–12 weeks.[25]

Drug info: Pegvisomant (Somavert®)

A genetically engineered competitive GH-receptor antagonist. Treatment for ≥ 12 mos results in normal IGF-1 levels in 97% of patients.[26] No change in pituitary tumor size has been observed.[27] Indications: failure of somatostatin in patient with GH secreting adenoma (patient is switched to pegvisomant, it is not added to regimen). **Side effects:** significant but reversible liver function abnormalities occur in < 1%. Serum GH typically increases for 5–6 months and then stabilizes, probably as a result of loss of negative feedback on IGF-1 production. Antibodies to GH occured in 17%, but tachyphylaxis was not observed

℞: 5–40 mg/d SQ (dose must be titrated to keep IGF-1 in the normal range, to avoid GH deficiency conditions).

53.1.6 Cushing's disease—management

Management algorithm

1. if pituitary MRI shows a mass: transsphenoidal surgery
2. if pituitary MR is negative (up to 40% of patients with Cushing's disease have negative MRI): perform inferior petrosal sinus (IPS) sampling (p. 880)
   a) if IPS sampling is positive: surgery
   b) if IPS sampling is negative: look for extra-pituitary source of ACTH (abdominal CT)
3. if pituitary surgery is performed but biochemical cure—see criteria (p. 903)—is not obtained with surgery:
   a) unlike acromegaly, a partial reduction is not helpful to the patient
   b) consider re-exploration if pituitary source is still suspected
   c) stereotactic radiosurgery or medical therapy (see below)
   d) adrenalectomy in appropriate patients (see below)

Transsphenoidal surgery

Transsphenoidal surgery is the treatment of choice for most (medical therapy is inadequate as initial therapy since there is no effective pituitary suppressive medication). Cure rates are ≈ 85% for microadenomas (i.e., tumors ≤ 1 cm dia), but are lower for larger tumors. Even with microadenomas, *hemihypophysectomy* on the side of the tumor is usually required for cure (the tumor is difficult to completely extirpate) with attendant increased risk of CSF leak. If this fails, consideration should then be for *total hypophysectomy*. Failure of total hypophysectomy prompts consideration for bilateral adrenalectomy (total hypophysectomy virtually eliminates risk of Nelson's syndrome following adrenalectomy—see below).

Stereotactic radiosurgery

Often normalizes serum cortisol levels. Useful for: recurrence after surgery, inaccessible tumors (e.g., cavernous sinus)[28]...

Adrenalectomy

Total bilateral adrenalectomy (TBA) corrects hypercortisolism in 96–100%[9] (unless there is an extra-adrenal remnant), but lifelong gluco- and mineralo-corticoid replacement are required and up to

53

30% develop Nelson's syndrome (p. 869) (incidence reduced by total hypophysectomy or possibly by pituitary XRT).

Indications: continued hypercortisolism with:

1. non-resectable PitNET/adenoma
2. failure of medical therapy to control symptoms after transsphenoidal surgery
3. life-threatening Cushing's disease (CD)
4. CD with no evidence of pituitary tumor; testing should include high-dose DMZ suppression test (p. 880) and/or inferior petrosal sinus sampling (p. 880)

Follow-up after TBA to rule out Nelson's syndrome: there is no standardized regimen. Suggestion: check serum ACTH levels q 3–6 months × 1 year, q 6 months × 2 years, q year thereafter. A pituitary MRI is done if an ACTH level is > 100 ng/L; otherwise, annual MRIs are sufficient[29] × 3 years and then if ACTH levels remain low, get an MRI every other year.

Medical therapy

For patients who fail surgical therapy or for whom surgery cannot be tolerated, medical therapy and/or radiation are utilized. Occasionally may be used for several weeks prior to planned surgery to control significant manifestations of hypercortisolism, e.g., diabetes, HTN, psychiatric disturbances… (p. 868).

Ketoconazole (Nizoral®)[11]: an antifungal agent that blocks adrenal steroid synthesis. The initial drug of choice. Over 75% of patients have normalization of urinary free cortisol and 17-hydroxycorticosteroid levels. **Side effects:** reversible elevations of serum hepatic transaminase (in 15%), GI discomfort, edema, skin rash. Significant hepatotoxicity occurs in 1 of 15,000 patients. See ▶ Table 8.2 for evidence of adrenal insufficiency.

℞ Start with 200 mg PO BID. Adjust dosage based on 24-hr urine free cortisol and 17-hydroxycorticosteroid levels. Usual maintenance doses 400–1200 mg daily in divided doses (maximum of 1600 mg daily).

Aminoglutethimide (Cytadren®)[11]: inhibits the initial enzyme in the synthesis of steroids from cholesterol. Normalizes urinary free cortisol in ≈ 50% of cases. **Side effects:** dose-dependent reversible effects include sedation, anorexia, nausea, rash and hypothyroidism (due to interference with thyroid hormone synthesis).

℞ Start with 125–250 mg PO BID. Effectiveness may diminish after several months and dose escalation may be needed. Generally do not exceed 1000 mg/d.

Metyrapone (Metopirone®): inhibits 11-β-hydroxylase (involved in one of the final steps of cortisol synthesis); may be used alone or in combination with other drugs. Normalizes mean daily plasma cortisol in ≈ 75%. **Side effects:** lethargy, dizziness, ataxia, N/V, primary adrenal insufficiency, hirsutism, and acne.

℞ Usual dose range is 750–6000 mg/d usually divided TID with meals. Initial effectiveness may diminish with time.

Mitotane (Lysodren®): related to the insecticide DDT. Inhibits several steps in glucocorticoid synthesis, and is cytotoxic to adrenocortical cells (adrenolytic agent). 75% of patients enter remission after 6–12 months of treatment, and the medication may sometimes be discontinued (however, hypercortisolism may recur). **Side effects:** may be limiting, and include anorexia, lethargy, dizziness, impaired cognition, GI distress, hypercholesterolemia, adrenal insufficiency (which may necessitate supernormal doses of glucocorticoids for replacement due to induced glucocorticoid degradation).

℞ Start with 250–500 mg PO q hs, and escalate dose slowly. Usual dose range is 4–12 g/d usually divided TID-QID. Initial effectiveness may diminish with time.

Cyproheptadine (Periactin®): a serotonin receptor antagonist that corrects the abnormalities of Cushing's disease in a small minority of patients, suggesting that some cases of "pituitary" Cushing's disease are really due to a hypothalamic disorder. Combined therapy with bromocriptine may be more effective in some patients. **Side effects:** sedation & hyperphagia with weight gain usually limit usefulness.

℞ Usual dosage range: 8–36 mg/d divided TID.

53.1.7 Thyrotropin (TSH)-secreting adenomas—management

General information

1. transsphenoidal surgery has been the traditional first-line treatment.[30] These tumors may be fibrous and difficult to remove[31]
2. for incomplete resection: post-op XRT is employed

3. if hyperthyroidism persists: medical therapy is added with agents including octreotide, bromocriptine (more effective for tumors that co-secrete PRL), and oral cholecystographic agents (which inhibit conversion of T4 to T3), e.g., iopanoic acid

Medical therapy

Normal and neoplastic anterior hypophyseal thyrotroph cells possess somatostatin receptors and most respond to octreotide (see below). Occasionally, beta-blockers or low-dose antithyroid drugs (e.g., Tapazole® (methimazole) ≈ 5 mg PO TID for adults) may additionally be required.

Octreotide (Sandostatin®)

Doses required are usually < than with acromegaly. TSH levels decline by > 50% in 88% of patients, and become normal in ≈ 75%. T4 and T3 levels decrease in almost all, with 75% becoming normal. Tumor shrinkage occurs in ≈ 33%.

   R Start with 50–100 mcg SQ q 8 hrs. Titrate to TSH, T4 and T3 levels.

53.1.8 Gonadotropin secreting adenoma

This pertains to the rare patient who is symptomatic from gonadotropin hypersecretion.

   Normal and neoplastic pituitary gonadotrophs have gonadotropin-releasing hormone (GnRH) receptors, and may respond to long-acting GnRH agonists (by down-regulating receptors) or GnRH antagonists, but significant reductions in tumor size does not occur.

53.2 Radiation therapy for PitNET/adenomas

53.2.1 General information

Conventional EBXRT usually consists of 40–50 Gy administered over 4–6 weeks.

   Stereotactic radiosurgery (p. 1908) for PitNET/adenomas.

53.2.2 Side effects

Radiation injury to the remaining normal pituitary results in hypocortisolism, hypogonadism, or hypothyroidism in 40–50% of patients after 10 years. It may also injure the optic nerve and chiasm (possibly causing blindness), cause lethargy, memory disturbances, cranial nerve palsies, and tumor necrosis with hemorrhage and apoplexy. Cure rates but also complications are higher after proton beam therapy.

53.2.3 Recommendation

Radiation therapy should *not* be routinely used following surgical removal. Follow patient with yearly MRI. Treat recurrence with repeat operation. Consider radiation if recurrence cannot be removed and tumor continues to grow.

53.2.4 Sellar radiation therapy for specific PitNET/adenoma types

XRT for nonfunctioning pituitary tumors

In one series of 89 *nonfunctioning* pituitary tumors ranging 0.5–5 cm diameter (mean = 2 cm) not totally resected because of involvement of cavernous sinus (or other inaccessible sites), half were treated with radiation therapy (XRT). The recurrence rate was neither lower (and was actually higher) nor later in the XRT group.[32] However, another series of 108 pituitary macroadenomas found the recurrence rates shown in ▶ Table 53.2 which tend to favor radiation therapy.

   When used, doses of 40 or 45 Gy in 20 or 25 fractions, respectively, is recommended.[34] The oncocytic variant of null cell pituitary tumors appears to be more radioresistant than the nononcocytic undifferentiated cell adenoma.[34]

Sellar radiation therapy for acromegaly

Not the preferred initial treatment. Works better with lower initial GH levels. In most patients, GH levels begin to fall during the first year after XRT, dropping by ≈ 50% after 2 years, and decrease gradually thereafter, reaching ≤ 10 ng/ml in 70% of patients after 10 years. It takes up to 20 years for 90%

53

Table 53.2 Recurrence rate of pituitary tumors removed transsphenoidally[a]

Extent of removal	Post-op XRT?	Recurrence rate
subtotal	no	50%
gross total		21%
subtotal	yes	10%
gross total		0

[a]108 macroadenomas, 6 mos to 14 years follow-up[33]

of patients to achieve GH levels < 5 ng/ml. During this latency period, patients are exposed to unacceptably high levels of GH (octreotide may be used while waiting). Patients are also still at risk for radiation side effects mentioned above. Options include: EBRT, stereotactic radiosurgery (about equally effective). Estimated cost: $20,000.

Sellar radiation therapy for Cushing's disease

XRT corrects hypercortisolism in 20–40%, and produces some improvement in another 40%. Improvement may not be seen for 1–2 yrs post treatment.

References

[1] Krisht AF. Giant invasive pituitary adenomas. Contemporary Neurosurgery. 1999; 21:1–6
[2] Lucas JW, Bodach ME, Tumialan LM, et al. Congress of Neurological Surgeons Systematic Review and Evidence-Based Guideline on Primary Management of Patients With Nonfunctioning Pituitary Adenomas. Neurosurgery. 2016; 79:E533–E535
[3] Greenman Y, Stern N. Non-functioning pituitary adenomas. Best Pract Res Clin Endocrinol Metab. 2009; 23:625–638
[4] Huang W, Molitch ME. Management of nonfunctioning pituitary adenomas (NFAs): observation. Pituitary. 2018; 21:162–167
[5] Dekkers OM, Hammer S, de Keizer RJ, et al. The natural course of non-functioning pituitary macroadenomas. Eur J Endocrinol. 2007; 156:217–224
[6] Arita K, Tominaga A, Sugiyama K, et al. Natural course of incidentally found nonfunctioning pituitary adenoma, with special reference to pituitary apoplexy during follow-up examination. J Neurosurg. 2006; 104:884–891
[7] Freda PU, Beckers AM, Katznelson L, et al. Pituitary incidentaloma: an endocrine society clinical practice guideline. J Clin Endocrinol Metab. 2011; 96:894–904
[8] Wilson CB. Endocrine-Inactive Pituitary Adenomas. Clinical Neurosurgery. 1992; 38:10–31
[9] Banasiak MJ, Malek AR. Nelson syndrome: comprehensive review of pathophysiology, diagnosis, and management. Neurosurgical Focus. 2007; 23
[10] Barrow DL, Mizuno J, Tindall GT. Management of Prolactinomas Associated with Very High Serum Prolactin Levels. Journal of Neurosurgery. 1988; 68:554–558
[11] Blevins LS. Medical Management of Pituitary Adenomas. Contemporary Neurosurgery. 1997; 19:1–6
[12] Molitch ME. Pregnancy and the hyperprolactinemic woman. New England Journal of Medicine. 1985; 312:1364–1370
[13] Landolt AM, Osterwalder V. Perivascular Fibrosis in Prolactinomas: Is it Increased by Bromocriptine? J Clin Endocrinol Metab. 1984; 58:1179–1183
[14] Barlas O, Bayindir C, Hepgul K, et al. Bromocriptine-induced cerebrospinal fluid fistula in patients with macroprolactinomas: report of three cases and a review of the literature. Surg Neurol. 1994; 41:486–489
[15] Cabergoline for Hyperprolactinemia. Medical Letter. 1997; 39:58–59
[16] Webster J, Piscitelli G, Polli A, et al. A Comparison of Cabergoline and Bromocriptine in the Treatment of Hyperprolactinemic Amenorrhea. New England Journal of Medicine. 1994; 331:904–909
[17] Schade R, Andersohn F, Suissa S, et al. Dopamine agonists and the risk of cardiac-valve regurgitation. N Engl J Med. 2007; 356:29–38
[18] Gillam MP, Molitch ME, Lombardi G, et al. Advances in the treatment of prolactinomas. Endocrine Reviews. 2006; 27:485–534
[19] Johnston DG, Hall K, Kendall-Taylor P, et al. Effect of dopamine agonist withdrawal after long-term therapy in prolactinomas. Studies with high-definition computerised tomography. Lancet. 1984; 2:187–192
[20] Schlechte JA. Long-term management of prolactinomas. Journal of Clinical Endocrinology and Metabolism. 2007; 92:2861–2865
[21] Melmed S. Medical progress: Acromegaly. N Engl J Med. 2006; 355:2558–2573
[22] Acromegaly Therapy Consensus Development Panel. Consensus Statement: Benefits Versus Risks of Medical Therapy for Acromegaly. American Journal of Medicine. 1994; 97:468–473
[23] Colao A, Attanasio R, Pivonello R, et al. Partial surgical removal of growth hormone-secreting pituitary tumors enhances the response to somatostatin analogs in acromegaly. Journal of Clinical Endocrinology and Metabolism. 2006; 91:85–92
[24] Cook DM. AACE Medical Guidelines for Clinical Practice for the diagnosis and treatment of acromegaly. Endocr Pract. 2004; 10:213–225
[25] Turner HE, Thornton-Jones V A, Wass JA. Systematic dose-extension of octreotide LAR: the importance of individual tailoring of treatment in patients with acromegaly. Clin Endocrinol (Oxf). 2004; 61:224–231
[26] van der Lely AJ, Hutson RK, Trainer PJ, et al. Long-term treatment of acromegaly with pegvisomant, a growth hormone receptor antagonist. Lancet. 2001; 358:1754–1759
[27] Pegvisomant (Somavert) for acromegaly. Medical Letter. 2003; 45:55–56
[28] Sheehan JM, Vance ML, Sheehan JP, et al. Radiosurgery for Cushing's disease after failed transsphenoidal surgery. J Neurosurg. 2000; 93:738–742
[29] Assie G, Bahurel H, Coste J, et al. Corticotroph tumor progression after adrenalectomy in Cushing's Disease: a reappraisal of Nelson's syndrome. Journal of Clinical Endocrinology and Metabolism. 2007; 49:381–386
[30] Clarke MJ, Erickson D, Castro MR, et al. Thyroid-stimulating hormone pituitary adenomas. J Neurosurg. 2008; 109:17–22

[31] Sanno N, Teramoto A, Osamura RY. Long-term surgical outcome in 16 patients with thyrotropin pituitary adenoma. J Neurosurg. 2000; 93:194–200

[32] Ebersold MJ, Quast LM, Laws ER, et al. Long-Term Results in Transsphenoidal Removal of Nonfunctioning Pituitary Adenomas. J Neurosurg. 1986; 64:713–719

[33] Ciric I, Mikhael M, Stafford T, et al. Transsphenoidal Microsurgery of Pituitary Macroadenomas with Long-Term Follow-Up Results. J Neurosurg. 1983; 59:395–401

[34] Breen P, Flickinger JC, Kondziolka D, et al. Radiotherapy for Nonfunctional Pituitary Adenoma: Analysis of Long-Term Tumor Control. Journal of Neurosurgery. 1998; 89:933–938

53

54 PitNET/Adenomas – Surgical Management, Outcome, and Recurrence Management

54.1 Surgical treatment for PitNET/adenomas

54.1.1 Medical preparation for surgery

General principles

1. stress dose steroids: given to all patients during and immediately after surgery
2. hypothyroidism: ideally, hypothyroid patients should have > 4 weeks of replacement to reverse hypothyroidism; however:
   a) ✘ do not replace thyroid hormone until the adrenal axis is assessed; giving thyroid replacement to a patient with hypoadrenalism can precipitate adrenal crisis. If hypoadrenal, begin cortisol replacement first, may begin thyroid hormone replacement after 24 hours of cortisol
   b) surgery is done frequently on patients with hypothyroidism and appears to be tolerated well in the vast majority of cases

Pre-op orders

1. for transsphenoidal approach: Polysporin® ointment (PSO) applied in both nostrils the night before surgery
2. antibiotics: e.g., Unasyn® 1.5 gm (1 gm ampicillin + 0.5 gm sulbactam) IVPB at MN & 6 AM
3. steroids, either:
   a) hydrocortisone sodium succinate (Solu-Cortef®) 50 mg IM at 11 PM & 6 AM. On call to OR: hang 1 L D5LR + 20 mEq KCl/l + 50 mg Solu-Cortef at 75 ml/hr
      OR
   b) hydrocortisone 100 mg PO at MN & IV at 6 AM
4. intra-op: continue 100 mg hydrocortisone IV q 8 hrs

54.1.2 Surgical approaches—overview

Practice guideline: Surgical approaches and technology for nonfunctioning PitNET/adenomas (NFPAs)

54

Level III[1] recommendations include:
- transsphenoidal surgery (microscopic or endoscopic) is recommended for relief of symptoms
- if microsurgery is used initially, endoscopic visualization afterwards is recommended since it frequently reveals additional resectable tumor
- for invasive NFPAs with significant suprasellar, frontal or temporal involvement: combined transsphenoidal and transcranial surgery is recommended
- intraoperative MRI: may improve overall gross total resection; however, it is not recommended for estimating residual tumor volume because of a variable false-positive rate

✘ There was insufficient evidence to recommend[1]:
- neuronavigation
- introduction of intrathecal saline or air to augment delivery of suprasellar tumor during transsphenoidal approach
- to prevent postop CSF leak: perioperative CSF diversion, or a specific dural closure technique

1. transsphenoidal: requires no brain retraction, no external scar (aside from where a fat graft is procured, if used), and is normally an extra-arachnoid approach unless the diaphragma sella is broached. Usually the procedure of choice. Indicated for microadenomas, macroadenomas without significant extension laterally beyond the confines of the sella turcica, patients with CSF rhinorrhea, and tumors with extension into sphenoid air sinus
   a) sublabial

b) trans-nares: for extremely small nares, an alotomy may be used to enlarge the exposure if necessary
2. transethmoidal approach[2(p 343–50)]
3. transcranial approaches:
   a) indications: most pituitary tumors are operated by the transsphenoidal technique (see above), even if there is significant suprasellar extension. However, a craniotomy may be indicated for the following[3]:
      • minimal enlargement of the sella with a large suprasellar mass, especially if the diaphragma sellae is tightly constricting the tumor (producing a "cottage loaf" tumor) and the suprasellar component is causing chiasmal compression[4(p 124)]
      • extrasellar extension into the middle fossa that is larger than the intrasellar component
      • unrelated pathology may complicate a transsphenoidal approach: rare, e.g., a parasellar aneurysm
      • unusually fibrous tumor that could not be completely removed on a previous transsphenoidal approach
      • recurrent tumor following a previous transsphenoidal resection
   b) choices of approach
      • subfrontal: provides access to both optic nerves. May be more difficult in patients with pre-fixed chiasm
      • frontotemporal (pterional): places optic nerve and sometimes carotid artery in line of vision of tumor. There is also incomplete access to intrasellar contents. Good access for tumors with significant unilateral extrasellar extension
      • ✖ subtemporal: usually not a viable choice. Poor visualization of optic nerve/chiasm and carotid. Does not allow total removal of intrasellar component

54.1.3 Transsphenoidal surgery

Booking the case: Transsphenoidal surgery

Also see defaults and disclaimers (p. 25) and pre-op orders (p. 896).
1. position: supine, horseshoe head rest or (especially if image-guided navigation is used) pin headholder
2. equipment:
   a) microscope
   b) C-arm (if used)
   c) image-guided navigation system (if used)
   d) endoscopy cart for cases performed endoscopically (surgeon preference)
3. instrumentation: transsphenoidal instrument set (usually includes speculum, curettes, long instruments including bipolars)
4. some surgeons use ENT to perform the approach and closure and for follow-up
5. post-op: ICU
6. consent (in lay terms for the patient—not all-inclusive):
   a) procedure: removal of pituitary tumor through the nose, possible placement of fat graft from abdomen
   b) alternatives: surgery through the skull (trans-cranial), radiation
   c) complications: CSF leak with possible meningitis, problems with pituitary hormones which may sometimes be permanent (which would require lifetime replacement therapy), injury to optic nerve with visual loss, injury to carotid artery with possible bleeding and/or stroke

54

Technique

General information
For pre- and post-op orders, see below.
Details of the surgery are beyond the scope of this text, see references.[4,5,6,7]

Intraoperative disasters
Usually related to loss of landmarks.[4] Can be minimized using intraoperative navigation or fluoroscopy to verify location.

- injury of carotid artery:
  - typically injured in lateral aspect of opening. Bone may be dehiscent over the ICA
  - signaled by profuse arterial bleeding
  - can usually be packed off, if fat/fascia graft from thigh or abdomen is available it may be used; otherwise use e.g., woven Surgicel®
  - the operation is halted, and a STAT post-op arteriogram must be done
  - if a pseudoaneurysm or site of injury is identified angiographically, it must be eliminated before a potentially lethal hemorrhage; accomplished either by endovascular techniques or by surgical trapping with clips above and below
- injury of basilar artery: with pulling on tissue adherent to the artery or reaching through sella and rongeuring
- opening through the clivus and erroneous biopsy of the pons
- opening through the floor of the frontal fossa with injury to the olfactory nerves and entry into inferior frontal lobes

Overview of the procedure

1. lumbar drain: may be used with some macroadenomas to inject fluid in order to help bring the tumor down (p. 896), also may be used for post-op CSF drainage (p. 899) following transsphenoidal repair of CSF fistula
2. medications (in addition to pre-op meds (p. 896)): intraoperatively 100 mg hydrocortisone IV bolus followed by 100 mg dripped in over 8 hrs
3. positioning
   a) elevate thorax 10–15°: reduces venous pressure
   b) head stabilization: if image-guided navigation is to be used, the head is placed in a Mayfield headholder, or a headband with registration array is attached and the head is placed on a horseshoe head rest. If no image guidance, a horseshoe headrest may be used
   c) position option 1: surgeon standing to right of patient
      - shoulder-roll
      - top of head canted slightly to left
      - neck position: For microscope: extend neck slightly with the head in either a Mayfield head-holder or on a horseshoe headrest. For endoscope: do not extend neck (more comfortable for holding instruments)
      - ET tube positioned down and to patient's *left* (to get it out of the way)
      - microscope: observer's eyepiece on the *left*
   d) position option 2: surgeon standing above patient's head: patient head pointing straight up towards ceiling, neck slightly extended
   e) abdomen or right thigh is prepped for possible fat graft if needed
4. C-arm fluoro: image-guided navigation can eliminate the need for fluoro. Orient the C-arm for a true lateral by aligning the mandibular rami and/or by superimposing the floor of the left and right frontal fossae. If this proves difficult, lay a Penfield 4 on the nasion oriented from lateral canthus to lateral canthus, then aim the fluoro to shoot "down the barrel" of the Penfield 4
5. after approach to floor of sella is complete (see below), outline the upper and lower boundaries of the sella using image navigation or fluoro using an instrument (e.g., suction tip)
6. opening the sellar floor:
   a) starting the opening: open *exactly* in the midline using the nasal septum as a landmark (NB: the septum of the sphenoid sinus is unreliable as a midline indicator, and often curves inferiorly towards one of the carotid arteries)
      - macroadenomas may have thinned the bone to the point that it just flakes off
      - otherwise, use a bayoneted chisel or high-speed diamond burr to start the opening
   b) use a Kerrison rongeur to expand the opening. ✖ CAUTION: stay away from the extreme lateral sella to avoid entering the cavernous sinus or injuring the carotid artery
7. coagulate the dura centrally in an "X" pattern (*NOT* "+" pattern) with bipolar cautery. Macroadenomas may cause yellowish discoloration of the dura directly over the tumor
8. consider aspirating through dura with a 20 gauge spinal needle to R/O large venous sinus (dura often has bluish discoloration), giant aneurysm (p. 1655), or empty sella
9. incise the dura in the "X" pattern in the midline with a #11 scalpel on a bayonetted handle
10. tumor removal for **macroadenoma**:
    a) gently bring tumor into the field with ring curettes, and remove with pituitary rongeurs or aspirate with suction. Some tumors are very fibrous and may be difficult to remove
    b) do not *pull* on the lateral component of the tumor with pituitary rongeur due to risk of injuring carotid artery

54

c) if the suprasellar component will not come down, it may be brought down by having the anesthesiologist inject 5 ml aliquots of saline into a previously placed lumbar drain while monitoring blood pressure and pulse[4 (p 135),8]

d) once the tumor is debulked internally, try to develop a plane between the tumor capsule and the pituitary. A good place to start looking is inferiorly where the dura can be separated from the tumor capsule and then followed on the surface. Sometimes the tumor capsule cannot be removed due to severe bleeding

e) complete tumor removal is often not possible, and the goal of the surgery then is "containment," with intractable post op re-growth treated with XRT

f) endoscopic techniques and image-guided navigation may be employed to assist in removal of macroadenomas

11. tumor removal for microadenoma

    a) if the side of the tumor is known, begin exploration of the gland on that side by making incision with #11 blade and using a dissector to try and locate the tumor (like a "grain of rice in a blueberry")

    b) for Cushing's disease, if no tumor is identified on pre-op MRI[9]:

- intraoperative ultrasound may help localize tumor in ≈ 70% of cases[10] (a specialized U/S probe is required)
- if IPS sampling showed a lateralizing ACTH gradient: start with a paramedian incision on the side of the higher ACTH gradient; if no adenoma is encountered, the contralateral paramedian and then midline incisions are used to explore the gland
- if IPS sampling and MRI do not suggest tumor location: the gland is explored sequentially with 2 paramedian incisions and then a midline incision
- if the adenoma cannot be found, a hemihypophysectomy is performed on the side of higher ACTH levels if IPS sampling shows a lateralizing gradient, or on the side with more suspicious tissue on frozen section. Total hypophysectomy is not routinely performed[9]

    c) most adenomas are purplish-gray and easily aspirated; however, some may be more fibrous. The normal pituitary gland is firm and rubbery (the adenohypophysis is orange-pink, the neurohypophysis is a whitish-gray), and normally does not curette very easily

    d) use image guidance or fluoro to determine approximate location of diaphragma sellae. Do not go cephalad to this to avoid a CSF leak, to avoid entering the circular venous sinus in the dura here, and to avoid trauma to the optic chiasm

12. after removal of macroadenoma, check depth of tumor bed on fluoro or image guidance, and make sure it correlates with approximate tumor volume on pre-op MRI

13. the sella may be packed in a number of ways,[7] one method:

    a) if CSF leak occurs: place muscle or fat in defect within sella. Some recommend against the use of muscle because it always putrefies.[4 (p 129)] Do not overpack to avoid recreating mass effect with the graft

    b) recreate the floor of the sella using nasal cartilage placed within the sella. Alternatively, a nonporous Medpor® polyethylene transsphenoidal sellar implant (Porex Surgical Products http://www.porexsurgical.com) may be used

    c) if CSF leak occurs pack sphenoid sinus with fat from abdomen (option: fat with fascia on surface)

    d) fibrin glue may optionally be used to help hold any of these components in place

    e) elaborate packing for closure is not mandatory if no CSF leak occurs during surgery

54

Approach to sphenoid sinus for microscopic removal

Often done by ENT co-surgeon. One method:

1. insert temporary speculum into nose. For this discussion, the right nares will be described

2. use endoscope to locate middle concha. Follow this posteriorly to identify os into sphenoid sinus, which is usually located posterior to and slightly above the posterior extent of the middle concha

3. inject local anesthetic with epinephrine to blanch mucosa

4. insert sickle knife into os with sharp side facing the septum (medially) and incise the mucosa as the knife is drawn outward

5. use a Freer to dissect the thusly created mucosal flaps off the medial septum (pull one up, the other down)

6. break through the posterior part of the septum so that both sides of the floor of the sphenoid sinus are exposed. Cartilage or bone from this step is saved to use later in reconstructing the floor of the sella if desired

7. open the floor of the sphenoid and take it all the way to the right os (you will probably not see the left os)

8. place the Hardy speculum or equivalent
9. strip mucosa off the walls of the sphenoid sinus using a Blakely and *slow* pulling motion

Endoscopic tumor removal

Advantages over microscopic removal: visualization is better, especially within tumor bed.

Disadvantages: most neurosurgeons have less facility with endoscopes compared to ENT surgeons. Lack of 3D visualization (may be overcome using 3D endoscopes). Need for single-handed technique (may be overcome by having assistant hold endoscope, or using an endoscope holder, e.g., Mitaka), need for a binasal approach if it is desired to use two hands for the actual surgery.

Recommendations (p.896): Either endoscopic or microscopic approach is acceptable; however, after microscopic approach it is recommended that an endoscope be used at the time of the same surgery to visualize additional resectable tumor.[1]

54.1.4 Perioperative complications

1. hormonal imbalance:
   a) acute post-op concerns:
      - alterations in ADH: transient abnormalities are common—see typical post-op patterns (p.902) – including DI. DI lasting > 3 mos is uncommon
      - cortisol deficiency → hypocortisolism → Addisonian crisis if severe
   b) long-term: hypopituitarism in ≈ 5% (retrospective series[11])
      - TSH deficiency → hypothyroidism → (rarely) myxedema coma if severe
      - adrenal insufficiency
      - deficiency of sex hormones → hypogonadotrophic hypogonadism
2. secondary empty sella syndrome (chiasm retracts into evacuated sella → visual impairment). Re-operation with gentle packing of fat into the sella may support the chiasm
3. hydrocephalus with coma[12]: may follow removal of tumors with suprasellar extension (trans-sphenoidally or transcranially). Consider ventriculostomy placement if hydrocephalus is present (even if not symptomatic). Possible etiologies:
   a) traction on the attached 3rd ventricle
   b) cerebral edema due to vasopressin release from manipulation of the pituitary and/or stalk
   c) tumor edema following resection
4. infection
   a) pituitary abscess[13,14]
   b) meningitis
5. CSF rhinorrhea (fistula): 3.5% incidence[15]
6. carotid artery rupture: rare. May occur intraoperatively (see above) or in delayed fashion after surgery, often ≈ day 10 post-op (due to breakdown of fibrin around carotid, or possibly due to rupture of a pseudoaneurysm created at surgery)
7. entry into cavernous sinus with possible injury of any structure within
8. nasal septal perforation

54.1.5 Frontotemporal (pterional) approach

A right-sided approach is usually employed (less risk to dominant hemisphere). Exceptions: when the left eye is the side of worse vision; if there is predominant left-sided tumor extension; if there is other pathology on the left (e.g., aneurysm).

Positioning is the same as for an ACoA aneurysm, as seen in ▶ Fig. 106.1, with the head turned 60° to the side. The frontal lobe is elevated, and the temporal tip is gently retracted posteriorly. Bridging veins to the temporal tip must be coagulated to avoid rupture, as for any pterional approach. The approach is similar to that for an ACoA aneurysm (i.e., more emphasis is placed on frontal lobe elevation than on temporal tip retraction), except that unlike ACoA aneurysm, exposure of the ICA is not needed because proximal control is not necessary.

The tumor capsule can usually be seen between the two optic nerves. The capsule is coagulated with bipolar cautery and is incised. The tumor is then debulked from within. By staying within the capsule, risk of injury to the pituitary stalk and optic chiasm is minimized. Significant amounts of tumor can be removed by aspiration if it is soft and suckable.

✖ Caution: the blood supply to the optic chiasm is from the inferior aspect. Skeletonizing the chiasm or attempting to tease away tumor adherent to it may worsen vision.

54

54.1.6 Postoperative management

"DI watch" (diabetes insipidus watch)

Following any surgery involving the pituitary gland, patients are at risk of developing DI (inadequate secretion of ADH) which can produce dangerous dehydration and hypernatremia (elevation of serum sodium [Na^+]). Therefore, these patients place on so-called "DI watch." One needs to be familiar with the 3 possible post-op patterns of ADH abnormalities (see typical patterns (p.902)). DI watch consists of:
1. strict intake & output (I's & O's) q 1 hr
2. urine specific gravity (USG) q 4° and any time urine output (UO) > 250 ml/hr
3. serum electrolytes q 6 hours: watching primarily [Na^+]

Diagnostic criteria for DI: UO > 250 ml/hr × 2 hrs, *and* SG < 1.005.
DI is not present if USG > 1.005. In DI, USG is usually < 1.003.

Post-op orders

1. strict intake & output (I's & O's) q 1 hr
2. urine specific gravity (USG) q 4° and any time urine output (UO) > 250 ml/hr X 2 hours
3. activity: BR with HOB @ 30°
4. diet: ice chips PRN, advance to clear liquids as tolerated. For transsphenoidal approach: patient is not to drink through a straw (to avoid negative pressure on sphenoid sinus with risk of promoting CSF fistula)
5. for transsphenoidal approach: no incentive spirometry (for same reason as no straw)
6. IVF
   a) basal IVF: IV D5 1/2 NS + 20 mEq KCl/L at appropriate rate (75–100 ml/hr)
   b) NB: patients normally receive IV fluids at the beginning of an operation to "fill the tank" to avoid hypotension as a result of muscle relaxation. It is normal for patients to have a post-op diuresis as they eliminate excess fluids. As long as the urine SG is > 1.003 and urine output (UO) is < 250 ml/hr, aggressive fluid administration is usually not warranted
   c) if UO > 250 ml/hr X 2 hrs and USG < 1.005, the patient probably has diabetes insipidus (DI). If this occurs, in addition to the basal IVF, replace UO that is over the IV basal rate ml for ml with ½ NS and consider starting medication (see "meds" below)
   d) if UO is high and patient is not clearly in DI, an option is to replace only ≈ 2/3 of UO > basal IV rate with ½ NS
7. meds
   a) antibiotics: continue antibiotics until nasal packing is removed
   b) steroids (some surgeons routinely use post-op steroids until the adequacy of endogenous steroids is established, especially with Cushing's disease, see below). If this is EITHER:
      • hydrocortisone 50 mg IM/IV q 6 hrs, on POD #2 change to prednisone 5 mg PO q 6 hrs × 1 day, then 5 mg PO BID, D/C on POD #6
         OR
      • hydrocortisone 50 mg IM/IV/PO BID, taper 10 mg/dose/day to physiologic dose of 20 mg q AM and 10 mg q PM until adrenal axis assessed
   c) if DI develops, attempt to keep up with fluid loss with oral and/or IV fluids (see above). If rate is too high to continue IV or PO replacement (> 300 cc/hr × 4 hrs or > 500 cc/hr × 2 hrs), check urine SG and if < 1.005 then give a vasopressin preparation (see below, or see ► Table 5.7). ✖ Caution: danger of overtreating in case of triphasic response (p.125). Use EITHER:
      • 5 U aqueous vasopressin (Pitressin®) IVP/IM/SQ q 6 hrs PRN
         OR
      • desmopressin (DDAVP®) injection SQ/IV titrated to UO. Usual adult dose: 0.5–1 ml (2–4 mcg) daily in 2 divided doses

      • ✖ AVOID tannate oil suspension (withdrawn from U.S. market in 1993), because it is a long acting preparation (and may overtreat) and has erratic absorption

      • THEN: (for transsphenoidal approach or when patient is taking po for transcranial approach) when nasal packs out, EITHER

54

intranasal DDAVP (100 mcg/ml): range 0.1–0.4 ml (10–40 mcg) intranasally BID (typically 0.2 ml BID) PRN

OR

- clofibrate (Atromid S®) 500 mg PO QID (does not always work)

8. labs: electrolytes with osmolarity q 6 hrs, 8 A.M. serum cortisol on post-op day 1
9. imaging: (this is one paradigm, but is not standard of care)
    a) non-contrast CT scan of the brain within 6-12 hours of surgery to look for acute complications (hematoma, hydrocephalus, pneumocephalus…)
    b) pituitary-MRI without and with contrast within 72 hours of surgery to assess degree of tumor removal
10. nasal packs (if used for transsphenoidal approach): remove on post-op day 3–6

Urinary output: patterns of postoperative diabetes insipidus

Manage diabetes insipidus (DI) as described above in post-op orders. Post-op DI generally follows one of three patterns[16]; see Diabetes insipidus for details (p. 124):
a) transient DI: lasts until ≈ 12–36 hrs post-op then normalizes
b) "prolonged" DI: lasts months, or rarely may be permanent
c) "**triphasic**" response (least common). 3 stages:
    1. DI (short duration): due to injury to posterior pituitary
    2. normalization or SIADH-like picture: due to release of ADH from neuron endings form hypothalamus. It is during this phase that there is a risk of severe iatrogenic hyponatremia from overtreatment initiated during the initial DI phase
    3. DI (long-term)

Discontinuation of steroids post-op

Simple management schemes
Options:
- taper and stop hydrocortisone 24–48 hrs post-op. Then, check 6 AM serum cortisol level 24 hrs after discontinuing hydrocortisone and interpret the results as shown in ▶ Table 54.1.[17]
- if there is any question about reserve, the patient can be discharged on hydrocortisone 50 mg PO q AM and 25 mg PO q 4 PM until adrenal reserve can be formally assessed (p. 902)

Table 54.1 Interpretation of 6 AM cortisol levels

6 AM cortisol	Interpretation	Management
≥9 mcg/dl	normal	no further tests or treatment
3–9 mcg/dl	possible ACTH deficiency	place patient on hydrocortisone[a] (p. 154)
≤3 mcg/dl	ACTH deficient	

[a]perform cosyntropin stimulation test (p. 880) 1 month post-op; D/C steroids if normal; if subnormal, then permanent replacement required

Assessment of postoperative ACTH (corticotropin) reserve
Simple assessment protocol for patients who go home on hydrocortisone and were not on it pre-op.
- taper hydrocortisone over 2–3 weeks down to 20 mg PO q AM and 10 mg q 4 PM (a little higher than maintenance to provide for some stress coverage) for several days
- then hold the PM dose and check an 8 AM serum cortisol the next day
- to avoid adrenal insufficiency in patients with incompetent reserve: as soon as the blood is drawn have the patient take their morning cortisol dose and resume regular dosing until the test results are available
- if this 8 AM cortisol shows any significant adrenal function, then taper the patient off hydrocortisone

Metyrapone (Metopirone®) test
This test more accurately assesses the hypothalamic-pituitary-adrenal axis and is useful if there is suspicion of reduced reserve of pituitary ACTH production. Metyrapone inhibits 11-β-hydroxylation in the adrenal cortex, reducing production of cortisol and corticosterone with concomitant increase of serum 11-deoxycortisol precursors and its 17-OHCS metabolites which appear in the urine. In response, a normal pituitary increases ACTH production.

1. all patients should have a cosyntropin stimulation test (p. 880) first to rule out primary adrenal insufficiency .
2. ✖ do not do this test if there is known primary adrenal insufficiency.
3. ✖ do not do this test as an outpatient.
4. test protocol
   a) give 2–3 grams metyrapone PO at midnight
   b) check serum 11-deoxycortisol level the next morning
   c) a normal response is a 11-deoxycortisol level > 7 mcg/dl
   d) CAUTION: in patients with very little reserve, the reduced cortisol may provoke adrenal insufficiency (this test is safer than the higher doses used for urinary 17-OHCS testing)

Postoperative CT/MRI scan

Immediate post-op imaging is often done to rule-out complications and to assess degree of removal (see post op orders (p. 901)). After that, it is recommended to wait 3-4 months post-op for routine follow-up imaging (usually MRI) as it may take this long for the maximal height of the pituitary gland to return to its baseline position (even with total tumor removal)[18]

54.2 Outcome following transsphenoidal surgery

54.2.1 General information

In a series of 108 macroadenomas, gross total removal was unusual in tumors with > 2 cm suprasellar extension.[15]

54.2.2 Visual deficit

In cases with compression of the optic apparatus, there can be significant improvements in vision following surgery.[15,19]

54.2.3 Biochemical outcome for hormonally active tumors

Prolactinomas

In a series of 108 macroadenomas, endocrinologic cure was attained in 25% of prolactin-secreting tumors.[15]

Acromegaly

Criteria of biochemical cure

The criteria for biochemical cure of acromegaly is not standardized. There may be a discord between IGF-1 levels and mean GH levels.[20] Many use a GH cutoff level; range of levels described: < 2.5–5 ng/ml. Others feel that an elevated IGF-1 represents lack of cure even if GH < 5. However, normal IGF-1 levels may not be mandatory.[21] Still others require a normal IGF-1 AND a normal response to an oral glucose suppression test (OGST) (p. 882).

Low GH levels that do not also suppress to < 1 ng/ml after an OGST are considered controlled but not cured (even with normal IGF-1 levels).[22] If asymptomatic, expectant management with close follow-up is recommended.[22]

Σ: Biochemical cure criteria for acromegaly after treatment

Biochemical cure criteria for acromegaly is not standardized. Recommendation[22]:
1. IGF-1 levels within age-matched reference range
2. basal (morning) serum GH level < 5 ng/ml, AND GH nadir < 1 ng/ml in OGST

Outcome with acromegaly

Transsphenoidal surgery results in biochemical cure in 85% of cases with adenomas < 10 mm diameter, no evidence of local invasion, and random GH levels < 40 ng/ml pre-op. Overall, ≈ 50% of *all*

54

acromegalics undergoing transsphenoidal surgery had a biochemical cure.[23] Only 30% of macroadenomas and very few with marked suprasellar extension have surgical cure. Patients not cured with surgery require lifelong medical suppression. These tumors may also recur years later after apparent cure. Patients should be monitored every 6–12 months for recurrence.[22]

Cushing's disease

There are numerous methodologies for determining biochemical cure for Cushing's disease. One difficulty is that exogenous steroids are often given post-op to avoid potential hypoadrenalism or Addisonian crisis or for nausea, and this can obscure the evaluation. Some options:
1. immediate post-op early morning cortisol levels[9]:
   a) all steroids are withheld post-op (including dexamethasone as an antiemetic) unless biochemical and/or clinical evidence of hypocortisolism (clinical signs: nausea, anorexia, H/A, arthralgias). ✱ Requires close monitoring and administration of steroids if symptoms develop
   b) serum ACTH and cortisol levels are drawn between 6 AM and 9 AM on post-op days 1 & 2
   c) early remission defined as a *lowest* cortisol level ≤ 140 nmol/L (≤ 5 mcg/dl)
      • 97% (31/32) patients with early remission had sustained remission with mean follow-up of 32 months
      • only 12.5% (1/8) without early remission showed evidence of sustained remission
      • this has been used to select patients for possible early re-exploration
      • early ACTH levels usually drop, but do not consistently become subnormal and are not reliable in predicting sustained remission[9]
2. provocative tests
   a) overnight low-dose dexamethasone suppression test: an AM cortisol level on post-op day 3 that is ≤ 8 mcg/dl after an overnight 1 mg dexamethasone suppression test is predictive of sustained remission in 97%[24]
   b) CRH stimulation test[25]
3. measurements usually conducted 3 days to 2 weeks post-op following 24 hours of steroid cessation after initial post-op coverage with glucocorticoids
   a) 24-hour urinary free cortisol
   b) serum cortisol: the criteria of a cortisol level < 50 nmol/l (< 1.8 mcg/dl)[26,27,28] is probably too stringent[9,29,30]
   c) serum ACTH

The overall remission rate since 1980 is 64–93%, with the highest rates (86–98%) in patients with noninvasive microadenomas identifiable on MRI.[9]

Following effective treatment, all of the following usually improve but may not normalize:
1. HTN and hyperglycemia: within ≈ 1 year
2. osteoporosis related to CD: over ≈ 2 years
3. psychiatric symptoms

Thyrotropin (TSH)-secreting adenomas

Following debulking, small amounts of residual tumor may continue to produce sufficient TSH for hyperthyroidism to persist.[31] Following surgery + XRT, only ≈ 40% achieve a cure (defined as no residual tumor at surgery or on imaging, and normal free T3 with TSH levels at or below normal).

54.3 Follow-up suggestions for PitNET/adenomas

54.3.1 Nonfunctioning PitNET/adenomas

Post treatment follow-up

Due to the lack of active hormonal products that can be followed with serial lab tests, follow-up relies primarily on serial imaging and monitoring for signs of mass effect from growing tumors (e.g., increasing visual field defects).

Practice guideline: Posttreatment follow-up evaluation for nonfunctioning PitNET/adenomas

Radiologic follow-up
Level III[32]
1. T1WI fat sat & T2WI MRI should be included in imaging of NFPAs after surgery or XRT
2. long-term surveillance for tumor regrowth or recurrence is recommended
3. patients with radiologically-proven gross total resection of NFPA require less frequent monitoring than those with subtotal resection
4. the first post-op imaging should be obtained 3–4 months post-op

Level inconclusive recommendations[32]
1. there is insufficient evidence to make recommendations for frequency of imaging or length of surveillance after surgery or XRT for NFPAs
2. there is insufficient evidence to make recommendations for the timing of the first post-XRT imaging

Endocrinologic follow-up
Level III[32]
1. evaluation for endocrinologic pituitary dysfunction is recommended after surgery and/or XRT for NFPAs
2. post-op adrenal function evaluation is recommended on post-op day 2, week 6, and 12 months
3. perioperative corticosteroid supplementation is recommended for patients with hypocortisolemia pre-op or on post-op day 2
4. post-op endocrinologic follow-up is not recommended beyond 1 year in patients with normal pituitary function
5. endocrinologic follow-up after surgical resection of NFPAs is recommended indefinitely in patients with abnormal pituitary function or those who undergo XRT of NFPAs
6. surveillance of serum sodium for 48 hours after surgery and on post-op days 7–8 is recommended to avoid symptomatic post-op hyponatremia

Level inconclusive recommendations[32]
1. there is insufficient information to make recommendations on the detection and treatment of post-op diabetes insipidus (DI)
2. there is insufficient evidence to make recommendations for frequency of endocrinologic evaluation after surgery or XRT for NFPAs

Ophthalmologic follow-up
Level III[32]
- ophthalmologic follow-up to assess visual fields and acuity is recommended after surgery and/or XRT for NFPAs

Level inconclusive recommendations[32]
- there is insufficient evidence to make recommendations on the frequency or duration of ophthalmologic follow-up

Integrated follow-up
Level inconclusive recommendations[32]
- there is insufficient evidence to make recommendations on integration of imaging, endocrinologic and ophthalmologic follow-up after surgery or XRT for NFPAs

54

54.4 Recurrent PitNET/adenomas

Recurrence incidence: ≈ 12%, with most recurring 4–8 years post-op (in the same series[15]).

For tumors demonstrating significant regrowth or symptoms following initial resection, consideration for re-resection may be given. Once the tumor is debulked, consideration should be given to XRT, either immediately following the second operation, or, if recurrence after a second operation then almost certainly after a third debulking.

References

[1] Kuo JS, Barkhoudarian G, Farrell CJ, et al. Congress of Neurological Surgeons Systematic Review and Evidence-Based Guideline on Surgical Techniques and Technologies for the Management of Patients With Nonfunctioning Pituitary Adenomas. Neurosurgery. 2016; 79:E536–E538

[2] Schmidek HH, Sweet WH. Operative Neurosurgical Techniques. New York 1982

[3] Wilson CB. Endocrine-Inactive Pituitary Adenomas. Clinical Neurosurgery. 1992; 38:10–31

[4] Powell M, Lightman SL. Management of Pituitary Tumours: A Handbook. New York 1996

[5] Hardy J. Transsphenoidal Hypophysectomy. J Neurosurg. 1971; 34:582–594

[6] Kern EB, Pearson BW, McDonald TJ, et al. The Transseptal Approach to Lesions of the Pituitary and Parasellar Region. Laryngoscope. 1979; 89S:1–34

[7] Spaziante R, de Divitiis E, Cappabianca P. Reconstruction of the Pituitary Fossa in Transsphenoidal Surgery: An Experience of 140 Cases. Neurosurgery. 1985; 17:453–458

[8] Zhang X, Fei Z, Zhang J, et al. Management of Nonfunctioning Pituitary Adenomas with Suprasellar Extension by Transsphenoidal Microsurgery. Surgical Neurology. 1999; 52:380–385

[9] Esposito F, Dusick JR, Cohan P, et al. Early morning cortisol levels as a predictor of remission after transsphenoidal surgery for Cushing's disease. Journal of Clinical Endocrinology and Metabolism. 2006; 91:7–13

[10] Watson JC, Shawker TH, Nieman LK, et al. Localization of Pituitary Adenomas by Using Intraoperative Ultrasound in Patients with Cushing's Disease and No Demonstrable Pituitary Tumor on Magnetic Resonance Imaging. Journal of Neurosurgery. 1998; 89:927–932

[11] Fatemi N, Dusick JR, Mattozo C, et al. Pituitary hormonal loss and recovery after transsphenoidal adenoma removal. Neurosurgery. 2008; 63:709–18; discussion 718-9

[12] Decker RE, Chalif DJ. Progressive Coma After the Transsphenoidal Decompression of a Pituitary Adenoma with Marked Suprasellar Extension: Report of Two Cases. Neurosurgery. 1991; 28:154–158

[13] Domingue JN, Wilson CB. Pituitary Abscesses. J Neurosurg. 1977; 46:601–608

[14] Robinson B. Intrasellar Abscess After Transsphenoidal Pituitary Adenectomy. Neurosurgery. 1983; 12:684–686

[15] Ciric I, Mikhael M, Stafford T, et al. Transsphenoidal Microsurgery of Pituitary Macroadenomas with Long-Term Follow-Up Results. J Neurosurg. 1983; 59:395–401

[16] Verbalis JG, Robinson AG, Moses AM. Postoperative and Post-Traumatic Diabetes Insipidus. Front Horm Res. 1985; 13:247–265

[17] Watts NB, Tindall GT. Rapid assessment of corticotropin reserve after pituitary surgery. JAMA. 1988; 259:708–711

[18] Teng MM, Huang CI, Chang T. The pituitary mass after transsphenoidal hypophysectomy. AJNR Am J Neuroradiol. 1988; 9:23–26

[19] Cohen AR, Cooper PR, Kupersmith MJ, et al. Visual Recovery After Transsphenoidal Removal of Pituitary Adenoma. Neurosurgery. 1985; 17:446–452

[20] Turner HE, Thornton-Jones V A, Wass JA. Systematic dose-extension of octreotide LAR: the importance of individual tailoring of treatment in patients with acromegaly. Clin Endocrinol (Oxf). 2004; 61:224–231

[21] Ayuk J, Clayton RN, Holder G, et al. Growth hormone and pituitary radiotherapy, but not serum insulin-like growth factor-I concentrations, predict excess mortality in patients with acromegaly. Journal of Clinical Endocrinology and Metabolism. 2004; 89:1613–1617

[22] Cook DM. AACE Medical Guidelines for Clinical Practice for the diagnosis and treatment of acromegaly. Endocr Pract. 2004; 10:213–225

[23] Davis DH, Laws ER, Ilstrup DM, et al. Results of Surgical Treatment of Growth Hormone-Secreting Pituitary Adenomas. Journal of Neurosurgery. 1993; 79:70–75

[24] Chen JC, Amar AP, Choi S, et al. Transsphenoidal microsurgical treatment of Cushing's disease: postoperative assessment of surgical efficacy by application of an overnight low-dose dexamethasone suppression test. Journal of Neurosurgery. 2003; 98:967–973

[25] Nishizawa S, Oki Y, Ohta S, et al. What can predict postoperative "endocrinological cure" in Cushing's disease? Neurosurgery. 1999; 45:239–244

[26] Trainer PJ, Lawrie HS, Verhelst J, et al. Transsphenoidal resection in Cushing's disease: undetectable serum cortisol as the definition of successful treatment. Clinical Endocrinology (Oxf). 1993; 38:73–78

[27] Rees DA, Hanna FW, Davies JS, et al. Long-term follow-up results of transsphenoidal surgery for Cushing's disease in a single centre using strict criteria for remission. Clinical Endocrinology (Oxf). 2002; 56:541–551

[28] Yap LB, Turner HE, Adams CB, et al. Undetectable postoperative cortisol does not always predict long-term remission in Cushing's disease: A single centre audit. Clinical Endocrinology (Oxf). 2002; 56:25–31

[29] Simmons NE, Alden TD, Thorner MO, et al. Serum cortisol response to transsphenoidal surgery for Cushing disease. Journal of Neurosurgery. 2001; 95:1–8

[30] Rollin GA, Ferreira NP, Junges M, et al. Dynamics of serum cortisol levels after transsphenoidal surgery in a cohort of patients with Cushing's disease. Journal of Clinical Endocrinology and Metabolism. 2004; 89:1131–1139

[31] Sanno N, Teramoto A, Osamura RY. Long-term surgical outcome in 16 patients with thyrotropin pituitary adenoma. J Neurosurg. 2000; 93:194–200

[32] Ziu M, Dunn IF, Hess C, et al. Congress of Neurological Surgeons Systematic Review and Evidence-Based Guideline on Posttreatment Follow-up Evaluation of Patients With Nonfunctioning Pituitary Adenomas. Neurosurgery. 2016; 79:E541–E543

54

Part XIII

Other Tumors and Tumor-like Conditions

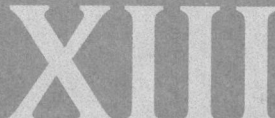

55 Metastases to the CNS

55.1 Cerebral metastases

55.1.1 General information

Key concepts

- brain metastases are the most common brain tumor seen clinically
- at the time of onset of neurologic symptoms, 70% will be multiple on MRI
- with solitary brain lesions in a patient with a history of cancer, biopsy should almost always be done since 11% of these lesions will not be mets
- although median survival with maximal treatment is only 8 months (similar to GBM), long-term survivors do occur

55.1.2 Metastases to the brain

Cerebral metastases are the most common brain tumor seen clinically, comprising slightly more than half of brain tumors (if one considers only imaging studies, they comprise ≈ 30%). In the U.S., the annual incidence of new cases of metastases is up to 170,000,[1] compared to 17,000 for primary brain tumors. 15–30% of patients with cancer (Ca) develop cerebral mets.[2] In patients with no Ca history, a cerebral met was the presenting symptom in 15%; of these, 43–60% will have an abnormal chest X-ray (**CXR**)[3,4] (showing either a bronchogenic primary or other mets to lung).

In 9% of cases, a cerebral met is the only detectable site of spread. Cerebral mets occur in only 6% of pediatric cancers.

The route of metastatic spread to the brain is usually hematogenous, although local extension can also occur.

Solitary mets
- CT (p. 914): at the time of *neurologic* diagnosis, 50% are solitary on CT[5,6]
- MRI: if the same patients have an MRI, < 30% will be solitary[7]
- on autopsy: mets are solitary in one–third of patients with brain mets, and 1–3% of solitary mets occur in the brainstem[8]

Increasing incidence of cerebral mets: may be due to a number of factors including:
1. increasing length of survival of cancer patients[9] as a result of improvements in treatment of systemic cancer
2. enhanced ability to diagnose CNS tumors due to availability of CT and/or MRI
3. many chemotherapeutic agents used systemically do not cross the blood-brain barrier (BBB) well, providing a "haven" for tumor growth there
4. some chemotherapeutic agents may transiently weaken the BBB and allow CNS seeding with tumor

55.1.3 Metastases of primary CNS tumors

Spread via CSF pathways

CNS tumors that more commonly spread via CSF pathways include the following (when these tumors spread to the spinal cord, they are often called "drop mets"):
1. high grade gliomas (p. 667) (10–25%)
2. embryonal tumors, primarily medulloblastoma (p. 750)
3. ependymoma (p. 724) (11%)
4. choroid plexus tumors (p. 739)
5. pineal region tumors
   a) germ cell tumors (p. 831)
   b) pineocytoma (p. 762) and pineoblastoma (p. 764)
6. rarely:
   a) oligodendrogliomas (p. 662) (≈ 1%)

55

b) hemangioblastomas (p.822)
c) primary CNS melanoma (p.830)

Extraneural spread

Although most CNS tumors do not spread systemically, there is some potential for extraneural spread with the following tumors:
1. medulloblastoma: the most common primary responsible for extraneural spread. May spread to lung, bone marrow, lymph nodes, abdomen
2. meningioma: rarely goes to heart or lungs
3. malignant astrocytomas rarely metastasize systemically
4. ependymomas
5. pineoblastomas
6. meningeal sarcomas
7. choroid plexus tumors
8. tumors that spread through CSF pathways (see above) may spread via a CSF shunt (e.g., to peritoneum with VP shunt or hematogenously with a VA shunt); however, this risk is probably quite small[10]

55.1.4 Location of cerebral mets

Intracranial metastases may be either parenchymal ($\approx$ 75%) or may involve the leptomeninges in a carcinomatous meningitis (p.920). 80% of solitary metastases are located in the cerebral hemispheres.

The highest incidence of parenchymal mets is posterior to the Sylvian fissure near the junction of temporal, parietal, and occipital lobes (presumably due to embolic spread to terminal MCA branches).[11] Many tend to arise at the gray/white-matter interface.

The cerebellum is a common site of intracranial mets, and is the location in 16% of cases of solitary brain mets. It is the most common p-fossa tumor in adults, thus "a solitary lesion in the posterior fossa of an adult is considered a metastasis until proven otherwise." Spread to the posterior fossa may be via the spinal epidural venous plexus (Batson's plexus) and the vertebral veins.

55.1.5 Primary cancers in patients with cerebral metastases

General information

Accurately ascertaining the source of cerebral metastases in the U.S. is difficult because of lack of detailed coding.[12] In over 2,700 adults with a primary cancer undergoing autopsy at Sloan-Kettering, the sources of cerebral metastases are shown in ▶ Table 55.1. Sources of brain metastases in pediatrics is shown in ▶ Table 55.2.

In adults, lung and breast Ca together account for > 50% of cerebral mets.

55

Table 55.1 Sources of cerebral mets in adults (autopsy data)

Primary	%
lung Ca	44
breast	10
kidney (renal cell)[a]	7
GI (colorectal)	6
melanoma[b]	3
undetermined	10

[a]an uncommon tumor that metastasizes frequently to brain (in 20–25% of cases)
[b]16% in older series[13]

Table 55.2 Sources of cerebral mets in peds

neuroblastoma
rhabdomyosarcoma
Wilm's tumor

In patients with a metastatic brain tumor as the initial presentation (i.e., undiagnosed primary) in 5–10% of cancers, and compared to patients with a known primary, there is about the same number of brain lesions, but there was an increased frequency of extracranial mets.[14] In up to 26% of cases, the primary tumor was never identified.[14]

The autopsy incidence of cerebral mets for various types of primary cancers at Sloan-Kettering Cancer Center is shown in ▸ Table 55.3.

Table 55.3 Autopsy incidence of cerebral mets for given primary cancers

Primary	% with cerebral mets
lung	21
breast	9
melanoma	40
lymphoma	1
• Hodgkin's	0
• non-Hodgkin's	2
GI	3
• colon	5
• gastric	0
• pancreatic	2
GU	11
• kidney (renal)	21
• prostate[a]	0
• testes	46
• cervix	5
• ovary	5
osteosarcoma	10
neuroblastoma	5
head and neck	6

[a]uncommon, but does occur

Lung cancer

The lungs are the most common source of cerebral mets, and these are usually multiple. The lung primary may be so small as to render it occult.

Necropsy demonstrates cerebral mets in up to 50% of patients with small-cell lung Ca (SCLC) and non-squamous, non-small-cell lung Ca.[15]

Cigarette smoking is responsible for 88% of all types of lung cancer combined (odds ratio for developing any type of lung cancer with cigarette smoking is 13.4), 91% of squamous cell (OR = 18.8), 89% of small cell (OR = 14.3), 95% of large cell (OR = 34.3), and 82% of adenocarcinoma (OR = 7.9).[16]

Small-cell lung cancer (SCLC)

AKA "oat cell" Ca. A neuroendocrine tumor. 95% arise in proximal airways, usually in mainstem or lobar bronchi. Typically younger (27–66 years) than other lung Ca. Median survival: 6–10 months. Considered a systemic disease. Staged in 1 of 2 categories:
1. limited: confined to an area of the chest that can be encompassed by a single radiation port
2. extensive: metastasis outside the thorax or intrathoracic disease that cannot be contained in a single radiation port

Although SCLC comprises only ≈ 20% of primary lung cancers, it is more likely to produce cerebral mets than other bronchogenic cell types (brain mets are found in 80% of patients who survive 2 yrs after diagnosis of SCLC).[9]

Treatment
Very radiosensitive.

No identified brain mets: prophylactic cranial irradiation (PCI) with WBXRT reduces the incidence of symptomatic brain mets and increases survival (disease-free & overall).[17,18] Typically 25 Gy in 10 fractions.

Brain mets: surgical resection considered for immediately life-threatening large lesions, XRT is used otherwise. Multiple SCLC brain lesions: XRT (initial treatment 30 Gy in 10 fractions) + chemotherapy.

Treatment of primary: usually not resected. Treated with chemotherapy ± XRT.

Recurrent brain mets after failure of initial treatment: 20 Gy in 10 fractions.

Non-small-cell lung cancer (NSCLC)

Includes: adenocarcinoma (the most common NSCLC), large cell, squamous cell, bronchoalveolar. Retrospective analysis of patients with NSCLC completely resected from the lung found a 6.8% first recurrence rate in the brain.[15] Staged with typical TNM system. Prognosis better than SCLC.

Treatment of lung primary:

1. grades I, II, IIIA: resection
2. higher grades (e.g., distal mets, excluding single brain met): XRT + chemotherapy

Staging studies for known lung primary

1. PET scan: can detect small malignancies. Useful in NSCLC to determine eligibility of resection of primary. Not useful in initial evaluation of SCLC
2. chest CT: usually includes adrenals and liver (thus abdomen and pelvis CT not necessary)
3. bone scan
4. brain: CT or MRI

When metastatic lung cancer is the suspected source of a newly diagnosed brain lesion, the lung lesion should be biopsied (if technically feasible) to rule out SCLC before obtaining tissue from the cerebral mass because XRT is the primary treatment for SCLC brain metastases.

Melanoma

General information

Melanoma: the 5th most common cancer in men, 7th in women. Incidence is increasing. Most common sites of origin of melanoma metastases: skin, retina, brain—primary CNS melanoma (p. 830)—nail bed. The primary site cannot be identified in up to ≈ 14% of cases.[19] Extremely difficult to locate primary sites: intraocular, GI mucosa.

Brain mets are found in 10–70% of patients with metastatic melanoma in clinical studies, and in 70–90% on autopsy of patients who died from melanoma. Patients with melanoma who have neurosurgical lesions typically presented 14 months after primary lesion was identified. Once cerebral mets of melanoma are detected, median survival is ≤ 6 months[20,21,22] and the mets contributed to the death in 94% of cases.[23] A small group with survival > 3 yrs had a single surgically treated met in the absence of other visceral lesions.

Evaluation

Metastatic melanoma to the brain classically causes pia/arachnoid involvement on imaging. Hemorrhagic involvement is common.

CT: lesions may be slightly hyperdense to brain on unenhanced CT due to melanin. Enhancement is less constant than for other mets (e.g., bronchogenic Ca).

MRI: decreased signal on T2WI surrounded by intense halo of edema. Enhancing T1WI lesions in a patient with melanoma is highly suggestive of melanoma metastases.

Systemic work-up: systemic disease determines ultimate survival after treatment of melanoma mets to the brain in 70% of patients. ∴ search for systemic mets should be done, including: CT of chest/abdomen/pelvis & bone scan. PET scan may be more sensitive for detecting metastatic spread than CT when there are clinical signs that the tumor has spread[24]; *except for the brain*, where brain MRI is more sensitive than CT or PET.

Treatment

Suggested algorithm for patients with metastatic melanoma to the brain (adapted,[25] see ▸ Fig. 55.1).

Patients with **Karnofsky performance scale (KPS) score** (p. 1640) < 70 are likely to be poor surgical candidates.

55

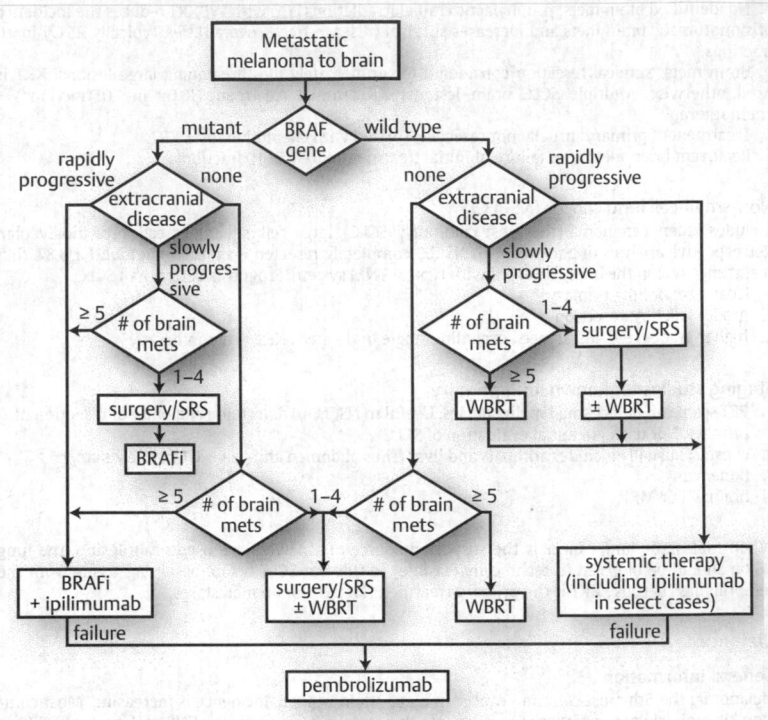

Fig. 55.1 Suggested algorithm for patients with metastatic melanoma to the brain (adapted[25]).
Abbreviations: BRAFi = BRAF inhibitors, SRS = stereotactic radiosurgery (p. 1903), WBRT = whole brain radiation therapy.

Some key points:
1. patients with rapidly progressive systemic disease: treat the systemic disease with chemotherapy first, before dealing with the brain mets
2. patients without systemic disease and 1–4 mets are candidates for surgery if all mets are accessible and can all be removed[26] (this is a general principle for brain mets, not just for melanoma). SRS is an alternative

▶ **Surgical indications**
1. patients with 1–4 CNS metastases that can be completely resected when systemic disease is absent or slowly progressive: long-term survival is possible
2. patients with intracranial mets that cannot be completely removed or with uncontrolled systemic disease may be surgical candidates for the following:
   a) for symptomatic relief: e.g., lesion causing painful pressure
   b) life-threatening lesion: e.g., large p-fossa lesion with 4th ventricle compression
   c) for hemorrhagic lesion causing symptoms by mass effect from the clot

▶ **Whole-brain radiation therapy (WBRT).** Melanoma is typically radioresistant. WBRT provides 2–3 month survival benefit and may be considered for palliation in patients with multiple mets that preclude complete excision or SRS.

▶ **Stereotactic radiosurgery (SRS).** Considered for ≤4 lesions, all ≤3 cm in diameter, that are surgically inaccessible, with limited or quiescent systemic involvement. Relative contraindications: hemorrhagic lesions, lesions with significant mass effect surrounding edema.

▶ **Chemotherapy**

1. alkylating agents:
   a) dacarbazine, formerly the gold-standard treatment for melanoma. About equally as effective as its newer orally administered analog temozolomide (Temodar®). Response rate: 10–20%
   b) Fotemustine appeared promising in phase II trials but only 6% responded in phase III (vs. 0% for dacarbazine)[27]

2. immunotherapy:
   a) ipilimumab (Yervoy®): monoclonal antibody against cytotoxic T lymphocyte antigen-4 (CTLA-4) antigen. More effective in patients who do not require corticosteroids
   b) interleukin-2 (IL-2): has shown minimal activity in brain mets, and trials have usually excluded patients with untreated or uncontrolled brain mets due to risk of cerebral edema and hemorrhage from capillary leak[28,29,30]

3. BRAF inhibitors (BRAFi): inhibits BRAF kinase (a protein that participates in regulation of cell division and differentiation), useful in tumors with BRAF oncogene mutation (as opposed to BRAF wildtype) which is common in melanoma
   a) dabrafenib: phase II trial (NCT01266967)[31]
   b) vemurafenib: promising results in heavily treated patients. Phase II trial (NCT01378975)[32]

4. anti-PD-1 drug (monoclonal antibody to PD-1 programmed cell death receptor): pembrolizumab (Keytruda) approved for advanced or unresectable melanoma not responding to other drugs[33]

Outcome

1. in a patient with a single brain met (any type) and good Karnofsky performance score (> 70) and no evidence of extracranial disease, surgery + XRT had a median survival of 40 weeks vs. 15 weeks for XRT alone[34,35]

2. for melanoma, retrospective studies have shown a benefit of treatment with either surgery or SRS only when all brain lesions are completely treated (selection bias possible in these studies)[35, 36,37,38]

3. predictors of poor outcome in melanoma:
   a) > 3 brain mets[21]
   b) development of brain mets after the diagnosis of extracranial disease[21]
   c) elevated lactate dehydrogenase > 2 × normal[22]
   d) presence of bone metastases[22]
   e) multiple brain mets and extensive visceral disease[39]

Renal-cell carcinoma

AKA hypernephroma. Usually associated with spread to lungs, lymph nodes, liver, bone (high affinity for bone), adrenals, and contralateral kidney before invading the CNS (thus, this tumor rarely presents as isolated cerebral metastases). Look for hematuria, abdominal pain, and/or abdominal mass on palpation or CT. Response to XRT is only ≈ 10%.

Esophageal cancer

Median survival is 4.2 months based on a review of 26 cases.[40] Solitary brain met with good Karnofsky score and surgical treatment may indicate a better prognosis.

55.1.6 Clinical presentation

As with most brain tumors, signs and symptoms are usually slowly progressive compared to those from vascular events (ischemic or hemorrhagic infarcts), which tend to be sudden in onset and slowly resolve, or electrical events (seizures), which tend to be sudden in onset and rapidly resolve. Metastases may also present acutely by hemorrhaging, causing an intraparenchymal hematoma (IPH). There are no findings that would allow differentiation of a metastatic tumor from a primary neoplasm on clinical grounds.

Signs and symptoms include:

1. those due to increased ICP from mass effect and/or blockage of CSF drainage (hydrocephalus):
   a) headache (H/A): the most common presenting symptom, occurs in ≈ 50%
   b) nausea/vomiting

2. focal deficits:
   a) due to compression of brain parenchyma by mass and/or peritumoral edema (e.g., monoparesis without sensory disturbance)
   b) due to compression of cranial nerve

55

3. seizures: occur only in ≈ 15% of cases
4. mental status changes: depression, lethargy, apathy, confusion
5. hemorrhage (p. 1612): producing IPH, often with H/A and sudden onset of focal deficit, obtundation may occur with large hemorrhages
6. symptoms suggestive of a TIA (dubbed "tumor TIA") or stroke, may be due to:
   a) occlusion of a vessel by tumor cells
   b) hemorrhage into the tumor, especially common with metastatic melanoma, choriocarcinoma,
      and renal-cell carcinoma[41]; see Hemorrhagic brain tumors (p. 1612). May also occur due to
      decreased platelet count

55.1.7 Evaluation

Imaging studies (CT or MRI)

Metastases usually appear as "non-complicated" masses (i.e., round, well circumscribed), often arising at the gray/white junction (▶ Fig. 55.2). Characteristically, profound white matter edema ("fingers of edema") reach deep into the brain from the tumor, usually more pronounced than that seen
with primary (infiltrating) brain tumors. When multiple lesions are present (on CT or MRI of brains
with multiple mets) Chamber's rule applies: "Whoever counts the most mets is right." Mets usually
enhance, and must be considered in the differential diagnosis of a ring-enhancing lesion.

MRI is more sensitive than CT, especially in the posterior-fossa (including brain stem). Detects
multiple mets in up to ≈ 20% of patients who appear to have single mets on CT.[2]

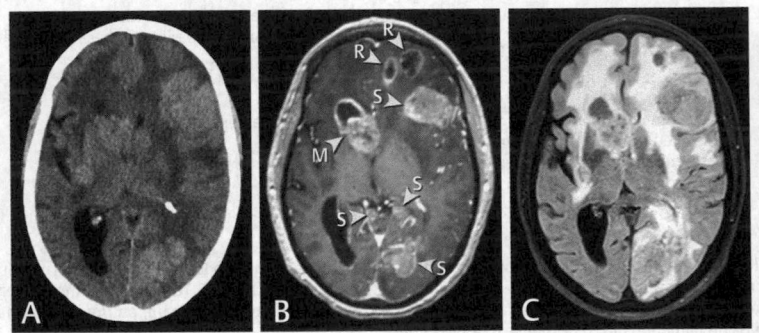

Fig. 55.2 Cerebral metastases.
65-year-old woman with small cell cancer of the lung metastatic to the brain.
Image: A: axial non-contrast head CT obtained at admission. B: axial MRI T1 + contrast, showing multiple metastatic
lesions (*yellow arrowheads*) (which were also present in the cerebellum, not shown), some are solid (S), some are
ring enhancing (R), and some are mixed (M). C: axial T2 MRI demonstrating characteristic extensive white-matter
"fingers of edema."

Lumbar puncture

Relatively contraindicated when there is a cerebral mass (may be considered once mass lesion has
been ruled out). May be most useful in diagnosing carcinomatous meningitis (p. 920), and may be of
limited help in diagnosing CNS lymphoma.

Metastatic work-up with suspected brain metastases

When metastatic disease is suspected based on imaging, a search for a primary site and assessment
for other metastatic lesions may be considered since it may provide alternative sites for tissue for
histologic diagnosis, and it may guide treatment (e.g., widely disseminated metastases may preclude
aggressive therapy). It is also undertaken to look for a primary and other metastases when biopsy is
consistent with brain metastases.

Metastatic work-up should include:
1. CT of the chest (more sensitive than CXR), abdomen and pelvis. Evaluates for primary and additional mets (to lung, adrenals, liver... CT has superseded CXR)
2. radionuclide bone scan: for patients with bone pain or bone lesions or for tumors that tend to produce osseous metastases (especially: prostate, breast, kidney, thyroid & lung)
3. mammogram in women
4. prostate specific antigen (PSA) in men
5. PET scan: can detect small malignancies

Cancer of unknown primary site (CUP): If the metastatic work-up (see above) is negative, the pathology of a metastatic brain lesion as determined by biopsy may implicate specific primary sites.

Small-cell carcinoma metastatic to the brain is most likely from the lung. These tumors stain positive for neuroendocrine stains (p. 632).

Adenocarcinoma: lung is the most common primary. Other sources: GI (mostly colon), breast. The primary site may remain occult even after extensive evaluation in up to 88%.[42] Immunostaining has been tried to identify the primary site but has not been found to be widely useful.

55.1.8 Management

General information

With optimal treatment, median survival of patients with cerebral mets is still only ≈ 26–32 weeks, therefore management is mostly palliative. Also see Outcome (p. 919) for comparison of various treatments.

Confirming the diagnosis

NB: 11% of patients with abnormalities on brain CT or MRI with a history of cancer (within past 5 yrs) do not have cerebral metastases.[34] Differential diagnoses include: primary brain tumor (glioblastoma, low grade astrocytoma), abscess, and nonspecific inflammatory reaction. If non-surgical treatment (e.g., chemotherapy or XRT) is being contemplated, the diagnosis should first be confirmed by biopsy in almost all cases.

Management decisions

Prognostication

This is critical since many treatment decisions depend on overall prognosis.

RTOG RPA: Radiation Therapy Oncology Group recursive partitioning analysis classification[43] (see ▶ Table 55.4). Conclusion: the specific tumor type, length of time since diagnosis, etc. are not as important prognostically as the Karnofsky Performance Scale (KPS) score (p. 1640).

The applicability of RPA to melanoma mets to the brain is controversial (it has been both validated[44] and disputed[38]).

RPA Class 3 patients have been shown to be unlikely to benefit from any of numerous treatment modalities studied. Class 1 are more likely to benefit. Most patients are Class 2, for whom benefit is unclear.

55

Table 55.4 Radiation Therapy Oncology Group recursive partitioning analysis (RPA) classification for patients with brain mets (from 1200 patients with ≥ 1 brain mets undergoing XRT)[43]

RPA class	Description	Median survival (mos)[a]
1	• KPS[b] ≥ 70 and • age < 65 years and • controlled[c] or absent primary tumor with the brain the only site of metastasis	7
2	• all others (i.e., not RPA class 1 or 3)	4
3	• KPS < 70	2

[a]for patients undergoing XRT
[b]KPS = Karnofsky Performance Scale score (p. 1640)
[c]controlled = stable disease over 3 months observation

Management algorithm

▶ Table 55.5 shows a summary of management suggestions (details appear in following sections).

Also, surgical excision may be considered for patients with completely resectable brain mets who are candidates for chemotherapy with interleukin-2 (IL-2) for systemic disease (e.g., for renal-cell Ca or melanoma) since there are case reports of significant cerebral edema associated with use of this drug in the presence of cerebral mets.

Table 55.5 Management suggestions for cerebral metastases[a]

Clinical situation		Management
unknown primary or unconfirmed diagnosis		stereotactic biopsy for ≈ all patients if surgical excision is not a consideration
uncontrolled widespread systemic cancer & obviously short life expectancy and/or poor performance status, KPS (p. 1640) ≤ 70		(biopsy as indicated above) + WBXRT or no treatment
metastases known to be extremely radiosensitive (lymphoma, small cell lung cancer, germ cell tumor, multiple myeloma)		XRT
Stable systemic disease & KPS > 70		
solitary met	symptomatic or threatening, and safely resectable[b] lesion	surgical excision[c, d] + WBXRT[e] or surgical excision[c, d] + SRS[e]
	asymptomatic, small, or not safely resectable[b]	WBXRT ± SRS boost
multiple mets	single large lesion that is life threatening or producing mass effect	surgery for the large lesion + WBXRT for the rest
	≤ 3 lesions: symptomatic & can all be removed	surgery + WBXRT or SRS + WBXRT
	≤ 3 lesions: cannot all be removed	WBXRT or SRS + WBXRT
	> 3 lesions: with no mass effect requiring surgery	WBXRT[45]

[a] adapted Pollock et al.[46] and the 2019 Congress of Neurological Surgeons Systematic Review and Evidence-Based Guidelines[47,48]
[b] safely resectable lesion implies surgery can be performed without undue risk of worsening neurologic condition (including hemiparesis, aphasia...) that would lower KPS and thereby shorten longevity
[c] surgery + WBXRT is superior to WBXRT alone (Level 1); surgery + SRS is superior to SRS alone (Level 3)[47]
[d] surgical excision: class III data suggests gross total resection is superior to subtotal resection in RPA class I patients, and that with single mets that en bloc resection reduses the risk of leptomeningeal disease compared to piecemeal resection[47]
[e] NB: used alone for patients with 1-3 mets, SRS is better for survival and neurocognition but is worse for local and distant control compared to WBXRT
Abbreviations: KPS = Karnofsky Performance Scale score (p. 1640); SRS = stereotactic radiosurgery; WBXRT = whole brain radiation therapy.

Medical management

Initial treatment

1. **antiseizure medications**: e.g., Keppra® (levetiracetam) starting with 500 mg PO or IV q 12 hours. Generally not indicated for posterior fossa lesions due to low epileptogenicity with these.
   Guidelines: ASMs showed a nonstatistically significant reduction of early seizures, and had no benefit for seizures at 3 months or for survival.[49,50] Guideline conclusions: no compelling data for prophylactic ASM pre-op or post-op.
   Non-guideline opinion: use is more justifiable in patients who actually have a seizure.
2. corticosteroids: many symptoms are due to peritumoral edema (which is primarily vasogenic), and respond to steroids within 24–48 hrs. This improvement is not permanent, and prolonged steroid administration may produce side effects; see Possible deleterious side effects of steroids (p. 626).
   Guidelines: steroids are recommended for temporary relief of symptoms due to increased ICP or edema related to mets (Level 3).[51] There is insufficient evidence to make recommendations for use with asymptomatic lesions without mass effect.[51]

Dexamethasone is the drug of choice (Level 3)[51]

R for mild-to-moderate symtoms in a patient who is not already on steroids: dexamethasone (Decadron®) 4–8 mg/d (Level 3)[51] usually given in divided doses. Higher doses are not more effective and side effects are more common[52]

R for severe symptoms consider higher dose of 16 mg/d (Level 3).[51]

Regardless of regimen used, taper steroids as rapidly as tolerated to the lowest effective dose for symptom control(Level 3).[51]

3. H2 antagonists (e.g., ranitidine 150 mg PO q 12 hrs) or proton pump inhibitor (omeprazole)

Chemotherapy

See discussion of Limitations of chemotherapy in the brain (p.627). If multiple lesions of known small-cell Ca are detected on cerebral imaging, treatment of choice is radiation plus chemotherapy.

Radiation therapy

General information

NB: not all brain lesions in cancer patients are mets (see above).

In patients not considered for surgery, steroids and radiation may be palliative. H/A are usually reduced, and in ≈ 50% of cases symptoms improve or completely resolve.[53] This does not result in local control for the majority of these patients and they frequently succumb from progressive brain disease.

"Radiosensitivity" of various metastatic tumors to whole brain radiation therapy (WBXRT) are shown in ▶ Table 55.6.

The usual dose is 30 Gy in 10 fractions given over 2 weeks. With this dose, 11% of 1-yr survivors and 50% of 2-yr survivors develop severe dementia.

Table 55.6 "Radiosensitivity" of brain metastases to WBXRT

Radiosensitivity	Tumor
Radiosensitive[34]	• small-cell lung Ca • germ cell tumors • lymphoma • leukemia • multiple myeloma
Moderately sensitive	• breast
Moderately resistant	• colon • non small-cell lung cancer
Highly resistant[a]	• thyroid • renal cell (10% respond) • malignant melanoma • sarcoma • adenocarcinoma

[a]SRS may be better than WBXRT for these

55

Prophylactic cranial irradiation

Prophylactic cranial irradiation after resection of small-cell lung carcinoma (SCLC) reduces relapses in brain, but does not affect survival.[54]

Post-op radiation therapy

WBXRT is usually recommended following craniotomy for metastatic disease,[55] especially with SCLC where "micro-metastases" are presumed to be present throughout brain. (**Note:** some centers do not routinely administer post-op WBXRT (except for very radiosensitive tumors such as SCLC) but instead follow patients with serial imaging studies and administer XRT only when metastases are documented.)

Optimal dose is controversial. Early reports recommended 30–39 Gy over 2–2.5 weeks (3 Gy fractions) with or without surgery.[56] This is acceptable in patients not expected to live long enough to get long-term radiation effects. Recent recommendations are for smaller daily fractions of 1.8–2.0 Gy to reduce neurotoxicity.[57] These low doses are also associated with a higher rate of recurrent brain metastases.[58] Since 50 Gy are needed to achieve > 90% control of micrometastases, some use

45–50 Gy WBXRT, plus a boost to the tumor bed to bring the total treatment up to 55 Gy, all with low fractions of 1.80–2.0 Gy.[59]

Stereotactic radiosurgery

Inconsistent in its ability to reduce tumor size. Some retrospective studies show results comparable to surgery.[60] Others do not.[61] Does not obtain tissue for histological analysis, and generally cannot be used for lesions > 3 cm. Also, see Stereotactic radiosurgery (p.919).

Surgical management

Solitary lesions

Indications favoring surgical excision of a solitary lesion:
1. primary disease quiescent
2. lesion accessible
3. lesion is symptomatic or life-threatening
4. primary tumor known to be relatively radioresistant (excision is rarely indicated for untreated brain metastases from SCLC because of its radiosensitivity)
5. for recurrent SCLC following XRT
6. diagnosis unknown: alternatively consider biopsy, e.g., stereotactic biopsy

Surgical resection in patients with progressive systemic disease and/or significant neurologic deficit is probably unjustified.[62] Also, in newly diagnosed cancer patients, craniotomy may delay systemic treatment for weeks and the ramifications of this need to be considered.

Multiple lesions

Patients with multiple metastases generally have much worse survival than those with solitary lesions.[57] Multiple metastases are usually treated with XRT without surgery. However, if total excision of *all* mets is feasible, then even multiple mets may be removed with survival similar to those having a single met removed[26] (also see ▶ Table 55.5 for summary). If only incomplete excision is possible (i.e., cannot remove all mets, or portions of 1 or more must be left behind) then there is no improvement in survival with surgery, and XRT alone is recommended. The mortality of removing > 1 met at a single sitting is not statistically significantly higher than removing a single met.

Situations where surgery may be indicated for multiple mets[63]:
1. one particular and accessible lesion is clearly symptomatic and/or life threatening (life-threatening lesions include p-fossa and large temporal lobe lesions). This is palliative treatment to reduce the symptom/threat from that particular lesion
2. multiple lesions that can all be completely removed (see above)
3. no diagnosis (e.g., no identifiable primary): consider stereotactic biopsy

Stereotactic biopsy

Considered for:
1. lesions not appropriate for open surgery. Includes cases with no definite diagnosis and:
   a) deep lesions
   b) multiple small lesions
2. patients not candidates for surgical resection
   a) poor medical condition
   b) poor neurologic condition
   c) active or widespread systemic disease
3. to ascertain a diagnosis
   a) when another diagnosis is possible: e.g., no other sites of metastases, long interval between primary cancer and detection of brain mets...
   b) especially if nonsurgical treatment modalities are planned (see above)

Intraoperative considerations for surgical removal

Most lesions present themselves on the surface of the brain or through the dura. For lesions not visible on the surface nor palpable immediately beneath the surface, intraoperative ultrasound or stereotactic techniques may be used to localize the lesion.

Metastases usually have a well defined border, thus a plane of separation from normal brain may be exploited, often allowing gross total removal.

55.1.9 Outcome

General information

▶ Table 55.7 lists factors associated with better survival regardless of treatment. Also, the prognosis gets worse as the number of mets increases.[46] Median survival even with best treatment in some studies is only ≈ 6 months. To put this into perspective, this is worse than with glioblastoma.

Table 55.7 Factors associated with better prognosis for brain mets (with any treatment)

- Karnofsky score[a] (KPS) > 70
- age < 60 yrs
- metastases to brain only (no systemic mets)
- absent or controlled primary disease
- > 1 yr since diagnosis of primary
- the fewer the number of brain mets
- female gender

[a]the KPS (p. 1640) is probably the most important predictor; those with a score of 100 had median survival > 150 weeks

Natural history

By the time that neurologic findings develop, median survival among untreated patients is ≈ 1 month.[64]

Steroids

Using steroids alone (to control edema) doubles survival[65] to 2 mos (**Note:** this is based largely on pre-CT era data, and the tumors were therefore probably larger than in current studies[66]).

Whole brain radiation therapy (WBXRT)

WBXRT + steroids increases survival to 3–6 mos.[26] 50% of deaths are due to progression of intracranial disease.

Surgery ± WBXRT

Recurrence of tumor was significantly less frequent and more delayed with the use of post-op WBXRT.[55] Length of survival was unchanged with supplemental use of WBXRT. There is also an additional loss of cognitive function in many cases, and patients are rarely independent after WBXRT.

In 33 patients treated with surgical resection of single mets and post-op WBXRT[67]: median survival was 8 months; with 44% 1-yr survival. If no evidence of systemic Ca, 1-yr survival is 81%. If systemic Ca is present (active or inactive), 1-yr survival is 20%. Patients with solitary mets and no evidence of active systemic tumor have the best prognosis.[53,62] With total removal, no recurrence nor new parenchymal mets occurred within 6 months, and the major cause of death was progression of Ca outside the CNS. A randomized trial verified the improved longevity and quality of survival of patients with solitary mets undergoing surgical excision plus WBXRT vs. WBXRT alone (40 weeks vs. 15 weeks median survival).[34] The surgical mortality was 4% (≈ same as 30-day mortality in the XRT-only group). More patients treated with WBXRT alone die of their brain mets than those who underwent surgery. Following total removal and post-op WBXRT, 22% of patients will have recurrent brain tumor at 1 year.[57] This is better than surgery without XRT (with reported failure rates of 46%[57] and 85%[58]).

Stereotactic radiosurgery (SRS)

There has not been a randomized study to compare surgery to SRS. *Retrospective* studies suggest that SRS may be comparable to surgery.[60,68] However, a prospective (non-randomized, retrospectively matched) study[61] found a median survival of 7.5 mos with SRS vs. 16.4 mos with surgery, and a higher mortality from cerebral disease in the SRS group (with the mortality due to the SRS treated lesions and not new lesions). A local control rate of ≈ 88% has been reported, with one study also recommending WBXRT following the SRS for better regional control.[69]

55

Actuarial control rates at 1 year following SRS + WBXRT were 75–80% and appear to be similar to surgery + WBXRT.[46] However, SRS was unreliable in reducing tumor size.

Multiple mets

Patients with multiple mets that were totally removed have a survival that is similar to those having single mets surgically removed[26] (see above).

Recurrent metastases

Surgery is recommended for intracranial recurrence after initial surgery or SRS (Level 3).[47]

55.1.10 Carcinomatous meningitis

General information

Carcinomatous meningitis (CM) AKA (lepto)meningeal carcinomatosis (LMC). Found in up to 8% of patients autopsied with systemic cancer. CM may be the presenting finding in up to 48% of patients with cancer (before the diagnosis cancer is known). Most common primaries: breast, lung, then melanoma.[70(p 610–2)] Always include *lymphomatous meningitis* in the differential diagnosis; see CNS lymphoma (p. 840).

Clinical

Simultaneous onset of findings in multiple levels of neuraxis. Multiple cranial nerve findings are frequent (in up to 94%, most common: VII, III, V, and VI), usually progressive. Most frequent symptoms: H/A, mental status changes, lethargy, seizure, ataxia. Non-obstructive hydrocephalus is also common. Painful radiculopathies can occur with "drop mets."

Diagnosis

Lumbar puncture
Perform only after mass lesion has been ruled out with cranial CT or MRI. Although the initial LP may be normal, CSF is eventually abnormal in > 95%.
   CSF should be sent for:
1. cytology to look for malignant cells (requires ≈ 10 ml for adequate evaluation for CM). Repeat if negative (45% positive on first study, 81% eventually positive after up to 6 LPs). May need to pass CSF through a millipore filter
2. bacterial and fungal cultures (including unusual organisms, e.g., cryptococcus)
3. tumor markers: carcinoembryonic antigen, alpha-fetoprotein
4. protein/glucose: elevated protein is the most common abnormality. Glucose may be as low as ≈ 40 mg% in about a third of patients

MRI
Contrast enhanced MRI is more sensitive in showing meningeal enhancement.[71]

CT
May show (mild) ventricular dilatation, enhancement of basal cisterns. Sulcal enhancement may also occur with involvement of the convexities.

Myelography
Spinal seeding ("drop mets") will produce filling defects on myelography.

Survival

Untreated: < 2 months. With radiation therapy + chemotherapy: median survival is 5.8 mos (range 1–29). Chemotherapy may be given intrathecally. About half of patients die of CNS involvement, and half die of systemic disease.

55.2 Spinal epidural metastases

55.2.1 General information

Key concepts

- suspected in a cancer patient with back pain that persists in recumbency
- occurs in ≈ 10% of all cancer patients
- 80% of primary sites: lung, breast, GI, prostate, melanoma, and lymphoma
- many treatments reduce pain. Surgery + XRT in selected cases increases chances of preserving ambulation & produces a modest improvement in survival
- if no neurologic compromise or bony instability, usual treatment: biopsy (CT- or fluoro-guided) followed by XRT (surgical indications ► Table 55.11)
- surgery not helpful for: total paralysis > 8 hrs, loss of ambulation > 24 hrs, and not recommended for prognosis < 3–4 months survival, poor medical condition (poor PFTs...), or radiosensitive tumor

Spinal epidural metastases (SEM) occur in up to 10% of cancer patients at some time,[72] and are the most common spinal tumor. 5–10% of malignancies present initially with cord compression.[73] For other etiologies of spinal cord compression, see items marked with a dagger (†) under Myelopathy (p. 1696).

Routes of metastasis to spine:
1. arterial
2. venous: via spinal epidural veins (Batson's plexus[74])
3. perinervous (direct spread)

The usual route of spread is hematogenous dissemination to the vertebral body with erosion back through pedicles and subsequent extension into the epidural space (i.e., *anterior* epicenter). Less commonly may initially metastasize to lateral or posterior aspect of canal. Most metastases (mets) are epidural, only 2–4% are intradural, and only 1–2% are intramedullary. Distribution between cervical, thoracic, and lumbar spine is proportional to the length of the segment, thus the thoracic spine is the most common site (50–60%).

55.2.2 Primary tumors that metastasize to the spine

► Table 55.8 shows primary tumor types that give rise to SEM. The majority are common primaries that tend to metastasize to bone (lung, breast, prostate, renal-cell, and thyroid). Rare tumors that

Table 55.8 Sources of spinal epidural metastases causing cord compression

Site of primary	Series A	Series B[a]	Series C[b]
lung	17%	14%	31%
breast	16%	21%	24%
prostate	11%	19%	8%
kidney (renal-cell)	9%		1%
unknown site	9%	5%	2%
sarcoma	8%		2%
lymphoma	6%	12%	6%
GI tract	6%		9%
thyroid	6%		
melanoma	2%		4%
others (including multiple myeloma)	13%	29%[c]	13%

[a]series B: retrospective study of 58 patients undergoing MRI evaluation for SEM[72]
[b]series C: 75 patients with SEM out of 140 patients evaluated prospectively for back pain[76]
[c]in series B, "other" includes GI, GU, skin, ENT, CNS

55

may go to bone include the myxoid subtype of liposarcoma[75] (17% of these patients develop bone mets, 5-year median survival is 16%).

55.2.3 Presentation

Pain: the most common initial symptom. Occurs in up to 95% of patients with SEM.[77,78] Types of pain:
1. local pain: typically aching, experienced at the level of involvement. Increased pain with *recumbency* (especially at night) is characteristic
2. radicular: tends to be sharp or shooting, referred into dermatome of the involved nerve root. Commonly bilateral in thoracic region
3. mechanical: usually exacerbated by movement

Neck-flexion, straight-leg-raising, coughing, sneezing, or straining may also aggravate the pain.

Motor or autonomic dysfunction: the second most common presentation. Up to 85% of patients have weakness at the time of diagnosis. Leg stiffness may be an early symptom. Bladder dysfunction (urinary urgency, hesitancy, or retention) is the most common autonomic manifestation; others include constipation or impotence.

Sensory dysfunction: anesthesia, hypesthesia, or paresthesias usually occur with motor dysfunction. Cervical or thoracic cord involvement may produce a sensory level.

Other presentations: pathologic fracture. Bone metastases can sometimes produce hypercalcemia (a medical emergency).

The greater the neurologic deficit when treatment is initiated, the worse the chances for recovery of lost function. 76% of patients have weakness by the time of diagnosis.[72] 15% are paraplegic on initial presentation, and <5% of these can ambulate after treatment. Median time from onset of symptoms to diagnosis is 2 months.[79]

Metastases to the upper cervical spine

For differential diagnosis, see Foramen magnum lesions (p.1649), and Axis (C2) vertebra lesions (p.1678).

Metastases to the C1–2 region comprise only ≈ 0.5% of spinal mets.[80] They typically present initially with suboccipital and posterior cervical pain, and as the lesion progresses patients develop a characteristic pain that makes it difficult to sit up (some will hold their heads in their hands to stabilize it). Possibly as a result of the capacious spinal canal at this level, only ≈ 11–15% of patients present with neurologic symptoms. 15% develop spinal cord compression,[81] and quadriplegia from atlantoaxial subluxation occurred in ≈ 6%.[81]

Anterior approaches for stabilization at this location are difficult. Pathologic fractures due to osteoblastic types of tumors (e.g., prostate, some breast) may heal with radiation treatment and immobilization. For others, good pain relief and stabilization may be achieved with radiation followed by posterior fusion.[81]

55.2.4 Evaluation and management of epidural spinal metastases

General information

There is no difference in outcome between lesions above or below the conus; thus spinal cord, conus medullaris, or cauda equina mets are considered together here as epidural spinal cord compression (ESCC). Features that help distinguish conus lesions from cauda equina are shown in ▸ Table 55.9.

Grading function

There is prognostic significance in the presenting neurologic condition. Grading scales such as that of Brice and McKissock (▸ Table 55.10) have been proposed, but are not widely used. The ASIA grading scale is more commonly applied.

Diagnostic tests

MRI in evaluating SEM
MRI without and with contrast is the diagnostic test of choice in most situations.

Table 55.9 Features distinguishing conus lesions from cauda equina lesions with metastases[82]

	Conus medullaris lesions	Cauda equina lesions
spontaneous pain	rare; when present, is usually bilateral & symmetric in perineum or thighs	may be most prominent symptom; severe; radicular type; in perineum, thighs & legs, back or bladder
sensory deficit	saddle; bilateral; usually symmetric; sensory dissociation	saddle; no sensory dissociation; may be unilateral & asymmetric
motor loss	*symmetric*; not marked; fasciculations may be present	*asymmetric*; more marked; atrophy may occur; fasciculations rare
autonomic symptoms (including bladder dysfunction, impotency...)	prominent early	late
reflexes	only ankle jerk absent (preserved knee jerk)	ankle jerk & knee jerk may be absent
onset	sudden and bilateral	gradual and unilateral

Table 55.10 Grading spinal cord function with spinal metastases (Brice & McKissock)[83]

Group	Grade	Description
1	mild	patient able to walk
2	moderate	able to move legs, but not antigravity
3	severe	slight residual motor and sensory function
4	complete	no motor, sensory, or sphincter function below level of lesion

MRI findings in spinal epidural metastases:
1. vertebral mets are slightly hypointense compared to normal bone marrow on T1WI, and are slightly hyperintense on T2WI
2. axial cuts typically show lesion involving the posterior vertebral body with invasion into one or both pedicles
3. when myelopathy or radiculopathy are present, there is usually tumor extension into the spinal canal (may not occur in lesions presenting only with local pain)
4. DWI images may help differentiate osteoporotic compression fracture from pathologic fracture[84]

Plain X-rays

Most spinal mets are osteolytic, but at least 50% of the bone must be eroded before plain X-rays will be abnormal.[85] Not very specific. Possible findings: pedicle erosion (defect in "owl's eyes" AKA "winking owl sign" on LS or thoracic spine AP view) or widening, pathological compression fracture, vertebral body (VB) scalloping, VB *sclerosis*, osteoblastic changes (may occur with prostate Ca, Hodgkin's disease, occasionally with breast Ca, and rarely with multiple myeloma).

Plain CT in evaluating SEM

Very good for bone detail. Often helpful for surgical planning. By itself, has low sensitivity for spinal cord compression by tumor. Sensitivity is increased with intrathecal contrast (CT-myelogram).

CT-myelogram (CT-myelo)

Indicated when MRI cannot be done (contraindications, unavailability...).
Advantages over MRI:
• Can obtain CSF (when performing LP to inject contrast) for cytological study
• Excellent bony detail
• Can be performed in patients with pacemaker/AICD, claustrophobia...

Disadvantages of myelography over MRI[72]:
Invasive
May require second procedure (C1–2 puncture) if there is a complete block (providers proficient in this technique are becoming fewer)

55

- Risk of neurologic deterioration from LP in patient with complete block
- Cannot detect lesions that do not cause bony destruction or distortion of the spinal subarachnoid space
- Up to 20% of patients with SEM have at least two sites of cord compression, MRI can evaluate region between two complete blocks, myelography cannot
- Cannot demonstrate paraspinal lesions
- Does not image spinal cord parenchyma

Positron emission tomography (PET) scan

PET scan using [18F]-fluorodeoxyglucose may be used for whole-body work-up for bone mets in patients with known cancer.[86] Sensitivity is high, but spatial resolution and specificity are low, so often must be used with CT and/or MRI.

Metastatic work-up for patients with suspected spine metastases

- CT of chest, abdomen and pelvis: assess tumor burden, staging, prognostication (which factors into decisions regarding surgery). Has superseded CXR to rule out lung lesion (primary or other mets)
- bone scan: looks for other sites of skeletal involvement
- serum prostate specific antigen (PSA) in males
- mammogram in females
- for multiple myeloma (p.930)
- careful physical exam of lymph nodes

Management algorithm

General information

Management is dependent on the degree and rapidity of neurologic involvement.[82] Patients may be categorized into one of the three groups that follows, which determines the subsequent steps. In a patient with suspected spine mets, the goals of management are:
- assessment of neurologic involvement and timeline of neurologic changes
- delineation of the degree of spinal involvement
- determination of a histologic diagnosis: this affects management
- preservation or restoration of neurologic function
- preservation or restoration spinal stability
- controlling pain

The tools that are employed in the assessment and stabilization phase are listed under diagnostic tests above. The section that follows discusses the rapidity with which they are implemented.

A metastatic work-up (p.924) is undertaken as time permits (a preliminary work-up, e.g., CXR and physical exam, may be all that can be initially obtained for patients in Group I, whereas more complete work-up can be done in others).

55

Group I—rapid progression or severe deficit

Group I characteristics

Signs/symptoms of new or progressive (hours to days) cord compression (e.g., urinary urgency, ascending numbness). These patients have a high risk of rapid deterioration and require immediate evaluation.

Management

1. dexamethasone (DMZ) (Decadron®): reduces pain in 85%, may produce transient neurologic improvement. Optimal dose is not known. No difference was found comparing 100 mg IV bolus to 10 mg.[87] Suggestion: 10 mg IV or PO q 6 hrs × 72 hrs, followed by lower dose of 4–6 mg q 6 hrs. Steroids may temporarily mask lymphoma (on imaging and at surgery); however, in this group the benefit of giving steroids usually outweighs this pitfall
2. radiographic evaluation
   a) *STAT MRI* (above)
   b) *plain X-rays* of entire spine: 67–85% will be abnormal (see above)

c) if time permits, plain CT scan through involved levels and at least 2 levels above and below to evaluate bone for surgical planning

d) **emergency** myelogram: indicated if MRI cannot be done (include possible C1–2 puncture on the consent). Start with a so-called "blockogram" to R/O complete block: instill small volume of contrast, e.g., iohexol (Omnipaque™) (p. 230) via LP and run the dye all the way up the spinal column; CSF is usually xanthochromic with complete block, see Froin's syndrome (p. 987)

- if there is not a complete block: withdraw 10 cc of CSF and send for *cytology*, protein & glucose. One may then inject more contrast to complete the study

- if complete block: do *not* remove CSF (pressure shifts via LP caused neurologic deterioration in ≈ 14% of patients with complete block,[88] whereas there was no deterioration after C1–2 puncture). In some cases, contrast can be "squeezed" past a "complete" block by injecting 5–10 ml of room air through a millipore filter.[89] Alternatively, perform a lateral C1–2 puncture (p. 1819) and instill water soluble contrast to delineate the superior extent of the lesion

- with myelography, epidural lesions classically produce hourglass deformity with smooth edges if block is incomplete, or paintbrush effect (feathered edges) if block is complete, unlike the sharp margins (capping or meniscus sign) of intradural extramedullary lesion, or fusiform cord widening of intramedullary tumors

- *bone scan* if time permits. Abnormal in ≈ 66% of patients with spine mets

3. treatment based on results of radiographic evaluation

a) if no epidural mass: treat primary tumor (e.g., systemic **chemotherapy**). Local radiation therapy (XRT) to bony lesion if present. Analgesics for pain

b) if epidural lesion, either surgery *or* start XRT (usually 30–40 Gy in 10 treatments over 7–10 d with ports extending 2 levels above and below lesion). XRT is usually as effective as laminectomy with fewer complications; for further discussion see Treatment for SEM (p. 926). Thus, *surgery* instead of XRT is considered only for the indications shown in ▶ Table 55.11

c) **urgency** of treatment (surgery or XRT) is based on degree of block and rapidity of deterioration:

- if > 80% block or rapid progression of deficit: emergency treatment ASAP (if treating with XRT instead of surgery, continue DMZ next day at 24 mg IV q 6 hrs x 2 days, then taper during XRT over 2 wks)

- if < 80% block: treatment on "routine" basis (for XRT, continue DMZ 4 mg IV q 6 hrs, taper during treatment as tolerated)

Table 55.11 Indications for surgery for spinal metastases

Indications

1. unknown primary and no tissue diagnosis (CT guided needle biopsy is an option for accessible lesions). NB: lesions such as spinal epidural abscess can be mistaken for metastases[93]
2. spinal instability (see the Spine Instability Neoplastic Score (SINS) ▶ Table 55.12)
3. deficit due to spinal deformity or compression by bone rather than by tumor (e.g., due to compression fracture with collapse and retropulsed bone)
4. radio-resistant tumors (e.g., renal-cell carcinoma, melanoma…) or progression during XRT (usual trial: at least 48 hrs, unless significant or rapid deterioration)
5. recurrence after maximal XRT
6. rapid neurologic deterioration

Relative contraindications

1. very radiosensitive tumors (multiple myeloma, lymphoma…) not previously radiated
2. total paralysis (Brice and McKissock group 4) > 8 hours duration, or inability to walk (B&M group > 1) for > 24 hrs duration (after this, there is essentially no chance of recovery and surgery is not indicated)
3. expected survival: ≤ 3–4 months
4. multiple lesions at multiple levels
5. patient unable to tolerate surgery: for patients with lung lesions, check PFTs

55

Group II—mild and stable signs and symptoms

Group II characteristics

Mild and stable signs/symptoms of cord compression (e.g., isolated Babinski), or either plexopathy or radiculopathy without evidence of cord compression. Admit and evaluate within 24 hrs.

Management

1. for suspected ESCC, manage as in Group I except on less emergent basis. Use low dose dexamethasone (DMZ) unless radiographic evaluation shows > 80% block or if suspicion of lymphoma is high and tissue will be obtained relatively soon

2. for radiculopathy alone (radicular pain, weakness, or reflex changes in one myotome or sensory changes in one dermatome): if plain X-rays show bony lesion then 70–88% will have ESCC on myelography. If the plain film is normal, only 9–25% will have ESCC. Obtain MRI or myelogram and manage as for suspected ESCC

3. for plexopathy (brachial or lumbosacral): pain is the most common early symptom, distribution not limited to single dermatome, commonly referred to elbow or ankle. May mask coexistent radiculopathy (denervation of paraspinal muscles occurs in radiculopathy) or presence of proximal signs and symptoms (Horner syndrome in cervical region, ureteral obstruction in lumbar region). Management:

    a) MRI is initial diagnostic procedure (CT if MRI unavailable): C4 through T4 for brachial plexopathy, L1 through pelvis for lumbosacral plexopathy

    b) if CT shows bony lesion or paraspinal mass (with negative CT, plain films and bone scan are rarely helpful; however, if done, and plain X-ray shows malignant appearing bony lesion, or if bone scan shows vertebral abnormality, perform MRI or myelogram within 24 hrs) (give dexamethasone if ESCC suspected or MRI/myelogram delayed). Management as in Group I based on degree of block, XRT ports extended laterally to include any mass shown on CT

    c) if no bony nor paraspinal lesion on MRI/CT, primary treatment of plexus tumor; analgesics for pain

Group III—pain without neurologic involvement

Group III characteristics

Back pain without neuro signs/symptoms. Can be evaluated as outpatient over several days (modify based on ability of patient to travel, reliability, etc.).

Treatment for SEM

Treatment goals and outcome

No treatment for SEM significantly prolongs life, with the possible exception of surgery for renal cell carcinoma with a solitary spine metastasis.[90] Treatment goals are palliative: pain control, preservation of spinal stability, and maintenance of sphincter control and ability to ambulate.

The most important factor affecting prognosis, regardless of treatment modality, is ability to walk at the time of initiation of therapy. Loss of sphincter control is a poor prognosticator and is usually irreversible.

The main decision is between surgery + post-op XRT, or XRT alone. As yet, no chemotherapy has been found to be useful for SEM (may help with primary). Surgery alone appears least effective for pain control (36%, compared to 67% for surgery + XRT, and 76% for XRT alone).[91] Surgery has the attendant complications of anesthetic risk, post-op pain, wound problems in 11% (further complicated by radiation),[91] and mortality in 5–6% after laminectomy and 10% after anterior approach with stabilization.[92] Therefore, surgery appears best reserved for situations described in ▶ Table 55.11.

Medical therapy

Chemotherapy is ineffective for SEM.

Bisphosphonates reduce the risk of vertebral compression fractures (VCF) by ≈ 50%, but the effect seems to abate after ≈ 2–3 years.

Promising agents undergoing trials include: denosumab (Prolia®), a RANK ligand (RANKL) inhibitor (p. 1212) that may counteract RANKL, which is overexpressed in response to lytic bony metastases.[94] The efficacy seems better than the bisphosphonates.

Vertebroplasty/kyphoplasty

Vertebroplasty/kyphoplasty (p. 1212) reduces pain associated with pathologic fractures in up to 84%[95] with an associated increase in functional outcome.[96] Kyphoplasty appears to offer comparable pain relief to vertebroplasty with lower rates of cement leakage.[96]

Relative contraindication: spinal cord compression. Unless the diagnosis has already been verified, a biopsy should be taken through one of the pedicles prior to injecting PMMA.

Radiation therapy

Radiosensitive tumors: ▶ Table 55.6 lists radiosensitivity of metastatic tumors (to brain or spine). Other radiosensitive tumors that metastasize to the spine include: myxoid liposarcoma.[97]

Treatment[98]: Dose: range = 25–40 Gy. Typical plan: 30 Gy delivered in 3 Gy fractions over 10 days (2 working weeks) to ports extending at least 1 vertebral level above and below the extent of the lesion. Timing: for initial treatment, try to start XRT within 24 hours of diagnosis; for post-op XRT, within about 14 days following surgery.

There is a theoretical risk of radiation induced edema causing or accelerating neurologic deterioration. This has not been borne out by experimental studies with the usual small daily fractions utilized. Deterioration is more likely to be due to tumor progression.[99] The spinal cord is usually the dose limiting structure in treating SEM.

Increased doses are being made possible with the application of the added precision of stereotactic radiosurgery techniques to spinal metastases.[100]

Surgical treatment

See ▶ Table 55.11 for indications for surgery.

The Spine Instability Neoplastic Score (SINS)[101] ▶ Table 55.12 was originally devised to help medical oncologists and radiation oncologists determine when surgical consultation should be sought, and to help spine surgeons assess the stability of various types of metastatic spine involvement. The decision to recommend surgery is not solely determined by stability, and must take into account prognosis, tumor type, systemic tumor burden, medical condition of the patient...

The SINS ranges from 0 to 18, and is interpreted as shown in ▶ Table 55.13

Pre-op embolization by interventional radiologist may facilitate resection with less blood loss for highly vascular tumors such as: renal-cell, thyroid, and hepatocellular. Blood supply is through the

Table 55.12 Spine Instability Neoplastic Score (SINS)[101] (see ▶ Table 55.13 for interpretation of total score)

Category	Finding	Points	Score
Mobility of involved spinal segment	junctional (occiput-C2, C7-T2, T11-L1, L5-S1)	3	(0 - 3)
	mobile spine (C3-6, L2-4)	2	
	semi-rigid spine (T3-10)	1	
	rigid spine (S2-5)	0	
Pain	pain relieved with recumbency and/or pain with movement/loading of the spine	3	(0 | 1 | 3)
	occasional, non-mechanical pain	1	
	no pain	0	
Bone lesion type	lytic	2	(0 - 2)
	mixed lytic/blastic	1	
	blastic	0	
Radiographic spinal alignment	subluxation or translation	4	(0 | 2 | 4)
	de novo deformity (kyphosis and/or scoliosis)[a]	2	
	normal	0	
Vertebral body involvement (anterior and middle column)	>50% collapse	3	(0 - 3)
	<50% collapse	2	
	no collapse with >50% VB inolved	1	
	none of the above	0	
Posterior column involvement[b]	bilateral	3	(0 | 1 | 3)
	unilateral	1	
	none	0	
SINS; range: 0 (stable) to 18 (unstable) → TOTAL			(0 - 18)

[a] requires prior imaging or comparison of upright with recumbent imaging

[b] posterior column = facets, pedicles or CV joint (see Three column model of the spine, ▶ Fig. 72.1). Involvement = fracture or replacement by tumor

55

Table 55.13 Stability based on SINS ▶ Table 55.12

SINS	Stability
0-6	stable
7-12	"indeterminate" or possibly "impending instability"
13-18	unstable

intercostal arteries, and care must be taken to avoid embolizing vessels providing significant blood supply to the spinal cord, especially the artery of Adamkiewicz (p. 87).

Approaches

Laminectomy alone is *poor* for spinal metastases when the pathology is *anterior* to the cord because of poor access to the tumor and the destabilizing effect of laminectomy when metastatic involvement of the vertebral body is significant.[102,103]

Deterioration in one of the 3 major criteria (pain, continence, ambulation) occurred in 26% of patients treated with *laminectomy* alone, 20% of laminectomy + XRT, and 17% of XRT alone (roughly comparable). There is a 9% incidence of spinal instability[91] following laminectomy *without* stabilization.

In a randomized controlled trial by Patchell et al,[104] approaches directed at the location of the tumor (e.g., costotransversectomy, transthoracic approach…) with stabilization where necessary, produced better results than simple laminectomy, and surgery + XRT was superior to XRT alone (see ▶ Table 55.14). This study found a modest increase in survival, but more significant maintenance or regaining of lost ambulation. However, operative mortality with anterior decompression and stabilization was ≈ double (10%) that of laminectomy with (5%) or without (6%) stabilization in a literature review.[92]

Table 55.14 Comparing surgery + XRT to XRT alone[104]

Result	XRT	Surgery + XRT
Ambulatory after treatment	57%	84%
Days ambulatory after treatment	13	122
Ambulatory after treatment when nonambulatory before treatment	19%	62%
Mean survival (days)	100	126

Solitary spinal metastases with indolent tumors (e.g., renal cell Ca) may be candidates for attempted cure with en bloc resection (total spondylectomy).[105,106]

Laminectomy is still appropriate with isolated involvement of the posterior elements. For anterior pathology, if the posterior elements are intact, a transthoracic approach with corpectomy and stabilization (e.g., with methylmethacrylate and Steinmann pins,[107] or with cage graft and lateral plate) followed by XRT improves neurologic function in ≈ 75% and pain in ≈ 85%. A posterolateral approach (e.g., costotransversectomy) may be used for anterolateral tumor.[108] Combining a corpectomy and removal of the pedicle and posterior elements destabilizes the spine; therefore, posterior instrumentation prior to performing the corpectomy is required, followed by cage graft.[109,110,111,112,113,114,115] To access a VB via a costotransversectomy, the rib of the like numbered VB and the one below need to be removed.

55.3 Hematopoietic tumors

55.3.1 Multiple myeloma

General information

Multiple myeloma (MM) (sometimes referred to simply as myeloma) is a neoplasm of a single clone of plasma cells characterized by proliferation of plasma cells in bone marrow, infiltration of adjacent tissues with mature and immature plasma cells, and the production of an immunoglobulin, usually monoclonal IgG or IgA (referred to collectively as M-protein[116]). Circulating pre-myeloma cells lodge in appropriate microenvironments (e.g., in bone marrow) where they differentiate and expand. Although MM is often referred to in the context of "metastatic lesions" to bone, it is also sometimes considered a primary bone tumor. If only a single lesion is identified, then it is referred to as a plasmacytoma (see below).

Epidemiology

In the U.S., incidence is ≈ 1–2 per 100,000 in Caucasians, and is ≈ twice that in black people. MM accounts for 1% of malignancies, and 10% of hematologic cancers. The peak age of occurrence is 60–70 yrs of age, with < 2% of patients being < 40 yrs old. Slightly more common in males. Monoclonal gammopathy without MM occurs in ≈ 0.15% of the population, and in long-term follow-up, 16% of these develop MM with an annual rate of 0.18%.[117]

Presentation

General information

MM presents as a result of the following (italicized items are characteristic for MM):
1. proliferation of plasma cells: interferes with normal immune system function → increased *susceptibility to infection*
2. bone involvement
   a) bone marrow involvement → destruction of hematopoietic capacity → normocytic normo-chromic *anemia*, leukopenia, thrombocytopenia
   b) bone resorption
      • → weakening of the bone → *pathologic fractures* (see below)
      • → *hypercalcemia* (present initially in 25% of MM patients, see below)
   c) swelling or local tenderness of bone
   d) *bone pain*: characteristically induced by movement, and absent at rest
   e) spinal involvement
      • invasion of spinal canal in ≈ 10% of cases → spinal cord compression → myelopathy
      • nerve root compression (radiculopathy)
3. overproduction of certain proteins by plasma cells. May lead to:
   a) hyperviscosity syndrome
   b) cryoglobulinemia
   c) amyloidosis
   d) *renal failure*: multifactorial, but monoclonal light chains play a role

Skeletal disease

MM involvement is by definition multiple, and is usually restricted to sites of red marrow: ribs, sternum, spine, clavicles, skull, or proximal extremities. Lesions of the spine and/or skull are the usual reasons for presentation to the neurosurgeon.

Bone resorption in MM is not due simply to mechanical erosion by plasma cells. Increased osteoclastic activity has been observed.

Plasma cell tumors of the skull involving the cranial vault usually do not produce neurologic symptoms. Cranial nerve palsies can arise from skull base involvement. Orbital involvement may produce proptosis (exophthalmos).

Neurologic involvement

Neurologic manifestations can occur as a result of:
1. tumor involvement of bone causing compression (see above)
   a) tumor in spine with compression of spinal cord or nerve roots
   b) tumor in skull with compression of brain or cranial nerves
2. deposition of amyloid within the flexor retinaculum of the wrist → carpal tunnel syndrome; the median nerve itself does not contain amyloid, and therefore responds well to surgical division of the transverse carpal ligament (p. 550)
3. diffuse progressive sensorimotor polyneuropathy: occurs in 3–5% of patients with MM
   a) about half are due to amyloidosis (p. 576)
   b) polyneuropathy can also occur without amyloidosis, especially in the rare osteosclerotic variant of MM
4. multifocal leukoencephalopathy has been described in MM[118]
5. hypercalcemia: may produce a dramatic encephalopathy with confusion, delirium, or coma. Neurologic symptoms of hypercalcemia associated with MM are more common than in hypercalcemia of other etiologies
6. very rare: intraparenchymal metastases[119]

55

Evaluation

The diagnostic criteria for MM is shown in ▶ Table 55.15. Tests that may be used in evaluating patients with MM or suspected MM include:

1. 24 hour urine for kappa Bence-Jones protein. A monoclonal immunoglobulin light chain (MW: 22–24 kDa) present in 75–80% of patients with MM (may also occur in other conditions). Typically kappa, occasionally lambda. Monoclonal proteins cannot be detected in the urine or serum of ≈ 1% of MM patients; two or more monoclonal bands are produced in ≈ 0.5–2.5% of patients with MM.[120]

2. bloodwork:
   a) SPEP with reflex IFE and FLC
      Explanation: serum protein electrophoresis (SPEP) looks for an M-spike (identifies monoclonal immunoglobulin gammopathies), if present (reflex) immunoelectrophoresis (IEP) AKA immunofixation (IFE) looks for IgG kappa band; free light chain (FLC) assay looks for K & λ light chains. These 3 assays together are highly sensitive for MM and related plasma cell disorders
   b) CBC: anemia eventually develops in most patients with MM as myeloma cells crowd out normal bone marrow cells. It is usually of moderate severity (Hgb ≈ 7–10 gm%) with a low reticulocyte count
   c) serum creatinine: for prognostication

3. skeletal radiologic survey. Characteristic X-ray finding: multiple, round, "punched-out" (sharply demarcated) lytic lesions in the bones typically involved (see above). Osteosclerotic lesions are seen in < 3% of patients with MM. Diffuse osteoporosis may also be seen

4. technetium-99 m nuclear bone scan is usually *negative* in untreated MM (due to rarity of spontaneous new bone formation) and is less sensitive than conventional radiographs. Therefore it is not usually helpful except perhaps to implicate etiologies other than MM to explain the observed findings. After treatment, bone scan may become positive as osteoblastic activity ensues ("flare" response)

5. bone marrow biopsy: virtually all MM patients have "myeloma cells" (mutated plasma cells). Although sensitive, this is not specific and other diagnostic criteria should be sought

Table 55.15 Criteria for diagnosis of MM[a]

1. Cytologic criteria
   a) marrow morphology: plasma cells and/or myeloma cells ≥ 10% of 1000 or more cells
   b) biopsy proven plasmacytoma

2. Clinical and laboratory criteria
   a) myeloma protein (M-component) in serum (usually > 3 gm/dl) or urine IEP
   b) osteolytic lesions on X-ray (generalized osteoporosis qualifies if marrow contains > 30% plasma or myeloma cells)
   c) myeloma cells in ≥ 2 peripheral blood smears

[a]diagnosis requires[121]: 1A & 1B, or 1A or 1B and 2A, 2B, or 2C

Treatment

Many aspects of treatment fall into the purvey of the oncologist (see review[117]). Some aspects pertinent to neurosurgical care include:

1. XRT (p. 917): MM is very radiosensitive. Focal XRT for pain due to readily identifiable bone lesions may allow pathologic fractures to heal and is effective in spinal cord compression due to tumor

2. mobilization: immobilization due to pain and fear of pathologic compression fractures leads to further detrimental increases in serum calcium and weakness

3. pain control: mild pain often responds well to salicylates (contraindicated in thrombocytopenia). Local XRT is also effective (see below)

4. percutaneous kyphoplasty (p. 1213) may be used for some spine lesions (preferred over vertebroplasty because of reduced potential of spreading neoplasm)

5. therapy for hypercalcemia: bisphosphonates usually improve symptoms related to this

6. bisphosphonates (p. 1364) inhibit bone resorption and rapidly reduces hypercalcemia. Pamidronate is currently preferred over older agents

7. bortezomib (Velcade®): the first proteasome inhibitor, indicated for treatment of refractory MM

Prognosis

Untreated MM has a 6-month median survival. Solitary plasmacytoma has a 50% 10-year survival. If there is an solitary site of involvement but M-protein is present (i.e., essentially a plasmacytoma except for the M-protein), elimination of the M-protein following XRT indicates a 50–60% chance of remaining free of MM; if the M-protein doesn't resolve, there is a high chance of developing MM.

55.3.2 Plasmacytoma

General information

A neoplasm of a single clone of plasma cells similar to multiple myeloma (see above) but meeting the following criteria:

1. there must be no other lesions on complete skeletal survey (*not* bone scan)
2. bone marrow aspirate must show no evidence of myeloma
3. and serum and urine electrophoresis should show no M-protein

MM will develop in 55–60% of patients with a solitary plasmacytoma in 5 years, and in 70–80% by 10 yrs.

Treatment

1. local XRT provides good local control rates
2. percutaneous kyphoplasty (p. 1213): preferred over vertebroplasty because of reduced potential of spreading neoplastic cells
3. surgery for instability

References

[1] Johnson JD, Young B. Demographics of brain metastasis. Neurosurg Clin N Am. 1996; 7:337–344

[2] Mintz AP, Cairncross JG. Treatment of a Single Brain Metastasis. The Role of Radiation Following Surgical Excision. Journal of the American Medical Association. 1998; 280:1527–1529

[3] Voorhies RM, Sundaresan N, Thaler HT. The Single Supratentorial Lesion: An Evaluation of Preoperative Diagnosis. J Neurosurg. 1980; 53:364–368

[4] Patchell RA, Posner JB. Neurologic Complications of Systemic Cancer. Neurol Clin. 1985; 3:729–750

[5] Zimm S, Galen L, Wampler GL, et al. Intracerebral Metastases in Solid-Tumor Patients: Natural History and Results of Treatment. Cancer. 1981; 48:384–394

[6] DeAngelis LM. Management of Brain Metastases. Cancer Invest. 1994; 12:156–165

[7] Davis PC, Hudgins PA, Peterman SB, et al. Diagnosis of Cerebral Metastases: Double-Dose Delayed CT versus Contrast-Enhanced MR Imaging. American Journal of Neuroradiology. 1991; 12:293–300

[8] Weiss HD, Richardson EP. Solitary Brainstem Metastasis. Neurology. 1978; 28:562–566

[9] Nugent JL, Bunn PA, Matthews MJ, et al. CNS Metastases in Small-Cell Bronchogenic Carcinoma: Increasing Frequency and Changing Pattern with Lengthening Survival. Cancer. 1979; 44:1885–1893

[10] Berger MS, Baumeister B, Geyer JR, et al. The Risks of Metastases from Shunting in Children with Primary Central Nervous System Tumors. J Neurosurg. 1991; 74:872–877

[11] Kindt GW. The Pattern of Location of Cerebral Metastatic Tumors. J Neurosurg. 1964; 21:54–57

[12] Gavrilovic IT, Posner JB. Brain metastases: epidemiology and pathophysiology. J Neurooncol. 2005; 75:5–14

[13] Vieth RG, Odom GL. Intracranial Metastases and their Neurosurgical Treatment. J Neurosurg. 1965; 23:375–383

[14] Agazzi S, Pampallona S, Pica A, et al. The origin of brain metastases in patients with an undiagnosed primary tumour. Acta Neurochir (Wien). 2004; 146:153–157

[15] Figlin RA, Piantadosi S, Feld R, et al. Intracranial Recurrence of Carcinoma After Complete Resection of Stage I, II, and III Non-Small-Cell Lung Cancer. N Engl J Med. 1988; 318:1300–1305

[16] Barbone F, Bovenzi M, Cavallieri F, et al. Cigarette smoking and histologic type of lung cancer in men. Chest. 1997; 112:1474–1479

[17] Auperin A, Arriagada R, Pignon JP, et al. Prophylactic cranial irradiation for patients with small-cell lung cancer in complete remission. Prophylactic Cranial Irradiation Overview Collaborative Group. N Engl J Med. 1999; 341:476–484

[18] Slotman B, Faivre-Finn C, Kramer G, et al. Prophylactic cranial irradiation in extensive small-cell lung cancer. N Engl J Med. 2007; 357:664–672

[19] Solis OJ, Davis KR, Adair LB, et al. Intracerebral Metastatic Melanoma: CT Evaluation. Comput Tomogr. 1977; 1:135–143

[20] Zakrzewski J, Geraghty LN, Rose AE, et al. Clinical variables and primary tumor characteristics predictive of the development of melanoma brain metastases and post-brain metastases survival. Cancer. 2011; 117:1711–1720

[21] Davies MA, Liu P, McIntyre S, et al. Prognostic factors for survival in melanoma patients with brain metastases. Cancer. 2011; 117:1687–1696

[22] Staudt M, Lasithiotakis K, Leiter U, et al. Determinants of survival in patients with brain metastases from cutaneous melanoma. Br J Cancer. 2010; 102:1213–1218

[23] Sampson JH, Carter JH, Friedman AH, et al. Demographics, Prognosis, and Therapy in 702 Patients with Brain Metastases from Malignant Melanoma. Journal of Neurosurgery. 1998; 88:11–20

[24] Swetter SM, Carroll LA, Johnson DL, et al. Positron emission tomography is superior to computed

55

tomography for metastatic detection in melanoma patients. Ann Surg Oncol. 2002; 9:646–653

[25] Carlino MS, Fogarty GB, Long GV. Treatment of Melanoma Brain Metastases: A New Paradigm. The Cancer Journal. 2012; 18:208–212

[26] Bindal RK, Sawaya R, Leavens ME, et al. Surgical treatment of multiple brain metastases. Journal of Neurosurgery. 1993; 79:210–216

[27] Avril MF, Aamdal S, Grob JJ, et al. Fotemustine compared with dacarbazine in patients with disseminated malignant melanoma: a phase III study. J Clin Oncol. 2004; 22:1118–1125

[28] Guirguis LM, Yang JC, White DE, et al. Safety and efficacy of high-dose interleukin-2 therapy in patients with brain metastases. J Immunother. 2002; 25:82–87

[29] Lochead R, McKhann G, Hankinson T, et al. High dose systemic interleukin-2 for metastatic melanoma in patients with treated brain metastases. Journal of Immunotherapy. 2004; 27

[30] Majer M, Jensen RL, Shrieve DC, et al. Biochemotherapy of metastatic melanoma in patients with or without recently diagnosed brain metastases. Cancer. 2007; 110:1329–1337

[31] ClinicalTrials.gov identifier: NCT 01266967. A Study of GSK 2118436 in BRAF Mutant Metastatic Melanoma to the Brain (Break MB). 2014. https://clinicaltrials.gov/ct2/show/results/NCT01266967

[32] ClinicalTrials.gov identifier: NCT 01378975. A Study of Vemurafenib in Metastatic Melanoma Patients With Brain Metastases. 2015. https://clinicaltrials.gov/ct2/show/NCT01378975?term=NCT01378975&rank=1&view=results

[33] U.S. Food and Drug Administration (FDA), . FDA approves Keytruda for advanced melanoma. 2014. https://wayback.archive-it.org/7993/20170112023823/http://www.fda.gov/NewsEvents/Newsroom/PressAnnouncements/ucm412802.htm

[34] Patchell RA, Tibbs PA, Walsh JW, et al. A Randomized Trial of Surgery in the Treatment of Single Metastases to the Brain. New England Journal of Medicine. 1990; 322:494–500

[35] Vecht CJ, Haaxma-Reiche H, Noordijk EM, et al. Treatment of single brain metastasis: radiotherapy alone or combined with neurosurgery? Ann Neurol. 1993; 33:583–590

[36] Sampson JH, Carter JH,Jr, Friedman AH, et al. Demographics, prognosis, and therapy in 702 patients with brain metastases from malignant melanoma. J Neurosurg. 1998; 88:11–20

[37] Fife KM, Colman MH, Stevens GN, et al. Determinants of outcome in melanoma patients with cerebral metastases. J Clin Oncol. 2004; 22:1293–1300

[38] Eigentler TK, Figl A, Krex D, et al. Number of metastases, serum lactate dehydrogenase level, and type of treatment are prognostic factors in patients with brain metastases of malignant melanoma. Cancer. 2011; 117:1697–1703

[39] Gupta G, Robertson AG, MacKie RM. Cerebral metastases of cutaneous melanoma. Br J Cancer. 1997; 76:256–259

[40] Song Z, Lin B, Shao L, et al. Brain metastases from esophageal cancer: clinical review of 26 cases. World Neurosurg. 2014; 81:131–135

[41] Kondziolka D, Bernstein M, Resch L, et al. Significance of Hemorrhage into Brain Tumors: Clinicopathological Study. J Neurosurg. 1987; 67:852–857

[42] Shildt RA, Kennedy PS, Chen TT, et al. Management of patients with metastatic adenocarcinoma of unknown origin: a Southwest Oncology Group study. Cancer Treatment Reports. 1983; 67:77–79

[43] Gaspar L, Scott C, Rotman M, et al. Recursive partitioning analysis (RPA) of prognostic factors in three Radiation Therapy Oncology Group (RTOG) brain metastases trials. Int J Radiat Oncol Biol Phys. 1997; 37:745–751

[44] Morris SL, Low SH, A'Hern RP, et al. A prognostic index that predicts outcome following palliative whole brain radiotherapy for patients with metastatic malignant melanoma. Br J Cancer. 2004; 91:829–833

[45] Nieder C, Andratschke N, Grosu AL, et al. Recursive partitioning analysis (RPA) class does not predict survival in patients with four or more brain metastases. Strahlenther Onkol. 2003; 179:16–20

[46] Pollock BE. Management of Patients with Multiple Brain Metastases. Contemporary Neurosurgery. 1999; 21:1–6

[47] Nahed BV, Alvarez-Breckenridge C, Brastianos PK, et al. Congress of Neurological Surgeons Systematic Review and Evidence-Based Guidelines on the Role of Surgery in the Management of Adults With Metastatic Brain Tumors. Neurosurgery. 2019; 84: E152–E155

[48] Ammirati M, Nahed BV, Andrews D, et al. Congress of Neurological Surgeons Systematic Review and Evidence-Based Guidelines on Treatment Options for Adults With Multiple Metastatic Brain Tumors. Neurosurgery. 2019; 84:E180–E182

[49] Forsyth PA, Weaver S, Fulton D, et al. Prophylactic anticonvulsants in patients with brain tumour. Can J Neurol Sci. 2003; 30:106–112

[50] Chen CC, Rennert RC, Olson JJ. Congress of Neurological Surgeons Systematic Review and Evidence-Based Guidelines on the Role of Prophylactic Anticonvulsants in the Treatment of Adults with Metastatic Brain Tumors. Neurosurgery. 2019; 84: E195–E197

[51] Ryken TC, Kuo JS, Prabhu RS, et al. Congress of Neurological Surgeons Systematic Review and Evidence-Based Guidelines on the Role of Steroids in the Treatment of Adults With Metastatic Brain Tumors. Neurosurgery. 2019; 84:E189–E191

[52] Vecht CJ, Hovestadt A, Verbiest HB, et al. Dose-effect relationship of dexamethasone on Karnofsky performance in metastatic brain tumors: a randomized study of doses of 4, 8, and 16 mg per day. Neurology. 1994; 44:675–680

[53] Horton J. Treatment of Metastases to the Brain. 1984

[54] Jackson DV, Richards F, Cooper MR, et al. Prophylactic Cranial Irradiation in Small Cell Carcinoma of the Lung: A Randomized Study. JAMA. 1977; 237:2730–2733

[55] Patchell RA, Tibbs PA, Regine WF, et al. Postoperative radiotherapy in the treatment of single metastases to the brain: a randomized trial. Journal of the American Medical Association. 1998; 280:1485–1489

[56] Kramer S, Hendrickson F, Zelen M, et al. Therapeutic Trials in the Management of Metastatic Brain Tumors by Different Time/Dose Fraction Schemes. Natl Cancer Inst Monogr. 1977; 46:213–221

[57] DeAngelis LM, Mandell LR, Thaler HT, et al. The Role of Postoperative Radiotherapy After Resection of Single Brain Metastases. Neurosurgery. 1989; 24:798–804

[58] Smalley SR, Schray MF, Laws ER, et al. Adjuvant Radiation Therapy After Surgical Resection of Solitary Brain Metastasis: Association with Pattern of Failure and Survival. International Journal of Radiation Oncology and Biological Physics. 1987; 13:1611–1616

[59] Shaw E. Comment on DeAngelis L M, et al.: The Role of Postoperative Radiotherapy After Resection of Single Brain Metastases. Neurosurgery. 1989; 24:804–805

[60] Sills AK. Current treatment approaches to surgery for brain metastases. Neurosurgery. 2005; 57:S24–32; discusssion S1-4

[61] Bindal AK, Bindal RK, Hess KR, et al. Surgery versus Radiosurgery in the Treatment of Brain Metastasis. Journal of Neurosurgery. 1996; 84:748–754

[62] Smalley SR, Laws ER, O'Fallon JR, et al. Resection for Solitary Brain Metastasis: Role of Adjuvant Radiation and Prognostic Variables in 229 Patients. Journal of Neurosurgery. 1992; 77:531–540

[63] Tobler WD, Sawaya R, Tew JM. Successful Laser-assisted Excision of a Metastatic Midbrain Tumor. Neurosurgery. 1986; 18:795–797

[64] Markesbery WR, Brooks WH, Gupta GD, et al. Treatment for Patients with Cerebral Metastases. Archives of Neurology. 1978; 35:754–756

55

[65] Ruderman NB, Hall TC. Use of Glucocorticoids in the Palliative Treatment of Metastatic Brain Tumors. Cancer. 1965; 18:298–306

[66] Posner JB. Surgery for Metastases to the Brain. N Engl J Med. 1990; 322:544–545

[67] Galicich JH, Sundaresan N, Thaler HT. Surgical Treatment of Single Brain Metastasis: Evaluation of Results by CT Scanning. Journal of Neurosurgery. 1980; 53:63–67

[68] Alexander E, Moriarty TM, Davis RB, et al. Stereotactic Radiosurgery for the Definitive Noninvasive Treatment of Brain Metastases. Journal of the National Cancer Institute. 1995; 87:34–40

[69] Fuller BG, Kaplan ID, Adler J, et al. Stereotactic Radiosurgery for Brain Metastases: The Importance of Adjuvant Whole Brain Irradiation. International Journal of Radiation Oncology and Biological Physics. 1992; 23:413–418

[70] Wilkins RH, Rengachary SS. Neurosurgery. New York 1985

[71] Sze G, Soletsky S, Bronen R, et al. MR Imaging of the Cranial Meninges with Emphasis on Contrast Enhancement and Meningeal Carcinomatosis. AJNR. 1989; 10:965–975

[72] Godersky JC, Smoker WRK, Knutzon R. Use of MRI in the Evaluation of Metastatic Spinal Disease. Neurosurgery. 1987; 21:676–680

[73] Livingston KE, Perrin RG. The neurosurgical management of spinal metastases causing cord and cauda equina compression. Journal of Neurosurgery. 1978; 49:839–843

[74] Batson OV. The Function of the Vertebral Veins and Their Role in the Spread of Metastases. Ann Surg. 1940; 112

[75] Schwab JH, Boland P, Guo T, et al. Skeletal metastases in myxoid liposarcoma: an unusual pattern of distant spread. Ann Surg Oncol. 2007; 14:1507–1514

[76] Rodichok LD, Ruckdeschel JC, Harper GR, et al. Early Detection and Treatment of Spinal Epidural Metastases: The Role of Myelography. Ann Neurol. 1986; 20:696–702

[77] Bach F, Larsen BH, Rhode K, et al. Metastatic spinal cord compression. Occurrence, symptoms, clinical presentations and prognosis in 398 patients with spinal cord compression. Acta Neurochirurgica (Wien). 1990; 107:37–43

[78] Helwig-Larsen S, Sorensen PS. Symptoms and signs in metastatic spinal cord compression: a study from first symptom until diagnosis in 153 patients. European Journal of Cancer. 1994; 30A:396–398

[79] Levack P, Graham J, Collie D, et al. Don't wait for a sensory level: listen to the symptoms: a prospective audit of the delays in diagnosis of malignant cord compression. Clinical Oncology (Royal College of Radiologists). 2002; 14:472–480

[80] Sherk HH. Lesions of the Atlas and Axis. Clinical Orthopedics. 1975; 109:33–41

[81] Nakamura M, Toyama Y, Suzuki N, et al. Metastases to the upper cervical spine. Journal of Spinal Disorders. 1996; 9:195–201

[82] Portenoy RK, Lipton RB, Foley KM. Back Pain in the Cancer Patient: An Algorithm for Evaluation and Management. Neurology. 1987; 37:134–138

[83] Brice J, McKissock W. Surgical Treatment of Malignant Extradural Spinal Tumors. Br Med J. 1965; 1:1341–1344

[84] Li KC, Poon PY. Sensitivity and specificity of MRI in detecting spinal cord compression and in distinguishing malignant from benign compression fractures of vertebrae. Magnetic Resonance Imaging. 1988; 6:547–556

[85] Gabriel K, Schi D. Metastatic spinal cord compression by solid tumors. Seminars in Neurology. 2004; 24:375–383

[86] Francken AB, Hong AM, Fulham MJ, et al. Detection of unsuspected spinal cord compression in melanoma patients by 18F-fluorodeoxyglucose-positron emission tomography. European Journal of Surgical Oncology. 2005; 31:197–204

[87] Vecht CJ, Haaxma-Reiche H, van Putten WL, et al. Initial bolus of conventional versus high-dose dexamethasone in metastatic spinal cord compression. Neurology. 1989; 39:1255–1257

[88] Hollis PH, Malis LI, Zappulla RA. Neurological Deterioration After Lumbar Puncture Below Complete Spinal Subarachnoid Block. J Neurosurg. 1986; 64:253–256

[89] Lee Y-Y, Glass JP, Wallace S. Myelography in Cancer Patients: Modified Technique. AJR. 1985; 145:791–795

[90] Jung ST, Ghert MA, Harrelson JM, et al. Treatment of osseous metastases in patients with renal cell carcinoma. Clin Orthop Relat Res. 2003:223–231

[91] Findlay GFG. Adverse Effects of the Management of Malignant Spinal Cord Compression. J Neurol Neurosurg Psychiatry. 1984; 47:761–768

[92] Witham TF, Khavkin YA, Gallia GL, et al. Surgery insight: current management of epidural spinal cord compression from metastatic spine disease. National Clinics of Practical Neurology. 2006; 2:87–94

[93] Danner RL, Hartman BJ. Update of Spinal Epidural Abscess: 35 Cases and Review of the Literature. Rev Infect Dis. 1987; 9:265–274

[94] Mundy GR. Metastasis to bone: causes, consequences and therapeutic opportunities. Nat Rev Cancer. 2002; 2:584–593

[95] Fourney DR, Schomer DF, Nader R, et al. Percutaneous vertebroplasty and kyphoplasty for painful vertebral body fractures in cancer patients. Journal of Neurosurgery. 2003; 98:21–30

[96] Bouza C, Lopez-Cuadrado T, Cediel P, et al. Balloon kyphoplasty in malignant spinal fractures: a systematic review and meta-analysis. BMC Palliat Care. 2009; 8. DOI: 10.1186/1472-684X-8-12

[97] Reitan JB, Kaalhus O. Radiotherapy of liposarcomas. Br J Radiol. 1980; 53:969–975

[98] Faul CM, Flickinger JC. The use of radiation in the management of spinal metastases. Journal of Neuro-Oncology. 1995; 23:149–161

[99] Rubin P. Extradural Spinal Cord Compression by Tumor: Part I. Experimental Production and Treatment Trials. Radiology. 1969; 93:1243–1248

[100] Rock JP, Ryu S, Yin FF, et al. The evolving role of stereotactic radiosurgery and stereotactic radiation therapy for patients with spine tumors. J Neurooncol. 2004; 69:319–334

[101] Fisher CG, DiPaola CP, Ryken TC, et al. A novel classification system for spinal instability in neoplastic disease: an evidence-based approach and expert consensus from the Spine Oncology Study Group. Spine (Phila Pa 1976). 2010; 35:E1221–E1229

[102] Onimus M, Schraub S, Bertin D, et al. Surgical Treatment of Vertebral Metastasis. Spine. 1986; 11:883–891

[103] Cooper PR, Errico TJ, Martin R, et al. A Systematic Approach to Spinal Reconstruction After Anterior Decompression for Neoplastic Disease of the Thoracic and Lumbar Spine. Neurosurgery. 1993; 32:1–8

[104] Patchell RA, Tibbs PA, Regine WF, et al. Direct decompressive surgical resection in the treatment of spinal cord compression caused by metastatic cancer: a randomized trial. Lancet. 2005; 366:643–648

[105] Fourney DR, Abi-Said D, Rhines LD, et al. Simultaneous anterior-posterior approach to the thoracic and lumbar spine for the radical resection of tumors followed by reconstruction and stabilization. Journal of Neurosurgery. 2001; 94:232–244

[106] Sakaura H, Hosono N, Mukai Y, et al. Outcome of total en bloc spondylectomy for solitary metastasis of the thoracolumbar spine. Journal of Spinal Disorders. 2004; 17:297–300

[107] Sundaresan N, Galicich JH, Lane JM, et al. Treatment of Neoplastic Epidural Cord Compression by Vertebral Body Resection and Stabilization. Journal of Neurosurgery. 1985; 63:676–684

[108] Overby MC, Rothman AS. Anterolateral Decompression for Metastatic Epidural Spinal Cord Tumors: Results of a Modified Costotransvectomy Approach. Journal of Neurosurgery. 1985; 62:344–348

55

[109] Shaw B, Mansfield FL, Borges L. One-Stage Postero-lateral Decompression and Stabilization for Primary and Metastatic Vertebral Tumors in the Thoracic and Lumbar Spine. Journal of Neurosurgery. 1989; 70:405–410

[110] Akeyson EW, McCutcheon IE. Single-stage posterior vertebrectomy and replacement combined with posterior instrumentation for spinal metastasis. Journal of Neurosurgery. 1996; 85:211–220

[111] Fourney DR, Abi-Said D, Lang FF, et al. Use of pedicle screw fixation in the management of malignant spinal disease: experience in 100 consecutive cases. Journal of Neurosurgery. 2001; 94:25–37

[112] Wang JC, Boland P, Mitra N, et al. Single-stage posterolateral transpedicular approach for resection of epidural metastatic spine tumors involving the vertebral body with circumferential reconstruction: results in 140 patients. Journal of Neurosurgery (Spine). 2004; 1:287–298

[113] Hunt T, Shen FH, Arlet V. Expandable cage placement via a posterolateral approach in lumbar spine reconstructions: technical note. Journal of Neurosurgery (Spine). 2006; 5:271–274

[114] Snell BE, Nasr FF, Wolfla CE. Single-stage thoracolumbar vertebrectomy with circumferential reconstruction and arthrodesis: surgical technique and results in 15 patients. Neurosurgery (Operative Neurosurgery). 2006; 58:263–269

[115] Sciubba DM, Gallia GL, McGirt MJ, et al. Thoracic kyphotic deformity reduction with a distractible titanium cage via an entirely posterior approach. Neurosurgery. 2007; 60:223–231

[116] Keren DF, Alexanian R, Goeken JA, et al. Guidelines for Clinical and Laboratory Evaluation of Patients with Monoclonal Gammopathies. Arch Pathol Lab Med. 1999; 123:106–107

[117] Bataille R, Harousseau J-L. Multiple Myeloma. New England Journal of Medicine. 1997; 336:1657–1664

[118] McCarthy J, Proctor SJ. Cerebral Involvement in Multiple Myeloma. Case Report. J Clin Pathol. 1978; 31:259–264

[119] Norum J, Wist E, Dahil IM. Cerebral Metastases from Multiple Myeloma. Acta Oncol. 1991; 30:868–869

[120] Foerster J, Lee GR, Bithell TC, et al. Multiple Myeloma. In: Wintrobe's Clinical Hematology. 9th ed. Philadelphia: Lea and Febiger; 1993:2219–2249

[121] Costa G, Engle RL, Schilling A, et al. Melphalan and Prednisone: An Effective Combination for the Treatment of Multiple Myeloma. American Journal of Medicine. 1973; 54:589–599

56 Other Tumors, Cysts, and Tumor-Like Lesions

56.1 Other tumors

56.1.1 Olfactory neuroblastoma (ONB)

General information

Formerly called esthesioneuroblastoma, originally described in 1924, AKA olfactory esthesioneuroblastoma, AKA esthesioneurocytoma, AKA olfactory placode tumor.[1] A rare nasal neoplasm with an incidence 0.4 per 1,000,000 people.[2] Believed to arise from the olfactory neural crest cells in the upper nares, it is considered to be malignant. These tumors occur over a wide age range (3 to 90 years), with a bimodal peak between the second and third decade and a second peak in the sixth and seventh decades.

Imaging

MRI: isointense with brain on T1-weighted imaging and intermediate to high signal intensity on T2-weighted imaging and enhance heterogeneously with gadolinium. Signal characteristics may mimic meningioma. For higher stage lesions, the cribriform plate may be eroded; better seen on thin cut CT. The most important factor determining resectability is intracranial extension. Magnetic resonance aids in the distinction between extradural tumor, dural invasion, or parenchymal brain invasion. None of these are specific to this tumor.

Differential diagnosis

Includes SNUC, nasal melanoma, nasal squamous cell carcinoma, and meningioma.

Diagnosis

Endoscopic biopsy is typically performed in the otolaryngology office prior to surgery.

A clinical oncology exam should be performed, and if there is suspicion for metastatic disease a PET scan, which is sensitive for metastatic disease, should be ordered.

Clinical classification systems

The modified Kadish system[3] (which added category D to the original Kadish system[4]) is shown in ▶ Table 56.1. This classification appears to correlate with survival.[3] Alternative systems by Biller et al[5] and Dulguerov and Calcaterra[6] (see ▶ Table 56.1) attempt to subdivide the Kadish C classification; however, the more popular modified Kadish system is more frequently used.

Table 56.1 Clinical classification systems for olfactory neuroblastoma

Modified Kadish[3]	Biller et al[5]	Dulguerov and Calcaterra[6]
A: Confined to Nasal Cavity	T1: Nasal/Paranasal Sinuses	T1: Nasal/Paranasal Sinuses
B: Extends to Paranasal Sinus	T2: Periorbital/Anterior Fossa Extension	T2: Erosion of Cribriform Plate
C: Local Extension (orbit or cribriform plate)	T3: Brain Involvement, Resectable Margins	T3: Periorbital/Anterior Fossa Extension
D: Distant Metastasis	T4: Unable to Obtain Negative Margins —Unresectable	T4: Brain Involvement

56

Pathologic grading

Hyams grading, a system used to define all upper respiratory tract carcinomas, is utilized to assess nuclear pleomorphism, mitotic activity, rosette presence, and necrosis, and summates these to produce Hyams 1–4 classification.[7] It has been shown in meta-analysis, as well as in large series, that Hyams grade 1 and 2 predict benign disease course, as compared to Hyams 3 and 4, which predict poor disease course. It is recommended that grading be performed in all cases.[8,9]

Treatment

Primary treatment is controversial. Some institutions believe in upfront combined radiation therapy and chemotherapy prior to craniofacial resection. However, most practice initial surgery, which classically consisted of endoscopic resection with negative margins for Kadish A and B lesions, and craniofacial resection (bifrontal craniotomy with associated lateral rhinotomy) for Kadish C and D lesions. However, with the advent of endoscopic techniques, the lateral rhinotomy is often replaced with a purely endoscopic approach, unless there is inferior lateral orbital or maxillary involvement, in which case the lateral rhinotomy is frequently used. Finally, some institutions are now managing Kadish stages purely endoscopically, unless they are unable to get negative margins at the time of surgery, in which case conversion to an open approach is performed or SRS is performed; however, this is controversial.

Outcome

Median overall survival is typically 7.2 ± 0.7 years.[8]

Mean progression free survival is 4.8 ± 0.7 years. The 5 and 10 year survivals are 63% and 40%.[8]

Population-based analysis of the Surveillance Epidemiology and End Results (SEER) database confirms that Kadish staging, lymph node involvement, and age at diagnosis have significant prognostic value.[10] These findings have been confirmed in a large meta-analysis recently published by Kane et al in 2010.[9] Furthermore, higher Hyams grading (grades 3 and 4) correlate with a poorer prognosis.[8,9]

Salvage treatment: For patients with recurrent disease, this typically occurs in 2 patterns: that of intracranial recurrence or those with distant metastasis.[11,12] Intracranial recurrence is typically treated with repeat transcranial resection; however, stereotactic radiosurgery is a viable option.[11,12,13] In patients with distant metastasis, those with cervical lymph node metastasis should undergo modified radical neck dissection to understand the extent of the disease. This typically leads to chemotherapy, of which platinum based therapies remain the standard of therapy at this time.[11,14,15]

56.1.2 Epidermoid and dermoid tumors

General information

AKA epidermoid or dermoid cysts.

Both are usually developmental, benign tumors that may arise when retained ectodermal implants are trapped by two fusing ectodermal surfaces. The growth rate of these tumors is linear, like skin (rather than exponential, as with neoplastic tumors).

They may occur in the following locations:
1. calvaria: skull involvement (p.973) occurs when ectodermal rests are included in the developing cranium, epidural extension may occur with growth
2. intracranial: the most common sites include
   a) suprasellar: commonly produce bitemporal hemianopsia and optic atrophy, and only occasionally pituitary (endocrine) symptoms (including DI)
   b) Sylvian fissure: may present with seizures
   c) cerebellopontine angle (CPA): may produce trigeminal neuralgia, especially in young patient
   d) basilar-posterior fossa: may produce lower cranial nerve findings, cerebellar dysfunction, and/or corticospinal tract abnormalities
   e) within the ventricular system: occur within the 4th ventricle more commonly than any other
3. scalp
4. within the spinal canal:
   a) most arise in the thoracic or upper lumbar spine
   b) epidermoids of the lower lumbar spine may occur iatrogenically following LP; see Lumbar puncture (p.1811)
   c) dermoids of the spinal canal are usually associated with a dermal sinus tract (p.286) and may produce recurrent bouts of spinal meningitis.

Comparison of dermoids and epidermoids

Distinguishing features between the two tumors are shown in ▶ Table 56.2.

Table 56.2 Comparison of epidermoids and dermoid

Feature	Epidermoid	Dermoid
frequency	0.5–1.5% of brain tumors	0.3% of brain tumors
lining	stratified squamous epithelium	also include dermal appendage organs (hair follicles and sebaceous glands)
contents	keratin, cellular debris, cholesterol, occasional hair	same as epidermoids, plus hair and sebum
location	more common laterally (e.g., CP angle)	more commonly near midline
associated anomalies	tend to be isolated lesions	associated with other congenital anomalies in up to 50% of cases
meningitis	may have recurrent episodes of chemical meningitis (p. 342)	may have repeated bouts of bacterial meningitis

Epidermoid cysts

General information

Key concepts

- usually arise from ectoderm trapped within or displaced into the CNS
- predilection for: CP angle, 4th ventricle, suprasellar region, spinal cord
- sometimes AKA cholesteatoma (not to be confused with cholesterol granuloma)
- grow at linear rate (unlike exponential rate of true neoplasms)
- imaging: CSF-like mass (hi-signal on DWI MRI is the best test to differentiate)
- may produce chemical meningitis
- treatment: surgical excision. XRT has no role

AKA cholesteatoma (not cholesterol granuloma [see below]), AKA pearly tumor, AKA ectodermal inclusion cyst (see ▶ Table 56.2 for comparison to dermoids). Although epidermoids and cholesteatomas are histologically identical (both arise from epithelium entrapped in an abnormal location, epidermoids are intradural, cholesteatomas are extradural), the term cholesteatoma is most often used to describe the lesion in the middle ear where the entrapped epithelium usually arises from chronic middle ear infections which lead to a retraction pocket (rarely, may instead be congenital).

▶ **May arise from any of the following[16]:**
1. displaced dorsal midline ectodermal cell rests trapped during neural tube closure between gestational weeks 3–5
2. multipotential embryonic cell rests
3. epithelial cell rests carried to the CPA with the developing otic vesicle
4. epidermal cells displaced into CNS, e.g., by LP—see Lumbar puncture (p. 1811)—or repeated percutaneous cranial subdural taps[17]

Epidemiology
Epidermoids comprise 1% of intracranial tumors,[18] and ≈ 7% of CPA tumors. Peak age of occurrence: 40 years. No gender difference.

Histology
Epidermoids are lined by stratified squamous epithelium, and contain keratin (from desquamated epithelium),[19] cellular debris, and cholesterol. Growth occurs at a linear rate like normal skin, unlike the exponential growth of true neoplasms.[20] The cyst contents may be liquid or may have a flaky consistency. They tend to spread along normal cleavage planes and surround vital structures (cranial nerves, ICA…). Bony destruction occurs in a minority, usually with larger tumors. Rare degeneration to squamous cell cancer[21] primarily in cases of repeated recurrences after multiple surgeries.

Distinction from cholesterol granuloma
Epidermoid cysts are sometimes mistakenly equated with cholesterol granulomas,[22] possibly because of the similarity between the terms cholesteatoma and cholesterol granuloma. However,

56

these are distinct lesions.[23] Cholesterol granulomas usually occur following chronic inflammation (usually in pneumatized portions of the temporal bone: petrous apex, mastoid air cells, middle ear space). Some differences are delineated in ▶ Table 56.3.

Table 56.3 Characteristics of epidermoid & cholesteatoma vs. cholesterol granuloma

Feature	Epidermoid	Cholesteatoma	Cholesterol granuloma
origin	ectodermal cells in abnormal location		chronic inflammatory cells surrounding cholesterol crystals (? from breakdown of RBC membranes)
	(within CNS, intra-dural)	(within ear, extradural)	
precursor	usually congenital, occasionally acquired, e.g., after LP (p. 1815)	usually acquired (following chronic infection ? due to epithelial cells from tympanic membrane), occasionally congenital	chronic middle ear infection or idiopathic hemotympanum
symptoms	vary depending on location	chronic hearing loss, ear drainage, pain, or numbness around ear	usually involve vestibular or cochlear dysfunction
imaging (may not reliably distinguish among these)	CT: low density; no enhancement; bone erosion in only 33% MRI: T1WI: intensity slightly > CSF; T2WI: tumor & CSF similar high intensity		CT: homogeneous & isodense; rim enhancement; extensive destruction of petrous bone MRI: increased signal on both T1WI and T2WI
gross appearance	pearly white		brown (from hemosiderin)
microscopic pathology[24]	hyperkeratotic cyst lined with stratified squamous epithelium		fibroblastic proliferation, hemosiderin-laden macrophages, cholesterol clefts, giant cell reaction
ideal treatment	aggressive near-total excision		subtotal resection followed by drainage & restoration of pneumatization[25]

Presentation

1. may present as any mass lesion in the same location
2. CPA lesions can produce V, VII, or VIII neuropathies
3. symptoms of hydrocephalus: hydrocephalus may be obstructive or communicating due to chemical meningitis
4. recurrent episodes of chemical meningitis caused by rupture of the cyst contents, which may lead to hydrocephalus
   a) symptoms include fever and meningeal irritation
   b) CSF shows pleocytosis, hypoglycorrhachia, elevated protein, and negative cultures. Cholesterol crystals may be seen and can be recognized by their amorphous birefringent appearance

Imaging

MRI (▶ Fig. 56.1): epidermoids mimic CSF on T1WI (low signal, may be slightly > CSF) and T2WI (high signal). Other tumors are also high signal on T2WI, but most enhance with contrast on T1WI (epidermoids do not enhance). An epidermoid may pass from the posterior fossa through the incisura to the middle fossa.

Diffusion weighted imaging (DWI) is the best test to differentiate epidermoids from CSF (e.g., as in similar appearing arachnoid cyst). Epidermoids show intense signal on DWI as a result of restriction of water movement.

Treatment

Caution when removing epidermoid cysts to minimize spilling contents as they are quite irritating and may cause severe chemical meningitis (see above). Berger[16] advocates intraoperative irrigation with hydrocortisone (100 mg/L of LR) to reduce the risk of post-op communicating hydrocephalus. Perioperative IV steroids and copious saline irrigation during surgery may provide similar results. The tumor is not in the cyst wall, and the surgical plan is generally to remove as much as possible

56

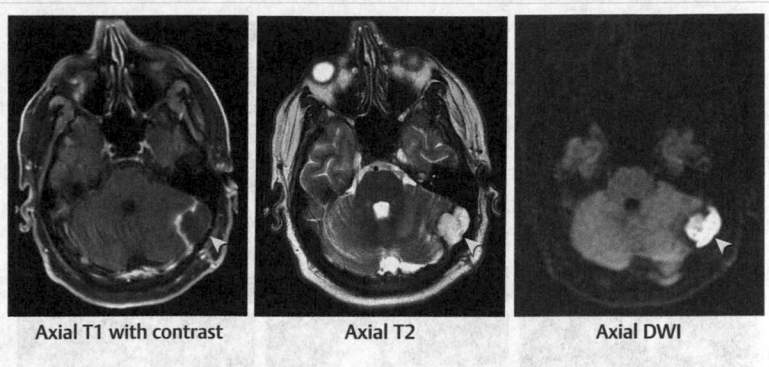

| Axial T1 with contrast | Axial T2 | Axial DWI |

Fig. 56.1 Epidermoid (*yellow arrowheads*) of the left posterior fossa on MRI. Note: the epidermoid is bright on the DWI, whereas an arachnoid cyst would be dark (as is the CSF).

but to leave capsule adherent to critical structures such as brainstem and blood vessels as the morbidity of removal is high and a small residual does not preclude satisfactory outcome.

In spite of adequate removal, it is not unusual to see persistent brainstem distortion on post-op imaging.[23] Post-op radiation is not indicated as the tumor is benign and XRT does not prevent recurrence.[26]

Dermoid cysts

Much of the description is covered above (p. 936). Imaging findings are shown in ▶ Fig. 56.2

56.1.3 Paraganglioma (WHO grade 1)

General information

AKA chemodectoma (obsolete), AKA glomus tumor. A WHO grade 1 neuroendocrine tumor that arises from specialized neural crest cells associated with autonomic ganglia, comprised of uniform cells with neural differentiation conglomerated into compact nests (Zellballen) surrounded by a capillary network.

Paragangliomas in the *CNS* are rare, and they primarily occur in the cauda equina/filum terminale or jugulotympanic regions. Outside the CNS, paragangliomas are often designated by a name that confers the site of origin, as shown in ▶ Table 56.4.

These tumors arise from paraganglion cells (not chemoreceptor cells as previously thought; therefore the term chemodectoma is rarely used). Slow growing tumors (<2 cm in 5 years). Histologically benign (<10% associated with lymph node involvement or distant spread). Most contain secretory granules on EM (mostly epinephrine and norepinephrine, and these tumors may occasionally secrete these catecholamines with risk of life-threatening HTN and/or cardiac arrhythmias).

Glomus tumors may occur in 2 patterns:
1. familial: non multicentric. Up to 50%
2. nonfamilial: may be multicentric (metachronous) 5%

Pheochromocytoma

General information

Located in the adrenal gland. May be sporadic, or as part of familial syndrome (von Hippel-Lindau disease (p. 646), MEN 2A and 2B, and neurofibromatosis). Consider genetic testing if age at diagnosis is <50 years for mutations of VHL and other genetic abnormalities (RET, SDHS, SDHB, SDHC[27]).

56

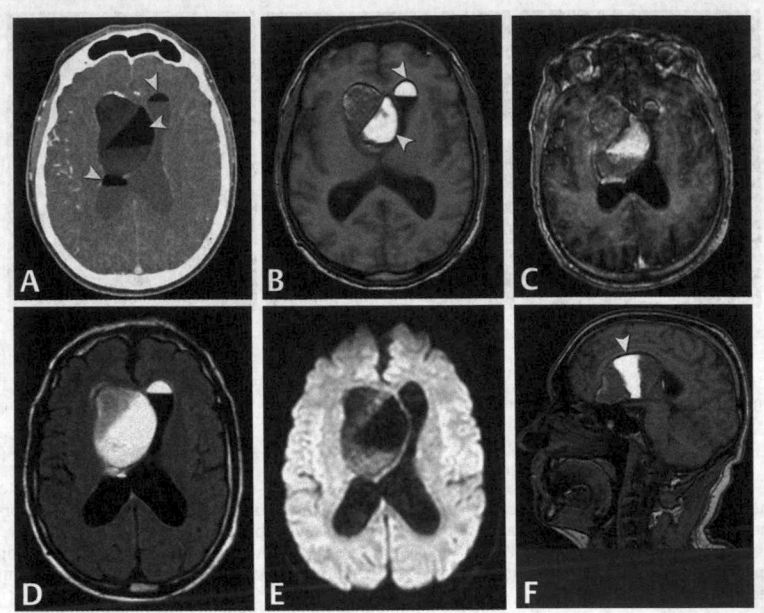

Fig. 56.2 Intraventricular dermoid cyst.
At surgery, the cyst was filled with cholesterol crystals, fat (*yellow arrowheads*), and hair.
Image: A: Axial CTA. B: Axial T1 noncontrast MRI. C: Axial T1 + contrast MRI (note the lack of significant enhancement with contrast). D: Axial FLAIR MRI. E: Axial DWI MRI. F: Sagittal T1 noncontrast MRI.

Table 56.4 Paraganglioma designation based on site of origin

Site	Designation
carotid bifurcation (most common)	carotid body tumors
auricular branch of vagus (middle ear)	glomus tympanicum
superior vagal ganglion (jugular foramen)	glomus jugulare
inferior vagal (nodose) ganglion (nasopharynx at skull base) (least common)	glomus intravagale (AKA glomus vagale)
adrenal medulla & sympathetic chain	pheochromocytoma

56

Laboratory studies

1. fractionated plasma metanephrines: 96% sensitivity, 85% specificity.[28] More sensitive than serum catecholamines with sporadic elevations. Pheochromocytoma is ruled out if plasma normetanephrine (NMN) < 112 pg/ml and metanephrine (MN) < 61 pg/ml. Highly suspicious if NMN > 400 pg/ml or MN > 236 pg/ml
2. 24 hr urine collection for: total catecholamines (epinephrine and norepinephrine) and metanephrines (88% sensitivity, 99.7% specificity[29]). **Note:** testing for vanillylmandelic acid (VMA) is no longer done as it does not measure fractionated metanephrines.
3. where elevation is found, a clonidine suppression test can be done. Normal response consists of a fall in plasma catecholamines to ≤ 50% of baseline and below 500 pg/ml (there will be a reduction in essential hypertension, but no change with pheochromocytoma or other tumor production)

Imaging
Indicated when laboratory tests confirm pheochromocytoma.

MRI with contrast is preferred over CT.

CT may be used when MRI is contraindicated, but is less sensitive, especially for lesions < 1 cm diameter.

123I-MIBG (iodine-123-meta-iodobenzylguanidine) scintigraphy detects extra-adrenal pheochromocytomas with 83–100% sensitivity, 95–100% specificity. If not available, 131I-MIBG may be used with 77–90% sensitivity, 95–100% specificity.

Carotid body tumors

General information
Possibly the most common paraganglioma (pheochromocytoma may possibly be more common). Approximately 5% are bilateral; the incidence of bilaterality increases to 26% in familial cases (these are probably autosomal dominant).

Clinical
Usually present as painless, slow growing mass in upper neck. Large tumors may → cranial nerve involvement (especially vagus and hypoglossal). May also cause stenosis of ICA → TIAs or stroke.

Evaluation
1. carotid angiogram: demonstrates predominant blood supply (usually external carotid, with possible contributions from vertebral and thyrocervical trunk). May also detect bilateral lesions. Characteristic finding: splaying of bifurcation
2. MRI (or CT): evaluates extent, and assesses for intracranial extension

Treatment
Resection reported to carry a high complication rate, including stroke (8–20%) and cranial nerve injury (33–44%). Mortality rate is 5–13%.

Glomus tumors

General information
Glomus tumors may be subdivided into glomus jugulare and glomus tympanicum tumors. Glomus jugulare tumors arise from the jugular bulb (in the jugular foramen at the junction of the sigmoid sinus and jugular vein). Glomus tympanicum tumors are centered higher than glomus jugulare. Glomus tumors are rare (0.6% of all head and neck tumors), yet the glomus tympanicum is the most common neoplasm of the middle ear. Glomus jugulare tumors (GJT) arise from glomus bodies, usually in the area of the jugular bulb, and track along vessels. May have finger-like extension into the jugular vein (which may embolize during resection).[30] Most are slow growing, although rapidly growing tumors do occur.

Vascular supply: very vascular. Main feeders of GJT are from the external carotid (especially inferior tympanic branch of ascending pharyngeal artery, and branches of posterior auricular, occipital, and internal maxillary), with additional feeders from petrous portion of the ICA. Glomus tympanicum tumors feed from the auricular artery.

Epidemiology
Female:male ratio is 6:1. Bilateral occurrence is almost nonexistent.

Pathology
General information
Histologically indistinguishable from carotid body tumors. May invade locally, both through temporal bone destruction and especially along pre-existing pathways (along vessels, eustachian tube, jugular vein, carotid artery). Intradural extension is rare. Malignancy, although rare, may occur. These tumors rarely metastasize.

Secretory properties
These tumors usually possess secretory granules (even the functionally inactive tumors) and may actively secrete catecholamines (similar to pheochromocytomas, occur in only 1–4% of GJT[31]). Norepinephrine will be elevated in functionally active tumors since glomus tumors lack the methyltransferase needed to convert this to epinephrine. Alternatively, serotonin and kallikrein may be released,

56

and may produce a carcinoid-like syndrome (bronchoconstriction, abdominal pain and explosive diarrhea, violent H/A, cutaneous flushing, hypertension, hepatomegaly, and hyperglycemia).[32] During surgical manipulation, these tumors may also release histamine and bradykinin, causing hypotension and bronchoconstriction.[33]

Clinical
Symptoms
Patients commonly present with hearing loss and pulsatile tinnitus. Dizziness is the third most common symptom. Ear pain may also occur.

Signs
Hearing loss may be conductive (e.g., due to obstruction of the ear canal) or sensorineural, due to invasion of the labyrinth often with accompanying vertigo (the eighth nerve is the most common cranial nerve involved). Various combinations of palsies of cranial nerves IX, X, XI, and XII occur—see Jugular foramen syndromes (p. 102)—with occasional VII palsy (usually from involvement within the temporal bone). Ataxia and/or hydrocephalus can occur with massive lesions that cause brainstem compression. Occasionally patients may present with symptoms due to secretory products (see below).

Otoscopic exam → pulsatile reddish-blue mass behind eardrum (occasionally, lamentably biopsied by ENT physician with possible ensuing massive blood loss).

Differential diagnosis
See Cerebellopontine angle (CPA) lesions (p. 1647). The major differential is neurilemmomas (vestibular schwannomas), both enhance on CT. A cystic component and extrinsic compression of the jugular bulb are characteristic of neurilemmomas. Angiography will differentiate difficult cases.

Evaluation
Neurophysiologic testing
Audiometric and vestibular testing should be performed.

Imaging
1. CT or MRI used to delineate location and extent of tumor; CT is better for assessing bony involvement of the skull base
2. angiography: confirms diagnosis (helping to rule out vestibular schwannoma), and ascertains patency of contralateral jugular vein in event that jugular on side of tumor must be sacrificed; jugular bulb and/or vein are usually partially or completely occluded

Endocrine/laboratory studies
See also details (p. 940).

Classification
A number of classification schemes have been proposed. The modified Jackson classification is shown in ► Table 56.5.

Table 56.5 Modified Jackson classification of glomus tumors[34]

Type	Description	Intracranial extension
I	small; involves jugular bulb, middle ear & mastoid	none
II	extends under IAC	possible
III	extends into petrous apex	possible
IV	extends beyond petrous apex into clivus or infratemporal fossa	possible

Treatment
Surgical resection is usually simple and effective for small tumors confined to the middle ear. For larger tumors that invade and destroy bone, the relative role of surgery and/or radiation is not fully determined. With large tumors, surgery carries the risk of significant cranial nerve palsies.

Medical management
General information
For tumors that actively secrete catecholamines, medical therapy is useful for palliation or as adjunctive treatment before embolization or surgery. Alpha and beta blockers given before embolization or surgery blocks possibly lethal blood pressure lability and arrhythmias. Adequate blockade takes ≈ 2–3 weeks of alpha blocker and at least 24 hours of beta blocker therapy; in emergency, 3 days of treatment may suffice.

Alpha blockers
Reduce BP by preventing peripheral vasoconstriction.
1. phenoxybenzamine (Dibenzyline®): long acting; peak effect 1–2 hrs. Start with 10 mg PO BID and gradually increase to 40–100 mg per day divided BID
2. phentolamine (Regitine®): short acting. Usually used IV for hypertensive crisis during surgery or embolization.
   R: 5 mg IV/IM (peds: 1 mg) 1–2 hrs pre-op, repeat PRN before and during surgery

Beta blockers
Reduces catecholamine-induced tachycardia and arrhythmias (may also prevent hypotension that might occur if only alpha blockade is used). These drugs are not always needed, but when used 6 NB: these drugs must *not* be started before starting alpha-blockers (to prevent hypertensive crisis and myocardial ischemia).
1. propranolol (Inderal®): R: oral dose is 5–10 mg q 6 hrs. IV dose for use during surgery is 0.5–2 mg slow IVP
2. labetalol (Normodyne®) (p. 131): may have some efficacy in blocking α1 selective and β non-selective (potency < propranolol)

Serotonin, bradykinin, histamine release blockers
These agents may provoke bronchoconstriction that does not respond to steroids, but may respond to inhaled β-agonists or inhaled anticholinergics. Somatostatin may be used to inhibit release of serotonin, bradykinin, or histamines. Since this drug has a short half-life, it is preferable to give octreotide (p. 890) 100 mcg sub-Q q 8 hrs.

Radiation therapy
XRT may relieve symptoms and stop growth in spite of persistence of tumor mass. 40–45 Gy in fractions of 2 Gy has been recommended.[35] Lower doses of ≈ 35 Gy in 15 fractions of 2.35 Gy appear as effective and have fewer side effects.[36] Generally used as primary treatment only for large tumors or in patients too elderly or infirmed to undergo surgery. Some surgeons pretreat 4–6 mos preoperatively with XRT to decrease vascularity[37] (controversial).

Embolization
1. generally reserved for large tumors with favorable blood supply (i.e., vessels that can be selectively embolized with no danger of particles passing through to normal brain)
2. post-embolization tumor swelling may compress brainstem or cerebellum
3. may be used preoperatively to reduce vascularity. Performed 24–48 hours pre-op (not used prior to that, because of post-embolization edema)
4. caution with actively secreting tumors that may release vasoactive substances (e.g., epinephrine) upon infarction from the embolization
5. may also be used as primary treatment (± radiation) in patients who are not surgical candidates. In this case, XRT is only palliative, as tumor will develop new blood supply
6. absorbable (Gelfoam®) and non-absorbable (Ivalon®) materials have been used

Surgical treatment
General information
The tumor is primarily extradural, with extremely vascular surrounding dura.

Suboccipital approach may cause dangerous bleeding and usually results in incomplete resection. Team approach by a neurosurgeon in conjunction with a neuro-otologist (and possibly head and neck surgeon) has been advocated.[38] This approach utilizes an approach to the skull base through the neck.

ECA feeders are ligated early, followed rapidly by draining veins (to prevent systemic release of catecholamines).

Sacrifice of the jugular vein (JV) is tolerated if the contralateral JV is patent (often, the ipsilateral JV will already be occluded).

Surgical complications and outcome

The most common complications are CSF fistula, facial nerve palsy, and varying degrees of dysphagia (from dysfunction of lower cranial nerves). Dysfunction of any of the cranial nerves VII thru XII can occur, and a tracheostomy should be performed if there is any doubt of lower nerve function, and a gastrostomy feeding tube may be needed temporarily or permanently. Lower cranial nerve dysfunction also predisposes to aspiration, the risk of which is also increased by impaired gastric emptying and ileus that may occur due to reduced cholecystokinin (CCK) levels post-op. Excessive blood loss can also occur.

Even after gross total tumor removal, recurrence rate may be as high as one third.[37,39]

56.2 Cyst like lesions

56.2.1 Colloid cyst

General information

> ## Key concepts
>
> - slow-growing benign tumor comprising < 1% of intracranial tumors
> - classically occurs in the anterior 3rd ventricle, blocking foramina of Monro bilaterally → obstructive hydrocephalus involving only the lateral ventricles (≈ pathognomonic)
> - enhances minimally or not at all on CT/MRI
> - natural history: risk of *sudden* death has been described, but is controversial. A small number of patients will present with acute obstructive hydrocephalus and progress to death despite appropriately rapid intervention
> - treatment, when indicated, is surgical. Main options: microsurgery (transcallosal, transcortical/transventricular (only if hydrocephalus)), ventriculoscopic

AKA neuroepithelial cysts. Most commonly found in the third ventricle in the region of the foramina of Monro, but may be seen elsewhere, e.g., in septum pellucidum.[40]

Epidemiology

Estimated incidence is 3.2 per 1,000,000 per year,[41] with a prevalence of about 1 in 5800.[42] They comprise 0.5-1.5% of all intracranial tumors.[41] Usual age of diagnosis: 20–50 yrs.

There is evidence that some cases are part of familial clusters which appear to have primarily mother-to-daughter transmission.[42]

Pathogenesis

Origin: unknown. Implicated structures include: paraphysis (evagination in roof of third ventricle, rudimentary in humans), diencephalic ependyma in the recess of the postvelar arch, ventricular neuroepithelium.

Comprised of a fibrous epithelial-lined wall filled with either mucoid or dense hyloid substance. A slow growing, benign tumor.

Clinical signs and symptoms

Presenting symptoms or indications neuroimaging in patients found to have a colloid cyst in one series are shown in ▶ Table 56.6. 46% of their symptomatic patients were found to have hydrocephalus which is responsible for the most common presenting symptoms (H/A, N/V, blurred vision, ataxia, and cognitive decline).[43] A small number of patients will present with acute obstructive hydrocephalus (estimates vary from 3-35%) and despite rapid institution of CSF diversion and accompanying critical care will progress to death in 5-38%[43] (see "Sudden death" below).

Most cysts < 1 cm diameter do not produce hydrocephalus and are asymptomatic.

▶ **Sudden death.** A high rate of sudden death has been reported with colloid cysts (20% in pre-CT era[44]), but is probably overestimated. One prevailing obsolete theory was that these tumors are mobile and thus could shift position and acutely block CSF flow with resultant herniation. More

Table 56.6 Presenting symptoms or indication for neuroimaging in 163 patients with colloid cyst[43]

Feature	Symptomatic (n=65)	Incidental[a] (n=98)
headache	58 (89%)	24 (25%)
nausea/vomiting	15 (23%)	5 (5%)
vision change	14 (22%)	2 (2%)
dizziness/ataxia	13 (20%)	6 (6%)
cognitive decline	9 (14%)	11 (11%)
syncope	6 (9%)	5 (5%)
seizure	4 (6%)	2 (2%)
bradycardia	4 (6%)	0
sensory change	3 (5%)	1 (1%)
memory decline	3 (5%)	0
urinary incontinence	2 (3%)	0
trauma	1 (2%)	27 (28%)
general medical	1 (2%)	12 (12%)
weakness	1 (2%)	3 (3%)
general neurological	0	8 (8%)
stroke	0	8 (8%)
cancer staging	0	6 (6%)
intoxication	0	2 (2%)
other	0	1 (1%)

[a]Most colloid cysts in the incidental group were discovered during routine neuroimaging for unrelated conditions (trauma, stroke, nonspecific H/A, ALS...).

careful analysis reveals that nearly all patients have progressive symptoms preceding what is then seen as a precipitious deterioration. Changes in CSF dynamics resulting from procedures (LP, ventriculography...) may have also contributed in some cases.[45] Another proposed mechanism is disturbance of hypothalamic-mediated cardiovascular reflex control.[45]

Given that sudden death, while infrequent, may occur with colloid cysts, and that the literature is rife with references to this, it is imperative that the existence of this small possibility should be expounded to the patient (and this discussion should be documented) and treatment decisions should involve patient input.

Evaluation

Imaging (MRI or CT) demonstrates the tumor usually located in the anterior 3rd ventricle (▶ Fig. 56.3). Here, it often blocks both foramina of Monro causing almost pathognomonic hydrocephalus involving only the lateral ventricles (sparing the 3rd and 4th). Differential diagnosis includes basilar artery aneurysms, hamartomas, primary or secondary neoplasm, and xanthogranulomas.[46]

MRI: usually the optimal imaging technique. However, there are cases where cysts are isointense on MRI and CT is superior[47] (scrutinize the midline T1WI MRI images). When the lesion is identifiable, MRI clearly demonstrates the location of the cyst and relation to nearby structures, usually obviating an angiogram. MRI appearance: variable. Usually hyperintense on T1WI, hypointense on T2WI. Some data suggests that symptomatic patients are more likely to display T2 hyperintense cysts on MRI, indicating higher water content which may reflect a propensity for continued cyst expansion.[48] Enhancement: minimal, sometimes involving only capsule.

CT scan: findings are variable. Most are hyperdense (however, iso- and hypodense colloid cysts occur), and about half enhance slightly. Density may correlate with viscosity of contents; hyperdense cysts were harder to drain percutaneously.[49] CT is usually not quite as good as MRI, especially with isodense cysts. These tumors calcify only rarely.

✖ LP: *contraindicated* prior to placement of shunt due to risk of herniation.

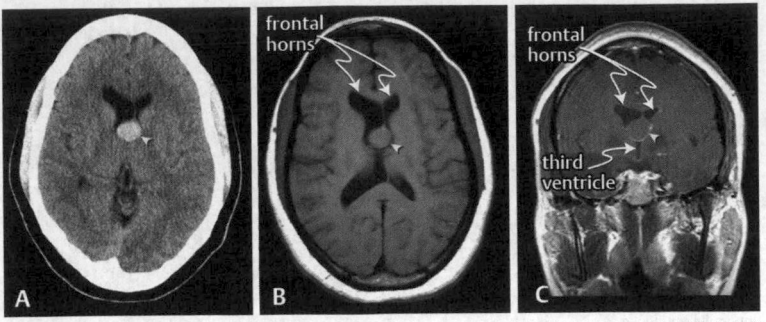

Fig. 56.3 Colloid cyst (*yellow arrowheads*) of the third ventricle.
Image: A: axial noncontrast CT scan. B: axial noncontrast T1 FLAIR MRI. C: coronal T1 contrast enhanced MRI showing relation to the normal sized 3rd ventricle and the frontal horns of the lateral ventricles (in this patient, the right lateral ventricle is enlarged, the left is not). Note: the colloid cyst does not enhance.

Treatment – general information and management options

General information

Optimal treatment remains controversial. Initially, shunting without treating the cyst was advocated.[50] The nature of the obstruction (both foramina of Monro) requires *bilateral* ventricular shunts (or, unilateral shunt with fenestration of the septum pellucidum). Presently, one form or another of direct surgical treatment of the tumor is usually recommended for some or all of the following reasons:

1. to prevent shunt dependency
2. to reduce the possibility of tumor progression
3. the mechanism of sudden neurologic deterioration may be due to factors such as cardiovascular instability from hypothalamic compression and not due to hydrocephalus

Management options

A meta-analysis of 1278 patients comparing endoscopic and various microsurgical techniques found that the microsurgical group had a significantly greater extent of resection (96.8% vs. 58.2%), lower rates of recurrence (1.48% vs. 3.91%), and lower rates of reoperation than the endoscopic group (0.38% vs. 3.0%). Both groups had similar rates of mortality (1.4% vs. 0.6%) and shunt dependency (6.2% vs. 3.9%). Overall, the complication rate was lower in the endoscopic group than in the microsurgical group (10.5% vs. 16.3%). Within the microsurgery group, the transcallosal approach had a lower overall morbidity rate (14.4%) than the transcortical approach (24.5%).[51]

Using natural history for treatment decisions

A review of 58 asymptomatic patients (average age 57 years) with incidentally discovered colloid cysts of the third ventricle with mean follow up of 79 months demonstrated the incidence of symptomatic worsening at 2-, 5-, and 10-year follow-up to be 0%, 0%, and 8%, respectively. Of the 34 patients who obtained follow up imaging, 32 demonstrated no change in cyst size or ventricular caliber. The average age of these patients was significantly higher than that of the patients undergoing surgery for symptomatic lesions (57 vs. 41) and thus may reflect a patient cohort with differing natural histories.[52]

NB: Many "asymptomatic" patients may have headaches at diagnosis. Careful evaluation of headache etiology (i.e., posttraumatic, migrainous, tension, etc.) should be undertaken to determine whether the headaches are due to the colloid cyst or if the cyst is asymptomatic.

Pollock et al[48] reviewed 155 patients with newly diagnosed colloid cysts, performing a recursive partitioning analysis, and divided patients into three classes as shown in ▶ Table 56.7.

Additionally, a significantly greater number of Class III patients had hyperintense cyst contents on T2 weighted imaging (44% vs. 13%), and symptomatic patients were more likely to have increased T2 signal (44% vs. 8%) compared to their asymptomatic counterparts. The authors suggest that asymptomatic patients with low T2 signal-containing cysts may reflect a group with low potential for cyst expansion and development of cyst-related symptoms (even in the presence of ventriculomegaly); thus they may represent a population that may be safely managed in a nonoperative fashion.[48] Nevertheless, most surgeons would recommend surgery for a patient with ventriculomegaly and symptoms such as headache even if they may not be definitely related.

Table 56.7 Classes of colloid cyst based on recursive partitioning analysis

Class	Characteristic			Symptomatic patients (% of total)	Treatment options
	Age (years)	Cyst diameter	Ventricles		
I	any	≤ 10 mm	normal	12%	May be monitored clinically and with serial imaging (CT or MRI)
II	> 50	≤ 10 mm	ventriculomegaly	50%	If asymptomatic, may be monitored clinically and with serial imaging (CT or MRI)
III	any	> 10 mm	normal	85%	Surgical removal is recommended
	≤ 50	any	ventriculomegaly		
	> 50	> 10 mm	ventriculomegaly		

Surgical treatment

Surgical options
Also see Approaches to the third ventricle.
1. transcallosal approaches: not dependent on dilated ventricles. Higher incidence of venous infarction or forniceal injury (see below)
2. transcortical approach: higher incidence of post-op seizures (≈ 5%). Not feasible with normal sized ventricles (e.g., in patient with VP shunt)
3. stereotactic drainage: see below
4. ventriculoscopic removal: see below

Transcallosal approach
Access to the 3rd ventricle via either the foramen of Monro or by interfornicial approach. Since colloid cysts tend to occur exactly at the foramen of Monro, it is *rarely* necessary to enlarge the foramen to locate the tumor. See Transcallosal approach to lateral or third ventricle (p. 1758).

Endoscopic (ventriculoscopic) resection
Ventriculoscopic resection has been shown to have a a reduced incidence of operative morbidity and overall surgical treatment cost (including reduced length of stay) when compared to microsurgery.[53] It is argued that this should be the initial procedure of choice, with craniotomy reserved for treatment failures).[54] However, endoscopic resection is associated with a significantly increased incidence of residual coagulated cyst-wall remnants compared to microsurgery. It remains to be seen whether this will ulitimatley result in an increased rate of reoperation, and how that will impact the overall patient outcome and costs.

Stereotactic drainage of colloid cysts
May be useful,[55] especially in patients with normal ventricles from shunting, but the contents may be too viscous,[56] and the tough capsule may make blind penetration difficult. Total or even subtotal aspiration may not require further treatment in some patients; however, recurrence rate is higher than with surgical removal.[57]

Early morbidity was relatively high from this procedure (not widely reported in literature), possibly from vascular injury or mechanical trauma; this has improved. May be more feasible with intraoperative ventriculography[58] or with a

Two features that correlate with *unsuccessful* stereotactic aspiration[59]:
1. high viscosity: correlates with hyperdensity on CT (low viscosity correlated with hypo- or isodense CT appearance; no MRI finding correlated with viscosity)
2. deflection of the cyst from tip of aspirating needle due to small size

56

Stereotactic technique[60]:
1. insertion point of stereotactic needle is just anterior to right coronal suture
2. start with sharp-tipped 1.8 mm probe, and advance to 3–5 mm beyond target site (to accommodate for displacement of cyst wall)
3. use a 10 ml syringe and apply 6–8 ml of negative aspiration pressure
4. if this does not yield any material, repeat with a 2.1 mm probe
5. although complete cyst evacuation is desirable, if this cannot be accomplished an acceptable goal of aspiration is re-establishment of patency of the ventricular pathways (may be verified by injecting 1–2 cc of iohexol)

56.2.2 Pineal cysts (PCs)

General information

Usually an incidental finding (i.e., not symptomatic), seen on ≈ 4% of MRIs[61] or on 25–40% of autopsies[62] (many are microscopic). The most common ones are intra-pineal glial-lined cysts with diameter < 1 cm. Etiology is obscure; PCs are nonneoplastic, and may be due to ischemic glial degeneration or due to sequestration of the pineal diverticulum. They have been regarded as benign, but the natural history is not known with certainty.[63] PCs may contain clear, slightly xanthochromic, or hemorrhagic fluid. In rare cases, they may enlarge, and like other pineal region masses, may become symptomatic by causing hydrocephalus by aqueductal compression,[64] gaze paresis[65] including Parinaud's syndrome (p. 101), or hypothalamic symptoms.

Positional H/As have been attributed to PCs; the theory is that the cyst could intermittently compress the vein of Galen and/or Sylvian aqueduct.[66] This remains unproven since asymptomatic compression of the vein of Galen and the quadrigeminal plate has been demonstrated on MRI.[67]

Imaging

May escape detection on CT because the cyst fluid density is often similar to CSF. MRI T1WI (▶ Fig. 56.4) shows round or ovoid abnormality in region of pineal recess, signal varies with protein content (isointense or slightly hyperintense). T2WI occasionally shows increased intensity.[63] Gadolinium occasionally enhances the cyst wall with a maximum thickness of 2 mm. Irregularities of the wall with nodular enhancement suggests the lesion is not a benign pineal cyst.

Epidermoid-dermoid cysts may also occur in the pineal region, and are larger and have different signal characteristics on MRI.

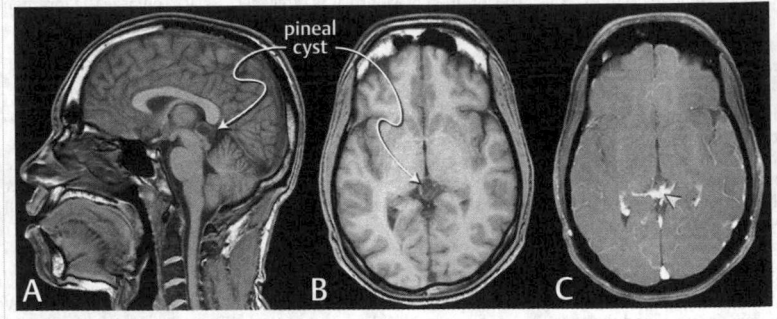

Fig. 56.4 Pineal cyst.
Dimensions: 1.5 cm AP, 1 cm height, 1.2 cm mediolateral. *Yellow arrowhead* marks contrast enchancement, probably representing the pineal gland.
Image: MRI, A: sagittal T1 noncontrast, B: axial T1 noncontrast, C: axial T1 with contrast.

Management

▶ **Asymptomatic PCs.** Asymptomatic PCs < 2 cm diameter with typical appearance (wall: ≤ 2 mm thick and no irregularities or nodular enhancement): are generally considered not to grow, but the natural history is not known with certainty. Risk of growing is ≈ 4% with 6 months median follow up in adults,[68] and 11% in children with 10 months median follow-up.[69] Based on this, it seems a little hard to justify not providing initial follow-up to reassure the patient and the practitioner.

A reasonable approach might consist of a 3-month follow-up MRI after the initial scan to check for rapid growth (as might occur with a neoplasm) and then if stable, annual imaging studies for an arbitrary period (some suggest 1 year[68]; 3 years is probably reasonable) to assure stability.

▶ **Symptomatic lesions or those that show changes on MRI.** Surgery to relieve symptoms and/or to obtain a diagnosis.

▶ **Hydrocephalus.** Surgical options include:
1. CSF diversion: recommended only for lesions with appearance of typical PC as it does not obtain tissue for pathology. May not relieve gaze disturbance from direct pressure on tectal plate
   a) CSF shunt
   b) endoscopic third ventriculostomy (ETV) (p. 1828). A few cases of regression of PCs after ETV have been reported[70]
2. aspiration only (stereotactic or endoscopic): may not get enough tissue for diagnosis
3. cyst excision (open or endoscopic): relieves symptoms and establishes diagnosis. Low morbidity[71]

56.2.3 Rathke's cleft cyst

General information

Rathke's cleft cysts (RCC) AKA pars intermedia cysts, are slow-growing nonneoplastic lesions that are thought to be remnants of Rathke's pouch (p. 151). They are primarily intrasellar, suprasellar extension is common, purely suprasellar presentation is rare.[72] RCC are found incidentally in 13–23% of necropsies.[73] Since the adenohypophysis arises from proliferation of the anterior wall of Rathke's pouch, RCCs and PitNET/adenomas have a similar lineage and rarely they are found together.[74] RCC are often discussed in contrast to craniopharyngiomas (**CP**) (see above). Some features are compared in ▶ Table 56.8. Recurrence after treatment is common.

Table 56.8 Comparison of craniopharyngioma to Rathke's cleft cyst

Feature	Craniopharyngioma	Rathke's cleft cyst
site of origin	anterior superior margin of pituitary	pars intermedia of pituitary
cell lining	stratified squamous epithelium	single layer cuboidal epithelium
cyst contents	cholesterol crystals	may be clear or may resemble motor oil
surgical treatment	total removal is the goal	partial excision and drainage[75]
cyst wall	thick	thin

Clinical presentation

Some symptom may be a result of mass effect; however, other symptoms may be related to inflammation that is associated with some RCCs.
• most are asymptomatic, discovered incidentally on imaging obtained for unrelated reasons
• headache occurs in 44–81% of symptomatic RCCs,[76] with sudden onset of severe H/A in up to 16%[77]
• 30–60% develop endocrine disturbance,[76] often with hypogonadism in males (producing fatigue and decreased libido), menstrual irregularities and galatorrhea in premenopausal females or panhypopituitarism in postmenopausal females. Diabetes insipidus is more common with symptomatic RCCs (up to 37%) than with pituitary adenomas (possibly due to associated inflammation)
• visual field deficit is present in 11–67%[76]

Evaluation

General workup
Workup for these lesions is the same as for sellar/suprasellar masses (p. 874) in general.
1. up to 60% have pituitary dysfunction. Endocrine workup (p. 876)is as for any sellar mass
2. visual field evaluation (p. 874)

56

Imaging

RCCs are typically midline, without stalk deviation.

CT: RCCs usually appear as low-density cystic lesions. One half show capsular enhancement. RCCs infrequently can erode the skull base.

MRI appearance is variable (▶ Fig. 56.5).[75] Typically high signal on T2WI. On T1WI they may be hyperintense (correlates with RCCs having proteinaceous mucinous contents) or hypointense (seen with RCCs containing clear low protein fluid). An intracystic nodule that is high signal on T1WI low signal on T2WI is described in > 75% of RCs.[78] Rule of thumb: a sellar lesion with a nodule is usually an RCC. There is no internal enhancement.

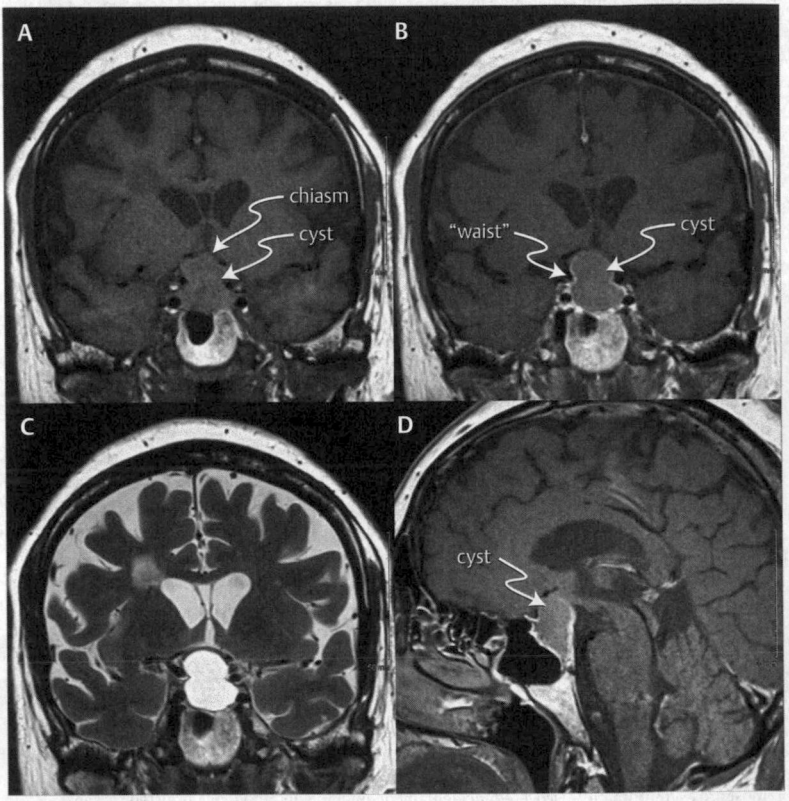

Fig. 56.5 Rathke cleft cyst.
Note: enhancment of the cyst wall but no enhancement within the cyst. The diaphragma sella creates a "waist" in the cyst where it extends into the suprasellar cistern. The optic chiasm drapes over the top of the cyst (not well visualized in this MRI).
Image: MRI. A: noncontrast T1 coronal, B: contrast enhanced T1 coronal, C: noncontrast T2 coronal, D: contrast enhanced T1 sagittal.

Natural history

Among 61 incidentally discovered RCCs, 69% showed no growth over 9 years.[79] In another series of 94 cases, only 5% increased in size and 16% actually decreased in size with 27 months mean follow-up.[80]

Management

Incidental (i.e., asymptomatic) lesions are followed with serial imaging.

Symptomatic RCCs are usually drained, most transsphenoidally, either microscopically or endo-scopically, usually combined with cyst fenestration.

▶ **Reduction of recurrence rate.** Methods to reduce recurrence include techniques that promote persistence of continued drainage by maintaining patency of the fenestration. There is not sufficient evidence to recommend one method over another. Techniques include:
1. mucosal coupling: the epithelium of the RCC and the mucosa of the sphenoid sinus are connected[81]
2. stenting of the fenestration, e.g., with a bioabsorbable steroid eluting stent (e.g., PROPEL® Mini (Intersect ENT, Menlo Park, CA, USA) mometasone furoate (a synthetic antiinflammatory cortico-steroid) implant, 370 mcg)
3. reduced recurrence rate has been quoted with complete cyst wall removal; however, the inci-dence of post-op endocrine dysfunction may be higher with this approach[76]
4. ✖ there is no strong evidence to support the use of hydrogen peroxide or alcohol irrigation in an effort to reduce the recurrence rate.

Surgical outcome

Complete cyst decompression occurs in the vast majority of cases (up to 97%[79]), with improved vision in 83–97%[79,82] in those presenting with visual disturbance. Headache improves in 71%, and endocrinopathies improve in 33–94%
  Morbidity:
1. CSF leak in ≈ 10% (higher rates with extension outside the sella)
2. diabetes insipidus (DI): permanent DI occurs in up to 9% after cyst drainage, and from to 19–69% with cyst wall resection[76]
3. other risks seen with any transspehonoidal operation: internal carotid artery injury

Recurrence of cyst: reported rate is as high as 42%, but 16–18% may be more typical over 2–5 years. Higher rates of recurrence may be associated with: purely suprasellar location, inflammation and reactive metaplasia in the cyst wall, cyst infection, and use of a fat graft within the cyst cavity.

56.3 Empty sella syndrome

56.3.1 General information

Empty sella syndrome (ESS) can be "primary," "secondary," or congenital.
  MRI is the imaging modality of choice (▶ Fig. 56.6). The sellar contents will follow imaging charac-teristics of CSF. The pituitary infundibulum may be seen traversing the sella (**infundibulum sign,**[83]

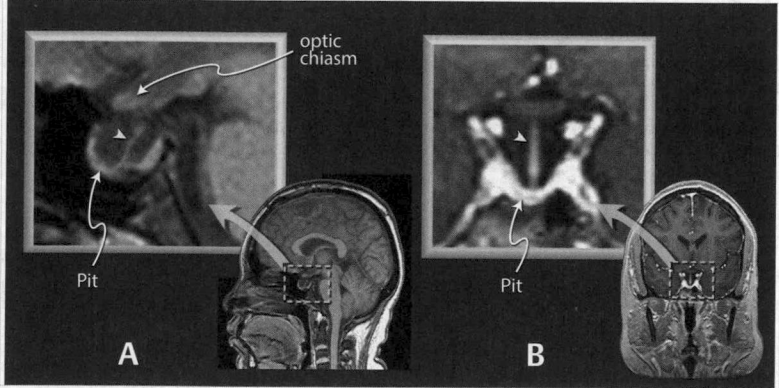

Fig. 56.6 Empty sella.
The infundibulum (AKA pituitary stalk) (*yellow arrowheads*) traverses the sella (infundibulum sign) to the pituitary gland, which is compressed against the floor of the sella.
Image: unenhanced T1 MRI, A: sagittal. B: coronal. Broken lines in inset shows from where the details are taken.
Abbreviation: Pit = pituitary gland.

which distinguishes empty sella from an intrasellar arachnoid cyst which displaces the infundibulum).

56.3.2 Primary empty sella syndrome

General information

Occurs in the absence of prior treatment of a pituitary tumor (medical, surgical, or XRT). Herniation of the arachnoid membrane into the sella turcica[84] which can act as a mass, probably as a result of repeated CSF pulsation. The pituitary gland may become compressed against the floor, and in the long term the sella itself can become enlarged (see Sella turcica (p. 227) for normal dimensions).

Frequent association: female sex (female:male ratio = 5:1), obesity, and HTN. The frequency of intrasellar arachnoid herniation is higher in patients with pituitary tumors and in those with increased intracranial pressure for any reason—including pseudotumor cerebri (p. 955)—than in the general population.

These patients usually present with symptoms that do not suggest an intrasellar abnormality including: headache (the most common symptom), dizziness, seizures... Occasionally patients may develop CSF rhinorrhea,[85] deterioration of vision (acuity or field deficit resulting from kinking of optic chiasm due to herniation into the sella), or amenorrhea-galactorrhea syndrome.

Clinically evident endocrine disturbances are rare with primary ESS; however, up to 30% have abnormal pituitary function tests, most commonly reduced growth hormone secretion following stimulation. Mild elevation of prolactin (PRL) and reduction of ADH may occur, probably from compression of the stalk. These patients show a normal PRL rise with TRH stimulation (whereas patients with prolactinomas do not).

Treatment

Surgical treatment is usually not indicated, except in the case of CSF rhinorrhea. In this setting, it is necessary to determine if there is increased ICP, and if so, if there is an identifiable cause. Simple shunting for hydrocephalus runs the risk of producing tension pneumocephalus from air drawn in through the former leak site. This may necessitate transsphenoidal repair with simultaneous external lumbar drainage, to be converted to a permanent shunt shortly thereafter. Hyperprolactinemia may be treated, e.g., with bromocriptine (p. 888) if it interferes with gonadal function.

56.3.3 Secondary empty sella syndrome

Entities associated with secondary empty sella syndrome:
1. following trauma[86]
2. after successful transsphenoidal removal or XRT for a pituitary tumor[86]
3. any cause of increased intracranial pressure, including: pseudotumor cerebri (p. 955), Chiari malformation

Often presents with visual deterioration due to herniation of the optic chiasm into the empty sella. There may be hypopituitarism from the underlying cause.

Visual deterioration may be treated with chiasmapexy (propping up the chiasm), usually by transsphenoidal approach and packing the sella with fat, muscle or cartilage. Usually done endoscopically.[87] Chiasmapexy appears to be better for improving visual field deficits than loss of visual acuity.[88]

References

[1] Berger L, Luc G, Richard D. L'Esthesioneuroepitheliome Olfactif. Bull Assoc Franc Etude Cancer. 1924; 13:410–421

[2] Theilgaard SA, Buchwald C, Ingeholm P, et al. Esthesioneuroblastoma: a Danish demographic study of 40 patients registered between 1978 and 2000. Acta Otolaryngol. 2003; 123:433–439

[3] Chao KS, Kaplan C, Simpson JR, et al. Esthesioneuroblastoma: the impact of treatment modality. Head Neck. 2001; 23:749–757

[4] Kadish S, Goodman M, Wang CC. Olfactory neuroblastoma. A clinical analysis of 17 cases. Cancer. 1976; 37:1571–1576

[5] Biller HF, Lawson W, Sachdev VP, et al. Esthesioneuroblastoma: surgical treatment without radiation. Laryngoscope. 1990; 100:1199–1201

[6] Dulguerov P, Calcaterra T. Esthesioneuroblastoma: the UCLA experience 1970-1990. Laryngoscope. 1992; 102:843–849

[7] Hyams V. Tumors of the upper respiratory tract and ear. Washington, D.C.: Armed Forces Institute of Pathology; 1988

[8] Van Gompel JJ, Giannini C, Olsen KD, et al. Long-term outcome of esthesioneuroblastoma: hyams grade predicts patient survival. J Neurol Surg B Skull Base. 2012; 73:331–336

[9] Kane AJ, Sughrue ME, Rutkowski MJ, et al. Posttreatment prognosis of patients with esthesioneuroblastoma. J Neurosurg. 2010; 113:340–351

[10] Gardner G, Robertson JH. Hearing Preservation in Unilateral Acoustic Neuroma Surgery. Ann Otol Rhinol Laryngol. 1988; 97:55–66

[11] Dias FL, Sa GM, Lima RA, et al. Patterns of failure and outcome in esthesioneuroblastoma. Arch Otolaryngol Head Neck Surg. 2003; 129:1186–1192

[12] Gore MR, Zanation AM. Salvage Treatment of Local Recurrence in Esthesioneuroblastoma: A Meta-analysis. Skull Base. 2011; 21:1–6

[13] Van Gompel JJ, Carlson ML, Pollock BE, et al. Stereotactic radiosurgical salvage treatment for locally recurrent esthesioneuroblastoma. Neurosurgery. 2013; 72:332–9; discussion 339-40

[14] Foote RL, Morita A, Ebersold MJ, et al. Esthesioneuroblastoma: the role of adjuvant radiation therapy. Int J Radiat Oncol Biol Phys. 1993; 27:835–842

[15] Kim HJ, Cho HJ, Kim KS, et al. Results of salvage therapy after failure of initial treatment for advanced olfactory neuroblastoma. J Craniomaxillofac Surg. 2008; 36:47–52

[16] Berger MS, Wilson CB. Epidermoid Cysts of the Posterior Fossa. J Neurosurg. 1985; 62:214–219

[17] Gutin PH, Boehm J, Bank WO, et al. Cerebral convexity epidermoid tumor subsequent to multiple percutaneous subdural aspirations. Case report. J Neurosurg. 1980; 52:574–577

[18] Guidetti B, Gagliardi FM. Epidermoids and Dermoid Cysts. J Neurosurg. 1977; 47:12–18

[19] Fleming JFR, Botterell EH. Cranial Dermoid and Epidermoid Tumors. Surg Gynecol Obstet. 1959; 109:57–79

[20] Alvord EC. Growth Rates of Epidermoid Tumors. Annals of Neurology. 1977; 2:367–370

[21] Link MJ, Cohen PL, Breneman JC, et al. Malignant squamous degeneration of a cerebellopontine angle epidermoid tumor. Case report. J Neurosurg. 2002; 97:1237–1243

[22] Sabin HI, Bardi LT, Symon L. Epidermoid Cysts and Cholesterol Granulomas Centered on the Posterior Fossa: Twenty Years of Diagnosis and Management. Neurosurgery. 1987; 21:798–803

[23] Altschuler EM, Jungreis CA, Sekhar LN, et al. Operative Treatment of Intracranial Epidermoid Cysts and Cholesterol Granulomas: Report of 21 Cases. Neurosurgery. 1990; 26:606–614

[24] Friedman I. Epidermoid Cholesteatoma and Cholesterol Granuloma: Experimental and Human. Ann Otol Rhinol Laryngol. 1959; 68:57–79

[25] Chang P, Fagan PA, Atlas MD, et al. Imaging destructive lesions of the petrous apex. Laryngoscope. 1998; 108:599–604

[26] Keville FJ, Wise BL. Intracranial Epidermoid and Dermoid Tumors. J Neurosurg. 1959; 16:564–569

[27] van Nederveen FH, Gaal J, Favier J, et al. An immunohistochemical procedure to detect patients with paraganglioma and phaeochromocytoma with germline SDHB, SDHC, or SDHD gene mutations: a retrospective and prospective analysis. Lancet Oncol. 2009; 10:764–771

[28] Kudva YC, Sawka AM, Young WF,Jr. Clinical review 164: The laboratory diagnosis of adrenal pheochromocytoma: the Mayo Clinic experience. Journal of Clinical Endocrinology and Metabolism. 2003; 88:4533–4539

[29] de Jong WH, Eisenhofer G, Post WJ, et al. Dietary influences on plasma and urinary metanephrines: implications for diagnosis of catecholamine-producing tumors. Journal of Clinical Endocrinology and Metabolism. 2009; 94:2841–2849

[30] Chretien PB, Engelman K, Hoye RC, et al. Surgical Management of Intravascular Glomus Jugulare Tumor. Am J Surg. 1971; 122:740–743

[31] Jackson CG, Harris PF, Glasscock MEI, et al. Diagnosis and Management of Paragangliomas of the Skull Base. Am J Surg. 1990; 159:389–393

[32] Farrior JB, Hyams VJ, Benke RH, et al. Carcinoid Apudoma Arising in a Glomus Jugulare Tumor: Review of Endocrine Activity in Glomus Jugulare Tumors. Laryngoscope. 1980; 90:110–119

[33] Jensen NF. Glomus Tumors of the Head and Neck: Anesthetic Considerations. Anesth Analg. 1994; 78:112–119

[34] Jackson CG, Glasscock ME, Nissen AJ, et al. Glomus Tumor Surgery: The Approach, Results, and Problems. Otolaryngol Clin North Am. 1982; 15:897–916

[35] Kim J-A, Elkon D, Lim M-L, et al. Optimum Dose of Radiotherapy for Chemodectomas of the Middle Ear. International Journal of Radiation Oncology and Biological Physics. 1980; 6:815–819

[36] Cummings SW, Beale FA, Garrett PG, et al. The Treatment of Glomus Tumors in the Temporal Bone by Megavoltage Radiation. Cancer. 1984; 53:2635–2640

[37] Spector GJ, Fierstein J, Ogura JH. A Comparison of Therapeutic Modalities of Glomus Tumors in the Temporal Bone. Laryngoscope. 1976; 86:690–696

[38] Schmidek HH, Sweet WH. Operative Neurosurgical Techniques. New York 1982

[39] Hatfield PM, James AE, Schulz MD. Chemodectomas of the Glomus Jugulare. Cancer. 1972; 30:1164–1168

[40] Ciric I, Zivin I. Neuroepithelial (Colloid) Cysts of the Septum Pellucidum. J Neurosurg. 1975; 43:69–73

[41] Hernesniemi J, Leivo S. Management outcome in third ventricular colloid cysts in a defined population: a series of 40 patients treated mainly by transcallosal microsurgery. Surg Neurol. 1996; 45:2–14

[42] Giantini-Larsen A M, Garton ALA, Villamater FN, et al. Familial colloid cysts: not a chance occurrence. J Neurooncol. 2022; 157:321–332

[43] Beaumont TL, Limbrick DD,Jr, Rich KM, et al. Natural history of colloid cysts of the third ventricle. J Neurosurg. 2016; 125:1420–1430

[44] Guner M, Shaw MDM, Turner JW, et al. Computed Tomography in the Diagnosis of Colloid Cyst. Surg Neurol. 1976; 6:345–348

[45] Ryder JW, Kleinschmidt BK, Keller TS. Sudden Deterioration and Death in Patients with Benign Tumors of the Third Ventricle Area. J Neurosurg. 1986; 64:216–223

[46] Tatter SB, Ogilvy CS, Golden JA, et al. Third ventricular xanthogranulomas clinically and radiologically mimicking colloid cysts. Report of two cases. J Neurosurg. 1994; 81:605–609

[47] Mamourian AC, Cromwell LD, Harbaugh RE. Colloid Cyst of the Third Ventricle: Sometimes More Conspicuous on CT Than MR. American Journal of Neuroradiology. 1998; 19:875–878

[48] Pollock BE, Schreiner SA, Huston J,3rd. A theory on the natural history of colloid cysts of the third ventricle. Neurosurgery. 2000; 46:1077–81; discussion 1081-3

[49] El Khoury C, Brugieres P, Decq P, et al. Colloid cysts of the third ventricle: are MR imaging patterns predictive of difficulty with percutaneous treatment? AJNR Am J Neuroradiol. 2000; 21:489–492

[50] Torkildsen A. Should Extirpation be Attempted in Cases of Neoplasm in or Near the Third Ventricle of the Brain? Experiences with a Palliative Method. J Neurosurg. 1948; 5:249–275

[51] Sheikh AB, Mendelson ZS, Liu JK. Endoscopic versus microsurgical resection of colloid cysts: a systematic review and meta-analysis of 1,278 patients. World Neurosurg. 2014; 82:1187–1197

[52] Pollock BE, Huston J,3rd. Natural history of asymptomatic colloid cysts of the third ventricle. Journal of Neurosurgery. 1999; 91:364–369

[53] Beaumont TL, Limbrick DD, Patel B, et al. Surgical management of colloid cysts of the third ventricle: a single-institution comparison of endoscopic and microsurgical resection. J Neurosurg. 2022:1–9

[54] Apuzzo MLJ. Comment on Garrido E, et al.: Cerebral Venous and Sagittal Sinus Thrombosis After Transcallosal Removal of a Colloid Cyst of the Third Ventricle: Case Report. Neurosurgery. 1990; 26

[55] Bosch DA, Rahn T, Backlund EO. Treatment of Colloid Cyst of the Third Ventricle by Stereotactic Aspiration. Surg Neurol. 1978; 9:15–18

[56] Rivas JJ, Lobato RD. CT-Assisted Stereotaxic Aspiration of Colloid Cysts of the Third Ventricle. J Neurosurg. 1985; 62:238–242

[57] Mathiesen T, Grane P, Lindquist C, et al. High Recurrence Rate Following Aspiration of Colloid Cysts in the Third Ventricle. Journal of Neurosurgery. 1993; 78:748–752

[58] Musolino A, Fosse S, Munari C, et al. Diagnosis and Treatment of Colloid Cysts of the Third Ventricle by Stereotactic Drainage. Report on Eleven Cases. Surg Neurol. 1989; 32:294–299

[59] Kondziolka D, Lunsford LD. Stereotactic Management of Colloid Cysts: Factors Predicting Success. J Neurosurg. 1991; 75:45–51

[60] Hall WA, Lunsford LD. Changing Concepts in the Treatment of Colloid Cysts. An 11-Year Experience in the CT Era. J Neurosurg. 1987; 66:186–191

[61] Di Costanzo A, Tedeschi G, Di Salle F, et al. Pineal Cysts: An Incidental MRI Finding? Journal of Neurology, Neurosurgery and Psychiatry. 1993; 56:207–208

[62] Hasegawa A, Ohtsubo K, Mori W. Pineal Gland in Old Age: Quantitative and Qualitative Morphological Study of 168 Human Autopsy Cases. Brain Research. 1987; 409:343–349

[63] Torres A, Krisht AF, Akouri S. Current Management of Pineal Cysts. Contemporary Neurosurgery. 2005; 27:1–5

[64] Maurer PK, Ecklund J, Parisi JE, et al. Symptomatic Pineal Cysts: Case Report. Neurosurgery. 1990; 27:451–454

[65] Wisoff JH, Epstein F. Surgical Management of Symptomatic Pineal Cysts. Journal of Neurosurgery. 1992; 77:896–900

[66] Klein P, Rubinstein LJ. Benign Symptomatic Glial Cysts of The Pineal Gland: A Report of Seven Cases and Review of the Literature. Journal of Neurology, Neurosurgery and Psychiatry. 1989; 52:991–995

[67] Mamourian AC, Towfighi J. Pineal Cysts: MR Imaging. American Journal of Neuroradiology. 1986; 7:1081–1086

[68] Nevins EJ, Das K, Bhojak M, et al. Incidental Pineal Cysts: Is Surveillance Necessary? World Neurosurg. 2016; 90:96–102

[69] Jussila MP, Olsen P, Salokorpi N, et al. Follow-up of pineal cysts in children: is it necessary? Neuroradiology. 2017; 59:1265–1273

[70] Di Chirico A, Di Rocco F, Velardi F. Spontaneous regression of a symptomatic pineal cyst after endoscopic third-ventriculostomy. Childs Nerv Syst. 2001; 17:42–46

[71] Berhouma M, Ni H, Delabar V, et al. Update on the management of pineal cysts: Case series and a review of the literature. Neurochirurgie. 2015; 61:201–207

[72] Wenger Markus, Simko Marian, Markwalder Regula, et al. An entirely suprasellar Rathke's cleft cyst: case report and review of the literature. Journal of Clinical Neuroscience. 2001; 8:564–567

[73] Maggio WW, Cail WS, Brookeman JR, et al. Rathke's Cleft Cyst: Computed Tomographic and Magnetic Resonance Imaging Appearances. Neurosurgery. 1987; 21:60–62

[74] Nishio S, Mizuno J, Barrow DL, et al. Pituitary Tumors Composed of Adenohypophysial Adenoma and Rathke's Cleft Cyst Elements: A Clinicopathological Study. Neurosurgery. 1987; 21:371–377

[75] Voelker JL, Campbell RL, Muller J. Clinical, Radiographic, and Pathological Features of Symptomatic Rathke's Cleft Cysts. Journal of Neurosurgery. 1991; 74:535–544

[76] Han SJ, Rolston JD, Jahangiri A, et al. Rathke's cleft cysts: review of natural history and surgical outcomes. J Neurooncol. 2014; 117:197–203

[77] Benveniste RJ, King WA, Walsh J, et al. Surgery for Rathke cleft cysts: technical considerations and outcomes. J Neurosurg. 2004; 101:577–584

[78] Byun WM, Kim OL, Kim D. MR imaging findings of Rathke's cleft cysts: significance of intracystic nodules. AJNR Am J Neuroradiol. 2000; 21:485–488

[79] Aho CJ, Liu C, Zelman V, et al. Surgical outcomes in 118 patients with Rathke cleft cysts. J Neurosurg. 2005; 102:189–193

[80] Sanno N, Oyama K, Tahara S, et al. A survey of pituitary incidentaloma in Japan. Eur J Endocrinol. 2003; 149:123–127

[81] Kino H, Akutsu H, Tanaka S, et al. Endoscopic endonasal cyst fenestration into the sphenoid sinus using the mucosa coupling method for symptomatic Rathke's cleft cyst: a novel method for maintaining cyst drainage to prevent recurrence. J Neurosurg. 2019:1–11

[82] Lillehei KO, Widdel L, Astete CA, et al. Transsphenoidal resection of 82 Rathke cleft cysts: limited value of alcohol cauterization in reducing recurrence rates. J Neurosurg. 2011; 114:310–317

[83] Haughton VM, Rosenbaum AE, Williams AL, et al. Recognizing the empty sella by CT: the infundibulum sign. AJR Am J Roentgenol. 1981; 136:293–295

[84] Kaufman B. The "empty" sella turcica - A manifestation of the intrasellar subarachnoid space. Radiology. 1968; 90:931–941

[85] Perani D, Scotti G, Colombo N, et al. Spontaneous CSF rhinorrhea through the lamina cribrosa associated with primary empty sella. Italian Journal of Neurological Sciences. 1984; 5:167–172

[86] Lee WM, Adams JE. The Empty Sella Syndrome. J Neurosurg. 1968; 28:351–356

[87] Alvarez Berastegui G R, Raza SM, Anand VK, et al. Endonasal endoscopic transsphenoidal chiasmapexy using a clival cranial base cranioplasty for visual loss from massive empty sella following macroprolactinoma treatment with bromocriptine: case report. J Neurosurg. 2015:1–7

[88] Fouad W. Review of empty sella syndrome and its surgical mangement. Alexandria Journal of Medicine. 2011; 47:139–147

56

57 Pseudotumor Cerebri Syndrome (PTCS)

57.1 General information

Key concepts

- increased ICP in the absence of a mass, hydrocephalus, CNS infection, or malignant hypertension
- primarily a neuro-ophthalmological (due to visual loss) and neurologic (due to H/A) condition
- a preventable cause of (often permanent) blindness from optic nerve atrophy
- may be primary (idiopathic intracranial hypertension) or secondary (to other conditions)
- more common in women of childbearing age who are either obese (BMI ≥ 30 kg/m^2) or who have recently gained weight than in the general population
- diagnostic criteria for pseudotumor cerebri syndrome (PTCS):
  - papilledema
  - ICP elevation ≥ 25 cm CSF on a properly performed LP
  - normal CSF analysis (no pleocytosis, elevated protein, hypoglycorrhachia, abnormal cytology, or other indication of infection or malignancy)
  - no focal neurologic deficit. Allowed exception: abducens (CN VI) palsy
  - no intracranial mass, infection, hydrocephalus, or hypertensive encephalopathy
  - normal neuroimaging. Allowed exceptions: slit-like ventricles and/or findings associated with increased intracranial pressure (empty sella (p. 951), transverse sinus stenosis, or intraorbital findings including flattening of the posterior globe (p. 587), dilated optic nerve sheath (p. 587) ...)
- pseudotumor cerebri syndrome without papilledema (p. 958) (PTCSWOP) is a variant with less risk to vision and more refractory H/A. May not be the same condition
- symptoms: headache is present in > 90% of patients. However, class I evidence suggests that H/A does not correlate with opening pressure (OP) on LP
- risk of blindness correlates best with progressive visual field constriction (enlarging blind spot is characteristic) diagnosed on visual field testing, and is not reliably correlated to duration of symptoms, degree of papilledema, H/A, Snellen visual acuity, or number of recurrences
- recommended work-up:
  - ✓ brain MRI (without and with contrast) to include craniocervical junction (to R/O Chiari malformation)
  - ✓ brain MRV to evaluate dural sinuses for patients who are male or not obese, or who have progression of visual deficit despite treatment
  - ✓ LP: measure opening pressure (OP) in lateral decubitus position, and send CSF at a minimum for cell count, protein and glucose, cytology and culture (aerobic, anaerobic, fungal, and TB)
  - ✓ BP (blood pressure) to R/O hypertensive encephalopathy
  - ophthalmologic eval. Priorities: ✓ visual fields and ✓ papilledema
    Secondarily: ✓ acuity, color vision, intraocular pressure, EOM testing for abducens palsy
  - assess for common associated conditions: obstructive sleep apnea, hypervitaminosis A or use of retinoids, iron deficiency anemia...
- long-term treatment depends on weight loss and appropriate H/A treatment
- neurosurgical involvement is generally restricted to
  - acute intervention for threatened vision (in cases of fulminant PTCS (p. 967))
  - treating surgical conditions that are not PTSC (tumors, subdural hematomas, hydrocephalus, cerebral hemorrhages...)
  - in a shunted patient, diagnosing and correcting overshunting if present
  - in limited circumstances: treating refractory H/A accompanied by increased ICP, preferably under advisement of a multidisciplary panel if available
- nonsurgical treatment:
  - weight loss: the only disease modifying treatment. 6-15% weight loss usually resolves papilledema. Dietary consultation and/or bariatric surgery may help
  - medical management: provides modest improvement. Acetazolamide (Diamox®) is initial drug of choice. Alternative: Topamax
- procedural interventions: not recommended unless vision threatened. Primarily:
  - optic nerve sheath fenestration (ONSF): best for visual loss without H/A
  - CSF shunt: better than ONSF for refractory H/A associated with visual loss

57

- stenting for bilateral focal transverse sinus stenosis: controversial. Requires antiplatelet drugs X ≈ 6 mos afterwards, which precludes other procedures (e.g., ONSF, shunting, LP...) during that time. Possible indications: a gradient > 8 mmHg (some say 5) across the stenosis in the presence of refractory increased ICP

First described in 1897 by Heinrich Quincke,[1] who called it "serous meningitis."

The nomenclature has varied widely over the years, and terms used include[2]: otitic hydrocephalus, pseudotumor cerebri (which was abandoned for a time and is now embraced), idiopathic intracranial hypertension (IIH) and the repudiated term which should be avoided "benign intracranial hypertension" (because loss of vision and reduced quality of life from debilitating headaches are not benign).

The following taxonomy has been endorsed in the U.S.[3] and abroad[4]:

▶ **Pseudotumor cerebri syndrome (PTCS).** A group of conditions characterized by increased intracranial pressure with no evidence of intracranial mass, hydrocephalus, infection (e.g., meningitis, especially chronic ones such as fungal meningitis), or hypertensive encephalopathy (see ▶ Table 57.3 for diagnostic criteria) which encompasses:
1. idiopathic intracranial hypertension (IIH) AKA primary pseudotumor cerebri. Includes: patients with obesity, recent weight gain, polycystic ovarian syndrome and thin children
2. secondary pseudotumor cerebri. Underlying causes include: conditions that increase intracranial venous pressure (dural venous sinus thrombosis, jugular vein thrombosis, superior vena cava syndrome...), certain medications and medical conditions (see below)

Either primary or secondary PTSC patients may have either:
1. papilledema (p. 586): this is considered "pseudotumor cerebri syndrome" or
2. "pseudotumor cerebri syndrome without papilledema (p. 958)" (PTCSWOP) which may be diagnosed in patients without papilledema (Frisen stage 0 ▶ Table 33.1) meeting PTCSWOP criteria in ▶ Table 57.3

57.2 Epidemiology

1. female:male ratio reported ranges from 2:1 to 8:1 (no gender difference in juvenile form)
2. obesity (BMI > 30 kg/m²) is reported in 11–90% of cases and is not as prevalent in men with PTCS[5]
3. incidence among obese women of childbearing years[6,7]: 19–21/100,000 (compared to incidence in general population[2]: 1–2/100,000). Also occurs in patients with recent weight gain (5-15% weight gain in the past year)[8]
4. peak incidence in 3rd decade (range: 1–55 years). 37% of cases are in children, 90% of these are age 5–15 years
5. PTCS is rare in age < 3 years or > 60 years: in these age groups other causes of increased ICP should be strongly considered[3]
6. frequently self limited: recurrence rate: 9–43%
7. severe visual deficits develop in 4–12%, unrelated to duration of symptoms, degree of papilledema, headache, visual obscuration, and number of recurrences.[9] Perimetry is the best means to detect and follow visual loss

57.3 Natural history

Spontaneous resolution may occur, sometimes within months, but usually after ≈ 1 year. Papilledema persists in ≈ 15%. *Permanent* visual loss occurs in 2–24% (depending on criteria used and degree to which it is sought). Persistent H/A may occur. PTCS recurs in ≈ 10% after initial resolution.[10]

57.4 Associated conditions

57.4.1 General information

Some cases of PTCS are idiopathic (IIH), i.e., primary. The remainder are secondary to another condition, e.g., transverse sinus thrombosis, hypervitaminosis A... (see below). Many conditions cited as being associated with PTCS may be coincidental. Four criteria suggested to establish a cause-effect relationship are shown in ▶ Table 57.1.[11]

Table 57.1 Criteria for causality of PTCS by another condition[11]

1. meets Dandy's criteria (▶ Table 57.4)
2. the condition should be proven to increase ICP
3. treatment of the condition should improve the PTCS
4. properly controlled studies should show an association between the condition and PTCS

▶ Table 57.2 shows a scale[12] to rank the likelihood of association between various conditions and PTCS that is somewhat dated.

Table 57.2 Conditions that may be associated with PTCS (modified[12])

Proven association

Meets 4 criteria from ▶ Table 57.1

- obesity. Recent weight gain (5-15% weight gain in the year prior to the diagnosis of PTCS was associated with increased risk of PTCS)[8]

Likely association

Meets 3 criteria from ▶ Table 57.1

- drugs: keprone, lindane
- hypervitaminosis A or use of retinoids

Probable association

Meets 2 criteria from ▶ Table 57.1

- steroid withdrawal[a]
- thyroid replacement in children
- ketoprofen & indomethacin in Bartter syndrome
- hypoparathyroidism
- Addison's disease[a]
- uremia
- iron deficiency anemia
- drugs: tetracycline, nalidixic acid, Danazol, lithium, amiodarone, phenytoin, nitrofurantoin, ciprofloxacin, nitroglycerin

Possible association

Meets 1 criteria from ▶ Table 57.1

- menstrual irregularity
- oral contraceptive use[b]
- Cushing's syndrome
- vitamin A deficiency
- minor head trauma
- Behçet syndrome

Unlikely association

Meets none of the criteria in ▶ Table 57.1

- hyperthyroidism
- steroid use
- immunization

Unsupported association

- pregnancy
- menarche

[a]may respond to steroids
[b]may be associated with dural sinus thrombosis, see text

Other conditions not included in this list that meet minimal criteria but are unconfirmed in case-control studies[2] include:

1. other drugs: isotretinoin (Accutane®), trimethoprim-sulfamethoxazole, cimetidine, tamoxifen, fluoroquinones[13]
2. systemic lupus erythematosus (SLE)
3. obstructive sleep apnea (OSA): hypercarbia increases ICP

Conditions that may be related by virtue of increased pressure in the dural sinuses (see below):
1. otitis media with petrosal extension (so-called otitic hydrocephalus)
2. radical neck surgery with resection of the jugular vein
3. hypercoagulable states

57.4.2 Venous hypertension and sinovenous abnormalities

Venous hypertension has often been proposed as a unifying underlying cause of PTCS. Abnormalities of the dural sinuses, including thrombosis, stenosis,[14] obstruction, or elevated pressure (reaching levels as high as 40 mm Hg) have been demonstrated in a number of studies. While these findings may underlie a number of cases, in many cases they may actually be epiphenomena (e.g., venous hypertension may be due to compression of the transverse sinuses by elevated intracranial pressure[15]), and it is unlikely that such abnormalities will explain all cases.

Bilateral sinovenous stenosis was seen (using 3D gadolinium-enhanced MRI venography) in 27 of 29 patients with PTCS and in only 4 of 59 controls.[14]

57.4.3 CSF fistula (leaks)

A subgroup of PTCS patients also have CSF fistula.[16] It is possible that the fistula arises as a result of chronic increased ICP (many years) causing erosion of the skull base and dural defects.[17] CSF fistula may actually protect against papilledema in patients with PTCS,[18] and cases have been reported where repair of the fistula results in increased ICPs to levels similar to PTCS without CSF fistula.[17] Furthermore, fistula repair has a higher rate of failure if the elevated ICP is not also treated.[17]

57.5 Diagnostic criteria

Diagnostic criteria are summarized in ▶ Table 57.3. Details of the criteria components appear in following sections.

Modified[21] Dandy's criteria[22] are still referenced especially in research articles (e.g., the IIHTT[21]), and are shown in ▶ Table 57.4.

▶ **Pseudotumor cerebri syndrome without papilledema (PTCSWOP).** May be diagnosed in patients without papilledema (Frisen stage 0 ▶ Table 33.1) meeting criteria in ▶ Table 57.3. Diagnoing PTCSWOP can be difficult, and subtle findings should be ruled out by an experienced trained observer.[23] Papilledema may not be discernible in the presence of optic atrophy.

This may not be the same disease entity as PTCS[3] Compared to patients with papilledema, PTCSWOP patients typically have:
1. lower opening pressure on LP: mean: 30.9 cm CSF (which is still abnormally elevated), vs. 37.3 in those with papilledema
2. higher incidence of photopsia (flashes of light)
3. higher incidence of non-physiologic visual field constriction[23] which tend not to progress over time[23,24]
4. lower incidence of abducens palsy
5. higher incidence of normal visual fields on presentation[23]
6. H/A that are more refractory to treatment[23,25]
7. preserved venous pulsation on funduscopy[23]

57.6 Clinical findings

57.6.1 Symptoms

See references.[11,26,27,28]
1. headache (H/A), see details (p. 960)
   a) the most common symptom, reported in > 90%[29] (range: 76–99%)
   b) results in significant disability and reduced quality of life[30]
2. tinnitus: 52-61%. The causal relationship with PTCS has been demonstrated by resolution of these symptoms with reduction of CSF pressure. Usually pulse synchronous. Described as rushing noise. May be unilateral (in these, tinnitus may be reduced by ipsilateral jugular vein compression + ipsilateral head rotation)
3. visual loss, see details (p. 961)
   • transient visual obscuration (TVO): 68-72%

Table 57.3 Diagnostic criteria for pseudotumor cerebri syndrome (PTCS)[3]

Criteria	PTCS		PTCS without papilledema	
	Definite	Probable	Definite	Suggested
papilledema[a]	+	+	-	-
normal neurologic exam[b]	+	+	+	+
normal neuroimaging[c]	+	+	+	+
normal CSF composition[d]	+	+	+	+
OP > 25 cm CSF on LP[e]	+	-	+	+
abducens nerve palsy (p. 598) [f]			+	-
≥ 3 neuroimaging criteria[g]			-	+

[a] (see text (p. 960) for description) may be asymmetric or (uncommonly) unilateral. NB: papilledema may not be reliably diagnosable in the presence of optic atrophy

[b] exception: cranial nerve abnormalities (usually VI or VII). For other deficits (e.g., encephalopathy, focal deficit...) other diagnoses should be sought

[c] MRI (or CT if MRI cannot be done) without and with contrast. May show findings of increased ICP (see g below), but must show normal brain parenchyma without hydrocephalus, mass or structural lesion, and
• for typical patient (specifically: obese (BMI ≥ 30 kg/m^2) female adult or adolescent[19]):
  no abnormal meningeal enhancement
• for others (men, non-obese women, prepubescent children, and patients with progressive visual loss despite therapy):
  no abnormal meningeal enhancement and normal MRV
NB: meningeal enhancement may occasionally be seen shortly after an LP

[d] none of the following: pleocytosis, elevated protein, hypoglycorrhachia, abnormal cytology or other indication of infection or malignancy

[e] opening pressure on a properly performed LP (p. 962) (see text):
in adults, or children who are not sedated or obese: ≥ 25 cm CSF,
in children who are sedated or obese: ≥ 28 cm CSF

[f] unilateral or bilateral, may be complete or incomplete. Produces esotropia (inward eye deviation)

[g] ≥ 3 neuroimaging criteria suggestive of increased ICP:
1. empty sella ► Fig. 56.6 (85% of PTCS had partial or complete empty sella)[20]
2. flattening of the posterior globe (► Fig. 33.1)
3. optic nerve sheath distension (► Fig. 33.1) with or without a tortuous optic nerve
4. transverse venous sinus (TVS) stenosis (but not thrombosis) is present in most cases of PTCS[3] (see MRV (p. 964) for details)

Table 57.4 Modified modified Dandy's criteria for PTCS

• signs & symptoms of increased ICP
• no localizing signs (other than possible Cr. N VI palsy[a] in an otherwise awake and alert patient)
• increased CSF pressure without chemical or cytological CSF abnormalities
• normal neuroimaging (especially no intracranial mass) aside from small ventricles and findings of increased ICP

[a] abducens palsy may result from ↑ ICP (p. 598)

• blurry vision: 32%
• afferent visual pathway injury: often reversible but may be permanent
4. diplopia: 18–30%. More common in adults, usually horizontal due to VI nerve palsy
5. less common or uncharacteristic symptoms
   a) neck stiffness (30–50%) or neck pain (42%)
   b) ataxia: 4–11%
   c) acral paresthesias: 25%
   d) back pain: 53%
   e) nausea: 32% (actual vomiting is less common)
   f) retrobulbar eye pain on eye movements
   g) arthralgia: 11–18%
   h) dizziness: 32-52%
   i) fatigue
   j) reduced olfactory acuity

NB: Worsening of any of the above symptoms with postural changes that increase ICP (bending over, Valsalva maneuver…) is characteristic in PTCS.

▶ **Headache in PTCS.** According to The International Classification of Headache Disorders, 3rd edition (ICHD-3),[31 (p 99)] H/A attributable to PTCS is a H/A in a patient with a nonvascular intracranial disorder known to cause H/A (here: increased ICP documented by OP ≥ 25 cm on LP) that is not better accounted for by another ICHD-3 diagnosis, and fulfills at least 2 of the following*
1. H/A developed in temporal relation to PTCS or led to its discovery
2. H/A worsens in parallel to worsening of PTCS (i.e., increasig ICP) and/or improves in parallel to improvement of PTCS (e.g., by reducing ICP)
3. H/A are typical for PTCS

* This definition has been challenged, since recent Class I evidence in a study of 165 PTCS patients with papilledema and mild vision loss[29] found:
1. there are no typical H/A characteristics for PTCS. H/A phenotype in PTCS changes over time, and is often mixed. 93% of patients with H/A in the IIHTT had features consistent with definitie or probable migraine (68%) or tension H/A (25%). Non-migraine H/A phenotypes may be exacerbated by increased ICP
2. H/A in PTCS did not correlate with opening pressure, BMI, papilledema grade or use of acetazolamide. 62% of patients continued to have H/A after successful treatment of increased CSF pressure[32]
3. ★ despite the fact that patients and providers perceive that H/As are linked to CSF pressure and that lowering CSF pressure will improve H/A control, evidence demonstrates that H/A and CSF pressure are clinically independent features of PTCS

NB: the findings in patients recruited to the study may not be generalizable e.g., to a patient who presents to the E/R with H/A and an occluded shunt.

Medication overuse headache (MOH): medication overuse (which can lead to medication overuse H/A) was found in 37% of H/A patients in the IIHTT.[29] MOH diagnostic criteria[31 (p 122)]:
1. H/A occurring ≥ 15 days/month in a patient with pre-existing primary H/A, developing as a result of regular overuse of H/A medication ≥ 10 days/month (for opioids, combined preparations, ergotamines or triptans) or ≥ 15 days/month (for NSAIDs, APAP, ASA)
2. regular overuse for > 3 months
3. not better accounted for by another ICHD-3 diagnosis

MOH usually (but not always) resolve after medication overuse stops.

57.6.2 Signs

General information

- signs are generally restricted to the visual system (see below)
- ✖ paradoxically *absent*: altered level of consciousness in spite of high ICP
- the presence of a focal neurologic deficit, or any unexplained cranial nerve deficit (except for abducens palsy) should prompt a search for an alternative diagnosis to PTCS
- the infantile form of PTCS may have only enlarging OFC, is frequently self-limited, and usually requires only follow-up without specific treatment

Eye findings in PTCS

Ophthalmologic consultation is generally recommended, especially in questionable cases.
1. papilledema
   a) the sine qua non of PTCS
   b) if papilledema is absent, PTCS without papilledema (PTCSWOP) may be diagnosed if the diagnostic criteria for that are met (▶ Table 57.3 [3,23,33])
   c) findings: optic disc elevation, blurring of the disc margin, peripilary halo, obscuration by nerve fiber layer of blood vessels crossing the disc margin, venous distension, and overlying of peripapillary hemorrhages, exudates, or cotton-wool spots[3]
   d) usually bilateral, may be asymmetric, infrequently unilateral[34]
   e) may be mild (subtle nerve fiber elevation)
   f) may be absent in cases of optic atrophy or resolved prior optic disc swelling[3]

g) other etiologies that must be ruled out include: optic neuritis, anterior ischemic optic neuropathy, neuroretinitis, pseudopapilledema (p. 588) (includes optic nerve head drusen)
2. abducens nerve (Cr. N. VI) palsy: 20%; a false localizing sign (p. 598). The esotropia ranges from < 5 prism diopters dysconjugate angle in primary gaze to > 50[10]
3. ★ visual field defect: correlates with visual loss more closely than other findings (see below)
4. visual acuity: relatively insensitive assessment of visual function in PTCS (see below)
5. loss of color vision: not sensitive for early papilledema-related optic atrophy

57.6.3 Visual loss in PTCS

General information

Prevalence in PTCS: 48–68% (lower numbers generally come from population-based samples).

Visual loss in PTCS may occur early or late, and is not reliably correlated to duration of symptoms, papilledema, H/A, visual acuity (as tested with a standard Snellen eye chart), or number of recurrences. Visual loss is usually gradual and spares central vision until late in the course[35] and thus may not be noticed by the patient until profound. In some cases visual loss can be sudden.

Visual field deficits are the most sensitive means for detecting visual loss in PTCS.

Pathomechanics

Increased ICP is transmitted along the optic nerve sheath → circumferential compression of the retinal ganglion cell axons at the level of the lamina cribrosa.[10]

Manifestations

1. transient visual obscurations (TVO): graying or blacking out of vision. Lasts ≈ 1 second. Uni- or bilateral. Typically occur with eye movement, bending over, or Valsalva maneuver. Directly proportional to severity of papilledema. Frequency of TVOs parallels ICP elevation, but doesn't correlate with permanent visual loss
2. ★ visual field deficits: the most sensitive measure of visual impairment in PTCS, found in 96% of 50 patients in one prospective series.[36] Visual field defects are diagnosed by perimetry (p. 589) (e.g., Goldmann or Humphrey). Automated perimetry can be quantified (to generate a measurement for comparison) as the perimetric mean deviation (PMD) (p. 589)
   a) enlarged blind spots are the classic field defect in PTCS, but are rarely noticed by the patient until there is encroachment on macular vision (fixation)[35]
   b) early changes[35]: constriction of fields usually with nasal quadrant defect ("nasal step") and arcuate defects (a curved visual defect) neither of which cross the horizontal meridian
   c) late: central vision is affected. Findings include: concentric constrictions, enlarged blind spot, cecocentral scotomas…[35]
3. less common visual symptoms[37]: blurry vision (32%), diplopia (18%) (usually horizontal, may be due to abducens palsy)

57.7 Differential diagnosis

1. true mass lesions: tumor, cerebral abscess, subdural hematomas, rarely gliomatosis cerebri may be undetectable on CT and will be misdiagnosed as PTCS
2. hydrocephalus: typically ventricles are enlarged. Patients generally have obtundation, lethargy, vomiting… Some patients with reduced cerebral compliance may develop increased ICP without ventriculomegaly
3. cranial venous outflow impairment (some authors include these in IIH,[38] others do not)
   a) dural sinus thrombosis (p. 1594)
   b) congestive heart failure
   c) superior vena cava syndrome
   d) unilateral or bilateral jugular vein or sigmoid sinus[39] obstruction
   e) hyperviscosity syndromes
   f) Masson's vegetant intravascular hemangioendothelioma[40]: an uncommon, usually benign lesion that may rarely involve the neuraxis (including intracranial occurrence). Not definitely neoplastic. Organizing thrombi develop endothelialized projections into the vessel lumen. Must be distinguished from other conditions such as angiosarcoma
4. Chiari I malformation (CIM) (see Chiari-pseudotumor cerebri syndrome (p. 301))
   a) CIM may produce clinical findings similar to PTCS

57

b) 6-21% of PTCS patients have tonsillar descent ≥ 5 mm below the FM on MRI[38,41,42]
c) ≈ 5% of patients with CIM have papilledema[10]
d) if severe, LP is contraindicated
e) in some cases, tonsillar descent may be a result of intracranial hypotension (p. 421) (low CSF pressure) possibly as a result of a spinal CSF leak[43]

5. infection (CSF will be abnormal in most of these): encephalitis, arachnoiditis, meningitis (especially basal meningitis or granulomatous infections, e.g., syphilitic meningitis, chronic cryptococcal meningitis, chronic brucellosis, cat scratch disease (in rare cases may produce neuroretinitis[44])
6. inflammatory conditions: e.g., neurosarcoidosis (p. 198), SLE
7. vasculitis: e.g., Behçet's syndrome
8. metabolic conditions: e.g., lead poisoning
9. **malignant hypertension**: (DBP ≥ 120 mm Hg or SBP ≥ 180 mm Hg[45]). May produce H/A and bilateral optic disc edema, which can be indistinguishable from papilledema. May also produce hypertensive encephalopathy (p. 202). Check BP in all PTCS suspects
10. meningeal carcinomatosis
11. Guillain-Barré syndrome (p. 193): CSF protein is usually elevated
12. glaucoma: visual field defects of PTCS mimic those of glaucoma except that glaucoma does not typically have an enlarged blind spot[35]
13. following head trauma

57.8 Evaluation

57.8.1 Overview

Investigations that may help confirm the diagnosis, or rule out conditions that may mimic PTCS, or identify underlying causes of secondary PTCS:
1. history to identify other possible causes of increased ICP (► Table 57.2)
2. VS: check BP to R/O malignant HTN (which can cause optic disc edema, see above)
3. ophthalmologic evaluation. Includes: dilated funduscopic exam for papilledema (see below) and formal visual field testing (to rule-out visual loss)
4. routine serum labs: CBC (to rule-out anemia), electrolytes, PT/PTT
5. imaging:
   a) cerebral MRI without and with contrast for all patients (see details below). CT without and with contrast is performed if MRI is not an option
   b) contrast MRV (p. 964): obtain in atypical patients (pre-pubertal children, males, non-obese females) or in patients with progressive visual loss despite therapy. In practice, this is usually ordered along with the initial MRI
6. LP: measure opening pressure (**OP**) with unsedated patient in the lateral decubitus position (see below), and obtain CSF for laboratory analysis (no proven benefit of large volume tap)
7. evaluation for obstructive sleep apnea (hypercarbia increases ICP)
8. W/U for systemic conditions (e.g., sarcoidosis or SLE if other findings are suggestive, e.g., cutaneous nodules, hypercoagulable state…)

57.8.2 Ophthalmologic evaluation

A thorough exam consists of all of the following. The first 2 items are the most critical.
1. **dilated funduscopic exam** for papilledema ± fundus photographs
2. **visual field testing** may be done at bedside initially by a proficient examiner, however formal testing using quantitative perimetry with evaluation of size of blind spot and determination of perimetric mean deviation (PMD) (p. 589) should be done as soon as practical
3. visual acuity testing
4. color vision testing
5. intraocular pressure measurement

57.8.3 Lumbar puncture

If contraindications to LP (p. 1811) have been ruled out on neuroimaging, perform an LP to 1) measure opening pressure and, 2) to obtain CSF for analysis. The benefit of removing a large volume of CSF (≥ 20 ml) is uncertain.[3]

Opening pressure (OP): key requirements for a properly performed LP to diagnose PTCS:

1. position: lateral decubitus position (requisite for diagnosis,[3]) measurement is most accurate in this position without knee flexion. Other positions may increase ICP:
   a) prone position: typically used for LP under fluoroscopy, may ↑ intra-thoracic pressure → decrease venous return from the brain → increased ICP
   b) sitting position: increases measured pressure due to column of CSF above the needle
   c) if the LP needle has to be inserted with the patient prone or sitting, once CSF is coming through the needle, replace the stylet and reposition the patient to the lateral decubitus and then remove the stylet to accurately measure OP
   d) knee flexion may increase ICP (controversial in children[46])
2. avoid sedation which may cause hypoventilation → hypercapnia → increased ICP)[47]
3. keep the base of the manometer level with the right cardiac atrium
4. avoid valsalva maneuver[48] (including patient crying or forced knee-chest position)
5. magnitude: the higher the OP, the more likely that it is pathologically elevated.[37] Suggested cutoffs:
   • OP < 25 cm CSF: normal
   • ★ OP ≥ 25 cm CSF: required for diagnosis of PTCS by criteria,[3] however there is some dissent
   • OP ≥ 30 cm CSF: almost universally accepted as abnormally elevated
   • in prepubertal children: OP ≥ 28 cm CSF (or ≥ 25 cm if the child is not sedated and not obese) meets diagnostic criteria[3]
   NB: OP on LP is a snapshot of CSF pressure. Diurnal variations in CSF pressure may occasionally cause a falsely low (i.e., normal) reading. ∴ If clinical suspicion is high, an LP at a different time of day or continuous ICP monitoring may be required
6. CSF analysis to rule out infection (especially chronic, e.g., fungus, TB, or Lyme disease), inflammation (e.g., sarcoidosis, SLE), or neoplasm (e.g., carcinomatous meningitis). Minimum:
   a) protein/glucose
   b) cell count
   c) routine and fungal cultures
   d) cytology if suspicion of carcinomatous meningitis

57.8.4 MRI of the brain

Intraparenchymal abnormalities are usually absent or minimal.

Slit ventricles are common (however, the incidence may be no higher in PTCS than in age-matched controls[49]).

Tonsillar ectopia (Chiari I) is more prevalent in PTCS than controls (see above)

Most findings are those of increased ICP (not specific just for PTCS):
a) empty sella (p.951) in 30–70%. Includes partially empty sella or decreased pituitary height
b) dural sinuses stenosis: (MRV is more sensitive—see below for findings)
c) Meckel's cave enlargement[50] ► Fig. 57.1 or compression[51] which may depend on the patency of the opening (porus trigeminus)

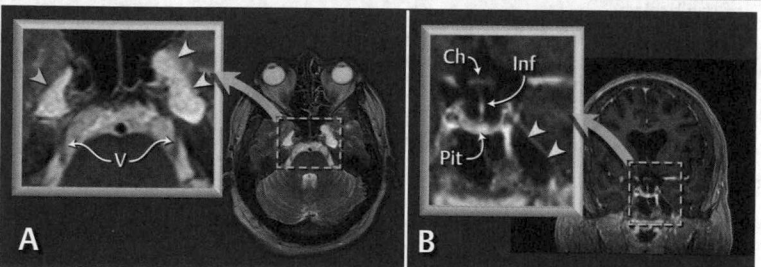

Fig. 57.1 Dilated Meckel's cave.
Image: MRI A: axial T2, B: coronal T1. Meckel's cave is mildly dilated on the right (*blue arrowhead*), and markedly dilated on the left (*yellow arrowheads*). The patient also has an empty sella demonstrating the "infundibulum sign" (see also ► Fig. 56.6).
Abbreviations: Ch = optic chiasm; Inf = infundibulum (pituitary stalk); Pit = pituitary gland; V = trigeminal nerve (Cr.N. V) as it crosses the CPA cistern.

57

d) intraorbital findings consistent with increased ICP include[10]:
  a) flattening of the posterior globe/sclera: (▶ Fig. 33.1) occurs in 80%
  b) enhancement of the prelaminar optic nerve (the prelaminar layer is essentially the middle layer of the retina): in 50%
  c) distention of the perioptic subarachnoid space (optic nerve sheath): (▶ Fig. 33.1) in 45%
  d) vertical tortuosity of the orbital optic nerve: in 40% (the intraorbital optic nerve normally has a slight "S" shape)
  e) intraocular protrusion of the prelaminar optic nerve head: in 30%

57.8.5 MRV (magnetic resonance venography)

MR venography (MRV) has largely replaced conventional venography to rule out dural sinus or venous thrombosis or AV fistula.

Indications: atypical PTCS patients (i.e., patients who are not both obese and female) or those with progressive visual loss despite therapy. If the first MRV is negative or equivocal and the suspicion of sinus thrombosis is high, a CT venogram, catheter angiogram or second MRV is indicated.

Sequences: maximum intensity projection (MIP) reconstructions from gadolinium-enhanced MRV is recommended, since time-of-flight MRV tends to overestimate stenosis.[52]

Findings: attenuation/stenosis (but not thrombosis) of dural venous sinuses is present in most cases of PTCS.[3] Includes bilateral transverse venous sinus (TVS) stenosis or stenosis of a dominant TVS (normal transverse sinuses are often asymmetric, with the right usually larger/dominant) (▶ Fig. 57.2). Bilateral TVS stenosis is uncommon in healthy individuals[53]

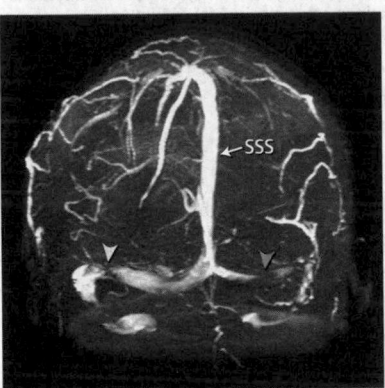

Fig. 57.2 Transverse sinus stenosis.
Image: coronal gadolinium MRV showing focal high-grade stenosis within the distal third of the dominant (larger) right transverse sinus (*yellow arrowhead*) and a longer area of stenosis in the non-dominant left transverse sinus (*blue arrowhead*). Abbreviation: SSS = superior sagittal sinus.

CT of the brain

MRI and MRV are preferred. Brain CT scan is less sensitive, but may be used if MRI is not an option. CT without and with IV contrast is usually adequate to R/O intracranial mass as a possible cause of intracranial hypertension. CT venography (CVT) may evaluate dural sinus compression.

57.9 Treatment and management

57.9.1 Treatment goals

* protect vision
* minimize headache morbidity

57.9.2 Interventional options

Overview

Initial management: usually consists of attempt at weight loss and pharmacologic therapy. However some patients will have acute (fulminant (p.967)) or progressive or persistent symptoms and require more aggressive intervention. Treatment options are shown below, management guidelines follow (p.967).

▶ **Treatment options.** This is only a catalogue of options. For *guidelines* on how to use them, see the list (p. 967) that follows.[37]
1. weight loss
2. medical treatment
    a) fluid and salt restriction, usually combined with carbonic anhydrase inhibitors
    b) carbonic anhydrase inhibitors and other diuretics: slow CSF production (see below)
    c) headaches should be characterized by phenotype and treated accordingly (p. 960) by a practitioner experienced in H/A management
    d) ✖ corticosteroids are not recommended due to the lack of sound clinical evidence.[37] Prolonged use may also exacerbate weight gain and increase the risk of venous thrombosis
3. treat obstructive sleep apnea (OSA) if present (hypercarbia increases ICP): e.g., CPAP
4. *surgical therapy* only for cases refractory to above, or where visual loss is progressive or is severe initially or unreliable patient
    a) CSF diversion (shunts): see below
    b) optic nerve sheath fenestration (p. 966) (ONSF)
    c) procedures that may be reserved for very specific situations
        • serial LPs: remove up to 30 ml to halve OP, perform qod until OP < 20 cm CSF, then decrease to q wk. Using large gauge needle (e.g., 18 Ga) may help promote a (desirable) post-LP CSF leak into subcutaneous tissues. LPs may be difficult in obese patients. Not recommended routinely.[37]
        Side effects: include sciatica from nerve root irritation, acquired cerebellar tonsillar herniation (p. 456), spinal H/A (from intracranial hypotension), back pain, risk of spinal hematoma (epidural or subdural)
        • decompressive craniectomy, usually subtemporal decompression (p. 967)
5. endovascular procedures (p. 966): transverse sinus stenting

Weight loss

This is the only disease-modifying therapy for PTCS. Patients with BMI ≥ 30 kg/m^2 should be counseled regarding weight management in a sensitive manner. The amount of weight loss required to arrest PTCS is not known. 15% weight loss was required in one cohort,[54] 6% weight loss resulted in 3 Frisen papilledema grade improvement (▶ Table 33.1) in a smaller study.[55]

NB: resolution of PTCS is too slow for acutely threatened vision. Also, symptoms often recur if the weight is regained.
• dieting: uncontrolled studies[56] suggest that this is effective, but it is difficult to accomplish and maintain
• bariatric surgery: gastric bypass, laparoscopic banding… may help

Diuretics

1. carbonic anhydrase (CA) inhibitors:
    a) *acetazolamide* (Diamox®): has been extensively studied.[21,57,58,59] Conclusion: when combined with a low-sodium weight-reduction diet, acetazolamide provides a modest improvement in papilledema, ICP and QOL,[21] but its use is often limited by side effects.[37] Has not been shown to be effective for treating H/A alone.
    ℞ start at 125–250 mg PO q 8–12 hrs, or long-acting Diamox Sequels® 500 mg PO BID. Increase by 250 mg/day until symptoms improve, side effects occur. 1 gm/d is usually tolerated,[60] 3 gm/d is a usual upper limit but doses up to 4 gm/day may be needed[59] (usually in very obese patients)
    Duration: no consensus. Expert opinion: treat for up to 2 years
    Side effects: at high doses: acral paresthesias, nausea, metabolic acidosis, altered taste, renal calculi, drowsiness, diarrhea. Rare: Stevens-Johnson syndrome, toxic epidermal necrolysis, agranulocytosis.
    ✖ contraindications: allergy to sulfa or a history of renal calculi. Use under advisement of high-risk obstetrician during pregnancy due to claims of teratogenicity (which are disputed)
    b) topiramate (Topamax®): antiseizure medication with secondary inhibition of CA. ℞ start at 50 mg/d,[61] with weekly dose escalation by 25-50 mg/d up to 100-150 mg/d.[61] May help weight reduction by suppressing appetite
    Side effects: Similar to acetazolamide, but can be used in sulfa allergic patients, may reduce the efficacy of oral contraceptives, potentially teratogenic. Has significant adverse cognitive effects (see topiramate for seizures (p. 498)).
    c) methazolamide has been used in place of acetazolamide. May also be teratogenic

57

2. *furosemide* (Lasix®): used by some as an alternative, role is uncertain
   a) start: 160 mg per day in adults, adjust per symptoms and eye exam (not to CSF pressure)
   b) if ineffective, double (320 mg/day)
   c) monitor K⁺ levels and supplement as needed

Shunts

The literature regarding shunt type is mainly observational and case series based. When considering shunting, complications (shunt infection or obstruction, shunt migration, low pressure H/A (p. 462), subdural hematoma (p. 464), mortality (low risk but not negligible)…) should be taken into account.
1. ventriculoperitoneal (VP) shunt is recommended due to reported lower revision rate[25,62]
   a) navigational techniques may facilitate ventricular catheter placement in the presence of small or slit-like ventricles (which are common in PTCS[63])
   b) a programmable valve with an antisiphon device should be considered to help manage and avoid low pressure H/A
2. lumbar shunt: usually lumboperitoneal; see insertion technique (p. 1830). Often more difficult in obese patients. May need a horizontal-vertical valve (p. 458) to prevent H/A from intracranial hypotension. Alternative: lumbopleural shunt. Visual loss has been reported in patients with functioning LP shunts.[64] Other potential complications include: back pain, radiculopathy, tonsillar herniation (secondary Chiari malformation) and scoliosis (p. 456). Contraindicated in the presence of lumbar spinal arachnoiditis
3. cisterna magna shunt: has been described, not commonly used. May shunt to vascular system
▶ **Important facts about shunts in PTCS**
- shunts are very effective for *acute* treatment of H/A in PTCS (95% have relief in the 1st month)[25]
- some patients will achieve long-term relief, however, at 3 years, ≈ 50% of PTCS patients will have recurrenc of severe H/A despite a working shunt[25]
- patients without papilledema had a higher rate of recurrence of H/A (75% by 3 years)[25]
- 80% of shunts require revision by 36 months[25]

Optic nerve sheath fenestration (ONSF)

See references.[65,66,67]

A surgical procedure usually performed by an ophthalmologist to create a window (fenestration) or series of slits in the optic nerve sheath immediately posterior to the globe. This may help by allowing egress of CSF thereby reducing pressure on the optic nerve within the sheath, and may also cause scarring that prevents Performed via medial transconjunctival approach (50%), a superomedial lid crease incision (31%) a lateral orbitotomy (10%).[68]

Generally better for protection of vision and reversal of papilledema than for other symptoms (fails to improve H/A in 33-50%[69]). No reported mortality. May reverse or stabilize visual deterioration[70] and sometimes (but not always) lowers ICP (by continued CSF filtration) and may protect the contralateral eye (if not, contralateral ONSF must be performed). Has succeeded in cases where visual loss progressed after LP shunting,[64] possibly due to poor communication between orbital and intracranial subarachnoid spaces. **Potential adverse effects:** includes pupillary dysfunction, peripapillary hemorrhage, chemosis, chorioretinal scarring,[71] diplopia (usually self-limited) from medial rectus disruption, worsening of vision (central retinal artery occlusion is a risk). Needs to be repeated in up to 6%.[10]

Endovascular procedures

Transverse sinus stenting. Transverse sinus (TVS) stenosis is a common epiphenomenon of increased ICP and in many cases may be a result of and not the cause of the increase. Endovascular placement of a stent across the stenosis to re-expand the lumen has been reported to improve symptoms after other measures fail. Stenting requires antiplatelet therapy afterwards (usually for > 6 months), which may preclude other intervention (e.g., shunting) if it fails. Most studies are observational and case series. Current guidelines consider the role of neurovascular stenting as not yet established[37]; however, since their publication there has been a recent trend to move to unilateral TVS stenting for PTCS patients with persistent increased ICP and papilledema who have failed to respond adequately to medical therapy who have bilateral TVS stenosis with an elevated TVS pressure gradient (a gradient > 8 mm Hg across the stenosis has been arbitrarily recommended,[72,73] some use 5 as the cutoff).[37,74]

In a series of 32 PTCS patients,[75] 90% had a pressure gradient > 8 mmHg, with bilateral TVS narrowing. Following stenting, papilledema was eliminated in 96% and 81% were able to discontinue acetazolamide. 6% had to have a repeat procedure.

57

Decompressive craniectomy

Usually subtemporal decompression, or less frequently suboccipital decompression.

Subtemporal decompression: older treatment advocated by Dandy. Fell out of favor (possibly because of risk of post-op seizures and painful bulging at decompression site), but may still have a place in the armamentarium[76] (e.g., patient with slit ventricles and in whom lumbar-peritoneal shunting is not feasible). Steps:

1. "silver-dollar size" craniectomies (approximately 1 inch = 25.4 mm) under the temporalis muscle to the floor of the middle fossa are made (usually bilaterally) through a linear incision. Kessler et al[76] used larger 6–8 cm diameter unilateral craniectomies; this larger craniectomy may explain their high incidence (62%) of H/A and tense bulging decompression site necessitating CSF diversion
2. the dura is opened
3. the brain is covered with an absorbable sponge (e.g., Gelfoam®)
4. the fascia and muscle are closed in a watertight fashion
5. a short course of antiseizure medications is used due to risk of post-op seizures

57.9.3 Guidelines for management

Adapted from the UK Guidelines[37] (there are currently no U.S. guidelines).

General measures

1. weight loss (p. 965): the only known disease-modifying intervention. Should be attempted in all patients with BMI ≥ 30 kg/m²
2. ophthalmologic evaluation: at a minimum, dilated exam for papilledema and visual field assessment. Then, when possible, thorough ophthalmologic evaluation (p. 962) should be done
3. stop possible offending drugs: e.g., vitamin A
4. brain imaging within 24 hours:
   - MRI or CT: to rule-out surgical conditions including subdural hematoma, hydrocephalus, Chiari malformation, true mass (tumor, hemorrhage)…
   - venography: MRV or CTV. Primarily for "atypical patients" (patients who are male or not obese) or patients who have progression of visual deficit despite treatment
5. properly performed LP (p. 962) (after brain imaging rules out contraindications to LP (p. 1811), which include Chiari malformation, obstructive hydrocephalus…) or shunt tap (in patients with shunt)
   a) indications:
      1. patients who have not yet been diagnosed with PTCS
      2. patients with clinical signs of infection (meningitis, shunt infection…)
      3. patients with refractory H/A due to documented elevated CSF pressure (p. 968)
   b) objectives of LP/shunt tap:
      1. measure CSF pressure
      2. obtain CSF for analysis: routine labs. Also include CSF culture if clinical suspicion of infection
6. follow newly diagnosed patient at least two years with repeat imaging (e.g., MRI) to R/O occult tumor
7. see sections immediately below for guidelines pertaining to specific scenarios

For visual loss with PTCS

By definition of PTCS, these patients have papilledema. In addition to general measures (above):
1. ★ **fulminant PTCS**. Suggested definition: < 4 weeks between symptom onset to severe loss of acuity or visual field, and worsening of vision over a few days.[77] Severe visual is not always defined, but likely includes PMD (p. 589) more negative than about -7. Occurs in ≈ 2-3% of PTSC patients.[77] Necessitates rapid intervention to protect vision:
   a) immediate
      1. lumbar drain: when definitive treatment (shunting or ONSF) will not occur within 24 hrs, temporize by using a lumbar drain to decrease ICP
      2. start acetazolamide or topamax (see below)
   b) optic nerve sheath fenestration or CSF diversion (shunting or revision of existing shunt) ASAP. These measures work well in the short term
   c) start or continue efforts at weight loss to modify the underlying disease

Shunting may relieve both H/A and papilledema simultaneously. ONSF may be more effective in relieving visual problems (the failure rate may be lower than the shunt malfunction rate) but is not as good for the H/A.

2. mild *stable* visual loss (no immediate threat to vision)
   a) start or continue efforts at weight loss to modify the underlying disease
   b) consider medical therapy
      * acetazolamide (p. 965) plus low-sodium weight-reduction diet. Provides modest visual field improvement compared to diet alone in patients with mild visual loss,[78] and at 6 months improved QOL measures.[79] Caution re metabolic acidosis, kidney stones, pregnancy… (see acetazolamide (p. 965))
        or
      * topiramate (p. 965): may help by reducing CSF production (carbonic anhydrase effect) and by suppressing appetite which may aid weight loss
   c) evaluate H/A phenotype (including medication overuse H/A), treat accordingly
   d) ophthalmological follow-up: based on papilledema grade and visual field status as shown in ▶ Table 57.5
   e) shunt or ONSF for significant visual deterioration on follow-up

Table 57.5 Recommended ophthalmologic follow-up schedule[a] [37]

Papilledema grade	Visual field status			
	Normal	Abnormal & improving	Abnormal & stable	Abnormal & worsening
Atrophic[b]			4-6 mos	≤ 4 wks
Mild	6 mos	3-6 mos	3-4 mos	≤ 4 wks
Moderate	3-4 mos	1-3 mos	1-3 mos	≤ 2 wks
Severe		1-3 mos	≤ 4 weeks	≤ 7 days

[a] once papilledema resolves, follow-up is not necessary except for asymptomatic patients who require longer follow-up since they will not be aware if there is recurrence
[b] atrophic papilledema: visible optic nerve head pallor due to nonviable optic nerve axons. Precludes diagnosis of papilledema

For H/A with PTCS and no visual loss (or mild/stable visual loss)

"Despite significant headache morbidity in IIH, there are no randomized controlled trials to guide headache management in IIH."[37] In addition to general measures (above):

1. rule-out overshunting (p. 462) in patients with shunts (low-pressure H/A, thickened meninges on imaging…). Consider revision if present
2. LP or shunt tap only for clinical suspicion of infection
3. a multidisciplinary approach involving a practitioner with expertise in H/A management is recommended to assess H/A phenotype (including medication overuse H/A) and to direct treatment specific for that phenotype
4. medication: judicious use of *non-opioid* medical therapy to treat H/A in the short-term (for the first few weeks) may help. Medication overuse headache (p. 960) (MOH) can occur with long-term use and is treated by elimination of overuse[80]
5. greater occipital nerve block: may be considered, but effectiveness is controversial
6. ✖ *not* recommended for H/A alone (without visual loss):
   * medication to ↓ ICP: acetazolamide has not been shown to be effective for H/A alone (see above)
   * CSF shunting or shunt revision*:[37] limited evidence of efficacy. 68% continue to have H/A at 6 months, and 79% at 2 years, 28% develop low pressure H/A.[81] Failure of shunting may be attributable to inadequate medical treatment of a migrainous component or medication overuse H/A
   * optic nerve sheath fenestration (ONSF)
   * serial LPs are not recommended for H/A alone[37]
   * neurovascular stenting is not recommended for H/A[37]

* Shunting or shunt revision may be indicated for refractory H/A, and then only after elevated ICP is documented (e.g., on ICP monitoring) and preferably under advisement of a multidisciplinary team (neurologist, ophthalmologist, sleep medicine, and neurosurgeon)

For pseudotumor cerebri syndrome without papilledema (PTCSWOP)

For PTCSWOP (p. 958),
1. "risk of visual loss has not been identified and does not seem to develop over the disease course."[37] Caution: papilledema may not be reliably discerned if optic atrophy is present
2. counselling as appropriate for weight management (p. 965) as with PTCS
3. H/A should be managed as with PTCS (see above)
4. ✖ surgical intervention (shunting, shunt revision, or ONSF) to control increased ICP should not be considered unless advised by a multidisciplinary team

Asymptomatic PTCS patients

Treatment of asymptomatic PTCS patients is controversial and challenging as there is no reliable predictor for visual loss. Close follow-up with serial formal visual field evaluation is necessary. Intervention is recommended in unreliable patients, or whenever visual fields deteriorate. It is possible to lose vision without H/A or papilledema.

For PTCS in children and adolescents

1. may be seen with withdrawal of steroids used for asthma
2. search for and correction of underlying etiology (offending drugs listed above, hypercalcemia, cancer…)
3. acetazolamide has been used with success

For PTCS in pregnancy

1. women who first present with PTCS during pregnancy: resolution of PTCS following delivery is common
2. weight management to maintain weight gain that is appropriate for the gestational age of the fetus as recommended by the ACOG[82]
3. no specific mode of delivery should be recommended based on the diagnosis of PTCS
4. women who become pregnant during therapy:
   a) 1st trimester: observation, limitation of weight gain, serial LPs.
      ✖ Acetazolamide should be avoided because of teratogenicity in rodents
   b) 2nd & 3rd trimester: acetazolamide has been used safely, but involvement of high-risk obstetrician specialist is advised
   c) topiramate should not be used in pregnancy
5. if acute vision loss is threatened, serial lumbar punctures (p. 965) may be used to temporize until CSF diversion or ONSF can be performed

For pseudopapilledema

Pseudopapilledema (p. 588) (associated with drusen, etc.) in the absence of intracranial hypertension needs no intervention.[10] Reassurance and H/A management are recommended.

References

[1] Quincke HI. Meningitis serosa. Sammlung Klinischer Vorträge. 1893; 67
[2] Radhakrishnan K, Ahlskog JE, Garrity JA, et al. Idiopathic intracranial hypertension. Mayo Clinic Proceedings. 1994; 69:169–180
[3] Friedman DI, Liu GT, Digre KB. Revised diagnostic criteria for the pseudotumor cerebri syndrome in adults and children. Neurology. 2013; 81:1159–1165
[4] Johnston I, Owler B, Pickard J. The Pseudotumor Cerebri Syndrome: Pseudotumor Cerebri, Idiopathic Intracranial Hypertension, Benign Intracranial Hypertension and Related Conditions. Cambridge, England: Cambridge University Press; 2007
[5] Digre KB, Corbett JJ. Pseudotumor Cerebri in Men. Arch Neurol. 1988; 45:866–872
[6] Durcan FJ, Corbett JJ, Wall M. The Incidence of Pseudotumor Cerebri: Population Studies in Iowa and Louisiana. Arch Neurol. 1988; 45:875–877

[7] Radhakrishnan K, Ahlskog JE, Cross SA, et al. Idiopathic Intracranial Hypertension (Pseudotumor Cerebri): Descriptive Epidemiology in Rochester, Minn, 1976 to 1990. Archives of Neurology. 1993; 50:78–80
[8] Daniels AB, Liu GT, Volpe NJ, et al. Profiles of obesity, weight gain, and quality of life in idiopathic intracranial hypertension (pseudotumor cerebri). Am J Ophthalmol. 2007; 143:635–641
[9] Rush JA. Pseudotumor Cerebri: Clinical Profile and Visual Outcome in 63 Patients. Mayo Clin Proc. 1980; 55:541–546
[10] Bejjani GK, Cockerham KP, Pless M, et al. Idiopathic intracranial hypertension. Contemporary Neurosurgery. 2002; 24:1–8
[11] Giuseffi V, Wall M, Siegel PZ, et al. Symptoms and disease associations in idiopathic intracranial hypertension (pseudotumor cerebri): a case-control study. Neurology. 1991; 41:239–244

57

[12] Digre KB. Epidemiology of idiopathic intracranial hypertension. 1992

[13] Sodhi M, Sheldon CA, Carleton B, et al. Oral fluoro-quinolones and risk of secondary pseudotumor cerebri syndrome: Nested case-control study. Neurology. 2017; 89:792–795

[14] Farb RI, Vanek I, Scott JN, et al. Idiopathic intracranial hypertension: The prevalence and morphology of sinovenous stenosis. Neurology. 2003; 60:1418–1424

[15] King JO, Mitchell PJ, Thomson KR, et al. Manometry combined with cervical puncture in idiopathic intracranial hypertension. Neurology. 2002; 58:26–30

[16] Schlosser RJ, Woodworth BA, Wilensky EM, et al. Spontaneous cerebrospinal fluid leaks: a variant of benign intracranial hypertension. Ann Otol Rhinol Laryngol. 2006; 115:495–500

[17] Chaaban MR, Illing E, Riley KO, et al. Spontaneous cerebrospinal fluid leak repair: a five-year prospective evaluation. Laryngoscope. 2014; 124:70–75

[18] Aaron G, Doyle J, Vaphiades MS, et al. Increased intracranial pressure in spontaneous CSF leak patients is not associated with papilledema. Otolaryngol Head Neck Surg. 2014; 151:1061–1066

[19] Friedman DI, Jacobson DM. Idiopathic intracranial hypertension. Journal of Neuro-Ophthalmology. 2004; 24:138–145

[20] Yuh WT, Zhu M, Taoka T, et al. MR imaging of pituitary morphology in idiopathic intracranial hypertension. J Magn Reson Imaging. 2000; 12:808–813

[21] The NORDIC Idiopathic Intracranial Hypertension Study Group Writing Committee, Wall M, McDermott MP, et al. Effect of acetazolamide on visual function in patients with idiopathic intracranial hypertension and mild visual loss: the idiopathic intracranial hypertension treatment trial. JAMA. 2014; 311:1641–1651

[22] Smith JL. Whence pseudotumor cerebri? J Clin Neuroophthalmol. 1985; 5:55–56

[23] Digre KB, Nakamoto BK, Warner JE, et al. A comparison of idiopathic intracranial hypertension with and without papilledema. Headache. 2009; 49:185–193

[24] Kathol RG, Cox TA, Corbett JJ, et al. Functional visual loss. Follow-up of 42 cases. Arch Ophthalmol. 1983; 101:729–735

[25] McGirt MJ, Woodworth G, Thomas G, et al. Cerebrospinal fluid shunt placement for pseudotumor cerebri-associated intractable headache: predictors of treatment response and an analysis of long-term outcomes. J Neurosurg. 2004; 101:627–632

[26] Ahlskog JE, O'Neill BP. Pseudotumor Cerebri. Ann Int Med. 1982; 97:249–256

[27] Round R, Keane JR. The minor symptoms of increased intracranial hypertension: 101 patients with benign intracranial hypertension. Neurology. 1988; 38:1461–1464

[28] Markey KA, Mollan SP, Jensen RH, et al. Understanding idiopathic intracranial hypertension: mechanisms, management, and future directions. Lancet Neurol. 2016; 15:78–91

[29] Friedman DI, Quiros PA, Subramanian PS, et al. Headache in Idiopathic Intracranial Hypertension: Findings From the Idiopathic Intracranial Hypertension Treatment Trial. Headache. 2017; 57:1195–1205

[30] Digre KB, Bruce BB, McDermott MP, et al. Quality of life in idiopathic intracranial hypertension at diagnosis: IIH Treatment Trial results. Neurology. 2015; 84:2449–2456

[31] Headache Classification Committee of the International Headache Society (IHS) The International Classification of Headache Disorders, 3rd edition. Cephalalgia. 2018; 38:1–211

[32] Friedman DI, Rausch EA. Headache diagnoses in patients with treated idiopathic intracranial hypertension. Neurology. 2002; 58:1551–1553

[33] Wang SJ, Silberstein SD, Patterson S, et al. Idiopathic intracranial hypertension without papilledema: a case control study in a headache center. Neurology. 1998; 51:245–249

[34] Sher NA, Wirtschafter J, Shapiro SK, et al. Unilateral Papilledema in 'Benign' Intracranial Hypertension (Pseudotumor Cerebri). JAMA. 1983; 250:2346–2347

[35] Rowe FJ, Sarkies NJ. Assessment of visual function in idiopathic intracranial hypertension: a prospective study. Eye (Lond). 1998; 12 (Pt 1):111–118

[36] Wall M, George D. Idiopathic Intracranial Hypertension: A Prospective Study of 50 Patients. Brain. 1991; 114:155–180

[37] Mollan SP, Davies B, Silver NC, et al. Idiopathic intracranial hypertension: consensus guidelines on management. J Neurol Neurosurg Psychiatry. 2018; 89:1088–1100

[38] Johnston I, Hawke S, Halmagyi M, et al. The Pseudotumor Syndrome: Disorders of Cerebrospinal Fluid Circulation Causing Intracranial Hypertension Without Ventriculomegaly. Archives of Neurology. 1991; 48:740–747

[39] Powers JM, Schnur JA, Baldree ME. Pseudotumor Cerebri due to Partial Obstruction of the Sigmoid Sinus by a Cholesteatoma. Arch Neurol. 1986; 43:519–521

[40] Wen DY, Hardten DR, Wirtschafter JD, et al. Elevated Intracranial Pressure from Cerebral Venous Obstruction by Masson's Vegetant Intravascular Hemangioendothelioma. Journal of Neurosurgery. 1991; 75:787–790

[41] Banik R, Lin D, Miller NR. Prevalence of Chiari I malformation and cerebellar ectopia in patients with pseudotumor cerebri. J Neurol Sci. 2006; 247:71–75

[42] Aiken AH, Hoots JA, Saindane AM, et al. Incidence of cerebellar tonsillar ectopia in idiopathic intracranial hypertension: a mimic of the Chiari I malformation. AJNR Am J Neuroradiol. 2012; 33:1901–1906

[43] Mukherjee S, Kalra N, Warren D, et al. Chiari I malformation and altered cerebrospinal fluid dynamics-the highs and the lows. Childs Nerv Syst. 2019; 35:1711–1717

[44] Cunningham ET, Koehler JE. Ocular bartonellosis. Am J Ophthalmol. 2000; 130:340–349

[45] Whelton PK, Carey RM, Aronow WS, et al. 2017 ACC/AHA/AAPA/ABC/ACPM/AGS/APhA/ASH/ASPC/NMA/PCNA Guideline for the Prevention, Detection, Evaluation, and Management of High Blood Pressure in Adults: Executive Summary: A Report of the American College of Cardiology/American Heart Association Task Force on Clinical Practice Guidelines. Hypertension. 2018; 71:1269–1324

[46] Avery RA, Mistry RD, Shah SS, et al. Patient position during lumbar puncture has no meaningful effect on cerebrospinal fluid opening pressure in children. J Child Neurol. 2010; 25:616–619

[47] Avery RA, Shah SS, Licht DJ, et al. Reference range for cerebrospinal fluid opening pressure in children. N Engl J Med. 2010; 363:891–893

[48] Neville L, Egan RA. Frequency and amplitude of elevation of cerebrospinal fluid resting pressure by the Valsalva maneuver. Can J Ophthalmol. 2005; 40:775–777

[49] Jacobson DM, Karanjia PN, Olson KA, et al. Computed Tomography Ventricular Size has no Predictive Value in Diagnosing Pseudotumor Cerebri. Neurology. 1990; 40:1454–1455

[50] Aaron GP, Illing E, Lambertsen Z, et al. Enlargement of Meckel's cave in patients with spontaneous cerebrospinal fluid leaks. Int Forum Allergy Rhinol. 2017; 7:421–424

[51] Degnan AJ, Levy LM. Narrowing of Meckel's cave and cavernous sinus and enlargement of the optic nerve sheath in Pseudotumor Cerebri. J Comput Assist Tomogr. 2011; 35:308–312

[52] Farb RI, Vanek I, Scott JN, et al. Idiopathic intracranial hypertension: the prevalence and morphology of sinovenous stenosis. Neurology. 2003; 60:1418–1424

[53] Kelly LP, Saindane AM, Bruce BB, et al. Does bilateral transverse cerebral venous sinus stenosis exist in patients without increased intracranial pressure? Clin Neurol Neurosurg. 2013; 115:1215–1219

[54] Sinclair AJ, Burdon MA, Nightingale PG, et al. Low energy diet and intracranial pressure in women

57

with idiopathic intracranial hypertension: prospective cohort study. BMJ. 2010; 341. DOI: 10.1136/bmj.c2701

[55] Johnson LN, Krohel GB, Madsen RW, et al. The role of weight loss and acetazolamide in the treatment of idiopathic intracranial hypertension (pseudotumor cerebri). Ophthalmology. 1998; 105:2313–2317

[56] Newberg B. Pseudotumor Cerebri Treated by Rice/Reduction Diet. Arch Intern Med. 1974; 133:802–807

[57] Ball AK, Howman A, Wheatley K, et al. A randomised controlled trial of treatment for idiopathic intracranial hypertension. J Neurol. 2011; 258:874–881

[58] Piper RJ, Kalyvas AV, Young AM, et al. Interventions for idiopathic intracranial hypertension. Cochrane Database Syst Rev. 2015. DOI: 10.1002/14651858.CD003434.pub3

[59] Smith SV, Friedman DI. The Idiopathic Intracranial Hypertension Treatment Trial: A Review of the Outcomes. Headache. 2017; 57:1303–1310

[60] ten Hove MW, Friedman DI, Patel AD, et al. Safety and Tolerability of Acetazolamide in the Idiopathic Intracranial Hypertension Treatment Trial. J Neuroophthalmol. 2016; 36:13–19

[61] Celebisoy N, Gokcay F, Sirin H, et al. Treatment of idiopathic intracranial hypertension: topiramate vs acetazolamide, an open-label study. Acta Neurol Scand. 2007; 116:322–327

[62] Kalyvas AV, Hughes M, Koutsarnakis C, et al. Efficacy, complications and cost of surgical interventions for idiopathic intracranial hypertension: a systematic review of the literature. Acta Neurochir (Wien). 2017; 159:33–49

[63] Hahn FJ, McWilliams FE. The Small Ventricle in Pseudotumor Cerebri: Demonstration of the Small Ventricle in Benign Intracranial Hypertension. CT. 1978; 2:249–253

[64] Kelman SE, Sergott RC, Cioffi GA, et al. Modified Optic Nerve Decompression in Patients with Functioning Lumboperitoneal Shunts and Progressive Visual Loss. Ophthalmology. 1991; 98:1449–1453

[65] Brourman ND, Spoor TC, Ramocki JM. Optic Nerve Sheath Decompression for Pseudotumor Cerebri. Arch Ophthalmol. 1988; 106:1384–1390

[66] Sergott RC, Savino PJ, Bosley TM. Modified Optic Nerve Sheath Decompression Provides Long-Term Visual Improvement for Pseudotumor Cerebri. Arch Ophthalmol. 1988; 106:1384–1390

[67] Corbett JJ, Nerad JA, Tse D, et al. Optic Nerve Sheath Fenestration for Pseudotumor Cerebri: The Lateral Orbitotomy Approach. Arch Ophthalmol. 1988; 106:1391–1397

[68] Sobel RK, Syed NA, Carter KD, et al. Optic Nerve Sheath Fenestration: Current Preferences in Surgical Approach and Biopsy. Ophthalmic Plast Reconstr Surg. 2015; 31:310–312

[69] Banta JT, Farris BK. Pseudotumor cerebri and optic nerve sheath decompression. Ophthalmology. 2000; 107:1907–1912

[70] Kelman SE, Heaps R, Wolf A, et al. Optic Nerve Decompression Surgery Improves Visual Function in Patients with Pseudotumor Cerebri. Neurosurgery. 1992; 30:391–395

[71] Spoor TC, Ramocki JM, Madion MP, et al. Treatment of Pseudotumor Cerebri by Primary and Secondary Optic Nerve Sheath Decompression. Am J Ophthalmol. 1991; 112:177–185

[72] Ahmed RM, Wilkinson M, Parker GD, et al. Transverse sinus stenting for idiopathic intracranial hypertension: a review of 52 patients and of model predictions. AJNR Am J Neuroradiol. 2011; 32:1408–1414

[73] Cappuzzo JM, Hess RM, Morrison JF, et al. Transverse venous stenting for the treatment of idiopathic intracranial hypertension, or pseudotumor cerebri. Neurosurg Focus. 2018; 45. DOI: 10.3171/2018.5.FOCUS18102

[74] Higgins JN, Owler BK, Cousins C, et al. Venous sinus stenting for refractory benign intracranial hypertension. Lancet. 2002; 359:228–230

[75] Reid Kate, Winters HStephen, Ang Timothy, et al. Transverse Sinus Stenting Reverses Medically Refractory Idiopathic Intracranial Hypertension. Frontiers in Ophthalmology. 2022; 2. DOI: 10.3389/fopht.2022.885583

[76] Kessler LA, Novelli PM, Reigel DH. Surgical treatment of benign intracranial hypertension–subtemporal decompression revisited. Surg Neurol. 1998; 50:73–76

[77] Thambisetty M, Lavin PJ, Newman NJ, et al. Fulminant idiopathic intracranial hypertension. Neurology. 2007; 68:229–232

[78] Wall M, Kupersmith MJ, Kieburtz KD, et al. The idiopathic intracranial hypertension treatment trial: clinical profile at baseline. JAMA Neurol. 2014; 71:693–701

[79] Bruce BB, Digre KB, McDermott MP, et al. Quality of life at 6 months in the Idiopathic Intracranial Hypertension Treatment Trial. Neurology. 2016; 87:1871–1877

[80] deSouza RM, Toma A, Watkins L. Medication overuse headache - An under-diagnosed problem in shunted idiopathic intracranial hypertension patients. Br J Neurosurg. 2015; 29:30–34

[81] Sinclair AJ, Kuruvath S, Sen D, et al. Is cerebrospinal fluid shunting in idiopathic intracranial hypertension worthwhile? A 10-year review. Cephalalgia. 2011; 31:1627–1633

[82] Committee on Obstetric Practice, . Weight Gain During Pregnancy. 2013. https://www.acog.org/clinical/clinical-guidance/committee-opinion/articles/2013/01/weight-gain-during-pregnancy

58 Tumors and Tumor-Like Lesions of the Skull

58.1 Skull tumors

58.1.1 General information

See Skull lesions (p.1661) for differential diagnosis and evaluation (including non-neoplastic lesions). Considering only tumors, the differential diagnosis includes:

1. benign tumors
   a) osteoma: see below
   b) hemangioma: see below
   c) dermoid and epidermoid tumors: see below
   d) chondroma: occur mainly in conjunction with the basal synchondroses
   e) meningioma involving the skull
   f) aneurysmal bone cyst
2. malignant tumors: malignancy is suggested by a single large or multiple (>6) small osteolytic lesions with margins that are ragged, undermined, and lacking sclerosis[1]
   a) bone metastases to the skull. Common ones include:
      - prostate
      - breast
      - lung
      - kidney
      - thyroid
      - lymphoma
      - multiple myeloma/plasmacytoma (p.928)
      - direct extension of head and neck tumors, e.g., squamous cell carcinoma of the scalp
   b) chondrosarcoma
   c) osteogenic sarcoma
   d) fibrosarcoma

58.1.2 Osteoma

General information

Osteomas are the most common primary bone tumor of the calvaria. They are benign, slow-growing lesions that occur commonly in the cranial vault, mastoid and paranasal air sinuses, and the mandible. Lesions within air sinuses may present as recurrent sinusitis. More common in females, highest incidence is in 6th decade. Triad of Gardner's syndrome: multiple cranial osteomas (of calvaria, sinuses, and mandible), colonic polyposis, and soft-tissue tumors.

See Localized increased density or hyperostosis of the calvaria (p.1664) for differential diagnosis.

Pathology

Consists of osteoid tissue within osteoblastic tissue, surrounded by reactive bone. Difficult to distinguish from fibrous dysplasia (p.975).

Radiographic evaluation

Skull X-ray: round, sclerotic, well-demarcated, homogeneous dense projection. Usually arise from outer table of skull (inner table less common). May be compact or spongy (spongy osteoma may be radiolucent). Unlike meningiomas, diploë are preserved and vascular channels are not increased.

Osteomas are "hot" on nuclear bone scan.

Treatment

Asymptomatic lesions may simply be followed. Surgery may be considered for cosmetic reasons, or if pressure on adjacent tissues produces discomfort. Lesions involving only the outer table may be removed, leaving the inner table intact.

58.1.3 Hemangioma

General information

Comprise ≈ 7% of skull tumors.[1] These benign tumors commonly occur in the skull (discussed here) and spine (p. 992). Two types: cavernous (most common) and capillary (rare).

Radiographic evaluation

Skull X-ray: characteristically shows a circular lucency with honeycomb or trabecular pattern (seen in ≈ 50% of cases) or radial trabeculations producing a sunburst pattern (seen in ≈ 11% of cases).[1] Sclerotic margins are evident in only ≈ 33%.

CT: hypodense lesion with sclerotic spaced trabeculations. Nonenhancing.

Bone scan: typically hot.

Treatment

Accessible lesions may be cured by en bloc excision or curettage. The gross appearance is of a hard, blue-domed mass beneath the pericranium. Radiation may be considered for inaccessible tumors.

58.1.4 Epidermoid and dermoid tumors of the skull

General information

See also epidermoids and dermoids in general (p. 973).

Dermoids and epidermoids are benign inclusion cysts of ectoderm that may involve skull and underlying dural venous structures or brain. They may become infected. Primary skull involvement is rare and occurs when ectodermal rests are entrapped in the developing skull, which causes these tumors to arise within the diploë and expand both inner and outer tables. Because they are not neoplastic, they grow at a linear rate (instead of exponential). Usually midline.

Epidermoid tumors contain only the outer layer of skin, and are therefore lined with stratified squamous epithelium and the resultant byproduct, keratin.

Dermoid tumors contain all elements of skin including hair follicles (which may produce hair in the tumor) and dermal glands (sebaceous glands (apocrine) and sweat glands (eccrine)).[2]

Teratomas are true neoplasms and may also contain bone, cartilage, teeth, and nails.

Presentation

These lesions may present as a result of mass effect from continued growth.

They may rupture (more common with dermoids than epidermoids), and can cause chemical meningitis (from the irritating properties of fat and or keratin), or, if infected, bacterial meningitis.

Radiographic evaluation

1. skull X-ray: these osteolytic lesions have well-defined, sclerotic margins
2. some imaging is required to evaluate possible intracranial involvement
   a) CT: the lesions are hypodense (keratin contains fats), and non-enhancing
   b) MRI: like CSF they are low intensity on T1WI and high signal on T2WI, but unlike CSF they are high signal on DWI > MRI (p. 938)

Treatment

Treatment is surgical. Radiation and chemotherapy are not indicated.

When possible, the goal is to avoid rupture during removal in order to avoid chemical and/or bacterial meningitis.

Bone margins are curetted. Search must be made for a tract leading to the intracranial cavity which must be followed if found. Preparation for dural sinus repair must be made for lesions overlying the sagittal sinus (including torcular Herophili).

Endoscopic surgery may be an option for some skull base lesions.

58

58.1.5 Langerhans cell histiocytosis

Formerly called histiocytosis X (or eosinophilic granuloma, when solitary). May occur in the skull as a result of direct invasion of craniofacial bone and skull base, or from meninges (p. 846).

58.1.6 Squamous cell carcinoma of the scalp involving the skull

It is not unusual for plastic surgeons to request neurosurgical assistance in managing squamous cell carcinoma of the scalp that involves the calvaria over the convexity. For first time surgical intervention (i.e., non-recurrence) without resectable mass or frank invasion through the inner table of the bone, neurosurgical management usually involves burring down the outer table in the area of involvement until normal appearing bone is encountered, taking care not to penetrate the inner table.

58.2 Non-neoplastic skull lesions

58.2.1 General information

Includes:
1. osteopetrosis (p. 1689)
2. Paget's disease of the skull
3. hyperostosis frontalis interna (see below)
4. fibrous dysplasia (p. 975)

58.2.2 Hyperostosis frontalis interna

General information

See differential diagnosis (p. 1664). Hyperostosis frontalis interna (HFI) is a benign irregular nodular thickening of the inner table of the frontal bone that is almost always bilateral. The midline is spared at the insertion of the falx. Unilateral cases have been reported,[3] and in these cases one must R/O other etiologies such as meningioma, calcified epidural hematoma, osteoma, fibrous dysplasia, an epidural fibrous tumor,[4] or Paget's disease.

Epidemiology

The incidence of HFI in the general population is ≈ 1.4–5%.[3] HFI is more common in women (female: male ratio may be as high as 9:1) with an incidence of 15–72% in elderly women. A number of possible associated conditions have been described (most are unproven), the majority of which are metabolic, earning it the alias of metabolic craniopathy. Associated conditions include:
1. Morgagni's syndrome (AKA Morgagni-Stewart-Morel syndrome): headache, obesity, virilism, and neuropsychiatric disorders (including mental retardation)
2. endocrinologic abnormalities
   a) acromegaly (p. 870)[5] (elevated growth hormone levels)
   b) hyperprolactinemia[5]
3. metabolic abnormalities
   a) hyperphosphatemia
   b) obesity
4. diffuse idiopathic skeletal hyperostosis (DISH) (p. 1373)

Clinical

HFI may present without symptoms as an incidental finding on radiographic evaluation for other reasons. Many signs and symptoms have been attributed to HFI, including: hypertension, seizures, headache, cranial nerve deficits, dementia, irritability, depression, hysteria, fatigability, and mental dullness. The incidence of headache may be statistically higher in patients with HFI than in the general population.[6]

Evaluation

Blood tests to R/O some of the above noted conditions may be indicated in appropriate cases: check growth hormone, prolactin, phosphate, alkaline phosphatase (to R/O Paget's disease).

Plain skull X-ray shows thickening of the frontal bone with characteristic sparing of the midline. Spread to parietal and occipital bone occasionally occurs.

CT demonstrates the lesion, which usually causes 5–10 mm of bone thickening, but as much as 4 cm has been reported.

Bone scan: usually shows moderate uptake in HFI (generally not as intense as with bone mets). Also, indium-111 leukocyte scan (commonly used to detect occult infection) will show accumulation in HFI (a false positive).[7,8]

Treatment

In spite of a large number of published descriptive works in the medical literature, primarily in the early and mid-20th century, little has been written about treatment of cases where symptoms are suspected to be due to HFI. In one report, removal of the thickened bone was accomplished without evidence of dural adhesions, and with improvement in the presenting hysteria.[3]

Surgical technique

One technique described consists of using the craniotome to excise the thickened portion of the bone (a plain skull X-ray may be used to make a template), and then the thickened bone is thinned down with a high-speed drill, and the bone flap is then replaced. Alternatively, a cranioplasty with methylmethacrylate or custom-made implant fabricated using CT data may be performed.

58.2.3 Fibrous dysplasia

General information

Key concepts

- non-neoplastic condition where bone is replaced by expansile fibrous connective tissue
- malignant transformation to osteosarcoma or other sarcoma occurs in < 1%
- common sites of involvement: ribs, proximal femur, craniofacial bone
- associated endocrinopathies are common: includes precocious puberty or growth hormone excess
- may be monostotic, polyostotic, or part of McCune-Albright syndrome (triad: café au lait spots, endocrinopathy (e.g., precocious puberty) and polyostotic fibrous dyslpasia)
- common presentation: may be incidental, cosmetic, hearing loss, rarely visual loss
- treatment:
  - observation is often the best initial management. Prophylactic surgery for optic nerve compression is not justified due to the typical slow progression and the high risk of visual loss with surgery
  - medical therapy may include calcitonin, bisphosphonates, ? RANK ligand inhibitors
  - treat endocrinopathies (reduces morbidity including visual loss with GH excess)
  - ✖ XRT is not recommended

Fibrous dysplasia (FD) is a non-neoplastic benign condition in which normal bone is replaced by fibrous connective tissue and immature woven bone that is weaker than normal bone and tends to expand. Most lesions occur in the ribs, proximal femur or craniofacial bones (especially the maxilla). Frequent femoral neck fractures can lead to a varus deformity (so-called "shepherd's crook deformity")

Molecular genetics: FD is not heritable. It results from somatic activating mutations in the α subunit of the stimulatory G protein encoded by the GNAS locus at 20q13.2-q13.3.

Types of involvement

Localization of involvement
3 patterns of involvement
1. monostotic fibrous dysplasia (MFD): most common. The most frequent site of involvement is the zygomatic-maxillary complex
2. polyostotic fibrous dysplasia (PFD): 25% with this form have > 50% of the skeleton involved with associated fractures and skeletal deformities
3. PFD as part of McCune-Albright syndrome (and its variants). Triad:
   a) café au lait spots which tend to occur on one side of the midline and tend to be more jagged than those seen in neurofibromatosis (p.638) and fewer in number

    b) endocrinopathy: including precocious puberty (primarily in females) and growth hormonesecretion

    c) polyostotic fibrous dysplasia (PFD)

Skull involvement occurs in 27% of MFD. In PFD and MAS, craniofacial involvement occurs in 90% of cases and the anterior skull base is involved inn > 95%.[9]

3 forms of fibrous dysplasia lesions

1. cystic (the lesions are not actually cysts in the strict sense): widening of the diplöe usually with thinning of the outer table and little involvement of the inner table. Typically occurs high in calvaria

2. sclerotic: usually involves skull base (especially sphenoid bone) and facial bones

3. mixed: appearance is similar to cystic type with patches of increased density within the lucent lesions

Epidemiology

True incidence is unknown since many cases are asymptomatic. FD constitutes ≈ 7% of benign bone lesions.[10] MFD is probably more common than PFD, but the actual ratio depends on the screening methodology. MAS is more common in females.

Clinical

Clinical manifestations of craniofacial fibrous dysplasia lesions include:

1. incidental finding (i.e., asymptomatic)

2. local pain or tenderness: the lesions are not tender, but overlying stretched periosteum may be. Associated aneurysmal bone cysts (ABCs) may be painful

3. local swelling (rarely: marked distortion resembling aneurysmal bone cyst)

4. changes due to facial deformity/asymmetry
    a) cosmetic: frontal bossing, hypertelorism
    b) orbital involvement may cause: proptosis, vertical dystopia (asymmetry in vertical alignment of the eyes), visual loss (p. 976)
    c) nasal congestion
    d) mandibular involvement: asymmetry which may produce malocclusion

5. may predispose to pathologic fractures when FD lesions occur in long bones

6. cranial nerve-related manifestations:
    a) hearing loss: temporal bone involvement may obliterate the external auditory canal or may restrict movement of middle ear ossicles. Temporal bone involvement occurs in > 70% of cases of craniofacial PFD and MAS and is uncommon in MFD[11]
    b) visual loss: an uncommon but recognized sequela of FD as a result of compression of the optic nerve in the optic canal, more common in children
    c) trigeminal neuralgia[12]
    d) facial nerve palsy: rare. Compression typically occurs within Fallopian canal and/or IAC

7. seizures: rare presentation

8. serum alkaline phosphatase is elevated in about 33%, calcium levels are normal

9. darkened hair pigmentation overlying skull lesions

10. spontaneous scalp hemorrhages

11. rarely associated with Cushing's syndrome, acromegaly

Evaluation

A major objective is to determine if the patient has a single lesion (MFD) or multiple lesions as in PFD or MAS.

1. history:
    • onset and nature of symptoms
    • rapidity of progression
    • history of pathologic fractures (clue for other FD lesions)
    • indications of endocrinopathies: age of menarche in females (R/O precious puberty), growth abnormalities (R/O growth hormone excess)

2. physical exam: look for and ask about skin discoloration (café-au-lait spots)

3. diagnostic studies:
    • skeletal survey (total body X-rays) or bone scan if additional lesions are suspected

- non-contrast head CT with thin cuts (▶ Fig. 58.1): characteristic ground glass appearance of craniofacial FD on X-rays and CT is due to the thin spicules of woven bone. With age, lesions morph into a mixed radio-dense/radio-lucent appearance. In prepubertal patients with PFD or MAS a homogeneous radio-dense appearance is more common.
- panorex and/or dental films when there is involvment around the teeth

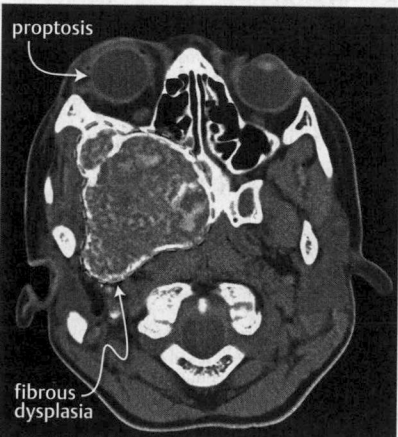

proptosis

fibrous dysplasia

Fig. 58.1 Fibrous dysplasia of the right middle cranial fossa (outlined by *blue broken line*).
Image: axial CT scan, bone window.

Natural history

FD lesions are usually slowly progessive.
   Rapid progression may occur:
- infrequently, in PFD or MAS prior to puberty. Progression usually slows when skeletal maturity is reached.
- malignant transformation: occurs in < 1% of cases.[11] Typically to osteosarcoma, but other sarcomas are possible (fibrosarcoma, chondrosarcoma…)
- associated expansile lesions:
   ○ aneurysmal bone cyst (ABC)
   ○ mucocele: when the ostium to a sinus becomes occluded by fibrous overgrowth
- osteomyelitis: often difficult to cure in the presence of FD

The most disfiguring and symptomatic lesions occur in patients with poorly controlled excess growth hormone (GH).[13] Therefore excess GH should be managed aggressively
   Craniofacial FD may be categorized as[11]:
1. quiescent: no progression. Typically with smaller lesions
2. non-aggressive: slow growing
3. aggressive: rapid growth, associated pain, pathologic fractures, malignant transformation…

Management

58

Observation is often the best first management option. Delay surgery until skeletal maturity (around age 10–12 years) if possible.
   Cure may be possible with smaller lesions in MFD but is unlikely with PFD or MAS. Local procedures (mostly orthopedic) are used for appendicular deformities or bone pain that is refractory to other treatment. Incompletely resected lesions are subject to regrowth.
   Consult an endocrinologist if there is any suspicion of endocrinopathy.
   Biopsy of an accessible lesion by the appropriate surgical specialist should be considered when the diagnosis is in doubt.[11] Bleeding may be brisk due to vascularity. Biopsy does not promote growth of the lesion. Histology does not predict biological behavior.
   Quiescent craniofacial lesions without complaints of facial deformity may be monitored with annual evaluations which should include: patient reported symptoms, neurologic exam including

sensory testing, photographs and facial CT for the first 2 visits and then less frequently based on prior CT results and clinical findings.

Non-aggressive or quiescent lesions producing bothersome facial disfigurement may be treated by a craniofacial surgeon. If practical, it is best to wait until the patient reaches skeletal maturity.

When optic canal involvement is documented, annual ophthalmological exams should be conducted. The diagnosis of optic neuropathy is made when there is a visual defect or if 2 out of 3 exams (contrast sensitivity, color vision and funduscopic exam) are abnormal. Optic neuropathy in FD is more common in patients with growth hormone excess.[13,14] Evidence suggest aggressive management of GH excess reduces the risk of optic neuropathy.

When there is temporal bone involvement, regular otolaryngology exams (including microscopy for EAC stenosis) should be performed to maintain patency of EAC (from bone, cerumen or the rare cholesteatoma). Annual audiology evaluations are recommended during periods of active lesion growth.

Pain is a common complaint, and is more prevalent in the lower extremities than with craniofacial involvement. It does not correlate with disease burden.

Calcitonin may be used for widespread lesions with bone pain and/or high serum alkaline phosphatase levels.

Bisphosphonates (e.g., alendronate, pamidronate or zoledronic acid): mixed results for craniofacial pain control and growth rate reduction in FD.

RANK ligand inhibitors e.g., denosumab: uncertain role in FD.[15]

✖ Radiation therapy is not recommended (risk of XRT induced tumors).

▶ **Neurosurgical involvement.** May be required for skull lesions producing refractory pain or neurologic symptoms or for rapidly growing associated lesions (e.g., ABC). Calvarial lesions may be treated with curettage and cranioplasty. Once the dysplastic bone is disconnected from the skull, the loss of vascular supply usually renders it inactive. Skull base lesions often require a multidisciplinary approach.

Acute visual deterioration associated with an expansile lesion near the optic canal should be treated with high-dose glucocorticoids and rapid surgical decompression.[14] However, vision is usually preserved despite optic canal narrowing with FD,[9] and visual loss may follow injudicious surgical intervention due to the intolerance of the optic nerve to surgical trauma. Rule out other possible explanations for visual loss before operating.

Image guidance may be helpful when drilling down exuberant bone to decompress the optic canal. Copious irrigation (e.g., with irrigating drill) is critical to avoid thermal damage. Endoscopic techniques may be useful adjuncts, but the distorted anatomy requires an experienced practitioner.

References

[1] Thomas JE, Baker HL. Assessment of Roentgenographic Lucencies of the Skull: A Systematic Approach. Neurology. 1975; 25:99–106

[2] Smirniotopoulos J G, Chiechi MV. Teratomas, dermoids, and epidermoids of the head and neck. Radiographics. 1995; 15:1437–1455

[3] Hasegawa T, Ito H, Yamamoto S, et al. Unilateral Hyperostosis Frontalis Interna: Case Report. Journal of Neurosurgery. 1983; 59:710–713

[4] Willison CD, Schochet SS, Voelker JL. Cranial Epidural Fibrous Tumor Associated with Hyperostosis: A Case Report. Surgical Neurology. 1993; 40:508–511

[5] Fulton JD, Shand J, Ritchie D, et al. Hyperostosis frontalis interna, acromegaly and hyperprolactinemia. Postgrad Med J. 1990; 66:16–19

[6] Bavazzano A, Del Bianco PL, Del Bene E, et al. A statistical evaluation of the relationships between headache and internal frontal hyperostosis. Research & Clinical Studies in Headache. 1970; 3:191–197

[7] Floyd JL, Jackson DE, Carretta R. Appearance of Hyperostosis Frontalis Interna on Indium-111 Leukocyte Scans: Potential Diagnostic Pitfall. J Nucl Med. 1986; 27:495–497

[8] Oates E. Spectrum of Appearance of Hyperostosis Frontalis Interna on In-111 Leukocyte Scans. Clin Nucl Med. 1988; 13:922–923

[9] Lee JS, FitzGibbon E, Butman JA, et al. Normal vision despite narrowing of the optic canal in fibrous dysplasia. N Engl J Med. 2002; 347:1670–1676

[10] Parekh SG, Donthineni-Rao R, Ricchetti E, et al. Fibrous dysplasia. J Am Acad Orthop Surg. 2004; 12:305–313

[11] Lee JS, FitzGibbon EJ, Chen YR, et al. Clinical guidelines for the management of craniofacial fibrous dysplasia. Orphanet J Rare Dis. 2012; 7 Suppl 1:S2–S2

[12] Finney HL, Roberts TS. Fibrous dysplasia of the skull with progressive cranial nerve involvement. Surg Neurol. 1976; 6:341–343

[13] Cutler CM, Lee JS, Butman JA, et al. Long-term outcome of optic nerve encasement and optic nerve decompression in patients with fibrous dysplasia: risk factors for blindness and safety of observation. Neurosurgery. 2006; 59:1011–7; discussion 1017–8

[14] Boyce AM, Glover M, Kelly MH, et al. Optic neuropathy in McCune-Albright syndrome: effects of early diagnosis and treatment of growth hormone excess. J Clin Endocrinol Metab. 2013; 98:E126–E134

[15] Boyce AM, Chong WH, Yao J, et al. Denosumab treatment for fibrous dysplasia. J Bone Miner Res. 2012; 27:1462–1470

59 Tumors of the Spine and Spinal Cord

59.1 Spine tumors – general information

15% of primary CNS tumors are intraspinal (the intracranial:spinal ratio for astrocytomas is 10:1; for ependymomas it is 3–20:1).[1] There is disagreement over the prevalence, prognosis, and optimal treatment. Most primary CNS spinal tumors are benign (unlike the case with intracranial tumors). Most present by compression rather than invasion.[2]

59.2 Compartmental locations of spinal tumors

May be classified into 3 groups based on the compartment involved. Although metastases may be found in each area, they are most commonly extradural. Frequencies quoted below are from a general hospital, extradural lesions are less common in neurosurgical clinics because many of these tumors are managed by oncologists without requiring neurosurgical involvement.
1. extradural (ED) (55%): arise outside cord in vertebral bodies or epidural tissues
2. intradural extramedullary (ID-EM) (40%): arise in leptomeninges or roots. Primarily meningiomas and neurofibromas (together = 55% of ID-EM tumors)
3. intramedullary spinal cord tumors (IMSCT) (p. 984), 5%: arise in SC substance. Invade and destroy tracts and gray matter

▶ **Spinal lymphoma.** Lymphoma may occur in any of or all 3 compartments.
1. epidural
   a) metastatic or secondary lymphoma: the most common form of spinal lymphoma. Spinal involvement occurs in 0.1–10% of patients with non-Hodgkin's lymphoma
   b) primary spinal epidural non-Hodgkin's lymphoma: rare. Completely epidural with no bony involvement. The existence of this entity is controversial, and some investigators feel that it represents extension of undetected retroperitoneal or vertebral body lymphoma. May have a better prognosis than secondary lymphoma[3]
2. intramedullary
   a) secondary (p. 986) (metastatic)
   b) primary: very rare (see below)

59.3 Differential diagnosis: spine and spinal cord tumors

59.3.1 General information

See also Myelopathy (p. 1696) for a list including not only tumors but also *nonneoplastic* causes of spinal cord dysfunction (e.g., spinal meningeal cyst, epidural hematoma, transverse myelitis…).

59.3.2 Extradural spinal cord tumors (55%)

Arise in vertebral bodies or epidural tissues
1. metastatic: comprise the majority of ED tumors
   a) most are osteolytic (cause bony destruction): see Spinal epidural metastases (p. 921). Common ones include:
      • lymphoma: most cases represent spread of systemic disease (secondary lymphoma); some cases may be primary (see below)
      • lung
      • breast
      • prostate
   b) metastases that may be osteoblastic:
      • in men: prostate Ca is the most common
      • in women: breast Ca is the most common
2. primary spinal tumors (very rare)
   a) chordomas (p. 825)
   b) osteoid osteoma (p. 990)
   c) osteoblastoma (p. 990)
   d) **aneurysmal bone cyst (ABC):** an expansile tumor-like osteolytic lesion consisting of a highly vascular honeycomb of blood-filled cavities separated by connective tissue septa, surrounded by a

59

thin cortical bone shell which may expand. Comprise 15% of spine tumors.[4] Etiology is controversial. May arise from preexisting tumor (including: osteoblastoma, giant cell tumor, fibrous dysplasia, chondrosarcoma) or following acute fracture. In the spine, there is a tendency to involve primarily the posterior elements. Peak incidence is in the second decade of life. Treatment usually consists of intralesional curettage. High recurrence rate (25–50%) if not completely excised

e) chondrosarcoma: a malignant tumor of cartilage. Lobulated tumors with calcified areas
f) osteochondroma (AKA chondroma AKA osteocartilaginous exostosis): benign tumors of bone that arise from mature hyaline cartilage. Most common during adolescence. An enchondroma is a similar tumor arising within the medullary cavity
g) vertebral hemangioma (p. 992)
h) **giant cell tumors (GCT)** of bone (p. 995) : AKA osteoclastoma
i) giant cell (reparative) granuloma: AKA solid variant of ABC.[5] Related to GCT. Occurs primarily in mandible, maxilla, hands and feet, but there are case reports of spine involvement.[5,6] Not a true neoplasm—more of a reactive process. Treatment: curettage. Recurrence rate: 22–50%, treated with re-excision
j) brown tumor of hyperparathyroidism
k) osteogenic sarcoma: rare in spine

3. miscellaneous
a) plasmacytoma (p. 931)
b) multiple myeloma (p. 928)
c) **unifocal Langerhans cell histiocytosis (LHC), formerly eosinophilic granuloma**: osteolytic defect with progressive vertebral collapse; LHC is one cause of **vertebra plana** (p. 1679) . C-spine is the most commonly affected region. Individual LHCs associated with systemic conditions (Letterer-Siwe or Hand-Schüller-Christian disease) are treated with biopsy and immobilization. Collapse or neurologic deficit from compression may require decompression and/or fusion. Low-dose XRT may also be effective[7,8]
d) Ewing's sarcoma: aggressive malignant tumor with a peak incidence during the second decade of life. Spine mets are more common than primary spine lesions. Treatment is mostly palliative: radical excision followed by XRT (very radiosensitive) and chemotherapy[9]
e) chloroma: focal infiltration of leukemic cells
f) angiolipoma: ≈ 60 cases reported in literature
g) neurofibromas (p. 982): most are intradural, but some are extradural, usually dilate neural foramen (dumbbell tumors)
h) Masson's vegetant intravascular hemangioendothelioma (p. 961) [10]

59.3.3 Intradural extramedullary spinal cord tumors (40%)

1. meningiomas: usually intradural, but may be partly or, in 15%, wholly extradural; see below
2. neurofibromas: usually intradural, but may be partly or wholly extradural
3. many lipomas are extramedullary with intramedullary extension
4. miscellaneous: only ≈ 4% of spinal metastases involve this compartment

59.3.4 Intramedullary spinal cord tumors (5%)

1. astrocytoma (p. 985): 30%
2. ependymoma (p. 984): 30%, including myxopapillary ependymoma (p. 985)
3. miscellaneous: 30%, includes:
a) malignant glioblastoma
b) dermoid. In addition to the general population, dermoids present in a delayed fashion following ≈ 16% of myelomeningocele (MM) closures.[11] An iatrogenic etiology has been debated[12]; however, a case of a congenital dermoid in a newborn with MM[13] indicates that the origin is not always from incompletely excised dermal elements at the time of MM closure
c) epidermoid
d) teratoma
e) lipoma
f) hemangioblastoma (p. 986)
g) neuroma (very rare intramedullary)
h) syringomyelia (not neoplastic)
4. extremely rare tumors
a) lymphoma
b) oligodendroglioma
c) cholesteatoma

d) intramedullary metastases: comprises only ≈ 2% of spinal mets
e) solitary fibrous tumors of the spinal cord: recognized in 1996. Probable mesenchymal origin. May also occur extramedullary (less common). Treatment is complete surgical excision. Prognosis is unclear[14]

59.4 Intradural extramedullary spinal cord tumors

59.4.1 Spinal meningiomas

See reference.[15]

Epidemiology

Peak age: 40–70 years. Female:male ratio = 4:1 overall, but the ratio is 1:1 in the lumbar region. 82% thoracic, 15% cervical, 2% lumbar. 90% are completely intradural, 5% are extradural, and 5% are both intra- and extradural. 68% are lateral to the spinal cord, 18% posterior, 15% anterior. Multiple spinal meningiomas occur rarely.

Clinical

Symptoms (▶ Table 59.1.)
Signs prior to surgery (only 1 of 174 patients was intact)[15]:
1. motor
   a) pyramidal signs only: 26%
   b) walks with aid: 41%
   c) antigravity strength: 17%
   d) flexion-extension with gravity removed: 6%
   e) paralysis: 9%
2. sensory
   a) radicular: 7%
   b) long tract: 90%
3. sphincter deficit: 51%

Table 59.1 Symptoms of spinal meningiomas

Symptom	At onset	At time of first surgery
local or radicular pain	42%	53%
motor deficits	33%	92%
sensory symptoms	25%	61%
sphincter disturbance		50%

Outcome

Recurrence rate with complete excision is 7% with a minimum of 6 years follow-up (relapses occurred from 4 to 17 years post-op).[15]

59.4.2 Spinal schwannomas

General information

Key concepts

59

- slow growing benign tumors
- most (75%) arise from the dorsal (sensory) rootlets
- early symptoms are often radicular
- recurrence is rare after total excision (except in neurofibromatosis)

Incidence: 0.3–0.4/100,000/yr. Most occur sporadically and are solitary, but they may also be associated with neurofibromatosis (p. 637), primarily type 2 (NF2), but can occur with type 1.

Configurations

Most are entirely intradural, but 8–32% may be completely extradural[16,17]; 1–19% are a combination, 6–23% are dumbbell, and 1% are intramedullary.

▶ **Dumbbell tumors.** Definition: tumors that develop an "hourglass" shape as a result of an anatomic barrier encountered during growth. Not all dumbbell tumors are schwannomas, e.g., neuroblastoma (p. 637). Most have a contiguous intraspinal, foraminal (usually narrower), and extraforaminal components (widening of the neural foramen is a characteristic finding, can be recognized even on plain films, and speaks to the longstanding benign nature of the lesion). The waist may also be due to a dural constriction.

Asazuma et al[18] classification system for dumbbell spinal schwannomas is shown in ▶ Fig. 59.1.

Type I tumors are intradural and extradural and are restricted to the spinal canal. The constriction occurs at the dura.

Type II are all extradural, and are subclassified as: IIa = do not extend beyond the neural foramen, IIb = inside spinal canal + paravertebral, IIc = foraminal + paravertebral.

Type IIIa are intradural and extradural foraminal, IIIb are intradural and extradural paravertebral.

Type IV are extradural and intravertebral. Type V are extradural and extralaminar with laminar invasion. Type VI show multidirectional bone erosion.

Craniocaudal spread: IF and TF designate the number of intervertebral foramina and transverse foramina involved, respectively (e.g., IF stage 2 = 2 foramens).

Schwannomas involving C1 & C2: May involve vertebral arteries and require additional caution.

Clinical

Patients typically present with local pain.

Neurologic deficits develop late. Tumors may cause radiculopathy (from nerve root compression), myelopathy (from spinal cord compression), radiculomyelopathy (from compression of both), or cauda equina syndrome (for tumors below conus medullaris).

Pathology

Composed of Antoni A (compact, interwoven bundles of long, spindly Schwann cells) and Antoni B tissue (sparse areas of Schwann cells in a loose eosinophilic matrix).

Surgical approaches

See reference.[19]

Posterior approaches: Types I, IIa, IIIa, some upper cervical IIIb, and some VI are generally amenable to a posterior approach. IIa and IIIa usually require total facetectomy for complete removal.[18] Reconstruction with instrumentation may be needed if substantial posterior disruption occurs.

Strategy for large tumors: a nerve stimulator can be used to identify a "safe zone" where the capsule can be incised without going through nerve tissue. Then the tumor is debulked internally. It is often not possible to separate tumor from nerve as the tumor passes into the neural foramen. Here it is not unusual to end up with a thin capsule of tumor attached to strands of nerve, and this typically results in satisfactory function.

Anterior and combined anterior/posterior approaches: Asazuma et al[18] recommend a combined approach for Type IIb, IIc, and IIIb lesions where the extraforaminal extension is large (viz. beyond the vertebral arteries). Reconstruction with instrumentation was required for some tumors (≈ 10% of all patients treated) which were type IV (2 patients), IIIb (1 pt), and VI (1 pt).

Nerve sacrifice

It is usually possible to preserve some fascicles of the nerve root, although sometimes section of the entire nerve root is required. New deficits may not occur, especially with large tumors, since involved fascicles are often nonfunctional, and adjacent roots may compensate. The risk for motor deficit is higher for schwannomas than for neurofibromas, for cervical vs. lumbar tumors, and for cervical tumors with extradural extension.

Outcome

Recurrence is rare following gross total excision, except in the setting of NF2.

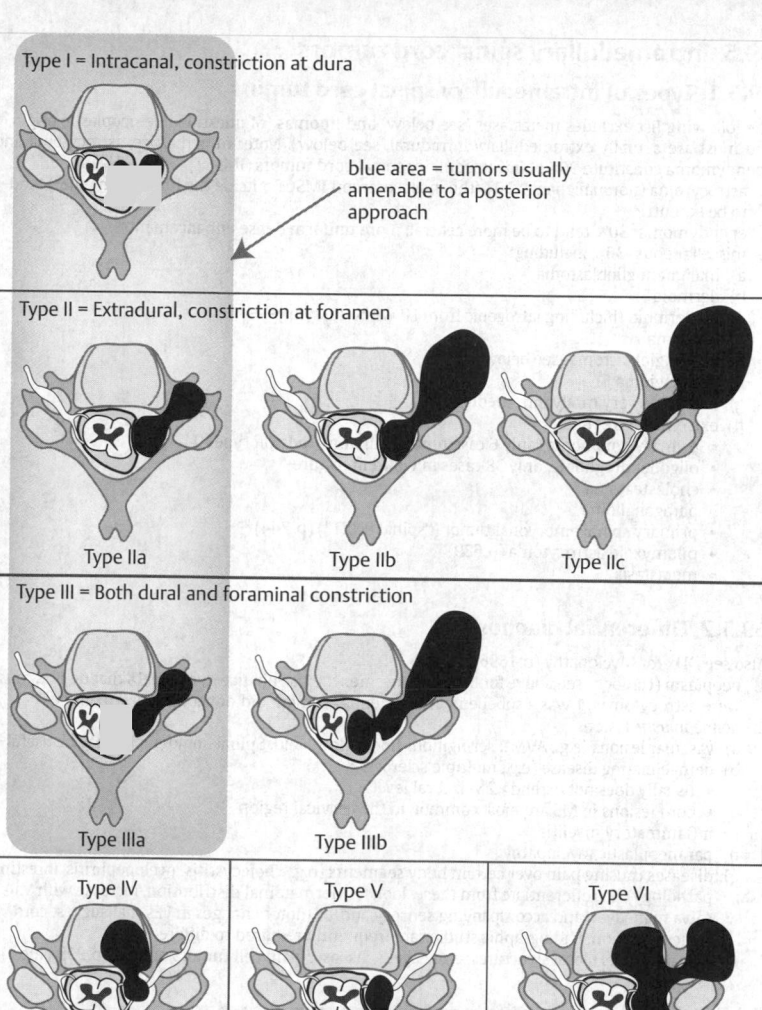

Fig. 59.1 Classification of dumbbell spinal tumors. (Modified with permission from Asazuma T, Yoshiaki T, Hirofumi M, et al. Surgical strategy for cervical dumbbell tumors based on a three-dimensional classification. Spine 2003;29(1):E10–4.)

59

59.5 Intramedullary spinal cord tumors

59.5.1 Types of intramedullary spinal cord tumors

The following list excludes metastases (see below) and lipomas (of questionable neoplastic origin,[20] and most are actually extramedullary intradural, see below). **Note:** in pediatrics, astrocytoma and ependymoma constitute 90% of intramedullary spinal cord tumors (IMSCT).

1. astrocytoma (nonmalignant): 30% (the most common IMSCT outside the filum terminale[2]) tend to be eccentric
2. ependymoma: 30%, tend to be more central, more uniform dense enhancement
3. miscellaneous: 30%, including:
   a) malignant glioblastoma
   b) dermoid
   c) epidermoid (including iatrogenic from LP without stylet)[21,22]
   d) teratoma
   e) hemangioblastoma (see below)
   f) hemangioma
   g) neuroma (very rarely intramedullary)
   h) extremely rare tumors
      - primary lymphoma (only 6 case reports, all non-Hodgkin type[23])
      - oligodendroglioma, only 38 cases in world literature[24]
      - cholesteatoma
      - paraganglioma
      - primary spinal embryonal tumor ("spinal PNET") (p.744) [25]
      - pilomyxoid astrocytoma (p.689)
      - metastasis

59.5.2 Differential diagnosis

Also see DDx for Myelopathy (p.1696).

1. neoplasm (tumor): (see above for list). Enhancement: 91% enhance[26]; of the 9% that do not, most were astrocytomas, 1 was a subependymoma; enhancement did not correlate with grade
2. *nonneoplastic* lesions
   a) vascular lesions (e.g., AVM): serpiginous linear flow-void. Spinal angiography may be useful[2]
   b) demyelinating disease (e.g., multiple sclerosis):
      - usually does not extend > 2 vertebral levels
      - cord lesions in MS are most common in the cervical region
   c) inflammatory myelitis
   d) paraneoplastic myelopathy
   e) diseases causing pain over certain body segments (e.g., cholecystitis, pyelonephritis, intestinal pathology). To differentiate from these, look for dermatomal distribution, increase with Valsalva maneuver, and accompanying sensory and/or motor changes in LEs that suggest cord/radicular lesion. Radiographic studies are frequently required to differentiate
   f) diseases of vertebral structures, e.g., Paget's disease, giant cell tumors of bone (p.995), etc.

59.5.3 Specific types of intramedullary spinal cord tumors

Ependymoma

General information

Key concepts

- the most common glioma of lower cord, conus, and filum (most ependymomas in conus and filum are myxopapillary ependymomas). More common in adults
- evaluation: includes imaging the entire neuraxis (usually with enhanced MRI: cervical, thoracic, lumbar, and brain) because of potential for seeding through CSF
- associated cysts are common
- treatment: surgical excision (most are encapsulated)

See WHO diagnostic criteria (p. 732). The most common glioma of the lower spinal cord, conus and filum (see below). Slow-growing. Benign. Slight male predominance; slight peak in 3rd to 6th decade. Over 50% in filum, next most common location is cervical. Histologically: papillary, cellular, epithelial, or mixed (in filum, myxopapillary ependymoma is most common, see below). Cystic degeneration in 46%. May expand spinal canal in filum.[27] Usually encapsulated and minimally vascular (papillary: may be highly vascular; may cause SAH). Symptoms present > 1 yr prior to diagnosis in 82% of cases.[28]

Myxopapillary ependymoma

Myxopapillary ependymomas are a subtype of ependymoma that tend to occur at the conus medullaris, the filum terminale or cauda equina (▶ Fig. 59.2). They are WHO grade 1. Usually solitary. Histology: papillary, with microcystic vacuoles, mucosubstance; connective tissue. No anaplasia, but CSF dissemination occurs rarely (can seed intracranially following removal of spinal tumor[29]). Denovo intracranial lesions also occur rarely. Rare reports of systemic mets.[1] Outside the CNS, may occur in sacrococcygeal subcutaneous tissues from heterotopic rests of ependymal cells.[30]

Surgical removal of filum tumors consists of coagulating and dividing the filum terminale just above and below the lesion—see Distinguishing features of the filum terminale intraoperatively (p. 292)—and excising it in total. The filum is first cut *above* the lesion to prevent retraction upwards.

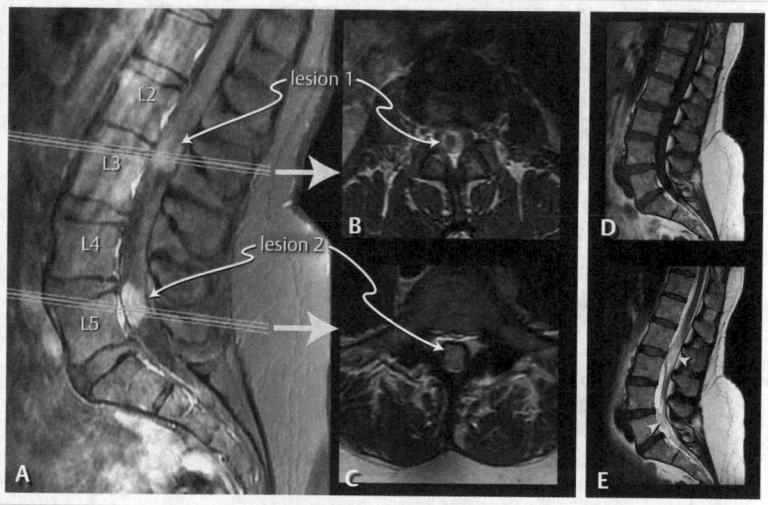

Fig. 59.2 Myxopapillary ependymoma. Two myxopapillary ependymomas of the lumbar spine.
Image: contrast T1 MRI, A: midline sagittal, B: axial slice through upper lesion located near the conus, C: axial slice through lower lesion located in the cauda equina. D: unenhanced sagittal T1 image, the lesions are isointense with their surroundings. E: lesions (*yellow arrowheads*) are fairly easily identified on this noncontrast T2WI sagittal image.

Astrocytoma

Uncommon in first year. Peak: 3rd–5th decade. Male:female = 1.5:1. The ratio of low-grade:high-grade = 3:1 in all ages.[27] Occurs at all levels, thoracic most common, then cervical. 38% are cystic; cyst fluid usually has high protein.

Dermoid and epidermoid

Epidermoids are rare before late childhood. Slight female predominance. Cervical and upper thoracic rare; conus common. Usually ID-EM, but conus/cauda equina may have IM component (completely IM lesions rare).

59

Lipoma

May occur in conjunction with spinal dysraphism, see Lipomyeloschisis (p. 284). The following considers lipomas that occur in the absence of spinal dysraphism.

Peak occurrence: 2nd, 3rd, and 5th decade. Technically hamartomas. No sex predominance. Usually ID-EM (a sub-type is truly IM and essentially replaces the cord[31]), cervicothoracic region is the most common location. NB: unlike other IMSCTs, most common symptom is ascending mono- or paraparesis (c.f. pain). Sphincter disturbance is common with low lesions. Local subcutaneous masses or dimples are frequent. Malis recommends early subtotal removal at about 1 year of age in asymptomatic patient.[31] Superficial extrasacral removal is inadequate, as patients then develop dense scarring intraspinally leading to fairly rapid severe neurological damage with poor salvage-ability even after the definitive procedure.

Hemangioblastoma

(▶ Fig. 59.3). Usually non-infiltrating, well demarcated, may have cystic caps. 80% of patients with spinal hemangioblastoma will have von Hippel-Lindau disease (p. 646). Cannot incise nor core because of vascularity. Requires microsurgical approach similar to AVM, possibly with intraoperative hypotension.

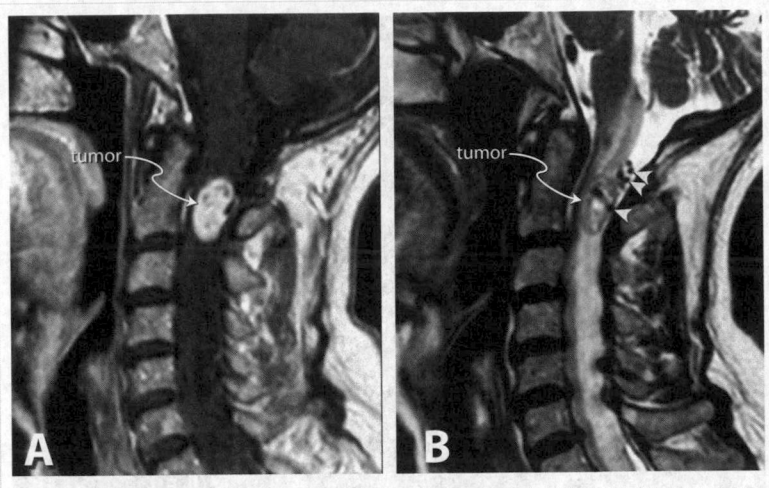

Fig. 59.3 Intramedullary hemangioblastoma of the cervical spinal cord.
Sagittal MRI. A: T1 with contrast. B: T2.
Flow voids appear dark on the T2 image, with several of them denoted by *yellow arrowheads*.

Metastases

Most spinal mets are extradural. Intramedullary metastases are rare,[32] accounting for 3.4% of symptomatic metastatic spinal cord lesions.[33] Primaries include: small-cell lung Ca,[34] breast Ca, malignant melanoma, lymphoma and colon Ca.[33,35] Ca rarely presents first as an intramedullary spinal met.

59.5.4 Presentation

1. pain: the most common complaint. Almost always present in filum tumors (exception: lipomas).[21] Possible pain patterns:
   a) radicular: increases with Valsalva maneuver and spine movement. Suspect SCT if dermatome is unusual for disc herniation
   b) local: stiff neck or back, Valsalva maneuver increases pain.
      ★ *Pain during recumbency ("nocturnal pain") is classic for SCT*

    c) medullary (as in syrinx): oppressive, burning, dysesthetic, non-radicular, often bilateral, unaffected by Valsalva maneuver

2. motor disturbances
    a) weakness is 2nd or 3rd most common complaint. Usually follows sensory symptoms temporally
    b) children present most frequently with gait disturbances
    c) syringomyelic syndrome: suggests IMSCT. Findings: UE segmental weakness, decreased DTR, dissociative anesthesia (see below)
    d) long-tract involvement → clumsiness and ataxia (distinct from weakness)
    e) atrophy, muscle twitches, fasciculations

3. non-painful sensory disturbances
    a) dissociated sensory loss: decreased pain and temperature, preserved light touch, as in Brown-Séquard syndrome (p. 1135). There is disagreement whether this is common[2] or uncommon[36] in IMSCT. ± non-radicular dysesthesias (early), with upward extension[37]
    b) paresthesias: either radicular or "medullary" distribution

4. sphincter disturbances
    a) usually urogenital (anal less common) → difficulty evacuating, retention, incontinence, and impotence. Early in conus/cauda equina lesions, especially lipomas (pain not prominent)
    b) sphincter dysfunction common in age < 1 yr due to frequency of lumbosacral lesions (dermoids, epidermoids, etc.)

5. miscellaneous symptoms:
    a) scoliosis or torticollis
    b) SAH
    c) visible mass over spine

Time course of symptoms

Onset usually insidious, but abruptness occurs (benign lesions in children occasionally progress in hours). The onset is often erroneously attributed to coincidental injury. Temporal progression has been divided into 4 stages[38]:
1. pain only (neuralgic)
2. Brown-Séquard syndrome
3. incomplete transectional dysfunction
4. complete transectional dysfunction

Note: 78% (of 23) ependymomas, 74% (of 42) gliomas, all 7 dermoids, and 50% (of 8) lipomas reached the latter 2 stages before diagnosis (not affected by location in cross-sectional nor longitudinal dimension of SC (excludes conus lesions—more frequently diagnosed in 1st stage) (a pre-CT study)).

59.5.5 Diagnosis

It is usually difficult to distinguish IMSCT, ID-EM, and ED on clinical grounds.[2] Schwannomas often start with radicular symptoms that later progress to cord involvement. Most IMSCTs are located posteriorly in cord, which may cause sensory findings to predominate early.[20]

Diagnostic studies

MRI: mainstay of diagnosis. Ependymomas enhance intensely and are often associated with hemorrhage and cysts. Cord edema may mimic a cyst.
    Plain radiographs: vertebral body destruction, enlarged intervertebral foramina, or increases in interpedicular distances suggests ED SCT.
    Lumbar puncture: Elevated protein is the most common abnormality[1] seen in ≈ 95%. The reported range with primary IMSCTs is 50–2,240 mg%. Glucose is normal except with meningeal tumor. SCT can cause complete block, indicated by:
- Froin's syndrome: clotting (due to fibrinogen) and xanthochromia of CSF
- Queckenstedt's test (failure of jugular vein compression to increase CSF pressure, which it normally does in the absence of block)
- barrier to flow of myelographic contrast media

Myelography (p. 925): classically shows fusiform cord widening (may be normal early). Distinct from ED tumors, which produce hourglass deformity (with incomplete block) or paintbrush effect (with complete block), or ID-EM tumors, which produce a capping effect with a sharp cutoff (meniscus sign).

CT: some IMSCTs enhance with IV contrast. Myelo-CT distinguishes IMSCT from ID-EM (poor in differentiating IMSCT subtypes).

Spinal angiography: rarely indicated, except in hemangioblastoma (may be suspected on myelography or MRI by linear serpiginous structures). MRI often obviates this test.

59.5.6 Management

General information

Asymptomatic lesions may be followed since there is significant risk of neurologic deficit with surgery. For symptomatic lesions, surgery should be performed as soon as possible (generally not as an emergency) after diagnosis since surgical results correlate with the preoperative neurologic condition, and it makes no sense to follow the patient as they develop progressive neurologic deficit[39] (some of which may be irreversible).

Astrocytomas: For low grade lesions, if a plane can be developed between the tumor and spinal cord (when it can, it usually consists of a thin gliotic layer traversed by small blood vessels and adhesions[20]), an attempt at total excision is an option.[40] For high-grade astrocytomas or for low-grade astrocytomas without a plane of separation, biopsy alone or biopsy plus limited excision is recommended.[40]

For high-grade lesions, post-op XRT (± chemotherapy) is recommended.[40] XRT is not supported following radical resection of low grade gliomas.[40]

Ependymomas: Gross total removal should be attempted. XRT is not recommended following gross total removal.[40]

59.5.7 Technical surgical considerations

Key concepts

In the surgical removal of IMSCT
- in almost all cases, IMSCTs should be debulked from within using ultrasonic aspirator or laser (to minimize manipulation of neural tissue), and no attempt should be made initially to develop a plane between tumor and spinal cord (even for ependymoma, which of the 3 most common IMSCTs is the only one that actually has such a plane)
- ★ the key to removing IMSCTs is knowing when to stop. If MEPs or D-waves are being monitored, it is suggested that tumor removal should be discontinued if the amplitudes drop to ≤ 50% of baseline

1. position: usually prone, well padded and also securely taped to avoid undesirable movement if MEP monitoring is to be used. Other options include: lateral oblique, sitting
2. if a cystic component is suspected, partial aspiration with a 25 Ga needle once the spinal cord is exposed will decrease the pressure (do not try to completely aspirate the contents because that can make it more difficult to locate the tumor).[41] If the cyst forms a "cap" at either end of the tumor, the dura does not need to be opened over the cyst, since drainage can be accomplished with removal of tumor
3. adjunctive options include:
   a) electrophysiologic monitoring (p. 989)
   b) intraoperative ultrasound: also controversial,[42] favored by some experts. Astrocytomas usually isoechoic with spinal cord, whereas ependymomas are usually hyperechoic
4. a myelotomy is performed either in the midline or just to one side of the dorsal midline to avoid the posteromedian vein. Alternatively, if the tumor is known to be very superficial off the midline (which may be confirmed by ultrasound), entry may be made there. Tumors may cause distortion and displacement of the midline—look for dorsal root entry zones on both sides to identify the midline as the midpoint between root entry zones
5. 6–0 silk sutures may be placed through the pial edge to gently retract the spinal cord open. Standard sized (i.e., non-micro) bayonet forceps can be used to gently spread tissues
6. copious irrigation is used whenever bipolar cautery is employed on the tumor/spinal cord in order to minimize transference of heat to the spinal cord. Monopolar cautery should not be used[41]

7. either laser or ultrasonic aspiration (USA) is used to debulk tumor from within until the glial-tumor interface is reached. Charring from laser may make it more difficult to recognize the glial-tumor interface than USA, and the laser tends to be slower when debulking larger tumors
8. watertight dural closure is critical

▶ **Electrophysiologic monitoring.** Intraoperative electrophysiologic monitoring (SSEP and motor evoked potentials [MEPs][43] and D-waves) is an aid in determining when to stop.

SSEPs almost always degrade with the initial myelotomy and do not correlate well with motor outcome[44] (which is critical),[42,45] and postoperative motor deficit may occur in spite of unaltered intraoperative SSEPs.[43,44] Conversely, SSEPs may be lost without motor deficit.

MEPs are useful, but since they can only be obtained intermittently they do not give real-time warning of a developing problem, and they often cause violent muscle contractions which can be disruptive to delicate surgery. There is a risk of seizures with transcranial MEPs, however none of 322 monitored patients undergoing *spinal cord* surgery had a seizure.[46]

Direct waves (D-waves): a single transcranial stimulus of 80-100 mA of 0.5-1 mS duration with a frequency 0.5-2 Hz produces a response that can be recorded by an electrode in the epidural or sub-dural space of the spinal cord.[47] They may be monitored continuously and since they do not need averaging they can alert the surgeon immediately when deterioration starts to occur.[48] They can determine the level of a deficit by moving the electrode to different levels, but they cannot determine laterality and cannot be used below T12 (due to too few corticospinal tract fibers) or in children less than ≈ 4 years age (due to incomplete maturation of motor pathways).[48] Deterioration to < 50% of baseline is highly correlated with severe post-op deficit.

59.5.8 Prognosis

No well-designed studies give long term functional results with microsurgery, laser, and radiotherapy. Better results occur with lesser initial deficits.[20] Recurrence depends on totality of removal, and on growth pattern of the specific tumor.

Ependymoma: total extirpation improves functional outcome, and myxopapillary ependymomas fare better than the "classic" type.[28] Best functional outcome occurs with modest initial deficits, symptoms < 2 years duration,[49] and total removal. Survival is independent of extent of excision.

Astrocytomas: radical removal is rarely possible (a cleavage plane is unusual even with a microscope). Long term functional results are poorer than with ependymomas. There is 50% recurrence rate in 4–5 yrs.

59.6 Primary bone tumors of the spine

59.6.1 General information

Types of tumors.
1. metastatic: the most common malignancy of spine
   a) common osteolytic metastatic tumors (p. 921) include:
      - lung
      - breast
      - prostate
      - lymphoma: most cases represent spread of systemic disease (secondary lymphoma); however, some may be primary (p. 979)
      - plasmacytoma (p. 928)
      - multiple myeloma (p. 928)
      - Langerhans cell histiocytosis: see differentiating features (p. 980)
   b) metastases that may be osteoblastic:
      - in men: prostate Ca is the most common
      - in women: breast Ca is the most common
   c) Ewing's sarcoma (p. 980)
   d) chloroma: focal infiltration of leukemic cells
2. primary spinal tumors (very rare)
   a) benign
      - vertebral hemangioma (p. 980)
      - osteoid osteoma (p. 990)
      - osteoblastoma (p. 990)
      - aneurysmal bone cyst (p. 979): cavity of highly vascular honeycomb surrounded by a thin cortical shell which may expand
      - osteochondroma (chondroma) (p. 980)

59

- giant cell tumors of bone (p.995): AKA osteoclastoma. Almost always benign with pseudo-malignant behavior
b) malignant
  - chondrosarcoma (p.980)
  - chordomas (p.825)
  - osteogenic sarcoma: rare in spine

59.6.2 Osteoid osteoma and osteoblastoma

General information

Key concepts

- both are benign bone tumors
- histologically identical, differentiation depends on size (≤ 1 cm = osteoid osteoma, > 1 cm = osteoblastoma)
- can occur in the spine and may cause neurologic symptoms (esp. osteoblastoma)
- high cure rate with complete excision

Two types of benign osteoblastic lesions of bone: osteoid osteoma (OO) and benign osteoblastoma (BOB), see ► Table 59.2. They are indistinguishable histologically, and must be differentiated based on size and behavior.

Characteristically cause night pain and pain relieved by aspirin (see Clinical below).

Table 59.2 Comparison of osteoid osteoma and benign osteoblastoma[50]

	Osteoid osteoma	Benign osteoblastoma
percent of primary bone tumors	3.2%	
percent of primary vertebral tumors	1.4%	
percent that occur in spine	10%	35%
size limitations	≤ 1 cm	> 1 cm
growth pattern	confined, self limiting	more extensive, may extend into spinal canal
potential for malignant change?	no	rare
location within spine (83 patients)		
• % in cervical spine	27%	25%
• % in thoracic spine		35%
• % in lumbar region	59%	35%
location within vertebra (81 patients)		
• lamina only	33%	16%
• pedicle only	15%	32%
• articular facet only	19%	0
• vertebral body (VB) only	7%	5%
• transverse process only	6%	8%
• spinous process	5%	5%
• >1 element of neural arch	6%	19%
• combined posterior elements & VB	0	11%

Osteoblastoma is a rare, benign, locally recurrent tumor with a predilection for spine that may rarely undergo sarcomatous change (to osteosarcoma,[51] only a handful of known cases of this). More vascular than OO.[52]

Differential diagnosis

Lesions with similar symptoms and increased uptake on radionuclide bone scan:
1. benign osteoblastoma

2. osteoid osteoma: more pronounced sclerosis of adjacent bone than BOB
3. osteogenic sarcoma: rare in spine
4. aneurysmal bone cyst (p.979): typically trabeculae in central, lucent region
5. unilateral pedicle/laminar necrosis

Clinical

See ▶ Table 59.3 for signs and symptoms. Tenderness confined to vicinity of the lesion occurs in ≈ 60%. 28% of patients with BOB presented with myelopathy. OO presented with neurologic deficit in only 22%.

Table 59.3 Signs and symptoms in 82 patients[50]

Finding	Osteoid osteoma	Benign osteoblastoma
pain on presentation	100%	100%
pain increased by motion	49%	74%
pain increased by Valsalva	17%	36%
nocturnal pain	46%	36%
pain relieved by aspirin	40%	25%
radicular pain	50%	44%
scoliosis	66%	36%
neurologic abnormalities	22%	54%
myelopathy	0	28%
weakness	12%	51%
atrophy	9%	15%

Evaluation

Bone scans are a very sensitive means for detecting these lesions. Once localized, CT or MRI may better define the lesion in that region.

Caution regarding needle biopsy: if the lesion turns out to be osteosarcoma, the contaminated needle tract can result in worse prognosis.

Osteoid osteoma

Radiolucent area with or without surrounding density, often isolated to pedicle or facet. May not show up on tomograms.

Osteoblastoma

Most are expansile, destructive lesions, with 17% having moderate sclerosis. 31% have areas of ↑ density, 20% surrounded by calcified shell. Often a contralateral spondylolysis.[51]

Treatment

In order to obtain a cure, these lesions must be *completely* excised. The role of radiation therapy is poorly defined in these lesions, but is probably ineffective.[51]

Osteoid osteoma

Cortical bone may be hardened and thickened, with granulomatous mass in underlying cavity.

Osteoblastoma

Hemorrhagic, friable, red to purple mass well circumscribed from adjacent bone. Complete excision → complete pain relief in 93%. Curettage only → pain relief, with more likely recurrence. Recurrence rate with total excision is ≈ 10%.

59.6.3 Osteosarcoma

The most common primary bone cancer. More common in children, usually occurring near the ends of long bones, but also in the mandible, pelvis, and rarely in the spine.[53] Spinal osteosarcoma usually

59

occurs in the lumbosacral region in males in their 40s, sometimes arising from areas of osteoblastoma or Paget's disease. If a percutaneous biopsy reveals osteosarcoma, the contaminated needle tract can increase the difficulty of subsequent surgery. Poor prognosis, median survival = 10 months.[53]

59.6.4 Vertebral hemangioma

General information

> ### Key concepts
>
> - the most common primary spine tumor
> - benign, but a small number behave aggressively
> - rarely symptomatic (< 1.2%), symptoms typically from compression fracture, and, rarely, neural compression from bone expansion or soft tissue mass
> - MRI: small lesions are hyperintense on T1WI and T2WI. Larger ones may be hypointense. CT or X-ray: striations (corduroy pattern) or "honeycomb" or polka dot pattern. Bone scan: usually do not have increased uptake
> - treatment: incidental lesions require no treatment or routine follow-up. Biopsy when mets or malignancy are a strong consideration. Treatment options (when indicated): XRT, embolization, vertebroplasty (better than kyphoplasty), surgery

Vertebral hemangiomas (VH), AKA spinal hemangioma, cavernous hemangioma (of the vertebral body), or hemangiomatous angioma. Benign lesions of the spine. The most common primary tumor of the spine (10–12% of primary spinal bone tumors). Estimated incidence: 9–12%,[54,55] with a 10-12% prevalence in the general population.[54] 70% are solitary, 30% are multiple (up to 5 levels may be involved, often noncontiguous). Lumbar and lower thoracic spine are the most common locations; cervical and sacral lesions are rare. Lesions involve only the vertebral bodies in ≈ 25%, posterior spinal arch in ≈ 25%, and both areas in ≈ 50%. Rarely, aggressive hemangiomas may compromise neural structures (▶ Fig. 59.7).

Occasional cases of purely extradural lesions have been described.[56] Intramedullary spinal cord lesions are even less common.[57] Typically found in post-pubertal females.

Malignant degeneration does not occur. Mature thin-walled blood vessels of varying sizes replace normal marrow, producing hypertrophic sclerotic bony trabeculations oriented in a rostral-caudal direction in one of two forms: cavernous (venous) or capillary (difference in subtype carries no prognostic significance).

Presentation

1. incidental (i.e., asymptomatic) lesions
2. symptomatic: only 0.9–1.2% are symptomatic. There may be a hormonal influence (unproven) that may cause symptoms to increase with pregnancy (could also be due to increased blood volume and/or venous pressure)[58] or to vary with the menstrual cycle and may explain why symptoms rarely occur before puberty
   a) pain: occasionally VH may present with pain localized to the level of involvement with no radiculopathy. However, pain is more often due to other pathology (compression fracture, herniated disc, spinal stenosis…) rather than the VH itself
   b) progressive neurologic deficit: this occurs rarely, and usually takes the form of thoracic myelopathy. Deficit may be caused by the following mechanisms
      - subperiosteal (epidural) growth of tumor into the spinal canal
      - expansion of the bone (cortical "blistering") with widening of the pedicles and lamina producing a "bony" spinal stenosis
      - compression by vessels feeding or draining the lesion
      - compression fracture of the involved vertebra (very rare)[59]
      - spontaneous hemorrhage producing spinal epidural hematoma[60] (also very rare)
      - spinal cord ischemia due to "steal"

Imaging

Typical imaging features of VH are shown in ▶ Table 59.4.[61]

Table 59.4 Typical features of VH[61]

Typical features of VH include:
1. lesion limited primarily to vertebral body
2. vertical striation/honeycomb appearance/polka-dot sign on CT
3. hypointense on T1 and hyperintense on T2 MRI
4. enhancement on contrast MRI
5. restriction to 1 vertebral level, and when soft tissue mass invades the spinal canal, the soft tissue mass is < 1 vertebral body in length

Plain X-rays: classically show coarse vertically oriented striations (corduroy pattern) or a "honeycomb" appearance. At least ≈ one-third of the VB must be involved to produce these findings on plain X-ray (see ▶ Fig. 59.4 for demonstration of this finding on sagittal CT).

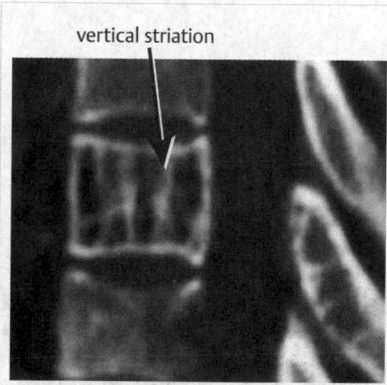

vertical striation

Fig. 59.4 Vertebral hemangioma.
Image: sagittal CT, bone window. Note the vertical striations ("corduroy pattern").

Bone scan: findings on multiphase^{99}Tx-MDP bone scintigraphy and PET scan are highly variable and are therefore not helpful.[62] If the lesion is "cold" (does not light up), it is likely not a metastasis.

MRI: small hemangiomas are focal, round, and hyperintense on T1WI and T2WI (▶ Fig. 59.5). More extensive lesions can be hypointense. MRI may help distinguish lesions that tend not to evolve (mottled increased signal on T1WI and T2WI, possibly due to adipose tissue) from those that tend to be symptomatic (isointense on T1WI, hyperintense on T2WI). Axial MRI may show "salt & pepper" appearance. VHs enhance due to high vascularity.

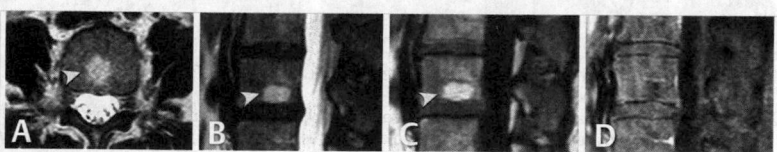

A   B   C   D

Fig. 59.5 Small round vertebral hemangioma (*yellow arrowheads*).
Image: MRI scans, A: axial T2, B:sagittal T2, C: sagittal T1, D: sagittal T1 with contrast (note lack of enhancement of the lesion).

59

CT: diagnostic procedure of choice for the bony involvement. Sagittal images may show vertical striations representing thickened trabeculae (▶ Fig. 59.4) while axial images show multiple high density dots within the bone ("Polka-dot sign"[63]) representing cross-sections through the trabeculae (▶ Fig. 59.6). NB: similar-appearing features may be seen in osteoporosis.

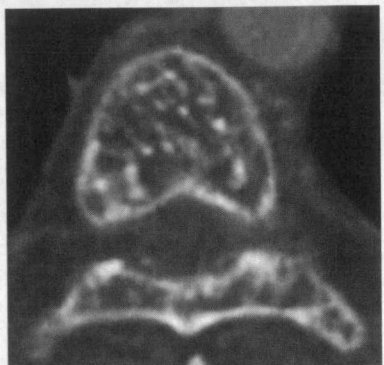

Fig. 59.6 Large vertebral hemangioma.
Image: axial CT bone window demonstrating "polka-dot sign."

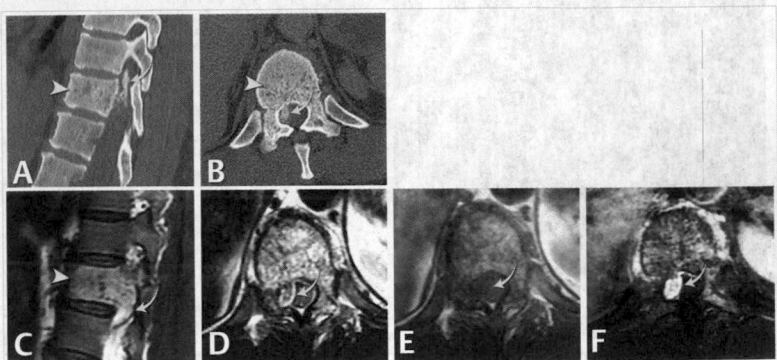

Fig. 59.7 Aggressive vertebral hemangioma.
Image: CT scan, A: sagittal through left side of spinal canal, B: axial.
MRI, C: sagittal T2 through left side of spinal canal, D: axial T2, E: axial T1, F: axial T1 + contrast.
Note the mottling of the VBs (*yellow arrowheads*), the extension of the lesion into the spinal canal (*curved blue arrow*), and the intense contrast enhancement.

Management

Management guidelines:

1. asymptomatic VH with typical features (▶ Table 59.4) without concern for malignancy: no treatment or routine follow-up is required[54,61]
2. biopsy: may be indicated in cases where malignancy (including metastases) is a concern or when there are atypical features on imaging (see typical features, ▶ Table 59.4).[61] In spite of their highly vascular nature, the risk of bleeding complications with CT guided biopsy is extremely low. An alternative to biopsy would be serial imaging, but the literature is sparse on this topic
3. those presenting with pain or neurologic deficit
   a) **radiation therapy** : VH are radiosensitive and undergo sclerotic obliteration. With aggressive VH, there is a risk of vertebral collapse following XRT[64]
      1. as a stand-alone treatment: for lesions causing pain without neuro deficit, XRT provided complete relief in 60-87.5%, and partial relief in nearly all.[65,66] Improvement in pain may be delayed up to years.
      With signs/symptoms of mild myelopathy (e.g. ASIA impairment scale ▶ Table 68.13 group D), some studies have shown clinical improvement with XRT. One review recommended a median total dose of 34 Gy, with a median single doses of 2.0 Gy.[66] Radiographic evidence of response may[66] or may not[54] occur

2. as an adjunct following incomplete resection to decrease recurrence.[67] Total dosage should be ≤ 40 Gy to reduce the risk of radiation myelopathy

b) **embolization**: can provide immediate relief of pain, and may be used alone[68] or as a pre-op surgical adjunct to reduce operative blood loss. Risks: spinal cord infarction if major radicular artery—e.g., artery of Adamkiewicz (p. 87)—is embolized, and it may increase the risk of future fracture (not statistically significant). The decision whether to embolize pre-op is up to the surgeon[68,69,70,71]

c) **vertebroplasty** (p. 1212): has been used for painful VH or following XRT. May be better than kyphoplasty for VH because kyphoplasty destroys the trabecular bone, but no direct comparisons have been made. May be performed at the same time as CT-guided biopsy.[72,73] Not known to be effective for VH with neurologic deficit, but may be used as an adjunct to surgery[74,75]

d) **surgery**: generally regarded as the primary treatment for VH producing severe or rapidly progressive neurologic deficit, or for painful lesions that fail to respond to above measures. Recurrence rate is low (see below) and resolution of symptoms is high. When needed, surgery can stabilize the spine with fusion. Surgery may be discussed with the patient as an option for treatment of VH presenting only with pain if the comparative risk profile is preferred over the other options above, especially for lesions with high risk of instability

Surgical treatment

For surgical indications, see above. Recommendations for surgical management are shown in ▶ Table 59.5.

Intralesional resection results in a low recurrence rate (3% with 3.9 years mean follow-up) (i.e., the increased risk with en bloc resection is not warranted),[76] and resolution of symptoms is high. Pre-operative embolization is a viable option.

Major risks of surgery: blood loss, destabilization of the spine requiring fusion, neurologic deficit (during surgery, or postoperatively usually from epidural hematoma).

With subtotal resection, recurrence rate is 20-30% at 2 years, which was decreased to 7% using post-op XRT.[54,69] Surgery often requires fusion due to the common involvement of the anterior and middle columns of the thoracic or lumbar spine.[69,76,77,78]

Table 59.5 Recommendations for surgical management of VH[a] [54]

VH involvement	Approach	Post-op XRT?
posterior elements only	radical excision via posterior approach	not for total excision
VB involvement with anterior canal compression (with or without ST in canal)	anterior corpectomy with strut graft	
VB involved but no expansion, ST in lateral canal	laminectomy with removal of soft-tissue	follow serial CT, give XRT if VB expansion or ST expansion
extensive involvement of anterior and posterior vertebral elements with circumferential bone expansion, no ST compression	laminectomy	either XRT, or close follow-up with CT and XRT for ST recurrence or progressive VB expansion
extensive anterior and posterior involvement with ST in anterior canal	anterior corpectomy with strut graft	

[a]abbreviations: XRT = radiation treatment; ST = soft-tissue component of VH; VB = vertebral body.

59.6.5 Giant cell tumors of bone

AKA osteoclastoma (cells arise from osteoclasts). In the same general category as aneurysmal bone cysts. Typically arise in adolescence. Most common in knees and wrists. Those that come to the attention of the neurosurgeon generally arise in the skull (especially the skull base, and in particular the sphenoid bone), or in the vertebral column (≈ 4% occur in sacrum).

Pathology

Lytic with bony collapse. Almost always benign with pseudomalignant behavior (recurrence is common, and pulmonary mets can occur).

59

Evaluation

Soft tissues are best evaluated with MRI. Spine CT is critical to assess degree of bony destruction and for surgical planning purposes.

Work-up includes chest CT because of possibility of pulmonary mets.

Treatment

Intratumoral curettage, possibly aided by pre-op embolization. Recurrence rate with this treatment (even if resection is subtotal) is only ≈ 20%. Role of XRT is controversial[7] because of the possibility of malignant degeneration (therefore use XRT only for non-resectable recurrence).

Osteoclast inhibiting drugs have met with some success following subtotal resection:

1. bisphosphonates: e.g., pamidronate (p. 1364)
2. RANKL inhibitors: e.g., denosumab (Prolia®) (p. 926))

For gross residual disease after resection, re-resection is a consideration.

Cryosurgery with liquid nitrogen has been employed in long bones. Its use is limited in neurosurgical cases because of risk of injury to adjacent neural structures (brain, spinal cord) and cryotherapy induced fractures, although it has been described for use in the sacrum.[79]

Close follow-up is required due to propensity for recurrence. MRI or CT initially q 3 months is suggested.

References

[1] Kopelson G, Linggood RM, Kleinman GM, et al. Management of Intramedullary Spinal Cord Tumors. Radiology. 1980; 135:473–479

[2] Adams RD, Victor M. Intraspinal Tumors. In: Principles of Neurology. 2nd ed. New York: McGraw-Hill; 1981:638–641

[3] Lyons MK, O'Neill BP, Kurtin PJ, et al. Diagnosis and Management of Primary Spinal Epidural Non-Hodgkin's Lymphoma. Mayo Clinic Proceedings. 1996; 71:453–457

[4] Liu JK, Brockmeyer DL, Dailey AT, et al. Surgical management of aneurysmal bone cysts of the spine. Neurosurg Focus. 2003; 15

[5] Suzuki M, Satoh T, Nishida J, et al. Solid variant of aneurysmal bone cyst of the cervical spine. Spine. 2004; 29:E376–E381

[6] Neviaser JS, Eisenberg SH. Giant cell reparative granuloma of the cervical spine; case report. Bulletin of the Hospital for Joint Diseases. 1954; 15:73–78

[7] Dunn EJ, Davidson RI, Desai S, et al. Diagnosis and Management of Tumors of the Cervical Spine. In: The Cervical Spine. 2nd ed. Philadelphia: JB Lippincott; 1989:693–722

[8] Menezes AH, Sato Y. Primary Tumors of the Spine in Children - Natural History and Management. Concepts Pediatr Neurosurg. 1990; 10:30–53

[9] Grubb MR, Currier BL, Pritchard DJ, et al. Primary Ewing's Sarcoma of the Spine. Spine. 1994; 19:309–313

[10] Porter DG, Martin AJ, Mallucci CL, et al. Spinal Cord Compression Due To Masson's Vegetant Intravascular Hemangioendothelioma: Case Report. Journal of Neurosurgery. 1995; 82:125–127

[11] Scott RM, Wolpert SM, Bartoshesky LE, et al. Dermoid tumors occurring at the site of previous myelomeningocele repair. Journal of Neurosurgery. 1986; 65:779–783

[12] Storrs BB. Are dermoid and epidermoid tumors preventable complications of myelomeningocele repair? Pediatr Neurosurg. 1994; 20:160–162

[13] Ramos E, Marlin AE, Gaskill SJ. Congenital dermoid tumor in a child at initial myelomeningocele closure: an etiological discussion. J Neurosurg Pediatrics. 2008; 2:414–415

[14] Metellus P, Bouvier C, Guyotat J, et al. Solitary fibrous tumors of the central nervous system: clinicopathological and therapeutic considerations of 18 cases. Neurosurgery. 2007; 60:715–22; discussion 722

[15] Solero CL, Fornari M, Giombini S, et al. Spinal meningiomas: review of 174 operated cases. Neurosurgery. 1989; 25:153–160

[16] Seppala MT, Haltia MJ, Sankila RJ, et al. Long-term outcome after removal of spinal schwannoma: a clinicopathological study of 187 cases. J Neurosurg. 1995; 83:621–626

[17] Conti P, Pansini G, Mouchaty H, et al. Spinal neurinomas: retrospective analysis and long-term outcome of 179 consecutively operated cases and review of the literature. Surg Neurol. 2004; 61:34–43; discussion 44

[18] Asazuma T, Toyama Y, Maruiwa H, et al. Surgical strategy for cervical dumbbell tumors based on a three-dimensional classification. Spine. 2004; 29: E10–E14

[19] Gottfried ON, Binning MJ, Schmidt MH. Surgical Approaches to Spinal Schwannomas. Contemporary Neurosurgery. 2005; 27:1–8

[20] Stein B. Intramedullary Spinal Cord Tumors. Clin Neurosurg. 1983; 30:717–741

[21] Stern WE. Localization and Diagnosis of Spinal Cord Tumors. Clin Neurosurg. 1977; 25:480–494

[22] DeSousa AL, Kalsbeck JE, Mealey J, et al. Intraspinal Tumors in Children. A Review of 81 Cases. J Neurosurg. 1979; 51:437–445

[23] Hautzer NW, Aiyesimoju A, Robitaille Y. Primary Spinal Intramedullary Lymphomas: A Review. Ann Neurol. 1983; 14:62–66

[24] Alvisi C, Cerisoli M, Giuloni M. Intramedullary Spinal Gliomas: Long Term Results of Surgical Treatment. Acta Neurochirurgica. 1984; 70:169–179

[25] Kumar R, Reddy SJ, Wani AA, et al. Primary spinal primitive neuroectodermal tumor: case series and review of the literature. Pediatr Neurosurg. 2007; 43:1–6

[26] White JB, Miller GM, Layton KF, et al. Nonenhancing tumors of the spinal cord. J Neurosurg Spine. 2007; 7:403–407

[27] Dorwart RH, LaMasters DL, Watanabe TJ, et al. Tumors. In: Computed Tomography of the Spine and Spinal Cord. San Anselmo: Clavadal Press; 1983:115–131

[28] Mork SJ, Loken AC. Ependymoma: A Follow-Up Study of 101 Cases. Cancer. 1977; 40:907–915

[29] Tzerakis N, Georgakoulias N, Kontogeorgos G, et al. Intraparenchymal myxopapillary ependymoma: case report. Neurosurgery. 2004; 55

[30] Helwig EB, Stern JB. Subcutaneous sacrococcygeal myxopapillary ependymoma. A clinicopathologic study of 32 cases. Am J Clin Pathol. 1984; 81:156–161

[31] Malis LI. Intramedullary Spinal Cord Tumors. Clin Neurosurg. 1978; 25:512–539

59

[32] Smaltino F, Bernini FP, Santoro S. Computerized Tomography in the Diagnosis of Intramedullary Metastases. Acta Neurochirurgica. 1980; 52:299–303

[33] Edelson RN, Deck MDF, Posner JB. Intramedullary Spinal Cord Metastases. Neurology. 1972; 22:1222–1231

[34] Murphy KC, Feld R, Evans WK, et al. Intramedullary Spinal Cord Metastases from Small Cell Carcinoma of the Lung. J Clin Onc. 1983; 1:99–106

[35] Jellinger K, Kothbauer P, Sunder-Plassmann, et al. Intramedullary Spinal Cord Metastases. J Neurol. 1979; 220:31–41

[36] Stein B. Surgery of Intramedullary Spinal Cord Tumors. Clin Neurosurg. 1979; 26:473–479

[37] Sebastian PR, Fisher M, Smith TW, et al. Intramedullary Spinal Cord Metastasis. Surg Neurol. 1981; 16:336–339

[38] Nittner K, Olivecrona H, Tonnis W. Handbuch der Neurochirurgie. New York: Springer-Verlag; 1972:1–606

[39] Post KD, Stein BM, Schmidek HH, et al. Surgical Management of Spinal Cord Tumors and Arteriovenous Malformations. In: Operative Neurosurgical Techniques. 3rd ed. Philadelphia: W.B. Saunders; 1995:2027–2048

[40] Nadkarni TD, Rekate HL. Pediatric Intramedullary Spinal Cord Tumors: Critical Review of the Literature. Child's Nervous System. 1999; 15:17–28

[41] Greenwood J. Surgical Removal of Intramedullary Tumors. J Neurosurg. 1967; 26:276–282

[42] Albright AL. Pediatric Intramedullary Spinal Cord Tumors. Child's Nervous System. 1999; 15:436–437

[43] Morota N, Deletis V, Constantini S, et al. The Role of Motor Evoked Potentials During Surgery for Intramedullary Spinal Cord Tumors. Neurosurgery. 1997; 41:1327–1336

[44] Kothbauer P, Deletis V, Epstein FJ. Intraoperative Spinal Cord Monitoring for Intramedullary Surgery: An Essential Adjunct. Pediatric Neurosurgery. 1997; 26:247–254

[45] Albright AL. Intraoperative Spinal Cord Monitoring for Intramedullary Surgery: An Essential Adjunct? Pediatric Neurosurgery. 1998; 29

[46] Ulkatan S, Jaramillo AM, Tellez MJ, et al. Incidence of intraoperative seizures during motor evoked potential monitoring in a large cohort of patients undergoing different surgical procedures. J Neurosurg. 2017; 126:1296–1302

[47] Kothbauer KF. Intraoperative neurophysiologic monitoring for intramedullary spinal-cord tumor surgery. Neurophysiol Clin. 2007; 37:407–414

[48] Park JH, Hyun SJ. Intraoperative neurophysiological monitoring in spinal surgery. World J Clin Cases. 2015; 3:765–773

[49] Guidetti B, Mercuri S, Vagnozzi R. Long-Term Results of the Surgical Treatment of 129 Intramedullary Spinal Gliomas. J Neurosurg. 1981; 54:323–330

[50] Janin Y, Epstein JA, Carras R, et al. Osteoid Osteomas and Osteoblastomas of the Spine. Neurosurgery. 1981; 8:31–38

[51] Amacher AL, Eltomey A. Spinal Osteoblastoma in Children and Adolescents. Childs Nervous System. 1985; 1:29–32

[52] Lichtenstein L, Sawyer WR. Benign Osteoblastoma. J Bone Joint Surg. 1964; 46A:755–765

[53] Shives TC, Dahlin DC, Sim FH, et al. Osteosarcoma of the spine. J Bone Joint Surg Am. 1986; 68:660–668

[54] Fox MW, Onofrio BM. The natural history and management of symptomatic and asymptomatic vertebral hemangiomas. J Neurosurg. 1993; 78:36–45

[55] Healy M, Herz DA, Pearl L. Spinal Hemangiomas. Neurosurgery. 1983; 13:689–691

[56] Richardson RR, Cerullo LJ. Spinal Epidural Cavernous Hemangioma. Surgical Neurology. 1979; 12:266–268

[57] Cosgrove GR, Bertrand G, Fontaine S, et al. Cavernous Angiomas of the Spinal Cord. Journal of Neurosurgery. 1988; 68:31–36

[58] Tekkök IH, Açikgöz B, Saglam A, et al. Vertebral Hemangioma Symptomatic During Pregnancy - Report of a Case and Review of the Literature. Neurosurgery. 1993; 32:302–306

[59] Graham JJ, Yang WC. Vertebral Hemangioma with Compression Fracture and Paraparesis Treated with Preoperative Embolization and Vertebral Resection. Spine. 1984; 9:97–101

[60] Kosary IA, Braham J, Shacked I, et al. Spinal Epidural Hematoma due to Hemangioma of Vertebra. Surgical Neurology. 1977; 7:61–62

[61] Wang B, Zhang L, Yang S, et al. Atypical Radiographic Features of Aggressive Vertebral Hemangiomas. J Bone Joint Surg Am. 2019; 101:979–986

[62] Gaudino S, Martucci M, Colantonio R, et al. A systematic approach to vertebral hemangioma. Skeletal Radiol. 2015; 44:25–36

[63] Persaud T. The polka-dot sign. Radiology. 2008; 246:980–981

[64] Tarantino R, Donnarumma P, Nigro L, et al. Surgery in extensive vertebral hemangioma: case report, literature review and a new algorithm proposal. Neurosurg Rev. 2015; 38:585–92; discussion 592

[65] Asthana AK, Tandon SC, Pant GC, et al. Radiation therapy for symptomatic vertebral haemangioma. Clin Oncol (R Coll Radiol). 1990; 2:159–162

[66] Heyd R, Seegenschmiedt M H, Rades D, et al. Radiotherapy for symptomatic vertebral hemangiomas: results of a multicenter study and literature review. Int J Radiat Oncol Biol Phys. 2010; 77:217–225

[67] Jiang L, Liu XG, Yuan HS, et al. Diagnosis and treatment of vertebral hemangiomas with neurologic deficit: a report of 29 cases and literature review. Spine J. 2014; 14:944–954

[68] Premat K, Clarencon F, Cormier E, et al. Long-term outcome of percutaneous alcohol embolization combined with percutaneous vertebroplasty in aggressive vertebral hemangiomas with epidural extension. Eur Radiol. 2017; 27:2860–2867

[69] Piper K, Zou L, Li D, et al. Surgical Management and Adjuvant Therapy for Patients With Neurological Deficits From Vertebral Hemangiomas: A Meta-Analysis. Spine (Phila Pa 1976). 2020; 45:E99–E110

[70] Yao KC, Malek AM. Transpedicular N-butyl cyanoacrylate-mediated percutaneous embolization of symptomatic vertebral hemangiomas. J Neurosurg Spine. 2013; 18:450–455

[71] Acosta FL,Jr, Sanai N, Chi JH, et al. Comprehensive management of symptomatic and aggressive vertebral hemangiomas. Neurosurg Clin N Am. 2008; 19:17–29

[72] Boschi V, Pogorelic Z, Gulan G, et al. Management of cement vertebroplasty in the treatment of vertebral hemangioma. Scand J Surg. 2011; 100:120–124

[73] Saracen A, Kotwica Z. Vertebroplasty (PVP) is effective in the treatment of painful vertebral hemangiomas. Acta Orthop Belg. 2018; 84:105–107

[74] Hu W, Kan SL, Xu HB, et al. Thoracic aggressive vertebral hemangioma with neurologic deficit: A retrospective cohort study. Medicine (Baltimore). 2018; 97. DOI: 10.1097/MD.0000000000012775

[75] Blecher R, Smorgick Y, Anekstein Y, et al. Management of symptomatic vertebral hemangioma: follow-up of 6 patients. J Spinal Disord Tech. 2011; 24:196–201

[76] Goldstein CL, Varga PP, Gokaslan ZL, et al. Spinal hemangiomas: results of surgical management for local recurrence and mortality in a multicenter study. Spine (Phila Pa 1976). 2015; 40:656–664

[77] Vasudeva VS, Chi JH, Groff MW. Surgical treatment of aggressive vertebral hemangiomas. Neurosurg Focus. 2016; 41. DOI: 10.3171/2016.5.FOCUS16169

[78] Kato S, Kawahara N, Murakami H, et al. Surgical management of aggressive vertebral hemangiomas causing spinal cord compression: long-term clinical follow-up of five cases. J Orthop Sci. 2010; 15:350–356

[79] Marcove RC, Sheth DS, Brien EW, et al. Conservative surgery for giant cell tumors of the sacrum. The role of cryosurgery as a supplement to curettage and partial excision. Cancer. 1994; 74:1253–1260

59

Part XIV

Head Trauma

XIV

60 Head Trauma – General Information, Grading, Initial Management

60.1 Head trauma – general information

60.1.1 Introduction

56–60% of patients with GCS score ≤8 have 1 or more other organ system injured.[1] 25% have "surgical" lesions. There is a 4–5% incidence of associated spine fractures with significant head injury (mostly C1 to C3).

When a detailed history is unavailable, remember: the loss of consciousness may have *preceded* (and possibly have caused) the trauma. Therefore, maintain an index of suspicion for e.g., aneurysmal SAH, hypoglycemia, etc. in the differential diagnosis of the causes of trauma and associated coma.

Brain injury from trauma results from two distinct processes:
1. primary brain injury: occurs at time of trauma (cortical contusions, lacerations, bone fragmentation, diffuse axonal injury, and brainstem contusion)
2. secondary injury: develops subsequent to the initial injury. Includes injuries from intracranial hematomas, edema, hypoxemia, ischemia (primarily due to elevated intracranial pressure (ICP) and/or shock), vasospasm

Since impact damage cannot be influenced by the treating neurosurgeon, intense interest has focused on reducing secondary injuries, which requires good general medical care and an understanding of intracranial pressure (p. 1036).

60.1.2 Delayed deterioration

≈ 15% of patients who do not initially exhibit signs of significant brain injury may deteriorate in a delayed fashion, sometimes referred to as patients who "talk and deteriorate," or when more lethal, patient who "talk and die."[2] Etiologies:
1. ≈ 75% will exhibit an intracranial hematoma
    a) may be present on initial evaluation and can then worsen
    b) may develop in a delayed fashion
        • delayed epidural hematoma (EDH) (p. 1075)
        • delayed subdural hematoma (SDH) (p. 1081)
        • delayed traumatic contusions (p. 1072)
2. posttraumatic diffuse cerebral edema (p. 1026)
3. hydrocephalus
4. tension pneumocephalus
5. seizures
6. metabolic abnormalities, includes:
    a) hyponatremia
    b) hypoxia: etiologies include pneumothorax, MI, CHF…
    c) hepatic encephalopathy
    d) hypoglycemia: including insulin reaction
    e) adrenal insufficiency
    f) drug or alcohol withdrawal
7. vascular events
    a) dural sinus thrombosis (p. 1594)
    b) carotid (or rarely, vertebral) artery dissection (p. 1578)
    c) SAH: due to rupture of aneurysm (spontaneous or posttraumatic) or carotid-cavernous fistula (CCF) (p. 1519)
    d) cerebral embolism: including fat embolism syndrome (p. 1013)
8. meningitis
9. hypotension (shock)

60.2 Grading

Despite many (valid) criticisms, the initial post-resuscitation Glasgow Coma Scale (GCS) score (▶ Table 18.1) remains the most widely used and perhaps best replicated scale employed for the assessment of head trauma. Problems with this type of scale include that it is an ordinal scale that is non parametric (i.e., does not represent precise measurements of discrete quantities), it is non-linear, and it is not an interval scale, so that for example, a decrease of 2 points in one parameter is not necessarily equal to a decrease in 2 points of another.[3] Thus, performing mathematical manipulations (e.g., adding components, or calculating mean values), while often done, is not statistically sound.[4]

▶ **Stratification.** There are a number of schemes to stratify the severity of head injury. Any such categorization is arbitrary and will be imperfect. A simple system based only on GCS score is as follows:
- GCS 14–15 = mild
- GCS 9–13 = moderate
- GCS ≤ 8 = severe

More elaborate systems (e.g., ▶ Fig. 60.1 [3]) may incorporate factors in addition to the GCS.

Minimal	Mild	Moderate	Severe
• GCS = 15 • No loss of consciousness (LOC) • No amnesia	GCS = 14 **OR**	GCS = 9–13 **OR**	GCS = 3–8
	GCS = 15 plus EITHER • Brief LOC (< 5 mins) • OR Impaired alertness or memory	LOC ≥ 5mins **OR**	Critical† GCS = 3–4
		Focal neurologic deficit	

Concussion

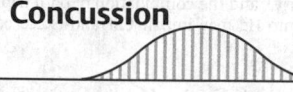

* Abbreviations: LOC = loss of consciousness, GCS = Glasgow Coma Scale score.
† "Critical" designation is used by some to indicate the most severe injuries (GCS=3-4).

Fig. 60.1 Sample stratification scheme for head injury severity.[3]

60.3 Transfer of trauma patients

It is sometimes necessary for a neurosurgeon to accept a trauma patient in transfer from another institution that is not equipped to handle major neurologic injuries, or to transfer patients to other facilities for a variety of reasons. ▶ Table 60.1 lists factors that should be assessed and stabilized (if

Table 60.1 Factors to assess in head injured patients

Clinical concern	Items to check	Steps to remedy
hypoxia or hypoventilation	ABG, respiratory rate	intubate any patient who has hypercarbia, hypoxemia, or is not localizing
hypotension or hypertension	BP, Hgb/Hct	transfuse patients with significant loss of blood volume
anemia	Hgb/Hct	transfuse patients with significant anemia
seizures	electrolytes, ASM levels	correct hyponatremia or hypoglycemia; administer ASMs when appropriate[a]
infection or hyperthermia	WBC, temperature	LP if meningitis is possible and no contraindications (p.1811)
spinal stability	spine X-rays	spine immobilization (spine board, cervical collar & sandbags...); patients with locked facets should be reduced if possible before transfer

[a]see Seizures (p.480), as well as Posttraumatic seizures (p.504)

60

possible) prior to transfer. These items should also be evaluated in trauma patients about whom a neurosurgeon is consulted in his or her own E/R, as well as in patients with other CNS abnormalities besides trauma (e.g., SAH).

60.4 Management in E/R

60.4.1 General measures

Blood pressure and oxygenation

Practice guideline: BP and oxygenation

Level II[5]: monitor BP and avoid hypotension (SBP < 90 mm Hg)
Level III[5]: monitor oxygenation and avoid hypoxia (PaO$_2$ < 60 mm Hg or O$_2$ saturation < 90%)

Hypotension

Hypotension (shock) is rarely attributable to head injury except:
- in terminal stages (i.e., with dysfunction of medulla and cardiovascular collapse)
- where enough blood has been lost from scalp wounds to cause hypovolemia (exsanguination)
- in infancy, where enough blood can be lost intracranially or into the subgaleal space to cause shock

Hypotension (defined as a single SBP < 90 mm Hg) doubles mortality, hypoxia (apnea or cyanosis in the field, or PaO$_2$ < 60 mm Hg on ABG) also increases mortality,[6] and the combination of both triples mortality and increases the risk of bad outcome. SBP < 90 mm Hg may impair CBF and exacerbate brain injury and should be avoided (p. 1050).

Early use of paralytics and sedation (prior to ICP monitoring)

Practice guideline: Early sedation and paralysis

Level III[7]: sedation and neuromuscular blockade (NMB) can be helpful for transporting the head-injured patient, but they interfere with the neuro exam
Level III[7]: NMB should be used when sedation alone is inadequate

The routine use of sedatives and paralytics in neurotrauma patients may lead to a higher incidence of pneumonia, longer ICU stays, and possibly sepsis.[8] These agents also impair neurologic assessment.[7,9] Use should therefore be reserved for cases with clinical evidence of intracranial hypertension (see ▶ Table 60.2), for intubation, or where use is necessary for transport or to permit evaluation of the patient (e.g., to get a combative patient to hold still for a CT scan).[10]

Table 60.2 Clinical signs of IC-HTN[a]

1. pupillary dilatation (unilateral or bilateral)
2. asymmetric pupillary reaction to light
3. decerebrate or decorticate posturing (usually contralateral to blown[b] pupil)
4. progressive deterioration of the neurologic exam not attributable to extracranial factors

[a]Items 1–3 represent clinical signs of herniation. The most convincing clinical evidence of IC-HTN is the witnessed evolution of 1 or more of these signs. IC-HTN may produce a bulging fontanelle in an infant.
[b]"blown pupil": fixed & dilated pupil

60

Intubation and hyperventilation

Indications for *intubation* in trauma; also see **Practice guideline: Intubation – indications** (p. 1003):
1. depressed level of consciousness (patient cannot protect airway): usually GCS ≤ 7
2. need for hyperventilation (HPV): see below
3. severe maxillofacial trauma: patency of airway tenuous or concern for inability to maintain patency with further tissue swelling and/or bleeding
4. need for pharmacologic paralysis for evaluation or management

Practice guideline: Intubation—indications

Level III[11]: secure the airway (usually by endotracheal intubation) in patients with GCS ≤ 8 who are unable to maintain their airway or who remain hypoxic despite supplemental O_2

Cautions regarding intubation:
1. if basal skull fracture through cribriform plate is possible, avoid nasotracheal intubation (to avoid intracranial entry of tube). Use orotracheal intubation
2. prevents assessment of patient's ability to verbalize[9] e.g., for determining Glasgow Coma Scale score. This ability should be noted (none, unintelligible, inappropriate, confused, or oriented) prior to intubation
3. risk of pneumonia: see **Practice guideline: Antibiotics for intubation** (p. 1003) regarding antibiotics

Practice guideline: Antibiotics for intubation

Level II[12]: periprocedural antibiotics for endotracheal intubation reduce the risk of pneumonia, but do not alter length of stay or mortality

Hyperventilation (HPV)

Practice guideline: Early/prophylactic hyperventilation

Level II[13]: prophylactic hyperventilation ($PaCO_2 \leq 25$ mm Hg) is not recommended
  Level III
• hyperventilation (HPV) before ICP monitoring is established should be reserved as a temporizing measure[13] for patients with signs of transtentorial herniation (see ► Table 60.2) or progressive neurologic deterioration not attributable to extracranial causes[7]
• HPV should be avoided during the first 24 hrs after TBI (when CBF is often dangerously decreased)[13]

1. since HPV may exacerbate cerebral ischemia, **HPV should not be used prophylactically** (p. 1052)
2. prior to ICP monitoring, HPV should only be used briefly when CT or clinical signs of IC-HTN are present[10] (see ► Table 60.2 for clinical signs)
   a) when appropriate indications are met: HPV to $PaCO_2 = 30$–$35\,mm$ Hg
   b) HPV should not be used to the point that $PaCO_2 < 30$ mm Hg (this further reduces CBF but does not necessarily reduce ICP)
3. acute alkalosis increases protein binding of calcium (decreases ionized Ca^{++}). Patients being *hyperventilated* may develop ionized hypocalcemia with tetany (despite normal total [Ca])

60

Mannitol in E/R

Practice guideline: Early use of mannitol

Level III[7,14]: the use of mannitol before ICP monitoring is established should be reserved for patients who are adequately volume-resuscitated with signs of transtentorial herniation (see ▶ Table 60.2) or progressive neurologic deterioration not attributable to extracranial causes

Indications in E/R, see also more details (p. 1053):
1. evidence of intracranial hypertension (see ▶ Table 60.2)
2. evidence of mass effect (focal deficit, e.g., hemiparesis)
3. sudden deterioration prior to CT (including pupillary dilatation)
4. after CT, if a lesion that is associated with increased ICP is identified
5. after CT, if going to O.R.
6. to assess "salvageability": in patient with no evidence of brainstem function, look for return of brainstem reflexes

Contraindications:
1. prophylactic administration is *not* recommended due to its volume-depleting effect. Use only for appropriate indications (see above)
2. hypotension or hypovolemia: hypotension can negatively influence outcome.[10] Therefore, when intracranial hypertension (IC-HTN) is present, first utilize sedation and/or paralysis, and CSF drainage. If further measures are needed, fluid resuscitate the patient before administering mannitol. Use hyperventilation in hypovolemic patients until mannitol can be given
3. relative contraindication: mannitol may slightly impede normal coagulation
4. CHF: before causing diuresis, mannitol transiently increases intravascular volume. Use with caution in CHF, may need to pre-treat with furosemide (Lasix®)

R: bolus with 0.25–1 gm/kg over < 20 min (for average adult: ≈ 350 ml of 20% solution). Peak effect occurs in ≈ 20 minutes (p. 1053) (for follow-up dosing).

Prophylactic antiseizure medications (ASMs)

Practice guideline: Prophylactic antiseizure medications after TBI

Level II[15,16,17]: prophylactic phenytoin, carbamazepine, phenobarbital, or valproate[18] do not prevent late PTS

Level II: ASMs[17] (e.g., phenytoin, valproate, or carbamazepine[15,16,18]) may be used to decrease the incidence of early PTS (within 7 days of TBI) in patients at high risk of seizures after TBI (see ▶ Table 60.3); however, this does not improve outcome

Routine use of prophylactic antiseizure medications (ASMs) in traumatic brain injury (TBI) is ineffective in preventing the late development of posttraumatic seizures (PTS) i.e., epilepsy, and has been shown to not be useful except in certain circumstances.[15,16]

Table 60.3 Conditions with increased risk of posttraumatic seizures

1. acute subdural, epidural, or intracerebral hematoma (SDH, EDH or ICH)
2. open-depressed skull fracture with parenchymal injury
3. seizure within the first 24 hrs after injury
4. Glasgow Coma Scale score < 10
5. penetrating brain injury
6. history of significant alcohol abuse
7. ± cortical (hemorrhagic) contusion on CT

See details on using (p. 506) and discontinuing (p. 506) prophylactic ASMs following TBI.
▶ Table 60.3 reiterates the markers for patients at increased risk of early PTSs.

60.4.2 Neurosurgical exam in trauma

General information

It is not possible to outline a physical exam that is universally applicable. Major trauma must be assessed rapidly, often under chaotic circumstances, and must be individualized based on patient's medical stability, type of injury, degree of combativeness, use of pharmacologic paralytics (p. 1002), the needs of other caregivers attending to other organ injuries, the need to triage in the event of multiple patients requiring simultaneous attention…

The following describes some features that should be assessed under certain circumstances with the understanding that this *must be individualized*. This addresses only craniospinal injuries, and assumes that general systemic injuries (internal bleeding, myocardial and/or pulmonary contusion…) as well as orthopedic injuries (long bone and pelvic fractures…) will be treated by other members of a "trauma team." Although organized here in outline form, the most efficient order of examination is usually dictated by circumstances unique to each situation.

General physical condition (oriented towards neuro assessment)

1. visual inspection of cranium:
   a) evidence of basal skull fracture (p. 1064):
      • raccoon's eyes (AKA Panda bear sign): periorbital ecchymoses
      • Battle's sign: postauricular ecchymoses (around mastoid air sinuses)
      • CSF rhinorrhea/otorrhea (p. 418)
      • hemotympanum or laceration of external auditory canal
   b) check for facial fractures
      • Le Fort fractures (p. 1067): palpate for instability of facial bones, including zygomatic arch
      • orbital rim fracture: palpable step-off
   c) periorbital edema, proptosis
2. cranio-cervical auscultation
   a) auscultate over carotid arteries: bruit may indicate carotid dissection
   b) auscultate over globe of eye: bruit may indicate traumatic carotid-cavernous fistula CCF; see Carotid-cavernous fistula (p. 1519)
3. physical signs of trauma to spine: bruising, deformity
4. evidence of seizure: single, multiple, or continuing (status epilepticus)

Neurologic exam

1. cranial nerve exam
   a) optic nerve function (p. 1014)
      • if conscious: serial quantitation of vision in each eye is important.[19] A Rosenbaum near vision card is ideal (see inside back cover), otherwise use any printed material. If patient cannot see this, check if they can count fingers. Failing this, check for hand motion vision and lastly light perception. Children may develop transient cortical blindness lasting 1–2 days, usually after a blow to the back of the head
      • if unconscious: check for afferent pupillary defect (p. 592), best demonstrated with swinging flashlight test (p. 591). Indicates possible optic nerve injury
      • funduscopic exam: check for papilledema, pre-retinal hemorrhages, retinal detachment, or retinal abnormalities suggestive of anterior optic nerve injury. If a detailed exam is required, pharmacologic dilatation with mydriatics (p. 593) may be employed; however, this precludes pupillary exam for a variable period of time, and should be undertaken advisedly
   b) pupil: size in ambient light; reaction to light (direct & consensual)
   c) VII: check for peripheral VII palsy (p. 1064) (facial asymmetry of unilateral upper and lower facial muscles)
   d) VI: abducens palsy (p. 598) following trauma may occur as a result of ↑ ICP or with clival fractures (p. 1065)

60

2. level of consciousness/mental status
   a) Glasgow coma scale for quantitating level of consciousness in poorly responsive patient (see
      ► Table 18.1)
   b) check orientation in patient able to communicate
3. motor exam (assesses motor tracts from motor cortex through spinal cord)
   a) if patient is cooperative: check motor strength in all 4 extremities
   b) if uncooperative: check for appropriate movement of all 4 extremities to noxious stimulus
      (differentiate voluntary movement from posturing or stereotypical spinal cord reflex). This
      also assesses sensation in an unresponsive patient
   c) if any doubt about integrity of spinal cord: also check "resting" tone of anal sphincter on rectal
      exam, evaluate voluntary sphincter contraction if patient can cooperate, check anal wink with
      pinprick, and assess bulbocavernosus reflex (p.1130) (see Neurological assessment, for
      details)
4. sensory exam
   a) cooperative patient:
      • check pinprick on trunk and in all 4 extremities, touch on major dermatomes (C4, C6, C7,
        C8, T4, T6, T10, L2, L4, L5, S1, sacrococcygeal)
      • check posterior column function: joint position sense of LEs
   b) uncooperative patient: check for central response to noxious stimulus (e.g., grimace, vocaliza-
      tion…, as opposed to flexion-withdrawal, which could be a spinal cord mediated reflex)
5. reflexes
   a) muscle stretch ("deep tendon") reflexes if patient is not thrashing: e.g., preserved reflex indi-
      cates that a flaccid limb is due to CNS injury and not nerve root injury (and vice versa)
   b) check plantar reflex for upgoing toes (Babinski sign)
   c) in suspected spinal cord injury: the anal wink and bulbocavernosus reflex are checked on the
      rectal exam (see above)

60.5 Radiographic evaluation of TBI in the E/R

60.5.1 General information

An unenhanced (i.e., non-contrast) CT scan of the head usually suffices for patients seen in the emergency department presenting after TBI or with a new neurologic deficit. Enhanced CT or MRI may be
appropriate after the unenhanced CT in some circumstances, but are not usually required emergently (exceptions include: suspected ischemic stroke, significant brain edema on non-contrast CT
suggesting a neoplasm that cannot be demonstrated without contrast).

Other tests: angiography may be needed acutely in certain circumstances, primarily in penetrating head trauma. Skull X-rays are usually inadequate for primary evaluation, but may be helpful in
certain situations, for example with some retained foreign bodies.

Spine imaging: victims of TBI are often at risk for concomitant spine injuries. Spine imaging is
covered in brief below and in detail under Spine Trauma.

See also special considerations in concussion (p.1023).

60.5.2 Indications for initial brain CT

► **Initial imaging inconcussion** (p.1019) **or mild TBI.** There is not uniform agreement about when
to obtain an admitting imaging study (usually a noncontrast head CT scan) with mild TBI and concussion. Some recommendations for adults are provided below. For patients ≤ 16 years see Pediatric
head injuries (p.1099). Also see Initial imaging for moderate to severe TBI (p.1008) for indications
for CT in severe TBI and for specific conditions excluded from the mTBI guidelines (e.g., penetrating
skull trauma).

The American College of Emergency Physicians (ACEP) guidelines (p.1007) [20] for initial imaging
for mTBI in patients ≥ 16 years age is based on previously published rules (including the Canadian CT
Head Rule (p.1007) for GCS = 13-15, and the New Orleans Criteria (► Table 60.5) for GCS = 15, which
are included below for completeness since they are validated and in common use). The ACEP guidelines have not been validated.

Practice guideline: initial head CT with mTBI (ACEP policy)

Noncontrast head CT for patients ≥ 16 years age with GCS = 14-15 following non-penetrating TBI are indicated only if one or more of the following is present

Level I[20]: For patients with LOC or posttraumatic amnesia

- headache
- vomiting
- age > 60 years
- intoxication (alcohol or drugs)
- short-term memory deficits
- physical signs of trauma above the clavicle
- posttraumatic seizure
- GCS < 15
- focal neurologic deficit
- coagulopathy (including anticoagulants/antiplatelet drugs)*

Level II[20]: For patients without LOC or posttraumatic amnesia

- focal neurologic deficit
- vomiting
- severe headache
- age ≥ 65 years
- signs of basal skull fracture (includes hemotympanum, "raccoon's eyes" (p. 1065), CSF rhinorrhea or otorrhea, Battle's sign (p. 1065))
- GCS < 15
- coagulopathy (including anticoagulants/antiplatelet drugs)*
- dangerous mechanism of injury: pedestrian hit by motor vehicle, ejection from automobile, fall from height > 3 feet or > 5 stairs

*data regarding the risk of adverse outcome in anticoagulated patients after mTBI is limited and of low quality[21]

Canadian CT Head Rule (CCTHR) for mild TBI (GCS = 13-15) (▶ Table 60.4)[22] is a validated[23] decision rule that may be used to determine if an initial head CT is indicated for mild TBI (Glasgow Coma Scale score (GCS) = 13-15) in patients ≥ 16 years age who have a witnessed loss of consciousness, amnesia or confusion after a TBI who do not have exclusionary criteria listed in the table footnote.

★ The CCTHR is 100% sensitive for injuries requiring neurosurgical intervention.[23]

Table 60.4 Canadian CT Head Rule (CCTHR)[22]

Head CT is indicated for patients ≥ 16 years age with GCS = 13-15 from witnessed TBI, only if one or more of any of the following are present*:

High-risk criteria ("CT is mandatory"[22])(presence of any 1 often requires neurosurgical intervention)

- GCS < 15 at 2 hours post injury
- suspected open or depressed skull fracture
- signs of basal skull fracture (includes hemotympanum, "raccoon's eyes" (p. 1065), CSF rhinorrhea or otorrhea, Battle's sign (p. 1065))
- 2 or more episodes of vomiting
- age ≥ 65 years

Medium risk criteria (presence of any 2 often have clinically important findings on CT)

- amnesia before injury > 30 minutes
- dangerous mechanism of injury: pedestrian hit by motor vehicle, ejection from automobile, fall from height > 3 feet or > 5 stairs

* exclusionary criteria for the CCTHR (i.e., these patients were not studied): age < 16, coagulopathy including anticoagulants/antiplatelet drugs, seizure, penetrating skull trauma, focal neurologic deficit, unstable vital signs, return for reassessment of the same injury, pregnancy.

NB: intoxication (drugs or alcohol) reduces the sensitivity of the CCTHR to 70%[24]

60

New Orleans Criteria (NOC) for head CT(▶ Table 60.5)[25] may be used for GCS = 15. It may be more sensitive than the CCTHR for showing clinically significant CT findings (99% vs. 87.3%), but it is less specific (5.6% vs. 39.7%).

Table 60.5 New Orleans Criteria[25] for head CT scan

Head CT scan is indicated for patients with TBI and GCS = 15 only if one or more of the following are present:
1. headache
2. vomiting
3. age ≥ 60 years
4. drug or alcohol intoxication
5. persistent anterograde amnesia (short-term memory deficits)
6. visible trauma above the clavicle
7. seizure

▶ **Indications for imaging in pediatrics with mTBI[26]** : See Pediatric head injuries (p. 1099).

▶ **Initial imaging for moderate to severe TBI**
1. brain CT is indicated in TBI with any of the following risk factors:
   a) GCS ≤ 14
   b) unresponsiveness
   c) depressed level of consciousness not clearly due to EtOH, drugs, metabolic abnormalities, postictal state, etc.
   d) coagulopathy including anticoagulants/antiplatelet drugs
   e) seizure
   f) penetrating skull trauma
   g) focal neurologic deficit
   h) unstable vital signs
   i) polytrauma
   j) suspected nonaccidental trauma (i.e., child abuse)
   k) patients intoxicated with alcohol or other drugs (due to unrealiability of clinical assessment)
   l) deteriorating neurologic status
2. assessment prior to general anesthesia for other procedures (during which neurologic exam cannot be followed in order to detect delayed deterioration)

60.5.3 CT findings in trauma

The main emergent conditions to rule out (and brief descriptions):
1. blood (hemorrhages or hematomas):
   a) extra-axial blood: surgical lesions are usually ≥ 1 cm maximal thickness
      • epidural hematoma (EDH) (p. 1072): usually biconvex and often due to arterial bleeding. Unlike SDH, EDH may cross dural barriers such as the the falx or tentorium (▶ Fig. 64.2)
      • subdural hematoma (SDH) (p. 1000): usually crescentic, usually due to venous bleeding. May cover larger surface area than EDH (dural adherence to inner table limits extension of EDH). Chronology of SDH: acute = high density, subacute ≈ isodense, chronic ≈ low density
   b) subarachnoid blood: trauma is the most common cause of subarachnoid hemorrhage (SAH). Unlike aneurysmal SAH (aSAH) (p. 1453) where blood is typically thickest near the circle of Willis, traumatic SAH (tSAH) (▶ Fig. 60.2) usually appears as high density spread thinly over the convexity, filling sulci (▶ Fig. 60.2) or basal cisterns. However, when the history of trauma is not clear, a CTA (or catheter arteriogram) may be indicated to R/O a ruptured aneurysm (that might have precipitated the trauma in some cases)
   c) intracerebral hemorrhage (ICH): increased density in brain parenchyma
   d) hemorrhagic contusion (p. 1071): often "fluffy" inhomogeneous high-density areas within brain parenchyma, usually adjacent to bony prominences (frontal and occipital poles, sphenoid wing). Typically less well-defined than primary ICH
   e) intraventricular hemorrhage (p. 1454): present in ≈ 10% of severe head injuries.[27] Associated with poor outcome; may be a marker for severe injury rather than the cause of the poor outcome. Use of intraventricular rt-PA has been reported for treatment[28]
2. hydrocephalus: enlarged ventricles may sometimes develop following trauma

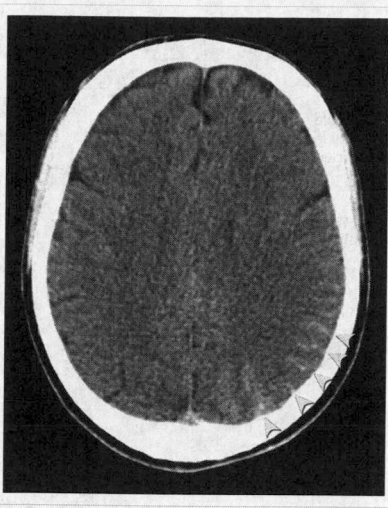

Fig. 60.2 Traumatic subarachnoid hemorrhage (tSAH) in a 22-year-old patient following an assault, demonstrating an example of tSAH (*yellow arrowheads*) overlying the high left convexity.
Image: noncontrast axial CT, brain windows.

3. cerebral swelling: obliteration of basal cisterns (p. 1109), compression of ventricles and sulci...
4. evidence of cerebral anoxia: loss of gray-white interface, signs of swelling
5. skull fractures (best appreciated using bone windows):
   a) basal skull fractures (including temporal bone fracture)
   b) orbital blow-out fracture
   c) calvarial fracture (CT may miss some linear nondisplaced skull fractures especially if the fracture is in the same plane as the CT slice)
      • linear vs. stellate
      • open vs. closed
      • diastatic (separation of sutures)
      • depressed vs. nondepressed: CT helps assess need for surgery
6. ischemic infarction (stroke): findings are usually minimal or subtle if < 24 hrs since stroke (DWI MRI is the test of choice for this)
7. pneumocephalus: may indicate skull fracture (basal or open convexity)
8. shift of midline structures (due to extra- or intra-axial hematomas or asymmetric cerebral edema): midline shift (p. 1110) can be associated with altered levels of consciousness

▶ **Marshall CT classification of TBI.** The Marshall CT classification (▶ Table 60.6 [29] has 6 categories of TBI severity based on the presence or absence of the factors shown below on a non-contrast head CT. The Marshall score was devised for descriptive purposes, the "Rotterdam score" ▶ Table 60.7 [30] is a stronger predictor of outcome.

1. intracranial abnormalities
2. CT evidence of increased ICP as demonstrated by
   a) midline shif (MLS) > 5 mm and/or
   b) compression of basal cisterns
3. presence or absence of mass lesions (contusions/hemorrhages)
4. planned evacuation of mass lesions

▶ **Rotterdam score for TBI.** The Marshall score was devised for descriptive purposes, and while it was subsequently shown to correlate with outcome parameters, including mortality, outcome prediction is stronger with the specific CT findings identified by recursive partitioning analysis in the "Rotterdam score" (▶ Table 60.7) which is calculated from a non-contrast head CT obtained within 4 hours of injury. There is evidence that the *worst* CT scan obtained during the admission has greater predictive value.[31]

The points from ▶ Table 60.7 are summed, and the predicted 6-month mortality is shown in ▶ Table 60.8.

60

Table 60.6 Marshall CT classification of TBI severity[29]

Category	Description	Mortality[30]
I - diffuse injury	• no visible pathology	6.4%
II - diffuse injury	• MLS[a] = 0 to 5 mm • basal cisterns remain visible • no high or mixed density lesions ≥ 25 cm³ estimated volume[b], may include bone fragments & foreign bodies	11%
III - diffuse injury (swelling)	• MLS = 0 to 5 mm • basal cisterns compressed or completely effaced[c] • no high or mixed density lesions ≥ 25 cm³	29%
IV - diffuse injury (shift)	• MLS > 5 mm • no high or mixed density lesions ≥ 25 cm³	44%
V - evacuated mass lesion	• any lesion evacuated surgically	30%
VI - non-evacuated mass lesion	• high or mixed density lesions ≥ 25 cm³ • not surgically evacuated	34%

[a]"MLS" = midline shift (p. 1110)
[b]to estimate volume of mass on CT (p. 1616)
[c]to assess the basal cisterns (p. 1109)

Table 60.7 "Rotterdam score" for CT findings in TBI

Feature		Points	Score
basal cisterns (p. 1109)	normal	0	(0 - 2)
	compressed	1	
	absent	2	
midline shift (MLS) (p. 1110)	0–5 mm	0	(0 - 1)
	>5 mm	1	
epidural mass lesion	absent	0	(0 - 1)
	present	1	
intraventricular blood or traumatic SAH (tSAH)	absent	0	(0 - 1)
	present	1	
add 1 point[a]			+1
Rotterdam score → TOTAL			(1 - 6)

[a]one point is added to all scores to bring the range from 1 to 6 in a nod to the original Marshall score

Table 60.8 Mortality associated with total "Rotterdam scores"[a]

Score	Mortality number & %
1	0/36 (0%)
2	41/600 (6.8%)
3	122/773 (16%)
4	121/465 (26%)
5	138/261 (53%)
6	69/114 (61%)

[a]6-month mortality

60.5.4 Follow-up CT

Routine follow-up CT (when there is no indication for urgent follow-up CT, see below):
1. it is our practice to perform a "stability scan" (a repeat head CT) with ≈ 24 hours (usually about 6-12 hours) for patients who are clinically stable but had findings on initial head CT of: traumatic SAH, small SDH or EDH, intraparenchymal contusions
2. for patients with *severe* head injuries:
   a) for *stable* patients, follow-up CTs are usually obtained between day 3 to 5 (some recommend at 24 hrs also) and again between day 10 to 14
   b) some recommend routine follow-up CT several hours after the "time zero" CT (i.e., initial CT done within hours of the trauma) to rule out delayed EDH (p. 1075), SDH (p. 1081), or traumatic contusions (p. 1071) [32]
3. for patients with mild to moderate head injuries:
   a) for those with an abnormal initial CT, the CT scan is usually repeated prior to discharge
   b) stable patients with mild head injury and normal initial CT do not require follow-up CT

Urgent follow-up CT: performed for neurological deterioration (loss of ≥ 2 points on the GCS, development of hemiparesis or new pupillary asymmetry), persistent vomiting, worsening H/A, seizures or unexplained rise in intracranial pressure (**ICP**) in patients with an ICP monitor.

60.5.5 Spine films

1. cervical spine: must be cleared radiographically from the cranio-cervical junction down through and including the C7–1 junction. Spinal injury precautions (cervical collar…) are continued until the C-spine is cleared. The steps in obtaining adequate films are outlined in *Spine injuries*, Radiographic evaluation and initial C-spine immobilization (p. 1141)
2. thoracic and lumbosacral LS-spine films should be obtained based on physical findings and on mechanism of injury (rarely for isolated TBI, especially in a patient who can tell you if they have spine tenderness on palpation); see *Spine injuries*, Radiographic evaluation and initial C-spine immobilization (p. 1141)

60.5.6 Skull X-rays

Practice guideline: Skull X-rays (SXR) in evaluating mTBI

Level II[20]: skull X-rays (SXR) are not recommended for evaluating mTBI

A skull fracture increases the probability of a surgical intracranial injury (ICI) (in a comatose patient it is a 20-fold increase, in a conscious patient it is a 400-fold increase[33,34]). However, significant ICI can occur with a normal skull X-ray (SXR) (SXR was normal in 75% of minor head injury patients found to have intracranial lesions on CT, attesting to the insensitivity of SXRs[35]). SXRs affect management of only 0.4–2% of patients in most reports.[36]

A skull X-ray (SXR) may be helpful in the following:
1. if a CT scan cannot be obtained, an SXR may identify significant findings such as pineal shift, pneumocephalus, air-fluid levels in the air sinuses, skull fracture (depressed or linear)… (however, sensitivity for detecting ICI is very low)
2. with penetrating injuries: helps by visualization of radio-opaque objects

60.5.7 MRI scans in trauma

Usually not appropriate for acute head injuries. This is due to longer acquisition time, less access to patients during study, increased difficulty in supporting patients (requires special non-magnetic ventilators, cannot use most IV pumps…), and MRI is less sensitive than CT for detecting acute blood.[37] There were no *surgical* lesions demonstrated on MRI that were not evident on CT in one study.[38] There may be some additional benefit in combining CT with an MRI performed directly in the emergency department.[39]

MRI may be helpful later after the patient is stabilized, e.g., to evaluate brainstem injuries, small white matter changes,[40] e.g., punctate hemorrhages in the corpus callosum seen in diffuse axonal injury (p. 1026)… Spinal MRI is indicated in patients with spinal cord injuries.

Rapid sequence MRI may be useful for follow-up in pediatrics to minimize radiation exposure.

60

60.5.8 Arteriogram in trauma

Cerebral arteriogram (p. 1096): useful with non missile penetrating trauma.

60.6 E/R management for minor or moderate head injury

60.6.1 Indications for admission to the hospital vs. observation at home

▶ **Patients who may be discharged with observation at home.** Patients with mild TBI (GCS = 14–15) who meet criteria in ▶ Table 60.9 may be managed with observation at home with written head-injury discharge instructions, e.g., as illustrated in ▶ Table 60.10.

For those not meeting discharge criteria, see sample admitting orders (p. 1012).

Table 60.9 Criteria for observation at home

1. head CT scan not indicated (see indications (p. 1006)), or CT scan normal if indicated[41]
2. initial GCS ≥ 14
3. patient is now neurologically intact (amnesia for the event is acceptable)
4. there is a responsible, sober adult that can observe the patient
5. patient has reasonable access to return to the hospital E/R if needed
6. no "complicating" circumstances (e.g., no suspicion of domestic violence, including child abuse)

Table 60.10 Sample discharge home instructions for head injuries

Seek medical attention for any of the following:
1. a change in level of consciousness (including difficulty in awakening)
2. abnormal behavior
3. increased headache
4. slurred speech
5. weakness or loss of feeling in an arm or leg
6. persistent vomiting
7. enlargement of one or both pupils (the black round part in the middle of the eye) that does not get smaller when a bright light is shined on it
8. seizures (also known as convulsions or fits)
9. significant increase in swelling at injury site

Do not take sedatives or pain medication stronger than acetaminophen (paracetamol in some countries) for 48 hours. Do not take aspirin or other anti-inflammatory medications because of interference with platelet function and theoretical increased risk of bleeding

---

60.6.2 Admitting orders for minor head injury (GCS ≥ 14)

1. activity: BR with HOB elevated 30–45°
2. neuro checks q 2 hrs (q 1 hr if more concerned; consider ICU for these patients). Contact physician for neurologic deterioration
3. NPO until alert; then clear liquids, advance as tolerated
4. isotonic IVF (e.g., NS + 20 mEq KCl/L) run at maintenance (p. 1050): ≈ 100 cc/hr for average size adult (peds: 2000 cc/m²/d). **Note:** the concept of "running the patient dry" is obsolete
5. mild analgesics: acetaminophen (PO, or PR if NPO), codeine or tramadol if necessary
6. anti-emetic: give infrequently to avoid excessive sedation, avoid phenothiazine anti-emetics (which lower the seizure threshold); e.g., use trimethobenzamide (Tigan®) 200 mg IM q 8 hrs PRN for adults

60.6.3 Admitting orders for moderate head injury (GCS 9–13)

1. orders as for minor head injury (see above) except patient is kept NPO in case surgical intervention is needed (including ICP monitor)
2. for GCS = 9–12 admit to ICU. For GCS = 13, admit to ICU if CT shows any significant abnormality (hemorrhagic contusions unless very small, rim subdural...)
3. patients with normal or near-normal CTs should improve within hours. Any patient who fails to reach a GCS of 14–15 within 12 hrs should have a repeat CT at that time[42]

60.7 Patients with associated severe systemic injuries

60.7.1 Intra-abdominal injuries

Diagnostic peritoneal lavage (DPL) looking for bloody fluid or FAST (focused abdominal sonogram for trauma) are often used by trauma surgeons to assess for intra-abdominal hemorrhage. If negative and the patient is hemodynamically stable, the patient should be taken for cranial CT (with DPL—if the initial fluid is not bloody, the remainder of the lavage fluid may be collected for quantitative analysis as the head CT is being done).

Patients with grossly positive DPL or positive FAST and/or hemodynamic instability may need to be rushed to the O.R. for emergent laparotomy by trauma surgeons without benefit of cerebral CT. Neurosurgical management is difficult in these patients, and must be individualized. These guidelines are offered:

✖ CAUTION: many patients with severe trauma may be in DIC (either due to systemic injuries, or directly related to severe head injury possibly because the brain is rich in thromboplastin[43]). Operating on patients in DIC is usually disastrous (p.175). At the least, check a PT/INR/PTT

1. if GCS > 8 (which implies at least localizing)
   a) operative neurosurgical intervention is probably not required
   b) utilize good neuroanesthesia techniques (elevate head of bed, judicious administration of IV fluids, avoiding prophylactic hyperventilation…)
   c) obtain a head CT scan immediately post-op
2. if patient has focal neurologic deficit, an exploratory burr hole should be placed in the O.R. simultaneously with the treatment of other injuries. Placement is guided by the pre-op deficit (p.1014)
3. if there is severe head injury (GCS ≤ 8) without localizing signs, or if initial burr hole is negative, or if there is no pre-op neuro exam, then
   a) measure the ICP: insert a ventriculostomy catheter (if the lateral ventricle cannot be entered after 3 passes, it may be completely compressed or it may be displaced, and an intraparenchymal fiberoptic monitor or subarachnoid bolt should be used)
      • normal ICP: unlikely that a surgical lesion exists. Manage ICP medically and, if an IVC was inserted, with CSF drainage
      • elevated ICP (≥ 2 mm Hg): inject 3–4 cc of air into ventricles through IVC, then obtain portable intraoperative AP skull X-ray (intraoperative pneumoencephalogram) to determine if there is any midline shift. If there is mass effect with ≥ 5 mm of midline shift, explore surgically[44] with burr hole(s) on the side opposite the direction of shift. If no mass effect, intracranial hypertension is managed medically and with CSF drainage
   b) routine use of exploratory burr holes for children with GCS = 3 has been found not to be justified[45]

60.7.2 Fat embolism syndrome

General information

Most often seen after a long bone fracture (usually femoral, but may include clavicular, tibial, and even isolated skull fracture). Although almost all patients have pulmonary fat emboli at autopsy, the syndrome is usually mild or subclinical, only ≈ 10–20% of cases are severe, and the fulminant form leading to multiple organ failure is rare. Clinical findings usually appear within 12–72 hrs of injury, and do not always include the complete classic clinical triad of:

• acute respiratory failure (including hypoxemia, tachypnea, dyspnea) with diffuse pulmonary infiltrates (usually seen as bilateral fluffy infiltrates). May be the only manifestation of fat emboli in up to 75% of cases
• global neurologic dysfunction: may include confusion (PaO_2 usually not low enough to account for these changes[46]), lethargy, seizures
• petechial rash: seen ≈ 24–72 hrs after the fracture, usually over thorax

Other possible findings include:
• pyrexia
• retinal fat emboli

There is no specific test for fat embolism syndrome (FES). The following have been proposed, but have poor sensitivity and specificity: fat globules in the urine (positive in ≈ one–third[47]) and serum, serum lipase activity. In cases of unexplained neurologic or pulmonary abnormalities, it may be possible to diagnose FES if on bronchoalveolar lavage[48] > 5% of cells in the washings staining for neutral

60

fat with red oil 0. Nonspecific tests include ABG (findings: hypoxemia, hypocarbia from hyperventilation, respiratory alkalosis).

Treatment

Pulmonary support with oxygen, and mechanical ventilation if necessary including use of PEEP. The use of steroids is controversial. Ethyl alcohol (to decrease serum lipase activity) and heparin have not been shown to be of benefit. Early operative fixation of long bone fractures may reduce the incidence of FES.[49]

Outcome

Usually related more to the underlying injuries. Although FES itself is usually compatible with good recovery, 10% mortality is usually quoted.

60.7.3 Indirect optic nerve injury

General information

≈ 5% of head trauma patients manifest an associated injury to some portion of the visual system. Approximately 0.5–1.5% of head trauma patients will sustain indirect injury (as opposed to penetrating trauma) to the optic nerve, most often from an ipsilateral blow to the head (usually frontal, occasionally temporal, rarely occipital).[19] The optic nerve may be divided into 4 segments: intraocular (1 mm in length), intraorbital (25–30 mm), intracanalicular (10 mm), and intracranial (10 mm). The intracanalicular segment is the most common one damaged with closed head injuries. Funduscopic abnormalities visible on initial exam indicates anterior injuries (injury to the intraocular segment (optic disc) or the 10–15 mm of the intraorbital segment immediately behind the globe where the central retinal artery is contained within the optic nerve), whereas posterior injuries (occurring posterior to this but anterior to the chiasm) take 4–8 weeks to show signs of disc pallor and loss of the retinal nerve fiber layer.

Treatment

See reference.[19]

No prospective study has been carried out. Optic nerve decompression has been advocated for indirect optic nerve injury; however, the results are not clearly better than expectant management with the exception that documented *delayed* visual loss appears to be a strong indication for surgery. Transethmoidal is the accepted route, and is usually done within 1–3 weeks from the trauma.[50] The use of "megadose steroids" may be appropriate as an adjunct to diagnosis and treatment.

60.7.4 Posttraumatic hypopituitarism

Trauma is a rare cause of hypopituitarism. It may follow closed head injury (with or without basilar skull fracture) or penetrating trauma.[51] In 20 cases in the literature[52] all had deficient growth hormone and gonadotropin, 95% had corticotropin deficiency, 85% had reduced TSH, 63% had elevated PRL. Only 40% had transient or permanent DI.

60.8 Exploratory burr holes

60.8.1 General information

In a trauma patient, the clinical triad of altered mental status, unilateral pupillary dilatation with loss of light reflex, and contralateral hemiparesis is most often due to upper brainstem compression by uncal transtentorial herniation which, in the majority of trauma cases, is due to an extraaxial intracranial hematoma. Furthermore, the prognosis of patients with traumatic herniation is poor. Outcome may possibly be improved slightly by increasing the rapidity with which decompression is undertaken; however, an upper limit of salvageability is probably still only ≈ 20% satisfactory outcome.

Burr holes are primarily a *diagnostic tool*, as bleeding cannot be controlled and most acute hematomas are too congealed to be removed through a burr hole. However, if the burr hole is positive, it is possible that modest decompression may be performed, and then the definitive craniotomy can be undertaken incorporating the burr hole(s).

With widespread availability of quickly accessible CT scanning, exploratory burr holes are infrequently indicated.

60.8.2 Indications

1. clinical criteria: based on deteriorating neurologic exam. Indications in E/R (rare): patient dying of rapid transtentorial herniation (see below) or brainstem compression that does not improve or stabilize with mannitol and hyperventilation.[53]
   a) indicators of transtentorial herniation/brainstem compression:
      - sudden drop in Glasgow Coma Scale (GCS) score
      - one pupil fixes and dilates
      - paralysis or decerebration develops (usually contralateral to blown pupil)
   b) recommended situations where criteria should be applied:
      - neurologically stable patient undergoes *witnessed* deterioration as described above
      - awake patient undergoes same process in transport, and changes are well documented by competent medical or paramedical personnel
2. other criteria
   a) some patients needing emergent surgery for systemic injuries (e.g., positive peritoneal lavage + hemodynamic instability) where there is not time for a brain CT (p. 1013)

60.8.3 Management

Controversial. The following should serve only as guidelines:
1. if patient fits the above criteria (emergent operation for systemic injuries or deterioration with failure to improve with mannitol and hyperventilation), and CT scan cannot be performed and interpreted immediately, then treatment should not wait for CT scan
   a) in general, if the O.R. can be immediately available, burr holes are preferably done there (equipped to handle craniotomy, better lighting and sterility, dedicated scrub nurse…), especially in older patients (> 30 yrs) not involved in MVAs (see below). This may more rapidly diagnose and treat extraaxial hematomas in herniating patients, although no difference in outcome has been proven
   b) if delay in getting to the O.R. is foreseen, emergency burr holes in the E/R should be performed
2. placement of burr hole(s) as outlined under Technique below

60.8.4 Technique

Position

Shoulder roll, head turned with side to be explored up. Three pin skull-fixation used if concern about possible aneurysm or AVM (to allow for retractors and increased stability) or if additional stability is desired (e.g., with unstable cervical fractures); otherwise a horse-shoe head-holder suffices and saves time and makes it easier to turn the head to access to the other side if needed.

Choice of side for initial burr hole

Start with a temporal burr hole (see below) on the side:
1. ipsilateral to a blown pupil. This will be on the correct side in > 85% of epidurals[54] and other extra-axial mass lesions[55]
2. if both pupils are dilated, use the side of the *first* dilating pupil (if known)
3. if pupils are equal, or it is not known which side dilated first, place on side of obvious external trauma
4. if no localizing clues, place hole on *left* side (to evaluate and decompress the dominant hemisphere)

Approach

Burr holes are placed along a path that can be connected to form a "trauma flap" if a craniotomy becomes necessary (▶ Fig. 60.3). The "trauma flap" is so-called because it provides wide access to most of the cerebral convexity permitting complete evacuation of acute blood clot and control of most bleeding.
First outline the trauma flap with a skin marker:
1. start at the zygomatic arch < 1 cm anterior to the tragus (spares the branch of the facial nerve to the frontalis muscle and spares the anterior branch of the superficial temporal artery (STA))
2. proceed superiorly and then curve posteriorly at the level of top of the pinna
3. 4–6 cm behind the pinna it is taken superiorly
4. 1–2 cm ipsilateral to the midline (sagittal suture) curve anteriorly to end behind the hairline

60

Burr hole locations

- temporal burr hole (1 in ► Fig. 60.3)
  - ○ over middle cranial fossa typically on side of dilated pupil (if there is one) just superior to the zygomatic arch. Provides access to middle fossa (the most common site of epidural hematoma) and usually allows access to most convexity subdural hematomas, as well as proximity to middle meningeal artery in region of pterion
  - ○ if no epidural hematoma, the dura is opened if it has bluish discoloration (suggests subdural hematoma (SDH)) or if there is a strong suspicion of a mass lesion on that side
- if completely negative, usually perform temporal burr hole on contralateral side in the same location (not shown)
- if negative and if a CT cannot now be done and the OR immediately available from there, proceed to
  - ○ ipsilateral frontal burr hole (2 in ► Fig. 60.3), if negative proceed to
  - ○ parietal region (3 in ► Fig. 60.3), if negative proceed to
  - ○ posterior fossa (4 in ► Fig. 60.3)

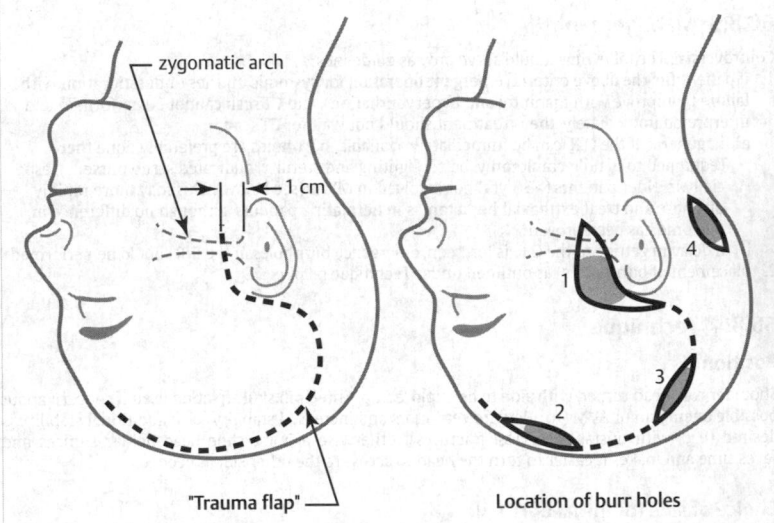

Fig. 60.3 Exploratory burr hole placement illustrating the technique to place the burr holes (blue circles) along an imaginary skin incision (broken line) that could be converted to a "trauma flap" - excluding burr hole 4 (adapted[55,56]).

Literature

In 100 trauma patients undergoing transtentorial herniation or brainstem compression as outlined above,[55] exploratory burr holes (bilateral temporal, frontal, and parietal, done in the O.R.) were positive in 56%. Lower rates in younger patients (< 30 yrs) and those in MVAs (as opposed to falls or assaults). SDH was the most common extraaxial mass lesion (alone and unilateral in 70%, bilateral in 11%, and in combination with EDH or ICH > 9%).

When burr holes were positive, the first burr hole was on the correct side 86% of the time when placed as suggested above. Six patients had significant extraaxial hematomas missed with exploratory burr holes (mostly due to incomplete burr hole exploration). Only 3 patients had the above neurologic findings as a result of intraparenchymal hematomas.

Outcome

Mean follow-up: 11 mos (range: 1–37). 70 of the 100 patients died. No morbidity or mortality was directly attributable to the burr holes. Four patients with good outcome and 4 with moderate disability had positive burr holes.

References

[1] Saul TG, Ducker TB. Effect of Intracranial Pressure Monitoring and and Aggressive Treatment on Mortality in Severe Head Injury. J Neurosurg. 1982; 56:498–503

[2] Reilly PL, Adams JH, Graham DI. Patients with Head Injury Who Talk and Die. Lancet. 1975; 2:375–377

[3] Stein SC, Narayan RK, Wilberger JE, et al. Classification of Head Injury. In: Neurotrauma. New York: McGraw-Hill; 1996:31–41

[4] Price DJ. Is Diagnostic Severity Grading for Head Injuries Possible? Acta Neurochirurgica. 1986; Suppl 36:67–69

[5] Brain Trauma Foundation, Povlishock JT, Bullock MR. Blood pressure and oxygenation. J Neurotrauma. 2007; 24:S7–13

[6] Chesnut RM, Marshall LF, Klauber MR, et al. The Role of Secondary Brain Injury in Determining Outcome from Severe Head Injury. J Trauma. 1993; 34:216–222

[7] The Brain Trauma Foundation. The American Association of Neurological Surgeons. The Joint Section on Neurotrauma and Critical Care. Initial management. J Neurotrauma. 2000; 17:463–469

[8] Hsiang JK, Chesnut RM, Crisp CD, et al. Early, Routine Paralysis for Intracranial Pressure Control in Severe Head Injury: Is It Necessary? Critical Care Medicine. 1994; 22:1471–1476

[9] Marion DW, Carlier PM. Problems with Initial Glasgow Coma Scale Assessment Caused by Prehospital Treatment of Patients with Head Injuries: Results of a National Survey. J Trauma. 1994; 36:89–95

[10] Bullock R, Chesnut RM, Clifton G, et al. Guidelines for the Management of Severe Head Injury. 1995

[11] The Brain Trauma Foundation. The American Association of Neurological Surgeons. The Joint Section on Neurotrauma and Critical Care. Resuscitation of blood pressure and oxygenation. J Neurotrauma. 2000; 17:471–478

[12] Brain Trauma Foundation, Povlishock JT, Bullock MR. Infection prophylaxis. J Neurotrauma. 2007; 24:S26–S31

[13] Brain Trauma Foundation, Povlishock JT, Bullock MR. Hyperventilation. J Neurotrauma. 2007; 24: S87–S90

[14] Brain Trauma Foundation, Povlishock JT, Bullock MR. Hyperosmolar therapy. J Neurotrauma. 2007; 24:S14–S20

[15] Bullock R, Chesnut RM, Clifton G, et al. The role of anti-seizure prophylaxis following head injury. In: Guidelines for the Management of Severe Head Injury.The Brain Trauma Foundation (New York), The American Association of Neurological Surgeons (Park Ridge, Illinois), and The Joint Section of Neurotrauma and Critical Care; 1995

[16] Chang BS, Lowenstein DH. Antiepileptic drug prophylaxis in severe traumatic brain injury. Report of the Quality Standards Subcommittee of the American Academy of Neurology. Neurology. 2003; 60:10–16

[17] Brain Trauma Foundation, Povlishock JT, Bullock MR. Antiseizure prophylaxis. J Neurotrauma. 2007; 24:S83–S86

[18] The Brain Trauma Foundation. The American Association of Neurological Surgeons. The Joint Section on Neurotrauma and Critical Care. Role of antiseizure prophylaxis following head injury. J Neurotrauma. 2000; 17:549–553

[19] Kline LB, Morawetz RB, Swaid SN. Indirect Injury of the Optic Nerve. Neurosurgery. 1984; 14:756–764

[20] Jagoda AS, Bazarian JJ, Bruns JJ,Jr, et al. Clinical policy: neuroimaging and decisionmaking in adult mild traumatic brain injury in the acute setting. Ann Emerg Med. 2008; 52:714–748

[21] Fuller GW, Evans R, Preston L, et al. Should adults with mild head injury who are receiving direct oral anticoagulants undergo computed tomography scanning? A systematic review. Ann Emerg Med. 2019; 73:66–75

[22] Stiell IG, Wells GA, Vandemheen K, et al. The Canadian CT Head Rule for patients with minor head injury. Lancet. 2001; 357:1391–1396

[23] Stiell IG, Clement CM, Rowe BH, et al. Comparison of the Canadian CT Head Rule and the New Orleans Criteria in patients with minor head injury. JAMA. 2005; 294:1511–1518

[24] Easter JS, Haukoos JS, Claud J, et al. Traumatic intracranial injury in intoxicated patients with minor head trauma. Acad Emerg Med. 2013; 20:753–760

[25] Haydel MJ, Preston CA, Mills TJ, et al. Indications for computed tomography in patients with minor head injury. N Engl J Med. 2000; 343:100–105

[26] Scorza KA, Raleigh MF, O'Connor FG. Current concepts in concussion: evaluation and management. Am Fam Physician. 2012; 85:123–132

[27] Le Roux PD, Haglund MM, Newell DW, et al. Intraventricular Hemorrhage in Blunt Head Trauma: An Analysis of 43 Cases. Neurosurgery. 1992; 31:678–685

[28] Grabb PA. Traumatic intraventricular hemorrhage treated with intraventricular recombinant-tissue plasminogen activator: technical case report. Neurosurgery. 1998; 43:966–969

[29] Marshall LF, Marshall SB, Klauber MR, et al. The diagnosis of head injury requires a classification based on computed axial tomography. J Neurotrauma. 1992; 9:S287–S292

[30] Maas AI, Hukkelhoven CW, Marshall LF, et al. Prediction of outcome in traumatic brain injury with computed tomographic characteristics: a comparison between the computed tomographic classification and combinations of computed tomographic predictors. Neurosurgery. 2005; 57:1173–82; discussion 1173–82

[31] Huang JH, Ranalli N, Zager EL. Comment on Maas A I, et al.: Prediction of outcome in traumatic brain injury with computed tomographic characteristics: A comparison between the computed tomographic classification and combinations of computed tomographic predictors. Neurosurgery. 2005; 57

[32] Young HA, Gleave JRW, Schmidek HH, et al. Delayed Traumatic Intracerebral Hematoma: Report of 15 Cases Operatively Treated. Neurosurgery. 1984; 14:22–25

[33] Jennett B, Teasdale G. Management of Head Injuries. Philadelphia: Davis; 1981

[34] Dacey RG, Alves WM, Rimel RW, et al. Neurosurgical Complications After Apparently Minor Head Injury: Assessment of Risk in a Series of 610 Patients. Journal of Neurosurgery. 1986; 65:203–210

[35] Ingebrigtsen R, Romner B. Routine Early CT-Scan is Cost Saving After Minor Head Injury. Acta Neurol Scand. 1996; 93:207–210

[36] Masters SJ, McClean PM, Arcarese JS, et al. Skull X-Ray Examination After Head Trauma. N Engl J Med. 1987; 316:84–91

[37] Snow RB, Zimmerman RD, Gandy SE, et al. Comparison of Magnetic Resonance Imaging and Computed Tomography in the Evaluation of Head Injury. Neurosurgery. 1986; 18:45–52

[38] Wilberger JE, Deeb Z, Rothfus W. Magnetic Resonance Imaging After Closed Head Injury. Neurosurgery. 1987; 20:571–576

[39] Kesterson L, Benzel EC, Marchand EP, et al. Magnetic Resonance Imaging in Acute Cranial and Cervical Spine Trauma. Neurosurgery. 1990; 26

[40] Levin HS, Amparo EG, Eisenberg HM, et al. Magnetic Resonance Imaging After Closed Head Injury in Children. Neurosurgery. 1989; 24:223–227

[41] Stein SC, Ross SE. The Value of Computed Tomographic Scans in Patients with Low-Risk Head Injuries. Neurosurgery. 1990; 26:638–640

[42] Stein SC, Ross SE. Moderate Head Injury: A Guide to Initial Management. J Neurosurg. 1992; 77:562–564

[43] Kaufman HH, Hui K-S, Mattson JC, et al. Clinicopathological Correlations of Disseminated Intravascular Coagulation in Patients with Head Injury. Neurosurgery. 1984; 15:34–42

[44] Becker DP, Miller JD, Ward JD, et al. The Outcome from Severe Head Injury with Early Diagnosis and Intensive Management. J Neurosurg. 1977; 47:491–502

60

[45] Johnson DL, Duma C, Sivit C. The Role of Immediate Operative Intervention in Severely Head-Injured Children with a Glasgow Coma Scale Score of 3. Neurosurgery. 1992; 30:320–324

[46] Fabian TC, Hoots AV, Stanford DS, et al. Fat Embolism Syndrome: Prospective Evaluation in 92 Fracture Patients. Crit Care Med. 1990; 18:42–46

[47] Dines DE, Burgher LW, Okazaki H. The Clinical and Pathologic Correlation of Fat Embolism Syndrome. Mayo Clin Proc. 1975; 50:407–411

[48] Chastre J, Fagon JY, Soler P, et al. Bronchoalveolar Lavage for Rapid Diagnosis of the Fat Embolism Syndrome in Trauma Patients. Ann Intern Med. 1990; 113:583–588

[49] Riska EB, Myllynen P. Fat Embolism in Patients with Multiple Injuries. J Trauma. 1982; 22:891–894

[50] Niho S, Niho M, Niho K. Decompression of the Optic Canal by the Transethmoidal Route and Decompression of the Superior Orbital Fissure. Can J Ophthalmol. 1970; 5:22–40

[51] Vance ML. Hypopituitarism. New England Journal of Medicine. 1994; 330:1651–1662

[52] Edwards OM, Clark JDA. Post-Traumatic Hypopituitarism: Six Cases and a Review of the Literature. Medicine. 1986; 65:281–290

[53] Mahoney BD, Rockswold GL, Ruiz E, et al. Emergency Twist Drill Trephination. Neurosurgery. 1981; 8:551–554

[54] McKissock W, Taylor JC, Bloom WH, et al. Extradural Hematoma: Observations on 125 Cases. Lancet. 1960; 2:167–172

[55] Andrews BT, Pitts LH, Lovely MP, et al. Is CT Scanning Necessary in Patients with Tentorial Herniation? Neurosurgery. 1986; 19:408–414

[56] Mayfield FH, McBride BH, Coates JB, et al. Differential Diagnosis and Treatment of Surgical Lesions. In: Neurological Surgery of Trauma. Washington D.C.: Office of the Surgeon General; 1965:55–64

61 Concussion, High-Altitude Cerebral Edema, Cerebrovascular Injuries

61.1 Concussion

61.1.1 General information

Key concepts

- a traumatic biomechanically induced complex pathophysiologic process affecting the brain with no identifiable structural abnormalities on imaging studies
- concussion is a subset of mild TBI (mTBI) and is therefore not equivalent to mTBI
- indicators of concussion: posttraumatic alterations in any of: orientation, balance, speed of reaction, and/or impaired verbal learning and memory in a patient with GCS 13–15[1]
- does not require loss of consciousness (LOC) or even a direct blow to the head
- grading scales have been abandoned in favor of experienced assessment assisted by various "sideline" tools, ideally with baseline (pre-injury) metrics for comparison

Concussion occurs in a subset of patient with mild traumatic brain injury (mTBI; ▶ Fig. 60.1). It is considered "mild" because it is usually not life-threatening by itself. While most victims recover completely, effects of concussion can be serious, and in some instances, may be lifelong.

Much of the discussion in this chapter relates to concussion in sports, which is the largest source of data on the subject, and generalization to other types of trauma must be done circumspectly.

There has been a move away from concussion grading scales. The current recommendation is for the diagnosis to be determined by an experienced examiner with the assistance of various assessment tools, ideally with the availability of pre-injury baseline metrics for comparison.

Concussion can occur without a direct blow to the head, e.g., with violent shaking of the torso and head. Concussion symptoms can present soon after an insult or in a delayed fashion.

The subject may not be aware that they have sustained a concussion.

61.1.2 Epidemiology

Incidence: 1.6–3.8 million concussions occur per year in the United States from sports and recreational activities. It is estimated that 50% of concussions go unreported.[2]

61.1.3 Concussion genetics

There is no clear evidence to support a genetic predisposition to concussion. Apolipoprotein E4, Apo E G-219T promoter and tau exon 6 have been studied in small retrospective and prospective trials without definitive association.[2,3]

61.1.4 Concussion—definition

There is no universally accepted definition for concussion.[4] Of the many contemporary definitions,[2,3,4,5,6,7] most key elements are contained in the Concussion in Sport Group 2012 consensus definition[3] summarized below. However, opinions differ e.g., whether there is any long-term effect of concussion or if that necessitates a different diagnosis.

▶ **Definition.** Concussion is a complex pathophysiological process affecting the brain resulting in alteration of brain function, that is induced by nonpenetrating biomechanical forces, without identifiable abnormality in standard structural imaging.

The Concussion in Sport Group[3] elaborates on this definition as follows:
- results in a graded set of neurological symptoms that may or may not involve loss of consciousness (LOC)
- symptom onset is usually rapid, short-lived and resolves spontaneously. Manifestations may include transient deficits in balance, coordination, memory/cognition, strength, or alertness

- may result in neuropathological changes, but the acute clinical symptoms largely reflect a functional disturbance rather than a structural injury
- resolution of the clinical and cognitive features typically follows a sequential course

61.1.5 Concussion versus mTBI

- concussion and mTBI are not interchangeable. Concussion may be thought as a subcategory of mTBI on the less severe end of the brain injury spectrum, though with similar clinical symptoms[2,5,6,8] (see ► Fig. 60.1)
- a major difference between the two is that mTBI may demonstrate abnormal structural imaging (such as cerebral hemorrhage/contusion) and concussion, by definition, must have normal imaging studies. mTBI is part of an injury severity spectrum primarily based on GCS score. TBI is evaluated 6 hours after injury and differentiated into mild, moderate and severe; see Grading (p. 1000). Concussion is evaluated directly after the insult and based on a clinical diagnosis aided by a multitude of standardized assessment tools. To include concussion under the full spectrum of traumatic brain injury then it must fall at the low end of mTBI and overlap with the subset of "minimal" injury. Most mTBIs with negative imaging can be considered concussions, but the majority of sports concussions cannot be classified as mTBI[5,8]

61.1.6 Risk factors for concussion

- history of previous concussion increases risk for further concussion
- being involved in an accident: bicyclist, pedestrian or motor vehicle collision
- combat soldier
- victim of physical abuse
- falling (especially pediatrics or elderly)
- males are diagnosed with sports-related concussion more than females (due to increased number of male participation in sports studied) but females have a higher risk overall when compared to males who play in the same sport (i.e., soccer and basketball)[7]
- articipating in sports with high risk of concussion:
  - American football
  - Australian rugby
  - ice hockey
  - boxing
  - ★ soccer is the highest risk for females
- (for contrast, sports with the lowest risk of concussion: baseball, softball, volleyball & gymnastics)
- BMI > 27 kg/m^2 and less than 3 hours of training per week increases the risk of sports-related concussion[7]

61.1.7 Diagnosis

Triggers

Findings suggestive of concussion are listed in ► Table 61.1. The diagnosis of concussion should be considered when any of these findings occur following trauma. In pre-verbal children, findings may include those in ► Table 61.2.

General diagnostic information

Clinical evaluation

No physiologic measure has been identified that can detect the underlying changes that lead to the manifestations of concussion. Therefore the diagnosis relies on: self-reporting of abnormal function (symptoms), observed physiologic abnormalities (signs) including assessment of cognitive dysfunction,[11] sometimes with the assistance of imaging tests to rule out a structural substrate.

A clinical diagnosis of concussion is made if there are abnormal findings in balance, coordination, memory/cognition, strength, reaction speed, or alertness after a traumatic insult to the head. Findings include confusion, amnesia, headache, drowsiness or LOC (LOC is *not* a requirement for diagnosing concussion,[6] patients themselves may be unaware whether or not they experienced LOC[4]). Frequent neurobehavioral features of concussion are shown in ► Table 61.1. In children who may not be able to verbalize their symptoms, evidence of concussion may include findings in ► Table 61.2. Positive imaging findings would necessitate a more severe diagnosis such as cerebral contusion.

Table 61.1 Possible findings in concussion[2,9,10]

Physical	Cognitive	Emotional	Sleep
• vacant stare or befuddled expression • dazed or stunned • headache or pressure sensation in the head • nausea • vomiting • fatigue • "seeing stars" • photophobia • phonophobia • ringing in the ears (tinnitus) • delayed verbal & motor responses: • difficulty focusing attention • inability to perform normal activities • speech alterations: slurred or incoherent, disjointed or incomprehensible statements • incoordination stumbling • any period of LOC, paralytic coma, unresponsiveness to stimuli	• feeling like being in a fog • slow to answer questions or follow instructions • easy distractibility • disorientation (e.g., walking in the wrong direction) • unaware of date, time or place • memory deficits: amnesia for the event • repeatedly asking same question that has been answered	• exaggerated emotionality: inappropriate crying • distraught appearance • irritability • nervousness	• drowsiness • insomnia • hypersomnia • difficulty falling asleep or staying asleep

Table 61.2 Concussion findings in children

listlessness and easy fatigability, change in sleeping patterns
irritability
appearing dazed
balance impairment
excessive crying
change in eating habits
loss of interest in favorite toys

Approach

• take a concussion specific symptom survey including inquiries about: H/A, N/V, light sensitivity, tinnitus, feeling like being in a fog, sleep disturbances
• history of diagnoses that might have an impact on the assessment or on a current concussion
  ○ history of prior concussions
  ○ H/A history
  ○ ADD/HD
  ○ learning disabilities
  ○ medications (prescribed and other) that might affect alertness or cognition
• perform a good general neurological exam
• include a concussion specific neuro exam
  ○ check orientation
  ○ assess for amnesia and impaired verbal memory
  ○ balance: Romberg test (look for significant sway or breaking stance), single leg stance
  ○ eye movements: optokinetic nystagmus (OKN), smooth pursuit
  ○ simultaneous task performance: e.g., snap fingers while walking
• include assessment aides ("sideline tools") as appropriate (see below)

Assessment aids

• there is no single validated assessment tool to diagnose concussion.[4] It is primarily a *clinical* diagnosis that is ideally made by certified healthcare providers who are familiar with the patient based on a detailed history and physical examination and a continuum of evaluation from the sideline to the clinic (diagnosis is ideally made within 24 hours of injury)[2,3,4,5,6,7].

- diagnosis may be aided by concussion assessment tools such as the SCAT3, ImPACT™.
  ✖ No test has shown high validity on independent testing, and no test should be used as the sole method of diagnosing concussion or for determining suitability for return to play. Athletes have also learned to "game" some baseline tests to avoid removal from play after possible concussion
- SCAT3 (Sports Concussion Assessment Tool – 3rd Edition)[12]: Derived from the 2012 Zurich Conference.[3] The SCAT has become the most commonly used standardized tool for sideline assessment of sport concussion. The sensitivity and specificity of concussion assessment tools change over the course of a concussion so a tool designed for sideline use (i.e., SCAT3) is not appropriate for office use
  - SCAT3™ is a trademarked tool developed by the Concussion in Sports Group for use only by medical professionals for assessing sports-related concussion
  - it can be found at http://bjsm.bmj.com/content/47/5/259.full.pdf
  - to be used in athletes of 13 years or older (for 12 and younger, use Child SCAT3[13])
  - is a multimodal assessment tool with 8 sections that includes self-reported symptoms and evaluation of functional domains such as cognition, memory, balance, gait and motor skills
  - takes 8–10 min to administer
  - a "normal" SCAT3 does *not* rule out concussion
  - it has not been validated
- other types of sports concussion assessment tools (many can be viewed on YouTube):
  - neurocognitive testing (may take up to 20 minutes to administer)
  - SAC (Standardized Assessment of Concussion)[14]: a neurocognitive test that includes tests of immediate memory, delayed recall, serial 7's, digit span
  - ImPACT™ (Immediate Post-Concussion Assessment and Cognitive Testing): a widely used commercially produced computer test (https://www.impacttest.com). Independent validation studies have yielded conflicting results and results can diverge from observations[15]
  - PCSS (Post-Concussive Symptom Scale)
  - CSI (Concussion Symptom Inventory)
  - BESS (Balance Error Scoring System): the subject stands in each of various standardized positions for 20 seconds each, and the number of errors are recorded (breaking stance, opening eyes, taking hands off hip…).
  - SOT (Sensory Organization Test)
  - "Concussion Quick Check" app for mobile devices produced by the AAN
  - King-Devick eye movement testing: only takes 2–3 minutes to administer. On printed cards or tablet computer (http://kingdevicktest.com/for-concussions/)
- formal neuropsychological testing: it is recommended that this be reserved for patients with prolonged cognitive symptoms
- concussion serum biomarkers: no moiety has been identified that can reliably diagnose concussion on serum or saliva testing. Neuron-specific enolase, S100, and cleaved tau protein have been studied for prognostication after mTBI and concussion. S100 has demonstrated only a 33.3% sensitivity for postconcussive symptoms and 93% sensitivity for an Extended Glasgow Outcome Scale (▶ Table 98.4) score < 5 at 1 month. Another study involving pediatric patients with mTBI showed no difference in levels of neuron-specific enolase or S100B in asymptomatic and symptomatic children. A prospective study found no significant correlation between cleaved tau protein and postconcussive syndrome in patients with mTBI[16]

On-site/sideline evaluation

Any individual suspected of having a concussion (displaying ANY findings in ▶ Table 61.1) should be removed from the activity (for athletes, stopped from playing) and assessed by a licensed healthcare provider trained in the evaluation and management of concussions with attention to excluding a cervical spine injury.[2,3] If no provider is available, return to the activity is not permitted and urgent referral to a physician should be arranged.

After ruling out emergency issues, the provider should perform a concussion assessment (may employ standardized tools such as SCAT3™ or other methodologies).

The patient should not be left alone, and serial evaluations for signs of deterioration should be made over the following few hours.

For return to play guidelines, see below.

61.1.8 Indications for imaging or other diagnostic testing in concussion

There is no imaging modality that is diagnostic for concussion. Imaging in concussion is typically used to rule out more serious traumatic injuries, or sometimes to "clear" a patient of occult intracranial pathology before general anesthesia for other injuries. Typically CT, or sometimes MRI, is utilized.

▶ **CT scan (or sometimes MRI) in concussion.** CT scans should not be performed routinely for mTBI. Validated decision rules (p. 1019) should be employed to determine when imaging is indicated.

▶ **Other studies (imaging and electrodiagnostic)**
- diffusion tensor imaging (DTI) MRI: used to quantify white matter tract integrity throughout the brain with 4 types of analysis methods—voxel analysis, region of interest (ROI) analysis, histogram analysis, and tractography. There is no strong consensus regarding the best method for utilizing DTI for diagnosis or prognosis in the *individual* patient but multiple studies have shown *group* differences in DTI parameters between mTBI and control patients[8]
- functional MRI (fMRI): consists of 2 types (task-based fMRI and resting state fMRI) and is based on the blood oxygen level dependent (BOLD) effect, in which specialized MRI sequences measure/detect regions of increased oxygen rich blood flow to areas of upregulated neuronal activity. Both task-based and resting state fMRI modalities have shown *group* differences between mTBI and control patients (specifically in frontal lobe dysfunction), but further studies need to be completed on both a single time point and longitudinal basis before these techniques can be widely adopted for individual diagnosis and therapeutic guidance[8]
- imaging studies that are currently used primarily in concussion research: positron emission tomography (PET), single photon emission CT (CT-SPECT), MR-spectroscopy (MRS)
- quantitative EEG (qEEG): digitized EEGs are analyzed for relative energy at different frequencies to assess brain activity, patterns of cortical activation and neuronal networks. Post-concussion studies are compared to baseline. Thus far, there are no qEEG features (or other EEG findings for that matter) that are specific and sensitive for concussed patients[17]

61.1.9 Acute pathophysiology

Biomechanical force results in unregulated ionic flux (K^+ efflux, Na^+/Ca^{2+} influx) and unrestricted hyperacute glutamate release from sublethal mechanoporation of lipid membranes at the cellular level. This triggers voltage/ligand gated ion channels causing a cortical spreading depression-like state that is thought to be the substrate behind immediate postconcussive symptoms. Subsequently, ATP-dependent ionic pumps are extensively upregulated to restore cellular homeostasis causing widespread intracellular energy reserve depletion and an increase in ADP. Cells then pass into a state of impaired metabolism (energy crisis) that can last up to 7–10 days and may be associated with alterations in CBF. This impaired metabolic state is associated with vulnerability to repeat injury as well as behavioral and spatial learning impairments. Cells also undergo cytoskeletal damage, axonal dysfunction, and altered neurotransmission with the as yet unproven impression that each of these pathologic processes correlate with a separate symptomology (see ▶ Table 61.3).[18]

Table 61.3 Physiologic perturbations and their proposed corresponding symptomology[18]

Pertubation	Symptom
ionic influx →	migraine headache, photophobia, phonophobia
energy crisis →	vulnerability to second injury
axonal injury →	impaired cognition, slowed processing, slowed reaction time
impaired neurotransmission →	impaired cognition, slowed processing, slowed reaction time
protease activation, altered cytoskeletal proteins, cell death →	chronic atrophy, persistent impairments

61.1.10 Post concussion syndrome (PCS)

Occurs in 10%-15% of concussed individuals. As with most concussion related pathologies, there are multiple definitions of PCS. An amalgam of some definitions is as follows: Patients having ≥ 3 symptoms including headache, fatigue, dizziness, irritability, difficulty concentrating, memory difficulty, insomnia, and intolerance to stress, emotion, or alcohol, and symptoms must begin within 4 weeks of injury and remain for ≥ 1 month after onset of symptoms.[16,19] In one retrospective study, the following conclusions were reached[19]:
- > 80% of PCS patients had at least 1 previous concussion
- average number of previous concussions was 3.4

- median duration of PCS was 6 months
- 50% of patients were < 18 years of age
- LOC does not increase the risk for PCS

61.1.11 Prevention of concussion

- AAN guidelines conclude that protective headgear in rugby is "highly probable" to decrease the incidence of concussion.[7] However, the AMSSM (American Medical Society for Sports Medicine) hold that there is no clear evidence that soft or hard helmets reduce the severity or incidence of concussion (in football, lacrosse, hockey, soccer, and rugby).[2,3] Biomechanical studies have shown helmets reduced impact forces on the brain but this has not translated into concussion prevention.[3]
- there is insufficient data to determine whether one type of football helmet protects better than another in preventing concussions[3,7]
- no significant evidence that a mouthpiece protects against concussion[3,7]

61.1.12 Management of concussion and post-concussion syndrome

Return to Play (RTP)

- no system of return to play (RTP) guidelines has been rigorously tested and proven to be scientifically sound
- after sustaining a concussion, athletes should not return to play the same day.[2,3,4,5,6,7] Prohibited by some state laws
- ✖ a symptomatic player should not return to competition
- if there is any uncertainty: "When in doubt, sit them out"
- evaluation should proceed in a stepwise fashion. A player needs to be completely asymptomatic both at rest and with provocative exercise before full clearance is given.[3] There is no standardized RTP protocol. Each player's progression should be individualized.[2] Generally, the athlete's level of activity should be gradually increased over 24-hour increments from light aerobic activity to full contact practice. The athlete is evaluated after each progression. If postconcussive symptoms occur then the player is dropped back to the previous asymptomatic level and then allowed another attempt at progression after a 24-hour rest period. 80–90% of concussions resolve within 7–10 days. This recovery time may be longer for children or adolescents[3]
- the CDC endorses a graded 5-step return to play for student athletes[20] as shown in ▶ Table 61.4. The athlete should move to the next step only if they have no new symptoms. If symptoms return or new ones develop, then medical attention should be sought and after clearance the student can return to the previous step.

Contraindications for return to play are shown in ▶ Table 61.5.

Table 61.4 5-step return to play progression

Step	Description
Baseline	athlete is back to regular school activities without symptoms
1	light aerobic activity: only to increase heart rate for 5–10 minutes. No weight lifting
2	moderate activity: increase heart rate with body or head movement. May include moderate intensity weight training (less time and intensity than their typical routine)
3	heavy, non-contact activity: may include running, high-intensity stationary biking, regular weight training, non-contact sports-specific drills
4	practice & full contact: in controlled practice
5	competition

Table 61.5 Cerebral contraindications for return to contact sports

1. persistent postconcussion symptoms
2. permanent CNS sequelae from head injury (e.g., organic dementia, hemiplegia, homonymous hemianopsia)
3. hydrocephalus
4. spontaneous SAH from any cause
5. symptomatic (neurologic or pain producing) abnormalities about the foramen magnum (e.g., Chiari malformation)

Management of post-concussive syndrome

An extremely complicated topic, partly because of potential for litigation and the fact that symptoms are often vague and nonspecific and there may be no objective findings to corroborate subjective symptoms.

Most symptoms from concussion resolve within 7–10 days and do not require treatment. The most common exception to this is posttraumatic headache, the most common subtype being acute posttraumatic migraine.

Typical symptoms include: H/A, dizziness, insomnia, exercise intolerance, depression, irritability, anxiety, memory loss, difficulty concentrating, fatigue, light or noise hypersensitivity.

Patients with protracted symptoms may require more directed treatment.

- psychological and neuropsychological involvement is often employed
- pharmacologic treatment: there are no evidence-based studies of the utility of medications for post-concussive symptoms (aside from H/A)
- intractable headaches: occurs in ≈ 15% of concussions
  - expert neurology consultation is usually required for difficult-to-control headaches
  - the first line drugs are OTC medications
  - triptans are usually employed for nonresponders
  - third line drugs includ Ketorolac or DHE-45 (dihydroergotamine)
  - steroids may be beneficial for some
  - avoid: narcotics, butalbital/caffeine preparations (Fioricet, Esgic…), beta blockers, and calcium channel blockers

61.1.13 Second impact syndrome (SIS)

A rare condition described primarily in athletes who sustain a second head injury while still symptomatic from an earlier one. Classically, the athlete walks off the field under their own power after the second injury, only to deteriorate to coma within 1–5 minutes and then, due to vascular engorgement, develops malignant cerebral edema that is refractory to all treatment and progresses to herniation. Mortality: 50–100%.

A syndrome compatible with SIS was first described by Schneider[21] in 1973, and was later dubbed the "second impact syndrome of catastrophic head injury" in 1984.[22] Although it is contended that SIS is rare (if it exists at all) and may be overdiagnosed,[23] its apparent predilection for teens and children still warrants extra precaution following concussion.

61.1.14 Chronic traumatic encephalopathy (CTE)

There is limited evidence-based research involving the pathophysiology and natural history of CTE. Thought to be a distinct neurodegenerative disease (tauopathy) associated with repetitive brain trauma, not limited to athletes with reported concussions, and can only be diagnosed postmortem with a pathology-confirmed analysis. Small studies have shown that there is a variable age of onset with variable behavioral, mood, and cognitive deficits present at the time of death (92% symptomatic at time of death).[10,16]

See section about CTE (p. 1112) for further details.

61.2 Other TBI definitions and concepts

61.2.1 Contusion

A contusion is a TBI with CT findings that may include:

- high attenuation areas (AKA "hemorrhagic contusions" AKA traumatic intraparenchymal hemorrhages) (▶ Fig. 61.1): usually produce less mass effect than their apparent size. Most common in areas where sudden deceleration of the head causes the brain to impact on bony prominences (e.g., frontal and occipital bones, sphenoid wing, petrous bone). Contused areas may progress (or "blossom" in neuroradiological jargon) to frank parenchymal hematomas. Surgical decompression (p. 1071) may be considered if herniation threatens.
- low attenuation areas: representing associated edema

61.2.2 Contrecoup injury

In addition to the injury to the brain directly under the point of impact, the brain may rebound after the impact and be thrust against the skull at a point diagonally opposite the blow (▶ Fig. 61.1), the so-called contrecoup (French: "counter blow") injury. This may produce contusions typically located subjacent to bony prominences listed above.

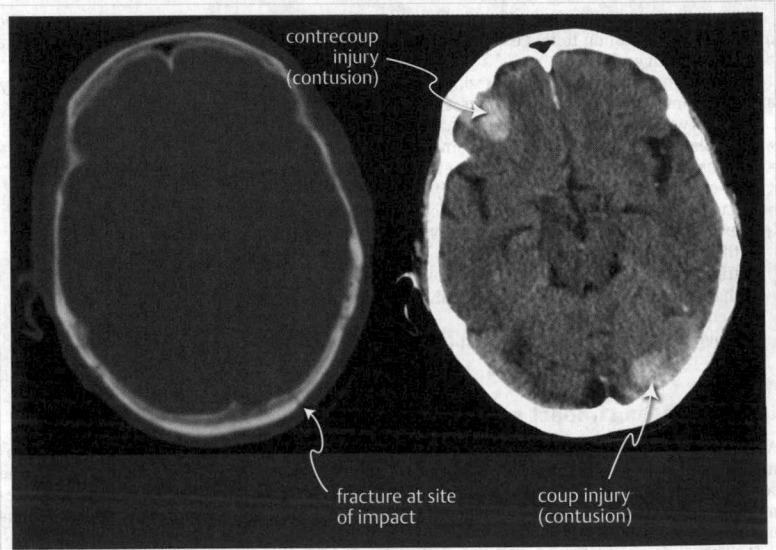

Fig. 61.1 Coup contrecoup injury in patient who fell, striking their occiput on the ground sustaining a skull fracture in the left occipital bone with a "coup injury" to the left cerebellum and a "contrecoup injury" to the right frontal lobe.
Image: axial CT scan of the brain, bone window on left, brain window on right.

61.2.3 Posttraumatic brain swelling

This term encompasses two distinct processes:
1. increased cerebral blood volume: may result from loss of cerebral vascular autoregulation. This hyperemia may sometimes occur with extreme rapidity, in which case it has sometimes been referred to as diffuse or "malignant cerebral edema,"[24] which carries close to 100% mortality and may be more common in children. Management consists of aggressive measures to maintain ICP < 22 mm Hg and CPP > 60-70 mm Hg.[25] (whether 60 or 70 is the optimal minimum for CPP is unclear). See ICP treatment threshold (p. 1047)
2. true cerebral edema: classically at autopsy these brains "weep fluid."[26] Both vasogenic and cytotoxic cerebral edema (p. 90) can occur within hours of head injury[26,27] and when indicated may be treated with decompressive craniectomy (p. 1071)

61.2.4 Diffuse axonal injury (DAI) (AKA diffuse axonal shearing)

A *primary* lesion of rotational acceleration/deceleration head injury.[28] In its severe form, hemorrhagic foci occur in the corpus callosum and dorsolateral rostral brainstem with microscopic evidence of diffuse injury to axons (axonal retraction balls, microglial stars, and degeneration of white matter fiber tracts). Often cited as the cause of prolonged loss of consciousness in patients rendered immediately comatose following head injury in the absence of a space occupying lesion on CT[29] (although DAI may also be present with subdural[30] or epidural hematomas[31]).

May be diagnosed clinically when loss of consciousness (coma) lasts > 6 hours in absence of evidence of intracranial mass or ischemia.

DAI may be graded clinically as shown in ▶ Table 61.6, or histologically as in ▶ Table 61.7.

Table 61.6 Clinical grading of diffuse axonal injury (DAI)

DAI grade	Description
mild	coma > 6–24 hrs, followed by mild-to-moderate memory impairment, mild-to-moderate disabilities
moderate	coma > 24 hrs, followed by confusion & long-lasting amnesia. Mild-to-severe memory, behavioral, and cognitive deficits
severe	coma lasting months with flexor and extensor posturing. Cognitive, memory, speech, sensorimotor, and personality deficits. Dysautonomia may occur

Table 61.7 Histologic grading of diffuse axonal injury (DAI)[32]

DAI grade	Description
grade I	axonal injury in the white matter of the cerebral hemisphere, corpus callosum, brainstem and, less commonly, cerebellum
grade II	focal lesion[a] in the corpus callosum in addition to above
grade III	focal lesion[a] in the dorsolateral quadrant(s) of the rostral brainstem in addition to above

[a]focal lesions often can only be perceived microscopically

61.3 Posttraumatic hearing loss

61.3.1 Etiologies

It is well known that posttraumatic hearing loss can follow temporal bone fractures (p. 1064). Other etiologies have been more difficult to elucidate.[33] This section does not include iatrogenic trauma.

1. conductive hearing loss: injury distal to the cochlea. Classically associated with longitudinal temporal bone fractures. Hearing loss may be due to:
    a) disruption of the ossicular chain
    b) hemotympanum: may be diagnosed with otoscopic exam
2. sensorineural hearing loss. Hearing loss may be due to:
    a) injury to inner ear structures, e.g., cochlea
        1. injuries due to temporal bone fractures
        2. hypothesized "labyrinthine concussion" or "cochlear concussion" in cases without fracture
    b) injury to Cr.N. VIII
3. "central" hearing loss. Injuries to brain or brainstem structures including: inferior colliculi,[34] superficial siderosis of the brainstem following TBI, injury to bilateral frontal lobes and the left middle temporal gyrus[33]
4. mixed hearing loss: injury to any combination of the above

61.3.2 Epidemiology

▶ **Hearing loss with temporal bone fractures.** Hearing loss after temporal bone trauma in children occurs in > 80% of cases, and resolves in 75% without treatment.[35] Less common in adults, occuring in about 40% of head trauma.

▶ **Hearing loss without temporal bone fractures.** Estimate of the lower limit of incidence in a prospective study of mild TBI is 0.9%,[36] with an estimated upper limit ranging from 18-58% primarily from retrospective studies.[33]

61.3.3 Clinical

Hearing loss is usually readily apparent to a conscious patient. It may be accompanied by tinnitus which does not have prognostic significance.

In the comatose patient, the diagnosis is often delayed or not made at all. Brainstem auditory evoked potentials may[37] or may not[34] be helpful in detection.

Dizziness and dysequilibrium may go unnoticed by the patient until they begin ambulating, but may be diagnosed clinically by the presence of nystagmus with the direction (the rapid phase) usually away from the affected ear.[35]

Determining the type of hearing loss is useful as surgical repair for conductive hearing loss can be helpful and may be performed any time, whereas sensorineural hearing loss is usually not responsive to treatment.[35]

Peripheral facial nerve palsy should be identified as it is essentially the only indication for possible *early* surgical intervention (p.1064).

61.4 High-altitude cerebral edema

Acute high-altitude sickness (AHAS) is a systemic disorder that affects individuals usually within 6–48 hrs after ascent to high altitudes. Acute mountain sickness (AMS) is the most common form of AHAS, with symptoms of nausea, headache, anorexia, dyspnea, insomnia, and fatigue,[38] and is often assessed using the Lake Louise system.[39] The incidence is ≈ 25% at 7,000 feet and ≈ 50% at 15,000 feet. Other symptoms of AHAS include edema of feet and hands, and pulmonary edema (HAPE = high-altitude pulmonary edema). Ocular findings include retinal hemorrhages,[40] nerve fiber layer infarction, papilledema and vitreous hemorrhage.[41] Cerebral edema (HACE = high-altitude cerebral edema), usually associated with pulmonary edema, may occur in severe cases of AHAS. Symptoms of HACE include: severe headache, mental dysfunction (hallucinations, inappropriate behavior, reduced mental status), and neurologic abnormalities (ataxia, paralysis, cerebellar findings).

The unproven "tight-fit" hypothesis postulated that individuals with less compliant CSF systems (smaller ventricles and CSF spaces) were more vulnerable to AMS.[42] A small study of 10 volunteers[43] analyzing CT scans before ascent and symptoms showed a trend that supports the hypothesis.

Prevention: gradual ascent, 2–4 day acclimatization at intermediate altitudes (especially to include sleeping at these levels), avoidance of alcohol or hypnotics.

Treatment of cerebral edema: immediate descent and oxygen (6–12 L/min by NC or face-mask) are recommended. Dexamethasone 8 mg PO or IV followed by 4 mg q 6 hrs may help temporize.

61.5 Traumatic cervical artery dissections

61.5.1 General information

Cervical arterial dissections are a subset of cervical cerebrovascular injuries as shown below.
Cervical cerebrovascular injuries:
* penetrating injury (p.1219)
* traumatic dissection: the subject of this chapter
  o due to blunt trauma
  o due to stretching: e.g., from neck hyperextension or therapeutic spinal manipulation
  o iatrogenic: dissection caused by intimal tear from angiography catheters
* traumatic compression or occlusion
  o kinking from malalignment: e.g., with cervical fracture-dislocation
  o compression by bone fragments: e.g., by fractures through foramen transversarium

This chapter deals with traumatic cervical artery dissections. There is significant overlap with spontaneous cerebrovascular arterial dissections (p.1576); however, features that are more pertinent to posttraumatic dissections are covered here.

Optimal screening, diagnostic and treatment methods are controversial. A 13% mortality rate is considered low. Nearly one-third of patients are not treatable.

61.5.2 Epidemiology

Incidence: 1–2% of blunt trauma patients[44] (among those who stayed > 24 hrs in a trauma hospital the incidence was 2.4%[44]). In pediatric patients identified with BCVI, 69% were located in the intracranial ICA, 23% in the extracranial ICA, and 6% in the VA.[45]

61.5.3 Risk factors

Traumatic risk factors for blunt cerebrovascular injury (BCVI) are shown in ► Table 61.8. Risk factors not directly related to the type of trauma include fibromuscular dysplasia, where dissections may follow minor injuries because of increased susceptibility of the vessels. BCVI can occur even in the absence of identifiable risk factors.[44]

Table 61.8 Traumatic factors with high risk for BCVI[46,47]

- severe cervical hyperextension with rotation or hyperflexion
- high energy transfer mechanism associated with:
  - displaced mid face fracture: Le Fort fracture type II or III (p. 1067)
  - basilar skull fracture involving carotid canal
- TBI consistent with DAI and GCS < 6
- cervical vertebral body or transverse foramen fracture, subluxation, or ligamentous injury at any level
- any fracture involving C1–3
- near hanging with anoxic brain injury
- clothesline-type injury or seat belt abrasion with significant cervical swelling, pain, or mental status changes

61.5.4 Presentation

Signs and symptoms of BCVI are shown in ► Table 61.9.

Table 61.9 Signs & symptoms of BCVI[47]

- arterial hemorrhage from neck/nose/mouth (? go to O.R.)
- cervical bruit in pt < 50 yrs old
- expanding cervical hematoma
- focal neurologic deficit: TIA, Horner syndrome, hemiparesis, VBI
- neurologic deficit inconsistent with head CT
- stroke on CT or MRI

61.5.5 Evaluation of patients with risk factors or signs/symptoms of BCVI

► **Imaging findings.** Briefly, imaging findings with dissection may include: filling defect/luminal stenosis (► Fig. 61.2), occlusion, extravassation of contrast outside the normal lumen. See detailed list (p. 1578).

Dissection is graded as shown in ► Table 61.10 (AKA the "Denver grading scale").

► **Imaging protocol.** The following is an adaptation of the guidelines of the Western Trauma Association flow chart[47] (including footnotes!) into an outline format. Their recommendations are based on observational studies and expert opinion (no Class I data was available).

NB: CTAs on scanners with ≥ 16 detectors (16-slice multidetector CT angiography (16MD-CTA)) have an accuracy near 99%[49] & equivalent predictive value to catheter cerebral angiogram. MRA[50,51] and ultrasound[52,53] are not considered adequate for BCVI screening. If 16MD-CTA is not available, then catheter angiography is recommended.

1. 16MD-CTA should be obtained as follows:
   a) emergently in patients with signs/symptoms of BCVI (► Table 61.9)
   b) *asymptomatic* patients with risk factors (► Table 61.8) for BCVI:
      - if the presence of BCVI would alter therapy (e.g., no contraindication to heparin) then 16MD-CTA should be done within 12 hours if possible
      - if heparin is contraindicated due to associated injuries, timing of 16MD-CTA is determined by patient stability
2. if the 16MD-CTA is equivocal, or if it is negative but clinical suspicion remains high: a catheter arteriogram should be done (otherwise, if negative: stop)
3. if the 16MD-CTA or catheter arteriogram is abnormal (see positive findings (p. 1578)):
   a) determine the BCVI grade (► Table 61.10)[48]
   b) proceed with grade-based management (see below)

61.5.6 Management of documented BCVI

Antiplatelet therapy is as effective in preventing stroke as anticoagulation for cerebrovascular dissection.[54,55]

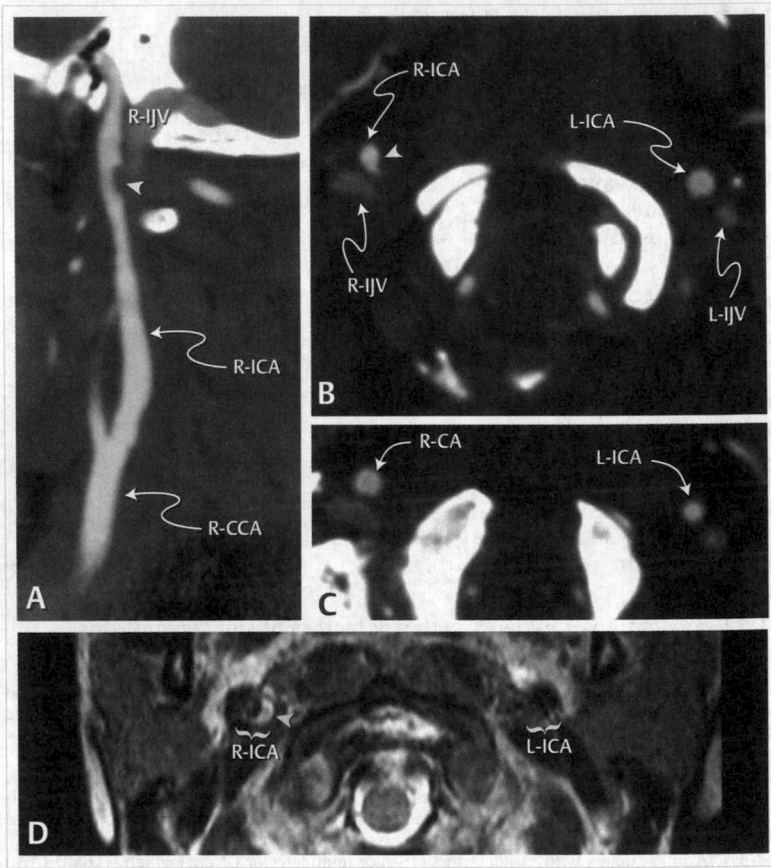

Fig. 61.2 Denver grade II focal dissection (*yellow arrowheads*) with 25% luminal stenosis of the right internal carotid artery at the level of C1 in a 27-year-old woman following a motor vehicle accident in which she also sustained atlanto-occipital dislocation that was subsequently operated.
Image: CTA, A: sagittal, B: axial through the dissection (note that the right ICA is not round, unlike the left ICA), C: axial just above the dissection to illustrate that the right ICA has returned to a round configuration which it also had below the dissection (not shown), D: T2 axial MRI through the dissection showing the "crescent sign" (*blue arrowhead*) with hematoma in the wall of the right ICA with narrowing of the lumen.
Abbreviations: CCA = common carotid artery, ICA = internal carotid artery, IJV = internal jugular vein, L = left, R = right.

Table 61.10 BCVI grading scale[48] ("Denver grading scale")

Grade	Description
I	luminal irregularity with < 25% stenosis
II	≥ 25% luminal stenosis or intraluminal thrombus or raised intimal flap
III	pseudoaneurysm
IV	occlusion
V	transection with free extravasation

▶ **Grade specific therapy.** Using the Denver BCVI grade (▶ Table 61.10):
- Grade I & II
  - most resolve on their own
  - even though there might be a slight benefit of heparin over aspirin for low grade injuries, due to the low overall risk the general trend is to treat these with aspirin
- Grade III
  - anticoagulate with heparin. Rationale: heparin & aspirin are roughly equivalent for Grade III; however, most will need to be restudied in 7–10 days and heparin is easier to stop for an angio
  - repeat angiogram or 16MD-CTA 7–10 days post-injury. See below for subsequent management
- Grade IV: endovascular occlusion to prevent embolization
- Grade V: highly lethal injury
  - accessible lesions should be considered for urgent surgical repair (anecdotal)
  - inaccessible lesions (the majority): incomplete transection may be amenable to endovascular stenting with concurrent antithrombotics; complete transections should be ligated (or occluded endovascularly)

For Grade III repeat 16MD-CTA or catheter angiography 7–10 days post injury to assess healing.[56] Results:
1. lesion healed: discontinue anticoagulation
2. non-healed lesions:
   a) consider endovascular stenting "with caution" for severe luminal narrowing or expanding pseudoaneurysm (controversial: results have been mixed – favorable[54] and unfavorable[57])
   b) transition from heparin to aspirin (75–150 mg/d) alone
   c) repeat 16MD-CTA or catheter angiography 3 months post injury (rationale: most heal with canalization in 6 wks). Results:
      1. healed lesion: consider discontinuing aspirin
      2. non-healed: optimal drug and duration is not known. Recommendation[47]: lifelong anti-platelet therapy with either aspirin or clopidogrel. Dual therapy is used for acute coronary syndromes and following angioplasty (± stenting) but is not recommended in patients who have had a stroke or TIA[58]

Heparinization:
When anticoagulation is employed, perform a baseline PTT and then begin heparin drip 15 U/kg/hr IV. Repeat PTT after 6 hours, and titrate to PTT = 40–50 seconds.

Trauma contraindications to anticoagulation: patients that are actively bleeding, have potential for bleeding, or in whom the consequences of bleeding are severe. Specific examples include: liver and spleen injuries, major pelvic fractures, and intracranial hemorrhage.

Dissection-related anticoagulation risks include: extension of the medial hemorrhage (with possible SAH), and intracerebral hemorrhage (conversion of pale infarct to hemorrhagic).

61.5.7 Carotid artery blunt injuries

General information

See general information related to cerebral arterial dissections and spontaneous dissections (p.1576). For evaluation and management, see above.

This section considers blunt (i.e., nonpenetrating) specifically related to ICA dissection. Neck hyperextension with lateral rotation is a common mechanism of injury, and is thought to stretch the ICA over the transverse processes of the upper cervical spine. In posttraumatic dissection, ischemic symptoms are the most common.[59]

Etiologies:
1. following MVAs: the most common etiology
2. attempted strangulation[60]
3. spinal manipulation therapy: VA dissections are more common than ICA

Most carotid dissections start ≈ 2 cm distal to the ICA origin.

Clinical

The risk of stroke increases with increasing grade for ICA injuries (▶ Table 61.11). This is not true for VA injuries.

Initially, there may be no neurologic sequelae; however, progressive thrombosis, intramural hemorrhage, or embolic phenomenon may develop in a delayed fashion. The distribution of time delays following trauma to time of presentation is shown in ▶ Table 61.12 (the majority are evident within the first 24 hours).

Table 61.11 Risk of stroke with ICA dissection

Grade[a]	Description	Stroke risk
I	stenosis < 25%	3%
II	stenosis > 25%	11%
III	pseudoaneurysm	44%
IV	occlusion	uniformly lethal

[a]for grading, see ▶ Table 61.10

Table 61.12 Time to presentation after non-penetrating trauma

Time	% of cases
0–1 hours	6–10
1–24 hours	57–73
after 24 hours	17–35

Management

See Management of documented BCVI (p. 1029).

Outcome

Natural history is not well known. Many patients with minor symptoms may not present and presumably do well. In one series, 75% of patients returned to normal, 16% had a minor deficit, and 8% had a major deficit or died.[61]

Grade I injuries: 70% heal with or without heparin. 25% will persist. 4–12% will progress to more severe grade. Data suggests that anticoagulation reduces the risk of progression.[46]

Grade II: ≈ 70% progress to more severe grade even with heparin therapy.

Grades III & IV: most persist.

61.5.8 Vertebral artery blunt injuries

General information

See anatomy of vertebral artery segments (p. 80).

Blunt vertebral artery injury (BVI) is very rare, being found in 0.5–0.7% of patients with blunt injuries with aggressive screening.[62] It may produce vertebrobasilar insufficiency (VBI) or posterior circulation stroke. Fractures through the foramen transversarium, facet fracture-dislocation, or vertebral subluxation are frequently identified in patients with BVI[46,63,64] (overall incidence increases to 6% in the presence of cervical fracture or ligamentous injury[62]).

Etiologies

While motor vehicle accidents are the most common mechanism of injury, any trauma that can injure the C-spine can cause BVI (diving accidents, spinal manipulation…).
1. automobile accidents
2. spinal manipulation therapy (SMT): including chiropractic[65] or similar, which comprise 11 of 15 case reports reviewed by Caplan et al.[66] VA dissections were independently associated with SMT within 30 days in multivariate analysis (odds ratio = 6.62, 95% CI 1.4 to 30)[67]
3. sudden head turning
4. direct blows to the back of the neck[66]

Stroke from BVI

The Denver grade of the dissection in BVI does not correlate with risk of stroke or mortality (as it does with ICA dissection).[68] Unlike with carotid injuries, there is rarely a premonitory "warning" TIA. Time from injury to stroke: mean 4 days (range: 8 hours-12 days).

Evaluation

When BVI is identified, it is critical to assess the status of the contralateral VA.

Practice guideline: Vertebral artery blunt injuries

Evaluation
Level I[69]
- Patients meeting the "Denver Screening Criteria" (symptoms shown in ▶ Table 61.9 or risk factors shown in ▶ Table 61.8) should undergo 16MD-CTA to screen for BVI

Level III[69]
- Catheter angiogram is recommended in select patients after blunt cervical trauma if 16MD-CTA is not available, especially if concurrent endovascular intervention is a consideration.
- MRI is recommended for BVI after blunt cervical trauma in patients with incomplete SCI or vertebral subluxation injuries.

Treatment

Practice guideline: Vertebral artery blunt injuries

Treatment
Level III[69]
- No specific guidelines were made among treatment options (anticoagulation, antiplatelet therapy, or no treatment)
- The role of endovascular therapy for BVI has not been defined

Strokes were more frequent in patients with BVI who were not treated initially with IV heparin despite an asymptomatic BVI.[46] However, based on historical controls, it is not clear if either screening or treatment improves overall outcome.[62]

Recommendations: treat all BVI with aspirin. Restudy chronic occlusion in 3 months.

Treatment options include endovascular stenting when amenable. This can restore near-normal flow, but long-term results are lacking.[70] Also, stenting requires ≥ ≈ 3 months of antiplatelet therapy which is contraindicated in some situations.

Outcome

Overall mortality with unilateral BVI ranges from 8–18%[68] which is lower than with ICA dissections (17–40%). Bilateral VA dissection appears highly fatal.

References

[1] Carney N, Ghajar J, Jagoda A, et al. Concussion guidelines step 1: systematic review of prevalent indicators. Neurosurgery. 2014; 75 Suppl 1:S3–15

[2] Harmon KG, Drezner JA, Gammons M, et al. American Medical Society for Sports Medicine position statement: concussion in sport. Br J Sports Med. 2013; 47:15–26

[3] McCrory P, Meeuwisse WH, Aubry M, et al. Consensus statement on concussion in sport: the 4th International Conference on Concussion in Sport held in Zurich, November 2012. Br J Sports Med. 2013; 47:250–258

[4] Scorza KA, Raleigh MF, O'Connor FG. Current concepts in concussion: evaluation and management. Am Fam Physician. 2012; 85:123–132

[5] McCrory P, Meeuwisse WH, Echemendia RJ, et al. What is the lowest threshold to make a diagnosis of concussion? Br J Sports Med. 2013; 47:268–271

[6] Putukian M, Raftery M, Guskiewicz K, et al. Onfield assessment of concussion in the adult athlete. Br J Sports Med. 2013; 47:285–288

[7] Giza CC, Kutcher JS, Ashwal S, et al. Summary of evidence-based guideline update: evaluation and management of concussion in sports: report of the Guideline Development Subcommittee of the American Academy of Neurology. Neurology. 2013; 80:2250–2257

[8] Yuh EL, Hawryluk GW, Manley GT. Imaging concussion: a review. Neurosurgery. 2014; 75 Suppl 4: S50–S63

[9] Kelly JP, Rosenberg JH. Diagnosis and Management of Concussion in Sports. Neurology. 1997; 48:575–580

[10] Putukian M, Kutcher J. Current concepts in the treatment of sports concussions. Neurosurgery. 2014; 75 Suppl 4:S64–S70

[11] Carney N, Ghajar J, Jagoda A, et al. Executive summary of Concussion guidelines step 1: systematic review of prevalent indicators. Neurosurgery. 2014; 75 Suppl 1:S1–S2

[12] SCAT3. Br J Sports Med. 2013; 47

[13] Child SCAT3. Br J Sports Med. 2013; 47

[14] McCrea M, Kelly JP, Kluge J, et al. Standardized Assessment of Concussion in Football Players. Neurology. 1997; 48:586–588

[15] Broglio StevenP, Ferrara MichaelS, Macciocchi Stephen N, et al. Test-Retest Reliability of Computerized Concussion Assessment Programs. Journal of Athletic Training. 2007; 42:509–514

[16] Saigal R, Berger MS. The long-term effects of repetitive mild head injuries in sports. Neurosurgery. 2014; 75 Suppl 4:S149–S155

[17] Papathanasiou ES, Cronin T, Seemungal B, et al. Electrophysiological testing in concussion: A guide to clinical applications. Journal of Concussion. 2018; 2:1–11

[18] Giza CC, Hovda DA. The new neurometabolic cascade of concussion. Neurosurgery. 2014; 75 Suppl 4:S24–S33

[19] Tator CH, Davis H. The postconcussion syndrome in sports and recreation: clinical features and demography in 138 athletes. Neurosurgery. 2014; 75 Suppl 4:S106–S112

[20] Centers for Disease Control and Prevention. Brain Injury Basics - Returning to Sports and Activities. 2015. http://www.cdc.gov/headsup/basics/return_to_sports.html

[21] Schneider RC. Head and Neck Injuries in Football. Baltimore: Williams & Wilkins; 1973

[22] Saunders RL, Harbaugh RE. Second Impact in Catastrophic Contact-Sports Head Trauma. Journal of the American Medical Association. 1984; 252:538–539

[23] McCrory PR, Berkovic SF. Second Impact Syndrome. Neurology. 1998; 50:677–683

[24] Bruce DA, Alavi A, Bilaniuk L, et al. Diffuse Cerebral Swelling Following Head Injuries in Children: The Syndrome of "Malignant Brain Edema". J Neurosurg. 1981; 54:170–178

[25] Carney N, Totten AM, O'Reilly C, et al. Guidelines for the Management of Severe Traumatic Brain Injury, Fourth Edition. Neurosurgery. 2017; 80:6–15

[26] Kimelberg H. Current Concepts of Brain Edema. Journal of Neurosurgery. 1995; 83:1051–1059

[27] Bullock R, Maxwell W, Graham D. Glial Swelling Following Cerebral Contusion: An Ultrastructural Study. Journal of Neurology, Neurosurgery, and Psychiatry. 1991; 54:427–434

[28] Gennarelli TA, Thibault LE, Adams JH, et al. Diffuse Axonal Injury and Traumatic Coma in the Primate. Ann Neurol. 1982; 12:564–574

[29] Adams JH, Graham DI, Murray LS, et al. Diffuse Axonal Injury Due to Nonmissile Head Injury in Humans: An Analysis of 45 Cases. Ann Neurol. 1982; 12:557–563

[30] Sahuquillo-Barris J, Lamarca-Ciuro J, Vilalta-Castan J, et al. Acute Subdural Hematoma and Diffuse Axonal Injury After Severe Head Trauma. J Neurosurg. 1988; 68:894–900

[31] , Lamarca-Ciuro J, Vilalta-Castan J, et al. Epidural Hematoma and Diffuse Axonal Injury. Neurosurgery. 1985; 17:378–379

[32] Adams JH, Doyle D, Ford I, et al. Diffuse axonal injury in head injury: definition, diagnosis and grading. Histopathology. 1989; 15:49–59

[33] Chen JX, Lindeborg M, Herman SD, et al. Systematic review of hearing loss after traumatic brain injury without associated temporal bone fracture. Am J Otolaryngol. 2018; 39:338–344

[34] Hu CJ, Chan KY, Lin TJ, et al. Traumatic brainstem deafness with normal brainstem auditory evoked potentials. Neurology. 1997; 48:1448–1451

[35] Patel A, Groppo E. Management of temporal bone trauma. Craniomaxillofac Trauma Reconstr. 2010; 3:105–113

[36] Spinos P, Sakellaropoulos G, Georgiopoulos M, et al. Postconcussion syndrome after mild traumatic brain injury in Western Greece. J Trauma. 2010; 69:789–794

[37] Jani NN, Laureno R, Mark AS, et al. Deafness after bilateral midbrain contusion: a correlation of magnetic resonance imaging with auditory brain stem evoked responses. Neurosurgery. 1991; 29:106–8; discussion 108-9

[38] Montgomery AB, Mills J, Luce JM. Incidence of Acute Mountain Sickness at Intermediate Altitude. Journal of the American Medical Association. 1989; 261:732–734

[39] Roach RC, Bartsch P, KHackett PH, et al. The Lake Louise Acute Mountain Sickness scoring system. Burlington: Queen City Printers; 1993

[40] Butler FK, Harris DJ, Reynolds RD. Altitude Retinopathy on Mount Everest, 1989. Ophthalmology. 1992; 99:739–746

[41] Frayser R, Houston CS, Bryan AC, et al. Retinal Hemorrhage at High Altitude. New England Journal of Medicine. 1970; 282:1183–1184

[42] Ross RT. The random nature of cerebral mountain sickness. Lancet. 1985; 1:990–991

[43] Wilson MH, Milledge J. Direct measurement of intracranial pressure at high altitude and correlation of ventricular size with acute mountain sickness: Brian Cummins' results from the 1985 Kishtwar expedition. Neurosurgery. 2008; 63:970–4; discussion 974-5

[44] Stein DM, Boswell S, Sliker CW, et al. Blunt cerebrovascular injuries: does treatment always matter? Journal of Trauma. 2009; 66:132–43; discussion 143-4

[45] Dewan MC, Ravindra VM, Gannon S, et al. Treatment Practices and Outcomes After Blunt Cerebrovascular Injury in Children. Neurosurgery. 2016; 79:872–878

[46] Biffl WL, Moore EE, Elliott JP, et al. The devastating potential of blunt vertebral artery injuries. Ann Surg. 2000; 231:672–681

[47] Biffl WL, Cothren CC, Moore EE. Western Trauma Association critical decisions in trauma: Screening for and treatment of blunt cerebrovascular injuries. Journal of Trauma. 2009; 67:1150–1153

[48] Biffl WL, Moore EE, Offner PJ, et al. Blunt carotid arterial injuries: implications of a new grading scale. J Trauma. 1999; 47:845–853

[49] Eastman AL, Chason DP, Perez CL, et al. Computed tomographic angiography for the diagnosis of blunt cervical vascular injury: is it ready for primetime? Journal of Trauma. 2006; 60:925–9; discussion 929

[50] Miller PR, Fabian TC, Croce MA, et al. Prospective screening for blunt cerebrovascular injuries: analysis of diagnostic modalities and outcomes. Annals of Surgery. 2002; 236:386–93; discussion 393-5

[51] Biffl WL, Ray CE,Jr, Moore EE, et al. Noninvasive diagnosis of blunt cerebrovascular injuries: a preliminary report. Journal of Trauma. 2002; 53:850–856

[52] Cogbill TH, Moore EE, Meissner M, et al. The spectrum of blunt injury to the carotid artery: a multicenter perspective. Journal of Trauma. 1994; 37:473–479

[53] Mutze S, Rademacher G, Matthes G, et al. Blunt cerebrovascular injury in patients with blunt multiple trauma: diagnostic accuracy of duplex Doppler US and early CT angiography. Radiology. 2005; 237:884–892

[54] Edwards NM, Fabian TC, Claridge JA, et al. Antith-rombotic therapy and endovascular stents are effective treatment for blunt carotid injuries: results from longterm followup. Journal of the American College of Surgeons. 2007; 204:1007–13; discussion 1014-5

[55] Markus HS, Hayter E, Levi C, et al. Antiplatelet treatment compared with anticoagulation treatment for cervical artery dissection (CADISS): a randomised trial. Lancet Neurol. 2015; 14:361–367

[56] Biffl WL, Ray CE,Jr, Moore EE, et al. Treatment-related outcomes from blunt cerebrovascular injuries: importance of routine follow-up arteriography. Annals of Surgery. 2002; 235:699–706; discussion 706-7

[57] Cothren CC, Moore EE, Ray CE,Jr, et al. Carotid artery stents for blunt cerebrovascular injury: risks exceed benefits. Archives of Surgery. 2005; 140:480–5; discussion 485-6

[58] Hermosillo AJ, Spinler SA. Aspirin, clopidogrel, and warfarin: is the combination appropriate and effective or inappropriate and too dangerous? Annals of Pharmacotherapy. 2008; 42:790–805

[59] Anson J, Crowell RM. Cervicocranial Arterial Dissection. Neurosurgery. 1991; 29:89–96

[60] Biller J, Hingtgen WL, Adams HP, et al. Cervicocephalic Arterial Dissections: A Ten-Year Experience. Arch Neurol. 1986; 43:1234–1238

[61] Hart RG, Easton JD. Dissections of Cervical and Cerebral Arteries. Neurol Clin North Am. 1983; 1:255–282

[62] Berne JD, Norwood SH. Blunt Vertebral Artery Injuries in the Era of Computed Tomographic Angiographic Screening: Incidence and Outcomes From 8292 Patients. Journal of Trauma. 2009. DOI: 10.1097/TA.0b013e31818888c7

[63] Louw JA, Mafoyane NA, Small B, et al. Occlusion of the vertebral artery in cervical spine dislocations. J Bone Joint Surg Br. 1990; 72:679–681

[64] Willis BK, Greiner F, Orrison WW, et al. The incidence of vertebral artery injury after midcervical spine fracture or subluxation. Neurosurgery. 1994; 34:435–41; discussion 441-2

[65] Mas JL, Henin D, Bousser MG, et al. Dissecting Aneurysm of the Vertebral Artery and Cervical Manipulation: A Case Report with Autopsy. Neurology. 1989; 39:512–515

[66] Caplan LR, Zarins CK, Hemmati M. Spontaneous Dissection of the Extracranial Vertebral Arteries. Stroke. 1985; 16:1030–1038

[67] Smith WS, Johnston SC, Skalabrin EJ, et al. Spinal manipulative therapy is an independent risk factor for vertebral artery dissection. Neurology. 2003; 60:1424–1428

[68] Fusco MR, Harrigan MR. Cerebrovascular dissections: a review. Part II: blunt cerebrovascular injury. Neurosurgery. 2011; 68:517–30; discussion 530

[69] Harrigan MR, Hadley MN, Dhall SS, et al. Management of vertebral artery injuries following nonpenetrating cervical trauma. Neurosurgery. 2013; 72 Suppl 2:234–243

[70] Lee YJ, Ahn JY, Han IB, et al. Therapeutic endovascular treatments for traumatic vertebral artery injuries. Journal of Trauma. 2007; 62:886–891

62 Neuromonitoring in Head Trauma

62.1 General information

This section considers neuromonitoring instrumentation that can be done primarily at the patient's bedside, and therefore does not include CT perfusion studies, PET scans…. The bulk of neuromonitoring literature deals with intracranial pressure (ICP). Other parameters that can be monitored include: jugular venous oxygen monitoring (p. 1045), regional CBF (p. 1046), brain tissue oxygen tension (p. 1045), and brain metabolites (pyruvate, lactate, glucose…) (p. 1046).

The role of adjunctive monitoring is currently unknown. Unanswered questions include: should neuromonitoring be disease specific (e.g., is SAH different from TBI), which monitors provide additional unique information, what are the critical values of the monitored entity, and what interventions should be undertaken to correct abnormalities?

62.2 Intracranial pressure (ICP)

62.2.1 Background

Intracranial pressure (ICP) is discussed in this section on trauma because of the close relationship between elevated ICP and brain damage from head injury. However, factors involved in diagnosing and treating intracranial hypertension (IC-HTN) also may pertain (with modifications) to brain tumors, dural sinus thrombosis, etc.

62.2.2 Cerebral perfusion pressure (CPP) and cerebral autoregulation

Secondary brain injury (i.e., following the initial trauma) is attributable in part to cerebral ischemia (see Secondary injury (p. 1000)). The critical parameter for brain function and survival is not actually ICP, rather it is adequate cerebral blood flow (CBF) to meet $CMRO_2$ demands (see discussion of CBF & $CMRO_2$ (p. 1536)). CBF is difficult to quantitate, and can only be measured continuously at the bedside with specialized equipment and difficulty.[1] However, CBF depends on cerebral perfusion pressure (CPP), which is related to ICP (which is more easily measured) as shown in Eq (62.1).

{cerebral perfusion pressure} = {mean arterial pressure*} − {intracranial pressure}

or, expressed in symbols $\hfill$ (62.1)

CPP = MAP* − ICP

*note: the actual pressure of interest is the mean carotid pressure (MCP) which may be approximated as the MAP with the transducer zeroed ≈ at the level of the foramen of Monro.[2]

As ICP becomes elevated, CPP is reduced at any given MAP. Normal adult CPP is > 50 mm Hg. Cerebral autoregulation is a mechanism whereby over a wide range, large changes in systemic BP produce only small changes in CBF. Due to autoregulation, CPP would have to drop below 40 in a normal brain before CBF would be impaired.

In the head injured patient, older recommendations were to maintain CPP ≥ 70 mm Hg (due to increased cerebral vascular resistance) & ICP < 20 mm Hg.[3] However, recent evidence suggests that elevated ICP (≥ 22 mm Hg) may be more detrimental than changes in CPP (as long as CPP is > 60-70 mm Hg[4])[5] (higher levels of CPP were not protective against significant ICP elevations[6]).

62.2.3 ICP principles

The following are approximations to help simplify understanding ICP (these are only models, and as such are not entirely accurate):
1. *normal* intracranial constituents (and approximate volumes):
   a) brain parenchyma (which also contains extracellular fluid): 1400 ml
   b) cerebral blood volume (CBV): 150 ml
   c) cerebrospinal fluid (CSF): 150 ml
2. these volumes are contained in an inelastic, completely closed container (the skull)
3. pressure is distributed evenly throughout the intracranial cavity (in reality, pressure gradients exist[7,8])

4. the modified **Monro-Kellie doctrine**[9] states that the sum of the intracranial volumes (CBV, brain, CSF, and other constituents (e.g., tumor, hematoma...)) is constant, and that an increase in any one of these must be offset by an equal decrease in another. If the pressure from one intracranial constituent increases (as when that component increases in volume), it causes the pressure inside the skull (ICP) to increase. This increased ICP will act to force one or more of the other constituents out through the foramen magnum (FM) (the only true effective opening in the intact skull) or though a craniectomy defect (after decompressive craniectomy surgery) until a new ICP equilibrium is established. The craniospinal axis can buffer small increases in volume with no change or only a slight increase in ICP. If the expansion continues, then the new equilibrium will be at a higher ICP. The result:

a) at pressures slightly above normal, if there is no obstruction to CSF flow (obstructive hydro-cephalus), CSF can be displaced from the ventricles and subarachnoid spaces and exit the intracranial compartment via the FM

b) intravenous blood can also be displaced through the jugular foramina via the IJVs

c) as ICP continues to rise above the intracranial arterial pressure, arterial blood (part of CBV) is displaced and further entry of arterial blood into the cranium is impaired. When ICP reaches the mean arterial pressure, arterial blood will be unable to enter the skull through the FM, producing complete cessation of blood flow to the brain, with resultant massive infarction

d) increased brain edema, or an expanding mass (e.g., hematoma) can push brain parenchyma downward into the foramen magnum (cerebral herniation) although brain tissue cannot actually exit the skull

62.2.4 Normal ICP

The normal range of ICP varies with age. Values for pediatrics are not well established. Guidelines are shown in ▶ Table 62.1.

Table 62.1 Normal ICP

Age group	Normal range (mm Hg)
adults and older children[a]	<10–15
young children	3–7
term infants[b]	1.5–6

[a]the age of transition from "young" to "older" child is not precisely defined
[b]may be subatmospheric in newborns[10]

62.2.5 Intracranial hypertension (IC-HTN)

General information

Traumatic IC-HTN may be due to any of the following (alone or in various combinations):

1. cerebral edema
2. hyperemia: the normal response to head injury.[11] Possibly due to vasomotor paralysis (loss of cerebral autoregulation). May be more significant than edema in raising ICP (p. 1084) [12]
3. traumatically induced masses
   a) epidural hematoma
   b) subdural hematoma
   c) intraparenchymal hemorrhage (hemorrhagic contusion)
   d) foreign body (e.g., bullet)
   e) depressed skull fracture
4. hydrocephalus due to obstruction of CSF absorption or circulation
5. hypoventilation (causing hypercarbia → vasodilatation)
6. systemic hypertension (HTN)
7. venous sinus thrombosis
8. increased muscle tone and Valsalva maneuver as a result of agitation or posturing → increased intrathoracic pressure → increased jugular venous pressure → reduced venous outflow from the head
9. sustained posttraumatic seizures (status epilepticus)

A *secondary increase in ICP* is sometimes observed 3–10 days following the trauma, and may be associated with a worse prognosis.[13] Possible causes include:

1. delayed hematoma formation
   a) delayed epidural hematoma (p. 1075)
   b) delayed acute subdural hematoma (p. 1081)
   c) delayed traumatic intracerebral hemorrhage[14] (or hemorrhagic contusions) with perilesional edema: usually in older patients, may cause sudden deterioration. May become severe enough to require evacuation (p. 1072)
2. cerebral vasospasm[15]
3. severe adult respiratory distress syndrome (ARDS) with hypoventilation
4. delayed edema formation: more common in pediatric patients
5. hyponatremia

Clinical presentation—Cushing's triad

The classic clinical presentation of IC-HTN (regardless of cause) is Cushing's triad which is shown in ▶ Table 62.2. However, the full triad is only seen in ≈ 33% of cases of IC-HTN.

Patients with significant ICP elevation due to trauma, brain masses (tumor), or hydrocephalus (but paradoxically not with pseudotumor cerebri) will usually be obtunded.

Table 62.2 Cushing's triad with elevated ICP

1. hypertension
2. bradycardia
3. respiratory irregularity

CT scan and elevated ICP

Whereas CT findings may be correlated with a risk of IC-HTN, no combination of CT findings has been shown to allow accurate estimates of actual ICP. 60% of patients with closed head injury and an abnormal CT will have IC-HTN.[16] (**Note:** "abnormal" CT: demonstrates hematomas (EDH, SDH or ICH), contusions,[16] compression of basal cisterns (p. 1109), herniation or swelling[17,18]).

Only 13% of patients with a *normal* CT scan will have IC-HTN.[16] However, patients with a normal CT AND 2 or more risk factors identified in ▶ Table 62.3 will have ≈ 60% risk of IC-HTN. If only 1 or none are present, ICP will be increased in only 4%.

Table 62.3 Risk factors for IC-HTN with a normal CT

- age > 40 yrs
- SBP < 90 mm Hg
- decerebrate or decorticate posturing on motor exam (unilateral or bilateral)

62.2.6 ICP monitoring

Indications for ICP monitoring

Practice guideline: Indications for ICP monitoring

For salvageable patients with severe traumatic brain injury (GCS ≤ 8 after cardiopulmonary resuscitation)
Level II[18]: with an abnormal admitting brain CT (note: abnormal" CT: demonstrates hematomas (EDH, SDH or ICH), contusions,[16] compression of basal cisterns (p. 1109), herniation, or swelling[17,18])
Level III[18]: with a *normal* admitting brain CT, but with ≥ 2 of the following risk factors for IC-HTN:

- age > 40 yrs
- SBP < 90 mm Hg
- decerebrate or decorticate posturing on motor exam (unilateral or bilateral)

1. ★ neurologic criteria: see **Practice guideline: Indications for ICP monitoring** (p. 1038)
   a) some centers monitor patients who don't follow commands. Rationale: patients who follow commands (GCS ≥ 9) are at low risk for IC-HTN, and one can follow sequential neurologic

exams in these patients and institute further evaluation or treatment based on neurologic deterioration
   b) some centers monitor patients who don't localize, and follow neuro exam on others
2. multiple systems injured with altered level of consciousness (especially where therapies for other injuries may have deleterious effects on ICP, e.g., high levels of PEEP or the need for large volumes of IV fluids or the need for heavy sedation)
3. with traumatic intracranial mass (EDH, SDH, depressed skull fracture…)
   a) a physician may choose to monitor ICP in some of these patients[17,19]
   b) post-op, subsequent to removal of the mass
4. non-traumatic indications for ICP monitoring: some centers monitor ICP in patients with acute fulminant liver failure with an INR > 1.5 and Grade III of IV coma. A *subarachnoid bolt* may be inserted after administration of factor VII 40 mcg/kg IV over 1–2 minutes (the bolt is inserted as soon as possible (usually within 15 minutes and no more than 2 hours after administration)) without significant risk of hemorrhage.[20] All patients were treated with hypothermia; other ICP treatment measures were used for refractory IC-HTN

Contraindications (relative)

1. "awake" patient: monitor usually not necessary, can follow neuro exam
2. coagulopathy (including DIC): frequently seen in severe head injury. If an ICP monitor is essential, take steps to correct coagulopathy (FFP, platelets…) and consider *subarachnoid bolt* or *epidural monitor* (an IVC or intraparenchymal monitor is contraindicated). See recommended range of PT or INR (p. 164).

Duration of monitoring

D/C monitor when ICP is normal × 48–72 hrs after withdrawal of ICP therapy. Caution: IC-HTN may have delayed onset (often starts on day 2–3, and day 9–11 is a common second peak, especially in peds). Also see delayed deterioration (p. 1000). Avoid a false sense of security imparted by a normal early ICP.

Complications of ICP monitors

General information
See ▶ Table 62.4 for a summary of complication rates for various types of monitors.[3]
1. infection: see below
2. hemorrhage[3]: overall incidence is 1.4% for all devices (see ▶ Table 62.4 for breakdown). The Angioma Alliance definition of hemorrhage (p. 1527) [23] is recommended. Risk of significant hematoma requiring surgical evacuation is ≈ 0.5–2.5%[16,24,25]
3. malfunction or obstruction: with fluid coupled devices, higher rates of obstruction occur at ICPs > 50 mm Hg
4. malposition: 3% of IVCs require operative repositioning

Infection with ICP monitors
Colonization of the monitoring device is much more common than clinically significant infection (ventriculitis or meningitis). See ▶ Table 62.4 for colonization rates. Fever, leukocytosis and CSF

Table 62.4 Complication rates with various types of ICP monitors

Monitor type	Bacterial colonization[a]	Hemorrhage	Malfunction or obstruction
IVC	ave: 10–17% range[21,22]: 0–40%	1.1%	6.3%
subarachnoid bolt	ave: 5% range: 0–10%	0	16%
subdural	ave: 4% range: 1–10%	0	10.5%
parenchymal	ave: 14% (two reports, 12% & 17%)	2.8%	9–40%

[a]some studies report this as infection, but do not distinguish between clinically significant infection and colonization of ICP monitor

pleocytosis have low predictive value (CSF cultures are more helpful). Range of reported infection rates: 1–27%.[26]

Practice guideline: Infection prophylaxis with ICP monitors

Level III[27]: neither prophylactic antibiotics nor routine ventricular catheter exchange is recommended to reduce infection
    Level III[5 (p 100)]: antimicrobial-impregnated catheters may be considered to prevent EVD related infections

Identified risk factors for infection include[26,28,22,29]:
1. intracerebral, subarachnoid or intraventricular hemorrhage
2. ICP > 20 mm Hg
3. duration of monitoring: contradictory results in literature. One prospective study in 1984 found an increased risk with monitor duration > 5 days (infection risk reaches 42% by day #11).[24,28] Another found no correlation with monitoring duration.[30] A retrospective analysis[22] found a non-linear increase of risk during the first 10–12 days, after which the rate diminished rapidly
4. neurosurgical operation: including operations for depressed skull fracture
5. irrigation of system
6. leakage around IVCs
7. open skull fractures (including basilar skull fractures with CSF leak)
8. other infections: septicemia, pneumonia

Factors *not* associated with increased incidence of infection:
1. insertion of IVC in neuro intensive care unit (instead of O.R.)
2. previous IVC
3. drainage of CSF
4. use of steroids

Treatment of infection
Removal of device if at all possible (if continued ICP monitoring is required consideration may be given to inserting a monitor at another site) and appropriate antibiotics.

Types of monitors

1. intraventricular catheter (IVC): AKA external ventricular drainage (EVD), connected to an external pressure transducer via fluid-filled tubing. The standard by which others are judged (also below; **note**: other options for IVCs utilize transducers tipped with fiberoptic or strain gauge devices, which are located within the intraventricular catheter; in this discussion, "IVC" does not refer to this type)
   a) advantages:
      - most accurate (can be recalibrated to minimize measurement drift)[31]
      - lower cost
      - in addition to measuring pressure, allows therapeutic CSF drainage (may help reduce ICP directly, and may drain particulate matter, e.g., blood breakdown products after SAH, that could occlude arachnoid granulations[32])
   b) disadvantages
      - may be difficult to insert into compressed or displaced ventricles
      - obstruction of the fluid column (e.g., by blood clot, or by coaptation of the ependymal lining on the catheter as the ventricle collapses with drainage) may cause inaccuracy
      - some effort is required to check and maintain function, e.g., IVC problems (p. 1042) and IVC trouble shooting (p. 1043)
      - transducer must be consistently maintained at a fixed reference point relative to patient's head (must be moved as HOB is raised/lowered)
2. intraparenchymal monitor (e.g., Camino labs or Honeywell/Phillips[33,34]): similar to IVC but more expensive. Some are subject to measurement drift,[35,36] others may not be[37]

3. *less accurate* monitors
   a) subarachnoid screw (bolt): risk of infection 1%, rises after 3 days. At high ICPs (often when needed most) surface of brain may occlude lumen → false readings (usually lower than actual, may still show ≈ normal waveform)
   b) subdural: may utilize a fluid coupled catheter (e.g., Cordis Cup catheter), fiberoptic tipped catheter, or strain gauge tipped catheter
   c) epidural: may utilize a fluid coupled catheter, or fiberoptic tipped catheter (e.g., Ladd fiberoptic). Accuracy is questionable
   d) in infants, one can utilize an open anterior fontanelle (AF):
      • fontanometry[38]: probably not very accurate
      • applanation principle: may be used in suitable circumstances (viz.: if the fontanelle is concave with the infant upright, and convex when flat or head down) to estimate the ICP within 1 cm H_2O.[10] The infant is placed supine, and the AF is visualized and palpated while the head is raised and lowered. When the AF is flat, the ICP equals atmospheric pressure, and ICP can be estimated in cm H_2O as the distance from the AF to the point where the venous pressure is 0 (for a recumbent infant, the midpoint of the clavicle usually suffices). If the AF is not concave with the infant erect, then this method cannot be used, because either the ICP exceeds the distance from the AF to the venous zero point, or the scalp may be too thick

Conversion factors between mm Hg and cm H_2O are shown in Eq (62.2) and Eq (62.3) (the density of mercury is 13.6 times that of water, and CSF is fairly close to water).

$$1 \text{ mm Hg [torr]} = 1.36 \text{ cm } H_2O \tag{62.2}$$

$$1 \text{ cm } H_2O = 0.735 \text{ mmHg [torr]} \tag{62.3}$$

Intraventricular catheter (IVC)

Insertion technique

For technique to place catheter in frontal horn, see Kocher's point (p. 1821). The right side is usually used unless specific reasons to use the left are present (e.g., blood clot in right lateral ventricle which might occlude IVC).

Set-up

▶ Fig. 62.1 shows a typical external ventricular drainage (EVD) system/ventriculostomy ICP monitor. Not every system will have the same components (some may have less and some may have more). Note that the effect of having an opening on the top of the drip chamber (through an air-filter) is the same as having the drip nozzle open to air, and therefore as long as this filter is not wet or plugged the pressure in the IVC is regulated by the height of the nozzle (as read on the pressure scale; note that the "0" is level with the nozzle).

The external auditory canal (EAC) is often used as a convenient external landmark for "0" (approximates the level of the foramen of Monro). In ▶ Fig. 62.1 the drip chamber is illustrated at 8 cm above the EAC.

Normal functioning of the IVC system

The system should be checked for proper functioning at least every 2–4 hours, and any time there is a change in: ICP (increase or decrease), neuro exam, or CSF output (for systems open to drainage).
1. check for presence of good waveform with respiratory variations and transmitted pulse pressures
2. IVCs: to check for patency, open the system to drain and lower the drip chamber below level of head and observe for 2–3 drops of CSF (normally do not allow more than this to drain)
3. for systems open to drainage:
   a) volume of CSF in drip chamber should be indicated every hour with a mark on a piece of tape on the drip chamber, and the volume should increase with time unless ICP is less than the

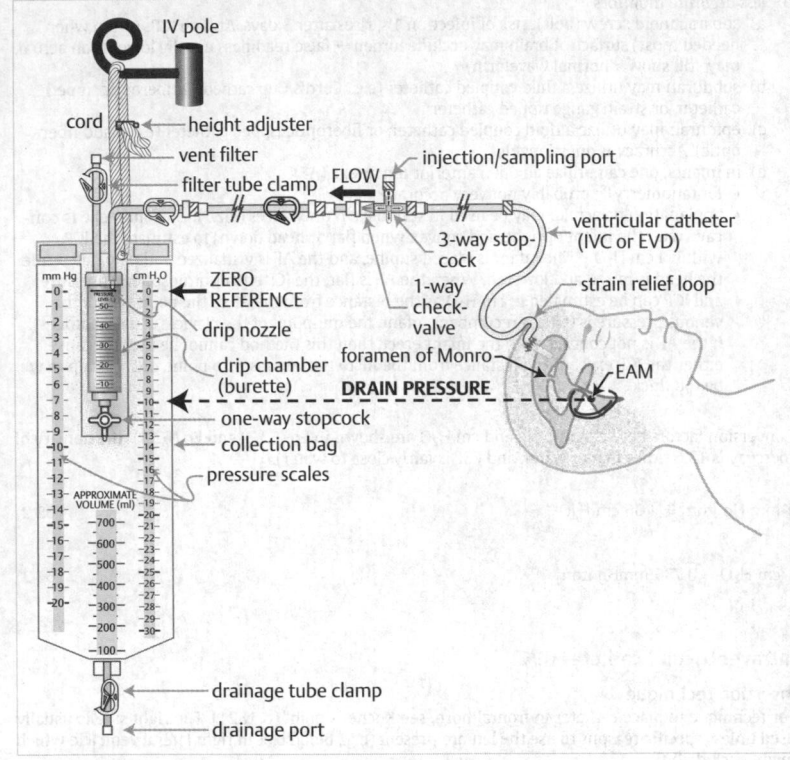

Fig. 62.1 Medtronic® ventricular drainage system/ICP monitor.

height of the drip chamber (in practice, under these circumstances the system would usually not be left open to drainage).

NB: the maximum expected output from a ventriculostomy would be ≈ 450–700 ml per day in a situation where none of the produced CSF is absorbed by the patient. This is not commonly encountered. A typical amount of drainage would be ≈ 75 ml every 8 hrs

b) drip chamber should be emptied into drainage bag regularly (e.g., q 4 or 8 hours) and any time the chamber begins to get full (record volume)

4. in cases where there is a question whether the monitor is actually reflecting ICP, lowering the HOB towards 0° should increase ICP. Gentle pressure on both jugular veins simultaneously should also cause a gradual rise in ICP over 5–15 seconds that should drop back down to baseline when the pressure is released

IVC problems

The following represents some of the error or pitfalls that commonly occur with external ventricular drainage. Some also apply to ICP monitoring in general.

1. air filter on drip chamber gets wet (prevents air from passing through filter)
   a) result: fluid cannot drain freely into drip chamber (the pressure is no longer regulated by the height of the drip nozzle)
      • if the outflow from the drip chamber is clamped, then no flow at all is possible

- if the clamp on the drip chamber outlet is open, then the pressure is actually regulated by the height of the nozzle in the *collection bag* and not the nozzle in the drip chamber
    b) solution: if a fresh filter is available, then replace the wet one. Otherwise one must improvise (with the risk of exposing the system to contamination): e.g., replace the wet filter with a filter from an IV set, or with a sterile gauze taped over the opening
2. air filter on collection bag gets wet: this will make it difficult to empty the drip chamber into the bag
    a) this is not usually an urgent problem unless the drip chamber is full and the collection bag is distended tensely with air
    b) the filter will dry out with time and will usually start to work again
    c) if it is necessary to empty the drip chamber before the filter is dry, then use sterile technique to insert a needle into the bag drainage port and decompress the bag of fluid and air
3. improper connections: a pressurized irrigation bag with or without heparinized solution should *never* be connected to an ICP monitor
4. changing position of head of bed: must move drip chamber up or down to keep it level with the same external landmarks (e.g., level of auditory canal):
    a) when open to drainage, this will assure the correct pressure will be maintained
    b) when opened to pressure transducer, will maintain correct zero
5. when open to drain, pressure reading from transducer is not meaningful: the pressure cannot exceed the height of the drip chamber in this situation (because at that point, fluid will drain off), and the opening to the "atmosphere" in the drip chamber will dampen the waveform
6. drip chamber falls to floor:
    a) overdrainage, possible seizures and/or subdural hematoma formation
    b) solution: securely tape chamber to pole, bed-rail…, check position regularly

IVC troubleshooting
See also IVC problems above.

▶ **IVC no longer works:**
1. manifestation of problem:
    a) dampening or loss of normal waveform
    b) no fluid drains into drip chamber (applies only when catheter has been opened to drain)
2. possible causes:
    a) occlusion of catheter proximal to transducer
        - slide clamp closed or stopcock closed
        - catheter occluded by brain particles, blood cells, protein
    b) IVC pulled out of ventricle
        - test: temporarily lower drip nozzle and watch for 2–3 drops CSF
        - solution:
            verify all clamps are open, and
            flush no more than 1.5 ml of non-bacteriostatic saline (AKA preservative-free saline) with very gentle pressure into ventricular catheter (NB: in elevated ICP the compliance of the brain is abnormally low and small volumes can cause large pressure changes).
            Note. If no return then brain or clot is probably plugging catheter. If it is known that the ventricles are ≈ completely collapsed then the IVC may be OK and CSF should still drain over time. Otherwise this is a non-functioning catheter, and if a monitor/drain is still indicated then a new catheter may need to be inserted (CT may be considered first if the status of the ventricles is not known). If catheter is clotted by intraventricular hemorrhage, rt-PA may sometimes be used (p. 1626) [39]

▶ **ICP waveform dampened.** Possible causes:
1. occlusion of catheter proximal to transducer: see above
2. IVC pulled out of ventricle: no fluid will drain
3. air in system:
    - solution: allow CSF to drain and expel air
    - caution: do not allow excessive amount of CSF to drain (may allow obstruction of catheter, subdural formation…). Do not inject fluid to flush air into brain
4. following decompressive craniectomy: due to the fact that the catheter is no longer in a closed space, this is a normal finding in this setting

Types of ICP waveforms

Normal waveforms

The normal ICP waveform (as occurs with normal blood pressure and in the absence of IC-HTN) as illustrated in ▶ Fig. 62.2 is rarely seen since ICP is usually monitored only when it is elevated. The origin of the variations seen in the normal tracing is somewhat in dispute. One explanation describes these two types of waveforms[40]:

1. small pulsations transmitted from the systemic blood pressure to the intracranial cavity
   a) large (1–2 mm Hg) peak corresponding to the arterial systolic pressure wave, with a small dicrotic notch
   b) this peak is followed by smaller and less distinct peaks
   c) followed by a peak corresponding to the central venous "A" wave from the right atrium
2. blood pressure pulsations are superimposed on slower respiratory variations. During expiration, the pressure in the superior vena cava increases, which reduces venous outflow from the cranium, causing an elevation in ICP. This may be reversed in mechanically ventilated patients, and is opposite to that in the lumbar subarachnoid space, which follows the pressure in the *inferior* vena cava

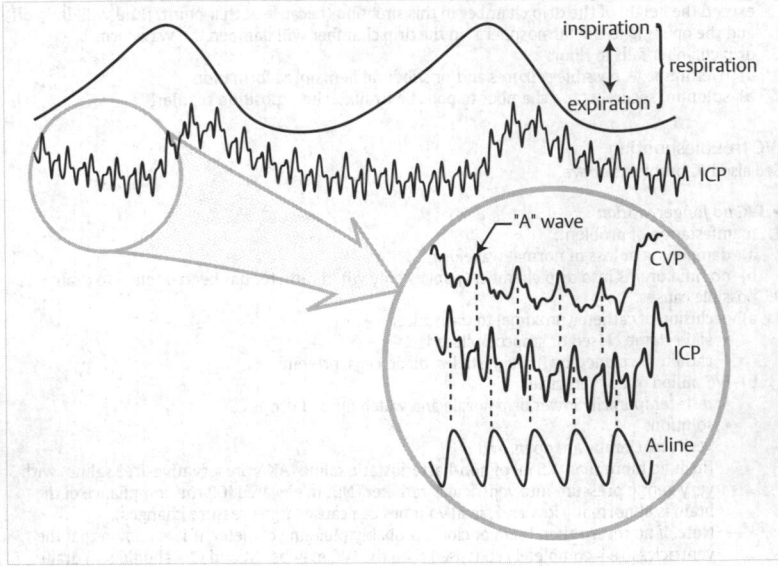

Fig. 62.2 Normal ICP waveform.

Pathological waveforms

As ICP rises and cerebral compliance decreases, the venous components disappear and the arterial pulses become more pronounced. In right atrial cardiac insufficiency, the CVP rises and the ICP waveform takes on a more "venous" or rounded appearance and the venous "A" wave begins to predominate.

A number of "pressure waves" that are more or less pathologic have been described. Currently, this classification is not considered to be of great clinical utility, with more emphasis being placed on recognizing and successfully treating elevations of ICP. Plateau waves will rarely be seen because they are usually aborted at the onset by instituting treatments outlined herein (p. 1046). A brief description of some of these waveforms is included here for general information[41]:

1. Lundberg A waves AKA plateau waves (of Lundberg, ▶ Fig. 62.3): ICP elevations ≥ 50 mm Hg for 5–20 minutes. Usually accompanied by a simultaneous increase in MAP (it is debated whether the latter is cause or effect)

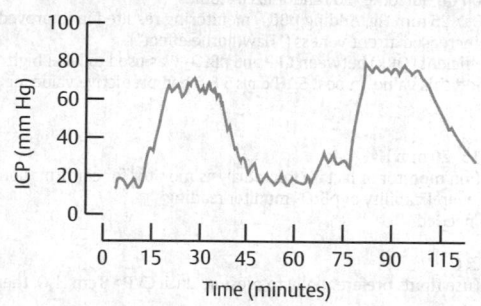

Fig. 62.3 **Plateau waves** (Lundberg A waves).

2. Lundberg B waves AKA pressure pulses: amplitude of 10–20 mm Hg is lower than A waves. Variation with types of periodic breathing. Last 30 secs–2 mins
3. Lundberg C waves: frequency of 4–8/min. Low amplitude C waves (AKA Traube-Hering waves) may sometimes be seen in the normal ICP waveform. High amplitude C-waves may be pre-terminal, and may sometimes be seen on top of plateau waves

62.3 Adjuncts to ICP monitoring

62.3.1 Jugular venous oxygen monitoring

Indications for SjVOs or $PbtO_2$ monitoring include the need for augmented hyperventilation (pCO_2 = 20–25) to control ICP. Parameters related to oxygen content of the blood in the jugular veins are global in nature and are insensitive to focal pathology. Requires retrograde placement of catheter near to the origin of the internal jugular vein at the base of the skull. Parameters that can be measured:

1. jugular venous oxygen saturation ($SjVO_2$): measured continuously with special fiberoptic catheter. Normal $SjVO_2$: ≥ 60%. Desaturations to < 50% suggest ischemia. Multiple desaturations (< 50%) or sustained (≥ 10 minutes) or profound desaturation episodes are associated with poor outcome.[42,43] Sustained desaturations should prompt an evaluation for correctable etiologies: kinking of jugular vein, anemia, increased ICP, poor catheter position, CPP < 60 mm Hg, vasospasm, surgical lesion, $PaCO_2$ < 28 mm Hg. High $SjVO_2$ > 75% may indicate hyperemia or infarcted tissue and is also associated with poor outcome[44]
2. jugular vein oxygen content (CVO_2). Requires intermittent sampling of blood
3. arterial-jugular venous oxygen content difference ($AVdO_2$)[45]: $AVdO_2$ > 9 ml/dl (vol%) probably indicates global cerebral ischemia,[46,47] while values < 4 ml/dl indicate cerebral hyperemia[48] ("luxury perfusion" in excess of the brain's metabolic requirement[47])

62.3.2 Brain tissue oxygen tension monitoring ($PbtO_2$)

Indications for SjVOs or $PbtO_2$ monitoring include the need for augmented hyperventilation (pCO_2 = 20–25) to control ICP. Monitored e.g., with Licox® probe. The likelihood of death increases with longer times of brain tissue oxygen tension ($p_{Bt}O_2$) < 15 mm Hg or even a brief drop of $PbtO_2$ < 6.[49] Initial $pBtO_2$ < 10 mm Hg for > 30 minutes correlates with increased risk of death or bad outcome.[50] Also, see **Practice guideline: Brain oxygen monitoring** (p. 1047).

Probe placement:

1. TBI: assumed to be a diffuse process, often placed on *least* injured side
2. SAH: placed in vascular distributions at greatest risk of vasospasm
   a) ACA (with ACA or AComA aneurysm): standard frontal placement (≈ 2–3 cm off midline on appropriate side)
   b) MCA (with ICA or MCA aneurysm): 4.5–5.5 cm off midline
   c) ACA-MCA watershed area: 3 cm lateral to midline
3. ICH: usually placed near the site of the hemorrhage

Effect of $pBtO_2$ monitoring/intervention on outcome: no randomized studies
1. in TBI[51]: goal was to maintain $pBtO_2 > 25$ mm Hg. Adding $pBtO_2$ monitoring resulted in improved outcome. May have been result of increased attentiveness ("Hawthorne effect")
2. in SAH[52]: a moving correlation coefficient (ORx) between CPP and $pBtO_2$ was used to label high ORx as disturbed autoregulation, and this value on post SAH days 5 & 6 had predictive value for delayed infarction

Management suggestions for $pBtO_2 < 15$–20 mm Hg:
1. consider jugular venous O_2 saturation monitor or lactate microdialysis monitor for confirmation
2. consider CBF study to determine generalizability of $pBtO_2$ monitor reading
3. treatment: proceed to each tier as needed
   a) tier 1
      • keep body temperature < 37.5 C
      • increase CPP to > 60 mm Hg (use fluids preferentially to pressors until CVP > 8 cm H_2O, then use pressors)
   b) tier 2
      • increase FiO_2 to 60%
      • increase $paCO_2$ to 45–50 mm Hg
      • transfuse PRBCs until Hgb > 10 g/dl
   c) tier 3
      • increase FiO_2 to 100%
      • consider increasing PEEP to increase PaO_2 if FiO_2 is at 100%
      • decrease ICP to < 10 mm Hg (drain CSF, mannitol, sedation...)

62.3.3 Bedside monitoring of regional CBF (rCBF)

Thermal diffusion flowmetry permits continuous rCBF monitoring by assessing thermal convection due to tissue blood flow. The probe tip is inserted into the *white matter* of the brain. Commercially available systems include Hemedex® monitoring system (Codman) utilizing the QFLOW 500® probe, which is ✖ not MRI compatible.
   Probe placement: issues similar to those discussed for $pBtO_2$ (see above).
   Readout:
1. K value (thermal conduction): range for white matter is 4.9–5.8 mW/cm-°C (the monitor suppresses CBF readings if the K value is outside this range)
   a) K < 4.9: the probe tip is probably out of the brain tissue or white matter—the probe should be *advanced* 1–2 mm
   b) K > 5.8: the tip is probably too deep, near a blood vessel, or in the ventricle or epidural or subdural space—the probe should be *retracted* 1–2 mm
2. CBF
   a) normal white matter: 18–25 ml/100 g-min
      • white matter CBF < 15: may indicate vasospasm or ischemia
      • white matter CBF < 10: may indicate infarction
   b) normal gray matter: 67–80 ml/100 g-min

Observational data: in a small study of SAH (n=5) and TBI (n=3)[53] there was good correlation between rCBF and $pBtO_2$ 91% of the time. Monitoring was not possible 36% of the time due to patient fever (wherein the system prevents monitoring).

62.3.4 Cerebral microdialysis

Compounds assayed include: lactate, pyruvate, lactate/pyruvate ratio, glucose, glutamate, urea and electrolytes including K^+ & calcium. Some observational data:
1. lactate levels increase during episodes of $SjVO_2$ desaturation[54]
2. decreased extracellular glucose was associated with increased mortality[55]

62.4 Treatment measures for elevated ICP

62.4.1 General information

This section presents a general protocol for treating documented (or sometimes clinically suspected) intracranial hypertension (IC-HTN). Guidelines promulgated by the Brain Trauma Foundation[3,56,57,58] are generally followed. Unless otherwise stated, guidelines are for adult patients (≥ 18 years of age).

62.4.2 Treatment thresholds

Intracranial pressure treatment thresholds

The optimal ICP at which to begin treatment is not known. Various cutoff values are used at different centers above which treatment measures for intracranial hypertension (IC-HTN) are initiated. Although 15, 20, and 25 have been quoted, the Brain Trauma Foundation guideline is ICP > 22 mm Hg[5] as shown in **Practice guideline: ICP treatment threshold** (p. 1047). ✖ Caution: patients can herniate even at ICP < 20[59] (depends on location of intracranial mass).

Rationale: ICP above 22 mm Hg was associated with increased mortality.[60] It is also possible that control may be better by treating early rather than waiting and trying to control higher ICPs or when plateau waves occur.[61]

Practice guideline: ICP treatment threshold

Level II[60 (p 172)]: treatment for IC-HTN should be initiated for **ICP > 22 mm Hg**

Level III[62]: the need for treatment should be based on ICP in combination with clinical examination & brain CT findings

Cerebral perfusion pressure (CPP)

The optimal value for CPP has yet to be determined. The threshold for ischemia is in the range of CPP < 50–60 mm Hg. **Practice guideline: Cerebral perfusion pressure issues** (p. 1047) outlines current recommendations regarding CPP.

Practice guideline: Cerebral perfusion pressure issues

Level II[63]: ✖ avoid aggressive use of fluids and pressors to maintain CPP (because of risk of adult respiratory distress syndrome (ARDS))

Level II[5]: the recommended target for **CPP is > 60-70 mm Hg** (whether 60 vs. 70 is optimal is unclear)

Level III[63]: ✖ avoid CPP < 50 mm Hg

Level III[63]: ancillary monitoring of CBF, oxygenation or metabolism assists CPP management

Brain oxygenation parameters

Suggestions for treatment thresholds are shown in **Practice guideline: Brain oxygen monitoring** (p. 1047). It remains to be determined which interventions are useful to achieve this, and whether this improves outcome.

Practice guideline: Brain oxygen monitoring

Level III[64]: jugular venous O_2 saturation < 50% or brain tissue oxygen tension (PbtO$_2$) < 15 mm Hg are treatment thresholds

62.4.3 ICP management protocol

Quick reference summary

▶ Table 62.5 summarizes a protocol for control of IC-HTN (below for details).

Dosages are given for an average adult, unless specified as mg/kg. Treatment may be initiated prior to insertion of a monitor if there is acute neurologic deterioration or clinical signs of IC-HTN, but continued treatment requires documentation of persistent IC-HTN.

For persistent IC-HTN consider "second tier" therapies (p. 1051).

Table 62.5 Summary of measures to control IC-HTN[a] Goals: ICP < 22 mm Hg, and CPP ≥ 60-70 mm Hg[5,60]

Step	Rationale/Remedy
GENERAL MEASURES (should be utilized routinely)	
elevate HOB to 30–45°	↓ ICP by enhancing venous outflow, but also reduces mean carotid pressure → no net change in CBF
keep neck straight, avoid neck constrictions (tight trach tape, tight cervical collar...)	constriction of jugular venous outflow causes ↑ ICP
avoid arterial hypotension (SBP < 90 mm Hg)	• hypotension reduces CBF • R: normalize intravascular volume, use pressors if needed
control hypertension if present	• R: nicardipine if not tachycardic • R: beta-blocker if tachycardic (labetalol, esmolol...) • ✖ avoid overtreatment → hypotension
avoid hypoxia (PaO$_2$ < 60 mm Hg or O$_2$ sat < 90%)	hypoxia may cause further ischemic brain injury R: maintain airway and adequate oxygenation
ventilate to normocarbia (PaCO$_2$ = 35–40 mm Hg)	✖ avoid prophylactic hyperventilation (p. 1052)
light sedation: e.g., codeine 30–60 mg IM q 4 hrs PRN	(same as heavy sedation, see below)
controversial: prophylactic hypothermia. If used, hold at target temp > 48 hrs	hypothermia → ↓ CMRO$_2$ – efficacy not rigorously proven (p. 1052)
unenhanced head CT scan for ICP problems[b]	rule out surgical condition
SPECIFIC MEASURES FOR IC-HTN	
proceed to successive steps if documented IC-HTN persists – each step is ADDED to the previous measure	
heavy sedation (e.g., fentanyl 1–2 ml or MSO4 2–4 mg IV q 1 hr) and/or paralysis (e.g., vecuronium 8–10 mg IV)	reduces elevated sympathetic tone and HTN induced by movement, tensing abdominal musculature...
drain 3–5 ml CSF if IVC present	reduces intracranial volume
hyperventilate to PaCO$_2$ = 30–35 mm Hg ("blows off" CO$_2$)	CO$_2$ is a potent vasodilator. Hyperventilation → ↓ PaCO$_2$ → ↓ CBV → ↓ ICP ✖ hyperventilation also → ↓ CBF
mannitol 0.25–1 gm/kg, then 0.25 gm/kg q 6 hrs, increase dose if IC-HTN persists & serum osmol ≤ 320 (NB: skip this step if hypovolemia or hypotension)	mannitol → initially ↑ plasma volume & ↑ serum tonicity which draws fluid out of brain → ↓ intracranial volume, may also improve rheologic properties of blood. ✖ mannitol is an osmotic diuretic, and eventually → ↓ plasma volume
if there is "osmotic room" (i.e., serum osmol < 320) bolus with 10–20 ml of 23.4% hypertonic saline (HS)	some patients refractory to mannitol will respond to HS
augmented hyperventilation to ↓ PaCO$_2$ to 25–30 mm Hg	due to risk of cerebral ischemia from ↓ CBF, monitor SjVO$_2$ (p. 1045) or CBF if possible
If IC-HTN persists, consider unenhanced head CT[b] & EEG[c]. Proceed to "second tier" therapy (p. 1051)	

[a] see text for details (p. 1050). As IC-HTN subsides, carefully withdraw treatment
[b] if IC-HTN persists, and especially for a sudden unexplained rise in ICP or loss of previously controlled ICP, give strong consideration to repeating cranial CT to rule out a surgical condition, i.e., "clot" (SDH, EDH, or ICH) or hydrocephalus
[c] EEG to rule out subclinical status epilepticus, which is a rare cause of sustained IC-HTN

Acute ICP crisis

An *acute* increase in ICP in a previously controlled patient may be due to:

1. **paroxysmal sympathetic hyperactivity** (PSH) AKA paroxysmal autonomic instability with dystonia (PAID)[65] : AKA neurostorming, AKA diencephalic seizures, AKA midbrain dysregulatory syndrome... A consensus conference[66] promulgated an assessment tool for determining the likelihood of PSH (see reference for details) which among other things includes points for:
   a) temperature > 37 °C (with increasing points up to ≥ 39 °C)
   b) pulse ≥ 100 beats/min (with increasing points up to ≥ 140)
   c) respiratory rate ≥ 18 (with increasing points up to ≥ 30)
   d) systolic BP ≥ 140 (with increasing points up to ≥ 180)
   e) diaphoresis

f) posturing

g) episodes that are paroxysmal in nature

h) sympathetic hyperactivity in response to normally non-noxious stimuli

i) episodes on ≥ 3 consecutive days

2. increased CO_2 (a potent vasodilator in the brain) e.g., by mucus plugging of part of the bronchial system, pulmonary embolism

3. development of new, or exansion of existing, intracranial hemorrhage (SDH, EDH, ICH...) monitor artifact

▶ **Management.** Temporary measures which may be used to quickly treat an acute ICP crisis are shown in ▶ Table 62.6.

Table 62.6 Measures to treat an acute ICP crisis[a]

Step	Rationale
Verify basics: check airway, neck position/compression... (see general measures in ▶ Table 62.5). For resistant or sudden IC-HTN, consider STAT unenhanced head CT	
be sure patient is sedated and paralyzed (▶ Table 62.5)	(▶ Table 62.5)
drain 3–5 ml CSF if IVC present	↓ intracranial volume
mannitol[b] 1 gm/kg IV bolus or 10–20 ml of 23.4% saline	↑ plasma volume → ↑ CBF → ↓ ICP, also ↑ serum osmolality → ↓ extracellular brain water
hyperventilate with Ambu® bag (✖ do not reduce $PaCO_2 < 25$ mm Hg)	"blow off" (reduce) $PaCO_2$ → ↓ CBV → ↓ ICP. ✖ CAUTION: due to reduced CBF, use for no more than several minutes (p. 1052)
pentobarbital[c] 100 mg slow IV or thiopental 2.5 mg/kg IV over 10 minutes	sedates, ↓ ICP, treats seizures, may be neuroprotective ✖ also myocardial depressant → ↓ MAP

[a]for measures to treat ICP that is trending up over a longer period, see ▶ Table 62.5 or information below under ICP management protocol details
[b]skip this step and go to hyperventilation if hypotensive, volume depleted, or if serum osmolality > 320 mOsm/L
[c]the availability of pentobarbital in the U.S. has been reduced, and other sedatives (p. 1056) may need to be substituted

62.4.4 ICP management protocol details

Goals of therapy

1. keep ICP ≤ 22 mm Hg (prevents "plateau waves" from compromising cerebral blood flow (CBF) and causing cerebral ischemia and/or brain death[32])

2. keep CPP ≥ 60-70 mm Hg.[5] The primary goal is to control ICP, CPP should simultaneously be supported by maintaining adequate MAP.[67] NB: exercise caution when considering aggressive measures to elevate CPP due to the risk of adult respiratory distress syndrome (ARDS)[5]

Surgical treatment

1. traumatic intracranial masses should be treated as indicated. See surgical indications for subdural (p. 1076), epidural (p. 1074) or intraparenchymal (p. 1071) hematoma or posterior fossa mass lesions (p. 1089)

2. decompressive craniectomy may be considered for IC-HTN that cannot be controlled medically

3. as a last resort, patients with severe hemorrhagic contusions ("pulped brain") showing progressive deterioration may benefit from surgical excision of portions of the contused brain tissue, especially if not eloquent brain (p. 1051). NB: even severely contused brain may contain significant viable brain tissue

General care

Major goals

1. avoid hypoxia ($pO_2 < 60$ mm Hg)

2. avoid hypotension (SBP ≤ 90 mm Hg): 67% positive-predictive value (PPV) for poor outcome (79% PPV when combined with hypoxia)[68]

Details of general treatment measures

1. prophylaxis against steroid ulcers (if steroids are used) and Cushing's (stress) ulcers (seen in severe head injury and in increased ICP, accompanied by hypergastrinemia)[69,70,71,72,73] for all patients including peds; see Prophylaxis for stress ulcers (p. 134).
   a) elevating gastric pH: titrated antacid and/or H2 antagonist (e.g., ranitidine 50 mg IV q 8 hrs) or proton pump inhibitor. See possible increased mortality as a result of increased gastric pH (p. 135)
   b) sucralfate
2. aggressive control of fever (fever is a potent stimulus to increase CBF, and may also increase plateau waves)[32]
3. arterial line for BP monitoring and frequent ABGs
4. CVP or PA line if high doses of mannitol are needed (goal: keep patient euvolemic)
5. IV fluids
   a) choice of fluids:
      - isolated head injury: IVF of choice is isotonic (e.g., NS + 20 mEq KCl/L)
      - avoid hypotonic solutions (e.g., lactated ringers) which may impair cerebral compliance[74]
   b) fluid volume:
      - provide adequate fluid resuscitation to avoid hypotension
      - normalization of intravascular fluid volume is not detrimental to ICP
      - although fluid restriction reduces the amount of mannitol needed to control ICP,[75] the concept of "running patients dry" is obsolete[76]
      - if mannitol is required, patient should be maintained at euvolemia
      - also exercise caution in restricting fluids following SAH; see Cerebral salt wasting (p. 122)
      - if injuries to other systems are present (e.g., perforated viscus), they may dictate fluid management
   c) pressors (e.g., dopamine) are preferable to IV fluid boluses in head injury

Measures to lower ICP

General measures that should be routine

1. positioning:
   a) elevate HOB 30–45° (see below)
   b) keep head midline (to prevent kinking jugular veins)
2. light sedation: codeine 30–60 mg IM q 4 hrs PRN, or lorazepam (Ativan®) 1–2 mg IV q 4–6 hrs PRN
3. avoid hypotension (SBP < 90 mm Hg): normalize intravascular volume, support with pressors if needed
4. control HTN; in ICH, aim for patient's baseline, see Initial management of ICH (p. 1619)
5. prevent hyperglycemia: (aggravates cerebral edema) usually present in head injury,[77,78] may be exacerbated by steroids
6. intubation: for GCS ≤ 8 or respiratory distress. Consider premedicating with IV lidocaine (see below) and antibiotics (p. 1003)
7. avoid hyperventilation: keep $PaCO_2$ at the low end of eucapnia (35 mm Hg)
8. prophylactic hypothermia: non-statistically significant trend suggests reduced mortality.[79] Maintain target temperature for > 48 hours

Measures to use for documented IC-HTN

First, check General measures that should be routine above. Proceed to each step if IC-HTN persists.

1. heavy sedation and/or paralysis when necessary (also assists treatment of HTN) e.g., when patient is agitated, or to blunt the elevation of ICP that occurs with certain maneuvers such as moving the patient to CT table. Caution: with heavy sedation or paralysis, the ability to follow the neurologic exam is lost (follow ICPs)
   a) for heavy sedation (intubation recommended to avoid respiratory depression → elevation of $PaCO_2$ → ↑ ICP): e.g., one of the following:
      - morphine (MSO_4): ℞ 2–4 mg/hr IV drip
      - fentanyl: ℞ 1–2 ml IV q 1 hr (or 2–5 mcg/kg/hr IV drip)
      - sufentanil: ℞ 10–30 mcg test dose, then 0.05 -2 mcg/kg/hr IV drip
      - midazolam (Versed®): ℞ 2 mg test dose, then 2–4 mg/hr IV drip
      - propofol drip (p. 110): 0.5 mg/kg test dose, then 20–75 mcg/kg/min IV drip ✖ avoid high-dose propofol (do not exceed 83 mcg/kg/min)
      - "low dose" pentobarbital (adult: 100 mg IV q 4 hrs; peds: 2–5 mg/kg IV q 4 hrs)
   b) paralysis (intubation mandatory): e.g., vecuronium 8–10 mg IV q 2–3 hrs

2. CSF drainage (when IVC is being utilized to measure ICP): 3–5 ml of CSF should be drained with the drip chamber at ≤ 10 cm above EAC. Works immediately by removal of CSF (reducing intracranial volume) and possibly by allowing edema fluid to drain into ventricles[80] (latter point is controversial)

3. "osmotic therapy" when there is evidence of IC-HTN:
   a) *mannitol* (also see below) 0.25–1 gm/kg bolus (over < 20 mins) followed by 0.25 gm/kg IVP (over 20 min) q 6 hrs PRN ICP > 22. Recent literature suggests that 1.4 gm/kg initial dose is more effective. May "alternate" with:
   furosemide (Lasix®) (also see below): adult 10–20 mg IV q 6 hrs PRN ICP > 22. Peds: 1 mg/kg, 6 mg max IV q 6 hrs PRN ICP > 22
   b) keep patient euvolemic to slightly hypervolemic
   c) if IC-HTN persists and serum osmolarity is < 320 mOsm/L, increase mannitol up to 1 gm/kg, and shorten the dosing interval
   d) if ICP remains refractory to mannitol, consider hypertonic saline, either continuous 3% saline infusion or as bolus of 10–20 ml of 23.4% saline
   (D/C after ≈ 72 hours to avoid rebound edema)
   e) hold osmotic therapy if serum osmolarity is ≥ 320 mOsm/L (higher tonicity may have no advantage and risks renal dysfunction; see below) or SBP < 100

4. hyperventilation (HPV) to $PaCO_2$ = 30–35 mm Hg (for details, see below)
   a) ✖ do not use prophylactically
   b) ✖ avoid aggressive HPV ($PaCO_2 ≤ 25$ mm Hg) at all times
   c) use only for
      • short periods for acute neurologic deterioration
      • or chronically for documented IC-HTN unresponsive to sedation, paralytics, CSF drainage, and osmotic therapy
   d) avoid HPV during the first 24 hrs after injury if possible

5. ✖ steroids: the routine use of glucocorticoids is not recommended for treatment of patients with head injuries (see below)

"Second tier" therapy for persistent IC-HTN

If IC-HTN remains refractory to the above measures, and especially if there is loss of previously controlled ICP, strong consideration should be given to repeating a head CT to rule out a surgical condition before proceeding with "second tier" therapies which are either effective but with significant risks (e.g., high-dose barbiturates), or are unproven in terms of benefit on outcome. Also consider an EEG to rule out subclinical status epilepticus (seizures that are not clinically evident); see treatment measures for status epilepticus (p. 512); some medications are effective for both seizures and IC-HTN, e.g., pentobarbital, propofol…

1. high dose barbiturate therapy (p. 1055): initiate if ICP remains > 20–25 mm Hg
2. hyperventilate to $PaCO_2$ = 25–30 mm Hg. Monitoring $SjVO_2$, $AVdO_2$, and/or CBF is recommended (see below)
3. hypothermia[81,82]: patients must be monitored for a drop in cardiac index, thrombocytopenia, elevated creatinine clearance, and pancreatitis. Avoid shivering which raises ICP[82]
4. decompressive surgery:
   a) decompressive craniectomy removal of portion of calvaria.[83] Controversial (may enhance cerebral edema formation[84] and enlargement of hemorrhagic contusions[85]). Craniectomy decreased ICP to < 20 mm Hg in 85%[86] regardless of pupillary response to light, timing of craniectomy, brain shift, and age. Outcomes were improved when IC-HTN responded.[18,86,87] The RESCUEicp trial[88] showed increased survival at 6 months, and it also resulted in higher rates of vegetative state. Early decompressive craniectomy may be considered in patients undergoing emergent surgery (for fracture, EDH, SDH…).[89] Flap must be at least 12 cm in diameter, and duraplasty is mandatory. Also, see Hemicraniectomy for malignant MCA territory infarction (p. 1589)
   b) removal of large areas of contused hemorrhagic brain (makes room immediately; removes region of disrupted BBB). If contused, consider temporal tip lobectomy (no more than 4–5 cm on dominant side, 6–7 cm on non-dominant) (total temporal lobectomy[90] is probably too aggressive) or frontal lobectomy. Has not shown great therapeutic promise
5. lumbar drainage: showing some promise. Watch for "cerebral sag"
6. hypertensive therapy

Adjunctive measures

1. *lidocaine*: 1.5 mg/kg IVP (watch for hypotension, reduce dose if necessary) at least one minute before endotracheal intubation or suctioning. Blunts the rise in ICP as well as tachycardia and

systemic HTN (based on patients with brain tumors undergoing intubation under light barbiturate-nitrous oxide anesthesia; extrapolation to trauma patients is unproven)[91]
2. high frequency (jet) ventilation: consider if high levels of positive end-expiratory pressure (PEEP) are required[92] (NB: patients with reduced lung compliance, e.g., pulmonary edema, transmit more of PEEP through lungs to thoracic vessels and may raise ICP). PEEP ≤ 10 cm H_2O does not cause clinically significant increases in ICP.[93] Higher levels of PEEP > 15–20 are not recommended. Also, rapid elimination of PEEP may cause a sudden increase in circulating blood volume which may exacerbate cerebral edema and also elevate ICP

Details of some measures employed in treating increased ICP

Elevating head of bed (HOB)
Seemingly simple, but there is still some controversy. Early data obtained from dog studies indicated that keeping the HOB at 30–45° optimized the trade-off between the following two factors as the HOB is elevated: reducing ICP (by enhancing venous outflow and by promoting displacement of CSF from the intracranial compartment to the spinal compartment) and reducing the arterial pressure (and thus CPP) at the level of the carotid arteries. Some studies showed a deleterious effect from elevating the HOB and were used to justify nursing these patients with HOB flat.[2]

Recent data[94] indicate that although mean carotid pressure (MCP) is reduced, the ICP is also reduced and the CBF is unaffected by elevating the HOB to 30°. The onset of action of raising the HOB is immediate.

Prophylactic hypothermia

Practice guideline: Prophylactic hypothermia

Level III[79]: prophylactic hypothermia:
• improves the chances of having a moderate to good outcome—4–5 on the Glasgow Outcome Score; see ► Table 98.4—at the end of the follow-up period when target temperatures of 32–35 °C (91.4–95 °F) were used (**note**: no clear relationship was found for cooling duration or rewarming rate)
• showed a non-significant trend suggesting that it lowers *mortality* when the target temperature is maintained for > 48 hrs (**note**: the actual target temperature and rewarming rate did not influence mortality)

Hyperventilation
Intra-arterial carbon dioxide ($PaCO_2$) is the most potent cerebrovascular vasodilator, the effect of which is probably mediated by changes in pH caused by the rapid diffusion of CO_2 across the BBB.[95] Hyperventilation (HPV) lowers ICP by reducing $PaCO_2$ which causes cerebral vasoconstriction, thus reducing the cerebral (intracranial) blood volume (CBV).[96] Of concern, vasoconstriction also lowers cerebral blood flow (CBF) which could produce focal ischemia in areas with preserved cerebral autoregulation as a result of shunting.[97,98] However, ischemia does not necessarily follow as the O_2 extraction fraction (OEF) may also increase, up to a point.[99]

Practice guideline: Hyperventilation for ICP management[a]

Level I[100]: in the absence of IC-HTN, chronic prolonged hyperventilation (HPV) ($PaCO_2$ ≤ 25 mm Hg) should be avoided
  Level II[101]: prophylactic hyperventilation (HPV) ($PaCO_2$ ≤ 25 mm Hg) is not recommended
  Level III:
• HPV may be necessary for brief periods when there is acute neurologic deterioration, or for longer periods if there is IC-HTN refractory to sedation, paralysis, CSF drainage and osmotic diuretics[100]
• HPV should be avoided ≤ 24 hrs after head injury[101]
• if HPV is used, jugular venous oxygen saturation ($SjVO_2$) (p. 1045) or $PbtO_2$ (p. 1045) should be measured to monitor brain O_2 delivery[101]

[a]See also **Practice guideline: Early/prophylactic hyperventilation** (p. 1003).

✖ Hyperventilation (HPV) is to be used in moderation only in specific situations[3] (see below). Prophylactic HPV may actually be associated with a *worse* outcome[102] (**note**: prophylactic HPV implies cases where there are no clinical signs of IC-HTN and where IC-HTN unresponsive to other measures has not been documented by ICP monitoring). When indicated, use HPV only to PaCO$_2$ = 30–35 mm Hg (see Caveats for hyperventilation below). CBF in severe head trauma patients is already about half of normal during the first 24 hrs after injury (typically < 30 cc/100 g/min during the first 8 hours, and may be < 20 during the first 4 hours in patients with the worst injuries).[103,104,105,106] In one study, the use of HPV to PaCO$_2$ = 30 mm Hg within 8–14 hrs of severe head injury did not impair global cerebral metabolism,[99] but focal changes were not studied. Hyperventilation to PaCO$_2$ < 30 mm Hg further reduces CBF, but does not consistently reduce ICP and may cause loss of cerebral autoregulation.[47] If carefully monitored, there may be occasion to use this. There are no studies showing any improvement in outcome with aggressive HPV (PaCO$_2$ ≤ 25 mm Hg) which can cause diffuse cerebral ischemia.[47] A summary of the ranges of PaCO$_2$ and the recommendations is shown in ▶ Table 62.7.

Reducing PaCO$_2$ from 35 to 29 mm Hg lowers ICP 25–30% in most patients. Onset of action: ≤ 30 seconds. Peak effect at ≈ 8 mins. Duration of effect is occasionally as short as 15–20 mins. Effect may be blunted by 1 hour (based on patients with intracranial tumors), after which it is difficult to return to normocarbia without rebound elevation of ICP.[107,108] Thus, HPV must be weaned slowly.[32]

Table 62.7 Summary of recommendations for PaCO$_2$ following head trauma (see text for details)

PaCO$_2$ (mm Hg)	Description
35–40	**normocarbia**. Use routinely
30–35	**hyperventilation**. Do not use prophylactically. Use only as follows: briefly for clinical evidence of IC-HTN (neurologic deterioration) or chronically for documented IC-HTN unresponsive to other measures
25–30	**augmented hyperventilation**. A second tier treatment. Use only when other methods fail to control IC-HTN. Additional monitoring recommended to R/O cerebral ischemia
< 25	**aggressive hyperventilation**. No documented benefit. Significant potential for ischemia

Indications for hyperventilation (HPV)

1. HPV for brief periods (minutes) at the following times
   a) prior to insertion of ICP monitor: if there are clinical signs of IC-HTN (▶ Table 60.2)
   b) after insertion of a monitor: if there is a sudden increase in ICP and/or acute neurologic deterioration, HPV may be used while evaluating patient for a treatable condition (e.g., delayed intracranial hematoma)
2. HPV for longer periods: when there is documented IC-HTN unresponsive to sedation, paralytics, CSF drainage (when available), and osmotic diuretics
3. HPV may be appropriate for IC-HTN resulting primarily from hyperemia (p. 1084)

Caveats for hyperventilation

1. avoid during the first 5 days after head injury if possible (especially first 24 hrs)
2. do not use prophylactically (i.e., without appropriate indications, see above)
3. if documented IC-HTN is unresponsive to other measures, hyperventilate only to PaCO$_2$ = 30–35 mm Hg
4. if prolonged HPV to PaCO$_2$ of 25–30 mm Hg is deemed necessary, consider monitoring SjVO$_2$, AVdO$_2$, or CBF to rule out cerebral ischemia (p. 1045)
5. do not reduce PaCO$_2$ < 25 mm Hg (except for very brief periods of a few minutes)

Mannitol

Practice guideline: Mannitol in severe traumatic brain injury

Level II[109,110]: mannitol is effective for control of IC-HTN after severe TBI (**note**: current information did not allow recommendations regarding hypertonic saline to be made[110])
• intermittent boluses may be more effective than continuous infusion
• effective doses range from 0.25–1 gm/kg body weight
• avoid hypotension (SBP < 90 mm Hg) which may result from the diuretic effect of mannitol, which can lead to ↓ circulating fluid volume

Level III[109]:
- indications: signs of transtentorial herniation or progressive neurological deterioration not attributable to systemic pathology
- euvolemia should be maintained (hypovolemia should be avoided) by fluid replacement. An indwelling urinary catheter is essential
- serum osmolarity should be kept < 320 mOsm when there is concern about renal failure

No controlled clinical trial has been conducted to show the benefits of mannitol over placebo.[3] The exact mechanism(s) by which mannitol provides its beneficial effects is still controversial, but probably includes some combination of the following
1. lowering ICP
    a) immediate plasma expansion[111,112,113]: reduces the hematocrit and blood viscosity (improved rheology) which increases CBF and O_2 delivery. This reduces ICP within a few minutes, and is most marked in patients with CPP < 70 mm Hg
    b) osmotic effect: increased serum tonicity draws edema fluid from cerebral parenchyma. Takes 15–30 minutes until gradients are established.[111] Effect lasts 1.5–6 hrs, depending on the clinical condition[3,114,115]
2. supports the microcirculation by improving blood rheology (see above)
3. possible free radical scavenging[116]

With bolus administration, onset of ICP lowering effect occurs in 1–5 minutes; peaks at 20–60 minutes. When urgent reduction of ICP is needed, an initial dose of 1 gm/kg should be given over 30 minutes. When long-term reduction of ICP is intended, the infusion time should be lengthened to 60 minutes[117] and the dose reduced (e.g., 0.25–0.5 gm/kg q 6 hrs). A large previous dose reduces the effectiveness of subsequent doses[75]; thus it is desirable to *use the smallest effective dose* (small frequent doses may be preferable, e.g., 0.25 mg/kg q 2–3 hrs; also results in fewer peaks as mannitol "troughs" are smoothed out). Titrating to ICP (instead of dosing at regular intervals) results in less mannitol being given.[75,118] The effectiveness of mannitol may be synergistically enhanced when combined with the use of loop acting diuretics (e.g., furosemide, see below),[119] and alternating these medications has been suggested.[75]

Cautions with mannitol
1. mannitol opens the BBB, and mannitol that has crossed the BBB may draw fluid into the CNS (this may be minimized by repeated bolus administration vs. continuous infusion[112,120]) which can aggravate vasogenic cerebral edema.[121] Thus, when it is time to D/C mannitol, it should be tapered to prevent ICP rebound[117]
2. caution: corticosteroids + phenytoin + mannitol may cause hyperosmolar nonketotic state with high mortality[32]
3. excessively vigorous bolus administration may → HTN and if autoregulation is defective → increased CBF which may promote herniation rather than prevent it[122]
4. high doses of mannitol carries the risk of acute renal failure (acute tubular necrosis), especially in the following[11,123]: serum osmolarity > 320 mOsm/L, use of other potentially nephrotoxic drugs, sepsis, pre-existing renal disease
5. large doses prevents diagnosing DI by use of urinary osmols or SG (p. 126)
6. because it may further increase CBF,[124] the use of mannitol may be deleterious when IC-HTN is due to hyperemia (p. 1084)

Furosemide
The use of furosemide (Lasix®) has been advocated, but little data exists to support this.[3] Loop acting diuretics may reduce ICP[125] by reducing cerebral edema[126] (possibly by increasing serum tonicity) and may also slow the production of CSF.[127] They also act synergistically with mannitol[128] (above).

℞: 10–20 mg IV q 6 hrs, may be alternated with mannitol such that the patient receives one or the other q 3 hrs. Hold if serum osmolarity > 320 mOsm/L.

Hypertonic saline (HS)

May reduce ICP in patients refractory to mannitol,[129,130] although no improvement in outcome over mannitol has been demonstrated.[130,131] Potentially deleterious effect on stroke penumbra in animal studies. Studies[132,133] are not adequate to make recommendations regarding use.[110]

℞: Continuous infusion: 3% saline at 25–50 ml/hr may be given through a peripheral IV. Bolus: 10–20 ml of 7.5–23.4% saline must be given through a central line. HS should be discontinued after ≈ 72 hours to avoid rebound edema.[130] Hold if serum osmolarity > 320 mOsm/L.

Steroids

Practice guideline: Glucocorticoids in severe head injury

Level I[134]: the use of glucocorticoids (steroids) is not recommended for improving outcome or reducing ICP in patients with severe TBI (except in patients with known depletion of endogenous adrenal hormones[135,136]). High-dose methylprednisolone is associated with increased mortality and is contraindicated[134]

Although glucocorticoids reduce vasogenic cerebral edema (e.g., surrounding brain tumors) and may be effective in lowering ICP in pseudotumor cerebri, they have little effect on cytotoxic cerebral edema, which is the more prevalent derangement following trauma; see Cerebral edema (p. 90).

Significant side effects may occur with steroids,[137] including coagulopathies, hyperglycemia[138] with its undesirable effect on cerebral edema—see Possible deleterious side effects of steroids (p. 626)—and increased incidence of infection (due to immunosuppression). High-dose methylprednisolone is associated with increased mortality.[139]

Non-glucocorticoid steroids (e.g., 21-aminosteroids, AKA lazaroids, including tirilazad[140,141]) and the synthetic glucocorticoid triamcinolone[142] have also failed to show overall benefit.

High-dose barbiturate therapy

Practice guideline: Barbiturates in severe head injury

Level II[143]: ✖ prophylactic use of barbiturates for burst suppression EEG is not recommended

Level II[143]: high-dose barbiturates are recommended for IC-HTN refractory to maximal medical and surgical ICP-lowering therapy. Patients should be hemodynamically stable before and during treatment

Theoretical benefits of barbiturates in head injury derive from vasoconstriction in normal areas (shunting blood to ischemic brain tissue), decreased metabolic demand for O_2 (CMRO$_2$) with accompanying reduction of CBF, free radical scavenging, reduced intracellular calcium, and lysosomal stabilization.[144] There is little question that barbiturates lower ICP, even when other treatments have failed,[145] but regarding outcome, studies have shown both benefits[146,147] and lack of same.[148,149] A subgroup of patients with preserved vasoreactivity may benefit from the use of barbiturates[150]; and when reserved for use in patients who failed to respond sufficiently to other measures, barbiturates have been shown to lower ICP.[151] Patients that do respond have a lower mortality (33%) than those in whom ICP control could not be accomplished (75%).[147]

The limiting factor for therapy is usually *hypotension* due to barbiturate-induced reduction of sympathetic tone[152 (p 354)] (causing peripheral vasodilatation) and direct mild myocardial depression. Hypotension occurs in ≈ 50% of patients in spite of adequate blood volume and use of dopamine.[153]

NB: the ability to follow the neurologic exam is lost with high-dose barbiturates, and one must follow ICP.

"Barbiturate coma" vs. high-dose therapy: If barbiturates are given until there is burst suppression (p. 249) on EEG, this is considered true "barbiturate coma." This results in near maximal reductions in CMRO$_2$ and CBF.[3] However, most regimens should technically be called "high dose intravenous therapy" since they simply try to establish target serum barbiturate levels (e.g., 3–4 mg% for pentobarbital), even though there is poor correlation between serum level, therapeutic benefit, and systemic complications.[3]

Adjunctive measures to administration of high-dose barbiturates:
1. consider a Swan-Ganz (PA) catheter placed during the first hour of loading dose
2. high-dose barbiturates often causes paralytic ileus: therefore NG tube to suction & IV hyperalimentation are usually needed
3. continuous EEG monitor may be employed (a double "banana" EEG montage is often used to cover a wide area) and the drug is titrated to 2–5 bursts per minute (▶ Fig. 14.1)

Indications

The use of barbiturates should be reserved for situations where the ICP cannot be controlled by the previously outlined measures,[147] as there is evidence that *prophylactic* barbiturates do not favorably alter outcome, and are associated with significant side effects, mostly hypotension,[153] that can cause neurologic deterioration.

Choice of agents

A number of agents have been studied; however, there are inadequate data to recommend one drug over another. The most information is available on pentobarbital (see below). Alternative agents which have not been as well studied: thiopental (see below), phenobarbital (p. 493) & propofol (p. 1057).

Drug info: Pentobarbital (Nembutal®)

Pentobarbital has a fast onset (full effects within ≈ 15 minutes), short duration of action (3–4 hrs), and a half–life of 15–48 hrs.

The neuro exam cannot be assessed on pentobarbital. It is a myocardial suppressant, therefore watch for hypotension. GI motility is reduced or absent, some use trickle tube feeds during pentobarbital thrapy.

Protocols for pentobarbital therapy in adults

There are many protocols. A simple one from a randomized clinical trial[151]:
1. loading dose:
   a) pentobarbital 10 mg/kg IV over 30 minutes
   b) then 5 mg/kg q 1 hr × 3 doses
2. maintenance: 1 mg/kg/hr

A more elaborate protocol:
1. *loading dose*: pentobarbital 10 mg/kg/hr IV over 4 hrs as follows:
   a) *FIRST HOUR*: 2.5 mg/kg slow IVP q 15 min × 4 doses (total: 10 mg/kg in first hr), follow BP closely
   b) *next 3 hours*: 10 mg/kg/hr continuous infusion (put 2500 mg in 250 ml of appropriate IVF, run at **K** ml/hr × 3 hrs (**K** = patient's weight in kg))
2. maintenance: 1.5 mg/kg/hr infusion (put 250 mg in 250 ml IVF and run at 1.5 × **K** ml/hr)
3. check serum pentobarbital level 1 hr after loading dose completed; usually 3.5–5.0 mg%
4. check serum pentobarbital level q day thereafter
5. if level ever > 5 mg% and ICP acceptable, reduce dose
6. baseline brainstem auditory evoked response (BAER) early in treatment. May be omitted on clinical grounds. Repeat BAER if pentobarbital level ever > 6 mg%. Reduce dose if BAER deteriorates (NB: hemotympanum may interfere with BAER)
7. goal: ICP < 24 mm Hg and pentobarbital level 3–5 mg%. Consider discontinuing pentobarbital due to ineffectiveness if ICP still > 24 with adequate drug levels × 24 hrs
8. if ICP < 20 mm Hg, continue treatment × 48 hrs, then taper dose. Backtrack if ICP rises

Sample orders if continuous EEG monitoring is available:
1. pentobarb concentration: 3000/mg/600 ml NS
2. loading dose: 5–15 mg/kg over 1 hour
3. maintenance dose:
   a) 0.4–4 mg/kg/hour
   b) titrate up or down by 0.5–1 mg/kg/hour steps to maintain 2–5 bursts/minute (some use 4–12 bursts/minute)
   c) absolute maximum dose: 10 mg/kg/hr

Neuro function takes ≈ 2 days off pentobarbital to return (► Table 62.8). If it is desired to perform a brain death exam, the pentobarbital level needs to be ≈ ≤ 10 mcg/ml before the exam is valid.

Table 62.8 CNS effects of various pentobarbital levels[a]

Degree of CNS depression	mg%	mcg/ml
level for valid brain death exam	≤ 1	≤ 10
sedated, relaxed, easily aroused	0.05–0.3	0.5–3
heavy sedation, difficult to arouse, respiratory depression	2	20
"coma" level (burst suppression occurs in most patients)	5	50

[a]levels reported are for intolerant patients; there is significant variability between patients, and tolerant patients may not be sedated even at levels as high as 100 mcg/ml

Drug info: Thiopental (Pentothal®)

May be useful when a rapidly acting barbiturate is needed (e.g., intra-op) or when large doses of pentobarbital are not available. One of many protocols is as follows (note: thiopental has not been as well studied for this indication, but is theoretically similar to pentobarbital[154,155]):

1. loading dose: thiopental 5 mg/kg (range: 3–5) IV over 10 minutes → transient burst suppression (< 10 minutes) and blood thiopental levels of 10–30 mcg/ml. Higher doses (≈ 35 mg/kg) have been used in the absence of hypothermia to produce longer duration burst suppression for cardiopulmonary bypass
2. follow with continuous infusion of 5 mg/kg/hr (range: 3–5) for 24 hours
3. may need to rebolus with 2.5 mg/kg as needed for ICP control
4. after 24 hours, fat stores become saturated, reduce infusion to 2.5 mg/kg/hr
5. titrate to control ICP or use EEG to monitor for electrocerebral silence
6. "therapeutic" serum level: 6–8.5 mg/dl

Drug info: Propofol (Diprivan®)

Level II[143]: propofol may control ICP after several hours of dosing, but it does not improve mortality or 6 month outcome. ✖ Caution: high-dose propofol (total dose > 100 mg/kg for > 48 hrs) can cause significant morbidity (see propofol infusion syndrome).

℞: 0.5 mg/kg test dose, then 20–75 mcg/kg/min infusion. Increase by 5–10 mcg/kg/min q 5–10 minutes PRN ICP control (do not exceed 83 mcg/kg/min = 5 mg/kg/hr).

Side effects: include propofol infusion syndrome (p. 140). Use with caution at doses > 5 mg/kg/hr or at any dose for > 48 hrs.

References

[1] Sioutos PJ, Orozco JA, Carter LP, et al. Continuous Regional Cerebral Cortical Blood Flow Monitoring in Head-Injured Patients. Neurosurgery. 1995; 36:943–950

[2] Rosner MJ, Coley IB. Cerebral Perfusion Pressure, Intracranial Pressure, and Head Elevation. J Neurosurg. 1986; 65:636–641

[3] Bullock R, Chesnut RM, Clifton G, et al. Guidelines for the Management of Severe Head Injury. 1995

[4] Unterberg AW, Kienning KL, Hartl R, et al. Multimodal Monitoring in Patients with Head Injury: Evaluation of the Effects of Treatment on Cerebral Oxygenation. J Trauma. 1997; 42:S32–S37

[5] Carney N, Totten AM, O'Reilly C, et al. Guidelines for the Management of Severe Traumatic Brain Injury, Fourth Edition. Neurosurgery. 2017; 80:6–15

[6] Juul N, Morris GF, Marshall SB, et al. Intracranial Hypertension and Cerebral Perfusion Pressure: Influence on Neurological Deterioration and Outcome in Severe Head Injury. Journal of Neurosurgery. 2000; 92:1–6

[7] Yano M, Ikeda Y, Kobayashi S, et al. Intracranial Pressure in Head-Injured Patients with Various Intracranial Lesions is Identical Throughout the Supratentorial Intracranial Compartment. Neurosurgery. 1987; 21:688–692

[8] Takizawa H, Gabra-Sanders T, Miller JD. Analysis of Changes in Intracranial Pressure and Pressure-Volume Index at Different Locations in the

Craniospinal Axis During Supratentorial Epidural Balloon Inflation. Neurosurgery. 1986; 19:1–8

[9] Mokri B. The Monro-Kellie hypothesis: applications in CSF volume depletion. Neurology. 2001; 56:1746–1748

[10] Welch K. The Intracranial Pressure in Infants. Journal of Neurosurgery. 1980; 52:693–699

[11] Mendelow AD, Teasdale GM, Russell T, et al. Effect of Mannitol on Cerebral Blood Flow and Cerebral Perfusion Pressure in Human Head Injury. Journal of Neurosurgery. 1985; 63:43–48

[12] Bruce DA, Alavi A, Bilaniuk L, et al. Diffuse Cerebral Swelling Following Head Injuries in Children: The Syndrome of "Malignant Brain Edema". J Neurosurg. 1981; 54:170–178

[13] Unterberg A, Kiening K, Schmiedek P, et al. Long-Term Observations of Intracranial Pressure After Severe Head Injury. The Phenomenon of Secondary Rise of Intracranial Pressure. Neurosurgery. 1993; 32:17–24

[14] Young HA, Gleave JRW, Schmidek HH, et al. Delayed Traumatic Intracerebral Hematoma: Report of 15 Cases Operatively Treated. Neurosurgery. 1984; 14:22–25

[15] Taneda M, Kataoka K, Akai F, et al. Traumatic Subarachnoid Hemorrhage as a Predictable Indicator of Delayed Ischemic Symptoms. Journal of Neurosurgery. 1996; 84:762–768

[16] Narayan RK, Kishore PRS, Becker DP, et al. Intracranial Pressure: To Monitor or Not to Monitor? A Review of Our Experience with Severe Head Injury. Journal of Neurosurgery. 1982; 56:650–659

[17] The Brain Trauma Foundation. The American Association of Neurological Surgeons. The Joint Section on Neurotrauma and Critical Care. Indications for intracranial pressure monitoring. J Neurotrauma. 2000; 17:479–491

[18] Brain Trauma Foundation, Povlishock JT, Bullock MR. Indications for intracranial pressure monitoring. J Neurotrauma. 2007; 24:S37–S44

[19] Bullock R, Chesnut RM, Clifton G, et al. Indications for intracranial pressure monitoring. In: Guidelines for the Management of Severe Head Injury. The Brain Trauma Foundation (New York), The American Association of Neurological Surgeons (Park Ridge, Illinois), and The Joint Section of Neurotrauma and Critical Care; 1995

[20] Le TV, Rumbak MJ, Liu SS, et al. Insertion of intracranial pressure monitors in fulminant hepatic failure patients: early experience using recombinant factor VII. Neurosurgery. 2010; 66:455–8; discussion 458

[21] Smith RW, Alksine JF. Infections Complicating the Use of External Ventriculostomy. J Neurosurg. 1976; 44:567–570

[22] Holloway KL, Barnes T, Choi S, et al. Ventriculostomy Infections: The Effect of Monitoring Duration and Catheter Exchange in 584 Patients. Journal of Neurosurgery. 1996; 85:419–424

[23] Al-Shahi Salman R, Berg MJ, Morrison L, et al. Hemorrhage from cavernous malformations of the brain: definition and reporting standards. Angioma Alliance Scientific Advisory Board. Stroke. 2008; 39:3222–3230

[24] Paramore CG, Turner DA. Relative Risks of Ventriculostomy Infection and Morbidity. Acta Neurochirurgica. 1994; 127:79–84

[25] Maniker AH, Vaynman AY, Karimi RJ, et al. Hemorrhagic complications of external ventricular drainage. Operative Neurosurgery. 2006; 59:419–425

[26] Lozier AP, Sciacca RR, Romanoli M, et al. Ventriculostomy-related infection: a critical review of the literature. Neurosurgery. 2002; 51:170–182

[27] Brain Trauma Foundation, Povlishock JT, Bullock MR. Infection prophylaxis. J Neurotrauma. 2007; 24:S26–S31

[28] Mayhall CG, Archer NH, Lamb VA, et al. Ventriculostomy-related infections. A prospective epidemiologic study. New England Journal of Medicine. 1984; 310:553–559

[29] Lyke KE, Obasanjo OO, Williams MA, et al. Ventriculitis complicating use of intraventricular catheters in adult neurosurgical patients. Clinical Infectious Diseases. 2001; 33:2028–2033

[30] Winfield JA, Rosenthal P, Kanter R, et al. Duration of intracranial pressure monitoring does not predict daily risk of infectious complications. Neurosurgery. 1993; 33:424–431

[31] Brain Trauma Foundation, Povlishock JT, Bullock MR. Intracranial pressure monitoring technology. J Neurotrauma. 2007; 24:S45–S54

[32] Ropper AH. Raised Intracranial Pressure in Neurologic Disease. Sem Neurology. 1984; 4:397–407

[33] Sundbarg G, Nordstrom C-H, Messetter K, et al. A Comparison of Intraparenchymatous and Intraventricular Pressure Recording in Clinical Practice. J Neurosurg. 1987; 67:841–845

[34] Crutchfield JS, Narayan RK, Robertson CS, et al. Evaluation of a Fiberoptic Intracranial Pressure Monitor. Journal of Neurosurgery. 1990; 72:482–487

[35] Ostrup RC, Luerssen TG, Marshall LF, et al. Continuous Monitoring of Intracranial Pressure with a Miniaturized Fiberoptic Device. Journal of Neurosurgery. 1987; 67:206–209

[36] Piek J, Bock WJ. Continuous Monitoring of Cerebral Tissue Pressure in Neurosurgical Practice - Experience with 100 Patients. Intens Care Med. 1990; 16:184–188

[37] Gopinath SP, Robertson CS, Contant CF, et al. Clinical Evaluation of a Miniature Strain-Gauge Transducer for Monitoring Intracranial Pressure. Neurosurgery. 1995; 36:1137–1141

[38] Salmon JH, Hajjar W, Bada HS. The Fontogram: A Noninvasive Intracranial Pressure Monitor. Pediatrics. 1977; 60:721–725

[39] Grabb PA. Traumatic intraventricular hemorrhage treated with intraventricular recombinant-tissue plasminogen activator: technical case report. Neurosurgery. 1998; 43:966–969

[40] Hamer J, Alberti E, Hoyer S, et al. Factors Influencing CSF Pulse Waves. J Neurosurg. 1977; 46:36–45

[41] Lundberg N. Continuous Recording and Control of Ventricular Fluid Pressure in Neurosurgical Practice. Acta Psych Neurol Scand. 1960; 36S:1–193

[42] Cruz J. On-Line Monitoring of Global Cerebral Hypoxia in Acute Brain Injury. Relationship to Intracranial Hypertension. Journal of Neurosurgery. 1993; 79:228–233

[43] Sheinberg M, Kanter MJ, Robertson CS, et al. Continuous Monitoring of Jugular Venous Oxygen Saturation in Head-Injured Patients. Journal of Neurosurgery. 1992; 76:212–217

[44] Cormio M, Valadka AB, Robertson CS. Elevated jugular venous oxygen saturation after severe head injury. J Neurosurg. 1999; 90:9–15

[45] Robertson CS, Narayan RK, Gokaslan ZL, et al. Cerebral Arteriovenous Oxygen Difference as an Estimate of Cerebral Blood Flow in Comatose Patients. Journal of Neurosurgery. 1989; 70:222–230

[46] Gotoh F, Meyer JS, Takagi Y. Cerebral Effects of Hyperventilation in Man. Archives of Neurology. 1965; 12:410–423

[47] Obrist WD, Langfitt TW, Jaggi JL, et al. Cerebral Blood Flow and Metabolism in Comatose Patients with Acute Head Injury. Relationship to Intracranial Hypertension. Journal of Neurosurgery. 1984; 61:241–253

[48] Pickard JD, Czosnyka M. Management of Raised Intracranial Pressure. Journal of Neurology, Neurosurgery, and Psychiatry. 1993; 56:845–858

[49] Valadka AB, Gopinath SP, Contant CF, et al. Relationship of brain tissue PO2 to outcome after severe head injury. Crit Care Med. 1998; 26:1576–1581

[50] van den Brink WA, van Santbrink H, Steyerberg EW, et al. Brain oxygen tension in severe head injury. Neurosurgery. 2000; 46:868–76; discussion 876-8

[51] Stiefel MF, Spiotta A, Gracias VH, et al. Reduced mortality rate in patients with severe traumatic brain injury treated with brain tissue oxygen monitoring. Journal of Neurosurgery. 2005; 103:805–811

[52] Jaeger M, Schuhmann MU, Soehle M, et al. Continuous monitoring of cerebrovascular autoregulation after subarachnoid hemorrhage by brain tissue oxygen pressure reactivity and its relation to delayed cerebral infarction. Stroke. 2007; 38:981–986

[53] Jaeger M, Soehle M, Schuhmann MU, et al. Correlation of continuously monitored regional cerebral blood flow and brain tissue oxygen. Acta Neurochirurgica (Wien). 2005; 147:51–6; discussion 56

[54] Goodman JC, Valadka AB, Gopinath SP, et al. Extracellular lactate and glucose alterations in the brain after head injury measured by microdialysis. Critical Care Medicine. 1999; 27:1965–1973

[55] Vespa PM, McArthur D, O'Phelan K, et al. Persistently low extracellular glucose correlates with poor outcome 6 months after human traumatic brain injury despite a lack of increased lactate: a microdialysis study. Journal of Cerebral Blood Flow and Metabolism. 2003; 23:865–877

[56] Bullock R, Chesnut RM, Clifton G, et al. Guidelines for the Management of Severe Head Injury. J Neurotrauma. 1996; 13:639–734

[57] Bullock R, Chesnut R, Ghajar J, et al. Guidelines for the management of severe traumatic brain injury. Journal of Neurotrauma. 2000; 17:449–454

[58] Brain Trauma Foundation, Povlishock JT, Bullock MR. Blood pressure and oxygenation. J Neurotrauma. 2007; 24:S7–13

[59] Marshall LF, Barba D, Toole BM, et al. The oval pupil: clinical significance and relationship to intracranial hypertension. J Neurosurg. 1983; 58:566–568

[60] Brain Trauma Foundation. Guidelines for the management of severe traumatic brain injury. 2016. https://braintrauma.org/uploads/03/12/Guidelines_for_Management_of_Severe_TBI_4th_Edition.pdf

[61] Saul TG, Ducker TB. Effect of Intracranial Pressure Monitoring and and Aggressive Treatment on Mortality in Severe Head Injury. J Neurosurg. 1982; 56:498–503

[62] Brain Trauma Foundation, Povlishock JT, Bullock MR. Intracranial pressure thresholds. J Neurotrauma. 2007; 24:S55–S58

[63] Brain Trauma Foundation, Povlishock JT, Bullock MR. Cerebral perfusion thresholds. J Neurotrauma. 2007; 24:S59–S64

[64] Brain Trauma Foundation, Povlishock JT, Bullock MR. Brain oxygen monitoring and thresholds. J Neurotrauma. 2007; 24:S65–S70

[65] Blackman JA, Patrick PD, Buck ML, et al. Paroxysmal autonomic instability with dystonia after brain injury. Arch Neurol. 2004; 61:321–328

[66] Baguley IJ, Perkes IE, Fernandez-Ortega J F, et al. Paroxysmal sympathetic hyperactivity after acquired brain injury: consensus on conceptual definition, nomenclature, and diagnostic criteria. J Neurotrauma. 2014; 31:1515–1520

[67] Bouma GJ, Muizelaar JP. Relationship between Cardiac Output and Cerebral Blood Flow in Patients with Intact and Impaired Autoregulation. Journal of Neurosurgery. 1990; 73:368–374

[68] The Brain Trauma Foundation. The American Association of Neurological Surgeons. The Joint Section on Neurotrauma and Critical Care. Hypotension. J Neurotrauma. 2000; 17:591–595

[69] Larson DE, Farnell MB. Upper Gastrointestinal Hemorrhage. Mayo Clin Proc. 1983; 58:371–387

[70] Grosfeld JL, Shipley F, Fitzgerald JF, et al. Acute Peptic Ulcer in Infancy and Childhood. Am Surgeon. 1978; 44:13–19

[71] Curci MR, Little K, Sieber WK, et al. Peptic Ulcer Disease in Childhood Reexamined. J Ped Surg. 1976; 11:329–335

[72] Krasna IH, Schneider KM, Becker JM. Surgical Management of Stress Ulcerations in Childhood. J Ped Surg. 1971; 6:301–306

[73] Chan K-H, Lai ECS, Tuen H, et al. Prospective Double-Blind Placebo-Controlled Randomized Trial on the Use of Ranitidine in Preventing Postoperative Gastroduodenal Complications in High-Risk Neurosurgical Patients. Journal of Neurosurgery. 1995; 82:413–417

[74] Shackford SR, Zhuang J, Schmoker J. Intravenous Fluid Tonicity: Effect on Intracranial Pressure, Cerebral Blood Flow, and Cerebral Oxygen Delivery in Focal Brain Injury. J Neurosurg. 1992; 76:91–98

[75] Garretson HD, McGraw CP, O'Connor C, et al. Effectiveness of Fluid Restriction, Mannitol and Furosemide in Reducing ICP. In: Intracranial Pressure V. Berlin: Springer-Verlag; 1983:742–745

[76] Ward JD, Moulton RJ, Muizelaar PJ, et al. Cerebral Homeostasis. In: Neurosurgical Critical Care. Baltimore: Williams and Wilkins; 1987:187–213

[77] De Salles AAF, Muizelaar JP, Young HF. Hyperglycemia, Cerebrospinal Fluid Lactic Acidosis, and Cerebral Blood Flow in Severely Head-injured Patients. Neurosurgery. 1987; 21:45–50

[78] Kaufman HH, Bretaudiere J-P, Rowlands BJ, et al. General Metabolism in Head Injury. Neurosurgery. 1987; 20:254–265

[79] Brain Trauma Foundation, Povlishock JT, Bullock MR. Prophylactic hypothermia. J Neurotrauma. 2007; 24:S21–S25

[80] Cao M, Lisheng H, Shouzheng S. Resolution of Brain Edema in Severe Brain Injury at Controlled High and Low ICPs. J Neurosurg. 1984; 61:707–712

[81] Metz C, Holzschuh M, Bein T, et al. Moderate Hypothermia in Patients with Severe Head Injury: Cerebral and Extracerebral Effects. Journal of Neurosurgery. 1996; 85:533–541

[82] Hypothermia after Cardiac Arrest Study Group. Mild therapeutic hypothermia to improve the neurologic outcome after cardiac arrest. New England Journal of Medicine. 2002; 346:549–556

[83] Polin RS, Shaffrey ME, Bogaev CA, et al. Decompressive Bifrontal Craniectomy in the Treatment of Severe Refractory Posttraumatic Cerebral Edema. Neurosurgery. 1997; 41:84–94

[84] Cooper PR, Hagler H, Clark W, et al. Intracranial Pressure IV. New York: Springer Verlag; 1980:277–279

[85] Cepeda S, Castano-Leon AM, Munarriz PM, et al. Effect of decompressive craniectomy in the postoperative expansion of traumatic intracerebral hemorrhage: a propensity score-based analysis. J Neurosurg. 2019:1–13

[86] Aarabi B, Hesdorffer DC, Ahn ES, et al. Outcome following decompressive craniectomy for malignant swelling due to severe head injury. J Neurosurg. 2006; 104:469–479

[87] Timofeev I, Kirkpatrick PJ, Corteen E, et al. Decompressive craniectomy in traumatic brain injury: outcome following protocol-driven therapy. Acta Neurochir Suppl. 2006; 96:11–16

[88] Hutchinson PJ, Kolias AG, Timofeev IS, et al. Trial of Decompressive Craniectomy for Traumatic Intracranial Hypertension. N Engl J Med. 2016; 375:1119–1130

[89] Holland M, Nakaji P. Craniectomy: Surgical indications and technique. Operative Techniques in Neurosurgery. 2004; 7:10–15

[90] Nussbaum ES, Wolf AL, Sebring L, et al. Complete Temporal Lobectomy for Surgical Resuscitation of Patients with Transtentorial Herniation Secondary to Unilateral Hemispheric Swelling. Neurosurgery. 1991; 29:62–66

[91] Hamill JF, Bedford RF, Weaver DC, et al. Lidocaine before Endotracheal Intubation: Intravenous or Laryngotracheal? Anesthesiology. 1981; 55:578–581

[92] Hurst JM, Saul TG, DeHaven CB, et al. Use of High Frequency Jet Ventilation during Mechanical Hyperventilation to Reduce ICP in Patients with Multiple Organ System Injury. Neurosurgery. 1984; 15:530–534

[93] Cooper KR, Boswell PA, Choi SC. Safe Use of PEEP in Patients with Severe Head Injury. J Neurosurg. 1985; 63:552–555

[94] Feldman Z, Kanter MJ, Robertson CS, et al. Effect of Head Elevation on Intracranial Pressure, Cerebral Perfusion Pressure, and Cerebral Blood Flow in

Head-Injured Patients. J Neurosurg. 1992; 76:207–211

[95] Raichle ME, Plum F. Hyperventilation and cerebral blood flow. Stroke. 1972; 3:566–575

[96] Grubb RL, Raichle ME, Eichling JO, et al. The Effects of Changes in PaCO2 on Cerebral Blood Volume, Blood Flow, and Vascular Mean Transit Time. Stroke. 1974; 5:630–639

[97] Darby JM, Yonas H, Marion DW, et al. Local 'Inverse Steal' Induced by Hyperventilation in Head Injury. Neurosurgery. 1988; 23:84–88

[98] Fleischer AS, Patton JM, Tindall GT. Monitoring Intraventricular Pressure Using an Implanted Reservoir in Head Injured Patients. Surg Neurol. 1975; 3:309–311

[99] Diringer MN, Yundt K, Videen TO, et al. No Reduction in Cerebral Metabolism as a Result of Early Moderate Hyperventilation Following Severe Traumatic Brain Injury. Journal of Neurosurgery. 2000; 92:7–13

[100] Bullock R, Chesnut RM, Clifton G, et al. The use of hyperventilation in the acute management of severe traumatic brain injury. In: Guidelines for the Management of Severe Head Injury.The Brain Trauma Foundation (New York), The American Association of Neurological Surgeons (Park Ridge, Illinois), and The Joint Section of Neurotrauma and Critical Care; 1995

[101] Brain Trauma Foundation, Povlishock JT, Bullock MR. Hyperventilation. J Neurotrauma. 2007; 24: S87–S90

[102] Muizelaar JP, Marmarou A, Ward JD, et al. Adverse Effects of Prolonged Hyperventilation in Patients with Severe Head Injury: A Randomized Clinical Trial. Journal of Neurosurgery. 1991; 75:731–739

[103] Bouma GJ, Muizelaar JP, Choi SC, et al. Cerebral Circulation and Metabolism After Severe Traumatic Brain Injury: The Elusive Role of Ischemia. Journal of Neurosurgery. 1991; 75:685–693

[104] Bouma GJ, Muizelaar JP, Stringer WA, et al. Ultra Early Evaluation of Regional Cerebral Blood Flow in Severely Head Injured Patients using Xenon Enhanced Computed Tomography. Journal of Neurosurgery. 1992; 77:360–368

[105] Fieschi C, Battistini N, Beduschi A, et al. Regional Cerebral Blood Flow and Intraventricular Pressure in Acute Head Injuries. Journal of Neurology, Neurosurgery, and Psychiatry. 1974; 37:1378–1388

[106] Schroder ML, Muizelaar JP, Kuta AJ. Documented Reversal of Global Ischemia Immediately After Removal of an Acute Subdural Hematoma. Neurosurgery. 1994; 80:324–327

[107] James H, Langfitt T, Kumar V, et al. Treatment of Intracranial Hypertension; Analysis of 105 Consecutive Continuous Recordings of ICP. Acta Neurochirurgica. 1977; 36:189–200

[108] Lundberg N, Kjallquist A. A Reduction of Increased ICP by Hyperventilation, a Therapeutic Aid in Neurological Surgery. Acta Psych Neurol Scand (Suppl). 1958; 139:1–64

[109] Bullock R, Chesnut RM, Clifton G, et al. The use of mannitol in severe head injury. In: Guidelines for the Management of Severe Head Injury.The Brain Trauma Foundation (New York), The American Association of Neurological Surgeons (Park Ridge, Illinois), and The Joint Section of Neurotrauma and Critical Care; 1995

[110] Brain Trauma Foundation, Povlishock JT, Bullock MR. Hyperosmolar therapy. J Neurotrauma. 2007; 24:S14–S20

[111] Barry KG, Berman AR. Mannitol Infusion. Part III. The Acute Effect of the Intravenous Infusion of Mannitol on Blood and Plasma Volume. New England Journal of Medicine. 1961; 264:1085–1088

[112] James HE. Methodology for the Control of Intracranial Pressure with Hypertonic Mannitol. Acta Neurochirurgica. 1980; 51:161–172

[113] McGraw CP, Howard G. The Effect of Mannitol on Increased Intracranial Pressure. Neurosurgery. 1983; 13:269–271

[114] Cruz J, Miner ME, Allen SJ, et al. Continuous Monitoring of Cerebral Oxygenation in Acute Brain Injury: Injection of Mannitol During Hyperventilation. Journal of Neurosurgery. 1990; 73:725–730

[115] Marshall LF, Smith RW, Rauscher LA, et al. Mannitol Dose Requirements in Brain-Injured Patients. Journal of Neurosurgery. 1978; 48:169–172

[116] Takagi H, Saito T, Kitahara T, et al. The Mechanism of the ICP Reducing Effect of Mannitol. In: ICP V. Berlin: Springer-Verlag; 1993:729–733

[117] Node Y, Yajima K, Nakazawa S, et al. A Study of Mannitol and Glycerol on the Reduction of Raised Intracranial Pressure on Their Rebound Phenomenon. In: Intracranial Pressure V. Berlin: Springer-Verlag; 1983:738–741

[118] Smith HP, Kelly DL, McWhorter JM. Comparison of Mannitol Regimens in Patients with Severe Head Injury Undergoing Intracranial Monitoring. Journal of Neurosurgery. 1986; 65:820–824

[119] Pollay M, Roberts PA, Fullenwider C, et al. The Effect of Mannitol and Furosemide on the Blood-Brain Osmotic Gradient and Intracranial Pressure. In: Intracranial Pressure V. Berlin: Springer-Verlag; 1983:734–736

[120] Cold GE. Cerebral Blood Flow in Acute Head Injury: The Regulation of Cerebral Blood Flow and Metabolism During the Acute Phase of Head Injury, and Its Significance for Therapy. Acta Neurochirurgica. 1990; Suppl 49:1–64

[121] Kaufmann AM, Cardoso ER. Aggravation of Vasogenic Cerebral Edema by Multiple Dose Mannitol. Journal of Neurosurgery. 1992; 77:584–589

[122] Ravussin P, Abou-Madi M, Archer D, et al. Changes in CSF Pressure After Mannitol in Patients With and Without Elevated CSF Pressure. Journal of Neurosurgery. 1988; 69:869–876

[123] Feig PU, McCurdy DK. The Hypertonic State. New England Journal of Medicine. 1977; 297:1444–1454

[124] Muizelaar JP, Lutz HA, Becker DP. Effect of Mannitol on ICP and CBF and Correlation with Pressure Autoregulation in Severely Head-Injured Patients. J Neurosurg. 1984; 61:700–706

[125] Cottrell JE, Robustelli A, Post K, et al. Furosemide-and Mannitol-Induced Changes in Intracranial Pressure and Serum Osmolality and Electrolytes. Anesthesiology. 1977; 47:28–30

[126] Tornheim PA, McLaurin RL, Sawaya R. Effect of Furosemide on Experimental Cerebral Edema. Neurosurgery. 1979; 4:48–52

[127] Buhrley LE, Reed DJ. The Effect of Furosemide on Sodium-22 Uptake into Cerebrospinal Fluid and Brain. Exp Brain Res. 1972; 14:503–510

[128] Marion DW, Letarte PB. Management of Intracranial Hypertension. Contemporary Neurosurgery. 1997; 19:1–6

[129] Doyle JA, Davis DP, Hoyt DB. The use of hypertonic saline in the treatment of traumatic brain injury. J Trauma. 2001; 50:367–383

[130] Ogden AT, Mayer SA, Connolly ES. Hyperosmolar agents in neurosurgical practice: The evolving role of hypertonic saline. Neurosurgery. 2005; 57:207–215

[131] Vialet R, Albanese J, Thomachot L, et al. Isovolume hypertonic solutes (sodium chloride or mannitol) in the treatment of refractory posttraumatic intracranial hypertension: 2 mL/kg 7.5% saline is more effective than 2 mL/kg 20% mannitol. Crit Care Med. 2003; 31:1683–1687

[132] Shackford SR, Bourguignon PR, Wald SL, et al. Hypertonic saline resuscitation of patients with head injury: a prospective, randomized clinical trial. J Trauma. 1998; 44:50–58

[133] Qureshi AI, Suarez JI, Castro A, et al. Use of hypertonic saline/acetate infusion in treatment of cerebral edema in patients with head trauma: experience at a single center. J Trauma. 1999; 47:659–665

[134] Brain Trauma Foundation, Povlishock JT, Bullock MR. Steroids. J Neurotrauma. 2007; 24:S91–S95

[135] Bullock R, Chesnut RM, Clifton G, et al. The role of glucocorticoids in the treatment of severe head injury. In: Guidelines for the Management of Severe Head Injury.The Brain Trauma Foundation

(New York), The American Association of Neurological Surgeons (Park Ridge, Illinois), and The Joint Section of Neurotrauma and Critical Care; 1995

[136] The Brain Trauma Foundation. The American Association of Neurological Surgeons. The Joint Section on Neurotrauma and Critical Care. Role of steroids. J Neurotrauma. 2000; 17:531–535

[137] Braughler JM, Hall ED. Current Application of "High-Dose" Steroid Therapy for CNS Injury: A Pharmacological Perspective. J Neurosurg. 1985; 62:806–810

[138] Lam AM, Winn HR, Cullen BF, et al. Hyperglycemia and Neurologic Outcome in Patients with Head Injury. J Neurosurg. 1991; 75:545–551

[139] Roberts I, Yates D, Sandercock P, et al. Effects of intravenous corticosteroids on death within 14 days in 10,008 adults with clinically significant head injury (MRC CRASH trial): randomized placebo controlled trial. Lancet. 2004; 364

[140] Doppenberg EMR, Bullock R. Clinical neuroprotection trials in severe traumatic brain injury: lessons from previous studies. Journal of Neurotrauma. 1997; 14:71–80

[141] Marshall LF, Maas AL, Marshall SB, et al. A multicenter trial on the efficacy of using tirilazad mesylate in cases of head injury. Journal of Neurosurgery. 1998; 89:519–525

[142] Grumme T, Baethmann A, Kolodziejczyk D, et al. Treatment of patients with severe head injury by triamcinolone: a prospective, controlled multicenter clinical trial of 396 cases. Research in Experimental Medicine. 1995; 195:217–229

[143] Brain Trauma Foundation, Povlishock JT, Bullock MR. Anesthetics, analgesics, and sedatives. J Neurotrauma. 2007; 24:S71–S76

[144] Lyons MK, Meyer FB. Cerebrospinal Fluid Physiology and the Management of Increased Intracranial Pressure. Mayo Clin Proc. 1990; 65:684–707

[145] Shapiro HM, Wyte SR, Loeser J. Barbiturate Augmented Hypothermia for Reduction of Persistent Intracranial Hypertension. Journal of Neurosurgery. 1979; 40:90–100

[146] Marshall LF, Smith RW, Shapiro HM. The Outcome with Aggressive Treatment in Severe Head Injuries. Part II: Acute and Chronic Barbiturate Administration in the Management of Head Injury. J Neurosurg. 1979; 50:26–30

[147] Rea GL, Rockswold GL. Barbiturate Therapy in Uncontrolled Intracranial Hypertension. Neurosurgery. 1983; 12:401–404

[148] Ward JD, Becker DP, Miller JD, et al. Failure of Prophylactic Barbiturate Coma in the Treatment of Severe Head Injury. J Neurosurg. 1985; 62:383–388

[149] Schwartz M, Tator C, Towed D, et al. The University of Toronto Head Injury Treatment Study: A Prospective Randomized Comparison of Pentobarbital and Mannitol. Can J Neurol Sci. 1984; 11:434–440

[150] Nordstrom C-H, Messeter K, Sundbarg G, et al. Cerebral Blood Flow, Vasoreactivity, and Oxygen Consumption During Barbiturate Therapy in Severe Traumatic Brain Lesions. J Neurosurg. 1988; 68:424–431

[151] Eisenberg HM, Frankowski RF, Contant CF, et al. High-Dose Barbiturate Control of Elevated Intracranial Pressure in Patients with Severe Head Injury. J Neurosurg. 1988; 69:15–23

[152] Gilman AG, Goodman LS, Gilman A. Goodman and Gilman's The Pharmacological Basis of Therapeutics. New York 1980

[153] Ward JD, Becker DP, Miller JD, et al. Failure of Prophylactic Barbiturate Coma in the Treatment of Severe Head Injury. J Neurosurg. 1985; 62:383–388

[154] Boarini DJ, Kassell NF, Coester HC. Comparison of Sodium Thiopental and Methohexital for High-Dose Barbiturate Anesthesia. J Neurosurg. 1984; 60:602–608

[155] Spetzler RF, Martin N, Hadley MN, et al. Microsurgical Endarterectomy Under Barbiturate Protection: A Prospective Study. J Neurosurg. 1986; 65:63–73

62

63 Skull Fractures

63.1 Types of skull fractures

Classified as either closed (simple fracture) or open (compound fracture).

Diastatic fractures extend into and separate sutures. More common in young children.[1]

63.2 Linear skull fractures over the convexity

90% of pediatric skull fractures are linear and involve the calvaria.

▶ Table 63.1 shows some differentiating features to distinguish linear skull fractures from vessel grooves and skull suture lines.

By themselves, linear skull fractures over the convexity rarely require surgical intervention.

Table 63.1 Differentiating linear skull fractures from normal *plain* film findings

Feature	Linear skull fracture	Vessel groove	Suture line
density	dark black	gray	gray
course	straight	curving	follows course of known suture lines
branching	usually none	often branching	joins other suture lines
width	very thin	thicker than fracture	jagged, wide

63.3 Depressed skull fractures

For special considerations in pediatrics, see Depressed skull fractures (p. 1101) in pediatrics section.

63.3.1 Indications for surgery

See **Practice guideline: Surgical management of depressed skull fractures** (p. 1062). Some additional observations regarding surgery to elevate a depressed skull fracture in an adult:
1. consider surgery for depressed skull fractures with deficit referable to underlying brain
2. ✖ more conservative treatment is recommended for fractures overlying a major dural venous sinus (**note:** exception: depressed fractures overlying and depressing one of the dural sinuses may be dangerous to elevate, and if the patient is neurologically intact, and no indication for operation (e.g., CSF leak mandates surgery) may be best managed conservatively).

Practice guideline: Surgical management of depressed skull fractures

Indications for surgery
Level III[2]:
1. open (compound) fractures
   a) surgery for fractures depressed > thickness of calvaria and those not meeting criteria for non-surgical management listed below
   b) nonsurgical management may be considered if
      • there is no evidence (clinical or CT) of dural penetration (CSF leak, intradural pneumocephalus on CT...)
      • and no significant intracranial hematoma
      • and depression is < 1 cm
      • and no frontal sinus involvement
      • and no wound infection or gross contamination
      • and no gross cosmetic deformity
2. closed (simple) depressed fractures: may be managed surgically or nonsurgically

Timing of surgery
Level III[2]: early surgery to reduce risk of infection

Surgical methods
Level III[2]:
1. elevation and debridement are recommended
2. option: if there is no evidence of wound infection, primary bone replacement
3. antibiotics should be used for all compound depressed fractures

There is no evidence that elevating a depressed skull fracture will reduce the subsequent development of posttraumatic seizures,[3] which are probably more related to the initial brain injury.

63.3.2 Surgical treatment for depressed skull fractures

General information

Booking the case: Craniotomy: for depressed skull fracture

Also see defaults & disclaimers (p. 25).
1. position: (depends on location of the fracture)
2. post-op: ICU
3. blood: type & screen (for severe fractures: type and cross 2 U PRBC)
4. consent (in lay terms for the patient—not all-inclusive):
   a) procedure: surgery in the area of the skull fracture to bone fragments that may have been displaced, to repair the covering of the brain, to remove any foreign material that can be identified and any permanently damaged brain tissue (i.e., dead brain tissue), remove any blood clot and stop any bleeding identified, possible placement of intracranial pressure monitor. If a large opening has to be left in the skull, it may require surgery to correct in a number of months (3 or more)
   b) alternatives: nonsurgical management
   c) complications: usual craniotomy complications (p. 25), plus any permanent brain injury that has already occurred is not likely to recover, seizures may occur (with or without the surgery), hydrocephalus, infection (including delayed infection/abscess)

Technical considerations of surgery

Surgical goals
See reference,[4] modified.
1. debridement of skin edges
2. elevation of bone fragments
3. repair of dural laceration
4. debridement of devitalized brain
5. reconstruction of the skull
6. skin closure

Techniques
1. with open (compound) contaminated fractures, it may be necessary to excise depressed bone. In these cases or when air sinuses are involved, to minimize the risk of infecting the flap, some surgeons follow the patient for 6–12 months to rule out infection before performing a cosmetic cranioplasty. There has been no documented increase in infection with replacement of bone fragments; soaking the fragments in povidone-iodine has been recommended[4]
2. elevating the bone may be facilitated by drilling burr holes around the periphery and either using rongeurs or craniotome to excise the depressed portion
3. in cases where laceration of a major dural sinus is suspected and surgery is mandated, adequate preparation must be made for dural sinus repair[5]; NB: the SSS is often to the right of the sagittal suture (p. 61)
   a) prepare for massive blood loss

b) have small Fogarty catheter ready to temporarily occlude sinus
c) have dural shunt ready (Kapp-Gielchinsky shunt, if available, has an inflatable balloon at both ends)
d) prep out saphenous vein area for vein graft
e) bone fragments that may have lacerated sinus should be removed last

63.4 Basal skull fractures

63.4.1 General information

Most basal (AKA basilar) skull fractures (BSF) are extensions of fractures through the cranial vault.

Severe basilar skull fractures may produce shearing injuries to the pituitary gland.

BSF, especially those involving the clivus, may be associated with traumatic aneurysms. This rarely occurs in pediatrics.[6]

63.4.2 Some specific basal skull fracture types

Temporal bone fractures

General information

The major concerns with temporal bone fractures are: hearing loss, facial nerve injury and CSF leak. Temporal bone fractures were traditionally categorized into two basic types (or a mixture of the two) (this system originated with cadaveric studies[7]):

- **longitudinal fracture**: more common (70–90%). Usually results from a lateral blow to the head.[8] Typically passes through the petro-squamosal suture, parallel to and through EAC. Often but not always passing anterior to the inner ear structures and also sparing the VII and VIII nerves. It may cause a conductive hearing loss by disrupting the ossicular chain and and/or by producing hemotympanum. Can often be diagnosed on otoscopic inspection of the EAC
- **transverse fracture**: perpendicular to EAC. Commonly associated with a blow to the back of the head.[8] Extends from the jugular foramen through the petrous pyramid to the foramen spinosum and foramen lacerum, often passing through the cochlea and may place stretch on the geniculate ganglion, resulting in deficits of the VIII nerve and VII, respectively, with sensorineural hearing loss in 50%[8]

▶ **Alternative classification.** The traditional classification above correlates poorly with clinically relevant issues of hearing loss, facial nerve injury and CSF leak.[9] It is now favored to classify temporal bone fractures based on CT scan assessment of involvement of the **otic capsule** (containing the cochlea, vestibule and semicircular canals (SCC))[10]:

- **otic-capsule sparing** (OCS)
- **otic-capsule violating** (OCV)

Posttraumatic facial palsy
General information

Posttraumatic unilateral peripheral facial nerve palsy occurs in 15-20% of longitudinal petrous bone fractures, and in 50% of transverse fractures.[8]

Management of posttraumatic facial palsy

Management is often complicated by multiplicity of injuries (including head injury requiring endotracheal intubation) making it difficult to determine the time of onset of facial palsy. Guidelines:

1. regardless of time of onset:
   a) steroids (glucocorticoids) are often utilized (efficacy unproven[8])
   b) consultation with ENT physician is usually indicated
2. immediate onset of unilateral peripheral facial palsy (i.e., within a few hours of injury): facial EMG (AKA electroneuronography[11] or ENOG) takes at least 72 hrs to become abnormal (∴ generally performed no earlier than 2-3 days, and no later than 2-3 weeks).[8] These cases are often followed and are possible candidates for surgical VII nerve decompression if no improvement occurs with steroids (timing of surgery is controversial, but is usually not done emergently)
3. delayed onset of unilateral peripheral facial palsy (may be days to weeks): follow serial ENOGs, if continued nerve deterioration occurs while on steroids, and activity on ENOG drops to less than 10% of the contralateral side, surgical decompression may be considered (controversial, thought to improve recovery from ≈ 40% to ≈ 75% of cases)

Posttraumatic hearing loss

Can be conductive or sensorineural (see above). See section 61.3 for causes of posttraumatic hearing loss other than temporal bone fractures.

Clival fractures

See reference.[12]

3 categories (75% are longitudinal or transverse):
1. longitudinal: may be associated with injuries of vertebrobasilar vessels, including:
   a) dissection or occlusion: may cause brainstem infarction
   b) traumatic aneurysms
2. transverse: may be associated with injuries to the anterior circulation
3. oblique

Clival fractures are highly lethal. May be associated with:
1. cranial nerve deficits: especially III through VI; bitemporal hemianopsia
2. CSF leak
3. diabetes insipidus
4. delayed development of traumatic aneurysms[13]

Occipital condyle fractures

These are considered in the section on Spine fractures (p. 1156).

63.4.3 Radiographic diagnosis

BSF appear as linear lucencies through the skull base.

CT scan with multiplanar projections is the most sensitive means for directly demonstrating BSF. Plain skull X-rays and clinical criteria (see below) may also be able to make the diagnosis.

Indirect radiographic findings (on CT or plain films) that suggest BSF include: pneumocephalus (diagnostic of BSF in the absence of an open fracture of the cranial vault), air/fluid level within or opacification of air sinus with fluid (suggestive).

63.4.4 Clinical diagnosis

Some of these signs may take several hours to develop. Signs include:
1. CSF otorrhea or rhinorrhea
2. hemotympanum or laceration of external auditory canal
3. postauricular ecchymoses (Battle's sign)
4. periorbital ecchymoses (raccoon's eyes) in the absence of direct orbital trauma, especially if bilateral
5. cranial nerve injury:
   a) VII and/or VIII: usually associated with temporal bone fracture
   b) olfactory nerve (Cr. N. I) injury: often occurs with anterior fossa BSF and results in anosmia, this fracture may extend to the optic canal and cause injury to the optic nerve (Cr. N. II)
   c) VI injury: can occur with fractures through the clivus (see below)

63.4.5 Management

NG tubes

✖ Caution: cases have been reported with BSF where an NG tube has been passed intracranially through the fracture[14,15,16] and is associated with fatal outcome in 64% of cases. Possible mechanisms include: a cribriform plate that is thin (congenitally or due to chronic sinusitis) or fractured (due to a frontal basal skull fracture or a comminuted fracture through the skull base).

Suggested contraindications to blind placement of an NG tube include: trauma with possible basal skull fracture, ongoing or history of previous CSF rhinorrhea, meningitis with chronic sinusitis.

Prophylactic antibiotics/vaccination

The routine use of prophylactic antibiotics is controversial. This remains true even in the presence of a CSF fistula; see CSF fistula (cranial) (p. 415). However, most ENT physicians recommend treating fractures through the nasal sinuses as open contaminated fractures, and they use broad spectrum antibiotics (e.g., ciprofloxacin) for 7–10 days.

If there is a CSF leak, **pneumococcal vaccine** is recommended for most patients (p. 341).

Treatment of the BSF

Most do not require treatment by themselves. However, conditions that may be associated with BSF that may require specific management include:
1. "traumatic aneurysms" (p. 1491)[17]
2. posttraumatic carotid-cavernous fistula (p. 1519)
3. CSF fistula: operative treatment may be required for persistent CSF rhinorrhea; see CSF fistula (cranial) (p. 415)
4. meningitis or cerebral abscess: may occur with BSF into air sinuses (frontal or mastoid) even in the absence of an identifiable CSF leak. May even occur many years after the BSF was sustained; see Post craniospinal trauma meningitis / posttraumatic meningitis (p. 340)
5. cosmetic deformities
6. posttraumatic facial palsy (see below)

63.5 Craniofacial fractures

63.5.1 Frontal sinus fractures

General information

Frontal sinus fractures account for 5–15% of facial fractures.

In the presence of a frontal sinus fracture, intracranial air (pneumocephalus) on CT, even without a clinically evident CSF leak, must be presumed to be due to dural laceration (although it could also be due to a basal skull fracture, below).

Anesthesia of the forehead may occur due to supratrochlear and/or supraorbital nerve involvement.

The risks of posterior wall fractures are not immediate, but may be delayed (some even by months or years) and include:
1. brain abscess
2. CSF leak with risk of meningitis
3. cyst or mucocele formation: injured frontal sinus mucosa has a higher predilection for mucocele formation than other sinuses.[18] Mucoceles may also develop as a result of frontonasal duct obstruction due to fracture or chronic inflammation. Mucoceles are prone to infection (mucopyocele), which can erode bone and expose dura with risk of infection

Anatomic considerations of the frontal sinus

The frontal sinus begins to appear around age 2 yrs, and becomes radiographically visible by age 8 as it extends above the superior orbital rim.[19] The sinus is lined with respiratory epithelium, the mucous secretion of which drains through the frontonasal duct medially and inferiorly into the middle nasal meatus.

Surgical considerations

Indications
Linear fractures of the anterior wall of the frontal sinus are treated expectantly.

Indications for exploration of posterior wall fractures are *controversial*.[20] Some argue that a few mm of displacement, or that CSF fistula that resolves may not require exploration. Others vehemently disagree.

Technique
In the presence of a traumatic forehead laceration, the frontal sinus may be exposed through judicious incorporation of the laceration in a forehead incision. Without such a laceration, either a bicoronal (souttar) skin incision or a butterfly incision (through the lower part of the eyebrows, crossing the midline near the glabella) is used.

In the presence of pneumocephalus, if no obvious dural laceration is found, the dural undersurface of the frontal lobes should be checked for leaks. Extradural inspection and repair is rarely indicated; the act of lifting the dura off the floor of the frontal fossa in the region of the ethmoid sinuses often creates lacerations.[21] Intradural repair is accomplished using a graft (fascia lata is most desirable; periosteum is thinner but is often acceptable) which is held in place with sutures and must extend all the way back to the ridge of the sphenoid wing (fibrin glue may be a helpful adjunct).

A periosteal flap is placed across the floor of the frontal fossa to help isolate the dura from the frontal sinus and to prevent CSF fistula.

Dealing with frontal sinus

✖ Simple packing of the sinus (with bone wax, Gelfoam®, muscle, or fat) increases the possibility of infection or mucocele formation.

The rear wall of the sinus is removed (so-called cranialization of the frontal sinus). The sinus is then exenterated (mucosa is stripped from sinus wall down to the nasofrontal duct, the mucosa is inverted over itself in the region of the duct and is packed down into the duct, and temporalis muscle plugs are then packed into the frontonasal ducts[20]), and the bony wall of the sinus is drilled with a diamond burr to remove tiny remnants of mucosa found in the surface of bone that may proliferate and form a mucocele.[18] If there is any remnant of sinus, it may then be packed with abdominal fat that fills all corners of the cavity. Post-op risks related to frontal sinus injury include: infection, mucocele formation, and CSF leak.

63.5.2 Le Fort fractures

Complex fractures through inherently weak "cleavage planes" resulting in an unstable segment ("floating face"). Shown in ▶ Fig. 63.1 (usually occur as variants of this basic scheme).
- Le Fort I: *transverse* AKA transmaxillary fracture. Fracture line crosses pterygoid plate and maxilla just above the apices of the upper teeth. May enter maxillary sinus(es)
- Le Fort II: *pyramidal*. Fracture extends upward across inferior orbital rim and orbital floor to medial orbital wall, then across nasofrontal suture. Often from downward blow to the nasal area
- Le Fort III: *craniofacial dislocation*. Involves zygomatic arches, zygomaticofrontal suture, nasofrontal suture, pterygoid plates, and orbital floors (separating maxilla from cranium). Requires significant force, and is therefore often associated with other injuries, including brain injuries

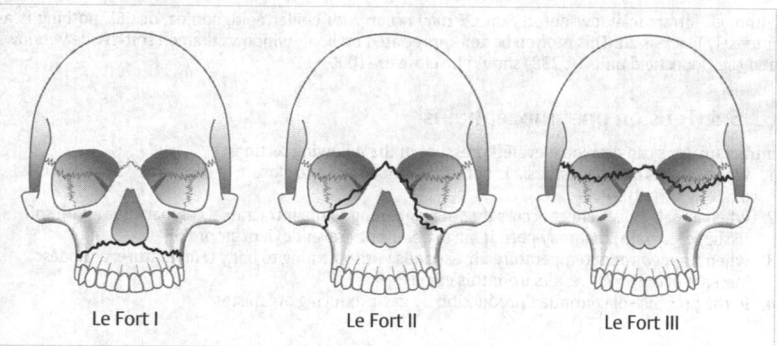

Le Fort I   Le Fort II   Le Fort III

Fig. 63.1 Le Fort fractures.

63.6 Pneumocephalus

63.6.1 General information

AKA (intra)cranial aerocele, AKA pneumatocele, is defined as the presence of intracranial gas. It is critical to distinguish this from tension pneumocephalus which is gas under pressure (see below). The gas may be located in any of the following compartments: epidural, subdural, subarachnoid, intraparenchymal, intraventricular.

63.6.2 Etiologies of pneumocephalus

Anything that can cause a CSF leak can produce associated pneumocephalus (p. 418).

1. skull defects
   a) post neurosurgical procedure
      - craniotomy: risk is higher when patient is operated with surgery in the sitting position[22]
      - shunt insertion[23,24]
      - burr hole drainage of chronic subdural hematoma[25,26]: incidence is probably < 2.5%[26] although higher rates have been reported
   b) posttraumatic
      - fracture through air sinus (frontal, ethmoid…): including basal skull fracture
      - open fracture over convexity (usually with dural laceration)
   c) congenital skull defects: including defect in tegmen tympani[27]
   d) neoplasm (osteoma,[28] epidermoid,[29] pituitary tumor): usually caused by tumor erosion through floor of sella into sphenoid sinus
2. infection
   a) with gas-producing organisms
   b) mastoiditis
3. post invasive procedure:
   a) lumbar puncture
   b) ventriculostomy
   c) spinal anesthesia[30]
4. spinal trauma (LP could be included here as well)
5. barotrauma[31]: e.g., with scuba diving (possibly through a defect in the tegmen tympani)
6. may be potentiated by a CSF drainage device in the presence of a CSF leak[32]

63.6.3 Presentation

H/A in 38%, N/V, seizures, dizziness, and obtundation.[33] An intracranial succussion splash is a rare (occurring in ≈ 7%) but pathognomonic finding. Tension pneumocephalus may additionally cause signs and symptoms just as any mass (may cause focal deficit or increased ICP).

63.6.4 Differential diagnosis (things that can mimic pneumocephalus)

Although intracranial low-density on CT may occur with epidermoid, lipoma, or CSF, nothing is as intensely black as air. This is often better appreciated on bone-windows than on soft-tissue windows and the Hounsfield units (p. 238) should be close to -1000.

63.6.5 Tension pneumocephalus

Intracranial gas can develop elevated pressure in the following settings:
1. when nitrous oxide anesthesia is not discontinued prior to closure of the dura[34]; see nitrous oxide, N_2O (p. 109)
2. when a "ball-valve" effect occurs due to an opening to the intracranial compartment with soft tissue (e.g., brain) that may permit air to enter but prevent exit of air or CSF
3. when trapped room temperature air expands with warming to body temperature: a modest increase of only ≈ 4% results from this effect[35]
4. in the presence of continued production by gas-producing organisms

63.6.6 Diagnosis

Pneumocephalus is most easily diagnosed on CT,[36] which can detect quantities of air as low as 0.5 ml. Air appears dark black (darker than CSF) and has a Hounsfield coefficient of -1000. One characteristic finding with bilateral pneumocephalus is the Mt. Fuji sign in which the two frontal poles appear peaked and are surrounded by and separated by air, resembling the silhouette of the twin peaks of Mt. Fuji[26] (see ► Fig. 63.2). Intracranial gas may also be evident on plain skull X-rays.

Since simple pneumocephalus usually does not require treatment, it is critical to differentiate it from tension pneumocephalus, which may need to be evacuated if symptomatic. It may be quite difficult to distinguish the two; brain that has been compressed e.g., by a chronic subdural hematoma may not expand immediately post-op and the "gas gap" may mimic the appearance of gas under pressure.

63.6.7 Treatment

When pneumocephalus is due to gas-producing organisms, treatment of the primary infection is initiated and the pneumocephalus is usually followed.

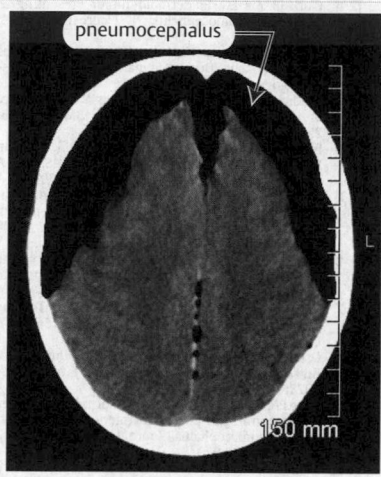

pneumocephalus

150 mm

Fig. 63.2 Mt. Fuji sign with bilateral pneumocephalus. Image: axial noncontrast CT scan.

Treatment of non-infectious simple pneumocephalus depends on whether or not the presence of a CSF leak is suspected. If there is no leak the gas will be resorbed with time, and if the mass effect is not severe it may simply be followed. If a CSF leak is suspected, management is as with any CSF fistula; see CSF fistula (cranial) (p.415).

Treatment of significant or symptomatic post-op pneumocephalus by breathing 100% O_2 via a nonrebreather mask increases the rate of resorption[37] (100% FiO_2 can be tolerated for 24–48 hours without serious pulmonary toxicity[38]).

Tension pneumocephalus producing significant symptoms must be evacuated. The urgency is similar to that of an intracranial hematoma. Dramatic and rapid improvement may occur with the release of gas under pressure. Options include placement of new twist drill or burr holes, or insertion of a spinal needle through a pre-existing burr hole (e.g., following a craniotomy).

References

[1] Mealey J, Section of Pediatric Neurosurgery of the American Association of Neurological Surgeons. Skull Fractures. In: Pediatric Neurosurgery. 1st ed. New York: Grune and Stratton; 1982:289–299

[2] Bullock MR, Chesnut RM, Ghajar J, et al. Surgical management of depressed cranial fractures. Neurosurgery. 2006; 58:S56–S60

[3] Jennett B. Epilepsy after Non-Missile Head Injuries. 2nd ed. London: William Heinemann; 1975

[4] Raffel C, Litofsky NS, Cheek WR, et al. Skull fractures. In: Pediatric Neurosurgery: Surgery of the Developing Nervous System. 3rd ed. Philadelphia: W.B. Saunders; 1994:257–265

[5] Kapp JP, Gielchinsky I, Deardourff SL. Operative Techniques for Management of Lesions Involving the Dural Venous Sinuses. Surgical Neurology. 1977; 7:339–342

[6] Buckingham MJ, Crone KR, Ball WS, et al. Traumatic Intracranial Aneurysms in Childhood: Two Cases and a Review of the Literature. Neurosurgery. 1988; 22:398–408

[7] Gurdjian ES, Lissner HR. Deformations of the skull in head injury studied by the stresscoat technique, quantitative determinations. Surg Gynecol Obstet. 1946; 83:219–233

[8] Patel A, Groppo E. Management of temporal bone trauma. Craniomaxillofac Trauma Reconstr. 2010; 3:105–113

[9] Ishman SL, Friedland DR. Temporal bone fractures: traditional classification and clinical relevance. Laryngoscope. 2004; 114:1734–1741

[10] Little SC, Kesser BW. Radiographic classification of temporal bone fractures: clinical predictability using a new system. Arch Otolaryngol Head Neck Surg. 2006; 132:1300–1304

[11] Esslen E, Miehlke A. Electrodiagnosis of Facial Palsy. In: Surgery of the Facial Nerve. 2nd ed. Philadelphia: W. B. Saunders; 1973:45–51

[12] Feiz-Erfan I, Ferreira MAT, Rekate HL, et al. Longitudinal clival fracture: A lethal injury survived. BNI Quarterly. 2001; 17

[13] Meguro K, Rowed DW. Traumatic aneurysm of the posterior inferior cerebellar artery caused by fracture of the clivus. Neurosurgery. 1985; 16:666–668

[14] Seebacher J, Nozik D, Mathieu A. Inadvertent Intracranial Introduction of a Nasogastric Tube. A Complication of Severe Maxillofacial Trauma. Anesthesia. 1975; 42:100–102

[15] Wyler AR, Reynolds AF. An Intracranial Complication of Nasogastric Intubation: Case Report. J Neurosurg. 1977; 47:297–298

[16] Baskaya MK. Inadvertent Intracranial Placement of a Nasogastric Tube in Patients with Head Injuries. Surgical Neurology. 1999; 52:426–427

[17] Benoit BG, Wortzman G. Traumatic Cerebral Aneurysms: Clinical Features and Natural History. J Neurol Neurosurg Psychiatry. 1973; 36:127–138

[18] Donald PJ. The Tenacity of the Frontal Sinus Mucosa. Otolaryngol Head Neck Surg. 1979; 87:557–566

[19] El-Bary THA. Neurosurgical Management of the Frontal Sinus. Surgical Neurology. 1995; 44:80–81

63

[20] Robinson J, Donald PJ, Pitts LH, et al. Management of Associated Cranial Lesions. In: Craniospinal Trauma. New York: Thieme Medical Publishers, Inc.; 1990:59–87

[21] Lewin W. Cerebrospinal Fluid Rhinorrhea in Closed Head Injuries. Br J Surgery. 1954; 17:1–18

[22] Lunsford LD, Maroon JC, Sheptak PE, et al. Subdural Tension Pneumocephalus: Report of Two Cases. J Neurosurg. 1979; 50:525–527

[23] Little JR, MacCarty CS. Tension Pneumocephalus After Insertion of Ventriculoperitoneal Shunt for Aqueductal Stenosis: Case Report. J Neurosurg. 1976; 44:383–385

[24] Pitts LH, Wilson CB, Dedo HH, et al. Pneumocephalus Following Ventriculoperitoneal Shunt: Case Report. J Neurosurg. 1975; 43:631–633

[25] Caron J-L, Worthington C, Bertrand G. Tension Pneumocephalus After Evacuation of Chronic Subdural Hematoma and Subsequent Treatment with Continuous Lumbar Subarachnoid Infusion and Craniostomy Drainage. Neurosurgery. 1985; 16:107–110

[26] Ishiwata Y, Fujitsu K, Sekino T, et al. Subdural Tension Pneumocephalus Following Surgery for Chronic Subdural Hematoma. J Neurosurg. 1988; 68:58–61

[27] Dowd GC, Molony TB, Voorhies RM. Spontaneous Otogenic Pneumocephalus: Case Report and Review of the Literature. Journal of Neurosurgery. 1998; 89:1036–1039

[28] Mendelson DB, Hertzanu Y, Firedman R. Frontal Osteoma with Spontaneous Subdural and Intracerebral Pneumatacele. J Laryngol Otol. 1984; 98:543–545

[29] Clark JB, Six EG. Epidermoid Tumor Presenting as Tension Pneumocephalus. J Neurosurg. 1984; 60:1312–1314

[30] Roderick L, Moore DC, Artru AA. Pneumocephalus with Headache During Spinal Anesthesia. Anesthesiology. 1985; 62:690–692

[31] Goldmann RW. Pneumocephalus as a Consequence of Barotrauma: Case Report. JAMA. 1986; 255:3154–3156

[32] Black PM, Davis JM, Kjellberg RN, et al. Tension Pneumocephalus of the Cranial Subdural Space: A Case Report. Neurosurgery. 1979; 5:368–370

[33] Markham TJ. The Clinical Features of Pneumocephalus Based on a Survey of 284 Cases with Report of 11 Additional Cases. Acta Neurochirurgica. 1967; 15:1–78

[34] Raggio JF, Fleischer AS, Sung YF, et al. Expanding Pneumocephalus due to Nitrous Oxide Anesthesia: Case Report. Neurosurgery. 1979; 4:261–263

[35] Raggio JF. Comment on Black P M, et al.: Tension Pneumocephalus of the Cranial Subdural Space: A Case Report. Neurosurgery. 1979; 5

[36] Osborn AG, Daines JH, Wing SD, et al. Intracranial Air on Computerized Tomography. J Neurosurg. 1978; 48:355–359

[37] Gore PA, Maan H, Chang S, et al. Normobaric oxygen therapy strategies in the treatment of postcraniotomy pneumocephalus. Journal of Neurosurgery. 2008; 108:926–929

[38] Klein J. Normobaric pulmonary oxygen toxicity. Anesthesia and Analgesia. 1990; 70:195–207

64 Traumatic Hemorrhagic Conditions

64.1 Posttraumatic parenchymal injuries

64.1.1 Cerebral edema

Surgical decompression is occasionally an option; see **Practice guideline: Posttraumatic cerebral edema** (p.1071).

Practice guideline: Posttraumatic cerebral edema

Indications and timing for surgery

Level III[1]: bifrontal decompressive craniectomy within 48 hrs of injury is a treatment option for patients with diffuse, medically refractory posttraumatic cerebral edema and associated IC-HTN

64.1.2 Diffuse injuries

Patients with severe diffuse injuries occasionally may be considered for decompressive craniectomy; see **Practice guideline: Diffuse injuries** (p.1071).

Practice guideline: Diffuse injuries

Indications for surgery

Level III[1]: decompressive craniectomy is an option for patients with refractory IC-HTN and diffuse parenchymal injury with clinical and radiographic evidence for impending transtentorial herniation

64.2 Hemorrhagic contusion

64.2.1 General information

AKA traumatic intracerebral hemorrhage (TICH). The definition is not uniformly agreed upon. Often considered as high density areas on CT (some exclude areas < 1 cm diameter[2]). TICH usually produce much less mass effect than their apparent size. Most commonly occur in areas where sudden deceleration of the head causes the brain to impact on bony prominences (e.g., temporal, frontal, and occipital poles) in coup or contrecoup fashion.

TICH often enlarge and/or coalesce with time as seen on serial CTs. They also may appear in a delayed fashion (see below). Surrounding low density may represent associated cerebral edema. CT scans months later often show surprisingly minimal or no encephalomalacia.

64.2.2 Treatment

Practice guideline: Surgical management of TICH

- Level III[1]: Indications for surgical evacuation for TICH:
  - progressive neurological deterioration referable to the TICH, medically refractory IC-HTN, or signs of mass effect on CT
  - or TICH volume > 50 cm³ cc or ml
  - or GCS = 6–8 with frontal or temporal TICH volume > 20 cm³ with midline shift (MLS) ≥ 5 mm (p.1110) and/or compressed basal cisterns on CT (p.1109)
- nonoperative management with intensive monitoring and serial imaging: may be used for TICH without neurologic compromise and no significant mass effect on CT and controlled ICP

64.2.3 Delayed traumatic intracerebral hemorrhage (DTICH)

TICH demonstrated in patients on imaging that was not evident on initial admitting CT scan.

Incidence of DTICH in patients with GCS ≤ 8: ≈ 10%[3,4] (reported incidence varies with resolution of CT scanner,[5] timing of scan, and definition). Most DTICH occur within 72 hrs of the trauma.[4] Some patients seem to be doing well and then present with an apoplectic event (although DTICH accounted only for 12% of patients who "talk and deteriorate"[6]).

Factors that contribute to formation of DTICH include local or systemic coagulopathy, hemorrhage into an area of necrotic brain softening, and coalescence of extravasated microhematomas.[7]

Treatment is the same as for TICH (see above).

Outcome for patients with DTICH described in the literature is generally poor, with a mortality ranging from 50–75%.[7]

64.3 Epidural hematoma

64.3.1 General information

Incidence of epidural hematoma (EDH): 1% of head trauma admissions (which is ≈ 50% the incidence of acute subdurals). Ratio of male:female = 4:1. Usually occurs in young adults, and is rare before age 2 yrs or after age 60 (perhaps because the dura is more adherent to the inner table in these groups).

Dogma was classically that a skull fracture disrupts the anterior branch of the middle meningeal artery as it exits its canal in the temporal bone to enter the skull, causing arterial bleeding that gradually dissects the dura from the inner table resulting in a delayed deterioration. Alternate hypothesis: dissection of the dura from the inner table occurs first, followed by bleeding into the space thus created.

Source of bleeding: 85% = arterial bleeding (the middle meningeal artery is the most common source of middle fossa EDHs). Many of the remainder of cases are due to bleeding from middle meningeal vein or dural sinus.

70% occur laterally over the hemispheres with their epicenter at the pterion, the rest occur in the frontal, occipital, and posterior fossa (5–10% each).

64.3.2 Presentation with EDH

"Textbook" presentation (< 10%-27% have this classic presentation[8]):
- brief posttraumatic loss of consciousness (LOC): from initial impact
- followed by a "lucid interval" for several hours
- then, obtundation, contralateral hemiparesis and ipsilateral pupillary dilatation as a result of mass effect from hematoma

Deterioration usually occurs over a few hours, but may take days and rarely, weeks (the longer intervals may be associated with venous bleeding).

Other presenting findings: H/A, vomiting, seizure (may be unilateral), hemi-hyperreflexia + unilateral Babinski sign, and elevated CSF pressure (LP is seldom used any longer). Bradycardia is usually a late finding. In peds, EDH should be suspected if there is a 10% drop in hematocrit after admission.

Contralateral hemiparesis is not uniformly seen, especially with EDH in locations other than laterally over the hemisphere. Shift of the brainstem away from the mass may produce compression of the opposite cerebral peduncle on tentorial notch which can produce *ipsilateral* hemiparesis (so called Kernohan's phenomenon or Kernohan's notch phenomenon),[9] a false localizing sign.

60% of patients with EDH have a dilated pupil, 85% of which are *ipsilateral.*

No initial loss of consciousness occurs in 60%. No lucid interval in 20%. NB: a lucid interval is not pahtognomonic for EDH and may also be seen in other conditions (including subdural hematoma).

64.3.3 Differential diagnosis

- subdural hematoma (see below for differentiating radiographic features)
- a posttraumatic disorder described by Denny-Brown consisting of a posttraumatic "lucid interval" followed by bradycardia, brief periods of restlessness and vomiting, without intracranial hypertension or mass. Children especially may have H/A, and may become drowsy and confused. Theory: a form of vagal syncope. CT must be done to rule out EDH

64.3.4 Evaluation

Plain skull X-rays

Usually not helpful. No fracture is identified in 40% of EDH. In these cases the patient's age was almost always < 30 yrs.

CT scan in EDH

"Classic" CT appearance occurs in 84% of cases: high density biconvex (lenticular) shape adjacent to the skull (▶ Fig. 64.1). In 11% the side against the skull is convex and that along the brain is straight, and in 5% it is crescent shaped (resembling subdural hematoma).[10] EDH may cross dural barriers (viz. falx or tentorium) (▶ Fig. 64.2) distinct from SDH, which is limited to one side, however EDH are usually limited by skull sutures which SDH are not. EDH usually has uniform density, sharply defined edges on multiple cuts, high attenuation (undiluted blood), is contiguous with inner table, and is

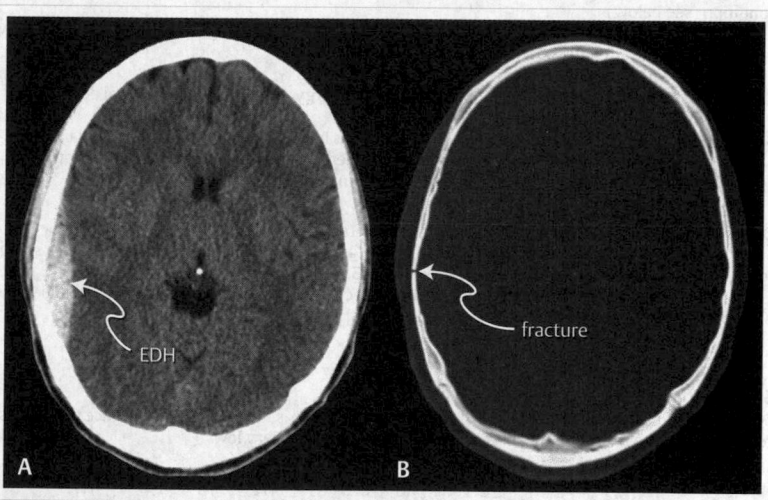

Fig. 64.1 Epidural hematoma, right side.
Epidural hematoma (EDH) appears as biconvex (lenticular) shaped hyperdensity adjacent to inner table of skull.
Note the underlying skull fracture seen on bone windows.
Image: axial CT scan. A: brain window. B: bone window.

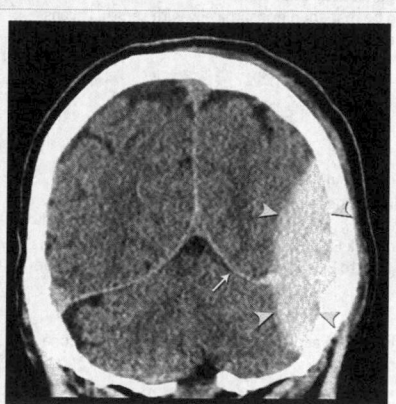

Fig. 64.2 Epidural hematoma, left side.
Image: coronal CT illustrating an EDH (*yellow arrowheads*) crossing the tentorium (*white arrow*), which in addition to its biconvex shape, helps distinguish this from a subdural hematoma (SDH).

usually confined to small segment of calvaria. Mass effect is frequent. Occasionally, an epidural may be isodense with brain and may not show up unless IV contrast is given,[10] although other clues are often present (e.g., inward displacement of the cortical ribbon). Mottled density may occur, and in some cases is associated with a hyperacute EDH.[11]

64.3.5 Treatment of EDH

General management

Prepare for surgery if indications below are met. Prompt surgery if signs of local mass effect, signs of herniation (increasing drowsiness, pupil changes, hemiparesis…) or cardiorespiratory abnormalities.

Management includes: admit to ICU with q 1 hour neuro checks, NPO. Reverse coagulopathies.

Medical

CT may detect small EDHs and can be used to follow them. However, in most cases, EDH is a surgical condition (see below).

Nonsurgical management may be attempted in patients not meeting surgical indications below, which generally limited to:
1. small (≤ 1 cm maximal thickness) subacute or chronic EDH[12]
2. minimal neurological signs/symptoms (e.g., slight lethargy, mild H/A) without focal deficit and without evidence of herniation
3. ✖ although medical management of p-fossa EDHs has been reported, these are more dangerous (see below) due to small volume of p-fossa and vulnerability of brainstem to compression by even modest hematoma expansion. Surgery is recommended

Optional: for persistent headache a short course of steroids (1–3 days) may help, then taper.

Follow-up CT: early after admission (e.g., 6 hours) and then any time the patient becomes symptomatic, or in 1–2 wks if clinically stable. Repeat in 1–3 mos (to document resolution).

In 50% of cases there will be a slight transient increase in size between days 5–16, and some patients required emergency craniotomy when signs of herniation occurred.[13]

Surgical

Surgical indications and timing
See also Practice guideline (p. 1074). EDH in pediatric patients is riskier than adults since there is less room for clot. The threshold for surgery in pediatrics should be very low.

Practice guideline: Surgical management of EDH

Indications for surgery
Level III[14]:
1. EDH volume* > 30 cm³ should be evacuated regardless of GCS.
2. EDH with all of the following characteristics can be managed nonsurgically with serial CT scans and close neurological observation in a neurosurgical center:
   a) volume* < 30 cm³
   b) and thickness < 15 mm
   c) and midline shift (MLS) < 5 mm (p. 1110)
   d) and GCS > 8
   e) and no focal neurologic deficit

*The estimated volume of a lens = (1.6 to 2) × r^2t = (0.4 to 0.5) × d^2t
≈ (H × AP × T)/2 (that is 1/2 the products of the height times the length in the AP dimension times the thickness T).

Helpful benchmarks: for the volume of a 1.5 cm thick EDH to be < 30 cc it would have to have a diameter (not radius) < 6.3–7 cm. For a 1 cm thick EDH to be < 30 cc, it would have to have a diameter < 7.7–8.6 cm.

Timing of surgery
Level III[14]: it is strongly recommended that patients with an acute EDH and GCS < 9 and anisocoria undergo surgical evacuation ASAP

Booking the case: Craniotomy for acute EDH/SDH

Also see defaults & disclaimers (p. 25).
1. position: (depends on location of bleed, usually supine)
2. blood: type & screen (for severe SDH: T & C 2 U PRBC)
3. post-op: ICU
4. consent (in lay terms for the patient—not all-inclusive):
   a) procedure: surgery through the skull to remove blood clot, stop any bleeding identified, possible placement of intracranial pressure monitor
   b) alternatives: nonsurgical management
   c) complications: usual craniotomy complications (p. 25) plus further bleeding which may cause problems (especially in patients taking blood thinners, antiplatelet drugs including aspirin, or those with coagulation abnormalities or previous bleeds) and may require further surgery, any permanent brain injury that has already occurred is not likely to recover, hydrocephalus

Surgical technical issues

Evacuation is performed in the OR unless the patient herniates in E/R and access to OR is not within acceptable timeframe (see Exploratory burr holes (p. 1014)). Objectives:
1. clot removal: lowers ICP and eliminates focal mass effect. Blood is usually thick coagulum, thus exposure must be large enough provide access to most of clot. Craniotomy permits more complete evacuation of hematoma than e.g., burr holes[14]
2. hemostasis: attempt to locate and neutralize the source of the hematoma (e.g., middle meningeal artery), coagulate bleeding soft tissue (dural veins & arteries). Requires an exposure larger than e.g., burr holes
3. prevent reaccumulation: some bleeding or oozing typically occurs post op, and the dura is now detached from inner table facilitates recurrence of EDH. Strategies to prevent:
   a) apply bone wax to intra-diploic bleeders
   b) dural tack-up sutures: small sutures (e.g., 4-0 braided nylon) from the dura to small drill holes in the bone along the edges of the craniotomy and a central "tenting" suture through drill holes in the flap
   c) perforating the bone flap with a drill and placing a subgaleal drain which is maintained for several days or until output is scant

64.3.6 Mortality with EDH

Overall: 20–55% (higher rates in older series). Optimal diagnosis and treatment within a few hours results in 5–10% estimated mortality (12% in a recent CT era series[15]). Mortality in patients without lucid interval is double that for patients with a lucid interval. Bilateral Babinski's or decerebration pre-op → worse prognosis. Death is usually due to respiratory arrest from uncal herniation causing injury to the midbrain.

20% of patients with EDH on CT also have ASDH at autopsy or operation. Mortality with both lesions concurrently is higher, reported range: 25–90%.

64.3.7 Special cases of epidural hematoma

Delayed epidural hematoma (DEDH)

Definition: an EDH that is not present on the initial CT scan, but is found on subsequent CT. Comprise 9–10% of all EDHs in several series.[16,17]

Theoretical risk factors for DEDH include the following (NB: many of these risk factors may be incurred *after* the patient is admitted following a negative initial CT):
1. lowering ICP either medically (e.g., osmotic diuretics) and/or surgically (e.g., evacuating contralateral hematoma) which reduces tamponading effect
2. rapidly correcting shock (hemodynamic "surge") may cause DEDH[18]
3. coagulopathies

DEDH tend to occur in patients with severe head injury and associated systemic injuries. However, DEDH have also been infrequently reported in *mild* head injury (GCS > 12) .[19] Presence of a skull fracture has been identified as a common feature of DEDH.[19]

Key to diagnosis: high index of suspicion. Avoid a false sense of security imparted by an initial "nonsurgical" CT. 6 of 7 patients in one series improved or remained unchanged neurologically despite enlarging EDH (most eventually deteriorate). 1 of 5 with an ICP monitor did not have a heralding increase in ICP. May develop once an intracranial lesion is surgically treated, as occurred in 5 of 7 patients within 24 hrs of evacuation of another EDH. 6 of 7 patients had known skull fractures in the region where the delayed EDH developed,[17] but none of 3 had a skull fracture in another report.[18]

Posterior fossa epidural hematoma

Comprise ≈ 5% of EDH.[20,21] More common in 1st two decades of life. Although as many as 84% have occipital skull fractures, only ≈ 3% of children with occipital skull fractures develop p-fossa EDH. The source of bleeding is usually not found, but there is a high incidence of tears of the dural sinuses. Cerebellar signs are surprisingly lacking or subtle in most. See surgical indications (p. 1090). Overall mortality is ≈ 26% (mortality was higher in patients with an associated intracranial lesion).

64.4 Acute subdural hematoma

64.4.1 General information

The magnitude of impact damage (p. 1000), as opposed to secondary damage, is usually much higher in acute subdural hematoma (ASDH) than in epidural hematomas, which generally makes this lesion much more lethal. There is often associated underlying brain injury, which may be less common with EDH. Symptoms may be due to compression of the underlying brain with midline shift, in addition to parenchymal brain injury and possibly cerebral edema.[22,23]

Two common causes of traumatic ASDH:

1. accumulation around parenchymal laceration (usually frontal or temporal lobe). There is usually severe underlying primary brain injury. Often no "lucid interval." Focal signs usually occur later and are less prominent than with EDH
2. surface or bridging vessel torn from cerebral acceleration-deceleration during violent head motion. With this etiology, primary brain damage may be less severe, a lucid interval may occur with later rapid deterioration

ASDH may also occur in patients receiving anticoagulation therapy,[24,25] usually with, but sometimes without, a history of trauma (the trauma may be minor). Receiving anticoagulation therapy increases the risk of ASDH 7-fold in males and 26-fold in females.[24]

64.4.2 CT scan in ASDH

Acute subdurals are usually hyperdense compared to brain (possible exceptions: patients with low hematocrit, SDH that admix with CSF as they form). Edema in the adjacent brain may be present.

Locations of ASDH:

• convexity (the most common). Usually appears as a crescentic mass of increased density adjacent to inner table (▶ Fig. 64.3), compared to a convexity epidural hematoma which is usually biconvex (▶ Fig. 64.1).
• interhemispheric (p. 1079) (▶ Fig. 64.6)
• layering on the tentorium (tentorial subdural, ▶ Fig. 64.4)
• in p-fossa (p. 1089)

▶ **Differences in convexity EDH from SDH.** SDH is typically more diffuse, less uniform, usually *crescentic* over brain surface, often less dense (possibly from mixing with CSF). SDH cannot cross intradural barriers such as the falx and tentorium, whereas an EDH can.

▶ **SDH changes with time on CT.** The density of subdural hematomas on CT scans changes with time as blood breaks down and transforms from thick coagulum to low viscosity fluid (see

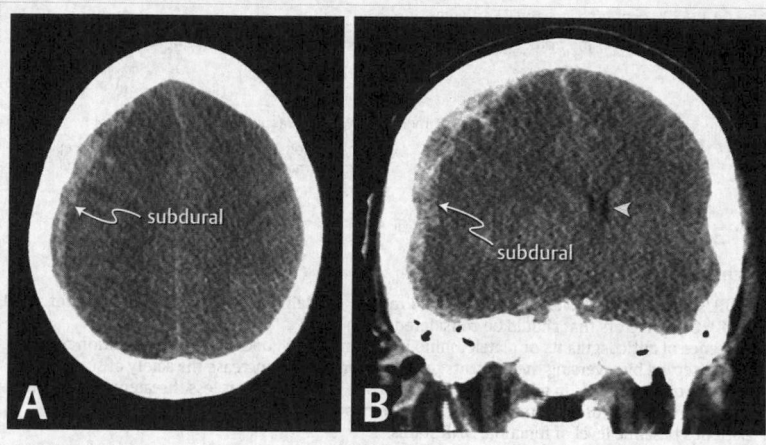

Fig. 64.3 Acute (convexity) subdural hematoma, right side.
Note the characteristic high-density crescentic shape of the hematoma. The lateral ventricles (*yellow arrowhead*) have been shifted to the patient's left.
Image: noncontrast CT scan, brain window. A: axial, B: coronal.

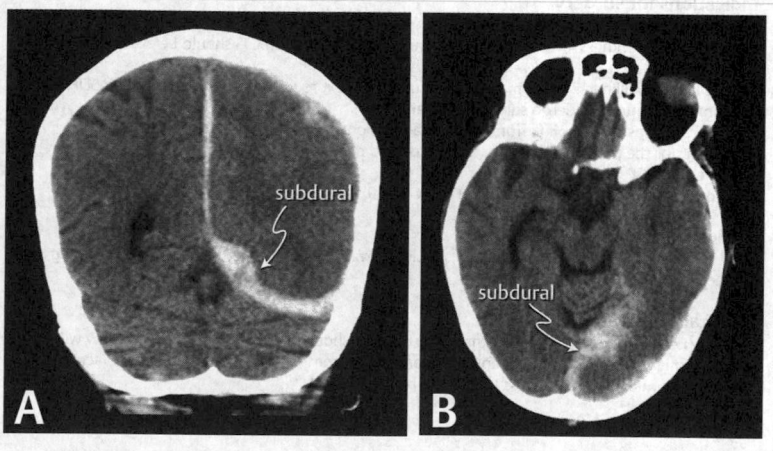

Fig. 64.4 Tentorial subdural hematoma, left side.
Image: noncontrast CT scan in the same patient, brain window. A: coronal, B: axial.

▶ Table 64.1 and ▶ Fig. 64.5, times are approximate, and vary from patient to patient). Acute SDH are usually hyperdense to brain, and become isodense after ≈ 2 wks where the only clues may be apparent obliteration of sulci or inward displacement of cortical surface from inner table of skull and lateralizing shift (the latter may be absent if the SDH are bilateral). Subsequently, the SDH becomes hypodense to brain and is considered a chronic subdural hematoma (p. 1081). Membrane formation begins by about 4 days after injury.[26]

Table 64.1 ASDH density changes on CT with time

Category	Time frame	Density on CT relative to brain
acute	1 to 3 days	hyperdense
subacute	4 days to 2 or 3 wks	≈ isodense
chronic	usually > 3 wks and < 3–4 mos	hypodense (approaching density of CSF)
	after about 1–2 months	may become lenticular shaped (similar to epidural hematoma) with density > CSF, < fresh blood

64.4.3 Treatment

Indications for surgery

Level III surgical indications are shown in **Practice guideline: Surgical management of ASDH** (p. 1078). Other factors that should be considered:

1. presence of anticoagulants or platelet inhibitors: patients in good neurologic condition may be better served by reversing these agents prior to operating (to increase the safety of surgery)
2. location of hematoma: in general, an SDH high over the convexity is less threatening than a temporal/parietal SDH of the same volume that also has MLS
3. patient's baseline level of function, DNR status…
4. while the guidelines suggest evacuating SDH < 10 mm thick in some circumstances, clots that are smaller than this may not be causing problems but may simply be an epiphenomenon

Practice guideline: Surgical management of ASDH

Indications for surgery
Level III[27]:
1. ASDH with thickness > 10 mm or midline shift (MLS) > 5 mm (on CT) should be evacuated regardless of GCS
2. ASDH with thickness < 10 mm and MLS < 5 mm (see text regarding the evacuation of ASDH < 10 mm thick) should undergo surgical evacuation if:
   a) GCS drops by ≥ 2 points from injury to admission
   b) and/or the pupils are asymmetric or fixed and dilated
   c) and/or ICP is > 20 mm Hg
3. monitor ICP in all patients with ASDH and GCS < 9

Timing of surgery
Level III[27]: ASDH meeting surgical criteria should be evacuated ASAP (for issues regarding timing of surgery, see text)

Surgical methods
Level III[27]: ASDH meeting the above criteria for surgery should be evacuated via craniotomy with or without bone flap removal and duraplasty (a large craniotomy flap is often required to evacuate the thick coagulum and to gain access to possible bleeding sites).

Timing of surgery

Timing of surgery for ASDH is a matter of controversy. As a general principle, when surgery for ASDH is indicated it should be done as soon as possible.

"Four hour rule"
This "rule" was based on a 1981 series of 82 patients with ASDH,[28] which held that:
1. patients operated within 4 hrs of injury had 30% mortality, compared to 90% mortality if surgery was delayed > 4 hrs
2. functional survival (Glasgow Outcome Scale ≥ 4, see ▶ Table 98.4) rate of 65% could be achieved with surgery within 4 hrs
3. other factors related to outcome in this series included:

a) post-op ICP: 79% of patients with functional recovery had post-op ICPs that didn't exceed 20 mm Hg, whereas only 30% of patients who died had ICP < 20 mm Hg
b) initial neuro exam
c) age was *not* a factor in this study (ASDH tend to occur in older patients than EDH)

However, a subsequent study of 101 patients with ASDH found a delay to surgery (delays > 4 hours from the injury) showed a nonstatistically-significant trend where mortality increased from 59% to 69% and functional survival decreased (Glasgow Outcome Scale ≤ 4, see ▶ Table 98.4) from 26% to 16%.[29]

Booking the case: Acute subdural hematoma

64

Same as for acute epidural hematoma (p. 1075).

Technical considerations

One may start with a small linear dural opening to effect clot removal and enlarge it as needed and only if brain swelling seems controllable. The actual bleeding site is often not identified at the time of surgery.

64.4.4 Morbidity and mortality with ASDH

Mortality range: 50–90% (a significant percentage of this mortality is from the underlying brain injury, and not the ASDH itself).

Mortality is traditionally thought to be higher in aged patients (60%), and is 90–100% in patients on anticoagulants.[25]

In a series of 101 patients with ASDH, functional recovery was 19%.[29] Postoperative seizures occurred in 9%, and did not correlate with outcome. The following variables were identified as strongly influencing outcome:

• mechanism of injury: the worst outcome was with motorcycle accidents, with 100% mortality in unhelmeted patients, 33% in helmeted
• age: correlated with outcome only > 65 yrs of age, with 82% mortality and 5% functional survival in this group (other series had similar results[30])
• neurologic condition on admission: the ratio of mortality to functional survival rate related to the admission Glasgow Coma Scale (**GCS**) is shown in ▶ Table 64.2
• postoperative ICP: patients with peak ICPs < 20 mm Hg had 40% mortality, and no patient with ICP > 45 had a functional survival

Of all the above factors, only the time to surgery and postoperative ICP can be directly influenced by the treating neurosurgeon.

Table 64.2 Outcome as related to admission GCS

Admission GCS	Mortality	Functional survival
3	90%	5%
4	76%	10%
5	62%	18%
6 & 7	51%	44%

64.4.5 Special cases of acute subdural hematoma

Interhemispheric subdural hematoma

General information

Subdural hematoma along the falx between the two cerebral hemispheres (older term: interhemispheric scissure) (▶ Fig. 64.6).

May occur in children,[31] possibly associated with child abuse.[32]

In adults, may be the consequence of[33]:

• head trauma in 79–91%

64

- ruptured aneurysm[34] in ≈ 12%
- surgery in the vicinity of the corpus callosum
- spontaneously: rare, mostly with the use of anticoagulation

Incidence is unknown. Spontaneous cases should be investigated for possible underlying aneurysm. Occasionally may be bilateral, sometimes may be delayed (see below)

Most often are asymptomatic, or may present with the so-called "falx syndrome"—paresis or focal seizures contralateral to the hematoma. Other presentations: gait ataxia, dementia, language disturbance, oculomotor palsies.

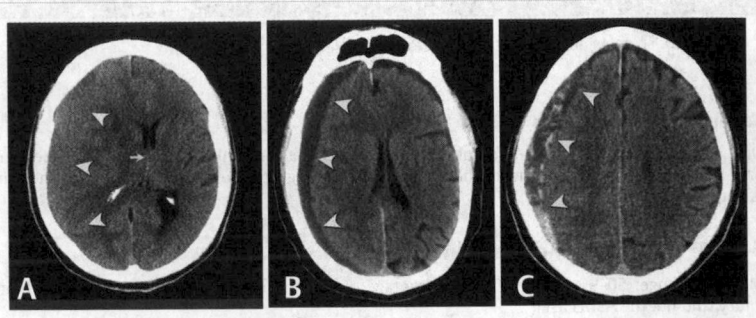

Fig. 64.5 Changes in subdural hematomas over time.
Right-sided convexity subdural hematomas (*yellow arrowheads*) in 3 different patients.
Image: axial CT scans. A: subacute subdural (isodense to brain and can barely be seen. Note absence of sulci on the ipsilateral side and the right-to-left midline shift (blue arrow) are clues to its presence), B: chronic SDH (low density), C: this subdural is often read as "acute on chronic SDH" (note the higher density areas mixed with lower density).

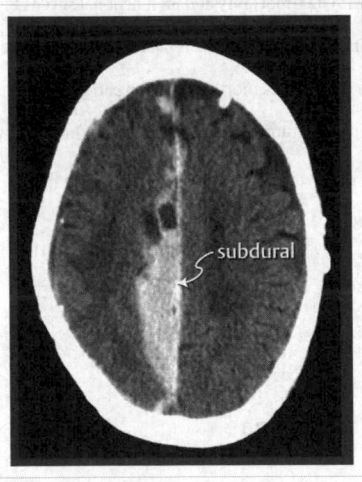

Fig. 64.6 Interhemispheric subdural hematoma on the right side of the falx in a 76-year-old male on anticoagulants.
Image: axial noncontrast CT scan.

Treatment

Controversial. Small asymptomatic cases may be managed expectantly. Surgery should be considered for progressive neurological deterioration with larger lesions. Approached through a parasagittal craniotomy. ✖ Surgery for these lesions can be treacherous—there is risk of venous infarction and one often finds they are dealing with a superior sagittal sinus injury.

Outcome

Reported mortality: 25–42%. Mortality is higher in the presence of altered levels of consciousness. Mortality rate may actually be lower (24%) than with all-comers.[33] This is significantly lower than SDH in other sites (see above).

Delayed acute subdural hematoma (DASDH)

DASDHs have received less attention than delayed epidural or intraparenchymal hematomas. Incidence is ≈ 0.5% of operatively treated ASDHs.[7]

Definition: ASDH not present on an initial CT (or MRI) that shows up on a subsequent study. Indications for treatment are the same as for ASDH. Neurologically stable patients with a small DASDH and medically controllable ICP are managed expectantly.

64

Infantile acute subdural hematoma

General information

Infantile acute subdural hematoma (IASDH) is often considered a special case of SDH. Roughly defined as an acute SDH in an infant due to minor head trauma without initial loss of consciousness or cerebral contusion,[35] possibly due to rupture of a bridging vein. The most common trauma is a fall backwards from sitting or standing. The infants will often cry immediately and then (usually within minutes to 1 hour) develop a generalized seizure. Patients are usually < 2 yrs old (most are 6–12 mos, the age when they first begin to pull themselves up or walk).[36]

These clots are rarely pure blood, and are often mixed with fluid. 75% are bilateral or have contralateral subdural fluid collections. It is speculated that IASDH may represent acute bleeding into a preexisting fluid collection.[36]

Skull fractures are rare. In one series, retinal and preretinal hemorrhages were seen in all 26 patients.[35]

Treatment

Treatment is guided by clinical condition and size of hematoma. Minimally symptomatic cases (vomiting, irritability, no altered level of consciousness and no motor disturbance) with liquefied hematoma may be treated with percutaneous subdural tap, which may be repeated several times as needed. Chronically persistent cases may require a subduroperitoneal shunt.

More symptomatic cases with high density clot on CT require craniotomy. A subdural membrane similar to those seen in adult chronic SDH is not unusual.[36] *Caution:* these patients are at risk of developing intraoperative hypovolemic shock.

Outcome

8% morbidity and mortality rate in one series.[35] Much better prognosis than ASDH of all ages probably because of the absence of cerebral contusion in IASDH.

64.5 Chronic subdural hematoma

64.5.1 General information

Originally termed "pachymeningitis hemorrhagica interna" by Virchow[37] in 1857. Chronic subdural hematomas (CSDH) generally occur in the elderly, with an average age of ≈ 63 yrs; exception: subdural collections of infancy (p. 1087). Head trauma is identified in < 50% (sometimes rather trivial trauma can produce these lesions). Other risk factors: alcohol abuse, seizures, CSF shunts, coagulopathies (including therapeutic anticoagulation[25]), and patients at risk for falls (e.g., with hemiplegia from previous stroke). CSDHs are bilateral in ≈ 20–25% of cases.[38,39]

Hematoma thickness tends to be larger in older patients due to a decrease in brain weight and increase in subdural space with age.[40]

Classically CSDHs contain dark "motor oil" fluid which does not clot.[41] When the subdural fluid is clear (CSF), the collection is termed a subdural hygroma (p. 1085).

64.5.2 Pathophysiology

Many CSDHs probably start out as acute subdurals. Blood within the subdural space evokes an inflammatory response. Within days, fibroblasts invade the clot and form neomembranes on the inner (cortical) and outer (dural) surface. This is followed by ingrowth of neocapillaries, enzymatic fibrinolysis, and liquefaction of bpslood clot. Fibrin degradation products are reincorporated into new clots and inhibit hemostasis. The course of CSDH is determined by the balance of plasma effusion and/or rebleeding from the neomembranes on the one hand and reabsorption of fluid on the other.[42,43]

64.5.3 Presentation

Patients may present with minor symptoms of headache, confusion, language difficulties (e.g., word-finding difficulties or speech arrest, usually with dominant hemisphere lesions), or TIA-like symptoms (p. 1685). Or, they may develop varying degrees of coma, hemiplegia, or seizures (focal, or less often generalized). Often, the diagnosis may be unexpected prior to imaging.

The Markwalder scale (▶ Table 64.3[44] is similar to other scales used for grading neurologic status of patients with CSDH, and is sometimes used for research purposes.

Table 64.3 Markwalder neurologic grading scale for CSDH[44]

Grade	Neurologic condition
0	• neurologically normal
1	• alert & oriented • mild symptoms (e.g., H/A) • no neurologic deficit or minimal neurologic deficit (e.g., reflex asymmetry)
2	• drowsy or disoriented • variable neurologic deficit (e.g., hemiparesis)
3	• stuporous but responds appropriately to noxious stimulus • severe focal signs (e.g., hemiplegia)
4	• comatose • no motor response to noxious stimulus • decerebrate or decorticate posturing

64.5.4 Imaging

Chronic subdurals most often appear on CT as hypodense crescentic extra-axial collections (see ▶ Fig. 64.5 panel B).

64.5.5 Treatment

Management overview

1. seizure prophylaxis: used by some. It may be safe to discontinue after a week or so if there are no seizures. If a late seizure occurs with or without prior use of ASMs, longer-term therapy is required
2. coagulopathies (including anticoagulation & antiplatelet therapy) should be reversed
3. treatment of the hematoma
   a) indications:
      • symptomatic lesions (usually > 1 cm maximal thickness). Symptoms include: focal deficit, mental status changes, seizures, severe H/A...
      • or progressive increase in size on serial imaging (CT or MRI scans)
   b) treatment options:
      • surgical evacuation of the hematoma: numerous methods employed (see below)
      • endovascular embolization of the middle meningeal artery (p. 1935)

Surgical options

Despite the fact that CSDH is one of the most common neurosurgical conditions, there is no consensus regarding optimal treatment. For details of techniques (burr holes, use of subdural drain...) see below.

1. placing two burr holes, and irrigating through and through with tepid saline until the fluid runs clear
2. single "large" burr hole with irrigation and aspiration: see below
3. single burr hole drainage with placement of a subdural drain, maintained for 24–48 hrs (removed when output becomes negligible)
4. twist drill craniostomy: see below (note that small "twist drill" drainage *without* subdural drain has higher recurrence rate than e.g., burr holes)

5. craniotomy with excision of subdural membrane (may be necessary in cases which persistently recur after above procedures, possibly due to seepage from the subdural membrane). Still a safe and valid technique.[45] No attempt should be made to remove the deep membrane adherent to the surface of brain

Techniques that promote continued drainage after the immediate procedure and that may thus reduce residual fluid and prevent reaccumulation:
1. use of a subdural drain: (see below)
2. using a generous burr hole under the temporalis muscle: (see below)
3. bed-rest restriction with the head of the bed flat (1 pillow is permitted) with mild overhydration for 24–48 hours post-op (or if a drain is used, until 24–48 hours after it is removed). May promote expansion of the brain and expulsion of residual subdural fluid. Allowing patients to sit up to 30–40° immediately post-op was associated with higher radiographic recurrence rate (2.3% for those kept flat, vs. 19% for those who sat up) but usually did not require reoperation[46]
4. some advocate continuous lumbar subarachnoid infusion when the brain fails to expand; however, there are possible complications[47]

Booking the case: Craniotomy: for chronic subdural hematoma

Also see defaults & disclaimers (p. 25).
1. position: (usually supine), horseshoe headrest
2. post-op: ICU
3. consent (in lay terms for the patient—not all-inclusive):
   a) procedure: surgery through the skull to remove blood clot, stop any bleeding identified, place a drainage tube to allow further fluid to drain after surgery for a day or so
   b) alternatives: nonsurgical management
   c) complications: usual craniotomy complications (p. 25) plus further bleeding which may cause problems (especially in patients taking blood thinners, antiplatelet drugs including aspirin, or those with coagulation abnormalities or previous bleeds) and may require further surgery, hydrocephalus

Twist drill craniostomy for chronic subdurals

This method is thought to decompress the brain more slowly and avoids the presumed rapid pressure shifts that occur following other methods, which may be associated with complications such as intraparenchymal (intracerebral) hemorrhage. May even be performed at the bedside under local anesthesia. There was no difference in outcome compared to burr holes.[48]

A 0.5 cm incision is made in the scalp in the rostral portion of the hematoma, and then a twist drill hole is placed at a 45° angle to the skull, aimed in the direction of the longitudinal axis of the collection. If the drill does not penetrate the dura, this is done with an 18 Ga spinal needle. A ventricular catheter is inserted into the subdural space, and is drained to a standard ventriculostomy drainage bag maintained 20 cm *below* the level of the craniostomy site[49,50,51] (below). The patient is kept flat in bed (see above). Serial CTs assess the adequacy of drainage. The catheter is removed when at least ≈ 20% of the collection is drained and when the patient shows signs of improvement, which occurs within a range of 1–7 days (mean of 2.1 days). Some include a low pressure shunt valve in the system to prevent reflux of fluid or air.

Burr holes for chronic subdural hematomas

To prevent recurrence, the use of *small* burr holes (without a subdural drain) is not recommended. A generous (> 2.5 cm in diameter—it is recommended that one actually measure this) subtemporal craniectomy should be performed, and bipolar coagulation is used to shrink the edges of the dura and subdural membrane back to the full width of the bony opening (do not try to separate these two layers as this may promote bleeding). This allows continued drainage of fluid into the temporalis muscle where it may be resorbed. A piece of Gelfoam® may be placed over the opening to help prevent fresh blood from oozing into the opening.

Subdural drain

Use of a subdural drain is associated with a decrease in need for repeat surgery from 19% to 10%.[48,52] If a subdural drain is used, a closed drainage system is recommended. Difficulties may occur with ventriculostomy catheters because the holes are small and are restricted to the tip region (so-designed to keep choroid plexus from plugging the catheter when inserted into the ventricles when used as intended as a CSF shunt), especially with thick "oily" fluid (on the positive side, slow drainage may be desirable). The drainage bag is maintained ≈ 50–80 cm below the level of the head.[44,51] An alternative is a small Jackson-Pratt® drain using "thumb-print" indentation of the suction bulb, which provides good drainage with a self-contained one-way valve (however, there may be a risk of excessive negative pressure with overcompression of the bulb). Drainage for 48 hours was as effective as 96 hours.[48]

Post-op, the patient is kept flat (see above). Prophylactic antibiotics may be given until ≈ 24–48 hrs following removal of the drain, at which time the HOB is gradually elevated. CT scan prior to removal of the drain (or shortly after removal) may be helpful to establish a baseline for later comparison in the event of deterioration.

There is a case report of administration of urokinase through a subdural drain to treat reaccumulation of clot following evacuation.[53]

64.5.6 Outcome

General information

There is clinical improvement when the subdural pressure is reduced to close to zero, which usually occurs after ≈ 20% of the collection is removed.[51]

Patients who have high subdural fluid pressure tend to have more rapid brain expansion and clinical improvement than patients with low pressures.[44]

Residual subdural fluid collections after treatment are common, but clinical improvement does not require complete resolution of the fluid collection on CT. CTs showed persistent fluid in 78% of cases on post-op day 10, and in 15% after 40 days,[44] and may take up to 6 months for complete resolution. Recommendation: do *not* treat persistent fluid collections evident on CT (especially before ≈ 20 days post-op) unless it increases in size on CT or if the patient shows no recovery or deteriorates.

76% of 114 patients were successfully treated with a single drainage procedure using a twist drill craniostomy with subdural ventricular catheter, and 90% with one or two procedures.[49] These statistics are slightly better than twist drill craniostomy with aspiration alone (i.e., no drain).

Complications of surgical treatment

Although these collections often appear innocuous, severe complications may occur, including:
1. seizures (including intractable status epilepticus)
2. intracerebral hemorrhage (ICH): occurs in 0.7–5%.[54] Very devastating in this setting: one–third of these patients die and one third are severely disabled (also, see below)
3. failure of the brain to re-expand and/or reaccumulation of the subdural fluid
4. tension pneumocephalus
5. subdural empyema: may also occur with untreated subdurals[55]

In 60% of patients ≥ age 75 yrs (and in no patients < 75 yrs), rapid decompression is associated with hyperemia in the cortex immediately beneath the hematoma, which may be related to the complications of ICH or seizures.[54] All complications are more common in elderly or debilitated patients.

Overall mortality with surgical treatment for CSDH is 0–8%.[54] In a series of 104 patients treated mostly with craniostomy,[56] mortality was ≈ 4%, all of which occurred in patients > 60 yrs old and were due to accompanying disease. Another large personal series reported 0.5% mortality.[57] Worsening of neurologic status following drainage occurs in ≈ 4%.[56]

64.6 Spontaneous subdural hematoma

64.6.1 General information

Occasionally patients with no identifiable trauma will present with severe H/A with or without associated findings (nausea, seizures, lethargy, focal findings including possible ipsilateral hemiparesis[58]…) and CT or MRI discloses a subdural hematoma that may be acute, subacute or chronic in appearance. The onset of symptoms is often sudden.[58]

64.6.2 Risk factors

Risk factors identified in a review of 21 cases in the literature[59] include:
1. hypertension: present in 7 cases
2. vascular abnormalities: arteriovenous malformation (AVM), aneurysm[60]
3. neoplasm
4. infection: including meningitis, tuberculosis
5. substance abuse: alcoholism, cocaine[61]
6. hypovitaminosis: especially vitamin C deficiency[37]
7. coagulopathies, including:
   a) iatrogenic (anticoagulation e.g., with warfarin)
   b) Ginkgo biloba (GB) extract: EGb761 and LI1379. Contains ginkgolides (especially Type B), which are inhibitors of platelet activating factor (PAF) at high concentrations[62]; also cause vasodilation and decreased blood viscosity. There have been case reports showing temporal relationship of hemorrhage to intake of GB,[63] especially at higher doses over long periods of time. However, no consistent alteration was demonstrable in 29 measurable coagulation/clotting variables after 7 days[64] (bleeding time was mildly prolonged in some case reports[63,65]). Some individuals may possibly be more susceptible to the supplement, and there may be as-yet uncharacterized interactions with other entities (such as alcohol, aspirin...), but studies so far have been unrevealing[66]
   c) factor XIII deficiency (protransglutaminase).[67,68] In peds: history may include report of bleeding from umbilical cord at birth. Check factor XIII levels as coagulation parameters may be normal or only slightly elevated
8. seemingly innocuous insults (e.g., bending over) or injuries resulting in no direct trauma to the head (e.g., whiplash injuries)
9. intracranial hypotension: spontaneous (p. 421), or following epidural anesthesia, lumbar puncture, or VP shunt[69,70]

64.6.3 Etiology

The bleeding site was determined in 14 of the 21 cases, and was *arterial* in each, typically involving a cortical branch of the MCA in the area of the Sylvian fissure[59] where there is a large number of branches to a wide cortical area.

Possible mechanisms for arterial rupture in idiopathic acute subdural hematoma (ASDH) include tears occurring secondary to sudden head movements or trivial head trauma of the following[71,72]:
1. small artery at perpendicular branch point off a cortical artery
2. small artery connecting the dura and cortex
3. adhesions between cortical artery and dura

64.6.4 Treatment

Same as for traumatic SDH. If symptomatic and/or > ≈ 1 cm thick, surgical evacuation is the treatment of choice. For subacute to chronic subdurals, burr hole evacuation is usually adequate (see above). For acute SDH, a craniotomy is usually required, and should expose the Sylvian fissure to identify bleeding point(s). Microsurgical repair of arterial wall has been described.[72]

64.7 Traumatic subdural hygroma

64.7.1 General information

From the Greek hygros, meaning wet. AKA traumatic subdural effusion, AKA hydroma. Excess fluid in the subdural space (may be clear, blood tinged, or xanthochromic and under variable pressure) is almost always associated with head trauma, especially alcohol-related falls or assaults.[73] Skull fractures were found in 39% of cases. Distinct from chronic subdural hematoma, which is usually associated with underlying cerebral contusion, and usually contains darker clots or brownish fluid ("motor oil" fluid), and may show membrane formation adjacent to inner surface of dura (hygromas lack membranes).

"Simple hygroma" refers to a hygroma without significant accompanying conditions. "Complex hygroma" refers to hygromas with associated significant subdural hematoma, epidural hematoma, or intracerebral hemorrhage.

64.7.2 Pathogenesis

Mechanism of formation of hygroma is probably a tear in the arachnoid membrane with resultant CSF leakage into the subdural compartment. Hygroma fluid contains pre-albumin, which is also found in CSF but not in subdural hematomas. The most likely locations of arachnoid tears are in the Sylvian fissure or the chiasmatic cistern. Another possible mechanism is post-meningitis effusion (especially influenza meningitis).

May be under high pressure. May increase in size (possibly due to a flap-valve mechanism) and exert mass effect, with the possibility of significant morbidity. Cerebral atrophy was present in 19% of patients with simple hygromas.

64.7.3 Presentation

▶ Table 64.4 shows clinical findings of subdural hygromas. Many present without focal findings. Complex hygromas usually present more acutely and require more urgent treatment.

Table 64.4 Major clinical features of traumatic subdural hygromas[73]

Type of hygroma	Simple	Complex	Total
number of patients	66	14	80
spontaneous eye opening	74%	57%	71%
disorientation or stupor	65%	57%	64%
mental status change without focal signs	52%	50%	51%
neurological plateau with deficit or delayed deterioration	42%	7%	36%
seizures (usually generalized)	36%	43%	38%
hemiparesis	32%	21%	30%
neck stiffness	26%	14%	24%
anisocoria (maintained light reflex)	15%	7%	14%
headache	14%	14%	14%
alert (no mental status change)	8%	0%	6%
hemiplegia	6%	14%	8%
comatose (responsive to pain only)	3%	43%	10%

64.7.4 Imaging

On CT, the density of the fluid is similar to that of CSF (▶ Fig. 64.7 panel A).
Signal characteristics on MRI follow those of CSF.

▶ **Differentiating a hygroma from a chronic subdural hematoma on imaging.** This may be very difficult. Clues:
1. the fluid in hygromas should be almost identical to CSF on CT (chronic SDH will tend to be slightly higher density) and MRI
2. **"cortical vein sign"**: hygromas typically expand the subarachnoid space and it may be possible to see a vein bridging from the cortex (which has been displaced inward) to the arachnoid membrane (which is now pressed up against the inner table of the skull) (▶ Fig. 64.7). In contrast, SDH will generally compress the arachnoid membrane against the brain and there will not be bridging veins. This sign is infrequently observed, and is best demonstrated on some MRI sequences or CT angiogram

64.7.5 Treatment

Asymptomatic hygromas do not require treatment. Recurrence following simple burr hole drainage is common. Many surgeons maintain a subdural drain for 24–48 hrs post-op. Recurrent cases may require either a craniotomy to locate the site of CSF leak (may be very difficult), or a subdural-peritoneal shunt may be placed.

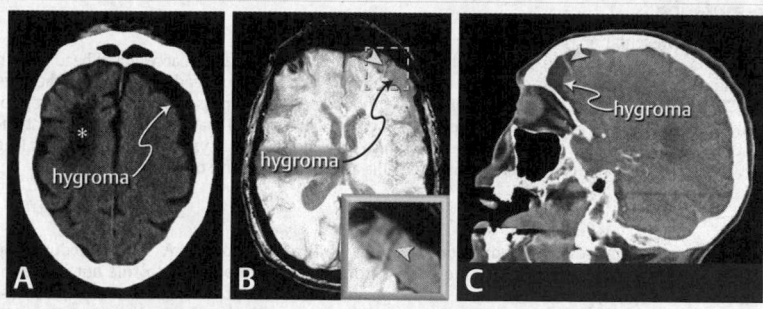

Fig. 64.7 Subdural hygroma over the left convexity.
Image: A: Axial CT scan (note previous stroke on the right (*asterisk*)), B: MRI SWI axial (inset shows magnified detail of area indicated by *broken blue line*), C: CTA sagittal.
Note: the "cortical vein sign" (bridging cortical vein) (*yellow arrowhead* in B & C, not seen in A).

64.7.6 Outcome

Outcome may be more related to accompanying injuries than to the hygroma itself.

5 of 9 patients with complex hygromas and subdural hematoma died. For simple hygromas, morbidity was 20% (12% for decreased mental status without focal findings, 32% if hemiparesis/plegia was present).

64.8 Extraaxial fluid collections in children

64.8.1 Differential diagnosis

1. benign subdural collection in infants (see below)
2. chronic *symptomatic* extraaxial fluid collections or effusions (see below)
3. cerebral atrophy: should not contain xanthochromic fluid with elevated protein
4. "external hydrocephalus": ventricles often enlarged, fluid is CSF (p. 433)
5. normal variant of enlarged subarachnoid spaces and interhemispheric fissure
6. acute subdural hematoma: high density (fresh blood) on CT (occasionally these will appear as low density collections in children with low hematocrits). Will usually be unilateral (the others above are usually bilateral). These lesions may occur as birth injuries, and typically present with seizures, pallor, tense fontanelle, poor respirations, hypotension, and retinal hemorrhages
7. "craniocerebral disproportion" (head too large for the brain)[74]: extracerebral spaces enlarged up to 1.5 cm in thickness and filled with CSF-like fluid (possibly CSF), ventricles at upper limits of normal, deep sulci, widened interhemispheric fissure, normal intracranial pressure. Patients are developmentally normal. May be the same as benign extra-axial fluid of infancy (see below). Making this diagnosis with certainty is difficult in first few months of life

64.8.2 Benign subdural collections of infancy

General information

Benign subdural collections (or effusions) of infancy,[75,76] are perhaps better characterized by the term benign extra-axial fluid collections of infancy, since it is difficult to distinguish whether they are subdural or subarachnoid.[77] They appear on CT as peripheral hypodensities over the frontal lobes in infants. Imaging may also show dilatation of the interhemispheric fissure, cortical sulci,[78] and Sylvian fissure. Ventricles are usually normal or slightly enlarged, with no evidence of transependymal absorption. Brain size is normal. Transillumination is increased over both frontal regions. The fluid is usually clear yellow (xanthochromic) with high protein content. The etiology of these is unclear; some cases may be due to perinatal trauma. They are more common in term infants than preemies. Must be differentiated from external hydrocephalus (p. 433).

Presentation

Mean age of presentation is ≈ 4 months.[77]

May show: signs of elevated intracranial pressure (tense or large fontanelle, accelerated head growth crossing percentile curves), developmental delay usually as a result of poor head control due to the large size (Carolan et al feel that developmental delay without macrocrania runs counter to the concept of "benign" collections[77]), frontal bossing, jitteriness. The poor head control may lead to positional flattening. Other symptoms, such as seizures (possibly focal) are indicative of symptomatic collections (see below). Large collections in the absence of macrocrania are more suggestive of cerebral atrophy.

Treatment

Most cases gradually resolve spontaneously, often within 8–9 months. A single subdural tap (p. 1811) for diagnostic purposes (to differentiate from cortical atrophy and to rule out infection) may be done, and may accelerate the rate of disappearance. Repeat physical exams with OFC measurements should be done at ≈ 3–6 month intervals. Head growth usually parallels or approaches normal curves by ≈ 1–2 yrs of age, and by 30–36 months orbital-frontal head circumference (OFC) approaches normal percentiles for height and weight. They usually catch up developmentally as OFCs normalize.

64.8.3 Symptomatic chronic extraaxial fluid collections in children

General information

Variously classified as hematomas (chronic subdural hematoma), effusions, or hygromas, with differing definitions associated with each. Since the appearance on imaging and the treatment is similar, Litofsky et al proposed that they all be classified as extraaxial fluid collections.[79] The difference between these lesions and "benign" subdural effusions (see above) may simply be the degree of clinical manifestation.

Etiologies

The following etiologies were listed in a series of 103 cases[79]:
1. 36% were thought to be the result of trauma (22 were victims of child abuse)
2. 22% followed bacterial meningitis (post-infectious)
3. 19 occurred after placement or revision of a shunt (p. 464)
4. no cause could be identified in 17 patients

Other causes include[74]:
1. tumors: extracerebral or intracerebral
2. post-asphyxia with hypoxic brain damage and cerebral atrophy
3. defects of hemostasis: vitamin K deficiency…

Signs and symptoms

Symptoms include: seizure (26%), large head (22%), vomiting (20%), irritability (13%), lethargy (13%), headache (older children), poor feeding, respiratory arrest…

Signs include: full fontanelle (30%), macrocrania (25%), fever (17%), lethargy (13%), hemiparesis (12%), retinal hemorrhages, coma, papilledema, developmental delay…

Evaluation

CT/MRI usually shows ventricular compression and obliteration of the cerebral sulci, unlike with benign subdural collections. The "cortical vein sign" (p. 434) helps distinguish this from external hydrocephalus.

Treatment

Options include:
1. observation: follow-up with serial OFC measurements, ultrasound, and CT/MRI
2. serial percutaneous subdural taps (p. 1811): some patients require as many as 16 taps.[80] Some series show good results and others show low success rate[81,82]

3. burr hole drainage: may include long-term external drainage. Simple burr hole drainage may not be effective with severe craniocephalic disproportion since the brain will not expand to obliterate the extra-axial space
4. subdural-peritoneal shunt: unilateral shunt is usually adequate even for bilateral effusions[79,82,83] (recent recommendations: no study is required to demonstrate communication between the 2 sides[79,84]). An extremely low pressure system should be utilized. The general practice is to remove the shunt after 2–3 months of drainage (once the collections are obliterated) to reduce the risk of associated mineralization of the dura and arachnoid and possible risk of seizures (these shunts are easily removed at this time, but may be more difficult to remove at a later date)[85]

Other recommendations:

At least one percutaneous tap should be performed to rule out infection.

Many authors recommend observation for the patient with no symptoms or with only enlarging head and developmental delay.

64.9 Traumatic posterior fossa mass lesions

64.9.1 General information

Less than 3% of head injuries involve traumatic mass lesions of the posterior fossa.[86] Epidural hematomas (p.1072) constitute the majority of these. The small remainder is comprised of subdural hematoma (see below and ▶ Fig. 64.8) and intraparenchymal hematoma[87]. Any of these can cause hydrocephalus[86] typically by displacing and compressing the 4th ventricle or its outlets. Until hydrocephalus develops, these hematomas may not produce elevated ICP using conventional monitoring techniques.

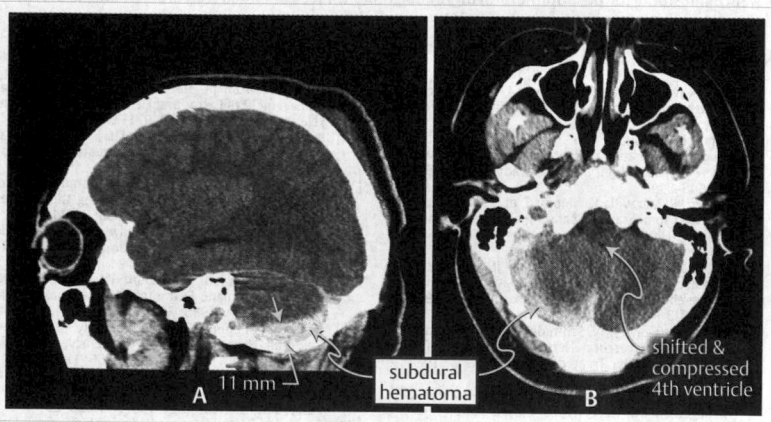

Fig. 64.8 Right-sided posterior fossa subdural hematoma.
Image: A: sagittal CT scan through the right cerebellar hemisphere. B: axial CT scan.

64.9.2 Posterior fossa subdural hematoma

Rare (comprise < 3% of TBIs[88]).

Based on case reports and retrospective series, the prognosis is poor (63% poor outcomes[88]).

64.9.3 Management

See **Practice guideline: Surgical management of traumatic posterior fossa mass lesions** (p.1090) for surgical management recommendations.

Practice guideline: Surgical management of traumatic posterior fossa mass lesions

Indications for surgery

Level III[89]: symptomatic posterior fossa mass lesions or those with mass effect on CT should be surgically removed. **Note:** mass effect on CT: defined as dislocation, compression or obliteration of the 4th ventricle; compression or loss of basal cisterns (p. 1109) or the presence of obstructive hydrocephalus

• asymptomatic lesions without mass effect on CT may be managed with close observation and serial imaging

Timing of surgery

Level III[89]: p-fossa mass lesions meeting surgical criteria should be evacuated ASAP due to the potential for rapid deterioration

Surgical methods

Level III[89]: suboccipital craniectomy (not replacing the bone) as opposed to craniotomy, is the recommended procedure because post-op bleeding or swelling is poorly tolerated in the small confines of the posterior fossa

Most parenchymal hemorrhages managed nonsurgically were < 3 cm in diameter.
Other options for surgical intervention[88]:
• bilateral suboccipital decompression: consider for patients with GCS < 9 or if mass effect is present on the initial CT
• resection of posterior arch of C1: suggested if tonsillar herniation is evident
• ventriculostomy for post op monitoring/management: recommended if hydrocephalus is present

References

[1] Bullock MR, Chesnut RM, Ghajar J, et al. Surgical management of traumatic parenchymal lesions. Neurosurgery. 2006; 58:S25–S46

[2] Lipper MH, Kishore PRS, Girevendulis AK, et al. Delayed Intracranial Hematoma in Patients with Severe Head Injury. Neuroradiology. 1979; 133:645–649

[3] Cooper PR, Maravilla K, Moody S, et al. Serial Computerized Tomographic Scanning and the Prognosis of Severe Head Injury. Neurosurgery. 1979; 5:566–569

[4] Gudeman SK, Kishore PR, Miller JD, et al. The Genesis and Significance of Delayed Traumatic Intracerebral Hematoma. Neurosurgery. 1979; 5:309–313

[5] Young HA, Gleave JRW, Schmidek HH, et al. Delayed Traumatic Intracerebral Hematoma: Report of 15 Cases Operatively Treated. Neurosurgery. 1984; 14:22–25

[6] Rockswold GL, Leonard PR, Nagib M. Analysis of Management in Thirty-Three Closed Head Injury Patients Who "Talked and Deteriorated". Neurosurgery. 1987; 21:51–55

[7] Cohen TI, Gudeman SK, Narayan RK, et al. Delayed Traumatic Intracranial Hematoma. In: Neurotrauma. New York: McGraw-Hill; 1996:689–701

[8] McKissock W, Taylor JC, Bloom WH, et al. Extradural Hematoma: Observations on 125 Cases. Lancet. 1960; 2:167–172

[9] Kernohan JW, Woltman HW. Incisura of the Crus due to Contralateral Brain Tumor. Arch Neurol Psychiatr. 1929; 21

[10] Tsai FY, Teal JS, Hieshima GB. Neuroradiology of Head Trauma. Baltimore: University Park Press; 1984

[11] Greenberg JJ, Cohen WA, Cooper PR. The "hyperacute" extraaxial intracranial hematoma: computed tomographic findings and clinical significance. Neurosurgery. 1985; 17:48–56

[12] Kaye EM, Cass PR, Dooling E, et al. Chronic Epidural Hematomas in Childhood: Increased Recognition and Nonsurgical Management. Pediat Neurol. 1985; 1:255–259

[13] Pang D, Horton JA, Herron JM, et al. Nonsurgical Management of Extradural Hematomas in Children. J Neurosurg. 1983; 59:958–971

[14] Bullock MR, Chesnut RM, Ghajar J, et al. Surgical management of acute epidural hematomas. Neurosurgery. 2006; 58:S7–15

[15] Rivas JJ, Lobato RD, Sarabia R, et al. Extradural Hematoma: Analysis of Factors Influencing the Courses of 161 Patients. Neurosurgery. 1988; 23:44–51

[16] Piepmeier JM, Wagner FC. Delayed Post-Traumatic Extracerebral Hematoma. J Trauma. 1982; 22:455–460

[17] Borovich B, Braun J, Guilburd JN, et al. Delayed Onset of Traumatic Extradural Hematoma. Journal of Neurosurgery. 1985; 63:30–34

[18] Bucci MN, Phillips TW, McGillicuddy JE. Delayed Epidural Hemorrhage in Hypotensive Multiple Trauma Patients. Neurosurgery. 1986; 19:65–68

[19] Riesgo P, Piquer J, Botella C, et al. Delayed Extradural Hematoma After Mild Head Injury: Report of Three Cases. Surgical Neurology. 1997; 48:226–231

[20] Zuccarello M, Pardatscher K, Andrioli GC, et al. Epidural hematomas of the posterior cranial fossa. Neurosurgery. 1981; 8:434–437

[21] Roda JM, Giminez D, Perez-Higueras A, et al. Posterior Fossa Epidural Hematomas: A Review and Synthesis. Surgical Neurology. 1983; 19:419–424

[22] Aoki N, Oikawa A, Sakai T. Symptomatic Subacute Subdural Hematoma Associated with Cerebral Hemispheric Swelling and Ischemia. Neurol Res. 1996; 18:145–149

[23] Nishio M, Akagi K, Abekura M, et al. [A Case of Traumatic Subacute Subdural Hematoma Presenting Symptoms Arising from Cerebral Hemisphere Edema]. No Shinkei Geka. 1998; 26:425–429

[24] Wintzen AR, Tijssen JGP. Subdural Hematoma and Oral Anticoagulation Therapy. Annals of Neurology. 1982; 39:69–72

[25] Kawamata T, Takeshita M, Kubo O, et al. Management of Intracranial Hemorrhage Associated with Anticoagulant Therapy. Surgical Neurology. 1995; 44:438–443

[26] Munro D, Merritt HH. Surgical Pathology of Subdural Hematoma: Based on a Study of One Hundred and Five Cases. Arch Neurol Psychiatry. 1936; 35:64–78

[27] Bullock MR, Chesnut RM, Ghajar J, et al. Surgical management of acute subdural hematomas. Neurosurgery. 2006; 58:S16–S24

[28] Seelig JM, Becker DP, Miller JD, et al. Traumatic Acute Subdural Hematoma: Major Mortality Reduction in Comatose Patients Treated within Four Hours. N Engl J Med. 1981; 304:1511–1518

[29] Wilberger JE, Harris M, Diamond DL. Acute Subdural Hematoma: Morbidity, Mortality, and Operative Timing. J Neurosurg. 1991; 74:212–218

[30] Howard MA, Gross AS, Dacey RG, et al. Acute Subdural Hematomas: An Age-Dependent Clinical Entity. J Neurosurg. 1989; 71:858–863

[31] Houtteville JP, Toumi K, Theoron J, et al. Interhemispheric subdural hematoma: seven cases and review of the literature. British Journal of Neurosurgery. 1988; 2:357–367

[32] Duhaime A-C, Gennarelli TA, Thibault LE, et al. The Shaken Baby Syndrome: A Clinical, Pathological, and Biomechanical Study. J Neurosurg. 1987; 66:409–415

[33] Rapana A, Lamaida E, Pizza V, et al. Inter-hemispheric scissure, a rare location for a traumatic subdural hematoma, case report and review of the literature. Clinical Neurology and Neurosurgery. 1997; 99:124–129

[34] Fein JM, Rovit RL. Interhemispheric subdural hematoma secondary to hemorrhage from a calloso-marginal artery aneurysm. Neuroradiology. 1970; 1:183–186

[35] Aoki N, Masuzawa H. Infantile Acute Subdural Hematoma. J Neurosurg. 1984; 61:273–280

[36] Ikeda A, Sato O, Tsugane R, et al. Infantile Acute Subdural Hematoma. Childs Nerv Syst. 1987; 3:19–22

[37] Scott M. Spontaneous Nontraumatic Subdural Hematomas. JAMA. 1949; 141:596–602

[38] Robinson RG. Chronic Subdural Hematoma: Surgical Management in 133 Patients. Journal of Neurosurgery. 1984; 61:263–268

[39] Wakai S, Hashimoto K, Watanabe N, et al. Efficacy of Closed-System Drainage in Treating Chronic Subdural Hematoma: A Prospective Comparative Study. Neurosurgery. 1990; 26:771–773

[40] Fogelholm R, Heiskanen O, Waltimo O. Influence of Patient's Age on Symptoms, Signs, and Thickness of Hematoma. Journal of Neurosurgery. 1975; 42:43–46

[41] Weir BK, Gordon P. Factors Affecting Coagulation, Fibrinolysis in Chronic Subdural Fluid Collection. Journal of Neurosurgery. 1983; 58:242–245

[42] Labadie EL, Sawaya R. Fibrinolysis in the Formation and Growth of Chronic Subdural Hematomas. In: Fibrinolysis and the Central Nervous System. Philadelphia: Hanley and Belfus; 1990:141–148

[43] Drapkin AJ. Chronic Subdural Hematoma: Pathophysiological Basis of Treatment. Br J Neurosurgery. 1991; 5:467–473

[44] Markwalder T-M, Steinsiepe KF, Rohner M, et al. The course of chronic subdural hematomas after burr-hole craniotomy and closed-system drainage. J Neurosurg. 1981; 55:390–393

[45] Hamilton MG, Frizzell JB, Tranmer BI. Chronic Subdural Hematoma: The Role for Craniotomy Reevaluated. Neurosurgery. 1993; 33:67–72

[46] Abouzari M, Rashidi A, Rezaii J, et al. The role of postoperative patient posture in the recurrence of traumatic chronic subdural hematoma after burr-hole surgery. Neurosurgery. 2007; 61:794–7; discussion 797

[47] Caron J-L, Worthington C, Bertrand G. Tension Pneumocephalus After Evacuation of Chronic Subdural Hematoma and Subsequent Treatment with Continuous Lumbar Subarachnoid Infusion and Craniostomy Drainage. Neurosurgery. 1985; 16:107–110

[48] Liu W, Bakker NA, Groen RJ. Chronic subdural hematoma: a systematic review and meta-analysis of surgical procedures. J Neurosurg. 2014; 121:665–673

[49] Camel M, Grubb RL. Treatment of Chronic Subdural Hematoma by Twist-Drill Craniostomy with Continuous Catheter Drainage. Journal of Neurosurgery. 1986; 65:183–187

[50] Hubschmann OR. Twist Drill Craniostomy in the Treatment of Chronic and Subacute Hematomas in Severely Ill and Elderly Patients. Neurosurgery. 1980; 6:233–236

[51] Tabaddor K, Shulman K. Definitive Treatment of Chronic Subdural Hematoma by Twist-Drill Craniostomy and Closed-System Drainage. J Neurosurg. 1977; 46:220–226

[52] Lind CR, Lind CJ, Mee EW. Reduction in the number of repeated operations for the treatment of subacute and chronic subdural hematomas by placement of subdural drains. Journal of Neurosurgery. 2003; 99:44–46

[53] Arginteanu MS, Byun H, King W. Treatment of a recurrent subdural hematoma using urokinase. Journal of Neurotrauma. 1999; 16:1235–1239

[54] Ogasawara K, Koshu K, Yoshimoto T, et al. Transient Hyperemia Immediately After Rapid Decompression of Chronic Subdural Hematoma. Neurosurgery. 1999; 45:484–489

[55] Dill SR, Cobbs CG, McDonald CK. Subdural Empyema: Analysis of 32 Cases and Review. Clin Inf Dis. 1995; 20:372–386

[56] Ernestus R-I, Beldzinski P, Lanfermann H, et al. Chronic Subdural Hematoma: Surgical Treatment and Outcome in 104 Patients. Surgical Neurology. 1997; 48:220–225

[57] Sambasivan M. An Overview of Chronic Subdural Hematoma: Experience with 2300 Cases. Surgical Neurology. 1997; 47:418–422

[58] Talalla A, McKissock W. Acute 'Spontaneous' Subdural Hemorrhage: An Unusual Form of Cerebrovascular Accident. Neurology. 1971; 21:19–25

[59] Hesselbrock R, Sawaya R, Means ED. Acute Spontaneous Subdural Hematoma. Surg Neurol. 1984; 21:363–366

[60] Korosue K, Kondoh T, Ishikawa Y, et al. Acute Subdural Hematoma Associated with Nontraumatic Middle Meningeal Artery Aneurysm: Case Report. Neurosurgery. 1988; 22:411–413

[61] Keller TM, Chappell ET. Spontaneous acute subdural hematoma precipitated by cocaine abuse: case report. Surgical Neurology. 1997; 47:12–4; discussion 14-5

[62] Koch E. Inhibition of platelet activating factor (PAF)-induced aggregation of human thrombocytes by ginkgolides: considerations on possible bleeding complications after oral intake of Ginkgo biloba extracts. Phytomedicine. 2005; 12:10–16

[63] Rowin J, Lewis SL. Spontaneous bilateral subdural hematomas associated with chronic Ginkgo biloba ingestion. Neurology. 1996; 46:1775–1776

[64] Kohler S, Funk P, Kieser M. Influence of a 7-day treatment with Ginkgo biloba special extract EGb 761 on bleeding time and coagulation: a randomized, placebo-controlled, double-blind study in healthy volunteers. Blood Coagul Fibrinolysis. 2004; 15:303–309

[65] Vale S. Subarachnoid haemorrhage associated with Ginkgo biloba. Lancet. 1998; 352

[66] Wolf HR. Does Ginkgo biloba special extract EGb 761 provide additional effects on coagulation and bleeding when added to acetylsalicylic acid 500 mg daily? Drugs R D. 2006; 7:163–172

[67] Albanese A, Tuttolomondo A, Anile C, et al. Spontaneous chronic subdural hematomas in young adults with a deficiency in coagulation factor XIII. Report of three cases. Journal of Neurosurgery. 2005; 102:1130–1132

[68] Vural M, Yarar C, Durmaz R, et al. Spontaneous Acute Subdural Hematoma and Chronic Epidural Hematoma in a Child with F XIII Deficiency. Journal of Emergency Medicine. 2008. DOI: 10.1016/j.jemermed.2007.11.041

[69] de Noronha RJ, Sharrack B, Hadjivassiliou M, et al. Subdural haematoma: a potentially serious consequence of spontaneous intracranial hypotension. Journal of Neurology, Neurosurgery, and Psychiatry. 2003; 74:752–755

64

[70] Chung SJ, Lee JH, Kim SJ, et al. Subdural hematoma in spontaneous CSF hypovolemia. Neurology. 2006; 67:1088–1089

[71] McDermott M, Fleming JF, Vanderlinden RG, et al. Spontaneous arterial subdural hematoma. Neurosurgery. 1984; 14:13–18

[72] Matsuyama T, Shimomura T, Okumura Y, et al. Acute subdural hematomas due to rupture of cortical arteries: a study of the points of rupture in 19 cases. Surgical Neurology. 1997; 47:423–427

[73] Stone JL, Lang RGR, Sugar O, et al. Traumatic Subdural Hygroma. Neurosurgery. 1981; 8:542–550

[74] Strassburg HM. Macrocephaly is Not Always Due to Hydrocephalus. J Child Neurol. 1989; 4:S32–S40

[75] Briner S, Bodensteiner J. Benign Subdural Collections of Infancy. Pediatrics. 1980; 67:802–804

[76] Robertson WC, Chun RWM, Orrison WW, et al. Benign Subdural Collections of Infancy. J Pediatr. 1979; 94

[77] Carolan PL, McLaurin RL, Towbin RB, et al. Benign Extraaxial Collections of Infancy. Pediatric Neurosciences. 1986; 12:140–144

[78] Mori K, Handa H, Itoh M, et al. Benign Subdural Effusion in Infants. J Comput Assist Tomogr. 1980; 4:466–471

[79] Litofsky NS, Raffel C, McComb JG. Management of Symptomatic Chronic Extra-Axial Fluid Collections in Pediatric Patients. Neurosurgery. 1992; 31:445–450

[80] McLaurin RL, Isaacs E, Lewis HP. Results of Nonoperative Treatment in 15 Cases of Infantile Subdural Hematoma. Journal of Neurosurgery. 1971; 34:753–759

[81] Herzberger E, Rotem Y, Braham J. Remarks on Thirty-Three Cases of Subdural Effusions in Infancy. Arch Dis Childhood. 1956; 31:44–50

[82] Moyes PD. Subdural Effusions in Infants. Can Med Assoc J. 1969; 100:231–234

[83] Aoki N, Miztani H, Masuzawa H. Unilateral Subdural-Peritoneal Shunting for Bilateral Chronic Subdural Hematomas in Infancy. J Neurosurg. 1985; 63:134–137

[84] Aoki N. Chronic Subdural Hematoma in Infancy. Clinical Analysis of 30 Cases in the CT Era. Journal of Neurosurgery. 1990; 73:201–205

[85] Johnson DL. Comment on Litofsky N S, et al.: Management of Symptomatic Chronic Extra-Axial Fluid Collections in Pediatric Patients. Neurosurgery. 1992; 31

[86] Karasawa H, Furuya H, Naito H, et al. Acute hydrocephalus in posterior fossa injury. J Neurosurg. 1997; 86:629–632

[87] d'Avella D, Servadei F, Scerrati M, et al. Traumatic intracerebellar hemorrhage: clinicoradiological analysis of 81 patients. Neurosurgery. 2002; 50:16–25; discussion 25-7

[88] de Amorim RL, Stiver SI, Paiva WS, et al. Treatment of traumatic acute posterior fossa subdural hematoma: report of four cases with systematic review and management algorithm. Acta Neurochir (Wien). 2014; 156:199–206

[89] Bullock MR, Chesnut RM, Ghajar J, et al. Surgical management of posterior fossa mass lesions. Neurosurgery. 2006; 58:S47–S55

65 Gunshot Wounds and Non-Missile Penetrating Brain Injuries

65.1 Gunshot wounds to the head

65.1.1 General information

Gunshot wounds to the head (GSWH) account for the majority of penetrating brain injuries, and comprise ≈ 35% of deaths from brain injury in persons < 45 yrs old. GSWH are the most lethal type of head injury, ≈ two-thirds die at the scene, and GSWH ultimately are the proximal cause of death in > 90% of victims.[1]

65.1.2 Primary injury

Primary injury from GSWH results from a number of factors including:
1. injury to soft tissue
   a) direct scalp and/or facial injuries
   b) soft tissue and bacteria may be dragged intracranially, the devitalized tissue may also then support growth of the bacteria
   c) pressure waves of gas combustion may cause injury if the weapon is close
2. comminuted fracture of bone: may injure subjacent vascular and/or cortical tissue (depressed skull fracture). May act as secondary missiles
3. cerebral injuries from missile
   a) direct injury to brain tissue in path of bullet, exacerbated by
      • fragmentation of bullet
      • ricochet off bone
      • deviations of the bullet from a straight path as it travels: tumbling (forward rotation – pitch), yaw (rotation about vertical axis), rotation (spin), nutation (similar to precession or wobble)
      • deformation of bullet at impact: e.g., mushrooming
   b) injury to tissue by shock waves, cavitation
4. coup + contrecoup injury from missile impact on head (may cause injuries distant from bullet path)

Because of the complexities of ballistics (some of which are described above) there is often more damage distally than at the entry site even though the bullet slows (losing kinetic energy).
   Extent of primary injury is related to *impact velocity*:
• *impact* velocity > 100 m/s: causes explosive intracranial injury that is uniformly fatal (NB: impact velocity is less than muzzle velocity)
• non-bullet missiles (e.g., grenade fragments) are considered low velocity
• low *muzzle* velocity bullets (≈ < 250 m/s): as with most handguns. Tissue injury is caused primarily by laceration and maceration along a path slightly wider than missile diameter
• high *muzzle* velocity bullets (≈ 600–750 m/s): from military weapons and hunting rifles. Causes additional damage by shock waves and temporary cavitation (tissue pushed away from the missile causes a conical cavity of injury that may exceed bullet diameter many-fold, and causes low-pressure region which may draw surface debris into the wound)

65.1.3 Secondary injury

Cerebral edema occurs similar to closed head injury. ICP may rise rapidly within minutes (higher ICPs result from higher impact velocities). Cardiac output may also fall initially. Together, ↑ ICP and ↓ MAP adversely affect cerebral perfusion pressure.
   Other common complicating factors include: DIC, intracranial hemorrhage from lacerated blood vessels.

65.1.4 Late complications

Late complications include:
1. cerebral abscess: migration of bullet may be a tip-off (see below). Usually associated with retained contaminated material (bullet, bone, skin...) but may also result from persistent communication with nasal sinuses
2. traumatic aneurysm (p. 1491) [2]: typically in distal ACA (▶ Fig. 89.1)
3. seizures
4. fragment migration
    a) migration of a bullet: often indicates abscess[3] or, less commonly, a hematoma cavity. May also migrate within the ventricles
    b) intraventricular fragments may migrate and cause obstructive hydrocephalus[4]
5. lead toxicity (p. 1219): more of an issue with bullet in disc space

65.1.5 Evaluation

Physical exam

Exam should describe visible entrance and exit wounds. In through-and-through missile wounds of the skull, the entrance wound is typically smaller than the exit wound due to bullet mushrooming. Entrance wounds may be especially small with direct contact of the muzzle to the head. At surgery or autopsy, the entrance wound will typically show bevelling of the inner table, whereas exit wounds have a bevelled outer table.

Imaging

AP and lateral skull X-rays
This is one situation where skull X-rays still may provide useful information, as they are less susceptible to artifact from the bullet than the CT scan. Helps to localize metal and bone fragments, and to help identify entrance/exit sites (omit if time not available)

Head CT scan without contrast
The main assessment tool. Demonstrates location of bone and metal. Delineates bullet trajectory: assesses if bullet passed through ventricles and how many quadrants of the hemisphere have been traversed. Shows amount of blood in brain and assesses intracranial hematomas (epidural, subdural or intraparenchymal).

Angiography in GSWH
Rarely performed emergently. When done, usually performed on ≈ day 2–3.
 Indications for angiography[5]:
• unexpected delayed hemorrhage
• a trajectory that would likely involve named vessels in a salvageable patient
• large intraparenchymal hemorrhages in a salvageable patient

65.1.6 Management

Initial management

General measures
1. CPR as required; endotracheal intubation if stuporous or airway compromised
2. additional injuries (e.g., chest wounds) identified and treated appropriately
3. usual precautions taken for spine injury
4. fluids as needed to replace estimated blood loss which may be variable: exercise restraint to avoid excessive hydration (to minimize cerebral edema)
5. pressors to support MAP during and after fluid resuscitation

Treatment specific to the injury
Neurological assessment as rapidly as possible and as thoroughly as time permits.
 The Glasgow Coma Scale is still the most widely used grading system and allows better comparison between series than specialized scales for GSWHs.

Decision by experienced neurosurgeon regarding the ultimate treatment of the patient will determine appropriate steps to be taken. Patients with little CNS function (in the absence of shock) are unlikely to benefit from craniotomy; supportive measures are indicated in most of these cases with (for possibility of organ donation, opportunity for family to adjust to situation, and requirements for observation period to determine actual brain death).

In patients considered for further treatment, rapid deterioration at any point with signs of herniation requires immediate surgical intervention. As time permits, the following should be undertaken:

1. initial steps
   a) control bleeding from scalp and associated wounds (hemostats on scalp vessels)
   b) shave scalp to identify entrance/exit sites, and to save time in the O.R.
2. medical treatment (similar to closed head injury)
   a) assume ICP is elevated:
      - elevate HOB 30–45° with head midline (avoids kinking jugular veins)
      - mannitol (1 gm/kg bolus) as blood pressure tolerates
      - hyperventilate to $PaCO_2$ = 30–35 mm Hg if indications are met (p. 1053)
      - steroids: (unproven efficacy) 10 mg dexamethasone IVP
   b) prophylaxis against GI ulcers: H2 antagonist (e.g., ranitidine 50 mg IVPB q 8 hrs) or proton pump inhibitor, NG tube to suction
   c) begin antiseizure medications (does not reduce incidence of late seizures)
   d) antibiotics: generally used although no controlled study demonstrates efficacy in preventing meningitis or abscess. Most organisms are sensitive to penicillinase resistant agents, e.g., *nafcillin*, recommended for ≈ 5 days
   e) tetanus toxoid administration

Surgical treatment

Indications for surgery are controversial. Some authors suggest that better outcome might occur with more aggressive management, and that poor outcome may be a self-fulfilling prophecy.[6] Patients with minimal neurologic function, e.g., fixed pupils, decorticate or decerebrate posturing… (when not in shock and with good oxygenation) should *not* be operated upon, because the chance of meaningful recovery is close to zero. Patients with less severe injuries should be considered for urgent operation.

Goals of surgery

1. debridement of devitalized tissue: less tissue is injured in civilian GSWH, but elevated ICP post-op may imply more vigorous debridement was needed, especially of non-eloquent brain (e.g., temporal tips)
2. evacuation of hematomas: subdural, intraparenchymal…
3. removal of *accessible* bone fragments
4. retrieval of bullet fragment for forensic purposes (note: everyone who handles the fragments may be subpoenaed to testify as to the "chain of evidence"). Large intact fragments should be sought as they tend to migrate (**note**: risk of infection and seizures due to retained bullet fragments is not high in civilian GSWH; therefore only accessible fragments should be sought and removed)
5. obtaining hemostasis
6. watertight dural closure (usually requires graft)
7. separation of intracranial compartment from air sinuses traversed by bullet
8. identification of entry and exit wounds for forensic purposes; see Evaluation (p. 1094)

Surgical technique

Some key points of surgical technique[7 (p 2098–104)]:
- positioning and draping should make both entry and exit wounds accessible
- devitalized tissue around the entry & exit wounds should be excised
- fractured bone should be excised by a circumferential craniectomy (craniotomy may be used in some civilian GSWH; the entry site within the craniotomy should be rongeured or drilled back to clean bone)
- air sinuses that are traversed should have the mucosa exenterated, and are then packed with muscle, and covered with a graft (e.g., periosteum or fascia lata) to separate them from intracranial compartment
- the dura is opened in a stellate fashion

- pulped brain is removed from within using suction and bipolar in an enlarging cone until healthy tissue is encountered (further injury to deep midline structures should be avoided, here, stay within bullet tract)
- contralateral fragments with no exit wound should only be removed if accessible
- intraventricular fragments can present significant risk. Ventriculoscopy (if available) may be well suited for removing these
- dural closure should be watertight; grafts of pericranium, temporalis fascia, or fascia lata grafts may be used; avoid dura substitutes
- cranioplasty should be delayed 6–12 months to reduce risk of infection
- a post-op CSF fistula that persists > 2 weeks should be repaired

ICP monitoring

ICP is often elevated after surgical debridement[6] and monitoring may be warranted.

Outcome

Prognostic factors:

1. level of consciousness is the most important prognostic factor: ≈ 94% of patients who are comatose with inappropriate or absent response to noxious stimulus on admission die, and half the survivors are severely disabled[8]
2. as initially espoused by Cushing, the path of the bullet is also an important prognosticator. Especially *poor prognosis* is associated with:
   a) bullets that cross the midline
   b) bullets that pass through the geographic center of the brain
   c) bullets that enter or traverse the ventricles
   d) the more lobes traversed by the bullet
3. hematomas seen on CT are poor prognostic findings
4. suicide attempts are more likely to be fatal

65.2 Non-missile penetrating trauma

65.2.1 General information

This section deals with penetrating injuries to the brain (and to some extent to the spinal cord) excluding missile injuries, i.e., gunshot wounds (p. 1093). Includes trauma from: knives, arrows, lawn darts… Injury to neural tissue tends to be more limited than with missiles because many of the associated injurious aspects of the missile are absent (p. 1093).

65.2.2 Arrow injuries

As a result of the lower velocity (e.g., 58 m/s) compared to firearms and the sharp tip, injury is usually limited to tissue directly incised by the arrowhead.[9]

65.2.3 Cases with foreign body still embedded

In penetrating trauma, it is usually not appropriate to remove any protruding part of the foreign body until the patient is in the operating room, unless it cannot be avoided. If possible, it is helpful to have another identical object for comparison in planning extrication of the embedded object.[10] To minimize extending the trauma to the CNS, the protruding object should be stabilized in some way during transportation and evaluation. Intraoperatively, devices such as the Greenberg retractor may be used to stabilize the object during preparation and the initial approach.

65.2.4 Indications for pre-op angiography

1. object passes in region of large named artery
2. object passes near dural sinuses
3. visible evidence of arterial bleeding: angiography is not appropriate if hemorrhage cannot be controlled

65.2.5 Surgical techniques

It is impossible to give details to cover every situation. Some guidelines:
1. empiric antibiotic coverage is appropriate; see Meningitis post craniospinal trauma (p. 340). Take cultures from the wound and the foreign body to guide later antibiotic therapy
2. optimal control can usually be gained by performing a craniotomy up to and if possible around the object, such that removing the bone flap will not disturb the object. The last remnants of bone may then be removed with a rongeur
3. if at all possible open the dura before removing the object, since removal with the dura closed does not allow adequate control of any bleeding from the brain
4. removal of the object ideally should follow the entry trajectory if possible
5. although gunshot wounds are not sterile as once thought, they are probably less contaminated than penetrating wounds. One should debride any easily accessible impacted bone and other extracranial tissue and material along the track

65.2.6 Post-op care

1. a course of antibiotics are usually appropriate since infection is common
2. consider a post-op arteriogram to rule out traumatic aneurysm

References

[1] Kaufman HH. Civilian Gunshot Wounds to the Head. Neurosurgery. 1993; 32:962–964
[2] Kaufman HH, Moake JL, Olson JD, et al. Delayed Intracerebral Hematoma due to Traumatic Aneurysm caused by a Shotgun Wound: A Problem in Prophylaxis. Neurosurgery. 1980; 6:181–184
[3] DesChamps GT, Jr, Morano JU. Intracranial bullet migration - a sign of brain abscess: case report. J Trauma. 1991; 31:293–295
[4] Sternbergh WC, Jr, Watts C, Clark K. Bullet within the fourth ventricle. Case report. J Neurosurg. 1971; 34:805–807
[5] Miner ME. Comment on Benzel E C, et al.: Civilian Craniocerebral Gunshot Wounds. Neurosurgery. 1991; 29

[6] Kaufman HH, Makela ME, Lee KF, et al. Gunshot Wounds to the Head: A Perspective. Neurosurgery. 1986; 18:689–695
[7] Youmans JR. Neurological Surgery. Philadelphia 1990
[8] Benzel EC, Day WT, Kesterson L, et al. Civilian Craniocerebral Gunshot Wounds. Neurosurgery. 1991; 29:67–72
[9] Karger B, Sudhues H, Kneubuehl BP, et al. Experimental arrow wounds: ballistics and traumatology. J Trauma. 1998; 45:495–501
[10] Salvino CK, Origitano TC, Dries DJ, et al. Transoral Crossbow Injury to the Cervical Spine: An Unusual Case of Penetrating Cervical Spine Injury. Neurosurgery. 1991; 28:904–907

65

66 Pediatric Head Injury

66.1 Epidemiology of pediatric head injury and comparison to adults

75% of children hospitalized for trauma have a head injury. Although most pediatric head injuries are mild and involve only evaluation or brief hospital stays, CNS injuries are the most common cause of pediatric traumatic death.[1] The overall mortality for all pediatric head injuries requiring hospitalization has been reported between 10–13%,[2] whereas the mortality associated with severe pediatric head injury presenting with decerebrate posturing has been reported as high as 71%.[3]

Differences between adult and pediatric head injury:
1. epidemiology:
   a) children often have milder injuries than adults
   b) lower chance of a surgical lesion in a comatose child than in an adult[4]
2. types of injury: injuries peculiar to pediatrics
   a) birth injuries: skull fractures, cephalhematoma (see below), subdural or epidural hematomas, brachial plexus injuries (p. 579)
   b) perambulator/walker injuries
   c) nonaccidental trauma (p. 1103) (NAT) (formerly child abuse): shaken baby syndrome…
   d) injuries from skateboarding, scooters…
   e) injuries related to the easier penetrability of the pediatric skull: e.g., recreational lawn darts
   f) cephalhematoma: see below
   g) leptomeningeal cysts, AKA "growing skull fractures" (p. 1100)
   h) retroclival hematoma (p. 1102)
3. response to injury
   a) responses to head injury of older adolescents are very similar to those of adults
   b) "malignant cerebral edema": acute onset of severe cerebral swelling (probably due to hyperemia[5,6]) following some head injuries, especially in young children (may not be as common as previously thought[7])
   c) posttraumatic seizures: more likely to occur within the first 24 hrs in children than in adults (p. 505) [8]

66.2 Management

66.2.1 Imaging studies

The PECARN algorithm[9] identified children with mTBI (GCS = 14–15) having a very low risk of clinically-significant brain injuries resulting in these recommendations regarding CT scan:
1. children < 2 years of age
   a) GCS = 14 or other signs of altered mental status or palpable skull fracture: CT recommended
   b) occipital or parietal or temporal scalp hematoma, or history of LOC ≥ 5 seconds, or severe mechanism of injury, or not acting normally according to the parent: CT vs. observation based on physician experience, multiple vs. isolated findings, worsening signs or symptoms after observation in E/R, and ≤ 3 months, parental preference
   c) all others: CT not recommended
2. children ≥ 2 years age
   a) GCS = 14 or other signs of altered mental status, or signs of basilar skull fracture: CT recommended
   b) history of LOC, or history of vomiting, or severe mechanism of injury, or severe H/A: CT vs. observation based on physician experience, multiple vs. isolated findings, worsening signs or symptoms after observation in E/R, parental preference
   c) all others: CT not recommended

Practice guideline: Imaging in minor pediatric head injury

- Level B[10]: CT scans should not be routinely used for children with mild TBI.
- Level B[10]: validated clinical decision rules (such as the PECARN algorithm described above) should be used to identify children at low risk for clinically significant TBI in whom CT is not indicated.
- Level B[10]: brain MRI imaging should not routinely be used in the acute evaluation of suspected or diagnosed mTBI*

*Rapid sequence MRI in nonsedated patients has been successfully used[11] but was not included in the guidelines

66.2.2 Home observation

Practice guideline: Home observation in minor pediatric head injury

Recommendations*: a child with GCS = 14–15 and normal CT scan can be considered for home observation if neurologically stable (these patients are at near zero risk of having an occult brain injury).
*Based mostly on prospective trials (not randomized) or large case series.
Definitions: pediatrics = ages 1 month–17 years of age. Minor head injury: GCS ≥ 13 (excludes: suspicion or proof of child abuse, patients requiring hospitalization for other reasons).

66.3 Outcome

As a group, children fare better than adults with head injury.[12] However, very young children do not do as well as the school-age child.[13]

All aspects of neuropsychological dysfunction following head injury may not always be related to the trauma, as children who get injured may have pre-existing tendencies that increased their propensity to get hurt[14] (this is controversial[15]).

66.4 Cephalhematoma

66.4.1 General information

Accumulation of blood under the scalp. Occurs almost exclusively in children.
Two types:
1. subgaleal hematoma: may occur without bony trauma, or may be associated with linear nondisplaced skull fracture (especially in age < 1 yr). Bleeding into loose connective tissue separates galea from periosteum. May *cross sutures*. Usually starts as a small localized hematoma, and may become huge (with significant loss of circulating blood volume in age < 1 year, transfusion may be necessary). Inexperienced clinicians may suspect CSF collection under the scalp which does not occur. Usually presents as a soft, fluctuant mass. These do *not* calcify
2. subperiosteal hematoma (some refer to this as cephalhematoma): most commonly seen in the newborn (associated with parturition, may also be associated with neonatal scalp monitor[16,17]). Bleeding elevates periosteum, extent is *limited by sutures*. Firmer and less ballotable than subgaleal hematoma[18 (p 312)]; scalp moves freely over the mass. 80% reabsorb, usually within 2–3 weeks. Occasionally may calcify

Infants may develop jaundice (hyperbilirubinemia) as blood is resorbed, occasionally as late as 10 days after onset.

66.4.2 Treatment

Treatment beyond analgesics is almost never required, and most usually resolve within 2–4 weeks. Avoid the temptation of percutaneously aspirating these because the risk of infection exceeds the risk of following them expectantly, and in the newborn removal of the blood may make them anemic. Follow serial hemoglobin and hematocrit in large lesions. If a subperiosteal hematoma persists > 6 weeks, obtain a skull film. If the lesion is calcified, surgical removal may be indicated for cosmetic reasons (although with most of these the skull will return to normal contour in 3–6 months).[18(p 315)]

66.5 Skull fractures in pediatric patients

66.5.1 General information

This section deals with some special concerns of skull fractures in pediatrics. Also see Child abuse (p. 1103).

66.5.2 Posttraumatic leptomeningeal cysts (growing skull fractures)

General information

Posttraumatic leptomeningeal cysts (PTLMC) (sometimes just traumatic leptomeningeal cysts), AKA growing skull fractures, are not to be confused with arachnoid cysts (AKA leptomeningeal cysts, which are not posttraumatic). PTLMC consists of a fracture line that widens with time. Although usually asymptomatic, the cyst may cause mass effect with neurologic deficit.

PTLMCs were first described in 1816,[19] and are *very* rare, occurring in 0.05–0.6% of skull fractures.[20,21] Usually requires both a widely separated fracture AND a dural tear. Mean age at injury: < 1 year; over 90% occur before age 3 years[22] (formation may require the presence of a rapidly growing brain[23]), although rare adult cases have been described[19,24,25] (a total of 5 cases in the literature as of 1998[19]). PTLMCs rarely occur > 6 mos out from the injury. Some children may develop a skull fracture that seems to grow during the initial few weeks that is *not* accompanied by a subgaleal mass, and that heals spontaneously within several months; the term "pseudogrowing fracture" has been suggested for these.[26]

Presentation

Most often presents as scalp mass (usually subgaleal), although there are reports of presentation with head pain alone.[24]

Diagnosis

Radiographic findings: progressive widening of fracture and scalloping (or saucering) of edges.

Screening for development of PTLMC

If early growth of a fracture line with no subgaleal mass is noted, repeat skull films in 1–2 months before operating (to rule out pseudogrowing fracture). In young patients with separated skull fractures (the width of the initial fracture is rarely mentioned), consider obtaining follow-up skull film 6–12 mos post-trauma. However, since most PTLMCs are brought to medical attention when the palpable mass is noticed, routine follow-up X-rays may not be cost-effective.

Treatment

Treatment of true PTLMC is surgical, with dural closure mandatory. Since the dural defect is usually larger than the bony defect, it may be advantageous to perform a craniotomy around the fracture site, repair the dural defect, and replace the bone.[25] Pseudogrowing fractures should be followed with X-rays and operated only if expansion persists beyond several months or if a subgaleal mass is present.

66.5.3 Depressed skull fractures in pediatrics

See reference.[27]

General information

Most common in frontal and parietal bones. One third are closed, and these tend to occur in younger children (3.4 ± 4.2 yrs. vs. 8.0 ± 4.5 yrs for compound fractures) as a result of the thinner, more deformable skull. Open fractures tended to occur with MVAs, closed fractures tended to follow accidents at home. Dural lacerations are more common in compound fractures.

Simple depressed skull fractures

There was no difference in outcome (seizures, neurologic dysfunction or cosmetic appearance) in surgical vs. nonsurgical treatment in 111 patients < 16 yrs of age. In the younger child, remodelling of the skull as a result of brain growth tends to smooth out the deformity.

Indications for surgery for pediatric simple depressed skull fracture:
1. definite evidence of dural penetration
2. persistent cosmetic defect in the older child after the swelling has subsided
3. ± focal neurologic deficit related to the fracture (this group has a higher incidence of dural laceration, although it is usually trivial)

"Ping-pong ball" fractures

See reference.[28]

A green-stick type of fracture → caving in of a focal area of the skull as in a crushed area of a ping-pong ball. Usually seen only in the newborn due to the plasticity of the skull.

Indications for surgery

No treatment is necessary when these occur in the temporoparietal region in the absence of underlying brain injury as the deformity will usually correct as the skull grows.
* radiographic evidence of intraparenchymal bone fragments
* associated neurologic deficit (rare)
* signs of increased intracranial pressure
* signs of CSF leak deep to the galea
* situations where the patient will have difficulty getting long-term follow-up

Technique

Frontally located lesions may be corrected for cosmesis by making a small linear incision behind the hairline, opening the cranium adjacent to the depression, and pushing it back out e.g., with a Penfield #3 dissector.

66.5.4 Dural sinus thrombosis/compression in pediatric skull fractures

▶ **The issue.** There is concern that a cerebral dural (venous) sinus thrombosis (DST) and/or compression may be associated with a skull fracture in the vicinity of dural venous sinuses, and that outcome in these cases will be worse if not treated with anticoagulation. Therefore there is a trend to evaluate pediatric patients with skull fractures for DST using CTV (which often involves additional radiation) or MRV, with the possible need for anesthesia.

▶ **The data.** DST is rare in pediatrics. Incidence: 0.67 per 100,000 children per year.[29]

DST is found in 4% of patients with *penetrating* head trauma.

Anticoagulation is recommended in children with DST (Level II[30]) to reduce the incidence of thrombus propagation, venous infarction and poor outcome.[31]

In a series of 2224 pediatric patients with skull fractures following *blunt* trauma, 41 patients (2%) had venous imaging (most because of proximity of the fracture to a dural sinus), 8 of those (20%) had DST, 14 (34%) had extrinsic sinus compression, 3 patients with DST developed venous infarcts.[29]

▶ **Recommendation.** For pediatric patients with skull fractures following *blunt* trauma, venous imaging (CTV or MRV) is recommended only when venous hypertension or venous infarction is suspected and anticoagulation is considered.[29]

66.6 Retroclival hematoma

66.6.1 General information

> **Key concepts**
>
> * rare. Predilection for pediatrics, where it usually occurs with trauma (e.g., MVA)
> * significant because it may be associated with atlantooccipital dislocation (AOD)
> * usually managed conservatively with brace (e.g., halo or SOMI)
> * outcome is usually good. Death can occur usually from other causes

66

A rare disorder. May occur following trauma, especially with violent hyperflexion or hyperextension of the neck usually in association with motor vehicle accidents. Predilection for pediatrics, possibly due to the higher ratio of head to body weight, flatter occipital condyles, and increased ligamentous laxity in children. It may also occur without trauma, more likely in adults e.g., with pituitry apoplexy, anticoagulation, subarachnoid hemorrhage…[32]

Blood can be epidural (anterior to the tectorial membrane (p.67)) or subdural (posterior to tectorial membrane) or a combination, and may originate from fracture or ligamentous disruption.[33]

May be associated with:
* atlantooccipital dislocation (p.1153) [34,35]
* occipital condyle fracture (p.1156)
* disruption of the apical odontoid ligament (p.69)
* fracture of the clivus
* odontoid fracture

66.6.2 Presentation

Neurologic findings may be due to stretching, compression, or contusion of adjacent brain parenchyma or nerves.[33]

Cranial nerve involvement reported includes:
* abducens (VI): the most commonly involved cranial nerve. May be unilateral or bilateral[33]
* optic (II)
* oculomotor (III)
* trigeminal (V)
* facial (VII)
* glossopharyngeal (IX)
* hypoglossal (XII)
* spinal accessory nerve (XI)

Other presentations include:
* hemiparesis
* quadriparesis
* hydrocephalus[34]
* occipitocervical instability

66.6.3 Evaluation

Noncontrast MRI is the imaging modality of choice. Demonstrates the hematoma (acutely may be best seen on T2WI), DWI assesses for stroke, and STIR images (p.241) to look for signal changes indicative of ligamentous injury (▶ Fig. 66.1).

CT including coronal reconstructions is useful to look for occipital condyle fractures, avulsion of the apical igament, and to assess the atlantooccipital interval (p.1154) (surrogate marker for atlantooccipital dislocation (p.1153))

Evaluation e.g., with CTA for concurrent blunt cerebrovascular injury (p.1029) may be appropriate in some instances (especially if stroke is suspected or demonstrated on MRI).

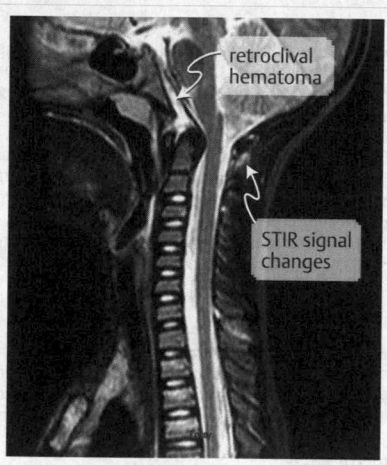

Fig. 66.1 Retroclival epidural hematoma.
6-year-old with atlantooccipital dislocation (AOD) following motor vehicle accident.
Sagittal STIR MRI.

66.6.4 Management

Most cases are managed conservatively, usually with a brace (halo/vest, SOMI...).
Indications for surgical interventions include:
- fusion: may be considered as follows
  - strong indication: ligamentous instability e.g., atlantooccipital dislocation meeting AOD surgical criteria (p. 1156)
  - soft indication: cranial nerve deficits
- evacuation of hematoma: indicated on rare occasion for symptomatic brainstem compression[36]
- ventriculostomy/shunt: indicated for hydrocephalus

66.6.5 Outcome

The hematoma generally resolves in 2–11 weeks.[33]
Conservative management results in good outcomes with minimal long-term neurologic deficits in the majority of cases.
Death occurs infrequently, and usually from other causes in patients who are neurologically devastated on admission.[33]

66.7 Nonaccidental trauma (NAT)

66.7.1 General information

AKA child abuse. At least 10% of children < 10 yrs of age that are brought to E/R with alleged accidents are victims of NAT.[37] The incidence of accidental head trauma of significant consequence below age 3 is low, whereas this is the age group in which battering (abuse) is highest.[38]
There are no findings that are pathognomonic for child abuse. Factors which raise the index of suspicion include:
1. retinal hemorrhage (see below)
2. bilateral chronic subdural hematomas in a child < 2 yrs of age (p. 1088)
3. skull fractures that are multiple (see below) or those that associated with intracranial injury
4. significant neurological injury with minimal signs of external trauma
5. multiple injuries of different ages in multiple locations

66.7.2 Shaken baby syndrome

Vigorous shaking of a child produces violent whiplash-like angular acceleration-decelerations of the head (the infant head is relatively large in proportion to the body, and the neck muscles are comparatively weak),[39] which may lead to significant brain injury. Some researchers believe that shaking alone may be inadequate to produce the severe injuries seen, and that impact is often also involved.[40]

Characteristic findings include retinal hemorrhages (see below), subdural hematomas (bilateral in 80%) and/or subarachnoid hemorrhage (SAH). There are usually few or no external signs of trauma (including cases with impact, although findings may be apparent at autopsy). In some cases there may be finger marks on the chest, multiple rib fractures and/or pulmonary compression ± parenchymal lung hemorrhage. Deaths in these cases are almost all due to uncontrollable intracranial hypertension. There may also be injury to the cervicomedullary junction.[41]

66.7.3 Retinal hemorrhage (RH) in child abuse

"In a traumatized child with multiple injuries and an inconsistent history, the presence of RH is pathognomonic of battering."[38] However, RH may also occur in the absence of any evidence of child abuse. 16/26 battered children < 3 yrs of age had RH on funduscopy, whereas 1/32 non-battered traumatized children with head injury had RH (the single false positive: traumatic parturition, where the incidence of RH is 15–30%).

Differential diagnosis of etiologies of retinal hemorrhage:
1. child abuse (including "shaken baby syndrome," see above)
2. benign subdural effusion in infants (p. 1087)
3. acute high altitude sickness (p. 1028)
4. acute increase in ICP: e.g., with a severe seizure (may be similar to Purtscher's retinopathy—see below)
5. Purtscher's retinopathy[42]: loss of vision following major trauma (chest crush injuries, airbag deployment[43]...), pancreatitis, childbirth or renal failure, among others. Posterior pole ischemia with cotton-wool exudates and hemorrhages around the optic disc due to microemboli of possibly fat, air, fibrin clots, complement-mediated aggregates, or platelet clumps. No known treatment

66.7.4 Skull fractures in child abuse

A series comparing 39 cases of skull fracture from documented child abuse to 95 cases of probable accidental injury[37] showed the following:
1. the parietal bone was the most common site of fracture in both groups (≈ 90%)
2. depression of skull fractures was frequently missed clinically due to overlying hematoma
3. clinical features in patients with skull fractures did not reliably differentiate child abuse from trauma (retinal hemorrhages (RH) were seen in 1 child abuse and 1 accidental trauma patient: note that RH is more common in "shaken child" syndrome which is not commonly associated with skull fractures)
4. 3 characteristics more frequently seen after child abuse than after other trauma:
   a) multiple fractures
   b) bilateral fractures
   c) fractures that cross sutures

References

[1] Ward JD, Narayan RK, Wilberger JE, et al. Pediatric Head Injury. In: Neurotrauma. New York: McGraw-Hill; 1996:859–867

[2] Zuccarello M, Facco E, Zampieri P, et al. Severe Head Injury in Children: Early Prognosis and Outcome. Childs Nerv Syst. 1985; 1:158–162

[3] Bruce DA, Raphaely RC, Goldberg AI, et al. Pathophysiology, Treatment and Outcome following Severe Head Injury in Children. Childs Brain. 1979; 5:174–191

[4] Alberico AM, Ward JD, Choi SC, et al. Outcome After Severe Head Injury: Relationship to Mass Lesions, Diffuse Injury, and ICP Course in Pediatric and Adult Patients. Journal of Neurosurgery. 1987; 67:648–656

[5] Bruce DA, Alavi A, Bilaniuk L, et al. Diffuse Cerebral Swelling Following Head Injuries in Children: The Syndrome of "Malignant Brain Edema". J Neurosurg. 1981; 54:170–178

[6] Humphreys RP, Hendrick EB, Hoffman HJ. The Head Injured Child Who "Talks and Dies". Child's Nervous System. 1990; 6:139–142

[7] Muizelaar JP, Marmarou AM, DeSalles AA, et al. Cerebral Blood Flow in Severely Head-Injured Children: Part I. Relationship with GCS Score, Outcome, ICP, and PVI. Journal of Neurosurgery. 1989; 71:63–71

[8] Hahn YS, Fuchs S, Flannery AM, et al. Factors Influencing Posttraumatic Seizures in Children. Neurosurgery. 1988; 22:864–867

66

[9] Kuppermann N, Holmes JF, Dayan PS, et al. Identification of children at very low risk of clinically-important brain injuries after head trauma: a prospective cohort study. Lancet. 2009; 374:1160–1170

[10] Lumba-Brown A, Yeates KO, Sarmiento K, et al. Centers for Disease Control and Prevention Guideline on the Diagnosis and Management of Mild Traumatic Brain Injury Among Children. JAMA Pediatr. 2018; 172. DOI: 10.1001/jamapediatrics.2018.2853

[11] Young JY, Duhaime AC, Caruso PA, et al. Comparison of non-sedated brain MRI and CT for the detection of acute traumatic injury in children 6 years of age or less. Emerg Radiol. 2016; 23:325–331

[12] Luerson TG, Klauber MR, Marshall LF. Outcome from Head Injury Related to Patient's Age: A Longitudinal Prospective Study of Adult and Pediatric Head Injury. Journal of Neurosurgery. 1988; 68:409–416

[13] Kriel RL, Krach LE, Panser LA. Closed Head Injury: Comparison of Children Younger and Older Than 6 Years of Age. Pediatr Neurol. 1989; 5:296–300

[14] Bijur PE, Haslum M, Golding J. Cognitive and Behavioral Sequelae of Mild Head Injury in Children. Pediatrics. 1990; 86:337–344

[15] Pelco L, Sawyer M, Duffielf G, et al. Premorbid Emotional and Behavioral Adjustment in Children with Mild Head Injury. Brain Inj. 1992; 6:29–37

[16] Listinsky JL, Wood BP, Ekholm SE. Parietal Osteomyelitis and Epidural Abscess: A Delayed Complication of Fetal Monitoring. Pediatr Radiol. 1986; 16:150–151

[17] Kaufman HH, Hochberg J, Anderson RP, et al. Treatment of Calcified Cephalhematoma. Neurosurgery. 1993; 32:1037–1040

[18] Matson DD. Neurosurgery of Infancy and Childhood. 2nd ed. Springfield: Charles C Thomas; 1969

[19] Britz GW, Kim K, Mayberg MR. Traumatic Leptomeningeal Cyst in an Adult: A Case Report and Review of the Literature. Surgical Neurology. 1998; 50:465–469

[20] Ramamurthi B, Kalyanaraman S. Rationale for Surgery in Growing Fractures of the Skull. J Neurosurg. 1970; 32:427–430

[21] Arseni CS. Growing Skull Fractures of Children. A Particular Form of Post-Traumatic Encephalopathy. Acta Neurochirurgica. 1966; 15:159–172

[22] Lende R, Erickson T. Growing Skull Fractures of Childhood. J Neurosurg. 1961; 18:479–489

[23] Gadoth N, Grunebaum M, Young LW. Leptomeningeal Cyst After Skull Fracture. Am J Dis Child. 1983; 137:1019–1020

[24] Halliday AL, Chapman PH, Heros RC. Leptomeningeal Cyst Resulting from Adulthood Trauma: Case Report. Neurosurgery. 1990; 26:150–153

[25] Iplikciglu AC, Kokes F, Bayar A, et al. Leptomeningeal Cyst. Neurosurgery. 1990; 27:1027–1028

[26] Sekhar LN, Scarff TB. Pseudogrowth in Skull Fractures of Childhood. Neurosurgery. 1980; 6:285–289

[27] Steinbok P, Flodmark O, Martens D, et al. Management of Simple Depressed Skull Fractures in Children. Journal of Neurosurgery. 1987; 66:506–510

[28] Loeser JD, Kilburn HL, Jolley T. Management of depressed skull fracture in the newborn. Journal of Neurosurgery. 1976; 44:62–64

[29] Hersh DS, Shimony N, Groves ML, et al. Pediatric cerebral venous sinus thrombosis or compression in the setting of skull fractures from blunt head trauma. J Neurosurg Pediatr. 2018; 21:258–269

[30] Roach ES, Golomb MR, Adams R, et al. Management of stroke in infants and children: a scientific statement from a Special Writing Group of the American Heart Association Stroke Council and the Council on Cardiovascular Disease in the Young. Stroke. 2008; 39:2644–2691

[31] Moharir MD, Shroff M, Stephens D, et al. Anticoagulants in pediatric cerebral sinovenous thrombosis: a safety and outcome study. Ann Neurol. 2010; 67:590–599

[32] Guillaume D, Menezes AH. Retroclival hematoma in the pediatric population. Report of two cases and review of the literature. J Neurosurg. 2006; 105:321–325

[33] Nguyen HS, Shabani S, Lew S. Isolated traumatic retroclival hematoma: case report and review of literature. Childs Nerv Syst. 2016. DOI: 10.1007/s00381-016-3098-y

[34] Papadopoulos SM, Dickman CA, Sonntag VK, et al. Traumatic atlantooccipital dislocation with survival. Neurosurgery. 1991; 28:574–579

[35] Vera M, Navarro R, Esteban E, et al. Association of atlanto-occipital dislocation and retroclival haematoma in a child. Childs Nerv Syst. 2007; 23:913–916

[36] Marks SM, Paramaraswaren R N, Johnston RA. Transoral evacuation of a clivus extradural haematoma with good recovery: a case report. Br J Neurosurg. 1997; 11:245–247

[37] Meservy CJ, Towbin R, McLaurin RL, et al. Radiographic Characteristics of Skull Fractures Resulting from Child Abuse. AJR. 1987; 149:173–175

[38] Eisenbrey AB. Retinal Hemorrhage in the Battered Child. Childs Brain. 1979; 5:40–44

[39] Caffey J. On the Theory and Practice of Shaking Infants. Its Potential Residual Effects of Permanent Brain Damage and Mental Retardation. Am J Dis Child. 1972; 124:161–169

[40] Duhaime A-C, Gennarelli TA, Thibault LE, et al. The Shaken Baby Syndrome: A Clinical, Pathological, and Biomechanical Study. J Neurosurg. 1987; 66:409–415

[41] Hadley MN, Sonntag VKH, Rekate HL, et al. The Infant Whiplash-Shake Injury Syndrome: A Clinical and Pathological Study. Neurosurgery. 1989; 24:536–540

[42] Buckley SA, James B. Purtscher's retinopathy. Postgrad Med J. 1996; 72:409–412

[43] Shah GK, Penne R, Grand MG. Purtscher's retinopathy secondary to airbag injury. Retina. 2001; 21:68–69

67 Head Injury – Long-Term Management, Complications, Outcome

67.1 Airway management

Practice guideline: Airway management

- Timing of tracheostomy (Level II[1]): early tracheostomy reduces the number of days of mechanical ventilation but does not affect mortality or incidence of pneumonia
- Timing of extubation (Level III[1]): early extubation for patients meeting extubation criteria does not increase the risk of pneumonia

67.2 Deep-vein thrombosis (DVT) prophylaxis

Also see further details about thromboembolism (p.176) in neurosurgical patients. The risk of developing DVT is ≈ 20% in untreated severe TBI.[2] See also **Practice guideline: DVT prophylaxis in severe TBI** (p.1106).

Practice guideline: DVT prophylaxis in severe TBI

Level III[3]:
- unless contraindicated, graduated compression stockings or intermittent compression boots are recommended until patients are ambulatory
- low molecular weight heparin (LMWH) (p.172) or low-dose unfractionated heparin in conjunction with mechanical measures lowers the DVT risk, but a trend suggests they increase the risk of expansion of intracranial hemorrhage (note: there is insufficient evidence to support use of one pharmacologic agent over another, or to define the optimal dose or timing of agents[3])

67.3 Nutrition in the head-injured patient

67.3.1 Summary of recommendations (see text for details)

Practice guideline: Nutrition

Level II[4]: full caloric replacement should be attained by post-trauma day 7

Σ: Nutrition goals following TBI

1. by post-trauma day 7, replace the following (enterally or parenterally):
   a) non-paralyzed patients: 140% of predicted basal energy expenditure (BEE)
   b) paralyzed patients: 100% of predicted BEE
2. provide ≥ 15% of calories as protein
3. nutritional replacement should begin within 72 hrs of head injury in order to achieve goal #1 by day 7
4. the enteral route is preferred (IV hyperalimentation is preferred if higher nitrogen intake is desired or if there is decreased gastric emptying)

67.3.2 Caloric requirements

Rested comatose patients with isolated head injury have a metabolic expenditure that is 140% of normal for that patient (range: 120–250%).[5,6,7,8] Paralysis with muscle blocker or barbiturate coma reduced this excess expenditure in most patients to ≈ 100–120% of normal, but some remained elevated by 20–30%.[9] Energy requirements rise during the first 2 weeks after injury, but it is not known for how long this elevation persists. Mortality is reduced in patients who receive full caloric replacement by day 7 after trauma[10] (a beneficial effect with an earlier goal of replacement by 3 days posttrauma was not found[11]). Since it generally takes 2–3 days to get nutritional replacement up to speed whether the enteral or parenteral route is utilized,[8] it is recommended that nutritional supplementation begin within 72 hrs of head injury.

67.3.3 Enteral vs. IV hyperalimentation

Caloric replacement that can be achieved is similar between enteral or parenteral routes.[12] The enteral route is preferred because of reduced risk of hyperglycemia, infection, and cost.[13] IV hyperalimentation may be utilized if higher nitrogen intake is desired or if there is decreased gastric emptying. No significant difference in serum albumin, weight loss, nitrogen balance, or final outcome was found between enteral and parenteral nutrition.[12]

Estimates of basal energy expenditure (BEE) can be obtained from the Harris-Benedict equation,[14] shown in Eq (67.1), (67.2), and (67.3), where W is weight in kg, H is height in cm, and A is age in years.

$$\text{Males}: \quad \text{BEE} = 66.47 + 13.75 \times W + 5.0 \times H - 6.76 \times A \tag{67.1}$$

$$\text{Females}: \quad \text{BEE} = 655.1 + 9.56 \times W + 1.85 \times H - 4.68 \times A \tag{67.2}$$

$$\text{Infants}: \quad \text{BEE} = 22.1 + 31.05 \times W + 1.16 \times H \tag{67.3}$$

67.3.4 Enteral nutrition

Isotonic solutions (such as Isocal® or Osmolyte®) should be used at full strength starting at 30 ml/hr. Check gastric residuals q 4 hrs and hold feedings if residuals exceed ≈ 125 ml in an adult. Increase the rate by ≈ 15–25 ml/hr every 12–24 hrs as tolerated until the desired rate is achieved.[15] Dilution is not recommended (may slow gastric emptying), but if it is desired, dilute with normal saline to reduce free water intake.

  Cautions:
- NG tube feeding may interfere with absorption of phenytoin; see phenytoin (PHT, Dilantin®) (p.488).
- reduced gastric emptying may be seen following head-injury[16] (NB: some may have temporarily elevated emptying) as well as in pentobarbital coma; patients may need IV hyperalimentation until the enteric route is usable. The technique of hypocaloric feeding[17] (AKA "trophic feed," "trickle feed," among others)through an enteral feeding tube (e.g., Dobhoff tube) at a rate variously defined as at 10–20 ml/hr may be tolerated and may reduce mucosal atrophy while providing a portion of nutritional requirements. Others have described better tolerance of enteral feedings using jejunal administration[18]

67.3.5 Nitrogen balance

A normal subject fed a protein-free diet for 3 days will excrete 85 mg of nitrogen/kg/d. These losses increase with injury. The rise in urinary N is due primarily to an increase in urea (comprises 80–90% of urinary N). This is thought to represent an increase in mobilization and breakdown of amino acids, which are felt to originate mainly from skeletal muscle.[19] Some of this represents a primary reaction to injury in which certain vital organs seem to be maintained at the expense of less active organs, and a significantly higher nitrogen balance cannot be achieved by increasing the amount of calories supplied as protein beyond a certain level.[12,15] Catabolism of protein yields 4 kcal/g (the same as for carbohydrates, compared to 9 kcal/g for fat), and in the non-injured adult normally supplies only ≈ 10% of energy needs.[20]

As an estimate, for each gram of N excreted (mostly in the urine; however, some is also lost in the feces), 6.25 gm of protein have been catabolized. It is recommended that at least 15% of calories be supplied as protein. The percent of calories consumed (PCC) derived from protein can be calculated from Eq (67.4), where N is nitrogen in grams, and BEE is the basal energy expenditure[5] (see Eq (67.1), (67.2), and (67.3)).

$$\text{PCC (from protein)} = \frac{N \text{ (gm N)} \times \frac{6.25 \text{ gm protein}}{\text{gm N}} \times \frac{4.0 \text{ kcal}}{\text{gm protein}}}{\text{BEE}} \times 100 \qquad (67.4)$$

Thus, to supply PCC (protein) = 15% once the BEE is known, use Eq (67.5). Some enteral formulations include Magnacal® (PCC = 14%) and TraumaCal® (PCC = 22%).

$$N \text{ (gm N)} = 0.006 \times \text{BEE} \qquad (67.5)$$

67.4 Posttraumatic hydrocephalus

67.4.1 General information

Hydrocephalus was found in 40% of 61 patients with severe head injury (GCS = 3–8) and in 27% of 34 patients with moderate head injury (GCS = 9–13).[21] Hydrocephalus developed by 4 weeks after injury in 58% and by 2 months in 70%.[21] There was no statistically significant relationship between posttraumatic hydrocephalus and age, the presence of SAH, or type of lesion (focal or diffuse). Post-traumatic hydrocephalus was associated with worse outcome.[21]

Hydrocephalus after traumatic subarachnoid hemorrhage

Incidence of clinically **symptomatic** hydrocephalus within 3 months of traumatic subarachnoid hemorrhage (tSAH) is ≈ 12%.[22] In this series of 301 tSAH patients, multivariate analysis showed the risk of developing hydrocephalus increased with age, intraventricular hemorrhage, blood thickness ≥ 5 mm, and diffuse distribution of blood (vs. focal distribution). There was no correlation with gender, admission GCS score, basal location of tSAH, or use of decompressive craniectomy.[22] NB: this is potentially confusing; univariate analysis shows the risk of hydrocephalus increases with increasing severity of TBI.

67.4.2 Differentiating true hydrocephalus from hydrocephalus ex vacuo

Delayed ventricular enlargement months to years after TBI may instead be due to atrophy (hydrocephalus ex vacuo) secondary to diffuse axonal injury, and may not represent true hydrocephalus. It may not be possible to accurately differentiate these two conditions, and the decision to shunt may therefore be difficult (similar to the dilemma in patients with NPH vs. atrophy).

67.4.3 Indications for surgical treatment

Factors favoring hydrocephalus, for which shunt should be considered:
1. elevated pressure on 1 or more LPs
2. papilledema on funduscopic exam
3. symptoms of headache/pressure
4. findings of "transependymal absorption" (p. 441) on CT or T2WI MRI
5. ± patients whose neurologic recovery seems worse than expected
6. provocative tests e.g., to test CSF Ro (p. 444) have been recommended[23]

Patients with enlarged ventricles who are asymptomatic and are doing well following their head injury should be managed expectantly.

67.5 Outcome from head trauma

67.5.1 Age

In general, the degree of recovery from closed head injury is better in infants and young children than in adults. In adults, decerebrate posturing or flaccidity with loss of pupillary or oculovestibular reflex is associated with a poor outcome in most cases; these findings are not as ominous in pediatrics.

67.5.2 Outcome prognosticators

General information

The frequency of poor outcome from closed head injury is increased with persistent ICP > 20 mm Hg after hyperventilation, increasing age, impaired or absent pupillary light response or eye movement, hypotension (SBP < 90), hypercarbia, hypoxemia, or anemia.[24] This is probably due at least in part to the fact that some of these are markers for significant injury to other body systems. One of the most important predictors for poor outcome is the presence of a mass lesion requiring surgical removal.[25] High ICP during the first 24 hrs is also a poor prognosticator.

Obliteration of basal cisterns on CT

The status of the basal cisterns (BCs) is evaluated on axial CT scan at the level of the midbrain (▶ Fig. 67.1) where they are divided into 3 limbs[26] (1 posterior limb = quadrigeminal cistern, 2 lateral limbs = posterior portion of the ambient cisterns). **Note:** "basal cisterns" in the trauma literature are a subset of the perimesencephalic cisterns (p. 1497). Possible findings:
1. open: all 3 limbs open
2. partially closed: 1 or 2 limbs obliterated
3. completely closed: 3 limbs obliterated

Compression or absence of the BCs carries a threefold risk of increased ICP, and the status of the BCs correlates with outcome.[26]

In a study of 218 patients with GCS ≤ 8, the BCs were classified on initial CT (within 48 hrs of admission) as: absent, compressed, normal, or not visualized (quality of CT too poor to tell).[27] The relationship of the BCs to outcome is shown in ▶ Table 67.1.

18 patients had a shift of brain structures > 15 mm associated with absent BCs; all of them died. The status of the BCs were more important within each GOS score than across scores. Also, see ▶ Table 64.4 for further information on CT.

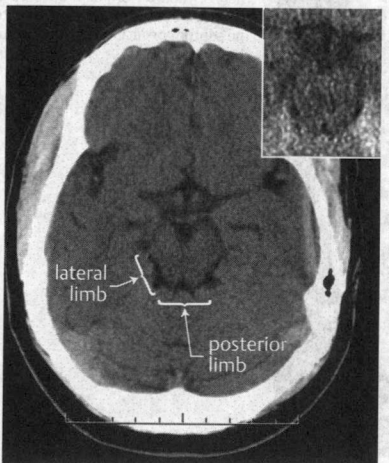

Fig. 67.1 Basal cisterns.
Axial brain CT demonstrating *open* basal cisterns (inset: example of ≈ complete obliteration of BCs).

lateral limb

posterior limb

Table 67.1 Correlation of GOS[a] with basal cisterns

Basal cisterns	Outcome[a]				
	Mortality	Vegetative	Severe disability	Moderate disability	Good
	(GOS 1)	(GOS 2)	(GOS 3)	(GOS 4)	(GOS 5)
normal	22%	6%	16%	21%	35%
compressed	39%	7%	18%	17%	19%
absent	77%	2%	6%	4%	11%
not-visualized	68%	0%	11%	9%	12%

[a]GOS = Glasgow outcome scale, see ▶ Table 98.4

Midline shift (MLS)

The presence of MLS correlates with a worse outcome. For the purpose of standardizing measurements in trauma, MLS is defined at the level of the foramen of Monro[26] as shown in ▶ Fig. 67.2, and is calculated using Eq (67.6).

$$\text{midline shift (MLS)} = \frac{BPD}{2} - SP \qquad (67.6)$$

where the midline shift is found by dividing the biparietal diameter (BPD) (the width of intracranial compartment at this location) by 2, and subtracting SP (the distance from the inner table to the septum pellucidum on the side of the shift). Measurements may be inaccurate if the vertical axis of the patient's head is not parallel to the long axis of the CT scanner.

Midline shift may be associated with altered levels of consciousness (p. 320).

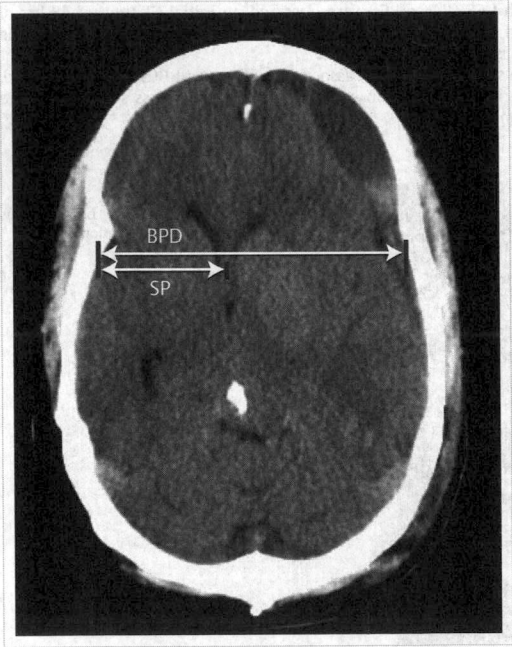

Fig. 67.2 Measurement of midline shift.
Axial noncontrast CT of a brain with a left-sided acute-on-chronic subdural hematoma.
Abbreviations: BPD = biparietal diameter (distance from inner table to inner table at the level of the foramen of Monro); SP = septum pellucidum (distance from the inner table to the septum pellucidum on the side of the shift).

Apolipoprotein E (apoE) ε4 allele

The presence of this genotype portends a worse prognosis following traumatic brain injury.[28] Furthermore, the incidence of severe brain injury in individuals with the apoE-4 allele greatly exceeds the rate of the allele in the general population.[29] This allele is also a risk factor for Alzheimer's disease (see below) as well as for chronic traumatic encephalopathy (p. 1112) .

67.6 Late complications from traumatic brain injury

67.6.1 General information

Long term complications include:
1. posttraumatic seizures (p. 505)
2. communicating hydrocephalus: incidence ≈ 3.9% of severe head injuries
3. posttraumatic syndrome (or postconcussive syndrome): see below
4. hypogonadotropic hypogonadism (p. 1014) [30]
5. chronic traumatic encephalopathy (p. 1112)
6. Alzheimer's disease (AD): head injury (especially if severe) promotes the deposition of amyloid proteins, especially in individuals possessing the apolipoprotein E (apoE) ε4 allele,[29] which may be related to the development of AD[31,32,33]

67.6.2 Postconcussive syndrome

General information

Variously defined collection of symptoms (see below) that is usually considered as a possible sequelae to minor head trauma (although some of these features can certainly be seen following more serious head trauma). Loss of consciousness is *not* a prerequisite to the development of the syndrome.

Controversy exists over the relative contribution of actual organic dysfunction vs. psychological factors (including conversion reaction, secondary gain which may be for attention, financial reward, drug seeking…). Furthermore, the presence of some of these symptoms can undoubtedly lead to the development of others (e.g., headache can cause difficulty concentrating and thus poor job performance and thence depression).

Presentation

A paradox has been noted by clinicians that the complaints following minor head injury seem out of proportion when considered in the context of the frequency of complaints after serious head injury. It has also been noted that patients with early posttraumatic complaints generally improve with time, whereas the late development of symptoms is often associated with a more protracted and fulminant course.

Symptoms commonly considered part of this syndrome include the following (with headache, dizziness and memory difficulties being the most frequent):
1. somatic
   a) headache
   b) dizziness or light-headedness
   c) visual disturbances: blurring is a common complaint
   d) anosmia
   e) hearing difficulties: tinnitus, reduced auditory acuity
   f) intolerance to light (photophobia) and/or loud (or even moderate) noise (phonophobia)
   g) balance difficulties
2. cognitive
   a) difficulty concentrating
   b) dementia: more common with multiple brain injuries than with a single concussion (p. 1112)
      • loss of intellectual ability
      • memory problems: usually impairs short-term memory more than long-term
   c) impaired judgment
3. psychosocial
   a) emotional difficulties: including depression, mood swings (emotional lability), euphoria/giddiness, easy irritability, lack of motivation, abulia
   b) personality changes
   c) loss of libido

d) disruption of sleep/wake cycles, insomnia
e) easy fatigability
f) increased rate of job loss and divorce (may be related to any of above)

Virtually any symptom can be ascribed to the condition. Other symptoms that may be described by patients which are generally not included in the definition:
1. fainting (vaso-vagal episodes): may need to rule out posttraumatic seizures, as well as other causes of syncope
2. altered sense of taste
3. dystonia[34]

Treatment

Treatment for symptoms attributed to this syndrome tends to be more supportive and reassuring than anything else. Often times these patients obtain treatment from primary care physicians, neurologists, physiatrists, and/or psychiatrists/psychologists. Neurosurgical involvement in the continuing care for these patients is usually at the discretion of the individual physician based on his or her practice patterns. Recovery follows a highly variable course.

Early follow-up care (consisting mainly of reassurance, providing information and neuropsychological assessment and counselling) was found to reduce post-concussion symptoms at 6 months in patients with posttraumatic amnesia lasting ≥ 1 hour or those who required hospitalization, but had no benefit in those not requiring hospitalization or having amnesia < 1 hr.[35]

Some symptoms may need to be evaluated for possible correctable late complications (seizures, hydrocephalus, CSF leak...). Alves and Jane[36] perform a head CT, MRI, BAER and neuropsychological battery if symptoms after minor head injury persist > 3 months. An EEG may be appropriate in cases where there is a question of seizures. If all studies are negative, "the authors tell the patient (and the lawyer) that there is no objective evidence for disease and that psychiatric evaluation is warranted." Non-correctable abnormalities on these studies prompt reassurance that significant symptoms should subside by 1 year, and that no specific treatment, other than psychological counselling, is helpful.

67.6.3 Chronic traumatic encephalopathy

General information

Often described in retired boxers, chronic traumatic encephalopathy (CTE) encompasses a spectrum of symptoms that range from mild to a severe form AKA dementia pugilistica,[37] or punch drunk syndrome (among others). Symptoms involve motor, cognitive, and psychiatric systems. CTE is distinct from posttraumatic dementia (which may follow a single closed head injury) or from posttraumatic Alzheimer's syndrome. Although generally accepted, not all authorities agree that repeated concussions have any long-term sequelae.[38]

There are some similarities with Alzheimer's disease (AD), including the presence of neurofibrillary tangles having similar microscopic characteristics (the main difference is that they tend to be more superficial in CTE than in AD[39]) and the development of amyloid angiopathy with the attendant risk of intracerebral hemorrhage.[40] EEG changes occur in one-third to one-half of professional boxers (diffuse slowing or low-voltage records).

Neuropathology

Findings include:
1. cerebral and cerebellar atrophy
2. neurofibrillary degeneration of cortical and subcortical areas
3. deposition of β-amyloid protein
   a) forming diffuse amyloid plaques
   b) in a subset of CTE patients this involves the vessel walls giving rise to cerebral amyloid angiopathy

Clinical

Clinical features of CTE are shown in ▶ Table 67.2 [37] and include[37]:
1. cognitive: mental slowing and memory deficits (dementia)
2. personality changes: explosive behavior, morbid jealousy, pathological intoxication with alcohol, and paranoia
3. motor: cerebellar dysfunction, symptoms of Parkinson's disease, pyramidal tract dysfunction

Table 67.2 CTE of boxing[a]

Motor	Cognitive	Psychiatric
Early (≈ 57%)		
dysarthria tremors mild incoordination, especially non-dominant hand	decreased complex attention	emotional lability euphoria/hypomania irritability, suspiciousness ease of aggression & talkativeness
Middle (≈ 17%)		
parkinsonism increased dysarthria, tremors, and incoordination	slowed mental speed mild deficits in memory, attention & executive ability	magnified personality decreased spontaneity paranoid, jealous inappropriate violent outbursts
Late (< 3%)		
pyramidal signs prominent parkinsonism prominent dysarthria, tremors & ataxia	prominent slowness of thought/speech amnesia attention deficits executive dysfunction	cheerful/silly decreased insight paranoid, psychotic disinhibited, violent possible Klüver-Bucy

[a]in professional boxers with ≥ 20 bouts

Grading scales have been devised to rank patients as having probable, possible, and improbable CTE.

The chronic brain injury scale (CBIS) assesses involvement of motor, cognitive, and psychological axes as shown in ▸ Table 67.3.

Table 67.3 Chronic brain injury scale

Grade involvement of each of the following axes separately:	Scoring for each axis:
• motor • cognitive • psychological	• 0 = none • 1 = mild • 2 = moderate • 3 = severe
Sum total points	**Severity**
0	normal
1–2	mild
3–4	moderate
> 4	severe

Risk factors for dementia pugilistica in boxing:

See reference.[37]
- risk increases with length of boxing career, especially > 10 yrs
- age at retirement: risk goes up after age 28 yrs
- number of bouts: especially ≥ 20 (more important than the number of knock-outs)
- boxing style: increased risk among poorer performers, those known as sluggers rather than "scientific" boxers, those known to be hard to knock out or known to take a punch and keep going
- age at examination: long latency causes increased prevalence with age
- and possibly, the number of head blows
- risk increases in patients with the apolipoprotein E (apo E) ε4 allele (as in Alzheimer's disease) as shown in ▸ Table 67.4
- professional boxers (more risk than amateurs)

Neuro-imaging

The most common finding is cerebral atrophy. A cavum septum pellucidum (CSP) is observed in 13% of boxers.[41] CSP in this setting probably represents an acquired condition[42] and correlates with cerebral atrophy.

Table 67.4 Odds ratio for developing Alzheimer's disease

Head injury	Apo E ε4 allele	Odds ratio
–	–	1
–	+	2
+	–	1
+	+	10

References

[1] Brain Trauma Foundation, Povlishock JT, Bullock MR. Infection prophylaxis. J Neurotrauma. 2007; 24:S26–S31

[2] Kaufman HH, Slatterwhite T, McConnell BJ, et al. Deep vein thrombosis and pulmonary embolism in head-injured patients. Angiology. 1983; 34:627–638

[3] Brain Trauma Foundation, Povlishock JT, Bullock MR. Deep vein thrombosis prophylaxis. J Neurotrauma. 2007; 24:S32–S36

[4] Brain Trauma Foundation, Povlishock JT, Bullock MR. Nutrition. J Neurotrauma. 2007; 24:S77–S82

[5] Clifton GL, Robertson CS, Grossman RG, et al. The Metabolic Response to Severe Head Injury. Journal of Neurosurgery. 1984; 60:687–696

[6] Young B, Ott L, Norton J, et al. Metabolic and Nutritional Sequelae in the Non-Steroid Treated Head Injury Patient. Neurosurgery. 1985; 17:784–791

[7] Deutschman CS, Konstantinides FN, Raup S, et al. Physiological and Metabolic Response to Isolated Closed Head Injury. Journal of Neurosurgery. 1986; 64:89–98

[8] Bullock R, Chesnut RM, Clifton G, et al. Guidelines for the Management of Severe Head Injury. 1995

[9] Clifton GL, Robertson CS, Choi SC. Assessment of Nutritional Requirements of Head Injured Patients. Journal of Neurosurgery. 1986; 64:895–901

[10] Rapp RP, Young B, Twyman D, et al. The Favorable Effect of Early Parenteral Feeding on Survival in Head Injured Patients. Journal of Neurosurgery. 1983; 58:906–912

[11] Young B, Ott L, Twyman D, et al. The Effect of Nutritional Support on Outcome from Severe Head Injury. Neurosurgery. 1987; 67:668–676

[12] Hadley MN, Grahm TW, Harrington T, et al. Nutritional Support and Neurotrauma: A Critical Review of Early Nutrition in Forty-Five Acute Head Injury Patients. Neurosurgery. 1986; 19:367–373

[13] The Brain Trauma Foundation. The American Association of Neurological Surgeons. The Joint Section on Neurotrauma and Critical Care. Nutrition. J Neurotrauma. 2000; 17:539–547

[14] Harris JA, Benedict FG. Biometric Studies of Basal Metabolism in Man. Washington, D.C. 1919

[15] Clifton GL, Robertson CS, Contant CF, et al. Enteral Hyperalimentation in Head Injury. Journal of Neurosurgery. 1985; 62:186–193

[16] Ott L, Young B, Phillips R, et al. Altered Gastric Emptying in the Head-Injured Patient: Relationship to Feeding Intolerance. J Neurosurg. 1991; 74:738–742

[17] Preiser JC, van Zanten AR, Berger MM, et al. Metabolic and nutritional support of critically ill patients: consensus and controversies. Crit Care. 2015; 19. DOI: 10.1186/s13054-015-0737-8

[18] Grahm TW, Zadrozny DB, Harrington T. Benefits of Early Jejunal Hyperalimentation in the Head-Injured Patient. Neurosurgery. 1989; 25:729–735

[19] Gadisseux P, Ward JD, Young HF, et al. Nutrition and the Neurosurgical Patient. Journal of Neurosurgery. 1984; 60:219–232

[20] Duke JH, Jorgensen SB, Broell JR, et al. Contribution of protein to caloric expenditure following injury. Surgery. 1970; 68:168–174

[21] Poca MA, Sahuquillo J, Mataro M, et al. Ventricular enlargement after moderate or severe head injury: a frequent and neglected problem. Journal of Neurotrauma. 2005; 22:1303–1310

[22] Tian HL, Xu T, Hu J, et al. Risk factors related to hydrocephalus after traumatic subarachnoid hemorrhage. Surgical Neurology. 2008; 69:241–6; discussion 246

[23] Marmarou A, Foda MA, Bandoh K, et al. Posttraumatic ventriculomegaly: hydrocephalus or atrophy? A new approach for diagnosis using CSF dynamics. Journal of Neurosurgery. 1996; 85:1026–1035

[24] Miller JD, Butterworth JF, Gudeman SK, et al. Further Experience in the Management of Severe Head Injury. J Neurosurg. 1981; 54:289–299

[25] Stablein DM, Miller JD, Choi SC, et al. Statistical Methods for Determining Prognosis in Severe Head Injury. Neurosurgery. 1980; 6:243–248

[26] Bullock MR, Chesnut RM, Ghajar J, et al. Appendix II: Evaluation of relevant computed tomographic scan findings. Neurosurgery. 2006; 58

[27] Toutant SM, Klauber MR, Marshall LF, et al. Absent or Compressed Basal Cisterns on First CT Scan: Ominous Predictor of Outcome in Severe Head Injury. Journal of Neurosurgery. 1984; 61:691–694

[28] Friedman G, Froom P, Sazbon L, et al. Apolipoprotein E-e4 Genotype Predicts a Poor Outcome in Survivors of Traumatic Injury. Neurology. 1999; 52:244–248

[29] Nicoll JAR, Roberts GW, Graham DI. Apolipoprotein E e4 Allele is Associated with Deposition of Amyloid ß-Protein Following Head Injury. Nature Med. 1995; 1:135–137

[30] Clark JDA, Raggatt PR, Edward OM. Hypothalamic Hypogonadism Following Major Head Injury. Clin Endocrin. 1988; 29:153–165

[31] Mayeux R, Ottman R, Tang MX, et al. Genetic Susceptibility and Head Injury as Risk Factors for Alzheimer's Disease Among Community-Dwelling Elderly Persons and Their First Degree Relatives. Annals of Neurology. 1993; 33:494–501

[32] Roberts GW, Gentleman SM, Lynch A, et al. ß Amyloid Protein Deposition in the Brain After Severe Head Injury: Implications for the Pathogenesis of Alzheimer's Disease. Journal of Neurology, Neurosurgery, and Psychiatry. 1994; 57:419–425

[33] Mayeux R, Ottman R, Maestre G, et al. Synergistic Effects of Traumatic Head Injury and Apolipoprotein-e4 in Patients with Alzheimer's Disease. Neurology. 1995; 45:555–557

[34] Lee MS, Rinne JO, Ceballos-Bauman A, et al. Dystonia After Head Trauma. Neurology. 1994; 44:1374–1378

[35] Wade DT, Crawford S, Wenden FJ, et al. Does Routine Follow Up After Head Injury Help? A Randomized Controlled Trial. Journal of Neurology, Neurosurgery, and Psychiatry. 1997; 62:478–484

[36] Alves WM, Jane JA, Youmans JR. Post-Traumatic Syndrome. In: Neurological Surgery. 3rd ed. Philadelphia: W. B. Saunders; 1990:2230–2242

[37] Mendez MF. The Neuropsychiatric Aspects of Boxing. International Journal of Psychiatry in Medicine. 1995; 25:249–262

[38] Parkinson D. Evaluating Cerebral Concussion. Surgical Neurology. 1996; 45:459–462

[39] Hof PR, Bouras C, Buee L, et al. Differential Distribution of Neurofibrillary Tangles in the Cerebral Cortex of Dementia Pugilistica and Alzheimer's Disease Cases. Acta Neuropathol. 1992; 85:23–30

[40] Jordan BD, Kanik AB, Horwich MS, et al. Apolipoprotein E e4 and Fatal Cerebral Amyloid Angiopathy Associated with Dementia Pugilistica. Annals of Neurology. 1995; 38:698–699

[41] Jordan BD, Jahre C, Hauser WA, et al. CT of 338 Active Professional Boxers. Radiology. 1992; 185:509–512

[42] Jordan BD, Jahre C, Hauser WA. Serial Computed Tomography in Professional Boxers. J Neuroimaging. 1992; 25:249–262

67

Part XV

Spine Trauma

XV

68 Spine Injuries – General Information, Neurologic Assessment, Whiplash and Sports-Related Injuries, Pediatric Spine Injuries

68.1 Introduction

20% of patients with a major spine injury will have a second spinal injury at another level, which may be noncontiguous. These patients often have simultaneous but unrelated injuries (e.g., chest trauma, TBI…). Injuries directly associated with spinal cord injuries include arterial dissections (carotid and/or vertebral arteries).

68.2 Terminology

68.2.1 Spinal stability

Many definitions have been proposed. A conceptual definition of clinical stability from White and Panjabi[1]: the ability of the spine under physiologic loads to limit displacement so as to prevent injury or irritation of the spinal cord and nerve roots (including cauda equina), and to prevent incapacitating deformity or pain due to structural changes.

Biomechanical stability refers to the ability of the spine ex vivo to resist forces.

Predicting spinal stability is often difficult, and to this end various models have been developed, none of which is perfect. See models of stability for cervical spine injuries (p. 1182) and thoracolumbar fractures (p. 1200).

68.2.2 Level of injury

There is disagreement over what should be defined as "the level" of a spinal cord injury. Some define the "level" of a spinal cord injury as the lowest level of completely *normal* function (thus a patient would be termed a C5 quadriplegic even with minor C6 motor function). However, most sources define the "level" as the most caudal segment with motor function that is at least 3 out of 5 and if pain and temperature sensation is present.

68.2.3 Completeness of lesion

Categorization is important for treatment decisions and prognostication.

Incomplete lesion

Definition: any residual motor or sensory function more than 3 segments below the level of the injury.[2] Look for signs of preserved long-tract function.

Signs of incomplete lesion:
1. sensation (including position sense) or voluntary movement in the LEs in the presence of a cervical or thoracic spinal cord injury
2. "sacral sparing": preserved sensation around the anus, voluntary rectal sphincter contraction, or voluntary toe flexion
3. an injury does *not* qualify as incomplete with preserved sacral reflexes alone (e.g., bulbocavernosus)

Types of incomplete spinal cord injury:
1. central cord syndrome (p. 1132)
2. Brown-Séquard syndrome (cord hemisection) (p. 1135)
3. anterior cord syndrome (p. 1135)
4. posterior cord syndrome (p. 1136): rare

Complete lesion

No preservation of any motor and/or sensory function more than 3 segments below the level of the injury in the absence of spinal shock (see below). About 3% of patients with complete injuries on initial exam will develop some recovery within 24 hours. Recovery is essentially zero if the spinal cord injury remains complete beyond 72 hours.

Spinal shock

This term is often used in two completely different senses:
- 1st SENSE: hypotension (shock) that follows spinal cord injury (SBP usually ≈ 80 mm Hg). See Hypotension (p. 1139) for treatment. Caused by multiple factors:
  - a) interruption of sympathetics: implies spinal cord injury above T1
    - ○ loss of vasoconstrictors → vasodilatation (loss of vascular tone) below the level of injury
    - ○ leaves parasympathetics relatively unopposed causing *bradycardia*
  - b) loss of muscle tone due to skeletal muscle paralysis below level of injury results in venous pooling and thus a relative hypovolemia
  - c) blood loss from associated wounds → true hypovolemia
- 2nd SENSE: transient loss of all neurologic function (including segmental and polysynaptic reflex activity and autonomic function) below the level of the SCI[3,4] → flaccid paralysis and areflexia
  - a) duration: may abate in as little as 72 hours, but typically persists 1–2 weeks, occasionally several months
  - b) accompanied by loss of the bulbocavernosus reflex
  - c) spinal cord reflexes immediately above the injury may also be depressed on the basis of the Schiff-Sherrington phenomenon (primarily described in animal models)
  - d) when spinal shock resolves, there will be spasticity below the level of the lesion and return of the bulbocavernosus reflex
  - e) a poor prognostic sign

68.3 Whiplash-associated disorders

68.3.1 General information

"Whiplash" was initially a lay term, which is currently defined as a traumatic injury to the soft tissue structures in the region of the cervical spine (including: cervical muscles, ligaments, intervertebral discs, facet joints...) due to hyperflexion, hyperextension, or rotational injury to the neck in the absence of fractures, dislocations, or intervertebral disc herniation.[5] It is the most common non-fatal automobile injury.[6] Symptoms may start immediately, but more commonly are delayed several hours or days. In addition to symptoms related to the cervical spine, common associated complaints include headaches, cognitive impairment, and low back pain.

68.3.2 Clinical grading

A proposed clinical classification system of WAD is shown in ► Table 68.1.[7]

Table 68.1 Clinical grading of WAD severity

Grade		Description
Whip-lash	0	no complaints, no signs[a]
	1	neck pain or stiffness or tenderness, no signs
	2	above symptoms with reduced range of motion or point tenderness
	3	above symptoms with weakness, sensory deficit, or absent deep tendon reflexes
	4	above symptoms with fracture or dislocation[a]

[a]the definition of whiplash excludes these patients[5]

68.3.3 Evaluation and treatment

A consensus[8] regarding diagnosis and management of these injuries is shown in ► Table 68.2 and ► Table 68.3. Keep in mind that conditions such as occipital neuralgia may occasionally follow whiplash-type injuries and should be treated appropriately (► Table 68.3).

Table 68.2 Evaluation of WAD

Grade 1: patients with normal mental status and physical exam do not require plain radiographs on presentation

Grade 2 & 3 patients: C-spine X-rays, possibly with flexion-extension views. Special imaging studies (MRI, CT, myelography...) are not indicated

Grade 3 & 4: these patients should be managed as suspected spinal cord injury; see Initial management of spinal cord injury (p. 1138) and sections that follow

Table 68.3 Treatment of WAD[8a]

Whiplash is usually a benign condition requiring little treatment and usually resolves in days to a few weeks in most cases.

Recommendation	Grade		
	1	2	3
Range of motion exercises	should be started immediately for all		
Encourage early return to regular activities	immediately	ASAP	
Cervical collars and rest[b]	no	not for > 72 hrs	not for > 96 hrs
Passive modality therapies: heat, ice, massage, TENS, ultrasound, relaxation techniques, acupuncture, and work alteration	no	optional if symptoms last > 3 wks	
Medications: optional use of NSAIDs and nonnarcotic analgesics? (recommended for ≤ 3 wks)	no	yes	yes. Limited narcotics may also occasionally be needed
Surgery	no	no	only for progressive neurologic deficit or persisting arm pain

✖ **Not** recommended: cervical pillows and soft collars, bed rest, spray and stretch exercises, muscle relaxant medication, TENS, reflexology, magnetic necklaces, herbal remedies, homeopathy, OTC medications (except NSAIDs, see above), and intra-articular, intrathecal, or trigger point steroid injections

[a]excluding patients with fractures, dislocations, or spinal cord injuries
[b]soft foam collars are generally discouraged; if they are to be used, the narrow part should be placed in front to avoid neck extension[5]

68.3.4 Outcome

In a study of 117 patients < 56 years of age having WAD due to automobile accidents (excluding those with cervical fractures, dislocations, or injuries elsewhere in the body) conducted in Switzerland[9] (where all medical costs were paid by the state and there was no opportunity for litigation and no compensation for pain and suffering, although there was the possibility of permanent disability), the recovery rate was as shown in ▶ Table 68.4. Of the 21 patients with continued symptoms at 2 yrs, only 5 were restricted with respect to work (3 reduced to part-time work, 2 on disability). Patients with persistent symptoms were older, had more varied complaints on initial exam, had a more rotated or inclined head position at the time of impact, had a higher incidence of pretraumatic headaches, and had a higher incidence of certain pre-existing findings (such as radiologic evidence of cervical osteoarthritis). The amount of damage to the automobile and the speed of the cars had little relationship to the degree of injury, and outcome was not influenced by gender, vocation, or psychological factors.

Table 68.4 Recovery of patients with WAD

Time (mos)	Percent recovered
3	56%
6	70%
12	76%
24	82%

68.4 Pediatric spine injuries

68.4.1 General information

> **Key concepts**
>
> - until age ≈ 16, spinal cord injury is relatively infrequent
> - ligamentous injuries are more common than actual fractures due to flexibility of ligamentous
> - spine/spinal cord injuries that are somewhat unique to the pediatric population
>   a) atlantooccipital dislocation (AOD) (p. 1153): a retroclival hematoma should raise the index of suspicion for AOD
>   b) SCIWORA (p. 1196) (spinal cord injury without radiographic abnormality)
>   c) synchondrosis fractures: os odontoideum (p. 1175), C2 synchondrosis
>   d) atlantoaxial rotatory fixation/subluxation (p. 1158)
> - when AOD is a consideration, cervical CT is the imaging modality of choice to measure the con-dyle-C1 interval (CCI)
> - most stable fractures and ligamentous injuries may be treated nonsurgically. C2 synchondrosis fractures are ususally managed with halo traction
> - surgical challenges include: finding hardware small enough for young children, the small size of C-spine lateral masses, and difficulty thoroughly removing disc material and cartilage

68

Spinal cord injury is fairly uncommon in children; the ratio of head injuries to spinal cord injuries is ≈ 30:1 in pediatrics. Only ≈ 5% of spinal cord injuries occur in children. Due to ligamentous laxity together with a high head-to-body weight ratio, immaturity of paraspinal muscles and the underdevel-oped uncinate processes, these tend to involve ligamentous rather than bony injuries (e.g., SCIWORA (p. 1196)). There is also the potential for physeal (growth plate) separation in young children, which may have good potential to heal. The cervical spine is the most vulnerable segment (with subaxial injuries being fairly uncommon), with 42% of injuries occurring here, 31% thoracic, and 27% lumbar. The fatality rate is higher with pediatric spine injuries than with adults (opposite to the situation with head injury), with the cause of death more often related to other severe injuries than to the spinal injury.[10]

68.4.2 Pediatric cervical spine injuries and mimics

General information

See pediatric C-spine anatomy (p. 224). In the age group ≤ 9 yrs, 67% of cervical spine injuries occur in the upper 3 segments of the cervical spine (occiput-C2).[11]

Synchondroses

Normal synchondroses (p. 226) may be mistaken for fractures, especially the dentocentral synchond-rosis of the axis (p. 224) which may be mistaken for an odontoid fracture. Conversely, synchondroses are biomechanically weak links and actual fractures may occur through them (▶ Fig. 68.1).[12,13]
C2 is the most common vertebra injured in children.

▶ **Odontoid epiphysiolysis.** A fracture through the dentocentral synchondrosis (much of the litera-ture says neurocentral synchondrosis, but I believe that is incorrect). Mimics an odontoid type II fracture. 23% will develop neurologic deficit, and in 53% of these the SCI level occurs lower at the cervicothoracic junction.[14] Recommended treatment for fractures through synchondroses: the ten-dency for synchondroses to fuse suggests that emergency reduction followed by external immobili-zation should be attempted. For C2, a halo is recommended, with 80–90% success rate.[12,14] Internal immobilization/fusion should be reserved for persistent instability[13] after 3–6 months.[14]

Evaluation

General information

Practice guidelines for diagnostic workup are shown below (see Practice guideline: Evaluation of pediatric C-spine injuries (p. 1122)).

Retroclival hematoma (p. 1102) on imaging should prompt immobilization and evaluation for atlantooccipital dislocation (AOD).

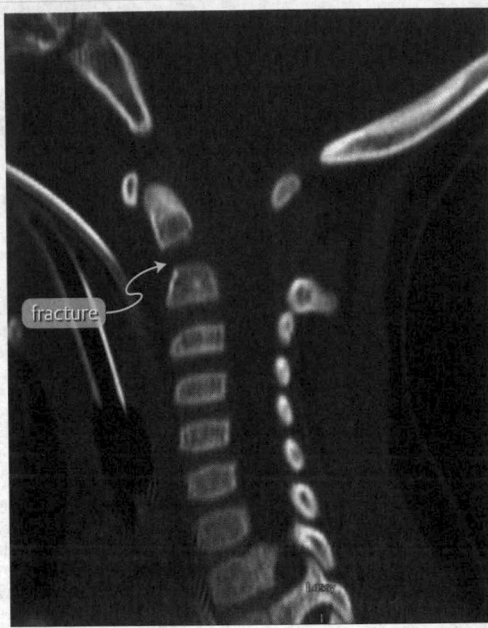

Fig. 68.1 Fracture through C2 dentocentral synchondrosis (odontoid epiphysiolysis). Sagittal cervical CT in 23-month-old injured in motor vehicle crash. Note anterior angulation of the odontoid process and several mm of separation from the main C2 vertebral body.

68

Practice guideline: Evaluation of pediatric C-spine injuries

Level I[15]
- Use CT to assess the condyle-C1 interval (CCI) (p. 1154) (AKA atlantooccipital interval) for pediatric patients with potential atlantooccipital dislocation (AOD)

Level II[15]:
- Do not perform C-spine imaging in children > 3 years of age with trauma who are:
  - alert
  - neurologically intact
  - without posterior midline cervical tenderness (with no distracting pain)
  - not hypotensive without explanation
  - not intoxicated
- Do not perform C-spine imaging in children < 3 years of age with trauma who meet all of the following conditions:
  - have a GCS > 13
  - are neurologically intact
  - have no cervical midline tenderness (without distracting injury)
  - are not intoxicated
  - do not have unexplained hypotension
  - were not in a motor vehicle collision, a fall > 10 feet, or non-accidental trauma (NAT) as the known or suspected mechanism of injury
- Obtain cervical spine X-rays or high-resolution cervical CT in pediatric trauma victims who do not meet either set of criteria above
- Obtain 3-position CT with C1–2 motion analysis to confirm and classify the diagnosis for children suspected of having atlantoaxial rotatory fixation (AARF)

Pseudospread of the atlas

Pseudospread of the atlas is defined as > 2 mm total overlap of the two C1 lateral masses on C2 on AP open-mouth view.[16] This could be misdiagnosed as a *Jefferson fracture* (p. 1162), which rarely occurs prior to the teen-ages (owing to lower weight of children, more flexible necks, increased plasticity of skull, and shock absorbing synchondroses of C1).

Pseudospread is probably a result of disproportionate growth of the atlas on the axis. It is present in most children 3 mos to 4 yrs of age. Prevalence is 91–100% during the second year of life. Youngest example at 3 mos, oldest at 5.75 yrs. Normal total offset is typically 2 mm during the first year, 4 mm during the second, 6 mm during the third, and decreasing thereafter. The maximum is 8 mm. Trauma is not a contributing factor.

Neck rotation can also sometimes simulate the appearance of a Jefferson fracture.

When suspicion of a Jefferson fracture is high: thin cut CT scan parallel to and through C1 can resolve the issue of whether or not there is a fracture.

Pseudosubluxation

Anterior displacement and/or significant angulation, usually of C2 (axis) on C3 (▶ Fig. 68.2) (occasionally C3 on C4) on lateral C-spine X-rays or sagittal imaging (CT or MRI) that may occur normally in children (up to age 10 yrs, sometimes persisting up to age 14[17]). When identified after trauma, this may be misinterpreted as a traumatic injury. Fractures and dislocations are unusual in children, and when they do occur, they resemble those in adults.

68

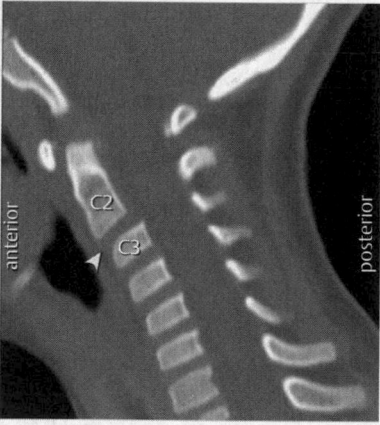

Fig. 68.2 Pseudosubluxation of C2 anteriorly on C3 (*yellow arrowhead*).
Image: sagittal cervical CT scan bone window in a 4-year-old girl.

Physiology: flexion and extension are initially centered at C2–3, this gradually moves down to C4–5 or C5–6 usually by age 10 yrs. C2 normally moves forward on C3 up to 2–3 mm in peds.[18] Forward displacement on neck flexion may be exacerbated by paraspinal spasm at lower levels.[19] It does not represent pathological instability.

10 cases reported between ages 4–6 yrs[20]: pain was not uncommon. In each case, either the head or neck was flexed (sometimes minimally); the pseudosubluxation corrected when X-ray was repeated with head in true neutral position. However, this does not rule out instability.

True subluxation may occur with:
1. fractures (e.g., hangman's fracture (p. 1165)) which allow the C2 VB to move forward without a corresponding displacement of the posterior elements of C2. This may be suspected on plain X-rays with C2-3 subluxation when the base of the C2 spinous process is 1.5 mm posterior to the posterior cervical line of Swischuk (▶ Fig. 12.1),[21] and is assumed to be present when ≥ 2 mm posterior.[17,21] CT scan is diaagnostic
2. injury to the C2-3 disc and posterior elements: may be demonstrable on STIR MRI (p. 241)

Treatment

Practice guideline: Treatment of pediatric C-spine injuries

Level III[15]:
- children < 8 yrs of age: when restrained, immobilize with thoracic elevation or an occipital recess (allows more neutral alignment due to the relatively large head)
- children < 7 yrs of age with injuries of the C2 synchondrosis (p. 226): closed reduction and halo immobilization
- patients with atlantoaxial rotatory subluxation/fixation (AARF):
  - acute AARF (< 4 weeks duration) that does not reduce spontaneously: reduction with manipulation or halter traction
  - chronic AARF (> 4 weeks duration): reduction with halter or tong/halo traction
  - recurrent or irreducible AARF: internal fixation and fusion
- for isolated cervical spine ligamentous injuries and unstable or irreducible fractures of dislocations with associated deformity: consider primary operative treatment
- for cervical spine injuries that fail non-operative management: operative treatment

Assessment tools for spinal stability used in adults have not been validated in the pediatric population.

68.5 Cervical bracing

68.5.1 Soft collars

Soft (sponge rubber) collar: does not immobilize the cervical spine to any significant degree. Its function is primarily to remind the patient to reduce neck movements.

68.5.2 Rigid cervical collars

Inadequate for stabilizing upper and mid-cervical spine and for preventing rotation.
    Common rigid collars:
- Miami J collar & Aspen collar: have removable pads
- Philadelphia collar: no removable pads. Feels hotter to wear

68.5.3 Poster braces

Distinguished from cervicothoracic orthoses (see below) by the lack of straps under the axilla. Includes the four poster brace. Generally good for preventing flexion at midcervical levels.

68.5.4 Cervicothoracic orthoses

Cervicothoracic orthoses (CTO) incorporate some form of body vest to immobilize the cervical spine. The following are presented in increasing degree of immobilization.
    Guilford brace: essentially a ring around the occiput and chin connected by two posts to anterior and posterior thoracic pads.
    SOMI brace: acronym for Sternal Occipital Mandibular Immobilizer. Good for bracing against flexion (especially upper cervical spine). Inadequate for hyper-extension type injuries because of weak occipital support. Has special forehead attachment to allow patient to eat comfortably without mandibular support.
    "Yale brace": a sort of extended Philadelphia collar. The most effective CTO for bracing against flexion-extension and rotation. Major shortcoming is poor prevention of lateral bending (only ≈ 50% reduced).

68.5.5 Halo-vest brace

Can immobilize the upper or lower cervical spine, not very good for mid-cervical spine (due to snaking of the midcervical spine). Unable to provide adequate distraction support following vertebral body resection when patient assumes upright position (i.e., it is *not* a portable cervical traction device). Overall reduction of flexion/extension as well as lateral bending is ≈ 90–95%, rotation is reduced by 98%. See placement (p. 1147).

68.6 Follow-up schedule

After initial management (surgical or nonsurgical) of cervical spine problems (stable or unstable), the follow-up schedule shown in ▶ Table 68.5 is suggested to permit recognition of problems in time for treatment[1] (start with 3 weeks and keep doubling the interval to 1 year).

Table 68.5 Sample follow-up cervical spine clinic visit schedule

Time post-op	Agenda
7–10 days	(for post-op patients only) wound check, D/C sutures/staples if used
4–6 weeks	AP & lateral C-spine X-ray in brace (no flexion/extension) to rule out instability or progression of fracture(s)
10–12 weeks	• AP & lateral C-spine X-rays with flexion/extension views out of brace • if X-rays show no instability or progression of fracture(s) and patient is doing well, begin weaning brace
6 months	• AP & lateral C-spine X-rays with flexion/extension views • some surgeons release patients at this time if they are doing well
1 year (optional)	• AP & lateral C-spine X-rays with flexion/extension views • release patient if they are doing well

68.7 Sports-related cervical spine injuries

68.7.1 General information

Any of the spine injuries described in this book can be sports-related. This section considers some injuries peculiar to sports.

Bailes et al[22] classified sports-related spinal cord injuries (SCI) as shown in ▶ Table 68.6. Type I injures may be complete or may have features of any of the incomplete SCI syndromes (often in mixed or partial forms). Type II injuries include spinal concussion, spinal neuropraxia (see below), and the burning hands syndrome (see below), all in the absence of radiographic abnormalities and all with complete resolution of symptoms. Patients should be carefully evaluated, and return to competition should not be allowed in the presence of neurologic deficit, radiographically demonstrated injury, certain congenital C-spine abnormalities, and possibly for "repeat offenders" (p. 1126). Type III injuries are the most common. Unstable injuries should be treated appropriately (p. 1194).

Table 68.6 Sports-related spinal cord injuries

Type	Description
I	permanent SCI
II	transient SCI without radiographic abnormality
III	radiologic abnormality without neurologic deficit

68.7.2 Football-related cervical spine injuries

General information

✖ Football players with suspected C-spine injury should not have their helmet removed in the field (p. 1138).

Terminology

The following terms probably originated as locker-room jargon for various cervical spine-related injuries usually sustained in playing football. Medical definitions have subsequently been retro-fitted to them. As a result, the precise definitions may not be uniformly agreed upon. Although the semantics may differ, it is more important from a diagnostic and therapeutic standpoint to distinguish nerve root injuries, brachial plexus injuries, and spinal cord injuries.

1. cervical cord neuropraxia[23] (CCN): sensory changes that may involve numbness, tingling or burning. May or may not be associated with motor symptoms of weakness or complete paralysis. Typically lasts < 15 mins (although may persist up to 48 hrs), involves all 4 extremities in 80% of cases. Narrowing of the sagittal diameter of the cervical spinal canal is felt to be a contributory

factor. With resumption of contact activities, recurrence rate is ≈ 56%, with higher risks of recurrence among those with narrower canal diameters. Evaluation should include cervical MRI. Torg[23] feels that uncomplicated cases of CCN (no spinal instability and no MRI evidence of cord defect or edema) have a low risk of permanent injury and does not recommend activity restrictions

2. "stinger" or "burner": distinct from the burning hands syndrome. Unilateral, burning dysesthetic pain radiating down one arm from the shoulder, sometimes associated with weakness involving the C5 or C6 nerve roots. Usually follows a tackle. May result from downward traction on the upper trunk of the brachial plexus (when the shoulder is forcefully depressed with the neck flexed to the contralateral side) or by direct nerve root compression in the neural foramina (not an SCI)

3. burning hands syndrome[24]: similar to a stinger, but bilateral. Probably represents an *SCI*; possibly a mild variant of a central cord syndrome (p. 1132)

4. other neurologic injuries include: vascular injury to carotid or vertebral arteries. Usually related to intimal dissection (p. 1220) following a direct blow to the neck or by extreme movements. Symptoms are those of a TIA or stroke

Spear tackler's spine

Rule changes in 1976 banned spearing (the practice of using the football helmet as a battering ram to tackle an opponent) and resulted in a reduction of the number of football-related occurrences of cervical spine fractures and quadriplegia.[25]

Four characteristics of spear tackler's spine:
1. cervical spinal stenosis
2. loss of normal cervical lordosis: as a result, the stress of axial loading is more likely to be imparted to the vertebral bodies, rather than being absorbed by the cervical musculature and ligaments, increasing the risk of burst fractures and quadriplegia
3. evidence of pre-existing traumatic abnormalities
4. documented spear tackler's technique

Suggested management:
The athlete is removed from competition until the cervical lordosis returns and the player learns to use other tackling techniques. This tackling technique has been banned since 1976.

68.7.3 Return to play and pre-participation guidelines

Return to play (RTP) and pre-participation evaluation guidelines related to the cervical spine are shown in ▶ Table 68.7 (modified[26]). These are just guidelines, and do not ensure safety. Clinical judgment must always be employed.

Table 68.7 C-spine-related contraindications for participation in contact sports[a]

Condition[b]			C.I.[c]
Congenital[d]			
1.	odontoid abnormalities (serious injury may result from atlanto-axial instability)		
	a.	complete aplasia (rare)	absolute
	b.	hypoplasia (seen in conjunction with achondroplasia and spondyloepiphyseal dysplasia)	absolute
	c.	os odontoideum (probably of traumatic origin)	absolute
2.	atlantooccipital fusion (partial or complete fusion of atlas to occiput): sudden onset of symptoms & sudden death have been reported		absolute
3.	Klippel-Feil anomaly (congenital fusion of 2 or more cervical vertebrae)[e]		
	a.	Type I: mass fusion of C-spine to upper T-spine	absolute
	b.	Type II: fusion of only 1 or 2 interspaces	
		● associated with limited ROM, occipitocervical anomalies, instability, disc disease or degenerative changes	absolute
		● associated with full ROM and none of the above	none

(continued)

Table 68.7 continued

Condition[b]	C.I.[c]
Acquired	
1. cervical spinal stenosis[f]	
a. asymptomatic	none
b. with one episode of cord neuropraxia	relative
c. cord neuropraxia + MRI evidence of cord defect or edema	absolute
d. cord neuropraxia + ligamentous instability, symptoms or neurologic findings > 36 hrs, or multiple episodes	absolute
2. spear tackler's spine (see text)	absolute
3. spina bifida occulta: rare, incidental X-ray finding	none
Posttraumatic upper cervical spine	
1. atlantoaxial instability (ADI > 3 mm adults, > 4 mm peds)	absolute
2. atlantoaxial rotatory fixation (may be associated with disruption of transverse ligament)	absolute
3. fractures	
a. healed, pain-free, full ROM, & no neurologic findings with any of the following fractures: nondisplaced Jefferson fracture; odontoid fracture; or lateral mass fracture of axis	none
b. all others	absolute
4. post-surgical atlantoaxial fusion	absolute
Posttraumatic subaxial cervical spine	
1. ligamentous injuries: > 3.5 mm subluxation, or > 11° angulation on flexion-extension views	absolute
2. fractures	
a. healed, stable fractures listed here with normal exam: VB compression fracture without posterior involvement; spinous process fractures	none
b. VB fractures with sagittal component or posterior bony or ligamentous involvement	absolute
c. comminuted fracture with displacement into spinal canal	absolute
d. lateral mass fracture producing facet incongruity	absolute
3. intervertebral disc injury	
a. healed herniated disc treated conservatively	none
b. S/P ACDF with solid fusion, no symptoms, normal exam, and full pain-free ROM	none
c. chronic herniated disc with pain, neuro findings or ↓ ROM, or acute herniated disc	absolute
4. S/P fusion	
a. stable one-level fusion	none
b. stable two-level fusion	relative
c. fusion > 2 levels	absolute

[a] organized contact sports includes[26]: boxing, football, ice hockey, lacrosse, rugby & wrestling
[b] see also cranial-related (and craniocervical) conditions (p. 1308) (e.g., Chiari I malformation...)
[c] C.I. = contraindications, classified as absolute, relative (i.e., uncertain) or none
[d] congenital abnormalities may have particular relevance to Special Olympics
[e] NB: Klippel-Feil may be associated with abnormalities in other organ systems (e.g., cardiac) which may impact on participation in contact sports (p. 289)
[f] Pavlov ratio (p. 1302) has a low positive predictive value for injuries in contact sports and is therefore not a useful screening test (i.e., an asymptomatic Pavlov ratio < 0.8 is not a contraindication to participation)

68.8 Neurological assessment

68.8.1 General information

Evaluation of the level of the lesion requires familiarity with the following concepts about the relationship between the bony spinal canal and the spinal cord and nerves (► Fig. 68.3).
1. since there are 8 pairs of cervical nerves and only 7 cervical vertebra
    a) cervical nerves 1 through 7 exit *above* the pedicles of their like-numbered vertebra
    b) C8 exits below the C7 pedicle
    c) thoracic, lumbar, and sacral nerves exit *below* the pedicles of their like-numbered vertebra

68

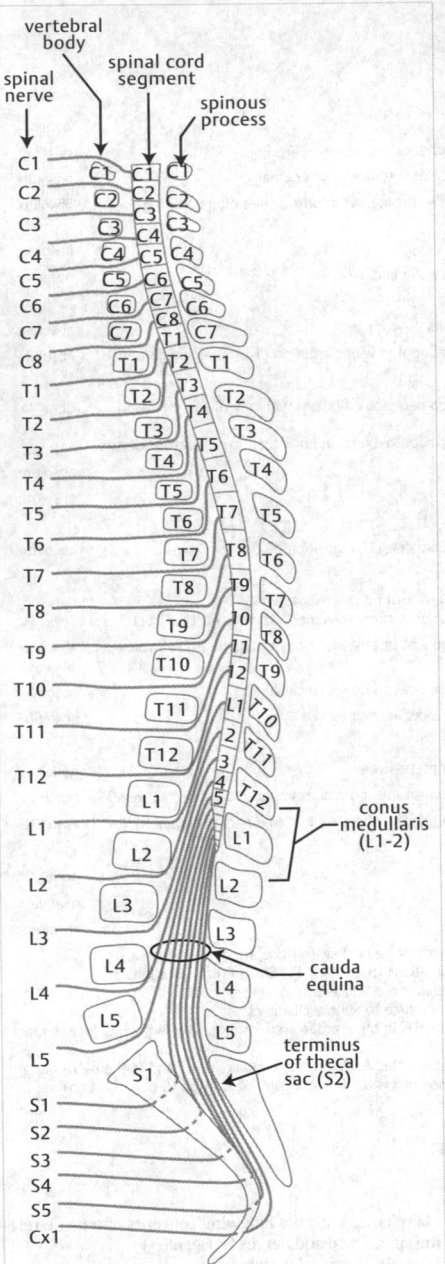

vertebral
body
spinal cord
segment
spinal
nerve
spinous
process

Fig. 68.3 Relationship between spinal cord, nerve roots, and bony spine.
The conus medullaris in the adult lies at about L1 or L2 of the spine (see text).
The lower extent of the thecal sac is typically around S2.
The C1 through C7 nerve roots exit *above* the pedicles of their like-numbered vertebra. Nerve roots of T1 and lower exit below the pedicles of their like-numbered vertebra.

conus
medullaris
(L1-2)

cauda
equina

terminus
of thecal
sac (S2)

2. due to disproportionately greater growth of the spinal column than the spinal cord during development, the following relationships of the spinal *cord* to the vertebral column exist:
   a) to determine which segment of the spinal cord underlies a given vertebra:
      - from T2 through T10: add 2 to the number of the spinous process
      - for T11, T12 and L1, remember that these overlie the 11 lowest spinal segments (L1 through L5, S1 through S5, and Coxygeal-1)
   b) the mean position of the conus medullaris (the lowest extent of the spinal cord) is attained during the first few months of life and doesn't change.[27] It is at the lower third of the L1 VB on MRI in adults (range: middle third of T12 to upper third of L3)[28]

68.8.2 Motor level assessment

General information

▶ Table 68.8 and ▶ Table 68.9 are for rapid assessment (see ▶ Table 30.5 and ▶ Table 30.7 for detailed tables of motor innervation).

Table 68.8 Key muscles for motor level classification (EXTREMITIES)

RIGHT grade	Segment	Muscle	Action to test	LEFT grade
0–5	C5	biceps	flex elbow	0–5
0–5	C6	wrist extensors	cock up wrist	0–5
0–5	C7	triceps	extend elbow	0–5
0–5	C8	flexor digitorum profundus	flex middle distal phalanx	0–5
0–5	T1	hand intrinsics	abduct little finger	0–5
0–5	L2	iliopsoas	flex hip	0–5
0–5	L3	quadriceps	straighten knee	0–5
0–5	L4	tibialis anterior	dorsiflex foot	0–5
0–5	L5	EHL	dorsiflex big toe	0–5
0–5	S1	gastrocnemius	plantarflex foot	0–5
50	← TOTAL POSSIBLE POINTS →			50
GRAND TOTAL: 100				

Table 68.9 Axial muscle evaluation[31]

Level	Muscle	Action to test
C4	diaphragm	tidal volume (TV), FEV1, and vital capacity (VC)
T2–9	intercostals	use sensory level, abdominal reflexes, & Beevor's sign
T9–10	upper abdominals	
T11–12	lower abdominals	

ASIA (American Spinal Injury Association) motor scoring system

A system[29,30] that may be rapidly applied to grade 10 key motor segments using the MRC Grading Scale (▶ Table 30.2) from 0–5 on the left and the right, for a total score of 100 possible points (see ▶ Table 68.8). NB: most muscles receive innervation from two adjacent spinal levels, the levels listed in ▶ Table 68.8 are the *lower* of the two. The standard considers a segment intact if the motor grade is fair (≥3). For additional information, see www.asia-spinalinjury.org.

More detailed motor evaluation

See ▶ Table 68.10.

68

Table 68.10 Skeletal muscles and their major spinal innervation (major contributing segment is shown in boldface)

Segment	Muscle	Action to test	Reflex
C1–4	neck muscles		
C3, 4, 5	diaphragm	inspiration, TV, FEV1, VC	
C5, 6	deltoid	abduct arm > 90°	
C5, 6	biceps	elbow flexion	biceps
C6, 7	extensor carpi radialis	wrist extension	supinator
C7, 8	triceps, extensor digitorum	elbow and finger extension	triceps
C8, T1	flexor digitorum profundus	grasp (flex distal phalanges)	
C8, T1	hand intrinsics	abduct little finger, adduct thumb	
T2–9	intercostals[a]		
T9,10	upper abdominals[a]	Beevor's sign[b]	abdominal cutaneous reflex[c]
T11, 12	lower abdominals[a]		
L2, 3	iliopsoas, adductors	hip flexion	cremasteric reflex[d]
L3, 4	quadriceps	knee extension	infrapatellar (knee jerk)
L4, 5	medial hamstrings, tibialis anterior	ankle dorsiflexion	medial hamstrings
L5, S1	lateral hamstrings, posterior tibialis, peroneals	knee flexion	
L5, S1	extensor digitorum, EHL	great toe extension	
S1, 2	gastrocs, soleus	ankle plantarflexion	Achilles (ankle jerk)
S2, 3	flex digitorum, flex hallucis		
S2, 3, 4	bladder, lower bowel, anal sphincter	clamp down during rectal exam	anal cutaneous reflex[e], bulbocavernosus & priapism

[a] also use sensory level to help evaluate these segments

[b] Beevor's sign: used to assess abdominal musculature for level of lesion. Patient lifts head off of bed by flexing neck; if lower abdominal muscles (below ≈ T9) are weaker than upper abdominal musculature, then umbilicus moves cephalad. Not helpful if both upper and lower abdominals are weak

[c] the abdominal cutaneous reflex: scratching one quadrant of abdomen with sharp object causes contraction of underlying abdominal musculature, causing umbilicus to migrate toward that quadrant. Upper abdominal reflex: T8–9. Lower abdominal reflex: T10–12. This is a cortical reflex (i.e., reflex loop ascends to cortex, and then descends to abdominal muscles). The presence of this response indicates an incomplete lesion for cord injuries above the lower thoracic level

[d] cremasteric reflex: L1–2 superficial reflex

[e] **anal-cutaneous reflex**: AKA anal wink. Normal reflex: mild noxious stimulus (e.g., pinprick) applied to skin in region of anus results in involuntary anal contraction. **Bulbocavernosus (BC) reflex**: see section 68.8.5

68.8.3 Sensory level assessment (dermatomes and sensory nerves)

ASIA standards.[29]

28 key points identified in ▶ Table 68.11 are scored separately for pinprick and light touch on the left & right side using the grading scale shown in ▶ Table 68.12, for a maximum possible total of 112 points for pinprick (left & right) and 112 points for light touch (left & right).

NB: regarding the "C4 cape" AKA "bib" region across the upper chest and back: sensory segments "jump" from C4 to T2 with the intervening levels distributed exclusively on the UEs (▶ Fig. 1.16). The location of this transition is not constant from person to person.

68.8.4 Rectal exam

1. external anal sphincter is tested by insertion of the examiner's gloved finger
   a) perceived sensation is recorded as present or absent. Any sensation felt by the patient indicates that the injury is sensory incomplete
   b) record resting sphincter tone and any voluntary sphincter contraction
2. bulbocavernosus (BC) reflex (p.1130); see also below: Absence suggests the presence of spinal shock, and it may not be possible to declare a suprasacral SCI as complete because there might be spinal shock which could transiently suppress spinal cord function

Table 68.11 Key sensory landmarks

Level	Dermatome
C2	occipital protuberance
C3	supraclavicular fossa
C4	top of acromioclavicular joint
C5	Lateral side of antecubital fossa
C6	thumb, dorsal surface, proximal phalanx
C7	middle finger, dorsal surface, proximal phalanx
C8	little finger, dorsal surface, proximal phalanx
T1	medial (ulnar) side of antecubital fossa
T2	apex of axilla
T3	third intercostal space (IS)
T4	fourth IS (nipple line)
T5	fifth IS (midway between T6 & T8)
T6	sixth IS (xiphoid process)
T7	seventh IS (midway between T6 & T8)
T8	eighth IS (midway between T6 & T10)
T9	ninth IS (midway between T8 & T10)
T10	tenth IS (umbilicus)
T11	eleventh IS (midway between T10 & T12)
T12	inguinal ligament at mid-point
L1	half the distance between T12 & L2
L2	mid-anterior thigh
L3	medial femoral condyle
L4	medial malleolus
L5	dorsum of foot at 3rd MTP (metatarsal phalangeal) joint
S1	lateral heel
S2	popliteal fossa in the mid-line
S3	ischial tuberosity
S4–5	perianal area (taken as 1 level)

Table 68.12 Sensory grading scale

Grade	Description
0	absent
1	impaired (partial or altered appreciation)
2	normal
NT	not testable

68.8.5 Bulbocavernosus (BC) reflex

A polysynaptic spinal cord mediated reflex relayed via S2–4 nerve roots. Contraction of anal sphincter in response to squeezing the glans penis in males, or to tugging on the Foley catheter in either sex is a normal response (must be differentiated from the movement of the Foley catheter balloon). Loss of the bulbocavernosus (BC) reflex can occur with:
1. spinal shock: the BC reflex may be lost with spinal shock as can occur with suprasacral injuries. Reportedly, the return of the BC reflex may be the earliest clinical indicator that spinal shock has subsided
2. injuries involving the cauda equina or conus medullaris

Presence of BC reflex used to be taken as an indication of an incomplete injury, but its presence alone is no longer considered to have a good prognosis for recovery.

68.8.6 Additional sensory exam

The following elements are considered optional but it is recommended that they be graded as absent, impaired, or normal:
1. position sense: test index finger and great toe on both sides
2. awareness of deep pressure/deep pain

68.8.7 ASIA impairment scale

The ASIA impairment scale*[29] is shown in ▶ Table 68.13 (a modified Frankel Neurological Performance scale[32]).

*NB: this scale indicates the completeness of spinal cord injury and is distinct from the other ASIA grading scales; see also motor and sensory scoring (p. 1129).

Table 68.13 ASIA impairment scale

Class	Description
A	complete: no motor or sensory function preserved
B	incomplete: sensory but no motor function preserved below the neurologic level (includes sacral segments S4–5)
C	incomplete: motor function preserved below the neurologic level (more than half of key muscles below the neurologic level have a muscle strength grade < 3)[a]
D	incomplete: motor function preserved below the neurologic level (more than half of key muscles below the neurologic level have a muscle strength grade ≥ 3)
E	normal: sensory & motor function returned to normal

[a]for muscle strength grading, see ▶ Table 30.2

68.9 Spinal cord injuries

68.9.1 Complete spinal cord injuries

See definition of complete vs. incomplete spinal cord injury (p. 1118).

In addition to loss of voluntary movement, sphincter control and sensation below the level of the injury, there may be priapism (p. 1140). Hypotension and bradycardia (p. 1119) (spinal shock) may also present.

68.9.2 Bulbar-cervical dissociation

Occurs as a result of spinal cord injury at or above ≈ C3 (includes SCI from atlantooccipital and atlantoaxial dislocation). Bulbar-cervical dissociation produces immediate pulmonary and, often, cardiac arrest. Death results if CPR is not instituted within minutes. Patients are usually quadriplegic and ventilator dependent (phrenic nerve stimulation may eventually allow independence from ventilator).

68.9.3 Incomplete spinal cord injuries

Central cord syndrome

General information

Key concepts

- disproportionately greater motor deficit in the upper extremities than lower
- usually results from hyperextension injury in the presence of osteophytic spurs
- surgery is often employed for ongoing compression, usually on a non-emergency basis except for rare cases of progressive deterioration

Originally described by Schneider et al[33] in 1954. Central cord syndrome (CCS) is the most common type of incomplete spinal cord injury syndrome. Usually seen following acute hyperextension injury in an older patient with pre-existing acquired stenosis as a result of bony hypertrophy (anterior spurs) and infolding of redundant ligamentum flavum (posteriorly), sometimes superimposed on congenital spinal stenosis. Translational movement of one vertebra on another may also contribute. A blow to the upper face or forehead is often disclosed on history, or is suggested on exam (e.g., lacerations or abrasions to face and/or forehead). This often occurs in relation to a motor vehicle accident or to a forward fall, often while intoxicated. Younger patients may also sustain CCS in sporting injuries; see burning hands syndrome (p. 1711). CCS may occur with or without cervical fracture or dislocation.[34] CCS may be associated with acute traumatic cervical disc herniation. CCS may also occur in rheumatoid arthritis.

Pathomechanics
Traditional dogma was that the centermost region of the spinal cord is a vascular watershed zone which renders it more susceptible to injury from compression or edema, and that the lateral corticospinal tract (CST) was somatotopically organized such that cervical fibers are located more medially than the fibers serving the lower extremities. This anatomical model has been convincingly challenged by Levi and Schwab,[35] who theorize that the proportionally greater effect on the upper extremities is due to the predominance of large-diameter motor axons subserving the upper extremities (especially the highly represented hands which is responsible for human manual dexterity), along with the fact that motor function of the lower extremities can be conveyed via other motor tracts including the rubrospinal and vestibulospinal tracts.

68

Presentation
The clinical syndrome is somewhat similar to that seen in syringomyelia[33]
1. motor: weakness of upper extremities with lesser effect on lower extremities
2. sensory: varying degrees of disturbance below level of lesion may occur
3. myelopathic findings: sphincter dysfunction (usually urinary retention)

Hyperpathia to noxious and non-noxious stimuli is also common, especially in the proximal portions of the upper extremities, and is often delayed in onset and extremely distressing to the patient.[36] Lhermitte's sign (p. 1712) occurs in ≈ 7% of cases.

Natural history
There is often an initial phase of improvement (characteristically: LEs recover first, bladder function next, UE strength then returns with finger movements last; sensory recovery has no pattern) followed by a plateau phase and then late deterioration.[37] 90% of patients are able to walk with assistance within 5 days.[38] Recovery is usually incomplete, and the amount of recovery is related to the severity of the injury and patient age.[39]

If CCS results from hematomyelia with cord destruction (instead of cord contusion), then there may be extension (upward or downward).

Evaluation
Findings: young patients tend to have disc protrusion, subluxation, dislocation or fractures.[38] Older patients tend to have multi-segmental canal narrowing due to osteophytic bars, discs, and inbuckling of ligamentum flavum.[38]

C-spine X-rays: may demonstrate congenital narrowing of AP diameter of spinal canal, superimposed osteophytic spurs, traumatic fracture-dislocation. Occasionally, AP narrowing alone without spurs may be seen.[34] Plain X-rays will fail to demonstrate canal narrowing due to thickening or inbuckling of ligamentum flavum, hypertrophy of facet joints, and poorly calcified spurs.[34]

Cervical CT scan: also helpful in diagnosing fractures and osteophytic spurs. Not as good as MRI for assessing status of discs, spinal cord, and nerves.

MRI: discloses compromise of anterior spinal canal by discs or osteophytes (when combined with plain C-spine X-rays or CT, it increases the ability to differentiate osteophyte from traumatic disc herniation). Also good for evaluating ligamentum flavum. T2WI may show spinal cord edema acutely,[40] and can detect hematomyelia. MRI is poor for identifying fractures.

Treatment
General information

Key concepts

- there is no role for surgery without ongoing compression or instability
- timing (for patient with ongoing spinal cord compression)
  - emergency surgery: documented *progressive deterioration* should be decompressed ASAP
  - early surgery (≤ 24 hrs) when possible for spinal instability or patients with long tract findings (p. 1149)
  - patients that are improving should be followed and decompression can be done electively (usually within 2–3 weeks) without an arbitrary waiting period

Practice guideline: Acute traumatic central cord injuries

Level III[39,41]
- ICU management of patients with acute traumatic central cord syndrome (ATCCS), especially for those with severe neurologic deficits (because of possible cardiac, pulmonary & BP disturbances)
- medical management to include the following: cardiac, hemodynamic, and respiratory monitoring and maintainence of MAP 85–90 mm Hg (use BP augmentation if necessary) for the 1st week after injury to improve spinal cord perfusion
- early reduction/stabilization of fracture-dislocation injuries
- surgical decompression of the compressed spinal cord, particularly if the compression is focal and anterior. Unresolved: the role of surgery in ATCCS with long segment cord compression or with spinal stenosis without bony injury[41] (see text for details)

Indications & timing of surgery
Surgical indications
1. continued compression of the spinal cord (e.g., by osteophytic spurs) that correlates with the level of deficit with any of the following:
   a) persistent significant motor deficit following a varying period of recovery (see below)
   b) deterioration of function
   c) continued significant dysesthetic pain
2. instability of the spine

Timing of surgery
Background: a perennial point of controversy. Early dogma was that early surgery for this condition is *contraindicated* because it worsened the deficit. In the absence of spinal instability, traditional management consisted of bed rest in a soft collar for ≈ 3–4 weeks, with consideration for surgery after this time, or else gradual mobilization in the same collar for an additional 6 weeks. However, the basis for this recommendation was at least in part derived from an early report of only 8 patients with CCS, 2 of which underwent surgery, with 1 being worse post-op (the operation consisted of laminectomy, opening the dura, sectioning the dentate ligament, and manipulation of the spinal cord in order to inspect the anterior spinal canal).[33]

▶ **Early surgery.** Early (usually considered < 24 hrs after injury) decompressive surgery (without cord manipulation) appears to be safe[42] in medically stable patients (see section 69.6 for discussion of timing). The strongest indications for *early* surgery for ATCCS are:
- the rare patient who is improving and then deteriorates.[43] However, great restraint must be used in avoiding what would be an inappropriate operation in many patients[44]
- additional presence of long tract findings: i.e., not a pure CCS, but a combination of other types of incomplete SCI

▶ **"Delayed surgery."** Defined as surgery after 24-26 hours following SCI.
For patients with ATCCS with significant persistent cord compression who consistently fail to progress after an initial period of improvement,[40] surgery is indicated often within 2–3 weeks following the trauma without an arbitrary waiting period. Better results occur with decompression within the first few weeks or months rather than very late (e.g., ≥ 1–2 years).[45 (p 1010)]

Some authorities contend that the worst time to operate on patients is starting 48 hours from the injury and lasting several days to a week due to swelling of the spinal cord which may render it fragile.

Technical considerations of surgery

The most rapid procedure to decompress the cord is often a multi-level laminectomy. This is frequently accompanied by dorsal migration of the spinal cord which may be seen on MRI.[37] With myelography, fused patients fare better than those that are just decompressed without fusion. Fusion may be accomplished posteriorly (e.g., with lateral mass screws and rods) at the time of decompression, or anteriorly (e.g., multi-level discectomy, or corpectomy with strut graft and anterior cervical plating) at the same sitting as the laminectomy or staged at a later date.

Prognosis

In patients with cord contusion without hematomyelia, ≈ 50% will recover enough LE strength and sensation to ambulate independently, although typically with significant spasticity. Recovery of UE function is usually not as good, and fine motor control is usually poor. Bowel and bladder control often recover, but bladder spasticity is common. Elderly patients with this condition generally do not fare as well as younger patients, with or without surgical treatment (only 41% over age 50 become ambulatory, versus 97% for younger patients[46]).

Anterior cord syndrome

68

General information

AKA anterior spinal artery syndrome. Cord infarction in the territory supplied by the anterior spinal artery. Some say this is more common than central cord syndrome.

May result from occlusion of the anterior spinal artery, or from anterior cord compression, e.g., by dislocated bone fragment, or by traumatic herniated disc.

Presentation

1. paraplegia, or (if higher than ≈ C7) quadriplegia
2. dissociated sensory loss below lesion:
   a) loss of pain and temperature sensation (spinothalamic tract lesion)
   b) preserved two-point discrimination, joint position sense, deep pressure sensation (posterior column function)[47]

Evaluation

It is vital to differentiate a non-surgical condition (e.g., anterior spinal artery occlusion) from a surgical one (e.g., anterior bone fragment). This requires one or more of: myelography, CT, or MRI.

Treatment

Surgical intervention is indicated for patients with evidence of cord compression (e.g., by large central disc herniation) or for spinal instability (ligamentous or bony).

Prognosis

The worst prognosis of the incomplete injuries. Only ≈ 10–20% recover functional motor control. Sensation may return enough to help prevent injuries (burns, decubitus ulcers…).

Brown-Séquard syndrome

General information

Spinal cord hemisection. First described in 1849 by Brown-Séquard.[48]

Etiologies

Usually a result of penetrating trauma, it is seen in 2–4% of traumatic spinal cord injuries.[49] Also may occur with radiation myelopathy, cord compression by spinal epidural hematoma, large cervical disc herniation[50,51,52] (rare), spinal cord tumors, spinal AVMs, cervical spondylosis, and spinal cord herniation (p. 1404).

Presentation

Classical findings (rarely found in this pure form):

1. motor: *ipsilateral* weakness below lesion (due to lateral corticospinal tract dysfunction). Neuro-anatomical correlate: motor fibers of the lateral corticospinal tract cross at the pyramidal decussation in the medulla
2. dissociated sensory loss
   a) *contralateral* loss of pain and temperature sensation inferior to lesion (lateral spinothalamic tract dysfunction) starting 1-2 levels *below* the lesion. Neuroanatomical correlate: pain & temperature fibers cross and ascend 1-2 levels in the dorsolateral fasciculus (zone of Lissauer) before entering the contralateral lateral spinothalamic tract
   b) *ipsilateral* loss of vibratory and joint position sense and touch and pressure (dorsal column dysfunction) starting *at the level* of the lesion. Neuroanatomical correlate: these fibers are transmitted by the dorsal columns of the spinal cord which ascend uncrossed until they decussate in the medial lemniscus in the medulla
   c) contralateral loss of crude touch due to disruption of the anterior spinothalamic tract. This may be partially mitigated to varying degrees by redundant fibers in the ipsilateral spinotectal tract

Prognosis

This syndrome has the best prognosis of any of the incomplete spinal cord injuries. ≈ 90% of patients with this condition will regain the ability to ambulate independently as well as anal and urinary sphincter control.

Posterior cord syndrome

AKA contusio cervicalis posterior. Relatively rare. Produces pain and paresthesias (often with a burning quality) in the neck, upper arms, and torso. There may be mild paresis of the UEs. Long tract findings are minimal.

References

[1] White AA, Panjabi MM. The Problem of Clinical Instability in the Human Spine: A Systematic Approach. In: Clinical Biomechanics of the Spine. 2nd ed. Philadelphia: J.B. Lippincott; 1990:277–378

[2] Waters RL, Adkins RH, Yakura J, et al. Profiles of Spinal Cord Injury and Recovery After Gunshot Injury. Clin Orthop. 1991; 267:14–21

[3] Atkinson PP, Atkinson JLD. Spinal Shock. Mayo Clinic Proceedings. 1996; 71:384–389

[4] Chesnut RM, Narayan RK, Wilberger JE, et al. Emergency Management of Spinal Cord Injury. In: Neurotrauma. New York: McGraw-Hill; 1996:1121–1138

[5] Hirsch SA, Hirsch PJ, Hiramoto H, et al. Whiplash Syndrome: Fact or Fiction? Orthop Clin North Am. 1988; 19:791–795

[6] Riley LH, Long D, Riley LHJr. The Science of Whiplash. Medicine. 1995; 74:298–299

[7] Spitzer WO, LeBlanc FE, Dupuis M, et al. Scientific Approach to the Assessment and Management of Activity-Related Spinal Disorders: A Monograph for Clinicians: Report of the Quebec Task Force on Spinal Disorders. Chapter 3: Diagnosis of the Problem (The Problem of Diagnosis). Spine. 1987; 12:S16–S21

[8] Spitzer WO, Skovron ML, Salmi LR, et al. Scientific Monograph of the Quebec Task Force on Whiplash-Associated Disorders: Redefining "Whiplash" and Its Management. Spine. 1995; 20:1S–73S

[9] Radanov BP, Sturzenegger M, Di Stefano G. Long-Term Outcome After Whiplash Injury. Medicine. 1995; 74:281–297

[10] Hamilton MG, Myles ST. Pediatric Spinal Injury: Review of 61 Deaths. Journal of Neurosurgery. 1992; 77:705–708

[11] Hamilton MG, Myles ST. Pediatric Spinal Injury: Review of 174 Hospital Admissions. Journal of Neurosurgery. 1992; 77:700–704

[12] Mandabach M, Ruge JR, Hahn YS, et al. Pediatric axis fractures: early halo immobilization, management and outcome. Pediatric Neurosurgery. 1993; 19:225–232

[13] Garton HJL, Park P, Papadopoulos SM. Fracture dislocation of the neurocentral synchondroses of the axis. Case illustration. Journal of Neurosurgery. 2002; (Spine 3) 96

[14] Fassett DR, McCall T, Brockmeyer DL. Odontoid synchondrosis fractures in children. Neurosurg Focus. 2006; 20

[15] Rozzelle CJ, Aarabi B, Dhall SS, et al. Management of pediatric cervical spine and spinal cord injuries. Neurosurgery. 2013; 72 Suppl 2:205–226

[16] Suss RA, Zimmerman RD, Leeds NE. Pseudospread of the Atlas: False Sign of Jefferson Fracture in Young Children. AJR. 1983; 140:1079–1082

[17] Shaw M, Burnett H, Wilson A, et al. Pseudosubluxation of C2 on C3 in polytraumatized children—prevalence and significance. Clin Radiol. 1999; 54:377–380

[18] Bailey DK. The Normal Cervical Spine in Infants and Children. Radiology. 1952; 59:712–719

[19] Townsend EH, Rowe ML. Mobility of the Upper Cervical Spine in Health and Disease. Pediatrics. 1952; 10:567–574

[20] Jacobson G, Bleeker HH. Pseudosubluxation of the Axis in Children. Am J Roentgenol. 1959; 82:472–481

[21] Swischuk LE. Anterior displacement of C2 in children: physiologic or pathologic? Radiology. 1977; 122:759–763

[22] Bailes JE, Hadley MN, Quigley MR, et al. Management of Athletic Injuries of the Cervical Spine and Spinal Cord. Neurosurgery. 1991; 29:491–497

[23] Torg JS, Corcoran TA, Thibault LF, et al. Cervical Cord Neuropraxia: Classification, Pathomechanics, Morbidity, and Management Guidelines. Journal of Neurosurgery. 1997; 87:843–850

[24] Maroon JC. "Burning Hands" in Football Spinal Cord Injuries. Journal of the American Medical Association. 1977; 238:2049–2051

[25] Cantu RC, Mueller FO. Catastrophic Spine Injuries in Football. J Spinal Disord. 1990; 3:227–231

[26] Torg JS, Ramsey-Emrhein JA. Management Guidelines for Participation in Collision Activities with Congenital, Developmental, or Post-Injury Lesions Involving the Cervical Spine. Clinics in Sports Medicine. 1997; 16:501–531

[27] Wilson DA, Prince JR. John Caffey award. MR imaging determination of the location of the normal conus medullaris throughout childhood. AJR Am J Roentgenol. 1989; 152:1029–1032

[28] Saifuddin A, Burnett SJ, White J. The variation of position of the conus medullaris in an adult population. A magnetic resonance imaging study. Spine (Phila Pa 1976). 1998; 23:1452–1456

[29] American Spinal Injury Association. International Standards for Neurological Classification of Spinal Cord Injury, Revised 2000. 6th ed. Chicago, IL: American Spinal Injury Association; 2000

[30] Ditunno JF,Jr. New spinal cord injury standards, 1992. Paraplegia. 1992; 30:90–91

[31] Lucas JT, Ducker TB. Motor Classification of Spinal Cord Injuries with Mobility, Morbidity and Recovery Indices. Am Surg. 1979; 45:151–158

[32] Frankel HL, Hancock DO, Hyslop G, et al. The Value of Postural Reduction in the Initial Management of Closed Injuries of the Spine with Paraplegia and Tetraplegia. Part I. Paraplegia. 1969; 7:179–192

[33] Schneider RC, Cherry G, Pantek H. The Syndrome of Acute Central Cervical Spinal Cord Injury. J Neurosurg. 1954; 11:546–577

[34] Epstein N, Epstein JA, Benjamin V, et al. Traumatic Myelopathy in Patients With Cervical Spinal Stenosis Without Fracture or Dislocation: Methods of Diagnosis, Management, and Prognosis. Spine. 1980; 5:489–496

[35] Levi AD, Schwab JM. A critical reappraisal of corticospinal tract somatotopy and its role in traumatic cervical spinal cord syndromes. J Neurosurg Spine. 2021:1–7

[36] Merriam WF, Taylor TKF, Ruff SJ, et al. A Reappraisal of Acute Traumatic Central Cord Syndrome. Journal of Bone and Joint Surgery. 1986; 68B:708–713

[37] Levi L, Wolf A, Mirvis S, et al. The Significance of Dorsal Migration of the Cord After Extensive Cervical Laminectomy for Patients with Traumatic Central Cord Syndrome. Journal of Spinal Disorders. 1995; 8:289–295

[38] Chen TY, Lee ST, Lui TN, et al. Efficacy of Surgical Treatment in Traumatic Central Cord Syndrome. Surgical Neurology. 1997; 48:435–440

[39] Section on Disorders of the Spine and Peripheral Nerves of the American Association of Neurological Surgeons and the Congress of Neurological Surgeons. Management of acute central spinal cord injuries. Neurosurgery. 2002; 50 Supplement:S166–S172

[40] Massaro F, Lanotte M, Faccani G. Acute Traumatic Central Cord Syndrome. Acta Neurol (Napoli). 1993; 15:97–105

[41] Aarabi B, Hadley MN, Dhall SS, et al. Management of acute traumatic central cord syndrome (ATCCS). Neurosurgery. 2013; 72 Suppl 2:195–204

[42] Molliqaj G, Payer M, Schaller K, et al. Acute traumatic central cord syndrome: a comprehensive review. Neurochirurgie. 2014; 60:5–11

[43] Fox JL, Wener L, Drennan DC, et al. Central spinal cord injury: magnetic resonance imaging confirmation and operative considerations. Neurosurgery. 1988; 22:340–347

[44] Ducker TB. Comment on Fox J L, et al.: Central spinal cord injury: magnetic resonance imaging confirmation and operative considerations. Neurosurgery. 1988; 22:346–347

[45] Rothman RH, Simeone FA. The Spine. Philadelphia 1992

[46] Penrod LE, Hegde SK, Ditunno JF. Age Effect on Prognosis for Functional Recovery in Acute, Traumatic Central Cord Syndrome. Archives of Physical Medicine and Rehabilitation. 1990; 71:963–968

[47] Schneider RC. The Syndrome of Acute Anterior Spinal Cord Injury. J Neurosurg. 1955; 12:95–122

[48] Brown-Sequard CE. De la transmission des impressions sensitives par la moelle epiniere. C R Soc Biol. 1849; 1

[49] Roth EJ, Park T, Pang T, et al. Traumatic Cervical Brown-Sequard and Brown-Sequard Plus Syndromes: The Spectrum of Presentations and Outcomes. Paraplegia. 1991; 29:582–589

[50] Rumana CS, Baskin DS. Brown-Sequard Syndrome Produced By Cervical Disc Herniation: Case Report and Literature Review. Surgical Neurology. 1996; 45:359–361

[51] Kobayashi N, Asamoto S, Doi H, et al. Brown-Sequard syndrome produced by cervical disc herniation: report of two cases and review of the literature. Spine J. 2003; 3:530–533

[52] Kim JT, Bong HJ, Chung DS, et al. Cervical disc herniation producing acute Brown-Sequard syndrome. J Korean Neurosurg Soc. 2009; 45:312–314

68

69 Management of Spinal Cord Injury

69.1 Spinal trauma management – general information

The major causes of death in spinal cord injury (SCI) are aspiration and shock.[1] Initial survey under ATLS protocol: assessment of airway takes precedence, then breathing, then circulation & control of hemorrhage ("ABC's"). This is followed by a brief neurologic exam.

NB: other injuries (e.g., abdominal injuries) may be masked below the level of SCI.

Any of the following patients should be treated as having an SCI until proven otherwise:
1. all victims of significant trauma
2. trauma patients with loss of consciousness
3. minor trauma victims with complaints referable to the spine (neck or back pain or tenderness) or spinal cord (numbness or tingling in an extremity, weakness, paralysis)
4. associated findings suggestive of SCI include
   a) abdominal breathing
   b) priapism (p. 1140)

Trauma patients are triaged as follows:
1. no history of significant trauma, completely alert, oriented, and free of drug or alcohol intoxication, with no complaints referable to the spine: most may be cleared clinically without the need for C-spine X-rays; see Radiographic evaluation (p. 1141)
2. significant trauma, but no strong evidence of spine or spinal cord injury: the emphasis here is in ruling out a bony lesion and preventing injury
3. patients with neurologic deficit: the emphasis here is to define the skeletal injury and to take steps to prevent further cord injury and loss of function and minimize or reverse the present deficit. The pros and cons of the high-dose methylprednisolone protocol (p. 1140) should be weighed if a neurologic deficit is identified

69.2 Management in the field

1. Spine immobilization prior to and during extrication from vehicle and transport to prevent active or passive movements of the spine.
   a) For possible C-spine injuries in football players, see ▶ Table 69.1 for the National Athletic Trainers' Association (NATA) guidelines for helmet removal. When CPR is necessary it takes precedence. Caution with intubation (see below)
   b) place patient on back-board
   c) sandbags on both sides of the head with a 3 inch strip of adhesive tape from one side of the back-board to the other across the forehead immobilizes the spine as well as a rigid orthosis[2] but allows movement of the jaw and access to the airway
   d) a rigid cervical collar (e.g., Philadelphia collar) may be used to supplement

---

Table 69.1 NATA helmet removal guidelines[a]

✖ NB: do not remove the helmet in the field.

- most injuries can be visualized with the helmet in place
- neurological exam can be done with the helmet in place
- the patient may be immobilized on a spine board with the helmet in place
- the facemask can be removed with special tools to access the airway
- hyperextension must be avoided following removal of the helmet and shoulder pads

In a controlled setting (usually after X-rays) the helmet and shoulder-pads are removed together as a unit to avoid neck flexion or extension

Possible indications for removal of helmet

- face mask cannot be removed in a reasonable amount of time
- airway cannot be established even with face mask removed
- life threatening hemorrhage under the helmet that can be controlled only by removal
- helmet & strap do not hold head securely so that immobilizing the helmet does not adequately immobilize the spine (e.g., poor fitting or damaged helmet)
- helmet prevents immobilization for transportation in an appropriate position
- certain situations where the patient is unstable (M.D. decision)

[a]for more details, see http://www.nata.org

2. maintain blood pressure, see below under Hypotension (p. 1139)
   a) pressors treat the underlying problem (SCI is essentially a traumatic sympathectomy). Dopamine is the agent of choice, and is preferred over fluids (except as necessary to replace losses); see Cardiovascular agents for shock (p. 133) for pressors. ✖ Avoid phenylephrine (see below)
   b) fluids as necessary to replace losses
   c) military anti-shock trousers (MAST): immobilizes lower spine, compensates for lost muscle tone in cord injuries (prevents venous pooling)
3. maintain oxygenation (adequate FIO_2 and adequate ventilation)
   a) if no indication for intubation: use NC or face mask
   b) intubation: may be required for airway compromise or for hypopnea. In SCI, hypopnea may be due to: paralyzed intercostal muscles, paralysis of diaphragm (phrenic nerve = C3, 4 & 5). Hypopnea may also be due to depressed LOC in TBI
   c) caution with intubation with uncleared C-spine
      • use chin lift (not jaw thrust) without neck extension
      • nasotracheal intubation may avoid movement of C-spine but patient must have spontaneous respirations
      • avoided tracheostomy or cricothyroidotomy if possible (may compromise later anterior cervical spine surgical approaches)
4. brief *motor* exam to identify possible deficits (also to document delayed deterioration); ask patient to:
   a) move arms
   b) move hands
   c) move legs
   d) move toes

69.3 Management in the hospital

69.3.1 Stabilization and initial evaluation

1. immobilization: maintain backboard/head-strap (see above) to facilitate transfers to CT table, etc. Log-roll patient to turn. Once studies are completed, remove patient from backboard ASAP (early removal from board reduces risk of decubitus ulcers)
2. *hypotension* (spinal shock): maintain SBP ≥ 90 mm Hg. Spinal cord injuries cause hypotension by a combination of factors (see Spinal shock (p. 1119)) which may further injure the spinal cord[3] or other organ systems
   a) pressors if necessary: dopamine is agent of choice (✖ avoid phenylephrine (Neosynephrine ®): non-inotropic and possible reflex increase in vagal tone → bradycardia)
   b) careful hydration (abnormal hemodynamics → propensity to pulmonary edema)
   c) atropine for bradycardia associated with hypotension
3. oxygenation (see above)
4. NG tube to suction: prevents vomiting and aspiration, and decompresses abdomen which can interfere with respirations if distended (paralytic ileus is common, and usually lasts several days)
5. indwelling (Foley) urinary catheter: for I's & O's and to prevent distension from urinary retention
6. DVT prophylaxis: see below
7. temperature regulation: vasomotor paralysis may produce poikilothermy (loss of temperature control), this should be treated as needed with cooling blankets
8. electrolytes: hypovolemia and hypotension cause increased plasma aldosterone which may lead to hypokalemia
9. more detailed neuro evaluation (p. 1127). Patients may be stratified using the ASIA impairment scale (▶ Table 68.13)
   a) focused history: key questions should center on:
      • mechanism of injury (hyperflexion, extension, axial loading...)
      • history suggestive of loss of consciousness
      • history of weakness in the arms or legs following the trauma
      • occurrence of numbness or tingling at any time following the injury
   b) palpation of the spine for point tenderness, a "step-off," or widened interspinous space
   c) motor level assessment
      • skeletal muscle exam (can localize dermatome)
      • rectal exam for voluntary anal sphincter contraction
   d) sensory level assessment

69

- sensation to pinprick (tests spinothalamic tract, can localize dermatome): be sure to test sensation in face also (spinal trigeminal tract can sometimes descend as low as ≈ C4)
- light (crude) touch: tests anterior cord (anterior spinothalamic tract)
- proprioception/joint position sense (tests posterior columns)

e) evaluation of reflexes
- muscle stretch reflexes: usually absent initially in cord injury
- abdominal cutaneous reflexes
- cremasteric reflex
- sacral: bulbocavernosus (p. 1130), anal-cutaneous reflex

f) examine for signs of autonomic dysfunction
- altered patterns of perspiration (abdominal skin may have low coefficient of friction above lesion, and may seem rough below due to lack of perspiration)
- bowel or bladder incontinence
- persistent penile erection in males (priapism) or clitoris (clitorism) in females indicates autonomic dysfunction. May be a sign of complete SCI, or of spinal shock

10. radiographic evaluation: see below
11. medical management specific to spinal cord injury:
   a) methylprednisolone (see below)
   b) experimental/investigational drugs: none of these agents shown to have unequivocal benefit in man: naloxone, DMSO, Lazaroid®. Tirilazad mesylate (Freedox®) was less beneficial than methylprednisolone[4]

69.3.2 General information

69

Practice guideline: Assessment of SCI in the hospital

Clinical assessment
Level III[5]: the ASIA international standards for neurological and functional assessment of spinal cord injury (SCI) is recommended (p. 1129)

Functional outcome assessment
Level II[5]: the Functional Impairment Measure™ (FIM™) is recommended (see ▶ Table 98.7)
   Level III[5]: the modified Barthel index is recommended (▶ Table 98.6)

Practice guideline: In-hospital critical care management of SCI

Level III[6]: monitor patients with acute SCI (especially those with severe cervical level injuries) in an ICU or similar monitored setting
   Level III[6]: cardiac, hemodynamic & respiratory monitoring after acute SCI is recommended
   Level III[7]: hypotension (SBP < 90 mm Hg) should be avoided or corrected ASAP
   Level III[7]: maintain MAP at 85–90 mm Hg for the first 7 days after SCI to improve spinal cord perfusion

69.3.3 Methylprednisolone

Practice guideline: Methylprednisolone in SCI

Level I[8]
- Methylprednisolone (MP) for the treatment of acute SCI is not recommended.
- GM-1 ganglioside (Sygen) for the treatment of acute SCI is not recommended.

MP is not FDA approved for use in treating acute SCI. There is no Class I or II evidence of benefit supporting this use of MP. Class III data had been used to advocate its use, but the benefits were likely due to random chance and/or selection bias.[8] Conversely, there is Class I, II and III level evidence that high dose steroids are associated with harmful side effects and even death.[8] Use of high-dose MP among spine surgeons has shown a steady decline[9]; however, it was still used by as many as 56% of respondents to one survey.[9]

69.3.4 Hypothermia for spinal cord injury

The position statement of the joint sections of the AANS and the CNS is that there is not enough evidence to recommend for or against local or systemic hypothermia for acute SCI, and that it should be noted that systemic hypothermia is associated with medical complications in TBI.[10]

69.3.5 Deep-vein thrombosis in spinal cord injuries

General information

Also see Thromboembolism in neurosurgery (p. 176). Incidence of DVT may be as high as 100% when 125I-fibrinogen is used.[11] Overall mortality from DVT is 9% in SCI patients.

Practice guideline: DVT in patients with cervical SCI

Prophylaxis
  Level I[12]:
• prophylactic treatment of venous thromboembolism (VTE) in patients with severe motor deficits due to SCI. Choices include:
  ○ LMW heparin, rotating beds, adjusted dose heparin, or some combination of these measures
  ○ or, low-dose heparin + pneumatic compression stockings or electrical stimulation

Level II[12]:
• early administration of VTE prophylaxis (within 72 hours)
• treat for 3 months
  ✖ low-dose heparin should not be used alone
  ✖ oral anticoagulation should not be used alone

Level III[12]:
• vena cava interruption filters should not be used for routine prophylaxis; they may be used for select patients who fail anticoagulation or are not candidates for anticoagulation

Diagnosis
  Level III[12]:
• duplex Doppler ultrasound, impedance plethysmography, venography, and the clinical examination are recommended as diagnostic tests for DVT in patients with SCI

Prophylaxis

A study of 75 patients found titrating dose of SQ heparin q 12 hrs to a PTT of 1.5 times control resulted in lower incidence of thromboembolic events (DVT, PE) than "mini-dose" heparin (5000 U SQ q 12 hrs) (7% vs. 31%).[13] Heparin can cause thrombosis or thrombocytopenia, and chronic therapy may produce osteoporosis (see heparin (p. 172)).

69.4 Radiographic evaluation and initial C-spine immobilization

69.4.1 Clinical criteria to rule out cervical spine instability

There is almost no chance of a significant occult cervical spine injury[14,15] in a trauma patient who met all of the criteria in the Practice Guideline below. (**Note:** Although reports of bony or ligamentous abnormalities have be described as possibly occurring in these patients, there has been no report of a patient who had neurologic injury as a result of these abnormalities.)

Practice guideline: Radiographic evaluation in awake, asymptomatic trauma patients

Level I[16] & Level II[17,18]: radiographic studies are not indicated in patients who meet all of the following (these are basically the NEXUS Low-Risk Criteria[19]):
- no mental status changes (and no evidence of alcohol or drugs). Note: altered mental status can include GCS ≤ 14; disorientation to person, place, time, or events; inability to remember 3 objects at 5 minutes; delayed response to external stimuli. Evidence of alcohol or drugs includes information from the history, physical findings (slurred speech, ataxia, odor of alcohol on the breath) or positive blood or urine tests
- no neck pain or posterior midline tenderness (and no distracting pain)
- no focal neurologic deficit (on motor or sensory exam)
- do not have significant associated injuries that detract/distract from their evaluation

The Canadian C-Spine Rule (CCR) was found to be more sensitive & specific than the NEXUS driteria,[20] and is a valid alternative used by some, but was not endorsed by the EAST (Eastern Association for the Surgery of Spine Trauma) as of 2009.[17]

Cervical immobilization may be discontinued without cervical spine imaging in these patients.

69

69.4.2 Cervical immobilization

General information

Cervical collars should be removed as soon as it can be determined that it is safe to do so. The benefits from early collar removal include: reduction of skin breakdown,[21] fewer days of mechanical ventilation,[22] shorter ICU stays,[22] reduction of ICP.[23,24]

Guidelines

Guidelines for "clearing" the cervical spine and removing the cervical collar are shown in **Practice guideline: Cervical immobilization in trauma patients** (p. 1142). A sample flow sheet is shown in

Practice guideline: Cervical immobilization in trauma patients

A cervical collar is not needed in trauma patients who meet these criteria
- Asymptomatic patients as in **Practice guideline: Radiographic evaluation in asymptomatic trauma patients** (p. 1142): patients who are alert, without neurologic deficit or distracting injury who have *no neck pain* or tenderness and full ROM of the cervical spine (Level II[17])
- Penetrating brain trauma: unless the trajectory suggests direct cervical spine injury (Level III[17])
- Level II[25] & Level III[17]: Patients who are awake *with* neck pain or tenderness and normal cervical CT scan after either (these tests are performed in the absence of an identifiable fracture or obviously unstable dislocation to rule out ligamentous or other soft-tissue injury that might be occult and unstable)
  - normal & adequate dynamic flexion-extension C-spine X-rays
  - or a normal cervical MRI is obtained. Note: AANS/CNS guidelines from 2002 recommended getting the MRI within 48 hours.[25] MRI is usually employed in this setting when the patient is unable to cooperate for flex-ext X-rays; see MRI findings and issues related to timing (p. 1145), etc.

In *obtunded* patients with normal cervical CT scan and gross movement of all 4 extremities
- ✗ flexion-extension C-spine X-rays should *not* be performed (Level II[17])
- options:
  - maintain cervical collar until a clinical exam can be performed[17]
  - remove the collar on the basis of the normal CT scan alone[17] (the incidence of ligamentous injury with negative CT is < 5%, and the incidence of clinically significant injury is unknown but is much < 1%[17])

- ○ obtain cervical MRI (AANS/CNS guidelines from 2002 recommended getting the MRI within 48 hours[25]) :
  - – Level III[17]: the risk and benefit of cervical MRI in addition to CT is unclear, and must be individualized
  - – Level II[17]: If the MRI is normal, the collar may be safely removed

69.4.3 Minimum radiographic evaluation

General information

There is controversy regarding what constitutes a minimum radiographic evaluation of the cervical spine in multiple trauma patient.

Asymptomatic patients—meeting criteria outlined in **Practice guideline: Radiographic evaluation in awake, asymptomatic trauma patients** (p.1142)—may be considered to have a stable cervical spine and *no* radiographic studies of the cervical spine are indicated.[17,25] Factors associated with increased risk of failing to recognize spinal injuries include: decreased level of consciousness (due to injury or drugs/alcohol), multiple injuries, technically inadequate X-rays (p.1221).[26]

Primary imaging recommendations

Practice guideline: Radiographic imaging in trauma patients who are obtunded or unevaluable | 69

Includes unresponsive patients or unreliable exam (altered mental status, distracting pain or injuries)
- Level I[18]
  - ○ high-quality computed tomography (CT) imaging is the modality of choice
    - ✘ if high-quality CT imaging is available, routine 3-view cervical spine X-rays are not recommended
  - ○ if high-quality CT imaging is not available, 3-view cervical spine X-rays (AP, lateral and open-mouth odontoid view) are recommended. Supplement with CT when available if needed to further define areas that are suspicious or poorly visualized on plain X-rays
- Level II[18]
  - ○ if high-quality CT imaging is normal but the index of suspicion is high, further management should fall to physicians trained in the diagnosis and treatment of spine injuries
- Level III[18]
  - ○ if high-quality CT imaging is normal, options include:
    - – continue cervical immobilization until asymptomatic
    - – obtain cervical MRI within 48 hours of injury and, if normal, D/C cervical immobilization*
    - – D/C cervical immobilization at the discretion of the treating physician
      - ✘ the routine use of dynamic imaging (flexion-extension) is of marginal benefit and is not recommended in this situation

* limited and conflicting Class II & III medical evidence

CT scan, while extremely sensitive for bony injuries, is not adequate for assessing soft tissues (e.g., traumatic disc herniation, spinal cord contusion...) or ligamentous injuries (may require flexion-extension X-rays (see below) and/or MRI).

When CT scan is not appropriate/available as the initial radiographic exam

When CT cannot be done, the following guidelines are offered:

See **X-rays,** C-Spine (p.222) for normal vs. abnormal findings. ▶ Table 69.2 lists some indicators that should alert the reviewer that there may be significant C-spine trauma (they do *not* indicate definite instability by themselves).

Table 69.2 Radiographic signs of C-spine trauma (modified[34])

Soft tissues

- retropharyngeal space > 7 mm, or retrotracheal space > 14 mm (adult) or 22 mm (peds), see ▶ Table 12.2 for details
- displaced prevertebral fat stripe
- tracheal deviation & laryngeal dislocation

Vertebral alignment

- loss of lordosis
- acute kyphotic angulation
- torticollis
- widened interspinous space (flaring)
- axial rotation of vertebra
- discontinuity in contour lines (p. 222)

Abnormal joints

- ADI: > 3 mm (adult) or > 4 mm (peds) (see ▶ Table 12.1 for details)
- narrowed or widened disc space
- widening of apophyseal joints

1. cervical spine: must be cleared radiographically from the cranio-cervical junction down through and including the C7–1 junction (incidence of pathology at C7–1 junction may be as high as 9%[27]):
   a) lateral portable C-spine X-ray while in rigid collar: this study by itself will miss ≈ 15% of injuries[28]
   b) if all 7 cervical vertebrae *AND* the C7–1 junction are adequately visualized and are normal, and if the patient has no neck pain or tenderness and is neurologically intact (neurologically intact implies patient is alert, not drugged/intoxicated, & able to report pain reliably), then remove the cervical collar and complete the remainder of the cervical spine series (AP and open-mouth odontoid (OMO) view). Lateral, AP, and OMO views together detect essentially all unstable fractures in neurologically intact patients[29] (although the AP view rarely provides unique information[30]). In a severely injured patient, limitation to an AP and lateral view usually suffices for the *acute* (but not complete) evaluation[31]
   c) if the above studies are normal, but there is neck pain, tenderness or neurologic findings (there may be a spinal cord injury even with normal plain films), or if the patient is unable to reliably verbalize neck pain or cannot be examined for neurologic deficit, then further studies are indicated, which may include any of the following:
      - oblique views (some authors include oblique views in a "minimal" evaluation,[31] others do not[29]): demonstrates the neural foramina (may be blocked with a unilateral locked facet (p. 1186)), shows a different projection of the uncinate processes than the AP view, and helps assess the integrity of the articular masses and lamina (the lamina should align like shingles on a roof)[31]
      - flexion-extension views: see below
      - CT scan: helpful in identifying bony injuries, especially in areas difficult to visualize on plain radiographs. However, CT cannot exclude significant soft-tissue or ligamentous injury[32]
      - MRI: utility is limited to specific situation (p. 1146) and the accuracy has not been determined
      - polytomograms: becoming less available
      - pillar view: devised to demonstrate the cervical articular masses en face (reserved for cases suspected of having articular mass fracture)[33]: the head is rotated to one side (requires that the upper cervical spine injury has been excluded by previous radiographs), the X-ray tube is off centered 2 cm from midline in the opposite direction and the beam is angled 25° caudad, centered at the superior margin of the thyroid cartilage
   d) if subluxation is present at any level and is ≤ 3.5 mm and the patient is neurologically intact (neurologically intact implies patient is alert, not drugged/intoxicated, and able to report pain reliably), then obtain flexion-extension films (see below)
      - if no pathologic movement, may discontinue cervical collar
      - even if no instability is demonstrated, may need delayed films once pain and muscle spasms have resolved to reveal instability
   e) if *lower* C-spine (and/or cervical-thoracic junction) are not well visualized
      - repeat lateral C-spine X-ray with caudal traction on the arms (if not contraindicated based on other injuries, e.g., to shoulders)

- if still not visualized, then obtain a "swimmer's" (Twining) view: the X-ray tube is positioned above the shoulder furthest from the film, and aimed towards the axilla closest to the film with the tube angled 10–15° toward the head while the arm is elevated above the head
- if still not visualized: CT scan through non-visualized levels (CT is poor for evaluating alignment and for fractures in the horizontal plane, thin cuts with reconstructions ameliorates this shortcoming)

f) see questions regarding stability of the subaxial spine (p. 1182)

g) patients with C-spine fractures or dislocations should have daily C-spine X-rays during initial traction or immobilization

2. thoracic and lumbosacral LS-spine: AP and lateral X-rays for all trauma patients who:
   a) were thrown from a vehicle, or fell ≥ 6 feet to the ground
   b) complain of back pain
   c) are unconscious
   d) are unable to reliably describe back pain or have altered mental status preventing adequate exam (including inability to verbalize regarding back pain/tenderness)
   e) have an unknown mechanism of injury, or other injuries that cast suspicion of spine injury

3. reminder: when abnormalities of questionable vintage are identified, a bone scan may be helpful to distinguish an old injury from an acute one (less useful in the elderly; in an adult, a bone scan will become "hot" within 24–48 hrs of injury, and will remain hot for up to a year; in the elderly, the scan may not become hot for 2–3 weeks and can remain so for over a year)

4. if a bony abnormality is identified or if there is a level of neurologic deficit ascribable to a specific spinal level, either a CT or MRI scan through that area should be done if possible

Flexion-extension cervical spine X-rays

69

Purpose: to disclose occult ligamentous instability.

Rationale: It is possible to have a purely ligamentous injury (p. 1186) involving the posterior ligamentous complex and/or intervertebral disc without any bony fracture. Lateral flexion-extension views help detect these injuries, and also evaluate other injuries (e.g., compression fracture) for stability. For patients with limited flexion due to paraspinal muscle spasm (sometimes resulting from pain), a rigid collar should be prescribed, and 2–3 weeks later after the pain decreases[35] the flexion-extension films should be repeated.

Options: a cervical MRI done within 48–72 hours of the trauma (may be more sensitive with STIR sequences (p. 241) or equivalent) may identify ligamentous or other soft-tissue injury, especially in patients who cannot cooperate for flexion-extension X-rays.

✖ Contraindications
- the patient must be cooperative and free of mental impairment (i.e., no head injury, street or prescription drugs, alcohol…)
- there should not be any subluxation > 3.5 mm at any level on neutral lateral C-spine X-rays, which is a marker for possible instability (p. 1186)
- patient must be neurologically intact (if there is any degree of spinal cord injury, proceed instead first with imaging studies, e.g., MRI)
- F/E X-rays are no longer recommended in obtunded patients due to a low yield, poor cost-effectiveness, and they may be dangerous[17]

Technique

The patient should be sitting, and is instructed to flex the head slowly, and to stop if it becomes painful. Serial X-rays are taken at 5–10° increments (or followed under fluoro with spot films at the end of movement), and if normal, the patient may be encouraged to flex further. This is repeated until evidence of instability is seen, or the patient cannot flex further because of pain or limitation of motion. The process is then repeated for extension.

Findings

Normal flexion-extension views demonstrate slight anterior subluxation distributed over all cervical levels with preservation of the normal contour lines (▶ Fig. 12.1). Abnormal findings include: translational movement > 3.5 mm of one level on another, "flaring" of the spinous processes (see exaggerated widening (p. 224)).

Emergent MRI (or myelogram)

General information

Indications for *emergent* MRI in spinal cord injury (SCI) are listed below.

When an MRI cannot be performed, a *myelogram* is required (employing intrathecal contrast with CT to follow) ✖ Caution: cervical myelogram in patients with cervical spine injuries usually requires C1–2 puncture to achieve adequate dye concentration in the cervical region without dangerous extension of the neck or tilting of the patient as required when dye is injected via LP. Furthermore, pressure shifts from LP exacerbates deficit in 14% of cases with complete block.[36]

Indications

1. incomplete SCI (to check for R/O soft tissue compressing cord) with normal alignment: to check for soft tissue compressing cord
2. neurologic deterioration (worsening deficit or rising level) including after closed reduction
3. neurologic deficit not explained by radiographic findings, including:
   a) fracture level different from level of deficit
   b) no bony injury identified: further imaging is done to R/O soft tissue compression (disc herniation, hematoma...) that would require surgery
   c) always keep in mind the possibility of arterial dissection in this setting (p. 1576)

MRI (non-emergent)

General information

MRI may be used to identify potentially unstable occult ligamentous or soft tissue injury. Note: abnormal signal on MRI is not always associated with instability on flexion-extension X-rays.[37] It has been recommended that this MRI should be done within 48 hours[25] or 72 hours[38] of injury. MRI is not reliable for identifying osseous injury.

Indications for non-emergent MRI (modified):

See reference.[39]
1. inconclusive cervical spine radiography, including questionable fractures
2. significant midline paraspinal tenderness and patient unable to have flexion-extension X-rays
3. obtunded or comatose patients

T2WI and STIR (p. 241) are the most helpful sequences. Significant abnormal findings:
1. ventral signal abnormalities with prevertebral swelling
2. dorsal signal abnormalities. Abnormal signal limited to the interspinous is probably not as unstable as when it extends into the ligamentum flavum.[39] These patients were treated with rigid collars or Minerva jackets for 1–3 months, and one that was felt to be very unstable underwent fusion
3. disc disruption indicated by abnormal signal intensity within the disc, increased disc height, or frank disc protrusions

69.5 Traction/reduction of cervical spine injuries

69.5.1 General information

Purpose

To reduce fracture-dislocations, maintain normal alignment and/or immobilize the cervical spine to prevent further spinal cord injury. Reduction decompresses the spinal cord and roots, and may facilitate bone healing.

Practice guidelines

Level III[40,41]

- early closed reduction of C-spine fracture-dislocation injuries with craniocervical traction to restore anatomic alignment in awake patients
- ✖ *not* recommended: closed reduction in patients with an additional rostral injury
- patients with C-spine fracture-dislocation who cannot be examined during attempted closed reduction, or before open posterior reduction, should undergo cervical MRI before attempted reduction (see note below). The presence of a significant herniated disc in this setting is a relative indication for anterior decompression (e.g., by an anterior cervical discectomy and fusion [ACDF]) before reduction
- cervical MRI is also recommended for patients who fail attempts at closed reduction (see note below)

Controversies

1. the rapidity with which reduction should be done[1]
2. whether MRI should be done prior to attempted closed reduction (prereduction MRI (p. 1147), will show disrupted or herniated discs in 33–50% of patients with facet subluxation. These findings do not seem to significantly influence outcome after closed-reduction in awake patients; ∴ the usefulness of prereduction MRI in this setting is uncertain)
   a) in intact patients, to R/O a condition that might cause worsening of neurologic condition with reduction (e.g., traumatic disc herniation)—must be balanced against risks of transferring patients to MRI
   b) in patients with neurologic deficit (complete or partial SCI)

✖ Contraindications

1. atlantooccipital dislocation (p. 1155): traction may worsen deficit. If immobilization with tongs/halo is desired, use no more than ≈ 4 lbs
2. types IIA or III hangman's fracture (p. 1165)
3. skull defect/fracture at anticipated pin site: may necessitate alternate pin site
4. use with caution in pediatric age group (do not use if age ≤ 3 yrs)
5. very elderly patients
6. demineralized skull: some elderly patients, osteogenesis imperfecta…
7. patients with an additional rostral injury
8. patients with movement disorders: constant motion may cause pin erosion through the skull

69.5.2 Application of tongs or halo ring

General information

Supplies: gloves, local anesthetic (typically 1% lidocaine with epinephrine), betadine ointment. Optional equipment: razor or hair clipper, scalpel.

Choice of device: a number of cranial "tongs" are available. Crutchfield tongs require predrilling holes in the skull. Gardner-Wells tongs are the most common tongs in use. If, after the acute stabilization, the later use of halo-vest immobilization is anticipated, a halo ring may be used for the initial cervical traction, and then converted to vest traction at the appropriate time (e.g., post-fusion).

Preparation: placed with patient supine on a gurney or bed. Option: shave hair around proposed pin sites (see below). Betadine skin prep, then infiltrate local anesthetic. Option: incise skin with scalpel (prevents pins from driving in surface contaminants).

Gardner-Wells tongs

Pin sites: the pins are placed in the temporal ridge (above the temporalis muscle), 2–3 finger-breadths (3–4 cm) above pinna. Place directly above external acoustic meatus for *neutral* position traction; 2–3 cm posterior for *flexion* (e.g., for locked facets); 2–3 cm anterior for *extension*. One pin has a central spring-loaded force-indicator. Tighten pins until the indicator protrudes 1 mm beyond the flat surface. Retighten pins daily until indicator protrudes 1 mm for 1 or 2 days only, then stop.

Halo ring

Supplies (in addition to above): optional paddle AKA "spoon" to support the head beyond the edge of the bed, traction adapter (called a "traction bail" from the circular handle on a baille, the old French word for bucket). Read all of this (including pointers) before starting

1. ring size: choose an appropriately sized ring that leaves a ≈ 1–2 cm gap between the scalp and the ring all the way around
2. ring position: generally placed at or just below the widest portion of the skull (the "equator"), but the front should be ≈ 1 cm above the orbital rim and the back should be ≈ 1 cm above the pinna.[42] To facilitate placement of the actual pins, the ring is usually temporarily stabilized with "pins" that have plastic discs where they contact the skull
3. pin sites: choose the threaded holes in the ring that place the pins as perpendicular to the skull as possible as follows
   a) anterior pins: above the *lateral* two–thirds of the orbit
   b) posterior pins: just behind the ears
   c) in pediatrics, additional pins may be placed to further distribute the load on the thinner skull
4. pin insertion: antibiotic ointment is usually places on the tips of the pins which are gradually brought close to the scalp which is then anesthetized with local anesthetic. Pins are then sequen-tially tightened, starting with any pin then going to the "kitty-corner" pin (diagonally opposite), then a third pin and finally its opposite. Most halos provide some type of torque wrench to per-mit approximately 8 in-lb of torque for most adults; 2–5 in-lb for peds
5. placement pointers
   a) the cervical collar is left in place until traction/immobilization is established
   b) try to place the halo as level from left to right as possible. Although compensation during vest placement can be made for a skewed ring, it looks bad
   c) prior to penetrating the forehead skin for anterior pins, have the patient close their eyes and hold them closed as the pins are advanced (this avoids "pinning the eyes open")
   d) ✖ avoid placing pins in the temporalis muscle or the temporal squamosa
   e) ✖ do not place pins above the medial third of the orbit to avoid the supraorbital and supra-trochlear nerves, and to reduce the risk of penetrating the relatively thin anterior wall of the frontal sinus

Application of traction

For traction, transfer to a bed with ortho headboard with the tongs or halo ring/traction bail in place. Tie a rope to the tongs/traction bail and feed through a pulley at the head of bed. Slight flexion or extension is achieved by changing the height of the pulley relative to the patient's long axis.

X-rays: check lateral C-spine X-rays *immediately* after application of traction, at regular intervals, after every change in weights and every move from bed. Check alignment and rule out overdistrac-tion at any level and atlantooccipital dislocation (p. 1153) (BDI should be ≤ 12 mm).

Weight: if there is no malalignment and traction is being used just to stabilize the injury and to compensate for ligamentous instability, use 5 lbs for the upper C-spine or 10 lbs for lower levels. See reducing locked facets (p. 1190) for information on that topic. The cervical collar may be removed once the patient is in traction with adequate reduction or stabilization.

Post-placement care

Pin tightening: pins are re-torqued in 24 hours. Some authors do one additional tightening the day after that. Avoid further tightenings thereafter which can penetrate the skull

Pin care: clean (e.g., half strength hydrogen peroxide), then apply povidone-iodine ointment. Frequency: in hospital: q shift. At home following discharge: twice daily. Alternatively, simple clean-ing with soap and water twice daily is acceptable.

Application of halo vest

For vest placement (i.e., patients not remaining in traction) once the halo ring is placed (see above) it needs to be attached to the vest by posts. The mechanism varies between manufacturers. If possible, have the patient in a cotton T-shirt prior to placing the vest (this may require cutting the neck opening to accommodate the ring).

The vest should be snug, but too tight so as to restrict respirations. Shoulder straps should be contacting the shoulders (the vest will tend to ride up when the patient is sitting). Most vests come with a wrench that is taped to the vest for emergency removal e.g., for cardiopulmonary resuscitation.

Reduction of locked facets

See Practice guideline: Initial closed reduction in fracture-dislocation cervical SCI (p. 1147) for background information and Reduction of locked facets (p. 1190) for technique.

Complications

1. skull penetration by pins. May be due to:
   a) pins torqued too tightly
   b) pins placed over thin bone: temporal squamosa or over frontal sinus
   c) elderly patients, pediatric patients, or those with an osteoporotic skull
   d) invasion of bone with tumor: e.g., multiple myeloma
   e) fracture at pin site
2. reduction of cervical dislocations may be associated with neurologic deterioration which is usually due to retropulsed disc[43] and requires immediate investigation with MRI or myelogram/CT
3. overdistraction from excessive weight (especially with upper cervical spine injuries), may also endanger supporting tissues
4. caution with C1–3 injury, especially with posterior element fracture (traction may pull fragments in towards canal)
5. infection:
   a) osteomyelitis in pin sites: risk is reduced with good pin care
   b) subdural empyema (p. 350): rare[44,45]

69.6 Timing of surgery following spinal cord injury

69.6.1 Early surgery for spinal cord compression

Background information

The theoretical benefit of decompression is to restore blood flow to potentially salvageable spinal cord tissue. Improvement with early surgery has been demonstrated in animal studies. Attempts to confirm the benefit of surgical decompression in humans within 24 hours of injury has shown conflicting results. There has been considerable variability in practices related to the timing of surgery. Guidelines[46] addressing optimal timing of surgery for SCI have been based on weak clinical evidence.

Recent study findings

A meta-analysis[47] of 4 prospective, multicenter SCI databases[4,48,49,50] that were rated as high quality resulted in these findings:
• surgical decompression within 24 hrs of SCI was associated with improvement at 1 year in: mean motor scores, light touch & pinprick sensory scores, and ASIA Impairment Scale (▶ Table 68.13) grades
• post-op changes in total motor scores decreased as time to decompression from injury increased during the first 24-36 hours, and plateaued after 24-36 hours following SCI
• in cervical SCI, the motor score improvement associated with early decompression is greater in the UEs extending cranially starting at or just inferior to the injury level, than it is in the LEs

▶ **Caveats regarding these findings.** Other areas not addressed but which may be ripe for study[51]:
• functional and quality of life outcomes (the above studies only looked at neurologic outcomes, i.e., improved scores in grading scales)
• the 24 hour cutoff for "early surgery" is arbitrary, and it is unknown if "ultra-early" (< 8-12 hrs following SCI) would be even better

69

69

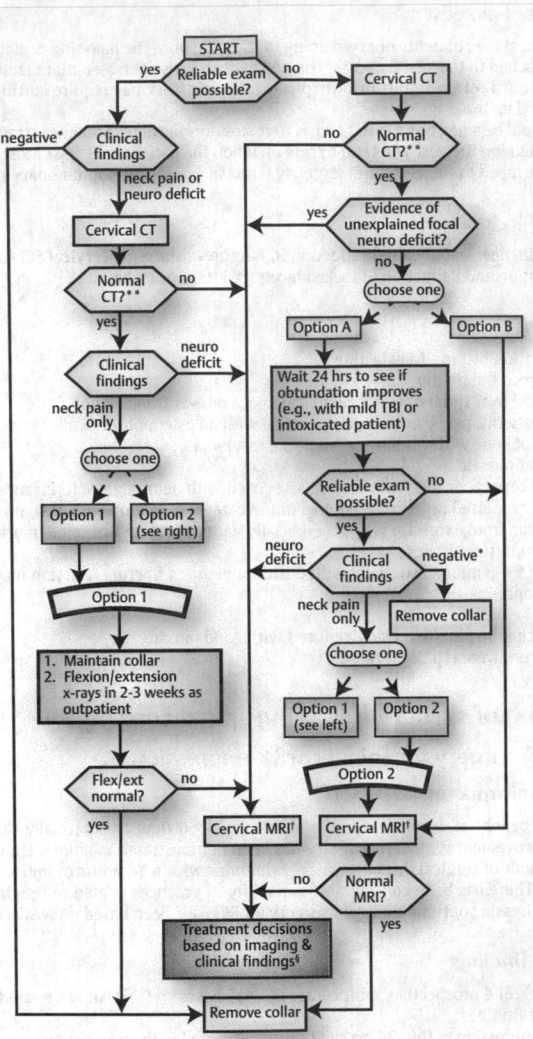

Fig. 69.1 Sample flowchart for "clearing" (i.e., removing) a rigid cervical collar after trauma.
* negative clinical findings (NEXUS criteria): no drugs/alcohol, TBI, confusion, distracting injury, neck pain or neuro-logic deficit
** CT 64 slice or higher Multi Detector CT (MDCT) is recommended. CT is not normal if fracture, dislocation or soft-tissue abnormality is demonstrated
† cervical MRI should be obtained within 48-72 hours of trauma because sensitivity decreases with time
§ treatment decision based on stability, neurologic/vascular involvement....

- these studies give no guidance as to what constitutes adequate decompression: e.g., is expansile duroplasty helpful?
- it is unknown if intrathecal pressure measurement would allow tailoring treatment measures (e.g., spinal cord perfusion pressure) to improve outcome
- if certain subgroups (e.g., central cord syndrome) don't benefit from early decompression
- it is unknown if complete SCI (i.e., ASIA A) benefits from early decompression
- is "after hours" early treatment (with its inherent limitations) more beneficial than waiting until the most proficient surgical team can be assembled for definitve treatment?

Cautious recommendations

Given the above limitations, it seems reasonable to state that:

∑: Surgery for SCI with ongoing compression

There is evidence that early decompression surgery (ideally within 24 hours, but possibly up to 36 hours, after injury) provides some benefit to neurologic function, and should be undertaken when feasible.

A Canadian study[52] found that this goal was attainable in < 50% of patients. Barriers to achieving this goal:
- patients who are medically unstable due to medical conditions or other injuries
- the time needed to obtain necessary diagnostic studies
- the time to transfer patients to centers that are capable of performing the needed surgery

69

69.6.2 Timing of surgery other than for decompression

Surgery for spinal *instability* as a result of fractures or ligamentous compromise when early surgery is not indicated should be performed within 72 hrs of injury whenever possible to permit earlier mobilization of the patient which is associated with lower rates of cardiac, respiratory and infectious complications.[53] As above, unavoidable delays may be encountered e.g., with medically unstable patients.

References

[1] Chesnut RM, Narayan RK, Wilberger JE, et al. Emergency Management of Spinal Cord Injury. In: Neurotrauma. New York: McGraw-Hill; 1996:1121–1138

[2] Podolsky SM, Baraff LJ, Simon RR, et al. Efficacy of Cervical Spine Immobilization Methods. J Trauma. 1983; 23:687–690

[3] Meguro K, Tator CH. Effect of Multiple Trauma on Mortality and Neurological Recovery After Spinal Cord or Cauda Equina Injury. Neurol Med Chir. 1988; 28:34–41

[4] Bracken MB, Shepard MJ, Holford TR, et al. Administration of Methylprednisolone for 24 or 48 Hours or Tirilazad Mesylate for 48 Hours in the Treatment of Acute Spinal Cord Injury. JAMA. 1997; 277:1597–1604

[5] Section on Disorders of the Spine and Peripheral Nerves of the American Association of Neurological Surgeons and the Congress of Neurological Surgeons. Clinical assessment after acute cervical spinal cord injury. Neurosurgery. 2002; 50 Supplement:S21–S29

[6] Section on Disorders of the Spine and Peripheral Nerves of the American Association of Neurological Surgeons and the Congress of Neurological Surgeons. Management of acute spinal cord injuries in an intensive care unit or other monitored setting. Neurosurgery. 2002; 50 Supplement:S51–S57

[7] Section on Disorders of the Spine and Peripheral Nerves of the American Association of Neurological Surgeons and the Congress of Neurological Surgeons. Blood pressure management after acute spinal cord injury. Neurosurgery. 2002; 50 Supplement:S58–S62

[8] Hurlbert RJ, Hadley MN, Walters BC, et al. Pharmacological therapy for acute spinal cord injury. Neurosurgery. 2013; 72 Suppl 2:93–105

[9] Schroeder GD, Kwon BK, Eck JC, et al. Survey of Cervical Spine Research Society members on the use of high-dose steroids for acute spinal cord injuries. Spine (Phila Pa 1976). 2014; 39:971–977

[10] Resnick DK, Kaiser MG, Fehlings M, et al. Hypothermia and human spinal cord injury: Position statement and evidence based recommendations from the AANS/CNS Joint Section on Disorders of the Spine and the AANS/CNS Joint Section on Trauma. 2007. http://www.spinesection.org/statement-detail/hypothermia-human-spinal-cord-injury

[11] Hamilton MG, Hull RD, Pineo GF. Venous Thromboembolism in Neurosurgery and Neurology Patients: A Review. Neurosurgery. 1994; 34:280–296

[12] Dhall SS, Hadley MN, Aarabi B, et al. Deep venous thrombosis and thromboembolism in patients with cervical spinal cord injuries. Neurosurgery. 2013; 72 Suppl 2:244–254

[13] Green D, Lee MY, Ito VY, et al. Fixed- vs Adjusted-Dose Heparin in the Prophylaxis of Thromboembolism in Spinal Cord Injury. JAMA. 1988; 260:1255–1258

[14] Bachulis BL, , Hynes GD, et al. Clinical indications for cervical spine radiographs in the traumatized patient. American Journal of Surgery. 1987; 153:473–478

[15] Harris MB, Waguespack AM, Kronlage S. 'Clearing' Cervical Spine Injuries in Polytrauma Patients: Is It Really Safe to Remove the Collar? Orthopedics. 1997; 20:903–907

[16] Section on Disorders of the Spine and Peripheral Nerves of the American Association of Neurological Surgeons and the Congress of Neurological Surgeons. Radiographic assessment of the cervical spine in asymptomatic trauma patients. Neurosurgery. 2002; 50 Supplement:S30–S35

[17] Como JJ, Diaz JJ, Dunham CM, et al. Practice management guidelines for identification of cervical spine injuries following trauma: update from the Eastern Association for the Surgery of Trauma Practice Management Guidelines Committee. Journal of Trauma. 2009; 67:651–659

[18] Ryken TC, Hadley MN, Walters BC, et al. Radiographic assessment. Neurosurgery. 2013; 72 Suppl 2:54–72

[19] Hoffman JR, Mower WR, Wolfson AB, et al. Validity of a set of clinical criteria to rule out injury to the cervical spine in patients with blunt trauma. National Emergency X-Radiography Utilization Study Group. N Engl J Med. 2000; 343:94–99

[20] Stiell IG, Clement CM, McKnight RD, et al. The Canadian C-spine rule versus the NEXUS low-risk criteria in patients with trauma. New England Journal of Medicine. 2003; 349:2510–2518

[21] Chendrasekhar A, Moorman DW, Timberlake GA. An evaluation of the effects of semirigid cervical collars in patients with severe closed head injury. American Surgeon. 1998; 64:604–606

[22] Stelfox HT, Velmahos GC, Gettings E, et al. Computed tomography for early and safe discontinuation of cervical spine immobilization in obtunded multiply injured patients. Journal of Trauma. 2007; 63:630–636

[23] Hunt K, Hallworth S, Smith M. The effects of rigid collar placement on intracranial and cerebral perfusion pressures. Anaesthesia. 2001; 56:511–513

[24] Mobbs RJ, Stoodley MA, Fuller J. Effect of cervical hard collar on intracranial pressure after head injury. ANZ J Surg. 2002; 72:389–391

[25] Section on Disorders of the Spine and Peripheral Nerves of the American Association of Neurological Surgeons and the Congress of Neurological Surgeons. Radiographic assessment of the cervical spine in symptomatic trauma patients. Neurosurgery. 2002; 50 Supplement:S36–S43

[26] Walter J, Doris P, Shaffer M. Clinical Presentation of Patients with Acute Cervical Spine Injury. Ann Emerg Med. 1984; 13:512–515

[27] Nichols CG, Young DH, Schiller WR. Evaluation of Cervicothoracic Junction Injury. Ann Emerg Med. 1987; 16:640–642

[28] Shaffer M, Doris P. Limitation of the Cross Table Lateral View in Detecting Cervical Spine Injuries: A Retrospective Analysis. Ann Emerg Med. 1981; 10:508–513

[29] MacDonald RL, Schwartz ML, Mirich D, et al. Diagnosis of Cervical Spine Injury in Motor Vehicle Crash Victims: How Many X-Rays Are Enough? J Trauma. 1990; 30:392–397

[30] Holliman C, Mayer J, Cook R, et al. Is the AP Radiograph of the Cervical Spine Necessary in Evaluation of Trauma? Ann Emerg Med. 1990; 19:483–484

[31] Harris JH. Radiographic Evaluation of Spinal Trauma. Orthopedic Clinics of North America. 1986; 17:75–86

[32] Tehranzedeh J, Bonk T, Ansari A, et al. Efficacy of Limited CT for Non-Visualized Lower Cervical Spine in Patients with Blunt Trauma. Skeletal Radiol. 1994; 23:349–352

[33] Miller MD, Gehweiler JA, Martinez S, et al. Significant new observations on cervical spine trauma. American Journal of Radiology. 1978; 130:659–663

[34] Clark WM, Gehweiler JA, Laib R. Twelve Significant Signs of Cervical Spine Trauma. Skeletal Radiol. 1979; 3:201–205

[35] Wales L, Knopp R, Morishima M. Recommendations for Evaluation of the Acutely Injured Spine: A Clinical Radiographic Algorithm. Ann Emerg Med. 1980; 9:422–428

[36] Hollis PH, Malis LI, Zappulla RA. Neurological Deterioration After Lumbar Puncture Below Complete Spinal Subarachnoid Block. J Neurosurg. 1986; 64:253–256

[37] Horn EM, Lekovic GP, Feiz-Erfan I, et al. Cervical magnetic resonance imaging abnormalities not predictive of cervical spine instability in traumatically injured patients. J Neurosurg Spine. 2004; 1:39–42

[38] Schuster R, Waxman K, Sanchez B, et al. Magnetic resonance imaging is not needed to clear cervical spines in blunt trauma patients with normal computed tomographic results and no motor deficits. Archives of Surgery. 2005; 140:762–766

[39] Benzel EC, Hart BL, Ball PA, et al. Magnetic resonance imaging for the evaluation of patients with occult cervical spine injury. Journal of Neurosurgery. 1996; 85:824–829

[40] Section on Disorders of the Spine and Peripheral Nerves of the American Association of Neurological Surgeons and the Congress of Neurological Surgeons. Initial closed reduction of cervical spine fracture-dislocation injuries. Neurosurgery. 2002; 50 Supplement:S44–S50

[41] Gelb DE, Aarabi B, Dhall SS, et al. Treatment of subaxial cervical spinal injuries. Neurosurgery. 2013; 72 Suppl 2:187–194

[42] Botte MJ, Byrne TP, Abrams RA, et al. Halo Skeletal Fixation: Techniques of Application and Prevention of Complications. Journal of the American Academy of Orthopaedic Surgeons. 1996; 4:44–53

[43] Robertson PA, Ryan MD. Neurological Deterioration After Reduction of Cervical Subluxation: Mechanical Compression by Disc Material. Journal of Bone and Joint Surgery. 1992; 74B:224–227

[44] Dill SR, Cobbs CG, McDonald CK. Subdural Empyema: Analysis of 32 Cases and Review. Clin Inf Dis. 1995; 20:372–386

[45] Garfin SR, Botte MJ, Triggs KJ, et al. Subdural Abscess Associated with Halo-Pin Traction. Journal of Bone and Joint Surgery. 1988; 70A:1338–1340

[46] Fehlings MG, Tetreault LA, Wilson JR, et al. A Clinical Practice Guideline for the Management of Patients With Acute Spinal Cord Injury and Central Cord Syndrome: Recommendations on the Timing (<\/=24 Hours Versus > 24 Hours) of Decompression Surgery. Global Spine J. 2017; 7:195S–202S

[47] Badhiwala JH, Wilson JR, Witiw CD, et al. The influence of timing of surgical decompression for acute spinal cord injury: a pooled analysis of individual patient data. Lancet Neurol. 2021; 20:117–126

[48] Grossman RG, Toups EG, Frankowski RF, et al. North American Clinical Trials Network for the Treatment of Spinal Cord Injury: goals and progress. J Neurosurg Spine. 2012; 17:6–10

[49] Fehlings MG, Vaccaro A, Wilson JR, et al. Early versus delayed decompression for traumatic cervical spinal cord injury: results of the Surgical Timing in Acute Spinal Cord Injury Study (STASCIS). PLoS One. 2012; 7. DOI: 10.1371/journal.pone.0032037

[50] Geisler FH, Coleman WP, Grieco G, et al. The Sygen multicenter acute spinal cord injury study. Spine (Phila Pa 1976). 2001; 26:S87–S98

[51] Ramakonar H, Fehlings MG. 'Time is Spine': new evidence supports decompression within 24 h for acute spinal cord injury. Spinal Cord. 2021. DOI: 10.1038/s41393-021-00654-0

[52] Glennie RA, Bailey CS, Tsai EC, et al. An analysis of ideal and actual time to surgery after traumatic spinal cord injury in Canada. Spinal Cord. 2017; 55:618–623

[53] Ruddell JH, DePasse JM, Tang OY, et al. Timing of Surgery for Thoracolumbar Spine Trauma: Patients With Neurological Injury. Clin Spine Surg. 2021; 34: E229–E236

70 Occipitoatlantoaxial Injuries (Occiput to C2)

70.1 Atlantooccipital dislocation (AOD)

70.1.1 General information

See Occipitoatlantoaxial-complex anatomy (p.67) for relevant anatomy.

Atlantooccipital dislocation (AOD), AKA craniocervical junction dislocation, AKA "internal decapitation" (in the lay press): disruption of the stability of the craniocervical junction (which results from *ligamentous* injuries). Probably underdiagnosed, may be present in ≈ 1% of patients with "cervical spine injuries"[1] (definition of cervical spine injuries not specified), found in 8–19% of fatal cervical spine injury autopsies.[2,3] More than twice as common in pediatrics as in adults, possibly owing to the flatter (i.e., less cupped) condyles in peds, the higher ratio of cranium-to-body weight, and increased ligamentous laxity. Most mortality results from anoxia due to respiratory arrest as a result of bulbar-cervical dissociation (BCD).

70.1.2 Clinical presentation

1. may be neurologically intact, therefore AOD must be ruled out in any major trauma
2. bulbar-cervical dissociation (p.1132)
3. may have lower cranial nerve deficits (as well as VI palsies) ± cervical cord injury
4. cruciate paralysis (p.1709)
5. worsening neurologic deficit with the application of cervical traction: check C-spine X-rays after applying traction, changing weights (see) (p.1148)

70.1.3 Radiographic evaluation

Numerous methodologies have been devised to radiographically diagnose AOD. Most utilize *surrogate markers* for the end-point of interest: viz. instability of the occipital-cervical junction. None are completely reliable.[4] Measurements on CT scans are more accurate than plain radiographs (landmarks are easier to identify, no magnification or rotation error) – however, normal values differ from plain radiographs. Some methods are shown in ► Table 70.1. Recommended methods: BAI-BDI method and the AOI method (the AOI method is a level I recommendation[5] for diagnosing AOD in pediatrics).

70

Table 70.1 Radiographic evaluation of atlantooccipital dislocation (AOD)

Method	Comments	Normal values	
		Plain X-ray	CT
BAI-BDI method[7a] Both BAI & BDI should be measured in adults.	**BAI[8]** (basion-axial interval) = distance from basion (inferior tip of the clivus) to rostral extension of posterior axial line (PAL) (the posterior cortical margin of the body of C2). AKA Harris line. Better for *anterior* or *posterior* AOD	Adults: -4 ≤ BAI ≤ 12 mm. Normal: BAI & BDI each ≤ 12 mm	May be used,[9] but was not reliably reproducible on CT[10]
		Peds: 0–12 mm (BAI should never be negative)	
	BDI (basion-dental interval) = distance from basion to the closest point on the tip of the dens. Better for *distracted* AOD	Adult: ≤ 12 mm (range: 2–15 mm) (mean: 7.5 ±þ4.3)	Adult: < 8.5 mm (range: 1.4–9 mm)[10]
		Peds: unreliable in age < 13 yrs because of variable age of ossification and fusion of the odontoid tip (os)	Peds[11b]: < 10.5 mm (95th percentile). With os[c]: < 9.5 mm. Without os[c]: < 11.5 mm

(continued)

Table 70.1 continued

Method	Comments	Normal values	
		Plain X-ray	CT
Atlantooccipital interval (AOI) AKA **CCI** (condyle-C1 interval) AKA **condylar gap**.[12] 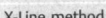	Distance between occipital condyle and superior articular surface of C1 measured on lateral X-ray or sagittal CT reconstructions thru O-C1 junction. Pang[13] averaged the interval between the condyle and C1 at 4 equidistant points on sagittal and 4 on coronal images (8 points total)	Adult[d]: ≤ 2 mm[12]	Adult: < 1.4 mm (95th percentile) (based on single measurement) [10]
		Peds: ≤ 5 mm (for all of 5 equally spaced measurements[14])	Peds: < 2.5 mm (single measure),[11] or < 4.0 mm (average of 8 measurements in 2 planes)[15]
Powers' ratio & Dublin measure 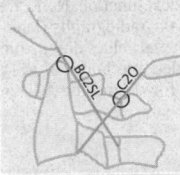 POWERS' RATIO - - - - DUBLIN MEASURE ———	**Powers' ratio**: cannot be used with fractures of C1 or foramen magnum. Only for *anterior* AOD (see text). Requires identification of 4 reference points: B = basion, A = anterior arch of C1, C = posterior arch of C1, O = opisthion[e]	Adult: < 1 (range: 0.5–1.2) (95th percentile = 0.6–0.9) (see text for details)	Same as plain X-ray[10]
		Peds: < 0.9[f]	
	Dublin measure[16] 25% sensitive[17]	Mandible to anterior atlas: ≤ 13 mm. Posterior mandible to dens: ≤ 20 mm	
X-Line method 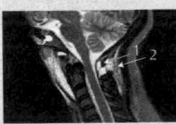	AKA occipital-axial lines method.[17] Requires identification of 6 reference points and 2 lines (sensitivity 75%).[17] Uses a 6 ft target-film distance in a sitting patient[18] which is not always practical in the E/R[19] • C2O line: from the posteroinferior corner of axis body to the opisthion[e]. Should intersect tangentially with the highest point on the C1 spinolaminar line • BC2SL line: from the basion to a point midway on the C2 spinolaminar line. Should intersect tangentially with the posterosuperior dens		
MRI	Abnormal MRI findings include: abnormal high signal on T2WI in the occipitoatlantal joints or in the posterior occipitoatlantal (O-C1) ligaments. Very sensitive (≈ 100%) but not specific for *unstable* AOD. The figure at left shows abnormal signal in the posterior O-C1 ligaments (arrow 1) and in the ligamentum flavum and soft tissues (arrow 2).		

[a]original study of lateral X-ray in a supine patient with a target-film distance of 40 in. (1 m). The sensitivity of the BAI-BDI method for AOD is good when all landmarks can be identified, but still may only be ≈ 75%[9]
[b]for this study, peds is defined up to the age of 10 years, by age ≈ 8–10 years the C-spine reaches adult proportions (not necessarily size)
[c]os = ossiculum terminale (p. 1175)
[d]the articular process of C1 is often obscured by the tip of the mastoid process on plain films
[e]the opisthion cannot be identified in ≈ 56% of lateral C-spine X-rays[8]
[f]could not be measured in many peds cases often due to lack of ossification (usually of posterior C1 arch)

▶ **Technical considerations for radiographic evaluation**
1. X-rays: verify that the film is a true lateral (e.g., check alignment of the two mandibular rami as well as of the posterior clinoids)
2. CT scan (bone windows)
   a) sensitivity, specificity, and positive/negative predictive values of most of these measures improve when sagittal CT views are used instead of plain radiographs[6] (relevant landmarks could be identified in > 99% of CTs, vs. 39–84% on X-ray)

b) indirect signs that may telegraph the presence of AOD include: blood in the basal cisterns and/or retroclival hematoma (p. 1102), on thin-cut axial CT there may be one or more slices showing no bone at all due to the gap between the occiput and C1

Practice guideline: Diagnosis of atlantooccipital dislocation

Level I[5]
• In pediatric patients, CT to assess the condyle-C1 interval (CCI) is recommended to diagnose AOD

Level III[5]
• In pediatric patients, CCI measured on CT has the highest sensitivity and specificity for AOD. The utility in adults has not been reported
• A lateral cervical spine X-ray is recommended to diagnose AOD. If it is desired to employ a radiologic method of measurement, the BAI-BDI method is recommended (see ▶ Table 70.1). Prevertebral soft tissue swelling in the upper cervical spine on an otherwise nondiagnostic X-ray should be followed with a cervical CT to rule out AOD

▶ **Powers' ratio.** Powers' ratio[1]: distance **BC** (basion to posterior arch of atlas) is divided by distance **AO** (opisthion to anterior arch of atlas), see ▶ Table 70.1. Interpretation is shown in ▶ Table 70.2.
    ✖ Cannot be used with any fracture involving the atlas or the foramen magnum, or with congenital anatomic abnormalities. Applies only to *anterior* AOD (i.e., not for posterior or distracted AOD).

Table 70.2 Powers' ratio

Ratio BC/AO	Interpretation	Comment
<0.9	normal	1 standard deviation below the lowest case of AOD
≥0.9 and <1	"gray zone" (indeterminate)	included 7% of normals and no cases of AOD
≥1	AOD	encompassed all AOD cases

▶ **Traynelis classification.**[20] Classifies the direction of the dislocation, as shown in ▶ Table 70.3.

Table 70.3 Traynelis directional classification of atlantooccipital dislocation* (AOD)[20]

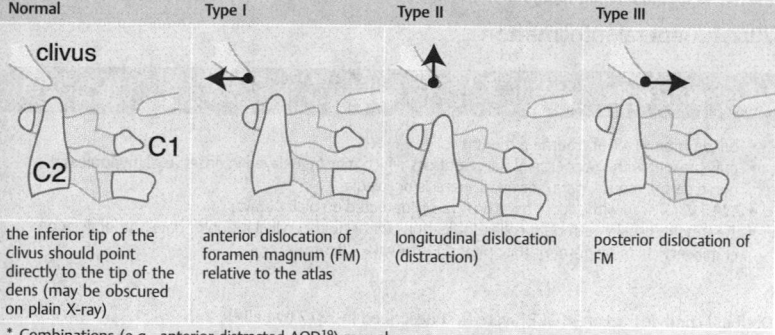

Normal	Type I	Type II	Type III
the inferior tip of the clivus should point directly to the tip of the dens (may be obscured on plain X-ray)	anterior dislocation of foramen magnum (FM) relative to the atlas	longitudinal dislocation (distraction)	posterior dislocation of FM

* Combinations (e.g., anterior-distracted AOD[19]) may also occur

70.1.4 Management

Initial management

If AOD is suspected, immediately immobilize the neck with halo orthosis or with sandbags.
✖ Cervical traction to reduce AOD is contraindicated because there is a 10% risk of neurologic deterioration.

70

Subsequent management

Controversial whether operative fusion vs. prolonged immobilization (4–12 months) with halo brace is required. However, posterior occipitocervical fusion is usually recommended (p. 1380).

(p. 1380)

Practice guideline: Treatment of atlantooccipital dislocation

Level III[5]
- internal fixation & arthrodesis (fusion) using one of a variety of methods
- ✖ CAUTION: cervical traction is not recommended in the management of AOD

Horn et al[9] suggest that patients be grouped and then managed as shown in ▸ Table 70.4.
In infants: reduce in the OR and fuse (usually with transarticular screws).

Table 70.4 Grading & management of AOD[9]

Grade	Definition	Management
I	no abnormal CT criteria[a] with only moderately abnormal MRI (high signal in posterior ligaments or occipitoatlantal joints)	external orthosis (halo or collar)
II	≥1 abnormal CT criteria[a] or grossly abnormal MRI findings in occipitoatlantal joints, tectorial membrane, or alar or cruciate ligaments	surgical stabilization

[a]CT criteria used: Power's ratio, BAI-BDI, X-line

70

70.1.5 Prognosis

The most important predictor of outcome is the severity of neurologic injuries at the time of presentation.[9] Among AOD patients who survived the initial injury, those with severe TBI and brainstem dysfunction or complete bulbar-cervical dissociation all had poor outcome.[9] Those with incomplete SCI or nonsevere TBI may improve.

70.2 Occipital condyle fractures

70.2.1 General information

Key concepts

- uncommon (0.4% of trauma patients)
- may present with lower cranial nerve deficits which may be delayed in onset (e.g., hypoglossal nerve palsy), mono-, para-, or quadriparesis or -plegia
- W/U: ✔ CT scan with reconstructions (rarely detected on plain X-rays)
- Treatment: usually with rigid collar. Indications for occipitocervical fusion or halo immobilization: craniocervical misalignment (occipital-C1 interval > 2.0 mm)

Occipital condyle fractures (OCF) were first described in 1817 by Bell.[21]
Rare. Incidence: 0.4% (in a series of 24,745 consecutive trauma patients surviving to the E/R[22])

70.2.2 Diagnosis

Clinical suspicion of occipital condyle fracture (OCF) should be raised by the presence of ≥1 of the following[23]:
- blunt trauma with high energy
- craniocervical injuries
- altered consciousness

- occipital pain or tenderness
- impaired cervical movement
- lower cranial nerve palsies
- retropharyngeal soft-tissue swelling

Practice guideline: Diagnosis of occipital condyle fractures

Level II[24]
- CT to establish the diagnosis of occipital condyle fracture (OCF)

Level III[24]
- MRI to assess the integrity of the ligaments of the craniocervical complex

70.2.3 Classification

A widely used classification system is that of Anderson & Montesano[25] as shown in ▶ Table 70.5.

Maserati et al[22] classified patients simply on the basis of whether craniocervical misalignment was present or absent on CT with reconstructions (they defined craniocervical misalignment as an occipital condyle-C1 interval > 2.0 mm). They felt other classification systems were superfluous as they did not affect outcome in their retrospective review (see Treatment below).

Table 70.5 Anderson & Montesano classification of occipital condyle fractures

Type	Description	Treatment
I	comminuted from impact: may occur from axial loading	± external immobilization (collar or halo)
II	extension of linear basilar skull fracture[26]	± external immobilization (collar or halo)
III	*avulsion* of condyle fragment (traction injury): may occur during rotation, lateral bending, or a combination of mechanisms. Considered unstable by many	external immobilization (collar or halo) X 6–8 weeks

70.2.4 Treatment

Controversial. Lower cranial nerve deficits often develop in untreated cases of OCF, and may resolve or improve with external immobilization. Anderson & Montesano Types I & II have been treated with or without external immobilization (cervical collar or, occasionally, halo) without obvious difference (▶ Table 70.5). External immobilization × 6–8 weeks is suggested for Type III fractures because of the higher risk of delayed deficits.

Treatment guidelines are also shown.

Practice guideline: Treatment of occipital condyle fractures

Level III[24]:
- For OCF with associated atlantooccipital ligamentous injury or evidence of instability: halo vest immobilization or occipitocervical stabilization (fusion).
- For bilateral OCFs, consider halo vest instead of a collar to provide increased immobilization.
- External cervical immobilization for all other OCFs.

70.2.5 Outcome

In a retrospective review of 100 patients with OCF,[22] 3 patients underwent occipitocervical fusion (p. 1773) for craniocervical misalignment (2) or unrelated C1–2 fracture (1). The remainder (without craniocervical misalignment) were treated with a rigid collar and delayed clinical & radiographic follow-up. None of their unoperated patients had neurologic deficit, and none developed delayed instability, malalignment, or neurologic deficit (regardless of their classification on the other systems in use).

70.3 Atlantoaxial (C1-2) subluxation/dislocation

70.3.1 General information

Lower morbidity and mortality than atlantooccipital dislocation.[27] See Occipitoatlantoaxial-complex anatomy (p.67) for relevant anatomy.

Types of atlantoaxial subluxation:
1. anterior subluxation (p.1160): more ominous
2. rotatory: (see below) usually seen in children after a fall or minor trauma
3. anterior subluxation (p.1160): more ominous. The most common type of C1-2 dislocation
4. posterior: rare. Usually from erosion of odontoid. Unstable. Requires fusion
5. distraction (p.1162): increased separation between C1 & C2 (BDI (p.1153) increases in the absence of AOD)

70.3.2 Atlantoaxial rotatory subluxation

General information

> ## Key concepts
>
> - typically seen in children
> - associations: trauma, RA, respiratory tract infections in peds (Grisel syndrome)
> - often presents with cock-robin head position (tilt, rotation, slight flexion)
> - classification: Fielding & Hawkins (► Table 70.6)
> - Tx: early traction is often successful. Treat infection in Grisel syndrome. Subluxation unreducible in traction may need transoral release then posterior fusion

Rotational deformity at the atlanto-axial junction is usually of short duration and easily corrected. Rarely, the atlantoaxial joint locks in rotation (AKA atlantoaxial rotatory *fixation*[28]). Usually seen in children. May occur spontaneously (with rheumatoid arthritis[29] or with congenital dens anomalies), following major or minor trauma (including neck manipulation or even with neck rotation while yawning[28]), or with an infection of the head or neck including upper respiratory tract (known as Grisel syndrome[30]: inflammation may cause mechanical and chemical injury to the facet capsules and/or transverse atlantal ligament (TAL)).

The vertebral arteries (VA) may be compromised in excessive rotation, especially if it is combined with anterior displacement.

Mechanism of subluxation

The dislocation may be at the occipito-atlantal and/or the atlanto-axial articulations.[31] The mechanism of the irreducibility is poorly understood. With an intact TAL, rotation occurs without anterior displacement. If the TAL is incompetent as a result of trauma or infection, there may also be anterior displacement with more potential for neurologic injury. Posterior displacement occurs only rarely due to incompetence of the odontoid.[28]

Classification

The Fielding and Hawkins classification[28] is shown in ► Table 70.6.

Clinical findings

Patients are usually young. Neurologic deficit is rare. Findings may include: neck pain, headache, torticollis—characteristic "cock robin" head position with ≈ 20° lateral tilt to one side, 20° rotation to the other, and slight (≈ 10°) flexion, see DDx (p.1677), reduced range of motion, and facial flattening.[28] Although the patient cannot reduce the dislocation, they can increase it with head rotation towards the subluxed joint with potential injury to the high cervical cord.

Table 70.6 Fielding & Hawkins classification of rotatory atlantoaxial subluxation[28]

Type	Description		AD[a] (mm)	Comment
	TAL[a]	Facet injury		
Type I **odontoid process** TAL C1 C2 ⊕ = pivot point	intact	bilateral	≤ 3	the most common. Dens acts as pivot
Type II	injured	unilateral	3.1–5	intact facet joint acts as pivot
Type III	injured	bilateral	> 5	rare. Very unstable. Risk of neurologic injury
Type IV	incompetence of the odontoid (e.g., fracture or erosion) with *posterior* displacement of C1			rare. Very unstable. High risk of neurologic injury

[a]AD = anterior displacement of C1 on C2, TAL = transverse atlantal ligament

70

Brainstem and cerebellar infarction and even death may occur with compromise of circulation through the VAs.[32]

Radiographic evaluation

X-rays : findings (may be confusing) include:
- pathognomonic finding on AP C-spine X-ray in severe cases: frontal projection of C2 with simultaneous oblique projection of C1.[33(p 124)] In less severe cases, the C1 lateral mass that is anterior appears larger and closer to the midline than the other
- asymmetry of the atlantoaxial joint that is not correctable with head rotation, which may be demonstrated by persistence of asymmetry on open mouth odontoid views with the head in neutral position and then rotated 10–15° to each side
- the spinous process of the axis is tilted in one direction and rotated to the other (may occur in torticollis of any etiology)

CT scan: demonstrates rotation of the atlas.[31]
MRI: may assess the competence of the transverse ligament.

Treatment

Grisel syndrome

Appropriate antibiotics for causative pathogen with traction (see below) and then immobilization for the subluxation as follows[30]: Fielding (▶ Table 70.6) Type I: soft collar, Type II: rigid collar or SOMI, Type III or IV: halo. After 6–8 weeks of immobilization, check stability with flexion-extension X-rays. Surgical fusion for residual instability.

Traction

If treated within the first few months,[34] the subluxation can usually be reduced with gentle traction (in children start with 7–8 lbs and gradually increase up to 15 lbs over several days, in adults start with 15 lbs and gradually increase up to 20). If the subluxation is present > 1 month, traction is less successful. Active left-right neck rotation is encouraged in traction.

If reducible, immobilization in traction or halo is maintained × 3 months[28] (range: 6–12 weeks).

Surgical fusion

Subluxation that cannot be reduced or that recurs following immobilization should be treated by surgical arthrodesis after 2–3 weeks of traction to obtain maximal reduction. The usual procedure is C1 to C2 fusion (p. 1778) unless other fractures or conditions are present.[28] Fusion may be performed even if the rotation between C1 & C2 is not completely reduced. For irreducible fixation, a staged procedure can be done with anterior transoral release of the atlantoaxial complex (the exposure is taken laterally to expose the atlantoaxial joints, which must be done carefully to avoid injury to the VAs, soft tissue is carefully removed from the joints and the atlantodental interval, no attempt at reduction was made at the time of this 1st stage), followed by gradual skull traction and then a second stage posterior C1–2 fusion.[34]

70.3.3 Anterior atlantoaxial subluxation (AAS)

General information

One third of patients with AAS have neurologic deficit or die.[27] For relevant anatomy, see Occipitoatlantoaxial-complex anatomy (p. 67).
Subluxation may be due to:
1. disruption (rupture) of the transverse atlantal ligament (TAL): the atlantodental interval (ADI) (see below) will be increased
   a) attachment points of the TAL may be weakened in rheumatoid arthritis (p. 1778)
   b) trauma: may cause anatomic or functional ligament disruption (see below)
2. incompetence of the odontoid process: ADI will be normal
   a) odontoid fracture
   b) congenital hypoplasia, e.g., Morquio syndrome (p. 1309)

Presentation

Neck pain is common. There are no specific patterns to the pain that are characteristic.

"V" shaped pre-dens space

Widening of the upper space between the anterior arch of C1 and the odontoid seen on lateral C-spine flexion X-ray.[35] It is not known if this increased mobility represents elongation or laxity of the transverse ligament and/or the posterior ligamentous complex. This may also be a normal finding in flexion in peds.

True subluxation will result in malalignment between C1 and C2. The key differentiating feature is whether the ADI is increased or normal, as indicated above.

Evaluation and classification

Diagnostic modalities

Both CT & MRI are recommended to evaluate fractures, TAL & its bony attachments.

Injury of the transverse atlantal ligament (TAL)
Assessing the integrity of the TAL

1. TAL disruption may be inferred *indirectly.* from
   a) rule of Spence (p. 223): if the total overhang (lateral mass displacement (LMD)) of both C1 lateral masses on C2 is ≥ 7 mm (NB: this rule is inaccurate and should not be used as the sole determinant)
   b) atlantodental interval (ADI) (p. 223): > 3 mm in adults, > 4 mm in peds
2. direct assessment: there is concern that indirect assessment above has low sensitivity (the rule of Spence missed 60% of TAL injuries detected on MRI[36]). MRI may be able to directly assess TAL integrity by imaging it. Possible findings: loss of continuity of the TAL, high signal within the TAL on gradient-echo MRI, blood separating the TAL from its insertion site on the medial tubercle. For subtypes of TAL injury, see below
3. CT may demonstrate bony injury in the regions of TAL insertion on C1 tubercles

Dickman classification of transverse atlantal ligament (TAL) disruption
See reference.[36]

Obtain high-resolution axial MRI using surface coils with fast-spin echo, gradient-echo T1WI & T2WI sequences.[36,37] Not recommended for patients < 14 years of age due to immaturity of the spine. Clinical use of this classification has not been fully validated.[38]

▶ **Dickman Type I.** Anatomic disruption. Tear of TAL itself without osseous component. Rare (the odontoid usually fractures before the TAL tears). Unlikely to heal. Requires surgical stabilization. Subtypes:
1. Type IA: midsubstance TAL disruption. Possible findings:
   1. loss of continuity of the TAL
   2. high signal within the TAL on gradient-echo MRI
2. Type IB: osteoperiosteal TAL disruption. Possible finding: blood separates the TAL from its insertion site on the medial tubercle

▶ **Dickman Type II.** Physiologic disruption. Detachment of the C1 tubercle (to which TAL is attached) (▶ Fig. 1.14) from the C1 lateral mass. May occur in comminuted C1 lateral mass fractures. 74% chance of healing with immobilization (halo recommended[36])

Treatment
- for TAL disruption: one approach is as follows[36,39]
  ○ fuse all Dickman Type I TAL injuries at diagnosis
  ○ fuse Dickman Type II TAL injuries that are still unstable after 3–4 months of immobilization
- fusion is also recommended with irreducible subluxations.
- if C1 is intact, a C1–2 fusion is usually adequate. If C1 is fractured, occipital cervical fusion may be needed
- for situations involving isolated C1 fractures, see below
- for odontoid fractures with intact TAL, see guideline (p. 1173)

70

70.3.4 Atlantoaxial distraction injuries

Rare. A purely distractive injury without disruption of the TAL or fracture of the odontoid process would require injury to the tectorial membrane, ascending and descending bands of the cruciate ligament, alar ligaments, and capsular and accessory C1-2 ligaments (see ► Fig. 1.12, ► Fig. 1.13, ► Fig. 1.14).[40]

70.4 Atlas (C1) fractures

70.4.1 General information

> **Key concepts**
>
> - the primary classification systems are the Jefferson and the Landell
> - no Level I or II data to determine optimal treatment
> - TAL (transverse atlantal ligament) integrity is a critical for stability
> - Tx: all but the most unstable injuries (viz.: anterior + posterior ring fractures with TAL disruption) can be managed with a trial period in a rigid collar for 3-4 months, with surgery reserved for treatment failures

Sir Geoffrey Jefferson described a four-point (burst) fracture of the C1 ring in 1920.[41] The term now includes any burst fracture of C1[42] (3 or 2-point fractures are more common[43] the latter usually through the C1 arches (thinnest part)). Usually from *axial* loading (a "blow-out" fracture).[44]

Acute C1 fractures account for 3–13% of cervical spine fractures.[45] 56% of 57 patients had isolated C1 fractures; 44% had combination C1–2 fractures; 9% had additional non-contiguous C-spine fractures. 21% had associated head injuries.[45]

In pediatrics, it is critical to differentiate a C1 fracture from the normal synchondroses (p.224) (a fracture may also occur through unfused synchondroses) and from pseudospread of the atlas (p.1123).

70.4.2 Clinical

Neurologic deficit is rare with isolated C1 fractures due to the large canal diameter at this level, plus the tendency for fragments to be forced outwards away from spinal cord. Possible clinical findings[39]:
1. neck pain is common and the patient will often guard against movement
2. prevertebral swelling may impinge on the esophagus and cause swallowing difficulties
3. pain in the distribution of the greater occipital nerve may occur from C2 root involvement (p.541)
4. associated vertebral artery dissection (p.1579) may produce symptoms of posterior circulation ischemia (diplopia, altered level of consciousness, lateral medullary syndrome...)
5. lower cranial nerve (IX-XII) palsies have also been reported

70.4.3 Evaluation

Modalities

Thin cut high-resolution CT is the diagnostic test of choice. It is critical to evaluate from C1 through C3 to delineate details of the C1 fracture and to assess for associated C2 injury.

MRI may be able to directly evaluate the integrity of the TAL,[36] but this may be difficult to assess in a number of cases (p.1161).

Stability

To reiterate: stability of the occipitoatlantoaxial complex is primarily due to ligaments, with little contribution from bony articulations. See Occipitoatlantoaxial-complex anatomy (p.67).

★ Integrity of the transverse (atlantal) ligament (TAL) is the most important determinant of stability in C1 fractures (see Assessing the integrity of the TAL (p.1161)).

70.4.4 Classification of C1 fractures

Representative examples of the Jefferson classification[41] are shown in ► Table 70.7 (Jefferson type III is the classic 4-point Jefferson fracture). The practice guidelines are based on the Landells classification[46] which is also illustrated in ► Table 70.7).

Table 70.7 Classification and management of isolated C1 (atlas) fractures

Landells class[46]	Illustration & Jefferson Classification[41]	Treatment recommendations[a] [38]
Type I posterior arch alone or anterior arch alone (single arch) 31–45% of C1 fractures	Jefferson I Jefferson II	rigid immobilization[b] X 8–12 weeks[c]
Type II anterior AND posterior arch ("burst fracture") 37–51%	Jefferson III	**TAL intact[d]** (i.e., stable) • rigid immobilization[b] X 10–12 weeks[c] **TAL disrupted[d]** (i.e., unstable) • halo[e] X 12 weeks • or surgical stabilization & fusion
Type III lateral mass fractures (comminuted) 13–37%	tubercle tubercle Jefferson IV	rigid immobilization[b] X 8–12 weeks[c]

[a]treatment recommendations are based on the text accompanying the 2013 practice guidelines.[42] To also consider subtypes of injuries to the TAL, see schema (p. 1164)
[b]there is insufficient evidence to recommend any of the following cervical immobilization devices over the other: rigid collar, SOMI (sternal-occipital-mandibular immobilizer), halo-vest[42]
[c]at the end of nonsurgical treatment, surgical fusion is recommended for late instability e.g., on flexion/extension C-spine X-rays[39,42]
[d]suggested criteria for TAL disruption include: LMD overhang ≥ 7 mm (rule of Spence (p. 1161), NB: this rule is inaccurate and should not be used as the sole determinant), atlantodental interval (ADI) (p. 223) > 5 mm in adults (this is the ADI used for the guidelines[42]; other authors use different cutoffs for the ADI, e.g., 3 mm[36]), or evidence of disruption or avulsion of the TAL on MRI
[e]although evidence is lacking, some prefer halo-vest for unstable C1 fractures[42]
Abbreviations: TAL = transverse atlantal ligament; LMD = lateral mass displacement.

70.4.5 Treatment decisions

Treatment guidelines

There is no Level I or II evidence for optimal treatment. Treatment recommendations depend primarily on the status of the TAL. Practice guidelines[42] are shown below, with associated treatment specifics, such as length of treatment, appearing in ▶ Table 70.7. For combination C1 & C2 injuries, see section 70.6.

> ### Practice guideline: Treatment of isolated atlas fractures
>
> Level III[42]
> - treatment is based on the fracture type and integrity of the transverse atlantal ligament (TAL)
> - if the TAL is intact[a]: cervical immobilization alone[b, c] (for Landells types I & III, nondisplaced fractures have been effectively treated with external immobilization)
> - if the TAL is disrupted[a]: either
>   a) cervical immobilization alone[b, c, d]
>   b) or surgical fixation and fusion
>
> [a]suggested criteria for TAL disruption include: LMD (overhang) ≥ 7 mm (rule of Spence (p. 1161) - NB: this rule is inaccurate and should not be used as the sole determinant), atlantodental interval (ADI) (p. 223) > 5 mm in adults (this is the ADI used for the guidelines[42]; other authors use different cutoffs, e.g., 3 mm for the ADI[36]), or evidence of disruption or avulsion of the TAL on MRI.
> [b]there is insufficient evidence to recommend any of the following cervical immobilization devices over the other: rigid collar, SOMI (sternal-occipital-mandibular immobilizer), halo-vest[42]
> [c]at the end of nonsurgical treatment, surgical fusion is recommended for late instability e.g., on flexion/extension C-spine X-rays[39,42]
> [d]although evidence is lacking, some prefer halo-vest when there is TAL disruption (unstable fractures)[42]
> Abbreviations: LMD = lateral mass displacement; TAL = transverse atlantal ligament.

Barrow Neurologic Institute (BNI) management guidelines for isolated C1 fractures

Based on the importance of TAL integrity and the assertion that pure ligamentous injuries of the TAL have a lower chance of healing than functional injuries resulting from fracture of the bone supporting the tubercle where the TAL is attached,[36] the following managment protocol was developed[39] (using the Dickman classification (p. 1161) and the lateral mass displacement (LMD)) (p. 223). It has been pointed out that the methodology of this protocol is not sufficient to classify the level above Class III medical evidence[42]; however, that is not very different from the level of recommendations in the current guidelines.

▶ **BNI treatment protocol for isolated C1 (atlas) fractures.** Evaluation: unless contraindicated, all patient's are evaluated with cervical MRI to assess the integrity of the TAL (p. 1161) and thin-cut cervical CT to assess the fracture. Lateral mass displacement (LMD) (p. 223) is measured in all cases.
1. Dickman Type I TAL disruption (pure ligamentous injury): surgical fusion
2. the following may be treated with immobilization for 3 months after which flexion/extension C-spine X-rays are obtained, and surgical fusion is performed if unstable
   a) TAL intact on MRI and LMD < 7 mm: cervical collar X 3 months
   b) Dickman Type II TAL disruption (bony avulsion) or LMD ≥ 7 mm: halo X 3 months

70.4.6 Surgical options

Fusion options when surgery is indicated:
1. unilateral ring or anterior C1 arch fractures: C1–2 fusion
2. multiple ring fractures or posterior C1 arch fractures: occipital-cervical fusion

Surgical options that do not involve arthrodesis:
1. posterior C1 screw placement
2. anterior transoral screw/plate placement

70.4.7 Outcome

In many series,[45,47] treatment without surgery results in satisfactory radiographic outcome when the TAL is not disrupted.

Even with a satisfactory X-ray result, 20–40% of patients have neck pain after rigid immobilization.[39]

Late complications may include basilar invagination as a result of telescoping of the odontoid through the splayed ring of C1 into the foramen magnum.

70.5 Axis (C2) fractures

70.5.1 General information

Acute fractures of the axis represent ≈ 20% of cervical spine fractures. Neurological injury is uncommon (occurs in < 10% of cases). Most injuries may be treated by rigid immobilization.

Steele's rule of thirds: each of the following occupies one–third of the area of the canal at the level of the atlas (C1): dens, space, spinal cord (▶ Fig. 110.2).[48]

70.5.2 Types of C2 fractures

1. odontoid fractures (p. 1171): type II odontoid fracture is the most common injury of the axis
2. hangman's fracture: see below
3. miscellaneous C2 fractures (p. 1177)

70.5.3 Hangman's fracture

General information

70

Key concepts

- bilateral fracture through the pars interarticularis of C2 with traumatic subluxation of C2 on C3, most often due to hyperextension + axial loading
- most are stable with no neurologic deficit
- classification: Levine system (▶ Table 70.8). Critical dividing line: disruption of C2–3 disc (Types II and higher) which may render the fracture unstable
- W/U: ✓ cervical CT with sagittal & coronal recons for all. ✓ Cervical MRI to assess C2–3 disc disruption (Levine II). ✓ CTA for dissection if fx passes thru foramen transversarium (consider for all C2 fractures—see ▶ Table 61.8)
- most do well with non-halo immobilization x 8–14 weeks. Exceptions: severe/unstable fractures (p. 1166) or those that do not remain aligned in brace

AKA traumatic spondylolisthesis of the axis (a term first used in 1964[49]).

Description: bilateral fracture through the pars interarticularis (isthmus) of the pedicle of C2 (▶ Fig. 70.1; the configuration of C2 is unique, and the distinction between the pars and the pedicle is ambiguous). There is often anterior subluxation of C2 on C3.

The term "hangman's fracture" (HF) was coined by Schneider et al,[50] although the mechanism of most modern HFs (hyperextension and *axial loading*, from MVAs or diving accidents) differs from that sustained in judicial hangings (where submental placement of the knot results in hyperextension and distraction[51]). Some cases may be due to forced flexion or compression of the neck while in extension.

Pediatrics: rare in children < 8 years old where the forces tend to fracture the incompletely fused odontoid, see epiphyseal fracture (p. 224). In pediatrics, consider pseudosubluxation in the differential diagnosis (p. 1123).

Usually *stable*. Deficit is rare. Nonunion is rare. 90% heal with immobilization only. Operative fusion is rarely needed. Fractures of C2 that do not go through the isthmus (p. 1177) are not true hangman's fractures and may require different management.

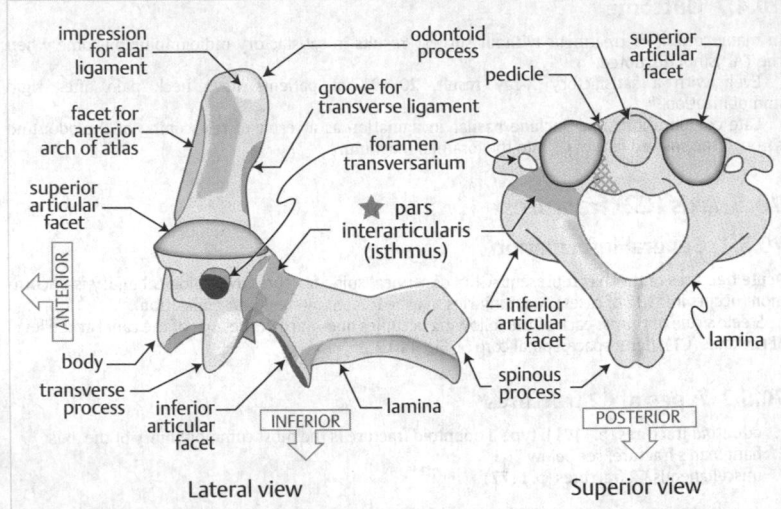

impression for alar ligament

facet for anterior arch of atlas

superior articular facet

ANTERIOR

body

transverse process

inferior articular facet

INFERIOR

lamina

odontoid process

groove for transverse ligament

pedicle

foramen transversarium

⭐ pars interarticularis (isthmus)

superior articular facet

inferior articular facet

spinous process

lamina

POSTERIOR

Lateral view

Superior view

Fig. 70.1 Anatomy of the axis (C2).
The pars interarticularis (shown in solid blue) is located between the inferior and superior articular facets. The pedicle (green cross-hatching) connects to the vertebral body.

70

Classification

Levine/Effendi classification
The system of Effendi et al[52] as modified by Levine[53] and others (▶ Table 70.8) is widely used in grading adult HF (not applicable to peds). Angulation is measured as the angle between the inferior endplates of C2 and C3. Anterior subluxation of C2 on C3 > 3 mm (Type II) is a surrogate marker for C2–3 disc disruption, which can be evaluated more directly with cervical MRI.

Grading system of Frances et al
The grading system[56] is shown in ▶ Table 70.9.
The methodology of measurements is depicted in ▶ Fig. 70.2.

Levine/Francis correlation
In a series of 340 axis fractures,[57] the most common fracture type was Type I in the Levine system (72%) and Grade I in the Francis system (65%); there was a close correlation as follows:
Levine Type I ≈ Francis Grade I
Levine Type III ≈ Francis Grade IV

Other fracture types
Not all fractures fit into one or both of these classification systems.[58] Example: coronally oriented fracture extending through the posterior C2 vertebral body.

Presentation

Most (≈ 95%) are neurologically intact, those few with deficits are usually minor (paresthesias, monoparesis...) and many recover within one month.[56] Almost all conscious patients will have cervical pain usually in the upper posterior cervical region, and occipital neuralgia is not uncommon.[59] There is a high incidence of associated head injury and there will be other associated C-spine injuries —e.g., C1 fracture (see above) or clay shoveler's fracture (p. 1183)—in ≈ one third, with most occurring in the upper 3 cervical levels. There are usually external signs of injury to the face and head associated with the hyperextending and axial force.

Table 70.8 Levine classification of hangman's fractures (modified Effendi system)[a]

Type	Description	Radiographic findings	Mechanism	Comment
I	vertical pars fx just posterior to the VB	≤3 mm subluxation of C2 on C3 & *no* angulation	axial loading & extension	stable on flexion/extension X-rays. Neurologic deficit rare
I A	fx lines on each side are not parallel. Fx may pass thru *foramen transversarium* on one side	fx line may not be visible on X-ray. *Anterior* C2 VB may be subluxed 2–3 mm anteriorly on C3 & the C2 VB may appear elongated	may be hyperextension + lateral bending	"atypical hangman's fracture."[54] Spinal canal may be narrowed. 33% incidence of paralysis
II	vertical fx thru pars. *Disruption of C2–3 disc* & posterior longitudinal ligament	subluxation of C2 on C3 > 3 mm and/or angulation[b]. Slight anterior compression of C3 possible	axial loading & extension with rebound flexion	may lead to early instability. Neurologic deficit rare. Usually reduces with traction
IIA	oblique fx (usually anterior-inferior to posterior superior) little subluxation (usually ≤3 mm) but more angulation (can be > 15°)		flexion distraction (posterior arch fails in tension)	rare (< 10%). Unstable. ✖ Traction → increased angulation & widening of disc space ∴ *do not use traction*
III	Type II + bilateral C2–3 facet capsule disruption. C2 posterior arch is free floating. Anterior longitudinal ligament may be disrupted or stripped off C3	facets of C2/C3 may be subluxed or locked	unclear, may be flexion (capsule disruption) followed by compression (isthmus fracture)	rare. Neurologic deficit may occur & may be fatal. Facet dislocation usually cannot be reduced by closed reduction. ✖ Traction may be dangerous (see text)

[a]Effendi et al,[52] Levine and Edwards,[53] Sonntag and Dickman,[27] and Levine[55]
[b]amount of angulation was not specified in original article, but > 10° has been suggested by some

Table 70.9 Francis grading[a] system for hangman's fracture

Grade	Angulation θ	Displacement
I	< 11°	d < 3.5 mm
II	> 11°	
III	< 11°	d > 3.5 mm and
IV	> 11°	d/b < 0.5
V		d/b > 0.5 (disc disruption)

[a]see ▶ Fig. 70.2 for illustration of θ, d & b

Evaluation

Cervical CT: with sagittal & coronal reconstructions should be done to fully assess the fracture.

CTA: should be done to evaluate the vertebral arteries if fracture extends through foramen transversarium (especially Levine Type IA) and in patients with symptoms suggestive of stroke. Some recommend CTA for all C2 fractures—see ▶ Table 61.8). Angiography or MRA may be done as an alternative to CTA.

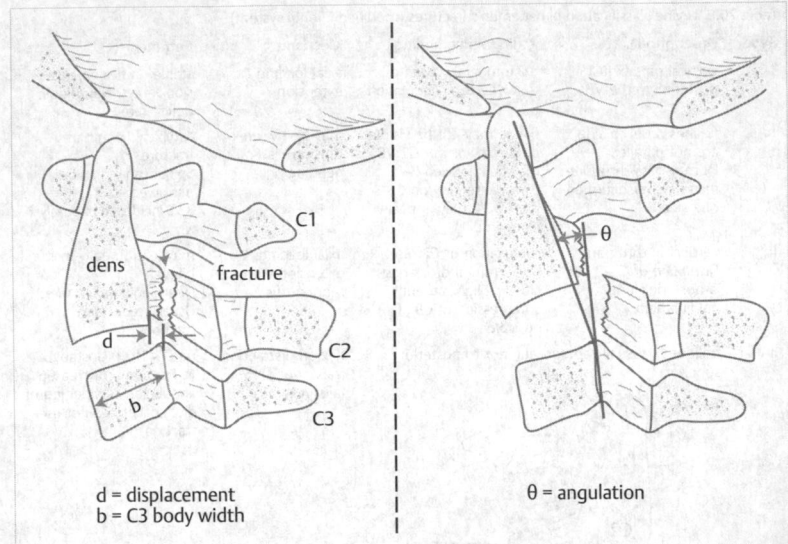

d = displacement
b = C3 body width

θ = angulation

Fig. 70.2 Parameters used in the Francis grading system for hangman's fractures.

★ **MRI**: cervical MRI should be done to look for C2–3 disc disruption (a marker for instability (▶ Fig. 70.3) (Levine grade II) which usually requires surgical stabilization). Findings include abnormal increased signal intensity on MRI (best seen on sagittal FLAIR images or T2WI) or significant distraction across the disc space.

X-rays: lateral C-spine X-rays show the fracture in 95% of cases. Also demonstrates C2 angulation and/or subluxation. Most fractures pass through the pars or the transverse foramen,[56] 7% go through the body of C2 (p.1177). Instability can usually be identified as marked anterior displacement of C2 on C3 (guideline[56]: unstable if displacement exceeds 50% of the AP diameter of C3 vertebral body), excessive angulation of C2 on C3, or by excessive motion on flexion-extension films.

Patients suspected of having Levine Type I fractures and are neurologically intact should have physician-supervised flexion-extension X-rays to rule out a reduced type II fracture.

Treatment

General information

Nonsurgical management produces adequate reduction in 97–100% and results in a fusion rate of 93–100%[27,60,61] if the external immobilization is adequately maintained for 8–14 weeks[62] (average time for healing is ≈ 11.5 weeks[56]). Specific treatment depends on the reliability of the patient and the degree of stability as described below. Most cases do well with non-halo immobilization.[61] Practice guidelines are shown here, and details follow.

Practice guideline: Management of isolated hangman's fracture

Level III[38,63]
- hangman's fractures may initially be managed with external immobilization in most cases (halo or collar)
- surgical stabilization should be considered in cases of:
  a) severe angulation of C2 on C3 (Levine II, Francis II & IV)
  b) disruption of the C2–3 disc space (Levine II, Francis V)
  c) or inability to establish or maintain alignment with external immobilization

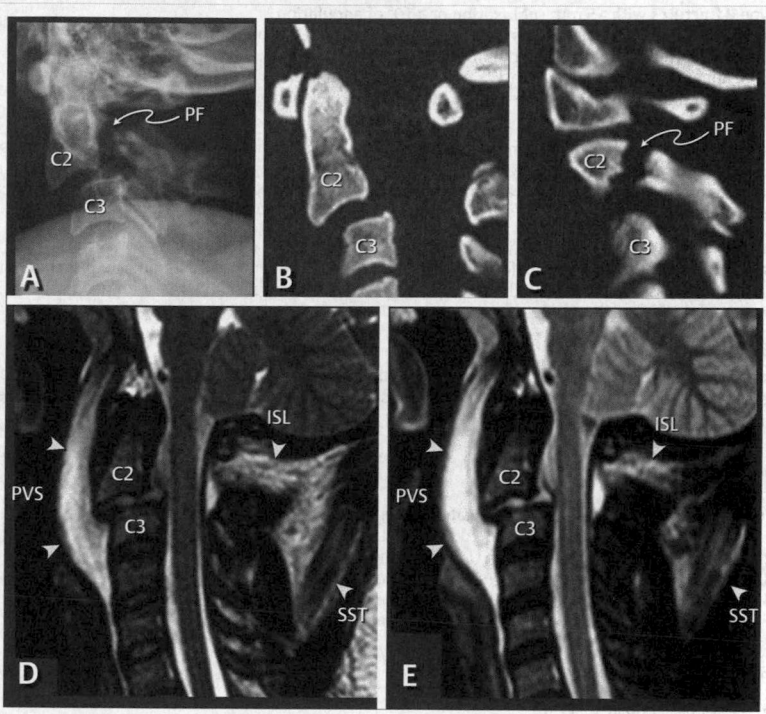

Fig. 70.3 Hangman's fracture Type II.
The amount of anterior displacement of C2 on C3 qualifies this as a Type II. Abnormal signal in the C2-3 disc on MRI indicates possible disc disruption.
Image: A: lateral C-Spine X-ray. B: sagittal midline CT scan, bone window. C: sagittal CT scan, left of midline through pars fracture, bone window. D: sagittal T2 MRI. E: sagittal STIR MRI.
Legend: PF = pars fracture. *Yellow arrowheads* indicate abnormal signal on MRI in the prevertebral space (PVS), inter-spinous ligament (ISL) between C2 and C3, and in the supraspinous tissues (SST).

Stable fractures (Levine Types I or IA, or Francis Grades I or II)

Treat with immobilization (Aspen or Philadelphia collar[64(p 2326)] or cervicothoracic orthosis (CTO) (e.g., SOMI) is usually adequate) × 3 months.[55] Halo-vest may be needed in unreliable patients or for combination C1–2 fractures. Schneider reported 50 cases of Type I fracture treated with non-halo fixation, only 1 was taken to surgery and was found to already be fused.

Unstable fractures

Levine Type II

Reduce with gentle *cervical traction* (most reduce with ≤ 30 lbs[55]) with the head in slight extension (preferably in halo ring) under close X-ray monitoring to prevent "iatrogenic hanging" in cases with ligamentous instability.[56] Place in halo vest × 3 months. Follow patients with serial X-rays. Stabilize surgically if fracture moves.

Type II fractures with ≤ 5 mm of subluxation and angulation < 10°

Once reduced, apply halo-vest and begin to mobilize (usually within 24 hrs of injury). Verify that immobilization is adequate in the halo with upright lateral C-spine X-ray, operate if inadequate. After 8–12 weeks, change to Philadelphia collar or CTO until fusion is definitely complete (usually 3–4 months).

Type II fractures with > 5 mm subluxation or ≥ 10° of angulation
Surgical fusion in these patients is recommended because of the following concerns:
1. risk of settling if immediately mobilized in halo-vest
2. healing with significant angulation may result in chronic pain
3. if not reduced, the gap may be too large for bony bridging using traction alone

Alternatively, cervical traction can be maintained for ≈ 4 weeks and then reduction should be reassessed 1 hour after removing weight from traction, and if stable, again 24 hours after mobilizing in a halo vest. If unstable, return to traction and repeat trial at 5 & 6 weeks. If still unstable at 6 weeks, surgical fusion is recommended.[55]

Levine Type IIA
✖ Traction will accentuate the deformity.[55] Fractures should be reduced by immediate placement in halo vest (bypassing traction) with extension and *compression* applied. Halo-vest immobilization × 3 months produces ≈ 95% union rate.

Levine Type III
✖ Reduction with traction may be dangerous with locked facets. ORIF is recommended.[27] MRI prior to surgery is recommended to assess the C2–3 disc. Can follow ORIF with halo-vest for the fracture, or can fuse at the same time as ORIF.

Surgical treatment
Indications
Few patients have indications for surgical treatment of HF, and include those with:
1. inability to reduce the fracture (includes most Levine Type III & some Type II)
2. failure of external immobilization to prevent movement at fracture site
3. traumatic C2–3 disc herniation with compromise of the spinal cord[65]
4. established non-union: evidenced by movement on flexion-extension film (p. 1145) [56]; all failures of nonoperative treatment had displacement > 4 mm[27]

Hangman's fractures likely to need surgery[57]:
1. Levine Type II or III
2. or Francis grade II, IV, or V
3. or if either:
   a) anterior displacement of C2 VB > 50% of the AP diameter of the C3 VB
   b) or if angulation produces widening of either the anterior or posterior borders of the C2–3 disc space > the height of the normal C3–4 disc below

Surgical options
For the infrequent patient who needs surgery for a hangman's fracture. The fracture is either transfixed (osteosynthesis) or fusion across the fracture must be done as outlined here:
1. fusion techniques:
   a) posterior approach:
      • C1–2 posterior wiring and fusion (e.g., using interspinous fusion technique of Dickman and Sonntag (p. 1783)) is an option only if all the following are intact: C2–3 disc, C2–3 joint capsules and posterior arch of C1. Rationale: this procedure unites C1 to the posterior fracture fragment of C2 which is still linked to C3 by the facet joints (posterior to the fracture), while the portion of C2 anterior to the fracture is still linked to C3 through the C2–3 disc. This technique preserves motion between C2 & C3.
      • C1–3 fusion using C1 lateral mass screws (p. 1780) & C3 lateral mass screws connected with rods (skipping C2)
      • occiput-C3 fusion: may be used if C1 is also damaged (skipping C1 & C2)
   b) anterior C2–3 discectomy[56] with fusion. Optional anterior plating or zero-profile graft/plate. Performed via a transverse anterior cervical incision midway between the angle of the jaw and the thyroid cartilage[60,65]
      • preserves more motion by excluding C1
      • this approach is also recommended for established nonunion[56]
      • not optimal for Levine Type III requiring ORIF for locked facets
      • also used when at least a partial reduction cannot be achieved
      • technique: for special considerations for approach to the C2–3 junction, see Anterior approaches to the cervical spine (p. 1771) (cannot be performed in some short & thick necks). The services of a head and neck surgeon for the approach is an option

2. osteosynthesis: screw placement from posterior approach through the C2 pedicle across the fracture fragment.[55 (p 443)] Not recommended for established nonunion. The fracture must be reduced before the screw holes are drilled[66] (the fracture may be reduced by patient positioning, and can be assisted by pulling posteriorly on the ring or C1 e.g., using a cable looped through C1[67]). Screw entry point and trajectory are similar to the technique for C2 pedicle screws (p. 1781). The posterior fracture fragment may be overdrilled with a 3.5 mm drill. A "top hat" or washer is placed in the hole and a 2.7 mm drill is used to drill the VB. Screw length: 30–35 mm for average adults. An alternative to overdrilling is to use a lag screw with 20 mm unthreaded portion (e.g., Depuy ASIF orthopedic screws are available in 4.5 mm diameter at 30 mm length with 16 mm unthreaded portion, which is close).

Treatment endpoint
Plain X-rays should show trabeculation across the fracture site or interbody fusion of C2 to C3. Flexion-extension lateral radiographs should show no movement at the fracture site.

70.5.4 Odontoid fractures

General information

Key concepts

- 10–15% of C-spine fx. Can occur in older patients with minor trauma (e.g., ground level fall), or in younger patients typically following MVA, falls from a height, skiing...
- classification: Anderson & D'Alonzo (▶ Table 70.10). Type II (at base) is the most common
- may be fatal at time of injury, most survivors are intact. Neck pain is common
- Treatment: surgery is considered for:
  ○ Type II if age > 50 yrs
  ○ Type IIA
  ○ or Type II & III if displacement ≥ 5 mm or if alignment cannot be maintained with halo

In young individuals, significant force is required to produce an odontoid fracture, usually sustained in a motor vehicle accident (MVA), a fall from a height, a skiing accident, diving head-first into shallow water, etc. In patients > 65 years of age, simple ground level falls (GLF) with head trauma may be sufficient to fracture the dens as a result of disproportionate reduction in bone density at the base of the odotoid relative to the rest of C2.[68] Odontoid fractures comprise ≈ 10–15% of all cervical spine fractures,[69] but are the most common cervical spine fracture in patients > 65 years old.[70] They are easily missed on initial evaluation, especially since significant associated injuries are frequent and may mask symptoms. Pathologic fractures can also occur, e.g., with metastatic involvement (p. 1679).

Flexion is the most common mechanism of injury, with resultant anterior displacement of C1 on C2 (atlantoaxial subluxation). Extension only occasionally produces odontoid fractures, usually associated with posterior displacement.

Classification

The Anderson and D'Alonzo[71] classification (▶ Fig. 70.4 and ▶ Table 70.10) is the most widely used.

▶ **Type I fractures.** Very rare. Result from avulsion of the odontoid tip due to traction on the alar ligament. Originally described as having an angulated orientation.[71] Once considered stable, they may not occur as an isolated fracture and may be a manifestation of atlantooccipital dislocation.[73] Also, it may be a marker for possible disruption of the transverse ligament,[74] which may result in atlanto-axial instability.

▶ **Type II odontoid fractures.** Nonunion rate is higher than with types I & III. Proposed explanations for this include:
1. the base of the odontoid has a watershed blood supply between arteries supplying the tip and those supplying the body[75]
2. paucity of cancellous bone and small surface area of the neck of the odontoid[76]
3. ligaments attached to the odontoid tend to distract and displace it

Table 70.10 Anderson and D'Alonzo classification of odontoid fractures

Type	Characteristics	Stability
I	through tip (above transverse ligament), rare	unstable[a]
II	through base of neck. The most common dens fracture	usually *unstable*
IIA	similar to type II, but with large bone chips at fracture site,[72] comprise ≈ 3% of type II odontoid fractures. Diagnosed by plain radiographs and/or CT	usually *unstable*
III	through body of C2 (usually involves marrow space). May involve superior articular surface	usually stable

[a]controversial, see text

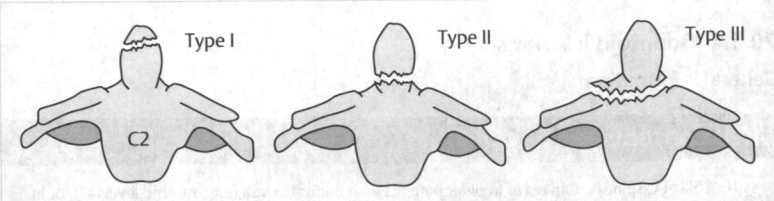

Fig. 70.4 Anderson and D'Alonzo classification of odontoid fractures (AP view).

Radiographic evaluation

A type III odontoid fracture may be misinterpreted as type II on sagittal CT (see "A" in ▶ Fig. 70.5) because the fracture may appear to lie just above the VB. The coronal view more readily demonstrates the relationship of the fracture to the VB.

On plain x-rays, type II fractures are usually better appreciated on AP view (including open mouth odontoid view).

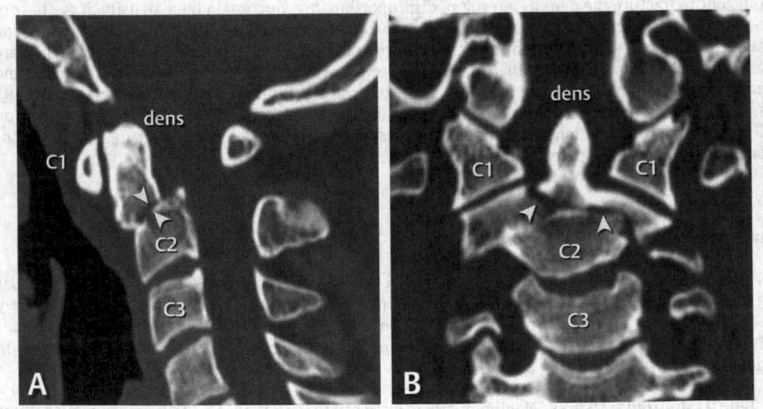

Fig. 70.5 Odontoid type III fracture (*yellow arrowheads*) with anterior displacement. Image: CT bone windows, A: midline sagittal, B: coronal.

Signs and symptoms

The frequency of fatalities at the time of the accident resulting directly from odontoid fractures is unknown, it has been estimated as being between 25–40%.[77] 82% of patients with Type II fractures in a review of 7 reports in the literature were neurologically intact, 8% had minor deficits of scalp or limb sensation, and 10% had significant deficit (ranging from monoparesis to quadriplegia).[78] Type III fractures are rarely associated with neurologic injury.

Common symptoms are high posterior cervical pain, sometimes radiating in the distribution of the greater occipital nerve (occipital neuralgia). Almost all patients with high posterior cervical pain will also have paraspinal muscle spasm, reduced range of motion of the neck, and tenderness to palpation over the upper cervical spine. A very suggestive finding is the tendency to support the head with the hands when going between the upright and supine position. Paresthesias in the upper extremities and slight exaggeration of muscle stretch reflexes may also occur. Myelopathy may develop in patients with nonunion (p. 1174).

Treatment

Practice guidelines

Practice guidelines are shown below. Details appear in the following sections.

Practice guideline: Management of isolated odontoid fractures

- Level II[38]: isolated Type II odontoid fractures in adults ≥ 50 years of age should be considered for surgical stabilization & fusion
- Level III[38]
  - Nondisplaced type I, II & III fractures may be managed initially with external cervical immobilization, recognizing that type II odontoid fractures have a higher rate of nonunion
  - Type II & III: consider surgical fixation for:
    a) dens displacement ≥ 5 mm
    b) or Type IIA fracture (comminution of fracture)
    c) or inability to maintain or achieve alignment with external immobilization
  - For surgical intervention, either an anterior or posterior approach may be used

70

Immobilization

For those not meeting surgical indications, 10–12 weeks of immobilization as suggested in ▶ Table 70.11 is recommended. There is no Class I medical evidence comparing immobilization options.

Halo vest: fusion rate = 72%,[79] appears superior to an SOMI. If a halo is used, obtain supine and upright lateral C-spine X-rays in the halo. If there is movement at the fracture site, then surgical stabilization is recommended.

Rigid collar[79,80]: fusion rate = 53%.

In patients who are poor surgical candidates, there is theoretical and anecdotal rationale to consider calcitonin therapy (p. 1211) in conjunction with a rigid cervical orthosis.[81]

Table 70.11 Immobilization for odontoid fractures

Fracture type	Option
Type I	collar, halo
Type II[a]	halo, collar[b]
Type IIA[a]	halo[a]
Type III[a]	collar[b], halo

[a]consider surgery for these, use indicated brace when surgery not deemed appropriate
[b]a CTO (cervicothoracic orthosis) provides better immobilization against flexion and rotation than a collar or an SOMI

Type I

So rare that meaningful analysis is difficult. If there is associated atlanto-axial instability, surgical fusion may at times be necessary.

Type II

General information

Treatment remains controversial. No agreement has been reached after many attempts to identify factors that will predict which type II fractures are most likely to heal with immobilization and which will require operative fusion. Critical review of the literature reveals a paucity of well-designed studies. A wide range of nonunion rates with immobilization alone (5–76%) is quoted: 30% is probably a reasonable estimate for overall nonunion rate, with 10% nonunion rate for those with displacement < 6 mm.[79] Possible key factors in predicting nonunion include:

1. degree of displacement: probably the most important factor
   a) some authors contend that displacement > 4 mm increases nonunion[71,82]
   b) some use ≥ 6 mm as the cutoff, citing a 70% nonunion rate[62] for these regardless of age or direction of displacement
2. age:
   a) children < 7 yrs old almost always heal with immobilization alone
   b) some feel that there is a critical age above which the nonunion rate increases, and the following ages have been cited: age > 40 yrs (possibly ≈ doubling the nonunion rate),[82] age > 55 yrs,[83] age > 65 yrs,[84] yet others do not support increasing age as a factor[79]

Indications for surgery for odontoid type II fractures

Given the above, there can be no hard and fast rules. The following is offered as a guideline (also, see above).

★ Surgical treatment (instead of external immobilization) is recommended for odontoid type II fractures in patients ≥ 7 years of age with any of the following:

1. displacement ≥ 5 mm
2. instability at the fracture site in the halo vest (see below)
3. age ≥ 50 years: increases nonunion rate (with halo) 21-fold[85]
4. nonunion (see ▶ Table 70.12 for radiographic criteria) including firm fibrous union,[86] especially if accompanied by myelopathy[59]
5. disruption of the transverse ligament: associated with delayed instability[36]

Surgical options

1. odontoid compression screw (p. 1779): appropriate for acute type II fractures with transverse ligament intact and attached
2. C1–2 arthrodesis (p. 1778): options include wiring/fusion, transarticular screws, halifax clamps…

Type IIA

Early surgery is recommended for all type IIA fractures.[72]

Type III

≈ 90% heal with external immobilization (and analgesics) if adequately maintained for 8–14 weeks.[62] Halo-vest brace is probably best,[80] fusion rate ≈ 100% in 1 series.[79] Rigid collar: fusion rate = 50–70%; if used, monitor the patient with frequent C-spine X-rays to rule out nonunion.

Surgical treatment options

See Atlantoaxial fusion (C1–2 arthrodesis) (p. 1778) and Anterior odontoid screw fixation (p. 1775) for surgical options and operative details.

Nonunion

The radiographic criteria for nonunion are shown in ▶ Table 70.12.

Table 70.12 Radiographic criteria of nonunion of odontoid fractures

- defect in the dens with contiguous sclerosis of both fragments (vascular pseudarthrosis)
- defect in the dens with contiguous resorption of both fragments (rarefying osteitis or atrophic pseudarthrosis)
- defect in the dens with definite loss of cortical continuity
- movement of dens fragment demonstrated on flexion-extension X-rays

The most common symptom of nonunion is continued high posterior cervical pain beyond the time that the brace is removed. Late myelopathy can develop in as many as 77% of mobile nonunions[77,87] as a result of motion and soft tissue proliferation around the unstable fracture site.

Os odontoideum

General information

A separate bone ossicle of variable size with *smooth* cortical borders separated from a foreshortened odontoid peg, occasionally may fuse with the clivus (▶ Fig. 70.6). May mimic Type 1 or 2 odontoid fracture. Etiology is debated with evidence to support both of the following (diagnosis & treatment do not depend on which etiologic theory is correct):

1. congenital: developmental anomaly (nonunion of dens to body of axis). However, does not follow known ossification centers (▶ Fig. 12.5) and has been demonstrated in 9 patients with previously normal odontoid processes[88]
2. acquired: postulated to represent an old nonunion fracture or injury to vascular supply of developing odontoid[88,89]

Two anatomic types:

1. orthotopic: ossicle moves with the anterior arch of C1
2. dystopic: ossicle is functionally fused to the basion. May sublux anterior to the C1 arch

True os odontoideum is rare. Ossiculum terminale: nonunion of the apex at the secondary ossification center, is more common.

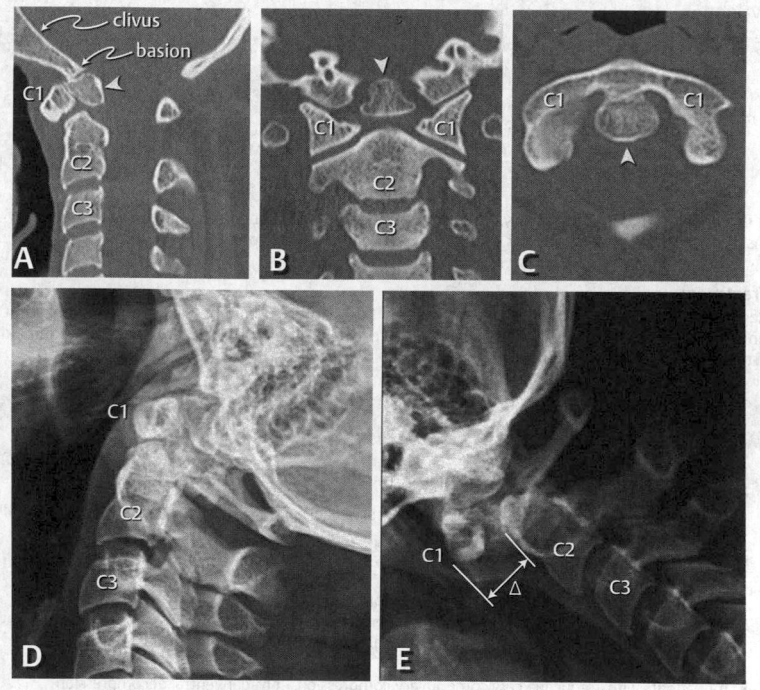

70

Fig. 70.6 Os odontoideum (*yellow arrowheads*).
Image: CT bone windows, A: sagittal; B: coronal, C: axial.
Lateral cervical spine X-rays, D: extension; E: flexion (note the forward displacement Δ of C1 upon flexion).

Presentation
Main groups identified in the literature[90]:
1. occipitocervical/neck pain
2. myelopathy: further subdivided[88]
   a) transient myelopathy: common following trauma
   b) static myelopathy
   c) progressive myelopathy
3. intracranial signs or symptoms: from vertebrobasilar ischemia
4. incidental finding

Most patients are neurologically intact and present with atlantoaxial instability, which may be discovered incidentally. Many symptomatic and asymptomatic patients have been reported with no new problems over many years of follow-up.[91] Conversely, cases of precipitous spinal cord injury after seemingly minor trauma have been reported.[92]

Σ: Natural history of os odontoideum

The natural history is variable, and predictive factors for deterioration, especially in asymptomatic patients, have not been identified.[93]

Evaluation

70

Practice guideline: Diagnosis of os odontoideum

Level III[94]
- recommended: the following plain C-spine X-rays: AP, open-mouth odontoid, lateral (static & flexion-extension) with or without tomography (CT or plain) and/or MRI of craniocervical junction

It is critical to R/O C1–2 instability. However, myelopathy does not correlate with the degree of C1–2 instability. An AP canal diameter < 13 mm does correlate with the presence of myelopathy.

Treatment
Regardless of whether os odontoideum is congenital or an old nonunion fracture, immobilization is unlikely to result in fusion. Therefore, when treatment is elected, surgery—usually atlantoaxial arthrodesis (p. 1778)—is required.

Practice guideline: Management of os odontoideum

Level III[94]
- patients without neurologic signs or symptoms:
  ○ may be followed with clinical & radiographic surveillance
  ○ or posterior C1–2 fusion may be done
- patients with neurologic signs or symptoms or C1–2 instability: posterior C1–2 internal fixation and fusion
- if surgery is done: if rigid internal instrumentation is not used, then post-op halo immobilization is recommended (e.g., following posterior wiring & fusion)
- for patients with irreducible cervicomedullary compression and/or evidence of associated occipitoatlantal instability: occipital-cervical fusion ± C1 laminectomy
- for patients with irreducible cervicomedullary compression, consider ventral decompression

70.5.5 Miscellaneous C2 fractures

Comprise ≈ 20% of C2 fractures.[27] Includes fractures of spinous process, lamina, facets, lateral mass or C2 vertebral body. Fractures of spinous process or lamina may be treated with Philadelphia collar or cervicothoracic orthosis (CTO). Fractures which compromise the anterior or middle columns (i.e., fractures of facets, C2 body, or lateral mass) require CTO or halo-vest if nondisplaced, or halo if displaced.

> ## Practice guideline: Management of fractures of the axis (C2) body
>
> Level III[38,63]:
> - fractures may initially be managed with external immobilization in most cases (halo or collar)
> - surgical stabilization should be considered in cases of:
>   a) severe ligamentous instability
>   b) or inability to establish or maintain alignment with external immobilization
> - evaluate for vertebral artery injury in cases of comminuted fracture of the axis body

70.6 Combination C1 & C2 injuries

70.6.1 General information

Combination C1–2 injuries are relatively common and may imply more significant structural and mechanical injury than isolated C1 or C2 fractures. The frequency of C2 fractures in C1–2 combination injuries is shown in ▶ Table 70.13. 5–53% of patients with Type II or III odontoid fractures and 6–26% of hangman's fractures have an associated C1 fracture.[95]

Table 70.13 Accompanying C2 injuries

Injury	%
Type II dens fracture	40
Type III dens fracture	20
hangman's fracture	12
other	28

70.6.2 Treatment

> ## Practice guideline: Treatment of combination atlas and axis fractures
>
> Level III[95]
> 1. recommended: base treatment primarily on the type of C2 injury
> 2. recommended: external immobilization of most C1–2 fractures
> 3. consider surgical stabilization for these situations. **Note**: loss of integrity of the C1 ring may necessitate modification of the surgical technique; these injuries are potentially unstable: see Axis (C2) fractures (p. 1165):
>   a) C1-Type II odontoid combination fractures with an ADI ≥ 5 mm
>   b) C1-hangman's combination fractures with C2–3 angulation ≥ 11°

Treatment options are summarized in ▶ Table 70.14.[95]

70

Table 70.14 Treatment options for combination C1–2 injuries

Injury	Treatment options
C1 + hangman's	
• stable	collar, halo, surgery[a]
• unstable (C2–3 angulation ≥ 11°)	halo, surgery
C1 + Type II odontoid fracture	
• stable (ADI[a] < 5 mm)	collar, halo, surgery
• unstable (ADI ≥ 5 mm)	halo, surgery
C1 + Type III odontoid fracture	halo
C1 + miscellaneous C2	collar, halo

[a]abbreviations: ADI = atlantodental interval; surgery = surgical fixation & fusion

70.6.3 Outcome

Only 1 nonunion (C1 + Type II odontoid, treated initially with halo). No new neuro deficits.

References

[1] Powers B, Miller MD, Kramer RS, et al. Traumatic Anterior Atlanto-Occipital Dislocation. Neurosurgery. 1979; 4:12–17

[2] Alker GJ, Leslie EV. High Cervical Spine and Craniocervical Junction Injuries in Fatal Traffic Accidents: A Radiological Study. Orthop Clin North Am. 1978; 9:1003–1010

[3] Bucholz RW, Burkhead WZ, Graham W, et al. Occult Cervical Spine Injuries in Fatal Traffic Accidents. J Trauma. 1979; 19:768–771

[4] Przybylski GJ, Clyde BL, Fitz CR. Craniocervical junction subarachnoid hemorrhage associated with atlanto-occipital dislocation. Spine. 1996; 21:1761–1768

[5] Theodore N, Aarabi B, Dhall SS, et al. The diagnosis and management of traumatic atlanto-occipital dislocation injuries. Neurosurgery. 2013; 72 Suppl 2:114–126

[6] Dziurzynski K, Anderson PA, Bean DB, et al. A blinded assessment of radiographic criteria for atlanto-occipital dislocation. Spine. 2005; 30:1427–1432

[7] Section on Disorders of the Spine and Peripheral Nerves of the American Association of Neurological Surgeons and the Congress of Neurological Surgeons. Diagnosis and management of traumatic atlanto-occipital dislocation injuries. Neurosurgery. 2002; 50 Supplement:S105–S113

[8] Harris JH, Carson GC, Wagner LK. Radiologic diagnosis of traumatic occipitovertebral dissociation: 1. Normal occipitovertebral relationships on lateral radiographs of supine subjects. AJR Am J Roentgenol. 1994; 162:881–886

[9] Horn EM, Feiz-Erfan I, Lekovic GP, et al. Survivors of occipitoatlantal dislocation injuries: imaging and clinical correlates. J Neurosurg Spine. 2007; 6:113–120

[10] Rojas CA, Bertozzi JC, Martinez CR, et al. Reassessment of the craniocervical junction: normal values on CT. AJNR Am J Neuroradiol. 2007; 28:1819–1823

[11] Bertozzi JC, Rojas CA, Martinez CR. Evaluation of the pediatric craniocervical junction on MDCT. AJR. American Journal of Roentgenology. 2009; 192:26–31

[12] Werne S. Studies in spontaneous atlas dislocation. Acta Orthop Scand Suppl. 1957; 23:1–150

[13] Pang D, Nemzek WR, Zovickian J. Atlanto-occipital dislocation: part 1–normal occipital condyle-C1 interval in 89 children. Neurosurgery. 2007; 61:514–21; discussion 521

[14] Kaufman RA, Carroll CD, Buncher CR. Atlantoccipital junction: standards for measurement in normal children. AJNR Am J Neuroradiol. 1987; 8:995–999

[15] Pang D, Nemzek WR, Zovickian J. Atlanto-occipital dislocation–part 2: The clinical use of (occipital) condyle-C1 interval, comparison with other diagnostic methods, and the manifestation, management, and outcome of atlanto-occipital dislocation in children. Neurosurgery. 2007; 61:995–1015; discussion 1015

[16] Dublin AB, Marks WM, Weinstock D, et al. Traumatic dislocation of the atlanto-occipital articulation (AOA) with short-term survival. With a radiographic method of measuring the AOA. J Neurosurg. 1980; 52:541–546

[17] Lee C, Woodring JH, Goldstein SJ, et al. Evaluation of traumatic atlantooccipital dislocations. AJNR Am J Neuroradiol. 1987; 8:19–26

[18] Wholey MH, Bruwer AJ, Baker HL. The lateral roentgenogram of the neck; with comments on the atlanto-odontoid-basion relationship. Radiology. 1958; 71:350–356

[19] Harris JH,Jr, Carson GC, Wagner LK, et al. Radiologic diagnosis of traumatic occipitovertebral dissociation: 2. Comparison of three methods of detecting occipitovertebral relationships on lateral radiographs of supine subjects. AJR Am J Roentgenol. 1994; 162:887–892

[20] Traynelis VC, Marano GD, Dunker RO, et al. Traumatic Atlanto-Occipital Dislocation. Case Report. Journal of Neurosurgery. 1986; 65:863–870

[21] Bell CL. Surgical Observations. Middlesex Hospital Journal. 1817; 4

[22] Maserati MatthewB, Stephens Bradley, Zohny Zohny, et al. Occipital condyle fractures: clinical decision rule and surgical management. Journal of Neurosurgery: Spine. 2009; 11:388–395

[23] Section on Disorders of the Spine and Peripheral Nerves of the American Association of Neurological Surgeons and the Congress of Neurological Surgeons. Occipital condyle fractures. Neurosurgery. 2002; 50 Supplement:S114–S119

[24] Theodore N, Aarabi B, Dhall SS, et al. Occipital condyle fractures. Neurosurgery. 2013; 72 Suppl 2:106–113

[25] Anderson PA, Montesano PX. Morphology and treatment of occipital condyle fractures. Spine. 1988; 13:731–736

[26] Jacoby CG. Fracture of the occipital condyle. AJR Am J Roentgenol. 1979; 132

[27] Sonntag VKH, Dickman CA, Rea GL, et al. Treatment of Upper Cervical Spine Injuries. In: Spinal Trauma: Current Evaluation and Management.American Association of Neurological Surgeons; 1993:25–74

[28] Fielding JW, Hawkins RJ. Atlanto-axial rotatory fixation. (Fixed rotatory subluxation of the atlanto-axial

joint). Journal of Bone and Joint Surgery. 1977; 59A:37–44

[29] Lourie H, Stewart WA. Spontaneous atlantoaxial dislocation: a complication of rheumatic disease. New England Journal of Medicine. 1961; 265:677–681

[30] Wetzel FT, La Rocca H. Grisel's syndrome. Clin Orthop. 1989:141–152

[31] Fielding JW, Stillwell WT, Chynn KY, et al. Use of computed tomography for the diagnosis of atlanto-axial rotatory fixation. Journal of Bone and Joint Surgery. 1978; 60A:1102–1104

[32] Schneider RC, Schemm GW. Vertebral artery insufficiency in acute and chronic spinal trauma. With special reference to the syndrome of acute central cervical spinal cord injury. Journal of Neurosurgery. 1961; 18:348–360

[33] Banna M. Spinal Fractures and Dislocations. In: Clinical Radiology of the Spine and the Spinal Cord. Rockville, Maryland: Aspen Systems Corporation; 1985:102–159

[34] Govender S, Kumar KP. Staged reduction and stabilisation in chronic atlantoaxial rotatory fixation. Journal of Bone and Joint Surgery. British Volume. 2002; 84:727–731

[35] Bohrer SP, Klein MD, Martin W. "V" shaped predens space. Skeletal Radiology. 1985; 14:111–116

[36] Dickman CA, Greene KA, Sonntag VK. Injuries involving the transverse atlantal ligament: classification and treatment guidelines based upon experience with 39 injuries. Neurosurgery. 1996; 38:44–50

[37] Dickman CA, Mamourian A, Sonntag VK, et al. Magnetic resonance imaging of the transverse atlantal ligament for the evaluation of atlantoaxial instability. J Neurosurg. 1991; 75:221–227

[38] Ryken TC, Hadley MN, Aarabi B, et al. Management of isolated fractures of the axis in adults. Neurosurgery. 2013; 72 Suppl 2:132–150

[39] Kakarla UK, Chang SW, Theodore N, et al. Atlas fractures. Neurosurgery. 2010; 66:60–67

[40] Carroll EA, Gordon B, Sweeney CA, et al. Traumatic atlantoaxial distraction injury: a case report. Spine (Phila Pa 1976). 2001; 26:454–457

[41] Jefferson G. Fractures of the atlas vertebra: report of four cases, and a review of those previously recorded. British Journal of Surgery. 1920; 7:407–422

[42] Ryken TC, Aarabi B, Dhall SS, et al. Management of isolated fractures of the atlas in adults. Neurosurgery. 2013; 72 Suppl 2:127–131

[43] Alker GJ, Oh YS, Leslie EV, et al. Postmortem Radiology of Head and Neck Injuries in Fatal Traffic Accidents. Radiology. 1975; 114:611–617

[44] Papadopoulos SM, Rea GL, Miller CA, et al. Biomechanics of Occipito-Atlanto-Axial Trauma. In: Spinal Trauma: Current Evaluation and Management. American Association of Neurological Surgeons; 1993:17–23

[45] Hadley MN, Dickman CA, Browner CM, et al. Acute Traumatic Atlas Fractures: Management and Long-Term Outcome. Neurosurgery. 1988; 23:31–35

[46] Landells CD, Van Peteghem PK. Fractures of the atlas: classification, treatment and morbidity. Spine. 1988; 13:450–452

[47] Levine AM, Edwards CC. Fractures of the atlas. J Bone Joint Surg Am. 1991; 73:680–691

[48] Spence KF, Decker S, Sell KW. Bursting atlantal fracture associated with rupture of the transverse ligament. J Bone Joint Surg. 1970; 52A:543–549

[49] Garber J. Abnormalities of the atlas and axis vertebrae: Congenital and traumatic. J Bone Joint Surg Am. 1964; 46A:1782–1791

[50] Schneider RC, Livingston KE, Cave AJE, et al. 'Hangman's Fracture' of the Cervical Spine. J Neurosurg. 1965; 22:141–154

[51] Wood-Jones F. The Ideal Lesion Produced by Judicial Hanging. Lancet. 1913; 1

[52] Effendi B, Roy D, Cornish B, et al. Fractures of the Ring of the Axis: A Classification Based on the Analysis of 131 Cases. J Bone Joint Surg. 1981; 63B:319–327

[53] Levine AM, Edwards CC. The Management of Traumatic Spondylolisthesis of the Axis. J Bone Joint Surg. 1985; 67A:217–226

[54] Starr JK, Eismont FJ. Atypical hangman's fractures. Spine. 1993; 18:1954–1957

[55] Levine AM, The Cervical Spine Research Society Editorial Committee. Traumatic Spondylolisthesis of the Axis: "Hangman's Fracture". In: The Cervical Spine. 3rd ed. Philadelphia: Lippincott-Raven; 1998:429–448

[56] Francis WR, Fielding JW, Hawkins RJ, et al. Traumatic Spondylolisthesis of the Axis. J Bone Joint Surg. 1981; 63B:313–318

[57] Greene KA, Dickman CA, Marciano FF, et al. Acute axis fractures. Analysis of management and outcome in 340 consecutive cases. Spine. 1997; 22:1843–1852

[58] Burke JT, Harris JH,Jr. Acute injuries of the axis vertebra. Skeletal Radiol. 1989; 18:335–346

[59] The Cervical Spine Research Society Editorial Committee. The Cervical Spine. Philadelphia 1989

[60] Tuite GF, Papadopoulos SM, Sonntag VKH. Caspar plate fixation for the treatment of complex hangman's fractures. Neurosurgery. 1992; 30:761–765

[61] Coric D, Wilson JA, Kelly DL. Treatment of Traumatic Spondylolisthesis of the Axis with Nonrigid Immobilization: A Review of 64 Cases. Journal of Neurosurgery. 1996; 85:550–554

[62] Sonntag VKH, Hadley MN. Nonoperative Management of Cervical Spine Injuries. Clin Neurosurg. 1988; 34:630–649

[63] Section on Disorders of the Spine and Peripheral Nerves of the American Association of Neurological Surgeons and the Congress of Neurological Surgeons. Isolated fractures of the axis in adults. Neurosurgery. 2002; 50 Supplement:S125–S139

[64] Youmans JR. Neurological Surgery. Philadelphia 1982

[65] Hadley MN. Comment on Tuite G F, et al.: Caspar plate fixation for the treatment of complex hangman's fractures. Neurosurgery. 1992; 30:761–765

[66] ElMiligui Y, Koptan W, Emran I. Transpedicular screw fixation for type II Hangman's fracture: a motion preserving procedure. European Spine Journal. 2010; 19:1299–1305

[67] Shin JJ, Kim SH, Cho YE, et al. Primary surgical management by reduction and fixation of unstable hangman's fractures with discoligamentous instability or combined fractures: clinical article. J Neurosurg Spine. 2013; 19:569–575

[68] Amling M, Hahn M, Wening VJ, et al. The microarchitecture of the axis as the predisposing factor for fracture of the base of the odontoid process. A histomorphometric analysis of twenty-two autopsy specimens. J Bone Joint Surg Am. 1994; 76:1840–1846

[69] Husby J, Sorensen KH. Fracture of the Odontoid Process of the Axis. Acta Orthop Scand. 1974; 45:182–192

[70] Iyer S, Hurlbert RJ, Albert TJ. Management of Odontoid Fractures in the Elderly: A Review of the Literature and an Evidence-Based Treatment Algorithm. Neurosurgery. 2018; 82:419–430

[71] Anderson LD, D'Alonzo RT. Fractures of the odontoid process of the axis. Journal of Bone and Joint Surgery. 1974; 56A:1663–1674

[72] Hadley MN, Browner CM, Liu SS, et al. New Subtype of Acute Odontoid Fractures (Type IIA). Neurosurgery. 1988; 22:67–71

[73] Scott EW, Haid RW, Peace D. Type I Fractures of the Odontoid Process: Implications for Atlanto-Occipital Instability: Case Report. Journal of Neurosurgery. 1990; 72:488–492

[74] Naim-ur-Rahman, Jamjoom ZA, Jamjoom AB. Ruptured transverse ligament: an injury that is often forgotten. British Journal of Neurosurgery. 2000; 14:375–377

[75] Schiff DC, Parke WW. The arterial supply of the odontoid process. Journal of Bone and Joint Surgery. 1973; 55A:1450–1456

[76] Govender S, Maharaj JF, Haffajee MR. Fractures of the odontoid process. Journal of Bone and Joint Surgery. British Volume. 2000; 82:1143–1147

[77] Crockard HA, Heilman AE, Stevens JM. Progressive myelopathy secondary to odontoid fractures:

70

clinical, radiological, and surgical features. Journal of Neurosurgery. 1993; 78:579–586

[78] Przybylski GJ. Management of Odontoid Fractures. Contemporary Neurosurgery. 1998; 20:1–6

[79] Hadley MN, Dickman CA, Browner CM, et al. Acute Axis Fractures: A Review of 229 Cases. J Neurosurg. 1989; 71:642–647

[80] Polin RS, Szabo T, Bogaev CA, et al. Nonoperative Management of Types II and III Odontoid Fractures: The Philadelphia Collar versus the Halo Vest. Neurosurgery. 1996; 38:450–457

[81] Darakchiev BJ, Bulas RV, Dunsker S. Use of Calcitonin for the Treatment of an Odontoid Fracture: Case Report. Journal of Neurosurgery. 2000; (Spine 1) 93:157–160

[82] Apuzzo MLJ, Heiden JS, Weiss MH, et al. Acute Fractures of the Odontoid Process. An Analysis of 45 Cases. J Neurosurg. 1978; 48:85–91

[83] Ekong CEU, Schwartz ML, Tator CH, et al. Odontoid Fracture: Management with Early Mobilization Using the Halo Device. Neurosurgery. 1981; 9:631–637

[84] Dunn ME, Seljeskog EL. Experience in the Management of Odontoid Process Injuries: An Analysis of 128 Cases. Neurosurgery. 1986; 18:306–310

[85] Lennarson PJ, Mostafavi H, Traynelis VC, et al. Management of type II dens fractures: a case-control study. Spine. 2000; 25:1234–1237

[86] Bohler J. Anterior Stabilization for Acute Fractures and Non-Unions of the Dens. J Bone Joint Surg. 1982; 64:18–28

[87] Paridis GR, Janes JM. Posttraumatic Atlanto-Axial Instability: The Fate of the Odontoid Process Fracture in 46 Cases. J Trauma. 1973; 13:359–367

[88] Fielding JW, Hensinger RN, Hawkins RJ. Os Odontoideum. J Bone Joint Surg. 1980; 62A:376–383

[89] Ricciardi JE, Kaufer H, Louis DS. Acquired Os Odontoideum Following Acute Ligament Injury. J Bone Joint Surg. 1976; 58A:410–412

[90] Clements WD, Mezue W, Mathew B. Os odontoideum: congenital or acquired? That's not the question. Injury. 1995; 26:640–642

[91] Spierings EL, Braakman R. The management of os odontoideum. Analysis of 37 cases. J Bone Joint Surg Br. 1982; 64:422–428

[92] Menezes AH, Ryken TC. Craniovertebral abnormalities in Down's syndrome. Pediatr Neurosurg. 1992; 18:24–33

[93] Section on Disorders of the Spine and Peripheral Nerves of the American Association of Neurological Surgeons and the Congress of Neurological Surgeons. Os odontoideum. Neurosurgery. 2002; 50 Supplement:S148–S155

[94] Rozzelle CJ, Aarabi B, Dhall SS, et al. Os odontoideum. Neurosurgery. 2013; 72 Suppl 2:159–169

[95] Section on Disorders of the Spine and Peripheral Nerves of the American Association of Neurological Surgeons and the Congress of Neurological Surgeons. Management of combination fractures of the atlas and axis in adults. Neurosurgery. 2002; 50 Supplement:S140–S147

70

71 Subaxial (C3 through C7) Injuries / Fractures

71.1 Classification systems

71.1.1 General information

Various systems have been proposed to help assess stability and/or guide management. The Allen-Ferguson system (p.1182) is based on the mechanism of injury. Attempts at quantifying biomechanical stability include the White and Panjabi system (p.1182) and the more recent subaxial injury classification (SLIC) (see below). Measurements for spine injuries are based on methods outlined by Bono et al.[1]

Practice guideline: Subaxial cervical spine injury classification

Level I[2]
- Use the Subaxial Injury Classification (SLIC) and severity scale for SCI (see below)
- Classify the stability and fracture pattern using the Cervical Spine Injury Severity Score (CSISS): the CSISS is somewhat complicated and may be better suited to clinical trials than daily practice (see reference[2])

71.1.2 Spine Trauma Study Group subaxial cervical spine injury classification (SLIC)

▶ **General information.** The subaxial injury classification (SLIC)[3] is shown in (▶ Table 71.1) and assesses injuries to the disco-ligamentous complex (DLC) in addition to neurologic and bony injuries. Inter-rater reliability intraclass correlation coefficient is 0.71.

Table 71.1 Subaxial injury classification (SLIC)[3]

Injury (rate *the most severe injury* at that level)		Points	Score
Morphology	no abnormality	0	(0 - 4)
	simple compression (compression fx, endplate disruption, sagittal or coronal plane VB fx)	1	
	burst fracture	2	
	distraction (perched facet, posterior element fx)	3	
	rotation/translation (facet dislocation, teardrop fx (p.1184), advanced compression injury, bilateral pedicle fx, floating lateral mass (p.1192). Guidelines: relative axial rotation ≥ 11°[4] or any translation not related to degenerative causes	4	
Discoligamentous complex (DLC)	intact	0	(0 - 2)
	indeterminate (isolated interspinous widening with < 11° relative angulation & no abnormal facet alignment, ↑ signal on T2WI MRI in ligaments...)	1	
	disrupted (perched or dislocated facet, < 50% articular apposition, facet diastasis > 2 mm, widened anterior disc space, ↑ signal on T2WI MRI through entire disc...)	2	
Neurologic status	intact	0	(0 - 3)
	root injury	1	
	complete spinal cord injury	2	
	incomplete spinal cord injury	3	
	● continuous cord compression with neuro deficit	+ 1	(+ 1)
SLIC score → TOTAL			(0 - 10)

71

▶ **DLC integrity.**[3] The DLC includes: anterior longitudinal ligament (the strongest component of the anterior DLC), posterior longitudinal ligament, ligamentum flavum, facet capsule (the strongest component of the posterior DLC), interspinous and supraspinous ligaments. The DLC is the hardest SLIC parameter to evaluate. Largely inferred indirectly from MRI findings. Healing is less predictable than bone healing in the adult. More data needs to be accrued before this parameter can be reliably quantified.

▶ **Management based on the total SLIC score is shown in** ▶ **Table 71.2.**

Table 71.2 Management based on total SLIC score

SLIC score	Management
1–3	non surgical
4	not specified
≥5	surgical

▶ **A given injury can be described using the SLIC as follows:**
1. spinal level
2. *SLIC morphology* (from ▶ Table 71.1): use the most severe injury type at this level
3. description of bony injury: e.g., fracture or dislocation of transverse process, pedicle, endplate, superior or inferior articular process, lateral mass…
4. *SLIC DLC status* (from ▶ Table 71.1) with descriptors: e.g., herniated disc…
5. *SLIC neurologic status* (from ▶ Table 71.1)
6. confounders: e.g., presence of ankylosing spondylitis, DISH, osteoporosis, previous surgery, degenerative disease…

71.1.3 Cervical spine injury classification on the basis of mechanism of trauma

A modification of the Allen-Ferguson system[5] divides cervical spine fracture-dislocations into 8 major groups based on the dominant loading force and neck position at the time of injury as shown in ▶ Table 71.3. Grades of severity within each group are described, and any of these fractures may also be associated with damage from rotatory loads.

Details on some of these fracture types are provided in the following sections.

Table 71.3 Examples of types of cervical spine injuries[a]

Major loading force	Acting alone	With compression	With distraction
Flexion (p. 1183)	unilateral or bilateral facet dislocation (p. 1186)	• anterior VB fx with kyphosis • disruption of interspinous ligament • teardrop fx (p. 1184)	• torn posterior ligaments (may be occult) • dislocated or locked facets (p. 1186)
Extension[b] (p. 1191)	fractured spinous process and possibly lamina[b]	fracture through lateral mass or facet[b], including horizontalization of facet (p. 1191)	disruption of ALL with retrolisthesis of superior vertebrae on inferior one[b]
Neutral position		burst fracture (p. 1183)	complete ligamentous disruption (very unstable)

[a]abbreviations: ALL = anterior longitudinal ligament; VB = vertebral body, fx = fracture; numbers in parentheses are page numbers for that topic
[b]any of the extension injuries may produce SCIWORA in young patients, or central cord syndrome in the presence of stenosis

71.1.4 Stability model of White and Panjabi

Guidelines for determination of clinical instability (p. 1118) of the subaxial cervical spine published by White and Panjabi[6(p 314)] are shown in ▶ Table 71.4. In general, all else being equal, compromise of anterior elements produces more instability in extension, whereas compromise of the posterior elements produces more instability in flexion (important in patient transfers and immobilization). NB: certain conditions such as ankylosing spondylitis (p. 1365) may cause an otherwise stable injury to be unstable.

Table 71.4 Panjabi and White criteria for instability of the mid & lower C-spine (Panjabi and White)[6]

Item	Points[a]	Score
anterior elements[b] destroyed or unable to function	2	(0 | 2)
posterior elements[b] destroyed or unable to function	2	(0 | 2)
positive stretch test[c]	2	(0 | 2)
spinal cord damage	2	(0 | 2)
nerve root damage	1	(0 | 1)
abnormal disc narrowing	1	(0 | 1)
developmentally narrow spinal canal, either • sagittal diameter < 13 mm, OR • Pavlov ratio[d] < 0.8	1	(0 | 1)
dangerous loading anticipated[e]	1	(0 | 1)

Evaluation of either one of the following 2 X-rays			
1) neutral position cervical spine X-rays OR	2) flexion-extension cervical spine X-rays		
• sagittal plane displacement > 3.5 mm or 20%	• sagittal plane translation > 3.5 mm or 20%	2	(0 | 2)
• relative sagittal plane angulation > 11°	• sagittal plane rotation > 20°	2	(0 | 2)
Range: 0 to 16; unstable if ≥ 5 → TOTAL			(0 - 16)

[a]if there is inadequate information for any item, add half of the value for that item to the total
[b]in the C-spine, posterior elements = anatomic components posterior to the posterior longitudinal ligament
[c]stretch test: apply incremental cervical traction loads of 10 lbs q 5 mins up to 33% body wt. (65 lbs max). Check X-ray and neuro exam after each change. Positive if increase in separation > 1.7 mm or increase angulation > 7.5° on X-ray or change in neuro exam. This test is contraindicated if obvious instability
[d]Pavlov ratio = the ratio of (distance from the midlevel of the posterior VB to the closest point on the spinolaminar line): (the AP diameter of the middle of the VB)
[e]e.g., heavy laborers, contact sports athletes, motorcyclists

71

Stretch test: The cervical stretch test may be helpful in cases where stability is difficult to determine based on other factors. It may also be useful in detecting instability in cases such as an athlete with no obvious bony or ligamentous disruption. It is performed by applying graduated cervical traction with the patient lying supine on an X-ray table. Serial neurologic exams and lateral radiographs are performed as outlined in the footnote of ▶ Table 71.4.

71.2 Clay shoveler's fracture

Avulsion of spinous processes (usually C7) first described in Perth, Australia (pathomechanics: during the throwing phase of shoveling, clay may stick to the shovel jerking the trapezius and other muscles which are attached to cervical spinous processes).[7] Can also occur with: whiplash injury,[8] injuries that jerk the arms upwards (e.g., catching oneself in falling), neck hyperflexion, or a direct blow to the spinous process.

This fracture is stable, and by itself poses little risk. If the patient is intact, they should have further study (flexion-extension C-spine X-rays or CT scan through the affected level) to R/O other occult fractures. A rigid collar is used PRN pain.

71.3 Vertical compression injuries

In order to apply a purely compressive force to the cervical spine without flexion or extension, reversal of the normal cervical lordosis is required, as may occur in a slightly flexed posture. Burst fractures are the most common result, with the possibility of retropulsion of bone into the spinal canal with neurologic deficit.

71.4 Flexion injuries of the subaxial cervical spine

71.4.1 General information

Constitute up to 15% of cervical spine trauma. Common causes include: MVAs, falls from a height, and diving into shallow water.[9]

71.4.2 Compression flexion injuries

The classic diving injury is the prototypical example. Posterior element fractures occur in up to 50% of compression flexion injuries.[10] Although flexion-compression injuries do distract the posterior elements to some degree, most do not produce posterior ligamentous injuries. Subtypes of compression-flexion fractures include: teardrop fractures (see below), quadrangular fractures (p. 1185).

Treatment: mild cervical compression fractures without neurologic deficit or retropulsion of bone into the spinal canal are usually treated with a rigid orthosis until X-rays show healing has occurred (usually 6–12 wks). Stability is assessed with flexion-extension views (p. 1145) before completely discontinuing the brace. More severe compression fractures heal in a halo brace with ≈ 90% rate of ankylosing fusion.

71.4.3 Teardrop fractures

General information

Originally described by Schneider & Kahn.[11] Results from hyperflexion or axial loading at the vertex of the skull with the neck flexed (eliminating the normal cervical lordosis)[12] (often mistakenly attributed to hyperextension because of the retrolisthesis). Two forces are involved: 1) compression of the anterior column, and 2) tension on DLC. There are varying degrees of severity. In its most severe form, the injury consists of complete disruption of all of the ligaments, the facet joints and the intervertebral disc[13] and ≥ 3 mm of posterior displacement of the body into the canal. As originally described, an important feature is displacement of the inferior margin of the fractured vertebral body posteriorly into the spinal canal.[11] Usually unstable.

Seen in ≈ 5% of patients in a large series of patients with X-ray evidence of cervical spine trauma.[14] Patients are often quadriplegic, although some may be intact and some may have anterior cervical cord syndrome (p. 1135).

Findings

Possible associated injuries and radiographic findings include[13,15] (► Fig. 71.1):
1. a small chip of bone (the "teardrop") just beyond the anterior inferior edge of the involved vertebral body (VB) on lateral cervical spine film
2. often associated with a fracture through the sagittal plane of the VB (sagittal split) which can almost always be seen on AP view (may be midline or off-center). Thin cut CT scan is more sensitive
3. a large triangular fragment of the anterior inferior VB
4. other fractures through the vertebral body may also occur
5. the fractured vertebra is usually displaced *posteriorly* on the vertebra below (also appreciated on oblique X-rays, ► Fig. 71.5). However, cases without retrolisthesis are also described[10]

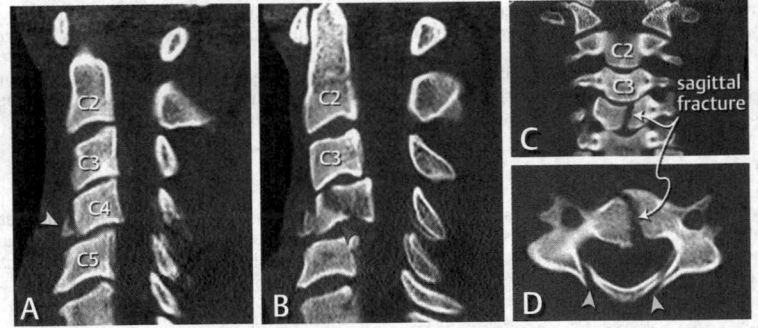

Fig. 71.1 Teardrop fracture of C4.
Image: CT bone windows, A: sagittal, showing the small chip of bone (the "teardrop") (*yellow arrowhead*) and the posteriorly displaced VB; B: sagittal (adjacent to A), showing a large triangular fragment of the C4 VB (*red arrowhead*); C: coronal; D: axial through the C4 VB, showing the sagittally oriented fracture (there are also bilateral lamina fractures [*blue arrowheads*]—not part of the criteria for a teardrop fracture).

6. the fractured body is often wedged anteriorly (kyphosis), and may also be wedged possibly laterally
7. disruption of the facet joints which may be appreciated as separation of the joints on lateral X-ray, often unmasked by cervical traction
8. prevertebral soft-tissue swelling, see for measurements (p. 224)
9. narrowing of the intervertebral disc below the fracture (indicating disruption)

Distinguishing between teardrop fracture and avulsion fracture

Rationale: Teardrop fractures must be distinguished from a simple avulsion fracture which may also result in a small chip of bone off the anterior inferior VB, usually pulled off by traction of the anterior longitudinal ligament (ALL) in hyperextension. Although there may be disruption of the ALL in these cases, it does not usually cause instability.

Methodology: In a patient with a small bone chip off of the inferior anterior VB, a "teardrop" fracture needs to be ruled out. Determine if the following criteria are met:

- neurologically intact (because of the need for cooperation, this includes mental status, and excludes the inebriated or concussed patient)
- size of bone fragment is small
- no malalignment of vertebral bodies
- no evidence of VB fracture in sagittal plane on AP C-spine X-rays or on CT
- no posterior element fracture on X-ray or CT
- no prevertebral soft tissue swelling (p. 224) at level of fragment
- and no loss of vertebral body height or disc space height

If the above criteria are met, obtain flexion-extension C-spine X-rays (p. 1145). If no abnormal movement, discharge patient in rigid collar (e.g., Philadelphia collar), and repeat the films in 4–7 days (i.e., after the pain has subsided to be certain that alignment is not being maintained by cervical muscle spasm from pain), D/C collar if 2nd set of films is normal.

If the patient does not meet the above criteria, treat them as an unstable fracture and obtain a CT scan through the fractured vertebra to evaluate for associated fractures (e.g., sagittal plane fracture that may not be apparent on plain X-ray).

MRI assesses the integrity of the disc and gives some information about the posterior ligaments.

Treatment of teardrop fracture

If the disc and ligaments are intact (determined by MRI) then an option is to employ a halo brace until the fragment is healed (perform flexion-extension X-rays after removing the halo to rule out persistent instability). Alternatively, surgical stabilization may be performed, especially if ligamentous or disc injury is seen on MRI. When the injury is primarily posterior due to disruption of the posterior ligaments and facet joints, and if there is no anterior compromise of the spinal canal, then posterior fusion suffices (p. 1195). Severe injuries with canal compromise often require a combined anterior decompression and fusion (performed first) followed by posterior fusion typically using lateral mass screws and rods.

71.4.4 Quadrangular fractures

See reference.[16]
Four features:

1. oblique vertebral body (VB) fracture passing from anterior-superior cortical margin to inferior endplate
2. posterior subluxation of superior VB on the inferior VB
3. angular kyphosis
4. disruption of disc and anterior and posterior ligaments

Treatment:
May require combined anterior and posterior fusion.

71.5 Distraction flexion injuries

71.5.1 General information

Ranges from hyperflexion sprain (mild, see below) to minor subluxation (moderate) to bilateral locked facets (severe, see below). Posterior ligaments are injured early and are usually evidenced by widening of the interspinous distance (p. 224).

71.5.2 Hyperflexion sprain

A purely ligamentous injury that involves disruption of the posterior ligamentous complex without bony fracture. May be missed on plain lateral C-spine X-rays if they are obtained in normal alignment; requires flexion-extension views (p. 1145). Instability may be concealed when films are obtained shortly after the injury if spasm of the cervical paraspinal muscles splints the neck and prevents true flexion.[17] For patients with limited flexion, a rigid collar should be prescribed, and if the pain persists 1–2 weeks later the films should be repeated (including flexion-extension).

Radiographic signs of hyperflexion sprain[18] (X-rays may also be normal):

1. kyphotic angulation
2. anterior rotation and/or slight (1–3 mm) subluxation
3. anterior narrowing and posterior widening of the disc space
4. increased distance between the posterior cortex of the subluxed vertebral body and the anterior cortex of the articular masses of the subjacent vertebra
5. anterior and superior displacement of the superior facets (causing widening of the facet joint)
6. fanning (abnormal widening) of the interspinous space on lateral C-spine X-ray, or increased interspinous distance on AP; see Interspinous distances (p. 224)

71.5.3 Subluxation

Cadaver studies have shown that horizontal subluxation > 3.5 mm of one vertebral body on another, or > 11° of angulation of one vertebral body relative to the next indicates ligamentous instability[19,20] (▶ Table 71.4). Thus, if subluxation of ≤ 3.5 mm on plain films is seen, and there is no neuro deficit, obtain flexion-extension films; see Flexion-extension cervical spine X-rays (p. 1145). If no abnormal movement, remove cervical collar.

71.5.4 Locked facets

General information

Severe flexion injuries can result in locked facets (AKA "sprung" facets AKA "jumped" facets) with reversal of the normal "shingled" relationship between facets (normally the inferior facet of the level above is posterior to the superior facet of the level below). Involves disruption of facet capsule. Facets may be fractured.

Facets that have not completely locked but have had significant ligamentous disruption allowing distraction with the tip of the inferior facet positioned on the apex of the superior facet below are known as "perched facets" (▶ Fig. 71.2).

Flexion + rotation → unilateral locked facets. Hyperflexion → bilateral locked facets.

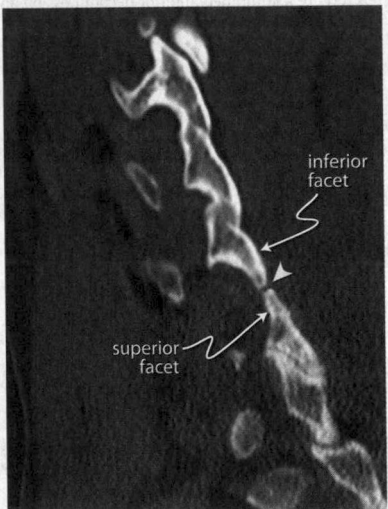

inferior facet

superior facet

Fig. 71.2 Perched facet (*yellow arrowhead*).
Image: sagittal CT through the facet joints in a patient with previous fusion above the perched facet level.

▶ **Unilateral locked facets.** Comprise 6–10% of cervical spine injuries.[21] 25% of patients are neurologically intact, 37% have root deficit, 22% have incomplete cord injuries, and 15% are complete quadriplegics.[22]

▶ **Bilateral locked facets.** Occurs with disruption of ligaments of apophyseal joints, ligamentum flavum, longitudinal and interspinous ligaments, and the anulus. Rare. Most common at C5–6 or C6–7. 65–87% have complete quadriplegia, 13–25% incomplete, ≤ 10% are intact. Adjacent fractures (VB, facet, lamina, pedicle…) occur in 40–60%.[5,23] Nerve root deficits may also occur.

Diagnosis

Both unilateral locked facets (ULF) and bilateral locked facets (BLF) will produce subluxation: BLF poduces anterolisthesis, ULF produces a *rotatory* subluxation and usually a milder anterolisthesis.

▶ **CT. Sagittal CT:** usually the optimal modality to identify locked facets. The inferior facet of the superior level will be located anterior to the superior facet of the inferior level (opposite of normal) (▶ Fig. 71.3).

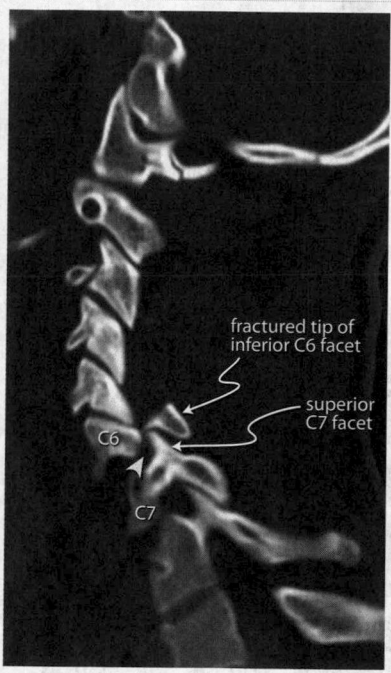

Fig. 71.3 Unilateral locked facet, left C6-7 (*yellow arrowhead*).
The C6 inferior facet is fractured with the tip displaced posteriorly.
Image: sagittal CT scan through the facet joints.

fractured tip of inferior C6 facet

superior C7 facet

C6

C7

71

Axial CT: "naked facet sign": the articular surface of the facet will be seen with the appropriate articulating mate either absent or on the wrong side of the facet (▶ Fig. 71.4). With ULF, CT also demonstrates the rotation of the level above anteriorly on the level below on the side of the locked facet.

▶ **C-spine X-rays. BLF:** Usually produces > 50% subluxation on lateral C-spine X-ray.
 ULF: Often missed on plain cervical spine X-rays because of relatively subtle findings.
✖ Beware of mimic (congenital absence of cervical pedicle - see below)
1. **AP X-ray:** spinous processes above the subluxation rotate to the same side as the locked facet (with respect to those below)
2. **lateral X-ray:** "bow-tie sign" (left & right facets at the level of the injury are side-by-side instead of the normal superimposed position[22]). Subluxation usually < 25% may be seen. Disruption of the posterior ligamentous complex may produce widening of the interspace between spinous processes

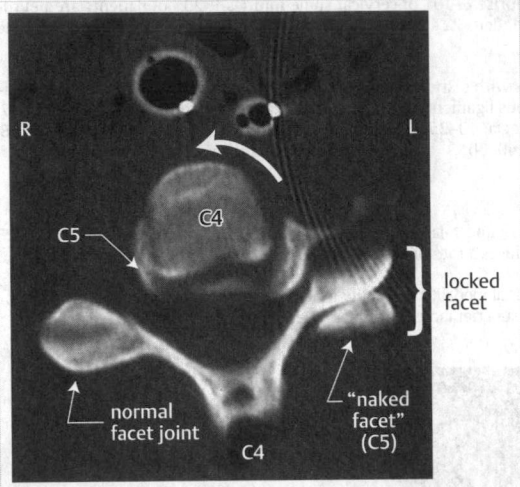

Fig. 71.4 Locked facet, left C4–5. (CT scan). Note the rotation of the C4 vertebral body on C5 (*curved arrow*).

3. **oblique X-ray:** (▶ Fig. 71.5) may demonstrate the locked facet which will be seen blocking the neural foramen (use ≈ 60° left anterior oblique (LAO) for left locked facet, 60° right anterior oblique (RAO) for right; e.g. with RAO the patient is angled with the right shoulder closer to the film)

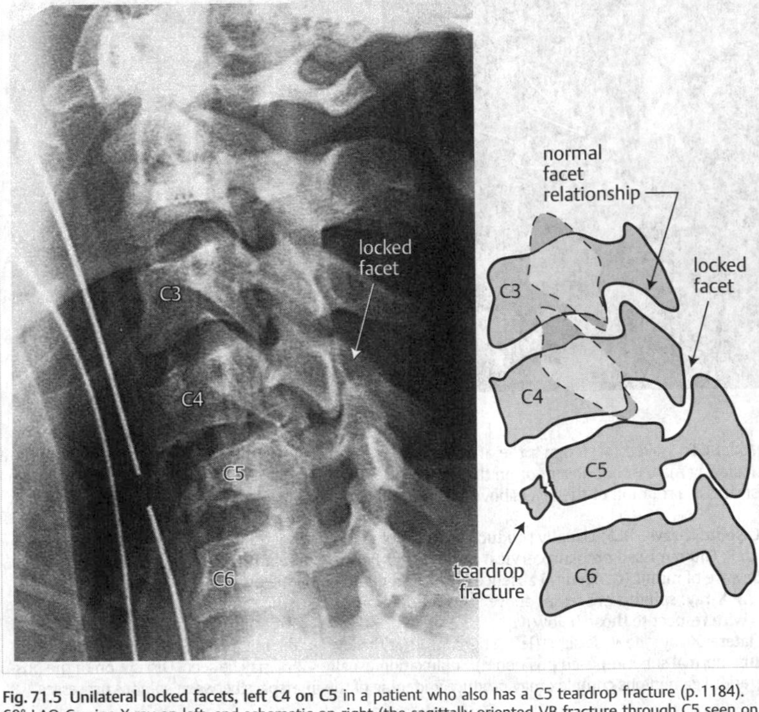

Fig. 71.5 Unilateral locked facets, left C4 on C5 in a patient who also has a C5 teardrop fracture (p. 1184). 60° LAO C-spine X-ray on left, and schematic on right (the sagittally oriented VB fracture through C5 seen on CT scan is not demonstrated). Note the anterior subluxation of C4 on C5, and the slight retrolisthesis of C5 on C6.

▶ **MRI.** Should be performed when possible to rule out traumatic disc herniation (found in 80% of BLF)[24] which may change the choice of approach (anterior vs. posterior) and is a contraindication to attempting closed reduction.

▶ **CTA.** Should be performed when possible because of the small chance of vertebral artery injury.

▶ ✖ **MIMIC: Congenital absence of a cervical pedicle.** Caution. This rare condition may mimic a unilateral locked facet (ULF) especially when discovered following trauma. C6 is the most common reported level.[25] The facet positions may be reversed from normal, as occurs in a locked facet.[26] It is almost always unilateral.[27]

A triad of findings has been described[28] (▶ Fig. 71.6):

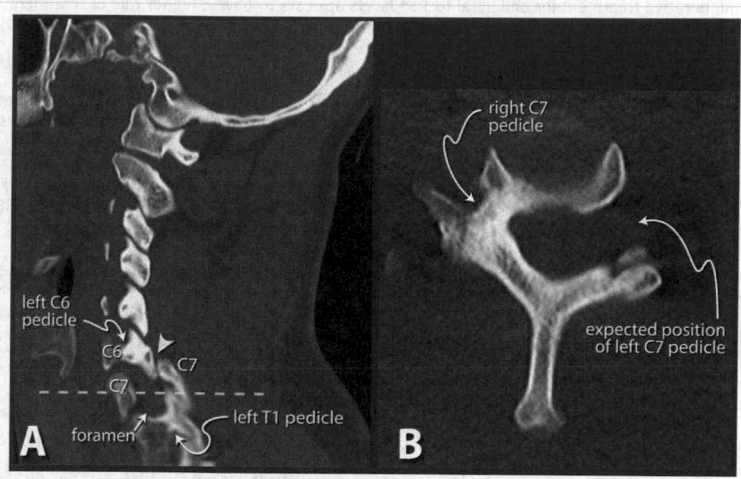

Fig. 71.6 Congenital absence of the left C7 pedicle.
The C6 inferior facet is positioned anterior to the superior C7 facet (*yellow arrowhead*) which mimics a unilateral locked left C6-7 facet. Note the neural foramen appears enlarged due to the absent pedicle (*short straight white arrow*).
Images: CT scan. A: Sagittal cut through the left facet joints. B: Axial CT cut at the level of the yellow broken line in A.

71

1. ipsilateral neural foramen appears enlarged. NB: this may falsely suggest the presence of a foraminal tumor such as a schwannoma
2. ipsilateral dorsally displaced dysplastic articular pillar and lamina. NB: the dysplastic reversed facet may mimic a locked facet[26]
3. ipsilateral dysplastic transverse process

Other clues for distinguishing this from ULF: there is no anterolisthesis in the lateral projection, and no deviation of the spinous processes from rotatory subluxation on the AP view.[27]

Most cases are asymptomatic. Symptoms that have been attributed to this include paresthesias or pain in the head, neck, shoulder, or arm. Surgery is unlikely to improve any symptoms.[27] It has been opined that the involved level may be less stable than normal, but no related serious spinal cord injuries have been reported.[27]

Treatment

Treatment options
Also see Practice guideline: Initial closed reduction in fracture-dislocation cervical SCI (p. 1147).

Unilateral locked facets: options include:
1. no treatment (i.e. leaving the facets locked): should generally be considered only for asymptomatic patients. May not be stable, and close follow-up is indicated with fusion recommended for failure
2. closed reduction with or without post-reduction fusion. May not be stable, and close follow-up is indicated with fusion recommended for failure
3. surgical intervention
   a) anterior approach: anterior cervical discectomy and fusion (ACDF) is the usual method. Cervical disc arthroplasty may be considered but is likely not as stable
   b) posterior approach: often open reduction and internal fixation
   c) combined anterior and posterior approach (360° fusion)

Nonoperative treatment for unilateral locked facets appears to have a higher rate of treatment failure, persistent pain, and neurologic deterioration than surgical treatment.[21]

Closed reduction of locked facets
✖ Contraindicated if traumatic disc herniation is demonstrated on MRI. Patients who cannot be assessed neurologically may be done using SSEP/MEP monitoring. Closed reduction was successful in 22% of 24 cases of ULF.[29] Two methods of closed reduction: traction or manipulation.
1. **traction:** more commonly employed in the U.S.
   a) initial weight (in lbs) ≈ 3 × cervical vertebral level, increase in 5–10 lb increments usually at 10–15 minute intervals until desired alignment is attained (assess neurologic exam (or SSEP/MEP) and lateral C-spine X-ray or fluoroscopy after each ≈ to avoid overdistraction)
   b) end points (i.e. do not add any more traction weight):
      • do not exceed 10 lbs per vertebral level (some say 5 lbs/level) under most circumstances. This is a guideline—you are trying to avoid overdistraction at the index level and at normal levels
      • distraction of perched/locked facet or desired reduction is achieved
      • if occipitocervical instability develops
      • if any disc space height exceeds 10 mm (overdistraction)
      • if any neurologic deterioration or deterioration of SSEP/MEP
   c) with unilateral locked facets, one may add gentle manual torsion *towards* the side of the locked facets. With bilateral locked facets, one may add gentle manual posterior tension (e.g. with a rolled towel under the occiput)
   d) once the facets are perched or distracted, gradual reduction of the weights will usually result in reduction—verify with X-ray (placing the neck in slight extension, e.g. with small shoulder roll, may help maintain the reduction)
2. **manipulation** (usually under anesthesia): less commonly employed,[22] more frequently used in Europe. Involves manually applying axial traction and sagittal angulation sometimes with rotation and direct pressure at the fracture level under fluoroscopy

Paraspinal muscle relaxation (but not enough to cause obtundation) may assist in reduction. Use IV diazepam (Valium®) and/or narcotic. General anesthesia may be used in difficult cases (with SSEP/MEP monitoring).
    Once reduction is achieved, the patient is left in 5–10 lbs of traction for stabilization.
    Disadvantage of closed reduction
1. fails to reduce ≈ 25% of cases of BLF
2. risks overdistraction at higher levels or worsening of other fractures
3. neurologic worsening following closed reduction may occur with traumatic disc herniation[23,30] and should be evaluated immediately with MRI and if confirmed treated with prompt discectomy
4. adds time and potentially pain to the patient's care, especially since many will go on to have surgical fusion anyway

Following closed reduction, the need for internal (operative) stabilization vs. external stabilization (i.e., bracing) may be addressed (see below).
    Open reduction and fixation is usually required if reduction is not achieved. Closed reduction is often more difficult with bilateral locked facets than with unilateral.

71

Open reduction of locked facets

1. **posterior approach:** the most common approach. Although rare, this still subjects the patient to risk of deterioration from traumatically herniated disc. Therefore a pre-op MRI should be done if possible. Often requires drilling of the tip of the superior aspect of the articular facet of the level below. A foraminotomy is recommended when there are root symptoms to visualize and decompress the root

2. **anterior approach:** this is used when there is a traumatic disc herniation at the level of the subluxation. By removing the disc at the subluxed level and exploring the anterior epidural space, the risk of worsening deficit due to a traumatic herniated disc is theoretically reduced. A unilateral locked facet may be reduced by placing Caspar pins in the VB and then under traction rotating the pin in the body above the dislocation towards the side of the locked facet. Reducing bilateral locked facets is more difficult from an anterior approach

3. **combined anterior/posterior (360°) approach:** using anterior plate and posterior lateral mass screws/rods may eliminate the need for post-op external immobilization

Stabilization

Surgical fusion is commonly performed after successful closed reduction, failed closed reduction, or following open reduction.

If there are fracture fragments about the articular surfaces, there may be satisfactory healing with halo vest immobilization (for 3 months) once closed reduction is achieved.[31] Frequent X-rays are needed to rule out redislocation.[32] Flexion-extension X-rays are obtained upon halo removal and surgery is required for continued instability. Up to 77% of patients with unilateral or bilateral facet dislocation (with or without facet fracture fragments) will have a poor anatomic result with halo vest alone (although late instability was uncommon), suggesting that surgery should be considered for all of these patients.[33] Surgical fusion is more clearly indicated in cases without facet fracture fragments (ligamentous instability alone may not heal) or if open reduction is required.

If surgery is indicated, an MRI should be done beforehand if possible. A posterior approach is preferred if there are no anterior masses (such as traumatic disc herniation or large osteophytic spurs), if subluxation of the bodies is > one–third the VB width (suggesting severe posterior ligamentous injury), or for fractures of the posterior elements. A posterior approach is mandatory if there is an unreducible dislocation. See also Options for posterior approach (p. 1195).

71

71.6 Extension injuries of the subaxial cervical spine

71.6.1 Extension injury without bony injury

Extension injuries can produce spinal cord injury (SCI) without evidence of bony injury. Injury patterns include central cord syndrome (p. 1132) usually in an older adult with cervical spondylosis, and SCIWORA (see below) usually in young children. Middle-aged adults with hyperextension dislocations that reduce spontaneously immediately may present with SCI and no bony abnormality on X-ray, but there may be rupture of the anterior longitudinal ligament (ALL) and/or intervertebral disc on MRI or autopsy. Extension forces may also be associated with carotid artery dissections (p. 1578).

71.6.2 Minor extension injuries

Results from extension acting alone. Includes spinous process and lamina fractures. By themselves, are stable.

71.6.3 Extension compression injury

This is the most common mechanism of lateral mass/facet fractures (see below).

71.6.4 Lateral mass and facet fractures of the cervical spine

General information

Often results from extension combined with compression.
For C3 through C6, there is risk of vertebral artery injury.

Classification of cervical lateral mass and facet fractures

4 patterns identified in lateral mass and facet fractures[34] are shown in ▶ Table 71.5.

Anterior subluxation of the fractured vertebra was observed in 77% of whole lateral-mass fractures.[34]

Horizontal facet or separation fracture of the articular mass

Extension combined with compression and rotation may produce fracture of one pedicle and ipsilateral lamina which permits the detached articular mass ("floating" lateral mass) to rotate forward to a more horizontal orientation[35] (horizontalization of the facet) (▶ Table 71.5). May be associated with rupture of the anterior longitudinal ligament (ALL) and fissure of the disc at one or two levels. Neuro deficit is common. Unstable.

Table 71.5 Classification of cervical lateral mass & facet fractures[34]

Designation	Diagram	Description
separation fracture		fractures through lamina and ipsilateral pedicle. Permits *horizontalization* of facet[35] (see text)
comminuted fracture		multiple fractures. Often associated with lateral angulation deformity
split fracture		coronally oriented vertical fracture in 1 lateral mass, with invagination of the superior articular facet of the level below
traumatic spondylolysis		*bilateral* horizontal fractures through pars interarticularis, separating anterior spinal elements from posterior

71

Failure of nonoperative treatment

A study of *CT scans* of 26 *unilateral* cervical facet fractures[36] identified the risk factors shown below for failure of nonoperative treatment (▶ Fig. 71.7 for illustration of the measurement definitions): where the fracture fragment (FF) height was defined as the maximum tip-to-tip cephalocaudal height on sequential sagittal reconstructions.

Nonoperative management is likely to fail if FF is:
1. >1 cm, or
2. >40% of LM (the height of the intact contralateral lateral mass at the same level, defined as the maximum tip-to-tip cephalocaudal height on the sagittal reconstructions)

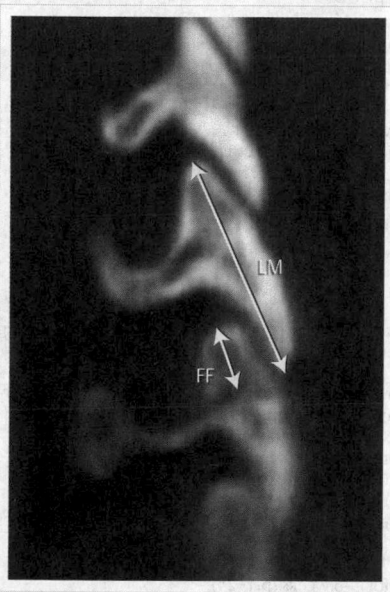

Fig. 71.7 Facet fracture fragment measurements. Sagittal CT through the facet joints. FF = fracture fragment height, LM = lateral mass height (measured on the *contralateral* side at the same level as the fracture, not as shown here which just illustrates the technique used to measure LM at a different level on the *same* side).

71

Surgical treatment of cervical lateral mass and facet fractures

Most cases can be treated with a posterior approach using fixation screws (lateral mass screws or pedicle screws[34]) and rods extending at least 1 level above and below the level of fracture (usually omitting a screw on the side of the fracture at the index level). Simultaneous neural decompression is performed when needed. Additional treatment with an anterior approach may be required for release of rigid deformity or for additional anterior column support.[34] Some separation fractures may be candidates for osteosynthesis (to preserve motion) using a cervical pedicle screw[34] that traverses the fracture.

An anterior approach is an alternative. Advantage: usually only 1 level needs to be fused. Disadvantages: decompression of compressing fragments cannot always be accomplished and requires disrupting an area that may not be compromised (if there is subluxation, the anterior column is probably compromised).

71.7 Treatment of subaxial cervical spine fractures

71.7.1 General information

> **Practice guideline: Treatment of subaxial cervical spine fractures or dislocations**
>
> Level III[37]
> - closed or open reduction of subaxial fractures or dislocations with the goal of decompression of the spinal cord and restoration of the spinal canal
> - stable immobilization either by internal fixation or by external immobilization to facilitate early patient mobilization and rehabilitation. If surgical treatment is employed, either anterior or posterior fixation is acceptable when a particular approach for decompression of the spinal cord is not required
> - treatment with prolonged bed rest in traction if more contemporary treatment options are not available
> - for patients with ankylosing spondylitis:
>   - routine use of CT and MRI is recommended even after minor trauma
>   - when surgical stabilization is required, posterior long segment instrumentation and fusion or a combined anterior/posterior procedure (360° fusion). Anterior stand-alone instrumentation and fusion procedures are associated with a failure rate of up to 50% in these patients

71.7.2 Management overview

Management of some specific types of C-spine fractures is covered in the corresponding preceding sections. For injuries not specifically addressed, general management principles are as follows[6]:
1. immobilize and reduce externally (if possible): may use traction × 0–7 days
2. determine if there is an indication for decompression as soon as practical (clinical conditions permitting), and decompress if needed. Although controversial, the following are generally accepted indications for *acute* decompression in patients without complete spinal cord injury:
   a) radiographic evidence of bone or foreign material in the spinal canal with associated spinal cord symptoms
   b) complete block on CT, myelogram, or MRI
   c) clinical judgment: e.g., a progressive incomplete spinal cord injury where the surgeon believes that decompression would be beneficial
3. ascertain stability of the injury (see ► Table 71.4)
   a) stable fractures: treat in non-halo orthosis for 1–6 weeks (p. 1124)
   b) unstable fractures: all of the following choices are appropriate, with little evidence (based on long-term spinal stability) to recommend one scheme over another in most cases
      - traction × 7 weeks, followed by orthosis × 8 weeks
      - halo × 11 weeks, followed by orthosis × 4 weeks
      - surgical fusion, followed by orthosis × 15 weeks
      - surgical fusion with internal immobilization (lateral mass screws & rods…) ± orthosis for short period of time (≈ several weeks)

71.7.3 Surgical treatment

In patients with complete spinal cord lesions

Operating on a patient with a complete cord injury (ASIA A and not in spinal shock) does not result in significant recovery of neurologic function.[38] If there is ongoing spinal cord compression and the bulbocavernosus reflex is absent, the patient may be in spinal shock. In this case, operate at the earliest time that is safe to do so at your institution. However, aggressive non-surgical reduction of traumatic subluxation should be pursued.

The primary goal of surgery in this setting is spinal stabilization, allowing the patient to be placed in a sitting position for improved pulmonary function, for psychological benefit, and to allow initiation of rehabilitation. Although the spine will fuse spontaneously in many cases (taking ≈ 8–12 weeks), surgical *stabilization* expedites the mobilization process and reduces the risk of delayed kyphotic angulation deformity. Early surgery may lead to further neurological injury, and should be delayed until the patient has stabilized medically and neurologically. In most cases, performing surgery within 4–5 days (if the patient is otherwise stable) is probably early enough to help reduce pulmonary complications.

In patients with incomplete lesions

Patients with incomplete cord injuries who have compromise of the spinal canal (by bone, disc, unreducible subluxation, or hematoma) and either do not improve with nonoperative therapy or deteriorate neurologically should undergo surgical decompression and stabilization.[38] This may facilitate some further return of spinal cord function. An exception may be the central cord syndrome (p.1132).

Anterior or posterior?

The choice of technique depends to a large degree on the *mechanism* of injury, as the treatment should tend to counteract the instability, and ideally should not compromise structures that are still functioning. Instrumentation (wires/cables, lateral mass screws & rods, clamps…) immobilizes the area of instability while bony fusion is occurring. In the absence of bony fusion, all mechanical devices will eventually fail, and so it becomes a "race" between fusion and instrument failure. Extensive injuries (including teardrop fractures (p.1184) and compression burst fractures) may require a combined anterior and posterior approach (staged, or in a single sitting; anterior decompression precedes posterior fusion).

Posterior immobilization and fusion

Indications: The procedure of choice for most *flexion* injuries. Useful when there is minimal injury to the vertebral bodies and in the absence of anterior compression of the spinal cord and nerves. Including: posterior ligamentous instability, traumatic subluxation, unilateral or bilateral locked facets, simple wedge compression fractures.

The most common technique consists of open or closed reduction, followed by lateral mass screws & rods (p.1164). Interlaminar Halifax clamps are an alternative.[39] Although successes have been reported using methylmethacrylate,[40] it does not bond to bone and weakens with age, and thus its use in the setting of traumatic injury is *discouraged*.[41]

Choice of posterior technique: If the anterior weight-bearing column is significantly damaged, or if there is absence or compromise of the lamina or spinous processes, then either a combined anterior-posterior approach is needed or posterior rigid instrumentation (e.g., lateral mass screw-plate or rod fixation) with fusion is recommended.[42]

Anterior approach

Does not depend on integrity of posterior elements to achieve stability.
  Indications:
1. fractured vertebral body with bone retropulsed into spinal canal (burst fracture)
2. most *extension* injuries
3. severe fractures of posterior elements that preclude posterior stabilization and fusion
4. may be used for traumatic subluxation of the cervical spine

Usually consists of:
1. corpectomy: decompresses the neural elements (if necessary) and removes fractured and structurally compromised bone
   a) decompression usually requires wide corpectomy, at least ≈ 16 mm (palpate anterior surface of vertebral body to determine width; note position of vertebral arteries on pre-op CT). NB: it is suggested to take the corpectomy no wider than 3 mm lateral to the medial edge of the longus colli muscle; this leaves ≈ 5 mm margin of safety to the foramen transversarium[43]
   b) if decompression is not needed, ≈ 12 mm corpectomy suffices (i.e., about the width of a half-inch cottonoid)
2. AND
   a) strut graft fusion: replaces the involved body or bodies with either:
      • bone (usually iliac crest, rib or fibula, either homologous or cadaveric)
      • or synthetic cage (e.g., titanium or PEEK)
   b) usually accompanied with compression plates
   c) usually followed with external immobilization
   d) corpectomy of > 1 level, or presence of injury to posterior elements is usually an indication for augmentation with posterior instrumentation

71

Complications of surgical treatment

1. hardware problems
   a) anterior cage problems
      - cage displacement/extrusion
      - cage subsidence/telescoping into endplate
      - vertebral body fracture
   b) problems with plating
      - screw pull-out, loosening, or breakage
      - fatigue fracture of plate
      - screw injury: nerve root, spinal cord, or vertebral artery
2. inadequate postoperative immobilization
   a) improper brace selected
   b) poor patient compliance with immobilization device
3. failure of graft to take (nonunion)
4. judgmental error
   a) failure to incorporate all unstable levels
   b) improper surgical approach

71.8 Spinal cord injury without radiographic abnormality (SCIWORA)

71.8.1 General information

Although spinal cord injuries are uncommon in children, there is a subgroup of these in which it is not possible to detect any bony or ligamentous abnormality on X-rays (including dynamic flexion-extension X-rays), CT scans, or myelograms. This was dubbed SCIWORA (an acronym for "Spinal Cord Injury Without Radiographic Abnormality").[44] However, with the increased use of MRI, a number of soft tissue findings and spinal cord abnormalities have been identified, some of which have prognostic signficance (see below).[45] A more appropriate name might now be Traumatic Spinal Myelopathy with Exclusively MRI Findings ("T-SMEMF") to denote that studies involving X-rays are negative by definition.

The age range of children with SCIWORA is 1.5–16 years; it has a much higher incidence in age ≤ 9 yrs.[46] This predilection for younger patients is attributed to the normally increased elasticity of their spinous ligaments and paravertebral soft-tissues.[44] The hypothesis is that the physiologic hypermobility of the young spine allows deformation to a degree that is beyond the tolerance of the spinal cord without causing fracture or discoligamentous instability. In addition to translational excursions, vertical stretching is also a possible mechanism of injury.[47] Other mechanisms include splitting of the growth zone of the vertebral body endplate and tearing of the anterior longitudinal ligament (ALL).[45]

There may be an increased risk of SCIWORA among young children with asymptomatic Chiari I malformation.[48]

Incidence: not accurately known, but probably 30-40% of children < 18 years of age with traumatic myelopathy have SCIWORA.[45]

71.8.2 Presentation of SCIWORA

54% of children with SCIWORA had a delay between injury (at which time some children experience transient numbness, paresthesias, Lhermitte's sign (p. 1712), or a feeling of total body weakness) and the onset of *objective* sensorimotor dysfunction ("latent period") ranging from 30 minutes to 4 days.

Four spinal cord injury patterns have been associated with SCIWORA[45]:

1. central cord syndrome (p. 1132)
2. Brown-Séquard syndrome (p. 1135)
3. partial cord syndrome: incomplete cord syndrome not consistent with either of the above
4. complete cord transection

Younger children tend to have upper cervical SCI, whereas older children skew towards the lower C-spine.

13% of SCIWORA cases involve the thoracic spine, almost exclusively from vehicular trauma.[45]

71.8.3 Radiographic evaluation

Practice guideline: Diagnosis of SCIWORA

Level III[49]
- MRI of the region of suspected injury
- radiographic screening of entire spine
- assess spinal stability with flexion-extension X-rays in the acute setting and at a late follow-up, even if MRI is negative for extraneural injury

✖ *not* recommended: spinal angiography or myelography

In addition to plain films and flexion-extension films (to identify overt instability which would require surgical fusion and would technically not be SCIWORA), should include MRI.

Possible MRI findings[45]:
1. extraneural findings. Fat-suppression sequences can enhance visualization of some findings. Includes: ALL rupture, loss of continuity of prevertebral soft-tissue low-signa stripe, splitting of the growth zone of the vertebral endplate, rupture of the PLL, intradiscal hemorrhages, hemorrhage in tectorial membrane, increased signal in the interspinous and interlaminar ligaments
2. neural findings: 5 patterns
   a) complete spinal cord disruption
   b) major cord hemorrhage: involves > 50% of cord cross-section. Severe deficit, poor prognosis for neurologic function
   c) minor cord hemorrhage: < 50% of cord cross-sectional involvement. Moderately severe deficit, fairly good prognosis for subtotal recovery
   d) edema only: T1 iso-intense or slightly hypo-intense, and T2 bright. Good prognosis
   e) no intraparenchymal abnormality: 35% of SCIWORA. Excellent chance of full recovery

There were no intraspinal space-occupying lesions in 13 patients studied with myelography/CT.[44]

71.8.4 Management

Practice guideline: Management of SCIWORA

Level III[49]
- external immobilization of the injured spinal segment for up to 12 weeks
- early discontinuation of external immobilization for patients who become asymptomatic and are confirmed to have no instability on flexion-extension X-rays
- avoidance of "high-risk" activities for up to 6 months after SCIWORA

Surgical intervention, including laminectomy, has shown no benefit in the few cases where it has been tried.[51]

Due to a 20% rate of repeat injury (some due to trivial trauma, and some without identifiable trauma) within 10 weeks of the original trauma when treated with only a rigid collar and restriction of contact sports (both for 2 months), more aggressive measures were initially recommended (▶ Table 71.6).

71

Table 71.6 Treatment protocol for SCIWORA (modified[50])

- admit patient to hospital (helps emphasize seriousness of injury)
- BR with rigid cervical collar until flexion-extension films are normal
- MRI of cervical spine to document presence of spinal cord injury
- detailed discussion with patient and family about seriousness of injury and rationale for treatment outlined here
- immobilization in Guilford brace for 3 months[a]
- prohibition of contact and noncontact sports
- regular follow-up visits for monitoring condition and compliance
- liberalize activities at 3 months if flexion-extension films are normal

[a]this represents an extremely conservative recommendation, a less restrictive recommendation is immobilization for 1–3 weeks[51]; see **Practice guideline: SCIWORA** (p. 1197).

References

[1] Bono CM, Vaccaro AR, Fehlings M, et al. Measurment techniques for lower cervical spine injuries: consensus statement of the Spine Trauma Study Group. Spine. 2006; 31:603–609

[2] Aarabi B, Walters BC, Dhall SS, et al. Subaxial cervical spine injury classification systems. Neurosurgery. 2013; 72 Suppl 2:170–186

[3] Vaccaro AR, Hulbert RJ, Patel AA, et al. The subaxial cervical spine injury classification system: a novel approach to recognize the importance of morphology, neurology, and integrity of the disco-ligamentous complex. Spine. 2007; 32:2365–2374

[4] White AA,3rd, Panjabi MM. Update on the evaluation of instability of the lower cervical spine. Instr Course Lect. 1987; 36:513–520

[5] Allen BL, Ferguson RL, Lehmann TR, et al. A Mechanistic Classification of Closed, Indirect Fractures and Dislocations of the Lower Cervical Spine. Spine. 1982; 7:1–27

[6] White AA, Panjabi MM. The Problem of Clinical Instability in the Human Spine: A Systematic Approach. In: Clinical Biomechanics of the Spine. 2nd ed. Philadelphia: J.B. Lippincott; 1990:277–378

[7] Hall RDM. Clay-Shoveller's Fracture. J Bone Joint Surg. 1940; 22:63–75

[8] Gershon-Cohen J, Budin E, Glauser F. Whiplash Fractures of Cervicodorsal Spinous Processes. JAMA. 1954; 155:560–561

[9] Abitbol J-J, Kostuik JP. The Cervical Spine Research Society Editorial Committee. Flexion Injuries to the Lower Cervical Spine. In: The Cervical Spine. 3rd ed. Philadelphia: Lippincott-Raven; 1998:457–464

[10] Fuentes J-M, Bloncourt J, Vlahovitch B, et al. La Tear Drop Fracture: Contribution à l'étude du Mécanisme et des Lésions Ostéo-Disco-Ligamentaires. Nirochirurgie. 1983; 29:129–134

[11] Schneider RC, Kahn EA, Arbor A. Chronic Neurologic Sequelae of Acute Trauma to the Spine and Spinal Cord. The Significance of Acute Flexion or Teardrop Cervical Fracture-Dislocation of the Cervical Spine. Journal of Bone and Joint Surgery. 1956; 38A

[12] Torg JS, Vegso JJ, Sennett B. The national football head and neck injury registry: 14-year report of cervical quadriplegia (1971-1984). Clinics in Sports Medicine. 1987; 6:61–72

[13] Harris JH, Edeiken-Monroe B, Kopaniky DR. A Practical Classification of Acute Cervical Spine Injuries. Orthopedic Clinics of North America. 1986; 17:15–30

[14] Gehweiler JA, Clark WM, Schaaf RE, et al. Cervical Spine Trauma: The Common Combined Conditions. Radiology. 1979; 130

[15] Gehweiler JA, Osborne RL. The Radiology of Vertebral Trauma. Philadelphia: W. B. Saunders; 1980

[16] Favero KJ, VanPeteghem PK. The Quadrangular Fragment Fracture: Roentgenographic Features and Treatment Protocol. Clinical Orthopedics. 1989; 239:40–46

[17] Webb JK, Broughton RBK, McSweeney T, et al. Hidden Flexion Injury of the Cervical Spine. Journal of Bone and Joint Surgery. 1976; 58B:322–327

[18] Fazl M, LaFebvre J, Willinsky RA, et al. Posttraumatic Ligamentous Disruption of the Cervical Spine, an Easily Overlooked Diagnosis: Presentation of Three Cases. Neurosurgery. 1990; 26:674–677

[19] White AA, Johnson RM, Panjabi MM, et al. Biomechanical Analysis of Clinical Stability in the Cervical Spine. Clin Orthop. 1975; 109:85–96

[20] White AA, Southwick WO, Panjabi MM. Clinical Instability in the Lower Cervical Spine - A Review of Past and Current Concepts. Spine. 1976; 1:15–27

[21] Dvorak M, Vaccaro AR, Hermsmeyer J, et al. Unilateral facet dislocations: Is surgery really the preferred option? Evid Based Spine Care J. 2010; 1:57–65

[22] Andreshak JL, Dekutoski MB. Management of Unilateral Facet Dislocations: A Review of the Literature. Orthopedics. 1997; 20:917–926

[23] Payer M, Schmidt MH. Management of traumatic bilateral locked facets of the subaxial cervical spine. Contemporary Neurosurgery. 2005; 27:1–4

[24] Rizzolo SJ, Piazza MR, Cotler JM, et al. Intervertebral disc injury complicating cervical spine trauma. Spine. 1991; 16:S187–S189

[25] Oh YM, Eun JP. Congenital absence of a cervical spine pedicle : report of two cases and review of the literature. J Korean Neurosurg Soc. 2008; 44:389–391

[26] Dimitrov DF, Bronec PR, Friedman AH. Congenitally absent C-7 pedicle presenting as a jumped locked facet. Case illustration. J Neurosurg. 2003; 99. DOI: 10.3171/spi.2003.99.2.0239

[27] van Dijk Azn R, Thijssen HO, Merx JL, et al. The absent cervical pedicle syndrome. A case report. Neuroradiology. 1987; 29:69–72

[28] Wiener MD, Martinez S, Forsberg DA. Congenital absence of a cervical spine pedicle: clinical and radiologic findings. AJR Am J Roentgenol. 1990; 155:1037–1041

[29] Shapiro SA. Management of unilateral locked facet of the cervical spine. Neurosurgery. 1993; 33:832–837

[30] Doran SE, Papadopoulos SM, Ducker TB, et al. Magnetic Resonance Imaging Documentation of Coexistent Traumatic Locked Facets of the Cervical Spine and Disc Herniation. Journal of Neurosurgery. 1993; 79:341–345

[31] Sonntag VKH. Management of Bilateral Locked Facets of the Cervical Spine. Neurosurgery. 1981; 8:150–152

[32] Glasser JA, Whitehall R, Stamp WG, et al. Complications Associated with the Halo Vest. Journal of Neurosurgery. 1986; 65:76–79

[33] Sears W, Fazl M. Prediction of Stability of Cervical Spine Fracture Managed in the Halo Vest and Indications for Surgical Intervention. Journal of Neurosurgery. 1990; 72:426–432

[34] Kotani Y, Abumi K, Ito M, et al. Cervical spine injuries associated with lateral mass and facet joint fractures: New classification and surgical treatment with pedicle screw fixation. European Spine Journal. 2005; 14:69–77

[35] Roy-Camille R, Saillant G. Osteosynthese des fractures du rachis cervical. Actualities Chir Orthop Hop R Poincarré Mason, Paris. 1970; 8:175–194

[36] Spector LR, Kim DH, Affonso J, et al. Use of computed tomography to predict failure of nonoperative treatment of unilateral facet fractures of the cervical spine. Spine (Phila Pa 1976). 2006; 31:2827–2835

[37] Gelb DE, Aarabi B, Dhall SS, et al. Treatment of subaxial cervical spinal injuries. Neurosurgery. 2013; 72 Suppl 2:187–194

[38] Sonntag VKH, Hadley MN. Nonoperative Management of Cervical Spine Injuries. Clin Neurosurg. 1988; 34:630–649

[39] Aldrich EF, Crow WN, Weber PB, et al. Use of MR Imaging-Compatible Halifax Interlaminar Clamps for Posterior Cervical Fusion. Journal of Neurosurgery. 1991; 74:185–189

[40] Branch CL, Kelly DL, Davis CH, et al. Fixation of Fractures of the Lower Cervical Spine Using Methylmethacrylate and Wire: Technique and Results in 99 Patients. Neurosurgery. 1989; 25:503–513

[41] Cooper PR. Comment on Branch C L, et al.: Fixation of Fractures of the Lower Cervical Spine Using Methylmethacrylate and Wire. Neurosurgery. 1989; 25:512–513

[42] McGuire RA, The Cervical Spine Research Society Editorial Committee. Cervical Spine Arthrodesis. In: The Cervical Spine. 3rd ed. Philadelphia: Lippincott-Raven; 1998:499–508

[43] Vaccaro A, Ring D, Seuderi G, et al. Vertebral artery location in relation to the vertebral body as determined by two-dimensional computed tomography evaluation. Spine. 1994; 19

[44] Pang D, Wilberger JE. Spinal Cord Injury without Radiographic Abnormalities in Children. Journal of Neurosurgery. 1982; 57:114–129

[45] Pang D. Spinal cord injury without radiographic abnormality in children, 2 decades later. Neurosurgery. 2004; 55:1325–42; discussion 1342-3

[46] Hamilton MG, Myles ST. Pediatric Spinal Injury: Review of 174 Hospital Admissions. Journal of Neurosurgery. 1992; 77:700–704

[47] Henrys P, Lyne ED, Lifton C, et al. Clinical review of cervical spine injuries in children. Clin Orthop Relat Res. 1977:172–176

[48] Bondurant CP, Oró JJ. Spinal Cord Injury without Radiographic Abnormality and Chiari Malformation. Journal of Neurosurgery. 1993; 79:833–838

[49] Rozzelle CJ, Aarabi B, Dhall SS, et al. Spinal cord injury without radiographic abnormality (SCIWORA). Neurosurgery. 2013; 72 Suppl 2:227–233

[50] Pollack IF, Pang D, Sclabassi R. Recurrent Spinal Cord Injury without Radiographic Abnormalities in Children. Journal of Neurosurgery. 1988; 69:177–182

[51] Madsen JR, Freiman T. Cervical Spinal Cord Injury in Children. Contemporary Neurosurgery. 1998; 20:1–5

71

72 Thoracic, Lumbar, and Sacral Spine Fractures

72.1 Assessment and management of thoracolumbar fractures

72.1.1 General information

A widely used model for thoracolumbar spine stability is the 3-column model of Denis (see below). See also the more recent TLICS system (p. 1206). Note: these systems are for *trauma*, see the Spine Instability Neoplastic Score (SINS) (▶ Table 55.12) for stability assessment in metastatic spine disease.

72.1.2 Three-column model

General information

Denis' 3-column model of the spine (▶ Fig. 72.1) attempts to identify *CT* criteria of instability of *thoracolumbar* spine fractures.[1] This model has generally good predictive value; however, any attempt to create "rules" of instability will have some inherent inaccuracy.

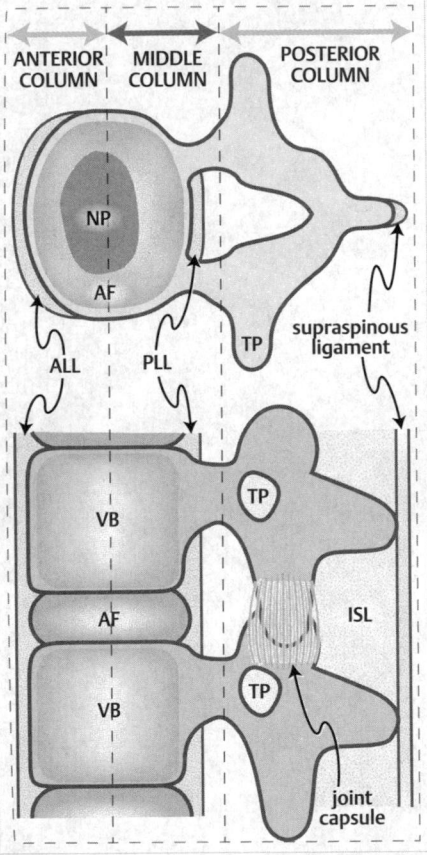

Fig. 72.1 Three-column model of the spine (Denis).
Image: top: viewed from above, bottom: viewed from the side.
Abbreviations: ALL = anterior longitudinal ligament; AF = anulus fibrosus; ISL = interspinous ligament; NP = nucleus pulposus; PLL = posterior longitudinal ligament; TP = transverse process; VB = vertebral body. (Adapted from Spine, Denis F, Vol. 8, pp. 317–31, 1983, with permission.)

72

Definitions

- **anterior column**: anterior half of disc and vertebral body (VB) (includes anterior anulus fibrosus (AF)) plus the anterior longitudinal ligament (ALL)
- **middle column**: posterior half of disc and vertebral body (includes posterior wall of vertebral body and posterior AF), and the posterior longitudinal ligament (PLL)
- **posterior column**: posterior bony complex (posterior arch) with interposed posterior ligamentous complex (supraspinous and interspinous ligament, facet joints and capsule, and ligamentum flavum (LF)). Injury to this column alone does *not* cause instability in flexion

Classification into major and minor injuries

Minor injuries

Involve only a part of a column and do not lead to acute instability (when not accompanied by major injuries). Includes:

1. fracture of transverse process: usually neurologically intact except in two areas:
    a) L4–5 → lumbosacral plexus injuries (there may be associated renal injuries, check U/A for blood)
    b) T1–2 → brachial plexus injuries
2. fracture of articular process or pars interarticularis
3. isolated fractures of the spinous process: in the TL spine: these are usually due to direct trauma. Often difficult to detect on plain X-ray
4. isolated laminar fracture: rare. Should be stable

Major injuries

The McAfee classification describes 6 main types of fractures.[2] A simplified system with four categories follows (also see ▶ Table 72.1):

Table 72.1 Column failure in the four major types of thoracolumbar spine injuries

Fracture type	Column		
	Anterior	Middle	Posterior
compression	compression	intact	intact, or distraction if severe
burst	compression	compression	intact
seat belt	intact or mild compression of 10–20% of anterior VB	distraction	
fracture-dislocation	compression, rotation, shear	distraction, rotation, shear	

Source: Adapted[1] with permission.

▶ **Type 1: Compression fracture.** Compression failure of anterior column only (▶ Fig. 72.2). Middle column *intact* (unlike the 3 other major injuries below) acting as a fulcrum

1. 2 subtypes:
    a) anterior: most common between T6–8 and T12–3
        - lateral X-ray: wedging of the VB anteriorly, no loss of height of posterior VB, no subluxation
        - CT: spinal canal intact. Disruption of anterior endplate
    b) lateral (rare)
2. clinical: no neurologic deficit

▶ **Type 2: Burst fracture.** See ▶ Fig. 72.3. Pure axial load → compression of vertebral body → compression failure of anterior and middle columns. Occur mainly at TL junction, usually between T10 and L2

1. 5 subtypes; L5 burst fractures (p.1206) may constitute a rare subtype
    a) fracture of both endplates: seen in lower lumbar region (where axial load → increased extension, unlike T-spine where axial load → flexion)
    b) fracture of superior endplate: the most common burst fracture. Seen at TL junction. Mechanism = axial load + flexion
    c) fracture of inferior endplate: rare
    d) burst rotation: usually midlumbar. Mechanism = axial load + rotation
    e) burst lateral flexion: mechanism = axial load + lateral flexion

72

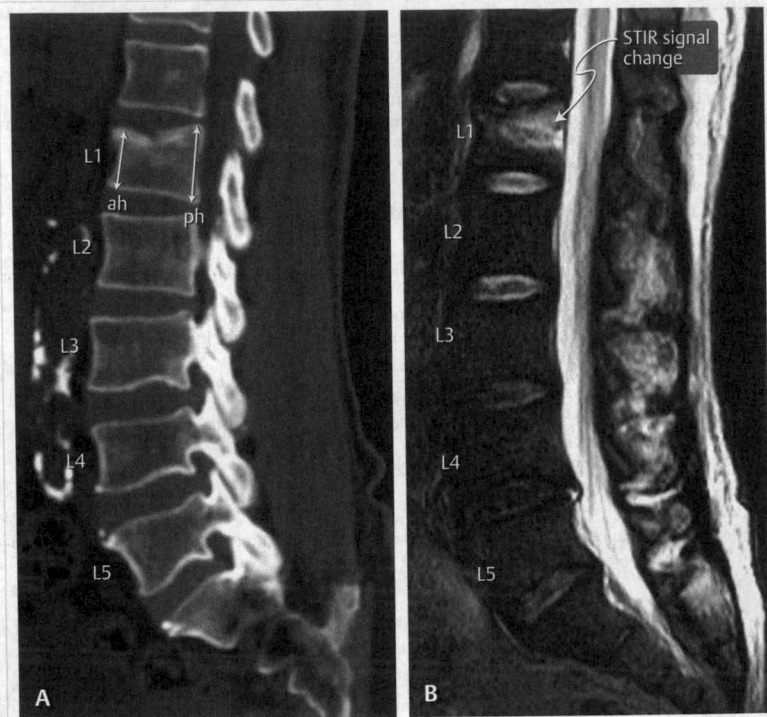

Fig. 72.2 L1 compression fracture.
Mild loss of anterior height with no involvement of middle or posterior columns.
STIR signal changes indicate the fracture is recent.
Yellow double arrows: "ah" = anterior height of the fractured vertebral body, "ph" = posterior height.
A: Sagittal (off midline) bone-window CT, B: Sagittal STIR MRI.

2. radiographic evaluation
    a) lateral X-ray: cortical fracture of posterior VB wall, loss of posterior VB height, retropulsion of bone fragment from endplate(s) into canal
    b) AP X-ray: increase of interpediculate distance (IPD), vertical fracture of lamina, splaying of facet joints: ↑ IPD indicates failure of *middle* column
    c) CT: demonstrates break in posterior wall of VB with retropulsed bone in spinal canal (average: 50% obstruction of canal area), increase in IPD with splaying of posterior arch (including facets)
    d) MRI: compromise of anterior canal by bone fragment; possible cord compression usually with fragments occupying > 50% of the canal diameter
    e) MRI or myelogram: compression in spinal canal
3. clinical: depends on level (thoracic cord more sensitive and less room in canal than conus region), the impact at the time of disruption, and the extent of canal obstruction
    a) ≈ 50% intact at initial examination (half of these recalled leg numbness, tingling, and/or weakness initially after trauma that subsided)
    b) of patients with deficits, only 5% had *complete* paraplegia
▶ **Type 3: Seat belt fracture.** Flexion across a fulcrum anterior to the anterior column (e.g., lap type seat belt) → compression of anterior column & distraction failure of both middle and posterior columns. May be bony or ligamentous. Current terminology: flexion-distraction injury (FDI)
1. 4 subtypes
    a) **Chance fracture** (first desribed by George Quentin Chance[3]): horizontal fracture, classically one level, purely through bone, splitting the spinous process, laminae, pedicles, and VB (▶ Fig. 72.4)

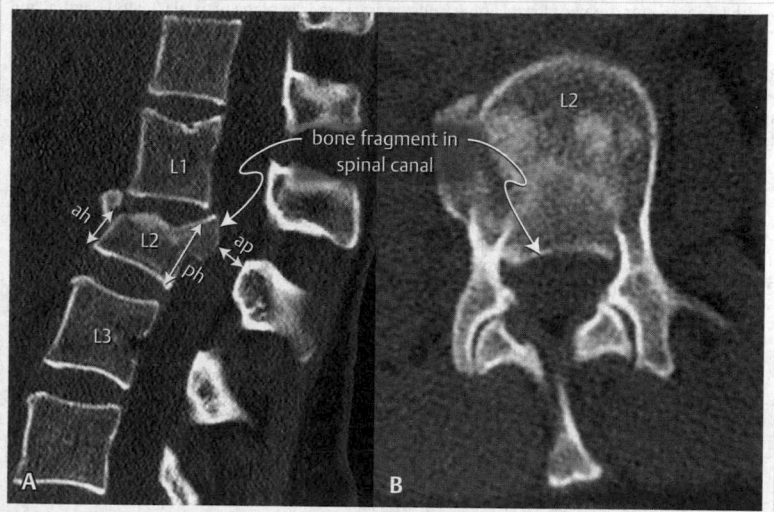

Fig. 72.3 L2 burst fracture.
Note the intact posterior elements (by definition in a burst fracture).
Yellow double arrows: "ap" = residual AP diameter of the canal, "ah" = anterior height of the fractured vertebral body, "ph" = posterior height.
CT scan, bone windows. A: Sagittal, B: Axial.

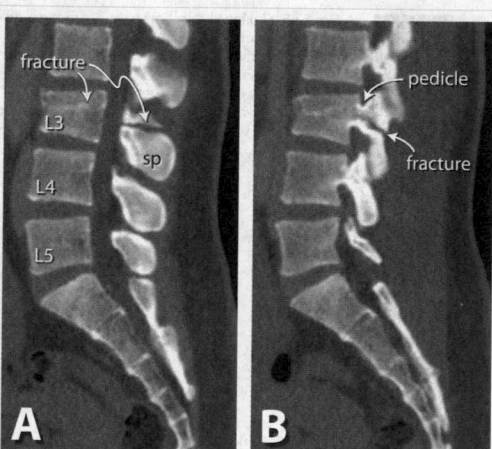

Fig. 72.4 L3 Chance fracture (Denis Type 3a).
Image: CT scan, bone windows. A: Sagittal midline, note the compression fracture through the vertebral body and the distraction fracture through the spinous process (sp); B: Parasagittal through right pedicle, showing the fracture extends through the pedicle.

72

   b) one level, through ligaments
   c) two level, through bone in middle column, through ligament in anterior and posterior columns
   d) two level, through ligament in all 3 columns
2. radiographic evaluation
   a) plain X-ray: ↑ interspinous distance, pars interarticularis fractures, and horizontal split of
      pedicles and transverse process. No subluxation

b) CT: axial cuts are poor for this type (most of fracture is in plane of axial CT cuts). Sagittal and coronal reconstructions demonstrate well. May disclose a pars fracture

c) MRI: T2 to check for canal compromise, STIR to check for ligamentous injury

3. clinical: no neurologic deficit

▶ **Type 4: Fracture-dislocation.** Failure of all 3 columns due to compression, tension, rotation or shear → subluxation or dislocation

1. radiographic evaluation

a) X-ray: occasionally, may be reduced when imaged. Look for other markers of significant trauma (multiple rib fractures, unilateral articular process fractures, spinous process fractures, horizontal laminar fractures, or increased signal on MRI)

b) CT scan: almost always indicated for assessment and surgical planning

c) MRI: assesses nerve involvement. Increased STIR or T2 signal in ligaments and/or disc can provide information about possible injury to those structures

2. 3 subtypes

a) flexion rotation: posterior and middle columns totally ruptured, anteriorly compressed → anterior wedging

- lateral X-ray: subluxation or dislocation. Preserved posterior VB wall. Increased interspinous distance

- CT: rotation and offset of VBs with ↓ canal diameter. Jumped facets

- clinical: 25% neurologically intact. 50% of those with deficits were complete paraplegics

b) shear: all 3 columns disrupted (including ALL)

- when trauma force is directed posterior to anterior (more common) VB above shears forward fracturing the posterior arch (→ free floating lamina) and the superior facet of the inferior vertebra

- clinical: all 7 cases were complete paraplegics

c) flexion distraction subtype of fracture-dislocation

- radiographically resemble seat belt type with addition of subluxation, or with compression of anterior column > 10–20% (▶ Fig. 72.5)

- clinical: neurologic deficit (incomplete in 3 cases, complete in 1)

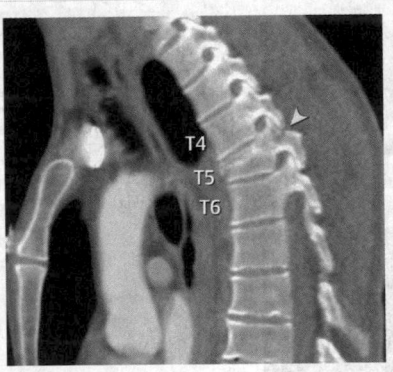

72

Fig. 72.5 Flexion distraction type of fracture dislocation (Denis Type 4c) of T5.
Image: CT scan, sagittal cut through the pedicles, bone windows.
Note the anterior compression fracture of > 10-20% through the vertebral body and the distraction fracture through the pedicle (*yellow arrowhead*).

Associated injuries

In addition to the above, associated injuries include: vertebral endplate avulsion, ligamentous injuries, and hip and pelvic fractures. Thoracolumbar fractures may be associated with hemodynamic instability as a result of hemothorax or aortic injury. Fractures of the transverse processes may be associated with abdominal trauma (e.g., renal injuries at L4–5).

Stability and treatment of thoracolumbar spine fractures

Minor injuries

Isolated thoracolumbar transverse process fractures (as demonstrated on spinal CT) do not require intervention or consultation of a spine service.[4,5]

Major spine injuries

Denis categorized the instability as:
- 1st degree: mechanical instability
- 2nd degree: neurological instability
- 3rd degree: both mechanical & neurological instability

Anterior column injury

Isolated anterior column injuries are usually stable and are treated as outlined in ▶ Table 72.2.
The following exceptions may be *unstable* (1st degree) and often require surgery[1,6]:

Table 72.2 Treatment of stable anterior or middle column thoracolumbar spine injuries

- treat initially with analgesics and recumbency (bed-rest) for comfort
- diminution of pain is a good indication to commence mobilization with or without external bracing (corset or Boston brace or extension TLSO × ≈ 12 weeks) depending on the degree of kyphosis
- vertebroplasty (± kyphoplasty) may be an option (p. 1212)
- serial X-rays to rule out progressive deformity

Unstable compression fractures

1. a single compression fracture with:
   a) loss of > 50% of height with angulation (particularly if the anterior part of the wedge comes to a point)
   b) excessive kyphotic angulation at one segment (various criteria are used, none are absolute. Values quoted: > 30°, > 40°)
2. 3 or more contiguous compression fractures
3. neurologic deficit (generally does not occur with pure compression fracture)
4. disrupted posterior column or more than minimal middle column failure
5. progressive kyphosis: risk of progressive kyphosis is increased when loss of height of anterior vertebral body is > 75%. Risk is higher for lumbar compression fractures than thoracic

Middle column failure

These are unstable (often requiring surgery) with the following exceptions, which should be stable (stable injuries may be treated as outlined in ▶ Table 72.2).

▶ **Stable middle column fractures**
- above T8 if the ribs and sternum are intact (provides anterior stabilization)
- below L4 if the posterior elements are intact
- Chance fracture (anterior column compression, middle column distraction) (▶ Fig. 72.4)
- anterior column disruption with minimal middle column failure

Posterior column disruption

Not *acutely* unstable unless accompanied by failure of the middle column (posterior longitudinal ligament and posterior anulus fibrosus). However, *chronic* instability with kyphotic deformity may develop (especially in children).

Seat belt type injuries without neurologic deficit

No immediate danger of neurologic injury. Treat most with external immobilization in extension (e.g., Jewett hyperextension brace or molded TLSO).

Fracture-dislocation

Unstable. Treatment options:
1. surgical decompression and stabilization: usually needed in cases with
   a) compression with > 50% loss of height with angulation
   b) or kyphotic angulation > 40° (or > 25%)
   c) or neurologic deficit
   d) or desire to shorten length of time of bedrest
2. prolonged bedrest: an option if none of the above are present

72

When vertebral body resection (vertebral corpectomy) is performed, options to access: transthoracic or transabdominal approach (or combined), transpedicular (for thoracic spine), lateral (retroperitoneal/retropleural) approach. Fracture and compression usually occurs at the superior margin of vertebral body, thus start resection at the *inferior* disc interspace. Followed by strut graft (cage or bone: iliac crest or fibula or tibia). Posterior instrumentation is usually required.

Burst fractures

Most thoracolumbar burst fractures occur at T12, L1 & L2.[7] Not all burst fractures are alike. Some burst fractures may eventually cause neurologic deficit (even if no deficit initially). Middle column fragments in canal endanger the neuro elements. Criteria have been proposed to differentiate mild burst fractures from severe ones. No system is uniformly accepted.

Surgical indications[1,8]: burst fracture with any of the following (see ▶ Fig. 72.3):
* anterior vertebral body height ≤ 50% of the posterior height
* residual canal diameter ≤ 50% of normal (note: retropulsed bone in the canal usually remodels over time to cause less compression, with either bracing or surgery and is therefore controversial as an isolated indication for surgery[9,10])
* kyphotic angulation ≥ 20°
* when the interpediculate distance (which is usually abnormally increased on the initial films) widens further on AP X-ray when standing in brace/cast
* neurologic deficit (incomplete)
* progressive kyphosis

Common surgical options for burst or severe compression fractures:
1. if instrumentation alone is needed
   a) can place pedicle screws in 2 levels above and 2 levels below the fracture
   b) if the index level (the fractured level) can be included (i.e., if the pedicles are intact enough to accept shorter screws), similar biomechanical stability can be achieved by placing screws at the index level and then just 1 above and 1 below[11]
2. if decompression of the spinal canal and/or anterior support is needed, corpectomy and strut graft (e.g., with expandable cage) with pedicle screws may be used. Approaches:
   a) from posterior approach e.g., laminectomy with transpedicular approach and impacting bone anteriorly out of canal with a mallet and reverse angled Scoville curette (here, open pedicle screws would be used), or
   b) lateral corpectomy and removal of bone from canal (here percutaneous pedicle screws may be used)

For those not undergoing surgery (i.e., when surgery is not required or is contraindicated), an option is to treat with recumbency from 1–6 weeks (the duration depending on pain and degree of deformity).[8] Avoid early ambulation → further axial loading (even in cast). When appropriate, begin ambulation in an orthosis (e.g., molded thoracolumbar sacral orthosis (TLSO) or a Jewett brace) and follow patient for 3–5 months with serial X-rays to detect progressive collapse or angulation which may need further intervention.

L5 burst fractures may be an exception to the usual management. They comprise only 2.2% of thoracolumbar fractures, and tend to be due to axial compression without rotation.[12] Disc herniation and delayed degeneration is common. Patients with neurologic deficit: surgery is recommended, impacting bone fragments anteriorly and removing herniated disc material, and fusing L4–S1 (with short L5 screws when possible). Vertebral body replacement from a posterior approach carries a risk of paralysis.[12]

72.1.3 Thoracolumbar injury classification and severity score (TLICS)

The TLICS system has been proposed to simplify classification and discussion of thoracolumbar fractures.[13,14] Points are assigned as shown in ▶ Table 72.3. The scores are summed, and management guidelines are given in ▶ Table 72.4.

Neurologic deficit, especially when partial, favors surgery. Note: this system is for trauma, see the Spine Instability Neoplastic Score (SINS) (▶ Table 55.12) for stability assessment in metastatic spine disease.

Table 72.3 Thoracolumbar injury classification & severity score (TLICS)[13,14]

Category	Finding	Points	Score
Radiographic findings	compression fx	1	(1 - 4)
	burst component or lateral angulation > 15°	2	
	translational/rotational injury	3	
	distraction injury	4	
Neurologic status	intact	0	(0 | 2 | 3)
	root injury	2	
	complete SCI (cord or conus medullaris)	2	
	incomplete SCI (cord or conus medullaris)	3	
	cauda equina syndrome	3	
Integrity of posterior ligamantous complex	intact	0	(0 | 2 | 3)
	undetermined	2	
	definite injury	3	
TLICS Score → TOTAL			(1 - 10)

Table 72.4 Management based on TLICS

TLICS	Management
≤ 3	nonoperative candidates
4	"gray zone" may be considered for operative or nonoperative management
≥ 5	surgical candidates

72.2 Surgical treatment

72.2.1 Ligamentotaxis

If the PLL is intact (may not be the case with middle column failure), distraction on the vertebral levels across the fractured level may be able to "pull" retropulsed fragments out of the canal and back towards their normal position (ligamentotaxis) although this is not assured.[15] Ligamentotaxis has a better chance of succeeding if performed within 48 hours of injury. From a posterior approach with laminectomy: intraoperative ultrasound may demonstrate residual canal fragments,[16] and if needed the fragments may be impacted anteriorly out of the canal, e.g., using tamps such as Sypert spinal impactors (Aesculap surgical instruments) or reverse cutting Scoville curettes. It is important not to overdistract to avoid neural injury.

72.2.2 Choice of surgical approach

The posterior approach is preferred when there is not a specific need to go from the front.

72.2.3 Burst fractures

Choice of approach

Surgical considerations: a posterior approach is preferred if there is a dural tear, whereas a burst fracture with partial deficit and canal compromise may be treated more effectively from an anterior approach.[2] A small progression in angular deformity may occur when posterior stabilization is performed alone (since the injury to the anterior column is not corrected), but by itself usually does not require intervention.

For a posterior approach

In an ideal situation (good bone quality, pedicle screw placement goes well (i.e., no fracture, no breach), and nonsmoking patient), one can fuse/rod one above and one below the fracture (using pedicle screws; longer constructs are needed with laminar hooks). With a short segment fusion like this, approximately 10° of lordosis will be lost with time; therefore, one should try to overcorrect a little to accommodate the anticipated settling. If the patient does not meet the above criteria (e.g.,

72

poor bone quality), an option is to "rod long, fuse short" (e.g., rod 2 levels above and below the fracture but fuse only 1 level above and below) and then to remove the hardware when the fusion is solid (e.g., at 8–12 months)—this avoids fusing a nonpathologic segment just to get a better anchor. Junctional deterioration to the point that further surgery is needed often occurs at 3 years when 4 segments are fused, as opposed to occurring at 8–9 years when only 3 levels are fused. Fusing across critical levels (i.e., thoracolumbar junction with T11 or L1 compression fractures) requires that the fusion incorporate 2–3 levels on each side of the junction (the forces of the long segment of the relatively immobile thoracic spine with the lumbar spine at the T-L junction increase the risk of nonunion).

For thoracic fractures that are not severe and do not require decompression, an option is to place pedicle screws and rods (which can be done percutaneously) without placing any graft. The concept is that the ribs anteriorly and the screws/rods posteriorly provide adequate stabilization while the fractured VB heals. The hardware can be removed electively once the fusion is solid (usually at 8–12 months). This is more commonly practiced in Europe than the U.S.

72.2.4 Wound infections

Postoperative wound infections with spinal instrumentation are usually due to *Staphylococcus aureus*. With titanium hardware, a reasonable initial attempt may be debridement of devitalized tissue (and any loose onlay bone graft) and thorough washout (typically with 3 L of antibiotic irrigation (e.g., 50,000 U of Bacitracin in 3 L of sterile irrigant) flushed into the wound using a pulsed lavage device—avoiding direct irrigation of any exposed dura) without removal of instrumentation, followed by antibiotics.[2] If this is inadequate, a repeat washout with a vascularized wound closure (e.g., with a reconstructive plastic surgeon) may succeed. If not, removal of instrumentation may occasionally be required.

72.3 Osteoporotic spine fractures

72.3.1 General information

Osteoporosis is defined as a condition of skeletal fragility as a result of low bone mass, microarchitectural deterioration of bone, or both[17] in the absence of a mineralization defect. It is found most commonly in postmenopausal white females, and is rare prior to menopause. Lifetime risk of symptomatic vertebral body (VB) osteoporotic compression fractures is 16% for women, and 5% for men. It affects 75 million people in the U.S., Europe, and Japan.[18] There are ≈ 700,000 VB compression fractures per year in the U.S.

These patients are often found to have significant VB compression fractures on plain films after presenting with back pain following a seemingly minor fall. CT often shows an impressive appearing amount of bone retropulsed into the canal.

72.3.2 Bone physiology

Bone is a dynamic tissue, constantly undergoing remodeling in a delicate balance between resorption by osteoclasts and new bone deposition by osteoblasts. Osteoporosis results from an imbalance in this process that favors resorption.

72.3.3 Risk factors

Factors that increase the risk of osteoporosis include:
1. weight < 58 kg
2. cigarette smoking[19]
3. low-trauma VB fracture in the patient or a first degree relative
4. drugs
   a) heavy alcohol consumption
   b) ASMs (especially phenytoin)
   c) warfarin
   d) chronic heparin use (p. 172)
   e) steroid use:
      • bone changes can be seen with 7.5 mg/d of prednisone for > 6 months
      • VB fractures occur in 30–50% of patients on prolonged glucocorticoids
5. postmenopausal female

6. males undergoing androgen deprivation therapy (e.g., for prostate Ca). Orchiectomy or ≥ 9 doses of gonadotropin-releasing hormone agonists had a 1.5 fold increase in risk of all fractures[20]
7. physical inactivity
8. low calcium intake
9. low serum levels of vitamin D (which decreases calcium absorption—see below). Lab: serum 25-hydroxyvitamin D [25(OH)D], AKA calcidiol is the best indicator of vitamin D status (▶ Table 72.6)
10. Cushing's disease for > 2 years duration

Factors that protect against osteoporosis include impact exercise and excess body fat.

72.3.4 Diagnostic considerations

To differentiate osteoporotic compression fractures from other pathologic fractures, see Pathologic fractures of the spine (p. 1679).

Pre-fracture diagnosis

1. measuring bone fragility directly is not possible
2. the best radiographic correlate with bone fragility is bone mineral density (BMD) determined using DEXA scan (see below)
3. patients with low-trauma fractures or fragility fractures are considered osteoporotic even if their BMD are greater than these cutoffs
4. measuring Hounsfield units on CT scans of lumbar VBs may be used (see below)
5. FRAX® tool (p. 1210)

▶ **CT scan.** Estimating BMD of lumbar VBs by CT may have advantages over DEXA scans:
• CT may reflect changes in BMD earlier than DEXA[21]
• CT can specifically assess S1 which DEXA does not[22]

Rule of thumb: Hounsfield units of a vertebral body < 100 correlates with significant risk of hardware failure.

▶ **DEXA scan (dual energy X-ray absorptiometry).** A DEXA scan (AKA DXA) is the preferred way to measure BMD which is expressed in g/cm².
1. proximal femur: BMD measurement in this location is the best predictor for future fractures
2. LS spine: DEXA typically measure BMD of L1–L4 individually and also calculates an aggregate. L1–4 is the most useful region to predict bone integrity for lumbar spinal fusions. Both AP *and* lateral views are needed since the AP often overestimates BMD because of superimposition of overlying posterior elements and aortic calcifications
3. forearm BMD may be used if hip or spine are unsuitable, but is not very accurate

Interpretation of DEXA scan results:
1. results are reported as
   a) T-score: norms for *healthy young adults* of the same gender
   b) Z-score: norms of subjects of *same age* and sex as the patient
2. the *lowest* T-score (of hip, lumbar spine or radius) is used for determination
3. diagnostic criteria: T-scores are not the same as standard deviations (SD) but they can be used that way.[23] With a normal distribution having a mean of 0, 68% of the population falls within 1 SD, 95% within 2 SD, and 99.7% within 3 SD.
   WHO classifications of BMD are shown in ▶ Table 72.5

72

Table 72.5 WHO classification of BMD based on DEXA T-score[23,24]

T-score	Description
T-score ≥ –1	normal
T-score < –1 and T-score > –2.5	osteopenia*
T-score ≤ –2.5	osteoporosis
T-score ≤ -2.5 *plus* fragility fracture	severe osteoporosis

* the International Society for Clinical Densitometry (ISCD) prefers the term "low mineral density"[23]

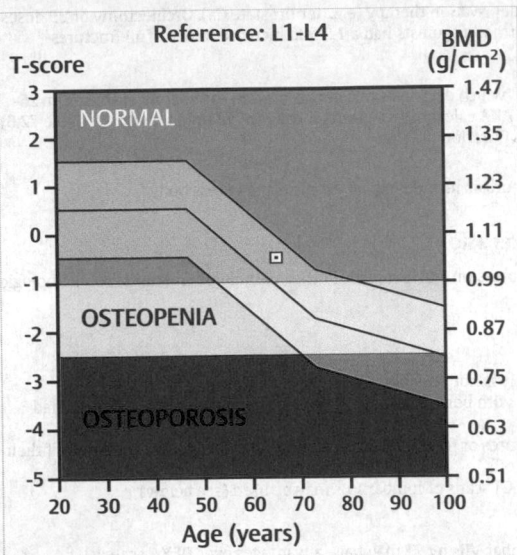

Fig. 72.6 **Bone mineral density (BMD) graph.** Example of a typical BMD graph generated from a DEXA scan.

Results are often depicted graphically as shown in ▶ Fig. 72.6.

▶ **FRAX® tool.** The FRAX® tool was developed for the WHO and uses femoral neck BMD (in g/cm^2) to calculate 10-year risk of hip fracture and also "major osteoporotic fracture" (fracture involving proximal femur, spine, proximal humerus, or distal radius).

Post-fracture considerations

1. other causes of pathologic fracture, especially neoplastic (e.g., multiple myeloma, metastatic breast cancer…) should be ruled out
2. younger patients with osteoporosis require evaluation for a remediable cause of osteoporosis (hyperthyroidism, steroid abuse, hyperparathyroidism, osteomalacia, Cushing's syndrome…)

72.3.5 Prevention of osteoporosis

High calcium intake during childhood may increase peak bone mass.

In adulthood: increased calcium intake is ineffective. Weight-bearing exercise in adulthood helps slow calcium loss from bones. Also effective: estrogen (see below), bisphosphonates (alendronate and risedronate), and raloxifene.

72.3.6 Treatment of osteoporosis

See references.[25,26,27,28]

Drugs that increase bone formation include:

1. parathyroid hormone analogues (PTAs): lifetime treatment limit of 2 years because the effectiveness diminishes and the risk of osteosarcoma (in rats) increases. Unlike drugs that reduce resorption, PTAs used intermittently (e.g., once daily) stimulate osteoblasts preferentially over osteoclasts with the result of laying down of new bone. FDA approved for patients at high risk of fracture who: are postmenopausal women, are men with hypogonadal osteoporosis, or either gender with osteoporosis due to systemic glucocorticoids. PTAs have been used off-label to treat patients with osteopenia/osteoporosis prior to spine instrumentation. Prior to treatment: check serum levels of intact parathyroid hormone (iPTH) and 25(OH)D. Do not use until any vitamin D

deficiency is corrected. Monitor Ca^{++} during therapy (transient rise in Ca^{++} is common, but persistent hypercalcemia has been reported[29])

✖ Contraindication: patients with increased risk of osteosarcoma (e.g., Paget's disease, unexplained elevation of alkaline phosphatase), prior radiation therapy involving the skeleton, young patients with open epiphyses, patients with hypercalcemia, ± patients on digoxin (these agents may increase calcium levels)

a) teriparatide (Forteo®, Bonsity®):
the bioactive 34 amino acid N-terminus segment of parathyroid hormone manufactured using recombinant DNA. Unknown if teriparatide reduces the risk of fractures in men
Rx: 20 mcg SQ daily. Total lifetime limit of all parathyroid analogues: 2 years

b) abaloparatide (Tymlos™):
a recombinant DNA copy of the entire human parathyroid hormone.
Rx: 80 mcg SQ daily. Total lifetime limit of all parathyroid analogues: 2 years

2. sodium fluoride: 75 mg/d increases bone mass but did *not* significantly reduce the fracture rate. 25 mg PO BID of a delayed-release formulation (Slow Fluoride®) reduced fracture rate but may make bone more fragile and could increase risk of hip fractures. Fluoride increases demand for Ca^{++}, therefore supplement with 800 mg/d Ca^{++} and 400 IU/d vitamin D. Not recommended for use > 2 yrs

Drugs that reduce bone resorption are less effective on cancellous bone (found mainly in the spine and at the end of long bones[26]). Improvement in spine bone mineral density accounts for only a small part of the observed reduction in the risk of vertebral fracture.[30] Medications include:

1. estrogen: cannot be used in men. Estrogen hormone replacement therapy (HRT) increases vertebral bone mass by > 5% and decreases rate of vertebral fractures by 50%. Also relieves post-menopausal symptoms and reduces risk of CAD. However, use is limited since HRT increases the risk of breast cancer[31] and breast cancer recurrence[32] as well as DVT

2. calcium: current recommendation for postmenopausal women: 1,000–1,500 mg/d taken with meals[33]

3. vitamin D or analogues: promote calcium absorption from the GI tract. Typically administered with calcium therapy (either calcium or vitamin D alone are less effective). Vitamin D 400–800 IU/d is usually sufficient. If urinary Ca^{++} remains low, high-dose vitamin D (50,000 IU q 7–10 d) may be tried. Since high-dose formulations have been discontinued in the U.S., analogues such as calcifediol (Calderol®) 50 mcg/d or calcitriol (Rocaltrol®) up to 0.25 mcg/d may be tried with Ca^{++} supplement. Serum levels of 25-hydroxyvitamin D [25(OH)D], AKA calcidiol is the best indicator of vitamin D status. The significance of vitamin D levels are shown in ▶ Table 72.6.[34] With high-dose vitamin D or analogues, monitor serum and urinary Ca^{++}

Table 72.6 Serum 25-hydroxyvitamin D (25(OH)D) levels

ng/ml[a]	nmol/L[a]	Interpretation
< 10–11	< 25–27.5	vit D deficiency → rickets (in peds) and osteomalacia (adults)
< 10–15	< 25–37.5	inadequate for bone and overall health
≥ 15	≥ 37.5	adequate for bone and overall health
consistently > 200	consistently > 500	potentially toxic → hypercalcemia & hyperphosphatemia

[a]1 ng/ml = 2.5 nmol/L

4. calcitonin: a hormone synthesized by the thyroid gland which decreases bone resorption by osteoclasts. May be derived from a number of sources, salmon is one of the more common ones. The skeletal response is maximal during the first 18–24 months of therapy. Benefit in preventing fractures is less well-established[28]

a) parenteral salmon calcitonin (Calcimar®, Miacalcin®): indicated for patients for whom estrogen is contraindicated. Expensive ($1,500–3,000/yr) and must be given IM or sub-Q. 30–60% of patients develop antibodies to the drug which negates its effect. R: 0.5 ml (100 U) of calcitonin (given with calcium supplements to prevent hyperparathyroidism) SQ q d

b) intranasal forms (Miacalcin nasal spray): less potent (works better in older women > 5 yrs post menopause). 200–400 IU/d given in one nostril (alternate nostrils daily) plus Ca^{++} 500 mg/d and vitamin D

5. bisphosphonates: carbon-substituted analogues of pyrophosphate have a high affinity for bone and inhibit bone resorption by destroying osteoclasts. Not metabolized. Remain bound to bone for several weeks

a) etidronate (Didronel®), a 1st generation drug. Not FDA approved for osteoporosis. May reduce rate of VB fractures, not confirmed on F/U. Possible increased risk of hip fractures due to inhibition of bone mineralization may not occur with 2nd & 3rd generation drugs listed below. ℞ 400 mg PO daily × 2 wks followed by 11–13 weeks of Ca^{++} supplementation

b) alendronate (Fosamax®): can cause esophageal ulcers. ℞ Prevention: 5 mg PO daily; treatment 10 mg PO daily; taken upright with water on an empty stomach at least 30 minutes before eating or drinking anything else. Once weekly dosing of 35 mg for prevention and 70 mg for treatment.[28,35] Taken concurrently with 1000–1500 mg/d Ca^{++} and 400/d IU of vitamin D

c) risedronate (Actonel®): ℞ Prevention or treatment: 5 mg PO daily, or 35 mg once/week[35] on an empty stomach (as for alendronate, see above)

6. estrogen analogues:
   a) tamoxifen (Nolvadex®), an estrogen antagonist for breast tissue but an estrogen agonist for bone, has a partial agonist effect on uterus associated with an increased incidence of endometrial cancer
   b) raloxifene (Evista®): similar to tamoxifen but is an estrogen antagonist for uterus.[36] Decreases the effect of warfarin (Coumadin®).
      ℞: 60 mg PO q d. **Supplied:** 60 mg tablets

7. RANK ligand (RANKL) inhibitors: RANKL binds to RANK receptors and stimulates precursor cells to mature into osteoclasts and inhibits their apoptosis.[37] Includes denosumab (Prolia®) 60 mg SQ q 6 months (found to be more effective than alendronate[38])

Treatment of osteoporotic vertebral compression fractures

Patients rarely have neurologic deficit. They are also usually fragile elderly women who usually do not tolerate large surgical procedures well, and the rest of their bones are also osteoporotic which are poor for internal fixation.

Management consists primarily of analgesics and bed rest followed by progressive mobilization, often in an external brace (often not tolerated well). Surgery is rarely employed. In cases where pain control is difficult to obtain or where neural compression causes deficit, limited bony decompression may be considered. Percutaneous vertebroplasty (see below) is a newer option.

Typical time course of conservative treatment:
1. initially, severe pain may require hospital or subacute care facility admission for adequate pain control utilizing
   a) sufficient pain medication
   b) bed rest for about 7–10 days (DVT prophylaxis recommended)
2. begin physical therapy (PT) after ≈ 7–10 days as patient tolerates (prolonged bed rest can promote "disuse osteoporosis")
   a) pain control as patient is mobilized may be enhanced by a *lumbar brace*, which may work by reducing movement that causes repetitive "microfractures"
   b) discharge from the hospital with lumbar brace for outpatient PT
3. pain subsides on the average after 4–6 weeks (range 2–12 weeks)

Vertebral body augmentation

Percutaneous vertebroplasty (PVP)

Transpedicular injection of polymethylmethacrylate (PMMA) AKA "methylmethacrylate cement" into the compressed bone with the following goals (note: PMMA injection is FDA approved for treatment of compression fractures due to osteoporosis or tumor, but not for trauma, as PMMA would prevent healing of the fracture):
1. to shorten the duration of pain (sometimes providing pain relief within minutes to hours). Remember: the natural history is that pain will eventually diminish in essentially all of these patients. Mechanism of pain relief may be due to stabilization of bone and/or thermal damage to pain sensing nerves by heat released during the exothermic curing of the cement
2. to try and stabilize the bone: may prevent progression of kyphosis

Randomized studies published in 2009 found no benefit in vertebroplasty over a sham procedure at 1 month[39] or at any time up to 6 months post-procedure.[40] NB: kyphoplasty (see below) was not studied; use with metastatic spine tumors was also not evaluated. Patient selection issues may make these results more or less applicable to a specific patient.

Kyphoplasty

Similar to PVP, except first, a balloon is inserted into the compressed VB through the pedicle. The balloon is inflated and then deflated and removed. PMMA is injected into the thusly created defect. Potential benefits of this over vertebroplasty: there may be some restoration of height, and there may be less tendency for PMMA extravasation/embolization (due to the cavity creation and the thicker PMMA used). In the (industry-sponsored) randomized non-blinded FREE study[41] there was a significant positive difference in pain reduction and quality of life improvement in the kyphoplasty group compared to the nonoperated group at 1 month that diminished by 1-year post-op.

Indications

1. painful osteoporotic compression fractures:
   a) usually do not treat fractures producing < 5–10% loss of height
   b) severe pain that interferes with patient activity
   c) failure to adequately control pain with oral pain medication
   d) ★ pain localized to fracture level
   e) acute fractures: procedure is not effective for healed fractures. In questionable cases, look for increased signal on STIR MRI (▶ Fig. 81.7 panel C) (also see below)
2. levels: FDA approved for use from T5 through L5; however, has been used off-label (primarily for tumor, e.g., multiple myeloma) from T1 through sacrum, and has been described (for tumor) in the cervical spine from an anterior approach
3. some symptomatic vertebral hemangiomas (p. 992) e.g., those causing vertebral collapse or neurologic deficit as a result of extension into the spinal canal (not for incidental hemangiomas): the first indication for PVP[42]
4. osteolytic metastases and multiple myeloma[43]: pain relief and stabilization
5. pathologic compression fractures[44] from metastases: PVP does not give as rapid pain relief as with osteoporotic compression fractures (it may actually be necessary to increase pain meds for 7–10 days post PVP)
6. intraoperative pedicle screw salvage when pedicle fractures or screws strip during pedicle screw placement. Fenestrated pedicle screws allow injection of cement directly into the VB through perforations in the screw

Contraindications

1. coagulopathy
2. completely healed fractures (no edema on MRI or cold on bone scan, no focal point tenderness)
3. active infections: sepsis, osteomyelitis, discitis and epidural abscess
4. spinal instability: requires more than cement in the VB to stabilize
5. focal neurologic deficit: may indicate herniated disc, retropulsed fragment in canal. Get CT or MRI to rule these out
6. relative contraindications:
   a) fractures > 80% loss of VB height, e.g., vertebra planum (▶ Fig. 72.7). Technically challenging and often not possible to inject more than a very small amount of cement

72

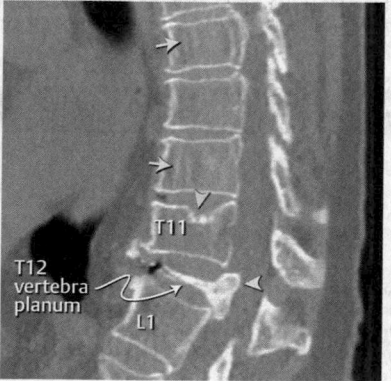

Fig. 72.7 Vertebra planum of T12.
Image: sagittal CT of thoracolumbar junction, bone window.
Near-complete collapse of T12 (vertebra planum) with bone retropulsed into the spinal canal (*yellow arrowhead*) in a 77-year-old woman with known osteoporosis (T-score = -3.6). Note vertical striations (some of which are indicated by *short green arrows*) indicative of osteoporosis and the mild superior endplate fracture of T11 (*blue arrowhead*).

b) significant canal compromise from tumor or retropulsed bone

c) partial or total destruction of the posterior VB wall: as with an acute burst fracture. Risk of cement leaking into spinal canal. Not an absolute contraindication, may be injected carefully with close fluoroscopic monitoring

7. iodine allergy: there is a small risk of a balloon rupturing with spill of the iodinated contrast used to fill the balloons prior to injecting the PMMA. Options include: iodine allergy prep (p. 232), use of gadolinium instead of iodinated contrast

Complications

Complication = rate: 1–9%. Lowest when used to treat osteoporotic compression fractures, higher with vertebral hemangiomas, highest with pathological fractures

1. methacrylate leakage:
   a) into soft tissues: usually of little consequence
   b) into spinal canal: symptomatic spinal cord compression is very rare
   c) into neural foramen: may cause radiculopathy
   d) into disc space
   e) venous: can get into spinal venous plexus or vena cava with ≈ 0.3–1% risk of clinically significant methacrylate pulmonary embolism (PE)[45]
2. radiculopathy: 5–7% incidence. Some cases may be due to heat released during cement curing. Often treated conservatively: steroids, pain meds, nerve block…
3. pedicle fracture
4. rib fracture
5. transverse process fracture
6. anterior penetration with needle: puncture of great vessels, pneumothorax…
7. increased incidence of future VB compression fractures at adjacent levels

Management of some associated developments

1. chest pain
   a) get rib X-rays
   b) VQ scan if indicated
2. patient starts coughing during injection: fairly common. May be reaction to rib pain or to odor of PMMA, may also indicate solvent in lungs. Stop injecting
3. back pain: take X-ray to rule out new fracture or PMMA in veins
4. neurologic symptoms: get CT scan

Pre-procedure evaluation

1. plain X-rays: minimum requirement, most practitioners get MRI or bone scan
2. CT: helps rule out *bony* compromise of spinal canal, which may indicate increased risk of leakage for PMMA into canal during procedure
3. MRI: not mandatory, may be helpful in some cases
   a) short tau inversion recovery (STIR) images (p. 241) demonstrate bone edema indicative of acute fractures (not as good for differentiating pathology)[46]
   b) MRI can also disclose neurologic compression by *soft* tissue (e.g., tumor)
4. patients with multiple compression fractures: consider getting bone scan and perform PVP in the VB near the level of pain that lights up the most (↑ activity on bone scan correlates strongly with good outcome from PVP)

Booking the case: Kyphoplasty

Also see default values (p. 25).

1. position: prone
2. anesthesia: may be done under general, or under MAC
3. equipment: 2 C-arms for bi-plane fluoro
4. implants:
   a) kyphoplasty set
   b) iodinated contrast from radiology to fill balloons
5. consent (in lay terms for the patient—not all-inclusive):
   a) procedure: insertion of a needle into the fractured/abnormal bone, sometimes getting a biopsy as well, and then inflating a balloon in the bone to try and bring it back to a more

normal size, and then injecting a liquid cement which will then harden inside the bone to strengthen it
b) alternatives: nonsurgical management, open surgery, in cases of tumor sometimes radiation therapy can be done
c) complications: leakage of cement which can compress nerves and may need to be removed surgically if possible, rib fracture (from positioning), injury to large blood vessel or lung by the needle, failure to achieve the desired pain relief

Procedure

1. pain medication
   a) remember, this procedure is done with the patient lying on their stomach and is usually performed on frail, elderly females who smoke. Therefore, use caution to avoid oversedation and respiratory compromise
   b) sedation and pain medication
   c) use of local anesthetic during needle placement
   d) additional pain medication just prior to injection
2. use bi-plane fluoro to pass needle through the pedicle to enter VB—see Percutaneous pedicle screws (p. 1797)—and place tip ≈ 1/2 to 2/3 of the way through the VB
3. test inject with contrast, e.g., iohexol (Omnipaque 300) (p. 230); do digital subtraction study if equipment is available. For kyphoplasty, the balloon is inflated at this time
   a) a little venous enhancement is acceptable
   b) if you visualize vena cava
      • do not pull needle back (the fistula has already been created)
      • push needle in a little further, or
      • push some gelfoam (soaked in contrast) through the needle, or
      • inject a very small amount of PMMA under visualization and allow it to set to block the fistula
4. inject PMMA (that has been opacified with tantalum or barium-sulfate) under fluoroscopic visualization until:
   a) 3–5 cc injected (minimal compression fractures accept more cement, sometimes up to ≈ 8 cc). No correlation between amount of PMMA injected and pain relief[43]
   b) PMMA approaches posterior VB wall. Stop if cement ever enters disc space, vena cava, pedicle, or spinal canal

Post-procedure

1. PVP is often an outpatient procedure, but sometimes overnight admission is used
2. watch for
   a) chest or back pain (may indicate rib fracture)
   b) fever: may be reaction to cement
   c) neurologic symptoms
3. activity
   a) gradual mobilization after ≈ 2 hours
   b) ± physical therapy
   c) ± short term use of external brace (most centers do not use)
4. institute medical treatment for osteoporosis: remember the patient with fragility fractures by definition has osteoporosis with risk of future fractures

72.4 Sacral fractures

72.4.1 General information

Uncommon. Usually caused by shear forces. Identified in 17% of patients with pelvic fractures[47] (∴ keep in mind that neurologic deficits in patients with pelvic fractures may be due to associated sacral fractures). Neurologic injuries occur in 22–60%.[47]

The sacrum below S2 is not essential to ambulation or support of the spinal column, but may still be unstable since pressure to the area may occur when supine or sitting.

72

72.4.2 Classification

Three characteristic clinical presentations based on zone of involvement[47,48] as shown in ▶ Table 72.7.

Table 72.7 Classification of sacral fractures

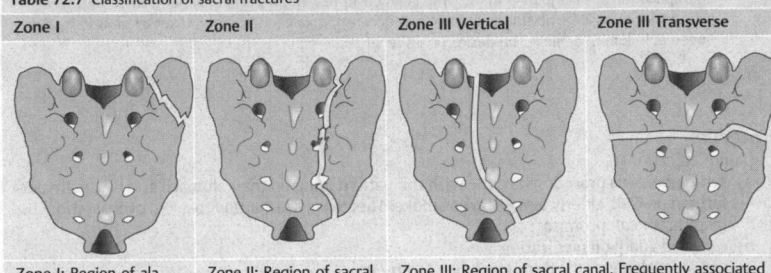

Zone I	Zone II	Zone III Vertical	Zone III Transverse
Zone I: Region of ala sparing the central canal and neural foramina. Occasionally associated with partial L5 root injury, possibly as a result of entrapment of the L5 root between the upwardly migrated fracture fragment and the transverse process of the L5 vertebra	Zone II: Region of sacral foramina (sparing the central canal). A vertical fracture which may be associated with unilateral L5, S1, and/or S2 nerve root involvement (producing sciatica). Bladder dysfunction is rare	Zone III: Region of sacral canal. Frequently associated with sphincter dysfunction (occurs only with bilateral root injuries) and saddle anesthesia. Subdivided[47]:	
		vertical: almost always associated with pelvic ring fracture	transverse (horizontal): rare. Often due to a direct blow to the sacrum as in a fall from a great height. Marked displacement of fracture fragment can produce severe deficit[a] (bowel & bladder incontinence)

[a]significant deficit is rare in fractures at or below S4

A rare U-shaped Zone III fracture consists of bilateral longitudinal fractures connected by a transverse fracture at S2–3 (a weak area) producing a disconnection between the lumbosacral spine and the pelvis (▶ Fig. 72.8). It often occurs from falls from a height (called a "suicide jumper's fracture" by Roy-Camille[49]) but may also be seen with sacral insufficiency fractures (which are more typically "H" shaped). It is unstable and often produces a kyphotic deformity. Nerve compression or transection is common, with concomitant loss of bowel and bladder control. 3 sub-types:

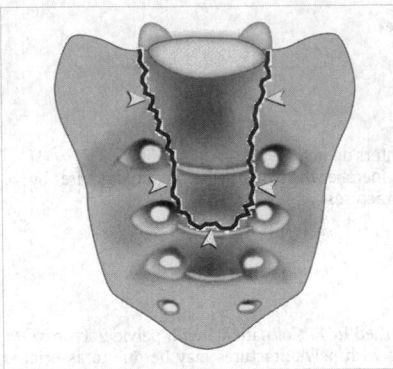

Fig. 72.8 U-shaped Zone III sacral fracture (*yellow arrowheads*).
Diagram of sacrum viewed from anterior perspective.

- Type 1: flexion fracture with anterior angulation of the upper fragment
- Type 2: flexion fracture with posterior displacement of the upper portion that perches almost horizontally on the lower fractur fragment
- Type 3: extension fracture with anterior displacement of the upper fragment

72.4.3 Treatment

In one series,[50] all 35 fractures were treated without surgery, and only 1 patient with a complete cauda equina syndrome did not improve. Others feel that surgery may have a useful role[47]:

1. operative reduction and internal fixation of unstable fractures may aid in pain control and promote early ambulation
2. decompression and/or surgical reduction/fixation may possibly improve radicular or sphincter deficits

Some observations[47]:

1. reduction of the ala may promote L5 recovery with Zone I fractures
2. Zone II fractures with neurologic involvement may recover with or without surgical reduction and fixation
3. horizontal Zone III with severe deficit: controversial. Reduction and decompression does not ensure recovery, which may occur with nonoperative management

▶ **U-shaped sacral fractures.** U-shaped sacral fractures are unstable and should be stabilized when possible. Percutaneous fixation may be performed with trans-iliac trans-sacral screws[51] (typically in conjunction with a surgeon experienced with pelvic stabilization). With this alone, the patient must be non-weight-bearing for 3 months. If this fixation is accompanied by posterior instrumented fusion from lumbar spine to pelvis (spino-pelvic AKA lumbo-pelvic fixation), the patient may begin weight-bearing immediately (▶ Fig. 72.9). If the anterior pelvis is also fractured, retrograde superior ramus screws AKA anterior column screws may be used to instrument that.

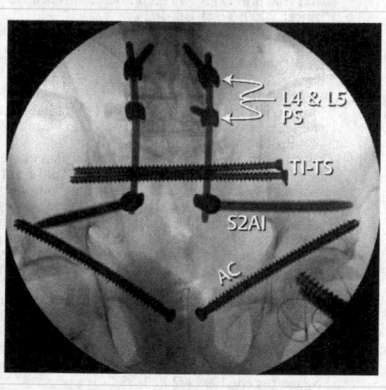

Fig. 72.9 Fixation of U-shaped Zone III sacral fracture.
AP X-ray. Abbreviations: AC = anterior column screws, PS = pedicle screws, S2A1 = S2-alar-iliac screws, TI-TS = trans-iliac trans-sacral screws.

72

References

[1] Denis F. The three column spine and its significance in the classification of acute thoracolumbar spinal injuries. Spine. 1983; 8:817–831

[2] Chedid MK, Green C. A Review of the Management of Lumbar Fractures With Focus on Surgical Decision-Making and Techniques. Contemporary Neurosurgery. 1999; 21:1–5

[3] Chance GQ. Note on a type of flexion fracture of the spine. Br J Radiol. 1948; 21. DOI: 10.1259/0007-128 5-21-249-452

[4] Homnick A, Lavery R, Nicastro O, et al. Isolated thoracolumbar transverse process fractures: call physical therapy, not spine. Journal of Trauma. 2007; 63:1292–1295

[5] Bradley LH, Paullus WC, Howe J, et al. Isolated transverse process fractures: spine service management not needed. Journal of Trauma. 2008; 65:832–6; discussion 836

[6] Hitchon PW, Jurf AA, Kernstine K, et al. Management options in thoracolumbar fractures. Contemporary Neurosurgery. 2000; 22:1–12

[7] Fredrickson BE, Yuan HA, Miller H. Burst Fractures of the Fifth Lumbar Vertebrae: A Report of Four Cases. Journal of Bone and Joint Surgery. 1982; 64A:1088–1094

[8] Hitchon PW, Torner JC, Haddad SF, et al. Management Options in Thoracolumbar Burst Fractures. Surgical Neurology. 1998; 49:619–627

[9] Klerk LWL, Fontijne PJ, Stijnen T, et al. Spontaneous remodeling of the spinal canal after conservative management of thoracolumbar burst fractures. Spine. 1998; 23:1057–1057

[10] Dai LY. Remodeling of the spinal canal after thoracolumbar burst fractures. Clinical Orthopaedics and Related Research. 2001; 382:119–119

[11] Baaj AA, Reyes PM, Yaqoobi AS, et al. Biomechanical advantage of the index-level pedicle screw in unstable thoracolumbar junction fractures. J Neurosurg Spine. 2011; 14:192–197

[12] Ramieri A, Domenicucci M, Cellocco P, et al. Neurological L5 burst fracture: posterior decompression

and lordotic fixation as treatment of choice. Eur Spine J. 2012; 21 Suppl 1:S119–S122

[13] Vaccaro AR, Zieller SC, Hulbert RJ, et al. The thoracolumbar injury severity score: a proposed treatment algorithm. Journal of Spinal Disorders Tech. 2005; 18:209–215

[14] Vaccaro AR, Lehman RA,Jr, Hurlbert RJ, et al. A new classification of thoracolumbar injuries: the importance of injury morphology, the integrity of the posterior ligamentous complex, and neurologic status. Spine. 2005; 30:2325–2333

[15] Bose B, Osterholm JL, Northrup BE, et al. Management of Lumbar Translocation Injuries: Case Reports. Neurosurgery. 1985; 17:958–961

[16] Blumenkopf B, Daniels T. Intraoperative Ultrasonography (IOUS) in Thoracolumbar Fractures. J Spinal Disord. 1988; 1:86–93

[17] Consensus Development Conference. Prophylaxis and Treatment of Osteoporosis. Am J Med. 1991; 90:107–110

[18] Johnell O, Kanis JA. An estimate of the worldwide prevalence and disability associated with osteoporotic fractures. Osteoporos Int. 2006; 17:1726–1733

[19] Daniell HW. Osteoporosis of the Slender Smoker: Vertebral Compression Fracture and Loss of Metacarpal Cortex in Relation to Postmenopausal Cigarette Smoking and Lack of Obesity. Arch Int Med. 1976; 136:298–304

[20] Shahinian VB, Kuo YF, Freeman JL, et al. Risk of fracture after androgen deprivation for prostate cancer. N Engl J Med. 2005; 352:154–164

[21] Mikula AL, Puffer RC, Jeor JDS, et al. Teriparatide treatment increases Hounsfield units in the lumbar spine out of proportion to DEXA changes. J Neurosurg Spine. 2019:1–6

[22] Zou D, Li W, Xu F, et al. Use of Hounsfield units of S1 body to diagnose osteoporosis in patients with lumbar degenerative diseases. Neurosurg Focus. 2019; 46. DOI: 10.3171/2019.2.FOCUS18614

[23] Choplin RH, Lenchik L, Wuertzer S. A Practical Approach to Interpretation of Dual-Energy X-ray Absorptiometry (DXA) for Assessment of Bone Density. Curr Radiol Rep. 2014; 2:1–12

[24] Kanis JA, Melton J, Christiansen C, et al. The Diagnosis of Osteoporosis. J Bone Miner Res. 1994; 9:1137–1141

[25] Choice of Drugs for Postmenopausal Osteoporosis. Medical Letter. 1992; 34:101–102

[26] Riggs BL, Melton LJ. The Prevention and Treatment of Osteoporosis. New England Journal of Medicine. 1992; 327:620–627

[27] Khosla S, Riggs BL. Treatment Options for Osteoporosis. Mayo Clinic Proceedings. 1995; 70:978–982

[28] Drugs for Prevention and Treatment of Postmenopausal Osteoporosis. Medical Letter. 2000; 42:97–100

[29] Thiruchelvam N, Randhawa J, Sadiek H, et al. Teriparatide induced delayed persistent hypercalcemia. Case Rep Endocrinol. 2014; 2014. DOI: 10.1155/2014/802473

[30] Cummings SR, Karpf DB, Harris F, et al. Improvement in spine bone density and reduction in risk of vertebral fractures during treatment with antiresorptive drugs. Am J Med. 2002; 112:281–289

[31] Rossouw JE, Anderson GL, Prentice RL, et al. Risks and benefits of estrogen plus progestin in healthy postmenopausal women: principal results From the Women's Health Initiative randomized controlled trial. JAMA. 2002; 288:321–333

[32] Holmberg L, Anderson H, , et al. HABITS (hormonal replacement therapy after breast cancer–is it safe?), a randomised comparison: trial stopped. Lancet. 2004; 363:453–455

[33] Office of Dietary Supplement - National Institutes of Health. Dietary supplement fact sheet: Calcium. 2018. https://dietary-supplements.info.nih.gov/factsheets/Calcium-HealthProfessional/

[34] Office of Dietary Supplement - National Institutes of Health. Dietary supplement fact sheet: Vitamin D. 2018. http://dietary-supplements.info.nih.gov/factsheets/vitamind.asp

[35] Once-A-Week Risedronate (Actonel). Medical Letter. 2002; 44:87–88

[36] Raloxifene for Postmenopausal Osteoporosis. Medical Letter. 1998; 40:29–30

[37] Bell NH. RANK ligand and the regulation of skeletal remodeling. Journal of Clinical Investigation. 2003; 111:1120–1122

[38] McClung MR, Lewiecki EM, Cohen SB, et al. Denosumab in postmenopausal women with low bone mineral density. New England Journal of Medicine. 2006; 354:821–831

[39] Kallmes DF, Comstock BA, Heagerty PJ, et al. A randomized trial of vertebroplasty for osteoporotic spinal fractures. New England Journal of Medicine. 2009; 361:569–579

[40] Buchbinder R, Osborne RH, Ebeling PR, et al. A randomized trial of vertebroplasty for painful osteoporotic vertebral fractures. New England Journal of Medicine. 2009; 361:557–568

[41] Wardlaw D, Cummings SR, Van Meirhaeghe J, et al. Efficacy and safety of balloon kyphoplasty compared with non-surgical care for vertebral compression fracture (FREE): a randomised controlled trial. Lancet. 2009; 373:1016–1024

[42] Deramond H, Depriester C, Galibert P, et al. Percutaneous Vertebroplasty with Polymethylmethacrylate. Radiol Clin North Am. 1998; 36:533–546

[43] Cotten A, Dewatre F, Cortet B, et al. Percutaneous vertebroplasty for osteolytic metastases and myeloma: effects of the percentage of lesion filling and the leakage of methyl methacrylate at clinical follow-up. Radiology. 1996; 200:525–530

[44] Fourney DR, Schomer DF, Nader R, et al. Percutaneous vertebroplasty and kyphoplasty for painful vertebral body fractures in cancer patients. Journal of Neurosurgery. 2003; 98:21–30

[45] Choe DH, Marom EM, Ahrar K, et al. Pulmonary embolism of polymethyl methacrylate during percutaneous vertebroplasty and kyphoplasty. American Journal of Roentgenology. 2004; 183:1097–1102

[46] Bendok BR, Halpin RJ, Rubin MN, et al. Percutaneous vertebroplasty. Contemporary Neurosurgery. 2004; 26:1–6

[47] Gibbons KJ, Soloniuk DS, Razack N. Neurological injury and patterns of sacral fractures. Journal of Neurosurgery. 1990; 72:889–893

[48] Denis F, Davis S, Comfort T. Sacral fractures: An important problem. Retrospective analysis of 236 cases. Clinical Orthopedics. 1988; 227:67–81

[49] Roy-Camille R, Saillant G, Gagna G, et al. Transverse fracture of the upper sacrum. Suicidal jumper's fracture. Spine (Phila Pa 1976). 1985; 10:838–845

[50] Sabiston CP, Wing PC. Sacral fractures: classification and neurologic implications. Journal of Trauma. 1986; 26:1113–1115

[51] Gray R, Molnar R, Suthersan M. A minimally invasive surgical technique for the management of U-shape sacral fractures. Spinal Cord Ser Cases. 2017; 3. DOI: 10.1038/scsandc.2017.45

73 Penetrating Spine Injuries and Long-Term Considerations of Spine Injuries

73.1 Gunshot wounds to the spine

73.1.1 General information

Most are due to assaults with handguns. Distribution: cervical 19–37%, thoracic 48–64%, and lumbo-sacral 10–29% (roughly proportional to lengths of each segment). Spinal cord injury due to civilian GSWs are primarily due to direct injury from the bullet (unlike military weapons which may create injury from shock waves and cavitation). Steroids are not indicated (p. 1140).

73.1.2 Indications for surgery

1. injury to the cauda equina (whether complete or incomplete) if nerve root compression is demonstrated[1]
2. neurologic deterioration: suggesting possibility of spinal epidural hematoma
3. compression of a nerve root
4. CSF leak
5. spinal instability: very rare with isolated GSW to the spine
6. to remove a copper jacketed bullet: copper can cause intense local reaction[2]
7. incomplete lesions: very controversial. Some series show improvement with surgery,[3] others show no difference from unoperated patients
8. debridement to reduce the risk of infection: more important for *military* GSW where there is massive tissue injury, not an issue for most civilian GSW except in cases where the bullet has traversed GI or respiratory tract
9. vascular injuries
10. surgery for late complications:
    a) migrating bullet
    b) lead toxicity[4] (plumbism): absorption of lead from a bullet occurs only when it lodges in joints, bursae, or *disc space*. Findings include: anemia, encephalopathy, motor neuropathy, nephropathy, abdominal colic
    c) late spinal instability: especially after surgery

73.2 Penetrating trauma to the neck

73.2.1 General information

Most often, injuries to the soft-tissues of the neck fall into the purvey of general/trauma surgeons and/or vascular surgeons. However, depending on local practice patterns, neurosurgeons may participate in care of these injuries, or they may get involved by virtue of associated spinal injuries (p. 1219).

The mortality rate for penetrating injury to the neck is ≈ 15%, with most early deaths due either to asphyxiation from airway compromise, or to exsanguination externally or into the chest or upper airways. Late death is usually due to cerebral ischemia or complications from spinal cord injury.

73.2.2 Vascular injuries

Venous injuries occur in ≈ 18% of penetrating neck wounds, and arterial injuries in ≈ 12%. Of the cervical arteries, the common carotid is most usually involved, followed by the ICA, the ECA, and then the vertebral artery. Outcome probably correlates most closely with neurologic condition on admission, regardless of treatment.

Vertebral artery (VA): the majority of injuries are penetrating. Due to the proximity of other vessels, the spinal cord and nerve roots, injuries are rarely isolated to the VA. 72% of documented VA injuries had no related physical findings on exam.[5]

73

73.2.3 Classification

Trauma surgeons have traditionally divided penetrating injuries of the neck into 3 zones,[6] and although definitions vary, the following is a general scheme[7]:

Zone I: inferiorly from the head of the clavicle to include the thoracic outlet.
Zone II: from the clavicle to the angle of the mandible.
Zone III: from the angle of the mandible to the base of the skull.

73.2.4 Evaluation

Neurologic examination: global deficits may be due to shock or hypoxemia due to asphyxiation. Cerebral neurologic deficits are usually due to vascular injury with cerebral ischemia. Local findings may be related to cranial nerve injury. Unilateral UE deficits may be due to nerve root or brachial plexus involvement. Median or ulnar nerve dysfunction can occur from compression by a pseudoaneurysm of the proximal axillary artery. Spinal cord involvement may present with complete injury, or with an incomplete spinal cord injury syndrome (p. 1132). Shock due to spinal cord injury is usually accompanied by bradycardia (p. 1119), as opposed to the tachycardia seen with hypovolemic shock.

Cervical spine X-rays: assesses trajectory of injury and integrity of C-spine.

Angiography: indicated in most cases if the patient is stable (especially for zone I or III injuries, and for zone II patients with no other indication for exploration, or for patients with penetration of the posterior triangle or wounds near the transverse processes where the VA may be injured). Patients actively hemorrhaging need to be taken to the OR without pre-op angiography. Angiographic abnormalities include:

1. extravasation of blood
   a) expanding hematoma into soft tissues: may compromise airway
   b) pseudoaneurysm
   c) AV fistula
   d) bleeding into airways
   e) external bleeding
2. intimal dissection, with
   a) occlusion, or
   b) luminal narrowing (including possible "string sign")
3. occlusion by soft tissue or bone

73.2.5 Treatment

Airway

Stable patients without airway compromise should not have "prophylactic" intubation to protect the airway. Immediate intubation is indicated for hemodynamically unstable patients or for airway compromise. Options:

* endotracheal: preferred
* cricothyroidotomy: if endotracheal intubation cannot be performed (e.g., due to tracheal deviation or patient agitation) or if there is evidence of cervical spine injury and manipulation of the neck is contraindicated, then cricothyroidotomy is performed with placement of a #6 or 7 cuffed endotracheal tube (followed by a standard tracheostomy in the OR once the patient is stabilized)
* awake nasotracheal: may be considered in the setting of possible spinal injury

Indications for surgical exploration

Surgical exploration has been advocated for all wounds that pierce the platysma and enter the anterior triangles of the neck[8]; however, 40–60% of these explorations will be negative. Although a selective approach may be based on angiography, false negatives have resulted in some authors recommending exploration of all zone II injuries.[9]

Surgical treatment for vascular injuries

Endovascular techniques may be suitable for select cases, especially for patients who are already in the endovascular suite for angiography. However, patients who are actively bleeding usually end up in the O.R. with an open procedure.

Carotid artery: choices are primary repair, interposition grafting, or ligation. Patients in coma or those with severe strokes caused by vascular occlusion of the carotid artery are poor surgical candidates for vascular reconstruction due to a high mortality rate ≥ 40%[7]; however, the outcome with ligation is worse. Repair of injuries is recommended in patients with no or only minor neurologic deficit. ICA ligation is recommended for bleeding that cannot be controlled and was used for extravasation of dye at the base of the skull in 1 patient.[10]

Vertebral artery: injuries are more often managed by ligation than by direct repair,[11] especially when bleeding occurs during exploration. Less urgent conditions (e.g., AV fistula) require knowledge of the patency of the contralateral VA and the ability to fill the ipsilateral PICA from retrograde flow through the BA before ligation can be considered (arteriographic anomalies contraindicate ligation in 15% of cases). Proximal occlusion may be accomplished with an anterior approach after the sternocleidomastoid is detached from the sternum. The VA is normally the first branch of the subclavian artery. Alternatively, endovascular techniques may be used, e.g., detachable balloons for proximal occlusion, or thrombogenic coils for pseudoaneurysms. Distal interruption may also be required, and this necessitates surgical exposure and ligation. Optimal management of a thrombosed injured VA in a foramen transversarium is unknown, and may require arterial bypass if ligation is not a viable option.

73.3 Delayed cervical instability

73.3.1 General information

Definition (adapted[12]): cervical instability (p.1118) that is not recognized until beyond 20 days after the injury. The instability itself may be delayed, or the recognition may be delayed.

73.3.2 Etiologies

Reasons for delayed cervical instability:
1. inadequate radiologic evaluation[13]
   a) incomplete studies (e.g., must see all the way down to C7–1 junction)
   b) suboptimal studies: motion artifact, incorrect positioning… Etiologies include: poor patient cooperation as a result of agitation/intoxication, portable films, poor technique…
2. abnormality missed on X-ray
   a) overlooked fracture, subluxation
   b) injury failed to be demonstrated despite sufficiently adequate X-rays[12]; see recommendations of extent of radiologic workup (p.1301)
      • type of fracture not demonstrated on the radiographs obtained
      • patient positioning (e.g., supine) may reduce some malalignment
      • spasm of cervical muscles may reduce and/or stabilize the injury
      • microfractures
3. inadequate models: some findings may be judged to be stable using certain models, but in the long-run may prove to be unstable (there is no perfect model for instability)

73.3.3 Indications for additional studies

Further studies or repeat X-rays several weeks after the trauma should be considered in patients with neurologic deficit, persistent pain, significant degenerative changes when the original films were suboptimal, subluxations < 3 mm, or when surgery is contemplated.[14]

73.4 Delayed deterioration following spinal cord injuries

Etiologies include:
1. posttraumatic syringomyelia (p.1411). Latency to symptoms: 3 mos–34 yrs
2. subacute progressive ascending myelopathy (SPAM): rare. Median time of occurrence: 13 days post injury (range: 4–86 days).[15] Signal changes extending to ≥ 4 levels above the original injury
3. unrecognized spinal instability[16]: mean delay in diagnosis was 20 days
4. tethered spinal cord: may be due to scar tissue at site of injury
5. delayed spinal epidural hematoma (SEH): most symptomatic SEH occur within 72 hours of surgery; however, longer delays have been reported[17]
6. apoptosis of neurons, oligodendrogliocytes, and astrocytes[18]: initiated during the acute phase, deterioration occurs during the chronic phase of SCI (months to years after SCI)
7. glial scar formation: mass effect as well as release of factors that may damage surviving neurons[19(p 43–5)]

73

73.5 Chronic management issues with spinal cord injuries

73.5.1 Overview

Most of the following topics are treated elsewhere in this handbook, but are pertinent to spinal cord injured (SCI) patients, and reference to the specific section is made.

- autonomic hyperreflexia: see below
- ectopic bone, includes para-articular heterotopic ossification: ossification of some joints that occurs in 15–20% of paralyzed patients
- osteoporosis and pathologic fracture (p. 1209)
- spasticity (p. 1845)
- syringomyelia (p. 1405)
- deep vein thrombosis (p. 1141): see below
- shoulder-hand syndrome: possibly sympathetically maintained

73.5.2 Respiratory management problems in spinal cord injuries

In attempting to wean high-level SCI patients from a ventilator, it may be helpful to change tube feedings to Pulmonaid® which lowers the CO_2 load.

Patients with cervical SCIs are more prone to pneumonia due to the fact that most of the effort in a normal cough originates in the abdominal muscles which are paralyzed.

73.5.3 Autonomic hyperreflexia

General information

Key concepts

- exaggerated autonomic response to normally innocuous stimuli
- in spinal cord injury, occurs only in patients with lesions above ≈ T6
- patients complain of pounding headache, flushing, and diaphoresis above lesion
- can be life-threatening, requires rapid control of hypertension and a search for an elimination of offending stimuli

73

AKA autonomic dysreflexia. Autonomic hyperreflexia[20,21] (AH) is an exaggerated autonomic response (sympathetic usually dominates) secondary to stimuli that would only be mildly noxious under normal circumstances. It occurs in ≈ 30% of quadriplegic and high paraplegic patients (reported range is as high as 66–85%), but does not occur in patients with lesions below T6 (only patients with lesions above the origin of the splanchnic outflow are prone to develop AH, and the origin is usually T6 or below). It is rare in first 12–16 weeks post-injury.

During attacks, norepinephrine (NE) (but not epinephrine) is released. Hypersensitivity to NE may be partially due to subnormal resting levels of catecholamines. Homeostatic responses include vasodilatation (above the level of the injury) and bradycardia (however, sympathetic stimulation may also cause tachycardia).

Stimuli sources

Stimulus sources causing episodes of autonomic hyperreflexia:
1. bladder: 76% (distension 73%, UTI 3%, bladder stones…)
2. colorectal: 19% (fecal impaction 12%, administering enema or suppository 4%)
3. decubitus ulcers/skin infection: 4%
4. DVT
5. miscellaneous: tight clothing or leg bag straps, procedures such as cystoscopy or debriding decubitus ulcers, case report of suprapubic tube

Presentation

1. paroxysmal HTN: 90%
2. anxiety
3. diaphoresis

4. piloerection
5. pounding H/A
6. ocular findings:
   a) mydriasis
   b) blurring of vision
   c) lid retraction or lid lag
7. erythema of face, neck, and trunk: 25%
8. pallor of skin below the lesion (due to vasoconstriction)
9. pulse rate: tachycardia (38%) or mild elevation over baseline, bradycardia (10%)
10. "splotches" over face and neck: 3%
11. muscle fasciculations
12. increased spasticity
13. penile erection
14. Horner syndrome
15. triad seen in 85%: cephalgia (H/A), hyperhidrosis, cutaneous vasodilatation

Evaluation

In the appropriate setting (e.g., a quadriplegic patient with an acutely distended bladder), the symptoms are fairly diagnostic.

Many features are also common to pheochromocytoma. Studies of catecholamine levels have been inconsistent; however, they can be mildly elevated in AH. The distinguishing feature of AH is the presence of hyperhidrosis and flushing of the face in the presence of pallor and vasoconstriction elsewhere on the body (which would be unusual for a pheochromocytoma).

Treatment

1. immediately elevate HOB (to decrease ICP), check BP q 5 min
2. treatment of choice: identify and eliminate the offending stimulus
   a) make sure bladder is empty (if catheterized check for kinks or sediment plugs). Caution: irrigating bladder may exacerbate AH (consider suprapubic aspiration)
   b) check bowels (avoid rectal exam, may exacerbate). Palpate abdomen or check abdominal X-ray (AH from this usually resolves spontaneously without manual disimpaction)
   c) check skin and toenails for ulceration or infection
   d) remove tight apparel
3. HTN that is extreme or that does not respond quickly may require treatment to prevent seizures and/or cerebral hemorrhage/hypertensive encephalopathy. Caution must be used to prevent hypotension following the episode. Agents used include: sublingual nifedipine[22] 10 mg SL, IV phentolamine—alpha cholinergic blocker (p. 943)—or nicardipine (p. 131).
4. consider diazepam (Valium®) 2–5 mg IVP (@ < 5 mg/min). Relieves spasm of skeletal and smooth muscle (including bladder sphincter). Is also anxiolytic

Prevention

Good bowel/bladder and skin care are the best preventative measures.

Prophylaxis in patients with recurrent episodes:

- *phenoxybenzamine* (Dibenzyline®): an alpha-blocker. Not helpful during the acute crisis. May not be as effective for alpha stimulation from sympathetic ganglia as with circulating catecholamines.[23] The patient may also develop hypotension after the sympathetic outflow subsides. Thus this is used only for resistant cases (note: will not affect sweating, which is mediated by acetylcholine).
  ℞ Adult: wide range quoted in literature: average 20–30 mg PO BID
- beta-blockers: may be necessary in addition to α-blockers to avoid possible hypotension from β_2-receptor stimulation (a theoretical concern)
- phenazopyridine (Pyridium®): a topical anesthetic that is excreted in the urine. May decrease bladder wall irritation; however, the primary cause of irritation should be treated if possible.
  ℞ Adult: 200 mg PO TID after meals. **Supplied:** 100, 200 mg tabs.
- "radical measures" such as sympathectomy, pelvic or pudendal nerve section, cordectomy, or intrathecal alcohol injection have been advocated in the past, but are rarely necessary and may jeopardize reflex voiding

73

- prophylactic treatment prior to procedures may employ use of anesthetics even in regions rendered anesthetic by the cord injury. Nifedipine 10 mg SL has also been used effectively for AH during cystoscopy and prophylactically[22]

References

[1] Robertson DP, Simpson RK. Penetrating Injuries Restricted to the Cauda Equina: A Retrospective Review. Neurosurgery. 1992; 31:265–270

[2] Messer HD, Cereza PF. Copper Jacketed Bullets in the Central Nervous System. Neuroradiology. 1976; 12:121–129

[3] Benzel EC, Hadden TA, Coleman JE. Civilian Gunshot Wounds to the Spinal Cord and Cauda Equina. Neurosurgery. 1987; 20:281–285

[4] Linden MA, Manton WI, Stewart RM, et al. Lead Poisoning from Retained Bullets. Pathogenesis, Diagnosis, and Management. Ann Surg. 1982; 195:305–313

[5] Reid JDS, Weigelt JA. Forty-Three Cases of Vertebral Artery Trauma. J Trauma. 1988; 28:1007–1012

[6] Monson DO, Saletta JD, Freeark RJ. Carotid Vertebral Trauma. J Trauma. 1969; 9:987–989

[7] Perry MO, Rutherford RB. Injuries of the Brachiocephalic Vessels. In: Vascular Surgery. 4th ed. Philadelphia: W.B. Saunders; 1995:705–713

[8] Fogelman MJ, Stewart RD. Penetrating Wounds of the Neck. Am J Surg. 1956; 91:581–596

[9] Meyer JP, Barrett JA, Schuler JJ, et al. Mandatory versus Selective Exploration for Penetrating Neck Trauma. A Prospective Assessment. Arch Surg. 1987; 122:592–597

[10] Ledgerwood AM, Mullins RJ, Lucas CE. Primary Repair vs Ligation for Carotid Artery Injuries. Arch Surg. 1980; 115:488–493

[11] Meier DE, Brink BE, Fry WJ. Vertebral Artery Trauma: Acute Recognition and Treatment. Arch Surg. 1981; 116:236–239

[12] Herkowitz HN, Rothman RH. Subacute Instability of the Cervical Spine. Spine. 1984; 9:348–357

[13] Walter J, Doris P, Shaffer M. Clinical Presentation of Patients with Acute Cervical Spine Injury. Ann Emerg Med. 1984; 13:512–515

[14] Delfini R, Dorizzi A, Facchinetti G, et al. Delayed Post-Traumatic Cervical Instability. Surgical Neurology. 1999; 51:588–595

[15] Planner AC, Pretorius PM, Graham A, et al. Subacute progressive ascending myelopathy following spinal cord injury: MRI appearances and clinical presentation. Spinal Cord. 2008; 46:140–144

[16] Levi AD, Hurlbert RJ, Anderson P, et al. Neurologic deterioration secondary to unrecognized spinal instability following trauma - a multicenter trial. Spine. 2006; 41:451–458

[17] Parthiban CJKB, Majeed SA. Delayed spinal extradural hematoma following thoracic spine surgery and resulting in paraplegia: a case report. 2008. http://www.jmedicalcasereports.com/content/2/1/141

[18] Liu XZ, Xu HM, Hu R, et al. Neuronal and glial apoptosis after traumatic spinal cord injury. Journal of Neuroscience. 1997; 17:5395–5406

[19] Liverman CT, Altevogt BM, Joy JE, et al. Spinal cord injury: progress, promise and priorities. Washington, D.C. 2005

[20] Erickson RP. Autonomic Hyperreflexia: Pathophysiology and Medical Management. Arch Phys Med Rehabil. 1980; 61:431–440

[21] Kewalramani LS, Orth MS. Autonomic Dysreflexia in Traumatic Myelopathy. Am J Phys Med. 1980; 59:1–21

[22] Dykstra DD, Sidi AA, Anderson LC. The Effect of Nifedipine on Cyctoscopy-Induced Autonomic Hyperreflexia in Patients with High Spinal Cord Injuries. J Urol. 1987; 138:1155–1157

[23] Sizemore GW, Winternitz WW. Autonomic Hyper-Reflexia - Suppression with Alpha-Adrenergic Blocking Agents. N Engl J Med. 1970; 282

Part XVI

Non-Traumatic Spine and Spinal Cord Conditions

XVI

74 Low Back Pain

74.1 Low back pain – general information

Key concepts

- low back pain is common, and in ≈ 85% of cases no specific diagnosis can be made[1]
- initial assessment is geared to detecting "red flags" (indicating potentially serious pathology), and in the absence of these, imaging studies and further testing of patients is usually not helpful during the first 4 weeks of low back symptoms
- relief of discomfort is usually best achieved with nonprescription pain medications and/or spinal manipulation
- while activities may need to be modified, bed rest beyond 4 days may be more harmful than helpful, and patients are encouraged to return to work or their normal daily activities as soon as possible
- 89–90% of patients with low back problems will improve within 1 month even without treatment (including patients with sciatica from disc herniation)

Σ: Simplified outline for initial management of acute LBP

(see details in text)
1. emergency: if any of these factors are present the patient should go to an emergency room
    a) progressive neurologic deficit (e.g., weakness)
    b) cauda equina syndrome (p. 1254) (includes bladder issues, saddle anesthesia...)
    c) intractable pain
2. absent these emergency conditions, conservative treatment measures should be employed during the first 4-6 weeks after onset of low back pain, and include
    a) manipulation therapy: e.g., PT or chiropractic
    b) analgesics (p. 1237) (with minimal opioid use)
    c) sometimes: interventional pain management (e.g., epidural steroid injections)
3. if the pain persists > 4 weeks, obtaining an MRI is appropriate option
4. referral to specialty care (i.e., spine surgeon) is appropriate if the MRI identifies a surgically treatable condition such as a herniated disc

74

Low back pain (LBP) is extremely prevalent, and is the second most common reason for people to seek medical attention.[2] After the common cold, it is the number two cause for loss of time at work. LBP accounts for ≈ 15% of all sick leave from work, and is the most common cause of disability for persons < 45 yrs of age.[3] Estimates of lifetime prevalence range from 60–90%, and the annual incidence is 5%.[4] Only 1% of patients will have nerve-root symptoms, and only 1–3% have lumbar disc herniation. The prognosis for most cases of LBP is good, and improvement usually occurs with little or no medical intervention.

74.2 Intervertebral disc

74.2.1 General information

The function of the intervertebral disc is to permit stable motion of the spine while supporting and distributing loads under movement. The intervertebral disc has been characterized as the largest nonvascularized structure in the human body, which imparts some unique attributes to it.

74.2.2 Anatomy

Anulus fibrosus (anulus may alternatively be spelled annulus, but fibrosus is the only correct spelling and is distinct from fibrosis)[5]: the multilaminated ligament that encompasses the periphery of the disc space. Attaches to the endplate cartilage and ring apophyseal bone. Blends centrally with the nucleus pulposus.

Nucleus pulposus: the central portion of the disc. A remnant of the notocord.

Capsule[5]: combined fibers of the anulus fibrosus and the posterior longitudinal ligament (this term is useful because these 2 structures may not be distinguishable on imaging studies).

74.2.3 Nomenclature for disc pathology

Historically, the terminology for lumbar disc pathology has been contentious and nonstandardized. A committee tasked to standardize the nomenclature has issued version 2.0 of their recommendations.[6] Some of these standardizations are useful primarily for consistency related to radiographic reports and for research, and may not be as useful for day-to-day clinical practice. A subset of the recommendations is shown in ▶ Table 74.1.

Degenerated disc: (see ▶ Table 74.1 for definition) some contend that these can cause radicular pain possibly by an inflammatory mechanism,[7] but this is not universally accepted.

Vacuum disc: gas in the disc space (empty space on imaging, e.g., as shown in ▶ Fig. 81.8 A), usually indicates disc degeneration, *not* infection. Levels with vacuum disc are often hypermobile and are therefore usually more amenable to surgical manipulation.

Table 74.1 Nomenclature for lumbar disc pathology[6]

Term	Description
anular tears AKA anular fissures	separations between anular fibers, avulsions of fibers from their VB insertions, or breaks through fibers that extend radially, transversely, or concentrically
degeneration	desiccation, fibrosis, narrowing of the disc space, diffuse bulging of the anulus beyond the disc space, extensive fissuring (numerous anular tears), mucinous degeneration of the anulus, defects & sclerosis of endplates, & osteophytes at the vertebral apophyses
degenerative disc disease	clinical syndrome of symptoms related to degenerative changes in the intervertebral disc (described above), also often considered to encompass degenerative changes outside the disc as well
bulging disc	generalized displacement of disc material (arbitrarily defined as > 50% or 180°) beyond the peripheral limits of the disc space. Not considered a form of herniation. May be a normal finding, not usually symptomatic
herniation	localized displacement of disc material (< 50% or 180°) beyond the limits of the intervertebral disc space
	focal: < 25% of the disc circumference
	broad-based: 25–50% of the disc circumference
	protrusion: the fragment does not have a "neck" that is narrower than the fragment in any dimension
	extrusion: the fragment has a "neck" that is narrower than the fragment in at least 1 dimension. 2 subtypes: a) sequestration: the fragment has lost continuity with the disc of origin (AKA free fragment) b) migration: the fragment is displaced away from the site of extrusion, regardless of whether sequestered or not
	intravertebral herniation (AKA Schmorl's node (p. 1266)): disc herniates in the cranio-caudal direction through the cartilaginous endplate into the VB

74

74.3 Clinical terms

▶ **Radiculopathy.** Dysfunction of a nerve root; signs and symptoms may include: pain in the distribution of that nerve root, dermatomal sensory disturbances, weakness of muscles innervated by that nerve root, and hypoactive muscle stretch reflexes of the same muscles.

▶ **Mechanical low back pain** (p. 1226). AKA "musculoskeletal" back pain (both non-specific terms). The most common form of low back pain. May result from strain of the paraspinal muscles and/or ligaments, irritation of facet joints… Excludes anatomically identifiable causes (e.g., tumor, disc herniation…).

▶ **Sciatica.** Pain along the course of the sciatic nerve, usually resulting from nerve root compromise (the sciatic nerve is composed of nerve roots L1 through S3).

74.4 Disability, pain, and outcome determinations

Disability scales for low back pain have been developed to assess outcomes for research purposes. Some widely used measures include:

1. visual analogue scale: used for any type of pain. The patient is asked to mark their pain level on a line divided into segments with sequential labels 0 (no pain) to 10 (the worst pain)
2. Oswestry disability index (ODI)[8]: a categorical ordinal scale that is used for low back pain. There are 4 English versions in wide use[9]; version 2.0[10] is recommended.[9]
   It consists of 10 questions related to activities of daily living. Each item is scored 0–5 (5 being the most disability) and the total is multiplied by 2% to obtain the final score (range: 0–100%). The interpretation of the final score is shown in ▶ Table 74.2. A score > 45% is essentially completely disabled. A score in the teens is very functional
3. Roland–Morris disability questionnaire[11]
4. Short Form 36 (SF36)[12]

Table 74.2 Oswestry disability index score

Score	Interpretation
0–20%	minimal disability: can cope with most daily activities
21–40%	moderate disability: pain and difficulty with sitting, lifting, and standing. The patient may be disabled from work
41–60%	severe disability: pain is the main problem, but other areas are affected
61–80%	crippled: back pain impinges on all aspects of the patient's life
81–100%	these patients are either bed-bound or else are exaggerating their symptoms

74.5 Differential diagnosis of low back pain

The differential diagnosis of low back pain (p. 1226) overlaps with that of myelopathy. In ≈ 85% of cases of LBP no specific diagnosis can be made[13]; however, serious and/or dangerous conditions can usually be reliably ruled out.

74.6 Initial assessment of the patient with back pain

74.6.1 Background

Initial assessment consists of a history and physical exam focused on identifying serious underlying conditions such as: fracture, tumor, infection, or cauda equina syndrome (p. 1254). Serious conditions presenting as low back problems are relatively rare.

74.6.2 History

The following information has been found to be helpful in identifying patients with serious underlying conditions such as cancer and spinal infection.[1]

1. age
2. history of cancer (especially malignancies that are prone to skeletal metastases: prostate, breast, kidney, thyroid, lung, lymphoma/myeloma)
3. unexplained weight loss
4. immunosuppression: from steroids, organ transplant medication, or HIV
5. prolonged use of steroids
6. duration of symptoms
7. responsiveness to previous therapy
8. pain that is worse at rest
9. history of skin infection: especially furuncle
10. history of IV drug abuse
11. UTI or other infection
12. pain radiating below the knee

13. persistent numbness or weakness in the legs
14. history of significant trauma. In a young patient: usually involves MVA, a fall from a height, or a direct blow to the back. In an older patient: minor falls, heavy lifting, or even a severe coughing episode can cause a fracture especially in the presence of osteoporosis
15. findings consistent with cauda equina syndrome (p. 1254):
    a) bladder dysfunction (usually urinary retention, or overflow incontinence) or fecal incontinence
    b) saddle anesthesia (p. 1254)
    c) unilateral or bilateral leg weakness or pain
16. psychological and socioeconomic factors (p. 1236) may influence the patient's report of symptoms, and one should inquire about:
    a) work status
    b) typical job tasks
    c) educational level
    d) pending litigation
    e) worker's compensation or disability issues
    f) failed previous treatments
    g) substance abuse
    h) depression
    i) domestic violence
    j) homelessness

▶ Table 74.3 shows the sensitivity and specificity of some features of the history for various conditions.

Table 74.3 Sensitivity and specificity of historical findings in patients with low back problems[1]

Condition	History	Sensitivity	Specificity
cancer	age ≥ 50 yrs	0.77	0.71
	previous cancer	0.31	0.98
	unexplained weight loss	0.15	0.94
	failure to improve after conservative therapy × 1 month	0.31	0.90
	any of the above	1.00	0.60
	pain > 1 month	0.50	0.81
spinal osteomyelitis	IV drug abuse, UTI, or skin infection	0.40	NA
compression fracture	age ≥ 50 yrs	0.84	0.61
	age ≥ 70 yrs	0.22	0.96
	trauma	0.30	0.85
	steroid use	0.06	0.995
HLD	sciatica	0.95	0.88
spinal stenosis	pseudoclaudication	0.60	NA
	age ≥ 50 yrs	0.90[a]	0.70
ankylosing spondylitis	positive response to 4 out of 5 of the following	0.23	0.82
	age at onset ≤ 40 yrs	1.00	0.07
	pain not relieved when supine	0.80	0.49
	morning back stiffness	0.64	0.59
	pain ≥ 3 mos duration	0.71	0.54

[a]estimate

74

74.6.3 Physical examination

Less helpful than the history in identifying patients who may be harboring conditions such as cancer, but may be more helpful in detecting spinal infections.

1. spinal infection (p. 380): findings that suggest this as a possibility (but are also common in patients without infection)
   a) fever: common in epidural abscess and vertebral osteomyelitis, less common in discitis
   b) vertebral tenderness
   c) very limited range of spinal motion
2. findings of possible neurologic compromise: the following physical findings will identify most cases of clinically significant nerve root compromise due to L4–5 or L5–1 HLD, which comprise > 90% of cases of radiculopathy due to HLD; limiting the exam to the following might not detect the much less common upper lumbar disc herniations, which may be difficult to detect on PE (p. 1263)
   a) dorsiflexion strength of ankle and great toe: weakness suggests L5 and some L4 dysfunction
   b) achilles reflex: diminished reflex suggests S1 root dysfunction
   c) light touch sensation of the foot:
      • diminished over medial malleolus and medial foot: suggests L4 nerve root involvement
      • diminished over dorsum of foot: suggests L5
      • diminished over lateral malleolus and lateral foot: suggests S1
   d) straight leg raising (SLR); also check for crossed SLR (p. 1252)

74.6.4 "Red flags" in the history and physical exam for low back problems

Based upon the above history and physical exam, the findings in ▶ Table 74.4 would suggest the possibility of a serious underlying condition as the cause of the low back problem. Also, thoracic region pain is relatively uncommon and should raise the index of suspicion.

Table 74.4 "Red flags" for patients with low back problems

Condition	Red flags
cancer or infection	1. age > 50 or < 20 yrs 2. history of cancer 3. unexplained weight loss 4. immunosuppression (see text) 5. UTI, IV drug abuse, fever, or chills 6. back pain not improved with rest
spinal fracture	1. history of significant trauma (see text) 2. prolonged use of steroids 3. age > 70 yrs
cauda equina syndrome or severe neurologic compromise	1. acute onset of urinary retention or overflow incontinence 2. fecal incontinence or loss of anal sphincter tone 3. saddle anesthesia 4. global or progressive weakness in the LEs

74.6.5 Special diagnostic tests

For patients without features suggesting a serious underlying condition, special diagnostic tests are not needed during the first month of symptoms. This covers approximately 95% of patients with low back problems.[1]

74.7 Radiographic evaluation

74.7.1 General information

Diagnosing lumbar spinal stenosis or herniated intervertebral disc is usually helpful only in potential surgical candidates.[14] This includes patients with appropriate clinical syndromes who have not responded satisfactorily to adequate non-surgical treatment over a sufficient period of time, and who have no medical contraindications to surgery. Radiologic confirmation of these diagnoses usually requires MRI, CT, myelography, or some combination (see below). NB: myelography,[15] CT,[16] or MRI[17] may also show bulging or herniated lumbar discs (HLD) or spinal stenosis in *asymptomatic* patients (e.g., 24% of asymptomatic patients have herniated discs on MRI and 4% have spinal stenosis; these numbers become 36% and 21% respectively in patients 60–80 years old).[18] Thus, these tests must be interpreted in light of clinical findings, and the anatomic level and side should correspond to the history, examination, and/or other physiologic data. Diagnostic radiology is of limited benefit as the initial evaluation in the majority of spinal disorders.[19]

In the absence of red flags for serious conditions, imaging studies are not recommended in the first month of symptoms.[1] For patients who have had previous back surgery, MRI with contrast is probably the best test. Myelography (with or without CT) is invasive and has increased risk of complications, and is therefore indicated only in situations where MRI cannot be done or is inadequate, and the possibility of surgery is anticipated.

Σ: Patients for whom radiographic imaging is recommended

Patients with:
1. suspected *benign* conditions with symptoms persisting > 4 weeks of great enough severity to consider surgery, including:
   a) back-related leg symptoms and clinically specific signs of nerve root compromise
   b) a history of neurogenic claudication (p. 1331) or other findings suggestive of lumbar spinal stenosis
   c) symptoms related to spinal deformity/imbalance, especially positional back pain that increases with time spent upright
2. red flags: physical examination or other test results suggesting other serious conditions affecting the spine (e.g., cauda equina syndrome, fracture, infection, tumor, or other mass lesions or defects)

Recommendations for use of MRI and discography to select patients for **fusion** are shown in the Practice Guideline (p. 1231).

Practice guideline: MRI and discography for patient selection for lumbar fusion*

1. **Level II**[20]:
   a) MRI is recommended as the initial diagnostic test
   b) normal appearing discs on MRI should not be considered for discography or treatment
   c) lumbar discography should not be used as a stand-alone test
   d) to consider a disc level for treatment, if discography is used, there should be a concordant pain response[a] and associated abnormalities on MRI[b]
2. **Level III**[20]: discography should be reserved for equivocal MRI findings, especially at levels adjacent to unequivocally abnormal levels

Notes:
   * see also recommendations on use of facet injections (p. 1239)
   [a] concordant pain response: pain identical or very similar to the patient's usual pain complaints (NB: discography can produce severe LBP in patients with no prior complaints[21,22])
   [b] abnormal disc morphology on MRI: loss of T2WI signal intensity ("black disc"), disc space collapse, Modic changes (see ▶ Table 81.5), and high-intensity zones (these findings also frequently occur in asymptomatic patients[23])

74

74.7.2 Plain lumbosacral X-rays

General information

Unexpected findings occurred in only 1 in 2500 adults < 50 years of age.[24] Diagnosis of surgical conditions of disc herniation and spinal stenosis cannot be made from plain films (although they may be inferred, further study would be required). Various congenital abnormalities of uncertain significance may be identified (e.g., spina bifida occulta), and evidence of degenerative changes (including osteophytes) are as frequent in symptomatic as in asymptomatic patients. Gonadal radiation is significant. Seldom indicated during pregnancy.

Recommendation

Not recommended for routine evaluation of patients with acute low back problems during the first month of symptoms unless a "red flag" is present (see below). Reserve LS X-rays for patients with a likelihood of having spinal malignancy, infection, inflammatory spondylitis, or clinically significant fracture. In these cases, plain X-rays are often just a starting point, and further study (CT, MRI…) may be indicated even if the plain X-rays are normal. "Red flags" for these conditions include the following:

* age > 70 yrs, or < 20 yrs
* systemically ill patients
* temp > 100 °F (or > 38 °C)
* history of malignancy
* recent infection
* patients with neurologic deficits suggesting possible cauda equina syndrome (p. 1254) (saddle anesthesia, urinary incontinence or retention, LE weakness)
* heavy alcohol or IV drug abusers
* diabetics
* immunosuppressed patients (including prolonged treatment with corticosteroids)
* recent urinary tract or spinal surgery
* *recent* trauma: any age with significant trauma, or > 50 yrs old with mild trauma
* unrelenting pain at rest
* persistent pain for more than ≈ 4 weeks
* unexplained weight loss

When spine X-rays are indicated, AP and lateral views are usually adequate.[25] Obliques and coned-down L5–1 views more than double the radiation exposure, and add information in only 4–8% of cases,[26] and can be obtained in specific instances where warranted (e.g., to diagnose spondylolysis when spondylolisthesis is found on the lateral film).

Specialized X-ray views

▶ **Flexion/extension lumbar spine X-rays.** Lateral X-rays taken with the patient in neutral position, then while flexing forward at the waist, then with hyperextension at the waist. May demonstrate "dynamic instability" (▶ Fig. 74.1) which may not be evident on static views (including CT and MRI obtained with the patient recumbent), and which may factor into decisions regarding fusion during lumbar spinal surgery.

▶ **Oblique X-rays.** Demonstrates spondylolysis as a fracture in the neck of the "Scotty dog." Utilized less frequently since CT scan demonstrates this with greater detail and accuracy (the pars defect is sometimes difficult to appreciate on MRI).

▶ **Standing scoliosis X-rays.** Primary indication is in preparation for surgical intervention (p. 1353).

74.7.3 Lumbosacral CT

If technically adequate images can be obtained (e.g., good quality scanner, images not obscured by artifact from patient movement or obesity), CT can demonstrate most spine pathology. For HLD, sensitivity is 80–95%, and specificity is 68–88%.[29,30] However, even some large disc herniations will be missed with plain CT. CT studies for HLD tend to be less satisfactory in the elderly. When MRI is an option, the main utility of CT is for imaging bone to assess fractures or to demonstrate details of bony anatomy for surgery.

Disc material has density (Hounsfield units) ≈ twice that of the thecal sac. Associated findings with herniated disc include:

* loss of epidural fat (normally seen as low density in the anterolateral canal)
* loss of normal "convexity" of thecal sac (indentation by herniated disc)

Advantages:
* excellent bony detail
* non-invasive
* outpatient evaluation
* evaluates paraspinal soft tissue (e.g., to rule out tumor, paraspinal abscess…)
* advantages over MRI: faster scanning (significant in patients who have difficulty lying still for a long time), less expensive, less claustrophobic, fewer contraindications, see Contraindications to MRI (p. 242)

74

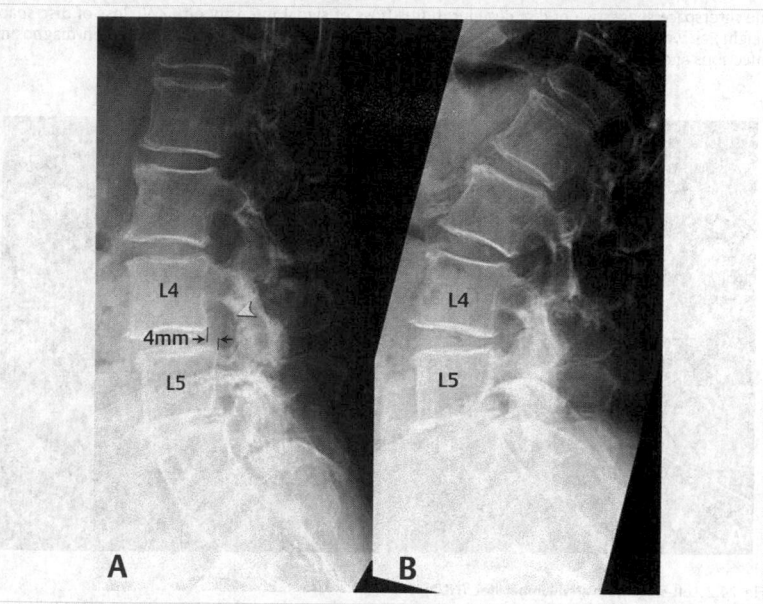

Fig. 74.1 Instability on lateral lumbar spine flexion/extension X-rays. Image: A: flexion, and B: extension, demonstrating dynamic instability at L4–5 with 4 mm of anterolisthesis of L4 on L5 in flexion that reduces in extension. This was not evident on lumbar MRI nor on neutral position lateral X-rays. Note the accompanying change in configuration of the neural foramen (*yellow arrowhead*) between the two views.

Disadvantages:
- involves ionizing radiation (X-rays)
- sensitivity is significantly lower than MRI or myelogram/CT

74.7.4 MRI

Unless contraindicated, noncontrast MRI is the initial diagnostic test of choice for diagnosing most cases of disc herniation and spinal stenosis. Specificity and sensitivity for HLD are on the same order as CT/myelography, which is better than myelography alone.[1,31,27]

Advantages:
- provides the most information about soft tissues (intervertebral discs, spinal cord, inflammation...) of any available diagnostic test
- provides information regarding tissue outside of the spinal canal, e.g., extreme lateral disc herniation (p. 1263), tumors...
- non-invasive and does not utilize ionizing radiation

Disadvantages:
- patients in severe pain or with claustrophobia may have difficulty holding still
- does not visualize bone well
- poor for studying blood early (e.g., spinal epidural hematoma)
- expensive
- interpretation with scoliosis is more difficult, may be partially compensated by contouring visualization plane through center of canal
- a number of contraindications to MRI: see Contraindications to MRI (p. 242)

Findings:

In addition to demonstrating herniated lumbar disc (HLD) outside of the disc interspace compressing nerve root or thecal sac (► Fig. 74.2), MRI can demonstrate signal changes of the disc within the interspace suggestive of *disc degeneration*[28] (loss of signal intensity on T2WI, loss of disc space height) as well as endplate changes (see Modic classification (p.1335)) and is useful in diagnosing infections and tumors.

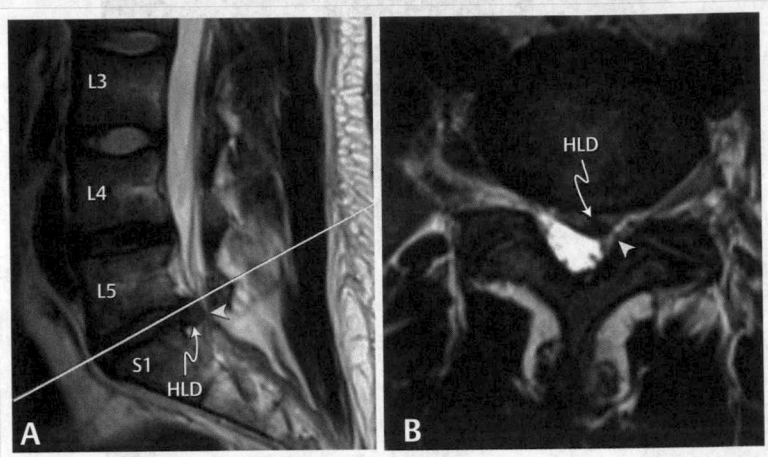

Fig. 74.2 Left-sided herniated lumbar disc (HLD).
Image: MRI, A: T2 sagittal, B: T2 axial images (the location and orientation of this slice is shown as the yellow line in A).
The *yellow arrowheads* indicate the location of compression of the nerve root en passant (the S1 nerve root).
Note that compared to the normal high density of the L2–3 and L3–4 discs, the lower density of the L4–5 and L5–S1 discs are consistent with disc degeneration. The L5-S1 disc has also lost some height.

74.7.5 Myelography

With water-soluble intrathecal contrast introduced via lumbar puncture, sensitivity (62–100%) and specificity (83–94%)[32,33,34,35] are similar to CT for detection of HLD. Usually combined with post-myelographic CT scan (myelogram/CT), which increases the sensitivity and especially the specificity.[36] A herniated disc in the large space between the thecal sac and posterior border of vertebral bodies at L5–1 (insensitive space) may not be seen on myelography alone (CT or MRI are usually better at demonstrating this).
  Advantages:
1. evaluates cauda equina better than noncontrast CT
2. provides "functional" information about degree of stenosis (a high-degree block will allow flow of dye only after certain position changes)
3. when combined with CT, may demonstrate some anatomy obscured by metal artifact on MRI in patients with prior instrumentation

Disadvantages:
1. may miss pathology outside of the dura (including far laterally herniated disc); sensitivity is improved with post-myelographic CT
2. invasive
   a) drugs e.g., warfarin must be stopped, and sometimes bridged to heparin
   b) with occasional side effects (post LP H/A, N/V, rare seizures)
3. iodine-allergic patients
   a) requires iodine allergy prep
   b) may still be risky (especially in severely iodine-allergic patients)

Findings:
  HLD produces extradural filling defect at the level of the intervertebral disc. Massive disc herniation or severe lumbar stenosis may produce a total or near-total block. In some cases of HLD, the

finding may be very subtle and may consist of a cut-off of the filling (with contrast) of the nerve root sleeve (compared to normal nerve(s) on contralateral side or at other levels). Another subtle finding may be a "dual shadow" on lateral view.

74.7.6 Bone scan for low back problems

Description: injection of a radiolabeled compound (usually technetium-99m) that is taken up by metabolically active bone. A gamma camera localizes regions of uptake. Total radiation dose is ≈ to a set of lumbar spine X-rays.[1] Contraindicated during pregnancy. Breast feeding must be briefly suspended following a bone scan due to presence of radiotracer in the breast milk.

A moderately sensitive test which may be used in evaluating low back pain when spinal tumor,[37] infection,[38] or occult fracture is suspected from "red flags" (see ▶ Table 74.4) on history or examination, or results of lab tests or plain X-rays. Not very specific, but may locate occult lesions and help differentiate these conditions from degenerative changes. A positive bone scan suggesting one of these conditions usually must be confirmed by other diagnostic tests or procedures (no studies have compared bone scans to CT or MRI).

Low yield in patients with longstanding low back problems and normal plain X-rays and laboratory tests (especially ESR or CRP).[37]

SPECT scans may provide additional information to a bone scan.

74.7.7 Discography

General information

Injection of water-soluble contrast agent directly into the nucleus pulposus of the intervertebral disc being studied by percutaneous needle access through Kambin's triangle (▶ Fig. 74.3) in an awake patient. Results of the test depend on volume of dye accepted into the disc, the pressure needed to inject the dye, the configuration of the dye (including leakage from the confines of the disc space) on radiographic imaging (plain X-rays produce the so-called "discogram"; CT scan is often also utilized following the injection), and reproduction of the patient's pain on injection. Some of the basis for performing a discogram is to identify levels that may produce "discogenic pain" or "painful disc syndrome" (p. 1235), a controversial point. When the pain produced mimics the patient's presenting pain, the pain is said to be "concordant."

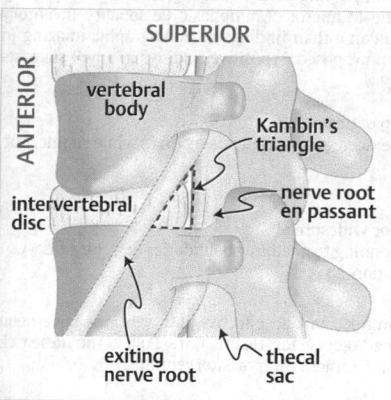

Fig. 74.3 **Kambin's triangle.**
Image: lateral diagramatic view of Kambin's triangle (*heavy broken line*), a right triangle bounded at the hypotenuse by the exiting nerve root, inferiorly by the superior endplate of the inferior vertebral body, and medially by the thecal sac.

74

Critique

Invasive. Interpretation is equivocal, and complications may occur (disc space infection, disc herniation, and significant radiation exposure with CT-discography). May be abnormal in asymptomatic patients[21,22] (as any of the above tests may be), but the false-positive rate is almost certainly not as high as reported in an older study (pain provoked in 100% of injections[21]).[39] See **Practice guideline: MRI and discography for patient selection for lumbar fusion** (p. 1231) for recommendations.

74.7.8 Thermography for low back problems

✖ Not recommended.[1] Did not accurately predict absence or presence of nerve root compression seen at surgery,[40] and may be positive in a significant percentage of asymptomatic patients.[41]

74.8 Electrodiagnostics for low back problems

If the diagnosis of radiculopathy seems likely on clinical grounds, electrophysiologic testing is not recommended.[1]

1. needle EMG (p. 255): can assess acute and chronic nerve root dysfunction, myelopathy and myopathy, and may be useful for patients with suspicion of other conditions (e.g., neuropathy) or when a reliable strength exam is not possible. Reduced recruitment may be seen within the first several days of onset; however, spontaneous activity (p. 255) takes 10–21 days to develop (∴ less helpful in the first ≈ 3 weeks). Also, not usually helpful with normal muscle strength exam. Accuracy is highly operator-dependent and improves with knowledge about imaging studies and clinical information.[42] See findings in radiculopathy (p. 256).
2. H-reflex (p. 255): measures sensory conduction through nerve roots. Use is limited to assessing S1 radiculopathy.[43] Correlates with Achilles reflex.
3. SSEPs (p. 250): assesses afferent fibers which travel in peripheral nerve and the posterior column of the spinal cord. May be abnormal in conditions affecting the dorsal columns with impaired joint position and proprioception (e.g., cervical spondylotic spinal myelopathy)
4. nerve conduction studies (including NCVs): helps identify acute and chronic entrapment neuropathies that may mimic radiculopathy
5. ✖ not recommended for assessing acute low back problems[1]
   a) F-wave response (p. 255): measures motor conduction through nerve roots, used to assess proximal neuropathies
   b) surface EMG: assesses acute and chronic recruitment patterns during static or dynamic tasks using surface (instead of needle) electrodes

74.9 Psychosocial factors

Although some patients with chronic LPB (> 3 months duration) may have started off with a diagnosable condition, psychological and socioeconomic factors (such as depression, secondary gain…) may come to play a significant role in perpetuating or amplifying pain. Psychological factors, especially elevated hysteria or hypochondriasis scales on the Minnesota Multiphasic Personality Inventory (MMPI) were found to be a better predictor of outcome than findings on radiographic imaging in one study.[42] A screening scale of 5 factors has been proposed[44] (positive findings in any 3 suggests psychological distress):

1. These items are potentially reliable[45]:
   a) pain on simulated axial loading: press on top of head
   b) inconsistent performance: e.g., difficulty tolerating straight leg raising (SLR) while supine, but no difficulty when sitting
   c) overreaction during the physical exam
2. These items may not be reliable[45]:
   a) inappropriate tenderness that is superficial or widespread
   b) motor or sensory abnormalities not corresponding to anatomic boundaries (e.g., for sensation: dermatomes, peripheral nerve distribution…)

However, the usefulness of this information is limited, and no effective interventions have been identified to address these factors. Therefore the Agency for Health Care Policy and Research (AHCPR) panel was unable to recommend specific assessment tools or interventions.[1]

74.10 Treatment

74.10.1 General information

An initial period of nonsurgical management (see below) is indicated except in the following circumstances where urgent surgery is indicated:

Situations where conservative treatment is not indicated:
• symptoms of cauda equina syndrome: urinary retention, saddle anesthesia… (p. 1254)
• progressive neurologic deficit, or profound motor weakness

• a relative indication for proceeding to urgent surgery without conservative management is severe pain that cannot be sufficiently controlled with adequate pain medication (rare)

If specific diagnoses such as herniated intervertebral lumbar disc or symptomatic lumbar stenosis are made, surgical treatment for these conditions may be considered if the patient fails to improve satisfactorily. In cases where no specific diagnosis can be made, management consists of conservative treatment and following the patient to rule out the possible development of symptoms suggestive of a more serious diagnosis that may not have initially been evident.

74.10.2 "Conservative" treatment

This term has regrettably come to be used for non-surgical management. With minor modification, similar approaches can be used for mechanical low back pain, as well as for acute radiculopathy from disc herniation.

Recommendations (based on AHCPR findings[1] in the absence of "red flags"; note: some key literature citations are given here, primarily those from the better studies that support the AHCPR panel recommendations. However, refer to Bigos et al[1] for full analysis and list of references):

1. activity modifications: no studies were found that met the panel's review criteria for adequate evidence. However, the following information was felt to be useful:
   a) bed rest: for 2–3 days maximum
      • the theoretical objective is to reduce symptoms by reducing pressure on the nerve roots and/or intradiscal pressures, which is lowest in the supine semi-Fowler position,[46] and also to reduce movements which are experienced as painful by the patient
      • deactivation from prolonged bed rest (> 4 days) appears to be worse for patients (producing weakness, stiffness, and increased pain) than a gradual return to normal activities[47]
      • recommendations: the majority of patients with low back problems will not require bed rest. Bed rest for 2–4 days may be an option for those with severe initial radicular symptoms; however, this may be no better than watchful waiting[48] and may be harmful[49]
   b) activity modification
      • the goal is to achieve a tolerable level of discomfort while continuing sufficient physical activity to minimize disruption of daily activities
      • risk factors: although there is not agreement on their exact role, the following were identified as having an increased incidence of low back problems. Jobs requiring heavy or repetitive lifting, total body vibration (from vehicles or industrial machinery), asymmetric postures, or postures sustained for long periods (including prolonged sitting)
      • recommendations: temporarily limit heavy lifting, prolonged sitting, and bending or twisting of the back. Establish activity goals to help focus attention on expected return to full functional status
   c) exercise (may be part of a *physical therapy* program):
      • during the 1st month of symptoms, low-stress aerobic exercise can minimize debility due to inactivity. In the first 2 weeks, utilize exercises that minimally stress the back: walking, bicycling, or swimming
      • conditioning exercises for trunk muscles (especially back extensors, and possibly abdominal muscles) are helpful if symptoms persist (during the first 2 weeks, these exercises may aggravate symptoms)
      • there is no evidence to support stretching of back muscles, or to recommend back-specific exercise machines over traditional exercise
      • recommended exercise quotas that are gradually escalated results in better outcome than having patients simply stop when pain occurs[50]
2. analgesics
   a) for the initial short-term period, acetaminophen (APAP) or NSAIDs (p. 144) may be used. In one study[51] of acute LBP, NSAIDs did not add any benefit to APAP + standard education (see below)
   b) stronger analgesics—mostly opioids (p. 146)—may be required for severe pain, primarily for severe radicular pain. For non-specific back pain, there was no earlier return to full activity than with NSAIDs or APAP.[1] Opioids should not be used > 2–3 weeks, at which time NSAIDs should be instituted unless contraindicated
3. muscle relaxants
   a) the therapeutic objective is to reduce pain by relieving muscle spasm. However, muscle spasms have not been proven to cause pain, and the most commonly used muscle relaxants have no peripheral effect on muscle spasm

74

b) probably more effective than placebo, but have not been shown to be more effective than NSAIDs, and their use in combination with NSAIDs has not been shown to be more effective than use of NSAIDs alone

c) potential for side effects: drowsiness (in up to 30%). Most manufacturers recommend use for < 2–3 weeks. Agents such as chlorzoxazone (Parafon Forte® and others) may be associated with risk of serious and potentially fatal hepatotoxicity[52]

4. education (may be provided as part of a *physical therapy* program):

a) explanation of the condition to the patient[53] in understandable terms, and positive reassurance that the condition will almost certainly subside[54] have been shown to be more effective than many other forms of treatment

b) proper posture, sleeping positions, lifting techniques… should be conveyed to the patient. Formal "back school" seems to be marginally effective.[55] There may be some early benefit, but long-term efficacy could not be shown.[56] The quality and expense of such programs varies widely[1]

5. spinal manipulation therapy (SMT): defined as manual therapy in which loads are applied to the spine using long or short lever methods with the selected joint being taken to its end range of voluntary motion, followed by application of an impulse loading (may be part of a *physical therapy* program)

a) may be helpful for patients with acute low back problems without radiculopathy when used in the first month of symptoms (efficacy after 1 month is unproven) for a period not to exceed 1 month. One study[51] found no added benefit to APA + standard education

b) there is insufficient evidence to recommend SMT in the presence of radiculopathy

c) SMT should not be used in the face of severe or progressive neurologic deficit until serious conditions have been ruled out

d) ✖ reports of arterial dissection: especially vertebral artery (p. 1579) and stroke, myelopathy & subdural hematoma with *cervical* SMT and cauda equina syndrome with lumbar SMT[57,58,59] and the uncertainty of benefits have led to the questioning of the use of SMT[57] (especially cervical)

6. epidural injections:

a) epidural (cortico)steroid injections (ESI): there is no evidence that this is effective in treating acute radiculopathy.[60] Most studies that show benefit are retrospective and noncontrolled. Prospective studies yield varied results.[61] Some improvement at 3 & 6 weeks may occur (but no functional benefit, and no change in the need for surgery), with no benefit at 3 months.[62] The response in chronic back pain is poor in comparison to acute pain. ESI may be an option for *short-term* relief of radicular pain when control on oral medications is inadequate or for patients who are not surgical candidates

b) there is no evidence to support the use of epidural injections of steroids, local anesthetics, and/or opioids for LBP without radiculopathy

c) reports on efficacy with conditions such as lumbar spinal stenosis are conflicting,[61] relief is almost uniformly temporary (4–6 weeks with initial injection, shorter times with subsequent ones)

74

✖ *Not* recommended by the AHCPR panel[1] for treatment of acute low back problems in the absence of "red flags" (▶ Table 74.4):

1. medications

a) oral steroids: no difference was found at 1 week and 1 year after randomization to receive 1 week therapy with oral dexamethasone or placebo[63]

b) colchicine: conflicting evidence shows either some[64] or no[65] therapeutic benefit. Side effects of N/V and diarrhea were common[1]

c) antidepressant medications: most studies of these medications were for chronic back pain. Some methodologically flawed studies failed to show benefits when compared to placebo for chronic (not acute) LBP[66]

2. physical treatments

a) TENS (transcutaneous electrical nerve stimulation): *not* statistically significantly better than placebo, and added no benefit to exercise alone[67]

b) traction (including pelvic traction): not demonstrated to be effective.[68] One possible explanation for lack of benefit is that due to the sizable paraspinal muscles and ligaments (as compared to the cervical spine) the amount of weight required to distract the intervertebral disc space is approximately ≥ 2/3 of the patient's body weight, which is painful and/or pulls the patient to the foot of the bed

c) physical agents and modalities: including heat (including diathermy), ice, ultrasound. Benefit is insufficiently proven to justify their cost; however, self-administered home programs for application of heat or cold may be considered. Ultrasound and diathermy should not be used in pregnancy

d) lumbar corsets and support belts: not proven beneficial for acute back problems. Prophylactic use has been advocated to reduce time lost from work by individuals doing frequent lifting as part of their job, but this is controversial[69]

e) biofeedback: has not been studied for acute back problems. Primarily advocated for chronic LBP, where effectiveness is controversial[70]

3. injection therapy

a) trigger point and ligamentous injections: the theory that trigger points cause or perpetuate LBP is controversial and disputed by many experts. Injections of local anesthetic are of equivocal efficacy (saline may be as effective[71]) and are mildly invasive

b) (zygapophyseal) facet joint injections: theoretical basis is that there exists a "facet syndrome" producing LBP which is aggravated by spine extension, with no nerve root tension signs (p. 1251). No studies have adequately investigated injections for pain < 3 months duration. For chronic LBP, neither the agent nor the location (intrafacet or pericapsular) made a significant difference in outcomes[72,73]

c) epidural injections in the absence of radiculopathy: see above

d) acupuncture: no studies were found that evaluated the use in acute back problems. All randomized clinical trials found were for patients with chronic LBP, and even the best studies were felt to be mediocre and contradictory. Meta-analysis found acupuncture was more effective in relieving chronic LBP than sham or no treatment,[74] but there was no comparison to other therapies

Practice guideline: Injection therapy for low back pain

Therapeutic recommendations

Level III[75]: lumbar epidural injections or trigger point injections are not recommended for long-term relief of chronic LBP. These techniques or facet injections may be used to provide temporary relief in select patients

Diagnostic recommendations

Level III[75]: lumbar facet injections
- may predict the response to radiofrequency facet ablation
- ✖ not recommended as a diagnostic tool to predict the response to lumbar fusion

74.10.3 Surgical treatment

Indications for surgery for herniated lumbar disc

See the section on **herniated lumbar discs** (p. 1256).

Indications for fusion for chronic LBP without stenosis or spondylolisthesis

Very controversial.

Practice guideline: Lumbar fusion for LBP without stenosis or spondylolisthesis

Level I[76]: lumbar fusion is recommended for carefully selected patients with disabling LBP due to one- or two-level degenerative disease without stenosis or spondylolisthesis (in the primary quoted study[77] patients had chronic LBP for ≥ 2 years and had radiologic evidence of disc degeneration at L4–5, L5–1, or both, and had failed best medical management).

Level III[76,78]: an intensive course of PT and cognitive therapy is recommended as an option for patients with LBP in whom conventional medical management has failed.

74

Practice guideline: Choice of fusion technique

Level II[79]: for ALIF or ALIF + instrumentation, the addition of a posterolateral fusion is not recommended (the demonstrated benefit does not outweigh the additional time and blood loss involved).

Level III[79]:

- either a posterolateral fusion or an interbody fusion (PLIF, TLIF, or ALIF) are options for patients with LBP due to DDD at 1 or 2 levels
- an interbody graft is an option to improve fusion rates and functional outcome (caution: the improvement in fusion rate and outcome is marginal, and interbody fusion is associated with an increased complication rate, especially with combined approaches, e.g., 360° fusion)

✖ the use of multiple approaches (anterior + posterior) is not recommended as a routine option for LBP without deformity

Surgical treatment options

The type of surgical procedure chosen is tailored to the specific condition identified. Examples are shown in ▶ Table 74.5. Discussion of some options is also provided below.

Table 74.5 Surgical options for low back problems

Condition	Surgical treatment options
"routine" HLD or initial recurrence of HLD	• standard discectomy and microdiscectomy are of similar efficacy • ✖ intradiscal procedures: nucleotome, laser disc decompression are not recommended (p. 1257)
foraminal or far lateral HLD	• partial or total facetectomy (p. 1265) • extracanal approach (p. 1265) • endoscopic techniques
lumbar spinal stenosis	• simple decompressive laminectomy • laminectomy plus fusion: may be indicated for patients with degenerative spondylolisthesis, stenosis and radiculopathy, adult degenerative scoliosis (ADS), or instability

Lumbar spinal fusion

Although there is no consensus on the indications,[80] lumbar spinal fusion (LSF) is most widely accepted as part of treatment for fracture-dislocation or instability resulting from tumor or infection.

For degenerative spine disease, practice parameters have been developed and are included herein. Pain associated with Modic type 1 changes (bone edema, see ▶ Table 81.5) may respond to stabilization procedures, the other Modic types do not exhibit this association. A substantial number of patients with herniated lumbar disc and radiculopathy who also have LBP will have relief of LBP.[81,82,83]

Practice guideline: Lumbar fusion for disc herniation

Level III[84]:

1. lumbar fusion is *not* routinely recommended following disc excision in patients with HLD or 1st time recurrent HLD causing radiculopathy
2. lumbar fusion is a potential adjunct to disc excision in cases of an HLD or recurrent HLD:
   a) with evidence of preoperative lumbar spinal deformity or instability
   b) in patients with chronic axial LBP associated with radiculopathy

Instrumentation as an adjunct to fusion

Practice guideline: Pedicle screw fixation

Level III[85]: pedicle screw fixation is recommended as a treatment option for patients with LBP treated with posterolateral fusion who are at high risk for fusion failure (routine use of pedicle screws is discouraged because of conflicting evidence of benefit, together with considerable evidence of increased cost and complications).

The use of instrumentation increases the fusion rate.[86] Hardware used in the absence of fusion will eventually fatigue (with one or more of the following: breakage of rods and/or screws, screw pullout, or spine fracture). Therefore, instrumentation must be viewed as a temporary internal stabilizing measure while awaiting the fusion process to complete.

74.11 Chronic low back pain

Rarely can an anatomic diagnosis be made in patients with chronic LBP ≥ 3 months duration.[87] Also, see Psychosocial factors (p.1236). Patients with chronic pain syndromes (CPS) refer to their problems with affective or emotional terms with a higher frequency than those with acute pain.[88] The amount of time that a patient has been out of work due to low back problems is related to the chances of the patient getting back to work as shown in ▶ Table 74.6.

Table 74.6 Chances of patients going back to work

Time out of work	Chances of getting back to work
<6 mos	50%
1 yr	20%
2 yrs	<5%

74.12 Coccydynia

74.12.1 General information

Pain and tenderness around the coccyx. A symptom, not a diagnosis. Typically, discomfort is experienced on sitting or on rising from sitting. More common in females, possibly due to a more prominent coccyx. The condition is unusual enough in males that in the absence of local trauma, strong consideration should be given to an underlying condition.

74.12.2 Etiologies

For differential diagnosis, see Acute low back pain (p.1706). Better accepted etiologies include[89]:
1. local trauma (may be associated with fracture or dislocation):
    a) 25% of patients give a history of a fall
    b) 12% had repetitive trauma (rowing machine, prolonged bicycle riding...)
    c) 12% started with parturition
    d) 5% started following a surgical procedure (half of which were in the lithotomy position)
2. idiopathic: excluding traumatic cases, no etiology can be identified in most cases
3. neoplasms
    a) chordoma
    b) giant cell tumor
    c) intradural schwannoma
    d) perineural cyst
    e) intraosseous lipoma
    f) carcinoma of the rectum
    g) sacral hemangioma[90]
    h) pelvic metastases (e.g., from prostate cancer)
4. prostatitis

74

Controversial etiologies include[89,91]:
1. local pressure over a prominent coccyx
2. referred pain:
   a) spinal disease
      • herniated lumbosacral disc
      • cauda equina syndrome
      • arachnoiditis
   b) pelvic/visceral disease
      • pelvic inflammatory disease (PID)
      • perirectal abscess
      • perirectal fistula
      • pilonidal cyst
3. inflammation of the various ligaments attached to the coccyx
4. neurosis or frank hysteria

Histological evaluation of the coccyx has not helped delineate the cause, even though avascular necrosis has been suggested.[92]

74.12.3 Evaluation

MRI: effective for detecting soft tissue masses, including presacral masses.

CT scan: no characteristic finding in coccydynia findings. Very sensitive for detecting bony pathology (fracture, destructive lesion…).

Sacrococcygeal films are often performed to rule out a bony destructive lesion. Often, the question of a fracture will be raised, and many times cannot be definitely ruled in or out based on this study. There may or may not be any significance to such a fracture.

Nuclear bone scans were not helpful in 50 patients with coccydynia.[89]

74.12.4 Treatment

Numerous treatments have been proposed, and some are offered here for historical purposes[89] (and to dissuade casual attempts to effect a "new" cure that in reality has already been tried):
1. plaster jackets
2. hot baths (sitz baths), heating pads
3. massage therapy
4. XRT
5. psychotherapy

Most cases resolve within ≈ 3 months of conservative management consisting of NSAIDs, mild analgesics, and measures to reduce pressure on the coccyx (e.g., a rubber ring ("doughnut") sitting cushion, lumbar supports to maintain sitting lumbar lordosis to shift weight from coccyx to posterior thighs).[93]

Management recommendations for refractory cases[89,93]:
1. local injection: 60% respond to corticosteroid + local anesthetic (40 mg Depo-Medrol® in 10 cc of 0.25% bupivacaine). Recommended as initial treatment; response should be achieved by 2 injections
2. manipulation of the coccyx: usually under general anesthesia. ≈ 85% successful when combined with local injection
3. ± physiotherapy (diathermy & ultrasound): found to be of benefit only in ≈ 16% (may be more effective with the addition of gentle manipulation of the coccyx *without* general anesthesia[94])
4. caudal epidural steroid injection
5. blockade or neurolysis (with chemicals or by cryoablation[95]) of the ganglion impar (AKA ganglion of Walther, the lowest ganglion of the paired paravertebral sympathetic chain, located just anterior to the sacrococcygeal junction): some success has been described with this technique (traditionally used for intractable sympathetic perineal pain of neoplastic etiology[96])
6. neurolytic techniques directed to S4, S5, and coccygeal nerves
7. coccygectomy (surgical removal of the mobile portion of the coccyx, followed by smoothening of the residual bony prominence on the sacrum): was required in ≈ 20% of patients in one series,[89] with a reported success rate of 90%. However, many practitioners do not view this as a highly effective treatment and feel that great restraint should be used in considering this form of therapy

74

74.12.5 Recurrence

Occurs in ≈ 20% of conservatively treated cases, usually within the first year. Repeat therapy was often successful in providing permanent relief. More aggressive treatment may be considered for refractory cases.

74.13 Failed back surgery syndrome

74.13.1 General information

Definition: failure to satisfactorily improve low back pain or radiculopathy following back surgery. These patients often require analgesics and are unable to return to work. The failure rate for lumbar discectomy to provide satisfactory long-term pain relief is ≈ 8–25%.[97] Pending legal or worker's compensation claims were the most frequent deterrents to a good outcome.[98]

74.13.2 Etiologies

Factors that may cause or contribute to the failed back syndrome:
1. incorrect initial diagnosis
   a) inadequate pre-op imaging
   b) clinical findings not correlated with abnormality demonstrated on imaging
   c) other causes of symptoms (sometimes in the presence of what was considered to be an appropriate lesion on imaging studies which may have been asymptomatic): e.g., trochanteric bursitis, diabetic amyotrophy…
2. continued nerve root or cauda equina compression caused by:
   a) residual compression (retained disc material, osteophytes…)
   b) recurrent pathology at same level: disc reherniation at the same level, usually have pain-free interval > 6 mos post-op (p. 1267); or restenosis (over many years[99]—was more common with midline fusions)
   c) adjacent level pathology: disc herniation or stenosis[99]
   d) compression of nerve root by peridural scar (granulation) tissue (see below)
   e) pseudomeningocele
   f) epidural hematoma
   g) conjoined nerve roots with compression at another level or in atypical location
   h) segmental instability: 3 patterns,[100] 1) lateral rotational instability, 2) post-op spondylolisthesis, 3) post-op scoliosis
3. permanent nerve root injury from the original disc herniation or from surgery, includes deafferentation pain which is usually constant and burning or ice cold
4. adhesive arachnoiditis: responsible for 6–16% of persistent symptoms in post-op patients[101] (see below)
5. discitis (p. 390): usually produces exquisite back pain 2–4 weeks post-op
6. spondylosis
7. other causes of back pain unrelated to the original condition: paraspinal muscle spasm, myofascial syndrome… Look for trigger points, evidence of spasm
8. post-op reflex sympathetic dystrophy (RSD) (p. 1259)
9. "non-anatomic factors": poor patient motivation, secondary gains, drug addiction, psychological problems (p. 1258)…

74.13.3 Arachnoiditis (AKA adhesive arachnoiditis)

General information

Inflammatory condition of the lumbar nerve roots. Actually a misnomer, since adhesive arachnoiditis is really an inflammatory process or fibrosis that involves all three meningeal layers (pia, arachnoid, and dura).

Etiologies/risk factors

Many putative "risk factors" have been described for the development of arachnoiditis, including[102]:
1. spinal anesthesia: either due to the anesthetic agents or to detergent contaminants on the syringes used for same
2. spinal meningitis: pyogenic, syphilitic, tuberculous

74

3. neoplasms
4. myelographic contrast agents: less common with currently available nonionic water-soluble contrast agents
5. trauma:
    a) post-surgical: especially after multiple operations
    b) external trauma
6. hemorrhage
7. idiopathic

Radiographic findings in arachnoiditis

NB: Radiographic evidence of arachnoiditis may also be found in *asymptomatic* patients.[102] Arachnoiditis must be differentiated from tumor: the central adhesive type (see below) may resemble CSF seeding of tumor, and myelographic block may mimic intrathecal tumor.

MRI

3 patterns on MRI[103,104]:
1. central adhesion (clumping) of the nerve roots into 1 or 2 central "cords"
2. "empty thecal sac" pattern: (▶ Fig. 74.4) roots adhere to meninges around periphery, giving the appearance of a thecal sac containing only CSF
3. thecal sac filled with inflammatory tissue, no CSF signal. Corresponds with myelographic block and *candle-dripping* appearance

Enhancement: acute arachnoiditis may enhance. Chronic arachnoiditis usually does not enhance with gadolinium as much as e.g., tumor.

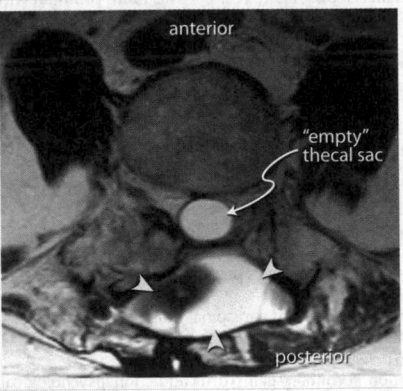

Fig. 74.4 "Empty thecal sac" appearance of arachnoiditis.
Axial T2 MRI through L4 in patient with adhesive arachnoiditis demonstrating nerve roots that are plastered against the posterior wall of the thecal sac and are thus not visible, giving the appearance of an empty thecal sac (bright oval).
The patient also has a pseudomeningocele (*yellow arrowheads*).

Myelogram

May demonstrate complete block, or clumping of nerve roots. One of many myelographic classification systems[105] for arachnoiditis is shown in ▶ Table 74.7.

Table 74.7 Myelographic classification of arachnoiditis

Type	Description
1	unilateral focal filling defect centered on the nerve root sleeve adjacent to disc space
2	circumferential constriction around thecal sac
3	complete obstruction with "stalactites" or "candle guttering," "candle-dripping," or "paint-brush" filling defects
4	infundibular cul-de-sac with loss of radicular striations

74.13.4 Peridural scar

General information

Although peridural scar tissue is frequently blamed for causing recurrent symptoms,[106,107] there has been no proof of correlation between the two.[108] Peridural fibrosis is an inevitable sequelae to lumbar disc surgery just as post-op fibrosis is a consequence of any surgical procedure. Even patients who are relieved of their pain following discectomy develop some scar tissue post-op.[109] Although it has been shown that if a patient has recurrent radicular pain following a lumbar discectomy there is a 70% chance that extensive peridural scar will be found on MRI,[108] this study also showed that on post-op MRIs at 6 months, 43% of patients will have extensive scar, but 84% of the time this will be *asymptomatic*.[110] Thus, one must use clinical grounds to determine if a patient with extensive scar on MRI is in the 16% minority of patients with radicular symptoms attributable to scar.[110]

See a discussion of measures to reduce peridural scarring (p. 1258).

Radiologic evaluation

General information

Patients with only persistent low back or hip pain without a strong radicular component, with a neurologic exam that is normal or unchanged from pre-op, should be treated symptomatically. Patients with signs or symptoms of recurrent radiculopathy (positive SLR is a sensitive test for nerve root compression), especially if these follow a period of apparent recovery, should undergo further evaluation.

It is critical to differentiate residual/recurrent disc herniation from scar tissue and adhesive arachnoiditis as surgical treatment has generally poor results with the latter two (see below).

MRI without and with IV gadolinium

Diagnostic *test of choice*. The best exam for detecting residual or recurrent disc herniation, and to reliably differentiate disc from scar tissue. Pre-contrast studies with T1WI and T2WI yield an accuracy of ≈ 83%, comparable to IV-enhanced CT.[111,112] With the addition of gadolinium, using the protocol below yields 100% sensitivity, 71% specificity, and 89% accuracy.[113] May also detect adhesive arachnoiditis (see above). As scar becomes more fibrotic and calcified with time, the differential enhancement with respect to disc material attenuates and may become undetectable at some point, ≈ 1–2 years post-op[112] (some scar continues to enhance for > 20 yrs).

Recommended MRI protocol

See reference.[113]

Get pre-contrast T1WI and T2WI. Give 0.1 mmol/kg gadolinium IV. Obtain T1WI images within 10 minutes (early post-contrast). No benefit from post-contrast T2WI.

Findings on unenhanced MRI

Signal from an HLD becomes more intense as the sequence is varied from T1WI → T2WI, whereas scar tissue becomes less intense with this transition. Indirect signs (also applicable to CT):
1. mass effect: a nerve root is displaced away from disc material, whereas it may be retracted toward scar tissue by adherence to it
2. location: disc material tends to be in contiguity with the disc interspace (best seen on sagittal MRI)

Findings on enhanced MRI

On early (≤ 10 mins post-contrast) T1WI images: scar enhances inhomogeneously, whereas disc does not enhance at all. A nonenhancing central area surrounded by irregular enhancing material probably represents disc wrapped in scar. Venous plexus also enhances, and may be more pronounced when it is distorted by disc material, but the morphology is easily differentiated from scar tissue in these cases.

On late (> 30 mins post-contrast) T1WI: scar enhances homogeneously, disc had variable or no enhancement. Normal nerve roots do not enhance even on late images.

CT scan without and with IV (iodinated) contrast

Unenhanced CT scan density measurements are unreliable in the postoperative back.[114] Enhanced CT is only fairly good in differentiating scar (enhancing) from disc (unenhancing with possible rim enhancement). Accuracy is about equal to *unenhanced* MRI.

Myelography, with post-myelographic CT

Postoperative myelographic criteria alone are unreliable for distinguishing disc material from scar.[102,115] With the addition of CT scan, neural compression is clearly demonstrated, but scar still cannot be reliably distinguished from disc.

Myelography (especially with post-myelographic CT) is very capable of demonstrating arachnoiditis[115] (see above).

Plain LS X-rays

Generally helpful only in cases of instability, malalignment, or spondylosis.[115] Flexion/extension views are most helpful when trying to demonstrate instability.

74.13.5 Treatment of failed back surgery syndrome

Postoperative discitis

For treatment of intervertebral disc-space infection, see Discitis (p.390).

Symptomatic treatment

Recommended for patients who do not have radicular signs and symptoms, or for most patients demonstrated to have scar tissue or adhesive arachnoiditis on imaging. As in other cases of non-specific LBP, treatment includes: short-term bed rest, analgesics (non-narcotic in most cases), anti-inflammatory medication (non-steroidal, and occasionally a short course of steroids), and physical therapy.

Surgery

Generally reserved for those with recurrent or residual disc herniation, segmental instability, or patients with a pseudomeningocele. Patients with post-op spinal instability should be considered for spinal fusion (p.1240).[100]

In most series with sufficient follow-up, success rates after reoperation are lower in patients with only epidural scar (as low as 1%) compared to those patients with disc and scar (still only ≈ 37%).[97] An overall success rate (> 50% pain relief for > 2 yrs) of ≈ 34% was seen in one series,[107] with better results in patients who were young and female, with good results following previous surgery, a small number of previous operations, employment prior to surgery, predominantly radicular (cf axial) pain, and absence of scar requiring lysis.

In addition to the absence of disc material, factors associated with poor outcome were: sensory loss involving more than one dermatome, and patients with past or pending compensation claims.[97,116]

Arachnoiditis:

Surgery for carefully selected patients with arachnoiditis (those with mild radiographic involvement (Types 1 & 2 in ▶ Table 74.7), and < 3 previous back operations)[105] has met with moderate success (although in this series, no patient returned to work). Approximate success rate in other series[117,118]: 50% failure, 20% able to work but with symptoms, 10–19% with no symptoms. Surgery consists of removal of extradural scar enveloping the thecal sac, removing any herniated disc fragments, and performing foraminotomies when indicated. Intradural lysis of adhesions is *not* indicated since no means for preventing reformation of scar has been identified.[118]

References

[1] Bigos S, Bowyer O, Braen G, et al. Acute Low Back Problems in Adults. Clinical Practice Guideline No.14. AHCPR Publication No. 95-0642. Rockville, MD: Agency for Health Care Policy and Research, Public Health Service, U.S. Department of Health and Human Services; 1994

[2] Cypress BK. Characteristics of Physician Visits for Back Symptoms: A National Perspective. Am J Public Health. 1983; 73:389–395

[3] Cunningham LS, Kelsey JL. Epidemiology of Musculoskeletal Impairments and Associated Disability. Am J Public Health. 1984; 74:574–579

[4] Frymoyer JW. Back Pain and Sciatica. N Engl J Med. 1988; 318:291–300

[5] Fardon DF, Milette PC. Nomenclature and classification of lumbar disc pathology. Recommendations of the Combined task Forces of the North American Spine Society, American Society of Spine Radiology, and American Society of Neuroradiology. Spine. 2001; 26:E93–E113

[6] Fardon DF, Williams AL, Dohring EJ, et al. Lumbar disc nomenclature: version 2.0: Recommendations of the combined task forces of the North American Spine Society, the American Society of Spine Radiology and the American Society of Neuroradiology. Spine J. 2014. http://www.thespinejournalonline.com/article/S1529-9430(14)00409-4/pdf. DOI: 10.1016/j.spinee.2014.04.022

[7] McCarron RF, Wimpee MW, Hudkins PG, et al. The Inflammatory Effect of Nucleus Pulposus: A Possible Element in the Pathogenesis of Low-Back Pain. Spine. 1987; 12:760–764

[8] Fairbank JC, Couper J, Davies JB, et al. The Oswestry low back pain disability questionnaire. Physiotherapy. 1980; 66:271–273

[9] Fairbank JC, Pynsent PB. The Oswestry Disability Index. Spine. 2000; 25:2940–52; discussion 2952

[10] Baker D, Pynsent P, Fairbank J, et al. The Oswestry Disability Index revisited. In: Back pain: New approaches to rehabilitation and education. Manchester: Manchester University Press; 1989:184–186

[11] Roland M, Morris R. A study of the natural history of back pain. Part I: development of a reliable and sensitive measure of disability in low-back pain. Spine (Phila Pa 1976). 1983; 8:141–144

[12] Grevitt M, Khazim R, Webb J, et al. The short form-36 health survey questionnaire in spine surgery. Journal of Bone and Joint Surgery. British Volume. 1997; 79:48–52

[13] Kelsey JL, White AA, Gordon SL. Idiopathic Low Back Pain: Magnitude of the Problem. 1982

[14] Deyo RA, Bigos SJ, Maravilla KR. Diagnostic Imaging Procedures for the Lumbar Spine. Ann Intern Med. 1989; 111:865–867

[15] Hitselberger WE, Witten RM. Abnormal Myelograms in Asymptomatic Patients. J Neurosurg. 1968; 28:204–206

[16] Wiesel SW, Tsourmas N, Feffer HL, et al. A Study of Computer-Assisted Tomography. I. The Incidence of Positive CAT Scans in an Asymptomatic Group of Patients. Spine. 1984; 9:549–551

[17] Jensen MC, Brant-Zawadzki MN, Obuchowski N, et al. Magnetic Resonance Imaging of the Lumbar Spine in People Without Back Pain. New England Journal of Medicine. 1994; 331:69–73

[18] Boden SD, Davis DO, Dina TS, et al. Abnormal Magnetic-Resonance Scans of the Lumbar Spine in Asymptomatic Subjects. J Bone Joint Surg. 1990; 72A:403–408

[19] Spitzer WO, LeBlanc FE, Dupuis M, et al. Scientific Approach to the Assessment and Management of Activity-Related Spinal Disorders: A Monograph for Clinicians: Report of the Quebec Task Force on Spinal Disorders. Chapter 3: Diagnosis of the Problem (The Problem of Diagnosis). Spine. 1987; 12: S16–S21

[20] Resnick DK, Choudhri TF, Dailey AT, et al. Part 6: Magnetic resonance imaging and discography for patient selection for lumbar fusion. Journal of Neurosurgery (Spine). 2005; 2:662–669

[21] Holt EP. The Question of Lumbar Discography. Journal of Bone and Joint Surgery. 1968; 50A:720–726

[22] Carragee EJ, Tanner CM, Khurana S, et al. The rates of false-positive lumbar discography in select patients without low back symptoms. Spine. 2000; 25:1373–80; discussion 1381

[23] Carragee EJ, Paragioudakis SJ, Khurana S. 2000 Volvo Award winner in clinical studies: Lumbar high-intensity zone and discography in subjects without low back problems. Spine. 2000; 25:2987–2992

[24] Nachemson AL. The Lumbar Spine: An Orthopedic Challenge. Spine. 1976; 1:59–71

[25] World Health Organization. A Rational Approach to Radiodiagnostic Investigations. 1983

[26] Scavone JG, Latschaw RF, Rohrer GV. Use of Lumbar Spine Films: Statistical Evaluation of a University Teaching Hospital. JAMA. 1981; 246:1105–1108

[27] Bosacco SJ, Berman AT, Garbarino JL, et al. A Comparison of CT Scanning and Myelography in the Diagnosis of Lumbar Disc Herniation. Clinical Orthopedics. 1984; 190:124–128

[28] Moufarrij NA, Hardy RW, Weinstein MA. Computed Tomographic, Myelographic, and Operative Findings in Patients with Suspected Herniated Lumbar Discs. Neurosurgery. 1983; 12:184–188

[29] Modic MT, Masaryk T, Boumphrey F, et al. Lumbar Herniated Disk Disease and Canal Stenosis: Prospective Evaluation by Surface Coil MR, CT, and Myelography. AJR. 1986; 147:757–765

[30] Jackson RP, Cain JE, Jacobs RR, et al. The Neuroradiologic Diagnosis of Lumbar Herniated Nucleus Pulposus: II. A Comparison of Computed Tomography (CT), Myelography, CT-Myelography, and Magnetic Resonance Imaging. Spine. 1989; 14:1362–1367

[31] Modic MT, Pavlicek W, Weinstein MA, et al. Magnetic Resonance Imaging of Intervertebral Disk Disease. Radiology. 1984; 152:103–111

[32] Aejmelaeus R, Hiltunen H, Härkönen M, et al. Myelographic Versus Clinical Diagnostics in Lumbar Disc Disease. Arch Orthop Trauma Surg. 1984; 103:18–25

[33] Herron LD, Turner J. Patient Selection for Lumbar Laminectomy and Discectomy with a Revised Objective Rating System. Clin Orthop. 1985; 199:145–152

[34] Kortelainen P, Puranen J, Koivisto E, et al. Symptoms and Signs of Sciatica and their Relation to the Localization of the Lumbar Disc Herniation. Spine. 1985; 10:88–92

[35] Hirsch C, Nachemson A. The Reliability of Lumbar Disk Surgery. Clin Orthop. 1963; 29

[36] Slebus FG, Braakman R, Schipper J, et al. Non-Corresponding Radiological and Surgical Diagnoses in Patients Operated for Sciatica. Acta Neurochirurgica. 1988; 94:137–143

[37] Schütte HE, Park WM. The Diagnostic Value of Bone Scintigraphy in Patients with Low Back Pain. Skeletal Radiol. 1983; 10:1–4

[38] Whalen JL, Brown ML, McLeod R, et al. Limitations of Indium Leukocyte Imaging for the Diagnosis of Spine Infections. Spine. 1991; 16:193–197

[39] Walsh TR, Weinstein JN, Spratt KF, et al. Lumbar Discography in Normal Patients. A Controlled, Prospective Study. Journal of Bone and Joint Surgery. 1990; 72A:1081–1088

[40] Mills GH, Davies GK, Getty CJM, et al. The Evaluation of Liquid Crystal Thermography in the Investigation of Nerve Root Compression due to Lumbosacral Lateral Spinal Stenosis. Spine. 1986; 11:427–432

[41] Harper CM, Low PA, Fealy RD, et al. Utility of Thermography in the Diagnosis of Lumbosacral Radiculopathy. Neurology. 1991; 41:1010–1014

[42] Spengler DM, Ouellette EA, Battié M, et al. Elective Discectomy for Herniation of a Lumbar Disc. Additional Experience with an Objective Method. Journal of Bone and Joint Surgery. 1990; 72A:230–237

[43] Braddom RL, Johnson EW. Standardization of H Reflex and Diagnostic Use in S1 Radiculopathy. Arch Phys Med Rehabil. 1974; 55:161–166

[44] Waddell G, McCulloch JA, Kummel E, et al. Nonorganic Physical Signs in Low Back Pain. Spine. 1980; 5:117–125

[45] McCombe PF, Fairbank JCT, Cockersole BC, et al. Reproducibility of Physical Signs in Low-Back Pain. Spine. 1989; 14:908–918

[46] Nachemson AL. Newest Knowledge of Low Back Pain. A Critical Look. Clin Orthop. 1992; 279:8–20

[47] Deyo RA, Diehl AK, Rosenthal M. How Many Days of Bed Rest for Acute Low Back Pain? A Randomized Clinical Trial. New England Journal of Medicine. 1986; 315:1064–1070

[48] Vroomen PCAJ, de Krom MCTFM, Wilmink JT, et al. Lack of Effectiveness of Bed Rest for Sciatica. New England Journal of Medicine. 1999; 340:418–423

[49] Allen C, Glasziou P, Del Mar C. Bed Rest: A Potentially Harmful Treatment Needing More Careful Evaluation. Lancet. 1999; 354:1229–1233

[50] Lindström I, Ohlund C, Eek C, et al. The Effect of Graded Activity on Patients with Subacute Low Back Pain: A Randomized Prospective Clinical Study with an Operant-Conditioning Behavioral Approach. Phys Ther. 1992; 72:279–293

[51] Hancock MJ, Maher CG, Latimer J, et al. Assessment of diclofenac or spinal manipulative therapy, or both, in addition to recommended first-line treatment for acute low back pain: a randomised controlled trial. Lancet. 2007; 370:1638–1643

[52] Chlorzoxazone Hepatotoxicity. Medical Letter. 1996; 38

[53] Deyo RA, Diehl AK. Patient Satisfaction with Medical Care for Low-Back Pain. Spine. 1986; 11:28–30

[54] Thomas KB. General Practice Consultations: Is There Any Point in Being Positive? Br Med J. 1987; 294:1200–1202

[55] Keijsers JFEM, Bouter LM, Meertens RM. Validity and Comparability of Studies on the Effects of Back

Schools. Physiother Theory Pract. 1991; 7:177–184

[56] Bergquist-Ullman M, Larsson U. Acute Low Back Pain in Industry. A Controlled Prospective Study with Special Reference to Therapy and Confounding Factors. Acta Orthop Scand. 1977; 170:1–117

[57] Di Fabio RP. Manipulation of the cervical spine: risks and benefits. Phys Ther. 1999; 79:50–65

[58] Ernst E. Life-threatening complications of spinal manipulation. Stroke. 2001; 32:809–810

[59] Stevinson C, Honan W, Cooke B, et al. Neurological complications of cervical spine manipulation. J R Soc Med. 2001; 94:107–110

[60] Cuckler JM, Bernini PA, Wiesel SW, et al. The Use of Epidural Steroids in the Treatment of Lumbar Radicular Pain. A Prospective, Randomized, Double-Blind Study. Journal of Bone and Joint Surgery. 1985; 67A:63–66

[61] Spaccarelli KC. Lumbar and Caudal Epidural Corticosteroid Injections. Mayo Clinic Proceedings. 1996; 71:169–178

[62] Carette S, Leclaire R, Marcoux S, et al. Epidural Corticosteroid Injections for Sciatica due to Herniated Nucleus Pulposus. New England Journal of Medicine. 1997; 336:1634–1640

[63] Haimovic IC, Beresford HR. Dexamethasone is Not Superior to Placebo for Treating Lumbosacral Radicular Pain. Neurology. 1986; 36:1593–1594

[64] Meek JB, Giudice VW, McFadden JW, et al. Colchicine Confirmed as Highly Effective in Disk Disorders. Final Results of a Double-Blind Study. J Neuro & Orthop Med & Surg. 1985; 6:211–218

[65] Schnebel BE, Simmons JW. The Use of Oral Colchicine for Low-Back Pain. A Double-Blind Study. Spine. 1988; 13:354–357

[66] Goodkin K, Gullion CM, Agras WS. A Randomized, Double-Blind, Placebo-Controlled Trial of Trazodone Hydrochloride in Chronic Low Back Pain Syndrome. J Clin Psychopharmacol. 1990; 10:269–278

[67] Deyo RA, Walsh NE, Martin DC, et al. A Controlled Trial of Transcutaneous Electrical Stimulation (TENS) and Exercise for Chronic Low Back Pain. N Engl J Med. 1990; 322:1627–1634

[68] Mathews JA, Hickling J. Lumbar Traction: A Double-Blind Controlled Study for Sciatica. Rheumatol Rehabil. 1975; 14:222–225

[69] van Poppel NNM, Koes BW, van der Ploeg T, et al. Lumbar Supports and Education for the Prevention of Low Back Pain in Industry: A Randomized Controlled Study. Journal of the American Medical Association. 1998; 279:1789–1794

[70] Bush C, Ditto B, Feuerstein M. A Controlled Evaluation of Paraspinal EMG Biofeedback in the Treatment of Chronic Low Back Pain. Health Psychol. 1985; 4:307–321

[71] Frost FA, Jessen B, Siggaard-Andersen J. A Control, Double-Blind Comparison of Mepivicaine Injection Versus Saline Injection for Myofascial Pain. Lancet. 1980; 1:499–501

[72] Carette S, Marcoux S, Truchon R, et al. A Controlled Trial of Corticosteroid Injections into Facet Joints for Chronic Low Back Pain. New England Journal of Medicine. 1991; 325:1002–1007

[73] Jackson RP. The Facet Syndrome. Myth or Reality? Clin Orthop Rel Res. 1992; 279:110–121

[74] Manheimer E, White A, Berman B, et al. Meta-analysis: acupuncture for low back pain. Ann Intern Med. 2005; 142:651–663

[75] Resnick DK, Choudhri TF, Dailey AT, et al. Part 13: Injection therapies, low-back pain, and lumbar fusion. Journal of Neurosurgery: Spine. 2005; 2:707–715

[76] Resnick DK, Choudhri TF, Dailey AT, et al. Part 7: Intractable low-back pain without stenosis or spondylolisthesis. Journal of Neurosurgery (Spine). 2005; 2:670–672

[77] Fritzell P, Hagg O, Wessberg P, et al. 2001 Volvo Award Winner in Clinical Studies: Lumbar fusion versus nonsurgical treatment for chronic low back pain: a multicenter randomized controlled trial from the Swedish Lumbar Spine Study Group. Spine. 2001; 26:2521–32; discussion 2532–4

[78] Ivar Brox J, Sorensen R, Friis A, et al. Randomized clinical trial of lumbar instrumented fusion and cognitive intervention and exercises in patients with chronic low back pain and disc degeneration. Spine. 2003; 28:1913–1921

[79] Resnick DK, Choudhri TF, Dailey AT, et al. Part 11: Interbody techniques for lumbar fusion. Journal of Neurosurgery (Spine). 2005; 2:692–699

[80] Turner JA, Ersek M, Herron L, et al. Patient Outcomes After Lumbar Spinal Fusions. Journal of the American Medical Association. 1992; 268:907–911

[81] Lewis PJ, Weir BKA, Broad R, et al. Long-Term Prospective Study of Lumbosacral Discectomy. J Neurosurg. 1987; 67:49–53

[82] Weinstein JN, Lurie JD, Tosteson TD, et al. Surgical vs nonoperative treatment for lumbar disk herniation: the Spine Patient Outcomes Research Trial (SPORT) observational cohort. JAMA. 2006; 296:2451–2459

[83] Sorensen ST, Bech-Azeddine R, Fruensgaard Søren, et al. Outcomes following discectomy for lumbar disc herniationin patients with substantial back pain. Journal of Neurosurgery (Spine). 2020; 33:623–626

[84] Resnick DK, Choudhri TF, Dailey AT, et al. Part 8: Lumbar fusion for disc herniation and radiculopathy. Journal of Neurosurgery (Spine). 2005; 2:673–678

[85] Resnick DK, Choudhri TF, Dailey AT, et al. Part 12: Pedicle screw fixation as an adjunct to posterolateral fusion for low-back pain. Journal of Neurosurgery (Spine). 2005; 2:700–706

[86] Lorenz M, Zindrick M, Schwaegler P, et al. A Comparison of Single-Level Fusions With and Without Hardware. Spine. 1991; 16:S455–S458

[87] Gatchel RJ, Mayer TG, Capra P, et al. Quantification of Lumbar Function, VI: The Use of Psychological Measures in Guiding Physical Functional Restoration. Spine. 1986; 11:36–42

[88] Morley S, Pallin V. Scaling the Affective Domain of Pain: A Study of the Dimensionality of Verbal Descriptors. Pain. 1995; 62:39–49

[89] Wray CC, Easom S, Hoskinson J. Coccydinia. Etiology and Treatment. Journal of Bone and Joint Surgery. 1991; 73B:335–338

[90] Lath R, Rajshekhar V, Chacko G. Sacral Hemangioma as a Cause of Coccydinia. Neuroradiology. 1998; 40:524–526

[91] Thiele GH. Coccydinia: Cause and Treatment. Dis Colon Rectum. 1963; 6:422–435

[92] Lourie J, Young S. Avascular Necrosis of the Coccyx: A Cause of Coccydinia? Case Report and Histological Findings in Sixteen Patients. Br J Clin Pract. 1985; 39:247–248

[93] Raj PP, Raj PP. Miscellaneous Pain Disorders. In: Pain Medicine: A Comprehensive Review. St. Louis: C V Mosby; 1996:492–501

[94] Boeglin ER. Coccydinia. Journal of Bone and Joint Surgery. 1991; 73B

[95] Loev MA, Varklet VL, Wilsey BL, et al. Cryoablation: A Novel Approach to Neurolysis of the Ganglion Impar. Anesthesiology. 1998; 88:1391–1393

[96] Plancarte R, Amescua C, Patt RB, et al. Superior Hypogastric Plexus Block for Pelvic Cancer Pain. Anesthesiology. 1990; 73:236–239

[97] Law JD, Lehman RAW, Kirsch WM, et al. Reoperation After Lumbar Intervertebral Disc Surgery. J Neurosurg. 1978; 48:259–263

[98] Davis RA. A Long-Term Outcome Analysis of 984 Surgically Treated Herniated Lumbar Discs. Journal of Neurosurgery. 1994; 80:415–421

[99] Caputy AJ, Luessenhop AJ. Long-Term Evaluation of Decompressive Surgery for Degenerative Lumbar Stenosis. Journal of Neurosurgery. 1992; 77:669–676

[100] Markwalder TM, Battaglia M. Failed Back Surgery Syndrome. Part 1: Analysis of the Clinical Presentation and Results of Testing Procedures for Instability of the Lumbar Spine in 171 Patients. Acta Neurochirurgica. 1993; 123:46–51

[101] Burton CV, Kirkaldy-Willis WH, Yong-Hing K, et al. Causes of Failure of Surgery on the Lumbar Spine. Clinical Orthopedics. 1981; 157:191–199

[102] Quencer RM, Tenner M, Rothman L. The Postoperative Myelogram: Radiographic Evaluation of Arachnoiditis and Dural/Arachnoidal Tears. Radiology. 1977; 123:667–669

[103] Ross JS, Masaryk TJ, Modic MT, et al. MR Imaging of Lumbar Arachnoiditis. American Journal of Neuroradiology. 1987; 8:885–892

[104] Delamarter RB, Ross JS, Masaryk TJ, et al. Diagnosis of Lumbar Arachnoiditis by Magnetic Resonance Imaging. Spine. 1990; 15:304–310

[105] Roca J, Moreta D, Ubierna MT, et al. The Results of Surgical Treatment of Lumbar Arachnoiditis. International Orthopedics. 1993; 17:77–81

[106] Martin-Ferrer S. Failure of Autologous Fat Grafts to Prevent Post Operative Epidural Fibrosis in Surgery of the Lumbar Spine. Neurosurgery. 1989; 24:718–721

[107] North RB, Campbell JN, James CS, et al. Failed Back Surgery Syndrome: 5-Year Follow-Up in 102 Patients Undergoing Repeated Operations. Neurosurgery. 1991; 28:685–691

[108] Ross JS, Robertson JT, Frederickson RCA, et al. Association Between Lumbar Peridural Scar and Recurrent Radicular Pain After Lumbar Discectomy: Magnetic Resonance Evaluation. Neurosurgery. 1996; 38:855–863

[109] Cooper PR. Comment on Ross J S, et al.: Association Between Peridural Scar and Recurrent Radicular Pain After Lumbar Discectomy. Neurosurgery. 1996; 38

[110] Sonntag VKH. Comment on Ross J S, et al.: Association Between Peridural Scar and Recurrent

[111] Bundschuh CV, Modic MT, Ross JS, et al. Epidural Fibrosis and Recurrent Disc Herniation in the Lumbar Spine: Assessment with Magnetic Resonance. AJNR. 1988; 9:169–178

[112] Sotiropoulos S, Chafetz NE, Lang P, et al. Differentiation Between Postoperative Scar and Recurrent Disk Herniation: Prospective Comparison of MR, CT, and Contrast-Enhanced CT. AJNR. 1989; 10:639–643

[113] Hueftle MG, Modic MT, Ross JS, et al. Lumbar Spine: Postoperative MR Imaging with Gd-DPTA. Radiology. 1988; 167:817–824

[114] Braun IF, Hoffman JC, Davis PC, et al. Contrast Enhancement in CT Differentiation between Recurrent Disk Herniation and Postoperative Scar: Prospective Study. AJR. 1985; 145:785–790

[115] Byrd SE, Cohn ML, Biggers SL, et al. The Radiologic Evaluation of the Symptomatic Postoperative Lumbar Spine Patient. Spine. 1985; 10:652–661

[116] Greenwood J, McGuire TH, Kimbell F. A Study of the Causes of Failure in the Herniated Intervertebral Disc Operation. An Analysis of Sixty-Seven Reoperated Cases. J Neurosurg. 1952; 9:15–20

[117] Jorgensen J, Hansen PH, Steenskov V, et al. A Clinical and Radiological Study of Chronic Lower Spinal Arachnoiditis. Neuroradiology. 1975; 9:139–144

[118] Johnston JDH, Matheny JB. Microscopic Lysis of Lumbar Adhesive Arachnoiditis. Spine. 1978; 3:36–39

74

75 Lumbar Disc Herniation and Radiculopathy

75.1 General information

75.2 Pathophysiology

Intervertebral discs may undergo degenerative changes (p. 1327); see ▶ Table 74.1 for description: this includes desiccation and fibrosis, which further leads to fissuring and tearing, which in turn increases the risk of herniation of disc material outside the normal confines of the disc space.

75.3 Herniation zones

75.3.1 General information

Lumbar disc herniations typically occur in one of several zones illustrated in ▶ Fig. 75.1.

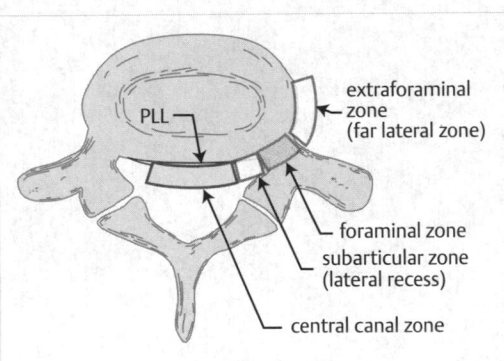

Fig. 75.1 Zones of lumbar disc herniation. Abbreviation: PLL = posterior longitudinal ligament.

PLL

extraforaminal zone (far lateral zone)

foraminal zone

subarticular zone (lateral recess)

central canal zone

75.3.2 Central and paramedial disc herniations

The posterior longitudinal ligament is strongest in the midline, and the posterolateral annulus may bear a disproportionate portion of the load exerted by the weight from above. This may explain why most posteriorly herniated lumbar discs (HLD) occur slightly off to one side (paramedian) within the central canal zone or in the subarticular zone (▶ Fig. 75.1). In the lumbar spine this characteristically compresses the nerve root en passant (that is, the nerve in the lateral recess just before it exits through the neural foramen of the level *below*; e.g., at L4–5 this would typically involve the L5 nerve root).

75

75.3.3 Extreme lateral disc herniation

Disc herniations in the foraminal zone or extraforaminal zone are often considered extreme lateral and often involve the nerve root *exiting* at that level (p. 1263).

75.4 Other disc herniation variants

1. intravertebral disc herniation (p. 1266): AKA Schmorl's node.
2. intradural disc herniation (p. 1266)
3. limbus fracture: traumatic separation of a segment of bone from the edge of the vertebral ring apophysis at the site of anular attachment. May accompany HLD

75.5 Clinical findings with hernaited lumbar disc

75.5.1 Characteristic findings on the history

- symptoms may start off with back pain, which after days or weeks gradually or sometimes suddenly yields to radicular pain often with reduction of the back pain
- precipitating factors: various factors are often blamed, but are rarely identified[1] with certainty
- pain relief upon flexing the knee and thigh (e.g., lying supine with a pillow under the knees)
- patients generally avoid excessive movements; however, remaining in any one position (sitting, standing, or lying) too long may also exacerbate the pain, sometimes necessitating position changes at intervals that range from every few minutes to 10–20 minutes. This is distinct from constant writhing in pain e.g., with ureteral obstruction
- "cough effect": ↑ pain with coughing, sneezing, or straining at the stool. Occurred in 87% of patients with HLD in one series[2]
- bladder symptoms: the incidence of voiding dysfunction is 1–18%.[3] (p 966) Most common: difficulty voiding, straining, or urinary retention. Reduced bladder sensation may be the earliest finding. The possible causes of this are sensory loss, or incomplete interruption of the preganglionic parasympathetic fibers. Later it is not unusual to see "irritative" symptoms including urinary urgency, frequency (including nocturia), increased post-void residual. Less common: enuresis, and dribbling incontinence[4]; NB: urinary symptoms may indicate cauda equina syndrome (p. 1254). Occasionally, radiculopathy from HLD may present only with bladder symptoms which may improve after surgery.[5] Discectomy may improve bladder function, but this cannot be assured

Back pain per se is usually a minor component (only 1% of patients with acute low back pain have sciatica[6]), and when it is the only presenting symptom, other causes should be sought; see Low back pain (p. 1226). Sciatica has such a high sensitivity for disc herniation, that the likelihood of a clinically significant disc herniation[7] in the absence of sciatica is ≈ 1 in 1000. Exceptions include a central disc herniation which may cause symptoms of lumbar stenosis (i.e., neurogenic claudication) or a cauda equina syndrome.

75

75.5.2 Physical findings in radiculopathy

General information

Nerve root impingement gives rise to a set of signs and symptoms present to variable degrees. Characteristic syndromes are described for the most common nerve roots involved; see Nerve root syndromes (p. 1253).

In a series of patients referred to neurosurgical outpatient clinics for radiating leg pain, 28% had motor loss (yet only 12% listed motor weakness as a presenting complaint), 45% had sensory disturbance, and 51% had reflex changes.[8]

Findings suggestive of nerve root impingement include the following. ► Table 75.1 shows the sensitivity and specificity of some findings on the exam among patients with sciatica.

1. signs/symptoms of radiculopathy (► Table 75.1)
   a) pain radiating down LE
   b) motor weakness
   c) dermatomal sensory changes
   d) reflex changes: mental factors may influence symmetry[9]
2. positive nerve root tension sign(s): including Lasègue's sign (see below)
3. tenderness over the sciatic notch

Table 75.1 Sensitivity and specificity of physical findings for HLD in patients with sciatica[10]

Test	Comment	Sensitivity	Specificity
ipsilateral SLR	positive result: pain at <60° elevation	0.80	0.40
crossed SLR	reproduction of contralateral pain	0.25	0.90
↓ ankle jerk	HLD usually at L5–1 (total absence increases specificity)	0.50	0.60
sensory loss	area of loss is poor in localizing level of HLD	0.50	0.50
↓ patellar reflex	suggests upper HLD	0.50	NA
Weakness			
knee extension (quadriceps)	HLD usually at L3–4	<0.01	0.99
ankle dorsiflexion (anterior tibialis)	HLD usually at L4–5	0.35	0.70
ankle plantarflexion (gastrocs)	HLD usually at L5–1	0.06	0.95
great toe extension (EHL)	HLD at L5–1 in 60%, at L4–5 in 30%	0.50	0.70

Nerve root tension signs

Includes[11]:

1. Lasègue's sign: AKA straight leg raising (SLR) test. Helps differentiate sciatica from pain due to hip pathology. Test: with patient supine, raise afflicted limb by the ankle until pain is elicited[12] (should occur at <60°, tension in nerve increases little above this angle). A positive test consists of leg pain or paresthesias in the distribution of pain (back pain alone does not qualify). The patient may also extend the hip (by lifting it off table) to reduce the angle. Although not part of Lasègue's sign, ankle dorsiflexion with SLR usually augments pain due to nerve root compression. SLR primarily tenses L5 and S1, L4 less so, and more proximal roots very little. Nerve-root compression produces a positive Lasègue's sign in ≈ 83% of cases[2] (more likely to be positive in patients < 30 yrs of age with HLD[13]). May be positive in lumbosacral plexopathy (p.571). Note: flexing both thighs with the knees extended ("long-sitting" or sitting knee extension) may be tolerated further than flexing the single symptomatic side alone

2. Cram test: with patient supine, raise the symptomatic leg with the knee slightly flexed. Then, extend the knee. Results similar to SLR

3. crossed straight leg-raising test AKA Fajersztajn's sign: SLR on the painless leg causes contralateral limb pain (a greater degree of elevation is usually required than the painful side). More specific but less sensitive than SLR (97% of patients undergoing surgery with this sign have confirmed HLD[14]). May correlate with a more *central* disc herniation

4. femoral stretch test,[15] AKA reverse straight leg raising: patient prone, examiner's palm at popliteal fossa, knee is maximally dorsiflexed. Often positive with L2, L3, or L4 nerve root compression (e.g., in upper lumbar disc herniation), or with extreme lateral lumbar disc herniation (may also be positive in diabetic femoral neuropathy or psoas hematoma); in these situations SLR (Lasègue's sign) is frequently negative (since L5 & S1 are not involved)

5. "bowstring sign": once pain occurs with SLR, lower the foot to the bed by flexing knee, keeping the hip flexed. Sciatic pain ceases with this maneuver, but hip pain persists

6. sitting knee extension test: with patient seated and both hips and knees flexed 90°, slowly extend one knee. Stretches nerve roots as much as a moderate degree of SLR

Other signs useful in evaluation for lumbar radiculopathy

1. FABER: an acronym for Flexion ABduction External-Rotation, AKA FABERE test (the terminal "E" is for extension), AKA Patrick's test (after Hugh Talbot Patrick). A test of hip motion. Method: the hip and knee are flexed and the lateral malleolus is placed on the contralateral knee. The ipsilateral knee is gently displaced downward towards the exam table. This stresses the hip joint and does not usually exacerbate true nerve root compression. Often markedly positive in the presence of hip joint disease—e.g., trochanteric bursitis (p.1332)—sacroiliitis or mechanical low-back pain

2. Trendelenburg sign: examiner observes pelvis from behind while patient raises one leg while standing. Normally the pelvis remains horizontal. A positive sign occurs when the pelvis tilts down toward the side of the lifted leg indicating weakness of the contralateral thigh abductors on the stance leg (primarily the gluteus medius, which is innervated by the superior gluteal nerve with contributions from L5 and some from L4 & S1)

75

3. crossed adductors: in eliciting patellar reflex (knee jerk (KJ)), the contralateral thigh adductors contract. In the presence of a hyperactive ipsilateral KJ it may indicate an upper motor neuron lesion; in the presence of a hypoactive ipsilateral KJ it may be a form of pathological spread, indicating nerve root irritability

4. Hoover sign[16]: to distinguish unilateral functional weakness of iliopsoas from organic weakness using synergistic contraction of the contralateral gluteus medius. The supine patient is asked to lift one leg off the bed against resistance from the examiner's hand. The examiner simultaneously places the palm of his/her other hand under the heel of the unlifted leg and gently lifts. Test 1: when the patient lifts the normal leg, if the paretic leg pushes down with more force than was exhibited on manual testing of the limb beforehand, the weakness is judged functional; if the force is equally weak the weakness is judged organic. Test 1 cannot be used if the hip extensor was normal beforehand. Test 2 (the better known test): the patient is asked to lift the weak leg. If the heel on the normal side lifts passively by the examiner, it suggests the weakness is functional (i.e., the patient is not trying). Not totally reliable[17,18]

5. abductor sign: an alternative to the Hoover test, to differentiate functional from organic weakness in the thigh abductors using synergistic contraction of the contralateral thigh abductors.[18] With the patient supine, the examiner places a hand on the lateral aspect of both legs. The patient is asked to abduct one leg, and then the other while the examiner applies resistance with his/her hand. The examiner mentally notes the response of the non-abducting LE. The results are as noted in ▶ Table 75.2

Table 75.2 Abductor sign

Abducting LE	Contralateral (nonabducting) LE	
	Organic weakness	Functional weakness
weak LE	maintains position	hyperadducts
normal LE	hyperadducts	maintains position

Nerve root syndromes

Due to the facts listed below, a herniated lumbar disc (HLD) usually spares the nerve root exiting at that interspace, and impinges on the nerve exiting from the neural foramen one level *below* (e.g., a L5–1 HLD usually causes S1 radiculopathy). This gives rise to the characteristic lumbar nerve root syndromes shown in ▶ Table 75.3.

Table 75.3 Lumbar disc syndromes

Syndrome	Level of herniated lumbar disc		
	L3–4	L4–5	L5–1
root usually compressed	L4	L5	S1
% of lumbar discs	3–10% (5% average)	40–45%	45–50%
reflex diminished	knee jerk[a] (Westphal's sign)	medial hamstring[b]	Achilles[a] (ankle jerk)
motor weakness	quadriceps femoris (knee extension)	tibialis anterior (foot drop) & EHL[c]	gastrocnemius (plantarflexion), ± EHL[c]
decreased sensation[d]	medial malleolus & medial foot	large toe web & dorsum of foot	lateral malleolus & lateral foot
pain distribution	anterior thigh	posterior LE	posterior LE, often to ankle

[a] Jendrassik maneuver may reinforce (see ▶ Table 30.2)
[b] medial hamstring reflex is unreliable (not always pure L5), may also stimulate adductors when eliciting
[c] see Weakness in ▶ Table 75.1 for breakdown
[d] sensory impairment is most common in the distal extremes of the dermatome[19]

Important applied anatomy in lumbar disc disease:

1. in the lumbar region, the nerve root exits *below* and in close proximity to the pedicle of its like-numbered vertebra
2. the intervertebral disc space is located well below the pedicle
3. not all patients have 5 lumbar vertebrae; see Localizing levels in spine surgery (p. 1719)

75

75.5.3 Cauda equina syndrome

Cauda equina syndrome (CES) is a clinical condition arising from dysfunction of multiple lumbar and sacral nerve roots within the lumbar spinal canal. To facilitate treatment, it is important to identify CES cases that are due to a surgially treatable condition. Since "no symptom or sign or combination can establish or exclude a diagnosis of CES,"[20,21] it has been recommended that MRI should be done as rapidly as possible.

▶ **Definition.** A 2009 review[22] found 17 different definitions for CES. For standardization, the following definition was proposed:

The diagnosis of cauda equina syndrome requires[22]:
1. one or more of the following:
   - bladder and/or bowel dysfunction
   - reduced sensation in the perineal region ("saddle anesthesia")
   - new onset of sexual dysfunction
2. possibly with neurologic deficit in the lower extremities (motor/sensory loss, reflex changes)

✖ It is recommended to avoid terms such as "complete", "incomplete", "true", "classic", "full blown", "partial"…[22]

Possible clinical findings in CES:
1. sphincter disturbance:
   a) urinary retention: the most consistent finding. Sensitivity ≈ 90% (at some point in time during course).[23,24] To evaluate acutely: have patient empty bladder and check post-void residual (by catheterization or with bladder ultrasound). Cystometrogram (when done) typically shows a hypotonic bladder with decreased sensation and increased capacity
   b) urinary and/or fecal incontinence[25]: some patients with urinary retention will present with overflow incontinence
   c) anal sphincter tone: assess resting tone and voluntary contraction. Diminished in 60–80%
2. "saddle anesthesia": the most common sensory deficit. Distribution: region of the anus, lower genitals, perineum, over the buttocks, posterior-superior thighs. Sensitivity ≈ 75%. Once total perineal anesthesia develops, patients tend to have permanent bladder paralysis[26]
3. significant motor weakness: usually involves more than a single nerve root (if untreated, may progress to paraplegia)
4. low back pain and/or sciatica (sciatica is usually bilateral, but may be unilateral or entirely absent; prognosis may be worse when absent or bilateral[24])
5. bilateral absence of Achilles reflex has been noted[27]
6. sexual dysfunction (usually not detected until a later time)

▶ **Categorization of CES.** Using MRI, a prospective series of 198 CES patients[21] classified them as:
1. scan positive CES: (24%) axial T2 MRI shows > 75% canal occlusion or no CSF signal. These patients were more likely to describe saddle anesthesia than the other groups
2. mixed scan results: (38%) radiographic evidence of nerve root compression or displacement not meeting criteria of scan positive CES (including crowding of cauda equina, nerve root compression or displacement)
3. scan negative CES: (31%) no nerve root compression or other radiographic explanation for CES symptoms. 96% did not have an explanatory diagnosis with 23 months mean follow-up. Etiologies included: stress incontinence, hyperactive bladder, spinal cord inflammation, spinal AVM, bladder inhibition due to pain or medication effects (Fowler's syndrome)

81% of patients referred to neurosurgery with CES have imaging that is normal or does not explain the symptoms (i.e., 81% do not have scan positive CES).[28]

Scan positive CES: usually due to compression of the cauda equina (the bundle of nerve root below the conus medullaris arising from the lumbar enlargement and conus). See ▶ Table 55.9 for features to help differentiate CES from a conus lesion.

Etiologies of CES includes (items with a dagger (†) typically produce scan postivie CES):
1. compression of cauda equina
   a) massive herniated lumbar disc†: see below
   b) tumor
      - e.g., metastatic disease to the spine with epidural extension causing compression†
      - intravascular lymphomatosis (B-cell lymphoma) (p. 842): a circulating lymphoma without solid mass. Often presents with CNS findings: dementia, enhancing meninges on MRI, lymphoma cells in CSF, and CES

c) free fat graft following discectomy[†][29]
d) trauma: fracture fragments compressing cauda equina[†]
e) spinal epidural hematoma[†]

2. infection: may cause neurologic deficit from
   a) compression: typically from spinal epidural abscess complicating discitis or vertebral osteomyelitis[†]
   b) a significant number of cases of CES from infection may be due to vascular compromise resulting from local *septic thrombophlebitis*. This may carry a worse prognosis as surgical decompression cannot correct this mechanism

3. neuropathy:
   a) ischemic
   b) inflammatory

4. ankylosing spondylitis (p. 1365): etiology is often obscure (i.e., compression may be absent)

▶ **CES associated with lumbar disc herniation.** May be due to massive herniated disc, usually midline, most common at L4–5, often superimposed on a preexisting condition (spinal stenosis, tethered cord…).[25]

Prevalence of CES

1. 0.0004 in all patients with LBP[7]
2. only ≈ 1–2% of HLD that come to surgery[7]

Time course: CES tends to develop either acutely, or (less typically) slowly (prognosis is worse in the acute onset group, especially for return of bladder function, which occurred in only ≈ 50%).[23] 3 patterns[30]:

• Group I—sudden onset of CES symptoms with no previous low back symptoms
• Group II—previous history of recurrent backache & sciatica, the current episode combined with CES
• Group III—presentation with backache & bilateral sciatica that later develop CES

Timing of discectomy in CES: controversial, and the point of contention in numerous lawsuits. In spite of early reports emphasizing rapid decompression,[27] other reports found no correlation between the time to surgery after presentation and the return of function.[23,24] Some evidence supports the goal of performing surgery within 48 hours of onet (although performing surgery within 24 hours if possible is considered desirable, there is no statistically significant proof that delaying up to 48 hours is detrimental).[31,32]

Operative issues: some advise a bilateral laminectomy[25] (but this is not mandatory). Occasionally, when it is difficult to remove a very tense midline disc herniation, transdural removal may be helpful.[27]

75.6 Radiographic evaluation

See Radiographic evaluation under Low back pain (p. 1706). 70% of herniated discs that migrate do so *inferiorly*.

75.7 Nonsurgical treatment

75.7.1 Natural history of lumbar disc herniation

The rationale underlying the use of nonsurgical treatment measures for herniated disc is to impart symptomatic relief while providing an opportunity for the body's natural healing mechanisms to reduce the pressure on the nerve root. Spontaneous reduction of the volume of herniate disc material occurs as a result of a number of processes mediated by the immune system which involves activated macrophages in conjunction with inflammatory cytokines, angiogenesis inducing factor and matrix degrading enzymes.[33]

As a result, over 85% of patients with acute disc herniation will have symptomatic resolution *without* surgical intervention in an average of 6 weeks[34] (70% within 4 weeks[35]). There is often, but not always, a corresponding improvement in the MRI appearance.

75.7.2 Conservative treatment methodologies

Treatments may appear to be effective because of the high spontaneous resolution rate (85%). To adequately power a study to prove that a particular treatment is more effective than the natural history would require extremely large enrollment and would be quite costly. While conservative treatment can help control pain, unfortunately, to date there is no high-quality study to show statistically significant benefit of any particular conservative treatment modality compared to the natural history for the relief of radicular symptoms.

Conservative treatment measures employed for herniated disc are essentially the same as those used for low back pain in general (see nonsurgical treatment measures (p. 1237)).

75.8 Surgical treatment

75.8.1 General information

Numerous studies have shown beneficial effects of surgery for herniated lumbar discs. The oft-misunderstood Spine Patient Outcomes Research Trial (SPORT) (p. 1262) failed in its primary objective; however, it did demonstrate significant benefits of surgery when it was indicated.

75.8.2 Indications for surgery

No predictive factors have been identified that can determine which patients are likely to improve on their own and which would be better served with surgery.

Surgical indications in patients with a radiographically identified herniated disc that correlates with findings on the history and physical exam:
1. failure of non-surgical management. Because of the high spontaneous resolution rate (see Natural history (p. 1255)) most clinicians advocate waiting ≈ 5 to 8 weeks from the onset of radiculopathy before considering surgery (assuming none of the emergent items listed below applies)
2. "EMERGENT SURGERY": (i.e., before the 5–8 weeks of symptoms have lapsed). Indications:
   a) cauda equina syndrome (CES): (see below)
   b) *progressive* motor deficit (e.g., foot drop). NB: paresis of unknown duration is a doubtful indication for surgery[1,36,37] (no study has documented that there is less motor deficit in surgically treated patients with this finding[38]). However, the acute development or progression of motor weakness is considered an indication for rapid surgical decompression
   c) "urgent" surgery may be indicated for patients whose pain remains intolerable in spite of adequate narcotic pain medication
3. ± patients who do not want to invest the time in non-surgical treatment if it is possible that they will ultimately require surgery (relief is more rapid with surgery than conservative management[39])

75.8.3 Surgical intervention

Booking the case: Lumbar discectomy

Also see defaults & disclaimers (p. 25).
1. position: prone
2. equipment: microscope (if used), minimally invasive retractors (if used)
3. consent (in lay terms for the patient—not all-inclusive):
   a) procedure: surgery through the back to go between the bones and remove the piece of disc that is pressing on the nerve(s)
   b) alternatives: nonsurgical management
   c) complications: usual spine surgery complications (p. 1220), plus the disc can herniate again in the same place in ≈ 6% of cases, it is possible that a fragment of disc can be missed at the time of surgery, there might not be the amount of pain relief desired (back pain does not respond as well to surgery as nerve-root pain)

75.8.4 Surgical options for lumbar radiculopathy

Once it is decided to treat surgically, options include:
1. trans-canal approaches
   a) standard open lumbar laminectomy and discectomy: 65–85% reported no sciatica one year post-op compared to 36% for conservative treatment.[40] Long-term results (> 1 year) were similar. 10% of patients underwent further back surgery during the first year[40]
   b) "microdiscectomy"[41,42]: similar to standard procedure, but a smaller incision is utilized. Advantages may be cosmetic, shortened hospital stay, lower blood loss. May be more difficult to retrieve some fragments.[43 (p 1319),44] Overall efficacy is similar to standard discectomy[45]
   c) sequestrectomy: removal of only the herniated portion of the disc without entering the disc space to remove disc material from there
2. intradiscal procedures (see below): a number of procedures have been devised over the years to percutaneously treat HLD by creating a cavity within the disc. Some have been abandoned for various reasons, not the least of which is the controversy regarding the validity of the underlying premise that this can work
   a) chemonucleolysis: using chymopapain to enzymatically dissolve the disc (no longer used)
   b) automated percutaneous lumbar discectomy: utilizes a nucleotome
   c) percutaneous endoscopic intradiscal discectomy: see below
   d) intradiscal endothermal therapy (IDET or IDTA): see below
   e) laser disc decompression

75.8.5 Intradiscal surgical procedures (ISP)

ISPs (see below for specific procedures) are among the most controversial procedures for lumbar spine surgery. The theoretical advantage is that epidural scarring is avoided, and that a smaller incision or even just a puncture site is used. This is also purported to reduce postoperative pain and hospital stay (often performed as an outpatient procedure). The conceptual problem with ISPs is that they are directed at removing disc material from the center of the disc space (which is not producing symptoms) and rely on the reduced intradiscal pressure to decompress the herniated portion of the disc from the nerve root. Only ≈ 10–15% of patients considered for surgical treatment of disc disease are candidates for an ISP. ISPs are usually done under local anesthetic in order to permit the patient to report nerve root pain to identify impingement on a nerve root by the surgical instrument or needle. Overall, ISPs are not recommended until rigorous controlled trials prove the efficacy.[10]

Indications utilized by proponents of intradiscal procedures:
1. type of disc herniation: appropriate only for "contained" disc herniation (i.e., outer margin of anulus fibrosus intact)
2. appropriate level: best for L4–5 HLD. May also be used at L3–4. Difficult but often workable (utilizing angled instruments or other techniques) at L5–1 because of the angle required and interference by iliac crest
3. not recommended in presence of severe neurologic deficit[46]

Results:
"Success" rate (≈ pain free and return to work when appropriate) reported ranges from 37–75%.[47,48,49]

Automated percutaneous lumbar discectomy: AKA nucleoplasty. Utilizes a nucleotome[50] to remove disc material from the center of the intervertebral disc space. 1-year success rate of 37%. Complications include cauda equina syndrome from improper nucleotome placement.[51] In another study, nucleoplasty (with or without IDET [see below]) for HLD showed only modest reduction in pain at 9 months.[52]

Laser disc decompression: Insertion of a needle into the disc, and introduction of a laser fiberoptic cable through the needle to allow a laser to burn a hole in the center of the disc[53,54] (with or without endoscopic visualization).

The 2014 North American Spine Society Coverage Committee[55] position statement:
"Laser spine surgery in the **cervical** or **lumbar** spine is NOT indicated at this time. Due to lack of high quality clinical trials concerning laser spine surgery with the cervical or lumbar spine, it cannot be endorsed as an adjunct to open, minimally invasive, or percutaneous surgical techniques."

Percutaneous endoscopic lumbar discectomy (PELD): This term refers to an essentially intradiscal procedure indicated primarily for contained disc herniations, although some small "noncontained" fragments may be treatable.[56] No large randomized study has been done to compare the technique to the accepted standard, open discectomy (with or without microscope). In one report[57] of 326 patients with L4–5 HLD, only 8 (2.4%) met study criteria (no previous operation, failure of conservative treatment, imaging study proving disc protrusion followed by discography to R/O "disc perforation") for PELD. Of these 8, only 3 were reported as having a good result. This study is not adequate for evaluating the technique.

Intradiscal endothermal therapy (IDET): AKA intradiscal (electro)thermal anuloplasty (IDTA). Efficacy: 23–60% at 1 year for treating "internal disc disruption"[58] (radial fissures in the nucleus pulposus extending into the anulus fibrosus) which is purported to account for 40% of patients with chronic low back pain of unknown etiology.[59]

75.8.6 Adjunctive treatment in lumbar laminectomy

Epidural steroids following discectomy

Perioperative epidural steroids after routine surgery for lumbar degenerative disease may result in a small reduction of post-op pain, length of stay, and the risk of not returning to work at 1 year, but most of the evidence originates from studies not using validated outcome assessment that favor positive results, and further study is recommended (various agents, dosages, co-administered drugs, and delivery methods were reported).[60] However, the combination of systemic steroids at the start of the case (Depo-Medrol® 160 mg IM and methylprednisolone sodium succinate (Solu-Medrol®) 250 mg IV) combined with infiltration of 30 ml of 0.25% bupivacaine (Marcaine®) into the paraspinal muscles at incision and closure, may reduce hospital stay and post-op narcotic requirements.[61]

75.8.7 Methods to reduce scar formation

Epidural free fat graft

The use of an autogenous free fat graft in the epidural space has been employed in an attempt to reduce post-op epidural scar formation. Opinion varies widely as to the effectiveness, some feel it is helpful, others feel it actually exacerbates scarring.[62] In some patients, no evidence of the graft will be found on reoperation years later. The fat graft can very rarely be a cause of nerve root compression[63] or cauda equina syndrome[29] within the first few days post-op, and there is a case report of compression 6 years following surgery.[64]

Other measures

Other measures include the placement of barrier films or gels. There are numerous products available, none has been shown to have reproducible benefit.

75.8.8 Risks of lumbar laminectomy

General information

Overall risk of mortality in large series[65,66]: 6 per 10,000 (i.e., 0.06%), most often due to septicemia, MI, or PE. Complication rates are very difficult to determine accurately,[40] but the following is included as a guideline.

Common complications

1. infection:
   a) superficial wound infection: 0.9–5%[67] (risk is increased with age, long-term steroids, obesity, ? DM): most are caused by *S. aureus*; see Laminectomy wound infection (p. 377) for management
   b) deep infection: < 1% (see below under Uncommon complications)
2. increased motor deficit: 1–8% (some transient)
3. unintended "incidental" durotomy (p. 1260) (the term "unintended durotomy" has been recommended in preference to "dural tear," see below): incidence is 0.3–13% (risk increases to ≈ 18% in redo operations).[68] Possible sequelae include those listed in ► Table 75.4
   a) CSF fistula (external CSF leak): the risk of a CSF fistula requiring operative repair is ≈ 10 per 10,000[65]
   b) pseudomeningocele: 0.7–2%[68] (may appear similar radiographically to spinal epidural abscess (SEA), but post-op SEA often enhances, is more irregular, and is associated with muscle edema)
4. recurrent herniated lumbar disc (same level either side) (p. 1267): 4% (with 10-year follow-up)[69]
5. postoperative urinary retention (POUR) (p. 1260): usually temporary, but may delay hospital discharge

75

Uncommon complications

1. direct injury to neural structures. For large disc herniations, consider a bilateral exposure to reduce risk

2. injury to structures anterior to the vertebral bodies (VB): injured by breaching the anterior longitudinal ligament (ALL) through the disc space, e.g., with pituitary rongeur. The depth of disc space penetration with instruments should be kept ≤ 3 cm, since 5% of lumbar discs had diameters as small as 3.3 cm.[70] Asymptomatic perforations of the ALL occur in up to 12% of discectomies. Breach of the ALL risks potential injuries to:

   a) great vessels[71]: risks include potentially fatal hemorrhage, and arteriovenous fistula which may present years later. Most such injuries occur with L4–5 discectomies. Only ≈ 50% bleed into the disc space intraoperatively, the rest bleed into the retroperitoneum. Emergent laparotomy or endovascular treatment[72] is indicated, preferably by a surgeon with vascular surgical experience, if available. Mortality rate is 37–67%
      - aorta: the aortic bifurcation is on the left side of the lower part of the L4 VB, and so the aorta may be injured above this level
      - below L4, the common iliac arteries may be injured
      - veins (more common than arterial injuries): vena cava at and above L4, common iliac veins below L4

   b) ureters

   c) bowel: at L5–1 the ileum is the most likely viscus to be injured

   d) sympathetic trunk

3. wrong site surgery: incidence in self-reporting survey was 4.5 occurrences per 10,000 lumbar spine operations.[73] Factors identified as potential contributors to the error: unusual patient anatomy, not performing localizing radiograph. 32% of responding neurosurgeons indicated that they removed disc material from the wrong level at some time in their career

4. rare infections:

   a) meningitis

   b) deep infection: < 1%. Including:
      - discitis (p. 390): 0.5%
      - spinal epidural abscess (SEA) (p. 381): 0.67%

5. cauda equina syndrome: may be caused by post-op spinal epidural hematoma (see below). Incidence was 0.21% in one series of 2842 lumbar discectomies[74] and 0.14% in a series of 12,000 spine operations.[75] Red flags: urinary retention, anesthesia that may be saddle or *bilateral* LE

6. postoperative visual loss (POVL)[76]: (see below)

7. complications of positioning:

   a) compression neuropathies: ulnar, peroneal nerves. Use padding over elbows and avoid pressure on posterior popliteal fossa

   b) anterior tibial compartment syndrome: due to pressure on anterior compartment of leg (reported with Andrew's frame). An orthopedic emergency that may require emergent fasciotomy

   c) pressure on the eye: corneal abrasions, damage to the anterior chamber

   d) cervical spine injuries during positioning due to relaxed muscles under anesthesia

8. post-op arachnoiditis (p. 1243): risk factors include epidural hematoma, patients who tend to develop hypertrophic scar, post-op discitis, and intrathecal injection anesthetic agents or steroids. Surgical treatment for this is disappointing. Intrathecal depo-medrol may provide short-term relief (in spite of the fact that steroids are a risk factor for the development of arachnoiditis).

9. thrombophlebitis and deep-vein thrombosis with risk of pulmonary embolism (PE)[65]: 0.1%; see Thromboembolism in neurosurgery (p. 176)

10. complex regional pain syndrome AKA reflex sympathetic dystrophy (RSD) (p. 525): reported in up to 1.2% of cases, usually after posterior decompression with fusion, often following reoperations[77] with onset 4 days to 20 weeks post-op. See also critique of RSD (p. 526). Treatment includes some or all of: PT, sympathetic blocks, oral methylprednisolone, removal of hardware if any

11. very rare: Ogilvie's syndrome (pseudo-obstruction ("ileus") of the colon). Usually seen in hospitalized/debilitated patients. May be related to narcotics, electrolyte deficiencies, possibly from chronic constipation. Also reported following spinal surgery/trauma, spinal/epidural anesthesia, spinal metastases, & myelography[78]

75

Postoperative urinary retention

Post-op urinary retention (ironically, abbreviated POUR) is very common, especially following lumbar spine surgery. It encompasses a subset of conditions associated with urinary retention (p.95) in general.

1. spinal cord or cauda equina compression: often (but not always) accompanied by other new neurologic deficit. When this is the result of surgery, it may be due to:
    a) nerve or spinal cord compression: in the post-op setting, possible sources include: hematoma, instrumentation (e.g., pedicle screws), bone graft material, fragments from bone fracture
    b) nerve or spinal cord injury during surgery
2. urinary tract infection (UTI)
3. immobility
4. narcotics
5. constipation

Management
Examine patient for: new sensory level, other neurologic deficit that is new compared to pre-op
1. STAT MRI or CT of the surgical site to rule out hematoma
2. U/A and urine culture and treat any identified UTI
3. treat constipation with stool softeners and/or laxatives as appropriate
4. preferably, teach patient how to perform clean intermittent catheterizations (CIC) q 4 hour and PRN. If this is not practical, send the patient home with a Foley (indwelling) urinary catheter
5. start Flomax (0.4 mg daily) if not contraindicated & send patient home on this
6. set up appointment with urology (typically 10–14 days post op) for a voiding trial. This is usually an early morning appointment at which time the urology service will remove the Foley catheter (if present) and check a post void residual (PVR) either with a bladder scan (ultrasound) or with a straight catheterization after a couple hours to assess urinary retention. Sometimes cystoscopy or urodynamics will be done at the same appointment

Unintended durotomy

Unintentional opening of the dura during spinal surgery has an incidence of 0–14%.[79]

Terminology: The terms "unintended durotomy," "incidental durotomy,"[79] or even just "dural opening," have been recommended in preference to "dural tear" which may imply carelessness[68] when none was present. Dural openings have been associated with one or more alleged complications or sequelae in medical malpractice suits involving surgery on the lumbar spine.

The injury: By itself, opening of the dura intentionally or otherwise is not expected to have a deleterious effect on the patient.[68,80] In fact, dural opening is often a standard part of the operation for intradural disc herniation,[81] tumors, etc. Although not frequent (for incidence, see above), unintended durotomy is not an unusual occurrence, and alone, is not considered an act of malpractice. However, it may result from an event or events that produce more serious injuries. These events and injuries should be dealt with on their own merits.

In the SPORT, there was a 9% incidence of unintended durotomy in patients undergoing first-time open laminectomy.[82] There were no long-term differences in nerve root injuries, mortality, additional operations, or outcome measures. Short-term differences included longer inpatient stay, increased blood loss, and duration of surgery.[82] In a Dartmouth study of 25 durotomy patients, there was no increase in post-op nerve root injury, wound infection, or wound hematoma in the durotomy group.[83]

Possible sequelae include those listed in ▶ Table 75.4. A CSF leak may produce "spinal headache" (p.1816) with its associated symptoms and if it breaches the skin it may be a risk factor for

Table 75.4 Possible sequelae of dural opening

Well documented

1. CSF leak
   a) contained: pseudomeningocele
   b) external: CSF fistula
2. herniation of nerve roots through opening
3. associated nerve root contusion, laceration, or injury to the cauda equina
4. CSF leak collapses the thecal sac and may increase blood loss from epidural bleeding

Less well documented
1. arachnoiditis 2. chronic pain 3. bladder, bowel, and/or sexual dysfunction

75

meningitis. Pain or sensory/motor deficits may be associated with injuries to nerve roots or delayed herniation of nerve roots through the dural opening.

Etiologies: Potential causes are many, and include[68]: unanticipated anatomic variations, adhesion of the dura to removed bone, slippage of an instrument, an obscured fold of dura caught in a rongeur or curette, thinning of the dura in cases of longstanding stenosis, and the possibility of a delayed CSF leak caused by perforation of the dura when it expands onto a surgically created spicule of bone.[84] The risk may be increased with anterior decompression for OPLL, with revision surgery, and with the use of high-speed drills.[79]

Treatment: If the opening is recognized at the time of surgery, watertight primary closure (with or without patch graft) should be attempted with nonabsorbable suture if at all possible to prevent pseudomeningocele and/or CSF fistula. A cottonoid placed over the opening prevents aspiration of nerve roots.[85] Care must be taken to avoid incorporating a nerve root into the closure. Most repairs will be accomplished with no complication or sequelae to the patient. When the opening is in the far (anterior) side of the dura, consideration may be given to intradural repair accessed through a posterior durotomy which is subsequently closed (this may risk additional injury to the nerve roots). Biocompatible fixatives (e.g., fibrin glue[79]) may be used to supplement primary closure.

Primary repair may be impossible in some situations (e.g., when the opening cannot be found or accessed, as is sometimes the case when it occurs on the nerve root sleeve) and alternatives here include placement of a fat or muscle graft over the suspected leak site, use of the patient's own blood for a "blood patch" (one technique is to have the anesthesiologist draw ≈ 5–10 ml of the patient's blood from an arm vein, keeping it in the syringe for several minutes until it starts to coagulate, and then to have the anesthesiologist inject the blood onto the dura), use of gelfoam, fibrin glue... Some recommend that the wound not be drained post-op, with a watertight closure of fascia, fat, and skin to add to the barrier. Others use a subcutaneous drain or epidural catheter. CSF diversionary procedures (e.g., through a drain inserted 1 or more levels away) may also be used.

Although bed rest × 4–7 days is often advocated to reduce symptoms and facilitate healing, when watertight closure has been achieved, normal post-op mobilization is not associated with a high failure rate (bed rest is recommended if symptoms develop).[79]

In one report of 8 patients with leaks that appeared post-op, reoperation was avoided when treated by resuturing the skin under local anesthesia, followed by bed rest in slight Trendelenburg position (to reduce pressure on the leakage site), broad-spectrum antibiotics and antibiotic ointment over the skin incision, and daily puncture and drainage of the subcutaneous collection.[86]

See other treatment measures for H/A associated with CSF leak (p. 1256).

Postoperative visual loss (POVL)

1. ischemic optic neuropathy[87]: the most common cause of the very uncommon postoperative loss of vision. Often bilateral. Usually associated with significant blood loss (median: 2 L), and/or prolonged operative time (≥ 6 hrs). All cases had anesthetic time > 5 hrs or blood loss > 1 L. Blood loss can cause hypotension (may cause release of endogenous vasoconstrictors in addition to reduced blood flow due to low hemodynamic pressure) and increased platelet aggregation. Is not due to direct pressure on the globe in most cases, and can occur at any age and even in otherwise healthy patients. No association with age, HTN, atherosclerosis, smoking, or DM.
   The blindness can be extensive and is often permanent. Prevention is critical since there is no known effective treatment.[88]
   a) posterior ischemic optic neuropathy (PION)[87]: may follow surgery (surgical PION). Risk factors as above, plus:
      • surgery in the *prone* position (can cause periorbital edema, and rarely, direct pressure on the orbit)
      • lack of tight glycemic control
      • use of Trendelenburg position
      • hemodilution or overuse of crystalloid vs. colloid (blood) fluid replacement
      • prolonged hypotension
      • cellular hypoxia
      • decreased renal perfusion
   b) 6 independent risk factors for POVL[88]
      • male gender: odds ratio (OR) = 2.53
      • obesity: by clinical assessment or BMI ≥ 30 OR = 2.83
      • use of Wilson frame: OR = 4.30
      • length of anesthesia: OR = 1.39 per hour
      • EBL: OR = 1.34 per liter
      • use of colloid as a percentage of nonblood replacement: less certain (small difference). OR = 0.67 per 5% colloid

75

c) anterior ischemic optic neuropathy (AION): divided into arteritic (as with giant cell arteritis (GCA)) and nonarteritic (common with DM)
2. central retinal artery occlusion
3. cortical blindness: from occipital lobe infarction possibly due to embolism

75.8.9 Post-op care

Post-op orders

The following are guidelines for postoperative orders for a lumbar laminectomy without intraoperative complications; variations between surgeons and institutions must be taken into consideration:
1. admit post-anesthesia care unit (PACU)
2. vital signs on the nursing unit: q 2° × 4 hrs, q 4° × 24°, then q 8°
3. activity: up with assist, advance as tolerated
4. nursing care
   - I's & O's
   - intermittent catheterization q 4–6° PRN no void
   - optional: TED hose (may reduce risk of DVT) or PCB
   - optional (if drain used): empty drain q 8° and PRN
5. diet: clear liquids, advance as tolerated
6. IV: D5 1/2 NS + 20 mEq KCl/l @ 75 ml/hr, D/C when tolerating PO well (after antibiotics D/C'd if prophylactic antibiotics are used)
7. meds
   - laxative of choice (LOC) PRN
   - sodium docusate (e.g., Colace®) 100 mg PO BID when tolerating PO (stool softener, does not substitute for LOC)
   - optional: prophylactic antibiotics if used at your institution
   - acetaminophen (Tylenol®) 325 mg 1–2 PO or PR q 6° PRN
   - narcotic analgesic
   - optional: steroids are used by some surgeons to reduce nerve-root irritation from surgical manipulation
8. labs
   - optional (if significant blood loss during surgery): CBC

Post-op check

In addition to routine, the following should be checked:
1. strength of lower extremities, especially muscles relevant to nerve root, e.g., gastrocnemius for L5–1 surgery, EHL for L4–5 surgery…
2. appearance of dressing: look for signs of excessive bleeding, CSF leak…
3. signs of cauda equina syndrome (p. 1254), e.g., by post-op spinal epidural hematoma
   a) loss of perineal sensation ("saddle anesthesia")
   b) inability to void: may not be unusual after lumbar laminectomy, more concerning if accompanied by loss of perineal sensation
   c) pain out of the ordinary for the post-op period
   d) weakness of multiple muscle groups

Any new neurologic deficit should prompt rapid evaluation for spinal epidural hematoma[75] (EDH). Delayed deficits may be due to EDH or epidural abscess. Post-op films in the recovery room can rule out graft or hardware malposition for fusions or instrumentation procedures, or changes in alignment. The diagnostic test of choice is MRI. If contraindicated or not available, CT/myelography may be indicated. An extradural defect immediately post-op suggests EDH.

75.8.10 Outcome of surgical treatment

In a series of 100 patients undergoing discectomy, at 1 year post-op 73% had complete relief of leg pain and 63% had complete relief of back pain; at 5–10 years the numbers were 62% for each category.[2] At 5–10 years post-op, only 14% felt that the pain was the same or worse than pre-op (i.e., 86% felt improved), and 5% qualified as having a failed back surgery syndrome (a heterogeneous, not precisely defined term, here meaning not returned to work, requiring analgesics, receiving worker's compensation, see Failed back surgery syndrome (p. 1243)). Other studies have confirmed that LBP improves in a significant number of patients with a HLD undergoing discectomy without fusion.[89,90]

Attempts to compare relative merits of conservative treatment vs. surgery have failed to yield meaningful answers due to severe methodologic flaws. This includes the Spine Patient Outcomes Research Trial (SPORT),[89,91] with methodologic flaws[39] that included large numbers of patient cross-overs from the surgical to the nonoperative arm, and thus SPORT more nearly approximated the current methodology of surgical selection than an actual RCT.[39] Earlier attempts at randomized trials also suffered from methodologic flaws.[1] Conclusions that can be drawn from these studies[39]: most patients with manageable or improving pain and less disability typically choose conservative treatment and most have improvement in symptoms, whereas patients with severe, persistent, or worsening pain and/or neurologic deficit are more likely to choose surgery with a resultant excellent outcome. Furthermore, surgery patients had more rapid symptom relief and did statistically significantly better on virtually all primary and secondary outcome measures throughout the 2-year SPORT.

In patients with a diminished knee-jerk or ankle-jerk pre-op, 35% and 43% (respectively) still had reduced reflexes 1 year post-op[8]; reflexes were lost post-op in 3% and 10% respectively. The same study found that motor loss was improved in 80%, aggravated in 3%, and was newly present in 5% post-op; and that sensory loss was improved in 69% and was worsened in 15% post-op.

Foot drop: severe or complete paralysis of ankle dorsiflexion occurs in 5–10% of HLD, and about 50% of cases recover with or without treatment. Discectomy does not improve the outcome, especially in cases of painless foot drop.[38]

See Recurrent disc herniation (p. 1267).

75.9 Herniated upper lumbar discs (levels L1–2, L2–3, and L3–4)

75.9.1 General information

L4–5 & L5–1 herniated lumbar discs (HLD) account for most cases of HLD (realistically ≈ 90%, possibly as high as 98%[7]). 24% of patients with HLD at L3–4 have a past history of an HLD at L4–5 or L5–1, suggesting a generalized tendency towards disc herniation. In a series of 1,395 HLDs, there were 4 at L1–2 (0.28% incidence), 18 at L2–3 (1.3%), and 51 at L3–4 (3.6%).[92]

75.9.2 Presentation

Typically presents with LBP, onset following trauma or strain in 51%. With progression, paresthesias and pain in the anterior thigh occur, with complaints of leg weakness (especially on ascending stairs).

75.9.3 Signs

Quadriceps femoris was the most common muscle involved, demonstrating weakness and sometimes atrophy.

Straight leg raising was positive in only 40%. Psoas stretch test was positive in 27%. Femoral stretch test may be positive (p. 1252).

50% had reduced or absent knee jerk; 18% had ankle jerk abnormalities; reflex changes were more common with L3–4 HLD (81%) than L1–2 (none) or L2–3 (44%).

75.10 Extreme lateral lumbar disc herniations

75.10.1 General information

Definition: herniation of a disc in the foraminal zone or the extraforaminal zone (▶ Fig. 75.1). Herniations in the foraminal zone are located anterior to the facet joint, and are also called foraminal disc herniations.

Foraminal disc herniations typically involve the nerve root exiting at that level (e.g., an L4–5 foraminal disc herniation will involve the L4 nerve root) (see ▶ Fig. 75.2). The dorsal root ganglion (DRG) containing the cell bodies of the sensory nerve is also located in the foramen within the nerve root sheath. Compression of the DRG by herniated disc material may be associated with a worse outcome.

Disc herniations in the extraforaminal zone occasionally involve the nerve root exiting at that level; however, disc herniation here and those herniating anterior to the spine may not result in any nerve root involvement.

Incidence (▶ Table 75.5): 3–10% of herniated lumbar discs (HLD) (series with higher numbers[93] include some HLD that are not truly extreme lateral).

75

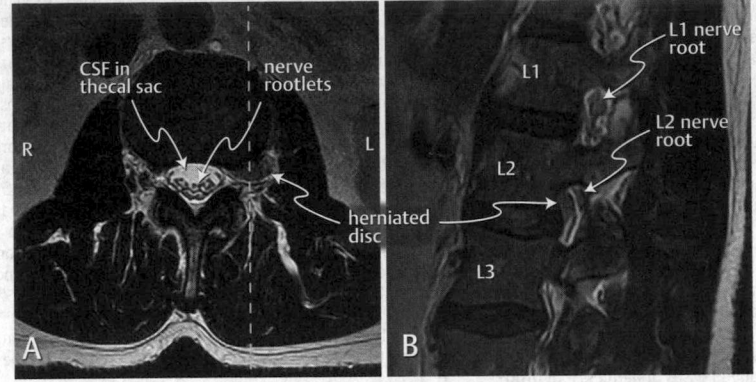

Fig. 75.2 Foraminal disc herniation.
Image: T2 MRI showing a large left-sided L2–3 disc herniation with a foraminal and an extraforaminal zone component.
A: axial cut through the L2–3 disc, B: parasagittal cut through the left neural foramina (slice location shown by green broken line) showing compression of the exiting left L2 nerve root. Note the normal left L1 nerve root.

Table 75.5 Incidence of extreme lateral HLD by level[a]

Disc level	No.	%
L1–2	1	1
L2–3	11	8
L3–4	35	24
L4–5	82	60
L5–S1	9	7

[a]series of 138 cases[93]

Occurs most commonly at *L4–5* and next at L3–4 (see ▸ Table 75.5), thus L4 is the most common nerve involved and L3 is next. With a clinical picture of an upper lumbar nerve root compression (i.e., radiculopathy with negative SLR), chances are ≈ 3 to 1 that it is an extremely lateral HLD rather than an upper lumbar disc herniation.

Differs from the more common central and subarticular zone HLD in that:
- the nerve root involved is usually the one exiting *at* that level (c.f. the root exiting at the level below)
- straight leg raising (SLR) (p.1252) is negative in 85–90% of cases ≥ 1 week after onset (excluding double herniations; ≈ 65% will be negative if double herniations are included); may have positive femoral stretch test
- pain is reproduced by lateral bending to the side of herniation in 75%
- higher incidence of extruded fragments (60%)
- higher incidence of double herniations on the same side at the same level (15%)
- pain tends to be more severe (may be due to the fact that the dorsal root ganglion may be compressed directly) and often has more of a burning dysesthetic quality

Presentation

Quadriceps weakness, reduction of patellar reflex, and diminished sensation in the L3 or L4 dermatome are the most common findings.

75.10.2 Differential diagnosis

1. lateral recess stenosis or superior articular facet hypertrophy
2. retroperitoneal hematoma or tumor

3. diabetic neuropathy (amyotrophy) (p. 572)
4. spinal tumor
    a) benign (schwannoma or neurofibroma)
    b) malignant tumors
    c) lymphoma
5. infection
    a) localized (spinal epidural abscess)
    b) psoas muscle abscess
    c) granulomatous disease
6. spondylolisthesis (with pars defect)
7. compression of conjoined nerve root
8. on MRI, enlarged foraminal veins may mimic extreme lateral disc herniation

75.10.3 Radiographic diagnosis

NB: if actively sought, many *asymptomatic* far-lateral disc herniations may be demonstrated on MRI or CT. Careful clinical correlation is usually required.

MRI: diagnostic test of choice. Sagittal views through the neural foramen may help demonstrate the disc herniation.[94] MRI may have ≈ 8% false positive rate due to presence of enlarged foraminal veins that mimic extreme lateral HLD.[95]

Myelography: myelography alone is rarely diagnostic (usually requires post-myelo CT).[96,97] Fails to disclose the pathology in 87% of cases due to the fact that the nerve root compression occurs distal to the nerve root sleeve (and therefore beyond the reach of the dye).[98]

CT scan[97]: reveals a mass displacing epidural fat and encroaching on the intervertebral foramen or lateral recess, compromising the emerging root. Or, may be lateral to foramen. Sensitivity is ≈ 50% and is similar with post-myelographic CT.[98] Post-discography CT[98,99] has also been able to demonstrate.

75.10.4 Surgical treatment

NB: compression of the dorsal root ganglion may result in a slower recovery from discectomy and overall less satisfying outcome than with the more commonplace paramedian disc herniation.

Foraminal discs

Usually requires mesial facetectomy to gain access to the region lateral to the dural sac without undue retraction on nerve root or cauda equina. Caution: total facetectomy combined with discectomy may result in a high incidence of instability (total facetectomy alone causes ≈ 10% rate of slippage), although other series found this risk to be lower (≈ 1 in 33[100,101]). An alternative technique is to remove just the lateral portion of the superior articular facet below.[102] Endoscopic techniques may be well suited for herniated discs in this location.[103] Even with a small amount of unroofing the foramen, it is often enough to adequately fish disc fragments out of the foramen with a nerve hook.

Discs herniated beyond (lateral to) the foramen

Numerous approaches may be used, including:
1. traditional midline hemilaminectomy: the ipsilateral facet must be partially or completely removed. The safest way to find the exiting nerve root is to take the laminectomy of the inferior portion of the upper vertebral level (e.g., L4 for a L4–5 HLD) high enough to expose the nerve root axilla, and then follow the nerve laterally through the neural foramen by removing the facet until the HLD is identified
2. lateral approach (i.e., extra-canal) through a paramedian incision.[104] Advantages: the facet joint is preserved (facet removal combined with discectomy may lead to instability), muscle retraction is easier. Disadvantages: unfamiliar approach for most surgeons and the nerve cannot be followed medial to lateral. A localizing X-ray is taken with a spinal needle. A 4–5 cm vertical skin incision is made 3–4 cm lateral to the midline on the side of the disc herniation. The incision is taken down to the thoracolumbar fascia and the subcutaneous tissue is dissected off the fascia. Above L4, one may palpate the groove between multifidus (medial) and longissimus (lateral), where the fascia is incised. The facet joint is palpated, and blunt dissection is used to gain access to the lateral facet joint and transverse processes above and below the level of the disc herniation. The correct level is confirmed on X-ray using a probe as a marker. The intertransversarius muscle and fascia are divided. Care must be taken to avoid mechanical and electrocautery injury to the nerve

75

and dorsal root ganglion (which lies immediately beneath the intertransverse ligament). The radicular artery, vein, and nerve root are located just beneath the transverse processes, usually slightly medial to this position. The nerve root hugs the pedicle of the level above as it exits the neural foramen (palpating this e.g., with a dental dissector helps locate it), and it may be splayed over the herniated disc fragment. If more medial exposure is necessary, the lateral facet joint may be resected. The HLD is removed. Additional removal of disc material from the disc space may be performed with down-biting pituitary rongeurs. Extracanal approach to L5–1 requires removal of part of the sacral ala in order to access the space caudal to the L5 transverse process

75.11 Lumbar disc herniations in pediatrics

Less than one percent of surgery for herniated lumbar disc is performed on patients between the ages of 10 and 20 yrs (one series at Mayo found 0.4% of operated HLD in patients < 17 yrs of age[105]). These patients often have few neurologic findings except for a consistently positive straight leg raising test.[106] Herniated disc material in youths tends to be firm, fibrous, and strongly attached to the cartilaginous endplate unlike the degenerated material usually extruded in adult disc herniation. Plain radiographs disclosed an unusually high frequency of congenital spine anomalies (transitional vertebra, hyperlordosis, spondylolisthesis, spina bifida…). 78% did well after their first operation.[105]

75.12 Intradural disc herniation

Herniation of a fragment of disc into the thecal sac, or into the nerve root sleeve (the latter sometimes referred to as "intraradicular" disc herniation) has been recognized with a reported incidence of 0.04–1.1% of disc herniations.[81,107] Although it may be suspected on the basis of pre-op MRI or myelography, the diagnosis is rarely made preoperatively.[107] Intraoperatively, it may be suggested by the appreciation of a tense firm mass within the nerve root sleeve or by the negative exploration of a level with obvious clinical signs and clear-cut radiographic abnormalities (after verifying that the correct level is exposed).

Surgical treatment:

Although a surgical dural opening may be utilized,[81] others have found this to be necessary in a minority of cases.[108]

75.13 Intravertebral disc herniation

75.13.1 General information

AKA Schmorl's node or nodule. Named for German pathologist Christian Georg Schmorl (1861–1932) the term was first used in 1971.[109] AKA Schmor's (no "l") nodule AKA Geipel hernia.[110] Disc herniation through the cartilaginous endplate into the cancellous bone of the vertebral body (VB) (AKA intraspongious disc herniation). Often an incidental finding on X-ray or MRI. Clinical significance is controversial. May produce low back pain initially that lasts ≈ 3–4 months after onset. Diffuse displacement (as may be seen in osteoporosis) is sometimes referred to as a balloon disc.[111]

75.13.2 Clinical findings

During the acute (symptomatic) phase, patients may exhibit LBP that is aggravated by weight bearing and movement. There may be tenderness to percussion or manual compression over the involved segment.

75.13.3 Radiographic findings

MRI: the extrusion of disc material into the VB is easily appreciated on sagittal images (▶ Fig. 75.3). It has been suggested[112] that acute (symptomatic) lesions may appear differentiated from chronic (asymptomatic) lesions by the presence of MRI findings of inflammation in the bone marrow immediately surrounding the node as outlined in ▶ Table 75.6.

CT: demonstrates defect in endplate and vertebral body since disc material has a significantly lower density than bone.

Plain X-ray: ≤ 33% may be seen on plain X-rays.[113] They may not be detectable acutely until sclerotic osseous bone casting develops.

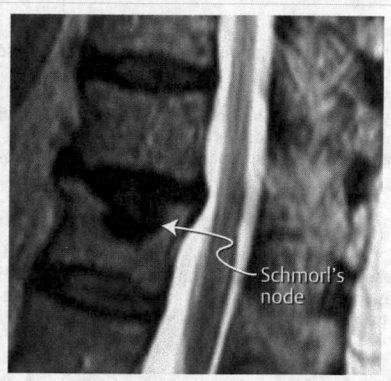

Fig. 75.3 Schmorl's node. Image: sagittal T2 MRI showing herniation of the intervertebral disc into the superior endplate of the vertebral body below the disc (Schmorl's node).
The lack of high intensity in the adjacent bone marrow on T2 MRI is compatible with a chronic condition.

Table 75.6 MRI signal intensity in bone marrow surrounding a Schmorl's node[a]

Lesion	T1WI	T2WI
symptomatic (acute)	low	high
asymptomatic (chronic)	high[b]	low[b]

[a]signal intensity in surrounding marrow
[b]the same as normal marrow

75.13.4 Treatment

Conservative treatment is indicated, usually consisting of non-steroidal anti-inflammatory drugs (NSAIDs). Occasionally stronger pain medication and/or lumbar bracing may be required. Surgery is rarely indicated.

75.13.5 Outcome

With conservative treatment, symptoms generally resolve within 3–4 months of onset (as with most vertebral body fractures).

75.14 Recurrent herniated lumbar disc

75.14.1 General information

Rates quoted in the literature range from 3–19% with the higher rates usually in series with longer follow-up.[114] In an individual series with 10-year mean F/U, the rate of recurrent disc herniation was 4% (same level, either side), one third of which occurred during the 1st year post-op (mean: 4.3 yrs).[69] A *second* recurrence at the same site occurred in 1% in another series[114] with mean F/U of 4.5 yrs. In this series,[114] patients presenting for a second time with disc herniation had a recurrence at the same level in 74%, but 26% had an HLD at another level. Recurrent HLD occurred at L4–5 more than twice as often as L5–1.[114]

It is often possible for a smaller volume of recurrent herniated disc to cause symptoms than in a "virgin back," due to the fact that the nerve root is often fixated by scar tissue and has little ability to deviate away from the fragment.[62]

75.14.2 Treatment

Initial recommended treatment is as with a first-time HLD. Nonsurgical treatment should be utilized in the absence of progressive neurologic deficit, cauda equina syndrome (CES), or intractable pain.

75

75.15 Surgical treatment

Disagreement occurs regarding optimal treatment. See **Practice guideline: Lumbar fusion for disc herniation** (p.1240).

Surgical outcome:

As with first-time HLD, the outcome from surgical treatment is worse in worker's compensation cases and in patients undertaking litigation, only ≈ 40% of these patients benefit.[114,115] A worse prognosis is also associated with: patients with < 6 mos relief after their first operation, cases where fibrosis without recurrent HLD is found at operation.

75.16 Spinal cord stimulation

One study actually showed a better response rate to spinal cord stimulation than to reoperation.[116] Since surgery for recurrent HLD carries a higher risk of dural and nerve root injury, and a lower success rate than first-time operations, this may be a viable option for some patients.

References

[1] Weber H. Lumbar Disc Herniation. A Controlled, Prospective Study with Ten Years of Observation. Spine. 1983; 8:131–140

[2] Lewis PJ, Weir BKA, Broad R, et al. Long-Term Prospective Study of Lumbosacral Discectomy. J Neurosurg. 1987; 67:49–53

[3] Wein AJ, Walsh PC, Retik AB, et al. Neuromuscular Dysfunction of the Lower Urinary Tract and Its Treatment. In: Campbell's Urology. 7th ed. Philadelphia: W.B. Saunders; 1998:953–1006

[4] Jones DL, Moore T. The Types of Neuropathic Bladder Dysfunction Associated with Prolapsed Lumbar Intervertebral Discs. Br J Urol. 1973; 45:39–43

[5] Ross JC, Jameson RM. Vesical Dysfunction Due to Prolapsed Disc. British Medical Journal. 1971; 3:752–754

[6] Frymoyer JW. Back Pain and Sciatica. N Engl J Med. 1988; 318:291–300

[7] Deyo RA, Rainville J, Kent DL. What Can the History and Physical Examination Tell Us About Low Back Pain? Journal of the American Medical Association. 1992; 268:760–765

[8] Blaauw G, Braakman R, Gelpke GJ, et al. Changes in Radicular Function Following Low-Back Surgery. J Neurosurg. 1988; 69:649–652

[9] Stam J, Speelman HD, van Crevel H. Tendon Reflex Asymmetry by Voluntary Mental Effort in Healthy Subjects. Archives of Neurology. 1989; 46:70–73

[10] Bigos S, Bowyer O, Braen G, et al. Acute Low Back Problems in Adults. Clinical Practice Guideline No.14. AHCPR Publication No. 95-0642. Rockville, MD: Agency for Health Care Policy and Research, Public Health Service, U.S. Department of Health and Human Services; 1994

[11] Scham SM, Taylor TKF. Tension Signs in Lumbar Disc Prolapse. Clin Orthop. 1971; 75:195–204

[12] Dyck P. Lumbar Nerve Root: The Enigmatic Eponyms. Spine. 1984; 9:3–6

[13] Spangfort EV. The Lumbar Disc Herniation. A Computer-Aided Analysis of 2,504 Operations. Acta Orthop Scand. 1972; 142:1–93

[14] Rothman RH, Simeone FA. The Spine. Philadelphia 1992

[15] Estridge MN, Rouhe SA, Johnson NG. The Femoral Stretch Test: A Valuable Sign in Diagnosing Upper Lumbar Disc Herniations. J Neurosurg. 1982; 57:813–817

[16] Hoover CF. A new sign for the detection of malingering and functional paresis of the lower extremities. Journal of the American Medical Association. 1908; 51:746–747

[17] Archibald KC, Wiechec F. A reappraisal of Hoover's test. Archives of Physical Medicine and Rehabilitation. 1970; 51:234–238

[18] Sonoo M. Abductor sign: A reliable new sign to detect unilateral non-organic paresis of the lower limb. Journal of Neurology, Neurosurgery and Psychiatry. 2004; 75:121–125

[19] Keegan JJ. Dermatome Hypalgesia Associated with Herniation of Intervertebral Disk. Arch Neurol Psychiatry. 1943; 50:67–83

[20] Todd NV, Dickson RA. Standards of care in cauda equina syndrome. Br J Neurosurg. 2016; 30:518–522

[21] Hoeritzauer Ingrid, Carson Alan, Statham Patrick, et al. "Scan-negative" cauda equina syndrome: A prospective cohort study. Neurology. 2020. DOI: 10.1212/wnl.0000000000011154

[22] Fraser S, Roberts L, Murphy E. Cauda equina syndrome: a literature review of its definition and clinical presentation. Arch Phys Med Rehabil. 2009; 90:1964–1968

[23] Kostuik JP, Harrington I, Alexander D, et al. Cauda Equina Syndrome and Lumbar Disc Herniation. Journal of Bone and Joint Surgery. 1986; 68A:386–391

[24] O'Laoire SA, Crockard HA, Thomas DG. Prognosis for Sphincter Recovery After Operation for Cauda Equina Compression Owing to Lumbar Disc Prolapse. British Medical Journal. 1981; 282:1852–1854

[25] Shapiro S. Cauda equina syndrome secondary to lumbar disc herniation. Neurosurgery. 1993; 32:743–6; discussion 746-7

[26] Scott PJ. Bladder Paralysis in Cauda Equina Lesions from Disc Prolapse. Journal of Bone and Joint Surgery. 1965; 47B:224–235

[27] Tay ECK, Chacha PB. Midline Prolapse of a Lumbar Intervertebral Disc with Compression of the Cauda Equina. Journal of Bone and Joint Surgery. 1979; 61B:43–46

[28] Hoeritzauer I, Wood M, Copley PC, et al. What is the incidence of cauda equina syndrome? A systematic review. J Neurosurg Spine. 2020:1–10

[29] Prusick VD, Lint DS, Bruder J. Cauda Equina Syndrome as a Complication of Free Epidural Fat-Grafting. Journal of Bone and Joint Surgery. 1988; 70A:1256–1258

[30] Tandon PN, Sankaran B. Cauda Equina Syndrome due to Lumbar Disc Prolapse. Indian J Orthopedics. 1967; 1:112–119

[31] Shapiro S. Medical Realities of Cauda Equina Syndrome Secondary to Lumbar Disc Herniation. Spine. 2000; 25:348–351

[32] Kostuik JP. Point of View: Comment on Shapiro, S: Medical Realities of Cauda Equina Syndrome Secondary to Lumbar Disc Herniation. Spine. 2000; 25

[33] Kato T, Haro H, Komori H, et al. Sequential dynamics of inflammatory cytokine, angiogenesis inducing factor and matrix degrading enzymes during spontaneous resorption of the herniated disc. J Orthop Res. 2004; 22:895–900

[34] Fager CA. Observations on Spontaneous Recovery from Intervertebral Disc Herniation. Surgical Neurology. 1994; 42:282–286

[35] Weber H, Holme I, Amlie E. The Natural Course of Acute Sciatica, with Nerve Root Symptoms in a

75

Double Blind Placebo Controlled Trial Evaluating the Effect of Piroxicam (NSAID). Spine. 1993; 18:1433–1438

[36] Weber H. The Effect of Delayed Disc Surgery on Muscular Paresis. Acta Orthop Scand. 1975; 46:631–642

[37] Saal JA, Saal JS. Nonoperative Treatment of Herniated Lumbar Intervertebral Disc with Radiculopathy: An Outcome Study. Spine. 1989; 14:431–437

[38] Marshall RW. The functional relevance of neurological recovery 20 years or more after lumbar discectomy. J Bone Joint Surg Br. 2008; 90:554–555

[39] McCormick PC. The Spine Patient Outcomes Research Trial results for lumbar disc herniation: a critical review. J Neurosurg Spine. 2007; 6:513–520

[40] Hoffman RM, Wheeler KJ, Deyo RA. Surgery for herniated lumbar discs: a literature synthesis. J Gen Intern Med. 1993; 8:487–496

[41] Williams RW. Microlumbar Discectomy: A Conservative Surgical Approach to the Virgin Herniated Lumbar Disc. Spine. 1978; 3:175–182

[42] Caspar W, Campbell B, Barbier DD, et al. The Caspar Microsurgical Discectomy and Comparison with a Conventional Lumbar Disc Procedure. Neurosurgery. 1991; 28:78–87

[43] Schmidek HH, Sweet WH. Operative Neurosurgical Techniques. New York 1982

[44] Fager CA. Lumbar Discectomy: A Contrary Opinion. Clinical Neurosurgery. 1986; 33:419–456

[45] Tulberg T, Isacson J, Weidenhielm L. Does Microscopic Removal of Lumbar Disc Herniation Lead to Better Results than the Standard Procedure? Results of a One-Year Randomized Study. Journal of Neurosurgery. 1993; 70:869–875

[46] Hoppenfeld S. Percutaneous Removal of Herniated Lumbar Discs. 50 Cases with Ten-Year Follow-Up Periods. Clin Orthop. 1989; 238:92–97

[47] Kahanovitz N, Viola K, Goldstein T, et al. A Multicenter Analysis of Percutaneous Discectomy. Spine. 1990; 15:713–715

[48] Davis GW, Onik G. Clinical Experience with Automated Percutaneous Lumbar Discectomy. Clin Orthop. 1989; 238:98–103

[49] Revel M, Payan C, Vallee C, et al. Automated Percutaneous Lumbar Discectomy Versus Chemonucleolysis in the Treatment of Sciatica. Spine. 1993; 18:1–7

[50] Maroon JC, Onik G, Sternau L. Percutaneous automated discectomy. A new method for lumbar disc removal. Technical note. Journal of Neurosurgery. 1987; 66:143–146

[51] Onik G, Maroon JC, Jackson R. Cauda Equina Syndrome Secondary to an Improperly Placed Nucleotome Probe. Neurosurgery. 1992; 30:412–415

[52] Cohen SP, Williams S, Kurihara C, et al. Nucleoplasty with or without intradiscal electrothermal therapy (IDET) as a treatment for lumbar herniated disc. J Spinal Disord Tech. 2005; 18 Suppl:S119–S124

[53] Yonezawa T, Onomura T, Kosaka R, et al. The System and Procedures of Percutaneous Intradiscal Laser Nucleotomy. Spine. 1990; 15:1175–1185

[54] Choy DSJ, Ascher PW, Saddekni S, et al. Percutaneous laser disc decompression: A new therapeutic modality. Spine. 1992; 17:949–956

[55] North American Spine Society Coverage Committee. Laser Spine Surgery. Burr Ridge, IL 2014. spine. org

[56] Mayer HM, Brock M. Percutaneous Endoscopic Discectomy: Surgical Technique and Preliminary Results Compared to Microsurgical Discectomy. J Neurosurgery. 1993; 78:216–225

[57] Kleinpeter G, Markowitsch MM, Bock F. Percutaneous Endoscopic Lumbar Discectomy: Minimally Invasive, But Perhaps Only Minimally Useful? Surgical Neurology. 1995; 43:534–541

[58] Karasek M, Bogduk N. Twelve-month follow-up of a controlled trial of intradiscal thermal anuloplasty for back pain due to internal disc disruption. Spine. 2000; 25:2601–2607

[59] Schwarzer AC, Aprill CN, Derby R, et al. The prevalence and clinical features of internal disc

[60] Ranguis SC, Li D, Webster AC. Perioperative epidural steroids for lumbar spine surgery in degenerative spinal disease. J Neurosurg Spine. 2010; 13:745–757

[61] Glasser RS, Knego RS, Delashaw JB, et al. The Perioperative Use of Corticosteroids and Bipuvicaine in the Management of Lumbar Disc Disease. Journal of Neurosurgery. 1993; 78:383–387

[62] Dunsker SB. Comment on Cobanoglu S, et al.: Complication of Epidural Fat Graft in Lumbar Spine Disc Surgery: Case Report. Surgical Neurology. 1995; 44:481–482

[63] Cabezudo JM, Lopez A, Bacci F. Symptomatic Root Compression by a Free Fat Transplant After Hemilaminectomy: Case Report. Journal of Neurosurgery. 1985; 63:633–635

[64] Cobanoglu S, Imer M, Ozylmaz F, et al. Complication of Epidural Fat Graft in Lumbar Spine Disc Surgery: Case Report. Surgical Neurology. 1995; 44:479–482

[65] Ramirez LF, Thisted R. Complications and Demographic Characteristics of Patients Undergoing Lumbar Discectomy in Community Hospitals. Neurosurgery. 1989; 25:226–231

[66] Deyo RA, Cherkin DC, Loeser JD, et al. Morbidity and mortality in association with operations on the lumbar spine. The influence of age, diagnosis, and procedure. Journal of Bone and Joint Surgery. 1992; 74A:536–543

[67] Shektman A, Granick MS, Solomon MP, et al. Management of Infected Laminectomy Wounds. Neurosurgery. 1994; 35:307–309

[68] Goodkin R, Laska LL. Unintended 'Incidental' Durotomy During Surgery of the Lumbar Spine: Medicolegal Implications. Surgical Neurology. 1995; 43:4–14

[69] Davis RA. A Long-Term Outcome Analysis of 984 Surgically Treated Herniated Lumbar Discs. Journal of Neurosurgery. 1994; 80:415–421

[70] Bilsky MH, Shields CB. Complications of Lumbar Disc Surgery. Contemporary Neurosurgery. 1995; 17:1–6

[71] DeSaussure RL. Vascular Injuries Coincident to Disc Surgery. Journal of Neurosurgery. 1959; 16:222–239

[72] Nam TK, Park SW, Shim HJ, et al. Endovascular treatment for common iliac artery injury complicating lumbar disc surgery : limited usefulness of temporary balloon occlusion. J Korean Neurosurg Soc. 2009; 46:261–264

[73] Jhawar BS, Mitsis D, Duggal N. Wrong-sided and wrong-level neurosurgery: a national survey. J Neurosurg Spine. 2007; 7:467–472

[74] Mclaren AC, Bailey SI. Cauda Equina Syndrome: A Complication of Lumbar Discectomy. Clinical Orthopedics. 1986; 204:143–149

[75] Porter RW, Detwiler PW, Lawton MT, et al. Postoperative Spinal Epidural Hematomas: Longitudinal Review of 12,000 Spinal Operations. BNI Quarterly. 2000; 16:10–17

[76] Lee LA, Roth S, Posner KL, et al. The American Society of Anesthesiologists Postoperative Visual Loss Registry: analysis of 93 spine surgery cases with postoperative visual loss. Anesthesiology. 2006; 105:652–659

[77] Sachs BL, Zindrick MR, Beasley RD. Reflex Sympathetic Dystrophy After Operative Procedures on the Lumbar Spine. Journal of Bone and Joint Surgery. 1993; 75A:721–725

[78] Feldman RA, Karl RC. Diagnosis and Treatment of Ogilvie's Syndrome After Lumbar Spinal Surgery. J Neurosurg. 1992; 76:1012–1016

[79] Hodges SD, Humphreys C, Eck JC, et al. Management of Incidental Durotomy Without Mandatory Bed Rest. Spine. 1999; 24:2062–2064

[80] Fink LH. Unintended 'incidental' durotomy. Surgical Neurology. 1996; 45

[81] Ciappetta P, Delfini R, Cantore GP. Intradural Lumbar Disc Hernia: Description of Three Cases. Neurosurgery. 1981; 8:104–107

75

[82] Desai A, Ball PA, Bekelis K, et al. SPORT: Does incidental durotomy affect longterm outcomes in cases of spinal stenosis? Neurosurgery. 2015; 76 Suppl 1:S57–63; discussion S63

[83] Desai A, Ball PA, Bekelis K, et al. Outcomes after incidental durotomy during first-time lumbar discectomy. J Neurosurg Spine. 2011; 14:647–653

[84] Horwitz NH, Rizzoli HV, Horwitz NH, et al. Herniated Intervertebral Discs and Spinal Stenosis. In: Postoperative Complications of Extracranial Neurological Surgery. Baltimore: Williams and Wilkins; 1987:1–72

[85] Eismont FL, Wiesel SW, Rothman RH. Treatment of Dural Tears Associated with Spinal Surgery. Journal of Bone and Joint Surgery. 1981; 63A:1132–1136

[86] Waisman M, Schweppe Y. Postoperative Cerebrospinal Fluid Leakage After Lumbar Spine Operations. Conservative Treatment. Spine. 1991; 15:52–53

[87] Hayreh SohanSingh. Ischemic optic neuropathy. Progress in Retinal and Eye Research. 2009; 28:34–62

[88] Postoperative Visual Loss Study Group. Risk factors associated with ischemic optic neuropathy after spinal fusion surgery. Anesthesiology. 2012; 116:15–24

[89] Weinstein JN, Lurie JD, Tosteson TD, et al. Surgical vs nonoperative treatment for lumbar disk herniation: the Spine Patient Outcomes Research Trial (SPORT) observational cohort. JAMA. 2006; 296:2451–2459

[90] Sorensen ST, Bech-Azeddine R, Fruensgaard Søren, et al. Outcomes following discectomy for lumbar disc herniationin patients with substantial back pain. Journal of Neurosurgery (Spine). 2020; 33:623–626

[91] Weinstein JN, Tosteson TD, Lurie JD, et al. Surgical vs nonoperative treatment for lumbar disk herniation: the Spine Patient Outcomes Research Trial (SPORT): a randomized trial. JAMA. 2006; 296:2441–2450

[92] Aronson HA, Dunsmore RH. Herniated Upper Lumbar Discs. J Bone Joint Surg. 1963; 45:311–317

[93] Abdullah AF, Wolber PGH, Warfield JR, et al. Surgical Management of Extreme Lateral Lumbar Disc Herniations: Review of 138 Cases. Neurosurgery. 1988; 22:648–653

[94] Osborn AG, Hood RS, Sherry RG, et al. CT/MR Spectrum of Far Lateral and Anterior Lumbosacral Disk Herniations. American Journal of Neuroradiology. 1988; 9:775–778

[95] Grenier N, Greselle J-F, Douws C, et al. MR Imaging of Foraminal and Extraforaminal Lumbar Disk Herniations. Journal of Computer Assisted Tomography. 1990; 14:243–249

[96] Godersky JC, Erickson DL, Seljeskog EL. Extreme Lateral Disc Herniation: Diagnosis by CT Scanning. Neurosurgery. 1984; 14:549–552

[97] Osborne DR, Heinz ER, Bullard D, et al. Role of CT in the Radiological Evaluation of Painful Radiculopathy After Negative Myelography. Neurosurgery. 1984; 14:147–153

[98] Jackson RP, Glah JJ. Foraminal and Extraforaminal Lumbar Disc Herniation: Diagnosis and Treatment. Spine. 1987; 12:577–585

[99] Angtuaco EJC, Holder JC, Boop WC, et al. Computed Tomographic Discography in the Evaluation of Extreme Lateral Disc Herniation. Neurosurgery. 1984; 14:350–352

[100] Garrido E, Connaughton PN. Unilateral Facetectomy Approach for Lateral Lumbar Disc Herniation. J Neurosurg. 1991; 74:754–756

[101] Epstein NE, Epstein JA, Carras R, et al. Far Lateral Lumbar Disc Herniations and Associated Structural Abnormalities. An Evaluation in 60 Patients of the Comparative Value of CT, MRI, and Myelo-CT in Diagnosis and Management. Spine. 1990; 15:534–539

[102] Jane JA, Haworth CS, Broaddus WC, et al. A Neurosurgical Approach to Far-Lateral Disc Herniation. Journal of Neurosurgery. 1990; 72:143–144

[103] Ditsworth DA. Endoscopic Transforaminal Lumbar Discectomy and Reconfiguration: A Posterolateral Approach into the Spinal Canal. Surgical Neurology. 1998; 49:588–598

[104] Maroon JC, Kopitnik TA, Schulhof LA, et al. Diagnosis and Microsurgical Approach to Far-Lateral Disc Herniation in the Lumbar Spine. Journal of Neurosurgery. 1990; 72:378–382

[105] Ebersold MJ, Quast LM, Bianco AJ. Results of Lumbar Discectomy in the Pediatric Patient. Journal of Neurosurgery. 1987; 67:643–647

[106] Epstein JA, Epstein NE, Marc J, et al. Lumbar Intervertebral Disk Herniation in Teenage Children: Recognition and Management of Associated Anomalies. Spine. 1984; 9:427–432

[107] Kataoka O, Nishibayashi Y, Sho T. Intradural Lumbar Disc Herniation: Report of Three Cases with a Review of the Literature. Spine. 1989:529–533

[108] Schisano G, Franco A, Nina P. Intraradicular and Intradural Lumbar Disc Herniation: Experience with Nine Cases. Surgical Neurology. 1995; 44:536–543

[109] Schmorl G, Junghanns H. The Human Spine in Health and Disease. New York: Grune & Stratton; 1971

[110] Deeg HJ. Schmorl's nodule. New England Journal of Medicine. 1978; 298

[111] Fardon DF, Milette PC. Nomenclature and classification of lumbar disc pathology. Recommendations of the Combined task Forces of the North American Spine Society, American Society of Spine Radiology, and American Society of Neuroradiology. Spine. 2001; 26:E93–E113

[112] Takahashi K, Miyazaki T, Ohnari H, et al. Schmorl's nodes and low-back pain. Analysis of magnetic resonance imaging findings in symptomatic and asymptomatic individuals. European Spine Journal. 1995; 4:56–59

[113] Hamanishi C, Kawabata T, Yosii T, et al. Schmorl's nodes on magnetic resonance imaging. Spine. 1994; 19:450–453

[114] Herron L. Recurrent Lumbar Disc Herniation: Results of Repeat Laminectomy and Discectomy. Journal of Spinal Disorders. 1994; 7:161–166

[115] Waddell G, Crummel EG, Solts WN, et al. Failed Lumbar Disc Surgery and Repeat Surgery Following Industrial Injuries. Journal of Bone and Joint Surgery. 1979; 61A:201–207

[116] Bell GK, Kidd D, North RB. Cost-effectiveness analysis of spinal cord stimulation in treatment of failed back surgery syndrome. J Pain Symptom Manage. 1997; 13:286–295

75

76 Thoracic Disc Herniation

76.1 General information

Key concepts

- comprise only 0.25% of herniated discs, and < 4% of operations for herniated disc
- usually occur at or below T8 (the more mobile portion of the thoracic spine)
- frequently calcified ∴ get CT through disc (may affect choice of surgical approach)
- primary indications for surgery: refractory pain, progressive myelopathy
- surgical treatment: laminectomy is usually not appropriate for midline or calcified herniated discs

Account for 0.25–0.75% of all protruded discs.[1] 80% occur between the 3rd and 5th decades. 75% are below T8 (the more mobile portion of the thoracic spine), with a peak of 26% at T11–12. 94% were centrolateral and 6% were lateral.[2] A history of trauma may be elicited in 25% of cases.

Most common symptoms: pain (60%), sensory changes (23%), motor changes (18%). With thoracic radiculopathy, pain and sensory disturbance is in a band-like distribution radiating anteriorly and inferiorly along the involved root's dermatome (paralleling a rib). Motor involvement is difficult to document.

76.2 Evaluation

1. MRI: noncontrast thoracic MRI is the mainstay of diagnosis. If MRI is contraindicated, a thoracic CT/myelogram is the second choice
2. CT scan: noncontrast thoracic CT scan should be routinely obtained to determine if it is a "soft disc" (noncalcified) (see ▶ Fig. 76.1) or a "hard disc" (calcified) (see ▶ Fig. 76.2) which can have a profound effect on the choice of approach and the removal technique. CT also delineates the bony detail which is helpful if instrumentation is needed.

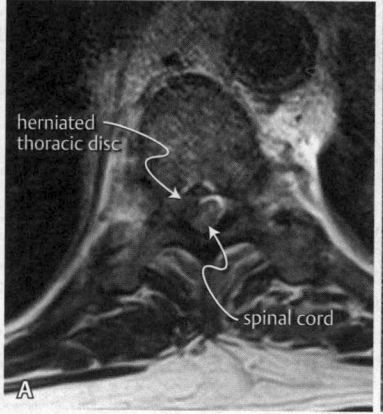
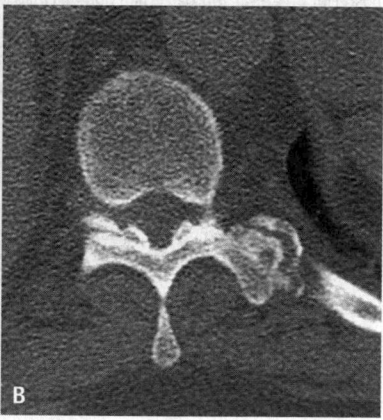

herniated thoracic disc

spinal cord

A   **B**

76

Fig. 76.1 "Soft" herniated thoracic disc. T10–11 right-sided.
Image: A: sagittal T2 MRI. B: CT scan through this disc shows it is not calcified (compare to ▶ Fig. 76.2).

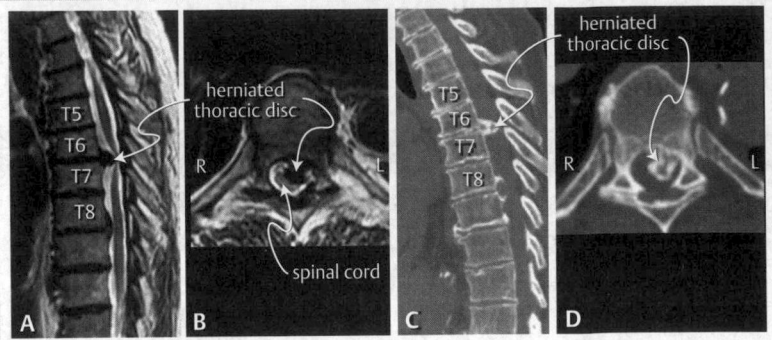

Fig. 76.2 Calcified herniated thoracic disc. T6–7 left-sided.
Image: A & B: T2 MRI (sagittal & axial respectively). C & D: unenhanced (bone window) CT (sagittal & axial respectively) showing the disc is calcified. All images from the same patient.

76.3 Indications for surgery

Herniated thoracic discs requiring surgery are rare.[2] Indications: refractory pain (usually radicular, bandlike) or progressive myelopathy. Uncommon: symptomatic syringomyelia originating at level of disc herniation.

76.4 Surgical approaches

Surgery for thoracic disc disease is challenging because of: the difficulty of anterior approaches, the proportionately tighter space between cord and canal compared to the cervical and lumbar regions, and the watershed blood supply which creates a significant risk of cord injury with attempts to manipulate the cord when trying to work anteriorly to it from a posterior approach. Herniated thoracic discs are calcified in 65% of patients considered for surgery[2] (more difficult to remove from a posterior or lateral approach than non-calcified discs).

Open surgical approaches[2,3]:
1. posterior (midline laminectomy): primary indication is for decompression of posteriorly situated intracanalicular pathology (e.g., metastatic tumor) especially over multiple levels. There is a high failure and complication rate when used for single-level anterior pathology (e.g., midline disc herniation)
2. posterolateral
   a) lateral gutter: laminectomy plus removal of pedicle
   b) transpedicular approach[4]
   c) costotransversectomy (see below)
   d) transfacet pedicle sparing
3. anterolateral (transthoracic): usually through the pleural space
4. lateral extracavitary (retrocoelomic)[5]: an approach posterior (external) to the pleural space

Thoracoscopic surgery is an alternative to open surgery.

76.5 Choosing the approach

76.5.1 General information

See anterior approaches to the thoracic spine (p. 1790).

Intraoperative SSEPs and MEPs may be helpful for patients with myelopathy.

For a laterally located herniated noncalcified thoracic disc (e.g., see ▶ Fig. 76.1) posterolateral approach with medial facetectomy is technically simple, and has generally good results. For a central disc herniation, especially when calcified (and therefore not as likely to be able to be pulled out from the side), or when myelopathy is present: transthoracic approach has the lowest incidence of cord injury with the best operative results (▶ Table 76.1).

Table 76.1 Results with various approaches for thoracic spine pathology[6]

Approach	Indication	Total no.	Outcome			
			Normal	Improved	Same	Worse
laminectomy	posteriorly located tumor	129	15%	42%	11%	32%
posterolateral (transpedicular)	radicular pain with lateral disc herniation; biopsy of tumor	27	37%	45%	11%	7%
lateral (costotransversectomy)	fair for midline disc; good ipsilateral access, poor access to opposite side	43	35%	53%	12%	0
transthoracic	best for midline lesions, especially for reaching both sides of cord	12	67%	33%	0	0

For centrally located anterior access: a transthoracic or lateral approach gives the best access. Some prefer a left-sided approach to avoid the vena cava, others prefer a right-sided approach because the heart does not impede access.

76.5.2 Costotransversectomy

Indications: in the past this was often used to drain tuberculous spine abscess. It may be used for lateral disc herniation, biopsy of VB or pedicle, limited unilateral decompression of spinal cord from tumor or bone fragments, or sympathectomy. Can be used at ≈ any T-spine level. Limitations: difficult to visualize anterior canal to access midline anterior pathology. Better for soft disc than for calcified central disc.

Involves resection of the transverse process and at least ≈ 4–5 cm of the posterior rib. A serious risk of this approach is interruption of a significant radicular artery which may compromise spinal cord blood supply; see Spinal cord vasculature (p.87). There is also a risk of pneumothorax, which is less grave.

Booking the case: Costotransversectomy

Also see defaults & disclaimers (p. 25).
1. position: prone, usually on chest rolls
2. equipment:
   a) microscope (not used for all cases)
   b) C-arm
3. implants: if post-op instability is anticipated, thoracic pedicle screws and possibly a cage (e.g., for fracture or tumor, not typically for disc herniation)
4. neuromonitoring: SSEP/MEP
5. blood availability: type and cross 2 U PRBC
6. consent (in lay terms for the patient—not all-inclusive):
   a) procedure: surgery through the back of the chest to remove a small piece of rib to permit removal of the herniated/calcified disc
   b) alternatives: nonsurgical management, surgery from the side through the chest
   c) complications: spinal cord injury with paralysis, lung complications including pneumothorax or hemothorax (blood or air outside lungs), possible seizures with MEPs

76

76.6 Surgical technique

The approach can be somewhat difficult due to the infrequent encounter with the anatomy by most neurosurgeons. Be prepared for a "deep, red hole, where everything initially looks the same and the bony anatomy is not easy to define." With patience and persistence and the help of an anatomic model in the O.R., the surgeon can get his/her bearings. One of the most helpful landmarks is following the NVB (or just the nerve root) medially to the neural foramen.

In the O.R., before the prep and skin incision, localizing X-rays are obtained; a spinal needle inserted between 2 spinous processes may be used as a marker.

Patient position: the approach is from the side of the pathology/symptoms; for central disc herniations a right-sided approach reduces risk of injury to artery of Adamkiewicz (located on the left in 80% (p.87)). Options:

1. lateral oblique, ≈ 30° elevated from straight prone, a "bean-bag" is good for stabilization. For a thin patient, the surgeon may stand in *front* of the patient (gives more horizontal angle of view—does not work as well with heavier patients due to mass of skin/muscle in the way laterally)
2. prone on chest rolls: the chest roll on the side of the pathology should be more medial to allow the shoulder and scapula to fall forward out of the way

Skin incision options:

1. curved paramedian skin incision: apex oriented away from the midline along the slight depression demarcating the junction of the lateral border of the paraspinal muscles with the ribs (≈ 6–7 cm lateral to midline) centered over the interspace of interest extending ≈ 3 vertebral bodies (VB) above and below. The incision is carried through the skin, subcutaneous fat, trapezius, and (for lower 6 thoracic levels, where most thoracic disc herniations occur) the latissimus dorsi, down to the ribs, and this musculocutaneous flap can be reflected medially as a unit
2. midline incision: need to extend 3–4 levels above and below the level of pathology to get an angle low enough to visualize posterior to the facet in order to access the posterior vertebral body. The inferior aspect can be curved laterally towards the side of pathology. Advantage: a laminectomy can more easily be performed if needed (if the angle does not provide adequate visualization, as a "bail-out" contingency, a facetectomy may be performed, and pedicle may even be removed to access inferior to the disc space. This usually permits easy decompression of the entire thecal sac. In the thoracic spine, stabilization is optional, and if chosen, unilateral pedicle screws and fusion are usually adequate)

Rib removal and thoracic exposure: for a simple biopsy or drainage of a small abscess, removal of only 1 rib may suffice. ★ The rib to be removed is from the level *inferior* to the disc space to be accessed[7] (e.g., remove the T5 rib to access T4–5 disc space). For most other pathologies, 2 or 3 ribs are often removed.[8] To access a VB, the like-numbered rib *and* the rib below are removed.

There are a number of ligaments attached to the rib: the intercostal neurovascular bundle (NVB) courses medial to the superior costotransverse ligament, which extends from the superior aspect of the rib to the transverse process of the level above. This ligament and the lateral costotransverse ligament are divided and the transverse process is rongeured off (the base of which lies on the lamina directly posterior to the pedicle). This exposes the rib anterior to the transverse process. The periosteum is incised on the rib from the angle of the rib to the costovertebral articulation, and by subperiosteal dissection around its circumference the pleura is dissected off the anterior surface of the rib. The NVB is dissected from the deep-inferior surface along with the periosteum. The rib is then transected laterally at the angle (≈ 5 cm lateral to the rib head) with rib shears, it is gripped with a clamp, and is rotated while the ligaments (including the radiate ligaments which attach the rib to both the VB above and the VB below the disc space at the superior and inferior costal facet, respectively, except T1, 11, & 12 which only articulate with their like-numbered VB) are *sharply* dissected off the rib which is then removed. The removed rib material may be used for fusion substrate except in cases of tumor or infection. The pleura is then dissected from the deep surface of the adjacent ribs and VB (taking care not to injure the segmental vessels and to dissect the sympathetic trunk off the VB with the pleura). The pleura is then retracted laterally with a malleable ribbon or Deaver retractor.

The intervertebral foramen of interest may be located by following the NVB of the rib *above* proximally, the intercostal nerve (the ventral ramus of the nerve root at that level) enters between the two pedicles. The dura may then be exposed by enlarging the neural foramen by removing part of the pedicles with a high-speed drill and Kerrison rongeurs.

Instrumentation/fusion are rarely required for simple discectomy. Instability due to fracture, tumor, or extensive resection (e.g., with total facet takedown) necessitates surgical stabilization, typically with pedicle screws/rods extending 2 levels above and 2 levels below. Prior to closure, check for air leak by filling the opening with saline and having the anesthesiologist apply a Valsalva maneuver. If an air leak is identified, a Cook catheter may be placed into the pleural space through the surgical exposure, or alternatively a chest tube is placed through a separate intercostal incision after the laminectomy wound is closed. A post-op CXR is obtained regardless of whether an air leak is identified.

76.6.1 Transpedicular approach

Drilling down the pedicle and removing a small amount of bone from the vertebral body, then pushing material from the epidural space into the defect created and removing it. Requires removal of just the rib head. Advantages: minimal risk of pneumothorax, more familiar anatomy. Disadvantages: requires instrumentation, especially if done bilaterally; the angle is not very oblique so visualization of epidural space is minimal; may need to be done bilaterally if there are extensive bilateral components to the pathology.

Booking the case: Transpedicular approach

Same as for costotransversectomy (p. 1273).

76.6.2 Transthoracic approach

Indications: thoracic disc disease with central fragment or calcified disc, burst fractures of the thoracic spine, etc.

Advantages[9]:
- excellent anterior exposure (especially advantageous for multiple levels)
- little compromise of stability (due to supporting effect of rib cage)
- low risk of mechanical cord injury

Disadvantages:
- requires thoracic surgeon (or familiarity with thoracic surgery)
- some risk of vascular cord injury (due to sacrifice of intercostal arteries)
- definitive diagnosis may not be possible if it is uncertain prior to procedure

Possible complications:
- pulmonary complications: pleural effusion, atelectasis, pneumonia, empyema, hypoventilation
- CSF-pleural fistula

Booking the case: Transthoracic spine surgery

Also see defaults & disclaimers (p. 25).
1. position: typically on the side, often on a beanbag
2. equipment:
   a) microscope (not used for all cases)
   b) C-arm
3. anesthesia: double lumen tube
4. implants: if post-op instability is anticipated, thoracic pedicle screws and possibly a cage (e.g., for fracture or tumor, not typically for disc herniation)
5. neuromonitoring: SSEP/MEP
6. blood availability: type and cross 2 U PRBC
7. some surgeons use chest surgeon for the approach, closure, and follow-up
8. consent (in lay terms for the patient—not all-inclusive):
   a) procedure: surgery through the chest with removal of a small piece of rib to permit removal of the herniated/calcified disc
   b) alternatives: nonsurgical management, surgery from the side or through the back
   c) complications: spinal cord injury with paralysis, pneumothorax, possible seizures with MEPs

76.6.3 Key technical points

1. the services of an experienced thoracic surgeon are usually engaged

2. position: true lateral (facilitates intra-op localizing X-rays); approached from the more involved side. For the upper thoracic *midline* region, some prefer right-side-up to eliminate thoracic aorta from obstructing exposure and to reduce the possibility of encountering the artery of Adamkiewicz,[10] while others prefer left-side-up to use the aorta as a landmark[9] (for levels below the cardiophrenic angle, a left-sided approach is preferred because the inferior vena cava is difficult to mobilize)
3. usually one rib is resected; most often the rib of the vertebra immediately *above* the disc space desired (facilitates exposure). Multiple ribs may be resected to increase exposure
4. when removing the vertebral body (VB) (corpectomy, e.g., for osteomyelitis, especially Pott's disease or for kyphoscoliosis)
   a) the posterior cortex of the VB must be pulled anteriorly (e.g., with angled curettes) to avoid mechanical cord trauma
   b) anterior fusion may be performed using the removed rib. If inadequate, fibula or iliac crest may be used
5. sizeable radicular arteries are spared. The intercostal nerve is used as a guide to the intervertebral foramen (nerve enters foramen superiorly and posteriorly)
6. the disc space is situated off the caudal aspect of the intervertebral foramen for most thoracic levels
7. one or two intervertebral arteries and veins usually have to be sacrificed; to minimize the risk of ischemic cord injury, cut them as close to the midline of the spine as possible (collaterals tend to lie on the lateral aspect of the spine)
8. the sympathetic chain is dissected off the VBs and is pushed posteriorly

76.6.4 Lateral retropleural approach

See reference.[5]

General information

An extra-coelomic approach does not violate the pleural space. If the parietal pleura is entered the procedure is essentially the same, but is considered a "trans-thoracic" approach.

Check a pre-op MRI or CT for the location of the aorta and to rule out aortic aneurysm which is a relative contraindication. For a herniated thoracic disc, a pre-op CT is necessay to determine if the disc is calcified (see ▶ Fig. 76.2), which alters the technique.

A dual lumen endotracheal tube is *not* required.

Indications

- thoracic corpectomy/discectomy. For herniated disc, this approach is indicated for a central disc herniation, or a calcified herniated disc that is situated anterior to the spinal cord. Pre-op CT is mandatory (see above)
- for some lateral interbody fusions (e.g., LLIF) at L1–2 and occasionally even at L2–3 if the ribs substantially overlie the disc space

Applied anatomy

External oblique (EO) muscle (mnemonic for direction of fibers: "hands in pocket" directed medially and inferiorly). The endothoracic fascia (ETF) can be dissected from the internal surface of the rib to allow the rib to be removed. Then the space between the ETF and the parietal pleura is entered (not the potential pleural space between the parietal and visceral pleura) to perform the operation. If the parietal pleura is violated during the approach, this can produce a pneumothorax. If the visceral pleura is also perforated, this can produce an air leak in addition to the pneumothorax.

Equipment

The same retractor (e.g., the Maxcess™ retractor by Nuvasive) used for lateral lumbar interbody fusion (p. 1802) may be used with blade extenders and an "egg beater" (lung retractor) center blade to retract the lungs. The retractor is "reversed" so that the center blade is positioned *anteriorly* and the table adapter arm is connected to the posterior "poker chip" on the retractor so that when the retractor is expanded in the AP direction, the lung retractor blade moves anteriorly and the lateral blades stay stationary.

The following additional instruments are needed:
- endo-Kitners (Kitners at the end of a "stick")

- Doyen rib separators
- Alexander periosteal elevator or Pennfield #1 dissector
- rib shears
- extra long instruments, including: e.g., long Midas Rex drill (21 cm attachment: 21TU with 21MH30 dissecting tool) or an angled drill (e.g., Midas Rex Clear View™) with diamond burr, and/ or BoneScalpel (with round tip), long suctions, Kerrison rongeurs…
- Intraoperative electrophysiologic spinal cord monitoring is usually used (typically SSEP & MEP).

Positioning and marking

The side of the approach is determined by the laterality of the disc herniation. If it is exactly midline, a left-sided approach is often preferrable because it is easier to retract the aorta than the vena cava.

Fluoro is used to position the patient in a true lateral position with the spinous processes midway between the pedicles at the surgical level and the patient is stabilized with adhesive tape.

A cross-hair localizer is used with fluoro to mark the skin at the anterior and posterior extent of the disc of interest. Mark the skin incision starting from the midposition of the disc and extending posteriorly along the direction of the ribs for 6–7 cm (by going a little more posterior than a perfectly lateral approach, the working distance is shortened and the angle is a little easier). Above ≈ T6 the scapula begins to get in the way, and it may need to be released a little by splitting the fibers of the latissiums dorsi.

Incision and approach

Make the skin incision along the surface of the rib overlying the disc space. The actual number of this rib is usually not important but it is typically 2 levels above the disc space in question (e.g., the T9 rib will be resected in approaching T10–11). Incise the external oblique (EO) over the center of the rib, and use a curette (e.g., Penfield #1 or Alexander) to separate the bone of the rib from the endo-thoracic fascia (ETF) deep to the rib. Sweeping a Doyen rib dissector beneath the rib can help complete the separation. Remove a section of the rib using rib shears (about 6 cm, get as far posterior as you can).

Separating the ETF from the outer surface of the parietal pleura (to enter the space between the ETF and the parietal pleura): during the process of separating the rib from the ETF, there is often an iatrogenically created opening through the ETF where this space can be entered (if not, carefully create an opening without violating the parietal pleura). Develop this potential space: begin to enlarge it using Kitners (some prefer endo-Kitners) and carefully insinuate a finger (moistening the glove helps) into this space after rib removal. If your finger moves freely, you have probably penetrated the parietal pleura and entered the pleural space (between the parietal and visceral pleura). In some cases it is not possible to develop this plane, in this case the pleural space is utilized, which works nearly as well (except at the diaphragm). Work the pleura and lung and (for lower T-spine) diaphragm anteriorly. Use a hand-held egg-beater retractor & follow the plane down to lateral VB, a sponge stick may help. Place the Maxcess retractor fitted with extensions oriented with the handles toward the abdomen with a short blade in the middle position for starters. Then replace it with an egg-beater blade. Connect the adapter arm to the "poker chip" furthest away from the posterior blade (so that posterior blade moves and not the side blades as you open the retractor). Take segmental artery(ies) as soon as they are seen (these usually cross in the middle of the VB).

Corpectomy

For a corpectomy, position blades of the retractor to span endplate to endplate (across the VB to be removed). Dissect the sympathetic chain anteriorly off the lateral VBs. If a segmental artery overlies the VB to be removed, it is coagulated and divided.

Discectomy for herniated thoracic disc
See reference.[11]

The head of the rib of the vertebral body below the the disc space overlies the posterior disc space (▶ Fig. 76.3) and must be removed (this is usually a different rib than the one from which the lateral part was removed earlier to access the retropleural space).

Once the rib head is removed, locate the pedicle of the lower VB. The disc space is just cranial to the pedicle. Locate the intervertebral (neural) foramen—the disc space is situated at the caudal aspect of the foramen. For herniated disc or other access to spinal canal/dura: you need to enlarge the neural foramen to be able to work, by drilling the cranial aspect of the pedicle of the level BELOW the disc space. If the pathology extends significantly posteriorly it may be necessary to remove part or all of the facet joint.

76

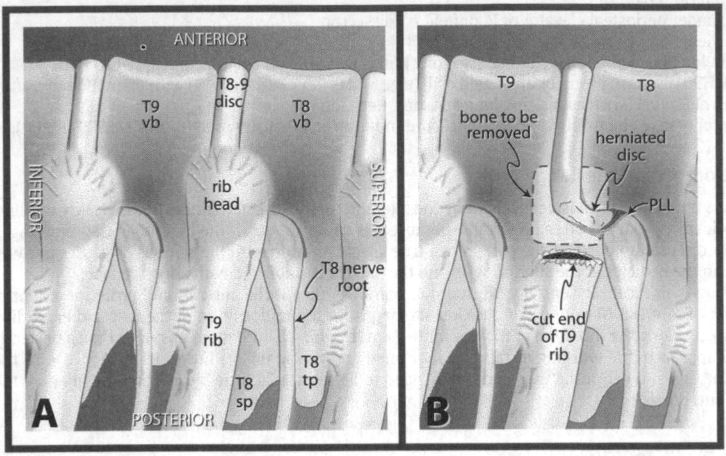

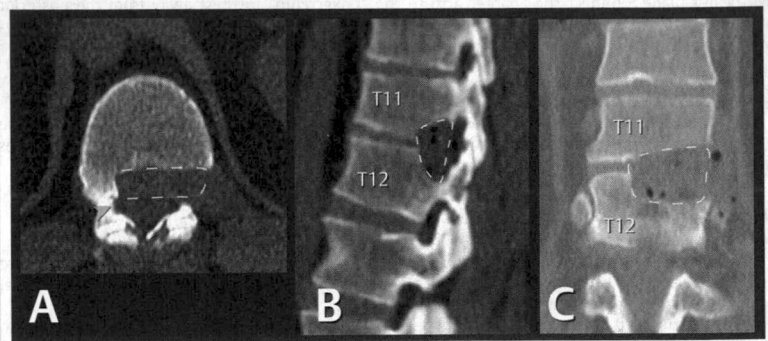

Fig. 76.3 Surgical view of lateral thoracic vertebral bodies from a left-sided approach (surgeon standing in back of the patient). A: anatomy. B: appearance after removal of rib head to access the T8–9 disc space.
Dashed lines depict bone that is removed (e.g., with a drill) for excision of a calcified thoracic disc (see ▶ Fig. 76.4 for post-op CT appearance).
Abbreviations: tp = transverse process; sp = spinous process; vb = vertebral body; PLL = posterior longitudinal ligament.

To remove a calcified thoracic disc, use e.g., the Midas Rex with 21 TU bit or Clear View™ diamond tip or the Misonix bone scalpel with the round burr to drill away bone from the posterior vertebral bodies above and a little below the disc space to a depth that is even with the medial aspect of the contralateral pedicle to expose the anterior spinal canal (▶ Fig. 76.4) and dura. Then hollow out the calcified disc with the drill until it is egg-shelled. Use a straight curette to push the egg-shell away from the dura into the defect now created in the vertebral bodies from whence it can then be removed.

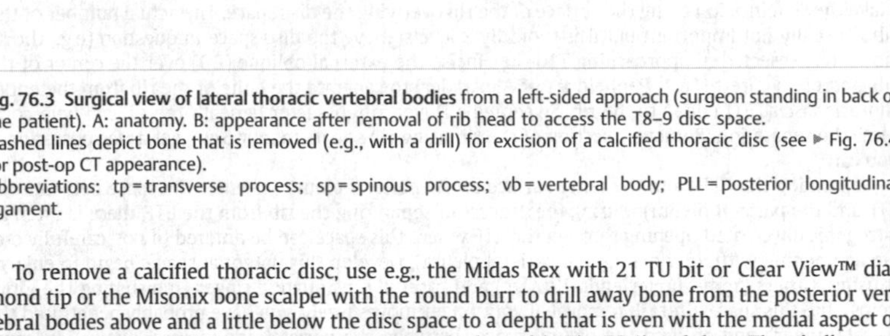

76

Fig. 76.4 Post-op CT bone windows following lateral (retrocoelomic) left-sided removal of a broad-based calcified T11–12 thoracic disc, illustrating the bone removed (*broken yellow lines*). A: axial. B: sagittal. C: coronal. Note the bony removal extends to the medial aspect of the right pedicle (*blue arrowhead*) in order to completely decompress the anterior spinal canal.

Closure and drains

An air leak may occur if the visceral pleura (lung lining) is violated. To rule this out, fill the wound with irrigation and have the anesthesiologist apply a Valsalva maneuver. Continuous bubbling (as opposed to initial bubbling that stops) signifies an air leak. In this case, if the leak is small, a medium hemovac in the pleural space may suffice; for large air leaks an actual chest tube is recommended and is connected to suction through a water seal.

If the parietal pleura (chest wall lining) alone is violated, an air leak will not result but a pneumothorax can occur. A medium hemovac or a pigtail catheter is usually adequate to treat this. Alternatively, a red-rubber catheter may be placed outside the parietal pleura, and the muscle closed around it. A Valsalva maneuver is performed by the anesthesiologist while the distal tip of the red rubber catheter is placed in water. As the lung expands a limited amount of bubbles will occur as the air is expelled from the pleural space (continuous bubbling means an air leak and requires a chest tube or equivalent). The red rubber catheter is then pulled out and a final stitch can be placed if necessary. Then the Valsalva can be released.

References

[1] El-Kalliny M, Tew JM, van Loveren H, et al. Surgical approaches to thoracic disk herniations. Acta Neurochirurgica. 1991; 111:22–32

[2] Stillerman CB, Chen TC, Couldwell WT, et al. Experience in the surgical management of 82 symptomatic herniated thoracic discs and review of the literature. Journal of Neurosurgery. 1998; 88:623–633

[3] Dohn DF. Thoracic Spinal Cord Decompression: Alternative Surgical Approaches and Basis of Choice. Clin Neurosurg. 1980; 27:611–623

[4] Le Roux PD, Haglund MM, Harris AB. Thoracic Disc Disease: Experience with the Transpedicular Approach in Twenty Consecutive Patients. Neurosurgery. 1993; 33:58–66

[5] Uribe JS, Smith WD, Pimenta L, et al. Minimally invasive lateral approach for symptomatic thoracic disc herniation: initial multicenter clinical experience. J Neurosurg Spine. 2012; 16:264–279

[6] Arce AC, Dohrmann GJ. Thoracic Disc Herniation. Surgical Neurology. 1985; 23:356–361

[7] Ahlgren BD, Herkowitz HN. A modified posterolateral approach to the thoracic spine. Journal of Spinal Disorders. 1195; 8:69–75

[8] O'Leary ST, Ganju A, Rauzzino MJ, et al. Costotransversectomy. In: Atlas of Neurosurgical Techniques. New York: Thieme Medical Publishers, Inc.; 2006:441–447

[9] Chou SN, Seljeskog EL. Alternative Surgical Approaches to the Thoracic Spine. Clin Neurosurg. 1972; 20:306–321

[10] Perot PL, Munro DD. Transthoracic Removal of Midline Thoracic Disc Protrusions Causing Spinal Cord Compression. J Neurosurg. 1969; 31:452–461

[11] Deviren V, Kuelling FA, Poulter G, et al. Minimal invasive anterolateral transthoracic transpleural approach: a novel technique for thoracic disc herniation. A review of the literature, description of a new surgical technique and experience with first 12 consecutive patients. J Spinal Disord Tech. 2011; 24:E40–E48

77 Cervical Disc Herniation

77.1 Cervical disc herniation – general information

Important applied anatomy in herniated cervical disc (HCD):
1. in the cervical region, the nerve root exits *above* the pedicle of its like-numbered vertebra (opposite to the situation in the lumbar spine, due to the fact that there are 8 cervical nerve roots and only 7 cervical vertebrae)
2. as each nerve root exits through its neural foramen, it passes in close relation to the undersurface of the like-numbered pedicle
3. the intervertebral disc space is located close to the inferior portion of the pedicle (unlike the lumbar region)

77.2 Cervical nerve root syndromes (cervical radiculopathy)

77.2.1 General information

Due to the facts listed above, an HCD usually impinges on the nerve exiting from the neural foramen *at* the level of the herniation (e.g., a C6–7 HCD usually causes C7 radiculopathy). This gives rise to the characteristic cervical nerve root syndromes shown in ▶ Table 77.1.

Table 77.1 Cervical disc syndromes

	Level of herniated cervical disc			
	C4–5	C5–6	C6–7	C7–1
% of cervical discs	2%	19%	69%	10%
compressed root	C5	C6	C7	C8
reflex diminished	deltoid & pectoralis	biceps & brachio-radialis	triceps	finger-jerk[a]
motor weakness	deltoid	forearm flexion	forearm ext (wrist drop)	hand intrinsics
paresthesia & hypesthesia	shoulder	upper arm, thumb, radial forearm	fingers 2 & 3, all fingertips	fingers 4 & 5

[a]not everyone has a finger flexor reflex. Description: gently lift the fingertips of the patient's pronated hand and tap the underside of the fingers with a reflex hammer. When present, fingers flex in response

77.2.2 Miscellaneous clinical facts

C4 radiculopathy is not common, and may produce nonradiating axial neck pain.

Left C6 radiculopathy (e.g., from C5–6 HCD) occasionally presents with pain simulating an MI (pseudo-angina).

C8 and T1 nerve root involvement may produce a partial Horner syndrome.

The most common scenario for patients with herniated cervical disc is that the symptoms were present upon awakening in the morning, without identifiable trauma or stress.[1]

Patients may offer (or may need to be asked) that placing the ipsilateral hand or forearm on the top of the head sometimes gives relief of pain due to a herniated cervical disc (so-called "cervical hand sign," ▶ Fig. 77.1).

77.3 Cervical myelopathy and SCI due to cervical disc herniation

Acute cord compression presenting with myelopathy or spinal cord injury (SCI) (including complete SCI and incomplete syndromes, especially **central cord syndrome** (p. 1132) and sometimes Brown-Séquard syndrome (p.1135) [2]) is well described in association with traumatic cervical disc herniation.[3] Less commonly, these findings may occur in non-traumatic cervical disc herniation.

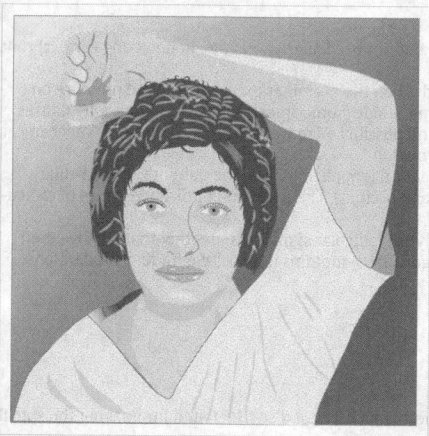

Fig. 77.1 "Cervical hand sign." A position that may provide some relief to patients with radiculopathy from cervical disc herniation.

77.4 Differential diagnosis

See Differential diagnosis (p. 1710).

77.5 Physical exam for cervical disc herniation

77.5.1 Overview

1. evaluation for radiculopathy
   a) lower motor neuron findings
      - weakness usually in one myotome group on one side
      - muscle bulk and tone: atrophy and fasciculations may be present
   b) sensation: with nerve root compression, sensory loss will follow a dermatomal pattern and will be in the same nerve root distribution as the weakness
   c) muscle stretch reflexes
   d) mechanical signs: reproduction of radicular symptoms with axial loading of the head
2. evidence of spinal cord involvement (myelopathy)
   a) upper motor neuron findings, usually in the lower extremities
      - weakness may occur without atrophy or fasciculations
      - spasticity: poor control of the legs when walking, scissoring of the legs
   b) sensation: any loss below the level of involvement will follow spinal cord patterns
      - complete loss
      - Brown-Séquard syndrome (p. 1135) pattern: ipsilateral vibratory and position sense loss and contralateral loss of pinprick
      - central cord syndrome: suspended sensory loss in upper extremities, less impaired below
      - pathologic reflexes: Hoffmann's reflex, Babinski sign, ankle clonus

77.5.2 Signs useful in evaluating cervical radiculopathy

General information

Almost all herniated cervical discs cause painful limitation of neck motion. Neck *extension* usually aggravates pain when cervical disc disease is present (a minority of patients instead exhibit pain with flexion). Some patients find relief in elevating the arm and cupping the back or the top of the head with the hand (abduction relief sign, see below for shoulder abduction test). Lhermitte's sign (p. 1712) (electrical shock-like sensation radiating down the spine) may be present; see DDx (p. 1712).

77

Miscellaneous

The following tests were found to be specific, but not particularly sensitive in detecting cervical root compression[4]:

1. Spurling's sign[5]: radicular pain reproduced when the examiner exerts downward pressure on vertex while tilting head towards symptomatic side (sometimes adding neck *extension*). Causes narrowing of the intervertebral foramen and possibly increases disc bulge. Used as a "mechanical sign" analogous to SLR for lumbar disc herniation
2. axial manual traction: 10–15 kg of axial traction is applied to a supine patient with radicular symptoms (pull up on patient's mandible and occiput). The reduction or disappearance of radicular symptoms is a positive finding
3. shoulder abduction test[6]: a sitting patient with radicular symptoms lifts their hand above their head. The reduction or disappearance of radicular symptoms is a positive finding. Moderately sensitive, fairly specific[7]

77.6 Radiologic evaluation

77.6.1 MRI

The study of choice for initial evaluation for herniated cervical disc (HCD) and for imaging the spinal cord.

Protocol:

1. sagittal T1WI
2. multiple echo cardiac gated sagittal images (Tr = 1560, Te = 25, 4th echo)
3. T2* GRE image: dark material adjacent to disc space is bone, disc is higher signal, CSF and flowing blood are high signal.

77.6.2 CT and myelogram/CT

Indications: when MRI cannot be done or when more bony detail than what MRI provides is required. Evaluates for ossification of the posterior longitudinal ligament (OPLL) when suspected.

Plain CT: is usually good at C5–6, is variable at C6–7 (due to artifact from patient's shoulders, depending on body habitus), and is usually poor at C7–1.

Myelogram/CT (water-soluble intrathecal contrast): invasive, on rare occasions requires overnight hospitalization. Accuracy is ≈ 98% for cervical disc disease.

77.6.3 Electrodiagnostics (EMG and NCV)

Compression may occur at the level of the dorsal (pre-ganglionic) sensory root (which, if occurs alone, produces a sensory-only radiculopathy) and/or at the ventral (motor) root. When motor exam is normal, EMG is unlikely to show abnormality. The AANEM practice parameter for cervical radiculopathy[8,9,10] reports sensitivity of 50–71% for the needle EMG examination and correlation between positive needle EMG and radiologic findings of 65–85%.

EMG can also be normal in sensory-only radiculopathy, which occasionally occurs in cervical spine, but not in lumbar spine. Since most muscles have at least dual innervation this poses a particular challenge for proximal cervical radiculopathies in which many muscles have the same shared innervation, e.g., biceps, deltoid, brachioradialis, infraspinatus, and supraspinatus are all innervated by C5–6.

For both cervical and lumbosacral radiculopathy, screening 6 muscles representing all root levels to include paraspinal muscles yields consistently high identification rates.[11]

For muscles to demonstrate fibrillations and positive waves there must be axonal loss in the motor nerve axons which innervate a muscle. Muscle demonstrates fibs and positive waves within 1 to 2 weeks following loss of innervation depending on the distance from the nerve to the muscle.

NCV is helpful when assessing for peripheral neuropathies, which may have symptoms similar to radiculopathy (e.g., carpal tunnel syndrome vs. C6 radiculopathy; ulnar neuropathy vs. C8 radiculopathy). A good physical exam can differentiate these entities in most cases.

Practice guideline: EDX guidelines for cervical radiculopathy[10]

1. Guideline: EMG needle examination:
   a) needle examination of at least 1 muscle innervated by C5, C6, C7, C8, and T1 spinal roots in a symptomatic limb
   b) cervical paraspinal muscles at 1 or more levels (except in patients with prior posterior approach cervical surgery)
   c) if abnormalities are identified, perform studies of 1 or 2 additional muscles innervated by the suspected root and different peripheral nerve
2. Guideline: At least 1 motor and 1 sensory nerve conduction study (NCS) in the clinically involved limb to determine if there is concomitant polyneuropathy or nerve entrapment. Motor and sensory NCS of median and ulnar nerves if symptoms and signs suggest CTS or ulnar neuropathy. If 1 or more NCS are abnormal or if clinical features suggest polyneuropathy, further evaluation may include NCS of other nerves in the ipsilateral and contralateral limb

77.7 Treatment

77.7.1 General information

Over 90% of patients with acute cervical radiculopathy due to cervical disc herniation can improve without surgery,[12] and regression of an extruded cervical disc has been demonstrated radiographically by CT and MRI.[13,14,15] The recovery period may be made more tolerable by adequate pain medication, anti-inflammatory medication (NSAIDs or short-course tapering steroids), and intermittent cervical traction (e.g., gradually escalating up to 10–15 lbs for 10–15 minutes, 2–3 × daily).

Surgery is indicated for those that fail to improve or those with progressive neurologic deficit while undergoing non-surgical management.

Management of myelopathy/central cord syndrome associated with acute cervical disc herniation is controversial, since the natural history is favorable in most cases. However, some patients have poor recovery and experience permanent deficits even with emergency surgery.[16]

77.7.2 Conservative management

Modalities include:
1. physical therapy, which may also include cervical traction
2. interventional pain management
   a) trigger point injections
   b) facet blocks
   c) epidural steroid injection: not used as often and with lumbar spine

77.7.3 Surgery

Surgical options

1. anterior cervical discectomy: see below
   a) without any prosthesis or fusion: rarely used today
   b) combined with interbody fusion: the most common approach
      • without anterior cervical plating
      • with anterior cervical plating or with zero profile
   c) with artificial disc AKA cervical disc arthroplasty
2. posterior approaches
   a) cervical laminectomy: not typically used for a herniated cervical disc, more common for cervical spinal stenosis, OPLL
      • without posterior fusion
      • with lateral mass fusion
   b) keyhole laminotomy: sometimes permits removal of disc fragment

77

For practice guidelines regarding intra-op electrophysiologic, see monitoring for surgery for cervical radiculopathy (p. 1304).

Anterior cervical discectomy with fusion (ACDF)

Without special modifications, a routine anterior approach is usually able to access levels C3–7. In patients with short thick necks, access may be even more limited. In some cases, with long thin necks, up to C2–3 or as low as C7–1 can be approached anteriorly.

Advantages over posterior (nonfused) approach:
1. safe removal of anterior osteophytes
2. fusion of disc space affords immobility (up to 10% incidence of subluxation with extensive posterior approach)
3. only viable means of directly dealing with centrally herniated disc

Disadvantages over posterior approach: immobility at fused level may increase stress on adjacent disc spaces. If a fusion is performed, some surgeons prescribe a rigid collar (e.g., Philadelphia collar) for 6–12 weeks. Multiple level ACDF can devascularize the vertebral body (or bodies) between discectomies.

Booking the case: ACDF

Also see defaults & disclaimers (p. 25).
1. position: supine, some use halter traction with this
2. equipment:
   a) microscope (not used by all surgeons)
   b) C-arm
3. implants: graft (e.g., PEEK, cadaver bone, titanium cage...) and anterior cervical plate (optional, especially on single level ACDF)
4. neuromonitoring: (optional) some surgeons use SSEP/MEP
5. consent (in lay terms for the patient—not all-inclusive):
   a) procedure: surgery through the front of the neck to remove the degenerated disc and bone spurs, and to place a graft where the disc was, and possibly place a metal plate on the front of the spine. Some surgeons take bone from the hip to replace the removed disc
   b) alternatives: nonsurgical management, surgery from the back of the neck, artificial disc (in some cases)
   c) complications: swallowing difficulties are common but usually resolve, hoarseness of the voice (< 4% chance of it being permanent), injury to: foodpipe (esophagus), windpipe (trachea), arteries to the brain (carotid), spinal cord with paralysis, nerve root with paralysis, possible seizures with MEPs

---

Technique

A summary of the steps: a 4–5 cm horizontal skin incision oriented along Langer's lines is centered on the anterior margin of the SCM in the mediolateral plane. Fluoroscopy is used for cranio-caudal localization, for C5–6 it is usually at the level of the cricoid cartilage. Many right-handed surgeons prefer operating from the right side of the neck, although the risk to the recurrent laryngeal nerve (RLN) is possibly lower with a left-sided approach (the RLN lies in a groove between the esophagus and trachea). The skin may be undermined off the platysma to permit a vertical incision in the platysma in the same orientation as its muscle fibers. Most just incise the platysma horizontally with Metzenbaum scissors.

Dissect in tissue plane medial to SCM. Sweep the omohyoid medially (to stay out of it and to protect the RLN). The trachea + esophagus are retracted medially. The carotid sheath + SCM are retracted laterally.

Verify the level with lateral C-spine X-ray with bayonetted spinal needle in the interspace. Bipolar cautery is used on the prevertebral fascia and medial edges of the longus colli muscles longitudinally in the midline. Self-retaining retractor blades are inserted underneath the fascia to retract the longus colli muscles laterally. The anesthesiologist deflates the cuff on the endotracheal tube and then re-inflates it using minimal leak technique to reduce the risk of compression injury from the retractor. The disc space is incised with a 15 scalpel blade. The discectomy is performed with curettes and pituitary rongeurs; a vertebral body spreader or Caspar pin distractor aids the exposure. The posterior longitudinal ligament (PLL) is opened, typically by insinuating a nerve hook through the fibers, and then expanding this opening initially with a 1 mm Kerrison rongeur and then with 2 mm Kerrison rongeurs. The subligamentous space is probed with a blunt nerve hook. The posterior osteophytes of the VB above and below are removed with a 2 mm Kerrison rongeur. Decompression of the roots is verified with the blunt nerve hook. A fusion is usually performed at this time by placing a graft in the interspace.

For redo operations (same or different levels): approach is usually from the same side as previous operation(s) since many patients have swallowing issues from the previous operation, and some may be due to partial recurrent laryngeal nerve injury, which can be subclinical and could result in a permanent need for a feeding tube if a contralateral injury occurs. If for some reason it is desired to go to the opposite side, an evaluation by an ENT physician is recommended, and should include scoping the patient to rule out subclinical vocal cord problems that could turn into major difficulties if bilateral.

Choice of graft material

Autologous bone (usually from iliac crest), non-autologous bone (cadaveric), bone substitutes (e.g., hydroxylapatite[17]) or synthetics (e.g., PEEK or titanium cage) filled with osteogenic material. Substitutes for autologous bone eliminate problems with the donor site (p. 1287), but may have a higher rate of absorption. There were cases of HIV transmission from cadaveric bone grafts in 1985; however, as a result of significant improvements in antibody testing and careful screening of donors, no further cases have been reported.

Anterior cervical plating

Recommendations for plating following ACDF are shown in **Practice guideline: Anterior cervical plating** (p. 1285).

Practice guideline: Anterior cervical plating

1-level ACDF: The addition of an anterior plate to an ACDF is recommended to reduce the pseudarthrosis rate and graft problems (Level D Class III) and to maintain lordosis (Level C Class II), but it does not improve clinical outcome alone (Level B Class II).[18]

2-level ACDF: Plating is recommended to improve arm pain. Plating does not improve other outcome parameters (Level C Class II).[18]

Use of bone morphogenetic proteins (BMP)

Practice guideline: Use of BMP in cervical interbody grafting

Current evidence does not support the *routine* use of rhBMP-2 for cervical arthrodesis (Level C Class II)[19] [italics added].

Note: Use with precautions (see text); may be indicated in cases with high risk of nonunion.

Use of BMP in anterior cervical discectomies is not FDA approved, but has been used off-label. Complication rates as high as 23–27% have been reported (including post-op swallowing or respiratory difficulties as a result of edema which is usually temporary) compared to 3% without BMP.[19] If used, it is recommended that a smaller dose be employed than in the lumbar spine (25% has been advocated) and to avoid contact of BMP with soft tissues in the neck.

Post-op check

In addition to routine, the following should be checked
1. evidence of airway obstruction—post-op wound hematoma: should be first consideration. Wound may need to be emergently opened at bedside (before getting to the OR) if airway is

compromised, see **Carotid endarterectomy,** disruption of arteriotomy closure, management (p. 1568). Also consider swelling from IJV thrombosis (rare) in differential diagnosis (see below)
  a) respiratory distress
  b) extreme difficulty swallowing: alternatively may indicate anterior extrusion of bone graft impinging upon esophagus (check lateral C-spine X-ray)
  c) tracheal deviation: may be visible or may be seen on AP C-spine X-ray
2. weakness of nerve root of level operated: e.g., biceps for C5–6, triceps for C6–7
3. long tract signs (Babinski sign…) which may indicate cord compression by spinal epidural hematoma
4. hoarseness: may indicate vocal cord paresis from recurrent laryngeal nerve injury: hold oral feeding until this can be further assessed

ACDF complications

General information
Common complications are listed below, see references[20,21] for more details. The most common complication following ACDFs: swallowing difficulties (p. 1287) (may be multifactorial).
1. exposure injuries
  a) perforation of viscus: minimize risk by blunt retraction until longus colli is separated from its attachment to vertebrae
     * pharynx
     * esophageal perforation (p. 1288): a rare but well-known complication
     * trachea
  b) vocal cord paresis: due to injury of the recurrent laryngeal nerve (RLN) or vagus. Incidence: 11% temporary (84% of temporary palsies resolve clinically by 6 months), 4% permanent paresis. Incidence may be higher in revision surgery. Symptoms include: hoarseness, breathiness, cough, aspiration, mass sensation, dysphagia, and vocal cord fatigue.[22] Avoid sharp dissection in paratracheal muscles. Some cases may be due to prolonged retraction against trachea and not to nerve division; to reduce this risk, after the self-retaining retractor is placed, have the anesthesiologist deflate the cuff on the ET tube and then inflate it to minimal leak pressure. More common with right-sided approaches, primarily in the lower cervical spine (C5–6 and below) where the RLN is more vulnerable[22]
  c) vertebral artery injury: thrombosis or laceration. 0.3% incidence.[21] Treatment alternatives include: packing, direct repair by temporary clipping with aneurysms clips and repair with 8–0 prolene[23] and endovascular trapping. Risks of treating hemorrhagic complications with packing include: recurrent bleeding, AV fistula, pseudoaneurysm, arterial thrombosis,[21] distal embolic stroke (primarily in cerebellum)
  d) carotid injury: thrombosis, occlusion, or laceration (usually by retraction)
  e) CSF fistula: usually difficult to repair directly. Place fascial graft beneath bone plug. Keep HOB elevated post-op. Consider: dural sealant (fibrin glue, DuraSeal®…), lumbar drain
  f) Horner syndrome: sympathetic plexus lies within longus coli, thus do not extend dissection far laterally into these muscles
  g) thoracic duct injury: in exposing lower cervical spine, primarily on left
  h) thrombosis of internal jugular vein[24]: rare. Carries 2–3% risk of PE.[25] Treatment options: anticoagulation (oral or IV) may lower the mortality,[26] SVC filter if anticoagulation is contraindicated,[27] percutaneous thrombectomy[28]
2. spinal cord or nerve root injuries
  a) spinal cord injury: especially risky in myelopathy due to narrowed canal. Minimize risk by penetrating the osteophyte at the lateral margin of interspace (however, this increases risk to nerve root)
  b) avoid hyperextension during intubation: use video laryngoscopy, or second choice, asleep fiberoptic bronchoscopy (awake fiberoptic intubation is rarely used)[29]
  c) bone graft must be shorter than interspace depth. Exercise caution in tapping graft into position
  d) sleep-induced apnea: rare but serious complications of C3–4 level operations.[30] May be associated with bradycardia & cardiorespiratory instability. Possibly due to disruption of the afferent component of the central respiratory control mechanism
3. bone fusion problems
  a) failure of fusion (pseudarthrosis): see below
  b) anterior (kyphotic) angulation deformity: may be as high as 60% with Cloward technique (may be reduced by collar immobilization). May develop in Hirsch technique with excessive bone removal

77

   c) graft extrusion: 2% incidence (rarely requires reoperation unless compression of cord posteriorly, or esophagus or trachea anteriorly occurs)

   d) donor site complications: hematoma/seroma, infection, fracture of ilium, injury to lateral femoral cutaneous nerve, persistent pain due to scar, bowel perforation

4. miscellaneous

   a) wound infection: incidence < 1%

   b) post-op hematoma: *see above*. Placing cervical collar in O.R. may delay recognition of immediate post-op hematoma

   c) dysphagia and hoarseness: common. Usually transient (*see below*)

   d) adjacent level degeneration: controversial whether this represents a sequela to altered biomechanics from surgery, or a predisposition to cervical spondylosis.[31] Many ($\approx$ 70%) are asymptomatic[32]

   e) postoperative discomfort:
- globus: the sensation of a lump in throat (see below)
- nagging discomfort in neck, shoulder, and very commonly in interscapular regions (may last several months). May correlate with amount of distraction of the disc space

   f) complex regional pain syndrome (CRPS) AKA reflex sympathetic dystrophy (**RSD**): rarely described in the literature,[33] possibly due to stellate ganglion injury; see discussion of RSD (p. 525)

   g) angioedema: massive edema of the tongue and neck.[34] A dramatic hypersensitivity reaction (not really a direct complication of ACDF, but superficially can mimic some findings of post-op hematoma. If limited to the tongue, the airway is not compromised. See treatment (p. 233)

   h) pneumothorax or hemothorax[35]: accessing C7–1 or lower may expose the pleural apex

Dysphagia following ACDF

Symptoms: Include: difficulty swallowing (solids, liquids including saliva), pain with swallowing (odynophagia), globus (sensation of a lump in throat), and compromise of ability to protect against aspiration. Food may stick in the throat (or feel as if it is stuck) and there may be coughing or choking.

   Incidence: Difficult to accurately quantify since definitions & surgical techniques vary, and selection biases produce wide ranges. Early dysphagia is common, with incidence as high as 60%[36] in a retrospective survey after noninstrumented fusion (dysphagia occurred in 23% in a control group undergoing unrelated lumbar spine surgery[36]), and 50% in a prospective study.[37] At 6 months, only $\approx$ 5% reported moderate or severe dysphagia.[37] Surgery at multiple levels increased the risk at 1 & 2 months.[37] Dysphagia decreases significantly in most cases by 6 months.[37]

   Etiologies: mild cases are usually self-limited and are related to a combination of retraction on esophagus, post-op inflammation, irritation following endotrachial intubation, and presence of hardware. More pronounced or prolonged dysphagia may be due to:
1. post-op hematoma. If severe, may cause tracheal obstruction (see above)
2. post-op edema, due in part to retraction of esophagus
3. effects of general anesthesia: e.g., irritation from ET tube. Accounts for up to 23% of early symptoms (dysphagia occurred in 23% in a control group undergoing unrelated lumbar spine surgery[36]). Usually subsides within $\approx$ 24–72 hours
4. recurrent laryngeal nerve dysfunction:
   a) temporary: usually due to traction on the nerve
   b) permanent: 1.3% at 12 months[37]
5. esophageal injury
   a) at time of surgery
   b) delayed: possibly from repetitive abrasion on hardware or from unrecognized esophageal injury at time of surgery[38]
6. cervical collar
   a) prevents patient from lowering jaw during swallow phase, which compromises effective glottic closure of airway
   b) may be too tight, thereby directly compressing the throat
7. protrusion of graft/hardware anterior to the vertebral bodies
   a) some protrusion is present with most anterior hardware. This may be minimized with "zero profile" instrumentation
   b) hardware failure (screw pullout, backout or breakage, plate loosening, pullout or migration)
   c) interbody graft migration: without anterior plate, or in conjunction with anterior plate displacement
8. excessive adhesions[39]

77

9. denervation of the pharyngeal plexus[39]
10. rare conditions: swelling from internal jugular vein (IJV) thrombosis, angioedema

Management:
1. initial management: rule out emergent/serious conditions (severe edema, hematoma with airway compromise, risk of aspiration)
   a) if there is significant stridor or dysphonia, especially if tracheal deviation is obvious, someone must stay with the patient as efforts are made to emergently take the patient to the O.R. for wound exploration & evacuation of hematoma if any. Consider opening the wound at the bedside if delays occur or if symptoms are severe; see Carotid endarterectomy, disruption of arteriotomy closure, management (p. 1568). Emergent anesthesia consultation for airway protection— alert them to the likelihood of deviated trachea, which challenges even the most expert at intubating
2. once emergent conditions are ruled out, early management is geared towards amelioration of symptoms
   a) advise patient to eat softer foods (temporarily avoiding steak or bread), to chew food well, to wash down dry foods with a drink. Reassure patient that most cases largely resolve within 6 months[37]
   b) treatment with dexamethasone 8-10 mg TID for 3 days will get most patients through this
   c) if significant symptoms persist > 2 weeks
      • ENT referral for evaluation that may include: laryngoscopy, FEES (flexible endoscopic evaluation of swallowing), to rule out vocal cord paralysis (from RLN injury (p. 1289)) or other etiologies
      • modified barium swallow (mBS)
3. persistent symptoms may be amenable to surgical intervention, including hardware removal and lysing of adhesions.[39] Management of esophageal perforation usually requires consultation with ENT (see below)

Esophageal perforation after anterior cervical spine surgery
Incidence: Data is imprecise due to reporting bias. It is also likely that minor injuries that heal spontaneously and go unrecognized may occur. Reported range: 0.02% to 1.52%. Incidence is higher when the surgery is performed for trauma.[40] Incidence may be higher with use of anterior cervical plate.
   Etiologies: Intraoperative injury (direct injury or from retractor), or delayed (from hardware failure & hardware erosion, graft extrusion...).
   Possible sequelae: Dysphagia, local infection, deep infection (including osteomyelitis), pseudarthrosis, pharyngoesophageal diverticulum, sepsis, mediastinitis, death in 4%.[40] Species reported with infection include: *Staphylococcus* (including MRSA), *Candida*, *Pseudomonas*, and *Streptococcus*.
   Delay to diagnosis: Mean = 717 days. Median = 44.5 days.[40]
• intraoperative recognized (often heralded by the appearance of mucous appearing in the operative field): zero delay to diagnosis
• early post-op: < 30 days post-op. Most are probably unrecognized intraoperative injuries
• delayed: as late as 18 years. Mostly hardware failure/erosion

Symptoms: Dysphagia (the most common), odynophagia, fever, neck swelling, and wound leakage.[40]
   Signs include: Fever, subcutaneous emphysema, sepsis ± shock
   Evaluation: Approximately 33% may not be detected on imaging or endoscopy.[41]
• swallow studies:
   ○ gastrograffin swallow: usually administered by radiologist to look for leak, or
   ○ (modified) barium swallow: usually curated by speech pathologist, can assess for leaks and also diagnose other swallowing pathologies
• esophagoscopy by ENT
• CT scan: assesses bony fusion (important to know since hardware often has to be removed) and may assist in making diagnosis
• MRI without and with contrast: assesses for epidural abscess, vertebral osteomyelitis (contrast T1WI)
• CXR

Management: Challenging. There is no consensus on optimal management. A multidisciplinary approach with head and neck surgeons together with the spine surgeon,[38] infectious disease specialist and, when needed, a cardiothoracic surgeon is suggested, with the following:

- primary closure: usually effective at the time of the original surgery if perforation is recognized then, or it is diagnosed within 24 hrs of the time of injury.[42] Not recommended once adjacent tissues become involved and/or when esophagus is inflamed (high risk of esophageal stricture)
- closure with muscle flap or possibly a pedicle flap: sternocleidomastoid muscle is most common. Other muscle flaps include: radial forearm, pectoralis, infrahyoid, omohyoid, latissisus dorsi, longus coli. Also described: omentum, jejunum
- removing all anterior hardware increases the chance of success.[40] If there is evidence that the fusion is not solid, posterior instrumentation may be necessary
- a wound drain is placed external to the esophagus, and can be used to check for extravasation of methylene blue administered orally to verify esophageal healing
- esophageal bypass: rarely required, high morbidity
- conservative management: usually used in conjunction with above. Use of conservative management alone is less common and is controversial. May be more viable if used early for small, contained defects (i.e., not involving mediastinitis[43]). Usually includes:
  - putting the esophagus at rest:
    - strict NPO
    - nutrition via one of the following: tube feeding (nasogastric tube, passed with caution and possibly in conjunction with endoscopy to pass tube at the level of the perforation), gastrostomy, jejunostomy, or parenteral nutrition
  - antibiotics

Outcome: Average number of esophageal repair attempts per patient: 1.54. 86% required just 1 operation. Average time to oral intake is 30 days (conservative management used alone averaged 68 days).[40] 4% mortality.

Recurrent laryngeal nerve paralysis

Heralded by breathy voice, hoarseness, or aspiration. Refer to ENT for endoscopy to determine if vocal cord is paralyzed and its position. 4 possible positions: 1) median, 2) paramedian, 3) intermediate, 4) lateral (cadaveric). Many patients can compensate for median or paramedian position.

Patients requiring intervention are usually treated with medialization techniques, either 1) injection, or 2) medialization thyroplasty using an implant. For injections, different materials may be selected for desired duration of effect. Early intervention may be employed with temporary materials. If no spontaneous recovery after 1 year, injection with Teflon is essentially permanent

Pseudarthrosis (or pseudoarthrosis) following ACDF

Pseudarthrosis may occur with or without supplemental anterior cervical plating.

Practice guideline: Assessment of subaxial fusion

>2 mm movement between spinous processes on dynamic (flexion-extension) cervical spine X-rays is recommended as a criterion for pseudarthrosis (Level B Class II); this measurement is unreliable when performed by the treating surgeon (Level C Class II).[44]

Visualization of bone trabeculation across the fusion on static films is a less reliable marker for fusion (Level D Class III) (2D reformatted CT increases the accuracy (Level D Class III)).[44]

77

Incidence: Difficult to assess because of lack of validated criteria. Estimate: 2–20%. Higher with dowel technique (Cloward) than with keystone technique of Bailey & Badgley or with interbody method of Smith-Robinson (10%) or with non-fusion advocated by Hirsch. One criterion: motion >2 mm between the tips of the spinous processes on lateral flexion/extension X-rays.[45,46] Other criteria that are specific but not sensitive: lucencies around the screws of an anterior plate, toggling of the screws on flexion/extension X-rays.

Presentation: Not uniformly associated with symptoms or problems.[45,47] Some patients may have chronic or recurrent neck pain, some may present with radicular symptoms. (NB: when DePalma's data is analyzed with patients reclassified as failures if neck and/or arm symptoms persist, the success rate of surgery is lower with pseudarthrosis.[48])

Management: Guidelines are shown in **Practice guideline: Management of anterior cervical pseudarthrosis** (p. 1290). No treatment is required for *asymptomatic* pseudarthrosis. Options for symptomatic patients include re-resection of the bone graft with repeat fusion[49] (some recommend using autologous bone if allograft was used; a plate may be considered if one was not used previously), cervical corpectomy with fusion,[49] or posterior cervical fusion.

Practice guideline: Management of anterior cervical pseudarthrosis

Revision of symptomatic pseudarthrosis should be considered (Level D Class III).[50] Posterior approaches may be associated with higher fusion rates on revision than anterior approaches (Level D Class III)[50]

Cervical disc arthroplasty

An alternative to fusion. Uses an artificial disc to preserve motion at the level of the discectomy. Some of the available cervical disc replacement (CDR) models are shown in ▶ Table 77.2.[51]

Table 77.2 Artificial cervical discs

Trade name	Manufacturer	Material	IAR[a]	Comment
Prestige®	Medtronic	MOM[a] (chrome cobalt stainless steel)	variable ball in trough	significant MRI artifact
Prestige® LP	Medtronic	MOM[a] (metal ceramic composite)	variable ball in trough	FDA approved for 1 or 2 levels
Bryan®	Medtronic	lubricated elastic nucleus sealed in a flexible membrane	variable in center of disc space	
ProDisc-C	Centinel Spine	metal-on-polyethylene	posterior part of inferior VB	midline keel inserts into VB; lots of MRI artifact
Mobi-C®	LDR Spine	metal-on-polyethylene	variable in center of disc space	FDA approved for 1 or 2 levels
PCM®	Nuvasive	metal-on-polyethylene	gliding motion	contoured to endplates
Secure-C®	Globus medical	metal-on-polyethylene	15° flex/ext, 10° lateral bending, unconstrained rotation	serrated keels with titanium spray coating

[a]Abbreviations: IAR = instantaneous axis of rotation; MOM = metal-on-metal; PCM = Porous-coated Motion.

Contraindications: described by the FDA have included: isolated axial neck pain, ankylosing spondylitis or pregnancy, rheumatoid arthritis, autoimmune disease, diffuse idiopathic skeletal hyperostosis, severe spondylosis with bridging osteophytes or ossification of the posterior longitudinal ligament, disc height loss > 50%, spinal infection, metal allergy to components of the prosthesis, severe osteoporosis/osteopenia, active malignancy, metabolic bone disease, trauma, segmental instability, 3 or more levels requiring treatment, insulin-dependent diabetes mellitus, human immunodeficiency virus, hepatitis B/C, morbid obesity, absence of motion (< 2 degrees), and posterior facet arthrosis.

Practice guideline: Cervical disc arthroplasty

Cervical arthroplasty is a recommended alternative to ACDF in selected patients for control of arm and neck pain (Level B Class II)[18]

Booking the case: Cervical disc arthroplasty

Also see defaults & disclaimers and/or more significant (p. 25).
1. position: supine, some use halter traction with this
2. equipment:
   a) microscope (not used by all surgeons)
   b) C-arm
3. implants: schedule vendor to provide desired artificial disc. Bail out implants (cages and plates) should also be available in case the artifical disc cannot be implanted
4. neuromonitoring: (optional) some surgeons use SSEP/MEP
5. consent (in lay terms for the patient—not all-inclusive):
   a) procedure: surgery through the front of the neck to remove the degenerated disc and bone spurs, and to place an artificial disc
   b) alternatives: nonsurgical management, surgical fusion (from the front or the back of the neck)
   c) complications: swallowing difficulties are common but usually resolve, hoarseness of the voice (<4% chance of it being permanent), injury to: foodpipe (esophagus), windpipe (trachea), arteries to the brain (carotid) with stroke, spinal cord with paralysis, nerve root with paralysis, possible seizures with MEPs (if used). The disc may eventually wear out and further surgery may be needed. It is possible that the artifical disc cannot be implanted, in which case a fusion may be necessary

Post-op orders:
1. no cervical collar (the goal is to preserve motion at the operated level)
2. NSAIDs around the clock for ≈ 2 weeks (this theoretically inhibits bone growth which helps avoid undesirable fusion at the operated level)

Technical pointers: The approach and spine work are similar to an ACDF (p. 1284), with the following modifications:
1. positioning: keep the neck in neutral position. Avoid neck extension which narrows the posterior disc space and can increase the difficulty of inserting the prosthesis
2. the height of the artificial disc should be snug, but should not distract the VBs because this can compromise the function of the disc flexing and extending (don't overstuff the disc space)
3. since you are not "jacking up" the disc space with a cage, you have to be extra-meticulous in the foraminal decompression
4. some surgeons wax all decorticated bone surfaces to prevent fusion
5. avoid aggressively removing cartilaginous endplates, or else fusion is more likely to occur
6. NSAIDs are often prescribed for at least 2 weeks post-op since they help inhibit bone growth

Posterior cervical decompression (cervical laminectomy)

Not necessary for unilateral radiculopathy (use either ACD or keyhole laminotomy). Consists of removal of cervical lamina (laminectomy) and spinous processes in order to convert the spinal canal from a "tube" to a "trough."
   Usually reserved for the following conditions:
1. multiple cervical discs or osteophytes (anterior cervical discectomy (ACD) is usually used to treat only 2, or possibly 3, levels without) with myelopathy
2. where the anterior pathology is superimposed on cervical stenosis, and the latter is more diffuse and/or more significant (p. 1296)
3. in professional speakers or singers where the 4% risk of permanent voice change due to recurrent laryngeal nerve injury with ACD may be unacceptable

Booking the case: Cervical laminectomy

Also see defaults & disclaimers (p. 25).
1. position: prone, some use pin headholder
2. equipment:
   a) C-arm
   b) high-speed drill
3. implants: cervical lateral mass screws and rods if fusion is being done

4. neuromonitoring: some surgeons use SSEP/MEP
5. consent (in lay terms for the patient—not all-inclusive):
   a) procedure: surgery through the back of the neck to remove the bone over the compressed spinal cord and nerves and possibly to place screws and rods to fuse the bones together
   b) alternatives: nonsurgical management, surgery from the front of the neck, posterior surgery without fusion, laminoplasty
   c) complications: nerve root weakness (C5 nerve root is the most common), may not relieve symptoms, further surgery may be needed, possible seizures with MEPs. If fusion is not done, there is a risk of progressive bone slippage, which would require further surgery

Posterior keyhole laminotomy

AKA "keyhole foraminotomy." First described in 1951.[52] A technique to decompress only individual nerve roots (but not the spinal cord) by creating a small "keyhole" in the lamina to access the nerve root.

Practice guideline: Cervical laminoforaminotomy

Cervical laminoforaminotomy is recommended as a surgical treatment option for symptomatic cervical radiculopathy caused by disc herniation or lateral recess narrowing (Level D Class III).[53]

Indications for keyhole approach (as opposed to anterior discectomy):
1. monoradiculopathy with posterolateral *soft* disc sequestration (small *lateral* osteophytic spurs may also be addressed). This approach does *not* provide adequate decompression with central or broad-based disc herniation or with stenosis of the spinal canal
2. radiculopathy in patients who are professional speakers or singers where the risk of recurrent laryngeal nerve injury is untenable (see above)
3. for lower (e.g., C7, C8, or T1) or upper (e.g., C3 or C4) cervical nerve root compression, especially in a patient with a short thick neck, an anterior approach is more difficult
4. in patients with a herniated disc when it is desired to avoid a fusion (as would be done with an anterior approach)

Booking the case: Cervical keyhole laminectomy

Also see defaults & disclaimers (p. 25).
1. position: prone, some use pin headholder
2. equipment:
   a) microscope (not used by all surgeons)
   b) C-arm
3. instrumentation: some surgeons use a tube retractor system
4. neuromonitoring: some surgeons use SSEP/MEP
5. consent (in lay terms for the patient—not all-inclusive):
   a) procedure: surgery through the back of the neck to remove the bone over the compressed nerve root and possibly remove fragment of herniated disc
   b) alternatives: nonsurgical management, surgery from the front of the neck, posterior surgery with fusion
   c) complications: nerve root injury; may not relieve symptoms, necessitating further surgery; possible seizures with MEPs

Technique

See references.[54,55,56]

Position:

a) prone, on chest rolls. Adhesive tape is used to retract shoulders down for any level below about C4–5. The head is stabilized on a horseshoe headrest or in a Mayfield head holder.

b) sitting position: generally abandoned. However, may be used with proper precautions (p. 1737)

"Open" keyhole foraminotomy

The desired level is localized with intra-op fluoroscopy before making the skin incision, a 2–3 cm midline incision is adequate. A unilateral exposure suffices. Periosteal elevators are used to dissect muscles off the lamina and facet joint in the subperiosteal plane. A Kocher clamp may be placed on the spinous process to permit confirmation of the correct level on intraoperative X-ray. A Scoville retractor or equivalent is employed.

A high-speed drill (e.g., with diamond burr) is used to make an opening in the medial one-third to one-half of the inferior facet of the vertebra above the desired disc space, extending slightly medially into the junction with the lamina. Once the inferior facet is penetrated, the superior facet of the inferior vertebral level will be visualized. This is also thinned with the drill (it is critical to remove the bone of the superior facet of the level below caudally to where it meets the pedicle). A small Kerrison rongeur may be used to slightly enlarge the laminectomy. An opening is made in the ligamentum flavum overlying the lateral aspect of the spinal cord dura. The nerve root can be identified as it exits from the thecal sac, and can be followed as it travels between the pedicles of the vertebrae above and below. Soft tissues (including ligamentum flavum) form fibrous bands across the dorsum of the nerve, and are removed to further expose the dura of the nerve root. The venous plexus around the nerve root is coagulated with bipolar cautery and then divided to mobilize the nerve. The nerve may then be gently moved a few millimeters rostrally using a micro nerve hook. The dura overlying the spinal cord should not be manipulated, and the disc space need not be entered. Inspection for free disc fragments should begin in the nerve root axilla using a probe (e.g., blunt nerve hook). Next, the space anterior to the root (the region of the disc) may be palpated. Any disc fragments that are dislodged are removed with a small pituitary rongeur. If the disc fragment is contained anterior to the posterior longitudinal ligament (PLL), the PLL may be incised in the region of the nerve root axilla with a #11 scalpel blade in a motion that is directed downward and laterally, away from the nerve root and spinal cord. The foraminotomy may be extended slightly laterally if the foramen still feels tight when probed. Small osteophytes can potentially be reduced using a small reverse-angled curette, although some surgeons believe that the need for this is obviated by the decompression provided by the keyhole opening. In some cases, simple posterior decompression of the nerve root (without removing a disc fragment) may be adequate to relieve compression. Spinal stability is usually preserved if less than half the facet joint is removed.

MIS keyhole foraminotomy

Positioning as described above.

1. skin incision
   a) use fluoro to locate the correct level for the incision
   b) incision 1 cm off midline on the side of the pathology at the level of the disc space
   c) remove adhesive plastic barrier (e.g., Ioban®) from around the opening to prevent pieces from being dragged into the incision
2. avoid using a guidewire to reduce the risk of penetrating the interlaminar space. STAY LATERAL and insert the thinnest dilator. Dock the dilator on the lateral mass and insert progressively sized dilators
3. use Bovie to expose lateral lamina and medial facet joint. Start laterally where bone is more easily felt and there is little danger of penetrating the interlaminar space and injuring the spinal cord
4. use a straight curette to expose the inferior edge of the superior lateral lamina and the medial facet joint
5. drill off the medial inferior facet, to expose the superior facet of the level below
6. drill the medial superior facet until you are flush with the superior aspect of the pedicle below
7. this completes the bony work, the soft tissue work proceeds as above under open keyhole foraminotomy

77

Outcome

A number of large series have reported good or excellent outcome in the range of 90–96%.[55]

References

[1] Mayfield FH. Cervical Spondylosis: A Comparison of the Anterior and Posterior Approaches. Clin Neurosurg. 1966; 13:181–188

[2] Kobayashi N, Asamoto S, Doi H, et al. Brown-Sequard syndrome produced by cervical disc herniation: report of two cases and review of the literature. Spine J. 2003; 3:530–533

[3] Dai Liyang, Jia Lianshun. Central Cord Injury Complicating Acute Cervical Disc Herniation in Trauma. Spine. 2000; 25:331–336

[4] Viikari-Juntura E, Porras M, Laasonen EM. Validity of Clinical Tests in the Diagnosis of Root Compression in Cervical Disc Disease. Spine. 1989; 14:253–257

[5] Spurling RG, Scoville WB. Lateral Rupture of the Cervical Intervertebral Discs: A Common Cause of Shoulder and Arm Pain. Surg Gynecol Obstet. 1944; 78:350–358

[6] Davidson RI, Dunn EJ, Metzmaker JN. The shoulder abduction test in the diagnosis of radicular pain in cervical extradural compressive miniradiculopathies. Spine. 1981; 6:441–446

[7] Rubinstein SM, Pool JJ, van Tulder MW, et al. A systematic review of the diagnostic accuracy of provocative tests of the neck for diagnosing cervical radiculopathy. European Spine Journal. 2006; 16:307–319

[8] Jablecki CK, Andary MT, Floeter MK, et al. Practice parameter: Electrodiagnostic studies in carpal tunnel syndrome. Report of the American Association of Electrodiagnostic Medicine, American Academy of Neurology, and the American Academy of Physical Medicine and Rehabilitation. Neurology. 2002; 58:1589–1592

[9] Campbell WW. Guidelines in electrodiagnostic medicine. Practice parameter for electrodiagnostic studies in ulnar neuropathy at the elbow. Muscle Nerve Suppl. 1999; 8:S171–S205

[10] American Association of Electrodiagnostic Medicine. Chapter 9: Practice parameter for needle electromyographic evaluation of patients with suspected cervical radiculopathy: Summary statement. Muscle and Nerve. 1999; 22:S209–S211

[11] Dillingham TR. Evaluating the patient with suspected radiculopathy. PM R. 2013; 5:S41–S49

[12] Saal J, Saal Y, Yurth E. Nonoperative Management of Herniated Cervical Intervertebral Disc with Radiculopathy. Spine. 1996; 21:1877–1883

[13] Maigne JY, Deligne L. Computed tomographic follow-up study of 21 cases of nonoperatively treated cervical intervertebral soft disc herniation. Spine (Phila Pa 1976). 1994; 19:189–191

[14] Mochida K, Komori H, Okawa A, et al. Regression of cervical disc herniation observed on magnetic resonance images. Spine (Phila Pa 1976). 1998; 23:990–5; discussion 996-7

[15] Bush K, Chaudhuri R, Hillier S, et al. The pathomorphologic changes that accompany the resolution of cervical radiculopathy. A prospective study with repeat magnetic resonance imaging. Spine (Phila Pa 1976). 1997; 22:183–6; discussion 187

[16] Joanes V. Cervical disc herniation presenting with acute myelopathy. Surgical Neurology. 2000; 54

[17] Senter HJ, Kortyna R, Kemp W. Anterior Cervical Discectomy with Hydroxylapatite Fusion. Neurosurgery. 1989; 25:39–43

[18] Matz PaulG, Ryken TimothyC, Groff MichaelW, et al. Techniques for anterior cervical decompression for radiculopathy. Journal of Neurosurgery: Spine. 2009; 11:183–197

[19] Ryken TimothyC, Heary RobertF, Matz PaulG, et al. Techniques for cervical interbody grafting. Journal of Neurosurgery: Spine. 2009; 11:203–220

[20] Tew JM, Mayfield FH. Complications of Surgery of the Anterior Cervical Spine. Clin Neurosurg. 1976; 23:424–434

[21] Taylor BA, Vaccaro AR, Albert TJ. Complications of Anterior and Posterior Surgical Approaches in the Treatment of Cervical Degenerative Disc Disease. Seminars in Spine Surgery. 1999; 11:337–346

[22] Netterville JL, Koriwchak MJ, Winkle M, et al. Vocal Fold Paralysis Following the Anterior Approach to the Cervical Spine. Ann Otol Rhinol Laryngol. 1996; 105:85–91

[23] Pfeifer BA, Freidberg SR, Jewell ER. Repair of Injured Vertebral Artery in Anterior Cervical Procedures. Spine. 1994; 19:1471–1474

[24] Karim A, Knapp J, Nanda A. Internal jugular venous thrombosis as a complication after an elective anterior cervical discectomy: case report. Neurosurgery. 2006; 59

[25] Ascher E, Salles-Cunha S, Hingorani A. Morbidity and mortality associated with internal jugular vein thromboses. Vasc Endovascular Surg. 2005; 39:335–339

[26] Sheikh MA, Topoulos AP, Deitcher SR. Isolated internal jugular vein thrombosis: risk factors and natural history. Vasc Med. 2002; 7:177–179

[27] Ascher E, Hingorani A, Mazzariol F, et al. Clinical experience with superior vena caval Greenfield filters. J Endovasc Surg. 1999; 6:365–369

[28] Tajima H, Murata S, Kumazaki T, et al. Successful interventional treatment of acute internal jugular vein thrombosis. AJR Am J Roentgenol. 2004; 182:467–469

[29] Holmes MG, Dagal A, Feinstein BA, et al. Airway Management Practice in Adults With an Unstable Cervical Spine: The Harborview Medical Center Experience. Anesth Analg. 2018; 127:450–454

[30] Krieger AJ, Rosomoff HL. Sleep-Induced Apnea. Part 2: Respiratory Failure After Anterior Spinal Surgery. J Neurosurg. 1974; 39:181–185

[31] Truumees E, Herkowitz HN. Adjacent Segment Degeneration in the Cervical Spine: Incidence and Management. Seminars in Spine Surgery. 1999; 11:373–383

[32] Gore DR, Sepic SB. Anterior Cervical Fusion for Degenerated or Protruded Discs. A Review of One Hundred and Fifty-Six Patients. Spine. 1984; 9:667–671

[33] Hawkins RJ, Bilco T, Bonutti P. Cervical Spine and Shoulder Pain. Clinical Orthopedics and Related Research. 1990; 258:142–146

[34] Krnacik MJ, Heggeness MH. Severe angioedema causing airway obstruction after anterior cervical surgery. Spine. 1997; 22:2188–2190

[35] Harhangi BS, Menovsky T, Wurzer HA. Hemothorax as a complication after anterior cervical discectomy: case report. Neurosurgery. 2005; 56

[36] Winslow CP, Winslow TJ, Wax MK. Dysphonia and dysphagia following the anterior approach to the cervical spine. Archives of Otolaryngology – Head and Neck Surgery. 2001; 127:51–55

[37] Bazaz R, Lee MJ, Yoo JU. Incidence of dysphagia after anterior cervical spine surgery: a prospective study. Spine. 2002; 27:2453–2458

[38] Dakwar E, Uribe JS, Padhya TA, et al. Management of delayed esophageal perforations after anterior cervical spinal surgery. J Neurosurg Spine. 2009; 11:320–325

[39] Fogel GR, McDonnell MF. Surgical treatment of dysphagia after anterior cervical interbody fusion. Spine J. 2005; 5:140–144

[40] Halani SH, Baum GR, Riley JP, et al. Esophageal perforation after anterior cervical spine surgery: a systematic review of the literature. J Neurosurg Spine. 2016; 25:285–291

[41] Gaudinez RF, English GM, Gebhard JS, et al. Esophageal perforations after anterior cervical surgery. J Spinal Disord. 2000; 13:77–84

[42] Kaman L, Iqbal J, Kundil B, et al. Management of esophageal perforation in adults. Gastroenterology Research. 2010; 3:235–244

[43] Hasan S, Jilaihawi AN, Prakash D. Conservative management of iatrogenic oesophageal perforations–a viable option. Eur J Cardiothorac Surg. 2005; 28:7–10

[44] Kaiser MichaelG, Mummaneni Praveen V, Matz PaulG, et al. Radiographic assessment of cervical subaxial fusion. Journal of Neurosurgery: Spine. 2009; 11:221–227

[45] Phillips FM, Carlson G, Emery SE, et al. Anterior Cervical Pseudarthrosis: Natural History and Treatment. Spine. 1997; 22:1585–1589

[46] Cannada LK, Scherping SC, Yoo JU, et al. Pseudoarthrosis of the cervical spine: a comparison of radiographic diagnostic measures. Spine (Phila Pa 1976). 2003; 28:46–51

[47] DePalma AF, Cooke AJ. Results of Anterior Interbody Fusion of The Cervical Spine. Clin Orthop. 1968; 60:169–185

[48] Puschak TJ, Anderson PA. Pseudarthrosis After Anterior Fusion: Treatment Options and Results. Seminars in Spine Surgery. 1999; 11:312–321

[49] Zdeblick TA, Hughes SS, Riew KD, et al. Failed anterior cervical discectomy and arthrodesis. Analysis and treatment of thirty-five patients. Journal of Bone and Joint Surgery. 1997; 79:523–532

[50] Kaiser MichaelG, Mummaneni Praveen V, Matz PaulG, et al. Management of anterior cervical pseudarthrosis. Journal of Neurosurgery: Spine. 2009; 11:228–237

[51] Yi S, Lee DY, Kim DH, et al. Cervical artificial disc replacement. Part 1: History, design, and overview of the cervical artificial disc. Neurosurgical Quarterly. 2008; 18

[52] Scoville WB, Whitcomb BB, McLaurin RL. The Cervical Ruptured Disc: Report of 115 Operative Cases. Trans Am Neurol Assoc. 1951; 76:222–224

[53] Heary RobertF, Ryken TimothyC, Matz PaulG, et al. Cervical laminoforaminotomy for the treatment of cervical degenerative radiculopathy. Journal of Neurosurgery: Spine. 2009; 11:198–202

[54] Aldrich F. Posterolateral Microdiscectomy for Cervical Monoradiculopathy Caused by Posterolateral Soft Cervical Disc Sequestration. Journal of Neurosurgery. 1990; 72:370–377

[55] Zeidman SM, Ducker TB. Posterior Cervical Laminoforaminotomy for Radiculopathy: Review of 172 Cases. Neurosurgery. 1993; 33:356–362

[56] Collias JC, Roberts MP, Schmidek HH, et al. Posterior Surgical Approaches for Cervical Disc Herniation and Spondylotic Myelopathy. In: Operative Neurosurgical Techniques. 3rd ed. Philadelphia: W.B. Saunders; 1995:1805–1816

78 Cervical Degenerative Disc Disease and Cervical Myelopathy

78.1 Cervical disc degeneration – general information

Cervical degenerative disc disease is generally discussed in terms of "cervical spondylosis," a term which is sometimes used synonymously with "cervical spinal stenosis." Spondylosis usually implies a more widespread age-related degenerative condition of the cervical spine including various combinations of the following:

1. congenital cervical spinal stenosis (the "shallow cervical canal"[1])
2. degeneration of the intervertebral disc producing a focal stenosis due to a "cervical bar," which is usually a combination of:
   a) osteophytic spurs ("hard disc" in neurosurgical jargon)
   b) and/or protrusion of intervertebral disc material ("soft disc")
3. hypertrophy of any of the following (which also contributes to canal stenosis):
   a) lamina
   b) dura
   c) articular facets
   d) ligaments, including
      • increased stenosis in extension is more common than with flexion (based on MRI studies[2] and cadaver studies), largely due to posterior inbuckling of ligamentum flavum[3]
      • posterior longitudinal ligament: may include ossification of the posterior longitudinal ligament (OPLL) (p. 1370).[4] May be segmental or diffuse. Often adherent to dura
      • ossification of the ligamentum flavum[5] (yellow ligament)
4. subluxation: due to disc and facet joint degeneration
5. altered mobility: severely spondylotic levels may be fused and are usually stable; however, there is often hypermobility at adjacent or other segments
6. telescoping of the spine due to loss of height of VBs and discs → "shingling" of laminae
7. alteration of the normal lordotic curvature[6] (NB: the amount of abnormal curvature did not correlate with the degree of myelopathy)
   a) reduction of lordosis: including
      • straightening
      • reversal of the curvature (kyphosis): may cause "bowstringing" of the spinal cord across osteophytes
   b) exaggerated lordosis (hyperlordosis): the least common variant (may also cause bowstringing)

78.2 Pathophysiology

Pathogenesis is controversial. Theories include the following alone or in combination:

1. direct cord compression between osteophytic bars and hypertrophy or infolding of the ligamentum flavum, especially if superimposed on congenital narrowing or cervical subluxations
2. ischemia due to compression of vascular structures[7] (arterial deprivation[8] and/or venous stasis[9])
3. repeated local cord trauma by normal movements in the presence of protruded discs and/or osteophytic (spondylotic) bars (cord and root injuries[10])
   a) cephalad/caudad movement with flexion extension[11]
   b) anterior/posterior traction on the cord by dentate ligaments[12] & nerve roots
   c) diameter of spinal canal varies during flexion and extension
      • increased stenosis is more common in extension (see above)
      • unstable segments may sublux (so-called pincer mechanism)[13]

Histologically,[14] there is degeneration of the central gray matter at the level of compression, degeneration of the posterior columns above the lesion (particularly in the anteromedial portion), and demyelination in the lateral columns (especially the corticospinal tracts) below the lesion. Anterior spinal tracts are relatively spared. There may be atrophic changes in the ventral and dorsal roots and neurophagia of anterior horn cells.

78.3 Epidemiology/Natural history

9% of individuals > 70 years of age had clinically significant cervical spinal stenosis (CSS) (including degenerative stenosis and OPLL) in a cadaveric study.[15]

23% of patients with CSS developed myelopathy with mean follow-up of 44 years.[16] This number is even lower in patients without radiculopathy or electrodiagnostic evidence of nerve root involvement (including prolonged SEPs and MEPs) on presentation (Class I).[16,17]

Patients with CSS without myelopathy who have T2 signal changes on MRI are at increased risk of developing myelopathy in the *long term* (> 1 year).[16]

Once myelopathy is detected, the time course of symptoms is highly variable and unpredictable. In ≈ 75% of cases of cervical spondylotic myelopathy (CSM), there is progression either in a stepwise fashion (in one–third) or gradually progressive (two–thirds).[18] In some series, the most common pattern was that of an initial phase of deterioration followed by a stabilization that typically lasts for years and may not change thereafter.[19,20] In these cases, the degree of disability may be established early in the course of CSM. Others disagree with such a "benign" outlook and cite that over 50% of cases continue to deteriorate with conservative treatment.[21] Sustained spontaneous improvement is probably rare.[22]

In patients < 75 years of age and mJOA score (p. 1299) > 12, the clinical condition remained stable in 3 years of follow-up (Class I)[17] (however, these patients can still have significant disability that can respond to surgery). Longstanding myelopathy with severe stenosis over many years may cause irreversible deficit due to necrosis in gray and white matter (Class III).[17]

78.4 Clinical

78.4.1 General information

Cervical spondylosis is a condition that may produce several types of clinical problems[23]:
1. myeloradiculopathy: some combination of
    a) radiculopathy: nerve root compression may cause nerve-root (radicular) complaints
    b) spinal cord compression may cause myelopathy (see stereotypical myelopathic syndromes (p. 1299))
2. pain and paresthesias in the head, neck, and shoulders with little or no suggestion of radiculopathy nor abnormal physical findings. This group is the most difficult to diagnose and treat, and often requires a good physician-patient relationship to decide if surgical treatment should be undertaken in an attempt to provide relief

Cervical spondylosis is the most common cause of myelopathy in patients > 55 yrs of age.[22] CSM is rare in patients < 40 years of age.

CSM develops in almost all patients with ≥ 30% narrowing of the cross-sectional area of the cervical spinal canal[24] (although some patients with more severe cord compression do not have myelopathy[25,26]).

Gait disturbance, often with LE weakness or stiffness, is a common early finding in CSM.[27] Ataxia may result from spinocerebellar tract compression. Early on, patients may experience difficulty running. Cervical pain and mechanical signs are uncommon in cases of pure myelopathy. See ▶ Table 78.1 for the frequency of symptoms in CSM in one series. In most cases the disability is mild, and the prognosis for these is good.

78.4.2 Motor

Findings can be due to cord (UMN) and/or root (LMN) compression. The earliest motor findings are typically weakness in the triceps and hand intrinsics.[29] There may be wasting of the hand muscles.[30] Slow, stiff opening and closing of the fists may occur.[31] Clumsiness with fine motor skills (writing, buttoning buttons…) is common.

There is often *proximal* weakness of the lower extremities (mild to moderate iliopsoas weakness occurs in 54%) and spasticity of the LEs.

78.4.3 Sensory

Sensory disturbance may be minimal, and when present is often not radicular in distribution. There may be a glove-distribution sensory loss in the hands.[32] A sensory level (i.e., a demarcation below which there is a sensory loss) may occur a number of levels below the area of cord compression.

78

Table 78.1 Frequency of symptoms in CSM (37 cases[28])

Finding	%
pure myelopathy	59
myelopathy + radiculopathy	41
reflexes	
• hyperreflexia	87
• Babinski	54
• Hoffman	13
sensory deficits	
• sensory level	41
• posterior column	39
• dermatomal arm	33
• paresthesias	21
• positive Romberg	15
motor deficits	
• arm weakness	31
• paraparesis	21
• hemiparesis	18
• quadriparesis	10
• Brown-Séquard	10
• muscle atrophy	13
• fasciculations	13
pain	
• radicular arm	41
• radicular leg	13
• cervical	8
spasticity	54
sphincter disturbance	49
cervical mechanical signs	26

LEs often exhibit loss of vibratory sense (in as many as 82%), and occasionally have reduced pin-prick sensation (9%) (almost always restricted to below the ankle). Compression of the spinocerebellar tract may cause difficulty running. Lhermitte's sign (p.1712) was present in only 2 of 37 cases. Some patients may present with a prominence of posterior column dysfunction (impaired joint position sense and 2-point discrimination).[33]

78.4.4 Reflexes

In 72–87%, reflexes are hyperactive at a varying distance below the level of stenosis. Clonus, Babinski's sign (p.91), or Hoffman's sign (p.91) may also be present. Dynamic Hoffman's sign[34] may be more sensitive: test for Hoffman's sign during multiple cervical flexion and extension movements as tolerated by the patient. 94% of asymptomatic individuals with Hoffman's reflex will have significant spinal cord compression on MRI.[35] Inverted radial reflex: flexion of the fingers in response to eliciting the brachioradialis reflex, said to be pathognomonic of CSM.[36]

A hyperactive jaw jerk indicates upper motor neuron lesion *above* the midpons, and distinguishes long tract findings due to pathology above the foramen magnum from those below (e.g., cervical myelopathy): not helpful if absent (a normal variant). Primitive reflexes (grasp, snout, rooting) are not reliable localizing signs (except perhaps the grasp reflex) of frontal lobe pathology.

78.4.5 Sphincter

Urinary urgency and frequency are common in CSM; however, these complaints are also protean in the aging population. Urinary incontinence is rare. Anal sphincter disturbances are uncommon.

78.4.6 Cervical spondylotic myelopathy syndromes

Clustering of CSM into these 5 clinical syndromes has been described[31]:

1. transverse lesion syndrome: involvement of corticospinal and spinothalamic tracts and posterior columns, with anterior horn cells *segmentally* involved. Most frequent syndrome, possibly an "end-stage" of the disease process
2. motor system syndrome: primarily corticospinal tract and anterior horn involvement with minimal or no sensory deficit. This creates a mixture of lower motor neuron findings in the upper extremities and upper motor neuron findings (myelopathy) in the lower extremities which can mimic ALS (see below). Reflexes may be hyperactive below the area of maximal stenosis (including the upper extremities), occasionally beginning several levels below the stenosis
3. central cord syndrome (p. 1132): motor and sensory involvement producing greater deficit in the UEs than the LEs. Results in so-called "numb-clumsy hand syndrome"[37]. Lhermitte's sign may be more common in this group
4. Brown-Séquard syndrome: often with asymmetric narrowing of the canal compressing the corticospinal tract producing upper motor neuron weakness ipsilateral to the side of greater narrowing, and posterior and lateral column compression producing contralateral impairment of pain, temperature and joint position sense
5. brachialgia and cord syndrome: primarily radiculopathy (UE pain and lower motor neuron weakness) with lesser associated long tract involvement (motor and/or sensory)

78.4.7 Grading

1. modified Japanese Orthopaedic Association scale (mJOA): a validated and reliable grading system, although it is non-specific. There are at least 3 slightly different versions of the mJOA scale in common use[38], the one by Benzel is the most widely used[38] (▶ Table 78.2)
2. Neck Disability Index[39]: a 10-question survey similar to the Oswestry Disability Index for the lumbar spine (see ▶ Table 74.2). Mild disability is defined as a score of 10–28%, moderate = 30–48%, severe = 50–68%, complete ≥ 72%
3. other commonly used scales (not tested for validity or reliability):
   a) Nurick[40] (see ▶ Table 83.2)
   b) Harsh

Table 78.2 Two examples of modified JOA (mJOA) scoring systems for cervical myelopathy[a]

Modality & anatomic region	Points	mJOA by Chiles et al.[29]		mJOA by Benzel et al.[41]	
		Description	Score	Description	Score
Motor dysfunction - Upper extremity (UE)	0	unable to feed self	(0 - 4)	unable to move hands	(0 - 5)
	1	unable to use knife & fork; can eat with spoon		unable to eat with a spoon, but able to move hands	
	2	can use knife & fork with much difficulty		unable to button shirt, able to eat with spoon	
	3	can use knife & fork with slight difficulty		able to button shirt with great difficulty	
	4	no deficit (normal)		able to button shirt with slight difficulty	
	5	—		no deficit (normal)	
Motor or sensorimotor dysfunction - Lower extremity (LE)	0	unable to walk	(0 - 4)	complete motor and sensory loss	(0 - 7)
	1	can walk on flat surface with walking aid		sensory preserved, no movement	
	2	can walk up and/or down stairs with handrail		leg movement, unable to walk	
	3	lack of smooth and stable gait		able to walk on flat surface with walking aid (e.g., cane, crutch...)	
	4	no motor deficit (normal)		able to walk up and/or down stairs using hand rail	

78

(continued)

Table 78.2 continued

Modality & anatomic region	Points	mJOA by Chiles et al.[29] Description	Score	mJOA by Benzel et al.[41] Description	Score
	5	—		moderate to marked instability, able to walk up and/or down stairs without hand rail	
	6			mild instability, smooth unaided gait	
	7			no deficit (normal)	
Sensory deficit - UE	0	severe sensory loss or pain	(0 - 2)	complete sensory loss of hand	(0 - 3)
	1	mild sensory loss		severe sensory loss or pain	
	2	no deficit (normal)		mild sensory loss	
	3	—		no deficit (normal)	
Sensory deficit - LE	0	severe sensory loss or pain	(0 - 2)	—	
	1	mild sensory loss			
	2	no deficit (normal)			
Sensory deficit - trunk	0	severe sensory loss or pain	(0 - 2)		
	1	mild sensory loss			
	2	no deficit (normal)			
Sphincter dysfunction	0	unable to void	(0 - 3)	no voluntary voiding	(0 - 3)
	1	marked voiding difficulty (retention)		marked difficulty micturating	
	2	some voiding difficulty (urgency or hesitation)		mild to moderate difficulty micturating	
	3	no deficit (normal)		no deficit (normal)	
mJOA score → TOTAL		range: 0–17 (normal)	(0 – 17)	range: 0–18 (normal)	(0 – 18)

[a]this table shows 2 different modified JOA scoring systems: the one by Chiles was used in formulating the 2009 AANS/CNS guidelines, the one by Benzel is the most commonly used mJOA.[38] They both differ from the original JOA score[42] by substituting "knife, fork, & spoon" for chopsticks

In an effort to standardize stratification of the severity of cervical myelopathy, the system shown in ▶ Table 78.3 has been proposed[43] (NB: in guidelines and other sections in this book, different definitions e.g., of "mild" may be used).

Table 78.3 Stratification of cervical spondylotic myelopathy

Descriptor	Nurick grade (▶ Table 83.2)	Benzel mJOA grade (▶ Table 78.2)[41]
mild	1 & 2	≥15
moderate	3 & 4	12-14
severe	5 & 6	≤11

78.5 Differential diagnosis

78.5.1 General information

See Myelopathy (p. 1696) for other possible causes. Some of these (e.g., spinal cord tumor, OPLL) may be demonstrated radiographically. Asymptomatic cervical spondylosis is very common.

12% of cases diagnosed as cervical spondylotic myelopathy are later found to be due to another disease process, which may include:
1. ALS: see below
2. demyelinating disease: especially neuromyelitis optica (NMO) (p. 1698), but also multiple sclerosis (MS). Spinal cord demyelination may mimic CSM. With MS, remissions and exacerbations are common, and patients tend to be younger

3. herniated cervical disc (soft disc): patients tend to be younger than with CSM. Course is more rapid
4. subacute combined system disease (p.1699): subnormal vitamin B12 level and possibly macrocytic anemia
5. hereditary spastic paraplegia: family history is key. Diagnosis of exclusion[44]
6. (spontaneous) intracranial hypotension (p.421)

78.5.2 Amyotrophic lateral sclerosis (ALS)

AKA (anterior horn) motor neuron disease; also see Amyotrophic lateral sclerosis (p.191). Can mimic the motor system syndrome of CSM (see above), and spinal cord compression may be seen on MRI in > 60% of patients with ALS.[45]

"Triad" of ALS:
1. atrophic weakness of hands and forearms (early)—LMN finding
2. mild LE spasticity—UMN finding
3. diffuse hyperreflexia—UMN finding

Inevitably, some cases of demyelinating disease will be misdiagnosed initially as CSM until some features suggestive of ALS occur (in one series of 1500 ALS patients, 4% underwent spine surgery (56% cervical, 42% lumbar, 2% thoracic)[45] before ALS was correctly diagnosed).

Features that may help differentiate ALS from CSM:
1. ALS: sensory changes are conspicuously *absent*. CSM: hand numbness may occur
2. bulbar symptoms (dysarthria, hyperactive jaw-jerk...): may occur in ALS,[46] absent in CSM
3. ALS: extensive weakness/muscle atrophy of hands, usually with fasciculations[47]
4. ALS: lower-motor neuron (LMN) findings in the tongue (visible fasciculations, or positive sharp waves on EMG) or in the LEs (e.g., fasciculations and atrophy) favor the diagnosis of ALS over CSM (however, LMN findings in the LEs may occur in CSM if there is coincidental lumbar radiculopathy)
5. CSM or herniated cervical disc: usually includes neck and shoulder pain, limitation of neck movement, sensory changes, and LMN findings restricted to 1 or 2 spinal cord segments

78.6 Evaluation

78.6.1 Plain X-rays

General information

Minimum evaluation consists of AP, lateral (neutral position), and open-mouth odontoid views. If desired, flexion-extension views and/or oblique views may be obtained but require specific orders.

When MRI is available, the additional information provided by plain cervical spine X-rays in patients with CSM is limited. In this setting, X-rays may be best for:
1. demonstrating dynamic instability with flexion-extension views (see below)
2. sagittal balance measured on standing lateral cervical spine X-rays may provide prognostic information[48]
3. X-rays may be able to compensate for the following MRI deficiencies, but cervical CT is much better
   a) differentiating calcified discs or bone spurs from "soft discs"
   b) differentiating OPLL from a thickened posterior longitudinal ligament
   c) bone abnormalities: fractures, bony lytic lesions

Cervical spinal stenosis

Cervical spinal stenosis can be inferred from plain X-rays. ★ NB: Canal diameter measured on X-ray is a surrogate marker for the actual item of interest: viz. spinal canal narrowing sufficient to produce spinal cord compression and thereby spinal cord symptoms. Since spinal cords can vary in size, this is not as accurate as directly assessing narrowing on MRI or CT/myelo, and MRI can also depict any intrinsic spinal cord signal abnormalities.

See Canal diameter (p.224) for normal dimensions and measurement techniques. Patients with CSM have an average minimal AP canal diameter of 11.8 mm,[49] and values ≤ 10 mm were likely to be associated with myelopathy.[50] Patients with an AP diameter < 14 mm may be at increased risk,[51] and CSM is rare in patients with a diameter > 16 mm, even with significant spurs.[22]

78

Cervical spinal stenosis is also suggested on plain films when the spinolaminar line is close to the posterior margin of the lateral masses.

Pavlov ratio (AKA Torg ratio[52,53]): the ratio of the AP diameter of the spinal canal at the mid-VB level to the VB at the same location. A ratio < 0.8 is sensitive for transient neuropraxia, but has been shown to have poor positive predictive value for CSM.

Oblique views

Oblique views can delineate foraminal compromise caused by osteophytic spurs.

Flexion-extension views

Lateral flexion/extension X-rays may provide valuable information by detecting dynamic instability (abnormalities that manifest with movement) that cannot be appreciated on (static) CT or MRI, including widening of the atlanto-dental interval on flexion (p. 223).

78.6.2 MRI

MRI provides information about the spinal canal, and can also show intrinsic cord abnormalities (demyelination, syringomyelia, spinal cord atrophy, edema…). MRI also rules out other diagnostic possibilities (Chiari malformation, spinal cord tumor…).

Bony structures and calcified ligaments are poorly imaged. These shortcomings and the difficulties in differentiating osteophytes from herniated discs on MRI are overcome with the addition of plain cervical spine films[54] or to better advantage with thin-section CT bone windows.

Findings that correlate with poor outcome (Class III)[55]:
1. *multilevel* T2WI hyperintensity within the spinal cord parenchyma
2. *single* level T2WI hyperintensity with corresponding T1WI hypointensity (single level T2WI hyperintensity without T1WI changes are of uncertain prognostic significance)
3. spinal cord atrophy (transverse area < 45 mm^2)

Other MRI findings seen with CSM:
1. reduced transverse area of the spinal cord (TASC) at the level of maximum compression. A "banana" shaped cord on axial images has a high correlation with the presence of CSM.[51] There is conflicting evidence whether the degree of canal stenosis predicts outcome.[55] Sagittal T2WIs tend to exaggerate the magnitude of spinal cord compression by osteophytes and/or discs, and therefore axial images and T1WIs also need to be considered in the evaluation. Narrowing is not specific for CSM: ≈ 26% of *asymptomatic* individuals > 64 years of age have spinal cord compression on MRI[56]
2. "snake eyes" (AKA "owl's eyes") within the spinal cord on axial T2WI (▶ Fig. 78.1) may be related to cystic necrosis of the cord[57] and may correlate with poor outcome (Class III)[55]

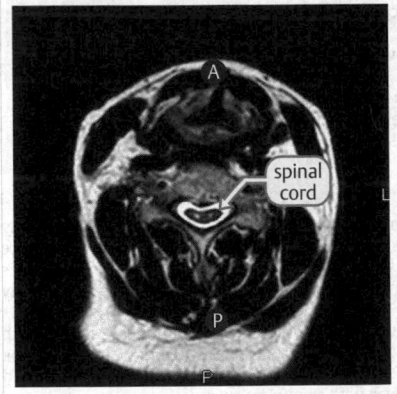

Fig. 78.1 "Snake eyes" (two foci of high signal) within a slightly flattened and mildly atrophic spinal cord on axial T2WI MRI.

spinal cord

78.6.3 CT and CT/myelogram

Plain CT scans may demonstrate a narrow canal, but do not provide adequate information regarding soft tissues (discs, ligaments, spinal cord, and nerve roots). However, bony detail may be invaluable in the surgical treatment of CSM.

Cervical myelography followed by high-resolution CT scanning provides sagittal and axial information (including spinal cord atrophy), and delineates bony detail better than MRI.[54] Unlike MRI, CT/myelogram is invasive (requires LP) and involves ionizing radiation and does not provide information about changes within the spinal cord parenchyma.

78.6.4 EMG

There are no EMG abnormalities with pure myelopathy (EMG does not detect upper motor neuron abnormalities). EMG can detect motor nerve root involvement, but has poor sensitivity in pure sensory cervical radiculopathy and is not reliable in predicting outcome from surgery for CSM (Class III).[55] EMG is most helpful in suspicious cases for eliminating etiologies such as peripheral neuropathy or ALS.

78.6.5 Sensory evoked potentials (SEPs)

SSEPs are of limited usefulness, although a normal pre-op SEP or normalization of SEPs in the early post-op period are associated with better outcome.[58]

Practice guideline: Pre-op SEPs in CSM

Pre-op SEPs should be considered if the additional prognostic information would help treatment decisions (Level B Class II)[58]

78.7 Treatment

78.7.1 Nonoperative management

Measures include: prolonged immobilization with rigid cervical bracing in an attempt to reduce motion and hence the cumulative effects of trauma on the spinal cord, modified activity to eliminate "high-risk" activities or bed rest, and anti-inflammatory medications.[59]

78.7.2 Surgical treatment

Indications for surgery

See **Practice guideline: Surgical vs. nonsurgical management** (p. 1303).

Practice guideline: Surgical vs. nonsurgical management

Myelopathy with mJOA (► Table 78.2) score > 12[a]: in the short-term (3 years) patients may be offered the option of surgical decompression or nonoperative management (prolonged immobilization in a rigid cervical collar, anti-inflammatory medications, and "low-risk" activities or bed rest (Level C Class II)).[60] **Note:** patients with mJOA scores > 12 (see ► Table 78.2) may derive significant improvement from surgery, and deterioration from this point may be ominous.

More severe myelopathy: should be treated with surgical decompression with benefits maintained at 5 and 15 years post-op (Level D Class III)[60]

Level B Class I[61]: Degenerative cervical *radiculopathy*: patients do better with anterior decompression ± fusion (compared to conservative management) for
- rapid relief (within 3–4 months) of arm & neck pain and sensory loss
- relief of longer term (≥ 12 months) symptoms of weakness of wrist extension, elbow extension, shoulder abduction, and internal rotation

[a] in this guideline, mJOA > 12 was considered "mild myelopathy"; however, mJOA 12–14 may more accurately be graded as moderate and mJOA ≥ 15 being mild (► Table 78.3 [43])

78

Intraoperative electrophysiologic monitoring

Practice guideline: Intraoperative electrophysiologic monitoring during surgery for CSM or radiculopathy

Use of intra-op EP monitoring during routine surgery for CSM or cervical radiculopathy is not recommended as an indication to alter the surgical plan or administer steroids since this paradigm has not been observed to reduce the incidence of neurologic injury (Level D Class III).[62]

Choice of approach

General information

The debate between anterior approaches (anterior cervical discectomy or corpectomy) and posterior approaches (decompressive cervical laminectomy or laminoplasty) dates back to the time that both became widely practiced.[23] General practice is to treat anterior disease at the disc level (e.g., osteophytic bar, herniated disc…) usually limited to ≤ 3 levels (or occasionally 4) with an anterior approach, and to use a posterior approach as the initial procedure in the situations outlined below. Considerations of spinal curvature may need to enter into the decision process.

Practice guideline: Choice of surgical approach for CSM

Level D Class III[63]:there was not enough evidence to recommend any of the following techniques over the other (in terms of short-term success in treating CSM): ACDF, anterior corpectomy and fusion, laminectomy (with or without fusion), and laminoplasty

Level D Class III[63]: laminectomy without fusion, however, is associated with a higher incidence of late kyphotic deformity with incidence = 14–47% (not all cases are symptomatic, not all cases need treatment: see text)

Posterior approach

Options include:
1. laminectomy: alone, or with arthrodesis (e.g., lateral mass fusion) Class III (this procedure was found to be effective, the class shows the strength of the evidence)[64])
2. laminoplasty (p. 1787) (Class III; this procedure was found to be effective, the class shows the strength of the evidence[65])
3. multilevel foraminotomies: usually not adequate for central canal stenosis

Situations where a posterior approach would generally be the initial approach:
1. congenital cervical stenosis where removing osteophytes will still not provide at least ≈ 12 mm of AP canal diameter
2. disease over ≥ 3 levels (although up to 4 may occasionally be dealt with anteriorly)
3. primary posterior pathology (e.g., infolding of ligamentum flavum)
4. some cases of OPLL (anterior approach has higher risk of dural tear)

Disadvantages of the posterior approach:
1. laminectomy *without* fusion
   a) degeneration and osteophytes continue to progress following surgery
   b) risk of subsequent subluxation or progressive kyphotic angulation ("swan neck" deformity) (facetiously dubbed "spina bifida neurosurgica")
      • quoted incidence: 14–47%[66,67,68] (risk may be minimized by careful preservation of facet joints)
      • not all cases need to be treated: in one series, 31% (18/58) developed post-op kyphosis, and 16% of these (3/18) required surgical stabilization[69]
      • the development of kyphotic deformity does not appear to diminish the clinical outcome[68] and does not correlate with neurologic deterioration when deterioration occurs[70]

2. more painful initially post-op and sometimes more prolonged rehabilitation
3. long-term complaints of a heaviness of the head possibly associated with atrophy of the paraspinal muscles
4. ✖ contraindicated with pre-existing swan neck deformity, and not recommended in the presence of reversal of the normal cervical lordosis (i.e., kyphotic curve)[41] where the spinal cord won't tend to move away from the anterior compression or in the presence of ≥ 3.5 mm subluxation or > 20° rotation in the sagittal plane[51] and caution must be exercised in hyperlordosis (see below)

Booking the case: Cervical laminectomy

Also see defaults & disclaimers (p. 25).
1. position: prone. For subaxial spine (ie. below C2), prone on radiolucent table with the head on a padded stabilizer (e.g., ProneView™) or on a padded horseshoe headrest. Take care to avoid any presure on the eyes. If C1–2 or occipital decompression is included in the operation, the head is commonly stabilized rigidly e.g., with Mayfield head holder
2. implants: for fusions, schedule with the vendor for the desired implants and associated instrumentation. If C1 is included, include smooth shank screws. If the occiput is included, include occipital plate
3. anesthesia: if there is myelopathy or severe stenosis, intubate using video laryngoscopy, or second choice, asleep fiberoptic bronchoscopy (awake fiberoptic intubation is rarely used)[71]
4. consent (in lay terms for the patient—not all-inclusive):
   a) procedure: surgery through the back to remove bone, ligament, and any other tissue that is pressing on the spinal cord and/or nerve(s). If a fusion is to be done, then typically this will be accomplished using screws and rods. SSEPs and MEPs are often monitored during surgery, and there is a risk of seizures with MEPs
   b) alternatives: nonsurgical management
   c) complications: usual spine surgery complications (p. 25), plus there might not be the amount of pain relief desired (neck pain does not respond as well to surgery as nerve-root pain). For subaxial fusions, approximately 50% of head rotation and flexion/extension will be lost. C1–2 contributes the other 50% of head rotation which will be lost if C1–2 is fused, and the occiput-C1 joint contributes the other 50% of neck flexion-extension and this will be lost if the occiput is fused to the cervical spine. Vascular injury of the vertebral artery may produce a stroke. Seizures may occur with MEPs

Anterior approach
Also shown to be effective (Class III[60]).
Instrumentation options: in terms of *fusion rates* for 2-level anterior operations (i.e., 2 disc spaces) (Class III)[63]:

$$\begin{array}{ccccc} \text{2-level ACDF} & & \text{1-level corpectomy} & & \text{1-level corpectomy} & & \text{2-level ACDF} \\ \text{with anterior plate} & = & \text{with plate} & > & \text{without plate}^* & > & \text{without plate} \end{array}$$

* however, the graft extrusion rate is higher for corpectomy than ACDF

Worsening of myelopathy has been reported in 2–5% of patients after anterior decompression[72,73] (intraoperative SSEP monitoring may reduce this rate[73]) and C5 radiculopathy may occur (see below).

78

Anterior cervical plating
Many instrumentation systems are available, with more similarities than differences. All include some method of preventing screw back-out. Some general pointers:
1. for single-level fusion, typical plate length is 22–24 mm
2. screw length: rule of thumb is 12 mm for females, 14 mm for males
3. do not completely tighten a single screw (to avoid kicking up plate) until the diagonally opposite screws are placed and loosely tightened
4. most systems have fixed and variable angle screws. Variable angle screws allow for load sharing with the graft (here is where a derivative of Wolff's law is often invoked: the weight sharing helps stimulate fusion). Avoid over-angling screws which may prevent the locking mechanism from properly engaging

5. optimal plate placement allows for contact of the plate with the VB at the screw locations. This may require
   a) contouring of plate to follow the lordosis of the C-spine
   b) reduction of anterior osteophytes

Posterior approach

For decompression, some recommend cervical laminectomy extending one or *two* levels beyond the stenosis above and below.[74,75] A C3–6 laminectomy is often considered a "standard" laminectomy. An "extended laminectomy" includes C7 and/or C2.

Curvature considerations: extending the laminectomy to include C2 and sometimes C1 has been recommended for patients with straightening of the cervical curvature.[6] In cases of *hyperlordosis*, posterior migration of the spinal cord following an extensive laminectomy may put increased tension on the nerve roots and blood vessels (with possible neurologic worsening), and a limited laminectomy just where the cord is compressed is often recommended (see below).

"Keyhole foraminotomies" or medial facetectomy with undercutting of the facets may be performed at levels involved with radiculopathy.

Position: choices are primarily: prone, lateral oblique, or sitting. Disadvantage of the prone position: difficulty elevating the head above the heart, resulting in venous engorgement with significant operative bleeding. Risks of the sitting position (p. 1737) include: spinal cord hypoperfusion[73] and air embolism (p. 1738). The lateral oblique position may introduce some distortion to the anatomy due to asymmetrical positioning.

The reported rate of post-op spinal deformity is 25–42%. Neurologic worsening has been reported in 2% in some series, higher in others. C5 radiculopathy may occur (see below).

To avoid significant destabilization of the cervical spine:

1. during the dissection, do not remove soft tissue overlying the facet joints (to preserve their blood supply)
2. take the laminectomy only as far lateral as the extent of the spinal canal, carefully preserving the facet joints[21] (use keyhole laminotomies where necessary)
3. avoid removing a total of one facet at any given level

Outcome

General information

Even excluding cases that are later proven to have demyelinating disease, the outcome from surgery for CSM is often disappointing. Once CSM is clinically apparent, complete remission almost never occurs. The prognosis with surgery is worse with increasing severity of involvement at the time of presentation[74] and with longer duration of symptoms (48% showed clinical improvement or cure if operated within 1 yr of onset, whereas only 16% responded after 1 yr[21]). The success of surgery is also lower in patients with other degenerative diseases of the CNS (ALS, MS…).

Progression of myelopathy may be arrested by surgical decompression. This is not always borne out, and some early series[40,20] showed similar results with conservative treatment as with laminectomy, which yielded improvement in 56%, no change in 25%, and worsening in 19%. Also, as discussed earlier, some cases of CSM develop most of the deficit early and then stabilize (p. 1297).

Some series show good results, with ≈ 64–75% of patients having improvement in CSM post-op.[28] However, other authors remain less enthusiastic. Utilizing a questionnaire in 32 post-op patients operated anteriorly, 66% had relief from radicular pain, while only 33% had improvement in sensory or motor complaints.[28] In one series, half of the patients had improvement in fine motor function of the hands, but the other half worsened postoperatively.[76] Spinal cord atrophy as a result of continued pressure or ischemia may be partly responsible for poor recovery. Bedridden patients with severe myelopathy rarely recover useful function.

Post-op C5 palsy (C5P)

Clinical thumbnail: new deltoid weakness (with or without biceps impairment) following decompressive cervical spine surgery with no worsening of myelopathy, with onset typically delayed 1–3 days post-op.

Diagnostic criteria: motor decline of deltoid muscle strength by ≥ 1 grade (see ▶ Table 30.3) within 6 weeks of surgery.[77]

General information: First described by Keegan in 1965.[78] Although post-op palsy may develop in other nerve roots, C5 is the most common.[79] Frequently not present immediately post-op. Most occur < 1 week post-op.[80] 92% are unilateral.[80] Etiology is not known with certainty, but traction on the nerve seems probable.

50% have motor involvement only (deltoid > biceps), 50% also have C5 dermatomal sensory loss and/or C5 dermatomal pain (shoulder). 82% have deltoid weakness alone.

Epidemiology: Although rates as high as 30% have been quoted,[81] pooled prevalence of 6% following cervical decompressive operations is more realistic.[81]

No demographic risk factor has been identified (including gender, smoking, diabetes, BMI…).[81]

No surgical risk factor has been identified (including the number of surgical levels, use of allograft…).[81] The incidence is higher after posterior surgery; however, posterior surgery is used more commonly than anterior surgery for myelopathy.[77] Association of C5 P with surgery for OPLL (p. 1370) has been alleged, but could not be confirmed.[81]

Radiologic risk factors: there is ≈ Level 2 evidence that decreased pre-operative C4–5 foraminal diameter along with spinal cord rotation is strongly associated with C5 P.[81] Lee et al.[82] found a 16-fold increase in post-op C5 P when the diameter of the C4–5 neural foramen was < 2 mm as measured on axial CT using the method[83] shown in ▶ Fig. 78.2.

Etiology: unresolved. Theories proposed to explain the nerve root injury include: mechanical, electrical, thermal (from high-speed drills), nerve root ischemia, reperfusion injury, bone graft displacement, increase in cervical lordosis… Most have been debunked. Based on current evidence, the leading contender for causation is tethering of the nerve root with subsequent traction from posterior migration of the cord after decompression.[81]

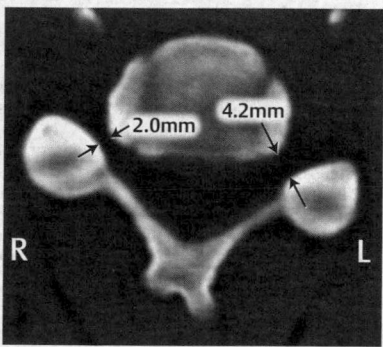

Fig. 78.2 Technique to measure cervical foraminal diameter.[83]
Image: axial CT bone window at the level of the C4–5 foramina.
The neural foramen diameter measures 2 mm on the right side, and 4.2 mm on the left.

Σ: C5 palsy following decompressive cervical spine surgery

This is likely not a single entity with a unique mechanism.[77,81] Posterior traction on the C5 nerve root has emerged as a likely common final pathway, but the precise manner in which this occurs is unknown and effective preventative measures have not been identified.

Applied anatomy: anatomical factors that may make the C5 nerve root more vulnerable to injury than other cervical roots: C5 has shorter rootlets, a more horizontal course to the neural foramen, the smallest cross-sectional area, is often at the apex of the decompression, and the C4–5 neural foramen has more profuse ligaments and the C4–5 zygophyseal joints protrude more anteriorly.[81]

Prevention: no effective preventative measures have been identified. In a series of 52 cases of post-op C5 palsy with intraoperative neuromonitoring, none had monitoring changes during surgery.[77] Performing a prophylactic bony C4–5 foraminotomy has shown mixed results[80] (some favorable,[84,85] others showing a trend towards increased prevalence of C5P[77,82]). The concept of an "extended foraminotomy" (removing the foraminal ligaments in addition to the bony decompression) has been proposed,[81] but requires study.

Prognosis: the chances of spontaneous recovery are generally good. 48% of mild cases resolved in < 3 months, whereas 52% of severe palsies persisted for up to 6 months.[77] Recovery occurred in 75% of the palsies after anterior approach, and in 89% after posterior approach.[77]

78

Management:
1. expectant management in most cases
2. while waiting for resolution, it is critical to keep the joints mobile to avoid contractures which can diminish the recovery if the nerve heals, and can also impede benefits of tendon transfers. Physical therapy and occupational therapy with attention to any fingers involved is vital
3. electrodiagnostic studies: perform EMG to look for evidence of reinnervation both for prognistication and to determine if intervention is indicated. May need serial EDX to follow
4. intervention: for patients with no reinnervation on EMG and that do not recover spontaneously, or for those developing contractures
   a) nerve transfers: work better in younger patients
   b) tendon transfers
   c) joint fusion: can place arm in a more functional position than dangling limply at the side

White cord syndrome

A very rare complication following spinal cord decompression performed for chronic compression (e.g., by degenerative changes, tumor…). Thought to be a reperfusion injury. Neurologic deficits are usually present *immediately* post-op, but delayed presentation has also been reported.[86] T2 MRI shows hyperintense changes consistent with edema and/or infarction. Anecdotal treatment recommendations (unvalidated opinion): steroids (e.g., dexamethasone 2 mg BID X 3 days, or high-dose methylprednisolone have been used), blood pressure augmentation (MAP > 85 mm Hg) and early physical therapy (PT).[86] Prognosis: improvement but not complete recovery is reported.

Late developments

Some patients who show early improvement will develop late deterioration (7–12 yrs after reaching a plateau),[51] with no radiographically apparent explanation in up to 20% of these cases.[87] In others, degeneration at levels adjacent to the operated segments may be demonstrated.

Adjacent segment disease (ASD): degeneration that develops at a motion segment adjacent to a previous fusion. Findings include: disc degeneration, stenosis, facet hypertrophy, scoliosis, listhesis, and instability. After ACDF, ASD occurred at a rate of 2.9% per year over 10 years' observation.[88] Estimate: 25% of patients will develop symptomatic adjacent level changes within 10 years of surgery.[88] This rate was higher with single-level fusion at C5–6 or C6–7 than it was with multilevel fusion, and natural progression of the disease was felt to be a significant contributor[88] (i.e., it was not all attributable to the fusion). Most cases of ASD observed radiographically are asymptomatic.

78.8 Coincident cervical and lumbar spinal stenosis

In 5%, lumbar and cervical stenoses are symptomatic simultaneously.[89]

Coincident symptomatic lumbar and cervical spinal stenosis is usually managed by first decompressing the cervical region, and later operating on the lumbar region (unless severe neurogenic claudication dominates the picture). It is also possible, in selected cases, to operate on both in a single sitting.[89,90]

78.9 Craniocervical junction and upper cervical spine abnormalities

78.9.1 Associated conditions

Also see Axis (C2) vertebra lesions (p.1678).

Abnormalities in this region are seen in a number of conditions including:
1. rheumatoid arthritis (p.1376)
2. traumatic & posttraumatic: including fractures of odontoid, occipital condyles…
3. ankylosing spondylitis (p.1365): may result in fusion of the entire spine, which spares the occipitoatlantal and/or atlantoaxial joints, which can lead to instability there
4. congenital conditions:
   a) Chiari malformations (p.295)
   b) Klippel-Feil syndrome (p.289)
   c) Down syndrome
   d) atlantoaxial dislocation (AAD)
   e) occipitalization of the atlas: seen in 40% of congenital AAD[91]

f) Morquio syndrome (a mucopolysaccharidosis): atlantoaxial subluxation occurs due to hypoplasia of the odontoid process and joint laxity
5. neoplasms: metastatic (p. 922) or primary
6. infection
7. following surgical procedures of the skull base or cervical spine: e.g., transoral resection of the odontoid

78.9.2 Types of abnormalities

Abnormalities include:
1. basilar impression/invagination: as with Paget's disease
2. atlantooccipital dislocation
3. atlantoaxial dislocation
4. occipitalization of the atlas, or thin or deficient posterior arch of atlas[92]

78.9.3 Treatment

Fractures of the occipital condyles, atlas, or axis are usually adequately treated with external immobilization; also see Occipital condyle fractures (p. 1156). Because traumatic occipitocervical dislocations are usually fatal, optimal treatment is not well defined. Occipitalization of the atlas may be treated by creating an "artificial atlas" from the base of the occiput and wiring to that.[92]

Indications and techniques are outlined in Atlantoaxial fusion (C1–2 arthrodesis) (p. 1778).

References

[1] Miller CA. Shallow Cervical Canal: Recognition, Clinical Symptoms, and Treatment. Contemp Neurosurg. 1985; 7:1–5
[2] Muhle C, Weinert D, Falliner A, et al. Dynamic changes of the spinal canal in patients with cervical spondylosis at flexion and extension using mangnetic resonance imaging. Investigative Radiology. 1998; 33:444–449
[3] Shedid D, Benzel EC, Benzel EC, et al. Cervical spondylosis anatomy: pathophysiology and biomechanics. Neurosurgery. 2007; 60:S1–1–11
[4] Nagashima C. Cervical Myelopathy due to Ossification of the Posterior Longitudinal Ligament. J Neurosurg. 1972; 37:653–660
[5] Miyazawa N, Akiyama I. Ossification of the ligamentum flavum of the cervical spine. J Neurosurg Sci. 2007; 51:139–144
[6] Batzdorf U, Batzdorf A. Analysis of Cervical Spine Curvature in Patients with Cervical Spondylosis. Neurosurgery. 1988; 22:827–836
[7] Taylor AR. Vascular Factors in the Myelopathy Associated with Cervical Spondylosis. Neurology. 1964; 14:62–68
[8] Bohlman HH, Emery JL. The pathophysiology of cervical spondylosis and myelopathy. Spine. 1988; 13:843–846
[9] Kim RC, Nelson JS, Parisi JE, et al. Spinal cord pathology. In: Principles and Practice of Neuropathology. St. Louis: C V Mosby; 1993:398–435
[10] Jeffreys RV. The Surgical Treatment of Cervical Myelopathy Due to Spondylosis and Disc Degeneration. Journal of Neurology, Neurosurgery, and Psychiatry. 1986; 49:353–361
[11] Adams CBT, Logue V. Studies in Cervical Spondylotic Myelopathy: I. Movement of the Cervical Roots, Dura and Cord, and their Relation to the Course of the Extrathecal Roots. Brain. 1971; 94:557–568
[12] Levine DN. Pathogenesis of Cervical Spondylotic Myelopathy. Journal of Neurology, Neurosurgery, and Psychiatry. 1997; 62:334–340
[13] Benzel EC. Biomechanics of Spine Stabilization. Rolling Meadows, IL: American Association of Neurological Surgeons Publications; 2001
[14] Ogino H, Tada K, Okada K, et al. Canal Diameter, Anteroposterior Compression Ratio, and Spondylotic Myelopathy of the Cervical Spine. Spine. 1983; 8:1–15
[15] Lee MJ, Cassinelli EH, Riew KD. Prevalence of cervical spine stenosis. Anatomic study in cadavers. J Bone Joint Surg Am. 2007; 89:376–380
[16] Bednarik J, Kadanka Z, Dusek L, et al. Presymptomatic spondylotic cervical myelopathy: an updated predictive model. Eur Spine J. 2008; 17:421–431
[17] Matz PaulG, Anderson PaulA, Holly LangstonT, et al. The natural history of cervical spondylotic myelopathy. Journal of Neurosurgery: Spine. 2009; 11:104–111
[18] Clarke E, Robinson PK. Cervical Myelopathy: A Complication of Cervical Spondylosis. Brain. 1956; 79:483–485
[19] Lees F, Aldren Turner JS. Natural History and Prognosis of Cervical Spondylosis. British Medical Journal. 1963; 2:1607–1610
[20] Nurick S. The Natural History and the Results of Surgical Treatment of the Spinal Cord Disorder Associated with Cervical Spondylosis. Brain. 1972; 95:101–108
[21] Cusick JF. Pathophysiology and Treatment of Cervical Spondylotic Myelopathy. Clinical Neurosurgery. 1989; 37:661–681
[22] Cooper PR. Cervical Spondylotic Myelopathy. Contemporary Neurosurgery. 1997; 19:1–7
[23] Mayfield FH. Cervical Spondylosis: A Comparison of the Anterior and Posterior Approaches. Clin Neurosurg. 1966; 13:181–188
[24] Yu YL, du Boulay GH, Stevens JM, et al. Computed Tomography in Cervical Spondylotic Myelopathy and Radiculopathy: Visualization of Structures, Myelographic Comparison, Cord Measurements and Clinical Utility. Neuroradiology. 1986; 28:221–236
[25] Epstein JA, Marc JA, Hyman RA, et al. Total Myelography in the Evaluation of Lumbar Disks. Spine. 1979; 4:121–128
[26] Houser OW, Onofrio BM, Miller GM, et al. Cervical Spondylotic Stenosis and Myelopathy: Evaluation with Computed Tomographic Myelography. Mayo Clinic Proceedings. 1994; 69:557–563
[27] Emery SE. Cervical spondylotic myelopathy: diagnosis and treatment. Journal of the American Academy of Orthopaedic Surgeons. 2001; 9:376–388
[28] Lunsford LD, Bissonette DJ, Zorub DS. Anterior Surgery for Cervical Disc Disease. Part 2: Treatment of Cervical Spondylotic Myelopathy in 32 Cases. J Neurosurg. 1980; 53:12–19
[29] Chiles BW, Leonard MA, Choudhri HF, et al. Cervical spondylotic myelopathy: Patterns of neurological

78

deficit and recovery after anterior cervical decompression. Neurosurgery. 1999; 44:762–769

[30] Ebara S, Yonenobu K, Fujiwara K, et al. Myelopathy hand characterized by muscle wasting: A different type of myelopathy hand in patients with cervical spondylosis. Spine. 1988; 13:785–791

[31] Crandall PH, Batzdorf U. Cervical Spondylotic Myelopathy. J Neurosurg. 1966; 25:57–66

[32] Voskuhl RR, Hinton RC. Sensory Impairment in the Hands Secondary to Spondylotic Compression of the Cervical Spinal Cord. Arch Neurol. 1990; 47:309–311

[33] MacFadyen DJ. Posterior Column Dysfunction in Cervical Spondylotic Myelopathy. Can J Neurol Sci. 1984; 11:365–370

[34] Denno JJ, Meadows GR. Early diagnosis of cervical spondylotic myelopathy. A useful clinical sign. Spine. 1991; 16:1353–1355

[35] Sung RD, Wang JC. Correlation between a positive Hoffmann's reflex and cervical pathology in asymptomatic individuals. Spine. 2001; 26:67–70

[36] Wiggins GC, Shaffrey CI. Laminectomy in the Cervical Spine: Indications, Surgical Techniques, and Avoidance of Complications. Contemporary Neurosurgery. 1999; 21:1–10

[37] Good DC, Couch JR, Wacasser L. "Numb, Clumsy Hands" and High Cervical Spondylosis. Surg Neurol. 1984; 22:285–291

[38] Kato S, Oshima Y, Oka H, et al. Comparison of the Japanese Orthopaedic Association (JOA) score and modified JOA (mJOA) score for the assessment of cervical myelopathy: a multicenter observational study. PLoS One. 2015; 10. DOI: 10.1371/journal.pone.0123022

[39] Vernon H, Mior S. The Neck Disability Index: a study of reliability and validity. Journal of Manipulative and Physiological Therapeutics. 1991; 14:409–415

[40] Nurick S. The Pathogenesis of the Spinal Cord Disorder Associated with Cervical Spondylosis. Brain. 1972; 95:87–100

[41] Benzel EC, Lancon J, Kesterson L, et al. Cervical laminectomy and dentate ligament section for cervical spondylotic myelopathy. Journal of Spinal Disorders. 1991; 4:286–295

[42] Yonenobu K, Abumi K, Nagata K, et al. Interobserver and intraobserver reliability of the Japanese Orthopaedic Association scoring system for evaluation of cervical compression myelopathy. Spine (Phila Pa 1976). 2001; 26:1890–4; discussion 1895

[43] Tetreault L, Kopjar B, Nouri A, et al. The modified Japanese Orthopaedic Association scale: establishing criteria for mild, moderate and severe impairment in patients with degenerative cervical myelopathy. Eur Spine J. 2017; 26:78–84

[44] Ungar-Sargon JY, Lovelace RE, Brust JC. Spastic paraplegia-paraparesis: A Reappraisal. Journal of Neurological Science. 1980; 46:1–12

[45] Yoshor D, Klugh A,3rd, Appel SH, et al. Incidence and characteristics of spinal decompression surgery after the onset of symptoms of amyotrophic lateral sclerosis. Neurosurgery. 2005; 57:984–9; discussion 984-9

[46] Campbell AMG, Phillips DG. Cervical Disk Lesions with Neurological Disorder. Differential Diagnosis, Treatment, and Prognosis. Br Med J. 1960; 2:481–485

[47] Rowland LP. Diagnosis of amyotrophic lateral sclerosis. Journal of Neurological Science. 1998; 160: S6–24

[48] Roguski M, Benzel EC, Curran JN, et al. Postoperative cervical sagittal imbalance negatively affects outcomes after surgery for cervical spondylotic myelopathy. Spine (Phila Pa 1976). 2014; 39:2070–2077

[49] Adams CBT, Logue V. Studies in Cervical Spondylotic Myelopathy: II. The Movement and Contour of the Spine in Relation to the Neural Complications of Cervical Spondylosis. Brain. 1971; 94:569–586

[50] Wolf BS, Khilnani M, Malis L. The Sagittal Diameter of the Bony Cervical Spinal Canal and its Significance in Cervical Spondylosis. J of Mount Sinai Hospital. 1956; 23:283–292

[51] Krauss WE, Ebersold MJ, Quast LM. Cervical Spondylotic Myelopathy: Surgical Indications and Technique. Contemporary Neurosurgery. 1998; 20:1–6

[52] Pavlov H, Torg JS, Robie B, et al. Cervical Spinal Stenosis: Determination with Vertebral Body Ratio Method. Radiology. 1987; 164:771–775

[53] Torg JS, Naranja RJ, Pavlov H, et al. The Relationship of Developmental Narrowing of the Cervical Spinal Canal to Reversible and Irreversible Injury of the Cervical Spinal Cord in Football Players. Journal of Bone and Joint Surgery. 1996; 78A:1308–1314

[54] Brown BM, Schwartz RH, Frank E, et al. Preoperative Evaluation of Cervical Radiculopathy and Myelopathy by Surface-Coil MR Imaging. American Journal of Neuroradiology. 1988; 9:859–866

[55] Mummaneni Praveen V, Kaiser MichaelG, Matz PaulG, et al. Preoperative patient selection with magnetic resonance imaging, computed tomography, and electroencephalography: does the test predict outcome after cervical surgery? Journal of Neurosurgery: Spine. 2009; 11:119–129

[56] Teresi LM, Lufkin RB, Reicher MA, et al. Asymptomatic degenerative disk disease and spondylosis of the cervical spine: MR imaging. Radiology. 1987; 164:83–88

[57] Mizuno J, Nakagawa H, Inoue T, et al. Clinicopathological study of "snake-eye appearance" in compressive myelopathy of the cervical spinal cord. Journal of Neurosurgery. 2003; 99:162–168

[58] Holly LangstonT, Matz PaulG, Anderson PaulA, et al. Clinical prognostic indicators of surgical outcome in cervical spondylotic myelopathy. Journal of Neurosurgery: Spine. 2009; 11:112–118

[59] Kadanka Z, Bednarik J, Vohanka S, et al. Conservative treatment versus surgery in spondylotic cervical myelopathy treated conservatively or surgically. European Spine Journal. 2000; 9:538–544

[60] Matz PaulG, Holly LangstonT, Mummaneni Praveen V, et al. Anterior cervical surgery for the treatment of cervical degenerative myelopathy. Journal of Neurosurgery: Spine. 2009; 11:170–173

[61] Matz PaulG, Holly LangstonT, Groff MichaelW, et al. Indications for anterior cervical decompression for the treatment of cervical degenerative radiculopathy. Journal of Neurosurgery: Spine. 2009; 11:174–182

[62] Resnick DanielK, Anderson PaulA, Kaiser MichaelG, et al. Electrophysiological monitoring during surgery for cervical degenerative myelopathy and radiculopathy. Journal of Neurosurgery: Spine. 2009; 11:245–252

[63] Mummaneni Praveen V, Kaiser MichaelG, Matz PaulG, et al. Cervical surgical techniques for the treatment of cervical spondylotic myelopathy. Journal of Neurosurgery: Spine. 2009; 11:130–141

[64] Anderson PaulA, Matz PaulG, Groff MichaelW, et al. Laminectomy and fusion for the treatment of cervical degenerative myelopathy. Journal of Neurosurgery: Spine. 2009; 11:150–156

[65] Matz PaulG, Anderson PaulA, Groff MichaelW, et al. Cervical laminoplasty for the treatment of cervical degenerative myelopathy. Journal of Neurosurgery: Spine. 2009; 11:157–169

[66] Hamanishi C, Tanaka S. Bilateral multilevel laminotomy with or without posterolateral fusion for cervical spondylotic myelopathy: relationship to type of onset and time until operation. Journal of Neurosurgery. 1996; 85:447–451

[67] Matsunaga S, Sakou T, Nakanisi K. Analysis of the cervical spine alignment following laminoplasty and laminectomy. Spinal Cord. 1999; 37:20–24

[68] Ryken TimothyC, Heary RobertF, Matz PaulG, et al. Cervical laminectomy for the treatment of cervical degenerative myelopathy. Journal of Neurosurgery: Spine. 2009; 11:142–149

[69] Guigui P, Benoist M, Deburge A. Spinal deformity and instability after multilevel cervical laminectomy for spondylotic myelopathy. Spine. 1998; 23:440–447

[70] Kaptain GJ, Simmons NE, Replogle RE, et al. Incidence and outcome of kyphotic deformity following

laminectomy for cervical spondylotic myelopathy. Journal of Neurosurgery. 2000; 93:199–204

[71] Holmes MG, Dagal A, Feinstein BA, et al. Airway Management Practice in Adults With an Unstable Cervical Spine: The Harborview Medical Center Experience. Anesth Analg. 2018; 127:450–454

[72] Yonenobu K, Hosono N, Iwasaki M, et al. Neurologic complications of surgery for cervical compression myelopathy. Spine. 1991; 16:1277–1282

[73] Epstein NE, Danto J, Nardi D. Evaluation of Intraoperative Somatosensory-Evoked Potential Monitoring During 100 Cervical Operations. Spine. 1993; 18:737–747

[74] Epstein J, Janin Y, Carras R, et al. A Comparative Study of the Treatment of Cervical Spondylotic Myeloradiculopathy: Experience with 50 Cases Treated by Means of Extensive Laminectomy, Foraminotomy, and Excision of Osteophytes During the Past 10 Years. Acta Neurochirurgica. 1982; 61

[75] Epstein NE, Epstein JA, The Cervical Spine Research Society Editorial Committee. Operative Management of Cervical Spondylotic Myelopathy: Technique and Result of Laminectomy. In: The Cervical Spine. 3rd ed. Philadelphia: Lippincott-Raven; 1998:839–848

[76] Gregorius FK, Estrin T, Crandall PH. Cervical Spondylotic Radiculopathy and Myelopathy. A Long-Term Follow-Up Study. Arch Neurol. 1976; 33:618–625

[77] Bydon M, Macki M, Kaloostian P, et al. Incidence and prognostic factors of C5 palsy: a clinical study of 1001 cases and review of the literature. Neurosurgery. 2014; 74:595–604; discussion 604-5

[78] Keegan JJ. The cause of dissociated motor loss in the upper extremity with cervical spondylosis. J Neurosurg. 1965; 23:528–536

[79] Kaneyama S, Sumi M, Kanatani T, et al. Prospective study and multivariate analysis of the incidence of C5 palsy after cervical laminoplasty. Spine (Phila Pa 1976). 2010; 35:E1553–E1558

[80] Sakaura H, Hosono N, Mukai Y, et al. C5 palsy after decompression surgery for cervical myelopathy: review of the literature. Spine. 2003; 28:2447–2451

[81] Jack A, Ramey WL, Dettori JR, et al. Factors associated with C5 palsy following cervical spine surgery:

A systematic review. Global Spine J. 2019; 9:881–894

[82] Lee HJ, Ahn JS, Shin B, et al. C4/5 foraminal stenosis predicts C5 palsy after expansive open-door laminoplasty. Eur Spine J. 2017; 26:2340–2347

[83] Matsunaga H, Inada M, Takeuchi M, et al. [Pathogenesis and prevention of C5 palsy after cervical laminoplasty]. Chubu Jpn Orthop Trauma Surg. 2007; 50:135–136

[84] Komagata M, Nishiyama M, Endo K, et al. Prophylaxis of C5 palsy after cervical expansive laminoplasty by bilateral partial foraminotomy. Spine J. 2004; 4:650–655

[85] Katsumi K, Yamazaki A, Watanabe K, et al. Can prophylactic bilateral C4/C5 foraminotomy prevent postoperative C5 palsy after open-door laminoplasty?: a prospective study. Spine (Phila Pa 1976). 2012; 37:748–754

[86] Singh RD, Arts MP, de Ruiter GCW. Delayed-onset white cord syndrome after anterior and posterior cervical decompression surgery for symptomatic ossification of spinal ligaments: illustrative cases. Journal of Neurosurgey: Case Lessons. 2021; 1:1–6

[87] Ebersold MJ, Pare MC, Quast LM. Surgical Treatment for Cervical Spondylitic Myelopathy. Journal of Neurosurgery. 1995; 82:745–751

[88] Hilibrand AS, Carlson GD, Palumbo MA, et al. Radiculopathy and myelopathy at segments adjacent to the site of a previous anterior cervical arthrodesis. J Bone Joint Surg Am. 1999; 81:519–528

[89] Epstein NE, Epstein JA, Carras R, et al. Coexisting Cervical and Lumbar Spinal Stenosis: Diagnosis and Management. Neurosurgery. 1984; 15:489–496

[90] Dagi TF, Tarkington MA, Leech JJ. Tandem Lumbar and Cervical Spinal Stenosis. J Neurosurg. 1987; 66:842–849

[91] Sinh G. Congenital Atlanto-Axial Dislocation. Neurosurg Rev. 1983; 6:211–220

[92] Jain VK, Mittal P, Banerji D, et al. Posterior Occipitoaxial Fusion for Atlantoaxial Dislocation Associated with Occipitalized Axis. Journal of Neurosurgery. 1996; 84:559–564

79 Spine Measurements

79.1 General information

This information is presented here because these measurements play a role in the diagnoses and management of scoliosis and degenerative disc disease discussed in the sections that follow. An invaluable free downloadable measurement manual is available.[1]

79.2 Scoliosis measurements

Scoliosis is defined as lateral curvature of the spine in the coronal (frontal) plane with Cobb angle (p. 1312) > 10° (curves ≤ 10° are considered "spinal asymmetry," not scoliosis).

Lordosis (curvature of the spine in the AP plane, convex anteriorly) is traditionally reported as negative numbers, **kyphosis** (curvature with convex posteriorly) as positive. However, when one is talking specifically about lordosis, the negative sign is often not explicitly shown. The spine is generally kyphotic between T1 and T12, and lordotic between L1 and L5 (▶ Fig. 79.2).

Apex (or apical) vertebra: the vertebra whose center is most laterally displaced from the central line ▶ Fig. 79.1. Curves are named for the convex side (the side towards which the curve bows out to): dextroscoliosis = convex to right, levoscoliosis = convex to left.

End vertebrae: the vertebrae at the top and bottom of the scoliotic curve with the greatest angle relative to the horizontal plane. Easily identified on imaging workstations by moving the measurement line up and down to determine which vertebra has the greatest angle.

Cobb angle: ▶ Fig. 79.1 the method used to measure the degree of scoliosis endorsed by the Scoliosis Research Society (SRS). Lippman-Cobb method: on a coronal X-ray, a line is drawn tangent to the superior endplate of the superior end vertebra, and a second line is drawn tangent to the inferior endplate of the inferior end vertebra ▶ Fig. 79.1. The Cobb angle is the angle between these 2 lines.

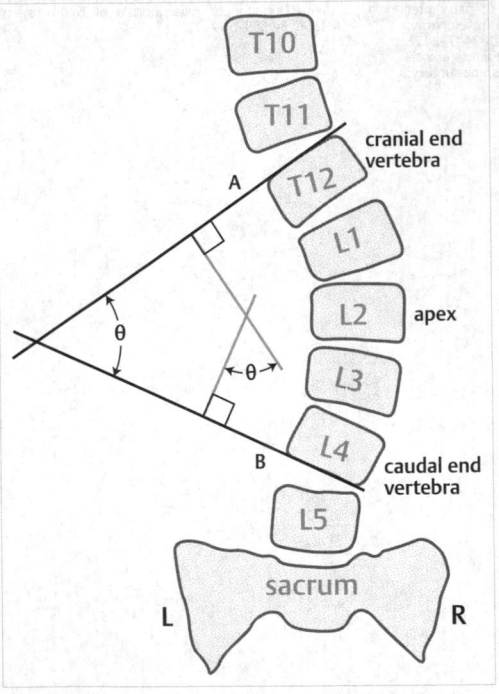

Fig. 79.1 Cobb measurement example. A dextroscolitic curve is illustrated (NB: on properly performed scoliosis X-rays left and right are reversed from conventional X-rays so that the left of the film is the patient's left) with apex at L2, end vertebrae of T12 and L4, and a Cobb angle of Θ° (the angle between lines A and B).

Most imaging workstation software will directly read out the angle between lines A & B. When working with printed films, it is often necessary to draw perpendiculars (shown as green lines) to bring the measurement location within the confines of the film.

On imaging workstations this can be measured using software. On X-ray films, a goniometer is used (if the lines meet too far off to the side of the X-ray, measurement is facilitated by drawing right angles to both of these lines and measuring the angle between these secondary lines which produces the same angle)[2]). Because of measurement variations, a Cobb angle change between X-rays of $\leq 5°$ is not considered to be significantly different.

79.3 Sagittal plane spine measurements

79.3.1 General information

In 1994 Dubousset[3] described the concept of "cone of economy" which is a range of spinal alignment in which a minimum of muscle activity is required to maintain balance. Classification of spinal deformity and quantification of severity helps guide appropriate treatment.[4,5]

Using validated outcome measures of disabilty, spinal alignment in the sagittal plane has been shown to be more important than coronal deformity.[6]

Some normal parameters that are useful for spine surgeons.
- lumbar lordosis: 10–40°[7]
- the absolute value of lumbar spinal lordosis should be about 30° greater than the absolute value of the thoracic kyphosis (e.g., a patient with thoracic kyphosis of 20° should have a lumbar lordosis of approximately -50°)[1]

79.3.2 Spino-pelvic alignment

Measurement methodology and pertinent information are shown in ► Table 79.1 and illustrated in ► Fig. 79.2 and ► Fig. 79.3. Basic measurements that can be correlated with pain reduction and quality of life measures:
- LL (lumbar lordosis)
- PI (pelvic incidence)
- PT (pelvic tilt)
- ± SVA (sagittal vertical axis): while helpful, the SVA may vary with patient-dependent compensatory mechanisms, e.g., flexing the knees, retroverting the pelvis... and since it is a linear measurement it requires calibration of the radiograph. The T1 pelvic angle (TPA) (p. 1314) appears to be more impervious to these issues[8]
- caveat: it is not reasonable or even desirable to realign every deformed spine exactly to values measured in healthy individuals[9]

With the exception of CSVL and CVA, the measurements shown in ► Table 79.1 are all taken from a *lateral* standing X-ray (► Fig. 79.2 and ► Fig. 79.3).

79.3.3 Distribution of lumbar lordosis in normal sagittal alignment

It is often asserted that the majority of the lumbar lordosis occurs from L4–S1, with ≈ 28% at L4–5 and ≈ 39% at L5–S1.[15,16] This is likely an oversimplification, as Roussouly et al.[17] have shown that normal individuals vary in the amount and distribution of the lumbar lordosis as well as in the location of the **inflection point** where the lumbar lordosis transitions to the thoracic kyphosis (which is not always at T12–L1 as is usually assumed), and they have identified 4 patterns in *normal* individuals (shown in ► Table 79.2).

Key points:
1. as sacral slope (SS) increases, the apex of the lordosis moves higher
2. patients with low SS (Types 1 & 2) have a flatter back (less lordosis) and less "reserve" when they develop lumbar spinal stenosis (less ability to compensate by retroverting the pelvis) and therefore they tend to present earlier for treatment
3. patients with higher SS (Types 3 & 4) have more reserve, but also higher chances of developing spondylolisthesis due to the steep angles

Importance of Roussouly classification: helps guide how the lumbar lordosis should be distributed. It can be especially helpful since PT is a compensatory mechanism and can change in response to pain, and LL can be altered by prior surgical fusions. ∴ In some cases it can be difficult to know the *native* SS and thence how the lumbar lordosis should be distributed and where the apex should be located to reduce the risk of PJK when planning surgery to correct sagittal imbalance. The Roussouly classification may help here: since PI typically varies from 40–60° and is fixed in a skeletally mature spine, and since SS = PI – PT, it follows that a low PI (< 55°) correlates with a low SS (i.e., Roussouly

Table 79.1 Spino-pelvic parameters: measurement methodology and pertinent information

Parameter	Description	Normal[a]	Alignment objective[a]	Comment
SVA (sagittal vertical axis) or (C7-SVA)	horizontal distance from the posterior edge of the S1 endplate to a plumb line dropped from the mid-C7 VB	<5 cm	<5 cm	numbers are positive if plumb line is anterior. Susceptible to variability depending on patient's stance, resting arms on equipment...
PT (pelvic tilt)	angle between the vertical reference line (VRL) and a line drawn from the midpoint of the femoral head[b] to the midpoint of the S1 endplate	10–25°[10]	<20°	PT above ≈ 20° indicates the patient is likely compensating for sagittal imbalance or pain (some authors consider up to 25° as normal)
PI (pelvic incidence)	angle between a point perpendicular to the S1 endplate and a line drawn from the midpoint of the femoral head[b] to the midpoint of the S1 endplate	≈ 50°	(see lumbar lordosis)	PI is fixed once skeletal maturity is reached.[c] For ease of measurement, PI = 90° − θ[2]
SS (sacral slope)	angle between the horizontal reference line (HRL) and the S1 endplate	36–42°		SS = PI − PT (by simple geometry)
LL (lumbar lordosis)	angle between the top of S1 and the top of L1	20–40°[7]	LL = PI ± 9°	LL should be within 9° of PI for "pelvic harmony"
TK (thoracic kyphosis)	angle between the top of T4 and the bottom of T12	41° ± 12°[11]		since T1 is often difficult to visualize, convention is to measure top of T4 to bottom of T12. Sometimes denoted as TK4
TPA (T1 pelvic angle)	angle between line drawn from center of T1 to center of femoral head and line from femoral head[b] to center of S1 endplate	20°[8]		may be less susceptible to influences than SVA from patient posture during X-ray
CSVL (central sacral vertical line)	on AP standing scoliosis X-ray: a line which bisects the sacrum perpendicular to a tangent drawn across the iliac crests[d]			positive numbers are to the right, negative to left
CVA (coronal vertical axis)	on AP standing scoliosis x-ray: the distance from the C7 plumb line to the CSVL	≤3 cm[12] or ≤4 cm[13] (higher values are regarded as coronal imbalance)	<3-4 cm	

[a] values shown may require modification based on age (p.1355)
[b] for measurements involving the femoral head (PT, PI, & TPA) if the two femoral heads are not superimposed, measure to a point that is midway between the centers of the two femoral heads
[c] PI is unaffected by posture or degenerative changes (i.e., patients cannot compensate by changing this). The higher the PI the higher the risk of progression of spondylolisthesis
[d] if the pelvic obliquity is > 2 cm due to leg-length inequality, use lifts under the foot on the lower side to level the pelvis (the CSVL may alternatively be drawn parallel to the lateral edge of the X-ray[14])

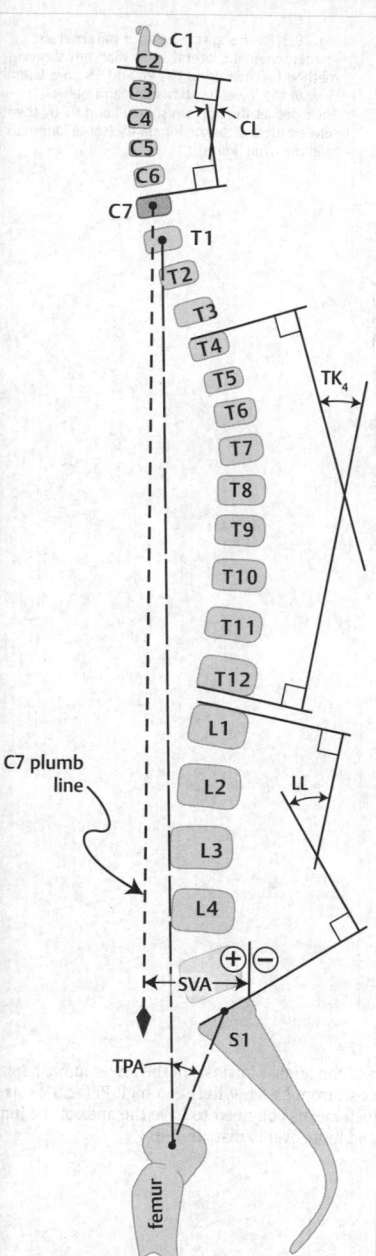

Fig. 79.2 Measuring curvature of spinal region.
Image: schematic lateral spine diagram showing
method for measuring CL (cervical lordosis), TK
(thoracic kyphosis), LL (lumbar lordosis), SVA (sagittal
vertical axis), and TPA (T1 pelvic angle) on a lateral full-
length spine X-ray.

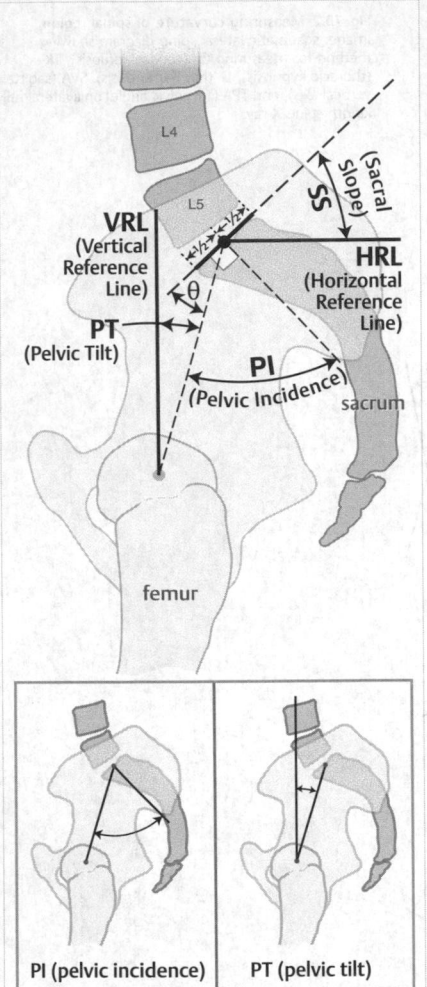

Fig. 79.3 Basic sagittal balance parameters.
Image: schematic lateral spine diagram showing method for measuring PT, PI, and SS on a lateral view of the lower lumbar spine and pelvis.
The insets at the bottom show PI and PT by themselves with less clutter for clarity (same landmarks as in the main figure).

Type 1 or 2) and you therefore need to put the apex of the lumbar lordosis in the lower lumbar spine (viz. lower L4 or center of L5) and most of the lordosis from L3-S1, whereas a high PI (> 55°) correlates with a high SS (i.e., Roussouly Type 3 or 4) which means you need to have the apex of the lumbar lordosis higher (viz. center of L4 or base of L3) and more evenly distributed.

Table 79.2 Roussouly classification of lumbar lordosis[a][17]

Type	Type 1	Type 2	Type 3	Type 4
Illustration				
Characteristic	SS < 35° apex[b] of LL in the center of L5 VB	SS < 35° apex[b] of LL at the base of L4 VB	SS = 35–45° apex[b] of LL at the center of L4 VB	SS > 45° apex[b] of LL at the base of L3 VB or higher
Implications	PI usually low. IP is low & posterior to S1P[c]. LL is distributed over only ≈ 3 lumbar levels	IP higher & is less posterior to S1P[c]. Entire spine is hypolordotic and hypokyphotic	well-balanced spine. IP at the T-L junction & just posterior to S1P[c]. LL is distributed over 4 levels (on average)	PI usually high. IP is almost exactly above S1P[c] or even anterior to it. LL is distributed over > 5 levels

[a] this classification is derived from measurements in NORMAL, unoperated subjects
[b] the red stars identify the location of the apex of the curve
[c] by "posterior to S1P" this means posterior to a vertical line (broken blue lines) passing through S1P = sacral promontory (black circles)
Abbreviations: IP = inflection point (the point where lumbar lordosis transitions to thoracic kyphosis (green circles), LL = lumbar lordosis, PI = pelvic incidence, SS = sacral slope, T-L = thoracolumbar, VB = vertebral body

References

[1] O'Brien MF, Kuklo TR, Blanke KM, et al. Radiographic Measurement Manual. 2008. http://www.oref.org/docs/default-source/default-document-library/sdsg-radiographic-measuremnt-manual.pdf?sfvrsn=2
[2] Ryan MD. Geometry for Dummies. 2nd ed. Indianapolis, Indiana: Wiley Publishing, Inc.; 2008
[3] Dubousset J, Weinstein SL. Three-dimensional analysis of the scoliotic deformity. In: The pediatric spine: Principles and practice. New York, NY: Raven Press; 1994:479–496
[4] Deukmedjian AR, Ahmadian A, Bach K, et al. Minimally invasive lateral approach for adult degenerative scoliosis: lessons learned. Neurosurg Focus. 2013; 35. DOI: 10.3171/2013.5.FOCUS13173
[5] Haque RM, Mundis GM, Jr, Ahmed Y, et al. Comparison of radiographic results after minimally invasive, hybrid, and open surgery for adult spinal deformity: a multicenter study of 184 patients. Neurosurg Focus. 2014; 36. DOI: 10.3171/2014.3.FOCUS1424
[6] Glassman SD, Bridwell K, Dimar JR, et al. The impact of positive sagittal balance in adult spinal deformity. Spine (Phila Pa 1976). 2005; 30:2024–2029
[7] Tuzun C, Yorulmaz I, Cindas A, et al. Low back pain and posture. Clin Rheumatol. 1999; 18:308–312
[8] Protopsaltis T, Schwab F, Bronsard N, et al. The T1 pelvic angle, a novel radiographic measure of global sagittal deformity, accounts for both spinal inclination and pelvic tilt and correlates with health-related quality of life. J Bone Joint Surg Am. 2014; 96:1631–1640
[9] Lafage R, Schwab F, Challier V, et al. Defining Spino-Pelvic Alignment Thresholds: Should Operative Goals in Adult Spinal Deformity Surgery Account for Age? Spine (Phila Pa 1976). 2016; 41:62–68
[10] Lafage V, Schwab F, Patel A, et al. Pelvic tilt and truncal inclination: two key radiographic parameters in the setting of adults with spinal deformity. Spine (Phila Pa 1976). 2009; 34:E599–E606
[11] Schwab F, Lafage V, Boyce R, et al. Gravity line analysis in adult volunteers: age-related correlation with spinal parameters, pelvic parameters, and foot position. Spine (Phila Pa 1976). 2006; 31:E959–E967
[12] Gao X, Wang L, Li S, et al. Predictors for Postoperative Loss of Lumbar Lordosis After Long Fusions Arthrodesis in Patients with Adult Scoliosis. Med Sci Monit. 2018; 24:531–538

79

[13] Lin JD, Osorio JA, Baum GR, et al. A new modular radiographic classification of adult idiopathic scoliosis as an extension of the Lenke classification of adolescent idiopathic scoliosis. Spine Deform. 2020. DOI: 10.1007/s43390-020-00181-7

[14] Lenke LG, Betz RR, Harms J, et al. Adolescent idiopathic scoliosis: a new classification to determine extent of spinal arthrodesis. J Bone Joint Surg Am. 2001; 83:1169–1181

[15] Bernhardt M, Bridwell KH. Segmental analysis of the sagittal plane alignment of the normal thoracic and lumbar spines and thoracolumbar junction. Spine (Phila Pa 1976). 1989; 14:717–721

[16] Troyanovich SJ, Cailliet R, Janik TJ, et al. Radiographic mensuration characteristics of the sagittal lumbar spine from a normal population with a method to synthesize prior studies of lordosis. J Spinal Disord. 1997; 10:380–386

[17] Roussouly P, Gollogly S, Berthonnaud E, et al. Classification of the normal variation in the sagittal alignment of the human lumbar spine and pelvis in the standing position. Spine (Phila Pa 1976). 2005; 30:346–353

80 Idiopathic Scoliosis

80.1 General information

Scoliosis is defined as lateral curvature of the spine in the coronal (frontal) plane with Cobb angle (p. 1312) > 10° (curves ≤ 10° are considered "spinal asymmetry," not scoliosis). Idiopathic scoliosis is often associated with vertebral body rotation and loss of thoracic kyphosis.

There are several distinct forms, which characteristically affect different age groups and are named for that age group:
1. congenital scoliosis: present at birth. Usually due to failure of vertebral segmentation or formation (p. 288)
2. infantile: 0–3 years. More common in males, with *levo*scoliosis. Potentially curable with Mehta (elongation derotation flexion) serial casting, ideally started before age 2 years (upper age limit is 4–5 years)
3. juvenile: 4–9 years
4. adolescent idiopathic scoliosis (AIS): 10–17 years. Overwhelming female dominance, almost all with *dextro*scoliosis. See below
5. adult idiopathic scoliosis (p. 1325) (AdIS): ≥ 18 years. Likely the chronological sequela of untreated AIS

Other forms of scoliosis that are not idiopathic: neuromuscular scoliosis, adult degenerative scoliosis, posttraumatic or post-infectious scoliosis, scoliosis associated with a tumor, syndromic scolioses (details in AIS below).

80.2 Adolescent idiopathic scoliosis (AIS)

80.2.1 General information

Key concepts

- idiopathic scoliosis most common in females ages 10–17 years, typically thoracic dextroscoliosis (convex to the right)
- a condition with benign natural history with regard to cardiopulmonary function, pain, & childbirth. The primary issue is deformity progression
- evaluation:
  - physical exam: to rule out other forms of scoliosis (syndromic, tumor...). AIS patients are neurologically intact
  - imaging:
    - standing scoliosis X-rays: 1) lateral, 2) neutral PA coronal, and, only if surgery is planned, 3) left bending coronal, 4) right bending coronal
      Categorize the scoliosis using the Lenke classification (p. 1321)
    - MRI: controversial. Trend is to do it routinely in patients requiring surgery, but also in cases of atypical patient (male, or thoracic levoscoliosis) or with neurologic deficit or findings of possible syndrome (café au lait spots...)
- treatment: based on skeletal maturity and magnitude of scoliosis
  - observation: for curves < 25° in patients who are still growing, or curves < 45–50° in patients who have completed their growth (skeletally mature)
  - bracing: *prevents progression* in AIS, does *not* correct scoliosis.
    Use for curves 25–40° in patients who are still growing (bracing makes no sense in skeletally mature patients), or skeletally immature patients with curve > 45° to tide them over until they can have surgery
  - Mehta casting for infantile scoliosis patients under age 4–5 years
  - surgery:
    - primarily for appropriate skeletally mature patients, mostly for main thoracic curve > 50° or thoracolumbar/lumbar curve > 40–45° (since these curves tend to progress): surgery consists of posterior scoliosis correction with fusion of structural (nonflexible) curves
    - for growing patients with early scoliosis: options include growing rods or vertebral body tethering

80

Definition: idiopathic scoliosis in children 10–17 years of age.

AIS is a diagnosis of exclusion. Incidence of underlying abnormalities: 6–25%.[1,2,3,4] Differential diagnoses to rule-out: connective tissue disorders, genetic syndromes (including neurofibromatosis), tumors (e.g., osteoid osteoma/osteoblastoma), Charcot-Marie-Tooth (p.568), Friederich's ataxia, Chiari malformation, syringomyelia, cerebral palsy, tethered cord, limb length discrepancy (false appearance of scoliosis)

▶ **Etiology.** Etiology remains unknown. It is probably due to a combination of genetic and environmental factors.

Heuter-Volkmann principle: reduced growth in areas of compressed cartilage (physes) in the curve concavity may result in progression of scoliosis through development of vertebral body wedging from asymmetric growth.

▶ **Epidemiology.** Overall population incidence: 2–3%. If a first-degree relative has scoliosis, incidence increases to 11%. There is a family history of scoliosis in ≈ 30%.

Female preponderance. The female:male prevalence ratio for curves 11–20° is 1.4:1, and it increases with increasing Cobb angles (for curves > 30° the ratio is 10:1). The majority are thoracic dextroscoliosis, with thoracic levoscoliosis being so rare that it should be investigated for an underlying cause (NB: thoracolumbar and lumbar idiopathic curves are typically levoscoliosis).

▶ **Natural history.** AIS is generally a benign condition.
- no difference in survival rate
- no difference in pulmonary function for AIS curves < 80°,[5] no significant pulmonary dysfunction with curves ≤ 100°
- back pain: incidence is higher, but intensity & frequency are similar to controls[6]
- body image: worse in scoliosis patients, but no difference in depression index
- curve progression:
  a) there is curve acceleration in the early adolescent phase of development[7]
  b) progression is more likely for thoracic curves > 50° (which generally progress at a rate of 0.5–2° per year into adulthood) or for lumbar curves > 40°
  c) main thoracic and double curves (see below for terms) are more likely to progress
  d) risk of progression is dependent on age at onset of scoliosis and magnitude of curve as shown in ▶ Table 80.1

Table 80.1 Risk of scoliosis curve progression*

Cobb angle of curve	Age of onset (years)		
	10–12	13–15	>16
<20°	25%	10%	0%
20–30°	60%	40%	10%
30–60°	90%	70%	30%
>60°	100%	90%	70%

* data from the Scoliosis Research Society

80.2.2 Evaluation

Physical exam

If scoliosis is mild, it may not be apparent on examination. The Adams forward bend test may help (see below). Obesity may conceal the presence of scoliosis on physical exam.[8]

Findings to assess:
1. findings directly related to the spine curvature:
   a) shoulder asymmetry (appearance of trapezius from posterior view and clavicle angles from anterior view)
   b) pelvic tilt
   c) leg length discrepancy
   d) Adams forward bend test: patient puts feet together, and bends forward at the waist with the knees straight and arms dangling (described by William Adams in 1865[9]). A rib hump may be seen on the *convex* side of a thoracic scoliotic curve (can differentiate scoliosis from postural

80

asymmetry which corrects on forward bending). An inclinometer (scoliometer) placed on the rib hump can help quantify the rotational deformity

   e) trunk shift: shift of the thorax to one side with respect to the pelvis. Manifests as asymmetric scapulae and/or waist asymmetry (space between the arm and the torso)

   f) breast asymmetry. Left breast/anterior chest wall usually more prominent and appear larger

2. neurologic exam: check abdominal cutaneous reflex, deep tendon reflexes, strength, sensory
3. evidence of underlying conditions: arachnodactyly, skin pigment changes (e.g., cafe au lait spots), tufts of hair or dimpling over the spine, findings of ligamentous laxity or striae that might suggest connective tissue disorder, high arched feet, claw toes, or asymmetric heel varus

Radiographic evaluation

▶ **Standing scoliosis X-rays** (p. 1353). Use includes measuring Cobb angle (p. 1312) of curves. Views for AIS (differs for adult idiopathic scoliosis (p. 1325)):

1. standing lateral (encompassing cervical, thoracic, and lumbar spines and pelvis)
2. standing neutral coronal PA (lower radiation to breast/gonads than AP view)

Only when surgery is indicated, for preoperative level selection, add "dynamic scoliosis X-rays" to determine the degree of curve rigidity preoperatively:

3. standing (or supine over bolster) coronal left lateral bending ("left bender")
4. standing (or supine over bolster) coronal right lateral bending ("right bender")

▶ **Assessing skeletal maturity.** Critical in the adolescent patient to guide decisions for bracing and timing of surgery. Options include:

1. Risser stage
   a) the U.S. system grades ossification and fusion of the iliac crest apophyses, which occurs from lateral to medial, as follows:
     • stage 0: no ossification center in the iliac crest apophysis
     • stage 1: apophysis < 25% of the iliac crest
     • stage 2: apophysis 25–50% of the iliac crest
     • stage 3: apophysis < 50–75% of the iliac crest
     • stage 4: apophysis > 75% of the iliac crest
     • stage 5: complete ossification and fusion of the iliac crest apophysis.
      NB: may appear similar to stage 0, but stage 0 is usually in age < 16 years in females or < 18 years in males, with open long bone growth plates (triradiate cartilage will be open for the majority of stage 0 and will always be closed for stage 5)
   b) grades 0 & 1 patients are growing rapidly. Scoliosis curve acceleration begins in stage 0. Grades 4 & 5 have stopped growing; see bracing recommendations based on Risser stage (p. 1324)
   c) the accuracy of Risser staging has recently been called into question and should not be used as the sole assessment of maturity[10]
2. Sanders simplified maturity scale[11]: uses an X-ray of the left hand, wrist, and distal forearm to correlate with the Tanner-Whitehouse-III RUS skeletal maturity assessment.[12] See bracing recommendations based on Sanders stage (p. 1324)
3. triradiate (hip) cartilage (TRC) closure[13]: scoliotic curves in patients with a closed TRC progressed an average of 3.12° compared to 6.86° with open TRC, and there is a higher risk for bracing failure in moderate curves with an open TRC.[14] TRC typically closes during peak height velocity

▶ **MRI.** Although controversial, universal preoperative MRI screening should be considered since clinical features do not reliably predict the presence of abnormalities.[1,3] Strong indications for MRI: early-onset scoliosis (age < 10 years), AIS in males,[2] atypical curves (thoracic levoscoliosis, kyphosis…), hyperkyphosis,[2] neurologic deficits.

80.2.3 AIS Classification (Lenke AIS Classification)

Classification goals include determining which curves need to be fused (i.e., immobile AKA structural curves), and which levels to choose as the stopping points for fusion.

80

▶ **Lenke classification.** The Lenke classification[15] is the de facto standard for classifying AIS. It describes a scoliotic spine using:

• a curve type (1–6) as summarized in ▶ Table 80.2 (see steps 1–4 below on how to determine the curve type)

Table 80.2 Lenke AIS classification[15]

Type	Proximal Thoracic (PT)	Main Thoracic (MT)	Thoracolumbar/Lumbar (TL/L)	Descriptive designator[a]
	apex: T3–5	apex: T6 thru T11–12 disc	apex: T12–L1 (TL) or L1–2 disc thru L4 (L)	
1	NS	**MAJOR**	NS	Main Thoracic (MT)
2	S†	**MAJOR**	NS	Double Thoracic (DT)
3	NS	**MAJOR**[c]	S†	Double Major (DM)
4	S†	**MAJOR**†[b]	**MAJOR**†[b]	Triple Major (TM)
5	NS	NS	**MAJOR**	Thoracolumbar/Lumbar (TL/L)
6	NS	S†	**MAJOR**[c]	Thoracolumbar/Lumbar - Main Thoracic (TL/L-MT)
Minor curve structural criteria†	Side bending residual Cobb ≥ 25° AND/OR			
	T2–5 kyphosis ≥ +20°	T10–L2 kyphosis ≥ +20°		

Abbreviations: NS = nonstructural (flexible), S = structural (major curves are structural by definition, minor structural curves are in cells labeled with †).

[a] the Descriptive designator may be confusing because the term "Main Thoracic (MT)" is also the name of a curve region, and the terms "Double Major" & "Triple Major" are used even though there is only one major curve.
[b] for Type 4, either MT or the TL/L curve may be the major curve. Use whichever has the larger Cobb angle (use MT if they are equal).
[c] to distinguish Type 3 from Type 6, the TL/L curve must be > 5° more than MT to be considered the major curve (i.e., Type 6), otherwise it is Type 3

- PLUS a lumbar spine modifier (A, B, or C) (see step 5 below)
- PLUS a thoracic sagittal plane modifier (–, N, or +) (see step 6 below)

▶ **Definitions.** Apex: in a given curve, the apex is the most horizontal and most laterally displaced VB or disc.

Major curve: the largest curve. There can be only one.[16] By definition, it is always structural.

Minor curves: the other 2 curves besides the major. Minor curves are either structural or non-structural.

Structural curve (non-flexible curve). Criteria:
1. the major curve: structural by definition
2. minor curve: (see "Minor curve structural criteria" in ▶ Table 80.2)

Non-structural curve: a minor scoliotic curve that does not meet the above criteria (i.e., it corrects to < 25° on side bending).

Fractional curve: the curve below the major curve. Often present in adult degenerative scoliosis.

Stable vertebra: the most proximal (cephalad) lower thoracic or lumbar VB most evenly bisected by the CSVL (p. 1314) (if this falls on a disc, use the next caudal VB).

Neutral vertebra: most cephalad vertebra below the apex of the major curve with neutral rotation (symmetric appearance of pedicle shadows within VB body).

Last substantially touched vertebra: most cephalad vertebra with the CSVL passing through or medial to the pedicle

▶ **Methodology.** Steps 1–4 below determine the curve type (type 1–6). Steps 5 & 6 determine the modifiers.

Step 1: measure the Cobb angle for all 3 curve regions which are:
1. PT (proximal thoracic): apex between T3–5. Cobb angle: _____°
2. MT (main thoracic): apex T6 thru T11–12 disc. Cobb angle: _____°
3. TL/L (thoracolumbar/lumbar): Cobb angle: _____°
   - TL (thoracolumbar): apex T12–L1
   - L (lumbar): apex L1–2 disc thru L4

Step 2: the **major curve** is the curve with the largest Cobb angle–it is always structural. It is *only* either MT or TL/L (never PT) as follows:
* if PT or MT is the largest curve: the major curve is designated **main thoracic** (even if PT is larger than MT)
* if TL/L is the largest curve: the major curve is TL/L
* if MT and TL/L have equal Cobb angles, then you have to complete steps 3 & 4 to identify the major curve because the curve could be Type 4

Step 3: classify the minor curves as structural or non-structural. Small minor curves (<25°) with kyphosis <20° are usually non-structural.[17] Structural minor curves meet criteria shown in the "Minor curve structural criteria" row of ▶ Table 80.2.

Step 4: determine the curve type (1–6). To simplify ▶ Table 80.2:
* if the major curve is MT, the type will be one of 1, 2, 3, or 4
  ○ Type 1: no structural minor curve
  ○ Type 2: PT structural minor curve
  ○ Type 3: TL/L structural minor curve
  ○ Type 4: both minor curves structural (PT & TL/L)*
* if the major curve is TL/L, the type will be one of 4, 5, or 6
  ○ Type 4: both minor curves structural (PT & MT)*
  ○ Type 5: no structural minor curve
  ○ Type 6: MT structural minor curve

* for Type 4, either MT or TL/L is the major curve (use whichever has the larger Cobb angle. If the Cobb angles are equal, use MT)

Step 5: Select a **lumbar modifier** (A, B, or C) based on where the CSVL (p. 1314) falls at the apex of the TL/L curve:
* A: little or no scoliosis & rotation of L-spine. CSVL falls between all lumbar pedicles up to the stable vertebra (p. 1322). Must have thoracic apex of major curve. If unsure whether CSVL touches medial aspect of lumbar apical vertebra, use modifier B.
  Subsequently, a modifier that affects level selection has been appended[18] for 1A & 2A curves: (L) if L4 tilts to the left, (R) if L4 tilts to the right (1AR curves, called "overhanging" curves, have a higher risk of adding on, necessitating a longer construct)
* B: moderate curve. CSVL touches apical lumbar vertebral body (or bodies if apex is at a disk space), but falls between medial border of lumbar concave pedicle and lateral margin of apical VB(s). Must have thoracic apex of major curve. If unsure whether CSVL touches lateral margin of apical VB(s), use modifier B
* C: large curve. CSVL lies medial to lateral aspect of lumbar apical VB(s) (i.e., does not touch apical VB[s]). May have a thoracic, thoracolumbar, and/or lumbar apex of major curve. If unsure whether CSVL touches lateral aspect of VB(s), use modifier B

Step 6: Determine the **sagittal thoracic modifier** (–, N, or +). In AIS, there tends to be thoracic hypokyphosis or even lordosis. To select the thoracic modifier, measure the **T5K angle** (the Cobb angle from the superior endplate of T5 to the inferior endplate of T12) on a lateral standing scoliosis X-ray. The thoracic modifier is:
* "–": (hypokyphosis) if T5K is <+10°
* "N": (normal) if T5K is between +10° and +40°
* "+" (hyperkyphosis) if T5K is >+40°

80.2.4 Treatment of AIS

Options: observation, bracing, or surgery.

Observation

Appropriate for curves <25° in patients who are still growing, or curves <45–50° in patients who have completed their growth. Most small curves (<20 degrees) don't progress. In growing children, close follow-up at 4–6 month intervals allows early initiation of bracing if progression occurs.

Bracing for (AIS)

Bracing in AIS is aimed at preventing progression, *not* correcting scoliosis.

✖ Contraindications:
1. bracing is not appropriate once the patient is skeletally mature
2. thoracic lordosis (a relative contraindication, a skilled orthotist can potentially make an appropriate orthosis)
3. insensate patients or insufficient neuromuscular function to draw away from pads
4. ± significant obesity: potentially decreased efficacy of brace in obesity, but can be effective[19]
5. using Sanders scale (p. 1321), patients likely to progress despite bracing:
   a) stage 2 (pre-adolescent slow): all digital epiphyses covered. Likely to fail if curve ≥ 20°
   b) stage 3 (adolescent rapid - early): most digits are capped; metacarpal epiphyses of digits #2–5 are wider than their metaphyses. Likely to fail if curve ≥ 30°

Indications:
- Scoliosis Research Society (SRS) recommendations: bracing for patients with: curves 25–40°, Risser stages (p. 1321) 0, 1, or 2 and who are premenarchal or < 1 year after menarche, or Sanders score ≤ 3
- bracing may also be used for:
  ○ skeletally immature patients with curve > 45° to tide them over until they can have surgery
  ○ 20° curve in younger patients (age < 10 years) or those with strong family history

Two basic types of braces:
- full-time TLSO: goal is to wear 18–23 hours/day. Includes: Boston, Wilmington, Rigo-Cheneau braces
- night-time TLSO: bends the patient. Goal is to wear 10 hours/night. Includes: Providence and Charleston braces

▶ **Bracing basics**
1. goal of bracing: to prevent progression, not to correct scoliosis
2. if leg-length discrepancy is > 2–2.5 cm, then correct with shoe lift prior to bracing
3. get X-ray in brace 3 weeks after delivery. Straps can usually be tightened after period of accommodation
4. discontinue brace when Risser stage (p. 1321) is ≥ 4 (for girls) or 5 (for boys) & < 1 cm growth in height over a 6-month period (recommend correlating with Sanders scale since Risser may be inaccurate), 2 years post-menarchal and Sanders 8[20]

▶ **Bracing results.** BRAIST trial[21]:
- 48% of braced patients and 72% of unbraced patients progressed to a curve ≥ 50°
- no QOL differences between braced and unbraced patients.
- number needed to treat to avoid surgery for curve progression = 3

Surgery for AIS

Goals: 1) halt ongoing progression, 2) correct as much deformity as possible.

▶ **Indications**

1. to halt ongoing progression in the following situations, since curves this size are expected to progress despite skeletal maturity
   a) main thoracic (MT) curve > 50°
   b) thoracolumbar/lumbar curve (TL, L) > 40–45°
2. risk factors for progression (not hard indications for surgery)
   a) apical vertebra rotated > 30%
   b) translational shift (TL or L)
   c) Mehta angle (the difference in angle between the two ribs attached to the apex vertebra) > 30°

▶ **Surgical options**

1. posterior spinal fusion: only for skeletally mature patients, or for appropriate level of maturity where it's safe and continued progression is anticipated while they complete growth that would be detrimental

2. for growing child (early-onset scoliosis)
   - growing rods: fuse only the cranial and caudal anchor points and then either lengthen rods with surgery every 6–9 months as child grows, or use MAGEC® rods (MAGnetic Expansion Control) to noninvasively lengthen the rods every 3 months using an external magnetic controller
   - vertebral body tethering: lateral bolts are placed thorascopically on the convexity side and are joined by a flexible non-elongating tether to inhibit growth (see Heuter-Volkmann principle (p. 1320)) and allow the concave side to "catch up." 40% revision rate at 2 years

▶ **Timing of fusion**

For fusions, an appropriate level of skeletal maturity is needed (e.g., closure of TRC (p. 1321)). A T1–T12 height of 22 cm is also desired.[22]

Risks of operating too early: continued growth risks crankshafting (continued anterior growth of the spine that results in twisting and worsening axial plane deformity) as well as adding-on or junctional deformity. This may be obviated with growing rods.

▶ **Surgical fusion goals**

1. correct scoliosis as much as possible ("perfect" correction is generally not possible nor mandatory), including de-rotation of rotated VBs
2. restore thoracic kyphosis
3. fuse all structural curves (i.e., the major curve plus structural minor curves).[15] NB: there is a move to attempt selective thoracic fusion on Lenke 3B and some 3C curves if they meet certain criteria which is controversial and beyond the scope of this book

80.3 Adult *idiopathic* scoliosis (AdIS)

80.3.1 General information

Adult *idiopathic* scoliosis (AdIS) is distinct from adult *degenerative* scoliosis. AdIS is the chronological sequela of untreated AIS. Factors differentiating AdIS from AIS include[23]:
- AdIS patients often present with back and/or LE pain
- coronal and/or sagittal malalignment is more common
- curves are less flexible, particularly the lumbosacral curve
- a degenerative lumbosacral fractional curve is often present as a result of degeneration
- when surgical fusion is indicated, it often requires inclusion of the sacrum or ilium

80.3.2 Radiographic evaluation

The radiographic evaluation differs from that used for AIS, and requires the following views:
1. standing lateral radiograph (encompassing cervical, thoracic, and lumbar spines and pelvis)
2. standing neutral coronal
3. *supine* coronal spine film (substituted for standing lateral bending views)

80.3.3 AdIS classification (Lenke AdIS classification)

The AdIS Classification[23] is analogous to the Lenke AIS Classification (p. 1321) [15] and has shown good interrater reliability. It awaits validation and utility studies.

The AdIS classification describes an adult spine with idiopathic scoliosis by:
- a curve type (1–6): the same as the Lenke AIS classification (▶ Table 80.2) except for the criteria for structural vs. nonstructural minor curves (as shown in ▶ Table 80.3)
- PLUS a lumbosacral modifier (NS or S):
  - NS: (nonstructural) lumbosacral supine Cobb < 20°
  - S: (structural) lumbosacral supine Cobb ≥ 20°
- PLUS a global alignment modifier (Aligned, Cor Malalign, Sag Malalign, Combined Malalign):
  - Aligned: SVA and CVA < 4 cm
  - Sag Malalign: (sagittal malalignment) SVA ≥ 4 cm
  - Cor Malalign: (coronal malalignment) CVA ≥ 4 cm or CVA ≤ –4 cm
  - Combined Malalign: (combined sagittal & coronal malalignment) SVA ≥ 4 cm and (CVA ≥ 4 cm or CVA ≤ –4 cm)

80

Table 80.3 Structural criteria for minor curves in the AdIS classification[23]

	Proximal Thoracic (PT)	Main Thoracic (MT)	Thoracolumbar/Lumbar (TL/L)
	apex: T3–5	apex: T6 thru T11–12 disc	apex: T12–L1 (TL) or L1–2 disc thru L4 (L)
Minor curve structural criteria	*Supine* Cobb ≥ 35° AND/OR		
	T2–5 kyphosis ≥ + 20°	T10–L2 kyphosis ≥ + 20°	

80.3.4 Treatment of AdIS

▶ **Indications for surgery**
1. increase in scoliosis over time
2. worsening pulmonary function
3. increasing pain

References

[1] Singhal R, Perry DC, Prasad S, et al. The use of routine preoperative magnetic resonance imaging in identifying intraspinal anomalies in patients with idiopathic scoliosis: a 10-year review. Eur Spine J. 2013; 22:355–359

[2] Lee CS, Hwang CJ, Kim NH, et al. Preoperative magnetic resonance imaging evaluation in patients with adolescent idiopathic scoliosis. Asian Spine J. 2017; 11:37–43

[3] Faloon M, Sahai N, Pierce TP, et al. Incidence of neuraxial abnormalities is approximately 8% among patients with adolescent idiopathic scoliosis: A meta-analysis. Clin Orthop Relat Res. 2018; 476:1506–1513

[4] Swarup I, Silberman J, Blanco J, et al. Incidence of intraspinal and extraspinal MRI abnormalities in patients with adolescent idiopathic scoliosis. Spine Deform. 2019; 7:47–52

[5] Johnston CE, Richards BS, Sucato DJ, et al. Correlation of preoperative deformity magnitude and pulmonary function tests in adolescent idiopathic scoliosis. Spine (Phila Pa 1976). 2011; 36:1096–1102

[6] Danielsson AJ, Nachemson AL. Childbearing, curve progression, and sexual function in women 22 years after treatment for adolescent idiopathic scoliosis: a case-control study. Spine (Phila Pa 1976). 2001; 26:1449–1456

[7] Sanders JO, Browne RH, McConnell SJ, et al. Maturity assessment and curve progression in girls with idiopathic scoliosis. J Bone Joint Surg Am. 2007; 89:64–73

[8] Goodbody CM, Sankar WN, Flynn JM. Presentation of Adolescent Idiopathic Scoliosis: The Bigger the Kid, the Bigger the Curve. J Pediatr Orthop. 2017; 37:41–46

[9] Fairbank J. Historical perspective: William Adams, the forward bending test, and the spine of Gideon Algernon Mantell. Spine (Phila Pa 1976). 2004; 29:1953–1955

[10] Minkara A, Bainton N, Tanaka M, et al. High Risk of Mismatch Between Sanders and Risser Staging in Adolescent Idiopathic Scoliosis: Are We Guiding Treatment Using the Wrong Classification? J Pediatr Orthop. 2020; 40:60–64

[11] Sanders JO, Khoury JG, Kishan S, et al. Predicting scoliosis progression from skeletal maturity: a simplified classification during adolescence. J Bone Joint Surg Am. 2008; 90:540–553

[12] Tanner JM, Healey MJR, Goldstein H, et al. Assessment of skeletal maturity and prediction of adult height (TW3 method). 3rd ed. London: W B Saunders; 2001

[13] Ryan PM, Puttler EG, Stotler WM, et al. Role of the triradiate cartilage in predicting curve progression in adolescent idiopathic scoliosis. J Pediatr Orthop. 2007; 27:671–676

[14] Karol LA, Virostek D, Felton K, et al. The Effect of the Risser Stage on Bracing Outcome in Adolescent Idiopathic Scoliosis. J Bone Joint Surg Am. 2016; 98:1253–1259

[15] Lenke LG, Betz RR, Harms J, et al. Adolescent idiopathic scoliosis: a new classification to determine extent of spinal arthrodesis. J Bone Joint Surg Am. 2001; 83:1169–1181

[16] Highlander Wiki. . https://highlander.fandom.com/wiki/There_can_be_only_one

[17] O'Brien MF, Kuklo TR, Blanke KM, et al. Radiographic Measurement Manual. 2008. http://www.oref.org/docs/default-source/default-document-library/sdsg-radiographic-measuremnt-manual.pdf?sfvrsn=2

[18] Miyanji F, Pawelek JB, Van Valin SE, et al. Is the lumbar modifier useful in surgical decision making?: defining two distinct Lenke 1A curve patterns. Spine (Phila Pa 1976). 2008; 33:2545–2551

[19] Karol LA, Wingfield JJ, Virostek D, et al. The Influence of Body Habitus on Documented Brace Wear and Progression in Adolescents With Idiopathic Scoliosis. J Pediatr Orthop. 2020; 40:e171–e175

[20] Cheung JPY, Cheung PWH, Luk KD. When Should We Wean Bracing for Adolescent Idiopathic Scoliosis? Clin Orthop Relat Res. 2019; 477:2145–2157

[21] Weinstein SL, Dolan LA, Wright JG, et al. Effects of bracing in adolescents with idiopathic scoliosis. N Engl J Med. 2013; 369:1512–1521

[22] Karol LA. Early definitive spinal fusion in young children: what we have learned. Clin Orthop Relat Res. 2011; 469:1323–1329

[23] Lin JD, Osorio JA, Baum GR, et al. A new modular radiographic classification of adult idiopathic scoliosis as an extension of the Lenke classification of adolescent idiopathic scoliosis. Spine Deform. 2020. DOI: 10.1007/s43390-020-00181-7

81 Lumbar and Thoracic Degenerative Disc Disease

81.1 Degenerative disc disease

81.1.1 Definition and background

A progressive deterioration of the structures of the spine not related to acute trauma. Since structures external to the disc are usually also involved, the term degenerative spine disease (DSD) may be more accurate but is not in general use. While spondylosis is a non-specific term which may include degenerative disc disease (DDD), "cervical spondylosis" usually refers to cervical stenosis (p. 1296).

The relationship of DDD to pain is not well established. Pain is most reliably linked to either:

1. neurogenic pain: due to compromise of neural spaces. Usually due to spinal stenosis, but may involve other factors such as spondylolisthesis, synovial cysts… (see below)
2. mechanical pain: may be provoked from muscles trying to compensate for the loss of spinal balance due to the degeneration, abnormal contact between bones (e.g. Baastrup's syndrome (p. 1332)), or possibly to focal excessive force on the spine itself (e.g., due to scoliosis or kyphosis)

The majority of this chapter deals with lumbar DDD. See Cervical Degenerative Disc Disease (p. 1296) for the cervical region. Symptomatic thoracic degenerative disc disease is uncommon.[1]

Most of the sequalae of lumbar DDD contribute to lumbar spinal stenosis.

81.1.2 Anatomic substrate

Changes in the intervertebral disc are a major factor in degenerative disc disease (DDD), and include:

1. age- and wear-related decrease in proteoglycan content of the disc
2. disc desiccation (loss of hydration)
3. tears develop in the annulus fibrosus (the outer fibrous ring) and progress to internal disruption of the lamellar architecture. Herniation of the nucleus pulposus (the inner gel-like center) may occur from increased pressure under mechanical loads
4. mucoid degeneration and ingrowth of fibrous tissue ensues (disc fibrosis)
5. subsequently disc resorption occurs
6. there is a loss of disc space height and increased susceptibility to injury
7. osteophytes form on the edges of the VB bordering the degenerated disc

81.1.3 Risk factors for degenerative disc (spine) disease

The risk of developing DSD is multifactorial and includes:

1. ★ the most powerful determinant in developing DSD in a study of identical twins was genetic influence, and possibly other unidentified factors.[2] Environmental factors studied (including sedentary vs. active lifestyles, occupation, cigarette smoking…) exerted only a modest influence, which may explain why conflicting findings for these have been reported
2. cumulative effects of microtrauma and macrotrauma to the spine
3. osteoporosis
4. cigarette smoking: several epidemiologic studies have shown that the incidence of back pain, sciatica, and spinal degenerative disease is higher among cigarette smokers than among non-smokers[3,4]
5. in the lumbar spine:
   a) stresses on the spine including effects of excess body weight
   b) loss of muscle tone (primarily abdominal and paraspinal muscles) resulting in increased dependence on the bony spine for structural support

81.2 Lumbar spinal stenosis

81.2.1 General information

Key concepts

- narrowing of the spinal spaces occupied by neural structures: central canal, neuroforamina, lateral recesses
- contributing factors: congenitally narrow spinal canal, hypertrophy of facets and ligamentum flavum, disc bulging, osteophytes, vertebral malalignment, and abnormal intraspinal structures such as synovial cysts
- most common at L4–5 and then at L3–4
- symptomatic stenosis typically produces neurogenic claudication (NC)—which classically is gradually progressive back and/or leg pain exacerbated by standing or walking that is relieved by sitting, lying down, or flexing forward at the waist
- NC is differentiated from vascular claudication which is usually relieved at rest regardless of position
- usually responds to decompressive surgery (sometimes also requiring fusion)

Spinal stenosis is narrowing of the one or more of the spinal spaces occupied by neural structures
1. central canal stenosis (see below)
2. foraminal stenosis (p. 1329)
3. lateral recess stenosis (p. 1329) (lumbar spine only)

First recognized as a distinct clinical entity producing characteristic symptoms in the 1950's and 60's.[5,6] Symptomatic lumbar stenosis is most common at L4–5, followed L3–4, L2–3, and lastly L5–1.[7] It is rare at L1–2.

Symptomatic lumbar spinal stenosis typically produces neurogenic claudication (p. 1331) (NC), consisting of back and/or lower extremity pain that is characteristically worse with standing or walking.

Contributing factors
1. narrow (central) spinal canal ("short pedicle syndrome") (see below) which renders the patient more susceptible to the following acquired changes
2. hypertrophy of facets
3. ligamentum flavum abnormalities:
   a) hypertrophy: very common
   b) ossification ▶ Fig. 81.1 (calcification): uncommon. More prevalent in East Asians, rare in Caucasians.[8] Often, but not always, associated with OPLL[9]
   c) infolding (buckling) caused by loss of disc space height

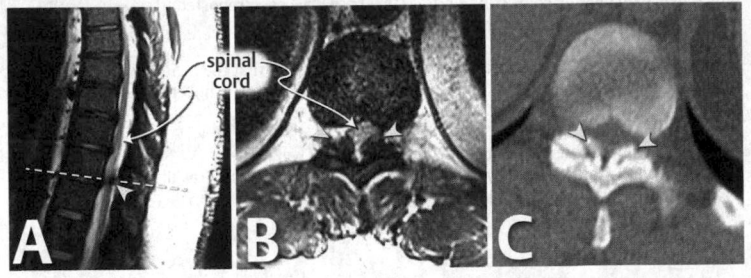

Fig. 81.1 Ossification of the ligamentum flavum (*yellow arrowheads*) located at T10–11 in 40-year-old patient with progressive myelopathy.
Image: A: sagittal T2 MRI, B: axial T2 MRI taken at the location of the broken line in A, C: axial CT through the same level.

4. disc space changes: disc bulging/herniation, osteophyte formation, collapse
5. malalignment of vertebral bodies (spondylolisthesis (p. 1337)): anterolisthesis, retrolisthesis, olisthesis
6. miscellaneous abnormal intraspinal structures: synovial/juxtafacet joint cysts (p. 1340), epidural lipomatosis (p. 1381) (most cases are not symptomatic despite the dramatic appearance)
7. other associated conditions: achondroplasia (see below), Paget's disease (p. 1362), ankylosing spondylitis (p. 1365), acromegaly

May be classified as[10]:

1. stable form of lumbar spinal stenosis: hypertrophy of facets and ligamentum flavum accompanied by disc degeneration and collapse
2. unstable form: have the above with superimposition of the following
   a) unisegmental degeneration: spondylolisthesis (p. 1337)
   b) multisegmental: degenerative scoliosis and/or sagittal imbalance

81.2.2 Neural spaces affected in lumbar spinal stenosis

Central canal stenosis

Narrowing of the central spinal canal area. When severe, it causes local compression of the nerve roots in the canal and/or to the exiting nerve roots and cauda equina (NB: in the cervical or thoracic spine, central stenosis may cause cervical spondylotic myelopathy (p. 1297) or thoracic myelopathy). Central canal stenosis may occur with:

- congenitally narrow canal: colloquially called "short pedicle syndrome." These patients become symptomatic more often and earlier than patients who have more "room" to begin with (see Normal LS spine measurements (p. 1333))
  1. as an anatomic variant: may be seen in otherwise healthy individuals
  2. may occur in certain syndromes: e.g., in *achondroplasia*, the most common form of skeletal dysplasia. Common spinal manifestations include thoracolumbar kyphosis and spinal stenosis, with about 33% requiring surgery for stenosis.[11] The animal model for a congenitally narrow canal is the dachshund ("wiener dog")
- acquired: as with degenerative changes including hypertrophy of facets, ligamentum flavum… (see above)
- symtomatic lumbar spinal stenosis is typically a combination of acquired stenosis superimposed on congenital narrowing

Lateral recess syndrome

The lateral recess is the "gutter" alongside the pedicle which the nerve root enters just proximal to its exit through the neural foramen (▶ Fig. 81.2). It is bordered anteriorly by the vertebral body, laterally by the pedicle, and posteriorly by the superior articular facet (SAF) of the inferior vertebral body. In the lateral recess, hypertrophy of the SAF compresses the nerve root en passant. L4–5 is the most commonly involved facet. Narrowing of the lateral recess is present in essentially all cases of central canal stenosis, but it can be symptomatic by itself.[12]

Foraminal stenosis

Narrowing of the neural foramen (▶ Fig. 81.3). May be the result of any combination of:

- foraminal disc protrusion/herniation
- vertebral malalignment: spondylolisthesis (p. 1337) with "uncovered" disc herniation (AKA "pseudodisc")
- facet hypertrophy
- disc space collapse: can cause compression by upward displacement of the superior articular facet (SAF) of the level below into the neural foramen
- juxtafacet joint cyst (p. 1340) (synovial cyst)
- hypertrophy of uncovertebral joints (cervical spine)

Axial loading (as when the patient is on their feet, or sitting straight up) exacerbates the narrowing. Commonly relieved by flexing forward at the waist.

The nerve root that is compressed is the one exiting through the foramen (i.e., the same number as the upper vertebra, e.g., for L4–5 foraminal stenosis the L4 nerve root is the one involved; see ▶ Fig. 81.3).

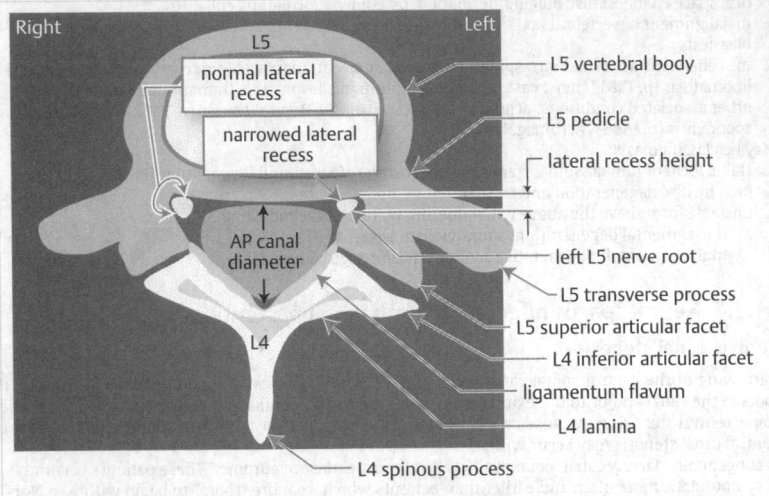

Fig. 81.2 Lateral recesses stenosis. Image: schematic axial CT through the L4–5 facet joint showing the lateral recesses (normal on patient's right, stenotic on left).

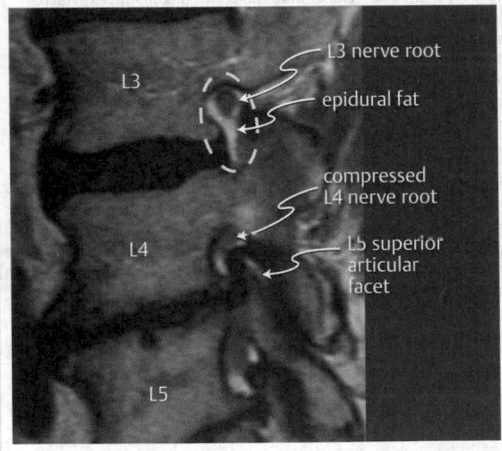

Fig. 81.3 Foraminal stenosis L4–5.
Image: T2 parasagittal MRI through the left lumbar neural foramina.
Note the normal "inverted teardrop" appearance of the L3–4 neural foramen (outlined in the *blue-dashed oval*).
In the L4–5 foramen, compression of the L4 nerve root by the superior articular facet of L5 is facilitated by hypertrophy of this facet and the collapsed L4–5 intervertebral disc. The compression worsens when the patient is upright.
For an example of foraminal stenosis by "pseudodisc" associated with spondylolisthesis, see ▶ Fig. 81.9.

Nerve compression is best appreciated on sagittal MRI through the foramen with loss of the normal "inverted teardrop" appearance of the foramen (can be seen on either T1WI or T2WI, both of which can highlight the fat that surrounds the nerve in a normal foramen—the fat is often absent in foraminal stenosis).

81.2.3 Clinical evaluation of lumbar spinal stenosis

Pain generators

1. spinal stenosis can lead to neural compromise, producing the following symptoms:
   a) radicular symptoms (more common in cervical spine than lumbar)

b) neurogenic claudication (lumbar) or spinal myelopathy (cervical or thoracic)
2. sagittal imbalance and scoliosis as a result of degenerative changes can place focal stress on specific spine structures which may be painful. Also, muscles used to compensate for the imbalance can cause pain from overuse fatigue
3. discogenic pain (controversial) may be less prevalent in the late stages of DDD. May contribute to "musculoskeletal low back pain" but the actual pain generators here are not definitively identified
4. DDD (including spinal stenosis and spondylolisthesis) may be asymptomatic, and the degenerative changes may be discovered incidentally

History

History is the most important part of the clinical evauation of lumbar spinal stenosis (LSS). The prototypical symptom of LSS is neurogenic claudication (see below) which usually presents as gradually progressive back and LE pain on walking and standing that is relieved by sitting or flexing at the waist. Sudden onset or excruciating pain is atypical for LSS. (see differential diagnosis below).

Neurologic exam

The neurologic exam is normal in ≈ 18% of cases (including normal muscle stretch reflexes and negative straight leg raising). Weakness in the anterior tibialis and/or extensor hallucis longus may occur in some cases of central canal stenosis at L4–5, or with foraminal stenosis of L5–1. Absent or reduced ankle jerks and diminished knee jerks are common[13]; however, this is also prevalent in the aged population. Forward flexion at the waist with ambulation is often observed. Pain may be reproduced by lumbar *extension* (having the patient bend backwards).

An important part of the exam is to rule out "mimics" that may be mistaken for LSS (e.g., sacroiliitis, trochanteric bursitis, vascular claudication...) but which will usually not respond to the same treatments for LSS, especially surgery (details below).

A herniated lumbar disc (HLD) produces pain on straight leg raising, and often has focal neurologic findings (weakness e.g., foot drop, loss of muscle stretch reflex, dermatomal sensory loss...).

The exam should assess: tenderness over the sacroiliac joints (as in sacroiliitis (p.1332)) or hip joints (as in bursitis), positive Patrick-FABERE test (p.1252) (as in primary hip pathology; see below)

81.2.4 Neurogenic claudication

Lumbar spinal stenosis characteristically presents with neurogenic claudication (NC) (claudicate: from Latin, claudico, to limp) AKA pseudoclaudication. Symptoms arise from compressive ischemia of the *nerves*, to be differentiated from vascular claudication (AKA intermittent claudication), which results from ischemia of exercising *muscles* due to vascular insufficiency of the muscles (see ▶ Table 81.1 for distinguishing characteristics).

NC is thought to arise from ischemia of lumbosacral nerve roots, as a result of increased metabolic demand from exercise together with vascular compromise of the nerve root due to pressure from surrounding structures. NC is only moderately sensitive (≈ 60%) but is highly specific for spinal stenosis.[13] Pain may not be the major complaint; instead, some patients may develop paresthesias or LE weakness with walking. Some may complain of muscle cramping, especially in the calves.

In contrast to e.g., a herniated lumbar disc (HLD) which usually produces acute severe nerve compression (radiculopathy) with abrupt onset of pain in a radicular distribution.

NC characteristics: unilateral or bilateral buttock, hip, thigh, or leg discomfort that is precipitated by standing or walking. Painful burning paresthesias of the lower extremities are also described. Valsalva maneuvers usually do not exacerbate the pain. Many patients report increased pain first thing in the morning that improves once they have been out of bed for varying periods (usually an hour more or less).

Relief from symptoms occurs with positions that decrease the lumbar lordosis which increases the diameter of the central canal (by reducing inward buckling of the ligamentum flavum) and distracts the facet joints (which enlarges the neural foramina). Favored positions include sitting, squatting, and recumbency. Patients may develop "anthropoid posture" (exaggerated waist flexion). "Shopping cart sign" patients often can walk farther if they can lean forward e.g., as on a grocery cart. Riding a bicycle is also often well tolerated.

The time course is usually gradually progressive over many months to years. As the condition progresses, the symptoms appear earlier with walking or standing and the ability to get relief from position changes tends to decrease. However, presentation with acute, unrelenting pain is not characteristic and other causes should be sought.

Table 81.1 Clinical features distinguishing neurogenic from vascular claudication[14]

Feature	Neurogenic claudication	Vascular claudication
distribution of pain	in distribution of nerve (dermatomal)	in distribution of muscle group with common vascular supply (sclerotomal)
sensory loss	dermatomal distribution	stocking distribution
inciting factors	variable amounts of exercise, also with prolonged maintenance of a given posture (65% have pain on standing at rest); coughing produces pain in 38%	reliably reproduced with fixed amount of exercise (e.g., distance ambulated) that decreases as disease progresses; rare at rest (27% have pain on standing at rest)
relief with rest	slow (often > 30 min), variable, usually positional (stooped posture or sitting often required, ★ *standing and resting is usually not sufficient*)	almost immediate; *not* dependent on posture (relief of walking-induced symptoms with standing is a key differentiating feature)
claudicating distance	variable day-to-day in 62%	constant day-to-day in 88%
discomfort on lifting or bending	common (67%)	infrequent (15%)
foot pallor on elevation	none	marked
peripheral pulses	normal; or if ↓ usually reduced only unilaterally	↓ or absent; femoral bruits are common
skin temp of feet	normal	decreased

▶ **What neurogenic claudication is NOT.** In general these features suggest an etiology other than lumbar spinal stenosis should be sought
1. pain that is sudden in onset: NC is gradually progressive. Sudden onset suggests trauma (includes disc herniation) or vascular event
2. valsalva maneuver (e.g., straining at the stool) usually does not exacerbate NC
3. migratory pain: NC is usually very reproducible, e.g., does not affect one lower extremity one day, and the other on another day
4. worsened by sitting: this suggests possible sacroiliitis
5. improved by walking: this suggests possible arthritis as an etiology
6. unremitting pain: typically, NC patients can get relief with certain positions. A possible exception is at very advanced stages (but then there is a history of previous ability to get relief, e.g., with sitting)

81.2.5 Differential diagnosis

Possible etiologies

Differential diagnosis that may mimic the pain from lumbar spinal stenosis:
1. vascular insufficiency (AKA vascular or intermittent claudication): see above
2. hip disease: trochanteric bursitis (see below), degenerative joint disease
3. radiculopathy, e.g., due to lumbar herniated disc. A HLD produces abrupt onset of pain, often unrelenting, worsened by Valsalva maneuvers (cough effect) and for some the pain increases on sitting
4. facet joint pain (controversial): may respond to medial branch block (therapeutic & diagnostic)
5. **sacroiliitis**: often associated with lumbar spinal stenosis, possibly due to alterations in gait. These patients are usually more uncomfortable sitting, and when doing so will lean to the side contralateral to the sacroiliitis, and when asked to point to the region of pain with one finger, patients will often point to ≤ 1 cm of the posterior superior iliac spine (PSIS) (a positive "Fortin Finger test"[15])
6. Baastrup's syndrome[16,17]: AKA arthrosis interspinosa. Radiographically: contact of adjacent spinous processes ("kissing spines") with enlargement, flattening and reactive sclerosis of apposing interspinous surfaces. Most common at L4–5. Produces localized midline lumbar pain & tenderness on back extension relieved by flexion, local anesthetic injection, or partial excision of the involved spinous processes
7. arachnoiditis: non-positional pain, unrelenting, often burning in quality
8. intraspinal tumor: eventually begins to produce neurologic findings

9. Type I spinal AVM (spinal dural AVM) (p. 1395): typically presents with LBP and progressive myeloradiculopathy or cauda equina syndrome in a middle aged male
10. diabetic neuritis: with this, the sole of the foot is usually very tender to pressure from the examiner's thumb and the pain is not positional (e.g., not relieved with sitting)
11. musculoskeletal pain
    a) nonspecific pain without ascribable pathology
    b) delayed onset muscle soreness (DOMS): onset usually 12–48 hours *after* beginning a new activity or changing activities (NC occurs during the activity). Symptoms typically peak within 2 days and subside over several days
12. inguinal hernia: typically produces groin pain (pain along inguinal ligament)
13. functional etiologies

Degenerative hip disease

Trochanteric bursitis (TBS) and degenerative arthritis of the hip are also included in the differential diagnosis of NC.[18,19] Although TBS may be primary, it can also be secondary to other conditions including lumbar stenosis, degenerative arthritis of the lumbar spine or knee, and leg length discrepancy. TBS produces intermittent aching pain over the lateral aspect of the hip. Although usually chronic, it occasionally may have acute or subacute onset. Pain radiates to lateral aspect of thigh in 20–40% (so called "pseudoradiculopathy"), but rarely extends to the posterior thigh or as far distally as the knee. There may be numbness and paresthesia-like symptoms in the upper thigh which are usually not dermatomal in distribution. Like NC, the pain may be triggered by prolonged standing, walking, and climbing, but unlike NC it is also painful to lie on the affected side. Localized tenderness over the greater trochanter can be elicited in virtually all patients, with maximal tenderness at the junction of the upper thigh and greater trochanter. Pain increases with weight bearing (and is often present from the very first step, unlike NC) and with certain hip movements, especially external rotation (over half the patients have a positive Patrick-FABERE test (p. 1252)), and rarely with hip flexion/extension. Treatment includes NSAIDs, local injection of glucocorticoid (usually with local anesthetic), physical therapy (with stretching and muscle-strengthening exercises), and local application of ice. No controlled studies have compared these modalities.

81.2.6 Imaging evaluation of lumbar spinal stenosis

X-rays

▶ **Lumbar spine X-rays.** May demonstrate bony abnormalities (however, CT scan is more sensitive and specific) such as spondylolisthesis, spondylolysis, congenitally narrow spinal canal. Also helpful for assessing existing fusion hardware. The AP diameter of canal is usually narrowed (congenitally or acquired) (see below) whereas the interpediculate distance (IPD) may be normal.[14] Oblique films may disclose pars defects, but this is better appreciated on CT.

Normal dimensions of the lumbar spine are shown in ▶ Table 81.2 for plain film and ▶ Table 81.3 for CT. Dimensions of the lateral recess on CT are shown in ▶ Table 81.4.

Table 81.2 Normal AP diameter of lumbar spinal canal on lateral *plain film* (from spinolaminar line to posterior vertebral body)[20]

average (normal)	22–25 mm
lower limits of normal	15 mm
severe lumbar stenosis	<11 mm

Table 81.3 Normal lumbar spine measurements on CT[21]

AP diameter	≥11.5 mm
interpediculate distance (IPD)*	≥16 mm
canal cross-sectional area	≥1.45 cm²
ligamentum flavum thickness[22]	≤4–5 mm
height of lateral recess (see below)	≥3 mm

* the interpediculate distance (IPD) may be normal even with a narrowed AP canal diameter[14]

Table 81.4 Dimensions of lateral recess on CT (bone windows)

Lateral recess height*	Degree of lateral recess stenosis
3–4 mm	borderline (symptomatic if other lesion co-exists, e.g., disc bulging)
<3 mm	suggestive of lateral recess syndrome
<2 mm	diagnostic of lateral recess syndrome

* see ▶ Fig. 81.2 for a diagram showing the lateral recess height

NB: these measurements are surrogate markers that attempt to answer the critical question: is there enough room for the neural structures in physiologic positions (which varies between individuals and between spine levels) which can usually be answered directly with more accuracy using MRI or CT-myelogram).

▶ **Lateral flexion-extension** (p. 1232) **X-rays.** These are invaluable for demonstrating dynamic instability (▶ Fig. 74.1, mobile spondylolisthesis) which may not be detectable on static imaging (MRI or CT).

▶ **Standing scoliosis X-rays.** Extremely important when a fusion is being considered (especially if >1 level is being fused) to assess coronal balance (scoliosis) and, especially, sagittal balance (see Adult degenerative scoliosis (p. 1352)).

CT scan

▶ **Unenhanced CT.** Excels in demonstrating bony anatomy, but is too insensitive to be relied upon for detecting spinal stenosis. CT also identifies calcification of structures such as the posterior longitudinal ligament (PLL), ligamentum flavum, calcified herniated discs, and can demonstrate vacuum disc (p. 1227). CT is the optimal modality for assessing pars fractures, bony fusion (spontaneous or iatrogenic) and fractures.

▶ **CT-myelogram.** Iodinated contrast (often referred to as "dye") is injected into the thecal sac via lumbar puncture, followed by X-rays (myelogram) and usually CT scan (CT-myelogram). Sensitivity for central canal stenosis approaches that of MRI, but is poor for foraminal stenosis since contrast normally does not extend very far into the neural foramen because the nerve root sheaths fuse with the epineurium of the nerve root. Most useful in patients with contraindications to MRI (such as non-MRI-compatible pacemaker), in patients with fusion hardware that significantly distorts the MRI images, or in patients with possible or definite intraspinal cysts to confirm the diagnosis or to determine if they communicate with the CSF space.

Lateral myelogram films often show "washboard pattern" (multiple anterior defects), AP films often show "wasp-waisting" (narrowing of dye column), may also show partial or complete block (especially in prone position). It may be difficult to perform LP if stenosis is severe (poor CSF flow and difficulty avoiding nerve roots with the LP needle).

MRI

Unenhanced lumbar MRI is the diagnostic test of choice. It demonstrates impingement on neural structures and loss of CSF signal on T2WI in the central canal (due facet and ligamentous hypertrophy, disc protrusion, spondylolisthesis...), lateral recess stenosis, foraminal stenosis as well as juxta-facet cysts, increased fluid in the facet joint... However, MRI is poor for visualizing bone and often needs to be complemented with additional X-rays and CT, particularly for surgical planning. For reference, a relatively normal axial MRI is shown in ▶ Fig. 81.4.

▶ **Abnormal findings.** Asymptomatic abnormalities are demonstrated in up to 33% of patients 50–70 years old without back-related symptoms.[7]

Possible findings with LSS include (▶ Fig. 81.5):
1. central canal stenosis with reduction or, when severe, complete loss of CSF signal on T2WI
2. the narrowed canal may assume a deltoid (AKA tricuspoid) shape
3. **redundant nerve roots** of the cauda equina: (▶ Fig. 81.5 panel C) originally described on myelography in the 1960s.[23] When the central lumbar canal becomes severely stenotic, the nerve roots of the cauda equina can no longer slide freely past the level of stenosis with normal body movements, and instead coil up proximally (or sometimes distally) to the stenosis. Stenosis of this severe of a degree is usually associated with symptoms of lumbar spinal stenosis.
4. narrowing of the neural foramina

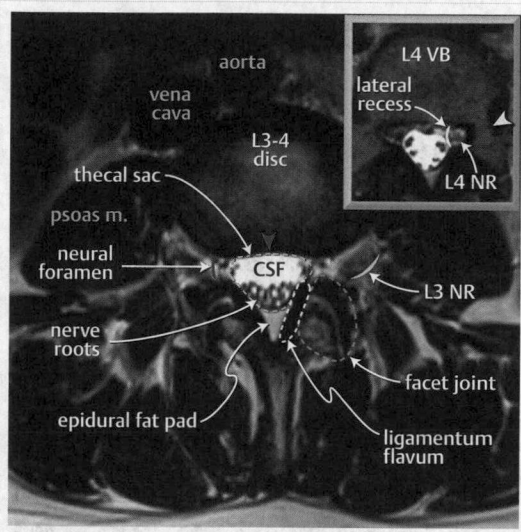

Fig. 81.4 Relatively normal axial lumbar MRI showing only mild-to-moderate degenerative changes for reference.

Image: main figure slice through L3–4 disc, inset slice through L4 VB at the level of the L4 pedicle (*yellow arrowhead*).

Broken lines outline: thecal sac (*pink*), ligamentum flavum (*yellow*), facet joint (*blue*) which is moderately hypertrophic in this patient with some excess fluid in the joint space.

Some key features: nerve roots appear as black "dots" that float down to the posterior canal in a patient lying supine in the scanner. Epidural fat is not as bright as CSF on T2WI. Inset shows adequate room in the lateral recess (*yellow crescent*) for the L4 nerve root (L4 NR).

5. narrowing of the lateral recess
6. Modic changes of the vertebral bodies may be seen (see below)

▶ **Vertebral body marrow changes (Modic changes).** VB bone marrow changes may be associated with degenerative or inflammatory processes. Modic's classification[25] based on MRI characteristics is shown in ▶ Table 81.5.

Table 81.5 Modic's classification of vertebral endplate changes on MRI

Modic type	Intensity changes		Description
	T1WI	T2WI	
1 ▶ Fig. 81.6	↓	↑	bone marrow edema associated with acute or subacute inflammation (signal characteristics mimic CSF/water). High signal seen on T2WI does not "drop out" (become low signal) on STIR images. Mnemonic: I (for type I) stands for "Inflammation" Back pain in this group may respond to fusion. Differential diagnosis includes discitis.
2 ▶ Fig. 81.7	↑	iso or ↑	fatty replacement of bone marrow. High signal "drops out" (becomes low signal) on STIR images (p. 241) (which are fat saturation) *(chronic changes)*
3	↓	↓	rare. Reactive subchondral osteo-sclerosis. No identified clinical relevance

81.2.7 Adjuncts to radiographic evaluation

1. when symptoms are suggestive of vascular claudication, tests to detect vascular insufficiency
   a) ankle-brachial index (ABI): using noninvasive means (such as ultrasound) to determine the ratio of ankle to brachial (arm) blood pressure (ABI < 0.9 is diagnostic of peripheral arterial disease in patients with claudication or other ischemic symptoms [95% sensitivity, 100% specificity][26])
   b) "Bicycle test": patients with NC can usually tolerate longer periods of exercise on a bicycle than patients with vascular claudication because the position in bicycling flexes the waist. Rarely used for spine disorders
2. EMG with NCV: are usually completely normal in patients with symptomatic lumbar spinal stenosis. May be helpful to exclude peripheral neuropathy when index of suspicion is high

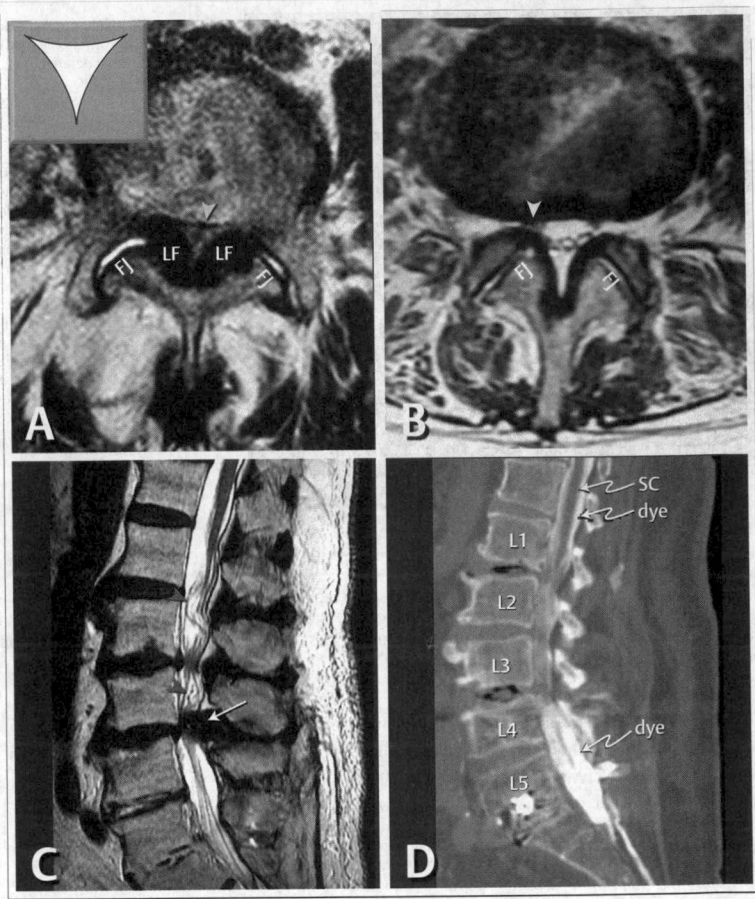

Fig. 81.5 MRI findings of lumbar spinal stenosis. Some illustrative findings (in different patients)
Image: A: axial T2 MRI showing severe central canal stenosis. There is complete loss of CSF signal, and the canal has
been narrowed to the shape of a deltoid curve (*blue arrowhead*) (inset: a deltoid curve[24]) by thickened ligamentum
flavum (LF), hypertrophied facet joints (FJ), and congenitally short pedicles.
B: axial T2 MRI showing significant lateral recess stenosis on the right, where the traversing nerve root (*yellow arrowhead*) is being compressed.
C: T2 sagittal MRI showing redundant nerve roots (*red arrowheads*) proximal to severe central canal stenosis (*white
arrow*).
D: sagittal CT/myelogram showing almost complete absence of contrast (*white*) from just above the L1–2 disc space
through just below the L3–4 disc space where it is the tightest. SC = spinal cord

3. bone density evaluation: most commonly a DEXA scan (p. 1209). Indicated when there is a concern about calcium-poor bone (osteopenia, or osteoporosis) contributing to the degenerative disc
   disease. Also indicated when instrumentation is contemplated when there is concern about calcium-poor bone (as may be suggested on X-rays or CT, or in patients with unexplained pathologic
   fractures, particulary in post-menopausal women)
4. facet blocks: typically performed by interventional pain management physicians. Some surgeons
   use relief of pain with a block as an indication to fuse a level

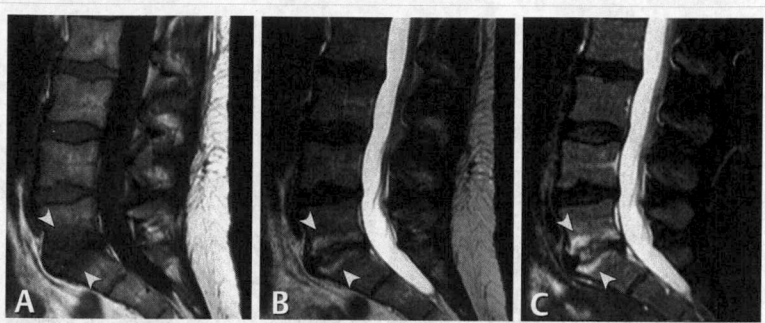

Fig. 81.6 Modic Type 1 changes (*yellow arrowheads*) in L5 & S1.
Image: sagittal lumbar MRI, A: T1WI, B: T2WI, C: STIR sequence.

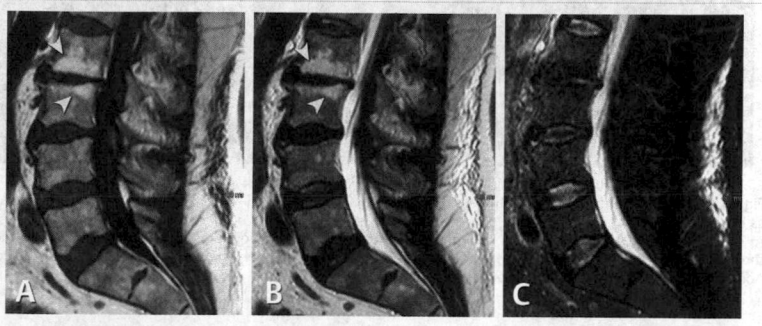

Fig. 81.7 Modic Type 2 changes (*yellow arrowheads*) in L2 & L3.
Image: sagittal lumbar MRI, A: T1WI, B: T2WI, C: STIR sequence.
NB: the high-signal associated with the Modic changes drop out on STIR (consistent with fat).

81.3 Spondylolisthesis

81.3.1 General information

Displacement (subluxation) of one vertebral body (VB) on another in any direction. Most commonly the superior VB is anterior to the inferior one (sometimes called **anterolisthesis** , when the superior VB is posterior, it is sometimes called "**retrolisthesis**"). **Olisthesis** is used by some to describe lateral displacement of one VB on another. Spondylolisthesis is most common at L5 on S1, the next most common is at L4–5. Discussion in this section focuses primarily on spondylolisthesis of the lumbar spine.

Disc herniation and nerve root compression with spondylolisthesis: it is rare for a herniated lumbar disc to occur at the level of the listhesis; however, the disc may "roll" out as it is uncovered and produce findings on axial MRI that may resemble a herniated disc which has been termed a "pseudodisc" (▶ Fig. 81.9). It is more common to see a true herniated disc at the level *above* the listhesis.

If the listhesis does cause nerve root compression, it tends to involve the nerve exiting below the pedicle of the anteriorly subluxed superior vertebra (e.g., if an L4–5 spondylolisthesis causes nerve root compression, it will generally involve the *L4* root). This is usually best seen on T2 sagittal MRI through the neuroforamen. The compression is usually due to upward displacement of the superior articular facet of the level below together with disc material, and symptoms typically resemble neurogenic claudication (p. 1331), although true radiculopathy may sometimes occur. There also may be a contribution from fibrous/inflammatory tissue from the nonunion.

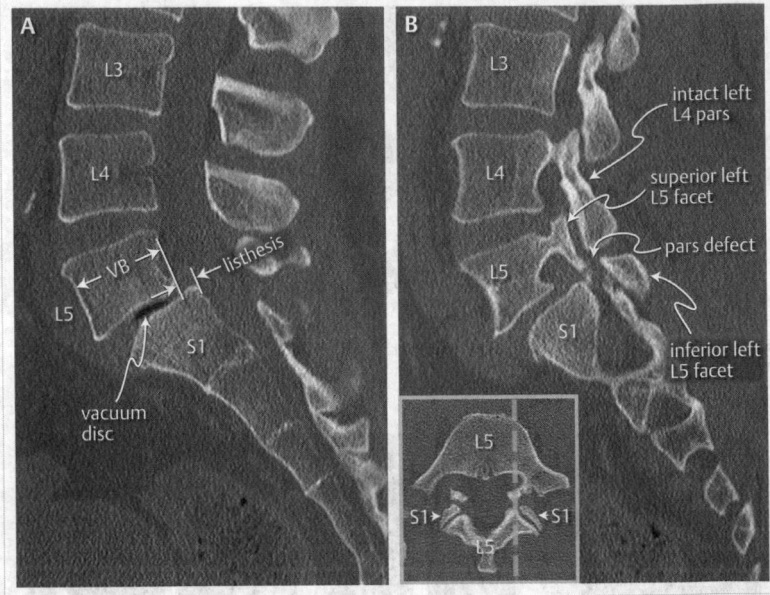

Fig. 81.8 Grade I spondylolisthesis with pars defect. Image: sagittal CT, L5–1 (with L5 pars defect). Same patient as in ▶ Fig. 81.9.
A: CT slice through the midline demonstrating measurement methodology for Meyerding grading. B: CT slice through the left facet joints and neural foramina (inset: slice location on axial CT) demonstrating left L5 pars defect. Additional findings include vacuum disc (p. 1227) in L5–1.

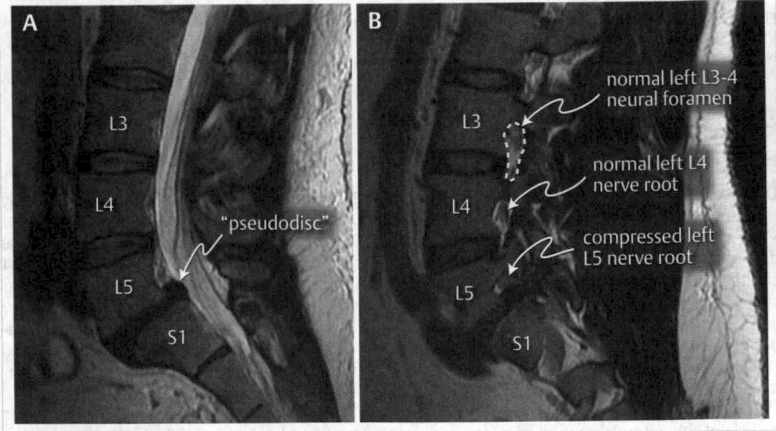

Fig. 81.9 Grade I spondylolisthesis. Image: sagittal MRI, L5–1. Same patient as in ▶ Fig. 81.8.
A: T2-weighted slice through the midline. B: T2-weighted slice through the left facet joints and neural foramina. Additional findings include compression of the left L5 nerve root by the L5–S1 "pseudodisc" (p. 1337).

Isthmic spondylolisthesis rarely produces central canal stenosis since only the anterior part of the vertebral body shifts forward. May present with radiculopathy or neurogenic claudication from compression in the neural foramen, with the nerve exiting under the pedicle at that level being the most vulnerable. May also present with low back pain. Many cases are asymptomatic.

81.3.2 Adolescent spondylolisthesis

In adolescents and teens, usually occurs in athletes subjected to repetitive hyperextension of the lumbar spine. Often associated with spondylolysis (▶ Fig. 81.10).

In girls, spondylolisthesis is frequently encountered in gymnasts and softball pitchers. In boys, it is common in American football, especially among placekickers (AKA kickers).

In these youngsters, a hiatus from sports for several months usually resolves the condition.

Surgery is sometimes performed for patients who are unwilling to interrupt their athletics.

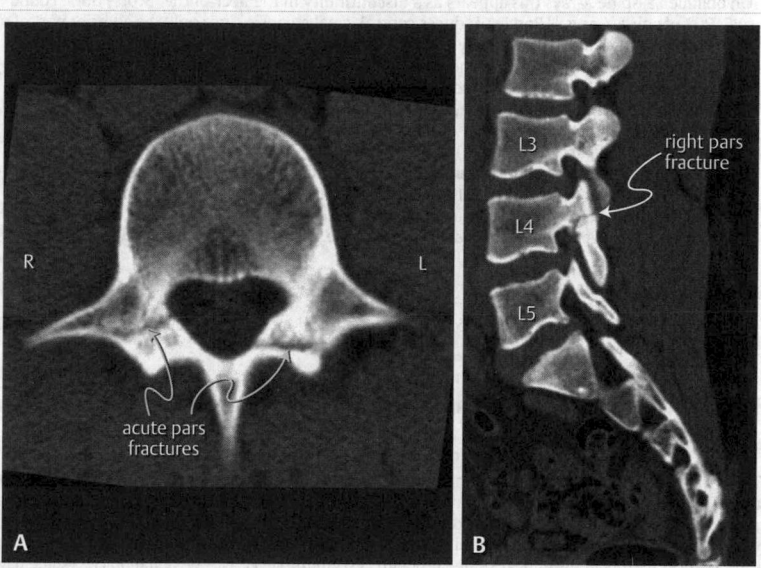

Fig. 81.10 Bilateral acute pars fractures in 16-year-old high-school football player (no spondylolisthesis). Image: A: Axial CT. B: Sagittal CT slice through right facet joints.

81.3.3 Grading spondylolisthesis

The Meyerding[27,28] grade of subluxation in the sagittal plane is widely used. Measurements are taken as in ▶ Fig. 81.8, and the percent subluxation is given by (81.1). Grading is shown in ▶ Table 81.6.

$$\% \text{ spondylolisthesis} = \frac{\text{listhesis}}{\text{VB}} \times 100\% \tag{81.1}$$

81.3.4 Types of spondylolisthesis

- Type 1: dysplastic: congenital. Upper sacrum or arch of L5 permits the spondylolisthesis. No pars defect. 94% are associated with spina bifida occulta. Some of these may progress (no way to accurately identify those that will progress)

Table 81.6 Spondylolisthesis grading (Meyerding grade[27])

Grade	% spondylolisthesis[a]
I	<25%
II	25–50%
III	50–75%
IV	75%–complete
spondyloptosis	>100%

[a]% of the AP diameter of the VB

- Type 2: isthmic spondylolisthesis AKA spondylolysis: a failure of the neural arch as a result of a defect in the pars interarticularis (literally the part between the superior and inferior facet joints). On oblique LS-spine X-rays this appears as a discontinuity in the neck of the "Scotty dog." Found in 5–20% of spine X-rays.[29] Rarely produces central canal stenosis since only the anterior part of the vertebral body shifts forward. May cause narrowing of the neural foramen. Three subtypes:
  a) lytic: fatigue fracture or insufficiency fracture of pars. In the pediatric age group may occur in athletes (especially gymnasts or football players); in some this may be an exacerbation of a pre-existing defect, in others it may be a result of repetitive trauma
  b) elongated but intact pars: possibly due to repetitive fractures and healing
  c) acute fracture of pars (▶ Fig. 81.10)
- Type 3: degenerative: due to long-standing intersegmental instability. Usually at L4–5. No break in the pars. Found in 5.8% of men and 9.1% of women (many of whom are asymptomatic)[29]
- Type 4: traumatic: due to fractures usually in areas other than the pars
- Type 5: pathologic: generalized or local bone disease, e.g., osteogenesis imperfecta

81.3.5 Natural history

Progression of spondylolisthesis may occur without surgical intervention, but is more common following surgery (p. 1344).[30]

81.4 Juxtafacet cysts of the lumbar spine

81.4.1 General information

The term juxtafacet cyst (JFC) was originated by Kao et al[31] in 1974 and includes both synovial cysts (those having a synovial lining membrane) and ganglion cysts (those lacking synovial lining) adjacent to a spinal facet joint or arising from the ligamentum flavum. Distinction between these two types of cysts may be difficult without histology (see below) and is clinically unimportant.[32]

JFC occur primarily in the lumbar spine (although cysts in the cervical[33,34,35] and thoracic[36] spine have been described). They were first reported in 1880 by von Gruker during an autopsy,[37] and were first diagnosed clinically in 1968.[38] The etiology is unknown (possibilities include: synovial fluid extrusion from the joint capsule, latent growth of a developmental rest, myxoid degeneration and cyst formation in collagenous connective tissue…), increased motion seems to have a role in many cysts, and the role of trauma in the pathogenesis is debated[34,39] but probably plays a role in a small number (≈ 14%).[40]

81.4.2 Pathology

Cyst walls are composed of fibrous connective tissue of varying thickness and cellularity. There are usually no signs of infection or inflammation. There may be a synovial lining[41] (synovial cyst) or it may be absent[42] (ganglion cyst). The distinction between the two may be difficult,[32] possibly owing in part to the fact that fibroblasts in ganglion cysts may form an incomplete synovial-like lining.[43] Proliferation of small venules is seen in the connective tissue. Hemosiderin staining may be present, and may or may not be associated with a history of trauma.[40]

81.4.3 Clinical

The average age was 63 years in one series[40] and 58 years in a review of 54 cases in the literature[41] (range: 33–87) with a slight female preponderance in both series. Most occur in patients with severe spondylosis and facet joint degeneration,[42] 25% had degenerative spondylolisthesis.[40] L4–5 is the most common level.[40,44] They may be bilateral. Pain is the most common symptom, and is usually radicular. Some JFC may contribute to canal stenosis and can produce neurogenic claudication (p. 1331)[45] or on occasion a cauda equina syndrome. Symptoms may be more intermittent in nature than with firm compressive lesions, such as HLD. A sudden exacerbation in pain may be due to hemorrhage within the cyst. Some JFC may be asymptomatic.[46]

81.4.4 Evaluation

Identifying a JFC pre-op helps the surgeon, as the approach differs slightly from that for HLD, and the cyst might otherwise be missed or unknowingly deflated and unnecessary time wasted afterwards trying to find a compressive lesion. Or, the unwitting surgeon may misinterpret the cyst as a "transdural disc extrusion" and needlessly open the dura. Pre-op diagnoses were incorrect in 30% of operated cases of JFC.[40]

Myelography: posterolateral filling defect (whereas most discs are situated anteriorly, an occasional fragment may migrate posterolaterally, whereas a JFC will always be posterolateral), often with a round extradural appearance.

CT scan: shows a low-density epidural cystic lesion typically with a posterolateral juxtaarticular location. Some have calcified rim,[46] and some may have gas within.[47] Erosion of bony lamina is occasionally seen.[44,48]

MRI (▶ Fig. 81.11): variable findings (may be due to differing composition of cyst fluid: serous vs. proteinaceous[49]). Unenhanced signal characteristics of non-hemorrhagic JFC may be similar to CSF. Hemorrhagic JFC are hyperintense. MRI usually misses bony erosion.

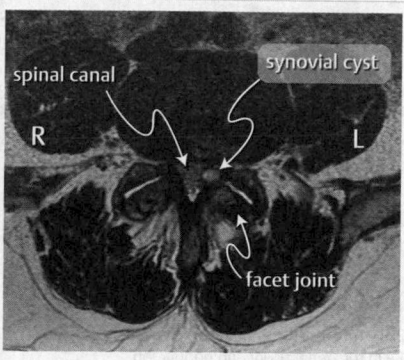

Fig. 81.11 Juxtafacet cyst.
Axial T2 MRI through L4–5 facet joints showing left-sided juxtafacet cyst.
Note fluid in facet joints suggesting degeneration and possibly increased motion.

Differential diagnosis

Also see **Differential diagnosis, Sciatica** (p. 1700). Differentiating JFC from other masses relies largely on the appearance and location. Other distinguishing features include:

1. neurofibroma: unlikely to be calcified
2. free fragment of HLD: not cystic in appearance
3. epidural or nerve root metastases: not cystic
4. dural subarachnoid root sleeve dilatation (p. 1400)
5. arachnoid cyst (from arachnoid herniation through a dural defect): not associated with facet joint, margins thinner than JFC[50]
6. perineural cysts (Tarlov cyst): arise in space between perineurium and endoneurium, usually on sacral roots,[51] occasionally show delayed filling on myelography. Usually associated with remodelling of adjacent bone

81.4.5 Treatment

Optimal treatment is not known. Cysts may resolve spontaneously (sympomatically and/or radiographically),[52] however, they are prone to recurrence. Intervention is indicated for persistent symptoms. Cyst aspiration or facet injection with steroids[53] has been described, but surgical excision of the cyst (often with fusion) is usually the definitive treatment.

Surgical treatment considerations: The cyst may be adherent to the dura. The cyst may also collapse during the surgical approach and may be missed. A JFC may serve as a marker for possible instability and should prompt an evaluation for the same. Some argue for performing a fusion since JFC may arise from instability; however, it appears that fusion is not required for a good result in many cases.[53] Therefore, consideration for fusion may be made on the basis of instability and not just by the mere presence of a JFC.

Minimally invasive spine surgery (MISS) may be used for removal.[54] A 15 mm entry incision is made 1.5 cm lateral to midline. Long-term follow-up is lacking.

Following surgical treatment, symptomatic JFCs may recur or may develop on the contralateral side.[40]

81.5 Degenerative scoliosis

One of the main differentiating features from juvenile scoliosis is that in degenerative scoliosis, the disc spaces are asymmetrically narrowed in the coronal plane and the vertebral bodies tend to maintain a more normal configuration (p. 1352).

81.6 Treatment of lumbar spinal stenosis

81.6.1 General information

In one study of 27 unoperated patients, 19 remain unchanged, 4 improved, and 4 worsened (mean follow-up: 49 months; range: 10–103 months).[55]

NSAIDs (acetaminophen may be as effective) and physical therapy are usually the initial measures of nonsurgical management. Unlike the cervical spine, traction is not usually helpful.

Brace therapy, e.g., with an LSO may be attempted. Guidelines are shown below.

Practice guideline: Brace therapy

Level II[56]:
- short-term use (1–3 weeks) of a rigid lumbar support is recommended for treatment of LBP of relatively short duration (<6 months)
- bracing in patients with LBP >6 months duration is *not* recommended because it has not been shown to have long-term benefit

Level III[56]:
- lumbar braces may reduce the number of sick days due to LBP among workers with a previous lumbar injury. Braces are *not* recommended for LBP in the general working population
- the use of pre-op bracing or transpedicular external fixation as tools to predict outcome for lumbar fusion is *not* recommended

---

Interventional pain management is an option for persistent pain. Modalities include epidural steroid injections (ESI), facet blocks (if helpful, rhizotomies—for longer relief—may be employed), trigger point injections, sacroiliac joint injections. ESI may provide temporary relief (usually days to weeks at most).

81.6.2 Management of isthmic spondylolisthesis

See reference.[29]

Some special management considerations for isthmic spondylolisthesis as a subset of spinal stenosis.

1. lesions with sclerotic borders are usually well-established with little chance of healing.
2. surgery is reserved for patients with neurologic deficit or incapacitating symptoms or progression of spondylolisthesis
3. lesions without sclerosis that show increased uptake on bone scan (indicating active lesion with potential for healing) or MRI high signal changes on T2WI[57] or STIR may heal in a rigid orthosis such as the **Boston brace** for ≥3 months
4. management of symptoms:
   a) LBP only: treat with NSAIDs, PT

b) LBP with myelopathy, radiculopathy, or neurogenic claudication: surgical treatment[58] (see ▶ Table 81.8 for surgical options)
5. in pediatrics: may be managed with TLSO and long course of PT (e.g., 6–9 months) for symptoms. Resumption of sports may be considered when symptoms subside, but recurrence should prompt elimination of athletics or consideration of surgery

81.6.3 Indications for surgery

Surgical intervention is undertaken when symptoms become severe in spite of conservative management. The goals of surgery are pain relief, halting progression of symptoms, and possibly reversal of some existing neurologic deficit. Most authors do not consider surgery unless the symptoms have been present > 3 months, and most patients who have surgery for this have symptoms of > 1 year duration.

81.6.4 Surgery

Surgical options

1. laminectomy: posterior (*direct*) decompression of central canal and neural foramina without or with fusion. Fusion options:
   a) posterolateral fusion ± pedicle screw/rod fixation
   b) interbody fusion: generally not done as a "stand-alone" (i.e., usually requires additional stabilization, options here include: pedicle screws, facet screws, facet dowels, spinous process clamp...)
      • posterior lumbar interbody fusion (PLIF) (p. 1801): usually bilateral graft placement
      • transforaminal lumbar interbody fusion (TLIF) (p. 1801): unilateral graft placement through a facet take-down on that side
2. procedures to increase disc space height and thereby *indirectly* decompress neural foramina without direct decompression
   a) anterior lumbar interbody fusion (ALIF) (p. 1795): through laparotomy
   b) lateral lumbar interbody fusion (p. 1802): some techniques trademarked as extreme lateral interbody fusion (XLIF™) or direct-lateral (DLIF™)
   c) axial lumbar interbody fusion (Ax-LIF): L5–1 only
3. limitation of extension by interspinous spacer: e.g., X-Stop® (see below)

Choosing which procedure to use

Items that factor into consideration when choosing which procedure to use include:
1. consider indirect decompression (lateral interbody fusion (e.g., XLIF® or DLIF®), ALIF, interspinous decompression (e.g., X-Stop):
   a) when foraminal stenosis appears to be the dominant problem (e.g., with loss of disc space height, facet hypertrophy, on the concave side of a scoliotic curve)
   b) previous spine surgery that might make exposure of the nerves more difficult or risky
   c) when the disc space is compressed (if the disc space height is normal, it is difficult to achieve indirect decompression by further distraction)
2. consider direct decompression (e.g., laminectomy)
   a) "pinpoint" (severe) central canal stenosis especially when disc height and neural foramina are well-preserved
   b) where a significant contributor to the compression is a focal, correctable lesion, e.g., herniated disc, synovial cyst, intraspinal tumor
   c) to avoid a fusion (in select cases)
3. consider motion-preservation surgery when a fusion is undertaken at a level and the adjacent level is already starting to show some degenerative changes that have not yet reached a surgical magnitude. Motion preservation at this adjacent segment theoretically shields it from some of the transmitted stresses from the fused level
4. situations where a fusion should be considered in addition to direct or indirect decompression of the nerves:
   a) spondylolisthesis (especially > Grade I)
   b) symptomatic sagittal imbalance or degenerative scoliosis
   c) dynamic instability on flexion/extension lateral lumbar spine X-rays
   d) expectation that the decompression will destabilize the spine (e.g., facet takedown for a TLIF)
   e) multiply recurrent herniated disc (when this is the third or more operation for the same disc)
   f) controversial: "black disc" on MRI with positive concordant discogram at this level: fusion without decompression has been advocated when there is no neural compression

When spondylolisthesis is present

Progression of spondylolisthesis may occur without decompression, but is more common following surgery.[30] However, lumbar instability following decompressive laminectomy is rare (only ≈ 1% of all laminectomies for stenosis will develop progressive subluxation). Fusion is rarely required to prevent progression of subluxation with degenerative stenosis.[59]

For Grade I and low Grade II spondylolisthesis, laminectomy without fusion may be considered. Stability (without need for instrumentation) is thought to be maintained if the pars is intact and > 50–66% of the facets are preserved during surgery and the disc space is not violated (maintains integrity of anterior and middle column). Younger or more active patients are at higher risk of subluxing. Patients with a tall (normal) disc space are also at higher risk of subluxing than those with collapsed disc space.

In a study of 40 patients 50–80 years of age with symptomatic Grade I spondylolisthesis (3–14 mm) without instability (defined as ≤ 3 mm movement on flexion/extension X-rays) followed for 5 years after laminectomy without fusion,[60] 15 patients (38%) underwent reoperation for pain related to instability. Radiographic risk factors for reoperation identified are shown in ▶ Table 81.7.

Table 81.7 Radiographic factors associated with reoperation in Grade I spondylolisthesis following initial laminectomy without fusion[60]

Radiographic factor	Diagram	Reoperation rate
disc height > 6.5 mm		45%
facet angle (FA)* > 50° FA = (RFA + LFA) / 2	 (PFL = posterior facet line, RFA & LFA = right & left facet angles)	39%
motion > 1.25 mm at spondylolisthesis level		54%
all 3 of the above		75%
none of the above		0%

* the facet angle (FA) is the average of the angles RFA and LFA, which are angles between a line drawn from the posterior to the anterior aspect of each facet to a line connecting the posterior aspect of both facets (PFL), that is: FA = (RFA + LFA) / 2

One approach is to obtain flexion/extension X-rays pre-op, and follow patients after decompression. The minority of patients who develop symptomatic slippage post-op may be treated by fusion, usually in conjunction with spinal instrumentation.

When surgery is indicated, ▶ Table 81.8 serves as a guide to the type of procedure.

Table 81.8 Surgical recommendations for spondylolisthesis

Nature of spondylolisthesis	Nature of problem	Type of procedure needed
degenerative	nerve root compression within confines of spinal canal	decompression (preserving facets)
	spinal stenosis at the level of spondylolisthesis	decompression; some advocate with intertransverse-process fusion[61]
	nerve root compression far lateral, outside confines of spinal canal	radical decompression (Gill procedure, see below) plus fusion
traumatic	(does not matter)	decompression plus fusion

Laminectomy/laminotomy—surgical technique

Posterior approach with removal of the spinous processes and lamina of affected levels (surgical "unroofing"), along with the associated ligamentum flavum. Individual nerve roots are palpated for compression within their neural foramen, with foraminotomies performed at appropriate levels. Doing a total L4 laminectomy for stenosis allows access to the L4–5 foramen, and the upper part of the L5–1 foramen. If, in addition, the inferior two-thirds of L3 are also removed, access is gained to the inferior pedicle of L3 and thus the L3–4 neural foramen. Undercutting the superior articular facet is often necessary to decompress the nerves in the lateral recess and neural foramen (p. 1329). Treatment of moderate stenosis at adjacent levels appears warranted as these levels have been shown to have a significant likelihood of becoming symptomatic later.[62]

Alternatively, laminotomies (as opposed to laminectomies) may be performed in cases where the central canal has a normal AP diameter, but the lateral canal gutter is stenotic.[63,64] Multilevel subarticular fenestrations are another slight variation on this theme.[65]

Position: either of the following is acceptable
1. prone: on a frame or chest rolls or knee-chest position to decompress the abdomen to decrease venous pressure and thus reduce bleeding
2. lateral decubitus position: if there is no laterality to symptoms, right lateral decubitus (left-side-up) is easier for most right-handed surgeons to use angled Kerrison rongeur parallel to nerve roots

Booking the case: Lumbar laminectomy

Also see defaults & disclaimers (p. 25).
1. position: prone
2. implants: for fusions, schedule with the vendor for the desired implants and associated instrumentation
3. consent (in lay terms for the patient—not all-inclusive):
   a) procedure: through the back to remove bone, ligament and any other tissue that is pressing on the nerve(s). If a fusion is to be done, then typically this will be accomplished using screws, rods, and small cages, as required
   b) alternatives: nonsurgical management
   c) complications: usual spine surgery complications (p. 25), plus there might not be the amount of pain relief desired (back pain does not respond as well to surgery as nerve-root pain). The surgery slightly weakens the spine, and as a result, about 15% of people will need a fusion at a later date

81

Minimally invasive spine surgery (MISS) decompression

Usually using ≈ 1" incisions and expandable retractors.
1. options include bilateral laminotomies (see above)
2. bilateral decompression through a unilateral laminotomy
   a) entry site: 3.5–4 cm off the midline to permit the needed angle
   b) when using a retractor with an "open side," orient the retractor with the open side facing laterally (e.g., with the Nuvasive Maxcess® place the handles medially) to permit the angle needed for contralateral decompression
   c) the laminectomy and facet takedown (usually for a TLIF) are done
   d) open the ligamentum flavum on the side you're working on, to visualize the posterior extent of the spinal canal, to permit finding the plane between the posterior part of the ligamentum flavum and the undersurface of the bone
   e) the ligamentum flavum is left in place on the contralateral side to protect the dura during drilling
   f) complete the decompression and disc removal on the side you're working on
   g) the undersurface of the bone (spinous process and contralateral lamina) are then drilled to decompress the contralateral side
   h) once the undersurface of the contralateral posterior canal has been drilled, the ligamentum flavum is removed with pituitary rongeurs. It is possible to even do a contralateral foraminotomy at this point (curved Kerrison rongeurs are very helpful for this)
   i) pedicle screws are placed through the open side, and then percutaneously through the contralateral side
   j) this is generally followed by a transforaminal lumbar interbody fusion (TLIF)

Interspinous process decompression/stabilization/fusion

Interspinous spacers (e.g., X-Stop™ (Medtronic)) limit extension at 1 or 2 levels (without fusion), preventing narrowing of the associated neural foramen, and may also off-load the facet joints and even the disc. "Success rate": 63% at 2 years. This device may be used as a stand-alone.

Interspinous plates (e.g., Aspen® (Lanx), Affix™ (Nuvasive), Spire® (Medtronic)) clamp across two spinous processes to fixate them (unlike X-Stop™ which just limits extension). The Aspen® clamps have a space for a graft which may optionally be used to promote fusion between the spinous processes. Interspinous plates may be used to augment other constructs, e.g., lateral interbody fusion,[66] but are *not* intended for stand-alone use. Biomechanical stability is reported to be similar to bilateral pedicle screws in flexion, and unilateral pedicle screws in lateral bending.[67]

Contraindications (includes exclusionary criteria from the IDE study):
1. instability at level considered for procedure: spondylolisthesis > Grade 1 or scoliosis with Cobb angle ≥ 25°
2. cauda equina syndrome
3. acute fracture of the spinous process
4. bilateral pars defects (disconnects spinous process from the anterior elements)
5. osteoporosis. Contraindications per the IDE: DEXA scan (p. 1209) with spine or hip T-score < –2.5 (i.e., more than 2.5 SD below the mean for normal adults) in the presence of ≥ 1 fragility fractures. Concerns: spinous process fracture at the time of insertion, or late subsidence due to microfractures. However, Kondrashov[68] interprets a T-score < –2.5 anywhere as indicative of osteoporosis (even without fragility fractures). Options here include:
   a) augmenting the spinous processes by injecting ≈ 0.5–1 cc of PMMA into each spinous process (SP) with a 13 Ga needle inserted ≈ halfway into the SP on lateral fluoro[68] prior to dilating the interspace or placing the X-Stop. Verify central position within SP on AP fluoro, and monitor injection on fluoro
   b) X-Stop[PK]® made of titanium and PEEK (the modulus of elasticity of PEEK is closer to bone than titanium is)
6. ankylosed level (i.e., already fused)
7. L5–1 level: the spinous process of S1 is usually too small (not usually an issue since symptomatic stenosis at L5–1 is rare)
8. age < 50 years: not studied in IDE investigation

Surgical pointers:
1. it is critical that the spacer sit in the anterior third of the spinous process
2. results may be better with the patient awake, under local anesthesia, lying on their side in a position that they feel is relieving their pain (thus opening up the critical levels). This may reduce the risk of undersizing the prosthesis

Post-op (based on manufacturer's recommendations):
1. to avoid spinous process stress fracture: build-up physical activity gradually
2. 1st 6 weeks post-op: no spine hyperextension, no heavy lifting. Minimize stair climbing
3. initially, walking (for < 1 hour) is recommended as long as it is comfortable
4. at 2 weeks post-op: cycling (stationary or bicycle) may be added
5. 6 months post-op: may add sports such as swimming, golf, racquetball, tennis, running, or jogging

Gill procedure

This procedure, and its modifications,[69] consist of radical decompression of nerve roots including removal of the loose posterior elements and total facetectomy. Currently, this is generally followed by fusion (posterolateral or interbody). Fusion rate may be enhanced with the use of internal fixation (e.g., transpedicular screw-rod fixation).[70]

Reduction of spondylolisthesis

Reduction of spondylolisthesis can be accomplished with instrumentation, and requires a fusion.
The risk of nerve root injury with reduction of grade I or II spondylolisthesis is low.
Reduction of high-grade (grade III or IV) spondylolisthesis carries a risk of radiculopathy (e.g., L5 radiculopathy in cases of L5–1 spondylolisthesis) in 50% of cases (some permanent) and may produce a cauda equina syndrome, probably from stretching nerve roots by distraction. Some have recommended intraoperative stimulation of nerve while performing EMG recording as the listhesis is gradually reduced, and stopping if the current required for stimulation increases 50% above baseline.

Isthmic spondylolisthesis (spondylolysis)—pars interarticularis defect

Instrumentation and/or fusion

Practice guideline: Fusion in patients with lumbar stenosis without spondylolisthesis

Level III[71]:
- in situ posterolateral fusion is *not* recommended following decompression in patients with lumbar stenosis in whom there is no evidence of preexisting spinal instability or likely iatrogenic instability due to facetectomy
- in situ posterolateral fusion is recommended in patients with lumbar stenosis in whom there is evidence of spinal instability
- the addition of pedicle-screw instrumentation is *not* recommended in conjunction with posterolateral fusion following decompression

Practice guideline: Fusion in patients with lumbar stenosis and spondylolisthesis

Level II[72]: posterolateral fusion is recommended for patients with stenosis and associated degenerative spondylolisthesis who require decompression.
Level III[72]: pedicle-screw fixation as an adjunct to posterolateral fusion should be considered in patients with stenosis and spondylolisthesis in cases where there is pre-op evidence of spinal instability or kyphosis at the level of the spondylolisthesis or when iatrogenic instability is anticipated (**note:** the definition of "instability" and "kyphosis" varies, and has not been standardized).

Fusion may accelerate degenerative changes at adjacent levels.
Some surgeons recommend fusion at levels of spondylolisthetic stenosis.[10,62,73] Patients with combined degenerative spondylolisthesis, stenosis, and radiculopathy may be reasonable candidates for fusion.[74]

Booking the case: Lumbar lami ± fusion for stenosis

Also see defaults & disclaimers (p. 25).
1. position: prone
2. implants: for fusions, schedule with the vendor for the desired implants and associated instrumentation
3. consent (in lay terms for the patient—not all-inclusive):
   a) procedure: through the back to remove bone, ligament, and any other tissue that is pressing on the nerve(s). If a fusion is to be done, then typically this will be accomplished using screws, rods, and small cages, as required
   b) alternatives: nonsurgical management
   c) complications: usual spine surgery complications (p. 25), plus there might not be the amount of pain relief desired (back pain does not respond as well to surgery as nerve-root pain). There can be problems with the implants, including breakage, migration (slippage), or undesirable positioning, which may require further surgery

81.7 Outcome

81.7.1 Morbidity/mortality

Risk of in-hospital mortality is 0.32%.[13] Other risks include: unintended durotomy (p. 1260) (0.32%[13] to ≈ 13%[59,75]), deep infection (5.9%), superficial infection (2.3%), and DVT (2.8%); see also Risks of lumbar laminectomy (p. 1258).

81.7.2 Nonunion

Risk factors for nonunion in fusion operations (does not necessarily correlate with success of operation):
1. cigarette smoking delays bone healing and increases the risk of pseudoarthrosis following spinal fusion procedures, especially in the lumbar spine[3]
2. number of levels: in lumbar fusions, fusing 2 levels resulted in increased nonunion rates compared to fusing 1 level[76]
3. NSAIDs: controversial
   a) short-term (≤ 5 days) post-op use: high-dose ketorolac (120–240 mg/d) was associated with increased risk of nonunion, but low-dose ketorolac (≤ 110 mg/d), and celecoxib (200–600 mg/d) were not[76]
   b) some feel that long-term NSAID use does lower fusion rate[77]

81.7.3 Success of operation

General information

Patients with a postural component to their pain had much better results (96% good result) than those without a postural component (50% good results), and the relief of leg pain was much more successful than relief of back pain.[78] Surgery is most likely to reduce LE pain and improve walking tolerance.[74]

Outcome studies

Spine Patient Outcomes Research Trial (SPORT) for lumbar stenosis

There have been many attempts to ascertain the benefit of surgery, including the $13.5 million SPORT. Shortcomings of the study include: allowing patients to decline randomization and entering them into an observational cohort which may introduce bias into the groups, patient crossovers between those randomized to surgery and those randomized to nonsurgical treatment (degrading the "intention to treat" analysis), no standardized surgical or nonsurgical technique, relatively low long-term follow-up (52% at 8 years), change in paradigm from analyzing intention-to-treat to an as-treated analysis.

Results indicated a strong benefit of surgery at 4-year follow-up[79] that appeared to diminish by 8 years in the randomized cohort but persisted in the observational cohort.[80]

Other long-term outcome studies

Literature review[13] with long-term follow-up found good or excellent outcome after surgery with a mean of 64% (range: 26–100%). A patient satisfaction survey indicated that 37% were much improved and 29% somewhat improved (total: 66%) post-op.[81] A prospective study found a success rate of 78–88% at 6 wks and 6 months, which dropped to ≈ 70% at 1 year and 5 yrs.[82] Success rates were slightly lower for lateral recess syndrome.

Reasons for surgical failure

Surgical failure may be divided into two groups:

1. patients with initial improvement who develop recurrent difficulties. Although short-term improvement after surgery is common,[79] many patients progressively deteriorate over time.[80,83] One study found a 27% recurrence of symptoms after 5-year follow-up[62] (30% due to restenosis at the operated level, 30% due to stenosis at a new level ("adjacent segment failure"); 75% of these patients respond to further surgery). Other etiologies include: development of herniated lumbar disc, development of late instability including kyphosis ("proximal junction kyphosis": PJK), coexisting medical conditions

2. patients who fail to have any post-op pain relief (early treatment failures). In one series of 45 such patients[84]:
    a) the most common finding was a lack of solid clinical and radiographic indications for surgery (e.g., non-radicular LBP coupled with modest stenosis)
    b) technical factors of surgery had less influence on outcome, with the most common finding being failure to decompress the lateral recess (which, in non-fusion cases, requires judicious medial facet resection or undercutting the superior articular facet)
    c) other diagnoses (e.g., arachnoiditis), missed diagnosis (e.g., spinal AVM)

References

[1] Yamamoto I, Matsumae M, Ikeda A, et al. Thoracic Spinal Stenosis: Experience with Seven Cases. Journal of Neurosurgery. 1988; 68:37–40

[2] Battie MC, Videman T, Gibbons LE, et al. 1995 Volvo Award in clinical sciences: determinants of lumbar disc degeneration. A study relating lifetime exposures and magnetic resonance imaging findings in identical twins. Spine. 1995; 20:2601–2612

[3] Hadley MN, Reddy SV. Smoking and the Human Vertebral Column: A Review of the Impact of Cigarette Use on Vertebral Bone Metabolism and Spinal Fusion. Neurosurgery. 1997; 41:116–124

[4] Fogelholm RR, Alho AV. Smoking and intervertebral disc degeneration. Medical Hypotheses. 2001; 56:537–539

[5] Verbiest H. A Radicular Syndrome from Developmental Narrowing of the Lumbar Canal. J Bone Joint Surg. 1954; 36B:230–237

[6] Epstein JA, Epstein BS, Lavine L. Nerve Root Compression Associated with Narrowing of the Lumbar Spinal Canal. J Neurol Neurosurg Psychiatry. 1962; 52:165–176

[7] Epstein NE. Symptomatic Lumbar Spinal Stenosis. Surgical Neurology. 1998; 50:3–10

[8] Xu R, Sciubba DM, Gokaslan ZL, et al. Ossification of the ligamentum flavum in a Caucasian man. J Neurosurg Spine. 2008; 9:427–437

[9] Miyazawa N, Akiyama I. Ossification of the ligamentum flavum of the cervical spine. J Neurosurg Sci. 2007; 51:139–144

[10] Duggal N, Sonntag VKH, Dickman CA. Fusion options and indications in the lumbosacral spine. Contemporary Neurosurgery. 2001; 23:1–8

[11] Schkrohowsky JG, Hoernschemeyer D G, Carson BS, et al. Early presentation of spinal stenosis in achondroplasia. J Pediatr Orthop. 2007; 27:119–122

[12] Ciric I, Mikhael MA, Tarkington JA, et al. The Lateral Recess Syndrome. J Neurosurg. 1980; 53:433–443

[13] Turner JA, Ersek M, Herron L, et al. Surgery for Lumbar Spinal Stenosis: Attempted Meta-Analysis of the Literature. Spine. 1992; 17:1–8

[14] Hawkes CH, Roberts GM. Neurogenic and Vascular Claudication. J Neurol Sci. 1978; 38:337–345

[15] Fortin JD, Falco FJ. The Fortin finger test: an indicator of sacroiliac pain. Am J Orthop (Belle Mead NJ). 1997; 26:477–480

[16] Kota GK, Kumar NKS, Thomas R. Baastrups Disease An Unusual Cause Of Backpain: A Case Report. 2005. http://ispub.com/IJRA/4/1/3268

[17] Filippiadis Dimitrios K, Mazioti Argyro, Argentos S, et al. Baastrup's disease (kissing spines syndrome): a pictorial review. Insights into Imaging. 2015; 6:123–128

[18] Shbeeb MI, Matteson EL. Trochanteric Bursitis (Greater Trochanter Pain Syndrome). Mayo Clinic Proceedings. 1996; 71:565–569

[19] Deen HG. Diagnosis and Management of Lumbar Disk Disease. Mayo Clinic Proceedings. 1996; 71:283–287

[20] Ehni G. Significance of the Small Lumbar Spinal Canal. J Neurosurg. 1969; 31:490–494

[21] Ullrich CG, Binet EF, Sanecki MG, et al. Quantitative Assessment of the Lumbar Spinal Canal by CT. Radiology. 1980; 134:137–143

[22] Post MJD. Computed Tomography of the Spine. Baltimore 1984

[23] Ehni G, Moiel RH, Bragg TG. The "redundant" or "knotted" nerve root: a clue to spondylotic cauda equina radiculopathy. Case report. J Neurosurg. 1970; 32:252–254

[24] Deltoid curve. 2021. https://en.wikipedia.org/wiki/Deltoid_curve

[25] Modic MT. Degenerative disorders of the spine. In: Magnetic Resonance Imaging of the Spine. New York: Yearbook Medical; 1989:83–95

[26] Sibley RC,3rd, Reis SP, MacFarlane JJ, et al. Noninvasive Physiologic Vascular Studies: A Guide to Diagnosing Peripheral Arterial Disease. Radiographics. 2017; 37:346–357

[27] Meyerding HW. Spondylolisthesis. Surgery, Gynecology and Obstetrics. 1932; 54:371–377

[28] Rothman RH, Simeone FA. The Spine. Philadelphia 1982

[29] Frymoyer JW. Back Pain and Sciatica. N Engl J Med. 1988; 318:291–300

[30] Tuite GF, Doran SE, Stern JD, et al. Outcome After Laminectomy for Lumbar Spinal Stenosis. Part II:

Radiographic Changes and Clinical Correlations. Journal of Neurosurgery. 1994; 81:707–715

[31] Kao CC, Winkler SS, Turner JH. Synovial Cyst of Spinal Facet. Case Report. Journal of Neurosurgery. 1974; 41:372–376

[32] Freidberg SR, Fellows T, Thomas CB, et al. Experience with Symptomatic Epidural Cysts. Neurosurgery. 1994; 34:989–993

[33] Cartwright MJ, Nehls DG, Carrion CA, et al. Synovial Cyst of a Cervical Facet Joint: Case Report. Neurosurgery. 1985; 16:850–852

[34] Onofrio BM, Mih AD. Synovial Cysts of the Spine. Neurosurgery. 1988; 22:642–647

[35] Goffin J, Wilms G, Plets C, et al. Synovial Cyst at the C1-C2 Junction. Neurosurgery. 1992; 30:914–916

[36] Lopes NMM, Aesse FF, Lopes DK. Compression of Thoracic Nerve Root by a Facet Joint Synovial Cyst: Case Report. Surgical Neurology. 1992; 38:338–340

[37] Heary RF, Stellar S, Fobben ES. Preoperative Diagnosis of an Extradural Cyst Arising from a Spinal Facet Joint: Case Report. Neurosurgery. 1992; 30:415–418

[38] Kao CC, Uihlein A, Bickel WH, et al. Lumbar Intraspinal Extradural Ganglion Cyst. Journal of Neurosurgery. 1968; 29:168–172

[39] Franck JI, King RB, Petro GR, et al. A Posttraumatic Lumbar Spinal Synovial Cyst. Case Report. Journal of Neurosurgery. 1987; 66:293–296

[40] Sabo RA, Tracy PT, Weinger JM. A Series of 60 Juxta-facet Cysts: Clinical Presentation, the Role of Spinal Instability, and Treatment. Journal of Neurosurgery. 1996; 85:560–565

[41] Liu CS, Williams KD, Drayer BP, et al. Synovial Cysts of the Lumbosacral Spine: Diagnosis by MR Imaging. American Journal of Neuroradiology. 1989; 10:1239–1242

[42] Silbergleit R, Gebarski SS, Brunberg JA, et al. Lumbar Synovial Cysts: Correlation of Myelographic, CT, MR, and Pathologic Findings. American Journal of Neuroradiology. 1990; 11:777–779

[43] Soren A. Pathogenesis and Treatment of Ganglion. Clin Orthop. 1966; 48:173–179

[44] Gorey MT, Hyman RA, Black KS, et al. Lumbar Synovial Cysts Eroding Bone. American Journal of Neuroradiology. 1992; 13:161–163

[45] Conrad M, Pitkethly D. Bilateral Synovial Cysts Creating Spinal Stenosis. Journal of Computer Assisted Tomography. 1987; 11:196–197

[46] Hemminghytt S, Daniels DL, Williams ML, et al. Intraspinal Synovial Cysts: Natural History and Diagnosis by CT. Radiology. 1982; 145:375–376

[47] Schulz EE, West WL, Hinshaw DB, et al. Gas in a Lumbar Extradural Juxtaarticular Cyst: Sign of Synovial Origin. Am J Radiol. 1984; 143:875–876

[48] Munz M, Tampieri D, Robitaille Y, et al. Spinal Synovial Cyst: Case Report Using Magnetic Resonance Imaging. Surgical Neurology. 1990; 34:431–434

[49] Martin D, Awwad E, Sundaram M. Lumbar Ganglion Cyst Causing Radiculopathy. Orthopedics. 1990; 13:1182–1183

[50] Budris DM. Intraspinal Lumbar Synovial Cyst. Orthopedics. 1991; 14:618–620

[51] Tarlov IM. Spinal Perineurial and Meningeal Cysts. Journal of Neurology, Neurosurgery, and Psychiatry. 1970; 33:833–843

[52] Mercader J, Gomez JM, Cardenal C. Intraspinal Synovial Cyst: Diagnosis by CT. Follow-Up and Spontaneous Remission. Neuroradiology. 1985; 27:346–348

[53] Kurz LT, Garfin SR, Unger AS, et al. Intraspinal Synovial Cyst Causing Sciatica. Journal of Bone and Joint Surgery. 1985; 67A:865–871

[54] Sehati N, Khoo LT, Holly LT. Treatment of lumbar synovial cysts using minimally invasive surgical techniques. Neurosurgical Focus. 2006; 20:E2–E6

[55] Johnsson KE, Rosén I, Udén A. The Natural Course of Lumbar Spinal Stenosis. Acta Orthop Scand. 1990; 61

[56] Resnick DK, Choudhri TF, Dailey AT, et al. Part 14: Brace therapy as an adjunct to or substitute for lumbar fusion. Journal of Neurosurgery: Spine. 2005; 2:716–724

[57] Sairyo K, Katoh S, Takata Y, et al. MRI signal changes of the pedicle as an indicator for early diagnosis of spondylolysis in children and adolescents: a clinical and biomechanical study. Spine. 2006; 31:206–211

[58] Weinstein JN, Lurie JD, Tosteson TD, et al. Surgical versus nonsurgical treatment for lumbar degenerative spondylolisthesis. New England Journal of Medicine. 2007; 356:2257–2270

[59] Silvers HR, Lewis PJ, Asch HL. Decompressive Lumbar Laminectomy for Spinal Stenosis. Journal of Neurosurgery. 1993; 78:695–701

[60] Blumenthal C, Curran J, Benzel EC, et al. Radiographic predictors of delayed instability following decompression without fusion for degenerative grade I lumbar spondylolisthesis. J Neurosurg Spine. 2013; 18:340–346

[61] Herkowitz HN, Kurz LT. Degenerative Lumbar Spondylolisthesis with Spinal Stenosis: A Prospective Study Comparing Decompression with Decompression and Intertransverse Process Arthrodesis. J Bone Joint Surg. 1991; 73A:802–808

[62] Caputy AJ, Luessenhop AJ. Long-Term Evaluation of Decompressive Surgery for Degenerative Lumbar Stenosis. Journal of Neurosurgery. 1992; 77:669–676

[63] Aryanpur J, Ducker T. Multilevel Lumbar Laminotomies for Focal Spinal Stenosis: Case Report. Neurosurgery. 1988; 23:111–115

[64] Aryanpur J, Ducker T. Multilevel Lumbar Laminotomies: An Alternative to Laminectomy in the Treatment of Lumbar Stenosis. Neurosurgery. 1990; 26:429–433

[65] Young S, Veeraoen R, O'Laoire SA. Relief of Lumbar Canal Stenosis Using Multilevel Subarticular Fenestrations as an Alternative to Wide Laminectomy: Preliminary Report. Neurosurgery. 1988; 23:628–633

[66] Wang JC, Haid RW,Jr, Miller JS, et al. Comparison of CD HORIZON SPIRE spinous process plate stabilization and pedicle screw fixation after anterior lumbar interbody fusion. J Neurosurg Spine. 2006; 4:132–136

[67] Wang JC, Spenciner D, Robinson JC. SPIRE spinous process stabilization plate: biomechanical evaluation of a novel technology. J Neurosurg Spine. 2006; 4:160–164

[68] Kondrashov Dimitriy. Personal communication. 2007

[69] Rombold C. Treatment of Spondylolisthesis by Posterolateral Fusion, Resection of the Pars Interarticularis, and Prompt Mobilization of the Patient: An End-Result Study of Seventy-Three Patients. J Bone Joint Surg. 1966; 48A:1282–1300

[70] Dickman CA, Fessler RG, MacMillan M, et al. Transpedicular Screw-Rod Fixation of the Lumbar Spine: Operative Technique and Outcome in 104 Cases. Journal of Neurosurgery. 1992; 77:860–870

[71] Resnick DK, Choudhri TF, Dailey AT, et al. Part 10: Fusion following decompression in patients with stenosis without spondylolisthesis. Journal of Neurosurgery (Spine). 2005; 2:686–691

[72] Resnick DK, Choudhri TF, Dailey AT, et al. Part 9: Fusion in patients with stenosis and spondylolisthesis. Journal of Neurosurgery (Spine). 2005; 2:679–685

[73] Ghogawala Z, Dziura J, Butler WE, et al. Laminectomy plus fusion versus laminectomy alone for lumbar spondylolisthesis. N Engl J Med. 2016; 374:1424–1434

[74] Bigos S, Bowyer O, Braen G, et al. Acute Low Back Problems in Adults. Clinical Practice Guideline No.14. AHCPR Publication No. 95-0642. Rockville, MD: Agency for Health Care Policy and Research, Public Health Service, U.S. Department of Health and Human Services; 1994

[75] Deburge A, Lassale B, Benoist M, et al. Le Traitment Chirurgical des Stenosis Lombaires et ses Resultats a Propos d'Une Serie de 163 Cas Operes. Rev Rheum Mal Osteoartic. 1983; 50:47–54

[76] Reuben SS, Ablett D, Kaye R. High dose nonsteroidal anti-inflammatory drugs compromise spinal fusion. Can J Anaesth. 2005; 52:506–512

[77] Thaller J, Walker M, Kline AJ, et al. The effect of non-steroidal anti-inflammatory agents on spinal fusion. Orthopedics. 2005; 28:299–303; quiz 304-5

[78] Ganz JC. Lumbar Spinal Stenosis: Postoperative Results in Terms of Preoperative Posture-Related Pain. Journal of Neurosurgery. 1990; 72:71–74

[79] Weinstein JN, Tosteson TD, Lurie JD, et al. Surgical versus nonoperative treatment for lumbar spinal stenosis four-year results of the Spine Patient Outcomes Research Trial. Spine (Phila Pa 1976). 2010; 35:1329–1338

[80] Lurie JD, Tosteson TD, Tosteson A, et al. Long-term outcomes of lumbar spinal stenosis: eight-year results of the Spine Patient Outcomes Research Trial (SPORT). Spine (Phila Pa 1976). 2015; 40:63–76

[81] Tuite GF, Stern JD, Doran SE, et al. Outcome After Laminectomy for Lumbar Spinal Stenosis. Part I: Clinical Correlations. Journal of Neurosurgery. 1994; 81:699–706

[82] Javid MJ, Hadar EJ. Long-Term Follow-Up Review of Patients Who Underwent Laminectomy for Lumbar Stenosis: A Prospective Study. Journal of Neurosurgery. 1998; 89:1–7

[83] Katz JN, Lipson SJ, Larson MG, et al. The Outcome of Decompressive Laminectomy for Degenerative Lumbar Stenosis. Journal of Bone and Joint Surgery. 1991; 73A:809–816

[84] Deen HG, Zimmerman RS, Lyons MK, et al. Analysis of Early Failures After Lumbar Decompressive Laminectomy for Spinal Stenosis. Mayo Clinic Proceedings. 1995; 70:33–36

82 Adult Spinal Deformity and Degenerative Scoliosis

82.1 Adult spinal deformity – general information

Key concepts

- adult spinal deformity (ASD) encompasses scoliosis, sagittal imbalance, and spondylolisthesis along with neural compression
- sagittal balance correlates with quality-of-life measures
- basic spine measurements employed: LL, PI, PT, TPA, ± SVA
- major alignment objectives (for age 50–60 years): LL = PI ± 9°, PT < 20°, SVA < 5 cm. Values change with advancing age (aging is a kyphosing process) – see text

Adult spinal deformity (ASD) is a broad term that refers to a wide spectrum of structural abnormalities of a mature spine. ASD encompass abnormalities in the coronal plane (scoliosis) as well as abnormalities in the sagittal plane.

The term "adult degenerative scoliosis" (**ADS**) (as distinguished from adolescent idiopathic scoliosis (AIS)) is often used interchangeably with ASD. Definition of adult degenerative scoliosis: spinal deformity with Cobb angle[1] > 10° in a skeletally mature individual.[2] ADS may be the result of childhood idiopathic scoliosis persisting into adulthood, or may be de novo. One of the main differentiating features from AIS is that in degenerative scoliosis, the disc spaces are asymmetrically narrowed in the coronal plane and the vertebral bodies tend to maintain a more normal configuration.

Deformity in ASD can be primarily due to asymmetric disc degeneration or secondary to hip pathology, osteoporosis, and asymmetric loads.[3] It subsequently involves posterior elements (including facet joints) and thereafter axial rotation, lateral olisthesis, and ligamentous laxity.[2,4] Progressive facet and discogenic degeneration may lead to segmental instability and subsequent central/foraminal stenosis secondary to ligamentum flavum hypertrophy and osteophyte formation[5] as well as spondylolisthesis.

While treatment goals include reduction of pain, symptomatic neural compression, and disability due to deformity, the methodology and biomechanics of ADS treatment differ greatly from treating AIS in the adolescent.

ADS tends to progress at an average rate of 3° per year (range: 1–6°).[4] Factors associated with higher rates of progression: Cobb angle > 30°, apical rotation > Grade II (on the Nash-Moe system,[6] which is falling into disuse), lateral listhesis > 6 mm, and an intercrest line through L5.[4] Factors *not* correlated with rate of progression: age and gender. Controversial associations: osteopenia.

82.2 Epidemiology

ASD is more prevalent in patients age > 60 years, but true prevalence is not well defined. More than 50% of adults hospitalized with spinal deformity are > 65 years of age.[7] Incidence of asymptomatic scoliosis ranges from 1.4%–32% and up to 68% in patients > 60.[8]

82.3 Clinical evaluation

Location, time, and duration of pain (leg vs. axial back) are important factors in the evaluation of a patient with ASD. These patients may also have symptoms of spinal stenosis (central or radicular), which may require concomitant decompression. The patient's ability to perform activities of daily living and medical co-morbidities (e.g., cardiac, osteoporosis, etc.) need to be taken into consideration for treatment planning.

Some patients present with obvious spinal deformity (scoliosis, forward flexion at the waist, walking with knees bent).

As with neurogenic claudication, patients tend to be more symptomatic when up on their feet. A significant amount of pain may be generated by attempting to correct for spinal imbalance by using paraspinal muscles as well as retroverting the pelvis (rotating it backward at the hips) and not fully extending the knees. All this extra muscle activity is fatiguing and begins to produce muscle pain in the back and thighs. Patients with ASD tend to be better in the morning when they are rested.

Unlike lumbar spinal stenosis in the absence of scoliosis, symptoms may not be relieved by flexion at the waist.[2] There may be some relief when supporting the trunk with the arms.

82.4 Diagnostic testing

▶ **MRI.** A non-contrast lumbar MRI is recommended for the evaluation of symptomatic spondylosis and ASD to determine extent of neural compression (in the central canal as well as neural foramen). If MRI cannot be done, a CT/myelogram is usually required. May be limited to the lumbar spine for simple degenerative changes limited to that region, thoracic images should be added for major reconstructions or suspicion of thoracic involvement (e.g., myelopathy with thoracic sensory level to pinprick).

A contrast MRI is indicated if there are findings of possible neoplasm or infection on the unenhanced MRI, and is sometimes obtained in patients who have had previous surgery.

▶ **CT.** CT scan provides unparalleled bony detail which is important in determining if there are any fusions (spontaneous or surgical), vacuum discs (which imply hypermobility), calcifications (in herniated discs, ligamentum flavum…), and for obtaining measurements for surgical instrumentation. A plain CT is usually not necessary if a CT/myelogram has been done.

▶ **DEXA (dual-energy X-ray absorptiometry).** Patients should be evaluated for osteopenia/osteoporosis prior to surgical planning. Medical treatment may be beneficial in the perioperative period.

Some surgeons use teriparatide (Forteo®) (p.1211) (off label) for 3 months to quickly increase osteoporotic bone strength for surgery.

▶ **Standing scoliosis X-rays.** Recommended for the evaluation of scoliosis, but also used for global and regional spinal balance (CT & MRI, which are obtained supine, do not provide equivalent information). Pre- and postoperative standing scoliosis X-rays help confirm that alignment objectives are achieved.

Images acquired consist of:
1. lateral image. Technical requirements:
   - X-ray must visualize from C7 down to the femoral heads
   - the patient needs to try to keep their knees straight (extended)
   - arms folded in front of the chest (the patient should not lean or hold on to anything)
2. coronal views. In addition to the lateral view, coronal views required depend on the situation as follows:
   a) for adult degenerative spine disease: standing coronal view
   b) for adolescent idiopathic scoliosis (AIS): standing coronal, standing coronal left bending & right bending[9]
   c) for *adult idiopathic* scoliosis (AdIS): standing coronal plus *supine* coronal view[10]

NB: by convention, coronal scoliosis X-rays are reversed from typical X-rays to coincide with the surgeon's view from the back, with the result that the patient's left is on the left side of the X-ray.

82.5 SRS-Schwab classification of adult degenerative spinal deformity

Adult degenerative scoliosis has been classified by the Scoliosis Research Society (SRS)[11] based on its regional/global radiographic features (a modification of previously established adolescent King/Moe and Lenke classifications) and most recently by spino-pelvic parameters as it relates to health-related quality of life,[12,13,14] and is shown here. Values listed may need to be adjusted for age (p.1355).

- Coronal Curve types
  - T: Thoracic only (with lumbar curve < 30°)
  - L: Thoracolumbar/lumbar only (with thoracic curve < 30°)
  - D: Double curve (both T and T/L curves > 30°)
  - N: No major coronal deformity (all coronal curves < 30°)
- Sagittal Modifiers
  - Pelvic harmony (PI minus LL)
    - 0: non-pathologic (PI–LL < 10°)
    - +: moderate deformity (10° < PI–LL < 20°)
    - ++: marked deformity (PI–LL > 20°)

- ○ Global alignment (SVA)
  - – 0: non-pathologic (SVA < 4 cm)
  - – +: moderate deformity (4 cm < SVA < 9.5 cm)
  - – ++: marked deformity (SVA > 9.5 cm)
- ○ Pelvic Tilt (PT)
  - – 0: non-pathologic (PT < 20°)
  - – +: moderate deformity (20° < PT < 30°)
  - – ++: marked deformity (PT > 30°)

82.6 Treatment/management

82.6.1 Goals

To improve quality-of-life measures, by reducing neuropathic and axial pain and correcting debilitating deformities. The aim is to do so using techniques that are tailored to the specific situation (neither too much nor too little) in a manner that provides the longest duration of improvement that is appropriate.

82.6.2 Options

1. observation
2. focal decompression
3. surgical correction of deformity and instability: the choice of the following is dependent on the specific deformity, pain generators, and patient factors (age, bone density, weight...)
   a) traditional open surgery: includes laminectomy, PLIF, TLIF, pedicle screw/rod fixation. Better for osteotomies than MIS
   b) MIS (minimally invasive (spine) surgery): may reduce approach-related morbidities. Includes percutaneous pedicle screw/rod fixation, MIS-TLIF, MIS-PLIF, lateral interbody fusion (XLIF, DLIF, OLIF), anterior column release (ACR), interspinous spacers/fusion
   c) hybrid (MIS + open)

Treatment options are based on clinical symptoms (axial back pain ± radiculopathy vs. radiculopathy alone) and degree of abnormalities in sagittal balance (need for open osteotomies or anterior column release ACR). In scoliosis, neuropathic symptoms most often originate from foraminal compromise on the concavity of the curve, but can be seen on the convexity in the setting of facet hypertrophy and may improve with indirect decompression and correction in the coronal plane. Significant central stenosis (neurogenic claudication) may require concomitant direct decompression in addition to deformity correction.

82.6.3 Correction of global spinal balance

Indications for surgery:

- axial back pain ± neuropathic symptoms (deleterious to ADLs)
  - ○ abnormal SVA
  - ○ ± CSVL (central sacral vertical line) abnormality
  - ○ or derangement of spino-pelvic parameters
- patient age, co-morbidities (e.g osteopenia, diabetes...), and anesthetic risk must be taken into consideration and can limit correction goal and amount of surgery that is safe

Summary of spino-pelvic alignment objectives (for ages other than 50–60 years, see ▶ Table 82.1)

- LL = PI ± 9°
- PT < 20°
- SVA < 5 cm

Table 82.1 Examples of some recommended upper limits of alignment parameters adjusted by age[15]

Age (years)	SVA (cm)	PI - LL	PT
< 35	-4.1	-10.5°	10.9°
50–60	5	9°	20°
> 75	7.8	16.7°	28.5°

In most instances, sagittal imbalance is due to a shortfall of lumbar lordosis (LL) relative to the pelvic incidence (PI) (i.e., LL is more than 9° below PI), which is designated as flat back syndrome. Possible causes of abnormally low LL include:

- degenerative changes
- prior fusion with inadequate LL for the patient's PI (surgical flat back)
- pain from nerve compression which may cause the patient to retrovert the pelvis (which opens the lateral recesses and neuroforamina) which decreases the LL (compensatory flat back). This may correct (partially or completely) with decompression of the nerves even without fusion

Pelvic tilt > 20° suggests the patient is trying to compensate by retroverting the pelvis (some authors accept up to 25° as normal).

The minimum amount of correction that the surgeon tries to achieve is therefore the amount that LL needs to increase to bring it within 9° of PI, and typically also adds in the amount that the patient is compensating (i.e., the amount that PT is greater than 20°), which yields the following approximation (applies when LL is more than 9° lower than PI, and PT is greater than 20°); see Eq (82.1):

$$\text{Increase in LL needed} \approx (PI - LL - 9°) + (PT - 20°) \tag{82.1}$$

▶ **Changes in sagittal balance with age.** Spino-pelvic alignment parameters that are widely quoted are valid for the age range of the majority of surgical patients with ASD (50–60 years) but are less representative of younger and especially older patients. It has been said that, "Aging is a kyphosing process." Higher HQOL scores in elderly individuals are associated with less lumbar lordosis and increased compensatory pelvic tilt.[15] There is a real risk that trying to achieve the same parameters in an elderly individual as for a younger person will result in "overcorrection." The ideal parameters are not known with certainty; some recommendations[15] are shown in ▶ Table 82.1.

▶ **Correcting thoracic hyperkyphosis.** The maximum measured kyphosis is the Cobb angle from the superior endplate of the proximal end-vertebra to the inferior endplate of the distal end-vertebra where an "*end vertebra*" is defined as the VB that is the most tilted from the horizontal apical vertebra. The stopping points for instrumentation are a point of controversy. In general:

1. the upper level of the fusion usually includes the proximal end vertebra[16]
2. to minimize the risk of distal junctional kyphosis (DJK), Lenke recommends that the distal stopping point for a construct when correcting thoracic hyperkyphosis is the *sagittal stable vertebra* (SSV) (▶ Fig. 82.1).[16] The SSV is the most proximal lumbar vertebral body substantially touched by the posterior sacral vertical line (PSVL), a vertical line drawn from the posterior-superior corner of the sacrum (some suggest that at least 50% of the VB should be in front of the PSVL to qualify as SSV[17]). This is in opposition to other paradigms that include: stopping at L1, or the first lordotic disc (the most proximal lumbar disc with endplates that converge posteriorly), or the distal end vertebra (which can be misidentified).

▶ **Coronal balance.** Measured on AP standing scoliosis X-ray. A "plumb line" is drawn straight down from the center of the C7 VB. If it falls > 4 cm from the midline of the sacrum (where the CSVL [▶ Table 79.1] is located), there is coronal imbalance (positive if the plumb line falls to the right of the CSVL, negative to the left).

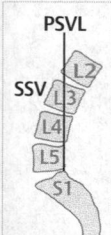

Fig. 82.1 PSVL & SSV.
The posterior sacral vertical line (PSVL) is drawn straight up from the posterior-superior sacrum. The sagittal stable vertebra (SSV) is the most proximal VB that the PSVL touches. In this figure, L3 is the SSV.

82.6.4 Classification of surgical osteotomies

Osteotomies are increasingly employed in surgery for spinal deformity correction as well as for other operations, e.g., spinal tumor excision. In an effort to standardize the nomenclature, Schwab et al[18] proposed the classification system shown in ▶ Table 82.2.

Table 82.2 Classification of surgical spinal osteotomies*[18]

Schwab grade & diagram	Description
1	resection of inferior facet and joint capsule. Requires mobile (non-fused) anterior column. Limited deformity correction (5–10°). AKA: Smith-Petersen osteotomy or opening wedge (with previously fused facets), chevron or extension osteotomy (with unfused facets).
2	resection of inferior and superior facets, ligamentum flavum, and possibly lamina, spinous process. Requires mobile (non-fused) anterior column. AKA: Ponte osteotomy.
3	partial wedge resection of the VB and the posterior elements with pedicles. 25–30° of correction at any given level. AKA: pedicle subtraction osteotomy (PSO), closing wedge osteotomy, transpedicular wedge resection.
4	a grade 3 plus inclusion of at least a portion of the endplate and 1 adjacent disc.

(continued)

Table 82.2 continued

Schwab grade & diagram	Description
5	complete removal of the vertebra and both adjacent discs (and rib resection in the thoracic region). AKA: vertebral column resection (VCR).
6	a grade 5 resection extended over multiple vertebral levels.

*modified with permission from Schwab F, Blondel B, Chay E, et al. The comprehensive anatomical spinal osteotomy classification. Neurosurgery 2014;74(1):112–20; discussion 120.

In addition to the posterior surgical component, Grades 2–6 may be supplemented with anterior work as well. Grades 5 & 6 are most commonly employed in the thoracic spine.

82.6.5 Surgical options for increasing lumbar lordosis

Various surgical techniques may be used to increase the lumbar lordosis to bring it within the desired specifications. If necessary, these techniques can be combined with procedures to decompress the neural elements (e.g., laminectomy). NB: in the normal spine, up to 30° of the total lumbar lordosis is made up by the combination of lordosis at L4–5 + L5–1; creating excessive lordosis at the upper lumbar levels to increase LL may be undesirable. A comparison of the approximate amount of lordosis that can be achieved with different techniques is shown in ▶ Table 82.3.

▶ **Transforaminal lumbar interbody fusion (TLIF) and posterior lumbar interbody fusion (PLIF).** Traditional operation. May be done open or MIS.

▶ **Lateral lumbar interbody fusion (LLIF).** e.g., XLIF™, DLIF™, OLIF™. Approach through psoas muscle (XLIF, DLIF) or anterior to psoas muscle (OLIF) through a lateral or anterolateral approach. Can distract the vertebral bodies by increasing the height of the disc space and thereby indirectly decompressing the neural elements. If bone quality is good, and there is no instability nor spondylolisthesis > Grade I, a stand-alone procedure (i.e., without screw instrumentation) may be an option if cage width of at least 22 mm in the AP dimension is used.

Table 82.3 Comparison of the amount of lumbar lordosis that can be obtained from various surgical techniques

Technique	Degrees of lumbar lordosis
TLIF/PLIF	<0 (i.e., kyphosis) up to 2°[19]
LLIF	1°[20]
ALIF	6°[19]
Schwab Grade 1 osteotomy (SPO)	5–10°[21]
Schwab Grade 1 osteotomy + ACR	16°[22]
Schwab Grade 3 osteotomy (PSO)	30–40°[22,23]

Abbreviations: TLIF = transforaminal lumbar interbody fusion; PLIF = posterior lumbar interbody fusion; LLIF = lateral lumbar interbody fusion; ALIF = anterior lumbar interbody fusion; SPO = Smith-Petersen osteotomy; ACR = anterior column release; PSO = pedicle subtraction osteotomy. For Schwab grading of osteotomies, see ▶ Table 82.2

▶ **Anterior column reconstruction (ACR).** AKA ALL release (ALLR). Involves division of the anterior longitudinal ligament (ALL) typically with placement of a "hyperlordotic" cage (20–30° lordosis) from an anterior or lateral approach. This is followed by posterior fixation, often combined with a Schwab Grade 1 or 2 osteotomy (especially for 30° cages) and posterior compression. It can increase LL up to 12° per ACR level and, depending on the level at which it is performed, improvement of SVA up to 3 cm.[22,24]

Risk of injury to great vessels, either directly (when cutting the ALL) or indirectly by elongating the anterior column. It is critical to evaluate the great vessels on axial MRI or CT or on angiogram and not to do the procedure if the vessels appear tightly approximated to the bodies or to osteophytes at that level.

▶ **Schwab Grade 2 osteotomy.** (▶ Fig. 82.2 **B**) can increase lordosis up to 10–12° per level. Involves removal of bilateral superior and inferior facets along with the ligamentum flavum and a portion of the lamina above and below. The created gap is then closed with compression of the posterior elements to give lordosis (resecting posterior elements and using the middle column as a fulcrum to elongate the anterior column).[25,26] Approximation: LL is increased 1° for every 1 mm of bone resected.[21,25]

The "Ponte procedure" consists of removal of multiple facets and was originally described for treating Scheuermann's kyphoscoliosis (p. 1374).[27]

▶ **Schwab Grade 3 osteotomy.** (▶ Fig. 82.2 **A**) AKA pedicle subtraction osteotomy (PSO). Involves removal of the posterior elements, including the ligmanetum flavum, lamina, and facets, widely followed by isolation and resection of pedicles bilaterally and wedge-shaped removal of the vertebral body just barely up to the ventral cortex. The created gap is then closed by compression of the posterior elements and subsequent greenstick fracture of the isolated ventral cortex.[23] Can increase LL by 30°–40° per level, improvement of SVA 5.5–13 cm per level.[22,23] A spine "shortening" procedure.

Technically challenging, often associated with high blood loss (average 3 L[28]) and increased risk of complications (including proximal junctional kyphosis (PJK) in 23%[28]) compared to a Grade 2 osteotomy. Generally reserved for spines that have previously been fused where it is not possible to get the amount of lordosis needed from the unfused levels.

Uses the anterior column as a fulcrum. Usually limited to levels *below* the conus medullaris (i.e., below L1–2) due to potential compression by inward buckling of the dura (L3 is the most common level). Intraoperative electrophysiologic monitoring is highly recommended. Relative contraindication: poor bone quality.

▶ **Anterior lumbar interbody fusion (ALIF).** Best for L5–S1 (where the great vessels tend not to interfere with the access, and where every degree of correction produces a more significant amount of improvement in SVA than at other levels as a result of being at the lowest point in the spine).

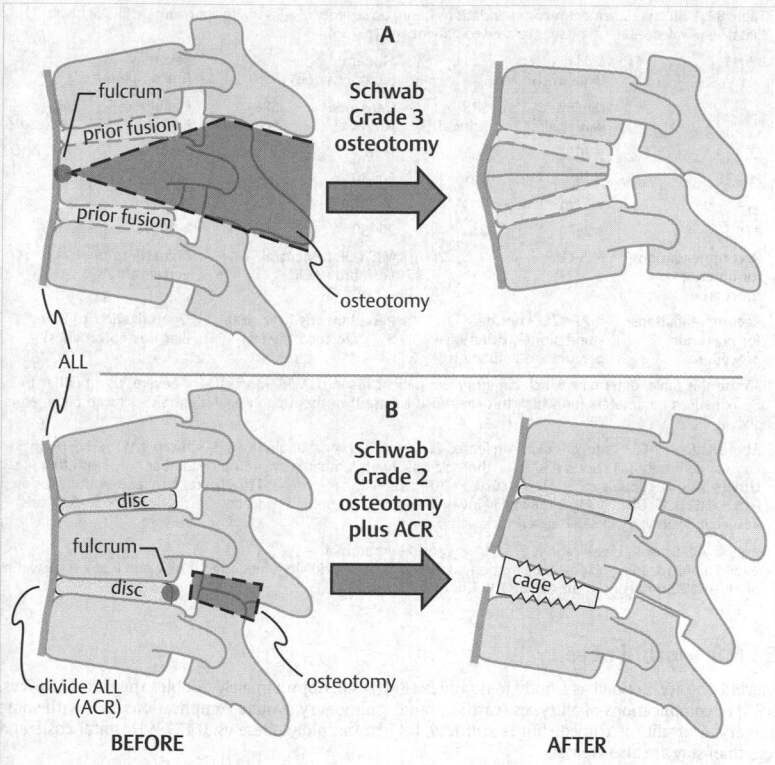

Fig. 82.2 Illustration of increasing lordosis via A: Schwab Grade 3 osteotomy (pedicle subtraction osteotomy) vs. B: a Grade 2 osteotomy (Ponte osteotomy) plus ACR.
Abbreviations: ACR = anterior column release; ALL = anterior longitudinal ligament.

82.6.6 Guidelines for MIS treatment for ASD

A simple algorithm for MIS management of sagittal imbalance based on spino-pelvic parameters and the approximate SRS-Schwab class is shown in ▶ Table 82.4.[29] See references[30,31] for a more detailed protocol.

82.6.7 Currently under investigation

When, and to what degree, does improvement in sagittal balance occur with simple decompression (possibly with a minimal fusion) as a result of the patient being able to stand up straighter with less pain?

Table 82.4 MIS management recommendations based on severity of ASD[29] with approximate SRS-Schwab Class[12] equivalence. See for issues related to patient age (p. 1355)

	Mild (balanced)		Moderate (compensated)		Severe (uncompensated)	
	Deukmedjian et al[29]	SRS-Schwab[12]	Deukmedjian et al[29]	SRS-Schwab[12]	Deukmedjian et al[29]	SRS-Schwab[12]
CCA	<30°	N	>30°	T, L, or D	>30°	T, L, or D
PI – LL	<20°	0 or +	20–30°	+ +	>30°	+ +
SVA	<5 cm	0	5–9 cm	+	>10 cm	+ +
PT[a]	<25°	0	25–30°	+	>30°	+ +
Recommendations for anterior procedure	MIS-LLIF		MIS-LLIF to neutral vertebra + ACR		MIS-LLIF to neutral vertebra ± ACR	
Recommendations for posterior procedure	If PT < 20° consider stand-alone[b], otherwise percutaneous fixation		Percutaneous fixation to S1 ± facetectomy(ies)		Open fixation to S2 or iliac + osteotomy(ies)	

To use this table, determine which category the patient fits into (Mild, Moderate, or Severe) using either the Deukmedjian parameters (on which this reference is based) or the roughly equivalent SRS-Schwab parameters shown

Abbreviations: ACR = anterior column release; CCA = Cobb coronal angle (for SRS-Schwab system, N = no major coronal deformity [all curves < 30°]; T = thoracic only [with lumbar curve < 30°]; L = lumbar only [with thoracic curve < 30°]; D = double curve [T & L curves > 30°]); LL = lumbar lordosis; LLIF = lateral lumbar interbody fusion (e.g., XLIF, DLIF, OLIF...); MIS = minimally invasive surgery; PI = pelvic incidence; PT = pelvic tilt; SRS = Scoliosis Research Society; SVA = sagittal vertical axis.

[a]in the SRS-Schwab classification, PT < 20° is considered normal
[b]stand-alone meaning no posterior fixation, assumes that bone quality is not osteoporotic and that a cage width of at least 22 mm is used (to reduce the risk of subsidence)

82.6.8 Morbid obesity

Morbid obesity, defined as a body mass index (BMI) > 40. Approximately doubles the risks (13.6% vs. 6.9%) of complications of all types (cardiac, renal, pulmonary, wound complications...)[32] with spine surgery. Mortality is tripled (but is still low, 0.41 in morbidly obese vs. 0.13).[32] Hospital costs and length of stay are also greater.

References

[1] Cobb JR. Outline for study of scoliosis. American Academy of Orthopedic Surgery. 1948; 5:261–275
[2] Silva FE, Lenke LG. Adult degenerative scoliosis: evaluation and management. Neurosurgical Focus. 2010; 28. DOI: 10.3171/2010.1.FOCUS09271
[3] Wiet RJ, Wiet RJ, Glasscock ME, et al. Dissection Manual. In: Surgical Anatomy of the Temporal Bone Through Dissection. Philadelphia: W.B. Saunders; 1980:677–725
[4] Pritchett JW, Bortel DT. Degenerative symptomatic lumbar scoliosis. Spine (Phila Pa 1976). 1993; 18:700–703
[5] Faldini C, Di Martino A, De Fine M, et al. Current classification systems for adult degenerative scoliosis. Musculoskelet Surg. 2013; 97:1–8
[6] Nash CL,Jr, Moe JH. A study of vertebral rotation. Journal of Bone and Joint Surgery. 1969; 51:223–229
[7] Drazin D, Shirzadi A, Rosner J, et al. Complications and outcomes after spinal deformity surgery in the elderly: review of the existing literature and future directions. Neurosurg Focus. 2011; 31. DOI: 10.3171/2011.7.FOCUS11145
[8] Schwab F, Dubey A, Gamez L, et al. Adult scoliosis: prevalence, SF-36, and nutritional parameters in an elderly volunteer population. Spine (Phila Pa 1976). 2005; 30:1082–1085
[9] Lenke LG, Betz RR, Harms J, et al. Adolescent idiopathic scoliosis: a new classification to determine extent of spinal arthrodesis. J Bone Joint Surg Am. 2001; 83:1169–1181

[10] Lin JD, Osorio JA, Baum GR, et al. A new modular radiographic classification of adult idiopathic scoliosis as an extension of the Lenke classification of adolescent idiopathic scoliosis. Spine Deform. 2020. DOI: 10.1007/s43390-020-00181-7
[11] Lowe T, Berven SH, Schwab FJ, et al. The SRS classification for adult spinal deformity: building on the King/Moe and Lenke classification systems. Spine (Phila Pa 1976). 2006; 31:S119–S125
[12] Schwab F, Ungar B, Blondel B, et al. Scoliosis Research Society-Schwab adult spinal deformity classification: a validation study. Spine (Phila Pa 1976). 2012; 37:1077–1082
[13] Liu Y, Liu Z, Zhu F, et al. Validation and reliability analysis of the new SRS-Schwab classification for adult spinal deformity. Spine (Phila Pa 1976). 2013; 38:902–908
[14] Ames CP, Smith JS, Scheer JK, et al. Impact of spinopelvic alignment on decision making in deformity surgery in adults: A review. J Neurosurg Spine. 2012; 16:547–564
[15] Lafage R, Schwab F, Challier V, et al. Defining Spino-Pelvic Alignment Thresholds: Should Operative Goals in Adult Spinal Deformity Surgery Account for Age? Spine (Phila Pa 1976). 2016; 41:62–68
[16] Cho KJ, Lenke LG, Bridwell KH, et al. Selection of the optimal distal fusion level in posterior instrumentation and fusion for thoracic hyperkyphosis: the sagittal stable vertebra concept. Spine (Phila Pa 1976). 2009; 34:765–770

[17] Yang J, Andras LM, Broom AM, et al. Preventing distal junctional kyphosis by applying the stable sagittal vertebra concept to selective thoracic fusion in adolescent idiopathic scoliosis. Spine Deform. 2018; 6:38–42

[18] Schwab F, Blondel B, Chay E, et al. The comprehensive anatomical spinal osteotomy classification. Neurosurgery. 2014; 74:112–20; discussion 120

[19] Hsieh PC, Koski TR, O'Shaughnessy B A, et al. Anterior lumbar interbody fusion in comparison with transforaminal lumbar interbody fusion: implications for the restoration of foraminal height, local disc angle, lumbar lordosis, and sagittal balance. J Neurosurg Spine. 2007; 7:379–386

[20] Le TV, Vivas AC, Dakwar E, et al. The effect of the retroperitoneal transpsoas minimally invasive lateral interbody fusion on segmental and regional lumbar lordosis. ScientificWorldJournal. 2012; 2012. DOI: 10.1100/2012/516706

[21] Smith-Petersen M N, Larson CB, Aufranc OE. Osteotomy of the spine for correction of flexion deformity in rheumatoid arthritis. Clin Orthop Relat Res. 1969; 66:6–9

[22] Manwaring JC, Bach K, Ahmadian AA, et al. Management of sagittal balance in adult spinal deformity with minimally invasive anterolateral lumbar interbody fusion: a preliminary radiographic study. J Neurosurg Spine. 2014; 20:515–522

[23] Mummaneni PV, Dhall SS, Ondra SL, et al. Pedicle subtraction osteotomy. Neurosurgery. 2008; 63:171–176

[24] Deukmedjian AR, Dakwar E, Ahmadian A, et al. Early outcomes of minimally invasive anterior longitudinal ligament release for correction of sagittal imbalance in patients with adult spinal deformity. ScientificWorldJournal. 2012; 2012. DOI: 10.1100/2 012/789698

[25] Cho KJ, Bridwell KH, Lenke LG, et al. Comparison of Smith-Petersen versus pedicle subtraction osteotomy for the correction of fixed sagittal imbalance. Spine (Phila Pa 1976). 2005; 30:2030–7; discussion 2038

[26] La Marca F, Brumblay H. Smith-Petersen osteotomy in thoracolumbar deformity surgery. Neurosurgery. 2008; 63:163–170

[27] Geck MJ, Macagno A, Ponte A, et al. The Ponte procedure: posterior only treatment of Scheuermann's kyphosis using segmental posterior shortening and pedicle screw instrumentation. J Spinal Disord Tech. 2007; 20:586–593

[28] Hyun SJ, Rhim SC. Clinical outcomes and complications after pedicle subtraction osteotomy for fixed sagittal imbalance patients: a long-term follow-up data. J Korean Neurosurg Soc. 2010; 47:95–101

[29] Deukmedjian AR, Ahmadian A, Bach K, et al. Minimally invasive lateral approach for adult degenerative scoliosis: lessons learned. Neurosurg Focus. 2013; 35. DOI: 10.3171/2013.5.FOCUS13173

[30] Haque RM, Mundis GM,Jr, Ahmed Y, et al. Comparison of radiographic results after minimally invasive, hybrid, and open surgery for adult spinal deformity: a multicenter study of 184 patients. Neurosurg Focus. 2014; 36. DOI: 10.3171/2014.3.FOCUS1424

[31] Mummaneni PV, Shaffrey CI, Lenke LG, et al. The minimally invasive spinal deformity surgery algorithm: a reproducible rational framework for decision making in minimally invasive spinal deformity surgery. Neurosurg Focus. 2014; 36. DOI: 10.3171/2 014.3.FOCUS1413

[32] Kalanithi PA, Arrigo R, Boakye M. Morbid obesity increases cost and complication rates in spinal arthrodesis. Spine (Phila Pa 1976). 2012; 37:982–988

82

83 Special Conditions Affecting the Spine

83.1 Paget's disease of the spine

83.1.1 Pathophysiology

Paget's disease (PD) (AKA osteitis deformans) is a disorder of osteoclasts (possibly virally induced) causing increased rate of bone resorption with reactive osteoblastic overproduction of new, weaker, woven bone, producing characteristic "mosaic pattern."

Initially there is a "hot" phase with elevated osteoclastic activity and increased intraosseous vascularity. Osteoblasts lay down a soft, nonlamellar bone. Later a "cool" phase occurs with disappearance of the vascular stroma and osteoblastic activity leaving sclerotic, radiodense, brittle bone[1] ("ivory bone").

83.1.2 Malignant degeneration

A misnomer, since the malignant changes actually occur in the reactive osteoblastic cells. About 1% (reported range: 1–14%) degenerate into sarcoma (osteogenic sarcoma, fibrous sarcoma, or chondrosarcoma),[2 (p 2642)] with the possibility of systemic (e.g., pulmonary) metastases. Malignant degeneration is much less common in the spine than in the skull or femur.

83.1.3 Epidemiology

Prevalence: ≈ 3% of population > 55 years old in the U.S. and Europe, much lower in Asia.[3] Slight male predominance. Family history of Paget's disease is found in 15–30% of cases (accuracy is poor since most are asymptomatic).

83.1.4 Common sites of involvement

Affinity for axial skeleton, long bones, and skull. In approximate descending order of frequency: pelvis, thoracic and lumbar spine, skull, femur, tibia, fibula, and clavicles.

83.1.5 Neurosurgical involvement

PD may present to the neurosurgeon as a result of:
1. back pain: usually not as a direct result of vertebral bone involvement (see below)
2. spinal cord and/or nerve root symptoms
   a) compression of the spinal cord or cauda equina (relatively rare)
   b) spinal nerve root compression
   c) vascular steal due to reactive vasodilatation adjacent to involved areas
3. with skull involvement:
   a) compression of cranial nerves as they exit through bony foramina: 8th nerve is most common producing deafness or ataxia (p. 1688)
   b) skull base involvement → basilar invagination
4. to ascertain diagnosis in unclear bone lesions of the spine or skull

83.1.6 Presentation

General information

Only ≈ 30% of pagetic sites are symptomatic,[4] the rest are discovered incidentally. The overproduction of weak bone may produce bone pain (the most common symptom), predilection for fracture and compressive syndromes: cranial nerve (p. 1688), spinal nerve root... Painless bowing of a long bone may be the first manifestation. A number of patients present due to pain from joint dysfunction related to PD.

The overwhelming majority of pagetic lesions are asymptomatic[5 (p 1413)] with lesions detected on radiographs or bone scan obtained for other reasons or as part of a work-up for an elevated alkaline phosphatase. Although the most common complaint in patients with Paget's disease is of back pain, this is attributable to pagetic involvement alone in only ≈ 12%[6]; in the remainder it is secondary to other factors, some of which are described below.

Symptoms that may be related to Paget's disease itself

Symptoms from the following are slowly progressive (usually present for > 12 mos; rarely < 6 mos):
1. neural compression
   a) causes of compression
      * due to expansion of woven bone
      * due to osteoid tissue
      * pagetic extension into ligamentum flavum and epidural fat[7]
   b) sites of compression
      * spinal cord (see below)
      * nerve root in neural foramen
2. osteoarthritis of facet joints (Paget's disease may precipitate osteoarthritis[6])

Symptoms from the following tend to progress more rapidly:
1. malignant (sarcomatous) change of involved bone (rare, see above)
2. pathologic fracture (pain usually sudden in onset)
3. neurovascular (compromise of vascular supply to nerves or spinal cord) by
   a) compression of blood vessels (arterial or venous)
   b) pagetic vascular steal (see below)

Spinal cord symptoms

Myelopathy or cauda equina syndrome may be due to spinal cord compression or from vascular effects (occlusion, or "steal" due to reactive vasodilatation of nearby blood vessels[5(p 1415)]). Only ≈ 100 cases had been described as of 1981.[8] Characteristically, 3–5 adjacent vertebrae are involved,[9(p 2307)] whereas monostotic involvement is usually asymptomatic.[10] In case reports in the literature, progressive quadri- or paraparesis was the most common presentation.[11] Sensory changes are usually the first manifestation, progressing to weakness and sphincter disturbance. Pain was the only symptom in a neurologically intact patient in only 5.5%.

A rapid course (averaging 6 wks) with a sudden increase in pain is more suggestive of malignant degeneration.

83.1.7 Evaluation

1. lab work (serum markers may be normal in monostotic involvement):
   a) serum alkaline phosphatase: usually elevated (this enzyme is involved in bone synthesis and so may *not* be elevated in purely lytic Paget's disease[5(p 1416)]); mean 380 ± 318 IU/L (normal range: 9–44).[6] Bone-specific alkaline phosphatase may be more sensitive and may be useful in monostotic involvement[3]
   b) calcium: usually normal (if elevated, one should R/O hyperparathyroidism)
   c) urinary hydroxyproline: hydroxyproline is found almost exclusively in cartilage. Due to the high turnover of bone, urinary hydroxyproline is often increased in PD with a mean of 280 ± 262 mg/24 hrs (normal range 18–38)[6]
2. bone scan: lights up in areas of involvement in most, but not all[6] cases
3. plain X-rays:
   a) localized enlargement of bone: a finding unique to PD (not seen in other osteoclastic diseases, such as prostatic bone mets)
   b) cortical thickening
   c) sclerotic changes
   d) osteolytic areas (in skull → osteoporosis circumscripta; in long bones → "V" shaped lesions)
   e) spinal Paget's disease often involves *several contiguous levels*. Pedicles and lamina are thickened, vertebral bodies are usually dense and compressed with increased width. Intervening discs are replaced by bone
4. CT: hypertrophic changes at the facet joints with coarse trabeculations

83.1.8 Treatment

Medical treatment for Paget's disease

General information

There is no cure for Paget's disease. Medical treatment is indicated for cases that are not rapidly progressive where the diagnosis is certain, for patients who are poor surgical candidates, and pre-op if excessive bleeding cannot be tolerated. Medical therapy reverses some neurologic deficit in 50% of cases,[12] but generally requires prolonged treatment ($\approx$ 6–8 months) before improvement occurs, and may need to be continued indefinitely due to propensity for relapses. Medications used include the following.

Calcitonin derivatives

Parenteral salmon calcitonin (Calcimar®)[12]: reduces osteoclastic activity directly, osteoblastic hyperactivity subsides secondarily. Relapse may occur even while on calcitonin. Side effects include nausea, facial flushing, and the development of antibodies to salmon calcitonin (these patients may benefit from a more expensive synthetic human preparation (Cibacalcin®) starting at 0.5 mg SQ q d[13]).

℞ 50–100 IU (medical research council units) SQ q d × 1 month, then 3 injections per week for several months.[3] If used pre-op to help decrease bony vascularity, $\approx$ 6 months of treatment is ideal. Doses as low as $\approx$ 50 IU 3 × per week may be used indefinitely post-op or as a sole treatment (alkaline phosphatase and urinary hydroxyproline decline by 30–50% in > half of patients in 3–6 months, but they rarely normalize).

Bisphosphonates

These drugs are pyrophosphate analogues that bind to hydroxyapatite crystals and inhibit reabsorption. They also alter osteoclastic metabolism, inhibit their activity, and reduce their numbers. They are retained in bone until it is resorbed. Oral absorption of all is poor (especially in the presence of food). Bone formed during treatment is lamellar rather than woven.

Etidronate (Didronel®) (AKA EHDP): reduces normal bone mineralization (especially at doses ≥ 20 mg/kg/d), producing mineralization defects (osteomalacia) which may increase the risk of fracture but which tend to heal between courses.[14] Contraindicated in patients with renal failure, osteomalacia, or severe lytic lesions of an LE. ℞ 5–10 mg/kg PO daily (average dose: 400 mg/d, or 200–300 mg/d in frail elderly patients) for 6 months, may be repeated after a 3–6 month hiatus if biochemical markers indicate relapse.

Tiludronate (Skelid®): unlike etidronate, does not appear to interfere with bone mineralization at recommended doses. Side effects: abdominal pain, diarrhea, N/V. ℞ 400 mg PO qd with 6–8 ounces of plain water > 2 hrs before or after eating × 3 months. Available: 200 mg tablets.

Pamidronate (Aredia®): much more potent than etidronate. May cause a transient acute flu-like syndrome. Oral dosing is hindered by GI intolerance, and IV forms may be required. Mineralization defects do not occur in doses < 180 mg/course. ℞ 90 mg/d IV × 3 days, or as weekly or monthly infusions.

Alendronate (Fosamax®): does not produce mineralization defects (p. 1212).

Clodronate (Ostac®, Bonefos®): ℞ 400–1600 mg/d PO × 3–6 months. 300 mg/d IV × 5 days (may be available outside the U.S.).

Risedronate (Actonel®): does not interfere with bone mineralization in recommended doses.[1] ℞: 30 mg PO q d with 6–8 oz. of water at least 30 minutes before the first meal of the day.

Surgical treatment

General information

In general, conservative treatment of fractures in PD are associated with a high rate of delayed union.

Surgical indications for spinal Paget's disease

1. rapid progression: indicating possible malignant change or spinal instability
2. spinal instability: severe kyphosis or compromise of canal by bone fragments from pathologic fracture. Although the collapse is usually gradual, sudden compression may occur
3. uncertain diagnosis: especially to R/O metastatic disease (osteoblastic lesions)
4. failure to improve with medications

Surgical considerations

1. profuse bleeding is common: if significant bleeding would present an unusual problem, treat for as long as feasible pre-op with a bisphosphonate or calcitonin (see above)
   a) use bone wax to help control bleeding
   b) hemostasis may be difficult

2. to treat resultant spinal stenosis: decompressive laminectomy is the standard procedure in the thoracic region.[11] However, if most of the pathology is anterior, consideration should be given to anterior approach
3. bone is often thickened, and may be fused with obliteration of interspace landmarks. A high-speed drill is usually helpful
4. post-op medical treatment may be necessary to prevent recurrences[12]
5. osteogenic sarcoma
   a) surgery and chemotherapy are used, cure is less likely than in primary osteosarcoma of non-pagetic origin
   b) biopsy proven of the scalp requires en-bloc excision of scalp and tumor

Surgical outcome

See reference.[11]

In 65 patients treated with decompressive laminectomy, 55 (85%) had definite but variable degrees of improvement. Patients who had only minimal improvement were often ones with malignant changes. One patient was worse after surgery, and the operative mortality was 7 patients (10%). Survival with malignant degeneration is < 5.5 mos after admission.

83.2 Ankylosing and ossifying conditions of the spine

83.2.1 Ankylosing spondylitis

General information

Key concepts

- prototypical spondyloarthritidy, now referred to as radiographic axial spondyloarthritis
- seronegative (absence of rheumatoid factor), associated with HLA-B27
- begins in SI joints (sine qua non of involvement) progressing rostrally
- clinical: morning back stiffness, kyphotic deformity, limited chest expansion
- X-ray findings: "bamboo spine," Andersson lesions, progressive thoracic kyphosis
- fragile rigid spine highly susceptible to fracture and SCI even after low-energy trauma
- surgical indications: severe deformity, neurologic involvement or unstable fracture

Historically known as Marie-Strümpell disease and Bechterew disease, ankylosing spondylitis (AS) is an HLA-B27–associated inflammatory disease and the prototype of a group of diseases known as the spondyloarthrithides (SpA). Common features are inflammatory back pain, negative serology for rheumatoid factor and absence of rheumatoid nodules, and asymmetric oligoarthritis predominantly of lower extremities. Currently referred to in the literature as Radiographic axial Spondyloarthritis (RaxSpA), AS is believed to be the late stage of a single disease entity, with axial Spondyloarthritis (axSpA) distinguished by definitive evidence of sacroiliitis on plain radiographs. Other conditions under this rubric include: psoriatic arthropathy, Reiter's disease, juvenile spondyloarthropathy... AS has in the past also been known as rheumatoid spondylitis, or rheumatoid arthritis of the spine, but use of these terms is discouraged because of the lack of rheumatoid factor. The spine is the primary skeletal site involved, usually starting in the sacroiliac joints and lumbar spine and progressing rostrally.

Enthesopathy: nongranulomatous inflammatory changes at the entheses (attachment points of ligaments, tendons, or capsules on bones; the locus of involvement in AS) stimulates replacement of ligaments by bone, ultimately resulting in osteoporotic VBs, calcified intervertebral discs (sparing the nucleus pulposus), and ossified ligaments, producing square-appearing VBs with bridging syndesmophytes, the so-called "bamboo spine" or "poker spine" (▶ Fig. 83.1). Extra-articular manifestations (EAMs) include: anterior uveitis, inflammatory bowel disease (IBD), and psoriasis.

Neurosurgical involvement usually results from the following:

1. cauda equina syndrome (**CES-AS**) : the etiology of CES in AS is frequently unclear, but is usually *not* due to stenosis or compressive lesion. Onset is slow and insidious and there is a high incidence of dural ectasia.[16] Any patient with AS and neurologic deficit should be assumed to have CES until proven otherwise. Without treatment most patients' neurological status continues to deteriorate[16]

83

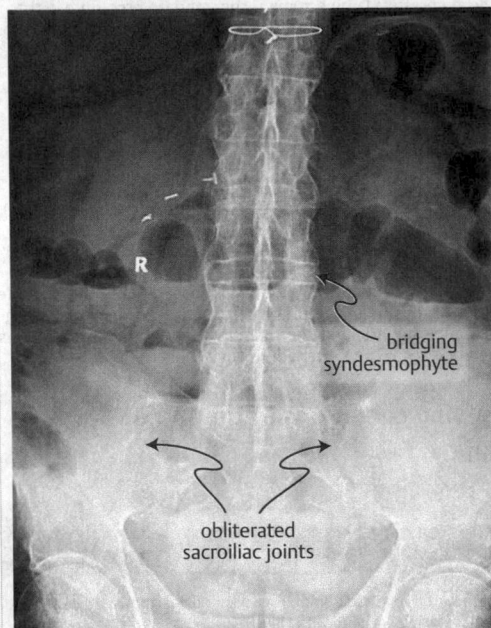

Fig. 83.1 AP lumbar/pelvic X-ray in patient with ankylosing spondylitis demonstrating "Bamboo spine" (bridging syndesmophytes) and sclerosing obliteration of sacroiliac joints.

2. rotatory subluxation: at occipitoatlantal and atlantoaxial joints. May occur as these are typically the last mobile segments of the spine. Incidence is much less than with rheumatoid arthritis
3. myelopathy secondary to bow-stringing of the cord: laminectomy may aggravate this
4. acute spinal cord injury (**SCI**): risk of SCI or CES due to fracture is increased in AS. The ankylosed spine may fracture even following minimal trauma, and this creates long lever arms that can be very unstable compared to the same fracture in a normal spine.[17] Injuries are more common in the lower cervical spine. Delayed deterioration may be due to spinal epidural hematoma[18]
5. Andersson lesion: discovertebral lesion that results from inflammation or fracture, mechanical stresses prevent lesion from fusion resulting in pseudarthrosis[19]
6. spinal deformity: classically progressive kyphotic deformity
7. spinal stenosis: rare
8. basilar impression

Epidemiology

Incidence in the general population is ≈ 0.44–7.3 cases per 100,000.[20] Traditionally reported male female ratio 3:1; however, this may stem from underdiagnosis in women, and more rapid progression of spinal ankylosis in men.[20] Peak incidence: 17–35 yrs of age. More than 90% of patients with AS are HLA-B27–positive (only 8% of people without AS have this antigen), but only 2% of people with HLA-B27 develop clinical AS. Although AS is not hereditary, first-degree relatives are at increased risk.

Clinical

▶ **Symptoms.** Typical initial presentation is with nonradiating low back pain, morning back stiffness, hip pain and swelling (due to large joint arthritis), exacerbated by inactivity and improved with exercise.[21]

▶ **Signs.** Patrick's test (p.1252) is usually positive. Compressing the pelvis with the patient in the lateral decubitus position produces pain.

Schober test (measure distraction between skin marks on the back before and after forward flexion to detect reduced mobility of the spine due to fusion). Is not specific for inflammatory spondylopathies[22] but may be helpful for monitoring ongoing physical therapy.

Diagnosis

Diagnosis by an experienced rheumatologist is the closest thing to a gold standard.[23] The Assessment of SpondyloArthritis International Society (ASAS) recently presented its recommendations for a modified Berlin Algorithm[23] as a potentially useful tool for rheumatologists in diagnosing AS. SI joint involvement is the sine qua non for definite diagnosis. Diagnosis is very involved, and includes: chronic low back pain, buttock pain, sacroiliitis, family history, psoriasis, an inflammatory bowel disease or an arthritis followed in ≤ 1 month with urethritis, cervicitis or acute diarrhea, an enthesopathy, and a family history, and positive X-rays.

The (obsolete) New York Criteria was an early attempt to establish diagnostic benchmarks, and is shown here (▶ Table 83.1) to provide an insight into some of the findings, but should no longer be used for definitive diagnosis.

Table 83.1 Modified New York Criteria for AS[24]—not to be used for diagnosis (obsolete)

Diagnosis (see criteria below)
Definite AS: radiologic criterion + ≥ 1 clinical criterion
Probable AS: radiological criteria without clinical criteria, or 3 clinical criteria without radiological criteria
Clinical criteria
low back pain > 3 months, improved by exercise, not relieved by rest
limitation of lumbar spine motion in both sagittal and frontal planes
limitation of chest expansion relative to normal values for age and sex
Radiological criterion
sacroiliitis

Radiographic evaluation

Plain X-rays. Vital for diagnosis and follow-up. Sacroiliac (SI) joint involvement (on AP pelvic X-rays or on oblique views through the plane of the SI joints) is one of the earliest findings, and the often symmetric osteoporosis followed by sclerosis is characteristic. Bridging syndesmophytes between VBs creates the so-called "Bamboo spine" appearance (see above) which is also classic (▶ Fig. 83.1). X-ray of the entire spine is recommended since multiple, non-contiguous (and often unsuspected) fractures are not unusual.

CT. Useful for diagnosis of cervical fracture not apparent on plain radiographs, and in preoperative assessment of bony anatomy.

MRI. Can rule out spinal epidural hematoma and the occasional herniated disc. May demonstrate dural ectasia in cases of CES-AS syndrome. Andersson lesions: pathologic changes at ligament insertion sites (MRI signal abnormalities at front and back of the endplates) are characteristic. Erosive changes due to pseudarthrosis at the disc space can mimic discitis (high signal on T1WI & T2WI with enhancement).

Bone scan. Ratio of uptake of SI joint to sacrum > 1.3:1 is suggestive of AS.

Differential diagnosis

- early on, AS may resemble rheumatoid arthritis. However, in AS nodules do not form in joints, and rheumatoid factor is absent in the serum
- metastatic prostate Ca in elderly male patients with sacroiliac pain and blastic changes compatible with sacroiliitis
- Forestier's disease (p. 1373) and DISH (p. 1373): these overlapping conditions produce exuberant bony overgrowth anterior and lateral to the disc without degeneration and ossification of the disc as occurs in AS. Both spare the facets and SI joints, do not produce flexion deformity, and tend to occur in men > 50 yrs old (older than typical AS)[25]

83

4. psoriasis, reactive arthritis (Reiter's syndrome), enteropathic (IBD-related) arthritis: the spondy-litis with these tends to be milder and less uniform, and SI joint involvement is *asymmetrical*. Cutaneous findings (erythema nodosum, and pyoderma gangrenosum) are absent in AS.[26]

Natural history

Progression of the disease is slow, and patients usually remain functionally active. Thoracic kyphosis with compensatory increase in cervical and lumbar lordosis is common. The shift in center of gravity together with spine stiffness and fragility predisposes to frequent falls and possible spine injuries. Eventually can progress to involvement of costovertebral joints resulting in restrictive lung disease pattern. AS patients are also predisposed to development of fibrotic lung disease in late stages.

The fragility of the spine and the loss of moveable segments increases the susceptibility to spine fractures. Fractures in AS often extend somewhat horizontally through all 3 columns of the spine (called a chalkstick fracture) (▸ Fig. 83.2), and do not follow typical fracture patterns of the non-spondylosed spine. These fractures are often very unstable (see below).

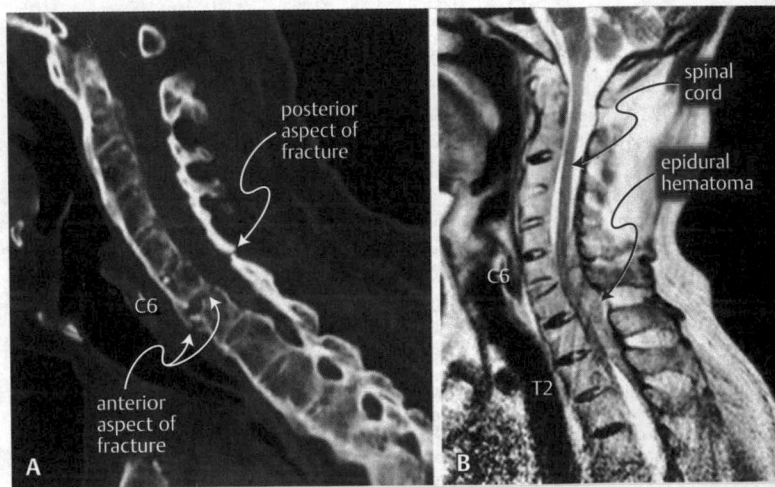

Fig. 83.2 Chalkstick fracture C6–7 with associated epidural hematoma in patient with ankylosing spondylitis. A: sagittal cervical CT, bone window. B: sagittal cervical T2 MRI showing associated epidural hematoma.

Treatment

General information

Combined ASAS/EULAR recommendations for management of AS are the most comprehensive cur-rently available (copy available at ASAS website). Multidisciplinary, coordinated by a rheumatolo-gist.[27] Goal of treatment is long-term quality of life through symptomatic control and prevention of progressive structural damage. NSAIDs are first-line pharmacological management.[27] Management of the disease itself may involve TNF inhibitors in patients with persistently high disease activity.[27]

Surgical treatment

General information

The most common surgical intervention is orthopedic total hip arthroplasty.[27]

Cervical fracture

The cervical spine is the most frequent fracture site in AS patients.[28] Patients often cannot distin-guish acute fracture pain from chronic inflammatory pain; therefore there should be a low threshold to obtain imaging. It is imperative to determine pre-injury alignment because application of a C-collar may cause hyperextension injury.[29] Gentle, low-weight traction with the force vector directed anteriorly and superiorly may be used for initial stabilization.[30,31] Halo vest or surgery for unstable fracture pattern.

Surgical indications:
- irreducible deformity
- deteriorating neurological status in the presence of epidural hematoma (see ▶ Fig. 83.2) or other source of compression[32]
- unstable fracture. Most 3-column fractures are very unstable as a result of long lever arms of fused segments above and below. Halo-vest immobilization is becoming less frequently employed for this

Procedures: Decompressive laminectomy if evidence of spinal cord compression.[32] Given poor bone quality and extended lever arms, good fusion bed and a construct extending multiple levels above and below the fracture are critical.[33] Proximally, lateral mass screws up to C3, possible pedicle screw in C2, and pedicle screws in thoracic spine for distal fixation.[33] 360° fusion may provide optimal stabilization in some cases (where feasible).

Thoracolumbar fracture
The majority occur at thoracolumbar junction.[33] Can be divided into 3 types[34]:
1. shearing injury: typically acute, resembling a Chance fracture (p. 1202). In AS this is a highly unstable 3-column injury[34] (due to the long lever arms on both sides of the fracture)
2. wedge compression: typically chronic
3. pseudarthrosis: typically subacute previously missed fracture

Wedge compression or pseudarthrosis; rule out posterior element involvement to determine if fracture is unstable.[33] Stable fracture can be treated with external orthosis. Unstable fractures, consider thicker rods or more rigid rod material to account for increased forces across fracture, and PMMA augmentation to prevent screw pullout.

Kyphotic deformity
ASAS/EULAR recommendations include corrective osteotomy for severe disabling deformity.[27] Can be accomplished via open wedge osteotomy, polysegmental wedge osteotomy, or closed wedge osteotomy (lowest complication rate).[35] Cervical deformity is most commonly addressed with wedge osteotomy at C7 and T1 given absence of vertebral artery in foramen transversarium at these levels. Current trend in literature is to address deformity simultaneously with acute fracture fixation.[31,32]

Cauda equina syndrome
Although evidence is limited, in the absence of demonstrable neural compression, a lumboperitoneal (LP) shunt may provide the best chance of improving neurologic dysfunction or halting progression of neurologic deficit.[36]

Surgical considerations
- anesthesia team should be aware of kyphotic deformity and fracture location: intubation using video laryngoscopy, or second choice, asleep fiberoptic bronchoscopy (awake fiberoptic intubation is rarely used)[37] to prevent hyperextension of the neck and exacerbation of neurologic injury[33]
- extensive pre-op evaluation: fracture pattern, posterior ligamentous restraint, neurologic compression and function, preexisting bone quality[33]
- surgical positioning modified to account for preexisting deformity; support in all regions to prevent hyperextension and exacerbation of neurologic injury[33]
- graft material: iliac crest bone graft (ICBG) is the gold standard; however, the donor site is often a significant pain source potentially limiting mobilization and increasing likelihood of stasis sequelae (e.g., DVT), consider allograft[32]
- extensive knowledge of lateral mass and pedicle anatomy to ensure adequate hardware placement despite distorted bony anatomy and obscuring of typical landmarks[32]
- post-op immobilization via halo-vest or TLSO[33]
- expedited mobilization out-of-bed as AS patients are predisposed to pulmonary complications[33]
- plastic surgery to help manage skin necrosis and wound closure[33]

83.2.2 Ossification of the posterior longitudinal ligament (OPLL)

General information

> ### Key concepts
>
> - fibrosis followed by calcification and then ossification of the posterior longitudinal ligament. The process may involve the dura
> - more common in Asian population
> - most patients have only mild subjective complaints
> - 50% of patients have impaired glucose tolerance. Respiratory compromise may result from ossification of the costotransverse and costovertebral ligaments
> - surgery is best for moderate neuro involvement (Nurick grade 3 & 4)

The age of patients with OPLL ranges from 32–81 years (mean = 53), with a slight male predominance. The prevalence increases with age. Duration of symptoms averages ≈ 13 months. It is more prevalent in the Japanese population (2–3.5%).[38,39]

Pathophysiology

The pathologic basis of OPLL is unknown, but there is an increased incidence of ankylosing hyperostosis which suggests a hereditary basis.

OPLL begins with hypervascular fibrosis in the PLL which is followed by focal areas of calcification, proliferation of periosteal cartilaginous cells and finally ossification.[40] The process frequently extends *into* the dura. Eventually active bone marrow production may occur. The process progresses at varying rates among patients, with an average annual growth rate of 0.67 mm in the AP direction and 4.1 mm longitudinally.[41]

When hypertrophied or ossified, the posterior longitudinal ligament may cause myelopathy (due to direct spinal cord compression or ischemia) and/or radiculopathy (by nerve root compression or stretching).

Changes within the spinal cord involve the posterolateral gray matter more than white matter, suggesting an ischemic basis for the neurologic involvement.

Distribution

Average involvement: 2.7–4 levels. Frequency of involvement:
1. cervical: 70–75% of cases of OPLL. Typically begins at C3–4 and proceeds distally, often involving C4–5 and C5–6 but usually sparing C6–7
2. thoracic: 15–20% (usually upper, ≈ T4–6)
3. lumbar: 10–15% (also usually upper, ≈ L1–3)

Pathologic classification

See reference.[42]
1. segmental: 39%. Confined to space behind vertebral bodies, does not cross disc spaces
2. continuous: 17%. Extends from VB to VB, spanning disc space(s)
3. mixed: 25%. Combines elements of both of the above with skip areas
4. other variants: 5%. Includes a rare type of OPLL that is contiguous with the endplates and is confined to the disc space (involves focal hypertrophy of the PLL with punctate calcification)

In the thoracic spine, 2 variants have been described:
1. beak: segmental OPLL with a focal protrusion posterior to the disc space
2. flat: continuous or flat OPLL

Clinical

Most patients are asymptomatic, or have only mild subjective complaints. This is probably explained by the protective effect of the fusion resulting from OPLL and the very gradual compression.

Natural history: 17% of patients without myelopathy developed myelopathy in one study[43] over 17.6 years mean follow-up. At 30 years 29% of patients developed myelopathy.[43]

Evaluation

Evaluation overview
Recommended radiographic evaluation of the spine consists of noncontrast MRI, noncontrast CT, and flexion/extension cervical spine X-rays. If MRI cannot be done, then a CT/myelogram combined with flexion/extension X-rays is recommended.

Plain X-rays
Often fail to demonstrate OPLL. Flexion/extension views may be helpful by assessing stability.

MRI
OPLL may be suspected on MRI by the appearance of large CSF filling defects anterior to the spinal cord. OPLL appears as a hypointense area and is difficult to appreciate until it reaches ≈ 5 mm thickness. On T1WI it blends in with the hypointensity of the ventral subarachnoid space. On T2WI it remains hypointense while the CSF becomes bright (Panel A, ► Fig. 83.3). Sagittal images may be very helpful in providing an overview of the extent of cord compression, and T2WI may demonstrate intrinsic spinal cord abnormalities (myelomalacia), which may be associated with a worse outcome.

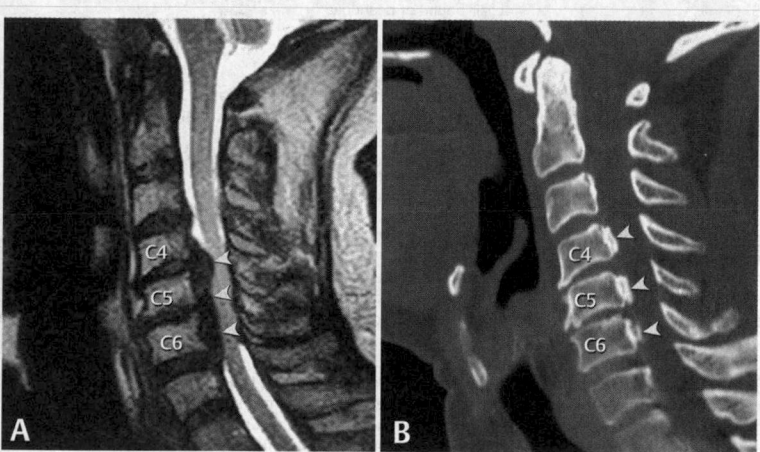

Fig. 83.3 Imaging of segmental OPLL (*yellow arrowheads*).
A: sagittal T2 MRI, OPLL appears dark and here is causing spinal cord compression. B: sagittal noncontrast CT.

CT
Shows calcification extremely well (Panel B, ► Fig. 83.3). Does not show spinal cord. When obtained in conjunction with MRI, provides a detailed static evaluation.

CT/myelogram
Myelography with post-myelographic CT (especially with 3D reconstructions) is probably best at demonstrating and accurately diagnosing OPLL.

Treatment

Treatment decisions
Based on clinical grade[42] as follows:
  Class I: radiographic evidence without clinical signs or symptoms. Most patients with OPLL are asymptomatic.[39] Conservative management unless severe
  Class II: patients with myelopathy or radiculopathy. Minimal or stable deficit may be followed expectantly. Significant deficit or evidence of progression warrants surgical intervention

- **Class IIIA**: moderate to severe myelopathy. Usually requires surgical intervention
- **Class IIIB**: severe to complete quadriplegia. Surgery is considered for incomplete quadriplegics showing progressive slow worsening. Rapid deterioration or complete quadriplegia, advanced age, or poor medical condition are all associated with worse outcome

In moderate grade patients (Nurick grades 3 & 4)[44] (see ▶ Table 83.2), surgery provided a statistically significant reduction in deterioration. There was no difference between surgery and conservative treatment in mild grade (Nurick 1 or 2), and surgery was ineffective in severe grade (Nurick 5).[43]

Table 83.2 Nurick grade of disability from cervical spondylosis[44]

Grade	Description
0	signs or symptoms of root involvement without myelopathy
1	myelopathy, but no difficulty in walking
2	slight difficulty in walking, able to work
3	difficulty in walking but not needing assistance, unable to work full-time
4	able to walk only with assistance or walker
5	chair-bound or bedridden

Pre-op assessment

Appropriate cardiorespiratory assessment should be made knowing that:
1. respiratory compromise may result from ossification of the costotransverse and costovertebral ligaments
2. 50% of patients have impaired glucose tolerance with the attendant risks associated with diabetes

Technical considerations for surgery

Severe OPLL increases the risk of spinal cord injury during neck positioning for intubation. To minimize, video laryngoscopy (or second choice: awake nasotracheal intubation) should be used.

An anterior approach is generally favored, although laminectomy may be acceptable. SSEP monitoring has been recommended by some.[40] Distraction should be avoided until the spinal cord has been decompressed from the OPLL.

Some authors advocate complete removal of bone from the dura, while others feel it is permissible to leave a thin rim of bone adherent to the dura. Care must be taken in removing bone because it tends to blend imperceptibly with dura and the next thing one may see is bare spinal cord.

Depending on the distance of vertical involvement, vertebral corpectomy with strut grafting may be required. Internal plate fixation is often used as an adjunct. Postoperative immobilization for at least 3 months is employed with rigid collars for single level ACDF or 1–2 level corpectomies, or halo-vest traction for corpectomies > 2 levels.

Results with surgery

The incidence of pseudarthrosis after vertebral corpectomy and strut graft ranges from 5–10% and increases with the number of levels fused.

In one series there was a 10% incidence of transient worsening of neurologic function following anterior surgery[41] which may have been related to distraction.

The risk of dural tear with CSF leak following an anterior approach depends on the aggressiveness with which bone is removed from the dura, and ranges ≈ 16–25%.

Other risks of anterior approaches, e.g., esophageal injury (p. 1286), also pertain.

83.2.3 Ossification of the anterior longitudinal ligament (OALL)

OALL of the cervical spine and/or hypertrophic anterior cervical osteophytes may produce dramatic radiographic findings and minimal clinical symptoms. Distinct from Forestier's disease (see below). Cervical involvement may produce dysphagia.[45]

83.2.4 Forestier disease/diffuse idiopathic skeletal hyperostosis (DISH)

Key concepts

- a rheumatologic disease of uncertain etiology
- Forestier disease refers to spine involvement, DISH includes extraspinal manifestations
- lack of SI joint involvement helps distinguish this from ankylosing spondylitis
- usually asymptomatic, but may present with spine stiffness, globus pharyngis (lump in the throat), dysphagia, or dyspnea
- W/U: ✓ speech therapy consult for dysphagia evaluation (usually includes ✓ modified barium swallow (mBS)), ✓ CT of cervical spine, ± ✓ digital video esophagoscopy
- treatment is indicated for significant swallowing difficulties (often with weight loss) related to the osteophytes on mBS, aspiration, or dyspnea
- surgery consists of drilling off osteophytes with high-speed drill
- pre- & post-op speech therapy is recommended. Dysphagia may transiently worsen post-op, a temporary PEG feeding tube may be required

In 1950 Forestier[46] described this ankylosing disease limited to the spine, distinct from ankylosing spondylitis. Resnick et al.[47] coined the term diffuse idiopathic skeletal hyperostosis (DISH) to include extraspinal involvement. AKA spondylitis ossificans ligamentosa, AKA ankylosing hyperostosis, among others. Some use the terms Forestier disease (or syndrome) and DISH interchangeably.

A rheumatologic disease of unknown etiology characterized by flowing osteophytic formation of the spine in the absence of degenerative, traumatic, or post-infectious changes. Affects Caucasians and males more commonly, and is usually seen in patients in their mid-60 s.

Distinguishing features from ankylosing spondylitis (p. 1365) (AS), DISH: spares the SI joints (primary distinguishing feature), has an older age of onset, does not produce kyphosis, on X-ray has a thick bulge over the entire VB (AS has a predilection for the VB adjacent to the disc space).

97% of cases occur in the thoracic spine, also in the lumbar spine in 90%, cervical spine in 78%, and all three segments in 70%. Sacroiliac joints are *spared*, unlike ankylosing spondylitis (AS) (p. 1365). As with AS, unfused levels may be very unstable.

Risk factors for DISH include: elevated body mass index,[48] elevated serum uric acid,[48] diabetes mellitus,[48] and elevated growth hormone or insulin levels.[49]

Usually does not produce clinical symptoms. Patients may have early morning stiffness and mild limitations of activities. Cervical involvement may present with dysphagia (p. 1373) or globus pharyngis (the subjective sensation of a lump in the throat, not to be confused with globus hystericus, which refers to the sensation of a lump in the throat where there is no identifiable pathology) due to compression of the esophagus between the osteophytes and the rigid laryngeal structures[50] (part of Forestier's disease[51]).

Plain X-rays and CT scan demonstrate the bony pathology.

▶ **Dysphagia due to esophageal compression by osteophytes** (▶ Fig. 83.4). Evaluation should also include speech therapy consult for dysphagia, (modified) barium swallow study to help localize the site of obstruction, and DVE (digital video esophagoscopy) to rule out intrinsic esophageal disease. Pre- and post-op speech therapy for swallowing therapy is recommended as these patients have not been swallowing normally for years and tend to have continued difficulties even after osteophyte reduction. Surgery may be considered in cases that do not respond satisfactorily to dietary modifications in patients who are losing weight or are having recurrent episodes of choking or (aspiration) pneumonia.

An anterior cervical approach and utilization of a high-speed drill with careful protection of soft-tissue structures (esophagus, carotid sheath) without need for discectomy nor spine stabilization has been recommended.[50] Patients need to be made aware that post-op they may be *worse* (from manipulation of esophagus and possibly disruption of some of the autonomic innervation of the esophagus) and that there is a significant chance they will need a (temporary) gastrostomy feeding (PEG) tube, and that they should not proceed with surgery unless they are willing to undergo PEG tube placement if it is indicated in the judgment of the surgeon and/or his consultants. Improvement sometimes takes up to 1 year to occur.

83

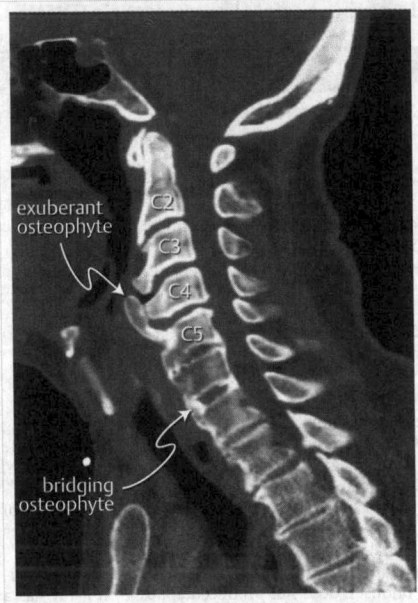

Fig. 83.4 Cervical osteophyte causing dysphagia.
DISH with exuberant anterior osteophytes C3 through C5 in a patient with dysphonia, dyspnea, and 17-lb weight loss due to dysphagia. All symptoms resolved with surgical reduction of exuberant osteophytes.
Image: sagittal cervical CT, bone window.

83.3 Scheuermann's kyphosis

83.3.1 General information

Key concepts

- criteria: anterior wedging of at least 5° of ≥ 3 adjacent thoracic vertebral bodies
- presentation: usually pain (when thoracic kyphosis (TK) > 50–60°) or cosmetic deformity
- workup: standing scoliosis X-rays, neuro exam, ± MRI
- surgical treatment: usually reserved for TK > 70°

AKA: Scheuermann's kyphoscoliosis, Scheuermann juvenile kyphosis, juvenile kyphosis, Scheuermann disease, juvenile osteochondrosis of the spine, vertebral epiphysitis. Originally dubbed "osteochondritis deformans juvenilis dorsi" by Danish orthopedic surgeon Holger Werfel Scheuermann in 1920.[52]

83.3.2 Epidemiology

Prevalence: 1–8% of the population.[53]
    Usually diagnosed between ages 11–17 years.
    Possible slight male predominance, but there is conflicting information regarding gender predilection.
    There is a genetic predisposition based on studies of monozygotic vs. dizygotic twins.[54]

83.3.3 Etiology

The underlying cause is unknown.
    The pathophysiology appears to be disorganization in the growth plate with increased growth of the posterior vertebral body with respect to the anterior VB. Hueter-Volkmann law may apply

compression of the cartilaginous endplate (physes) at the anterior vertebral body inhibits *longitudinal* growth (this law may also apply in adolescent idiopathic scoliosis unilaterally in the VB).

83.3.4 Classification

- Type I: involves only the thoracic spine. Apex usually ≈ T7/T8
- Type II (adult variant): 25% of cases. Involves thoracolumbar spine.[55] Scoliosis is present in 88%
- the term "lumbar Scheuermann's disease" has been proposed for a lumbar variant

83.3.5 Presentation

50–75% of patients will have pain, which tends to occur during teenage years. Younger patients have more pain than older ones (only ≈ 25% will develop pain after skeletal maturity). Pain is uncommon if the curve remains < 50–60°.

Adolescents: may also present as a result of the cosmetic deformity associated with progressive kyphosis, which may be mistaken for "slouching" (postural kyphosis is usually < 60°).

83.3.6 Evaluation

1. standing scoliosis X-rays
2. careful neurologic exam
3. MRI: may be considered to rule out hemivertebrae and thoracic disc herniation

83.3.7 Radiographic findings

Sørenson criteria[56(p 19)]: 3 contiguous vertebrae with ≥ 5° of kyphotic deformity (anterior wedge) per level.

Associated findings may include:
1. endplate irregularities
2. anterior narrowing of disc space
3. Schmorl's nodes (p. 1266)
4. scoliosis in ≈ 25%
5. spondylolysis (p. 1340) in 50%[57]: likely due to the increased lumbar lordosis that compensates for the increased thoracic kyphosis

83.3.8 Treatment

Bracing

Bracing may be considered:
1. in young (adolescent) asymptomatic patients with mild-to-moderate curve, defined as:
   - Type 1 Scheuermann's: TK ≤ 40–50°
   - Type 2 Scheuermann's: thoracolumbar kyphosis < 55°
2. ✖ it is not logical to brace a skeletally mature spine

Brace types:
1. Milwaukee brace: often used, especially when the apex is above T8 and for overweight patients
2. TLSO with cowhorns

Whatever brace is chosen, it must be worn at least 23 hrs/day for 1–2 years.

Other treatments

When pain is the main issue:
1. NSAIDs: especially in adults
2. physical therapy: reduced pain in 16–32%[58]

Surgical indications

Surgery is generally indicated for:
1. thoracic kyphosis > 70° (some authors recommend > 80°)

2. unacceptable cosmetic appearance
3. refractory pain
4. progressive kyphosis
5. neurologic deficit: very uncommon. Obtain MRI to rule out thoracic disc herniation

Surgical considerations

Optimal surgical procedure is not known. Well accepted: posterior fusion with multiple osteotomies (Ponte AKA Schwab type 2 (▶ Table 82.2) osteotomies).

Treat osteoporosis if present.
Don't overcorrect: limit correction to ≤ 50% of the original deformity.
Consider wiring the spinous processes at the cranial and caudal levels. Don't overexpose.
Lumbar hyperlordosis usually corrects spontaneously after correction of thoracic kyphosis.

Levels to include:
- cranial level: the top of the kyphosis
- distal level:
  ○ the level below the first lordotic disc as determined on lateral X-ray
  ○ Cho et al[59] recommend including the sagittal stable vertebra (SSV), defined as the most proximal lumbar vertebral body touched by the vertical line from the posterior-superior corner of the sacrum on standing scoliosis X-rays
- fusion should be balanced on either side of the apex of the curve, and a plumb line from C7 should pass through the middle of the last fused VB
- the most common levels fused: from T2 to L2 or L3

83.4 Rheumatoid arthritis

83.4.1 General information

More than 85% of patients with moderate or severe rheumatoid arthritis (RA) have radiographic evidence of C-spine involvement.[60]

The grading system of Ranawat et al[60] for myelopathy as shown in ▶ Table 83.3 is used in RA as well as some other etiologies of myelopathy.

Table 83.3 Ranawat classification of myelopathy

Class	Description
I	no neural deficit
II	subjective weakness + hyperreflexia + dysesthesia
III	objective weakness + long tract signs III A = ambulatory III B = quadriparetic & non-ambulatory

83.4.2 Cervical spine involvement in RA

Common involvement
1. upper cervical spine: involved in 44–88% of RA cases[61] (often found together):
   a) anterior atlantoaxial subluxation: the most common manifestation of RA in the cervical spine found in up to 25% of patients with RA (see below)
   b) basilar impression (BI): upward translocation of the odontoid process, found in ≈ 8% of patients with RA (p. 1380)
   c) C1–2 pannus: chronic inflammatory granulation tissue that forms around the odontoid (▶ Fig. 83.5)
2. subaxial C-spine (i.e., below C2) subluxation (p. 1380)

Less common involvement of the cervical spine in RA
1. posterior subluxation of the atlantoaxial joint: must have either associated fracture of or near total arthritic erosion of odontoid
2. vertebral artery insufficiency secondary to changes at the cranio-cervical junction[62]

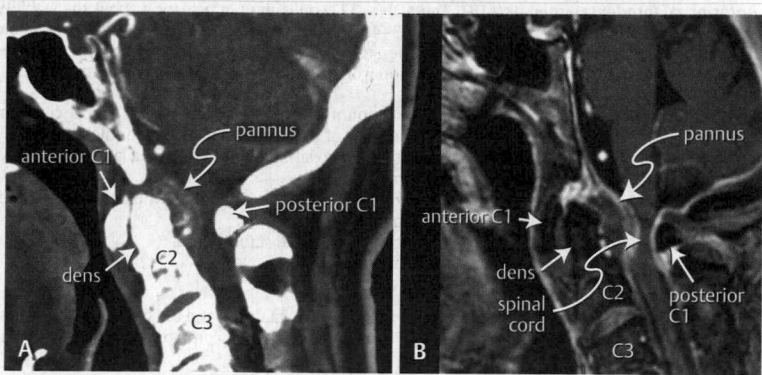

83

Fig. 83.5 C2 pannus.
Image: A: sagittal CT of cervical spine, soft tissue window. B: sagittal enhanced T1 cervical MRI.
Note the spinal cord being compressed between the pannus and the anteriorly displaced posterior arch of C1 shown on the MRI.

83.4.3 Atlantoaxial subluxation (AAS) in RA

General information

Inflammatory involvement of the atlantoaxial synovial joints causes erosive changes in the odontoid process (anteriorly at the synovial joint with the C1 arch, and posteriorly at the synovial joint with the transverse ligament) and decalcification and loosening of the insertion of the transverse ligament on the atlas. These changes lead to instability, allowing a scissoring effect with anterior subluxation of C1 on C2. AAS occurs in ≈ 25% of patients with RA.[62] Mean time between onset of RA symptoms to the diagnosis of AAS in 15 patients: 14 years.[63]

Clinical

Signs and symptoms of AAS are shown in ▶ Table 83.4.

AAS is usually slowly progressive. Mean age at onset of AAS symptoms: 57 years.

Pain is experienced locally (upper cervical and suboccipital regions, often from compression of C2 nerve root) or is referred (to mastoid, occipital, temporal, or frontal regions).

VBI may occur from VA involvement (p. 1591).

Table 83.4 Signs and symptoms of AAS[a] (15 patients with AAS[63])

Finding	%
pain	
• local	67
• referred	27
hyperreflexia	67
spasticity	27
paresis	27
sensory disturbance	20

[a]other possible findings not reported in this series: clumsiness, neurogenic bladder, Babinski sign

Radiographic evaluation

General information

The magnitude of AAS usually increases with neck flexion.

▶ **Anterior atlantodental interval (ADI).** The ADI (p. 223) only gives information about the stability of the C1–2 joint. The normal ADI in adults is < 3–4 mm.[64,65] Widening of the ADI suggests possible incompetence of the transverse ligament. However, the ADI *does not correlate* with the risk of neurologic injury[66,67] and is not predictive of progression from asymptomatic AAS to symptomatic AAS.

▶ **Posterior atlantodental interval (PADI).** The amount of room available for the spinal cord can vary for any given ADI depending on the AP diameter of the spinal canal and the thickness of any pannus. The PADI (p. 223) and the AP diameter of the subaxial canal measured on a lateral C-spine X-ray correlates with the presence and severity of paralysis.[66]

The PADI also predicts neurologic recovery following surgery. Patients with paralysis from AAS showed no recovery if the pre-op PADI was < 10 mm.[66]

PADI ≤ 14 mm has been proposed as an indication for surgical stabilization.

Lateral C-spine X-ray

Both the ADI and PADI (see above) are surrogate markers for instability and for spinal cord compression. With the availability of MRI, the ability to directly assess spinal cord compression has diminished the usefulness of these measurements.

MRI

MRI is the optimal test to evaluate the source and magnitude of upper cord or medullar compression. Demonstrates location of odontoid process, extent of pannus, and effects of subluxation.

CT scan

In addition to providing information that is invaluable for surgical planning, CT gives detailed information about the degree of bone destruction which can help in assessing stability. Bony erosion at the insertion sites of the transverse ligament on the C1 tubercles (▶ Fig. 1.14) is a marker for potential instability due to incompetence of the ligament.

Treatment

General information

Requires knowledge of the following information:

1. natural history: AAS in most patients progresses, with a small percentage either stabilizing or fusing spontaneously. In one series[68] with 4.5 years mean follow-up, 45% of patients with 3.5–5 mm subluxation progressed to 5–8 mm, and 10% of these progressed to > 8 mm
2. once myelopathy occurs, it may be irreversible
3. the worse the myelopathy, the higher the risk for sudden death
4. the chances of finding myelopathy are significantly increased once the subluxation reaches ≥ 9 mm[69]
5. associated cranial settling further decreases the tolerance for AAS
6. the life expectancy of patients with RA is 10 years less than the general population[68]
7. the morbidity and mortality of surgical treatment (see below)
8. pannus often recedes after surgical fusion. This may be enhanced with the use of tumor necrosis factor alpha (TNF-α) inhibitors such as etanercept (Enbrel) or adalimumab (Humira), or monoclonal antibodies against TNF-α, e.g., infliximab (Remicade)

When to treat?

1. symptomatic patients with AAS: almost all require surgical treatment (C1–2 fusion in most cases). For management, see below. Some surgeons do not operate if the maximal dens-C1 distance is < 6 mm
2. asymptomatic patients: controversial
   a) some authors feel surgical fusion is not necessary in asymptomatic patient if the dens-C1 distance is below a certain cutoff. Recommendations for this cutoff have ranged from 6 to 10 mm,[70] with 8 mm commonly cited (an unvalidated delineation)
   b) these patients are often placed in a rigid cervical collar, e.g., while outside the home, even though it is generally acknowledged that a collar probably does not provide significant support or protection
   c) NB: some cases of sudden death in previously asymptomatic RA patients may be due to AAS and may then be erroneously attributed to cardiac arrhythmias, etc.[71]

Surgical management

It is necessary to either reduce the subluxation or to decompress the upper cord before doing a C1–2 or occipital-C1–2 fusion.

Menezes assesses all subluxed patients for reducibility using MRI-compatible halo cervical traction as follows: start with 5 lbs, and gradually increase over a period of a week. Most cases reduce within 2–3 days. If not reduced after 7 days then it is probably not reducible. Only ≈ 20% of cases are not reducible (most of these have odontoid > 15 mm above foramen magnum).

Most require posterior stabilization, either of C1 to C2, or of occiput to C2. The latter is used when fusion is combined with decompression (posterior laminectomy of C1 with posterior enlargement of the foramen magnum). See Atlantoaxial fusion (C1–2 arthrodesis) (p. 1778).

Posterior fusion alone does not provide adequate relief if the subluxation is irreducible, or if pannus causes significant compression (however, there may be some reduction of pannus after fusion, especially with TNF-α inhibitors (p. 1378)). In these cases, odontoidectomy either transoral or transnasal endoscopic may be indicated. Performing the posterior stabilization and decompression first allows some patients to avoid a second operation, and permits the remainder to undergo the anterior approach without becoming destabilized. Still, some surgeons do the odontoidectomy first[70] (requires the patient to remain in traction until the fusion).

Reminder: the patient must be able to open the mouth greater than ≈ 25 mm in order to perform transoral odontoidectomy without splitting the mandible.

Posterior fusion

See Atlantoaxial fusion (C1–2 arthrodesis) (p. 1778) for technique. In RA, erosion and osteoporosis weakens the C1 arch, and extra care is needed to avoid fracturing it.

83.4.4 Surgical morbidity and mortality

Because of the frequency of simultaneous involvement of other systems in RA, including pulmonary, cardiac, and endocrine, operative mortality ranges from 5–15%.[70]

The non-fusion rate for C1–2 wiring and fusion has been reported as high as 50%,[72] typical rates are lower (with 18% of patients in one series developing a fibrous union[70]). The most common site of failure of osseous fusion is the interface between the bone graft and the posterior arch of C1.[73]

83.4.5 Postoperative care

The patient is usually mobilized almost immediately post-op in halo vest traction (some use an optional period of maintained traction before mobilization). Impaired healing in RA dictates that the halo be worn until fusion is well-established, as seen on X-ray (usually 8–12 weeks). Sonntag evaluates the patient with flexion-extension lateral C-spine X-rays by disconnecting the halo ring from the vest.

83.4.6 Basilar impression in rheumatoid arthritis

General information

AKA atlantoaxial impaction. Erosive changes in the lateral masses of C1 → telescoping of the atlas onto the body of C2 causing ventral migration of C1 with resultant ↓ in AP diameter of the spinal canal. There is concomitant upward displacement of the dens. The posterior arch of C1 often protrudes superiorly through the foramen magnum. All of these factors lead to compression of the pons and medulla. Rheumatoid granulation tissue behind the odontoid also contributes to the brainstem compression. Vertebral artery and/or anterior spinal artery compression may also cause neurologic dysfunction.

The degree of erosion of C1 correlates with the extent of odontoid invagination.

Clinical

See ▶ Table 83.5 for signs & symptoms.

Pain may occur as a result of compression of the C1 and/or C2 nerve roots. Compression of the medulla can cause cranial nerve dysfunction.

Motor exam usually difficult because of severe polyarticular degeneration and associated pain. Sensory findings (all non-localizing): diminished vibratory, position, and light touch.

83

Table 83.5 Symptoms and signs of BI (45 patients with RA[61])

Finding	%
headache (occipital pain)	100
progressive difficulty ambulating	80
hyperreflexia + Babinski	80
limb paresthesias	71
trigeminal nerve anesthesia[a]	38
neurogenic bladder	31
lower cranial nerve dysfunction • glossopharyngeal • vagus • hypoglossal	22
miscellaneous findings • internuclear ophthalmoplegia • vertigo • diplopia • downbeat nystagmus • sleep apnea • spastic quadriparesis	

[a]all of these patients had odontoid invagination > 10 mm above the foramen magnum

Radiographic evaluation

See Basilar invagination & basilar impression (BI) (p.228) for radiographic criteria of BI. Erosion of the tip of the odontoid, commonly seen in RA, obviates use of any measurement that is based on the location of the tip of the odontoid.[74] For this reason, other measures have been developed, including the Clark station,[73] Redlund-Johnell criteria,[75] and Ranawat criteria.[60] Since even these methods will miss up to 6% of cases of BI in RA,[74] it is recommended that suspicious cases be investigated further (e.g., with CT and/or MRI).

MRI: optimal for demonstrating brainstem impingement, poor for showing bone. Cervicomedullary angle: the angle between a line drawn through the long axis of the medulla on a sagittal MRI and a line drawn through the cervical spinal cord. The normal CMA is 135–170°. A CMA < 135° correlates with signs of cervicomedullary compression, myelopathy, or C2 radiculopathy.[76]

CT: primarily done to assess bony anatomy (erosion, fractures…).

CTA should be performed when surgery is contemplated, to show detail of VA anatomy.

Myelography (water-soluble) with CT: also good for delineating bony pathology.

Treatment

See also Craniocervical junction and upper cervical spine abnormalities (p.1308).

Cervical traction

May attempt with Gardner-Wells tongs. Begin with ≈ 7 lbs, and slowly increase up to 15 lbs. Some may require several weeks of traction to reduce.

Surgery

Reducible cases: posterior occipitocervical fusion ± C1 decompressive laminectomy.

Irreducible cases: requires transoral resection of odontoid. May perform before posterior fusion (but then must be kept in traction while waiting for posterior fusion).

83.4.7 Subaxial subluxation in rheumatoid arthritis

The direct effects of RA on the subaxial spine involves the facet joints posteriorly. Degenerative disc disease, which is generally a late manifestation in RA, is not the result of synovitis.[77] Involvement is most common at C2–3 and C3–4.

83.5 Down syndrome

83.5.1 General information

Down syndrome is associated with ligamentous laxity of the spine. This has implications whenever a fusion is contemplated, as adjacent segment failure with kyphosis is very common. Ligamentous laxity may also result in atlantoaxial subluxation (**AAS**).

83.5.2 Atlantoaxial subluxation (AAS) in Down syndrome

General information

Not all cases of AAS are unstable (an unstable spine, by definition, needs treatment).

Incidence of AAS in Down syndrome (DS) is 20%,[78] but only 1–2% of DS patients have *symptomatic* AAS.[79] AAS in DS appears to be due to laxity of the transverse atlantal ligament (TAL). This laxity may decrease with age as the TAL stiffens.

Management

Controversial. There have been position statements[80] and rebuttals.[79,81]

Recommendations (modified[82]); ADI = atlantodental interval (p.223), PADI = posterior atlantodental interval (p.223):

1. children who have been screened and do not have AAS: no further screening after age 10 years (since AAS does not develop later; the cutoff age is controversial)
2. os odontoideum: surgical fusion
3. symptomatic AAS
   a) symptoms may include: gait difficulties, neck pain, limited neck motion, torticollis, clumsiness, sensory deficits, and other symptoms of myelopathy
   b) for ADI > 4.5 mm or PADI < 14 mm or spinal cord damage on cervical MRI: surgical fusion
4. asymptomatic AAS seen on lateral C-spine X-ray:
   a) for ADI ≤ 4.5 mm *and* PADI ≥ 14 mm: no need for further testing
   b) for ADI > 4.5 mm or PADI < 14 mm: cervical MRI
      • if the MRI shows spinal cord damage: surgical fusion
      • if MRI shows no spinal cord damage: surgical fusion is optional. If fusion is not done, prohibit high-risk activities and restudy in 1 year

83.6 Spinal epidural lipomatosis (SEL)

83.6.1 General information

Hypertrophy of histologically normal unencapsulated epidural fat. Most commonly seen with prolonged exogenous steroid therapy (in 75% of cases[83]) usually moderate to high dosage for years,[84] but may also be associated with: Cushing's disease, Cushing's syndrome, obesity,[85] hypothyroidism, hyperprolactinemia or with use of protease inhibitors as part of antiretroviral therapy for HIV.[86] SEL may also be idiopathic.[87] Male:female = 3:1.[84]

Back pain usually precedes all other symptoms. Progressive LE weakness and sensory changes are common. Sphincter disturbance occurs but is rare. SEL is most common in the thoracic spine (≈ 60% of cases); the rest are in the lumbar spine (no cases reported in cervical spine).

Prevalence: SEL was found in 2.5% of lumbar MRIs.[86]

★ It is often very difficult to differentiate cases with increased epidural fat (even to the point that CSF may be obliterated at the levels of involvement) that is not causing symptoms from those where the exuberant fat is responsible for the findings.

83.6.2 Evaluation

CT: density of adipose tissue is extremely low (-80 to -120 Hounsfield units),[88] which distinguishes SEL from most other lesions (except lipoma, which is also comprised of fat).

MRI: (▶ Fig. 83.6) signal follows fat (high signal on T1WI, intermediate on T2WI). On T2WI, epidural fat may be mistaken for CSF, but is usually subtly less bright than CSF, and does not drop out on T1WI as CSF does. Suggested diagnostic criteria: epidural adipose should be > 7 mm thick to be considered SEL.[85,89]

83

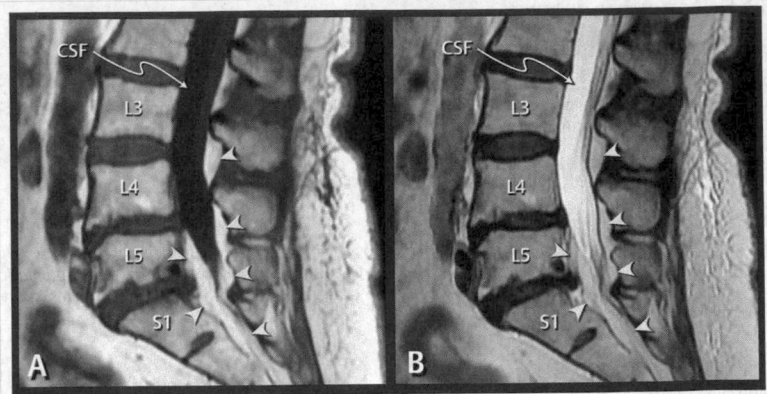

Fig. 83.6 Epidural lipomatosis (*yellow arrowheads*).
Image: lumbar sagittal MRI, A: T1WI, B: T2WI (note: epidural fat is not as bright white as CSF on T2WI).
Note: complete loss of CSF at the L5–S1 disc space level due to epidural fat.

83.6.3 Treatment

Symptomatic patients who are overweight and/or on steroids may get relief without surgery by weaning off steroids and losing weight.[90]

Surgery is indicated for symptomatic patients in whom the above interventions are unsuccessful or not feasible. An effort to normalize cortisol levels in those with endogenous hypercortisolism (Cushing's disease…) should be made before laminectomy is performed. Due to potential complications and slow growth of the lipomatous tissue and the difficulty of being certain that the epidural fat is the source of significant symptoms, the decision to operate should be made with caution.

Surgery usually consists of laminectomy with removal of adipose tissue. Occasionally repeat surgery is needed for reaccumulation.

83.6.4 Outcome

Surgery usually results in significant improvement.[89] Idiopathic cases may fare better than those due to steroid excess. Cauda equina compression responds better than thoracic myelopathy.

Complication rates may be higher than expected in part due to medical comorbidities. Fessler et al[91] reported 22% 1-year mortality.

83.7 Miscellaneous conditions affecting the spine

83.7.1 Bertolotti's syndrome

Bertolotti's syndrome is a common anomaly (prevalence = 4–8%) of the lumbar spine in which a (usually) unilateral hypertrophied transverse process (TP) of the caudal-most lumbar vertebra articulates or fuses with the sacrum and/or ilium.[92,93]

It is controversial whether this pseudoarticulation is a potential cause of low back pain.

The anomalous joint may contribute to instability and degeneration at the suprajacent level.[94,93]

May be associated with radicular symptoms, possibly by compression or inflammatory involvement of the nerve (usually L5) exiting through the foramen.

▶ **Diagnosis.** Imaging studies include lumbar spine X-ray, lumbar CT Scan (▶ Fig. 83.7), lumbar MRI and sometimes bone scintigraphy. At one time local steroid injections into the transitional articulation were employed in the evaluation; however, pain relief did not correlate highly with successful surgical outcome.[95]

▶ **Treatment.** Local steroid injections into the transitional articulation may provide pain relief, but did not reliably correlate with successful outcome with surgical treatment.[95]

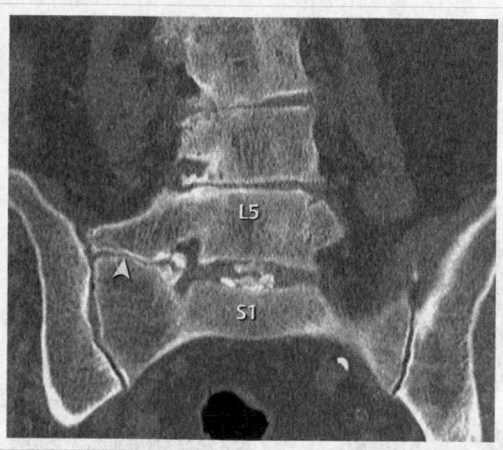

Fig. 83.7 Bertolotti's syndrome. Image: coronal lumbar CT scan, bone window, showing accessory joint (*yellow arrowheads*) on the right between L5 and S1.

In one series,[95] pain relief was obtained in 9 of 11 patients from surgical resection of the accessory bone. Fusion may be employed to eliminate motion or when instability is a concern.

83.7.2 Spinal epidural hematoma (SEH)

General information

Rare. Varying etiologies have been reported,[96] a significant number of cases are associated with anti-coagulation therapy.[97] NSAIDs may also be a risk factor.[98] Etiologies include:
1. traumatic: including following LP or epidural anesthesia,[96,99,100,101] fracture (see below), spinal surgery[102] or chiropractic manipulation.[103] Occurs predominantly in a patient who is: anticoagulated,[104] thrombocytopenic, or has bleeding diathesis or a vascular lesion
2. spontaneous[105]: rare. Etiologies: hemorrhage from spinal cord AVM (p. 1395), from vertebral hemangioma (p. 992), or tumor. Again, often in anticoagulated patients

May occur at any level of the spine; however, thoracic is most common. Most often located posterior to spinal cord (except for hematomas following anterior cervical procedures), facilitating removal via laminectomy.[97]

Traumatic spinal epidural hematoma (TSEH) associated with spine fracture

In one series,[106] among 74 trauma patients who underwent emergent spinal MRI, ≈ half of the patients with spine fractures also had TSEH. Treatment was based solely on the fracture, and the outcome in patients with neurologic deficits was no worse in the group with TSEH than in the group without.

Presentation

The clinical picture of *spontaneous* spinal epidural hematoma is fairly consistent but nonspecific. Usually starts with severe back pain with radicular component. It may occasionally follow straining, and is less commonly preceded by major straining or back trauma. Spinal neurologic deficits follow, usually progressing over hours, occasionally over days. Motor weakness may go unnoticed when patients are bedridden with pain.

Evaluation

MRI is the imaging modality of choice. Findings are illustrated in ▶ Fig. 83.8 in a patient with a spontaneous SEH and in ▶ Fig. 83.9 in a patient with posttraumatic SEH.

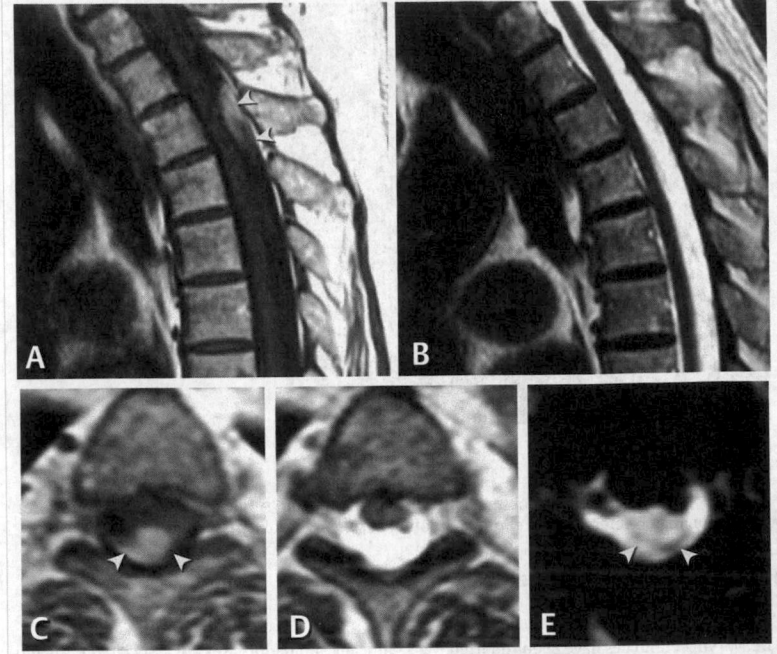

Fig. 83.8 Spontaneous spinal epidural hematoma (*yellow arrowheads*) located posterior to the thoracic spinal cord in a 73-year-old male on warfarin with no history of trauma.
Image: Thoracic MRI, A: sagittal T1, B: sagittal T2, C: axial T1, D: axial T2 with default windowing, E: axial T2 windowed to show the hematoma.
Note: the hematoma is difficult to appreciate on T2 imaging (B & D) without altering the windowing from the typical default values (as in C).

Treatment

With spontaneous SEH, recovery of neurologic deficit without surgery is rare (only a handful of case reports in the literature[98]), therefore optimal treatment is immediate decompressive laminectomy in those patients who can tolerate surgery.[97] In one series, most patients who recovered underwent decompression within 72 hrs of onset of symptoms.[107] In another, decompression within 6 hours was associated with better outcome.[102]

High-risk patients: for medically high-risk patients (e.g., acute MI on anticoagulation, surgical mortality and morbidity is extremely high, and this must be considered when making the decision of whether or not to operate. In patients not operated, anticoagulants should be stopped, and reversed if possible; see Correction of coagulopathies or reversal of anticoagulants (p. 174). Consider use of high-dose methylprednisolone to minimize cord injury; see Methylprednisolone under spinal cord injury (p. 1140). Percutaneous needle aspiration may be a consideration in high-risk patients.

83.7.3 Spinal subdural hematoma

Rare. May be posttraumatic (including iatrogenic causes) or may occur spontaneously. Spinal subdural hematomas (SSH) that occur spontaneously or following lumbar puncture usually occur in patients with coagulopathies (primary or iatrogenic).[108]

Conservative treatment is possible in nontraumatic SSHs with minimal neurologic impairment.[108]

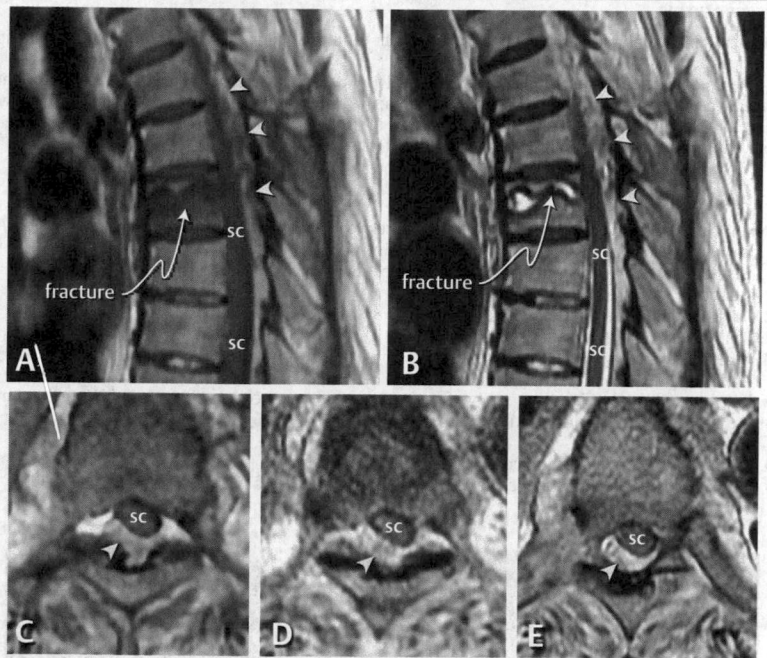

Fig. 83.9 Posttraumatic spinal epidural hematoma (*yellow arrowheads*) located posterior to the thoracic spinal cord in a 76-year-old male with DISH taking clopidogrel after sustaining a Chance thoracic fracture following a fall. Image: Thoracic MRI, A: sagittal T1, B: sagittal T2, C: axial T1, D: axial T2, E: axial T2FSE (fast spin echo). sc = spinal cord.

83.7.4 Spinal cord infarction

General information

Spinal cord infarction is uncommon in industrialized countries with the virtual elimination of syphilitic endarteritis. Most often involves the territory of the anterior spinal artery, sparing posterior columns. Most commonly ≈ T4 level (watershed zone).

Etiologies

1. atherosclerosis of radicular artery in elderly patient with hypotension is now the major cause of this rare condition
2. clamping aorta during surgery (e.g., for abdominal aortic aneurysm [AAA])
3. trauma: including herniated thoracic or cervical disc, fracture with bone compressing the anterior spinal cord especially when accompanied by kyphotic angulation
4. hypotension (relative or absolute) during surgery in the sitting position in the presence of spinal stenosis.[109] May be improved by avoiding absolute hypotension, intubation using video laryngoscopy, or second choice, asleep fiberoptic bronchoscopy (awake fiberoptic intubation is rarely used),[37] intraoperative SSEP monitoring and inducing hypertension if changes occur with positioning, avoidance of sitting position, and avoiding hyperflexion, hyperextension, and traction
5. aortic dissection
6. embolization of spinal arteries
7. syphilitic endarteritis

83

Presentation

Onset: unlike cerebral infarcts, spinal cord infarcts tend to produce pain in addition to neurologic findings.

Neurologic findings are similar to spinal cord injury by any means. When the anterior spinal artery (p.87) is involved (which is common), an acute anterior spinal cord syndrome (p.1135) may develop (findings: motor paralysis below the level of the injury, loss of pain & temperature with preserved vibratory and position sense and loss of sphincter control).

Evaluation

When the source is not obvious (e.g., immediately following clamping of the aorta during AAA repair) the etiology of the infarct must be sought, including:

1. search for vascular abnormalities: arterial dissections (aorta for thoracic infarcts, vertebral for cervical), AVMs
2. looking for an infectious etiology
3. ruling out spinal cord compression
4. rule out hypercoagulable state

▶ **Imaging.** MRI is the diagnostic study of choice. Imaging sequences should include DWI to demonstrate ischemic tissue as increased signal (restricted diffusion) (▶ Fig. 83.10).

Diagnostic tests:
- routine bloodwork plus blood cultures to look for septicemia
- labs for hypercoagulable state (see e.g., Etiologies for stroke in young adults (p.1541)

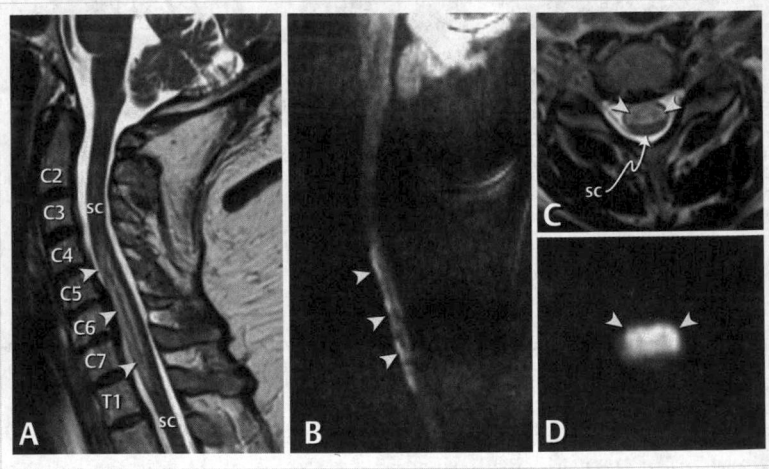

Fig. 83.10 Spinal cord infarction: increased MRI signal in the anterior spinal cord from C4 to T1 in a 55-year-old woman indicated by *yellow arrowheads*. No abnormality was seen on T1WI with or without contrast (not shown). Diagnosis suspected but unproven.
Image: cervical MRI, A: sagittal T2, B: sagittal DWI, C: axial T2, D: axial DWI.
Abbreviation: sc = spinal cord.

Management

Neurosurgical intervention is generally limited to cases of spinal cord compression or spinal instability.

83.7.5 Pneumorrhachis

General information

AKA pneumatorrhachis, intraspinal pneumocele, spinal pneumatosis and spinal emphysema.[110]
Definition: air within the spinal canal (intracranial air is called pneumocephalus). Classified as external pneumorrhachis (epidural) or internal pneumorrhachis (subdural or subarachnoid).[110,111] A rare condition most commonly seen in association with trauma (including surgery or certain invasive diagnostic testing) or with primary diseases of the respiratory tract.

83

Etiologies

1. trauma (penetrating - usually associated with external pneumorrhachis, or blunt - usually internal pneumorrhachis associated with pneumocephalus)
   a) spine fracture[110,111]
   b) pneumocephalus: spinal air from this is usually in the subarachnoid space and is more common with skull base fractures[110,111]
   c) pneumothorax
   d) pneumomediastinum
   e) iatrogenic
      • following thoracic spine surgery
      • epidural anesthesia[110,111]
      • after LP (e.g., diagnostic LP, or LP for myelography…)
      • following lumbar discectomy[112]
      • intentional injection of air: historically used diagnostically (so-called air myelogram)
2. non-traumatic
   a) pneumomediastinum[110,111]: 5.8% have associated pneumorrhachis,[113] (more common when all mediastinal compartments are involved)
   b) elevated intrathoracic pressure: e.g., acute exacerbation of coughing in bronchial asthma, emesis in diabetic ketoacidosis, CPR, and in foreign body aspiration causing airway obstruction[110]
   c) regional necrotizing fasciitis (rare)
   d) bronchial-subarachnoid fistula (AKA thoracoarachnoid fistula)[110,111,114]
   e) emphysematous pyelonephritis[115]
   f) opportunistic pneumonia in immunocompromised patients[116]

Presentation

Many cases are asymptomatic,[110,111] especially external pneumorrhachis. Reported findings have included:
1. new-onset radicular pain (cervical or lumbar)[110,111]
2. cauda equina syndrome[117]
3. positional headache[114]
4. transient unilateral lower extremity paresis[118]
5. unilateral distal upper extremity hypesthesia[111]

Evaluation

Non-contrast CT scan is probably the most sensitive test for detecting pneumorrhachis as well as air in other body compartments, but cannot reliably distinguish external from internal pneumorrhachis. Air shows up as dense black (see ▶ Fig. 83.11).
MRI is superior at delineating the anatomic boundaries of intraspinal air.[110,111]
Plain X-rays may detect large collections of air.[111]

Treatment

Air associated with asymptomatic pneumorrhachis in an otherwise stable patient will undergo spontaneous reabsorption over the course of a few days (particularly with external pneumorrhachis), possibly expedited by the delivery of hyperbaric oxygen.[110,111]

83

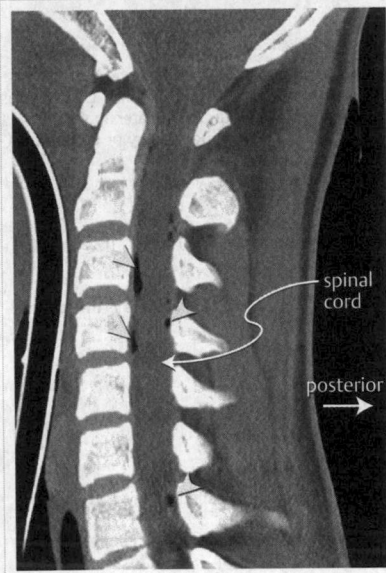

Fig. 83.11 Pneumorrhachis in a polytrauma patient who also had pneumocephalus.
Air (*yellow arrowheads*) appears as densely black areas anterior and posterior to the spinal cord.
Image: non-contrast sagittal CT of the cervical spine.

Antibiotics are not indicated in the absence of spinal infection (meningitis) or extraspinal indications.

Surgical indications:
1. intracranial hypo-/hypertension refractory to medical management
2. significant or persistent CSF leak[110,111,112]
3. evidence of unidirectional ball valve (termed tension pneumorrhachis)[119] near at-risk nervous tissue
4. herniation or serious injury of adjacent structures (e.g., lung) into the spinal cord

Surgical considerations:
1. surgical intervention is often directed at the underlying etiology, and may require a multidisciplinary approach
2. inhalational nitrous oxide diffuses into air-filled spaces, causing expansion of existing cavitary air, and further raising the CSF pressure which can worsen coexistent pneumocephalus
3. techniques that add pressure to the nasopharynx or oropharynx are contraindicated for similar reasons
4. intermittent positive-pressure ventilation with hyperbaric oxygen therapy has been recommended[110]

Outcome

While pneumorrhachis may be associated with an increased morbidity and mortality risk (particularly internal pneumorrhachis in the setting of severe trauma[117]), the appropriate evaluation and management of this often self-limiting condition results in reversal of symptomatology and no permanent deficit in most cases.

83.7.6 Airport screening and spinal implants

Patients often ask or may be advised about the issue of airport or other screening procedures in the presence of spinal implants.

- archway metal detectors do not detect any current era (titanium alloy) spinal implants regardless of the quantity or location (anterior or posterior, cervical, lumbar or thoracic) or patient's BMI[120]
- hand-held "wand" metal detectors may detect the following (this may be important e.g., for patients that are screened with a wand after triggering the archway detector from non-spinal sources)
  - all posterior instruments (cervical, lumbar, thoracic)[120]
  - anterior instruments only in the cervical spine[120]
- full-body scanners (utilizing "back-scatter" of low-dose ionizing radiation) cannot detect implants deeper than a few millimeters below the skin surface

83.7.7 Catheter tip granuloma

General information

Catheter-associated inflammatory masses (CIMs), AKA catheter tip granulomas, are a recognized complication that may be associated with a number of intrathecal devices. An inflammatory reaction at the tip of the catheter produces a mass[121] arising from the arachnoid layer of the meninges[122] composed of macrophages, plasma cells, eosinophils, and lymphocytes.[123] CIMs are usually intra-dural and extramedullary, but may rarely be extradural or intramedullary.[124]

Granulation tissue has been associated with intrathecal drug delivery systems (IDDS) utilizing opioids, especially morphine,[125] but also other agents including hydromorphone, fentanyl, trama-dol,[126] sufentanil,[127] methadone, baclofen,[128] clonidine,[129] and ziconiotide. Non-drug delivery devices have also been implicated, including: lumbar shunts,[130] ventricular shunts,[131,132] and spinal cord stimulators.[133]

Epidemiology

Reported incidence range of CIMs: 0.1–5% of intrathecal drug systems.[134,135] The average time for development of a CIM after initiation of infusion therapy is 39.5 ± 13.5 months.[136] However, granulo-mas can also occur within months of catheter placement.[136]

Etiology

The exact mechanism remains unknown. Granuloma formation is thought to be related to the migra-tion of inflammatory cells from the meningeal vasculature and not dependent on opioid receptor activation.[137] Although the mass is typically sterile, bacterial infections have been implicated, sug-gesting CIMs be evaluated for the presence of aerobic and anaerobic bacteria.[138] Factors such as drug concentration, CSF flow rate, drug distribution, drug flow rate (with low flow rates thought to be more likely to increase risk), anatomic variance that disrupts CSF flow, prior history of granuloma, and duration of infusion have all been noted to predispose a patient to granuloma formation.[139] The association between drug dose and concentration delivered is considered the most contributory to granuloma formation.[136] No relation between catheter tip location or catheter material and CIM for-mation has been identified to date.

Signs and symptoms

For patients receiving intrathecal opioids, the most common presentation is an increase in pain, pos-sibly related to decreased opioid release due to granuloma obstruction.[140] This is often misinter-preted as opioid tolerance; a yearly increase in opioid dose should be regarded as a warning sign.[136] New radicular pain in the dermatomal level corresponding to the catheter tip also warrants investi-gation. Other signs and symptoms reflective of spinal cord dysfunction include myelopathy, paraes-thesias, bowel and bladder dysfunction, radicular pain, paralysis, paraplegia, paresis, and generalized weakness or lower extremity muscle weakness.

Diagnosis

Gadolinium-contrasted MRI with thin slices is the gold standard for diagnosis. However, routine screening is not cost-effective given the low incidence.[134] Granuloma appears: isointense on T1 with rim enhancement (▶ Fig. 83.12); hyperintense on T2. If MRI is not an option, CT myelogram may be used.

Addition of a CT scan allows for correlation of catheter tip and the mass, as the catheter tip material may obstruct direct visualization on MRI.[139]

The differential on imaging may also include abscess or tumor.

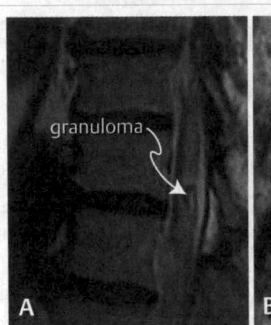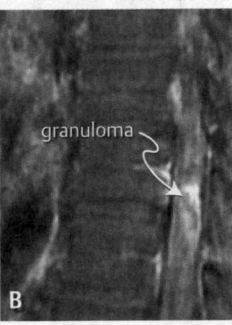

Fig. 83.12 Catheter tip granuloma. Image: sagittal thoracic MRI, A: T1 noncontrast, B: T1 with gadolinium contrast.

Management

Treatment of catheter granulomas is highly influenced by a patient's clinical status, size of the granuloma, and prior history of CIMs.

The following are treatment guidelines by expert panels at the Polyanalgesic Consensus Conferences (PACC) in 2007 and 2012.[135,139]

If a patient requires frequent increases in medication dose or concentration, or presents with changes in neurological status (motor, sensory, or proprioceptive function), obtain an MRI with gadolinium contrast or a CT myelogram. The flow chart in ▶ Fig. 83.13 outlines the management guidelines.

Conservative management (changing drug or concentration…) is also used for asymptomatic patients (i.e., an incidentally discovered granuloma). Granuloma regression has been demonstrated over time.

The patient should be awake during withdrawal or removal of a catheter. If paresthesias or resistance is encountered, an open surgical removal should be performed.

Prevention

Preclinical evidence suggests that adding clonidine to opioid infusions decreases the risk of granuloma formation.[122] However, case reports have challenged translation to humans. Evidence for nonopioid alternatives, such as ziconotide[139] have been indeterminate, with some case reports demonstrating regression[141] and others showing persistence of inflammation[142] after substitution.

According to the PACC, decreasing the dose and concentration may be among the most effective ways to prevent or delay onset of granuloma formation.[135] One study demonstrated almost 50% reduction in relative risk of CIM formation by reducing the dose and concentration of morphine from the recommended maximum of 15 mg/day and 20 mg/mL to 10 mg/day and 15 mg/mL.[143] Bolus dosing instead of continuous infusion may further limit continuous exposure and reduce the risk.[139]

Previous recommendations to place the catheter tip below the conus have not proven to be clinically significant.[139] However, consensus is to place the tip as close to the pain level as possible to minimize dilution of the drug by diffusion to achieve similar concentration of drug at the target with lower doses. Experts have anecdotally recommended dorsal placement of catheters given a larger CSF space and because granuloma formation would be easier to treat surgically.[135]

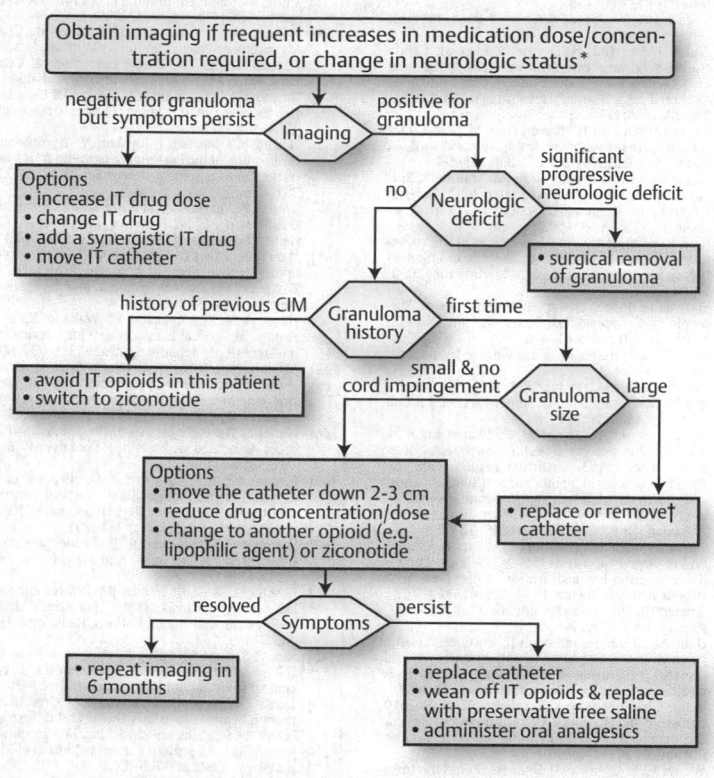

Fig. 83.13 A management algorithm for catheter tip granulomas.
Adapted from Deer TR, Prager J, Levy R, et al. Polyanalgesic Consensus Conference–2012: Consensus on diagnosis, detection, and treatment of catheter-tip granulomas (inflammatory masses). Neuromodulation 2012;15(5):483–496.
* changes in neurological status include motor, sensory, or proprioceptive function. Imaging consists of enhanced MRI or CT/myelogram.
Abbreviations: CIM = catheter-associated inflammatory mass; IT = intrathecal.
† the algorithm does not indicate what to do if the catheter is removed

References

[1] Walpin LA, Singer FR. Paget's Disease: Reversal of Severe Paraparesis Using Calcitonin. Spine. 1979; 4:213–219

[2] Youmans JR. Neurological Surgery. Philadelphia 1990

[3] Delmas PD, Meunier PJ. The Management of Paget's Disease of Bone. New England Journal of Medicine. 1997; 336:558–566

[4] Meunier PJ, Salson C, Mathieu L, et al. Skeletal Distribution and Biochemical Parameters of Paget's Disease. Clinical Orthopedics. 1987; 217:37–44

[5] Rothman RH, Simeone FA. The Spine. Philadelphia 1992

[6] Altman RD, Brown M, Gargano F. Low Back Pain in Paget's Disease of Bone. Clin Orthop. 1987; 217:152–161

[7] Hadjipavlou A, Shaffer N, Lander P, et al. Pagetic Spinal Stenosis with Extradural Pagetoid Ossification. Spine. 1988; 13:128–130

[8] Douglas DL, Duckworth T, Kanis JA, et al. Spinal Cord Dysfunction in Paget's Disease of Bone: Has Medical Treatment a Vascular Basis? J Bone Joint Surg. 1981; 63B:495–503

[9] Wilkins RH, Rengachary SS. Neurosurgery. New York 1985

[10] Dinneen SF, Buckley TF. Spinal Nerve Root Compression due to Monostotic Paget's Disease of a Lumbar Vertebra. Spine. 1987; 12:948–950

[11] Sadar ES, Walton RJ, Gossman HH. Neurological Dysfunction in Paget's Disease of the Vertebral Column. J Neurosurg. 1972; 37:661–665

[12] Chen J-R, Rhee RSC, Wallach S, et al. Neurologic Disturbances in Paget Disease of Bone: Response to Calcitonin. Neurology. 1979; 29:448–457

[13] Human Calcitonin for Paget's Disease. Medical Letter. 1987; 29:47–48

83

[14] Tiludronate for Paget's Disease of Bone. Medical Letter. 1997; 39:65–66

[15] Risedronate for Paget's Disease of Bone. Medical Letter. 1998; 40:87–88

[16] Ahn NU, Ahn UM, Nallamshetty L, et al. Cauda equina syndrome in ankylosing spondylitis (the CES-AS syndrome): meta-analysis of outcomes after medical and surgical treatments. J Spinal Disord. 2001; 14:427–433

[17] Caron T, Bransford R, Nguyen Q, et al. Spine fractures in patients with ankylosing spinal disorders. Spine (Phila Pa 1976). 2010; 35:E458–E464

[18] Farhat SM, Schneider RC, Gray JM. Traumatic Spinal Epidural Hematoma Associated with Cervical Fractures in Rheumatoid Spondylitis. Journal of Trauma. 1973; 13:591–599

[19] Bron JL, de Vries MK, Snieders MN, et al. Discovertebral (Andersson) lesions of the spine in ankylosing spondylitis revisited. Clin Rheumatol. 2009; 28:883–892

[20] Stolwijk C, Boonen A, van Tubergen A, et al. Epidemiology of spondyloarthritis. Rheum Dis Clin North Am. 2012; 38:441–476

[21] Calin A. Early diagnosis of ankylosing spondylitis. Lancet. 1977; 2

[22] Rae PS, Waddell G, Venner RM. A Simple Technique for Measuring Lumbar Spinal Flexion. J R Coll Surg Edin. 1984; 29:281–284

[23] van den Berg R, de Hooge M, Rudwaleit M, et al. ASAS modification of the Berlin algorithm for diagnosing axial spondyloarthritis: results from the SPondyloArthritis Caught Early (SPACE)-cohort and from the Assessment of SpondyloArthritis international Society (ASAS)-cohort. Annals of the Rheumatic Diseases. 2013; 72:1646–1653

[24] van der Linden S, Valkenburg HA, Cats A. Evaluation of diagnostic criteria for ankylosing spondylitis. A proposal for modification of the New York criteria. Arthritis Rheum. 1984; 27:361–368

[25] Bennett GJ. Ankylosing Spondylitis. Clinical Neurosurgery. 1991; 37:622–635

[26] Qubti MA, Flynn JA, Imboden JB, et al. Ankylosing spondylitis & the arthritis of inflammatory bowel disease. In: Current rheumatology diagnosis & treatment. 1st ed. New York: McGraw-Hill; 2004

[27] Braun J, van den Berg R, Baraliakos X, et al. 2010 update of the ASAS/EULAR recommendations for the management of ankylosing spondylitis. Ann Rheum Dis. 2011; 70:896–904

[28] Westerveld LA, Verlaan JJ, Oner FC. Spinal fractures in patients with ankylosing spinal disorders: a systematic review of the literature on treatment, neurological status and complications. Eur Spine J. 2009; 18:145–156

[29] Clarke A, James S, Ahuja S. Ankylosing spondylitis: inadvertent application of a rigid collar after cervical fracture, leading to neurological complications and death. Acta Orthop Belg. 2010; 76:413–415

[30] Detwiler KN, Loftus CM, Godersky JC. Management of Cervical Spine Injuries in Patients with Ankylosing Spondylitis. Journal of Neurosurgery. 1990; 72:210–215

[31] Schneider PS, Bouchard J, Moghadam K, et al. Acute cervical fractures in ankylosing spondylitis: an opportunity to correct preexisting deformity. Spine (Phila Pa 1976). 2010; 35:E248–E252

[32] Kanter AS, Wang MY, Mummaneni PV. A treatment algorithm for the management of cervical spine fractures and deformity in patients with ankylosing spondylitis. Neurosurg Focus. 2008; 24. DOI: 10.3171/FOC/2008/24/1/E11

[33] Chaudhary SB, Hullinger H, Vives MJ. Management of acute spinal fractures in ankylosing spondylitis. ISRN Rheumatol. 2011; 2011. DOI: 10.5402/2011/150484

[34] Trent G, Armstrong GW, O'Neil J. Thoracolumbar fractures in ankylosing spondylitis. High-risk injuries. Clin Orthop Relat Res. 1988; 227:61–66

[35] Van Royen BJ, De Gast A. Lumbar osteotomy for correction of thoracolumbar kyphotic deformity in ankylosing spondylitis. A structured review of three methods of treatment. Ann Rheum Dis. 1999; 58:399–406

[36] Dinichert A, Cornelius JF, Lot G. Lumboperitoneal shunt for treatment of dural ectasia in ankylosing spondylitis. J Clin Neurosci. 2008; 15:1179–1182

[37] Holmes MG, Dagal A, Feinstein BA, et al. Airway Management Practice in Adults With an Unstable Cervical Spine: The Harborview Medical Center Experience. Anesth Analg. 2018; 127:450–454

[38] Tsuyama N. Ossification of the Posterior Longitudinal Ligament of the Spine. Clinical Orthopedics. 1984; 184:71–84

[39] Nakanishi T, Mannen T, Toyokura Y. Asymptomatic Ossification of the Posterior Longitudinal Ligament of the Cervical Spine. J Neurol Sci. 1973; 19:375–381

[40] Epstein N. Diagnosis and Surgical Management of Ossification of the Posterior Longitudinal Ligament. Contemporary Neurosurgery. 1992; 14:1–6

[41] Harsh GR, Sypert GW, Weinstein PR, et al. Cervical Spine Stenosis Secondary to Ossification of the Posterior Longitudinal Ligament. Journal of Neurosurgery. 1987; 67:349–357

[42] Hirabayashi K, Watanabe K, Wakano K, et al. Expansive Cervical Laminoplasty for Cervical Spinal Stenotic Myelopathy. Spine. 1983; 8:693–693

[43] Matsunaga S, Sakou T, Taketomi E, et al. Clinical course of patients with ossification of the posterior longitudinal ligament: a minimum 10-year cohort study. J Neurosurg. 2004; 100:245–248

[44] Nurick S. The Pathogenesis of the Spinal Cord Disorder Associated with Cervical Spondylosis. Brain. 1972; 95:87–100

[45] Epstein NE, Hollingsworth R. Ossification of the Cervical Anterior Longitudinal Ligament Contributing to Dysphagia: Case Report. Journal of Neurosurgery. 1999; 90 (Spine 2):261–263

[46] Forestier J, Rotes-Querol J. Senile ankylosing hyperostosis of the spine. Ann Rheum Dis. 1950; 9:321–330

[47] Resnick D, Shaul SR, Robins JM. Diffuse idiopathic skeletal hyperostosis (DISH): Forestier's disease with extraspinal manifestations. Radiology. 1975; 115:513–524

[48] Kiss C, Szilagyi M, Paksy A, et al. Risk factors for diffuse idiopathic skeletal hyperostosis: a case-control study. Rheumatology. 2002; 41:27–30

[49] Denko CW, Boja B, Moskowitz RW. Growth promoting peptides in osteoarthritis and diffuse idiopathic skeletal hyperostosis–insulin, insulin-like growth factor-I, growth hormone. Journal of Rheumatology. 1994; 21:1725–1730

[50] Burkus JK. Esophageal Obstruction Secondary to Diffuse Idiopathic Skeletal Hyperostosis. Orthopedics. 1988; 11:717–720

[51] McCafferty RR, Harrison MJ, Tamas LB, et al. Ossification of the Anterior Longitudinal Ligament and Forestier's Disease: An Analysis of Seven Cases. Journal of Neurosurgery. 1995; 83:13–17

[52] Scheuermann HW. The classic: kyphosis dorsalis juvenilis. Clin Orthop Relat Res. 1977:5–7

[53] Ali RM, Green DW, Patel TC. Scheuermann's kyphosis. Curr Opin Pediatr. 1999; 11:70–75

[54] Damborg F, Engell V, Andersen M, et al. Prevalence, concordance, and heritability of Scheuermann kyphosis based on a study of twins. J Bone Joint Surg Am. 2006; 88:2133–2136

[55] Blumenthal SL, Roach J, Herring JA. Lumbar Scheuermann's. A clinical series and classification. Spine (Phila Pa 1976). 1987; 12:929–932

[56] Sorensen KH, la Cour Anna(née Claessen). Scheuermann's Juvenile Kyphosis: Clinical Appearances, Radiography, Aetiology, and Prognosis. Copenhagen, Denmark: Munksgaard (Blackwell Munksgaard); 1964

[57] Ogilvie JW, Sherman J. Spondylolysis in Scheuermann's disease. Spine (Phila Pa 1976). 1987; 12:251–253

[58] Weiss HR, Dieckmann J, Gerner HJ. Effect of intensive rehabilitation on pain in patients with Scheuermann's disease. Stud Health Technol Inform. 2002; 88:254–257

[59] Cho KJ, Lenke LG, Bridwell KH, et al. Selection of the optimal distal fusion level in posterior instrumentation and fusion for thoracic hyperkyphosis:

[60] Ranawat CS, O'Leary P, Pellicci P, et al. Cervical Spine Fusion in Rheumatoid Arthritis. Journal of Bone and Joint Surgery. 1979; 61A:1003–1010

[61] Menezes AH, VanGilder JC, Clark CR, et al. Odontoid upward migration in rheumatoid arthritis. An analysis of 45 patients with "cranial settling". J Neurosurg. 1985; 63:500–509

[62] Rana NA, Hancock DO, Taylor AR. Atlanto-Axial Subluxation in Rheumatoid Arthritis. J Bone Joint Surg. 1973; 55B:458–470

[63] Hildebrandt G, Agnoli AL, Zierski J. Atlanto-Axial Dislocation in Rheumatoid Arthritis: Diagnostic and Therapeutic Aspects. Acta Neurochirurgica. 1987; 84:110–117

[64] Hinck VC, Hopkins CE. Measurement of the Atlanto-Dental Interval in the Adult. Am J Roentgenol Radium Ther Nucl Med. 1960; 84:945–951

[65] Meijers KAE, van Beusekom GT, Luyendijk W, et al. Dislocation of the Cervical Spine with Cord Compression in Rheumatoid Arthritis. J Bone Joint Surg. 1974; 56B:668–680

[66] Boden SD, Dodge LD, Bohlman HH, et al. Rheumatoid arthritis of the cervical spine. A long-term analysis with predictors of paralysis and recovery. Journal of Bone and Joint Surgery. 1993; 75:1282–1297

[67] Collins DN, Barnes CL, FitzRandolph RL. Cervical spine instability in rheumatoid patients having total hip or knee arthroplasty. Clin Orthop Relat Res. 1991:127–135

[68] Smith PH, Benn RT, Sharp J. Natural History of Rheumatoid Cervical Luxations. Ann Rheum Dis. 1972; 31:431–439

[69] Weissman BNW, Aliabadi P, Weinfeld MS, et al. Prognostic Features of Atlantoaxial Subluxation in Rheumatoid Arthritis Patients. Radiology. 1982; 144:745–751

[70] Papadopoulos SM, Dickman CA, Sonntag VKH. Atlantoaxial Stabilization in Rheumatoid Arthritis. J Neurosurg. 1991; 74:1–7

[71] Mikulowski P, Wollheim FA, Rotmil P, et al. Sudden death in rheumatoid arthritis with atlanto-axial dislocation. Acta Medica Scandinavica. 1975; 198:445–451

[72] Kourtopoulos H, von Essen C. Stabilization of the Unstable Upper Cervical Spine in Rheumatoid Arthritis. Acta Neurochirurgica. 1988; 91:113–115

[73] Clark CR, Goetz DD, Menezes AH. Arthrodesis of the Cervical Spine in Rheumatoid Arthritis. J Bone Joint Surg. 1989; 71A:381–392

[74] Riew KD, Hilibrand AS, Palumbo MA, et al. Diagnosing basilar invagination in the rheumatoid patient. The reliability of radiographic criteria. Journal of Bone and Joint Surgery. 2001; 83-A:194–200

[75] Redlund-Johnell I, Pettersson H. Radiographic measurements of the cranio-vertebral region. Designed for evaluation of abnormalities in rheumatoid arthritis. Acta Radiologica: Diagnosis. 1984; 25:23–28

[76] Bundschuh C, Modic MT, Kearney F, et al. Rheumatoid arthritis of the cervical spine: surface-coil MR imaging. AJR. American Journal of Roentgenology. 1988; 151:181–187

[77] Kim DH, Hilibrand AS. Rheumatoid arthritis in the cervical spine. Journal of the American Academy of Orthopaedic Surgeons. 2005; 13:463–474

[78] Martel W, Tishler JM. Observations on the spine in mongoloidism. American Journal of Roentgenology, Radium Therapy and Nuclear Medicine. 1966; 97:630–638

[79] Pueschel SM. Should children with Down syndrome be screened for atlantoaxial instability? Archives of Pediatrics and Adolescent Medicine. 1998; 152:123–125

[80] American Academy of Pediatrics Committee on Sports Medicine and Fitness. Atlantoaxial instability in Down syndrome: subject review. Pediatrics. 1995; 96:151–154

[81] Cohen WI. Atlantoaxial instability. What's next? Archives of Pediatrics and Adolescent Medicine. 1998; 152:119–122

[82] Brockmeyer D. Down syndrome and craniovertebral instability. Topic review and treatment recommendations. Pediatr Neurosurg. 1999; 31:71–77

[83] George WE, Wilmot M, Greenhouse A, et al. Medical Management of Steroid-Induced Epidural Lipomatosis. N Engl J Med. 1983; 308:316–319

[84] Fassett DR, Schmidt MH. Spinal epidural lipomatosis: a review of its causes and recommendations for treatment. Neurosurg Focus. 2004; 16

[85] Kumar K, Nath RK, Nair CPV, et al. Symptomatic Epidural Lipomatosis Secondary to Obesity: Case Report. J Neurosurg. 1996; 85:348–350

[86] Theyskens NC, Paulino Pereira N R, Janssen SJ, et al. The prevalence of spinal epidural lipomatosis on magnetic resonance imaging. Spine J. 2017; 17:969–976

[87] Haddad SF, Hitchon PW, Godersky. Idiopathic and Glucocorticoid-Induced Spinal Epidural Lipomatosis. J Neurosurg. 1991; 74:38–42

[88] Roy-Camille R, Mazel C, Husson JL, et al. Symptomatic spinal epidural lipomatosis induced by a long-term steroid treatment. Review of the literature and report of two additional cases. Spine. 1991; 16:1365–1371

[89] Robertson SC, Traynelis VC, Follett KA, et al. Idiopathic spinal epidural lipomatosis. Neurosurgery. 1997; 41:68–75

[90] Beges C, Rousselin B, Chevrot A, et al. Epidural lipomatosis. Interest of magnetic resonance imaging in a weight-reduction treated case. Spine. 1994; 19:251–254

[91] Fessler RD, Johnson DL, Brown FD, et al. Epidural lipomatosis in steroid-treated patients. Spine. 1992; 17:183–188

[92] Brault JS, Smith J, Currier BL. Partial lumbosacral transitional vertebra resection for contralateral facetogenic pain. Spine (Phila Pa 1976). 2001; 26:226–229

[93] Ugokwe KT, Chen TL, Klineberg E, et al. Minimally invasive surgical treatment of Bertolotti's Syndrome: case report. Neurosurgery. 2008; 62: ONSE454–5; discussion ONSE456

[94] Mitra R, Carlisle M. Bertolotti's syndrome: a case report. Pain Pract. 2009; 9:152–154

[95] Santavirta S, Tallroth K, Ylinen P, et al. Surgical treatment of Bertolotti's syndrome. Follow-up of 16 patients. Archives of Orthopaedic and Trauma Surgery. 1993; 112:82–87

[96] Tekkok IH, Cataltepe K, Tahta K, et al. Extradural Hematoma After Continuous Extradural Anesthesia. Brit J Anaesth. 1991; 67:112–115

[97] Harik SI, Raichle ME, Reis DJ. Spontaneous Remitting Spinal Epidural Hematoma in a Patient on Anticoagulants. N Engl J Med. 1971; 284:1355–1357

[98] Silber SH. Complete Nonsurgical Resolution of a Spontaneous Spinal Epidural Hematoma. Am J Emergency Med. 1996; 14:391–393

[99] Shnider SM, Levinson G. Neurologic Complications of Regional Anesthesia. In: Anesthesia for Obstetrics. 2nd ed. Baltimore: Williams and Wilkins; 1987:319–320

[100] Sage DJ. Epidurals, Spinals and Bleeding Disorders in Pregnancy: A Review. Anaesth Intens Care. 1990; 18:319–326

[101] Gustafsson H, Rutberg H, Bengtsson M. Spinal Hematoma Following Epidural Analgesia: Report of a Patient with Ankylosing Spondylitis and a Bleeding Diathesis. Anaesthesia. 1988; 43:220–222

[102] Porter RW, Detwiler PW, Lawton MT, et al. Postoperative Spinal Epidural Hematomas: Longitudinal Review of 12,000 Spinal Operations. BNI Quarterly. 2000; 16:10–17

[103] Domenicucci M, Ramieri A, Salvati M, et al. Cervicothoracic epidural hematoma after chiropractic spinal manipulation therapy. Case report and review of the literature. J Neurosurg Spine. 2007; 7:571–574

[104] Dickman CA, Shedd SA, Spetzler RF, et al. Spinal Epidural Hematoma Associated with Epidural Anesthesia: Complications of Systemic Heparinization in Patients Receiving Peripheral Vascular Thrombolytic Therapy. 1990; 72

[105] Packer NP, Cummins BH. Spontaneous Epidural Hemorrhage: A Surgical Emergency. Lancet. 1978; 1:356–358

[106] Bennett DL, George MJ, Ohashi K, et al. Acute traumatic spinal epidural hematoma: imaging and neurologic outcome. Emerg Radiol. 2005; 11:136–144

[107] Rebello MD, Dastur HM. Spinal Epidural Hemorrhage: A Review of Case Reports. Neurol India. 1966; 14:135–145

[108] Domenicucci M, Ramieri A, Ciappetta P, et al. Non-traumatic Acute Spinal Subdural Hematoma. Journal of Neurosurgery. 1999; (Spine 1) 91:65–73

[109] Epstein NE, Danto J, Nardi D. Evaluation of Intraoperative Somatosensory-Evoked Potential Monitoring During 100 Cervical Operations. Spine. 1993; 18:737–747

[110] Oertel MF, Korinth MC, Reinges MH, et al. Pathogenesis, diagnosis and management of pneumorrhachis. Eur Spine J. 2006; 15 Suppl 5:636–643

[111] Hadjigeorgiou GF, Singh R, Stefanopoulos P, et al. Traumatic pneumorrhachis after isolated closed head injuries: An up-to-date review. J Clin Neurosci. 2016; 34:44–46

[112] Karavelioglu E, Eser O, Haktanir A. Pneumocephalus and pneumorrhachis after spinal surgery: case report and review of the literature. Neurol Med Chir (Tokyo). 2014; 54:405–407

[113] Behr G, Mema E, Costa K, et al. Proportion and Clinical Relevance of Intraspinal Air in Patients With Pneumomediastinum. AJR Am J Roentgenol. 2018; 211:321–326

[114] Kazimirko DN, Parker EE, Joyner DA, et al. An unusual cause of acute headache: subarachnoid free air secondary to spontaneous bronchopleuro-durosubarachnoid fistula from a Pancoast tumor. Radiol Case Rep. 2016; 11:238–241

[115] Gomez CA, Vela-Duarte D, Veldkamp PJ. Infectious Pneumorrhachis Due to Emphysematous Pyelonephritis. JAMA Neurol. 2017; 74:1374–1375

[116] Saleem N, Parveen S, Odigwe C, et al. Pneumomediastinum, pneumorrhachis, and subcutaneous emphysema in Pneumocystis jiroveci pneumonia in AIDS. Proc (Bayl Univ Med Cent). 2016; 29:188–190

[117] Paik NC, Lim CS, Jang HS. Cauda equina syndrome caused by epidural pneumorrhachis: treatment with percutaneous computed tomography-guided translaminar trephination. Spine (Phila Pa 1976). 2013; 38:E440–E443

[118] Payne R, Sieg EP, Choudhary A, et al. Pneumorrhachis Resulting in Transient Paresis after PICC Line Insertion into the Ascending Lumbar Vein. Cureus. 2016; 8. DOI: 10.7759/cureus.833

[119] Kieser DC, Cawley DT, Tavolaro C, et al. Delayed post-operative tension pneumocephalus and pneumorrhachis. Eur Spine J. 2018; 27:231–235

[120] Chinwalla F, Grevitt MP. Detection of modern spinal implants by airport metal detectors. Spine (Phila Pa 1976). 2012; 37:2011–2016

[121] Blount JP, Remley KB, Yue SK, et al. Intrathecal granuloma complicating chronic spinal infusion of morphine. Report of three cases. J Neurosurg. 1996; 84:272–276

[122] Yaksh TL, Horais KA, Tozier NA, et al. Chronically infused intrathecal morphine in dogs. Anesthesiology. 2003; 99:174–187

[123] Allen JW, Horais KA, Tozier NA, et al. Time course and role of morphine dose and concentration in intrathecal granuloma formation in dogs: a combined magnetic resonance imaging and histopathology investigation. Anesthesiology. 2006; 105:581–589

[124] Jhas S, Tuli S. Intrathecal catheter-tip inflammatory masses: an intraparenchymal granuloma. J Neurosurg Spine. 2008; 9:196–199

[125] Bejjani GK, Karim NO, Tzortzidis F. Intrathecal granuloma after implantation of a morphine pump: case report and review of the literature. Surg Neurol. 1997; 48:288–291

[126] De Andres J, Tatay Vivo J, Palmisani S, et al. Intrathecal granuloma formation in a patient receiving long-term spinal infusion of tramadol. Pain Med. 2010; 11:1059–1062

[127] Gupta A, Martindale T, Christo PJ. Intrathecal catheter granuloma associated with continuous sufentanil infusion. Pain Med. 2010; 11:847–852

[128] Deer TR, Raso LJ, Garten TG. Inflammatory mass of an intrathecal catheter in patients receiving baclofen as a sole agent: a report of two cases and a review of the identification and treatment of the complication. Pain Med. 2007; 8:259–262

[129] Toombs JD, Follett KA, Rosenquist RW, et al. Intrathecal catheter tip inflammatory mass: a failure of clonidine to protect. Anesthesiology. 2005; 102:687–690

[130] Vural M, Ozkara E, Adapinar B, et al. A late and extreme complication of lumboperitoneal shunt. Spine J. 2015; 15:e7–12

[131] de Oliveira RS, Amato MC, Brassesco MS, et al. Clinical and cytogenetic analysis of an intracranial inflammatory myofibroblastic tumor induced by a ventriculoperitoneal shunt. J Neurosurg Pediatr. 2009; 4:372–377

[132] Millward CP, Perez da Rosa S, Williams D, et al. Foreign body granuloma secondary to ventriculo-peritoneal shunt: a rare scenario with a new insight. Pediatr Neurosurg. 2013; 49:236–239

[133] Scranton RA, Skaribas IM, Simpson RK,Jr. Spinal stimulator peri-electrode masses: case report. J Neurosurg Spine. 2015; 22:70–74

[134] Deer TR. A prospective analysis of intrathecal granuloma in chronic pain patients: a review of the literature and report of a surveillance study. Pain Physician. 2004; 7:225–228

[135] Deer T, Krames ES, Hassenbusch S, et al. Management of intrathecal catheter-tip inflammatory masses: an updated 2007 consensus statement from an expert panel. Neuromodulation. 2008; 11:77–91

[136] Duarte RV, Raphael JH, Southall JL, et al. Intrathecal inflammatory masses: is the yearly opioid dose increase an early indicator? Neuromodulation. 2010; 13:109–113

[137] Allen JW, Horais KA, Tozier NA, et al. Opiate pharmacology of intrathecal granulomas. Anesthesiology. 2006; 105:590–598

[138] Miele VJ, Price KO, Bloomfield S, et al. A review of intrathecal morphine therapy related granulomas. Eur J Pain. 2006; 10:251–261

[139] Deer TR, Prager J, Levy R, et al. Polyanalgesic Consensus Conference–2012: consensus on diagnosis detection, and treatment of catheter-tip granulomas (inflammatory masses). Neuromodulation. 2012; 15:483–95; discussion 496

[140] Bloomfield S, Hogg J, Ortiz O, et al. Analysis o breakthrough pain in 50 patients treated with intrathecal morphine infusion therapy. Development of tolerance or infusion system malfunction Stereotact Funct Neurosurg. 1995; 65:142–146

[141] Codipietro L, Maino P. Aseptic arachnoiditis in a patient treated with intrathecal morphine infusion: symptom resolution on switch to ziconotide Neuromodulation. 2015; 18:217–20; discussion 220

[142] Tomycz ND, Ortiz V, McFadden KA, et al. Management of symptomatic intrathecal catheter-associated inflammatory masses. Clin Neurol Neurosurg 2012; 114:190–195

[143] Duarte RV, Raphael JH, Southall JL, et al. Intrathecal granuloma formation as result of opioid delivery systematic literature review of case reports and analysis against a control group. Clin Neuro Neurosurg. 2012; 114:577–584

84 Special Conditions Affecting the Spinal Cord

84.1 Spinal vascular malformations

84.1.1 General information

Often also referred to by the term spinal AVMs, which technically refers to a subset of spinal vascular malformations (SVMs). Incidence of SVM is about 4% of primary intraspinal masses. 80% occur between age 20 and 60 years.[1](p 1850–3)

84.1.2 Classification

For a review of the history of classification systems, see the excellent review by Black.[2]
There are three current-era classification systems.

The "American/English/French Connection" classification

References for classification: include[2,3,4,5,6,7,8,9,10]
1. **Type I:** dural AVM, AKA AV-fistula (AVF) or dural AV-fistula (dAVF). The most common type (80%) of SVM in the adult.[11] Fed by a radicular artery, which forms an AV shunt (fistula) at the dural root sleeve (located in the intervertebral foramen)[8] and drains into an engorged vein that connects to the venous system on the *posterior* cord. Usually in lumbar or lower thoracic spine. Slow flow. High pressure in the draining veins causes venous congestion of the cord. MRI characteristically shows spinal cord edema and flow voids and/or serpiginous vessels on the surface of the cord (panel A in ► Fig. 84.1). Cord involvement may be distant to the fistula. Symptoms: LBP and progressive myeloradiculopathy or cauda equina syndrome (due to venous congestion) with urinary retention usually in middle-aged patients, 90% males. Up to 35% have pain. 15–20% are associated with other AVMs (cutaneous or other). Rarely bleed
   a) Type IA: single arterial feeder
   b) Type IB: two or more arterial feeders
2. intradural AVMs (high flow): 75% present with acute onset of symptoms, usually from hemorrhage (SAH or intramedullary)
   a) **Type II:** AKA spinal glomus AVM. Intramedullary. True AVM of the spinal cord. 15–20% of all SVMs. Compact nidus fed by medullary arteries with the AV shunt contained at least partially within the spinal cord or pia. May be associated with feeding artery aneurysms. Worse prognosis than dural AVM.[8] Fed by 1, or at most 2–3 feeders 80% of the time
   b) **Type III:** AKA juvenile spinal AVM. Essentially an enlarged glomus AVM which occupies the entire cross-section of the cord and invades the vertebral body which may cause scoliosis
   c) **Type IV**[7]: intradural perimedullary AVM (also called arteriovenous fistulae (AVF)). Direct fistula between artery supplying spinal cord (usually anterior spinal artery, often the artery of Adamkiewicz (► Fig. 84.2)) and draining veins. Typically occur in younger patients than Type I, and may present catastrophically with hemorrhage into the subarachnoid space.[12] ► Table 84.1 shows the 3 subtypes[9]
3. miscellaneous spinal vascular lesions:
   a) spinal cord cavernomas
   b) spinal cord venous angiomas: extremely rare. Difficult to visualize angiographically
   c) vertebral body hemangiomas (p.992)

Hôpital Bicêtre classification

See reference.[13]
1. AVMs
2. fistulae: micro- or macrofistulae
3. genetic classification of spinal cord

AV shunts
a) genetic hereditary lesions: macrofistulae and hereditary hemorrhagic telangiectasias
b) genetic nonhereditary lesions: multiple lesions with metameric or myelomeric associations
c) single lesions: incomplete associations of categories a or b

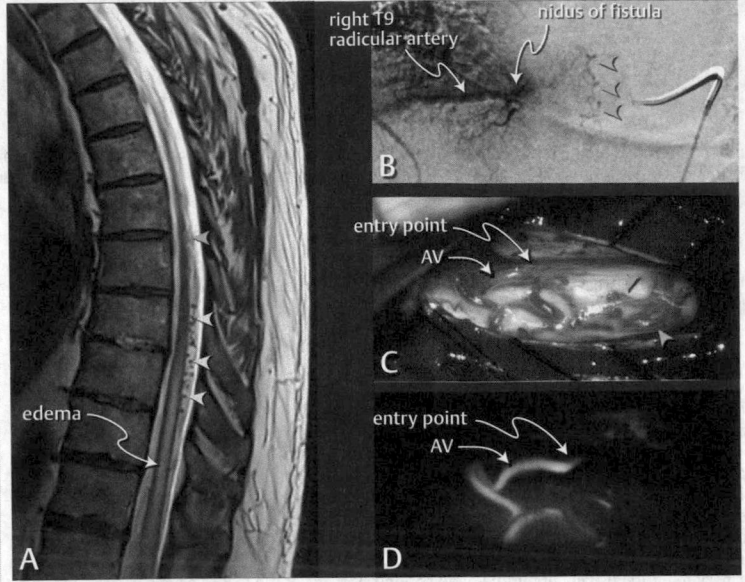

Fig. 84.1 Type I thoracic spinal dural AVF.
Image: A: T2 sagittal MRI of the thoracic spine. Note characteristic flow voids (*yellow arrowheads*) and spinal cord edema (high signal within the spinal cord parenchyma). Serpiginous vessels can also be appreciated on the spinal cord (*green arrowheads*).
B: spinal arteriogram, AP, right T9 radicular artery injection. The nidus is located in the nerve root sleeve.
C: intraoperative photograph. The dura is tented open with sutures. The patient's head is to the left. "Entry point" indicates where the arteriolized vein (AV) enters the dura where the posterior rootlets exit.
D: intraoperative indocyanine green (ICG) angiogram (same view as panel C) which shows the suspected vessel enhancing early after ICG injection (before other veins), confirming the identification of the major feeding vein.

Spetzler et al classification

See reference.[14]

This system reincorporated vascular spinal neoplasms.
1. neoplastic vascular lesions
   a) hemangioblastoma
   b) cavernous malformation
2. spinal aneurysms (rare)
3. arteriovenous lesions
   a) AVFs
      - extradural
      - intradural: dorsal or ventral
   b) AVMs
      - extradural-intradural
      - intradural
      - intramedullary
      - intramedullary-extramedullary
      - conus medullaris

84.1.3 Presentation

85% present as progressive neuro deficit (back pain associated with progressive sensory loss and LE weakness over months to years). Yet, SVMs account for < 5% of lesions presenting as spinal cord "tumors." 10–20% of SVMs present as sudden onset of myelopathy, usually in patients < 30 yrs o

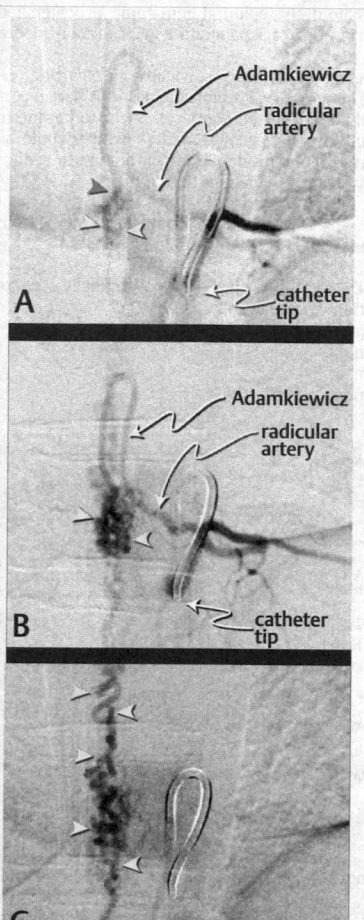

A

B

C

Fig. 84.2 Type IV thoracic spinal dural AVF.
Image: spinal angiogram, AP view. A: early injection, the artery of Adamkiewicz is faintly seen. The fistula is located in the general region of the green arrowhead, and early venous filling (*yellow arrowheads*) is beginning to be visible. B: moments later, more filling of the engorged veins (*yellow arrowheads*) is seen. C: venous phase, showing further retrograde filling of serpiginous veins.

Table 84.1 Merland's subclassification of *Type IV* (perimedullary) AV fistulas[a]

Subtype	Arterial supply	AVF	Venous drainage
I	single (thin ASA)	single, small	slowly ascending perimedullary venous system
II	multiple (dilated ASA & PSA)	multiple, medium	
III		single, giant	giant venous ectasia, rapid metameric venous drainage

[a]ASA = anterior spinal artery; AVF = arteriovenous fistula; PSA = posterior spinal artery

age,[15,16] secondary to hemorrhage (causing SAH, hematomyelia, epidural hematoma, or watershed infarction). Coup de poignard of Michon = sudden excruciating back pain with SAH (clinical evidence of SVM).

Foix-Alajouanine syndrome (subacute necrotic myelopathy): acute or subacute neurologic deterioration in a patient with an SVM without evidence of hemorrhage. Presents as spastic → flaccid paraplegia, with ascending sensory level and loss of sphincter control. Initially thought to be due to spontaneous thrombosis of the AVM causing subacute necrotizing myelopathy[17] which would be irreversible. However, more recent evidence suggests that the myelopathy may be due to venous hypertension with secondary ischemia, and there may be improvement with treatment.[18]

84

▶ **Clinical.** Auscultation over spine reveals a bruit in 2–3% of cases. Cutaneous angioma over back is present in 3–25%; Valsalva maneuver may enhance the redness of the angioma.[16]

▶ **Clinical grading.** The Aminoff-Logue disability (ALD) scale[15] (▶ Table 84.2) was originally used for rating disability of gait and micturition (bladder function) related to spinal dAVF.

The scale has subsequently been validated for prognostication[19] as follows:
- ALD score 0–3: 78% chance of substantial improvement.
- ALD score 4–5: 29% chance of substantial improvement.
- ALD score 6–8: 11% chance of substantial improvement.

Table 84.2 Aminoff-Logue disability scale[15] for spinal dural AVF

Characteristic		Points	Score
Gait disturbance	none	0	
	leg weakness or abnormal gait, activity not restricted	1	
	as above + restricted activity	2	(0 - 5)
	1 stick (cane) required for walking	3	
	2 sticks (canes) required for walking	4	
	unable to stand, confined to bed/wheelchair	5	
Micturition (bladder function)	normal	0	
	hesitancy, frequency, urgency	1	(0 - 3)
	occasional urinary incontinence or retention	2	
	total urinary incontinence or retention	3	
Aminoff-Logue disability scale score (range: 0–8) → TOTAL			(0 – 8)

84.1.4 Evaluation

Spinal angiography: necessary for treatment planning. Best performed at centers that do this study regularly.

For Type I dural AVMs, the fistula occurs in the nerve root sleeve. Before it can be considered negative, angiography must encompass all dural feeders of the neuraxis, which includes:
1. ICAs: because of the artery of Bernasconi & Cassinari (p.77)
2. every radicular artery including the artery of Adamkiewicz (p.87)
3. internal iliac arteries: for sacral feeders

MRI: detects some SVMs with greater sensitivity and safety than angiography,[20] but is inadequate for treatment planning. 82% show extramedullary flow voids (▶ Fig. 84.1 panel A). Spinal cord edema is common. Cord enhancement (from venous congestion or venous infarction) is variable. Negative MRI does not rule out diagnosis.

Myelography: generally superseded by MRI. Classically shows serpiginous intradural filling defects. If done, patient should be imaged prone *and* supine (to avoid missing a dorsal AVM). ✖ There is a risk of significant bleeding if the myelography needle punctures a dilated artery or vein.

84.1.5 Treatment

Type I (dural AVFs): usually require treatment. The goal is to interrupt the feeding *vein* close to the nidus which is located in the nerve root sleeve, therefore the vein should be sacrificed close to where it enters the dura of the thecal sac. Some are amenable to endovascular techniques using glue, in which case the proximal draining vein must be taken as well. Localization of the nidus at surgery is facilitated by placing a coil in the feeding artery at the time of angiography, which is then easily located on fluoroscopy at the time of surgery. Once identified, the vein is coagulated *and* divided. Some dAVF have extradural venous feeders as well. Conventional intraoperative angiography and indocyanine green (ICG) angiography (▶ Fig. 84.1 panel D) assist in confirming the elimination of the dAVF. If you don't completely eliminate a dural fistula (spinal or intracranial) it will come back!

Type II (spinal glomus AVMs): may be amenable to interventional neuroradiologic procedures including embolization,[21] especially type IIA (single feeder). However, recurrence may be higher with endovascular treatment than surgery, and surgery is often preferred for Type IIB (≥2 feeders). Surgical strategy: similar to intracranial AVMs, except that the parenchyma cannot be retracted, bleeding is rarely life-threatening, and en passant arteries must be preserved to avoid devastating deficits. Intraoperative ICG angio is often helpful. The nidus is compact, and the hemosiderin ring around the nidus on MRI often represents a plane that can be exploited.

Type III (juvenile spinal AVMs): the natural history is probably better than the prognosis with any type of treatment.

Type IV (perimedullary fistulae): suggested management[10] is shown in ▶ Table 84.3.

Table 84.3 Suggested management for Type IV arteriovenous fistulae[10]

Subtype	Diagnosis	Embolization	Surgery
Subtype I	difficult; ? reliability of MRI[a]; tomomyelography; angiotomomyelography	difficult	easy on filum terminale; difficult on conus medullaris
Subtype II	easy: MRI or myelography	incomplete occlusion	on posterolateral AVFs
Subtype III		effective	difficult, dangerous

[a]due to inaccuracy, do not delay angiogram to get MRA, etc.

84.2 Spinal cord cavernous malformations

May be intramedullary (▶ Fig. 84.3) or epidural (rare) (▶ Fig. 84.4).

Intramedullary lesions: indication for surgery is similar to brainstem cavernous malformations.

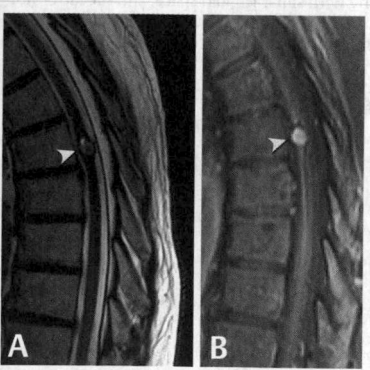

Fig. 84.3 Spinal cavernous malformation of the thoracic spine (*yellow arrowheads*).
Image: MRI of the thoracic spine. A: Noncontrast T2 sagittal, B: Contrast-enhanced T1 sagittal.

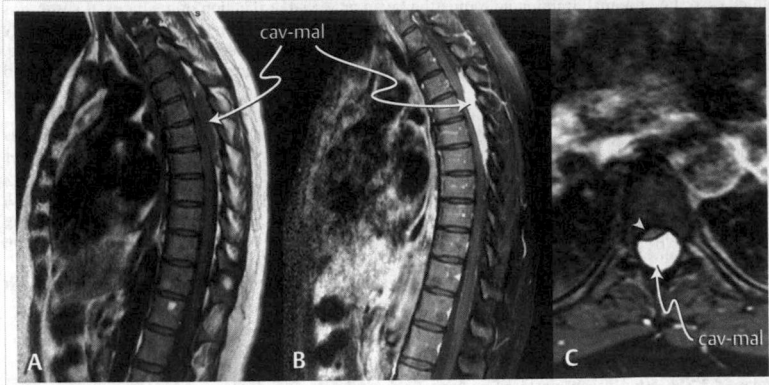

Fig. 84.4 Epidural cavernous malformation ("cav-mal") of the thoracic spine (pathologically confirmed). Image: MRI of the thoracic spine. A: Noncontrast T1 sagittal, B: Contrast-enhanced T1 sagittal, C: Contrast-enhanced axial T1. Note the compressed spinal cord (*yellow arrowhead*).

84.3 Abnormalities involving spinal meninges

84.3.1 Spinal meningeal cysts

General information

Spinal meningeal cysts (SMC): diverticula of the meningeal sac, nerve root sheath, or arachnoid. Some may have familial tendency.

Terminology in literature is confusing. One classification system is shown in ▶ Table 84.4. Previously AKA Tarlov perineural cysts, spinal arachnoid cysts, and extradural diverticula, pouches, or cysts. Some may develop following trauma, or inflammation.

- Type I SMCs above the sacrum usually have a pedicle adjacent to entrance of dorsal nerve root
- Type II SMCs: formerly called Tarlov cysts and were differentiated from nerve root diverticula because the former were defined as communicating with subarachnoid space, and the latter not. However, intrathecal contrast CT (ICCT) shows that both communicate. Often multiple. Occur on dorsal roots anywhere, but are most prominent and symptomatic in sacrum (▶ Fig. 84.5). Seen in 1.5–4.6% of MRIs[23]
- Type III SMCs: may also be multiple and asymptomatic. More common along posterior subarachnoid space. Attributed to proliferation of arachnoid trabeculae

Table 84.4 Types of spinal meningeal cysts[22]

Type	Description
Type I	extradural meningeal cysts without spinal nerve root fibers
IA	"extradural meningeal/arachnoid cyst"
IB	(occult) "sacral meningocele"
Type II	extradural meningeal cysts with spinal nerve root fibers ("Tarlov perineural cyst," "spinal nerve root diverticulum")
Type III	spinal intradural meningeal cysts ("intradural arachnoid cyst")

Presentation

Usually asymptomatic (i.e., incidental finding). May cause radiculopathy by pressure on adjacent nerve root (may or may not cause symptoms of nerve root from which it actually arises). Symptom complex depends on size of SMC, and proximity to spinal cord and nerve roots.

1. Type I SMCs: in thoracic and cervical region, may present with acute myelopathy (spasticity and sensory level); lumbar region → LBP and radiculopathy; sacral region → sphincter disturbance

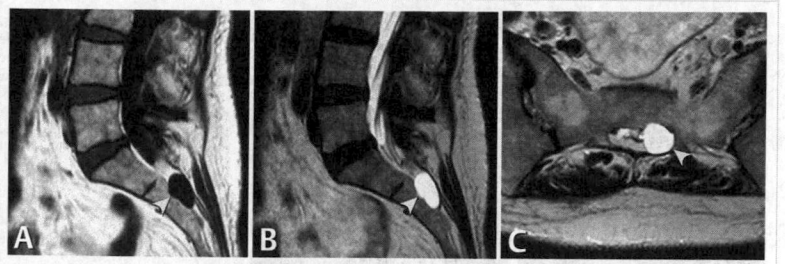

Fig. 84.5 Spinal meningeal cyst just below S2 (*yellow arrowheads*).
Image: MRI, A: Sagittal T1, B: Sagittal T2, C: Axial T2.
NB: the signal characteristics of the cyst follows that of CSF in all sequences (including STIR, not shown). There is bony remodeling around the cyst (best appreciated on CT, not shown).

2. Type II SMCs: most remain asymptomatic,[24,25] although cases of positional coccydynia, sacral pain, and radiculopathy as well as sphincter disturbance have been reported. A ball-valve mechanism may be the mechanism of symptom production in some cases.[25] There are case reports of Tarlov cysts presenting with back pain and radicular pain after spontaneous SAH,[23,26] with symptomatic relief following CT-guided aspiration of blood from the cyst.[23] Spontaneous hemorrhage into the cyst may occur[26]
3. Type III SMCs: may also be multiple and asymptomatic; more common along posterior subarachnoid space

Evaluation

MRI to identify the mass. If desired, water-soluble ICCT scan may be used to evaluate communication of the cyst with subarachnoid space or when MRI is conraindicated.
1. Type I SMCs: all 18 cases had bony erosion (demonstrated by canal widening, pedicle erosion, foraminal enlargement, or vertebral body scalloping)
2. Type III SMCs: may also cause bony erosion; appear on myelogram as intradural defect, may not appear on ICCT if they communicate with subarachnoid space, which causes them to blend with adjacent subarachnoid space

Treatment

1. Type I SMCs: close ostium between cyst and subarachnoid space. Cysts above the sacrum, can usually be dissected from dura; occasionally fibrous adhesions prevent this
2. Type II SMCs: no pedicle, thus either partially resect and oversew cyst wall, or excise cyst and involved nerve root. Simple aspiration is not recommended due to a high rate of recurrence.[27] Other treatment modalities include: NSAIDs, shunting, decompressive laminectomy, cyst excision, and microsurgical cyst fenestration.[28,29] All treatment should be taken under advisement as the failure rate may be considerable and complications of recalcitrant CSF leak are not uncommon
3. Type III SMCs: excise completely unless dense fibrous adhesions prevent this, in which case marsupialize cyst. Tend to recur if incompletely excised

84.3.2 Spinal arachnoid cysts & spinal arachnoid webs (SAWs)

These two conditions may or may not be distinct entities, and may be on a continuum (SAWs may be incomplete or disrupted arachnoid cysts[30]). The cyst walls or the web are sometimes difficult to appreciate on MRI.

Spinal arachnoid cyst

Unlike a spinal arachnoid web, which typically has distinct borders (► Fig. 84.6) on MRI, and there is no open communcation with the rest of the subarachnoid space. Intrathecal contrast may slowly seep through the cyst wall and therefore demonstrate delayed filling.[30]

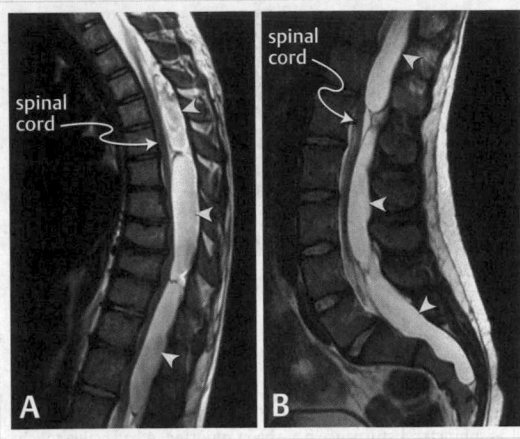

Fig. 84.6 **Spinal arachnoid cysts.** 17-year-old male with multiple spinal arachnoid cysts in the thoracic and lumbar spine (*yellow arrowheads*: each point to an individual cyst).
Image: T2 sagittal MRI. A: thoracic, B: lumbar.

Spinal arachnoid web

Epidemiology: rare (< 50 reported cases as of 2021[31]). High male predominance. All reported cases were in the thoracic spine (usually between T2 and T8),[31] 95% were dorsal to the spinal cord.

Risk factors: patients should be queried regarding history of SAH, spinal infections, or trauma as possible risk factors.

Presentation: focal thoracic pain is the most common symptom, followed by lower extremity symptoms and then myelopathy.[31] Upper extremity symptoms (numbness and paresthesias) were surprisingly common.

Imaging: MRI may show a "scalpel sign," an indentation or displacement of the spinal cord (▶ Fig. 84.7).[30] Usually lacks distinct borders. Syringomyelia is present in over two-thirds of symptomatic cases.[32] Increased signal within the cord on T2 MRI was present in 53% of cases.[31]

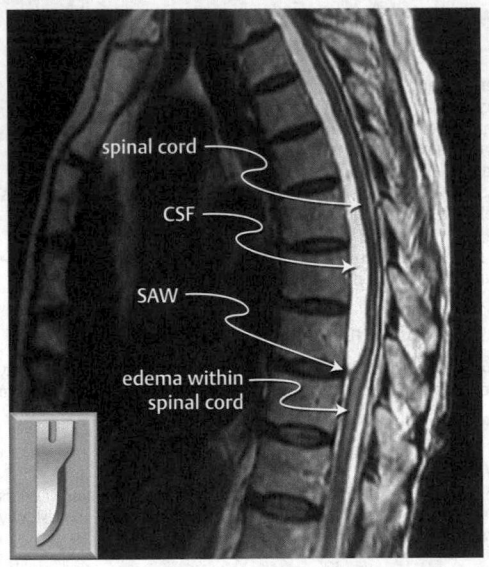

Fig. 84.7 **Spinal arachnoid web** showing the "scalpel sign."
Image: T2 sagittal MRI, showing an atypical presentation where the web is anterior to the spinal cord.
Abbreviations: SAW = spinal arachnoid web. CSF is cerebrospinal fluid proximal to the block caused by the arachnoid web.
Inset: illustration of a #15 scalpel blade to show whence the "scalpel sign" takes its name.

Surgery: surgical intervention consists of laminectomy with lysing of the web. Intraoperative ultrasound can help with the localization and can confirm improvement in the CSF flow after web lysis.

Outcome: myelopathic symptoms showed a non-statistically significant trend towards post-op improvement. Thoracic pain was not altered with surgery. Sensory disturbances in the thoracic spine and upper extremities showed a statistically significant *increase* post-op.[31]

84.3.3 Pseudomeningocele

May occur following trauma or surgery. Infrequently occurs spontaneously.

MRI: signal characteristics of cyst contents should follow those of CSF (► Fig. 84.8).

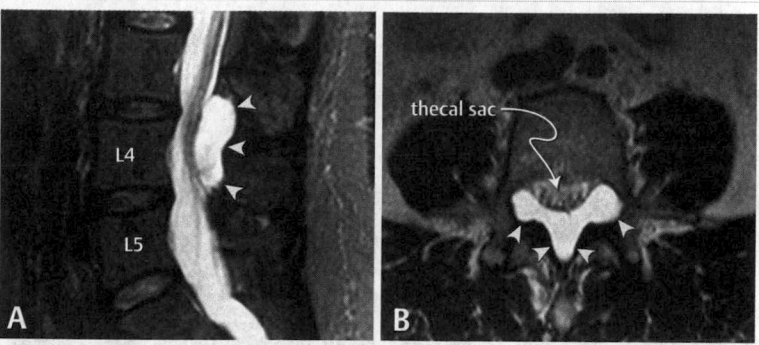

Fig. 84.8 Spontaneous pseudomeningocele (*yellow arrowheads*) posterior to L4.
Image: MRI: A: sagittal STIR, B: axial T2.
At surgery, the pseudomeningocele was entered, revealing a small rent in the dura with a few nerve roots adherent to the dura near the opening.

84.3.4 Hirayama disease

General information

AKA monomelic amyotrophy AKA juvenile muscular atrophy of the upper extremity. Rare. Characterized by insidious painless wasting of the distal UE muscles (usually asymmetric) predominantly affecting the C8-T1 innervated muscles, sparing sensation. Typically affects males in the age range of 15-20 years,[33] usually starting in the right UE and then extending into the contralateral side in 50%. Atrophy progresses slowly and typically stabilizes after several years.

Etiology

Initially considered to be an idiopathic motor neuron disease, there is mounting evidence that the etiology in many cases may be asymmetric compression of the spinal cord by the dura separating from the posterior bony spinal canal in flexion[34] leading to necrosis of the anterior horn cells in the lower cervical cord.

Evaluation

Imaging: Unenhanced cervical MRI may show spinal cord atrophy and may or may not show intrinsic cord signal changes. Diagnosis may be assisted by obtaining sagittal cervical enhanced fat-suppressed and T1 axial MRI images in neutral and flexed position and measuring the LDS (laminodural space) at the point of widest separation of the dura from the posterior spinal canal on the sagittal images, and the AP and transverse diameter at that same level.[35] The ratio of maximal LDS to the AP canal decreased by 0.46 from neutral to flexion, and the change of the ratio of the cord AP/transverse diameter increased by 0.118. Enhanced MRI in flexion often shows an enhancing epidural venous plexus in the posterior canal.

Electrodiagnostics: generally rule out other neurodegenerative diseases such as motor neuron disease. Nerve conduction velocities, SNAPs and distal motor latencies are normal. Half the patients had reduction of CMAPs only in the ulnar nerves. Most patients exhibited findings of segmental injury to the anterior horn cells of the lower cervical spine with spontaneous firing and prolonged motor unit potentials (MUPs).[33]

Treatment

Treatment starts with a cervical collar to limit flexion, and may eventually require multilevel cervical fusion (± coagulation of posterior epidural veins) to permanently limit flexion.

84.3.5 Spinal cord herniation (idiopathic)

General information

Rare. Spinal cord herniates though a defect in the dura usually located anteriorly or anterolaterally between T2–8.[36] Bone erosion anterior to the dural defect may occasionally be seen (▶ Fig. 84.9). Frequently associated with a calcified disc fragment, which theoretically may have gradually eroded through the dura.

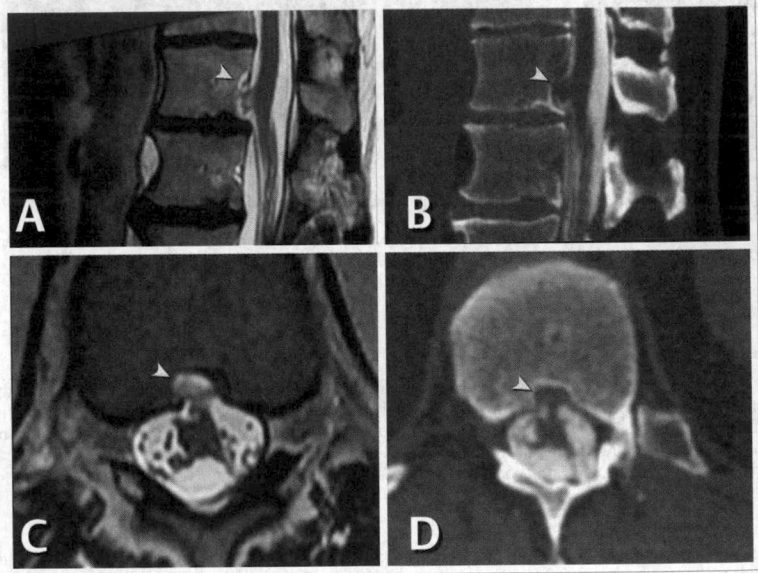

Fig. 84.9 Spontaneous spinal cord herniation at T12.
Image: T2 MRI, A: sagittal, C: axial. CT/myelogram, B: sagittal, D: axial.
Yellow arrowheads indicate the bone defect in the posterior T12 vertebral body into which the spinal cord herniates.

Differential diagnosis

Main differential diagnosis is with dorsal arachnoid cyst (p. 1696). Both result in increased subarachnoid space posterior to the spinal cord, and a ventral kinking of the cord. Contiguous CSF pulsation artifact on MRI can be seen with cord herniation, whereas an arachnoid cyst tends to interrupt this.

Presentation

Commonly presents as an incomplete Brown-Séquard syndrome (with relative sparing of posterior columns). Symptoms may be due to distortion of the spinal cord, but vascular injury may also play a role.

Surgery

Requires a lateral or anterolateral approach (p. 1790) to access the anterior spinal canal while minimizing spinal cord manipulation. The dural defect is widened which usually results in reduction of the spinal cord herniation. A sling of dural substitute can then be slid anterior to the cord to prevent reherniation.

84

84.4 Syringomyelia

84.4.1 General information

> **Key concepts**
>
> - AKA syrinx. Cystic cavitation of the spinal cord
> - 70% are associated with Chiari I malformation, 10% with basilar invagination. May also be posttraumatic or associated with etiologies such as tumor, infection…
> - symptoms: progressive neurologic deterioration over months to years, usually affecting UE more prominently (similar to central cord syndrome (p. 1132))
> - workup: MRI entire neuraxis (including brain to R/O Chiari malformation and hydrocephalus) without and with contrast (to look for associated neoplasm). If MRI cannot be done, workup is challenging
> - diameter > 5 mm + associated edema predict a more rapid deterioration
> - indications for surgery: progressive symptoms or progressive enlargement
> - preferred treatment is directed at correcting the causative pathophysiology, but this is often not possible and cyst shunting is then indicated

AKA syrinx. Cystic cavitation of the spinal cord. Other terms not precisely defined include: hydrosyringomyelia, communicating or noncommunicating syringomyelia.

Syringobulbia: Rostral extension into brainstem (usually medulla). May present with (bilateral) perioral tingling and numbness, due to compression of the spinal trigeminal tracts as the fibers decussate.

84.4.2 Etiologies

Primary syringomyelia

This term is used differently by different authors.[37] Herein, refers to syrinx in the absence of an identifiable cause.

Secondary syringomyelia

Most cases are thought to be secondary to partial obstruction of the spinal subarachnoid space.[37] Unanswered question: Why then do patients with varying degrees of degenerative cervical spinal stenosis generally not get syringomyelia?

Etiologies include:

1. Chiari I malformation (p. 295): the most common cause of syrinx
2. postinflammatory
   a) postinfectious
      - granulomatous meningitides (TB and fungal)
      - postoperative meningitis, especially after intradural procedure
   b) chemical or other sterile inflammations
      - rarely after SAH
      - after myelography: especially with older oil-based agents no longer in use

3. posttraumatic syringomyelia (p.1411): (✖ the concept of syrinx developing as a coalescence of foci of traumatic hematomyelia is obsolete)
   a) with severe posttraumatic kyphotic deformity: e.g., with retropulsed bone, scarring…
   b) severe injury to spinal cord and/or its coverings. Blood may be a contributing factor
4. postsurgical: has been identified many years after uncomplicated intradural neoplasm removal (e.g., neurofibromas)
5. basilar arachnoiditis:
   a) idiopathic
   b) postinfectious: see above
6. basilar impression (p.228) with constriction at the foramen magnum
7. associated with spinal tumors: this is distinct from a tumor cyst
8. other conditions that interfere with unencumbered CSF flow through the spinal canal
   a) spinal arachnoid cyst (p.1401): typically has distinct borders
   b) spinal arachnoid web (p.1402) (SAW): MRI may show "scalpel sign"
9. associated with disc protrusion
10. cerebellar ectopia
11. Dandy Walker syndrome (p.270)

84.4.3 Epidemiology

See reference.[38]
Prevalence of non-posttraumatic syringomyelia: 8.4 cases/100,000 population. Usually presents between ages 20–50.
Associated clinical syndromes are shown in ▶ Table 84.5.

Table 84.5 Conditions associated with syringomyelia

Condition	%[a]
Chiari type 1 malformation	70
basilar invagination	10
intramedullary spinal cord tumors	4

[a]percent of cases of syringomyelia

84.4.4 Pathophysiology

Major theories of formation of the cyst:
1. hydrodynamic ("water-hammer") theory of Gardner: systolic pulsations are transmitted with each heartbeat from the intracranial cavity to the central canal. Has been essentially disproven using MRI[39]
2. Williams' ("craniospinal dissociation") theory: maneuvers that raise CSF pressure (Valsalva, coughing…) cause "hydrodissection" through the spinal cord tissue. May be more common in noncommunicating syringomyelia
3. Heiss-Oldfield theory: occlusion at the foramen magnum causes CSF pulsations during cardiac systole to be transmitted through the Virchow-Robin spaces, which increases the extracellular fluid, which coalesces to form a syrinx[38] (i.e., through the cord parenchyma)

84.4.5 Clinical

Presentation: highly variable. Usually progresses over months to years, with a more rapid deterioration early that gradually slows.[38] Initially, pain, weakness, atrophy, and loss of pain & temperature sensation in the upper extremities (with cervical syrinx) are common. Myelopathy that progresses slowly over years ensues.

▶ **Characteristic syndromes.** Findings are nonspecific for intramedullary spinal cord pathology:
1. sensory loss (similar to central cord syndrome) with a suspended ("cape") dissociated sensory loss (loss of pain and temperature sensation with preserved touch and joint position sense → painless ulcerations from unperceived injuries and/or burns)
2. pain: commonly cervical and occipital. Dysesthetic pain often occurs in the distribution of the sensory loss.[38] Many patients experience neurologic deficits but do not develop pain
3. weakness: lower motor neuron weakness of the hand and arm

▶ **Other findings with syringomyelia.** Neuropathic (or neurogenic) arthropathy (Charcot joint) including the elbow (most common), shoulder & hands.[40] Rare (seen in < 5% of patients with syrinx). Pathogenesis: 1) neurotrauma theory[41] – loss of pain & temperature sensation leads to insensate injuries, or 2) neurovascular theory[42] – disruption of the neurovascular reflex produces hyperemia and active bone resorption by osteoclasts. Profound joint destruction may occur (especially in the shoulder), as can hypertrophy (primarily in the elbows and wrists). In most cases the syrinx is asymmetric to one side which correlates with the side of the Charcot joint(s).[40] With a Charcot shoulder, if a syrinx is present, it is the likely cause although other etiologies need to be ruled out, viz.: diabetes (the most common cause), infection, tumor. Treatment of the syrinx (e.g., treating Chiari malformation if present, or shunting the syrinx) may reduce progression.

84

84.4.6 Evaluation

MRI: Test of choice. Defines anatomy in sagittal as well as axial plane (▶ Fig. 84.10). Include cervical & thoracic spine (without & with contrast to R/O neoplasm) and brain to include craniocervical junction (to R/O Chiari malformation and hydrocephalus). Syringomyelic cavities may be complex, with noncommunicating channels (more common with posttraumatic syrinx).

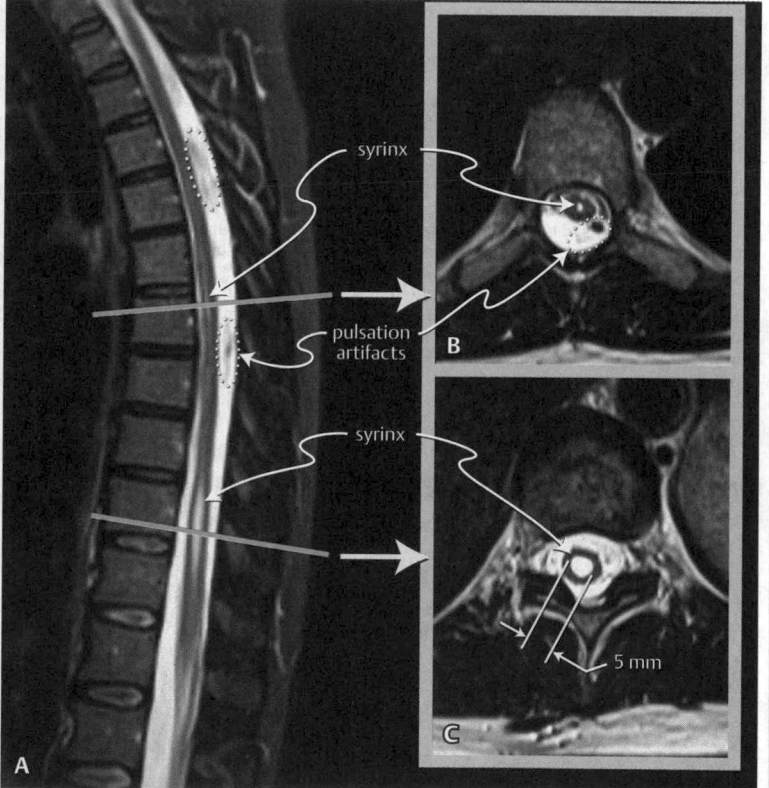

Fig. 84.10 Syringomyelia in thoracic spine.
Image: T2 MRI. A: Sagittal, B & C: axial slices through upper (B) and lower (C) areas of syrinx (B). Note: several areas of pulsation artifact are circled in dotted lines. The fact that the diameter of the lower portion of the cyst is > 4 mm disqualifies this as a residual central spinal canal (see text).

CT: low attenuation area within cord seen on either plain CT or myelogram/CT (with water-soluble contrast).

Myelogram: rarely used alone (usually performed in conjunction with CT). When used alone: often normal (false negative), some → complete block at level of syrinx; iodine contrast studies may show fusiform widening of spinal cord, whereas air contrast studies may show collapse of the cord.[43] Dye may slowly leach into the cyst.

EMG: no characteristic findings, but may be useful to R/O other conditions that may be responsible for symptoms (e.g., peripheral neuropathy causing paresthesias).

84

84.4.7 Distinguishing from similar entities

1. tumor cyst
   a) especially with intramedullary spinal cord gliomas. Tumors may secrete fluid, or may cause microcysts that eventually coalesce. Most (but not all) intramedullary tumors will enhance with IV contrast on MRI
   b) tumor cyst fluid is usually highly proteinaceous, syrinx fluid usually has the same MRI characteristics as CSF (NB: true syrinx can occur with tumor)
2. central spinal canal
   a) residual (▶ Fig. 84.11) central spinal canal: the central canal is present within the spinal cord at birth and normally gradually involutes with age.[44] Persistence of the canal is a normal variant. Characteristic imaging features of a central canal:
      • linear or fusiform on sagittal MRI
      • ≤ 4 mm in maximal width
      • may be singular, or there may be several discontinuous regions in the rostral-caudal direction
      • perfectly round in cross-section and centrally located on axial MRI
      • if IV contrast is given, there should be no enhancement
   b) simple dilatation of the central canal with ependymal cell lining has sometimes been called hydromyelia, but this usage is ambiguous
3. ventriculus terminalis: (▶ Fig. 84.12) an ependymal lined CSF containing intramedullary cyst usually located at the conus, sometimes called the "fifth ventricle" ("fifth ventricle" is also used for other entities, including: pseudomeningocele, cavum septum pelucidum (p. 1657)).[45] It communicates with the central canal. It is normal in utero during development, and usually regresses. Has rarely been reported to enlarge on serial imaging.[45,46] May be asymptomatic or may present with progressive neurologic deficit, or rarely, cauda equina syndrome.[47] Imaging of the neuraxis (brain and entire spine) is recommended to rule-out other pathology (e.g., Chiari malformation…).[45] Surgical treatment is indicated for symptomatic cysts or those that enlarge on serial MRIs. Surgical options include: fenestration, cyst-subarachnoid shunt, or percutaneous MRI-guided aspiration

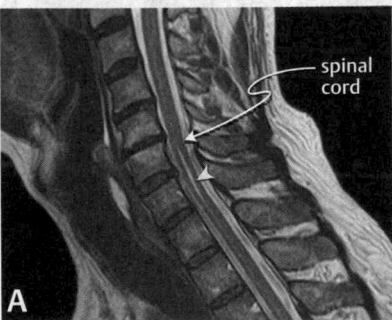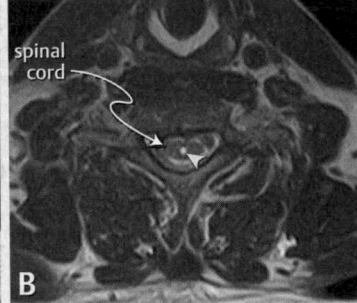

Fig. 84.11 Central spinal canal (*yellow arrowheads*).
Image: T2 MRI of the cervical spine, A: sagittal, B: axial.
Note: this qualifies as a central canal as it is round, centrally located, and has a maximal diameter of 3 mm which is less than the maximal 4 mm.

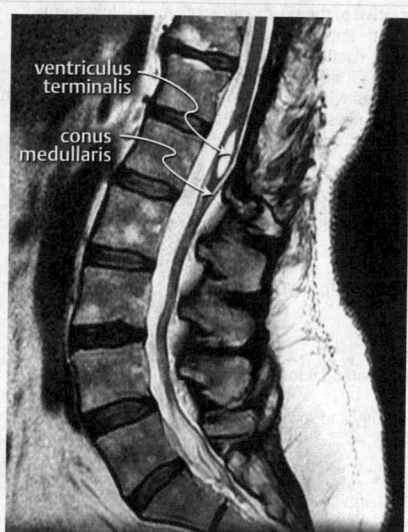

Fig. 84.12 Ventriculus terminalis.
Image: T2 sagittal MRI of the lumbar spine.

84.4.8 Management

Incidental syrinx

For an incidentally discovered syrinx (i.e., asymptomatic and no neurologic deficit):
1. obtain a contrast MRI to rule out enhancement (indicative of tumor)
2. if no enhancement and no symptoms referrable to the syrinx are present, obtain a follow-up MRI in 3 months (without contrast, unless a contrasted MRI was not previously done in which case order without and with contrast)
3. if the syrinx is stable at 3 months
   a) for lesions meeting the criteria of a central canal (p. 1408), no routine follow-up is indicated
   b) for those not consistent with central canal, repeat MRIs annually for 2–3 years if no change in symptoms, if stable then if desired, repeat MRI every 2–3 years
4. for any of the above, repeat the MRI for concerning symptoms

Surgical treatment

Intervention is considered for symptomatic lesions (not all are symptomatic) including neuropathic arthropathy (p. 1407). For a small syrinx (e.g., < 5 mm diameter), if an underlying cause of the syrinx is not identified (e.g., tumor), it is unlikely that the syrinx is symptomatic and direct treatment can be very difficult without risking causing more harm than good.
  Options include:
1. when possible, treat the underlying pathophysiology to re-establish subarachnoid CSF flow. Use syrinx draining procedures as second choice when this is not feasible
   a) posterior decompression: procedure of choice when posterior anomalies (e.g., Chiari malformation) are present
   b) decompression if feasible if a site of compression, blockage, or tethering is identified
2. syrinx shunts:
   a) indications: syrinx diameter > 3–4 mm with:
      1. no identifiable cause
      2. or blockages that cannot be circumvented due to thick adhesions (e.g., diffuse arachnoiditis following tuberculous or chemical meningitis)
      3. or blockage extending over many levels
   b) syrinx catheter options

- **K** tube (outflow catheter is angulated relative to the syrinx catheter). Available systems include Medtronic #23069 or Heyer-Schulte-Pudenz system
- **T** tube (outflow catheter is at a right angle). Available systems include:

Edwards-Barbaro syringoperitoneal shunt (▶ Fig. 84.13; distributed by Integra™): T-shaped proximal end ≈ 5FR diameter & 3.5 cm total length, supplied with optional valveless Foltz reservoir, which may be incorporated to permit percutaneous needle access to the system

Medtronic #44520 T-tube: the proximal limbs that go into the syrinx are 8 cm in total length and can be trimmed to desired length

c) choices of distal sites include
- peritoneum[48] (difficult to access from cervical region syrinx)
- pleural cavity: advantage is that the negative pleural pressure can facilitate drainage of these cysts which are typically low pressure
- subarachnoid space: requires normal CSF flow in subarachnoid space, therefore cannot be used in arachnoiditis. A K tube is better suited than a T tube

d) outcome/complications
- complication rate: 16%
- clinical stabilization rate: 54% at 10 yrs
- may produce traction on spinal cord with potential for further injury
- prone to obstruction: 50% at 4 yrs
- does not correct underlying pathophysiology and so syrinx may recur

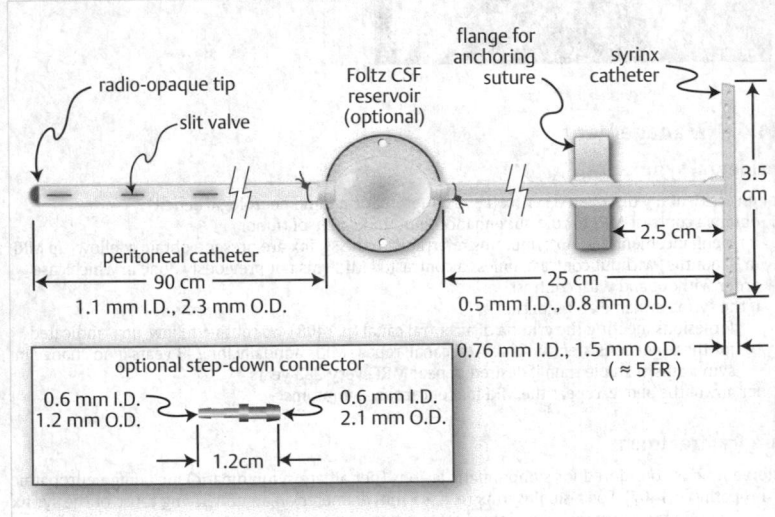

Fig. 84.13 **Edwards-Barbaro syringo-peritoneal shunt** (Integra™).

3. subarachnoid-subarachnoid bypass shunts[49]: 1 or more silastic drainage tubes placed intradurally with one end above and the other end below the site of CSF flow blockage to allow CSF flow around a site of blockage. Anchored with suture. 60% (of 20 patients) improved, 20% were stable, and 20% deteriorated (mean follow-up: 48 months)

4. ✖ no longer recommended
   a) for syrinx associated with Chiari malformation: plugging the obex with muscle, teflon, or other material; removing the inferior cerebellar tonsils
   b) syringostomy: usually fails to remain patent, therefore using a stent or a shunt (syringosubarachnoid or syringoperitoneal) is recommended
   c) cordectomy: usually only for posttraumatic syrinx in ASIA A SCI patients with ascending syrinx[50,51]
   d) percutaneous aspiration of the cyst[52]

► **Technical considerations**

1. intraoperative ultrasound is often helpful for:
   a) localizing the cyst
   b) assessing for septations (to avoid shunting only part of cyst)
2. if Chiari malformation is not present, consider syringosubarachnoid shunt as the initial procedure. If this fails, then a syringoperitoneal or syringopleural shunt may be inserted
3. Rhoton suggests performing the myelotomy in the dorsal root entry zone (DREZ), between the lateral and posterior columns (instead of the midline as with a tumor) because this is consistently the thinnest part and there is usually already an upper extremity proprioceptive deficit from the syrinx.[53 (p 1317)] There is ≈ 10% incidence of posterior column dysfunction with shunting
4. with syringosubarachnoid shunts, be sure the distal shunt tip is subarachnoid (and not just subdural) or else it will not function
5. for syringopleural shunt: to avoid having to reposition the patient to place the distal catheter, the pleural opening can be made *posteriorly*, subadjacent to one of the ribs as described for ventriculopleural shunt (p. 1827). You need to go about 5–6 cm lateral to the midline to access the rib and avoid the paraspinal muscles, which usually requires you to tunnel the catheter inferior to the inferior scapular pole. Over the posterior thorax the ribs are closer together and less mobile than they are anteriorly so access can be more challenging
6. for peritoneal terminus of shunt: the proximal shunt may be placed in the syrinx with the patient in the prone position, and the peritoneal end of the catheter may be tunneled to an intermediate position in the flank in the midaxillary line where it can be coiled into a small subcutaneous pouch, which can be temporarily closed with staples and dressed with Tegaderm. After the spinal incision is closed, the patient can be undraped and rotated to the supine position, the Tegaderm is removed, the abdomen and the flank incision are prepped, the staples are removed, and the catheter is retrieved from the sub-Q pocket and tunneled to the peritoneal opening that is made at this time. A small bump (rolled sheet…) to elevate the flank may be employed in both parts of the operation to facilitate access to the pouch

84.4.9 Outcome

Assessing treatment results is difficult due to rarity of the condition, variability of natural history (which may arrest spontaneously), and too short follow-up.[54] Enthusiasm for direct treatment (shunts, fenestration…) is low among neurosurgeons because of the perceived poor response and risk of iatrogenic neurologic worsening. However, this may remain as the only option for a deteriorating patient and positive outcomes do occur.[55]

84.5 Posttraumatic syringomyelia

84.5.1 General information

Posttraumatic syringomyelia (PTSx) may follow significant spinal trauma (with or without clinical spinal cord injury). Includes penetrating injury or non-penetrating "violent" trauma to the spinal cord (injuries such as post-spinal anesthesia or following thoracic disc herniation are not included).

84.5.2 Epidemiology

Often a late presentation following spinal cord injury, and therefore incidence is higher in series with longer follow-up. Incidence is increasing as a result of longer survival following spinal cord injury and improved detection with proliferation of MRI scans. Range: ≈ 0.3–3% of cord injured patients (see ► Table 84.6).

Table 84.6 Incidence of posttraumatic syringomyelia

Type of injury	No./risk[a]	Incidence
all spinal cord injuries	30/951	3.2%
complete quadriplegia	14/177	7.9%
incomplete quadriplegia	4/181	4.5%
complete paraplegia	4/282	1.7%
incomplete paraplegia	4/181	2.2%
[a]number occurring over number at risk in 951 patients followed for 11 years[56]		

In a large number of patients followed via multicenter cooperative data bank, there were fewer cases of syrinx following cervical injuries than following thoracic injuries[57] (may be artifactual since patients with lower lesions may be more aware of ascending levels).

Latency following spinal cord injury:

1. latency to symptoms: 3 mos to 34 yrs (mean 9 yrs) (earlier in complete cord lesions than incomplete: mean 7.5 vs. 9.9 yrs)
2. latency to diagnosis: up to 12 yrs (mean 2.8 yrs) after onset of new symptoms

84.5.3 Clinical

The presentation of patients with PTSx is shown in ▶ Table 84.7. The late appearance of *upper* extremity symptoms in a paraplegic patient should raise a high index of suspicion of posttraumatic syringomyelia.[58]

Hyperhidrosis may be the only feature of *descending* syringomyelia in patients with complete cord lesions.[60] For the differential diagnosis, see Delayed deterioration following spinal cord injuries (p. 1221).

Table 84.7 Presentation (in 30 SCI patients with syrinx[56])

Symptom	Initial	At time of diagnosis
pain[a]	57%	70%
numbness	27%	40%
increased motor deficit	23%	40%
increased spasticity	10%	23%
increased sweating (hyperhidrosis)	3%	13%
autonomic dysreflexia	3%	3%
no symptoms	7%	7%
Signs	**Frequency**	
ascending sensory level	93%	
depressed tendon reflexes	77%	
increased motor deficits	40%	

[a]pain is often quite severe, and unrelieved with analgesics[59]

84.5.4 Evaluation

One end of the cavity is often found at a site of spinal column fracture or abnormal angulation.

84.5.5 Management

General information

Many authors advocate early surgical drainage of cysts as a means of reducing increased delayed deficit.[61] Some authors feel that aside from disturbing sensory symptoms, motor loss was infrequent and therefore conservative management is indicated in most cases.[62]

Medical

Managed non-surgically: 31% remained stable, 68% progressed over yrs (longer F/U in latter).

Surgical

There is probably no benefit in operating on a patient with a small syrinx.[56]

Surgical options

Same as in communicating syringomyelia, with the following differences:

1. cord transection (cordectomy)[63]: an option in *complete* injuries only
2. plugging the obex is probably *not* indicated (controversial in congenital syrinx)

Outcome

In 9 PTSx patients treated with syringosubarachnoid shunt[56]: pain relieved in all 9 (1 only slightly), motor recovery in 5/8, improved tendon reflex in 1/10. Some post-op complications in 9 patients included: 1 incomplete lesion became complete, 1 sensorimotor deterioration, transient pain in 3.

Most results are good for radicular symptoms, with dubious efficacy for autonomic symptoms or spasticity.

References

[1] Youmans JR. Neurological Surgery. Philadelphia 1982

[2] Black P. Spinal vascular malformations: an historical perspective. Neurosurg Focus. 2006; 21

[3] Di Chiro G, Doppman J, Ommaya AK. Selective arteriography of arteriovenous aneurysms of spinal cord. Radiology. 1967; 88:1065–1077

[4] Djindjian R. Embolization of angiomas of the spinal cord. Surg Neurol. 1975; 4:411–420

[5] Kendall BE, Logue V. Spinal epidural angiomatous malformations draining into intrathecal veins. Neuroradiology. 1977; 13:181–189

[6] Oldfield EH, Di Chiro G, Quindlen EA, et al. Successful treatment of a group of spinal cord arteriovenous malformations by interruption of dural fistula. J Neurosurg. 1983; 59:1019–1030

[7] Heros RC, Debrun GM, Ojemann RG, et al. Direct spinal arteriovenous fistula: a new type of spinal AVM. Case report. J Neurosurg. 1986; 64:134–139

[8] Rosenblum B, Oldfield EH, Doppman JL, et al. Spinal Arteriovenous Malformations: A Comparison of Dural Arteriovenous Fistulas and Intradural AVM's in 81 Patients. Journal of Neurosurgery. 1987; 67:795–802

[9] Gueguen B, Merland JJ, Riche MC, et al. Vascular Malformations of the Spinal Cord: Intrathecal Perimedullary Arteriovenous Fistulas Fed by Medullary Arteries. Neurology. 1987; 37:969–979

[10] Mourier KL, Gobin YP, George B, et al. Intradural Perimedullary Arteriovenous Fistulae: Results of Surgical and Endovascular Treatment in a Series of 35 Cases. Neurosurgery. 1993; 32:885–891

[11] Strugar J, Chyatte D. In Situ Photocoagulation of Spinal Dural Arteriovenous Malformations Using the Nd:YAG Laser. J Neurosurg. 1992; 77:571–574

[12] Bederson JB, Spetzler RF. Pathophysiology of Type I Spinal Dural Arteriovenous Malformations. BNI Quarterly. 1996; 12:23–32

[13] Rodesch G, Hurth M, Alvarez H, et al. Classification of spinal cord arteriovenous shunts: proposal for a reappraisal-the Bicetre experience with 155 consecutive patients treated between 1981 and 1999. Neurosurgery. 2002; 51:374–9; discussion 379-80

[14] Spetzler RF, Detwiler PW, Riina HA, et al. Modified classification of spinal cord vascular lesions. J Neurosurg. 2002; 96:145–156

[15] Aminoff MJ, Logue V. The prognosis of patients with spinal vascular malformations. Brain. 1974; 97:211–218

[16] Tobin WD, Layton DD. The Diagnosis and Natural History of Spinal Cord Arteriovenous Malformations. Mayo Clin Proc. 1976; 51:637–646

[17] Wirth FP, Post KD, Di Chiro G, et al. Foix-Alajouanine Disease. Spontaneous Thrombosis of a Spinal Cord Arteriovenous Malformation: A Case Report. Neurology. 1970; 20:1114–1118

[18] Criscuolo GR, Oldfield EH, Doppman JL. Reversible Acute and Subacute Myelopathy in Patients with Dural Arteriovenous Fistulas: Foix-Alajouanine Syndrome Reconsidered. Journal of Neurosurgery. 1989; 70:354–359

[19] Fugate JE, Lanzino G, Rabinstein AA. Clinical presentation and prognostic factors of spinal dural arteriovenous fistulas: an overview. Neurosurg Focus. 2012; 32. DOI: 10.3171/2012.1.FOCUS11376

[20] Barnwell SL, Dowd CF, Davis RL, et al. Cryptic Vascular Malformations of the Spinal Cord: Diagnosis by Magnetic Resonance Imaging and Outcome of Surgery. J Neurosurg. 1990; 72:403–407

[21] Anson JA, Spetzler RF. Interventional Neuroradiology for Spinal Pathology. Clinical Neurosurgery. 1991; 39:388–417

[22] Nabors MW, Pait TG, Byrd EB, et al. Updated Assessment and Current Classification of Spinal Meningeal Cysts. J Neurosurg. 1988; 68:366–377

[23] Kong WK, Cho KT, Hong SK. Symptomatic Tarlov cyst following spontaneous subarachnoid hemorrhage. J Korean Neurosurg Soc. 2011; 50:123–125

[24] Acosta FL,Jr, Quinones-Hinojosa A, Schmidt MH, et al. Diagnosis and management of sacral Tarlov cysts. Case report and review of the literature. Neurosurg Focus. 2003; 15. DOI: 10.3171/foc.2003.15.2.15

[25] Langdown AJ, Grundy JR, Birch NC. The clinical relevance of Tarlov cysts. J Spinal Disord Tech. 2005; 18:29–33

[26] Cho KT, Nam K. Perineural cyst with intracystic hemorrhage following aneurysmal subarachnoid hemorrhage: A case report. Medicine (Baltimore). 2019; 98. DOI: 10.1097/MD.0000000000014184

[27] Voyadzis JM, Bhargava P, Henderson FC. Tarlov cysts: a study of 10 cases with review of the literature. J Neurosurg. 2001; 95:25–32

[28] Mummaneni PV, Pitts LH, McCormack BM, et al. Microsurgical treatment of symptomatic sacral Tarlov cysts. Neurosurgery. 2000; 47:74–8; discussion 78-9

[29] Guo D, Shu K, Chen R, et al. Microsurgical treatment of symptomatic sacral perineurial cysts. Neurosurgery. 2007; 60:1059–65; discussion 1065-6

[30] Reardon MA, Raghavan P, Carpenter-Bailey K, et al. Dorsal thoracic arachnoid web and the "scalpel sign": a distinct clinical-radiologic entity. AJNR Am J Neuroradiol. 2013; 34:1104–1110

[31] Laxpati N, Malcolm JG, Tsemo GB, et al. Spinal arachnoid webs: Presentation, natural history, and outcomes in 38 patients. Neurosurgery. 2021; 89:917–927

[32] Nisson PL, Hussain I, Hartl R, et al. Arachnoid web of the spine: a systematic literature review. J Neurosurg Spine. 2019:1–10

[33] Guo XM, Qin XY, Huang C. Neuroelectrophysiological characteristics of Hirayama disease: report of 14 cases. Chin Med J (Engl). 2012; 125:2440–2443

[34] de Carvalho M, Swash M. Monomelic neurogenic syndromes: a prospective study. J Neurol Sci. 2007; 263:26–34

[35] Boruah DK, Prakash A, Gogoi BB, et al. The Importance of Flexion MRI in Hirayama Disease with Special Reference to Laminodural Space Measurements. AJNR Am J Neuroradiol. 2018; 39:974–980

[36] Darbar A, Krishnamurthy S, Holsapple JW, et al. Ventral thoracic spinal cord herniation: frequently misdiagnosed entity. Case reports. Spine. 2006; 31:E600–E605

[37] Batzdorf U. Primary spinal syringomyelia. Invited submission from the joint section meeting on disorders of the spine and peripheral nerves, March 2005. J Neurosurg Spine. 2005; 3:429–435

[38] Heiss JD, Oldfield EH. Pathophysiology and treatment of syringomyelia. Contemporary Neurosurgery. 2003; 25:1–8

[39] Oldfield EH, Muraszko K, Shawker TH, et al. Pathophysiology of syringomyelia associated with Chiari I malformation of the cerebellar tonsils. Implications for diagnosis and treatment. J Neurosurg. 1994; 80:3–15

[40] Deng X, Wu L, Yang C, et al. Neuropathic arthropathy caused by syringomyelia. J Neurosurg Spine. 2013; 18:303–309

84

84

[41] Johnson JT. Neuropathic fractures and joint injuries. Pathogenesis and rationale of prevention and treatment. J Bone Joint Surg Am. 1967; 49:1–30

[42] Brower AC, Allman RM. Pathogenesis of the neurotrophic joint: neurotraumatic vs. neurovascular. Radiology. 1981; 139:349–354

[43] Williams B, Terry AF, Jones F, et al. Syringomyelia as a Sequel to Traumatic Paraplegia. Paraplegia. 1981; 19:67–80

[44] Yasui K, Hashizume Y, Yoshida M, et al. Age-related morphologic changes of the central canal of the human spinal cord. Acta Neuropathol (Berl). 1999; 97:253–259

[45] Severino R, Severino P. Surgery or not? A case of ventriculus terminalis in an adult patient. J Spine Surg. 2017; 3:475–480

[46] Woodley-Cook J, Konieczny M, Spears J. The Slowly Enlarging Ventriculus Terminalis. Pol J Radiol. 2016; 81:529–531

[47] Brisman JL, Li M, Hamilton D, et al. Cystic dilation of the conus ventriculus terminalis presenting as an acute cauda equina syndrome relieved by decompression and cyst drainage: case report. Neurosurgery. 2006; 58. DOI: 10.1227/01.neu.0000197486.6 5781.88

[48] Suzuki M, Davis C, Symon L, et al. Syringoperitoneal Shunt for Treatment of Cord Cavitation. J Neurol Neurosurg Psychiatry. 1985; 48:620–627

[49] Hayashi T, Ueta T, Kubo M, et al. Subarachnoid-subarachnoid bypass: a new surgical technique for posttraumatic syringomyelia. J Neurosurg Spine. 2013; 18:382–387

[50] Klekamp J, Batzdorf U, Samii M, et al. Treatment of syringomyelia associated with arachnoid scarring caused by arachnoiditis or trauma. J Neurosurg. 1997; 86:233–240

[51] Lee TT, Alameda GJ, Camilo E, et al. Surgical treatment of post-traumatic myelopathy associated with syringomyelia. Spine (Phila Pa 1976). 2001; 26: S119–S127

[52] Booth AE, Kendall BE. Percutaneous Aspiration of Cystic Lesions of the Spinal Cord. J Neurosurg. 1970; 33:140–144

[53] Schmidek HH, Sweet WH. Operative Neurosurgical Techniques. New York 1982

[54] Logue V, Edwards MR. Syringomyelia and its Surgical Treatment. J Neurol Neurosurg Psychiatry. 1981; 44:273–284

[55] Phillips TW, Kindt GW. Syringoperitoneal shunt for syringomyelia: a preliminary report. Surgical Neurology. 1981; 16:462–466

[56] Rossier AB, Foo D, Shillito J, et al. Posttraumatic Cervical Syringomyelia. Brain. 1985; 108:439–461

[57] Vernon JD, Chir B, Silver JR, et al. Posttraumatic Syringomyelia. Paraplegia. 1982; 20:339–364

[58] Griffiths ER, McCormick CC. Posttraumatic Syringomyelia (Cystic Myelopathy). Paraplegia. 1981; 19:81–88

[59] Shannon N, Symon L, Logue V, et al. Clinical Features, Investigation and Treatment of Posttraumatic Syringomyelia. J Neurol Neurosurg Psychiatry. 1981; 44:35–42

[60] Stanworth PA. The Significance of Hyperhidrosis in Patients with Posttraumatic Syringomyelia. Paraplegia. 1982; 20:282–287

[61] Dworkin GE, Staas WE. Posttraumatic Syringomyelia. Arch Phys Med Rehabil. 1985; 66:329–331

[62] Watson N. Ascending Cystic Degeneration of the Cord After Spinal Cord Injury. Paraplegia. 1981; 19:89–95

[63] Durward QJ, Rice GP, Ball MJ, et al. Selective Spinal Cordectomy: Clinicopathological Correlation. J Neurosurg. 1982; 56:359–367

Part XVII

Subarachnoid Hemorrhage and Aneurysms

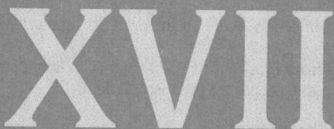

XVII

85 Aneurysms – Introduction, Grading, Special Conditions

85.1 Introduction and overview

85.1.1 Definitions

Subarachnoid hemorrhage: blood in the subarachnoid space (i.e., between the arachnoid membrane and the pia mater).

Aneurysm: (from the Greek aneurusma "dilatation"). An outpouching in the wall of an artery. May be focal (as in saccular AKA berry aneurysm) or fusiform. May be congenital or developmental. Etiologies:

1. congenital
2. developmental
   a) flow-related: generally at branch points of arteries, usually due to shear forces at these locations. Obsolete theory that this is due to underlying weakness of the media layer of the arterial wall at that location. Risk is increased in high flow states (e.g., chronic hypertension, drug-related e.g., cocaine, feeding vessels of AVMs…)
   b) mycotic (p. 1492): due to infection
   c) posttraumatic (p. 1491)
   d) conditions with abnormalities of blood vessels, including: autosomal dominant polycystic kidney disease (ADPKD) (p. 1455), vasculopathy (e.g., fibromuscular dysplasia (p. 209)), connective tissue disorders (Marfan syndrome (p. 1576), Ehlers-Danlos…)

Dissecting aneurysm (p. 1576): results from a tear in the arterial lining which allows blood to enter the arterial wall. Usually traumatically induced.
Pseudoaneurysm (p. 1576) (false aneurysm): a blood clot adjacent to a rent in the arterial wall.

85.1.2 Miscellaneous facts about SAH

1. may be posttraumatic or spontaneous. Trauma is the most common cause
2. most cases of spontaneous SAH are due to aneurysmal rupture
3. peak age for aneurysm SAH (aSAH) is 55–60 yrs, ≈ 20% of cases occur between ages 15–45 yrs[1]
4. 30% of aSAHs occur during sleep
5. sentinel headaches that precede the aSAH-associated ictus have been reported by 10–50% of patients and most commonly occur within 2–8 weeks before overt SAH.[2,3,4]
6. headache is lateralized in 30%, most to the side of the aneurysm
7. SAH is complicated by:
   a) intracerebral hemorrhage in 20–40%
   b) intraventricular hemorrhage (p. 1454) in 13–28%
   c) subdural blood in 2–5%.
   When the subdural blood is over the convexity, it is usually due to PComA aneurysm. With an interhemispheric subdural hematoma, it is usually due to a distal anterior intracerebral artery (DACA) aneurysm (p. 1475)
8. soft evidence suggests that rupture incidence is higher in spring and autumn
9. patients ≥ 70 yrs of age have a higher proportion with a severe neurologic grade[5]
10. seizures may occur in up to 20% of patients after SAH, most commonly in the first 24 hours, and are associated with ICH, HTN, and aneurysm location (MCA & acomm)[6,7]

85.1.3 Outcome of aneurysmal SAH

1. 10–15% of patients die before reaching medical care
2. mortality is 10% within first few days
3. 30-day mortality rate was 46% in one series,[8] and in others over half the patients died within 2 weeks of their SAH[9]
4. median mortality rate in epidemiological studies from U.S. has been 32% vs. 44% in Europe and 27% in Japan (may be an underestimate based on underreported prehospital death)[10]
5. causes of mortality
   a) 25% die as a result of medical complications of SAH[11]

- neurogenic pulmonary edema (p. 1439)
- neurogenic stress cardiomyopathy (p. 1438) (AKA neurogenic stunned myocardium)
  b) about 8% die from progressive deterioration from the initial hemorrhage[12(p 27)]
6. among patients surviving the initial hemorrhage treated without surgery, rebleeding (p. 1437) is the major cause of morbidity and mortality. The risk is ≈ 15–20% within 2 weeks. The goal of early surgery (p. 1462) is to reduce this risk
7. of those reaching neurosurgical care, vasospasm (p. 1439) kills 7%, and causes severe deficit in another 7%[13]
8. about ≈ 30% of survivors have moderate to severe disability,[14] with rates of persistent dependence estimated between 8–20% in population-based studies[10]
9. ≈ 66% of those who have successful aneurysm clipping never return to the same quality of life as before the SAH[14,15]
10. patients ≥ 70 yrs of age fare worse for each neurologic grade.[5] A multivariate analysis revealed age and WFNS grade to be most predictive of long-term outcome, regardless of treatment modality[16]
11. the severity of clinical presentation is the strongest prognostic indicator

85.2 Etiologies of SAH

Etiologies of subarachnoid hemorrhage (SAH) include[17]:
1. trauma: the most common cause of SAH.[18,19] In all of the following discussion, only non-traumatic (i.e., "spontaneous") SAH will be considered
2. "spontaneous SAH"
   a) ruptured intracranial aneurysms (p. 1454): **75–80%** of spontaneous SAHs
   b) cerebral arteriovenous malformation (AVM): 4–5% of cases. AVMs more commonly cause ICH & IVH than SAH (p. 1505)
   c) certain vasculitides that involve the CNS, see Vasculitis and vasculopathy (p. 203)
   d) rarely due to tumor (many case reports[20,21,22,23,24,25,26,27,28,29,30,31])
   e) cerebral artery dissection (may also be posttraumatic)
      - carotid artery (p. 1578)
      - vertebral artery (p. 1579): may cause intraventricular blood (especially 4th and 3rd ventricle)
   f) rupture of a small superficial artery
   g) rupture of an infundibulum (p. 1423)
   h) coagulation disorders:
      - iatrogenic or bleeding dyscrasias
      - thrombocytopenia
   i) dural sinus thrombosis
   j) spinal AVM (p. 1395): usually cervical or upper thoracic
   k) cortical subarachnoid hemorrhage
   l) pretruncal nonaneurysmal SAH (p. 1496) (perimesencephalic hemorrhage)
   m) rarely reported with some drugs: e.g., cocaine (p. 215)
   n) sickle cell disease
   o) pituitary apoplexy (p. 865)
   p) no cause can be determined in 14–22% (p. 1494)

85.3 Incidence of aneurysmal SAH (aSAH)

Estimated annual rate of aSAH in the United States: 9.7–14.5 per 100,000 population.[32,33] Reported rates are lower in South and Central America,[34] and higher in Japan and Finland.[35] Incidence of SAH increases with age (avg. age of onset > 50[33,36,37,38]); tends to be higher in women (1.24 times higher than men),[34] and appears to be higher in African Americans and Hispanics (compared to Caucasians).[32,39,40]

85.4 Risk factors for aSAH

See references.[17,41]
1. behavioral
   - hypertension
   - cigarette smoking[42]
   - alcohol abuse

- sympathomimetic drugs such as cocaine (p. 215), amphetamines (including "crystal meth")
- exercise/sports: weight training,[43] especially when performed with valsalva maneuver, carries a low risk of precipitating bleeding from a pre-existing aneurysm
2. gender and race (see above)
3. history of cerebral aneurysm
   - ruptured aneurysm
   - unruptured aneurysm (esp. those that are symptomatic, larger in size, and located in posterior circulation)
   - morphology: bottleneck shape[44] and increased ratio of size of aneurysm to parent vessel have been associated with increased risk of rupture[45,46]
4. family history of aneurysms (at least 1 first-degree family member and especially if ≥ 2 are affected)
5. genetic syndromes
   - autosomal dominant polycystic kidney disease (p. 1455)
   - type IV Ehlers-Danlos syndrome
6. pregnancy: controversial. Studies have found evidence for increased risk while others have not (p. 1425)

85.5 Clinical features

85.5.1 Symptoms of SAH

Sudden onset of severe H/A (see below), usually with vomiting, syncope (apoplexy), neck pain (meningismus), and photophobia. If there is LOC, patient may subsequently recover consciousness.[47] Focal cranial nerve deficits may occur (e.g., third nerve palsy from aneurysmal compression of the third cranial nerve, causing diplopia and/or ptosis). Low back pain may develop due to irritation of lumbar nerve roots by dependent blood.

85.5.2 Headache

The most common symptom, present in up to 97% of cases. Usually severe (classic description: "the worst headache of my life") and sudden in onset (paroxysmal). The H/A may clear and the patient may not seek medical attention (referred to as a **sentinel hemorrhage** or headache, or warning headache; they occur in 30–60% of patients presenting with SAH). If severe or accompanied by reduced level of consciousness, most patients present for medical evaluation. Patients with H/A due to minor hemorrhages will have blood on CT or LP. However, warning headaches may also occur without SAH and may be due to aneurysmal enlargement or to hemorrhage confined within the aneurysmal wall.[48] Warning H/A are usually sudden in onset, milder than that associated with a major rupture, and may last a few days.

Differential diagnosis of severe, acute, paroxysmal headache (25% will have SAH[49]):
1. subarachnoid hemorrhage: including "warning headache" or sentinel H/A (see above)
2. benign "thunderclap headaches" (BTH) or crash migraine.[50] Severe global headaches of abrupt onset that reach maximal intensity in < 1 minute, accompanied by vomiting in ≈ 50%. They may recur, and are presumably a form of vascular headache. Some may have transient focal symptoms. There are no clinical criteria that can reliably differentiate these from SAH[51] (although seizures and diplopia, when they occurred, were always associated with SAH). There is no subarachnoid blood on CT or LP (CT and/or CTA should probably be performed on at least the first presentation to R/O SAH). Earlier recommendations to angiogram these individuals[52] have since been tempered by experience[53,54]
3. reversible cerebral vasoconstrictive syndrome (RCVS)[55] (AKA benign cerebral angiopathy or vasculitis[56]): severe H/A with paroxysmal onset, ± neurologic deficit, and string-of-beads appearance on angiography of cerebral vessels that usually clears in 1–3 months. More than 50% report prior use of vasoconstrictive substances (cocaine, marijuana, nasal decongestants, ergot derivatives, SSRIs, interferon, nicotine patches) sometimes combined with binge drinking. May also occur post-partum. Complications occurred in 24% including:
   a) usually during the 1st week: SAH, ICH, seizures, RPLS
   b) usually during the 2nd week: ischemic events (TIA, stroke)
4. airplane headache: usually sudden, often (but not exclusively) with onset during take-off (less common) or landing of aircraft. Short-lasting (by definition: ≤ 30 minutes after completion of ascent or descent[57]; however, in one series 76% of H/A otherwise typical for airplane H/A lasted > 30 minutes[58]), usually unilateral, primarily orbitofrontal (occasionally with spread to parietal

region). Typically jabbing or stabbing in quality. Ipsilateral nasal congestion, a stuffy feeling of the face, or tearing may occur in < 5%.[57] Pathogenesis may be related to obstructed drainage of sinuses ("aerosinusitis" or barosinusitis); however, a vascular mechanism may be possible. H/A may respond to triptans (19%) or acetaminophen (5%).[58]

5. **benign orgasmic cephalgia**: a severe, throbbing, sometimes "explosive" H/A with onset just before or at the time of orgasm (distinct from pre-orgasmic headaches which intensify with sexual arousal[59]). In a series of 21 patients[60] neurologic exam was normal in all, and angiography done in 9 was normal. 9 had a history of migraine in the patient or a family member. No other symptoms developed in 18 patients followed for 2–7 yrs. Recommendations for evaluation are similar to that for thunderclap headaches above

85.5.3 Signs

Meningismus (see below), hypertension, focal neurologic deficit (e.g., oculomotor palsy, hemiparesis), obtundation or coma (see below), ocular hemorrhage (see below).

Meningismus

Nuchal rigidity (especially to flexion) often ensues in 6 to 24 hrs. Patients may have a positive Kernig sign (flex thigh to 90° with knee bent, then straighten knee, positive sign if this causes pain in hamstrings) or Brudzinski sign (flex the supine patient's neck, involuntary hip flexion is a positive sign).

Coma following SAH

Coma may follow SAH because of any one or a combination of the following[61]:
1. increased ICP
2. damage to brain tissue from intraparenchymal hemorrhage (may also contribute to increased ICP)
3. hydrocephalus
4. diffuse ischemia (may be secondary to increased ICP)
5. seizure
6. reduced CBF (p. 1438) low blood flow (e.g., due to reduced cardiac output)

Ocular hemorrhage

Three types of ocular hemorrhage (OH) may be associated with SAH. They occur alone or in various combinations in 20–40% of patients with SAH.[62]
1. subhyaloid (preretinal) hemorrhage: seen funduscopically in 11–33% of cases as bright red blood near the optic disc that obscures the underlying retinal vessels. May be associated with a higher mortality rate[63]
2. (intra)retinal hemorrhage: may surround the fovea
3. hemorrhage within the vitreous humor (Terson syndrome). First described by the French ophthalmologist Albert Terson. Occurs in 4–27% of cases of aneurysmal SAH,[64,65,66] usually bilateral. May occur with other causes of increased ICP including ruptured AVMs. Funduscopy reveals vitreous opacity. The location of the origin of the vitreous hemorrhage differs in various reports (subhyaloid, epiretinal, subinternal limiting membrane).[67] May be more common with anterior circulation aneurysms (especially ACoA), although 1 study found no correlation with location.[65] Also rarely reported with SDH and traumatic SAH. Often missed on initial examination. When sought, usually present on initial exam; however, it may develop as late as 12 days post SAH, and may be associated with rebleeding.[65] The mortality rate may be higher in SAH patients with vitreous hemorrhage than in those without. Patients should be followed for complications of OH (elevated intraocular pressure, retinal membrane formation → retinal detachment, retinal folds[68]). Most cases clear spontaneously in 6–12 mos. Vitrectomy should be considered in patients whose vision fails to improve[66] or if more rapid improvement is desired.[69] The long-term prognosis for vision is good in ≈ 80% of cases with or without vitrectomy[69]

The pathomechanics of OH are controversial. OH was originally attributed to extension of the blood from the subarachnoid space into the vitreous, but no communication exists between these two spaces. In actuality may be due to compression of the central retinal vein and the retinochoroidal anastomoses by elevated CSF pressure,[66] causing venous hypertension and disruption of retinal veins.

85.6 Work-up of suspected SAH

85.6.1 Overview

1. tests to diagnose SAH
   a) non-contrast high-resolution CT scan: very sensitive and specific (see below)
   b) if CT is negative: LP in suspicious cases. Very sensitive, but only 65–80% specific (see below)
   c) with CT, the concern is a false negative test (missing a SAH), and with LP the concern is a false positive (a bloody tap mimicking a SAH). However, the combination of a negative CT and a negative LP is extremely strong in ruling out SAH[70]
2. tests to identify *source* of SAH. Options: CTA, MRA, or catheter angiography. The choice needs to take into account the patient's age, renal function, and even best guess of where an aneurysm might be located
   a) MRA (p. 243). Pros: no radiation, and 2D-TOF MRA does not use contrast. Cons: poor sensitivity for aneurysm detection early after SAH (see below)
   b) CTA vs. digital subtraction catheter angiogram (DSA): one needs to balance the risk of the procedure and ease of obtaining it against the information expected to be obtained
      • total iodine load in a healthy adult should be < 90 gm in 24 hours. In older patients and/or possible compromised renal function, this volume should be less. CTA typically uses 65–75 cc of contrast with ≈ 300 mg iodine/ml, or ≈ 21 gm iodine. The amount of contrast with a cerebral arteriogram varies. However, if an angiogram is needed after a CTA, in most cases you do not have to wait 24 hours
      • if there is concern about renal function (e.g., serum creatinine > 100 mcmol/L) hydrate the patient and optionally give Mucomyst® (p. 232)
      • catheter angiography (DSA) may be necessary after a positive CTA to better delineate the anatomy, or to determine dominant filling and cross flow, or in highly suspicious cases with a negative CTA (see below). While CTA permits reliable assessment of feasibility of endovascular treatment in most cases,[71] DSA is still necessary in some
3. if CTA/angiogram is negative: see SAH of unknown etiology (p. 1494)

85.6.2 Laboratory/radiographic findings

CT scan

▶ **Sensitivity and specificity.** High-quality non-contrast CT (no motion artifact, 3rd generation or newer high-resolution CT scanner) is very sensitive to intracranial SAH. Sensitivity decreases with time as the blood dissipates.
• within 6 hrs of SAH: sensitivity is 98–100%, specificity 100%, negative predictive value 99.4%, positive predictive value 100% (in 240 adults with new acute H/A peaking in ≤ 1 hr[72])
• sensitivity of CT < 12 hrs after SAH: ≈ 98%
• after 12 hrs, the sensitivity is too low to rely on noncontrast CT alone to exclude the potentially lethal diagnosis of ruptured aneurysm. But it can be helpful if positive
   ○ sensitivity of CT < 24 hrs of SAH: ≈ 93%
   ○ CT < 72 hrs of SAH: ≈ 80%
   ○ CT 1 week after SAH: ≈ 50%

▶ **Findings.** Blood appears as high density (white) within subarachnoid spaces (▶ Fig. 85.1). Subtle hints for SAH: look for blood in the occipital horns of the lateral ventricles and the dependent portions of the Sylvian fissures.
CT also assesses:
1. ventricular size: acute hydrocephalus after aneurysmal rupture (p. 1426) occurs in 21%[73]
2. hematoma: intracerebral hemorrhage or large amount of subdural blood with mass effect may need emergent evacuation (most common with MCA aneurysms)
3. amount of blood in cisterns and fissures: important prognosticator for vasospasm (p. 1441) and can identify pretruncal nonaneurysmal hemorrhage (p. 1496)
4. CT can predict aneurysm location based on the pattern of blood in ≈ 78% of cases (but mostly for MCA and AComA aneurysms)[74]
   a) blood predominantly in anterior interhemispheric fissure (± blood in lateral ventricles) (▶ Fig. 88.1) or within the gyrus rectus suggests AComA aneurysm
   b) blood predominantly in 1 Sylvian fissure is compatible with PComA or MCA aneurysm on that side (▶ Fig. 85.1)
   c) blood predominantly in the prepontine or peduncular cistern suggests a basilar apex or SCA aneurysm

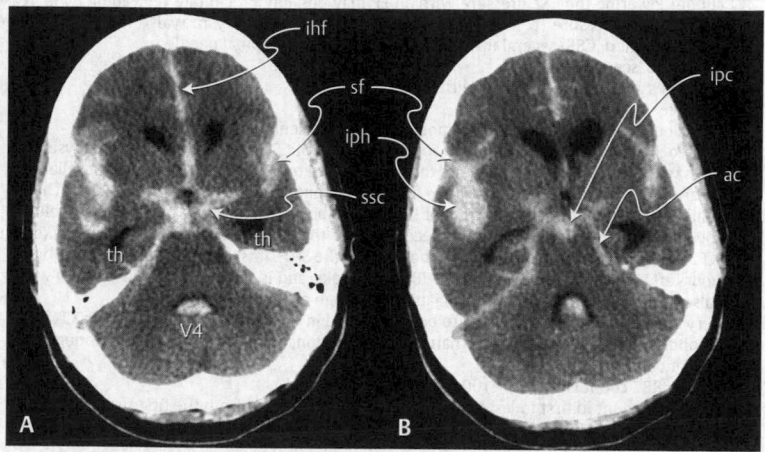

Fig. 85.1 SAH on CT. Image: axial CT scan in patient with SAH (and intraparenchymal hematoma) from a ruptured right middle cerebral artery aneurysm.
Image: A: CT slice through the suprasellar cistern (ssc) showing a classic SAH pattern, with blood in the ssc, interhemispheric fissure (ihf) & Sylvian fissures (sf).
B: CT slice slightly above the ssc showing SAH in the interpeduncular cistern (ipc), the ambient cisterns (ac) as well as intraparenchymal hematoma (iph) from the aneurysmal rupture.
Note the dilated temporal horns (th) suggesting early hydrocephalus and blood in the 4th ventricle (V4).

85

d) blood predominantly within ventricles (p. 1454)
- blood primarily in 4th and 3rd ventricle (▶ Fig. 88.2): suggests lower posterior fossa source, such as PICA aneurysm (p. 1480) or VA dissection
- blood primarily in the 3rd ventricle suggests a basilar apex aneurysm

5. with multiple aneurysms, CT may help identify which one bled by the location of blood (see above). See also other "clues" (p. 1490)
6. ✖ CT is not sensitive for infarct in the first 24 hours after infarct (see CT scan with acute ischemic infarct (p. 1559))

▶ **Differential diagnosis of SAH on CT.** Things that can mimic the appearance of SAH on CT include:
1. pus: as in meningitis
2. following contrast administration: sometimes IV, and especially intrathecal
3. occasionally the pachymeningeal thickening seen in spontaneous intracranial hypotension (p. 421)

CT angiography (CTA)

CTA (p. 238), a 64-slice CTA is 98% sensitive and 100% specific for detecting aneurysms > 3 mm diameter,[75] and in a prospective study detected 97% of aneurysms, and was deemed as safe and effective when used as the initial and sole imaging study for ruptured and unruptured cerebral aneurysms.[76] CTA shows a 3-dimensional image (as can modern catheter angiography), which can help differentiate adherent vessels from those arising from the aneurysm. CTA also demonstrates the relation to nearby bony structures which can be important in surgical planning. CTA may also be used for evaluation of vasospasm.[77]

Lumbar puncture

The most sensitive test for SAH, approaching 100%, with a negative predictive value of 100% for SAH. However, false positives—e.g., with traumatic taps (Differentiating SAH from traumatic tap (p. 1814))—occur with enough frequency that the specificity may be in the range of 80%[78] and possibly as low as 65%.[75] Skipping the LP and going right to CTA is controversial with arguments both for[79] and against.[80] The LP is more helpful to *rule-out* SAH if CSF has no blood.

✖ Caution: lowering the CSF pressure with an LP may possibly precipitate rebleeding by increasing the transmural pressure (p. 1427) (the pressure across the aneurysm wall). Therefore remove only a small amount of CSF (several ml) and use a small (≤ 20 Ga) spinal needle.

Findings (also, see ▶ Table 23.4):

1. opening pressure: usually elevated with SAH
2. appearance:
   a) non-clotting bloody fluid that does not clear with sequential collection tubes
   b) xanthochromia (XTC): yellow coloration (▶ Fig. 85.2) of CSF supernatant due to the lysis of RBCs which releases heme pigments that break down to bilirubin. XTC is the most reliable means of differentiating traumatic tap from SAH in patients with a negative head CT. The minimum amount of time required for bilirubin to become detectable in the CSF, as well as the minimum amount of blood that needs to enter the CSF to produce XTC remains unknown. XTC is usually not apparent until 2–4 hours after the SAH. It is present in almost 100% by 12 hours after the bleed, and remains in 70% at 3 weeks, and is still detectable in 40% at 4 weeks. False positives: XTC may occur with jaundice or high protein levels in the CSF.
   Very bloody specimens may need to be centrifuged in the lab to be able to look for XTC. Spectrophotometry is more sensitive than visual inspection, but may not be specific enough to warrant widespread use[81,82]
3. cell count: RBC count is usually > 100,000 RBCs/mm³ in SAH
4. compare RBC count in first to last tube: a reduction of RBC count from the first tube to the last tube of 70% with < 500 RBC/mm³ in the final tube has been suggested to be diagnostic of a traumatic tap[83] (controversial (p. 1814))
5. protein: elevated due to blood breakdown products
6. glucose: normal or reduced (RBCs may metabolize some glucose with time)

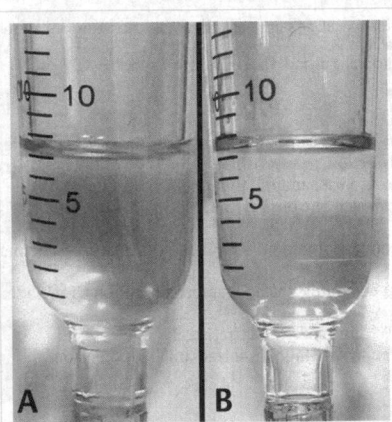

Fig. 85.2 Xanthochromic CSF in A, compared to normal CSF in B.

MRI

Not sensitive for SAH acutely within the first 24–48 hrs[84] (too little met-Hb), especially with thin layers of blood. Better after ≈ 4–7 days (excellent for subacute to remote SAH, > 10–20 days). FLAIR MRI is the most sensitive imaging study for detecting blood in the subarachnoid space. May be helpful in determining which of multiple aneurysms bled (p. 1490).[85]

Magnetic resonance angiography (MRA)

Compared to catheter DSA, sensitivity is 87% and specificity is 92% for detecting intracranial aneurysms (IAs). Sensitivity is significantly worse for aneurysms < 3 mm diameter.[86,87,88]

MRA's ability to detect IAs depends on aneurysm size, rate and direction of blood flow in the aneurysm relative to the magnetic field, and aneurysmal thrombosis and calcification. MRA may be most useful as a screening test in high-risk patients, including patients with two first-degree relatives with IAs, especially those who are also smokers or hypertensive themselves.[89]

Catheter angiogram

General information

Injection of radio-opaque (iodinated) contrast ("dye") into selective vessels using a catheter typically inserted into the femoral artery at the upper thigh, while taking serial X-rays to obtain a "video-like" representation of the vasculature.

The gold standard for evaluation of cerebral aneurysms. Current state of the art uses digital subtraction angiography (DSA). Demonstrates source (usually aneurysm) in ≈ 80–85%; remainder are so-called "SAH of unknown etiology" (p. 1494). Shows if radiographic vasospasm is present— **clinical** vasospasm (p. 1439) almost never occurs < 3 days following SAH—and assesses primary feeding arteries, collateral flow in case of a need for arterial sacrifice.

General principles:

1. study the vessel of highest suspicion first (in case patient's condition should change, necessitating discontinuation of procedure)
2. continue to do complete 4-vessel angiogram (even if aneurysm(s) have been demonstrated) to rule out additional aneurysms and assess collateral circulation
3. if there is an aneurysm or suspicion of one, obtain additional views to help delineate the neck and orientation of the aneurysm (see index for specific aneurysm)
4. ★ if no aneurysm is seen, before an arteriogram can be considered negative, must:
   a) visualize *both PICA origins*: 1–2% of aneurysms occur at PICA origin. Both PICAs can usually be visualized with one VA injection if there is enough flow to reflux down the contralateral VA. Occasionally it is necessary to see more of the contralateral VA than what refluxes to PICA and selective catheterization may be required
   b) *flow contrast through the ACoA*: if both ACAs fill from one side, this is usually satisfactory. It may be necessary to perform a cross compression AP study with carotid injection (first, rule out plaque in the carotid to be compressed), or use a higher injection rate to facilitate flow through the ACoA
   c) if an infundibulum (see below) co-localizes to the SAH, it may be unwise to label the case as angiogram-negative, and exploration is recommended by some[90]

Infundibulum

A funnel-shaped initial segment of an artery, to be distinguished from an aneurysm. Found in 7–13% of otherwise normal arteriograms,[91,92] with a higher incidence in cases of multiple or familial aneurysms. Bilateral in 25%.[92] Most commonly found at the origin of the PComAs, but they rarely occur at other sites. Criteria for differentiating infundibula from aneurysms are shown in ▶ Table 85.1. Infundibula may represent incomplete remnants of previous fetal vessels.[93(p 272)]

Although they may bleed,[90,95,96,97] there is less risk of rupture than with a saccular aneurysm (no

Table 85.1 Criteria of an infundibulum

1. triangular in shape
2. mouth (widest portion) < 3 mm[a] [94]
3. vessel at apex

[a] a widely accepted but probably arbitrary dimension

infundibulum < 3 mm in size bled[98] in the cooperative study). However, infundibula have been documented to progress to an aneurysm (i.e., they are preaneurysmal) which may bleed (13 case reports in the literature as of 2009). Recommended treatment: at the time of surgery for another reason, consider treating an infundibulum with wrapping, or placing in an encircling clip, or sacrificing the artery if it can be done safely (infundibula lack a true neck).

Angiographic findings

1. general features to take note of when analyzing an aneurysm on angiogram (special considerations for specific aneurysms are covered in designated sections)
   a) size of aneurysm dome:
      - MRI or CT helps with this since the aneurysm may be partially thrombosed and the portion that is patent and fills with contrast and is therefore visualized on angiogram may be much smaller than the actual size
      - large aneurysms (≥ 15 mm dia.) are associated with lower rates of complete occlusion by endovascular coiling[99,100]
   b) neck size
      - narrow necks < 5 mm are ideal for coiling[101]

- broad necks ≥ 5 mm are associated with increased risk of incomplete occlusion and recanalization with coiling[100]
- stent or balloon-assisted coiling may be needed for wide-necked aneurysms. Stents should be avoided if possible (p. 1923)

c) dome:neck ratio ≥ 2 is associated with higher rate of successful coil occlusion[101]

2. for basilar bifurcation aneurysms (p. 1482)

85.7 Grading SAH

85.7.1 General information

Four grading scales are in common use. The two most widely quoted grading scales, the Hunt-and-Hess and the WFNS, are presented below.

85.7.2 Hunt and Hess grade

See ▶ Table 85.2 and ▶ Table 85.3 for grading system. Grades 1 and 2 were operated upon as soon as an aneurysm was diagnosed. Grade ≥ 3 managed until the condition improved to Grade 2 or 1. Exception: life-threatening hematoma or multiple bleeds (which were operated on regardless of grade).

Analysis of data from the International Cooperative Aneurysm Study revealed that with normal consciousness, Hunt and Hess (H&H) grades 1 and 2 had identical outcome, and that hemiparesis and/or aphasia had no effect on mortality.

Mortality:

Admission Hunt and Hess Grade 1 or 2: 20%.

Patients taken to O.R. (for any procedure) at H&H Grade 1 or 2: 14%.

Major cause of death in Grade 1 or 2 is rebleed.

Signs of meningeal irritation increases surgical risk.

Table 85.2 Hunt and Hess classification[a] of SAH[102]

Grade	Description
1	asymptomatic, or mild H/A and slight nuchal rigidity
2	Cr. N. palsy (e.g., III, VI), moderate to severe H/A, nuchal rigidity
3	mild focal deficit, lethargy, or confusion
4	stupor, moderate to severe hemiparesis, early decerebrate rigidity
5	deep coma, decerebrate rigidity, moribund appearance

Add one grade for serious systemic disease (e.g., HTN, DM, severe atherosclerosis, COPD) or severe vasospasm on arteriography.

[a]original paper did not consider patient's age, site of aneurysm, or time since bleed; patients were graded on admission and pre-op

Table 85.3 Modified classification[103] adds the following

Grade	Description
0	unruptured aneurysm
1 a	no acute meningeal/brain reaction, but with fixed neuro deficit

85.7.3 World Federation of Neurosurgical Societies / World Federation of Neurological Surgeons (WFNS) grading of SAH

Due to lack of data on the significance of features such as headache, nuchal rigidity, and major focal neurologic deficit, the WFNS Committee on a Universal SAH Grading Scale[104,105] developed the grading system shown in ▶ Table 85.4. It employs the Glasgow Coma Scale (▶ Table 18.1) (GCS) to grade the level of consciousness, and uses the presence or absence of major focal neurologic deficit to distinguish grade 2 from grade 3.

Table 85.4 WFNS SAH grade[104]

WFNS grade	GCS score[a]	Major focal deficit[b]
0[c]		
1	15	–
2	13–14	–
3	13–14	+
4	7–12	+ or –
5	3–6	+ or –

[a]GCS = Glasgow Coma Scale, see ▶ Table 18.1
[b]aphasia, hemiparesis or hemiplegia (+ = present, – = absent)
[c]intact (unruptured) aneurysm

85.8 Pregnancy and intracranial hemorrhage

85.8.1 General information

Intracranial hemorrhage (subarachnoid or intraparenchymal) is a rare occurrence during pregnancy (estimated range of incidence: 0.01–0.05% of all pregnancies[106]) and yet is responsible for 5–12% of maternal deaths during pregnancy.

Intracranial hemorrhage of pregnancy (ICHOP) commonly occurs in the setting of eclampsia, and is more commonly intraparenchymal[107] and may be associated with loss of cerebrovascular autoregulation PRES (p.202).[108] HELLP syndrome (hemolysis, elevated liver enzymes, and low platelet count) is a severe variant of pre-eclampsia.[109] Symptoms of eclampsia with or without ICHOP include H/A, mental status changes, and seizures.

It has been asserted that risk of aneurysmal SAH does not appear to be increased in pregnancy, delivery, and puerperium.[110,111] A literature review of 154 reported cases of ICHOP-related SAH revealed that 77% were aneurysmal and 23% were from ruptured AVM (other series show the percentage of AVMs range from 21–48%). Mortality is ≈ 35% for aneurysmal and ≈ 28% for AVM hemorrhage (the latter being higher than in non-gravid patients). There is an increasing tendency for bleeding with advancing gestational age for both aneurysms and AVMs (earlier it had been asserted that this held true for aneurysms only[112]).

Patients with ICHOP having AVMs tend to be younger than those with aneurysm, paralleling the occurrence in the general population. One major oft-quoted study showed an increased risk of hemorrhage from AVMs during pregnancy[113] (citing an 87% hemorrhage rate); however, another investigation disputes this assertion,[114] and found the risk of hemorrhage to be 3.5% during the pregnancy in patients with no history of hemorrhage, or 5.8% in those with previous hemorrhage. Another study evaluated risk of aneurysm rupture during pregnancy and delivery from the Nationwide Inpatient data and calculated the rupture risk during pregnancy and delivery to be 1.4% and 0.05%, respectively.[115] Literature review[106] found that the risk of recurrent hemorrhage following ICHOP from aneurysm or AVM during the remainder of the pregnancy was 33–50%.

85.8.2 Management modifications for pregnant patients

Modifications of evaluation and treatment techniques may be necessary for the pregnant patient.
1. neuroradiologic studies
   a) CAT scan: with shielding of the fetus, CAT scanning of the brain produces minimal radiation exposure to the child
   b) MRI:
      - generally felt to have low potential for complications; however, many centers will not do MRI during first trimester.
      - gadolinium-based contrast agents (GBCAs) are teratogenic in animals in high repeated doses. It has not been studied in human pregnancy. A cohort of 26 women who received GBCAs during the first trimester showed no evidence of teratogenicity or mutagenicity.[116] There have also been no reported issues related to nephrogenic systemic fibrosis (p.243). GBCAs are FDA Class C drugs—not recommended for use during pregnancy, but may be used if benefits outweigh potential risks.
   c) angiography: with shielding of the fetus, radiation exposure is minimal. Iodinated contrast agents pose little risk to the fetus. The mother should be well hydrated during and after the study[106]

2. antiseizure medications: see Pregnancy and antiseizure medications (p. 500)
3. diuretics: the use of mannitol in pregnancy should be avoided to prevent fetal dehydration and maternal hypovolemia with uterine hypoperfusion
4. antihypertensives: nitroprusside should not be used in pregnancy
5. nimodipine is potentially teratogenic in animals, the effect on humans is unknown. It should be used only when the potential benefit justifies the risk

85.8.3 Neurosurgical management

The currently recommended treatment of a ruptured aneurysm in the pregnant patient is immediate surgical treatment to avoid rebleeding and ischemic complications due to vasospasm. A meta-analysis has demonstrated that mother and fetus both benefit from surgical treatment—with maternal mortality decreasing from 63% to 11% and fetal mortality decreasing from 27% to 5%.[106,117] Successful endovascular treatment for aSAH has been reported, but fetal exposure to radiation is a concern. The absorbed fetal dose has been estimated to range from 0.17 to 2.8 mGy, corresponding to a fetal risk of a hereditary disease at birth and a cumulative risk for a fatal cancer by age 15, which are both substantially lower than those which naturally occur.[118] Because endovascular treatment requires heparin for systemic anticoagulation, it carries the risk of hemorrhagic implications when labor spontaneously begins during or around the time of embolization.

85.8.4 Obstetric management following ICHOP

Several reports have indicated that the fetal and maternal outcome is no different for vaginal delivery vs. C-section, and is probably more dependent on whether the offending lesion has been treated. However, there are no formal studies to help guide the optimal treatment of pregnant women with aSAH. One strategy[117] is to perform an emergent C-section, followed by aneurysm treatment, if the fetus is mature enough for survival outside the uterus. If the fetus is < 24 weeks, treat the aneurysm and maintain the pregnancy. If the fetus is between 24–28 weeks, a strategy should be tailored according to the maternal and fetal status. C-section may be used for fetal salvage for a moribund mother in the third trimester. During vaginal delivery, the risk of rebleeding may be reduced by the use of caudal or epidural anesthesia, shortening the second stage of labor, and low forceps delivery if necessary.

85.9 Hydrocephalus after SAH

85.9.1 Hydrocephalus after traumatic SAH

See also posttraumatic hydrocephalus (p. 1108).

85.9.2 Acute hydrocephalus

General information

The frequency of hydrocephalus (HCP) on the initial CT after SAH depends on the defining criteria used, with a reported range of 9–67%.[119] A realistic range is ≈ 15–20% of SAH patients, with 30–60% of these showing no impairment of consciousness.[119,120] 3% of those *without* HCP on initial CT develop HCP within 1 week.[119]

Factors felt to contribute to acute HCP include blood interfering with CSF flow through the Sylvian aqueduct, 4th ventricle outlet, or subarachnoid space, and/or with reabsorption at the arachnoid granulations.

Findings associated with acute HCP include[120]

1. increasing age
2. admission CT findings: intraventricular blood, diffuse subarachnoid blood, and thick focal accumulation of subarachnoid blood (intraparenchymal blood did *not* correlate with chronic HCP, and patients with a normal CT had a low incidence)
3. hypertension: on admission, prior to admission (by history), or post-op
4. by location:
   a) posterior circulation aneurysms have a higher incidence of HCP
   b) MCA aneurysms correlate with low incidence of HCP
5. miscellaneous: hyponatremia, patients who were not alert on admission, use of preoperative antifibrinolytic agents, and low Glasgow outcome score

Treatment

About half the patients with acute HCP and impaired consciousness improved spontaneously.[119] Patients in poor grade (H&H IV–V) with large ventricles may be symptomatic from the HCP and consideration should be given to ventriculostomy which caused improvement in ≈ 80% of patients in whom it was used.[119] There may be an increased risk of aneurysm rebleeding in patients undergoing ventriculostomy shortly after SAH[119,121,122] especially if performed early and if ICP is lowered precipitously. The risk of aneurysm rebleeding with EVD has been studied in retrospective case series with mixed results.[123,124,125] The mechanism is controversial, but may be due to an increase in the transmural pressure (the pressure across the aneurysm wall which equals the difference between arterial pressure and ICP).

When a ventriculostomy is used, it is recommended to keep ICP in the range of 15–25 mm Hg[126] and to avoid rapid pressure reduction (unless absolutely necessary) to decrease the risk of IVC-induced aneurysmal rebleeding. One paradigm is to keep the EVD open with the drip chamber nozzle 15–20 cm above the tragus.

85

Practice guideline: Acute hydrocephalus associated with aSAH

Level B[41]: CSF diversion (EVD or lumbar drain) for acute symptomatic hydrocephalus associated with aSAH.

85.9.3 Chronic hydrocephalus

Practice guideline: Chronic hydrocephalus associated with aSAH

- Level B[41]: permanent CSF diversion (shunt) for symptomatic chronic hydrocephalus following aSAH.
- Level C[41]: Weaning an EVD over > 24 hours does not appear to reduce the need for permanent CSF diversion.
- Level C[41]: Routine fenestration of the lamina terminalis is not recommended as it does not reduce the need for permanent CSF diversion.

Chronic hydrocephalus (chronic HCP) is due to pia-arachnoid adhesions or permanent impairment of the arachnoid granulations. Acute HCP does not inevitably lead to chronic HCP. 8–45% (reported range[127]) of all ruptured aneurysm patients, and ≈ 50% of those with acute HCP following SAH need permanent CSF diversion. A number of studies have attempted to identify factors predictive of aSAH-associated shunt-dependent chronic hydrocephalus. Intraventricular blood increases this risk.[127] There is controversy as to whether the use of ventriculostomy for acute HCP increases[128] or possibly even decreases[127] the incidence of shunt dependency. There may be a positive association between Fisher grade and the likelihood of requiring CSF diversion for chronic hydrocephalus.[129] In addition, Hoh et al[130] found age (2% increase/year), comorbidity score (presence of DM, HTN, alcohol abuse), admission type, insurance type (increased with Medicaid and private payer), and hospital aneurysm volume (high > low) to be predictive of shunt placement in ruptured aneurysm patients. Treatment type (clip versus coil) has also been studied with no clear advantage for one modality over the other (p. 1457).

The method of determining which patients require shunt placement has also been studied in a single center RCT.[131] There was no difference in the rate of shunt placement between those who underwent rapid weaning (< 24 hrs) versus gradual weaning (96 hrs) of the EVD (63.4% rapid versus 62.5% gradual).

References

[1] Biller J, Toffol GJ, Kassell NF, et al. Spontaneous Subarachnoid Hemorrhage in Young Adults. Neurosurgery. 1987; 21:664–667

[2] Okawara SH. Warning Signs Prior to Rupture of an Intracranial Aneurysm. Journal of Neurosurgery. 1973; 38:575–580

85

[3] de Falco FA. Sentinel headache. Neurol Sci. 2004; 25 Suppl 3:S215–S217

[4] Polmear A. Sentinel headaches in aneurysmal subarachnoid haemorrhage: what is the true incidence? A systematic review. Cephalalgia. 2003; 23:935–941

[5] Yamashita K, Kashiwagi S, Kato S, et al. Cerebral Aneurysms in the Elderly in Yamaguchi, Japan. Analysis of the Yamaguchi Data Bank of Cerebral Aneurysm From 1985 to 1995. Stroke. 1997; 28:1926–1931

[6] Ohman J. Hypertension as a risk factor for epilepsy after aneurysmal subarachnoid hemorrhage and surgery. Neurosurgery. 1990; 27:578–581

[7] Sundaram MB, Chow F. Seizures associated with spontaneous subarachnoid hemorrhage. Can J Neurol Sci. 1986; 13:229–231

[8] Broderick JP, Brott TG, Tomsick T, et al. Intracerebral Hemorrhage More Than Twice as Common as Subarachnoid Hemorrhage. J Neurosurg. 1993; 78:188–191

[9] Sarti C, Tuomilehto J, Salomaa V, et al. Epidemiology of Subarachnoid Hemorrhage in Finland from 1983 to 1985. Stroke. 1991; 22:848–853

[10] Nieuwkamp DJ, Setz LE, Algra A, et al. Changes in case fatality of aneurysmal subarachnoid haemorrhage over time, according to age, sex, and region: a meta-analysis. Lancet Neurol. 2009; 8:635–642

[11] Solenski NJ, Haley EC, Kassell NF, et al. Medical complications of aneurysmal subarachnoid hemorrhage: a report of the multicenter, cooperative aneurysm study. Participants of the Multicenter Cooperative Aneurysm Study. Critical Care Medicine. 1995; 23:1007–1017

[12] Sahs AL, Nibbelink DW, Torner JC. Aneurysmal Subarachnoid Hemorrhage: Report of the Cooperative Study. Baltimore-Munich 1981

[13] Kassell NF, Sasaki T, Colohan ART, et al. Cerebral Vasospasm Following Aneurysmal Subarachnoid Hemorrhage. Stroke. 1985; 16:562–572

[14] Hop JW, Rinkel GJ, Algra A, et al. Case-Fatality Rates and Functional Outcome After Subarachnoid Hemorrhage: A Systematic Review. Stroke. 1997; 28:660–664

[15] Drake CG. Management of Cerebral Aneurysm. Stroke. 1981; 12:273–283

[16] Park J, Woo H, Kang DH, et al. Critical age affecting 1-year functional outcome in elderly patients aged >/= 70 years with aneurysmal subarachnoid hemorrhage. Acta Neurochir (Wien). 2014; 156:1655–1661

[17] Wirth FP. Surgical Treatment of Incidental Intracranial Aneurysms. Clin Neurosurg. 1986; 33:125–135

[18] Greene KA, Marciano FF, Johnson BA, et al. Impact of Traumatic Subarachnoid Hemorrhage on Outcome in Nonpenetrating Head Injury. Journal of Neurosurgery. 1995; 83:445–452

[19] Taneda M, Kataoka K, Akai F, et al. Traumatic Subarachnoid Hemorrhage as a Predictable Indicator of Delayed Ischemic Symptoms. Journal of Neurosurgery. 1996; 84:762–768

[20] Dagi TF, Maccabe JJ. Metastatic Trophoblastic Disease Presenting as a Subarachnoid Hemorrhage. Surg Neurol. 1980; 14:175–184

[21] Memon MY, Neal A, Imami R, et al. Low Grade Glioma Presenting as Subarachnoid Hemorrhage. Neurosurgery. 1984; 14:574–577

[22] Miller RH. Spontaneous Subarachnoid Hemorrhage: A Presenting Symptom of a Tumor of the Third Ventricle. Surg Clin N Amer. 1961; 41:1043–1048

[23] Glass B, Abbott KH. Subarachnoid Hemorrhage Consequent to Intracranial Tumors. Arch Neurol Psych. 1955; 73:369–379

[24] Gleeson RK, Butzer JF, Grin OD. Acoustic Neurinoma Presenting as Subarachnoid Hemorrhage. J Neurosurg. 1978; 49:602–604

[25] Yasargil MG, So SC. Cerebellopontine Angle Meningioma Presenting as Subarachnoid Hemorrhage. Surg Neurol. 1976; 6:3–6

[26] Smith VR, Stein PS, MacCarty CS. Subarachnoid Hemorrhage Due to Lateral Ventricular Meningiomas. Surg Neurol. 1975; 4:241–243

[27] Ernsting J. Choroid Plexus Papilloma Causing Spontaneous Subarachnoid Hemorrhage. J Neurol Neurosurg Psychiatry. 1955; 18:134–136

[28] Simonsen J. Fatal Subarachnoid Hemorrhage Originating in an Intracranial Chordoma. Acta Pathol Microbiol Scand. 1963; 59:13–20

[29] Latchaw JP, Dohn DF, Hahn JF, et al. Subarachnoid Hemorrhage from an Intracranial Meningioma. Neurosurgery. 1981; 9:433–435

[30] Fortuna A, Palma L, Ferrante L, et al. Repeated Subarachnoid Hemorrhage with Vasospasm Secondary to Tuberculum Sella Meningioma. J Neurosurg Sci. 1977; 21:251–256

[31] Ellenbogen RG, Winston KR, Kupsky WJ. Tumors of the Choroid Plexus in Children. Neurosurgery. 1989; 25:327–335

[32] Labovitz DL, Halim AX, Brent B, et al. Subarachnoid hemorrhage incidence among Whites, Blacks and Caribbean Hispanics: the Northern Manhattan Study. Neuroepidemiology. 2006; 26:147–150

[33] Shea AM, Reed SD, Curtis LH, et al. Characteristics of nontraumatic subarachnoid hemorrhage in the United States in 2003. Neurosurgery. 2007; 61:1131–7; discussion 1137-8

[34] de Rooij NK, Linn FH, van der Plas JA, et al. Incidence of subarachnoid haemorrhage: a systematic review with emphasis on region, age, gender and time trends. J Neurol Neurosurg Psychiatry. 2007; 78:1365–1372

[35] Bederson JB, Awad IA, Wiebers DO, et al. Recommendations for the management of patients with unruptured intracranial aneurysms. A statement for healthcare professionals from the Stroke Council of the American Heart Association. Circulation. 2000; 102:2300–2308

[36] Ingall T, Asplund K, Mahonen M, et al. A multinational comparison of subarachnoid hemorrhage epidemiology in the WHO MONICA stroke study. Stroke. 2000; 31:1054–1061

[37] Mahindu A, Koivisto T, Ronkainen A, et al. Similarities and differences in aneurysmal subarachnoid haemorrhage between eastern Finland and northern Sydney. J Clin Neurosci. 2008; 15:617–621

[38] Vadikolias K, Tsivgoulis G, Heliopoulos I, et al. Incidence and case fatality of subarachnoid haemorrhage in Northern Greece: the Evros Registry of Subarachnoid Haemorrhage. Int J Stroke. 2009; 4:322–327

[39] Broderick JP, Brott T, Tomsick T, et al. The risk of subarachnoid and intracerebral hemorrhages in blacks as compared with whites. N Engl J Med 1992; 326:733–736

[40] Eden SV, Heisler M, Green C, et al. Racial and ethnic disparities in the treatment of cerebrovascular diseases: importance to the practicing neurosurgeon. Neurocrit Care. 2008; 9:55–73

[41] Connolly ES,Jr, Rabinstein AA, Carhuapoma JR, et al. Guidelines for the management of aneurysmal subarachnoid hemorrhage: a guideline for healthcare professionals from the American Heart Association/american Stroke Association. Stroke 2012; 43:1711–1737

[42] Bonita R. Cigarette Smoking, Hypertension and the Risk of Subarachnoid Hemorrhage: A Population Based Case-Control Study. Stroke. 1986; 17:831–835

[43] Haykowsky MJ, Findlay JM, Ignaszewski AP. Aneurysmal subarachnoid hemorrhage associated with weight training: three case reports. Clin J Sport Med. 1996; 6:52–55

[44] Hoh BL, Sistrom CL, Firment CS, et al. Bottleneck factor and height-width ratio: association with ruptured aneurysms in patients with multiple cerebral aneurysms. Neurosurgery. 2007; 61:716–22 discussion 722-3

[45] Dhar S, Tremmel M, Mocco J, et al. Morphology parameters for intracranial aneurysm rupture risk assessment. Neurosurgery. 2008; 63:185–96; discussion 196-7

[46] Rahman M, Smietana J, Hauck E, et al. Size ratio correlates with intracranial aneurysm rupture status: a prospective study. Stroke. 2010; 41:916–920

[47] Mohr JP, Caplan LR, Melski JW, et al. The Harvard cooperative stroke registry: A prospective study. Neurology. 1978; 28:754–762

[48] Verweij RD, Wijdicks EFM, van Gijn J. Warning Headache in Aneurysmal Subarachnoid Hemorrhage: A Case-Control Study. Arch Neurol. 1988; 45:1019–1020

[49] Linn FHH, Wijdicks EFM, van der Graaf Y, et al. Prospective Study of Sentinel Headache in Aneurysmal Subarachnoid Hemorrhage. Lancet. 1994; 344:590–593

[50] Fisher CM. Painful States: A Neurological Commentary. Clin Neurosurg. 1984; 31:32–35

[51] Linn FHH, Rinkel GJE, van Gijn J. Headache Characteristics in Subarachnoid Hemorrhage and Benign Thunderclap Headache. Journal of Neurology, Neurosurgery, and Psychiatry. 1998; 65:791–793

[52] Day JW, Raskin NH. Thunderclap Headache: Symptom of Unruptured Cerebral Aneurysm. Lancet. 1986; 2:1247–1248

[53] Wijdicks EFM, Kerkhoff H, van Gijn J. Long-Term Follow-Up of 71 Patients with Thunderclap Headache Mimicking Subarachnoid Hemorrhage. Lancet. 1988; 2:68–70

[54] Markus HS. A Prospective Follow-Up of Thunderclap Headache Mimicking Subarachnoid Hemorrhage. J Neurol Neurosurg Psychiatry. 1991; 54:1117–1118

[55] Ducros A, Boukobza M, Porcher R, et al. The clinical and radiological spectrum of reversible cerebral vasoconstriction syndrome. A prospective series of 67 patients. Brain. 2007; 130:3091–3101

[56] Snyder BD, McClelland RR. Isolated benign cerebral vasculitis. Arch Neurol. 1978; 35:612–614

[57] Headache Classification Committee of the International Headache Society (IHS). The International Classification of Headache Disorders, 3rd edition (beta version). Cephalalgia. 2013; 33:629–808

[58] Bui SebastianBao Dinh, Petersen Torben, Poulsen Jeppe Nørgaard, et al. Headaches attributed to airplane travel: A Danish survey. The Journal of Headache and Pain. 2016; 17:1–5

[59] Frese A, Eikermann A, Frese K, et al. Headache associated with sexual activity: demography, clinical features, and comorbidity. Neurology. 2003; 61:796–800

[60] Lance JW. Headaches Related to Sexual Activity. Journal of Neurology, Neurosurgery, and Psychiatry. 1976; 39:1226–1230

[61] Ogilvy CS, Rordorf G, Bederson JB, et al. Mechanisms and Treatment of Coma After Subarachnoid Hemorrhage. In: Subarachnoid Hemorrhage: Pathophysiology and Management. Park Ridge, IL: American Association of Neurological Surgeons; 1997:157–171

[62] Manschot WA. Subarachnoid Hemorrhage. Intraocular Symptoms and Their Pathogenesis. Am J Ophthalmol. 1954; 38:501–505

[63] Tsementzis SA, Williams A. Ophthalmological Signs and Prognosis in Patients with a Subarachnoid Hemorrhage. Neurochirurgia. 1984; 27:133–135

[64] Vanderlinden RG, Chisholm LD. Vitreous Hemorrhages and Sudden Increased Intracranial Pressure. J Neurosurg. 1974; 41:167–176

[65] Pfausler B, Belcl R, Metzler R, et al. Terson's Syndrome in Spontaneous Subarachnoid Hemorrhage: A Prospective Study in 60 Consecutive Patients. Journal of Neurosurgery. 1996; 85:392–394

[66] Garfinkle AM, Danys IR, Nicolle DA, et al. Terson's Syndrome: A Reversible Cause of Blindness Following Subarachnoid Hemorrhage. Journal of Neurosurgery. 1992; 76:766–771

[67] Friedman SM, Margo CE. Bilateral Subinternal Limiting Membrane Hemorrhage with Terson Syndrome. American Journal of Ophthalmology. 1997; 124:850–851

[68] Keithahn MAZ, Bennett SR, Cameron D, et al. Retinal Folds in Terson Syndrome. Ophthalmology. 1993; 100:1187–1190

[69] Schultz PN, Sobol WM, Weingeist TA. Long-Term Visual Outcome in Terson Syndrome. Ophthalmology. 1991; 98:1814–1819

[70] Edlow JA, Wyer PC. Evidence-based emergency medicine/clinical question. How good is a negative cranial computed tomographic scan result in excluding subarachnoid hemorrhage? Ann Emerg Med. 2000; 36:507–516

[71] van der Jagt M, Flach HZ, Tanghe HL, et al. Assessment of feasibility of endovascular treatment of ruptured intracranial aneurysms with 16-detector row CT angiography. Cerebrovascular Diseases. 2008; 26:482–488

[72] Perry JJ, Stiell IG, Sivilotti ML, et al. Sensitivity of computed tomography performed within six hours of onset of headache for diagnosis of subarachnoid haemorrhage: prospective cohort study. BMJ. 2011; 343. DOI: 10.1136/bmj.d4277

[73] Milhorat TH. Acute Hydrocephalus After Aneurysmal Subarachnoid Hemorrhage. Neurosurgery. 1987; 20:15–20

[74] Karttunen AI, Jartti PH, Ukkola VA, et al. Value of the quantity and distribution of subarachnoid haemorrhage on CT in the localization of a ruptured cerebral aneurysm. Acta Neurochirurgica (Wien). 2003; 145:655–61; discussion 661

[75] Meurer W, Walsh B. CTA of the brain is a reasonable option to consider to help rule out subarachnoid hemorrhage in select patients. 2014. https://www.aaem.org/UserFiles/CTAtoHelpRuleOurSubarachnoidHemorrhage.pdf

[76] Hoh BL, Cheung AC, Rabinov JD, et al. Results of a prospective protocol of computed tomographic angiography in place of catheter angiography as the only diagnostic and pretreatment planning study for cerebral aneurysms by a combined neurovascular team. Neurosurgery. 2004; 54:1329–40; discussion 1340-2

[77] Chaudhary SR, Ko N, Dillon WP, et al. Prospective evaluation of multidetector-row CT angiography for the diagnosis of vasospasm following subarachnoid hemorrhage: a comparison with digital subtraction angiography. Cerebrovascular Diseases. 2008; 25:144–150

[78] Bonita R, Thomson S. Subarachnoid hemorrhage: epidemiology, diagnosis, management, and outcome. Stroke. 1985; 16:591–594

[79] Probst MA, Hoffman JR. Computed Tomography Angiography of the Head Is a Reasonable Next Test After a Negative Noncontrast Head Computed Tomography Result in the Emergency Department Evaluation of Subarachnoid Hemorrhage. Ann Emerg Med. 2016; 67:773–774

[80] Chin N, Sarko J. Tried and True and Still the Best: Lumbar Puncture, Not Computed Tomography Angiogram, for the Diagnosis of Subarachnoid Hemorrhage. Ann Emerg Med. 2016; 67:774–775

[81] Perry JJ, Sivilotti ML, Stiell IG, et al. Should spectrophotometry be used to identify xanthochromia in the cerebrospinal fluid of alert patients suspected of having subarachnoid hemorrhage? Stroke. 2006; 37:2467–2472

[82] Gangloff A, Nadeau L, Perry JJ, et al. Ruptured aneurysmal subarachnoid hemorrhage in the emergency department: Clinical outcome of patients having a lumbar puncture for red blood cell count, visual and spectrophotometric xanthochromia after a negative computed tomography. Clin Biochem. 2015; 48:634–639

[83] Gorchynski J, Oman J, Newton T. Interpretation of traumatic lumbar punctures in the setting of possible subarachnoid hemorrhage: who can be safely discharged? Cal J Emerg Med. 2007; 8:3–7

[84] Consensus Conference. Magnetic Resonance Imaging. JAMA. 1988; 259:2132–2138

[85] Hackney DB, Lesnick JE, Zimmerman RA, et al. MR Identification of Bleeding Site in Subarachnoid Hemorrhage with Multiple Intracranial Aneurysms. J Comput Assist Tomogr. 1986; 10:878–880

[86] Ross JS, Masaryk TJ, Modic MT, et al. Intracranial Aneurysms: Evaluation by MR Angiography. American Journal of Neuroradiology. 1990; 11:449–456

85

85

[87] Ronkainen A, Hernesniemi J, Puranen M, et al. Familial Intracranial Aneurysms. Lancet. 1997; 349:380–384

[88] White PM, Wardlaw JM, Easton V. Can noninvasive imaging accurately depict intracranial aneurysms? A systematic review. Radiology. 2000; 217:361–370

[89] Broderick JP, Brown RD,Jr, Sauerbeck L, et al. Greater rupture risk for familial as compared to sporadic unruptured intracranial aneurysms. Stroke. 2009; 40:1952–1957

[90] Coupe NJ, Athwal RK, Marshman LA, et al. Subarachnoid hemorrhage emanating from a ruptured infundibulum: case report and literature review. Surgical Neurology. 2007; 67:204–206

[91] Saltzman GF. Infundibular Widening of the Posterior Communicating Artery Studied by Carotid Angiography. Acta Radiol. 1959; 51:415–421

[92] Wollschlaeger G, Wollschlaeger PB, Lucas FV, et al. Experience and Results with Post-Mortem Cerebral Angiography Performed as Routine Procedure of the Autopsy. Am J Roentgenol Radium Ther Nucl Med. 1967; 101:68–87

[93] Osborn AG. Diagnostic Cerebral Angiography. Philadelphia: Lippincott, Williams and Wilkins; 1999

[94] Yoshimoto T, Suzuki J. Surgical Treatment of an Aneurysm on the Funnel-Shaped Bulge of the Posterior Communicating Artery. Journal of Neurosurgery. 1974; 41:377–379

[95] Archer CR, Silbert S. Infundibula May Be Clinically Significant. Neuroradiology. 1978; 152:247–251

[96] Trasi S, Vincent LM, Zingesser LH. Development of Aneurysm from Infundibulum of Posterior Communicating Artery with Documentation of Prior Hemorrhage. American Journal of Neuroradiology. 1981; 2:368–370

[97] Leblanc R, Worsley KJ, Melanson D, et al. Angiographic Screening and Elective Surgery of Familial Cerebral Aneurysms. Neurosurgery. 1994; 35:9–18

[98] Locksley HB. Report on the Cooperative Study of Intracranial Aneurysms and Subarachnoid Hemorrhage: Section V - Part II: Natural History of Subarachnoid Hemorrhage, Intracranial Aneurysms, and Arteriovenous Malformations - Based on 6368 Cases in the Cooperative Study. J Neurosurg. 1966; 25:321–368

[99] Henkes H, Fischer S, Weber W, et al. Endovascular coil occlusion of 1811 intracranial aneurysms: early angiographic and clinical results. Neurosurgery. 2004; 54:268–80; discussion 280-5

[100] Henkes H, Fischer S, Mariushi W, et al. Angiographic and clinical results in 316 coil-treated basilar artery bifurcation aneurysms. Journal of Neurosurgery. 2005; 103:990–999

[101] Debrun GM, Aletich VA, Kehrli P, et al. Selection of cerebral aneurysms for treatment using Guglielmi detachable coils: the preliminary University of Illinois at Chicago experience. Neurosurgery. 1998; 43:1281–95; discussion 1296-7

[102] Hunt WE, Hess RM. Surgical Risk as Related to Time of Intervention in the Repair of Intracranial Aneurysms. J Neurosurg. 1968; 28:14–20

[103] Hunt WE, Kosnik EJ. Timing and Perioperative Care in Intracranial Aneurysm Surgery. Clin Neurosurg. 1974; 21:79–89

[104] Drake CG. Report of World Federation of Neurological Surgeons Committee on a Universal Subarachnoid Hemorrhage Grading Scale. J Neurosurg. 1988; 68:985–986

[105] Teasdale GM, Drake CG, Hunt W, et al. A universal subarachnoid hemorrhage scale: report of a committee of the World Federation of Neurosurgical Societies. J Neurol Neurosurg Psychiatry. 1988; 51

[106] Dias MS, Sekhar LN. Intracranial Hemorrhage from Aneurysms and Arteriovenous Malformations during Pregnancy and the Puerperium. Neurosurgery. 1990; 27:855–866

[107] Crawford S, Varner MW, Digre KB, et al. Cranial Magnetic Resonance Imaging in Eclampsia. Obstet Gynecol. 1987; 70:474–477

[108] Postma IR, Slager S, Kremer HP, et al. Long-term consequences of the posterior reversible encephalopathy syndrome in eclampsia and preeclampsia: a review of the obstetric and nonobstetric literature. Obstet Gynecol Surv. 2014; 69:287–300

[109] Rimaitis K, Grauslyte L, Zavackiene A, et al. Diagnosis of HELLP Syndrome: A 10-Year Survey in a Perinatology Centre. Int J Environ Res Public Health. 2019; 16. DOI: 10.3390/ijerph16010109

[110] Hirsch KG, Froehler MT, Huang J, et al. Occurrence of perimesencephalic subarachnoid hemorrhage during pregnancy. Neurocrit Care. 2009; 10:339–343

[111] Tiel Groenestege A T, Rinkel GJ, van der Bom JG, et al. The risk of aneurysmal subarachnoid hemorrhage during pregnancy, delivery, and the puerperium in the Utrecht population: case-crossover study and standardized incidence ratio estimation. Stroke. 2009; 40:1148–1151

[112] Robinson JL, Hall CJ, Sedzimir CB. Subarachnoid Hemorrhage in Pregnancy. J Neurosurg. 1972; 36:27–33

[113] Robinson JL, Hall CS, Sedzimir CB. Arteriovenous Malformations, Aneurysms, and Pregnancy. J Neurosurg. 1974; 41:63–70

[114] Horton JC, Chambers WA, Lyons SL, et al. Pregnancy and the Risk of Hemorrhage from Cerebral Arteriovenous Malformations. Neurosurgery. 1990; 27:867–872

[115] Kim YW, Neal D, Hoh BL. Cerebral aneurysms in pregnancy and delivery: pregnancy and delivery do not increase the risk of aneurysm rupture. Neurosurgery. 2013; 72:143–9; discussion 150

[116] De Santis M, Straface G, Cavaliere AF, et al. Gadolinium periconceptional exposure: pregnancy and neonatal outcome. Acta Obstet Gynecol Scand. 2007; 86:99–101

[117] Kataoka H, Miyoshi T, Neki R, et al. Subarachnoid hemorrhage from intracranial aneurysms during pregnancy and the puerperium. Neurol Med Chir (Tokyo). 2013; 53:549–554

[118] Marshman LA, Rai MS, Aspoas AR. Comment to "Endovascular treatment of ruptured intracranial aneurysms during pregnancy: report of three cases". Arch Gynecol Obstet. 2005; 272. DOI: 10.1007/s00404-004-0707-x

[119] Hasan D, Vermeulen M, Wijdicks EFM, et al. Management Problems in Acute Hydrocephalus After Subarachnoid Hemorrhage. Stroke. 1989; 20:747–753

[120] Graff-Radford N, Torner J, Adams HP, et al. Factors Associated With Hydrocephalus After Subarachnoid Hemorrhage. Arch Neurol. 1989; 46:744–752

[121] Kusske JA, Turner PT, Ojemann GA, et al. Ventriculostomy for the Treatment of Acute Hydrocephalus Following Subarachnoid Hemorrhage. Journal of Neurosurgery. 1973; 38:591–595

[122] van Gijn J, Hijdra A,, Wijdicks EFM, et al. Acute Hydrocephalus After Aneurysmal Subarachnoid Hemorrhage. Journal of Neurosurgery. 1985; 63:355–362

[123] Hellingman CA, van den Bergh WM, Beijer IS, et al. Risk of rebleeding after treatment of acute hydrocephalus in patients with aneurysmal subarachnoid hemorrhage. Stroke. 2007; 38:96–99

[124] Pare L, Delfino R, Leblanc R. The relationship of ventricular drainage to aneurysmal rebleeding. Neurosurg. 1992; 76:422–427

[125] McIver JI, Friedman JA, Wijdicks EF, et al. Preoperative ventriculostomy and rebleeding after aneurysmal subarachnoid hemorrhage. J Neurosurg. 2002; 97:1042–1044

[126] Voldby B, Enevoldsen EM. Intracranial Pressure Changes Following Aneurysm Rupture. 3. Recurrent Hemorrhage. Journal of Neurosurgery. 1982; 56:784–789

[127] Auer LM, Mokry M. Disturbed Cerebrospinal Fluid Circulation After Subarachnoid Hemorrhage and Acute Aneurysm Surgery. Neurosurgery. 1990; 26:804–809

[128] Connolly ES, Kader AA, Frazzini VI, et al. The Safety of Intraoperative Lumbar Subarachnoid Drainage for Acutely Ruptured Intracranial Aneurysm: Technical Note. Surgical Neurology. 1997; 48:338–344

[129] Koh KM, Ng Z, Low SY, et al. Management of ruptured intracranial aneurysms in the post-ISAT era: outcome of surgical clipping versus endovascular coiling in a Singapore tertiary institution. Singapore Med J. 2013; 54:332–338

[130] Hoh BL, Kleinhenz DT, Chi YY, et al. Incidence of ventricular shunt placement for hydrocephalus with clipping versus coiling for ruptured and unruptured cerebral aneurysms in the Nationwide Inpatient Sample database: 2002 to 2007. World Neurosurg. 2011; 76:548–554

[131] Klopfenstein JD, Kim LJ, Feiz-Erfan I, et al. Comparison of rapid and gradual weaning from external ventricular drainage in patients with aneurysmal subarachnoid hemorrhage: a prospective randomized trial. J Neurosurg. 2004; 100:225–229

86 Critical Care of Aneurysm Patients

86.1 Initial management of SAH

86.1.1 General information

Practice guideline

Practice guideline: Initial management of aneurysmal SAH

Level I[1]:
- administer oral nimodipine to all patients with aneurysmal SAH. The value of other calcium channel blockers is uncertain
- maintain euvolemia and normal circulating blood volume

Level II[1]:
- control of HTN: the ideal BP to reduce the risk of rebleeding has not been established. A reasonable target is to maintain systolic blood pressure (SBP) < 160 mm Hg

Initial management concerns

1. rebleeding: the major concern during the initial stabilization. Risk factors: female gender, high-grade SAH, large aneurysm, SBP > 175 mm Hg
2. hydrocephalus: hydrocephalus developing precipitously may be obstructive (due to blockage of CSF flow by blood clot). Ventriculomegaly early after SAH as well as at later stages is often due to communicating hydrocephalus (p. 1426) (due to toxic effect of blood breakdown products on arachnoid granulations)
3. delayed cerebral ischemia (DCI) which can produce delayed ischemic neurologic deficit (DIND), usually attributed to vasospasm (p. 1439). Typically does not occur until several days following SAH
4. hyponatremia with hypovolemia (p. 1435)
5. DVT and pulmonary embolism (p. 176)
6. seizures (p. 1436)
7. augmenting cerebral O_2 delivery (see below)
8. determining source of bleeding: should be investigated early with CTA or catheter angiography. The timing and choice of study takes into consideration the patient's condition (unstable or pre-morbid patients are not candidates), the feasibility of early treatment (ideal), and the likelihood of endovascular therapy (based on patient's age and predicted aneurysm location as well as availability)

Cerebral O_2 delivery (DO_2)

DO_2 (Cerebral O_2) delivery is given by equation (86.1)

$$DO_2 = CBF \times C_aO_2 \tag{86.1}$$

where C_aO_2 (arterial O_2 content) is given by

$$C_aO_2 = S_aO_2 \times Hgb \times 1.34 \tag{86.2}$$

where S_aO_2 is the arterial O_2 saturation, and CBF (cerebral blood flow) is given by (86.3)

$$CBF = CPP/CVR = (MAP - ICP)/CVR \tag{86.3}$$

where CPP = cerebral perfusion pressure, MAP = mean arterial pressure, ICP = intracranial pressure, CVR = cerebrovascular resistance, so that the expanded equation is:

$$DO_2 = (MAP - ICP)/CVR \times S_aO_2 \times Hgb \times 1.34 \tag{86.4}$$

Methods that may be used to augment DO_2 can be gleaned from these equations
1. optimizing CBF (usually consists of increasing CBF) (refer to (86.3))

a) ✖ avoid induced hypertension:
- when cerebral autoregulation is intact, increasing CPP has little effect on increasing CBF over most of the physiologic range (see ► Fig. 92.1) because of a compensatory increase in CVR
- no evidence shows that increasing BP consistently increases CBF (the HIMALAIA study[2] for DCI was terminated prematurely because of lack of effect on CBF and slow recruitment)
- even if induced HTN increased CPP, this risks rebleeding with an unsecured aneurysm

b) ✖ avoid hypotension as this negatively impacts CBF. If pressors are needed to maintain BP (caution: avoid pressors in hypovolemic patients):
- if heart rate is low: use norepinephrine
- if heart rate is not low: use phenylephrine

c) maintaining euvolemia
- avoid hypovolemia: the majority of patients become hypovolemic in the first 24 hrs after aSAH. Hypovolemia can → hypotension and is associated with vasospasm
- avoid prophylactic hypervolemia: has deleterious effects (e.g., CHF) and does not increase CBF, reduce the incidence of vasospasm, or improve clinical outcome

d) maintaining normal ICP: i.e., avoiding intracranial hypertension (increased ICP)

e) reducing CVR:
- improving blood rheology: effectively reduces CVR. RBC aggregability increases after SAH[3]
- nimodipine: class II evidence. Does not reduce vasospasm, does not improve mortality, does improve outcome in survivors
- intra-arterial verapamil (by endovascular interventionalist)
- EG-1962: NEWTON-2 trial comparing it to oral nimodipine, results pending (clinicaltrials. gov, trial identifier: NCT02790632)

2. elevate O_2 saturation: for patients at risk of DCI the goal is 100%, for all other patients aim for ≥ 92%

3. hemoglobin (Hgb): optimal Hgb is still controversial
a) increasing Hgb increases oxygen carrying capacity of blood (see (86.2)); however, this increases blood viscosity[4] which effectively increases CVR
b) evidence of transfusing vs. withholding blood in aSAH is lacking. SAHaRA trial (clinicaltrials. gov, trial identifier: NCT03309579) will be completed in September 2024
c) current recommended Hgb: 8–10
d) SANGUINATE™: bovine Hgb modified to decrease immunogenicity, extravasation, and renal toxicity.[5] Still being studied to determine effect on DCI in aSAH

86.1.2 Monitors/tubes

1. arterial-line: for patients who are hemodynamically unstable, stuporous or comatose, those with difficult to control hypertension, or those requiring frequent labs (e.g., ventilator patients)

2. airway management
a) intubation: intubate patients who are comatose (GCS < 8)
b) intubation vs. noninvasive ventilation (NIV) (CPAP or BiPAP): if O_2 sats are < 92% (or < 100% in patiens at risk for DCI) on room air or with 2 L NC:
- NIV is preferred: patient should be fully awake, calm & cooperative
- consider intubation if a patient with a primary diagnosis of CNS pathology needs sedation to tolerate NIV mask
- BiPAP makes it easier for patient to exhale than with CPAP
- NIV does not prevent hyperventilation

3. maintaining euvolemia:
a) use dynamic indices to assess preload and response to fluid bolus. Stroke volume variation (SVV) & stroke volume (SV) (the area under the arterial waveform calculated by ICU monitors) and use responses to fluid bolus to determine fluid status
b) ✖ rarely used pulmonary-artery catheter (PA-catheter, AKA Swann-Ganz catheter): measures central venous pressure (CVP). Device safety and efficacy is debatable.[6] CVP is unreliable (in isolation) in determining volume status

4. cardiac rhythm monitor: arrhythmias may occur following SAH (p.1438)

5. intraventricular catheter (IVC) AKA external ventricular drain (EVD). Possible indications:
a) patients developing acute hydrocephalus following SAH or in those with significant intraventricular blood (allows measurement of ICP as well as drainage of blood-laden CSF). IVC causes symptomatic improvement in almost two-thirds.[7] May increase the risk of rebleeding (p.1427); however, the risk of untreated hydrocephalus is probably higher[8]

b) H&H grade ≥ 3 (except good grade 3 patients). If a high-grade patient improves with an IVC, the prognosis may be more favorable. If ICP is elevated, management includes the use of mannitol; see Treatment measures for elevated ICP (p. 1046).

86.1.3 Admitting orders

1. admit to ICU (monitored bed)
2. VS with neuro checks q 1 hr
3. activity: BR with HOB at 30°. SAH precautions (i.e., low level of external stimulation, restricted visitation, no loud noises)
4. nursing
   a) strict I's & O's
   b) daily weights
   c) knee-high TED hose and pneumatic compression boots (PCB)
   d) indwelling Foley catheter if patient is lethargic, incontinent, or unable to void in urinal or bedpan. Consider temperature-sensing catheter for strict fever control
5. diet: NPO (in preparation for surgery or endovascular intervention)
6. IV fluids: early aggressive fluid therapy to head off cerebral salt wasting
   a) NS + 20 mEq KCl/L at ≈ 2 ml/kg/hr (typically 140–150 ml/hr)
   b) consider Plasma-Lyte or other isotonic balanced crystalloid solutions (see below) (caution in patients with hypermagnesemia, hyperkalemia, AKI/CKI)
7. medications (avoid IM medications to reduce pain)
   a) prophylactic antiseizure medications: often used, but controversial (see post-SAH seizures (p. 1436)). If elected one option, ℞ levetiracetam (Keppra®) 500 or 1000 mg BID (PO or IV) while aneurysm is unsecured and for ≈ 1 week thereafter
   b) sedation (not oversedation): e.g., with propofol (for intubated patients)
   c) analgesics: fentanyl (lowers ICP & unlike morphine, does not cause histamine release) 25–100 mcg (0.5–2 ml) IVP, q 1–2 hrs PRN
   d) dexamethasone (Decadron®): may help with H/A and neck pain. Effect on edema controversial. Usually given pre-op prior to craniotomy
   e) stool softener in patients able to take PO (docussate 100 mg PO BID)
   f) anti-emetics: e.g., Zofran® (ondansetron) 4 mg IV over 2–5 minutes, may repeat in 4 & 8 hours, and then q 8 hours for 1–2 days. Avoid phenothiazines (e.g., Phenergan) which may lower seizure threshold (especially in patients who have had a seizure)
   g) calcium channel blockers (p. 1444): nimodipine (Nimotop®) 60 mg PO/NG q 4 hrs initiated within 96 hrs of SAH (some use 30 mg q 2 hrs to avoid periodic dips in BP). IV administration is equally as effective[9] where available. Oral nimodipine should be administered to all patients with aSAH
   h) H_2 blockers (e.g., ranitidine) or proton pump inhibitors (e.g., Prevacid® (lansoprazole) 30 mg PO or IV q d): to reduce risk of stress ulceration
   i) ✖ these agents impair coagulation and are *used with caution*: ASA, dextran,[10] heparin, and repeated administration of hetastarch (Hespan®)[11,12] over a period of days
   j) ✖ statins: meta-analysis[13] and multicenter randomized phase 3 trial of simvastatin[14] found no clinical benefit
8. oxygenation (for intubation criteria, see above)
   a) goals: $pO_2 > 100$ mm Hg. O_2 saturation: in patients at risk for vasospasm, strive for 100%, aim for 92% saturation in all others
   b) in non-intubated patient: O_2 2 L per NC PRN (based on ABG) and if tolerated. To achieve above goals, increase FiO_2 and mean airway pressure (PEEP)
   c) in ventilated patient:
      • CO_2: strive for normocarbia. Avoid prophylactic hyperventilation → hypocarbia → cerebral vasoconstriction (may exacerbate vasospasm). Monitor $ETCO_2$ and correlate it with p_aCO_2 from ABG
      • Avoid arterial hyperoxia ($p_aO_2 > 300$ mm Hg) because of theoretical risk of vasoconstriction
9. temperature (normothermia): medications (Tylenol) and cooling measures (e.g., ice packs, Arctic Sun external cooling device) to reduce and prevent fever are encouraged, as fever has been shown to be independently associated with worse cognitive and functional outcome in survivors of aSAH[15,16,17]
10. HTN: SBP 120–160 mm Hg is a guideline with unclipped aneurysm (see Blood pressure and volume management (p. 1435)). Use calcium channel blocker (nifedipine, or clevidipine). ✖ Avoid SBP > 175 mm Hg (risk of aneurysm rupture). ✖ Avoid vasodilators (NTG, nipride…) (risk of increased CBV → increased ICP)

11. labs
    a) ABG, electrolytes, CBC, PT/PTT on admission
    b) ABG, electrolytes, CBC q day (ABG q 6 hrs if patient unstable, electrolytes q 12 hrs if hypona-
       tremia develops, see Hyponatremia following SAH (p. 1435)
    c) serum and urine osmolality if urine output high or low; see Syndrome of inappropriate anti-
       diuretic hormone secretion (SIADH) (p. 117)
    d) hemoglobin and hematocrit: some studies suggest that higher hemoglobin values are associ-
       ated with improved outcomes after aSAH.[18,19] However, liberal RBC transfusion has been
       associated with worse outcomes in aSAH.[20,21] The optimal hemoglobin goal after aSAH is not
       yet known, and may depend on the presence or absence of vasospasm
    e) serum glucose: effective glucose control after aSAH can significantly reduce the risk of poor
       outcome[22]
    f) CXR daily until stable: patients undergoing triple-H therapy can develop dangerous pulmo-
       nary edema as they "fall off" the Starling curve with volume expansion. Patients with SAH
       are also rarely at risk for neurogenic pulmonary edema (p. 1439) [23]
    g) if available, transcranial Doppler to monitor MCA, ACA, ICA, VA, and BA velocities and Linde-
       gaard ratio (p. 1443) q Mon, Wed, & Fri

86

86.1.4 Blood pressure and volume management

General information

With an unsecured (unclipped or uncoiled) aneurysm, gentle volume expansion with slight hemodilution and mild elevation of blood pressure may help prevent or minimize the effects of vasospasm[24]
and cerebral salt wasting. However, extreme hypertension must be avoided (to reduce risk of rebleeding). Hypervolemia is to be avoided since it does not mitigate vasospasm and increases
complications.[25]

Initial blood pressure

Ideal blood pressure is controversial, and must take patient's baseline into consideration. The magnitude of blood pressure control to reduce the risk of rebleeding has not been established, but a
decrease in systolic blood pressure to < 160 mm Hg is reasonable. SBP > 175 mm Hg is a risk factor for
rebleeding.

If blood pressure is labile, nicardipine (p. 131) or clevidipine (p. 131) should be used in conjunction with an arterial line. Clevidipine performed well in pilot study with aSAH (CLASH study[26]). Consider clevidipine over nicardipine when volume overload from nicardipine (75 ml/hr) is of concern.
Labetalol is a 2nd line drug option.

Avoid hypotension as it may exacerbate ischemia.

Long-acting drugs (e.g., ACE inhibitors) should be started in patients requiring continued therapy
but cannot be titrated for acute management. In patients who were normotensive prior to SAH with
easily controlled hypertension, ACE inhibitors may be used PRN in conjunction with a beta-blocker,
e.g., labetalol (p. 131).

86.1.5 Hyponatremia following aneurysmal subarachnoid hemorrhage (aSAH)

Background

Hyponatremia follows aSAH in 10–30%[1] of cases.

The neurologic effects of hyponatremia (p. 117) may mimic delayed ischemic neurologic deficit
from vasospasm. Hyponatremic patients have ≈ 3 times the incidence of delayed cerebral infarction
after SAH than normonatremic patients[27] and have longer hospital stays.[28]

Risk factors for hyponatremia after SAH include: history of diabetes, CHF, cirrhosis, adrenal insufficiency, or the use of any of the following drugs: NSAIDs, acetaminophen, narcotics, thiazide
diuretics.[29]

The etiology of hyponatremia may be multifactorial and may differ in specific cases. Etiologies
include:

cerebral salt wasting (CSW) (p. 122): a result of natriuresis and diuresis. CSW is the cause of hyponatremia in the majority of aSAH patients.[30] Extracellular fluid volume (which is more difficult to
measure) is low in CSW and is normal or elevated in SIADH

SIADH (p. 118): the observed increase in ADH after aSAH may be secondary to hypovolemia

86.1.6 Post-SAH seizures

General information

No RCT has been performed to help guide decisions on prophylaxis or treatment of seizures. There is also conflicting evidence on whether onset seizures are predictive of late seizures or post-SAH epilepsy.[31,32,33] As such, there is no consensus amongst practitioners regarding the need for ASMs, the best ASM to use, which patients should receive prophylactic ASMs, nor the optimal dose or duration of treatment. Guidelines (p.1436) appear below.

Epidemiology

▶ **Incidence.** The incidence of seizure-like episodes varies widely between observational studies. One literature review[34] reported that 4–26% of SAH patients had onset seizures, 1–28% had early seizures (within first 2 weeks), and 1–35% had late seizures (after 2 weeks).[35] Additionally, nonconvulsive status epilepticus has been reported in 3–18% of SAH patients, and should be considered in patients with a poor neurological exam or in the setting of neurological deterioration.[36,37]

▶ **Risk factors for post-SAH seizures**[1,34,35,36,38,39,40,41]
- increasing age (> 65 years)
- MCA aneurysm
- volume of subarachnoid blood/thickness of clot
- associated intracerebral or subdural hematoma
- poor neurological grade
- rebleeding
- cerebral infarction
- vasospasm
- hyponatremia
- hydrocephalus
- hypertension
- treatment modality, see coiling vs. clipping (p.1457)

Outcome

The association between seizures and functional outcome remains unclear. One study[36] showed that an in-hospital seizure was independently predictive of one-year mortality (65% with seizures vs. 23% without seizures), but others have shown no association with a poorer prognosis.[34,40,42] Two large, retrospective, single-institution studies of patients with aSAH found that nonconvulsive status epilepticus is a very strong predictor of poor outcome.[1,37,43]

ASMs

Studies have assessed neurological outcome following short- and long-term phenytoin use, with higher doses and longer duration associated with poorer outcomes.[44,45] When compared to phenytoin, Keppra is associated with a higher rate of short-term seizure recurrence,[46] but improved long-term outcomes and fewer side effects.[35,47] Although use of prophylactic ASM for aSAH is controversial, a generalized seizure may be devastating in the presence of a tenuous aneurysm. As such, ASMs are often given in the acute setting. One option: ℞ levetiracetam (Keppra®) 500 or 1000 mg BID (PO or IV) while aneurysm is unsecured and for ≈ 1 week thereafter

Practice guideline: Post-SAH seizures

- Level II[1]: prophylactic antiseizure medications may be considered in the immediate posthemorrhagic period
- Level III[1]: the routine long-term use of antiseizure medications is not recommended
- Level II[1]: long-term antiseizure medications may be considered with known risk factors for delayed seizure disorder (e.g., prior seizure, intracerebral hematoma, intractable hypertension, infarction, or MCA aneurysm)

86.2 Rebleeding

86.2.1 General information

Approximately 3000 North Americans die each year from rebleeding of ruptured cerebral aneurysms.[48] For untreated ruptured aneurysms, the maximal frequency of rebleeding is in the 1st day (between 4% and 13.6%),[49,50,51,52] with more than 1/3 of rebleeds occurring within 3 hours and 1/2 within 6 hours of symptoms onset.[53] After the first day, the subsequent risk is 1.5% daily for 13 d. Overall, 15–20% rebleed within 14 d, 50% will rebleed within 6 months, thereafter the risk is ≈ 3%/yr with a mortality rate of 2%/yr.[54] (**Note:** to understand the calculation of long-term *cumulative* risk for aneurysmal rupture, see Annual and lifetime risk of hemorrhage and recurrent hemorrhage (p.1506); that discussion is related to AVMs but the same concepts pertain to aneurysms). 50% of deaths occur in the 1st month.

There is a risk of rebleeding during any period that the aneurysm is untreated. As such, early treatment of the ruptured aneurysm can reduce risk of rebleeding[55] (see Timing of aneurysm surgery (p.1461)). In addition, higher Hunt and Hess grades,[56] larger aneurysm size, and poorly controlled blood pressure (> 160 mm Hg) have also been associated with an increased risk of rebleeding.[51,52,57]

Preoperative ventriculostomy—e.g., for acute post-SAH hydrocephalus (p.1427)—and possibly lumbar spinal drainage (p.1464) increase the risk of rebleeding.

The risk of rebleeding in SAH of unknown etiology and with AVMs, as well as the risk of bleeding with incidental multiple unruptured aneurysms, are all similar at ≈ 1%/yr; may actually be less in SAH of unknown etiology (p.1494).[58]

86.2.2 Prevention of rebleeding

The optimal method of preventing rebleeding is early coiling or surgical clipping. Bed rest and hyperdynamic therapy do *not* prevent rebleeding.[59]

86.2.3 Antifibrinolytic therapy

The role of clot lysis in early rebleeding is uncertain.

Practice guideline: Antifibrinolytic therapy

Level II[1]: for patients with aneurysmal SAH where there is an unavoidable delay in treatment of the aneurysm, and in whom there is a significant risk of rebleeding and no compelling medical contraindications, up to 72 hours of therapy with tranexamic acid or aminocaproic acid is reasonable

Drug info: Tranexamic acid (Cyklokapron®)

Reduces the risk of early rebleeding.[50]

R: 1 gm IV as soon as diagnosis of SAH is verified (if patient is to be transported to another facility for definitive care, the dose is given before the patient is transported), followed by 1 gm q 6 hours until the aneurysm is occluded; this treatment did not exceed 72 hours.

Drug info: Epsilon-aminocaproic acid (Amicar®)

Epsilon-aminocaproic acid (EACA), an antifibrinolytic agent, competitively inhibits activation of plasminogen to plasmin. Existing plasmin is neutralized by endogenous antiplasmins. EACA does reduce the risk of rebleeding. However, the incidence of hydrocephalus and delayed ischemic deficits (vasospasm) have been shown to be higher with prolonged use.[60] There may also be a lag of 24–48 hrs before effectiveness occurs.[61]

Because of the increased rate of cerebral infarction, EACA was found not to reduce early mortality, and its use was discouraged.

Reevaluation in a non-randomized study,[62] excluding grade IV and V patients, suggests that the problems with EACA may be minimized by use of an IV loading dose (to eliminate the lag-period to effectiveness) and by limiting the duration of use until the patient can undergo early surgery. A more recent investigation[63] showed a significant decrease in rebleeding in EACA-treated patients versus non-EACA patients (2.7 vs. 11.4%). There was a 76% reduction in mortality attributable to rebleeding, a 13% increase in favorable outcome in good-grade (Hunt Hess I–III) EACA-treated patients, and a 6.8% increase in poor-grade patients (Hunt Hess IV/V), but these results did not reach statistical significance. Although there was an 8-fold increase in DVT in the EACA group, there was no increase in pulmonary embolism. Additionally, there was no difference in ischemic complications between groups.

℞ [63]: EACA 4 g IV loading dose, followed by 1 g/h with cessation of infusion 4 hours before angiography for a maximum duration of 72 hours after SAH.

86.3 Neurogenic stress cardiomyopathy (NSC)

86.3.1 General information

> **Key concepts**
>
> - impaired cardiac function (reduced ejection fraction) not attributable to underlying coronary artery disease or myocardial abnormalities. May be reversible
> - cardiac enzymes (troponin) tend to be lower than expected for the degree of myocardial impairment, distinguishes NSC from acute MI
> - putative mechanism in SAH: catecholamine surge (possibly in myocardial sympathetic nerves) as a result of hypothalamic stimulation or injury from SAH
> - possible sequelae: hypotension, CHF, arrhythmias... all of which may further exacerbate cerebral ischemia
> - peak incidence: 2 days to 2 weeks post-SAH
> - risk factors: Hunt and Hess grade > 3
> - treatment: may include dobutamine (for SBP < 90 and low SVR) and/or milrinone (for SBP > 90 and increased SVR)

Older terms: reversible postischemic myocardial dysfunction,[64] neurogenic stunned myocardium. Classically seen in patients following cardiac surgery, and attributed to a defect in troponin-I (TnI).[65] Some patients develop myocardial hypokinesis following SAH.[66] Stroke volume and cardiac output are reduced. May mimic an MI on echocardiography and on EKG (see below), but troponin levels are typically lower (often < 2.8 ng/ml) than would be predicted for the observed level of myocardial impairment.[67] Hypotension does not always occur since the reduced cardiac output (CO) may be offset by an increase in SVR. However, the reduced CO may impair the ability to tolerate barbiturates administered for cerebral protection due to their myocardial suppressant effect. The reduced CO may also impede successful use of hyperdynamic therapy for vasospasm.

Peak incidence: 2 days to 2 weeks post-SAH. The condition reverses completely in most cases within about 5 days as normal myocardial cells replace those with defective TnI. However, ≈ 10% of patients may progress on to an actual MI.

SAH risk factors include higher Hunt Hess grade (> 3),[68,69,70,71] female gender,[71,72] smoking status and age.[68] Intraoperative TEE monitoring may be a useful guide for titrating pressors.

86.3.2 Arrhythmias and EKG changes

EKG changes occur in > 50% of cases of SAH and include: broad or inverted T-waves, Q-T prolongation, S-T segment elevation or depression, U-waves, premature atrial or ventricular contraction, SVT V-flutter or V-fib,[73] bradycardia. In some cases EKG abnormalities may be indistinguishable from an acute MI.[74,75]

86.3.3 Possible mechanism

Elevation of intracranial pressure secondary to aSAH is thought to cause sympathetic activation resulting in hypercontraction of cardiac myocytes and subsequent myocardial injury.[68] A related theory invokes hypothalamic ischemia resulting in increased sympathetic tone, whereby the hypo-thalamic ischemia results in increased sympathetic tone and the resultant catecholamine surge may produce subendocardial ischemia[76] or coronary artery vasospasm.[66] The catecholamine surge appears to be more focal (i.e., in the heart) than systemic.

86.3.4 Treatment

Interventions that have been studied for increasing cardiac output in NSC[77,78]:
1. milrinone: used when SBP > 90 mm Hg and normal SVR, or when the patient is on chronic beta-blockers
2. dobutamine: more effective with hypotension (SBP < 90 mm Hg) and low SVR
3. other options: stellate ganglion block, magnesium

86.4 Neurogenic pulmonary edema

86.4.1 General information

A rare condition associated with a variety of intracranial pathologies, including:
- subarachnoid hemorrhage
- generalized seizures
- head injury

86.4.2 Pathophysiology

Two possibly synergistic mechanisms. Sudden increased ICP or hypothalamic injury may produce a salvo of sympathetic discharge causing redistribution of blood to the pulmonary circulation, result-ing in elevation of pulmonary capillary wedge pressures (PCWP) and increased permeability. Sec-ondly, the associated surge of catecholamines directly disrupts the capillary endothelium which increases alveolar permeability.

86.4.3 Treatment

Supportive, using measures such as positive pressure ventilation with low levels of PEEP (p. 1052) and treatment to normalize ICP.

A PA-catheter is usually helpful.

There may be some efficacy in using a dobutamine infusion[79] supplemented with furosemide as needed. The theoretical advantage of dobutamine over previously attempted alpha- and beta-blockers is that dobutamine does not reduce cerebral perfusion.

86.5 Vasospasm (AKA cerebrovascular vasospasm)

86.5.1 General information

Key concepts

- delayed cerebral ischemia (DCI) symptoms and/or cerebral arterial narrowing on angiography that follows some cases of SAH (usually), trauma, or other insults
- time course: almost never before day 3 post-SAH, peak incidence 6–8 days post-SAH, rarely starts after day 17. Main time of risk: 3–14 days post-SAH
- risk factors: higher SAH grade, more blood on CT
- results in pathologic changes within the vessel walls (not just vasoconstriction)
- diagnosis: may be clinical, angiographic, or with transcranial Doppler
- treatment: none are curative. Mainstays of treatment:
  - euvolemia and hemodynamic augmentation (formerly "triple H" therapy)
  - neuroendovascular intervention: angioplasty or intra-arterial verapamil

Cerebral vasospasm is a condition that is most commonly seen following some cases of aneurysmal subarachnoid hemorrhage (SAH), but may also follow other intracranial hemorrhages (e.g., intraven-tricular hemorrhage from AVM,[80] and SAH of unknown etiology), head trauma (with or without

SAH),[81] brain surgery, lumbar puncture, hypothalamic injury, infection, and may be associated with preeclampsia (p. 202). The concept of vasospasm was originated in 1951 by Ecker.[82] Vasospasm has two not-necessarily reconcilable definitions (see below):
1. clinical vasospasm: see below
2. radiographic vasospasm: see below

86.5.2 Definitions

Delayed cerebral ischemia (DCI) and early brain injury (EBI)

There has been a move away from thinking of the deleterious effects of SAH in terms of vasospasm, and the concepts of DCI and EBI are coming to the fore.[83]

DCI: Delayed development of a neurological deficit, decline in Glasgow coma scale of at least 2 points, and/or cerebral infarction unrelated to aneurysm treatment or other causes. DCI is an umbrella term that encompasses a number of clinical entities including symptomatic vasospasm, delayed ischemic neurological deficit (DIND), and asymptomatic delayed cerebral infarction.[84]

EBI: In addition to direct mechanical damage from the SAH, EBI also refers to a number of other factors including the transient increase in ICP, reduction of CBF, apoptosis, and edema formation.

Clinical vasospasm

Sometimes referred to as delayed ischemic neurologic deficit (DIND), or symptomatic vasospasm. A *delayed* ischemic neurologic deficit following SAH. Clinically characterized by confusion or decreased level of consciousness sometimes with focal neurologic deficit (speech or motor). The diagnosis is one of exclusion, and sometimes cannot be made with certainty.

See clinical findings (p. 1440).

Radiographic vasospasm (AKA angiographic vasospasm)

Arterial narrowing demonstrated on cerebral angiography, often with slowing of contrast filling. The diagnosis is solidified by previous or subsequent angiograms showing the same vessel(s) with normal caliber. In some cases a DIND corresponds to a region of vasospasm seen angiographically. The incidence of angiographic vasospasm following SAH is around 50% (range: 20–100%).[85]

86.5.3 Characteristics of cerebral vasospasm

Clinical findings

Findings usually develop gradually, and may progress or fluctuate. May include:
1. non-localizing findings
   a) new or increasing H/A
   b) alterations in level of consciousness (lethargy...)
   c) disorientation
   d) meningismus
2. focal neurological signs may occur including cranial nerve palsies[86,87] and focal motor deficits. Also, symptoms may cluster into one of the following "syndromes" (vasospasm incidence is higher in the distribution of the ACA than in that of the MCA):
   a) anterior cerebral artery (ACA) syndrome: frontal lobe findings predominate (abulia, grasp/suck reflex, urinary incontinence, drowsiness, slowness, delayed responses, confusion, whispering). Bilateral anterior cerebral artery distribution infarcts are usually due to vasospasm following an AComm aneurysm rupture
   b) middle cerebral artery (MCA) syndrome: hemiparesis, monoparesis, aphasia (or apractagnosia of non-dominant hemisphere—inability to use objects or perform skilled motor activities, due to lesions in the lower occipital or parietal lobes; subtypes: ideomotor apraxia and sensory apraxia)

Incidence

1. radiographic cerebral vasospasm (CVS) is identified in 20–100% of arteriograms performed around the 7th day following SAH, whereas clinical vasospasm associated with radiographic CVS occurs in only ≈ 30% of patients with SAH[88]
2. radiographic CVS may occur in the absence of clinical deficit, and vice-versa

Severity

1. CVS is a significant cause of morbidity and mortality in patients surviving SAH long enough to reach medical care, exceeded only by the direct effects of aneurysmal rupture as well as re-bleeding[89,90]
2. CVS ranges in severity from mild reversible dysfunction, to severe permanent deficits secondary to ischemic infarction in up to 60% of SAH patients,[91] extensive enough to be fatal in 7% of SAHs[88,91]
3. earlier onset of CVS is associated with greater deficit

Time course of vasospasm

1. onset: almost never before day 3 post-SAH[92]
2. maximal frequency of onset during days 6–8 post-SAH (however, rarely can occur as late as day 17). Typical at-risk period is quoted as days 3–14[93]
3. clinical CVS is almost always resolved by day 12 post-SAH. Once radiographic CVS is demonstrated, it usually resolves slowly over 3–4 weeks
4. onset is usually insidious, but ≈ 10% have an abrupt and severe deterioration

Correlated findings

1. risk is higher in conditions where arterial blood at high pressure contacts the vessels at the base of the brain. CVS rarely occurs in the setting of intraparenchymal or pure intraventricular hemorrhage (e.g., from AVM) or in SAH with distribution limited to the cerebral convexity
2. blood clots are especially spasmogenic when in direct contact with the proximal 9 cm of the ACA and the MCA
3. not all patients with SAH develop CVS, and CVS can follow other insults besides SAH, such as mass resection,[94] meningitis,[95] and amygdalohippocampectomy.[96] Can even be associated with sexual intercourse[97] and over-consumption of black licorice[98]
4. the Hunt and Hess grade on admission correlates with the risk of CVS (▶ Table 86.1)

86

Table 86.1 Correlation of DIND with Hunt and Hess grade

Hunt and Hess grade	% DIND (clinical vasospasm)
1	22%
2	33%
3	52%
4	53%
5	74%

5. the amount of blood on CT correlates with the severity of CVS[99,100] (▶ Table 86.2; also holds true for traumatic SAH[101]). There is less utility in these scales with the increasing availability of non-invasive monitoring for vasospasm (e.g., transcranial Doppler)

Table 86.2 Modified[105] grading system of Fisher[99] (correlation between the amount of blood on CT and the risk of vasospasm)

Modified Fisher scale group	Blood on CT[a]	Symptomatic vasospasm
0	no SAH or IVH	
1	focal or diffuse thin SAH, no IVH	24%
2	focal or diffuse thin SAH, with IVH	33%
3	focal or diffuse thick SAH, no IVH	33%
4	focal or diffuse thick SAH, with IVH	40%

[a]measurements made in the greatest longitudinal & transverse dimension on a printed EMI CT scan (no scaling to actual thickness) performed within 5 d of SAH in 47 patients; falx never contributed more than 1 mm thickness to interhemispheric blood

6. higher incidence with increasing age of patient
7. a history of active cigarette smoking is an independent risk factor[102]
8. history of preexisting hypertension
9. there is good but not perfect correlation between the site of major blood clots on CT, the focality of delayed ischemic neurological deficits, and the visualization of angiographic CVS in corresponding arteries
10. pial enhancement on CT ≈ 3 days after SAH (with IV contrast administration) may correlate with higher risk of CVS (indicates increased permeability of BBB),[103] but this is controversial[104]
11. for patients undergoing early surgery, if there is little SAH left on a CT done 24 hours post-op, there is little risk of vasospasm
12. antifibrinolytic therapy reduces *rebleeding*, but increases the risk of hydrocephalus and vasospasm (p. 1437)[60]
13. angiographic dye can exacerbate CVS
14. hypovolemia

86.5.4 Pathogenesis

Pathogenesis is still poorly understood.

In humans, CVS is a chronic condition with definite long-term changes in the morphology of the involved vessels. Much of CVS is poorly understood because of lack of a good animal model (humans show a mild acute phase, and most animal studies fail to demonstrate a chronic phase).

Pathological changes observed within the vessel wall are outlined in ▶ Table 86.3.

Table 86.3 Pathological changes in vasospasm

Time	Vessel layer	Pathologic change
day 1–8	adventitia	↑ inflammatory cells (lymphocytes, plasma cells, mast cells) and connective tissue
	media	muscle necrosis and corrugation of elastica
	intima	thickening with endothelial swelling and vacuolization, opening of interendothelial tight junctions[106,107]
day 9–60	intima	proliferation of smooth muscle cells → progressive intimal thickening

▶ **Direct mediators.** Vasospasm is caused by smooth muscle contraction, due to either impaired vasodilatory mediators, overactive vasoconstrictive mediators, or more likely, both.
- the formed components of blood have each been shown to contribute to vasospasm
  - oxyhemoglobin in pure form can cause contraction of cerebral arteries when contacting the abluminal surface of the vessel
  - hemoglobin scavenges nitric 0xide, a powerful vasorelaxant[108]
  - platelet-derived growth factor induces vascular proliferation → vascular stiffening and impaired ability to dilate[109]
- endothelial dysfunction: theories include decreased production of nitrous oxide and prostacyclins, and overproduction of endothelin-1
- vessel innervation by the sympathetic nervous system. Interruption of sympathetic innervation prevents vasospasm in rats[110]

▶ **Proposed mechanisms of vasospasm include**
- contraction of the smooth muscle in the media of the vessel wall, as a result of:
  - vasoconstrictors within the hemorrhagic arterial blood[111] (see below)
  - vasoactive substances released into the CSF[112,113]
  - neuronal mechanisms via nervi vasorum (nerves in the vessel wall)
    - increased vasoconstrictor tone (possibly due to denervation supersensitivity)
    - loss of vasodilator tone
    - time-dependent relative imbalance favoring vasoconstrictor over vasodilator innervation[114]
    - sympathetic hyperactivity: e.g., due to hypothalamic injury from elevated ICP[115]
  - impairment of endothelial derived relaxant factor (EDRF): vascular endothelium plays an obligatory role in vasodilatation caused by several pharmacologic agents by releasing a relaxant substance called EDRF[116]
- proliferative vasculopathy
- immunoreactive process

- inflammatory process
- mechanical phenomenon
  - stretching of arachnoid fibers
  - direct compression by blood clot
  - platelet aggregation[111]

86.5.5 Diagnosis of cerebral vasospasm

General information

Diagnosis requires appropriate clinical criteria, and ruling out other conditions that can produce delayed neurologic deterioration, as shown in ▶ Table 86.4.

Table 86.4 Diagnosis of clinical vasospasm[117]

- delayed onset or persisting neuro deficit
- onset 4–20 days post-SAH
- deficit appropriate to involved arteries
- rule out other causes of deterioration
  - rebleeding
  - hydrocephalus
  - cerebral edema
  - seizure
  - metabolic disturbances: hyponatremia...
  - hypoxia
  - sepsis
- ancillary tests (see text)
  - transcranial Doppler
  - CBF studies

86

Ancillary tests for vasospasm

In addition to angiographically demonstrating vasospasm:
- transcranial Doppler (TCD): see below
- alterations in intracranial pulse wave[118]
- CTA: specific for vasospasm, but may overestimate the degree of stenosis[119]
- MRA: may be useful for management of vasospasm (not a practical alternative to conventional angiography)[120]
- continuous quantitatively analyzed EEG monitoring in the ICU:
  - a decline of the percent of alpha activity (defined here as 6–14 Hz) called "relative alpha" (RA) from a mean of 0.45 to 0.17 predicted the onset of vasospasm earlier than TCD or angiographic changes[121]
  - a decline of total EEG power (amplitude) was 91% sensitive for predicting vasospasm[122]
- alterations in cerebral blood flow (CBF):
  - MRI: DWI and PWI may detect early ischemia (p. 243)
  - CT perfusion study (p. 238)
  - xenon CT: may detect large global changes in CBF, but too insensitive to detect focal blood flow changes,[123,124] and does not correlate with increased TCD velocities, positron emission tomography (PET),[125] or SPECT scans (nonquantitative, and takes longer than xenon studies)

Transcranial Doppler (TCD)

A noninvasive method of semiquantitatively measuring velocity of blood flow in a specific artery through the skull (in regions of thinner bone – insonation windows) utilizing ultrasound phase shift.

Narrowing of the arterial lumen as occurs in vasospasm elevates the blood flow velocity, which may be detected with TCD.[126,127,128] Detectable changes may precede clinical symptoms by up to 24–48 hrs. Findings are often more helpful when baseline studies performed before vasospasm is likely to have begun are available.

Typical values are shown for the MCA in ▶ Table 86.5. Also, daily increases of > 50 cm/sec may suggest vasospasm. There is less correlation between velocities and vasospasm in the anterior cerebral arteries (ACA). Distinguishing vasospasm from hyperemia (which increases blood flow velocities in both the MCA and the ICA) is facilitated by using the ratio of these velocities (the so-called Lindegaard ratio) also shown in ▶ Table 86.5.

Once values become elevated, it often takes several weeks to go back down.

Table 86.5 Interpretation of transcranial Doppler for vasospasm

Mean MCA velocity (cm/sec)	MCA:ICA (Lindegaard) ratio	Interpretation
<120	<3	normal
120–200[a]	3–6	mild vasospasm[a]
>200	>6	severe vasospasm

[a]velocities in this range are specific for vasospasm but are only ≈ 60% sensitive

Table 86.6 PPV & NPV of various tests for cerebral vasospasm

Test		PPV (%)	NPV (%)
TCD	MCA	83–100	29–98
	ACA	41–100	37–80
	ICA	73	56
	PCA	37	78
	BA	63	88
	VA	54	82
CTA		43–100	37–100
CTP		71–100	27–99

Comparison of diagnostic modalities

Determining the sensitivities and specificities for the tests shown in ▶ Table 86.6 has allowed calculation of the positive predictive values (PPV) and negative predictive values (NPV) as listed.[84]

86.5.6 Treatment for vasospasm

General information

See management protocol (p. 1446).

Numerous treatments for cerebral arterial vasospasm (CVS) have been evaluated.[129,130] Vasospasm in humans does not respond to the large variety of drugs that reverse experimental vasospasm in animal models.

Prevention of vasospasm

To date, there is no effective prophylactic intervention for CVS.[1] Vasospasm can often be mitigated by preventing post-SAH hypovolemia and anemia by employing hydration and blood transfusion. Although *early* aneurysm treatment (clipping or coiling) does not prevent CVS (in fact, manipulation of vessels may increase the risk), it facilitates treatment of CVS by eliminating the risk of rebleeding (permitting safe use of hypertension as needed) and surgical removal of clot (see below) may reduce the incidence of CVS; see Timing of aneurysm surgery (p. 1461) for discussion of early surgery. *Prophylactic* (i.e., before vasospasm has been diagnosed) hyperdynamic therapy—triple H therapy (p. 1447)—is not indicated (it may cause complications and does not provide any benefit).[25]

Vasospasm treatment options

Treatment options fall into the following categories:
1. direct pharmacological arterial dilatation
   a) smooth muscle relaxants:
      - calcium channel blockers (generally accepted for standard usage): nimodipine does not counteract vasospasm, but does improve neurologic outcomes (p. 1447)
      - endothelin receptor antagonists (experimental or research technique with potential for future application): ET_A antagonists (clazosentan) and $ET_{A/B}$ antagonists[131,132]
      - Ryanodine receptor blocker: Dantrolene. Mediates intracellular calcium release from the sarcoplasmic reticulum. One of the few drugs shown to both prevent and reverse vasospasm[133,134]
      - Magnesium: MASH-2 study showed no improvement in clinical outcome[135]

b) sympatholytics (technique that is accepted for use but not necessarily standard or available at all centers)

c) intra-arterial papaverine[136,137]: short-lived (see below)

d) αICAM-1 inhibition (antibody to intracellular adhesion molecule; technique that is accepted for use but not necessarily standard or available at all centers)

2. direct mechanical arterial dilatation: balloon angioplasty (see below)

3. indirect arterial dilatation: utilizing hyperdynamic therapy (generally accepted for standard usage; see below)

4. surgical treatment to dilate arteries: cervical sympathectomy (technique *not* generally used or no longer accepted)[138]

5. removal of potential vasospasmogenic agents
   a) removal of blood clot: does not completely prevent vasospasm
      • mechanical removal at the time of aneurysm surgery[139,140]
      • subarachnoid irrigation with thrombolytic agents at the time of surgery or post-op through cisternal catheters[141,142,143,144] (must be initiated within ≈ 48 hrs of clipping) or intrathecally.[145] Hazardous with incompletely clipped aneurysm[144]
   b) CSF drainage: via serial lumbar punctures, continuous ventricular drainage, or postoperative cisternal drainage[146]

6. protection of the CNS from ischemic injury: calcium channel blockers (p. 1444)—generally accepted for standard usage

7. improvement of the rheologic properties of intravascular blood to enhance perfusion of ischemic zones; also an endpoint of hyperdynamic therapy (p. 1446); generally accepted for standard usage
   a) includes: plasma, albumin, low molecular weight dextran (technique *not* generally used or no longer accepted), perfluorocarbons (experimental or research technique with potential for future application), mannitol (p. 1464)
   b) the optimal hematocrit is controversial, but ≈ 30–35% is a good compromise between lowered viscosity without overly reducing O_2 carrying capacity (hemodilution is used to lower Hct; phlebotomy is not used)

8. statins: no benefit was detected with simvastatin[14]

9. extracranial-intracranial bypass around zone of vasospasm (technique *not* generally used or no longer accepted)[147,148]

Vasodilatation by angioplasty

Catheter-directed balloon angioplasty of vessels demonstrated to be in vasospasm[149,150]: available only in centers with interventional neuroradiologists. Risks of the procedure: arterial occlusion, arterial rupture, displacement of aneurysm clip,[151,152] arterial dissection. Only feasible in large cerebral vessels (distal arteries not accessible). Clinical improvement occurs in ≈ 60–80%. Improvements in vessel diameter and neuro deficits have been observed in most studies.[153]

Prophylactic transluminal balloon angioplasty (TBA): phase II prospective trial failed to show primary end point benefit (Glasgow Outcome Score), but fewer patients developed vasospasm.[154]

Criteria for TBA:

1. failure of hyperdynamic therapy
2. ruptured aneurysm is repaired
3. optimal results when performed within 12 hours of onset of symptoms
4. may be done immediately post-clipping for vasospasm that was observed pre-op
5. controversial: asymptomatic vasospasm seen on the contralateral side during angioplasty for ipsilateral vasospasm. Some would balloon the asymptomatic side, but others cite the complication rate and would observe
6. ✖ recent cerebral infarction (stroke): a contraindication to TBA. Prior to TBA, perform CT or MRI to rule out

Vasodilatation by intra-arterial drug injection

Vasodilatation by intra-arterial drug (IAD) injection produces effects that are shorter-lived and less profound at their peak than with angioplasty. While IAD can be repeated, this requires multiple arterial catheterizations. IAD is also of value to help open up vessels to allow placement of the angioplasty balloon, and for vessels inaccessible to angioplasty balloons.

Agents currently used for chemical spasmolysis (p. 1925):

1. verapamil: the primary drug employed
2. nicardipine: a dihydropiridine calcium channel blocker which acts preferentially on vascular smooth muscle more than cardiac smooth muscle. Restores vessels to at least 60% of normal

86

diameter. 70% of those treated had no stroke on CT. May cause a drop in SBP, but not > 30%.[155] R intra-arterial therapy: 10–40 mg per procedure. Three retrospective case series have reported vessel dilation and transient improvement in neuro deficits.[153]

3. papaverine
4. nitroglycerine

86.5.7 Vasospasm management

Pertinent guidelines

> ### Practice guideline: Management of cerebral vasospasm/DCI after aneurysmal SAH
>
> - Level I[1]: maintain euvolemia and normal circulating blood volume
> - Level I[1]: induce hypertension unless BP is elevated at base-line or if precluded by cardiac stents
> - Level II[1]: endovascular angioplasty and/or selective intra-arterial vasodilator therapy is reasonable for patients not responding rapidly to or candidates for hypertensive therapy

Specific measures for vasospasm/DCI after aSAH

Patients with clinical suspicion of vasospasm (DIND), or with transcranial Doppler (TCD) *increases* of > 50 cm/sec or with absolute velocities > 200 cm/sec:

1. general care measures
   a) serial neuro exams: while important, sensitivity for CVS/DCI is limited in poor-grade patients[1]
   b) activity: bed rest, HOB elevated to ≈ 30°
   c) TED hose and/or sequential compression boots
   d) strict I & O measurements
2. diagnostic measures (primarily to rule out other causes of deficit)
   a) STAT non-contrast CT to rule out hydrocephalus, edema, infarct, or rebleed
   b) option: perfusion CT or MRI (if available)
   c) STAT bloodwork
      - electrolytes to rule out hyponatremia[156]
      - CBC to assess rheology and rule out sepsis or anemia
      - ABG to rule out hypoxemia
   d) repeat TCD if available to detect changes indicative of vasospasm
3. monitors
   a) A-line to monitor BP
   b) PA catheter to monitor PCWP and cardiac output when possible (central line to monitor CVP when PA catheter cannot be placed)
   c) insert ICP monitor if ICP felt to be problematic, treat elevated ICP with mannitol or CSF drainage before institution hemodynamic augmentation (caution: the diuresis from mannitol in treating ICP may produce hypovolemia; also, exercise caution in lowering ICP with unsecured aneurysm)
4. treatment measures
   a) continue nimodipine therapy. Give via NG tube if patient is unable to swallow
   b) administer O_2 to keep pO_2 > 70 mm Hg
5. ensure euvolemia: patients with SAH often develop hypovolemia early in their course.[27,157,158]
   a) primary IV fluid is crystalloid, usually isotonic (e.g., NS)
   b) blood (whole or PRBC) when Hct drops < 40%
   c) colloid: plasma fraction or 5% albumin (at 100 ml/hr) to maintain 40% Hct (if Hct is > 40%, use crystalloids[159])
   d) mannitol 20% at 0.25 gm/kg/hr as a drip may improve rheologic properties of blood in the microcirculation (avoid hypovolemia from resultant diuresis)
   e) replace urinary output (**U.O.**) with crystalloid (if Hct < 40%, then use 5% albumin, usually @ ≈ 20–25 ml/hr)
   f) avoid hetastarch (Hespan®) (p. 1434) and dextran, which impair coagulation

6. monitoring labs
   a) ABG and H/H daily
   b) serum and urine electrolytes and osmolalities q 12 hr (creatinine elevations may indicate peripheral ischemia from vasopressors)
   c) CXR daily
   d) frequent EKG
7. initiate hyperdynamic therapy (see below) unless BP is elevated at baseline (or cardiac stents preclude it) for 6 hours
8. if no response to 6 hrs of hyperdynamic therapy, or if Doppler or perfusion CT or MRI suggests vasospasm, patient is taken to angiography to confirm presence of vasospasm and for interventional neuroradiologic treatment (intra-arterial verapamil, angioplasty…)

▶ **Hemodynamic augmentation.** Many older treatment schemes for CVS included so-called "triple-H" therapy (for: Hypervolemia, Hypertension, and Hemodilution).[160] This has given way to "hemodynamic augmentation" consisting of maintenance of euvolemia and induced arterial hypertension.[161] While potentially confusing, this has now sometimes been referred to as triple-H therapy.[1]

Inducing HTN may be risky with an unclipped ruptured aneurysm. Once the aneurysm is treated, initiating therapy before CVS is apparent may minimize morbidity from CVS.[24,162]

Use fluids to maintain euvolemia.

Administer pressors to increase SBP in 15% increments until neurologically improved or SBP of 220 mm Hg is reached. Agents include:
- dopamine (p. 133)
  ○ start at 2.5 mcg/kg/min (renal dose)
  ○ titrate up to 15–20 mcg/kg/min
- levophed
  ○ start at 1–2 mcg/min
  ○ titrate every 2–5 minutes: double the rate up to 64 mcg/min, then increase by 10 mcg/min
- neosynephrine (phenylephrine): does not exacerbate tachycardia
  ○ start at 5 mcg/min
  ○ titrate every 2–5 minutes: double the rate up to 64 mcg/min, then increase by 10 mcg/min up to a max of 10 mcg/kg
- dobutamine: positive inotrope
  ○ start at 5 mcg/kg/min
  ○ increase dose by 2.5 mcg/kg/min up to a maximum of 20 mcg/kg/min

Complications of hemodynamic augmentation:
- intracranial complications[163]
  ○ may exacerbate cerebral edema and increase ICP
  ○ may produce hemorrhagic infarction in an area of previous ischemia
- extracranial complications
  ○ pulmonary edema in 17%
  ○ 3 rebleeds (1 fatal)
  ○ MI in 2%
  ○ complications of PA catheter[164]:
    – catheter related sepsis: 13%
    – subclavian vein thrombosis: 1.3%
    – pneumothorax: 1%
    – hemothorax: may be promoted by coagulopathy from dextran[163]

86.6 Post-op orders for aneurysm clipping

- admit PACU, transfer to ICU (neuro unit if available) when stable
- VS: q 15 min × 4 hrs, then q 1 hr. Temperature q 4 hrs × 3 d, then q 8 hrs. Neuro check q 1 hr
- activity: bed rest (BR) with HOB elevated 20–30°
- knee-high TED hose and pneumatic compression boots
- I & O q 1 hr (if no Foley: straight cath q 4 hrs PRN bladder distension)
- incentive spirometry q 2 hrs while awake (*do not use following transsphenoidal surgery*)
- IVF: NS + 20 mEq KCl/L @ 90 ml/hr

For extubated patients:
- diet: NPO except minimal ice chips and meds as ordered
- O_2: 2 L per NC

86

For intubated patients:
- diet: NPO. NG tube to intermittent suction. May clamp for 1 hour after meds given
- ventilator orders

For all patients:
- meds:
  a) H2 antagonist, e.g., ranitidine 50 mg IVPB q 8 hrs
  b) Keppra® (levetiracetam): 500 mg PO or IV q 12 hours. Maintain therapeutic ASM levels for 2–3 months post-op for most supratentorial craniotomies
  c) Cardene® drip: titrate to keep SBP < 160 mm Hg and/or DBP < 100 mm Hg (use cuff pressures, may use A-line pressures if they correlate with cuff pressures)
  d) analgesics: fentanyl (unlike morphine, does not cause histamine release. Lowers ICP) 25–100 mcg (0.5–2 ml) IVP, q 1–2 hrs PRN
  e) acetaminophen (Tylenol®) 650 mg PO/PR q 4 hrs PRN temperature T > 100.5 °F (38 C)
  f) mini-dose heparin or enoxaparin (for DVT prophylaxis; no difference in heparin-induced thrombocytopenia with these 2 agents[165])
  g) calcium channel blockers; see admitting orders (p. 1434): nimodipine (Nimotop®) 60 mg PO/ NG q 4 hrs or 30 mg q 2 hrs to avoid dips in BP. May be given IV where available
  h) continue prophylactic antibiotics if used (e.g., cefazolin [Kefzol®] 500–1000 mg IVPB q 6 hrs x 24 hrs, then D/C)
- if available, transcranial Doppler (p. 1443) to monitor MCA, ACA, ICA, VA, and BA velocities and Lindegaard ratio (typical protocol is 3 × per week)
- labs:
  a) CBC once stabilized in ICU and q d thereafter
  b) renal profile once stabilized in ICU and q 12 hrs thereafter
  c) ABG once stabilized in ICU and q 12 hrs × 2 days, then D/C (also check ABG after any ventilator change if patient is on ventilator)
- call M.D. if any deterioration in crani checks, for T > 101 °F (38.5 °C), sudden increase in SBP, SBP < 120, U.O. < 60 ml/2 hrs

References

[1] Connolly ES,Jr, Rabinstein AA, Carhuapoma JR, et al. Guidelines for the management of aneurysmal subarachnoid hemorrhage: a guideline for healthcare professionals from the American Heart Association/american Stroke Association. Stroke. 2012; 43:1711–1737

[2] Gathier CS, van den Bergh WM, van der Jagt M, et al. Induced Hypertension for Delayed Cerebral Ischemia After Aneurysmal Subarachnoid Hemorrhage: A Randomized Clinical Trial. Stroke. 2018; 49:76–83

[3] Mori K, Arai H, Nakajima K, et al. Hemorheological and Hemodynamic Analysis of Hypervolemic Hemodilution Therapy for Cerebral Vasospasm After Aneurysmal Subarachnoid Hemorrhage. Stroke. 1996; 26:1620–1626

[4] Daniel MK, Bennett B, Dawson AA, et al. Haemoglobin concentration and linear cardiac output, peripheral resistance, and oxygen transport. Br Med J (Clin Res Ed). 1986; 292:923–926

[5] Dhar R, Misra H, Diringer MN. SANGUINATE (PEGylated Carboxyhemoglobin Bovine) Improves Cerebral Blood Flow to Vulnerable Brain Regions at Risk of Delayed Cerebral Ischemia After Subarachnoid Hemorrhage. Neurocrit Care. 2017; 27:341–349

[6] Dalen JE, Bone RC. Is it time to pull the pulmonary artery catheter? JAMA. 1996; 276:916–918

[7] Milhorat TH. Acute Hydrocephalus After Aneurysmal Subarachnoid Hemorrhage. Neurosurgery. 1987; 20:15–20

[8] Redekop G, Ferguson G, Carter LP, et al. Intracranial Aneurysms. In: Neurovascular Surgery. New York: McGraw-Hill; 1995:625–648

[9] Kronvall E, Undren P, Romner B, et al. Nimodipine in aneurysmal subarachnoid hemorrhage: a randomized study of intravenous or peroral administration. Journal of Neurosurgery. 2009; 110:58–63

[10] Nearman HS, Herman ML. Toxic Effects of Colloids in the Intensive Care Unit. Crit Care Med. 1991; 7:713–723

[11] Bianchine JR. Intracranial Bleeding During Treatment with Hydroxyethyl Starch - Letter in Reply. New Engl J Med. 1987; 317

[12] Trumble ER, Muizelaar JP, Myseros JS. Coagulopathy with the Use of Hetastarch in the Treatment of Vasospasm. Journal of Neurosurgery. 1995; 82:44–47

[13] Vergouwen MD, de Haan RJ, Vermeulen M, et al. Effect of statin treatment on vasospasm, delayed cerebral ischemia, and functional outcome in patients with aneurysmal subarachnoid hemorrhage: a systematic review and meta-analysis update. Stroke. 2010; 41:e47–e52

[14] Kirkpatrick PJ, Turner CL, Smith C, et al. Simvastatin in aneurysmal subarachnoid haemorrhage (STASH): a multicentre randomised phase 3 trial. Lancet Neurol. 2014; 13:666–675

[15] Fernandez A, Schmidt JM, Claassen J, et al. Fever after subarachnoid hemorrhage: risk factors and impact on outcome. Neurology. 2007; 68:1013–1019

[16] Zhang G, Zhang JH, Qin X. Fever increased in-hospital mortality after subarachnoid hemorrhage. Acta Neurochir Suppl. 2011; 110:239–243

[17] Badjatia N, Fernandez L, Schmidt JM, et al. Impact of induced normothermia on outcome after subarachnoid hemorrhage: a case-control study. Neurosurgery. 2010; 66:696–700; discussion 700-1

[18] Naidech AM, Drescher J, Ault ML, et al. Higher hemoglobin is associated with less cerebral infarction, poor outcome, and death after subarachnoid hemorrhage. Neurosurgery. 2006; 59:775–9; discussion 779-80

[19] Naidech AM, Jovanovic B, Wartenberg KE, et al. Higher hemoglobin is associated with improved

[20] Kramer AH, Gurka MJ, Nathan B, et al. Complications associated with anemia and blood transfusion in patients with aneurysmal subarachnoid hemorrhage. Crit Care Med. 2008; 36:2070–2075

outcome after subarachnoid hemorrhage. Crit Care Med. 2007; 35:2383–2389

[21] Smith MJ, Le Roux PD, Elliott JP, et al. Blood transfusion and increased risk for vasospasm and poor outcome after subarachnoid hemorrhage. J Neurosurg. 2004; 101:1–7

[22] Schlenk F, Vajkoczy P, Sarrafzadeh A. Inpatient hyperglycemia following aneurysmal subarachnoid hemorrhage: relation to cerebral metabolism and outcome. Neurocrit Care. 2009; 11:56–63

[23] Ciongoli AK, Poser CM. Pulmonary Edema Secondary to Subarachnoid Hemorrhage. Neurology (NY). 1972; 22:867–870

[24] Solomon RA, Fink ME, Lennihan L. Prophylactic Volume Expansion Therapy for the Prevention of Delayed Cerebral Ischemia After Early Aneurysm Surgery. Arch Neurol. 1988; 45:325–332

[25] Egge A, Waterloo K, Sjoholm H, et al. Prophylactic hyperdynamic postoperative fluid therapy after aneurysmal subarachnoid hemorrhage: a clinical, prospective, randomized, controlled study. Neurosurgery. 2001; 49:593–605; discussion 605-6

[26] Varelas PN, Abdelhak T, Corry JJ, et al. Clevidipine for acute hypertension in patients with subarachnoid hemorrhage: a pilot study. Int J Neurosci. 2014; 124:192–198

[27] Wijdicks EFM, Vermeulen M, Hijdra A, et al. Hyponatremia and Cerebral Infarction in Patients with Ruptured Intracranial Aneurysms: Is Fluid Restriction Harmful? Ann Neurol. 1985; 17:137–140

[28] Kao L, Al-Lawati Z, Vavao J, et al. Prevalence and clinical demographics of cerebral salt wasting in patients with aneurysmal subarachnoid hemorrhage. Pituitary. 2009; 12:347–351

[29] Harbaugh RE. Aneurysmal Subarachnoid Hemorrhage and Hyponatremia. Contemporary Neurosurgery. 1993; 15:1–5

[30] Harrigan MR. Cerebral salt wasting syndrome: A Review. Neurosurgery. 1996; 38:152–160

[31] Butzkueven H, Evans AH, Pitman A, et al. Onset seizures independently predict poor outcome after subarachnoid hemorrhage. Neurology. 2000; 55:1315–1320

[32] Byrne JV, Boardman P, Ioannidis I, et al. Seizures after aneurysmal subarachnoid hemorrhage treated with coil embolization. Neurosurgery. 2003; 52:545–52; discussion 550-2

[33] Panczykowski D, Pease M, Zhao Y, et al. Prophylactic Antiepileptics and Seizure Incidence Following Subarachnoid Hemorrhage: A Propensity Score-Matched Analysis. Stroke. 2016; 47:1754–1760

[34] Lin CL, Dumont AS, Lieu AS, et al. Characterization of perioperative seizures and epilepsy following aneurysmal subarachnoid hemorrhage. J Neurosurg. 2003; 99:978–985

[35] Marigold R, Gunther A, Tiwari D, et al. Antiepileptic drugs for the primary and secondary prevention of seizures after subarachnoid haemorrhage. Cochrane Database Syst Rev. 2013; 6. DOI: 10.1002/14651858.CD008710.pub2

[36] Claassen J, Mayer SA, Kowalski RG, et al. Detection of electrographic seizures with continuous EEG monitoring in critically ill patients. Neurology. 2004; 62:1743–1748

[37] Dennis LJ, Claassen J, Hirsch LJ, et al. Nonconvulsive status epilepticus after subarachnoid hemorrhage. Neurosurgery. 2002; 51:1136–43; discussion 1144

[38] Ohman J. Hypertension as a risk factor for epilepsy after aneurysmal subarachnoid hemorrhage and surgery. Neurosurgery. 1990; 27:578–581

[39] Ukkola V, Heikkinen ER. Epilepsy after operative treatment of ruptured cerebral aneurysms. Acta Neurochir (Wien). 1990; 106:115–118

[40] Choi KS, Chun HJ, Yi HJ, et al. Seizures and Epilepsy following Aneurysmal Subarachnoid Hemorrhage: Incidence and Risk Factors. J Korean Neurosurg Soc. 2009; 46:93–98

[41] Kotila M, Waltimo O. Epilepsy after stroke. Epilepsia. 1992; 33:495–498

[42] Rhoney DH, Tipps LB, Murry KR, et al. Anticonvulsant prophylaxis and timing of seizures after aneurysmal subarachnoid hemorrhage. Neurology. 2000; 55:258–265

[43] Little AS, Kerrigan JF, McDougall CG, et al. Nonconvulsive status epilepticus in patients suffering spontaneous subarachnoid hemorrhage. J Neurosurg. 2007; 106:805–811

[44] Chumnanvej S, Dunn IF, Kim DH. Three-day phenytoin prophylaxis is adequate after subarachnoid hemorrhage. Neurosurgery. 2007; 60:99–102; discussion 102-3

[45] Naidech AM, Kreiter KT, Janjua N, et al. Phenytoin exposure is associated with functional and cognitive disability after subarachnoid hemorrhage. Stroke. 2005; 36:583–587

[46] Murphy-Human T, Welch E, Zipfel G, et al. Comparison of short-duration levetiracetam with extended-course phenytoin for seizure prophylaxis after subarachnoid hemorrhage. World Neurosurg. 2011; 75:269–274

[47] Szaflarski JP, Sangha KS, Lindsell CJ, et al. Prospective, randomized, single-blinded comparative trial of intravenous levetiracetam versus phenytoin for seizure prophylaxis. Neurocrit Care. 2010; 12:165–172

[48] Kassell NF, Drake CG. Review of the Management of Saccular Aneurysms. Neurol Clin. 1983; 1:73–86

[49] Kassell NF, Torner JC. Aneurysmal rebleeding: a preliminary report from the Cooperative Aneurysm Study. Neurosurgery. 1983; 13:479–481

[50] Hillman J, Fridriksson S, Nilsson O, et al. Immediate administration of tranexamic acid and reduced incidence of early rebleeding after aneurysmal subarachnoid hemorrhage: a prospective randomized study. J Neurosurg. 2002; 97:771–778

[51] Naidech AM, Janjua N, Kreiter KT, et al. Predictors and impact of aneurysm rebleeding after subarachnoid hemorrhage. Arch Neurol. 2005; 62:410–416

[52] Ohkuma H, Tsurutani H, Suzuki S. Incidence and significance of early aneurysmal rebleeding before neurosurgical or neurological management. Stroke. 2001; 32:1176–1180

[53] Tanno Y, Homma M, Oinuma M, et al. Rebleeding from ruptured intracranial aneurysms in North Eastern Province of Japan. A cooperative study. J Neurol Sci. 2007; 258:11–16

[54] Winn HR, Richardson AE, Jane JA. The Long-Term Prognosis in Untreated Cerebral Aneurysms. I. The Incidence of Late Hemorrhage in Cerebral Aneurysm: A 10-Year Evaluation of 364 Patients. Ann Neurol. 1977; 1:358–370

[55] Kassell NF, Torner JC, Haley EC,Jr, et al. The International Cooperative Study on the Timing of Aneurysm Surgery. Part 1: Overall Management Results. J Neurosurg. 1990; 73:18–36

[56] Inagawa T, Kamiya K, Ogasawara H, et al. Rebleeding of Ruptured Intracranial Aneurysms in the Acute Stage. Surg Neurol. 1987; 28:93–99

[57] Matsuda M, Watanabe K, Saito A, et al. Circumstances, activities, and events precipitating aneurysmal subarachnoid hemorrhage. J Stroke Cerebrovasc Dis. 2007; 16:25–29

[58] Jane JA, Kassell NF, Torner JC, et al. The Natural History of Aneurysms and AVMs. J Neurosurg. 1985; 62:321–323

[59] Biller J, Godersky JC, Adams HP. Management of Aneurysmal Subarachnoid Hemorrhage. Stroke. 1988; 19:1300–1305

[60] Kassell NF, Torner JC, Adams HP. Antifibrinolytic Therapy in the Acute Period Following Aneurysmal Subarachnoid Hemorrhage: Preliminary Observations from the Cooperative Aneurysm Study. J Neurosurg. 1984; 61:225–230

[61] Glick R, Green D, Ts'ao C-H, et al. High Dose e-Aminocaproic Acid Prolongs the Bleeding Time and Increases Rebleeding and Intraoperative Hemorrhage in Patients with Subarachnoid Hemorrhage. Neurosurgery. 1981; 9:398–401

86

[62] Leipzig TJ, Redelman K, Horner TG. Reducing the Risk of Rebleeding Before Early Aneurysm Surgery: A Possible Role for Antifibrinolytic Therapy. Journal of Neurosurgery. 1997; 86:220–225

[63] Starke RM, Kim GH, Fernandez A, et al. Impact of a protocol for acute antifibrinolytic therapy on aneurysm rebleeding after subarachnoid hemorrhage. Stroke. 2008; 39:2617–2621

[64] Braunwald E, Kloner RA. The Stunned Myocardium: Prolonged Postischemic Ventricular Dysfunction. Circulation. 1982; 66:1146–1149

[65] Murphy AM, Kögler H, Georgakopoulos D, et al. Transgenic Mouse Model of Stunned Myocardium. Science. 2000; 389:491–495

[66] Yuki K, Kodama Y, Onda J, et al. Coronary Vasospasm Following Subarachnoid Hemorrhage as a Cause of Stunned Myocardium. Journal of Neurosurgery. 1991; 75:308–311

[67] Bulsara KR, McGirt MJ, Liao L, et al. Use of the peak troponin value to differentiate myocardial infarction from reversible neurogenic left ventricular dysfunction associated with aneurysmal subarachnoid hemorrhage. Journal of Neurosurgery. 2003; 98:524–528

[68] Malik AN, Gross BA, Rosalind Lai PM, et al. Neurogenic Stress Cardiomyopathy After Aneurysmal Subarachnoid Hemorrhage. World Neurosurg. 2015; 83:880–885

[69] Hravnak M, Frangiskakis JM, Crago EA, et al. Elevated cardiac troponin I and relationship to persistence of electrocardiographic and echocardiographic abnormalities after aneurysmal subarachnoid hemorrhage. Stroke. 2009; 40:3478–3484

[70] Kilbourn KJ, Levy S, Staff I, et al. Clinical characteristics and outcomes of neurogenic stress cardiomyopathy in aneurysmal subarachnoid hemorrhage. Clin Neurol Neurosurg. 2013; 115:909–914

[71] Tung P, Kopelnik A, Banki N, et al. Predictors of neurocardiogenic injury after subarachnoid hemorrhage. Stroke. 2004; 35:548–551

[72] Mayer SA, Lin J, Homma S, et al. Myocardial injury and left ventricular performance after subarachnoid hemorrhage. Stroke. 1999; 30:780–786

[73] Harries AD. Subarachnoid Hemorrhage and the Electrocardiogram: A Review. Postgrad Med J. 1981; 57:294–296

[74] Beard EF, Robertson JW, Robertson RCL. Spontaneous Subarachnoid Hemorrhage Simulating Acute Myocardial Infarction. Am Heart J. 1959; 58:755–759

[75] Gascon P, Ley TJ, Toltzis RJ, et al. Spontaneous Subarachnoid Hemorrhage Simulating Acute Transmural Myocardial Infarction. Am Heart J. 1983; 105:511–513

[76] Marion DW, Segal R, Thompson ME. Subarachnoid hemorrhage and the heart. Neurosurgery. 1986; 18:101–106

[77] DiDomenico RJ, Park HY, Southworth MR, et al. Guidelines for acute decompensated heart failure treatment. Annals of Pharmacotherapy. 2004; 38:649–660

[78] Naidech A, Du Y, Kreiter KT, et al. Dobutamine versus milrinone after subarachnoid hemorrhage. Neurosurgery. 2005; 56:21–27

[79] Knudsen F, Jensen HP, Petersen PL. Neurogenic Pulmonary Edema: Treatment with Dobutamine. Neurosurgery. 1991; 29:269–270

[80] Maeda K, Kurita H, Nakamura T, et al. Occurrence of Severe Vasospasm Following Intraventricular Hemorrhage from an Arteriovenous Malformation. Journal of Neurosurgery. 1997; 87:436–439

[81] Martin NA, Doberstein C, Zane C, et al. Posttraumatic Cerebral Arterial Spasm: Transcranial Doppler Ultrasound, Cerebral Blood Flow, and Angiographic Findings. J Neurosurg. 1992; 77:575–583

[82] Ecker A, Riemenschneider PA. Arteriographic Demonstration of Spasm of the Intracranial Arteries: With Special Reference to Saccular Aneurysms. J Neurosurg. 1951; 8:660–667

[83] Etminan N. Aneurysmal subarachnoid hemorrhage–status quo and perspective. Transl Stroke Res. 2015; 6:167–170

[84] Washington CW, Zipfel GJ. Detection and monitoring of vasospasm and delayed cerebral ischemia: a review and assessment of the literature. Neurocrit Care. 2011; 15:312–317

[85] Dorsch N. A clinical review of cerebral vasospasm and delayed ischaemia following aneurysm rupture. Acta Neurochir Suppl. 2011; 110:5–6

[86] Wedekind C, Hildebrandt G, Klug N. A case of delayed loss of facial nerve function after acoustic neuroma surgery. Zentralbl Neurochir. 1996; 57:163–166

[87] Kudo T. Postoperative oculomotor palsy due to vasospasm in a patient with a ruptured internal carotid artery aneurysm: a case report. Neurosurgery. 1986; 19:274–277

[88] Kassell NF, Sasaki T, Colohan ART, et al. Cerebral Vasospasm Following Aneurysmal Subarachnoid Hemorrhage. Stroke. 1985; 16:562–572

[89] Awad IA, Carter LP, Spetzler RF, et al. Clinical Vasospasm After Subarachnoid Hemorrhage: Response to Hypervolemic Hemodilution and Arterial Hypertension. Stroke. 1987; 18:365–372

[90] Broderick JP, Brott TG, Duldner JE, et al. Initial and recurrent bleeding are the major causes of death following subarachnoid hemorrhage. Stroke. 1994; 25:1342–1347

[91] Alaraj A, Wallace A, Mander N, et al. Outcome following symptomatic cerebral vasospasm on presentation in aneurysmal subarachnoid hemorrhage: coiling vs. clipping. World Neurosurg. 2010; 74:138–142

[92] Weir B, Grace M, Hansen J, et al. Time Course of Vasospasm in Man. J Neurosurg. 1978; 48:173–178

[93] Pasqualin A. Epidemiology and pathophysiology of cerebral vasospasm following subarachnoid hemorrhage. J Neurosurg Sci. 1998; 42:15–21

[94] Bejjani GK, Sekhar LN, Yost AM, et al. Vasospasm after cranial base tumor resection: pathogenesis, diagnosis, and therapy. Surg Neurol. 1999; 52:577–83; discussion 583-4

[95] Popugaev KA, Savin IA, Lubnin AU, et al. Unusual cause of cerebral vasospasm after pituitary surgery. Neurol Sci. 2011; 32:673–680

[96] Mandonnet E, Chassoux F, Naggara O, et al. Transient symptomatic vasospasm following anteromesial temporal lobectomy for refractory epilepsy. Acta Neurochir (Wien). 2009; 151:1723–1726

[97] Valenca MM, Valenca LP, Bordini CA, et al. Cerebral vasospasm and headache during sexual intercourse and masturbatory orgasms. Headache. 2004; 44:244–248

[98] Chatterjee N, Domoto-Reilly K, Fecci PE, et al. Licorice-associated reversible cerebral vasoconstriction with PRES. Neurology. 2010; 75:1939–1941

[99] Fisher CM, Kistler JP, Davis JM. Relation of Cerebral Vasospasm to Subarachnoid Hemorrhage Visualized by CT Scanning. Neurosurgery. 1980; 6:1–9

[100] Kistler JP, Crowell RM, Davis KR, et al. The Relation of Cerebral Vasospasm to the Extent and Location of Subarachnoid Blood Visualized by CT. Neurology. 1983; 33:424–426

[101] Taneda M, Kataoka K, Akai F, et al. Traumatic Subarachnoid Hemorrhage as a Predictable Indicator of Delayed Ischemic Symptoms. Journal of Neurosurgery. 1996; 84:762–768

[102] Lasner TM, Weil RJ, Riina HA, et al. Cigarette Smoking-Induced Increase in the Risk of Symptomatic Vasospasm After Aneurysmal Subarachnoid Hemorrhage. Journal of Neurosurgery. 1997; 87:381–384

[103] Fox JL, Ko JP. Cerebral Vasospasm: A Clinical Observation. Surg Neurol. 1978; 10

[104] Davis JM, Davis KR, Crowell RM. Subarachnoid Hemorrhage Secondary to Ruptured Intracranial Aneurysm: Prognostic Significance of Cranial CT. AJNR. 1980; 1:17–21

[105] Frontera JA, Claassen J, Schmidt JM, et al. Prediction of symptomatic vasospasm after subarachnoid hemorrhage: the modified fisher scale. Neurosurgery. 2006; 59:21–7; discussion 21-7

[106] Sasaki T, Kassell NF, Zuccarello M, et al. Barrier Disruption in the Major Cerebral Arteries During the Acute Stage After Experimental Subarachnoid Hemorrhage. Neurosurgery. 1986; 19:177–184

[107] Sasaki T, Kassell NF, Yamashita M, et al. Barrier Disruption in the Major Cerebral Arteries Following Experimental Subarachnoid Hemorrhage. J Neurosurg. 1985; 63:433–440

[108] Pluta RM, Thompson BG, Afshar JK, et al. Nitric oxide and vasospasm. Acta Neurochir Suppl. 2001; 77:67–72

[109] Borel CO, McKee A, Parra A, et al. Possible role for vascular cell proliferation in cerebral vasospasm after subarachnoid hemorrhage. Stroke. 2003; 34:427–433

[110] Svendgaard NA, Brismar J, Delgado TJ, et al. Subarachnoid Hemorrhage in the Rat: Effect on the Development of Vasospasm of Selective Lesions of the Catecholamine Systems in the Lower Brain Stem. Stroke. 1985; 16:602–608

[111] Honma Y, Clower BR, Haining JL, et al. Comparison of Intimal Platelet Accumulation in Cerebral Arteries in Two Experimental Models of Subarachnoid Hemorrhage. Neurosurgery. 1989; 24:487–490

[112] Allen GS, Gross CJ, French LA, et al. Cerebral Arterial Spasm. Part 5: In Vitro Contractile Activity of Vasoactive Agents Including Human CSF on Human Basilar and Anterior Cerebral Artery. J Neurosurg. 1976; 44:596–600

[113] Sasaki T, Asano T, Takakura K, et al. Nature of the Vasoactive Substance in CSF from Patients with Subarachnoid Hemorrhage. J Neurosurg. 1984; 60:1186–1191

[114] Tew J, Tsai S-H, Greenberg M, et al. Disturbance of Cerebrovascular Innervation After Experimental Subarachnoid Hemorrhage. Baltimore 1987

[115] Wilkins RH. Cerebral Vasospasm. Contemp Neurosurg. 1988; 10:4:1–6

[116] Nakagomi T, Kassell NF, Sasaki T, et al. Effect of Subarachnoid Hemorrhage on Endothelium-Dependent Vasodilatation. J Neurosurg. 1987; 66:915–923

[117] Findlay JM. Current Management of Cerebral Vasospasm. Contemporary Neurosurgery. 1997; 19:1–6

[118] Cardoso ER, Reddy K, Bose D. Effect of Subarachnoid Hemorrhage on Intracranial Pulse Waves in Cats. J Neurosurg. 1988; 69:712–718

[119] Greenberg ED, Gold R, Reichman M, et al. Diagnostic accuracy of CT angiography and CT perfusion for cerebral vasospasm: a meta-analysis. AJNR Am J Neuroradiol. 2010; 31:1853–1860

[120] Tamatani S, Sasaki O, Takeuchi S, et al. Detection of delayed cerebral vasospasm, after rupture of intracranial aneurysms, by magnetic resonance angiography. Neurosurgery. 1997; 40:748–53; discussion 753–4

[121] Vespa PM, Nuwer MR, Juhász C, et al. Early Detection of Vasospasm After Acute Subarachnoid Hemorrhage Using Continuous EEG ICU Monitoring. Electroencephalography & Clinical Neurophysiology. 1997; 103:607–615

[122] Labar DR, Fisch BJ, Pedley TA, et al. Quantitative EEG Monitoring for Patients with Subarachnoid Hemorrhage. Electroencephalography & Clinical Neurophysiology. 1991; 78:325–332

[123] Weir B, Menon D, Overton T. Regional Cerebral Blood Flow in Patients with Aneurysms: Estimation by Xenon 133 Inhalation. Can J Neurol Sci. 1978; 5:301–305

[124] Knuckney NW, Fox RA, Surveyor I, et al. Early Cerebral Blood Flow and CT in Predicting Ischemia After Cerebral Aneurysm Rupture. J Neurosurg. 1985; 62:850–855

[125] Powers WJ, Grubb RL, Baker RP, et al. Regional Cerebral Blood Flow and Metabolism in Reversible Ischemia due to Vasospasm: Determination by Positron Emission Tomography. J Neurosurg. 1985; 62:539–546

[126] Seiler RW, Grolimund P, Aaslid R, et al. Cerebral Vasospasm Evaluated by Transcranial Ultrasound Correlated with Clinical Grade and CT-Visualized Subarachnoid Hemorrhage. J Neurosurg. 1986; 64:594–600

[127] Lindegaard KF, Nornes H, Bakke SJ, et al. Cerebral Vasospasm After Subarachnoid Hemorrhage Investigated by Means of Transcranial Doppler Ultrasound. Acta Neurochirurgica. 1988; 42:81–84

[128] Sekhar LN, Wechsler LR, Yonas H, et al. Value of Transcranial Doppler Examination in the Diagnosis of Cerebral Vasospasm After Subarachnoid Hemorrhage. Neurosurgery. 1988; 22:813–821

[129] Wilkins RH. Attempted Prevention or Treatment of Intracranial Arterial Spasm: A Survey. Neurosurgery. 1980; 6:198–210

[130] Wilkins RH. Attempts at Prevention or Treatment of Intracranial Arterial Spasm: An Update. Neurosurgery. 1986; 18:808–825

[131] Foley PL, Caner HH, Kassell NF, et al. Reversal of Subarachnoid Hemorrhage-Induced Vasoconstriction with an Endothelin Receptor Antagonists. Neurosurgery. 1994; 34:108–113

[132] Zuccarello M, Soattin GB, Lewis AI, et al. Prevention of Subarachnoid Hemorrhage-Induced Cerebral Vasospasm by Oral Administration of Endothelin Receptor Antagonists. Journal of Neurosurgery. 1996; 84:503–507

[133] Muehlschlegel S, Rordorf G, Sims J. Effects of a single dose of dantrolene in patients with cerebral vasospasm after subarachnoid hemorrhage: a prospective pilot study. Stroke. 2011; 42:1301–1306

[134] Majidi S, Grigoryan M, Tekle WG, et al. Intra-arterial dantrolene for refractory cerebral vasospasm after aneurysmal subarachnoid hemorrhage. Neurocrit Care. 2012; 17:245–249

[135] Mees SanneM Dorhout, Algra Ale, Vandertop WPeter, et al. Magnesium for aneurysmal subarachnoid haemorrhage (MASH-2): a randomised placebo-controlled trial. The Lancet. 2012; 380:44–49

[136] Kaku Y, Yonekawa Y, Tsukahara T, et al. Superselective Intra-Arterial Infusion of Papaverine for the Treatment of Cerebral Vasospasm After Subarachnoid Hemorrhage. Journal of Neurosurgery. 1992; 77:842–847

[137] Kassell NF, Helm G, Simmons N, et al. Treatment of Cerebral Vasospasm with Intra-Arterial Papaverine. Journal of Neurosurgery. 1992; 77:848–852

[138] Hori S, Suzuki J. Early Intracranial Operations for Ruptured Aneurysms. Acta Neurochirurgica. 1979; 46:93–104

[139] Mitzukami M, Kawase T, Tazawa T. Prevention of Vasospasm by Early Operation with Removal of Subarachnoid Blood. Neurosurgery. 1982; 10:301–306

[140] Nosko M, Weir BKA, Lunt A, et al. Effect of Clot Removal at 24 Hours on Chronic Vasospasm After Subarachnoid Hemorrhage in the Primate Model. J Neurosurg. 1987; 66:416–422

[141] Findlay JM, Weir BKA, Steinke D, et al. Effect of Intrathecal Thrombolytic Therapy on Subarachnoid Clot and Chronic Vasospasm in a Primate. J Neurosurg. 1988; 69:723–735

[142] Findlay JM, Weir BKA, Kanamaru K, et al. Intrathecal Fibrinolytic Therapy After Subarachnoid Hemorrhage: Dosage Study in a Primate Model and Review of Literature. Can J Neurol Sci. 1989; 16:28–40

[143] Findlay JM, Weir BKA, Gordon P, et al. Safety and Efficacy of Intrathecal Thrombolytic Therapy in a Primate Model of Cerebral Vasospasm. Neurosurgery. 1989; 24:491–498

[144] Findlay JM, Kassell NF, Weir BKA, et al. A Randomized Trial of Intraoperative, Intracisternal Tissue Plasminogen Activator for the Prevention of Vasospasm. Neurosurgery. 1995; 37:168–178

[145] Mizoi K, Yoshimoto T, Fujiwara S, et al. Prevention of Vasospasm by Clot Removal and Intrathecal Bolus Injection of Tissue-Type Plasminogen Activator: Preliminary Report. Neurosurgery. 1991; 28:807–813

[146] Ito U, Tomita H, Yamazaki S, et al. Enhanced Cisternal Drainage and Cerebral Vasospasm in Early Aneurysm Surgery. Acta Neurochirurgica. 1986; 80:18–23

[147] Benzel EC, Kesterson L. Extracranial-Intracranial Bypass Surgery for the Management of Vasospasm After Subarachnoid Hemorrhage. Surg Neurol. 1988; 30:231–234

86

[148] Batjer H, Samson D. Use of Extracranial-Intracranial Bypass in the Management of Symptomatic Vasospasm. Neurosurgery. 1986; 19:235–246

[149] Hieshima GB, Higashida RT, Wapenski J, et al. Balloon Embolization of a Large Distal Basilar Artery Aneurysm: Case Report. J Neurosurg. 1986; 65:413–416

[150] Zubkov YN, Nikiforov BM, Shustin VA. Balloon Catheter Technique for Dilatation of Constricted Cerebral Arteries After Aneurysmal Subarachnoid Hemorrhage. Acta Neurochirurgica. 1984; 70:65–79

[151] Newell DW, Eskridge JM, Mayberg MR, et al. Angioplasty for the Treatment of Symptomatic Vasospasm Following Subarachnoid Hemorrhage. J Neurosurg. 1989; 71:654–660

[152] Linskey ME, Horton JA, Rao GR, et al. Fatal Rupture of the Intracranial Carotid Artery During Transluminal Angioplasty for Vasospasm Induced by Subarachnoid Hemorrhage. J Neurosurg. 1991; 74:985–990

[153] Kimball MM, Velat GJ, Hoh BL. Critical care guidelines on the endovascular management of cerebral vasospasm. Neurocrit Care. 2011; 15:336–341

[154] Zwienenberg-Lee M, Hartman J, Rudisill N, et al. Effect of prophylactic transluminal balloon angioplasty on cerebral vasospasm and outcome in patients with Fisher grade III subarachnoid hemorrhage: results of a phase II multicenter, randomized, clinical trial. Stroke. 2008; 39:1759–1765

[155] Tejada JG, Taylor RA, Ugurel MS, et al. Safety and feasibility of intra-arterial nicardipine for the treatment of subarachnoid hemorrhage-associated vasospasm: initial clinical experience with high-dose infusions. AJNR. American Journal of Neuroradiology. 2007; 28:844–848

[156] Wise BL. SIADH After Spontaneous Subarachnoid Hemorrhage: A Reversible Cause of Clinical Deterioration. Neurosurgery. 1978; 3:412–414

[157] Maroon JC, Nelson PB. Hypovolemia in Patients with Subarachnoid Hemorrhage: Therapeutic Implications. Neurosurgery. 1979; 4:223–226

[158] Wijdicks EFM, Vermeulen M, ten Haaf JA, et al. Volume Depletion and Natriuresis in Patients with a Ruptured Intracranial Aneurysm. Ann Neurol. 1985; 18:211–216

[159] Vermeulen LC, Ratko TA, Erstad BL, et al. The University Hospital Consortium Guidelines for the Use of Albumin, Nonprotein Colloid, and Crystalloid Solutions. Archives of Internal Medicine. 1995; 155:373–379

[160] Origitano TC, Wascher TM, Reichman OH, et al. Sustained Increased Cerebral Blood Flow with Prophylactic Hypertensive Hypervolemic Hemodilution ("Triple-H" Therapy) After Subarachnoid Hemorrhage. Neurosurgery. 1990; 27:729–740

[161] Dankbaar JW, Slooter AJ, Rinkel GJ, et al. Effect of different components of triple-H therapy on cerebral perfusion in patients with aneurysmal subarachnoid haemorrhage: a systematic review. Crit Care. 2010; 14. DOI: 10.1186/cc8886

[162] Solomon RA, Fink ME, Lennihan L. Early Aneurysm Surgery and Prophylactic Hypervolemic Hypertensive Therapy for the Treatment of Aneurysmal Subarachnoid Hemorrhage. Neurosurgery. 1988; 23:699–704

[163] Shimoda M, Oda S, Tsugane R, et al. Intracranial Complications of Hypervolemic Therapy in Patients with a Delayed Ischemic Deficit Attributed to Vasospasm. Journal of Neurosurgery. 1993; 78:423–429

[164] Rosenwasser RH, Jallo JI, Getch CC, et al. Complications of Swan-Ganz Catheterization for Hemodynamic Monitoring in Patients with Subarachnoid Hemorrhage. Neurosurgery. 1995; 37:872–876

[165] Kim GH, Hahn DK, Kellner CP, et al. The incidence of heparin-induced thrombocytopenia Type II in patients with subarachnoid hemorrhage treated with heparin versus enoxaparin. Journal of Neurosurgery. 2009; 110:50–57

87 SAH from Cerebral Aneurysm Rupture

87.1 Epidemiology of cerebral aneurysms

The incidence of cerebral aneurysms is difficult to estimate. Range of autopsy prevalence of aneurysms: 0.2–7.9% (variability depends on use of dissecting microscope, hospital referral and autopsy pattern, overall interest...). Estimated prevalence of incidental aneurysms range from 1–5% of the population,[1,2,3,4,5] and detection is increased with widespread use of CT and MRI.[6] Ratio of ruptured: unruptured (incidental) aneurysm is 5:3 to 5:6 (rough estimate is 1:1, i.e., 50% of these aneurysms rupture).[7] Unruptured intracranial aneurysms are more common in women (≈ 3:1 ratio)[8,9] and in the elderly,[10] and only 2% of aneurysms present during childhood.[11] When present in children, they tend to occur more frequently in males (2:1) and to a greater degree in the posterior circulation (40–45%).[12,13]

87.2 Etiology of cerebral aneurysms

The exact pathophysiology of the development of aneurysms is still controversial. In contrast to extracranial blood vessels, there is less elastic in the tunica media and adventitia of cerebral blood vessels, the media has less muscle, the adventitia is thinner, and the internal elastic lamina is more prominent.[14,15] This, together with the fact that large cerebral blood vessels lie within the subarachnoid space with little supporting connective tissue,[16(p 1644)] may predispose these vessels to the development of saccular aneurysms. Aneurysms tend to arise in areas where there is a curve in the parent artery, in the angle between it and a significant branching artery, and point in the direction that the parent artery would have continued had the curve not been present.[17]

The etiology of aneurysms may be:
1. congenital predisposition (e.g., defect in the muscular layer of the arterial wall, referred to as a medial gap)
2. "atherosclerotic" or hypertensive: presumed etiology of most saccular aneurysms, probably interacts with congenital predisposition described above
3. embolic: as in atrial myxoma
4. infectious—so called "mycotic aneurysms" (p. 1492)
5. traumatic: see Traumatic aneurysms (p. 1491)
6. associated with other conditions (see below)

87.3 Location of cerebral aneurysms

Saccular aneurysms, AKA berry aneurysms are usually located on major named cerebral arteries at the apex of branch points, which is the site of maximum hemodynamic stress in a vessel.[18] More peripheral aneurysms do occur, but tend to be associated with infection (mycotic aneurysms) or trauma. Fusiform aneurysms are more common in the vertebrobasilar system. Dissecting aneurysms should be categorized with arterial dissection (p. 1577).

Saccular aneurysms location:
1. 85–95% in carotid system, with the following 3 most common locations:
   a) ACoA (single most common): 30% (ACoA & ACA more common in males)
   b) PComA: 25%
   c) middle cerebral artery (MCA): 20%
2. 5–15% in posterior circulation (vertebro-basilar)
   a) ≈ 10% on basilar artery: basilar bifurcation, AKA basilar tip, is the most common, followed by BA-SCA, BA-VA junction, AICA
   b) ≈ 5% on vertebral artery: VA-PICA junction is the most common
3. 20–30% of aneurysm patients have multiple aneurysms (p. 1490) [19]

87.4 Natural history of cerebral aneurysms

This is an overview. Many of these items will be addressed in detail in following sections.
1. major rupture (see below): typically into the subarachnoid space (subarachnoid hemorrhage (SAH)). Possible other sites include: ventricles, brain parenchyma, subdural space... (see below)
   a) for previously ruptured aneurysms, this is the risk of rebleeding (p. 1437)
   b) see for unruptured aneurysms (p. 1486)

87

2. spontaneous thrombosis of an aneurysm is a rare occurrence[20,21,22] (estimate in autopsy series is 9–13%[22]). However, thrombosed aneurysms may re-open,[23,24] and delayed rupture may occur sometimes even years later
3. aneurysms can also cause symptoms without a major rupture (e.g., cranial neuropathies, hemiparesis, endocrine disturbances, proptosis, strokes…): see below
4. some incidental aneurysms may lie "dormant" and be amenable to observation (see unruptured aneurysms (p. 1486))

87.5 Presentation of cerebral aneurysms

87.5.1 Major rupture

The most frequent presentation. This may produce:
1. subarachnoid hemorrhage (SAH) (p. 1437): the most common sequela of aneurysmal rupture. The following may occur with or without SAH
2. intracerebral hemorrhage: occurs in 20–40% (more common with aneurysms distal to the Circle of Willis, e.g., MCA aneurysms)
3. intraventricular hemorrhage: occurs in 13–28%[25] (see below)
4. hemorrhage into vascular space (producing an arteriovenous fistula), e.g., with cavernous carotid artery aneurysms (p. 1489)
5. subdural blood occurs in 2–5%

▶ **Intraventricular hemorrhage.** See also other etiologies of intraventricular hemorrhage (IVH) (p. 1671).

IVH occurs in 13–28% of ruptured aneurysms in clinical series (higher in autopsy series)[25] and appears to carry a worse prognosis (64% mortality).[25] The size of the ventricles on admission was the most important prognosticator (large vents being worse). Patterns that may occur:
1. distal PICA aneurysms: may rupture directly into 4th ventricle through the foramen of Luschka[26]
2. AComA aneurysm: it has been asserted that IVH occurs from rupture through the lamina terminalis into the anterior 3rd or lateral ventricles; however, this is not always borne out at the time of surgery
3. distal basilar artery or carotid terminus aneurysms: may rupture through the floor of the 3rd ventricle (rare)

87.5.2 Presentation other than major rupture

General information

May be thought of as possible "warning signs."
1. mass effect: usually associated with enlargement of the aneurysm. May be gradual as with giant aneurysms, or acute often associated with minor enlargement
   a) giant aneurysms: including brainstem compression producing hemiparesis and cranial neuropathies
   b) cranial neuropathy (average latency from symptom to SAH was 110 days; **note:** the average latency quoted for some of these symptoms comes from a retrospective study of patients presenting with SAH who were identified as having a warning symptom[27]) (see below)
   c) intra- or suprasellar aneurysm producing endocrine disturbance[28] due to pituitary gland or stalk compression
2. minor hemorrhage: warning or sentinel hemorrhage; see Headache (p. 1418). This group had the shortest latency (10 days) between symptom and SAH (**note:** the average latency quoted for some of these symptoms comes from a retrospective study of patients presenting with SAH who were identified as having a warning symptom[27])
3. small infarcts or transient ischemia due to distal embolization (including amaurosis fugax, homonymous hemianopsia…)[29]: average latency from symptom to SAH was 21 days
4. seizures: at surgery, an adjacent area of encephalomalacia may be found.[29] The seizures may arise as a result of localized gliosis and do not necessarily represent aneurysmal expansion as there is no data to indicate an increased risk of hemorrhage in this group
5. headache[29] without hemorrhage: abates after treatment in most cases
   a) acute: may be severe and "thunderclap" in nature,[30] some describe as "worst headache of my life." Has been attributed to aneurysmal expansion, thrombosis, or intramural bleeding,[31] all without rupture

b) present for ≥ 2 weeks: unilateral in about half (often retro-orbital or periorbital), possibly due to irritation of overlying dura. Diffuse or bilateral in the other half, possibly due to mass effect → increased ICP

6. incidentally discovered (i.e., asymptomatic, e.g., those found on angiography, CT, or MRI obtained for other reasons)

Cranial neuropathies from aneurysmal compression

1. oculomotor (3rd nerve) palsy (ONP): occurs in ≈ 9% of PComA aneurysms[32] (ruptured and unruptured), less common with basilar apex aneurysm. Symptoms of ONP may include:
   a) extraocular muscle palsy (eye deviates "down and out" → diplopia)
   b) ptosis
   c) dilated unreactive pupil (p. 591): ★ non-pupil-sparing third nerve palsy is the classic finding of 3rd nerve compression
2. visual loss due to[29]
   a) compressive optic neuropathy with ophthalmic artery aneurysms: characteristically produces nasal quadrantanopsia
   b) chiasmal syndromes due to ophthalmic, AComA, or basilar apex aneurysms
3. facial pain syndromes in the ophthalmic or maxillary nerve distribution that may mimic trigeminal neuralgia can occur with intracavernous or supraclinoid aneurysms[29,33]

▶ **Note.** The development of a third nerve palsy in a patient with an unruptured aneurysm is a medical emergency as it probably results from aneurysmal expansion and may portend impending rupture.

87.6 Conditions associated with aneurysms

87.6.1 Overview

1. autosomal dominant polycystic kidney disease (see below)
2. fibromuscular dysplasia (**FMD**): prevalence of aneurysms in renal FMD is 7%, in aortocranial FMD 21%
3. arteriovenous malformations (AVM) including moyamoya disease; see AVMs and aneurysms (p. 1507)
4. connective tissue disorders[34]:
   a) Ehlers-Danlos, especially type IV (deficient collagen type III) which also has a high rate of arterial dissection, including with angiography or coiling
   b) Marfan syndrome (p. 1576)
   c) pseudoxanthoma elasticum
5. multiple other family members with intracranial aneurysms. Familial intracranial aneurysm syndrome (FIA): 2 or more relatives, third-degree or closer, harbor radiographically proven intracranial aneurysms. Also, see Familial aneurysms (p. 1490)
6. coarctation of the aorta[35]
7. hereditary hemorrhagic telangiectasia[36] (Osler-Weber-Rendu syndrome)
8. atherosclerosis[37]
9. bacterial endocarditis
10. multiple endocrine neoplasia type I[38]
11. neurofibromatosis type I[39]

87.6.2 Autosomal dominant polycystic kidney disease

General information

Adult polycystic kidney disease is seen in 1 of every 500 autopsies, and approximately 500,000 people in the U.S. carry the mutant gene for autosomal dominant polycystic kidney disease (ADPKD; there is also an autosomal recessive polycystic kidney disease). Renal function is usually normal during the first few decades of life, with progressive chronic renal failure ensuing. HTN is a common sequelae. Transmission is autosomal dominant, with 100% penetrance by 80 yrs of age.[40] Cystic disease of other organs may occur (viz.: liver in ≈ 33%, and occasionally lung, pancreas).[41]

The first association between ADPKD and cerebral aneurysms is attributed to Dunger in 1904. Reported prevalence of intracranial aneurysms with ADPKD: 10–30%,[42] with 15% being a reasonable estimate.[43] Most were located on the MCA, with multiple aneurysms present in 31%.[44] In addition to

87

the increased incidence of aneurysms, there appears to be an increased risk of rupture,[45] with 64% occurring before age 50. As a result, patients with ADPKD carry a 10–20-fold increased risk of SAH compared to the general population.[46] Aneurysms are rarely detectable before age 20 years. The average rate of rupture of incidental aneurysms is ≈ 2%/yr (p. 1437).

Recommendations

Using the above statistics, together with the life expectancy of patients with ADPKD and other estimations (of operative morbidity and mortality, etc.), the result of decision analysis is that arteriography *not* be routinely employed in patients older than 25 years.[42] However, patients with symptoms possibly due to unruptured aneurysms, and those with SAH, should undergo angiography and subsequent treatment of any aneurysms discovered (especially those > 1 cm diameter). A decision analysis study[43] determined that screening with *MRA* was beneficial compared to treating patients once they became symptomatic. Repeat MRA screening may be effectively repeated as follows:
1. every ≈ 2–3 years for a young patient with ADPKD with either
   a) a history of aneurysms, or
   b) a kindred of ADPKD with aneurysms
2. every 5–20 years for a patient with ADPKD in a kindred of ADPKD with no history of aneurysms[43]

87.7 Treatment options for aneurysms

87.7.1 General information

The optimal treatment for an aneurysm depends on the age and condition of the patient, the anatomy of the aneurysm and associated vasculature, the ability of the surgeon and the availability of endovascular treatment options, and must be weighed against the natural history (p. 1453) of the condition. Also, treatment of the aneurysm facilitates treatment of cerebrovascular vasospasm (p. 1439), should it occur.

In general, the appropriateness of endovascular treatment should be assessed initially in treating ruptured and unruptured aneurysms (not all will be amenable).

87.7.2 Therapies that do not directly address the aneurysm

The hope here is that the aneurysm will not bleed and that it will thrombose (see above).
1. continue medical management initiated on admission: i.e., control of HTN, continue calcium-channel blockers, stool softeners, activity restrictions…
2. treatment options generally *not* used
   a) antifibrinolytic therapy (e.g., ε-aminocaproic acid (EACA)): ✘ NB: *NOT USED*. Reduces rebleeding, but increases the incidence of arterial vasospasm and hydrocephalus[47]
   b) serial LPs: an historical treatment,[48] may increase the risk of aneurysmal re-rupture

87.7.3 Endovascular techniques to treat the aneurysm

1. thrombosing the aneurysm:
   a) "coiling" with Guglielmi electrolytically detachable coils (see below)
   b) Onyx HD 500 has been used for wide-necked or giant ICA aneurysms.[49] Out of 22 patients, there was 1 parent ICA stenosis and 2 ICA occlusions caused by Onyx migration
   c) "flow diversion" with "covered stents" (p. 1924) (tightly woven stents) which promotes thrombosis of the aneurysm
2. trapping: effective treatment requires distal AND proximal arterial interruption, usually by endovascular techniques,[50] occasionally by direct surgical means (ligation or clip occlusion), or some combination. May also incorporate vascular bypass (e.g., EC-IC bypass) to maintain flow distal to trapped segment[51]
3. proximal ligation (so-called hunterian ligation after Hunter ligated the popliteal artery proximal to a peripheral aneurysm in 1784[52]): useful for giant aneurysms.[53,54] For non-giant aneurysms provides little benefit and adds the risk of thromboembolism (which may be reduced by occluding the CCA rather than the ICA[54]). May also elevate the risk of developing aneurysms in the contralateral circulation[55]

87.7.4 Surgical treatment options for aneurysms

1. clipping: the *surgical* gold standard. Surgical placement of a clip across the neck of the aneurysm to exclude the aneurysm from the circulation (see below) without occluding normal vessels
2. wrapping or coating the aneurysm: although this should never be the goal of surgery, situations may arise in which there is little else that can be done (e.g., fusiform basilar trunk aneurysms, aneurysms with significant branches arising from the dome, or part of the neck within the cavernous sinus)
   a) with muscle: the first method used to surgically treat an aneurysm[56] (the patient described died from rebleeding)
   b) with cotton or muslin: popularized by Gillingham.[57] An analysis of 60 patients showed that 8.5% rebled in ≤ 6 mos, and the annual rebleeding rate was 1.5% thereafter[58] (similar to the natural history)
   c) with plastic resin or other polymer: may be slightly better than muscle or gauze.[59] One study with long follow-up found no protection from rebleeding during the first month, but thereafter the risk was slightly lower than the natural history.[59] Other studies show no difference from natural course[60]
   d) teflon and fibrin glue[61]

87.7.5 Treatment decisions: coiling vs. clipping

General information

The use of endovascular treatment for aneurysms has increased, with coil embolization being the most common endovascular modality (see above for other options). From 2002–2008, the rate of aneurysm coiling in the U.S. and U.K. increased from 17 and 35% to 58 and 68%, respectively.[62,63] There is considerable controversy and debate as to the best therapeutic approach for aneurysms ruptured and unruptured). Impediments to resolving the debate include methodological shortcomings of published studies, the fact that endovascular methods are still rapidly evolving, which renders many studies obsolete before completion, and the critical need for long-term follow-up of endovascular results.

This section reviews some of the available information comparing surgical treatment to coil embolization.

Ruptured intracranial aneurysms

To date, four randomized controlled trials have been published comparing functional outcome after coil embolization versus surgical clip ligation for ruptured intracranial aneurysms: the "Finnish study,"[64] ISAT 2002,[65] the "Chinese Study,"[66] and BRAT 2012.[67] ▶ Table 87.1 summarizes the treatment data from the 4 RCTs.

Table 87.1 Summary of rebleeding, complete occlusion, and retreatment rates as a function of treatment modality (clip vs. coil) for the 4 randomized controlled trials

	Rebleed[a]: Clip	Rebleed[a]: Coil	Complete occlusion: Clip	Complete occlusion: Coil	Retreatment: Clip	Retreatment: Coil
Finnish	0%	0%	73.7%[b]	50%[b]	7%	23.1%
ISAT	1.0%	2.6%	82%	66%	4.2%	15.1%
ISAT$_5$[c]	0.3%*	0.9%*	n/a	n/a	———	———
ISAT$_{10}$[c]	0.4%	1.6%	n/a	n/a	———	———
Chinese	3.3%	3.2%	83.7%*	64.9%*	———	———
BRAT[d]	0.8%[e]	0%	85%	58%	4.5%*	10.6%*
BRAT$_3$[d]	0%	0%	87%	52%	5%*	13%*

* statistically significant difference (p < 0.05)
[a]Rebleeding from target aneurysm after first procedure
[b]Result achieved after treatment during first hospitalization
[c]ISAT$_5$ & ISAT$_{10}$ refer to the 5- and 10-year follow-up studies. Rebleeding results for these studies refer to recurrent SAH after the 1st year of follow-up
[d]BRAT$_3$ refers to the 3-year follow-up study. BRAT & BRAT$_3$ are "as-treated" results
[e]Both rebleeding events occurred during the initial hospitalization

87

▶ **ISAT.** The largest trial, the International Subarachnoid Hemorrhage Aneurysm Trial (ISAT), enrolled 2143 patients and ran from 1997 to 2002, and was stopped prematurely because of a significant outcome difference between the 2 groups favoring endovascular coil embolization. Despite the limitations of ISAT (see below), the findings have often been generalized to all patients with aneurysms, resulting in a dramatic change in management.

Results: At 1 year, there was an absolute reduction of risk of having a poor outcome (i.e., ▶ Table 98.5, modified Rankin Scale score > 2) by 7% with coiling (24%) compared to open surgery (31%; p=0.0019). Although not statistically significant, rebleeding in the first year after treatment was higher for coiling (2.6%) than clipping (1.0%). As such, the durability of coil embolization and its ability to prevent subsequent rebleeding of the treated aneurysm were questioned. Additionally, ISAT had many important shortcomings, as detailed in ▶ Table 87.2.

Table 87.2 Methodological shortcomings of ISAT

1. only 20% of 9559 patients presenting with SAH were randomized[a]
   a) selection could introduce bias
   b) more nonrandomized patients underwent MS than EDC
   c) guidelines not provided for which patients to consider for EDC
2. most study centers were located in Europe, Australia & Canada
3. the expertise of the surgeons and the interventionalists were not reported and were not necessarily comparable
4. the following features are not entirely representative of SAH patients at large
   a) 80% of patients were in good clinical condition (H&H grade 1 or 2)
   b) 93% of aneurysms were ≤ 10 mm diameter
   c) 97% were in the anterior circulation
5. rebleeding rate: after EDC (2.4%) or MS (1.0%) was high for both groups, and the difference could be more significant beyond the 1-year follow-up provided

[a]most SAH patients were referred specifically for MS or EDC. The only patients who were randomized were those for whom a panel decided it was not clear which procedure would be superior. Outcomes were not provided for non-randomized patients

Following the initial report, medium-term follow-up results have been published.[68] In the endovascular cohort, there were 10 episodes of rebleeding from the treated aneurysm after 1 year, in 8,447 person-years of follow-up. In the surgical cohort, 3 patients rebled from the treated aneurysm after 1 year, in 8,177 person-years of follow-up (one of these patients had declined surgery after randomization and underwent coiling instead). There was a non-significant increased risk of rebleeding from the treated aneurysm in the endovascular cohort (p=0.06), by an intention-to-treat analysis, but a significant difference when analysis was by actual treatment (p=0.02). The probability of death at 5 years was significantly lower in the coiled group (11%) than in the clipping group (14%; p=0.03). However, when patients who died before treatment are excluded from this analysis, the statistical difference is no longer present (p=0.1).[69] The probability of independent survival for those patients alive at 5 years was no different between groups (83% coil; 82% clip).

The 10-year results have been reported for the U.K. cohort from the initial trial.[70] Similar to the 5-year results, the proportion of patients with a good outcome did not differ between the two groups, but the probability of being alive with a good outcome compared with death or dependence was significantly better for the endovascular group. Thirteen patients in the endovascular group rebled from the target aneurysm (1 per 641 patient-years) compared to 4 in the surgical group (1 per 2,048 patient-years). Although the risk of rebleeding was higher in the endovascular group, the overall risk was small and the risk of death or dependency from a rebleed did not differ between the groups.

A follow-up study, ISAT II (multicenter RCT), is currently being conducted to help elucidate differences in outcomes between treatment modalities.[71]

▶ **Chinese study**[66]. 192 patients with aSAH randomized to coiling or clipping. Surgical clipping increased the risk of symptomatic vasospasm (OR 1.24), and there were significantly more new cerebral infarctions in the clipping group (21.7 vs. 12.8%). Incidence of complete aneurysm occlusion was significantly lower in the coiling group (64.9 vs. 83.7%). Rebleeding rates were similar in both groups (≈ 3%). At 1 year, there was no significant difference in probability of mortality (coiling: 10.6%, clipping: 15.2%). Furthermore, there was no significant difference in probability of a good outcome (coiling: 75%, clipping: 67.9%).

▶ **BRAT**[67]. Initiated at Barrow Neurologic Institute in 2002. Designed to reflect "real-world" practices of ruptured aneurysm treatment in North America. Randomly assigned in an alternate fashion every patient with SAH who agreed to participate. A large number of patients allocated endovascular treatment crossed over to the surgical arm because patients could be enrolled regardless of whether the aneurysm was amenable to both treatment modalities (75 crossed over from coil to surgery; 4 crossed over from surgery to coil). Proportion of patients with a poor outcome (i.e., mRS > 2) was 33.7% in the surgical group versus 23.2% in the endovascular group (p=0.02, intention-to-treat analysis). An "as-treated" analysis yielded similar results (33.9 vs. 20.4%, p=0.01). There were 2 episodes of rebleeding following treatment—one assigned to and treated with clipping and the other assigned to coil, but treated with surgical clipping. Twelve patients (2.9%) required retreatment during the initial hospitalization (9 surgical and 3 coil patients). Overall, during the 1st year, there was a significant increased probability of retreatment in patients actually treated with coiling compared with those actually treated by clipping (10.6% of coil vs. 4.49% of surgical patients, p=0.03).

At 3 years,[72] there was no significant difference in poor outcome between coiling (30%) and clipping (35.8%). Subgroup analysis: there were no differences in mRS scores between treatment groups at any time point among patients with anterior circulation aneurysms (83%). However, among posterior circulation aneurysms (17%), mRS scores were significantly better after endovascular management than after surgical treatment at every time point. Of note, with the exception of basilar tip aneurysms, the randomization of the posterior circulation aneurysms was unexpectedly skewed (large majority of SCA and PICA were clipped, whereas majority of PCA, vertebral, and basilar were coiled). The lack of anatomical parity between the treatment groups makes it difficult to draw strong conclusions. In addition, the degree of aneurysm obliteration (87 vs. 52%), rate of aneurysm recurrence, and rate of retreatment (5 vs. 13%) were significantly better in the group treated with clipping as compared to coiling. However, no rebleeding occurrences were documented in the 2nd or 3rd year of BRAT.

87

► **Meta-analyses.** Lanzino et al[73] conducted a meta-analsysis on the 3 prospective controlled studies (Finnish, ISAT, BRAT). Pooled data showed poor outcome at 1 year to be lower in the embolization group and no difference in mortality between groups; rebleeding rates within the first month were higher in coiled patients. However, the results were largely skewed by ISAT data.

Li et al[74] conducted a meta-analysis on the 4 RCTs (see above) and 23 observational studies. The result of the RCT analysis with regard to poor outcome at 1 year paralleled that by Lanzino et al. However, there was no difference in poor outcome between groups in the nonrandomized controlled trial analysis. Additional subgroup analysis showed a higher incidence of rebleeding after coiling (≈ 2–3 vs. 1%), corresponding to a better complete occlusion rate of clipping (84 vs. 66.5%). Procedural complication rates and 1-year mortality did not differ significantly between the groups.

► **Vasospasm.** Whether coiling or clipping has an independent correlation with symptomatic vasospasm is debatable. One meta-analysis[75] suggested a trend toward less symptomatic vasospasm after coiling as compared to clipping. However, the analysis had multiple limitations—the two treatment groups were not comparable (age, clinical grade, aneurysm location); there were differences in study design and definitions of vasospasm; and there was a lack of angiographic diagnosis of vasospasm. In the Chinese RCT (above) symptomatic vasospasm and consequent cerebral infarction were more common in the clipping group. Li et al[74] found vasospasm was more common after clipping (48.8 vs. 43.1%); however, ischemic infarction did not differ significantly. Treatment choice may also alter the spasm pattern: on one study,[76] patients who underwent clipping developed localized vasospasm around the rupture site, whereas those treated with coiling demonstrated progressive distal vasospasm over time (possibly related to treatment-specific effects on CSF circulation).

► **Shunt-dependent hydrocephalus.** One study showed a lower incidence of shunt-dependent hydrocephalus in the surgical treatment group (19.9 vs. 47.1%),[77] but many others have failed to show this relationship.[74,78,79,80,81,82,83,84,85,86] A suggestion that fenestration of the lamina terminalis at the time of surgery may decrease shunt-dependent chronic hydrocephalus was refuted by a meta-analysis[87] of 11 non-randomized studies (hydrocephalus rates of 10% with fenestration compared to 15% without).

► **Seizures.** A literature review[88] of seizures after aSAH reported a rate of ≈ 2% following either neurosurgical clipping or endovascular coiling. In contrast, ISAT showed endovascular intervention had lower seizure rates (13.3% to 3.3%) compared to surgical clipping (2.2–5.2%) in the first year. As such, there is no consensus as to whether treatment modality independently impacts seizure and/or epilepsy occurrence.

Factors to consider (clipping vs. coiling)
  health care environment / equipment available
  skill set and experience of the neurosurgeon and interventionalist

- ○ greater annual numbers of aneurysms treated by individual practitioners were significantly related to decrease in morbidity[89]
- anatomy and location of the aneurysm
  - ○ favorable dome/neck ratio versus wide neck aneurysms
  - ○ MCA aneurysms may be difficult to coil because of a branch near the neck
  - ○ basilar apex: favors coiling
  - ○ associated IPH/SDH: surgery allows both evacuation of hemorrhage and treatment of aneurysm
  - ○ symptoms due to mass effect: clipping[90,91] may be better than coiling. In 13 patients with PComA aneurysms and oculomotor nerve (3rd nerve) palsy (**ONP**), 6 of 7 patients clipped vs. 2 of 6 with coiling recovered completely.[32] Partial ONP improved with either treatment, but complete ONP recovered in 3 of 4 patients clipped vs. 0 of 3 coiled[32]
- patient age
  - ○ younger age: lower risk of surgery, and lower lifetime risk of recurrence than with coiling
- clinical state/comorbidities
  - ○ good outcome seen in 63% clip vs. 46% coil in poor-grade (WFNS IV/V) patients (contrary to findings in practice guidelines[92]); therefore, microsurgery and endovascular treatment, when selected primarily according to angiographic features, were equally likely to achieve good outcome[93]
  - ○ patients on anticoagulation (e.g., Plavix) favor endovascular treatment

87

Practice guideline: Aneurysm treatment decisions

Level C[92]: Treatment decisions should be multidisciplinary (made by experienced cerebrovascular and endovascular specialists) based on characteristics of the patient and aneurysm.

Level C[92]: Microsurgical clipping may receive increased consideration in patients presenting with large (> 50 ml) intraparenchymal hematomas and middle cerebral artery aneurysms (▶ Fig. 85.1).

Level C[92]: Endovascular coiling may receive increased consideration in the elderly (> 70 yo), in those presenting with poor-grade WFNS classification (IV/V) aSAH, and in those with aneurysms of the basilar apex

Level B[92]: For patients with ruptured aneurysms judged to be technically amenable to both endovascular coiling and neurosurgical clipping, endovascular coiling should be considered

Unruptured intracranial aneurysms

As with ruptured aneurysms, there is controversy over the best treatment method for unruptured intracranial aneurysms (IUAs), and additional uncertainty surrounds the question of which IUA need to be treated (vs. observed). Darsaut et al[94] found that practitioners do not agree regarding management of IUAs, even when they share a background in the same specialty, similar capabilities in aneurysm management, or years of practice.

There are no prospective randomized studies of treatment interventions vs. conservative management,[95] or studies comparing treatment options to each other. Most data are either from personal series or are retrospective.

▶ **Surgical clipping.** One summary of 260 patients (including a retrospective multicenter analysis) shows no surgical mortality, and morbidity of 0–10.3% (6.5% major and 8% minor morbidity in the multicenter study).[5] Findings from one meta-analysis of 733 patients who underwent surgical clipping showed a mortality rate of 1% and major morbidity rate of 4%.[96] A larger meta-analysis of 2,460 patients revealed mortality and morbidity rates of 2.6% and 10.9%, respectively.[97]

The ISUIA investigators found surgical mortality to be 2.3% at 30 days, and 3.8% at 1 year.[98] Additionally, they found a combined morbidity and mortality at 1 year of 12.6% for those without previous hemorrhage and 10.1% for those with previous subarachnoid hemorrhage from another aneurysm. For patients treated with surgical clipping, morbidity and mortality were greatest in those with aneurysms that were large or in the posterior circulation, and in patients older than age 50. In comparison, the combined morbidity and mortality for the 451 patients treated with an endovascular procedure was 9.1% at 30 days and 9.5% at 1 year. Predictors of adverse outcome included aneurysm size and posterior circulation aneurysms. Additionally, the presence of calcification (independent of aneurysm size) has been shown to increase the likelihood of poor outcome.[99]

▶ **Comparison of clipping to coil embolization.** Early retrospective studies have shown a lower incidence of in-hospital death and discharge to skilled nursing facilities with endovascular therapy compared to those treated surgically.[100,101] A recent retrospective study conducted at a single center showed early outcome and lower complication rate favoring clipping, but the results did not remain significant long-term.[102] A meta-analysis[103] showed that clipping resulted in significantly higher disability as compared to coiling (OR 2.38–2.83). However, subgroup analysis by outcome-measurement time revealed clipping to be associated with greater risk of disability in the short-term (< 6 months) but not in the long-term (> 6 months). In addition, mortality (in-hospital and overall), hemorrhage, and infarction were no different between groups. Despite inclusion of a large number of studies and patients, it is very challenging to draw any conclusion from the meta-analysis, as all the studies were observational (i.e., low levels of evidence), and the analysis did not stratify outcomes based on size and/or location of aneurysms.

Lawson et al[104] compared natural history rupture risk to national treatment risk for coiling and clipping (taken from the Nationwide Inpatient Sample from 2002–2008). Overall mortality rate for clipping and coiling was 2.66% and 2.17%, respectively. Poor outcome was significantly greater for clipping (4.75%) versus coiling (2.16%). Data regarding the homogeneity of the two groups regarding aneurysm size or location was not available. Treatment risk curves were generated and compared against natural history actuarial risk curves calculated from four prominent studies.[9,105,106,107] Overall, the analysis demonstrated rationale for clipping small, unruptured aneurysms in patients < 61–70 years and coiling small unruptured aneurysms in patients < 70–80 years.

Additional studies have focused on the effect of age on outcomes. Mahaney et al[108] showed that procedural and in-hospital morbidity and mortality increased with age in patients treated with surgery, but remained relatively constant with endovascular treatment. Poor neurological outcome from aneurysm or procedure-related morbidity and mortality did not differ between management groups for patients 65 years old and younger, but was significantly higher in the surgical group for patients older than 65 years. Surgery appeared to show a surgical benefit in patients < 50 years old at 1 year. Others have suggested an overall benefit of endovascular treatment over surgical clipping, which becomes more pronounced with age.[109]

▶ **Cost.** Several studies have compared total hospital costs for treatment of unruptured aneurysms with mixed results. Halkes et al[110] and Hoh et al[111] found endovascular treatment to be associated with higher total hospital costs. A later study by Hoh et al[112] found that on a national level, surgical clipping was associated with higher costs. A long-term outcome study[113] showed that clipping was associated with higher initial costs, but overall costs at 2 and 5 years were similar to coiling (due to higher number of follow-up angiograms and outpatient costs). More recently, total hospital cost was shown to be lower for clipping, despite higher fixed-direct and fixed-indirect costs.[114] This is a function of much higher variable costs (i.e., the cost of coils and devices) overcoming any substantial cost reduction due to shorter length of stay in patients treated endovascularly.

▶ **Miscellaneous.** *Oculomotor nerve palsy:* Complete recovery of oculomotor nerve palsy associated with PComA aneurysms is more common with surgical clipping than with endovascular treatment (87 % vs. 44%).[115]

Pregnancy: No studies have directly compared clipping versus coiling. Clipping may be preferred by some[116]; see pregnancy and SAH (p. 1425).

37.8 Timing of aneurysm surgery

37.8.1 Background

Historically, there was controversy between so-called "early surgery" (generally, but not precisely defined as ≤ 48–96 hrs post-SAH) and "late surgery" (usually ≥ 10–14 days post-SAH). The current consensus is that there should be intervention for a ruptured aneurysm (clipping or coiling) as promptly as possible to secure the aneurysm and prevent rebleeding. In a review of all patients with SAH treated by clipping or coiling in the Nationwide Inpatient Sample between 2002–2010, treatment at non-teaching hospitals and older age (> 80 yo) were associated with delays in time to aneurysm clipping, but these associations were not seen when endovascular treatment was performed.[117] Increased time to procedure (> 3 days) was significantly associated with an increased likelihood of moderate to severe neurological deficit. Ultra-early (< 24 h after SAH) coiling of ruptured aneurysms has also been associated with improved clinical outcomes (mRS 0–2) compared to coiling at > 24 hours in poor-grade SAH patients (Hunt and Hess (H&H) grade IV/V).[118] This does not rule out a selection bias, however. Additionally, the increased morbidity and mortality associated with surgical intervention on patients who present subacutely with evidence of vasospasm on imaging, may be better suited for endovascular intervention.

Early surgery advocated for the following reasons:
1. if successful, virtually eliminates the risk of rebleeding, which occurs most frequently in the period immediately following SAH (p.1437)
2. facilitates treatment of vasospasm which peaks in incidence between days 6–8 post-SAH (never seen before day 3) by allowing induction of arterial hypertension and volume expansion without danger of aneurysmal rupture
3. allows lavage to remove potentially vasospasmogenic agents from contact with vessels, including use of thrombolytic agents (p.1444)
4. although operative mortality is higher, overall patient mortality is lower[119]

Arguments against early surgery in favor of late surgery include
1. inflammation and brain edema are most severe immediately following SAH
   a) this necessitates more brain retraction
   b) at the same time this softens the brain, making retraction more difficult (retractors have more tendency to lacerate the more friable brain)
2. the presence of solid clot that has not had time to lyse impedes surgery
3. the risk of intraoperative rupture is higher with early surgery
4. incidence of vasospasm possibly increased after early surgery from mechanotrauma to vessels

Factors that favor choosing early surgery include:
1. good medical condition of patient
2. good neurologic condition of patient (H&H grade ≤ 3)
3. large amounts of subarachnoid blood, increasing the likelihood and severity of subsequent vasospasm (p.1447), ▶ Table 86.2. Having the aneurysm clipped permits use of hyperdynamic therapy for vasospasm
4. conditions that complicate management in face of unclipped aneurysm: e.g., unstable blood pressure; frequent and/or intractable seizures
5. large clot with mass effect associated with SAH
6. early rebleeding, especially multiple rebleeds
7. indications of imminent rebleeding (see below)

Factors that favor choosing delayed surgery (10–14 days post-SAH) include:
1. poor medical condition and/or advanced age of patient (age may not be a separate factor related to outcome, when patients are stratified by H&H grade[120])
2. poor neurologic condition of patient (H&H grade ≥ 4): *controversial.* Some say the risk of rebleeding and its mortality argues for early surgery even in bad-grade patients,[121] since denying surgery on clinical grounds may result in withholding treatment from some patients who would do well (54% of H&H grade IV and 24% of H&H grade V patients had favorable outcome in one series[120]). Some data show no difference in surgical complications in good- and bad-grade patients with anterior circulation aneurysms[122]
3. aneurysms difficult to clip because of large size, or difficult location necessitating a lax brain during surgery (e.g., difficult basilar bifurcation or mid-basilar artery aneurysms, giant aneurysms)
4. significant cerebral edema seen on CT
5. the presence of active vasospasm

87.8.2 Conclusions

Practice guideline: Timing of intervention for ruptured aneurysm

Level B[92]: Surgical clipping or endovascular coiling of a ruptured aneurysm causing aSAH should be performed as early as feasible in the majority of patients to reduce the risk of rebleeding.

87.8.3 Imminent aneurysm rupture

Findings that may herald impending aneurysm rupture and may therefore increase the need for expedient intervention include:
1. progressing cranial nerve palsy e.g., development of 3rd nerve palsy with PComA aneurysm; traditionally regarded as an indication for urgent treatment (p.1454)
2. increase in aneurysm size on repeat angiography
3. beating aneurysm sign[123]: pulsatile changes in aneurysm size between cuts or slices on imaging (may be seen on angiography, MRA, or CTA)

87.9 General technical considerations of aneurysm surgery

87.9.1 General information

The goal of aneurysm surgery is to prevent rupture or further enlargement of the aneurysm, while at the same time preserving all normal vessels and minimizing injury to brain tissue and cranial nerves. This is usually accomplished by excluding the aneurysm from the circulation with a clip across its neck. Placing the clip too low on the aneurysm neck may occlude the parent vessel, while too distal placement may leave a so-called "aneurysmal rest," which is not benign since it may enlarge (see below).

See Intraoperative aneurysm rupture (p.1466) for general measures to reduce the risk of this complication during surgery.

87

87.9.2 Aneurysmal rest

When a portion of the aneurysm neck is not occluded by a surgical clip, it is referred to as an aneurysmal rest. A "dog-ear" occurs when a clip is angled to leave part of the neck at one end, and obliterates the neck at the other. Rests are not innocuous, even if only 1–2 mm, because they may later expand and possibly rupture years later, especially in younger patients.[124] The incidence of rebleeding was 3.7% in one study, with an annual risk of 0.4–0.8% during the observation period of 4–13 yrs.[125] Patients should be followed with serial angiography, and any increase in size should be treated by reoperation or endovascular techniques if possible.

Booking the case: Craniotomy for aneurysm

Also see defaults & disclaimers (p.25).
1. position: (depends on location of aneurysm), radiolucent head-holder
2. intraoperative angiography (optional)
3. equipment: microscope (with ICG capability if used)
4. blood: type and cross 2 U PRBC
5. post-op: ICU
6. consent (in lay terms for the patient—not all-inclusive):
   a) procedure: surgery through the skull to place a permanent clip on the base of the aneurysm to prevent future bleeding, intraoperative angiogram, possible placement of external (ventricular) drain, possible lumbar drain
   b) alternatives: nonsurgical management, endovascular treatment only for aneurysms that are candidates
   c) complications: usual craniotomy complications (p.25) plus (the following are not really complications of surgery but are possible developments) post-op vasospasm, hydrocephalus, formation of new aneurysms

87.9.3 Surgical exposure

General information

To avoid excessive brain retraction, surgical exposure requires sufficient bony removal and adequate brain relaxation (see below).

Brain relaxation

More critical for ACoA and basilar tip than for easier-to-reach aneurysms such as PComA or MCA....
Techniques include:
1. hyperventilation
2. CSF drainage: provides brain relaxation and a field dry of CSF, and removes blood & blood break-down products along with the CSF. ✖ CSF drainage *before* opening the dura is associated with an increased risk of aneurysmal rebleeding (p. 1437)
   a) ventriculostomy: risks include seizures, bleeding from catheter insertion, infection (ventriculitis, meningitis), possible increased risk of vasospasm
      • placed pre-op in cases of acute post-SAH hydrocephalus (p. 1426)
      • placed intra-op
   b) lumbar spinal drainage (see below)
   c) intraoperative drainage of CSF from cisterns
3. diuretics: mannitol and/or furosemide. Although proof is lacking, lowering ICP by this or any means may theoretically increase the risk of rebleeding[126]

Lumbar spinal drainage

See section 110.4.

May be inserted with Tuohy needle following induction of anesthesia (to minimize BP elevation), prior to final positioning. CSF is gradually withdrawn by the anesthesiologist *only* after the dura is opened (to minimize chances of intraoperative aneurysmal bleeding); usually a total of 30–50 cc are removed in ≈ 10 cc aliquots.

Risks include[127]: aneurysmal rebleeding (≤ 0.3%), back pain (10%, may be chronic in 0.6%), catheter malfunction preventing CSF drainage (< 5%), catheter fracture or laceration resulting in retained catheter tip in the spinal subarachnoid space, post-op CSF fistula, spinal H/A (may be difficult to distinguish from post-craniotomy H/A), infection, neuropathy (from nerve root impingement with needle), epidural hematoma (spinal and/or intracranial).

Cerebral protection during surgery

Pathophysiology of cerebral ischemia

The cerebral metabolic rate of oxygen consumption ($CMRO_2$) (p. 1537) arises from neurons utilizing energy for two functions: 1) maintenance of cell integrity (homeostasis) which normally accounts for ≈ 40% of energy consumption, and 2) conduction of electrical impulses. Occlusion of an artery produces a central core of ischemic tissue where the $CMRO_2$ is not met. The oxygen deficiency precludes aerobic glycolysis and oxidative phosphorylation. ATP production declines and cell homeostasis cannot be maintained, and within minutes irreversible cell death occurs; a so-called cerebral infarction. Surrounding this central core is the penumbra, where collateral flow (usually through leptomeningeal vessels) provides marginal oxygenation which may impair cellular function without immediate irreversible damage. Cells in the penumbra may remain viable for hours.

Cerebral protection by increasing the ischemic tolerance of the CNS

1. drugs that mitigate the toxic effects of ischemia without reducing $CMRO_2$
   a) calcium channel blockers: nimodipine, nicardipine, flunarizine
   b) free radical scavengers: superoxide dismutase, dimethylthiourea, lazaroids, barbiturates, Vitamin C
   c) mannitol: although not a cerebral protectant per se, it may help re-establish blood flow to compromised parenchyma by improving the microvascular perfusion by transiently increasing CBV and decreasing blood viscosity
2. reduction of $CMRO_2$
   a) by reducing the electrical activity of neurons: titrating these agents to a isoelectric EEG reduces $CMRO_2$ by up to a maximum of ≈ 50%
      • barbiturates: in addition to reducing $CMRO_2$, they also redistribute blood flow to ischemic cortex, quench free radicals, and stabilize cell membranes. For dosing of thiopental, see below
      • isoflurane (p. 109): shorter acting and less myocardial depression than with barbiturates
   b) by reducing the maintenance energy of neurons: no drugs developed to date can accomplish this, only hypothermia has any effect on this. Below mild hypothermia, extracerebral effects must be monitored (p. 1051)

- mild hypothermia (core temperatures down to 33 °C): in a multicenter RCT,[128] mild hypothermia was demonstrated to be safe, but did not improve the neurological outcome after craniotomy among good-grade (Hunt and Hess I–III) patients with aSAH
- moderate hypothermia: 32.5–33 °C has been used for head injury
- deep hypothermia to 18 °C permits the brain to tolerate up to 1 hour of circulatory arrest
- profound hypothermia to < 10 °C allows several hours of complete ischemia (the clinical usefulness of this has not been substantiated)

Adjunctive cerebral protection techniques used in aneurysm surgery

1. systemic hypotension
   a) usually used during final approach to aneurysm and during manipulation of aneurysm for clip application
   b) theoretical goals
      - to reduce turgor of aneurysm facilitating clip closure, especially with atherosclerotic neck
      - to decrease transmural pressure (p. 1427) to reduce the risk of intraoperative rupture
   c) one retrospective study[129] suggests that a decrease in MAP > 50% is associated with poor outcome. However, after adjustment for age, this association was no longer statistically significant. Because of the potential danger of hypoxic injury to brain and other organs (including areas of impaired autoregulation as well as normal areas), some surgeons avoid this method
2. "focal" hypotension: using temporary aneurysm clips (specially designed with low closing force to avoid intimal injury) placed on parent vessel (small perforators will not tolerate temporary clips without injury)
   a) used in conjunction with methods of cerebral protection against ischemia
   b) may be combined with systemic hypertension to increase collateral flow
   c) the proximal ICA can tolerate an hour or more of occlusion in some cases, whereas the perforator-bearing segments of the MCA and the basilar apex may tolerate clipping for only a few minutes
   d) in addition to the risk of ischemia, there is the risk of intravascular thrombosis and subsequent release of emboli upon removal of the clip
3. circulatory arrest, utilized in conjunction with deep hypothermia
   a) candidates include patients with large aneurysms that contain significant atherosclerosis and/or thrombosis that impedes clip closure and a dome that is adherent to vital neural structures
4. blood glucose: intraoperative hyperglycemia has been associated with long-term decline in cognition and gross neurologic function[130] and should be avoided

Systematic approach to cerebral protection

See reference.[131]

The following factors may mandate the use of temporary clips (and associated techniques of cerebral protection): giant aneurysm, calcified neck, thin/fragile dome, adherence of dome to critical structures, vital arterial branches near the aneurysm neck, intraoperative rupture. Aside from giant aneurysms, most of these factors may be difficult to identify pre-op. Therefore, Solomon provides some degree of cerebral protection to all patients undergoing aneurysm surgery.

1. spontaneous cooling is permitted during surgery, which usually results in a body temperature of 34 °C by the time that dissection around the aneurysm begins
2. if temporary clipping is utilized
   a) if a long segment of the ICA is being trapped, administer 5,000 U IV heparin to prevent thrombosis and subsequent emboli
   b) < 5 mins temporary clip occlusion: no further intervention
   c) up to 10 or 15 mins occlusion: administer IV brain protection anesthesia (e.g., thiopental, propofol, and/or etomidate) and titrate to burst suppression (p. 249) on EEG
      - administration of IV brain protection anesthesia to burst suppression has been shown to significantly decrease infarction rate with temporary clipping within this time range[132]
      - intermittent reperfusion has been shown to be advantageous in some studies,[132] while in others findings have been contradictory[133,134]
   d) > 20 mins occlusion: not tolerated (except possibly ICA proximal to PComA), terminate operation if possible and plan repeat operation utilizing
      - deep hypothermic circulatory arrest (see above)
      - endovascular techniques
      - bypass grafting around the segment to be occluded

87

87.9.4 Intraoperative and postoperative angiography

Due to the fact that unexpected findings (aneurysmal rest, unclipped aneurysm, or major vessel occlusion) were seen on 19% of post-op angiograms (the only predictive factor identified was a new post-op deficit, which signaled major vessel occlusion), the routine use of some confirmatory test is recommended. May also be applied to AVM surgery. Options include:

1. post-op angiography[135]: correctable problems identified with this option require a return to the operating room, and some potentially reversible deficits may be too late to recover by that time
2. intraoperative options
    a) catheter angiography using traditional iodinated contrast and fluoroscopy. Requires use of radiolucent headholder. Typically the introducer sheath is placed in the femoral artery at the time of initial pre-op angio, and is left in place for intraoperative use. Requires the services of an angiographer if the surgeon does not do this
    b) visualize the vessels during surgery (has largely supplanted intra-op catheter angiography)
        1. indocyanine green (ICG)[136,137,138]: can be visualized under normal light, or sometimes to better advantage when illuminated with near-infrared light. Use is restricted to surface vessels. May be less reliable with giant or wide-neck aneurysms or with thick-walled atherosclerotic vessels.
        Adult dose: may give 25 mg diluted to 5 ml with sterile water as rapid IV bolus. PDR advises do not exceed maximum of 2 mg/kg (adult or child).
        2. fluorescein video angiography[138]

87.9.5 Some drugs useful in aneurysm surgery

Drug info: Propofol (Diprivan®)

May be used to achieve burst suppression[139] with shorter duration of action than other barbiturates. Results are preliminary, further investigation is needed to demonstrate the degree of neuroprotection. Has been reported at doses 170 mcg/kg/min for neuroprotection[140] (if tolerated) but this may be risky. May also be used as a continuous drip for sedation (p. 140), and for ICP management (p. 1049). Reverses rapidly upon discontinuation (usually within 5–10 minutes).

Side effects: possible anaphylactic reaction with angioneurotic edema (angioedema) of the airways,[141] see propofol infusion syndrome (p. 140).

87.9.6 Intraoperative aneurysm rupture

Epidemiology

Reported rates of intraoperative aneurysm rupture (IAR) range from ≈ 18% in the cooperative study (1963–1978)[142] to ≈ 36% in a pre-microscope series[143] (NB: this series had an unexplained high IAR rate of 61% with the microscope) and 40% in a more recent series.[144] Although rupture rate may be higher in early surgery than with late surgery,[144] other series found no difference.[145]

Morbidity and mortality for patients experiencing significant IAR is ≈ 30–35% (vs. ≈ 10% in the absence of this complication), although IAR may primarily affect outcome when it occurs during induction of anesthesia or opening of dura.[144]

See aneurysm rupture during coiling (p. 1924).

Prevention of intraoperative rupture

Presented as a list here to be incorporated into general operative techniques.

1. prevent hypertension from catecholamine response to pain:
    a) ensure deep anesthesia during headholder pin placement and skin incision
    b) consider local anesthetic (without epinephrine) in headholder pin-sites and along incision line
2. minimize increases in transmural pressure: reduce MAP to slightly below baseline just prior to dural opening
3. reduce shearing forces on aneurysm during dissection by minimizing brain retraction:
    a) radical removal of sphenoid wing for circle of Willis aneurysms

b) reduce brain volume by a number of mechanisms: diuretics (mannitol, furosemide), CSF drainage through lumbar subarachnoid drain placed preoperatively and opened by the anesthesiologist at the time of dural incision, hyperventilation

4. reduce risk of large tear in aneurysm fundus or neck:
   a) utilize sharp dissection in exposing aneurysm and in removing clot from around aneurysm
   b) whenever possible, completely mobilize and inspect aneurysm before attempting clip application

Details of intraoperative rupture

Rupture can occur during any of the three following stages of aneurysm surgery[146]:

1. initial exposure (predissection)
   a) rare. Brain can become surprisingly tight even when bleeding seems to be into open subarachnoid space. Usually carries poor prognosis
   b) possible causes:
      • vibration from bone work: dubious
      • increasing transmural pressure upon opening the dura
      • hypertension from catecholamine response to pain (see above)
   c) management tactics:
      • have anesthesiologist radically drop BP
      • control bleeding (with anterior circulation aneurysms) by placing temporary clip across ICA as it exits from cavernous sinus, or if not possible then compress ICA in patient's neck through drapes
      • if necessary to gain control, resect portions of frontal or temporal lobe

2. dissection of the aneurysm: accounts for the majority of IARs, two basic types:
   a) tears caused by blunt dissection
      • tends to be profuse, proximal to the neck, and difficult to control
      • do not attempt definitive clipping unless adequate exposure has been achieved (which is usually not the case with these tears)
      • temporary clipping: this step is often necessary in this situation; after the temporary clip is in place return the MAP to normal and administer neuroprotective agent (e.g., propofol)
      • once the temporary clip is in place, it is better to take a few extra moments to improve the exposure and apply a well-placed permanent clip instead of hastily clipping and trying to restore circulation
      • microsutures may need to be placed to close any portion of the tear that extends onto the parent vessel
   b) laceration by sharp dissection
      • tend to be small, often distally on fundus, and usually easily controlled by a single suction
      • may respond to gentle tamponade with a small cottonoid
      • may shrink down with repeated low current strokes with the bipolar (avoid the temptation to use continuous high current)

3. clip application: bleeding at this point is usually due to either
   a) inadequate exposure of aneurysm: clip blade may penetrate unseen lobe of aneurysm. Similar to tears caused by blunt dissection (see above). Bleeding worsens as clip blades become approximated
      • prompt opening and removal of clip at the first hint of bleeding may minimize the extent of the tear
      • utilize 2 suckers to determine if definitive clipping can be done, or what is more common, to allow temporary clipping (see above)
   b) poor technical clip application: tends to abate as clip blades become approximated. Inspect the blade tips for the following:
      • to be certain that they span the breadth of the neck. If not, a second longer clip is usually applied parallel to the first, which may then be advanced
      • to verify that they are closely approximated. If not, tandem clips may be necessary, and sometimes multiple clips are needed

87.9.7 Aneurysm recurrence after treatment

Incompletely treated aneurysms may increase in size and/or bleed. This includes aneurysms that are clipped or coiled where there is still aneurysm filling, as well as a persistent aneurysm rest or a neck (p. 1463). While most aneurysm rests appear to be stable, there is a small subset that may enlarge or rupture.[147]

87

Additionally, even an aneurysm that has been completely obliterated may recur, and therefore one has to consider the durability of treatment. The risk of recurrence of a completely clipped aneurysm is ≈ 1.5% at 4.4 years.[147]

87.9.8 Follow-up after aneurysm treatment

Based on the above, together with the small risk of de novo aneurysm formation,[147] there is a trend to indefinitely follow patients with known aneurysms. One suggested follow-up schedule is shown in ► Table 87.3.

Table 87.3 Follow-up schedule for treated aneurysms

Perform indicated study at the following times after treatment	
Coiled aneurysms	*Clipped* aneurysms
Study: gad-MRA[a] or CTA[b]	Study: CTA
6 mos	1 year
1.5 years	5 years
3.5 years	every 10 years thereafter
? every 5–10 years (as with clipped aneurysms)	

[a]gad-MRA indicates gadolinium MRA, which is more sensitive here than TOF-MRA (p. 243). Use the same modality for each follow-up to facilitate accurate comparison
[b]gad-MRA is usually preferred after coiling because of dense artifact from coils on CTA

References

[1] Jellinger K. Pathology of intracerebral hemorrhage. Zentralbl Neurochir. 1977; 38:29–42

[2] Jakubowski J, Kendall B. Coincidental aneurysms with tumours of pituitary origin. J Neurol Neurosurg Psychiatry. 1978; 41:972–979

[3] Vlak MH, Algra A, Brandenburg R, et al. Prevalence of unruptured intracranial aneurysms, with emphasis on sex, age, comorbidity, country, and time period: a systematic review and meta-analysis. Lancet Neurol. 2011; 10:626–636

[4] Brown RD,Jr, Broderick JP. Unruptured intracranial aneurysms: epidemiology, natural history, management options, and familial screening. Lancet Neurol. 2014; 13:393–404

[5] Wirth FP. Surgical Treatment of Incidental Intracranial Aneurysms. Clin Neurosurg. 1986; 33:125–135

[6] Menghini VV, Brown RD,Jr, Sicks JD, et al. Incidence and prevalence of intracranial aneurysms and hemorrhage in Olmsted County, Minnesota, 1965 to 1995. Neurology. 1998; 51:405–411

[7] Fox JL. Intracranial Aneurysms. New York: Springer-Verlag; 1983

[8] Chason JL, Hindman WM. Berry aneurysms of the circle of Willis; results of a planned autopsy study. Neurology. 1958; 8:41–44

[9] Wiebers DO, Whisnant JP, Huston J,3rd, et al. Unruptured intracranial aneurysms: natural history, clinical outcome, and risks of surgical and endovascular treatment. Lancet. 2003; 362:103–110

[10] Inagawa T, Hirano A. Autopsy study of unruptured incidental intracranial aneurysms. Surg Neurol. 1990; 34:361–365

[11] Almeida GM, Pindaro J, Plese P, et al. Intracranial Arterial Aneurysms in Infancy and Childhood. Childs Brain. 1977; 3:193–199

[12] Storrs BB, Humphreys RP, Hendrick EB, et al. Intracranial aneurysms in the pediatric age-group. Childs Brain. 1982; 9:358–361

[13] Meyer FB, Sundt TM,Jr, Fode NC, et al. Cerebral aneurysms in childhood and adolescence. J Neurosurg. 1989; 70:420–425

[14] Fang H, Wright IS, Millikan CH. A Comparison of Blood Vessels of the Brain and Peripheral Blood Vessels. In: Cerebral Vascular Diseases. New York Grune and Stratton; 1958:17–22

[15] Wilkinson IMS. The Vertebral Artery: Extracranial and Intracranial Structure. Archives of Neurology 1972; 27:392–396

[16] Youmans JR. Neurological Surgery. Philadelphia 1990

[17] Rhoton AL. Anatomy of Saccular Aneurysms. Surgical Neurology. 1981; 14:59–66

[18] Ferguson GG. Physical Factors in the Initiation Growth, and Rupture of Human Intracranial Saccular Aneurysms. Journal of Neurosurgery. 1972; 37:666–677

[19] Nehls DG, Flom RA, Carter LP, et al. Multiple Intracranial Aneurysms: Determining the Site of Rupture. J Neurosurg. 1985; 63:342–348

[20] Davila S, Oliver B, Molet J, et al. Spontaneous Thrombosis of an Intracranial Aneurysm. Surgical Neurology. 1984; 22:29–32

[21] Kumar S, Rao VRK, Mandalam KR, et al. Disappearance of a Cerebral Aneurysm: An Unusual Angiographic Event. Clin Neurol Neurosurg. 1991 93:151–153

[22] Sobel DF, Dalessio D, Copeland B, et al. Cerebral Aneurysm Thrombosis, Shrinkage, Then Disappearance After Subarachnoid Hemorrhage. Surgical Neurology. 1996; 45:133–137

[23] Spetzler RF, Winestock D, Newton HT, et al. Disappearance and Reappearance of Cerebral Aneurysm in Serial Arteriograms: Case Report. Journal of Neurosurgery. 1974; 41:508–510

[24] Atkinson JLD, Lane JI, Colbassani HJ, et al. Spontaneous Thrombosis of Posterior Cerebral Artery Aneurysm with Angiographic Reappearance. Journal of Neurosurgery. 1993; 79:434–437

[25] Mohr G, Ferguson G, Khan M, et al. Intraventricular Hemorrhage from Ruptured Aneurysm: Retrospective Analysis of 91 Cases. Journal of Neurosurgery. 1983; 58:482–487

[26] Yeh HS, Tomsick TA, Tew JM. Intraventricular Hemorrhage due to Aneurysms of the Distal Posterior Inferior Cerebellar Artery. J Neurosurg. 198 62:772–775

[27] Okawara SH. Warning Signs Prior to Rupture of a Intracranial Aneurysm. Journal of Neurosurger 1973; 38:575–580

87

[28] White JC, Ballantine HT. Intrasellar Aneurysms Simulating Hypophyseal Tumors. Journal of Neurosurgery. 1961; 18:34–50

[29] Raps EC, Galetta SL, Solomon RA, et al. The Clinical Spectrum of Unruptured Intracranial Aneurysms. Archives of Neurology. 1993; 50:265–268

[30] Day JW, Raskin NH. Thunderclap Headache: Symptom of Unruptured Cerebral Aneurysm. Lancet. 1986; 2:1247–1248

[31] Verweij RD, Wijdicks EFM, van Gijn J. Warning Headache in Aneurysmal Subarachnoid Hemorrhage: A Case-Control Study. Arch Neurol. 1988; 45:1019–1020

[32] Chen PR, Amin-Hanjani S, Albuquerque FC, et al. Outcome of oculomotor nerve palsy from posterior communicating artery aneurysms: comparison of clipping and coiling. Neurosurgery. 2006; 58:1040–6; discussion 1040-6

[33] Sano H, Jain VK, Kato Y, et al. Bilateral Giant Intracavernous Aneurysms: Technique of Unilateral Operation. Surgical Neurology. 1988; 29:35–38

[34] ter Berg HW, Bijlsma JB, Veiga Pires JA, et al. Familial association of intracranial aneurysms and multiple congenital anomalies. Arch Neurol. 1986; 43:30–33

[35] Bigelow NH. The association of polycystic kidneys with intracranial aneurysms and other related disorders. Am J Med Sci. 1953; 225:485–494

[36] Maher CO, Piepgras DG, Brown RD,Jr, et al. Cerebrovascular manifestations in 321 cases of hereditary hemorrhagic telangiectasia. Stroke. 2001; 32:877–882

[37] Longstreth WT, Koepsell TD, Yerby MS, et al. Risk Factors for Subarachnoid Hemorrhage. Stroke. 1985; 16:377–385

[38] Schievink WI. Genetics and aneurysm formation. Neurosurg Clin N Am. 1998; 9:485–495

[39] Schievink WI, Riedinger M, Maya MM. Frequency of incidental intracranial aneurysms in neurofibromatosis type 1. Am J Med Genet A. 2005; 134A:45–48

[40] Beeson PB, McDermott W. Cecil's Textbook of Medicine. Philadelphia 1979

[41] Brown RA. Polycystic disease of the kidneys and intracranial aneurysms. The etiology and interrelationship of these conditions: review of recent literature and report of seven cases in which both conditions coexisted. Glasgow Med J. 1951; 32:333–348

[42] Levey AS, Pauker SG, Kassirer JP. Occult Intracranial Aneurysms in Polycystic Kidney Disease: When is Cerebral Angiography Indicated? N Engl J Med. 1983; 308:986–994

[43] Butler WE, Barker FG, Crowell RM. Patients with Polycystic Kidney Disease Would Benefit from Routine Magnetic Resonance Angiographic Screening for Intracerebral Aneurysms: A Decision Analysis. Neurosurgery. 1996; 38:506–516

[44] Chauveau D, Pirson Y, Verellen-Dumoulin C, et al. Intracranial aneurysms in autosomal dominant polycystic kidney disease. Kidney International. 1994; 45:1140–1146

[45] Schievink WI, Prendergast V, Zabramski JM. Rupture of a Previously Documented Small Asymptomatic Intracranial Aneurysm in a Patient with Autosomal Dominant Polycystic Kidney Disease. Journal of Neurosurgery. 1998; 89:479–482

[46] Schievink WI, Torres VE, Piepgras DG, et al. Saccular Intracranial Aneurysms in Autosomal Dominant Polycystic Kidney Disease. J Am Soc Nephrol. 1992; 3:88–95

[47] Kassell NF, Torner JC, Adams HP. Antifibrinolytic Therapy in the Acute Period Following Aneurysmal Subarachnoid Hemorrhage: Preliminary Observations from the Cooperative Aneurysm Study. J Neurosurgery. 1984; 61:225–230

[48] Aring CD. Treatment of Aneurysmal Subarachnoid Hemorrhage. Arch Neurol. 1990; 47:450–451

[49] Weber W, Siekmann R, Kis B, et al. Treatment and follow-up of 22 unruptured wide-necked intracranial aneurysms of the internal carotid artery with Onyx HD 500. AJNR. American Journal of Neuroradiology. 2005; 26:1909–1915

[50] Fox AJ, Vinuela F, Pelz DM, et al. Use of Detachable Balloons for Proximal Artery Occlusion in the Treatment of Unclippable Cerebral Aneurysm. J Neurosurg. 1987; 66:40–46

[51] Bey L, Connolly S, Duong H, et al. Treatment of Inoperable Carotid Aneurysms with Endovascular Carotid Occlusion After Extracranial-Intracranial Bypass Surgery. Neurosurgery. 1997; 41:1225–1234

[52] Drake CG. Giant Intracranial Aneurysms: Experience with Surgical Treatment in 174 Patients. Clin Neurosurg. 1979; 26:12–95

[53] Drake CG. Ligation of the Vertebral (Unilateral or Bilateral) or Basilar Artery in the Treatment of Large Intracranial Aneurysms. Journal of Neurosurgery. 1975; 43:255–274

[54] Swearingen B, Heros RC. Common Carotid Occlusion for Unclippable Carotid Aneurysms: An Old but Still Effective Operation. Neurosurgery. 1987; 21:288–295

[55] Drapkin AJ, Rose WS. Serial Development of 'de Novo' Aneurysms After Carotid Ligation: Case Report. Surgical Neurology. 1992; 38:302–308

[56] Dott NM. Intracranial Aneurysms: Cerebral Arteriography, Surgical Treatment. Trans Med Chir Soc Edin. 1933; 40:219–234

[57] Gillingham FJ. The Management of Ruptured Intracranial Aneurysms. Hunterian Lecture. Ann R Coll Surg Engl. 1958; 23:89–117

[58] Todd NV, Tocher JL, Jones PA, et al. Outcome Following Aneurysm Wrapping: A 10-Year Follow-Up Review of Clipped and Wrapped Aneurysms. Journal of Neurosurgery. 1989; 70:841–846

[59] Cossu M, Pau A, Turtas S, et al. Subsequent Bleeding from Ruptured Intracranial Aneurysms Treated by Wrapping or Coating: A Review of the Long-Term Results in 47 Cases. Neurosurgery. 1993; 32:344–347

[60] Minakawa T, Koike T, Fujii Y, et al. Long Term Results of Ruptured Aneurysms Treated by Coating. Neurosurgery. 1987; 21:660–663

[61] Pellissou-Guyotat J, Deruty R, Mottolese C, et al. The Use of Teflon as Wrapping Material in Aneurysm Surgery. Neurol Res. 1994; 16:224–227

[62] Gnanalingham KK, Apostolopoulos V, Barazi S, et al. The impact of the international subarachnoid aneurysm trial (ISAT) on the management of aneurysmal subarachnoid haemorrhage in a neurosurgical unit in the UK. Clin Neurol Neurosurg. 2006; 108:117–123

[63] Smith GA, Dagostino P, Maltenfort MG, et al. Geographic variation and regional trends in adoption of endovascular techniques for cerebral aneurysms. J Neurosurg. 2011; 114:1768–1777

[64] Koivisto T, Vanninen R, Hurskainen H, et al. Outcomes of early endovascular versus surgical treatment of ruptured cerebral aneurysms. A prospective randomized study. Stroke. 2000; 31:2369–2377

[65] Molyneux A, Kerr R, Stratton I, et al. International Subarachnoid Aneurysm Trial (ISAT) of neurosurgical clipping versus endovascular coiling in 2143 patients with ruptured intracranial aneurysms: a randomized trial. J Stroke Cerebrovasc Dis. 2002; 11:304–314

[66] Li ZQ, Wang QH, Chen G, et al. Outcomes of endovascular coiling versus surgical clipping in the treatment of ruptured intracranial aneurysms. Journal of international medical research. 2012; 40:2145–2151

[67] McDougall CG, Spetzler RF, Zabramski JM, et al. The Barrow Ruptured Aneurysm Trial. J Neurosurg. 2012; 116:135–144

[68] Molyneux AJ, Kerr RS, Birks J, et al. Risk of recurrent subarachnoid haemorrhage, death, or dependence and standardised mortality ratios after clipping or coiling of an intracranial aneurysm in the International Subarachnoid Aneurysm Trial (ISAT): long-term follow-up. Lancet Neurol. 2009; 8:427–433

[69] Bakker NA, Metzemaekers JD, Groen RJ, et al. International subarachnoid aneurysm trial 2009: endovascular coiling of ruptured intracranial

87

aneurysms has no significant advantage over neurosurgical clipping. Neurosurgery. 2010; 66:961–962

[70] Molyneux AJ, Birks J, Clarke A, et al. The durability of endovascular coiling versus neurosurgical clipping of ruptured cerebral aneurysms: 18 year follow-up of the UK cohort of the International Subarachnoid Aneurysm Trial (ISAT). Lancet. 2015; 385:691–697

[71] Darsaut TE, Jack AS, Kerr RS, et al. International Subarachnoid Aneurysm Trial - ISAT part II: study protocol for a randomized controlled trial. Trials. 2013; 14. DOI: 10.1186/1745-6215-14-156

[72] Spetzler RF, McDougall CG, Albuquerque FC, et al. The Barrow Ruptured Aneurysm Trial: 3-year results. J Neurosurg. 2013; 119:146–157

[73] Lanzino G, Murad MH, d'Urso PI, et al. Coil embolization versus clipping for ruptured intracranial aneurysms: a meta-analysis of prospective controlled published studies. AJNR Am J Neuroradiol. 2013; 34:1764–1768

[74] Li H, Pan R, Wang H, et al. Clipping versus coiling for ruptured intracranial aneurysms: a systematic review and meta-analysis. Stroke. 2013; 44:29–37

[75] de Oliveira JG, Beck J, Ulrich C, et al. Comparison between clipping and coiling on the incidence of cerebral vasospasm after aneurysmal subarachnoid hemorrhage: a systematic review and meta-analysis. Neurosurg Rev. 2007; 30:22–30; discussion 30-1

[76] Jones J, Sayre J, Chang R, et al. Cerebral vasospasm patterns following aneurysmal subarachnoid hemorrhage: an angiographic study comparing coils with clips. J Neurointerv Surg. 2015; 7:803–807

[77] Dorai Z, Hynan LS, Kopitnik TA, et al. Factors related to hydrocephalus after aneurysmal subarachnoid hemorrhage. Neurosurgery. 2003; 52:763–9; discussion 769-71

[78] Gruber A, Reinprecht A, Bavinzski G, et al. Chronic shunt-dependent hydrocephalus after early surgical and early endovascular treatment of ruptured intracranial aneurysms. Neurosurgery. 1999; 44:503–9; discussion 509-12

[79] Bae IS, Yi HJ, Choi KS, et al. Comparison of Incidence and Risk Factors for Shunt-dependent Hydrocephalus in Aneurysmal Subarachnoid Hemorrhage Patients. J Cerebrovasc Endovasc Neurosurg. 2014; 16:78–84

[80] de Oliveira JG, Beck J, Setzer M, et al. Risk of shunt-dependent hydrocephalus after occlusion of ruptured intracranial aneurysms by surgical clipping or endovascular coiling: a single-institution series and meta-analysis. Neurosurgery. 2007; 61:924–33; discussion 933-4

[81] Varelas P, Helms A, Sinson G, et al. Clipping or coiling of ruptured cerebral aneurysms and shunt-dependent hydrocephalus. Neurocrit Care. 2006; 4:223–228

[82] Dehdashti AR, Rilliet B, Rufenacht DA, et al. Shunt-dependent hydrocephalus after rupture of intracranial aneurysms: a prospective study of the influence of treatment modality. J Neurosurg. 2004; 101:402–407

[83] Mura J, Rojas-Zalazar D, Ruiz A, et al. Improved outcome in high-grade aneurysmal subarachnoid hemorrhage by enhancement of endogenous clearance of cisternal blood clots: a prospective study that demonstrates the role of lamina terminalis fenestration combined with modern microsurgical cisternal blood evacuation. Minim Invasive Neurosurg. 2007; 50:355–362

[84] Jartti P, Karttunen A, Isokangas JM, et al. Chronic hydrocephalus after neurosurgical and endovascular treatment of ruptured intracranial aneurysms. Acta Radiol. 2008; 49:680–686

[85] Sethi H, Moore A, Dervin J, et al. Hydrocephalus: comparison of clipping and embolization in aneurysm treatment. J Neurosurg. 2000; 92:991–994

[86] Hoh BL, Kleinhenz DT, Chi YY, et al. Incidence of ventricular shunt placement for hydrocephalus with clipping versus coiling for ruptured and unruptured cerebral aneurysms in the Nationwide Inpatient Sample database: 2002 to 2007. World Neurosurg. 2011; 76:548–554

[87] Komotar RJ, Hahn DK, Kim GH, et al. Efficacy of lamina terminalis fenestration in reducing shunt-dependent hydrocephalus following aneurysmal subarachnoid hemorrhage: a systematic review. Clinical article. J Neurosurg. 2009; 111:147–154

[88] Lanzino G, D'Urso PI, Suarez J. Seizures and anticonvulsants after aneurysmal subarachnoid hemorrhage. Neurocrit Care. 2011; 15:247–256

[89] Brinjikji W, Rabinstein AA, Lanzino G, et al. Patient outcomes are better for unruptured cerebral aneurysms treated at centers that preferentially treat with endovascular coiling: a study of the national inpatient sample 2001-2007. AJNR Am J Neuroradiol. 2011; 32:1065–1070

[90] Leivo S, Hernesniemi J, Luukkonen M, et al. Early surgery improves the cure of aneurysm-induced oculmotor palsy. Surgical Neurology. 1996; 45:430–434

[91] Feely M, Kapoor S. Third nerve palsy due to posterior communicating artery aneurysm: the importance of early surgery. Journal of Neurology, Neurosurgery and Psychiatry. 1987; 50:1051–1052

[92] Connolly ES,Jr, Rabinstein AA, Carhuapoma JR, et al. Guidelines for the management of aneurysmal subarachnoid hemorrhage: a guideline for healthcare professionals from the American Heart Association/american Stroke Association. Stroke. 2012; 43:1711–1737

[93] Sandstrom N, Yan B, Dowling R, et al. Comparison of microsurgery and endovascular treatment on clinical outcome following poor-grade subarachnoid hemorrhage. J Clin Neurosci. 2013; 20:1213–1218

[94] Darsaut TE, Estrade L, Jamali S, et al. Uncertainty and agreement in the management of unruptured intracranial aneurysms. J Neurosurg. 2014; 120:618–623

[95] Bederson JB, Awad IA, Wiebers DO, et al. Recommendations for the management of patients with unruptured intracranial aneurysms. A statement for healthcare professionals from the Stroke Council of the American Heart Association. Circulation 2000; 102:2300–2308

[96] King JT,Jr, Berlin JA, Flamm ES. Morbidity and mortality from elective surgery for asymptomatic unruptured, intracranial aneurysms: a meta-analysis. J Neurosurg. 1994; 81:837–842

[97] Raaymakers TW, Rinkel GJ, Limburg M, et al. Mortality and morbidity of surgery for unruptured intracranial aneurysms: a meta-analysis. Stroke 1998; 29:1531–1538

[98] The International Study Group of Unruptured Intracranial Aneurysms Investigators (ISUIA). Unruptured Intracranial Aneurysms - Risk of Rupture and Risks of Surgical Intervention. New England Journal of Medicine. 1998; 339:1725–1733

[99] Bhatia S, Sekula RF, Quigley MR, et al. Role of calcification in the outcomes of treated, unruptured intracerebral aneurysms. Acta Neurochir (Wien) 2011; 153:905–911

[100] Johnston SC, Zhao S, Dudley RA, et al. Treatment of unruptured cerebral aneurysms in California. Stroke. 2001; 32:597–605

[101] Johnston SC, Dudley RA, Gress DR, et al. Surgical and Endovascular Treatment of Unruptured Cerebral Aneurysms at University Hospitals. Neurology. 1999; 52:1799–1805

[102] Birski M, Walesa C, Gaca W, et al. Clipping versus coiling for intracranial aneurysms. Neurol Neurochir Pol. 2014; 48:122–129

[103] Hwang JS, Hyun MK, Lee HJ, et al. Endovascular coiling versus neurosurgical clipping in patients with unruptured intracranial aneurysm: a systematic review. BMC Neurol. 2012; 12. DOI: 10.1186/471-2377-12-99

[104] Lawson MF, Neal DW, Mocco J, et al. Rationale for treating unruptured intracranial aneurysms: actuarial analysis of natural history risk versus treatment risk for coiling or clipping based on

14,050 patients in the Nationwide Inpatient Sample database. World Neurosurg. 2013; 79:472–478

[105] Juvela S, Porras M, Poussa K. Natural history of unruptured intracranial aneurysms: probability of and risk factors for aneurysm rupture. J Neurosurg. 2000; 93:379–387

[106] Tsutsumi K, Ueki K, Morita A, et al. Risk of rupture from incidental cerebral aneurysms. J Neurosurg. 2000; 93:550–553

[107] Ishibashi T, Murayama Y, Urashima M, et al. Unruptured intracranial aneurysms: incidence of rupture and risk factors. Stroke. 2009; 40:313–316

[108] Mahaney KB, Brown RD,Jr, Meissner I, et al. Age-related differences in unruptured intracranial aneurysms: 1-year outcomes. J Neurosurg. 2014; 121:1024–1038

[109] Brinjikji W, Rabinstein AA, Lanzino G, et al. Effect of age on outcomes of treatment of unruptured cerebral aneurysms: a study of the National Inpatient Sample 2001-2008. Stroke. 2011; 42:1320–1324

[110] Halkes PH, Wermer MJ, Rinkel GJ, et al. Direct costs of surgical clipping and endovascular coiling of unruptured intracranial aneurysms. Cerebrovasc Dis. 2006; 22:40–45

[111] Hoh BL, Chi YY, Dermott MA, et al. The effect of coiling versus clipping of ruptured and unruptured cerebral aneurysms on length of stay, hospital cost, hospital reimbursement, and surgeon reimbursement at the university of Florida. Neurosurgery. 2009; 64:614–9; discussion 619-21

[112] Hoh BL, Chi YY, Lawson MF, et al. Length of stay and total hospital charges of clipping versus coiling for ruptured and unruptured adult aneurysms in the Nationwide Inpatient Sample database 2002 to 2006. Stroke. 2010; 41:337–342

[113] Lad SP, Babu R, Rhee MS, et al. Long-term economic impact of coiling vs clipping for unruptured intracranial aneurysms. Neurosurgery. 2013; 72:1000–11; discussion 1011-3

[114] Duan Y, Blackham K, Nelson J, et al. Analysis of short-term total hospital costs and current primary cost drivers of coiling versus clipping for unruptured intracranial aneurysms. J Neurointerv Surg. 2015; 7:614–618

[115] Khan SA, Agrawal A, Hailey CE, et al. Effect of surgical clipping versus endovascular coiling on recovery from oculomotor nerve palsy in patients with posterior communicating artery aneurysms: A retrospective comparative study and meta-analysis. Asian J Neurosurg. 2013; 8:117–124

[116] Kataoka H, Miyoshi T, Neki R, et al. Subarachnoid hemorrhage from intracranial aneurysms during pregnancy and the puerperium. Neurol Med Chir (Tokyo). 2013; 53:549–554

[117] Attenello FJ, Reid P, Wen T, et al. Evaluation of time to aneurysm treatment following subarachnoid hemorrhage: comparison of patients treated with clipping versus coiling. J Neurointerv Surg. 2015. DOI: 10.1136/neurintsurg-2014-011642

[118] Luo YC, Shen CS, Mao JL, et al. Ultra-early versus delayed coil treatment for ruptured poor-grade aneurysm. Neuroradiology. 2015; 57:205–210

[119] Milhorat TH, Krautheim M. Results of Early and Delayed Operations for Ruptured Intracranial Aneurysms in Two Series of 100 Consecutive Patients. Surgical Neurology. 1986; 26:123–128

[120] Le Roux PD, Elliott JP, Newell DW, et al. Predicting Outcome in Poor-Grade Patients with Subarachnoid Hemorrhage: A Retrospective Review of 159 Aggressively Managed Cases. Journal of Neurosurgery. 1996; 85:39–49

[121] Disney L, Weir B, Grace M, et al. Factors Influencing the Outcome of Aneurysm Rupture in Poor Grade Patients: A Prospective Series. Neurosurgery. 1988; 23:1–9

[122] Le Roux PD, Elliot JP, Newell DW, et al. The Incidence of Surgical Complications is Similar in Good and Poor Grade Patients Undergoing Repair of Ruptured Anterior Circulation Aneurysms: A Retrospective Review of 355 Patients. Neurosurgery. 1996; 38:887–897

[123] Malek AM, Halbach VV, Holmes S, et al. Beating aneurysm sign: angiographic evidence of ruptured aneurysm tamponade by intracranial hemorrhage. Case illustration. J Neurosurg. 1999; 91

[124] Lin T, Fox AJ, Drake CG. Regrowth of Aneurysm Sacs from Residual Neck Following Aneurysm Clipping. J Neurosurg. 1989; 70:556–560

[125] Feuerberg I, Lindquist M, Steiner L. Natural History of Postoperative Aneurysm Rests. Journal of Neurosurgery. 1987; 66:30–34

[126] Rosenorn J, Westergaard L, Hansen PH. Mannitol-Induced Rebleeding from Intracranial Aneurysm: Case Report. Journal of Neurosurgery. 1983; 59:529–530

[127] Connolly ES, Kader AA, Frazzini VI, et al. The Safety of Intraoperative Lumbar Subarachnoid Drainage for Acutely Ruptured Intracranial Aneurysm: Technical Note. Surgical Neurology. 1997; 48:338–344

[128] Todd MM, Hindman BJ, Clarke WR, et al. Mild intraoperative hypothermia during surgery for intracranial aneurysm. New England Journal of Medicine. 2005; 352:135–145

[129] Hoff RG, , Mettes S, et al. Hypotension in anaesthetized patients during aneurysm clipping: not as bad as expected? Acta Anaesthesiol Scand. 2008; 52:1006–1011

[130] Pasternak JJ, McGregor DG, Schroeder DR, et al. Hyperglycemia in patients undergoing cerebral aneurysm surgery: its association with long-term gross neurologic and neuropsychological function. Mayo Clin Proc. 2008; 83:406–417

[131] Solomon RA. Methods of Cerebral Protection During Aneurysm Surgery. Contemporary Neurosurgery. 1995; 16:1–6

[132] Lavine SD, Masri LS, Levy ML, et al. Temporary occlusion of the middle cerebral artery in intracranial aneurysm surgery: time limitation and advantage of brain protection. J Neurosurg. 1997; 87:817–824

[133] Ogilvy CS, Carter BS, Kaplan S, et al. Temporary vessel occlusion for aneurysm surgery: risk factors for stroke in patients protected by induced hypothermia and hypertension and intravenous mannitol administration. J Neurosurg. 1996; 84:785–791

[134] Samson D, Batjer HH, Bowman G, et al. A clinical study of the parameters and effects of temporary arterial occlusion in the management of intracranial aneurysms. Neurosurgery. 1994; 34:22–8; discussion 28-9

[135] Macdonald RL, Wallace C, Kestle JRW. Role of Angiography Following Aneurysm Surgery. Journal of Neurosurgery. 1993; 79:826–832

[136] Raabe A, Nakaji P, Beck J, et al. Prospective evaluation of surgical microscope-integrated intraoperative near-infrared indocyanine green videoangiography during aneurysm surgery. Journal of Neurosurgery. 2005; 103:982–989

[137] Dashti R, Laakso A, Niemela M, et al. Microscope-integrated near-infrared indocyanine green videoangiography during surgery of intracranial aneurysms: the Helsinki experience. Surgical Neurology. 2009; 71:543–50; discussion 550

[138] Lane B, Bohnstedt BN, Cohen-Gadol AA. A prospective comparative study of microscope-integrated intraoperative fluorescein and indocyanine videoangiography for clip ligation of complex cerebral aneurysms. J Neurosurg. 2015; 122:618–626

[139] Ravussin P, de Tribolet N. Total Intravenous Anesthesia with Propofol for Burst Suppression in Cerebral Aneurysm Surgery: Preliminary Report of 42 Patients. Neurosurgery. 1993; 32:236–240

[140] Batjer HH, Samson DS, Bowman M. Comment on Ravussin R and de Tribolet N: Total Intravenous Anesthesia with Propofol for Burst Suppression in Cerebral Aneurysm Surgery: Preliminary Report of 42 Patients. Neurosurgery. 1993; 32

[141] Couldwell WT, Gianotta SL, Zelman V, et al. Life-Threatening Reactions to Propofol. Neurosurgery. 1993; 33:1116–1117

[142] Graf CJ, Nibbelink DW, Sahs AL, et al. Randomized Treatment Study: Intracranial Surgery. In: Aneurysmal Subarachnoid Hemorrhage - Report of the

87

Cooperative Study. Baltimore: Urban and Schwarzenburg; 1981:145–202

[143] Pertuiset B, Pia HW, Langmaid C. Intraoperative Aneurysmal Rupture and Reduction by Coagulation of the Sac. In: Cerebral Aneurysms - Advances in Diagnosis and Therapy. Berlin: Springer-Verlag; 1979:398–401

[144] Schramm J, Cedzich C. Outcome and Management of Intraoperative Aneurysm Rupture. Surgical Neurology. 1993; 40:26–30

[145] Kassell NF, Boarini DJ, Adams HP, et al. Overall Management of Ruptured Aneurysm: Comparison of Early and Later Operation. Neurosurgery. 1981; 9:120–128

[146] Batjer H, Samson DS. Management of Intraoperative Aneurysm Rupture. Clin Neurosurg. 1988; 36:275–288

[147] David CA, Vishteh AG, Spetzler RF, et al. Late angiographic follow-up review of surgically treated aneurysms. Journal of Neurosurgery. 1999; 91:396–401

88 Aneurysm Type by Location

88.1 Anterior communicating artery aneurysms

88.1.1 General information

The single most common site of aneurysms presenting with SAH.[1] May also present with diabetes insipidus (DI) or other hypothalamic dysfunction.

88.1.2 CT scan

SAH in these aneurysms results in blood in the anterior interhemispheric fissure (▶ Fig. 88.1) in essentially all cases, and is associated with intracerebral hematoma in 63% of cases.[2] Intraventricular hematoma is seen in 79% of cases, with the blood entering the ventricles from the intracerebral hematoma in about one–third of these. Acute hydrocephalus was present in 25% of patients (late hydrocephalus, a common sequela of SAH, was not studied).

Frontal lobe infarcts occur in 20%, usually several days following SAH.[2] One of the few causes of the rare finding of bilateral ACA distribution infarcts is vasospasm following hemorrhage from rupture of an ACoA aneurysm. This results in prefrontal lobotomy-like findings of apathy and abulia.

88

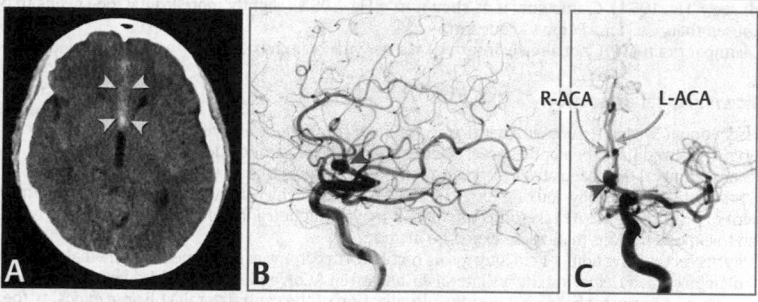

Fig. 88.1 ACoMA aneurysm (*red arrowheads*) measuring 10 X 11 X 8 mm in a 62-year-old woman with a "sentinel hemorrhage" (p.1418) (WFNS Grade 1 ▶ Table 85.4).
Image: A: noncontrast axial CT scan of the brain showing blood in the anterior interhemispheric fissure (*yellow arrowheads*). B: catheter angiogram, left ICA injection, lateral view. C: catheter angiogram, left ICA injection, AP view, showing both ACAs fill from left-sided injection (demonstrating the ACoMA cross-fills). On right ICA injection (not shown), only the right ACA filled (indicating left ACA is dominant).
Abbreviations: ACA = anterior cerebral artery, ICA = internal carotid artery.

88.1.3 Angiographic considerations

Essential to evaluate contralateral carotid, to determine if both ACAs fill the aneurysm. If the aneurysm fills with one side only, it is desirable to inject the other side while cross-compressing the side that fills the aneurysm to see if collateral flow is present. Also, determine if either carotid fills both ACAs, or if each ACA fills from the ipsilateral carotid injection (may permit trapping, see below).

▶ **If additional views are needed to better demonstrate aneurysm.** Try oblique 25° away from injection side, center beam 3–4 cm above lateral aspect of ipsilateral orbital rim, orient X-ray tube in Towne's view. A submental vertex view may also visualize the area but the image may be degraded by the large amount of interposed bone.

88.1.4 Surgical treatment

Approaches

General information
1. *pterional approach*: the usual approach (see below)
2. subfrontal approach: especially useful for aneurysms pointing superiorly when there is a large amount of frontal blood clot (allows clot removal during approach)
3. anterior interhemispheric approach[3]: ✘ contraindicated for anteriorly pointing aneurysms as the dome is approached first and proximal control cannot be obtained (see below)
4. transcallosal approach

Pterional approach
Side of craniotomy:
A *right* pterional craniotomy is used with the following exceptions (for which a left pterional crani is used):
1. large ACoA aneurysm pointing to right: left crani exposes neck before dome
2. dominant left A1 feeder to aneurysm (with no filling from right A1): left crani provides proximal control
3. additional left-sided aneurysm

See Pterional craniotomy (p. 1748) for positioning, etc. (use shoulder roll, rotate head 60° from vertical; see ▶ Fig. 106.1). Craniotomy is as shown in ▶ Fig. 106.3 (slightly more frontal lobe needs to be exposed than, e.g., for a PComA aneurysm).
Lumbar drain (if IVC not already inserted) assists with brain relaxation.

Microsurgical dissection

Dissect down Sylvian fissure with gentle retraction of frontal lobe away from base of skull. Olfactory nerve visualized first, then optic nerve. Open arachnoid over carotid and optic cistern and drain CSF. Elevate temporal tip, coagulate any bridging temporal tip veins that are present, and expose ICA.

Follow the ICA distally, looking for A1 (the exposure of which allows temporary clipping in the event of rupture). If the A1 take-off is too high, it may be hidden and would require excessive retraction to expose. Options to increase exposure include
1. gyrus rectus resection: a 1 cm long gyrus rectus corticectomy is performed[4] just medial to the olfactory tract. Helps find the ipsilateral A1 and often ACoA and A2. This is also helpful for down-pointing aneurysms because it permits visualization of the contralateral A1 before exposing the dome of the aneurysm (for proximal control). May lead to neuropsychiatric deficits. A subpial resection is performed with preservation of the small arterial branch that is consistently located here
2. fronto-temporal-orbital-zygoma removal
3. splitting the Sylvian fissure: about 50% of experts do this routinely
4. ventricular drainage

Once found, A1 is followed until the ipsilateral A2 is identified. Then the contralateral A2 is identified and is followed proximally until the contralateral A1 is exposed. The AComA is usually encountered in the process.

Critical branches to preserve: recurrent artery of Heubner; small ACoA perforators (may be adherent to aneurysm dome). If the aneurysm cannot be clipped, it may be trapped by clipping both ends of the ACoA *only* if each ACA fills from the carotid on its own side.

Post clipping, some authors recommend fenestrating the lamina terminalis in an effort to reduce the need for post-op shunting.

Anterior interhemispheric approach
See reference.[3]
Involves minimal brain retraction.
More suitable for an aneurysm that points straight up, but even with this proximal control is poor.
Position: supine with the neck extended ≈ 15°. A transverse skin incision is made in a skin crease in the lower forehead. The authors[3] describe using a 1.5 inch trephine craniotomy in the midline just superior to the glabella. Alternatively, better advantage of the dural opening may be possible with a

more rectangular opening. The dural flap is hinged on the superior sagittal sinus. The depth of the aneurysm is ≈ 6 cm from the dura. Proximal control of the A1 branch of the ACA is difficult with this approach.

88.2 Distal anterior cerebral artery aneurysms

88.2.1 General information

Aneurysms of the distal anterior cerebral artery (DACA) (i.e., the ACA distal to the ACoA) are usually located at the origin of the frontopolar artery, or at the bifurcation of the pericallosal and calloso-marginal arteries at the genu of the corpus callosum. Aneurysms located more distally are usually posttraumatic, infectious (mycotic), or due to tumor embolus.[5] DACA aneurysms are often associated with intracerebral hematoma or interhemispheric subdural hematoma[6] since the subarachnoid space is limited here. Conservative treatment of DACA aneurysms is often associated with poor results. Unruptured DACA aneurysms have a higher incidence of bleeding than unruptured aneurysms in other locations. These aneurysms are fragile and adherent to the brain, which predisposes to frequent premature intraoperative rupture.

On arteriography, if both ACAs fill from a single-sided carotid injection, it may be difficult to make the important determination as to which ACA feeds the aneurysm. Multiple aneurysms are commonly associated with DACA aneurysms.

88.2.2 Treatment

Mycotic aneurysms should be treated as outlined (p. 1492).

Aneurysms up to 1 cm from the ACoA may be approached through a standard pterional craniotomy with partial gyrus rectus resection.

Aneurysms > 1 cm distal to the ACoA up to the genu of the corpus callosum, including those of the pericallosal/callosomarginal bifurcation, may be approached surgically by a basal frontal interhemispheric approach[7] via a frontal craniotomy using a bicoronal skin incision. The patient is positioned supine with the neck slightly extended, positioned vertically or just a few degrees to the left. A right-sided craniotomy is preferred in most instances (exception: aneurysm dome buried in the right cerebral hemisphere making retraction hazardous), but should cross to the contralateral side by a couple centimeters. It must be taken all the way to the floor of the frontal fossa to permit exposure of the anterior cerebral artery for proximal control. The craniotomy extends ≈ 8 cm above the supraorbital ridge in order to provide leeway in circumnavigating veins bridging to the superior sagittal sinus. The dural flap is based on the superior sagittal sinus. If the sinus needs to be mobilized, it may be divided low anteriorly.

ACA aneurysms distal to the genu of the corpus callosum may also be approached by an interhemispheric approach using a unilateral skin incision. For these, the patient's neck is not extended, and a parasagittal craniotomy is used that doesn't need to be as low on the frontal fossa. The cingulate gyri may be difficult to separate, and care must be taken because excessive retraction may pull the cingulate gyrus off the dome of the aneurysm and produce premature rupture.

Ideally, A2 proximal to the aneurysm should be identified initially for proximal control and then followed distally to the aneurysm. When this is not possible, dissection should follow distal ACA branches proximally toward the aneurysm, taking care not to disturb the aneurysm. Often, a portion of the cingulate gyrus may need to be removed and sometimes up to 1–2 cm of the anterior corpus callosum may need to be divided.

Surgical complications: Prolonged retraction on the cingulate gyrus may produce akinetic mutism that is usually temporary. The pericallosal arteries are small in caliber and may be atherosclerotic, which together increases the risk of occlusion of the parent artery with the aneurysm clip.

88.3 Posterior communicating artery aneurysms

88.3.1 General information

May occur at either end of PComA; that is at the junction with the PCA, or more commonly at the junction with the carotid (typically points laterally, posteriorly, and inferiorly). May impinge on the third nerve in either case and cause third nerve palsy (ptosis, mydriasis, "down and out" deviation) that is *not* pupil-sparing in 99% of cases. Surgical clipping may be more advantageous than endovascular coiling to treat oculomotor nerve palsies caused by PComA aneurysms.[8,9]

88

88.3.2 Angiographic considerations

Vertebral artery (**VA**) injection is necessary to help evaluate the PComA artery:
1. if the PComA is patent: determine if there is a "fetal circulation" where the posterior circulation is fed only through the PComA
2. determine if the aneurysm fills from VA injection

If additional views are needed to better demonstrate aneurysm

Try paraorbital oblique 55° away from injection side, center beam 1 cm posterior to inferior portion of lateral rim of ipsilateral orbit, orient X-ray tube 12° cephalad.

88.3.3 Surgical treatment

Pterional approach

See Pterional craniotomy (p.1748) for positioning, etc. For the more common aneurysm at the ICA-PComA junction, rotate head 15–30° from vertical (▶ Fig. 106.1). Craniotomy is as shown in ▶ Fig. 106.3 (less frontal lobe needs to be exposed than for an ACoA aneurysm).

Microsurgical dissection

Ultimately, the major vector of retraction will be on tip of temporal lobe (less on frontal lobe than in ACoA aneurysm), but the initial approach will be more anterior to reduce risk of intraoperative rupture.
1. dissect down Sylvian fissure, retract frontal lobe and come down on optic nerve
2. cautiously elevate temporal tip (aneurysm may be adherent to temporal tip and/or to tentorium), coagulate bridging temporal tip veins if necessary
3. incise arachnoid membrane along the optic nerve from *anterior* to posterior
4. open arachnoid and drain CSF to gain relaxation
5. start to dissect carotid at anterior margin (at junction with optic nerve) and work towards the posterior margin of carotid where the aneurysm is located (isolating the carotid gives proximal control)

The aneurysm dome usually points laterally, posteriorly, and inferiorly, and is encountered before and usually blocks visualization of the PComA. The aneurysm frequently projects behind the tentorial edge, which then obscures the dome.

Critical branches to preserve: anterior choroidal artery, posterior communicating artery (PComA). If necessary, the PComA may be sacrificed (e.g., included in clip) without deleterious effect in most cases if there is not a fetal circulation.

88.4 Carotid terminus (bifurcation) aneurysms

88.4.1 Angiographic considerations

▶ **If additional views are needed to better demonstrate aneurysm.** Try oblique 25° away from injection side, center beam 3–4 cm above lateral aspect of ipsilateral orbital rim, orient X-ray tube in Towne's view. Also may try submentovertex view.

88.4.2 Surgical considerations

See Pterional craniotomy (p.1748) for positioning, etc. (rotate head 30° from vertical, see ▶ Fig. 106.1). Craniotomy is as shown in ▶ Fig. 106.3.

88.5 Middle cerebral artery (MCA) aneurysms

88.5.1 General information

The following considers MCA aneurysms of the M1-M2 junction (referred to as "trifurcation" region, although this is not a true trifurcation (p.75)).

88.5.2 Surgical treatment

Approaches

1. transsylvian approach through a *pterional craniotomy*: this is the most commonly used approach
2. superior temporal gyrus approach[10]:
   a) advantages: minimizes brain retraction, possible reduced vasospasm from manipulation of proximal vessels
   b) disadvantages: proximal control difficult, slightly larger bone flap, possible increased risk of seizures

Craniotomy vs. craniectomy

Primary decompressive craniectomy (vs. craniotomy) for poor-grade MCA aneurysm SAH (WFNS IV/ V) with associated IPH (> 30 cc) has not been shown to provide any survival benefit and is not associated with improved outcome.[11]

Pterional approach

See Pterional craniotomy (p. 1748) for positioning, etc. (rotate head 45° from vertical, ▶ Fig. 106.1).

Craniotomy

Craniotomy is as shown in ▶ Fig. 106.3. Less frontal lobe needs to be exposed than for, e.g., an ACoA aneurysm (distance "B" in ▶ Fig. 106.3 only needs to be ≈ 1 cm). The height "H" of the bony opening should be ≈ 5–6 cm (larger than for circle of Willis aneurysms).

88

Microsurgical dissection

Dissect down Sylvian fissure with major vector of retraction on tip of temporal lobe (less on frontal lobe than in ACoA aneurysm). Open arachnoid and drain CSF. Elevate temporal tip, coagulate bridging temporal tip veins, and expose the ICA for proximal control in the event of rupture.

Follow the ICA distally by splitting the Sylvian fissure to expose the M1 (again, for proximal control). Although exposure for proximal control is helpful to have as a contingency, one may be able to avoid temporary clipping of the MCA in the event of intraoperative rupture by controlling bleeding with a large suction, and subsequent clip placement (since the blood flow through the MCA is not as voluminous as through the ICA, and the surgical access to these aneurysms is usually fairly unrestricted).

Critical branches to preserve: distal MCA branches, recurrent perforators from the origin of the major MCA branches.

88.6 Cavernous carotid artery aneurysms (CCAAs)

88.6.1 General information

Most CCAAs develop on the horizontal segment of the cavernous ICA. They may occur spontaneously, but may also follow trauma (p. 1491).

88.6.2 Presentation

Aneurysms on the portion of the ICA within the cavernous sinus (cavernous carotid artery aneurysms [CCAAs]) have a unique risk profile among intracranial aneurysms. When CCAAs rupture, they usually produce a Type A (high flow) carotid–cavernous fistula (CCF) (p. 1519).

Exceptions (wherein CCICA rupture results in findings other than CCF):
1. giant aneurysms that straddle the carotid ring thereby having an intracranial component (presence may be revealed by "waisting" of the aneurysm at the ring on angiography[12]) may produce subarachnoid hemorrhage (SAH).[13,14]
2. epistaxis from rupture into sphenoid sinus usually with traumatic CCAAs (p. 1491) (which are generally pseudoaneurysms) associated with skull fracture. Triad: epistaxis, blindness, and orbital fracture[15] (or other basilar skull fracture)

88.7 Supraclinoid aneurysms

See reference.[16]

88.7.1 Applied anatomy

The carotid artery exits the cavernous sinus and enters the subarachnoid space at the dural constriction known as the carotid ring (AKA clinoidal ring) (see ▶ Fig. 2.4). The supraclinoid portion of the carotid artery may be divided into the following segments[17]:
1. ophthalmic segment: the largest portion of the supraclinoid ICA. Lies between the take-off of the ophthalmic artery and the posterior communicating artery (PCoA) origin. The proximal portion of this (including the origin of the ophthalmic artery) is often obscured by the anterior clinoid process. Branches include:
   a) ophthalmic artery: usually originates from the supracavernous ICA just after the ICA enters the subarachnoid space; see variants (p.78). Enters the optic canal positioned inferolateral to the optic nerve
   b) superior hypophyseal artery: the largest of several perforators supplying the dura of the cavernous sinus and the superior pituitary gland and stalk
2. communicating segment: from the PCoA origin to the origin of the anterior choroidal artery (AChA)
3. choroidal segment: from the AChA origin to the terminal bifurcation of the ICA

88

88.7.2 Ophthalmic segment aneurysms (OSAs)

See reference.[18]

General information

Ophthalmic segment aneurysms (OSAs) include (NB: nomenclature varies among authors):
1. ophthalmic artery aneurysms
2. superior hypophyseal artery aneurysms:
   a) paraclinoid variant: usually does not produce visual symptoms
   b) suprasellar variant: when giant, may mimic pituitary tumor on CT

Presentation (excluding incidental discovery)

Ophthalmic artery aneurysms

Arise from the ICA just distal to the origin of ophthalmic artery. They project dorsally or dorsomedially towards the lateral portion of the optic nerve.
   Presentation:
1. ≈ 45% present as SAH
2. ≈ 45% present as visual field defect:
   a) as the aneurysm enlarges it impinges on the lateral portion of the optic nerve → inferior temporal fiber compression → ipsilateral *monocular superior nasal quadrantanopsia*
   b) continued enlargement → upward displacement of the nerve against the falciform ligament (or fold) → superior temporal fiber compression → *monocular inferior nasal quadrantanopsia*
   c) in addition to near-complete loss of vision in the involved eye, compression of the optic nerve near the chiasm may also produce a superior temporal quadrant defect in the *contralateral* eye (junctional scotoma AKA anterior chiasmal syndrome from injury to the anterior knee of Wilbrand (nasal retinal fibers that course anteriorly for a short distance after they decussate in the contralateral optic nerve[19,20])
3. ≈ 10% present as both

Superior hypophyseal artery aneurysms

Originate in the small subarachnoid pocket medial to the ICA near the lateral aspect of the sella. The direction of enlargement is dictated by the size of this pocket and the height of the lateral sellar wall resulting in two variants: paraclinoid & suprasellar.
   Suprasellar variant may actually grow to a size large enough to compress the pituitary stalk and cause hypopituitarism and "classic" chiasmal visual symptoms (bilateral temporal hemianopsia).

Angiographic considerations

A notch can often be observed in the anterior, superior, and medial aspects of giant ophthalmic artery aneurysms due to the optic nerve.[21]

▶ **If additional views are needed to better demonstrate aneurysm.** Try oblique 25° away from injection side, center beam 3–4 cm above lateral aspect of ipsilateral orbital rim, orient X-ray tube in Towne's view. Try submentovertex view.

88.7.3 Surgical treatment

See reference.[16]

Ophthalmic artery aneurysms

If necessary, the ophthalmic artery may be sacrificed without worsening of vision in the vast majority. Clipping a contralateral ophthalmic artery aneurysm is not technically difficult, and is not uncommonly required as OSAs are often multiple.

The aneurysm arises from the superomedial aspect of the ICA just distal to the ophthalmic artery origin, and projects superiorly.

Cutting the falciform fold early decompresses the nerve, and helps minimize worsening of visual deficit from surgical manipulation.

For unruptured aneurysms, drill off anterior clinoid via an extradural approach before opening dura to approach neck; for ruptured aneurysms, this may not be as safe.

In most cases, a side-angled clip can be placed parallel to the parent artery along the neck of the aneurysm.

Superior hypophyseal artery aneurysms

If necessary, the superior hypophyseal artery on one side may be clipped without demonstrable deleterious effect (due to bilateral supply to stalk and pituitary). Clipping a contralateral superior hypophyseal aneurysm is not really feasible.

With a usual pterional approach, the carotid artery is usually encountered first, and with large aneurysms is usually bowed laterally towards the surgeon. Clinoidal removal is usually required. The entire ICA wall may appear to be involved, and it may necessitate temporary ICA clipping (with cerebral protection) to reconstitute the ICA using encircling clips parallel to the parent vessel.

88.8 Posterior circulation aneurysms

88.8.1 General information

See also basilar tip aneurysms (p. 1482). Clinical syndrome of SAH in the posterior fossa is indistinguishable from that due to anterior circulation aneurysms except for possible increased tendency towards respiratory arrest and subsequent neurogenic pulmonary edema (p. 1439).[22] Vasospasm following posterior fossa SAH may be more likely to cause midbrain symptoms than vasospasm due to SAH elsewhere.

88.8.2 Hydrocephalus

In Yamaura's series,[23] 12% of patients required external ventricular drainage (EVD) following posterior fossa SAH to remove bloody CSF causing hydrocephalus, and 20% eventually required permanent ventricular shunt.

88.8.3 Vertebral artery aneurysms

General information

Traumatic vertebral artery aneurysms (VAA) (AKA dissecting aneurysms) are more common than non-traumatic VAAs. The following discussion concerns non-traumatic VAA.

Most VAAs arise at the VA-PICA junction. Other sites: VA-AICA, VA-BA.

Angiographic considerations

Angiography of VAA should assess the contralateral VA for patency in case of the need to trap the aneurysm. Allcock test (vertebral artery injection with carotid compression) may be used to assess patency of circle of Willis. Test occlusion with a balloon catheter can determine if patient will tolerate occlusion (a double-lumen balloon will even allow measurement of distal back pressure).

Treatment

Options:
1. direct aneurysmal clipping
2. endovascular coil embolization: may not be as effective as clipping for relief of symptoms due to brainstem or cranial nerve compression
3. choices for unclippable and uncoilable aneurysms (e.g., fusiform, giant, or dissecting aneurysms) include:
   a) proximal (hunterian) VA ligation[24] which must be *distal* to the PICA origin to prevent severe morbidity or mortality[25]
   b) occlusion of the VA distal to the PICA origin (usually done endovascularly)
   c) midcervical VA occlusion (allows collateral flow through suboccipital muscular branches) e.g., endovascular Amplatzer plug

88.8.4 PICA aneurysms

General information

For PICA anatomy, see ▶ Fig. 2.7. For arteriogram, see ▶ Fig. 2.8.

A PICA aneurysm should be suspected with a CT showing blood predominantly in the 4th ventricle[26] (▶ Fig. 88.2 panel A). The dome of distal PICA aneurysms may adhere to the foramen of Luschka and rupture fills the ventricles often with little subarachnoid blood visible on CT.

Comprise ≈ 3% of cerebral aneurysms. 3 common sites:
1. VA-PICA junction[27] (PICA origin aneurysm): saccular aneurysms occur most commonly at the distal (superior) angle (▶ Fig. 88.2 panel B). The level is as varied as the PICA origin, and ranges from as low as the foramen magnum to as high as the pontomedullary junction. Most VA-PICA aneurysms lie in the anterolateral portion of the medullary cistern,[28] anterior to the first dentate ligament.[29] However, the PICA origin may sometimes lie in the midline or across it
2. PICA aneurysms distal to the VA-PICA junction: tend to be fragile and often develop multiple hemorrhages in a relatively short period, ∴ should be treated promptly, even when discovered incidentally
3. fusiform aneurysms (p.1579) of the VA involving PICA: usually the result of prior arterial dissection

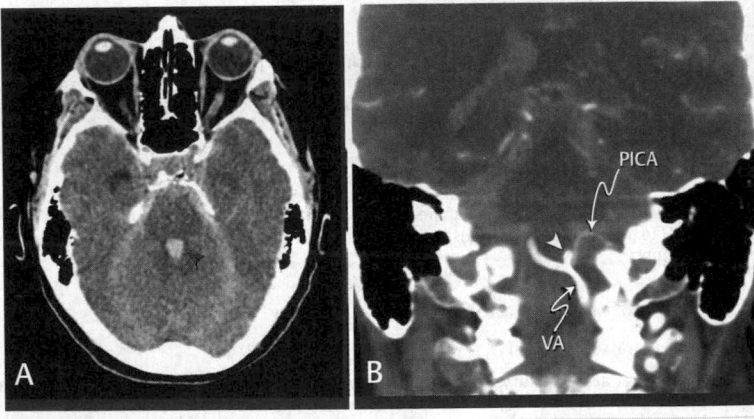

Fig. 88.2 PICA origin aneurysm (*yellow arrowhead*) 5 X 3 mm diameter at the origin of the left PICA presenting with SAH demonstrating a disproportionate amount of blood in the 4th ventricle (*red arrowhead*).
Image: A: noncontrast axial CT scan of the brain at the level of the 4th ventricle. B: CT angiogram, coronal view.
Abbreviations: VA = vertebral artery, PICA = posterior inferior communicating artery.

Surgical clipping of VA-PICA junction (PICA origin) saccular aneurysms

One approach to the VA-PICA junction is via a low extreme-lateral p-fossa approach. However, if the aneurysm is too far anterior to the brainstem, it may be totally out of vision or reach. Also, since these aneurysms usually project posteriorly and superiorly, the critical PICA will be directly in harm's way. Direct lateral approach more directly exposes the aneurysm[30] through a lateral subocci-pital transcondylar approach.

Position: options include sitting position—less frequently used, see Sitting position (p.1737)—or lateral oblique ("park bench").

▶ **Lateral oblique position. Position:** side of involved PICA is up, thorax elevated ≈ 15°. Head in line with the thorax, neck slightly flexed, and slightly rotated 20° toward the floor (away from the side of the aneurysm). Upper shoulder depressed with adhesive tape. Lumbar spinal subarachnoid catheter placed, allows CSF drainage once dura is opened.

Skin incision: Options:

Avoid opening too far laterally, otherwise the muscle mass impedes surgeon's vision.[31 (p 1747)]

1. From just above superior nuchal line to C2 vertebra[28]
   a) paramedian vertical incision
   b) midline vertical incision (hockey stick)
2. "sigmoid" incision starting 2 cm medial to mastoid notch, and curving to midline at level of C1 arch[32]

Craniectomy: lateral exposure of bone to the base of the mastoid, medially crossing the midline. Need not be quite as high as the transverse sinus. The foramen magnum is removed to its lateral margin. Removing the posterior arch of C1 from midline to the sulcus arteriosus (under VA) may help with proximal VA exposure[32] but is not usually necessary.[33]

Dural opening: K-shaped dural opening with a linear incision across the band at the foramen magnum (some patients have a sinus known as the arcuate sinus here that may require vascular clips).

Approach: gain proximal control of the VA where it first becomes intradural (in case of aneurys-mal rupture). Retract cerebellum superiorly (caution: aneurysm dome may be adherent). Follow VA up from point where it enters dura; PICA origin then encountered usually just at neck of aneurysm (PICA origin may be confused for continuation of VA). Dissection must spare branches of pharyngeal filaments of spinal accessory nerve and lower filaments of vagus. May place temporary clip on VA proximal to PICA. Permanent clip usually placed between the fibers of IX & X above and XI below. It is better to leave a small residual aneurysm than to risk compromising PICA.[33]

Postoperative care: when neuropraxia of the lower cranial nerves is likely (in cases of difficult dissection or traction applied during clipping) the patient is kept intubated overnight. Patients who do not tolerate extubation at this point are immediately reintubated and elective tracheostomy is scheduled. Tracheostomy is maintained until the neuropraxia resolves.

Surgical clipping of distal PICA aneurysms

Aneurysms distal to the lateral medullary segment are approached through a craniectomy that extends across the midline.

88.8.5 Vertebrobasilar junction aneurysms

General information

Saccular aneurysms located where the two vertebral arteries join often form at the location of a basi-lar artery fenestration (basilar fenestration aneurysm).

Angiographic considerations

CT-angiogram may be helpful as an adjunct because it can opacify both vertebral arteries simultane-ously (not generally feasible with catheter angiogram).

Surgical approaches

1. suboccipital approach: for most; performed in lateral oblique position
2. subtemporal-transtentorial approach if the vertebrobasilar junction is high; performed in supine position

Suboccipital approach in lateral oblique position

NB: the side of approach must be chosen based on angiogram, as the extreme tortuosity of the VAs may cause the aneurysm of one VA to lie on the contralateral side of the brainstem.

Position: thorax elevated ≈ 15°. Head in line with the thorax, neck slightly flexed, and slightly rotated away from side of aneurysm. Upper shoulder depressed with adhesive tape. Spinal subarachnoid catheter placed for CSF drainage, opened only once dura is opened.

88.8.6 Basilar bifurcation aneurysms

General information

AKA basilar tip aneurysms. The most common posterior circulation aneurysm. Comprise ≈ 5% of intracranial aneurysms. Considered inoperable until Drake reported 4 cases in 1961,[34] with larger series reported later.[35]

Presentation

Most present with SAH indistinguishable from SAH due to anterior circulation aneurysmal rupture. Enlargement of the aneurysm prior to rupture may rarely compress the optic chiasm → bitemporal field cut (mimicking pituitary tumor), or occasionally may compress the third nerve as it exits from the interpeduncular fossa → oculomotor nerve palsy.[22]

CT/MRI scan

May occasionally be seen on CT or MRI as round mass in region of suprasellar cistern. With SAH, tend to see blood in interpeduncular cistern with some reflux into 4th (and to a lesser extent, 3rd and lateral) ventricle. Occasionally may mimic pretruncal nonaneurysmal SAH (p. 1496).

Angiography

Dome usually points superiorly. Should evaluate flow through posterior communicating arteries (may require Allcock test) in case trapping is required. Need to assess the height of the basilar bifurcation in relation to the dorsum sella (see below).

Critical angiographic features to assess: On angiogram or CTA:
1. general features (p. 1423)
2. orientation: determines whether surgery is an option. Posteriorly pointing aneurysms obscure perforators which may be adherent to the aneurysm, making surgery more difficult
3. patency of PCAs & SCAs
4. patency and size of PComAs:
   a) Diameter of PComA > 1 mm is needed to support collateral flow (expert opinion)
   b) to determine if the P1's can be sacrificed.
   c) PComA patency and size is important for endovascular treatment as a potential route for deployment of horizontally oriented stent extending from P1 to contralateral P1,[36,37]
   d) which can facilitate temporary clipping, or sacrifice, or placement of stents.
5. height of the aneurysm relative to the posterior clinoid process which will affect the selection of surgical approach[38,39] (the range of height of the posterior clinoid is 4–14 mm[39])
   a) supraclinoidal: aneurysm neck > 5 mm superior to posterior clinoid process
   b) clinoidal: aneurysm neck within 5 mm of posterior clinoid process
   c) infraclinoidal: aneurysm neck > 5 mm inferior to posterior clinoid process

Surgical treatment

Timing

Initial experience tended to favor allowing basilar tip aneurysms to "cool-down" for ≈ 10–14 days after SAH before attempting surgery to permit cerebral edema to subside. More recently, early surgery for these aneurysms has been advocated as for anterior circulation aneurysms (p. 1461).[40] However, some surgeons still recommend waiting ≈ 1 week,[41] and most would agree that if there are obvious technical difficulties because of size, configuration, or location of the aneurysm, early surgery may not be appropriate. Also, if during the craniotomy it becomes apparent that cerebral edema is impairing the exposure, the operation should be aborted and attempted again at a later date.

Approaches

1. right subtemporal craniotomy (classical approach of Drake): approached through the incisura or division of the tentorium. Most basilar tip aneurysms are probably best approached via pterional approach (see below) except for posteriorly pointing aneurysms
    a) advantages:
        - less distance to basilar tip
        - may be better than pterional approach for aneurysms projecting posteriorly or posteroinferiorly[41]
    b) disadvantages:
        - requires temporal lobe retraction (minimized with lumbar drainage, mannitol, and possibly zygomatic arch section[42])
        - poor visualization of contralateral P1 segment and thalamoperforators
2. pterional approach (described by Yasargil): transsylvian (see below)
    a) advantages:
        - little or no retraction on temporal lobe (unlike subtemporal approach)
        - better visualization of both P1 segments and thalamoperforators
        - other aneurysms, e.g., of the anterior circulation, can be dealt with at the same sitting
    b) disadvantages:
        - increases reach to aneurysm by ≈ 1 cm compared to subtemporal
        - requires wide splitting of the Sylvian fissure
        - operating field is narrower than subtemporal approach
        - perforators arising from the posterior aspect of P1 may not be visible
3. modified pterional craniotomy: may allow transsylvian or subtemporal approach.[41] The craniotomy is taken further posteriorly than a standard pterional craniotomy
4. orbitozygomatic approach: allows access to portions of the basilar artery below the bifurcation. May be augmented by removal of the top of the clivus

Optional resection of the temporal tip will increase exposure of either approach. Unlike most anterior circulation aneurysms, securing proximal control is very difficult.

If the basilar bifurcation is high above the dorsum sella, then more retraction is required on a subtemporal approach than for a normal bifurcation height (near the dorsum sella). A high bifurcation is dealt with on a transsylvian approach by opening the Sylvian fissure more widely, or by a subfrontal approach through the 3rd ventricle via the lamina terminalis.[43] A low bifurcation may require splitting the tentorium behind the 4th nerve.

Pterional approach
See reference.[44]

Risks include: oculomotor palsy in ≈ 30% (most are minimal and temporary).
Approach is from the *right* unless:

1. additional left-sided aneurysm (e.g., PComA aneurysm) which could be treated simultaneously by a left-sided approach
2. aneurysm points to the right
3. aneurysm is located to the left of midline (the operation is more difficult when the aneurysm is even just 2–3 mm contralateral to the craniotomy)[41]
4. patient has right hemiparesis or left oculomotor palsy

See Pterional craniotomy (p. 1748) for general information. Rotate the head ≈ 30° off the vertical so that the malar eminence points directly upward (▶ Fig. 106.1). Slight neck flexion is used for low-lying aneurysms, slight extension for high ones. Craniotomy is as shown in ▶ Fig. 106.3, with aggressive removal of the sphenoid wing. The sphenoid wing and the orbital roof may be reduced with a drill. The posterior clinoid can be removed to improve exposure.

Approach
The Sylvian fissure is split until the take-off of the proximal M1 from the carotid terminus is identified. The approach is medial to the ICA (between the ICA and optic nerve) when this space is ≥ 5–10 mm. If the ICA is close to the optic nerve, an approach lateral to the ICA may be used, aided by medial retraction of the ICA/M1 segment (▶ Fig. 106.4). Here, the exposure is limited by the height of the M1 branch above the skull base, and if the basilar tip height above the skull base greatly exceeds this, clipping via this approach is not feasible.[23]

The 3rd nerve is identified. Also the PComA and the anterior choroidal artery (AChA) are located as they arise from the posterior surface of the ICA (to differentiate between them: the PComA origin is proximal to that of the AChA, PComA courses perpendicular to Liliequist's membrane, whereas AChA courses obliquely into the crural cistern). The PComA is followed posteriorly through Liliequist's membrane, which is opened, revealing the prepontine cistern. The PComA is followed until it joins the PCA at the P1/P2 junction. If PComA is absent, follow the third nerve back to find where it emerges between PCA and SCA. P1 is followed proximally to the basilar bifurcation region where the contralateral P1 and both SCAs are identified. Caudal dissection of Liliequist's membrane exposes the interpeduncular cistern with proximal BA (this exposure is critical for proximal control of BA in the event of aneurysmal rupture).

Thalamoperforating arteries (ThPAs) arise from the distal PComA and proximal PCA, and often compromise the access. Early poor results with clipping of basilar tip aneurysms have been attributed to sacrificing these vessels, which produces lacunar infarcts in the thalamus, midbrain, subthalamic, and pretectal regions. If hypoplastic, the PComA may be divided between clips to improve exposure (preserving the ThPAs which will then arise from the stumps). Similarly, a hypoplastic P1 may be divided if the PCA fills from the PComA. If the ThPAs make it impossible to clip the aneurysm, some may have to be sacrificed, which is best done at their origin. Fortunately, there are some anastamoses[45] and thus they are not entirely end-arteries as originally thought.

Outcome

88

If the aneurysm cannot be treated with endovascular technique, then the surgical option can be considered. Overall mortality is 5%, and morbidity is 12% (mostly due to injury to perforating vessels).[46]

88.8.7 Basilar trunk aneurysms

Most aneurysms of the basilar trunk are fusiform in morphology. Surgical access for these is extremely difficult.

References

[1] Locksley HB. Report on the Cooperative Study of Intracranial Aneurysms and Subarachnoid Hemorrhage: Section V. J Neurosurg. 1966; 25:219–239

[2] Yock DH, Larson DA. CT of Hemorrhage from Anterior Communicating Artery Aneurysms, with Angiographic Correlation. Radiology. 1980; 134:399–407

[3] Yeh H, Tew JM. Anterior Interhemispheric Approach to Aneurysms of the Anterior Communicating Artery. Surg Neurol. 1985; 23:98–100

[4] VanderArk GD, Kempe LG, Smith DR. Anterior Communicating Aneurysms: The Gyrus Rectus Approach. Clin Neurosurg. 1974; 21:120–133

[5] Olmsted WW, McGee TP. The Pathogenesis of Peripheral Aneurysms of the Central Nervous System: A Subject Review from the AFIP. Radiology. 1977; 123:661–666

[6] Fein JM, Rovit RL. Interhemispheric subdural hematoma secondary to hemorrhage from a callosomarginal artery aneurysm. Neuroradiology. 1970; 1:183–186

[7] Becker DH, Newton TH. Distal Anterior Cerebral Artery Aneurysm. Neurosurgery. 1979; 4:495–503

[8] Tan H, Huang G, Zhang T, et al. A retrospective comparison of the influence of surgical clipping and endovascular embolization on recovery of oculomotor nerve palsy in patients with posterior communicating artery aneurysms. Neurosurgery. 2015; 76:687–94; discussion 694

[9] Khan SA, Agrawal A, Hailey CE, et al. Effect of surgical clipping versus endovascular coiling on recovery from oculomotor nerve palsy in patients with posterior communicating artery aneurysms: A retrospective comparative study and meta-analysis. Asian J Neurosurg. 2013; 8:117–124

[10] Heros RC, Ojemann RG, Crowell RM. Superior Temporal Gyrus Approach to Middle Cerebral Artery Aneurysms: Technique and Results. Neurosurgery. 1982; 10:308–313

[11] Zhao B, Zhao Y, Tan X, et al. Primary decompressive craniectomy for poor-grade middle cerebral artery aneurysms with associated intracerebral hemorrhage. Clin Neurol Neurosurg. 2015; 133:1–5

[12] White JA, Horowitz MB, Samson D. Dural Waisting as a Sign of Subarachnoid Extension of Cavernous Carotid Aneurysms: A Follow-Up Case Report. Surgical Neurology. 1999; 52:607–610

[13] Hamada H, Endo S, Fukuda O, et al. Giant Aneurysm in the Cavernous Sinus Causing Subarachnoid Hemorrhage 13 Years After Detection: A Case Report. Surgical Neurology. 1996; 45:143–146

[14] Lee AG, Mawad ME, Baskin DS. Fatal Subarachnoid Hemorrhage from the Rupture of a Totally Intracavernous Carotid Artery Aneurysm: Case Report. Neurosurgery. 1996; 38:596–599

[15] Maurer JJ, Mills M, German WJ. Triad of unilateral blindness, orbital fractures and massive epistaxis after head injury. J Neurosurg. 1961; 18:937–949

[16] Day AL. Clinicoanatomic Features of Supraclinoid Aneurysms. Clinical Neurosurgery. 1988; 36:256–274

[17] Gibo H, Lenkey C, Rhoton AL. Microsurgical Anatomy of the Supraclinoid Portion of the Internal Carotid Artery. Journal of Neurosurgery. 1981; 55:560–574

[18] Day AL. Aneurysms of the Ophthalmic Segment: A Clinical and Anatomical Analysis. Journal of Neurosurgery. 1990; 72:677–691

[19] Berson EL, Freeman MI, Gay AJ. Visual Field Defects in Giant Suprasellar Aneurysms of Internal Carotid. Arch Ophthalmol. 1966; 76:52–58

[20] Donaldson LC, Eshtiaghi A, Sacco S, et al. Junctional Scotoma and Patterns of Visual Field Defects Produced by Lesions Involving the Optic Chiasm. J Neuroophthalmol. 2022; 42:e203–e208

[21] Heros RC, Nelson PB, Ojemann RG, et al. Large and Giant Paraclinoid Aneurysms: Surgical Techniques, Complications, and Results. Neurosurgery. 1983; 12:153–163

[22] Drake CG. The Treatment of Aneurysms of the Posterior Circulation. Clin Neurosurg. 1979; 26:96–144

[23] Yamaura A. Surgical Management of Posterior Circulation Aneurysms - Part I. Contemporary Neurosurg. 1985; 7:1–6

[24] Friedman AH, Drake CG. Subarachnoid hemorrhage from intracranial dissecting aneurysm. J Neurosurg. 1984; 60:325–334

[25] Yamada K, Hayakawa T, Ushio Y, et al. Therapeutic Occlusion of the Vertebral Artery for Unclippable Vertebral Aneurysm. Neurosurgery. 1984; 15:834–838

[26] Yeh HS, Tomsick TA, Tew JM. Intraventricular Hemorrhage due to Aneurysms of the Distal Posterior Inferior Cerebellar Artery. J Neurosurg. 1985; 62:772–775

[27] Fox JL. Intracranial Aneurysms. New York: Springer-Verlag; 1983

[28] Hammon WM, Kempe LG. The Posterior Fossa Approach to Aneurysms of the Vertebral and Basilar Arteries. J Neurosurg. 1972; 37:339–347

[29] Drake CG. The Surgical Treatment of Vertebral-Basilar Aneurysms. Clin Neurosurg. 1969; 16:114–169

[30] Sen CN, Sekhar LN. An Extreme Lateral Approach to Intradural Lesions of the Cervical Spine and Foramen Magnum. Neurosurgery. 1990; 27:197–204

[31] Youmans JR. Neurological Surgery. Philadelphia 1982

[32] Heros RC. Lateral Suboccipital Approach for Vertebral and Vertebrobasilar Artery Aneurysms. J Neurosurg. 1986; 64:559–562

[33] Getch CC, O'Shaughnessy B A, Bendok BR, et al. Surgical management of intracranial aneurysms involving the posterior inferior cerebellar artery. Contemporary Neurosurgery. 2004; 26:1–7

[34] Drake CG. Bleeding Aneurysms of the Basilar Artery: Direct Surgical Management in Four Cases. J Neurosurg. 1961; 18:230–238

[35] Drake CG. Further Experience with Surgical Treatment of Aneurysms of the Basilar Artery. J Neurosurg. 1968; 29:372–392

[36] Cross DT,3rd, Moran CJ, Derdeyn CP, et al. Neuroform stent deployment for treatment of a basilar tip aneurysm via a posterior communicating artery route. AJNR. American Journal of Neuroradiology. 2005; 26:2578–2581

[37] Wanke I, Gizewski E, Forsting M. Horizontal stent placement plus coiling in a broad-based basilar-tip aneurysm: an alternative to the Y-stent technique. Neuroradiology. 2006; 48:817–820

[38] Friedman RA, Pensak ML, Tauber M, et al. Anterior petrosectomy approach to infraclinoidal basilar artery aneurysms: the emerging role of the neuro-otologist in multidisciplinary management of basilar artery aneurysms. Laryngoscope. 1997; 107:977–983

[39] Aziz KM, van Loveren HR, Tew JM,Jr, et al. The Kawase approach to retrosellar and upper clival basilar aneurysms. Neurosurgery. 1999; 44:1225–34; discussion 1234-6

[40] Peerless SJ, Hernesniemi JA, Gutman FB, et al. Early Surgery for Ruptured Vertebrobasilar Aneurysms. Journal of Neurosurgery. 1994; 80:643–649

[41] Chyatte D, Philips M. Surgical Approaches for Basilar Artery Aneurysms. Contemporary Neurosurgery. 1991; 13:1–6

[42] Pitelli SD, Almeida GGM, Nakagawa EJ, et al. Basilar Aneurysm Surgery: The Subtemporal Approach with Section of the Zygomatic Arch. Neurosurgery. 1986; 18:125–128

[43] Canbolt A, Önal Ç, Kiris T. A High-Position Basilar Top Aneurysm Apprached via Third Ventricle: Case Report. Surgical Neurology. 1993; 39:196–199

[44] Yasargil MG, Antic J, Laciga R, et al. Microsurgical Pterional Approach to Aneurysms of the Basilar Bifurcation. Surg Neurol. 1976; 6

[45] Marinkovic SV, Milisavljevic MM, Kovacevic MS. Anastomoses Among the Thalamoperforating Branches of the Posterior Cerebral Artery. Archives of Neurology. 1986; 43:811–814

[46] Drake CG. Management of Cerebral Aneurysm. Stroke. 1981; 12:273–283

88

89 Special Aneurysms and Non-Aneurysmal SAH

89.1 Unruptured aneurysms

89.1.1 General information

Unruptured intracranial aneurysms (UIA) include incidental aneurysms (those that do not produce any symptoms and are discovered incidentally) and aneurysms that produce symptoms other than those due to hemorrhage (e.g., pupillary dilatation due to third nerve compression). UIA merit consideration for treatment since the outcome from SAH with or without surgery is poor even under the best of circumstances. About 65% of patients die from the first SAH,[1] and even in patients with no neurologic deficit after aneurysm rupture, only 46% fully recover, and only 44% return to their former jobs.[2] However, the risk of aneurysmal rupture without intervention should be weighed against the risks of surgical clipping or endovascular treatment. Estimated prevalence of incidental aneurysms is 5–10% of the population.[2]

89.1.2 Presentation

See items other than those listed under "rupture" in Presentation of aneurysms (p. 1454).

89.1.3 Natural history

Risk of bleeding from UIA differs from aneurysms that have ruptured. True risk is not known with certainty. Early studies found annual bleeding rate of 6.25%, whereas later reports estimate lifetime risk for a 20-year-old with a UIA to be 16%, which drops off to 5% for a 60-year-old.[2] The average annual rupture rate is closer to ≈ 1%.[3] The International Study of Unruptured Aneurysms (ISUIA)[4] was the first large-scale, prospective study evaluating the natural history of unruptured aneurysms as well as the risks of treatment of unruptured aneurysms. The authors concluded that rupture rate was related to size and location of the aneurysm, and that risk is increased with previous aSAH from a separate aneurysm (see below). However, there were important limitations of ISUIA (see ► Table 89.1).

Table 89.1 Main methodological limitations of ISUIA study

- patients were not randomized to surgery (vs. no surgery), and there were substantial differences between treated and untreated groups
- follow-up was < 5 years in 50% of patients
- selection bias: low recruitment numbers from each center

Σ: The natural history of unruptured intracranial aneurysms

There appear to be 2 distinct types: those that rupture, and those that tend to remain stable. Most UIAs seen in the clinic fall into the latter group.

Spontaneous thrombosis of unruptured aneurysms (p. 1454) may occur rarely.

Retrospective and prospective studies have assessed the natural history of unruptured aneurysms. Overall, several variables have been identified as risk factors for rupture:

1. patient factors
   a) history of previous aSAH from a separate aneurysm[4,5]
   b) multiple aneurysms[6,7]
   c) age: there is conflicting evidence, as some studies have found an inverse relationship between age and rupture risk,[7,8] while others have found an increased risk of rupture for those aged 40 or older,[9] or no effect of age on rupture risk[10]
   d) medical conditions:
      - hypertension[7]
      - smoking[8]

e) geographic location: North America/Europe < Japan < Finland[11]

f) gender?: risk of rupture was greater amongst women compared to men in one study, but only approached statistical significance[9]

g) family history?: in the Familial Intracranial Aneurysm study,[12] rupture rate in patients with unruptured aneurysm and first-degree relative with intracranial aneurysm was 17x higher than that for patients with unruptured intracranial aneurysm in ISUIA (after matching for aneurysm size and location), although conclusions are limited secondary to small number of ruptures in the study. Other studies have failed to demonstrate an increased risk in this subgroup

2. aneurysm characteristics

a) size: risk of rupture appears critically dependent on aneurysm diameter

1. the annual risk of rupture of aneurysms < 10 mm was estimated to be 0.05%/year by ISUIA,[4] whereas a number of other studies have demonstrated a rupture risk closer to ≈ 1%/year[5,8,13,14,15]

2. the prospective Small Unruptured Intracranial Aneurysm Verification Study[7] (SUAVe) found the rupture risk of aneurysms < 5 mm is ≈ 0.5%/year which is not trivial. Risk was higher with age < 50 years (hazard ratio (HR) 5.23%), diameter ≥ 4 mm (HR 5.86%), HTN (HR 7.93%), and multiple aneurysms (HR 4.87%), but risk was not increased by previous aSAH

3. a more recent retrospective review demonstrated the majority (62%) of ruptured aneurysms to be < 7 mm, with most of these being anterior communicating artery aneurysms.[16] Some speculate that this may be due to a shrinkage of aneurysms following rupture

4. larger aneurysms (10–25 mm) are estimated to have ≈ 3–18%/year risk, while giant aneurysms (≥ 25 mm) have a risk of ≈ 8–50%/year

b) location: ISUIA showed an increase in rupture risk for PComA and posterior circulation aneurysms.[16] Ishibashi et al[5] also demonstrated increased risk amongst posterior circulation aneurysms. Conversely, some studies found an increased risk of rupture with anterior communicating aneurysms[8,16,17]

c) morphology: presence of a daughter sac,[15] bottleneck shape,[18] and increased ratio of size of aneurysm to parent vessel have all been associated with increased risk of rupture[19,20]

Estimation of absolute risk of aneurysm rupture in a patient based on a combination of risk factors is complex. The PHASES scoring system[11] estimates 5-year rupture risk and was derived by pooling patient data from six prospective studies.[5,7,8,15,21,22] The PHASES predictors are shown in ▶ Table 89.2,

Table 89.2 Components of the PHASES aneurysm rupture risk score[11]

Predictor		Points	Score
(P) Population	North American, European (other than Finnish)	0	(0 | 3 | 5)
	Japanese	3	
	Finnish	5	
(H) Hypertension	no	0	(0 | 1)
	yes	1	
(A) Age	< 70 years	0	(0 | 1)
	≥ 70 years	1	
(S) Size	< 7 mm	0	(0 | 3 | 6 | 10)
	7–9 mm	3	
	10–19.9 mm	6	
	20 mm	10	
(E) Earlier rupture from another aneurysm	no	0	(0 | 1)
	yes	1	
(S) Site of aneurysm	ICA	0	(0 | 2 | 5)
	MCA	2	
	ACA, PComA, or posterior circulation (vertebral, basilar, cerebellar, & posterior cerebral arteries)	5	
PHASES score → TOTAL			(0 - 23)

Abbreviations: ICA = internal carotid artery, MCA = middle cerebral artery, ACA = anterior cerebral artery, PComA = posterior communicating artery.

and the predicted 5-year cumulative risk of aneurysm rupture based on the PHASES score is summarized in ▶ Table 89.3. Further study is needed to externally validate the methodology.

Table 89.3 Predicted 5-year cumulative risk of aneurysm rupture based on PHASES score[11]

PHASES score	5-year risk of aneurysm rupture
2	0.4%
3	0.7%
4	0.9%
5	1.3%
6	1.7%
7	2.4%
8	3.2%
9	4.3%
10	5.3%
11	7.2%
12	17.8%

89.1.4 Management

Cumulative rupture risk

The calculation of the cumulative lifetime risk of aneurysm rupture uses the same mathematical concepts as for AVMs (p. 1506), with the appropriate parameters plugged into the equation.

Decision analysis

Decision analysis is a means of mathematically modeling outcomes of various decision options using probabilities and assigning "desirability factors" to the outcomes. This analysis requires data about the natural history (see above), *life expectancy*, and morbidity and mortality of SAH and aneurysm surgery. Although it is only a model, it does yield some insights in some complicated decisions.

In one such study,[23] using the values shown in ▶ Table 89.4, the result obtained was that a life expectancy of 12 more years is the break-even point, i.e., if the patient is not expected to live for 12 more years, then non-surgical management is a better choice than surgery (this result involves numerous assumptions and estimations; e.g., 5% "risk aversiveness" (intermediate) relates to patient's fears of immediate surgical risk vs. risk of rupture spread over many years). Another analysis of various scenarios for a 50-year-old female found that treatment was cost-effective for UIAs that were symptomatic, ≥ 10 mm diameter, or with a previous history of SAH.[24]

Table 89.4 Data used in decision analysis of management of unruptured aneurysms[23]

	Typical value	Range
annual risk of rupture[a]	1%	0.5–2%
3 month mortality of SAH	55%	50–60%
serious morbidity after SAH	15%	10–20%
surgical morbidity & mortality	2% & 6%	4–10%

[a]this is an intermediate risk for aneurysms 6–10 mm diameter (NB: size may change; small aneurysms may grow)

Management recommendations

Decisions are based on natural history data balanced against the effectiveness and morbidity and mortality of intervention (surgery/endovascular), with recommendations being based mainly on expert opinion, given that high-level evidence is lacking. Size, patient age, and location are important factors in determining whether to treat and by which means to treat an unruptured aneurysm (in a patient without prior SAH). In addition, treatment should be recommended for patients with a history of aSAH, strong family history, symptomatic aneurysms, and for enlargement or change in configuration of the aneurysm.[25] Numerous recommendations have been made for a critical size above which an unruptured aneurysm should be considered for surgery, and have included 3 mm,[26] 5 mm,[27] 7 mm,[28] and 9 mm.[29] The most recent American Heart Association guidelines did not advocate for repair of small incidental aneurysms (< 10 mm) in patients with no history of subarachnoid hemorrhage,[25] but this report was prior to more recent prospective trials. In addition, the patient's expected longevity must also be taken into account, and therefore special consideration for treatment should be given to young patients in this group. In all treatment decisions, coexisting medical conditions must also be borne in mind.

A number of scales have been developed to try and guide treatment for UIAs. The unruptured intracranial aneurysm treatment score (UIATS)[30] was found to recommend overtreatment based on some practice patterns.[31]

One proposed strategy[32] in management is summarized here:

1. large and/or symptomatic aneurysms (especially in young patients) → intervention
2. patients < 60 years old:
   a) < 7 mm
      • anterior circulation, NO risk factors → medical management or intervention
      • PComA/posterior circulation, symptomatic aneurysm, strong family hx → intervention
   b) > 7 mm → intervention (surgery or endovascular based on size, location)
3. patients > 60 years old:
   a) < 7 mm
      • no family hx and asymptomatic → medical management
      • + risk factors → intervention
   b) 7–12 mm
      • anterior circulation → medical management or intervention
      • PComA/posterior circulation → intervention
   c) > 12 mm → intervention

89

Recommended follow-up for UIAs treated conservatively

Σ: Recommended F/U for UIAs treated conservatively

Annual follow-up with MRA/CTA is recommended for most incidental UIAs that are not treated. Intervention is indicated for *any* documented growth. If no growth, may consider repeat imaging at a reduced frequency after an arbitrary number of years of stability.

Background: The morbidity from catheter arteriograms is probably too high to recommend them for this purpose. CTA is more accurate than MRA, but involves iodine contrast and radiation. A TOF-MRA (not gadolinium-MRA) has no known risks and does not involve radiation, but has lower spatial resolution.

Unfortunately, most aneurysms rupture without demonstrable enlargement on follow-up. Aneurysms do not grow at a constant rate, and it may take several years to appreciate a millimeter of increased size on MRA.

Studies have identified risk factors for growth, including size,[33,34,35,36] location (MCA, basilar bifurcation),[35,36] > 1 aneurysm,[34,35] family history of SAH,[35] and smoking.[33]

Risk of rupture in the setting of growth is hard to estimate, given most aneurysms that increase in size are subsequently treated. In one study, the rupture rate was 2.4%/year for aneurysms showing growth (vs. 0.2%/year in those without growth).[33] In another study of 18 Japanese patients, rupture risk after growth was 18.5%/year.[37]

Unruptured cavernous carotid aneurysms (CCAAs)

Life-threatening complications are rare. When cavernous carotid artery aneurysms (CCAAs) rupture, they usually produce a high-flow (Type A) carotid-cavernous fistula (CCF) (p. 1519). For exceptions, see section 88.6. Most CCAAs develop on the horizontal segment of the cavernous ICA.

▶ **Presentations of unruptured CCAAs.** The natural history is not precisely known.

1. CCAAs may be discovered incidentally
   a) on arteriography for other reason
   b) on brain MRI
   c) on head CT or CTA
2. symptomatic presentations (other than rupture):

a) usually present with:
- headache
- cavernous sinus syndrome (p. 1689): primarily produces diplopia (due to ophthalmoplegia). Classically the third nerve palsy from an enlarging CCAA will *not* produce a dilated pupil because the sympathetics which dilate the pupil are also paralyzed[38 (p 1492)]
- those that expand through the carotid ring into the subarachnoid space may cause monocular blindness from strangulation of the optic nerve[39]

b) rarely, pain (retro-orbital or pain mimicking trigeminal neuralgia[40,41])

c) *giant* CCAAs may produce emboli[42]

▶ **Treatment.** The natural history is not precisely known.
Emergent treatment is indicated for cases with epistaxis or SAH.
Indications for treatment for unruptured CCAAs:

1. symptomatic: patients with intolerable pain or visual problems[43] (urgent treatment for severe eye pain or threat to vision)
2. giant CCAAs: especially those that straddle the clinoidal ring (subarachnoid extension of CCAAs may be indicated by "waisting" of the aneurysm on angiography[44])
3. aneurysms that enlarge on serial imaging
4. controversial: incidental CCAA on the same side as a stenotic carotid artery for which carotid endarterectomy is indicated. There has been no evidence that doing the endarterectomy increases the risk of rupture, and, as indicated above, most ruptures are not life-threatening and so generally the carotid disease should be treated on its own merits

▶ **Treatment options for CCAAs.** Treatment of small incidental intracavernous CCAAs is not generally indicated.[25]

For other unruptured CCAAs, options include detachable coils (p. 1456) in an attempt to thrombose the aneurysm. This results in reduction of mass effect in ≈ 50%. Open surgical treatment is rarely appropriate. Aneurysms that rupture and produce a carotid-cavernous fistula may be treated by endovascular occlusion (p. 1519).

89.2 Multiple aneurysms

Multiple aneurysms are present in 15–33.5% of cases of SAH.[2] In one study of multiple factors, hypertension was found to be the most important one associated with multiplicity.[45]

When a patient presents with SAH and is found to have multiple aneurysms, the following may be clues as to which aneurysm has bled:

1. epicenter (center of greatest concentration) of blood on CT or MRI[46,47]
2. area of focal vasospasm on angiogram
3. irregularities in the shape of the aneurysm (so-called "Murphy's teat")
4. if none of the above help, then suspect the largest aneurysm
5. NB: in one series, the most common cause of post-op bleeding in 93 patients with multiple aneurysms was felt to be from rebleeding of the original aneurysm that ruptured that was actually *missed* on initial angiogram[48]

89.3 Familial aneurysms

89.3.1 General information

The role of inheritance in the development of intracranial aneurysms (IA) is well established for disorders such as polycystic kidney disease, and connective tissue disorders such as Ehlers-Danlos type IV, Marfan syndrome, and pseudoxanthoma elasticum (p. 1455). Overall, it is not uncommon for patients with aSAH to have a family history. In one study of patients with subarachnoid hemorrhage,[49] 9.4% had a first-degree relative with aSAH or intracranial aneurysm and 14% had a second degree relative with these diagnoses. In families with two or more affected members, the age adjusted prevalence of intracranial aneurysm among first-degree relatives was 9.2% in those aged 30 years or older.[50,51]

Additional cases of IAs in identical twins,[52,53] as well as familial aggregations of IAs without a recognized inherited disorder, have also been reported but are felt to be rare (it has been estimated that < 2% of IAs are familial[54]). Most reported cases consist of only 2 family members with IAs, and these are most commonly siblings.[55] In fact, siblings of an affected aSAH patient have a higher risk of aneurysm than do children of an affected patient.[32] Analysis of case reports reveals that when IAs occur in siblings they tend to occur at identical or mirror image sites, and in comparison to sporadic

IAs, familial IAs tend to rupture at a smaller size and at a younger age, and that the incidence of anterior communicating artery aneurysms is lower.[56] It has been postulated that IAs occurring in siblings may represent a distinct population of IAs.[57]

Natural history

See natural history (risk of hemorrhage) (p. 1487).

89.3.2 Screening recommendations

The indications and best method for investigation of asymptomatic relatives of a patient found to harbor an intracranial aneurysm are controversial. Negative studies do not guarantee that at a later date an aneurysm will not be discovered that either subsequently developed or expanded, or was simply not detected on the initial study.[58,59,60] Cerebral angiography is the most sensitive study; however, the risk and expense may not justify its use as a screening test in many cases. Furthermore, there is some evidence that aneurysms that rupture tend to do so shortly after their formation,[29] which would reduce the value of screening.

89.3.3 Genetics

A large meta-analysis identified 19 single nucleotide polymorphisms associated with sporadic intracranial aneurysms.[61] The strongest associations were found on chromosomes 9 (CDKN2B; antisense inhibitor gene), 8 (SOX17; transcription regulator gene), and 4 (EDNRA gene).

Screening with either MRA or CTA is typically recommended for first-degree relatives (especially siblings) of affected family members *when two or more* members of the family have an intracranial aneurysm or aSAH.[32] The overall need for screening second-degree relatives is less clear. Screening of first-degree relatives is not typically recommended if only one family member is affected.[25,59] In patients with coarctation of the aorta, screening is typically recommended. Finally, patients with ADPKD who have a family history of intracranial aneurysm or aSAH should be screened. Findings suspicious for intracranial aneurysms should be followed-up with four-vessel arteriography to confirm suspected lesions (MRA has a high false-positive rate of ≈ 16%[50]) and to rule out additional aneurysms.

89.4 Traumatic aneurysms

89.4.1 General information

Traumatic aneurysms (**TAs**) comprise < 1% of intracranial aneurysms.[62,63] Most are actually false aneurysms, AKA pseudoaneurysms (a rupture of all the vessel wall layers with the "wall" of the aneurysm being formed by surrounding cerebral structures[64]). They may occur rarely in childhood. The mechanism of injury usually falls into one of the following groups[65]:

▶ **Those arising from penetrating trauma.** Usually from gunshot wounds, although penetration with a sharp object (which is less common) may be more prone to cause traumatic aneurysms.[66]

▶ **Those arising from closed head injury.** More common. Theories of pathogenesis include traction injury to the vessel wall or entrapment within a fracture. Tend to occur either:
1. peripherally
   a) distal anterior cerebral artery aneurysms (▶ Fig. 89.1): secondary to impact against the falcine edge
   b) distal cortical artery aneurysms: often associated with an overlying skull fracture, sometimes a growing skull fracture
2. at the skull base, usually involving the ICA in one of the following sites:
   a) petrous portion (virtually always associated with basal skull fractures)
   b) cavernous carotid artery (virtually always associated with basal skull fractures):
      • aneurysm enlargement may cause a progressive cavernous sinus syndrome
      • rupture may lead to a posttraumatic carotid-cavernous fistula (p. 1519) or to massive epistaxis in the presence of a sphenoid sinus fracture[67,68,69]
   c) supraclinoid carotid artery

▶ **Iatrogenic.** Following surgery in or around the skull base, the sinuses, or orbits (including following transsphenoidal surgery[70]). The first such case was described in 1950.

89

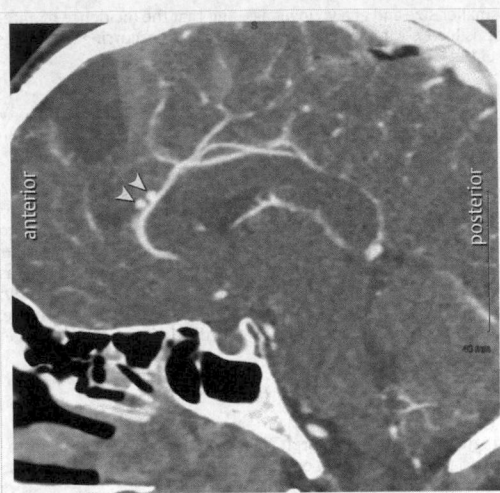

Fig. 89.1 Two traumatic aneurysms in a patient < 2 weeks following a gunshot wound to the head.
The aneurysms (*yellow arrowheads*) are arising from distal branches of the anterior cerebral artery, a typical location.
Image: sagittal CT angiogram.

89.4.2 Presentation

1. delayed intracranial hemorrhage (subdural, subarachnoid, intraventricular, or intraparenchymal): the most common presentation. TAs tend to have a high rate of rupture
2. recurrent epistaxis
3. progressive cranial nerve palsy
4. enlarging skull fracture
5. may be incidental finding on CT scan
6. severe headache

89.4.3 Treatment

Although there are case reports of spontaneous resolution, treatment is usually recommended. ICA aneurysms at the skull base should undergo trapping or endovascular embolization. Peripheral lesions should be treated surgically with clipping of aneurysm neck, excision of the aneurysm, coiling, or wrapping if no other method is feasible.

89.5 Mycotic aneurysms

89.5.1 General information

The name *"mycotic"* originated with Osler in whose time the term referred to any infectious process[71] rather than the current usage which implies a fungal etiology. Currently accepted terminology favors infectious aneurysm (or bacterial aneurysm). Infectious aneurysms can, however, also occur with fungal infections.[72] Tend to form in distal (often unnamed) vessels.

89.5.2 Epidemiology and pathophysiology

1. comprise ≈ 4% of intracranial aneurysms
2. occurs in 3–15% of patients with subacute bacterial endocarditis (SBE)
3. most common location: distal MCA branches (75–80%)
4. at least 20% have or develop multiple aneurysms
5. increased frequency in immunocompromised patients (e.g., AIDS) and drug users
6. most probably start in the adventitia (outer layer) and spread inward

89.5.3 Evaluation

Blood cultures and LP may identify the infectious organism. ▶ Table 89.5 shows typical pathogens recovered. Patients with suspected infectious aneurysm(s) should undergo echocardiography to look for signs of endocarditis.

Table 89.5 Pathogens implicated in mycotic aneurysms[73 (p 933-40)]

Organism	%	Comment
streptococcus	44%	S. viridans (classic cause of SBE)
staphylococcus	18%	S. aureus (cause of acute bacterial endocarditis)
miscellaneous	6%	(pseudomonas, enterococcus, corynebacteria...)
multiple	5%	
no growth	12%	
no info	14%	
total	99%	

89.5.4 Treatment

These aneurysms usually have fusiform morphology and are usually very friable; therefore, surgical treatment is difficult and/or risky. Most cases are treated acutely with antibiotics, which are continued 4–6 weeks. Serial angiography (at 7–10 days and 1.5, 3, 6, and 12 months, even if aneurysms seem to be getting smaller, they may subsequently increase[74] and new ones may form) helps document effectiveness of medical therapy (serial MRA may be a viable alternative in some cases). Aneurysms may continue to shrink following completion of antibiotic therapy.[75] Delayed clipping may be more feasible; indications include:

1. patients with SAH
2. increasing size of aneurysm while on antibiotics[76] (controversial, some say not mandatory[75])
3. failure of aneurysm to reduce in size after 4–6 weeks of antibiotics[76]

Patients with SBE requiring valve replacement should have bioprosthetic (i.e., tissue) valves instead of mechanical valves to eliminate the need for risky anticoagulation.

89.6 Giant aneurysms

89.6.1 General information

Definition: > 2.5 cm (≈ 1 inch) diameter. Two types: saccular (probably an enlarged "berry" aneurysm) and fusiform. Comprise 3–5% of intracranial aneurysms; peak age of presentation 30–60 years; female:male ratio = 3:1.

Drake's series of 174 giant aneurysms[77]: 35% presented as hemorrhage, with 10% showing some evidence of remote bleeding. The bleeding rate is 8–50%/year (p. 1487).

May also present as TIAs (by reducing flow or by emboli) or as a mass. About one-third have a neck amenable to clipping.

89.6.2 Evaluation

General information

Drake contended that even after thorough radiographic evaluation, actual operative visualization is the only way to definitively assess the aneurysm and its branches. 3D-CTA can add substantial information that rivals and may exceed direct visualization.

Angiogram

Often underestimates the size of the lesion secondary to thrombosed regions of the aneurysm that do not fill with contrast. CT or MRI is required to visualize the thrombosed portion.

89

CT scan

Frequently have a significant amount of edema surrounding the aneurysm. May see contrast enhancement of the brain surrounding the aneurysm; probably due to increased vascularity secondary to inflammatory reaction to the aneurysm.

MRI scan

Turbulence within → complicated signal on T1WI. Pulsation artifact (linear distortion radiation through aneurysm) on MRI helps differentiate giant aneurysms from solid or cystic lesions.

89.6.3 Treatment

Options include:
1. direct surgical clipping: usually possible in only ≈ 50% of cases
2. vascular bypass of aneurysm with subsequent clipping
3. trapping
4. proximal arterial ligation (hunterian ligation)
   a) for vertebral-basilar aneurysms[78]: results in improvement of cranial nerve deficit in ≈ 95% of patients. A reasonable alternative in the presence of an adequately sized contralateral VA that unites with the VA to be ligated
5. wrapping (p. 1457)
6. endovascular treatment

89.7 Cortical subarachnoid hemorrhage

Cortical SAH (cSAH) appears as SAH over the convexity. Trauma is the most common cause.
Etiologies of cSAH[79]:
- trauma: the most common etiology
- pial AVMs
- dural AV fistulas
- cerebrovascular arterial dissection
- dural or cortical venous thrombosis
- vasculitis
- reversible cerebral vasoconstriction syndrome (RCVS), AKA Call-Fleming syndrome,[80] a group of disorders sharing the cardinal clinical and angiographic features of reversible segmental multifocal cerebral vasoconstriction with severe headaches, focal ischemia, and/or seizures. Over 95% experience "thunderclap headaches".[81] Risk factors: postpartum (sometimes called postpartum cerebral angiopathy), use of certain drugs (vasoactive substances, cannabis (marijuana), SSRIs...). More common in women. CT may demonstrate SAH restricted to a cortical sulcus.[82] CTA or DSA may show beading of vessels.[82] Symptoms are usually self-limiting, nimodipine may help
- posterior reversible encephalopathy syndrome (PRES) (p. 202)
- cerebral amyloid angiopathy (CAA) (p. 1612)
- coagulopathies
- brain tumors (primary or metastatic)

89.8 SAH of unknown etiology

89.8.1 General information

Incidence: traditionally quoted as 20–28% of all SAH, but this includes data from older series (some did not perform true pan-angiography, and/or CT was not available to R/O intracerebral hemorrhage). Recent estimates of incidence: 7–10%. This is a heterogeneous category, and a better term might be "angiogram-negative SAH"; see requirements to be met before considering an arteriogram to be negative (p. 1423). The quantity of blood on CT may predict the chances of an arteriogram disclosing a cerebral aneurysm.[83,84,85,86]

Patients with angiogram-negative SAH tend to be younger, less hypertensive, and more commonly male than those with positive angiography.[84]

Possible causes of SAH with a negative angiogram include:

▶ **Aneurysm that fails to be demonstrated in initial angiogram:**
1. inadequate angiography, causes include:

a) incomplete angio: (p.1423)
- must see both PICA origins (1–2% of aneurysms occur here)
- need to cross-fill through the ACoA (p.1423)

b) degradation of images due to
- poor patient cooperation (e.g., from agitation). Either sedate patient (use caution in non-intubated patients) or repeat the study at a later time when patient is more cooperative
- poor-quality equipment providing substandard images

2. obliteration of aneurysm by the hemorrhage
3. thrombosis of the aneurysm after SAH (p.1456)
4. aneurysm too small to be visualized[87]: although "microaneurysms" may be a source of SAH, their natural history and optimal treatment are unknown
5. lack of filling of aneurysm due to vasospasm (of parent artery or of aneurysmal orifice)

▶ **Nonaneurysmal SAH from source that fails to show up on angiography.** See for etiologies of SAH other than aneurysm (p.1417) (many of which may not be demonstrated on angiography), including:

1. angiographically occult (or cryptic) vascular malformation (p.1524)
2. pretruncal nonaneurysmal SAH: see below

89.8.2 Risk of rebleeding

Overall rebleed rate is 0.5%/yr, which is lower than with aneurysmal SAH or rebleeding from AVMs. There is also a smaller risk of delayed cerebral ischemia (vasospasm). Neurological outcome is likewise better.

89.8.3 Management

General measures

These patients are still at risk for the same complications of SAH as with aneurysmal SAH: vasospasm, hydrocephalus, hyponatremia, rebleeding, etc. (p.1432) and should be managed as any SAH (p.1432). Some subgroups may be at lower risk for complications and may be managed accordingly (e.g., below).

Repeat angiography

Yield of positive second angiogram after technically adequate negative study: 1.8–9.8%[88] in early (pre-CT) studies, 2–24% quoted more recently.[87,89,90] CT scan findings are helpful in the decision to repeat angiography.[91] 70% of cases with diffuse SAH and thick layering of blood in the anterior interhemispheric fissure were associated with an ACoA aneurysm that showed up on repeat angiography.[85] The absence of blood on CT (performed within 4 days of SAH), or thick blood in the perimesencephalic cisterns alone (see below) were unlikely to be associated with a missed aneurysm.

Recommendations regarding repeat angio:
. repeat angio after ≈ 10–14 days (allows vasospasm & some clot to resolve; **note:** between 5 and 10 days there is decreased chance of seeing an aneurysm because of vasospasm; angiography at ≈ day 10 permits surgery to be done if needed ≈ at day 14, which is about the earliest time after the "no-op" window of day 3–12)
   a) technically adequate 4-vessel angiogram is negative, and evidence for SAH is strong
   b) original angio was incomplete or if there are suspicious findings
. if CT localizes blood clot to particular area, place special attention to this area on repeat angio
. do not repeat angio for classic pretruncal SAH (see below) or if no blood on CT
. patients are usually kept in the hospital 10–14 days while waiting for repeat angio (to watch for and manage complication of SAH or rebleeding)

Third arteriogram:
   If the first two arteriograms are negative, and the history is suggestive of aneurysmal SAH, a third arteriogram 3–6 months after SAH has ≈ 1% chance of showing a source of bleeding.

89

Other studies

1. imaging studies of the brain: MRI (with MRA if available) or CT (with angio-CT if available). This may visualize an aneurysm that fails to show up on angiography, and may identify other sources of SAH such as angiographically occult vascular malformation (p. 1524), tumor…
2. tests to rule out spinal AVM: a rare cause of intracerebral SAH (p. 1395)
   a) spinal MRI: cervical, thoracic, and lumbar
   b) spinal angiography: too difficult and risky to be justified in most cases of angio-negative SAH. Consider in cases with high suspicion of spinal source

Surgical exploration

Advocated by some for cases of SAH with CT findings compatible with an aneurysmal source in which a suspicious area is demonstrated angiographically[87] with careful explanation to the patient and family of the possibility of negative operative findings.

89.9 Pretruncal nonaneurysmal SAH (PNSAH)

89.9.1 General information

Formerly perimesencephalic nonaneurysmal SAH.[92] The suggestion to change the name to pretruncal nonaneurysmal SAH was proposed because neuroimaging has shown the true anatomic localization of the blood to be in front of the brainstem (truncus cerebri) centered in front of the pons rather than perimesencephalic.[93] The existing literature on PNSAH is somewhat limited by the lack of a rigorous anatomic definition, with criteria of blood pattern differing amongst studies. Blood often extends into the interpeduncular or premedullary cisterns. It has also sometimes been referred to as the "Dutch disease" due to the initial profusion of information in that literature.

A distinct entity considered to be a benign condition with good outcome and less risk of rebleeding and vasospasm than in other patients with SAH of unknown etiology[94] (no rebleeding occurred in 37 patients with PNSAH and 45 months mean follow-up,[95] nor in 169 patients with 8–51 months follow-up[90]; vasospasm has been reported in only 3 patients and may have been related to cerebral angiography rather than the PNSAH, and although it is low, the incidence of angiographic vasospasm may be higher than originally thought[96]).

The actual etiology has yet to be determined (there are 3 case reports of patients explored surgically with no abnormal findings[90] and one case where a pontine abnormality resembling a capillary telangiectasia was demonstrated on MRI[97]), but it may be secondary to rupture of a small perimesencephalic vein or capillary.[96] Studies have shown an association with abnormal venous anatomy including primitive variants of the basal vein of Rosenthal,[98,99] which some authors have hypothesized results in hemorrhage secondary to central cerebral venous hypertension.[100,101] Other proposed etiologies include a ruptured perforating artery, cavernous malformation, intraluminal basilar dissection, and capillary telangiectasia.[102]

89.9.2 Presentation

Patients may present with severe paroxysmal H/A, meningismus, photophobia, and nausea. Loss of consciousness is rare. These patients are usually not critically ill (all were grade 1 or 2 [H&H or WFNS grading scale]); however, complications such as hyponatremia or cardiac abnormalities may still occur. Preretinal hemorrhages and sentinel H/A have not occurred. CT and/or MRI demonstrate characteristic findings (see below) although it may initially be missed on CT,[96] and LP may yield bloody CSF. By definition, all have negative angiography.

89.9.3 Epidemiology

PNSAH has been reported to comprise 20–68% of cases of angiogram-negative SAH[94,103] (depending on the timing of CT, adequacy of angiography, and the definition of PNSAH). However, the true incidence is probably more in the range of 50–75%.[90]

The reported age range is 3–70 years (mean: 50 yrs),[90] 52–59% are male, and pre-existing HT was present in 3–20% of patients.

89.9.4 Relevant anatomy

Posterior fossa cisterns:

The perimesencephalic cisterns include: interpeduncular, crural, ambient, and quadrigeminal cisterns. The prepontine cistern lies immediately anterior to the pons.

Lilequist's membrane (LM)[104]: Basically considered to separate the interpeduncular cistern from the chiasmatic cistern[105] (it forms a competent barrier in only 10–30% of the population). In further detail, the superior leaflet of LM (diencephalic membrane) separates the interpeduncular cistern from the chiasmatic cistern medially and from the carotid cisterns laterally.[106,107] The inferior leaflet (the mesencephalic membrane) separates the interpeduncular from the prepontine cistern.

The diencephalic membrane is thicker and is more often competent, effectively isolating the chiasmatic cistern. However, the carotid cisterns often communicate with the crural cisterns and in turn with the interpeduncular cistern.[107]

Thus, blood in the carotid or prepontine cistern is compatible with a low-pressure pretruncal source of bleeding; however, blood in the chiasmatic cistern should raise concern about aneurysmal rupture.

89.9.5 Diagnostic criteria

Without knowledge of the actual substrate of PNSAH, the following suggested diagnostic criteria must be viewed as empiric (adapted[90]): (an example of a typical CT scan is shown in ▶ Fig. 89.2)

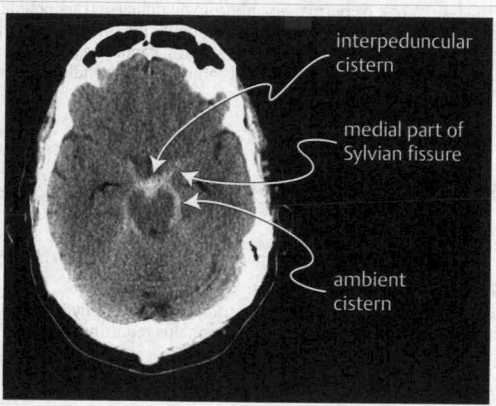

interpeduncular cistern

medial part of Sylvian fissure

ambient cistern

Fig. 89.2 Pretruncal (perimesencephalic) nonaneurysmal SAH in a 67-year-old male.
Image: axial noncontrast CT scan of the brain.

89

1. CT or MRI scan performed ≤ 2 days from ictus meeting the criteria shown in ▶ Table 89.6 (later scans render the diagnosis unreliable, e.g., washout could cause an aneurysmal SAH to fit the criteria). These criteria imply that blood should be contained inferior to Lilequist's membrane (LM) (i.e., perimesencephalic and/or prepontine cisterns). Extension into the suprasellar cistern is common. Significant amounts of blood penetrating LM to the chiasmatic, Sylvian, or interhemispheric cisterns should be viewed with suspicion

2. a negative high-quality 4-vessel cerebral angiogram[108] (radiographic vasospasm is common, and does not preclude the diagnosis nor does it mandate repeat angiography). NB: ≈ 3% of patients with a ruptured basilar bifurcation aneurysm meet the criteria of ▶ Table 89.6,[109] and therefore an *initial* arteriogram is mandatory

Table 89.6 CT or MRI criteria for PNSAH[96,110]

1. epicenter of hemorrhage immediately anterior to brainstem (interpeduncular or prepontine cistern)
2. there may be extension into anterior part of ambient cistern or basal part of the Sylvian fissure
3. absence of complete filling of anterior interhemispheric fissure
4. no more than minute amounts of blood in lateral portion of Sylvian fissure
5. absence of frank intraventricular hemorrhage (small amounts of blood sedimenting in the occipital horns of the lateral ventricles is permissible)

3. appropriate clinical picture: no loss of consciousness, no sentinel H/A, SAH grade 1 or 2 (H&H or WFNS grading scale) (p. 1424), and absence of drug use. Variance from this should raise suspicion of alternate pathogenesis

A more stringent set of anatomic criteria (▶ Table 89.7) showed excellent inter-observer agreement (97.2%) in PNSAH. Additionally, no aneurysms were identified on catheter angiography when the anatomical criteria were met.[111]

Table 89.7 Alternative anatomic CT criteria for PNSAH[111]

- epicenter of bleeding located immediately anterior to and in contact with the brainstem in the prepontine, interpeduncular, or posterior suprasellar cistern
- blood limited to the prepontine, interpeduncular, suprasellar, crural, ambient, and/or quadrigeminal cisterns and/or cisterna magna
- NO extension of blood into the Sylvian or interhemispheric fissures
- intraventricular blood limited to incomplete filling of the fourth ventricle and occipital horns of the lateral ventricles
- no intraparenchymal blood

89.9.6 Repeat angiography

Controversial. Angiography carries ≈ 0.2–0.5% risk of permanent neurologic deficit in this population.[90] Most experts agree that repeat angiography is not indicated in patients meeting the criteria of PNSAH[89,108] (although others recommend repeat angiography in all surgical candidates[87,112]). One should probably repeat the study if any uncertainty exists or if there is a history of a condition associated with increased risk of cerebral aneurysms.[96]

89.9.7 Treatment

Optimal treatment is not known with certainty. The low risk of rebleeding and delayed ischemia suggests that extreme measures are not indicated. The following recommendations are made[90,96] (period not specified):
1. symptomatic treatment
2. cardiac monitoring
3. electrolyte monitoring for hyponatremia
4. follow patient clinically (and if appropriate, with repeat imaging studies) to rule out hydrocephalus (transient ventricular enlargement is common; however, hydrocephalus requiring shunting is rare (only ≈ 1%)[90])
5. ✖ *not* recommended
   a) hyperdynamic therapy
   b) calcium channel blockers: use has not been investigated in PNSAH, but is probably not warranted due to low incidence of vasospasm and should be discontinued when normal angiographic findings are documented[96]
   c) activity restrictions (except in cases of increasing H/A with mobilization)
   d) antiseizure medications
   e) reduction of blood pressure below normal
   f) surgical exploration

89.9.8 Long-term implications

In one study,[113] 160 patients with PNSAH were contacted for "long term" follow-up (mean 7.5 years, range 1–23). There were no new episodes of SAH in this cohort. Furthermore, the mortality was not elevated above that of the general population. Based on this, the authors concluded that no restrictions should be placed on these patients by physicians or health or life insurance providers.

Absent any long-term prospective study, there is no consensus. Routine repeated vascular workup is not the standard of care. If it is desired to reassess the patient for some specific reason, catheter angiography is almost certainly not indicated (due to the risks and the low yield); here, CTA might be considered. Avoiding HTN, as for the general population, seems reasonable.

References

[1] Tew JM, Thompson RA, Green JR. Guidelines for Management and Surgical Treatment of Intracranial Aneurysms. In: Controversies in Neurology. New York: Raven Press; 1983:139–154

[2] Wirth FP. Surgical Treatment of Incidental Intracranial Aneurysms. Clin Neurosurg. 1986; 33:125–135

[3] Jane JA, Kassell NF, Torner JC, et al. The Natural History of Aneurysms and AVMs. J Neurosurg. 1985; 62:321–323

[4] The International Study Group of Unruptured Intracranial Aneurysms Investigators (ISUIA). Unruptured Intracranial Aneurysms - Risk of Rupture and Risks of Surgical Intervention. New England Journal of Medicine. 1998; 339:1725–1733

[5] Ishibashi T, Murayama Y, Urashima M, et al. Unruptured intracranial aneurysms: incidence of rupture and risk factors. Stroke. 2009; 40:313–316

[6] Yasui N, Suzuki A, Nishimura H, et al. Long-Term Follow-Up Study of Unruptured Intracranial Aneurysms. Neurosurgery. 1997; 40:1155–1160

[7] Sonobe M, Yamazaki T, Yonekura M, et al. Small unruptured intracranial aneurysm verification study: SUAVe study, Japan. Stroke. 2010; 41:1969–1977

[8] Juvela S, Poussa K, Lehto H, et al. Natural history of unruptured intracranial aneurysms: a long-term follow-up study. Stroke. 2013; 44:2414–2421

[9] Lee EJ, Lee HJ, Hyun MK, et al. Rupture rate for patients with untreated unruptured intracranial aneurysms in South Korea during 2006-2009. J Neurosurg. 2012; 117:53–59

[10] Mahaney KB, Brown RD,Jr, Meissner I, et al. Age-related differences in unruptured intracranial aneurysms: 1-year outcomes. J Neurosurg. 2014; 121:1024–1038

[11] Greving JP, Wermer MJ, Brown RD,Jr, et al. Development of the PHASES score for prediction of risk of rupture of intracranial aneurysms: a pooled analysis of six prospective cohort studies. Lancet Neurol. 2014; 13:59–66

[12] Broderick JP, Brown RD,Jr, Sauerbeck L, et al. Greater rupture risk for familial as compared to sporadic unruptured intracranial aneurysms. Stroke. 2009; 40:1952–1957

[13] Juvela S, Porras M, Poussa K. Natural history of unruptured intracranial aneurysms: probability of and risk factors for aneurysm rupture. J Neurosurg. 2000; 93:379–387

[14] Tsutsumi K, Ueki K, Morita A, et al. Risk of rupture from incidental cerebral aneurysms. J Neurosurg. 2000; 93:550–553

[15] Morita A, Kirino T, Hashi K, et al. The natural course of unruptured cerebral aneurysms in a Japanese cohort. New England Journal of Medicine. 2012; 366:2474–2482

[16] Orz Y, AlYamany M. The impact of size and location on rupture of intracranial aneurysms. Asian J Neurosurg. 2015; 10:26–31

[17] Joo SW, Lee SI, Noh SJ, et al. What Is the Significance of a Large Number of Ruptured Aneurysms Smaller than 7 mm in Diameter? J Korean Neurosurg Soc. 2009; 45:85–89

[18] Hoh BL, Sistrom CL, Firment CS, et al. Bottleneck factor and height-width ratio: association with ruptured aneurysms in patients with multiple cerebral aneurysms. Neurosurgery. 2007; 61:716–22; discussion 722-3

[19] Dhar S, Tremmel M, Mocco J, et al. Morphology parameters for intracranial aneurysm rupture risk assessment. Neurosurgery. 2008; 63:185–96; discussion 196-7

[20] Rahman M, Smietana J, Hauck E, et al. Size ratio correlates with intracranial aneurysm rupture status: a prospective study. Stroke. 2010; 41:916–920

[21] Wiebers DO, Whisnant JP, Huston J,3rd, et al. Unruptured intracranial aneurysms: natural history, clinical outcome, and risks of surgical and endovascular treatment. Lancet. 2003; 362:103–110

[22] Wermer MJ, van der Schaaf I C, Velthuis BK, et al. Yield of short-term follow-up CT/MR angiography for small aneurysms detected at screening. Stroke. 2006; 37:414–418

[23] van Crevel H, Habbema JDF, Braakman R. Decision Analysis of the Management of Incidental Intracranial Saccular Aneurysms. Neurology. 1986; 36:1335–1339

[24] Johnston SC, Gress DR, Kahn JG. Which Unruptured Cerebral Aneurysms Should be Treated? A Cost-Utility Analysis. Neurology. 1999; 52:1806–1815

[25] Bederson JB, Awad IA, Wiebers DO, et al. Recommendations for the management of patients with unruptured intracranial aneurysms. A statement for healthcare professionals from the Stroke Council of the American Heart Association. Circulation. 2000; 102:2300–2308

[26] Solomon RA, Correll JW. Rupture of a Previously Documented Asymptomatic Aneurysm Enhances the Argument for Prophylactic Surgical Intervention. Surg Neurol. 1988; 30:321–323

[27] Ausman JI, Diaz FG, Malik GM, et al. Management of Cerebral Aneurysms: Further Facts and Additional Myths. Surg Neurol. 1989; 32:21–35

[28] Ojemann RG. Management of the Unruptured Intracranial Aneurysm. N Engl J Med. 1981; 304:725–726

[29] Wiebers DO, Whisnant JP, Sundt TM, et al. The Significance of Unruptured Intracranial Saccular Aneurysms. J Neurosurg. 1987; 66:23–29

[30] Etminan N, Brown RD,Jr, Beseoglu K, et al. The unruptured intracranial aneurysm treatment score: a multidisciplinary consensus. Neurology. 2015; 85:881–889

[31] Ravindra VM, de Havenon A, Gooldy TC, et al. Validation of the unruptured intracranial aneurysm treatment score: comparison with real-world cerebrovascular practice. J Neurosurg. 2018; 129:100–106

[32] Brown RD,Jr, Broderick JP. Unruptured intracranial aneurysms: epidemiology, natural history, management options, and familial screening. Lancet Neurol. 2014; 13:393–404

[33] Villablanca JP, Duckwiler GR, Jahan R, et al. Natural history of asymptomatic unruptured cerebral aneurysms evaluated at CT angiography: growth and rupture incidence and correlation with epidemiologic risk factors. Radiology. 2013; 269:258–265

[34] Burns JD, Huston J,3rd, Layton KF, et al. Intracranial aneurysm enlargement on serial magnetic resonance angiography: frequency and risk factors. Stroke. 2009; 40:406–411

[35] Miyazawa N, Akiyama I, Yamagata Z. Risk factors for growth of unruptured intracranial aneurysms: follow-up study by serial 0.5-T magnetic resonance angiography. Neurosurgery. 2006; 58:1047–53; discussion 1047-53

[36] Matsubara S, Hadeishi H, Suzuki A, et al. Incidence and risk factors for the growth of unruptured cerebral aneurysms: observation using serial computerized tomography angiography. J Neurosurg. 2004; 101:908–914

[37] Inoue T, Shimizu H, Fujimura M, et al. Annual rupture risk of growing unruptured cerebral aneurysms detected by magnetic resonance angiography. J Neurosurg. 2012; 117:20–25

[38] Wilkins RH, Rengachary SS. Neurosurgery. New York 1985

[39] Day AL. Clinicoanatomic Features of Supraclinoid Aneurysms. Clinical Neurosurgery. 1988; 36:256–274

[40] Raps EC, Galetta SL, Solomon RA, et al. The Clinical Spectrum of Unruptured Intracranial Aneurysms. Archives of Neurology. 1993; 50:265–268

[41] Sano H, Jain VK, Kato Y, et al. Bilateral Giant Intracavernous Aneurysms: Technique of Unilateral Operation. Surgical Neurology. 1988; 29:35–38

[42] Hamada H, Endo S, Fukuda O, et al. Giant Aneurysm in the Cavernous Sinus Causing Subarachnoid Hemorrhage 13 Years After Detection: A Case Report. Surgical Neurology. 1996; 45:143–146

89

89

[43] Kupersmith MJ, Hurst R, Berenstein A, et al. The Benign Course of Cavernous Carotid Artery Aneurysms. Journal of Neurosurgery. 1992; 77:690–693

[44] White JA, Horowitz MB, Samson D. Dural Waisting as a Sign of Subarachnoid Extension of Cavernous Carotid Aneurysms: A Follow-Up Case Report. Surgical Neurology. 1999; 52:607–610

[45] Ostergaard JR, Hog E. Incidence of Multiple Intracranial Aneurysms. J Neurosurg. 1985; 63:49–55

[46] Hackney DB, Lesnick JE, Zimmerman RA, et al. MR Identification of Bleeding Site in Subarachnoid Hemorrhage with Multiple Intracranial Aneurysms. J Comput Assist Tomogr. 1986; 10:878–880

[47] Karttunen AI, Jartti PH, Ukkola VA, et al. Value of the quantity and distribution of subarachnoid haemorrhage on CT in the localization of a ruptured cerebral aneurysm. Acta Neurochirurgica (Wien). 2003; 145:655–61; discussion 661

[48] Hino A, Fujimoto M, Iwamoto Y, et al. False localization of rupture site in patients with multiple cerebral aneurysms and subarachnoid hemorrhage. Neurosurgery. 2000; 46:825–830

[49] Kissela BM, Sauerbeck L, Woo D, et al. Subarachnoid hemorrhage: a preventable disease with a heritable component. Stroke. 2002; 33:1321–1326

[50] Ronkainen A, Hernesniemi J, Puranen M, et al. Familial Intracranial Aneurysms. Lancet. 1997; 349:380–384

[51] Ronkainen A, Miettinen H, Karkola K, et al. Risk of harboring an unruptured intracranial aneurysm. Stroke. 1998; 29:359–362

[52] Fairburn B. "Twin" Intracranial Aneurysms Causing Subarachnoid Hemorrhage in Identical Twins. Br Med J. 1973; 1:210–211

[53] Schon F, Marshall J. Subarachnoid Hemorrhage in Identical Twins. J Neurol Neurosurg Psychiatry. 1984; 47:81–83

[54] Toglia IU, Samii AR. Familial Intracranial Aneurysms. Dis Nerv Syst. 1972; 33:611–613

[55] Norrgard O, Angquist K-A, Fodstad H, et al. Intracranial Aneurysms and Heredity. Neurosurgery. 1987; 20:236–239

[56] Lozano AM, Leblanc R. Familial Intracranial Aneurysms. J Neurosurg. 1987; 66:522–528

[57] Andrews RJ. Intracranial Aneurysms: Characteristics of Aneurysms in Siblings. New England Journal of Medicine. 1977; 279

[58] Brisman R, Abbassioun K. Familial Intracranial Aneurysms. J Neurosurg. 1971; 34:678–682

[59] Schievink WI, Limburg M, Dreisen JJR, et al. Screening for Unruptured Familial Intracranial Aneurysms: Subarachnoid Hemorrhage 2 Years After Angiography Negative for Aneurysms. Neurosurgery. 1991; 29:434–438

[60] Vanninen RL, Hernesnieni JA, Puranen MI, et al. Magnetic Resonance Angiographic Screening for Asymptomatic Intracranial Aneurysms: The Problem of False Negatives: Technical Case Report. Neurosurgery. 1996; 38:838–841

[61] Alg VS, Sofat R, Houlden H, et al. Genetic risk factors for intracranial aneurysms: a meta-analysis in more than 116,000 individuals. Neurology. 2013; 80:2154–2165

[62] Benoit BG, Wortzman G. Traumatic Cerebral Aneurysms: Clinical Features and Natural History. J Neurol Neurosurg Psychiatry. 1973; 36:127–138

[63] Parkinson D, West M. Traumatic Intracranial Aneurysms. Journal of Neurosurgery. 1980; 52:11–20

[64] Morard M, de Tribolet N. Traumatic Aneurysm of the Posterior Inferior Cerebellar Artery: Case Report. Neurosurgery. 1991; 29:438–441

[65] Buckingham MJ, Crone KR, Ball WS, et al. Traumatic Intracranial Aneurysms in Childhood: Two Cases and a Review of the Literature. Neurosurgery. 1988; 22:398–408

[66] Kieck CF, de Villiers JC. Vascular Lesions due to Transcranial Stab Wounds. J Neurosurg. 1984; 60:42–46

[67] Handa J, Handa H. Severe Epistaxis caused by Traumatic Aneurysm of Cavernous Carotid Artery. Surg Neurol. 1976; 5:241–243

[68] Maurer JJ, Mills M, German WJ. Triad of unilateral blindness, orbital fractures and massive epistaxis after head injury. J Neurosurg. 1961; 18:937–949

[69] Ding MX. Traumatic Aneurysm of the Intracavernous Part of the Internal Carotid Artery Presenting with Epistaxis. Case Report. Surgical Neurology. 1988; 30:65–67

[70] Ahuja A, Guterkman LR, Hopkins LN. Carotid Cavernous Fistula and False Aneurysm of the Cavernous Carotid Artery: Complications of Transsphenoidal Surgery. Neurosurgery. 1992; 31:774–779

[71] Bohmfalk GL, Story JL, Wissinger JP, et al. Bacterial Intracranial Aneurysm. Journal of Neurosurgery. 1978; 48:369–382

[72] Horten BC, Abbott GF, Porro RS. Fungal Aneurysms of Intracranial Vessels. Archives of Neurology. 1976; 33:577–579

[73] Schmidek HH, Sweet WH. Operative Neurosurgical Techniques. New York 1982

[74] Pootrakul A, Carter LP. Bacterial Intracranial Aneurysm: Importance of Sequential Angiography. Surgical Neurology. 1982; 17:429–431

[75] Morawetz RB, Karp RB. Evolution and Resolution of Intracranial Bacterial (Mycotic) Aneurysms. Neurosurgery. 1984; 15:43–49

[76] Bingham WF. Treatment of Mycotic Intracranial Aneurysms. Journal of Neurosurgery. 1977; 46:428–437

[77] Drake CG. Giant Intracranial Aneurysms: Experience with Surgical Treatment in 174 Patients. Clin Neurosurg. 1979; 26:12–95

[78] Drake CG. Ligation of the Vertebral (Unilateral or Bilateral) or Basilar Artery in the Treatment of Large Intracranial Aneurysms. Journal of Neurosurgery. 1975; 43:255–274

[79] Cuvinciuc V, Viguier A, Calviere L, et al. Isolated acute nontraumatic cortical subarachnoid hemorrhage. AJNR Am J Neuroradiol. 2010; 31:1355–1362

[80] Call GK, Fleming MC, Sealfon S, et al. Reversible cerebral segmental vasoconstriction. Stroke. 1988; 19:1159–1170

[81] Mehdi A, Hajj-Ali RA. Reversible cerebral vasoconstriction syndrome: a comprehensive update. Curr Pain Headache Rep. 2014; 18. DOI: 10.1007/s11916-014-0443-2

[82] Ducros A. Reversible cerebral vasoconstriction syndrome. Lancet Neurol. 2012; 11:906–917

[83] Hayward RD, O'Reilly GVA. Intracerebral Hemorrhage: Accuracy of Computerized Transverse Axial Scanning in Predicting the Underlying Etiology. Lancet. 1976; 1:1–6

[84] Cioffi F, Pasqualin A, Cavazzani P, et al. Subarachnoid Hemorrhage of Unknown Origin: Clinical and Tomographical Aspects. Acta Neurochirurgica. 1989; 97:31–39

[85] Iwanaga H, Wakai S, Ochiai C, et al. Ruptured Cerebral Aneurysms Missed by Initial Angiographic Study. Neurosurgery. 1990; 27:45–51

[86] Farres MT, Ferraz-Leite H, Schindler E, et al. Spontaneous Subarachnoid Hemorrhage with Negative Angiography: CT Findings. Journal of Computer Assisted Tomography. 1992; 16:534–537

[87] Tatter SB, Crowell RM, Ogilvy CS. Aneurysmal and Microaneurysmal 'Angiogram Negative' Subarachnoid Hemorrhage. Neurosurgery. 1995; 37:48–55

[88] Nishioka H, Torner JC, Graf CJ, et al. Cooperative Study of Intracranial Aneurysms and Subarachnoid Hemorrhage: III. Subarachnoid Hemorrhage of Undetermined Etiology. Arch Neurol. 1984 41:1147–1151

[89] Kaim A, Proske M, Kirsch E, et al. Value of Repeat Angiography in Cases of Unexplained Subarachnoid Hemorrhage (SAH). Acta Neurol Scand. 1996 93:366–373

[90] Schwartz TH, Solomon RA. Perimesencephalic Nonaneurysmal Subarachnoid Hemorrhage: Review of the Literature. Neurosurgery. 1996 39:433–440

[91] Rinkel GJE, van Gijn J, Wijdicks EFM. Subarachnoid Hemorrhage Without Detectable Aneurysm: A Review of the Causes. Stroke. 1993; 24:1403–1409

[92] van Gijn J, van Dongen KJ, Vermeulen M, et al. Perimesencephalic Hemorrhage. A Nonaneurysmal and Benign Form of Subarachnoid Hemorrhage. Neurology. 1985; 35:493–497

[93] Schievink WI, Wijdicks EFM. Pretruncal Subarachnoid Hemorrhage: An Anatomically Correct Description of the Perimesencephalic Subarachnoid Hemorrhage. Stroke. 1997; 28

[94] van Calenbergh F, Plets C, Goffin J, et al. Nonaneurysmal Subarachnoid Hemorrhage: Prevalence of Perimesencephalic Hemorrhage in a Consecutive Series. Surgical Neurology. 1993; 39:320–323

[95] Rinkel GJE, Wijdicks EFM, Vermeulen M, et al. Outcome in Perimesencephalic (Nonaneurysmal) Subarachnoid Hemorrhage: A Follow-Up Study in 37 Patients. Neurology. 1990; 40:1130–1132

[96] Wijdicks EFM, Schievink WI, Miller GM. Pretruncal Nonaneurysmal Subarachnoid Hemorrhage. Mayo Clinic Proceedings. 1998; 73:745–752

[97] Wijdicks EFM, Schievink WI. Perimesencephalic Nonaneurysmal Subarachnoid Hemorrhage: First Hint of a Cause? Neurology. 1997; 49:634–636

[98] Buyukkaya R, Yildirim N, Cebeci H, et al. The relationship between perimesencephalic subarachnoid hemorrhage and deep venous system drainage pattern and calibrations. Clin Imaging. 2014; 38:226–230

[99] Sabatino G, Della Pepa GM, Scerrati A, et al. Anatomical variants of the basal vein of Rosenthal: prevalence in idiopathic subarachnoid hemorrhage. Acta Neurochir (Wien). 2014; 156:45–51

[100] Sangra MS, Teasdale E, Siddiqui MA, et al. Perimesencephalic nonaneurysmal subarachnoid hemorrhage caused by jugular venous occlusion: case report. Neurosurgery. 2008; 63:E1202–3; discussion E1203

[101] Mathews MS, Brown D, Brant-Zawadzki M. Perimesencephalic nonaneurysmal hemorrhage associated with vein of Galen stenosis. Neurology. 2008; 70:2410–2411

[102] Lansberg MG. Concurrent presentation of perimesencephalic subarachnoid hemorrhage and ischemic stroke. J Stroke Cerebrovasc Dis. 2008; 17:248–250

[103] Rinkel GJE, Wijdicks EFM, Hasan D, et al. Outcome in Patients with Subarachnoid Hemorrhage and Negative Angiography According to Pattern of Hemorrhage on Computed Tomography. Lancet. 1991; 338:964–968

[104] Liliequist B. The Subarachnoid Cisterns: An Anatomic and Roentgenologic Study. Acta Radiol (Stockh). 1959; 185:1–108

[105] Yasargil MG. Microneurosurgery. New York: Thieme-Stratton Inc.; 1985

[106] Matsuno H, Rhoton AL, Peace D. Microsurgical Anatomy of the Posterior Fossa Cisterns. Neurosurgery. 1988; 23:58–80

[107] Brasil AVB, Schneider FL. Anatomy of Liliequist's Membrane. Neurosurgery. 1993; 32:956–961

[108] Adams HP, Gordon DL. Nonaneurysmal Subarachnoid Hemorrhage. Annals of Neurology. 1991; 29:461–462

[109] Pinto AN, Ferro JM, Canhao P, et al. How Often is a Perimesencephalic Subarachnoid Hemorrhage CT Pattern Caused by Ruptured Aneurysms? Acta Neurochirurgica. 1993; 124:79–81

[110] Rinkel GJE, Wijdicks EFM, Vermeulen M, et al. Nonaneurysmal Perimesencephalic Subarachnoid Hemorrhage: CT and MR Patterns that Differ from Aneurysmal Rupture. American Journal of Neuroradiology. 1991; 12:829–834

[111] Wallace AN, Vyhmeister R, Dines JN, et al. Evaluation of an anatomic definition of non-aneurysmal perimesencephalic subarachnoid hemorrhage. J Neurointerv Surg. 2015. DOI: 10.1136/neurintsurg-2015-011680

[112] Cloft HJ, Kallmes DF, Dion JE. A Second Look at the Second-Look Angiogram in Cases of Subarachnoid Hemorrhage. Radiology. 1997; 205:323–324

[113] Greebe P, Rinkel GJ. Life expectancy after perimesencephalic subarachnoid hemorrhage. Stroke. 2007; 38:1222–1224

89

Part XVIII

Vascular Malformations

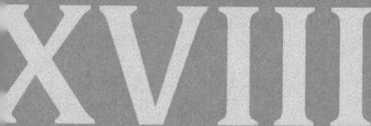

90 Vascular Malformations

90.1 Vascular malformations – general information and classification

This designation encompasses a number of non-neoplastic vascular lesions of the CNS. The four types originally described by McCormick in 1966 are shown in ▶ Table 90.1.[1]

Possible additional categories:

1. direct fistula AKA arteriovenous fistula (AV- fistula, *not* AVM). Single or multiple dilated arterioles that connect directly to a vein *without* a nidus. These are high-flow, high-pressure. Low incidence of hemorrhage. Usually amenable to interventional neuroradiological procedures. Examples include:
   a) vein of Galen malformation (aneurysm) (p. 1518)
   b) dural AVM (p. 1514)
   c) carotid-cavernous fistula (p. 1519)
2. mixed or unclassified angiomas: 11% of AOVM[2]

Table 90.1 4 classic types of vascular malformation

Type	Prevalence (%)
arteriovenous malformation (AVM)[a]	44–60
cavernous malformation (p. 1525)	19–31
capillary telangiectasia (p. 1525)	4–12
developmental venous anomaly (DVA) (p. 1512)—formerly venous angioma	9–10

[a]Sometimes referred to as "pial AVM" to distinguish it e.g., from dural AVM

90.2 Arteriovenous malformation (AVM)

90.2.1 General information

Key concepts

- dilated arteries and veins with dysplastic vessels. Arterial blood flows directly between them with no capillary bed and no intervening neural parenchyma (brain) in the nidus
- may be congenital, many are acquired
- AVMs are medium-to-high pressure and high-flow
- usually presents with hemorrhage, less often with seizures
- risk of 1st-time hemorrhage is ≈ 1%/yr. Prognostic factors that alter this risk are uncertain
- risk of recurrent ICH is 5%/year. Increasing age, deep venous drainage, feeding artery aneurysms and female gender may elevate this risk
- 5-year risk of 1st seizure is 8% for unruptured AVM. 5-year risk of epilepsy after a 1st seizure is 58%
- aneurysms on feeding arteries are common and are often the source of the hemorrhage
- demonstrable on angiography, MRI, or CT (especially with contrast)
- main treatment options (when expectant management not elected):
  - surgical excision: often curative. Surgical risk can be estimated by Spetzler-Martin grade (p. 1509)
  - stereotactic radiosurgery (SRS): obliterates 70–80% of AVMs over 1–3 years. Usually reserved for deep lesions < 3 cm dia
  - endovascular embolization: curative in select cases. Usually used as an adjunct to surgery or SRS, for high-risk angiographic entities, or to palliate high-flow symptoms

90.2.2 Description

A collection of dysplastic dilated blood vessels (neither arteries nor veins) wherein arterial blood flows directly into draining veins without the normal interposed capillary beds. AVMs are usually congenital, tend to enlarge somewhat with age, and often progress from low-flow juvenile lesions at birth to medium-to-high-flow high-pressure lesions in adulthood. AVMs appear grossly as a "tangle" of vessels, often with a fairly well-circumscribed center (the nidus) which contains no brain parenchyma, with draining "red veins" (usually on the surface) containing oxygenated blood under higher pressure than in normal veins.

May be classified as:
1. parenchymal AVMs (discussed below). Subclassified as:
   a) pial
   b) subcortical
   c) paraventricular
   d) combined
2. pure dural AVM (p. 1514)
3. mixed parenchymal and dural (rare)

90.2.3 Epidemiology

Prevalence: usually quoted as 0.14%. Asymptomatic prevalence on brain MRIs: 0.05%.[3]
   Incidence of detected asymptomatic or symptomatic AVMs: ≈ 1.3 per 100,000 person-years.[3]
   Slight male preponderance.
A few types are known to be hereditary. Other types are part of known hereditary syndromes: 15–20% of patients with Osler-Weber-Rendu syndrome (hereditary hemorrhagic telangiectasia) (p. 1524) have cerebral AVMs (the most common genetic cause of AVMs).
   Comparison to aneurysms: the average age of patients diagnosed with AVMs is ≈ 33 yrs, which is ≈ 10 yrs younger than for aneurysms.[4] 64% of AVMs are diagnosed before age 40 (cf. 26% for aneurysms).

90

90.2.4 Presentation

1. hemorrhage (most common): 58%[3] (compared to 92% for aneurysms) (see below)
2. seizures: 34%[3]
3. remainder: 8%
   a) mass effect: e.g., trigeminal neuralgia due to CPA AVM
   b) ischemia: by steal
   c) H/A: rare. AVMs may occasionally be associated with migraines. Occipital AVMs may present with visual disturbance (typically hemianopsia or quadrantanopsia) and H/A that are indistinguishable from migraine[5]
   d) bruit: especially with dural AVMs (p. 1514)
   e) increased ICP
   f) findings limited almost exclusively to peds, usually with large midline AVMs that drain into an enlarged vein of Galen ("vein of Galen malformation" (p. 1518)):
      • hydrocephalus with macrocephaly: due to compression of Sylvian aqueduct by enlarged vein of Galen or to increased venous pressure
      • congestive heart failure with cardiomegaly
      • prominence of forehead veins (due to increased venous pressure)

90.2.5 Hemorrhage

General information

Most data are from observational research studies, so the true natural history in unselected patients is not known.[6] Peak age for hemorrhage is between 15 and 20 yrs.[7] See Pregnancy & intracranial hemorrhage (p. 1425) for a discussion of that topic.
   Morbidity and mortality from AVM hemorrhage: data varies widely. With each bleed, an estimate is 10% mortality, 30–50% morbidity[8] (neurological deficit). ICH from AVMs tend to be more benign than primary ICH.[3]

Hemorrhage location with AVMs

1. intraparenchymal (ICH): 82% (the most common site of bleeding)[9]

2. intraventricular hemorrhage:
    a) usually accompanied by ICH as the result of rupture of the ICH into the ventricle
    b) pure IVH (with no ICH) may indicate an intraventricular AVM
3. subarachnoid: SAH may also be due to rupture of an aneurysm on a feeding artery (common with AVMs)
4. subdural: uncommon. May be the source of a spontaneous SDH (p. 1088)

Annual risk of hemorrhage

A subject of much study and conflicting results.

The oft-quoted annual risk is 2%[10] to 4%.[4] Based on the largest meta-analysis, the unselected annual risk of hemorrhage is 2.3% per year.[11] Factors that may influence the annual risk include the following.

▶ **Previous rupture.** The strongest prognosticator for future hemorrhage. 1.3% per year for unruptured AVMs, and 4.3% for (repeat) hemorrhage for ruptured AVMs at diagnosis.[11] The risk of rebleeding is highest within the first year (historically, results are conflicting).

▶ **Age** *at diagnosis.* 30% increase in risk per decade[11] (historically, results are conflicting).

▶ **Drainage pattern.** AVMs with exclusively deep venous drainage: 1.6–2.4-fold increase in annual risk.[11]

▶ **AVM size.** Conflicting information—an association is not found in larger cohorts. The contention was that small AVMs tend to present more often as hemorrhage than do large ones.[12,13] Small AVMs were thought to have higher pressure in the feeding arteries.[13]

▶ **Hemorrhage rate related to Spetzler-Martin grade.** Controversial. The S-M scale was devised for assessing *surgical risk* (not hemorage). Some studies show increased risk of hemorrhage with Spetzler-Martin (S-M) grade (p. 1509) 4–5 AVMs[14] (high grade), others studies show the opposite effect.

▶ **Combined risk factors.** A bingo sheet showing risk of bleeding based on history of prior bleeding, venous drainage pattern, and nidus location using data from Stapf et al is shown in ▶ Table 90.2 as an illustration (some results are conflicting).

Table 90.2 Annual average hemorrhage rates for various AVM subgroups[15]

Venous drainage	Nidus location	No prior hemorrhage	Prior hemorrhage
No deep venous drainage	Not deep	0.9%	4.5%
	Deep	3.1%	14.8%
Deep venous drainage	Not deep	2.4%	11.4%
	Deep	8.0%	34.4%

Lifetime risk of hemorrhage/recurrent hemorrhage

The risk of bleeding over the remainder of one's life is given by Eq (90.1); (this analysis assumes a constant risk of bleeding, ignoring influences of a previous bleed, AVM location, changes in risk with aging or pregnancy, etc.).

$$\text{risk of bleeding (at least once)} = 1 - (\text{annual risk of not bleeding})^{\text{expected years of remaining life}} \quad (90.1)$$

where the annual risk of not bleeding is equal to 1 – the annual risk of bleeding. For example, if a 3% annual risk of bleeding is used as an average, and the remaining life expectancy is 25 years, the result is as illustrated in Eq (90.2).

$$\text{risk of bleeding (at least once in 25 years)} = 1 - 0.97^{25} = 0.53 = 53\% \quad (90.2)$$

A simple first approximation to Eq (90.1) for an annual 3% risk of bleeding is given by Eq (90.3).

$$\text{risk of bleeding (at least once)} \approx 105 - \text{age in years} \quad (90.3)$$

▶ Table 90.3 shows the risk for various ages using Eq (90.1) (longevity is taken from insurance life-tables).

Table 90.3 Lifetime risk of hemorrhage[a]

Age at presentation	Estimated years to live[b]	Lifetime risk of hemorrhage		
		For 1% annual risk[c]	For 2% annual risk	For 3% annual risk
0	76	53%	78%	90%
15	62	46%	71%	85%
25	52	41%	65%	79%
35	43	35%	58%	73%
45	34	29%	50%	64%
55	25	22%	40%	53%
65	18	16%	30%	42%
75	11	10%	20%	28%
85	6	5.8%	11%	17%

[a]modified from reference[16]
[b]based on 1992 Preliminary Life tables prepared by Metropolitan Life Insurance Company
[c]1% annual risk is also presented because it may be applicable for incidental aneurysms (p.1486)

90.2.6 Seizures

The mechanism of seizure generation is unknown. The younger the patient at the time of diagnosis, the higher the risk of developing convulsions (▶ Table 90.4). AVM features with increased risk of seizures: temporal location, cortical involvement, nidus diameter > 3 cm.[3] Patients presenting with hemorrhage have 22% risk of developing epilepsy in 20 yrs.

Table 90.4 Risk of seizures with AVMs

Age at diagnosis (years)	20-year risk of developing seizures
10–19	44%
20–29	31%
30–60	6%

90.2.7 AVMs and aneurysms

7% of patients with AVMs have aneurysms. 75% of these are located on a major feeding artery (probably from increased flow).[12] These aneurysms may be classified into 1 of 5 types shown in ▶ Table 90.5. Aneurysms also may form within the nidus or on draining veins. When treating tandem AVMs and aneurysms, the symptomatic one is usually treated first (when feasible, both may be treated at the same operation).[17] If it is not clear which bled, the odds are that it was the aneurysm. Although a significant number (≈ 66%) of related aneurysms will regress following removal of the AVM, this does not always occur. In one series, none of the 9 associated aneurysms ruptured or enlarged following AVM removal.[17]

Table 90.5 Categories of aneurysms associated with AVMs[a] [17]

Type	Aneurysm location
I	proximal on ipsilateral major artery feeding AVM
IA	proximal on major artery related but contralateral to AVM
II	distal on superficial feeding artery
III	proximal or distal on deep feeding artery ("bizarre")
IV	on artery unrelated to AVM

[a]excludes intranidal and venous aneurysms

90.2.8 Evaluation

General information

Various imaging modalities provide information that are additive when analyzed in combination.

Definitive diagnosis and aspects of treatment planning are obtained with catheter angiography.

Cross-section-based modalities (CT, CTA, MRI, MRA) provide important information about adjacent brain that is not obtained with catheter angiography.

MRI and MRA approach CT/CTA in detecting AVMs in the setting of ICH, but MRI/MRA may not show important angiogenic features demonstrable on CTA.

CT

Unenhanced brain CT is the best study to rule out acute hemorrhage (>90% sensitivity). It can miss some AVMs, but can demonstrate calcifications within the lesion or increased density of the nidus. Adding a contrast CT will show enhancement within the vessels, and can delineate the nidus (dense central area of an AVM).

CT angiography (CTA)

Pros: excellent spatial resolution, fast, minimally invasive, fewer contraindications than MRI/MRA.

Cons: involves ionizing radiation, iodine carries risk of allergic reaction in sensitized individuals and risk of renal injury.

In patients with ICH, sensitivity for detecting AVM is 84–100% and specificity is 77–100%[3,18] (comparable to catheter angiography).

MRI

Characteristics of AVM on MRI:

1. flow void on T1WI or T2WI within the AVM
2. feeding arteries
3. draining veins
4. increased intensity on partial flip-angle (to differentiate signal dropout on T1WI or T2WI from calcium)
5. significant edema around the lesion may indicate a tumor that has bled rather than an AVM
6. T2* GRE (gradient echo sequences) or susceptibility-weighted imaging (SWI) help demonstrate surrounding hemosiderin, which suggests a previous significant hemorrhage
7. a complete ring of low density (due to hemosiderin) surrounding the lesion suggests AVM over neoplasm

Magnetic resonance angiography (MRA)

Cons: both time-of-flight and contrast bolus MRA are more limited in detecting small vessels (<1 mm dia), aneurysms, small AVMs (nidus <10 mm), and venous outflow anatomy, all of which assume greater importance in treatment planning.

Catheter angiography

Characteristics of AVM on angiography:

1. tangle of vessels
2. large feeding artery
3. large draining veins
4. draining veins are visualized in the same images as arteries (arterial phase)

Most but not all AVMs show up on angiography. Few cavernous malformations and venous angiomas do (see Angiographically occult vascular malformations (p. 1524)).

AVM grading scales

Surgical grading scales for AVMs

This section presents AVM grading scales (Spetzler-Martin and Lawton-Young) for use with surgical treatment. For treatment with stereotactic radiosurgery, Virginia Radiosurgery AVM Scale (VRAS) (▶ Table 115.3) is preferable.

Spetzler-Martin (S-M) grade of AVMs

The Spetzler-Martin grading scale is the most widely used and highly validated classification for estimating *the risk of surgical resection* of an AVM.[3,19] Often requires catheter angiography and cross-sectional imaging (CT or MRI) to determine the grade.

S-M Grade = sum of points from ▶ Table 90.6, ranges from 1 to 5. A separate grade 6 is reserved for untreatable lesions (by any means: surgery, SRS...), resection of these would almost unavoidably be associated with disabling deficit or death. May not be applicable to pediatrics (juvenile AVMs are immature and the margins are less well defined; AVMs mature at ≈ age 18 yrs and tend to become more compact).

Table 90.6 Spetzler-Martin AVM grading system[21]

Graded feature	Criteria	Points	Score
Size[a]	small (<3 cm)	1	(1 - 3)
	medium (3–6 cm)	2	
	large (>6 cm)	3	
Eloquence of adjacent brain[b]	non-eloquent	0	(0 - 1)
	eloquent	1	
Pattern of venous drainage[c]	superficial only	0	(0 - 1)
	deep	1	
Spetzler-Martin grade → TOTAL			(1 - 5)

[a]largest diameter of nidus on non-magnified angiogram (is related to and therefore implicitly includes other factors relating to difficulty of AVM excision, e.g., number of feeding arteries, degree of steal, etc.)
[b]eloquent brain[22]: sensorimotor, language, and visual cortex; hypothalamus and thalamus; internal capsule; brainstem; cerebellar peduncles; deep cerebellar nuclei
[c]considered superficial if all drainage is through cortical venous system; considered deep if any or all is through deep veins (e.g., internal cerebral vein, basal vein, or pre-central cerebellar vein)

90

Based on the Spetzler-Martin grade: 100 consecutive cases operated by an expert (Spetzler) had the outcomes shown in ▶ Table 90.7 (no deaths). The majority of AVMs presenting to academic medical centers are S-M grade III.[20]

Table 90.7 Surgical outcome by Spetzler-Martin grade operated on by Spetzler

Grade	No.	No deficit		Minor deficit[a]		Major deficit[b]		Poor outcome[c]
1	23	23	(100%)	0		0		4%
2	21	20	(95%)	1	(5%)	0		10%
3	25	21	(84%)	3	(12%)	1	(4%)	18%
4	15	11	(73%)	3	(20%)	1	(7%)	31%
5	16	11	(69%)	3	(19%)	2	(12%)	37%

[a]minor deficit: mild brainstem deficit, mild aphasia, mild ataxia
[b]major deficit: hemiparesis, increased aphasia, homonymous hemianopsia
[c]pooled analysis published in 2011[23]

★ Spetzler has since published this 3-tiered management recommendation scheme[23]:
- Class A (S-M Grade I & II): surgical resection
- Class B (S-M Grade III): multimodality treatment (also see Lawton-Young scale below)
- Class C (S-M Grade IV & V): follow clinically and repeat angiogram every 5 years. Treatment only for progressive neurologic deficit, steal-related symptoms, or aneurysms identified on surveillance angiograms

Lawton-Young supplementary grading scale for AVMs

The Lawton-Young (L-Y) supplementary grading scale[24] is a validated scale[25] that enhances the S-M grade. The full weighted model (combining the S-M & L-Y grade) is shown in the reference.[24] The simplified model is shown in ▶ Table 90.8 and the L-Y score is the sum of the points. The accuracy of the L-Y model was almost as good as the full weighted model, and either one was better than the S-M grade at predicting changes in modified Rankin Scale (mRS) score (▶ Table 98.5) postoperatively. This model is derived only using operated AVMs, and tended to be more helpful when there was a

Table 90.8 Lawton-Young supplementary grading scale[24]

Graded feature		Points	Score
Patient age	< 20 years	1	(1 - 3)
	20–40 years	2	
	> 40 years	3	
Presentation	ruptured	0	(0 - 1)
	unruptured	1	
Pattern of venous drainage	compact nidus	0	(0 - 1)
	diffuse nidus	1	
L-Y score → TOTAL			(1 - 5)

mismatch with the S-M grade: a S-M grade III with a low L-Y score behaved more like a S-M II AVM, whereas a S-M grade III AVM with a high L-Y grade AVM behaved more like a S-M grade IV.[3]

90.2.9 Management

1. for patients presenting with nontraumatic ICH with clinical or radiologic suspicion for underlying cause, CTA, MRA, & catheter angiography can be useful to evaluate for AVM (Level II[3])
2. the initial hemorrhage should be managed in accordance with 2015 AHA ICH management guidelines (p. 1619) (covers HTN, seizures, correction of coagulopathy…)
   • surgical evacuation of an ICH should be undertaken if indicated regardless of whether or not there is an AVM. Small superficial AVMs can be removed at the time of emergency surgery
   • the resection of larger, deep AVMs may be deferred for 2–6 weeks to allow a reduction of brain swelling and better evaluation of the residual AVM angiographically and surgically
3. for AVMs that have ruptured:
   • surgical resection of low S-M grade AVMs with low L-Y scores, and some S-M grade IV AVMs with low L-Y scores should be considered
   • surgical resection of high S-M grade AVMs is risky, but if the patient has a fixed neurologic deficit that is unlikely to worsen with surgery, it may be a consideration[3]
4. management of unruptured AVMs has been contentious, and an attempt to determine the best course, the ARUBA (A Randomized trial of Unruptured Brain AVM) study[26] has been roundly criticised[27] for its design and premature closure due to endpoint satisfaction. Its conclusion that medical management alone was superior to medical management + intervention (surgery, SRS, embolization, or a combination) is not uniformly supported

90.2.10 Treatment

General information

Options and some pros and cons of each include:
1. surgery: (see below) the treatment of choice for AVMs. When surgical risk is unacceptably high, alternative procedures (e.g., SRS) may be an option:
   a) pros: eliminates risk of bleeding almost immediately. Seizure control improves
   b) cons: invasive, risk of surgery, cost (high initial cost of treatment may be offset by effectiveness or may be increased by complications)
   c) surgical excision: best suited for S-M grades I & II. S-M grades IV & V are high risk for poor outcome
2. radiation treatment:
   a) ✖ conventional radiation: effective in only ≤ 20% of cases.[28,29] Therefore not considered effective therapy
   b) stereotactic radiosurgery (SRS): accepted for some small (≤ 2.5–3 cm nidus), deep AVMs. See Stereotactic radiosurgery for AVMs (p. 1906)
      • pros: done as an outpatient, non-invasive, gradual reduction of AVM flow, no recovery period. Previous radiation makes AVM tissue more amenable to resection, reducing surgical morbidity.[30] Seizure control improves (usually in patients with reduction or obliteration of nidus)[3]
      • cons: the therapeutic response takes 1–3 years (the so-called "latency period"). During that time, the risk of bleeding is about the same as the natural history (1–3%/year). Limited to lesions with nidus ≤ 3 cm. Obliteration rate (70–80%) less than with surgery. Delayed side effects include: radiation necrosis, brain edema, & cyst formation. Permanent neurological changes occur in 2–3%[3]

3. endovascular techniques: e.g., (AVM embolization (p. 1926))
    a) pros: facilitates surgery[31] or (controversial) SRS
    b) cons: sometimes inadequate by itself to permanently obliterate AVMs, induces acute hemody-namic changes, may require multiple procedures, embolization prior to SRS reduces the oblit-eration rate from 70% (without embolization) to 47% (with embolization)[32]
4. combination techniques: e.g., embolization to shrink nidus, then stereotactic radiosurgery

Considerations to take into account in managing AVMs:
1. associated aneurysms: on feeding vessels, draining veins, or intranidal
2. flow: high or low
3. age of patient
4. history of previous hemorrhage
5. size and compactness of nidus
6. availability of interventional neuroradiologist
7. general medical condition of the patient

Surgical treatment for AVMs

Pre-op medical management
Before direct surgical treatment, patient should ideally be pre-treated with propranolol 20 mg PO QID for 3 days to minimize post-op normal perfusion pressure breakthrough (postulated cause of postoperative bleeding and edema,[33] see below). Labetalol has also been used perioperatively to keep MAP 70–80 mm Hg.[34]

Booking the case: Craniotomy for AVM

90

Also see defaults & disclaimers (p. 25).
1. position: (depends on location of AVM), radiolucent headholder
2. pre-op embolization (by neuroendovascular interventionalist): typically 24–48 hours pre-op
3. intraoperative angiography (optional)
4. equipment
    a) microscope (with ICG capability if used)
    b) image-guided navigation: primarily for the bone flap placement
5. blood availability: type and cross 2 U PRBC
6. post-op: ICU
7. consent (in lay terms for the patient—not all-inclusive):
    a) procedure: surgery to open the skull and remove the abnormal tangle of blood vessels in the brain, intraoperative angiography
    b) alternatives: stereotactic radiosurgery, endovascular techniques (not considered definitive treatment for most AVMs, but often used as an adjunct)
    c) complications: usual craniotomy complications (p. 25) plus stroke (the main concern), bleed-ing intra-op (requiring transfusion) and post-op, neurologic deficit related to the area of AVM location, failure to be able to remove entire AVM, recurrence in future

Basic tenets of AVM surgery
1. wide exposure
2. isolate and occlude feeding (terminal) arteries before draining veins (lesions with a single drain-ing vein can become impossible to deal with if premature blockage of the draining vein occurs, e.g., by kinking, coagulation)
3. excision of whole nidus is necessary to protect against rebleeding (occluding feeding arteries is not adequate)
4. identify and spare en passant vessels and adjacent (uninvolved) arteries
5. dissect directly on nidus of AVM, work in sulci and fissures whenever possible
6. in lesions that are high-flow on angiography, consider preoperative embolization
7. lesions with supplies from multiple vascular territories may require staging
8. clip accessible aneurysms on feeding arteries

Delayed postoperative deterioration

May be due to any of the following:

1. normal perfusion pressure breakthrough[33]: characterized by post-op swelling or hemorrhage. Thought to be due to loss of autoregulation, although this theory has been challenged.[35] Risk may be reduced by pre-op medication (see above)
2. occlusive hyperemia[36]: in the immediate post-op period probably due to obstruction of venous outflow from adjacent normal brain, in a delayed presentation may be due to delayed thrombosis of draining vein or dural sinus.[37] Risk may be elevated by keeping the patient "dry" post-op
3. rebleeding from a retained nidus of AVM
4. seizures

90.2.11 Follow-up of treated AVMs

For AVMs that have been resected:

1. an intraoperative or early post-op angiogram should be done to confirm completed removal of the nidus
2. residual nidus should be treated with re-resection or other treatment
3. suggestion: when satisfactory complete angiographic obliteration of an AVM has been accomplished, follow-up with *catheter angiogram* (not CTA or MRA) at 1 & 5 years post treatment

Following radiosurgery, imaging is required.

1. MRI/MRA is commonly repeated at 6-month intervals through the latency period (CT/CTA is substituted if MRI is contraindicated)
2. if SRS-induced obliteration is demonstrated, a catheter angiogram should be done to confirm
3. long-term MRI or CT follow-up may be used to monitor for delayed effects (necrosis, cysts...)

While catheter angiography (CA) is the gold standard, it carries some risk. Post-treatment MRI may be considered, as it demonstrated an accuracy of 90% for AVMs < 2.8 cm^3 volume and 70% for AVMs > 2.8 cm^3 compared to CA.[38]

90.3 Developmental venous anomaly (DVA) (venous angioma)

90.3.1 General information

Key concepts

- a vascular malformation of the brain with normal intervening brain present
- functions as part of the venous drainage for that region of the brain
- low-flow, low-pressure
- characteristic imaging finding: caput medusae (starburst pattern)
- rarely symptomatic: seizures rare, hemorrhage even less common. Venous infarcts may occur
- commonly associated with a cavernous malformation (p. 1525) (cav mal) which is more likely to be the source of any symptoms
- direct treatment is rarely indicated due to the vital function of venous drainage, the risk of venous infarct with excision, and the rarity of symptoms

Developmental venous anomaly (DVA), formerly (developmental) venous angioma AKA venous malformation. A tuft of medullary veins that converge into an enlarged central trunk (draining vein or "collector vein") that drains either to a deep ependymal vein or into a dural venous sinus. Thought to be congenital abnormalities that arise as a result of a failure in the normal sequence of cerebral venous development.[39] The veins lack large amounts of smooth muscle and elastic. No abnormal arteries are found. There is neural parenchyma between the vessels. Most common in regions supplied by the MCA[40] or in the region of the vein of Galen. They may be associated with a cavernous malformation (p. 1525). Non-hereditary. No apparent gender predilection. DVAs are low-flow and low-pressure.

90.3.2 Presentation

Most are clinically silent, but rarely seizures and even less frequently hemorrhage may occur. Venous infarcts have been reported rarely and may arise from thrombosis of the draining vein.[41] If symptoms are present, look for an associated cavernous malformation which is more likely to be the source (T2* GRE or SWI MRI images may reveal cavernous malformations that might otherwise be occult).

90.3.3 Imaging
Recommendations

* contrast T1 MRI + MRV
* T2* GRE (gradient echo) or SWI: to look for hemosiderin staining (from cav mal)

General features

Classic finding: the appearance of the tuft of veins has been described as the caput medusae (other descriptive terms include: a hydra, spokes of a wheel, a spider, an umbrella, a mushroom, or a sunburst or starburst).[42 (p 1471)] Typically has a long draining vein (longer than a normal vein).

CT scan

Unenhanced CT: is usually negative. May show up as a hyperdense lesion if there is thrombosis or calcifications (► Fig. 90.1).

Enhanced CT: the wedge of veins comprising the caput medusae may be seen. The enlarged elongated draining vein is usually demonstrated.

90

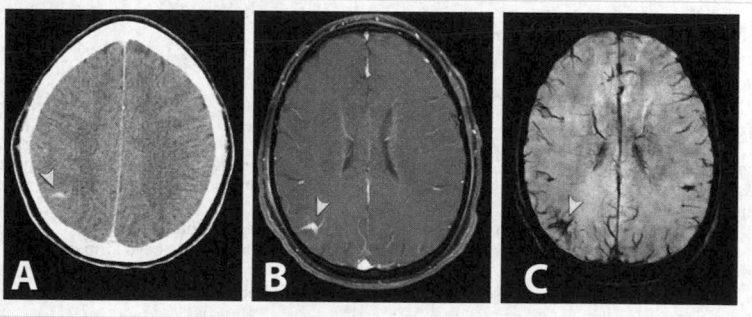

Fig. 90.1 Developmental venous anomaly, right parietal (*yellow arrowheads*). No hemosiderin staining nor associated cavernous malformation were identified in this patient.
The collecting vein drained into the torcular Herophili (not shown).
Image: A: CT scan axial noncontrast. B: MRI axial contrast T1. C: MRI axial susceptibility-weighted image (SWI).

MRI/MRV

Noncontrast T1WI & T2WI: if flow is high enough, flow voids may be seen, otherwise may be negative.

T1 contrast images: DVAs enhance intensely (findings as in enhanced CT, see above (► Fig. 90.1).

T2* GRE or SWI: hemosiderin from previous bleeds (usually from an associated cav mal) will show up as hypointense blooming.

MRV: usually shows the characteristic caput medusae (see above) & draining vein.

Angiogram

Usually not necessary to make the diagnosis. A DVA may occasionally be angiographically occult. Angiographic considerations[43] include:
* the caput medusae (see above): can usually be seen in the venous phase

- long draining vein: drains an excessive amount of brain tissue (it is theorized that venous restrictive disease may occur because of the length)
- the arterial phase should show no arteriovenous (AV) shunting (characteristic of an AVM), however, there are isolated reports of an associated AV shunt[41] (these fistulized DVAs—called mixed vascular malformations—may have a more ominous prognosis akin to an AVM)

90.3.4 Treatment

In general, these should not be treated, as they are rarely symptomatic and they represent the venous drainage of the brain in that vicinity. Due to the significant risk of venous infarction, surgery for the angioma itself is reserved only for documented bleeding or for intractable seizures that can definitely be attributed to the lesion. If surgery is indicated for an associated lesion (e.g., cavernous malformation), the angioma should be left alone.

90.4 Dural arteriovenous fistulae (DAVF)

90.4.1 General information

AKA dural AVMs (DAVM). Vascular abnormality in which an arteriovenous shunt is contained within the leaflets of the dura mater, exclusively supplied by branches of the internal/external carotid or vertebral arteries.[44] Because they are considered acquired rather than congenital lesions, the term fistula is preferred over malformation, although the latter term has also been used in the literature. Multiple fistulas may be found in up to 8% of cases.

Usually found adjacent to dural venous sinuses. Common locations:

1. transverse/sigmoid: the most common[45] (63% of cases) with a slight left-sided predominance,[46] with the epicenter of these almost invariably at the junction of the transverse and sigmoid sinuses
2. tentorial/petrosal
3. anterior fossa/ethmoidal
4. middle fossa/Sylvian
5. cavernous sinus (carotid-cavernous fistula (CCF))
6. superior sagittal sinus
7. foramen magnum

90.4.2 Etiology

Evidence suggests that most DAVFs are acquired, idiopathic lesions, and they have a well-recognized association with venous sinus thrombosis, although their exact pathogenesis is not fully understood. Theories include:

1. venous sinus occlusion awakens dormant embryonic dural arteriovenous channels[45]
2. venous hypertension/thrombosis promotes local angiogenesis and the de novo formation of DAVF[47]
3. the DAVF may arise first and itself result in venous sinus thrombosis[48]

90.4.3 Epidemiology

DAVFs comprise 10–15% of all intracranial AVMs.[46] 61–66% occur in females, and patients are usually in their 40s or 50s. They occur rarely in children, and when they do they tend to be complex, bilateral dural sinus malformations.[49]

90.4.4 Presentation

Common findings are listed in ▶ Table 90.9. Pulsatile tinnitus is the most common presenting symptom of a DAVF. Cortical venous drainage with resultant venous hypertension can produce IC-HTN, and this is the most common cause of morbidity and mortality and thus the strongest indication for DAVF treatment. DAVFs may also cause global cerebral edema or hydrocephalus due to poor cerebral venous drainage or by impairing the function of the arachnoid granulations, respectively. Other DAVF symptoms/signs include headaches, seizures, cranial nerve palsies, and orbital venous congestion.

Table 90.9 Clinical findings in 27 patients with dural AVMs in the lateral and/or sigmoid sinus[50]

Sign/symptom	No. (%)
pulsatile tinnitus	25 (92%)
occipital bruit	24 (89%)
headache	11 (41%)
visual impairment	9 (33%)
papilledema	7 (26%)

90.4.5 Evaluation

General information

Brain CT or MRI without contrast are often normal. CTA may reveal dilated tortuous vessels corresponding to enlarged arterial feeders or ectatic draining veins. MRA may reveal dilated pial vessels, early prominent venous sinus filling, sinus enlargement or occlusion, and white matter edema related to venous hypertension. Full 6-vessel cerebral angiography (bilateral ICAs, bilateral ECAs, bilateral vertebral arteries) is required to establish the diagnosis and to plan treatment.

Angiographic classification

Several classification systems have been described to characterize DAVFs. The Borden[51] (▶ Table 90.10) and the Cognard[52] (▶ Table 90.11) systems have emerged as the most commonly utilized contemporary grading schemes. Cortical venous drainage is the defining angiographic feature that distinguishes benign (low-grade) from aggressive (high-grade) fistulas. (Borden I, Cognard I, and Cognard IIa are low-grade, all others are high-grade.)

90

Table 90.10 Borden classification

Type	Features
I	DAVF drainage into a dural venous sinus or meningeal veins, with normal anterograde flow. Usually clinically benign.
II	DAVF draining anterograde into dural venous sinus, but with retrograde flow into cortical veins.
III	DAVF with direct retrograde flow from fistula into cortical veins, causing venous hypertension.
Above further subclassified into a: with single hole and b: multiple holes	

Table 90.11 Angiographic classification of dural AVMs[52a]

Venous drainage: sinus	
Type I	Type IIa

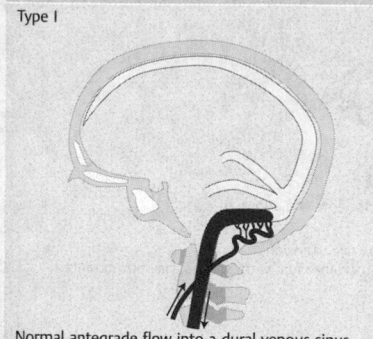

Normal antegrade flow into a dural venous sinus
Course: benign[b]

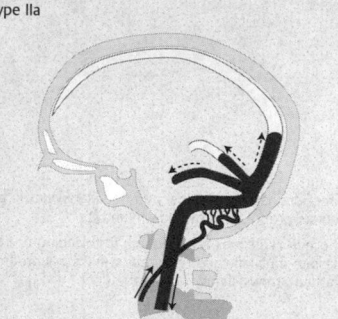

Drainage into a sinus with retrograde flow within the sinus[c]
Course: sinus reflux caused IC-HTN in 20%

(continued)

Table 90.11 continued

Venous drainage: sinus

Type IIb	Type IIa + b

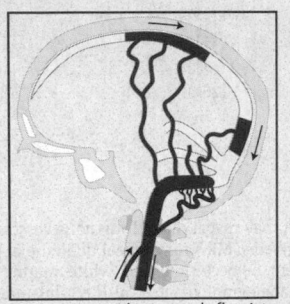

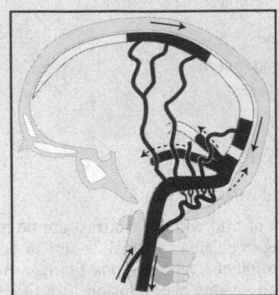

Drainage into a sinus with retrograde flow into cortical vein(s)
Course: reflux into veins induced hemorrhage in 10%

Drainage into a sinus with retrograde flow within the sinus[c] and cortical vein(s)
Course: aggressive in 66% with bleeding and/or IC-HTN

Venous drainage: directly into cortical veins[b]

Type III	Type IV

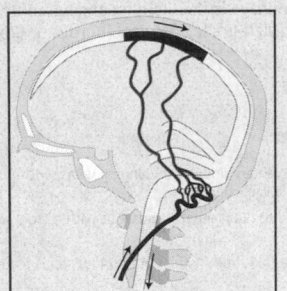

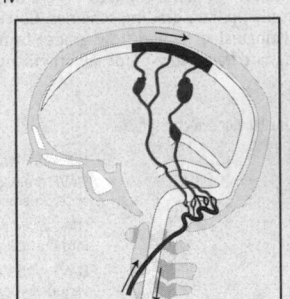

Direct drainage into a cortical vein without venous ectasia.
Course: hemorrhage occurs in 40%

Direct drainage into a cortical vein with venous ectasia
Course: hemorrhage occurs in 65%

Venous drainage: spinal in addition to all of the above

Type V

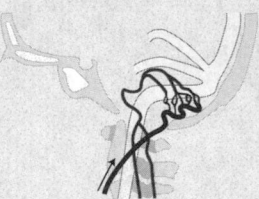

Direct drainage into spinal perimedullary veins in addition to all of the above
Course: progressive myelopathy in 50%

[a]those in red boxes are high risk for bleeding or intracranial hypertension
[b]despite a usually good prognosis, ≈ 2% will progress and therefore follow-up studies may be warranted
[c]dashed arrows signify retrograde flow

Borden classification system
The Borden classification[51] is shown in ▶ Table 90.10.

Cognard angiographic classification
The Cognard system[52] is shown in ▶ Table 90.11. This system is generally most applicable to DAVFs involving the transverse sinus.

Cognard found 54% had no cortical venous reflux (Types I and IIa) and usually exhibit benign behavior.

★ Key determinant: in the Cognard system, the pattern of venous drainage is the most critical factor. As a general rule, lesions with retrograde flow in the cortical veins (IIb, IIa + b, III & IV—red frames in ▶ Table 90.11) are high risk (for bleeding or intracranial hypertension…).

90.4.6 Natural history

The concept of benign vs. aggressive DAVF behavior based on the absence or presence, respectively, of cortical venous drainage was validated by data reported by University of Toronto group. Over a 3-year period, 98% of benign lesions (no cortical venous drainage) remained benign.[53] On the other hand, over a 4-year period, annual rates of hemorrhage, non-hemorrhagic neurologic deficit, and mortality were 8.1%, 6.9%, and 10.4%, respectively, for aggressive lesions (with cortical venous drainage).[54]

In a meta-analysis of 377 cases,[55] three DAVF locations were associated with particularly aggressive behavior (aggressive:benign ratio)—tentorial (31:1), middle fossa/Sylvian (2.5:1), anterior fossa/ethmoidal (2.1:1).

90.4.7 Management
General information

Lesions with cortical venous drainage should generally be treated. Lesions without cortical venous drainage should be followed radiographically and clinically (2% may evolve to develop cortical venous drainage). A change in a bruit (either worsening, or disappearance) should prompt restudy.
Indications for intervention:
1. presence of cortical venous drainage
2. neurologic dysfunction
3. hemorrhage
4. orbital venous congestion
5. refractory symptoms (headache, pulsatile tinnitus)

Manual carotid self-compression

Advocated by some, the thrombosis rate of ≈ 22% and clinical improvement rate of 33%[56] may mimic the natural course. Patients are advised to compress with the hand that would be affected by ischemia if it were to occur (e.g., with a left-sided DAVF, the right hand should be used to compress the left carotid artery). That way, the hand would fall away if ischemia develops. Recommendations vary, one option: start with 10 minutes once a day, gradually increase frequency and duration.

Endovascular embolization

May be performed transarterial or transvenous. Before the availability of liquid embolic agents (Onyx and NBCA), treatment was directed at the *venous* drainage (unlike pial AVMs) which had higher success, because the coils could be deployed to sacrifice the venous drainage very close to the point of arteriovenous shunting, resulting in thrombosis of the fistula. It is more difficult to deploy coils across the point of arteriovenous shunting from the arterial side, whereas the liquid embolic agents, particularly Onyx, can be injected at somewhat of a distance and pushed forward across the fistulous point. Whether a transarterial, transvenous, or combined approach is utilized depends on the unique angioarchitecture of the fistula.

Surgery

While endovascular approaches have emerged as the primary treatment for most DAVFs, certain fistula types are still best dealt with via open surgery as the first-line strategy.[57] Furthermore, surgery has been used to successfully treat DAVFs after previous partial, incomplete, or failed endovascular

90

treatment. Finally, surgery can be used adjunctively in a combined approach to provide direct access for embolization of DAVFs that are inaccessible by a purely endovascular route.

Preoperative embolization may facilitate surgical treatment[58] by lessening the risk of catastrophic hemorrhage, which may occur simply during the performance of the craniotomy.[50] The use of the craniotome is discouraged, as a sinus or venous laceration could produce a fatal hemorrhage. Contingencies for the rapid administration of blood products must be made (large-bore central lines). The scalp incision, craniotomy flap, and dural incision should be planned in a strategic manner to control and sequentially eliminate the blood supply to the lesion at each step, while maximizing the exposure as needed. Surgical options for the treatment of DAVFs include the following techniques[57]:

1. radical fistula excision
2. sinus skeletonization
3. disconnection of cortical venous drainage
4. ligation of the fistulous point and/or outflow vein
5. sinus packing
6. coagulation of arterial feeders to the lesion

While surgery vs. endovascular treatment can be considered for all DAVF locations, two locations generally remain more favorable for surgery:

1. anterior fossa/ethmoidal
2. tentorial DAVFs

The endovascular approach to these fistulas is difficult, whereas the surgical approach is often straightforward. Surgically-assisted embolization, whereby a craniotomy is performed followed by direct puncture for embolization of the target vessel, may be utilized in select cases.

Stereotactic radiosurgery

May be used post-embolization.[59] Pan et al[60] reported a complete obliteration rate of 58% of transverse/sigmoid fistulae treated with only radiosurgery (1650–1900 cGy), or with radiosurgery after surgery/embolization had failed to produce complete obliteration. 71% of the patients were cured of their symptoms.

With the continued improvement of endovascular technology over the past two decades, the role of radiosurgery for DAVF treatment has steadily decreased; however, it remains an option for those difficult lesions in which endovascular/surgical options have been exhausted.

90.5 Vein of Galen malformation

90.5.1 General information

Enlargement of the great cerebral vein of Galen (VOG) may occur in "vein of Galen malformations" (VOGM) (some refer to these as vein of Galen aneurysms). Congenital, develop before the 3-month embryo stage or secondarily to high flow from adjacent deep parenchymatous AVMs or pial fistulae. Most likely consist not of the vein of Galen but rather of the medial vein of the prosencephalon. Parenchymatous AVMs can be distinguished from true VOG malformations by retrograde filling of the internal cerebral vein in the former.[61]

True VOG malformations are predictably fed from the medial and lateral choroidal, circumferential, mesencephalic, anterior choroidal, pericallosal, and meningeal arteries.[61,62] Agenesis of the straight sinus may be an associated finding.

90.5.2 Presentation

Newborns tend to present with congestive heart failure in first few weeks of life (due to high blood flow)[63] and a cranial bruit. Hydrocephalus may result from obstruction of the Sylvian aqueduct by the enlarged VOG, or it may be caused by the increased venous pressure (which can also produce prominence of the scalp veins[64]).

Parenchymatous AVMs are usually diagnosed later in life due to neurological manifestations,[65] including focal neurologic deficit and hemorrhage.

90.5.3 Classification

Classified based on the location of the fistula[66,67]:

1. pure internal fistulae: single or multiple
2. fistulae between thalamoperforators and the VOG
3. mixed form: the most common
4. plexiform AVMs

90.5.4 Natural history

Untreated VOG malformations have a poor prognosis, with neonates having nearly 100% mortality, and 1–12-month-olds having ≈ 60% mortality, 7% major morbidity, and 21% being normal.[68]
Parenchymatous AVMs behave similarly to other AVMs.

90.5.5 Treatment

Hydrocephalus

Hydrocephalus associated with VOGM is obstructive, due to the varix. Although admonitions about shunting were common due to fear of precipitating a hemorrhage, when hydrocephalus is present the patient needs a shunt.

Vein of Galen malformations

Pediatric patients are often in poor medical condition, limiting the efficacy of operative treatment. Treatment options for these include embolization of the main feeding arteries. Prognosis is poor. Those presenting with hydrocephalus from aqueductal obstruction often do so at the end of the first year of life. Neurosurgical excision may be considered here, and the prognosis is better.
Repeated embolization while monitoring the venous drainage is employed.

Parenchymal AVM with enlarged VOG

The AVM is treated by the same methods as other AVMs (embolization, resection, or radiosurgery).

90.6 Carotid-cavernous fistula

90.6.1 General information

Key concepts

- direct (high flow, from ICA) or indirect (low flow, from meningeal branches)
- classic triad (more common with direct CCF): chemosis, pulsatile proptosis, ocular bruit
- risk of SAH is low. Major risk is to vision
- natural history of low-flow CCF is up to 50% spontaneous thrombosis

See also anatomy and venous inflow and outflow of the cavernous sinus (p. 86).
Carotid-cavernous fistula (CCF): divided into direct (Type A) and indirect (Types B–D)[69]:
1. Type A: direct high-flow shunts between the *internal* carotid artery and cavernous sinus:
   a) traumatic (including iatrogenic): occur in 0.2% of patients with craniocerebral trauma. Iatrogenic: may follow percutaneous trigeminal rhizotomy,[70] endovascular procedures...
   b) spontaneous: usually due to ruptured cavernous sinus ICA aneurysm. May also occur in patients with connective tissue disorders
2. indirect (dural): most are shunts: from dural arteries that are branches of the *external* carotid (not from ICA) (exception: Type B) – low flow
   a) Type B: from meningeal branches of the internal carotid artery (ICA)
   b) Type C: from meningeal branches of the external carotid artery (ECA)
   c) Type D: from meningeal branches of both the ICA and ECA

90.6.2 Presentation

1. orbital and/or retro-orbital pain
2. chemosis (arteriolization of conjunctiva)

3. pulsatile proptosis
4. ocular and/or cranial bruit
5. deterioration of visual acuity: may be due to hypoxic retinopathy as a result of reduced arterial pressure, increased venous pressure, and increased intraocular pressure
6. diplopia: abducens (VI) palsy is the most common
7. pupillary dilatation
8. ophthalmoplegia (usually unilateral, but may present initially as bilateral or may progress to bilateral)
9. increased intraocular pressure
10. neo-vascularization of the iris or retina
11. rarely: SAH

Indirect CCFs generally have a more gradual onset and milder presentation than direct.

90.6.3 Evaluation

CT or MRI: usually demonstrates proptosis. Serpiginous and engorged intraocular vessels including the superior ophthalmic vein (best seen on T2WI coronals—helps to differentiate from rectus muscles) and convexity of lateral wall of cavernous sinus.

Angiography: shunting of blood from ICA into cavernous sinus. Rapid opacification of petrosal sinus and/or ophthalmic vein may be seen.

1. Huber maneuver: lateral view, inject VA and manually compress affected carotid. Helps identify upper extent of fistula, multiple fistulous openings, and complete transection of ICA
2. Mehringer-Hieshima maneuver: inject contrast at a rate of 2–3 ml/s into affected carotid while compressing the carotid in the neck (below the catheter tip) to control flow to help demonstrate the fistula

90.6.4 Treatment

General information

20–50% of *low-flow* CCF spontaneously thrombose, and therefore one may observe these as long as visual acuity is stable and intra-ocular pressure is < ≈ 25. Symptomatic (e.g., progressive visual deterioration) high-flow CCFs rarely resolve spontaneously, and urgent treatment is usually indicated. Treatment is usually in the form of embolization by an interventional neuroradiologist or trapping between surgically placed clips.

Even if normal ocular motility cannot be achieved in the affected eye, preservation of vision is desirable because:

1. for some ocular motility abnormalities, surgical treatment may reduce diplopia
2. patient may be provided with frosted eyeglass lens which will eliminate diplopia but will maintain peripheral vision
3. in the rare event of injury to contralateral eye (trauma, central retinal artery occlusion...) there would be "reserve" vision in the eye with reduced motility (with loss of the other eye, there would not be diplopia)

Indications for treatment

1. proptosis
2. visual loss
3. cranial nerve VI palsy
4. intractable bruit
5. severely elevated intraocular pressure
6. increased filling of cortical veins on angiography

Endovascular treatment

Options include:

1. electrolytically detachable coils
2. Amplatzer™ Vascular Plug (AVP) (Abbott Laboratories): a self-expanding nitinol wire mesh

Routes available include:

1. transarterial through internal carotid. If this fails (e.g., wide aneurysm neck), the carotid artery may be occluded on either side of fistula to trap it (sacrifices carotid artery, therefore test occlusion must be done first to determine if patient can tolerate this; however, **note**: test occlusion with an open fistula may give a false-positive result because steal through the fistula may reduce CBF and cause neurologic symptoms not related to the occlusion acting alone). The distal occlusion needs to be proximal to the ophthalmic artery

2. transarterial through external carotid: useful only for dural fistulas

3. transvenous:
   a) traversing heart to enter jugular vein, then through petrosal sinus to cavernous sinus. Lower success rate (≈ 20%) than transarterial route
   b) via superior ophthalmic vein: entered where supra-optic vein enters orbit to become superior ophthalmic vein. If possible, it is best to wait for the vein to become arterialized by the high flow pressure. Reports of "disasters" due to injury to the fragile vein performed before arterialization took place may have been due to more primitive balloon catheters that were standard before current commercially produced versions were available (which are softer than the originals). Must avoid lacerating the vein inside the orbit, and avoid distal ligation of the vein without proximal occlusion (shunts even more blood into eye)

Choice of technique

With indirect fistulas, it is mandatory to place coils on the venous side (otherwise new feeders will be recruited).

Coils or clips may be used to occlude direct fistulas.

90.7 Sigmoid sinus diverticulum

Sigmoid sinus diverticulum (SSD, see ▶ Fig. 90.2) or sigmoid sinus dehiscence is found in 1.2% of asymptomatic patients.[71] However, these abnormalities may be found ipsilaterally in up to 23% of patients with pulsatile tinnitus, presumably due to turbulent flow which may occur in these abnormalities.[72] SSD are more common in women.

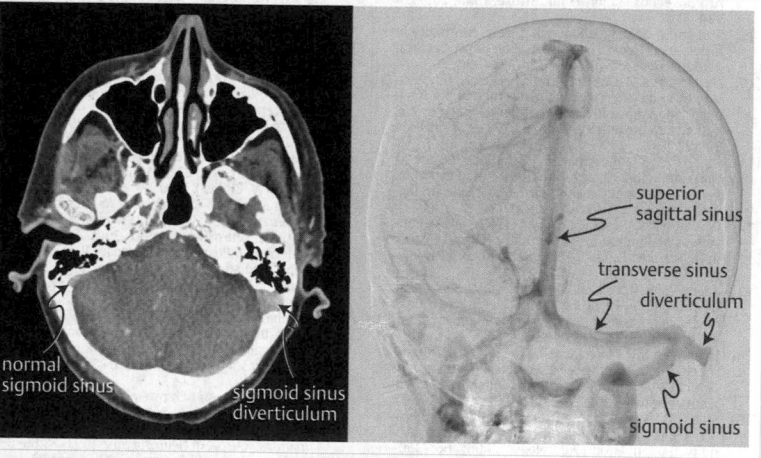

Fig. 90.2 Sigmoid sinus diverticulum.
Image: axial contrast head CT (left) and AP venous-phase angiogram (right) showing sigmoid sinus diverticulum on the patient's left side.

When treatments such as masking noise generators fail, surgical intervention can be considered. Surgical treatment options include:

- Endovascular coiling/stenting
- Transmastoid "resurfacing" (see below)
- Craniectomy with clip reconstruction

Transmastoid "resurfacing" consists of partial mastoidectomy, and subtotal obliteration of the area of the diverticulum (so-called sinus wall resurfacing[72,73,74]) with e.g., bone chips, fibrin glue, or muscle.

References

[1] McCormick WF. The Pathology of Vascular ('Arteriovenous') Malformations. J Neurosurg. 1966; 24:807–816

[2] Lobato RD, Perez C, Rivas JJ, et al. Clinical, Radiological, and Pathological Spectrum of Angiographically Occult Intracranial Vascular Malformations. J Neurosurg. 1988; 68:518–531

[3] Derdeyn CP, Zipfel GJ, Albuquerque FC, et al. Management of Brain Arteriovenous Malformations: A Scientific Statement for Healthcare Professionals From the American Heart Association/American Stroke Association. Stroke. 2017; 48:e200–e224

[4] Ondra SL, Troupp H, George ED, et al. The Natural History of Symptomatic Arteriovenous Malformations of the Brain: A 24-Year Follow-Up Assessment. J Neurosurg. 1990; 73:387–391

[5] Kupersmith MJ, Vargas ME, Yashar A, et al. Occipital arteriovenous malformations: visual disturbances and presentation. Neurology. 1996; 46:953–957

[6] Al-Shahi R, Warlow C. A systematic review of the frequency and prognosis of arteriovenous malformations of the brain in adults. Brain. 2001; 124:1900–1926

[7] Perret G, Nishioka H. Report on the Cooperative Study of Intracranial Aneurysms and Subarachnoid Hemorrhage: Arteriovenous Malformations. J Neurosurg. 1966; 25:467–490

[8] Hartmann A, Mast H, Mohr JP, et al. Morbidity of Intracranial Hemorrhage in Patients with Cerebral Arteriovenous Malformation. Stroke. 1998; 29:931–934

[9] Morgan M, Sekhon L, Rahman Z, et al. Morbidity of Intracranial Hemorrhage in Patients with Cerebral Arteriovenous Malformation. Stroke. 1998; 29

[10] Hernesniemi JA, Dashti R, Juvela S, et al. Natural history of brain arteriovenous malformations: a long-term follow-up study of risk of hemorrhage in 238 patients. Neurosurgery. 2008; 63:823–9; discussion 829-31

[11] Kim H, Al-Shahi Salman R, McCulloch CE, et al. Untreated brain arteriovenous malformation: patient-level meta-analysis of hemorrhage predictors. Neurology. 2014; 83:590–597

[12] Crawford PM, West CR, Chadwick DW, et al. Arteriovenous Malformations of the Brain: Natural History in Unoperated Patients. J Neurol Neurosurg Psychiatry. 1986; 49:1–10

[13] Spetzler RF, Hargraves RW, McCormick PW, et al. Relationship of Perfusion Pressure and Size to Risk of Hemorrhage from Arteriovenous Malformations. J Neurosurg. 1992; 76:918–923

[14] Jayaraman MV, Marcellus ML, Do HM, et al. Hemorrhage rate in patients with Spetzler-Martin grades IV and V arteriovenous malformations: is treatment justified? Stroke. 2007; 38:325–329

[15] Stapf C, Mast H, Sciacca RR, et al. Predictors of hemorrhage in patients with untreated brain arteriovenous malformation. Neurology. 2006; 66:1350–1355

[16] Kondziolka D, McLaughlin MR, Kestle JRW. Simple Risk Predictions for Arteriovenous Malformation Hemorrhage. Neurosurgery. 1995; 37:851–855

[17] Cunha MJ, Stein BM, Solomon RA, et al. The Treatment of Associated Intracranial Aneurysms and Arteriovenous Malformations. Journal of Neurosurgery. 1992; 77:853–859

[18] Josephson CB, White PM, Krishan A, et al. Computed tomography angiography or magnetic resonance angiography for detection of intracranial vascular malformations in patients with intracerebral haemorrhage. Cochrane Database Syst Rev. 2014. DOI: 10.1002/14651858.CD009372.pub2

[19] Hamilton MG, Spetzler RF. The Prospective Application of a Grading System for Arteriovenous Malformations. Neurosurgery. 1994; 34:2–7

[20] Hofmeister C, Stapf C, Hartmann A, et al. Demographic, morphological, and clinical characteristics of 1289 patients with brain arteriovenous malformation. Stroke. 2000; 31:1307–1310

[21] Spetzler RF, Martin NA. A Proposed Grading System for Arteriovenous Malformations. J Neurosurg 1986; 65:476–483

[22] Ogilvy CS, Stieg PE, Awad I, et al. AHA Scientific Statement: Recommendations for the management of intracranial arteriovenous malformations: a statement for healthcare professionals from a special writing group of the Stroke Council, American Stroke Association. Stroke. 2001; 32:1458–1471

[23] Spetzler RF, Ponce FA. A 3-tier classification of cerebral arteriovenous malformations. Clinical article. J Neurosurg. 2011; 114:842–849

[24] Lawton MT, Kim H, McCulloch CE, et al. A supplementary grading scale for selecting patients with brain arteriovenous malformations for surgery. Neurosurgery. 2010; 66:702–13; discussion 713

[25] Kim H, Abla AA, Nelson J, et al. Validation of the supplemented Spetzler-Martin grading system for brain arteriovenous malformations in a multicenter cohort of 1009 surgical patients. Neurosurgery 2015; 76:25–31; discussion 31-2; quiz 32-3

[26] Mohr JP, Parides MK, Stapf C, et al. Medical management with or without interventional therapy for unruptured brain arteriovenous malformation (ARUBA): a multicentre, non-blinded, randomised trial. Lancet. 2014; 383:614–621

[27] Magro E, Gentric JC, Darsaut TE, et al. Responses to ARUBA: a systematic review and critical analysis for the design of future arteriovenous malformation trials. J Neurosurg. 2017; 126:486–494

[28] Laing RW, Childs J, Brada M. Failure of Conventionally Fractionated Radiotherapy to Decrease the Risk of Hemorrhage in Inoperable Arteriovenous Malformations. Neurosurgery. 1992; 30:872–876

[29] Redekop G, Elisevich KV, Gaspar LE, et al. Conventional Radiation Therapy of Intracranial Arteriovenous Malformations: Long-Term Results. J Neurosurg. 1993; 78:413–422

[30] Sanchez-Mejia RO, McDermott MW, Tan J, et al. Radiosurgery facilitates resection of brain arteriovenous malformations and reduces surgical morbidity. Neurosurgery. 2009; 64:231–8; discussion 238–40

[31] Jafar JJ, Davis AJ, Berenstein A, et al. The Effect of Embolization with N-Butyl Cyanoacrylate Prior to Surgical Resection of Cerebral Arteriovenous Malformations. Journal of Neurosurgery. 1993; 78:60–69

[32] Andrade-Souza YM, Ramani M, Scora D, et al. Embolization before radiosurgery reduces the obliteration rate of arteriovenous malformations. Neurosurgery. 2007; 60:443–51; discussion 451-2

[33] Spetzler RF, Wilson CB, Weinstein P, et al. Normal Perfusion Pressure Breakthrough Theory. Clinical Neurosurgery. 1978; 25:651–672

[34] Orlowski JP, Shiesley D, Vidt DG, et al. Labetalol to Control Blood Pressure After Cerebrovascular Surgery. Crit Care Med. 1988; 16:765–768

[35] Young WL, Kader A, Prohovnik I, et al. Pressure Autoregulation Is Intact After Arteriovenous Malformation Resection. Neurosurgery. 1993; 32:491–497

[36] al-Rodhan NRF, Sundt TM, Piepgras DG, et al. Occlusive Hyperemia: A Theory for the Hemodynamic Complications Following Resection of Intracerebral Arteriovenous Malformations. J Neurosurg. 1993; 78:167–175

[37] Wilson CB, Hieshima G. Occlusive hyperemia: A new way to think about an old problem. J Neurosurg. 1993; 78:165–166

[38] O'Connor TE, Friedman WA. Magnetic resonance imaging assessment of cerebral arteriovenous malformation obliteration after stereotactic radiosurgery. Neurosurgery. 2013; 73:761–766

[39] Mullan S, Mojtahedi S, Johnson DL, et al. Embryological basis of some aspects of cerebral vascular fistulas and malformations. J Neurosurg. 1996; 85:1–8

[40] Steiger HJ, Tew JM. Hemorrhage and Epilepsy in Cryptic Cerebrovascular Malformations. Arch Neurol. 1984; 41:722–724

[41] Agazzi S, Regli L, Uske A, et al. Developmental venous anomaly with an arteriovenous shunt and a thrombotic complication. Case report. J Neurosurg. 2001; 94:533–537

[42] Wilkins RH, Rengachary SS. Neurosurgery. New York 1985

[43] Mullan S, Mojtahedi S, Johnson DL, et al. Cerebral venous malformation-arteriovenous malformation transition forms. J Neurosurg. 1996; 85:9–13

[44] Malik GM, Pearce JE, Ausman JI. Dural Arteriovenous Malformations and Intracranial Hemorrhage. Neurosurgery. 1984; 15:332–339

[45] Graeb DA, Dolman CL. Radiological and Pathological Aspects of Dural Arteriovenous Fistulas. J Neurosurg. 1986; 64:962–967

[46] Arnautovic KI, Krisht AF. Transverse-Sigmoid Sinus Dural Arteriovenous Malformations. Contemporary Neurosurgery. 2000; 21:1–6

[47] Houser OW, Campbell JK, Campbell RJ, et al. Arteriovenous malformation affecting the transverse dural venous sinus-an acquired lesion. Mayo Clin Proc. 1979; 54:651–661

[48] Aminoff MJ. Vascular anomalies in the intracranial dura mater. Brain. 1973; 96:601–612

[49] Ashour R, Aziz-Sultan MA, Soltanolkotabi M, et al. Safety and efficacy of onyx embolization for pediatric cranial and spinal vascular lesions and tumors. Neurosurgery. 2012; 71:773–784

[50] Sundt TM, Piepgras DG. The Surgical Approach to Arteriovenous Malformations of the Lateral and Sigmoid Dural Sinuses. J Neurosurg. 1983; 59:32–39

[51] Borden JA, Wu JK, Shucart WA. A proposed classification for spinal and cranial dural arteriovenous fistulous malformations and implications for treatment. Journal of Neurosurgery. 1995; 82:166–179

[52] Cognard C, Gobin YP, Pierot L, et al. Cerebral dural arteriovenous fistulas: clinical and angiographic correlation with a revised classification of venous drainage. Radiology. 1995; 194:671–680

[53] Davies MA, Saleh J, Ter Brugge K, et al. The natural history and management of intracranial dural arteriovenous fistulae. Part 1: benign lesions. Interv Neuroradiol. 1997; 3:295–302

[54] van Dijk JM, terBrugge KG, Willinsky RA, et al. Clinical course of cranial dural arteriovenous fistulas with long-term persistent cortical venous reflux. Stroke. 2002; 33:1233–1236

[55] Awad IA, Little JR, Akarawi WP, et al. Intracranial dural arteriovenous malformations: factors predisposing to an aggressive neurological course. J Neurosurg. 1990; 72:839–850

[56] Halbach V, Higashida R, Hieshima G, et al. Dural fistulas involving the transverse and sigmoid sinuses: results of the treatment in 28 patients. Radiology. 1987; 163:443–447

[57] Ashour R, Morcos JJ, Spetzler RF, et al. Surgical Management of Cerebral Dural Arteriovenous Fistulae. In: Comprehensive Management of Arteriovenous Malformations of the Brain and Spine. Cambridge: Cambridge University Press; 2015:144–170

[58] Barnwell SL, Halbach VV, Higashida RT, et al. Complex Dural Arteriovenous Fistulas: Results of Combined Endovascular and Neurosurgical Treatment in 16 Patients. J Neurosurg. 1989; 71:352–358

[59] Lewis AI, Tomsick TA, Tew JM. Management of Tentorial Dural Arteriovenous Malformations: Transarterial Embolization Combined with Stereotactic Radiation or Surgery. Journal of Neurosurgery. 1994; 81:851–859

[60] Pan DH, Chung WY, Guo WY, et al. Stereotactic radiosurgery for the treatment of dural arteriovenous fistulas involving the transverse-sigmoid sinus. J Neurosurg. 2002; 96:823–829

[61] Khayata MH, Casaco A, Wakhloo AK, et al. Vein of Galen malformations: intravascular techniques. In: Neurovascular Surgery. New York: McGraw-Hill; 1995:1029–1039

[62] Lasjaunias P, Rodesch G, Pruvost P, et al. Treatment of vein of Galen aneurysmal malformation. Journal of Neurosurgery. 1989; 70:746–750

[63] Cummings GR. Circulation in neonates with intracranial arteriovenous fistula and cardiac failure. American Journal of Cardiology. 1980; 45:1019–1024

[64] Strassburg HM. Macrocephaly is Not Always Due to Hydrocephalus. J Child Neurol. 1989; 4:S32–S40

[65] Clarisse J, Dobbelaere P, Rey C, et al. Aneurysms of the great vein of Galen. Radiological-anatomical study of 22 cases. Journal of Neuroradiology. 1978; 5:91–102

[66] Yasargil MG. AVM of the brain, clinical considerations, general and specific operative techniques, surgical results, nonoperated cases, cavernous and venous angiomas, neuroanesthesia. In: Microneurosurgery. Stuttgart: Georg Thieme; 1988:317–396

[67] Litvak J, Yahr MD, Ransohoff J. Aneurysms of the great vein of Galen and mid-line cerebral arteriovenous anomalies. Journal of Neurosurgery. 1960; 17:945–954

[68] Johnston IH, Whittle IR, Besser M, et al. Vein of Galen malformation: diagnosis and management. Neurosurgery. 1987; 20:747–758

[69] Barrow DL, Spector RH, Braun IF, et al. Classification and Treatment of Spontaneous Carotid-Cavernous Fistulas. J Neurosurg. 1985; 62:248–256

[70] Kuether TA, O'Neill OR, Nesbit GM, et al. Direct Carotid Cavernous Fistula After Trigeminal Balloon Microcompression Gangliolysis: Case Report. Neurosurgery. 1996; 39:853–856

[71] Schoeff S, Nicholas B, Mukherjee S, et al. Imaging prevalence of sigmoid sinus dehiscence among patients with and without pulsatile tinnitus. Otolaryngol Head Neck Surg. 2014; 150:841–846

[72] Song JJ, Kim YJ, Kim SY, et al. Sinus Wall Resurfacing for Patients With Temporal Bone Venous Sinus Diverticulum and Ipsilateral Pulsatile Tinnitus. Neurosurgery. 2015; 77:709–717

[73] Otto KJ, Hudgins PA, Abdelkafy W, et al. Sigmoid sinus diverticulum: a new surgical approach to the correction of pulsatile tinnitus. Otol Neurotol. 2007; 28:48–53

[74] Santa Maria PL. Sigmoid sinus dehiscence resurfacing as treatment for pulsatile tinnitus. J Laryngol Otol. 2013; 127 Suppl 2:S57–S59

90

91 Angiographically Occult Vascular Malformations

91.1 General information

91.1.1 Terminology

Terminology is controversial. The term "cryptic cerebrovascular malformations" was originally applied to angiographically and clinically silent lesions regardless of size.

Recommendation: use the term "**angiographically** occult (or cryptic) vascular malformations" (AOVM) to refer to cerebrovascular malformations that are not demonstrable on technically satisfactory catheter cerebral angiography (i.e., good quality films, with subtraction views, and the following as appropriate: magnification, angiotomography, rapid serial angiograms, or delayed films).[1] Many lesions have large patent vessels at surgery in spite of negative angiography.[2] Other imaging modalities (i.e., CT, MRI) may be able to reveal these lesions. Although often used interchangeably, the term "occult malformation" (omitting the word "angiographically") is suggested for use with lesions that also do not appear on these other imaging modalities.

91.1.2 Etiologies

The reasons for a vascular lesion being angiographically cryptic include:
1. lesions that have hemorrhaged
   a) the bleeding may obliterate the lesion: difficult to substantiate[3]
   b) the clot may temporarily compress the lesion[3] which may re-open after weeks to months as the clot dissolves
2. sluggish flow
3. small size of the abnormal vessels
4. may require very late angiographic films (i.e., delayed films) to visualize due to late filling

91.1.3 Epidemiology

Incidence of AOVM has been estimated as ≈ 10% of cerebrovascular malformations.[4] AOVMs were found at necropsy in 21 (4.5%) of 461 patients with spontaneous intracranial hemorrhage (**ICH**),[5] but refinements in angiography have occurred since this 1954 report.

The average age at diagnosis in one literature review[1] was 28 yrs.

91.1.4 Presentation

AOVM most often present with seizures or H/A. Less commonly they may present with progressive neurologic symptoms (usually as a result of spontaneous ICH).[6] They may also be discovered incidentally.

91.2 Osler-Weber-Rendu syndrome

91.2.1 General information

AKA hereditary hemorrhagic telangiectasia (HHT), AKA capillary telangiectasia: slightly enlarged capillaries with low flow. Cannot be imaged on any radiographic study. Usually incidentally found at necropsy without clinical significance (risk of hemorrhage is very low, except possibly in brainstem. Has intervening neural tissue[4] (unlike cavernous malformations). Usually solitary, but may be multiple when seen as a part of a syndrome: Osler-Weber-Rendu (see below), Louis-Barr (ataxia telangiectasia), Myburn-Mason, Sturge-Weber.

Associated cerebrovascular malformations (CVM) include: telangiectasias, AVMs (the most common CVM, seen in 5-13% of HHT patients[7]), venous angiomas, and aneurysms. Patients are also prone to pulmonary arteriovenous fistulas with associated risk of paradoxical cerebral embolism which predisposes to embolic stroke and cerebral abscess formation (p. 343).

91.2.2 Epidemiology

Rare autosomal dominant genetic disorder of blood vessels affecting ≈ 1 in 5,000 people. 95% have recurrent epistaxis.

91.2.3 Imaging

CT

May show a well-demarcated homogeneous or mottled high density[6] (high density due to hematoma, calcification, thrombosis, hemosiderin deposition, alterations in BBB, and/or increased blood volume[1]) with some form of contrast enhancement (around or within lesion) in 17 of 24 patients.[6] Surrounding edema or mass effect is rare (except in cases that have recently hemorrhaged).

MRI

May demonstrate previous hemorrhage(s)[8] (may be important when the presence of multiple occurrences affects therapeutic choices). T2WI finding: reticulated core of increased and decreased intensity, a prominent surrounding rim of reduced intensity may be present (due to hemosiderin-laden macrophages from previous hemorrhages). T2* GRE image demonstrates flow-related enhancement in ≈ 60% of cases, which allows signal dropout from flowing blood on other sequences to be differentiated from that due to calcium (and thus, bone) or air (limitations: hemosiderin causes signal dropout, and slow in-plane flow does not enhance).[9]

91.2.4 Treatment

Surgery is indicated mainly for evacuation of hematoma or diagnosis, especially when favorably located. Also consider surgery for recurrent hemorrhages (rupture has been reported even after normal angiography) or medically intractable seizures. Stereotactic radiosurgery has not had a satisfactorily high enough benefit-to-risk ratio to justify its use.[10]

91.3 Cavernous malformation

91.3.1 General information

91

Key concepts

- usually angiographically occult. MRI is the study of choice (open channels → flow void on T2WI, previous hemorrhage → "popcorn" pattern especially on gradient echo or SWI)
- low-flow. No intervening neural parenchyma. No arteries
- may be associated with developmental venous anomaly (DVA) (p. 1512) which participates in venous outflow and should be preserved
- may be sporadic, hereditary, or may follow XRT
- presentation: usually seizures. Hemorrhage: risk is difficult to predict
- treatment:
  a) ♦ surgery is the treatment of choice for symptomatic accessible lesions
  b) ✘ radiosurgery is controversial, and should be reserved for symptomatic, inaccessible, nonfamilial CMs

AKA: cavernous hemangioma, cavernoma, cavernous angioma, angioma, hemangioma, and in medical jargon "cav-mal." A well-circumscribed, benign vascular hamartoma consisting of irregular thick- and thin-walled sinusoidal vascular channels located within the brain but *lacking intervening neural parenchyma*,[4] large feeding arteries, or large draining veins. Usually 1–5 cm in size. May hemorrhage, calcify, or thrombose. Occur rarely in the spinal cord.[11] Caverns are filled with blood in various stages of thrombus formation/organization/dissolution. Frequently associated with venous angiomas (p. 1512). Capillary telangiectasias may be found adjacent to lesions and may represent a precursor. Stain positive for angiogenesis factor.[12] Lesions may arise de novo,[13] and may grow (although slower than hemangioblastomas), shrink, or remain unchanged with time.[14]

91.3.2 Pathology

Gross appearance resembles a mulberry (facetiously dubbed a "hemorrhoid of the brain"). Structural characteristics:
- comprised of dilated endothelial-lined capillary vessels (caverns) with defective tight junctions
- no identifiable arterial feeders on angiography

3. often associated with a developmental venous anomaly (DVA)
4. no functional brain tissue with the encapsulated core[4]

Light microscopy: stains for von Willebrand's factor. Smooth muscle layer is absent (except for some tiny portions). EM: shows abnormal gapping of the tight junctions between endothelial cells[15] (may permit leakage of blood) and sparse or poorly characterized subendothelial smooth muscle cells.[15]

91.3.3 Epidemiology

Cerebral cavernous malformations (CM) comprise 5–13% of CNS vascular malformations, and develop in 0.02–0.16% of the population (based on large autopsy[16] and MRI[17,18] series). 48–86% are supratentorial (with 5–10% in the basal ganglia), 4–35% brainstem.[19] Multiple in 23%[20] to 50%[21] of cases, and multiplicity may be more common in hereditary cases.[17,22]

Spinal CMs: CMs occur rarely in the spinal cord.

CMs may be sporadic, hereditary, or may follow XRT.[23]

XRT appears to be a risk factor[24] (e.g., following craniospinal XRT[25] for medulloblastoma), especially for spinal CMs. 42% of patients with spinal CMs also harbor ≥ 1 intracranial CM.[26]

91.3.4 Genetics

Many cases of hereditary CMs follow a Mendelian *autosomal dominant* pattern with variable expressivity.[27] There appear to be at least 3 gene loci (see ▶ Table 91.1).

Table 91.1 Subtypes of CCM

	CCM1	CCM2	CCM3
locus	7q11-q22	7p15-13	3q25.2-q27
gene	KRIT1	MGC4607 (malcavernin)	PDCD10
feature	more common in Hispanics		rate of new CM formation: 0.4–2.7 new CMs/year

91.3.5 Presentation/natural history

General information

Presentation[28,29,30,31]:
1. seizures: 50%[31]
2. hemorrhage: 25%.[31] Usually intraparenchymal (see box (p. 1527) for definition of hemorrhage)
3. other: 25%. Including focal neurologic deficit without evidence of recent hemorrhage (25%),[31] hydrocephalus, or as in incidental finding in 20–50%.[18,32]

Hemorrhage

Accurately determining the risk of hemorrhage has been elusive. Reported rates depend on study design (retrospective vs. prospective, natural history vs. surgical series),[33] the definition of hemorrhage used (clinical vs. radiographic) and whether one assumes the CMs have been present since birth.

A standardized definition of hemorrhage by the Angioma Alliance[34] (see box) has been proposed (since essentially all CMs have surrounding hemosiderin indicative of small leaks and CMs are prone to recurrent small hemorrhages that are rarely devastating, and to differentiate a bleed from the mere presence of intralesional thrombus).

Spelling this out in more concrete terms[35]: a hemorrhagic event is considered to have occurred with:
1. *extra*lesional hemorrhage: acute or subacute blood-degradation products outside the CM
2. intralesional hemorrhage: acute or subacute blood-degradation products
   a) in a previously identified CM: accompanied by lesion growth, mass effect, edema or corresponding symptoms
   b) at first imaging (i.e., in a newly identified CM with no prior imaging): accompanied by corresponding clinical symptoms

✖ A hemorrhage is not considered to have occurred with:
1. only lesion growth without signal change
2. presence of hemosiderin without signs of a recent hemorrhage
3. the appearance of blood-degradation products without lesion growth or edema or clinical symptoms

---

∑: Angioma Alliance definition of hemorrhage in cavernous malformations[34]

Acute or subacute symptoms (any of: headache, seizure, impaired consciousness, or new/worsened focal neurological deficit referable to the anatomic location of the CM) accompanied by radiological, pathological, surgical, or (rarely) only cerebrospinal fluid evidence of recent extra- or intralesional hemorrhage.

This definition does not include either an increase in CM diameter without other evidence of recent hemorrhage, nor the presence of a hemosiderin halo.

Neurologic impairment following initial hemorrhage from a CM tends to be less than with other types of vascular malformations.[36] Each hemorrhage carries about 20% risk of morbidity, and 5% mortality.

Risk of hemorrhage in cerebral CMs
risk of first-time hemorrhage among incidentally discovered CMs is very low (0.08%)[32]
the two factors most consistently associated with increased bleeding risk[31]:
○ CMs initially presenting with hemorrhage: hazard ratio for bleeding = 5.6
○ brainstem CMs: hazard ratio = 4.4
hemorrhage outside the boundaries of the CM (extralesional hemorrhage) increase the rehemorrhage rate[35]
younger age: the hazard ratio for rehemorrhage is increased for younger patients[37]
inconsistent findings reported for risk differences with female gender, CM size, and CM multiplicity
the annual risk of recurrent hemorrhage declines over time[37,38,39,40]: with rate during the first ≈ 2.5 years that decreases[33,37,41]
higher annual ICH rates are reported in familial CMs (4.3–6%) than in sporadic cases[42] but this could be artifactual[31]
pregnancy & parturition are not thought to be risk factors for hemorrhage[27,43,44]
the risk of hemorrhage from a CM may not be increased by platelet inhibitors[39] or anticoagulation,[45] but this is based on uncontrolled studies that likely avoided treatment of patients with recent hemorrhage
in a study of 185 Hispanic patients with CCM1 mutation, no significant association was identified with any cardiovascular risk factor including hypertension[46]
no relation of physical activity to hemorrhage from CMs has been identified[39] including aerobic exercise and noncontact sports.[47] Less is known about contact sports, high-altitude climbing, and scuba diving and spinal cord CMs[47]

Hemorrhage as a function of cavernous malformation classification. The Zabramski Classification[42] of CMs (with an additional category V denoting extralesional extension added by Nikoubashman et al.[35]) is shown in ► Table 91.2.
Using the standardized definition of hemorrhage, Nikoubashman et al. found no significant difference in hemorrhage rates for types I, II and V, whereas types III and IV differed significantly.[35] This yielded 3 levels of morphology-based risk stratification for CMs shown in b► Table 91.3.
Spinal CMs: data is limited. Annual hemorrhage rate of 2.1% has been reported.[49] 17% of patients with spinal CMs also have cerebral CMs, and 12% had a family history of CMs.[49]

Seizures

The 5-year risk of first-time seizure was 6% among CM patients presenting with symptoms vs. 4% for those with incidental CMs.[50]

Table 91.2 Zabramski classification of cavernous malformations[42] (modified from Clinical Radiology, 68, Nikou-bashman O, Wiesmann M, Tournier-Lasserve E, et al. Natural history of cerebral dot-like cavernomas. e453–e459, 2013, with permission from Elsevier[a 35]) - schematic diagrams

Type	T1WI	T2WI	Gradient echo
I subacute hemorrhage with a rim of hemosiderin laden macrophages & gliotic brain. AHR[b] = 29.8%	hyperintense core (methemoglobin)	hyper- or hypo-intense core (hemosiderin & ferritin) with hypointense halo	
II loculated areas of hemorrhage & thrombus of varying age with a rim of gliotic, hemosiderin stained brain; large lesions may have areas of calcifications. AHR[b] = 20.1%	reticulated core of mixed signal ("popcorn" appearance)	reticulated core of mixed signal with hypointense rim ("popcorn" appearance)	
III chronic resolved hemorrhage with hemosiderin staining within & around the CM. AHR[b] = 3.4%	iso- or hypo-intense	hypointense with a hypotintense rim that magnifies the size of the lesion	hypointense with more magnification than T2WI
IV (some lesions in this category were found to be telangiectasias). AHR[b] = 1.3%	poorly seen or not visualized	poorly seen or not visualized	punctate hypointense lesions (minute deposits of hemosiderin)
V[a] presenting with extralesional hemorrhage. AHR[b] = 23.1%			

[a] Type V is not part of the original Zabramski classification and was proposed by Nikoubashman et al.[35]); only parts of the CM may be visible within the hemorrhage
[b] AHR = annual hemorrhage rate found by Nikoubashman et al.[35] in patients age < 18 years

Table 91.3 Risk stratification based on CM morphology[35]

Description	Annual hemorrhage risk	Mean hemorrhage-free interval (months)	Clinical correlates
High risk (Zabramski I, II or V). CMs with acute or subacute blood-degradation products	23.4%	22.63	associated with acute or subacute clinical symptoms
Intermediate risk (Zabramski III). CMs without acute or subacute blood-degradation products	3.4%	27.88	may be symptomatic (especially seizures)
Lowest risk (Zabramski IV). Punctate lesions (visible ≈ only on gradient echo)	1.3%	37.78	asymptomatic unless they are hemorrhagic[48]

91.3.6 Evaluation

Guidelines

> **Practice guideline: Imaging recommendations for cavernous malformations**
>
> 1. **Level I**[31]: brain MRI for the diagnosis and follow-up of known or suspected CMs
> 2. **Level I**[31]: MRI should include gradient echo or susceptibility-weighted sequences
> 3. **Level III**[31]: catheter angiography is not recommended unless an AVM is suspected
> 4. **Level I**[31]: follow-up imaging should be done to assess new or worsened symptoms to guide treatment decisions. There is insufficient data to make recommendations regarding timing of routine surveillance imaging

CT

Not sensitive: CT misses many small lesions, some large ones, and even some that have bled.

Not specific: CT findings may overlap with low-grade tumors, hemorrhages, granulomas. Isolated multifocal calcifications may suggest the diagnosis. Contrast CT may be helpful when MRI cannot be done.

CT scans are usually more readily available than MRI, and can rule out emergent conditions such as significant hematoma, hydrocephalus, and mass effect.

MRI

Diagnostic test of choice. MRI with either *gradient-echo T2WI* or *susceptibility-weighted (SWI)* images is the most sensitive test due to high sensitivity to susceptibility artifact from blood breakdown products within and around CMs. Findings are similar to AOVM in general (mixed-signal core with low-signal rim—sometimes described as "popcorn" pattern; see above); see ▶ Fig. 91.1. The diagnosis is strongly suggested by finding multiple lesions with these characteristics and a positive family history.[21] A venous malformation may be seen adjacent to a solitary CM, but not with multiple CMs.[51] Diffusion tensor imaging/white matter tractography[52] and pre-op 3D-constructive interference in steady-state (CISS) MRI[53] may improve localization, approach, and post-op outcomes.

Gadolinium-contrasted MRI may be helpful for identifying possible associated DVAs or capillary telangiectasia or to exclude tumors in questionable cases.

In the absence of spine symptoms, routine imaging of the spine is not indicated in patients with cerebral CMs.[31]

91

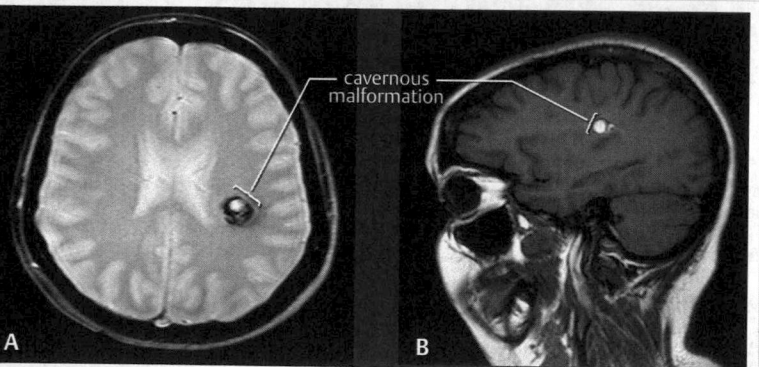

Fig. 91.1 Cavernous malformation of the left hemisphere.
Image: A: T2* GRE axial MRI showing classic "popcorn appearance."
B: T1 sagittal MRI showing hemosiderin ring around lesion (same patient as A).

Angiography

Does not demonstrate lesion. MRI appearance is nearly pathognomonic, and angiography is not necessary in classically appearing cases. Angiography may be needed to R/O other diagnoses in questionable cases.

Familial considerations

First-degree relatives of patients with more than one family member having a cavernous malformation should have MRI screening and appropriate genetic counseling (consult the guidelines[31] for details of testing & counseling).

91.3.7 Treatment/management

Overview

Management options:
1. observation
2. surgical excision
3. XRT or stereotactic radiosurgery

Even after many years, there is still conflicting data regarding optimal management of CMs. This has resulted in the somewhat confusing and conflicting treatment guidelines shown in (p. 1530)

Practice guideline: Treatment recommendations for cavernous malformations

1. **Level III**[31]: surgery is not recommended for asymptomatic CMs, especially those that are deep, or in eloquent areas or brainstem, or with multiple CMs
2. **Level II**[31]: consider surgery for: solitary asymptomatic CMs if easily accessible and not in eloquent brain, to prevent future hemorrhage, because of psychological burden, expensive & time-consuming follow-ups, to facilitate lifestyle or career decisions, or in patients who might need to be on anticoagulation
3. **Level II**[31]: consider early CM resection (≤ 6 weeks from hemorrhage) in patients with seizures, especially when medically refractory, if the CM is the likely cause of the seizure
4. **Level II**[31]: consider surgery in symptomatic easily accessible CMs (surgical morbidity & mortality is equivalent to living with the CM for 1–2 years after a first bleed)
5. **Level II**[31]: consider surgery after a second symptomatic bleed in a brainstem CM after reviewing the high risks of early post-op morbidity, mortality, and impact on quality of life
6. **Level II**[31]: consider surgery in deep CMs if symptomatic or after prior hemorrhage (surgical morbidity & mortality is equivalent to living with the CM for 5–10 years after a first bleed)
7. **Level II**[31]: surgical indications are weaker after a single, disabling bleed from a brainstem CM
8. **Level II**[31]: consider radiosurgery in solitary CMs with previous symptomatic hemorrhage if the CM is located in eloquent areas that have an unacceptably high risk with surgery
9. **Level III**[31]: radiosurgery is not indicated for CMs that are asymptomatic, or surgically accessible, or are part of familial CMs because of the concern about precipitating formation of additional CMs

---

Determining treatment response is difficult since no imaging study can prove elimination of the lesion. Therefore some have suggested that recurrent hemorrhage rate be followed as an endpoint.

No randomized prospective study has been done. No high-quality study has confirmed dramatic benefit or harm from surgical resection, and the few studies that showed some benefit appear to be biased.[31]

Recommendations

Incidental lesions

Asymptomatic, incidentally discovered CMs should be managed expectantly, (especially Zabramski types III & IV) with serial imaging studies for about 2–3 years (to rule out frequent subclinical bleeds) additional studies thereafter based on clinical grounds. Some experts recommend removal for single easily accessible incidental CMs in non-eloquent brain.[54] See (p. 1530) for practice guidelines.

✖ Since the radiographic appearance is almost pathognomonic, biopsy or excision solely to verify the diagnosis is rarely appropriate.

Patients presenting with intracererbal or intraventricular hemorrhage

Management should follow evidence-based guidelines (p. 1530) for these entities.

Brainstem CMs

Imaging findings in a brainstem (pontine) cavernous malformation are shown in ▶ Fig. 91.2.

Surgery is almost never indicated for brainstem CMs that have not bled. Operative management has been suggested for CMs with a history of > 2 prior hemorrhages and "pial/ependymal representa-

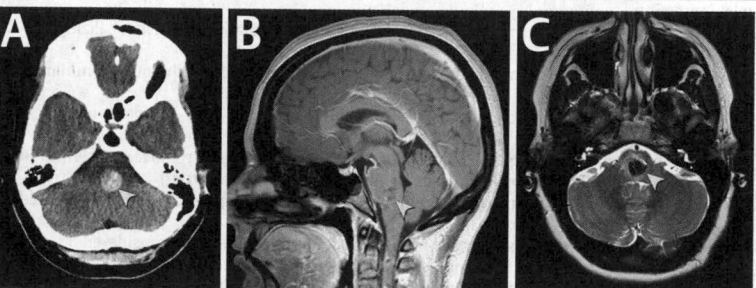

Fig. 91.2 Brainstem cavernous malformation (*yellow arrowheads*) in a 35-year-old presenting with diplopia and right hand paresthesias.
Image: A: Noncontrast CT scan, B: sagittal T1 MRI with contrast, C: axial T2 MRI.
The admitting CT scan (A) shows acute bleed. The contrast sagittal MRI (B) shows the subtle appearance of the lesion which appears identical on the non-contrast MRI (not shown), i.e., no enhancement. The axial T2 MRI (C) shows the signal dropout from the blood. This lesion and bleed did not present on the surface of the brainstem.

91

ion" on T1WI MRI.[55,56] See (p. 1530) for practice guidelines.

Bleeds that do not come to the surface cannot be removed without creating neurologic deficit worsening of neurologic outcome was 9% vs. 29% in superficial vs. deep brainstem CM resections, respectively[57]). The approach is chosen to expose the site where the bleed comes closest to the surface. CMs are frequently associated with a venous angioma (p. 1512) which must be preserved since it provides critical venous outflow. Outcome was worse with surgery through the floor of the 4th ventricle than with a lateral approach. Significant short-term neurologic deficit is expected in ≈ 50% with brainstem CM resection.[55]

Spinal cord CMs

Managed essentially the same as brainstem CMs.

Cranial nerve CMs

Many case reports and reviews document CMs of cranial nerves (rarely extra-axial) with various presentations.[58,59,60] Case reports suggest patients may benefit from early surgical decompression from hemorrhagic chiasmal cavernomas since they are at risk for recurrent micro-hemorrhages.[61]

Surgery

Indications

Surgical indications for intracranial CMs (see (p. 1530) for practice guidelines):
1. accessible lesions with
   a) focal deficit
   b) or symptomatic hemorrhage
   c) or seizures: seizure control is lower with longer seizure duration[62]

2. less accessible lesions that repeatedly bleed with progressive neurologic deterioration may be considered for excision, even in delicate regions such as the brainstem[63,64,65] or spinal cord

Surgical risks

The risk of surgery varies with CM location. Overall risk of death or nonfatal stroke after resection of *incidental* CM: 6%.[66] This risk is greater than the natural history (2.4% over 5 years), but is better than the risk of a recurrent hemorrhage after a first bleed (29.5% over 5 years). The risk for deep CMs (basal ganglia, insula, thalamus) is higher, with 5–18% morbidity and almost 2% mortality.[67] Brainstem CMs carry even higher risk (morbidity almost 50%) but most improve over time.[31]

Surgical technique

- goal of surgery is complete resection of the lesion. The rate of rehemorrhage is higher with incomplete resection
- stereotactic localization or intraoperative ultrasound are particularly helpful in localizing and increasing the chance for GTR
- choose a surgical corridor along the greated length of the CM (2-point technique) to minimize injury to adjacent brain
- in comparison to AVMs, a wide exposure is not needed
- initial dissection is directed at separating the lesion from the adjacent brain
- once the dissection is complete, the contents of the CM capsule may be removed piecemeal to minimize the parenchymal opening (especially important in the brainstem)
- with CMs that have bled, one usually encounters a cavity containing the CM and blood degradation products.[68]
- the hemosiderin stained rim is normally not removed, but removal can be considered if seizures are associated with the lesion if it is not located in eloquent brain (controversial). Some improvement in seizure control can occur even with resection limited to the CM alone[69]
- if there is an associated developmental venous anomalies (p. 1512) (DVA) it is not removed as it represents venous drainage of the area, and DVAs often regress following complete removal of the CM
- for deep CMs meeting surgical indications, surgical corridors are discussed in the references for for the thalamus[70] and for the brainstem[71]

Brainstem CMs

DTI may be helpful to identify splitting or displacement of critical tracts. The use of retractors is to be avoided; cottonoids and exploitation of hematoma cavity may be used to gain access. Unlike supratentorial CMs, brainstem CMs may be extremely adherent to brain parenchyma[65]. Bipolar cautery: use on low power with constant irrigation to reduce thermal injury. Unlike supratentorial CM with seizures, the adjacent hemosiderin-stained parenchyma is not removed.

Post-op follow-up

Follow-up MRI ≈ 3 months post-op is recommended. It never looks "normal" but can determine i removal was complete.

Stereotactic radiosurgery (SRS)

See references.[72,73,74,75,76,77] Controversial: results appear comparable to natural history. Some non controlled studies have shown a possible reduction in recurrent hemorrhage rate following a 2-yea latency period after SRS[75]; however, radiation-induced morbidity was significant.[78,79] Other serie have failed to show reduction.[80] Findings may reflect the natural history of CMs with temporal clus tering of hemorrhagic events with decrease in hemorrhage rates after 28 months.[37] SRS may pro mote development of new CMs in familial cases (controversial). See (p. 1530) for practice guidelines

91.3.8 Prognosis

When CMs can be completely removed, the risk of further growth or hemorrhage is essentially per manently eliminated[68] (however, recurrence of symptoms has been reported after partial and eve seemingly complete removal[65,81]).

For CMs treated surgically, patients need to be aware that post-op neurologic worsening is very com mon, especially with brainstem CMs.[82] Worsening may be transient,[83] but may take months to resolve.

91

References

[1] Cohen HCM, Tucker WS, Humphreys RP, et al. Angiographically Cryptic Histologically Verified Cerebrovascular Malformations. Neurosurgery. 1982; 10:704–714

[2] Shuey HM, Day AL, Quisling RG, et al. Angiographically Cryptic Cerebrovascular Malformations. Neurosurgery. 1979; 5:476–479

[3] Ropper AH, Davis KR. Lobar Cerebral Hemorrhages: Acute Clinical Syndromes in 26 Cases. Ann Neurol. 1980; 8:141–147

[4] Steiger HJ, Tew JM. Hemorrhage and Epilepsy in Cryptic Cerebrovascular Malformations. Arch Neurol. 1984; 41:722–724

[5] Russell DS. The Pathology of Spontaneous Intracranial Hemorrhage. Proceedings of the Royal Society of Medicine. 1954; 47:689–693

[6] Bitoh S, Hasegawa H, Fujiwara M, et al. Angiographically Occult Vascular Malformations Causing Intracranial Hemorrhage. Surg Neurol. 1982; 17:35–42

[7] Willemse RB, Mager JJ, Westermann CJ, et al. Bleeding risk of cerebrovascular malformations in hereditary hemorrhagic telangiectasia. J Neurosurg. 2000; 92:779–784

[8] Lemme-Plaghos L, Kucharczyk W, Brant-Zawalski M, et al. MRI of Angiographically Occult Vascular Malformations. AJNR. 1986; 7:217–222

[9] Needell WM, Maravilla KR. MR Flow Imaging in Vascular Malformations Using Gradient Recalled Acquisition. American Journal of Neuroradiology. 1988; 9:637–642

[10] Lindquist C, Guo W-Y, Kerlsson B, et al. Radiosurgery for Venous Angiomas. Journal of Neurosurgery. 1993; 78:531–536

[11] Cosgrove GR, Bertrand G, Fontaine S, et al. Cavernous Angiomas of the Spinal Cord. Journal of Neurosurgery. 1988; 68:31–36

[12] Uranishi R, Baev NI, Ng PY, et al. Expression of endothelial cell angiogenesis receptors in human cerebrovascular malformations. Neurosurgery. 2001; 48:359–67; discussion 367-8

[13] Detwiler PW, Porter RW, Zabramski JM, et al. De novo formation of a central nervous system cavernous malformation: implications for predicting risk of hemorrhage. Case report and review of the literature. J Neurosurg. 1997; 87:629–632

[14] Clatterbuck RE, Moriarity JL, Elmaci I, et al. Dynamic nature of cavernous malformations: a prospective magnetic resonance imaging study with volumetric analysis. J Neurosurg. 2000; 93:981–986

[15] Wong JH, Awad IA, Kim JH. Ultrastructural pathological features of cerebrovascular malformations: a preliminary report. Neurosurgery. 2000; 46:1454–1459

[16] Simard JM, Garcia-Bengochea, Ballinger WE, et al. Cavernous angioma: A review of 126 collected and 12 new clinical cases. Neurosurgery. 1986; 18:162–172

[17] Moriarity JL, Wetzel M, Clatterbuck RE, et al. The natural history of cavernous malformations: a prospective study of 68 patients. Neurosurgery. 1999; 44:1166–1173

[18] Morris Z, Whiteley WN, Longstreth WT, Jr, et al. Incidental findings on brain magnetic resonance imaging: systematic review and meta-analysis. BMJ. 2009; 339. DOI: 10.1136/bmj.b3016

[19] Gross BA, Batjer HH, Awad IA, et al. Cavernous malformations of the basal ganglia and thalamus. Neurosurgery. 2009; 65:7–18; discussion 18-9

[20] Moran NF, Fish DR, Kitchen N, et al. Supratentorial cavernous haemangiomas and epilepsy: a review of the literature and case series. Journal of Neurology, Neurosurgery, and Psychiatry. 1999; 66:561–568

[21] Rigamonti D, Drayer BP, Johnson PC, et al. The MRI Appearance of Cavernous Malformations (Angiomas). J Neurosurg. 1987; 67:518–524

[22] Perlemuter G, Bejanin H, Fritsch J, et al. Biliary obstruction caused by portal cavernoma: a study of 8 cases. Journal of Hepatology. 1996; 25:58–63

[23] Gastelum E, Sear K, Hills N, et al. Rates and characteristics of radiographically detected intracerebral cavernous malformations after cranial radiation therapy in pediatric cancer patients. J Child Neurol. 2015; 30:842–849

[24] Detwiler PW, Porter RW, Zabramski JM, et al. Radiation-induced cavernous malformation. J Neurosurg. 1998; 89:167–169

[25] Maraire JN, Abdulrauf SI, Berger S, et al. De novo development of a cavernous malformation of the spinal cord following spinal axis radiation. Case report. J Neurosurg. 1999; 90:234–238

[26] Cohen-Gadol AA, Jacob JT, Edwards DA, et al. Coexistence of intracranial and spinal cavernous malformations: a study of prevalence and natural history. J Neurosurg. 2006; 104:376–381

[27] Hayman LA, Evans RA, Ferrell RE, et al. Familial Cavernous Angiomas: Natural History and Genetic Study Over a 5-Year Period. Am J Med Genet. 1982; 11:147–160

[28] Robinson JR, Awad IA, Little JR. Natural history of the cavernous angioma. Journal of Neurosurgery. 1991; 75:709–714

[29] Del Curling O,Jr, Kelly DL,Jr, Elster AD, et al. An analysis of the natural history of cavernous angiomas. Journal of Neurosurgery. 1991; 75:702–708

[30] Kim DS, Park YG, Choi JU, et al. An analysis of the natural history of cavernous malformations. Surgical Neurology. 1997; 48:9–17; discussion 17-8

[31] Akers A, Al-Shahi Salman R, , et al. Synopsis of Guidelines for the Clinical Management of Cerebral Cavernous Malformations: Consensus Recommendations Based on Systematic Literature Review by the Angioma Alliance Scientific Advisory Board Clinical Experts Panel. Neurosurgery. 2017; 80:665–680

[32] Moore SA, Brown RD,Jr, Christianson TJ, et al. Long-term natural history of incidentally discovered cavernous malformations in a single-center cohort. J Neurosurg. 2014; 120:1188–1192

[33] Stapleton CJ, Barker FG,2nd. Cranial Cavernous Malformations: Natural History and Treatment. Stroke. 2018; 49:1029–1035

[34] Al-Shahi Salman R, Berg MJ, Morrison L, et al. Hemorrhage from cavernous malformations of the brain: definition and reporting standards. Angioma Alliance Scientific Advisory Board. Stroke. 2008; 39:3222–3230

[35] Nikoubashman O, Di Rocco F, Davagnanam I, et al. Prospective Hemorrhage Rates of Cerebral Cavernous Malformations in Children and Adolescents Based on MRI Appearance. AJNR Am J Neuroradiol. 2015; 36:2177–2183

[36] Cordonnier C, Al-Shahi Salman R, Bhattacharya JJ, et al. Differences between intracranial vascular malformation types in the characteristics of their presenting haemorrhages: prospective, population-based study. J Neurol Neurosurg Psychiatry. 2008; 79:47–51

[37] Barker FG,2nd, Amin-Hanjani S, Butler WE, et al. Temporal clustering of hemorrhages from untreated cavernous malformations of the central nervous system. Neurosurgery. 2001; 49:15–24; discussion 24-5

[38] Horne MA, Flemming KD, Su IC, et al. Clinical course of untreated cerebral cavernous malformations: a meta-analysis of individual patient data. Lancet Neurol. 2016; 15:166–173

[39] Flemming KD, Link MJ, Christianson TJ, et al. Prospective hemorrhage risk of intracerebral cavernous malformations. Neurology. 2012; 78:632–636

[40] Al-Shahi Salman R, Hall JM, Horne MA, et al. Untreated clinical course of cerebral cavernous malformations: a prospective, population-based cohort study. Lancet Neurol. 2012; 11:217–224

[41] Taslimi S, Modabbernia A, Amin-Hanjani S, et al. Natural history of cavernous malformation: Systematic review and meta-analysis of 25 studies. Neurology. 2016; 86:1984–1991

[42] Zabramski JM, Wascher TM, Spetzler RF, et al. The natural history of familial cavernous malformations: results of an ongoing study. J Neurosurg. 1994; 80:422–432

[43] Witiw CD, Abou-Hamden A, Kulkarni AV, et al. Cerebral cavernous malformations and pregnancy: hemorrhage risk and influence on obstetrical management. Neurosurgery. 2012; 71:626–30; discussion 631

[44] Kalani MY, Zabramski JM. Risk for symptomatic hemorrhage of cerebral cavernous malformations during pregnancy. J Neurosurg. 2013; 118:50–55

[45] Schneble HM, Soumare A, Herve D, et al. Antithrombotic therapy and bleeding risk in a prospective cohort study of patients with cerebral cavernous malformations. Stroke. 2012; 43:3196–3199

[46] Choquet H, Nelson J, Pawlikowska L, et al. Association of cardiovascular risk factors with disease severity in cerebral cavernous malformation type 1 subjects with the common Hispanic mutation. Cerebrovasc Dis. 2014; 37:57–63

[47] Joseph NK, Kumar S, Lanzino G, et al. The influence of physical activity on cavernous malformation hemorrhage. J Stroke Cerebrovasc Dis. 2020; 29. DOI: 10.1016/j.jstrokecerebrovasdis.2019.104629

[48] Nikoubashman O, Wiesmann M, Tournier-Lasserve E, et al. Natural history of cerebral dot-like cavernomas. Clin Radiol. 2013; 68:e453–e459

[49] Badhiwala JH, Farrokhyar F, Alhazzani W, et al. Surgical outcomes and natural history of intramedullary spinal cord cavernous malformations: a single-center series and meta-analysis of individual patient data: Clinic article. J Neurosurg Spine. 2014; 21:662–676

[50] Josephson CB, Leach JP, Duncan R, et al. Seizure risk from cavernous or arteriovenous malformations: prospective population-based study. Neurology. 2011; 76:1548–1554

[51] Abdulrauf SI, Kaynar MY, Awad IA. A comparison of the clinical profile of cavernous malformations with and without associated venous malformations. Neurosurgery. 1999; 44:41–6; discussion 46-7

[52] Chen X, Weigel D, Ganslandt O, et al. Diffusion tensor imaging and white matter tractography in patients with brainstem lesions. Acta Neurochirurgica (Wien). 2007; 149:1117–31; discussion 1131

[53] Zausinger S, Yousry I, Brueckmann H, et al. Cavernous malformations of the brainstem: three-dimensional-constructive interference in steady-state magnetic resonance imaging for improvement of surgical approach and clinical results. Neurosurgery. 2006; 58:322–30; discussion 322-30

[54] Scott. Annual meeting of the Congress of Neurological Surgeons. Orlando, FL 2008

[55] Gross BA, Batjer HH, Awad IA, et al. Brainstem cavernous malformations. Neurosurgery. 2009; 64: E805–18; discussion E818

[56] Dammann P, Abla AA, Al-Shahi Salman R, et al. Surgical treatment of brainstem cavernous malformations: an international Delphi consensus. J Neurosurg. 2021; 136:1220–1230

[57] Ferroli P, Sinisi M, Franzini A, et al. Brainstem cavernomas: long-term results of microsurgical resection in 52 patients. Neurosurgery. 2005; 56:1203–12; discussion 1212-4

[58] Deshmukh VR, Albuquerque FC, Zabramski JM, et al. Surgical management of cavernous malformations involving the cranial nerves. Neurosurgery. 2003; 53:352–7; discussion 357

[59] Albanese A, Sturiale CL, D'Alessandris Q G, et al. Calcified extra-axial cavernoma involving lower cranial nerves: technical case report. Neurosurgery. 2009; 64:135–6; discussion 136

[60] Itshayek E, Perez-Sanchez X, Cohen JE, et al. Cavernous hemangioma of the third cranial nerve: case report. Neurosurgery. 2007; 61. DOI: 10.1227/01.NEU.0000290916.63094.8E

[61] Crocker M, Desouza R, King A, et al. Cavernous hemangioma of the optic chiasm: a surgical review. Skull Base. 2008; 18:201–212

[62] von der Brelie C, Kuczaty S, von Lehe M. Surgical management and long-term outcome of pediatric patients with different subtypes of epilepsy associated with cerebral cavernous malformations. J Neurosurg Pediatr. 2014; 13:699–705

[63] Bicknell JM. Familial Cavernous Angioma of the Brain Stem Dominantly Inherited in Hispanics. Neurosurgery. 1989; 24:102–105

[64] Ondra SL, Doty JR, Mahla ME, et al. Surgical Excision of a Cavernous Hemangioma of the Rostral Brain Stem: Case Report. Neurosurgery. 1988; 23:490–493

[65] Zimmerman RS, Spetzler RF, Lee KS, et al. Cavernous Malformations of the Brain Stem. J Neurosurg 1991; 75:32–39

[66] Poorthuis M, Samarasekera N, Kontoh K, et al. Comparative studies of the diagnosis and treatment of cerebral cavernous malformations in adults: systematic review. Acta Neurochir (Wien). 2013 155:643–649

[67] Pasqualin A, Meneghelli P, Giammarusti A, et al. Results of surgery for cavernomas in critical supratentorial areas. Acta Neurochir Suppl. 2014 119:117–123

[68] Wascher TM, Spetzler RF, Carter LP, et al. Cavernous malformations of the brain stem. In: Neurovascular Surgery. New York: McGraw-Hill; 1995:541–555

[69] Ferroli P, Casazza M, Marras C, et al. Cerebral cavernomas and seizures: a retrospective study on 16 patients who underwent pure lesionectomy. Neuro Sci. 2006; 26:390–394

[70] Rangel-Castilla L, Spetzler RF. The 6 thalamic regions: surgical approaches to thalamic cavernous malformations, operative results, and clinical outcomes. J Neurosurg. 2015; 123:676–685

[71] Cavalcanti DD, Preul MC, Kalani MY, et al. Microsurgical anatomy of safe entry zones to the brainstem. Neurosurg. 2016; 124:1359–1376

[72] Kondziolka D, Lunsford LD, Flickinger JC, et al. Reduction of hemorrhage risk after stereotactic radiosurgery for cavernous malformations. Journal of Neurosurgery. 1995; 83:825–831

[73] Porter RW, Detwiler PW, Han PP, et al. Stereotactic radiosurgery for cavernous malformations: Kjellberg's experience with proton beam therapy in 9 cases at the Harvard Cyclotron. Neurosurgery 1999; 44:424–425

[74] Zhang N, Pan L, Wang BJ, et al. Gamma knife radio surgery for cavernous hemangiomas. Journal of Neurosurgery. 2000; 93:74–77

[75] Pollock BE, Garces YI, Stafford SL, et al. Stereotact radiosurgery for cavernous malformations. J Neurosurg. 2000; 93:987–991

[76] Wen R, Shi Y, Gao Y, et al. The Efficacy of Gamma Knife Radiosurgery for Cavernous Malformations: Meta-Analysis and Review. World Neurosurg. 2019 123:371–377

[77] Lunsford LD, Niranjan A, Kano H, et al. Leksell Stereotactic Radiosurgery for Cavernous Malformation. Prog Neurol Surg. 2019; 34:260–266

[78] Hasegawa T, McInerney J, Kondziolka D, et al. Long-term results after stereotactic radiosurgery for patients with cavernous malformations. Neurosurgery. 2002; 50:1190–7; discussion 1197-8

[79] Liu KD, Chung WY, Wu HM, et al. Gamma knife surgery for cavernous hemangiomas: an analysis of 125 patients. Journal of Neurosurgery. 2005; 10 Suppl:81–86

[80] Karlsson B, Kihlstrom L, Lindquist C, et al. Radiosurgery for cavernous malformations. Journal Neurosurgery. 1998; 88:293–297

[81] Bertalanffy H, Gilsbach JM, Eggert HR, et al. Micro surgery of deep-seated cavernous angiomas: repo of 26 cases. Acta Neurochirurgica. 1991; 108:91–9

[82] Weil SM, Tew JM Jr. Surgical management of brain stem vascular malformations. Acta Neurochir (Wien). 1990; 105:14–23

[83] Bartolomei J, Wecht DA, Chaloupka J, et al. Occipital lobe vascular malformations: prevalence of visual field deficits and prognosis after therapeutic intervention. Neurosurgery. 1998; 43:415–21; discussion 421-3

Part XIX

Stroke and Occlusive Cerebrovascular Disease

XIX

92 Stroke – General Information and Physiology

92.1 Definitions

Acute ischemic stroke (AIS) AKA cerebral infarction. Obsolete term: cerebrovascular accident (CVA).

▶ **TIA.** (Transient ischemic attack): transient neuronal dysfunction secondary to focal ischemia (of brain, spinal cord, or retina) without (permanent) acute infarction[1] (**note:** obsolete operational definitions used an arbitrary 24-hour cutoff for duration of symptoms).

10–15% of patients with TIA have a stroke within 3 months, 50% of which occur within 48 hours.

▶ **Stroke.** Permanent (i.e., irreversible) death of neurons caused by inadequate perfusion of a region of the brain or brainstem.

▶ **Watershed infarct.** Ischemic infarction in a territory located at the periphery of two bordering arterial distributions due to a disturbance in flow in one or both of the arteries.

92.2 Cerebrovascular hemodynamics

92.2.1 Cerebral blood flow (CBF) and oxygen utilization

▶ Table 92.1 shows typical CBF values and the corresponding neurophysiologic state. CBF < 20 is generally associated with ischemia and if prolonged will produce cell death.[2] However, this assumes normal metabolic rate and may be more applicable to global cerebral hypoperfusion.[3] There is a higher CBF threshold for loss of electrical excitability than that for cell death—this has led to the concept of the ischemic penumbra—nonfunctioning cells that are still viable.[2]

Table 92.1 Correlates of CBF

CBF (ml per 100 gm tissue/min)	Condition
>60 (approx)	hyperemia (CBF > tissue demand)
45–60	normal brain at rest
75–80	gray matter
20–30	white matter
<20: Ischemia	
16–18	EEG becomes flatline
15	physiologic paralysis
12	brainstem auditory evoked response (BAER) changes
10	alterations in cell membrane transport (cell death; stroke)

CBF is related to blood pressure as shown in Eq (92.1).

$$CBF = \frac{CPP}{CVR} = \frac{MAP - ICP}{CVR} \tag{92.}$$

where CPP = cerebral perfusion pressure (p. 1036), CVR = cerebrovascular resistance (see below), and MAP = mean arterial pressure.

92.2.2 Cerebrovascular resistance (CVR) and cerebral autoregulation

In the range of CPP ≈ 50–150 mm Hg, CVR (the resistance of the cerebral vascular bed to blood flow of normal brain tissue varies linearly to maintain an almost constant CBF (▶ Fig. 92.1). This phenomenon is called (cerebral) autoregulation. It is accomplished by alterations in blood vessel tone via a myogenic mechanism. Cerebral autoregulation can be disrupted in certain pathologic states.

CVR is affected by the $PaCO_2$ such that there is a linear increase in CBF with increasing $PaCO_2$ within the range of $PaCO_2$ = 20–80 mm Hg.

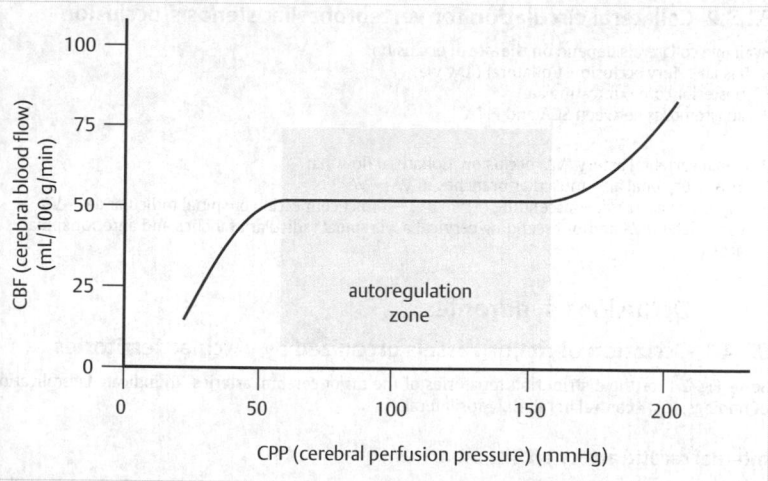

Fig. 92.1 Cerebral autoregulation.
The range of CPP where CBF is relatively constant is indicated by the yellow square.

92.2.3 Cerebral metabolic rate of oxygen consumption (CMRO$_2$)

CMRO$_2$ averages 3.0–3.8 ml/100 gm tissue/min. The ratio of CBF to CMRO$_2$ (the coupling ratio[4]) in the quiescent brain is 14:18. With focal cortical activity, local CBF increases ≈ 30% while CMRO$_2$ increases ≈ 5%.[5] CMRO$_2$ can be manipulated to some degree.

92.2.4 Cerebrovascular reserve and reactivity

May be evaluated with xenon-enhanced CT, CTP (p. 239), TCD, SPECT, or MRI.[6,7,8,9] Response of CBF to a vasodilator challenge with 1000 mg of IV acetazolamide (ACZ) (Diamox®) is classified as[8,9]:
- Type I: normal baseline CBF with 30–60% increase following ACZ challenge
- Type II: decreased baseline CBF with blunted response of < 10% increase or < 10 ml/100 g/min absolute increase after ACZ challenge
- Type III: decreased baseline CBF with paradoxical decrease of regional CBF following ACZ challenge, suggesting a steal phenomenon in regions with maximally dilated vasculature at baseline

92.3 Collateral circulation

92.3.1 Collateral circulation for ICA stenosis/occlusion

The effects of ICA stenosis/occlusion may be ameliorated by collateral blood flow. Potential alternate routes for blood to reach brain tissue include:
1. flow through the circle of Willis
    a) from contralateral ICA through anterior communicating a.
    b) from forward flow through the ipsilateral posterior communicating a.
2. retrograde flow through *ophthalmic a.* parasitizing blood from *both* ECAs via:
    a) facial a. → angular a. → dorsal nasal a. & medial palpebral a.
    b) maxillary a.
        - middle meningeal a. → lacrimal a.
        - vidian a. (a. of the pterygoid canal)
    c) transverse facial a. → lateral palpebral a.
    d) superficial temporal a. → supraorbital a.
3. proximal maxillary a. → anterior tympanic a. → caroticotympanic branch of ICA
4. cortical-cortical anastomoses
5. dural-leptomeningeal anastomoses

92

92.3.2 Collateral circulation for vertebrobasilar stenosis/occlusion

Available collaterals depend on the site of occlusion.

Basilar artery occlusion. Collateral flow via:
1. posterior communicating aa.
2. anastomoses between SCA and PICA

Proximal vertebral artery (VA) occlusion. Collateral flow via:
1. ECA → occipital a. → muscular branches of VA → VA
2. thyrocervical trunk → ascending cervical a. → direct connection or spinal radicular aa.→ VA
3. contralateral VA and/or ascending cervical a. via spinal radicular branches and anterior spinal artery

92.4 "Occlusion" syndromes

92.4.1 Occlusion of major vessels organized by vascular territories

See ► Fig. 2.1 for the distribution territories of the major cerebral arteries. To indicate lateralization of findings, {CL} = contralateral, {IL} = ipsilateral.

Internal carotid artery and its branches

Risk and extent of stroke is influenced by suddenness of occlusion, location of occlusion, and collateral circulation (see above).
1. statistics:
   a) acute ICA occlusion (all comers): 26–49% risk of stroke[10] (not all of these strokes are severe)
   b) annual stroke risk in 1,261 patients with symptomatic ICA occlusion: 7% overall, 5.9% ipsilateral to the occlusion (mean follow-up = 45.5 mos) (even with anticoagulation or antiplatelet drugs) (12 prospective studies[11])
   c) St. Louis Carotid Occlusion Study[12]: 2-year ipsilateral ischemic stroke rate in patients with symptomatic ICA occlusion = 5% in patients with normal O_2 extraction fraction (OEF) by PET scan, and 26% in patients with increased OEF
   d) stroke risk is less when one includes asymptomatic ICA occlusions (i.e., there are people walking around with ICA occlusion and no symptoms)
   e) in patients presenting with ICA territory stroke or TIA, complete ICA occlusion is found in 10–15%[12]
2. anterior cerebral artery: {CL} weakness of LE > UE
3. worst-case scenario of total ICA occlusion with no AComA or PComA flow and no collateral rescue: stroke in ACA and MCA territories (► Table 92.2)

Table 92.2 Total ICA occlusion

Deficit[a]	Complete (M1 occlusion)	Superior division	Inferior division
{CL} weakness of UE > LE	X	X	
{CL} weakness of lower face	X	X	
{CL} hemisensory loss (UE & LE)	X	X	
{CL} hemisensory loss of face (all modalities)	X	X	
{CL} neglect[b]	X	X	
{IL} gaze preference	X		
{CL} homonymous hemianopsia	X		X[c]
receptive aphasia[d] (Wernicke's area)	X		X
expressive aphasia[d] (Broca's area)	X	X	
Gerstmann syndrome (p. 99): with dominant parietal lobe infarct			

[a][CL] = contralateral, [IL] = ipsilateral. An "X" indicates that the deficit is present
[b]with involvement on side of nondominant hemisphere
[c]plus [CL] upper quadrantanopsia
[d]with involvement on the side of the dominant hemisphere

4. posterior cerebral artery
   a) unilateral occipital lobe infarction → homonymous hemianopsia with macular sparing (visual cortex of the macula receives dual blood supply from MCA and PCA)
   b) Balint syndrome
   c) cortical blindness (Anton syndrome)
   d) Weber syndrome
   e) alexia without agraphia
   f) thalamic pain syndrome (Dejerine-Roussy syndrome)
5. recurrent medial striate artery (of Heubner): expressive aphasia + *mild* hemiparesis (UE > LE, proximal muscles weaker than distal) - dense hemiparesis is not typical
6. anterior choroidal artery (AChA) syndrome: first described by Foix et al in 1925. The complete triad consists of {CL} hemiplegia, hemihypesthesia, and homonymous hemianopsia (mnemonic: 3 H's); however, incomplete forms are more common.[13] Occlusion is usually due to small vessel disease, and CT or MRI usually shows infarct in posterior limb of IC (just above temporal horn of lateral vent)[14] and white matter posterior and lateral to it. Occlusion is usually tolerated fairly well, and ligation of this artery was actually utilized in treatment of Parkinsonism sometimes without ill effect[15 (p 540)]—see Surgical treatment of Parkinson's disease (p. 1840)—but internal capsule infarct occurred in ≈ 15%.
7. artery of Percheron (p. 82): bilateral thalamic and mesencephalic infarctions[16]

Posterior circulation

1. vertebral artery
   a) medial medullary syndrome (Dejerine syndrome)
   b) lateral medullary syndrome (Wallenberg syndrome): see below
2. basilar artery
3. AICA: lateral pontine syndrome (Marie-Foix syndrome)
4. PICA: sometimes lateral medullary (Wallenberg) syndrome: see below
5. SCA: infarction of superior cerebellar vermis and superior cerebellum
6. anterior spinal artery

Lateral medullary syndrome (LMS)

AKA Wallenberg's syndrome, AKA PICA syndrome. Classically attributed to PICA occlusion, but in 80–85% of cases the *vertebral artery* is also involved.[17] No cases have been reported arising from brainstem hemorrhage. Onset is usually acute. The findings are listed in ► Table 92.3 (NB: *absence of pyramidal tract findings*, and *no change in sensorium*). The location of the lesion and medullary structures are shown in ► Fig. 92.2.

Table 92.3 Findings in lateral medullary syndrome[15 (p 547)]

GENERALIZED symptoms	Responsible lesion
• vertigo, N/V, nystagmus, diplopia, oscillopsia	vestibular nuclei & connections
• hiccups	?
IPSILATERAL to lesion	**Responsible lesion**
• facial pain, paresthesias, & impaired sensation	descending tract and nucleus V over half of face
• ataxia of limbs	(restiform body?)
• Horner syndrome	descending sympathetic tract
• dysphagia, diminished gag, hoarseness	exiting fibers of IX & X
• numbness of arm, trunk, or leg	cuneate & gracile nuclei
CONTRALATERAL to lesion	**Responsible lesion**
• impaired pain & temp sense over half of body	spinothalamic tract

► **Note.** This is essentially the only location where a lesion will produce sensory loss on one side of the face (ipsilateral to the lesion) and contralateral sensory loss in the body. All in the absence of pyramidal tract findings (i.e., overt weakness).

These patients sometimes develop severe cerebellar swelling that responds to neurosurgical decompression (the tissue aspirates easily).

92

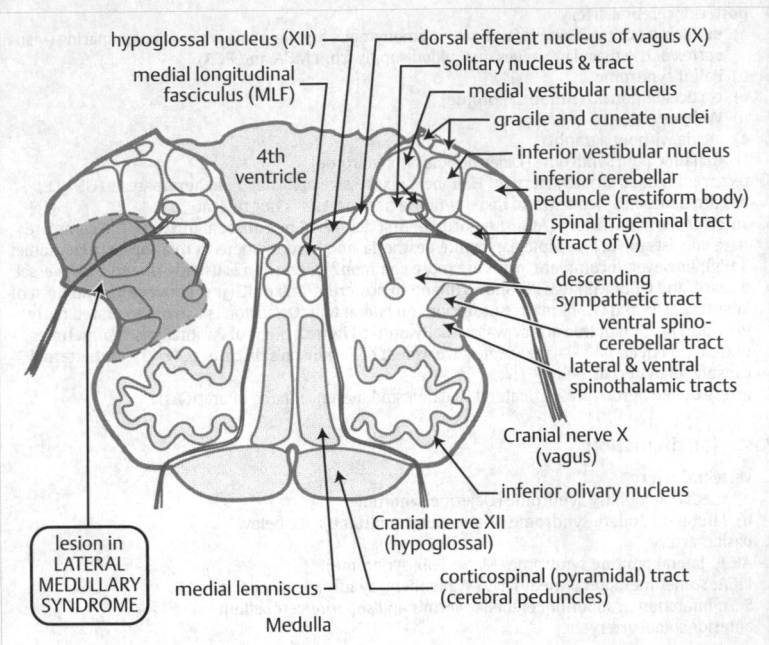

Fig. 92.2 **Typical lesion in lateral medullary syndrome.** Image: schematic cross-section through medulla (the lesion is indicated as shaded area).

In a patient presenting with LMS, one needs to rule out vertebral dissection (p. 1579), since this would be treated with heparin. MRI including fat-suppressed T1WI and MRA would detect dissection in most cases.

Prognosis: 12% of 43 patients died during the acute phase from respiratory and cardiovascular complications and 2 new posterior-fossa strokes occurred.[18] Recurrent vertebrobasilar territory stroke rate was 1.9% per year.[18]

92.4.2 Lacunar strokes

General information

Small infarcts in deep noncortical cerebrum or brainstem (▶ Table 92.4) resulting from occlusion of penetrating branches of cerebral arteries. Size of infarcts ranges from 3–20 mm (CT detects larger ones; better sensitivity in white matter).

Table 92.4 Typical locations for lacunar strokes *(in descending frequency)*

- putamen
- caudate
- thalamus
- pons
- internal capsule (IC)
- convolutional white matter

Small (3–7 mm) lacunes may be due to lipohyalinosis (vasculopathy due to HTN) of arteries < 200 microns (may also be cause of many ICHs); this vasculopathy is indicative of small vessel disease, unlikely to be prevented by carotid endarterectomy.

Clinically, diagnosis is virtually *excluded* by: aphasia, apractagnosia, sensorimotor stroke, monoplegia, homonymous hemianopsia (**HH**), severe isolated memory impairment, stupor, coma, LOC, or seizures.

L'etat lacunaire: multiple lacunes → chronic progressive neuro decline with one or more episodes of hemiparesis; results in invalidism, dysarthria, small-step gait (marche á petits pas), imbalance, incontinence, pseudobulbar signs, dementia. Many signs and symptoms are possibly due to NPH (unrecognized originally).

Lacunar syndromes

Major syndromes (see reference[19] for others):
1. pure sensory stroke or TIA: (the most common lacunar manifestation) usually isolated unilateral numbness of face, arm, and leg. Only 10% of TIA go on to stroke. Lacune in sensory (posteroventral) thalamus → CT detection is poor. Dejerine-Roussy = rare thalamic pain syndrome that may develop late
2. pure motor hemiparesis (PMH): (2nd most common lacunar manifestation) pure unilateral motor deficit of face, arm, and leg without sensory deficit, HH, etc. Lacune in posterior limb of IC, or in lower basis pontis where corticospinal (CS) tracts coalesce, or rarely in mid-cerebral peduncle
3. ataxic hemiparesis: contralateral PMH + cerebellar ataxia of affected limbs (if they can move). Lacune in basis pontis at junction of upper third and lower two–thirds → dysarthria, nystagmus, and unidirectional toppling possible. Differential severity in face, arm, and leg possible because CS fibers are dispersed by nuclei pontis (unlike compact pyramids and peduncle)
   a) variant: dysarthria-clumsy hand syndrome: lesion in same location or genu of IC. May be mimicked by a cortical infarct, but latter will have numb lips
4. PMH sparing the face: lacune in medullary pyramid; at onset, there may be vertigo and nystagmus (approaching lateral medullary syndrome)
   a) variant: thalamic dementia: central region of one thalamus + adjacent subthalamus → abulia, memory impairment + partial Horner (miosis + anhydrosis)
5. mesencephalothalamic syndrome: "top o' the basilar syndrome." Usually caused by embolus. Infarct typically butterfly-shaped & bilateral involving rostral brainstem and cerebral hemisphere regions fed by the distal basilar artery. Clinical: III palsy, Parinaud's syndrome (p. 101) & abulia, may have amnesia, hallucinations, and somnolence, usually without significant motor dysfunction
6. Weber's syndrome: Cr. N. III palsy with contralateral PMH (no sensory loss). Usually due to occlusion of interpeduncular branches of basilar artery → central midbrain infarction, disrupting cerebral peduncle and issuing fibers of III. May also be due to aneurysm of basilar bifurcation or BA-SCA junction
7. PMH with crossed VI palsy: lacune in paramedian inferior pons
8. cerebellar ataxia with crossed III palsy (*Claude* syndrome): lacune in dentatorubral tract (superior cerebellar peduncle)
9. hemiballism: classically, infarct or hemorrhage in subthalamic semilunar nucleus of Luys
10. lateral medullary syndrome: see below
11. locked-in syndrome: bilateral PMH from infarct at IC, pons, pyramid, or (rarely) cerebral peduncles

92.5 Stroke in young adults

92.5.1 General information

Only 3% of ischemic strokes occur in patients < 40 yrs of age.[20] Over 10% of ischemic strokes occur in patients ≤ 55 yrs.[21] Incidence: 10 per 100,000 persons age 35–44 yrs,[22] 73 per 100,000 for age < 55 yrs.[21]

92.5.2 Etiologies

The differential diagnosis is lengthy,[20] with *trauma* being the most common cause of strokes (22%) in patients under 45 yrs.[23] Most of the rest are covered by the small number of etiologies listed below (excludes: trauma, post-op stroke, SAH, and intracerebral hemorrhage).
1. atherosclerosis: 20%—less common than in older population (all 18 patients in one series had either ID-DM, or were males > 35 yrs with ≥ 1 risk factor (see below), most had TIAs earlier)
2. embolism with recognized source: 20%

92

a) cardiac origin is the most common (above), most have previously known cardiac disease:
- rheumatic heart disease
- prosthetic valve
- endocarditis
- mitral valve prolapse (MVP): present in 5–10% of young adults, in 20–40% of young adults with stroke (although one series found MVP in only 2% of stroke in young adults[22])
- a-fib
- left-atrial myxoma

b) fat embolism syndrome: neurologic manifestation is usually global neurologic dysfunction; see Fat embolism syndrome (p. 1013)

c) paradoxical embolism: e.g., ASD, pulmonary AVM including Osler-Weber-Rendu syndrome, patent foramen ovale (above)

d) amniotic fluid embolism: may occur typically in the post-partum period

3. vasculopathy: 10%
  a) inflammatory
   - Takayasu's
   - infective: TB, syphilis, ophthalmic zoster
   - amphetamine abuse
   - herpes zoster ophthalmicus (HZO): usually presents with delayed contralateral hemiplegia with a mean of ≈ 8 weeks following HZO[24]
   - mucormycosis: a nasal and orbital fungal infection primarily in diabetics and immunocompromised patients that causes an arteritis which may thrombose the orbital veins and ICA or ACA. Produces proptosis, ocular palsy, and hemiplegia
   - associated with systemic disease such as: SLE (lupus) (also see below under Coagulopathy); arteritis (especially periarteritis nodosa (p. 208)) when confined to CNS is usually multifocal and progressive, but may mimic stroke early; multiple sclerosis (MS); cancer; rheumatoid arthritis
  b) non-inflammatory
   - fibromuscular dysplasia (p. 209)
   - carotid or vertebral artery dissections (including posttraumatic)
   - moyamoya disease (p. 1601)
   - homocystinuria: a genetic defect in methionine metabolism that produces intimal thickening and fibrosis in almost all vessels with associated thromboembolic events (arterial and venous, including dural venous sinuses). Estimated risk of stroke is 10–16%. Patients have a Marfan syndrome-like physical appearance, malar blotches, mental retardation, and elevated levels of urinary homocysteine
   - pseudoxanthoma elasticum

4. coagulopathy: 10%. The following are associated with hypercoagulable states
  a) SLE: lupus anticoagulant → prolonged PTT incompletely corrects with 50/50 mix. Collagen vascular disease only rarely presents initially with stroke
  b) polycythemia or thrombocytosis
  c) sickle cell disease
  d) TTP (thrombotic thrombocytopenic purpura)
  e) antithrombin III deficiency (controversial—not seen in large series of young adults with stroke)
  f) protein C or protein S deficiency (familial): protein C attenuates hemostatic reactions, homozygous deficiency is fatal in the neonatal period. Heterozygous deficiency is associated with *thrombotic* strokes. A rare complication during initial therapy with warfarin is a drop in protein C before other coagulation factors resulting in a hypercoagulable state
  g) antiphospholipid-antibody syndrome (APLAS)[25,26]: causes venous and/or arterial thrombosis. The two best known antiphospholipid-antibodies are anticardiolipin antibodies (ACLA), and lupus anticoagulant (LAC). Once they become symptomatic, treatment is high-intensity warfarin therapy to an INR ≥ 3.[27] There is a dramatic increase in thrombotic events after discontinuing warfarin. Aspirin is useless
  h) following use of the street drug 3,4-methylenedioxymethamphetamine (MDMA, commonly known as ecstasy),[28] possibly independent of the hypercoagulable state that occurs with hyperthermia when insufficient fluids are consumed in conjunction with use of the drug

5. peripartum: 5% (usually within 2 wks of parturition)

6. miscellaneous causes: 35%
  a) uncertain etiology

b) oral contraceptives (BCP): associated with ninefold increased risk for stroke, many with prior migraine history

c) cerebral venous thrombosis (CVT) (p. 1594) including dural sinus thrombosis: incidence may be increased with use of BCP

d) migraine[29]: widely accepted, but difficult to assess objectively (incidence of stroke in these patients may be same as general population). *Rare.* Usually occurs in women, with a benign long-term course; recurs in < 3%. Possible mechanisms include: vasospasm, platelet dysfunction, and arteriopathy.[30] Strokes often occur during a migrainous attack[31] or shortly thereafter

e) cocaine abuse[32]: stroke may result from vasoconstriction, or from HTN in the presence of aneurysms or AVMs (frank vasculitis occurs[33] but is rare with cocaine, unlike amphetamines); strokes with alkaloidal cocaine ("crack") are ≈ equally divided between ischemic and hemorrhagic

f) posterior reversible encephalopathy syndrome (PRES) (p. 202)

92.5.3 Risk factors

In a retrospective "neighborhood control" study of 201 Australian patients aged 15–55 (mean = 45.5) with first-time strokes, the following risk factors were identified[21]:
1. diabetes: odds ratio = 12
2. HTN: odds ratio = 6.8
3. current cigarette smoking: odds ratio = 2.5
4. long-term heavy alcohol consumption: odds ratio = 15 (heavy alcohol ingestion within 24 hrs preceding the stroke was *not* a risk factor)

92.5.4 Evaluation

1. history & physical exam directed at uncovering systemic disease (see above) and modifiable risk factors (see above)
2. cardiology work-up including EKG and echocardiogram
3. bloodwork (include as appropriate):
   a) routine: electrolytes, CBC, platelet count and/or function, ESR (elevation may suggest SLE, arteritis, atrial myxoma... but a normal ESR does not rule out vasculitis), PT/PTT, VDRL (should be obtained in all young adults with stroke), fasting lipid profile
   b) for unexplained stroke: ANA, antithrombin III, protein C, protein S, homocysteine, factor V Leiden, PPD, sickle-cell screen, toxicology screen (blood and urine, to R/O drugs such as cocaine), SPEP, lupus anticoagulant, serum amino acid, tissue plasminogen-activator and -inhibitor
4. miscellaneous tests: U/A, CXR, CSF exam when indicated
5. cerebral angiography: not always necessary for patients with obvious systemic disease or strong evidence for cardiac embolism; may occasionally diagnose cerebral embolism if performed within 48 hrs of ictus

92.6 Atherosclerotic carotid artery disease

92.6.1 General information

Atherosclerotic plaques begin to form in the carotid artery at 20 yrs of age. In the extracranial cerebral circulation, plaques typically start on the back wall of the common carotid artery (CCA). As they enlarge, they encroach on the lumen of the ICA. Calcified hard plaques may not change with time. The risk of stroke correlates with the degree of stenosis and with certain types of plaque morphology, and is also increased in hypercoagulable states and with increased blood viscosity.

Plaque morphology

"Vulnerable" plaques are atherosclerotic plaques likely to cause thrombotic complications, or those that tend to progress rapidly. Criteria for vulnerable plaques include: intimal thickening, plaque fissure, lipid/necrotic core with thin fibrous cap, calcification, thrombus, intraplaque hemorrhage, and outward remodeling. Some of these features can be identified with high-resolution MRI.[34,35,36,37]

92.6.2 Presentation

General information

Carotid artery lesions are considered symptomatic if there are one or more lateralizing ischemic episodes appropriate to the distribution of the lesion. A lesion is considered to be *asymptomatic* if the patient only has non-specific visual complaints, dizziness, or syncope not associated with TIA or stroke.[38] The majority (80%) of carotid atherothrombotic strokes occur without warning symptoms.[39]

Asymptomatic carotid stenosis

Usually discovered as a carotid bruit. Asymptomatic bruit: prevalence increases with age (2.3% in ages 45–54 yrs, 8.2% at ≥ 75).[40] Accuracy of a bruit in predicting ICA stenosis: 50–83% (depending on cohort, criteria for stenosis...). Sensitivity is as low as 24%.[41]

Symptomatic carotid disease

May present as a TIA, RIND, or stroke with any of the following findings; see also ICA occlusion syndromes (p. 1538):
1. retinal insufficiency or infarction (central retinal artery is a branch of the ophthalmic artery): ipsilateral monocular blindness
   a) may be temporary: amaurosis fugax, AKA transient monocular blindness (TMB). Four types:
      • Type I: embolic. Described "like a black curtain coming down" in *one eye*. Complete loss of vision, usually lasts 1–2 minutes
      • Type II: flow-related. Retinal hypoperfusion → desaturation of color, usually described as a graying of vision
      • Type III: vasospastic. May occur with migraines
      • Type IV: miscellaneous. May occur with anticardiolipin antibodies
   b) blindness may be permanent
2. middle cerebral artery symptoms:
   a) contralateral motor or sensory TIA (arm and face worse than leg) with hyperreflexia and upgoing toe
   b) language deficits if dominant hemisphere involved

92.6.3 Evaluation of the extent of carotid disease

Overview

Symptomatic patients will usually be assessed as part of a stroke/TIA protocol.
   Check CBC with platelet count, fibrinogen, PT/PTT/INR (to R/O hypercoagulable state).
   Funduscopic exam may show Hollenhorst plaques (cholesterol crystal emboli) in the retina.
   Classification of patients based on the hemodynamics and also the embolic propensity of carotid lesions has thus far been too complex to be utilized in large studies. The tests described below place a great deal of emphasis on the greatest degree of stenosis, which is probably an oversimplification. Plaque composition and morphology is probably important.

Recommendations for screening for carotid stenosis

1. the U.S. Preventive Services Task Force (USPSTF) currently recommends against screening for carotid stenosis in the adult general population (grade D recommendation: moderate or high certainty that the service has no net benefit or that the harm outweighs the benefit)[42]
2. the AHA Primary Prevention of Stroke Guidelines does not recommend screening for asymptomatic carotid stenosis[43]
3. the American Society of Neuroimaging advised that screening should be considered only for age ≥ 65 years with 3 or more cardiovascular risk factors[44]
4. the Society of Vascular Surgery recommends ultrasonography screening for age ≥ 55 years with cardiovascular risk factors, such as HTN, diabetes, smoking, hypercholesterolemia, or known cardiovascular disease[45]

Assessment options

See also recommendations for which tests to use (p. 1547).

Angiography

The "gold standard" test is a catheter arteriogram. It cannot be justified as a *screening* test because it is invasive, and too costly and risky (recent data show < 1% risk of transient or permanent deficit (risk is 2–3 times higher in symptomatic patients than in asymptomatic)[46,47,48] in good hands). Also, unlike duplex Doppler and MRA, it does not provide any information about the thickness of the plaque. Different definitions of the degree of stenosis are employed; ▶ Table 92.5 compares the definitions used by the NASCET study[49] to those of the ECST.[50] For both, N is the linear diameter of the carotid artery at the site of greatest narrowing. The studies differ in the denominator, NASCET uses D (the diameter of the normal artery *distal* to the carotid bulb, taken at the first point at which the arterial walls become parallel), whereas the ECST uses B (the *estimated* carotid bulb diameter).

Table 92.5 Comparison of NASCET and ECST measurements of ICA stenosis[a]

	NASCET	ECST
	$1 - \dfrac{N}{D}$	$1 - \dfrac{N}{B}$
	Approximate equivalent degrees of ICA stenosis based on direct comparison (%)	
	30[b]	65[b]
	40[b]	70
	50	75
	60	80
	70	85
	80	91
	90	97

[a]adapted from Donnan GA, Davis SM, Chambers BR, et al. Surgery for the prevention of stroke. Lancet 351: 1372, 1998, with permission
[b]degrees of stenosis for which surgery was NOT of clear benefit for symptomatic stenosis (p. 1565)

For example, using the NASCET definition, the degree of stenosis is shown in Eq (92.2).

$$\% \text{ stenosis (NASCET)} = \left(1 - \frac{N}{D}\right) \times 100 \tag{92.2}$$

The relationship between the degree of narrowing based on the NASCET definition vs. that of the ECST has also been estimated by equation[51] as shown in Eq (92.3).

$$\% \text{ stenosis (by ECST)} = 0.6 \times \% \text{ stenosis (by NASCET)} + 40\% \tag{92.3}$$

Angiography also affords the opportunity to perform endovascular intervention if indicated.

Duplex Doppler ultrasound

B-mode image evaluates the artery in cross-sectional plane, and spectrum analysis shows blood flow. Performs poorly with a "string sign." Cannot scan above the angle of the mandible. Lower frequencies give greater depth of penetration, but signal definition is sacrificed (used in transcranial Doppler). Sensitivity: 88%, specificity: 76%.[52]

Magnetic resonance angiography (MRA)

May obviate the need for angiography in some cases of carotid stenosis, specifically in symptomatic patients with a focal "gap" of signal intensity loss with distal reappearance of signal.[53,54] Sometimes overestimates the degree of stenosis.[55] Sensitivity: 91%, specificity: 88% for extracranial carotid disease.[56] 2D TOF-MRA is adequate (contrast-MRA shows more, but is not necessary for surgical lesions[57]).

Can be performed at the time as MRI with stroke protocol in TIA/stroke patients, and also detects thrombus or dissection. As with Doppler, has difficulties distinguishing very severe stenosis from occlusion. Less operator-dependent than Doppler, but is more expensive and time-consuming. MRA is more difficult to perform if the patient is critically ill, unable to lie supine, or has claustrophobia, a pacemaker, or ferromagnetic implants. High-resolution MRI may also detect vulnerable plaques (p.1543).

Computed tomography angiography (CTA)

CTA involves ionizing radiation (X-rays) and IV iodinated contrast, limiting its use in patients with dye allergies and renal dysfunction. Results are comparable to MRA and Doppler. CTA can be performed within a few seconds and yields high-resolution images of all vessels from the aortic arch through the intracranial/extracranial vessels as well as the surrounding soft tissues (► Fig. 92.3). In a meta-analysis, sensitivity and specificity for detection of a 70% to 99% stenosis were 85% and 93%, respectively.[58] CTA is still evolving and may help detect vulnerable plaques (p.1543). Another potential advantage: ability to obtain CT-perfusion (p.239) studies at the same time.

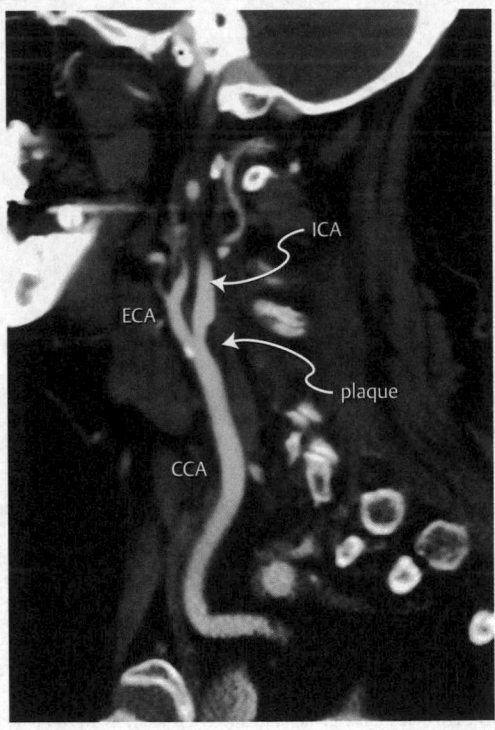

Fig. 92.3 CTA demonstrating soft ICA plaque.
Sagittal CTA through left carotid artery demonstrating soft plaque producing approximately 60% ICA stenosis.
Abbreviations: ICA = internal carotid artery; CCA = common carotid artery; ECA = external carotid artery.

Choice of imaging test/management decisions

Despite a great deal of research on the subject, there are no data to support a particular testing algorithm.[1] Doppler, CTA, or MRA are acceptable initial screening tests. In patients with an abnormal screening test, a common strategy is to obtain a second confirmatory noninvasive test to evaluate the carotid bifurcation before intervention. The combination of carotid ultrasound and MRA has proved cost-effective with good interobserver reliability.[59] If 2 noninvasive tests are discordant, catheter angiography should be considered before intervention.

92.6.4 Treatment

Treatment alternatives are primarily between the following.
1. "best medical management": see below
2. carotid endarterectomy (p. 1565)
3. endovascular techniques: combined angioplasty and stenting (± distal embolus protection)

Medical treatment

General information

What constitutes "best medical management" has not been precisely determined, and recommendations are constantly changing. Some or all of the following are utilized:
1. antiplatelet therapy (p. 169):
   a) usually aspirin (ASA): cyclooxygenase inhibitor (see below)
   b) P2Y12 receptor blockers: clopidogrel, ticlopidine, ticagrelor, prasugrel… either alone or in combination with ASA (see below)
   c) combination of extended-release dipyridamole and ASA (Aggrenox®) (no benefit from dipyridamole (Persantine®) alone)
2. antihypertensive therapy as appropriate
3. good control of diabetes if present
4. patients with asymptomatic a-fib should be treated with anticoagulation; see Cardiogenic brain embolism (p. 1590)
5. antilipid therapy if needed—statins
6. intervention to help patients to quit smoking

92

Antiplatelet therapy

Drug info: Aspirin

Irreversibly inhibits cyclooxygenase, preventing synthesis of vascular prostacyclin (a vasodilator and platelet inhibitor) and platelet thromboxane A2 (a vasoconstrictor and platelet activator). Platelets, lacking cellular organelles, cannot resynthesize cyclooxygenase, whereas the vascular tissues do so rapidly.[60] NB: < 1000 mg ASA per day probably does not help with high-grade stenosis where there is perfusion failure or flow failure. Some (but not all) studies show less effectiveness in women,[61] and no large study has shown that ASA prevents a second stroke in patients that have already had one.

℞: For angina, a bolus dose of 160–325 mg PO is followed by maintenance doses of 80–160 mg/d (lower doses appear to be as effective as higher doses).[62] Optimal dose for cerebrovascular ischemia continues to be debated. 325 mg PO q d reduces risk of stroke following TIA by 25–30%. Daily doses of 81 or 325 mg when compared to higher doses were associated with a lower rate of stroke, MI, and death (6.2% vs. 8.4%) following carotid endarterectomy.[63]

Drug info: Aspirin/ER-Dipyridamole (Aggrenox®)

Combination of extended-release dipyridamole and ASA (Aggrenox) is more effective than ASA alone for prevention of TIA, stroke, and myocardial infarction.[64,65,66] Aggrenox was not superior to clopidogrel, with increased hemorrhage with Aggrenox.[67] **Side effects:** H/A with initial therapy.

℞: 1 capsule PO BID. **Supplied:** fixed-dose capsules of aspirin 25 mg/extended-release with dipyridamole 200 mg.

Drug info: Clopidogrel (Plavix®)

A thienopyridine. Incidence of severe neutropenia (0.04%) is close to that of ASA (≈ 0.02%).[68] Interferes with platelet membrane function by inhibiting ADP-induced platelet fibrinogen binding and release of platelet granule contents, as well as subsequent platelet-platelet interactions. Produces a time- and dose-dependent irreversible inhibition of platelet aggregation and prolongation of bleeding time. May replace ASA if intolerance or resistance. Used in combination with ASA for some endovascular procedures. Although clopidogrel plus aspirin is recommended over aspirin for acute coronary syndromes, the MATCH[69] results do not suggest a similar benefit for stroke and TIA. Combination therapy significantly increased risk of hemorrhage.[69]

Pharmacokinetics: Dosed once daily. Requires several days to reach maximal effect (∴ a loading dose may be used, e.g., after an *acute* event such as an MI, or before stenting). Takes ≈ 5 days off the drug for platelet inhibition to reverse.

℞: 75 mg PO q d. Loading dose: 225 mg (3 pills) the first day of therapy. **Supplied:** 75 mg film-coated tablet.

Choice of antiplatelet agents

Individualization is recommend for antiplatelet agents for secondary stroke prevention. ASA is effective, and its low cost may help compliance. A small reduction of vascular events with Aggrenox may justify its expense from a broader healthcare perspective. Clopidogrel is appropriate for those intolerant or resistant to ASA. Clopidogrel plus ASA may be indicated in patients with recent cardiac ischemia or vascular stenting.[70]

Asymptomatic carotid artery stenosis

Key concepts

- natural history: reveals low stroke rate (2%/yr), half of which are not disabling
- large randomized trials have revealed moderate surgical benefit versus medical management for: asymptomatic stenosis > 60%
- treatment selection criteria depend on patient's age, gender, and comorbidities (and therefore life expectancy), and on perioperative complication rate

Practice guideline: Asymptomatic carotid stenosis

- Level I[71]: CEA is reasonable in asymptomatic patients with > 70% ICA stenosis if risk of perioperative stroke, MI, and death is low
- Level II[71]: It is reasonable to choose CEA over CAS when revascularization is indicated in older patients especially when the anatomy is unfavorable for endovascular intervention
- Level II[71]: It is reasonable to choose CAS over CEA when revascularization is indicated in patients with anatomy unfavorable for surgery
- Level II[71]: prophylactic CAS may be considered in highly selected patients with asymptomatic ICA stenosis (≥ 60% by angiography, > 70% by validated Doppler ultrasound), but the effectiveness compared to medical therapy alone is not well-established
- Level II[71]: In patients with high risk of complications by either CEA or CAS (includes: age > 80 years, NYHA heart failure class II or IV, LVEF < 30%, class III or OV angina pectoris, left main or multivessel CAD, need for cardiac surgery within 30 days, MI within 4 weeks, and severe chronic lung disease), the effectiveness of revascularization over medical therapy alone is not well-established

Abbreviations: CEA = carotid endarterectomy; CAS = carotid artery stenting.

92

Natural history

Prevalence of carotid stenosis > 50% in men and women > 65 years of age is 5–10%, with 1% having stenosis > 80%.[72,73,74]

Natural history studies reflect an annual stroke risk of 1–3.4% with asymptomatic carotid artery stenosis of 50–99% at 2–3 years.[75,76,77,78,79,80] A cohort study found similar cumulative rates of ipsilateral stroke over 10 years (9.3%, or 0.9%/year) and 15 years (16.6%, or 1.1%/year).[81]

Attempts to identify subgroups of patients with asymptomatic carotid stenosis at elevated stroke risk suggest that the rate of unheralded stroke ipsilateral to a hemodynamically significant extracranial carotid artery stenosis is 1–2% annually, with some data suggesting that the stroke rate may be higher with progressing stenosis or with more severe stenosis. Asymptomatic carotid stenosis is an important marker of concomitant ischemic cardiac disease.[75,76,77,80,81] In the REACH Study,[82] patients with asymptomatic carotid stenosis (n = 3164) had statistically significantly higher age- and sex-adjusted 1-year rates of transient ischemic attack, non-fatal stroke, fatal stroke, and cardiovascular death compared to patients without asymptomatic carotid stenosis (n = 30 329).

Surgery vs. medical management: the studies

ACST

See reference.[83]

> **Σ**
>
> The ACST[83] revealed a moderate benefit for immediate CEA vs. medical management in patients age < 75 with asymptomatic stenosis ≥ 60%.

Details: 3,120 patients with ≥ 60% stenosis by duplex ultrasound were randomized to immediate CEA (50% had CEA within 1 month, 88% within 1 year) or medical therapy at the discretion of the treating physician. Mean follow-up: 3.4 years. Exclusion criteria included: poor surgical risk, prior ipsilateral CEA, and probable cardiac emboli. Surgeons were required to have a perioperative morbidity and mortality rate of < 6%.

Net five-year risk for all stroke or perioperative stroke or death: 6.4% in the CEA group, vs. 11.8% in the medical group (p < 0.0001). Fatal or disabling stroke: 3.5 vs. 6.1%. Fatal stroke alone: 2.1 vs. 4.2%. Although men and women benefited, men benefited more. CEA did not demonstrate a statistically significant benefit for patients over the age of 75. Statistical benefit was not seen in the immediate CEA group until nearly two years after surgery, despite a relatively low perioperative morbidity and mortality rate of 3.1% (in contrast to patients with symptomatic stenosis (NASCET[84]) where benefit was seen much earlier).

ACAS

See reference.[85]

> **Σ**
>
> Large trial that randomized patients in good health with asymptomatic stenosis (calculated in the same manner as the NASCET study) ≥ 60% to CEA plus aspirin, or aspirin alone[85] found a reduced 5-year risk of ipsilateral stroke if CEA was performed with < 3% perioperative morbidity and mortality and is added to aggressive management of modifiable risk factors.

Details: CEA reduced 5-year stroke risk by 66% in males, 17% in females (not statistically significant), and 53% overall (males & females lumped together). CEA did *not* significantly protect against major stroke or death (P = 0.16) (half of the strokes were not disabling), and was somewhat protective against any stroke or death (P = 0.08). The study group was 95% Caucasian, and 66% were male. Excluded patients (age > 79 yrs, unstable CAD, uncontrolled HTN) may have been higher risk. Surgeons were carefully selected and the surgical morbidity (1.5%) and mortality (0.1%) was very low.

92

Surprisingly, ≈ half of the total morbidity (1.2%) was related to angiography. The implication is that for a generally healthy white male with ACAS > 60%, management with CEA (when performed by a surgeon with a low complication rate, as described) reduces his annual risk of all strokes from 0.5% to 0.17% (the reduction of risk for severe stroke is less). The benefit from CEA is realized within less than one year after the CEA. This is in contrast to the ACST trial (see above) and is most likely due to the lower perioperative event rate. The risk from mortality from other causes (including MI) is ≈ 3.9% per year. Combined stroke and death rates in community hospitals,[86] while improved over the last 20 yrs, remain higher at ≈ 6.3% than at centers used in this study.

Veteran's Administration Cooperative Study (VACS)
See reference.[84]

CEA reduces ipsilateral neurologic events, but did not reduce the rate of ipsilateral strokes nor death (most deaths were secondary to MI). This trial did not include women and was not powered to detect differences in outcome subgroups.

CASANOVA Study
See reference.[87]

No difference in outcome between CEA vs. aspirin (new stroke or death), but an unusual protocol lessened its statistical validity.[88]

Mayo Clinic Asymptomatic Carotid Endarterectomy (MACE) Study
See reference.[89]

There were no major strokes or deaths in either the medical or the endarterectomy group. Surgically treated patients were not given aspirin, and 26% had an MI compared to 9% in the aspirin-treated medical arm, reflecting the high incidence of concomitant CAD in patients with an asymptomatic carotid artery stenosis.

References

[1] Easton JD, Saver JL, Albers GW, et al. Definition and evaluation of transient ischemic attack. Stroke. 2009; 40:2276–2293

[2] Astrup J, Siesjö BK, Symon L. Thresholds in Cerebral Ischemia - The Ischemic Penumbra. Stroke. 1981; 12:723–725

[3] Powers WJ, Grubb RL, Darriet D, et al. Cerebral Blood Flow and Cerebral Metabolic Rate of Oxygen Requirements for Cerebral Function and Viability in Humans. J Cereb Blood Flow Metab. 1985; 5:600–608

[4] Raichle ME, Grubb RL, Gado MH, et al. Correlation Between Regional Cerebral Blood Flow and Oxidative Metabolism. In Vivo Studies in Man. Archives of Neurology. 1976; 33:523–526

[5] Henegar MM, Silbergeld DL. Pharmacology for Neurosurgeons. Part II: Anesthetic Agents, ICP Management, Corticosteroids, Cerebral Protectants. Contemporary Neurosurgery. 1996; 18:1–6

[6] Chimowitz MI, Furlan AJ, Jones SC, et al. Transcranial Doppler assessment of cerebral perfusion reserve in patients with carotid occlusive disease and no evidence of cerebral infarction. Neurology. 1993; 43:353–357

[7] Guckel FJ, Brix G, Schmiedek P, et al. Cerebrovascular reserve capacity in patients with occlusive cerebrovascular disease: assessment with dynamic susceptibility contrast-enhanced MR imaging and the acetazolamide stimulation test. Radiology. 1996; 201:405–412

[8] Rogg J, Rutigliano M, Yonas H, et al. The acetazolamide challenge: imaging techniques designed to evaluate cerebral blood flow reserve. AJR. American Journal of Roentgenology. 1989; 153:605–612

[9] Vagal AS, Leach JL, Fernandez-Ulloa M, et al. The acetazolamide challenge: techniques and applications in the evaluation of chronic cerebral ischemia. AJNR. American Journal of Neuroradiology. 2009; 30:876–884

[10] Allen JW. Proximal internal carotid artery branches: prevalence and importance for balloon occlusion test. Journal of Neurosurgery. 2005; 102:45–52

[11] Hankey GJ, Warlow CP. Prognosis of symptomatic carotid artery occlusion: an overview. Cerebrovascular Diseases. 1991; 1:245–256

[12] Grubb RLJr, Powers WJ, Derdeyn CP, et al. The Carotid Occlusion Surgery Study. Neurosurg Focus. 2003; 14

[13] Derex L, Ostrowsky K, Nighoghossian N, et al. Severe Pathological Crying After Left Anterior Choroidal Artery Infarction: Reversibility with Paroxetine Treatment. Stroke. 1997; 28:1464–1466

[14] Helgason C, Caplan LR, Goodwin J, et al. Anterior Choroidal Artery-Territory Infarction: Report of Cases and Review. Arch Neurol. 1986; 43:681–686

[15] Adams RD, Victor M. Principles of Neurology. 2nd ed. New York: McGraw-Hill; 1981

[16] Matheus MG, Castillo M. Imaging of acute bilateral paramedian thalamic and mesencephalic infarcts. AJNR. American Journal of Neuroradiology. 2003; 24:2005–2008

[17] Fisher CM, Karnes WE, Kubik CS. Lateral Medullary Infarction: The Pattern of Vascular Occlusion. J Neuropath Exp Neurol. 1961; 29:323–379

[18] Norrving B, Cronqvist S. Lateral medullary infarction: prognosis in an unselected series. Neurology. 1991; 41:244–248

[19] Fisher CM. Lacunar Strokes and Infarcts: A Review. Neurology (NY). 1982; 32:871–876

[20] Hart RG, Miller VT. Cerebral Infarction in Young Adults: A Practical Approach. Stroke. 1983; 14:110–114

[21] You RX, McNeil JJ, O'Malley HM, et al. Risk factors for stroke due to cerebral infarction in young adults. Stroke. 1997; 28:1913–1918

[22] Adams HP, Butler MJ, Biller J, et al. Nonhemorrhagic Cerebral Infarction in Young Adults. Arch Neurol. 1986; 43:793–796

[23] Hilton-Jones D, Warlow CP. The causes of stroke in the young. J Neurol. 1985; 232:137–143

[24] Verghese A, Sugar AM. Herpes zoster ophthalmicus and granulomatous angiitis: An ill-appreciated cause of stroke. J Am Geriatr Soc. 1986; 34:309–312

[25] Toschi V, Motta A, Castelli C, et al. High Prevalence of Antiphosphatidylinositol Antibodies in Young Patients with Cerebral Ischemia of Undetermined Cause. Stroke. 1998; 29:1759–1764

[26] Tanne D, Triplett DA, Levine SR. Antiphospholipid-protein antibodies and ischemic stroke: Not just cardiolipin anymore. Stroke. 1998; 29:1755–1758

[27] Khamashta MA, Cuadrado MJ, Mujic F, et al. The Management of Thrombosis in the Antiphospholipid-Antibody Syndrome. New England Journal of Medicine. 1995; 332:993–997

[28] Milroy CM, Clark JC, Forrest AR. Pathology of Deaths Associated with "Ecstasy" and "Eve" Misuse. J Clin Pathol. 1996; 49:149–153

[29] Welch KMA, Levine SR. Migraine-related stroke in the context of the International Headache Society Classification of head pain. Arch Neurol. 1990; 47:458–462

[30] Rothrock JF, Walicke P, Swenson MR, et al. Migrainous stroke. Arch Neurol. 1988; 45:63–67

[31] Spaccavento LJ, Solomon GD. Migraine as an etiology of stroke in young adults. Headache. 1984; 24:19–22

[32] Levine SR, Brust JCM, Futrell N, et al. Cerebrovascular Complications of the Use of the 'Crack' Form of Alkaloidal Cocaine. N Engl J Med. 1990; 323:699–704

[33] Kaye BR, Fainstat M. Cerebral Vasculitis Associated with Cocaine Abuse. JAMA. 1987; 258:2104–2106

[34] Cai JM, Hatsukami TS, Ferguson MS, et al. Classification of human carotid atherosclerotic lesions with in vivo multicontrast magnetic resonance imaging. Circulation. 2002; 106:1368–1373

[35] Saam T, Cai J, Ma L, et al. Comparison of symptomatic and asymptomatic atherosclerotic carotid plaque features with in vivo MR imaging. Radiology. 2006; 240:464–472

[36] Saam T, Hatsukami TS, Takaya N, et al. The vulnerable, or high-risk, atherosclerotic plaque: noninvasive MR imaging for characterization and assessment. Radiology. 2007; 244:64–77

[37] Nighoghossian N, Derex L, Douek P. The vulnerable carotid artery plaque: current imaging methods and new perspectives. Stroke. 2005; 36:2764–2772

[38] Moneta GL, Taylor DC, Nicholls SC, et al. Operative Versus Nonoperative Management of Asymptomatic High-Grade Internal Carotid Artery Stenosis. Stroke. 1987; 18:1005–1010

[39] Kistler JP, Furie KL. Carotid Endarterectomy Revisited. New England Journal of Medicine. 2000; 342:1743–1745

[40] Heyman A, Wilkinson WE, Heyden S, et al. Risk of stroke in asymptomatic persons with cervical arterial bruits: a population study in Evans County, Georgia. New England Journal of Medicine. 1980; 302:838–841

[41] Sonecha TN, Delis KT, Henein MY. Predictive value of asymptomatic cervical bruit for carotid artery disease in coronary artery surgery revisited. International Journal of Cardiology. 2006; 107:225–229

[42] U.S. Preventive Services Task Force. Screening for carotid artery stenosis: U.S. Preventive Services Task Force recommendation statement. Annals of Internal Medicine. 2007; 147:854–859

[43] Goldstein LB, Adams R, Alberts MJ, et al. Primary prevention of ischemic stroke. Stroke. 2006; 37:1583–1633

[44] Qureshi AI, Alexandrov AV, Tegeler CH, et al. Guidelines for screening of extracranial carotid artery disease. Journal of Neuroimaging. 2007; 17:19–47

[45] Society for Vascular Surgery. SVS Position Statement on Vascular Screening. 2011. https://vascular.org/news-advocacy/svs-position-statement-vascular-screening

[46] Connors JJ,3rd, Sacks D, Furlan AJ, et al. Training, competency, and credentialing standards for diagnostic cervicocerebral angiography, carotid stenting, and cerebrovascular intervention: a joint statement from the American Academy of Neurology, the American Association of Neurological Surgeons, the American Society of Interventional and Therapeutic Neuroradiology, the American Society of Neuroradiology, the Congress of Neurological Surgeons, the AANS/CNS Cerebrovascular Section,

and the Society of Interventional Radiology. Neurology. 2005; 64:190–198

[47] Willinsky RA, Taylor SM, TerBrugge K, et al. Neurologic complications of cerebral angiography: prospective analysis of 2,899 procedures and review of the literature. Radiology. 2003; 227:522–528

[48] Kaufmann TJ, Huston J,3rd, Mandrekar JN, et al. Complications of diagnostic cerebral angiography: evaluation of 19,826 consecutive patients. Radiology. 2007; 243:812–819

[49] The North American Symptomatic Carotid Endarterectomy Trial. Beneficial Effect of Carotid Endarterectomy in Symptomatic Patients with High-Grade Carotid Stenosis. New England Journal of Medicine. 1991; 325:445–453

[50] The European Carotid Surgery Trialists' Collaborative Group. Randomized Trial of Endarterectomy for Recently Symptomatic Carotid Stenosis: Final Results of the MRC European Carotid Surgery Trial (ECST). Lancet. 1998; 351:1379–1387

[51] Rothwell PM, Gibson RJ, Slattery J, et al. Equivalence of Measurements of Carotid Stenosis: A Comparison of Three Methods on 1001 Angiograms. Stroke. 1994; 25:2435–2439

[52] Buskens E, Nederkoorn PJ, Buijs-Van Der Woude T, et al. Imaging of carotid arteries in symptomatic patients: cost-effectiveness of diagnostic strategies. Radiology. 2004; 233:101–112

[53] Anson JA, Heiserman JE, Drayer BP, et al. Surgical Decisions on the Basis of Magnetic Resonance Angiography of the Carotid Arteries. Neurosurgery. 1993; 32:335–343

[54] Heiserman JE, Zabramski JM, Drayer BP, et al. Clinical Significance of the Flow Gap in Carotid Magnetic Resonance Angiography. Journal of Neurosurgery. 1996; 85:384–387

[55] Anderson CM, Saloner D, Lee RE, et al. Assessment of Carotid Artery Stenosis by MR Angiography: Comparison with X-Ray Angiography and Color-Coded Doppler Ultrasound. American Journal of Neuroradiology. 1992; 13:989–1003

[56] Debrey SM, Yu H, Lynch JK, et al. Diagnostic accuracy of magnetic resonance angiography for internal carotid artery disease: a systematic review and meta-analysis. Stroke. 2008; 39:2237–2248

[57] Babiarz LS, Romero JM, Murphy EK, et al. Contrast-enhanced MR angiography is not more accurate than unenhanced 2D time-of-flight MR angiography for determining > or =70% internal carotid artery stenosis. AJNR. American Journal of Neuroradiology. 2009; 30:761–768

[58] Koelemay MJ, Nederkoorn PJ, Reitsma JB, et al. Systematic review of computed tomographic angiography for assessment of carotid artery disease. Stroke. 2004; 35:2306–2312

[59] Kent KC, Kuntz KM, Patel MR, et al. Perioperative imaging strategies for carotid endarterectomy. An analysis of morbidity and cost-effectiveness in symptomatic patients. JAMA. 1995; 274:888–893

[60] Weksler BB, Pett SB, Alonso D, et al. Differential Inhibition by Aspirin of Vascular and Platelet Prostaglandin Synthesis in Atherosclerotic Patients. N Engl J Med. 1983; 308:800–805

[61] Grotta JC. Current Medical and Surgical Therapy for Cerebrovascular Disease. N Engl J Med. 1987; 317:1505–1516

[62] Théroux P, Fuster V. Acute Coronary Syndromes: Unstable Angina and Non-Q-Wave Myocardial Infarction. Circulation. 1998; 97:1195–1206

[63] Taylor DW, Barnett HJM, Haynes RB, et al. Low-Dose and High-Dose Acetylsalicylic Acid for Patients Undergoing Carotid Endarterectomy: A Randomized Controlled Trial. Lancet. 1999; 353:2179–2184

[64] Halkes PH, van Gijn J, Kappelle LJ, et al. Aspirin plus dipyridamole versus aspirin alone after cerebral ischaemia of arterial origin (ESPRIT): randomised controlled trial. Lancet. 2006; 367:1665–1673

[65] Diener HC, Cunha L, Forbes C, et al. European Stroke Prevention Study. 2. Dipyridamole and acetylsalicylic acid in the secondary prevention of stroke. Journal of Neurological Sciences. 1996; 143:1–13

[66] Verro P, Gorelick PB, Nguyen D. Aspirin plus dipyridamole versus aspirin for prevention of vascular

92

events after stroke or TIA: a meta-analysis. Stroke. 2008; 39:1358–1363

[67] Sacco RL, Diener HC, Yusuf S, et al. Aspirin and extended-release dipyridamole versus clopidogrel for recurrent stroke. New England Journal of Medicine. 2008; 359:1238–1251

[68] Clopidogrel for Reduction of Atherosclerotic Events. Medical Letter. 1998; 40:59–60

[69] Diener HC, Bogousslavsky J, Brass LM, et al. Aspirin and clopidogrel compared with clopidogrel alone after recent ischaemic stroke or transient ischaemic attack in high-risk patients (MATCH): randomised, double-blind, placebo-controlled trial. Lancet. 2004; 364:331–337

[70] Sacco RL, Adams R, Albers G, et al. Guidelines for prevention of stroke in patients with ischemic stroke or transient ischemic attack: a statement for healthcare professionals. Stroke. 2006; 37:577–617

[71] Brott TG, Halperin JL, Abbara S, et al. 2011 ASA/ACCF/AHA/AANN/AANS/ACR/ASNR/CNS/SAIP/SCAI/SIR/SNIS/SVM/SVS guideline on the management of patients with extracranial carotid and vertebral artery disease. Stroke. 2011; 42:e464–e540

[72] O'Leary DH, Polak JF, Kronmal RA, et al. Distribution and correlates of sonographically detected carotid artery disease in the Cardiovascular Health Study. The CHS Collaborative Research Group. Stroke. 1992; 23:1752–1760

[73] Fine-Edelstein J S, Wolf PA, O'Leary DH, et al. Precursors of extracranial carotid atherosclerosis in the Framingham Study. Neurology. 1994; 44:1046–1050

[74] Hillen T, Nieczaj R, Munzberg H, et al. Carotid atherosclerosis, vascular risk profile and mortality in a population-based sample of functionally healthy elderly subjects: the Berlin ageing study. Journal of Internal Medicine. 2000; 247:679–688

[75] Autret A, Pourcelot L, Saudeau D, et al. Stroke risk in patients with carotid stenosis. Lancet. 1987; 1:888–890

[76] Bogousslavsky J, Despland P-A, Regli F. Asymptomatic Tight Stenosis of the Internal Carotid Artery. Neurology. 1986; 36:861–863

[77] Chambers BR, Norris JW. Outcome in patients with asymptomatic neck bruits. New England Journal of Medicine. 1986; 315:860–865

[78] Hennerici M, Hulsbomer HB, Hefter H, et al. Natural history of asymptomatic extracranial arterial disease. Results of a long-term prospective study. Brain. 1987; 110 (Pt 3):777–791

[79] Mackey AE, Abrahamowicz M, Langlois Y, et al. Outcome of asymptomatic patients with carotid disease. Asymptomatic Cervical Bruit Study Group. Neurology. 1997; 48:896–903

[80] Meissner I, Wiebers DO, Whisnant JP, et al. The natural history of asymptomatic carotid artery occlusive lesions. JAMA. 1987; 258:2704–2707

[81] Nadareishvili ZG, Rothwell PM, Beletsky V, et al. Long-term risk of stroke and other vascular events in patients with asymptomatic carotid artery stenosis. Archives of Neurology. 2002; 59:1162–1166

[82] Aichner FT, Topakian R, Alberts MJ, et al. High cardiovascular event rates in patients with asymptomatic carotid stenosis: the REACH registry. European Journal of Neurology. 2009. DOI: 10.1111/j.1468-1331.2009.02614.x

[83] Halliday A, Mansfield A, Marro J, et al. Prevention of disabling and fatal strokes by successful carotid endarterectomy in patients without recent neurological symptoms: randomised controlled trial. Lancet. 2004; 363:1491–1502

[84] Hobson RW, Weiss DG, Fields WS, et al. Efficacy of Carotid Endarterectomy for Asymptomatic Carotid Stenosis. New England Journal of Medicine. 1993; 328:221–227

[85] The Executive Committee for the Asymptomatic Carotid Atherosclerosis Study. Endarterectomy for Asymptomatic Carotid Artery Stenosis. Journal of the American Medical Association. 1995; 273:1421–1428

[86] Mattos MA, Modi JR, Mansour MA, et al. Evolution of Carotid Endarterectomy in Two Community Hospitals: Springfield Revisited - Seventeen Years and 2243 Operations Later. J Vasc Surg. 1995; 21:719–728

[87] CASANOVA Study Group. Carotid Surgery Versus Medical Therapy in Asymptomatic Carotid Stenosis. Stroke. 1991; 22:1229–1235

[88] Mayberg MR, Winn HR. Endarterectomy for Asymptomatic Carotid Artery Stenosis. Resolving the Controversy. Journal of the American Medical Association. 1995; 273:1459–1461

[89] Mayo Asymptomatic Carotid Endarterectomy Study Group. Results of a randomized controlled trial of carotid endarterectomy for asymptomatic carotid stenosis. Mayo Clinic Proceedings. 1992; 67:513–518

93 Evaluation and Treatment for Acute Ischemic Stroke

93.1 Stroke management – general information (time = brain)

In the complete absence of blood flow, neuronal death occurs within 2–3 minutes from exhaustion of energy stores. However, in most strokes, there is a salvageable penumbra (tissue at risk) that retains viability for a period of time through suboptimal perfusion from collaterals. Local cerebral edema from the stroke results in compromise of these collaterals and progression of ischemic penumbra to infarction if flow is not restored and maintained. Prevention of this secondary neuronal injury drives the treatment of stroke and has led to the creation of designated Primary Stroke Centers that offer appropriate and timely triage and treatment of all potential stroke patients.

This section incorporates recommendations from the 2018 AHA Guidelines for Acute Ischemic Stroke.[1] "Class of Recommendation": Level I = strong, Level II = moderate to weak.

> ## Key concepts – move quickly (treatment benefits are time-dependent)
>
> Level I.[1]
> * history/physical exam: include a stroke scale (preferably NIHSS (p. 1554))
> * ✔ blood glucose (p. 1557): essential lab to obtain in case IV tPA is indicated
> * noncontrast brain CT: the usual initial diagnostic tool of choice (image in ≤ 20 mins)
>   ○ to rule out: hemorrhage (SAH, ICH, EDH, SDH), mass (tumor, abscess...)
>   ○ to calculate ASPECTS (p. 1559) (to identify candidates for thrombectomy)
> * CTA for patients with NIHSS score ≥ 10 (correlates with large vessel occlusion [LVO]) to identify candidates for thrombectomy (do not delay IV tPA to get CTA)
> * thrombectomy is the standard of care for eligible patients: cerebral ischemia (including infarct) caused by LVO of the ICA or M1 segment of the MCA, 1) when it can be initiated within 6 hours of symptom onset, or 2) if perfusion studies identify viable tissue 6–24 hours from onset
> * IV tPA (tissue plasminogen activator, alteplase)
>   ○ within 4.5 hours of onset when thrombectomy not being done *immediately* or for patients who are not thrombectomy candidates
>   ○ goal: "door-to-needle" (DTN) time ≤ 60 minutes

93

93.2 Rapid initial evaluation/management

Upon presentation of a patient with symptoms of a potential stroke.

history & physical exam: key components
a) onset or last known well (LKW) time (the last time the patient was seen to be normal): stroke on awakening ("wake-up stroke") may require additional considerations for management
b) current deficit and clinical presentation
c) ★ NIH Stroke Scale score (p. 1554) (or Canadian Neurological Scale) assessed and recorded (Level I[1])

laboratories:
a) ★ **blood glucose** (p. 1557) is the only essential lab to get immediately since it affects eligibility for IV tPA (Level I[1])
b) see Admitting orders (p. 1556) for subsequent detailed labs (including cardiac troponins...)

imaging:
a) ★ **STAT noncontrast head CT** scan: AHA goal: image the brain in ≤ 20 minutes of arrival in the E/R in ≥ 50% of eligible patients (Level I[1]). In most cases this provides the necessary information for management (Level I[1]). For details and findings, see section 93.5.1
  * rule out hemorrhage (ICH, SAH, subdural, epidural...) or other lesions (e.g., tumor).
  * determine Alberta stroke program early CT score (ASPECTS) (p. 1559)
b) a noninvasive intracranial vascular study (usually a CTA) is obtained in potential candidates for endovascular therapy (EVT) (viz. patients with large vessel occlusion (LVO)) who are best

identified by the NIHSS score[2]:
- NIHSS score ≥ 10: is 73% sensitive & 74% specific for LVO
- NIHSS score ≥ 6: is 87% sensitive and 52% specific for LVO

This study should not delay IV tPA if indicated; the CTA can be obtained ASAP after IV tPA. It is reasonable to image the extracranial carotid and vertebral circulations in addition to intracranial vessels in potential candidates for EVT to help determine patient eligibility and to plan the procedure (Level II[1]).

4. **intervention**: depending on results of above
   a) candidates for EVT (essentially mechanical thrombectomy or IA tPA) should be taken immediately to angio suite
   b) if there is going to be a delay, or if the patient is not eligible for EVT, IV tPA is given if indicated

93.3 NIH stroke scale (NIHSS)

Administer in order shown (▶ Table 93.1). Record initial performance only (do not go back).

Table 93.1 NIH Stroke scale[a]

Scale	Finding
1a. Level of consciousness (LOC)	
0	alert; keenly responsive
1	not alert, but arousable by minor stimulation to obey, answer, or respond
2	not alert, requires repeated stimulation to attend, or is obtunded and requires strong painful stimulation to make movements (not stereotyped)
3	comatose: responds only with reflex motor (posturing) or autonomic effects, or totally unresponsive, flaccid, and areflexic
1b. Level-of-consciousness questions	
Patient is asked the month and their age.	
0	answers both questions correctly: must be correct (no credit for being close)
1	answers one question correctly, or cannot answer because of: ET tube, orotracheal trauma, severe dysarthria, language barrier, or any other problem not secondary to aphasia
2	answers neither question correctly, or is: aphasic, stuporous, or does not comprehend the questions
1c. Level-of-consciousness commands	
Patient is asked to open and close the eyes, and then to grip and release the non-paretic hand. Substitute another 1-step command if both hands cannot be used. Credit is given for an unequivocal attempt even if it cannot be completed due to weakness. If there is no response to commands, demonstrate (pantomime) the task. Record only first attempt.	
0	performs both tasks correctly
1	performs one task correctly
2	performs neither task correctly
2. Best gaze	
Test only horizontal eye movement. Use motion to attract attention of aphasic patients.	
0	normal horizontal movements
1	partial gaze palsy (gaze abnormal in one or both eyes, but forced deviation or total gaze paresis are not present) or patient has an isolated cranial nerve III, IV, or VI paresis
2	forced deviation or total gaze paresis not overcome by oculocephalic (Doll's eyes) maneuver (do not do caloric testing)
3. Visual	
Visual fields (upper and lower quadrants) are tested by confrontation. May be scored as normal if patient looks at side of finger movement. Use ocular threat where consciousness or comprehension limits testing. Then test with double-sided simultaneous stimulation (DSSS).	
0	no visual field deficit
1	partial hemianopia (clear-cut asymmetry), or extinction to DSSS
2	complete hemianopia
3	bilateral hemianopia (blind, including cortical blindness)

(continued)

93

Table 93.1 continued

Scale	Finding

4. Facial palsy

Ask patient (or pantomime) to show their teeth, or raise eyebrows and close eyes. Use painful stimulus and grade grimace response in poorly responsive or non-comprehending patients.

0	normal symmetrical movement
1	minor paralysis (flattened nasolabial fold, asymmetry on smiling)
2	partial paralysis (total or near-total paralysis of lower face)
3	complete paralysis of one or both sides (absent facial movement in upper and lower face)

5. Motor Arm (5a = left, 5b = right)

Instruct patient to hold the arms outstretched, palms down (at 90° if sitting, or 45° if supine). If consciousness or comprehension impaired, cue patient by actively lifting arms into position while verbally instructing patient to maintain position.

0	no drift (holds arm at 90° or 45° for full 10 seconds)
1	drift (holds limbs at 90° or 45° position, but drifts before full 10 seconds but does not hit bed or other support)
2	some effort against gravity (cannot get to or hold initial position, drifts down to bed)
3	no effort against gravity, limb falls
4	no movement
9	amputation or joint fusion: explain

6. Motor leg (6a = left, 6b = right)

While supine, instruct patient to maintain the non-paretic leg at 30°. If consciousness or comprehension impaired, cue patient by actively lifting leg into position while verbally instructing patient to maintain position. Then repeat in paretic leg.

0	no drift (holds leg at 30° full 5 seconds)
1	drift (leg falls before 5 seconds, but does not hit bed)
2	some effort against gravity (leg falls to bed by 5 seconds)
3	no effort against gravity (leg falls to bed immediately)
4	no movement
9	amputation or joint fusion: explain

7. Limb ataxia

Looking for unilateral cerebellar lesion. Finger-nose-finger and heel-knee-shin tests are performed on both sides. Ataxia is scored only if clearly out of proportion to weakness. Ataxia is absent in the patient who cannot comprehend or is paralyzed.

0	absent
1	present in one limb
2	present in two limbs
9	amputation or joint fusion: explain

8. Sensory

Test with pin. When consciousness or comprehension impaired, score sensation normal unless deficit clearly recognized (e.g., clear-cut asymmetry of grimace or withdrawal). Only hemisensory losses attributed to stroke are counted as abnormal.

0	normal, no sensory loss
1	mild to moderate sensory loss (pinprick dull or less sharp on the affected side, or loss of superficial pain to pinprick but patient aware of being touched)
2	severe to total (patient unaware of being touched in the face, arm, and leg)

9. Best language

In addition to judging comprehension of commands in the preceding neurologic exam, the patient is asked to describe a standard picture, to name common items, and to read and interpret the standard text in the box below. The intubated patient should be asked to write:

- You know how.
- Down to earth.
- I got home from work.
- Near the table in the dining room.
- They heard him speak on the radio last night.

93

(continued)

Table 93.1 continued

Scale	Finding
0	normal, no aphasia
1	mild to moderate aphasia (some loss of fluency, word-finding errors, naming errors, paraphasias and/or impairment of communication by either comprehension or expression disability)
2	severe aphasia (great need for inference, questioning, and guessing by listener; limited range of information can be exchanged)
3	mute or global aphasia (no usable speech or auditory comprehension) or patient in coma (item 1a = 3)

10. Dysarthria

Patient may be graded based on information already gleaned during evaluation. If patient is thought to be normal, have them read (or repeat) the standard text shown in this box.
- MAMA
- TIP-TOP
- FIFTY-FIFTY
- THANKS
- HUCKLEBERRY
- BASEBALL PLAYER
- CATERPILLAR

0	normal speech
1	mild to moderate (slurs some words, can be understood with some difficulty)
2	severe (unintelligible slurred speech in the absence of, or out of proportion to, any dysphasia, or is mute/anarthric)
0	intubated or other physical barrier

11. Extinction and inattention (formerly neglect)

Sufficient information to identify neglect may already be gleaned during evaluation. If the patient has severe visual loss preventing visual DSSS, and the cutaneous stimuli are normal, the score is normal. Scored as abnormal only if present.

0	normal, no sensory loss
1	visual, tactile, auditory, spatial, or personal inattention or extinction to DSSS in one of the sensory modalities
2	profound hemi-inattention or hemi-inattention to more than one modality. Does not recognize own hand or orients to only one side of space.

A. Distal motor function (not part of NIHSS) (a = left arm, b = right)

Patient's hand is held up at the forearm by the examiner, and is asked to extend the fingers as much as possible. If patient cannot do so, the examiner does it for them. Do not repeat the command.

0	normal (no finger flexion after 5 seconds)
1	at least some extension after 5 seconds (any finger movement is scored)
2	no voluntary extension after 5 seconds

[a]based on the Cincinnati stroke scale.[3] Free online text version (https://www.ninds.nih.gov/sites/default/files/NIH_Stroke_Scale.pdf) or graphical version (https://www.ninds.nih.gov/sites/default/files/NIH_Stroke_Scale_-Booklet.pdf)

Higher NIHSS scores indicate more deficit and correlate with more proximal vascular lesion (larger vessel occlusion causes more widespread deficit).

93.4 General management for acute ischemic stroke (AIS)

93.4.1 Admitting orders

Orders are for TIA or stroke, but not SAH (p. 1432) nor intracerebral hemorrhage (ICH) (p. 1619). Entries from the 2018 AHA guidelines[1] are indicated by the corresponding level of the recommendation.

1. admit to ICU
2. frequent VS with crani checks (q 1 hr × 12 hrs, then if stable, q 2 hrs)
3. monitor cardiac rhythm
4. activity: bed rest

5. labs:
   a) routine: CBC + platelet count, electrolytes, PT/PTT/INR, U/A, ABG
   b) ★ only blood glucose (p. 1557) determination must precede initiation of IV tPA in all patients (Level I[1])
   c) usefulness of CXR in the absence of cardiovascular indications is unclear, and should not delay IV tPA (LevelI I[1])
   d) baseline EKG & cardiac troponins are recommended but should not delay IV tPA (Level I[1]). EKG changes occur in 5–10% of AIS; acute MIs in 2–3%
   e) "special" (when appropriate): RPR (to rule out neurosyphilis), ESR (to rule out giant cell arteritis), hepatic profile, cardiac (lipid) profile
   f) at 24 hrs: CBC, platelet count, cardiac (lipid) profile, EKG
6. oxygenation
   a) provide supplemental O_2 to maintain O_2 saturation > 94% (Level I[1])
   b) airway support and ventilator for decreased level of consciousness or for bulbar dysfunction that compromises the patient's ability to protect their airway (Level I[1])
   c) supplemental O_2 is not recommended in nonhypoxic patients (no benefit[1])
   d) hyperbaric oxygen is not recommended except for air embolism (no benefit[1])
7. diet: NPO
8. nursing care
   a) indwelling Foley (urinary) catheter if consciousness impaired or if unable to use urinal or bedpan; intermittent catheterization q 4–6 hrs PRN no void if Foley not used
   b) accurate I's & O's; notify M.D. for urine output < 20 cc/hr × 2 hrs by Foley, or < 160 cc in 8 hrs if no Foley
9. glucose:
   a) avoid hyperglycemia in the 1st 24 hours after AIS (worse outome). Goal: blood sugar 140–180 mg/dL (Level II[1])
   Rationale: hyperglycemia may extend ischemic zone (penumbra).[5]
   b) avoid hypoglycemia < 60 mg/dL (Level I[1])
   c) hyperglycemia and hypoglycemia may mimic AIS and should be treated if identified (tPA is not indicated for nonvascular conditions) (no benefit[1])
10. IV fluids: NS or 1/2 NS at 75–125 cc/hr for most patients (to eliminate dehydration if present)
    a) *avoid glucose*: (see above)
    b) avoid overhydration in cases of ICH, CHF, or SBP > 180
11. seizures:
    a) treat recurrent seizures the same as for other neurologic conditions (Level I[1])
    b) prophylactic seizure medication is not recommended (no benefit[1])
12. treat CHF and arrhythmias. MI or myocardial ischemia may present with neuro deficit
13. blood pressure (BP) management:
    a) for patients with HTN who are otherwise candidates for IV tPA: carefully lower SBP to < 185 mm Hg, and DBP to < 110 before giving IV-tPA (Level I[1]), and maintain < 180/105 for 24 hours after tPA (Level I[1])
    Otherwise, for general management, see Hypertension in stroke patients below.
    b) avoid hypotension and hypovolemia (Level I[1]): no specifics provided. Suggestion: for patients presenting with SBP < 110 or DBP < 70:
       • unless contraindicated (viz.: ICH, cerebellar infarct, or decreased cardiac output) give 250 cc NS over 1 hr, then 500 cc over 4 hrs, then 500 cc over 8 hrs
       • if fluid ineffective or contraindicated: consider pressors
    c) the benefit of drug-induced hypertension is not well-established in AIS (Level II[1])
14. osmotic therapy (mannitol 50 to 100 gm IV over 20 minutes or 3% saline): for clinical deterioration from cerebral edema associated with AIS (Level II[1])
15. patient temperature:
    a) fever > 38 °C: identify and treat the source, use antipyretics as needed (Level I[1])
    b) induced hypothermia: use is not well-established and should only be employed within approved clinical trials (Level II[1])
16. other medications
    a) corticosteroids (including dexamethasone)
       • ✖ not recommended for cerebral edema and/or increased ICP complicating stroke (potential harm[1])
       • exceptions: steroid-responsive vasculitis, e.g., giant cell arteritis (temporal arteritis), demonstration of associated brain tumor
    b) stool softener
    c) avoid diuretics unless volume overloaded

93

17. antiplatelet therapy key points (see below (p. 1558) for some additional details)
    a) ★ aspirin (ASA): recommended within 24–48 hrs after onset of IAS (Level II[1]). Doses used: 160–300 mg/d. If IV tPA was given, ASA is usually delayed until 24 hrs later, but can be started earlier for strong indications
    b) ★ patients with minor stroke: dual antiplatelet therapy (ASA + clopidogrel) for 21 days starting ≤ 24 hrs can reduce secondary stroke for up to 90 days (Level II[1])
    c) ASA is not a substitute for IV tPA or thrombectomy in eligible patients (no benefit[1])

93.4.2 Hypertension in stroke patients

General information

HTN may actually be needed to maintain CBF in the face of elevated ICP, and it usually resolves spontaneously. Therefore treat HTN cautiously and slowly to avoid rapid reduction and overshooting the target. Avoid treating mild HTN. Indications to treat HTN emergently include:
1. acute LV failure (rare)
2. acute aortic dissection (rare)
3. acute hypertensive renal failure (rare)
4. neurologic complications of HTN
    a) hypertensive encephalopathy
    b) conversion of a large pale (ischemic) infarct into a hemorrhagic infarct
    c) patients with ICH; some HTN is needed to maintain CBF, see Initial management of ICH (p. 1619)

Hypertension treatment algorithm

See reference,[4] modified.
Recommended lower limits for treatment endpoints are shown in ▶ Table 93.2.
1. if DBP > 140 (malignant hypertension): ≈ 20–30% reduction is desirable. Cardene infusion or IV

Table 93.2 Guidelines for lower limits of treatment endpoints for HTN in strokes

	No prior history of HTN	Prior history of HTN
do not lower SBP below	160–170 mm Hg	180–185 mm Hg
do not lower DBP below	95–105 mm Hg	105–110 mm Hg

labetalol are agents of choice; arterial-line monitor recommended; sympatholytics (e.g., trimethaphan) contraindicated (they reduce CBF)
2. SBP > 230 or DBP 120–140 × 20 mins: **labetalol** (p. 131) (unless contraindicated): start at 10 mg slow IVP over 2 mins, then double q 10 min (20, 40, 80, then 160 mg slow IVP) until controlled or total of 300 mg given. Maintenance: effective dose (from above) q 6–8 hrs PRN SBP > 180 or DBP > 110
3. SBP 180–230 or DBP 105–120: defer emergency treatment unless there is evidence of LV failure or if readings persist × 60 mins
    a) oral **labetalol** (p. 131) (unless contraindicated) dosed as follows:
        • for SBP > 210 or DBP > 110: 300 mg PO BID
        • for SBP 180–210 or DBP 100–110: 200 mg PO BID
    b) if labetalol contraindicated:
        nicardipine (p. 131)

93.4.3 Antiplatelet drugs in AIS – additional info

• IV tirofiban & eptifibatide: efficacy is not established pending further clinical trials (Level II[1])
• ✖ abciximab & other glycoprotein IIb/IIIa receptor antagonists are not recommended (potential harm[1])
• ticagrelor is not recommended over ASA in the acute treatment of minor stroke (no benefit[1])

93.4.4 Emergency surgery

Possible indications:
1. herniation from subdural hematoma

2. suboccipital craniectomy for progressive neurologic deterioration due to brainstem compression from cerebellar hemorrhage or infarction (see below)
3. decompressive craniectomy for malignant MCA territory stroke (see below)
4. carotid endarterectomy for high-grade carotid stenosis ipsilateral to *fluctuating* neuro deficit; see Emergency carotid endarterectomy (p.1570)

93.5 Imaging in acute ischemic stroke (AIS)

93.5.1 CAT scan findings with acute ischemic stroke (AIS)

Findings at various times after ischemic stroke

NB: These principles do *not* apply to small lacunar infarcts, nor to hemorrhagic strokes (ICH). NB: CT is normal in 8–69% of MCA strokes in the first 24 hours.[6]

▶ **Hyperacute (<6 hours after stroke).** Early signs of infarction involving large areas of the MCA territory correlate with poor outcome.[7] Early findings may include[8]:
1. hyperdense artery sign (see below): low sensitivity, but helpful if present
2. focal low attenuation within the gray matter*
3. loss of the gray-white interface*
4. attenuation of the lentiform nucleus
5. mass effect*
    a) early: effacement of the cerebral sulci (often subtle)[9]
    b) late: midline shift in large territory infarction
6. loss of the insular ribbon sign (hypodensity involving the insular cortex, susceptible to ischemia due to poor collaterals)
7. enhancement with IV contrast: occurs in only 33%. Stroke becomes isodense (called "masking" effect) or hyperdense with normal brain, and, rarely, may be the only indication of infarction[9]

These findings are probably due to increased water content resulting from the following: cellular edema arising from altered cell permeability, which produces a shift of sodium and water from the extracellular to the intracellular compartment, which also increases the extracellular osmotic pressure causing transudation of water from capillaries into the interstitium.[10]

▶ **24 hrs.** Most strokes can be identified as low density by this time.

▶ **1–2 wks.** Strokes are sharply demarcated. In 5–10% there may be a short window (at around day 7–10) where the stroke becomes isodense, called "fogging effect." IV contrast will usually demonstrate these.

▶ **3 wks.** Stroke approaches CSF density.

Mass effect. Common between day 1 to 25. Then atrophy is usually seen by ≈ 5 wks (2 wks at the earliest). Serial CT scans have shown that midline shift increases after ischemic stroke and reaches a maximum 2–4 days after the insult.

Calcifications. Over a long period of time (months to years) ≈ 1–2% of strokes calcify (in adults, it is probably a much smaller fraction than this; and in peds it is higher). Therefore, in an adult, calcifications almost rule out a stroke (consider AVM, low-grade tumor…).

Alberta stroke program early CT score (ASPECTS)

The ASPECTS[11] is derived from 2 noncontrast axial CT slices: one at the level of the thalamus, the second just rostral to the basal ganglia. The MCA is divided into 10 territories that each get 1 point: 3 subcortical structures (caudate, lentiform nucleus, & internal capsule), and 7 cortical territories: insular cortex (ribbon) and M1 through M6 (as shown in ▶ Fig. 93.1).

Starting with a normal score of 10, 1 point is subtracted for each of the territories that show signs of early ischemic change: viz. swelling (evidenced by compression of sulci or ventricles) or hypoattenuation (relative to other areas of the brain) involving ≥ 1/3 of the territory. A score ≤ 7 is associated with a worse outcome from stroke. Despite its limitations (only asseses MCA distribution infarcts, cortical territories are not equally weighted…), it is simple, has reasonably good interrater reliability, and can also be used on MRI.[12]

93

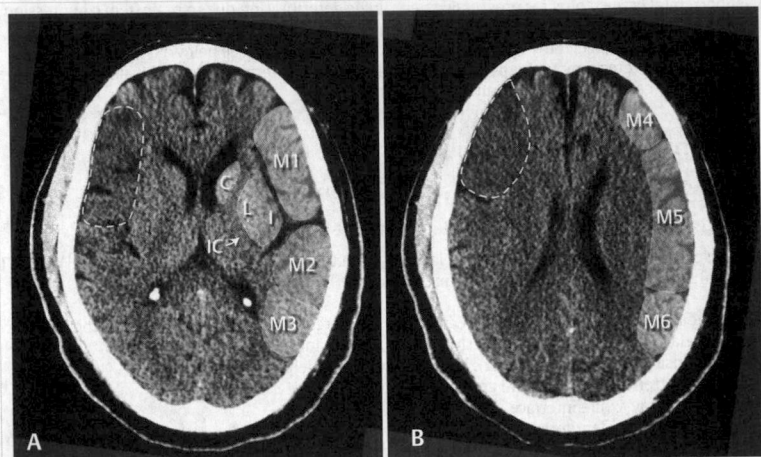

Fig. 93.1 ASPECTS (Alberta stroke program early CT score) with illustration in a 71-year-old male with acute right MCA infarct (demarcated by the yellow broken lines).
Image: noncontrast axial head CT, A: at level of the thalamus, B: just above the basal ganglia.
The 10 graded areas are shown as colored shapes on the patient's left side: C = caudate (head), IC = internal capsule, L = lentiform nucleus (BG), I = insular cortex, M1 through M6 = convexity cortical territories.
ASPECTS here is 8 (10 points minus 1 point for M1, minus 1 point for M4, but no point off for M5 because slightly less than 1/3 of M5 is involved).

Hyperdense artery sign

First described in the MCA in 1983.[13] The cerebral vessel (usually the MCA) appears as high density on unenhanced CT (▶ Fig. 93.2), indicating intra-arterial clot (thrombus or embolus).[14] Seen in 12% of 50 patients scanned within 24 hrs of stroke, and in 34% of 23 very early CTs done to R/O hemorrhage. Sensitivity for MCA occlusion is low, but specificity is high (although it may also be seen with carotid dissection, or (usually bilaterally) with calcific atherosclerosis or high hematocrit[14]). Does not have independent prognostic significance.[15]

Enhancement

CT enhancement with IV contrast in stroke: not routinely used in AIS
1. many enhance by day 6, most by day 10, some will enhance up to 5 wks
2. rule of 2's: 2% enhance at 2 days, 2% enhance at 2 mos
3. gyral enhancement: AKA "ribbon" enhancement. Common. Usually seen by 1 week (gray matter enhances > white). DDx includes inflammatory infiltrating lesions such as lymphoma, neurosarcoidosis... (due to breakdown of BBB)
4. rule of thumb: there should not be enhancement at the same time that there is mass effect

93.5.2 CT angio (CTA)

CTA (p.238) is useful for assessing the location and extent of vascular occlusion in acute ischemic stroke,[16] and may identify the bleeding source in subarachnoid hemorrhage. Findings can direct treatment towards endovascular options when a proximal or significant large vessel occlusion is seen.

To avoid delays in candidates for endovascular therapy, it is reasonable to proceed with CTA without waiting for serum creatinine if there is no history of renal impairment (Level II[1]).

93.5.3 CT perfusion

Theoretically identifies salvageable penumbra as a region of mismatch between CBF and CBV. Assumption: the infarcted core (with no salvageable tissue) has decreased CBF within a region

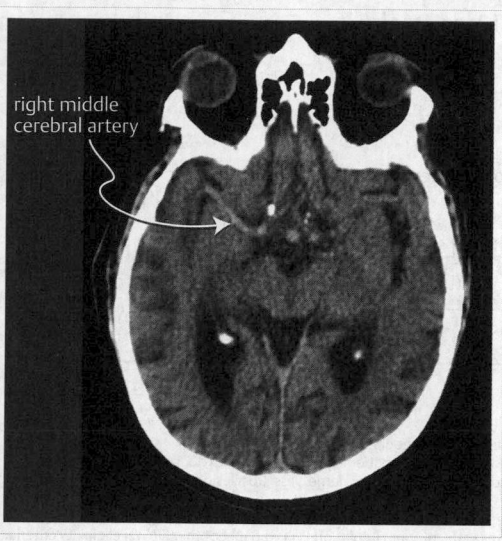

right middle cerebral artery

Fig. 93.2 Hyperdense artery sign.
Image: noncontrast axial CT scan.
The right middle cerebral artery (MCA) appears hyperdense in this 85-year-old patient with acute right MCA stroke. The left MCA is also slightly hyperdense.

decreased CBV (CBF/CBV match). A mismatched area (decreased CBV *without* a decrease in CBF) represents potentially salvageable penumbra.[17] Implication: thrombolytics and interventional treatment modalities without mismatch will likely increase morbidity and mortality without clinical benefit.

93.5.4 MRI

With newer, faster acquisition times, and with gradient echo sequences that are highly sensitive to hemorrhage, MRI is increasingly being utilized in the hyperacute setting and is at times replacing CT as the initial evaluation. More sensitive than CT (especially DWI-MRI (p.243), and particularly in the first 24 hrs after stroke), and especially with brainstem or cerebellar infarction. More contraindications (p.242) than CT.

Contrast MRI: not often used. 4 enhancement patterns[18]:

* intravascular enhancement: occurs in ≈ 75% of 1–3-day-old cortical infarcts, and is probably due to sluggish flow and vasodilatation (thus, it is not seen with complete occlusion). May indicate areas of brain at risk of infarction
* meningeal enhancement: especially involving the dura. Seen in 35% of cortical strokes 1–3 days old (not seen in deep cerebral or brainstem strokes). No angiographic nor CT equivalent
* transitional enhancement: above two types of enhancement coexist with early evidence of BBB breakdown; usually seen on days 3–6
* parenchymal enhancement: classically appears as a cortical or subcortical gyral ribbon enhancement. May not be apparent for the first 1–2 days, and gradually approaches 100% by 1 week. Enhancement may eliminate "fogging effect" (as on CT) which may obscure some strokes at ≈ 2 weeks on unenhanced T2WI

93.5.5 MRI perfusion

Similar to CT perfusion (p.239), areas of matched DWI and PWI abnormality are thought to represent infarcted tissue. PWI abnormalities that do not have a DWI correlate are thought to represent potentially salvageable penumbra.[19]

93

93.6 Management of TIA or stroke

93.6.1 Treatment options timeline

See ▶ Fig. 93.3.

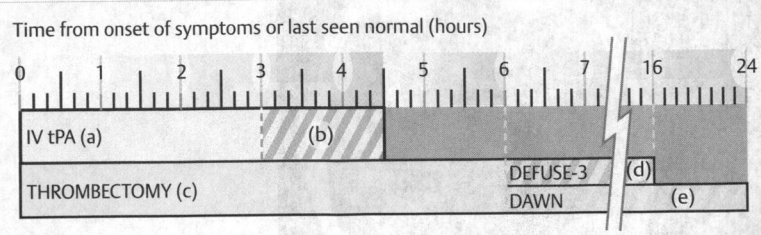

Fig. 93.3 Treatment options timeline.
(a) IV tPA: give to essentially all candidates within 4.5 hours of onset.
(b) 3–4.5 hrs: IV tPA reasonable but not studied in same patient population (see text).
(c) thrombectomy candidates: NIHHS score ≥ 6, ASPECTS ≥ 6, large vessel occlusion (LVO), puncture ≤ 6 hrs from onset.
(d) thrombectomy 6–16 hrs in candidates who meet other DAWN or DEFUSE-3 (p. 1562) eligibility (see text).
(e) thrombectomy 16–24 hrs in candidates with anterior circulation LVO who meet other DAWN eligibility criteria.

These times are applicable to anterior circulation strokes. Posterior circulation occlusions may be treated more aggressively.

The American Heart Association has recommended a goal of "door-to-needle" (DTN) time of ≤ 60 minutes in ≥ 50% of acute ischemic stroke patients being treated with tPA (Level I[1]), with a DTN of ≤ 45 minutes being a reasonable secondary goal (Level II[1]).

93.6.2 Endovascular therapy for stroke

Recent trials favor rapid endovascular intervention in acute ischemic stroke with proximal vessel occlusion, small infarct core, and moderate to good collateral circulation.[20,21,22,23]

The primary modality is mechanical clot retrieval (thrombectomy), although intra-arterial tPA may be used in select situations. See Endovascular intervention (p. 1932) for details.

Practice guideline: Mechanical thrombectomy for acute ischemic stroke (AIS)

Mechanical thrombectomy with stent retriever is recommended when all criteria met (Level I[1]):
- prestroke (modified Rankin Score (mRS), ▶ Table 98.5) of 0–1
- causative occlusion of ICA or M1 segment of MCA
- age ≥ 18 years
- NIHSS (p. 1554) score ≥ 6
- ASPECTS (p. 1559) ≥ 6
- treatment can be initiated (groin puncture) ≤ 6 hours of onset

Benefits uncertain, but mechanical thrombectomy may be reasonable for (Level II[1])
- carefully selected patients with causative occlusion of M2 or M3 segment of MCA, or anterior cerebral, vertebral, basilar, or posterior cerebral arteries
- or prestroke mRS > 1, ASPECTS < 6 and causative occlusion of ICA or M1 segment; however, additional randomized trials are needed
- when treatment can be initiated (groin puncture) ≤ 6 hours after onset

Mechanical thrombectomy is recommended for selected patients 6–16 hours from onset with large vessel occlusion (LVO) in the anterior circulation who meet other DAWN[a] or DEFUSE-3[a] eligibility criteria (Level I[1]).

Mechanical thrombectomy is reasonable in selected patients 16–24 hours from onset with anterior circulation LVO who meet other DAWN[a] eligibility criteria (Level II[1]).

The goal of thrombectomy should be reperfusion to a mTICI 2b/3 angiographic result (▶ Table 116.2) and to minimize the time to treatment in order to maximize the chances of good functional outcome (Level I[1]).

[a] DAWN[24] & DEFUSE-3[25] are the only randomized controlled trials that showed benefit of mechanical thrombectomy > 6 hours from onset. CTP, DW-MRI, or MRI perfusion can aid in patient selection when RCT eligibility criteria are strictly met. Trial elegibility can be found online at http://stroke.aha-journals.org/lookup/suppl/doi:10.1161/STR.0000000000000158/-/DC1

DEFUSE-3 used perfusion/core mismatch & maximum core size (< 70 ml) to select patients 6–16 hrs from onset. Proprietary software (such as iSchemaView's RAPID™) can quickly analyze scans to determine the mismatch.

DAWN: used clinical/imaging mismatch (combination of NIHSS score and imaging findings on CTP or DWI-MRI) to select patients 6–24 hrs from onset.

93.6.3 Thrombolytic therapy

General information

Tissue plasminogen activator (tPA) is an enzyme that is naturally found in vascular endothelial cells. It catalyzes the conversion of plasminogen to the fibrinolytic compound plasmin (the major enzyme involved in thrombolysis). tPA for clinical use is manufactured using recombinant DNA technology (rtPA, or just tPA).

Alteplase (Activase®, Actilyse®) is the primary agent used clinically. It is FDA-approved for the IV treatment of acute ischemic stroke (see below).

Tenecteplase (TNKase®), an alternative tPA, has not shown superiority or inferiority to alteplase,[26] and pending further investigation may be considered in patients with minor neurologic deficit and no major intracranial occlusion (Level II[1]).

Other agents: benefits are unproven, and their use is not recommended outside of clinical trials (no benefit[1]).

IV tissue plasminogen activator (IV tPA)

For this section, tPA refers to alteplase. For *intra-arterial* tPA see endovascular therapy (p. 1932).

The use of tPA administered within the first 3 hours of stroke onset has been shown to be safe and effective in multiple randomized controlled trials and by extensive community experience in numerous countries.[1] This window was extended to 4.5 hours in 2009 after ECASS-3,[27] but the study population differed (see Eligibility below).

Guidelines for the administration of IV tPA

Eligibility:
- age ≥ 18 years (although use in childhood stroke is increasing[28]
- time since last seen normal ≤ 4.5 hrs prior to administration
  (NB: the 3–4.5-hr window was not studied in patients ≥ 80 years of age, patients with severe stroke (NIHSS (p. 1554) score > 25), and patients with prior stroke + DM.[29] However, it may still be reasonable to treat these patients (Level II[1])
- tPA is reasonable in otherwise eligible patients with history of ≤ 10 cerebral microbleeds on MRI (Level II[1])
- AIS in adults with known sickle cell disease

Contraindications[1]:
- intracerebral hemorrhage (ICH): on admitting CT, or history of prior ICH
- patients with history of > 10 cerebral microbleeds showed an increased risk of ICH and the benefits of tPA are uncertain but treatment may be beneficial if there is substantial potential benefit (Level II[1])
- clinical presentation of SAH (even with negative CT)

93

4. known intracranial aneurysm or AVM
5. active internal bleeding
6. known bleeding diathesis, including but not limited to the following:
   a) full anticoagulation with LMWH within the previous 24 hours (possible harm[1])
   b) platelet count < 100,000/mm³ (given the low risk of unsuspected abnormal platelet counts or coagulation studies, it is reasonable that urgent tPA should not be delayed to wait for test results (Level II[1]))
7. serious head trauma, serious stroke, or intracranial surgery within past 3 months
8. SBP > 185 mm Hg, or DBP > 110 mm Hg that cannot be controlled despite use of nicardipine infusion or IV labetalol

✖ **Cautions:**
1. seizure witnessed at the time of onset of stroke symptoms
2. major surgery within the last 14 days
3. arterial puncture at non-compressible site within past 7 days
4. recent lumbar puncture
5. rapidly improving or minor symptoms. Note: IV tPA should not be delayed to monitor for further improvement (possible harm[1])
6. blood glucose > 400 mg/dl or < 50 mg/dl
7. history of GI or urinary tract hemorrhage within past 21 days
8. post myocardial infarction pericarditis

Additional issues relevant to giving IV tPA:
1. hypoattenuation on CT is not a criterion to withhold IV tPA[1]
2. hyperdense MCA sign is not a criterion to withhold IV tPA (no benefit[1])
3. routine use of MRI to exclude cerebral microbleeds before IV tPA is not recommended (no benefit[1])
4. use of imaging criteria to select candidates for IV tPA when the time of onset of symptoms is unknown is not recommended (no benefit[1])
5. do not delay IV tPA to obtain multimodal CT and/or MRI (possible harm[1])
6. for candidates for endovascular therapy, a noninvasive vascular study is recommended during the initial evaluation, but should not delay administration of IV tPA if indicated (Level I[1])
7. do not administer abciximab concurrently with tPA (potential harm[1])
8. rule out hypoglycemia and hyperglycemia (p. 1557)
9. be prepared to treat complications of tPA including: bleeding complications, angioedema (may require intubation) (Level I[1])
10. hypertension is aggressively controlled
11. the use of antithrombic therapy within the first 24 hours of IV tPA is uncertain. Use may be con sidered when there is substantial benefit (Level II[1])

Treatment protocol: Also, see Eligibility (p. 1563) & Contraindications (p. 1563) above.
℞ alteplase (Activase®): initiate < 4.5 hrs from onset of deficit or last known well (see indications contraindications above).
NINDS protocol: 0.9 mg/kg (up to a maximum of 90 mg total) given as follows: IV bolus 10% of th dose over 1 min, followed *immediately* by the remainder as a constant infusion over 60 minute (Level I[1]).
If there is an indication for anticoagulation, obtain a non-contrast CT 24 hours prior to startin anticoagulation since there is a risk of subclinical intracerebral hemorrhage.

ICH following IV tPA
There is an increased risk of symptomatic intracerebral hemorrhage (ICH) with the use of tPA (NIND study: 6.4% vs. 0.6% with placebo; ECASS II: 8.8% vs. 3.4%). In spite of this, the NINDS study found tha mortality in the tPA group was similar to controls at 3 mos (17% vs. 21%). The following factors wer associated with an increased risk of symptomatic ICH (with only a 57% efficiency rate of predictin ICH): severity of NIHSS score, or pre-treatment CT showing brain edema or mass effect. In one stud ICH did not influence outcome except in the rare instance when a massive hematoma occurred. Outcomes were still better in the treated group, and the conclusion is that these patients are sti reasonable candidates for tPA.[31] Since then, multicenter analyses have demonstrated that size infarction and elevated blood sugar are independent risk factors for symptomatic ICH.[32]
Management of post-tPA ICH:
1. discontinue tPA infusion and obtain STAT head CT

2. send labs: PT, aPTT, platelet count, fibrinogen, and type & cross
3. prepare to administer 6–8 units cryoprecipitate containing Factor VIII
4. prepare to administer 6–8 units of platelets
5. if emergent EVD placement or other interventional procedure is needed, consider the use of recombinant Factor VIIa (40–80 mg/kg) immediately beforehand (NB: this is only a temporizing measure and cryoprecipitate still needs to be given)

93.7 Carotid endarterectomy

93.7.1 Indications

Trials and results

▶ Table 93.3 shows the status of current studies for the surgical treatment of carotid stenosis (NB: some of the results may be contradictory).

Table 93.3 Summary of study findings for carotid endarterectomy (CEA)[a] (modified[33])

Stenosis	Relevant study	Recommendation	Risk reduction[b]
Symptomatic Narrowing			
70–99%	NASCET[34]	CEA	16.5 @ 2 yrs
>60%	ECST[35]	CEA	11.6 @ 3 yrs
50–69%	NASCET[36]	CEA[c]	10.1 @ 5 yrs
<30%	NASCET[36]	BMM	0.8 @ 5 yrs
<40%	ECST[37]	BMM	CEA worse @ 3 yrs
Asymptomatic Narrowing (p. 1548)			
>60%	ACST[38]	CEA if age <75 yrs	5.4% @ 5 yrs
>60%	ACAS,[39] ACST[d]	CEA[d]	6.3 @ 5 yrs
>50%	VACS	± CEA[e]	
<90%	CASANOVA	BMM[e]	

[a]abbreviations: NASCET = North American Symptomatic Carotid Endarterectomy Trial; ECST = European Carotid Surgery Trial; CASANOVA = Carotid Artery Stenosis with Asymptomatic Narrowing Operation Versus Aspirin; ACAS = Asymptomatic Carotid Atherosclerosis Study; ACST = Asymptomatic Carotid Surgery Trial; VACS = Veteran's Administration Cooperative Study; CEA = carotid endarterectomy; BMM = best medical management
[b]reduction in risk of all nonfatal strokes and death from any cause with CEA vs. BMM (e.g., with an absolute risk reduction of 16.5 at 2 yrs, for every 100 patients treated, 16.5 nonfatal strokes or deaths were prevented over a 2-yr period)
[c]surgery moderately beneficial (requires low complication rate)
[d]the overall health of the patient is critical
[e]results equivocal

93

The North American Symptomatic Carotid Endarterectomy Trial[34] (NASCET) found that for patients with a hemispheric or retinal TIA or a mild (non-disabling) stroke within 120 days and *ipsilateral high-grade* stenosis (> 70%), that carotid endarterectomy (CEA) reduced the rate of fatal and non-fatal strokes (by 17% at 18 months) and death from any cause (by 7% at 18 months) when compared to best medical management (when surgery was performed with perioperative risk of stroke or death of 5.8%). Results were twice as good for patients with stenosis from 90–99% than for those with 70–79%. Furthermore, with CEA the frequency of major functional impairment was reduced at years.[40] NB: see differences in techniques for measuring stenosis between NASCET and ECST ▶ Table 92.5).

See also **asymptomatic** patients (p. 1548).

Unresolved controversies

include:

- progressive STROKE ("stroke in evolution"): see Emergency carotid endarterectomy (p. 1570)
- abrupt occlusion: see Emergency endarterectomy (p. 1570)

3. tandem lesions (e.g., carotid siphon and bifurcation stenosis): although this topic remains contro-versial, CEA in patients with tandem lesions has not been associated with increased postopera-tive stroke rates.[41,42] Recent case series also report success with endovascular treatment
4. progressive retinal ischemia

93.7.2 Timing with respect to acute stroke

For patients with small fixed deficits or small infarcts on CT or MRI, the risk of early CEA is not increased.[41,43] In the pooled analysis of the three symptomatic CEA studies, patients randomized in the trials within 2 weeks of the last symptomatic event had greater benefit from CEA.[44] Data from Sundt (see below) indicates that a stroke is a risk factor for a complication only if it occurred within 7 days pre-op.

Since the introduction of tPA for the treatment of acute ischemic stroke, there have been reports on the successful treatment of residual critical ICA stenosis following tPA recanalization as early as 24 hours after administration of tPA in patients with small fixed deficit or small ischemic areas on MRI.[44,45]

93.7.3 Pre-op risk factors for CEA

> **Σ: Pre-op risk factors for CEA**
>
> The characteristics of patients who are high risk for complications from CEA have not been well defined, despite the perception that this group exists.

Identifying patients at high risk for complications after CEA has proven challenging. Typically, the exclusion criteria from studies are cited, but in most cases these are simply patients who were not included in the study because it was the investigators' perception that these patients might be "high risk." Therefore these risk factors are not validated. They are included here for completeness.

NASCET and ACAS: age > 80 years, prior ipsilateral CEA, prior contralateral CEA within 4 months, prior neck XRT, tandem lesion larger than target lesion, other conditions that could cause symptoms (atrial fibrillation, prior stroke with persistent major deficit, valvular heart disease), major organ fail-ure, uncontrolled hypertension or diabetes mellitus, and significant coronary artery disease.[46,47]

The SAPPHIRE Trial (Stenting and Angioplasty with Protection in Patients at High-Risk for Endar-terectomy): patients with clinically significant cardiac disease (CHF, abnormal stress test, or need for open-heart surgery), severe pulmonary disease, contralateral carotid occlusion, contralateral laryng-eal-nerve palsy, previous radical neck surgery or neck XRT, recurrent stenosis after endarterectomy, and age > 80 years.[48] The ARCHeR Trial (ACCULINK for Revascularization of Carotids in High-Risk patients) also included patients with tracheostomy, spinal immobility, and dialysis-dependent renal failure.[49]

93.7.4 Carotid endarterectomy—surgical considerations

Perioperative management

Pre-op management (carotid endarterectomy)
1. ASA 325 mg TID for at least 2 days, preferably 5 days pre-op[50] (NB: patients should be kept on their ASA for surgery, and if not on ASA they should be started, in order to reduce risks of MI and TIA[51])

Post-op management (carotid endarterectomy)
1. patient monitored in ICU with A-line
2. keep patient well hydrated (run IVF ≥ 100 cc/hr for most adults)
3. SBP ideally 110–150 mm Hg (higher pressures are permitted in patients with chronic severe HTN)
   a) BP frequently labile in first 24 hrs post-op, may be due to "new" pressure in carotid bulb; to prevent rebound hyper- or hypotension, avoid long-acting agents
   b) hypotension
      - check EKG – R/O cardiogenic shock
      - if mild, start with fluids (crystalloid or colloid)
      - phenylephrine (Neo-Synephrine®) for resistant hypotension

c) hypertension: nicardipine (Cardene®) (p. 131) is the agent of choice. Avoid rebound hypotension
4. avoid antiplatelet drugs for 24–48 hrs post-op (causes oozing); may start these 24–72 hrs post-op (note: ASA 325 mg + dipyridamole 75 mg TID have been shown *not* to reduce the rate of restenosis after endarterectomy[52])
5. optional: reverse half of heparin with protamine 10 minutes after closing arteriotomy

Post-op check (carotid endarterectomy)

In addition to routine, the following should be checked:
1. change in neurologic status due to cerebral dysfunction, including:
   a) pronator drift (R/O new hemiparesis)
   b) signs of dysphasia (especially for left-sided surgery)
   c) mimetic muscle symmetry (assesses facial nerve function)
2. pupil diameter and reaction (R/O stroke, Horner syndrome)
3. severe H/A (especially unilateral) > may indicate hyperperfusion syndrome
4. STA pulses (R/O external carotid occlusion)
5. tongue deviation (R/O hypoglossal nerve injury)
6. symmetry of lips (R/O weakness of lower lip depressors due to retraction of marginal mandibular branch of facial nerve against mandible, usually resolves in 6–12 wks, must differentiate from central VII palsy due to stroke)
7. check for hoarseness (R/O recurrent laryngeal nerve injury)
8. assess for hematoma in operative site: note any tracheal deviation, dysphagia

Post-op complications (carotid endarterectomy)

To justify CEA, the absolute upper limit of (significant) complication rate should be ≤ 3%.
1. overall in-hospital mortality: 1%[53]
2. disruption of arteriotomy closure: rare, but emergent (see below)
   a) evidenced by:
      • swelling of neck: rupture may produce a pseudoaneurysm
      • tracheal deviation (visible, palpable, or on CXR)
      • symptoms: dysphagia, air hunger or worsening hoarseness, difficulty swallowing
   b) dangers:
      • asphyxiation: most immediate danger
      • stroke
      • exsanguination (unlikely, unless skin closure is also disrupted)
   c) late (often delayed weeks to months): false aneurysm.[54] Risk = 0.33%. Presents as neck mass. Risk is increased with wound infection and possibly with patch graft as compared to endarterectomy alone[54,55,56]

93

3. stroke (cerebral infarction) intra-op or post-op rate[57]: 5%
   a) embolic (the most common cause of *minor* post-op neurologic deficit): source may be denuded media of endarterectomy
   b) intracerebral hemorrhagic (ICH) (breakthrough bleeding): occurs in < 0.6%.[58] Related to cerebral hyperperfusion in most[59,60] (see below). Usually occurs within first 2 weeks, often in basal ganglion 3–4 days post-op with hypertensive episode. Patients at greatest risk are those with severe stenosis and limited hemispheric collateral flow
   c) post-op ICA occlusion
      • most common cause of *major* post-op stroke, but may be asymptomatic
      • risk is reduced by attention to technical details at surgery[61 (p 249)]
      • some may be due to hypercoagulable state induced by heparin (predictable in patients whose platelet count drops while on heparin. No known therapy for this condition[61 (p 249-50)])
      • the endarterectomized surface is highly thrombogenic for 4 hrs following endarterectomy (Sundt recommends not reversing heparin)
      • in Sundt's series using patch graft[61 (p 229)]: 0.8% incidence, associated with major stroke in 33% and minor stroke in 20%
      • occlusion rate with primary closure: 4% in Sundt's experience, 2–5% in literature[61 (p 249)]

post-op TIAs: most due to ICA occlusion. Some may be due to microemboli. Hyperperfusion syndrome produces a 1% incidence of post-op TIAs[61 (p 229)]

seizures[62]: usually focal in onset with possible generalization, most occur late (post-op day 5–13) with an incidence of ≈ 0.4%[58] to 1%.[63] May be due to cerebral hyperperfusion,[58] emboli,[64] and/or intracerebral hemorrhage. Usually difficult to control initially, lorazepam and phenytoin are recommended (p. 213)

6. late restenosis: identifiable restenosis occurs in ≈ 25% by 1 yr, and half of these reduce luminal diameters by > 50%.[65] Restenosis within 2 yrs is usually due to fibrous hyperplasia, after 2 yrs it is typically due to atherosclerosis[66]

7. cerebral hyperperfusion syndrome (AKA normal pressure hyperperfusion breakthrough): classically thought to result from return of blood flow to an area that has lost autoregulation due to chronic cerebral ischemia typically from high-grade stenosis. Controversial.[60] Usually presents as ipsilateral vascular H/A or eye pain that subsides within several days[67] or with seizures (± PLEDs on EEG, more common with Halothane®, due to petechial hemorrhages[58]). May cause ICH.[68] Most complications occur several days post-op

8. hoarseness: the most common cause is laryngeal edema and *not* superior nor recurrent laryngeal nerve injury

9. cranial nerve injury: the most common complication after CEA with an incidence of up to 8–10%[69]
   a) hypoglossal nerve → tongue deviation towards the side of injury: incidence ≈ 1% (with mobilizing XII to allow displacement). Unilateral injury may cause speaking, chewing, and swallowing difficulties. Bilateral injuries can cause upper airway obstruction.[70] The presence of a unilateral palsy is a contraindication to doing contralateral endarterectomy until the first side recovers. May last as long as four months
   b) vagus or recurrent laryngeal nerve → unilateral vocal cord paralysis: 1% risk
   c) mandibular branch of facial nerve → loss of ipsilateral lip depressor

10. headache[58]

11. hypertension[71,72]: may develop 5–7 days post-op. Longstanding HTN may occur as a result of the loss of the carotid sinus baroreceptor reflex

Complication management

1. post-op TIAs
   a) if TIA occurs in recovery room, emergency CT (to R/O hemorrhage) and then angiogram recommended to assess for ICA or CCA occlusion (vs. emboli)
   b) if TIA occurs later, consider emergency ocular pneumoplethysmography; if abnormal → emergency surgery (if neurologically intact, pre-op angiogram is appropriate)[61]

2. fixed post-op deficit in distribution of endarterectomized carotid
   a) if deficit occurs immediately post-op (i.e., in PACU), recommend immediate re-exploration without delay for CT or angiogram[73] (case reports of no deficit when flow re-established in ≤ 45 mins). For later onset, workup is indicated. Technical considerations for emergency reoperation[61 (p 255)]:
      • isolate the 3 arteries (CCA, ECA, & ICA)
      • occlude CCA first, then ECA, and ICA last (to minimize emboli)
      • open arteriotomy, check backflow; if none, pass a No. 4 Fogarty catheter into ICA, gently inflate and withdraw (avoid intimal tears)
      • if good backflow established, close with patch graft
      • remove tortuous vessel loops and kinks before closing
   b) immediate management (unless ICH or SDH are likely) includes
      • fluids (e.g., Plasmanate®) to improve rheology and to elevate BP
      • pressors (e.g., phenylephrine) to elevate SBP to ≈ 180 mm Hg
      • oxygen
      • heparinization (may be controversial)
   c) theoretical benefits of radiographic evaluation include:
      • CT: identifies ICH or SDH that might require treatment other than re-exploration of the surgical site, elevating BP, etc.
      • angiogram: identifies whether ICA is occluded, or if deficit is from another cause (e.g., emboli from endarterectomy site) that would not benefit from re-exploration or possibly endovascular treatment

3. disruption of arteriotomy closure, management
   a) OPEN WOUND—if there is any stridor, it is critical to do this before trying to intubate (although ideally performed in O.R., the delay may be decisive). Evacuate clot (start with a sterile gloved finger) and stop bleeding, preferably without traumatizing the artery; a DeBakey clamp is optimal
   b) INTUBATION—high priority, may be difficult or impossible if trachea is deviated (open wound immediately). Preferably done by anesthesiologist in controlled setting (i.e., O.R.) unless there is acute airway obstruction
   c) call O.R. and have them prepare set-up for endarterectomy, and take patient to O.R.

93

93.7.5 Operative technique

Anesthesia and monitoring

Most (but not all) surgeons monitor some parameter of neurologic function during carotid endarterectomy, and will alter technique (e.g., insert a vascular shunt) if there is evidence of hemodynamic intolerance of carotid clamping (only occurs in ≈ 1–4%).

1. local/regional anesthesia: permits "clinical" monitoring of patient's neurologic function.[74,75] Disadvantages: patient movement during procedure (often exacerbated by sedation and alterations in CBF), lack of cerebral protection from anesthetic and adjunctive agents. The only prospective randomized study found no difference between local and general anesthesia.[76] The multicenter, randomized controlled General Anesthesia versus Local Anesthesia (GALA) Trial[77] found no significant differences in the prevention of stroke, MI, or death for either anesthetic technique. Subgroup analysis showed trends (not statistically significant) favoring local anesthesia for perioperative death, event-free survival at 1 year, and patients with contralateral occlusion. Local anesthesia was associated with a significant reduction of shunt insertion.[77] A Cochrane Database Review found no evidence from randomized trials to favor either anesthetic technique[78]

2. general anesthesia, possibly including barbiturates (thiopental boluses of 125–250 mg until 15–30-second burst suppression on EEG, followed by small bolus injections or constant infusion to maintain burst suppression[50])
   a) EEG monitoring
   b) SSEP monitoring
   c) measurement of distal stump pressure after CCA occlusion (unreliable), e.g., using a shunt if stump pressure < 25 mm Hg
   d) transcranial Doppler
   e) near-infrared spectroscopy

Position and incision

1. supine, neck slightly extended and rotated slightly (≈ 30°) away from the operative side
2. the incision curves gently and follows the anterior border of the sternocleidomastoid muscle, and curves posteriorly at the rostral end
3. keep the horizontal portion of the incision ≈ 1 cm away from the mandible to avoid injury to marginal mandibular branch of facial nerve (which lies in the inferior parotid gland and supplies lip depressor) due to retraction against mandible
4. retractors should not be placed deeper than the platysma to avoid injury to recurrent laryngeal nerve, which runs between the esophagus and trachea. Blunt retractors are used to avoid internal jugular vein injury

Dissection

1. the common facial vein (CFV) usually crosses the field over the carotid bifurcation, it is doubly ligated and divided. It leads to the internal jugular vein (IJV)
2. identifying the IJV is key, dissection is carried down between the carotid artery and the IJV
3. the *ansa hypoglossi* runs superficial to the ICA and serves as a useful guide to the *hypoglossal nerve* (XII) which should be identified since it is at greater risk when it is not seen. XII can arise anywhere from the carotid bifurcation to the angle of the mandible, although it is usually in the vicinity of the CFV. Mobilization can be facilitated by dividing the small artery (sternocleidomastoid branch of the ECA) and vein that cross over it[70]
4. the ansa hypoglossi can usually be spared, and if mobilized, allows medial retraction of the hypoglossal nerve out of harm's way. If it is necessary to divide the ansa it is done close to the hypoglossal nerve to be certain it is not a branch of the vagus and to minimize neurologic deficit (the ansa has an anterior cervical limb from the cervical plexus)
5. the superior thyroid artery is the first branch of the ECA, and helps differentiate ECA from the ICA (the ICA is located posterior to the ECA)
6. the carotid bulb may be anesthetized with ≈ 2–3 ml of 1% plain lidocaine using a 27 Ga needle. This may be done routinely, or, as some prefer only if hypotension and/or bradycardia occur during dissection (indicating IX nerve stimulation)
7. the ICA must be exposed beyond the extent of the plaque which can be determined by gentle palpation with a moistened finger and by visualization as the area where the artery turns from yellowish to its normal pinker color

93

Occlusion and arteriotomy

1. a vessel loop is placed around the ECA at least 2 cm above the bifurcation
2. a vessel loop is also placed around the ICA but is looped only once
3. umbilical tape with a choke is placed around the CCA 2–3 cm below the bifurcation
4. IV heparin (usually 5,000 IU) is given 1 minute prior to cross clamping
5. a temporary aneurysm clip is placed on the superior thyroid artery
6. the order of *occlusion* of the vessels is as follows (mnemonic: "ICE"):
   a) ICA (e.g., with temporary aneurysm clip)
   b) CCA (e.g., with a small DeBakey clamp)
   c) ECA (e.g., with temporary aneurysm clip)
7. during ICA clamping, mild hypertension is maintained by the anesthesiologist
8. shunt: some surgeons use some form of monitoring (EEG, BSAER, etc.) to determine if a shunt is needed—see Anesthesia and monitoring (p. 1569); yet others routinely use a shunt whenever possible without assessing the need
9. the arteriotomy is begun in the CCA with a #11 scalpel, and once the lumen is entered, Potts' scissors carry the incision through to the ICA beyond the plaque. Stay in the midline to facilitate arteriotomy closure

Plaque removal

1. the plaque usually cannot be completely removed from the CCA, and thus it is usually transected with Potts' scissors, taking care not to inadvertently incise the artery wall and to leave as smooth an edge as possible
2. in the ICA, great care must be made to avoid leaving an intimal flap which could become a nidus for an arterial dissection. If necessary the intima may be tacked down by suturing from the lumen out on both ends (using double-armed suture) and tying the knot outside the vessel

Arteriotomy closure and vessel release

1. arteriotomy may be performed with a running Prolene suture using either
   a) primary closure
   b) or a patch graft to increase the caliber of the vessel and reduce the risk of re-stenosis
   c) limited evidence suggests that carotid patch angioplasty may reduce the risk of perioperative arterial occlusion and re-stenosis. Synthetic patches (Dacron, PTFE) are preferred to autologous vein (risk of aneurysmal dilatation, thrombogenic surface)[79,80]
2. the order of releasing the vessels (reverse that of the clamping order):
   a) ECA
   b) CCA (allows air and debris to be washed into the ECA)
   c) ICA

93.7.6 Emergency carotid endarterectomy

General information

Emergency CEA indications include crescendo TIAs and stroke in evolution. The treatment paradigm of these conditions has shifted towards the use of interventional methods, such as thrombolysis and stenting, although there are no randomized controlled trial data to support that approach. A recent meta-analysis of emergent CEA has shown that the pooled stroke and stroke/death rates after CEA for crescendo TIA in 176 patients were 6.5% and 9.0%, respectively. For those with stroke in evolution the overall stroke and stroke/death rates in 114 patients were 16.9% and 20.0%, respectively.[81]

After retrospective analysis of 64 emergency endarterectomies[82] the guidelines given below were suggested. However, the efficacy of immediate surgical removal of obstruction is controversial and unproven. In one early study, over 50% of patients suffered fatal intracranial hemorrhage within 72 hours of emergency carotid endarterectomy.

Initial management of patient presenting with acute neuro deficit

1. obtain history directed at determining presence of previous stroke and other serious medical illness, and to try to differentiate from seizure
2. baseline neurological assessment including evaluation of STA pulses and carotid bruits
3. during evaluation: close control of BP. O_2 per NC. Labs + EKG; see Management of TIA or stroke (p. 1562). Consider hemodilution with LMD

4. CT to R/O ICH or infarction (early stroke will not be visible)
5. when carotid disease is suspected, and CT is negative for ICH or acute infarct, emergency angiography, MRI/MRA, or CTA is performed

Indications for emergency carotid endarterectomy

General information

In patients with acute neurological deficits, the need for rapid decision making often does not allow differentiating between TIA, stroke in evolution and acute stroke, nor in assessing the stability or fluctuating nature of the deficit.

Indications

1. stroke in evolution
2. crescendo TIAs: TIAs that abruptly increase in frequency to ≥ several per day
3. following intra-arterial thrombolysis, emergent/urgent CEA is indicated for residual critical carotid stenosis[45,83]

Contraindications

See also more details (p. 1563). Patients with depressed levels of consciousness or acute fixed deficits.

Surgical management

Again, most cases would now be managed initially with endovascular thrombolysis and stenting. Surgery would be considered if this is not an option.

1. for emergency surgery, it is essential that blood pressure be stable
2. in patients with complete occlusion, ICA is not occluded intra-op (to avoid breaking up thrombus, if present)
3. if thrombus is present
   a) attempt spontaneous extrusion using back pressure
   b) if this fails, attempt to remove with smoothened suction catheter
   c) if this fails, pass balloon embolectomy catheter as far as base of skull (caution: avoid injury to distal ICA that could cause CCF)
   d) obtain intra-op angiogram unless thrombus emerges and backflow is excellent
   e) plicate ICA (avoid creating a blind pouch at origin) if there is good backflow or if satisfactory angiography cannot be obtained

Surgical results

Highest correlation was with presenting neurologic status (▶ Table 93.4).

Table 93.4 Surgical results

Presenting deficit	Same or improved	Deaths
intact or mild	92%	0
moderate	80%	1 (7%)
severe	77%	3 (13%)

93.8 Carotid angioplasty/stenting

93.8.1 General information

Σ: Endarterectomy vs. stenting

There are no well-designed studies that convincingly show superiority of angioplasty/stenting over CEA in *average-risk* symptomatic patients, and the recommendation in these patients is to continue with the time-tested technique of CEA.

93

There is a paucity of randomized control trials[48,49,84,85,86,87] comparing carotid angioplasty/stenting with CEA, and many nonrandomized registries.[49,88,89,90,91,92,93,94,95,96]

However, data from multicenter randomized trials showing that carotid angioplasty/stenting is as safe over the short term or as efficacious over the long term as CEA in average-risk symptomatic patients are lacking. Published trials are heterogeneous (clinically and methodologically), too small to provide robust and convincing data, and limited in long-term follow-up. Only the SAPPHIRE study[48] comparing CEA with stenting (using a distal embolic protection device) for moderate to severe carotid stenosis with comorbidities that might increase the risk of CEA (high-risk patients), found that angioplasty/stenting was not inferior (risk within 3%, P = 0.004) to CEA (based on a composite primary end point of stroke, death, or MI within 30 days, or death from neurologic causes or ipsilateral stroke between 31 days and 1 year).[48] However, the study methodology has been criticized.[97,98,99]

A 2007 Cochrane review concluded that available data on carotid angioplasty/stenting are difficult to interpret and does not support a change in clinical practice away from recommending CEA as the treatment of choice for suitable carotid artery stenosis.[100]

93.8.2 Indications for angioplasty/stenting

Carotid stenting performed with adequate procedural quality levels should be considered instead of CEA in the presence of[101]:

1. severe vascular and cardiac comorbidities:
   a) congestive heart failure (New York Heart Association class III/IV) and/or known severe left ventricular dysfunction
   b) open heart surgery needed within 6 weeks
   c) recent myocardial infarction (< 24 hours and > 4 weeks)
   d) unstable angina (Canadian Cardiovascular Society class III/IV)
   e) contralateral carotid occlusion
2. specific conditions:
   a) contralateral laryngeal nerve palsy
   b) radiation therapy to the neck
   c) previous CEA with recurrent restenosis
   d) high cervical internal carotid/below the clavicle common carotid lesions
   e) severe tandem lesions
   f) age > 80 years
   g) severe pulmonary disease

The 2009 European Society for Vascular Surgery (ESVS) Guidelines state that carotid angioplasty/stenting is indicated in cases of: contralateral laryngeal nerve palsy, previous radical neck dissection or cervical XRT, prior CEA (re-stenosis), high bifurcation or intracranial extension of a carotid lesion provided that the peri-interventional stroke or death rate is not higher than that accepted for CEA (Class C recommendation).[79]

AHA Guidelines state that angioplasty/stenting might be a reasonable alternative to CEA in *asymptomatic high-risk* patients. However, they stress that it remains uncertain whether this group of patients should have either procedure.[102]

References

[1] Powers WJ, Rabinstein AA, Ackerson T, et al. 2018 Guidelines for the Early Management of Patients With Acute Ischemic Stroke: A Guideline for Healthcare Professionals From the American Heart Association/American Stroke Association. Stroke. 2018; 49:e46–e110

[2] Smith EE, Kent DM, Bulsara KR, et al. Accuracy of Prediction Instruments for Diagnosing Large Vessel Occlusion in Individuals With Suspected Stroke: A Systematic Review for the 2018 Guidelines for the Early Management of Patients With Acute Ischemic Stroke. Stroke. 2018; 49:e111–e122

[3] Brott T, Adams HP, Olinger CP, et al. Measurements of Acute Cerebral Infarction: A Clinical Examination Scale. Stroke. 1991; 20:864–870

[4] Brott T, Reed RL. Intensive care for acute stroke in the community hospital setting: The first 24 hours. Stroke. 1989; 20:694–697

[5] Pulsinelli WA, Levy DE, Sigsbee B, et al. Increased damage after ischemic stroke in patients with hyperglycemia with or without established diabetes mellitus. Am J Med. 1983; 74:540–544

[6] Moulin T, Cattin F, Crépin-Leblond T, et al. Early CT Signs in Acute Middle Cerebral Artery Infarction: Predictive Value for Subsequent Infarct Location and Outcome. Neurology. 1996; 47:366–375

[7] Marks MP, Holmgren EB, Fox AJ, et al. Evaluation of early computed tomographic findings in acute ischemic stroke. Stroke. 1999; 30:389–392

[8] Tomandl BF, Klotz E, Handschu R, et al. Comprehensive imaging of ischemic stroke with multisection CT. Radiographics. 2003; 23:565–592

[9] Wall SD, Brant-Zawadzki M, Jeffrey RB, et al. High Frequency CT Findings Within 24 Hours After Cerebral Infarction. American Journal of Radiology. 1982; 138:307–311

93

[10] Aarabi B, Long DM. Dynamics of Cerebral Edema. Journal of Neurosurgery. 1979; 51:779–784

[11] Barber PA, Demchuk AM, Zhang J, et al. Validity and reliability of a quantitative computed tomography score in predicting outcome of hyperacute stroke before thrombolytic therapy. ASPECTS Study Group. Alberta Stroke Programme Early CT Score. Lancet. 2000; 355:1670–1674

[12] Schroder J, Thomalla G. A Critical Review of Alberta Stroke Program Early CT Score for Evaluation of Acute Stroke Imaging. Front Neurol. 2016; 7. DOI: 10.3389/fneur.2016.00245

[13] Gacs G, Fox AJ, Barnett HJM, et al. CT Visualization of Intracranial Thromboembolism. Stroke. 1983; 14:756–762

[14] Tomsick TA, Brott TG, Olinger CP, et al. Hyperdense Middle Cerebral Artery: Incidence and Quantitative Significance. Neuroradiology. 1989; 31:312–315

[15] Manelfe C, Larrue V, von Kummer R, et al. Association of Hyperdense Middle Cerebral Artery Sign With Clinical Outcome in Patients Treated With Plasminogen Activator. Stroke. 1999; 30:769–772

[16] Sims JR, Rordorf G, Smith EE, et al. Arterial occlusion revealed by CT angiography predicts NIH stroke score and acute outcomes after IV tPA treatment. AJNR. American Journal of Neuroradiology. 2005; 26:246–251

[17] Nabavi DG, Cenic A, Craen RA, et al. CT assessment of cerebral perfusion: experimental validation and initial clinical experience. Radiology. 1999; 213:141–149

[18] Elster AD, Moody DM. Early Cerebral Infarction: Gadopentetate Dimeglumine Enhancement. Radiology. 1990; 177:627–632

[19] Barber PA, Darby DG, Desmond PM, et al. Prediction of stroke outcome with echoplanar perfusion- and diffusion-weighted MRI. Neurology. 1998; 51:418–426

[20] Campbell BC, Mitchell PJ, Kleinig TJ, et al. Endovascular therapy for ischemic stroke with perfusion-imaging selection. N Engl J Med. 2015; 372:1009–1018

[21] Goyal M, Demchuk AM, Menon BK, et al. Randomized assessment of rapid endovascular treatment of ischemic stroke. N Engl J Med. 2015; 372:1019–1030

[22] Berkhemer OA, Fransen PS, Beumer D, et al. A randomized trial of intraarterial treatment for acute ischemic stroke. N Engl J Med. 2015; 372:11–20

[23] Fransen PS, Beumer D, Berkhemer OA, et al. MR CLEAN, a multicenter randomized clinical trial of endovascular treatment for acute ischemic stroke in the Netherlands: study protocol for a randomized controlled trial. Trials. 2014; 15. DOI: 10.1186/1745-6215-15-343

[24] Nogueira RG, Jadhav AP, Haussen DC, et al. Thrombectomy 6 to 24 Hours after Stroke with a Mismatch between Deficit and Infarct. N Engl J Med. 2018; 378:11–21

[25] Albers GW, Marks MP, Kemp S, et al. Thrombectomy for Stroke at 6 to 16 Hours with Selection by Perfusion Imaging. N Engl J Med. 2018; 378:708–718

[26] Logallo N, Novotny V, Assmus J, et al. Tenecteplase versus alteplase for management of acute ischaemic stroke (NOR-TEST): a phase 3, randomised, open-label, blinded endpoint trial. Lancet Neurol. 2017; 16:781–788

[27] Lansberg MG, Bluhmki E, Thijs VN. Efficacy and safety of tissue plasminogen activator 3 to 4.5 hours after acute ischemic stroke: a metaanalysis. Stroke. 2009; 40:2438–2441

[28] Benedict SL, Ni OK, Schloesser P, et al. Intra-arterial thrombolysis in a 2-year-old with cardioembolic stroke. Journal of Child Neurology. 2007; 22:225–227

[29] Fisher M, Hachinski V. European Cooperative Acute Stroke Study III: support for and questions about a truly emerging therapy. Stroke. 2009; 40:2262–2263

[30] Toni D, Fiorelli M, Bastianello S, et al. Hemorrhagic transformation of brain infarct: Predictability in the first 5 hours from stroke onset and influence on clinical outcome. Neurology. 1996; 46:341–345

[31] The National Institute of Neurological Disorders and Stroke rt-PA Stroke Study Group. Intracerebral hemorrhage after intravenous t-PA therapy for ischemic stroke. Stroke. 1997; 28:2109–2118

[32] Paciaroni M, Agnelli G, Corea F, et al. Early hemorrhagic transformation of brain infarction: rate, predictive factors, and influence on clinical outcome: results of a prospective multicenter study. Stroke. 2008; 39:2249–2256

[33] Chassin MR. Appropriate Use of Carotid Endarterectomy. New England Journal of Medicine. 1998; 339:1468–1471

[34] The North American Symptomatic Carotid Endarterectomy Trial. Beneficial Effect of Carotid Endarterectomy in Symptomatic Patients with High-Grade Carotid Stenosis. New England Journal of Medicine. 1991; 325:445–453

[35] The European Carotid Surgery Trialists' Collaborative Group. Randomized Trial of Endartectomy for Recently Symptomatic Carotid Stenosis: Final Results of the MRC European Carotid Surgery Trial (ECST). Lancet. 1998; 351:1379–1387

[36] Barnett HJM, Taylor W, Eliasziw M, et al. Benefit of Carotid Endarterectomy in Patients with Symptomatic Moderate or Severe Stenosis. New England Journal of Medicine. 1998; 339:1415–1425

[37] The European Carotid Surgery Trialists' Collaborative Group. Endartectomy for Moderate Symptomatic Carotid Stenosis: Interim Results of the MRC European Carotid Surgery Trial. Lancet. 1996; 347:1591–1593

[38] Halliday A, Mansfield A, Marro J, et al. Prevention of disabling and fatal strokes by successful carotid endarterectomy in patients without recent neurological symptoms: randomised controlled trial. Lancet. 2004; 363:1491–1502

[39] The Executive Committee for the Asymptomatic Carotid Atherosclerosis Study. Endarterectomy for Asymptomatic Carotid Artery Stenosis. Journal of the American Medical Association. 1995; 273:1421–1428

[40] Haynes RB, Taylor DW, Sackett DL, et al. Prevention of Functional Impairment by Endarterectomy for Symptomatic High-Grade Stenosis. Lancet. 1994; 351:1379–1387

[41] Faries PL, Chaer RA, Patel S, et al. Current management of extracranial carotid artery disease. Vasc Endovascular Surg. 2006; 40:165–175

[42] Rouleau PA, Huston J,3rd, Gilbertson J, et al. Carotid artery tandem lesions: frequency of angiographic detection and consequences for endarterectomy. AJNR. American Journal of Neuroradiology. 1999; 20:621–625

[43] Bond R, Rerkasem K, Rothwell PM. Systematic review of the risks of carotid endarterectomy in relation to the clinical indication for and timing of surgery. Stroke. 2003; 34:2290–2301

[44] Rothwell PM, Eliasziw M, Gutnikov SA, et al. Endarterectomy for symptomatic carotid stenosis in relation to clinical subgroups and timing of surgery. Lancet. 2004; 363:915–924

[45] Bartoli MA, Squarcioni C, Nicoli F, et al. Early carotid endarterectomy after intravenous thrombolysis for acute ischaemic stroke. European Journal of Vascular and Endovascular Surgery. 2009; 37:512–518

[46] Nguyen LL, Conte MS, Reed AB, et al. Carotid endarterectomy: who is the high-risk patient? Seminars in Vascular Surgery. 2004; 17:219–223

[47] Kang JL, Chung TK, Lancaster RT, et al. Outcomes after carotid endarterectomy: is there a high-risk population? A National Surgical Quality Improvement Program report. Journal of Vascular Surgery. 2009; 49:331–8, 339 e1; discussion 338-9

[48] Yadav JS, Wholey MH, Kuntz RE, et al. Protected carotid-artery stenting versus endarterectomy in high-risk patients. New England Journal of Medicine. 2004; 351:1493–1501

93

[49] Gray WA, Hopkins LN, Yadav S, et al. Protected carotid stenting in high-surgical-risk patients: the ARCHeR results. Journal of Vascular Surgery. 2006; 44:258–268

[50] Spetzler RF, Martin N, Hadley MN, et al. Microsurgical Endarterectomy Under Barbiturate Protection: A Prospective Study. J Neurosurg. 1986; 65:63–73

[51] Mayo Asymptomatic Carotid Endarterectomy Study Group. Results of a Randomized Controlled Trial of Carotid Endarterectomy for Asymptomatic Carotid Stenosis. Mayo Clinic Proceedings. 1992; 67:513–518

[52] Harker LA, Bernstein EF, Dilley RB, et al. Failure of Aspirin plus Dipyridamole to Prevent Restenosis After Carotid Endarterectomy. Ann Int Med. 1992; 116:731–736

[53] McPhee JT, Hill JS, Ciocca RG, et al. Carotid endarterectomy was performed with lower stroke and death rates than carotid artery stenting in the United States in 2003 and 2004. Journal of Vascular Surgery. 2007; 46:1112–1118

[54] Branch CL, Davis CH. False Aneurysm Complicating Carotid Endarterectomy. Neurosurgery. 1986; 19:421–425

[55] McCollum CH, Wheeler WG, Noon GP, et al. Aneurysms of the Extracranial Carotid Artery. Am J Surg. 1979; 137:196–200

[56] Welling RE, Taha A, Goel T, et al. Extracranial Carotid Artery Aneurysms. Surgery. 1983; 93:319–323

[57] Brott TG, Labutta RJ, Kempczinski RF. Changing Patterns in the Practice of Carotid Endarterectomy in a Large Metropolitan Area. JAMA. 1986; 255:2609–2612

[58] Reigel MM, Hollier LH, Sundt TM, et al. Cerebral Hyperperfusion Syndrome: A Cause of Neurologic Dysfunction After Carotid Endarterectomy. J Vasc Surg. 1987; 5:628–634

[59] Piepgras DG, Morgan MK, Sundt TM, et al. Intracerebral Hemorrhage After Carotid Endarterectomy. Journal of Neurosurgery. 1988; 68:532–536

[60] Ascher E, Markevich N, Schutzer RW, et al. Cerebral hyperperfusion syndrome after carotid endarterectomy: predictive factors and hemodynamic changes. J Vasc Surg. 2003; 37:769–777

[61] Sundt TM. Occlusive Cerebrovascular Disease. Philadelphia: W. B. Saunders; 1987

[62] Kieburtz K, Ricotta JJ, Moxley RT. Seizures Following Carotid Endarterectomy. Arch Neurol. 1990; 47:568–570

[63] Sundt TM, Sharbrough FW, Piepgras DG, et al. Correlation of Cerebral Blood Flow and Electroencephalographic Changes During Carotid Endarterectomy. Mayo Clin Proc. 1981; 56:533–543

[64] Wilkinson JT, Adams HP, Wright CB. Convulsions After Carotid Endarterectomy. JAMA. 1980; 244:1827–1828

[65] Bernstein EF, Humber PB, Collins GM, et al. Life expectancy and late stroke following carotid endarterectomy. Ann Surg. 1983; 198:80–86

[66] Callow AD. Recurrent Stenosis After Carotid Endarterectomy. Arch Surg. 1982; 117:1082–1085

[67] Dolan JG, Mushlin AI. Hypertension, Vascular Headaches, and Seizures After Carotid Endarterectomy. Arch Intern Med. 1984; 144:1489–1491

[68] Caplan LR, Skillman J, Ojemann R, et al. Intracerebral Hemorrhage Following Carotid Endarterectomy: A Hypertensive Complication. Stroke. 1979; 9:457–460

[69] Sajid MS, Vijaynagar B, Singh P, et al. Literature review of cranial nerve injuries during carotid endarterectomy. Acta Chirurgica Belgica. 2007; 107:25–28

[70] Imparato AM, Bracco A, Kim GE, et al. The Hypoglossal Nerve in Carotid Arterial Reconstructions. Stroke. 1972; 3:576–578

[71] Skydell JL, Machleder HI, Baker JD, et al. Incidence and Mechanism of Postcarotid Endarterectomy Hypertension. Arch Surg. 1987; 122:1153–1155

[72] Lehv MS, Salzman EW, Silen W. Hypertension Complicating Carotid Endarterectomy. Stroke. 1970; 1:307–313

[73] Baker WH, Bergan JJ, Yao JST. Management of stroke during and after carotid surgery. In: Cerebrovascular Insufficiency. New York: Grune and Stratton; 1983:481–495

[74] Zuccarello M, Yeh H-S, Tew JM. Morbidity and Mortality of Carotid Endarterectomy under Local Anesthesia: A Retrospective Study. Neurosurgery. 1988; 23:445–450

[75] Lee KS, Courtland CH, McWhorter JM. Low Morbidity and Mortality of Carotid Endarterectomy Performed with Regional Anesthesia. Journal of Neurosurgery. 1988; 69:483–487

[76] Forssell C, Takolander R, Bergqvist D, et al. Local Versus General Anesthesia in Carotid Surgery. A Prospective Randomized Study. Eur J Vasc Surg. 1989; 3:503–509

[77] Lewis SC, Warlow CP, Bodenham AR, et al. General anaesthesia versus local anaesthesia for carotid surgery (GALA): a multicentre, randomised controlled trial. Lancet. 2008; 372:2132–2142

[78] Rerkasem K, Rothwell PM. Local versus general anaesthesia for carotid endarterectomy. Cochrane Database Syst Rev. 2008. DOI: 10.1002/14651858.CD000126.pub3

[79] Liapis CD, Bell PR, Mikhailidis D, et al. ESVS guidelines. Invasive treatment for carotid stenosis: indications, techniques. European Journal of Vascular and Endovascular Surgery. 2009; 37:1–19

[80] Bond R, Rerkasem K, AbuRahma AF, et al. Patch angioplasty versus primary closure for carotid endarterectomy. Cochrane Database Syst Rev. 2004. DOI: 10.1002/14651858.CD000160.pub2

[81] Karkos CD, Hernandez-Lahoz I, Naylor AR. Urgent carotid surgery in patients with crescendo transient ischaemic attacks and stroke-in-evolution: a systematic review. European Journal of Vascular and Endovascular Surgery. 2009; 37:279–288

[82] Walters BB, Ojemann RG, Heros RC. Emergency Carotid Endarterectomy. J Neurosurg. 1987; 66:817–823

[83] Mayo Asymptomatic Carotid Endarterectomy Study Group. Results of a randomized controlled trial of carotid endarterectomy for asymptomatic carotid stenosis. Mayo Clinic Proceedings. 1992; 67:513–518

[84] CAVATAS Investigators. Endovascular versus surgical treatment in patients with carotid stenosis in the Carotid and Vertebral Artery Transluminal Angioplasty Study (CAVATAS): a randomised trial. Lancet. 2001; 357:1729–1737

[85] Alberts MJ. Results of a multicenter prospective randomized trial of carotid artery stenting vs. carotid endarterectomy. Stroke. 2001; 32

[86] Mas JL, Chatellier G, Beyssen B, et al. Endarterectomy versus stenting in patients with symptomatic severe carotid stenosis. New England Journal of Medicine. 2006; 355:1660–1671

[87] Ringleb PA, Allenberg J, Bruckmann H, et al. 30 day results from the SPACE trial of stent-protected angioplasty versus carotid endarterectomy in symptomatic patients: a randomised non-inferiority trial. Lancet. 2006; 368:1239–1247

[88] CaRESS Steering Committee. Carotid Revascularization Using Endarterectomy or Stenting Systems (CaRESS) phase I clinical trial: 1-year results. Journal of Vascular Surgery. 2005; 42:213–219

[89] White CJ, Iyer SS, Hopkins LN, et al. Carotid stenting with distal protection in high surgical risk patients: the BEACH trial 30 day results. Catheterization and Cardiovascular Interventions. 2006; 67:503–512

[90] Safian RD, Bresnahan JF, Jaff MR, et al. Protected carotid stenting in high-risk patients with severe carotid artery stenosis. Journal of the American College of Cardiology. 2006; 47:2384–2389

[91] Hill MD, Morrish W, Soulez G, et al. Multicenter evaluation of a self-expanding carotid stent system with distal protection in the treatment of carotid stenosis. AJNR. American Journal of Neuroradiology. 2006; 27:759–765

[92] Fairman R, Gray WA, Scicli AP, et al. The CAPTURE registry: analysis of strokes resulting from carotid artery stenting in the post approval setting

93

timing, location, severity, and type. Annals of Surgery. 2007; 246:551–6; discussion 556-8

[93] Iyer SS, White CJ, Hopkins LN, et al. Carotid artery revascularization in high-surgical-risk patients using the Carotid WALLSTENT and FilterWire EX/EZ: 1-year outcomes in the BEACH Pivotal Group. Journal of the American College of Cardiology. 2008; 51:427–434

[94] Bosiers M, Peeters P, Deloose K, et al. Does carotid artery stenting work on the long run: 5-year results in high-volume centers (ELOCAS Registry). Journal of Cardiovascular Surgery. 2005; 46:241–247

[95] Theiss W, Hermanek P, Mathias K, et al. Pro-CAS: a prospective registry of carotid angioplasty and stenting. Stroke. 2004; 35:2134–2139

[96] Zahn R, Roth E, Ischinger T, et al. Carotid artery stenting in clinical practice results from the Carotid Artery Stenting (CAS)-registry of the Arbeitsgemeinschaft Leitende Kardiologische Krankenhausarzte (ALKK). Zeitschrift fur Kardiologie. 2005; 94:163–172

[97] Goldstein LB. New data about stenting versus endarterectomy for symptomatic carotid artery stenosis. Curr Treat Options Cardiovasc Med. 2009; 11:232–240

[98] Fayad P. Endarterectomy and stenting for asymptomatic carotid stenosis: a race at breakneck speed. Stroke. 2007; 38:707–714

[99] Naylor AR, Bell PR. Treatment of asymptomatic carotid disease with stenting: con. Seminars in Vascular Surgery. 2008; 21:100–107

[100] Ederle J, Featherstone RL, Brown MM. Percutaneous transluminal angioplasty and stenting for carotid artery stenosis. Cochrane Database Syst Rev. 2007. DOI: 10.1002/14651858.CD000515.pub3

[101] Cremonesi A, Setacci C, Bignamini A, et al. Carotid artery stenting: first consensus document of the ICCS-SPREAD Joint Committee. Stroke. 2006; 37:2400–2409

[102] Goldstein LB, Adams R, Alberts MJ, et al. Primary prevention of ischemic stroke. Stroke. 2006; 37:1583–1633

93

94 Cerebral Arterial Dissections and Moyamoya Disease

94.1 Cerebral Arterial Dissections

94.1.1 Cerebral arterial dissections – key concepts

> **Key concepts**
>
> - hemorrhage into the tunica media of an artery
> - may be spontaneous, posttraumatic, or iatrogenic (e.g., angiography-related), may be intracranial or extracranial
> - may present with pain (usually ipsilateral H/A or carotidynia), Horner syndrome (in carotid dissections), TIA/stroke, or SAH
> - extracranial dissections are usually treated medically (anticoagulation), intracranial dissections with SAH are treated surgically

This section primarily discusses "spontaneous" dissections. Cerebrovascular arterial dissections following blunt cervical trauma (p. 1028) are much more common.

94.1.2 Nomenclature

Some confusion has arisen because of inconsistent terminology in the literature. Although by no means standard, Yamaura[1] has suggested the following:

▶ **Dissection.** Extravasation of blood between the intima and media, creating luminal narrowing or occlusion.

▶ **Dissecting aneurysm.** Dissection of blood between the media and adventitia, or at the media, causing aneurysmal dilatation, which may rupture into the subarachnoid space.

▶ **Pseudoaneurysm.** Rupture of artery with subsequent encapsulation of the extravascular hematoma, may or may not produce luminal narrowing.

94.1.3 Pathophysiology

The lesion common to all dissections is hemorrhage outside of the vascular lumen due to pathological trans-intimal extravasation of blood from the true lumen into the vessel wall. The hematoma may either dissect the internal elastic membrane from the intima[2] causing narrowing of the true lumen, or it may dissect into the subadventitial plane producing an adventitial outpouching from the vessel wall (pseudoaneurysm). Rupture through the vessel wall producing SAH occurs occasionally.

Subintimal dissection is more common with intracranial dissections, whereas extracranial vessels (including the aorta) usually dissect at the media or between media and adventitia.

"Spontaneous" dissections have been associated with a large number of conditions, oftentimes the association is unproven. These conditions include:
- fibromuscular dysplasia (FMD): found in ≈ 15% of cases[3]
- cystic medial necrosis (or degeneration): originally thought to be a common finding, now thought to perhaps be linked to a higher likelihood of *fatal* dissection
- saccular aneurysm
- Marfan syndrome: autosomal dominant inherited disorder of connective tissue. Phenotypic manifestations are due to production of abnormal fibrillin, the main component of extracellular microfibrils, a component in the media of certain blood vessels, encoded by the FBN1 gene on chromosome 15q21
- Ehlers-Danlos syndrome
- atherosclerosis: only rarely implicated as an etiology. More likely to be a factor with subintimal dissection of *extra*cranial arteries

94

- Takayasu's disease
- medial degeneration
- syphilitic arteritis (more common in the past, associated with 60% of dissections before 1950)
- autosomal dominant polycystic kidney disease (p. 1455): associated with a higher incidence of cerebral aneurysms
- variant periarteritis nodosa
- allergic arteritis
- homocystinuria
- moyamoya disease (p. 1581) [4]
- strenuous physical activity

94.1.4 Epidemiology

Occurs primarily in middle-aged patients, with a mean age of ≈ 45 yrs (average age of traumatic dissections is slightly younger). More frequent in men.[1,3] Incidence is unknown, since oftentimes the condition produces mild, transient symptoms. Increased awareness of the condition has resulted in an increased rate of diagnosis. ICA dissection accounts for 1–2.5% of first strokes.[5] However, in middle-aged and young adults it comprises 10–25% of strokes.[6]

94.1.5 Sites of dissection

A review of 260 cases[1] (literature review + new cases) found the incidence by location shown in ▶ Table 94.1. The vertebral artery was the most common intracranial site. Previously, it was believed that the ICA was the most common site. This change may be due to the recent increased recognition of arterial dissections as a source of SAH (and vertebral dissections most often present as SAH). Multiple dissections occur in ≈ 10% (the most common: bilateral vertebrobasilar lesions).

Table 94.1 Spontaneous intracranial dissections by site[1]

Location	Left	Right	Total
vertebral	122	82	204
basilar		35	35
internal carotid	17	13	30
middle cerebral	16	10	26
anterior cerebral	10	3	13
posterior cerebral	7	9	16
PICA	4	10	14
Total	**176**	**127**	**338**

94.1.6 Clinical

Cerebral arterial dissections may cause symptoms by:
1. embolization secondary to:
   a) platelet aggregation stimulated by the exposed surfaces
   b) dislodged thrombus (formation of which is enhanced by reduced flow)
2. reduced distal flow secondary to:
   a) thrombosis due to reduced flow
   b) occlusion of the true lumen by the expansion of the mural hematoma
3. subarachnoid hemorrhage (atypical presentation, may be more common with posterior circulation dissection than with anterior circulation)[7]

The most common presentation in patients < 30 yrs of age was due to internal carotid dissection without SAH. In patients > 30 yrs, vertebrobasilar artery (VBA) dissection with SAH was the most common.[1]

Headache, usually severe, often predates neurologic deficit by days or weeks (p. 1492). See sections ICA (p. 1578) and vertebrobasilar (p. 1579) for specifics.

94

94.1.7 Evaluation

▶ **CT.** More useful for evaluating brain for infarction. Dissection can sometimes be visualized directly.[8]

▶ **CT angiogram (CTA).** Often obviates the need for cerebral angiography since CTA scanners with ≥ 16 detectors are equal in predictive value and have an accuracy near 99%.[9]

▶ **Angiography.** The definitive diagnostic study. However, diagnosis may be delayed if the dissection is misinterpreted as:
1. an unusual saccular aneurysm (the most common error)
2. atherosclerotic lesions: with dissections, the location is unusual, the lesion may be isolated, the age is usually younger, and the stenosis is smooth. Cervical ICA dissection typically spares the carotid bulb whereas cervical ICA atherosclerosis tends to involve the bulb.
3. vasospasm following SAH: however, the narrowing with vasospasm is delayed in onset vs. the changes with dissection which are present from the beginning.

Angiographic findings may include:
1. luminal stenosis: irregular stenosis over long segments of the artery often with focal areas of near-total stenosis ("string sign")
2. fusiform dilation with proximal or distal narrowing ("string and pearl" sign)
3. occlusion: artery usually tapers to a point
4. intimal flap: when seen, usually found at proximal end of dissection
5. may see proximal beading ("string of beads" configuration, indicative of FMD)
6. "double lumen sign": true vessel lumen and an intramural false lumen with an intimal flap. Usually with retention of contrast within the false lumen well into the venous phase. The only pathognomonic sign
7. wavy "ripple" appearance
8. severe kinking (frequently bilateral). With VBA lesions: dolichoectasia

A characteristic of arterial dissections is that they often change configuration on repeat angiography[10] (some resolve, and some worsen). NB: forceful intra-arterial contrast injection during the performance of angiography carries a potential for worsening the dissection.

▶ **MRI.** Probably not as accurate as CTA or angiography. Optimal MRI study is source *T1WI axial images with fat suppression* ("fat sat"), look for loss of visualization over several slices, with good visualization above and below. May visualize intimal flap and distinguish a dissection from a fusiform aneurysm.
Crescent sign: bright signal in wall of ICA (▶ Fig. 61.2) on T2WI axial images (hematoma in vessel wall).

94.1.8 Overall outcome

An early review of the literature found an 83% mortality within a few weeks of presentation with vertebrobasilar artery (VBA) dissection.[11] A later report tempered that grim prognosis.[12]
Based on a review of 260 cases,[1] an overall mortality of 26% was found. 70% had a favorable outcome (assessed using Glasgow Outcome scale, ▶ Table 98.4), 5% poor. Mortality was higher in ICA lesions (49%) than VBA lesions (22%). Mortality was 24% in the SAH group, and 29% in non-SAH cases.

94.1.9 Internal carotid dissection

See General information on arterial dissections (p.1576). Posttraumatic ICA dissection (p.1577) is much more common than spontaneous.
Some cases considered "spontaneous" may actually be due to trivial trauma, including violent coughing, nose blowing, and simple neck turning. Usually seen in young women.
In spontaneous dissection, the most common initial symptom is ipsilateral headache. Most of these (60%) are orbital or periorbital, but they may also be auricular or mastoid (39%), frontal (36%), temporal (27%). May also produce sudden onset of severe pain over carotid artery (carotidynia).[13]
Incomplete Horner syndrome (oculosympathetic palsy): ptosis and miosis without anhidrosis (due to involvement of plexus around the ICA, sparing the ECA plexus which innervates facial sweat

glands) may occur. Bruits may be heard by the examiner or by the patient. These and other clinical features are shown in ▶ Table 94.2.

May be a cause of some cases of infantile and childhood hemiplegia and hemiparesis.[14]

Table 94.2 Clinical features of spontaneous ICA dissection[3]

Feature	%
focal cerebral ischemia	76
headache	59
oculosympathetic palsy	30
bruit	25
amaurosis fugax	10
neck pain	9
syncope	4
scalp tenderness	2
neck swelling	2

94.1.10 Vertebrobasilar system artery dissection

Vertebral artery dissections

General information

See general information on cerebral arterial dissections (p. 1576). See also posttraumatic vertebrobasilar dissection (p. 1032).

Less common than carotid. Extracranial lesions outnumber intracranial.

Traumatic dissections tend to occur where the VA crosses bony prominences, e.g., at the C1–2 junction or where it enters the foramen transversarium (usually at C6). Spontaneous dissections tend to be intracranial and commonly occur on the *dominant* VA. Unlike cervical ICA dissections, which tend not to propagate intracranially through the carotid canal, high cervical VA dissections can readily propagate intracranially through the foramen magnum.

Spontaneous VA dissections have been associated with FMD, migraine, and oral contraceptives.[15] Unrecognized or forgotten trauma or sudden head motion may have occurred in some cases reported as spontaneous. Commonly occurs in young adults (mean age: 48 yrs). With spontaneous dissections, 36% of patients have dissections at other sites, 21% of cases have bilateral VA dissections.[16]

Dissecting aneurysms of the VA (possibly a distinct entity) are also described.[17,18,19] They tend to be fusiform, and may be amenable to clipping, and were associated with vertebral dissections in 5 of 7 cases reported in one series.[20] As of 1984, only ≈ 50 cases of dissecting aneurysms were published.[20]

Presentation

In spontaneous extradural dissections, neck pain is a prominent early finding in most patients, and is commonly located over the occiput and posterior cervical region. Generalized severe headache is also common. TIAs or stroke (usually lateral medullary syndrome (p. 1539)[21] or cerebellar infarction, especially in patients with occlusion of the third or fourth portion of the VA[22]). None of 5 patients developed new neurologic symptoms after the original stroke in an average of 21 months follow-up.[22] In 3 of these 5, VA dissection was bilateral.

Dissecting aneurysms may present with altered consciousness, and may cause SAH (seen in 6 of 30 cases of vertebrobasilar complex dissections).[20] Rebleeding occurs in 24–30% of those cases presenting with SAH,[16] making these lesions treacherous, with a very high mortality.[23,24]

Traumatic extradural dissections or pseudoaneurysms may have a similar presentation, but can also produce massive external hemorrhage or neck hematomas.[16]

Evaluation

See section under Cerebral arterial dissections, Evaluation (p. 1578).

▶ **Angiography.** Diagnosis by angiography may be difficult in many cases (the most common misdiagnosis is ruptured saccular aneurysm of unusual shape[25]).

94

In posttraumatic dissections, the most common finding is irregular stenosis of horizontal loops of distal extracranial VAs as they pass behind C1, often bilateral.

In 14 of 15 posttraumatic VA dissections, the lesion was located posterior to the atlas (distal extracranial 3rd segment), the single exception being a patient with direct trauma causing proximal VA involvement. This predilection is possibly explained by the fact that the first and third portions of the VA are movable, whereas the second and fourth are relatively immobilized by bone.

Treatment

Except for cases presenting with hemorrhage or large ischemic stroke, medical therapy should be started emergently. Classically consists of anticoagulation, with heparin acutely, followed by oral agents (e.g., Coumadin) probably for a total of 6 months. Recent preliminary study showed antiplatelet therapy was equally as effective.[26]

As with traumatic dissections, endovascular techniques are now assuming a more prominent role in management.

▶ **Indications for intervention.** Surgery or endovascular techniques (mostly stents, but also occlusion, angioplasty[16]) are required for dissections presenting with SAH (due to their propensity to rebleed) and is recommended for most intradural dissections. For extradural lesions it is indicated for dissections that progress (angiographically) or for persistent symptoms in spite of adequate medical therapy. Some less malignant lesions may be amenable to endovascular stenting.

▶ **Endovascular treatment.** Balloon-mounted, self-expandable, or covered stents have been used relatively infrequently to treat dissections of the internal carotid or vertebral arteries, with good technical results and low procedure-related complication rates.[27] Given the small number of patients treated and the fact that medical therapy is generally effective, the role of stenting for dissection remains to be defined. It should be reserved for patients in whom medical therapy is ineffective or contraindicated or when the dissection causes symptomatic flow-limiting stenosis.

▶ **Surgical treatment.** At the time of surgery, the site of dissection may be recognized by fusiform or tubular enlargement of the artery with discoloration due to blood within the arterial wall (the discoloration has been described as black, bluish, purple, purple-red, or brown[25]).

Surgical treatment of intradural dissection when endovascular techniques are not an option includes the following alternatives:

1. non-clippable aneurysms may be candidates for Hunterian occlusion of the VA proximal to the BA (either by microsurgical technique, or by endovascular techniques which may not be as precise). Some may not tolerate clipping the dominant VA, especially if the contralateral VA is hypoplastic. Conversely, some may tolerate bilateral VA occlusion.[28] Balloon test occlusion[16] is recommended
   a) if the dissection involves the PICA origin, then clip proximal to dissection. PICA then fills from retrograde flow, and the reversal of flow across the site of dissection should push the intima back against the wall
   b) if the dissection is proximal to PICA and doesn't involve PICA, then trap the aneurysm between clips. PICA fills by retrograde flow
   c) if the aneurysm begins distal to the PICA origin, occlude the VA[7] *distal* to the PICA takeoff[29]
2. combining VA clipping (non-clippable aneurysms may be candidates for Hunterian occlusion of the VA proximal to the aneurysm) with vascular bypass, options:
   a) side-to-side PICA-PICA anastomosis
   b) transplantation of the PICA origin to the VA outside the aneurysm
   c) occipital artery-to-PICA bypass
3. resection accompanied by autogenous interposition vein graft
4. non-occlusive surgical techniques
   a) clipping with specially designed clips for fusiform aneurysms (e.g., Sundt-Kees clip)
   b) wrapping: of dubious benefit

94.1.11 Vertebrobasilar system dissections excluding the VA

Basilar artery dissections tend to present with brainstem infarction and more rarely with SAH.[24] The prognosis is generally regarded as poor. Endovascular techniques may be able to treat some.

94.2 Moyamoya disease

94.2.1 General information

> ### Key concepts
>
> - progressive bilateral spontaneous occlusion or stenosis of terminal ICAs with compensatory capillary collaterals that look like a "puff of smoke" (Japanese: moyamoya) on angio
> - typical presentation: juvenile form → ischemic infarcts/TIAs (suspect diagnosis in any child presenting with TIAs). Adult form → hemorrhage
> - pathology: intimal thickening w/o inflammation, may also involve heart, kidneys. Associated aneurysms may be source of bleeding
> - evaluation: cerebral angiography is necessary to delineate degree of stenosis as well as to evaluate potential extracranial donor vessels for revascularization. Also identifies aneurysms
> - treatment:
>   a) medical treatment (antiplatelet drugs, anticoagulation, vasodilators...): not shown to be effective, although antiplatelet/anticoagulation is often used
>   b) surgical revascularization: reduces the incidence of strokes and TIAs, but benefit on reducing the rate of hemorrhage is unproven

Progressive spontaneous occlusion of one or usually both ICAs (usually at the level of the carotid siphon) and their major branches, with secondary formation of an anastomotic collateral capillary network at the base of the brain which has been termed "moyamoya," the Japanese word for something hazy like a "puff of cigarette smoke"[30] (which it fancifully resembles on angiography) (first described in 1957,[31] and named in 1969[30]). With progression, involvement includes the proximal MCAs and ACAs and on rare occasion the vertebrobasilar system. Associated aneurysms (see below) and rarely AVMs[32,33] may be observed.

Eventually the dilated capillary (moyamoya) vessels disappear with the development of collaterals from the ECA (meningeal collaterals are called "rete mirabile").

94.2.2 Pathophysiology

Primary moyamoya disease

The most common pathology is stenosis of the proximal anterior and middle cerebral arteries that is neither atherosclerotic nor inflammatory in origin. Exact etiology is unknown but some studies show elevated basic fibroblast growth factor in the dura and scalp arteries in patients with moyamoya.[34] The internal elastic lamina of affected vessels may be thinned or duplicated. Similar vascular changes may also occur in the heart, kidney, and other organs, suggesting it may be a systemic vascular disease.

Secondary moyamoya disease

AKA "quasi-moyamoya disease" or "moyamoya syndrome."[35] Angiographic findings of moyamoya associated with e.g.:
1. Graves' disease/thyrotoxicosis
2. history of cerebral inflammatory disease, including meningitis (especially tubercular (TB) meningitis and leptospirosis)
3. retinitis pigmentosa
4. vascular disorders: atherosclerosis, fibromuscular dysplasia, pseudoxanthoma elasticum
5. congenital disorders: Down syndrome, Marfan syndrome, Turner syndrome, neurofibromatosis type 1, tuberous sclerosis, Apert syndrome
6. hematologic disorders: Fanconi anemia, sickle cell disease (in the U.S. one of the more common associations) and sickle cell trait
7. following radiation therapy for skull base glioma in children[36]
8. head trauma
9. systemic lupus erythematosus (SLE)

94

Associated aneurysms

Intracranial *aneurysms* are frequently associated with moyamoya disease (MMD). This may be a result of the increased flow through dilated collaterals, or it may be that patients with moyamoya may also have a congenital defect in the arterial wall that predisposes them to aneurysms. 3 types: 1) usual sites of aneurysms in the Circle of Willis, 2) in peripheral portions of cerebral arteries, e.g., posterior/anterior choroidal, Heubner's, and 3) within moyamoya vessels. The frequency of aneurysms in the vertebrobasilar system is ≈ 62%, which is much higher than in the general population.[37] Aneurysmal SAH may be the actual cause of some hemorrhages that were erroneously attributed to moyamoya vessels.

94.2.3 Epidemiology

Risk factors

A history of inflammation in the head & neck region has been implicated.

Demographics

Incidence in Japan is higher (0.35/100,000/yr) than in North America. Two peaks (may not be same disease): juvenile (highest peak), age < 10 yrs (mean 3); adult, 3rd & 4th decade. Slight female predominance (1.8:1). Some evidence for familial tendency (some Asian families have an incidence as high as 7%), genetics appears autosomal dominant with low penetrance. Associated with some HLA antigens (B40 in juvenile form; B54(20) in adult) and anti-double-stranded DNA antibody.

94.2.4 Presentation

Juvenile form

Moyamoya is associated with 6% of childhood strokes.[34] Ischemic presentation more common (81%); includes TIAs (41%) which may alternate sides (alternating hemiplegia is a suggestive clinical finding), RINDs, or infarct (40%). Neurologic events are often provoked by straining or by hyperventilation (e.g., during crying or blowing a wind instrument), which is thought to produce hypocapnea with reactive vasoconstriction.

Headache is the most common presenting symptom, but seizures, focal neurologic deficits, choreoathetotic movements and hemorrhages can also be presenting symptoms. The risk of hemorrhage is increased in stages 5 & 6 of MMD.

Adult form

Hemorrhage has been described as being more common (60%), but in a Stanford series[38] 89% presented with ischemia. Rupture of the fragile moyamoya vessels produces bleeding in the basal ganglia (BG), thalamus, or ventricles (from the ventricular wall) in 70–80% of hemorrhages. SAH may occur, usually due to rupture of associated aneurysms (see above). In the pre-CT era, the most common form of hemorrhage was thought to be SAH from the rupture of moyamoya vessels, but most cases were probably intraventricular blood or SAH from associated aneurysms.[39]

94.2.5 Natural history

Incidence of disease progression in one study was 20% in adult patients with MMD.[40] Female patients had a higher risk of disease progression than males.

Prognosis of untreated MMD is poor, with 73% rate of major deficit or death within 2 years of diagnosis in children, and similarly poor outlook in adults.[38]

94.2.6 Evaluation and diagnosis

Diagnostic criteria

Diagnosis of moyamoya requires bilateral symmetrical stenosis or occlusion of the terminal portion of the ICAs as well as the presence of dilated collateral vessels at the base of the brain.[34] (If unilateral the diagnosis is considered questionable,[41] and these cases may progress to bilateral involvement).

Other characteristic findings include:

1. stenosis/occlusion starting at termination of ICA and at origins of ACA and MCA

2. abnormal vascular network in region of BG (intraparenchymal anastomosis)
3. transdural anastomosis (rete mirabile), AKA "vault moyamoya." Contributing arteries: anterior facial, middle meningeal, ethmoidal, occipital, tentorial, STA
4. moyamoya collaterals may also form from internal maxillary artery via ethmoid sinus to fore-brain in frontobasal region

CT

Work-up in suspected cases typically begins with a non-enhanced head CT. Up to 40% of ischemic cases have normal CT. Low-density areas (LDAs) may be seen, usually confined to cortical and sub-cortical areas (unlike atherosclerotic disease or acute infantile hemiplegia which tend to have LDAs in basal ganglia as well). LDAs tend to be multiple and bilateral, especially in the PCA distribution (poor collaterals), and are more common in children.

MRI and MRA

MRA usually discloses the stenosis or occlusion of the ICA. Moyamoya vessels appear as flow voids on MRI (especially in basal ganglia) and a fine network of vessels on MRA, and are demonstrated better in children than adults. Parenchymal ischemic changes are commonly shown, usually in watershed areas.

Angiography

In addition to helping to establish the diagnosis, angiography also identifies suitable vessels for revascularization procedures and unearths associated aneurysms. The angiography-related compli-cation rate is higher than with atherosclerotic occlusive disease. Avoid dehydration prior to and hypotension during the procedure. Six angiographic stages of MMD that tend to progress up until adolescence and stabilize by age 20 are described in ▶ Table 94.3.[30]

Table 94.3 Six angiographic stages of MMD (Suzuki stages)[30]

Stage	Finding
1	stenosis of suprasellar ICA, usually bilateral
2	development of moyamoya vessels at base of brain. ACA, MCA, & PCA dilated
3	increasing ICA stenosis & prominence of moyamoya vessels (most cases diagnosed at this stage). Maximal basal moyamoya
4	entire circle of Willis and PCAs occluded, extracranial collaterals start to appear, moyamoya vessels begin to diminish
5	further progression of stage 4 with intensification of ECA collaterals & reduction of moyamoya associated vessels
6	total occlusion of ICA & major cerebral arteries and complete absence of moyamoya vessels

94

EEG

Non-specific in the adult. Juvenile cases: high-voltage slow waves may be seen at rest, predomi-nantly in the occipital and frontal lobes. Hyperventilation produces a normal buildup of monophasic slow waves (delta-bursts) that return to normal 20–60 seconds after hyperventilation. In > 50% of cases, after or sometimes continuous with buildup is a second phase of slow waves (this character-istic finding is called "rebuildup"), which are more irregular and slower than the earlier waves, and usually normalize in ≤ 10 minutes.[42]

Cerebral blood flow (CBF) studies

CBF is decreased in children with MMD, but relatively normal in adults. There is a shift of CBF from the frontal to the occipital lobes[43] probably reflecting the increasing dependency of CBF on the pos-terior circulation. Children with MMD have impaired autoregulation of CBF to blood pressure and CO_2 (with more impairment of vasodilatation in response to hypercapnia or hypotension than vaso-constriction in response to hypocapnia or hypertension).[44]

Xenon (Xe-133) CT can identify areas of low perfusion. Repeating the study after an acetazola-mide challenge (which causes vasodilatation) evaluates reserve capacity of CBF and can identify areas of "steal" which are at high risk of future infarction.

94.2.7 Treatment

General information

No medical or surgical treatment has been proven effective in reducing the rate of hemorrhage in the adult with MMD. However, multiple large case series have supported the efficacy of cerebral revascularization for reducing the incidence of ischemic strokes and TIAs.[35]

Asymptomatic moyamoya disease

Guidelines for management of asymptomatic moyamoya disease have not yet been established. A multicenter, nationwide survey in Japan focusing on asymptomatic moyamoya disease provided the following findings[45]: subtle findings of cerebral infarction and disturbed cerebral hemodynamics were detected in 20% and 40% of the involved hemispheres, respectively. Angiographic stage was more advanced in elderly patients. Of 34 medically-treated patients, 7 experienced TIA, ischemic stroke, or hemorrhage during a mean follow-up period of 43.7 months. Cerebral infarction or hemorrhage did not occur in the 6 patients who underwent surgical revascularization.

Medical treatment

Medical treatment with platelet inhibitors, anticoagulants, calcium channel blockers,[38] steroids, mannitol, low-molecular-weight dextran, and antibiotics have not proven to be of benefit. Steroids may be considered for involuntary movements and acutely during recurrent TIAs.

Surgical treatment

General information

Patients with mass effect from clot may be candidates for urgent decompression. Revascularization procedures, however, should be performed when the patient is stable under nonemergent conditions.

Perioperative management

During any surgical procedure:

1. avoid hyperventilation: due to increased sensitivity of collaterals, keep $PaCO_2$ 40–50 mm Hg to avoid ischemic infarction
2. avoid hypotension: maintain BP at normotensive levels
3. avoid alpha-adrenergic agents because of vasoconstrictive effects
4. cerebral protection: mild hypothermia (32–34 °C)[46] and barbiturates are routinely used
5. papaverine helps prevent vascular spasm

Postoperatively following STA-MAC bypass procedures:

1. avoid hypertension: may cause bleeding at anastomotic site and in areas of increased perfusion within the brain
2. avoid hypotension: may result in graft occlusion
3. aspirin is started on the post-op day #1
4. watch for evidence of CSF leak
5. monitor coag studies and correct abnormalities
6. cerebral arteriogram is recommended 2–6 months post-op

Suggested criteria for revascularization procedures

See reference.[35]

1. patients presenting with infarction or hemorrhage but are in good neurologic condition
2. infarction < 2 cm maximal diameter on CT, and all previous hemorrhages have completely resolved
3. angiographic stage is II–IV (see ▸ Table 94.3)
4. timing of operation: ≥ 2 months after most recent attack

Surgical revascularization options

Various methods to revascularize the ischemic brain, used primarily in children, include:

1. direct revascularization procedures:

a) results are superior to indirect revascularization procedures[47,48] if a donor and recipient vessel of sufficient caliber (≥ 1 mm outer dia) can be identified (may be difficult in the pediatric age group who are the most likely to benefit[49]). Otherwise, indirect revascularization procedures (see below) are options.

b) Among direct revascularization procedures, STA-MCA bypass[50] is the procedure of choice.

2. indirect revascularization procedures: usually reserved for younger patients (suggested cutoff age ≈ < 15 years). May be combined with STA-MCA bypass. Includes:

a) encephalomyosynangiosis (**EMS**): laying the temporalis muscle on the surface of the brain (may cause problems with muscle contractions during talking and chewing, and neural impulses on surface of brain)

b) encephaloduroarteriosynangiosis (**EDAS**)[51,52]: suturing the STA with a galeal cuff to a linear defect created in the dura. Variations on this technique include splitting the dura[53]

c) omental transposition[54]: either as a pedicle graft or as a vascularized free flap. Felt to have higher potential to revascularize ischemic tissue than above procedures, but there is greater risk of mass effect from the thickness of the omentum

3. the above indirect revascularization procedures improve blood flow in the MCA distribution, but not ACA circulation. This may be rectified by:

a) simple placement of frontal burr holes with opening of the underlying dura and arachnoid[55]

b) "ribbon EDAS" where a pedicle of galea is inserted into the interhemispheric fissure on both sides[56]

4. stellate ganglionectomy and perivascular sympathectomy: unproven that this increases CBF permanently

Outcome with surgical treatment

Neurologic status at time of treatment generally predicts long-term outcome.[34] The mortality rate in adults (≈ 10%) is higher than for juveniles (≈ 4.3%).[41] The cause of death was bleeding in 56% of 9 children and 63% of 30 adults. With treatment the prognosis is good in 58%.[39]

References

[1] Yamaura A. Nontraumatic Intracranial Arterial Dissection: Natural History, Diagnosis, and Treatment. Contemporary Neurosurgery. 1994; 16:1–6

[2] Goldstein SJ. Dissecting Hematoma of the Cervical Vertebral Artery: Case Report. J Neurosurg. 1982; 56:451–454

[3] Anson J, Crowell RM. Cervicocranial Arterial Dissection. Neurosurgery. 1991; 29:89–96

[4] Yamashita M, Tanaka K, Matsuo T, et al. Cerebral dissecting aneurysms in patients with moyamoya disease. Journal of Neurosurgery. 1983; 58:120–125

[5] Bogousslavsky J, Despland PA, Regli F. Spontaneous carotid dissection with acute stroke. Arch Neurol. 1987; 44:137–140

[6] Debette S, Leys D. Cervical-artery dissections: predisposing factors, diagnosis, and outcome. Lancet Neurol. 2009; 8:668–678

[7] Friedman AH, Drake CG. Subarachnoid hemorrhage from intracraniai dissecting aneurysm. J Neurosurg. 1984; 60:325–334

[8] Hodge C, Leeson M, Cacayorin E, et al. Computed Tomographic Evaluation of Extracranial Carotid Artery Disease. Neurosurgery. 1987; 21:167–176

[9] Eastman AL, Chason DP, Perez CL, et al. Computed tomographic angiography for the diagnosis of blunt cervical vascular injury: is it ready for primetime? Journal of Trauma. 2006; 60:925–9; discussion 929

[10] Kitanaka C, Tanaki J-I, Kuwahara M, et al. Nonsurgical Treatment of Unruptured Intracranial Vertebral Artery Dissection with Serial Follow-Up Angiography. Journal of Neurosurgery. 1994; 80:667–674

[11] Berger MS, Wilson CB. Intracranial dissecting aneurysms of the posterior circulation. Report of six cases and review of the literature. Journal of Neurosurgery. 1984; 61:882–894

[12] Pozzati E, Padovani R, Fabrizi A, et al. Benign Arterial Dissection of the Posterior Circulation. Journal of Neurosurgery. 1991; 75:69–72

[13] Welling RE, Taha A, Goel T, et al. Extracranial Carotid Artery Aneurysms. Surgery. 1983; 93:319–323

[14] Chang V, Newcastle NB, Harwood-Nash DCF, et al. Bilateral dissecting aneurysms of the intracranial

[15] Leys D, Lesoin F, Pruvo JP, et al. Bilateral Spontaneous Dissection of Extracranial Vertebral Arteries. J Neurol. 1987; 234:237–240

[16] Halbach VV, Higashida RT, Dowd CF, et al. Endovascular Treatment of Vertebral Artery Dissections and Pseudoaneurysms. Journal of Neurosurgery. 1993; 79:183–191

[17] Miyazaki S, Yamaura A, Kamata K, et al. A dissecting aneurysm of the vertebral artery. Surg Neurol. 1984; 21:171–174

[18] Hugenholtz H, Pokrupa R, Montpetit VJA, et al. Spontaneous dissecting aneurysm of the extracranial vertebral artery. Neurosurgery. 1982; 10:96–100

[19] Senter HJ, Sarwar M. Nontraumatic dissecting aneurysm of the vertebral artery. J Neurosurg. 1982; 56:128–130

[20] Shimoji T, Bando K, Nakajima K, et al. Dissecting Aneurysm of the Vertebral Artery. J Neurosurg. 1984; 61:1038–1046

[21] Okuchi K, Watabe Y, Hiramatsu K, et al. [Dissecting Aneurysm of the Vertebral Artery as a Cause of Wallenberg's Syndrome]. No Shinkei Geka. 1990; 18:721–727

[22] Caplan LR, Zarins CK, Hemmati M. Spontaneous Dissection of the Extracranial Vertebral Arteries. Stroke. 1985; 16:1030–1038

[23] Aoki N, Sakai T. Rebleeding from intracranial dissecting aneurysm in the vertebral artery. Stroke. 1990; 21:1628–1631

[24] Pozzati E, Andreoli A, Limoni P, et al. Dissecting Aneurysms of the Vertebrobasilar System: Study of 16 Cases. Surgical Neurology. 1994; 41:119–124

[25] Yamaura A, Watanabe Y, Saeki N. Dissecting Aneurysms of the Intracranial Vertebral Artery. Journal of Neurosurgery. 1990; 72:183–188

[26] Markus HS, Hayter E, Levi C, et al. Antiplatelet treatment compared with anticoagulation treatment for cervical artery dissection (CADISS): a randomised trial. Lancet Neurol. 2015; 14:361–367

94

[27] Pham MH, Rahme RJ, Arnaout O, et al. Endovascular stenting of extracranial carotid and vertebral artery dissections: a systematic review of the literature. Neurosurgery. 2011; 68:856–66; discussion 866

[28] Six EG, Stringer WL, Cowley AR, et al. Posttraumatic Bilateral Vertebral Artery Occlusion. Case Report. Journal of Neurosurgery. 1981; 54:814–817

[29] Yamada K, Hayakawa T, Ushio Y, et al. Therapeutic Occlusion of the Vertebral Artery for Unclippable Vertebral Aneurysm. Neurosurgery. 1984; 15:834–838

[30] Suzuki J, Takaku A. Cerebrovascular "moyamoya" disease. Disease showing abnormal net-like vessels in base of brain. Archives of Neurology. 1969; 20:288–299

[31] Takeuchi K, Shimuzi K. Hypogenesis of Bilateral Internal Carotid Arteries. No To Shinkei. 1957; 9:37–37

[32] Kayama T, Suzuki S, Sakurai Y, et al. A Case of Moyamoya Disease Accompanied by an Arteriovenous Malformation. Neurosurgery. 1986; 18:465–468

[33] Lichtor T, Mullan S. Arteriovenous Malformation in Moyamoya Syndrome: Report of Three Cases. Journal of Neurosurgery. 1987; 67:603–608

[34] Smith ER, Scott RM. Surgical management of moyamoya syndrome. Skull Base. 2005; 15:15–26

[35] Zipfel GJ, Fox DJ,Jr, Rivet DJ. Moyamoya disease in adults: the role of cerebral revascularization. Skull Base. 2005; 15:27–41

[36] Rajakulasingam K, Cerullo LJ, Raimondi AJ. Childhood Moyamoya Syndrome: Postradiation Pathogenesis. Childs Brain. 1979; 5:467–475

[37] Kwak R, Ito S, Yamamoto N, et al. Significance of Intracranial Aneurysms Associated with Moyamoya Disease (Part I): Differences Between Intracranial Aneurysms Associated with Moyamoya Disease and Usual Saccular Aneurysms - Review of the Literature. Neurol Med Chir. 1984; 24:97–103

[38] Chang SD, Steinberg GK. Surgical Management of Moyamoya Disease. Contemporary Neurosurgery. 2000; 22:1–9

[39] Ueki K, Meyer FB, Mellinger JF. Moyamoya Disease: The Disorder and Surgical Treatment. Mayo Clinic Proceedings. 1994; 69:749–757

[40] Kuroda S, Ishikawa T, Houkin K, et al. Incidence and clinical features of disease progression in adult moyamoya disease. Stroke. 2005; 36:2148–2153

[41] Nishimoto A. Moyamoya Disease. Neurol Med Chir. 1979; 19:221–228

[42] Kodama N, Aoki Y, Hiraga H, et al. Electroencephalographic Findings in Children with Moyamoya Disease. Archives of Neurology. 1979; 36:16–19

[43] Ogawa A, Yoshimoto T, Suzuki J, et al. Cerebral Blood Flow in Moyamoya Disease. Part 1. Correlation with Age and Regional Distribution. Acta Neurochirurgica. 1990; 105:30–34

[44] Ogawa A, Nakamura N, Yoshimoto T, et al. Cerebral Blood Flow in Moyamoya Disease. Part 2. Autoregulation and CO2 Response. Acta Neurochirurgica. 1990; 105:107–111

[45] Kuroda S, Hashimoto N, Yoshimoto T, et al. Radiological findings, clinical course, and outcome in asymptomatic moyamoya disease: results of multicenter survey in Japan. Stroke. 2007; 38:1430–1435

[46] Hypothermia after Cardiac Arrest Study Group. Mild therapeutic hypothermia to improve the neurologic outcome after cardiac arrest. New England Journal of Medicine. 2002; 346:549–556

[47] Matsushima Y, Inoue T, Suzuki SO, et al. Surgical Treatment of Moyamoya Disease in Pediatric Patients - Comparison between the Results of Indirect and Direct Vascularization. Neurosurgery. 1992; 31:401–405

[48] Ishikawa T, Houkin K, Kamiyama H, et al. Effects of Surgical Revascularization on Outcome of Patients with Pediatric Moyamoya Disease. Stroke. 1997; 28:1170–1173

[49] Fabi AY, Meyer FB. Moyamoya Disease. Contemporary Neurosurgery. 1997; 19:1–6

[50] Karasawa J, Kikuchi H, Furuse S, et al. Treatment of Moyamoya Disease with STA-MCA Anastomosis. Neurosurg. 1978; 49:679–688

[51] Matsushima Y, Fukai N, Tanaka K, et al. A new surgical treatment of moyamoya disease in children: A preliminary report. Surg Neurol. 1980; 15:313–320

[52] Matsushima Y, Inaba Y. Moyamoya Disease in Children and Its Surgical Treatment. Childs Brain. 1984 11:155–170

[53] Kashiwagi S, Kato S, Yasuhara S, et al. Use of Split Dura for Revascularization if Ischemic Hemispheres in Moyamoya Disease. Journal of Neurosurgery 1996; 85:380–383

[54] Karasawa J, Kikuchi H, Kawamura J, et al. Intracranial Transplantation of the Omentum for Cerebrovascular Moyamoya Disease: A Two-Year Follow-Up Study. Surg Neurol. 1980; 14:444–449

[55] Endo M, Kawano N, Miyasaka Y, et al. Cranial Bur Hole for Revascularization in Moyamoya Disease. Neurosurg. 1989; 71:180–185

[56] Kinugasa K, Mandai S, Tokunaga K, et al. Ribbon Encephalo-Duro-Arterio-Myo-Synangiosis for Moyamoya Disease. Surgical Neurology. 1994; 41:455–461

95 Other Vascular Occlusive Conditions

95.1 Totally occluded internal carotid artery

95.1.1 General information

10–15% of patients presenting with carotid territory stroke or transient ischemic attacks (TIA) are found to have carotid occlusion. This amounts to an estimated 61,000 first-ever strokes and 19,000 TIAs per year in the United States. Prevention of subsequent stroke in symptomatic patients with carotid artery occlusion remains a difficult challenge. The overall rate of subsequent stroke is 7% per year for all stroke and 5.9% per year for ischemic stroke ipsilateral to the occluded carotid artery.[1] These risks persist even despite treatment with antiaggregants and anticoagulants.[2] The prevalence of asymptomatic carotid occlusion is not known, and the incidence of ipsilateral stroke in never-symptomatic carotid occlusion is negligible.[3]

95.1.2 Presentation

3 patterns of stroke with total internal carotid artery occlusion:
1. whole hemisphere stroke
2. watershed infarct
3. **carotid stump syndrome**: continued cerebral or retinal symptoms following complete occlusion of the ipsilateral ICA.[4] Rare. Both hemodynamic and embolic mechanisms have been implicated[5]:
   a) hemodynamic: inadequacy of collaterals may lead to recurrent ischemic symptoms
   b) emboli formed in the turbulent flow at the ostium of the stump can reach MCA-supplied brain tissue via ECA-ICA anastamoses either directly or through reverse flow through the ophthalmic artery. Other pathways have also been described[6]

Treatment options include: stump excision[7] or endovascular treatment with stenting across the stump.[8] If there is ipsilateral ECA stenosis, either of these may be combined with ECA endarterectomy or angioplasty ± stenting. Most patients also receive post-treatment dual antiplatelet therapy.

In symptomatic patients[9]: hemiparetic TIA 53%, dysphasic TIA 34%, fixed neuro deficit 21%, crescendo TIAs 21%, amaurosis fugax 17%, acute hemiplegia 6%. 27% were asymptomatic in one series.[10]

95.1.3 Natural history

See reference.[11]

Patients with mild deficit and angiographically proven ICA occlusion have a stroke rate (in two series) of 3 or 5% per year (2 or 3.3% related to occluded side). In patients with acute ICA occlusion and profound neurological deficit, 2–12% make good recovery, 40–69% will have profound deficit, and 16–55% will have died by the time of follow-up.

95.1.4 Endovascular thrombolysis and stenting for acute carotid occlusion

Case reports and series of endovascular treatment of internal carotid artery occlusion have confirmed the feasibility of this technique. Intra-arterial thrombolysis within 6 hours of stroke onset may increase recanalization rates to 37–100% and clinical improvement to 53–94% without significant increase in hemorrhagic transformation when compared with intravenous thrombolytic therapy alone.[12,13,14,15,16,17] Although results appear promising, randomized controlled trials on cervical carotid thrombolysis and/or stenting are lacking.

95.1.5 Surgery

Options include: endarterectomy, Fogarty balloon catheter embolectomy (utilizing a No. 2 French catheter with 0.2-ml balloon gently passed 10–12 cm up ICA from small arteriotomy made distal to atheromatous plaque[18]), extracranial-intracranial bypass. Restored patency rate is inversely related to suspected duration of occlusion. Chronically occluded ICA has poor patency rate and little gain from re-opening.

95

Determining the exact time of occlusion is frequently impossible. One must often rely on clinical grounds; therefore an occasional chronic occlusion will be included.

Retrograde filling of ICA to petrous or cavernous segment from ECA (e.g., via ophthalmic) or from contralateral ICA is a good sign of operability.[9]

Surgical results[9]

32% (15/47 cases) immediate surgical failures (no or minimal back bleeding), at least 3 deaths. Among immediate successes no strokes and no TIAs. If operated < 2 days reported patency rate 70–100%, from 3–7 days 50–100%, 8–14 days 27–58%, 15–30 days 4–61%, over 1 month (2 series) 20–50%.

95.1.6 Guidelines

Emergency operations for acute neuro deficit associated with total occlusion should not be performed after about 2 hrs. Extremely poor neuro status (lethargy/coma) is a contraindication to surgery. Patients without persistent neuro deficit: operate ASAP. If the patient has recurrent TIAs (despite maximal medical therapy) following recent carotid occlusion, and no definite infarct on MRI, consider bypass surgery.

95.2 Cerebellar infarction

95.2.1 General information

Relatively rare (seen on only 0.6% of all CTs obtained for any reason[19]). Cerebellar infarcts may be classified as involving the PICA distribution (cerebellar tonsil and/or inferior vermis), superior cerebellar artery distribution (superior hemisphere or superior vermis), or other indeterminate patterns.[20] 80% of patients developing signs of brainstem compression will die, usually within hours to days.

95.2.2 Early clinical findings

In most cases the onset is sudden, without premonitory symptoms.[21] The first 12 hrs after onset were characterized by lack of progression. Early findings are due to the *intrinsic* cerebellar lesion (ischemic infarction or hemorrhage):

1. symptoms
   a) dizziness or vertigo
   b) nausea/vomiting
   c) loss of balance, often with a fall and inability to get up
   d) headache (infrequent in one series[21])
2. signs
   a) truncal and appendicular ataxia
   b) nystagmus
   c) dysarthria

95.2.3 Later clinical findings

Patients with cerebellar infarction may subsequently develop increased pressure within the posterior fossa (due to cerebellar edema or mass effect from clot), with brainstem compression (particularly posterior pons). Clinical findings generally increase between 12 and 96 hrs following onset. Compression of the Sylvian aqueduct can cause acute hydrocephalus with attendant increased ICP.

95.2.4 Imaging studies

CT scan: may be normal very early in these patients. There may be subtle findings of a tight posterior fossa: compression or obliteration of basal cisterns or 4th ventricle or hydrocephalus.

MRI: (including DWI) more sensitive for ischemia, especially in the posterior fossa.

95.2.5 Surgical indications

Surgical decompression (see below) should probably be done as soon as any of the following signs develop if there is no response to medical therapy.[22] It is important to recognize a lateral medullary syndrome (LMS) (p. 1539) which may often accompany a cerebellar infarct. With LMS, the signs are usually present from the onset (dysphagia, dysarthria, Horner syndrome, ipsilateral facial numbness, crossed sensory loss…), and are not accompanied by a change in sensorium. There is no place for surgical decompression in LMS since it represents primary brainstem ischemia and not compression

Findings proceed in the approximate following sequence if there is no intervention:
1. abducens (VI) nerve palsy
2. loss of ipsilateral gaze (compression of VI nucleus and lateral gaze center)
3. peripheral facial nerve paresis (compression of facial colliculus)
4. confusion and somnolence (may be partly due to developing hydrocephalus)
5. Babinski sign
6. hemiparesis
7. lethargy
8. small but reactive pupils
9. coma
10. posturing → flaccidity
11. ataxic respirations

95.2.6 Suboccipital craniectomy for cerebellar infarction

Unlike the situation with supratentorial masses causing herniation, there are several reports of patients in deep coma from direct brainstem compression who were operated upon quickly and made useful recovery.[22,23,24] See also Guidelines for patients with cerebellar hemorrhage (p. 1625).

The operation of choice is a suboccipital decompression to include enlargement of the foramen magnum. The dura is then opened and the infarcted cerebellar tissue usually exudes "like toothpaste" and is easily aspirated. Avoid using ventricular drainage alone as this may cause upward cerebellar herniation (p. 325) and does not relieve the direct brainstem compression.

95.3 Malignant middle cerebral artery territory infarction

95.3.1 General information

A distinct syndrome that occurs in up to 10% of stroke patients,[25,26] which carries a mortality of up to 80% (mostly due to severe postischemic cerebral edema → increased ICP → herniation).[26]

Patients usually present with findings of severe hemispheric stroke (hemiplegia, forced eye and head deviation) often with CT findings of major infarct within the first 12 hours. Most develop drowsiness shortly after admission. There is progressive deterioration during the first 2 days, and subsequent transtentorial herniation usually within 2–4 days of stroke. Fatalities are often associated with: severe drowsiness, dense hemiplegia, age > 45–50 yrs,[27] early parenchymal hypodensity involving > 50% of the MCA distribution on CT scan,[28] midline shift > 8–10 mm, early sulci effacement, and hyperdense artery sign (p. 1560)[27] in MCA.

Neurosurgeons may become involved in caring for these patients because aggressive therapies in these patients may reduce morbidity and mortality. Options include:
1. conventional measures to control ICP (with or without ICP monitor): mortality is still high in this group, and elevated ICP is not a common cause of initial neurologic deterioration in large hemispheric stroke
2. hemicraniectomy (decompressive craniectomy): see below
3. ✖ to date, the following treatments have not improved outcome: agents to lyse clot, hyperventilation, mannitol, or barbiturate coma

95.3.2 Hemicraniectomy for malignant MCA territory infarction

May reduce mortality to as low as 32% in nondominant hemisphere strokes[29] (37% in all comers[30]) with surprising reduction of hemiplegia, and in dominant hemisphere strokes, with only mild-moderate aphasia (better results occur with early surgery, especially if surgery is performed *before* any changes associated with herniation occur). Meta-analysis[31] of 3 randomized controlled trials found that hemicraniectomy within 48 hours after stroke onset resulted in decreased mortality and increased the number of patients with a favorable functional outcome.

Indications: No firm indications. Guidelines:
1. age < 70 years
2. more strongly considered in nondominant hemisphere (usually right)
3. clinical & CT evidence of acute, complete ICA or MCA infarcts and direct signs of impending or complete severe hemispheric brain swelling (severe post-admission neurologic deterioration is the usual event that triggers surgical intervention)

See also **Technique** (p. 1766).

95

95.4 Cardiogenic brain embolism

95.4.1 General information

About one stroke in six is cardioembolic. Emboli may be composed of fibrin-rich thrombi (e.g., mural thrombi due to segmental myocardial hypokinesis following MI or ventricular aneurysm), platelets (e.g., nonbacterial thrombotic endocarditis), calcified material (e.g., in aortic stenosis), or tumor particles (e.g., atrial myxoma).

▶ **Following acute myocardial infarction (AMI).** 2.5% of patients will have a stroke within 1–2 weeks of an AMI (the period when most emboli occur). The risk is higher with anterior wall MI (≈ 6%) vs. inferior wall MI (≈ 1%).

▶ **Atrial fibrillation (a-fib).** Nonrheumatic patients with a-fib have a 3–5-fold increased risk of stroke,[32] with a 4.5% rate of stroke per year without treatment.[33] The incidence of a-fib in the U.S. is 2.2 million. About 75% of strokes in patients with a-fib are due to left atrial thrombi.[34] Independent risk factors for stroke in patients with a-fib are: advanced age, prior embolism (stroke or TIA), HTN, DM, and echocardiographic evidence of left atrial enlargement or left ventricular dysfunction.[32]

CHADS2 scoring system (▶ Table 95.1) for risk of stroke with a-fib has been widely validated.[35] Points are totaled and risk is shown in ▶ Table 95.2. If CHADS2 score is ≥ 2, warfarin therapy is significantly protective for out-of-hospital death or hospitalization for stroke, MI, or hemorrhage (CI = 0.61–0.91).[36]

Table 95.1 CHADS2 scoring items

Item	Points
CHF (any history)	1
HTN (prior history)	1
Age > 75 yrs	1
Diabetes mellitus	1
Secondary prevention: in patients with prior ischemic stroke or TIA; most also include systemic embolic events	2

Table 95.2 Risk based on CHADS2 score

CHADS2 score	Annual stroke risk (%/year)
0	1.9
1	2.8
2	4
3	5.9
4	8.5
5	12.5
6	18.2

▶ **Prosthetic heart valves.** Patients with mechanical prosthetic heart valves on long-term anticoagulation have an embolism rate of 3%/year for mitral and 1.5%/year for aortic valves. With bioprosthetic heart valves and no anticoagulation, the risk is 2–4%/year.

▶ **Paradoxical embolism.** Paradoxical embolism can occur with a patent foramen ovale which is present in 10–18% of the general population, but in up to 56% of young adults with unexplained stroke.[37]

▶ **Endocarditis.** Blood cultures and TEE help evaluate.

95.4.2 Diagnosis of cardiogenic brain embolism

General information

No specific neurologic features can distinguish these patients. The diagnosis is suggested in imaging studies showing multiple intracranial ischemic strokes in different arterial distributions, the differential diagnosis includes: vasculitis, intracranial atherosclerosis (focal plaques, more common in Asian populations that consume Western diets), and intravascular lymphomatosis.

The diagnosis of cardiogenic brain embolism (CBE) as a cause of a stroke relies on demonstrating a potential cardiac source, the absence of cerebrovascular disease, and non-lacunar stroke.

Large areas of hemorrhagic transformation within an ischemic infarct may be more indicative of CBE due to thrombolysis of the clot and reperfusion of infarcted brain with subsequent hemorrhagic conversion. Hemorrhagic transformation most often occurs within 48 hrs of a CBE stroke, and is more common with larger strokes.

Detection of cardiac source

Most centers rely on echocardiography (without transesophageal ability). Using restricted criteria (i.e., excluding mitral valve prolapse), about 10% of patients with ischemic stroke will have potential cardiac source detected by echo, and most of these patients have other manifestations of cardiac disease. In stroke patients without clinical heart disease, only 1.5% will have a positive echo; the yield is higher in younger patients without cerebrovascular disease.[38]

EKG may detect atrial fibrillation, which may be seen in 6–24% of ischemic strokes and may be associated with a 5-fold increased risk of stroke (see below).

95.4.3 Treatment

CBE is essentially the only condition for which anticoagulation has been shown to significantly reduce the rate of further strokes.

One must balance the risk of recurrent emboli (12% of patients with a cardioembolic stroke will have a second embolic stroke within 2 weeks) against that of converting a pale infarct into a hemorrhagic one. No study has shown a clear benefit of *early* anticoagulation.

Recommendations for anticoagulation:
1. if anticoagulation is to be used, it should not be instituted within the first 48 hrs of a probable CBE stroke
2. CT should be obtained after 48 hrs following a CBE stroke and before starting anticoagulation (to R/O hemorrhage)
3. anticoagulation should not be used in the face of large infarcts
4. start heparin and warfarin simultaneously. Continue heparin for 3 days into warfarin therapy, see Anticoagulation (p. 163)
5. optimal range of oral anticoagulation to minimize subsequent embolism and/or hemorrhage has not been determined, but pending further data, an INR of 2–3 appears satisfactory
6. patients with asymptomatic a-fib have 66–86% reduction in stroke risk with warfarin (Coumadin®).[32,39] ASA is only about half as effective, but may be sufficient for those without associated risk factors (p. 1590) [32]

95.5 Vertebrobasilar insufficiency

95.5.1 General information

Signs and symptoms resulting from inadequate blood flow through the posterior cerebral circulation (vertebral arteries, basilar artery and their branches).

95.5.2 Symptoms

► Table 95.3 shows a mnemonic of the symptoms of vertebrobasilar insufficiency (VBI). Predicting the site of the lesion based only on clinical evaluation is very unreliable.

Diagnostic criteria for VBI are shown in ► Table 95.4.

Table 95.3 Mnemonic: "The 5 D's of VBI"

- "drop attack"
- diplopia
- dysarthria
- defect (visual field)
- dizziness

Table 95.4 Criteria for clinical diagnosis of VBI

Clinical diagnosis requires 2 or more of the following
- motor or sensory symptoms or both, occurring bilaterally in the same event
- diplopia: ischemia of upper brainstem (midbrain) near ocular nuclei
- dysarthria: ischemia of lower brainstem
- homonymous hemianopsia: ischemia of occipital cortex (NB: this is *binocular*, in contrast to amaurosis fugax which is monocular)

VBI may also be suspected in a patient with transient episodes of "dizziness" (vertigo that is otherwise unexplained, e.g., absence of orthostatic hypotension or benign positional vertigo) that are initiated by positional changes. VBI may sometimes be due to compression of the VA at the C1–2 level with:

1. head turning (see below)
2. os odontoideum (p. 1175)
3. anterior atlantoaxial subluxation: e.g., in rheumatoid arthritis (p. 1377)
4. with rotatory atlantoaxial subluxation (p. 1158)

95.5.3 Pathophysiology

Atheromatous and stenotic lesions of the posterior circulation occur most frequently at the VA origin.

VBI symptoms may be due to:

1. hemodynamic insufficiency (may be the most common etiology), including:
    a) subclavian steal: reversed flow in VA due to proximal stenosis of subclavian artery
    b) stenosis of both VAs or of one VA where the other is hypofunctional (e.g., hypoplastic, occluded, or terminates in PICA) causing reduced distal flow in face of inadequate collaterals (see below)
2. embolism from ulcerations
3. atherosclerotic occlusion of brainstem perforators
4. vertebrobasilar hypoplasia: reported as a possible etiology for cerebellar stroke.

95.5.4 Natural history

No clinical study accurately defines the natural history. The estimated stroke rate is 22–35% over 5 years, or 4.5–7% per year[40] (one study estimating 35% stroke rate in 5 years did not use angiography).

Risk of stroke after first VBI-TIA has been estimated as 22% for first year.[41]

95.5.5 Evaluation

Adequate investigation usually requires selective four-vessel angiography,[42] sometimes with provocative maneuvers (see e.g., Bow hunter's stroke (p. 1592)). CTA may also be useful.

95.5.6 Treatment

Anticoagulation is the mainstay of medical management. Alternatives include anti-platelet drugs such as ASA (efficacy of either remains unproven[40,42]).

Surgical treatment includes:

1. vertebral endarterectomy
2. transposition of VA to ICA (with or without carotid endarterectomy, with or without saphenous vein patch graft) or to thyrocervical trunk or to subclavian artery[43]
3. bypass grafting (e.g., occipital artery to PICA)
4. C1–2 posterior arthrodesis (p. 1778) may prevent potentially life-threatening stroke in cases of os odontoideum (p. 1176)

95.6 Bow hunter's stroke

95.6.1 General information

A special subset of VBI. The term was coined in 1978 by Sorensen.[44] Bow hunter's stroke (BHS) hemodynamic VBI induced by intermittent VA occlusion resulting from head rotation[45] (ischemi sequelae range from TIA (bow hunter's sign) to completed stroke). May occur with forced (e.g., with chiropractic neck manipulation[46]) or voluntary[47] head rotation.

Occlusion usually involves the VA *contralateral* to the direction of rotation, and usually occurs at the C1–2 junction (due to the immobility of the VA at this location).[48] However, other sites have also been reported.[49,50]

VA occlusion does not produce symptoms in most individuals due to collateral flow through the contralateral VA and/or the circle of Willis. Symptomatic occlusion usually involves the dominant VA,[51] but it may also occur with non-dominant VA[47]. Most cases of BHS occur in patients with an isolated posterior circulation (incompetent posterior communicating arteries).

BHS has also been postulated as one possible cause of SIDS.[52]

95.6.2 Contributing factors

1. external VA compression[50]
   a) spondylotic bone spurs: particularly in the foramen transversarium[53]
   b) tumors
   c) fibrous bands (e.g., proximal to entrance of VA into C6 foramen transversarium[49])
   d) infectious processes
   e) trauma
2. tethering of the VA
   a) at the transverse foramina of C1 & C2
   b) along the sulcus arteriosus proximal to where the VA enters the dura
3. defect in odontoid process[54]
4. atherosclerotic vascular disease

95.6.3 Diagnosis

General information

BHS should be suspected in patient with symptoms of VBI precipitated by head movement. This may be very difficult to differentiate from vertigo and nausea due to vestibular dysfunction (which can also be induced by head movement). (Rotation of the body keeping the head motionless should not cause symptoms from vestibular dysfunction and might help distinguish these conditions.[55])

Dynamic cerebral angiography (DCA)

✸ NB: significant consequences can be precipitated during DCA in patients with BHS.[48] The involved VA shows loss of flow as the head is rotated from the neutral position to the contralateral side. Carotid injections demonstrate patency of PComAs and the presence of any persistent fetal anastomoses.

CT angiogram (CTA)

Same precautions as with DCA (see above). Probably not the initial diagnostic study of choice. If the DCA is negative, CTA is not needed. If DCA is positive, CTA may be helpful to demonstrate the arterial relationship to the bony anatomy.

95.6.4 Treatment

Options include:
1. anticoagulation[55]
2. cervical collar: to remind patient not to turn their head
3. for VA compression at C1–2 (see ▶ Table 95.5 for a comparison):
   a) C1–2 fusion (p. 1781)
   b) VA decompression: C1 "hemilaminectomy" via a posterior approach[56]

Table 95.5 Comparison of surgical treatment for positional VA occlusion at C1–2

Procedure	Advantages	Disadvantages
C1–2 fusion	high success rate in eliminating symptoms	loss of 50–70% of neck rotation with possible discomfort
VA decompression	no loss of motion	33% continue to have symptoms[57]

95

4. for compression at other sites: elimination of the source of compression where possible (e.g., sectioning off offending fibrous band,[49] removal of osteophytic spurs[53]...)

Management recommendations: For compression at C1–2, it is suggested that VA decompression be performed as the initial treatment. This should be followed by DCA to verify maintenance of patency with head turning. Patients who fail clinically or on DCA should undergo C1–2 fusion.[48] Patients need to know pros and cons of each option.

95.7 Cerebral venous thrombosis

95.7.1 General information

Cerebral venous thrombosis (CVT) involves the dural sinuses and/or cerebral veins.

It is an uncommon condition that comprises 0.5–1% of strokes[58] and usually affects young people (78% occur in patients age < 50 years[59]). Estimated incidence: 1.32 per 100,000 person-years, with a higher incidence of 2.78 in women 31–50 years of age.

It has been observed that patients are usually either mildly symptomatic or extremely ill and unstable.

There are 3 types of CVT, any of which may produce venous infarctions:
1. dural sinus thrombosis (DST)
2. cortical venous thrombosis
3. deep venous thrombosis

95.7.2 Etiologies

Partial list of etiologies

Many conditions have been incriminated with CVT, some of which may be due to referral and ascertainment biases.[60] Some common ones are listed here[60,61 (p 1301)]:
1. infection
    a) usually local, e.g., otitis media[62,63] (leading to the now obsolete term otitic hydrocephalus), sinusitis, peritonsillar abscess, paranasal sinusitis[64]: in the pre-antibiotic era, CVT was most commonly associated with chronic suppurative infection
    b) meningitis
2. pregnancy & puerperium: see below
3. oral contraceptives† (birth control pills [BCP])[65]
4. dehydration and cachexia (marantic thrombosis): includes burns and cachexia of neoplastic disease
5. cardiac disease (including CHF)
6. ulcerative colitis (UC): 1% of UC patients have some thrombotic complication (not necessarily all intracranial), and this is the cause of ≈ 33% of deaths (usually pulmonary embolism, PE)
7. periarteritis nodosa
8. sickle cell trait
9. trauma: including closed head injury (see below)
10. iatrogenic: e.g., S/P radical neck surgery,[66] transvenous pacemaker placement, post-craniotomy, internal jugular vein catheterization
11. malignancy: including myeloproliferative disorders
12. hypercoagulable state (AKA thrombophilia or prothrombotic conditions)
    a) protein C deficiency† or resistance to activated protein C: hereditary factor V Leiden mutation may produce resistance to activated protein C.[67] Apparent protein C deficiency may be an artifact of dehydration in some cases
    b) antithrombin III deficiency†
    c) protein S deficiency†
    d) antiphospholipid antibodies†: associated with a variety of clinical syndromes including ischemic stroke, DVTs, thrombocytopenia, and systemic lupus erythematosus (SLE). The best known antibodies include
        • anticardiolipin antibodies†
        • lupus anticoagulant
    e) paroxysmal nocturnal hemoglobinuria (PNH)
    f) plasminogen deficiency
    g) prothrombin G20210A mutation of factor II†: causes a mild elevation of prothrombin
    h) systemic lupus erythematosus[68]
    i) factor VIII elevation[69]: may explain some cases of CVT in pregnancy (see below)

95

13. diabetes mellitus: especially with ketoacidosis
14. (hyper)homocystinuria (p. 208)
15. Behçet's syndrome (p. 208) [70]
16. rarely associated with lumbar puncture, associated with hereditary activated protein C resistance due to the factor V R506Q mutation (FV Leiden) in one report[71]

† Strongly associated with CVT (odds ratio ≥ 5)[60]

Pregnancy/puerperium

Highest risk is in the third trimester and for 6–8 weeks post-partum.[60] One series[72] found that no case of CVT occurred later than 16 days post-partum. Incidence ≈ 1/10,000 births. Etiology may be related to elevation of clotting factors (VII, X, and especially factor VIII[73]). Hypercoagulability increases post-partum due to volume depletion and trauma.

Trauma

A rare sequelae of closed head injury.[74] CVT occurs in ≈ 10% of combat injuries involving the brain. May occur in absence of skull fracture. CVT should be suspected in patients with fractures or missiles crossing sinus.

95.7.3 Relative frequency of venous structures involved

The relative frequency of involvement of dural sinuses and other veins with thrombotic issues
1. sinuses
   a) superior sagittal sinus (**SSS**) and left transverse sinus (**TS**) (70% each)
   b) multiple sinuses in 71%
   c) isolated inferior sagittal sinus: rare, first case report in 1997[75]
   d) straight sinus[76]
2. superficial cortical veins
3. deep venous system (e.g., internal cerebral vein)
4. cavernous sinus[77,78]: rare. Thrombophlebitis of the cavernous sinus may be caused by sphenoid sinusitis. MRI may show enlargement and abnormal enhancement of the cavernous sinus, increased signal of the petrous apex and clivus on T2WI, and narrowing of the cavernous portion of the ICA[78]

95.7.4 Pathophysiology

Venous thrombosis reduces venous outflow from the brain and diminishes effective blood flow to the involved area. This venous engorgement causes white matter edema. The increased venous pressure may also lead to infarction and/or hemorrhage. These processes may all elevate ICP. Thus, clinical findings may be due to elevated ICP, and focal findings may be due to edema and/or hemorrhage. Cerebral infarction due to venous stasis is called venous infarction.

95.7.5 Clinical

Clinical presentations of DST are shown in ▶ Table 95.6. There are no pathognomonic findings. Many signs and symptoms are due to elevated ICP as a result of impaired venous outflow and may present as a syndrome clinically indistinguishable from pseudotumor cerebri (p. 955). Others present as a result of focal brain injury from venous insufficiency or infarction/hemorrhage. Headache is the most common symptom.[79]

There is a high association of concurrent thromboembolic disease in other organs.

The anterior 1/3 of the SSS may occlude without neurologic sequelae. Posterior to this (especially posterior to the vein of Trolard), venous infarction is more likely to develop. Midportion SSS occlusion usually → increased muscle tone ranging from spastic hemi- or quadriparesis to decerebration. Posterior SSS thrombosis → field cuts or cortical blindness, or massive stroke with cerebral edema and death. Occlusion of the TS may occur without deficit unless the contralateral TS is hypoplastic, in which case presentation is similar to posterior SSS occlusion.

SSS occlusion alone will not cause cranial nerve findings except perhaps for visual obscuration and abducens (VI) nerve palsy from elevated ICP. Thrombosis in the jugular bulb may compress the nerves in the jugular foramen pars nervosa causing hoarseness, aphonia, difficulty swallowing, and breathlessness; see Vernet's syndrome (p. 102).[80]

95

Table 95.6 Presentation of dural sinus thrombosis[a]

Sign/symptom	Series A[b]	Series B[c]
H/A	100%	74%
N/V	75%	–
seizures	70%	29%
hemiparesis	70%	34%
papilledema	70%	45%
blurred vision	60%	–
altered consciousness	35%	26%

[a]other symptoms include: focal neurologic deficit, cranial nerve palsy, nystagmus[81]
[b]series A: 20 young females[72]
[c]series B: 38 cases from France[82]

95.7.6 Diagnosis of DST

General information

CT (especially CTV) & MRI/MRV are very sensitive and specific for identifying areas of clot.

Catheter angiography is better at demonstrating the presence of residual flow, and can identify areas of reversal of flow, and sometimes is able to demonstrate clot as a filling defect. Angiography is often used as a complementary test[83] when the diagnosis is suggested by CT or MRI.

Non-contrast CT

Low sensitivity. A wide range of accuracy is reported: 30–100% sensitivity & 83–100% specificity (a realistic range of sensitivity from reviews is ≈ 30%[60] to 75%[84] of cases of CVT). False positives may occur with high hematocrit. Hounsfield unit (p. 238) > 70 is highly specific for acute CVT.[84] Findings include:
1. hyperdense sinus (► Fig. 95.1) or cortical vein: high-density clots in cortical veins; has been dubbed the cord sign, which is pathognomonic for cerebral venous thrombosis; seen in only 2/3 of patients

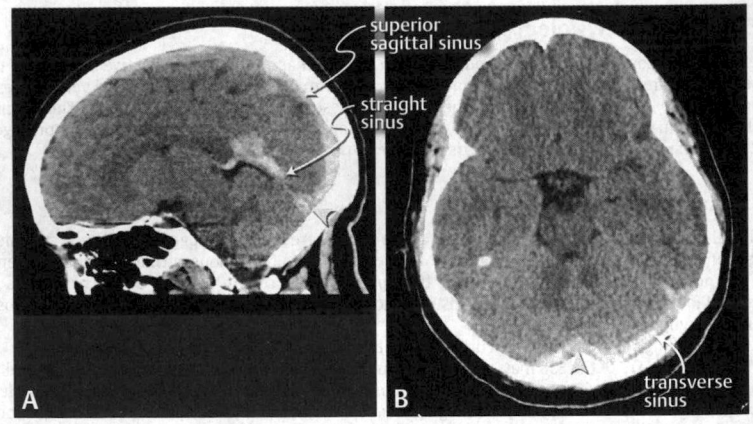

Fig. 95.1 Cerebral venous thrombosis.
Noncontrast CT scan, A: sagittal, B: axial.
Thrombus (white) is seen in the superior sagittal sinus, the straight sinus, the left transverse sinus extending slight into the right transverse sinus, and in the torcular Herophili (*yellow arrowheads*).

2. hemorrhage: 9–39% show some form of hemorrhage
   a) petechial "flame" hemorrhages (intraparenchymal): seen in 20% (suspect sinus thrombosis with intracerebral hemorrhages in unusual locations for aneurysm or "hypertensive" hemorrhage)
   b) SAH: in < 1% (usually over convexity)
   c) intraventricular
3. small ventricles: seen in 50%
4. thrombosis of superior sagittal sinus may produce a triangular-shaped high density within the sinus posteriorly near the torcular Herophili on axial CT images (delta sign (▶ Fig. 95.2, panel A) or "dense/filled delta sign" as opposed to the "empty delta" sign, see below & ▶ Fig. 95.2, panel B) (there is also confusion when an apparent "empty delta" sign is seen *without* contrast; this may occur when there is blood surrounding the SSS, e.g., following subarachnoid hemorrhage; this has been called a "false delta sign" or pseudodelta sign[85]). Recommendation: avoid the confusion of the variations on "delta signs" and describe the findings
5. venous infarct: infarct that doesn't follow arterial territories, especially near a dural sinus[86]
6. white matter edema
7. above changes occurring *bilaterally*

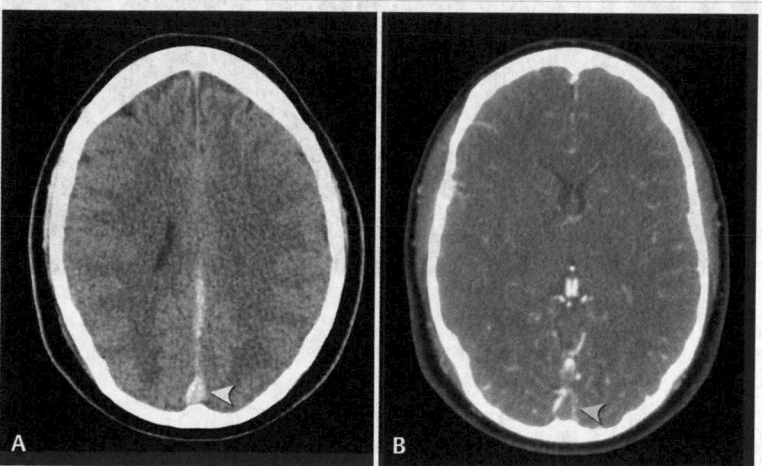

Fig. 95.2 Delta sign on axial CT scan in CVT.
A: non-contrast, demonstrating the "(full) delta sign" (*yellow arrowhead*) in the torcular Herophili.
B: IV contrast-enhanced, demonstrating the "empty delta sign" (*blue arrowhead*).

95

IV contrast CT

Findings of DST include:
1. with *contrast*, the dura around the sinus may enhance and become denser than clot in 35% of cases.[87] Near the torcular Herophili this produces what has been called the empty delta sign (▶ Fig. 95.2, panel B),[88] but sometimes this, too, is called the delta sign
2. gyral enhancement occurs in 32%
3. dense deep (white matter) veins (collateral flow)
4. intense tentorial enhancement (common)

CTV

CT venography is approximately equivalent to MRV in diagnosing CVT.[60]

MRI & MRA/MRV

MRI excels for diagnosis and follow-up. MRI shows absence of flow and clot burden and demonstrates parenchymal changes including venous infarcts (▶ Fig. 95.3, panel B). Can differentiate occluded sinus from congenital absence. Shows cerebral edema and non-acute hemorrhagic changes to better advantage than CT. Also may help estimate age of clots (▶ Table 95.7). Findings include the hyperintense vein sign (▶ Fig. 95.3, panel A).

MR angiography may increase the utility. MR venography (MRV) tends to overestimate the degree of occlusion.

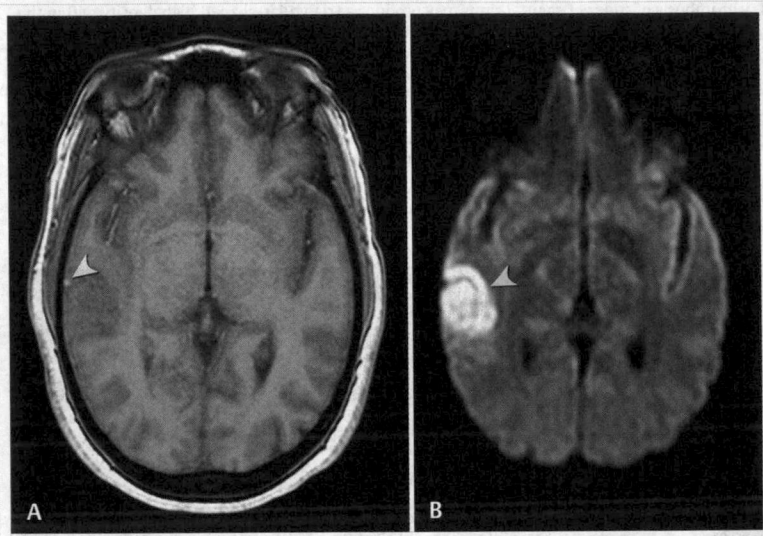

Fig. 95.3 MRI findings in CVT.
A: T1 axial showing hyperintense vein sign (*yellow arrowhead*).
B: DWI showing venous infarct (*blue arrowhead*) adjacent to the thrombosed vein.

Table 95.7 MRI appearance of thrombosed sinuses at various stages[60]

Age of clot in sinus	Hemoglobin state	Appearance of clotted sinus	
		T1WI	T2WI
acute (0–7 days)	deoxyhemoglobin	isointense	hypointense (black): can mimic flow void
subacute	methemoglobin	hyperintense (1st)	hyperintense (2nd)
late (recanalized)	paramagnetic products of above	black (flow void)	black (flow void)

Catheter angiography for CVT

Catheter angiography is close to MRI in sensitivity, and some still consider it to be the standard of diagnosis. MRI has some advantages over angiography (e.g., on angiography a hypoplastic transverse sinus may not visualize, or non-opacified blood entering a sinus may mimic a filling defect). Be sure to image all the way to the venous phase (requires extra vigilance).

Findings include:
1. non-filling of segments of sinuses, or filling defects in segments that are visualized
2. prolonged circulation time: present in 50% of cases (may need delayed films to see veins)
3. stumps and abnormal collateral pathways

LP

LP (lumbar puncture) is generally not indicated unless there is suspicion of meningitis. There are no specific CSF abnormalities, so LP is often not helpful. Opening pressure (OP) is increased in > 80%.[79] CSF may be bloody or xanthochromic.

Bloodwork

Routine blood studies (CBC, chemistry, PT & aPTT) should be performed (Level I[60]).

To detect prothrombotic conditions, useful tests include: protein C and S levels*, antithrombin deficiency*, antiphospholipid antibodies = anticardiolipin antibodies and lupus anticoagulant as well as tests for specific predisposing conditions (Factor II level, serum homocysteine level, paroxysmal nocturnal hemoglobinuria (PNH) panel, leukocyte alkaline phosphatase (Level II[60])).

* Tests for protein C & protein S, and antithrombin deficiency should be deferred until 2–4 weeks after completing anticoagulation (testing is of limited value on warfarin or in the acute setting since the acute process will cause numerous abnormalities in the clotting system (Level II[60])).

D-dimer: a fibrin degradation product, showed a sensitivity of 97.1%, specificity of 91.2%, a negative prdictive value of 99.6%, and a positive predictive value of 55.7%.[89] A normal D-dimer level by a sensitive radioimmunoassay or ELISA may help identify patients with a low probability of CVT (Level II[60]). However, if suspicion is high, further evaluation is indicated.

Ultrasound for DST

May be used in diagnosis of superior sagittal sinus thrombosis in the neonate.[90]

95.7.7 Management of CVT

General information

Driving principle: treat the underlying abnormality (if possible).

Management should be aggressive because recoverability of brain is probably greater than with arterial occlusive stroke. Management is challenging because measures that counteract thrombosis (e.g., anticoagulation) tend to increase the risk of hemorrhagic infarct (the risk of which is already increased), and measures that lower ICP tend to increase blood viscosity → increased coagulability.

The following is derived from the 2011 AHA Scientific Statement for the Diagnosis and Management of Cerebral Venous Thrombosis[60] and the 2018 Report of the Society of NeuroInterventional Surgery on Endovascular Strategies for Cerebral Venous Thrombosis.[84]

Key concepts: Evaluation and treatment of CVT

1. history & bloodwork: identify risk factors (p. 1594) and symptoms (▶ Table 95.6). Treat underlying conditions
2. initial diagnostic test in cases of suspected CVT: either brain CT + CTV head/neck, or brain MRI + MRV head/neck[84] (if normal, these tests do not rule out CVT). MRI/MRV is probably more sensitive than CT/CTV
3. catheter angiography may be helpful with inconclusive CTV or MRV when the clinical suspicion is high (Level II[60]). Be sure to obtain late images (venous phase)
4. if CVT is confirmed: treatment
   a) anticoagulation: start with dose-adjusted unfractionated heparin (UFW) or weight-based LMWH, followed by vitamin K antagonists (e.g., warfarin) (Level II[60]). ICH is *not* a contraindication
   b) indications for endovascular treatment (p. 1934) (chemical thrombolysis or thrombectomy):
      1. clinical deterioration despite anticoagulation
      2. contraindications to anticoagulation
      3. coma
      4. deep CVT
      5. intracerebral hemorrhage (ICH)
   c) decompressive hemicraniectomy indications: large lesions with herniation
   d) intracranial pressure monitoring and treatment: start with acetazolamide for elevated ICP
5. if CVT is not confirmed: diagnosis of alternative conditions
   a) brain tumor
   b) infection
   c) ischemic stroke
   d) posterior reversible encephalopathy syndrome (PRES) (p. 202)
   e) pseudotumor cerebri (p. 955)

95

Treatment specifics

1. general measures
   a) patients suspected of having infection should receive appropriate treatment: antibiotics, drainage of purulent collections… (Level I[60])
   b) seizures:
      - ASMs for a defined duration are recommended for a single seizure with (Level I[60]) or without (Level II[60]) parenchymal lesions to prevent futher seizures
      - ASMs are not recommended in the absence of seizures (potential harm[60])
   c) steroids: not recommended unless needed for other underlying disease (potential harm[60]) (reduces fibrinolysis, increases coagulation)
   d) control HTN
2. anticoagulation
   a) anticoagulation: start with dose-adjusted unfractionated heparin (UFW) or weight-based LMWH (Level II[60]). See dosing information (p. 172). Numerous studies show a lower mortality rate with heparin than without.[91,92,93] It remains the best treatment even when there is evidence of intracerebral hemorrhage (ICH) with the attendant risk of increasing the size of the hemorrhage.[83] There is no consensus on duration of treatment. Success rate may be higher if administered before patient becomes moribund
      ★ during pregnancy, full-dose LMWH is recommended over UFH (Level II[60])
   b) transition from heparin to vitamin K antagonists (e.g., warfarin)
3. monitor ICP if patient continues to deteriorate: ventriculostomy is preferred, but use caution in placing catheter if patient is on heparin
   a) hydrate aggressively as ICP tolerates
   b) measures to lower ICP: differ somewhat from treatment for traumatic ICP elevation
      - acetazolamide (Level II[60]): one of the few measures to treat elevated ICP that do not rely on venous outflow
      - elevate HOB
      - drain CSF
      - pentobarbital coma: also does not depend on venous outflow
      - hyperosmotic and/or loop diuretics: reserve for last because diuretics → hypertonicity → ↑ viscosity → ↑ coagulation. Replace fluid loss with isotonic IV fluids to prevent dehydration; i.e., goal is hypertonic euvolemia
   c) monitor patients with increased ICP for progressive visual loss and treat elevated ICP urgently if detected (Level I[60]). Treatment measures include: serial LPs, optic nerve sheath fenestration,[94] or VP shunt (Level II[60])
4. endovascular therapy (EVT) (p. 1934) for deterioration despite intensive anticoagulation (Level II[60]). There are no guidelines for how long to wait before declaring medical therapy a failure, decision takes into account how sick the patient is. Also, there is no information when to use DC vs. EVT. Modalities include chemical thrombolysis (direct injection of tPA into the sinus) and mechanical thrombectomy
5. decompressive craniectomy (DC): consider for neurologic deterioration due to mass effect or intracranial hemorrhage causing increased ICP (Level II[60]). Risky, but may be lifesaving. Early surgery (≤ 12 hrs from admission) & younger patients are predictors for a more favorable response to DC. If DC is elected, the options of heparinization and tPA cannot be employed for ≈ 2–3 days
6. long-term anticoagulation after resolution of acute phase with heparin (Level II[60]):
   a) spontaneous CVT: vitamin K antagonists (VKA) for 6–12 months, target INR = 2–3
   b) CVT with risk factors that have been eliminated: VKA for 3–6 months, target INR = 2–3
   c) recurrent CVT, VTE after CVT, or severe thrombophilia (e.g., homozygous prothrombin G20210A, homozygous factor V Leiden, protein C or S or antithrombin deficiency, antiphospholipid syndrome, or combined thrombophilic conditions): indefinite VKA, target INR = 2–3
   d) consider consultation with a physician with expertise in coagulation
   e) for CVT during pregnancy: continue full anticoagulation with LMWH during the pregnancy, and LMWH or VKA with a target INR = 2–3 for ≥ 6 weeks post-partum (for a total duration of therapy of 6 months) (Level I[60])

95.7.8 Prognosis

Morbidity & mortality:

Natural history (without treatment): reported mortality range is 14–40% (based on small sample sizes).[84]

With anticoagulation: ≈ 13% die or remain dependent.[84]

95

Poor prognosticators:
1. clinical status:
   a) coma[95]
   b) rapid neurologic deterioration,[95] focal signs
2. demographics
   a) age: extremes of age (infancy or elderly)[95]
   b) male gender
3. radiographic findings:
   a) hemorrhages, especially larger hemorrhages
   b) venous infarcts
4. deep venous involvement

▶ **Future pregnancies in patients with a history of CVT**
1. advise the patient that future pregnancy is *not* contraindicated. Consultation with a hematologist and/or maternal fetal medicine specialist is reasonable (Level II[60])
2. prophylaxis with LMWH during future pregnancies and the post-partum period for women with a history of CVT is recommended (Level II[60])

95.8 Extracranial-intracranial (EC/IC) bypass

95.8.1 The 1985 international EC/IC bypass study

The EC/IC bypass, pioneered by Donaghy and Yasargil in 1967,[96] plummeted in popularity[97] after publication of the international cooperative EC/IC bypass study[98] in 1985. The EC/IC trial randomized 1,377 patients with symptomatic ICA or MCA stenosis to either STA-MCA bypass or medical therapy with ASA. Despite a graft patency rate of 96%, surgical patients suffered more and earlier fatal and nonfatal strokes. Patients with severe MCA stenosis and those with persistent symptoms following ICA occlusion fared especially worse with bypass.

Critique: inclusion criteria failed to distinguish between hemodynamic vs. thromboembolic causes of stroke.[2,99,100] Ischemia secondary to thromboembolic events would not be expected to improve with flow augmentation, and inclusion of such patients in the surgical arm could therefore artificially lower the apparent efficacy of the procedure.

95.8.2 Current state of affairs

Imaging technologies introduced since the 1985 EC/IC trial can identify flow-dependent ischemia. Xenon-CT, TCD, SPECT, and MRI and CT perfusion may be used in combination with acetazolamide challenge to evaluate cerebrovascular reserve and reactivity (p. 1537).

As cerebral perfusion pressure decreases in severe atherosclerotic occlusive disease, cerebral autoregulation (p. 1536) is unable to maintain adequate CBF to meet metabolic demands. In this state of "misery perfusion," oxygen extraction fraction (OEF) of available blood flow will increase.[101,102] Abnormal OEF, as quantified by PET, is an independent predicator of subsequent stroke.[2] Patients with abnormal response to acetazolamide challenge (p. 239) and/or with elevated OEF are therefore potential candidates for cerebral revascularization.[2,100,103,104,105]

The Japanese EC-IC Bypass Trial (JET) and Carotid Occlusion Surgery Study (COSS) were designed to stratify candidates according to hemodynamic criteria.
● JET: 169 patients, study period of almost 4 years, 2-year follow-up. A significant reduction of the primary and secondary stroke was observed after surgery.
● COSS: halted after inclusion of 195 patients due to high 30-day event rate and no significant benefits on the overall outcome of the surgical patients. The high event rate (14.4%) was dramatically higher than that of the 1985 EC-IC bypass study. Furthermore, the COSS data demonstrated a clear postoperative reduction of ipsilateral ischemic events beyond the 30-day perioperative period.

Conclusion: EC-IC bypass remains an option in carefully selected patients with ischemic cerebrovascular disease, limited to interdisciplinary and specialized high-volume centers and within the framework of controlled studies.[106,107,108,109] Recently, the Japanese Adult Moyamoya Trail (JAM) reported the preventative effect of direct bypass against rebleeding in adult patients with moyamoya disease who had experienced intracranial hemorrhage.[110]

95

95.8.3 Indications for EC/IC bypass

1. symptomatic patients with misery perfusion (see above)[111]
2. aneurysms: certain aneurysms are not amendable to either direct microsurgical clipping or endovascular coiling due to extreme size, location, calcification or atherosclerosis, dissection, or the incorporation of perforators or major arteries. EC/IC bypass remains a highly viable adjunctive measure in patients requiring Hunterian occlusion of parent vessel or prolonged temporary occlusion for definite treatment.[112,113,114,115,116] Cerebrovascular reserve and need for bypass can be assessed preoperatively using balloon test occlusion (BTO) with hypotensive challenge
3. tumors encasing or invading major arteries
4. moyamoya disease (p. 1581) and moyamoya syndrome

95.8.4 Bypass types

The type of graft used depends on preoperative determination of amount of flow augmentation necessary, the size of the recipient graft, and the availability of donor vessel[117,118]:

1. pedicled arterial grafts: STA, occipital artery
   a) low-flow (15–25 ml/min)
   b) only one anastomosis required
   c) 95% graft patency in superficial temporal artery-middle cerebral artery (STA-MCA) bypasses
2. radial artery graft
   a) moderate to high flow (40–70 ml/min)
   b) advantages: physiological conduit for arterial blood; constant location makes it easy to harvest; lumen size closely approximates that of M2 or P1 and reduces flow mismatch with subsequent flow turbulence and graft thrombosis
   c) disadvantages: risk of vasospasm (reduced with pressure distension technique)
   d) > 90% graft patency at 5 years
3. saphenous vein graft
   a) high flow (70–140 ml/min)
   b) advantages: easy accessibility; longer length
   c) disadvantages: risk of thrombosis at distal anastomosis due to flow mismatch and turbulence; lower graft patency rates
   d) 82% graft patency at 5 years

95.8.5 Perioperative complications of EC/IC bypass

In addition to risks of surgery, risks of EC/IC bypass include: risk of stroke from temporary occlusion of a cortical vessel, cerebral hyperperfusion, and "watershed shift" phenomenon with the risk of cerebral hemorrhage from a sharp increase in focal CBF.[119]

95

References

[1] Hankey GJ, Warlow CP. Prognosis of symptomatic carotid artery occlusion: an overview. Cerebrovascular Diseases. 1991; 1:245–256

[2] Grubb RL,Jr, Derdeyn CP, Fritsch SM, et al. Importance of hemodynamic factors in the prognosis of symptomatic carotid occlusion. JAMA. 1998; 280:1055–1060

[3] Powers WJ, Derdeyn CP, Fritsch SM, et al. Benign prognosis of never-symptomatic carotid occlusion. Neurology. 2000; 54:878–882

[4] Lakshminarayan R, Scott PM, Robinson GJ, et al. Carotid stump syndrome: pathophysiology and endovascular treatment options. Cardiovasc Intervent Radiol. 2011; 34 Suppl 2:S48–S52

[5] Nagalapuram V, Tharumia Jagadeesan C, Ramasamy B. Carotid Stump Syndrome: An Uncommon Cause of Recurrent Ipsilateral Strokes. Cureus. 2021; 13. DOI: 10.7759/cureus.12688

[6] Finklestein S, Kleinman GM, Cuneo R, et al. Delayed stroke following carotid occlusion. Neurology. 1980; 30:84–88

[7] Kumar SM, Wang JC, Barry MC, et al. Carotid stump syndrome: outcome from surgical management. Eur J Vasc Endovasc Surg. 2001; 21:214–219

[8] Nano G, Dalainas I, Casana R, et al. Endovascular treatment of the carotid stump syndrome. Cardiovasc Intervent Radiol. 2006; 29:140–142

[9] Hafner CD, Tew JM. Surgical Management of the Totally Occluded Internal Carotid Artery. Surgery 1981; 89:710–717

[10] Satiani B, Burns J, Vasko JS. Surgical and Nonsurgical Treatment of Total Carotid Artery Occlusion. Am J Surg. 1985; 149:362–367

[11] Walters BB, Ojemann RG, Heros RC. Emergency Carotid Endarterectomy. J Neurosurg. 1987 66:817–823

[12] Sugg RM, Malkoff MD, Noser EA, et al. Endovascular recanalization of internal carotid artery occlusion in acute ischemic stroke. AJNR. American Journal of Neuroradiology. 2005; 26:2591–2594

[13] Nesbit GM, Clark WM, O'Neill OR, et al. Intracranial intraarterial thrombolysis facilitated by microcatheter navigation through an occluded cervical internal carotid artery. Journal of Neurosurgery. 1996 84:387–392

[14] Endo S, Kuwayama N, Hirashima Y, et al. Results of urgent thrombolysis in patients with major stroke and atherothrombotic occlusion of the cervical internal carotid artery. AJNR. American Journal of Neuroradiology. 1998; 19:1169–1175

[15] Srinivasan A, Goyal M, Stys P, et al. Microcatheter navigation and thrombolysis in acute symptomatic cervical internal carotid occlusion. AJNR. American Journal of Neuroradiology. 2006; 27:774–779

[16] Imai K, Mori T, Izumoto H, et al. Emergency carotid artery stent placement in patients with acute ischemic stroke. AJNR. American Journal of Neuroradiology. 2005; 26:1249–1258

[17] Jovin TG, Gupta R, Uchino K, et al. Emergent stenting of extracranial internal carotid artery occlusion in acute stroke has a high revascularization rate. Stroke. 2005; 36:2426–2430

[18] McCormick PW, Spetzler RF, Bailes JE, et al. Thromboendarterectomy of the Symptomatic Occluded Internal Carotid Artery. J Neurosurg. 1992; 76:752–758

[19] Tomaszek DE, Rosner MJ. Cerebellar Infarction: Analysis of Twenty-One Cases. Surgical Neurology. 1985; 24:223–226

[20] Hinshaw DB, Thompson JR, Haso AN, et al. Infarctions of the Brain Stem and Cerebellum: A Correlation of Computed Tomography and Angiography. Radiology. 1980; 137:105–112

[21] Sypert GW, Alvord EC. Cerebellar Infarction: A Clinicopathological Study. Archives of Neurology. 1975; 32:357–363

[22] Heros RC. Surgical Treatment of Cerebellar Infarction. Stroke. 1992; 23:937–938

[23] Heros RC. Cerebellar Hemorrhage and Infarction. Stroke. 1982; 13:106–109

[24] Chen H-J, Lee T-C, Wei C-P. Treatment of Cerebellar Infarction by Decompressive Suboccipital Craniectomy. Stroke. 1992; 23:957–961

[25] Moulin DE, Lo R, Chiang J, et al. Prognosis in Middle Cerebral Artery Occlusion. Stroke. 1985; 16:282–284

[26] Hacke W, Schwab S, Horn M, et al. Malignant Middle Cerebral Artery Territory Infarction: Clinical Course and Prognostic Signs. Archives of Neurology. 1996; 53:309–315

[27] Wijdicks EFM, Diringer MN. Middle Cerebral Artery Territory Infarction and Early Brain Swelling: Progression and Effect of Age on Outcome. Mayo Clinic Proceedings. 1998; 73:829–836

[28] von Kummer R, Meyding-Lamadé U, Forsting M, et al. Sensitivity and Prognostic Value of Early CT in Occlusion of the Middle Cerebral Artery Trunk. American Journal of Neuroradiology. 1994; 15:9–15

[29] Carter BS, Ogilvy CS, Candia GJ, et al. One-Year Outcome After Decompressive Surgery for Massive Nondominant Hemispheric Infarction. Neurosurgery. 1997; 40:1168–1176

[30] Schwab S, Steiner T, Aschoff A, et al. Early Hemicraniectomy in Patients With Complete Middle Cerebral Artery Infarction. Stroke. 1998; 29:1888–1893

[31] Vahedi K, Hofmeijer J, Juettler E, et al. Early decompressive surgery in malignant infarction of the middle cerebral artery: a pooled analysis of three randomised controlled trials. Lancet Neurol. 2007; 6:215–222

[32] Blackshear JL, Kopecky SL, Litin SC, et al. Management of Atrial Fibrillation in Adults: Prevention of Thromboembolism and Symptomatic Treatment. Mayo Clinic Proceedings. 1996; 71:150–160

[33] Atrial Fibrillation Investigators. Risk factors for stroke and efficacy of antithrombotic therapy in atrial fibrillation: Analysis of pooled data from five randomized controlled trials. Archives of Internal Medicine. 1994; 154:1449–1457

[34] Hart RG, Helperin JL. Atrial fibrillation and stroke: Revisiting the dilemmas. Stroke. 1994; 25:1337–1341

[35] Gage BF, Waterman AD, Shannon W, et al. Validation of clinical classification schemes for predicting stroke: results from the National Registry of Atrial Fibrillation. JAMA. 2001; 285:2864–2870

[36] Gage BF, Birman-Deych E, Kerzner R, et al. Incidence of intracranial hemorrhage in patients with atrial fibrillation who are prone to fall. American Journal of Medicine. 2005; 118:612–617

[37] Lechat P, Mas JL, Lascault G, et al. Prevalence of patent foramen ovale in patients with stroke. N Engl J Med. 1988; 318:1148–1152

[38] Cerebral Embolism Task Force. Cardiogenic Brain Embolism. Arch Neurol. 1989; 46:727–743

[39] Stroke Prevention in Atrial Fibrillation Study Group. Preliminary report of the stroke prevention in atrial fibrillation study. New England Journal of Medicine. 1990; 322:863–868

[40] Hopkins LN, Martin NA, Hadley MN, et al. Vertebrobasilar Insufficiency, Part 2: Microsurgical Treatment of Intracranial Vertebrobasilar Disease. J Neurosurg. 1987; 66:662–674

[41] Robertson JT. Current Management of Vertebral Basilar Occlusive Disease. Clin Neurosurg. 1983; 31:165–187

[42] Ausman JI, Shrontz CE, Pearce JE, et al. Vertebrobasilar Insufficiency: A Review. Arch Neurol. 1985; 42:803–808

[43] Diaz FG, Ausman JI, de los Reyes RA, et al. Surgical Reconstruction of the Proximal Vertebral Artery. J Neurosurg. 1984; 61:874–881

[44] Sorensen BF. Bow hunter's stroke. Neurosurgery. 1978; 2:259–261

[45] Fox MW, Piepgras DG, Bartleson JD. Anterolateral decompression of the atlantoaxial vertebral artery for symptomatic positional occlusion of the vertebral artery. Journal of Neurosurgery. 1995; 83:737–740

[46] Pratt-Thomas HR, Berger KE. Cerebellar and spinal injuries after chiropractic manipulation. Journal of the American Medical Association. 1947; 133:600–603

[47] Matsuyama T, Morimoto T, Sakaki T. Bow hunter's stroke caused by a nondominant vertebral artery occlusion: Case report. Neurosurgery. 1997; 41:1393–1395

[48] Lemole GM, Henn JS, Spetzler RF, et al. Bow hunter's stroke. BNI Quarterly. 2001; 17:4–10

[49] Mapstone T, Spetzler RF. Vertebrobasilar insufficiency secondary to vertebral artery occlusion from a fibrous band. Case report. Journal of Neurosurgery. 1982; 56:581–583

[50] George B, Laurian C. Impairment of vertebral artery flow caused by extrinsic lesions. Neurosurgery. 1989; 24:206–214

[51] Kuether TA, Nesbit GM, Clark WM, et al. Rotational Vertebral Artery Occlusion: A Mechanism of Vertebrobasilar Insufficiency. Neurosurgery. 1997; 41:427–433

[52] Pamphlett R, Raisanen J, Kum-Jew S. Vertebral artery compression resulting from head movement: a possible cause of the sudden infant death syndrome. Pediatrics. 1999; 103:460–468

[53] Okawara S, Nibbelink D. Vertebral artery occlusion following hyperextension and rotation of the head. Stroke. 1974; 5:640–642

[54] Ford FR. Syncope, vertigo and disturbances of vision resulting from intermittent obstruction of vertebral arteries due to defect in odontoid process and excessive mobility of second cervical vertebra. Bulletin of the Johns Hopkins Hospital. 1952; 91:168–173

[55] Tatlow WFT, Bammer HG. Syndrome of vertebral artery compression. Neurology. 1957; 7:331–340

[56] Shimizu T, Waga S, Kojima T, et al. Decompression of the vertebral artery for bow-hunter's stroke. Case report. J Neurosurg. 1988; 69:127–131

[57] Matsuyama T, Morimoto T, Sakaki T. Comparison of C1-2 posterior fusion and decompression of the vertebral artery in the treatment of bow hunter's stroke. J Neurosurg. 1997; 86:619–623

[58] Stam J. Thrombosis of the cerebral veins and sinuses. N Engl J Med. 2005; 352:1791–1798

[59] Bousser MG, Ferro JM. Cerebral venous thrombosis: an update. Lancet Neurol. 2007; 6:162–170

[60] Saposnik G, Barinagarrementeria F, Brown RD,Jr, et al. Diagnosis and management of cerebral venous thrombosis: a statement for healthcare professionals from the American Heart Association/American Stroke Association. Stroke. 2011; 42:1158–1192

[61] Wilkins RH, Rengachary SS. Neurosurgery. New York 1985

[62] Symonds CP. Otitic Hydrocephalus. Brain. 1931; 54:55–71

[63] Garcia RDJ, Baker AS, Cunningham MJ, et al. Lateral Sinus Thrombosis Associated with Otitis Media

95

and Mastoiditis in Children. Pediatr Infect Dis J. 1995; 14:617–623

[64] Dolan RW, Chowdry K. Diagnosis and Treatment of Intracranial Complications of Paranasal Sinus Infections. J Oral Maxillofac Surg. 1995; 53:1080–1087

[65] Shende MC, Lourie H. Sagittal Sinus Thrombosis Related to Oral Contraceptives: Case Report. J Neurosurg. 1970; 33:714–717

[66] Mahasin ZZ, Saleem M, Gangopadhyay K. Transverse Sinus Thrombosis and Venous Infarction of the Brain Following Unilateral Radical Neck Dissection. Journal of Laryngology and Otology. 1998; 112:88–91

[67] Martinelli I, Landi G, Merati G, et al. Factor V Gene Mutation is a Risk Factor for Cerebral Venous Thrombosis. Thromb Maemost. 1996; 75:393–394

[68] Flusser D, Abu-Shakra M, Baumgarten-Kleiner A, et al. Superior Sagittal Sinus Thrombosis in a Patient with Systemic Lupus Erythematosus. Lupus. 1996; 5:334–336

[69] Bugnicourt JM, Roussel B, Tramier B, et al. Cerebral venous thrombosis and plasma concentrations of factor VIII and von Willebrand factor: a case control study. Journal of Neurology, Neurosurgery, and Psychiatry. 2007; 78:699–701

[70] Bousser MG. Cerebral Vein Thrombosis in Behcet's Syndrome. Archives of Neurology. 1982; 39

[71] Wilder-Smith E, Kothbauer-Margreiter I, Lämmle B, et al. Dural Puncture and Activated protein C Resistance: Risk Factors for Cerebral Venous Sinus Thrombosis. Journal of Neurology, Neurosurgery, and Psychiatry. 1997; 63:351–356

[72] Estanol B, Rodriguez A, Conte G, et al. Intracranial Venous Thrombosis in Young Women. Stroke. 1979; 10:680–684

[73] Brenner B. Haemostatic changes in pregnancy. Thrombosis Research. 2004; 114:409–414

[74] Ferrera PC, Pauze DR, Chan L. Sagittal Sinus Thrombosis After Closed Head Injury. American Journal of Emergency Medicine. 1998; 16:382–385

[75] Elsherbiny SM, Grunewald RA, Powell T. Isolated Inferior Sagittal Sinus Thrombosis: A Case Report. Neuroradiology. 1997; 39:411–413

[76] Gerszten PC, Welch WC, Spearman MP, et al. Isolated Deep Cerebral Venous Thrombosis Treated by Direct Endovascular Thrombolysis. Surgical Neurology. 1997; 48:261–266

[77] Sofferman RA. Cavernous Sinus Thrombosis Secondary to Sphenoid Sinusitis. Laryngoscope. 1983; 93:797–800

[78] Kriss TC, Kriss VM, Warf BC. Cavernous Sinus Thrombophlebitis: Case Report. Neurosurgery. 1996; 39:385–389

[79] Ferro JM, Canhao P, Stam J, et al. Prognosis of cerebral vein and dural sinus thrombosis: results of the International Study on Cerebral Vein and Dural Sinus Thrombosis (ISCVT). Stroke. 2004; 35:664–670

[80] Kalbag RM, Kapp JP, Schmidek HH. Cerebral Venous Thrombosis. In: The Cerebral Venous System and its Disorders. Orlando: Grune and Stratton; 1984:505–536

[81] Lee SK, Kim BS, Terbrugge KG. Clinical Presentation, Imaging and Treatment of Cerebral Venous Thrombosis (CVT). Interv Neuroradiol. 2002; 8:5–14

[82] Bousser MG, Chiras J, Bories J, et al. Cerebral Venous Thrombosis - A Review of 38 Cases. Stroke. 1985; 16:199–213

[83] Perkin GD. Cerebral Venous Thrombosis: Developments in Imaging and Treatment. Journal of Neurology, Neurosurgery, and Psychiatry. 1995; 59:1–3

[84] Lee Seon-Kyu, Mokin Maxim, Hetts StevenW, et al. Current endovascular strategies for cerebral venous thrombosis: report of the SNIS Standards and Guidelines Committee. Journal of NeuroInterventional Surgery. 2018; 10. http://jnis.bmj.com/content/10/8/803.abstract

[85] Yeakley JW, Mayer JS, Patchell LL, et al. The Pseudodelta Sign in Acute Head Trauma. Journal of Neurosurgery. 1988; 69:867–868

[86] Ford K, Sarwar M. Computed tomography of dural sinus thrombosis. AJNR Am J Neuroradiol. 1981; 2:539–543

[87] Rao KCVG, Knipp HC, Wagner EJ. CT Findings in Cerebral Sinus and Venous Thrombosis. Radiology. 1981; 140:391–398

[88] Virapongse C, Cazenave C, Quisling R, et al. The empty delta sign: Frequency and significance in 76 cases of dural sinus thrombosis. Radiology. 1987; 162:779–785

[89] Kosinski CM, Mull M, Schwarz M, et al. Do normal D-dimer levels reliably exclude cerebral sinus thrombosis? Stroke. 2004; 35:2820–2825

[90] Lam AH. Doppler Imaging of Superior Sagittal Sinus Thrombosis. Journal of Ultrasound in Medicine. 1995; 14:41–46

[91] Levine SR, Twyman RE, Gilman S. The Role of Anticoagulation in Cavernous Sinus Thrombosis. Neurology. 1988; 38:517–522

[92] Villringer A, Garner C, Meister W, et al. High-Dose Heparin Treatment in Cerebral Sinus Thrombosis. Stroke. 1988; 19

[93] Einhäupl KM, Villringer A, Meister W, et al. Heparin Treatment in Sinus Venous Thrombosis. Lancet. 1991; 338:597–600

[94] Horton JC, Seiff SR, Pitts LH, et al. Decompression of the Optic Nerve Sheath for Vision-Threatening Papilledema Caused by Dural Sinus Occlusion. Neurosurgery. 1992; 31:203–212

[95] Stam J, Majoie CB, van Delden OM, et al. Endovascular thrombectomy and thrombolysis for severe cerebral sinus thrombosis: a prospective study. Stroke. 2008; 39:1487–1490

[96] Crowley RW, Medel R, Dumont AS. Evolution of cerebral revascularization techniques. Neurosurgical Focus. 2008; 24. DOI: 10.3171/FOC/2008/24/2/E3

[97] Amin-Hanjani S, Butler WE, Ogilvy CS, et al. Extracranial-intracranial bypass in the treatment of occlusive cerebrovascular disease and intracranial aneurysms in the United States between 1992 and 2001: a population-based study. Journal of Neurosurgery. 2005; 103:794–804

[98] EC/IC Study Group. Failure of EC-IC arterial bypass to reduce the risk of ischemic stroke. N Engl J Med 1985; 313:1191–1200

[99] Garrett MC, Komotar RJ, Merkow MB, et al. The extracranial-intracranial bypass trial: implications for future investigations. Neurosurgical Focus 2008; 24. DOI: 10.3171/FOC/2008/24/2/E4

[100] Garrett MC, Komotar RJ, Starke RM, et al. The efficacy of direct extracranial-intracranial bypass in the treatment of symptomatic hemodynamic failure secondary to athero-occlusive disease: a systematic review. Clinical Neurology and Neurosurgery. 2009; 111:319–326

[101] Baron JC, Bousser MG, Rey A, et al. Reversal of focal "misery-perfusion syndrome" by extra-intracranial arterial bypass in hemodynamic cerebral ischemia. A case study with 15O positron emission tomography. Stroke. 1981; 12:454–459

[102] Powers WJ, Press GA, Grubb RL,Jr, et al. The effect of hemodynamically significant carotid artery disease on the hemodynamic status of the cerebral circulation. Annals of Internal Medicine. 1987 106:27–34

[103] Grubb RL,Jr, Powers WJ, Derdeyn CP, et al. The Carotid Occlusion Surgery Study. Neurosurg Focus 2003; 14

[104] Kappelle LJ, Klijn CJ, Tulleken CA. Management of patients with symptomatic carotid artery occlusion. Clinical and Experimental Hypertension 2002; 24:631–637

[105] Kuroda S, Houkin K, Kamiyama H, et al. Long-term prognosis of medically treated patients with internal carotid or middle cerebral artery occlusion can acetazolamide test predict it? Stroke. 2001 32:2110–2116

[106] Hanggi D, Steiger HJ, Vajkoczy P, et al. EC-IC bypass for stroke: is there a future perspective? Acta Neurochir (Wien). 2012; 154:1943–1944

[107] Hanggi D, Steiger HJ, Vajkoczy P. The Role of MCA-STA Bypass Surgery After COSS and JET: The European Point of View. Acta Neurochir Suppl. 2014; 119:77–78

[108] Reynolds MR, Derdeyn CP, Grubb RL,Jr, et al. Extracranial-intracranial bypass for ischemic cerebrovascular disease: what have we learned from the Carotid Occlusion Surgery Study? Neurosurg Focus. 2014; 36. DOI: 10.3171/2013.10.FOCUS134 27

[109] Powers WJ, Clarke WR, Grubb RL,Jr, et al. Extracranial-intracranial bypass surgery for stroke prevention in hemodynamic cerebral ischemia: the Carotid Occlusion Surgery Study randomized trial. JAMA. 2011; 306:1983–1992

[110] Miyamoto S, Yoshimoto T, Hashimoto N, et al. Effects of extracranial-intracranial bypass for patients with hemorrhagic moyamoya disease: results of the Japan Adult Moyamoya Trial. Stroke. 2014; 45:1415–1421

[111] Guzman R, Lee M, Achrol A, et al. Clinical outcome after 450 revascularization procedures for moyamoya disease. Clinical article. J Neurosurg. 2009; 111:927–935

[112] Cantore G, Santoro A, Guidetti G, et al. Surgical treatment of giant intracranial aneurysms: current viewpoint. Neurosurgery. 2008; 63:279–89; discussion 289-90

[113] Mohit AA, Sekhar LN, Natarajan SK, et al. High-flow bypass grafts in the management of complex intracranial aneurysms. Neurosurgery. 2007; 60: ONS105–22; discussion ONS122-3

[114] O'Shaughnessy B A, Salehi SA, Mindea SA, et al. Selective cerebral revascularization as an adjunct in the treatment of giant anterior circulation aneurysms. Neurosurgical Focus. 2003; 14

[115] Schaller B. Extracranial-intracranial bypass to reduce the risk of ischemic stroke in intracranial aneurysms of the anterior cerebral circulation: a systematic review. Journal of Stroke and Cerebrovascular Diseases. 2008; 17:287–298

[116] Sekhar LN, Bucur SD, Bank WO, et al. Venous and arterial bypass grafts for difficult tumors, aneurysms, and occlusive vascular lesions: evolution of surgical treatment and improved graft results. Neurosurgery. 1999; 44:1207–23; discussion 1223-4

[117] Liu JK, Kan P, Karwande SV, et al. Conduits for cerebrovascular bypass and lessons learned from the cardiovascular experience. Neurosurgical Focus. 2003; 14

[118] Yoon S, Burkhardt JK, Lawton MT. Long-term patency in cerebral revascularization surgery: an analysis of a consecutive series of 430 bypasses. J Neurosurg. 2018:1–8

[119] Hayashi T, Shirane R, Fujimura M, et al. Postoperative neurological deterioration in pediatric moyamoya disease: watershed shift and hyperperfusion. J Neurosurg Pediatr. 2010; 6:73–81

Part XX

Intracerebral Hemorrhage

XX

96 Intracerebral Hemorrhage in Older Adults

96.1 Intracerebral hemorrhage – general information

Intracerebral hemorrhage (ICH) is a hemorrhage within the brain parenchyma. In the past it was commonly referred to as "hypertensive hemorrhage," but hypertension is a debatable etiology in many cases; see *Hypertension as a cause?* (p.1612). This section deals primarily with spontaneous intracerebral hemorrhage (sICH), i.e., not due to trauma, tumor, etc. Ongoing trials for this condition may be viewed at www.strokecenter.org/trials/.

Key concepts: intracerebral hemorrhage (ICH) in adults

- the second most common form of stroke (15–30% of strokes), but the most deadly
- unlike ischemic infarct: smooth progressive onset over minutes to hours, often with severe headache, vomiting, and alterations in level of consciousness
- unenhanced CT scan of the brain is the initial diagnostic study of choice
- the volume of the hematoma correlates highly with morbidity and mortality
- ICH enlarges in > 33% of cases within the first 3 hours of onset
- worse prognosis for patient on anticoagulants or with elevated cardiac troponins
- additional diagnostics (e.g., CTA, catheter angiogram, MRV…) if suspicion of underlying abnormality (e.g., AVM, dural sinus thrombosis, neoplasm…)
- hypertension (SBP > 150 mm Hg): reduce SBP to 140
- surgery
  a) supratentorial ICH: still controversial. Surgery does not improve neurologic outcome, but may reduce length of ICU stay and mortality
  b) cerebellar ICH with neurologic deterioration, or brainstem compression, or obstructive hydrocephalus from intraventricular clot: surgical evacuation ASAP (initial treatment with EVD is *not* recommended)

96.2 Epidemiology

96.2.1 Incidence

ICH is the second most common form of stroke (≈ 15–30% of all strokes) (earlier estimates: 10%[1]), and the most deadly. Approximately 12–15 cases per 100,000/yr. Early studies estimated an incidence equal to SAH, but more recent studies in the CT era show approximately twice the incidence as SAH[2] (pre-CT studies may have misclassified some ICH as ischemic stroke, and some cases of ICH that rupture into the subarachnoid space (occurs in ≈ 7%) may have been misclassified as SAH). After a decline in the 1970's, the incidence increased in the 1980s for those age ≥ 65 years.[3] Onset is usually during activity (rarely during sleep), which may be related to elevation of BP or increased CBF; see Etiologies (p.1610).

The diagnosis and management of ICH is a medical emergency. Over 20% of patients deteriorate by ≥ 2 GCS levels between the first EMS assessment and the E/R,[4] and 15–23% of patients deteriorate further within the first few hours in the hospital.[5]

96.2.2 Risk factors

The following are epidemiologic risk factors; see also others (p.1610).
1. age: the incidence increases significantly after age 55 years and doubles with each decade of age until age > 80 yrs where incidence is 25 times that during previous decade. Relative risk for age > 70 yrs is 7
2. gender: more common in men
3. race: in the U.S., ICH affects blacks more than whites. May be related to higher prevalence of poorly controlled HTN in blacks. Incidence may also be higher in Asians[6]
4. previous stroke (any type) increases risk to 23:1
5. alcohol consumption[6,7]:
  a) recent use: moderate or heavy alcohol consumption both within the 24 hours and the week preceding the ICH were independent risk factors for ICH[8] as shown in ▶ Table 96.1

b) chronic use: one study suggests that consuming > 3 drinks a day increases the risk of ICH by ≈ 7 times[9(p 15)]

c) ICH in patients with high ethanol consumption were more commonly lobar than the typical "hypertensive hemorrhages" in the basal ganglia[10]

6. cigarette smoking: increases the risk of SAH and ischemic infarction but probably does *not* increase the risk of ICH,[11,12] further clarification is needed

7. street drugs: cocaine, amphetamines, phencyclidine[13]

8. liver dysfunction: hemostasis may be impaired on the basis of thrombocytopenia, reduced coagulation factors, and hyperfibrinolysis[14] (may be responsible for the increased risk of ICH with chronic EtOH consumption)

Table 96.1 Relative risk of ICH with EtOH consumption

Period prior to ICH	Amount[a] (g EtOH)	Relative risk
24 hours	41–120	4.6
	> 120	11.3
1 week	1–150	2.0
	151–300	4.3
	> 300	6.5

[a]1 standard drink = 12 g EtOH

96.3 Locations of hemorrhage within the brain

96.3.1 General information

Common sites of spontaneous intracerebral hemorrhage (sICH) are shown in ► Table 96.2. Common arterial feeders of ICHs:

1. lenticulostriates: the source of putaminal hemorrhages (possibly secondary to microaneurysms of Charcot-Bouchard, see below)

2. thalamoperforators

3. paramedian branches of BA

4. intraventricular hemorrhage: occurs in ≈ 45% of sICH and is an independent risk factor for worse outcome.[5] May be primary, or more commonly, results from intraventricular extension

Table 96.2 Common sites for ICH (modified[15])

%	Location
50	striate body (basal ganglia); putamen most common; also includes: lenticular nucleus, internal capsule, globus pallidus
15	thalamus
10–15	pons (≈ 90% of these are genuinely hypertensive)
10	cerebellum
10–20	cerebral white matter
1–6	brainstem

96

96.3.2 Lobar hemorrhage

This term was popularized in 1980 after a report delineating 4 clinical syndromes associated with ICH in each of the cerebral lobes[16] (occipital, temporal, frontal, and parietal) as in contrast to hemorrhage of deep structures (e.g., basal ganglion, thalamus, and infratentorial structures).[16] Accounts for 10–32% of nontraumatic ICHs.[16] With large hemorrhages, it may be difficult to distinguish between lobar and deep ICH.

Lobar hemorrhages are more likely to be associated with structural abnormalities than deep hemorrhages (see below). They may also be more common in patients with high alcohol consumption (see above). Lobar hemorrhages may also have a more benign outcome than ganglionic-thalamic hemorrhages.[16]

Etiologies of lobar hemorrhage: Although many causes of ICH can produce lobar hemorrhages (see below for a detailed list), those that are more likely to produce lobar hemorrhages include:

1. extension of a deep hemorrhage

2. cerebral amyloid angiopathy (p. 1612): the most common cause of lobar ICH in elderly normotensive patients
3. trauma
4. hemorrhagic transformation of an ischemic infarct: see below
5. hemorrhagic tumor (p. 1612). Multiple lobar hemorrhages may occur with metastases
6. cerebrovascular malformation (especially AVM) (p. 1524)
7. rupture of an aneurysm: see below for circumstances likely to produce this
8. idiopathic

96.3.3 Internal capsule hemorrhages

There may be prognostic significance with regard to contralateral motor function if the hemorrhage is medial to and/or extending through the internal capsule (IC), or lateral to the IC and merely compressing it, making the clot more accessible to surgical treatment without damaging the IC.

96.4 Etiologies

1. "hypertension" (debatable as a cause or effect, see below) but is a risk factor
   a) acute hypertension (HTN): as may occur in eclampsia (see below) or with certain drugs, e.g., cocaine (p. 215)
   b) chronic HTN: possibly causes degenerative changes within blood vessels
2. possibly associated with acutely increased CBF (globally or focally),[17] especially to areas previously rendered ischemic:
   a) following carotid endarterectomy[18,19]
   b) following repair of congenital heart defects in children[20]
   c) previous stroke (embolic[21] or otherwise): hemorrhagic transformation may occur in up to 43% of strokes during the first month.[22] May follow dislodgment or recanalization of an arterial occlusion, although it has been demonstrated with persistent occlusion.[23] May occur as early as ≤ 24 hrs after a stroke in patients with a negative CT done within 6 hours.[24] Two types[22,25]:
      • type 1: diffuse or multifocal. Heterogeneous or mottled appearance within the boundaries of the stroke. Less hyperdense than primary ICH
      • type 2: extensive hematoma. Probably unifocal source. As hyperdense as primary ICH and may extend outside the original stroke boundaries. Unlike type 1, classically associated with anticoagulation therapy, and tends to occur in initial few days after stroke and is often associated with clinical worsening. May be difficult to distinguish from primary ICH, and may be frequently misdiagnosed as such[24]
   d) migraine: during[26] or following[27] a migraine attack (probably an exceedingly rare event)
   e) following surgery to remove an AVM: "normal perfusion pressure breakthrough." Some cases may be due to incomplete AVM excision
   f) physical factors: following strenuous physical exertion,[28] exposure to cold[29]...
3. vascular anomalies
   a) AVM: rupture; see Arteriovenous malformation (p. 1505)
   b) aneurysm rupture
      • saccular ("berry") aneurysms: (i) **aneurysms of the circle of Willis (COW)**: aneurysms that have become adherent to brain surface by fibrosis as a result of inflammation or previous hemorrhage may produce ICH when they rupture instead of the usual SAH; (ii) **aneurysms distal to the COW** (e.g., MCA aneurysms)
      • microaneurysms of Charcot-Bouchard (p. 1612)
   c) venous angioma rupture: significant ICH from these common lesions is a very rare event
4. "arteriopathies"
   a) cerebral amyloid angiopathy (p. 1612): usually → repeated lobar hemorrhages (see below)
   b) fibrinoid necrosis[1,30] (sometimes seen in cases of amyloid angiopathy)
   c) lipohyalinosis: subintimal lipid-rich hyaline material[31]
   d) cerebral arteritis (including necrotizing angiitis)
5. brain tumor (primary or metastatic): see below
6. coagulation or clotting disorders
   a) leukemia
   b) thrombocytopenia:
      • thrombotic thrombocytopenic purpura
      • aplastic anemia
   c) patients on anticoagulation therapy (p. 1613) constitute 12–20% of patients with ICH[5]

96

d) patients receiving thrombolytic therapy:
- for acute ischemic stroke: incidence of *symptomatic* ICH within 36 hrs of treatment with rtPA is 6.4% (vs. 0.6% in the placebo-treated group)[32]
- for acute MI or other thrombosis: incidence is ≈ 0.36–2%.[33,34,35] Risk is increased with higher doses than the recommended 100 mg of alteplase (Activase®, recombinant tissue plasminogen activator (rt-PA))[36] in older patients, in those with anterior MI or higher Killip class, and with bolus administration (vs. infusion).[37] When heparin was used adjunctively, higher doses were associated with higher risk of ICH.[38] ICH is thought to occur in those patients with some preexisting underlying vascular abnormality.[39] Immediate coronary angioplasty is safer than rt-PA when available[35]

e) aspirin therapy:
- one ASA qod was associated with increased risk of ICH,[40] with a rate of 0.2–0.8% per year[41]
- ASA 100 mg/d did not increase the risk of significant ICH in patients > 60 yrs with mild-to-moderate head injury (GCS ≥ 9)[42]

f) Vitamin E supplements[43]: associated with reduction of 1 ischemic stroke in 476 individuals, and increase of 1 ICH in 1,250 patients taking vitamin E

7. CNS infection:
   a) especially fungal, which damages blood vessels
   b) granulomas
   c) herpes simplex encephalitis: may initially produce low-density lesions that progress to hemorrhagic ones

8. venous or dural sinus thrombosis (p. 1594)

9. drug-related
   a) substance abuse
   - alcohol: consumption of > 3 drinks/day increases the risk of ICH ≈ 7-fold (p. 1608)
   - drug abuse: especially sympathomimetics (cocaine,[44,45] amphetamine[46])
   b) drugs that raise BP:
   - alpha-adrenergic agonists (sympathomimetics): including phenylephrine, ephedrine,[47] and pseudoephedrine[48,49]
   - ephedra alkaloids: sold as a dietary supplement (ma huang) to suppress appetite and increase energy. Associated in case reports with HTN, SAH, ICH, seizures, and death[50]

10. posttraumatic: often in a delayed fashion[51,52]; see **Hemorrhagic contusion** (p. 1071)

11. pregnancy-related: the risk of ICH in pregnancy and puerperium (up to 6 weeks postpartum) is ≈ 1 in 9,500 births[53]
    a) most commonly associated with eclampsia or preeclampsia: the mortality of eclampsia is ≈ 6% with ICH being the most frequent direct cause[54]; also see Pregnancy & intracranial hemorrhage (p. 1425)
    b) postpartum ICH (median 8 days, range 3–35 days) in the absence of eclampsia has been reported[55]; when associated with vasculopathy the term **postpartum cerebral angiopathy** has been used
    c) vascular findings:
    - some cases associated with isolated cerebral vasculopathy in the absence of systemic vasculitis[56]
    - some cases demonstrate vasospasm
    - some cases show findings (e.g., patchy enhancement in occipital lobes) suggestive of cerebrovascular dysautoregulation (p. 1536)
    - some cases show no vascular-related abnormalities

12. postoperative:
    a) following carotid endarterectomy (see above)
    b) following craniotomy:
    - at site of craniotomy[57]: risk factors identified: within residual astrocytoma after subtotal resection, following craniotomy for AVM (see above)
    - at site remote from craniotomy. In a series of 37 patients, unlike hematomas at the craniotomy site, the following were identified as *not* being related to risk of hemorrhage: HTN, coagulopathy, CSF drainage, underlying occult lesion following drainage of chronic SDH (p. 1082), and cerebellar hemorrhage following pterional craniotomy[58] (this author incriminated possibly rapid overdrainage of CSF), or following temporal lobectomy[59]

13. idiopathic[16]

96.4.1 Cerebellar hemorrhage etiologies

Etiologies are similar to ICH of any location; however, some nuances:

1. HTN is a factor in up to two-thirds of cerebellar hemorrhages

96

2. AVM is a consideration, aneurysm is very rare (possibly AICA aneurysm, but usually only in association with other high-flow lesions, e.g., AVM[60])
3. may be related to recent previous spinal or supratentorial surgery

96.4.2 Hypertension as a cause?

Hypertension (HTN) is controversial as cause of ICH since the incidence of both ICH and HTN increases with age (66% of patients > 65 yrs have HTN). The relative risk for ICH with HTN is 3.9–5.4, depending on the definition of HTN used.[61] Many patients with ICH are dramatically hypertensive on presentation; however, acute elevations of ICP from the hemorrhage may actually precipitate HTN (part of Cushing's triad, see ▶ Table 62.2). HTN is probably a risk factor primarily for pontine/cerebellar ICH and is probably not a factor in at least 35% of basal ganglion hemorrhages.

96.4.3 Microaneurysms of Charcot-Bouchard

AKA miliary aneurysms.[62] Occur primarily at bifurcation of small (< 300 mcm) perforating branches of lateral lenticulostriate arteries in basal ganglia (found in 46% of hypertensive patients over age 66, but only in 7% of controls[63]). Possibly the origin of some "hypertensive" ganglionic (putaminal) hemorrhages,[64] but this is controversial.

96.4.4 (Cerebral) amyloid angiopathy

Cerebral amyloid angiopathy (CAA) AKA congophilic angiopathy. Pathologic deposition of beta amyloid protein (appears as birefringent "apple-green" under polarized light when stained with congo red) within the media of small meningeal and cortical vessels (especially those in white matter) without evidence of systemic amyloidosis.[65] Some vessels may show fibrinoid necrosis of vessel wall.[66,67] There is a treatable subset of CAA with inflammation (see below).

CAA should be suspected in patients with *recurrent* hemorrhages (uncommon with "hypertensive hemorrhages" (p. 1608) [68]) that are *lobar* in location. Gradient-echo MRI may identify petechial hemorrhages (microbleeds) or hemosiderin deposits from small cortical hemorrhages.[69] Less likely in the case of basal ganglion or brainstem hemorrhages.[16]

Incidence increases with age: CAA is present in ≈ 50% of those over 70 years of age,[70] but most do not hemorrhage. CAA is probably responsible for ≈ 10% of cases of ICH. May be associated with genetic factors (including the apolipoprotein E ε4 allele[71]), and may be more prevalent in patients with Down syndrome. Although they are distinct diseases, there is some overlap between CAA and Alzheimer's disease; the amyloid in CAA is identical to that found in senile plaques of Alzheimer's disease. CAA may increase the risk of ICH by potentiating plasminogen[72] (may be of special relevance to patients receiving tissue plasminogen activator (t-PA) to treat MI or stroke).

Patients with CAA may present with a TIA-like prodrome (see below).

Among patients with lobar hemorrhage, those with the apoE ε4 allele typically have their first hemorrhage > 5 yrs earlier than noncarriers (73 ± 8 yrs vs. 79 ± 7 yrs).[71]

Diagnostic tests are useful mainly to rule out other conditions. The definitive diagnosis of CAA requires pathologic evaluation of brain tissue. Criteria for the diagnosis of CAA are shown in ▶ Table 96.3.[73]

A subset of CAA patients treatable with immunosuppressants have CAA-related inflammation (CAA-ri) as a result of an autoimmune response to the amyloid protein. These patients present with H/A, subacute cognitive impairment or seizures, with vasogenic edema on imaging. Anti-β-amyloid antibodies appear in the CSF, but currently no clinical test is available. To avoid resorting to brain biopsy, MRI criteria for probable CAA-ri have been developed: uni- or multi-focal asymmetric white matter hyperintensities that extend to subcortical in addition to the typical CAA findings of lobar-ICH, microbleeds, superficial siderosis... (82% sensitive, 97% specific).[74]

96.4.5 Hemorrhagic brain tumors

Although any brain tumor can hemorrhage, tumoral ICH is usually associated with malignancies. Tumors on occasion can also produce SAH or subdural hematomas.

Malignant tumors most commonly associated with ICH:
1. glioblastoma
2. lymphoma
3. metastatic tumors
   a) melanoma[75,76]: ≈ 40% hemorrhage
   b) choriocarcinoma[75,77,78]: ≈ 60% hemorrhage

Table 96.3 Criteria for the diagnosis of cerebral amyloid angiopathy (CAA)[73]

Diagnosis	Criteria
definite CAA	full postmortem exam showing all 3 of the following: a) lobar, cortical, or corticosubcortical hemorrhage b) severe CAA c) absence of another diagnostic lesion
probable CAA with supporting pathological evidence	clinical data & pathological tissue showing all 3 of the following: a) lobar, cortical, or corticosubcortical hemorrhage b) some degree of vascular amyloid deposition in specimen c) absence of another diagnostic lesion
probable CAA	clinical data and MRI findings showing all 3 of the following: a) age ≥ 60 yrs b) multiple hemorrhages restricted to the lobar, cortical, or corticosubcortical region c) absence of another cause of hemorrhage[a]
possible CAA	clinical data and MRI findings: a) age ≥ 60 yrs b) single lobar, cortical, or corticosubcortical hemorrhage without another cause[a], or multiple hemorrhages with a possible but not a definite cause[a], or with some hemorrhages in an atypical location (e.g., brainstem)

[a]e.g., excessive anticoagulation (INR > 3.0), head trauma, ischemic stroke, CNS tumor, cerebrovascular malformation, vasculitis, or blood dyscrasia

c) renal cell carcinoma
d) bronchogenic carcinoma: although only ≈ 9% hemorrhage, this tumor is such a frequent source of cerebral mets that it therefore is a more common source of tumoral ICH

Malignant tumors that hemorrhage less commonly include:
1. medulloblastoma[79,80,81,82] (most commonly in children)
2. gliomas[83,84]

Some *benign* brain tumors that have been associated with ICH include:
1. meningiomas have been associated with intratumoral, subdural, and nearby parenchymal hemorrhage.[85,86,87,88] Tendency to bleed is similar for angioblastic variety as for other highly vascular meningiomas
2. PitNET/adenoma: see Pituitary apoplexy (p.865)
3. oligodendroglioma (relatively benign): rarely presents with hemorrhage,[89] classically after years of causing seizures
4. hemangioblastoma[90]
5. vestibular schwannoma[91,92,93]
6. cerebellar astrocytoma[94]

96.4.6 Anticoagulation preceding ICH

10% of patients on warfarin (Coumadin®) develop a significant bleeding complication per year (not all are intracranial), including ICH (65% mortality in this group). The risk of ICH in patients treated with warfarin for a-fib varies between 0–0.3% per year[41] (historically, this was as high as ≈ 1.8% in older studies[95] from the 1960s and 1970s), but when an elderly subgroup (mean age 80 yrs) was analyzed, this rate was 1.8% per year.[41] ICH was the only cause of fatal bleeding complications of warfarin therapy in one series where the cumulative risk of a fatal hemorrhage was 1% at 1 year and 2% at 3 yrs.[96]

The risk of hemorrhagic complications was increased with the length and also the variability of the PT, and during the first three months of anticoagulation.[96] Patients with cerebral amyloid angiopathy (CAA) (see above) are also at increased risk of ICH following administration of antiplatelet drugs or anticoagulants.[73]

96.5 Clinical

96.5.1 General information

In general, the neurologic deficit with ICH is characterized by a smooth progressive onset over minutes to hours, unlike embolic/ischemic stroke where deficit is maximal at onset. With ICH, severe

96

headache, vomiting, and alterations in level of consciousness may be more common (H/A may not be more prevalent than in embolic stroke, but it is often a first and prominent symptom[16]).

96.5.2 Prodrome

TIA-like symptoms may precede lobar hemorrhages[97,98] in patients with CAA, and may occur in up to ≈ 50% of patients for whom a complete history is obtainable. Unlike typical TIAs, these usually consist of numbness, tingling, or weakness (corresponding to the area where the hemorrhage will subsequently occur) that gradually spreads in a manner reminiscent of a Jacksonian-march and may spill-over vascular territories (probably an electrical phenomenon rather than an ischemic event). This is suggestive of but not pathognomonic for the subsequent development of lobar ICH.

96.5.3 Concomitants of specific lesions in ICH

Putaminal hemorrhage

The most common site for ICH. Smooth gradual deterioration in 62% (maximal deficit at onset in 30%); never fluctuating. Contralateral hemiparesis, may progress to hemiplegia or even coma or death. H/A in 14% at onset. No H/A at any time in 72%. Papilledema and subhyaloid preretinal hemorrhage are rare.

Thalamic hemorrhage

Classically, contralateral hemisensory loss. Also hemiparesis when the internal capsule is involved. Extension into upper brainstem → vertical gaze palsy, retraction nystagmus, skew deviation, loss of convergence, ptosis, miosis, anisocoria, ± unreactive pupils. H/A in 20–40%. Motor deficit similar to putaminal hemorrhage, but contralateral sensory deficit widespread and striking. Hydrocephalus may occur from compression of CSF pathways.

In 41 patients, when hemorrhage > 3.3 cm on CT, all died. Smaller hematomas usually caused permanent disability.

Cerebellar hemorrhage

See ▶ Fig. 96.1. May include any combination of the following:
1. symptoms of increased ICP (lethargy, N/V, HTN with bradycardia…) due to hydrocephalus, which may occur as a result of:
   a) compression of the 4th ventricle → obstruction of CSF
   b) extension of the hemorrhage into the ventricular system
2. direct compression of brainstem may produce:
   a) facial palsy: due to pressure on the facial colliculus
   b) these patients classically become comatose without first having hemiparesis, unlike many supratentorial etiologies

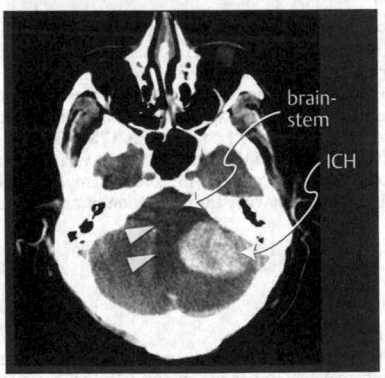

Fig. 96.1 Spontaneous left cerebellar hemisphere ICH in 73-year-old male.
Axial CT showing ICH producing brainstem compression and obliteration of the 4th ventricle. The patient had hydrocephalus. There is also edema (low-density) in the cerebellar vermis and brainstem (*yellow arrowheads*) most likely due to ischemia.

Lobar hemorrhage

Syndromes associated with hemorrhage in the 4 cerebral lobes[16] ($\approx$ 50% have H/A as a first and prominent symptom):

1. frontal lobe (the most distinctive of the syndromes): frontal H/A with contralateral hemiparesis, usually in the arm with mild leg and facial weakness
2. parietal lobe: contralateral hemisensory deficit and mild hemiparesis
3. occipital lobe: ipsilateral eye pain and contralateral homonymous hemianopsia, some may spare superior quadrant
4. temporal lobe: on dominant side, produces fluent dysphasia with poor auditory comprehension but relatively good repetition

96.5.4 Delayed deterioration

General information

Deterioration after the initial hemorrhage is usually due to any combination of the following:

1. rebleeding: see below
2. edema: see below
3. hydrocephalus: higher risk with intraventricular extension or posterior fossa ICH
4. seizures
5. increased ICP

Rebleeding or extension of bleed

Early rebleeding: Rebleeding (more so in basal ganglion hemorrhages than in lobar hemorrhages) has been documented during the first hour by "ultra-early" scanning and repeating CT scans. Rebleeding is usually accompanied by clinical deterioration.[99] The incidence of hematoma enlargement decreases with time, 33–38% in 1–3 hrs,[100] 16% in 3–6 hrs, and 14% between 24 hrs of onset and a second CT within 24 hrs of the first.[101] Risk of early rebleeding is increased in patients with a "spot sign" on CTA (p. 1616). Patients with enlarging hematomas were more likely to have larger hematomas and/or coagulopathy, and had a worse outcome.[101] Rebleeding may still occur following surgical evacuation of clot even with satisfactory intraoperative hemostasis. Hemostatic agents (p. 1619) (e.g., NovoSeven®) may reduce this risk.

Late rebleeding: Quoted rates for late rebleeding from ICH range from 1.8–5.3% (depending on length of follow-up).[102] Diastolic BP was significantly higher in the group with recurrent hemorrhage, with a 10%/yr risk for DBP > 90 mm Hg vs. < 1.5% for DBP ≤ 90 (mean F/U of 67 months).[102] Other risk factors include diabetes and tobacco and alcohol abuse.[103] Recurrent hemorrhages may indicate underlying vascular malformations or amyloid angiopathy (lobar rebleeding is likely to be due to amyloid angiopathy[103]).

Edema

Edema and ischemic necrosis around the hemorrhage may cause delayed deterioration.[1] Although necrosis from mass effect of the clot contributes a small part to the edema, experiments indicate that by itself, the mass effect is insufficient to account for the amount of edema that occurs. It is believed that an edemogenic toxin is released from the clot. Experiments with various components of blood clots have disclosed that thrombin in concentrations that could be released from the clot causes increased permeability of the blood-brain barrier, and is also a potent vasoconstrictor. This is the leading suspect as the major cause of delayed edema and deterioration. Also see Cerebral edema (p. 90).

96.6 Evaluation

96.6.1 Overview

Practice guideline: Initial diagnosis & assessment in spontaneous ICH

Level I[5]:
- obtain a baseline severity score
- rapid imaging with noncontrast CT (or MRI) to differentiate from ischemic stroke

96

Level II[5]:
- consider CTA & contrast CT to identify patients at risk for hematoma expansion
- consider CT venogram, contrast CT, contrast MRI, MRA, and/or catheter angiogram as appropriate when clinical or imaging suspicion of underlying abnormality (vascular or neoplastic)

96.6.2 CT scan

General information

Noncontrast head CT scan is the usual initial imaging procedure of choice. It is rapid, has few contra-indications, and easily demonstrates blood as high-density within the brain parenchyma immediately after hemorrhage.

Although mass effect is common, the tendency for the hemorrhage to dissect through brain tissue often results in less mass effect than would be anticipated from the size of the clot.

Volume measurements on CT scan

ICH volume carries prognostic significance. It can be measured volumetrically using computer algorithms available on some CT scanners, or it can very simply be approximated by the ellipsoid method[104] as shown in Eq (96.1), where AP, LAT, and HT are the *diameters* of the clot in each of the 3 dimensions (anteroposterior, lateral, and height). This estimate was originally developed for AVMs, based on the principle that the volume of an ellipsoid is approximately half of that of a parallele-piped into which it is placed[105] and is simpler than other slightly more accurate estimation methods.[106] An illustration of the measurements is shown in ▶ Fig. 96.2. To estimate the height of a lesion when only axial images are available (as on some CTs), count the number of images on which the lesion is seen, and multiply by the slice thickness of the CT cuts[104,106,107] (this information is usually indicated on the images), or subtract the table position of the highest cut that shows the clot from the table position of the lowest cut showing the clot.

$$\text{ellipsoid volume} \approx \frac{AP \times LAT \times HT}{2} \qquad (96.1)$$

On average, the size of the clot decreases ≈ 0.75 mm/day, and the density decreases by ≈ 2 CT units/day, with little change for the first 2 wks.

96.6.3 CT angiography (CTA)

Not necessary to identify ICH. However, CTA is very sensitive and specific in detecting vascular lesions (e.g., AVM or aneurysm). May also demonstrate the "spot sign"[108]: a small enhancing focus within an acute ICH (see ▶ Fig. 96.2 panel C) which correlated with increased risk of hematoma expansion.

CTA has supplanted catheter angiography in most situations. Indications for CTA include:
- subarachnoid hemorrhage
- findings suggestive of cerebral venous thrombosis (p. 1594) (CVT): increased attenuation in dural sinuses or cortical veins
- enlarged vessels/flow voids or rim calcifications suggestive of AVM
- also see entry under Management guidelines (p. 1620) below

96.6.4 MRI

Usually *not* the procedure of choice for initial study. Disadvantages compared to CT scan:
1. does not show blood well within the first few hours (gradient echo and SWI are the best sequences)
2. difficult to ventilate or access patient during the study
3. slower and more expensive, not available in as many E/Rs
4. contraindications e.g., claustrophobia in awake patients, as well as others that may not be known at the time of initial evaluation (e.g., shrapnel in the eye, non-MRI-compatible pacemaker or spinal cord stimulator...)

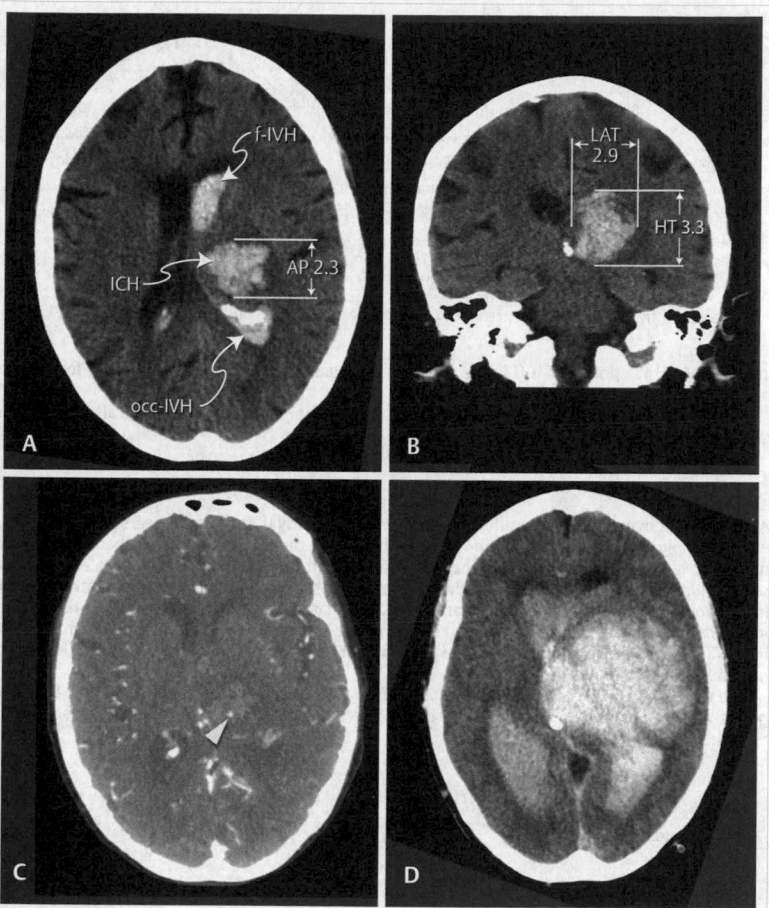

Fig. 96.2 Spontaneous left thalamic ICH in 71-year-old female.
A: axial CT showing ICH with ventricular extension (f-IVH = intraventricular hemorrhage in frontal horn of left lateral ventricle, occ-IVH = IVH in occipital horn).
B: coronal CT.
Estimated ICH volume = (2.3 cm X 2.9 cm X 3.3 cm)/2 = 11 cc.
C: CTA done immediately after CT shown in A & B, demonstrating a "spot sign" (*yellow arrowhead*) within the ICH.
D: Repeat CT scan done 1 hour later showing massive enlargement of ICH.
AP = AP dimension of ICH in cm, LAT = mediolateral dimension, HT = height.

May be useful later, e.g., to help diagnose cerebral amyloid angiopathy (CAA) (p. 1612).

The appearance of ICH on MRI is very complicated. It is highly dependent on the age of the clot[109] s summarized in (▶ Table 96.4).

6.6.5 Catheter cerebral angiography

For diagnosing ICH itself, angiography cannot reliably differentiate the mass effect due to an ICH from that due to an ischemic infarct or tumor.[110] May demonstrate AVMs and aneurysms when they are associated with the ICH. The yield may be increased by delaying the study.[16] May demonstrate vascular blush in some cases of tumor. Normal arteriography cannot eliminate cerebral amyloid

Table 96.4 Variation of brain MRI signal characteristics of intraparenchymal blood over time (modified[109])

Phase	Approximate time after onset	Hemoglobin (Hgb) state	T1 MRI[a]	T2 MRI[a]	Mnemonic[b]
hyperacute	0–6 hrs[c]	oxy-Hgb (intracellular)	I	B (slight ↑)	I be
acute	6–72 hrs	deoxy-Hgb (intracellular)	I (or slight ↑)	D	iddy
early subacute	3–7 d	met-Hgb (intracellular)	B	D	biddy
late subacute	7–14 d	met-Hgb (extracellular[d])	B	B	baby
chronic	>2 weeks[e]	hemosiderin (intracellular)	D (slight ↑)	D	doodoo

[a] B = bright (hyperintense compared to brain), D = dark (hypointense), I = isointense
[b] silly/easy-to-remember mnemonic made from I, B, or D in the preceding columns
[c] some authors consider up to about 24 hrs as hyperacute
[d] when RBCs lyse, the Hgb becomes extracellular
[e] the center of the clot may be isointense on T1 and slightly hyperintense on T2

angiopathy as the etiology of ICH in the elderly.[111] CTA has supplanted most indications for catheter angiography.

Indications for CTA/catheter angiography in ICH: see entry under Nonsurgical management guidelines (p. 1620).

96.6.6 ICH score

A caveat about overreliance on grading systems, especially early in the course, bears discussion. In an effort to apply evidence-based methodology to the care of the ICH patient, a number of prognostic models have been developed. While they are helpful, their development may have been biased by self-fulfilling prophecies based on withdrawal of medical support in the face of apparently devastating neurologic injury. The American Heart Association statement on "Palliative and End-of-Life Care in Stroke"[112] discusses palliative care, and it is recommended that in the absence of known preexisting DNR wishes, the decision to withdraw support not be made until at least the second full day of hospitalization after ICH (Level II[5]).

The widely used ICH score[113] assigns points based on 5 features as indicated in ▶ Table 96.5. The points are then summed for the "ICH score." The associated 30-day mortality is tabulated in ▶ Table 96.6.

Table 96.5 ICH Score[113]

Graded feature	Criteria	Points	Score
GCS (Glasgow coma scale score; ▶ Table 18.1)	3–4	2	(0 - 2)
	5–12	1	
	13–15	0	
Age[a]	≥80 yrs	1	(0 - 1)
	<80 yrs	0	
Location	infratentorial	1	(0 - 1)
	supratentorial	0	
ICH volume see Eq (96.1)	≥30 cc	1	(0 - 1)
	<30 cc	0	
Intraventricular blood	yes	1	(0 - 1)
	no	0	
ICH Score → TOTAL			(0 – 6)

[a] possible bias since treatment decisions in elderly patients may have differed from younger patients

96

Table 96.6 Mortality based on ICH Score

ICH Score[a]	30-day mortality	N[b]
0	0%	26
1	13%	32
2	26%	27
3	72%	32
4	97%	29
5	100%	6
6	? 100%[c]	0

[a] from ► Table 96.5
[b] N is the number of patients with that score
[c] no patient in the study had a score of 6, but "it is expected this would be associated with a high rate of mortality"[113]

96.7 Initial management of ICH

96.7.1 History checklist

The following checklist is presented to assist in gathering historical information important in evaluating & managing the adult with spontaneous ICH (modified)[5]:

1. time course of symptoms: time of initial onset (or when last seen normal)
2. initial symptoms and progression
3. seizure
4. hypertension history
5. drugs:
   a) sympathomimetics:
      • amphetamines, cocaine
      • appetite suppressants or nasal decongestants (pseudoephedrine)
   b) dietary supplements: especially ephedra alkaloids (ma huang)
   c) anticoagulants: warfarin (Coumadin®), dabigatran (Pradaxa®), apixaban (Eliquis®)...
   d) antiplatelet drugs: aspirin (patients often forget taking low-dose 81 mg), Plavix, NSAIDS
   e) oral contraceptive (birth control pills): questionable association
   f) history of alcohol abuse
6. past medical history
   a) coagulopathies
   b) history of dementia: ICH may be associated with cerebral amyloid angiopathy (p. 1612)
   c) liver disease: may be associated with coagulopathy
   d) previous stroke
   e) history of known vascular abnormalities (AVM, venous angioma...)
   f) tumor: known history of cancer, especially those that tend to go to brain (lung, breast, GI, renal, melanoma...) or associated with coagulopathy (leukemia)
7. recent surgery: especially carotid stenting or endarterectomy, procedures requiring heparin...
8. recent childbirth and/or eclampsia or preeclampsia
9. history of recent trauma

96.7.2 Initial laboratory tests

1. CBC (including platelet count), electrolytes (including BUN/creatinine and glucose): hyperglycemia is associated with worse prognosis
2. PT/INR & aPTT
3. cardiac-specific troponins: elevation is associated with worse outcome
4. toxicology screen (urine or serum): mainly for cocaine and/or sympathomimetics
5. pregnancy test in women of childbearing potential

96.7.3 Nonsurgical management outline

The following assumes the diagnosis has already been made, usually on CT scan. There is not uniform agreement on many management aspects. The following is offered as a guide.
1. patients should initially be managed in an ICU or dedicated stroke unit by personnel experienced in critical care (Level I[5])

96

2. hypertension (HTN) may contribute to further bleeding, especially within the first hour.[99] However, some HTN may be needed to maintain perfusion. See practice guideline (p. 1621)
3. intubate if stuporous or comatose
4. maintain normothermia: treatment of fever after ICH may be reasonable (Level II[5]) (NB: a causal relation between fever and worse outcome and/or increase in ICH is not established; mild hypothermia is considered investigational)
5. antiseizure medications
   a) seizures (clinical and subclinical) are treated with appropriate ASMs
   b) ✖ prophylactic ASMs: not recommended
   c) ASM options
      • Keppra has a very favorable therapeutic/toxic profile. Dose 500 mg BID
      • OR phenytoin (p. 488) (Dilantin®): load with 17 mg/kg slow IV over 1 hour, follow with 100 mg q 8 hrs
6. hemostatic issues:
   a) INR (or PT), PTT & platelet count (PC), platelet function assay (PFA)
      • correct coagulopathies, see Correction of coagulopathies or reversal of anticoagulants (p. 174)
      • platelets: correct thrombocytopenia or platelet-inhibiting drugs as discussed below
   b) ✖ bleeding time: obsolete, not generally helpful
   c) for hemostasis management issues, see practice guideline (p. 1621)
7. steroids: ✖ not recommended for ICH[5] (exception: if underlying tumor is identified)
8. treat intracranial hypertension presumptively: mannitol and/or furosemide as tolerated, also helps with HTN; for more, see Treatment measures for elevated ICP (p. 1046). If significant problems from suspected increased ICP, consider ICP monitor
9. external ventricular drain (EVD): for hydrocephalus (✖ but not for hydrocephalus associated with cerebellar hemorrhage – see below), some cases of intraventricular blood, or to manage ICP (see below). ✖ R/O coagulopathy before placing
10. follow electrolytes and osmolarity:
    a) monitor for hyponatremia (possible SIADH (p. 118))
    b) maintain euglycemia: avoid hyper- or hypoglycemia (Level I[5])
11. **cardiac:** systematic screening for myocardial ischemia or infarction is recommended. EKG & cardiac enzymes should be checked routinely (Level II[5])
12. swallowing: formal screening for dysphagia before initiating oral intake is recommended (Level I[5])
13. **CTA or catheter angiography:** primarily to R/O underlying vascular malformation, aneurysm (a less common cause of ICH) & tumor (which is usually better diagnosed on contrast CT or MRI)
    a) if urgent surgery is indicated (e.g., for herniation), the delay in obtaining an angiogram may be detrimental and it may be best deferred to post-op
    b) ★ indications: angiography is not routinely recommended for patients > 45 yrs of age with preexisting hypertension *and* ICH in thalamus, putamen, or posterior fossa because there was a 0% yield out of 29 patients in this group[114] and low yield in all patients with isolated deep ICH.[115] It may be considered for:
       • patients > 45 yrs with a history of HTN and a *lobar* ICH: angiography had a 10% yield,[114] with the ratio of AVM:aneurysm ≈ 4.3:1
       • patients with intraventricular hemorrhage (without parenchymal hematoma): the yield c angiography was ≈ 65%,[114] primarily AVM
    c) an underlying lesion may be obliterated by ICH, especially acutely. If initial angio is negative repeat after CT shows resorption of clot (≈ in 2–3 mos). If still negative, follow CT or MRI q 4 6 mos for ≈ 1 year to R/O tumor.[1] Delaying the initial angiogram for several weeks may increase the yield and is also an option[16]
    d) MRI/MRA has only ≈ 90% sensitivity for detecting structural abnormalities in this setting, and so a negative study cannot completely exclude this possibility[114]
    e) the yield of angiography in ICH would be expected to be lower in patients at increased risk ICH: patients on warfarin (Coumadin®), chronic alcoholics, patients with amyloid angiopathy...

Practice guideline: Blood pressure management in patients with ICH

1. patients with SBP 150–200 mm Hg and no contraindication to acute BP management: lowering SBP to 140[a] is safe (Level I[5]) and improves functional outcome (Level II[5])
2. patients with SBP > 200 mm Hg: it is reasonable to consider aggressive reduction of BP with continuous IV infusion and monitoring of BP (Level II[5])

[a] since the publication of these guidelines,[5] the INTERACT-II[116] & ATACH-2[117] trials have shown that rebleeding occurs despite blood pressure control, and that reducing SBP < 140 mm Hg is associated with increased incidence of adverse renal events[117] probably from hypoperfusion

Practice guideline: Seizure & ASM management in patients with ICH

1. treat clinical seizures, or seizures on EEG in patients with altered mental status (Level I[5])
2. continuous EEG monitoring is probably indicated when depression of mental status is out of proportion to the degree of brain injury (Level II[5])
3. prophylactic ASMs are not recommended (Level III[5])

Practice guideline: Hemostasis & coagulopathy in patients with ICH

1. for severe coagulation factor deficiency or severe thrombocytopenia: replace deficient factors or administer platelets (Level I[5])
2. patients on vitamin K antagonists (VKA) (e.g., warfarin) with elevated INR:
   a) withhold VKA (Level I[5])
   b) replace vitamin K-dependent clotting factors (Level I[5])
   c) correct the INR (Level I[5])
      • consider prothrombin complex concentrate (PCC) (p. 174) over FFP because PCC may have fewer complications, and corrects INR faster & closer to normal (Level II[5])
      • ✘ not recommended: rFVIIa (doesn't replace all clotting factors & may not restore clotting in vivo despite normalization of INR, & thromboembolic complications also occur) (Level III[5])
   d) administer IV vitamin K (Level I[5])
3. patients on dabigatran (Pradaxa®)[a], rivaroxaban (Xarelto®)[a], or apixaban (Eliquis®)[a]: consider treatment with activated PCC factor eight bypassing activity (FEIBA), other PCCs or vFVIIa (Level II[5]); consider dialysis for dabigatran (Level II[5])
4. patients on heparin: consider reversal with protamine sulfate (Level II[5])
5. patients on antiplatelet drugs: platelet transfusion is of uncertain benefit (Level II[5])
6. ✘ not recommended: rFVIIa in unselected ICH patients (no clear clinical benefit) (Level III[5])

[a] subsequent to publication of these guidelines,[5] the following reversal agents have become available and may be considered (not part of guidelines): idarucizumab (p. 173) for dabigatran, andexanet alfa (p. 175) for rivaroxaban or apixaban

Practice guideline: Prophylaxis & treatment of thromboembolism in patients with ICH

1. intermittent pneumatic compression device beginning the day of admission to prevent DVT (Level I[5]). ✘ not recommended: graduated compression device to prevent DVT or improve outcome (Level III[5])

96

2. after documentation of cessation of bleeding: consider low-dose sub-Q heparin (LMW or unfractionated) to prevent DVT in patients with lack of mobility after 1–4 days from ICH (Level II[5])
3. for patients with symptomatic DVT or PE: systemic anticoagulation or IVC filter placement is probably indicated (Level II[5]). The choice of modality should consider the time from ICH, ICH stability, cause of ICH, & overall patient condition (Level II[5])

▶ **Thrombocytopenia or platelet inhibiting drugs**
1. thrombocytopenia: in general situations platelet transfusions are recommended only for PC < 50 K, but ICH is so serious that it is suggested to keep PC > 100K (if this is difficult to attain, aim for platelet count > 75K)
2. benefit of platelet transfusion in patients receiving platelet-inhibiting drugs (e.g., aspirin or Plavix®) is uncertain
3. when needed: start with 6 units of platelets; see Platelets (p. 161)

▶ **NovoSeven® (recombinant-activated coagulation factor VII [rFVIIa]). ✗** Use in ICH is not recommended.[5] FDA-approved for various bleeding diatheses (including hemophiliacs with antibodies to factor VIII or IX). Initial results appeared promising for ICH[118]; however, further study could not show clear benefit in noncoagulopathic patients, and thromboembolic complications also occurred.

96.7.4 Anticoagulation following ICH

> ### Practice guideline: Resumption of anticoagulation in patients following ICH
>
> 1. for nonvalvular a-fib: long-term anticoagulation with warfarin should probably be avoided after warfarin-associated lobar ICH because of relatively high risk of recurrence (Level II[5])
> 2. for strong indications, consider anticoagulation after nonlobar sICH or antiplatelet monotherapy after any sICH (Level II[5])
> 3. optimal timing to resume treatment is uncertain
>   • avoidance of oral anticoagulant (OAC) use for at least 4 weeks after OAC-associated ICH in patients without mechanical heart valves may decrease the risk of recurrent ICH (Level II[5])
>   • if indicated, aspirin monotherapy can probably be resumed in the days following ICH although optimal timing is uncertain (Level II[5])
> 4. substitution of dabigatran, rivaroxaban, or apixaban for warfarin in patients with a-fib in an effort to reduce the risk of recurrent ICH is uncertain (Level II[5])
> 5. data regarding use of statins after ICH is insufficient to make recommendations (Level II[5])

96

Patients with ICH who subsequently require anticoagulation (e.g., for embolic ischemic stroke or for mechanical heart valve) pose a management dilemma. In the case of embolic disease, the fear of converting an ischemic infarct to a hematoma or increasing the size of a small ICH with continued anticoagulation has traditionally outweighed the possible benefit of protection from further embolization. However, an anecdotal (retrospective uncontrolled) report of 12 such patients found no incidence of increased intracranial bleeding with either continued anticoagulation (6 patients) or resumption of anticoagulation after a hiatus (several days in 4 patients, 5 days in 1, and 14 days in 1).[119] In another study,[120] none of 35 patients who had resumption of warfarin had recurrent intracranial hemorrhage (ICH, SAH, or subdural hematoma). While this does not prove that anticoagulation is safe after ICH, it does demonstrate that if there is a strong indication for anticoagulation, and if there is not an acceptable alternative (e.g., Greenfield filter for DVT (p. 179)), that anticoagulation in this setting is not always met with disastrous results.

The probability of having an ischemic stroke at 30 days following cessation of warfarin for a median of 10 days using Kaplan-Meier survival estimates are approximately 2.9% for patients who had originally been treated with warfarin for prosthetic heart valves, 2.6% for those treated for atrial fibrillation and 4.8% for those treated for cardioembolic stroke.[120] These numbers may be gross underestimates as many patients died within 2 weeks, and follow-up imaging was scant[121]; another study[122] showed a much higher rate of 20%; see Cardiogenic brain embolism (p. 1590) for more details.

Antiplatelet therapy after ICH is not associated with a substantially increased risk of recurrent ICH[123] (prospective cohort study).

Recommendations

A-fib: long-term anticoagulation should be *avoided* after ICH.[124]

Mechanical heart valves: 1–2 weeks off anticoagulation (to observe ICH, or to evacuate an SDH or clip an aneurysm).[120,125] Patients with deep hemispheric ICH at high risk for thromboembolic stroke may benefit from resumption of long-term anticoagulation.[124]

Patients requiring hemodialysis after ICH: heparin-free dialysis may be used.

96.8 Ventriculostomy (IVC) with ICH

Indications for Ventriculostomy (IVC) AKA external ventricular drainage (EVD) (also see guidelines below)
1. acute hydrocephalus:
   a) due to compression of CSF pathways: e.g., thalamic ICH compressing the 3rd ventricle (not recommended for cerebellar ICH (Level III[5]), see (p. 1623))
   b) associated with intraventricular blood: clot may cause obstructive hydrocephalus, and intraventricular blood alone is a risk factor for communicating hydrocephalus due to toxic effect on CSF resorptive mechanisms. IVCs may get blocked by clot, and intraventricular rtPA has been used to help maintain patency, but the overall benefit is uncertain[5]
2. for ICP management

Practice guideline: ICP monitoring & treatment in patients with ICH

1. EVD is reasonable for patients with hydrocephalus, especially with reduced level of consciousness (Level II[5]) (✖ not for cerebellar ICH – see text)
2. patients with GCS ≤ 8, or evidence of transtentorial herniation or significant IVH or hydrocephalus: consider ICP monitoring and treatment. A goal of CPP 50–70 mm Hg may be reasonable depending on the status of cerebral autoregulation (Level II[5])
3. ✖ corticosteroids are not recommended for treatment of increased ICP (Level III[5])
4. intraventricular rtPA appears to have a low complication rate, but the overall safety and benefit are uncertain (Level III[5])

96.9 Surgical treatment

96.9.1 General information

The first successful evacuation of an intracerebral hematoma was reported by MacEwan in 1888.[126] The patient recovered completely from an upper-extremity monoplegia. Ever since then, surgical treatment of ICH has been fraught with controversy. See (p. 1623).

96

Practice guideline: Surgical treatment in patients with ICH

1. cerebellar hemorrhage with neurologic deterioration, or brainstem compression and/or obstructive hydrocephalus from intraventricular clot:
   a) surgical removal of the clot should be done ASAP (Level I[5]); see Cerebellar hemorrhage (p. 1614) for details
   b) ✖ initial treatment with EVD instead of surgical evacuation is not recommended (Level III[5])
2. supratentorial ICH: the usefulness of surgery is not well-established (Level II[5]). Potential exceptions & additional considerations:
   a) early ICH evacuation is not clearly superior to evacuation when the patient deteriorates (Level II[5])
   b) deteriorating patients: ICH evacuation may be considered as a life-saving measure (Level II[5])
   c) patients in coma, or large ICH with significant midline shift, or elevated ICP refractory to medical management: decompressive craniectomy (DC) with or without ICH evacuation may reduce mortality (Level II[5])
   d) minimally invasive ICH evacuation with stereotactic or endoscopic aspiration with or without thrombolytics is of uncertain effectiveness (Level II[5])

Booking the case: Craniotomy for ICH

Also see defaults & disclaimers (p. 25).
1. position: (depends on location of bleed)
2. equipment:
   a) microscope (not used for all cases)
   b) image-guided navigation (typically used for minimally invasive ICH removal)
3. post-op: ICU
4. consent (in lay terms for the patient—not all-inclusive):
   a) procedure: surgery through the skull to remove blood clot, stop any bleeding identified, possible placement of external (ventricular) drain
   b) alternatives: nonsurgical management
   c) complications: usual craniotomy complications (p. 25) plus further bleeding which may cause problems (especially in patients taking blood thinners, antiplatelet drugs including aspirin, or those with coagulation abnormalities or previous bleeds) and may require further surgery, areas of the brain that have already been damaged by the bleeding are not likely to recover, hydrocephalus (buildup of fluid in the brain) may occur with or without surgery and may require a temporary drainage tube or a permanent shunt

96.9.2 Indications for surgery

General information

Considerable controversy persists regarding indications for surgery. Surgery may lower morbidity from rebleeding (especially if an aneurysm or AVM is identified as the cause of the ICH), edema, or necrosis from mass effect of hematoma (unproven), but rarely causes neurologic improvement. Meta-analyses[127,128] yield inconclusive or conflicting results and could not identify whether there was a favorable effect of surgery, the types of ICH and patients that are likely to benefit, and the relative effectiveness of the various available surgical options.

Randomized prospective studies (RPS) in the current CT/surgical era

One RPS[129] found lower mortality for patients with GCS 7–10 treated surgically (**note**: only 20% of these patients were operated on < 8 hrs from the bleed, and the mean time for all patients to operation was 14.5 hours (range: 6–48 hrs), which may be long). However, survivors in this group were all severely disabled (none were independent).

Another[130] found no benefit from surgery for *putaminal* hemorrhages, also with poor outcomes in all patients.

International STICH[131]: enrolled 1,033 patients. Study shortcomings: possible selection bias (the responsible neurosurgeon had to be uncertain of the benefits of medical vs. surgical treatment), "early surgery" had a somewhat long median time to treatment of 30 hours, and 26% of medically treated patients crossed over and had surgery at a mean of 60 hours (late). Given these limitations, the conclusion was that for supratentorial ICH there was no benefit of early surgery (although there may have been some benefit in the subgroup with a hematoma within 1 cm of the cortical surface). This trial may be more accurately considered to be a comparison of early vs. delayed surgery in patients subjectively judged to need surgery by the investigator.

Conclusion

The decision to operate therefore must be individualized based on patient's neurologic condition, size and location of hematoma, patient's age, and the patient's expressed preferences (e.g., by a "living will") and the family's wishes concerning "heroic" measures in the face of catastrophic illness. Also, see (p. 1623).

Guidelines for considering surgery vs. medical management

(For separate indications for surgery for *cerebellar* hemorrhage, see below.)
1. NON-SURGICAL: factors that may favor medical management
   a) minimally symptomatic lesions: e.g., alert patient with subtle hemiparesis (especially patient with GCS > 10[129])

b) situations with little chance of good outcome
- high ICH score (p. 1618), which overlaps with the following
- massive hemorrhage with significant neuronal destruction (see below)
- large hemorrhage in dominant hemisphere
- poor neurologic condition: e.g., comatose with posturing (i.e., GCS ≤ 5), loss of brainstem function (fixed pupils, posturing…)
- ≈ age > 75 yrs: do not do well with surgery for this

c) severe coagulopathy or other significant underlying medical disorder(s): in the event of herniation, rapid decompression surgery may be considered in spite of the risks

d) basal ganglion (putaminal) or thalamic hemorrhage: surgery is no better than medical management, and both have little to offer[130,132] (see below)

2. SURGICAL: factors that may favor rapid surgical removal of the blood clot

a) lesions with marked mass effect, edema, or midline shift on imaging (removal is considered due to the potential for herniation)

b) lesions where the symptoms (e.g., hemiparesis/plegia, aphasia, or sometimes just confusion or agitation…) appear to be due to increased ICP or to mass effect (i.e., compression) from the clot or surrounding edema. Symptoms attributable directly to brain injury from the hemorrhage are unlikely to be reversed by surgical evacuation

c) volume: surgery for *moderate volume* hematomas (i.e., ≈ 10–30 cc, Eq (96.1)) may be more appropriate than with:
- ✖ small clot (< 10 cc): mass effect from clot + edema is usually not significant enough to require surgery
- ✖ large clot (> 30 cc): associated with poor outcome (only 1 of 71 patients could function independently at 30 days[133])
- ✖ massive hemorrhage > 60 cc with GCS ≤ 8: 91% 30-day mortality[133]
- ✖ massive hemorrhage > 85 cc (the volume of a sphere with a diameter of 5.5 cm): no patient survived, regardless of treatment in one series[134]

d) persistent elevated ICP in spite of therapy (failure of medical management). Evacuating clot definitely lowers ICP, but the effect on outcome is uncertain

e) rapid deterioration (especially with signs of brainstem compression) regardless of location in a patient considered to be salvageable

f) favorable location, for example:
- lobar (as opposed to deep hemispheric): in spite of optimistic results in a non-randomized study done in 1983 indicating good outcomes in patients with deep hemorrhages treated with early surgery,[64] a later randomized study failed to confirm this benefit[130]
- cerebellar: see below
- external capsule
- non-dominant hemisphere

g) young patient (especially age ≤ 50 yrs): they tolerate surgery better than elderly patients, and, unlike elderly patients with brain atrophy, they also have less room in the head to accommodate the mass effect of clot + edema

h) early intervention following hemorrhage: surgery after 24 hrs from onset of symptoms or deterioration may be of less benefit[129]

Management of cerebellar hemorrhage

96

recommendations[5]:
. cerebellar hematoma ≤ 3 cm diameter: treat conservatively
. cerebellar hematoma > 3 cm with either hydrocephalus or clinical signs of brainstem compression: surgical evacuation ASAP (level I[5])
. patients with absent brainstem reflexes and flaccid quadriplegia: intensive therapy is not indicated. **Note:** some authors contend that the loss of brainstem reflexes from direct compression may not be irreversible,[135] and that cerebellar hemorrhage represents a surgical emergency (and that the above criteria would thus deny potentially helpful surgery to some, see discussion of cerebellar infarction and decompression (p. 1588))
. patients with hydrocephalus from ventricular obstruction: ✖ initial treatment with an intraventricular catheter (IVC) without ICH evacuation is not recommended. IVC can only be inserted if there is no coagulopathy. Risk of upward cerebellar herniation (p. 325).

Endoscopic treatment of intraventricular hemorrhage

Endoscopic treatment of intraventricular hemorrhage is of uncertain efficacy (Level II[5]).

96.9.3 Surgical considerations

General recommendations

1. send specimens (hematoma, abnormal-looking tangle of blood vessels if present, and possibly biopsy walls of hematoma cavity) to pathology for analysis[136] (to rule out tumor, AVM, amyloid angiopathy...)
2. surgical options:
   a) "standard approach": craniotomy with evacuation of the clot under direct vision (with or without microscope)
   b) stereotactic aspiration with thrombolytic agents has also been used; see **Stereotactic surgery**, evacuation of intracerebral hemorrhage (p. 1838), including surgery using an "exoscope" through a tube
   c) endoscopic surgery[137]

Surgical techniques for cerebellar hemorrhage

1. position: lateral oblique (p. 1738) with the involved side up
2. if rapidity is crucial, a midline skin incision is preferred because it can be taken down quickly with little fear of encountering a vertebral artery
3. craniectomy (without bone replacement) is preferred over craniotomy to accommodate post-op swelling
4. a prophylactic Frazier burr hole is recommended to allow rapid treatment if post-op hydrocephalus develops—see placement (p. 1742) and use (p. 1745), or a ventricular catheter may be placed to monitor ICP and allow CSF drainage post-op
5. in cases where there has been rupture into the ventricular system, the surgical microscope should be used to follow the clot to the fourth ventricle, which is then cleared of clot

Intraventricular tissue plasminogen activator (tPA)

Intraventricular tPA may help lyse clot and maintain intraventricular catheter (IVC) patency or reopen a clotted IVC. However, the CLEAR III trial[138] showed no benefit of using 1 mg tPA vs. saline for the primary endpoint of mRS score (▶ Table 98.5) ≤ 3 at 6 mos for patients with < 30 ml clot (lower mortality at 6 mos was offset by a larger number of survivors with mRS = 5). ✖ In cases of suspected aneurysm, AVM, or other vascular malformation, it cannot be used until the source of bleeding has been neutralized.[139,140]

℞: 2–5 mg of tPA[139,141,142] in NS is administered through an intraventricular catheter (IVC) every ? hours for up to 4 days. The IVC is closed for 2 hours after injection.[142]

96.10 Outcome

Thalamic hemorrhages that tend to destroy the internal capsule (IC) are more likely to produce hemiplegia than hemorrhages lateral to the IC that compress but do not disrupt the IC.

Mortality: The chief cause of death (in a series testing the effects of dexamethasone) is cerebral herniation,[143] occurring mainly during the first week and mostly in patients with initial Glasgow Coma Scale scores ≤ 7. The in-hospital death rate decreased overall during the 1980s but increased for patients ≥ 65 years of age.[3]

Quoted mortality rates vary widely, and depend on size and location of clot, age, and medical condition of the patient, and etiology of the hemorrhage. Overall, the 30-day mortality rate is ≈ 44% for ICH,[2] which is similar to that for SAH (≈ 46%). Patients with lobar hemorrhages (p. 1614) tend to fare better than deep ICH (basal ganglion, thalamus...) with only ≈ 11% mortality in 26 patients.? Patients on anticoagulation for a-fib fare worse than those who are not.[144]

References

[1] Ojemann RG, Heros RC. Spontaneous Brain Hemorrhage. Stroke. 1983; 14:468–475

[2] Broderick JP, Brott TG, Tomsick T, et al. Intracerebral Hemorrhage More Than Twice as Common as Subarachnoid Hemorrhage. J Neurosurg. 1993; 78:188–191

[3] Chyatte D, Easley K, Brass LM. Increasing Hospital Admission Rates for Intracerebral Hemorrhage During the Last Decade. Journal of Stroke and Cerebrovascular Diseases. 1997; 6:354–360

[4] Moon JS, Janjua N, Ahmed S, et al. Prehospital neurologic deterioration in patients with intracerebral hemorrhage. Crit Care Med. 2008; 36:172–175

[5] Hemphill JC,3rd, Greenberg SM, Anderson CS, et al. Guidelines for the Management of Spontaneous Intracerebral Hemorrhage: A Guideline for Health care Professionals From the American Heart Association/American Stroke Association. Stroke. 2015; 46:2032–2060

96

[6] Gorelick PB, Kelly MA, Feldman E. Ethanol. In: Intracerebral Hemorrhage. Armonk, New York: Futura Publishing Co.; 1994:195–208

[7] Camargo CA. Moderate alcohol consumption and stroke: The epidemiological evidence. Stroke. 1989; 20:1611–1626

[8] Juvela S, Hillbom M, Palomäki H. Risk Factors for Spontaneous Intracerebral Hemorrhage. Stroke. 1995; 26:1558–1564

[9] Feldman E. Intracerebral Hemorrhage. Armonk, NY 1994

[10] Monforte R, Estruch R, Graus F, et al. High Ethanol Consumption as Risk Factor for Intracerebral Hemorrhage in Young and Middle-Aged People. Stroke. 1990; 21:1529–1532

[11] Shinton R, Beevers G. Meta-analysis of relation between cigarette smoking and stroke. British Medical Journal. 1989; 298:789–794

[12] Fogelholm R, Murros K. Cigarette Smoking and Risk of Primary Intracerebral Hemorrhage: A Population-Based Case-Control Study. Acta Neurol Scand. 1993; 87:367–370

[13] Gorelick PB. Stroke from alcohol and drug abuse. A current social peril. Postgrad Med. 1990; 88:171–178

[14] Niizuma H, Shimizu Y, Nakasato N, et al. Influence of Liver Dysfunction on Volume of Putaminal Hemorrhage. Stroke. 1988; 19:987–990

[15] Schmidek HH, Sweet WH. Operative Neurosurgical Techniques. New York 1982

[16] Ropper AH, Davis KR. Lobar Cerebral Hemorrhages: Acute Clinical Syndromes in 26 Cases. Ann Neurol. 1980; 8:141–147

[17] Caplan L. Intracerebral Hemorrhage Revisited. Neurology. 1988; 38:624–627

[18] Caplan LR, Skillman J, Ojemann R, et al. Intracerebral Hemorrhage Following Carotid Endarterectomy: A Hypertensive Complication. Stroke. 1979; 9:457–460

[19] Bernstein M, Fleming JFR, Deck JHN. Cerebral Hyperperfusion After Carotid Endarterectomy: A Cause of Cerebral Hemorrhage. Neurosurgery. 1984; 15:50–56

[20] Humphreys RP, Hoffman HJ, Mustard WT, et al. Cerebral hemorrhage following heart surgery. J Neurosurg. 1975; 43:671–675

[21] Fisher CM, Adams RD. Observations on Brain Embolism with Special Reference to the Mechanism of Hemorrhagic Infarction. J Neuropathol Exp Neurol. 1951; 10:92–93

[22] Hornig CR, Dorndorf W, Agnoli AL. Hemorrhagic Cerebral Infarction: A Prospective Study. Stroke. 1986; 17:179–185

[23] Okada Y, Yamaguchi T, Minematsu K, et al. Hemorrhagic Transformation in Cerebral Embolism. Stroke. 1989; 20:598–603

[24] Bogousslavsky J, Regli F, Uske A, et al. Early Spontaneous Hematoma in Cerebral Infarct: Is Primary Cerebral Hemorrhage Overdiagnosed? Neurology. 1991; 41:837–840

[25] Cerebral Embolism Study Group. Cardioembolic stroke, early anticoagulation, and brain hemorrhage. Archives of Internal Medicine. 1987; 147:626–630

[26] Raabe A, Krug U. Migraine associated bilateral intracerebral hemorrhages. Clinical Neurology and Neurosurgery. 1999; 101:193–195

[27] Cole A, Aube M. Late-Onset Migraine with Intracerebral Hemorrhage: A Recognizable Syndrome. Neurology. 1987; 37S1

[28] Lee K-C, Clough C. Intracerebral Hemorrhage After Break Dancing. N Engl J Med. 1990; 323:615–616

[29] Caplan LR, Neely S, Gorelick P. Cold-Related Intracerebral Hemorrhage. Arch Neurol. 1984; 41

[30] Rosenblum WI. Miliary Aneurysms and 'Fibrinoid' Degeneration of Cerebral Blood Vessels. Hum Pathol. 1977; 8:133–139

[31] Fisher CM. Pathological Observations in Hypertensive Cerebral Hemorrhage. J Neuropathol Exp Neurol. 1971; 30:536–550

[32] The National Institute of Neurological Disorders and Stroke rt-PA Stroke Study Group. Tissue plasminogen activator for acute ischemic stroke. New England Journal of Medicine. 1995; 333:1581–1587

[33] Aldrich MS, Sherman SA, Greenberg HS. Cerebrovascular Complications of Streptokinase Infusion. JAMA. 1985; 253:1777–1779

[34] Maggioni AP, Franzosi MG, Santoro E, et al. The risk of stroke in patients with acute myocardial infarction after thrombolytic and antithrombotic treatment. New England Journal of Medicine. 1992; 327:1–6

[35] Grines CL, Browne KF, Marco J, et al. A Comparison of Immediate Angioplasty with Thrombolytic Therapy for Acute Myocardial Infarction. New England Journal of Medicine. 1993; 328:673–679

[36] Public Health Service. Approval of Thrombolytic Agents. FDA Drug Bulletin. 1988; 18:6–7

[37] Mehta SR, Eikelboom JW, Yusuf S. Risk of intracranial hemorrhage with bolus versus infusion thrombolytic therapy: a meta-analysis. Lancet. 2000; 356:449–454

[38] Tenecteplase (TNKase) for thrombolysis. Medical Letter. 2000; 42:106–108

[39] DaSilva VF, Bormanis J. Intracerebral Hemorrhage After Combined Anticoagulant-Thrombolytic Therapy for Myocardial Infarction: Two Case Reports and a Short Review. Neurosurgery. 1992; 30:943–945

[40] The Steering Committee of the Physician's Health Study Group. Preliminary Report: Findings from the Aspirin Component of the Ongoing Physician's Health Study. N Engl J Med. 1988; 318:262–264

[41] Blackshear JL, Kopecky SL, Litin SC, et al. Management of Atrial Fibrillation in Adults: Prevention of Thromboembolism and Symptomatic Treatment. Mayo Clinic Proceedings. 1996; 71:150–160

[42] Spektor S, Agus S, Merkin V, et al. Low-dose aspirin prophylaxis and risk of intracranial hemorrhage in patients older than 60 years of age with mild or moderate head injury: a prospective study. J Neurosurg. 2003; 99:661–665

[43] Schurks M, Glynn RJ, Rist PM, et al. Effects of vitamin E on stroke subtypes: meta-analysis of randomized controlled trials. BMJ. 2010; 341

[44] Lowenstein DH, Collins SD, Massa SM, et al. The Neurologic Complications of Cocaine Abuse. Neurology. 1987; 37S1

[45] Levine S. Cocaine and stroke. Current concepts of cerebrovascular disease. Stroke. 1987; 22:25–29

[46] Harrington H, Heller A, Dawson D, et al. Intracerebral Hemorrhage and Oral Amphetamines. Arch Neurol. 1983; 40:503–507

[47] Bruno A, Nolte KB, Chapin J. Stroke associated with ephedrine use. Neurology. 1993; 43:1313–1316

[48] Stoessl AJ, Young GB, Feasby TE. Intracerebral hemorrhage and angiographic beading following ingestion of catecholaminergics. Stroke. 1985; 16:734–736

[49] Phenylpropanolamine and other OTC alpha-adrenergic agonists. Medical Letter. 2000; 42

[50] Haller CA, Benowitz NL. Adverse cardiovascular and central nervous system events associated with dietary supplements containing ephedra alkaloids. New England Journal of Medicine. 2000; 343:1833–1838

[51] Gudeman SK, Kishore PR, Miller JD, et al. The Genesis and Significance of Delayed Traumatic Intracerebral Hematoma. Neurosurgery. 1979; 5:309–313

[52] Young HA, Gleave JRW, Schmidek HH, et al. Delayed Traumatic Intracerebral Hematoma: Report of 15 Cases Operatively Treated. Neurosurgery. 1984; 14:22–25

[53] Wang KC, Chen CP, Yang YC, et al. Stroke complicating pregnancy and the puerperium. Zhonghua Yi Xue Za Zhi (Taipei). 1999; 62:13–19

[54] Salerni A, Wald S, Flannagan M. Relationships Among Cortical Ischemia, Infarction, and Hemorrhage in Eclampsia. Neurosurgery. 1988; 22:408–410

[55] Witlin AG, Mattar F, Sibai BM. Postpartum stroke: a twenty-year experience. Am J Obstet Gynecol. 2000; 183:83–88

[56] Geocadin RG, Razumovsky AY, Wityk RJ, et al. Intracerebral hemorrhage and postpartum cerebral vasculopathy. J Neurol Sci. 2002; 205:29–34

[57] Kalfas IH, Little JR. Postoperative Hemorrhage: A Survey of 4992 Intracranial Procedures. Neurosurgery. 1988; 23:343–347

[58] Papanastassiou V, Kerr R, Adams C. Contralateral Cerebellar Hemorrhagic Infarction After Pterional Craniotomy: Report of Five Cases and Review of the Literature. Neurosurgery. 1996; 39:841–852

[59] Toczek MT, Morrell MJ, Silverberg GA, et al. Cerebellar Hemorrhage Complicating Temporal Lobectomy: Report of Four Cases. Journal of Neurosurgery. 1996; 85:718–722

[60] Menovsky T, Andre Grotenhuis J, Bartels RH. Aneurysm of the anterior inferior cerebellar artery (AICA) associated with high-flow lesion: report of two cases and review of literature. J Clin Neurosci. 2002; 9:207–211

[61] Brott T, Thalinger K, Hertzberg V. Hypertension as a Risk Factor for Spontaneous Intracerebral Hemorrhage. Stroke. 1986; 17:1078–1083

[62] Wakai S, Nagai M. Histological Verification of Microaneurysms as a Cause of Cerebral Hemorrhage in Surgical Specimens. Journal of Neurology, Neurosurgery, and Psychiatry. 1989; 52:595–599

[63] Newton TH, Potts DG. Radiology of the Skull and Brain. Saint Louis 1971

[64] Kaneko M, Tanaka K, Shimada T, et al. Long-Term Evaluation of Ultra-Early Operation for Hypertensive Intracerebral Hemorrhage in 100 Cases. J Neurosurg. 1983; 58:838–842

[65] Gilles C, Brucher JM, Khoubesserian P, et al. Cerebral Amyloid Angiopathy as a Cause of Multiple Intracerebral Hemorrhages. Neurology. 1984; 34:730–735

[66] Mandybur TI. Cerebral Amyloid Angiopathy: The Vascular Pathology and Complications. Journal of Neuropathology and Experimental Neurology. 1986; 45:79–90

[67] Vonsattel JP, Myers RH, Hedley-White ET, et al. Cerebral Amyloid Angiopathy Without and With Cerebral Hemorrhages: A Comparative Histological Study. Annals of Neurology. 1991; 30:637–649

[68] Kase CS, Kase CS, Caplan LR. Cerebral Amyloid Angiopathy. In: Intracerebral Hemorrhage. Boston: Butterworth-Heinemann; 1994:179–200

[69] Greenberg SM, Briggs ME, Hyman BT, et al. Apolipoprotein E e4 Is Associated With the Presence and Earlier Onset of Hemorrhage in Cerebral Amyloid Angiopathy. Stroke. 1996; 27:1333–1337

[70] Vinters HV, Gilbert JJ. Amyloid Angiopathy: Its Incidence and Complications in the Aging Brain. Stroke. 1981; 12

[71] Greenberg SM, Rebeck GW, Vonsattel JPV, et al. Apolipoprotein E e4 and Cerebral Amyloid Hemorrhage Associated with Amyloid Angiopathy. Annals of Neurology. 1995; 38:254–259

[72] Kingston IB, Castro MJ, Anderson S. In Vitro Stimulation of Tissue-Type Plasminogen Activator by Alzheimer Amyloid Beta-Peptide Analogues. Nature Med. 1995; 1:138–142

[73] Greenberg SM, Edgar MA. Cerebral Hemorrhage in a 69-Year Old Woman Receiving Warfarin. Case Records of the Massachusetts General Hospital. Case 22-1996. New England Journal of Medicine. 1996; 335:189–186

[74] Auriel E, Charidimou A, Gurol ME, et al. Validation of Clinicoradiological Criteria for the Diagnosis of Cerebral Amyloid Angiopathy-Related Inflammation. JAMA Neurol. 2016; 73:197–202

[75] Scott M. Spontaneous Intracerebral Hematoma caused by Cerebral Neoplasms. J Neurosurg. 1975; 42:338–342

[76] Dublin AB, Norman D. Fluid-Fluid Level in Cystic Cerebral Metastatic Melanoma. J Comput Assist Tomogr. 1979; 3:650–652

[77] Acosta-Sison H. Extensive Cerebral Hemorrhage Caused by the Rupture of a Cerebral Blood Vessel due to a Chorionepithelioma Embolus. Am J Ob Gyn. 1956; 71

[78] Weir B, MacDonald N, Mielke B. Intracranial Vascular Complications of Choriocarcinoma. Neurosurgery. 1978; 2

[79] Weinstein ZR, Downey EF. Spontaneous Hemorrhage in Medulloblastomas. AJNR. 1983; 4:986–988

[80] McCormick WF, Ugajin K. Fatal Hemorrhage into a Medulloblastoma. J Neurosurg. 1967; 26:78–81

[81] Chugani HT, Rosemblat AM, Lavenstein BL, et al. Childhood Medulloblastoma Presenting with Hemorrhage. Childs Brain. 1984; 11:135–140

[82] Zee CS, Segall HD, Miller C, et al. Less Common CT Features of Medulloblastoma. Radiology. 1982; 144:97–102

[83] Oldberg E. Hemorrhage into Gliomas. Arch Neurol Psych. 1933; 30:1061–1073

[84] Richardson RR, Siqueira EB, Cerullo LJ. Malignant Glioma: Its Initial Presentation as Intracranial Hemorrhage. Acta Neurochirurgica. 1979; 46:77–84

[85] Nakao S, Sato S, Ban S, et al. Massive Intracerebral Hemorrhage Caused by Angioblastic Meningioma. Surg Neurol. 1977; 7:245–247

[86] Modesti LM, Binet EF, Collins GH. Meningiomas causing Spontaneous Intracranial Hematomas. Neurosurg. 1976; 45:437–441

[87] Goran A, Ciminello VJ, Fisher RG. Hemorrhage into Meningiomas. Arch Neurol. 1965; 13:65–69

[88] Cabezudo-Artero, Areito-Cebrecos, Vaquero-Crespo J. Hemorrhage Associated with Meningioma. J Neurol Neurosurg Psych. 1981; 44

[89] Little JR, Dial B, Belanger G, et al. Brain Hemorrhage from Intracranial Tumor. Stroke. 1979 10:283–288

[90] Wakai S, Inoh S, Ueda Y, et al. Hemangioblastoma Presenting with Intraparenchymatous Hemorrhage. J Neurosurg. 1984; 61:956–960

[91] McCoyd K, Barron KD, Cassidy RJ. Acoustic Neurinoma Presenting as Subarachnoid Hemorrhage. Neurosurg. 1974; 41:391–393

[92] Gleeson RK, Butzer JF, Grin OD. Acoustic Neurinoma Presenting as Subarachnoid Hemorrhage. Neurosurg. 1978; 49:602–604

[93] Yonemitsu T, Niizuna H, Kodama N, et al. Acoustic Neurinoma Presenting as Subarachnoid Hemorrhage. Surg Neurol. 1983; 20:125–130

[94] Vincent FM, Bartone JR, Jones MZ. Cerebellar Astrocytoma Presenting as a Cerebellar Hemorrhage in a Child. Neurology. 1980; 30:91–93

[95] Kawamata T, Takeshita M, Kubo O, et al. Management of Intracranial Hemorrhage Associated with Anticoagulant Therapy. Surgical Neurology. 1995 44:438–443

[96] Fihn SD, McDonell M, Martin D, et al. Risk Factors for Complications of Chronic Anticoagulation: a Multicenter Study. Annals of Internal Medicine. 1993; 118:511–520

[97] Smith DB, Hitchcock M, Philpot PJ. Cerebral Amyloid Angiopathy Presenting as Transient Ischemic Attacks: Case Report. Journal of Neurosurgery. 1985; 63:963–964

[98] Greenberg SM, Vonsattel JP, Stakes JW, et al. The Clinical Spectrum of Cerebral Amyloid Angiopathy: Presentations without Lobar Hemorrhage. Neurology. 1993; 43:2073–2079

[99] Broderick JP, Brott TG, Tomsick T, et al. Ultra-Early Evaluation of Intracerebral Hemorrhage. J Neurosurg. 1990; 72:195–199

[100] Brott T, Broderick J, Kothari R, et al. Early hemorrhage growth in patients with intracerebral hemorrhage. Stroke. 1997; 28:1–5

[101] Fujii Y, Tanaka R, Takeuchi S, et al. Hematoma Enlargement in Spontaneous Intracerebral Hemorrhage. Journal of Neurosurgery. 1994; 80:51–57

[102] Arakawa S, Saku Y, Ibayashi S, et al. Blood Pressure Control and Recurrence of Hypertensive Brain Hemorrhage. Stroke. 1998; 29:1806–1809

[103] Gonzalez-Duarte A, Cantu C, Ruiz-Sandoval J et al. Recurrent Primary Cerebral Hemorrhage: Frequency, Mechanisms, and Prognosis. Stroke 1998; 29:1802–1805

[104] Stocchetti N, Croci M, Spagnoli D, et al. Mass volume measurement in severe head injury: accuracy and feasibility of two pragmatic methods. J Neurol Neurosurg Psychiatry. 2000; 68:14–17

[105] Pasqualin A, Barone G, Cioffi F, et al. The relevance of anatomic and hemodynamic factors to a classification of cerebral arteriovenous malformations. Neurosurgery. 1991; 28:370–379

[106] Bullock MR, Chesnut RM, Ghajar J, et al. Appendix I: Post-traumatic mass volume measurements in traumatic brain injury. Neurosurgery. 2006; 58

[107] Kothari RU, Brott T, Broderick JP, et al. The ABCs of measuring intracerebral hemorrhage volumes. Stroke. 1996; 27:1304–1305

[108] Wada R, Aviv RI, Fox AJ, et al. CT angiography "spot sign" predicts hematoma expansion in acute intracerebral hemorrhage. Stroke. 2007; 38:1257–1262

[109] Bradley WG. MR Appearance of Hemorrhage in the Brain. Radiology. 1993; 189:15–26

[110] Taveras JM, Gilson JM, Davis DO, et al. Angiography in Cerebral Infarction. Radiology. 1969; 93:549–558

[111] Toffol GJ, Biller J, Adams HP, et al. The Predicted Value of Arteriography in Nontraumatic Intracerebral Hemorrhage. Stroke. 1986; 17:881–883

[112] Holloway RG, Arnold RM, Creutzfeldt CJ, et al. Palliative and end-of-life care in stroke: a statement for healthcare professionals from the American Heart Association/American Stroke Association. Stroke. 2014; 45:1887–1916

[113] Hemphill JC,3rd, Bonovich DC, Besmertis L, et al. The ICH score: a simple, reliable grading scale for intracerebral hemorrhage. Stroke. 2001; 32:891–897

[114] Zhu XL, Chan MSY, Poon WS. Spontaneous Intracranial Hemorrhage: Which Patients Need Diagnostic Cerebral Angiography? A Prospective Study of 206 Cases and Review of the Literature. Stroke. 1997; 28:1406–1409

[115] Laissy JP, Normand G, Monroc M, et al. Spontaneous Intracerebral Hematomas from Vascular Causes: Predictive Value of CT Compared with Angiography. Neuroradiology. 1991; 33:291–295

[116] Qureshi AI, Palesch YY, Martin R, et al. Interpretation and Implementation of Intensive Blood Pressure Reduction in Acute Cerebral Hemorrhage Trial (INTERACT II). J Vasc Interv Neurol. 2014; 7:34–40

[117] Qureshi AI, Palesch YY, Barsan WG, et al. Intensive Blood-Pressure Lowering in Patients with Acute Cerebral Hemorrhage. N Engl J Med. 2016; 375:1033–1043

[118] Mayer SA, Brun NC, Begtrup K, et al. Recombinant activated factor VII for acute intracerebral hemorrhage. N Engl J Med. 2005; 352:777–785

[119] Pessin MS, Estol CJ, Lafranchise F, et al. Safety of Anticoagulation After Hemorrhagic Infarction. Neurology. 1993; 43:1298–1303

[120] Phan TG, Koh M, Wijdicks EF. Safety of discontinuation of anticoagulation in patients with intracranial hemorrhage at high thromboembolic risk. Archives of Neurology. 2000; 57:1710–1713

[121] Hacke W. The dilemma of reinstituting anticoagulation for patients with cardioembolic sources and intracranial hemorrhage: how wide is the strait between skylla and karybdis? Archives of Neurology. 2000; 57:1682–1684

[122] Bertram M, Bonsanto M, Hacke W, et al. Managing the therapeutic dilemma: patients with spontaneous intracerebral hemorrhage and urgent need for anticoagulation. Journal of Neurology. 2000; 247:209–214

[123] Viswanathan A, Rakich SM, Engel C, et al. Antiplatelet use after intracerebral hemorrhage. Neurology. 2006; 66:206–209

[124] Eckman MH, Rosand J, Knudsen KA, et al. Can patients be anticoagulated after intracerebral hemorrhage? A decision analysis. Stroke. 2003; 34:1710–1716

[125] Wijdicks EF, Schievink WI, Brown RD, et al. The dilemma of discontinuation of anticoagulation therapy for patients with intracranial hemorrhage and mechanical heart valves. Neurosurgery. 1998; 42:769–773

[126] MacEwen W. An Address on the Surgery of the Brain and Spinal Cord. British Medical Journal. 1888; 2:302–309

[127] Hankey GJ, Hon C. Surgery for Primary Intracerebral Hemorrhage: Is It Safe and Effective? A Systematic Review of Case Series and Randomized Trials. Stroke. 1997; 28:2126–2132

[128] Teernstra OP, Evers SM, Kessels AH. Meta analyses in treatment of spontaneous supratentorial intracerebral haematoma. Acta Neurochir (Wien). 2006; 148:521–8; discussion 528

[129] Juvela S, Heiskanen O, Poranen A, et al. The Treatment of Spontaneous Intracerebral Hemorrhage: A Prospective Randomized Trial of Surgical and Conservative Treatment. J Neurosurg. 1989; 70:755–758

[130] Batjer HH, Reisch JS, Plaizier LJ, et al. Failure of Surgery to Improve Outcome in Hypertensive Putaminal Hemorrhage: A Prospective Randomized Trial. Arch Neurol. 1990; 47:1103–1106

[131] Mendelow AD, Gregson BA, Fernandes HM, et al. Early surgery versus initial conservative treatment in patients with spontaneous supratentorial intracerebral haematomas in the International Surgical Trial in Intracerebral Haemorrhage (STICH): a randomised trial. Lancet. 2005; 365:387–397

[132] Waga S, Miyazaki M, Okada M, et al. Hypertensive Putaminal Hemorrhage: Analysis of 182 Patients. Surgical Neurology. 1986; 26:159–166

[133] Broderick JP, Brott TG, Duldner JE, et al. Volume of intracerebral hemorrhage. A powerful and easy-to-use predictor of 30-day mortality. Stroke. 1993; 24:987–993

[134] Volpin L, Cervellini P, Colombo F, et al. Spontaneous intracerebral hematomas: A new proposal about the usefulness and limits of surgical treatment. Neurosurgery. 1984; 15:663–666

[135] Heros RC. Surgical Treatment of Cerebellar Infarction. Stroke. 1992; 23:937–938

[136] Hinton DR, Dolan E, Sima AF. The Value of Histopathological Examination of Surgically Removed Blood Clot in Determining the Etiology of Spontaneous Intracerebral Hemorrhage. Stroke. 1984; 15:517–520

[137] Auer LM, Deinsberger W, Niederkorn K, et al. Endoscopic Surgery Versus Medical Treatment for Spontaneous Intracerebral Hematoma: A Randomized Study. Journal of Neurosurgery. 1989; 70:530–535

[138] Hanley DF, Lane K, McBee N, et al. Thrombolytic removal of intraventricular haemorrhage in treatment of severe stroke: results of the randomised, multicentre, multiregion, placebo-controlled CLEAR III trial. Lancet. 2017; 389:603–611

[139] Findlay JM, Grace MGA, Weir BKA. Treatment of Intraventricular Hemorrhage with Tissue Plasminogen Activator. Neurosurgery. 1993; 32:941–947

[140] Engelhart HH, Andrews CO, Slavin KV, et al. Current management of intraventricular hemorrhage. Surg Neurol. 2003; 60:15–21; discussion 21-2

[141] Grabb PA. Traumatic intraventricular hemorrhage treated with intraventricular recombinant-tissue plasminogen activator: technical case report. Neurosurgery. 1998; 43:966–969

[142] Rohde V, Schaller C, Hassler WE. Intraventricular recombinant tissue plasminogen activator for lysis of intraventricular hemorrhage. Journal of Neurology, Neurosurgery and Psychiatry. 1995; 58:447–451

[143] Poungvarin N, Bhoopat W, Viriyavejakul A, et al. Effects of Dexamethasone in Primary Supratentorial Intracerebral Hemorrhage. N Engl J Med. 1987; 316:1229–1233

[144] Ruff CT, Giugliano RP, Braunwald E, et al. Comparison of the efficacy and safety of new oral anticoagulants with warfarin in patients with atrial fibrillation: a meta-analysis of randomised trials. Lancet. 2014; 383:955–962

97 ICH in Young Adults and Pediatrics

97.1 ICH in young adults

97.1.1 General information

In a review of 72 patients age 15–45 yrs suffering nontraumatic ICH,[1] a presumed cause was found in 76% (▶ Table 97.1).

AVM: lobar hemorrhages in this age group are highly suggestive of AVM. Of 40 lobar hemorrhages, 37.5% were determined to be from AVMs.[1]

Pregnancy/postpartum: 3 patients had labor or postpartum hemorrhages (p.1611); see also Pregnancy & intracranial hemorrhage (p.1425).

Herpes simplex encephalitis: may produce hemorrhagic changes on CT, especially in the temporal lobes; see Herpes simplex encephalitis (p.397).

Drug abuse: especially with sympathomimetics such as cocaine (p.1611) should also be considered in young adults.

Leukemia: ICH may be the initial presentation of leukemia in a young adult (may be due to metastases (chloroma) or to thrombocytopenia).

Table 97.1 Causes of spontaneous ICH in young adults[1]

Etiology	%
ruptured AVM	29.1
arterial hypertension	15.3
ruptured saccular aneurysm	9.7
sympathomimetic drug abuse	6.9
tumor[a]	4.2
acute EtOH intoxication	2.8
preeclampsia/eclampsia	2.8
superior sagittal sinus thrombosis	1.4
moyamoya	1.4
cryoglobulinemia	1.4
undetermined	23.6

[a]hemangioma, ependymoma, metastatic choriocarcinoma...see Hemorrhagic brain tumors (p.1612)

97.1.2 Outcome

Overall in-hospital survival (including those treated medically) was 87.5%.

97.2 Intracerebral hemorrhage in the newborn

97.2.1 General information

Occurs primarily in premature infants. Alternate terms: subependymal hemorrhage (SEH), germinal matrix hemorrhage (GMH), periventricular-intraventricular hemorrhage (PIVH). Intraventricular hemorrhage (IVH) arises from extension of SEH through ependymal lining of ventricle and occurs in 80% of cases of SEH.[2]

97.2.2 Etiology

The highly vascular germinal matrix is part of the primordial tissue of the developing brain and is the source of future neurons and glial cells. It is located just beneath the ependymal lining of the lateral ventricles, and undergoes progressive involution until 36 weeks gestational age (GA). Thus the matrix may persist out of utero in premature infants. A disproportionate amount of the total CBF perfuses the periventricular circulation through these capillaries which are immature and fragile and have impaired autoregulation.[3,4] The site of hemorrhage is age-dependent. Between 24–28 weeks GA they occur over the body of the caudate nucleus and at 29 weeks GA or greater they arise over the head of the caudate nucleus.[5]

97.2.3 Pathogenesis of PIVH in the pre-term infant

The metabolically active GM is susceptible to hypotension and hypoperfusion, which can lead to infarction. The GM is a vulnerable watershed zone supplied by Heubner's artery (from the anterior cerebral artery), terminal branches of the lateral striate arteries (off the middle cerebral artery), and the anterior choroidal artery (off the internal carotid or middle cerebral artery).

1. postnatal hypoxia due to respiratory distress syndrome related to hyaline membrane disease, pneumothorax, and/or anemia can deprive the metabolically active GM of oxygen. This ischemia to the endothelial cells lining the capillaries makes them vulnerable to infarction and then disruption
2. hypercapnia maximally dilates the thin-walled vessels of the GM. If this is followed by sudden increases in perfusion the result can be rupture of the vessels
3. increased venous pressure from any cause (labor and delivery, positive pressure ventilation, stimulation, endotracheal suctioning, myocardial failure from ischemia) can result in increased venous pressure in the GM leading to hemorrhage
4. dehydration followed by rapid resuscitation with hyperosmolar solutions increases the intravascular volume by osmotically encouraging the movement of fluid from tissues into the intravascular space. With associated increases in systemic blood pressure the GM capillaries are at increased risk of rupture

97.2.4 Risk factors for PIVH

Increased cerebral perfusion pressure (CPP) with the associated increased cerebral blood flow (CBF) and hypoxia are the common denominators for most risk factors for PIVH. The elevated pressure may cause the hemorrhage by rupturing the fragile vessels of the germinal matrix, possibly already damaged by previous insults of high or fluctuating CBF and hypoxia.

Risk factors for PIVH include[6]:

1. those associated primarily with increased CBF or CPP:
   a) asphyxia: including hypercapnia (see above)
   b) rapid volume expansion
   c) seizures
   d) pneumothorax
   e) cyanotic heart disease (including PDA)
   f) infants being mechanically ventilated having RDS and fluctuating CBF velocity documented by Doppler flow meter[7]
   g) anemia
   h) decreased blood glucose
   i) arterial catheterization
   j) blood pressure fluctuations
2. younger gestational age (GA)
3. low birth weight
4. acute amnionitis
5. failure to give antenatal steroids (p. 1632) during the 48 hours prior to pre-term delivery[8] (i.e., to women at risk of delivering low-birth-weight infants)
6. APGAR's < 4 at 1 minute and < 8 at 5 minutes
7. acidosis
8. coagulopathies
9. general anesthesia for C-section
10. extracorporeal membrane oxygenation (ECMO): due to heparinization in addition to increased CPP
11. maternal cocaine abuse[9]
12. maternal aspirin use

97.2.5 Epidemiology

Incidence

Depends on the method used for detection (many PIVHs are asymptomatic) and the population being evaluated. 540,000 pre-term infants are born in the United States annually. 85,000 are very

97

pre-term (<32 weeks GA) and 385,000 are late pre-term (34–36 weeks GA). 63,000 very-low-birth-weight (<1500 grams) infants are born each year. Of the preemies weighing <1500 gm birth weight, 20–25% will suffer from a PIVH.[10],[11]

In a 1978 study, PIVH was found by CT in 43% (20/46) of preemies with birth-weight <1500 gm.[12] Mortality in infants with PIVH was 55%, compared to 23% in those without PIVH.[12] Ultrasound (U/S) detected PIVH in 90% of 113 preemies <34 weeks gestation[13] (49% were grade III or IV, see ▶ Table 97.2 for grading).

Table 97.2 Grading subependymal hemorrhage[12]

Grade	Description
I	subependymal
II	IVH without ventricular dilatation
III	IVH with ventricular dilatation
IV	IVH with parenchymal hemorrhage

Abbreviation: IVH = intraventricular hemorrhage.

Timing

The timing of PIVH has a bimodal distribution. A substantial number occur within 6 hours of birth with 50% occurring within 12 hours of birth.[14],[15] At postnatal days 3–4, a second peak occurs. Only 5% of bleeds will develop after postnatal day 4. Progression of hemorrhage has been documented in 10–20% of infants.[15] Early-onset PIVH is more likely to progress and has a higher mortality.[16]

97.2.6 Prevention

Numerous studies have been conducted to find a method of directly reducing the incidence of PIVH among premature infants. Many are controversial. Optimal resuscitation and neonatal care, with an emphasis on measures which minimize cerebral blood flow fluctuations, are key.

1. good prenatal care and avoiding pre-term labor
2. antenatal corticosteroids: administration of one course of antenatal corticosteroids to women at risk of having premature birth infants reduces neonatal mortality, respiratory distress syndrome, and PIVH.[17] Multiple courses of antenatal corticosteroids did not improve outcomes and were associated with decreased head circumference, weight, and length at birth[18]
3. indomethacin: results in cerebral vasoconstriction and reduces the responsiveness of CBF to changes in CO_2, lowers CBF and increases arterial oxygenation reducing patent ductus arteriosus (PDA). However, use is possibly associated with increased risk of intestinal perforation
4. antenatal vitamin K given IM >4 hrs prior to delivery decreases PIVH from 33% to 5%
5. sluicing umbilical cord blood and delaying umbilical cord clamping by 30–120 seconds in *premature* babies increased hematocrit and decreased PIVH in 5 of 7 studies[19]
6. using surfactant to reduce RDS
7. minimizing external stimulation (some centers use fentanyl drips)
8. steroids to stabilize the GM vessels

97.2.7 Clinical

Grading

The most commonly used grading system of Papile et al (▶ Table 97.2) is based on MRI, CT, or U/S findings, as illustrated in ▶ Fig. 97.1.

There is a direct correlation between younger gestational age (GA) and the severity of PIVH. In infants 24–26 weeks GA, 32% will have a Grade III PIVH and 19% will have a Grade IV PIVH, whereas in infants 31–32 weeks GA, 11% will have a Grade III PIVH and 5% will have a Grade IV PIVH.[20]

Presentation

Asymptomatic PIVH

Most PIVHs are clinically unsuspected (especially with smaller hemorrhages) and are discovered incidentally on surveillance U/S. Symptomatic PIVH may present acutely or subacutely (see below).

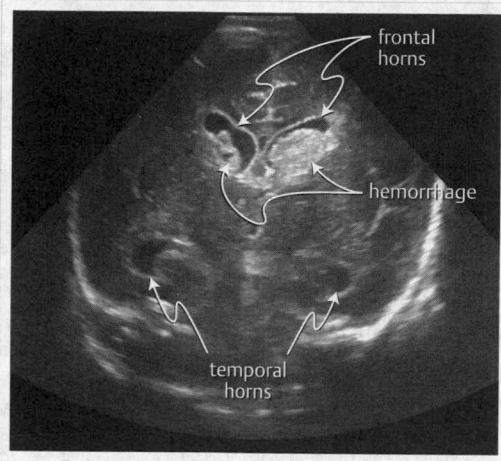

frontal horns

hemorrhage

temporal horns

Fig. 97.1 Grade IV bilateral germinal matrix hemorrhages in premature infant 27 weeks gestational age. Temporal horns of lateral ventricles are slightly dilated.
Coronal ultrasound through anterior fontanelle.

Retrospectively, these PIVHs may have been suggested by a fall in Hct or delays in neurologic development. Silent PIVHs have a 78% 6-month survival, vs. 20% for PIVH showing signs.

Subacute presentation

Usually smaller or more slowly developing hemorrhages. Clinically may present as irritability, reduced motor activity, or abnormal eye movements.

Acute presentation

1. changes in muscle tone or activity: usually decerebrate or decorticate posturing, sometimes flaccid paralysis
2. seizures: often subclinical
3. tense fontanelle
4. hypotension
5. respiratory and cardiac irregularities: apnea & bradycardia ("A's and B's")
6. unreactive pupils and/or loss of extraocular muscle movements
7. Hct drop > 10%

Hydrocephalus

General information

20–50% of infants with PIVH will develop either transient or progressive hydrocephalus (HCP). Grades III and IV are more often associated with progressive ventricular dilatation than are lower grades (however, HCP may develop even after low-grade PIVH[21]). Younger gestational age infants may be at *lower* risk.

Post-PIVH hydrocephalus usually occurs 1–3 weeks after the hemorrhage. Probably caused by cellular debris and/or the toxic effects of blood breakdown products on the arachnoid granulations (communicating HCP), or by an adhesive arachnoiditis in the posterior fossa, or, rarely, by compression or blockage of critical pathways, e.g., at the Sylvian aqueduct (obstructive HCP). In a case of HCP following intra-uterine PIVH, aqueductal gliosis was found at autopsy.[22]

Differential diagnosis of ventriculomegaly in PIVH

When ventriculomegaly is detected, it needs to be differentiated from the following:

1. transient ventriculomegaly: occurs in the first few days after PIVH. This may not cause elevated ICP. As implied, it is self-limited
2. progressive ventriculomegaly: occurs in 20–50% of cases (true hydrocephalus)
3. "hydrocephalus ex vacuo": due to loss of brain tissue or maldevelopment. Is not progressive on serial U/S. OFCs may fall below normal due to lack of growing brain as stimulus for head growth

97

Possible presentations

Abnormally increasing OFC (crossing percentile curves faster than body weight), lethargy, apnea and bradycardia, vomiting. There is progressive dilatation of the ventricular system on serial U/S or CT or MRI evaluations.

97.2.8 Pathophysiologic effects of PIVH

Deleterious effects of PIVH on the brain are due to[23]:
1. destruction of the germinal matrix and glial precursors
2. direct injury to neural tissue from hematoma: once hemorrhage resorbs may leave patient with porencephaly or cystic lesions
3. pressure of hematoma on nearby brain tissue reducing CBF even to parts of the same hemisphere distant from the hemorrhage[24]
4. diffuse decreased CBF following the hemorrhage[25] due to elevated ICP
5. injury from the same hypoxic event that precipitated the PIVH
6. decreased CPP leads to periventricular leukomalacia (PVL) and cerebral infarction
7. periventricular hemorrhagic infarction
8. hydrocephalus (see above): numerous deleterious effects on the CNS
9. seizures: repeated or prolonged seizures may be deleterious to neuronal function

97.2.9 Diagnosis

Ultrasound (U/S)

Performed through the open fontanelles.[13] Accuracy $\approx$ 88% (91% sensitivity, 85% specificity).[26] U/S is invaluable because:
1. it demonstrates the size of the ventricles, the location and size of the hematoma, and the thickness of the cortical mantle
2. it may be brought to the infant's bedside (obviating transportation)
3. it is non-invasive
4. it is not adversely affected by occasional infant movements (eliminating the need for sedation)
5. there is no exposure to ionizing radiation (radiation from diagnostic imaging in children has long-term risks for cancer[27] and damage to the lens)
6. it may be followed serially with relative ease

CT scan

Sometimes necessary when U/S is not readily available, or in complicated cases where anatomy is difficult to deduce from U/S images. Many ICUs have portable CT scans available which obviates need for patient transport.

Rapid-sequence MRI

Pros: Eliminates the risk of ionizing radiation associated with CT scan.
Cons: Requires moving the infant from the neonatal ICU to the radiology suite.

97.2.10 Treatment

General measures

General measures are directed at optimizing CPP without further excessive elevation of CBF by carefully maintaining normal MAP and normalizing pCO_2, and by treating active hydrocephalus as needed (see above).

While daily LPs can control the deleterious effects of posthemorrhagic HCP, they do not reduce the frequency of long-term HCP (requiring permanent shunting). Ventricular size must be monitored with serial U/S.

Medical treatment

1. not very effective. Treated patients fared worse in several studies
2. osmotic agents: isosorbide, glycerol. Effects are short-lived
3. ✖ diuretic therapy: has been used, but a large study showed increased nephrocalcinosis and biochemical abnormalities, resulting in a borderline increase in the risk for motor impairment at

one year.[28] The results were so compelling, the data-monitoring committee terminated the study prematurely. Furosemide and acetazolamide therapy was deemed neither safe nor effective in treating post-hemorrhagic ventricular dilatation and cannot therefore be recommended[29]

Surgical/interventional treatment for the clot

Due to poor operative results, surgical evacuation of an intracerebral hemorrhage in the newborn is not indicated with the possible exception of a posterior fossa hemorrhage causing brainstem compression that does not respond to medical treatment.[30] Supportive measures are usually in order.

Intervention for intraventricular blood

General information

34% of infants < 1500 g require shunt/reservoir drainage after failed medical management. Grade III and IV PIVH: > 70% of cases develop progressive ventricular dilatation, and 32–47% of this subset will ultimately require shunting.[31]

Indications for intervention

Intervention for intraventricular blood is indicated in the setting of progressive ventriculomegaly with the OFC crossing percentile curves and clinical evidence of increased ICP (split sutures, tense fontanelle…).

Serial lumbar punctures

Used at many facilities for hemorrhages with intraventricular extension and communicating hydrocephalus (the usual type of HCP that occurs with PIVH).[32]

This should be undertaken with the knowledge that meta-analysis[33] showed that sequential lumbar or ventricular taps of ≈ 10 ml/kg/tap for prophylaxis or treatment of progressive hydrocephalus offers no clear benefit over conservative treatment, and had an infection rate of 5–9%. In rare cases, LPs may succeed in temporizing progressive HCP for a few weeks until the infant is large enough for shunt placement.

Infants < 800 gm may not tolerate LPs because of desaturation when lying on their side, or the LP itself may be difficult. In these patients, consider 1–2 ventricular taps to at least obtain fluid for analysis (in some cases nothing further needs to be done).

Serial ventricular taps

May be a viable short-term option for those infants who cannot tolerate LPs or in whom there is obstruction to CSF flow in the lumbar subarachnoid space (e.g., due to spinal subdural hematoma from previous LP). However, it is not desirable for long-term use because of repeated trauma to brain (risk of porencephaly) and risk of intracerebral, intraventricular, or subdural hemorrhage.

If continued taps are likely (i.e., large hemorrhage, or rapid recurrence of intracranial hypertension as determined by palpation of fullness of anterior fontanelle (AF) following several taps), the acceptable options include:

1. continuing serial LPs (see below)
2. percutaneous ventricular taps: not recommended for more than a few treatments as it causes porencephaly
3. placement of a temporary ventricular access device (TVAD)—a *ventricular catheter* connected to a subgaleal *reservoir* (e.g., a Rickham reservoir, or a low profile McComb reservoir[34]). These can be inserted safely at the bedside, obviating the need for transport to the O.R.[35]
   a) temporary ventricular access: the reservoir can be used for serial percutaneous taps. Usually tapped QD or QOD (see below). Use a 27 Ga butterfly needle, clean with at least 3 betadine stick swabs, withdraw ≈ 10 ml and send for culture. Reported infection rate: 8–12%[36]
   b) ventricular-subgaleal shunt: the side-port of the reservoir is left uncapped. A subgaleal pocket must be created at the time of surgery. Fluid is reabsorbed from this potential space. First performed in 1893 by Mikulicz-Radecki (1850–1905). Use has been reported up to 35 days.[37] Infection rate: ≈ 6%
   c) the reservoir may be converted to VP shunt if and when appropriate. Not recommended in infants < 1100 gms due to very high infection rate
4. external ventricular drainage (EVD): similar to reservoir placement, but with possibility of inadvertent dislodgment (13%) and comparable infection rate (6%)

97

5. early VP shunting: high infection rate, peritoneal cavity not suitable in many cases, e.g., due to necrotizing enterocolitis (NEC), paucity of subcutaneous tissue through which to pass shunt tube… Not recommended for infants < 2000 gms

Temporary ventricular access device (TVAD)
Advantages of TVAD
1. avoids shunt in unhealthy children at risk of infection, skin breakdown, or other operative/anesthetic complications
2. clears protein and cellular debris (more favorable for subsequent shunting)
3. avoids repeated penetration of brain with risk of porencephaly
4. provides port for infusion of medication (e.g., antibiotics) PRN
5. avoids cumbersome, easily dislodged EVD with infection risk 6% on average of 13 days of EVD
6. up to 25% of patients will recover and avoid permanent shunt placement[38,39]

Disadvantages of TVAD
1. requires services of a neurosurgeon (not always available)
2. increases risk of infection of subsequent permanent shunt from 5% to 13%[40]
3. inherent risks of surgery including hemorrhage, infection, ventriculitis, meningitis, CSF leak
4. risks of overdrainage including subdural hematoma, impaired skull growth

Technical considerations for serial taps (via ventricular reservoir or LP)
8–20 cc of fluid are removed initially, and this is repeated daily (or more often if AF become very tense before 24 hours elapse) for several days, and then usually varies from 5–20 cc qod to 15 cc TID depending on response. The frequency and volume of the taps are modified based on:
1. fullness of AF: attempt to keep AF from becoming tense
2. appearance of ventricles on serial U/S: strive to prevent progressive enlargement, reduction in size can usually be achieved
3. follow OFC: should not cross percentile curves (need to differentiate from the so-called "catch-up phase" of brain growth which may occur once the infant overcomes their overall medical problems and is able to adequately utilize nutrition[41,42]; serial U/S will show rapid brain growth without progressive ventriculomegaly in cases of catch-up brain growth)
4. CSF protein concentration: controversial. Diminishes with serial taps. Some feel that as long as it is ≥ 100 mg/dl it is unlikely that significant spontaneous resorption will occur and continued serial taps will probably be needed
5. NB: removal of this volume of fluid may cause electrolyte disturbances, primarily hyponatremia; ∴ follow serum electrolytes on a regular basis

Follow with serial U/S on day 3–5, and then weekly for several weeks, and then bi-weekly. A baseline CT scan is often obtained prior to placement of a permanent shunt.

Insertion of VP shunt or conversion of sub-Q reservoir to VP shunt
Indications and requirements:
1. symptomatic hydrocephalus (p. 1633) and/or progressive ventriculomegaly
2. infant is extubated (and thus off ventilator)
3. infant weighs ≥ 2000 grams (some prefer ≥ 2500 grams)
4. no evidence of NEC (might create problems with peritoneal end of catheter)
5. CSF protein ideally < 100 mg/dl (because of concerns about plugging of the shunt, or causing ileus or malabsorption of the fluid—which was not seen with high-protein fluid shunted from the subdural space[43]—and also to see if patient will start reabsorbing CSF on their own)

Technical recommendations:
1. do not tap reservoir for at least 24 hrs before inserting a new ventricular catheter (allows ventricles to expand to facilitate catheterization)
2. obtain U/S the day prior to conversion
3. use a low- or very-low-pressure system (if CSF protein is high, consider a valveless system), upgrade later in infancy if necessary
4. avoid placing shunt hardware in areas on which these debilitated infants tend to lie (to prevent skin breakdown with hardware exposure)

97

97.2.11 Outcome

Short-term

Preemies with PIVH have higher mortality than matched preemies without PIVH.

The incidence of mortality and progression of hemorrhage is higher the earlier the hemorrhage occurs. The more severe the hemorrhage, the higher the mortality and the higher the risk of HCP (► Table 97.3).

Table 97.3 Short-term outcome of PIVH (≈ 250 cases[2])

Severity of hemorrhage	Deaths (%)	Progressive hydrocephalus (%)
mild	0	0–10
moderate	5–15	15–25
severe	50–65	65–100

Long-term

The effect of low-grade PIVH on long-term neurodevelopment has not been studied well. Most investigators feel that higher grades of PIVH are associated with greater degrees of handicaps than matched controls.

In one study of 12 infants with Grade II PIVH treated with serial LPs and in the 7 with progressive ventriculomegaly with VP shunt followed for a mean of 4.5 years, all were ambulatory and 75% had IQ within normal range.[44]

A recent study of very-low-birth-weight infants showed that children 18–22 months of age with severe PIVH and shunts had significantly lower scores on the Bayley Scales of Infant Development IIR compared with children with no PIVH and children with equal grades of PIVH who did not require a shunt.[45]

97.3 Other causes of intracerebral hemorrhage in the newborn

1. birth trauma may result in subdural hemorrhage, tentorial hemorrhage, parenchymal hemorrhage, and/or subarachnoid blood. This is usually detected by imaging (U/S or CT) when an infant develops seizures, apnea, bradycardia, or, rarely, focal neurological deficits. It rarely requires surgical intervention
2. choroid plexus hemorrhage can result in IVH. In some cases HCP can develop and require shunt placement
3. hemorrhagic stroke has been identified in 6.2 per 100,000 live births.[46] The usual presentation was with encephalopathy (100%) and seizures (65%). 75% of the strokes were idiopathic. Other identified etiologies were thrombocytopenia and a single case of a cavernous malformation. Risk factors for perinatal hemorrhagic stroke include: male gender, fetal distress, emergent C-section, prematurity, and post-maturity
4. tumors in the neonate can present with hemorrhage
5. vascular malformations of any form can present in the neonate with hemorrhage, although this is uncommon. Vein of Galen malformations are diagnosed in the neonate in about 40% of cases.[47] Most of these infants present with fulminant congestive heart failure and 50% have ventriculomegaly

97

References

[1] Toffol GJ, Biller J, Adams HP. Nontraumatic Intracerebral Hemorrhage in Young Adults. Arch Neurol. 1987; 44:483–485
[2] Volpe JJ. Neonatal Intraventricular Hemorrhage. N Engl J Med. 1981; 304:886–891
[3] Lou HC, Lassen NA, Friis-Hansen B. Impaired Autoregulation of Cerebral Blood Flow in the Distressed Newborn Infant. J Pediatr. 1979; 94:118–121
[4] Milligan DWA. Failure of Autoregulation and Intraventricular Hemorrhage in Preterm Infants. Lancet. 1980; 1:896–898
[5] Hambleton G, Wigglesworth JS. Origin of intraventricular haemorrhage in the preterm infant.

Archives of Disease in Childhood. 1976; 51:651–659
[6] Dykes FD, Lazzara A, Ahmann P, et al. Intraventricular Hemorrhage: A Prospective Evaluation of Etiopathologies. Pediatrics. 1980; 66:42–49
[7] Perlman JM, McMenamin JB, Volpe JJ. Fluctuating Cerebral Blood-Flow Velocity in Respiratory Distress Syndrome. N Engl J Med. 1983; 309:204–209
[8] Wirtschafter DD, Danielsen BH, Main EK, et al. Promoting antenatal steroid use for fetal maturation: results from the California Perinatal Quality Care Collaborative. Journal of Pediatrics. 2006; 148:606–612

[9] Volpe JJ. Effect of Cocaine Use on the Fetus. New England Journal of Medicine. 1992; 327:399–407

[10] Murphy BP, Inder TE, Rooks V, et al. Posthaemorrhagic ventricular dilatation in the premature infant: natural history and predictors of outcome. Archives of Disease in Childhood. Fetal and Neonatal Edition. 2002; 87:F37–F41

[11] Sheth RD. Trends in incidence and severity of intraventricular hemorrhage. Journal of Child Neurology. 1998; 13:261–264

[12] Papile LA, Burstein J, Burstein R, et al. Incidence and Evolution of Subependymal and Intraventricular Hemorrhage: A Study of Infants with Birth Weights Less Than 1,500 Gm. J Pediatr. 1978; 92:529–534

[13] Bejar R, Curbelo V, Coen RW, et al. Diagnosis and Follow-Up of Intraventricular and Intracerebral Hemorrhages by Ultrasound Studies of Infant's Brain Through the Fontanelles and Sutures. Pediatrics. 1980; 66:661–673

[14] Tsiantos A, Victorin L, Relier JP, et al. Intracranial Hemorrhage in the Prematurely Born Infant. J Pediatr. 1974; 85:854–859

[15] Perlman JM, Volpe JJ. Cerebral Blood Flow Velocity in Relation to Intraventricular Hemorrhage in the Premature Newborn Infant. J Pediatr. 1982; 100:956–959

[16] Ment LR, Oh W, Philip AG, et al. Risk factors for early intraventricular hemorrhage in low birth weight infants. Journal of Pediatrics. 1992; 121:776–783

[17] Crowley P, Chalmers I, Keirse MJ. The effects of corticosteroid administration before preterm delivery: an overview of the evidence from controlled trials. British Journal of Obstetrics and Gynaecology. 1990; 97:11–25

[18] Murphy KE, Hannah ME, Willan AR, et al. Multiple courses of antenatal corticosteroids for preterm birth (MACS): a randomised controlled trial. Lancet. 2008; 372:2143–2151

[19] Rabe H, Reynolds G, Diaz-Rossello J. Early versus delayed umbilical cord clamping in preterm infants. Cochrane Database Syst Rev. 2004. DOI: 10.1002/14651858.CD003248.pub2

[20] Volpe JJ. Neurology of the Newborn. 4th ed. Philadelphia: W. B. Saunders; 2008

[21] Fishman MA, Dutton RY, Okumura S. Progressive Ventriculomegaly following Minor Intracranial Hemorrhage in Premature Infants. Dev Med Child Neurol. 1984; 26:725–731

[22] Hill A, Rozdilsky B. Congenital Hydrocephalus Secondary to Intra-Uterine Germinal Matrix/Intraventricular Hemorrhage. Dev Med Child Neurol. 1984; 26:509–527

[23] James HE, Bejar R, Merritt A, et al. Management of Hydrocephalus Secondary to Intracranial Hemorrhage in the High Risk Newborn. Neurosurgery. 1984; 14:612–618

[24] Volpe JJ, Herscovitch P, Perlman JM, et al. Positron Emission Tomography in the Newborn: Extensive Impairment of Regional Cerebral Blood Flow with Intraventricular Hemorrhage and Hemorrhagic Intracerebral Involvement. Pediatrics. 1983

[25] Ment LR, Duncan CC, Ehrenkranz RA, et al. Intraventricular Hemorrhage in the Preterm Neonate: Timing and Cerebral Blood Flow Changes. J Pediatr. 1984; 104:419–425

[26] Trounce JQ, Fagan D, Levene MI. Intraventricular Hemorrhage and Periventricular Leucomalacia: Ultrasound and Autopsy Correlation. Arch Dis Child. 1983; 61:1203–1207

[27] Brenner DJ. Estimating cancer risks from pediatric CT: going from the qualitative to the quantitative. Pediatric Radiology. 2002; 32:228–3; discussion 242–4

[28] International PHVD Drug Trial Group. International randomised controlled trial of acetazolamide and furosemide in posthaemorrhagic ventricular dilatation in infancy. Lancet. 1998; 352:433–440

[29] Whitelaw A, Kennedy CR, Brion LP. Diuretic therapy for newborn infants with posthemorrhagic ventricular dilatation. Cochrane Database Syst Rev. 2001. DOI: 10.1002/14651858.CD002270

[30] Rom S, Serfontein GL, Humphreys RP. Intracerebellar Hematoma in the Neonate. J Pediatr. 1978; 93:486–488

[31] Murphy BP, Inder TE, Rooks V, et al. Posthaemorrhagic ventricular dilatation in the premature infant: natural history and predictors of outcome. Archives of Disease in Childhood. Fetal and Neonatal Edition. 2002; 87:F37–F41

[32] Kreusser KL, Tarby TJ, Kovnar E, et al. Serial Lumbar Punctures for at Least Temporary Amelioration of Neonatal Posthemorrhagic Hydrocephalus. Pediatrics. 1985; 75

[33] Whitelaw A. Repeated lumbar or ventricular punctures in newborns with intraventricular hemorrhage. Cochrane Database Syst Rev. 2001

[34] Benzel EC, Reeves JP, Nguyen PK, et al. The treatment of hydrocephalus in preterm infants with intraventricular haemorrhage. Acta Neurochirurgica (Wien). 1993; 122:200–203

[35] Marlin AE, Rivera S, Gaskill SJ. Treatment of posthemorrhagic ventriculomegaly in the preterm infant: Use of the subcutaneous ventricular reservoir. Concepts in Pediatric Neurosurgery. 1988; 8:15–22

[36] Hudgins RJ, Boydston WR, Gilreath CL. Treatment of posthemorrhagic hydrocephalus in the preterm infant with a ventricular access device. Pediatr Neurosurg. 1998; 29:309–313

[37] Tubbs RS, Smyth MD, Wellons JC,3rd, et al. Alternative uses for the subgaleal shunt in pediatric neurosurgery. Pediatr Neurosurg. 2003; 39:22–24

[38] Fulmer BB, Grabb PA, Oakes WJ, et al. Neonatal ventriculosubgaleal shunts. Neurosurgery. 2000; 47:80–3; discussion 83-4

[39] Rahman S, Teo C, Morris W, et al. Ventriculosubgaleal shunt: a treatment option for progressive posthemorrhagic hydrocephalus. Child's Nervous System. 1995; 11:650–654

[40] Wellons JC, Shannon CN, Kulkarni AV, et al. A multicenter retrospective comparison of conversion from temporary to permanent cerebrospinal fluid diversion in very low birth weight infants with posthemorrhagic hydrocephalus. J Neurosurg Pediatr 2009; 4:50–55

[41] Bridgers SL, Ment LR. Absence of Hydrocephalus despite Disproportionately Increasing Head Size After the Neonatal Period in Preterm Infants with Known Intraventricular Hemorrhage. Childs Brain 1981; 8:423–426

[42] Sher PK, Brown SA. A Longitudinal Study of Head Growth in Preterm Infants: II. Differentiation between 'Catch-Up' Head-Growth and Early Infantile Hydrocephalus. Dev Med Child Neurol. 1975; 17:711–718

[43] Aoki N, Miztani H, Masuzawa H. Unilateral Subdural-Peritoneal Shunting for Bilateral Chronic Subdural Hematomas in Infancy. J Neurosurg. 1985; 63:134–137

[44] Krishnamoorthy K, Kuehnle KJ, Todres ID, et al. Neurodevelopmental Outcome of Survivors with Posthemorrhagic Hydrocephalus. Ann Neurol. 1984; 15:201–204

[45] Adams-Chapman I, Hansen NI, Stoll BJ, et al. Neurodevelopmental outcome of extremely low birth weight infants with posthemorrhagic hydrocephalus requiring shunt insertion. Pediatrics. 2008; 121 e1167–e1177

[46] Armstrong-Wells J, Johnston SC, Wu YW, et al. Prevalence and predictors of perinatal hemorrhagic stroke: results from the Kaiser Pediatric Stroke Study. Pediatrics. 2009; 123:823–828

[47] Alexander MJ, Spetzler RF. Pediatric Neurovascular Disease. New York: Thieme Medical Publishers, Inc; 2006

Part XXI

Outcome Assessment

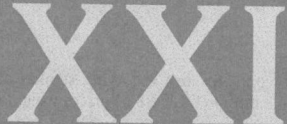

98 Outcome Assessment

98.1 Cancer

▶ **Karnofsky performance scale (KPS).** ▶ Table 98.1 (after David A. Karnofsky), often used for grading functional status in patients with cancer. A KPS score < 70 (particularly with brain tumors) often identifies patients with a worse prognosis for any given treatment.

Table 98.1 Karnofsky performance status scale (modified[1,2])

Score	Criteria	General category
100	normal: no complaints, no evidence of disease	Able to carry on normal activity and work. No special care is needed
90	able to carry on normal activity: minor signs or symptoms	
80	normal activity with effort: some signs or symptoms	
70	cares for self: unable to carry on normal activity or to do active work	Unable to work. Able to live at home, care for most personal needs. Variable assistance is required
60	requires occasional assistance: cares for most of needs	
50	requires considerable assistance and frequent care	
40	disabled: requires special care and assistance	Unable to care for self. Requires equivalent of institutional or hospital care. Disease may be rapidly progressing
30	severely disabled: hospitalized; death not imminent	
20	very sick: hospitalized; active supportive care needed	
10	moribund: fatal processes are progressing rapidly	
0	dead	

WHO performance score. ▶ Table 98.2, the WHO Performance score[3] (AKA The Eastern Cooperative Oncology Group (ECOG) score, AKA Zubrod score [after C. Gordon Zubrod]), ranges from 0 to 5, with 0 indicating perfect health and 5 death. The advantage over the Karnofsky scale is its simplicity.

Table 98.2 WHO performance scale

Grade	Description
0	Fully active, no performance restriction as a result of disease.
1	Restricted in physically strenuous activity. Ambulatory. Able to do light work, e.g., light house work, desk work.
2	Unable to perform any work activities. Ambulatory. Up & about > 50% of waking hours.
3	Only able to perform limited self-care. Wheelchair-confined > 50% of waking hours.
4	Completely disabled. Unable to perform self-care. Totally bed- or chair-confined.
5	Dead

98.2 Head injury

The **Ranchos Los Amigos scale** (▶ Table 98.3) is often used in rating *disability* following head injury. The Glasgow outcome scale[4] and the augmented Glasgow Outcome Scale - Extended (GOSE) (▶ Table 98.4) are frequently employed in *outcome* assessment. For the GOSE, the use of a structured interview is recommended to enhance the consistency of ratings.

98.3 Cerebrovascular events

98.3.1 General information

Several outcome grading scales have come to be favored for use following strokes or SAH. Each emphasizes different aspects of outcome. The Barthel Index (▶ Table 98.6) places weight on activities

Table 98.3 Ranchos Los Amigos cognitive scale

Level	Meaning
I	no response to pain, touch, sight, or sound
II	generalized reflex responses to pain
III	**Localized response** blinks to strong light, turns towards/away from sound, responds to physical discomfort, inconsistent responses to commands
IV	**Confused—Agitated** alert, very active, agitated, aggressive, or bizarre behaviors. Performs motor activities but behavior is non-purposeful, extremely short attention span
V	**Confused—Non-agitated** gross attention to environment, easily distracted, requires continual redirection, difficulty learning new tasks, agitated by excess stimulation. May converse socially but with inappropriate verbalizations
VI	**Confused—Appropriate** inconsistent orientation to time and place. Retention span and recent memory impaired. Begins to recall past, consistently follows simple commands, goal-directed behavior with assistance
VII	**Automatic—Appropriate** performs daily routine in highly familiar environment in a non-confused but automatic "robot-like" fashion. Skills deteriorate in unfamiliar environment. Lacks realistic planning for future
VIII	**Purposeful—Appropriate**

Table 98.4 Glasgow outcome scale extended[5] and original[4]

Glasgow Outcome Scale - Extended (GOSE)[5]		Score	Glasgow Outcome Scale (original)[4]
death		1	death—most deaths ascribable to primary head injury occur within 48 hrs
vegetative		2	persistent vegetative state—unresponsive & speechless. After 2–3 weeks, may open eyes & have sleep/wake cycles
severe disability	low severe disability: dependent for daily support for physical and/or mental disability, but can be left alone at home > 8 hrs	3	severe disability (conscious but disabled)—dependent for daily support (may be institutionalized, but this is not a criterion)
	upper severe disability: as with #3, but cannot be left alone at home > 8 hrs	4	moderate disability (disabled but independent)—travel by public transportation, can work in sheltered setting (exceeds mere ability to perform "activities of daily living")
moderate disability	low moderate disability: some disability (e.g., aphasia, hemiparesis, seizures, memory deficits...). Independent at home, but dependent outside. Unable to return to work	5	good recovery—resumption of normal life despite minor deficits ("return to work" not reliable)
	upper moderate disability: as with #5 but able to return to work even if special arrangement is needed	6	—
good recovery	lower good recovery: resumption of normal life with capacity to work, even if pre-injury status is not achieved, but no disabling deficits	7	—
	upper good recovery: as with #7, but with disabling deficits	8	—

of daily living (ADLs), while others, such as the modified Rankin Scale[6] (▶ Table 98.5) assess levels of independence, include a comparison to previous activity levels, and show fairly good interobserver consistency.[7] While it does measure functional status, the modified Rankin is not sensitive to subtle neurologic deficits such as dysphasia or visual field defects.

Table 98.5 The modified* Rankin Scale

Grade	Description
0	no symptoms at all
1	no significant disability despite symptoms: able to carry out all usual duties & activities
2	slight disability: unable to carry out all previous activities. Able to look after own affairs without assistance
3	moderate disability: requiring some help, but able to walk without assistance
4	moderately severe disability: unable to walk without assistance, and unable to attend to own bodily needs without assistance
5	severe disability: bedridden, incontinent, and requiring constant nursing care and attention

*the original Rankin scale[8]: did not have Grade 0, Grade 1 did not include the words "despite symptoms" and "& activities," and it defined Grade 2 as "unable to carry out some of previous activities..."

Table 98.6 The Barthel index

Item	Original Barthel Index			Modified Barthel Index				
	Unable to perform task	Needs assistance	Fully independent	CODE 1	CODE 2	CODE 3	CODE 4	CODE 5
				Unable to perform task	Attempts task but unsafe	Moderate help required	Minimal help required	Fully independent
Personal hygiene	0	0	5	0	1	3	4	5
Self-bathing	0	0	5	0	1	3	4	5
Feeding	0	5	10	0	2	5	8	10
Toilet	0	5	10	0	2	5	8	10
Stair climbing	0	5	10	0	2	5	8	10
Dressing	0	5	10	0	2	5	8	10
Bowel control	0	5	10	0	2	5	8	10
Bladder control	0	5	10	0	2	5	8	10
Ambulation	0	5–10	15	0	3	8	12	15
Wheelchair[a]	0	0	5	0	1	3	4	5
Chair/bed transfers	0	5–10	15	0	3	8	12	15
Total (range)	0	→→	100	0	→→→→			100

[a]score only if unable to walk and patient trained in wheelchair management

98.3.2 Scales

▶ **Modified Rankin scale** (▶ Table 98.5)
▶ **Barthel index** (▶ Table 98.6). The original Barthel index[9,10] assigns one of three scores to 10 ratable ADLs, and then the individual scores are summed. The modified Barthel index (MBI) with a 5-step scoring system appears to have greater sensitivity.[11] The total ranges from 0 to 100 (a score of 100 implies functional independence, not necessarily normality).

Of all the factors, independence in bathing was the most difficult. Abilities on the Barthel index tend to return in a fairly consistent order, and so most patients with the same score will have similar patterns of disability.

98.4 Spinal cord injury

▶ **Functional Independence Measure™ (FIM™)**.[12,13,14] Developed to provide uniform evaluation of disability for spinal cord injuries. Rates 18 items shown in ▶ Table 98.7 (13 motor, 5 cognitive) on the 7-level scale shown in ▶ Table 98.8.

The FIM™ has high internal consistency and is a good indicator of burden of care.[15,16]

Table 98.7 The Functional Independence Measure™ (FIM)

Classification	Item	Score*
Motor		
self-care	eating	(1 - 7)
	grooming	(1 - 7)
	bathing	(1 - 7)
	dressing—upper body	(1 - 7)
	dressing—lower body	(1 - 7)
	toileting	(1 - 7)
sphincter control	bladder management	(1 - 7)
	bowel management	(1 - 7)
mobility	bed, chair, wheelchair	(1 - 7)
	toilet	(1 - 7)
	tub, shower	(1 - 7)
locomotion	walk or wheelchair	(1 - 7)
	stairs	(1 - 7)
Cognitive		
communication	comprehension	(1 - 7)
	expression	(1 - 7)
social cognition	social interaction	(1 - 7)
	problem solving	(1 - 7)
	memory	(1 - 7)
FIM™ → TOTAL		(18 – 126)

* Score 1–7 as shown in ▶ Table 98.8

Table 98.8 The 7 FIM™ rating levels of disability

Degree of dependency	Level of function	Score
no helper	complete independence	7
	nodified independence	6
modified dependence on a helper	supervision	5
	minimal assist (≥ 75% independent)	4
	moderate assist (≥ 50% independent)	3
complete dependence on a helper	maximal assist (≥ 25% independence)	2
	total assist (< 25% independence)	1

98

References

[1] Karnofsky DA, Burchenal JH, Macleod CM. Evaluation of Chemotherapy Agents. New York: Columbia University Press; 1949:191–205

[2] Karnofsky D, Burchenal JH, Armistead GC, et al. Triethylene melamine in the treatment of neoplastic disease. Archives of Internal Medicine. 1951; 87:477–516

[3] Oken MM, Creech RH, Tormey DC, et al. Toxicity and response criteria of the Eastern Cooperative Oncology Group. Am J Clin Oncol. 1982; 5:649–655

[4] Jennett B, Bond M. Assessment of Outcome After Severe Brain Damage: A Practical Scale. Lancet. 1975; i:480–484

[5] Wilson JT, Pettigrew LE, Teasdale GM. Structured interviews for the Glasgow Outcome Scale and the extended Glasgow Outcome Scale: guidelines for their use. J Neurotrauma. 1998; 15:573–585

[6] UK-TIA Study Group. The UK-TIA Aspirin Trial: Interim Results. British Medical Journal. 1988; 296:316–320

[7] van Swieten JC, Koudstaal PJ, Visser MC. Interobserver agreement for the assessment of handicap in stroke patients. Stroke. 1988; 19:604–607

[8] Rankin J. Cerebral Vascular Accidents in Patients Over the Age of 60. 2. Prognosis. Scott Med J. 1957; 2:200–215

[9] Mahoney FI, Barthel DW. Functional Evaluation: The Barthel Index. Maryland State Med J. 1965; 14:61–65

[10] Wade DT, Hewer RL. Functional abilities after stroke: Measurement, natural history and prognosis. Journal of Neurology, Neurosurgery, and Psychiatry. 1987; 50:177–182

[11] Shah S, Vanclay F, Cooper B. Improving the sensitivity of the Barthel Index for stroke rehabilitation. J Clin Epidemiol. 1989; 42:703–709

[12] Forer S, Granger C, et al. Functional Independence Measure. Buffalo, NY: The Buffalo General Hospital, State University of New York at Buffalo; 1987

[13] Ditunno JF,Jr. New spinal cord injury standards, 1992. Paraplegia. 1992; 30:90–91

[14] Ditunno JF,Jr. Functional assessment measures in CNS trauma. J Neurotrauma. 1992; 9:S301–S305

[15] Dodds TA, Martin DP, Stolov WC, et al. A validation of the functional independence measurement and its performance among rehabilitation inpatients. Arch Phys Med Rehabil. 1993; 74:531–536

[16] Linacre JM, Heinemann AW, Wright BD, et al. The structure and stability of the Functional Independence Measure. Arch Phys Med Rehabil. 1994; 75:127–132

Part XXII

Differential Diagnosis

XXII

99 Differential Diagnosis by Location or Radiographic Finding – Intracranial

99.1 Diagnoses covered outside this chapter

See ▶ Table 99.1.

Table 99.1 Differential diagnoses by location or radiographic finding, intracranial—covered outside this chapter

DDx
chordomas (p. 825)
extra-axial fluid (peds) (p. 1087)
gyral enhancement (p. 1560)
hydrocephalus (p. 433)
pineal region tumors (p. 758)
pneumocephalus (p. 1067)
schizencephaly (p. 309)

99.2 Posterior fossa lesions

99.2.1 Cerebellar lesions

General information

The following addresses *intra*-axial p-fossa abnormalities (for extra-axial lesions, see below).

Adult

Single lesion
▶ **Note.** Rule of thumb: "the differential diagnosis of a solitary intraparenchymal lesion in an adult p-fossa is metastasis, metastasis, metastasis, until proven otherwise."
1. tumors:
   a) metastasis
   b) hemangioblastoma (p. 822): the most common PRIMARY intra-axial p-fossa tumor in adults (7–12% of p-fossa tumors). Very vascular nodule, often has cyst. Almost all p-fossa tumors are relatively avascular on angiography *except* these (look for serpentine signal voids especially in the periphery of the lesion on MRI,[1] much less common in cavernous hemangioma)
   c) cerebellar (pilocytic) astrocytoma (p. 693): may be solid or cystic, tends to occur in younger adults
   d) brainstem glioma: an isolated glioblastoma in the posterior fossa of an adult is a reportable rarity
   e) choroid plexus tumor: usually infratentorial in adults (p. 1665)
   f) cerebellar liponeurocytoma (p. 721)
2. infectious: abscess
3. vascular
   a) cavernous hemangioma
   b) hemorrhage
   c) infarction: cerebellar stroke may be associated with H/A and/or pain in suboccipital region or upper neck
      • embolic
      • thrombotic/plaque-related
      • vertebral artery dissection: much less common than carotid dissection (p. 1579)
      • vertebrobasilar hypoplasia (p. 1592)
4. Lhermitte-Duclos (p. 716): Focal or diffuse. Nonenhancing. Characteristic tiger stripes. Widens folia (cf. most neoplasms which destroy folial pattern)

Multiple lesions
1. metastases
2. hemangioblastoma (possibly as part of von Hippel-Lindau) (p. 646)

99

3. abscesses
4. cavernous hemangiomas

Pediatric

Also see Pediatric brain tumors (p.621).

Early data: 67% of childhood brain tumors occur in p-fossa, and astrocytomas were the most common there. Currently: p-fossa tumors comprise 54–60% of childhood brain tumors (breakdown listed below). 4 types account for ≈ 95% of infratentorial tumors in patients ≤ 18 yrs of age.[2] The 3 most common are equal in incidence (expressed as percent of p-fossa tumors pooled from 1,350 pediatric brain tumors[3]):

1. medulloblastoma (p.744): 27%
   a) most start in *roof* of 4th ventricle (fastigium), and most are solid
   b) differentiating medulloblastoma (MB) from ependymoma:
      • 4th ventricle drapes around medulloblastoma ("banana sign") from the anterior aspect, cf. ependymoma which tends to grow into 4th ventricle from floor. Ependymoma may grow through foramen of Luschka and/or Magendie
      • ependymomas tend to be inhomogeneous on T1WI MRI (unlike MB)
      • the exophytic component of ependymomas tends to be high signal on T2WI MRI (with MB this is only mildly hyperintense)
      • calcifications: common in ependymomas, but only in < 10% of MB
2. cerebellar (pilocytic) astrocytoma (p.693): 27%. Most start in cerebellar hemisphere. Often cystic with enhancing mural nodule
3. brainstem gliomas (p.695): 28%. Usually present with multiple cranial nerve palsies and long tract findings
4. ependymoma (p.724): usually arise in *floor* of 4th ventricle
5. choroid plexus papilloma (p.739): majority of patients are < 2 yrs old
6. atypical teratoid/rhabdoid tumor (AT/RT) (p.754)
7. metastasis: neuroblastoma, rhabdomyosarcoma, Wilms tumor…
8. PHACES syndrome: acronym for a group of findings including Posterior fossa malformations, cervicofacial Hemangioma, Arterial anomalies of the head and neck, Coarctation of the aorta and cardiac defects, Eye anomalies, and Sternal cleft. Ratio girls:boys = 9:1. Thought to begin during gestation weeks 8–10

99.2.2 Cerebellopontine angle (CPA) lesions

Lesions in general

Vestibular schwannoma, meningioma, and epidermoid account for most. For those lesions that may be cystic, see below.

1. vestibular schwannoma: (80–90% of CPA lesions); see below for differentiating from meningioma (p.1648)
2. meningioma: (5–10%); see below for differentiating from vestibular schwannoma (p.1648)
3. ectodermal inclusion tumors (p.937)
   a) epidermoid (cholesteatoma): 5–7%. High signal on DWI MRI (p.937). Tumor passing from the posterior fossa to the middle fossa though the incisura is highly suggestive of epidermoid
   b) dermoid
4. metastases
5. neuroma from cranial nerves other than VIII (also see below for some differentiating features)
   a) trigeminal neuroma: expands towards Meckel's cave
   b) facial nerve neuroma[4]: may arise in any portion of the VII nerve, with a predilection for the geniculate ganglion.[5] Even in these tumors, hearing loss tends to precede facial paresis. Hearing loss may be sensorineural from VIII nerve compression from tumors arising in the proximal portion of VII (cisternal or internal auditory canal (IAC) segment), or it may be conductive from erosion of the ossicles by tumors arising in the second (tympanic, or horizontal) segment of VII. Facial palsy (peripheral) (p.607) may also develop, usually late[4]
   c) neurinoma of lowest 4 cranial nerves (IX, X, XI, XII)
6. arachnoid cyst (p.260)
7. neurenteric cyst (p.313): rare.[6] May secrete mucin
8. cholesterol granuloma (distinct from epidermoid) (p.937)
9. lipoma
10. aneurysm: PICA, AICA, vertebrobasilar
11. dolichobasilar ectasia

99

12. cysticercosis
13. extensions of:
    a) brainstem or cerebellar glioma
    b) PitNET/adenoma
    c) craniopharyngioma
    d) chordoma & tumors of skull base
    e) 4th ventricle tumors (ependymoma, medulloblastoma)
    f) choroid plexus papilloma: from 4th ventricle through foramen of Luschka
    g) glomus tumor
        • glomus jugulare
        • glomus tympanicum
    h) primary tumors of temporal bone (e.g., sarcoma or carcinoma)

Cystic lesions of the CPA

CPA lesions from the above list that may be cystic or have a cystic component[6]:
1. arachnoid cyst: same intensity as CSF on all MRI sequences, homogeneous
2. epidermoid cyst (▶ Fig. 56.1): ★ high signal on DWI MRI differentiates this from arachnoid cyst
3. dermoid cyst: high-intensity areas on T1WI similar to fat; usually midline
4. cystic schwannoma
5. cholesterol granuloma: ★ ≈ only lesion that is high signal on T1WI (due to blood breakdown products; exception: the rare "white" epidermoid). Also high signal on T2WI. Usually extradural, especially near petrous apex. Bone destruction is common
6. neurenteric cyst: nonenhancing. Low intensity on DWI MRI
7. choroidal cyst
8. cysticercosis: enhancing nodule (scolex)

Differentiating neuromas of V, VII, and VIII cranial nerves

All 3 of these tumors may present in the CPA and may cross from posterior fossa to middle fossa, but they tend to do so in different manners. Vestibular schwannomas show "transhiatal" extension by passing through the tentorial hiatus medially. Most trigeminal neuromas show "transapicopetrosal" extension by crossing into the middle fossa via the petrous apex (although some show transhiatal extension). When facial neuromas cross, they tend to spread across the midpetrosal bone, which is characteristic for facial neuromas.[4] When a facial neuroma enlarges the IAC, unlike a vestibular schwannoma, it tends to erode the anterosuperior aspect of the IAC.

Differentiating vestibular schwannoma from CPA meningioma

1. vestibular schwannoma (VS) (AKA acoustic neuroma):
   a) clinical: progressive unilateral hearing loss, usually with tinnitus. Progression results in unsteadiness, with true vertigo being rare. The facial nerve is more resistant to stretching, and thus facial nerve signs and symptoms occur late. Trigeminal nerve involvement may occur with tumors > 3 cm (check corneal reflex), with tic douloureux-like symptoms being unusual
   b) imaging: often heterogeneous signal and nonuniform enhancement. Medium-size tumors look like ice cream in a cone (IAC is the cone). Rarely calcified. Except for very small tumors, IAC is frequently enlarged. Look for an acute angle between the tumor and the petrous bone (meningiomas usually have an obtuse angle)
2. meningiomas: may mimic VSs with these differences:
   a) clinical: since they often arise from the superior anterior edge of the IAC, early facial nerve involvement is more common, and hearing loss is usually *late*. Trigeminal neuralgia-like pain is more common than with VSs
   b) imaging: homogeneous signal and enhancement. The tumor may enter the IAC but it tends not to enlarge it. IAC often eccentric in tumor. Tumor is flat against petrous bone with an obtuse angle to the bone. *Calcification and bony hypertrophy* may occur (which occasionally *narrows* the IAC).

99.2.3 Petrous apex lesions

1. infection/inflammatory:
   a) osteomyelitis: may produce Gradenigo's syndrome (p.601)
   b) cholesterol granuloma (bright on T1WI; epidermoid cysts, ▶ Fig. 56.1 are bright on DWI, neither enhance)

2. vascular lesions: aneurysm
3. neoplastic:
   a) squamous cell cancer
   b) glomus tumor
   c) chondrosarcoma: will displace the carotid from medial to lateral (almost every other tumor in this region encases the carotid)

99.2.4 Foramen magnum lesions

Differential diagnosis

See Foramen magnum lesions (p. 1649) for *nonneoplastic* lesions. Most foramen magnum (FM) region tumors are extra-axial. This includes:
1. extra-axial tumors
   a) meningioma: the anterior lip of the foramen magnum is the second most common site of origin of posterior fossa meningiomas. Meningiomas (p. 817) comprise 38–46% of FM tumors[7,8] and most are intradural
   b) Chordoma (p. 825): a mass behind the dens compressing the spinal cord is a chordoma until proven otherwise
   c) neurilemmoma
   d) epidermoid
   e) chondroma
   f) chondrosarcoma
   g) metastases
2. exophytic component of a brainstem tumor
3. non-neoplastic lesions
   a) aneurysms or ectasia of the vertebral artery
   b) odontoid process in cases of basilar invagination (p. 228)
   c) pannus from involvement of the odontoid with rheumatoid arthritis or old nonunion of fracture
   d) synovial cyst of the quadrate ligament of the odontoid[9]

Presentation

In the pre-imaging era (i.e., before CT & MRI) these lesions were often diagnosed relatively late due to the unusual associated clinical syndromes and the rarity of visualizing this region on myelography.

Clinical findings

Symptoms:
1. sensory
   a) craniocervical pain: usually an early symptom, commonly in neck and occiput. Aching in nature. ↑ with head movement
   b) sensory findings: usually occur later. Numbness and tingling of the fingers
2. motor
   a) spastic weakness of the extremities: weakness usually starts in the ipsilateral UE, then the ipsilateral LE, then the contralateral LE, and finally the contralateral UE ("rotating paralysis")

Signs:
1. sensory
   a) dissociated sensory loss: loss of pain and temperature contralateral to lesion with preservation of tactile sensation
   b) loss of position and vibratory sense, greater in the upper than the lower extremities
2. motor
   a) spastic weakness of the extremities
   b) atrophy of the intrinsic hand muscles: a lower motor nerve finding
   c) cerebellar findings may rarely be present with extensive intracranial extension
3. long tract findings
   a) brisk muscle stretch reflexes (hyperreflexia, spasticity)
   b) loss of abdominal cutaneous reflexes
   c) neurogenic bladder: usually a very late finding

99

4. ipsilateral Horner syndrome: due to compression of cervical sympathetics
5. nystagmus: classically downbeat nystagmus (p.586), but other types can occur

It had been postulated that long tract findings were due to direct compression at the cervicomedullary junction, and that lower motor nerve findings in the upper extremities were due to central necrosis of the gray matter as a result of compression of arterial blood supply. Anatomic study suggests that it is actually *venous* infarction at lower cervical levels (C8–1) that is responsible for the lower motor neuron findings.

99.3 Multiple intracranial lesions on CT or MRI

1. neoplastic
   a) primary
      - multicentric gliomas; ≈ 6% of gliomas are multicentric, more common in neurofibromatosis, see Multiple gliomas (p.667)
      - tuberous sclerosis (including giant cell astrocytomas); (usually periventricular)
      - multiple meningiomas
      - lymphoma
      - PNET
      - multiple neuromas (usually in neurofibromatosis, including bilateral vestibular schwannomas)
   b) metastatic: usually cortical or subcortical, surrounded by prominent vasogenic edema (p.911). More common tumors include:
      - lung
      - breast
      - melanoma: may be higher density than brain on unenhanced CT
      - renal cell
      - gastrointestinal tumors
      - genitourinary tract tumors
      - choriocarcinoma
      - testicular
      - atrial myxoma
      - leukemia
2. infection: mostly abscess or cerebritis. Most commonly due to:
   a) pyogenic bacteria
   b) toxoplasmosis: common in AIDS patients (p.404)
   c) fungal
      - cryptococcus
      - mycoplasma
      - coccidiomycosis
      - aspergillosis
      - candidiasis
   d) echinococcus
   e) schistosomiasis
   f) paragonimiasis
   g) herpes simplex encephalitis (HSE): usually temporal lobe (p.397)
3. inflammatory
   a) demyelinating disease
      - MS: usually in white matter, periventricular, with little mass effect, margins are usually very sharp. Ring-enhancing lesions can occur with tumefactive demyelinating lesions (p.187)
      - progressive multifocal leukoencephalopathy (PML): primarily in white matter. No enhancement. Patients are usually very sick
   b) gummas
   c) granulomas
   d) amyloidosis
   e) sarcoidosis
   f) vasculitis or arteritis
   g) collagen vascular disease, including:
      - periarteritis nodosa (PAN) (p.208)
      - systemic lupus erythematosus (SLE)
      - granulomatous arteritis
4. vascular
   a) multiple aneurysms (congenital or atherosclerotic)

b) multiple hemorrhages, e.g., associated with DIC or other coagulopathies (including anticoagulant therapy)
c) venous infarctions, especially in dural sinus thrombosis (p. 1594)
d) moyamoya disease (p. 1581)
e) subacute hypertension (as in malignant HTN, eclampsia…) → symmetric confluent lesions with mild mass effect and patchy enhancement, usually in occipital subcortical white matter
f) multiple strokes
   • lacunar strokes (l'etat lacunaire)
   • multiple emboli (e.g., in atrial fibrillation, mitral valve prolapse, SBE, air emboli)
   • sickle cell disease
   • vasculitis
   • intravascular lymphomatosis (p. 842)
5. hematomas and contusions
   a) traumatic (multiple hemorrhagic contusions, multiple SDH)
   b) multiple "hypertensive" hemorrhages (amyloid angiopathy, etc.)
6. intracranial calcifications (p. 1665)
7. miscellaneous
   a) radiation necrosis
   b) foreign bodies (e.g., post gunshot wound)
   c) periventricular low densities
      • Binswanger's disease
      • transependymal absorption of CSF (e.g., in active hydrocephalus)

▶ **Evaluation.** Deciding which of the following tests are needed to evaluate a patient with multiple intracranial lesions must be individualized for the appropriate clinical setting.
1. cardiac echo: to R/O SBE that could shed septic emboli
2. "metastatic workup" (p. 914) including:
   a) CT of chest/abdomen/pelvis with and without contrast: has become a relatively standard part of the metastatic workup. It has largely supplanted CXR, lower GI (barium enema), and IVP. Rationale:
      • Chest: R/O primary bronchogenic Ca or pulmonary metastases of another Ca. Can demonstrate mediastinal lymphadenopathy. Also to R/O pulmonary abscess that could shed septic emboli
      • Assesses for possible primary lesions: e.g., kidneys, GI, prostate
      • Evaluates for metastases to liver, adrenal, and even spine
   b) mammogram in women
   c) PSA in men

99.4 Ring-enhancing lesions on CT/MRI

99.4.1 Abscess vs. tumor

See ▶ Fig. 99.1 and ▶ Fig. 99.2. Tumor: the enhancing ring may be incomplete and irregular. Abscess: ring is usually complete, often thinner and smoother than with tumor. Abscess: usually brighter than tumor on DWI MRI.

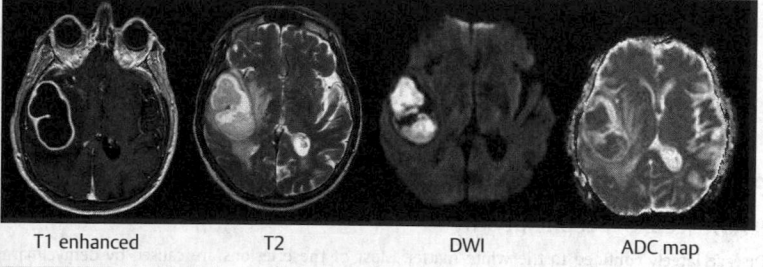

| T1 enhanced | T2 | DWI | ADC map |

Fig. 99.1 **Cerebral abscess**, right side. Image: MRI. NB: contents are bright on DWI.

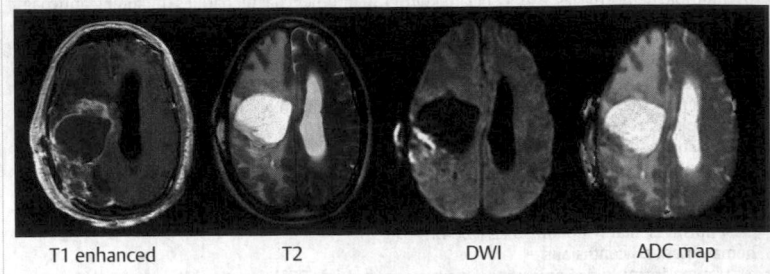

| T1 enhanced | T2 | DWI | ADC map |

Fig. 99.2 Glioblastoma, right side. Image: MRI. NB: dark on DWI.

MR spectroscopy (MRS) (p. 244) should theoretically be ideal for differentiating tumor from abscess (abscess should show reduced NAA, Cr and choline, and "atypical peaks" may be present), but in practice is often not conclusive.

99.4.2 Short list

Multiple lesions: metastases or abscess are much more likely than astrocytoma.
In adults, the main differential (short list) is:
1. high-grade glioma (glioblastoma)
2. metastasis
3. abscess
4. lymphoma should also always be tacked on as a possibility

99.4.3 Long list

Mnemonic: "Magic Dr" (metastasis (including lymphoma), abscess, glioma, infarct, contusion, demyelination, radiation).
1. astrocytoma: usually glioblastoma (GBM)
2. metastases (p. 908): especially lung
3. abscess (p. 343):
   a) may see visible growth over several days on serial imaging
   b) pyogenic abscesses are often (but not always) associated with fever and rapidly progressing neurologic deficit
   c) Nocardia abscesses (p. 366) are often *multiloculated* and are usually associated with a lung lesion
4. others
   a) lymphoma (primary brain lymphoma or metastatic systemic lymphoma): wall is thicker than abscess.[10] Incidence is increasing (p. 843)
   b) radiation necrosis
   c) resolving intracerebral hematoma: on T1 gradient echo sequence, a continuous ring suggests hematoma, an interrupted ring suggests malignancy
   d) cystic lesions with enhancing wall or mural nodule (see also intracranial cysts):
      • cysticercosis cyst, see Neurocysticercosis (p. 404)
      • hemangioblastoma
      • pilocytic astrocytoma
      • cystic acoustic neuroma
   e) trauma
   f) recent infarct
   g) thrombosed giant aneurysm

99.5 White matter lesions

99.5.1 Leukoencephalopathy

Disease largely confined to the white matter. Most of these lesions are caused by demyelinating disease.

Appear as white matter low density on CT or low signal on T1WI MRI, and high-intensity on T2WI. Usually does not enhance. Unlike a stroke, changes tend to spare the cortex. Conditions such as metabolic derangements, leuko-araiosis, etc. tend to produce fairly symmetric findings.

Differential diagnosis:
1. anoxia/ischemia
2. demyelinating disease
   a) MS
   b) ADEM (p. 190)
3. intoxication: cyanide, organic solvents, carbon monoxide
4. vitamin deficiencies: B12 with subacute combined degeneration
5. infectious, especially viral:
   a) progressive multifocal leukoencephalopathy (PML) (p. 354)
   b) herpes varicella-zoster leukoencephalitis (p. 399)
   c) HIV infection (AIDS): perivascular pattern of demyelination
   d) cytomegalovirus infection
   e) Creutzfeldt-Jakob disease: small and perivascular demyelination
6. metabolic derangements: hyponatremia (p. 114), excessively rapid correction of hyponatremia (causing osmotic myelinolysis)
7. hereditary: metachromatic leukodystrophy, adult-onset Schilder's disease
8. leuko-araiosis (p. 1670)
9. multiple myeloma (p. 928)
10. low-grade (WHO grade 2 infiltrating) glioma

99.5.2 Corpus callosum lesions

1. lymphoma
2. MS plaque
3. tumefactive demyelinating lesions (p. 190)
4. lipoma
5. diffuse axonal injury from trauma

99.6 Sellar, suprasellar, and parasellar lesions

99.6.1 General information

May enlarge, erode, or destroy the sella turcica. Considerations in adults (adenoma is the most common enhancing pituitary lesion) are different than for children (adenomas are rare, craniopharyngioma and germinoma are more common). Includes (modified[11]):

99.6.2 Tumors/pseudotumors

Tumors having epicenter within the sella

Pituitary tumor:
1. adenohypophyseal tumors
   a) pituitary neuroendocrine tumor (p. 854) (PitNET) AKA pituitary adenoma
      • microadenoma: < 1 cm diameter
      • macroadenoma: ≥ 1 cm diameter
      • invasive adenoma (p. 855): Includes aggressive tumors of Nelson's syndrome (p. 869)
   b) pituitary carcinoma (p. 855)
2. neurohypophyseal tumors (tumors of the posterior pituitary)
   a) metastases: the most common tumor found in the posterior pituitary (presumably due to rich blood supply): breast and lung are most common primaries[12]
   b) pituicytoma (p. 853): the most common tumor arising from neurohypophysis/pituitary stalk (i.e., primary)
   c) astrocytoma: arising from stalk or posterior pituitary

Pituitary "pseudotumor":
hyperplasia (enlargement)
   a) thyrotroph hyperplasia due to primary hypothyroidism[13] (see ▶ Table 52.2) causing chronic pituitary stimulation by TRH. Typically: free T4 is low or normal, TSH ↑↑, symmetrical sellar mass on MRI

b) gonadotroph hyperplasia: due to primary hypogonadism

c) somatotroph hyperplasia: due to ectopic GH-RH secretion

d) pregnancy: during pregnancy, the number of lactotrophs increases by 40% in response to elevated estrogen levels (lactotroph hyperplasia). The mean height of the gland on MRI during pregnancy is 9.6–10 mm, immediately postpartum it is 10–12 mm, and it returns to its pregravid size ≈ 6 months postpartum[14]

2. pituitary enlargement may occur in intracranial hypotension (p. 421)

3. the pituitary gland of young women of childbearing potential is normally slightly enlarged

Juxtasellar or suprasellar tumors or masses: any of these lesions may extend into the sella

1. craniopharyngioma (p. 849): in this region, these account for 20% of tumors in adult, 54% in peds

2. Rathke cleft cyst (p. 949)

3. meningioma (parasellar, tuberculum sellae, or diaphragma sellae): to differentiate tuberculum sellae meningioma from pituitary macroadenoma on MRI (▶ Fig. 99.3), 3 characteristics of meningioma are (1) bright homogeneous enhancement with gadolinium (cf. heterogeneous, poor enhancement with macroadenoma), (2) suprasellar epicenter (vs. sellar), and (3) tapered extension of intracranial dural base[15] (*dural tail*). Also, the *sella is usually not enlarged*, and even large suprasellar meningiomas rarely produce endocrine disturbances.[16] The pituitary stalk is sometimes being pushed posteriorly by a meningioma. Tuberculum sellae meningiomas may be associated with sphenoid pneumosinus dilatans[17] (enlargement of the underlying sphenoid sinus without bone erosion) as shown in ▶ Fig. 46.7

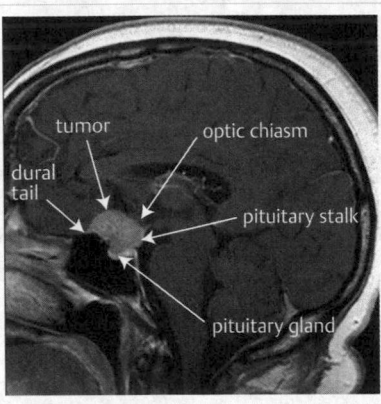

Fig. 99.3 Tuberculum sellae meningioma that could be mistaken for a PitNET/adenoma.
Image: contrast-enhanced T1WI sagittal MRI.

tumor

optic chiasm

dural tail

pituitary stalk

pituitary gland

4. pituitary tumor (mostly adenomas) with extrasellar extension: tends to push carotids laterally (unlike meningioma which may encase carotid), more symmetric than meningioma

5. germ cell tumors (GCT) (p. 831): choriocarcinoma, germinoma, teratoma, embryonal carcinoma, endodermal sinus tumor. In females, suprasellar GCTs are more common; in males pineal region is more common

a) *suprasellar* GCT: triad of diabetes insipidus, visual deficit, and panhypopituitarism.[18] May also present with obstructive hydrocephalus

b) simultaneous suprasellar and pineal lesions is diagnostic of GCT (so-called synchronous germ cell tumors (p. 831))

6. glioma

7. hypothalamic glioma

8. optic nerve or chiasm (optic glioma) (p. 694)

9. metastasis

10. chordoma

11. parasitic infections: cysticercosis

12. epidermoid cyst

13. suprasellar arachnoid cyst: see Arachnoid cysts (p. 280)

14. sarcoidosis (p.198): hypothalamic involvement is a more likely site as a cause of anterior and/or posterior pituitary insufficiency
15. bone abnormalities
    a) giant cell tumor (p.992)
    b) chondromyxoid fibroma
    c) brown tumor of hyperparathyroidism
    d) bone spur
    e) extramedullary hematopoiesis[19]

99.6.3 Vascular lesions

a) aneurysm: ACoA, ICA (p.1612) (cavernous carotid or suprasellar variant of superior hypophyseal artery aneurysm), ophthalmic, basilar bifurcation. Giant aneurysms may produce mass effect, and some may be mistaken for a PitNET/adenoma (see ▶ Fig. 99.4)
b) carotid-cavernous fistula (CCF) (p.1519)

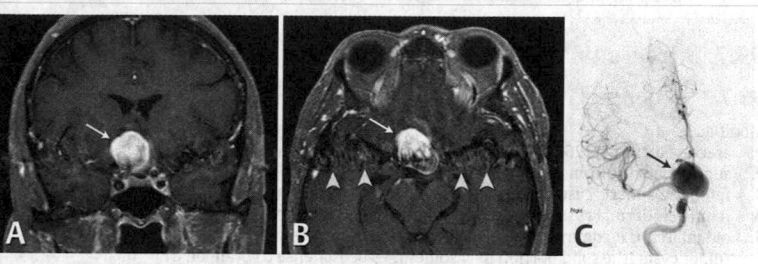

Fig. 99.4 Giant right ICA aneurysm that could be mistaken for a PitNET/adenoma.
Image: MRI T1 + contrast, A: coronal, B: axial; C: AP R ICA arteriogram.
The aneurysm is indicated by the long arrows. Pulsation artifact (*yellow arrowheads* in B) may be a tip-off that this is an aneurysm.

99.6.4 Inflammatory

a) (autoimmune) hypophysitis (see below):
   • distinguishing imaging characteristics are shown in ▶ Table 99.2
   • the most important clinical feature: pregnancy
   • the most important laboratory feature: diabetes insipidus (if DI is present, it is unlikely to be an adenoma)
b) pituitary granuloma[20]

Table 99.2 Imaging characteristics of hypophysitis vs. adenoma[21]

Feature	Hypophysitis	Adenoma
Enlargement	symmetric	asymmetric
Pituitary stalk	thickened, nontapering	not thickened, tapering, deviated
Sellar floor[a]	spared	may be eroded
Enhancement	intense, may be heterogeneous	less intense, usually homogeneous
Mean size at time of presentation	3 cm³	10 cm³
Posterior pituitary bright spot[b]	lost	preserved in 97%

[a] on CT scan
[b] the normal hyperintensity of the posterior pituitary on T1WI MRI (p.882) [22]

9.6.5 Empty sella syndrome

primary (p.952)
secondary: following pituitary tumor resection (p.952)

99

99.6.6 Hypophysitis

AKA autoimmune hypophysitis (AH)

Two main forms:

1. lymphocytic (adeno)hypophysitis[21] AKA lymphoid adenohypophysitis: the more commonly encountered form. Inflammation of the pituitary stalk with lymphocytic infiltrate. Well-established autoimmune etiology, although the antigens have not been identified. Primarily affects women in late pregnancy or early postpartum period, and classically presents with sudden onset of diabetes insipidus
2. granulomatous hypophysitis: more aggressive. No gender bias. No association with pregnancy. May be autoimmune, but pathogenesis not definitely known

Because AH often mimics a nonsecretory pituitary macroadenoma (enhancing sellar mass on imaging, with negative endocrine tests), many of these lesions undergo surgical resection instead of what may be more appropriate medical therapy (e.g., steroids,[23] or discontinuing possible offending agents such as ipilimumab[24]).

For distinguishing imaging characteristics, see ▶ Table 99.2.

99.7 Intracranial cysts

99.7.1 In general

Modified[25]:

1. arachnoid cysts (p.260): Typically lined with meningothelial cells
2. suprasellar cyst from dilated 3rd ventricle
3. interhemispheric cyst from porencephaly
4. neuroectodermal cysts (glioependymal cysts): intraparenchymal, located near ventricles
5. old infarct: if it communicates with a ventricle it is called a porencephalic cyst
6. tumor cysts (the solid portion may sometimes be isodense to brain on CT):
   a) ganglioglioma (p.707): usually solid but may appear cystic on CT
   b) pilocytic astrocytoma (p.691): usually has enhancing mural nodule
   c) neurilemmomas may be cystic
   d) supratentorial ependymomas (p.724) are often cystic
7. infectious
   a) abscess
   b) cysticercosis: see Neurocysticercosis (p.404)
   c) hydatid cyst: see Echinococcosis (p.408)
8. pineal cysts (p.948)
9. colloid cyst (p.944)
10. Rathke's cleft cyst (p.949)
11. giant aneurysm
12. on CT, a low-density non-enhancing tumor can mimic a cyst
13. chronic subdural hematoma or hygroma may mimic a cyst
14. posterior fossa: (for cysts of the CPA) (p.1648). Includes:
    a) cyst associated with Dandy-Walker malformation (p.270). Cerebellar vermis is usually hypoplastic (or, less commonly, completely absent). Hydrocephalus often present
    b) epidermoid (p.936)
    c) enlarged (mega) cisterna magna (p.271) may mimic a cyst. No mass effect on cerebellum
    d) cerebellar hemangioblastoma (p.648): often has an enhancing mural nodule
    e) arachnoid cyst of posterior fossa: usually associated with mass effect on cerebellum
    f) neurenteric cyst (p.313)
    g) pilocytic astrocytoma of the cerebellum (p.689): usually has an enhancing mural nodule
15. intraventricular cysts include: arachnoid cysts (p.260), cysticercosis cyst

99.7.2 Midline cavities

Three potential supratentorial midline cavities in the center of the brain and differentiating features are shown in ▶ Table 99.3.

99

Table 99.3 Features of midline brain cavities[26]

Cavity	Anatomy	Frequency	Clinical significance
cavum septum pellucidum (CSP) (see text)	located between leaflets of septum pellucidum	100% of preemies, 97% of newborns, 10% of adults	may be a normal variant, but has been linked to several neurodevelopmental & psychiatric disorders
cavum vergae (see text)	directly posterior to, and often communicating with CSP. Bounded posteriorly by the splenium of the corpus callosum	relatively uncommon	possible association with neurologic abnormalities[a]
cavum velum interpositum	due to separation of crura of fornix between thalami above the 3rd ventricle	present in 60% of children < 1 yr of age, and in 30% between 1 and 10 yrs	no known association with pathologic conditions

[a]including developmental delay, macrocephaly, Apert's syndrome, abnormal EE

99.7.3 Cavum septi pellucidi (CSP) and cavum vergae (CV)

The septum pellucidum (Latin: translucent wall) is a membrane that separates the two lateral ventricles. It is absent in septo-optic dysplasia (p.276). Embryologically it starts as two thin parallel leaves (the septi pellucidi) with fluid between them (the cavum septi pellucidi or cavity of the septum pellucidum) (CSP) (A, ▶ Fig. 99.5) along with its posterior extension, the cavum vergae (CV) (B, ▶ Fig. 99.5) (first described by Andrea Verga). Archaic terms are "5th ventricle" for the CSP and "6th ventricle" for the CV.

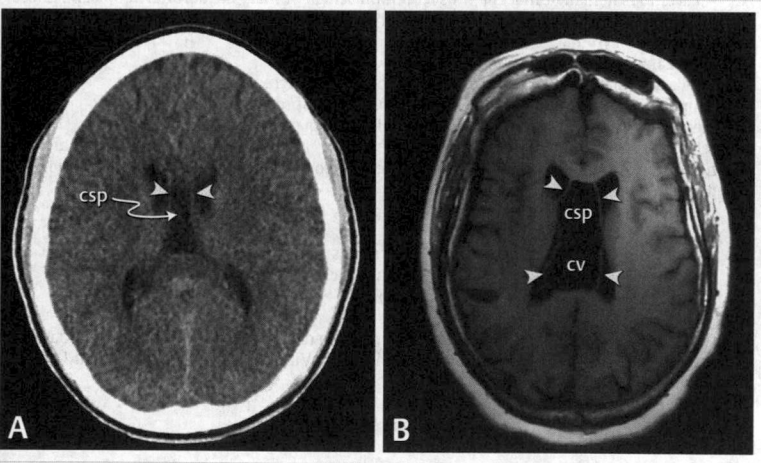

Fig. 99.5 Cavum septi pellucidi and cavum vergae (in 2 diferent patients). Image: A: Axial noncontrast CT shows a cavum septi pellucidi (csp) by itself (which was not previously present but developed in a 16-year-old female following a gunshot wound to the brain). B: Axial T1 MRI demonstrating a cavum vergae (cv), situated posterior to a csp in a 40-year-old woman. The leaflets of the septi pellucidi are indicated by the *yellow arrowheads*.

The leaflets comprising the walls of the CSP and the CV begin to fuse together at ≈ 24 weeks gestation and both are usually completely obliterated by the time of a full-term birth or shortly thereafter. As a result, CSP is present in ≈ all preemies. The CSP and the CV fuse from posterior to anterior, therefore persistence of the CV is almost always accompanied by CSP (together called "cavum septi pellucidi et vergae").

Persistence of the CSP is found in up to 10% of the adult population, and can be a normal variant representing an asymptomatic developmental anomaly. However, sometimes it is associated with neurodevelopmental disruption. It has been *loosely* associated with psychiatric conditions including bipolar disorder, Tourette's syndrome, obsessive-compulsive disorder, and schizophrenia, among others.[27] CSP may also result from trauma possibly as a result of tears in the membrane, and has been associated with TBIs especially in professional boxers[28] suffering from chronic traumatic encephalopathy (p. 1112), and motor vehicle trauma.[27]

The compartment is usually isolated, although some communicate with the 3rd ventricle.

99.8 Orbital lesions

99.8.1 General information

4 compartments of the orbit:
1. ocular (AKA globe, AKA bulbar)
2. optic nerve sheath
3. intraconal
4. extraconal

CT remains a strong imaging modality within the orbit (less susceptible to motion artifact than MRI because of the speed, images bony structures to good advantage). MRI adds info for related extraorbital structures (iptic chiasm, hypothalamus…).

99.8.2 Orbital lesions in adults

Orbital pseudotumor is the most common.
1. neoplastic
    a) discrete tumors that may occur adjacent to but not envelop the optic nerve sheath
        • cavernous hemangioma: the most common *benign* primary intraorbital neoplasm. Choroidal hemangioma is seen in Sturge-Weber syndrome
        • fibrohistiocytoma
        • hemangiopericytoma
    b) capillary hemangioma: produces infantile proptosis. Regresses spontaneously
    c) lymphangioma: produces infantile proptosis. Does *not* regress
    d) melanoma: the most common primary ocular malignancy of adulthood
    e) retinoblastoma: congenital, malignant primary retinal tumor. 40% are bilateral, 90% are calcified (often a key differentiating feature; does not portend benignity as with other lesions). CT may show retinal detachment
    f) lymphoma of the orbit: causes painless proptosis. The 3rd most common cause of proptosis
    g) intraorbital meningioma
    h) primary tumors of the optic nerve & its coverings
        • optic pathway glioma (p. 694): fusiform nerve enlargement usually > 1 cm in length
        • optic nerve sheath tumor (schwannoma)
2. congenital
    a) Coats disease: telangiectatic vascular malformation of retina which leaks a lipid exudate causing retinal detachment. May mimic retinoblastoma. Vitreous is hyperintense on MRI on both T1WI and T2WI due to lipid
    b) persistent hyperplastic primary vitreous
    c) retinopathy of prematurity (retrolental fibroplasia)
3. infectious
    a) toxocara endophthalmitis
4. inflammatory/collagen vascular disease: usually bilateral
    a) scleritis
    b) pseudotumor of the orbit: the most common intraconal lesion. Usually unilateral (p. 600)
    c) sarcoidosis: usually affects the conjunctiva and lacrimal gland and spares connective tissues and intraorbital muscles
    d) Sjögren's syndrome
5. vascular
    a) enlargement of the superior orbital vein: may occur in thrombosis of cavernous sinus or in carotid-cavernous fistula
    b) dural AVM

6. miscellaneous
   a) drusen: degenerated subretinal epithelial pigmented deposits in the posterior globe that may resemble calcified masses on CT. Often associated with age-related macular degeneration (AMD)
   b) thyroid ophthalmopathy: Graves' disease (hyperthyroidism & swelling of EOMs → *painless* proptosis). 80% of cases are bilateral. The ophthalmopathy is independent of the level of thyroid hormone (possibly an autoimmune process). NB: a swollen inferior rectus muscle may resemble an orbital tumor if seen only on lower CT cut through the orbit
   c) EOM enlargement can also occur with steroid use or occasionally with obesity
   d) fibrous dysplasia (p. 975)
   e) optic nerve sheath dilatation: this and other intraorbital findings (p. 964) may occur with increased intracranial pressure

99.8.3 Orbital tumors in pediatrics

1. dermoid cyst: 37%. The most common lesion in children
2. hemangioma: 12%. Most regress spontaneously without surgery
3. rhabdomyosarcoma: 9%. The most common malignant tumor of the orbit
4. optic nerve glioma: 6%
5. lymphangioma: < 7%. Imaging resembles hemangioma. But will not regress spontaneously, requires surgery. Proptosis may worsen after a URI. May bleed into itself (chocolate cysts)

99.9 Dural sinus lesions

This section considers lesions within the dural sinuses (e.g., superior sagittal sinus, transverse sinus…) and not external compression of the sinus by a mass.

1. dural sinus thrombus (p. 1594): acute thrombus is hyperdense on CT, and hyperintense on T1 MRI
2. tumor: especially parasagittal meningiomas (p. 808) (up to 50% invade the superior sagittal sinus)
3. focal sinus stenosis: e.g., transverse sinus stenosis (p. 964) is common in pseudotumor cerebri (bilateral stenosis was seen in 93%). This may be causative in some cases of pseudotumor, but it may be a result of increased CSF pressure in some. Transverse sinuses are normally asymmetric, with the right usually larger/dominant
4. giant arachnoid granulation: most common in the transverse sinus in the middle or lateral third with a slight left-sided prevalence, the superior sagittal sinus is the next most common location (▶ Fig. 99.6).[29] Typically > 1 cm diameter. May erode into the inner table of the skull. The arachnoid granulation does not enhance (but there is often a linear central enhancing vessel, presumably a vein) and does not show diffusion restriction on DWI MRI

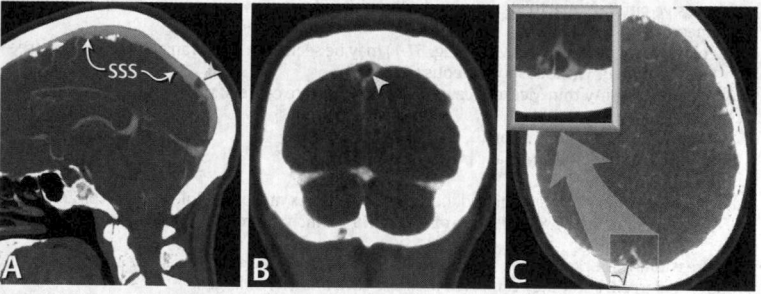

Fig. 99.6 Giant arachnoid granulation (*yellow arrowheads*) in the posterior portion of the superior sagittal sinus (SSS) appearing as a filling defect in the SSS.
Image: A: sagittal CTV, B: coronal CTV, C: axial CTA (inset shows an enlargement of the lesion in the SSS which demonstrates the enhancing central vessel [retouched photo to accentuate the visibility of the vessel]). This was an incidental finding in a patient who had a contraindication to MRI.

99

99.10 Cavernous sinus lesions

Modified[30]:
1. primary tumors (rare)
   a) meningiomas[31]
   b) neurinomas
2. tumors from adjacent areas that may extend into cavernous sinus (head and neck cancers may track intracranially along cranial nerves, especially V)
   a) meningiomas
   b) neurinomas
   c) chordomas
   d) chondromas
   e) chondrosarcomas
   f) pituitary tumors[32]
   g) nasopharyngeal carcinomas
   h) olfactory neuroblastoma (p. 935)
   i) nasopharyngeal angiofibromas
   j) metastatic tumors
3. inflammation: e.g., Tolosa-Hunt (p. 600)
4. infection: mucormycosis (phycomycosis) (p. 599). Usually in diabetics
5. vascular
   a) cavernous carotid aneurysm
   b) carotid-cavernous fistula (p. 1519)
   c) cavernous sinus thrombosis

99.11 Meckel's cave abnormalities

99.11.1 Etiologies

Also see anatomy of Meckel's cave (p. 1858). Some of these may rarely cause trigeminal neuralgia or atypical facial pain (p. 1857) that may mimic trigeminal neuralgia (e.g., trigeminal neuroma,[33] arachnoid cyst[34]).

▶ **Enlargement of Meckel's cave**
1. neoplasms
   a) nerve sheath tumors: trigeminal neuroma is the most common neoplasm
   b) meningioma
   c) tumors of the head and neck with perineural extension along the trigeminal nerve
   d) extension of PitNET/adenoma
   e) epidermoid[35]
   f) metastases: including lymphoma
   g) invasive pituitary macroadenomas invading through cavernous sinus into Meckel's cave
2. non-neoplastic
   a) enlargement of Meckel's cave: (▶ Fig. 57.1) may be seen with intracranial hypertension (see below) (with or without spontaneous CSF leak[36])
   b) arachnoid cyst within Meckel's cave (▶ Fig. 99.7): a rare cause of trigeminal neuralgia[34]
   c) vascular
      1. peristent trigeminal artery
      2. aneurysms of the internal carotid artery
      3. trigeminal AVM
   d) infectious/inflammatory: sarcoid, herpes, petrous apex mucocele, Tolosa-Hunt (p. 600),[37] idiopathic inflammatory sensory neuropathy (IIHS) (which can mimic a schwannoma)[38]

▶ **Compression of Meckel's cave.** Increased ICP can distend Meckel's cave if the porus trigeminu (p. 1858) is enlarged, but it may compress Meckel's cave if it isn't enlarged.
   It can also be compressed by tumors or aneurysms external to the cave.

99.11.2 Evaluation

▶ **MRI.** Recommended MRI protocol: imaging in 3 planes with T1, T2 short-tau inversino recove (STIR) and gadolinium enhanced T1 images with fat suppression. The contrast study rules out mos neoplasms that are potential causes.

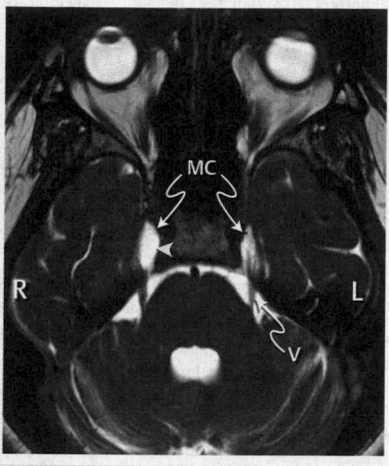

Fig. 99.7 Arachnoid cyst of Meckel's cave.
Image: axial FIESTA MRI in a 44-year-old patient with bilateral dilatation of Meckel's cave, with trigeminal symptoms on the right. The trigeminal nerve can be seen trifurcating within Meckel's cave on the left, whereas on the right the nerve is compressed against the lateral wall of the cave by what appears to be an arachnoid cyst (*yellow arrowhead*).
Abbreviations: MC = Meckel's cave; V = trigeminal nerve (Cr.N. V) as it crosses the CPA cistern.

Other MRI findings of increased ICP (p. 963) should be sought, and include: empty sella ▶ Fig. 56.6, ± infundibulum sign), dilated optic nerve sheath (▶ Fig. 33.1), flattening of the posterior lobe, empty sella, dilated optic nerve sheath, flattening of the posterior globes.

Ophthalmology consultation. If increased intracranial pressure is suspected, ophthalmology consultation should be obtained to rule out papilledema, visual field deficit and Cr.N. VI palsy. If any of these findings are present in the absence of a mass, hydrocephalus or evidence of infection, a workup for pseudotumor cerebri (p. 962) may need to be undertaken (including lumbar puncture).

Percutaneous biopsy through the foramen ovale. In questionable cases, a percutaneous biopsy through the foramen ovale may be performed.[38,39]

99.12 Skull lesions

99.12.1 General information

The most common *benign* tumors of skull are osteoma and hemangioma. Osteogenic sarcoma is the most common *malignancy*. See also specific skull tumors (p. 972).

Evaluating roentgenographic skull lucencies

There is enough overlap of features to prevent any systematic means of determining the etiology of all or even most radiographic skull lucencies. The following features should be noted for any lucency; some are more helpful than others (modified[40]):

- multiplicity (single or multiple?): except for multiple venous lakes, the presence of 6 or more defects is usually indicative of a malignancy
  origin (intradiploic, full-thickness, inner or outer table only):
  a) most vault lesions originate intradiploically, so limitation to this space may merely signify early recognition of a lesion
  b) expansion of the diploë with bulging of one or both tables almost always signifies a benign lesion
  c) full-thickness lesions affecting both tables congruently usually indicates malignancy, whereas non-congruent erosion is more common with benign lesions
  edges (smooth or ragged):
  a) smooth edges, whether regular, distinct, or indistinct: no predictive value
  b) irregular margins (especially ragged undermined edges): more suggestive of infection (osteomyelitis) or malignancy
  c) sharply demarcated, full-thickness punched-out defects: suggest myeloma

99

4. presence of peripheral sclerosis: circumferential bony sclerosis suggests benignity (may indicate slow expansion and longstanding nature). The ring of sclerosis is generally narrow except in fibrous dysplasia
5. presence or absence of peripheral vascular channels: presence is highly suggestive of benign lesions (seen in ≈ 66% of venous lakes and ≈ 50% of hemangiomas)
6. pattern within the lucency:
   a) ★ hemangiomas classically show *honeycomb* or *trabecular* pattern (seen in ≈ 50% of cases) or *sunburst* pattern (seen in ≈ 11% of cases)
   b) fibrous dysplasia (p.975) may show well-defined islands of bone, or a grossly mottled appearance with randomly arranged cystic and dense areas
7. location on the cranial vault (high vs. low): poor correlation with benign vs. malignant lesions
8. pain: Langerhans cell histiocytosis lesions are often *tender*

NB: keep in mind that skull lesions may have an intracranial component. CT scanning is good for assessing bone (MRI is poor for this); however, CT may miss small intracranial lesions tucked within the convexity of the calvaria due to bone-hardening artifact (MRI has better sensitivity in this setting).

Nuclear bone scan may be a helpful adjunctive test (see specific lesion for findings).

Biopsy: indicated for questionable skull lesions. If the bone has not been destroyed by soft tissue, biopsy may be accomplished with a Craig needle, and the specimen may need decalcification by the pathologist before histologic evaluation can be completed.

99.12.2 Radiolucent lesion or bone defect in skull (AKA lytic lesions)

1. congenital or developmental
   a) epidermoid (cholesteatoma): *sclerotic* edge
   b) congenital: encephalocele, meningoencephalocele, dermal sinus
   c) fibrous dysplasia (p.974). A benign condition in which normal bone is replaced by fibrous connective tissue. Tends to occur higher in calvaria. 3 types:
      • cystic: widening of the diplöe usually with thinning of the outer table and little involvement of the inner table. Typically involves calvaria
      • sclerotic: usually involves skull base (especially sphenoid bone) and facial bones
      • mixed: appearance is similar to cystic type with patches of increased density within the lucent lesions
   d) hemangioma or AVM of bone or scalp
   e) pacchionian depression: arachnoid granulations (older terms: Pacchioni's granulation (after Italian anatomist Antonio Pacchioni) or pacchionian bodies) resorb CSF into vascular system and occasionally cause a bony lucency, usually near the superior sagittal sinus
   f) Albright's syndrome
   g) congenital foramina: "holes" in skull traversed by emissary veins
   h) parietal thinning: usually a bilateral process
   i) frontal fenestrae
   j) venous lakes
   k) cerebral herniations: AKA occipital pacchionian granulations
2. traumatic
   a) surgical defect: burr hole, craniectomy
   b) fracture
   c) posttraumatic leptomeningeal cyst (p.1100)
   d) following trauma in children[41]
3. inflammatory
   a) osteomyelitis: including tuberculosis[42]
   b) sarcoidosis
   c) syphilis
4. neoplastic
   a) hemangioma: fine, honeycombed matrix. Classic X-ray finding: "starburst" appearance due to radiating bone spicules (may occur in as few as ≈ 11% of cases[40])
   b) intracranial tumor with erosion
   c) lymphoma, leukemia
   d) meningioma
   e) metastasis: usually hot on bone scan
   f) multiple myeloma, plasmacytoma (p.929). Usually cool on bone scan
   g) sarcoma or fibrosarcoma of bone

h) skin tumor with invasion (rodent ulcer)
i) neuroblastoma
j) lipoma
k) epidermoid (may also be considered congenital, thus also see above)
. miscellaneous
a) Langerhans cell histiocytosis (p.846). Perfectly round *non-sclerotic* punched-out lesion, may be single (formerly called eosinophilic granuloma) or multiple, tender
b) Paget's disease (when seen as a zone of osteolysis without osteoblastic sclerosis on skull films, this is defined as osteoporosis circumscripta). Usually "hot" on bone scan
c) aneurysmal bone cyst: rare. Arises in diploë and expands both tables, which become thin but remain intact
d) brown tumor of hyperparathyroidism

9.12.3 Diffuse demineralization or destruction of the skull

Includes "salt and pepper skull."
. common
a) hyperparathyroidism, primary or secondary
b) metastatic carcinoma or neuroblastoma
c) multiple myeloma
d) osteoporosis
. uncommon
a) Paget's disease (osteoporosis circumscripta)

9.12.4 "Hair-On-End" appearance in skull

. common
a) congenital hemolytic anemia (e.g., thalassemia, sickle cell, hereditary spherocytosis, pyruvate kinase deficiency)
. uncommon
a) hemangioma
b) cyanotic congenital heart disease (with secondary polycythemia)
c) iron deficiency anemia
d) metastases: especially neuroblastoma, thyroid carcinoma
e) multiple myeloma
f) meningioma
g) osteosarcoma
h) polycythemia vera

9.12.5 Diffuse increased density, hyperostosis, or calvarial thickening

common
a) anemia (sickle cell, iron deficiency, thalassemia, hereditary spherocytosis)
b) fibrous dysplasia
   • leontiasis ossea ("lion-like facies"): a form of polyostotic fibrous dysplasia
c) hyperostosis interna generalisata
d) osteoblastic metastases (especially prostate, breast)
e) Paget's disease (begins with lytic zone and diploic thickening)
f) treated hydrocephalus
uncommon
a) chronic phenytoin therapy
b) Engelman's disease (progressive diaphyseal dysplasia)
c) fluorosis
d) hypervitaminosis D
e) hypoparathyroidism, pseudohypoparathyroidism
f) meningioma
g) osteogenesis imperfecta
h) osteopetrosis (p.1689)
i) secondary polycythemia
j) syphilitic osteitis
k) tuberous sclerosis

99

99.12.6 Focal increased density of skull base

1. common
   a) fibrous dysplasia
   b) meningioma
2. uncommon
   a) mastoiditis
   b) nasopharyngeal carcinoma
   c) osteoblastic metastasis
   d) osteoma of the outer table or diploë
   e) chondroma
   f) sarcoma of bone (e.g., osteosarcoma, chondrosarcoma)
   g) sphenoid sinusitis

99.12.7 Generalized increased density of skull base

1. common
   a) fibrous dysplasia
   b) Paget's disease
2. uncommon
   a) severe anemia (e.g., thalassemia, sickle cell)
   b) Engelman's disease (progressive diaphyseal dysplasia)
   c) fluorosis
   d) hyperparathyroidism, primary or secondary (treated)
   e) hypervitaminosis D
   f) idiopathic hypercalcemia
   g) meningioma
   h) osteopetrosis (p. 1689)

99.12.8 Localized increased density or hyperostosis of the calvaria

1. common
   a) anatomic variation (e.g., sutural sclerosis)
   b) fibrous dysplasia
   c) osteoma (p. 972)
   d) meningioma
   e) hyperostosis frontalis interna (p. 974)
   f) osteoblastic metastases (especially: prostate, breast)
   g) Paget's disease (begins with lytic zone and diploic thickening)
   h) cephalohematoma
   i) depressed skull fracture
2. uncommon
   a) osteosarcoma
   b) chronic osteomyelitis, tuberculosis
   c) tuberous sclerosis
   d) osteoid osteomas: radiolucent nidus with surrounding zone of dense sclerosis
   e) osteoblastoma
   f) ossifying fibromas: predilection for frontotemporal region
   g) radiation necrosis

99.13 Other abnormalities of the skull

99

99.13.1 Pneumocele

Pneumocele: enlargement of an air sinus often with bone erosion. Pneumosinus dilatans, in contras
generally denotes enlargement of an air sinus *without* bone erosion (▶ Fig. 46.7), as may occur wi
tuberculum sellae (p. 809) or planum sphenoidale (p. 809) meningiomas.

Pneumoceles occur primarily in the maxillary antrum. Etiology is unknown, and may involve
trap-valve mechanism, ruptured mucocele, or possibly congenital.

Presentation of pneumocele or pneumosinus dilatans:

1. headache
2. neuralgia

3. facial asymmetry
4. frontal bossing (with frontal pneumosinus dilatans)
5. exophthalmous
6. CSF fistula (leak)
7. treatment for maxillary pneumocele: opening the sinus into the nasal cavity via endoscopic approach. Watch for encephalocele.

99.13.2 Frontal bossing

Protuberance of the frontal bone. Forehead appears prominent. May be associated with an exaggerated brow ridge.

Etiologies include:
1. hydrocephalus (p.427) in a young child
2. acromegaly (p.870)
3. fibrous dysplasia (p.975)
4. extramedullary hematopoiesis (p.179)
5. achondroplasia
6. Hurler syndrome

99.14 Combined intracranial/extracranial lesions

Lesion causing mass outside skull with intracranial component.
1. intra-axial: rule of thumb—"there is no intra-axial lesion that grows out of skull"; however, untreated fungating malignant gliomas may do this
2. extra-axial:
   a) meningioma
      • may arise in diploë, grows outward and inward
      • intracranial meningioma can grow through bone by destroying it
      • intracranial meningioma can induce hyperostosis that causes extracranial mass
   b) metastatic disease (e.g., GI carcinoma, and especially prostate Ca)
   c) bone (skull) lesion:
      • hemangioma
      • epidermoid
      • fibrous dysplasia (rare)
      • giant cell tumor (rare)
      • Ewing's sarcoma (rare in skull)
      • aneurysmal bone cyst (5% occur in skull, occipital bone most common)

99.15 Intracranial hyperdensities

Differential diagnosis of an intracranial structure that is hyperdense with respect to brain (i.e., appear "whiter" than brain) on non-contrast CT:
1. acute blood
2. calcium
3. vessels with low flow
4. melanoma: may be slightly hyperdense to brain due to melanin

99.16 Intracranial calcifications

99.16.1 Single intracranial calcifications

1. benign ("physiologic")
   a) choroid plexus: (▶ Fig. 99.8) calcifications usually bilateral (see below)
   b) arachnoid granulation
   c) diaphragma sellae
   d) dural: common locations include falx (falcine) (▶ Fig. 99.8), tentorial, sagittal sinus
   e) habenular commissure
   f) petroclinoid or interclinoid ligaments
   g) pineal: (▶ Fig. 99.8) 55% of patients > 20 yrs of age have a calcified pineal gland visible on plain skull X-ray

99

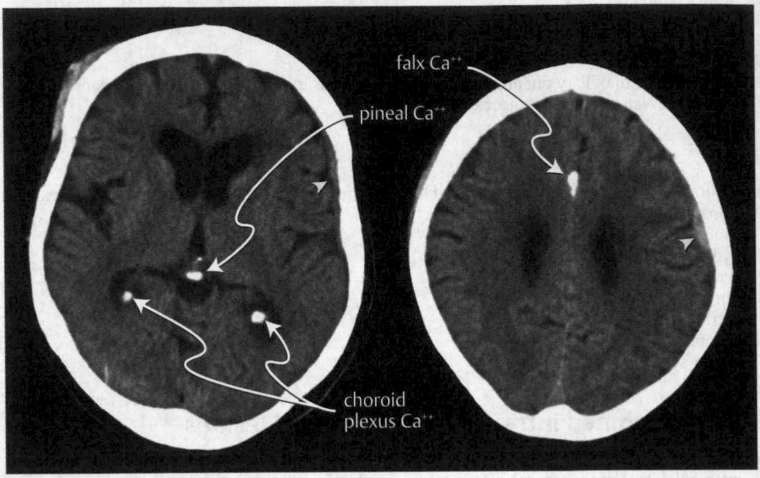

Fig. 99.8 **Benign intracranial calcifications** in an 81-year-old woman who also has small subdural hematomas (*yellow arrowheads*).
Abbreviations: Ca^{++} = calcifications.
Image: axial noncontrast CT scans at two different positions.

2. infection
    a) cysticercosis cyst: single or multiple, see Neurocysticercosis (p. 404)
    b) encephalitis, meningitis, cerebral abscess (acute and healed)
    c) granuloma (torulosis and other fungi)
    d) hydatid cyst
    e) tuberculoma
    f) paragonimiasis
    g) rubella
    h) syphilitic gumma
3. vascular
    a) aneurysm, including:
        • vein of Galen aneurysm
        • giant aneurysm
    b) arteriosclerosis (especially carotid artery in siphon region)
    c) hemangioma, AVM, Sturge-Weber syndrome
4. neoplastic: calcifications usually suggest a more benign process
    a) meningioma (p. 803)
    b) craniopharyngioma
    c) choroid plexus papilloma
    d) ependymoma
    e) glioma (especially oligodendroglioma, also astrocytoma)
    f) ganglioglioma
    g) lipoma of corpus callosum
    h) pinealoma
    i) hamartoma of tuber cinereum
5. miscellaneous
    a) hematoma: ICH, EDH, or SDH. Calcifications usually only when chronic
    b) idiopathic
    c) tuberous sclerosis (p. 644)

99

99.16.2 Multiple intracranial calcifications

1. common
   a) choroid plexus: the most common site for physiologic calcification (in lateral ventricles where it is usually bilateral and symmetric; rare in 3rd & 4th ventricles). Increases in frequency and extent with age (prevalence: 75% by 5th decade). Rare under age 3. Under age 10, consider possible choroid plexus papilloma. Involvement in the temporal horns is often associated with neurofibromatosis
   b) basal ganglia (BG): slight bilateral BG calcifications on CT are common, especially in the elderly. Considered a normal radiographic variant by some. They may be idiopathic, secondary to conditions such as hypoparathyroidism or long-term antiseizure medication use, or part of rare conditions such as Fahr's disease (see below). BG calcifications > 0.5 cm dia are possibly associated with cognitive impairment and a high prevalence of psychiatric symptoms (including bipolar and obsessive-compulsive disorders, but no patients had schizophreniform disorders)[43]
2. uncommon
   a) Fahr's disease: progressive idiopathic calcification of medial portions of basal ganglia, sulcal depths of cerebral cortex, and dentate nuclei[44]
   b) hemangioma, AVM, Sturge-Weber syndrome, von Hippel-Lindau disease
   c) basal cell nevus syndrome (falx, tentorium)
   d) Gorlin's syndrome. Associated findings: mandibular cysts, rib and vertebral deformities, short metacarpals. Medulloblastoma seen in several patients
   e) deposition of calcium in the media of medium-sized blood vessels without compromise of the lumen. Usually asymptomatic. May become symptomatic by the time the involvement is significant enough to be visible on plain X-ray in a young person
   f) cytomegalic inclusion disease
   g) encephalitis (e.g., measles, chickenpox, neonatal herpes simplex)
   h) hematomas (SDH or EDH, chronic)
   i) neurofibromatosis (choroid plexi)
   j) toxoplasmosis
   k) tuberculomas; tuberculous meningitis (treated)
   l) tuberous sclerosis
   m) hypoparathyroidism (including post-thyroidectomy cases[45]) and pseudohypoparathyroidism
   n) multiple tumors (e.g., meningiomas, gliomas, metastases)
   o) cysticercosis cyst: may be single or multiple, see Neurocysticercosis (p. 404)

99.17 Intraventricular lesions

99.17.1 General information

Intraventricular tumors represent only ≈ 10% of CNS neoplasms. A clue to differentiating a tumor located within the ventricle from an intraparenchymal tumor invaginating into the ventricle is a "cap" of CSF surrounding an intraventricular tumor on CT or MRI.

99.17.2 Differential diagnosis

Percentages quoted here are from a series of 73 patients with an intraventricular lesion on CT seen at UCSF[46]).

.   astrocytoma: (20%) the most common lesion. Hydrocephalus (HCP) is present in 73%. Hyperdense on non-contrast CT (NCCT) in 77%.
    Locations in descending order of frequency:
    a) frontal horn
    b) 3rd ventricle
    c) atrium (AKA trigone)
    d) 4th ventricle

.   colloid cyst (p. 944): (14%) essentially seen only in anterior 3rd ventricle at foramen of Monro (other sites have been described but are exceedingly rare). 50% are hyperdense on NCCT. MRI appearance is variable, and may occasionally be missed. Little or no enhancement on CT/MRI. DDx includes xanthogranuloma

99

3. meningioma: (12%) most in atrium, rarely in frontal horn. All hyperdense with dense uniform enhancement. May be calcified. Most have dense tumor blush on angiogram, most supplied from anterior choroidal artery, posterior choroidal less common. Thought to arise from arachnoidal cells within the choroid plexus

4. ependymoma (p.724): (10%) most in 4th ventricle, may occur in body of lateral ventricle. Often hyperdense on CT because of high cellularity

5. craniopharyngioma: (7%) primarily in 3rd ventricle. Most have punctate calcification. Squamous epithelial rests in region of lamina terminalis are felt to give rise to this uncommon variety of craniopharyngioma

6. medulloblastoma: (5%) often fill 4th ventricle. Hyperdense on CT with homogeneous enhancement

7. cysticercosis: (5%) may involve any ventricle or may be panventricular (NB: incidence related to geographic location)

8. choroid plexus papilloma: (5%) most common in lateral ventricle (may be bilateral), but also may be seen in 4th and occasionally in 3rd. Non-obstructive HCP may occur (possible CSF over-production). Intense blush on angiogram

9. epidermoid: (4%) mostly in 4th ventricle. Hypodense on CT with no enhancement (tend to follow CSF signal). The most common 4th ventricular low-density lesion in the U.S.

10. dermoid: (3%) common in 4th ventricle. May see free-floating fat in ventricles suggestive of cyst rupture. Tendency to form in midline

11. choroid plexus carcinoma: (3%) common in atrium of lateral ventricle. May extend into adjacent brain parenchyma with edema and shift. Intense blush on angio. NB: very rare lesion

12. subependymoma (p.735): (3%) 4th ventricle or frontal horn. Typically isodense on CT with *minimal or no enhancement* (▶ Fig. 41.12). May have calcification or cystic degeneration (more common in ependymoma). Most commonly in floor of 4th ventricle near obex

13. ependymal cyst: (3%) common in lateral ventricle. Absence of communication demonstrated by water-soluble contrast cisternography

14. arachnoid cyst: (1%) lateral ventricle. Absence of communication demonstrated by water-soluble contrast cisternography

15. arteriovenous malformation (AVM): (3%)

16. teratoma: (1%) Located in anterior 3rd ventricle. Partially calcified with foci of fat density. Marked enhancement

17. central neurocytoma (p.719)

18. metastases: breast and lung reported[47]

19. chordoid glioma of the 3rd ventricle[48]

Additional lesions not included in this list: intraventricular arachnoid cyst (p.260) (uncommon) cysticercosis

99.17.3 Features to help identify type of intraventricular lesions

By location within ventricular system

▶ Table 99.4 shows the breakdown of lesion type by location within the ventricular system.

By location and age within lateral ventricle

See reference.[49]

See ▶ Table 99.5. This study excluded tumors that were clearly arising in the 3rd ventricle or were predominantly parenchymal with intraventricular extension.

The teratoma and both PNETs occurred in age < 1 year, and all showed calcifications. Only one CP occurred above age 5 years.

In adults > 30 years of age, the only tumors found in the trigone were meningiomas. Subependymomas (p.735) were the *only* nonenhancing intraventricular tumor in this age group.

By location within 3rd ventricle

1. anterior 3rd ventricle
   a) colloid cyst
   b) sellar mass
   c) sarcoidosis
   d) aneurysm

Table 99.4 Type of intraventricular lesions by location[46] (numbers are patients out of 73[a])

3rd ventricle		4th ventricle		Lateral ventricle					
				Atrium		**Body**		**Frontal horn**	
colloid cyst	10	medulloblast.	4	meningi-oma	8	ependymoma	3	astrocytoma	7
craniopharyng.	5	ependymoma	4	astrocy-toma	3	ch. plexus papil.[b]	1	meningioma	1
astrocytoma	4	epidermoid	3	ch. plexus papil.	1	ch. plexus carc.	1	subepen-dym.	1
teratoma	1	cysticercosis	2	ch. plexus carc.	1	ependym. cyst	1	dermoid	1
ch. plexus papil.	1	astrocytoma	1	arachnoid cyst (p. 260)	1	AVM	1		
cysticercosis	1	subependym.	1	ependym. cyst	1				
dermoid	1								
ch. plexus carc.	1								
AVM	1								

[a] 1 patient had cysticercosis diffusely throughout ventricles
[b] 1 patient with bilateral lateral ventricle papillomas

Table 99.5 Lateral ventricle tumor type by location & age

Age (yrs)	Location within lateral ventricle[a]		
	Foramen of Monro region	**Trigone**	**Body**
0–5	0	8 CPP	2 PNETs 1 teratoma
6–30	5 SEGAs 2 pilocytic astrocytomas 1 CPP 1 meningioma 1 oligodendroglioma	1 ependymoma 1 oligodendroglioma	1 mixed glioma 1 ependymoma 1 pilocytic astrocytoma
>30	2 metastases	8 meningiomas	2 glioblastomas 1 lymphoma 1 metastasis 6 subependymomas

[a] abbreviations: CPP = choroid plexus papillomas, PNET = primitive neuroectodermal tumor, SEGA = subependymal giant cell astrocytoma

e) hypothalamic glioma
f) histiocytosis
g) meningioma
h) optic glioma
2. posterior third ventricle
a) pinealoma (dysgerminoma)
b) meningioma
c) arachnoid cyst (p. 260)
d) vein of Galen aneurysm

99

By enhancement

All lesions enhanced except: cysts (ependymal and arachnoid), dermoids, and epidermoids.

Subependymomas (p. 735): there are differences of opinion of the tendency for these to enhance. Jelinek et al[49] found that they were the only consistently nonenhancing tumors at the foramen of Monro or in the body of the ventricles (3rd ventricular colloid cysts were excluded).

By multiplicity

Multiple lesions are more suggestive of: neurocysticercosis, metastases, or ruptured epidermoid cyst.

99.18 Periventricular lesions

99.18.1 Periventricular solid enhancing lesions (in decreasing frequency)

1. lymphoma; CNS involvement from systemic, or rarely primary brain (p. 840): must be included in differential diagnosis of any solid enhancing periventricular brain tumor. Very radiosensitive.
2. ependymoma (usually invaginates)
3. metastatic Ca: especially malignant melanoma or choriocarcinoma
4. ventriculitis
5. medulloblastoma (in peds), AKA cerebellar sarcoma in adults
6. pineal tumor (dysgerminoma type): usually midline, young patient
7. occasionally, glioblastoma can present like this

99.18.2 Periventricular low density on CT, or high signal on T2WI MRI

1. increased extracellular or intracellular water content (edema)
   a) in hydrocephalus: transependymal CSF absorption (p. 431)
   b) necrosis from infarction
   c) edema from tumor
2. uncommon late variants of adrenoleukodystrophy
3. vascular disorders
   a) subacute arteriosclerotic encephalopathy (Binswanger's disease)[50,51]
   b) cerebral embolism
   c) vasculitis
   d) amyloid angiopathy
   e) low flow states
4. demyelination: including multiple sclerosis
5. leukoaraiosis[52]: a term coined to describe white matter disease with symmetric (or nearly so) periventricular white matter changes on CT or MRI. May be asymptomatic or may present with findings including dementia. May be related to:
   a) Binswanger's encephalopathy
   b) watershed infarction[53]
   c) normal aging[54]: increases each decade after age 60, usually patchy
   d) hypoxia
   e) hypoglycemia[55]
6. heterotopias: islands of gray matter in abnormal locations
7. following radiation therapy (XRT)

99.19 Meningeal thickening/enhancement

99.19.1 Dural enhancement (intracranial)

Visible beneath the inner table of the skull. Unlike leptomeningeal enhancement, does not follow the gyral convolutions. May be either focal or diffuse[56]:
1. focal
   a) adjacent to meningioma: so called "dural tail" (▶ Fig. 46.4 panel D)
   b) pleomorphic xanthoastrocytoma (PXA): also can have "dural tail"
2. diffuse dural enhancement[57]: associated with extraaxial neoplastic processes in ≈ 65%. Clinically: H/A, multiple cranial nerve palsies, seizures
   a) intracranial hypotension (p. 421): diffuse pachymeningeal enhancement on cerebral MRI
   b) infection: bacterial meningitis
   c) primary CNS tumors: medulloblastoma, malignant meningioma
   d) sarcoidosis
   e) following craniotomy
   f) metastases (mostly carcinomas). May cause dural thickening as well:
      • dural metastases

- leptomeningeal carcinomatosis (carcinomatous meningitis) (p. 920)
- lymphoma[58]
g) neurosarcoidosis
h) following subdural hemorrhage[59]
i) idiopathic

99.19.2 Leptomeningeal enhancement

See reference.[56]
1. thin linear enhancement that closely follows the gyri
2. small nodules attached to the brain

99.20 Ependymal and subependymal enhancement

Some overlap with periventricular enhancement. Ependymal enhancement often heralds a serious condition.[60] Main DDx is tumor vs. infectious process.
1. ventriculitis or ependymitis: ependymal enhancement occurs in 64% of cases of pyogenic ventriculitis[61]
   a) infection may occur in the following settings:
      - following shunt surgery
      - after intraventricular surgery
      - with indwelling prosthetic devices (e.g., Ommaya reservoir)
      - with use of intrathecal chemotherapy
      - with meningitis
      - with viral ependymitis
      - in some cases of CMV encephalitis in immunocompromised patients
      - granulomatous involvement: esp. in immunocompromised patients; e.g., tuberculosis, *Mycobacterium*, syphilis
   b) infections may be[60]
      - bacterial (pyogenic) ventriculitis
      - tuberculous ventriculitis
      - cystic lesions suggest cysticercosis
2. carcinomatous meningitis: typically also produces meningeal enhancement (p. 920)
3. multiple sclerosis: usually more *peri*ventricular (in the white matter)
4. tumors
   a) lymphoproliferative disorders
      - CNS lymphoma (p. 840)
      - leukemia
   b) ependymoma
      - with tumor spread
      - transient enhancement reported in a child with ependymoma in the absence of tumor spread[62]
   c) metastasis
   d) germ cell tumors
5. tuberous sclerosis: subependymal hamartomas appear as nodules which occasionally enhance (p. 644). These gradually calcify with age
6. in the presence of appropriate constitutional symptoms: rare causes of linear enhancement include: neurosarcoidosis, Whipple's disease, metastatic multiple myeloma (usually nodular)

In immunocompromised patients, the enhancement pattern may help distinguish between the following (which tend to occur in this population[60]):
1. thin linear enhancement: suggests virus (CMV or varicella-zoster)
2. nodular enhancement: suggests CNS lymphoma
3. band enhancement: less specific (may occur with virus, lymphoma, or tuberculosis (TB))

99

99.21 Intraventricular hemorrhage

Etiologies:
1. most occur as a result of extension of intraparenchymal hemorrhages
   a) in the adult:
      - spontaneous ICH: especially thalamic or putaminal hemorrhages (p. 1614)
      - associated with AVM

b) in newborns: extension of subependymal hemorrhage (p. 1630)
2. *pure* intraventricular hemorrhage (IVH) is usually the result of a rupture of
   a) aneurysm: accounts for ≈ 25% of IVH in adults, and is second only to extension of intracerebral hemorrhage as the most common cause. IVH occurs in 13–28% of ruptured aneurysms in clinical series.[63] More common with the following aneurysms: AComA, distal basilar artery or carotid terminus, VA or distal PICA (for patterns) (p. 1454)
   b) vertebral artery dissection (p. 1577) (or dissecting aneurysms)
   c) intraventricular AVM
   d) intraventricular tumor
   e) SAH outside the ventricles refluxing into foramina of Luschka and/or Magendie

99.22 Medial temporal lobe lesions

May be responsible for seizures, especially "uncal fits" (temporal lobe seizures).
1. hamartoma: nonenhancing
2. mesial temporal sclerosis (p. 482): should see atrophy of the parenchyma in this area with dilatation of the temporal horn of the lateral ventricle
3. glioma: look for mass effect. Usually unilateral. Enhancement suggests higher grade than low grade
4. (autoimmune) limbic encephalitis: an inflammatory disease of the medial temporal lobes that may present with temporal lobe seizures or rapid onset of neuropsychiatric symptoms that may respond to immunotherapy.[64] May be a paraneoplastic condition, however, disease-causing antibodies are identified in many cases. Diagnostic criteria[65]:
   a) rapid onset (< 3 months) of short-term memory deficit, seizures, or psychiatric symptoms consistent with limbic system involvement (e.g., anxiety, depression, behavioral changes)
   b) *bilateral* abnormalities highly restricted to medial temporal lobes on T2 FLAIR MRI (▶ Fig. 99.9) or 18-fluorodeoxyglucose (^{18}F-FDG) PET scan
   c) one or both of:
      1. CSF pleocytosis: WBCs > 5/mm^3
      2. EEG: epileptic or slow-wave activity involving the temporal lobes
   d) reasonable exclusion of alternative causes
   e) if one of the first 3 criteria is not met, the diagnosis may only be made with identification of antibodies against cell-surface, synaptic, or onconeural proteins
5. acute ischemic stroke involving the posterior cerebral artery
6. encephalitis: including
   a) *herpes simplex encephalitis* (p. 397) : comprises 25% of cases of encephalitis with temporal lobe involvement. Differentiating features: bilateral involvement is characteristic (but may be *unilateral*), often hemorrhagic, crosses into insula ("transsylvian sign"), spares basal ganglia

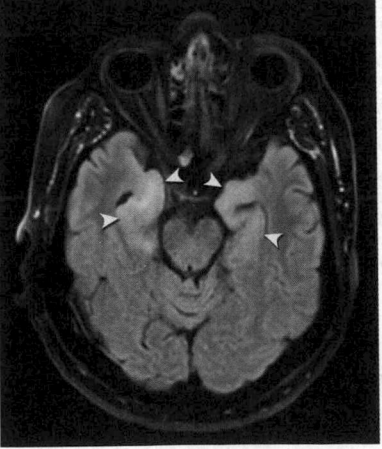

Fig. 99.9 Limbic encephalitis.
Image: axial T2 FLAIR MRI. Finding: increased signal in bilateral medial temporal lobes (*yellow arrowheads*).

b) varicella-zoster
c) TB
d) neurosyphilis

99.23 Basal ganglion abnormalities

1. generally symmetric abnormalities
   a) calcification (p. 1667)
   b) Wilson's disease (hepatolenticular degeneration): autosomal recessive disease causing accumulation of copper in tissues
   c) Huntington's disease (or chorea): caused by > 40 trinucleotide CAG repeats in the Huntington gene (4p16.3) which leads to the production of the protein huntingtin. Cell loss in caudate nucleus can be seen on CT or MRI
   d) manganese (p. 185): symmetrical high-signal abnormalities on T1WI primarily in the globus pallidus with essentially no findings on T2WI or T2* GRE (almost pathognomonic)
   e) globus pallidus (low density on CT):
      • severe carbon monoxide intoxication
      • cyanide poisoning
      • hypoxia
   f) putamen
      • hypoglycemia: affects corpus striatum (caudate and putamen)
2. stroke

99.24 Thalamic lesions

Astrocytomas are the most common tumors.

1. common neoplasms
   a) adults
      • astrocytoma, IDH-mutant, grade 3
      • glioblastoma, IDH-wildtype
      • metastasis
      • primary CNS lymphoma
   b) pediatrics
      • astrocytoma, IDH-mutant, grade 2
      • astrocytoma, IDH-mutant, grade 3
      • glioblastoma, IDH-wildtype
      • pilocytic astrocytoma
2. uncommon neoplasms
   a) adults
      • astrocytoma, IDH-mutant, grade 2
      • neurocytoma
      • oligodendroglioma
      • pilocytic astrocytoma
      • hamartoma
   b) pediatrics
      • germinoma
      • oligodendroglioma
      • PNET
      • subependymal giant cell tumor
3. non-neoplastic (pediatric and adult)
   a) cavernous angioma
   b) granuloma
   c) heterotopias
   d) AVM
   e) infarct

99.25 Intranasal/intracranial lesions

Lesions within the nose that may communicate with the intracranial cavity:
1. infectious
   a) tuberculosis

  b) syphilis
  c) Hansen's disease (leprosy)
  d) fungal infections, especially:
    • aspergillosis
    • mucormycosis: seen primarily in diabetics or immunocompromised patients (p.599)
    • *Sporothrix schenckii*
    • *Coccidioides*
  e) Wegener's granulomatosis (p.207): necrotizing granulomatous vasculitis of the upper and lower respiratory tracts with glomerulonephritis and nasal destruction[66]
  f) lethal midline granuloma (p.207): a locally destructive lymphomatoid infiltrative disease that may not have true granulomas, and may also cause local nasal destruction. However, renal and tracheal involvement do not occur as in Wegener's granulomatosis
  g) polymorphic reticulosis: may be a nasal lymphoma. Possibly the same disease as lethal midline granuloma (see above)
2. mucocele: a retention cyst of an air sinus that results from an occluded ostium and may cause expansive erosion of the involved sinus. Often enhances with IV contrast (MRI or CT), and may contain mucus or pus
3. neoplasms
  a) carcinoma of the nasal sinus
    • squamous cell
    • glandular
    • nasopharyngeal carcinomas: may be related to Epstein-Barr Virus (EBV) infection
    • sinonasal undifferentiated carcinoma (SNUC)[67]: distinct from lymphoepithelioma (less keratinizing). Rare, aggressive carcinoma (more lethal variant of squamous cell carcinoma) with poor prognosis. Incidence may be higher with prior XRT and in woodworkers and nickel factory workers. May invade adjacent structures, those relevant to neurosurgeons: frontal fossa and cavernous sinus. No relation to EBV. Treatment: tri-modal therapy (XRT, chemotherapy, and salvage surgery)
  b) olfactory neuroblastoma (p.935) (formerly esthesioneuroblastoma). A very rare malignant tumor arising from crest cells of the nasal vault, often with intracranial invasion. Presents with epistaxis (76%), nasal obstruction (71%), tearing (14%), pain (11%), diplopia, proptosis, anosmia, and endocrinopathies[68]
  c) metastatic tumors: very rare, possibly with renal cell carcinoma
  d) benign tumors
    • frontal meningioma: rarely erodes into nasal cavity
    • rhabdomyoma
    • benign hemangiopericytoma
    • cholesteatoma
    • chordoma
4. congenital lesions
  a) **encephalocele**: a nasal polypoid mass in a *newborn* should be considered an encephalocele until proven otherwise. Classifications:
    • cranial vault
    • frontal ethmoidal
    • basal
    • posterior fossa
  b) nasal glioma: non-neoplastic glial tissue located within the nose, often conceptually and diagnostically confused with an encephalocele (▶ Table 99.6). The term "glioma" is a misnomer, and nasal glial heterotopia is preferred. Does not communicate with the subarachnoid space

99

Table 99.6 Encephalocele vs. nasal glioma

Finding	Encephalocele	Nasal glioma
pulsatile?	frequently (may not be if small)	no
changes with Valsalva maneuver	swells (Furstenberg sign)	no change
presence of hypertelorism	suggests encephalocele	does not correlate
attachment to CNS	stalk	none, or minimal
probe	can be passed lateral	cannot be passed lateral

References

[1] Ho VB, Smirniotopoulos JG, Murphy FM, et al. Radiologic-Pathologic Correlation: Hemangioblastoma. American Journal of Neuroradiology. 1992; 13:1343–1352

[2] Laurent JP, Cheek WR. Brain Tumors in Children. J Pediatr Neurosci. 1985; 1:15–32

[3] Section of Pediatric Neurosurgery of the American Association of Neurological Surgeons. Pediatric Neurosurgery. New York 1982

[4] Inoue Y, Tabuchi T, Hakuba A, et al. Facial Nerve Neuromas: CT Findings. Journal of Computer Assisted Tomography. 1987; 11:942–947

[5] Tew JM, Yeh HS, Miller GW, et al. Intratemporal Schwannoma of the Facial Nerve. Neurosurgery. 1983; 13:186–188

[6] Enyon-Lewis NJ, Kitchen N, Scaravilli F, et al. Neurenteric Cyst of the Cerebellopontine Angle. Neurosurgery. 1998; 42:655–658

[7] George B, Lot G, Boissonnet H. Meningioma of the Foramen Magnum: A Series of 40 Cases. Surgical Neurology. 1997; 47:371–379

[8] George B, Lot G, Velut S. Tumors of the Foramen Magnum. Neuro-Chirurgie. 1993; 39:1–89

[9] Onofrio BM, Mih AD. Synovial Cysts of the Spine. Neurosurgery. 1988; 22:642–647

[10] O'Neill BP, Illig JJ. Primary Central Nervous System Lymphoma. Mayo Clinic Proceedings. 1989; 64:1005–1020

[11] Davis DO. Sellar and Parasellar Lesions. Clinical Neurosurgery. 1970; 17:160–188

[12] Kovacs K. Metastatic cancer of the pituitary gland. Oncology. 1973; 27:533–542

[13] Atchison JA, Lee PA, Albright L. Reversible Suprasellar Pituitary Mass Secondary to Hypothyroidism. JAMA. 1989; 262:3175–3177

[14] Laway BA, Mir SA. Pregnancy and pituitary disorders: Challenges in diagnosis and management. Indian J Endocrinol Metab. 2013; 17:996–1004

[15] Taylor SL, Barakos JA, Harsh GR, et al. Magnetic Resonance Imaging of Tuberculum Sellae Meningiomas: Preventing Preoperative Misdiagnosis as Pituitary Macroadenoma. Neurosurgery. 1992; 31:621–627

[16] Symon L, Rosenstein J. Surgical Management of Suprasellar Meningioma. Journal of Neurosurgery. 1984; 61:633–641

[17] Mai A, Karis J, Sivakumar K. Meningioma with pneumosinus dilatans. Neurology. 2003; 60

[18] Hoffman HJ, Ostubo H, Hendrick EB, et al. Intracranial Germ-Cell Tumors in Children. Journal of Neurosurgery. 1991; 74:545–551

[19] Aarabi B, Haghshenas M, Rakeii V. Visual failure caused by suprasellar extramedullary hematopoiesis in beta thalassemia: case report. Neurosurgery. 1998; 42:922–5; discussion 925–6

[20] Daniels DL, Williams AL, Thornton RS, et al. Differential Diagnosis of Intrasellar Tumors by Computed Tomography. Radiology. 1981; 141:697–701

[21] Gutenberg A, Larsen J, Lupi I, et al. A radiologic score to distinguish autoimmune hypophysitis from nonsecreting pituitary adenoma preoperatively. AJNR. American Journal of Neuroradiology. 2009; 30:1766–1772

[22] Kucharczyk W, Davis DO, Kelly WM, et al. Pituitary adenomas: high-resolution MR imaging at 1.5 T. Radiology. 1986; 161:761–765

[23] Miyake I, Takeuchi Y, Kuramoto T, et al. Autoimmune hypophysitis treated with intravenous glucocorticoid therapy. Internal Medicine. 2006; 45:1249–1252

[24] Carpenter KJ, Murtagh RD, Lilienfeld J, et al. Ipilimumab-induced hypophysitis: MR imaging findings. American Journal of Neuroradiology. 2009; 30:1751–1753

[25] Harsh GR, Edwards MSB, Wilson CB. Intracranial Arachnoid Cysts in Children. J Neurosurg. 1986; 64:835–842

[26] Miller ME, Kido D, Horner F. Cavum Vergae: Association With Neurologic Abnormality and Diagnosis by Magnetic Resonance Imaging. Archives of Neurology. 1986; 43:821–823

[27] Silk T, Beare R, Crossley L, et al. Cavum septum pellucidum in pediatric traumatic brain injury. Psychiatry Res. 2013; 213:186–192

[28] Rocky V. 1990. https://en.wikipedia.org/wiki/Rocky_V

[29] De Keyzer B, Bamps S, Van Calenbergh F, et al. Giant arachnoid granulations mimicking pathology. A report of three cases. Neuroradiol J. 2014; 27:316–321

[30] Sekhar LN, Moller AR. Operative Management of Tumors Involving the Cavernous Sinus. J Neurosurg. 1986; 64:879–889

[31] Knosp E, Perneczky A, Koos WT, et al. Meningiomas of the Space of the Cavernous Sinus. Neurosurgery. 1996; 38:434–444

[32] Knosp E, Steiner E, Kitz K, et al. Pituitary Adenomas with Invasion of the Cavernous Sinus Space: A Magnetic Resonance Imaging Classification Compared with Surgical Findings. Neurosurgery. 1993; 33:610–618

[33] Tancioni F, Gaetani P, Villani L, et al. Neurinoma of the trigeminal root and atypical trigeminal neuralgia: case report and review of the literature. Surg Neurol. 1995; 44:36–42

[34] Hanakita S, Oya S, Matsui T. Trigeminal neuralgia caused by an arachnoid cyst in Meckel's cave: A case report and literature review. Surg Neurol Int. 2021; 12. DOI: 10.25259/SNI_734_2020

[35] Ohta H, Ottomo M, Nakamura T, et al. [A case of epidermoid tumor inside the Meckel's cave]. No Shinkei Geka. 1997; 25:943–947

[36] Aaron GP, Illing E, Lambertsen Z, et al. Enlargement of Meckel's cave in patients with spontaneous cerebrospinal fluid leaks. Int Forum Allergy Rhinol. 2017; 7:421–424

[37] Malhotra A, Tu L, Kalra VB, et al. Neuroimaging of Meckel's cave in normal and disease conditions. Insights Imaging. 2018; 9:499–510

[38] Janjua RM, Wong KM, Parekh A, et al. Management of the great mimicker: Meckel cave tumors. Neurosurgery. 2010; 67:416–421

[39] Sindou M, Chavez JM, Saint Pierre G, et al. Percutaneous biopsy of cavernous sinus tumors through the foramen ovale. Neurosurgery. 1997; 40:106–10; discussion 110-1

[40] Thomas JE, Baker HL. Assessment of Roentgenographic Lucencies of the Skull: A Systematic Approach. Neurology. 1975; 25:99–106

[41] Horning GW, Beatty RM. Osteolytic Skull Lesions Secondary to Trauma. Journal of Neurosurgery. 1990; 72:506–508

[42] Le Roux PD, Griffin GE, Marsh HT, et al. Tuberculosis of the Skull – A Rare Condition: Case Report and Review of the Literature. Neurosurgery. 1990; 26:851–856

[43] Lopez-Villegas D, Kulisevsky J, Deus J, et al. Neuropsychological Alterations in Patients with Computed Tomography-Detected Basal Ganglia Calcification. Archives of Neurology. 1996; 53:251–256

[44] Ang LC, Alport EC, Tchang S. Fahr's Disease Associated with Astrocytic Proliferation and Astrocytoma. Surgical Neurology. 1993; 39:365–369

[45] Bhimani S, Sarwar M, Virapongse C, et al. Computed Tomography of Cerebrovascular Calcifications in Postsurgical Hypoparathyroidism. J Comput Assist Tomogr. 1985; 9:121–124

[46] Morrison G, Sobel DF, Kelley WM, et al. Intraventricular Mass Lesions. Radiology. 1984; 153:435–442

[47] D'Angelo VA, Galarza M, Catapano D, et al. Lateral ventricle tumors: Surgical strategies according to tumor origin and development - a series of 72 cases. Neurosurgery. 2005; 56:ONS36–ONS45

[48] Brat DJ, Scheithauer BW, Staugaitis SM, et al. Third ventricular chordoid glioma: a distinct clinicopathologic entity. J Neuropathol Exp Neurol. 1998; 57:283–290

[49] Jelinek J, Smirniotopoulos JG, Parisi JE, et al. Lateral ventricular neoplasms of the brain: Differential diagnosis based on clinical, CT, and MR findings. AJNR. 1990; 11:567–574

99

[50] Kinkel WR, Jacobs L, Polachini I, et al. Subcortical Arteriosclerotic Encephalopathy (Binswanger's Disease). Arch Neurol. 1985; 42:951–959

[51] Roman GC. Senile Dementia of the Binswanger Type: A Vascular Form of Dementia in the Elderly. JAMA. 1987; 258:1782–1788

[52] Hachinski VC, Potter P, Merskey H. Leuko-Araiosis. Arch Neurol. 1987; 44:21–23

[53] Steingart A, Hachinski VC, Lau C, et al. Cognitive and Neurologic Findings in Subjects With Diffuse White Matter Lucencies on Computed Tomographic Scan (Leuko-Araiosis). Arch Neurol. 1987; 44:32–35

[54] Zatz LM, Jernigan TL, Ahumada AJ. White Matter Changes in Cerebral Computed Tomography Related to Aging. J Comput Assist Tomogr. 1982; 6:19–23

[55] Janota I, Mirsen TR, Hachinski VC, et al. Neuropathologic Correlates of Leuko-Araiosis. Arch Neurol. 1989; 46:1124–1128

[56] Paakko E, Patronas NJ, Schellinger D. Meningeal Gd-DTPA enhancement in patients with malignancies. J Comput Assist Tomogr. 1990; 14:542–546

[57] River Y, Schwartz A, Gomori JM, et al. Clinical significance of diffuse dural enhancement detected by magnetic resonance imaging. J Neurosurg. 1996; 85:777–783

[58] Estevez M, Chu C, Pless M. Small B-cell lymphoma presenting as diffuse dural thickening with cranial neuropathies. J Neurooncol. 2002; 59:243–247

[59] Sze G, Soletsky S, Bronen R, et al. MR Imaging of the Cranial Meninges with Emphasis on Contrast Enhancement and Meningeal Carcinomatosis. AJNR. 1989; 10:965–975

[60] Guerini H, Helie O, Leveque C, et al. [Diagnosis of periventricular ependymal enhancement in MRI in adults]. J Neuroradiol. 2003; 30:46–56

[61] Fukui MB, Williams RL, Mudigonda S. CT and MR imaging features of pyogenic ventriculitis. AJNR Am J Neuroradiol. 2001; 22:1510–1516

[62] Butler WE, Khan A, Khan SA. Posterior fossa ependymoma with intense but transient disseminated enhancement but not metastasis. Pediatr Neurosurg. 2002; 37:27–31

[63] Mohr G, Ferguson G, Khan M, et al. Intraventricular Hemorrhage from Ruptured Aneurysm: Retrospective Analysis of 91 Cases. Journal of Neurosurgery. 1983; 58:482–487

[64] Budhram A, Leung A, Nicolle MW, et al. Diagnosing autoimmune limbic encephalitis. CMAJ. 2019; 191: E529–E534

[65] Graus F, Titulaer MJ, Balu R, et al. A clinical approach to diagnosis of autoimmune encephalitis. Lancet Neurol. 2016; 15:391–404

[66] Brandwein S, Esdaile J, Danoff D, et al. Wegener's Granulomatosis: Clinical Features and Outcome in 13 Patients. Arch Intern Med. 1983; 143:476–479

[67] Jeng YM, Sung MT, Fang CL, et al. Sinonasal undifferentiated carcinoma and nasopharyngeal-type undifferentiated carcinoma: two clinically, biologically, and histopathologically distinct entities. Am J Surg Pathol. 2002; 26:371–376

[68] Hlavac PJ, Henson SL, Popp AJ. Esthesioneuroblastoma: Advances in Diagnosis and Treatment. Contemporary Neurosurgery. 1998; 20:1–5

100 Differential Diagnosis by Location or Radiographic Finding – Spine

100.1 Diagnoses covered outside this chapter

See ▶ Table 100.1.

Table 100.1 Differential diagnoses by location or radiographic finding, spine—covered outside this chapter

DDx
chordomas (p. 825)
lateral disc herniation (p. 1264)
spinal cord tumors (p. 979)
spinal epidural abscess (p. 382)
spinal stenosis
• lumbar (p. 1332)
synovial cyst (spinal) (p. 1341)
thoracic outlet syndrome (p. 581)

100.2 Atlantoaxial subluxation

1. incompetence of the transverse atlantal ligament (TAL): results in *increased* atlanto-dental interval (ADI) (p. 223)
   a) rheumatoid arthritis: erosion of insertion points of the TAL (p. 1377)
   b) traumatic
      • disruption (tear) of the TAL (rare)
      • avulsion of the insertion points of the TAL (as in comminuted C1 fx)
   c) congenital laxity of the TAL:
      • Down syndrome: 20% incidence (p. 1381) [1]
      • may be associated with neurofibromatosis
   d) retropharyngeal infections: chronic tonsillitis (p. 1158), Grisel syndrome
   e) chronic steroid use
2. incompetence of the odontoid process: ADI is *normal*
   a) odontoid fractures (p. 1171)
   b) os odontoideum (p. 1175)
   c) erosion of the odontoid due to rheumatoid arthritis (RA) (p. 1376)
   d) neoplastic erosion of the odontoid:
      • metastases to the upper cervical spine (p. 922)
      • other tumors of the axis
   e) Morquio syndrome: hypoplasia of the dens (p. 1308)
   f) congenital absence/dysplasia of the odontoid
   g) following transoral odontoidectomy: creates severe ligamentous instability (p. 1771)
   h) local infection

▶ **Note.** Chronic atlantoaxial subluxation (AAS) seen in conditions such as rheumatoid arthritis or Down syndrome may be significant yet asymptomatic. Treatment decisions in this group are difficult. Acute AAS is more commonly symptomatic and may be life-threatening.

100.3 Abnormalities in vertebral bodies

See also lesions unique to the craniocervical junction & upper cervical spine (p. 1308).
   For abnormalities unique to the axis (C2), see below.
1. neoplasms; see more extensive list (p. 570)
   a) metastases: prostate, breast, lung, renal cell, thyroid, lymphoma, & myeloma commonly go to bone. Four patterns (≈ all are *low intensity* on T1WI):
      • focal lytic (most common): T1WI = hypointense, T2WI = hyperintense

100

- focal sclerotic: hypointense on T1WI and T2WI
- diffuse homogeneous: T1WI = hypointense, T2WI = hyperintense or heterogeneous
- diffuse heterogeneous: mixed signal intensities on T1WI & T2WI
  b) primary bone tumors; see more extensive discussion (p.989)
  - vertebral hemangioma
  - osteoblastoma
2. infection: osteomyelitis/discitis
3. fatty infiltrate or replacement of bone marrow: with age, hematopoietic red marrow of VBs is gradually replaced by yellow marrow in a splotchy pattern at a slower rate than in many other locations, e.g., distal appendicular bones.[2] T1WI: yellow marrow (MRI characteristics similar to subcutaneous fat) is hyperintense to red marrow (caution: bright areas on T1WI may be fat, or may be a normal area next to a low-intensity met). T2WI: yellow marrow is bright
4. degenerative changes (Modic changes), see ▶ Table 81.2
5. metabolic
   a) Paget's disease: plain X-rays → enlargement of VBs with cortical thickening usually involving **several contiguous levels** (p.1363)
   b) osteoporosis: reduced bone density. Vertebral compression fractures may be seen
   c) ankylosing spondylitis (p.1365): osteoporotic VBs, calcified intervertebral discs (sparing the nucleus pulposus), and ossified ligaments → square VBs with bridging syndesmophytes ("bamboo spine"). Starts in sacroiliac joints & lumbar spine

100.4 Axis (C2) vertebra lesions

1. tumors: rare. Possibilities include those that involve the spine at any location. Some factors pertinent to this location[3]:
   a) primary bone
   - chondroma
   - chondrosarcoma: rare in the craniovertebral junction. Lobulated tumors with calcified areas
   - chordoma: slow-growing radioresistant malignancy (p.827)
   - osteochondroma (chondroma)
   - osteoblastoma (p.990)
   - osteoid osteoma (p.990): more common in posterior elements than VB[4]
   - giant-cell tumors of bone: typically arise in adolescence. Lytic with bony collapse[5]
   b) metastatic: including
   - typical metastases that spread hematogenously to bone, including: breast cancer, prostate cancer, malignant melanoma, paraganglioma, renal cell carcinoma
   - extension of regional tumors: nasopharyngeal tumors, craniopharyngioma
   c) meningioma
   d) neurofibroma
   e) miscellaneous
   - plasmacytoma
   - multiple myeloma
   - Langerhans cell histiocytosis: osteolytic defect with progressive vertebral collapse. Occasionally occur in C2[6]
   - Ewing's sarcoma: malignant. Peak incidence during 2nd decade of life
   - aneurysmal bone cyst[7]
2. infection: osteomyelitis of the axis
3. pannus from old nonunion of fracture or from rheumatoid arthritis (**RA**)
4. erosive changes in the odontoid process with RA (p.1377)

100.5 Mass posterior to the odontoid process

1. RA pannus. Involvement of the c-spine in RA typically begins early in the disease process and often parallels the extent of peripheral disease correlating with the degree of hand and wrist erosion
2. retro-odontoid pseudotumor (ROP)[8] in patients without RA. AAS may play a role in developing ROP. ROP unassociated with AAS can be seen in patients without RA but is rare. All cases reported were seen in the elderly and most have severe OA changes at the atlanto-axial joint
3. calcium pyrophosphate deposition (CPPD) disease (formerly referred to as pseudogout)
4. psoriatic arthritis
5. chondrocalcinosis

100

100.6 Pathologic fractures of the spine

100.6.1 General information

Fractures due to metastatic involvement are hypointense on T1WI and hyperintense on T2WI. Benign VB collapse should be isointense to normal VBs on all sequences[9,10] and the VB should look homogeneous. On T2WI or STIR images, the cortex of the VB (which should be a dark border around the VB due to low water content of cortical bone) should be intact.

100.6.2 Etiologies

1. osteoporosis
2. neoplasm: short list
   a) metastases: common sources of spine mets: lung, breast, prostate, myeloma
   b) Langerhans cell histiocytosis (p. 846): may cause vertebra plana (see below)
   c) lymphoma
   d) hemangioma (p. 992)
3. infection
4. avascular necrosis of the vertebral body
   a) Calve-Kummel-Verneuil disease (see below)
   b) with steroid use

100.6.3 Vertebra plana

Criteria:
1. uniform collapse of vertebral body into flat thin disc
2. increased density of vertebra
3. spares neural arches
4. normal disc and intervertebral disc space
5. intervertebral vacuum cleft sign (pathognomonic)
6. no kyphosis

Etiologies include:
1. Langerhans cell histiocytosis
2. Calve-Kummel-Verneuil disease: avascular necrosis of the vertebral body. Occurs in 2–15-year-olds
3. hemangioma

100.7 Spinal epidural masses

See items marked with a dagger (†) under Myelopathy (p. 1696).

100.8 Destructive lesions of the spine

100.8.1 Etiologies

1. neoplastic; see Differential diagnosis: spine & spinal cord **tumors** (p. 979) for more:
   a) metastatic tumors with a predilection for bone: prostate, breast, renal cell, lymphoma, thyroid, lung…; see Spinal epidural metastases (p. 921)
   b) primary bone tumors: chordomas (p. 825), osteoid osteoma (p. 990), hemangioma (p. 992)
2. infection:
   a) vertebral osteomyelitis: occurs mostly in IV drug abusers, patients with diabetes mellitus, and hemodialysis patients. May have associated spinal epidural abscess. Also see Vertebral osteomyelitis (p. 386)
   b) discitis (p. 390)
3. chronic renal failure: some patients develop a destructive spondyloarthropathy that resembles infection[11,12]
4. ankylosing spondylitis (p. 1365): bamboo spine (square VBs with bridging syndesmophytes)
5. lesions producing *posterior* scalloping of VB (mnemonic: AMEN)
   Acromegaly or achondroplasia
   Marfan syndrome or mucopolysaccharidosis

100

Ehlers-Danlos
Neurofibromatosis
also: dural ectasia
6. lesions producing *anterior* scalloping of VB
   a) aortic aneurysm
   b) lymphoma
   c) spinal TB

100.8.2 Differentiating factors

Of the many lytic or destructive lesions that involve the vertebra, destruction of the disc space is highly suggestive of *infection*, which often involves at least two adjacent vertebral levels. Although tumors may involve adjacent vertebral levels and cause collapse of disc height, the disc space is usually not destroyed[13] (possible exceptions include: some vertebral plasmacytomas, a reported metastatic cervical carcinoma, and there may occasionally be destruction of the disc in ankylosing spondylitis[14]). Unlike pyogenic infections, the disc may be relatively resistant to tuberculous involvement in Pott's disease (▶ Fig. 21.1).[15] Also, since metastatic tumor involvement usually produces widespread bony involvement, it is less likely with involvement of a single bone.

100.9 Vertebral hyperostosis

1. Paget's disease (p. 1362): classic "ivory bone" with cortical thickening ("picture frame" appearance on plain X-rays). Consider Paget's with a *dense* vertebra on X-ray in an older patient, commonly involving several contiguous vertebrae
2. osteoblastic metastases
   a) in men: prostate
   b) in women: breast
   c) lymphoma
3. osteoid osteoma and osteoblastoma (p. 990)
4. bone island (AKA enostosis)[16]: cortical bone (histologically normal) within cancellous bone (abnormal location). Some consider it a hamartoma. Usually asymptomatic, most common in long bones and pelvis. Low signal on MRI (like cortical bone). High density on CT and plain radiographs. Usually cold on bone scan

100.10 Sacral lesions

100.10.1 Tumors

1. metastases: the most common sacral neoplasm
2. primary neoplasms of the sacrum are uncommon and include:
   a) giant cell tumor (p. 1701)
   b) chordoma
   c) teratoma:
      • adults: pre-sacral or sacro-coccygeal teratomas may arise from cells sequestered from Hensen's node in the caudal embryo. Rarely cause neurologic involvement (distinguishing this from chordoma). Sacrum may be normal in up to 50% (abnormal in almost all chordomas). Treatment is complete removal, usually by general surgeon
      • peds: malignant pre-sacral teratoma is a rare tumor seen primarily in female children

100.10.2 Infection

Most infections of the sacrum or sacroiliac joint are due to contiguous spread from a suppurative focus.

100.10.3 Arthritic disorders

1. ankylosing spondylitis (p. 1367): involves SI joint almost by definition
2. osteoarthritis

100

100.10.4 Sacral fractures

May be due to:
1. trauma
2. repetitive stress
3. sacral insufficiency (p. 1705)

100.10.5 Congenital

Sacral agenesis (caudal regression syndrome): rare (prevalence: 0.005–0.01%; higher (0.1–0.2%) in children of diabetic mothers (16–20% of children with sacral agenesis have diabetic mothers)). Increased incidence of associated spinal abnormalities including: syrinx, tethered cord, lipoma, and lipomyelomeningocele.
1. Four types:
   a) Type 1: partial unilateral agenesis, localized to the sacrum or coccyx
   b) Type 2: partial bilaterally symmetric defects in the sacrum. Iliac bones articulate with S1, and distal segments of the sacrum and coccyx fail to develop
   c) Type 3: total sacral agenesis + iliac bones articulate with the lowest segment of the lumbar spine present
   d) Type 4: total sacral agenesis + iliac bones fused posteriorly along the midline
2. in cases of total sacral agenesis (types 3 & 4), MR findings include: absence of the sacrum and coccyx and variable absence of a portion of the lumbar spine, with a characteristic club-shaped configuration of the conus medullaris

100.10.6 Miscellaneous

Osteitis condensans ilii: increased density in ilium, usually asymptomatic (incidental) finding. Occasionally may produce low back pain or tenderness.

100.11 Enhancing nerve roots

1. tumor
   a) meningeal carcinomatosis
   b) lymphoma
2. infection: especially CMV (often seen in AIDS patients)
3. inflammatory
   a) Guillain-Barré
   b) arachnoiditis
   c) sarcoid

100.12 Nodular enhancing lesions in the spinal canal

1. neurofibromatosis (NFT)
2. tumor
   a) drop mets
   b) neurofibroma
   c) schwannoma

100.13 Intraspinal cysts

- spinal meningeal cysts (p. 1400)
- cystic neurofibroma
- ependymoma: may be cystic. In filum terminale: myxopapillary ependymoma (p. 985)
- syringomyelia (p. 1405)
- dilated central canal (p. 1405)

100.14 Diffuse enhancement of nerve roots/cauda equina

(as distinct from nodular enhancement, see above)
- Guillain-Barré (p. 193)

100

2. meningitis
3. cytomegalovirus (CMV) (especially in AIDS)
4. lymphoma
5. sarcoid (look for hilar adenopathy)

References

[1] Martel W, Tishler JM. Observations on the spine in mongoloidism. American Journal of Roentgenology, Radium Therapy and Nuclear Medicine. 1966; 97:630–638

[2] Lakhkar BN, Aggarwal M, Jose J. Pictorial essay: MR appearances of osseous spine tumors. Indian J Radiol Imaging. 2002; 12:383–390

[3] Piper JG, Menezes AH. Management Strategies for Tumors of the Axis Vertebra. Journal of Neurosurgery. 1996; 84:543–551

[4] Molloy S, Saifuddin A, Allibone J, et al. Excision of an osteoid osteoma from the body of the axis through an anterior approach. Eur Spine J. 2002; 11:599–601

[5] Honma G, Murota K, Shiba R, et al. Mandible and Tongue-Splitting Approach for Giant Cell Tumor of Axis. Spine. 1989; 14:1204–1210

[6] Osenbach RK, Youngblood LA, Menezes AH. Atlanto-Axial Instability Secondary to Solitary Eosinophilic Granuloma of C2 in a 12-Year-Old Girl. Case Report. J Spinal Disord. 1990; 3:408–412

[7] Verbiest H, The Cervical Spine Research Society Editorial Committee. Benign Cervical Spine Tumors: Clinical Experience. In: The Cervical Spine. 2nd ed. Philadelphia: J.B. Lippincott; 1989:723–774

[8] Yu SH, Choi HJ, Cho WH, et al. Retro-Odontoid Pseudotumor without Atlantoaxial Subluxation or Rheumatic Arthritis. Korean J Neurotrauma. 2016; 12:180–184

[9] Li KC, Poon PY. Sensitivity and specificity of MRI in detecting spinal cord compression and in distinguishing malignant from benign compression fractures of vertebrae. Magnetic Resonance Imaging 1988; 6:547–556

[10] Yuh WTC, Zachar CK, Barloon TJ, et al. Vertebra compression fractures: distinction between benign and malignant causes with MR imaging. Radiology 1989; 172:215–218

[11] Kuntz D, Naveau B, Bardin T, et al. Destructive spondyloarthropathy in hemodialyzed patients: A new syndrome. Arthritis Rheum. 1984; 27:369–375

[12] Alcalay M, Goupy M-C, Azais I, et al. Hemodialysis is not Essential for the Development of Destructive Spondyloarthropathy in Patients with Chronic Renal Failure. Arthritis Rheum. 1987; 30:1182–1186

[13] Borges LF. Case Records of the Massachusetts General Hospital: Case 24-1989. New England Journal of Medicine. 1989; 320:1610–1618

[14] Cawley MD, Chalmers TM, Kellgren JH, et al. Destructive Lesions of Vertebral Bodies in Ankylosing Spondylitis. Ann Rheum Dis. 1972; 31:345–348

[15] Rothman RH, Simeone FA. The Spine. Philadelphia 1992

[16] Greenspan A. Bone island (enostosis): current concept–a review. Skeletal Radiol. 1995; 24:111–115

101 Differential Diagnosis (DDx) by Signs and Symptoms – Primarily Intracranial

101.1 Diagnoses covered outside this chapter

See ▶ Table 101.1.

Table 101.1 Differential diagnoses by signs and symptoms, primarily intracranial—covered outside this chapter

DDx
abducens palsy (p. 598)
anisocoria (p. 591)
chordomas (p. 825)
chronic meningitis (p. 341)
coma (p. 319)
Creutzfeldt-Jakob disease (p. 403)
diabetes insipidus (p. 124)
dizziness (p. 603)
facial nerve palsy (Bell's palsy) (p. 607)
giant cell arteritis (p. 203)
gyral enhancement (p. 1560)
hemiplegia/hemiparesis—see spine section (p. 1703)
internuclear ophthalmoplegia (p. 596)
Meniere disease (p. 604)
multiple sclerosis (p. 188)
ophthalmoplegia
• painful (p. 599)
• painless (p. 600)
papilledema (p. 586)
Parinaud's syndrome (p. 101)
Parkinson's disease (p. 185)
pneumocephalus (p. 1067)
prolactin elevation (▶ Table 52.4)
pseudotumor cerebri (p. 961)
retinal hemorrhage (p. 1104)
sarcoidosis (p. 199)
seizures
• new onset, adult (p. 503)
• new onset, peds (p. 504)
• nonepileptic (p. 507)
• status epilepticus (p. 511)
schizencephaly (p. 309)
torticollis (p. 1844)
trigeminal neuralgia (p. 1859)
vertigo (p. 603)

101.2 Encephalopathy

Many etiologies are similar to that for coma (p. 319). EEG may be helpful in distinguishing some etiologies (p. 249).
   a rare cause may be (spontaneous) intracranial hypotension (p. 421)
   hypertensive encephalopathy from malignant hypertension

101.3 Syncope and apoplexy

101.3.1 General information

Syncope may be defined as one or more episodes of brief loss of consciousness (LOC) with prompt recovery (this term is considered by many to signify a vasovagal episode). The uncommonly used term lipothymia may be less likely to imply an etiology. Prevalence may be as high as ≈ 50% (higher in the elderly). Apoplexy is traditionally considered a form of hemorrhage, usually intracerebral. The recovery from apoplexy would therefore usually be slower than for syncope.

101.3.2 Etiologies

(Adapted.[1,2]) NB: in a large number of cases no cause can be determined.

1. vascular: a few myotonic jerks may be seen in cerebral ischemia
   a) cerebrovascular
      • subarachnoid hemorrhage (most commonly aneurysmal)
      • intracerebral hemorrhage
      • brainstem infarction
      • pituitary apoplexy (p.865) (rare)
      • vertebrobasilar insufficiency (VBI) (p.1591)
      • rarely with migraine
   b) cardiovascular
      • Stokes-Adams attacks: disorder of AV-node conduction in the heart resulting in syncope with bradycardia
      • carotid sinus syncope: minimal stimulation (e.g., tight shirt collar, syncope while shaving…) causes reflex bradycardia with hypotension, more common in patients with carotid vascular disease. Bedside carotid massage with ECG and BP monitor may diagnose[2]
      • cardiac standstill: seen rarely in patients with glossopharyngeal neuralgia (p.1873)
      • vasodepressor syncope (the common faint), AKA vasovagal response, and recently AKA neurocardiogenic syncope[3]: the most common cause of transient LOC. Hypotension usually with any of the following autonomic manifestations: pallor, nausea, heavy perspiration, pupillary dilatation, bradycardia, hyperventilation, salivation. Usually benign. Most common in age < 35 yrs
      • orthostatic hypotension: drop in SBP ≥ 25 mm Hg on standing
      • triggered syncope: includes micturition syncope, tussive syncope, weight-lifting syncope… (most involve elevation of intrathoracic pressure)
2. infectious
   a) meningitis
   b) encephalitis
3. seizure (p.480): in general, there are involuntary movements and confusion afterwards, lasts at least several minutes. Todd's paralysis may follow and usually resolves slowly over a period of a few hours. There may be irritative special-sense phenomena (visual, auditory, or olfactory hallucinations)
   a) generalized
   b) complex partial
   c) akinetic seizure
   d) drop attack (loss of posture without LOC): seen in Lennox-Gastaut
4. metabolic: hypoglycemia (may produce seizure, usually generalized)
5. miscellaneous
   a) intermittent ventricular obstruction: the classic example is a colloid cyst of the 3rd ventricle (p.944), but this mechanism is questionable
   b) narcoleptic cataplexy: narcolepsy is characterized by somnolence and sudden attacks of weakness (cataplexy) when awake. Easy arousal and lack of post-ictal drowsiness distinguishes cataplexy from a seizure. The somnolence is treated with CNS stimulants (such as amphetamines or modafinil (Provigil®) 200 mg PO q AM), and cataplexy is treated with antidepressants
   c) psychogenic
6. intracranial hypotension: typically when assuming upright position. May be spontaneous (p.421), or may follow LP, CSF shunt, spinal surgery with CSF leak
7. unknown: in ≈ 40% of cases no cause can be diagnosed

101.3.3 Practical approach to syncope
Introduction

The core of diagnosis and management are the H&P, orthostatic vital signs, and the ECG, with a combined diagnostic yield of 50%[4] covering:
1. reflex-mediated such as vasovagal or Valsalva/stress-induced: 36-62%
2. cardiac valvular etiology or arrhythmia: 10–30%
3. orthostatic due to autonomic dysregulation, dehydration, or polypharmacy: 2–24%
4. cerebrovascular due to stroke: ≈ 1%
5. seizure

Evaluation

1. history: includes
   a) medication list: look for drugs that may cause orthostatic hypotension, especially blood pressure medication, beta-blockers
   b) precipitating factors: e.g., change in position, sensitivity to tight collars…
   c) premonitory factors: e.g., sweating and tremulousness may signify hypoglycemia, bradycardia is associated with vasovagal events, tonic-clonic movements may occur with a seizure
   d) post-ictal emergence: usually rapid after a simple faint, slower after seizure which may also exhibit Todd's paralysis (p. 480)
2. cardiovascular etiologies: Testing is also guided by H&P, vital signs & ECG:
   a) cardiac arrhythmia evaluation: 12-lead ECG & 24-hour Holter monitor, and may lead to electrophysiologic (EP) testing/intervention[4,5]
   b) abnormal orthostatics warrant a formal tilt-table test
   c) history of cardiomyopathy or CAD merits an echocardiogram and formal stress testing. These results determine the need for cardiac catheterization
3. neurologic etiologies: comprise < 1% of cases.[6] In the absence of clinical evidence of a neurologic etiology, neurodiagnostic testing (EEG, CT scan, MRI/MRA, carotid Doppler) has a diagnostic yield of 2–6%. ∴ These tests are warranted only when clinically indicated[5] (seizures, altered consciousness, gradually resolving Todd's paralysis, known history of cerebrovascular compromise). Tests include:
   a) unenhanced brain CT: rules out most acute neurosurgical etiologies (bleed, hydrocephalus, edema that may be associated with tumor)
   b) MRI without and with enhancement in cases with unexplained CT findings, or with a negative CT but high suspicion of a CNS etiology
   c) seizure evaluation: when symptoms suggest possible seizure:
      • EEG: usually a sleep-deprived EEG. Not very sensitive
      • 24-hour video EEG monitoring: in cases with high index of suspicion of seizures or nonepileptic seizures

Management

Admission and inpatient management are warranted for patients with diagnosed cardiac or neurologic syncope, either by suggestive history (family history of sudden death, syncope during exertion, witnessed seizure) or diagnostic testing (arrhythmia, severe orthostatic changes, hemodynamic instability).[4,7]

101.4 Transient neurologic deficit

For apoplexy, etc., see Syncope and apoplexy (p. 1684).
The first three etiologies listed below cover most cases of transient neurologic deficit:
1. transient ischemic attack (TIA) (p. 1536): temporary neurologic dysfunction as a result of ischemia. Maximum deficit usually at onset. Most resolve in < 20 mins
2. migraine: unlike TIA, tends to progress in a march-like fashion over several minutes. May or may not be followed by headache; see Migraine (p. 183)
3. seizure: may be followed by Todd's paralysis (p. 480)
4. TIA-like syndrome
   a) "tumor TIA": a transient deficit in a patient with a tumor, may be clinically indistinguishable from an ischemic TIA. Intravascular lymphomatosis may mimic TIAs (p. 842)
   b) TIA-like symptoms may occur as a prodrome (p. 1614) to a lobar intracerebral hemorrhage[8,9] in cases of cerebral amyloid angiopathy (CAA). Unlike typical TIAs, these usually consist of

numbness, tingling, or weakness that gradually spreads in a manner reminiscent of a Jacksonian march and may cross over vascular territories. Caution: antiplatelet drugs and anticoagulation may increase the risk of hemorrhage in patients with CAA (p. 1612)

c) chronic subdural hematoma: may cause recurrent TIA-like symptoms of the involved hemisphere[10] (including transient aphasia with dominant hemisphere involvement, hemisensory or motor abnormalities). The duration of symptoms tends to be longer than the typical TIA.[10] Postulated mechanisms include:

- electrical basis: the possibility of epileptic activity (e.g., due to irritation of the cortex by blood breakdown products) has not been supported in the literature; however, spreading depression of Leao has been considered[11]
- impairment of venous outflow by compression of surface veins
- compromised regional cerebral perfusion by indirect shifting of the anterior and posterior cerebral arteries[12]
- transient ICP elevations → variations in cerebral perfusion pressure

101.5 Ataxia/balance difficulties

1. cerebellar origin: usually with involvement of UEs in addition to LEs
   a) cerebellar tumors
   b) cerebellar hemorrhage
   c) acute cerebellar ataxia: usually follows viral infection in a child < 3 years. Usually self-limited with good prognosis for complete recovery
2. spinal cord: usually worse with eyes closed (loss of proprioceptive input)
   a) spinal stenosis
   b) neoplastic cord compression
   c) syringomyelia (may be part of Chiari malformation)
3. degenerative
   a) ataxia-telangiectasia syndrome
   b) ataxia oculomotor apraxia
   c) Friedreich's ataxia
   d) spinocerebellar degeneration
4. metabolic/nutritional
   a) vitamin B_{12} deficiency
   b) drugs
      - ASMs (especially phenytoin or carbamazepine)
      - alcohol: acutely with intoxication and chronic
      - heavy metal poisoning: primarily lead (wrist drop is more common)
5. conditions that may mimic ataxia
   a) weakness
   b) peripheral neuropathy
   c) dizziness: including orthostatic hypotension; see Dizziness and vertigo (p. 603)
6. peripheral neuropathy:
   a) ataxia can occur with Guillain-Barré syndrome (p. 193), especially Miller Fisher variant (p. 194)
   b) balance difficulties are common with chronic inflammatory demyelinating polyneuropathy (CIDP) (p. 195)

101.6 Wide-based gait

Definition: gait with feet spread > 2–4 inches apart.
   This symptom may have intracranial or spinal etiology (myelopathy).
1. idiopathic normal pressure hydrocephalus (iNPH) (p. 438). Often accompanied by magnetic gait (p. 439). Memory disturbance is common
2. cerebellar ataxia. Poor placement of feet. Look for other cerebellar signs: dysdiadochokinesia (impairment of rapid alternating movements), dysmetria, nystagmus...
3. sensorimotor peripheral neuropathy: due to loss of input of joint position sense. Worsens with loss of visual input (closing eyes, as in Romberg's test)
4. vestibular ataxia: Meniere disease, labyrinthitis. Associated with N/V, nystagmus, hearing loss...
5. myelopathy: due to cervical or thoracic spinal cord dysfunction (compression, or intrinsic spinal cord disease, see myelopathy (p. 1696)). Usually accompanied by other long tract signs: reflex abnormalities (Babinski, clonus, hyperreflexia), decreased vibratory and/or joint position sense

(posterior columns). With cervical spinal cord involvement, upper extremity findings may also occur (typically numb/clumsy hands). Asymmetric spinal cord involvement may produce Brown-Sequard syndrome (p. 1135): dissociated sensory loss (contralateral loss of pain and temperature with ipsilateral loss of vibratory sense and proprioception) with ipsilateral weakness

6. ✖ Parkinson disease (p. 184): wide-based gait is *not* typical. Classically: short shuffling steps, intermittent freezing. Associated with resting tremor, bradykinesia, cogwheeling, reduced arm swing...

101.7 Diplopia

1. cranial nerve palsy of any one or combination of III, IV (rare), or VI
   a) multiple cranial nerve palsies (p. 1687)
   b) VI palsy (p. 598): can occur with increased intracranial pressure, e.g., in pseudotumor cerebri (p. 955), sphenoid sinusitis...; see other causes of abducens palsy (p. 344)
   c) isolated muscle paresis of III suggests nuclear lesion or myasthenia gravis
2. intraorbital mass compressing extraocular muscles
   a) orbital pseudotumor (p. 600)
   b) meningioma
3. Graves' disease: hyperthyroidism + ophthalmopathy (p. 1658)
4. myasthenia gravis
5. giant cell arteritis (p. 204)
6. botulism: due to toxin from *Clostridium botulinum* (in adults: ingested or in wound). N/V, abdominal cramps, and diarrhea often precede neurologic symptoms. Neurologic involvement is typically symmetric. Dry mouth & cranial nerve palsies (diplopia, ptosis, loss of accommodation, and pupillary light reflex) are followed by descending weakness. Bulbar paresis (dysarthria, dysphagia, dysphonia, flaccid facial muscles) follows. Muscles of the trunk/extremities and respiration progressively weaken in a descending fashion. Sensory disturbances are absent. Sensorium usually remains clear
7. following head trauma: includes injury to EOMs, orbital hematoma, VI palsy from increased ICP

101.8 Anosmia

1. abrupt onset of anosmia
   a) severe upper respiratory infection with damage to the neuroepithelium: the most common cause
   b) head trauma: second most common cause. Anosmia occurs in 7–15% of patients with significant head trauma
2. gradual onset of anosmia
   a) allergic rhinitis and sinus disease[13]: third most common cause of anosmia (anosmia in this setting may be intermittent)
   b) intracranial neoplasms: olfactory groove meningioma (see Foster Kennedy syndrome (p. 100)), olfactory neuroblastoma (p. 935)
   c) may also be associated with Alzheimer's disease
   d) olfactory sense diminishes with age: ≈ 50% of patients 65–85 years of age have some loss of sense of smell
   e) metabolic abnormalities: vitamin deficiency
   f) physical blockage of nasal passages: nasal polyps...
   g) endocrine abnormalities: diabetes...
   h) chemical: alcohol abuse, exposure to solvents,[14] cocaine (ischemic infarction of olfactory mucosa from vasoconstriction)
3. congenital anosmia: Kallmann syndrome (anosmia with hypogonadotrophic hypogonadism[15])

101.9 Multiple cranial nerve palsies (cranial neuropathies)

101.9.1 Framework

The differential diagnosis is legion. The following is a framework (modified[16]):
1. congenital
   a) Möbius syndrome: AKA congenital facial diplegia. Facial plegia is complete in ≈ 35% (in rest, affects upper face more than lower face, unlike central or peripheral facial palsy), associated

with abducens palsy in 70%, external ophthalmoplegia in 25%, ptosis in 10%, lingual palsy in 18%

b) congenital facial diplegia may be part of facioscapulohumeral or myotonic muscular dystrophy

2. infectious

a) chronic meningitis:
- spirochetal, fungal, mycoplasma, viral (including AIDS)
- mycobacterial AKA tuberculous (TB) meningitis: 6th nerve involved first and most frequently. CSF shows lymphocytic pleocytosis and hypoglycorrhachia. Smears are usually negative and multiple cultures are needed to diagnose

b) stage II Lyme disease (p. 607). Facial nerve weakness is common, sometimes bilateral (Lyme disease is the most common cause of facial diplegia in endemic areas). Other cranial nerve involvement is rare

c) neurosyphilis: rare nowadays except with AIDS. Diagnosed by serologic testing

d) fungal infection
- cryptococcal meningitis (p. 409): CSF analysis for cryptococcal antigen and India ink prep can detect
- aspergillosis: may extend to the orbit from sinuses and involve cranial nerves
- mucormycosis (phycomycosis) (p. 1541): produces cavernous sinus syndrome, usually occurs in diabetics

e) cysticercosis: especially with basal form; see Neurocysticercosis (p. 404)

3. traumatic: especially with basal skull fractures. Lower cranial nerve palsies may occur (sometimes delayed in onset) with occipital condyle fractures (p. 1156) or atlantooccipital dislocation (p. 1153)

4. neoplastic (brainstem compression and intrinsic lesions usually also produce long tract findings early). Also see Jugular foramen syndromes (p. 102)

a) chordoma (p. 827)

b) sphenoid-ridge meningioma

c) neoplasms of the temporal bone (often in conjunction with chronic otitis media and otalgia): adenoid cystic carcinoma, adenocarcinoma, mucoepidermoid carcinoma

d) glomus jugulare tumors: often affects nerves IX, X, and XI. May cause pulsatile tinnitus; see Paraganglioma (p. 939)

e) carcinomatous or lymphomatous meningitis (p. 920): CSF pleocytosis and elevated protein. Palsies are painless or associated with diffuse headache. Sensory palsies are common, resulting in deafness and blindness

f) invasive PitNET/adenomas involving the cavernous sinus (p. 864): extraocular cranial neuropathies tend to develop after visual field deficits in these tumors, and are less common when compared to other intracavernous solid tumors[17]

g) primary CNS lymphoma (p. 843)

h) multiple myeloma involving the skull base (p. 929)

i) intrinsic brainstem tumors: gliomas, ependymoma, metastases...

5. vascular

a) aneurysm: intracranial or cavernous sinus (p. 1489)

b) brainstem stroke: usually also produces long tract findings (p. 101)
- Weber's syndrome: Cr N III (usually pupil-sparing) + contralateral hemiparesis
- Millard-Gubler syndrome: Cr N VI + VII + contralateral hemiparesis

c) vasculitis: Wegener's granulomatosis usually affects eighth nerve in addition to others

6. granulomatous

a) sarcoidosis: ≈ 5% have CNS involvement, usually as fluctuating single or multiple cranial neuropathies (facial nerve is most common, and may be indistinguishable from Bell's palsy). CSF pleocytosis (p. 208) is common

7. inflammatory

8. neuropathies

a) Guillain-Barré syndrome (GBS) (p. 193): cranial nerve involvement includes facial diplegia, oropharyngeal paresis. Peripheral neuropathy usually presents with ascending weakness, proximal muscle weakness > distal, and absent deep tendon reflexes

b) Miller Fisher variant GBS: ataxia, areflexia & ophthalmoplegia. Serum marker: anti-GQ1b antibodies

c) idiopathic cranial polyneuropathy: subacute onset of constant facial pain, usually retro-orbital. Frequently precedes sudden onset of cranial nerve palsies, usually involving III, IV, & VI, less frequently V, VII, and lower nerves (IX through XII). Olfactory and auditory nerves are usually spared. Acute and chronic inflammation of unknown etiology similar to Tolosa-Hunt and orbital pseudotumor. Steroids reduce pain and expedite recovery

9. entrapment in abnormal bone
   a) hyperostosis cranialis interna: a rare autosomal dominant abnormality of the bone of the base of the skull causing recurrent facial palsy and other cranial nerve palsies[18]
   b) osteopetrosis: see below
   c) Paget's disease (p. 1362) involving the skull: 8th nerve involvement (deafness) is most common. Optic nerve atrophy, and palsies of oculomotor, facial, IX, XI, olfactory nerves and others may also occur[19]
   d) fibrous dysplasia (p. 974)

101.9.2 Specific syndromes

Facial diplegia

Items culled from the above list that have facial diplegia (p. 607) as a prominent finding:
1. congenital: Möbius syndrome, congenital facial diplegia
2. infectious: Lyme disease
3. neuropathies: Guillain-Barré syndrome
4. isolated 4th ventricle (p. 607): compression at the facial colliculus
5. granulomatous: sarcoidosis

Cavernous sinus syndrome

Multiple cranial nerve palsies (involving any of the cavernous sinus cranial nerves: III, IV, V1, V2, VI) that primarily produce diplopia (due to ophthalmoplegia). Classically the third nerve palsy (e.g., from an enlarging cavernous carotid artery aneurysm) will *not* produce a dilated pupil because the sympathetics which dilate the pupil are also paralyzed.[20(p 1492)] Facial pain or altered facial sensation may occur.

See list of lesions that may produce cavernous sinus syndrome (p. 1660).

Osteopetrosis

AKA "marble bone disease" (there is also some confusion with the term osteosclerosis; osteosclerosis fragilis generalisata is the obsolete term for osteopetrosis). A rare group of genetic disorders of defective osteoclastic resorption of bone resulting in increased bone density, may be transmitted either as autosomal dominant or recessive.[21] The dominant form is usually benign and is seen in adults and adolescents. The recessive ("malignant") form is often associated with consanguinity, and is similar to hyperostosis cranialis interna (see above), but in addition to the proclivity for the skull, it also involves ribs, clavicles, long bones, and pelvis (long-bone involvement results in destruction of marrow and subsequent anemia). Cranial nerves involved primarily include optic (optic atrophy and blindness are the most common neurologic manifestation), facial, and vestibulo-acoustic (with deafness); trigeminal nerve may also be involved. There may also be extensive intracranial calcifications, hydrocephalus, intracranial hemorrhage, and seizures.

Bilateral optic nerve decompression via a supraorbital approach may improve or stabilize vision.[21]

101.10 Binocular blindness

- **Bilateral occipital lobe dysfunction**
  1. bilateral posterior cerebral artery flow impairment
     a) top of the basilar syndrome
     b) increased intracranial pressure
        • hydrocephalus with shunt malfunction
        • pseudotumor cerebri (p. 956)
        • cryptococcal meningitis: decreased visual acuity (p. 409)
  2. trauma: bilateral occipital lobe injury (e.g., contrecoup injury)

- **Other etiologies**
  1. seizures: epileptic blindness
  2. migraine: cortical spreading depression

3. posterior ischemic optic neuropathy (p. 1261): usually in the setting of shock, rarely following spine surgery in the prone position
4. bilateral vitreous hemorrhage: e.g., with SAH (Terson syndrome (p. 1419))
5. functional: conversion reaction, hysterical blindness…

101.11 Monocular blindness

Due to a lesion anterior to the optic chiasm.
1. Amaurosis fugax: often described as a "shade coming down" over one eye
   a) TIA: usually due to occlusion of the retinal artery (p. 1544)
   b) giant cell arteritis (GCA) (p. 203): usually due to ischemia of optic nerve or tracts (less commonly due to retinal artery occlusion)[22]
2. trauma: optic nerve injury
3. ruptured carotid cavernous aneurysm: resultant carotid-cavernous fistula increases intraocular pressure by impeding venous return
4. intraorbital pathology: tumors
5. injury within the globe: retinal detachment, ocular trauma
6. unilateral vitreous hemorrhage: e.g., with SAH (Terson's syndrome)

101.12 Exophthalmos

101.12.1 General information

Alternate spelling: exophthalmus.
  Definition: abnormal protrusion of the eyeball. Some authors reserve the term exophthalmos for cases due to endocrinopathies and use proptosis (of the eye) for other causes, but these terms are widely used interchangeably.
  Clinical criteria (there are other criteria that may be used): anterior displacement of the globe > 18 mm (Hertal exophthalmometry can be used to measure clinically – requires intact lateral orbital bone).
  CT/MRI criteria: proptosis is diagnosed when > 2/3 of the globe lies anterior to a line drawn from lateral orbit to medial canthus. For most accurate results, eyes should be open and fixated on a point in the primary gaze position. NB: most routine CT scans do not include the orbits to reduce the radiation to the eye.

101.12.2 Pulsatile

1. carotid-cavernous fistula (CCF) (p. 1519)
2. transmitted intracranial pulsation due to defect in orbital roof
   a) seen unilaterally e.g., in neurofibromatosis type 1 (p. 638)
   b) post-op following procedures that remove orbital roof or wall
3. vascular tumors

101.12.3 Non-pulsatile

1. tumor
   a) intraorbital tumor: may be due to mass effect from tumor or to compromised venous drainage from the orbit
      • optic glioma (p. 694)
      • optic sheath neuroma
      • lymphoma
      • optic sheath meningioma[23]
      • orbital involvement with multiple myeloma (p. 929)
      • orbital invasion by invasive PitNET/adenoma (p. 963)
      • in peds: metastatic neuroblastoma
      • in peds: Langerhans cell histiocytosis (p. 846) as part of Hand-Schüller-Christian (triad: DI, exophthalmos, and lytic bone lesions (particularly of cranium))
   b) due to hyperostosis from a sphenoid ridge meningioma
2. Graves' disease (hyperthyroidism + exophthalmos) (p. 1658): even though the exophthalmos is usually bilateral with this (80%), thyroid disease is still the most common cause of *unilateral* proptosis[24]
3. enlargement of periorbital fat[25]

4. infection: orbital cellulitis (usually has concomitant sinusitis)
5. inflammatory: orbital pseudotumor. Usually unilateral (p. 600)
6. hemorrhage
   a) traumatic
   b) spontaneous
7. 3rd nerve palsy: can cause up to 3-mm proptosis from relaxation of the rectus muscles
8. cavernous sinus occlusion (may affect both eyes)
   a) cavernous sinus thrombosis (p. 1595)
   b) cavernous sinus tumor obstructing venous outflow
9. pseudo-exophthalmos
   a) congenital macrophthalmos (bull's eye)
   b) lid retraction: e.g., in Graves' disease (p. 1691)
   c) coronal craniosynostosis can cause a "relative" proptosis (p. 266)

101.13 Ptosis

AKA blepharoptosis. Drooping of the upper eyelid.

Distinguished from pseudoptosis (lid droop not resulting from weakness of levator palpebrae superioris (LPS)), which can be due to enophthalmos (globe displaced posteriorly, e.g., with orbital floor blow-out fracture), microphthalmia, blepharospasm, Duane syndrome.

Etiologies of ptosis:
1. congenital: most are simple (autosomal dominant inheritance), complicated ptosis is associated with other findings (e.g., ptosis with ophthalmoplegia)
2. traumatic: injury to eyelid, orbital roof fracture…
3. neurogenic:
   a) third nerve palsy (p. 596)
      • involvement of main trunk of third nerve: can occur intradurally or within cavernous sinus. Ptosis may be an early sign of pituitary tumor expansion (apoplexy) (p. 865)
      • involvement of the superior division of the third nerve within the orbit
   b) Horner syndrome (p. 594): ptosis here is partial (may be a pseudoptosis since weakness is in tarsal muscles, not LPS), and the lower eyelid will be higher than the uninvolved contralateral lower eyelid
4. myogenic ptosis
   a) botulinum toxin injection (e.g., Botox®)
   b) myasthenia gravis
5. mechanical ptosis
   a) tumors: neurofibroma, hemangioma, malignant melanoma, mets…
   b) extension of mucocele of frontal sinus
6. pharmacologic (drugs). Partial list:
   a) corticosteroids: including topical
   b) alcohol
   c) opium

101.14 Pathologic lid retraction

1. hyperthyroidism (p. 1659)
2. psychiatric: schizophrenia…
3. steroids
4. Parinaud's syndrome (p. 101)

101.15 Macrocephaly

Macrocephaly means increased size of the head.[26] Although sometimes used synonymously, the term macrocrania by convention refers to a head circumference > 98th percentile.[27 (p 203)] Also, not to be confused with macrencephaly AKA megalencephaly (see below). In a pediatric practice the 3 most common etiologies in decreasing order of frequency: familial (parents have big heads), benign subdural fluid collections of infancy (p. 1087), and hydrocephalus.
1. with ventricular enlargement
   a) (hydrostatic) hydrocephalus (HCP), see for etiologies (p. 426)
      • communicating
      • obstructive

   b) hydranencephaly (p. 309)
   c) constitutional ventriculomegaly: ventricular enlargement of no known etiology with normal neurologic function
   d) hydrocephalus ex vacuo: loss of cerebral tissue (more often associated with *micro*cephaly, e.g. with TORCH infections)
   e) vein of Galen aneurysms: see below
2. with normal or mildly enlarged ventricles
   a) "external hydrocephalus": prominent subarachnoid spaces and basal cisterns; see External hydrocephalus (AKA benign external hydrocephalus) (p. 433)
   b) subdural fluid
      • hematoma
      • hygroma
      • effusion benign and symptomatic
      • benign subdural collections of infancy (p. 1087)
   c) cerebral edema: some consider this to be a form of pseudotumor cerebri[26]
      • toxic: e.g., lead encephalopathy (from chronic lead poisoning)
      • endocrine: hypoparathyroidism, galactosemia, hypophosphatasia, hypervitaminosis A, adrenal insufficiency...
   d) familial (hereditary) macrocrania: parents also have large heads, the brains eventually "catch up"
   e) idiopathic
   f) megalencephaly (AKA macrencephaly): an enlarged brain (p. 312)
   g) neurocutaneous disorders (p. 637): usually due to increased volume of brain tissue (megalencephaly, see above).[26] Seen especially in neurofibromatosis and congenital hypermelanosis (Ito's syndrome). Less common in tuberous sclerosis and Sturge-Weber. Also seen in the rare hemimegalencephaly syndrome
   h) arachnoid cyst (AKA subependymal or subarachnoid cyst)[26]: a duplication of the ependyma or arachnoid layer filled with CSF. Usually reach maximal size by 1 month of age and do not enlarge further. Treatment is required in ≈ 30% due to rapid enlargement or growth beyond first month. Cyst may be shunted or fenestrated. Prognosis with true arachnoid cyst is generally good (unlike porencephalic cyst) if no increased ICP or progressive macrocephaly during 1st year of life
   i) arteriovenous malformation: especially vein of Galen "aneurysm" (p. 1518). Auscultate for cranial bruit. With vein of Galen aneurysms, macrocephaly may be due to HCP from obstruction of the Sylvian aqueduct.[26] With other malformations, macrocrania may be due to increased pressure in venous system without HCP
   j) brain tumors without hydrocephalus: brain tumors are rare in infancy, and most cause obstructive HCP. Tumors that occasionally present without HCP include astrocytomas. May also be seen in the rare diencephalic syndrome, see tumor of anterior hypothalamus (p. 695)
   k) "gigantism syndromes"
      • Soto's syndrome: associated with advanced bone age on X-ray, and multiple dysplastic features of face, skin, and bones
      • exomphalomacroglossia-gigantism (EMG) syndrome: hypoglycemia (from abnormalities in islets of Langerhans), large birth weight, large umbilicus or umbilical hernia, and macroglossia
   l) "craniocerebral disproportion" (p. 1087)[26]: may be the same as benign extra-axial fluid of infancy
   m) achondroplastic dwarf: cranial structures are enlarged but the skull base is small, giving rise to a prominent forehead and an OFC ≥ 97th percentile for age, hypoplasia of midface, and stenosis at foramen magnum. Head growth follows different curve than normal (OFC ≥ 97th percentile for age is not unusual and does not necessitate shunting)
   n) Canavan's disease: AKA spongy degeneration of the brain, an autosomal recessive disease of infancy prevalent among Ashkenazi Jews. Produces symmetrical low attenuation of hemispheric white matter on CT[28] and macrocephaly
   o) neurometabolic diseases: usually due to deposition of metabolic substances in the brain. Seen in Tay-Sachs gangliosidosis, Krabbe disease...
3. due to thickening of the skull
   a) anemia: e.g., thalassemia
   b) skull dysplasia: e.g., osteopetrosis (p. 1689)

101.16 Tinnitus

101.16.1 General information

May be either subjective (heard only by patient) or objective (e.g., cranial bruit, can be heard by examiner as well, usually with a stethoscope placed over the cranium, orbit, or carotid arteries in the neck). Objective tinnitus is almost always due to vascular turbulence (from increased flow or partial obstruction).

101.16.2 Pulsatile tinnitus

Most cases are due to vascular lesions.
1. pulse-synchronous:
   a) carotid-cavernous fistula (p. 1519)
   b) AVM:
      • cerebral (pial) AVM
      • dural AVM (p. 1514)
   c) glomus jugulare tumor (p. 941)
   d) cerebral aneurysm: (rare) possibly with turbulent flow in giant aneurysm
   e) hypertension
   f) hyperthyroidism
   g) pseudotumor cerebri (p. 955)
   h) transmitted bruit: from heart (e.g., aortic stenosis), carotid artery stenosis (especially external carotid)
   i) dehiscent jugular bulb or high-riding jugular bulb: normal venous variant
   j) rarely with posterior fossa tumors: CP-angle tumors e.g., vestibular schwannoma or meningi-oma, vascular intraparenchymal tumors e.g., hemangioblastoma (especially in CPA)
   k) lesions that can present with a red tympanic membrane
      • aberrant carotid artery in middle ear
      • persistent stapedial artery: rare. Arises from aberrant ICA or from junction of horizontal and vertical petrous ICA. Foramen spinosum is absent on the affected side. Enlargement of anterior tympanic segment of seventh nerve canal
      • glomus tympanicum tumor (p. 941)
   l) sigmoid sinus diverticulum
2. non-pulse-synchronous: asymmetrical enlargement of sigmoid sinus and jugular vein may pro-duce a low-grade hum

Workup for pulsatile tinnitus:
1. MRI without and with enhancement: to look for tumors, e.g., glomus jugulare
2. angiogram: include internal and external carotid injections
3. tests that are usually *not* helpful and should not be ordered routinely:
   a) carotid ultrasound: nonspecific, not sensitive
   b) MRI/MRV: may miss small dural fistulas and do not give details needed for treatment for large ones

101.16.3 Non-pulsatile tinnitus

1. occlusion of external ear: cerumen, foreign body
2. middle ear infection (otitis media)
3. otosclerosis
4. stapedial muscle spasms: as occurs in hemifacial spasm
5. CP-angle tumors: including vestibular schwannoma (p. 777)
6. Meniere disease (p. 604)
7. labyrinthitis
8. endolymphatic sac tumors: e.g., as in von Hippel-Lindau disease (p. 648)
9. drugs
   a) salicylates: aspirin, bismuth subsalicylate (Pepto Bismol®)
   b) quinine
   c) aminoglycoside toxicity: streptomycin, tobramycin (tinnitus precedes hearing loss)

101.17 Facial sensory changes

1. circumoral paresthesias
   a) hypocalcemia
   b) syringobulbia
2. unilateral facial sensory changes
   a) trigeminal nerve neuroma
   b) vestibular schwannoma (VS): to involve Cr. N. V a VS has to be > 2 cm in diameter; see symptoms from 5th nerve compression under vestibular schwannoma (p. 778)
   c) compression of the spinal trigeminal tract (large compressive lesions may cause bilateral alteration of facial sensation) that chiefly manifests in diminution of pain and temperature sense with little effect on touch sense.[29] The tract usually extends down into the spinal cord as far as ≈ the C2 vertebral level (although it may occasionally extend down to C4)

101.18 Language disturbance

1. aphasia:
   a) injury to speech areas of brain: the classic nosology is likely an oversimplification in view of more recent models of speech (e.g., dual stream model)
      • Wernicke's aphasia (p. 90): classically produces *fluent* aphasia (normal sentence length & intonation, devoid of meaning)
      • Broca's aphasia (p. 90): faltering, dysarthric
      • conduction aphasia (p. 90): fluent spontaneous speech and paraphasias, but patients understand spoken or written words, and are aware of their deficit
   b) transitory aphasia following a seizure; see Todd's paralysis (p. 480)
   c) primary progressive aphasia of adulthood: idiopathic & degenerative
2. akinetic mutism: seen with bilateral frontal lobe dysfunction (e.g., with bilateral ACA distribution infarction due to vasospasm from AComA aneurysm rupture or with large bilateral frontal lesions; may actually be abulia) or with bilateral cingulate gyrus lesions
3. cerebellar mutism (p. 100) (AKA muteness of cerebellar origin)[30,31]
4. following transcallosal surgery: as a result of bilateral cingulate gyrus retraction or thalamic injury together with section of the midportion of the corpus callosum[32]

References

[1] Cardoso ER, Peterson EW. Pituitary Apoplexy: A Review. Neurosurgery. 1984; 14:363–373

[2] Kapoor WN. Evaluation and Management of the Patient with Syncope. Journal of the American Medical Association. 1992; 268:2553–2560

[3] Barron SA, Rogovski Z, Hemli Y. Vagal Cardiovascular Reflexes in Young Persons with Syncope. Annals of Internal Medicine. 1993; 118:943–946

[4] Miller TH, Kruse JE. Evaluation of syncope. American Family Physician. 2005; 72:1492–1500

[5] Linzer M, Yang EH, Estes NA,3rd, et al. Diagnosing syncope. Part 1: Value of history, physical examination, and electrocardiography. Clinical Efficacy Assessment Project of the American College of Physicians. Annals of Internal Medicine. 1997; 126:989–996

[6] Sarasin FP, Louis-Simonet M, Carballo D, et al. Prospective evaluation of patients with syncope: a population-based study. American Journal of Medicine. 2001; 111:177–184

[7] Brignole M, Alboni P, Benditt D, et al. Guidelines on management (diagnosis and treatment) of syncope. European Heart Journal. 2001; 22:1256–1306

[8] Smith DB, Hitchcock M, Philpot PJ. Cerebral Amyloid Angiopathy Presenting as Transient Ischemic Attacks: Case Report. Journal of Neurosurgery. 1985; 63:963–964

[9] Greenberg SM, Vonsattel JP, Stakes JW, et al. The Clinical Spectrum of Cerebral Amyloid Angiopathy: Presentations without Lobar Hemorrhage. Neurology. 1993; 43:2073–2079

[10] Kaminski HJ, Hlavin ML, Likavec MJ, et al. Transient Neurologic Deficit Caused by Chronic Subdural Hematoma. American Journal of Medicine. 1992; 92:698–700

[11] Moster M, Johnston D, Reinmuth O. Chronic Subdural Hematoma with Transient Neurologic Deficits: A Review of 15 Cases. Annals of Neurology 1983; 14:539–542

[12] McLaurin R. Contributions of Angiography to the Pathophysiology of Subdural Hematomas. Neurology. 1965; 15:866–873

[13] Apter AJ, Mott AE, Frank ME, et al. Allergic rhinitis and olfactory loss. Annals of Allergy, Asthma, and Immunology. 1995; 75:311–316

[14] Emmett EA. Parosmia and hyposmia induced by solvent exposure. British Journal of Industrial Medicine. 1976; 33:196–196

[15] Lieblich JM, Rogol AD, White BJ, et al. Syndrome of anosmia with hypogonadotropic hypogonadism (Kallmann syndrome): clinical and laboratory studies in 23 cases. American Journal of Medicine. 1982 73:506–519

[16] Beal MF. Multiple Cranial-Nerve Palsies - A Diagnostic Challenge. N Engl J Med. 1990; 322:461–463

[17] Krisht AF. Giant invasive pituitary adenomas. Contemporary Neurosurgery. 1999; 21:1–6

[18] Manni JJ, Scaf JJ, Huygen PLM, et al. Hyperostosis cranialis interna: A new hereditary syndrome with cranial-nerve entrapment. New England Journal of Medicine. 1990; 322:450–454

[19] Chen J-R, Rhee RSC, Wallach S, et al. Neurologic disturbances in Paget Disease of Bone: Response to Calcitonin. Neurology. 1979; 29:448–457

[20] Wilkins RH, Rengachary SS. Neurosurgery. New York 1985

[21] Al-Mefty O, Fox JL, Al-Rodhan N, et al. Optic Nerve Decompression in Osteopetrosis. Journal of Neurosurgery. 1988; 68:80–84

[22] Salvarani C, Cantini F, Boiardi L, et al. Polymyalgia rheumatica and giant-cell arteritis. New England Journal of Medicine. 2002; 347:261–271

[23] Clark WC, Theofilos CS, Fleming JC. Primary Optic Sheath Meningiomas: Report of Nine Cases. Journal of Neurosurgery. 1989; 70:37–40

[24] Gibson RD. Measurement of proptosis (exophthalmos) by computerised tomography. Australasian Radiology. 1984; 28:9–11

[25] Peyster RG, Ginsberg F, Silber JH, et al. Exophthalmos caused by excessive fat: CT volumetric analysis and differential diagnosis. AJR. American Journal of Roentgenology. 1986; 146:459–464

[26] Strassburg HM. Macrocephaly is Not Always Due to Hydrocephalus. J Child Neurol. 1989; 4:S32–S40

[27] Section of Pediatric Neurosurgery of the American Association of Neurological Surgeons. Pediatric Neurosurgery. New York 1982

[28] Rushton AR, Shaywitz BA, Duncan CC, et al. Computed Tomography in the Diagnosis of Canavan's Disease. Ann Neurol. 1981; 10:57–60

[29] Carpenter MB. Core Text of Neuroanatomy. 2nd ed. Baltimore: Williams and Wilkins; 1978

[30] Rekate H, Grubb R, Aram D, et al. Muteness of Cerebellar Origin. Archives of Neurology. 1985; 42:637–638

[31] Ammirati M, Mirzai S, Samii M. Transient Mutism Following Removal of a Cerebellar Tumor: A Case Report and Review of the Literature. Child's Nervous System. 1989; 5:12–14

[32] Apuzzo MLJ. Surgery of Masses Affecting the Third Ventricular Chamber: Techniques and Strategies. Clinical Neurosurgery. 1988; 34:499–522

102 Differential Diagnosis (DDx) by Signs and Symptoms – Primarily Spine and Other

102.1 Diagnoses covered outside this chapter

See ▸ Table 102.1.

Table 102.1 Differential diagnoses by signs and symptoms, spine and other—covered outside this chapter

DDx
ankylosing spondylitis (p. 1367)
bladder dysfunction (p. 93)
brachial plexopathy (p. 570)
carpal tunnel syndrome (p. 547)
cervical stenosis (p. 1300)
lateral disc herniation (p. 1265)
meralgia paresthetica (p. 561)
myopathy
spinal cord tumors (p. 979)
spinal epidural abscess (p. 381)
spinal stenosis
• lumbar (p. 1332)
synovial cyst (spinal) (p. 1341)
thoracic outlet syndrome (p. 581)
torticollis (p. 1844)
urinary retention (p. 95)

102.2 Myelopathy

Items marked with a dagger (†) may present as a *spinal epidural mass*.

▸ **Congenital**

1. (Arnold)-Chiari malformation (p. 303): Type I often presents in early adulthood
2. tethered cord: often may not present until after some trauma
3. syringomyelia: may be congenital or posttraumatic in quadriplegics, usually presents with a central cord syndrome—see Syringomyelia (p. 1405)—or progressive myelopathy
4. neurenteric cyst (p. 313)
5. cord compression that occurs with some mucopolysaccharidoses: e.g., Morquio syndrome (due to atlantoaxial subluxation), Hurler syndrome
6. hereditary spastic paraplegia: family history is key. Diagnosis of exclusion[1]

▸ **Acquired**

1. cervical or thoracic spinal stenosis: often degenerative disease superimposed on congenitally narrow canal (congenital narrowing is frequent in achondroplasia)
2. traumatic: including spinal shock, hematomyelia, spinal epidural hematoma (see vascular below), barotrauma, electrical injuries, compression by bone fracture†. May follow minor trauma in the setting of spinal stenosis
3. herniated intervertebral disc†: myelopathy more common in thoracic region, radiculopathy more common in cervical region (long tract signs are rare with herniated cervical disc)
4. kyphosis
5. extramedullary hematopoiesis† (p. 179): hypertrophy of marrow → cord compression. Primarily in chronic anemias (e.g., thalassemia major)
6. bony compression secondary to incompetence of odontoid process or transverse atlantal ligament†. May be congenital, traumatic (p. 1171), neoplastic, or inflammatory (especially rheumatoid arthritis)

7. epidural lipomatosis† (p. 1381): hypertrophy of epidural fat most often due to years of exogenous steroid therapy.[2] Rarely symptomatic
8. ossification of the posterior longitudinal ligament (OPLL) (p. 1370) [3]
9. vertebral Paget's disease† (p. 1362)
10. idiopathic spinal cord herniation (p. 1404) [4,5]: rare. Thoracic spinal cord herniates through an anterior dural defect frequently producing a Brown-Séquard syndrome or spastic paraparesis
11. spinal arachnoid cyst (p. 1401)
12. spinal arachnoid web (p. 1402)
13. Hirayama disease (p. 1403): a rare condition characterized by insidious, usually asymmetric painless wasting of the distal UE muscles typically affecting males in the age range of 15-20 years. May be caused by asymmetric compression of the spinal cord by the dura separating from the posterior bony spinal canal in flexion
14. superficial siderosis: rare. Hemosiderin deposition on the surface of the brain, cranial nerves, and spinal cord causes neurodegeneration. Triad: hearing loss, ataxia, and myelopathy. May follow trauma, surgical procedures, dural laceration, CNS tumors. Some success reported in treating with deferiprone (Ferriprox®), a lipid-soluble iron chelator that crosses the BBB[6]
15. arachnoiditis ossificans: a rare condition involving calcification of the arachnoid membrane.[7] In the T-spine, may occur as ossified plaques or in a cylindrical form surrounding the spinal cord. May be difficult to detect on MRI and myelography. Plain unenhanced CT may be optimal for diagnosis

▶ **Neoplastic**

1. spine/spinal cord tumors† (p. 979) (for details)
    a) extradural (55%):
        • primary tumors (rare) include: neurofibromas, chordomas, osteoid osteoma, aneurysmal bone cyst, vertebral hemangioma[8]
        • if age > 40 yrs, suspect extradural lymphoma (primary or secondary) or leukemic deposits (chloroma), especially with pre-existing diagnosis of hematopoietic or lymphatic disorder
        • epidural metastases (p. 921) become increasingly common after age 50 yrs. Occurs in up to 10% of cancer patients. 5–10% of malignancies present initially with cord compression
    b) intradural-extramedullary (40%): meningiomas, neurofibromas
    c) intradural-intramedullary: primary cord tumors (p. 980) (ependymoma, astrocytoma) and, rarely, intramedullary mets
2. carcinomatous meningitis (p. 920): neurologic deficit usually cannot be localized to a single level
3. paraneoplastic syndrome (p. 569): including effects on spinal cord or on peripheral nerves

▶ **Vascular**

1. hematoma/hemorrhage
    a) spinal epidural hematoma† (p. 1383): usually associated with anticoagulation therapy[9]
        • traumatic: following LP or epidural anesthesia (p. 1383)
        • spontaneous[10]: rare. Includes hemorrhage from spinal cord AVM (p. 1383) or from vertebral hemangioma (p. 1395)
    b) spinal subarachnoid hemorrhage: as is the case with spinal epidural hematoma (p. 1383), this may also be posttraumatic (e.g., following LP[11,12]) or secondary to spinal cord AVM
    c) spinal subdural hematoma
    d) hematomyelia
2. spinal cord infarction (p. 1385): uncommon. Usually involves the anterior spinal artery, sparing posterior columns. Usually ≈ T4 level (watershed zone).
    a) atherosclerosis of radicular artery in elderly patient with hypotension
    b) clamping aorta during surgery (e.g., for abdominal aortic aneurysm)
    c) hypotension (relative or absolute) during surgery in the sitting position in the presence of spinal stenosis[13]
    d) aortic dissection: especially thoracic spinal levels
    e) vertebral artery dissection: especially cervical spinal levels
    f) embolization of spinal arteries
3. spinal cord vascular malformations† (p. 1395): 10–20% present as sudden onset of myelopathy, usually in patients < 30 yrs,[14] myelopathy may be secondary to:
    a) mass effect from AVM: spinal AVMs account for < 5% of lesions presenting as cord "tumors"
    b) rupture → SAH, hematomyelia, or epidural hematoma
    c) watershed infarction due to "steal"
    d) spontaneous thrombosis (necrotizing myelopathy of Foix-Alajouanine disease (p. 1398) [15]): presents as spastic → flaccid paraplegia, with ascending sensory level
4. radiation myelopathy: due to microvascular occlusion (p. 1901)

5. secondary to iodinated contrast material used for mesenteric or aortic angiography. Especially when angiogrammed in presence of hypotension, where cardiac output is shunted away from viscera and into spinal radicular arteries. Treatment: place patient sitting, remove ≥ 100 ml of CSF via LP and replace with equal amount of saline over 30 mins[16]

▶ Autoimmune

1. post-viral (or post-vaccination): may actually be etiology of autoimmune process (i.e., transverse myelitis). Viral prodrome present in ≈ 37% of cases of ATM. Viral infection is usually most damaging to gray matter (e.g., poliomyelitis)

▶ Demyelinating

1. acute (idiopathic) transverse myelitis (ATM) (p. 195). Peak incidence during first 2 decades of life. Abrupt onset of LE weakness, sensory loss, back pain, and sphincter disturbance indistinguishable from spinal cord compression. Thoracic region most common. CT and myelogram are normal. MRI may demonstrate. CSF → pleocytosis and hyperproteinemia

2. multiple sclerosis (**MS**): diagnosed in only 7% of patients presenting as acute transverse myelopathy. Although more common in young adults, MS can occur at any time in life. Myelopathy of MS is usually insidious, and is usually incomplete (i.e., some sparing). Affects myelin, thus sparing gray matter. Abdominal cutaneous reflexes are almost always absent in MS

3. **neuromyelitis optica (NMO)** (AKA Devic syndrome): an idiopathic inflammatory, demyelinating process characterized by acute bilateral optic neuritis and transverse myelitis extending ≥ 3 vertebral levels[17] (▶ Fig. 102.1). These processes evolve separately over a period of months to years. Brain lesions are uncommon but can involve the brainstem, thalamus, and corpus callosum.[18] Callosal lesions are longitudinally oriented (unlike in MS where they are ovoid and horizontally oriented).[19] Spinal cord edema may become so severe as to cause complete block on myelography.

   NMO is no longer considered a variant of MS, supported by the discovery of circulating antibodies (NMO-IgG)[20] against aquaporin-4[21] (the dominant water channel of the CNS primarily located on the foot processes of astrocytes[22]). Mean age of onset: 41.1 years.[23] Strong female predominance. Prevalence in Caucasians is 0.4 per 100,000, and is higher in those of Asian or Indian descent.[24] Seropositivity is not required for the diagnosis, but is associated with a higher incidence of co-existing autoimmune disorder and more severe clinical attacks. Seronegative patients have a higher incidence of simultaneous optic neuritis and transverse myelitis with a shorter time to

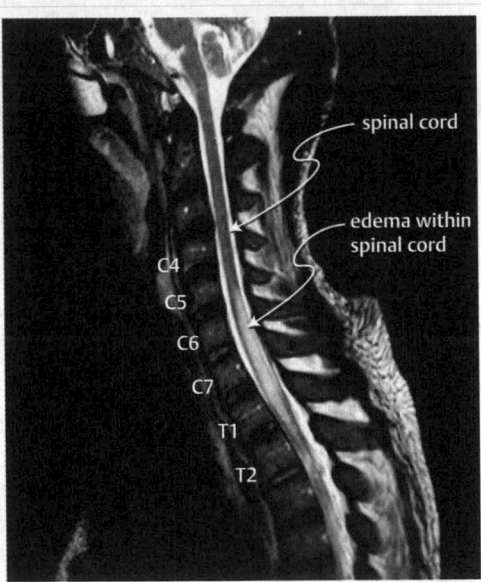

Fig. 102.1 Neuromyelitis optica. Image: T2 sagittal cervical MRI. Spinal cord edema extends from C5 to T2.

spinal cord

edema within spinal cord

C4
C5
C6
C7
T1
T2

diagnosis.[25] Unlike MS, only partial recovery occurs after acute attacks. Relapse is common: 60% after 1 year, 90% after 3 years.[26]

Acute treatment includes high-dose IV methylprednisolone or rescue plasma exchange (7 total exchanges)

▶ **Metabolic/toxic**

1. (subacute) combined system disease (CSD) (AKA subacute combined columnal degeneration): due to vitamin B_{12} (cyanocobalamin) deficiency

   Vitamin B_{12} is a water-soluble vitamin found in meats and dairy products. Its absorption in the distal duodenum is facilitated by intrinsic factor, a small polypeptide secreted by gastric parietal cells.[27] B_{12} is involved in neurologic function, production of RBCs, DNA synthesis, conversion of methylmalonic acid to succinyl coenzyme A, and conversion of homocysteine to methionine[28]

   a) etiologies of vitamin B_{12} deficiency:
      • dietary deficiency of B_{12}: non meat-eaters may have insufficient intake.
      • chronic autoimmune gastritis: reduces available intrinsic factor which leads to intestinal malabsorption of B_{12} in the distal ileum
      • other gastric disorders: low gastric pH, e.g., in Zollinger-Ellison syndrome, can inhibit attachment of intrinsic factor to ileal receptors
      • chronic use of metformin (> 4 months), proton pump inhibitors (> 12 months), or histamine H_2 blockers (> 12 months)

   b) clinical manifestations of B_{12} deficiency include:
      • pernicious anemia: a macrocytic megaloblastic anemia
      • combined system disease (CSD): myelopathy involving primarily the posterior columnbs. Onset is gradual and uniform. Begins with symmetrical paresthesias in feet or hands (posterior column involvement) → leg stiffness, weakness, and proprioceptive deficits with unsteadiness that is worse in the dark → spasticity → paraplegia → bowel and bladder dysfunction. Dementia (confusion, memory impairment, irritability…) occurs in advanced cases due to cerebral white matter changes. Visual disturbances with or without optic atrophy may be due to optic nerve demyelination

   c) labs:
      • CBC: most (but not all) patients will have a *macrocytic* (megalocytic) anemia (folic acid deficiency also produces megaloblastic anemia. Folic acid corrects the anemia, even with CSD, but *not* the neurologic deficits which may actually worsen)
      • serum vitamin B_{12} (cobalamin): levels < 150 pg/ml are diagnostic. However, normal B_{12} levels do not R/O B_{12} deficiency[28]
      • if B_{12} levels are low, or if they are normal but the patient has macrocytic anemia or neurologic symptoms, then check for elevated serum methylmalonic acid (also check homocysteine to R/O folate deficiency)
      • **Schilling test**: determines the cause of the B_{12} deficiency even if B_{12} injections have already been given (radiolabeled cyanocobalamin is given orally, followed by a parenteral flushing dose of nonradioactive vitamin, and the percentage of radioactivity is measured in the urine over 24 hours, performed once without and then once with added intrinsic factor, and then once following antibiotic therapy)

   d) imaging: T2WI MRI may demonstrate increased signal within the white matter of the spinal cord, predominantly in the posterior columns but may also be seen in spinothalamic tracts

   e) treatment: B_{12} injections q 1–3 months or large doses of oral preparations[29] (other transport systems independent of intrinsic factor result in absorption of ≈ 1% of orally administered B_{12}, doses of 300–100,000 mcg result in absorption of more than the daily requirement of 1–2.5 mcg)

2. toxins: e.g., local anesthetics used for spinal anesthesia rarely cause myelopathy

▶ **Infectious**

. (para) spinal abscess, AKA **spinal epidural abscess** or epidural empyema (p. 381) †: often history of *Staphylococcus* infection, usually a skin furuncle. Vertebral osteomyelitis often accompanies.[30] Produces local tenderness, back pain, fever, elevated ESR

. vertebral osteitis/osteomyelitis (p. 386) †

. pyogenic discitis†: spontaneous or following procedures (p. 390)

. HIV- or AIDS-related myelopathy: similar to B_{12} deficiency. Spastic weakness & ataxia. Can cause vacuolization of spinal cord. "Tropical (spastic) paraparesis of AIDS" also seen in HTLV-I infection[31]

. tuberculosis: Pott's disease, see Tuberculous vertebral osteomyelitis (p. 387)

. spinal meningitis with pachymeningitis

. viral:
   a) herpes varicella-zoster: rarely causes necrotizing myelopathy

102

b) herpes simplex type 2: may cause ascending myelitis
c) cytomegalovirus: may cause transverse myelitis
8. syphilitic involvement: may cause tabes dorsalis, syphilitic meningomyelitis, or spinal vascular syphilis. Diagnosed by serum and CSF serology
9. parasitic cysts†
10. some forms of Creutzfeldt-Jakob disease (CJD) (p. 399) with predominant initial muscle wasting may mimic spinal cord disease or ALS

▶ **Peripheral neuromuscular disorder**
1. Guillain-Barré syndrome (GBS) (p. 193): rapidly ascending weakness (mimics cord compression) with areflexia and near-normal sensation
2. chronic dysimmune neuropathies: presumed to be immune-mediated[32]
   a) chronic inflammatory demyelinating polyneuropathy (CIDP) (p. 194): similar to GBS but can progress over a longer period of time
   b) multifocal motor neuropathy (MMN): a rare almost purely motor neuropathy affecting only lower motor neurons (unlike ALS which also affects upper motor neurons) characterized by asymmetric muscle wasting, cramping & LE twitching. May mimic ALS, but is treatable (with IVIg or immunosuppression)
3. myopathies: including steroid myopathy (usually affects proximal > distal muscles)

▶ **Motor neuron diseases**
1. amyotrophic lateral sclerosis (ALS) (p. 191): upper and lower motor neuron disease. *Slight* spasticity of LEs (extreme spasticity is rare), atrophic weakness of the hands and forearms, fasciculations in the UEs, absence of sensory changes (including lack of pain), sphincter control usually preserved
2. primary lateral sclerosis: age > 50. No LMN signs. Slower progression than ALS (years to decades). Pseudobulbar palsy (p. 186) is common[33]

† Items with dagger may also present as a spinal epidural mass.

102.3 Sciatica

102.3.1 General information

Definition: pain in the distribution of the sciatic nerve.
 Anatomy: the sciatic nerve is comprised of components of nerve roots of L4–S3 containing fiber from the anterior and posterior divisions of the lumbosacral plexus. The nerve passes out of the pelvis through the greater sciatic foramen along the back of the thigh. In the lower third of the thigh it divides into the tibial and common peroneal nerves.

102.3.2 Etiologies

The most common cause of sciatica is *radiculopathy* due to a herniated lumbar disc.[34] The differential diagnosis is similar to that for myelopathy (see above) but also includes:
1. congenital:
   a) meningeal cyst (perineural cyst); see Spinal meningeal cysts (p. 1400)
   b) conjoined nerve root (p. 293): initially dismissed as a possible cause of radiculopathy, but current thinking recognizes that these may be symptomatic possibly by tethering
2. acquired:
   a) spinal stenosis/spondylosis/spondylolysis/spondylolisthesis
   b) juxtafacet cyst: includes synovial cyst and ganglion cyst (p. 1340)[35]: detection is increasing with the use of MRI
   c) nerve root sheath cyst: may be congenital or acquired. May arise near axilla of nerve root and cause compression of adjacent roots. Treatment: excise cyst and oversew the ostium
   d) arachnoiditis ossificans (p. 1697): rare. In the lumbar region may occur as columnar, cylindrical, or irregularly shaped masses.[36] May produce low back pain, radiculopathy, or cauda equina syndrome
   e) heterotopic ossification around the hip[37]
   f) injection injuries from misplaced IM injections
   g) compartment syndrome of the posterior thigh
   h) injury complicating total hip arthroplasty[38]
   i) radiation injury following treatment of nearby tumors

3. infectious:
   a) discitis (p. 390): usually causes excruciating pain with any movement
   b) Lyme disease (p. 364)
   c) herpes zoster: a rare cause of radiculopathy.[39] Lumbosacral dermatomes are involved in ≈ 10–15% of zoster cases. Pain is usually independent of position. Typical herpetic skin lesions usually follow onset of pain by 3–5 days. 1–5% develop motor weakness (usually in arms or trunk). Sacral zoster can cause detrusor paralysis, producing urinary retention. 55% of those with motor symptoms have good recovery, 30% have fair to good recovery

4. neoplastic:
   a) spine tumors: multiple myeloma (p. 928), metastases (p. 928)
   b) bone or soft-tissue tumors along the course of the sciatic nerve: may result in erroneous laminectomy for herniated lumbar disc.[40] Pain is usually *insidious* in onset, and *not positional* (see below)
      • intra-abdominal or pelvic neoplasm
      • tumors of the thigh
      • tumors in the popliteal fossa or calf

5. inflammatory:
   a) trochanteric bursitis (p. 1333): may produce pseudoradiculopathy. Rarely extends to the posterior thigh or as far distally as the knee
   b) myositis ossificans of the biceps femoris muscle[41]

6. vascular:
   a) sciatica may be mimicked by intermittent (i.e., vascular) claudication
   b) psoas hematoma: usually in patient on anticoagulant. Sometimes drainage is required

7. referred pain of nonspinal origin: not dermatomal. Nerve root tension signs (p. 1333) are usually negative. Includes:
   a) pyelonephritis
   b) renolithiasis, including ureteral obstruction
   c) cholecystitis
   d) appendicitis
   e) endometritis/endometriosis
   f) posterior perforating duodenal ulcer
   g) inguinal hernia, especially if incarcerated
   h) aortic dissection (p. 1705)

8. piriformis syndrome (PS): controversial. Piriformis muscle originates on anterior S2–4 VBs, sacrotuberous ligament and passes through the greater sciatic notch to attach to the greater trochanter of the femur. It is innervated by L5–1. It is the principal *external* rotator of the extended hip. It may irritate or compress the sciatic nerve (AKA pseudosciatica, can mimic symptoms of a herniated disc). The superior gluteal nerve is spared as it has a take-off proximal to the muscle. Conversely, PS may occur secondary to lower lumbar radiculopathy. Produces pain in the sciatic distribution and weakness of external rotation and abduction of the hip. Signs: Freiberg test (pain with forced internal rotation of the hip with thigh extension) or the Pace test (pain on resisted abduction/external rotation of the hip). No well-designed studies of treatments. Advocated therapies include: PT, stretching, injection of the muscle localized by digital rectal exam taking care not to inject the sciatic nerve itself & piriformis muscle section. Sometimes long-lasting relief can follow injection with local anesthetic. Use of botulinum toxin (Botox®) injections has been described

9. more peripheral involvement (i.e., neuropathy) that may be confused with radiculopathy. Including:
   a) femoral neuropathy mistaken for L4 radiculopathy (see below)
   b) proximal sacral plexus lesion mistaken for S1 radiculopathy (see below)
   c) diabetic neuropathy (p. 572) including diabetic amyotrophy
   d) tumors (see below)

102.3.3 Extraspinal tumors causing sciatica

★ Pain characteristics: pain is almost always insidious in onset.[40] It may be intermittent initially, but eventually all patients develop pain that is constant, progressive, and unaffected by position or rest.[40] Significant night pain is described in ≈ 80%.

Straight leg raising was positive in most, but in more than half the pain was localized to a specific point along the course of the nerve, distal to the sciatic notch.[40] Conservative treatment brings either no or only temporary relief.

Approximately 20% will have a previous history of tumor (usually neurofibromatosis or previous malignancy). Malignancies include[40]: metastatic lesions, primary bone sarcomas (chondrosarcoma...), soft-tissue sarcomas (liposarcoma...). Benign tumors include: lipoma, neurofibroma, schwannoma, aneurysmal bone cyst of the sacrum, giant cell tumor of the sacrum, tenosynovial giant cell tumor.

In two-thirds of cases, a detailed medical history and physical exam allowed localization and even determined the nature (bone tumor vs. soft-tissue) of the lesion.[40] Radiographs that show the entire pelvis and the proximal femur will demonstrate almost all tumors in these locations.[40,42]

102.3.4 Features differentiating radiculopathy in sciatica

General information

Sciatica may result from nerve root involvement within the spinal canal (e.g., with lumbar disc herniation). Clinically this produces a nerve root syndrome; see Nerve root syndromes (p. 1253). Spinal imaging studies (MRI, myelogram/CT) will usually detect nerve root compression here.

L4 involvement

Femoral neuropathy is often mistakenly identified as an L4 radiculopathy. Distinguishing features are shown in ▶ Table 102.2.

Table 102.2 Distinguishing femoral neuropathy from L4 radiculopathy

Feature	Femoral neuropathy	L4 radiculopathy
Sensory loss		
distribution (▶ Fig. 1.16)	anterior thigh	dermatome from ≈ knee to medial malleolus, spares anterior thigh
Muscle weakness		
iliopsoas	weak	normal
thigh adductors	normal (innervated by obturator nerve)	may be weak
quadriceps	weak	weak

L5 involvement

Peroneal nerve palsy may be mistaken for L5 radiculopathy (p. 1706).

S1 involvement

Outside the spinal canal, S1 can also be involved as it enters the sacral plexus, e.g., by a pelvic tumor. In plexus lesions, EMG will show sparing of the paraspinal muscles (nerves to paraspinal muscles exit in the region of the neural foramen) and the gluteus maximus and medius (superior and inferior gluteal nerves take off just distal to the paraspinal nerves).

102.4 Acute paraplegia or quadriplegia

102.4.1 General information

Entities causing spinal cord compression usually present as: paraplegia or -paresis (or quadriplegia -paresis), urinary retention (may require bladder ultrasound or checking a post-void residual to detect), and impaired sensation below level of compression. May develop over hours or days. Reflexes may be hyper- or hypoactive. There may or may not be a Babinski sign. Excluding trauma, the most common cause is compression by tumor or bone.

102.4.2 Etiologies

Some overlap with myelopathy.
1. in infancy (may produce "floppy infant syndrome")
   a) spinal muscular atrophy (the most severe form is called Werdnig-Hoffmann disease and is usually fatal within months): a rare autosomal recessive congenital disease of childhood with

degeneration of anterior horn cells. Only rarely evident at birth (where it presents as a paucity of movement), produces weakness, areflexia, muscle and tongue fasciculations with normal sensation. Usually starts in proximal muscles and muscles of respiration. Severe cases progress over the first year or two to quadriplegia.

Disease progression was halted in 60% of cases associated with mutation of the SMN1 gene on chromosome 5 (which codes for survival motor neuron (SMN) protein) with intrathecal administration of Spinraza™ (nusinersen),[43] an orphan drug that costs $125,000 U.S. per injection or $750,000 per year.

102

b) spinal cord injury during parturition: a rare sequela of breech delivery
c) congenital myopathies: e.g., infantile acid maltase deficiency (Pompe disease)
d) infantile botulism: ileus, hypotonia, weakness, mydriasis, *Clostridium botulinum* bacteria and toxin in feces

2. traumatic spinal cord injury
   a) major trauma: diagnosis is usually evident
   b) minor trauma: may cause cord injury in setting of spinal stenosis which may → central cord syndrome (p. 1132)
   c) atlantoaxial dislocation: from major trauma or due to instability from tumor or rheumatoid arthritis

3. congenital
   a) extradural spinal cord compression by bone secondary to cervical hemivertebra (symptoms not present at birth, may develop decades later, occasionally after minor trauma)
   b) cervical stenosis (p. 1301) (usually with superimposed spondylosis): quadriplegia or central cord syndrome may follow minor trauma
   c) achondroplasia: spinal stenosis (animal model: dachshund)
   d) syringomyelia: usually presents with central cord syndrome

4. metabolic
   a) combined system disease* (p. 1699)
   b) thallium poisoning: usually causes sensory and autonomic symptoms, quadriplegia and dysarthria may be seen in severe cases
   c) central pontine myelinolysis (p. 119)

5. infectious
   a) epidural spinal infection (abscess or empyema)*
   b) post-viral (or post-vaccination): may be a transverse myelitis*

6. peripheral neuromuscular disorder*
   a) Guillain-Barré syndrome (p. 194): classically an *ascending* paralysis, but paraparesis mimicking a spinal cord lesion is an unusual variant[44]
   b) myopathies

7. neoplastic*: spinal cord tumors

8. autoimmune*

9. vascular
   a) acute pontomedullary infarction: age usually > 50 yrs. Patient is quadriplegic, alert, with bulbar palsies (eye movement abnormalities, impaired gag and speech)
   b) spinal cord infarction*: including AVM, radiation myelopathy…

10. miscellaneous compressive*: including epidural hematoma, bony compression, epidural lipomatosis

11. functional: hysteria, malingering

12. bilateral cerebral hemisphere lesion (involving both motor strips): e.g., post-cerebral irradiation or parasagittal lesion. Will not have sensory *level*

For items with asterisk, see Myelopathy (p. 1696) for details.

102.5 Hemiparesis or hemiplegia

102.5.1 General information

May be produced by anything that interrupts the corticospinal tract from its origin in the pyramidal cells of Betz in the motor strip (p. 56) down to the cervical spine. This results in upper motor neuron paralysis (see ▶ Table 30.4), which should also produce long tract findings, including Babinski sign ipsilateral to hemiplegia.

102

102.5.2 Etiologies

▶ **Lesions of the cerebral hemisphere in the region of the contralateral motor strip.** Large lesions may also involve the sensory cortex producing reduced sensation ipsilateral to the hemiparesis
1. tumor (neoplasm): primary or metastatic
2. traumatic: epidural or subdural hematoma, hemorrhagic contusion of the brain, compression by depressed skull fracture
3. vascular:
   a) infarction
      • ischemic: embolic, low flow (due to atherosclerosis, arterial dissection…)
      • hemorrhagic: intracerebral hemorrhage, aneurysmal SAH…
   b) TIA (p.1536)
4. infection: cerebritis, abscess

▶ **Lesions of the contralateral internal capsule.** Produces pure motor hemiplegia without sensory loss. Most common etiology is ischemic lacunar infarct

▶ **Lesions of the brainstem.** Ischemic infarct, hemorrhage, tumor

▶ **Lesions of the cervicomedullary junction.** Foramen magnum lesions (p.1649)

▶ **Unilateral spinal cord lesions.** Above ≈ C5 ipsilateral to the weakness producing a Brown-Séquard syndrome (p.1135) with contralateral sensory loss to pain and temperature. See etiologies (p.1135)

▶ **Hypoglycemia.** Can sometimes be associated with hemiparesis that clears after administration of glucose

▶ **Note.** In a patient with unexplained hemiparesis/hemiplegia, especially after trauma, consider carotid dissection

102.6 Ascending paralysis

1. Guillain-Barré syndrome (p.193)
2. tick-borne paralysis: usually asymmetrical
3. spinal infection: e.g., spinal epidural abscess (p.381)
4. in a patient with prior spinal cord injury below
   a) early after spinal cord injury (≤ 4 weeks): ascending hematomyelia (blood within spinal cord), spinal cord edema. An argument for surgical decompression and rigid fusion early after spinal cord injury was to reduce the risk of acute ascending myelopathy[45]
   b) delayed after spinal cord injury: posttraumatic syringomyelia (p.1411), arachnoiditis

102.7 Descending paralysis

1. botulism: key features in addition to descending paralysis are oculomotor weakness (ophthalmoplegia), miosis (pupillary constriction), and constipation
2. myasthenia gravis: can also produce ophthalmoplegia

102.8 Low back pain

102.8.1 General information

The following considers primarily low back pain (LBP) *without* radiculopathy or myelopathy, although some overlap occurs. Trauma is usually obvious and is not discussed here. See Sciatic (p.1700) for differential diagnosis of that condition and also Low back pain and radiculopathy (p.1226) for evaluation.

102.8.2 Acute low back pain

Similar to list for myelopathy (p.1696). Most cases are non-specific (e.g., lumbosacral sprain), only 10–20% can be given a precise pathoanatomical diagnosis[46]:

▶ **Patients writhing in pain.** Should be evaluated for an intra-abdominal or vascular condition (e.g., pain of aortic dissection is typically described as a "tearing" pain): patients with neurogenic LBP tend to remain as still as possible, possibly needing to change positions at intervals

▶ **Unrelenting pain at rest:**
1. spinal tumor (intradural or extradural) (p.1235)
   a) primary or metastatic spine tumor: suspected in patients with pain duration > 1 month, unrelieved by bed rest, failure to improve with conservative therapy, unexplained weight loss, age > 50 yrs[47]
   b) nocturnal back pain relieved by aspirin is suggestive of osteoid osteoma or benign osteoblastoma (p.990) [48]
2. infection (especially in IV drug abusers, diabetics, post-spinal surgery, immunosuppressed patients, or those with pyelonephritis or UTI post-GU surgery). Fever is somewhat insensitive for spinal infections. Spine tenderness to percussion has 86% sensitivity with bacterial infections, but a low specificity of 60%.[47] Types of infections include:
   a) discitis
   b) spinal epidural abscess: should be considered in patients with back pain, fever, spine tenderness, or skin infection (furuncle)
   c) vertebral osteomyelitis
3. inflammatory
4. sacroiliitis: may produce pain and tenderness over one or both SI joints. Pelvic X-rays may show sclerosis of one or both sacroiliac joints.
   a) bilateral & symmetric
      • ankylosing spondylitis (p.1365): morning back stiffness, no relief at rest, improvement with exercise.[49] Usually seen in males with symptom onset before age 40 yrs. Positive Patrick's test (p.1252) and pain on compressing the pelvis with the patient in the lateral decubitus position
      • Reiter syndrome (after Hans Reiter, a German bacteriologist): a reactive arthritis (usually 1–3 weeks following certain bacterial infections) with involvement of at least one other non-joint area (urethritis, uveitis/conjunctivitis, skin lesions, mucosal ulcerations...). 75% are HLA-B27–positive
      • may occur in Crohn's disease
   b) bilateral & asymmetric
      • psoriatic arthritis
      • rheumatoid arthritis: adult & juvenile forms
   c) unilateral
      • gout
      • osteoarthritis
      • infection

▶ **Evolving neurologic deficit.** (**Cauda equina syndrome:** perineal anesthesia, urinary incontinence or urgency or retention, progressive weakness) all require emergent diagnostic evaluation to rule out treatable conditions such as:
1. spinal epidural abscess (p.381)
2. spinal epidural hematoma (p.1383)
3. spinal tumor (intradural or extradural) (p.979)
4. massive central disc herniation (p.1254)

▶ **Pathologic fracture.** Acute pain in patients at risk for osteoporosis or with known Ca should prompt evaluation for pathologic fractures
1. lumbar compression fracture: see Osteoporotic spine fractures (p.1208)
2. sacral insufficiency fracture[50]: especially in rheumatoid arthritis patients on chronic steroids, often with no antecedent history of trauma. May cause back pain and/or radiculopathy. Often missed on plain films, best seen on CT, but may also be detected on bone scan

▶ **Coccydynia** (p.1241). Pain and tenderness around the coccyx

▶ **Tears in the anulus fibrosus.** ("Anular tears")[51] (NB: also present in 40% of asymptomatic patients between 50 and 60 yrs of age, and 75% between 60 and 70 yrs[52])

▶ **Rarely following subarachnoid hemorrhage.** (SAH) due to irritation of lumbar nerve roots and dura: usually accompanied by other signs of SAH (p.1417)

▶ **Myalgia.** May be a side effect of "statins" (drugs used to lower serum concentration of LDL cholesterol) with or without elevation of serum creatinine phosphokinase, sometimes with accompanying weakness and rarely with severe rhabdomyolysis and myoglobinuria leading to renal failure (risk may be increased with renal or hepatic dysfunction, advanced age, hypothyroidism, or serious infection)[53]

▶ **Drug-induced:**
1. statins: see above under Myalgia
2. phosphodiesterase type 5 (PDE5) inhibitors used for erectile dysfunction: all may be associated with LBP, but the incidence is higher with tadalafil,[54] etiology unknown. Usually occurs 12–24 hours post-dose and resolves by 48 hours. Most respond to simple analgesics

102.8.3 Subacute low back pain

10% of patients with LBP have symptoms that persist > 6 weeks.
Differential diagnosis includes causes of acute LBP (above) and also:
1. continued pain at rest should prompt evaluation for spinal osteomyelitis (especially with fever and elevated ESR) or neoplasm if not already done
2. plain spine X-rays may show possibly causative conditions, although many or all of the following may also be seen in *asymptomatic* patients:
   a) spondylolisthesis (p. 1337)
   b) spinal osteophytes
   c) lumbar stenosis
   d) **Schmorl's node** or **nodule** (p. 1266): disc herniation through cartilaginous endplate into vertebral body (NB: may also be seen in 19% of asymptomatic patients[55])

Chronic low back pain

After 3 months, only ≈ 5% of patients with LBP will continue to have persistent symptoms. A structural diagnosis is possible in only ≈ 50% of these patients. These patients account for 85% of the cost in lost work and compensation.[46]
Differential diagnosis includes causes of acute and subacute LBP listed above, as well as:
1. degenerative conditions
   a) degenerative spondylolisthesis (p. 1340)
   b) spinal stenosis (affecting the spinal canal)
   c) lateral recess syndrome
2. spondyloarthropathies
   a) ankylosing spondylitis: look for erosive changes adjacent to SI joint and positive test for HLA-B27 antigen
   b) Paget's disease of the spine: vertebral involvement is very common in patients with Paget's disease
3. osteitis condensans ilii: increased density in ilium, usually asymptomatic (incidental) finding. Occasionally may produce low back pain or tenderness. Usually found in women who have been pregnant
4. psychological overlay: including secondary gain (financial, emotional...)

102.9 Foot drop

102.9.1 General information

> ### Key concepts
>
> - weak anterior tibialis (foot extension) innervated by deep peroneal nerve (L4, 5)
> - most common etiologies: L4/L5 radiculopathy, common peroneal nerve palsy
> - in a patient with foot drop, check posterior tibialis (foot inversion) and gluteus medius (internal rotation of flexed hip)—both are spared in peroneal nerve palsy and both should be involved with L4/L5 radiculopathy
> - EMG can assist in localization and prognostication

Definition: weakness of anterior tibialis (primarily L4 and to a lesser extent L5), often accompanied by a weak extensor digitorum longus and extensor hallucis longus (primarily L5 with some S1 contribution), all of which are innervated by the *deep peroneal nerve*.

102.9.2 Underlying substrates of foot drop

The most common dilemma is to distinguish foot drop due to radiculopathy from that due to peroneal nerve palsy (usually common peroneal nerve). With common peroneal nerve (CPN) palsy, there is *sparing* of posterior tibialis (foot inversion, innervated by posterior tibial nerve) and gluteus medius (internal rotation of the thigh with the hip flexed, innervated by superior gluteal nerve, primarily L5 with some L4, the takeoff is shortly after the roots exit from neural foramen). With L4 or L5 root lesions these muscles will also be weak; see ▶ Fig. 102.2.

Flail foot results from paralysis of dorsiflexors *plus* plantarflexors, e.g., in sciatic nerve dysfunction as can occur during surgery for hip fracture-dislocation[56] or injection injuries (IM injections should be given superiorly and laterally to a line drawn between the posterior superior iliac spine and the greater trochanter of the hip). NB: the peroneal division of the sciatic nerve tends to be more vulnerable to injury than the tibial division.

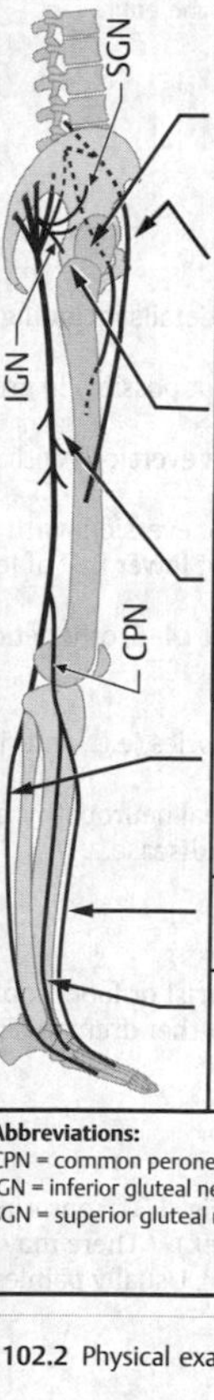

Muscle to check	Rationale	Finding: exam
Thigh adductors (adductors longus, brevis, and magnus) (**L2**, **L3**): innervated by the **obturator nerve**	Involvement indicates that the lesion includes more than sciatic nerve/L5 root (e.g., paravertebral mass, cauda equina lesion if bilateral findings)	Weakness when adducting thigh while supine with knee extended
Quadriceps femoris innervated by the **femoral nerve**	(Same as above)	Weakness of knee extension (L2, **L3**, **L4**)
Muscles innervated by **L5 branches** that exit the lumbar plexus very close to the neural foramina	Involvement indicates very proximal lesion (e.g., nerve root or very proximal (paravertebral) lumbar plexus)[a]	Weakness of: 1. gluteus medius (**L4**, **L5**, S1): internally rotate thigh 2. gluteus maximus (**L5**, **S1**, 2): dig heel into bed while supine
L5 innervated muscles (**via sciatic nerve**) proximal to the take off of the common peroneal nerve (CPN)[b]	If muscles listed above are intact, involvement of muscles to the right localizes the lesion to sciatic nerve above L5 root, injury to sciatic nerve at the greater sciatic notch	1. Slight weakness of biceps femoris (lateral hamstrings) (L5, **S1**, 2): flex the knee (with thigh flexed) 2. Gastrocnemius weakness (foot plantarflexion) unless injury only to peroneal division of sciatic nerve[b]
Muscles innervated by (posterior) **tibial nerve**	Sparing of these with foot drop indicates lesion distal to take off of common peroneal nerve (foot drop with weak foot inversion may be L4 or 5 radiculopathy)	Weakness of tibialis posterior (**L4**, **L5**): invert foot (foot should be plantarflexed to eliminate anterior tibialis)
Anterior tibialis innervated by **deep peroneal nerve**	Involvement does not narrow down etiology until other muscles are examined	Weakness of ankle dorsiflexion (foot drop)
Muscles innervated by **superficial peroneal nerve**	Preservation of these with foot drop localizes the lesion to the deep peroneal nerve	Weakness of the peroneus longus and brevis (L5, S1): evert the foot

Abbreviations:
CPN = common peroneal nerve
IGN = inferior gluteal nerve
SGN = superior gluteal nerve

[a]Note: EMG can differentiate root lesion from plexus by detecting involvement of paraspinal muscles, which occurs in root but not in plexus lesions because dorsal rami exit proximal to plexus

[b]The peroneal division of the sciatic nerve is more vulnerable to injury than the tibial division for several reasons. It is thus not unusual to see isolated peroneal nerve injuries above the knee, e.g. from hip dislocation or fractures, stab wounds, injection injuries...

Fig. 102.2 Physical exam to localize the lesion in a patient with LE weakness.

Table 102.3 Localization of lesion with foot drop

Lesion	Motor deficit[a]					Sensory changes
	anterior tibialis (L4, 5 ankle dorsiflexion)	peroneus longus/ brevis (L5, S1 foot eversion)	tibialis posterior (L4, 5 foot inversion)	biceps femoris (L5, S1, 2 knee flexion)	gastro-cnemius (S1, 2 plantar-flexion)	
deep peroneal nerve	x					minimal, or great toe web space
superficial peroneal nerve		x				lateral distal leg and dorsum of foot
common peroneal nerve (CPN)	x	x				all of the above
L4 or L5 radiculopathy	x	x	x			dermatomal (▶ Fig. 1.16)
peroneal division of sciatic nerve[b]	x	x	x	x		as with common peroneal
main trunk of sciatic nerve	x	x	x	x	x	lateral distal leg and entire foot

[a]x denotes that the indicated muscle is involved (i.e., weak)
[b]see footnote (b) under ▶ Fig. 102.2

102.9.3 Etiologies of foot drop

Three major categories: 1) muscular, 2) neurologic, 3) anatomic.
1. peripheral nerve palsies (more common). See ▶ Table 102.3 and ▶ Fig. 102.2.
   a) peroneal nerve injury (also, see Common peroneal nerve palsy (p. 563) for details including etiologies). Branches that may be involved:
      • deep peroneal nerve: isolated foot drop with minimal sensory loss (except possibly in great toe web space)
      • superficial peroneal nerve: weakness of peroneus longus and brevis (foot eversion) with *no* foot drop. Sensory loss: lateral aspect of lower half of leg and foot
      • common peroneal nerve: combination of above, i.e., foot drop + weak foot eversion, with sparing of tibialis posterior (foot inversion). Sensory loss: lateral aspect of lower half of leg and foot
   b) L5 radiculopathy (or, less commonly, L4). The most common cause is HLD at L4–5, other etiologies include: lumbar spinal stenosis at L4–5, sacral ala fracture (p. 1215)
      • results in pain and/or sensory changes in L5 (or L4) dermatome
      • weakness with radiculopathy tends to be more pronounced in distal muscles (e.g., anterior tibialis) than in proximal (e.g., gluteus maximus)
      • *painless* foot drop is unlikely to be due to radiculopathy; consider peroneal neuropathy, diabetic neuropathy, lesion anywhere along pyramidal tract, motor neuron disease…
   c) lumbar plexus injury
   d) lumbosacral plexus neuropathy (p. 571)
   e) injury to lateral trunk of sciatic nerve
   f) peripheral neuropathy: weakness tends to be greater distally, producing wrist or foot drop. Classic example: Charcot-Marie-Tooth (p. 568) (CMT), findings tend to be rather dramatic in spite of the fact that it often doesn't seem to bother the patient very much
   g) early in the course of motor neuron disease (ALS)
   h) heavy metal poisoning
2. central nervous system causes (foot drop here is usually painless)
   a) cortical lesion (UMN): parasagittal lesions in region of motor strip (see ▶ Fig. 1.3) (sensation will be spared if the lesion does not extend posteriorly to the sensory cortex).[57] There may be a Babinski sign or hyperactive Achilles reflex (so-called "spastic foot drop"). Usually painless
   b) spinal cord injury: including cervical spinal myelopathy
3. non-neurogenic causes
   a) muscular dystrophy
   b) lead toxicity: in children may cause foot drop with no sensory loss
   c) anterior compartment syndrome

102.9.4 Clinical

Loss of dorsiflexion causes foot slap with the front of the foot when the heel strikes the ground while walking. Also during the swing phase of gait the front of the foot may snag the ground (especially on uneven surfaces) which may cause tripping; thus patients develop steppage gait (exaggerated thigh & knee flexion) on the affected side. Associated weakness of tibialis posterior, when present (e.g., with L5 radiculopathy) destabilizes the ankle, permitting eversion which also predisposes to falls and to ankle fractures. Chronic foot drop may produce Achilles tendon contracture with talipes equinus.

Wasting of the extensor digitorum brevis may be seen.

102.9.5 Evaluation

1. bloodwork: glucose, ESR
2. EMG: can help differentiate L5 radiculopathy from peroneal nerve palsy, plexus lesion (▶ Fig. 102.2), or motor neuron disease (p. 191) (for details). EMG is not reliable until symptoms have been present at least ≈ 3 weeks
3. For suspected radiculopathy: MRI (or CT/myelogram if MRI is not possible)

102.10 Weakness/atrophy of the hands/UEs

102.10.1 Hand/UE weakness or atrophy with relatively preserved function in the LEs

1. cervical spondylosis (p. 1296): often causes sensory disturbance
2. cervical radiculopathy (p. 1280)
3. amyotrophic lateral sclerosis (ALS): no sensory involvement. One of the few causes of clinically prominent *fasciculations*. See details of ALS (p. 1700), other distinguishing features (p. 1700), fibrillations (p. 531)
4. spinal cord pathology
   a) central cord syndrome (p. 1132): typically causes more impairment (weakness, sensory disturbance) in the UE than the LE
   b) syringomyelia (p. 1405): usually burning dysesthesias of the hands with dissociated sensory loss
5. brachial plexus injury (p. 579)
6. brachial plexus neuropathy (p. 570) (includes Parsonage-Turner syndrome (p. 570))
7. peripheral nerve problems, including:
   a) carpal tunnel syndrome (p. 546)
   b) ulnar neuropathy (p. 553)
   c) other peripheral nerve entrapment syndromes (p. 541)
8. foramen magnum lesions (p. 1649): can cause (Bell's) cruciate paralysis[58] due to compression above the pyramidal decussation (located in the inferior medulla oblongata), which produces bilateral UE weakness and possibly atrophy of the hands with sparing of the LEs[59] (in the differential diagnosis for central cord syndrome). Compression on only one side may produce the similarly named but clinically different hemiplegia cruciata (spastic palsy of one UE and the contralateral LE)[59]
9. thoracic outlet syndrome (p. 581)
10. botulism (p. 1687)
11. Hirayama disease (p. 1403): due to asymmetric compression of the spinal cord by the dura in flexion
12. pharyngeal-cervical-brachial variant of Guillain-Barré syndrome (p. 194)

102.10.2 Atrophy of the first dorsal interosseous muscle

Etiologies: either C8/T1 nerve root or ulnar nerve involvement (may be either focal or diffuse). There are 4 main differential diagnoses:
1. ulnar neuropathy: check median nerve to see if findings extend to a nearby but separate nerve
   a) at the elbow (p. 558)
   b) at Guyon's canal (p. 558)
2. nerve root involvement:
   a) cervical radiculopathy: C8 or T1

b) nerve root avulsion (p. 255): weakness + sensory loss with normal SNAP on EMG, usually with a history of precipitating trauma
3. lower brachial plexus involvement
   a) thoracic outlet syndrome (p. 581)
   b) Pancoast tumor (p. 570)
4. neurodegenerative disorders
   a) amyotrophic lateral sclerosis (ALS) (p. 1301) (AKA motor neuron disease)
   b) multifocal motor neuropathy (MMN) (p. 1700): a chronic dysimmune motor neuropathy with asymmetric muscle wasting, cramping, & LE twitching

102.11 Radiculopathy, upper extremity (cervical)

See Weakness/atrophy of the hands/UEs (p. 1709). In addition to those items:
1. primary shoulder pathology: characteristically, pain is aggravated by active and/or passive shoulder movement. In general, shoulder pathology does not produce pain referred to the neck
   a) rotator cuff tear
   b) bicipital tendonitis: tenderness over biceps tendon
   c) subacromial bursitis: there may be tenderness over the AC joint
   d) adhesive capsulitis
   e) impingement syndrome: the "empty can test" is usually positive (each arm held out in front, 30° lateral to straight forward, thumbs pointing down, as in emptying out a soda can. Examiner pushes down on the patient's hands while the patient resists. Test is positive if it reproduces pain)
2. shoulder pain is very common in polymyalgia rheumatica (p. 206), typically worsens with movement
3. interscapular pain: a common location for referred pain with cervical radiculopathy, may also occur with cholecystitis or some shoulder pathologies
4. MI: some cases of cervical radiculopathy (especially left C6) may present with symptoms that are suggestive of an acute myocardial infarction
5. complex regional pain syndrome AKA reflex sympathetic dystrophy (p. 525): may be difficult to distinguish from cervical radiculopathy. Stellate ganglion blocks may help.[60]

102.12 Neck pain (cervical pain)

This section deals primarily with axial neck-pain without radicular features. For radicular features, see Radiculopathy, upper extremity (cervical) above.
1. cervical spondylosis (including facet arthritis)
2. cervical sprain: including whiplash-associated disorder
3. fracture of the cervical spine: with upper cervical spine fractures (e.g., odontoid), patients characteristically hold their head in their hands, especially when going from recumbent to upright position
   a) traumatic
   b) pathologic (tumor invasion, rheumatoid arthritis)
4. occipital neuralgia (p. 541)
5. herniated cervical disc:
   a) lateral herniated disc: if symptomatic, tends to produce more radicular symptoms in the UE than actual neck pain
   b) central disc herniation: if symptomatic, tends to produce myelopathy, does not produce any neck pain whatsoever in many cases
6. abnormalities of the craniocervical junction:
   a) Chiari type 1 malformation (p. 295)
   b) atlantoaxial subluxation
7. **fibromyalgia**: idiopathic chronic pain syndrome characterized by widespread nonarticular musculoskeletal pain, nodularity, and stiffness[61,62] without pathologic inflammation. Possible link to neuroendocrine dysfunction.[63] Afflicts 2% of the population,[62] female:male ratio is 7:1. No diagnostic laboratory study. May be associated with psychiatric illness and multiple non-specific somatic complaints including malaise, fatigue, impaired sleep, GI complaints, and cognitive impairment
8. **Eagle syndrome** (first described by otolaryngologist Watt Weems Eagle in 1937): AKA stylohyoid syndrome. Elongation of the styloid process (defined as length > 3 cm[64]) (▶ Fig. 102.3) and/or calcification of the stylohyoid ligament. Symptoms may be due to compression of adjacent nerves

(e.g., IX, V, chorda tympani, or sympathetic plexus on carotid sheath), or pain from fracture or inflammation.[64] Palpation over the styloid process may reproduce symptoms. Surgical resection can ameliorate the pain. Two variants:
a) typical variant: history of tonsillectomy. Pharyngeal pain, dysphagia, and otalgia
b) second variant: AKA carotid artery-styloid process syndrome. Carotidynia radiating into ipsilateral eye and vertex

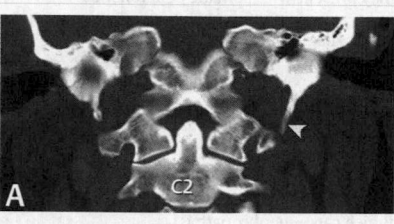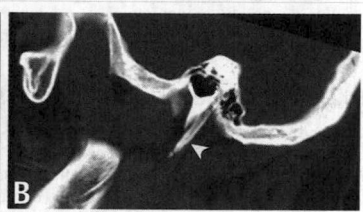

Fig. 102.3 Eagle syndrome.
Image: CT bone window showing elongated left styloid process (*yellow arrowheads*). A: coronal, B: sagittal.

9. crystal deposition diseases: gout, pseudogout, hydroxyapatite (HA), or calcium pyrophosphate dihydrate (CPPD) crystal deposition diseases. May appear as a crown-like density encompassing the odontoid process (crowned-dens syndrome)[65] representing calcifications in the transverse ligament, seen best on cervical CT. May be treated with a short course of prednisolone (e.g., 15 mg/d) followed by NSAIDs

102.13 Burning hands/feet

1. spinal cord syndromes:
   a) central cord syndrome (CCS) (p. 1132)
   b) burning hands syndrome (p. 1126): a possible variant of CCS, described in football-related cervical spine injury
   c) numb-clumsy hand syndrome (p. 1299): seen in cervical myelopathy
2. complex regional pain syndrome (CRPS) (p. 525) AKA reflex sympathetic dystrophy
3. peripheral neuropathy
   a) diabetic amyotrophy (p. 572) AKA Bruns-Garland syndrome
4. erythermalgia AKA erythromelalgia: a rare disorder characterized by erythema, edema, increased skin temperature, and burning pain of the hands and/or feet. Usually refractory to medical management, although some success is reported with epidural bupivacaine,[66] lidocaine patches,[67] or cold soaks
   a) primary erythermalgia: etiology is idiopathic
   b) secondary erythermalgia: associated with autoimmune and rheumatologic factors
5. vascular:
   a) occlusive arterial disease: atherosclerosis, Raynaud's syndrome
   b) venous insufficiency

102.14 Glove/stocking sensory disturbance

Sensory loss in a stocking distribution is more common than a glove or glove-stocking sensory loss.

Sensory level: there is a subjective and often an objective sensory level in a limb distal to which there is impairment. This differs from a *dermatomal* sensory disturbance which produces issues that follow one or more dermatomes (areas of sensory disturbance oriented along the long axis of the limb, as shown in the blue and white portions of ▶ Fig. 1.16) or a mononeuropathy (i.e., involvement of a single peripheral nerve) which produces patches of sensory loss corresponding to the distribution of a peripheral nerve (as shown in the colored portions of ▶ Fig. 1.16), neither of which is circumferential.

Symptoms may include any combination of: numbness, tingling, burning dysesthesias, hyperesthesia and aching sensation.

Etiologies
1. vascular insufficiency: this usually involves the lower extremities only
2. polyneuropathy: most cases start in the feet and gradually progress upwards
   a) large fiber polyneuropathy: can be diagnosed with EMG
   b) small fiber polyneuropathy: does not show up on an EMG. The small nerves involved do not produce imbalance or muscle weakness. May be associated with diabetes mellitus (the most common), autoimmune disorders (e.g., Sjögren or sarcoidosis), paraproteinemia, amyloid angiopathies, sodium channelopathies. It may present with somatic or autonomic symptoms.[68]
   If it is felt to be necessary, skin biopsy can aid in diagnosis

102.15 Muscle pain/tenderness

1. fibromyalgia: see above
2. myopathy
3. statin-induced myopathy: can vary from mild (with symptoms of muscle aches, symptoms usually abate rapidly after discontinuation of the statin, although occasionally up to 2 months may be required) to severe (with rhabdomyolysis which can → nephropathy)
4. diffuse severe sensitivity to light touch is often a marker of nonorganic pain[69]

102.16 Lhermitte's sign

102.16.1 General information

Technically, a symptom (not a sign). Electrical shock-like sensation radiating down the spine usually provoked by neck flexion (shocks radiating up the spine are sometimes referred to as reverse Lhermitte's sign). Classically attributed to MS, but may occur in any pathology involving primarily the posterior columns of the spinal cord (see below).

102.16.2 Etiologies

1. multiple sclerosis (MS) (p. 187)
2. cervical spondylosis (cervical spondylotic myelopathy (p. 1297))
3. subacute combined degeneration (p. 1699): check for vitamin B_{12} deficiency
4. cervical cord tumor
5. cervical disc herniation
6. radiation myelopathy (p. 1901)
7. Chiari type I malformation (p. 295)
8. central cord syndrome (p. 1132)
9. SCIWORA (spinal cord injury without radiographic abnormality) (p. 1196)

102.17 Swallowing difficulties

1. mechanical: the term globus describes a sensation of a lump in the throat. Odynophagia is pain on swallowing, which may occur without dysphagia
   a) ossification of the anterior longitudinal ligament (OALL) (p. 1372)
   b) diffuse idiopathic skeletal hyperostosis (DISH) (AKA Forestier disease) (p. 1373): An enthesopathy
   c) post-op following ACDF
      • it is normal to have a little swelling and fullness early post-op
      • may be increased with multiple levels and with anterior plating
      • as a complication from post-op hematoma
2. neurologic

References

[1] Ungar-Sargon JY, Lovelace RE, Brust JC. Spastic paraplegia-paraparesis: A Reappraisal. Journal of Neurological Science. 1980; 46:1–12

[2] George WE, Wilmot M, Greenhouse A, et al. Medical Management of Steroid-Induced Epidural Lipomatosis. N Engl J Med. 1983; 308:316–319

[3] Nagashima C. Cervical Myelopathy due to Ossification of the Posterior Longitudinal Ligament. J Neurosurg. 1972; 37:653–660

[4] Marshman LAG, Hardwidge C, Ford-Dunn SZ, et al. Idiopathic Spinal Cord Herniation: Case Report and Review of the Literature. Neurosurgery. 1999; 44:1129–1133

[5] Darbar A, Krishnamurthy S, Holsapple JW, et al. Ventral thoracic spinal cord herniation: frequently misdiagnosed entity. Spine. 2006; 31:E600–E605

[6] Levy M, Llinas RH. Update on a patient with superficial siderosis on deferiprone. AJNR Am J Neuroradiol. 2012; 33:E99–100

[7] Lucchesi AC, White WL, Heiserman JE, et al. Review of Arachnoiditis Ossificans with a Case Report. BNI Quarterly. 1998; 14:4–9

[8] Fox MW, Onofrio BM. The natural history and management of symptomatic and asymptomatic vertebral hemangiomas. J Neurosurg. 1993; 78:36–45

[9] Harik SI, Raichle ME, Reis DJ. Spontaneous Remitting Spinal Epidural Hematoma in a Patient on Anticoagulants. N Engl J Med. 1971; 284:1355–1357

[10] Packer NP, Cummins BH. Spontaneous Epidural Hemorrhage: A Surgical Emergency. Lancet. 1978; 1:356–358

[11] Brem SS, Hafler DA, Van Uitert RL, et al. Spinal Subarachnoid Hematoma: A Hazard of Lumbar Puncture Resulting in Reversible Paraplegia. N Engl J Med. 1981; 303:1020–1021

[12] Rengachary SS, Murphy D. Subarachnoid Hematoma Following Lumbar Puncture Causing Compression of the Cauda Equina. J Neurosurg. 1974; 41:252–254

[13] Epstein NE, Danto J, Nardi D. Evaluation of Intraoperative Somatosensory-Evoked Potential Monitoring During 100 Cervical Operations. Spine. 1993; 18:737–747

[14] Tobin WD, Layton DD. The Diagnosis and Natural History of Spinal Cord Arteriovenous Malformations. Mayo Clin Proc. 1976; 51:637–646

[15] Wirth FP, Post KD, Di Chiro G, et al. Foix-Alajouanine Disease. Spontaneous Thrombosis of a Spinal Cord Arteriovenous Malformation: A Case Report. Neurology. 1970; 20:1114–1118

[16] Rothman RH, Simeone FA. The Spine. Philadelphia 1982

[17] Wingerchuk DM, Lennon VA, Pittock SJ, et al. Revised diagnostic criteria for neuromyelitis optica. Neurology. 2006; 66:1485–1489

[18] Pittock SJ, Lennon VA, Krecke K, et al. Brain abnormalities in neuromyelitis optica. Arch Neurol. 2006; 63:390–396

[19] Nakamura M, Misu T, Fujihara K, et al. Occurrence of acute large and edematous callosal lesions in neuromyelitis optica. Mult Scler. 2009; 15:695–700

[20] Lennon VA, Wingerchuk DM, Kryzer TJ. A serum autoantibody marker of neuromyelitis optica: distinction from multiple sclerosis. Lancet. 2004; 364:2106–2112

[21] Wingerchuk DM. Neuromyelitis optica: new findings on pathogenesis. Int Rev Neurobiol. 2007; 79:665–688

[22] Jacob A, McKeon A, Nakashima I, et al. Current concept of neuromyelitis optica (NMO) and NMO spectrum disorders. J Neurol Neurosurg Psychiatry. 2013; 84:922–930

[23] Mealy MA, Wingerchuk DM, Greenberg BM, et al. Epidemiology of neuromyelitis optica in the United States: a multicenter analysis. Arch Neurol. 2012; 69:1176–1180

[24] Asgari N, Lillevang ST, Skejoe HP, et al. A population-based study of neuromyelitis optica in Caucasians. Neurology. 2011; 76:1589–1595

[25] Jarius S, Ruprecht K, Wildemann B, et al. Contrasting disease patterns in seropositive and seronegative neuromyelitis optica: A multicentre study of 175 patients. J Neuroinflammation. 2012; 9. DOI: 10.118 6/1742-2094-9-14

[26] Wingerchuk DM, Hogancamp WF, O'Brien PC, et al. The clinical course of neuromyelitis optica (Devic's syndrome). Neurology. 1999; 53:1107–1114

[27] Pruthi RK, Tefferi A. Pernicious Anemia Revisited. Mayo Clinic Proceedings. 1994; 69:144–150

[28] Langan RC, Goodbred AJ. Vitamin B12 Deficiency: Recognition and Management. Am Fam Physician. 2017; 96:384–389

[29] Elia M. Oral or Parental Therapy for B12 Deficiency. Lancet. 1998; 352:1721–1722

[30] Altrocchi PH. Acute Spinal Epidural Abscess vs Acute Transverse Myelopathy: A Plea for Neurosurgical Caution. Arch Neurol. 1963; 9:17–25

[31] Sheremata WA, Berger JR, Harrington WJ, et al. Human T Lymphotropic Virus Type I-Associated Myelopathy: A Report of 10 Patients Born in the United States. Archives of Neurology. 1992; 49:1113–1118

[32] Busby M, Donaghy M. Chronic dysimmune neuropathy. A subclassification based upon the clinical features of 102 patients. Journal of Neurology. 2003; 250:714–724

[33] Rowland LP. Diagnosis of amyotrophic lateral sclerosis. Journal of Neurological Science. 1998; 160: S6–24

[34] Deen HG. Diagnosis and Management of Lumbar Disk Disease. Mayo Clinic Proceedings. 1996; 71:283–287

[35] Gritza T, Taylor TKF. A Ganglion Arising from a Lumbar Articular Facet Associated with Low Back Pain and Sciatica. J Bone Joint Surg. 1970; 52:528–531

[36] Kitigawa H, Kanamori M, Tatezaki S, et al. Multiple Spinal Ossified Arachnoiditis. A Case Report. Spine. 1990; 15:1236–1238

[37] Thakkar DH, Porter RW. Heterotopic Ossification Enveloping the Sciatic Nerve Following Posterior Fracture-Dislocation of the Hip: A Case Report. Injury. 1981; 13:207–209

[38] Johanson NA, Pellici PM, Tsairis P, et al. Nerve Injury in Total Hip Arthroplasty. Clinical Orthopedics. 1983; 179:214–222

[39] Burkman KA, Gaines RW, Kashani SR, et al. Herpes Zoster: A Consideration in the Differential Diagnosis of Radiculopathy. Arch Phys Med Rehabil. 1988; 69:132–134

[40] Bickels J, Kahanovitz N, Rupert CK, et al. Extraspinal Bone and Soft-Tissue Tumors as a Cause of Sciatica. Clinical Diagnosis and Recommendations: Analysis of 32 Cases. Spine. 1999; 24:1611–1616

[41] Jones BV, Ward MW. Myositis Ossificans in the Biceps Femoris Muscles Causing Sciatic Nerve Palsy: A Case Report. Journal of Bone and Joint Surgery. 1980; 62B:506–507

[42] Thompson RC, Berg TL. Primary Bone Tumors of Pelvis Presenting as Spinal Disease. Orthopedics. 1996; 19:1011–1016

[43] FDA. Highlights of prescribing information (Spinraza™). 2016. https://www.accessdata.fda.gov/drugsatfda_docs/label/2016/209531lbl.pdf

[44] Ropper AH. Unusual clinical variants and signs in Guillain-Barré syndrome. Arch Neurol. 1986; 43:1150–1152

[45] Yablon IG, Ordia J, Mortara R, et al. Acute ascending myelopathy of the spine. Spine (Phila Pa 1976). 1989; 14:1084–1089

[46] Frymoyer JW. Back Pain and Sciatica. N Engl J Med. 1988; 318:291–300

[47] Deyo RA, Rainville J, Kent DL. What Can the History and Physical Examination Tell Us About Low Back Pain? Journal of the American Medical Association. 1992; 268:760–765

[48] Janin Y, Epstein JA, Carras R, et al. Osteoid Osteomas and Osteoblastomas of the Spine. Neurosurgery. 1981; 8:31–38

[49] Calin A, Porta J, Fries JF, et al. Clinical History as a Screening Test for Ankylosing Spondylitis. Journal of the American Medical Association. 1977; 237:2613–2614

[50] Crayton HE, Bell CL, De Smet AA. Sacral Insufficiency Fractures. Sem Arth Rheum. 1991; 20:378–384

[51] McCarron RF, Wimpee MW, Hudkins PG, et al. The Inflammatory Effect of Nucleus Pulposus: A Possible Element in the Pathogenesis of Low-Back Pain. Spine. 1987; 12:760–764

[52] Hirsch C, Schajowicz F. Studies on Structural Changes in the Lumbar Annulus Fibrosus. Acta Orthop Scand. 1952; 22:184–231

[53] Choice of lipid-regulating drugs. Medical Letter. 2001; 43:43–48

[54] Seftel AD, Farber J, Fletcher J, et al. A three-part study to investigate the incidence and potential etiologies of tadalafil-associated back pain or myalgia. Int J Impot Res. 2005; 17:455–461

[55] Jensen MC, Brant-Zawadzki MN, Obuchowski N, et al. Magnetic Resonance Imaging of the Lumbar Spine in People Without Back Pain. New England Journal of Medicine. 1994; 331:69–73

[56] Bonney G. Iatrogenic Injuries of Nerves. Journal of Bone and Joint Surgery. 1986; 68B:9–13

[57] Eskandary H, Hamzel A, Yasamy MT. Foot Drop Following Brain Lesion. Surgical Neurology. 1995; 43:89–90

[58] Bell HS. Paralysis of both arms from injury of the upper portion of the pyramidal decussation: "cruciate paralysis". Journal of Neurosurgery. 1970; 33:376–380

[59] Yayama T, Uchida K, Kobayashi S, et al. Cruciate paralysis and hemiplegia cruciata: report of three cases. Spinal Cord. 2006; 44:393–398

[60] Hawkins RJ, Bilco T, Bonutti P. Cervical Spine and Shoulder Pain. Clinical Orthopedics and Related Research. 1990; 258:142–146

[61] Goldenberg DL. Fibromyalgia Syndrome. Journal of the American Medical Association. 1987; 257:2782–2787

[62] Wolfe F, Smythe HA, Yunus MB, et al. The American College of Rheumatology 1990 Criteria for the Classification of Fibromyalgia: Report of the Multicenter Criteria Committee. Arthritis Rheum. 1990; 33:160–172

[63] Adler GK, Kinsley BT, Hurwitz S, et al. Reduced Hypothalamic-Pituitary and Sympathoadrenal Responses to Hypoglycemia in Women with Fibromyalgia Syndrome. Am J Med. 1999; 106:534–543

[64] Raina D, Gothi R, Rajan S. Eagle syndrome. Indian J Radiol Imaging. 2009; 19:107–108

[65] Goto S, Umehara J, Aizawa T, et al. Crowned Dens syndrome. J Bone Joint Surg Am. 2007; 89:2732–2736

[66] Stricker LJ, Green CR. Resolution of refractory symptoms of secondary erythermalgia with intermittent epidural bupivacaine. Reg Anesth Pain Med. 2001; 26:488–490

[67] Davis MD, Sandroni P. Lidocaine patch for pain of erythromelalgia. Arch Dermatol. 2002; 138:17–19

[68] Levine TD. Small Fiber Neuropathy: Disease Classification Beyond Pain and Burning. J Cent Nerv Sys Dis. 2018; 10. DOI: 10.1177/1179573518771703

[69] Sobel JB, Sollenberger P, Robinson R, et al. Cervical nonorganic signs: A new clinical tool to assess abnormal illness behavior in neck pain patients. Archives of Physical Medicine and Rehabilitation. 2000; 81:170–175

Part XXIII

Procedures, Interventions, Operations

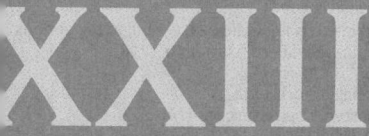

103 Intraoperative Dyes, O.R. Equipment, Surgical Hemostasis, and Bone Extenders

103.1 Introduction

This section provides information useful in the O.R. that applies to a number of different topics. Some items that are pertinent to only one topic will be found in their respective sections instead (e.g. transsphenoidal tumor removal is found in the section on pituitary tumors).

REMEMBER: before performing any invasive procedure, know the patient's coagulation status (history of anticoagulant and/or antiplatelet function medications, and if indicated: PT, PTT, INR, platelet count and platelet function assay, FDP…).

103.2 Intraoperative dyes

This section covers visible dyes that may be useful in the O.R. For radio-opaque dyes, see Contrast agents in neuroradiology (p.230). There is little information available in the literature regarding the intrathecal (IT) use of the following agents:

Indigo carmine: a blue dye which has been used intrathecally to locate CSF leaks. There are few published reports, and no accounts of adverse effects. In 1933 it was reported[1] that IT injection o 5 ml of 0.6% indigo carmine solution produced blue-green discoloration of the CSF draining through a fistula into the nose within 15 minutes, lasting for 5 hours, with no indication of toxicity. It i excreted in the urine (and not in mucous membranes). The consensus is that it should be relatively safe for IT use, but the manufacturer did not recommend this application.

✖ Methylene blue: methylene blue is probably *cytotoxic* and appears to become fixed to neura tissue. It should therefore *not* be used as a stain in neurosurgical operations or diagnostic tests. CNS damage (some permanent) occurred in 14 patients given an IT injection of a 1% solution. Symptom included: paraparesis, quadriplegia, multiple cranial nerve involvement (including anosmia and optic atrophy), dementia, and hydrocephalus.[2]

Fluorescein: although intrathecal injection (e.g., to look for CSF leak) has been used by ENT sur geons with apparently acceptable results, there is a risk of seizures. 2.5% fluorescein is diluted 1:10 with CSF or saline and ≈ 6 ml is injected into the spinal subarachnoid space (or 0.5 ml of 5% fluores cein mixed with 5–10 ml of CSF[3]).

Fluorescein has also been used *IV* (adult dose: 1 amp IV) to help mark areas of the brain wher there is breakdown of the blood-brain barrier (BBB), e.g., in tumors (p.628); however, fluorescein i eventually excreted in mucus, urine, etc., and just about everything turns orange. It has also bee used to perform intraoperative "visible angiograms" during the removal of AVMs.

Indigocyanine green (ICG): used for intraoperative angiography (p.1466).

103.3 Operating room equipment

103.3.1 Operating microscope—observer's eyepiece

For spine cases, the ideal location of the observer eyepiece is usually directly opposite the surgeon For intracranial work, the observer's (assistant's) eyepiece is placed to the *right* of the operator', except in the following cases where it is placed to the left:
1. transsphenoidal surgery (when the surgeon stands to the patient's right)
2. *right* posterior fossa craniotomy in the lateral oblique (suboccipital) position

103.3.2 Head stabilization

General information

Options include:
1. non-pin head stabilization: when absolute head fixation is not indicated, the following options avoid some of the complications associated with pin-based head fixation (p.1717):
   a) horse-shoe head rest
   b) doughnut: gel type, or one can be fashioned using a stockinette
   c) Prone-view® for prone position e.g., during posterior spine surgery

2. pin-based head-fixation: the Mayfield head-holder or head frame is the most common, devised by Dr. Frank Henderson Mayfield (1908–1991)

Pin-based head-fixation

Indications for pin stabilization:

1. ✖ not recommended for use in age < 3 years, use pediatric pins with care in ages 3–10 years (this age cutoff is not based on scientific evidence, most reported complications occur in age > 3 years)
2. craniotomies:
   a) most intracranial vascular operations: a radiolucent head-holder should be used if intraoperative angiogram is to be performed
   b) often for tumor operations, especially if there is need for a self-retaining retractor system that attaches to the Mayfield head-holder (e.g., Budde halo)
   c) when intraoperative image-guidance (IG) systems are used (an alternative here is to use mask-based or strap-on registration array holders)
3. cervical spine: often used for posterior cervical operations (laminectomies, instrumentation, fusions…)

Application of pin head holder:

1. "skull block" (p. 1733) (blockade of scalp innervation) may be administered prior to pin placement. Critical for awake craniotomies (for the wake-up), and for vascular cases and cases with increased ICP where the block blunts the precipitous increase in blood pressure[4,5] that may otherwise accompany pinning, which may → increased ICP. For technique, see Typical sequence of anesthesia (p. 1733).
2. plan pin placement
   a) the manufacturer recommends that the pins be placed within a band-like area similar to a "sweatband" worn just above the orbits and the pinna
   b) avoid placing pins on the thin temporal squamosa, and use with caution over the frontal sinus[6]
   c) the single pin is typically placed anteriorly when the patient is in the supine position (▶ Fig. 106.1); for a posterior fossa approach in the prone position, if the craniotomy is on one side, the single pin is placed on that side (▶ Fig. 105.2)
   d) most current head clamps have a dual pin "rocker" opposite the single pin, and this should be placed equidistant from the centerline for maximal stability
3. appropriately sized sterile pins (usually coated with antibiotic ointment) are placed in the head-holder (disposable pins have largely superseded reusable pins):
   a) ✖ children < 3 yrs of age: increased risk of calvarial penetration or depressed skull fractures. A padded cerebellar head rest should be used instead[6,7]
   b) children ≥ 3 yrs of age and < 10 yrs of age: pediatric skull pins should be employed. These pins have a "shoulder" (▶ Fig. 103.1) to ensure shorter depth of skull penetration. NB: with a thick scalp these pins may not adequately contact the skull
4. NB: before doing the following, make sure that the single pin that has the spring loaded pressure adjustment is backed out enough so that there is room to tighten it after this step is completed). The ends of the Mayfield clamp are squeezed together, allowing the linear ratchet and pawl to slide, until the pins are initially seated in the skull
5. the knob housing the tension spring and gauge is tightened (each ring = 20 lbs)
   a) adults: tighten until the third ring (60 lbs) is visible (▶ Fig. 103.1); up to 80 lbs has been described
   b) pediatrics: less pressure should be applied, 30–40 lbs has been suggested.[6] Even with pediatric pins & decreased pressure, complications may occur, consider horseshoe headrest

Complications of pin head-fixation:

1. malposition of pins:
   a) through unintended anatomic structures: pinna, orbit, superficial temporal artery, shunt hardware, prior craniotomy defect
   b) poor fixation by not properly placing pins close to "equator" resulting in movement during surgery (with risk of cervical spine injury, injury to structures being operated on due to the sudden movement, loss of image-guided registration) and possible skin laceration
2. skin penetration by pins: can cause injury to intracranial structures, or infection including delayed abscess, epidural hematoma[6]…
   a) overtightening of pins

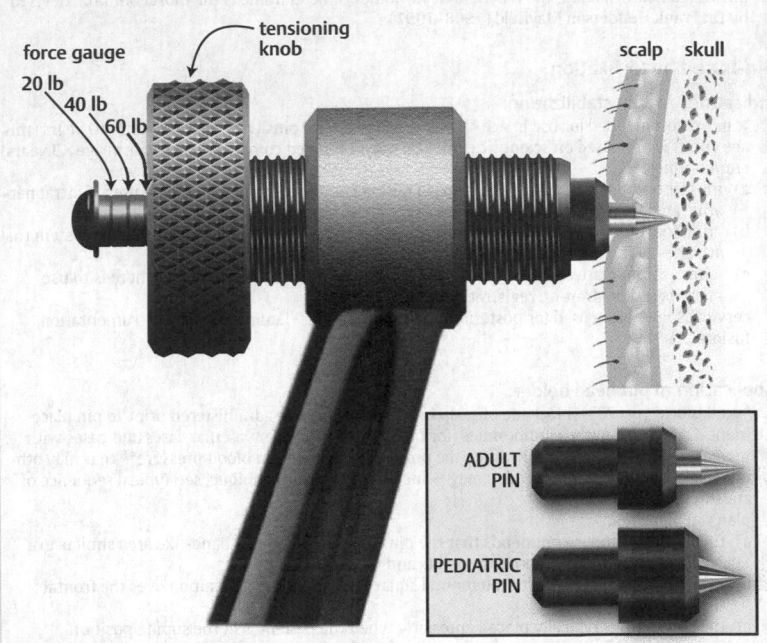

Fig. 103.1 Mayfield head-holder.
Image: detail of the tension knob of a Mayfield-head holder that has been tightened to 60 lbs of force (3 rings showing).
Inset shows disposable pins, highlighting the shorter exposed metal points of the "pediatric pin" (for ages approximately 3–10 years) compared to the adult pin.

b) incorrect pin selection: see above
c) soft skull: in elderly patients, poorly calcified skulls, pediatric patients[6]
3. skin necrosis: especially with pediatric pins due to the "shoulder" of the pins
4. skull fracture: including "ping-pong ball" fractures in young children
5. slippage of any of the joints or connections to the O.R. table
6. clamp breakage[8,9]: inspect the head-holder for cracks prior to each application, store properly and maintain per the manufacturer's specifications
7. bleeding from pin site: usually when the head-holder is removed. If bleeding does not stop after a minute or so of pressure, a suture or surgical staple may be used

103.4 Surgical hemostasis

103.4.1 Basic options

1. thermocoagulation
   a) electrical coagulation:
      • monopolar (Bovie) cautery: electric current passes through the patient to a grounding pad. Because of possible transmission through electrically and thermally sensitive neural structures, this modality is not used directly on the brain or in proximity to named nerves (including cranial nerves) & nerve roots
      • bipolar cautery: current passes only between the tips of the cautery device. Used for precise coagulation. When used directly on or near to the brain or nerves, the current setting is typically reduced from that employed for general use

   b) thermal units: e.g., AccuTemp® disposable eye cautery units (particularly useful to coagulate dura when inserting a ventriculostomy in the ICU)
   c) laser: especially neodymium:yttrium-aluminum-garnet (Nd:YAG) laser
2. mechanical
   a) bone wax: originated by Sir Victor Horsely. Stops bone bleeding. NB: *Inhibits bone formation* so its use is limited in spinal fusions
   b) ligature: less commonly used in neurosurgery than other specialties
   c) "silver clips" (e.g., HemoClips®)
3. chemical hemostasis: see below

103.4.2 Chemical hemostasis

See review[10] for more information. Some key points:
1. gelatin sponge (Gelfoam®): no intrinsic coagulating effect. Absorbs 45 times its weight in blood which causes it to expand and tamponade bleeding. Absorbable. May be combined with thrombin as patties or as powder (e.g., FLOSEAL®, SurgiFlo®)
2. oxidized cellulose (Oxycel®) and oxidized regenerated cellulose (Surgicel®): absorbable. Acidic material that reacts with blood to form a reddish brown "pseudoclot." Bactericidal to over 20 different organisms. May retard bone growth. Oxycel® interferes with epithelialization more than Surgicel®
3. microfibrillar collagen (Avitene®): promotes adhesion and aggregation of platelets. Loses effectiveness in severe thrombocytopenia (< 10,000/ml). May be used on bone bleeding. Remove excess material to reduce risk of infection
4. thrombin (Thrombostat®): does not depend on any intermediate physiological agent. Caution: although thrombin may cause significant edema when placed on brain where the pia has been disrupted, practical experience indicates this is uncommon

103.5 Dural substitutes

Indications: incompetent dura due to any of a number of causes: trauma, tumor, infection, surgery....
   Dura consists primarily of collagen and elastin.[11]
   Options:
autologous grafts (from the patient). Common donor sites include:
a) fascia lata
b) galea/pericranium (when doing a craniotomy)
allograft: some are designed to be absorbable, some are non-absorbable
a) reconstituted materials: processed collagen...
b) processed intact natural materials: e.g., ovine (sheep) or bovine (cattle) pericardium, porcine intestinal mucosa...
c) synthetic materials: e.g.,Polyesterurethane, PLGA (Polyglactin 910) and PDO (Polydioxanone)...
d) biosynthetic materials: e.g., cellulose produced by Gluconacetobacter xylinus

Examples of some commercially available dural substitutes are shown in ► Table 103.1.

103.6 Localizing levels in spine surgery

Identifying the correct level in spine surgery may be extremely challenging in certain situations. With the proliferation of minimally invasive spine techniques and the associated reduction in the structures that are directly visualized, the reliance on intraoperative imaging or navigation to determine the spinal level has increased.
   Potential pitfalls which increase the chances of error, including:
● pre-op, pathology is usually identified on MRI, and there can be challenges in translating MRI images to imaging available in the O.R.
   a) thoracic lesions: pre-op MRI usually counts from the top (C2) down, and in surgery it is often necessary to count from the bottom (S1) up, the count could be off if there are not 5 lumbar vertebrae and 12 pairs of ribs
   b) lumbar spine: a well-developed S1–2 disc or an L5 vertebra fused to the sacrum can confuse the count (see below)
● not all patients have 12 ribs, or 5 "lumbar" vertebrae. In the modal (most common) human spine, there are 24 presacral vertebrae; however, some individuals have 23 and others have 25

103

Table 103.1 Characteristics of some commercially available dural allograft substitutes

Trade name (manufacturer)	Material	Abs[a]	Sut[b]	Seal[c]	Description
Biodesign Dural Graft (Cook Medical)	collagen (porcine small intestinal submucosa derived)	+	+	*	thin; lower amount of elastin than dermis derived products
Biodesign Duraplasty Graft (Cook Medical)	collagen (porcine small intestinal submucosa derived)	+	–	*	
Cerafix® (Acera Surgical)	PLGA (polyglactin 910) and PDO (polydioxanone)	+	–	–	porous, fully synthetic, fully resorbable material; mimics architecture of extracellular matrix
DuraFlex™ Suturable Graft (Integra)	bovine pericardium	+	–	*	non-crosslinked collagen; manufactured using the Tutoplast® Tissue Sterilization Process
DuraGen® Plus (Integra)	collagen (bovine derived)	+	–	+	porous monolayer crosslinked collagen
DuraGen® Classic Matrix (Integra)	collagen (bovine derived)	+	–	–	
DuraGen® Secure (Integra)	collagen (bovine derived)	+	–	–	has additional cellulose microlayer used to keep graft in place; applied dry
DuraGen® Suturable (Integra)	collagen (bovine derived)	+	+	–	thick, porous bilayer collagen
Durepair® Regeneration Matrix (Medtronic)	collagen (bovine derived)	+	+	–	thin; uniquely uses type III fetal bovine tissue in addition to type I collagen without crosslinking
DuraMatrix® Onlay (Stryker)	collagen (bovine dermis derived)	+	+	*	thin; highly conformable; lower liquid permeability than other similar products
DuraMatrix® Onlay PLUS (Stryker)	collagen (bovine dermis derived)	+	–	*	thick; non-porous, multi-layered with lower liquid permeability than other similar products
DuraMatrix® Suturable (Stryker)	collagen (bovine dermis derived)	+	+	*	thick; bovine collagen reinforced with additional crosslinking
Durepair® Regeneration Matrix (Medtronic)	collagen (bovine derived)	+	+	–	thin; uniquely uses type III fetal bovine tissue in addition to type I collagen without crosslinking
Tutopatch® (Tutogen Medical)	bovine pericardium	+	+	+	thin; retains a structure similar to non-processed collagen
Neuro-Patch® (B. Braun)	polyester urethane	–	+	+	thin; microporous fleece with high liquid tightness
SYNTHECEL® Dura Repair (DePuy Synthes)	bionanocellulose	–	–	–	thin; porous; made of biosynthesized cellulose and water; entirely non-animal derived

[a] Abs: + indicates absorbable, – indicates non-absorbable.
[b] Sut: + indicates suturable. Most other allografts may be **anchored** using tensionless sutures; a tapered (not cutting) needle is recommended.
[c] Seal: – means the manufacturer states dural sealants should not be used with this product, * means no information is provided regarding sealants.

(variations include: 11 or 13 rib-bearing vertebrae, or a lumbosacral transitional vertebra; the terminology of a "lumbarized S1 vertebra" or a "sacralized L5 vertebra" is imprecise and confusing). An HLD at the ultimate disc space (usually L5–1) most often impinges on the 25th nerve root (however, in the variant cases, it may actually impinge on the 24th or 26th root)[12]

3. patients may have variant or ambiguous anatomy (e.g., a well-developed S1–2 disc space, an enlarged L1 transverse process mimicking a 12th rib…)
4. some "landmarks" used for localizing levels are unreliable or changeable (e.g., mobile spondylolisthesis)
5. plain radiographs/fluoroscopy have difficulty imaging the upper thoracic and sometimes the lower cervical spine
   a) on lateral imaging, the shoulders often obscure lower cervical/upper thoracic levels
   b) on AP imaging, the pronounced kyphosis of this region requires cranio-caudal angulation of the X-ray beam, which throws off imaging at other levels
6. spinous processes of lumbar and especially thoracic levels are below the corresponding VB
7. changes may occur between the time of the pre-op imaging and the surgery

Aids in determining spinal levels:
1. image-guided systems, when available
2. built-in or portable intra-op MRI or CT (e.g., Airo® CT by Mobius marketed by BrainLab), or CT-like modalities (e.g., O-arm™ by Medtronic, ARCADIS® C-arm by Siemens), or image-guided spine technology
3. ★ pre-op plain X-rays:
   a) for lumbar pathology: lumbar AP & lateral
   b) for thoracic pathology: lumbar + thoracic AP & lateral (to verify there are 12 thoracic vertebrae and 5 lumbar vertebrae)
4. on lateral lumbar spine X-rays, the top of the iliac crests are even with the L4 spinous process or the L4–5 interspinous space
5. on sagittal MRI there are generally no numbering cues, but on axial MRI, the sacral ala are reliably identifiable and this can be used to identify L5–1 disc space
6. counting methods (if possible, using more than 1 method is highly recommended)
   a) counting up from T12 or L5 on fluoro: be sure there are 12 ribs. You can "bridge" from lumbar or lower thoracic spine to higher thoracic levels using an instrument on the patient as a marker, or you can count up to a given level (e.g., T9) and then while a hemostat is placed at this level on the fluoro screen, under real-time fluoro the machine is slowly moved up the spine and the hemostat is moved along with T9 (to count up from L5, verify there are 5 lumbar (i.e., non-rib-bearing) presacral vertebrae). Radiation safety: avoid live fluoro as much as possible
   b) AP view: starting at T12 (lowest rib) or from L5
   c) lateral view: starting at the L5 and counting up
   d) counting down from T1 (first rib) on AP fluoro: the fluoro machine may need to be angled caudally from the anterior position because of the thoracic kyphosis. Sometimes counting pedicles helps
   e) by palpation: with thoracotomy, in the upper T-spine you can palpate the ribs from the inside from T1 and count down. The rib inserts at the upper end of the thoracic vertebra near the junction with the VB above (e.g., the T5 rib joins T5 close to the T4–5 disc space)

03.7 Bone graft

03.7.1 Use of bone graft extenders/substitutes as an adjunct to fusion

Practice guideline: Bone graft extenders and substitutes

Level I[13]: autologous bone or recombinant human bone morphogenetic protein (rhBMP-2) bone graft substitute is recommended in the setting of an ALIF in conjunction with a threaded titanium cage

Level III[13]:
- rhBMP-2 in conjunction with hydroxyapatite and tricalcium phosphate may be substituted for autograft in some cases of posterolateral fusion
- calcium phosphate is recommended as a bone graft extender, especially when combined with autologous bone

103.7.2 Assessing surgical lumbar fusion

See **Practice guideline: Radiographic assessment of fusion** (p. 1722).

103

Practice guideline: Radiographic assessment of fusion

Level I[14]: static X-rays alone are *not* recommended

Level II[14]:
- in the *absence* of rigid instrumentation, lack of motion between vertebrae on lateral flexion/extension X-rays is highly suggestive of successful fusion
- ✖ technetium-99 bone scanning is *not* recommended

Level III[14]: radiographic techniques, often in combination, may be used when failed lumbar fusion is suspected, including: static and flexion/extension X-rays, CT scan

Practice guideline: Correlation between fusion and outcome

Level III[15]: the correlation between fusion and clinical outcome is not strong, and in any given situation fusion status may be unrelated to outcome

103.7.3 Bone graft properties

General information

For spine fusions, components of bone graft that are important for fusion:
1. osteoinduction: recruitment of mesenchymal cells and the stimulation of these cells to develop into osteoblasts and osteoclasts
2. osteogenesis: formation of new bone by host or graft mesenchymal stem cells transformed into osteoblasts
3. osteoconduction: the structure of the graft that acts as a scaffold upon which new bone and blood vessels form
4. mechanical stability: the structural anatomical biomechanical support provided, e.g., following discectomy, corpectomy, or resection of vertebral tumor

▶ Table 103.2 summarizes the properties of various bone graft materials (adapted[16,17,18]). See the sections that follow for more details.

Table 103.2 Characteristics of bone graft materials[a] (see text for details)

Material	Mechanical stability	Osteogenic	Osteo-inductive	Osteo-conductive
Cancellous autograft	±	++++	++	++++
Cortical autograft	+++	+	+	+
Vascularized autograft	+++	+++	++	+++
Allograft	+	–	±	+
Bone marrow aspirate	–	+	±	+
Demineralized bone matrix (DBM)	–	–	+	+
Bone morphogenetic protein (BMP)	–	–	++++	–
Collagen	–	–	–	–
Ceramics	+	–	–	+++

[a] Key: – no effect, ± minimal or no effect, + mild, ++ moderate, +++ strong, ++++ very strong effect

Autograft

Common donor sites: iliac crest, rib,[19] fibula, bone removed during decompression. Characteristics:
1. PROS: no histocompatibility or disease transmission issues
2. CONS:
   a) persistent post-op donor site pain: occurs in as many as 34% of patients (the severity of which was graded as "unacceptable" in 3%)[20]
   b) increased surgical risks of:
      - blood loss
      - wound infection
      - fracture
      - cosmetic deformity
      - increased operative time to procure
      - numbness from nerve injury (e.g., cluneal nerves see below)
      - hematoma
3. subtypes
   a) cancellous bone: provides all graft components except mechanical stability
   b) cortical bone:
      - provides superior and immediate mechanical strength
      - has diminished osteoinduction and osteoconduction capacity
   c) corticocancellous bone: e.g., tricortical iliac crest wedge. Contains all bone graft components
   d) vascularized autograft:
      - technically challenging
      - best suited for areas that are scarred, irradiated, or that span long segments
   e) autologous bone marrow:
      - source of osteoprogenitor cells and osteoinductive substrates
      - diminished donor site risks
      - no osteoconductive nor structural properties

Allograft

Acquired through organ procurement agencies. Primarily frozen or freeze-dried. Donor sites include: ilium, tibia, fibula, femur, rib.
1. PROS: eliminates risks associated with harvesting autograft
2. CONS:
   a) small but real risk of disease transmission
   b) provides only osteoconduction (lacks osteoinduction and osteogenesis)
   c) availability may vary from time to time
3. subtypes
   a) tricortical block, bicortical plug, or unicortical dowel
   b) corticocancellous: matchsticks, crushed
   c) cancellous: cubes, block, crushed, bone powder
4. uses: allografts are acceptable for structural grafts such as in anterior spinal interbody fusion, where compressive forces are applied to the graft. However, for onlay grafts such as for posterior cervical fusion, the lack of osteoinductive and osteogenetic properties is a critical shortcoming

Demineralized bone matrix (DBM)

Prepared by acid extraction, reducing antigenicity, but preserving some osteoconductive and variable osteoinductive properties.
1. available as putty, gel, chips, granules, or powder
2. primarily used as an adjunct to other grafting materials
3. CONS:
   a) increased cost
   b) variable efficacy between preparations and batches of the same preparation
   c) no mechanical or structural properties

Bone morphogenetic proteins (BMP)

Biological compounds that are a group of cytokines which induce the transformation of mesenchymal stem cells into osteoblasts (osteoinduction) with the potential to induce ectopic bone formation. There are ≈ 20 different proteins from the transforming growth factor-β family. Produced using recombinant DNA technology.

1. a carrier matrix is required to retain the soluble factor at the graft site (i.e., to prevent the BMP from diffusing into adjacent tissues, thereby reducing the desired effect and possibly inducing bone growth at undesired foci)
2. FDA approved in U.S. only for ALIF. Other uses are "off label"
3. available preparations: rhBMP-2 (Infuse® by Medtronic)
4. PROS: increases fusion rates
5. CONS:
   a) expensive
   b) ectopic bone formation, bone resorption (so-called osteolysis) or remodelling at the graft site[21]
   c) in anterior cervical spine surgery: neck swelling with airway compromise, hematoma, painful seroma[21]
6. contraindications include:
   a) patients with active malignancy or those undergoing treatment for a malignancy
   b) should not be used in the vicinity of a resected tumor
   c) patients who are skeletally immature

Collagen

Used primarily as a carrier for other osteoinductive, osteoconductive, or osteogenetic materials and as a composite with other graft extenders
1. PROS: contributes to vascular ingrowth, mineral deposition, and growth factor binding
2. CONS:
   a) minimal structural support
   b) potential immunogenicity

Ceramics

Includes tricalcium phosphate, calcium carbonate, & hydroxyapatite.
1. PROS: no risk of disease transmission
2. CONS: only recommended for use as bone graft extenders (i.e., must be combined with autograft bone marrow aspirate, BMP...)

103.7.4 Bone growth stimulators

Introduction

Electical current, electromagnetic fields, and ultrasound have been shown to influence osteogenesi (p. 1722) and therby bone growth and healing, possibly as a result of affecting some combination c the following: calcium influx through voltage-gated channels,[22] modulation of gene expression in connective tissues with a resultant increase in production of various bone morphogenetic protein (BMP) (p. 1723).[23]

There are a number of commercially available bone growth stimulators (BGS) for spine fusion that can be implanted internally (at the time of surgery), or, more commonly, worn externally afte surgery in accordance to specific protocols established by the manufacturer for each device.

Since there is controversy regarding the criteria for determination of spinal fusion, and with th correlation of fusion with good outcome (some patients without fusion have good outcome), the effi cacy and cost-effectiveness of BGS are unknown.

Available technologies

BGS technologies typically employed in spine fusions include:
- DCS: direct current stimulation using electrodes implanted at the time of surgery
- CCS: capacitance coupling stimulation using 2 electrodes placed on the skin over a fusion site
- PEMFS: pulsed electromagnetic field stimulation using coils typically embedded in a brace

Indications & contraindications

According to the National Coverage Determination (NCD),[24] electrical Osteogenic Stimulators (BG are effective in increasing the fusion rate as an adjunct to spinal fusion surgery in patients at high risk for pseudoarthrosis shown in the practice guideline below.

Technologies recommended for payer coverage[25] for spine fusion include: DCS, CCS, & PEMFS.

Technologies with insufficient information to recommend payer coverage for spine fusion includ LIPUS (low-intensity pulsed ultrasound) and CMF (combined magnetic field = DC field & AC field).

Practice guideline: Nationally covered indications for bone growth stimulators in spine fusions

- previously failed spinal fusion at the same site
- fusion involving 3 or more vertebrae

Other factors that the NASS Coverage Policy[25] recommended for consideration for BGS include the presence of one or more of the following: diabetes, inflammatory arthritis requiring long-term corticosteroids, immunocompromise (e.g., chemotherapy and radiation therapy to the spine, hypogammaglobulinemia, granulocytopenia, acquired immune deficiency syndrome, chronic granulomatous disease), systemic vascular disease, osteopenia or osteoporosis, cigarette smokers who cannot stop smoking in preparation for surgery.

In addition to those not qualifying for BGS based on the above, BGS is *not* indicated: in patients with malignancy, as an adjunct for primary bone healing for spinal fractures, or as a nonsurgical treatment for established pseudarthrosis.

The safety of BGS in the following situations is not fully known: pregnancy, infection, patients with cardiac pacemakers or defibrillators (consult a cardiologist), skeletally immature patients (children).

With implanted BGS: MRI procedures must follow specific guidelines related to magnet strength and spatial gradient (confer with your MRI facility).

Specific recommendations for the type of BGS in the *lumbar* spine[25]:
- DCS & CCS: for posterolateral fusion using autograft + extender
- PEMFS: for lumbar interbody fusion

103.7.5 Bone graft procurement

Iliac crest

Anterior iliac bone graft

Should be obtained at least $\approx$ 3–4 cm lateral to the anterior superior iliac spine (ASIS) to avoid the lateral femoral cutaneous nerve and to reduce the risk of avulsion fractures of the remaining ilium. When a tricortical graft is taken, keep the dissection in the subperiosteal plane and avoid electrocautery on the medial (inner) surface when detaching the iliacus muscle to avoid injury to the ilioinguinal, iliohypogastric, and lateral femoral cutaneous nerves.

Posterior iliac crest bone graft

May be used to obtain corticocancellous strips or plates for onlay bone grafts, or tricortical grafts which may be used as strut grafts or for C1–2 arthrodesis.

They are taken from the medial 6–8 cm of the iliac crest (▶ Fig. 103.2) to avoid the superior cluneal nerves (which cross the posterior iliac crest $\approx$ 8 cm lateral to the posterior superior iliac spine) with resultant buttock numbness or the development of painful neuromas. A vertical incision just medial to the posterior superior iliac spine usually works well.

The spine may sometimes be found on corpulent patients by locating the "dimple of Venus" (fossae lumbales laterales—indentation sometimes visible superior to the gluteal cleft, directly superficial to the sacroiliac joint) and incising slightly lateral to it. Avoid mistaking the sacrum for the iliac spine.

The gluteus maximus is dissected off the lateral surface subperiosteally. To avoid fractures extending into the iliac crest, a wide osteotome should be used to create a "stop cut"; alternatively, a sagittal saw may be used. Avoid penetration through the inner cortical surface of the crest so as not to enter the pelvis and possibly cause an intra-abdominal hematoma. Another potential complication is fracture extension into the greater sciatic notch with possible injury to the gluteal arteries and sciatic nerve among others. Once the graft is removed and cancellous bone is gouged out, the exposed bone surfaces should be waxed and closed system drainage should be used to reduce the risk of local hematoma formation.

Fibula

Autogenous fibular graft provides a high arthrodesis rate,[26] but may be associated with significant morbidity, and so may be best reserved for salvage procedures.[27] Preserve the proximal fibular head to avoid injury to the peroneal nerve. At least 7 cm of distal fibula should be maintained to preserve ankle stability.[19]

103

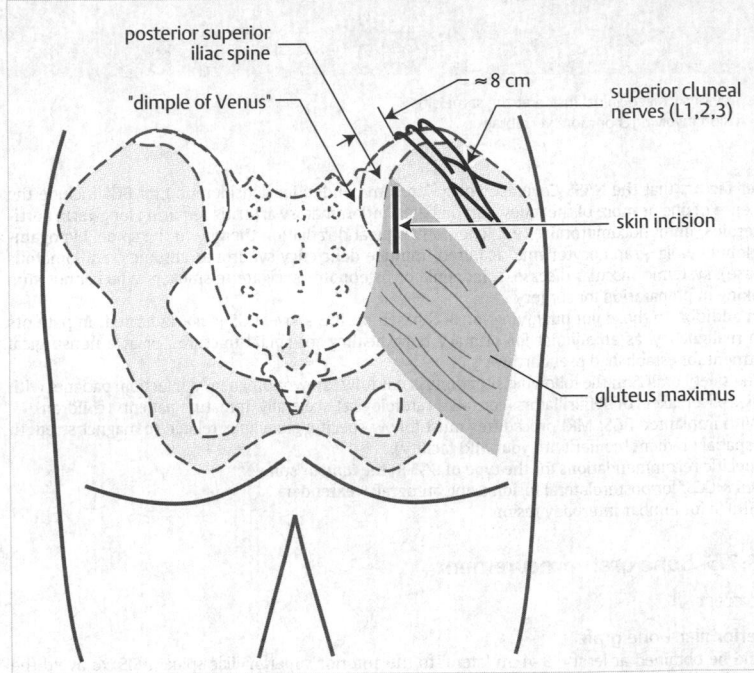

Fig. 103.2 Posterior iliac crest bone donor site.

References

[1] Fox N. Cure in a Case of Cerebrospinal Rhinorrhea. Arch Otolaryngol. 1933; 17:85–87

[2] Evans JP, Keegan HR. Danger in the Use of Intrathecal Methylene Blue. Journal of the American Medical Association. 1960; 174:856–859

[3] Calcaterra TC. Extracranial Repair of Cerebrospinal Rhinorrhea. Ann Otol Rhinol Laryngol. 1980; 89:108–116

[4] Pinosky ML, Fishman RL, Reeves ST, et al. The effect of bipuvicaine skull block on the hemodynamic response to craniotomy. Neurosurgical Anesthesia. 1996; 83:1256–1261

[5] el Gohary M, Gamil M, Girgis K, et al. Scalp nerve blocks in children undergoing a supratentorial craniotomy: A randomized controlled study. Asian Journal of Scientific Research. 2009; 2:105–112

[6] Vitali AM, Steinbok P. Depressed skull fracture and epidural hematoma from head fixation with pins for craniotomy in children. Child's Nervous System. 2008; 24:917–23; discussion 925

[7] Agrawal D, Steinbok P. Simple technique of head fixation for image-guided neurosurgery in infants. Child's Nervous System. 2006; 22:1473–1474

[8] Lee TH, Kim SJ, Cho do S. Broken Mayfield head clamp. J Korean Neurosurg Soc. 2009; 45:306–308

[9] Taira T, Tanikawa T. Breakage of Mayfield head rest. Journal of Neurosurgery. 1992; 77:160–161

[10] Arand AG, Sawaya R. Intraoperative Chemical Hemostasis. Neurosurgery. 1986; 18:223–233

[11] Patin DJ, Eckstein EC, Harum K, et al. Anatomic and biomechanical properties of human lumbar dura mater. Anesth Analg. 1993; 76:535–540

[12] Wigh RE. Classification of the Human Vertebral Column: Phylogenic Departures and Junctional Anomalies. Medical Radiography and Photography 1980; 56:2–11

[13] Resnick DK, Choudhri TF, Dailey AT, et al. Part 16 Bone graft extenders and substitutes. Journal of Neurosurgery: Spine. 2005; 2:733–736

[14] Resnick DK, Choudhri TF, Dailey AT, et al. Part 4 Radiographic assessment of fusion. Journal of Neurosurgery (Spine). 2005; 2:653–657

[15] Resnick DK, Choudhri TF, Dailey AT, et al. Part 5 Correlation between radiographic and functional outcome. Journal of Neurosurgery (Spine). 2005; 2:658–661

[16] Whang PG, Wang JC. Bone graft substitutes for spinal fusion. Spine J. 2003; 3:155–165

[17] Giannoudis PV, Dinopoulos H, Tsiridis E. Bone substitutes: an update. Injury. 2005; 36 Suppl 3:S20–S27

[18] Shen FH, Samartzis D, An HS. Cell technologies for spinal fusion. Spine J. 2005; 5:231S–239S

[19] Galler RM, Sonntag VKH. Bone graft harvest. BN Quarterly. 2003; 19:13–19

[20] Heary RF, Schlenk RP, Sacchieri TA, et al. Persistent iliac crest donor site pain: independent outcome assessment. Neurosurgery. 2002; 50:510–6; discussion 516-7

[21] Vaidya R, Sethi A, Bartol S, et al. Complications in the use of rhBMP-2 in PEEK cages for interbody spinal fusions. J Spinal Disord Tech. 2008; 21:557–56

[22] Brighton CT, Wang W, Seldes R, et al. Signal transduction in electrically stimulated bone cells. J Bone Joint Surg Am. 2001; 83-A:1514–1523

[23] Wang Z, Clark CC, Brighton CT. Up-regulation of bone morphogenetic proteins in cultured murine bone cells with use of specific electric fields. J Bone Joint Surg Am. 2006; 88:1053–1065

[24] Centers for Medicare and Medicaid Services. National Coverage Determination (NCD) for Osteogenic Stimulators (150.2). 2005. https://www.cms.gov/medicare-coverage-database/details/ncd-details.aspx?NCDId=65&ncdver=2&DocID=150.2&bc=gAAAABAAAAAA

[25] North American Spine Society Coverage Committee. Electrical stimulation for bone healing. Burr Ridge, IL 2016

[26] Gore DR. The arthrodesis rate in multilevel anterior cervical fusions using autogenous fibula. Spine. 2001; 26:1259–1263

[27] Kim CW, Abrams R, Lee G, et al. Use of vascularized fibular strut grafts as a salvage procedure for previously failed spinal arthrodesis. Spine. 2001; 19:2171–2175

103

104 Craniotomies – General Information and Cortical Mapping

104.1 Craniotomy – general information

104.1.1 Cranial perforators

Perforators are one means used to create burr holes which enable the surgeon to access the brain for intracranial procedures. Many brands of perforators are designed with a slip clutch that disengages the drill and stops the outer shaft from spinning and entering the skull once the central part of the drill penetrates the inner table. While these clutches are generally reliable and immensely helpful there is a possibility of malfunction such that the outer shaft continues to rotate and if it penetrates the inner table, the entire drill can plunge into the brain. In 8 months of 2005 the FDA received reports of 200 injuries as a result of the drill failing to disengage.[1] The FDA released a number of recommendations to reduce the risk of injury,[1] excerpts of which are shown here:

- select the appropriate perforator based on the skull thickness (pediatric vs. adult)
- keep the perforator perpendicular to the skull throughout the drilling process
- do not rock, rotate, or change the angle of the device during drilling
- avoid using excessive pressure on the drill. Brace the hand holding the drill on the other hand, which should rest on the patient's skull, and thereby prevent plunging if the drill completely penetrates the skull
- use caution when:
  - drilling through areas of irregular bone contour, curvature, or variations in thickness
  - drilling on skulls of infants/children, the elderly, or any other patient who might have softer bone consistency (including osteogenesis imperfecta…)
  - perforating bone in an area where the bone might be diseased or incompetent or have loose fragments

104.1.2 Intraparenchymal cyst aspiration

When a cystic tumor or intracerebral hemorrhage is being operated on, an attempt should be made to insert a ventricular needle into the lesion and aspirate some but not all of the cyst contents. This often produces significant decompression. Avoid evacuating all of the contents; otherwise the lesion might be difficult to find. The needle may then be left in place to allow localization of the lesion (or the needle track can be followed, which may occasionally be difficult).

104.1.3 Intraoperative brain swelling

Background

Under certain circumstances during surgery, the brain may start to severely swell out of the craniotomy wound. Etiologies of this emergency situation include:
1. extraparenchymal bleeding: from a vessel or intraoperative aneurysm rupture, remotely situated epidural/subdural hematoma
2. intracerebral hemorrhage
3. venous outflow obstruction
4. vasodilatation induced by hypercarbia
5. severe diffuse cerebral edema following stroke or traumatic brain injury (TBI)

Management

First efforts should be aimed at ruling out and correcting the aforementioned causes as well as some adjunctive measures. Most maneuvers are similar to those used in controlling an ICP crisis. During the process, it is critical to try to avoid having the brain compress itself against the craniotomy bone edges, which can lacerate the cortex and can also further compromise cortical veins, which impair venous outflow, causing more brain edema and swelling, which accelerates the vicious cycle.
1. elevate the head of the patient (e.g., with reverse Trendelenburg of the O.R. table)
2. make sure the jugular veins are not kinked: this may require rotating the head by loosening the pivot that connects the table adapter to the Mayfield head-holder and rotating the head to a more neutral position

3. rule out hypercarbia: make sure the endotracheal tube is not kinked, check the patient's end-tidal pCO_2
4. measures to lower ICP and protect the brain
   a) give mannitol 1 gm/kg IV bolus
   b) drain CSF if an option: from adjacent cistern or lumbar drain
   c) tap and drain a ventricle e.g., using an EVD or a ventricular needle
   d) have anesthesiologist hyperventilate to a pCO_2 of 30–35 mm Hg
   e) have anesthesiologist induce burst suppression (e.g., with barbiturates, or propofol…)
   f) apply sterile ice water on the brain
5. emergently intubate patients who are undergoing awake craniotomy
6. consider intraoperative CT or ultrasound if rapidly available to rule out hematoma (intracerebral, EDH, SDH) which could potentially be immediately evacuated
7. during the above steps, place a moist sponge on the surface of the brain and gently but firmly apply evenly distributed pressure to push the brain back into the wound
8. if all else is failing, the craniotomy flap can be enlarged as much as possible to create a decompressive craniotomy. Enlarging the skin incision to do so is preferable to having too small a bony opening, which risks brain compression/laceration against the edges. The skin is closed without the bone flap and without dural closure as in a decompressive craniectomy (p. 1765)
9. a last-ditch life-saving measure for continued uncontrollable swelling which is to be taken under advisement with eloquent cortex: use a gloved hand to sweep the herniating brain out of the wound (i.e., remove it from the patient)

104.1.4 Craniotomy pre- and post-op management

Risks

Many risks cannot be generalized for all craniotomies and are specific to various tumors, aneurysms, etc. General information:
1. postoperative hemorrhage
   a) overall risk of postoperative hemorrhage[2,3]: 0.8–1.1%. The most common indication for craniotomy in these series was for meningioma, followed by trauma, aneurysm, and then intrinsic supratentorial tumors. 43–60% of the hematomas were intraparenchymal, 28–33% epidural, 5–7% subdural, 5% intrasellar, 8% mixed, 11% confined to superficial wound. Overall mortality was 32%
   b) hematoma may occur at the surgical site or in remote locations, e.g., intracerebellar hemorrhage after pterional[4] and temporal[5] craniotomies
2. in craniotomy for brain tumor[6]:
   a) risk of anesthetic complications: 0.2%
   b) increased neurologic deficit in first 24 hours post-op: ≈ 10%
   c) wound infection: 2%
3. postoperative headache (p. 1731)

Pre-op orders

1. for tumor: if patient on steroids, give ≈ 50% higher dose 6 hrs before and on-call to O.R. (stress doses); if not on steroids give dexamethasone 10 mg PO 6 hrs before and on-call to O.R. (in A.M., give with a sip of water)
2. antiepileptic medication
   a) if there is a history of seizures:
      • if already on antiseizure medications (ASMs) continue same doses
      • if not on ASMs, load with Keppra 500 mg or oral PHT (may give 300 mg PO q 4 hrs × 3 doses (total 900 mg) to load orally)
   b) if no history of seizures:
      • if surgery does not require a cortical incision (e.g., aneurysm) then ASMs are generally not used
      • if a cortical incision is anticipated, option to load with ASMs as above
3. prophylactic antibiotics: (optional) ideally 30–60 minutes before incision. For most antibiotics, it is given in the O.R. before the skin incision. For antibiotics that take a long time to infuse (e.g., vancomycin) it may help to order it to be given "on call to O.R."
4. DVT prophylaxis: pneumatic compression boots or knee-high TED® hose

104

Post-op orders

Guidelines (individualize as appropriate) for patient to be extubated
1. admit PACU, transfer to ICU (neuro unit if available) when stable
2. VS: q 15 min x 4 hrs, then q 1 hr. Temperature q 4 hrs x 3 d, then q 8 hrs. Neuro check q 1 hr
3. activity: bed rest (BR) with HOB elevated 20–30°
4. knee-high TED hose or pneumatic compression boots
5. I & O q 1 hr (if no Foley: straight cath q 4 hrs PRN bladder distension)
6. incentive spirometry q 2 hrs while awake (*do not use following transsphenoidal surgery*)
7. diet: NPO except minimal ice chips and meds as ordered
8. IVF: NS + 20 mEq KCl/L @ 90 ml/hr
9. O$_2$: 2 L per NC
10. meds:
    a) dexamethasone (Decadron®): if not on chronic steroids, give 4 mg IV q 6 hrs. Otherwise give stress doses based on patient's current dose and length of treatment
    b) H2 antagonist, e.g., ranitidine 50 mg IVPB q 8 hrs
    c) Anti-epileptic drug (ASM) especially when cerebral cortex is violated: typically Keppra® (levetiracetam): 500 mg PO or IV q 12 hours. If there is no prior history of seizure, typically discontinue after ≈ 1 week
    d) Cardene® drip: titrate to keep SBP < 160 mm Hg and/or DBP < 100 mm Hg (use cuff pressures, may use A-line pressures if they correlate with cuff pressures)
    e) codeine 30–60 mg IM q 3–4 hrs PRN H/A
    f) acetaminophen (Tylenol®) 650 mg PO/PR q 4 hrs PRN temperature > 100.5 °F (38 °C)
    g) continue prophylactic antibiotics if used: (e.g., cefazolin (Kefzol®) 500–1000 mg IVPB q 6 hrs x 24 hrs, then D/C)
11. labs:
    a) CBC once stabilized in ICU and q d thereafter
    b) renal profile once stabilized in ICU and q 12 hrs thereafter
    c) ABG once stabilized in ICU and q 12 hrs x 2 days, then D/C (also check ABG after any ventilator change if patient on ventilator)
12. call M.D. if any deterioration in crani checks, for T > 101 °F (38.5 °C), sudden increase in SBP, SBP < 120, U.O. < 60 ml/2-hrs
13. post-op CT: non-contrast post-op head CT is performed if the patient does not return to baseline neurologic function within a reasonable amount of time; also, performed routinely at many institutions following all craniotomies

104.1.5 Postoperative deterioration

General information

When the postoperative neurologic status is worse than pre-op, especially in a patient who deteriorates after initially doing well following surgery, emergency evaluation and treatment is indicated.
Possible etiologies:
1. hematoma (p. 1729)
   a) intracerebral hemorrhage (ICH): at or remote from surgical site
   b) epidural hematoma
   c) subdural hematoma
2. cerebral infarction
   a) arterial
   b) venous infarction: especially with surgery on or around the venous sinuses (p. 1761)
3. postoperative seizure: may be due to inadequate antiseizure medication levels, and may be exacerbated by any of the above (see below for management)
4. acute hydrocephalus
5. pneumocephalus; also see Pneumocephalus (p. 1067):
   a) tension pneumocephalus: see Tension pneumocephalus (p. 1068)
   b) simple pneumocephalus: the simple presence of air in the cranium can cause neurologic symptoms even if not under tension (as would commonly occur following the now outdated pneumoencephalogram). Symptoms include: lethargy, confusion, severe headache, nausea & vomiting, seizures. Air may be located over the cerebral convexities, in the p-fossa, and/or in the ventricles and usually resorbs with symptomatic improvement in 1–3 days

6. edema: may improve with steroids
   a) worsening of cerebral edema: moderate post-op worsening of cortical function of immediately adjacent brain is not unexpected in many operations, and is usually transient. However, reversible etiologies (such as subdural hematoma (SDH)) must be ruled out
   b) traction or manipulation of cranial nerves may cause dysfunction that may be temporary. Division of cranial nerves can cause permanent dysfunction
7. persistent anesthetic effect (including paralytics): unlikely in a patient who deteriorates after initially doing well post-op. Consider reversing medication given during surgery (caution re: hypertension and agitation), e.g., naloxone, flumazenil (p. 320), or reversal of pharmacologic muscle block (p. 143)
8. vasospasm: following SAH or may be due to manipulation of blood vessels

Postoperative seizure management

1. intubate if patient does not rapidly regain consciousness, is not protecting airway, or has labored respirations
2. CT scan: rule out hematoma (intracerebral or extra-axial) or hydrocephalus
3. antiseizure medications:
   a) draw blood for appropriate antiseizure medication level
   b) bolus with additional antiseizure medications: do not wait for levels

104.1.6 Postoperative headache

General information

Also see the "syndrome of the trephined" (p. 1763).

Persistent headache (H/A) is well described following posterior fossa craniectomy (incidence range: 0–83%[7]). The time course in one series[8] was: 23% at 3 mos, 16% at 1 yr, and 9% at 2 yrs.

Persistent H/A may also be observed following supratentorial craniotomy[9] (prevalence 1 year after anterior temporal lobectomy for seizures: 12%[9]).

These H/A have been attributed to traction on the dura when the bone is not replaced, tension on the dura due to tight dural closure, temporalis or nuchal muscle dissection, nerve entrapment in the closing sutures or in the healing scar (especially the greater occipital nerve following suboccipital craniotomies), intradural blood and/or bone dust, and CSF leak.[9]

Prevention

No single method or group of methods has been successful in completely eliminating the complaint of post-op H/A.[10,11] Until further research can further advance the understanding of the cause and prevention of these H/A, it seems reasonable to employ the following measures as much as possible in an attempt to minimize these debilitating symptoms: restoring function of the temporalis or suboccipital musculature, rigid fixation of bone flaps, cranioplasty for large craniectomies, meticulous tension-free dural closure (using duraplasty when necessary), and keeping intradural blood clot and bone dust to the minimum possible.[12] Cranioplasty following posterior fossa surgery for vestibular schwannoma reduced the incidence of post-op H/A from 17% to 4%.[13]

Treatment

Initially, symptomatic treatment is indicated. Referral to a H/A specialist may be appropriate when it becomes apparent that the H/A are not resolving spontaneously after ≈ 3 months.[12]

104.2 Intraoperative cortical mapping (brain mapping)

104.2.1 General information

Indications: typically used to locate the motor strip, sensory cortex, or speech centers intraoperatively for surgery in and around these eloquent areas. Localization of these areas based on visible anatomy alone is unreliable. These techniques are typically employed in seizure surgery as well as in treating lesions in areas of eloquent brain.

Some techniques require an awake patient, with the surgery done under local anesthesia with sedation. Motor and sensory cortex can also be localized in anesthetized patients using SSEPs (see below).

104.2.2 Phase reversal method for localizing primary sensory and motor cortex

General information

Utilizes intraoperative SSEPs to localize primary sensory and motor cortex in patients under general anesthesia (as opposed to using brain mapping techniques in awake patients).[14,15]

Technique

See anesthesia requirements for intraoperative EP monitoring (p. 112). A strip grid is placed on the surface of the brain perpendicular to the anticipated orientation of the central sulcus. SSEP stimulation is performed while recording through the strip grid. Phase reversal of the N20/P20 peak between a pair of electrodes in the strip grid indicates that those electrodes straddle the central sulcus (▶ Fig. 104.1) with primary motor cortex located anteriorly, and sensory cortex posteriorly. The grid is then repositioned and the test is run again to verify the findings.

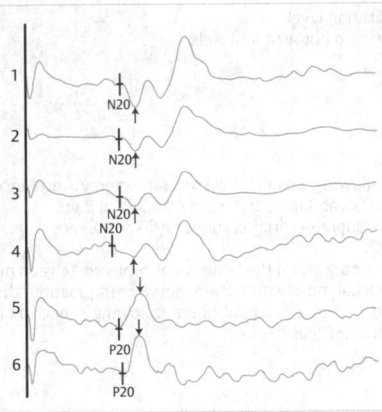

Fig. 104.1 Phase reversal.
Intra-op 6-electrode recording strip placed on the brain during SSEP recording. Phase reversal of the negative N20 peak (*arrows*) to a positive P20 peak between electrodes #4 & 5 indicates that electrodes #4 & 5 straddle the central sulcus.

104.2.3 Awake craniotomy

General information

Usually employed for brain mapping, especially for speech areas. Numerous techniques and protocols have been described. Typically, the patient is temporarily anesthetized with short-acting agent (inhalational and/or injectable). This is supplemented with local anesthetic. The craniotomy is performed and the patient is allowed to wake up while the brain is exposed to permit neurophysiologic testing during surgery. If (short-acting) paralytics are used, it is critical to reverse these agents 15–30 minutes prior to applying the electrical stimulation and that a train-of-four muscle twitch can be elicited.

Booking the case: Awake craniotomy

Also see defaults & disclaimers (p. 25) and pre-op counselling (see below).
1. position: depends on lesion location, with pin headholder (for image-guided navigation if used)
2. equipment:
   a) microscope if needed e.g., for tumor dissection
   b) image-guided navigation system (if used)
   c) ultrasonic aspirator (for tumors)
3. anesthesia: pre-op consult for "awake craniotomy" & skull block
4. consult neurology or neuropsychology to be available during surgery for intra-op neurologic testing for "awake craniotomy"

5. EEG techs to perform intra-op EEG and provide brain stimulator
6. post-op: ICU
7. consent (in lay terms for the patient—not all-inclusive):
    a) procedure: surgery on the brain to be performed with periods where the patient will be woken up for testing (plus whatever else is planned, e.g., removal of tumor, removal of seizure source...)
    b) alternatives: the same surgery under general anesthesia, nonsurgical management (for some diagnoses, e.g., tumor, radiation therapy)
    c) complications: (usual craniotomy complications (p. 25): stroke, bleeding, coma, death, infection, seizures), difficulty accurately mapping the desired areas of the brain

104

Indications

1. surgery in eloquent brain (near motor strip (Brodmann's area 4 in ▶ Fig. 1.1) or speech/language centers or thalamus) including tumors and epileptic foci
2. removal of brainstem tumors
3. some seizure surgery to look for seizure focus

Contraindications to awake craniotomy

1. patients unlikely to be able to cooperate: very young or very elderly patients, confused patients, those with significant speech deficits already present or language barrier

Patient counselling pre-op

Patients need to be aware of what the sequence of events will be and what will be expected of them. It may be helpful to have them practice reading some typical material that will be used in the O.R. Patients over age ≈ 40 usually need reading glasses to see written material, and they should have their own available in the O.R., although the temples (earpieces) usually can't be accommodated. The patient should be advised that there may be some pain involved.

Patient positioning for surgery

Significantly more time must be spent on patient positioning to ensure that they will be as comfortable as possible without moving. Extra padding is employed. Access to the patient's face is necessary for the anesthesiologist and the neurophysiologist.

Typical sequence for anesthesia

See reference.[16]

1. in the pre-op holding area, load with Precedex® (dexmedetomidine) 0.5 mcg/kg IV over 20 minutes followed by intra-op infusion at 0.4–1.0 mcg/kg/hr
2. induction of anesthesia utilizes propofol 3 mg/kg IV followed by laryngeal mask airway (LMA) placement
3. skull block[17]: injection of local anesthetic (e.g., 30 ml of 0.5% bupivacaine) to permit the skin incision and also rigid head fixation with pins (as required for image navigation devices, and situations where no head movement can be tolerated during surgery) without pain at the time of the wake-up. Injection at 4 regions on each side as shown in ▶ Fig. 104.2:
    ❶ supraorbital & supratrochlear nerves: 2 ml injected 1.5 cm above the supraorbital foramen above the medial third of the orbit. NB: if you are going to use surface matching to register the patient for image guidance (e.g., BrainLab or Stealth), injecting here may deform the skin and affect the registration accuracy. Consider injecting a lower volume of higher concentration agent (e.g., 2% lidocaine)
    ❷ auriculotemporal nerve: 5 ml injected 1.5 cm anterior to the tragus. ✖ Caution: to avoid anesthetizing the facial nerve, inject just deep to the subcutaneous tissue
    ❸ postauricular branches of the greater auricular nerve: 2 ml 1.5 cm posterior to the antitragus
    ❹ greater, lesser, & third occipital nerves: inject 5 ml with a 22 gauge spinal needle at the mastoid process and proceed along the nuchal ridge until the midline is reached
4. start inhalational anesthesia with 0.5 MAC desflurane with the patient breathing spontaneously while the scalp incision, craniotomy, and dural opening are performed (the dura is pain-sensitive, the brain is not)

104

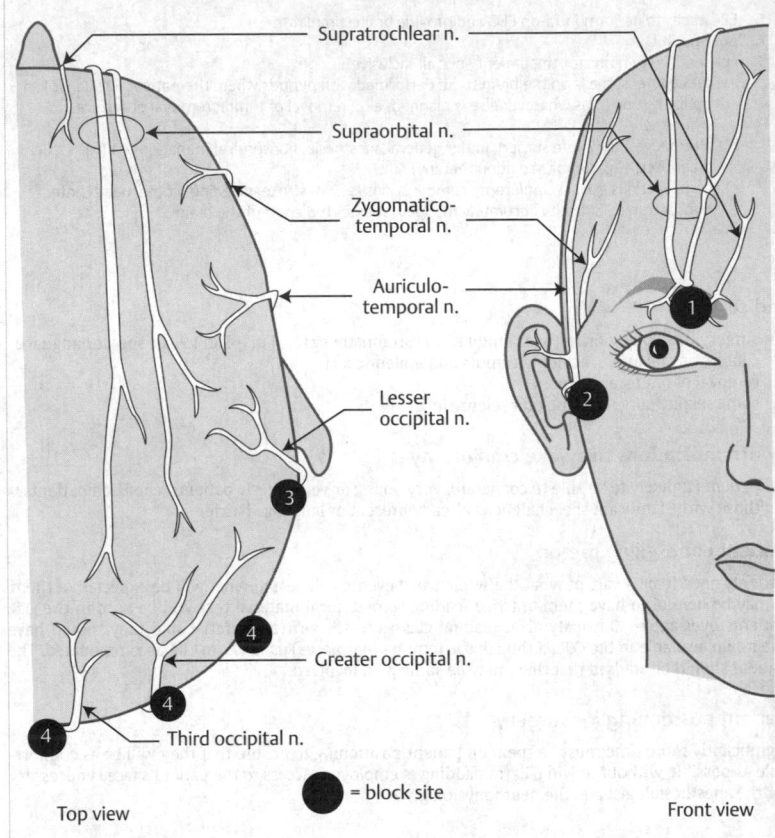

Fig. 104.2 Infiltration sites for skull block.

5. as the dural opening is begun, the desflurane is turned off and a remifentanil infusion of 0.1–0.2 mcg/kg/min IV is started
6. by the time the dural opening is completed, the desflurane has usually worn off and the LMA can be removed
7. remifentanil is then titrated for pain control
8. neurophysiologic testing can usually be performed at this time (e.g., below)
9. the operation may often be carried to completion with the patient awake, although once the intracranial part of the operation is completed, more pain relief may be desired and general anesthesia may be needed for pain control or agitation (LMA may suffice here)

104.2.4 Speech mapping

General information

Typical settings for a constant current generator using a bipolar electrode are shown in ▶ Table 104.1. If a voltage-based unit is used, start at 1 volt and increase.

Table 104.1 Settings for constant current generator

Control	Setting[a]
frequency	50–60 Hz
waveform	biphasic square wave
duration	2–4 mS peak-to-peak
mode	repeat
polarity	normal
current	varies between 2–16 mA

[a]not all settings are present on all models

104

Techniques for language mapping

There are numerous methodologies. One protocol for cortical mapping:

1. requires awake craniotomy
2. once the temporal lobe is exposed, a recording electrode strip is placed on the brain surface
3. using a bipolar stimulator, start with a low current (e.g., 2 mA) and begin stimulating an area of the cortex for 3–5 seconds, and observe for afterdischarges (akin to a focal seizure) on the recording strip. If no afterdischarges, increase the current in 2-mA increments up to a maximum of ≈ 10 mA. If afterdischarges occur, back off by 1–2 mA and then test that area for speech changes as follows
4. stimulate cortex while patient names objects shown on picture cards (automatic verbalization, such as counting, is robust and may persist). Observe for effects including[18]:
   a) total speech arrest[18]: on the dominant hemisphere typically in the pars opercularis or precentral gyrus, but also in frontal operculum and temporoparietal region. On the non-dominant hemisphere, this occurred only in the pars opercularis.
   b) able to speak but unable to name[18,19] (dysnomia): in dominant hemisphere, typically in posterior inferior frontal gyrus, and posterior temporal and inferior parietal regions
   c) semantic errors: posterior middle temporal gyrus, anterior supramarginal gyrus, and inferior frontal gyrus
   d) phonological paraphrasias, neologisms, and circumlocution: superior temporal sulcus
   e) NB: subcortical fiber mapping may identify white matter tracts that participate in language processing (see reference[19])
5. repeat the above steps at the next area (first finding threshold for afterdischarges and then stimulating while testing)

References

[1] FDA. Cranial Perforators with an Automatic Clutch Mechanism, Failure to Disengage: FDA Safety Communication. 2015. http://wayback.archive-it.org/7993/20170722215717/https://www.fda.gov/MedicalDevices/Safety/AlertsandNotices/ucm464596.htm
[2] Kalfas IH, Little JR. Postoperative Hemorrhage: A Survey of 4992 Intracranial Procedures. Neurosurgery. 1988; 23:343–347
[3] Palmer JD, Sparrow OC, Iannotti FI. Postoperative Hematoma: A 5-Year Survey and Identification of Avoidable Risk Factors. Neurosurgery. 1994; 35:1061–1065
[4] Papanastassiou V, Kerr R, Adams C. Contralateral Cerebellar Hemorrhage After Pterional Craniotomy: Report of Five Cases and Review of the Literature. Neurosurgery. 1996; 39:841–852
[5] Toczek MT, Morrell MJ, Silverberg GA, et al. Cerebellar Hemorrhage Complicating Temporal Lobectomy: Report of Four Cases. Journal of Neurosurgery. 1996; 85:718–722
[6] Mahaley MS, Mettlin C, Natarajan N, et al. National Survey of Patterns of Care for Brain-Tumor Patients. J Neurosurg. 1989; 71:826–836
[7] Driscoll CL, Beatty CW. Pain After Acoustic Neuroma Surgery. Otolaryngologic Clinics of North America. 1997; 30:893–903
[8] Harner SG, Beatty CW, Ebersold MJ. Headache After Acoustic Neuroma Excision. American Journal of Otolaryngology. 1993; 14:552–555

[9] Kaur A, Selwa L, Fromes G, et al. Persistent Headache After Supratentorial Craniotomy. Neurosurgery. 2000; 47:633–636
[10] Catalano PJ, Jacobowitz O, Post KD. Prevention of Headache After Retrosigmoid Removal of Acoustic Tumors. American Journal of Otology. 1996; 17:904–908
[11] Lovely TJ, Lowry DW, Jannetta PJ. Functional Outcome and the Effect of Cranioplasty After Retromastoid Craniectomy for Microvascular Decompression. Surgical Neurology. 1999; 51:191–197
[12] Long DM. Comment on Kaur A et al.: Persistent Headache After Supratentorial Craniotomy. Neurosurgery. 2000; 47
[13] Harner SG, Beatty CW, Ebersold MJ. Impact of cranioplasty on headache after acoustic neuroma removal. Neurosurgery. 1995; 36:1097–9; discussion 1099-100
[14] Gregori EM, Goldring S. Localization of Function in the Excision of Lesions from the Sensorimotor Region. Journal of Neurosurgery. 1984; 61:1047–1054
[15] Woolsey CN, Erickson TC, Gibson WE. Localization in Somatic Sensory and Motor Areas of Human Cerebral Cortex as Determined by Direct Recording of Evoked Potentials and Electrical Stimulation. Journal of Neurosurgery. 1979; 51:476–506
[16] Dreier JD, Williams B, Mangar D, et al. Patients selection for awake neurosurgery. HSR Proc. 2009; 1:19–27

[17] Pinosky ML, Fishman RL, Reeves ST, et al. The effect of bipuvicaine skull block on the hemodynamic response to craniotomy. Neurosurgical Anesthesia. 1996; 83:1256–1261

[18] Penfield W, Roberts L. Speech and Brain Mechanisms. Princeton, NJ: Princeton University Press; 1959:103–137

[19] Chang EF, Raygor KP, Berger MS. Contemporary model of language organization: an overview for neurosurgeons. J Neurosurg. 2015; 122:250–261

104

105 Posterior Fossa Craniotomies

105.1 Indications

To gain access to the cerebellum, cerebellopontine angle (CPA), to one vertebral artery, posterior brainstem, 4th ventricle, pineal region, or using extreme lateral posterior fossa approach to the antero-lateral brainstem. See paramedian (p. 1740) and midline (p. 1742) suboccipital craniectomies for details.

105.2 Position

105.2.1 Options

Position options include:
1. sitting position (p. 1737)
2. lateral oblique (p. 1738) ("park bench"): patient three-quarters oblique (almost prone). Often used for access to cerebellar hemisphere lesion
3. semi-sitting
4. supine with shoulder roll, head almost horizontal
5. prone
6. Concorde position: often used for access to midline (e.g., 4th ventricle). Prone, thorax elevated 20°, neck flexed and tilted slightly away from the side on which the surgeon will be standing

105.2.2 Sitting position

Used less frequently than in the past because of associated complications and acceptable alternative positions (except for some specific circumstances). However, some experts feel that the risks of the sitting position have been greatly overstated.[1] The presence of a ventricular CSF shunt is considered to be a contraindication to the use of the sitting position by some.

Advantages

1. improved drainage of blood and CSF out of surgical site
2. enhanced venous drainage which helps reduce venous bleeding and also ICP
3. easy ventilation due to unencumbered chest
4. patient's head may be kept exactly midline, aiding operator orientation and reducing risk of kinking of vertebral arteries

Disadvantages/risks

1. possible air embolism (see below)
2. fatigue of operator's hands
3. increased surgical risks from placement of CVP catheter (required to treat possible AE): e.g., pneumothorax with subclavian vein catheterization, thrombosis
4. risk of post-op hematoma at the operative site may be increased because potential venous bleeders may remain occult while the patient is sitting, but may manifest when patient returns to a horizontal position post-op. However, one study found no such increased incidence[2]
5. risk of post-op subdural hematoma: 1.3% of p-fossa cases[3]
6. possible brachial plexus injury: prevent this by not allowing patient's arms to hang at the side. Instead, fold them across abdomen
7. midcervical quadriplegia[4,5]: presumably due to flexion myelopathy.[6,7,8] The combination of the sitting position with hypotension[9] or neck flexion with possible compression of the anterior spinal artery, ± cervical bar, and elevation of the head thus reducing the arterial pressure may all contribute
8. sciatic nerve injury (piriformis syndrome)[10]: prevent this by flexing patient's knees (reduces tension on sciatic nerve)
9. extent of post-op pneumocephalus is more pronounced, and may increase the risk of tension pneumocephalus[11]; see Pneumocephalus (p. 1067)
10. venous pooling of blood in the LEs under anesthesia may cause relative hypovolemia and should be counteracted by binding the LEs prior to positioning
11. decreased cerebral blood flow due to lower hemodynamic arterial pressure[12]

► **Air embolism (AE).** A potentially fatal complication of any operation when an opening to air occurs in a non-collapsible vein (e.g., diploic vein or a dural sinus) when there is a negative pressure in the vein (e.g., when the head is elevated above the heart).[13] Air is entrained in the vein and can become trapped in the right atrium of the heart, which may impair venous return, causing hypotension. AE has also been described with endovascular procedures.[14] AE may also produce cardiac arrhythmias. Paradoxical air embolism can occur in the presence of a patent foramen ovale[15] or pulmonary AV fistula, and may produce ischemic cerebral infarction.

Greater negative pressures occur in the sitting position due to the extreme elevation of the head, but AE can occur in any operation with the head elevated higher than the heart. Incidence: a wide range has been quoted in the literature, and depends on the monitoring method used: ≈ 7–25% incidence with the sitting position using Doppler monitoring is an estimate.[3]

For operations with a *significant* risk of AE, a right atrial CVP line is recommended (to aspirate air), and monitoring for air embolism; options include: transesophageal echo (the most sensitive), precordial Doppler monitoring. (Although technically the risk of air embolism includes *any* case where the head is higher than the right cardiac atrium, practically it is limited to cases where the head of the bed is ≈ > 30° which is mostly limited to the sitting position for posterior fossa tumors.)

Diagnosis and treatment:

AE should be suspected in any operative case in which the surgical site is higher than the heart when there is any unexplained hypotension or decrease in EtCO$_2$.[18]

- transesophageal echocardiography (TEE). Bubbles can be seen on the 2D echo display
  pros: considered the most sensitive monitoring modality
  cons: significant false-positive rate, expensive, invasive, requires experience and vigilance
- precordial Doppler U/S: probe may be placed over 2nd to 4th intercostal space either to right or left of sternum, or posteriorly between the scapula and spine. AE is heralded by a change in sonic intensity and character at first by a superimposed irregular high-pitched swishing sound, and then as more air is entrained so called "mill wheel" or machinery sounds dominate
  pros: the most sensitive of the non-invasive techniques
  cons: difficult in morbidly obese patients and in certain patient positions (e.g., prone or lateral), interference from other sounds in the O.R., requires vigilance

The earliest indication of AE may be a rise in the end-tidal nitrogen (requires mass-spectrometer on monitor), then a fall in the end-tidal pCO$_2$ occurs. Machinery sounds in the precordial Doppler also suggest AE. Hypotension may develop. Measures shown in ► Table 105.1 should be immediately instituted.

Table 105.1 Treatment for air embolism

1. find and occlude site of air entry, or else rapidly pack wound with sopping wet sponges/laps and wax bone edges
2. Durant's maneuver[16]: lower patient's head if at all possible (Trendelenburg) and rotate patient *LEFT* side down (attempt to trap air in right atrium)
3. jugular venous compression (bilateral best; second choice: right only)
4. aspirate air from right atrium via CVP catheter
5. ventilate patient with 100% O$_2$
6. discontinue nitrous oxide if used (may expand AE)[17]
7. use pressors and volume expanders to maintain BP
8. PEEP is *ineffective* in preventing or treating AE; may increase the risk of paradoxical AE[13]

105.2.3 Lateral oblique position

AKA "park bench" position.

- axillary roll for the down-side arm (see ► Fig. 105.1) (or position the patient so that the down-side arm extends over the edge of the table and is held in place by a sling formed by the Mayfield table attachment with copious padding)
- upper arm supported on pillows or towels (avoid using a Mayo stand, which restricts the ability to laterally tilt the O.R. table during surgery)
- adhesive tape to gently pull down on the upper shoulder
- bring the patient's back as close to the side edge of the table as possible (usually limited by the travel of the head clamp) to bring the patient closer to the surgeon
- elevate thorax 10–15°
- see Head positioning (p. 1739)
- optional spinal drainage (usually for large tumors)

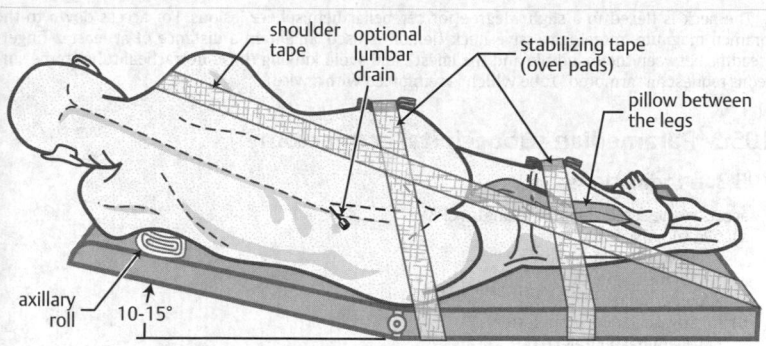

Fig. 105.1 Lateral oblique ("park bench") position.

- some surgeons prefer the LE that contacts the table to be slightly flexed at the hip & knee to stabilize the patient, others prefer the uppermost LE to be flexed to allow the patient to "fall forward" a little more at the hips. Place a pillow between the legs
- secure patient with adhesive tape over pads so that the table can be "airplaned" (rolled) during the operation

For access to the porus acusticus or more caudally

(E.g., for vestibular schwannomas; not necessary for microvascular decompression for trigeminal neuralgia.)

Get the shoulders out of the way by flexing the neck as much as possible while maintaining patent airway (aided by use of non-kinking wire-reinforced ET tube, so-called **"armored tube"**). The upper shoulder is retracted caudally by adhesive tape (avoid excess traction which may injure brachial plexus).

Head positioning

A Mayfield head-holder (p. 1717) is placed with the single pin on the side of the lesion, slightly anterior to a true-lateral on the skull (▸ Fig. 105.2). In an adult, it is tightened until the third ring (60 lbs) is just visible on the spring-loaded indicator.

Tip the vertex of the head slightly towards the floor by bringing the downside ear towards the ipsilateral shoulder.

The head is rotated 20–30° face-down from the horizontal (▸ Fig. 105.2).

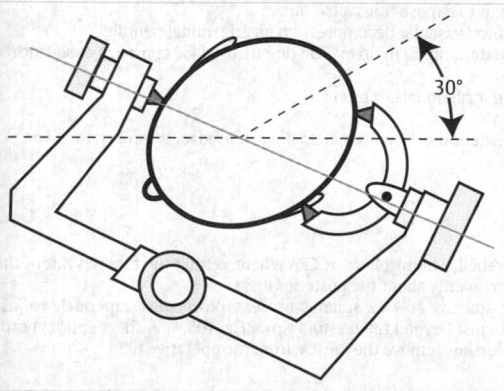

Fig. 105.2 Head-holder placement and rotation of head for a right suboccipital craniectomy (looking down on top of patient's head).

The neck is flexed to a slight degree for cerebellar hemisphere lesions. For access down to the foramen magnum, more aggressive neck flexion is used (maintain a distance of at least 2 finger-breadths between the mandible and the chest), and avoid kinking the endotracheal tube (some surgeons request an "armored" tube which is reinforced with a wire).

105.3 Paramedian suboccipital craniectomy

105.3.1 Indications

1. access to the cerebellopontine angle (CPA)
   a) CPA tumors, including:
      - vestibular schwannoma
      - CPA meningioma
      - epidermoid
   b) microvascular decompression
      - trigeminal neuralgia
      - hemifacial spasm
      - miscellaneous: geniculate neuralgia, glossopharyngeal neuralgia
2. lesions of one cerebellar hemisphere (typically lesions < 2.5 cm diameter):
   a) tumors: metastases, hemangioblastomas…
   b) hemorrhage within cerebellar hemisphere
3. access to vertebral artery
   a) aneurysms: PICA, vertebrobasilar junction
   b) vertebral endarterectomy
4. access to anterolateral brainstem tumors (extreme lateral p-fossa approach)
   a) foramen magnum tumors, including: chordomas, meningiomas

105.3.2 Position, skin incision, craniectomy, approach…

See list of alternatives (p. 1737). See lateral oblique position (p. 1738).

105.3.3 Skin incision

Linear (paramedian) incisions

A vertical linear paramedian incision provides adequate exposure for lesions < 2.5 cm diameter and involves less trauma to overlying muscles, and may be easier to get watertight closure than with midline incision.

For lesions in the cerebellar hemisphere: a linear vertical incision approximately midway between the midline and the mastoid notch may be used.

Access to CPA (for microvascular decompressions and *small* CPA tumors): a slightly curved retro-mastoid incision placed 5 mm medial to the mastoid notch (a palpable landmark) is used (▶ Fig. 105.3):

1. "5–6-4" incision (incision placed 5 mm medial to mastoid notch, extending from 6 cm above notch to 4 cm below). High enough to expose transverse sinus:
   a) for approach to fifth nerve: microvascular decompression for trigeminal neuralgia
2. "5–5-5" incision (5 mm medial, extending 5 cm up to 5 cm down), used for approach to seventh/eighth nerve complex:
   a) microvascular decompression for hemifacial spasm
   b) small vestibular schwannoma
3. "5–4-6" incision (5 mm medial, extending 4 cm up to 6 cm down): used for approach to lower cranial nerves:
   a) glossopharyngeal neuralgia

"Hockey-stick" incision

Useful for lesions > 2.5 cm in the cerebellar hemisphere or CPA where getting the muscles out of the way will facilitate maneuvering instruments about the posterior fossa.

Incision is made in the midline starting at ≈ C2 spinous process, proceeding superiorly to just above the inion, and then laterally to just beyond the mastoid tip (▶ Fig. 105.4). A short optional caudal curve may be made laterally to further remove the muscle from the operative field.

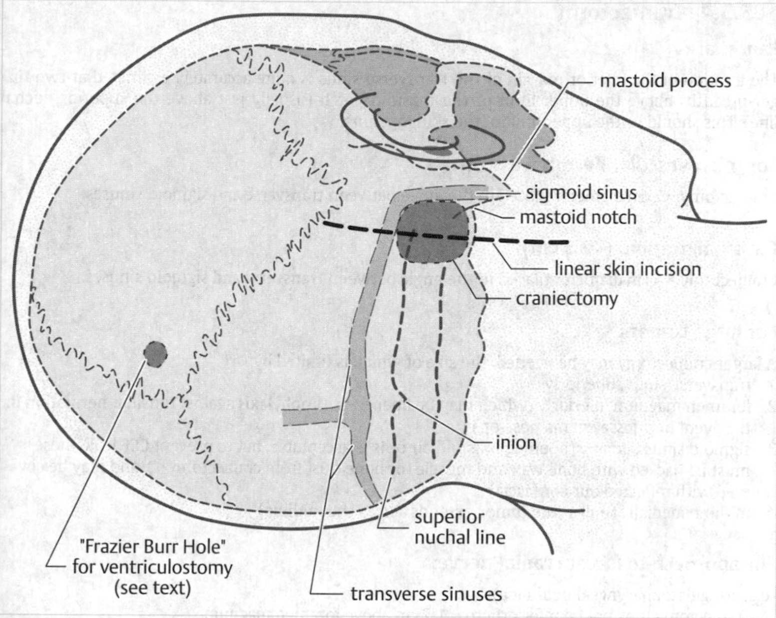

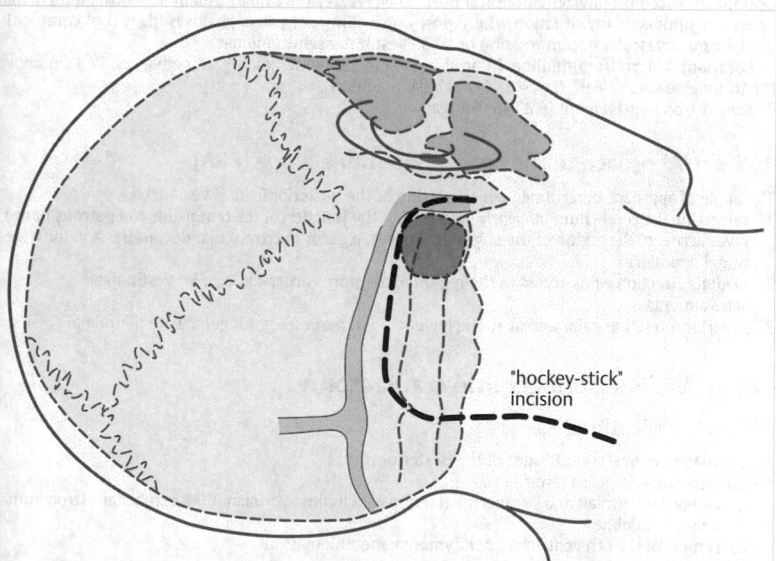

Fig. 105.3 Retromastoid suboccipital craniectomy.

mastoid process
sigmoid sinus
mastoid notch
linear skin incision
craniectomy
inion
superior nuchal line
transverse sinuses
"Frazier Burr Hole" for ventriculostomy (see text)

Fig. 105.4 "Hockey-stick" skin incision.

"hockey-stick" incision

105.3.4 Craniectomy

Landmarks

The location of the inferior margin of the transverse sinus is quite accurately estimated at two fin-ger-breadths above the upper limit of the mastoid notch (usually just above the superior nuchal line). This should be the upper limit of the skull opening.

For microvascular decompression

Craniectomy ≈ 2 cm diameter placed in the angle between transverse and sigmoid sinuses.

For small tumors (<2.5 cm)

Craniectomy ≈ 4 cm diameter placed in the angle between transverse and sigmoid sinuses.

For large tumors

A larger craniectomy may be needed, the size of which is limited by:
1. transverse sinus superiorly
2. foramen magnum inferiorly (which may be opened as prophylaxis against tonsillar herniation in the event of p-fossa edema post-op)
3. sigmoid sinus laterally (opening mastoid air cells is acceptable, but to prevent CSF leak, these must be packed with bone wax and muscle (or bone dust from craniectomy[19]), and may be cov-ered with reflected dura or fascia)
4. midline medially (unless the tumor extends across the midline)

For approach to lower cranial nerves

(e.g., for glossopharyngeal neuralgia).
Craniectomy is extended inferiorly to ≈ 1/2 cm above foramen magnum.

Burr hole for emergency ventriculostomy

Optionally placed prophylactic occipital burr hole (**Frazier burr hole**) usually for intraparenchymal cerebellar tumors or any situation where post-op swelling or hydrocephalus is likely (not commonly used for microvascular decompression or small vestibular schwannomas).
Location: 3–4 cm from midline. In adults, 6–7 cm above the inion[20]; in pediatrics, 2–3 cm above the transverse sinus[21 (p 429)] (i.e., ≈ 3–4 cm above the inion).
See Post-op management (p. 1745) for use.

105.3.5 Approach to the cerebellopontine angle (CPA)

The angle of approach determines which portion of the posterior fossa is visualized.
1. retracting the cerebellum *inferiorly* (working in the junction of the tentorium and petrous bone) gives access to the region of the trigeminal nerve, e.g., for microvascular decompression for trige-minal neuralgia
2. *medial* retraction gains access to the region of the porus acusticus, e.g., for vestibular schwannomas
3. *superior* retraction gains access to the lower cranial nerves, e.g., for geniculate neuralgia

105.4 Midline suboccipital craniectomy

105.4.1 Indications

Access to the midline or both sides of the posterior fossa
1. midline posterior fossa lesions
   a) cerebellar vermian and paravermian lesions, including: vermian AVM, cerebellar astrocytoma near the midline
   b) tumors of the 4th ventricle: ependymoma, medulloblastoma
   c) pineal region tumors
   d) brainstem lesions: brainstem vascular lesions (e.g., cavernous angioma)
2. decompressive craniectomies: e.g., for Chiari malformation
3. cerebellar hemisphere tumors: metastases, hemangioblastoma, pilocytic astrocytoma...

105.4.2 Position

See positioning (p. 1737). For midline lesions the Concorde position (p. 1737) is usually used.

105.4.3 Skin/fascia incision

Midline incision from ≈ 6 cm above inion to ≈ C2 spinous process. Take the incision a little higher if a Frazier burr hole is to be done (can then utilize the same skin incision). The skin incision should leave the muscles and fascia intact. It is often difficult to place Raney clips on the skin in this region. To facilitate water-tight closure, the fascia is "T'd" at the top, leaving a cuff of tissue on the occiput just above the superior nuchal line.

105.4.4 Craniectomy

105

Craniectomy implies removal of bone (often piecemeal) with no intention of replacing it. The advantage to not replacing the bone is that if there is post-op swelling, the inelastic bone flap may cause more pressure to be transmitted to the brainstem. A down-side to not replacing the bone is that local pain and/or "syndrome of the trephined" (p. 1763) may be more common. The bone opening is usually taken down to foramen magnum.

C1 removal: for cerebellar hemisphere tumors, many remove the posterior arch of C1 (caution re: vertebral arteries on superior aspect of C1). For 4th ventricular tumors, consider removing the arch of the tonsils extend below the foramen magnum.[22]

105.4.5 Approach

A "Y"-shaped durotomy is often used. If the lesion has a cystic component, aspiration through a ventricular needle is used to partially decompress it.

105.4.6 Approaches to the 4th ventricle

Applied anatomy[23]:
- 9 lobules of the cerebellar vermis: lingula, central lobule, culmen, declive, folium, tuber, pyramid, uvula, and nodule
- the tonsils are part of the cerebellar hemispheres. The 2 tonsils generally meet in the midline and must be separated to access the inferior 4th ventricle
- roof of the 4th ventricle
  - fastigium: the apex of the roof of the 4th ventricle and the dividing point between the superior and inferior portion of the 4th ventricle
  - the roof of the superior portion of the 4th ventricle is comprised primarily of the superior medullary velum and the medial surface of the superior cerebellar peduncles
  - the roof of the inferior portion of the 4th ventricle is formed by the tela choroidea and the inferior medullary velum. Key point: the roof of the inferior 4th ventricle is devoid of any known functional neural structures
- floor of the 4th ventricle
  - rostral two-thirds is the posterior aspect of the pons. Anatomical feature: the facial colliculus – a slight protuberance due to the internal genu (p. 607) of the facial nerve (Cr. N. VII)
  - caudal one-third is the posterior medulla oblongata
  - at the apex of the floor is the inferior terminus of the Sylvian aqueduct
  - the obex (where the 4th ventricle becomes the central spinal canal) is at the caudal end (deep and anterior to the foramen of Magendie)

General information:
- position, skin incision, craniectomy: as in Midline suboccipital craniectomy (p. 1742) using the Concorde position (p. 1737)
- the posterior arch of C1 does not need to be removed unless the tonsils extend inferior to the foramen magnum[22]
- options:
  - neuromonitoring: SSEP/MEP, BAER
  - temporary pacemaker in case of bradycardia due to brainstem manipulation
  - image-guided navigation: if used, fiducials placed before pre-op imaging and kept in place until surgery usually helps with registration

- complications:
  - hydrocephalus: incidence as high as 30%[24,25]; average is probably lower[22]
  - cerebellar mutism (p. 100): develops in up to 30%[24,25,26]
  - other complications[26]: dysarthria: 30%, dysphagia: 33%

Two main approaches to the 4th ventricle[23]:
1. transvermian approach (splitting the cerebellar vermis in the midline)
   - overview: the inferior vermis is incised and the two halves are retracted to opposite sides
   - split the vermis to the smallest extent possible (usually up to the fastigium, but not into the superior medullary velum)
   - the nodule, tela choroidea, and inferior medullary velum also need to be incised to access the 4th ventricle
   - superior exposure is limited by the superior medullary velum
   - PROS: wider and slighly more rostral exposure than telovelar approach
   - CONS: risk of caudal vermis syndrome (truncal ataxia, dysequilibrium, oscillation of head and trunk, nystagmus), cerebellar mutism, injury to dentate nucleus (more severe dysequilibrium)
2. telovelar approach (TVA)[22,23]
   - overview: exposes the 4th ventricle through the cerebello-medullary fissure without incising the vermis or cerebellar hemisphere
   - PROS: no functioning nerve tissue is harmed in the approach – which may reduce the risk of cerebellar dysfunction, including cerebellar mutism (p. 100); improved access to the lateral recess of the 4th ventricle
   - CONS: narrower corridor than with a widely split vermis; limited access to deep or large tumors involving the rostral third of the 4th ventricle; limited access to contralateral floor of the 4th ventricle (TVA can be done bilaterally to circumvent this limitation[23])
   - technique:
     - the uvula is exposed by separating the two tonsils
     - on the side where the approach is planned, dissect between the tonsil and the adjacent uvula
     - the tonsil is retracted to the side of the approach and the uvula is retracted to the opposite side to expose the tela choroidea and inferior medullary velum
     - PICA is usually seen clearly at this time & should be protected (along with its branches)
     - the inferior aspect of large tumors can often be seen protruding through the foramen of Magendie under the thin inferior medullary velum and tela choroidea
     - the tela choroidea and inferior medullary velum are opened to one side of the vermis and the vermis is retracted as a whole
     - the floor of the 4th ventricle (brainstem) is protected by sliding a cottonoid up along the floor

105.5 Extreme lateral posterior fossa approach

Allows access to anterolateral region of brainstem. Differs from above in that the skin incision is designed to get the bulk of the skin and muscle flap out of the way.

Key: remove the lip of the foramen magnum as far laterally as possible, best done with a diamond drill.

105.6 Cranioplasty for suboccipital craniectomy

Methylmethacrylate cranioplasty as part of the closure following suboccipital crani for vestibular schwannoma reduced the incidence of post-op H/A from 17% to 4%.[27]

105.7 Post-op considerations for p-fossa craniotomies

105.7.1 Post-op check

In addition to routine, the following should be checked:
1. respirations: rate, pattern (see Intubation below)
2. follow closely for hypertension (see below)
3. evidence of CSF leak through wound

105.7.2 Post-op management

Intubation

Post-op intubation for 24–48 hours is sometimes maintained on a precautionary basis: many complications often have respiratory arrest as the initial manifestation (see below), and the patient may deteriorate precipitously from this point. There is a trade-off as the stimulus of the endotracheal tube may exacerbate hypertension and patient agitation, and so sedation is often required, which may obscure the neuro exam and depress respirations. If the patient wakes up extremely well from an uncomplicated p-fossa crani and it is not late at night, most surgeons will extubate.

Hypertension

Hypertension should be avoided at all costs to prevent bleeding from tenuous vessels (e.g., nicardipine or clevedipine should be prepared prior to termination of the operation, and should be hanging and ready to titrate to keep SBP ≥ 160 mm Hg during the reversal of anesthesia and post-op).

Physician should be called for any sudden changes in BP post-op (may indicate elevated pressure in posterior fossa, see below).

105

105.7.3 Post-op complications

Posterior fossa edema and/or hematoma

In the posterior fossa, a small amount of mass effect can be rapidly fatal due to the paucity of room and the immediate transmission of pressure directly to the brainstem. It can also occlude CSF circulation through the aqueduct and cause *acute hydrocephalus* with the attendant risk of tonsillar herniation. Increased pressure in the p-fossa is usually heralded by sudden increases in BP or changes in respiratory pattern (pupillary reflexes, level of consciousness, and ICP are *not* affected until late). See p.1745) for emergency treatment measures.

Emergency treatment for p-fossa swelling

★ Rapid intubation, ventricular tap (through previously placed burr hole, if possible, see text), and reoperation are indicated. The wound should be opened immediately wherever patient is (recovery room, ICU, floor…). CT scanning may cost valuable minutes; it is rarely appropriate to delay treatment for this (must be judged on an individual basis).

To expedite ventricular taps, a prophylactic occipital burr hole (Frazier burr hole) is often placed during posterior fossa surgery to permit drainage of CSF from the lateral ventricles in the event of acute hydrocephalus from blockage of the 4th ventricle or aqueduct. If acute hydrocephalus develops (e.g., from a hematoma), an emergent percutaneous ventricular tap with ventricular needle (or, if not available, spinal needle) is performed, passing the needle through the burr hole aiming for the middle of the forehead. In the presence of acute hydrocephalus, CSF should be encountered at a depth of 4–5 cm. A final insertion depth of 10 cm is usually used. NB: this maneuver may provide a few more minutes while preparing for the definitive treatment of re-opening the wound; however, hydrocephalus may not initially be present since it takes some time to develop.

Suboccipital pseudomeningocele

An "internal" CSF fistula. Incidence following suboccipital craniectomy: 8[28]–28%.[29]

May be asymptomatic, but also may be associated with H/A, nausea/vomiting, local pain/tenderness. Some are soft and compressible, others may be tense.

Indications for operation:
1. external leak (CSF fistula, see below)
2. threatening integrity of incision
3. cosmetic deformity
4. causing symptoms

Treatment options (up to 67% require permanent CSF drainage[30]):
1. noninvasive measures: expectant management, fluid restriction, head wrapping, keeping HOB elevated, acetazolamide. Steroids may be used if aseptic meningitis is suspected

2. percutaneous aspiration: "tap and wrap."[21 (p 436)],[31] Risks introducing bacteria, causing infection
3. direct surgical exploration with multilayer re-closure[21 (p 436)]
4. lumbar drain: effective only if pseudomeningocele communicates with the subarachnoid space.
   ✖ May produce acute posterior fossa syndrome (H/A, nausea, vomiting, ataxia…)[28] especially if the pseudomeningocele doesn't communicate. Symptoms usually resolve with prompt discontinuation of lumbar drainage.[28],[29] Other potential complications: vagal nerve palsy, tonsillar herniation, subdural hematoma, kinking of PCA → stroke. Drainage options:
   a) external drain (temporary)
   b) lumboperitoneal shunt (permanent)
5. ventricular drainage
   a) EVD (temporary)
   b) shunt (permanent)

105

CSF fistula

Occurs in 5–17% of cases. A potential source of meningitis, thus CSF leak must be treated immediately.

Etiologies: controversial. May include:
1. abnormal CSF hydrodynamics (i.e., hydrocephalus). Maneuvers to stem the leak will likely fail until the CSF is shunted or hydrodynamics normalize
2. poor wound closure: probably blamed more often than it is the actual cause
3. subarachnoid scarring

May be associated with meningitis (aseptic or infectious), multiple operations. Formation may be facilitated by coughing/sneezing, postural changes, one-way ball-valve mechanism due to a tissue flap.

An external CSF leak may occur through:
1. the skin incision
2. via the eustachian tube; see possible routes of egress following suboccipital vestibular schwannoma removal (p. 794):
   a) through the nose (CSF rhinorrhea)
   b) down the back of the throat
3. the ear (CSF otorrhea) in cases with perforated TM

Treatment
Initial treatment measures to temporize in the hope that CSF hydrodynamics will normalize and/or that the leak site will scar closed within a few days:
1. elevate the HOB
2. lumbar subarachnoid drainage
3. if the leak occurs through the skin incision:
   a) reinforce the incision with sutures, e.g., running locked 3–0 nylon after preparation of the skin with antimicrobial and local anesthetic
   b) alternatively, the incision may be painted with several coats of collodion
If persistent, a CSF fistula requires surgical correction, see CSF fistula (cranial); for general information (p. 415), see CSF fistula following suboccipital removal of vestibular schwannoma (p. 796).

Fifth or seventh nerve injuries

Causes diminished corneal reflex with potential corneal ulceration; initially managed with isotonic eye drops (e.g., Natural Tears®) q 2–4 hrs & PRN, or with a moisturizing insert (e.g., Lacricert®) day, and at night with an eye patch or taping eyelid shut.

Miscellaneous

Supratentorial intracerebral hemorrhage has been described, and may result from transient hypertension.[32]

References

[1] Fager CA. Comment on Zeidman S M and Ducker T B: Posterior Cervical Laminoforaminotomy for Radiculopathy: Review of 172 Cases. Neurosurgery. 1993; 33

[2] Kalfas IH, Little JR. Postoperative Hemorrhage: A Survey of 4992 Intracranial Procedures. Neurosurgery. 1988; 23:343–347

[3] Standefer MS, Bay JW, Trusso R. The Sitting Position in Neurosurgery. Neurosurgery. 1984; 14:649–658

[4] Kurze T. Microsurgery of the Posterior Fossa. Clinical Neurosurgery. 1979; 26:463–478

[5] Hitselberger WE, House WF. A Warning Regarding the Sitting Position for Acoustic Tumor Surgery. Arch Otolaryngol. 1980; 106

[6] Wilder BL. Hypothesis: The Etiology of Midcervical Quadriplegia After Operation with the Patient in the Sitting Position. Neurosurgery. 1982; 11:530–531

[7] Iwasaki Y, Tashiro K, Kikuchi S, et al. Cervical Flexion Myelopathy: A "Tight Dural Canal Mechanism". Journal of Neurosurgery. 1987; 66:935–937

[8] Haisa T, Kondo T. Midcervical Flexion Myelopathy After Posterior Fossa Surgery in the Sitting Position: Case Report. Neurosurgery. 1996; 38:819–822

[9] Epstein NE, Danto J, Nardi D. Evaluation of Intraoperative Somatosensory-Evoked Potential Monitoring During 100 Cervical Operations. Spine. 1993; 18:737–747

[10] Brown JA, Braun MA, Namey TC. Piriformis Syndrome in a 10-Year-Old Boy as a Complication of Operation with the Patient in the Sitting Position. Neurosurgery. 1988; 23:117–119

[11] Lunsford LD, Maroon JC, Sheptak PE, et al. Subdural Tension Pneumocephalus: Report of Two Cases. J Neurosurg. 1979; 50:525–527

[12] Tindall GT, Craddock A, Greenfield JC. Effects of the Sitting Position on Blood Flow in the Internal Carotid Artery of Man During General Anesthesia. Journal of Neurosurgery. 1967; 26:383–389

[13] Grady MS, Bedford RF, Park TS. Changes in Superior Sagittal Sinus Pressure in Children with Head Elevation, Jugular Venous Compression, and PEEP. J Neurosurg. 1986; 65:199–202

[14] Gupta R, Vora N, Thomas A, et al. Symptomatic cerebral air embolism during neuro-angiographic procedures: incidence and problem avoidance. Neurocrit Care. 2007; 7:241–246

[15] Black S, Cucchiara RF, Nishimura RA, et al. Parameters Affecting Occurrence of Paradoxical Air Embolism. Anesthesiology. 1989; 71:235–241

[16] Ely EW, Hite RD, Baker AM, et al. Venous air embolism from central venous catheterization: a need for increased physician awareness. Crit Care Med. 1999; 27:2113–2117

[17] Munson ES, Merrick HC. Effect of Nitrous Oxide on Venous Air Embolism. Anesthesiology. 1966; 27:783–787

[18] Mirski MA, Lele AV, Fitzsimmons L, et al. Diagnosis and treatment of vascular air embolism. Anesthesiology. 2007; 106:164–177

[19] Symon L, Pell MF. Cerebrospinal Fluid Rhinorrhea Following Acoustic Neurinoma Surgery: Technical Note. J Neurosurg. 1991; 74:152–153

[20] Schmidek HH, Sweet WH. Operative Neurosurgical Techniques. New York 1982

[21] Matson DD. Neurosurgery of Infancy and Childhood. 2nd ed. Springfield: Charles C Thomas; 1969

[22] Tomasello F, Conti A, Angileri FF, et al. Telo-velar approach to fourth-ventricle tumours: how I do it. Acta Neurochir (Wien). 2015; 157:607–610

[23] Tanriover N, Ulm AJ, Rhoton AL,Jr, et al. Comparison of the transvermian and telovelar approaches to the fourth ventricle. J Neurosurg. 2004; 101:484–498

[24] Zaheer SN, Wood M. Experiences with the telovelar approach to fourth ventricular tumors in children. Pediatr Neurosurg. 2010; 46:340–343

[25] Han S, Wang Z, Wang Y, et al. Transcerebellomedullary fissure approach to lesions of the fourth ventricle: less is more? Acta Neurochir (Wien). 2013; 155:1011–1016

[26] Mei C, Morgan AT. Incidence of mutism, dysarthria and dysphagia associated with childhood posterior fossa tumour. Childs Nerv Syst. 2011; 27:1129–1136

[27] Harner SG, Beatty CW, Ebersold MJ. Impact of cranioplasty on headache after acoustic neuroma removal. Neurosurgery. 1995; 36:1097–9; discussion 1099-100

[28] Manley GT, Dillon W. Acute posterior fossa syndrome following lumbar drainage for treatment of suboccipital pseudomeningocele. Report of three cases. J Neurosurg. 2000; 92:469–474

[29] Roland PS, Marple BF, Meyerhoff WL, et al. Complications of lumbar spinal fluid drainage. Otolaryngol Head Neck Surg. 1992; 107:564–569

[30] Culley DJ, Berger MS, Shaw D, et al. An Analysis of Factors Determining the Need for Ventriculoperitoneal Shunts After Posterior Fossa Tumor Surgery in Children. Neurosurgery. 1994; 34:402–408

[31] Stein BM, Tenner MS, Fraser RAR. Hydrocephalus Following Removal of Cerebellar Astrocytomas in Children. Journal of Neurosurgery. 1972; 36:763–768

[32] Haines SJ, Maroon JC, Jannetta PJ. Supratentorial Intracerebral Hemorrhage following Posterior Fossa Surgery. J Neurosurg. 1978; 49:881–886

105

106 Supratentorial Craniotomies

106.1 Pterional craniotomy

106.1.1 Indications

1. aneurysms
   a) all aneurysms of anterior circulation
   b) basilar tip aneurysms
2. direct surgical approach to cavernous sinus
3. suprasellar tumors
   a) PitNET/adenoma (when there is a large suprasellar component)
   b) craniopharyngioma

106.1.2 Technique

Position, skin incision, craniectomy, approach...

1. supine, ipsilateral shoulder roll if head turned > 30° (see below)
2. elevate thorax 10–15°: reduces venous distension
3. flex knees
4. Mayfield 3 pin head-holder: applied between true AP and true lateral (so that it is ≈ horizontal when head is rotated to the necessary position, see ▶ Fig. 106.1)
5. neck extended 15°: allows gravity to retract frontal lobe away from skull base
6. head rotated from vertical as shown in ▶ Fig. 106.1

Room arrangement

1. microscope: observer tube to operator's *right* for either right or left pterional crani

Skin incision

See ▶ Fig. 106.2. From zygomatic arch 1 cm in front of tragus (to avoid frontalis branch of facial nerv and frontal branch of superficial temporal artery), curving slightly anteriorly, staying behind hairlin to widow's peak, optional additional curve beyond midline to aid in skin retraction. Over temporali muscle, incise skin down to but not through temporalis fascia.

The temporalis muscle may be incised caudal to the skin incision (i.e., closer to zygomatic arch) this minimizes the muscle mass that needs to be retracted inferiorly and yet keeps the scar behin the hairline (note: there is a greater risk of frontalis weakness with this technique than if the tempo ralis muscle is incised in-line with the skin incision).

Burr holes

Two burr holes are sufficient; made as far caudally as possible to minimize the amount of bone to b rongeured off to gain access to the floor of the middle cranial fossa. One burr hole is made at th posterior insertion of the zygomatic arch ("A" in ▶ Fig. 106.3); this burr hole may be placed slightl forward when exposure is centered over structures around the ACoA (e.g., suprasellar tumor). Th second burr hole ("Z") is made at the intersection of the zygomatic bone (near the frontozygomati suture), the superior temporal line, and the supraorbital ridge. The hole should be as low as possib on the orbit; aim the drill slightly superiorly to avoid actually entering the orbit. The dura is dis sected off the inner table with a Penfield #3 dissector.

Craniotomy

The resulting bone flap is centered over the depression of the sphenoid ridge. Approximately 33% the craniotomy is anterior to the anterior margin of temporalis muscle insertion, ≈ 66% is posterior.

With the craniotome, starting at the frontal burr hole the craniotomy is taken anteriorly acros the anterior margin of the superior temporal line, staying as low as possible on the orbit (to obvia having to rongeur bone, which is unsightly on the forehead). The distance "B" from the medial exter of the craniotomy to the frontal burr hole is 3 cm for anterior circulation aneurysms. For th approaches to skull base (e.g., Dolenc approach), distance "B" is larger and takes the opening to ≈ th

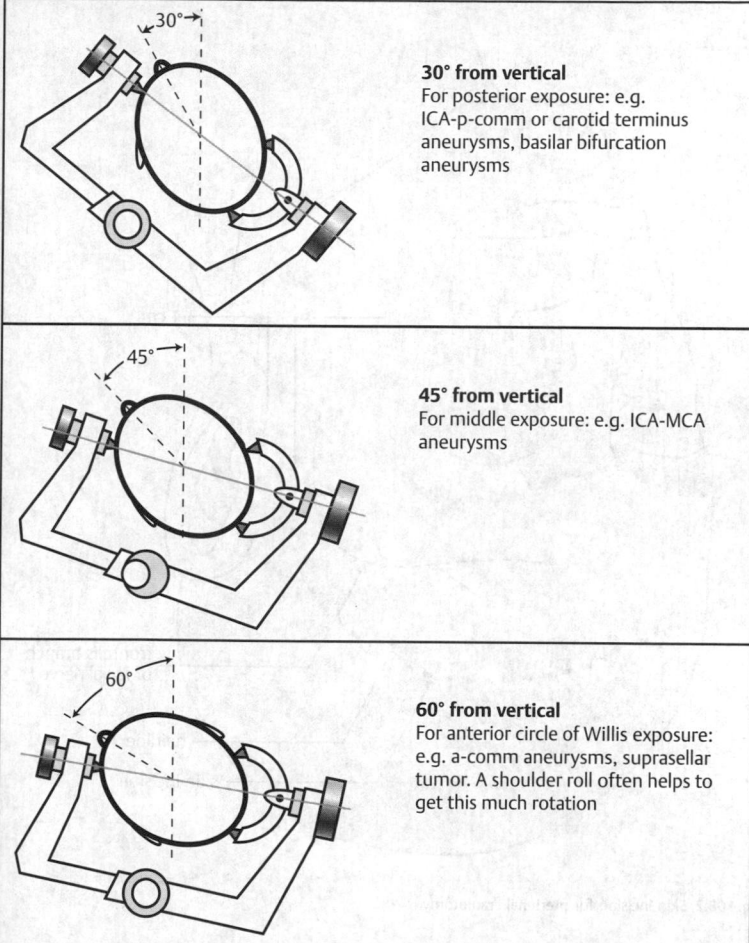

30° from vertical
For posterior exposure: e.g.
ICA-p-comm or carotid terminus
aneurysms, basilar bifurcation
aneurysms

45° from vertical
For middle exposure: e.g. ICA-MCA
aneurysms

60° from vertical
For anterior circle of Willis exposure:
e.g. a-comm aneurysms, suprasellar
tumor. A shoulder roll often helps to
get this much rotation

Fig. 106.1 Head position for pterional craniotomy depending on exposure required. The blue line indicates the approximate center line.

mid-orbit. Then from point "B," a sharp superior turn is made and the opening is taken back to point "A." The height ("H") of the craniotomy needs to be only ≈ 3 cm for aneurysms of the Circle of Willis, and slightly larger (≈ 5 cm) for middle cerebral artery aneurysms. Minimal exposure of temporal cortex is necessary for aneurysms of the skull base region. For large flaps (e.g., for tumors), "H" is made larger to expose more temporal lobe.

From the frontal burr hole, the craniotomy is then taken posteriorly towards the depression corresponding to the sphenoid wing until the drill hangs up.

The craniotomy from the posterior burr hole is taken forward towards the depression corresponding to the sphenoid wing until the drill hangs up.

The bone between the two points where the drill hangs up is scored with the craniotome, and then the bone is fractured at this point. A rongeur is used to remove as much sphenoid wing as possible.

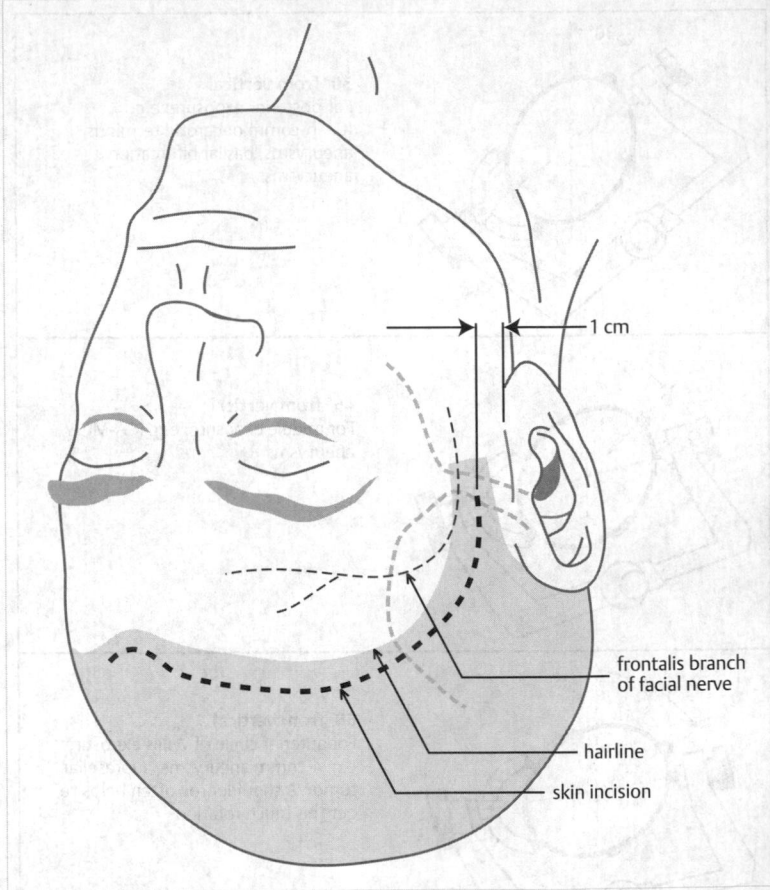

1 cm

frontalis branch
of facial nerve

hairline

skin incision

Fig. 106.2 Skin incision for pterional craniotomy.

Dural flap

Curvilinear, centered over sphenoid wing, retracted inferiorly with dural stitch.

Dissection

For some anterior circulation aneurysms (e.g., MCA aneurysms) and for the Yasargil approach basilar tip aneurysms, the Sylvian fissure needs to be split. This can be accomplished by workir from the lateral aspect of the fissure medially, or by starting at the point where the carotid arte penetrates the fissure and working laterally. The latter method may be easier when prolific vei overlie the junction of the frontal and temporal lobe. There are no arteries that cross the Sylvian fi sure, and so if the correct plane is maintained, no arteries need to be sacrificed.

▶ Fig. 106.4 shows a theoretical exposure of the circle of Willis possible through a pterional cr niotomy. This diagram is semi-schematic, and in reality dissection would be directed either anter orly (e.g., to expose ACoA) or posteriorly (e.g., for basilar tip aneurysms) but not both.

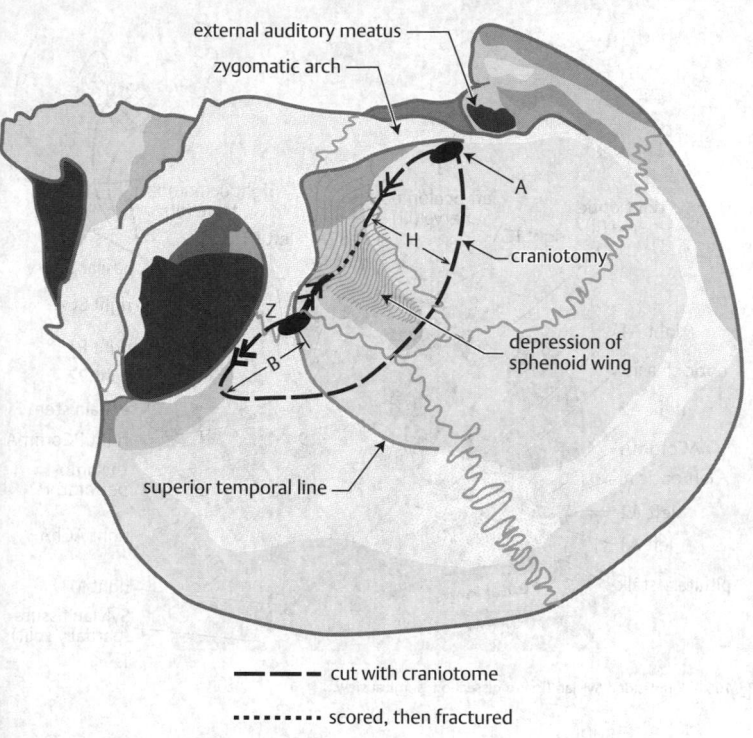

——— cut with craniotome

········· scored, then fractured

Fig. 106.3 Skull landmarks for right pterional craniotomy.

06.2 Temporal craniotomy

06.2.1 Indications

temporal lobe biopsy: herpes simplex encephalitis
temporal lobectomy: for resection of seizure focus, decompression post-trauma...
hematoma (epidural or subdural) overlying temporal lobe
tumors of the temporal lobe
small, laterally located vestibular schwannomas[1]
access to the floor of the middle cranial fossa (including foramen ovale/Meckel's cave, the labyrinthine and upper tympanic portion of the facial nerve)
access to medial temporal lobe e.g., for amygdalo-hippocampectomy (p.1893) or for mesial temporal sclerosis (p.482)

06.2.2 Technique

see ▶ Fig. 106.5. Two basic methods for temporal craniotomy:
small craniotomy or craniectomy through a linear skin incision: good for cortical biopsy or draining chronic subdural hematoma. Also permits access to floor of middle fossa. Simple quick closure
question-mark skin incision with standard craniotomy flap: useful for temporal lobe exposure for tumor or acute hematoma

106

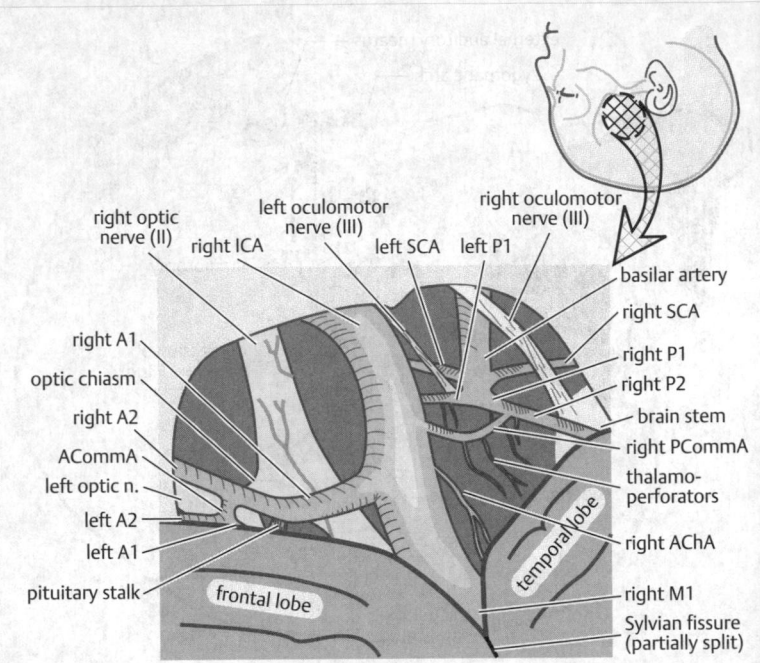

Fig. 106.4 Right-sided Sylvian fissure dissection, surgical view.

106.2.3 Position, skin incision, craniectomy, approach...

1. patient supine with shoulder roll (to assist in rotating neck to get head almost horizontal)
2. elevate thorax 10–15°: reduces venous distension
3. flex knees slightly
4. Mayfield 3 pin head-holder: true AP with single pin anteriorly
5. head rotated almost horizontal to floor: avoid over-extending to prevent kinking neck veins

106.2.4 Craniotomies

Small craniectomy

Linear skin incision completely within the extent of the temporalis muscle. To access the temporal ti place the incision midway between the lateral canthus and external auditory canal (EAC); extend from the zygomatic arch upward for ≈ 6 cm. For small, laterally located vestibular schwannomas, th incision is made 0.5 cm anterior to the EAC, extending ≈ 7–8 cm above the zygomatic arch.[1] To drain subdural, place the incision just anterior to the tragus and start it 1–2 cm above the zygomatic arch f ≈ 6 cm (modified based on the location of the epicenter of the subdural). Take the incision down temporalis fascia with the knife, and incise the fascia and muscle with Bovie cautery. Spread with se retaining retractors, and make a burr hole. Enlarge with rongeurs and/or Kerrison punches.

Standard craniotomy

Question-mark skin incision

See ▶ Fig. 106.5. Used for access to the temporal lobe including tip (a reverse question mark incisi may be used to gain access to the middle and posterior temporal lobe).

1. the pinna is either sutured inferiorly out of the way before draping, or it can be folded under th drapes which may be stapled to the skin

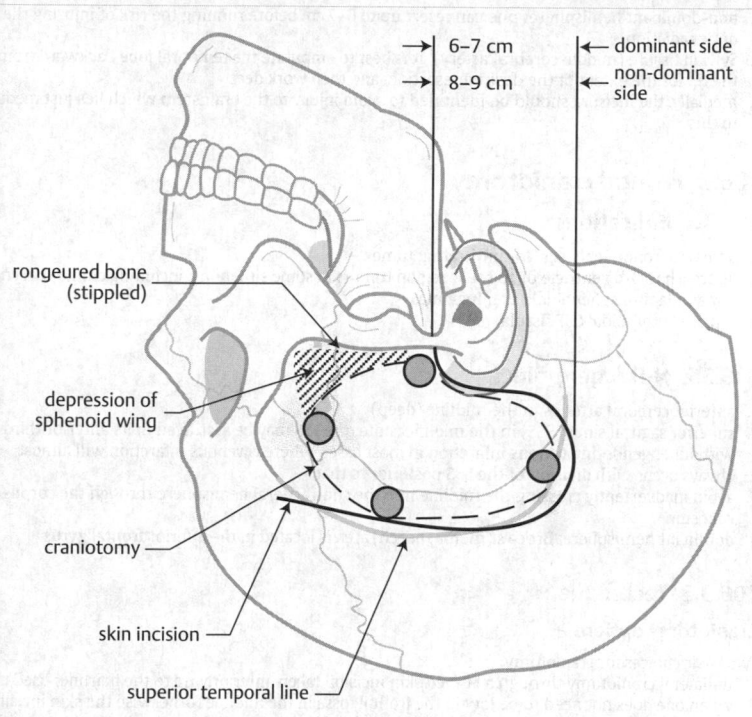

Fig. 106.5 Temporal craniotomy (exposing entire temporal lobe).

2. the lower limb extends from the zygomatic arch just anterior to the tragus (to avoid the superficial temporal artery)
3. curve as far posteriorly as ≈ 6–7 cm on the dominant side, or ≈ 8–9 cm on the non-dominant side at the level of the top of the pinna (these dimensions allow access to the "safe" area of temporal tip for lobectomy)
4. then superiorly to the level of the superior temporal line
5. then anteriorly towards the forehead, stopping at the hairline

Burr hole placement
1. at the posterior insertion of the zygomatic arch
2. at upper anterior junction of zygomatic arch
3. one or two burr holes along posterior and superior aspect of the skin incision

Craniotomy
Connect the burr holes with the craniotome, keeping as low as possible in the middle fossa to minimize the amount of bone that must be rongeured. The remaining bone is rongeured down to the floor of the middle fossa (cross-hatched area in ▸ Fig. 106.5).

Temporal lobectomy
◆ Danger points:
1. dominant hemisphere: Wernicke's speech area. Although variable (see Temporal lobectomy (p. 1893)), one can usually safely resect up to 4–5 cm from temporal tip without use of mapping techniques to localize speech

2. non-dominant hemisphere: one can resect up to 6–7 cm before running the risk of injuring the optic radiation
3. Sylvian fissure (middle cerebral artery): it is best to amputate the temporal lobe backward from the tip for the extent of the desired resection, and then work deep
4. medially, the incisura should be identified to avoid injury to the brainstem which lies just medial to this

106.3 Frontal craniotomy

106.3.1 Indications

1. access to frontal lobe: e.g., for infiltrating tumor
2. approach to 3rd ventricle or to sellar region tumors in some situations, including craniopharyngiomas, planum sphenoidale meningiomas
3. repair of ethmoidal CSF fistula

106.3.2 ✖ Danger points

1. anterior cerebral arteries in the midline (deep)
2. superior sagittal sinus (SSS) in the midline (note: the SSS may be sacrificed in its anterior third without engendering venous infarction in most cases, whereas venous infarction will almost always occur with division of the SSS posterior to that)
3. avoid inadvertently crossing the midline into the contralateral hemisphere through the corpus callosum
4. dominant hemisphere: Broca's (motor speech) area is located in the inferior frontal gyrus

106.3.3 Technique

Craniotomy options

Two basic choices for craniotomy:
1. unilateral craniotomy through a curved skin incision taken anteriorly up to the hairline: used when one does not need to be low in the frontal fossa in the midline (otherwise the skin incision would have to be taken far into forehead) and when there is no need to cross the midline
2. large bifrontal skin incision from "ear-to-ear" (souttar skin incision[2]) allowing low approach to one or both frontal fossa

Unilateral frontal craniotomy

▶ Fig. 106.6. Skin incision starts < 1 cm anterior to the tragus, and does not need to go all the way down to the zygomatic arch. It curves superiorly and slightly posteriorly before being taken to the midline frontally.

Burr holes

1. at the junction of the superior temporal line and the orbital rim
2. just posterior to the depression of the sphenoid wing (behind the pterion)
3. anteriorly just behind the hairline to avoid having a burr hole under the forehead (which causes an unsightly depression)
4. superiorly

Bilateral frontal craniotomy

1. "ear-to-ear" or souttar skin incision
   a) just behind hairline with a slight widow's peak at the front
   b) does not need to go all the way to the zygomatic arch, it just needs to be ≈ as low as the orbital roof
   c) unlike pterional craniotomy, usually do not need to incise the temporalis muscle and fascia. Dissect the flap off the muscle/fascia
   d) if a periosteal flap is likely to be needed, it sometimes helps not to incise the periosteum at the same time as the skin incision. Then, the periosteum can be incised behind the skin incision to yield a longer periosteal graft than would have otherwise been obtained

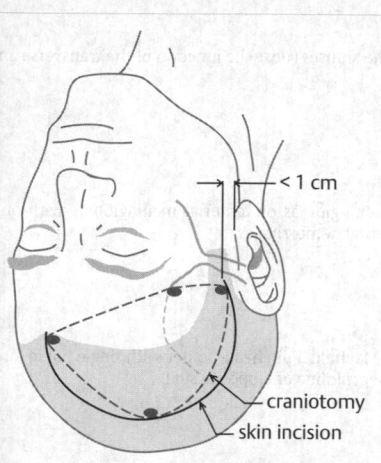

Fig. 106.6 Unilateral frontal craniotomy.

< 1 cm

craniotomy

skin incision

106

2. burr holes: to avoid burr hole defects on the forehead, the bone flap can be created with two burr holes straddling the SSS close to the skin incision, and two burr holes laterally
3. the SSS may be divided low, near the orbital roof, with little risk
4. if the frontal sinus is entered, it is dealt with as outlined under Frontal sinus fractures (p. 1066)

106.4 Petrosal craniotomy

106.4.1 Indications

1. lesions of the petrous apex (e.g., petroclival meningiomas)
2. lesions of the clivus (e.g., chordomas) with both posterior fossa and supratentorial components

106.4.2 Advantages

Spares sinus and otologic apparatuses. Minimizes cerebellar and temporal lobe retraction.

106.4.3 Technique

See reference.[3]

Position

1. patient supine, ipsilateral shoulder roll
2. elevate thorax 10°: reduces venous distension
3. flex knees
4. Mayfield 3 pin head-holder: close to true AP with single pin on forehead
5. head positioned to place petrous base at highest point of field:
   a) head rotated 40–60° from vertical
   b) head abducted towards contralateral shoulder
   c) neck extended 15°: allows gravity to retract frontal lobe away from skull base

Skin incision

Reverse question mark starting from zygomatic arch 1 cm anterior to tragus, arcing posteriorly over ear, descending to 0.5–1 cm medial to mastoid notch.
Temporalis muscle and periosteum reflected anteriorly and inferiorly.

Craniotomy

Four burr holes are utilized, two on each side of the sinuses (near the junction of the transverse and sigmoid sinuses).

106.5 Occipital craniotomy

106.5.1 Indications

Occipital lobe tumors including posterior falx meningiomas or tentorial meningiomas with only supratentorial component. Occipital lobe intracerebral hemorrhages.

106.5.2 Positions

Supine

Shoulder roll on affected side; elevate thorax 15°. Mayfield 3 pin head-holder with single pin in forehead off to the side of the crani, double pin just over midline on opposite side.

Lateral oblique

1. affected side up, can operate either
   a) from behind patient similar to p-fossa crani for CPA lesion
      OR
   b) from top of table
2. alternative approach: affected side down. Useful in lesions adjacent to the falx; see **Interhemispheric approach** (p. 1762)

References

[1] Brackmann DE, Sekhar LN, Janecka IP. The Middle Fossa Approach. In: Surgery of Cranial Base Tumors. New York: Raven Press; 1993:367–377

[2] Souttar HS. New methods of surgical access to the brain. British Medical Journal. 1928; 1:295–300

[3] Al-Mefty O, Fox JL, Smith RR. Petrosal Approach to Petroclival Meningiomas. Neurosurgery. 1988; 22:510–517

107 Approaches to the Lateral and Third Ventricles, Decompressive Craniectomies, and Cranioplasty

107.1 Approaches to the lateral ventricle

Surgical approaches to the trigone[1]

Classic review[2(p 561–74)] summarized:

1. atrium (AKA trigone); numerous approaches include[1]:
   a) middle temporal gyrus: through the dilated temporal horn
   b) lateral temporal parietal
   c) superior parietal occipital
   d) transcallosal (see below)
   e) transtemporal horn: access to temporal horn is via lobectomy of the temporal tip
   f) occipital lobe incision or occipital lobectomy: recommended only if patient has homonymous hemianopsia pre-op
2. frontal horn
   a) middle frontal gyrus
3. midventricular body
   a) transcallosal
   b) middle frontal gyrus: usually prevents access to vascular supply until most of the tumor is removed (especially for tumors supplied primarily by posterior choroidal artery)
4. temporal horn
   a) middle temporal gyrus
   b) transtemporal horn

107.2 Approaches to the third ventricle

107.2.1 General information

Classic references review the microsurgical anatomy[3] and surgical approaches,[4] and are briefly summarized below.

Alternative approaches for lesions of the anterior 3rd ventricle[5]:

1. transcortical: approach is through the lateral ventricle and is feasible only in the presence of hydrocephalus; especially useful if the tumor extends from the 3rd ventricle into one of the lateral ventricles. Risk of seizures is 5% (higher than with transcallosal) (p. 1762).
2. transcallosal: may be preferable in the absence of hydrocephalus (see below)
   a) anterior transcallosal: good visualization of both walls of 3rd ventricle; risk of bilateral fornicial damage
   b) posterior transcallosal: allows approach to quadrigeminal plate or pineal region; risk of damage to deep veins
3. subfrontal: allows four different approaches
   a) subchiasmatic: between optic nerve and optic chiasm
   b) optico-carotid: through the triangular space bordered by optic nerve medially, carotid artery laterally, and ACA posteriorly
   c) lamina terminalis: above the optic chiasm[6]
   d) transsphenoidal: requires removal of tuberculum sellae, planum sphenoidale, and anterior wall of the sella turcica
4. transsphenoidal
5. subtemporal
6. stereotactic: may be useful for aspiration of colloid cysts; see Stereotactic drainage of colloid cysts (p. 947)

107.2.2 General principles of tumor removal

summarized.[4] During the approach, deep veins should be preserved at all costs, even if it means stretching them to the point that they may rupture.

It is helpful to place a suture through the tumor capsule to act as a tether.

The tumor should first be removed from within the capsule; techniques include aspiration, and then opening the capsule and debulking from within. The capsule may then be collapsed and

107

dissected from adherent structures. If the capsule adhesions seem unyielding, the most likely cause is incomplete intracapsular evacuation.

Vessels on the surface of the tumor should be presumed to be supplying normal brain, and should be dissected off the capsule once it is completely emptied.

107.2.3 Transcallosal approach to lateral or third ventricle

General information

Performed through an interhemispheric approach to the corpus callosum (CC) via a parietal craniotomy, usually right-sided in a left-hemisphere-dominant patient.

Indications

Primarily for tumors or lesions of the lateral or 3rd ventricle, including:
1. colloid cysts
2. craniopharyngiomas
3. cysticercosis cysts
4. thalamic glioma
5. AVM

Booking the case: Transcallosal surgery

Also see defaults & disclaimers (p. 25).
1. position: supine with pin head-holder
2. equipment:
   a) microscope
   b) image-guided navigation system
3. post-op: ICU
4. consent (in lay terms for the patient—not all-inclusive):
   a) procedure: operation between the two halves of the brain to remove lesion
   b) alternatives: non-surgical management, surgery through the surface of the brain (transcortical), radiation therapy for some diagnoses
   c) complications: stroke, "disconnection syndrome" (uncommon) (p. 1893), hydrocephalus with possible need for a shunt, memory deficits

Technique

See references.[3,4,7]

General information

▶ Fig. 107.1. Image-guided navigation is very helpful in ascertaining the correct trajectory which permits minimizing the size of the callosotomy, and helps distinguish the corpus callosum from the cingulate gyri.

Position

Supine with neck flexed. Thorax elevated 20°. Spinal drain *not* used. Keep the head perfectly vertical to minimize disorientation that can easily occur with this approach. Alternatively, gravity retraction may be employed either by tilting the head slightly to the right (causing the right hemisphere to fall away) or by using the lateral position.

Skin incision

Either of the following may be used:
1. inverted "U" with the top just left of midline, extending from 6 cm anterior to the coronal suture to 2 cm behind the coronal suture, taking the sides for 7–8 cm
2. souttar skin incision

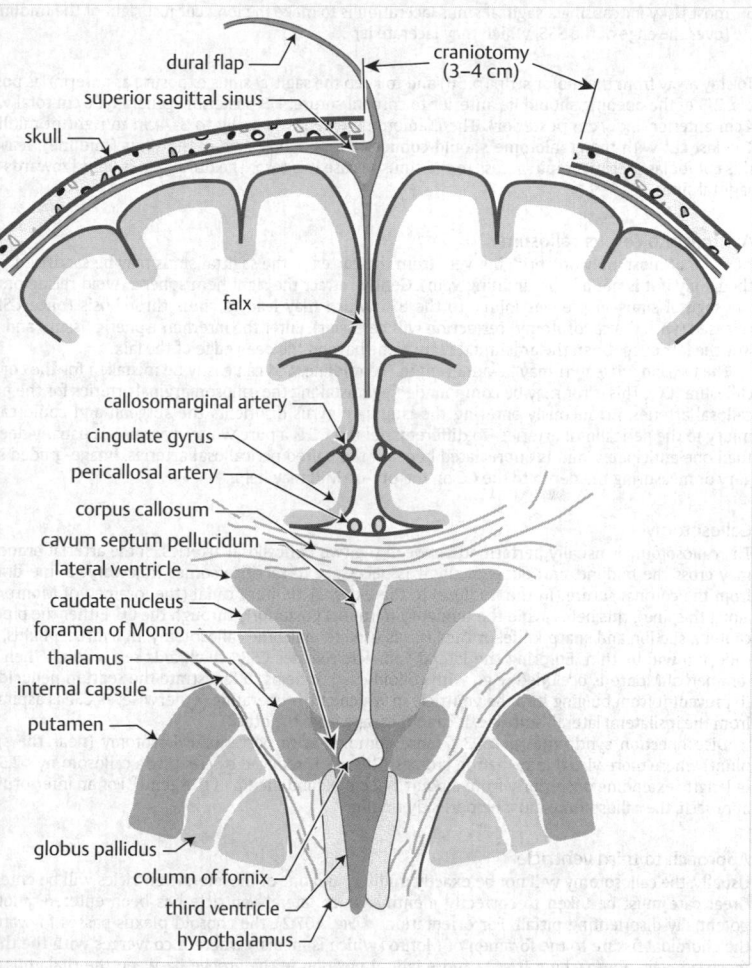

Fig. 107.1 Transcallosal approach to the third ventricle: frontal view.

Labels on figure (top to bottom, left side):
- dural flap
- superior sagittal sinus
- skull
- craniotomy (3–4 cm)
- falx
- callosomarginal artery
- cingulate gyrus
- pericallosal artery
- corpus callosum
- cavum septum pellucidum
- lateral ventricle
- caudate nucleus
- foramen of Monro
- thalamus
- internal capsule
- putamen
- globus pallidus
- column of fornix
- third ventricle
- hypothalamus

Craniotomy

Pre-op angiography is recommended to plan the position of the flap to avoid sacrificing large cortical veins. MRI may also suffice for this.[8] There tend to be fewer veins bridging from the cortex to the superior sagittal sinus (SSS) anterior to the coronal suture; therefore, this is often a good location to enter the interhemispheric fissure. The bone flap is either trapezoidal or triangular in shape, for adequate exposure it is *critical* to go all the way to the SSS. Several techniques may be used. NB: the SSS is often to the right of the sagittal suture (p. 61).

- to expose the SSS, straddle the SSS with paired burr holes anteriorly and posteriorly, dissect the dura from the inner table between pairs, and make the longitudinal cut on the *left* of midline. Disadvantage: removing the midline bone puts the SSS at greater risk of injury and makes it more difficult to control lacerations
- one can make the long cut well to the right of midline, and then under direct vision rongeur off the bone to the SSS. Safe, but leaves a large bone gap that may need to be filled (e.g., with methyl methacrylate) and is time-consuming

3. most risky for causing a sagittal sinus laceration is to make the long cut just right of the midline (over the edge of the SSS, which may lacerate it)

To stay away from the motor strip (p. 56) and to keep the sagittal sinus exposure as anterior as possible, 2/3 of the opening should lie anterior to coronal suture, 1/3 posterior (generally: 6 cm total with 4 cm anterior and 2 cm posterior). The craniotomy extends laterally to 3–4 cm to right of midline. The last cut with the craniotome should connect the burr holes along the sinus (midline); leaving this cut for last permits rapid access to the sinus in case it is torn. The dural flap is based towards the sagittal sinus.

Approach to corpus callosum

None, or at most, only one bridging vein from the cortex to the sagittal sinus may be sacrificed (and then, only if it is not a large draining vein). Gently retract the right hemisphere. Avoid retractors on the sagittal sinus to prevent injury to the SSS which may lead to sinus thrombosis (once CSF is released (with the callosotomy) retraction will be easier). Enter the interhemispheric fissure and follow the falx deep. Open the arachnoid membrane beyond the deep edge of the falx.

The two cingulate gyri may be adherent in the midline, and can easily be mistaken for the corpus callosum (CC). This error may be compounded by mistaking the callosomarginal arteries for the pericallosal arteries. Erroneously entering the cingulate gyrus disorients the surgeon and could cause injury to the pericallosal arteries. To differentiate: the CC is a pure white structure, is usually deeper than one anticipates, and is appreciated beneath the paired pericallosal arteries. Image-guided surgery or measuring the depth to the CC on the pre-op MRI may help.

Callosotomy

The callosotomy is usually performed between the two pericallosal arteries. Some arterial branches may cross the midline, and occasionally it is necessary to sacrifice some. Trajectory: a line drawn from the coronal suture (in the midline) to the external auditory canal (the foramen of Monro lies along this line); this helps avoid the tendency to tunnel posteriorly through the CC. Either the bipolar cautery, suction and sharp knife, or the laser is used to make the callosotomy. In hydrocephalus, the callosum will be thin. Entering the lateral ventricle releases CSF, which aids retraction. When the foramen of Monro is occluded (e.g., with colloid cyst), it helps to fenestrate the septum pellucidum to prevent it from bulging into the ventricle in which one is operating (otherwise, as CSF is aspirated from the ipsilateral lateral ventricle, it cannot escape from the other).

Disconnection syndrome (p. 1893): more common with posterior callosotomy (near the splenium) where more visual information crosses. The risk is reduced by creating a callosotomy < 2.5 cm in length, extending posteriorly from a point 1–2 cm behind the tip of the genu.[9] For an interfornicial approach, the callosotomy must be perfectly midline.

Approach to third ventricle

Usually, the callosotomy will not be exactly midline, and one of the lateral ventricles will be entered. Great care must be taken to correctly identify which lateral ventricle has been entered, another potentially disorienting pitfall. For orientation (▶ Fig. 107.2), the choroid plexus passes forward in the choroidal fissure to the foramen of Monro (which is medial) where it converges with the thalamostriate vein approaching from a more lateral position in the groove between the thalamus and caudate. The septal and caudate veins approach the foramen from anterior. With colloid cysts, the foramen of Monro may be hard to recognize initially as it will be plugged with the cyst, which can resemble the ependymal lining of the ventricle, but on close inspection is usually slightly grayer (the choroid plexus enters the posterior aspect of the foramen).

Another possible pitfall upon incising the CC is entering a cavum septum pellucidum (p. 1657). The give-away here is that *no* landmarks will be visible.

Alternative approaches to third ventricle

1. interfornicial[9]: go *above* body of fornix, approaches *roof* of 3rd ventricle. Well suited for lesions of the mid- and posterior 3rd ventricle. Callosotomy should be as close to midline as possible
2. from lateral ventricle through the foramen of Monro: with hydrocephalus, the foramen of Monro is usually dilated. If the foramen is too small for adequate access to the 3rd ventricle, one can
   a) return to the interfornicial approach (see above) or
   b) enlarge the foramen of Monro only if absolutely necessary. Either by:
      • opening the foramen laterally

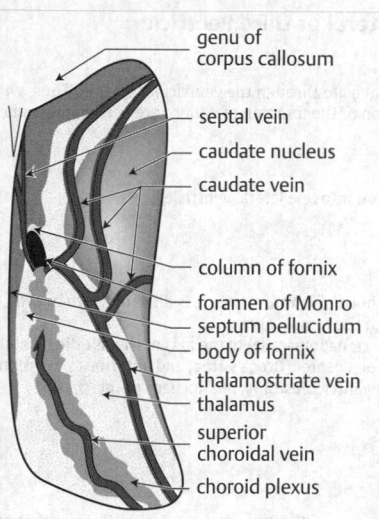

genu of
corpus callosum

septal vein

caudate nucleus

caudate vein

column of fornix

foramen of Monro

septum pellucidum

body of fornix

thalamostriate vein

thalamus

superior
choroidal vein

choroid plexus

Fig. 107.2 Right foramen of Monro viewed from above through right lateral ventricle.[3]

107

- the "subchoroidal" approach, making the incision posteriorly (sacrificing the thalamostriate vein) which is reportedly well tolerated[4,10]
- last resort: incising the anterosuperior margin of the foramen through the column of one fornix.[9] Caution: if the other fornix is non-functional for any reason, this would produce a bilateral forniceal lesion and may (but not definitely[9]) result in loss of short-term memory and ability for new learning

Colloid cyst removal

It is critical to debulk and empty a cystic lesion, such as a colloid cyst, before delivering it from the 3rd ventricle through the foramen of Monro. This will minimize the retraction and manipulation of the fornix. Inserting a needle and aspirating may work. The partially emptied cyst is grasped with a micro-pituitary and is delivered into the lateral ventricle through the foramen of Monro. One should only attempt to deliver the empty capsule through the foramen of Monro (p.1757). There is usually a stalk attaching the lesion to the roof of the 3rd ventricle, this is coagulated with bipolar cautery and divided.

For other tumors, if the tumor is too large to fit through the foramen of Monro, it should be gutted from within.

Complications

1. venous infarction, may be due to:
   a) sacrifice of critical cortical draining veins: plan the flap to avoid this with preoperative angiography, or with sagittal T2WI MRI images[11]
   b) superior sagittal sinus (SSS) thrombosis.[12] Factors that may contribute to sinus injury include[8]:
      - injury from retractor: avoid placing retractor on sinus (deformation of midline should not exceed 5 mm)
      - over-retraction of the dural sinus flap or on SSS itself (lateral deformation should be < 2 cm)
      - injury during the opening of the bone in the region of the sinus
      - over-use of bipolar coagulation in the region of the SSS
      - hypercoagulable state of the patient, including dehydration
2. transient mutism as a result of bilateral cingulate gyrus retraction or thalamic injury in conjunction with section of the midportion of the callosum[11]

107.2.4 Transcortical approach to lateral or third ventricle

Indications

In the absence of hydrocephalus, it is difficult to navigate through the ventricular system. Thus, with normal sized ventricles, the 3rd ventricle and region of the foramen of Monro are better approached transcallosally (p. 1758).
1. tumors of the atrium of the lateral ventricle
2. tumors of the roof of the 3rd ventricle
3. 3rd ventricular tumors with significant extension into one lateral ventricle

Approaches

1. posterior parietal
2. middle temporal gyrus: useful when temporal horn of lateral ventricle is dilated due to hydrocephalus caused by the tumor; access is through the temporal horn
3. middle frontal gyrus approach: a 4-cm incision is made parallel to the axis of the middle frontal gyrus, above and anterior to the expressive speech center (Broca's area) and anterior to the motor strip[4]; about the same point as used for frontal ventriculostomy, see Kocher's point (p. 1821)

107.3 Interhemispheric approach

107.3.1 Indications

For lesions abutting on midline, deep to surface, but superficial to corpus callosum (lesions that can "fall away" from midline). Similar to transcallosal approach above, except that the pathology can be placed on the down-side, which allows gravity to retract the hemisphere and thus minimizes pressure necrosis injury from mechanical retractors.

107.3.2 Technique

Position

True lateral (prevents getting lost from unusual angles). Head tilted slightly up.

Approach

Similar to transcallosal (p. 1758). Need to be sure that lateral portion of craniotomy extends at least 4 cm from midline to minimize the necessity of retraction of brain against bone.

107.4 Cranioplasty

107.4.1 Indications/contraindications

General indications

1. cosmetic restoration of external skull appearance and symmetry
2. relief of symptoms due to craniotomy defect (p. 1731)
    a) pain or tenderness: especially at the bone edges
    b) syndrome of the trephined: *nonfocal* (see below)
    c) focal deficit related to the defect: e.g., sinking skin syndrome (see below)
    d) seizures originating in the brain beneath the defect
3. protection from trauma (blunt or penetrating) in area of post-craniotomy or posttraumatic skull defect
4. reduction of irritation of the brain as a result of pressure on and deformity of the surface of the brain. Reducing this irritation may improve seizure control if this is an issue
5. cognitive deficits: may improve following cranioplasty (especially with large defects)[13]

Onset of symptoms may be delayed months to years after the craniectomy.

Contraindications

1. infection: especially at the craniectomy site, but also at distal sites because of the fear of seeding the cranioplasty flap
2. brain protruding beyond the confines of the skull
3. untreated hydrocephalus: this is complicated because treating hydrocephalus may require repairing the bone defect, usually in combination with a shunt

Syndrome of the trephined

Symptoms first described in the French literature during World War I. The term "syndrome of the trephined" was coined by Grant & Norcross,[14] at that time the description consisted of nonfocal symptoms including: headache (present in 54%[15]) and sometimes pulsatile pain (usually localized to the area of the skull defect), vertigo (24%), amnesia, inability to concentrate, insomnia, fatigue, depression... Similar in many ways to postconcussive syndrome (p.1111).

Since then the definition has been liberally expanded to include delayed focal neurologic symptoms,[16] tinnitus,[17] and even "any symptoms reversible with cranioplasty."[18]

The symptoms sometimes change with posture.[19]

Other syndromes related to the bone defect

For those purists who want to restrict the use of the term "syndrome of the trephined" to nonfocal symptoms described above, the following syndromes have been proposed.

Sinking skin flap syndrome[20]: neurologic deficit related to brain immediately underlying the skull defect when the scalp is displaced inward by atmospheric pressure. Deficits may include contralateral hemiparesis (more common in UE than LE due to location of UE motor neurons over the convexity; see ▶ Fig. 1.3), contralateral visual and somatosensory deficit, speech/language deficit (with dominant hemisphere defects). Not all patients with a sunken flap develop a deficit.

Motor trephine syndrome[16]: limited to contralateral hemiparesis. Mean delay to onset: 5 months.

107.4.2 Etiology of symptoms

Possible explanation for symptoms related to the bone defect:
1. atmospheric pressure exerted directly on the surface of the brain including compression of cortical veins
   - changes in cerebral blood flow (CBF)
   - impaired cerebral glucose metabolism
   - local alteration in CSF flow
2. globally altered CSF flow dynamics
3. scar tissue adhering to the dura and/or brain
4. acute angulation of scalp at bone edges stimulating pain fibers causing local pain
5. pulsations (CSF and/or blood) causing irritation of (pain-sensitive) dura

The effects of barometric pressure are modified by:
1. scalp elasticity
2. size of the bone defect
3. amount of skull curvature at defect site
4. changes in CSF pressure with: postural changes (incorrectly referred to as "siphoning," in reality is a reduction in pressure of a fluid column (hydrostatics)), coughing/straining, hydrocephalus

107.4.3 Timing of cranioplasty

brain swelling: enough time needs to have lapsed so that any brain swelling that was present has subsided to the point that the brain is no longer protruding beyond the normal confines of the intracranial space (you don't want to be "pushing brain" back into the skull with the cranioplasty flap). This sometimes requires shunting hydrocephalus if present
contamination status of wound
   ○ skull defect from clean wounds (following decompressive craniectomy, post-craniotomy brain swelling...): recent studies found no significant difference in *infection* between early and late (variously defined) cranioplasty (contaminated cases were not included).[21,22] However, one series reported an increased risk of infection for repair of a decompressive craniectomy within 14 days.[23]

107

Clean surgical cases without brain swelling (e.g., repair of defect after removing skull hemangioma): there appears to be little risk of infection with immediate cranioplasty

- ○ contaminated wound (open fracture, fractures that traverse the nasal sinuses, penetrating trauma, infection…): classic teaching was to delay cranioplasty using allograft (a "foreign body" e.g., PEEK implant) at least 6 months to reduce the risk of infection. Some authors even recommended waiting > 1 year.[24] More contemporary practice seems to be to wait ≈ 3–6 months after the craniectomy if there are no signs of infection

- extenuating circumstances: consideration may be made to shorten the delay before cranioplasty e.g., if the patient is having significant symptoms related to the absent area of bone (e.g., "syndrome of the trephined" or "sinking skin flap" syndrome)

107.4.4 Material

Options for material include:

1. the patient's own bone. Bone that is removed at the time of craniectomy that has been preserved for future implantation. This is generally not employed in contaminated cases (penetrating trauma, infection…). Storage options:
   a) in a "pocket" created in the patient's subcutaneous abdominal fat
   b) in preservative (e.g., RPMI (p. 1766)) and stored in ultralow-temperature freezer
2. materials that can be formed by the surgeon
   a) polymethylmethacrylate (PMMA): created by mixing methylmethacrylate powder with a liquid methylmethacrylate monomer in the O.R., which is molded to desired shape, and allowed to set (harden) before being attached to the skull with plates, sutures, or wire. The seting reaction is exothermic, and to prevent heat injury to the underlying brain, insulate the brain with wet surgical sponges and irrigate copiously during the setting process, or preferably, once the material is reasonably firm it can be removed from the operative site to complete the setting
   b) mesh: may be made of titanium or tantalum. Options include:
      - standard flat mesh. Can be molded to a limited degree. Usually better for smaller defects, e.g., < 5 cm diameter
      - preformed mesh (e.g., SmartMesh by KLS Martin, or CranioCurve® by Zimmer Biomet): mesh implants that are contoured to average skull shapes and common craniectomy configurations
3. pre-fabricated custom bone flaps: commercially manufactured using 3-D printing based on thin-cut CT scans of the defect and, if available, utilizing a "mirror image" of the intact contralateral side as a model for the desired contour
   a) polymethylmethacrylate (PMMA)
   b) PEEK (poly-ether-ether-ketone)
   c) titanium
   d) tantalum
   e) acrylic
4. split-thickness calvaria

When synthetic material is used, the flap should be perforated with a dozen or so drill holes to prevent the accumulation of fluid (either underneath the flap, or between the flap and the skull).

107.4.5 Complications

Complications include:
a) infection: ≈ 8% risk[21]
b) hematoma: under the cranioplasty flap (epidural or subdural)
c) seizures
d) brain injury
e) bone flap resorption (BFR): when using autologous bone (the patient's own bone). Reported range: 3–51%.[25] When BFR occurs, the rate of resorption is about 3%/year.[25] Risk factors have bee postulated, including length of time to reimplantation[26] but so far only younger age has been shown to correlate with increased incidence of BFR[25]
f) hydrocephalus
g) implant dislodgement

Risk of complication is increased with bifrontal bone defects.[27,28,29]

107.4.6 Technique

General information

The following pertains primarily to cranioplasty following a decompressive craniotomy.

Surgical objectives

a) separate the temporalis muscle from where it has scarred onto the dura
b) avoid CSF leak by not violating the dura (or pseudo-dura) or by closing any opening that is identified
c) repair the bone defect with a bone flap (see above for material options)
d) replace the temporalis muscle outside the bone graft and, if necessary, tack it into position

Risks

a) infection
b) post-op hematoma: epidural more likely than subdural
c) CSF leak

107

Surgical details

The following pertains in particular to decompressive craniectomy defect which extends from the parietal and frontal regions to include varying amounts of bone overlying the middle fossa.

* re-incise the previous skin incision, being careful to stay on bone where possible and, where the incision is not over bone, by using, e.g., a hemostat under the skin to prevent the scalpel from intracranial penetration
* starting at a point near the superior-most aspect of the defect, begin to separate the scalp flap from where it is scarred to the dura or pseudodora for a short distance (a couple of centimeters or so) inside the bone edges. This is usually easier if a barrier (e.g., silastic sheet) was placed at the time of the craniectomy. A Langenbeck periosteal elevator may work in areas where the planes separate easily, a #10 scalpel used with the sharp side of the blade pointing up may be used where scarring is more tenacious
* work around the defect in both directions towards the base of the flap, which is where the caudal aspect of the temporalis muscle crosses the edge of the defect to the outside of the skull
* as long as the tissue is thin (i.e., scar only, no temporalis muscle) use monopolar (Bovie) cautery along the bone as close as possible to the bone edge to expose the bone
* when you get to the point where the anterior and posterior aspect of the temporalis muscle pedicle is identified, you can begin to separate the muscle from where it is scarred to the dura/pseudodora and lift it off the dura along with the scalp
* during the process, some or all of the temporalis muscle will be detached from the dura and the overlying scalp (some surgeons intentionally detach it completely). Later in the case, the muscle may be tacked down to the bone flap (e.g., through perforation holes) or to the underside of the scalp
* the cup end of a Penfield #1 dissector may be used to free the scar tissue off the bone edge around the entire defect. The dissector need only expose down to the deep edge of the inner table, without separating the scar from the inner table (which could facilitate epidural bleeding/hematoma formation)
* if the flap is not already perforated, on the back table, the flap is multiply drilled to provide a route of drainage for epidural blood
* the bone flap is placed in the defect. If it is riding up at any point, the soft tissue and any irregularities my be corrected with a drill and/or rongeur
* the flap is secured in position, usually with titanium plates and screws
* a subgaleal drain is brought out through a separate stab incision and closure is performed in the usual manner

107.5 Decompressive craniectomy

107.5.1 Indications

Indications (controversial) include:

* malignant middle cerebral artery occlusion syndrome (p. 1589) primarily for nondominant hemisphere. Use on dominant side is more controversial

2. traumatic intracranial hypertension
   a) as an adjunct for persistent intracranial hypertension when other ICP control measures fail (p. 1100) [30]
   b) early in the management: may be considered for patients undergoing emergent surgery (for fracture, EDH, SDH…) [31]
3. uncontrollable brain swelling during craniotomy (p. 1729)
4. reported in children with refractory nontraumatic intracranial hypertension [32] (e.g., infection, infarction, Reye's syndrome…)

107.5.2 Potential complications

1. bleeding
2. herniation of the brain through the opening, compressing and lacerating the brain on the bone edges (risk may be reduced by making generous craniectomy)
3. post-op injury to the brain from inadvertent external pressure applied to the now relatively less protected brain
4. post-op fluid collections: hygromas or hematomas at the operative site, on the contralateral side, or interhemispheric

107.5.3 Techniques

General considerations

1. it is necessary to open the dura
2. options for the removed bone flap
   a) discard it: this may be the best option when the bone flap has been contaminated as a result of an open traumatic scalp laceration
   b) place it in a separate subcutaneous pouch in the patient's abdomen for later retrieval and reimplantation into the skull. This is especially helpful if the patient's own skull is preferred and the patient is not at the facility where the cranioplasty to replace the bone is likely to be performed (the patient takes the flap with them)
   c) store it externally for future reimplantation: saturate with sterile preservative solution (e.g., RPMI medium 1640; www.invitrogen.com/GIBCO) and then place within sterile storage (e.g., intestinal bags which are then placed in a sterile plastic container) and store in an ultralow-temperature freezer (approximately -80 °C)
   d) for non-contaminated situations (e.g., stroke): reimplantation can be considered after 6–12 weeks
3. bone openings need to be large (e.g., > 12 cm diameter, [33] often > 15 cm)

Hemicraniectomy

1. some prefer use of a Mayfield head-holder placed low (▶ Fig. 107.3) to give greater access [31] (not feasible with severe comminuted skull fractures)
2. AP axis of head is placed horizontal to floor (unless C-spine not cleared or if neck too immobile—one may compensate for this by rotating table)
3. skin incision: two options
   a) ▶ Fig. 107.4 A starts at widow's peak, similar to trauma flap (p. 1015), but with increased exposure by taking it posteriorly close to the inion, then turning sharply anteriorly and hugging the ear to preserve blood supply

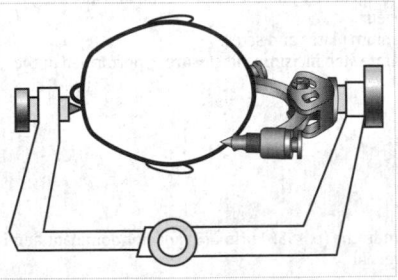

Fig. 107.3 Position of head and head-holder for right hemicraniectomy (looking down on top of patient's head).

b) ▶ Fig. 107.4 **B** "T" incision. Less risk of flap ischemia. The "T" joins the midline incision behind the coronal suture to preserve the STA[31]

c) burr holes (▶ Fig. 107.5): a burr hole is made just above the posterior root of the zygomatic arch, a second one may be made just behind the frontal insertion of the zygomatic arch, inferior to the superior temporal line

d) bone flap: proceed posteriorly from the posterior zygomatic arch using the footplated craniotome. Posteriorly, stay ≈ 1 cm superior to asterion to avoid the transverse sinus. The flap is taken 1 cm beyond the lambdoid suture, and then up towards the sagittal suture, crossing the lambdoid suture again (this leaves a small amount of bone posteriorly on which the head can rest post-op). An anterior turn is made 1 cm short of the sagittal suture to avoid the superior sagittal sinus, and the sagittal suture is paralleled. The coronal suture is crossed and the drill is taken as low as possible in the frontal fossa near the midline. Staying as low as possible, the orbital roof is followed posteriorly towards the second burr hole. The burr holes are then connected

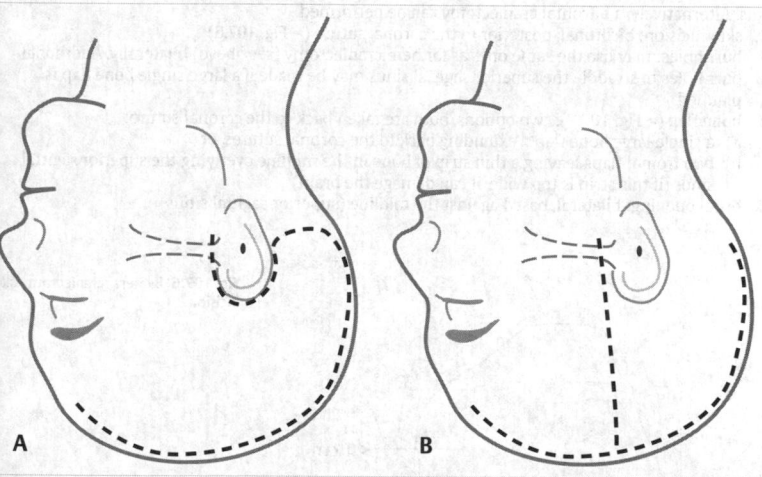

107

A B

Fig. 107.4 Two options for skin incision for hemicraniectomy (see text).

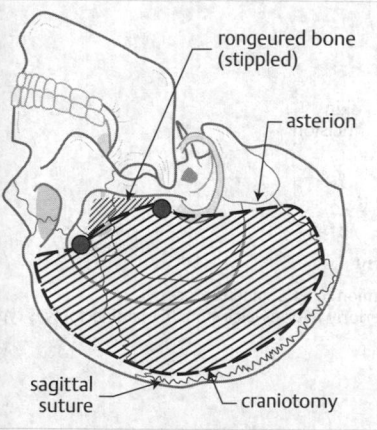

rongeured bone (stippled)

asterion

sagittal suture

craniotomy

Fig. 107.5 Hemicraniectomy bone flap.

e) some bone may need to be rongeured to expose the floor of the middle fossa (stippled area in ▶ Fig. 107.5)

f) dural opening: based inferiorly, taken to 1 cm short of the craniotomy edge. Dural releasing incisions may be made at intervals up to the bone margin to avoid strangulation of the brain on the dural edge

g) duraplasty
  • onlay: 2-cm-wide strips of dural substitute can then be placed partway under the dural edge around the periphery to isolate the brain from the undersurface of the skin flap where there will be a gap in the dura
  • some authors suture a dural graft in place

h) the dural flap is then replaced on top of the brain and dural substitute strips, and is not sutured

Bilateral craniectomy

The above procedure can be performed bilaterally; however, it is difficult to position the head to do this. Alternatively, a bifrontal craniectomy can be performed.
1. skin incision: bicoronal, posterior to the coronal suture (▶ Fig. 107.6)
2. burr holes: may use the same ones as for hemicraniectomy (see above) bilaterally. Additional burr holes to straddle the superior sagittal sinus may be made if a large single bone flap is planned
3. bone flap (▶ Fig. 107.7): two options, both are taken back to the coronal suture:
    a) a single large bone flap[34] extending back to the coronal sutures, or
    b) two frontal flaps leaving a thin strip of bone in the midline overlying the superior sagittal sinus (if this strip is too wide, it can damage the brain)
4. dural opening: bilateral, based against the midline (superior sagittal sinus)

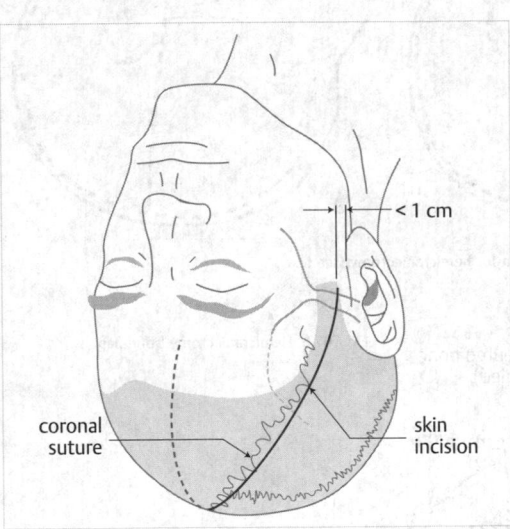

Fig. 107.6 Bilateral craniectomy skin incision.

< 1 cm

coronal suture

skin incision

Posterior fossa decompressive craniectomy

1. skin incision: midline skin incision from above inion to ≈ C2 spinous process
2. bone opening: laterally to sigmoid sinuses, superiorly to transverse sinus. C1 laminectomy is typically performed as well[32]
3. dural opening: "Y"-shaped incision

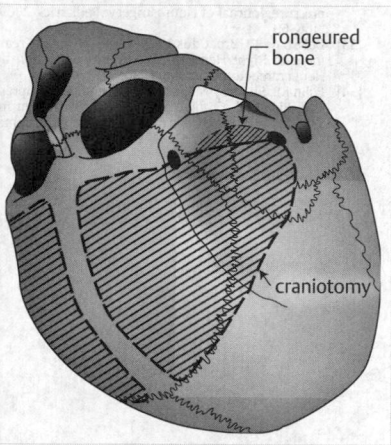

Fig. 107.7 Bilateral craniectomy skull flap shown with 2 separate frontal flaps (the preserved midline bone strip over the superior sagittal sinus is optional).

107

References

[1] Rowe R. Surgical approaches to the trigone. Contemporary Neurosurgery. 2005; 27:1–5

[2] Schmidek HH, Sweet WH. Operative Neurosurgical Techniques. New York 1982

[3] Yamamoto I, Rhoton AL, Peace DA. Microsurgery of the Third Ventricle: Part 1. Neurosurgery. 1981; 8:334–356

[4] Rhoton AL, Yamamoto I, Peace DA. Microsurgery of the Third Ventricle: Part 2. Operative Approaches. Neurosurgery. 1981; 8:357–373

[5] Carmel PW. Tumors of the Third Ventricle. Acta Neurochirurgica. 1985; 75:136–146

[6] Klein HJ, Rath SA. Removal of Tumors of the III Ventricle Using Lamina Terminalis Approach: Three Cases of Isolated Growth of Craniopharyngiomas in the III Ventricle. Child's Nervous System. 1989; 5:144–147

[7] Shucart WA, Stein BM. Transcallosal Approach to the Anterior Ventricular System. Neurosurgery. 1978; 3:339–343

[8] Apuzzo MLJ. Comment on Garrido E, et al.: Cerebral Venous and Sagittal Sinus Thrombosis After Transcallosal Removal of a Colloid Cyst of the Third Ventricle: Case Report. Neurosurgery. 1990; 26

[9] Apuzzo MLJ, Chikovani OK, Gott PS, et al. Transcallosal, Interforniceal Approaches for Lesions Affecting the Third Ventricle: Surgical Considerations and Consequences. Neurosurgery. 1982; 10:547–554

[10] Hirsch JF, Zouaoui A, Renier D, et al. A new surgical approach to the third ventricle with interruption of the striothalamic vein. Acta Neurochirurgica. 1979; 47:135–147

[11] Apuzzo MLJ. Surgery of Masses Affecting the Third Ventricular Chamber: Techniques and Strategies. Clinical Neurosurgery. 1988; 34:499–522

[12] Garrido E, Fahs GR. Cerebral Venous and Sagittal Sinus Thrombosis After Transcallosal Removal of a Colloid Cyst of the Third Ventricle: Case Report. Neurosurgery. 1990; 26:540–542

[13] Paredes I, Castano-Leon AM, Munarriz PM, et al. Cranioplasty after decompressive craniectomy. A prospective series analyzing complications and clinical improvement. Neurocirugia (Astur). 2015; 26:115–125

[14] Grant FC, Norcross NC. Repair of Cranial Defects by Cranioplasty. Annals of Surgery. 1939; 110:488–512

[15] Grantham EC, Landis HP. Cranioplasty and the post-traumatic syndrome. Journal of Neurosurgery. 1948; 5:19–22

[16] Stiver SI, Wintermark M, Manley GT. Reversible monoparesis following decompressive hemicraniectomy for traumatic brain injury. Journal of Neurosurgery. 2008; 109:245–254

[17] Mokri B. Orthostatic headaches in the syndrome of the trephined: resolution following cranioplasty. Headache. 2010; 50:1206–1211

[18] Fodstad H, Love JA, Ekstedt J, et al. Effect of cranioplasty on cerebrospinal fluid hydrodynamics in patients with the syndrome of the trephined. Acta Neurochirurgica (Wien). 1984; 70:21–30

[19] Joseph V, Reilly P. Syndrome of the trephined. Journal of Neurosurgery. 2009; 111:650–652

[20] Yamaura A, Sato M, Meguro K, et al. [Cranioplasty following decompressive craniectomy–analysis of 300 cases (author's transl)]. No Shinkei Geka. Neurological Surgery. 1977; 5:345–353

[21] Yadla S, Campbell PG, Chitale R, et al. Effect of early surgery, material, and method of flap preservation on cranioplasty infections: a systematic review. Neurosurgery. 2011; 68:1124–9; discussion 1130

[22] Xu H, Niu C, Fu X, et al. Early cranioplasty vs. late cranioplasty for the treatment of cranial defect: A systematic review. Clin Neurol Neurosurg. 2015; 136:33–40

[23] Morton RP, Abecassis IJ, Hanson JF, et al. Predictors of infection after 754 cranioplasty operations and the value of intraoperative cultures for cryopreserved bone flaps. J Neurosurg. 2016; 125:766–770

[24] Rish BL, Dillon JD, Meirowsky AM, et al. Cranioplasty: a review of 1030 cases of penetrating head injury. Neurosurgery. 1979; 4:381–385

[25] Park SP, Kim JH, Kang HI, et al. Bone Flap Resorption Following Cranioplasty with Autologous Bone: Quantitative Measurement of Bone Flap Resorption and Predictive Factors. J Korean Neurosurg Soc. 2017; 60:749–754

[26] de Franca SA, Nepomuceno TB, Paiva WS, et al. Cranial autologous bone flap resorption after a cranioplasty: A case report. Surg Neurol Int. 2018; 9. DOI: 10.4103/sni.sni_388_17

[27] Gooch MR, Gin GE, Kenning TJ, et al. Complications of cranioplasty following decompressive craniectomy: analysis of 62 cases. Neurosurgical Focus. 2009; 26. DOI: 10.3171/2009.3.FOCUS0962

[28] De Bonis P, Frassanito P, Mangiola A, et al. Cranial repair: how complicated is filling a "hole"? J Neurotrauma. 2012; 29:1071–1076

[29] Coulter IC, Pesic-Smith JD, Cato-Addison WB, et al. Routine but risky: a multi-centre analysis of the

outcomes of cranioplasty in the Northeast of England. Acta Neurochir (Wien). 2014; 156:1361–1368

[30] Bullock MR, Chesnut RM, Ghajar J, et al. Surgical management of traumatic parenchymal lesions. Neurosurgery. 2006; 58:S25–S46

[31] Holland M, Nakaji P. Craniectomy: Surgical indications and technique. Operative Techniques in Neurosurgery. 2004; 7:10–15

[32] Aghakhani Nozar, Durand Philippe, Chevret Laurent, et al. Decompressive craniectomy in children with nontraumatic refractory high intracranial pressure. Journal of Neurosurgery: Pediatrics. 2009; 3:66–69

[33] Delashaw JB, Broaddus WC, Kassell NF, et al. Treatment of Right Hemispheric Cerebral Infarction by Hemicraniectomy. Stroke. 1990; 21:874–881

[34] Polin RS, Shaffrey ME, Bogaev CA, et al. Decompressive Bifrontal Craniectomy in the Treatment of Severe Refractory Posttraumatic Cerebral Edema. Neurosurgery. 1997; 41:84–94

108 Spine, Cervical

108.1 Anterior approaches to the cervical spine

1. anterior odontoid screw (p.1775)
2. C1–3 (upper cervical spine):
   a) transoral approach: including odontoidectomy (p.1771)
   b) extrapharyngeal approaches: use nasotracheal intubation (so that the mandible can be completely closed) through the contralateral nares. The head is slightly extended and is rotated 15° to the contralateral side. Avoid any oral tubes
      • medial extrapharyngeal approach: medial to carotid sheath. Provides a more anterior position than the lateral retropharyngeal approach. Structures encountered: branches of external carotid artery, upper laryngeal nerves, hypoglossal nerve
      • lateral retropharyngeal approach: only the spinal accessory nerve is encountered
3. C3–7: standard anterior cervical discectomy approach
   a) For 1 or 2 level ACDF or 1 level corpectomy, a horizontal incision is usually employed
   b) For more levels, a vertically oriented incision may be preferred to facilitate access

108.2 Transoral approach to anterior craniocervical junction

108

108.2.1 General information

Primarily useful for midline *extradural* lesions (approach to intradural lesions has been described,[1] but the use has been extremely limited because of difficulties obtaining watertight closure and increased risk of meningitis). Refinements in techniques and equipment (e.g., flexible reinforced oral endotracheal tube, McGarver or Crockard retractor, operating microscope, and suturing transnasal red-rubber catheters to the uvula to aid in retraction) allow access from as high as the inferior third of the clivus to as low as C3 (and sometimes C4[2]) vertebral body without need for tracheostomy or splitting of the tongue. Additional access can be achieved with use of extended techniques, including splitting of the hard & soft palate, tongue splitting, and transmandibular approach.

108.2.2 Transoral odontoidectomy

Indications

Anterior extradural compression of the cervicomedullary junction as with pannus from rheumatoid arthritis, irreducible basilar invagination, tumors of C2, infection.

Stabilization

75% of patients undergoing transoral removal of the odontoid process required posterior fusion afterwards[3] due to ligamentous instability.[4,5] While the stabilization intuitively seems like it should be done first, it is often done following the decompression at the same sitting or at a soon-to-follow date. Some reasons for decompressing before stabilization:
1. positioning the patient for fusion may cause neurologic compromise if there is cord compression
2. a post-op MRI can be done to determine if enough decompression was achieved from the odontoidectomy. If not, a laminectomy can be done at the same time as the posterior stabilization
3. the amount of destabilization may not be known until after the odontoidectomy—in some cases a C1–2 fusion may suffice[5]

Stabilization usually entails posterior occipitocervical fusion. Occasionally fusion may be limited to C1–2 or C1–3 without the occiput. It is also possible to place an anterior strut between the body of C2 and the clivus, or between C2 and C1. Fibula is recommended. Metal instrumentation should be avoided.

Pre-op preparation

• make sure that the patient can open the mouth at least 25 mm. If not, then other approaches such as translabiomandibular should be considered

2. for conditions resulting in malalignment or basilar invagination, cervical traction for 1 or more days is sometimes required
3. radiographic evaluation
    a) cervical MRI without and with contrast to define the soft tissue pathology
    b) CT of the craniocervical junction with sagittal and coronal reconstruction
    c) CTA to assess the position and involvement of the vertebral arteries. Measuring the distance between the VAs provides useful information

Booking the case: Transoral approach

Also see defaults & disclaimers (p. 25).
1. position: supine with pin head-holder
2. equipment
    a) microscope
    b) high-speed drill with long bits
    c) C-arm
    d) image-guided navigation system (if used)
3. instruments
    a) transoral set (usually includes oral retractor such as Crockard, Dingman, Dickman-Sonntag...)
    b) long instruments: microdiscectomy instruments often work
4. anesthesia: intubation using video laryngoscopy, or second choice, asleep fiberoptic bronchoscopy[6]
5. some surgeons use ENT to perform the approach and closure and for follow-up
6. consent (in lay terms for the patient—not all-inclusive):
    a) procedure: transoral resection of odontoid, placement of halo-vest immobilization, MEP monitoring (MEP should be consented specifically due to risk of seizures). Need for posterior stabilization at the same setting or in the immediate future
    b) alternatives: nonsurgical management, radiation therapy for some diagnoses
    c) complications: CSF leak with possible meningitis, spinal cord injury, wound breakdown, breathing problems (may require tracheostomy), seizures with MEP, swallowing difficulties (may require PEG tube, usually temporary). The patient should not undergo the operation if they would not be willing to have a PEG tube placed if it is indicated in the opinion of the operating surgeon and/or their consultants

Technical considerations

Some key points (see references for details[2,3,7]):

Video laryngoscopy, or second choice, asleep fiberoptic bronchoscopy are now the intubation methods of choice (awake fiberoptic intubation is rarely used).[6] Nasotracheal (NT) is used by some but at the narrow upper part of the exposure the NT tube tends to get in the way.

SSEP and MEP monitoring are used in appropriate cases.

Positioning: 3-point fixation with a Mayfield head-holder is typically used. The patient is supine with no *neck rotation* (distorts the anatomical relationships and may bring one VA closer to the midline). Tilt the whole patient or the table towards the surgeon. 10–15° neck extension improves the exposure. Alternatively, the surgeon can stand above the patient who is kept perfectly supine.

A specialized retractor (e.g., Crockard transoral retractor) or a conventional Dingman retractor is placed. Verify that the tongue is not being compressed against the teeth.

Landmark: the tubercle of the atlas can be palpated through the posterior pharynx to locate the midline and for craniocaudal orientation.

The mucosa of the posterior pharynx is infiltrated with 1% lidocaine with epinephrine. Some authors culture the oropharynx to obtain drug sensitivities of organisms for use in the event of infection. Some advocate liberal topical use of 1% hydrocortisone ointment to the mucosa of the oropharynx and posterior tongue at the beginning and also during the operation to reduce intra-op and post-op swelling. Others feel it has no effect, and IV Decadron is used by some.

A 3-cm-long vertical midline incision is made.

To reduce the risk of C1 spreading and allowing basilar invagination, C1 ring-sparing surgery may be attempted by removing only the inferior half to two-thirds of the anterior C1. When C1 ring sparing is not done, the central 3 cm of the atlas is removed with a high-speed drill.

108

There is ≈ about 20–25 mm working distance between the two vertebral arteries at their point of closest approximation where they enter the foramen transversarium at the inferior aspect of the lateral mass of C2.

The odontoid is hollowed out ("like a canoe") using a high-speed drill, checking progress on lateral fluoro at frequent intervals. Once the bone has been reduced to a thin shell, it can be fractured in towards the hollowed-out portion using curettes. The superior tip of the odontoid is particularly challenging due to the apical ligament.

Closure: a two-layer closure is preferred by some. Others recommend a single-layer closure incorporating deep muscle, superficial muscle, and mucosa.[2] If the dura has been violated, a fascial patch is secured with tissue adhesive and a lumbar subarachnoid drain is placed in the O.R. and maintained at low pressure for 3–4 days. An NG tube is placed under direct visualization to avoid injury or penetration of the mucosal closure.

Posterior stabilization

Transoral odontoidectomy produces instability in most cases (sometimes delayed).[4,5]

For basilar invagination or occipitocervical instability, an occipitocervical fusion (p. 1773) is recommended.[7]

For C1–2 instability alone, a posterior C1–2 arthrodesis may be performed (p. 1778).[7]

Possible complications

1. dural tear with CSF leak and risk of meningitis
2. vertebral artery injury
3. spinal cord injury

Post-op care

1. NG feeding or IV hyperalimentation is used initially (in anticipation of oropharyngeal swelling (lasts 2–3 days) and to avoid disruption of the mucosal closure)
2. intubation is maintained until the swelling subsides. Initial removal of the endotracheal tube over a tube changer facilitates reintubation if needed; the tube changer can be removed if no problem develops after 1 hour[7]
3. if the NG tube comes out, it should only be replaced under direct vision (usually by ENT physician) to avoid injury/penetration of the mucosal incision
4. halo-vest immobilization is maintained until the posterior fusion is performed
5. for staged procedures when the fusion is being done at a later date, a post-op MRI should be done to assess the degree of decompression. If further decompression is needed, then a laminectomy can be added to the posterior fusion

108.3 Occipitocervical fusion

The patient will lose about 30% of neck flexion mobility with an occipital to C1 fusion.

Indications for occipitocervical fusion[8]:
1. traumatic occipitoatlantal dislocation
2. absence of a complete arch of C1. **Note:** Alternatively, C1–2 lateral mass fusion (with or without lateral mass screws) (p. 1779) may be used in cases b and c if only the posterior arch of C1 is compromised
   a) congenital
   b) post-decompression
   c) posttraumatic: "bursting" C1 fracture (bilateral or multiple C1 ring fractures). NB: some feel that this may be satisfactorily treated with halo immobilization until the atlas fracture heals (as they almost all do) followed by C1 to C2 wiring/fusion.[9]
3. congenital anomalies of the occipitocervical joints
4. upward migration of the odontoid into the foramen magnum
5. marked irreducible shifts of C1 or C2

Disadvantages of occipitocervical fusion:
1. loss of movement at the occipitoatlantal junction further reduces the range of motion as follows[10]:
   a) flexion/extension: reduced by ≈ 30% (13° occurs at occiput–C1 junction)
   b) lateral rotation: 10° is lost
   c) lateral bending: 8° is lost
2. non-union rate is higher than with C1–2 fusion alone[11]

Options:
1. keel plate (placed centrally over the thickest portion of the occipital bone) connected via rods to cervical screws (C2 pedicle screws and C3 lateral mass screws): reduced range of motion (ROM) to 17% of normal in a cadaver study[12] (for technique, see below)
2. occipital condyle (OC)–C1 polyaxial screws[13]: see below
3. occipital–C1 (AKA atlantooccipital) transarticular screws (see below)
4. looped rod wired to the occiput via wire cables placed through holes drilled in the occiput. Reduced ROM only to 31% of normal[12]

108.3.1 Keel plate occipital-cervical fusion

Pre-op planning:
1. CT scan through C2
   a) to rule out aberrant position of foramen transversarium
   b) to measure diameter of pedicles (may be best done on coronal sections due to the fact that the axial images are not usually oriented along path of pedicle) and estimate length of screws to be used
   c) to verify trajectory of screws
2. measure thickness of occipital bone to determine screw-length for occipital screws

108

Technique:
1. occipital keel screws/plate
   a) a drill, tap, and screwdriver with flexible shafts or universal joints are usually needed because of interference from patient's skin
   b) midline holes are preferred since occipital bone is thickest here
   c) drill with drill guide set to 8 mm, check depth with probe, if the inner cortex has not been breached, increase the drill depth by 2 mm, drill to the new depth, check depth again, and continue the process increasing the drill length by 2 mm at a time until the inner cortex is breached or 14–16 mm is reached. Use a screw length equal to the depth that was drilled
   d) SCREWS occipital screws are cortical screws (narrow pitch) and the distal tip is **blunt** (to avoid dural injury).
      Typical dimensions: 4.5 mm diameter, 8–12 mm length
2. C2 pedicle screws (p. 1784)
3. C3 lateral mass screws (p. 1784) (if used)

108.3.2 Occipital condyle to C1 polyaxial screw fusion

See references.[13,14]
   Utilizes polyaxial screws placed in the occipital condyles that are then connected to screws placed at lower levels (see below) via connecting rods.
1. PROS compared to occipital plate/keel instrumentation:
   a) circumvents problem of poor occipital bone purchase which may occur with keel plates
   b) can be used even following posterior fossa craniectomy
   c) greater surface area for fusion
   d) avoids risk of intracranial injury from occipital screws
2. CONS: due to condylar variability, not all patients are candidates
3. biomechanics: compared to occipital plate, similar stiffness in flexion-extension and axial rotation, increased stiffness to lateral bending[15]

Pre-op planning: CT scan occiput through C2.
   Technique:
   ✖ Structures to avoid include: hypoglossal nerve in hypoglossal canal (just above the occipital condyles (OC)), carotid and vertebral arteries, jugular bulb. Image guidance can be helpful.
1. occipital condyle screws
   a) ENTRY 4–5 mm lateral to the foramen magnum, 1–2 mm rostral to the atlantooccipital joint (no need to expose the entire condyle—it is only necessary to expose as far laterally as the posterior condylar emissary vein which is best left alone but if necessary may be safely coagulated in most cases[13])
   b) TRAJ 12–22° medial (mean: 17°), 5° maximal superior angulation
   c) SCREWS 3.5 mm diameter polyaxial screws; bicortical purchase obtained using 20–24 mm length (mean: 22 mm)

2. condyle screws are connected with 3 mm diameter rods to either:
   a) C1 lateral mass screws (p. 1781) and C2 pars screws (p. 1784), or
   b) C1–2 transarticular screws (p. 1779)

108.3.3 Occipital–C1 (AKA atlantooccipital) transarticular screws

See references.[16,17]
1. PROS: no compromise of C1–2 joint
2. CONS: steep trajectory requires additional incision at level of C–T junction
3. ENTRY midpoint of posterior C1 lateral mass
4. TRAJ 10–20° medially, aiming cranially to TARGET middle of occipital condyle
5. SCREWS 28–32 mm cannulated lag screws
6. biomechanics: ≈ equal to occipital plate–C1 lateral mass fusion[18]
7. clinical data: 2 cases reported, 2 year F/U, no complication

108.3.4 Post-op immobilization/bracing

1. for severe C1 fractures, or those with impaired bone healing capacity (elderly or unreliable patients, smokers…) a halo-vest is recommended × 8–12 weeks
2. otherwise, if C1 is not badly damaged, a collar that limits flexion (e.g., Miami-J collar) suffices × 8–12 weeks

108

108.4 Anterior odontoid screw fixation (OSF)

108.4.1 Introduction

50% of axial rotation of the head occurs at the C1–2 complex. Stability of the C1–2 joint depends primarily on the integrity of the odontoid process and the atlantal transverse ligament (p. 69) (which is the most important structure holding the odontoid process in position against the anterior arch of C1).

Odontoid screw fixation (OSF) treats odontoid fractures by restoring the structural integrity of the odontoid process (osteosynthesis) without sacrificing normal mobility. Other treatment methods, e.g., C1–2 fusion, significantly reduce rotational mobility (although subaxial articulations will compensate to some degree over time).

108.4.2 Evaluation

A full set of C-spine X-rays is needed (including an open-mouth odontoid view in addition to AP, lateral, and flexion/extension views). MRI is recommended to rule out disruption of atlantal transverse ligament. Cervical axial CT with coronal and sagittal reconstructions are also recommended to demonstrate the orientation of the fracture path and to verify the integrity of the posterior elements.

108.4.3 Indications

See guidelines for management of isolated odontoid fractures. (p. 1173)

In general, a reducible odontoid Type II fracture (and Type III fractures where the fracture line is in the cephalad portion of the body of C2 in an elderly patient who may not fuse as well with immobilization as a younger patient[19]). Absolute requirement: the transverse ligament *must be* intact.

108.4.4 Contraindications

1. fractures of the C2 vertebral *body* (except cephalad Type III fracture)
2. disruption of transverse atlantal ligament (TAL): see Atlantoaxial transverse ligament (TAL) injuries (p. 1778). May be directly demonstrated on MRI. Indirect evidence: if the sum of the overhang of the lateral masses of C1 on C2 exceeds 7 mm (rule of Spence (p. 1161) - NB: this rule is inaccurate and should not be used as the sole determinant)
3. large odontoid fracture gap
4. irreducible fracture
5. age of fracture: controversial. Fusion rates in fracture > 18 months old was 25%.[20] Fracture < 6 months old have ≈ 90% fusion rate[20]

6. patients with short, thick necks and/or barrel chest: makes it difficult to achieve the proper angle. May be circumvented by the instrumentation distributed by Richard-Nephew which utilizes a cannulated flexible drill, tap, and screwdriver
7. pathologic odontoid fracture
8. fracture line in oblique orientation to frontal plane (shearing forces can cause malalignment during screw tightening)

Booking the case: Odontoid screw fixation

See defaults & disclaimers (p. 25).
1. position: supine head on horseshoe headrest, halter traction
2. anesthesia: video laryngoscopy, or second choice, asleep fiberoptic bronchoscopy are the intubation methods of choice (awake fiberoptic intubation is rarely used).[6] Do NOT use a wire-reinforced endotracheal tube
3. equipment: **2 C-arms** for biplane fluoro, or image guidance system
4. instrumentation:
   a) some surgeons use specialized instrumentation (e.g., Apfelbaum set). Alternatively the following may be used
   b) ACDF surgical set
   c) retractor: a tubular retractor (e.g., METRx® by Medtronic) works well, a radiolucent tube may be advantageous
   d) consider having posterior cervical fusion instrumentation available (e.g., for C1–2 fusion (p. 1778) ± occipital plate as appropriate) in case the odontoid screw has to be aborted
5. implants: 4 mm diameter cannulated screws, lag screws & conventional screws, 40–50 mm lengths will cover most situations. These may be found in cannulated screw sets e.g., as used by orthopedic surgeons for minor fractures or in specialty sets such as Medtronic UCSS (Universal Cannulated Screw Set)
6. consent (in lay terms for the patient—not all-inclusive):
   a) procedure: surgery to place screw(s) from the front of the neck across the fractured odontoid bone. Possible posterior approach in case the anterior approach cannot be completed
   b) alternatives: nonsurgical management in a collar (which has a low chance of success in certain situations, e.g., age ≥ 50, displacement ≥ 5 mm), fusion (C1–2 or occiput–C2 or other, as appropriate) which will result in some loss of motion
   c) complications: screw breakage/pullout, failure to fuse which might require additional surgery (which will reduce neck motion), some of the usual risks of anterior cervical spine approaches (p. 1286) (swallowing difficulties, injury to esophagus, trachea, carotid artery, recurrent laryngeal nerve palsy..., but generally not including spinal cord, nerve root, or vertebral artery injury). The patient should not undergo the operation if they would not be willing to have a PEG tube placed if it is indicated in the opinion of the operating surgeon and/or their consultants
   d) consider consenting patient for posterior C1–2 fusion in case the odontoid screw has to be aborted

108.4.5 Technique summary

Preparation

Various instrumentation systems have been developed to facilitate the procedure. The following describes some of the basic elements that are not specific to any one instrumentation (see reference by Apfelbaum[21] for details of his instrumentation distributed by Aesculap Instrument Corporation, South San Francisco, CA).

Two C-arm fluoroscopy machines are mandatory for bi-plane imaging (simultaneous AP and lateral views). Some surgeons prefer placing 2 screws if there is enough bone to accommodate them; however, this may also reduce the amount of bone surface that can heal and the fusion rate appears to be the same.[22]

Anesthetic considerations

The anesthesiologist is positioned at the *foot* of the table. Video laryngoscopy, or second choice, asleep fiberoptic bronchoscopy are now the intubation methods of choice (awake fiberoptic intubation is rarely used).[6] Do NOT use a wire-reinforced endotracheal tube since the wire interferes with the AP imaging.

Position

Supine. The neck is placed in *extension* (critical to performing the procedure) either with Holter traction and a small shoulder roll with the head on a gel donut (a strip of tape across the forehead stabilizes the head), or a radiolucent head-holder may be used. Place the *lateral* fluoro unit first, then the AP unit slides into the "C" of the lateral unit. Lateral fluoroscopy is used to assess reduction of the fracture fragment, and the head is repositioned to try and achieve reduction. If there is retrolisthesis of the odontoid, the neck may need to be slightly less extended. A radiolucent mouth gag is placed to hold the mouth open for AP transoral imaging (a small tape roll works well). Abort the procedure if AP and lateral fluoroscopic views do not adequately image the odontoid.

Once the patient is positioned, place a guidewire alongside the neck and verify with fluoro that the screw passing through C2 into the odontoid tip will project to a point that is not inside the patient's chest (if that cannot be corrected with repositioning of the head, then the operation should be aborted).

Approach

A Cloward-type of horizontal skin incision at ≈ C5–6 (the entry site can be localized by placing a guidewire adjacent to the patient's neck and taking a lateral fluoro as noted above) and approach identical to anterior cervical discectomy are used (all the way to exposing the longus colli muscles (p. 1284)). A Kittner is used to dissect superiorly anterior to the longus colli muscles in the loose areolar tissue up to C2. A self-retaining retractor (e.g., Caspar retractor, not distractor) with a superior retractor blade attached may be used (or a hand-held retractor, preferably radiolucent, may be used). Alternatively, a retractor tube system[23] (e.g., METRx® by Medtronic, which manufactures a specialized extra-angled bevelled tube for this procedure) may be used. The bovie is used to remove the soft tissue over the inferior front of C2.

Procedure

Localization: lateral fluoro is used to place the tip of an awl *as far anteriorly as possible* on the inferior endplate of C2 (▶ Fig. 108.1; common errors: 1) entering too far posterior along the inferior

108

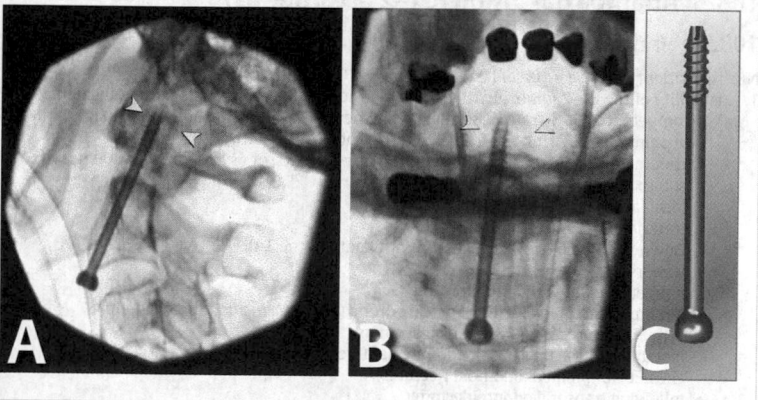

Fig. 108.1 Anterior odontoid screw.
Final radiographs, A: lateral, B: AP. The edges of the odontoid tip fragment are indicated by *yellow arrowheads*. C: illustration of a lag screw as used in this case.

margin of C2, which results in the guidewire ending up toward the back of the dens, 2) entering too far anterior which pre-disposes to the screw breaking out through the anterior cortex of C2). AP fluoro is used to place the awl in the exact center of the C2 body in the medio-lateral dimension. The awl is used to make a pilot hole at this location.

Guidewire placement, drilling, tapping, and ultimately screw placement are performed while monitoring the progress on frequent fluoro images, aiming for the exact middle of the dens on AP fluoro, and aiming toward the apex of the odontoid fracture fragment on lateral fluoro.

Drilling is performed under fluoro all the way *through* the apical cortex of the dens to avoid cracking the dens with the screw (the area just distal to the apex of the dens is safe).

Screw placement. If there is a minimal gap a fully threaded cannulated screw may be used. If there is a gap between the odotoid tip fragment and the body of the odontoid, a cannulated lag screw (a screw with an unthreaded proximal shaft, ▶ Fig. 108.1–C) is preferred. If a lag screw is not available, one can overdrill (i.e., using a larger diameter drill bit) the part of the path through the body of C2 up to the fracture and then use a fully threaded screw, which will slip through the overdrilled hole and still have a lag effect on the fracture fragment. If a second side-by-side screw is used, it may be fully threaded. In chronic nonunion cases, prior to advancing the screw, a bifaced curette may be inserted within the fracture space to freshen the fracture site. The screw(s) should be drawn up tightly to the inferior edge of C2. The challenge is to turn the screw enough to draw the fragment closer to the body to narrow the gap without turning it so much that it strips the bone in the fragment and the operation is for naught. ▶ Fig. 108.1 shows the final position of an anterior odontoid screw.

At the end of the procedure confirm integrity of the transverse ligament by carefully flexing the neck under lateral fluoro.

Postoperative immobilization

The immediate post-op strength of the odontoid + screw is only ≈ 50% of the normal odontoid. Therefore, a cervical brace is recommended for 6 weeks[19] (although some authors don't use one[21]). If the patient has significant osteoporosis, a halo brace is recommended.

Results

Healing takes ≈ 3 months (or longer with chronic nonunion). With fractures < 6 months old, the union rate was 95%. Chronic nonunions > 6 months old have a significant risk of hardware failure (screw breakage or pull-out), with a bony union rate of 31%, and 38% rate of presumed fibrous union.[21] Thus, in cases of chronic nonunion > 6 months old, C1–2 arthrodesis is probably a better choice unless the need to maintain motion is worth the risk of needing a second operation if the one fails.

The average technical complication rate is ≈ 6% (2% screw malposition, 1.5% screw breakout).

108.5 Atlantoaxial fusion (C1–2 arthrodesis)

108.5.1 Indications

NB: The patient will lose ≈ 50% of head rotation with C1–2 fusion.
1. instability of the C1–2 joints (usually with associated **atlantoaxial dislocation**), including:
   a) incompetence of the transverse atlantal ligament (TAL) (most result from damage to the insertion point of the TAL on the medial tubercles of C1 (▶ Fig. 1.14):
      - rheumatoid arthritis (p. 1378): symptomatic patients, or asymptomatic patients with subluxation ≥ 8 mm
      - local infection
      - traumatic disruption of the TAL
      - Down syndrome (p. 1381) patients with laxity of the TAL
      - tumors
   b) incompetence of the odontoid process
      - odontoid fractures meeting surgical criteria (p. 1174), including (in patients ≥ 7 years of age) Type II fractures with ≥ 5 mm displacement
        instability at the fracture site despite halo-vest traction
        chronic nonunion of odontoid fractures
      - following transoral odontoidectomy
      - tumors destroying the odontoid process
2. hangman's fractures that require surgical stabilization
3. vertebrobasilar insufficiency with head turning (p. 1592) (bow hunter's sign)

108.5.2 Technical considerations

Some cases require incorporation of the occiput in addition to C1–2.
  Surgical options include:

▶ **Rigid instrumentation:**
1. C1–2 fusion using polyaxial screws connected by rods:
    a) C1: screws placed in lateral masses. May be used in cases where the posterior arch of C1 is compromised
    b) C2 screw options:
        • screws may be placed in pedicles (pars)
        • screws may be placed in lateral masses
        • crossed C2 laminar screws[24]
2. C1–2 posterior transarticular facet screws (TAS)[25,26,27]

▶ **Posterior cervical wiring and fusion.** With the development of rigid fixation, these techniques are used less frequently. While they are poor in limiting rotation, they are effective in limiting flexion. And since the Dickman and Sonntag technique is effective in limiting extension, it has recently been used to offload C1 lateral mass screws which have a tendency to break at the bone interface (point of entry to the bone) of C1
1. interspinous fusion technique of Dickman and Sonntag (p. 1783)
2. not presented here:
    a) Brooks fusion[28] (the Smith-Robinson technique as modified by Griswold[29]): C1 to C2 sublaminar wires with 2 wedge bone grafts
    b) Gallie fusion[30 (p 1477–93)] and its modifications: midline wire under the arch of C1 with an "H" bone graft

▶ **Halifax clamps with fusion.**[31] These clamps are effective in minimizing movement in flexion, but are less stable in extension or with rotation

▶ **Odontoid compression screw fixation** (p. 1775). Essentially only for odontoid Type II fractures < months old with intact transverse ligament (p. 1775).[32] Preserves more mobility than C1–2 fusion

▶ **Combined anterolateral and posterior bone grafting.**[32]
▶ **Combining anterior (transoral) decompression with posterior fusion.** Indicated when a significant anterior mass is present, causing neural compression and/or making passage of sublaminar wires at C1 unsafe

108.5.3 Techniques of atlantoaxial fusion

Positioning

The patient is placed in a halo ring (with a gap in the back and secured to the table using a Mayfield adapter) or Mayfield pin fixation and is then placed prone on the O.R. table on chest rolls. The table will usually need to be positioned in a maximal reverse-Trendelenburg position to bring up the surgical area. The patient's feet are allowed to rest on a padded footplate on the table to prevent the patient from sliding down. Lateral intraoperative X-rays are taken after patient positioning.

Incision and approach

A midline skin incision is made from just below the inion to the spinous process of C5 or C6.

C1–2 transarticular facet screws (TAS)

May be used as an adjunct to posterior C1–2 wiring and bone graft—e.g., technique of Dickman and Sonntag (p. 1783)—to achieve immediate stabilization without the need for postoperative external orthosis, or in cases where the posterior arch of C1 is fractured or absent. ✖ A major risk of the procedure is vertebral artery (VA) injury. Therefore many practitioners have adopted C1 lateral mass screws (p. 1780).

Selection of candidates

May be appropriate in elderly patients or those with rheumatoid arthritis, in whom there may be slow fusion, or for those who have failed a previous attempt at C1–2 wiring/fusion. Also in young individuals who have ligamentous laxity.

All patients must have thin-cut CT scans from the occipital condyles through C3 with sagitta reconstruction through the C1–2 facet on both sides to look for the presence of a vertebral artery ir the intended path of the screw. Also, risk of VA injury can be reduced using CT scans reconstructed along the planned trajectory of the screw (aiming from a point 4 mm above the inferior C2 facet to a point in the anterior C1 button on CT[33]).

Technique summary
A number of instrumentation sets are available for the procedure, and each has its own nuances. The following is intended to primarily cover the basic procedure common to most or all (see reference by Apfelbaum[21] for details with that system).

▶ **Position.** Patient prone, with the head clamped in a Mayfield head-holder with a slight military tuck of the chin. Lateral C-arm fluoroscopy is used for the procedure, and some have advocated biplane fluoro.

▶ **Approach.** Utilize a standard midline posterior laminectomy approach from occiput to the C3 spinous process. The lamina of C2 and the posterior arch of C1 are exposed to the lateral aspect of the C2 inferior articular facet. The lateral extent of the spinal canal is defined using a small angled curette. The C1–2 facet is curetted to facilitate arthrodesis and permits observation of the drill as i crosses the joint.

▶ **Screw placement and fusion.** ENTRY 1–2 mm superior to the C2–3 facet on the midline axis c the pars interarticularis. The trajectory is determined fluoroscopically using a Kirschner wire (K wire) placed on the side of the neck as a guide, aiming it through the C2 inferior articular proces: pars interarticularis, superior articular process and across the C1–2 articulation into the lateral mas of C1. This helps establish the appropriate entry site for the drill guide through a separate sta wound, usually around the T1–2 level, 2–3 cm off the midline.

TRAJ A pilot hole is then drilled using visual guidance to maintain a straight parasagittal course (helps to stand on 1 or 2 footstools to eliminate some of the parallax error) and fluoroscopic guidanc to maintain the trajectory towards the C1 lateral mass. An assistant can reduce any atlanto-axi translational malalignment using a towel clip on C1 or C2 just prior to the drill crossing the C1– facet joint. To minimize the risk of VA injury, keep the drill as far dorsally as possible within the par interarticularis. The pilot hole is then tapped and a fully threaded titanium screw is placed. If bris arterial bleeding (not bone bleeding) occurs after drilling or tapping the first side, the VA may hav been injured. The screw may still be placed but the contralateral hole and screw should *not* b placed. A post-op arteriogram is then performed to assess for propagating thrombus or dissectio Barring any contraindications, the procedure is repeated on the contralateral side. After screw plac ment, then posterior bone fusion—e.g., technique of Dickman and Sonntag (p. 1783)—is performed.

▶ **Post-operative care.** External immobilization is optional. Some surgeons do not feel it is manda tory as they consider the screws to supply adequate internal immobilization.

Results
A fusion rate of up to 99% with no complications has been reported.[25] Injury to the vertebral arter is the main potential complication.

C1–2 screw fixation

Placement of polyaxial mini screws in C1 (lateral mass, originated by Goel and Laheri[34] in 1994 ar promulgated in 2001 by Harms and Melcher[35] or posterior arch lateral mass (PALM)[36,37]) and C pedicle with rod fixation.

Advantages over C1–2 transarticular screws (see above):
1. the more superior and medial trajectory should reduce the risk of VA injury[35]
2. may be used in the presence of C1–2 subluxation
3. may be usable in certain cases of aberrant VA course
4. in selected cases, this can be used for temporary fixation without fusion (since joint spaces remain intact) and the hardware may be removed after an appropriate time to reclaim motion i the C1–2 articulation

Booking the case: C1–2 lateral mass fusion

Also see defaults & disclaimers (p. 25) and pre-op assessment (see below).
1. position: prone, pin head-holder
2. anesthesia: intubation using video laryngoscopy, or second choice, asleep fiberoptic broncho-scopy (awake fiberoptic intubation is rarely used)[6]
3. equipment: C-arm or (optional) image-guided navigation system
4. implants:
   a) mini-polyaxial screws (smooth shank screws needed if C1 lateral mass screws are a possibility)
   b) cable for interspinous graft: C1 ring must be intact (optional, but recommended)
   c) have occipital plates and instrumentation available in case of inability to place C1 screws, thereby enabling occipital-cervical fusion as a bail-out option
5. consent (in lay terms for the patient—not all-inclusive):
   a) procedure: surgery to place screws & rods from the back of the neck to stabilize and usually to fuse the top 2 bones of the neck
   b) alternatives: nonsurgical management in a collar, in some cases screws may be temporary and no fusion would be done
   c) complications: screw breakage/pullout, failure to fuse which might require additional surgery, loss of some neck bending motion is expected (≈ 20% is typical)

108

Surgical technique (excerpted highlights)
See references.[35,38]

Applied anatomy: there is no true neural foramen at C1–2, the C2 nerve root lies on the posterior surface of the capsule of the C1–2 articular joint.

Pre-op assessment
It is mandatory to know the position of the VA on both sides (and in particular, the location of both foramina transversarium of C1), and the following bony information (requires thin-cut CT scan):
1. craniocaudal thickness (height) of the posterior arch of C1 (in case the arch needs to be drilled to facilitate screw placement)
2. to determine screw length: distance from the planned entry point (see below) to the planned exit target (midposition of the anterior part of the superior C1 VB)
3. to estimate mediolateral angle for screws

C1 lateral mass screws
This is one option for C1 lateral mass screws. For the PALM technique, see below.
1. NB: if fusion is to accompany screw placement (i.e., permanent screw placement), strong consideration should be given to supplemental interspinous fusion, if not contraindicated (p. 1783) to prevent fatigue breakage of C1 screws where they penetrate the lateral mass
2. dissect over the superior surface of the C2 pars interarticularis to reach the posterior aspect of the C1–2 joint. Expose approximately the lateral half of the C1–2 joint (allows the C2 root to be retracted inferiorly and medially). Use a Penfield #4 dissector to palpate the medial aspect of the joint to accurately locate the entry point for the C1 lateral mass screws in the midpoint. Bleeding is controlled with bipolar cautery and/or Gelfoam-thrombin.
3. C1 lateral mass screws ENTRY visualization commonly requires caudal & medial retraction of the C2 dorsal root ganglion (occasionally this may not be feasible[38]; sacrificing the C2 root may be required but this can lead to post-op pain and numbness[39]; technique is to divide the *preganglionic* nerve fibers and to close the dural defect[38]). The screw entry point is the midpoint of the inferior part of the C1 lateral mass (for both mediolateral and craniocaudal directions). An awl or a 1- to 2-mm high-speed drill is used to mark the position to prevent slippage while drilling the hole. Drilling a portion of the inferior arch of C1 is sometimes needed to allow screw placement (✖ CAUTION: the thickness of the arch in the craniocaudal dimension varies widely, and the horizontal segment of the VA lies immediately above—use pre-op CT for planning)
TRAJ averages ≈ 17° medially, ≈ 22° rostrally, TARGET the superior aspect of the anterior tubercle of C1 on lateral fluoro (see ▶ Fig. 108.2)
C1 SCREWS 3.5 or 4 mm diameter, length is determined from pre-op fine-cut CT to obtain bicortical purchase (✖ CAUTION: the ICA may be as close as 1 mm to the ideal exit site of the screw[40] ∴ some authors use only unicortical purchase). The screw needs to be proud to bring it up to the level of the C2 screw (it may actually be necessary to have the C1 screw protruding 1–2 mm more

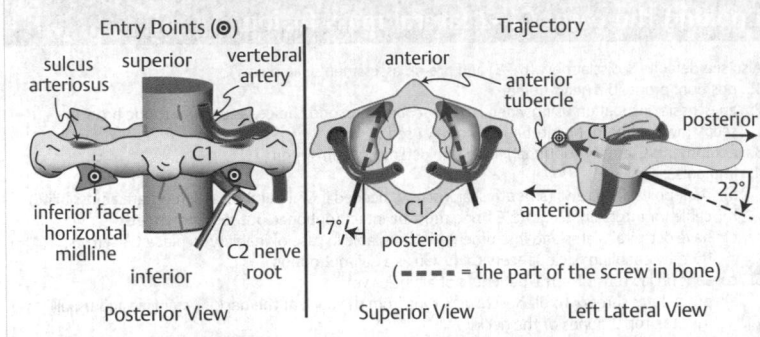

Fig. 108.2 Screw entry point and trajectory for C1 lateral mass screws.

than the C2 screw in order to allow rod attachment[38]), and it should have an unthreaded portion (smooth shank) to minimize irritation of the C2 nerve, which could produce occipital neuralgia (unfortunately, most of the screws have only ≈ 10 mm smooth shank which is usually not long enough so some threads will contact the C2 nerve root)

6. C2 pedicle (pars) screws are placed as usual (see C2 pedicle (pars) screws (p. 1784))
7. if a fusion is to be performed: the posterior arch of C1 and the C2 lamina are decorticated with a drill. Onlay fusion substrate is then placed, taking care not to compress the dura. Optional adjunct: intra-articular decortication and packing bone within the C1–2 joint

Posterior arch lateral mass (PALM) C1 screws

C1 lateral mass polyaxial screws that enter through the arch as an alternative to entering the lateral mass directly. A slight variation results in "C1 pedicle screws".[41] May be used in patients who do not have a diminutive posterior C1 arch (the average C1 pedicle height ranges from 3.95–4.8 mm[41]; even then a small inferior breach should not be harmful). Advantages: reduces the amount of C1 lateral mass dissection needed with less bleeding, obviates the need to sacrifice the C2 nerve root which is required in some cases of direct lateral mass screws, avoids having exposed C1 screw that tends to break at the bone interface.[36,37]

1. the position of the VA must be known. To protect it during drilling, it can be dissected subperiosteally from the sulcus arteriosus (▶ Fig. 108.3) on the superior surface of C1 and lifted gently off the bone with a dissector[36]
2. ENTRY the posterior arch of C1, various localizing options include
   • centered over C2 screw if already placed
   • in line with the center of the C2 facet[36,41]
   • 2 cm from midline, 2 mm from inferior border of posterior arch[42]

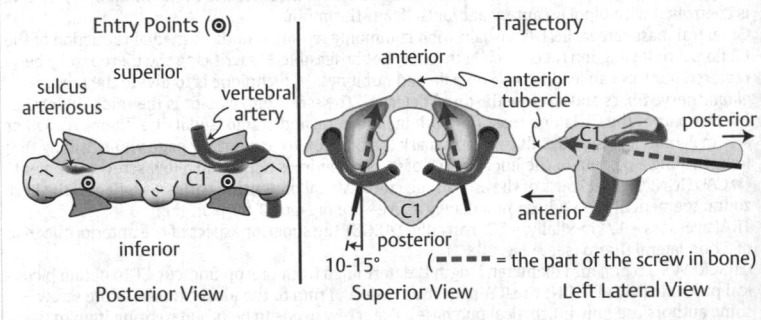

Fig. 108.3 Screw entry point and trajectory for C1 PALM screws.

3. TRAJ 10–15° medial (similar to above); craniocaudal direction is determined using lateral fluoro-scopy to parallel the C1 arch[41]
4. SCREWS 3.5 mm diameter; length to bring the tip just behind the front of the C1 anterior tubercle
5. C2 pedicle (pars) screws are placed as usual if not already done (see C2 pedicle (pars) screws (p.1784))

Post-op care
Optional: cervical collar (soft or rigid, as preferred) for 4–6 weeks.

Interspinous fusion technique of Dickman and Sonntag

A single bicortical graft is used, with multistranded cable passed sublaminar to C1 only. The bone graft is wedged between C1 and C2 (trapping it between loops of cable),[43,44] see ▶ Fig. 108.4. Currently, this technique is infrequently used as the primary fixation for C1–2 fusion (unless technical difficulties prevent e.g., C1–2 lateral mass fusion). However, it may be most useful for limiting flexion and extension to offload C1 lateral mass screws to reduce the risk of screw breakage.[45]

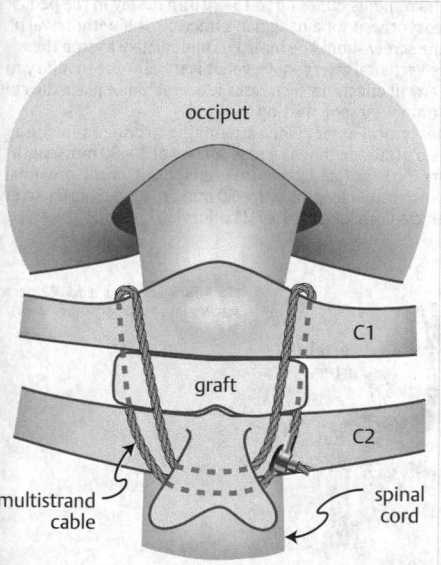

Fig. 108.4 Dickman and Sonntag C1–2 inter-spinous fusion.
Illustrated with multistrand cable system, e.g., Medtronic ATLAS™ (formerly Songer Cable).

108

Cannot be used if the posterior ring of C1 or C2 is not intact.

Bone graft. Autologous bone is preferred. Bone is often taken from the posterior iliac crest (p.1725). A tricortical graft of ≈ 4 cm length and > 1 cm height is obtained. The top edge is removed to create a bicortical graft of ≈ 1 cm height.

108.6 C2 screws

108.6.1 Options

pedicle screws (pars interarticularis screws): directed medially (see below)
lateral mass screws: directed laterally. Length is sized to fall short of foramen transversarium
C1–2 transarticular screws (p.1779): associated with more risk of VA injury

4. translaminar screws[46,47]: 1 year stability appears to be less than C2 pedicle screws when used for subaxial fusions, but was ≈ as effective for axial fusions (C1–2 or C1–3).[48] May be useful as a "bail out" for subaxial fusions when the C2 pars diameter is too small for pedicle screws[49]

108.6.2 C2 pedicle (pars) screws

Check CT scan or MRI to rule out aberrant location of vertebral artery or unusual location of foramen transversarium before placing C2 pedicle screws. Some find image-guided navigation systems to be helpful.

Technique:

1. ENTRY palpate the medial and superior aspect of the pars with a Penfield 4 dissector (► Fig. 108.5). Enter at the estimated center of the surface projection of the C2 pars at the mid-point mediolaterally[35] in the superomedial quadrant of the surface of the C2 isthmus
2. TRAJ **20–30° medially** (through the central axis of the C2 pedicle),[50] 25° superiorly (on lateral fluoroscopy, place the screw parallel to the pars) (► Fig. 108.6). To assist with trajectory, expose the proximal upper and medial border of the C2 pars interarticularis, and use a Penfield 4 to palpate during drilling (► Fig. 108.5)
3. drill a shallow entry point, then drill with drill-stop set at 12 mm, monitoring progress at intervals under fluoro and palpating with probe, and if no breakout, then complete drilling by gradually increasing drilling depth by 2-mm increments either up to 15–20 mm to stay in the pedicles or up to ≈ 30 mm depth to perform osteosynthesis for a hangman's fracture. ✖ If withdrawal of the drill is followed by brisk bleeding, the screw should be inserted immediately to stop the bleeding. This bleeding may be from the vertebral artery; however, it is usually due to injury to the venous plexuses, and will not have any ill effects. In such cases it is best to not place the contralateral screw and to obtain an angiogram very soon post-op
4. SCREWS **3.5 mm dia.** Screw length is not critical except when attempting to bridge a fracture gap (osteosynthesis) e.g., with a hangman's fracture in which case screws of 20–30 mm length are placed to avoid penetrating anterior C2 cortex (lag screws are used for this, or the proximal bone can be overdrilled); for most purposes screw lengths of 15–20 mm are used. Shorter screws (15–16 mm length) can still grip the pedicle with lower risk of VA injury

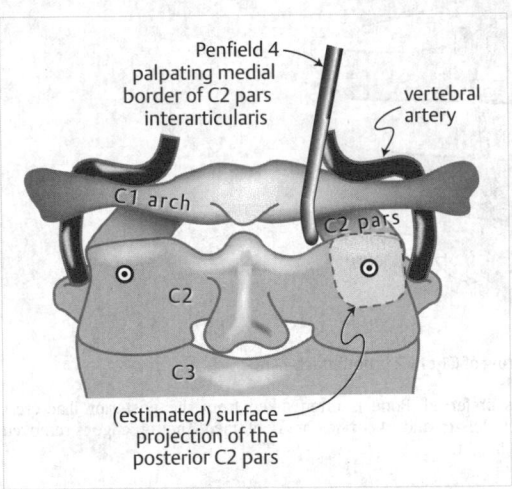

Fig. 108.5 Entry point for C2 pedicle screw placement (posterior view).

Penfield 4 palpating medial border of C2 pars interarticularis

vertebral artery

C1 arch

C2 pars

C2

C3

(estimated) surface projection of the posterior C2 pars

108.6.3 C3–6 fixation

Lateral mass screws

Generally applicable to C3–6. The lateral masses of the thoracic spine are usually too small and not strong enough[51] for these screws. C7 is a transitional level, and lateral mass screws may sometimes be used. Occasionally even T1 may be amenable (see below).

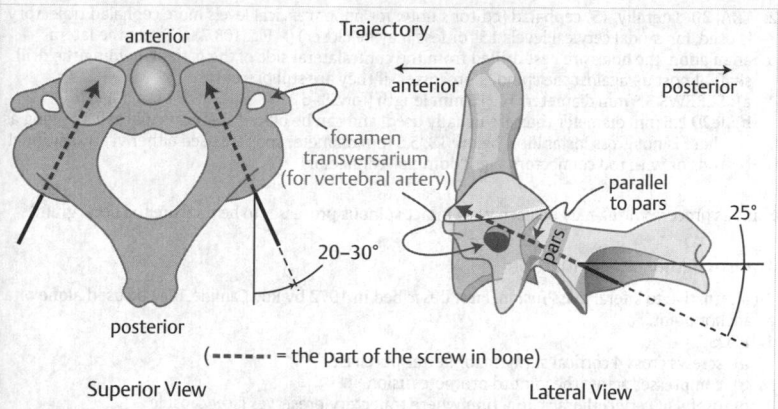

Fig. 108.6 Screw trajectory for C2 pedicle screws.

108

Technique:

A number of methods have been promulgated with various screw entry points and trajectories, some are shown in ▶ Table 108.1). Comparing 3 techniques,[52] there was a lower risk of nerve injury with the following (method of An[53]):

1. ENTRY[53] 1 mm medial to the midpoint of the lateral mass (▶ Fig. 108.7). In the craniocaudal direction, the midpoint is used. A Penfield 4 may be used to palpate the medial wall of the pars to help determine entry point and trajectory

Table 108.1 Comparison of methods for lateral mass screw placement for C3–6

Method	Entry point		Trajectory angle	
	Mediolateral	Craniocaudal	Mediolateral	Craniocaudal
An	1 mm medial to midpoint	midpoint	30° lateral	15° cephalad
Magerl	2 mm medial to midpoint	2 mm cranial to midpoint	20–25° lateral	parallel to facet joint[a]
Roy-Camille	midpoint	midpoint	0–10° lateral	0°

[a]angle can be determined by inserting probe into the joint

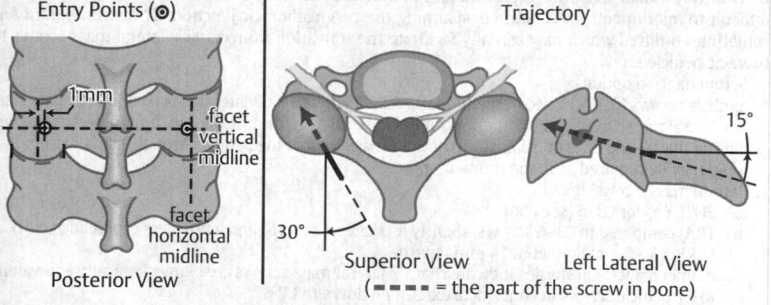

Fig. 108.7 Screw entry point and trajectory for C3–6 lateral mass screws (method of An).

2. TRAJ 30° laterally, 15° cephalad (editor's note: for upper cervical levels more cephalad trajectory is used, for caudal cervical levels 15° or less may be closer) (▶ Fig. 108.7).[53] To get the lateral angulation, the holes are best drilled from the contralateral side of the patient, holding the drill shaft almost up against the spinous processes (if they are still present)
    a) SCREWS 3.5 mm diameter, 14–16 mm length (for C3–6)
    b) ROD 3.5 mm diameter rods are usually used, and can be placed as far caudally as T3 as long as there is not gross instability (below T3, 5.5 mm diameter rods are used either via transitional rods or with rod connectors, e.g., "domino" connector)

Spinous process wiring may be used with intact spinous processes to help secure the bone graft.[51]

Transarticular screw fixation

An alternative to lateral mass fusion. First described in 1972 by Roy Camille. May be used alone or as an anchor point.
1. PROS:
    a) screws cross 4 cortical surfaces for better purchase
    b) compresses across the joint to promote fusion
    c) useful at cervicothoracic junction where trajectory preserves facet capsule
    d) lower implant profile
2. CONS: cannot correct deformity
3. ENTRY midpoint of lateral mass
4. TRAJ perpendicular to joint, neutral to 5° lateral (to avoid VA and exiting root)
5. biomechanics: stability equivalent to lateral mass screws[54]
6. clinical: 25 patients (81 screws), 71 anchor, 10 fixation, 3.5 years F/U: solid fusion, no complications[55]

Translaminar cervical screw fixation

May be used in cervical or thoracic spine.[56,57]
1. indications: salvage technique when anatomy precludes pedicle screws
2. PROS:
    a) avoids complications related to pedicle screws
    b) no need for fluoroscopy (reduces radiation exposure)
3. CONS: requires intact posterior elements (cannot do with laminectomy)
4. ENTRY contralateral spinolaminar junction (at base of spinous process)
5. TARGET junction of the transverse process and the superior facet contralateral to the entry point
6. SCREWS 3.5–4.5 mm × 26 mm polyaxial screw
7. biomechanics: no data
8. clinical: 7 patients (C–T fixation), 14 months F/U, no hardware complications. Inconsequential ventral penetration in 5%[56]

108.6.4 C7 screws

C7 is a transitional level, the lateral masses and/or pedicles may be relatively small and therefore difficult to instrument. For constructs spanning the cervicothoracic junction, C7 instrumentation is sometimes omitted which may actually facilitate the transition from cervical lateral mass screws to thoracic pedicle screws.
    Screw fixation options:
1. pedicle screws (p.1791): recommended especially when the C7 lateral mass is of inadequate size for lateral mass screws.[53] Placement with fluoroscopy may be difficult due to shoulder artifact on lateral fluoro, and direct visualization of the medial wall of the pedicle through a small laminotomy may be required as in the thoracic spine
2. lateral mass screws[50]:
    a) ENTRY as for C3–6 (see above)
    b) TRAJ compared to C3–6 screws, slightly less lateral at ≈ 15° and a little less cephalad at ≈ 10°
    c) SCREWS 3.5 mm diameter, 14 mm length
    d) biomechanics: lab studies indicate that C7 lateral mass screws are biomechanically equivalent to C7 pedicle screws in constructs extending down to C7[58]
3. C7 transfacet screw[59]:
    a) PROS: reduced risk to spinal cord and nerve roots

   b) CONS: disrupts C7–1 facet capsule, so T1 must be included in fusion. Short screws result in low pullout strength ∴ may be best used as an intermediate anchor point and not a construct endpoint

   c) ENTRY 1–2 mm medial and superior to center of facet

   d) TRAJ 30° inferiorly and 20° laterally, TARGET goal is bicortical purchase

   e) SCREWS 3.5 mm diameter × 8–10 mm polyaxial screws

   f) biomechanics: equivalent to C7–1 pedicle screws[60]

   g) clinical: 10 patients, long cervicothoracic fixation, 6 months F/U, 3 patients with solid fusion

108.6.5 Cervical laminoplasty

General information

A procedure similar to laminectomy except that the decompressed posterior elements are not removed, and no fusion between vertebral levels is attempted. Pros & cons:

1. post-op range of motion is reduced 30–50% in extension, lateral bending, and rotation[61] which is better than laminectomy + fusion, but not as good as with laminectomy alone
2. lower incidence of post-op kyphosis than with laminectomy
3. preserving the lamina might protect against some posterior trauma
4. contraindications: laminoplasty is not appropriate with
   a) cervical instability
   b) cervical kyphosis
5. disappointments
   a) does not reduce the incidence of post-op C5 palsy (p. 1306)
   b) does not mitigate against "bow-stringing" of the spinal cord in patients with high cervical lordosis (high Ishihara index)

108

Surgical techniques

The neck is positioned in slight flexion to open the interlaminar spaces.

A midline skin incision is used, dissection through this relatively avascular plane reduces blood loss. The interspinous ligament is preserved between levels and is divided above the uppermost and below the lowermost laminoplasty levels.

Methods for the laminoplasty include:

unilateral ("open door")[62]: a partial-thickness trough is cut along one side at the junction between the lamina and lateral mass, and a complete cut is made on the other side. The fully cut side is pried open, creating a greenstick fracture on the partial-thickness cut side, and bone graft spacers (e.g., small discs sliced from iliac crest or cadaver rib) are inserted to maintain a gap on the open side (usually at every-other level). Plates (e.g., Centerpiece™ laminoplasty plates by Medtronic, or small cranial fixation plates) are placed (also at every other level)

midline enlargement ("French door"): partial-thickness troughs are made on both sides, and a compete opening is made in the midline. The central opening is then pried apart creating greenstick fractures on both sides, and spacers are placed to maintain the opening. More symmetric decompression. Midline osteotomy is riskier than lateral troughs.

108.7 Anterior cervical vertebral body screw-plate fixation

Plate should be contoured to directly contact the front of the VBs being instrumented.

Typically, fixed-angle screws are used in the lowest level, and variable-angle screws are used at levels above. However, practices vary.

For the most rostral and most cranial screw holes, the plate should be sized such that the edge of the VB would just barely be visible when looking through the hole.

Screw length: Typical lengths vary from 12 mm (usually in women) to 16 mm. As a guide, if Caspar distraction pins (distributed by Aesculap Implant Systems) are used during the operation, the pin thread length can be used as a rough guide in estimating desired screw length based on how close the pins come to the posterior VB. Caspar pins are available in 12, 14, 16, & 18 mm tip lengths (14 mm is common, but you should verify the thread length on the pins you are using). Since the screws in the plate are usually angled, an additional 1–2 mm can be accommodated.

108.8 Zero profile interbody devices

These anteriorly placed devices incorporate holders for screw placement into an interbody cage without need for a separate anterior plate. Most often used in cervical spine.

1. PROS:
   a) are often easier to place adjacent to a previously placed anterior plate (because the plate will often cover too much of the VB to provide enough room for another plate on the same VB)
   b) avoids plates that are not parallel to the long axis of the spine
   c) posterior migration of the cage is prevented once the screws are placed
2. CONS: biomechanical stability is less than that with a plate (4-screw devices are more stable than 3-screw devices)

References

[1] Crockard HA, Sen CN. The Transoral Approach for the Management of Intradural Lesions at the Craniovertebral Junction: Review of 7 Cases. Neurosurgery. 1991; 28:88–98

[2] Hadley MN, Spetzler RF, Sonntag VKH. The Transoral Approach to the Superior Cervical Spine. A Review of 53 Cases of Extradural Cervicomedullary Compression. Journal of Neurosurgery. 1989; 71:16–23

[3] Menezes AH, VanGilder JC. Transoral-Transpharyngeal Approach to the Anterior Craniocervical Junction. Journal of Neurosurgery. 1988; 69:895–903

[4] Dickman CA, Locantro J, Fessler RG. The Influence of Transoral Odontoid Resection on Stability of the Craniocervical Junction. J Neurosurg. 1992; 77:525–530

[5] Dickman CA, Crawford NR, Brantley AGU, et al. Biomechanical Effects of Transoral Odontoidectomy. Neurosurgery. 1995; 36:1146–1153

[6] Holmes MG, Dagal A, Feinstein BA, et al. Airway Management Practice in Adults With an Unstable Cervical Spine: The Harborview Medical Center Experience. Anesth Analg. 2018; 127:450–454

[7] Mummaneni PV, Haid RW. Transoral odontoidectomy. Neurosurgery. 2005; 56:1045–50; discussion 1045-50

[8] Fielding JW. The Status of Arthrodesis of the Cervical Spine. J Bone Joint Surg. 1988; 70A:1571–1574

[9] Lipson SJ. Fractures of the Atlas Associated with Fractures of the Odontoid Process and Transverse Ligament Ruptures. J Bone Joint Surg. 1977; 59A:940–943

[10] White A, Panjabi M, White AA. Kinematics of the Spine. In: Clinical Biomechanics of the Spine. 2nd ed. Philadelphia: J.B. Lippincott; 1990:85–126

[11] Roberts A, Wickstrom J. Prognosis of Odontoid Fractures. J Bone Joint Surg. 1972; 54A

[12] Bambakidis NC, Feiz-Erfan I, Horn EM, et al. Biomechanical comparison of occipitoatlantal screw fixation techniques. J Neurosurg Spine. 2008; 8:143–152

[13] Uribe JS, Ramos E, Vale F. Feasibility of occipital condyle screw placement for occipitocervical fixation: a cadaveric study and description of a novel technique. Journal of Spinal Disorders and Techniques. 2008; 21:540–546

[14] La Marca F, Zubay G, Morrison T, et al. Cadaveric study for placement of occipital condyle screws: technique and effects on surrounding anatomic structures. J Neurosurg Spine. 2008; 9:347–353

[15] Uribe JS, Ramos E, Youssef AS, et al. Craniocervical fixation with occipital condyle screws: biomechanical analysis of a novel technique. Spine. 2010; 35:931–938

[16] Grob D. Transarticular screw fixation for atlanto-occipital dislocation. Spine. 2001; 26:703–707

[17] Feiz-Erfan I, Gonzalez LF, Dickman CA. Atlantooccipital transarticular screw fixation for the treatment of traumatic occipitoatlantal dislocation. Technical note. J Neurosurg Spine. 2005; 2:381–385

[18] Gonzalez LF, Crawford NR, Chamberlain RH, et al. Craniovertebral junction fixation with transarticular screws: biomechanical analysis of a novel technique. Journal of Neurosurgery. 2003; 98:202–209

[19] Morone MA, Rodts GR, Erwood S, et al. Anterior Odontoid Screw Fixation: Indications, Complication Avoidance, and Operative Technique. Contemporary Neurosurgery. 1996; 18:1–6

[20] Rao G, Apfelbaum RI. Odontoid screw fixation for fresh and remote fractures. Neurol India. 2005 53:416–423

[21] Apfelbaum RI. Screw Fixation of the Upper Cervical Spine: Indications and Techniques. Contemporary Neurosurgery. 1994; 16:1–8

[22] Sasso R, Doherty BJ, Crawford MJ, et al. Comparison of the One- and Two-Screw Technique. Spine. 1993 18:1950–1950

[23] Hott JS, Henn JS, Sonntag VKH. A new table-fixed retractor for anterior odontoid screw fixation: technical note. Journal of Neurosurgery. 2003; 98:118–120

[24] Wang MY. C2 crossing laminar screws: cadaveri morphometric analysis. Neurosurgery. 2006; 59 ONS84–8; discussion ONS84-8

[25] Grob D, Jeanneret B, Aeb M, et al. Atlanto-Axial Fusion with Transarticular Screw Fixation. Journal of Bone and Joint Surgery. 1991; 73B:972–976

[26] Stillerman CB, Wilson JA. Atlanto-Axial Stabilization with Posterior Transarticular Screw Fixation: Technical Description and Report of 22 Cases. Neurosurgery. 1993; 32:948–955

[27] Marcotte P, Dickman CA, Sonntag VKH, et al. Posterior Atlantoaxial Facet Screw Fixation. Journal of Neurosurgery. 1993; 79:234–237

[28] Brooks AL, Jenkins EB. Atlanto-Axial Arthrodesis by the Wedge Compression Method. J Bone Joint Surg; 1978; 60A:279–284

[29] Griswold DM, Albright JA, Schiffman E, et al Atlanto-Axial Fusion for Instability. J Bone Joint Surg. 1978; 60A:285–292

[30] Schmidek HH, Sweet WH. Operative Neurosurgical Techniques. New York 1982

[31] Aldrich EF, Crow WN, Weber PB, et al. Use of MR Imaging-Compatible Halifax Interlaminar Clamp for Posterior Cervical Fusion. Journal of Neurosurgery. 1991; 74:185–189

[32] Bohler J. Anterior Stabilization for Acute Fracture and Non-Unions of the Dens. J Bone Joint Surg 1982; 64:18–28

[33] Paramore CG, Dickman CA, Sonntag VKH. The Anatomical Suitability of the C1-2 Complex for Transarticular Screw Fixation. Journal of Neurosurgery 1996; 85:221–224

[34] Goel A, Laheri V. Plate and screw fixation for atlanto-axial subluxation. Acta Neurochir (Wien 1994; 129:47–53

[35] Harms J, Melcher RP. Posterior C1-C2 fusion with polyaxial screw and rod fixation. Spine. 2001 26:2467–2471

[36] Thomas JA, Tredway T, Fessler RG, et al. An alternate method for placement of C-1 screws. J Neurosu Spine. 2010; 12:337–341

[37] Moisi M, Fisahn C, Tkachenko L, et al. Posterior arc C-1 screw technique: a cadaveric comparison stud J Neurosurg Spine. 2017; 26:679–683

[38] Rocha R, Safavi-Abbasi S, Reis C, et al. Working are safety zones, and angles of approach for posterio C-1 lateral mass screw placement: a quantitati

anatomical and morphometric evaluation. J Neurosurg Spine. 2007; 6:247–254

[39] McCormick PC, Kaiser MG. Comment on Goel A et al.: Atlantoaxial fixation using plate and screw method: a report of 160 treated patients. Neurosurgery. 2002; 51

[40] Currier BL, Todd LT, Maus TP, et al. Anatomic relationship of the internal carotid artery to the C1 vertebra: A case report of cervical reconstruction for chordoma and pilot study to assess the risk of screw fixation of the atlas. Spine. 2003; 28:E461–E467

[41] Menger RP, Storey CM, Nixon MK, et al. Placement of C1 Pedicle Screws Using Minimal Exposure: Radiographic, Clinical, and Literature Validation. Int J Spine Surg. 2015; 9. DOI: 10.14444/2043

[42] Tan M, Wang H, Wang Y, et al. Morphometric evaluation of screw fixation in atlas via posterior arch and lateral mass. Spine (Phila Pa 1976). 2003; 28:888–895

[43] Papadopoulos SM, Dickman CA, Sonntag VKH. Atlantoaxial Stabilization in Rheumatoid Arthritis. J Neurosurg. 1991; 74:1–7

[44] Dickman CA, Sonntag VKH, Papadopoulos SM, et al. The Interspinous Method of Posterior Atlantoaxial Arthrodesis. J Neurosurg. 1991; 74:190–198

[45] Hott JS, Lynch JJ, Chamberlain RH, et al. Biomechanical comparison of C1-2 posterior fixation techniques. J Neurosurg Spine. 2005; 2:175–181

[46] Wright NM. Posterior C2 fixation using bilateral, crossing C2 laminar screws: case series and technical note. J Spinal Disord Tech. 2004; 17:158–162

[47] Jea A, Sheth RN, Vanni S, et al. Modification of Wright's technique for placement of bilateral crossing C2 translaminar screws: technical note. Spine J. 2008; 8:656–660

[48] Parker SL, McGirt MJ, Garces-Ambrossi G L, et al. Translaminar versus pedicle screw fixation of C2: comparison of surgical morbidity and accuracy of 313 consecutive screws. Neurosurgery. 2009; 64:343–8; discussion 348-9

[49] Wang MY. Comment on Parker, SL, McGirt, MJ et al., Translaminar versus pedicle screw fixation of C2: comparison of surgical morbidity and accuracy of 313 consecutive screws. Neurosurgery. 2009; 64. DOI: 10.1227/01.NEU.0000338955.36649.4F

[50] Dickman CA, Sonntag VKH, Marcotte PJ. Techniques of screw fixation of the cervical spine. BNI Quarterly. 1993; 9:27–39

[51] Chapman JR, Anderson PA, Pepin C, et al. Posterior Instrumentation of the Unstable Cervicothoracic Spine. Journal of Neurosurgery. 1996; 84:552–558

[52] Xu R, Haman SP, Ebraheim NA, et al. The Anatomic Relation of Lateral Mass Screws to the Spinal Nerves. A Comparison of the Magerl, Anderson and An Techniques. Spine. 1999; 24:2057–2061

[53] An HS, Gordin R, Renner K. Anatomic considerations for plate-screw fixation of the cervical spine. Spine. 1991; 16:S548–S551

[54] Miyanji F, Mahar A, Oka R, et al. Biomechanical differences between transfacet and lateral mass screw-rod constructs for multilevel posterior cervical spine stabilization. Spine (Phila Pa 1976). 2008; 33:E865–E869

[55] Takayasu M, Hara M, Yamauchi K, et al. Transarticular screw fixation in the middle and lower cervical spine. Technical note. Journal of Neurosurgery. 2003; 99:132–136

[56] Kretzer RM, Sciubba DM, Bagley CA, et al. Translaminar screw fixation in the upper thoracic spine. J Neurosurg Spine. 2006; 5:527–533

[57] Gardner A, Millner P, Liddington M, et al. Translaminar screw fixation of a kyphosis of the cervical and thoracic spine in neurofibromatosis. Journal of Bone and Joint Surgery. British Volume. 2009; 91:1252–1255

[58] Xu R, McGirt MJ, Sutter EG, et al. Biomechanical comparison between C-7 lateral mass and pedicle screws in subaxial cervical constructs. Presented at the 2009 Joint Spine Meeting. Laboratory investigation. J Neurosurg Spine. 2010; 13:688–694

[59] Horn EM, Theodore N, Crawford NR, et al. Transfacet screw placement for posterior fixation of C-7. J Neurosurg Spine. 2008; 9:200–206

[60] Horn EM, Reyes PM, Baek S, et al. Biomechanics of C-7 transfacet screw fixation. J Neurosurg Spine. 2009; 11:338–343

[61] Satomi K, Nishu Y, Kohno T, et al. Long-term follow-up studies of open-door expansive laminoplasty for cervical stenotic myelopathy. Spine (Phila Pa 1976). 1994; 19:507–510

[62] Hirabayashi K, Watanabe K, Wakano K, et al. Expansive Cervical Laminoplasty for Cervical Spinal Stenotic Myelopathy. Spine. 1983; 8:693–693

108

109 Spine, Thoracic and Lumbar

109.1 Anterior access to the thoracic spine

109.1.1 General information

The thoracic spinal cord does not tolerate anything more than *minimal* manipulation. Therefore, unless the pathology (e.g., tumor or herniated disc) has already displaced the cord to one side, it is necessary to go around the spinal cord to gain access to the space anterior to the cord.

Indications: calcified thoracic disc herniation, spontaneous spinal cord herniation, tumors involving thoracic vertebral bodies.

109.1.2 Anterior access to the cervicothoracic junction/upper thoracic spine (T1, T2)

Depending on the patient's body habitus, anterior access below C7 may not be possible through a traditional anterior cervical approach. A sternal splitting procedure may be used. Permits access down to T3 (occasionally as far as T5) from an anterior midline approach (access to this region with a lateral (transthoracic) approach is poor due to the small volume of the pulmonary apices).

▶ **Sternal splitting procedure.** The neck and thorax are prepped down to the umbilicus. A hockey stick incision may be used, the horizontal portion is the usual for an ACDF. The vertical limb is centered over the sternum. In most cases, the services of a CV surgeon are employed to split the sternum and divide the sternocleidomastoid. This approach does not violate the pericardium or pleura and a chest tube is not required (but is often used as a large-bore drain to prevent hemomediastinum, and also as a precaution in case the parietal pleura is cut during the exposure). Because of the depth of the approach, longer instruments than the routine 7-inch-length instruments used for an ACDF are required.

The exposed edges of the sternum may also be used to obtain cancellous bone for the graft.

109.1.3 Anterior access to mid- and lower thoracic spine

▶ **Transthoracic/retropleural approach.** If the pathology requires access that includes ≈ T10 and below, the attachment of the diaphragm increases the difficulty of a transthoracic approach, and a retrocoelmic approach (outside the pleural cavity) can facilitate surgery by allowing the diaphragm to be reflected off the VB.

Determining the level in the upper T-spine can be quite difficult intraoperatively. Counting up from the sacrum on an AP view using live fluoro will sometimes work when lateral spine X-rays can not penetrate the upper T-spine due to the shoulders. If the patient does not have exactly 12 rib and 5 lumbar vertebrae, this must be accounted for when counting levels. Image-guided navigation can also be helpful.

▶ **Laterality of approach.** If the pathology does not dictate use of one side over another:
1. advantages of right-sided thoracotomy: the heart, mediastinum, and brachiocephalic vein do not impede access
2. advantages of left-sided thoracotomy: aorta is easier to mobilize and retract than the vena cava

▶ **Position.** Lateral position on a bean-bag on the O.R. table with the break in the table under the level of pathology (remember to unbreak the table prior to instrumenting). Stabilize the patient using adhesive tape over surgical towels. An axillary roll is placed. Classically, a double-lumen endotracheal tube was recommended to permit deflating the lung on the side of the thoracotomy. The reality is that only minimal displacement of the lung is required to access the vertebral bodies, which permits continuous ventilation of both lungs with a normal single-lumen ET tube. The lung can be gently retracted with an "egg beater" retractor cushioned with a moistened sponge.

If a compression plate is going to be used, the goal is to be lateral on the VB; to achieve this, try to position it as far posterior as possible (rongeur off a little bit of the rib heads to facilitate this).

To increase the exposure, a rib may need to be resected. Generally, the level opened and the rib removed are one or two levels above the level of pathology (e.g., for T7 VB tumor, the T6 or T5 rib is removed).

109

109.1.4 Anterior access to thoracolumbar junction

▶ **Retroperitoneal approach.** Unless the pathology is predominantly right-sided, a left-sided approach is preferred because the spleen is easier to retract than the liver, and the aorta is easier to mobilize than the inferior vena cava. Flex the ipsilateral leg to relax the psoas muscle and thereby reduce traction on the ipsilateral lumbosacral plexus.

109.2 Thoracic pedicle screws

109.2.1 General information

referable to lateral mass screws because the transverse processes (which are analogous to the lateral masses in the cervical spine) of most thoracic vertebrae are not as strong.[1] Thoracic pedicles are typically very narrow in the lateral dimension (the width is usually a little larger at the cranial end) nd are very tall in the cranio-rostral direction.

Accurate placement of thoracic pedicle screws is generally more challenging than the lumbar spine. There are at least 4 methods to place these screws, and a combination of them may be used details follow this overview):

. intraoperative fluoro: for parts of the thoracic spine, biplane fluoro may be used as in percutaneous lumbar spine pedicle screw (p.1797) placement
   a) PROS:
      • allows percutaneous screw placement
      • generally good accuracy in screw placement
   b) CONS:
      • due to the dense bone of the shoulders, lateral fluoroscopy imaging from T1 to about T4 is usually difficult. For non-percutaneous cases, Steinman pins may be placed at the estimated entry points for the screws, and AP fluoro is used to fine-tune the position so that the screw enters the pedicle at the desired location
      • may increase radiation exposure to surgery team and patient
. anatomic ("freehand" (p.1792)) thoracic pedicle screw placement based on anatomic landmarks. Fluoroscopy is still usually performed after all screws are placed, and any screws with questionable position need to be reevaluated (usually removing the screw and re-probing) and possibly revised
   a) PROS:
      • as the number of levels (and therefore, screws) placed in a patient increases, may save time over other methods
      • the small facetectomies that are needed to visualize the facet joint of the level below can facilitate correction of spinal curves and provides a good fusion surface as well as fusion material
      • likely reduces radiation to the surgical team and the patient
      • excels in complex scoliosis cases with varying degrees of rotation at different levels (which can be taxing when relying on fluoroscopy)
   b) CONS: steep learning curve: this method probably takes the most practice to master
performing small laminotomies at each level where pedicles are not exposed by a laminectomy, and use position of pedicle either by visualization or by palpation of the medial and superior aspect of the pedicles with a dissector to get an approximation of the entry point and pedicle trajectory
   a) PROS: can permit accurate placement at essentially any level with potentially less radiation (depending on how often the surgeon checks screw position)
   b) CONS: takes a little time at each level, but overall this is comparable to other methods
image guidance using instruments that are fitted with specialized markers that are tracked realtime by "cameras" that project the drill and/or screw location on a CT or X-ray image viewed in the OR. Robotic screw placement simply automates the use of image guidance
   a) PROS:
      • reduces intraoperative radiation to surgical team, and to a lesser extent to the patient
      • allows percutaneous screw placement
      • easily deals with spine rotation
   b) CONS: accuracy may be compromised by movement of spinal segments relative to the registration array, or by technical errors. The surgeon must be vigilant for screw placement that is visually not appropriate based on anatomic knowledge

109

As in the lumbar spine, there are 2 options for craniocaudal trajectories (► Fig. 109.2:[2]
1. anatomic screw placement: parallel to the axis of the pedicle—provides a longer path for screw contact with bone but requires a multiaxial screw head
2. straightforward screw placement: parallel to the superior endplate. Allows fixed-head screws for spine derotation, therefore often used for pediatric scoliosis surgery. Provides 27% increase in pullout strength vs. the anatomic trajectory[3]

109.2.2 Fluoroscopy or laminotomy techniques for thoracic pedicle screw placement

1. ENTRY: several methods are used, including:
   a) making a small laminotomy ► Fig. 109.1 (typically with high-speed drill) to allow palpation of the medial and cephalad edges of the pedicle e.g., with a Penfield #4 dissector. This works very well for very small pedicles where a 1–2-mm error in estimating the pedicle position may cause the pedicle to be missed
   b) placing a small "dimple" and then a Steinman pin at the estimated entry points (see Freehand thoracic pedicle screw placement technique (p.1792) for entry points using anatomic landmarks which can be useful here for first approximation) and then using AP fluoro to fine-tune the position of the pins (see ► Fig. 109.1).

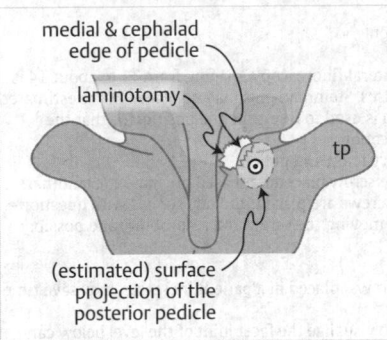

medial & cephalad edge of pedicle

laminotomy

tp

(estimated) surface projection of the posterior pedicle

Fig. 109.1 Entry point for thoracic *pedicle* screws (posterior view). tp = transverse process. A small laminotomy is shown on the right side to allow localization by palpating the medial and cephalad edge of the pedicle with a dissector.

2. TRAJ
   a) below T1: 5–10° *medially* and 10–20° *caudad*[1] (► Fig. 109.2). A thoracic Lenke probe may be used as a pedicle finder
   b) T1: if a *lateral mass* screw is placed at T1 (instead of a pedicle screw), aim almost straight down at the floor (with patient positioned horizontally, i.e., without Trendelenberg or reverse-Trendelenberg)
3. SCREWS Smaller pedicles (usually T1–4, especially in females) usually require the smallest screw diameter (typically 4.5 mm). Others may accommodate 5.5 mm. Typical length: 20–25 mm
4. ROD When connecting to a cervical rod, down to ≈ T3 you can use a 3.5 mm diameter cervical rod throughout (here, the stiffer cobalt-chrome rod may be advantageous over titanium) with some systems using a 4.35–4.5 diameter rod. Below T3, ≈ 5.5 mm diameter rods (or 6.35 mm for scoliosis surgery) are usually used either via a transitional rod (that tapers from the larger diameter to the smaller one) or using a domino connector to mate the two rods

109.2.3 Anatomic ("freehand") thoracic pedicle screw placement technique

Advantages and disadvantages

Possible advantages
- may speed up surgery especially when instrumenting a large number of levels
- reduces the amount of X-rays/fluoroscopy needed during surgery

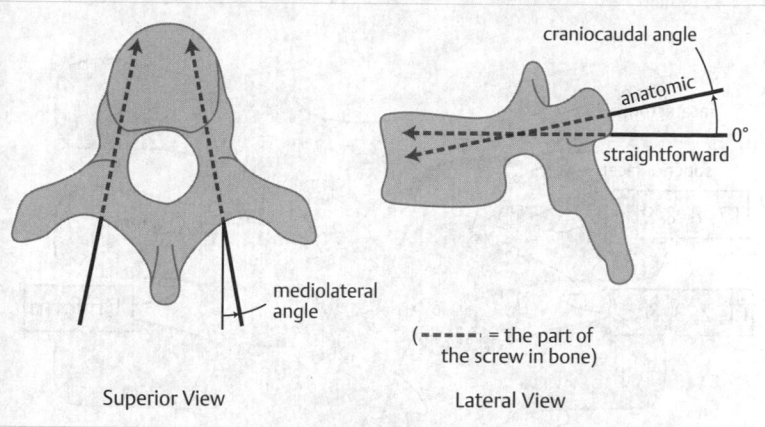

Fig. 109.2 Screw trajectory for thoracic *pedicle* screws. See text for mediolateral angle.

- avoids the challenges of getting fluoro aligned for each level in a scoliotic spine, especially when a rotational component is present
- not impeded in areas that are difficult to image on fluoroscopy (typically upper thoracic spine)
- accuracy as good as or better than other techniques.[4] Pedicle breach rates were highest bewteen T4 and T6[4]
- since facetectomies (removing part of the inferior facet) are usually employed, if an osteotome or bone scalpel (as opposed to a drill) is used, it provides bone for use in bone graft (facetectomties can also be performed in conjunction with other screw placement techniques)
- exposes bone (of facet joints) to assist in fusion
- releases joints which facilitates reduction of scoliosis

Possible disadvantages
- cannot be used if anatomy is distorted by previous fusions, congenital anomalies…
- steep learning curve: proficiency requires knowing detailed level-specific anatomy and acquiring a feel for pedicle cannulation. Necessitates performing numerous screw placements, usually with a mentor
- possible increased blood loss from increased exposure and facetectomies
- individual variability from the "average" may produce sub-optimal screw placement

Procedure – freehand pedicle screws

summary of key points/information[5]:
- complete exposure of entire posterior elements (lamina, pars interarticularis, facets, transverse process (tp)…) at every level (except the upper instrumented vertebra (UIV)) is mandatory
- intraoperative electrophysiologic monitoring: SSEP, MEP, triggered EMG
- inferior facetectomies: performed bilaterally at every level except the most superior (which is not being fused to the level above) to expose the superior facet of the level below. Make 2 cuts (► Fig. 109.3): vertical cut is parallel to spinal canal at the medial edge of facet joint (caution: in scoliosis, the spinal cord is at risk on the side of concavity), horizontal cut is at upper edge of inferior facet
- a series of steps are repeated without deviation with every screw placement:
  - make pilot hole at entry point (as indicated below)
  - insert curved pedicle finder with the tip directed laterally until 2 cm deep (do not force)
  - completely remove the pedicle finder, rotate it 180° and re-insert it down the same path just created, but now with the curve directed medially and insert it an additional centimeter, then remove it
  - palpate all 4 walls and the deep end with a thin ball probe, push it gently through the cancellous bone ("crunch through") until the tip strikes the cortical bone of the anterior vertebral body (sound and feel). Place a clamp where the probe enters the bone and…

109

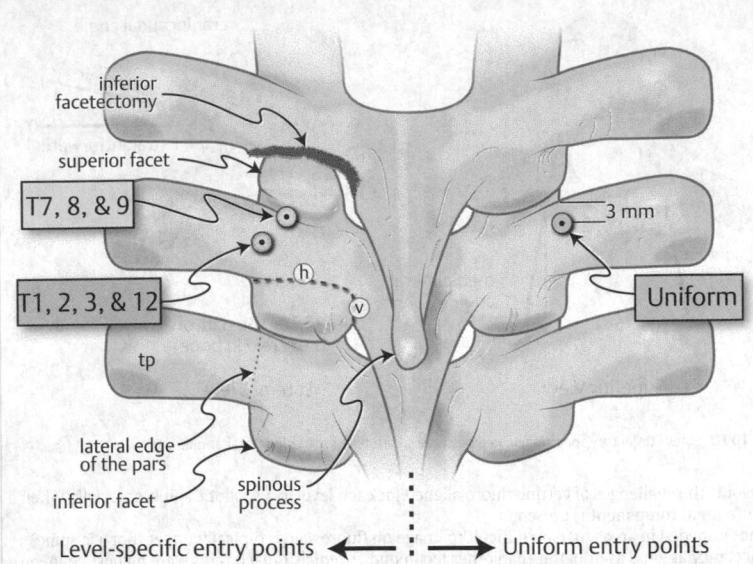

109

Level-specific entry points ◄┄┄┄► **Uniform entry points**

Fig. 109.3 Entry points for thoracic pedicle screws.
The left side illustrates level-specific entry points, and the right side shows uniform placement (see text).
Posterior view, stylized representation of generic thoracic level.
Mnemonic for level-specific entry points: "T1, 2, 3: mid tp (tp = transverse process). T7, 8, 9: top of the line (the "top of the line" being the superior border of the tp)."
Inferior facetectomy: red broken line shows cut lines for the (v) = vertical cut and (h) = horizontal cut. Facetectomy may also be used with the uniform entry point method.

- ○ measure the depth that the probe was inserted to determine maximum screw length; if the length is much shorter than expected, the probe may be hitting the lateral VB wall and consideration should be given to redirecting the screw more medially
- ○ tap the pedicle (i.e., cut the threads for the screw using a tap that is 0.5 mm smaller than the planned screw diameter)
- ○ probe 2nd time with a thin ball probe and palpate all 4 walls and the deep
- ○ place screw
- ○ run a set of motor evoked potentials on electrophysiologic monitoring
- ○ optional: after all screws are placed, stimulate each screw (e.g., with a Prass probe inserted into the screw head within the tulip of the pedicle screw) and determine the lowest current that produces an EMG response (triggered EMG): stimulation at < 6 mA (some surgeons prefer 8 mA) or a threshold that is 65% or more decreased from the average of the other screws indicates a possible medial pedicle breach and should prompt a re-evaluation of the screw (remove screw & re-probe the hole or obtain a fluoro image)[5]

ENTRY[5] (this describes "level-specific" entry points and trajectories. Alternatively, see uniform entry points & trajectories (p. 1795))
- • craniocaudal (illustrated on the left side of ► Fig. 109.3)
  - ○ T1, 2, 3, & 12: even with the middle of the transverse process
    (mnemonic: T1–2-3: "mid tp"); same for T12 (as with lumbar spine levels below it)
  - ○ T7, 8, & 9: even with the top of the transverse process
    (mnemonic: T7–8-9: "top of the line")
  - ○ for levels in between these 2 groups (viz. T4, 5, & 6), gradually move slightly superiorly at each level from mid-tp at T3 to the top of the tp at T7

- mediolateral (illustrated on the left side of ▶ Fig. 109.3). Tip: safe zone is *lateral* to the midpoint of the superior articular facet (SAF). Some use Lenke's "superior facet rule": enter 2–3 mm lateral to the SAF midline
  - T1, 2, & 3: even with the lateral edge of the pars
  - T7, 8, & 9: just lateral to midposition of the base of the superior articular facet (the most medial starting points)
  - T11, 12: at or just medial to lateral edge of pars
  - levels in between these groups: gradually transition the position

TRAJ: two methodologies
1. using anatomic landmarks: more commonly used than "angle technique" by most practitioners
   - advantage: angles are difficult to estimate, and using landmarks allows screws to be placed even in rotated, scoliotic spines
   - technique: the screw is inserted perpendicular to the surface of the superior articular facet (which is exposed during the facetectomies) while also "aiming" at the contralateral pedicle
2. angle technique: since estimating angles is difficult, this technique may be more helpful to conceptualize the general orientation
   - craniocaudal orientation (p. 1792)[6]:
     - for straightforward configuration: aim 0° relative to horizontal
     - for anatomic configuration: aim 10–15° caudal
   - mediolateral trajectory[6]: (▶ Fig. 109.2): the angle gradually becomes more medial as you progress from
     - T12 where the angle is slightly lateral (≈ –5°) to
     - T11 where it is ≈ 0° and as a rough approximation it increases by 2° per level above this to
     - T1 where the angle is ≈ 27° medial

SCREW
- length: the depth to the anterior cortex varies from 40–45 mm when measured along the axis of the pedicle (or 30–42 mm when measured parallel to the sagittal plane).[6] Typical thoracic screw length is 35–40 mm
- diameter: the narrowest pedicles in the mediolateral dimension are typically T4–7.[6] Screw diameter should be approximately 80% of the pedicle diameter

109.3 Uniform entry points for freehand pedicle screws

Alternatively, a uniform entry point for thoracic pedicle screws (instead of modifying the entry point based on level as described above) may be used, e.g., the method of Baaj et al,[7] illustrated on the right side of ▶ Fig. 109.3

ENTRY 3 mm inferior to the junction of the lateral edge of the superior facet and the transverse process.
TRAJ for a "straightforward" trajectory, the pedicle finder is oriented orthogonal to the curve of the spine in the sagittal plane.

109.4 Anterior access to the lumbar spine

109.4.1 Anterior lumbar interbody fusion (ALIF)

Relatively contraindicated in males because of risk of retrograde ejaculation in 1–2% (as high as 45% in some reviews). Other risks: injury to great vessels, especially with calcified arteries, in particular at L4–5.

Bowel prep the day before surgery may be used for complex cases.

Position: a general OR table is usually used. Place the iliac crests over the kidney rest or use a sacral bump to increase lordosis. Trendelenburg position allows gravity to retract the abdominal contents superiorly.

Aproach: retroperitoneal usually through a Pfannenstiel's abdominal incision. A vertical incision is an alternative. Avoid injuring the ureters.

As a result of the bifurcation of the great vessels (aorta and inferior vena cava) which ranges from just above to just below the L4–5 disc space, this approach is best suited for access to L5–1.

At L5–1, the anterior sacral artery runs down the midline of the VB and has to be sacrificed to do an ALIF.

Dissection: At L5–S1, bovie cautery should be avoided when exposing the anterior longitudinal ligament because of risk of injury to the (superior) hypogastric plexus which can cause retrograde ejaculation in males. A vertical midline incision of the prevertebral soft tissues is made and the tissues are swept to their respective side using periosteal elevators.

Discectomy: a rectangular opening in the ALL and anterior anulus is incised with a scalpel and the discectomy is performed as in an ACDF, using fluoroscopy to check the depth to avoid penetrating the PLL. Endplates are prepared using curettes and rasps to remove all cartilage from the endplates.

Implant: typical implant width is 35–38 mm for women, and 40–42 mm for men.

Complications: retrograde ejaculation in males occurs in 1–20% using a retroperitoneal approach. Venous thrombosis (usually of the common iliac veins) occurs in up to 10%.

109.5 Instrumentation/fusion pearls for the lumbar and lumbosacral spine

1. a lumbar fusion that includes L1 should not be terminated at L1 or T12
2. the taller the disc space the less likely that interbody grafts are well suited:
   a) the disc may not be significantly degenerated to require discectomy
   b) tall disc space means larger interbody implants which requires more retraction of nerve to insert (using a PLIF technique)
3. a long fusion should not be terminated at or near a vertebral level that is at the apex of scoliosis[8(p 382)]
4. laminectomy without fusion should be avoided at the apex of scoliosis
5. posterior midline fusion: early experience with midline fusions resulted in lumbar spinal stenosis as a late complication. Therefore, current fusion techniques include posterolateral fusion, interbody fusion (from anterior or posterior approach), facet fusion…

109.6 Lumbosacral pedicle screws

109.6.1 General information

Pedicle screw pull-out strength is determined in part by the major screw diameter which should be 70–80% of pedicle diameter (in adults, larger screws can break through the pedicle wall or can burst the pedicle; in peds, larger screws may be used as the pedicle can expand). The minor diameter determines the strength of the screw and should be ≥ 5.5 mm in the adult lumbar spine.

109.6.2 Placement techniques

There are at least 4 screw placement techniques
1. intraoperative fluoro: biplane fluoro facilitates this technique
   a) PROS:
      • allows percutaneous screw placement
      • generally good accuracy in screw placement
   b) CONS:
      • imaging may be difficult in some parts of the lumbar spine, especially in larger patients. In these cases, the Steinman pin method below can be used to supplement
      • may increase radiation exposure to surgery team and patient
2. Steinman pin method: Steinman pins are placed at the estimated entry points for the screws, and AP (and often lateral) fluoro is used to fine-tune the position so that the screw enters the pedicle at the desired location
3. freehand placement based on anatomic landmarks. Usually with X-ray verification after all screws are placed. Greatly facilitated at levels where a laminectomy has been performed since the medial pedicle is exposed and is easily palpated
   a) PROS: likely reduces radiation to the surgical team and the patient
   b) CONS: requires somewhat more experience than the other methods; distortion of landmarks e.g., by previous surgery can preclude using this method; since the methodology uses averages in anatomy, it can be unreliable for patients whose anatomy differs from average
4. image guidance using instruments that are fitted with specialized markers that are tracked realtime by "cameras" that project the drill and/or screw location on a CT or X-ray image viewed in the O.R.
   a) PROS:
      • reduces intraoperative radiation to surgical team, and to a lesser extent to the patient
      • allows percutaneous screw placement
   b) CONS: accuracy may be compromised by movement of spinal segments relative to the registration array, or by technical errors. The surgeon must be vigilant for screw placement that does not look appropriate based on the anatomy

109

109.6.3 Open lumbar pedicle screw technique (see below for percutaneous placement)

. ENTRY at the base of the transverse process, at the intersection of the center of the transverse process (in the rostral-caudal direction) and the sagittal plane through the lateral aspect of the superior facet. If a laminectomy has been performed at that level, the location of the pedicle is verified by palpation using a probe within the spinal canal, otherwise fluoroscopy is used. NB: degenerative changes include facet hypertrophy which can obscure these landmarks. At all but the superior-most level, it is ofen helpful to rongeur or drill off the hypertrophied part of the facet (avoid this at the superior level to reduce the risk of proximal junctional kyphosis)

. TRAJ
   a) the approximate mediolateral trajectory is shown in ▶ Table 109.1, and equals the lumbar vertebral number multiplied by 5° for each level from L1 to L5.[9] The angle of the screw in the rostral-caudal direction is determined by fluoroscopy, maintaining a course that is either parallel to the vertebral endplate (for "straightforward" trajectory), or parallel to the axis of the pedicle (anatomic trajectory) (▶ Fig. 109.2). Image-guided navigation may be used
   b) S1 craniocaudal trajectory: aim for the sacral promontory (the anterior superior edge of S1)
   c) S2 screws may be oriented laterally and superiorly (into the ala) and can be as long as 60 mm. Alternatively, they can be oriented medially

Table 109.1 Medial angles for lumbar pedicle screw

Level	Medial angle
L1	5° medially
L2	10° medially
L3	15° medially
L4	20° medially
L5 & S1[a]	25° medially
S2	40–45° *laterally*

[a]aim for sacral promontory

109

. SCREWS major screw diameter = 70–80% of pedicle diameter. Length should put tip 2/3 of the way across the VB (typical screw lengths: 40–55 mm) except for S1, which are usually only 35–40 mm long. Bicortical purchase or anterior VB penetration should be avoided (except for S1) to reduce the risk of injury to great vessels or abdominal viscera
   ROD Typically 5–6.5 mm diameter

-ray verification once pedicle screws are placed: on AP view if the screw tip crosses the midline to he contralateral side, there is likely to be a breach of the medial pedicle (sensitivity 0.87, specificity 97, accuracy 0.98),[10] and if the screw does not pass medial to the medial pedicle wall there is likely o be lateral pedicle/VB violation (sensitivity 0.94, specificity 0.90, accuracy 0.96[10]).

09.6.4 Percutaneous pedicle screws

he principles here are also employed in accessing the pedicles for e.g., vertebroplasty/kyphoplasty, ercutaneous biopsy of pathology in the pedicle and/or vertebral body.
   Basic principles:
   requires AP and lateral fluoro, or image guidance (e.g., "O-arm"). With fluoro, biplane fluoro (1 C-arm dedicated for AP view, another for lateral) expedites the procedure
   this method can be employed essentially from T1 through S1 as long as adequate AP & lateral imaging of the involved level is possible. Using fluoro for upper thoracic placement (e.g., above ≈ T5) is challenging (small pedicles, and the shoulders interfere with lateral X-ray)
   the skin entry site is lateral to the lateral edge of the pedicle. This permits the needle to pass through the pedicle in a medial direction into the VB. The degree of angulation and therefore the distance off the midline for the entry site depends on the vertebral level being accessed (thoracic pedicles are oriented in a more AP direction, lumbar pedicles angulate medially inward) as well as the amount of overlying muscle/fat

rocedure:
   for an average size patient, the skin entry points will be about 4.5–5 cm lateral to midline; for larger patients this moves a little further laterally. Local anesthetic is injected using a spinal

needle which is adjusted under fluoro to determine an approximate entry site for the Jamshidi needle in the craniocaudal plane. The skin is incised just enough to accommodate the tower that is attached to the pedicle screw (usually ≈ 1.5 cm)

2. a Jamshidi needle (or equivalent) is inserted and the tip is positioned just short of entering the pedicle on the lateral fluoro (on left in ▶ Fig. 109.4)
3. at this point, on the AP view the needle tip should be at or just barely lateral to the lateral edge o the pedicle near the equator of the pedicle ("3:00" position on the right pedicle, "9:00" position on the left)

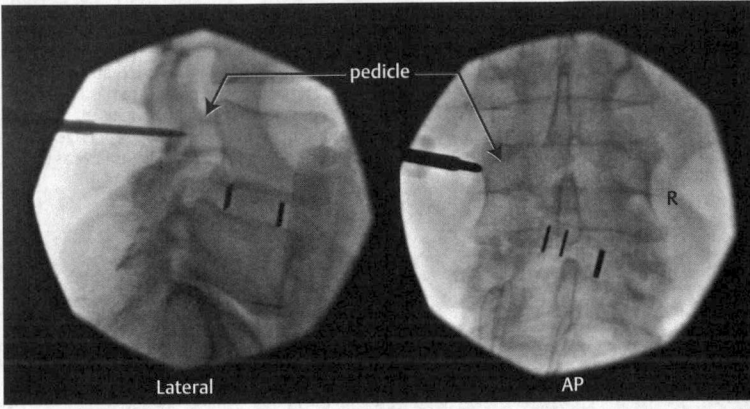

Fig. 109.4 Pedicle cannulation—entering pedicle.

4. the needle is advanced to just enter the pedicle on lateral fluoro; at this point it should be just within the pedicle margin on AP fluoro (as shown on the right in ▶ Fig. 109.4)
5. continue advancing the needle into the pedicle. Intermediate fluoro images can be obtained (e.g to monitor trajectory on the lateral fluoro), but the next critical landmark is when the needle tip is just traversing the junction of the pedicle and the VB on the lateral fluoro (i.e., just entering th VB, as shown on the left in ▶ Fig. 109.5). It should be close to but never more medial than the medial border of the pedicle on the AP view (as shown on right in ▶ Fig. 109.5). If this criterion i

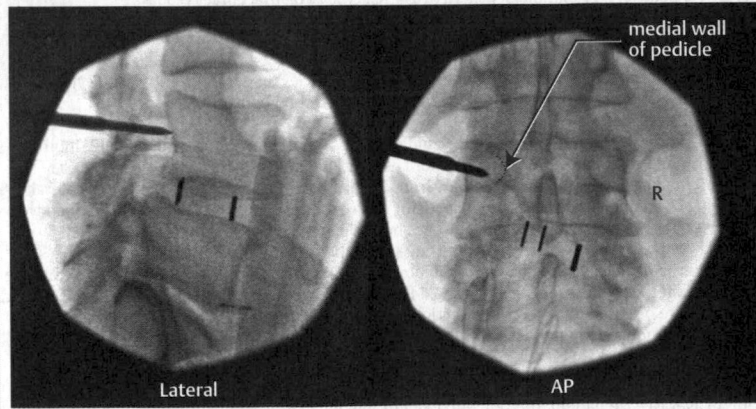

Fig. 109.5 Pedicle cannulation—entering the vertebral body.

maintained, the needle cannot breach the medial wall of the pedicle where it can threaten neural structures or compromise the purchase of the pedicle screw

5. after the needle tip is ≈ 1 cm into the VB, the stylet is removed and a guidewire is inserted through the needle for an additional 1–2 cm into the VB

7. the needle is removed taking great care not to dislodge the guidewire

8. in some cases, the cannulated screw with tower may be placed over the guidewire at this time, or the guidewire may be gently bent out of the way (without kinking it) for screw placement at a later step in the procedure

09.6.5 Pedicle-screw rod diameters

Approximate weight guidelines for pedicle-screw *rod* diameters are shown in ► Table 109.2.

Table 109.2 Minimum recommended titanium rod diameter for lumbar pedicle-screw fixation

Patient weight		Rod diameter (mm)
(lbs)	(kg)	
30–90	12–40	4.5
90–225	40–100	5.5
>225	>100	6.35 (1/4 inch)

09.6.6 Pedicle screw breach classification

CT is the diagnostic test of choice for evaluating pedicle screws for violation of bony margins (breach).[11] However, CT may distort the apparent screw location by as much as 25%.[4]

A number of breach grading scales have been proposed. Many are variations of 2 systems.

The Gertzbein system[12] measures *medial* pedicle breach from T8 to S1 and stratifies them as shown in ► Table 109.3. In the original study, medial violation > 4 mm was associated with neurologic deficit. There are nonvalidated opinions that 2 or 4 mm for medial breach, and 4 mm for lateral breach are "safe zones."[11]

109

Table 109.3 Gertzbein classification of pedicle screw medial breach[12]

Grade	Breach distance (mm)
0	no breach
1	<2
2	2–4
3	>4

Table 109.4 Heary classification of pedicle screw breach[13]

Grade	Breach
1	no breach
2	lateral with screw tip within VB
3	anterior or lateral breach of screw tip
4	medial or inferior breach
5	proximity to sensitive structures necessitates immediate revision

The Heary system[13] (► Table 109.4) takes into account the fact that sometimes a lateral breach is intentional (e.g., with small thoracic pedicles) and also that anterior breaches may have consequences. However, this system does not consider the degree of violation.

09.7 Lumbar cortical bone trajectory screw fixation

09.7.1 General information

AKA "Cortical Screws" (a trademarked name). Screws enter the bone of a lumbar vertebra posteriorly near the inferomedial border of the pedicle. They are directed superiorly and laterally, thereby passing close to 3 cortical margins, which purportedly provides a pull-out strength close to that of traditionally oriented pedicle screws.

Cortical screw threads are closer together (higher pitch) than pedicle screws to better grip cortical bone. Typical screw diameter (4.5–5.5 mm) is smaller than pedicle screws.

Limitations: Use is generally restricted to lumbar spine and S1 (L1 to S1). May be precluded if entry points are compromised by previous laminectomy. Use is more controversial with high-grade spondylolisthesis or scoliosis (especially if instrumentation needs to go higher than L1 or L2).

1. PROS:
   a) placement through a midline incision is somewhat easier compared to trying to aim medially from a more lateral entry point as with traditional pedicle screws (especially in obese patients)
   b) construct is medial to the segmental back muscles causing less injury to them
   c) may be used as rescue screws for failed pedicle screws
   d) may be used to extend a previous pedicle screw construct (may be placed in the same VB as traditional pedicle screw)
2. CONS:
   a) pull-out strength is probably slightly less than pedicle screws
   b) the bone that has to be left unviolated at the screw entry site may interfere with some of the decompression

109.7.2 Lumbar cortical bone trajectory screw technique

1. ENTRY (exceptions: the cranial-most screw and S1, see below)
   • craniocaudal: the entry point is even with the cranial margin of the neural foramen (on lateral fluoro). Mediolateral: 3–5 mm medial to lateral edge of the pars interarticularis.
   On AP fluoro, this is at the inferomedial border of the pedicle
   • there are 2 exceptions to this entry point
     ○ exception 1 – the cranial-most screw: enters 2–3 mm lower than the other screws (to avoid injuring the rostral facet joint that will not be part of the fusion)
     ○ exception 2 – S1 screw: enters midway between the L5–1 facet and the first dorsal foramen
   • practical method: find the "corner" where the lateral pars and inferior TP (transverse process) meet (▶ Fig. 109.6), move the drill tip 3 mm medial to that, and make a dimple with the drill (at the cranial-most level, also move 2–3 mm inferior)
   • pitfall: a severely hypertrophied facet of the level above may cover the entry point and may need to be partially removed

2. TRAJ
   • overview: ≈ 20° laterally, and 30–45° cephalad
   • practical method: with the drill tip in the entry dimple, bring the drill shaft medially to the spinous process (SP) and inferiorly to the bottom half of the SP (▶ Fig. 109.6). Aim for a point in the superior endplate approximately 1/3 of the way forward from the back of the VB on lateral fluoro
   • drill with a pistoning technique. When first learning the technique, check that when you reach the midposition of the pedicle on lateral fluoro you should be in the center of the pedicle on AP fluoro. Drill the entire length of the screw (no pedicle finders!). Probe with a narrow probe to rule out breach and to measure screw length. Holes should be tapped to the actual screw diameter (not undertapped) for the entire screw length (tap "line-to-line") to avoid fracturing the dense cortical bone
3. if needed, the laminectomy is done at this time, leaving a 3-mm cuff of bone around the screw entry points. Alternatively, modular screws (without the tulips attached) may be placed before the laminectomy
4. SCREWS
   • use specialized cortical screws (not pedicle screws)
   • typical screw diameter: 5 mm (range: 4.5 to 5.5).
   • typical length: 30–35 mm.
   • S1 screw: usually 6.6 mm diameter, length measured with a probe (usually ≈ 45 mm).
   • leave the cranial-most screw 2–3 mm proud
5. ROD typically 5–6.5 mm diameter

109.8 Translaminar lumbar screw fixation

1. indications:
   a) short-segment lumbar fusion
   b) posterior component in a 360° fixation combined with interbody fusion

109

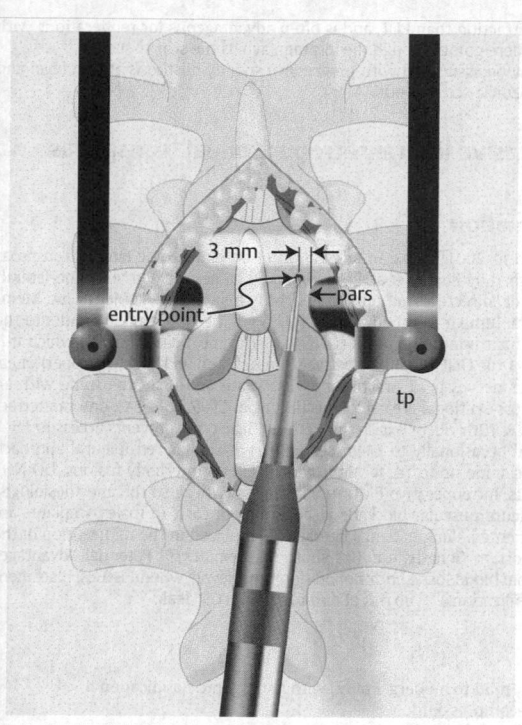

Fig. 109.6 Entry point for cortical bone trajectory screws (see text for differences for the most cranial level and S1).

The tip of the drill is positioned 3 mm medial to the lateral edge of the pars at the inferior edge of the tp.

Abbreviations: tp = transverse process; pars = pars interarticularis.

109

2. PROS:
   a) small incision, minimal soft tissue disruption
   b) decreased cost (fewer screws implanted)
   c) decreased blood loss
   d) adjacent facet joint spared
3. CONS:
   a) requires intact posterior elements (cannot use with laminectomy)
   b) cannot reduce
4. ENTRY skin incision 5–7 mm off midline, screw entry into bone in contralateral side of spinous process. Can be placed bilaterally
5. drill between the tables of the lamina across the center of the facet joint, terminating at the base of the transverse process
6. SCREWS 4.5 mm diameter fully threaded screws (no polyaxial head)
7. biomechanics: equivalent to bilateral pedicle screws.[14] Limited in extension[15]
8. clinical: 476 patients, 10 years mean F/U, 74% good outcomes[15]

109.9 Posterior lumbar interbody fusion (PLIF and TLIF)

Originally developed by Cloward[16] in 1943. Bilateral laminectomy and aggressive discectomy followed by the placement of bone grafts into the decorticated disc space. It has been advocated to reduce the movement in an abnormal "motion segment" (defined as the area between two vertebra). Relatively contraindicated with well-preserved disc-space height.

Many PLIFs when studied ≈ 1 year later show re-collapse of the disc space, which raises the question as to whether the PLIF has any benefit over simple discectomy. Areas of concern include: concerns regarding injury to nerves at the time of surgery or later due to retropulsion of bone graft.

Transforaminal lumbar interbody fusion (TLIF): a variation on a PLIF where the graft is placed from one side (via the "neural foramen") after complete removal of the facet joint on that side.

Requires much less nerve root retraction than PLIF, and is often advantageous for reoperations with primarily unilateral pathology where going through the foramen avoids the scar tissue.

Stand-alone PLIFs or TLIFs may be associated with progressive spondylolisthesis at that level and are usually supplemented with pedicle screws/rods.

109.10 Minimally invasive lateral retroperitoneal transpsoas interbody fusion

109.10.1 General information

First introduced by Luiz Pimenta in 2001[17,18] as an adaptation of an endoscopic lateral transpsoas approach to lumbar fusion described by Bergey et al.[19] Trademarked names include "extreme-lateral" (XLIF™, NuVasive, San Diego, CA) or "direct-lateral" lumbar interbody fusion (DLIF™, Medtronic, Memphis, TN); the generic term lateral lumbar interbody fusion (LLIF) will be used here. Variants to the approach include the oblique lumbar interbody fusion (OLIF™, Medtronic, Memphis, TN) which utilizes a pre-psoas approach (at L5–1 the OLIF is halfway between an ALIF and an LLIF). A retroperitoneal approach indirectly decompresses nerves by distracting the disc space and fuses the spine with an interbody cage that has a large cross-sectional area. Access is best from L1–5. For L1–2, one can retract the 12th rib, or go between 11th & 12th rib, or excise the 12th rib. Iliac crest prevents access to L5–1 (axial-LIF may be used here) and occasionally to L4–5 (see below). A similar retropleural approach may be employed in the thoracic spine up to T4. ✖ With *thoracic* lateral interbody fusions, DO NOT penetrate the contralateral anulus. Intraoperative EMG monitoring is critical, so the anesthesiologist needs to use only *short-acting* neuromuscular blockade at beginning of case. In males, implants are typically 55–60 mm in length (oriented along patient's lateral axis) if placed in the midposition of the VB, or 45 mm in the anterior portion (lengths are 10% shorter in females).[20] Potential advantages include less tissue trauma, minimal blood loss, shorter operation time, fewer wound issues, placement of a larger cage, early patient mobilization,[21,22] no risk of durotomy with CSF leak.

109.10.2 Indications

- central lumbar spinal stenosis (mild to moderate only) with neurogenic claudication
- foraminal stenosis (indirect decompression)
- spondylolisthesis grade 1 or 2
- axial low back pain associated with degenerative disc disease
- total disc replacement
- for correction of sagittal or coronal imbalance
- adjacent segment failure: LLIF is particularly attractive here because it obviates dealing with scar tissue and (often) hardware from previous surgery and which also reduces risk of durotomy
- burst fractures and tumors in the thoracolumbar area (corpectomy)
- to retrieve damaged or malpositioned lumbar disc replacement devices[23]
- adult spinal deformity: can be used to correct scoliosis and to increase lumbar lordosis especially when combined with release of the anterior longitudinal ligament (ALL release)[22]

109.10.3 Contraindications

1. cases requiring direct decompression: includes
   a) pathology within the spinal canal e.g., herniated disc, synovial cyst, where simply distracting the disc space is less likely to correct the pathology
   b) somewhat imprecisely defined "pinpoint" central canal stenosis (some cases may still respond)
2. tall disc spaces: disc space height > 12 mm usually implies that further distraction may be difficult to achieve. However, the interbody cage can still prevent compression at these levels when the patient stands up
3. prior retroperitoneal surgery on the planned side of LLIF (can still be done on contralateral side, sometimes may still be feasible on ipsilateral side) or extensive or complicated abdominal surgery (adhesions may preclude approach from either side)
4. pathology at L5–1: the technique usually cannot access L5–1 due to the interference from the ilium of the pelvis (an OLIF (oblique aproach) or ALIF may be an alternative)
5. may not be able to access L4–5 if the iliac crest extends more than ≈ halfway up the L4 VB. Sometimes it is necessary to position the patient on the O.R. table with the table flexed and a bump under the hip to see if the space will "open up" and permit access. Angled instruments can

usually permit acceptable access to the space anterior to the lumbar plexus if it is not located too far forward on the VB

6. anomalous vascular anatomy interfering with approach: check position of great vessels on pre-op imaging (CR or MRI)

7. relative contraindications:
   a) osteoporosis: may also be contraindication to lateral plates
   b) active infection (relatively contraindicated with any fusion technique)

109.10.4 Surgical technique (MIS retroperitoneal transpsoas approach)

1. Position
   a) lateral decubitus position with the top of the iliac crest just superior to the table break
   b) choice of side: if there is no reason not to do so, the left side is usually placed up. Factors that might influence which side is to be up:
      • right side up if access is needed to L4–5 and the iliac crest is higher on left and would inter-fere (use AP X-rays, lateral X-rays, and/or lumbar CT to evaluate)
      • previous retroperitoneal surgery would cause one to consider placing the contralateral side up
      • if scoliosis is present and the intent is to correct this, the concave side is usually up: this usually provides better access to L4–5 if it is an operative level. Also usually allows access to multiple levels through potentially fewer and smaller incisions because the corridors to each disc space tend to converge
      • if ACR is planned, a posterior location of the great vessels and especially the lack of any soft tissue between the vertebral body/osteophyte and the vessel would speak for using the contralateral side if that is more favorable (if not, ACR may not be advisable)
   c) true orthogonal position: the C-arm fluoroscopy is placed horizontal with 0° tilt, the patient position is then fine-tuned until the spinous process is exactly in the center between the pedicles on the AP view. If this is not possible due to rotation between levels, a relatively neu-tral level is chosen to start, and the O.R. table will need to be rotated slightly for each level as it is being worked on in order to make that level true lateral (centering spinous process). Adhesive tape is applied to maintain the patient in this position

2. lateral fluoroscopy is used to mark the index disc space transversely and the posterior third of the disc space vertically. An exception is at L4–5, where the vertical mark is at the middle of the disc space based on the anatomic safe zones[24]

3. retroperitoneal access through a single lateral skin incision and blunt dissection through abdomi-nal muscles and fascia (external oblique, internal oblique, transversalis)

4. transpsoas approach and retractor placement is achieved using sequential tubular dilators that are placed under the guidance of fluoroscopic imaging (or navigation) and using directional EMG monitoring (Neurovision™, NuVasive, San Diego, CA), allowing the dilator to be placed anterior to the main lumbar plexus

5. discectomy and preparation of the disc space without violation of the endplates (to reduce the risk of subsidence) are performed. Work straight up-and-down in the ventral-dorsal plane (to avoid injuring the ALL anteriorly or entering the spinal canal posteriorly)

6. interbody spacer is placed usually with the posterior edge in the posterior third of the disc space (as the EMG monitoring allows)

7. for anterior column release (MIS-ACR), additional steps have to be performed after discectomy, which include dissection/section of the ALL and placement of hyperlordotic cages (20 or 30 degrees), usually more anteriorly in the disc space than a routine cage. This is a technique for the advanced lateral access surgeon

109.10.5 Instrumented augmentation (pedicle screws or lateral plate)

Standalone cage

A standalone cage (i.e., no additional instrumentation) may be feasible in the following circumstances:

no osteoporosis

no instability on pre-op lateral flexion/extension X-rays

the ALL was not disrupted during LLIF surgery

a cage width of at least 22 mm in the AP dimension has been placed: the large surface area reduces the risk of subsidence

When these conditions are not met, additional instrumentation should be considered.

109

Lateral plate and screws

May be applied through the same exposure. May not be optimal in patients with osteoporosis or age > 55 due to increased risk of subsidence from weaker bone. Not as practical for multilevel LLIFs.

Posterior instrumentation

Posterior instrumentation (e.g., pedicle screws, including percutaneous placement) provides the most stabilization. Also, may be indicated if laminectomy is needed for direct decompression.

109.10.6 Complications

1. thigh numbness: incidence is ≈ 10–12%.[22,25] Due to injury to the genitofemoral nerve. Risk of direct injury in the quadrant anterior to the midline at L2–3 and in the anterior quadrant at L3–4 and L4–5.[24] A sensory nerve cannot be monitored with EMG. Usually transient, resolves in ≈ 2 weeks
2. thigh flexion weakness: due to psoas injury. Risk increases if > 2 levels are done. Usually transient, resolves in 1–8 weeks
3. femoral nerve or femoral/obturator nerve palsy as a result of nerve root/plexus injury.[26] 83% of cases show findings of axonotmesis (► Table 32.6) at 6 weeks.[27] Produces quadriceps weakness. Incidence is ≈ 2.6%.[27] Many cases are likely due to compression of the nerves within the psoas muscle when the muscle is retracted against the transverse processes; weakness is usually evident immediately post-op. Another possible etiology is psoas hematoma in which case the onset may be delayed 1–2 d. Prognosis: all 6 cases improved to 4/5 MRC strength by 12 months, some as early as 3 months (► Table 30.2).[27] Prior to recovery, patients may be able to ambulate with a brace
4. lumbar plexus injuries: the risk of direct injury to the lumbar plexus is reduced by staying at or anterior to "safe" working zones defined by Uribe et al[24] as follows (NB: it is often possible to work posterior to these zones using EMG monitoring to ascertain the proximity of the plexus, and conversely injuries can occur even in these safe zones).
    Safe zones:
    - L1–2 through L3–4: middle of the posterior quarter of the VB
    - L4–5: midpoint of the VB
5. contralateral femoral nerve injury
6. genitofemoral neuralgia
7. abdominal viscera perforation
8. vascular injury[28] including common iliac artery (at the L4–5 level) or aortic injury (above L4–5), common iliac vein or inferior vena cava
9. kidney-ureter injury
10. graft subsidence
11. unintended rupture of anterior longitudinal ligament
12. psoas/retroperitoneal hematoma ipsilateral/contralateral
13. abdominal wall paresis or hernia[29]
14. rhabdomyolysis (p. 136)
15. retrograde ejaculation (primarily with ACR and pre-psoas approaches)

109.10.7 Postoperative care

- for single-level lumbar LLIF: mobilize the patient in the immediate post-op period without a brace
- hip flexion pain on the approach side is anticipated during the immediate postoperative period
- transient hip flexion weakness related to psoas muscle manipulation is usually self-limited and improves by 8 weeks post-op
- in case of significant leg weakness (femoral nerve injury), a lumbar CT or MRI is indicated to rule out compression by a psoas hematoma, disc extrusion, or malposition of cage or screw. If compression is ruled out, patients can be followed by postoperative EMG at 6 weeks to define extent of injury (neuropraxia, axonotmesis, neuronotmesis), again at 3 months to evaluate if the expected interval improvement from neuropraxia has occurred and 5 months to follow up axonal growth[26]

109.10.8 Outcomes

- fusion rates range from 91–100%[30]
- outcomes scales (ODI and VAS leg and back) are significantly improved at follow-up[31]

109

Booking the case: Lateral interbody fusion

Also see defaults & disclaimers (p. 25) and pre-op orders (see below).
1. position: lateral decubitus, typically left-side up unless specified otherwise
2. equipment: C-arm
3. implants:
   a) interbody graft
   b) some stabilizing hardware is usually needed, especially if spondylolisthesis is present. Options:
   • pedicle screws: bilateral or unilateral
   • interspinous clamps
4. consent (in lay terms for the patient—not all-inclusive):
   a) procedure: surgery through the side to place a spacer between two of the vertebrae (back-bones) to make more space for the nerves and to stop painful movement, screws/plates etc., will then need to be placed either from the side through the same opening or sometimes from the back. In case the procedure cannot be done from the side due to the position of the lumbar plexus (uncommon, when it occurs it is usually an issue at L4–5), determine if patient wants to have a posterior procedure (e.g., TLIF) and put that on the consent. Be sure to notify the vendor of this possibility
   b) alternatives: nonsurgical management, open surgery through the back
   c) complications: thigh weakness (usually temporary), knee weakness (uncommon), thigh numbness, graft subsidence/migration, failure to achieve desired relief

109

109.11 Transfacet pedicle screws

109.11.1 General information

Screws placed directly across the lumbar facet joint into the pedicle of the level below. No rod is needed. Immobilizes only, does not provide any decompression, distraction, or fusion. Therefore not intended for use as a stand-alone. Can be placed percutaneously.

109.11.2 Indications

Placement is optimal for L3–4, L4–5, or L5–1. Difficulty increases in upper lumbar levels.
   May be used as adjunct to:
1. ALIF
2. LLIF (when lateral plate not used)
3. contralateral to TLIF (pedicle screws could be used on the side of the TLIF, or a spinous process clamp could be used)
4. axial-LIF (Ax-LIF)

109.11.3 Contraindications

A transfacet pedicle screw cannot be used where the facet has been removed (e.g., for a TLIF) or with a pars defect in the upper of the two levels to be fused.

109.11.4 Technique

1. placed percutaneously or via an open procedure usually in the prone position
2. approximate skin incision site: a single midline ≈ 1.5-cm vertical incision is used
   a) for L5–1 or L4–5: incision at L3 spinous process
   b) for L3–4: incision at L2 spinous process
3. use AP & lateral fluoro to guide trajectory
   a) AP fluoro: lay a guidewire on the patient's back and orient it to pass through the desired pedicle. Use a skin marker on the patient's back to mark the guidewire's trajectory
   b) lateral fluoro: initial bony target is the midpoint of the inferior facet of the upper level. The tip of the guidewire should contact the bone directly posterior to the inferior endplate of the upper level

109.12 Facet fusion

A bone dowel (e.g., TruFUSE® by MinSURG) is placed into a predrilled opening in the facet joint to promote fusion across the joint. Marketed as a possible stand-alone.

109.13 S2 screws

May be directed medially (analogous to pedicle screws), or more commonly, directed laterally and superiorly into the ala (S2 alar screws) (see below for S2-alar-*iliac* screws). In either case, bicortical purchase is necessary.

The main pitfall to avoid is penetrating the sacroiliac (SI) joint with the screw.

109.14 Iliac fixation

109.14.1 General information

Stronger fixation than S1 or S2 *alar* screws (S2 alar screws not to be confused with S2-alar-iliac screws (p. 1807)).

Primary indications for extending fixation to ilium (i.e., pelvis)
1. long constructs (any construct from S1 that extends above L2)
2. high-grade spondylolisthesis (Meyerding grade (p. 1339) ≥ 3)
3. S1 screw failure
4. pseudarthrosis of prior attempted L5–S1 fusion
5. sacral insufficiency

In the absence of sacroiliac joint fusion (autofusion or surgical fusion), the iliac screws or rods connecting to them will eventually break. The function of the iliac screws here is to assist the S1 screw during the early stages of the fusion.

3 main options
1. iliac screw (AKA iliac bolt)
2. "percutaneous" iliac bolt
3. S2-alar-iliac screws

If the sacroiliac joint (SIJ) is not fused, the screw or the rod will usually eventually break because of continued movement across the SIJ.

109.14.2 Iliac screws

Wide exposure is needed. On the initial few cases, the surgeon may be better served by exposing all the way to the posterosuperior aspect of the sciatic notch so that the screw trajectory can be aimed using a palpating finger.

An offset adapter is often required to connect to rods passing through pedicle screws in the level above.

ENTRY The classic entry point is the posterior superior iliac spine (PSIS) (▶ Fig. 109.7). A small amount of bone is removed just below and medial to the PSIS. This prevents the head of the screw from being too superficial, which may cause discomfort or skin breakdown.

TRAJ Overview: the screw trajectory aims towards the acetabulum to (ideally) pass approximately 1 cm superior to the sciatic notch. Placement is facilitated by 2 oblique fluoroscopy views:
1. obturator outlet view (AKA "teardrop view") (▶ Fig. 109.8 A): parallel to the iliac wing. On the teardrop view, stay within the hollow of the teardrop—the walls are cortical surfaces you don't want to violate. Also, avoid penetrating the cortex of the sciatic notch
2. iliac oblique view: perpendicular to the hemipelvis
SCREWS Length 50–80 mm (the screw should end just at or beyond the midpoint of the sciatic notch). Diameter: 6–8 mm.

109.14.3 Percutaneous iliac screw

Advantages

Compared to iliac screws
1. can line up with lumbar pedicle screws above without need for offset adapter

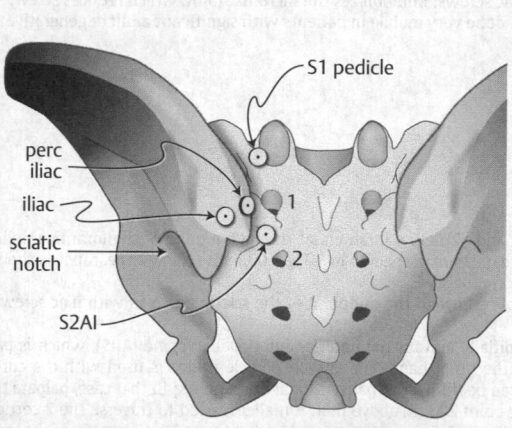

Fig. 109.7 Entry points for iliac fixation.
Entry points (*white circles with black central dots*) on the left side for S1 pedicle screws (depicted for reference, these are not iliac fixation screws), iliac screws (at the PSIS), percutaneous iliac screws, and S2-alar-iliac screws. Innominate bone and sacrum, dorsal view.
Key: 1 = 1st dorsal sacral foramen; 2 = 2nd dorsal sacral foramen; perc = percutaneous; S2AI = S2-alar-iliac.

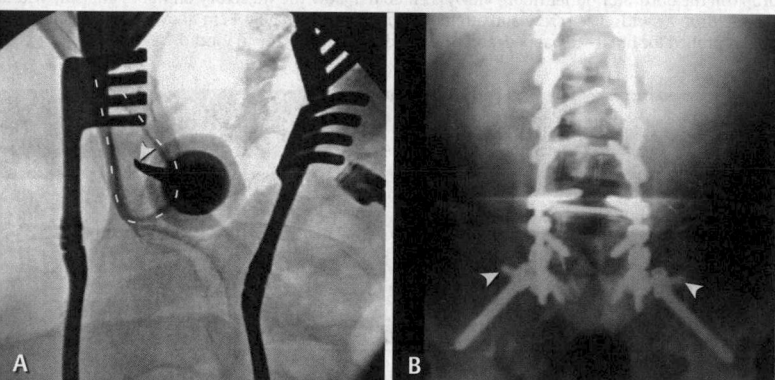

Fig. 109.8 Teardrop view and final AP X-ray for iliac screws.
A: Teardrop view (the teardrop is outlined as a broken yellow line). The pedicle finder (the tip is identified by the *yellow arrowhead*) is shown entering the teardrop.
B: A final AP X-ray. The offset connectors are identified with *blue arrowheads*.

2. less muscle dissection
3. less prominent on the surface of the skin
4. may be placed percutaneously

Technique

ENTRY The entry point is on the medial surface of the ilium (▶ Fig. 109.7).
TRAJ Same as for iliac screws.

109.14.4 S2-alar-iliac screws (S2AI screws)

Advantages

1. compared to iliac screws, same advantages as percutaneous iliac screws
   a) can line up with lumbar pedicle screws without need for offset adapter
   b) less muscle dissection
   c) less prominent on the surface of the skin

2. compared to percutaneous iliac screws: immobilizes the sacroiliac joint, which reduces screw/rod breakage (this joint may not be very mobile in patients with significant adult degenerative disc disease)

Technique

Options for placement include:
- fluoroscopy-assisted
- image navigation
- free-hand[32]

ENTRY midway between the S1 and S2 neural foramen, at the lateral edge of the foramina, inline with the S1 pedicle screw (if used) (schematic shown in ▶ Fig. 109.7; the X-ray appearance is shown in ▶ Fig. 109.9 panel A).

SCREWS Length 80–90 mm (at or beyond the midpoint of the sciatic notch as with iliac screws). Diameter: 6–8 mm.

TRAJ Fluoroscopic method: initially aim for the anterior inferior iliac spine (AIIS), which is palpated through the drapes with the other hand. The curved pedicle finder is used with the curve directed posteriorly.[32] The AIIS can be difficult to palpate in larger patients; in that case, palpate the greater trochanter and aim for a point 2–3 cm above that. A mallet is used to traverse the 2 cortical surfaces of the sacroiliac joint (SIJ) which are usually encountered at about 35-40 mm. Once the teardrop (on the obturator outlet fluoro view) is entered, follow the trajectory on fluoro and stay within the teardrop as with iliac screw and attempt to pass approximately 1 cm above the iliac notch. The hole is probed for breaches, tapped, and re-probed before the screw is placed.

109

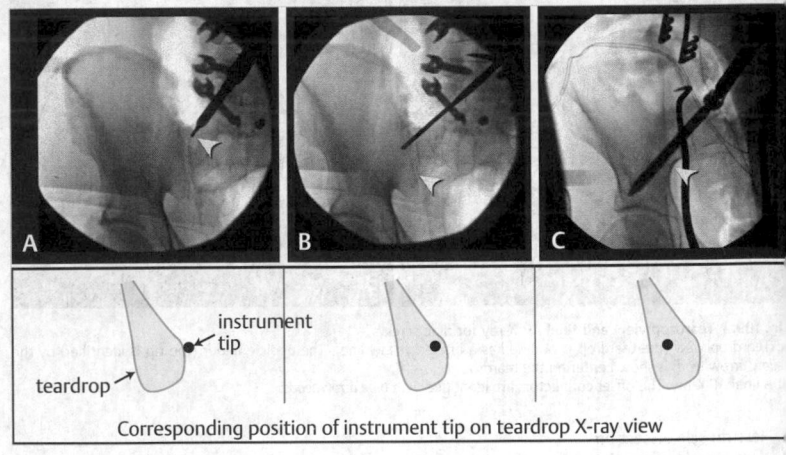

Fig. 109.9 S2-alar-iliac screws.
A: X-ray appearance of the entry point on AP view (*arrowhead* shows drill tip after drilling about 1 cm depth starting at the entry point shown in ▶ Fig. 109.7).
B: Pedicle finder crossing the sacroiliac joint (SIJ) (*arrowhead*).
C: Final screw placement on sciatic notch view. Note that the screw passes approximately 1 cm above the sciatic notch (*arrowhead*).
The lower panel shows corresponding location of the tip (*black circle*) of the pedicle finder on the teardrop view.

109.15 Post-op clinic visits—lumbar and/or thoracic spine fusion

109.15.1 Visit schedule

Patients are seen in the clinic at intervals depending on the preference of the surgeon. A typical follow-up schedule with studies routinely performed is shown in ▶ Table 109.5. For specific problems additional investigations are usually needed.

Table 109.5 Sample post-op lumbar fusion clinic visit schedule[a]

Time post-op	Agenda
7–10 d	wound check, D/C sutures/staples if used
6 wks	AP & lateral LS-spine X-ray in brace
10–12 wks	• AP & lateral LS-spine X-rays with flexion/extension views out of brace • if X-rays look good and patient is doing well, begin weaning brace
6 months	• AP & lateral LS-spine X-rays with flexion/extension views • some surgeons release patients at this time if they are doing well
1 year (optional)	• AP & lateral LS-spine X-rays with flexion/extension views • release patient if they are doing well

[a]the same schedule can be used for thoracic fusions with the difference that standing AP & lateral X-rays are done in place of flexion/extension views

109.15.2 Post-op X-rays

Items to check on post-op X-rays include:
1. alignment
2. position of grafts if used (e.g., interbody grafts)
3. integrity of hardware (look for screw or rod breakage, screw pull-out, rod disconnection)
4. lucencies around screws which may indicate motion and implies nonunion
5. any evidence of fusion (may be difficult, e.g., with synthetic interbody cages)
6. on flexion/extension films: look for motion across fused segments (sometimes absence of motion may be the only evidence of fusion on plain X-rays) and the development of abnormal motion at adjacent segments

109

References

[1] Chapman JR, Anderson PA, Pepin C, et al. Posterior Instrumentation of the Unstable Cervicothoracic Spine. Journal of Neurosurgery. 1996; 84:552–558

[2] Rosner MK, Polly DW,Jr, Kuklo TR, et al. Thoracic pedicle screw fixation for spinal deformity. Neurosurg Focus. 2003; 14

[3] Lehman RA,Jr, Polly DW,Jr, Kuklo TR, et al. Straightforward versus anatomic trajectory technique of thoracic pedicle screw fixation: a biomechanical analysis. Spine (Phila Pa 1976). 2003; 28:2058–2065

[4] Parker SL, McGirt MJ, Farber SH, et al. Accuracy of free-hand pedicle screws in the thoracic and lumbar spine: analysis of 6816 consecutive screws. Neurosurgery. 2011; 68:170–8; discussion 178

[5] Kim YJ, Lenke LG, Bridwell KH, et al. Free hand pedicle screw placement in the thoracic spine: is it safe? Spine (Phila Pa 1976). 2004; 29:333–42; discussion 342

[6] Zindrick MR, Wiltse LL, Doornik A, et al. Analysis of the morphometric characteristics of the thoracic and lumbar pedicles. Spine (Phila Pa 1976). 1987; 12:160–166

[7] Fennell VS, Palejwala S, Skoch J, et al. Freehand thoracic pedicle screw technique using a uniform entry point and sagittal trajectory for all levels: preliminary clinical experience. J Neurosurg Spine. 2014; 21:778–784

[8] Benzel EC. Biomechanics of Spine Stabilization. Rolling Meadows, IL: American Association of Neurological Surgeons Publications; 2001

[9] Dickman CA, Fessler RG, MacMillan M, et al. Transpedicular Screw-Rod Fixation of the Lumbar Spine: Operative Technique and Outcome in 104 Cases. Journal of Neurosurgery. 1992; 77:860–870

[10] Kim YJ, Lenke LG, Cheh G, et al. Evaluation of pedicle screw placement in the deformed spine using intraoperative plain radiographs: A comparison with computerized tomography. Spine. 2005; 30:2084–2088

[11] Puvanesarajah V, Liauw JA, Lo SF, et al. Techniques and accuracy of thoracolumbar pedicle screw placement. World J Orthop. 2014; 5:112–123

[12] Gertzbein SD, Robbins SE. Accuracy of pedicular screw placement in vivo. Spine (Phila Pa 1976). 1990; 15:11–14

[13] Heary RF, Bono CM, Black M. Thoracic pedicle screws: postoperative computerized tomography scanning assessment. J Neurosurg. 2004; 100:325–331

[14] Ferrara LA, Secor JL, Jin BH, et al. A biomechanical comparison of facet screw fixation and pedicle screw fixation: effects of short-term and long-term repetitive cycling. Spine. 2003; 28:1226–1234

[15] Aepli M, Mannion AF, Grob D. Translaminar screw fixation of the lumbar spine: long-term outcome. Spine (Phila Pa 1976). 2009; 34:1492–1498

[16] Cloward RB. The Treatment of Ruptured Lumbar Intervertebral Discs by Vertebral Body Fusion. Journal of Neurosurgery. 1953; 10:154–168

[17] Pimenta L. Lateral endoscopic transpsoas retroperitoneal approach for lumbar spine surgery. Belo Horizo te, Minas Gerais, Brazil 2001

[18] Ozgur BM, Aryan HE, Pimenta L, et al. Extreme Lateral Interbody Fusion (XLIF): a novel surgical technique for anterior lumbar interbody fusion. Spine J. 2006; 6:435–443

[19] Bergey DL, Villavicencio AT, Goldstein T, et al. Endoscopic lateral transpsoas approach to the lumbar spine. Spine (Phila Pa 1976). 2004; 29:1681–1688

[20] Hall LT, Esses SI, Noble PC, et al. Morphology of the lumbar vertebral endplates. Spine. 1998; 23:1517–22; discussion 1522-3

[21] Rodgers WB, Gerber EJ, Patterson J. Intraoperative and early postoperative complications in extreme lateral interbody fusion: an analysis of 600 cases. Spine (Phila Pa 1976). 2011; 36:26–32

[22] Dakwar E, Cardona RF, Smith DA, et al. Early outcomes and safety of the minimally invasive, lateral retroperitoneal transpsoas approach for adult degenerative scoliosis. Neurosurg Focus. 2010; 28. DOI: 10.3171/2010.1.FOCUS09282

[23] Pimenta L, Diaz RC, Guerrero LG. Charite lumbar artificial disc retrieval: use of a lateral minimally invasive technique. Technical note. J Neurosurg Spine. 2006; 5:556–561

[24] Uribe JS, Arredondo N, Dakwar E, et al. Defining the safe working zones using the minimally invasive lateral retroperitoneal transpsoas approach: an anatomical study. Journal of Neurosurgery (Spine). 2010; 13:260–266

[25] Knight RQ, Schwaegler P, Hanscom D, et al. Direct lateral lumbar interbody fusion for degenerative conditions: early complication profile. J Spinal Disord Tech. 2009; 22:34–37

[26] Ahmadian A, Deukmedjian AR, Abel N, et al. Analysis of lumbar plexopathies and nerve injury after lateral retroperitoneal transpsoas approach: diagnostic standardization. J Neurosurg Spine. 2013; 18:289–297

[27] Abel NA, Januszewski J, Vivas AC, et al. Femoral nerve and lumbar plexus injury after minimally invasive lateral retroperitoneal transpsoas approach: electrodiagnostic prognostic indicators and a roadmap to recovery. Neurosurg Rev. 2018; 41:457–464

[28] Assina R, Majmundar NJ, Herschman Y, et al. First report of major vascular injury due to lateral transpsoas approach leading to fatality. J Neurosurg Spine. 2014; 21:794–798

[29] Dakwar E, Vale FL, Uribe JS. Trajectory of the main sensory and motor branches of the lumbar plexus outside the psoas muscle related to the lateral retroperitoneal transpsoas approach. J Neurosurg Spine. 2011; 14:290–295

[30] Youssef JA, McAfee PC, Patty CA, et al. Minimally invasive surgery: lateral approach interbody fusion: results and review. Spine (Phila Pa 1976). 2010; 35: S302–S311

[31] Alimi M, Hofstetter CP, Cong GT, et al. Radiological and clinical outcomes following extreme lateral interbody fusion. J Neurosurg Spine. 2014; 20:623–635

[32] Shillingford JN, Laratta JL, Tan LA, et al. The Free-Hand Technique for S2-Alar-Iliac Screw Placement: A Safe and Effective Method for Sacropelvic Fixation in Adult Spinal Deformity. J Bone Joint Surg Am. 2018; 100:334–342

110 Miscellaneous Surgical Procedures

110.1 Percutaneous ventricular puncture

110.1.1 Indications

In pediatrics, may be used to remove hemorrhagic ventricular fluid following intraventricular hemorrhage, or to obtain CSF specimen in cases of suspected ventriculitis. May be used emergently in pediatrics or adults as a temporizing measure in patients herniating from obstructive hydrocephalus.

110.1.2 Peds

Clip hair. 5-minute Betadine® prep.

The right side is preferred. Enter through coronal suture just lateral to anterior fontanelle (AF) using a 20–22 Ga spinal needle. If a CT scan has been done, it may be used to help judge angulation (usually varies between contra- and ipsilateral medial canthus and intersection with EAM).

110.1.3 Adult

See reference.[1]

Only used emergently. Takes advantage of thin orbital roof in adult.

Prep conjunctiva and skin with antiseptic (e.g., ophthalmic Betadine). Elevate the eyelid and depress the globe. Using a 16–18 Ga spinal needle, penetrate the anterior third of orbital roof (1–2 cm behind orbital rim) with firm pressure (may need gentle tapping). Aim at coronal suture in the midline. The frontal horn should be about 3–4 cm deep.

110.2 Percutaneous subdural tap

110.2.1 Indications

Utilized in pediatrics. Used to be done for diagnostic purposes, but this has been supplanted by CT, MRI, & ultrasound. Currently, this procedure may be used emergently for decompression, to drain subdural collections, and to obtain fluid for diagnostic tests, such as culture (repeat taps may be used, but surgery should be considered after ≈ 5–6 taps).

110.2.2 Technique

Clip hair. Prep 5 minutes with povidone iodine (Betadine®). Using a short 20–21 Ga spinal needle (spinal needle is recommended because the stylet may reduce the risk of implanting epidermal cells into the CNS), penetrate the lateral margin of the anterior fontanelle (AF) or coronal suture at least 2 cm off midline. Remove the stylet and aspirate. With bilateral fluid collections, bilateral taps should be done.

110.3 Lumbar puncture

110.3.1 Contraindications

1. risk of tonsillar herniation (p. 1815)
   a) known or suspected intracranial mass (tumor, abscess, blood, cerebral edema…)
   b) non-communicating (obstructive) hydrocephalus
   c) relative contraindication: Chiari malformation, especially with a severe blockage of CSF circulation through the foramen magnum. This is less of a concern following satisfactory surgical decompression of Chiari malformation
2. infection in region desired for puncture: e.g skin ulceration. Choose another site if possible
3. coagulopathy
   a) platelet count < 50,000/mm^3 (p. 161)
   b) patient should not be on anticoagulants because of risk of epidural hematoma (p. 1383) or subarachnoid hemorrhage[2] with secondary cord compression

4. use caution in suspected aneurysmal SAH: excessive lowering of the CSF pressure increases the transmural pressure (pressure across the aneurysm wall) and may precipitate rerupture
5. caution in patients with complete spinal block: 14% will deteriorate after LP[3]

Elevated ICP and/or papilledema by themselves are *NOT* contraindications (e.g., LP is actually used diagnostically and as a treatment in pseudotumor cerebri, see below).

110.3.2 Technique

Background and anatomy

The spinal cord and column are the same length in a 3-month fetus. After that, the spinal column grows faster than the cord. As a result, the conus medullaris (the lower terminus of the spinal cord) is located rostral to the termination of the thecal sac in the adult, situated between the middle thirds of the vertebral bodies (VB) of L1 and L2 in 51–68% of adults (the most common location), T12–1 in ≈ 30%, and L2–3 in ≈ 10% (with 94% of cords terminating within the territory of L1 and L2 VB).[4] The thecal sac ends ≈ S2. The tips of the spinous processes as palpated on the surface are located caudal to the corresponding VB. The intercristal line (connecting the superior border of the iliac crests) crosses the spine at the L4 spinous process or between the L4 and L5 spinous processes in most adults.

Procedure

Position: the procedure is usually performed in the lateral decubitus position. As the needle is advanced, it is helpful to have the patient bring the knees up and to flex the neck in order to open up the spaces between the posterior elements of the spine.

For diagnostic LP, a 20 Ga spinal needle is often selected. Larger needles (e.g., 18 Ga) may be used e.g., with pseudotumor cerebri to encourage post-procedure drainage of CSF into the soft tissues of the back.

The back is prepped and draped to create a sterile working area.

Entry point: in an adult, use the L4–5 interspace in most cases (located at or just below the intercristal line) or 1 level higher (L3–4). Peds: L4–5 is preferred over L3–4.

The needle is always advanced with the *stylet in place* at least through the skin and some subcutaneous tissue to avoid introducing epidermal cells, which may cause iatrogenic *epidermoid tumors*; see Complications following LP (p. 1814). The needle is aimed slightly cranially (to parallel the spinous processes) and usually a little down towards the bed (aiming towards the umbilicus). If a Quincke LP (standard) needle is used, the bevel is turned parallel to the length of the spinal column to reduce the risk of post-LP H/A (p. 1817). In general, if bone is encountered it is more often due to deviation from a true midline trajectory rather than a failure to aim correctly in the rostral-caudal direction. The needle should be withdrawn to just below the skin surface before attempting a new trajectory.

If during insertion of the needle the patient experiences pain radiating down one LE, this usually indicates that a nerve root has been encountered. The needle should be withdrawn immediately and reinserted aiming more towards the side *contralateral* to the extremity that experienced the pain. The stylet is removed at intervals during the insertion to look for CSF (a distinct pop is sometimes felt as the needle penetrates the dura).

Once CSF flows, the needle is connected to a manometer through a 3-way stopcock, the pressure is measured and recorded (see below), and CSF is drained into sterile tubes (1–2 ml for each tube for laboratory analysis (see below). The practitioner should also note the color of the fluid (clear, blood-tinged, xanthochromic…) and the clarity (clear, cloudy, purulent…).

At the end of the procedure, the stylet should be replaced before the needle is withdrawn (to reduce post-LP H/A, see below).

Opening pressure: The opening pressure (OP) should be measured and recorded for every LP. To be meaningful, the patient should be lying down and as relaxed as possible (should not be in forced fetal position), with the bed flat. The variation of pressure with respirations is usually a good indication of a communicating fluid column (the fluctuation is in-phase with the respiratory pressures in the inferior vena cava, rising with inspiration and falling with expiration[5]). Normal values: in the left lateral decubitus position, average OP = 12.2 ± 3.4 cm H_2O (8.8 ± 0.9 mm Hg).[6] Also, see ► Table 23. for peds.

Queckenstedt's test: if a subarachnoid block is suspected (e.g., from spinal tumor), compress the jugular vein (JV) first on one side then on both sides (do not compress carotid arteries). If there is no block, the pressure will rise to 10–20 cm of fluid, and will drop to the original level within 10 seconds of release of the JV.[7(p 11)] Do *not* do JV compression if intracranial disease is suspected.

110.3.3 Laboratory analysis

Routinely, three tubes are sent for analysis as shown in ▶ Table 110.1. See ▶ Table 23.4 for interpreting the results of the laboratory analysis.

Table 110.1 Routine tests for CSF

Test	If there is *no* concern about possible traumatic tap	If there is concern about traumatic tap
cell count		Tube 1
gram stain + C & S (culture & sensitivity)	Tube 1	Tube 2
protein and glucose	Tube 2	Tube 3
cell count	Tube 3	Tube 4

If the tap is possibly traumatic (i.e., bloody), or if having an accurate cell count is essential (e.g., to R/O SAH) then 4 tubes are collected, and the first and last are sent for cell counts and are compared; see Traumatic tap (p. 1813).

If special cultures are required (e.g., acid-fast, fungal, viral) they are also specified on the tube for culture & sensitivity (C & S).

If CSF for cytology is desired (e.g., to R/O carcinomatous meningitis or CNS lymphoma), then at least 10 ml of CSF must be sent in one tube to pathology (where it is spun down and examined for cells).

110.3.4 Traumatic tap

General information

A traumatic tap (**TT**) (AKA bloody tap) occurs when the spinal needle damages a blood vessel with the result that (usually venous) blood either alone or admixed with CSF will be obtained.

TT has been defined as containing more than a certain number of RBCs per microliter, and different cutoffs have been used as a minimum: > 200, > 500, or > 1000 have been used.[8]

Incidence of TT varies depending on the study population and the cutoff used, and ranges from 8–30%.[8,9]

Suggestions for "mining useful data" from a bloody tap for the purpose of diagnosing elevated WBCs (as in bacterial meningitis) or diagnosing SAH appear in the sections below.

Estimating true WBC count in CSF with a traumatic tap

When many RBCs and WBCs are present in the CSF due to a TT, it is difficult to know if there is a true leukocytosis on the CSF. It may help to determine if the WBCs are elevated or if they are present in the same ratio as in the peripheral blood. In non-anemic patients, there should be ≈ 1–2 WBCs for every 1000 RBCs (as a correction[10(p 176)]: subtract 1 WBC for every 700 RBCs[10(p 176)]). In the presence of anemia or *peripheral* leukocytosis, use Fishman's formula[10(p 176)] shown in Eq (110.1) to estimate the original WBC count in the CSF *before* the TT,

$$WBC_{CSF\ Original} = WBC_{CSF} - \frac{WBC_{Blood} \times RBC_{CSF}}{RBC_{Blood}} \qquad (110.1)$$

where $WBC_{CSF\ Original}$ = WBC count in the CSF before the TT, WBC_{CSF} & RBC_{CSF} = WBC & RBC counts measured in the CSF, and WBC_{Blood} & RBC_{Blood} = WBC & RBC per mm^3 in the peripheral blood.

Estimating true total CSF protein content with a traumatic tap

If the hemogram and peripheral protein are normal, then have the cell count and protein content run on the *same tube*, and the correction is[10(p 176)]:

subtract 1 mg per 100 ml of protein for every 1000 RBC per mm^3

110

Differentiating SAH from traumatic tap

The sensitivity of detecting RBCs in CSF approaches 100%, and if it is assumed that 20% of LPs are traumatic (an approximation), then the specificity of a bloody tap for diagnosing the presence of blood in the CSF prior to the LP is only ≈ 80%.[11]

See typical findings in SAH (p.1422). Some features helpful in differentiating SAH from TT are shown in ► Table 110.2.

Table 110.2 Features distinguishing traumatic tap from SAH

Feature	Traumatic tap (TT)	SAH
RBC count	< 2000 RBC/mm³ [12] (< 500 RBC/mm³ had a 100% negative predictive value for SAH in one small study[13])	usually > 100,000 RBC/mm³
clearing of RBCs from 1st tube to last tube	declines as CSF drains (controversial - see text)	changes little as CSF drains
ratio of WBC:RBC	similar to the ratio in peripheral blood (above)	usually promotes a leukocytosis (elevated WBC count)
supernatant	clear	xanthochromic (p.1422)[a] (rarely in < 2 hrs, present in 70% by 6 hrs, and > 90% by 12 hrs after SAH)
clotting of fluid	usually clots if erythrocyte count > 200,000/mm³	usually does not clot
protein concentration	fresh bleeding elevates CSF protein from normal by only ≈ 1 mg per 1000 RBC	blood breakdown products elevate this more than TT (measured protein exceeds the sum of normal protein + 1 mg protein/ 1000 RBC)
repeat LP at higher level	usually clear	remains bloody
opening pressure	usually normal	usually elevated

[a]NB: other conditions can cause xanthochromia

► **Clearing of RBCs with TT.** It is commonly held that the reduction of RBC count in the last tube compared to the first tube is indicative of a TT. An older study recommended a reduction > 30% as the requirement,[14] and a smaller study (15 patients with SAH) recommended > 70% clearance as the cutoff.[13]

► **Xanthochromia.** Details and photo (p.1422). Although it can occur earlier, a minimum of 4 hrs is usually required to develop xanthochromia (XTC). It is present in ≈ 100% of bleeds at 12 hours, persists for ≈ 2 weeks. By 3 weeks it is found in about 70%, and may be detected as late as 4 weeks after the bleed.

► **Recommendations.** Conservative recommendation: clearing > 70% of RBCs from the first tube to the last with < 500 RBC/mm³ in the final tube is strongly supportive of a TT.[13]

The presence of XTC in the setting of bloody CSF virtually rules out a TT.

110.3.5 Complications following LP

General information

The overall risk of disabling or persistent symptoms (defined as severe H/A lasting > 7 days, cranial nerve palsies, major exacerbation of preexisting neurological disease, prolonged back pain, aseptic meningitis, and nerve root or peripheral nerve injuries) has been estimated at 0.1–0.5%.[15] Severe side effects, which include brainstem herniation, infection, subdural hematoma or effusion, and SAH, are rare.[16(p 171-2)]

Possible complications

1. tonsillar herniation
   a) acute herniation in the presence of mass lesion (see below)
   b) chronic tonsillar herniation (acquired Chiari 1 malformation): this has been reported after multiple traumatic LPs with presumed post-LP CSF leak[17]

2. infection (spinal meningitis)
3. "spinal headache": usually positional (diminishes with recumbency) (see below)
4. spinal epidural hematoma (p. 1383): usually seen only with coagulopathy
5. spinal epidural CSF collection: may be fairly common in patients with post-LP H/A. Usually resolves spontaneously
6. epidermoid tumor: risk may be increased by advancing LP needle without stylet (transplanting a core of epidermal tissue)[18,19,20]
7. impinging nerve root with needle: usually causes transient radicular pain. May cause permanent radiculopathy in rare instances
8. *intracranial* subdural hygroma or hematoma[21,22] (rare)
9. vestibulocochlear dysfunction[23]:
   a) subclinical (demonstrated on audiogram) or moderate reduction in hearing may occur, and seems to correlate with post-procedure CSF leakage. Most studies show reduction is at frequencies < 1000 Hz
   b) sudden hearing loss may occur. Perform audiogram to quantify loss. Treat with bedrest for several days, prednisone 60 mg/d tapered over 2–3 weeks
   c) pathogenesis: reduced CSF pressure may reduce perilymph pressure through the cochlear aqueduct (may be especially pronounced with a patent aqueduct),[24] producing endolymphatic hydrops
10. ocular abnormalities
    a) abducens palsy: almost invariably unilateral. Often delayed 5–14 days post-LP, usually recovers after 4–6 wks[25]
11. dural sinus thrombosis[26] (usually with underlying thrombophilia)

Risk of acute tonsillar herniation following lumbar puncture

The question of when to do LP first (to save time) and when to obtain CT scan first to R/O intracranial mass (for safety) before performing an LP is controversial.

110

Issues

The time delay to initiating antibiotics is the most important variable in the outcome of meningitis. Mortality increase 13% per hour delay in treatment.[27] Time may be more crucial in community-acquired meningitis, where a virulent organism typically infects an immune-intact host (or immune-susceptible hosts such as children or the elderly), than in post-op neurosurgical meningitis (usually a low-virulence organism, e.g., *Staph. aureus*, in a host where the BBB has been disrupted but the patient is otherwise immune-intact).

The theoretical risk in performing an LP with elevated intracranial pressure (e.g., from intracranial mass, obstructive hydrocephalus, Chiari malformation…) is that the lowering of spinal CSF pressure resulting from removal of CSF during the procedure or the leakage of CSF through the puncture site after the procedure may precipitate tonsillar herniation due to the resultant increased pressure gradient.

Starting antibiotics without first having a CSF specimen from an LP may prevent cultures from growing in the lab which then risks the difficulties inherent in managing partially treated meningitis, or a suboptimal choice of antibiotic medication.

Clinical evaluation for possible contraindication to LP is unreliable. Papilledema is one possible indication of increased ICP. Papilledema takes a minimum of 6 hrs to develop after the onset of increased ICP, and in most cases it requires up to 24 hrs to develop. Therefore, its absence does not ensure normal ICP. Furthermore, papilledema may be seen in conditions where there is not a contraindication to LP, e.g., pseudotumor cerebri (p. 955), where LP is one of the accepted treatments.

The ready availability of CT scans, often within the emergency department itself, may involve a delay of only a few minutes, if qualified personnel to interpret the study are also immediately available. However, in practice, obtaining a CT scan delayed subsequent treatment by an average of 1.6 hours[27] and increased mortality.

Historical information

Herniation following LP was more common prior to ≈ 1950, long before CT scans were available, where the procedure was performed even when some patients had clear evidence of ↑ ICP, large-bore spinal needles (12–16 gauge) were more commonly employed, and large quantities of CSF were removed for therapeutic purposes. In a 1969 report of 30 patients who deteriorated after LP,[28] 73% had localizing signs (hemiparesis, anisocoria…) and 30% had papilledema. None of 5 patients with cerebral abscess deteriorated after the first of multiple LPs.

In a series of 129 patients with ↑ ICP,[29] the complication rate reported was 6%; however, some of these complications were probably unrelated to LP, and many of these patients were in extremis. In 7 series totalling 418 patients, a complication rate of 1.2% was calculated.[29] The risk of LP is small[30] especially with a 20 gauge or smaller needle and removing only a few ml of CSF.

Σ: LP in acute bacterial meningitis (ABM)

Herniation as a result of LP is consistently reported only in patients with severe non-infectious proc-esses, often with accompanying signs of mass effect (localizing signs, papilledema...). Modified inter-national guidelines[27] list these contraindications to LP in cases of suspected acute bacterial meningitis: papilledema, focal neurologic signs & immunocompromised state.

Antibiotics and corticosteroids should be started immediately (the goal is within 30–60 minutes, but this has been achieved in only 35%) in cases of suspected ABM. If a CT scan is indicated before LP, treatment can be started before the LP. If the CT scan does not show a space-occupying lesion, LP may be performed. In the unlikely event that there is acute deterioration associated with the with-drawal of a few ml of CSF, the (anecdotal) recommendation is to immediately replace the fluid through the LP needle.

Post-LP (myelogram) H/A

General information
AKA "postspinal headache" or "spinal headache." May also follow procedures other than LP/myelo-gram, such as dural opening (p. 1260). Can also occur with spontaneous intracranial hypotension (p. 421) and following decompressive craniectomy.[31]

Clinical features
Important distinctive characteristic: H/A occurs when patient is erect, and is completely or partially (but significantly) relieved when recumbent. May be associated with nausea, vomiting, dizziness, or visual disturbances.

▶ **Time course.** Most post-LP headaches (PLPHA) have a delayed onset 24–48 hrs after the LP, and although they may occur weeks post-LP, most also develop within 3 days. The duration of PLPHA varies, with a mean of 4 days,[32] and reports of duration of months[33] and even > 1 year.[34]

Pathophysiology
Thought to be due to continued CSF leakage through the hole in the dura,[35] which reduces the CSF "cushion" of the brain. In the upright position, the pull of gravity on the brain produces traction on the blood vessels and any structures tethering the brain to the pain-sensitive dura. CSF may some-times be demonstrable in the *epidural* space.

Epidemiology following LP
Reported incidence range is 2–40% (typically ≈ 20%), higher after diagnostic LP than for epidural anesthesia.[32]

See also variables in LP that impact upon the risk of PLPHA (p. 1816) (e.g., incidence is lower with smaller-gauge spinal needle).
1. risk factors for post-LP H/A outside the control of the physician:
   a) age: incidence ↑ in younger patients
   b) sex: incidence ↑ in females
   c) prior headache history (including previous PLPHA)
   d) body size: ↑ with small body mass index = weight/height^2 [36]
   e) pregnancy
2. variables that have been shown to influence the incidence of PLPHA:
   a) needle size: larger needles carry increased risk[37]
   b) bevel orientation: orienting the bevel parallel to the longitudinally running fibers of the dura reduces the risk of PLPHA[38]
   c) replacing the stylet prior to needle removal lowers the incidence[36]
   d) the number of dural punctures (may not be totally under the physician's control)

110

3. variables that may or may not influence the incidence of PLPHA: needle type:
   a) Quincke needle: bevelled edge with cutting tip (the standard LP needle). Incidence of PLPHA with 20 and 22 gauge Quincke needles: 36%[39]
   b) atraumatic needles: a number of types are available (Sprotte, Whitacre...). Most are "pencil-pointed" and may produce a hole with a lower incidence of transdural leak.[40] Unproven[36]
4. factors found *not* to affect the incidence of PLPHA:
   a) the position of the patient after LP (does not seem to prevent PLPHA, but may delay the onset of symptoms[41,42])
   b) volume of fluid removed at the time of LP
   c) hydration following LP[36]

Treatment for H/A following LP

Initial "conservative" measures include:
1. flat in bed for at least 24 hrs
2. hydration (PO or IV)
3. analgesics for H/A
4. tight abdominal binder
5. deoxycortisone acetate 5 mg IM q 8 hrs[32]
6. caffeine sodium benzoate 500 mg in 2 cc IV q 8 hrs up to 3 d max (70% of patients had relief with 1 or 2 injections)[43]
7. high-dose steroids: report of success in a case of intracranial hypotension associated with spontaneous slit ventricles tapering down from a starting dose of dexamethasone 20 mg/day[44]
8. blood patch if refractory

▶ **Epidural blood patch.** For refractory post-lumbar puncture or post-myelogram H/A. Works in one application in over 90% of cases, may be repeated if ineffective.[33] Theoretical risks: infection, cauda equina compression, failure to relieve H/A.

▶ **Technique.** Summary: 10 ml of non-heparinized autologous blood injected into *epidural* space.
   Accessing epidural space (one of several techniques): proceed as routine LP. When ligaments are traversed, and needle tip is nearing spinal canal, stylet is removed. Then, either place drop of sterile saline in hub (hanging drop technique) and advance while watching for it to be drawn into needle as epidural space is entered, or gently try injecting air with small syringe (preferably glass, lower resistance) while advancing, when the epidural space is entered, resistance to injection disappears, but CSF cannot be aspirated.
   A venipuncture site is prepared aseptically. 10 ml of the patient's blood is withdrawn. After verifying CSF cannot be aspirated through the spinal needle, the blood is injected into the epidural space. After 30 minutes supine, patient may ambulate ad lib.

110.4 Lumbar catheter CSF drainage

110.4.1 General information

Insertion of a catheter into the lumbar subarachnoid space for the purpose of draining CSF. Usually connected to a closed drainage system similar to that for an EVD. Generally used for periods of only a few days or so.

110.4.2 Indications

1. to reduce CSF pressure at a site of CSF leak/fistula. Examples:
   a) dural breach during spine surgery or craniotomy (especially posterior fossa)
   b) for spontaneous CSF fistula (p. 418) (rare)
2. to reduce intracranial pressure in cases of *communicating* hydrocephalus: e.g., drain test for NPH, or when an infected shunt has been removed
3. to reduce CSF pressure to attempt to increase perfusion of the spinal cord: e.g., during surgery for abdominal aortic aneurysm, or following spinal cord injury

110.4.3 Contraindications

As with lumbar puncture (see above).

110

110.4.4 Insertion technique

Positioning, entry site, and trajectory are all similar to lumbar puncture (see above). Placing the patient in slight reverse Trendelenburg helps distend the lumbar thecal sac. Instead of a spinal needle, a specialized needle designed for inserting a catheter is used. A Tuohy needle is commonly used, it is a spinal needle with a slightly curved beveled tip (▶ Fig. 110.1) and a stylet to avoid coring tissue and displacing it into the spinal canal. The needle with stylet in olace is inserted with the bevel parallel to the fibers of the dura (rostro-caudal). As the needle is advanced, periodically the stylet is removed and if necessary the needle is aspirated with a syringe to see if CSF drains.[45] If not, the stylet is replaced and the needle is advanced. Once the tip is intrathecal (as evidenced by flow of CSF through the needle), the needle is rotated 90° (usually pointing rostrally – the direction of the needle curve is indicated by a small notch in the hub of the needle) and the catheter is threaded into the needle.

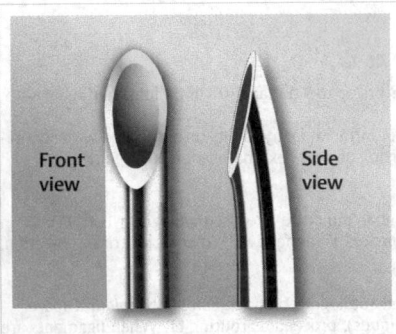

Fig. 110.1 Tuohy needle tip.
Diagram of the tip of a Tuohy needle.

Front view

Side view

✖ If the catheter does not thread, the needle must be withdrawn *together* with the catheter. Attempting to withdraw the catheter through the needle will shear off the catheter at the tip of the needle, leaving a portion of the catheter tube inside the patient.

110.4.5 Management

Nursing orders to maintain the catheter include:
1. instructions to regulate the CSF drainage. Most commonly, either:
   a) by pressure: accomplished by specifying a height of the drip chamber, usually at the level of the tragus or shoulder
   b) by withdrawing a specified amount of CSF per hour: usually 10–20 cc. This method reduces the risk of overdrainage if the drip chamber is too low
2. the risk of overdrainage (by either of the above methods) may be reduced by connecting the catheter to a volume-limiting drainage system (e.g., LimiTorr™ by Integra)
3. instructions for the exit site dressing: usually treated as an arterial-line

110.4.6 Complications

1. infection
2. overdrainage: usually as a result of the drainage bag being too low when using the pressure drainage method described above (either from falling to the floor, or not being raised when the patient sits or stands up) or from catheter disconnection. Can cause:
   a) subdural hematoma from tearing of bridging veins from downward displacement of the brain
   b) headache
3. pneumocephalus: usually from placing the drain height below the site of a fistula, and air is drawn in through the fistula tract
   a) tension pneumocephalus: usually with a ball-valve effect at the fistula site
4. catheter pull-out: frequently occurs simply as a result of patient movement in bed or with patient transfers

110

110.5 C1–2 puncture and cisternal tap

110.5.1 Indications

Situations where CSF specimen is required but access via LP is difficult or contraindicated (lumbar arachnoiditis, superficial infection, marked obesity, patients who cannot be turned on their sides…), or to instill contrast to demonstrate the rostral extent of a block documented by dye injected via LP. Spinal headache is less common with these procedures than with LP. C1–2 puncture is safer than cisternal tap.

✖ Contraindicated: in patient with Chiari malformation (often present in myelomeningocele) due to low-lying cerebellar tonsils and medullary kink.

Normal CSF values for glucose and protein differ only slightly from CSF obtained by lumbar puncture. Opening pressures averaged 18 cm of fluid with lateral puncture.

110.5.2 C1–2 puncture

AKA lateral cervical puncture. Equipment: LP tray (useful for the specimen tubes, extension tube for contrast injection under fluoroscopy, lidocaine, and spinal needle) with a standard 20 Ga spinal needle, contrast if needed (e.g., Iohexol®). It is preferred to perform the procedure under fluoro, but it has also been described without fluoroscopic guidance with a completely cooperative patient.[46]

Patient position: supine in bed without a pillow, with the head straight up. Avoid any head rotation which may bring the vertebral artery (VA) into the needle path.[47] Place head within lateral fluoroscopy unit (since this is rarely available, a C-arm fluoro positioned horizontally may be used).

If iodinated dye is being injected for myelography, the head should be elevated to prevent contrast from running into posterior fossa; in cases with cervical spine injury, one can put the entire bed in reverse Trendelenburg.

Entry point: 1 cm caudal and 1 cm posterior (dorsal) to the tip of the mastoid process. Needle insertion: use a 25 Ga needle to anesthetize the skin at the entry point. Under fluoro, advance a larger needle (e.g., 21 Ga) towards the C1–2 interspace while injecting local anesthetic: aim for a target in the middle of the posterior third of the bony spinal canal (or, alternatively, 2–3 mm anterior to the posterior margin of the bony canal) ("X" in ▶ Fig. 110.2). Leave this needle in as a marker.

110

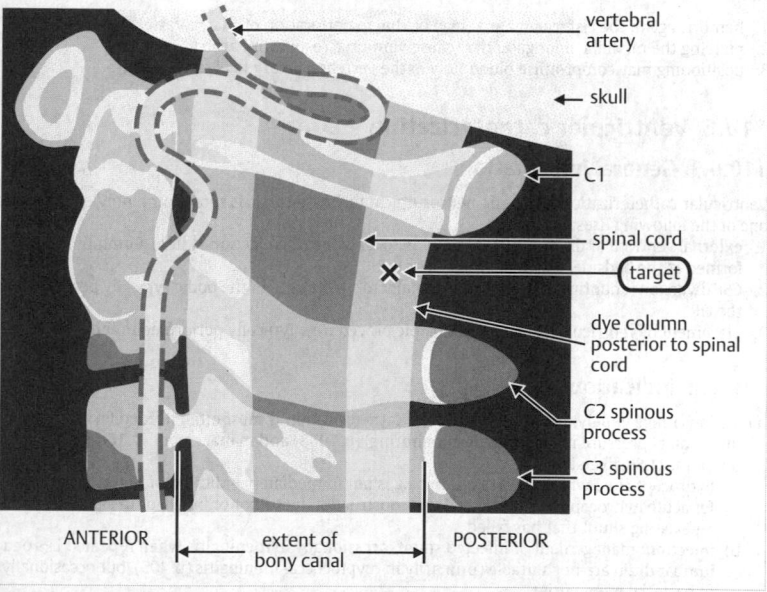

Fig. 110.2 C1–2 puncture target.[*]
[*] Left lateral view through upper C-spine: composite diagram of a myelogram and vertebral arteriogram illustrating the relative location of the spinal cord, CSF space, and VA. Only bony landmarks will be visible with fluoroscopy.

Insert the 20 Ga spinal needle parallel to the marker needle. Verify the course with fluoro. If fluoro is not used, insert the spinal needle at the entry point, and advance it parallel to the plane of the bed, perpendicular to the neck.[46] If the needle penetrates deeply without encountering bone or CSF, it is most likely that the tip is too far posterior. If bone is encountered, redirect the needle in the rostro-caudal plane.

Several "pops" may be felt, and the stylet should be removed after each to check for CSF return. The subarachnoid space is ≈ 5–6 cm deep to the skin surface in most adults.[48] The needle must be supported more than with a lumbar puncture.

To inject iodinated contrast, use e.g., ≈ 5 ml of 180 mgI/ml Iohexol® for cervical myelogram, watch dye on fluoro (should be able to see it in subarachnoid space).

Risks

Case report of a death from subdural hematoma due to puncture of an anomalous vertebral artery[49] (found in ≈ 0.4% of population). If the VA is penetrated, the needle is withdrawn and local pressure is applied. Penetration of the upper spinal cord/lower medulla (risk of serious neurologic sequelae, even from this, is small). Herniation (as with LP) when there is increased ICP.

110.5.3 Cisternal tap

Suboccipital access to the cisterna magna. Usually done with patient sitting, with neck slightly flexed.[50] Overlying hair should be shaved. Local anesthetic is infiltrated. A 22 gauge spinal needle is inserted exactly in the midline between the inion and the C2 spinous process, directed superiorly toward the glabella until the needle strikes the occiput or enters the cisterna magna. If the occiput is encountered, the needle is withdrawn slightly and reinserted, directed slightly inferiorly, and the process is repeated ("walking down the occiput") until the cisterna magna is entered (a "pop" will be felt).

The distance from the skin surface to the cisterna magna is 4–6 cm, and from the dura to the medulla is ≈ 2.5 cm. However, due to tenting of the dura, the needle may be very close to the medulla before entering the subarachnoid space.

Risks

1. hemorrhage in the cisterna magna: may be due to perforation of a large vessel[46]
2. piercing the medulla oblongata: may cause vomiting, respiratory arrest…
3. positioning may compromise blood flow in the vertebral artery in elderly patients

110.6 Ventricular catheterization

110.6.1 General information

Ventricular catheterization is a basic neurosurgical technique that is most commonly employed for one of the following uses:

1. external ventricular drain (EVD): drains CSF to an external collection system. Commonly performed at the bedside, usually in the ICU or E/R
2. CSF diversion (shunting): drains CSF internally to a distal site in the body. Typically performed in the OR
3. placement of ventriculoscope for endoscopic procedures. Typically performed in the OR

110.6.2 Indications

Indications range widely; however, ventricular catheterization is most often needed for:

1. intracranial pressure measurement (monitoring) (p. 1038) and management (p. 1046)
2. temporary CSF diversion
   a) hydrocephalus: when definitive shunting is not immediately indicated or practical. Typically for acute hydrocephalus associated with obstruction by tumor or blood, or in a patient with an existing shunt that has failed
   b) infection: management of infected shunt, occasionally in meningitis when repeated LPs or a lumbar drain are not suitable (primarily in cryptococcal meningitis (p. 409), but occasionally in bacterial meningitis)

3. intrathecal drug administration: for long-term use, a ventricular access device (p. 1831) is often preferred. Typically for chemotherapy (e.g., for CNS lymphoma) or sometimes for antibiotics (for ventriculitis complicating meningitis)

110.6.3 Procedure risks

The primary risks of the procedure are:
1. infection
2. bleeding: including bleeding along catheter tract (intraparenchymal), within the subdural/epidural or intraventricular space, or SAH in patients with an aneurysm (sometimes as a result of lowering ICP which can increase the transmural pressure (p. 1427)). Risk of any bleeding = 7%, clinically significant bleeding 0.8%[51]
3. malposition of catheter
4. catheter failure: occlusion by blood, debris (includes brain tissue, infectious debris…), or ependymal lining of ventricles if the ventricles completely collapse on the catheter, damage to catheter, catheter pullout

110.6.4 Coagulation

To reduce the risk of bleeding, coagulopathies need to be identified and corrected prior to the procedure. Ideally, patients should have an INR ≤ 1.6, platelet count > 100K, and no recent antiplatelet medication (can be screened by checking thromboelastogram (TEG)).

Elevated INR: for patients with an elevated INR (such as patients on warfarin), it has generally been recommended that placement of intraparenchymal catheters be delayed until the INR is ≤ 1.6 in order to reduce the risk of hemorrhage to an acceptable level.[52,53] However, intraparenchymal ICP monitors were placed without hemorrhagic or thrombotic complications in 11 patients with grade III/IV hepatic encephalopathy associated with fulminant hepatic failure who had an average INR of 3 when it was performed within 15–120 minutes after receiving 36.7 micrograms/kg IV of recombinant activated factor VII (rFVIIa).[54] All of these studies showed that ICP monitors were inserted in the study patients without hemorrhagic complications – but bear in mind that absence of proof is not proof of absence.

110.6.5 Common ventricular catheter insertion sites

1. ★ Kocher's point (coronal): localizes an entry point into the frontal horn of the lateral ventricle that passes anterior to the motor strip. The right side is usually used since that is more commonly the nondominant hemisphere. Often employed for ICP monitors, EVDs, shunts, ventriculoscopes…. Originally described as "about 2 cm from the central line and 3 cm from the precentral fissure."[55] A number of surface landmarks have been described to locate a point anterior to the motor strip that is in this general vicinity, and many of them refer to their target as "Kocher's point." Commonly cited landmarks:
   a) entry site: (► Fig. 110.3)
      • 2–3 cm from midline, which is approximately the mid-pupillary line with forward gaze
      • 1 cm anterior to the coronal suture, which is approximately 11 cm back from the nasion in an adult (to avoid the motor strip (p. 56))
   b) trajectory: direct catheter perpendicular to surface of brain,[56] which can be approximated by aiming in coronal plane toward the medial canthus of the ipsilateral eye and in the AP plane toward the EAM
   c) insertion length: advance catheter with stylet until CSF is obtained (should be < 5–7 cm depth; this may be 3–4 cm with markedly dilated ventricles). Advance catheter without stylet 1 cm deeper. ✘ CAUTION: if CSF is not obtained until very long insertion length (e.g., ≥ 8 cm) the tip is probably in a cistern (e.g., prepontine cistern) which is undesirable
2. ★ occipital-parietal region: commonly used for CSF shunt
   a) entry site: a number of means have been described, including:
      • Frazier burr hole: placed prophylactically before p-fossa crani for emergency ventriculostomy in event of post-op swelling. Location: 3–4 cm from midline, 6–7 cm above inion[57] (p 520) (caution: an error in locating the inion could put the catheter in an undesirable location if this method alone is used)
      • parietal boss: flat portion of parietal bone
      • follow point from mid-pupillary line parallel to sagittal suture until it intersects line extending posteriorly from the top of the pinna
      • ≈ 3 cm above and ≈ 3 cm posterior to top of pinna

110

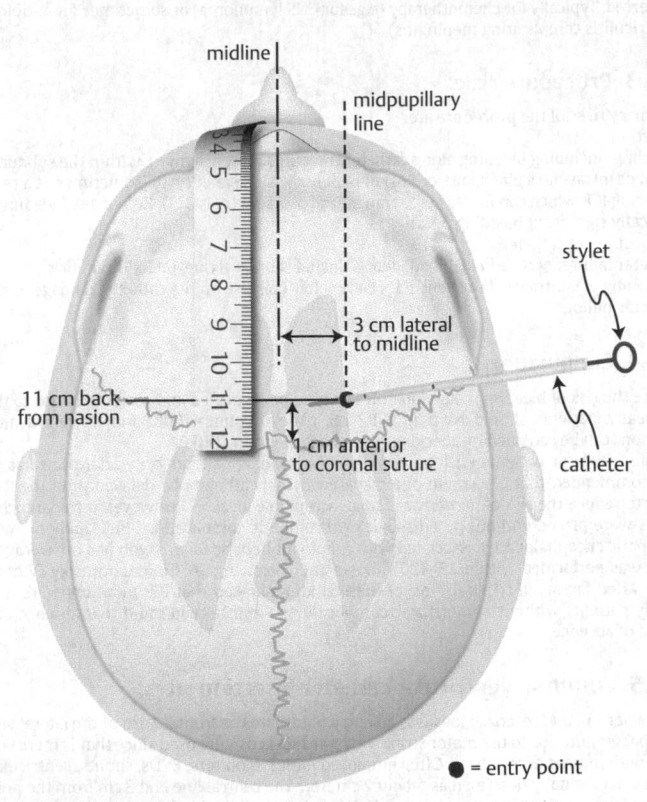

midline

midpupillary line

stylet

3 cm lateral to midline

11 cm back from nasion

1 cm anterior to coronal suture

catheter

● = entry point

Fig. 110.3 Kocher's point. Ventriculostomy landmarks for Kocher's point. See text for details.

110

b) trajectory: insert the catheter parallel to skull base:
  • initially aim for middle of forehead
  • if this fails, aim for ipsilateral medial canthus
c) insertion length: ideally, the tip should be just anterior to the foramen of Monro in the frontal horn.[58] Ventriculoscopic guidance (if available) increases the accuracy to a significant degree. In the absence of this:
  • intracranial length should be ≈ two-thirds of the length of the skull (this is short enough to prevent penetration of frontal brain parenchyma, but long enough to take tip beyond the foramen of Monro to prevent catheter from ending up in the temporal horn where choroid plexus increases the chance of obstruction)
  • in adults without macrocrania the inserted length is usually ≈ 12 cm when the burr hole is in line with the axis of the lateral ventricle[59] (lengths > 12 cm are rarely required). In hydrocephalic infants usually ≈ 7–8 cm is required
  • use the stylet for the initial ≈ 6 cm of insertion, then remove it and insert the remaining length (keeps the catheter straight during penetration of occipital parenchyma and

prevents the tip from dropping into the temporal horn where there is choroid plexus; also, the temporal horn may collapse and occlude the catheter when the HCP is resolved)

3. Keen's point (posterior parietal): (placement in trigone) 2.5–3 cm posterior and 2.5–3 cm superior to pinna (was the usual site of occurrence of cerebral abscesses arising from otitis media, and was often used to tap these)
4. Dandy's point: 2 cm from midline, 3 cm above inion (may be more prone to damage visual pathways than above)

110.6.6 Ventriculostomy/ICP monitor – bedside insertion technique

General information

Intraventricular catheter (IVC) AKA external ventricular drain (EVD) placement at the bedside has a number of unique challenges that differ from ventricular catheterization in the OR where supplies, anesthesia, assistance (and possibly image navigation) are normally available.

★ 3 things that have been reproducibly shown to reduce the risk of infection[60]:
1. tunneling the exit for the catheter > 2 cm
2. antibiotic impregnated ventricular catheter
3. shorter duration of presence of catheter

Informed consent

For procedures performed in the OR, see Booking the case (for shunts) (p.1831). The consent form for bedside ventricular catheterization should list the following which should be discussed with the patient or family when possible: infection, bleeding (stroke), and catheter malposition or failure. Often, patients requiring urgent placement of an EVD are unresponsive or unable to give informed consent, and an appropriate health care surrogate may not be available. In these situations, follow your specific institution's policy for emergency procedures.

110

Supplies

To enhance sterility and speed of the procedure, it is critical to have the required supplies immediately available. Many hospitals have an "EVD cart" with the supplies pre-stocked. A partial list is included here.
• ventricular catheter: an antibiotic impregnated catheter is recommended (see above)[60]
• ventriculostomy kit: these kits usually contain a cranial access kit with scalpel, prep solution, drapes, razor, local anesthetic, hand drill with bit
• ventricular catheter drainage collection system: connects to the ventricular catheter. Usually consists of a drainage bag, a calibrated drip chamber with adjustable height, ports for sampling CSF and for connection to a pressure transducer
• sterile gowns, gloves, masks
• adhesive tape to stabilize the patient's head
  optional: marker to tape to middle of forehead that can be palpated through the drape to help the surgeon easily find this location. Items that work well: a "red-dot" EKG lead sticker, or a cap from a TB syringe turned so the "cup" faces forward

Insertion technique

Unless contraindicated (e.g., right ventricular bleed), the right (non-dominant) side is preferred.
1. clip the hair around the planned incision site and the exit site for the tunneled catheter (avoid shaving which compromises the skin barrier against infection)
2. mark the skin at Kocher's point (► Fig. 110.3): approximately *11 cm back from the nasion*, and *2–3 cm (about 2 fingerbreadths) lateral to midline*
3. stabilize the head with adhesive tape
4. don sterile gown and gloves, face mask, and eye protection
5. prep with an acceptable surgical prep and drape
6. infiltrate local anesthetic
7. a 2.5-cm skin incision is centered over Kocher's point. It is usually straight and sagittally oriented (in case it needs to be incorporated in a craniotomy flap in the future)
8. elevate the periosteum: the back end of the scalpel is convenient for this
9. place a self-retaining retractor

10. make a twist drill hole at Kocher's point (if you can see the coronal suture through the skin incision, drill the hole 1 cm anterior to it)
11. perforate the dura with the tip of a needle, moving it side-to-side (the dural opening must be large enough for the catheter or monitor probe)
12. inserting a ventricular catheter
    - the ventricular catheter is initially inserted with the stylet in place
    - insert the catheter *perpendicular* to the skull surface[56] to a maximum intracranial depth of 5–7 cm (most catheters are marked at 5 and 10 cm). If there is midline shift (MLS) on the pre-op CT, aim slightly towards the side of the MLS. When the catheter tip enters the ventricle, a subtle "pop" can be palpated, and if the CSF is under pressure some CSF may drip out through the proximal catheter around the stylet. The stylet may be removed if there is any question if the catheter tip is in the ventricle. It may be necessary to put the patient in reverse Trendelenburg to get CSF to flow if the pressure is low. See also other maneuvers (p. 1824). With any ventricular enlargement, the ventricle should be entered by 3–4 cm depth (with normal size ventricles, this may be 4–5 cm). If a pop is felt, the catheter is inserted an additional 1/2 cm with the stylet. Then an additional 1 cm is inserted without the stylet. Verify CSF flow
      ✖ If no CSF is encountered by 7 cm, passing the catheter deeper will place it in an undesirable location (even if CSF is then obtained). At ≈ 9–11 cm the tip will often be in the pre-pontine cistern, a subarachnoid space, which is undesirable.
    - if unsuccessful after a maximum of three passes, then place a subarachnoid bolt or intraparenchymal monitor
    - the proximal end of the catheter is tunneled at least 2 cm[60] under the scalp using a sharp stylet before being brought out through the skin to reduce the risk of infection
    - luer lock adapter is attached to proximal end of catheter and is attached to collection system
13. for (Richmond) subarachnoid bolt: screw in until tip is flush with inner table
14. for intraparenchymal monitor, a path is "cleared" for a few cm into the brain parenchyma using the included blunt stylet. The monitor is then inserted and then backed out about ½ cm so that the tip does not butt up against brain tissue

110

▶ **Tricks of the trade: getting CSF with an IVC.** It is common to have difficulty obtaining CSF with ventricular catheterization. There are numerous maneuvers that may help. NB: the problem is almost never that you need to insert deeper! Possible problems and solutions include:
- malposition of catheter tip
  a) again, the problem is almost never that you need to insert deeper. Never exceed 7 cm
  b) mediolateral deviation: most of us tend to consistently aim too medial or too lateral. If you know your natural bias, reinsert the IVC aimed slightly in the opposite direction to compensate for this. If you don't know your bias, try reinserting the IVC slightly more medially or laterally
  c) re-check the pre-op CT for midline shift and adjust aim accordingly
- low ICP:
  ○ lower the head of the bed (HOB) (reverse Trendelenburg)
  ○ gently compress the veins of the neck for no more than 1 minute
- try irrigating no more than 1–2 cc of preservative-free saline into the IVC and see if it comes back out. This can work for
  ○ plugging of the IVC with blood or debris or "air lock"
  ○ collapsed or near-collapsed ventricles

Removal

Patients receiving anticoagulants need to have normal coagulation and platelet function before discontinuing the catheter to reduce the risk of intracranial hemorrhage. For heparin and LMW heparin stop the drug 24 hours prior to discontinuing the drain.

"Sump drainage"

The tip of a 25 gauge butterfly may be bent at a 90° angle, and inserted into a subcutaneous reservoir for (e.g., a ventricular access device (p. 1831), or the reservoir of a shunt with a *distal* occlusion) prolonged ventricular drainage.[61] In one series of 34 patients, this was used for prolonged periods (up to 44 days) with acceptably low infection rate.[62] The use of a one-way valve, continuous antibiotic (ampicillin and cloxacillin), and meticulous technique was credited for the lack of infection.

110.7 CSF diversionary procedures

110.7.1 Ventricular shunts

Booking the case: Ventricular shunt

Also see defaults & disclaimers (p. 25).
1. position: supine with shoulder roll
2. implants: need to specify shunt manufacturer and valve type (e.g., programmable, low-profile...)
   Uncommon components (e.g., ultra-low pressure, tumor filter) may need special order
3. equipment:
   a) C-arm for ventriculo-atrial shunts
   b) endoscopic display (e.g., if NeuroPen is used)
   c) image-guided navigation system (infrequently used)
4. consent (in lay terms for the patient—not all-inclusive):
   a) procedure: surgery to insert a permanent drainage tube from the brain to the abdomen, out-side of the lungs, vein near the heart (as appropriate) to drain excess cerebrospinal fluid
   b) alternatives: nonsurgical management (rarely effective for hydrocephalus), third ventriculos-tomy (for certain cases)
   c) complications: infection, suboptimal position which might require reoperation, failure to relieve hydrocephalus/symptoms, subdural hematoma, bleeding in the brain, shunts are mechanical devices and will eventually fail (break, block up, move...) and need repair/replace-ment (sometimes sooner rather than later). Abdominal shunts: risk of bowel injury (which could require further surgery)

Ventricular catheter

Kocher's point is currently used in most cases for insertion site of ventricular catheter; see Ventricu-lar catheterization (p. 1820) for technique. An alternative is an occipital burr hole aiming toward the frontal horn of the lateral ventricle.

An inverted "J"-shaped incision is used to keep hardware from lying directly under the skin inci-sion (minimizes risk of skin breakdown and also creates additional barrier to infection of subjacent hardware). CSF should be sent for culture at the time of insertion since it has been estimated that in ≈ 3% of patients the CSF is already infected. 4 mg of preservative-free gentamicin may be instilled into the ventricular catheter by the technique of barbotage (a technique to administer a drug while reducing the amount of drug lost in the dead space of the catheter: a portion of the antibiotic solu-tion is injected into the CSF, then a lesser amount of CSF is aspirated, a second portion is then injected and the process is repeated until all of the medication is administered).

If you think the catheter is in the ventricle, but you don't get CSF flow, it may be due to low pres-sure; you can compress the jugular veins or lower the head of the bed to try and induce CSF flow.

Connectors

If a connector must be used near the clavicle, place it rostral to (above) the clavicle. ✖ Avoid placing it caudal to the clavicle because this increases the risk of disconnection.

Distal catheter placement options

All things being equal, the general order of preference for distal catheter placement:
1. peritoneal cavity: intrinsic pressure ≈ 6–7 cm H_2O. See below
2. pleural space (p. 454): not for age ≤7 years (approximate). For technique, see below
3. right atrium or superior vena cava (p. 1828): intrinsic pressure ≈ 4–5 cm H_2O
4. infrequently used ("salvage" techniques) distal shunt sites
   a) gallbladder (p. 1828): intrinsic pressure ≈ 10–20 cm H_2O
   b) internal jugular vein (with the catheter pointing "upstream")
   c) superior sagittal sinus
   d) urinary bladder
   e) stomach (ventriculogastric shunt)

Peritoneal catheter placement

General information
Used for ventriculoperitoneal shunts, lumboperitoneal shunts...

For small children, use at least 30 cm length of intraperitoneal tubing to allow for continued growth (120 cm total length of peritoneal tubing was associated with a lower revision rate for growth without significant increase in other complications[63]). A silver clip is placed at the point where the catheter enters the peritoneum so that the amount of residual intraperitoneal catheter can be determined on later films (more important in growing children).

Distal slits on the peritoneal catheter may increase the risk of distal obstruction,[64] and some authors recommend that they be trimmed off. Wire-reinforced catheters should not be used because of excessively high rate of viscus perforation, and this tubing was designed to prevent kinking which is not a problem with modern shunts.

Open technique
A vertical incision lateral and superior to the umbilicus is one of several choices. The following layers should be identified as they are traversed to avoid confusing preperitoneal fat with omentum and erroneously placing the tip in the preperitoneal space:
1. subcutaneous fat
2. anterior sheath of the abdominis rectus muscle (anterior rectus sheath)
3. abdominis rectus muscle fibers: should be split longitudinally
4. posterior rectus sheath
5. preperitoneal fat (may be very well developed in a few individuals, but is essentially nonexistent in most)
6. peritoneum (usually closely adherent to the posterior rectus sheath)

Trocar technique
A trocar (e.g., Codman #82-4095 disposable split trocar (▶ Fig. 110.4), which is designed to place catheters with outer diameters up to 3.0 mm) may be used. Also very helpful in conjunction with laparascopic surgery.

✖ Contraindications: prior abdominal surgery, extremely overweight patients.
Technique:
1. place a Foley catheter to decompress the bladder prior to draping
2. 1 cm skin incision above and lateral to the umbilicus
3. tent-up the abdominal skin anteriorly (away from patient)
4. insert trocar with plastic stylet in place aiming toward the ipsilateral iliac crest
5. feel 2 "pops" of penetration: 1st = anterior rectus sheath, 2nd = posterior rectus sheath/peritoneum
6. remove the plastic stylet
7. feed the catheter through the central channel of the trocar. The peritoneal catheter should feed easily through trocar (if it doesn't, the tip of the trocar may be in the preperitoneal space, or pushing up against an organ, adhesion, etc.). You can check if a small amount of irrigation fluid runs into the peritoneum through the trocar (if not, placement may not be serviceable)
8. once the peritoneal catheter is in position, it is stabilized with bayonet pickups as the split trocar is withdrawn allowing the catheter to slide through the split opening in its side so that the catheter remains in place

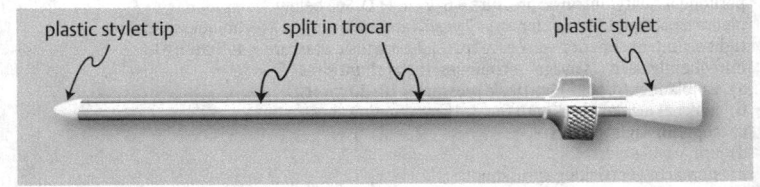

plastic stylet tip   split in trocar   plastic stylet

Fig. 110.4 Codman disposable split trocar.

VP shunt, post-op orders (adult)

1. flat in bed (to avoid overshunting and possible subdural hematoma) with gradual mobilization
2. if peritoneal end is new or revised, do not feed until bowel sounds resume (usually at least 24 hrs, due to ileus from manipulation of peritoneum)
3. shunt series (AP & lateral skull, and chest/abdominal X-ray) as baseline for future comparison (some surgeons obtain these films immediately post-op in case some immediate revision is indicated, e.g., ventricular catheter tip in temporal horn)

Pleural catheter placement

For ventriculopleural shunts, syringopleural shunts… see reference.[65] See also more details (p.454). In addition to the open technique described below, a trocar method (using the same trocar used for peritoneal catheters, ▶ Fig. 110.4) for introducing the pleural catheter has been described.[66]

✖ Use under advisement in age ≤ 7 years[67] due to reduced surface area for resorption of CSF which may result in high pleural fluid levels.

A 3 cm horizontal incision is made just below the level of the breast either in the midclavicular line or in the anterior axillary line. Divide the subcutaneous tissue, deep fascia, and pectoralis muscle. The external and internal intercostal muscles are divided along the *superior* margin of the inferior of the two ribs exposed (to avoid the neurovascular bundle running along the inferior margin of each rib). A self-retaining retractor between the ribs aids the exposure. The parietal pleura is visualized with the visceral pleura sliding underneath with each respiration. The pleura is not opened until the catheter is brought out subcutaneously at this incision. Have the anesthesiologist hold respirations, and nick the parietal pleura (or use a blunt-tip hemostat to pop through) to admit the catheter. Allow the lung to drop away and insert 20–40 cm of tubing into the pleural cavity. If the pleural opening is lax around the catheter, it can be snugged with a 4–0 absorbable suture. Have the anesthesiologist provide a Valsalva maneuver before cinching down the pleural suture, and again before closing the deep muscle layer. A chest tube is usually not required. A maneuver that may sometimes be helpful is to place a red-rubber catheter next to the shunt tube at the same time (to permit the escape of air from the pleural space). Begin closing, but prior to placing the last deep suture, have the anesthesiologist perform a Valsalva maneuver and allow air to escape through the red-rubber catheter (you can place the end in saline to see the bubbles). Once the bubbles stop, pull the red-rubber catheter and close the last stitch. If the bubbles don't stop, there is an air leak in the visceral pleura and a pigtail catheter or a chest tube connected to a Pleur-evac® should be used.

Right atrial catheter placement

General information

For ventriculo-atrial shunt…

Open method

The common facial vein (CFV) is located by making a diagonal cervical incision across the anterior border of the sternocleidomastoid at or just below the level of the angle of the mandible (the CFV may be as far as ≈ 2 cm below this point). The platysma is divided, and the CFV is located as it joins the internal jugular vein (IJV) at the level of the hyoid bone. The CFV is cannulated with the atrial tubing, and is secured with a snug ligature close to the junction with the IJV. If the CFV is not suitable, a purse-string suture is placed directly in the IJV, and the IJV is then opened in the center of the purse string and cannulated.

Percutaneous method

May be utilized in adults (and possibly peds). The IJV is catheterized using the Seldinger technique[68] with a guide-wire and needle through a stab incision at the anterior margin of the SCM. Fluoroscopy is used to place the tip of the wire at the desired location (see below). A No. 13 French peel-away introducer and dilator are then inserted over the wire, which is then bent at the skin edge and withdrawn[69] (for a pediatric case: may use a No. 7 French introducer with a 1.5 mm O.D. *lumboperitoneal* catheter for the distal atrial catheter). The atrial catheter is cut to the length of the wire distal to the bend, and the catheter is then threaded into the introducer. The position of the catheter tip should again be confirmed (e.g., with radio-opaque contrast under fluoroscopy). A short skin incision is then made starting at the point where the catheter penetrates the skin to permit subcutaneous tunneling of the tubing.

Location of distal tip

If the catheter repeatedly goes down the wrong vessel (e.g., the subclavian vein), a "J" guidewire may help. Also, rotating the head to a more neutral position sometimes works.

The ideal location of the distal tip is in the right atrium (unlike the location for central catheters in the superior vena cava (SVC)) so that the turbulent blood flow will reduce the risk of thrombus formation. The tip may enter the right atrium, but must not penetrate the tricuspid valve. A number of methods for optimal placement of the distal shunt tip may be employed, and include:

1. using an intraoperative chest X-ray to locate the tip between the level of T6–8 vertebra in an adult. In a growing child, initially insert to ≈ T10 level. This method is subject to error due to malalignment of the X-ray beam (parallax error)
2. place the tip near the level described above, then inject iodinated contrast, e.g., 20 ml of Omnipaque 180 (iohexol) (p. 230) under intraoperative fluoroscopy to locate the tip in right atrium
3. fill the catheter with normal or 3% saline and use the catheter as an EKG electrode. The P-wave changes from a downward to a biphasic morphology as the tip enters the atrium. A sharp upward deflection occurs as the tricuspid valve is approached.[70] Some recommend advancing the tip to maximal P-wave amplitude and then backing off a centimeter or two
4. fill the catheter with heparinized saline (1–5 U per cc NS) and measure the pressure as the tip is advanced,[71] leave tip just short of where atrial pressure tracing occurs
5. utilizing intraoperative echocardiography[72]

A growing patient is followed with annual CXRs. When the catheter tip is above ≈ T4, the catheter must be lengthened or converted to a VP shunt.

Gallbladder

Uncommonly used distal site. First described in 1958, there have been a number of publications,[73,74] with a 63% success rate in one series.[74] Relevant physiology[75]:

- gallbladder capacity: 30–60 cc. Can absorb up to 1500 cc of liquid per day
- pressure: resting internal pressure is 10–20 cm H_2O, which may counteract siphon effect of CSF. Post-prandial elevation of ICP up to 24 cm H_2O in children with ventriculogallbladder (VGB) shunts has been reported[76]
- bile: lytic properties increase protein breakdown and may prevent adhesions. Normally sterile, but it has been purported that ≈ 50% of patients > 50 years of age have unsterile bile

Classically inserted via open laparotomy through the dome of the gallbladder using a purse-string suture to attain water-tight closure, which often necessitates using a metal connector inserted in the shunt tubing to prevent constriction.

Challenges:

1. contraindications:
   - prior gallbladder disease or procedures
   - gallstones
2. technical difficulties: optimal purse-string placement and tension
3. risks:
   - leakage of bile into abdomen due to disconnection or laxity in purse-string
   - occlusion of shunt tubing by too tight of a purse-string
   - resultant cholelithiasis
4. placement in young children may result in catheter pull-out of gallbladder as child grows

A novel option has been described of percutaneous ultrasound-guided placement of an 8-French pigtail catheter into the gallbladder through the liver (transhepatic) – which is commonly done by interventional radiologists to drain bile or treat cholangitis – and connecting this to the ventricular catheter. This is less invasive, and decreases the risk of bile leakage, and if the catheter occludes, the tubing may be removed percutaneously without need for a laparotomy (which entails a 3% risk of major bile leak, and 3% risk of minor bile leak[77]). Risk of percutaneous technique is 1.7% risk of minor bleeding and 0.4% risk of major bleeding.

110.7.2 Third ventriculostomy

General information

See also indications and complications (p. 453).

Older techniques include a subfrontal approach, opening the chiasmatic and lamina terminalis cisterns, and making a 5–10 mm opening in the lamina terminalis. Stereotactic third ventriculostomy (using contrast ventriculography[78] or CT-guided) has also been described. Current technique, endoscopic third ventriculostomy (ETV), often with assistance of image guidance, consists of fenestrating the floor of the third ventricle using a ventriculoscope.

Ventriculoscopic technique (endoscopic third ventriculostomy (ETV))

1. equipment: requires a rigid endoscope (does not work well with flexible)
2. image-guided stereotactic technology helps immensely with the trajectory, but once you've entered the third ventricle, you must navigate by visual landmarks and cannot rely on image guidance because of the limitations of the accuracy
3. burr hole: 2–3 cm lateral to the midline just anterior to the coronal suture (Kocher's point)
4. pass through the foramen of Monro and fixate the sheath just within the third ventricle
5. the floor of the third ventricle is inspected and must be thin enough and translucent enough to permit visualization of the basilar artery and mammillary bodies. If these structures cannot be visualized then the procedure should be aborted
6. the location of the opening is chosen:
   a) in the midline (avoids PComA and PCA)
   b) in the region of the tuber cinereum (prominence of the base of the hypothalamus, extending ventrally into the infundibulum and pituitary stalk)
   c) posterior to the infundibular recess
   d) anterior to the mammillary bodies
   e) anterior to the tip of the basilar artery
7. an effective technique consists of "rubbing through" the floor of the third ventricle either with a probe or Decq forceps. Alternatively, hydrodissection or bipolar electrocautery may be used to thin down the lamina. ✖ Do not use laser due to possibility of injury to basilar artery![79]
8. the opening can be enlarged with the Decq forceps, or a 3 French Fogarty balloon or a double balloon (Fogarty or Neuroballoon™ catheter (Integra LifeSciences 7CBD10)). The balloon is inflated distal to the opening in the floor and is then withdrawn through the opening
9. the opening does not need to be large (unlike e.g., fenestrating an arachnoid cyst): ≈ 4–5 mm is usually adequate[80,81]
10. after penetrating through the floor of the third ventricle, make certain that you can see vessels (sometimes the arachnoid is not perforated, or there is a second membrane or webs of membranes that need to be lysed)
11. consider injection of diluted iohexol or other intrathecal contrast agent into the lateral/third ventricle (see ventriculogram) prior to removal of scope. CT of head 1 hour after surgery will show diffuse subarachnoid contrast in cisterns and over convexity if ETV successful
12. sagittal T2 weighted, thin-slice sequence will show drop-out of T2 signal at stoma of ETV

110

10.7.3 LP shunt placement

General information

Often placed without a mechanical valve (relies on the slits in the distal cather ("slit valves") and the narrow inner diameter of the lumbar drain tubing to limit flow rate).
Commercially available systems include:
- Integra Spetzler™ Lumbar Peritoneal Shunt Kit, a one-piece straight tube with slit valves on the peritoneal end. (NB: catheter length is only 80 cm, which may not be long enough for a morbidly obese adult. If more length is desired, a conventional peritoneal catheter can be connected to a lumbar drain using a step-down connector, as found in Edwards-Barbaro shunt kit (p. 1410)). If it is desired to inject contrast or to aspirate CSF to assess LP shunt patency post-op, one may optionally insert a Spetzler™ Lumbar Peritoneal Flushing Reservoir, a valveless reservoir (inlet and outlet tubing 0.7 mm inner diameter and 1.5 mm outer diameter). Separate in-line miter valves (low, medium, or high pressure) may optionally be inserted for added resistance.
- Medtronic Lumboperitoneal Shunt Kit, #44420 contains a specialized programmable Strata® NSC valve with small-diameter connectors on the inlet and outlet ports, which accommodates the smaller lumbar catheter and the *specialized* small inner-diameter peritoneal/pleural catheter contained in the kit (both catheters are 0.7 mm ID, the distal catheter is 120 cm long). The valve has a tappable reservoir as well as inlet and outlet occluders.

Insertion technique

See reference.[82]
1. position: lateral decubitus position, both knees flexed (right-side-up preferred)
2. prep back, flank, and abdomen
3. 1 cm skin incision over L4–5 or L5–1 (in obese patients, use larger skin incision carried down to fascia overlying spinous processes. This may also be superficially incised between spinous processes to aid insertion)
4. tilt table to 30° reverse-Trendelenburg to expand lumbar subarachnoid space
5. insert the 14 gauge Tuohy needle into subarachnoid space. When passing the needle, some surgeons orient it so that the opening in the needle tip is pointing laterally or medially in order that the tip penetrates the dura in line with the longitudinally running dural fibers. The needle is then rotated so that the opening is directed rostrally (caudal placement is also acceptable). Confirm there is CSF flow
6. remove the stylet, insert shunt tubing. For L4–5 insertion, insert a total of ≈ 17 cm of catheter into the needle. This will accommodate withdrawal of 9 cm when removing the needle, leaving about 8 cm within the canal, which minimizes conus medullaris irritation. The Spetzler one-piece shunt has 4 black tantalum-impregnated length markers: when the first marker is at the needle hub, the tip of the catheter is at the tip of the needle. The next 3 markers are at 5 cm intervals.
   NB: the catheter pliability varies among manufacturers. Some are too flaccid to push through the Tuohy needle; for these, inserting the provided guidewire helps, but can be challenging itself. To facilitate guidewire placement, first wet the catheter and guidewire and pass the wire into the catheter while holding the catheter so that it is dangling vertically, such that the guidewire goes straight down into the catheter
7. ✖ never pull the catheter out through the needle—the catheter is prone to shear off on the angulated tip of the Tuohy needle
8. the Tuohy needle is then withdrawn until the tip of the needle comes out of the tissue (the standard Tuohy needle is 9 cm long), usually accompanied by the 9 cm of catheter inside the needle. Once the needle tip is visible, pinch the catheter there to hold it against further withdrawal and continue to remove the needle over the catheter
9. make a flank incision, pass a tunneler from the flank to the back incision. Pass the catheter from the back to the flank through the tunneler. Withdraw the tunneler, leaving the catheter
10. abdominal placement:
    a) open: incision made through peritoneum. Place purse-string in peritoneal opening
    b) trocar method (p. 1826)
11. pass tunneler from abdominal incision to flank incision. Feed catheter from flank to abdomen. Withdraw tunneler over catheter
12. verify CSF flow. Place the catheter inside the peritoneum. For open technique: cinch and tie a purse-string snugly, but loose enough to allow the catheter to slide with gentle pushing
13. a snug-fitting retaining sleeve is placed around the catheter at all three incisions, and secured to subcutaneous tissue with non-absorbable suture

Insertion of programmable valve: in severely obese patients the valve will tend to twist within the subcutaneous tissue, which may make programming difficult or impossible. Some pointers regarding valve placement:
1. the valve must be fairly close to the surface of the skin to allow the programming magnet to work (Medtronic recommends ≤ 1 cm of thickness of tissue overlying the Strata NSC valve)
2. a technique to stabilize the valve is to use a linear skin the length of the valve with a dog-leg bend at both ends to allow the skin and a small amount of sub-Q tissue to be opened like a door. The valve is sutured *upside down* in all 4 corners to the underside of this flap so that when the flap is closed, the valve will be right-side-up under the skin
3. placing the valve over a rib (superficial to a rib, not directly on the rib) may provide some additional stability

Lumboperitoneal (LP) shunt evaluation

When problems develop, evaluation of function may be more difficult than with VP shunt. Evaluation may include:
1. abdominal X-rays: AP & lateral X-rays can rule out breakage or migration of a shunt component
2. noncontrast brain CT scan: can rule out complication such as subdural hematoma
3. LP: perform LP just above or below level of lumbar catheter. The pressure may be 0 or negative, and it may be necessary to aspirate CSF to confirm placement

a) can give indirect evidence of shunt function by measuring the CSF pressure, which should be low if the shunt is working (only helpful in cases where the shunt was placed for elevated CSF pressure, e.g., pseudotumor cerebri; not helpful in NPH)

b) "shunt-o-gram": inject contrast into subarachnoid space through LP needle
  • radionuclide (p. 459): inject radio-isotope via LP and look for subsequent tracer activity in peritoneal cavity
  • with water-soluble contrast[83]: inject 10 ml of iohexol and monitor the flow of contrast fluoroscopically as the patient is brought vertical. Coughing or Valsalva maneuver will accelerate the flow of contrast

4. shunt tap: if an antechamber has been installed, it is accessed after cleaning the skin with antiseptic using a 22 Ga or smaller needle placed perpendicular to the dome to prevent leakage. If there is no access chamber, it is sometimes possible to tap the tubing itself with a 27 gauge butterfly needle

110.8 Ventricular access device

110.8.1 General information

An indwelling ventricular catheter connected to a reservoir that is positioned under the scalp for the purpose of chronic access to the intrathecal space (usually the ventricular system), or sometimes other intracranial compartments such as tumor cysts. Sometimes referred to generically as an Ommaya® reservoir; however, this is actually a trade name.

110.8.2 Indications

1. administration of intrathecal (IT) antineoplastic chemotherapy:
   a) for CNS neoplasms, including: carcinomatous meningitis, methotrexate for CNS lymphoma or leukemia (p. 844)
   b) IT chemotherapy is often used for the following even in the absence of CNS involvement because of the high relapse rate in the CNS: acute lymphoblastic leukemia, lymphoblastic lymphoma, Burkitt's lymphoma
2. administration of intrathecal antibiotic for chronic meningitis
3. chronic removal of CSF from infants with intraventricular hemorrhage
4. for fluid aspiration from a chronic tumor cyst that is resistant to therapy (radiation or surgery)[84]

110

Booking the case: Ventricular access device

Also see defaults & disclaimers (p. 25).
1. position: supine
2. equipment
   a) endoscopic display (e.g., if NeuroPen is used)
   b) C-arm (optional) to verify position of ventricular catheter
   c) image-guided navigation system (if used)
3. implants: need to specify reservoir manufacturer
4. consent (in lay terms for the patient—not all-inclusive):
   a) procedure: surgery to insert a tube into the fluid space within the brain (ventricle) which is connected to a port under the skin so that fluids can be removed or injected (usually medication)
   b) alternatives: sometimes fluid can be removed and medication can be injected using a lumbar puncture (spinal tap). The effectiveness of this may not be the same as the operation being discussed here
   c) complications: infection, suboptimal position which might require reoperation, subdural hematoma, bleeding in the brain, this is a mechanical device and may eventually fail (break, block up...) and need repair/replacement

110.8.3 Technique of insertion

See reference.[85]

Preferably placed in the right frontal region, unless indicated otherwise (e.g., for tumor cyst). Usually placed under endotracheal general anesthesia, although local anesthesia occasionally may be used (e.g., for patients too ill to tolerate general anesthesia).

Patient position: supine, head midline, neck flexed 5°.

Incision: inverted "U," slightly larger than the reservoir (the original Ommaya® reservoir is 3.4 cm diameter), with the center over the coronal suture approximately 3 cm from midline, roughly centered near Kocher's point (p. 1821). A circle of pericranium of diameter equal to that of the reservoir is excised and saved. Alternatively, the pericranium may be flapped separately in the opposite direction (i.e., a right-side-up "U"), and closed over the reservoir to help secure it in position.

Make a burr hole over the coronal suture 3 cm off midline. A cruciate incision in the dura is made large enough to visualize the cortical surface, minimal cortical bipolar coagulation is used, and a pial/cortical incision is made to avoid surface vessels.

One may inject 15–20 cc of filtered air into the ventricles with a ventricular needle prior to the catheter insertion to guide the tip of the catheter with intraoperative lateral skull X-rays (intraoperative pneumoencephalogram). Alternatively, image guidance may be used with the same tracking systems that may be used for ventricular shunts. The trajectory is towards a point intersecting a plane 2 cm anterior to the EAM aiming minimally towards the midline (1–2°). Alternatively, one may aim perpendicular to the surface of the skull.[56] A total length of ≈ 7.25 cm of catheter is fixed to the base of the reservoir, which allows the catheter to lie on the floor of the anterior horn of the lateral ventricle in most adults. This location can be verified with intraoperative pneumoencephalography[8] or with ventriculoscopic techniques.

The excised pericranium is placed over the dura, and the reservoir is sutured to the pericranium. Note: the dome of the original Ommaya® reservoir has a low resistance, and may be easily collapsed if too much tension is placed on the overlying scalp. If early use of the reservoir is desired (i.e., within 48 hrs post-op), the skin closure should be performed with a running nonabsorbable suture (e.g., nylon) and coated with cyanoacrylate skin adhesive, and the surgical site can then be left without gauze dressing for easier access to the reservoir. A skin tattoo can be created over the center of the reservoir (to assist in localizing the reservoir for injection) using India ink and pricking the skin with a sterile needle.

110.8.4 Reservoir puncture

The scalp is prepped with antimicrobial scrub, and using sterile technique, a 25 gauge or smaller butterfly needle is introduced at an oblique angle, preferably with a non-coring needle. The original (Ommaya®) reservoir has firm plastic bottom surface which can be penetrated with the needle if too much force is applied.

110.9 Sural nerve biopsy

110.9.1 Indications & contraindications

Nerve biopsy plays an ever diminishing role in diagnosing peripheral neuropathies, to a significant degree as a result of increased sophistication of molecular biologic testing. In general, the yield of nerve biopsy is higher in cases of severe demyelinating, distal asymmetric, and multifocal neuropathy than in chronic, axonal, and symmetric types.[86,87]

Nerve biopsy should not be performed if a diagnosis and etiology can be established by less invasive tests, which may include: clinical exam, electrodiagnostics (NCV & EMG), blood tests, CSF analysis, or skin biopsy for quantitative epidermal nerve fiber density.

Indications (only class IV evidence was found[86]):
1. major indications: most helpful in
   • vasculitis (non-systemic vasculitic neuropathy)
   • diabetic neuropathy when superimposed chronic inflammatory demyelinating polyneuropathy (p. 195) (CIDP)[86] is suspected
2. minor indications (see reference for more extensive list[86])
   • infection: e.g., Hansen disease, HIV
   • may help distinguish between the two types of Charcot-Marie-Tooth syndrome (p. 568)
   • select hereditary neuropathies with negative appropriate genetic tests[87]
   • may show demyelination in diabetic amyotrophy (p. 572)

Contraindications:
• absolute contraindication: infection or skin breakdown at the biopsy site
• relative contraindications: situations where yield of the test is low

- the nerve is normal clinically and on nerve conduction testing with no abnormality on MRI or ultrasonography (an exception to this may be when there is a strong suspicion of vasculitis with predominantly motor features and asymmetric involvement)[87]
- evaluation of small-fiber neuropathy is rarely an indication for nerve biopsy. Skin biopsy can be done in this situation for quantification of intradermal nerve fiber density; and the test can be repeated in follow-up
- paraproteinemic neuropathies: IgM deposits in the nerve may predate serum IgM gammopathy
- if thorough and optimal nerve processing cannot be performed: in addition to fixed and frozen sections, the lab should be able to evaluate teased fibers, electron microscopy, and immunohistochemistry

110.9.2 Selection of nerve to be biopsied

Although a number of peripheral nerves may be biopsied, the sural nerve fulfills the criteria of being well studied, expendable with minimal deficit, easily accessible, and often involved in the pathologic process in question. However, being exclusively a sensory nerve, it would usually not be an appropriate choice for purely motor neuropathy.

Alternatively, the superficial peroneal nerve may be appropriate in select cases if a simultaneous muscle biopsy is indicated as the peroneus brevis is convenient.[87]

110.9.3 Risks of procedure

1. sensory loss in the sural nerve distribution (lateral foot) is expected, often does not persist for more than several weeks (unless the underlying disease process prevents recovery)
2. pain and paresthesias: tend to recover more than sensory loss
3. problems with wound healing: the ankle is a notorious region for poor circulation and the loss of sensation (from the disease or biopsy) may render the area subject to repeated trauma without the patient being aware. Furthermore, many patients with an undiagnosed systemic disease requiring a sural nerve biopsy will have poor wound healing (a significant number are also diabetic)
4. failure to make a diagnosis: although biopsy may be able to exclude some contingencies, it often does not make a specific diagnosis

110.9.4 Applied anatomy

The sural nerve is formed by the merging of the distal portion of the medial sural cutaneous nerve (one of the terminal branches of the tibial nerve) and the anastomotic ramus of the common peroneal nerve. It is entirely sensory except for some unmyelinated autonomic fibers. It supplies cutaneous sensation to the posterolateral third of the leg, the lateral heel and foot, and the little toe. At the level of the ankle it lies between the Achilles tendon and the lateral malleolus. This location is constant, superficial, and relatively protected from external trauma which might otherwise confuse the analysis.

110.9.5 Technique

Modified technique.[88(p 771-2)] Usually done under local anesthesia with sedation. Side to biopsy: if one leg shows more involvement, that is often the preferred side.

Position: under general anesththesia, patient prone. If patient is not under general anesthesia, use 3/4 oblique position (not prone) with a pillow between the legs. The leg to be biopsied is uppermost and is flexed 90° at the knee to relax tension on the nerve, the ankle is slightly everted. Compressing the calf (can be done using a sterile Penrose drain as a temporary tourniquet during surgery) distends the lesser saphenous vein (LSV) at the lateral malleolus (LM), which (when visible) reliably locates the sural nerve usually deep and anterior to the vein.

After prepping, drape the limb with a sterile stockinette or similar drape, infiltrate local anesthetic subcutaneously just posterior to the LM and proximally, paralleling the Achilles tendon for ≈ 10 cm. A 7–10 cm incision is made overlying the course of the LSV beginning usually just posterior to and ≈ 1 cm proximal to the LM. The vein can be seen through the translucent Scarpa's fascia. The fascia is incised over the vein, which is gently retracted to reveal the nerve, usually deep to the vein. A common pitfall is to go too deep, but the nerve is fairly superficial; it is not necessary to go through the thick fascia. If at any time you see tendons to the toes, you have gone too deep.

To differentiate the sural nerve from the LSV (which may resemble the nerve in some cases): the nerve has many branches at acute angles, especially proximal to the LM, vs. the vein which has

110

right-angle branches. If in doubt, a frozen section may be helpful to verify that the biopsied structure is a nerve in order to avoid potentially embarrassing explanations and the possible need to repeat the procedure.

After exposing at least 3–5 cm of the nerve, anesthetize the proximal portion with 0.5% lidocaine using a 27 Ga needle and cut it sharply just distal to the infiltration site. Cut the nerve with slight tension on it to allow the ends to retract deep to the skin incision to prevent the formation of a scar neuroma. Some pathologists request that the proximal end of the nerve be marked, e.g., with a suture.

Although a full thickness nerve biopsy is most common, a fascicular biopsy (partial nerve biopsy) may be performed to minimize the sensory deficit (NB: if the disease is patchy, the chances of a positive biopsy is decreased) by opening the epineurium for the length of the exposure and teasing out a fascicle with minimal branching.

If it is desired to obtain a biopsy of the sural nerve higher up for comparison, it may be accessed in the mid-upper calf between the heads of the gastrocnemius muscle. Here it may be as deep as ≈ 2 cm. Gently tugging on the exposed nerve in the ankle may help in localization.

A dissolvable subcuticular closure may be used. Generous padding should be placed over the incision to protect it from bumps (since many patients are numb from the pathology and/or surgery, there is increased risk of inadvertently traumatizing the wound). An elastic pressure dressing is applied after closure.

110.9.6 Nerve handling

For light microscopy, which suffices in most cases, immerse the nerve in formalin. For electron microscopy, glutaraldehyde is used. For biochemical and immunofluorescence studies, use rapid freezing.

110.9.7 Post-op care

Pressure dressing should be worn for protection for two weeks. The patient is allowed to walk but should restrict their activity for 2–3 days. If nonabsorbable sutures are used instead of subcuticular closure, they should be left in place 10–14 days.

110.10 Nerve blocks

Also see Occipital nerve block (p. 542).

110.10.1 Stellate ganglion block

General information

✖ Do not perform stellate ganglion block bilaterally (can cause bilateral laryngeal paralysis → respiratory compromise). The stellate ganglion is actually closer to C7 than C6, but risks at C7 are much higher (closer to pleura → pneumothorax, vertebral artery → arterial injection → seizures and/or hematoma, recurrent laryngeal nerve → unilateral vocal cord paralysis → hoarseness (common), brachial plexus → UE weakness). Other complications: intradural injection → spinal anesthesia, phrenic nerve block.

Technique

Position: patient supine with an interscapular roll, head tilted backward, mouth slightly open to relax the strap muscles.

Displace the SCM and carotid sheath laterally, and insert a 1.5 inch 22 Ga needle to contact Chassaignac's tubercle (anterior tubercle of transverse process of C6) AKA carotid tubercle (the most prominent in the C-spine), usually at the level of the cricoid cartilage, approximately 1.5–2 inches above clavicle.

Withdraw the needle 1–2 mm and aspirate to avoid intravascular injection. Inject small test dose, then full 10 ml of 0.5% bupivacaine (Marcaine®) or 20 ml of 1% lidocaine. Remove needle and elevate patient's head on pillow to facilitate spread.

Verify block by Horner syndrome, and anhidrosis and increased warmth of ipsilateral hand.

110.10.2 Lumbar sympathetic block

Technique

Patient prone on fluoro table. Use local anesthetic to allow insertion of 20–22 gauge spinal needles (10 to 12.5 cm long) at L2, L3, and L4 levels. Needle inserted 4.5–5 cm lateral to spinous process until transverse process contacted, then redirected caudally and inserted to a depth 3.5–4 cm deeper than transverse process. Final needle tip position should be just anterolateral to vertebral bodies. At each level, instill ≈ 8 ml of 1% lidocaine local after verifying that nothing can be aspirated.

Keep patient on bed rest for several hours, then ambulate with assist; watch for orthostatic hypotension due to vascular pooling in blocked lower extremity.

110.10.3 Intercostal nerve block

Indications

1. postthoracotomy pain
2. intercostal neuralgia
3. postherpetic neuralgia
4. pain from rib fractures

General principles

In order to obtain good anesthesia, the following should be noted:
1. a good site for injection is in the *posterior axillary line* (PAL) because
   a) this is proximal to the origin of the lateral cutaneous nerve (which originates ≈ in the anterior axillary line)
   b) this avoids the scapula for nerves above ≈ T7
   c) this reduces the risk of pneumothorax from injecting closer to the spine (the latter requires a longer needle path and there is increased difficulty palpating landmarks)
2. due to overlap, at least 3 intercostal nerves usually need to be blocked to achieve at least some area of anesthesia; it is usually necessary to block 1–2 intercostal nerves both above and below the affected dermatome
3. the intercostal nerves lie on the undersurface of the corresponding rib in close proximity to the pleura; the order of structures from top down is: rib, vein, artery, nerve

Technique

1. after raising a skin wheal at the desired level in the PAL, insert a 22 Ga or smaller needle directly against the rib
2. walk the needle down the rib millimeter by millimeter until the needle just slips under the rib; to avoid pleural puncture, do not advance the needle more than one-eighth inch deep to the anterior surface of the rib
3. aspirate to be certain that there is no air (from lung penetration) or blood (from entering the intercostal artery or vein)
4. if no air or blood returns, inject 3–5 ml of local anesthetic
5. if there is any question about lung penetration, obtain a portable CXR to R/O pneumothorax

110.11 Multistranded cable for spine fusion

Multistranded cable (usually titanium alloy or stainless steel) has replaced twisted wire and has itself been largely supplanted by rigid immobilization (spinal screws/rods) for internal immobilization of the spine. There are still some situations where cable has a role (most commonly in the cervical spine) usully supplementing rigid immobilization, such as C1–2 lateral mass fusion (p.1780). Systems include Medtronic ATLAS™ cable (formerly Songer cable), Synthes cable system.

ATLAS™ cable system: maximal cable tension for titanium alloy cables is 30 lbs, for stainless steel it is 60 lbs (these maximums are for the cables; actual tension depends on the quality of the bone).

References

[1] Navarro IM, Renteria JAG, Peralta VHR, et al. Transorbital Ventricular Puncture for Emergency Ventricular Decompression. J Neurosurg. 1981; 54:273–274

[2] Brem SS, Hafler DA, Van Uitert RL, et al. Spinal Subarachnoid Hematoma: A Hazard of Lumbar Puncture Resulting in Reversible Paraplegia. N Engl J Med. 1981; 303:1020–1021

[3] Hollis PH, Malis LI, Zappulla RA. Neurological Deterioration After Lumbar Puncture Below Complete Spinal Subarachnoid Block. J Neurosurg. 1986; 64:253–256

[4] Reimann AE, Anson BJ. Vertebral Level of Termination of the Spinal Cord with a Report of a Case of Sacral Cord. Anat Rec. 1944; 88

[5] Antoni N. Pressure Curves from the Cerebrospinal Fluid. Acta Medica Scandinavica. Supplementum. 1946; 170:439–462

[6] Bono F, Lupo MR, Serra P, et al. Obesity does not induce abnormal CSF pressure in subjects with normal cerebral MR venography. Neurology. 2002; 59:1641–1643

[7] Adams RD, Victor M. Principles of Neurology. 2nd ed. New York: McGraw-Hill; 1981

[8] Howard SC, Gajjar AJ, Cheng C, et al. Risk factors for traumatic and bloody lumbar puncture in children with acute lymphoblastic leukemia. JAMA. 2002; 288:2001–2007

[9] Shah KH, Edlow JA. Distinguishing traumatic lumbar puncture from true subarachnoid hemorrhage. J Emerg Med. 2002; 23:67–74

[10] Fishman RA. Cerebrospinal Fluid in Diseases of the Nervous System. Philadelphia: W. B. Saunders; 1980

[11] Bonita R, Thomson S. Subarachnoid hemorrhage: epidemiology, diagnosis, management, and outcome. Stroke. 1985; 16:591–594

[12] Perry JJ, Stiell IG, Sivilotti ML, et al. Sensitivity of computed tomography performed within six hours of onset of headache for diagnosis of subarachnoid haemorrhage: prospective cohort study. BMJ. 2011; 343. DOI: 10.1136/bmj.d4277

[13] Gorchynski J, Oman J, Newton T. Interpretation of traumatic lumbar punctures in the setting of possible subarachnoid hemorrhage: who can be safely discharged? Cal J Emerg Med. 2007; 8:3–7

[14] Rinkel GJE, van Gijn J, Wijdicks EFM. Subarachnoid Hemorrhage Without Detectable Aneurysm: A Review of the Causes. Stroke. 1993; 24:1403–1409

[15] Wiesel J, Rose DN, Silver AL, et al. Lumbar Puncture in Asymptomatic Late Syphilis. An Analysis of the Benefits and Risks. Archives of Internal Medicine. 1985; 145:465–468

[16] Fishman RA. Cerebrospinal Fluid in Diseases of the Nervous System. Philadelphia: W. B. Saunders; 1992

[17] Sathi S, Stieg PE. "Acquired" Chiari I Malformation After Multiple Lumbar Punctures: Case Report. Neurosurgery. 1993; 32:306–309

[18] Stern WE. Localization and Diagnosis of Spinal Cord Tumors. Clin Neurosurg. 1977; 25:480–494

[19] DeSousa AL, Kalsbeck JE, Mealey J, et al. Intraspinal Tumors in Children. A Review of 81 Cases. J Neurosurg. 1979; 51:437–445

[20] McDonald JV, Klump TE. Intraspinal Epidermoid Tumors Caused by Lumbar Puncture. Arch Neurol. 1986; 43:936–939

[21] Pavlin J, McDonald JS, Child B, et al. Acute Subdural Hematoma: An Unusual Sequela to Lumbar Puncture. Anesthesiology. 1979; 52:338–340

[22] Rudehill A, Gordon E, Rahu T. Subdural Hematoma: A Rare but Life Threatening Complication After Spinal Anesthesia. Acta Anaesthesiol Scand. 1983; 17:376–377

[23] Sundberg A, Wang LP, Fog J. Influence of hearing of 22 G Whitacre and 22 G Quincke needles. Anaesthesia. 1992; 47:981–983

[24] Michel O, Brusis T. Hearing Loss as a Sequel of Lumbar Puncture. Ann Otol Rhinol Laryngol. 1992; 101:390–394

[25] Kestenbaum A. Clinical Methods of Neuroophthalmologic Examination. 2nd ed. New York: Grune and Stratton; 1961

[26] Wilder-Smith E, Kothbauer-Margreiter I, Lämmle B, et al. Dural Puncture and Activated protein C Resistance: Risk Factors for Cerebral Venous Sinus Thrombosis. Journal of Neurology, Neurosurgery, and Psychiatry. 1997; 63:351–356

[27] Glimaker M, Johansson B, Grindborg O, et al. Adult bacterial meningitis: earlier treatment and improved outcome following guideline revision promoting prompt lumbar puncture. Clin Infect Dis. 2015; 60:1162–1169

[28] Duffy GP. Lumbar Puncture in the Presence of Raised Intracranial Pressure. Brit Med J. 1969; 1:407–409

[29] Korein J, Cravioto H, Leicach M. Reevaluation of Lumbar Puncture: A Study of 129 Patients with Papilledema or Intracranial Hypertension. Neurology. 1959; 9:290–297

[30] van de Beek D, de Gans J, Spanjaard L, et al. Clinical features and prognostic factors in adults with bacterial meningitis. N Engl J Med. 2004; 351:1849–1859

[31] Mokri B. Orthostatic headaches in the syndrome of the trephined: resolution following cranioplasty. Headache. 2010; 50:1206–1211

[32] DiGiovanni AJ, Dunbar BS. Epidural Injections of Autologous Blood for Postlumbar-Puncture Headache. Anesth and Analg. 1970; 49:268–271

[33] Seebacher J, Ribeiro V, Le Guillou JL, et al. Epidural Blood Patch in the Treatment of Post Dural Puncture Headache: A Double Blind Study. Headache. 1989; 29:630–632

[34] Lance JW, Branch GB. Persistent Headache After Lumbar Puncture. Lancet. 1994; 343

[35] Gass H, Goldstein AS, Ruskin R, et al. Chronic Postmyelogram Headache. Arch Neurol. 1971; 25:168–170

[36] Evans RW, Armon MD, Frohman MHS, et al. Assessment: prevention of post-lumbar puncture headaches: report of the therapeutics and technology assessment subcommittee of the American Academy of Neurology. Neurology. 2000; 55:909–914

[37] Tourtellotte WW, Henderson WG, Tucker RP, et al. A Randomized, Double Blind Clinical Trial Comparing the 22 Versus 26 Gauge Needle in the Production of the Post-Lumbar Puncture Syndrome in Normal Individuals. Headache. 1972; 12:73–78

[38] Mihic DN. Postspinal Headache and Relationship of Needle Bevel to Longitudinal Dural Fibres. Reg Anesth. 1985; 10:76–81

[39] Kuntz KM, Kokmen E, Stevens JC, et al. Post-Lumbar Puncture Headaches: Experience in 501 Consecutive Procedures. Neurology. 1992; 42

[40] Carson D, Serpell M. Choosing the Best Needle for Diagnostic Lumbar Puncture. Neurology. 1996; 47:33–37

[41] Hilton-Jones D, Harrad RA, Gill MW, et al. Failure of Postural Maneuvers to Prevent Lumbar Puncture Headache. J Neurol Neurosurg Psychiatry. 1982; 45:743–746

[42] Carbaat PAT, van Crevel H. Lumbar Puncture Headache: Controlled Study on the Preventive Effect of 24 Hours Bed Rest. Lancet. 1981; 1:1133–1135

[43] Sechzer PH, Abel L. Post-Spinal Anesthesia Headache Treated with Caffeine: Evaluation with Demand Method. Part 1. Cur Ther Res. 1978; 24:307–312

[44] Murros K, Fogelholm R. Spontaneous Intracranial Hypotension with Slit Ventricles. Journal of Neurology, Neurosurgery, and Psychiatry. 1983; 46:1149–1151

[45] Wynn MM, Mell MW, Tefera G, et al. Complications of spinal fluid drainage in thoracoabdominal aortic aneurysm repair: a report of 486 patients treated from 1987 to 2008. J Vasc Surg. 2009; 49:29–34 discussion 34–5

[46] Zivin JA. Lateral Cervical Puncture: An Alternative to Lumbar Puncture. Neurology. 1978; 28:616–618

110

[47] Penning L. Normal Movements of the Cervical Spine. AJR. 1978; 130:317–326

[48] Section of Pediatric Neurosurgery of the American Association of Neurological Surgeons. Pediatric Neurosurgery. New York 1982

[49] Rogers LA. Acute Subdural Hematoma and Death Following Lateral Cervical Spinal Puncture. J Neurosurg. 1983; 58:284–286

[50] Ward E, Orrison WW, Watridge CB. Anatomic Evaluation of Cisternal Puncture. Neurosurgery. 1989; 25:412–415

[51] Bauer DF, Razdan SN, Bartolucci AA, et al. Meta-analysis of hemorrhagic complications from ventriculostomy placement by neurosurgeons. Neurosurgery. 2011; 69:255–260

[52] Davis JW, Davis IC, Bennink LD, et al. Placement of intracranial pressure monitors: are "normal" coagulation parameters necessary? J Trauma. 2004; 57:1173–1177

[53] Bauer DF, McGwin G,Jr, Melton SM, et al. The relationship between INR and development of hemorrhage with placement of ventriculostomy. J Trauma. 2011; 70:1112–1117

[54] Le TV, Rumbak MJ, Liu SS, et al. Insertion of intracranial pressure monitors in fulminant hepatic failure patients: early experience using recombinant factor VII. Neurosurgery. 2010; 66:455–8; discussion 458

[55] Tillmanns H. Something about puncture of the brain. Sheffield, England 1908

[56] Ghajar JBG. A Guide for Ventricular Catheter Placement: Technical Note. J Neurosurg. 1985; 63:985–986

[57] Schmidek HH, Sweet WH. Operative Neurosurgical Techniques. New York 1982

[58] Becker DP, Nulsen FE. Control of Hydrocephalus by Valve-Regulated Venous Shunt: Avoidance of Complications in Prolonged Shunt Maintenance. J Neurosurg. 1968; 28:215–226

[59] Keskil SI, Ceviker N, Baykaner K, et al. Index for Optimum Ventricular Catheter Length: Technical Note. J Neurosurg. 1991; 75:152–153

[60] Fried HI, Nathan BR, Rowe AS, et al. The Insertion and Management of External Ventricular Drains: An Evidence-Based Consensus Statement : A Statement for Healthcare Professionals from the Neurocritical Care Society. Neurocrit Care. 2016; 24:61–81

[61] Mann KS, Yue CP, Ong GB. Percutaneous Sump Drainage: A Palliation for Oft-Recurring Intracranial Cystic Lesions. Surg Neurol. 1983; 19:86–90

[62] Chan KH, Mann KS. Prolonged Therapeutic External Ventricular Drainage: A Prospective Study. Neurosurgery. 1988; 23:436–438

[63] Couldwell WT, LeMay DR, McComb JG. Experience with Use of Extended Length Peritoneal Shunt Catheters. Journal of Neurosurgery. 1996; 85:425–427

[64] Cozzens JW, Chandler JP. Increased Risk of Distal Ventriculoperitoneal Shunt Obstruction Associated With Slit Valves or Distal Slits in the Peritoneal Catheter. Journal of Neurosurgery. 1997; 87:682–686

[65] McComb JG, Scott RM. Techniques for CSF Diversion. In: Hydrocephalus. Baltimore: Williams and Wilkins; 1990:47–65

[66] Richardson MD, Handler MH. Minimally invasive technique for insertion of ventriculopleural shunt catheters. J Neurosurg Pediatr. 2013; 12:501–504

[67] Venes JL, Shaw RK. Ventriculopleural shunting in the management of hydrocephalus. Childs Brain. 1979; 5:45–50

[68] Seldinger SI. Catheter replacement of the needle in percutaneous arteriography. A new technique. Acta Radiol. 1953; 39:368–376

[69] Harrison MJ, Welling BG, DuBois JJ. A new method for inserting the atrial end of a ventriculoatrial shunt. Technical note. Journal of Neurosurgery. 1996; 84:705–707

[70] Robertson JT, Schick RW, Morgan F, et al. Accurate Placement of Ventriculo-Atrial Shunt for Hydrocephalus under Electrocardiographic Control. Journal of Neurosurgery. 1961; 18:255–257

[71] Cantu RC, Mark VH, Austen WG. Accurate Placement of the Distal End of a Ventriculo-Atrial Shunt Catheter Using Vascular Pressure Changes. Journal of Neurosurgery. 1967; 27:584–596

[72] Szczerbicki MR, Michalak M. Echocardiograhic Placement of Cardiac Tube in Ventriculoatrial Shunt. Technical Note. Journal of Neurosurgery. 1996; 85:723–724

[73] Ketoff JA, Klein RL, Maukkassa KF. Ventricular cholecystic shunts in children. J Pediatr Surg. 1997; 32:181–183

[74] Girotti ME, Singh RR, Rodgers BM. The ventriculo-gallbladder shunt in the treatment of refractory hydrocephalus: a review of the current literature. Am Surg. 2009; 75:734–737

[75] Hasslacher-Arellano J F, Arellano-Aguilar G, Funes-Rodriguez J F, et al. [Ventriculo-gallbladder shunt: An alternative for the treatment of hydrocephalus]. Cir Cir. 2016; 84:225–229

[76] Frim DM, Lathrop D, Chwals WJ. Intraventricular pressure dynamics in ventriculocholecystic shunting: a telemetric study. Pediatr Neurosurg. 2001; 34:73–76

[77] Wise JN, Gervais DA, Akman A, et al. Percutaneous cholecystostomy catheter removal and incidence of clinically significant bile leaks: a clinical approach to catheter management. AJR Am J Roentgenol. 2005; 184:1647–1651

[78] Hoffman HJ. Technical Problems in Shunts. Monogr Neural Sci. 1982; 8:158–169

[79] McLaughlin MR, Wahlig JB, Kaufmann AM, et al. Traumatic Basilar Aneurysm After Endoscopic Third Ventriculostomy: Case Report. Neurosurgery. 1997; 41:1400–1404

[80] Grant JA, McLone DG. Third ventriculostomy: a review. Surg Neurol. 1997; 47:210–212

[81] Jones RF, Stening WA, Brydon M. Endoscopic third ventriculostomy. Neurosurgery. 1990; 26:86–91; discussion 91-2

[82] Spetzler R, Wilson CB, Schulte R. Simplified Percutaneous Lumboperitoneal Shunting. Surg Neurol. 1977; 7:25–29

[83] Ishiwata Y, Yamashita T, Ide K, et al. A new technique for percutaneous study of lumboperitoneal shunt patency. Journal of Neurosurgery. 1988; 68:152–154

[84] Rogers LR, Barnett G. Percutaneous aspiration of brain tumor cysts via the Ommaya reservoir system. Neurology. 1991; 41:279–282

[85] Leavens ME, Aldama-Luebert A. Ommaya Reservoir Placement: Technical Note. Neurosurgery. 1979; 5:264–266

[86] Sommer CL, Brandner S, Dyck PJ, et al. Peripheral Nerve Society Guideline on processing and evaluation of nerve biopsies. J Peripher Nerv Syst. 2010; 15:164–175

[87] Mellgren SI, Lindal S. Nerve biopsy-some comments on procedures and indications. Acta Neurol Scand Suppl. 2011; 124:64–70

[88] Dyck PJ, Thomas PK. Peripheral Neuropathy. 2nd ed. Philadelphia: W. B. Saunders; 1984

110

111 Functional Neurosurgery and Stereotactic Neurosurgery

111.1 Introduction

Functional neurosurgery (FN) involves the use of electrical stimulation, ablative therapy, or therapeutic infusions to mask or relieve symptoms of aberrant neurophysiology. Functional procedures may be performed in the brain, spinal cord, or on cranial or peripheral nerves and may be used in the treatment of:
1. movement disorders
2. neurovascular compression syndromes
3. autonomic dysfunction
4. psychiatric disease
5. pain (p.518)
6. epilepsy (p.1889)

Deep brain techniques (lesioning or stimulation) rely on stereotactic methods discussed below.

111.2 Stereotactic surgery

111.2.1 General information

The techniques of stereotactic surgery are utilized in some functional procedures (e.g., DBS) as well as for biopsies, cyst drainage, etc. The term stereotactic (Greek: stereo = 3-dimensional, tactic = to touch) surgery was initially used in animals, and was based on atlases of three-dimensional coordinates compiled from dissections. The term was then used for surgery performed in humans, usually for thalamic lesioning to treat parkinsonism (see Surgical treatment of Parkinson's disease (p.1840)) where the target site to be lesioned was located relative to landmarks with intraoperative pneumoencephalography or contrast ventriculography. Use of this procedure fell off dramatically in the late 1960s with the introduction of L-dopa for parkinsonism.[1]

Current techniques would be more appropriately termed *image-guided* stereotactic surgery. In the first part of the procedure, a CT scan or MRI (or occasionally, angiogram) is performed. For increased precision, "fiducial" markers or a stereotactic frame is attached to the patient's head during this image acquisition phase. Acceptable accuracy for biopsies can often be obtained using high resolution thin-cut imaging slices (usually with a 0 angle of the gantry), and then surface-matching algorithms in the guidance system will match the pre-op CT/MRI to the patient's head. This is not accurate enough for lesion generation or electrode placement.

The second part of the procedure usually takes place in an operating room. The patient is "registered" with the pre-op images, and then tracking cameras follow the movement of instruments with appropriate attachments to show in "real-time" the location of the instrument with respect to the pre-op image. An important limitation to be aware of is the fact that the pre-op images are "historical" and are not updated as the surgical procedure alters the anatomy of the patient. Even the administration of mannitol can cause brain shifts that may cause the target of the surgery to move away from its pre-op location by several millimeters.[2]

111.2.2 Indications for stereotactic surgery

1. biopsy (also, see below)
   a) deeply located cerebral lesions: especially near eloquent brain
   b) brainstem lesions: may be approached through the cerebral hemisphere[3]
   c) multiple small lesions (p.357) (e.g., in some AIDS patients)
   d) patient medically unable to tolerate general anesthesia for open biopsy
2. catheter placement
   a) drainage of deep lesions: colloid cyst, abscess
   b) indwelling catheter placement for intratumoral chemotherapy
   c) radioactive implants for interstitial radiation brachytherapy[4]
   d) shunt placement: for hydrocephalus (rarely used) or to drain cyst
3. electrode placement
   a) depth electrodes for epilepsy
   b) "deep brain stimulation" for chronic pain (requires electrophysiologic stimulation)

4. lesion generation
   a) movement disorders: parkinsonism (p. 1841), dystonia, hemiballismus
   b) treatment of chronic pain
   c) treatment of epilepsy (rarely used)
5. evacuation of intracerebral hemorrhage
   a) using an Archimedes' screw device[5,6]
   b) with adjunctive urokinase[7,8] or recombinant tissue-plasminogen activator (p. 1626) [9]
6. stereotactic "radiosurgery"—see Stereotactic radiosurgery & radiotherapy (p. 1902)
7. to localize a lesion for open craniotomy (e.g., AVM,[10] deep tumor)
   a) using a ventricular-type catheter
   b) using a blunt biopsy needle or introducer[11]
   c) systems using visible light laser beam for guidance
8. transoral biopsy of C2 (axis) vertebral body lesions[12]
9. "experimental" or unconventional applications
   a) stereotactic clipping of aneurysms[13]
   b) stereotactic laser surgery
   c) CNS transplantation[14]: e.g., for parkinsonism (p. 184)
   d) foreign body removal[15]

111.2.3 Stereotactic biopsy

General information

This section presents information regarding stereotactic brain biopsy (SBB) in general. For SBB in specific conditions, see the index entry for that condition. Biopsy may be through a small "cookie cutter" craniotomy, or through a smaller burr hole with a needle. Although it may be performed under local or general anesthesia, it is more commonly done under general.

Contraindications

1. coagulation disorders
   a) coagulopathies: bleeding diatheses, iatrogenic (heparin or coumadin)
   b) low platelet count (PC): PC < 50,000/ml is an absolute contraindication, it is desirable to get the PC ≥ 100,000
2. inability to tolerate general anesthesia and to cooperate for local anesthesia

Yield

The yield rate (i.e., the ability to make a diagnosis from an SBB) reported in large series in the literature ranges from 82–99% in nonimmunocompromised (NIC) patients, and is slightly lower in AIDS patients at 56–96%. Higher yield rates in AIDS may result from improved surgical technique and histologic evaluation.[16]

The yield rate is higher for lesions that enhance with contrast on CT or MRI (99% in NIC patients) than with lesions that do not enhance (74%).[17]

Complications

The most frequent complication is hemorrhage, although most are too small to have clinical impact. The risk of a major complication (mostly due to hemorrhage) in NIC patients ranges from 0–3% (with most < 1%), and 0–12% in AIDS.[17] Higher complication rates seen in AIDS patients in some series may be due to reduced platelet count or function, and to vessel fragility in primary CNS lymphoma. In NIC patients, multifocal high-grade gliomas had the highest complication rate.

Infection is an infrequent complication with needle biopsy.

111.3 Deep brain stimulation

111.3.1 General information

Deep brain stimulation (DBS): the use of electical stimulation through surgically implanted electrodes to produce neuromodulation of electrical signals for the purpose of symptom improvement. For many indications, DBS has supplanted ablative procedures in the brain. A variety of conditions may be treated including:

111

1. movement disorders
   a) Parkinson's disease: STN stimulation may be superior to best medical management[18,19] because of similar efficacy to levodopa with fewer side effects (primarily dyskinesias) (see below)
   b) dystonia (p. 1842)
   c) tremor (p. 1841)
2. epilepsy (p. 1891)
3. pain (p. 1886): response is variable, typically only 25–60% respond
4. potential uses
   a) psychiatric disorders (p. 1841): mainly
      - Tourette syndrome (p. 1842): GPi, STN, ALIC
      - obsessive-compulsive disorders (p. 1842): anterior capsule and STN stimulation[20] and, recently, targets more posterior & rostral[21]
      - depression (p. 1842): subgenual cingulate gyrus[22] and anterior capsule stimulation[23]
   b) obesity[24]
   c) drug addiction[25]
   d) hypertension (case report of lowering BP in a patient treated for pain[26])

111.3.2 Surgical treatment of Parkinson's disease

Historical background

Prior to the availability of effective medications, surgical procedures were developed to treat Parkinson's disease (PD). An early procedure was ligation of the anterior choroidal artery. Due to variability in distribution, destruction often extended beyond the desired confines of the pallidum and the results were too unpredictable (p. 1539). Anterodorsal pallidotomy became an accepted procedure in the 1950's, but long-term improvement was mainly in rigidity, while tremor and bradykinesia did not improve.[27] The ventrolateral thalamus subsequently became the preferred target. Lesions there were most effective in diminishing tremor. In actuality, the tremor was often not the most debilitating symptom, particularly since it is a resting tremor at first (it may become more pervasive later). Bradykinesia and rigidity were frequently more problematic for the patient. Furthermore, the procedure only reduces tremor in the contralateral half of the body, and bilateral thalamotomies were not recommended due to an unacceptably high risk of post-op dysarthria and gait disturbance. Use of thalamotomy fell off dramatically in the late 1960's with the introduction of L-dopa.[1]

Current trends

At some point most patients will experience problematic side effects and/or resistance to treatment with antiparkinsonian drugs. This, together with recent refinements in surgical techniques resulting in improved outcomes, has produced a resurgence of interest in the operative treatment of Parkinson's disease. Tissue transplantation (e.g., with adrenal medullary tissue) has been all but abandoned in the U.S.

Since 1987, a shift has taken place from lesioning to stimulation techniques. The subthalamic nucleus (STN) was an early target in PD. Deep brain stimulation (DBS) in the area of the globus pallidus pars interna (GPi)[28] or the ventral intermediate nucleus of the thalamus (Vim) can also relieve parkinsonian symptoms[29] without irreversibly destroying tissue. A randomized study showed similar efficacy between thalamotomy and DBS, but fewer side effects with DBS.[30]

Indications for surgical treatment of PD

1. patients refractory to medical therapy (including multiple agents). However, some investigators feel the response to surgery might be better if done early
2. primary indication (based on an opinion survey[31]): patients with levodopa-induced dyskinesias (especially those with associated painful muscle spasms). Initial results indicate that these are very responsive to pallidotomy
3. gait and postural instability[32] as well as falls and freezing (non-human primate data)[33] may respond to DBS of the pedunculopontine nucleus (PPN)
4. patients primarily with rigidity or bradykinesia (unilateral or bilateral), on-off fluctuations, or dystonia. Tremor may be present, but if it is the predominant symptom, then using the ventralis intermedius (VIM) nucleus of the thalamus as the target (for ablation (thalamotomy) or stimulation)[34] is a better procedure. VIM stimulation is also used to treat essential tremor[35]

Contraindications

1. patients with significant dementia: further cognitive impairment has been noted primarily in patients with cognitive deficits prior to treatment
2. patients with risk of intracerebral hemorrhage: those with coagulopathy, poorly controlled hypertension, those on anti-platelet drugs that cannot be withheld (may consider stereotactic radiosurgery lesions for these rare patients, see below)
3. patients with ipsilateral hemianopsia: due to the risk of post-op contralateral hemianopsia from optic tract injury, which would make the patient blind
4. age ≥ 85 yrs
5. patients with secondary parkinsonism (p. 185), i.e., *not* idiopathic Parkinson's disease: respond poorly, presumably due to different pathophysiology. Look for:
   a) signs of autonomic nervous system dysfunction (suggests Shy-Drager)
   b) EOM abnormalities (may occur in progressive supranuclear palsy (PSNP))
   c) long-tract signs
   d) cerebellar findings (as in olivo-ponto-cerebellar atrophy (OPCA))
   e) failure to improve with levodopa
   f) MRI: lacunar infarcts in basal ganglia (as in arteriosclerotic parkinsonism), or tumor in region of substantia nigra
   g) PET scanning (if available): decreased striatal metabolism detected by deoxyglucose PET scan (suggests striato-nigral degeneration (SND))
6. patients with normal dopamine transport (DaT) scan which may rule out PD as the cause of a tremor

Results

At present, the major focus of therapy has been on improvement of motor symptoms. Although 97% of patients showed at least some improvement (some poor results may derive from inclusion of some patients with secondary parkinsonism), in 17% the degree of improvement was graded as mild.

Significant reduction of levodopa-induced dyskinesias occurred in 90%. Bradykinesia improved in 85%, rigidity in 75%, and tremor in 57%. Other areas of improvement include: speech, gait, posture, and reduction of on-off phenomenon and freezing. Although symptoms may be ameliorated, overall functional improvement may not be remarkable.[36]

Although dosages of antiparkinsonian medication are often reduced, continued medical therapy is usually required, and no change is made for at least 2 months.

Indications are that beneficial surgical effects can last ≥ 5 years, with early failures possibly due to production of too small of a lesion, and late failures possibly due to progression of the disease.

Ongoing studies are investigating longer-term results, microelectrode recording, alternate lesioning targets, the role of early surgery... Until more information is available, one cannot make any statements about the optimal target, localizing method, etc.

111.3.3 Tremor

Tremor is the most common movement disorder (intention > postural > resting), with essential tremor affecting 5–10 million persons in the U.S. Thalamic stimulation may be useful for tremors that are refractory to medical treatment, including tremor-dominant Parkinson's disease, essential tremor,[37,38] cerebellar and posttraumatic tremor.[34]

Prior to being considered for surgical intervention, it should be determined that the patient has failed maximal medical therapy.

Side effects of Vim stimulation include: paresthesias, H/A, dysequilibrium, dysarthria, dystonia, and localized pain.

111.3.4 Psychiatric disorders

General principles/disorders

Surgical treatment of psychiatric disorders has a long and storied history. The first documented surgeries aimed at treating psychiatric disease occurred in the late 1800's. Psychosurgery fell out of favor due to negative public perception, the advent of effective anti-psychotic medications, and skepticism regarding surgical outcomes.

111

Most current applications of functional neurosurgery in psychiatric disease remain investigational. Several ongoing trials have shown promising preliminary results for severe refractive obsessive-compulsive disorder (OCD),[39] depression,[40] & Tourette syndrome[41] (see below).

Tourette syndrome (TS)

A disorder characterized by random, repeated, and stereotyped motor or vocal tics for > 1 year,[42] usually in several "bouts" per day. Onset is before age 18 years (mean age: 5 years). Male:female ratio is 4:1. The tics may be socially unappropriate, as such, are disabling. TS is often associated with OCD, ADHD, and other personality disorders.

Medical therapy has focused on blocking dopamine receptors, central adrenergic receptors, or on catecholamine-depleting agents.[43]

Surgical targets for TS have included the frontal lobes, the cingulate gyrus, the anterior limb of the internal capsule (ALIC), the limbic system, and the subthalamic zona incerta.[44] Current targets of interest for DBS include: GPi, STN, ALIC, and thalamus. Early results have been promising.[45]

Obsessive-compulsive disorder (OCD)

A debilitating psychiatric disorder characterized by anxiety-provoking intrusive thoughts (obsessions) that lead to stereotyped motor, cognitive acts, or rituals that are performed (compulsions) to relieve the associated anxiety.[46] Affects up to 2% of the population, and is the 10th leading cause of disability worldwide.[47,48] 12–20% of cases remain refractory to standard behavioral psychotherapy and medical treatment with serotonin reuptake inhibitors (SSRI) or atypical antipsychotics.[49]

DBS targets explored for OCD include the anterior limb of the internal capsule (ALIC), nucleus accumbens (NAc), ventral capsule/ventral striatum (VC/VS), subthalamic nucleus (STN), and inferior thalamic peduncle (ITP).[50,51] The FDA recently granted a humanitarian device exemption approving the use of VC/VS DBS for medically intractable OCD.

Major depressive disorder (MDD)

Major depressive disorder (MDD) is the fifth leading cause of non-fatal disability worldwide.[52] First-line treatment includes pharmacotherapy, psychotherapy, and forms of non-invasive brain stimulation such as transcranial magnetic stimulation and electroconvulsive therapy. Patients who fail conservative therapy may be candidates for functional neuromodulatory procedures.

Initial attempts at surgical treatment for chronic depression or MDD included nonspecific destructive surgeries such as the prefrontal leucotomy (lobotomy). After these procedures fell out of favor, more selective ablative procedures targeting the orbitofrontal cortex and the medial prefrontal cortex were attempted. Recently, DBS targets investigated for treatment of medically intractable depression include: the subcallosal cingulate gyrus, inferior thalamic peduncle, nucleus accumbens, and ventral capsule/striatum.[53,54,55] Several of these targets gained interest after patients undergoing DBS for OCD noted improved mood as a side effect.[56] Vagus nerve stimulation (VNS) has also been explored as an option after patients receiving VNS for seizures were noted to have improvement in depressive symptoms independent of seizure control.[57]

111.3.5 Dystonia

Pallidal stimulation is the primary surgical treatment for dystonia.[58] Response is better for primary dystonias, e.g., tardive dystonias than for secondary dystonias such as postanoxic, postencephalitic perinatal, and poststroke dystonias[58] (other targets need to be assessed).

For primary dystonias, the globus pallidus internus (GPi) is the most common primary target (▶ Fig. 111.1). Good results have also been reported with STN DBS. Dyskinetic cerebral palsy in children may also be treated with pallidal stimulation.[59]

111.3.6 Deep brain stimulation technique

Overview

1. medications (anti-tremor or anti-parkinsonian depending on the condition being treated) are withheld the morning of the procedure to bring out symptoms
2. a stereotactic frame is applied under local anesthetic parallel to the orbitomeatal line (which aligns somewhat with the AC-PC line (p. 58))

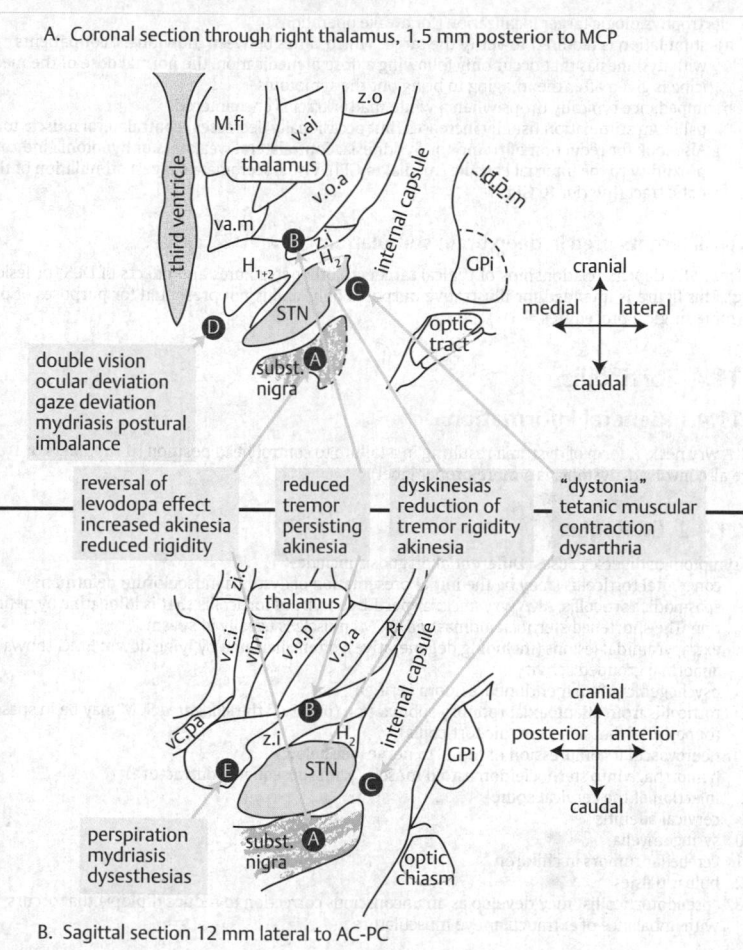

A. Coronal section through right thalamus, 1.5 mm posterior to MCP

double vision
ocular deviation
gaze deviation
mydriasis postural
imbalance

reversal of
levodopa effect
increased akinesia
reduced rigidity

reduced
tremor
persisting
akinesia

dyskinesias
reduction of
tremor rigidity
akinesia

"dystonia"
tetanic muscular
contraction
dysarthria

perspiration
mydriasis
dysesthesias

B. Sagittal section 12 mm lateral to AC-PC

Fig. 111.1 Illustration of some targets for functional brain surgery. Abbreviations: AC = anterior commissure; GPi = globus pallidus interna; H_1 = Forel's H_1 field; MCP = midcommissural point (halfway between AC & PC); PC = posterior commissure; STN = subthalamic nucleus; subst. nigra = substantia nigra; z.i = zona incerta.

3. radiologic target localization: (depends on the condition being treated)
   a) may utilize MRI or CT. MRI is the most common imaging modality, and may best demonstrate the desired anatomy, but is susceptible to geometric distortion. Therefore many centers also utilize CT to supplement MRI. T1WI images are commonly employed; however, some feel that optimal MRI imaging may be performed with gadolinium-enhanced axial and coronal projections using 1-mm slice intervals and an STIR or gradient echo acquisition protocol
   b) identify the AC-PC line on imaging
4. for some situations (e.g., GPi or STN targets for Parkinson's disease), there is a choice between awake and asleep placement of DBS electrodes, and the results appear fairly equivalent.[60] For some conditions, the patient must be awake to assess the response to stimulation

5. electrophysiologic target localization (for awake operations)
   a) stimulation is required to verify the target which varies between individuals. For patients with dyskinesias that occur only following a dose of medication, the normal dose of the medicine is given after the imaging to bring out the symptoms
   b) impedance typically drops when a white matter tract is encountered
   c) pallidum stimulation usually increases (but occasionally decreases) contralateral muscle tone. Also look for reduction of tremor or dyskinesia. Contralateral weakness or hypotonia indicates proximity to the internal capsule (medial to GPi). Visual scotomata suggest stimulation of the optic tract (inferior to GPi)

Typical targets used in deep brain stimulation

▶ Fig. 111.1 depicts relationships of typical targets to other structures and effects of DBS (or lesioning). This figure is intended for illustrative purposes only, and is not presented for purposes of performing surgical procedures.

111.4 Torticollis

111.4.1 General information

AKA wry neck. A form of dystonia resulting in a failure to control head position (if shoulders or trunk are also involved, dystonia is a more proper label).

111.4.2 Etiologies

A symptom of diverse causes. Differential diagnosis includes:
1. congenital torticollis (may be the initial presentation of dystonia musculorum deformans)
2. spasmodic torticollis, AKA wry neck: a specific subtype of torticollis that is idiopathic by definition. The shortened sternocleidomastoid (SCM) muscle is usually in spasm
3. extrapyramidal lesions (including degenerative): often alleviated by lying down; EMG shows abnormal grouped activity
4. psychogenic (often mentioned, seldom verified)
5. torticollis from atlantoaxial rotatory subluxation (p. 1158): the *elongated* SCM may be in spasm (opposite of that in spasmodic torticollis)
6. neurovascular compression of the 11th nerve (see below)
7. hemorrhage into sternocleidomastoid muscle (with subsequent contracture)
8. infection of the cervical spine
9. cervical adenitis
10. syringomyelia
11. cerebellar tumors in children
12. bulbar palsies
13. "pseudotorticollis" may develop as an unconscious correction to reduce diplopia that occurs with imbalance of extraocular eye musculature

111.4.3 Non-surgical treatment of torticollis

Should be attempted first, and includes:
1. relaxation training, including biofeedback
2. thorough neuropsychiatric evaluation
3. trans-epidermal neuro-stimulation (TENS) to the neck

111.4.4 Surgical procedures

Reserved for disabling, refractory cases. Includes:
1. dorsal cord stimulation
2. local injection of botulinum toxin: may work for retrocollis, is poor for lateral torticollis (must inject posterior cervicals and both SCM, and may cause temporary pharyngeal muscle dysfunction resulting in dysphagia), and is totally ineffective for anterocollis
3. selective rhizotomy and spinal accessory nerve section

111.4.5 Torticollis of 11th nerve origin

1. usually a horizontal type (manifests as horizontal head movement) which may be exacerbated when supine (unlike extrapyramidal torticollis)
2. contraction of SCM is usually accompanied by activity in contralateral agonist muscles
3. may be treated surgically. Procedures include
   a) sectioning of the anastomotic branches between the 11th nerve and the upper cervical posterior root (C1 anastomotic branch is sensory only)
   b) microvascular decompression of the 11th nerve (most cases caused by vertebral artery, but PICA compression is also described[61]). Relief takes several weeks post-op

111.5 Spasticity

111.5.1 General information

Spasticity results from lesions in upper motor neuron pathways, causing absence of inhibitory influence on alpha motor neurons (αMN) (alpha spasticity) as well as on gamma motor neurons (intrafusal fibers) (gamma spasticity). Result: uninhibited reflex arc between αMN and Ia afferents from muscle spindles, resulting in a hypertonic state of muscles with clonus, and sometimes with involuntary movements. Etiologies include: injury to cerebrum (e.g., stroke) or spinal cord (spasticity is an expected sequela of spinal cord injury rostral to the conus medullaris), multiple sclerosis, and congenital abnormalities (e.g., cerebral palsy, spinal dysraphism).

111.5.2 Clinical

General information

Increased resistance to passive movement, hyperactive muscle stretch reflexes, simultaneous activation of antagonistic muscle groups, may occur spontaneously or in response to minimal stimuli. Characteristic postures include scissoring of legs or hyperflexion of thighs. May be painful, or may disrupt patient's ability to sit in wheelchair, lie in bed, drive modified vehicles, sleep, etc. May also promote development of decubitus ulcers. A spastic bladder will have low capacity and will empty spontaneously.

Spasticity is often exacerbated by same type of stimuli that aggravate autonomic hyperreflexia; see Autonomic hyperreflexia (p.1222).

The onset of spasticity following spinal cord injury may be delayed for several days to months; the latency period is attributed to "spinal shock" (p.1119), during which time there is decreased tone and reflexes).[62] Onset of spasticity following spinal shock starts with increasing flexor synergistic activity over 3–6 mos, with more gradual increases of extensor synergy which ultimately predominates in most cases.

Some "beneficial" aspects of mild spasticity:
• maintains muscle tone and therefore bulk: provides support for patient when sitting in wheelchair, helps prevent decubitus ulcers over bony prominences
• muscle contractions may help prevent DVTs
• may be useful in bracing

Grading spasticity

The Ashworth scale (▶ Table 111.1) is commonly used for the clinical grading of the *severity* of spasticity. Assessment should be performed with patient supine and relaxed. Many attempts have been made to quantitate spasticity electrodiagnostically, the most reliable has been H-reflex measurement.

Table 111.1 Ashworth scores[63]

Ashworth score	Degree of muscle tone
1	no increase in tone (normal)
2	slight increase, a "catch" with flexion or extension
3	more marked increase, passive movements easy
4	considerable increase, passive movements difficult
5	affected part rigid in flexion or extension

111

111.5.3 Treatment

General information

Depends on extent of useful function (or potential for same) present in areas at and below the level where spasticity starts (complete spinal cord injuries usually have little function, whereas patients with MS may have significant function).

Non-surgical treatment of spasticity

1. "prevention": measures to decrease inciting stimuli (physical therapy to prevent joint damage, good skin & bladder care... see Autonomic hyperreflexia (p. 1222))
2. prolonged stretching (more than just range of motion): not only prevents joint and muscle contractures, but modulates spasticity
3. oral medications[64]; (see Surgical treatment (p. 1846) for intrathecal medications): few drugs are effective without significant undesirable side effects
   a) *diazepam* (Valium®): activates GABA-A receptors, increases presynaptic inhibition of αMN. Most useful in patients with complete spinal cord injuries.
      ℞ start with 2 mg PO BID-TID, increase by 2 mg per day q 3 days up to a max of 20 mg TID.
      Side effects: may cause sedation, weakness, decreased stamina (most of which may be minimized by gradual increases in dosage). Abrupt discontinuation may cause depression, seizures, withdrawal syndrome
   b) *baclofen* (Lioresal®): a GABA derivative that activates presynaptic GABA-B receptors of Ia muscle spindle afferents, causes presynaptic inhibition of αMN and decreases nociception. May be most useful in patients with spinal cord lesions (complete or incomplete).
      ℞ start with 5 mg PO BID-TID, increase in 5 mg increments q 3 days up to max of 20 mg QID.
      Side effects: sedation, lowers seizure threshold. Must be tapered to discontinue (abrupt discontinuation may result in seizures, rebound hyper-spasticity or hallucinations)
   c) *dantrolene* (Dantrium®): reduces depolarization induced Ca^{++} influx into sarcoplasmic reticulum of skeletal muscle; acts on all skeletal muscle (with no preferential effect on spasmogenic reflex arc).
      ℞ start with 25 mg PO q d, increase q 4–7 days to BID, TID, then QID, then by 25 mg per day up to max of ≈ 100 mg QID (may take 1 week at new steady state to see effect);
      Side effects: muscle weakness (may make ambulation impossible), sedation, idiosyncratic hepatitis (may be fatal; more common in patients on > 300 mg/d x > 2 mos) that is often preceded by anorexia, abdominal pain, N/V; D/C if no benefit is seen by ≈ 45 days; follow LFTs (SGPT or SGOT)
   d) progabide: activates both GABA-A and GABA-B receptors. Useful for patients with severe flexor spasms
   e) other agents that have not been successful include[62]: phenothiazines (reduce gamma spasticity, but only at high PO doses or parenterally), clonidine, tetrahydrocannabinol...
4. intramuscular injections: botulinum toxin (Botox®), phenol

Surgical treatment of spasticity – overview

Reserved for spasticity refractory to medical treatment, or where side effects of medications are intolerable. Generally either orthopedic (e.g., tendon release operations (tenotomies) of heel cord (Achilles tendon lengthening) or hamstrings, iliopsoas myotomies, adductor lengthening, derotational osteotomies...) or neurosurgical (e.g., nerve blocks, neurectomies, myelotomy, rhizotomies...).
   Neurosurgical treatment options:

1. nonablative procedures
   a) intrathecal (IT) baclofen: delivered via an implantable pump (see below)
   b) intrathecal morphine (tolerance and dependence may develop)
   c) electrical stimulation via percutaneously placed epidural electrodes[65]
2. ablative procedures, with *preservation* of potential for ambulation
   a) selective dorsal rhizotomy (p. 1851): divides *sensory* rootlets involved in spastic reflex arc
   b) motor point block[62] (intramuscular phenol neurolysis): preserves sensation and existing voluntary function. Especially useful in patients with incomplete myelopathies; time-consuming
   c) phenol nerve block: similar to motor point block, but used when spasticity more severe and complete block of muscle desired. Open phenol block used instead of percutaneous when nerve is mixed and sensory preservation is desired (also reduces post-block dysesthesias)[66]
   d) selective neurectomies[62]
      • sciatic neurectomy (may be done with RF lesion)[67]

- obturator neurectomy: useful if strong hip adductor spasticity that causes scissoring and wasted energy expenditure in ambulating
- pudendal neurectomy: useful if excessive detrusor dyssynergy interferes with bladder retraining

e) percutaneous radiofrequency foraminal rhizotomy[67]: small unmyelinated sensory fibers are more sensitive to RF lesions than larger myelinated A-alpha fibers of motor units.
Technique: start at S1 on one side, and work up to T12, then repeat on other side. At each level: verify needle position by stimulating with 0.1–0.5 V and watch for movement in appropriate myotome (tip should be extradural, avoid subarachnoid placement), ablate with 70–80 °C × 2 mins for S1, and 70 °C × 2 mins for L5 to T12 (to preserve motor function). If symptoms recur, may repeat with lesions at 90 °C × 2 mins

f) myelotomies[68]
- Bischof's myelotomy: divides anterior and posterior horns via laterally placed incision, disrupts reflex arc. No effect on α–spasticity
- midline "T" myelotomy: interrupts reflex arc from sensory to motor units without disrupting connections from corticospinal tract to anterior motor neurons. Slightly higher risk of losing motor function.
Technique: laminectomy from T11 to L1. Mobilize midline dorsal longitudinal vein and incise cord in midline from T12 at a depth of 3 mm to S1 at a depth of 4 mm (preserving S2–4 maintains bladder reflex pathways. Unilateral extension up to conus medullaris reduces bladder spasticity and increases capacity before reflex emptying occurs)

g) stereotactic thalamotomy or dentatotomy: may be useful in cerebral palsy.[69] Useful for unilateral dystonia, but cannot be used for bilateral dystonia as bilateral lesions would be required which jeopardizes speech, cognition… Effective only for dystonia *distal* to shoulders or hips, and should not be used if the condition is rapidly progressive

• ablative procedures, with *sacrifice* of potential for ambulation (in complete cord injuries, nonablative procedures are not indicated because there is no motor function to recover). Used after failure of percutaneous rhizotomy (see above) and "T" myelotomy (see above)

a) intrathecal injection of 6 ml of 10% phenol (by weight) in glycerin mixed with 4 ml of iohexol (Omnipaque® 300) (p. 230) for a final concentration of 6% phenol and ≈ 120 mg iodine/ml. Administered via LP at L2–3 interspace with patient in lateral decubitus position (most symptomatic side down) under fluoro until T12–1 nerve root sleeves are filled (sparing S2–4 for bladder function). Patient is maintained in this position × 20–30 mins and then kept sitting upright × 4 hrs[70] (absolute alcohol provides more permanent blocks, but is hypobaric and more difficult to control)

b) selective anterior rhizotomy: results in flaccid paralysis with denervation atrophy of muscles

c) neurectomies, often combined with tenotomies[67]

d) intramuscular neurolysis by phenol injection[67]

e) cordectomy[71]: most drastic measure, reserved for patients who do not respond to any other measure. Results in total flaccidity with loss of benefits from mild spasticity. Converts bladder from UMN to LMN control. Works well for progressive deficit from syringomyelia and for spasticity, but poor for "phantom" leg pain[72]

f) cordotomy: rarely used

intrathecal baclofen

See references.[73,74,75,76]

Selection criteria used in one study[75] are shown in ▶ Table 111.2. Other indications include: stroke,[77] cerebral palsy, TBI, dystonia, stiff-man syndrome.

Test doses: Incremental test doses of 50, 75, and then 100 mcg intrathecal baclofen (ITB) via lumbar puncture or temporary catheter were used,[75] randomly alternated with placebo, with dose escalation halted if a response to active drug occurred. The following parameters were evaluated at 0.5, 2, 4, 8, & 24 hrs post injection: pulse and respiratory rate, BP, hypertonia (Ashworth score, Table 111.1), reflexes, spasm score, voluntary muscle movement, and adverse effects (if any, including seizures). Pump implantation was offered if there was a 2-point reduction in the Ashworth score and muscle spasm score for ≥ 4 hrs after bolus injection of active drug without intolerable side effects. Usual daily dose for ITB is twice the test dose, typically 200 micrograms/d.

Alternatively, give 25 mcg IT in the O.R., and if the patient improves, insert subcutaneous pump.[64]

Pumps: available programmable systems include those manufactured by Medtronic, Inc., Minneapolis, MN: the Synchromed II Pump (▶ Fig. 111.2) with the N'Vision programmer, or the somewhat similarly shaped Synchromed EL which has a screen over the CAP to prevent inadvertent access.

Table 111.2 Selection criteria for baclofen pump

- age 18–65 yrs (older patients treated on compassionate use basis)
- able to give informed consent
- severe, chronic spasticity (≥ 12 mos duration) due to spinal cord lesion or MS
- spasticity refractory to oral drugs (including baclofen), or unacceptable side effects
- no CSF block (e.g., on myelography)
- positive response to IT baclofen at test dose ≤ 100 mcg and no response to placebo
- no implanted programmable device such as cardiac pacemaker[a]
- females of childbearing potential: not pregnant & using adequate contraception
- no hypersensitivity (allergy) to baclofen
- no history of stroke, impaired renal function, or severe hepatic or GI disease

[a]this study used a programmable IT pump

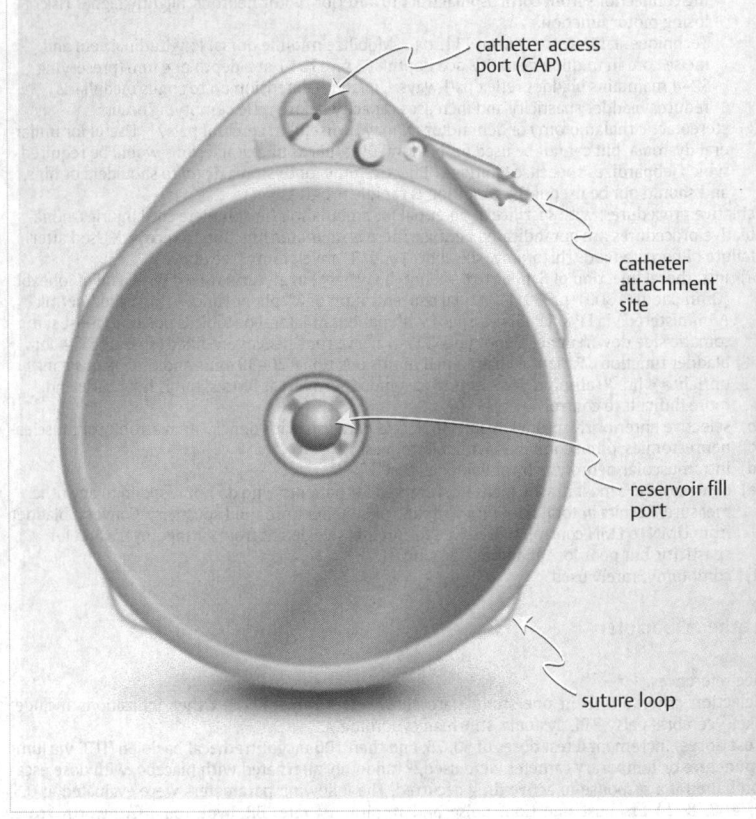

catheter access port (CAP)

catheter attachment site

reservoir fill port

suture loop

Fig. 111.2 Medtronic Synchromed II.

Insertion technique: IT catheter is typically inserted ≈ L2–3, and is threaded rostrally ≈ 3 leve[l] but should be no higher than T10 (risk of rostral progression of hypotonia). Record the cathet[er] length used (this is progammed into the Synchromed II and is important when injecting the port [or] withdrawing drug).

Post-op orders: Guidelines for postoperative orders following baclofen pump insertion

1. admit PACU, transfer to:
   a) floor if insertion follows test dosing or if patient has just been transitioned from stable PO dose
   b) ICU if there has been a hiatus in baclofen therapy
2. neuro checks q 2 hrs for 1st 24 hours
3. baclofen:
   a) for patients on oral or IV baclofen: continue baclofen at the previous dose via the same route (oral or IV) until the ITB takes effect (usually 2–4 hrs, full effect is delayed up to 24 hrs). The IV/PO drug is then tapered
   b) if there has been a hiatus in baclofen therapy: baclofen 20 mg PO QID
4. have 2 vials of IV physostigmine available and labeled "FOR EMERGENCY USE ONLY" for possible baclofen overdose

▶ **Device-related complications.** Shown in ▶ Table 111.3. The frequency of most is ≈ 1%, except catheter-related problems which had a rate of ≈ 30%[75]

Table 111.3 ITB pump complications[a]

1. mechanical problems
   a) pump underinfusion
   b) catheter problems: occlusion, kink, dislodgment, cut, break (including microleaks), or disconnection
2. wound complications
   a) pocket erosion
   b) incisional pain
   c) infection:
      1. infection at the pump site can be introduced at the time of insertion, or when accessing any of the ports, or from hematogenous spread from unrelated bacteremia
      2. infection of the catheter may be associated with meningitis
   d) seroma (may require aspiration)
   e) CSF collection

[a]device-related complications requiring a secondary invasive procedure

111

Pump site infection: If the patient is still receiving ITB (i.e., not going into baclofen withdrawal (p. 1849)) and not showing signs of sepsis or meningitis, start antibiotics and attempt to taper the IT baclofen over a few weeks if tolerated, supplementing as necessary with PO medication. Once the pump-delivered dose is negligible, the pump and catheter can be removed and antibiotics continued until the infection is convincingly cleared (typically 3-6 months), and then a new system can be implanted. For patients that are septic, the pump may need to be removed emergently and the ITB is managed as described below.

▶ **Baclofen overdose.** Etiologies: wrong concentration of drug (standard concentrations: 500, 1000 or 2000 mcg/cc, compounding pharmacies may make custom doses as high as 3000–5000 mcg/cc), programming error, not aspirating catheter access port (CAP) prior to injections.
Presentation: rostral progression of hypotonia, respiratory depression, coma, and seizures.
Attend to ABCs (airway/breathing/circulation). Intubate if necessary.
Pump-related measures:
1. empty pump reservoir to stop drug flow (record amount withdrawn)
2. administer physostigmine if not contraindicated:
   a) ℞ adult: 0.5–1.0 mg IM or IV @ rate ≤ 1 mg/min
      (may repeat q 10–30 minutes PRN)
   b) ℞ peds: 0.02 mg/kg IM or IV @ rate ≤ 0.5 mg/min
      (may repeat q 5–10 min up to 2 mg max)
3. withdraw 30–40 ml CSF either via LP or through catheter access port
4. notify the pump manufacturer

▶ **Intrathecal baclofen withdrawal.** ITB results in down-regulation of GABA-B receptors that cannot be compensated by PO baclofen or small doses of ITB.
Interruption of ITB therapy may occur as a result of: empty pump reservoir, pump battery failure, end of pump life (Synchromed II pumps shut off automatically after 5 years, audible alarms give ample warning to replace the pump), catheter migration/breakage/kinking/disconnection/occlusion, programming error, catheter tip granuloma (p. 1389) (less common with ITB than with opioid, see that section for management) or stiff-man syndrome (antibodies to glutamic acid decarboxylase which reduces available endogenous GABA).

If it is necessary to electively (or semi-electively) remove a pump system (e.g., for infection), the optimal scenario is to gradually taper the drug by reprogramming the pump and/or by filling the reservoir with solution of decreased baclofen concentration while supplementing with PO baclofen as needed and as tolerated.

The severity of withdrawal syndrome depends on dose of drug used (increased with higher dose) and duration of therapy (increased with longer therapy).

Syndromes arising from abrupt discontinuation of ITB:
1. mild withdrawal symptoms: return of spasticity and rigidity, tachycardia, piloerection (goosebumps) & pruritus (pruritus without a rash is very suggestive of ITB withdrawal)
2. moderate withdrawal symptoms: seizures & hallucinations
3. severe withdrawal symptoms (estimated incidence: 3–5%)[78]: increased rebound spasticity, rigidity, fever, labile BP, and reduced level of consciousness. If untreated, the severe syndrome can progress over 24–72 hours to rhabdomyolysis (with elevated creatine phosphokinase (CPK) and transaminase), hepatic and renal failure, DIC, and occasionally death. Differential diagnosis:
   - malignant hyperthermia (p. 112)
   - autonomic dysreflexia (p. 1222): exaggerated sympathetic response, classically presents with HTN + bradycardia in a patient with a spinal cord injury at T6 or above
   - neuroleptic malignant syndrome: caused by dopamine (DA) receptor blocking drugs or sudden cessation of DA agonists. Treat with DA agonists and IV dantrolene
   - sepsis
   - status epilepticus

Management of *abrupt* ITB withdrawal syndrome (adapted[78,79]):
1. ABCs (airway/breathing/circulation). Intubate if necessary
2. assess for noxious stimulation, infection, other drugs, progression of underlying disease
3. labs: CPK
4. primary goal is to reestablish ITB therapy at the same dose as soon as possible
5. assess pump/system as outlined in ▶ Table 111.4

Table 111.4 Assessing ITB infusion systems (adapted[79])

- interrogate the pump (with device programmer): alarm log for low reservoir, low battery, or end of service, check rotor log (rotor stops temporarily in MRI scanners)
- verify reservoir volume: aspirate entire volume of drug and compare to volume calculated by the programmer; discrepancies > 25% may signal mechanical faults. Refill reservoir with drug if empty (by experienced ITB practitioner)
- obtain AP & lateral X-rays to assess location of catheter tip and to look for breaks[a], kinks, or migration
- program the pump to administer a prescribed bolus, observe for decreased spasticity (takes up to 4 hours)
- aspirate 3–4 ml thru the catheter aspiration port (CAP) (see ▶ Fig. 111.2). Difficulty aspirating or bubbles are abnormal
- contrast study (either of the following can miss a microleak):
  - if abrupt onset: aspirate the CAP (if unsuccessful, do NOT inject dye because of danger of overdose), then inject iodinated contrast into the CAP either under fluoroscopy or while the patient is in the CT scanner (do not move the ptient between injectin & imaging). High rate of false negatives
  - insidious onset: an indium study can be done, it takes ≈ 24 hrs to get the radio-isotope. DPTA radio-isotope is injected into the reservoir fill port (see ▶ Fig. 111.2) - not into the CAP! (OK for it to mix with baclofen). Image with nuclear medicine camera (length of sudy depends on programmed flow rate). This test is expensive, takes a long time to complete (2–3 days from the time it is ordered) and has low sensitivity

[a]NB: in 2012 Medtronic replaced the radio-opaque catheter with a stronger Ascenda catheter which is radiolucent except for a small spot at the distal tip

6. early use of high-dose oral/enteral baclofen: ≥ 120 mg/d in 6–8 divided doses if the patient's condition permits (NB: PO baclofen is not reliable as the lone treatment for ITB withdrawal, and safety not established for age < 12 yrs)
7. attempt to restore ITB therapy at or near pre-withdrawal dosage by experienced physician by one of the following:
   a) using a programmed bolus through the pump
   b) injection via the catheter access port
   c) via LP
   d) via new externalized catheter
8. if restoration of ITB therapy is delayed and if symptoms persist
   a) move patient to ICU if not already there

b) parenteral benzodiazepine (BDZ) infusion: diazepam or midazolam. Titrate dose to reduce muscle rigidity, hyperthermia, BP lability, seizures. BDZs do not prevent baclofen withdrawal syndrome, but they may buy some time

c) cyproheptadine[80]: a serotonin antagonist. Start with 4 mg PO q 6 hrs

d) diphenhydramine 50 mg PO or IM, may repeat q 6 hrs for pruritus

e) dantrolene: may *not* be as effective as it is for malignant hyperthermia

f) rectal baclofen

9. surgical repair/replacement of defective components

Selective dorsal rhizotomy

General information

Key concepts: Selective dorsal rhizotomy (SDR)

- an ablative technique primarily used to reduce LE spasticity in children with cerebral palsy
- uses intraoperative stimulation and EMG to identify and divide a portion of the *sensory* lower-extremity rootlets involved in the spastic reflex arc (no motor roots are cut)
- optimal candidates: no consensus; consider for children > 2 yrs old with spastic diplegia (LEs > UEs) that hampers gait, preemie at birth or full term + brain MRI → no major abnormalities
- avoid pts with: dystonia, nonambulatory or unable to maintain antigravity posture, significant scoliosis or hip dislocation, orthopedic procedure within last 1 year or botox in last 3 months
- results in gait improvement in ambulatory patients at 5, 10, & 15 yrs. Physiotherapy is a must
- risks: scoliosis, urinary retention, CSF leak

Selective dorsal rhizotomy (SDR): uses intraoperative electrophysiological stimulation and EMG to eliminate a portion of sensory rootlets involved in "handicapping spasticity" (leaves all motor rootlets and those sensory rootlets subserving "useful spasticity" intact). Decreases the afferent limb of the pathologic reflex arc. No effect on α–spasticity. Ambulatory children with cerebral palsy have improved gait, has been used in nonambulatory children with improvement of spasticity (helps facilitate care) but they are still not able to ambulate afterwards.

111

Selection criteria

There is currently no consensus on the optimal candidate.[81] Factors to consider:

1. most often used in children > 2 years of age
2. some surgeons reserve SDR for patients who have failed IT baclofen
3. mild-to-moderate LE weakness with the ability to walk or maintain antigravity posture. On the GMFCS (▶ Table 111.5), most are Level II or III, some Level IV are candidates
4. spasticity hampers gait and/or development of motor skills
5. legs worse than arms
6. gestation (to be certain that you're dealing with CP and not some other entity)
   a) preemies < 33 weeks gestation at birth with spastic diplegia
   b) full-term children with spastic diplegia and brain MRI with no major structural abnormality (periventricular leucomalacia is common and is acceptable)

Table 111.5 Gross Motor Function Classification System – Expanded and Revised (GMFCS – E&R) (see reference[82] for full description and website[83] for helpful illustrations)

Level	Brief description
I	able to walk at home, school, & outdoors; climbs stairs without railing; speed, balance, and coordination are limited
II	able to walk in most settings & climb stairs holding railing; difficulty on long distances or uneven terrain, inclines, & crowded spaces
III	able to walk with hand-held mobility device in most indoor settings; climb stairs with railing + assist/supervision, use wheeled mobility for long distances
IV	assistance or powered mobility in most situations, may walk short distances with assist at home
V	wheeled mobility in all settings; limited ability to maintain antigravity postures and control leg & arm movements

7. avoid patients with dystonia (becomes evident by age 5 years, SDR does not work for this), significant scoliosis (relative contraindication – may be candidates with small conus exposure), hip dislocation, orthopedic procedure (e.g., tendon release) within the last year or botox injection within the last month
8. willing and able to undergo intense physical therapy post-op

Technique
1. EMG monitoring leads: muscles of LEs, pudendal, bladder, and anal sphincter
2. anesthesia techniques (p. 112) to maintain EMG
3. position: prone, in slight Trendelenburg to reduce loss of CSF
4. laminectomy or laminoplasty: more commonly used options (check pre-op MRI for the level of the conus)
   a) wide opening to expose cauda equina: e.g., L1–5. May be higher risk for developing scoliosis
   b) small opening over conus. In children < 10 years: ultrasound can be used through the skin to localize the conus in the OR. For age > 10 years, the laminectomy is made based on the location of the conus gleaned from the pre-op MRI (usually ≈ L1–2). May be harder to identify lower sacral roots (the ones you don't want to cut) which tend to be thinner and more medially situated
5. open the dura, identify sensory rootlets (dorsal to the dentate ligament), and place a thin barrier underneath (e.g., strip cut from a sterile glove) to keep them separated form the motor roots
6. L2 is identified by locating the root exiting the neural foramen between L2 & L3
7. stimulation: each dorsal root from L2 through S1 is stimulated before subdividing into separate rootlets. The root is elevated with hooked stimulator probes, the cathode probe is positioned cranial to the anode probe. Starting at 0.5 mA, progressively larger single-pulsed stimuli are applied (up to 4 mA max) until there is a response. Then this amplitude is used in a 1-second 50 Hz train and the response is graded as shown in ▶ Table 111.6

Table 111.6 EMG response grading to a 1-second train of stimuli for SDR[84]

Grade	EMG response
0	unsustained or single discharge isolated to that root
1+	sustained discharges from segmentally innervated muscles
2+	sustained discharges from segmentally innervated muscles and muscles from immediately adjacent segments
3+	sustained discharges from segmentally innervated muscles & muscles from distant segments
4+	sustained discharges from contralateral muscles ± sustained discharges from ipsilateral muscles

8. selective sectioning (adapted from Park,[84] see reference for details):
   a) roots with a 0 response are left intact
   b) roots with 3+ or 4+ response: separate into rootlets along natural planes, divide all but 1 rootlet (1 is left to avoid complete sensory loss)
   c) roots with 1+ or 2+ response: separate into rootlets, divide 50–65% of rootlets from that nerve - targeting the ones with the most activity if any (e.g., if there are 6 rootlets, cut 3 (50%) or 4 (66%)). Move the rootlets to be spared beneath the barrier to protect them
   d) spare sacral roots (to avoid bladder problems): in general, do not cut the S2 root (which has a single fascicle), or at most, cut ≤ 35% of S2.[85] Do not cut S3 or lower
   e) the L1 root is identified and 50% is cut without testing (Park feels L1 testing is unreliable[84])

▶ **Post-op care.** Most institutions have their own protocol. Patients are generally kept flat on bed rest for 48–72 hours.

Patients are started very early with PT.

NB: with reduction in spasticity, the patient's metabolic requirements often decrease substantially. The patient and caregivers must be aware of this and decrease calorie intake accordingly to avoid increases in body weight that could impair mobility because the UE & LE muscles may not be strong enough to compensate.

Outcome
Benefits are not immediately evident, it may take ≈ 2–3 months.
Ashworth scale (▶ Table 111.1) scores improve by 0.5–1.5.[86]

Benefits may be temporary, but functional gains of improved mobility, self-care, ambulation and quality of life (for patient and caregivers) can be shown at 5, 10, & 15 years.[87,88,89]

Patients with cerebral palsy plateau in motor development. Patients with SDR plateau later.

For inexplicable reasons, L1–5 dorsal rhizotomies often reduces spasticity in the UEs.

Complications

1. sensory loss or dysesthesia: transient (typically lasting ≤ 3 months): 2.5–40%[85]; permanent but not disabling sensory loss: 0–6%
2. transient urinary retention (1.25–24%[85]) or urinary incontinence (4.4%)
3. CSF leak: 3%
4. infection: 2%
5. motor weakness: must differentiate from underlying weakness unmasked from SDR. Cutting less of L4 to preserve more quadriceps tone may help (this does not increase strength, just the spasticity)
6. spinal deformity: scoliosis, spondylolisthesis. True incidence is unknown, patients with spastic CP have higher rates in general even without SDR.[90] Possible lower risk with limited laminectomy is uncertain

11.6 Sympathectomy

11.6.1 Cardiac sympathectomy (angina pectoris)

With the advances in percutaneous coronary artery techniques, cardiovascular surgery and drugs, cardiac sympathectomy for angina pectoris has found less application. However, it may still be useful in patients who have no further treatment options. Bilateral sympathectomy from the stellate ganglion through the T7 ganglia is required. Newer thoracoscopic techniques may revive some interest in this.

11.6.2 Upper extremity sympathectomy

General information

Various pathologies that may be indications for upper extremity sympathectomy are shown in Table 111.7.

Table 111.7 Indications for UE sympathectomy

- essential hyperhidrosis
- primary Raynaud's disease
- shoulder-hand syndrome
- intractable angina
- ± causalgia major (p. 525)

Hyperhidrosis

General information

Either essential (primary, or idiopathic) or secondary (etiologies include: hyperthyroidism, diabetes mellitus, pheochromocytoma, acromegaly, parkinsonism, CNS trauma, syringomyelia, hypothalamic tumors, menopause).[91]

Due to overactivity of eccrine sweat glands (found over entire body, highest concentration in palms and soles of feet). They produce a hypotonic secretion with saline as the primary constituent. These glands are under control of the sympathetic nervous system; however, the neurotransmitter is paradoxically acetylcholine (i.e., they are cholinergic, unlike most sympathetic end organs, which are adrenergic). Most eccrine sweat glands serve a thermoregulatory function; however, those on the palms and soles respond primarily to emotional stress.[91]

Essential hyperhidrosis is a generalized condition that usually manifests mostly in the palms. The prevalence is approximately 2.8% in the United States.[92]

Treatment

Mild cases are treated medically with

111

1. topical agents: astringents (potassium permanganate, tannic acid...) or antiperspirants (contact dermatitis usually limits use of these agents)
2. or systemically with anticholinergics: including atropine, propantheline bromide... (side effects of dry mouth and blurred vision usually limits use of these)
3. tap water iontophoresis: may produce keratinization of palmar epithelium

Severe cases refractory to medical therapy may be candidates for surgical sympathectomy (see below).

Surgical technique

Removal of only the second thoracic ganglion is probably adequate, and avoids a Horner syndrome in most. Techniques used include: anterior transthoracic, thoracic endoscopic,[93] percutaneous radio frequency, and supraclavicular. An approach via a midline posterior incision with a T3 costotransverse sectomy allows bilateral access.[91,94] The risk of significant complications is ≈ 5%, and they include pneumothorax, intercostal neuralgia, spinal cord injury, and Horner syndrome.

111.6.3 Upper thoracic sympathectomy

Approaches include
1. posterior paravertebral approach
2. axillary thoracotomy with transthoracic exposure of the sympathetic chain
3. supraclavicular, retropleural exposure
4. percutaneous radiofrequency technique[95,96]
5. video endoscopic approach[97]

111.6.4 Lumbar sympathectomy

Primary indication is for causalgia major of the lower extremity. Preoperative lumbar sympathetic blocks may be utilized to evaluate patient for response.

Removal of the L2 and L3 sympathetic ganglion is usually adequate to remove sympathetic tone from the lower extremities (occasionally L1 and sometimes T12 are also removed for causalgia of the thigh).

The most common approach is a retroperitoneal approach through a flank incision. The patient is placed in a lateral oblique position, and the skin incision is made from the anterior superior iliac spine to the tip of the 12th rib. The peritoneum is dissected from the muscular wall and is retracted anteriorly. The kidney and ureter are retracted anteriorly; injury to the ureter being a major risk of the operation. The sympathetic chain is identified on the lateral aspect of the vertebral bodies. The vena cava makes a right-sided approach more difficult as the aorta is easier to deal with on left-sided approaches.

References

[1] Gildenberg PL. Whatever Happened to Stereotactic Surgery? Neurosurgery. 1987; 20:983–987
[2] Bucholz RD, Yeh DD, Trobaugh J, et al. The correction of stereotactic inaccuracy caused by brain shift using an intraoperative ultrasound device. In: Lecture Notes in Computer Science. Berlin: Springer; 1997. DOI: 10.1007/BFb0029268
[3] Hood TW, Gebarski SS, McKeever PE, et al. Stereotactic Biopsy of Intrinsic Lesions of the Brain Stem. J Neurosurg. 1986; 65:172–176
[4] Coffey RJ, Friedman WA. Interstitial Brachytherapy of Malignant Brain Tumors Using Computed Tomography-guided Stereotaxis and Available Imaging Software: Technical Report. Neurosurgery. 1987; 20:4–7
[5] Backlund E-O, von Holst H. Controlled Subtotal Evacuation of Intracerebral Hematomas by Stereotactic Technique. Surgical Neurology. 1978; 9:99–101
[6] Tanikawa T, Amano K, Kawamura H, et al. CT-Guided Stereotactic Surgery for Evacuation of Hypertensive Intracerebral Hematoma. Appl Neurophysiol. 1985; 48:431–439
[7] Niizuma H, Otsuki T, Johkura H, et al. CT-Guided Stereotactic Aspiration of Intracerebral Hematoma –

Result of a Hematoma-Lysis Method Using Urokinase. Appl Neurophysiol. 1985; 48:427–430
[8] Niizuma H, Shimizu Y, Yonemitsu T, et al. Results of Stereotactic Aspiration in 175 Cases of Putaminal Hemorrhage. Neurosurgery. 1989; 24:814–819
[9] Schaller C, Rohde V, Meyer B, et al. Stereotactic Puncture and Lysis of Spontaneous Intracerebral Hemorrhage Using Recombinant Tissue-Plasminogen Activator. Neurosurgery. 1995; 36:328–335
[10] Sisti MB, Solomon RA, Stein BM. Stereotactic Craniotomy in the Resection of Small Arteriovenous Malformations. Journal of Neurosurgery. 1991; 75:40–44
[11] Moore MR, Black PM, Ellenbogen R, et al. Stereotactic Craniotomy: Methods and Results Using the Brown-Roberts-Wells Stereotactic Frame. Neurosurgery. 1989; 25:572–578
[12] Patil AA. Transoral Stereotactic Biopsy of the Second Cervical Vertebral Body: Case Report with Technical Note. Neurosurgery. 1989; 25:999–1002
[13] Kandel EI, Peresedov VV. Stereotaxic Clipping of Arterial Aneurysms and Arteriovenous Malformations. J Neurosurg. 1977; 46:12–23
[14] Backlund E-O, Granberg P-O, Hamberger B, et al. Transplantation of Adrenal Medullary Tissue

Striatum in Parkinsonism: First Clinical Trials. J Neurosurg. 1985; 62:169–173

15] Blacklock JB, Maxwell RE. Stereotactic Removal of a Migrating Ventricular Catheter. Neurosurgery. 1985; 16:230–231

16] Levy RM, Russell E, Yungbluth M, et al. The efficacy of image-guided stereotactic brain biopsy in neurologically symptomatic acquired immunodeficiency syndrome patients. Neurosurgery. 1992; 30:186–190

17] Nicolato A, Gerosa M, Piovan E, et al. Computerized Tomography and Magnetic Resonance Guided Stereotactic Brain Biopsy in Nonimmunocompromised and AIDS Patients. Surgical Neurology. 1997; 48:267–277

18] Deuschl G, Schade-Brittinger C, Krack P, et al. A randomized trial of deep-brain stimulation for Parkinson's disease. New England Journal of Medicine. 2006; 355:896–908

19] Weaver FM, Follett K, Stern M, et al. Bilateral deep brain stimulation vs best medical therapy for patients with advanced Parkinson disease: a randomized controlled trial. JAMA. 2009; 301:63–73

20] Mallet L, Polosan M, Jaafari N, et al. Subthalamic nucleus stimulation in severe obsessive-compulsive disorder. New England Journal of Medicine. 2008; 359:2121–2134

21] Greenberg BD, Malone DA, Friehs GM, et al. Three-year outcomes in deep brain stimulation for highly resistant obsessive-compulsive disorder. Neuropsychopharmacology. 2006; 31:2384–2393

22] Lozano AM, Mayberg HS, Giacobbe P, et al. Subcallosal cingulate gyrus deep brain stimulation for treatment-resistant depression. Biological Psychiatry. 2008; 64:461–467

23] Malone DA Jr, Dougherty DD, Rezai AR, et al. Deep brain stimulation of the ventral capsule/ventral striatum for treatment-resistant depression. Biological Psychiatry. 2009; 65:267–275

24] Halpern CH, Wolf JA, Bale TL, et al. Deep brain stimulation in the treatment of obesity. Journal of Neurosurgery. 2008; 109:625–634

25] Stelten BM, Noblesse LH, Ackermans L, et al. The neurosurgical treatment of addiction. Neurosurgical Focus. 2008; 25. DOI: 10.3171/FOC/2008/25/7/E5

26] Green AL, Wang S, Bittar RG, et al. Deep brain stimulation: a new treatment for hypertension? J Clin Neurosci. 2007; 14:592–595

27] Laitinen LV, Bergenheim AT, Hariz MI. Leksell's Posteroventral Pallidotomy in the Treatment of Parkinson's Disease. Journal of Neurosurgery. 1992; 76:53–61

28] Iacono RP, Lonser RR, Mandybur G, et al. Stimulation of the Globus Pallidus in Parkinson's Disease. Br J Neurosurg. 1995; 9:505–510

29] Limousin P, Pollack P, Benazzouz A, et al. Bilateral Subthalamic Nucleus Stimulation for Severe Parkinson's Disease. Movement Disorders. 1995; 10:672–674

30] Schuurman PR, Bosch DA, Bossuyt PM, et al. A comparison of continuous thalamic stimulation and thalamotomy for suppression of severe tremor. N Engl J Med. 2000; 342:461–468

31] Favre J, Taha JM, Nguyen TT, et al. Pallidotomy: A Survey of Current Practice in North America. Neurosurgery. 1996; 39:883–892

32] Stefani A, Lozano AM, Peppe A, et al. Bilateral deep brain stimulation of the pedunculopontine and subthalamic nuclei in severe Parkinson's disease. Brain. 2007; 130:1596–1607

33] Pereira EA, Muthusamy KA, De Pennington N, et al. Deep brain stimulation of the pedunculopontine nucleus in Parkinson's disease. Preliminary experience at Oxford. British Journal of Neurosurgery. 2008; 22 Suppl 1:S41–S44

34] Jankovic J, Cardoso F, Grossman RG, et al. Outcome After Stereotactic Thalamotomy for Parkinsonian, Essential, and Other Types of Tremor. Neurosurgery. 1995; 37:680–687

35] Pahwa R, Lyons KE, Wilkinson SB, et al. Long-term evaluation of deep brain stimulation of the thalamus. J Neurosurg. 2006; 104:506–512

[36] Sutton JP, Couldwell W, Lew MF, et al. Ventroposterior Medial Pallidotomy in Patients with Advanced Parkinson's Disease. Neurosurgery. 1995; 36:1112–1117

[37] Sydow O, Thobois S, Alesch F, et al. Multicentre European study of thalamic stimulation in essential tremor: a six year follow up. Journal of Neurology, Neurosurgery, and Psychiatry. 2003; 74:1387–1391

[38] Schuurman PR, Bosch DA, Merkus MP, et al. Long-term follow-up of thalamic stimulation versus thalamotomy for tremor suppression. Movement Disorders. 2008; 23:1146–1153

[39] Burdick A, Goodman WK, Foote KD. Deep brain stimulation for refractory obsessive-compulsive disorder. Front Biosci (Landmark Ed). 2009; 14:1880–1890

[40] Jimenez F, Velasco F, Salin-Pascual R, et al. Neuromodulation of the inferior thalamic peduncle for major depression and obsessive compulsive disorder. Acta Neurochir Suppl. 2007; 97:393–398

[41] Maciunas RJ, Maddux BN, Riley DE, et al. Prospective randomized double-blind trial of bilateral thalamic deep brain stimulation in adults with Tourette syndrome. J Neurosurg. 2007; 107:1004–1014

[42] Kurlan R. Clinical practice. Tourette's Syndrome. N Engl J Med. 2010; 363:2332–2338

[43] Leckman JF. Tourette's syndrome. Lancet. 2002; 360:1577–1586

[44] Temel Y, Visser-Vandewalle V. Surgery in Tourette syndrome. Mov Disord. 2004; 19:3–14

[45] Martinez-Fernandez R, Zrinzo L, Aviles-Olmos I, et al. Deep brain stimulation for Gilles de la Tourette syndrome: a case series targeting subregions of the globus pallidus internus. Mov Disord. 2011; 26:1922–1930

[46] Shah DB, Pesiridou A, Baltuch GH, et al. Functional neurosurgery in the treatment of severe obsessive compulsive disorder and major depression: overview of disease circuits and therapeutic targeting for the clinician. Psychiatry (Edgmont). 2008; 5:24–33

[47] Narrow WE, Rae DS, Robins LN, et al. Revised prevalence estimates of mental disorders in the United States: using a clinical significance criterion to reconcile 2 surveys' estimates. Arch Gen Psychiatry. 2002; 59:115–123

[48] Murray CJ, Lopez AD. Global mortality, disability, and the contribution of risk factors: Global Burden of Disease Study. Lancet. 1997; 349:1436–1442

[49] Eisen JL, Goodman WK, Keller MB, et al. Patterns of remission and relapse in obsessive-compulsive disorder: a 2-year prospective study. J Clin Psychiatry. 1999; 60:346–51; quiz 352

[50] Greenberg BD, Gabriels LA, Malone DA Jr, et al. Deep brain stimulation of the ventral internal capsule/ventral striatum for obsessive-compulsive disorder: worldwide experience. Mol Psychiatry. 2010; 15:64–79

[51] Sturm V, Lenartz D, Koulousakis A, et al. The nucleus accumbens: a target for deep brain stimulation in obsessive-compulsive- and anxiety-disorders. J Chem Neuroanat. 2003; 26:293–299

[52] Murray CJ, Lopez AD. Measuring the global burden of disease. N Engl J Med. 2013; 369:448–457

[53] Jimenez F, Velasco F, Salin-Pascual R, et al. A patient with a resistant major depression disorder treated with deep brain stimulation in the inferior thalamic peduncle. Neurosurgery. 2005; 57:585–93; discussion 585-93

[54] Lozano AM, Mayberg HS, Giacobbe P, et al. Subcallosal cingulate gyrus deep brain stimulation for treatment-resistant depression. Biol Psychiatry. 2008; 64:461–467

[55] Malone DA Jr, Dougherty DD, Rezai AR, et al. Deep brain stimulation of the ventral capsule/ventral striatum for treatment-resistant depression. Biol Psychiatry. 2009; 65:267–275

[56] Nuttin BJ, Gabriels LA, Cosyns PR, et al. Long-term electrical capsular stimulation in patients with obsessive-compulsive disorder. Neurosurgery. 2003; 52:1263–72; discussion 1272-4

111

[57] Elger G, Hoppe C, Falkai P, et al. Vagus nerve stimulation is associated with mood improvements in epilepsy patients. Epilepsy Res. 2000; 42:203–210

[58] Awan NR, Lozano A, Hamani C. Deep brain stimulation: current and future perspectives. Neurosurgical Focus. 2009; 27. DOI: 10.3171/2009.4.FOCUS0982

[59] Keen JR, Przekop A, Olaya JE, et al. Deep brain stimulation for the treatment of childhood dystonic cerebral palsy. J Neurosurg Pediatr. 2014; 14:585–593

[60] Chen T, Mirzadeh Z, Chapple KM, et al. Clinical outcomes following awake and asleep deep brain stimulation for Parkinson disease. J Neurosurg. 2018:1–12

[61] Shima F, Fukui M, Kitamura K, et al. Diagnosis and Surgical Treatment of Spasmodic Torticollis of 11th Nerve Origin. Neurosurgery. 1988; 22:358–363

[62] Merritt JL. Management of Spasticity in Spinal Cord Injury. Mayo Clin Proc. 1981; 56:614–622

[63] Ashworth B. Preliminary Trial of Carisoprodal in Multiple Sclerosis. Practitioner. 1964; 192:540–542

[64] Scott BA, Pulliam MW. Management of Spasticity and Painful Spasms in Paraplegia. Contemp Neurosurg. 1987; 9:1–6

[65] Richardson RR, Cerullo LJ, McLone DG, et al. Percutaneous Epidural Neurostimulation in Modulation of Paraplegic Spasticity. Acta Neurochirurgica. 1979; 49:235–243

[66] Garland DE, Lucie RS, Waters RL. Current use of open phenol block for adult acquired spasticity. Clin Ortho Rel Res. 1982; 165:217–222

[67] Herz DA, Looman JE, Tiberio A, et al. The Management of Paralytic Spasticity. Neurosurgery. 1990; 26:300–306

[68] Padovani R, Tognetti F, Pozzati E, et al. The Treatment of Spasticity by Means of Dorsal Longitudinal Myelotomy and Lozenge-Shaped Griseotomy. Spine. 1982; 7:103–109

[69] Gornall P, Hitchcock E, Kirkland IS. Stereotaxic Neurosurgery in the Management of Cerebral Palsy. Dev Med Child Neurol. 1975; 17:279–286

[70] Scott BA, Weinstein J, Chiteman R, et al. Intrathecal Phenol and Glycerin in Metrizamide for Treatment of Intractable Spasms in Paraplegia. J Neurosurg. 1985; 63:125–127

[71] McCarty CS. The Treatment of Spastic Paraplegia by Selective Spinal Cordectomy. J Neurosurg. 1954; 11:539–545

[72] Durward QJ, Rice GP, Ball MJ, et al. Selective Spinal Cordectomy: Clinicopathological Correlation. J Neurosurg. 1982; 56:359–367

[73] Albright AL, Cervi A, Singletary J. Intrathecal Baclofen for Spasticity in Cerebral Palsy. JAMA. 1991; 265:1418–1422

[74] Penn RD. Intrathecal Baclofen for Spasticity of Spinal Origin: Seven Years of Experience. J Neurosurg. 1992; 77:236–240

[75] Coffey RJ, Cahill D, Steers W, et al. Intrathecal Baclofen for Intractable Spasticity of Spinal Origin: Results of a Long-Term Multicenter Study. J Neurosurg. 1993; 78:226–232

[76] Albright AL, Barron WB, Fasick P, et al. Continuous Intrathecal Baclofen Infusion for Spasticity of Cerebral Origin. Journal of the American Medical Association. 1993; 270:2475–2477

[77] Meythaler JM, Guin-Renfroe S, Brunner RC, et al. Intrathecal baclofen for spastic hypertonia from stroke. Stroke. 2001; 32:2099–2119

[78] Coffey RJ, Edgar TS, Francisco GE, et al. Abrupt withdrawal from intrathecal baclofen: Recognition and management of a potentially life-threatening syndrome. Archives of Physical Medicine and Rehabilitation. 2002; 83:735–741

[79] Boster A, Nicholas J, Bartoszek MP, et al. Managing loss of intrathecal baclofen efficacy: Review of the literature and proposed troubleshooting algorithm. Neurol Clin Pract. 2014; 4:123–130

[80] Meythaler JM, Roper JF, Brunner RC. Cyproheptadine for intrathecal baclofen withdrawal. Archive of Physical Medicine and Rehabilitation. 2003; 84:638–642

[81] Grunt S, Fieggen AG, Vermeulen RJ, et al. Selection criteria for selective dorsal rhizotomy in children with spastic cerebral palsy: a systematic review of the literature. Dev Med Child Neurol. 2014; 56:302–312

[82] Palisano R, Rosenbaum P, Walter S, et al. Development and reliability of a system to classify gross motor function in children with cerebral palsy. Dev Med Child Neurol. 1997; 39:214–223

[83] Cerebral Palsy Alliance. Gross Motor Function Classification System (GMFCS). 2017. https://research.cerebralpalsy.org.au/what-is-cerebral-palsy/severity-of-cerebral-palsy/gross-motor-function-classification-system/

[84] Park TS, Johnston JM. Surgical techniques of selective dorsal rhizotomy for spastic cerebral palsy. Technical note. Neurosurg Focus. 2006; 21

[85] Steinbok P. Selective dorsal rhizotomy for spastic cerebral palsy: a review. Childs Nerv Syst. 2007; 23:981–990

[86] Armstrong RW. The first meta-analysis of randomized controlled surgical trials in cerebral palsy (2002). Dev Med Child Neurol. 2008; 50. DOI: 10.111/j.1469-8749.2008.00244.x

[87] Bolster EA, van Schie PE, Becher JG, et al. Long-term effect of selective dorsal rhizotomy on gross motor function in ambulant children with spastic bilateral cerebral palsy, compared with reference centiles. Dev Med Child Neurol. 2013; 55:610–616

[88] Josenby AL, Wagner P, Jarnlo GB, et al. Functional performance in self-care and mobility after selective dorsal rhizotomy: a 10-year practice-based follow-up study. Dev Med Child Neurol. 2012; 57:286–293

[89] Park TS, Edwards C, Liu JL, et al. Beneficial Effects of Childhood Selective Dorsal Rhizotomy in Adulthood. Cureus. 2017; 9. DOI: 10.7759/cureus.1077

[90] Balmer GA, MacEwen GD. The incidence and treatment of scoliosis in cerebral palsy. J Bone Joint Surg Br. 1970; 52:134–137

[91] Bay JW. Management of Essential Hyperhidrosis. Contemp Neurosurg. 1988; 10:1–5

[92] Strutton DR, Kowalski JW, Glaser DA, et al. US prevalence of hyperhidrosis and impact on individuals with axillary hyperhidrosis: results from a national survey. J Am Acad Dermatol. 2004; 51:241–248

[93] Kao M-C. Video Endoscopic Sympathectomy Using a Fiberoptic CO2 Laser to Treat Palmar Hyperhidrosis. Neurosurgery. 1992; 30:131–135

[94] Dohn DF, Sava GM. Sympathectomy for Vascular Syndromes and Hyperhidrosis of the Upper Extremities. Clinical Neurosurgery. 1978; 25:637–650

[95] Wilkinson HA. Percutaneous radiofrequency upper thoracic sympathectomy: A new technique. Neurosurgery. 1984; 15:811–814

[96] Wilkinson HA. Percutaneous Radiofrequency Upper Thoracic Sympathectomy. Neurosurgery. 1996; 38:715–725

[97] Lee KH, Hwang PYK. Video Endoscopic Sympathectomy for Palmar Hyperhidrosis. Journal of Neurosurgery. 1996; 84:484–486

112 Neurovascular Compression Syndromes

112.1 General information

Syndromes due to compression of cranial nerves at the root entry zone (REZ) (or in the case of motor nerves, root exit zone) typically by an adjacent artery. The REZ (AKA Obersteiner-Redlich zone) is the point where central myelin (from oligodendroglial cells) changes to peripheral myelin (from Schwann cells).

A neurovascular compression syndrome has been described for cranial nerves V, VII, VIII, IX, X, and XI as shown in ▶ Table 112.1.

Table 112.1 Neurovascular compression syndromes

Cranial nerve	Syndrome	Typical offending vessel
V	trigeminal neuralgia	superior cerebellar artery (SCA)
VII (facial nerve proper)	hemifacial spasm (p. 1870)	
VII (nervus intermedius)	geniculate neuralgia (p. 1873)	anterior inferior cerebellar artery (AICA)
VIII	disabling positional vertigo (p. 1873)	
IX	glossopharyngeal neuralgia (p. 1873)	posterior inferior cerebellar artery (PICA)
X	superior laryngeal neuralgia (p. 1874)	PICA or VA
XI	torticollis of XI nerve origin (p. 1845)	VA or (rarely) PICA

112.2 Trigeminal neuralgia

112.2.1 General information

Key concepts

- sharp, electric shock-like paroxysmal lancinating pain in the distribution of one or more branches of the trigeminal nerve on one side
- characterized by periods of remission and initial response to carbamazepine
- neurologic exam must be intact (only exception: mild sensory loss)
- 80–90% of cases are caused by compression of the trigeminal nerve at the root entry zone by the superior cerebellar artery. In MS patients, may be due to MS plaque (MS patients are usually less responsive to procedures)
- 75% will ultimately fail medical therapy and require a procedure (main options: microvascular decompression, percutaneous rhizotomy, or radiosurgery). Choice of modality depends on patient age, location of symptoms, prior treatment and the side effect profile of the treatment modality

Trigeminal neuralgia (TGN) (AKA tic douloureux): paroxysmal lancinating electric-like pain lasting a few seconds, often triggered by sensory stimuli, confined to the distribution of one or more branches of the trigeminal nerve (▶ Fig. 112.1) on one side of the face, with no neurologic deficit.

Atypical facial pain (AFP): this term is sometimes used to describe any other type of facial pain. Some of these conditions may mimic TGN, but have features inconsistent with TGN, such as: constant pain, hyperactive autonomic dysfunction, hypesthesia to pinprick. The term "atypical trigeminal neuralgia" should be avoided.

Rarely, TGN manifests as status trigeminus, a rapid succession of tic-like spasms triggered by seemingly any stimulus. IV carbamazepine (where available) or phenytoin may be effective for this.

112

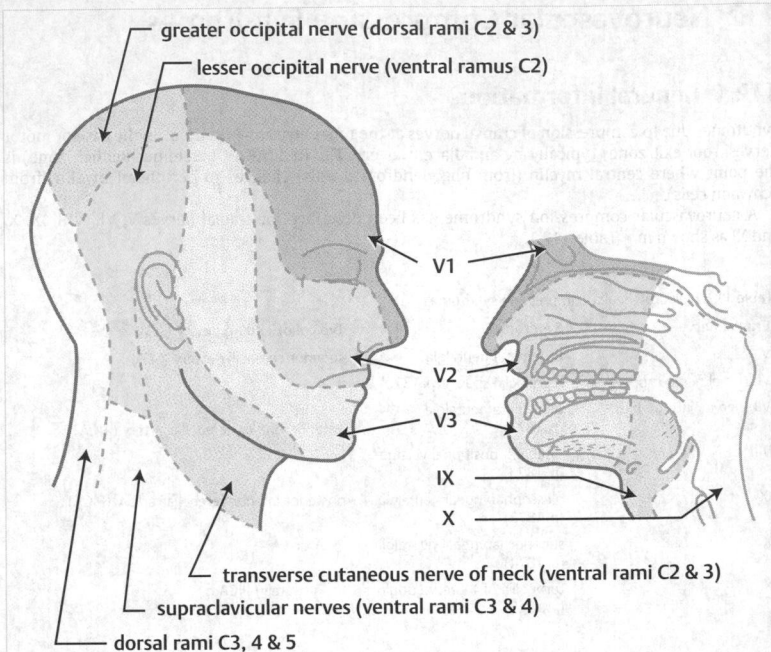

greater occipital nerve (dorsal rami C2 & 3)

lesser occipital nerve (ventral ramus C2)

V1

V2

V3

IX

X

transverse cutaneous nerve of neck (ventral rami C2 & 3)

supraclavicular nerves (ventral rami C3 & 4)

dorsal rami C3, 4 & 5

Fig. 112.1 Pain/temperature innervation of the head*.
* KEY: V = branches of the trigeminal nerve (V1 = ophthalmic nerve; V2 = maxillary nerve; V3 = mandibular nerve);
IX = glossopharyngeal nerve; X = vagus nerve.

112

112.2.2 Applied anatomy

The trigeminal nerve is a mixed motor and sensory cranial nerve. The major branch (portio major) penetrates the pons and conveys pain, touch, and temperature sensation (but not taste) of cutaneous and deep facial structures (the dermatomal distribution of sensation is shown in ► Fig. 112.1) as well as special visceral afferents (*not* motor fibers) subserving proprioception of mastication muscles.

The motor branch (portio minor) exits the pons immediately adjacent to the portio major, and controls 4 of the muscles of mastication and the tensor tympani, tensor palatini, mylohyoid, and the anterior belly of the digastric.

The nerve traverses the cerebellopontine angle cistern (where it can come into proximity of the superior cerebellar artery which can be a source of trigeminal neuralgia) as it crosses between the pons and Meckel's cave.

Meckel's cave is a space between two layers of dura (dura propria and periosteal layers) located in the anterior petrous apex (shown on MRI in ► Fig. 99.7) that normally measures ≈ 4 X 9 mm wide X 15 mm long.[1] It rests in a depression of the petrous bone (impressio trigemini) and houses the trigeminal cistern, a subarachnoid CSF containing space, which in turn contains the Gasserian ganglion (AKA semilunar ganglion) wherein the cell bodies of the sensory portion of the trigeminal nerve reside. The entrance to the cave is the porus trigeminus. Distal to the Gasserian ganglion, the trigeminal nerve trifurcates into the ophthalmic division (V1), mandibular division (V3), and the maxillary division (V2). V1 & V2 pass through the cavernous sinus to exit the skull through the superior orbital fissure (V1) and foramen rotundum (V2). V3 does not enter the cavernous sinus, and exits the skull through the foramen ovale. See abnormalities within Meckel's cave (p.1660), some of which can rarely cause trigeminal neuralgia.

112.2.3 Epidemiology

See ▸ Table 112.2. Annual incidence 4/100,000. There is no correlation with herpes simplex infection.[2] There is a tendency for spontaneous remission, with pain-free intervals of weeks or months being characteristic, regardless of treatment. 2% of patients with MS have TGN,[3] whereas ≈ 18% of patients with bilateral trigeminal neuralgia have MS.[4]

Table 112.2 Epidemiology of trigeminal neuralgia[5,6]

age (years)	typically > 50 (average 63)
female:male	1.8:1
Laterality	
right	60%
left	39%
both	1%
Division involved	
V1 only	2%
V2 only	20%
V3 only	17%
V1 & V2	14%
V2 & V3	42%
all three	5%

112.2.4 Pathophysiology

Probably due to ephaptic transmission in trigeminal nerve from large-diameter partially demyelinated A fibers to thinly myelinated A-delta and C (nociceptive) fibers. Pathogenesis may be due to:

1. vascular compression of the trigeminal nerve at the root entry zone (NB: compression may be seen in up to 50% of autopsies in patients without TGN[7]):
   a) most commonly (80%) by the SCA; see Neurovascular compression syndromes (p.1857) for more details
   b) persistent primitive trigeminal artery (p.83) [8]
   c) dolichoectatic basilar artery[9](p 1108)
2. posterior fossa tumor (see below)
3. in MS, plaque within brainstem may cause TGN that is often poorly responsive to microvascular decompression

In addition to the sensory division of the trigeminal nerve, other possible pain pathways include[10]: the motor branch of the 5th nerve (portio minor), or the 7th or 8th nerve.

112.2.5 Tumors and trigeminal neuralgia

In > 2000 patients with facial pain seen over 10 yrs, only 16 harbored tumor (< 0.8% incidence).[11] 5 tumors outside cranial vault included nasal carcinoma and skull base mets; all had hypalgesia and atypical facial pain (AFP). 6 middle fossa tumors included 2 meningiomas, 2 schwannomas (1 primary tumor of Gasserian ganglion), and 1 PitNET/adenoma. Posterior fossa tumors are the most likely to cause symptoms that most closely resemble true TGN; of these, vestibular schwannoma (VS) is most common. 2 of 7 VSs had tumors contralateral to the neuralgia (presumably due to brainstem shift). Patients with true TGN initially responded to carbamazepine, none with AFP did.

When facial pain is caused by tumor, especially with peripheral tumors, the pain is frequently atypical (usually constant), neurologic abnormalities are often present (usually sensory loss, although some are neurologically normal at first), and the age is often younger than typical TGN.

112.2.6 Differential diagnosis

See Craniofacial pain syndromes (p.519).

112

112.2.7 Evaluation

History and physical (in addition to routine):

1. history
   a) accurate description of pain localization to determine which divisions of trigeminal nerve need to be treated
   b) determine time of onset of TGN, trigger mechanisms
   c) ascertain presence and length of pain-free intervals (lack of any pain-free interval is atypical for TGN)
   d) determine duration, side effects, dosages, and responses to medications tried
   e) inquire about symptoms that may indicate the presence of conditions other than TGN: e.g., history of herpetic vesicles, excessive tearing of the eye (may indicate SUNCT (p. 520)), facial twitching (tic convulsif), tongue pain (glossopharyngeal neuralgia), sensory loss (tumor…), progressive relentless pain (tumor, herpes…), symptoms that suggest MS
2. physical exam: the exam should be normal in TGN, any neurologic deficit (except very mild sensory loss) in previously unoperated patient should prompt search for structural cause, e.g., tumor (see below). This exam also serves as a baseline for post-op comparison
   a) assess sensation in all 3 divisions of trigeminal nerve bilaterally (include corneal reflexes)
   b) assess masseter function (bite) and pterygoid function (on opening mouth, chin deviates to weak side)
   c) assess EOM function

112.2.8 Imaging

MRI is often used to evaluate these patients for possible intracranial tumors or MS plaques, especially in cases with atypical features. The yield in typical cases is low.

112.2.9 Medical therapy for trigeminal neuralgia

Drug info: Carbamazepine (Tegretol®)

Complete or acceptable relief in 69% (if 600–800 mg/d are tolerated and give no relief, diagnosis of TGN is suspect[3]). **Side effects:** Drowsiness. Rash in 5–10%. Possible Stevens-Johnson syndrome. Relative leukopenia is common (usually does not require discontinuing drug). See precautions under carbamazepine (**CBZ**, Tegretol®) (p. 491).

℞ 100 mg PO BID, increase by 200 mg/d up to maximum of 1200 mg/d divided TID. **Supplied:** See supply information (p. 491).

Drug info: Oxcarbazepine (Trileptal®)

Rapidly metabolized to carbamazepine, similar efficacy, often tolerated at higher doses than carbamazepine. **Side effects:** symptomatic hyponatremia.

℞ for trigeminal neuralgia: 300 mg PO BID, increase by 600 mg/d q week. Usual dose: 450–1200 mg. Maximum of 2400 mg/d. **Supplied:** 150, 300, 600 mg tablets; 500 mg/5-ml suspension.

Drug info: Baclofen (Lioresal®)

2nd DOC (not as effective as carbamazepine, but fewer side effects). Caution: teratogenic in rats. Avoid abrupt withdrawal (can cause hallucinations and seizures). May be more effective if used in conjunction with low-dose carbamazepine.

℞ Start low, 5 mg PO TID, increase q 3 d by 5 mg/dose; not to exceed 20 mg QID (80 mg/d); use smallest effective dose.

Drug info: Gabapentin (Neurontin®)

An antiseizure medication, may act synergistically with carbamazepine and baclofen. **Side effects:** include ataxia, sedation and rash.

℞ start with 100 mg PO BID, titrate to 5–7 mg/kg/day (3600 mg/d max).

12.2.10 Miscellaneous drugs

Also possibly effective:

1. phenytoin (Dilantin®): may be useful IV in patients in too much pain to open their mouths to take carbamazepine orally
2. capsaicin (Zostrix®): 1 gm applied TID for several days resulted in remission of symptoms in 10 of 12 patients (4 relapsed in < 4 mos, but remained pain-free for 1 yr after 2nd course)[12]
3. clonazepam (Klonopin®) (p.495): works in 25%
4. lamotrigine (Lamictal®)
5. amitriptyline (Elavil®): more commonly used for atypical facial pain
6. botulinum **toxin** (Botox®): reduces transmission of CGRP, producing a direct effect on the sensory nerve fibers
7. intranasal lidocaine spray (2 metered sprays of 0.1 ml of 8%, or 4 sprays of 4%) into the nostril on the affected side with the patient positioned supine with HOB 30–45° (and remaining in that position for 30 seconds) may provide temporary relief (approximately 4 hours) for V2 TGN by blocking V2 as it passes through the sphenopalatine ganglion (SPG) posterior to the middle turbinate[13]

12.2.11 Surgical therapy for trigeminal neuralgia

Indications for surgery

Reserved for cases refractory to medical management, or when side effects of medications exceed risks and drawbacks of surgery.

Surgical options

1. peripheral trigeminal nerve branch procedures to block or ablate the division involved with *pain*, or can be used to block the trigger[14]:
   a) means of blocking
      • local blocks (phenol, alcohol)
      • neurectomy of trigeminal branch involved
   b) nerve branches:
      • V1 (ophthalmic division) at the supraorbital, supratrochlear, or infraorbital nerves
      • V2 (maxillary division) at the foramen rotundum
      • V3 (mandibular division) block at the foramen ovale, or neurectomy of inferior dental nerve

   blocking the *trigger*: either via percutaneous rhizotomy or alcohol block
   percutaneous trigeminal rhizotomy (PTR): AKA percutaneous (stereotactic) rhizotomy (PSR) of trigeminal (Gasserian) ganglion (see below) (not truly a stereotactic procedure in the current sense of the word, therefore the term percutaneous trigeminal rhizotomy is preferred). Objective is to selectively destroy A-delta and C fibers (nociceptive) while preserving A-alpha and beta fibers (touch). Ideally, a retrogasserian lesion (not a ganglionic lesion). May also be used to block trigger. Lesioning techniques include (see below for comparison of techniques):
   a) *radiofrequency* rhizotomy (RFR) (originated by Sweet and Wespic[15]). Uses radiofrequency energy to thermocoagulate the pain fibers. Requires the patient to be awake at intervals during the procedure
   b) *glycerol* injection into Meckel's cave[16,17]: possibly lower incidence of sensory loss and anesthesia dolorosa than with radiofrequency lesion.[18] Water-soluble contrast cisternography was recommended in original description, may not be essential[19]
   c) mechanotrauma (percutaneous microcompression (PMC) rhizolysis): via inflation of No. 4 Fogarty catheter balloon.[20,21,22] Does not require the patient to be awake
   d) injection of sterile boiling water

4. Spiller-Frazier subtemporal extradural approach with retrogasserian rhizotomy (rarely used today). Original Spiller-Frazier technique involved avulsion of the nerve, which had an unacceptably high risk of bleeding. Subsequently, the same exposure was used with partial sectioning of the nerve or just mildly traumatizing the ganglion
5. intradural retrogasserian trigeminal nerve section (sensory portion ± motor root, see below): may be performed during MVD if no vascular compression is identified
6. cutting descending trigeminal tract in lower medulla (99.5% success): rarely used
7. microvascular decompression (MVD)[23]: (see below) microsurgical exploration of root entry zone, usually via posterior fossa craniectomy, and displacement of vessel impinging on nerve (if such a vessel is found). Usually with the placement of a non-absorbable "insulator" (Ivalon® sponge or shredded Teflon felt; see relative merits of Ivalon® vs. Teflon felt (p. 1872)
8. complete section of the nerve proximal to the ganglion via a p-fossa crani
9. stereotactic radiosurgery (p. 1864)
10. motor cortex stimulation[24]: (somewhat analogous to spinal cord stimulation for spinal or extremity pain). Better for neuropathic trigeminal pain (as distinct from trigeminal neuralgia)

Selection of surgical option

Some pearls that influence treatment option choices (expert opinion[25]):
1. V3 neuralgia: RF. Can selectively treat V3 without involving other divisions
2. V1 or V2: balloon compression. Causes numbness in all 3 divisions, but unlike the lesion with RF the corneal numbness is better tolerated and the corneal reflex is often preserved
3. bilateral pain: glycerol. It has the shortest duration of effect, which is an advantage if you think you may need to treat the other side at some point
4. SRS: due to latency until pain relief, suboptimal for patients who need immediate pain relief

Peripheral nerve ablation and neurectomies

Limited to pain or trigger points in territory of supraorbital/supratrochlear, infraorbital, or inferio dental nerves. Neurectomy may be a consideration especially for elderly patients who are not candi dates for MVD (neurectomy may be done under local anesthesia) with pain in the forehead (to avoi anesthesia of the eye, as could occur with RFR). Disadvantages include sensory loss in the distribu tion of the nerve and a high rate of pain recurrence due to nerve regeneration (usually in 18–3 months) which often responds to repeat neurectomy.[26] May also be used following PTR.

Supraorbital and supratrochlear nerve: See also information on supraorbital neuralgia (SON) c supratrochelar neuralgia (STN) (p. 521). SON may be treated with rhizotomy (e.g., with alcohol o radiofrequency) or with neurectomy. Alcohol injection is used with caution for STN because of ris of injury to the superior oblique muscle. For neurectomy, these nerves are exposed through a 2 cr incision parallel to and just above the medial portion of the eyebrow (never through the eyebrow a this can create an unsightly "bi-brow"; shaving the eyebrow is also discouraged since it occasionall does not grow back). The incision is carried down to the bone and the periosteum is elevated cau dally towards the supraorbital foramen or notch. The nerves will be visible on the undersurface the periosteal flap. The supraorbital nerve is freed in its foramen/notch, and is then avulsed b grasping it with a mosquito hemostat and twisting the clamp. The nerve avulses "like pulling worm out of a hole." The distal portion of the nerve should be located at the site where the perios teum was incised and it, too, should be avulsed. The process can be repeated for the more mediall situated supratrochlear nerve.

Other nerves: Not covered here, other nerve branches that may be cut or avulsed include: infra trochlear, lacrimal (the branch of V1 at the lateral edge of the orbit), infraorbital nerve, inferio alveolar, lingual and mental nerves.[27 (p 290)]

Percutaneous trigeminal rhizotomy (PTR)

Recommended for patients who: are poor risk for general anesthesia (elderly or those with increase risk for general anesthesia), wish to avoid "major" surgery, have unresectable intracranial tumor have MS, have impaired hearing on the other side, or have limited life expectancy (<5 yrs).[18] F "atypical facial pain," denervating the painful region of the face benefits <20% of patients, and wo sens 20%.[28] Recurrences are easily treated by repeat procedures. May be used to treat failures peripheral nerve ablation.

▶ **Choice of lesion technique.** Recurrence rates and incidence of dysesthesias are comparab among the various lesioning techniques. Incidence of intraoperative hypertension is less wi percutaneous microcompression (PMC) than with radiofrequency rhizotomy (RFR) lesion[22] (no reports of intracerebral hemorrhage).

RFR requires a patient who is able to cooperate; PMC can be done with the patient asleep. Paralysis of ipsilateral trigeminal motor root (e.g., pterygoids) is more common after PMC (usually temporary) than RFR, and so PMC should not be done if there is already contralateral paralysis from a previous procedure. See also description of technique (p. 1865).

Bradycardia may occur with any of the percutaneous rhizotomy techniques. It is usually not harmful, however, preparation for possible symptomatic bradycardia should routinely include:

1. place defibrillator leads on chest prior to beginning procedure
2. have atropine available (some surgeons administer atropine prophylactically[29])
3. have crash cart available

Complications with percutaneous radiofrequency (note: some "numbness" is actually expected in most successful PTRs and occurs in 98% of cases,[6] and is not considered a complication here):

1. mortality: only 17 deaths in over 22,000 procedures (includes less experienced neurosurgeons and patients often considered poor surgical risks)[3]
2. dysesthesias[6] (sometimes called "annoying paresthesias"): higher rate in more complete lesions
   a) minor: 9%
   b) major (requiring medical treatment): 2%
   c) anesthesia dolorosa (severe, constant, burning aching pain that is refractory to all treatment): 0.2–4%
3. meningitis[5]: 0.3%
4. alterations in salivation[30]: 20% (increased in 17%, decreased in 3%)
5. partial masseter weakness (usually not perceived by patient, ▶ Table 112.3)
6. oculomotor paresis (usually temporary, ▶ Table 112.3)
7. reduced hearing (secondary to paresis of tensor tympani, ▶ Table 112.3)
8. **neuroparalytic keratitis** (keratitis due to fifth nerve deficit which impairs sensation, ▶ Table 112.3)

Table 112.3 Complications with percutaneous radiofrequency

Complication	850 cases[40]		315 cases[30]
	straight electrode (N = 700)	curved electrode (N = 150)	
partial masseter weakness (usually not perceived by patient)	15–24%	7%	50%
oculomotor paresis (usually temporary)	2%	0	
reduced hearing (secondary to paresis of tensor tympani)	0	0	27%
neuroparalytic keratitis (keratitis due to fifth nerve deficit which impairs sensation)	4%	2%	0

9. intracranial hemorrhage: personal report of 7 cases (6 fatal) in > 14,000 procedures, probably due to transient HTN (SBP up to 300 torr)
10. alterations in lacrimation[30]: 20% (increased in 17%, decreased in 3%)
11. herpes simplex eruption: prescribe antiherpetic drug if patient develops symptoms, e.g., Acyclovir® (p. 399).
12. bradycardia and hypotension: 1% with RFR compared to up to 15% with glycerol injection
13. rare[31,32]:
    a) temporal lobe abscess
    b) aseptic meningitis
    c) intracerebral abscess: 0.1%
    d) trigeminal trophic syndrome (TTS)[33]: triad of unilateral crescentic nasal alar ulceration with anesthesia and paresthesia of the trigeminal dermatome (may present with severe pruritus and self-induced skin lesions from scratching). A result of trigeminal nerve injury. Treatment has included: carbamazepine, diazepam, amitriptyline, chlorpromazine, clonazepam or pimozide[34]
    e) complications related to needle placement[35]:
       • carotid-cavernous fistula (CCF): may occur with any percutaneous technique[36] (including balloon microcompression[37])

112

- blindness: from penetration of inferior orbital fissure[38]
- injury to other cranial nerves: II, III, IV, VI[39]

f) subarachnoid hemorrhage

g) seizures

Microvascular decompression (MVD)

See also more detailed information (p. 1867).

Recommended for patients with inadequate medical control of pain with > 5 years anticipated survival and able to tolerate a small craniotomy[18] (surgical morbidity increases with age). Relief is often long lived, persevering 10 yrs in 70%. Incidence of facial anesthesia is much less than with PTR, and anesthesia dolorosa does not occur. Mortality: < 1%. Incidence of aseptic meningitis (AKA hemogenic meningitis): 20%. 1–10% major neurologic morbidity. Failure rate: 20–25%.

1–2% of patients with MS will have a demyelinating plaque at the root entry zone; this usually does not respond to MVD, and one should attempt a PTR.

Stereotactic radiosurgery (SRS)

The first use of SRS by Leksell was for the treatment of TGN. Initially, this was reserved for refractory cases following multiple operations,[41] now becoming more widely practiced. SRS is the least invasive procedure. Generally recommended for patients with co-morbidities, high-risk medical illness, pain refractory to prior surgical procedures, or those on anticoagulants (anticoagulation does not have to be reversed to have SRS).

Treatment plan: 4–5 mm isocenter in the trigeminal nerve root entry zone identified on MRI. Use 70–80 Gy at the *center,* keeping the 80% isodose curve outside of the brainstem.

Results: Significant pain reduction after initial SRS: 80–96%,[42,43,44,45] but only ≈ 65% become pain free. Median latency to pain relief: 3 months (range: 1 d–13 months).[46] Recurrent pain occurs within three years in 10–25%. Patients with TN and multiple sclerosis are less likely to respond to SRS than those without MS. SRS can be repeated, but only after four months following the original procedure.

Favorable prognosticators: higher radiation doses, previously unoperated patient, absence of atypical pain component, normal pre-treatment sensory function.[47]

Side effects: Hypesthesia occurred in 20% after initial SRS, and in 32% of those requiring repeat treatment[46] (higher rates associated with higher radiation doses[43]).

Management of surgical treatment failures

90% of recurrences are in distribution of previously involved divisions; 10% are in new division and may represent progression of the underlying process. Some treatment failures are not persistent TN but rather represent trigeminal neuropathic pain (AKA trigeminal deafferentation pain).

PTR may be repeated in patients who have a recurrence with some preservation of facial sensation. Attempted repeat PTR is often productive, and failures can be managed as below.

MVD may be performed in patients failing PTR, but the success rate may be reduced[48] (91% for patients undergoing MVD first, vs. 43% for those having MVD following PTR; note: 91% may be an unrealistically high success rate, and taking patients that fail PTR may select for a more difficult sub group). Repeat MVD may also be performed, with attention given to possible slippage of the insulating sponge, or the fact that the true offending vessel may be "artificially" moved away from the nerve secondary to the surgical positioning.

SRS can be repeated, using the same dose, with reported significant reduction in pain in 89%, and complete relief in 58%.[46]

Intradural retrogasserian trigeminal nerve section

May be used as a measure of last resort in patients who have recurrent TGN following one or more PTRs in the presence of total facial anesthesia, or in patients undergoing posterior-fossa craniectomy for the purpose of MVD when no impinging vessel can be identified. In the latter case, partial rhizotomy is performed by sectioning 2/3 of the nerve, with resulting partial anesthesia. In the case of patients with facial anesthesia pre-op, consideration should be given to sectioning the motor division (portio minor) as an alternate pain pathway.[10]

112.2.12 Percutaneous trigeminal rhizotomy (PTR)

Due to concerns about hemorrhage, check coagulation profile (PT/PTT, consider bleeding time), and discontinue ASA and NSAIDs, preferably 10 days pre-op. Procedure may be performed in OR with fluoro, or in angiography suite in X-ray department.

Booking the case: Percutaneous trigeminal rhizotomy

(For any of the percutaneous methods: balloon, glycerol, RFR)
Also see defaults & disclaimers (p. 25) and pre-op orders (see below).
1. position: supine
2. anesthesia: MAC with sedation
3. equipment:
   a) lesion generator and needle kit for radiofrequency rhizotomy
   b) C-arm fluoroscopy (2 C-arms for balloon compression)
   c) calibrated inflatable balloons (as in kyphoplasty) for balloon rhizotomy
4. consent (in lay terms for the patient—not all-inclusive):
   a) procedure: put a needle into the cheek to numb the nerve to the face
   b) alternatives: medical treatment, surgery through the back of the skull (microvascular decompression), radiation (stereotactic radiosurgery)
   c) complications: facial numbness is anticipated, rarely: stroke, bleeding, blindness

Pre-op orders (RFR)

1. NPO after MN except meds
2. continue Tegretol® & other meds PO with sips of water
3. AM of procedure: IV NS @ KVO in arm contralateral to neuralgia
4. atropine 0.4 mg IM PRN (✖ contraindications include rapid a-fib)
5. non-disposable LP tray to accompany patient

Technique: Percutaneous trigeminal radiofrequency rhizotomy (RFR)

Adapted technique.[49]
NB: needle insertion and/or lesioning may cause HTN, consider monitoring BP. Use either a straight electrode (bare 5 mm for 1 division, 7.5 mm for 2 divisions, or 10 mm for total lesions) or a curved electrode.[40]

Electrode insertion
1. attach ground electrode to patient's upper arm
2. prep the cheek on the involved side with Betadine
3. entry point: under short-acting anesthetic agent—e.g., propofol (Diprivan®) (p. 140) or methohexital (Brevitol®) (p. 139)—insert electrode-needle 2.5–3 cm lateral to oral commissure
4. trajectory:
   a) palpate the buccal mucosa with a gloved finger inside the mouth (lateral to the teeth) and with the other hand pass the electrode medial to the coronoid process of the mandible (keeping the needle deep to the oral mucosa, i.e., outside the oral cavity), initially aiming towards the plane intersecting a point 3 cm anterior to EAM and the medial aspect of the pupil when the eye is directed forward. Be careful not to contaminate the field with the hand that was in the patient's mouth
   b) as insertion progresses, use fluoroscopy to direct the tip towards the intersection of the top of the petrous bone with the clivus (5–10 mm below floor of sella along clivus)
   c) upon entering foramen ovale the masseter often contracts, causing the jaw to briefly close. Remove the stylet, look for CSF to verify location (may not occur in re-do cases), and insert electrode through needle

In difficult cases, intraoperative fluoroscopy may assist in localizing the needle to Meckel's cave and to R/O e.g., entry into superior orbital fissure (which can cause blindness after lesioning), or entry into foramen spinosum (middle meningeal artery). If necessary to visualize (e.g., when there is difficulty entering), the foramen ovale is optimally seen on a submental X-ray by hyperextending neck 20° and rotating head 15–20° away from side of pain.[50]

Impedance measurements: from the tip of the electrode, when available, may help indicate location of needle tip. Impedance: CSF (or any fluid) low (≈ 40–120 Ω); connective tissue, muscle, or nerve is usually 200–300 Ω (may be up to 400 Ω); if > 400 Ω this likely indicates electrode is contacting periosteum or bone. After starting the lesion, impedance often goes down by 30 Ω transiently, and then as the lesioning continues it gradually returns to baseline or ≈ 20 Ω above it. If char develops on the electrode tip, the impedance will read higher than where it started.

112

Stimulation and repositioning

Once the foramen ovale is entered, the needle is positioned with the following guidelines: for V3 division lesion the curved electrode should be just short of the clivus and pointing down, for V2 it is at the clivus and directed up, for V1 it is 5 mm beyond clivus and pointing up. ✖ At no time should the needle tip extend > 8 mm beyond clival line (to avoid Cr. N. III or VI complications).

The patient is allowed to wake up and is stimulated through the electrode with the following settings: frequency = 50–75 Hz, 1 mS duration, start at 0.1 V amplitude and slowly increase (usually 0.2–0.5 V is adequate, higher voltages may indicate that the needle is not near the target and that stimulation is due to far-field currents; however, in previously lesioned patients up to 4 V may sometimes be necessary). If stimulation does not reproduce pain in the distribution of the patient's TGN, then the amplitude is returned to 0, the electrode is repositioned (straight electrode: advance needle < 5 mm at a time, until the tip is in the vicinity of the clival line; curved tip electrode: advance and/or rotate); then slowly elevate the voltage again from 0 and repeat the repositioning-stimulating process until stimulation reproduces the distribution of tic pain. If previous lesions have produced analgesia and the patient cannot feel the stimulating current, one may stimulate at 2 Hz and watch for masseter twitch (requires preserved motor root).

Lesioning

When stimulation produces pain in the involved distribution of the TGN, perform the first lesion under short-acting anesthesia at 60–70 °C × 90 sec. A facial flush may be noted.[50] After every lesion, perform a post-lesion assessment (see below). The goal is analgesia (but not anesthesia) in the areas of tic pain and hypalgesia in areas of trigger points. An average of three lesions are necessary at the first sitting, each ≈ 5 °C higher than the previous for 90 seconds. Anesthetic may not be needed after the first lesion if moderate analgesia has been produced by previous lesions.

Post-lesion assessment

After each lesion and at completion of procedure, assess:

1. sensitivity to pinprick and light touch in all three divisions of trigeminal nerve (grading: normal, hypalgesic, analgesic, anesthetic)
2. corneal reflex bilaterally
3. EOM function
4. masseter muscle strength (patient clenches teeth, palpate cheeks for contraction)
5. pterygoid muscle strength (ask patient to open mouth, chin deviates towards side of pterygoid weakness)

Post-op care (PTR)

Include in post-op orders:

1. ice pack to face on side of procedure for 4 hrs
2. soft diet
3. routine activity when alert
4. avoid narcotics (usually not necessary)
5. if corneal reflex impaired: risk of neuroparalytic keratitis. Natural tears 2 gtt q 2 hrs while awake to eye on affected side. Lacrilube® to eye & tape eye shut q hs

Prior to discharge from hospital, repeat post-lesion assessment (see above). Patients are then weaned off of carbamazepine as tolerated.

112.2.13 Percutaneous microcompression rhizolysis balloon (PMC)

Via inflation of No. 4 Fogarty catheter balloon.

Technique:

1. the needle is placed as with RFR (p. 1865).
2. aim for balloon placement in the medial foramen ovale (to avoid entering the middle fossa). After placing the balloon, insert the stylet to visualize where the balloon will go. Use Omnipaque 240 to fill the balloon
3. inflate to 1.4 atmospheres of pressure

112.2.14 Results

Results of various PTR techniques compared to microvascular decompression (MVD) are shown in ► Table 112.4. Recurrence rate is higher in patients with multiple sclerosis (50% at 3 yrs mean F/U).[5]

Table 112.4 Comparison of outcomes of percutaneous techniques to MVD

Parameter	Percutaneous techniques (PTR)			MVD
	RFR[a]	Glycerol	Balloon	
initial success rate[6,10]	91–99%	91%	93%	85–98%
medium-term recurrence rate	19% at 6 yrs[5]	54% at 4 yrs	21% at 2 yrs	15% in 5 yrs
long-term recurrence rate	80% at 12 yrs[30b]			30% at 10 yrs
facial numbness[6]	98%	60%	72%	2%

[a]abbreviations: RFR = radiofrequency rhizotomy; MVD = microvascular decompression; balloon = balloon microcompression

[b]this author included initial failures to PTR requiring repeat procedures during same hospitalization

112.2.15 Microvascular decompression (MVD) for trigeminal neuralgia

Indications

1. patients unable to achieve adequate medical control of trigeminal neuralgia with ≥ 5 yrs anticipated survival, without significant medical or surgical risk factors[18] (although a small p-fossa exploration is usually well-tolerated, surgical morbidity increases with age)
2. may be used in patients who do not fit the above criteria, but have intractable pain and fail PTR
3. patient with tic involving V1 for whom the risk of exposure keratitis due to corneal anesthesia would be unacceptable (e.g., already blind in contralateral eye) or patient wishing to avoid facial anesthesia for any reason
4. ✖ patients with MS are usually not considered candidates for MVD due to low response rate

Booking the case: Microvascular decompression

Also see defaults & disclaimers (p. 25) and pre-op preparation (see below).

1. position: park bench
2. equipment: microscope
3. implants: Ivalon sponge or shredded Teflon
4. intra-op monitoring: (optional) BAER, facial EMG (monitors VII and portio minor (motor) of VII), VIII (CNAP (compound nerve action potential) using Cueva electrode placed directly on VIII nerve referenced to ipsilateral earlobe)
5. consent (in lay terms for the patient—not all-inclusive):
   a) procedure: surgery behind the ear to move a blood vessel from the sensory nerve of the face, if no offending vessel can be identified then possible partial sectioning of the appropriate part of the trigeminal nerve with associated numbness)
   b) alternatives: needle procedures through the cheek (percutaneous rhizotomy), radiation (stereotactic radiosurgery)
   c) complications: (in addition to usual craniotomy complications (p. 25)), CSF leak, hearing loss (≈ 10%), facial numbness, pain near incision (occipital neuralgia or lesser occipital neuralgia), rarely: diplopia, facial paralysis, failure of the procedure

112

Technique

Also see Paramedian suboccipital craniectomy (p. 1740) for important pointers, including use of armored endotracheal tube.

Preoperative preparation

An MRI is recommended (with FIESTA sequence or equivalent, if available) to rule out mass lesion or vascular abnormality. Baseline BAER are performed by some[52] (see below for intra-op monitoring).

O.R. setup

Setup for lateral oblique suboccipital (posterior-fossa) craniotomy (p. 1738). Microscope: observer's eyepiece is placed on the side opposite to that of the tic.

Positioning
See reference.[53]
1. lateral oblique position (p. 1738), symptomatic side *up*, axillary roll
2. thorax elevated 10–15° to reduce venous pressure
3. 3-pin skull fixation. Head position:
   a) head rotation: head rotated 10–15° away from the affected side. Do not exceed 30° rotation
   b) lateral head tilt
      • for trigeminal neuralgia or VIII nerve approach: the head is parallel to the floor (if it is lower, nerves VII & VIII will obscure view of V)
      • for VII nerve or lower, the vertex is tilted 15° *down* from the horizontal
   c) flex neck: leave 2 fingerbreadths room between the chin and the sternum
4. upper shoulder retracted caudally with adhesive tape
5. option: lumbar spinal drain. Drain 20–30 cc during craniotomy, then drain off small amounts from time-to-time during the case to keep the field mostly dry, but occasionally letting CSF build up to bathe cranial nerves

Intraoperative monitoring
Option: intraoperative monitoring of facial EMG and BAER (assesses acoustic nerve).[52]

Approach
1. skin incision[53]: vertical incision 3–5 cm in length, 5 mm medial to mastoid notch, a small "5-6-4" incision (p. 1740); in thick or short-necked patients, a slightly longer incision that angles infero-medially is used. 75% of the incision is inferior to the transverse sinus, 25% superior
2. burr hole:
   a) 1 cm inferior and 1 cm medial to the asterion[54(p 60)]
   b) if the asterion is not easily identified or if there are concerns about the reliability of the asterion as a landmark for the junction of the transverse and sigmoid sinuses,[55] place the burr hole directly over the mastoid emissary vein which drains superolaterally into the sigmoid sinus
3. craniotomy: top of bone opening as close as possible to transverse sinus. The position of the transverse sinus can be approximated by a line drawn from the posterior base of the zygomatic process to the inion, or roughly ≈ 2 finger-breadths above the upper end of the mastoid notch. Lateral limit of bone opening is sigmoid sinus. A triangular bony opening with a leg along each sinus works well. Craniectomy diameter needs to be only ≈ 3 cm. Apply bone wax liberally (blocks off any possible opening into the mastoid air cells)
4. dural opening: either a curvilinear with each end at a sinus and the convexity *away* from the junction (Jannetta) or an inverted "T" (with one incision towards each sinus and the third towards junction of sinuses, lets you get as close as possible to the sinuses)
5. minimal or no retraction of cerebellum is usually required
6. allow CSF to drain before proceeding: this may require gentle advancement of a cottonoid in the CPA. A lumbar drain should be placed if CSF cannot be drained
7. follow the junction of tentorium with temporal bone deep. Place a retractor that both medially displaces the cerebellum *and* slightly "lifts" the cerebellum towards the surgeon (medial displacement alone is not as effective)
8. superior petrosal vein (SPV): drains to the superior petrosal sinus within the tentorial dura and often blocks access to Cr. N V (sometimes there is a venous complex of 2–3 veins). Coagulating and dividing the SPV is controversial,[56,57,58] with risks including cerebellar infarction, midbrain and pontine infarction (0–5%) and thus should be avoided if possible.[57,58] If the vein is torn, the dural side is tamponaded (sometimes up to 30 minutes is needed) while the free end is coagulated
9. V is deeper than the VII/VIII complex, which should not even be seen with this approach. If VII/VIII are seen, move the retractor superiorly as even gentle traction may cause hearing loss (▶ Fig. 1.11). In some cases the suprameatal tubercle (a small hillock of bone just posterior to Meckel's cave) may be large enough to obscure the site where the fifth nerve enters the cave and may need to be reduced with a diamond burr

Decompression of nerve
1. arachnoid overlying the fifth nerve is sharply divided (caution re Cr. N. IV, which follows the tentorial opening in the arachnoid rostral to the fifth nerve). Intra-op changes in BAER are often attributed to retraction of arachnoid that is tethered to the VII/VIII complex
2. the fifth nerve may be markedly atrophic if previous PTRs have been done

3. identify the smaller motor root (portio minor) of the fifth nerve
4. arteries and/or veins compressing V should be dissected off the nerve. NB: vessels located proximally are the most likely offenders; however, the dorsal root entry zone (which is the sensitive part of the nerve) may be variable in location and peripheral vessels may be culpable. The nerve should be inspected and freed of vessels from its origin at the brainstem all the way to its entrance into Meckel's cave.[53] Veins may be coagulated and then should be divided (to prevent recanalization)
5. the most common cause of compression is the superior cerebellar artery (SCA)
6. check the nerve at the junction with brainstem for any residual compression prior to the next step
7. insulating material is interposed between nerve and vessel to prevent re-compression. Options include:
    a) e.g., Ivalon® (polyvinyl formyl alcohol) sponge (Ivalon Surgical Products, 1040 OCL Parkway, Eudora, KS, 66025, U.S.A. distributed by Fabco in the U.S.A. (860) 536–8499, toll free: (888) 813–8214, http://fabco.net/catalog/ivalon-ophthalmic/) cut in a saddle shape. Note: if an Ivalon block is used instead of pre-packaged sterile pads, it must be rinsed thoroughly to remove formalin, then autoclaved. Ivalon should be hydrated in NS for 10 minutes prior to cutting it
    b) shredded Teflon felt; see merits of Ivalon® vs. Teflon or muscle (p. 1872)
8. Wilson recommends performing a partial sensory rhizotomy of the inferior one-half to two-thirds of the portio major for the following: cases where no vascular contact with the nerve or no deformity of the nerve is identified, in most cases of patients undergoing a repeat MVD, or for cases with duration of symptoms > 8–9 yrs, as this latter group tends to have a lower success rate with MVD alone[59]
9. if the procedure is for a failed MVD and it is desired to partially divide the nerve, the nerve is organized somatotopically with V1 fibers superiorly, and V3 inferiorly. If the goal is total elimination of pain pathways and there is concern about pain conduction through ancillary pathways, consider also dividing the motor root (portio minor)

Closure

. bone wax should be applied liberally to the exposed lateral bone edges (to paraphrase Dr. Jannetta[53] and Mr. Miyagi,[60] "Wax in, wax out.")
. irrigate gently with *warm* saline (avoid "jet" irrigation which can damage the VIII nerve)
. intra-op BAER decline may occur on dural closure and should prompt re-opening of the dura and checking for tension on the VIII nerve from a vessel or Telfa
. perform several Valsalva maneuvers to ensure watertight closure of dura
. the bone defect should be covered e.g., with burr hole cover to reduce chance of pain associated with uncovered craniectomy
. after fascial closure, Valsalva maneuver is performed again to ensure watertight closure
. use 4–0 running locked nylon to approximate skin in watertight fashion (avoid excessive tension)

Post-op care following MVD

Include in post-op orders

. admit to ICU
. arterial-line for continuous BP monitoring
. analgesics (e.g., codeine 30–60 mg IM q 3 hrs)
. anti-emetics (e.g., ondansetron 4 mg IV q 6 hrs)
. medication to aggressively treat HTN (viz. SBP > 160 mm Hg)

Post-op H/A, nausea, and pain

Patients routinely have H/A and nausea for 2–3 days (there tends to be less intracranial air and less "pneumoencephalogram sickness" if the park-bench position is used instead of the sitting position). However, *severe* H/A should prompt a STAT CT to R/O bleeding. If the CT is negative, severe H/A may be due to transient elevation of CSF pressure that occurs in some, and which usually responds to 1, or at most 2, LPs to halve the pressure. Aseptic meningitis usually responds to steroids. Some patients have continued but lessened tic douloureux pain for several days post-op; this usually subsides.[53]

Complications

The short list:
    cerebellar injury
    hearing loss
    CSF leak

The long list:
1. mortality: 0.22–2% in experienced hands (> 900 procedures)[61,62]
2. meningitis
   a) aseptic meningitis (AKA hemogenic meningitis): H/A, meningismus, mild fever, culture-negative CSF, pleocytosis. Incidence: ≈ 2% (up to 20% has been reported). Usually occurs 3–7 days post-op. Responds to LP + steroids
   b) bacterial meningitis: 0.9%
3. major neurologic morbidity: 1–10% (higher rates with less experienced surgeons), including:
   a) deafness: 1%
   b) vestibular nerve dysfunction
   c) facial nerve dysfunction
4. mild facial sensory loss: 25%
5. cranial nerve palsies[63]:
   a) fourth nerve (diplopia): 4.3% (only ≈ 0.1% are permanent)
   b) facial nerve: 1.6% (most are transient)
   c) eighth nerve (hearing loss): 3%
6. postoperative hemorrhage[64]: subdural, intracerebral (1%[6]), subarachnoid
7. seizures: including status epilepticus[64]
8. infarction[64]: including posterior cerebral artery distribution, brainstem
9. CSF leak: resolves with lumbar drainage in most cases
10. pneumonia: 0.6%

Outcome
1. success rate: 75–80% (rates may be lower in patients having prior destructive procedure); good but not total relief in an additional ≈ 10%
2. recurrence rate in large series is difficult to ascertain from literature; in a series of 40 patients followed 8.5 yrs mean[62]:
   a) major recurrence (recurrent tic not controlled by medications) rate: 31%
   b) minor recurrence (mild or controlled by medications) rate: 17%
   c) using Kaplan-Meier curve, expect 70% to be either pain-free or have minor recurrence by 8.5 years (or ≈ 80% at 5 years)
      • the risk for a *major* recurrence after MVD is 3.5% annually
      • the risk for a *minor* recurrence after MVD is 1.5% annually
   d) major recurrence rate is lower for patients having major arterial cross-compression of the nerve discovered at the time of surgery (patients with venous compression had much higher rate)
   e) this study found no correlation between previous destructive surgery and major recurrence rate (in 11 patients)

Some feel that the longer one waits before performing an MVD, the lower the success rate.

112.3 Hemifacial spasm

112.3.1 General information

Key concepts

- intermittent unilateral painless contractions of facial muscles
- typically caused by compression of VII nerve by AICA
- along with palatal myoclonus: the only movement disorder that persists in sleep
- responds well to microvascular decompression, but risk of hearing loss is ≈ 20%

Hemifacial spasm (HFS) is a condition of intermittent, painless, involuntary, spasmodic contraction of muscles innervated by the facial nerve in one side of the face only. May be limited to the upper or lower half of the face only, and excess lacrimation may be present. HFS usually begins with rare contractions of the orbicularis oculi, and slowly progresses to involve the entire half of the face and increases in frequency until the ability to see out of the affected eye is impaired.

HFS may be associated with trigeminal neuralgia, geniculate neuralgia; see **Tic convulsif** (p. 1873), or vestibular and/or cochlear[65] nerve dysfunction.

HFS is more common in women, is seen more often on the left, and usually presents after the teenage years. Auditory function testing reveals abnormal acoustic middle ear reflex in almost half of patients, indicating some degree of VIII compromise.[65]

Meige's syndrome: hemifacial spasm with oral movements.

► **Note.** HFS and palatal myoclonus are the only involuntary movement disorders that persist during sleep.[66]

112.3.2 Etiologies

1. vascular compression syndrome (see below): the most common etiology (much more common than with trigeminal neuralgia)
2. idiopathic
3. tumor compressing the nerve
4. can follow some cases of Bell's palsy
5. conditions that can mimic HFS
   a) blepharospasm (bilateral spasmodic closure of the orbicularis oculi muscles) which is more common in the elderly, and may be associated with organic brain syndrome. Blepharospasm is notorious for disappearing when the patient presents for medical evaluation (an effect of alerting), but may be elicited by asking the patient to gently close the eyes and then rapidly open them, following which a blepharospasm may occur. HFS usually involves more than the ocular muscles
   b) facial myokymia: continuous facial spasm which may be a manifestation of an intrinsic brainstem glioma or of multiple sclerosis. Often associated with other findings

112.3.3 Vascular compression

HFS is usually caused by compression of the facial nerve at the root exit zone (REZ) by a vessel, which is most often an artery (most commonly *AICA*[67] (either pre- or postmeatal[68]), but other vascular possibilities include an elongated PICA, SCA, a tortuous VA, the cochlear artery, a dolichoectatic basilar artery, AICA branches…), aneurysm, a vascular malformation, and rarely, veins have been implicated. In typical HFS (onset in the orbicularis oculi, and progressing downward over the face), the vessel impinges on the antero-caudal aspect of the VII/VIII nerve complex; in atypical HFS (beginning in the buccal muscles and progressing upward over the face), the compression is rostral or posterior to VII.[69]

Vessels contacting the REZ of the vestibular nerve may cause vertigo, whereas tinnitus or hearing loss may result from cochlear nerve REZ compression.

Infrequently, benign tumors or a cyst in the cerebellopontine angle, multiple sclerosis, adhesions, or osseous skull deformities will be the cause of HFS.

Evidence indicates that there is not cross (ephaptic) conduction at the compressed REZ, but that the facial motonucleus is involved secondarily as a result of the REZ compression, via a phenomenon similar to kindling.[70] In addition to the spasm, a 2nd electrophysiological phenomenon associated with HFS is synkinesis, where stimulation of one branch of the facial nerve results in delayed discharges through another branch (average latency: 11 mSec[71]).

112.3.4 Evaluation

In typical cases of HFS, the diagnostic work-up is negative.

Most patients should have MRI of the posterior fossa (CT scan is less sensitive here) to R/O tumors or AVMs.

Vertebral angiography is usually not performed if imaging is normal. The neurovascular compression responsible for HFS usually cannot be identified on angiography.

112.3.5 Treatment

Medical management

HFS is generally a surgical condition. Early, mild cases may be managed expectantly. Carbamazepine and phenytoin are generally ineffective, unlike the situation with the causally similar condition of trigeminal neuralgia. Local injection of botulinum toxin (Oculinum®) may be effective in treating HFS and/or blepharospasm.[72,73] Baclofen has been advocated but is not very effective.

112

Surgical management

General information

Many ablative procedures are effective for HFS (including sectioning of divisions of the facial nerve); however, this leaves the patient with some degree of facial paresis. The current procedure of choice for HFS is microvascular decompression (MVD), wherein the offending vessel is physically moved off of the nerve and a sponge (e.g., Ivalon®, polyvinyl formyl alcohol foam) is interposed as a cushion. Other cushions may not prove to be as satisfactory (muscle may disappear, and Teflon felt may thin[74]).

Most often, the offending vessel approaches the nerve at a right angle, and causes grooving in the nerve. Compression must occur at the root exit zone; decompression of vessels impinging distal to this area is usually ineffective.

Operative risks: see below.

Postoperatively, there may be episodes of mild HFS, but they usually begin to diminish 2–3 days following MVD. Severe spasm that does not abate suggests failure to achieve adequate decompression, and reoperation should be considered.

Surgical results of MVD depends on the duration of symptoms (shorter duration has better prognosis) as well as on the age of the patient (elderly patients do less well). Complete resolution of HFS occurred in 44 (81%) of 54 patients undergoing MVD; however, 6 of these patients had relapse.[7] 5 patients (9%) had partial improvement, and 5 (9%) had no relief.

112.3.6 Technique of MVD

Intraoperative brainstem auditory evoked potential (BAER),[76] or more applicable, direct VIII nerve monitoring,[77] may help prevent hearing loss during MVD for 7th or 8th nerve dysfunction. Furthermore, monitoring for the disappearance of the (delayed) synkinetic response may aid in determining when adequate decompression has been achieved (generally reserved for teaching institutions).[70]

For a diagram of the normal anatomy of the CPA, see ► Fig. 1.11. The facial nerve should not be manipulated, and one should avoid dissection around the VII and VIII nerves near the IAC.[78] Vessels must be preserved, especially the cochlear artery and small perforators.

Place gentle medial traction on the cerebellum (< 1 cm is recommended[78]), and incise the arachnoid membrane between the flocculus and the eighth nerve (to avoid tension on nerves that could cause post-op deficit). The IX nerve may be followed medially from the jugular foramen to locate the origin of the VII nerve (the origin of VII is 4 mm cephalad and 2 mm anterior to that of the IX nerve[79]).

112.3.7 Surgical results

Complete resolution of spasm occurs in ≈ 85–93%.[74,80,81,82,83] Spasm is diminished in 9%, and unchanged in 6%.[83] Of 29 patients with complete relief, 25 (86%) had immediate post-op resolution, and the remaining 4 patients took from 3 mos to 3 yrs to attain quiescence.

Recurrence

Return of symptoms after a period of complete resolution of HFS occurs in up to 10% of patients, 86% of recurrences happen within 2 yrs of surgery, and the risk of developing recurrence after 2 yrs of post-op relief is only ≈ 1%.[83]

Surgical complications

1. ipsilateral hearing loss: may occur from traction injury or a vasospasm
   a) total hearing loss occurs in ≈ 13% (range: 1.6–15%) (2.8% in one series,[65] 15% in another series[75])
   b) partial hearing loss: 6%
2. facial weakness
   a) transient: 18%
   b) permanent facial weakness: 6%[81]
3. ataxia in 1–6%
4. other complications that are minor or temporary include:
   a) aseptic meningitis (AKA hemogenic meningitis) in 8.2%
   b) hoarseness or dysphagia in 14%
   c) CSF rhinorrhea in 0.3%
   d) perioral herpes in 3%[78]

112.4 Geniculate neuralgia

112.4.1 General information

Geniculate neuralgia (GeN) AKA Hunt's neuralgia AKA nervus intermedius neuralgia: a very rare neuralgia affecting the nervus intermedius (the somatic sensory branch of the facial nerve primarily innervating mechanoreceptors of the hair follicles on the inner surface of the pinna and deep mechanoreceptors of nasal and buccal cavities and chemoreceptors in the taste buds on the anterior 2/3 of the tongue).

Symptoms: unilateral paroxysmal otalgia (lancinating pain experienced deep within the ear, often described as an "ice pick in the ear") radiating to the auricle, with occasional burning sensations around the ipsilateral eye and cheek, and prosopalgia (pain referred to deep facial structures, including orbit, posterior nasal, and palatal regions). During pain attacks, some patients have: salivation, bitter taste, tinnitus, or vertigo.

GeN occasionally has cutaneous trigger points in the anterior EAC and tragus, and pain may also be triggered by cold, noise, or swallowing.

Work-up includes neuro-otologic evaluation with audiometry and ENG. Some patients may require imaging (MRI or high-resolution CT) and angio (to R/O aneurysm).

112.4.2 Variants

Tic convulsif (AKA convulsive tic): GeN combined with hemifacial spasm, usually due to neurovascular compression of both the sensory and motor roots of the facial nerve,[84] most often by AICA. First described by Cushing in 1920.

GeN may be associated with herpetic infections of the geniculate ganglion (AKA herpetic ganglionitis, AKA Ramsay Hunt syndrome (RHS)) in which case herpetic lesions appear on pinna, in EAC, and possibly on TM. May include facial palsy, decreased auditory acuity, tinnitus or vertigo. Unlike idiopathic GeN, RHS is more chronic and less paroxysmal, tends to remit with time, and is usually refractory to carbamazepine. Idiopathic GeN tends to be more painful than RHS, and does not remit spontaneously.

112.4.3 Treatment

112

1. medical therapy
   a) mild cases may respond to carbamazepine, sometimes in combination with phenytoin
   b) may respond to valproate (Depakote®) 250 mg PO BID
   c) topical antibiotics for secondary infections of herpetic lesions
   d) local anesthetic to EAC
2. surgery: for severe cases where medical treatment fails or is not tolerated
   a) microvascular decompression together with division of the nervus intermedius (nerve of Wrisberg).[85] To find the nerve, a micro nerve hook is hooked around the VII nerve, the hook is rotated 90°, and the nerve is fished out from in front of VII. Operating under local anesthesia allows verification by stimulating nerve
   b) geniculate ganglion section[86]

112.5 Disabling positional vertigo

As described by Jannetta et al,[87] constant disabling positional vertigo or dysequilibrium, causing ≈ constant nausea. No vestibular dysfunction nor hearing loss (tinnitus may be present). One possible cause is vascular compression of the vestibular nerve which may respond to microvascular decompression

112.6 Glossopharyngeal neuralgia

112.6.1 Epidemiology

Incidence: 1 case for every 70 of trigeminal neuralgia.[88 (p 3604–5)]

112.6.2 Clinical

Severe, lancinating pain in the distribution of the glossopharyngeal and vagus nerves (throat & base of tongue most commonly involved, radiates to ear (otalgia), occasionally to neck), occasionally with salivation and coughing. Rarely: hypotension,[89] syncope,[90] cardiac arrest and convulsions may accompany. May be triggered by swallowing, talking, chewing. Trigger zones are rare.

112.6.3 Treatment

Pain may be reduced by application of locan anesthetic to tonsillar pillars and fossa. Usually, the persistence and severity of pain requires surgical intervention. One may either perform microvascular decompression, or nerve division via extra- or intra-cranial approach (latter may be required for permanent relief).

Intracranial approach: Section of preganglionic glossopharyngeal nerve (IX) and upper one–third or two fibers (whichever is larger) of vagus (X). IX is readily identified at its dural exit zone where it is separated from X by a dural septum. The upper third of X is usually composed of a single rootlet, or less commonly, multiple small rootlets. Initial post-op dysphagia usually resolves. Cardiovascular complications following vagal section have been reported, warrants close monitoring × 24 hrs.

112.7 Superior laryngeal neuralgia

A rare disorder characterized by severe pain in the distribution of the superior laryngeal nerve. Patients experience pain along the anterior cervical triangle with extension to the ipsilateral ear and eyes, intermittent hoarseness, and paralysis of the ipsilateral cricothyroid muscle on laryngoscopy.[91] Pain is usually worsened by swallowing, shouting, or by head turning. The etiology of this disorder may vary: can occur after trauma, iatrogenic injury (after surgery in the anterior neck such as carotid endarterectomy), or as a result of vascular compression by PICA or vertebral artery. It can be treated with superior laryngeal nerve blocks, nerve sectioning, or less commonly by microvascular decompression.

References

[1] Janjua RM, Al-Mefty O, Densler DW, et al. Dural relationships of Meckel cave and lateral wall of the cavernous sinus. Neurosurg Focus. 2008; 25. DOI: 10.3171/FOC.2008.25.12.E2

[2] Wepsic JG. Tic Douloureux: Etiology, Refined Treatment. N Engl J Med. 1973; 288:680–681

[3] Sweet WH. The Treatment of Trigeminal Neuralgia (Tic Douloureux). N Engl J Med. 1986; 315:174–177

[4] Brisman R. Bilateral Trigeminal Neuralgia. J Neurosurg. 1987; 67:44–48

[5] van Loveren H, Tew JM, Keller JT, et al. A 10-Year Experience in the Treatment of Trigeminal Neuralgia: Comparison of Percutaneous Stereotaxic Rhizotomy and Posterior Fossa Exploration. Journal of Neurosurgery. 1982; 57:757–764

[6] Taha JM, Tew JM. Comparison of Surgical Treatments for Trigeminal Neuralgia: Reevaluation of Radiofrequency Rhizotomy. Neurosurgery. 1996; 38:865–871

[7] Hardy DG, Rhoton AL. Microsurgical Relationships of the Superior Cerebellar Artery and the Trigeminal Nerve. J Neurosurg. 1978; 49:669–678

[8] Morita A, Fukushima T, Miyazaki S, et al. Tic Douloureux Caused by Primitive Trigeminal Artery or its Variant. J Neurosurg. 1989; 70:415–419

[9] Apfelbaum RI, Carter LP, Spetzler RF, et al. Trigeminal Neuralgia: Vascular Decompression. In: Neurovascular Surgery. New York: McGraw-Hill; 1995:1107–1117

[10] Keller JT, van Loveren H. Pathophysiology of the Pain of Trigeminal Neuralgia and Atypical Facial Pain: A Neuroanatomical Perspective. Clin Neurosurg. 1985; 32:275–293

[11] Bullitt E, Tew JM, Boyd J. Intracranial Tumors in Patients with Facial Pain. J Neurosurg. 1986; 64:865–871

[12] Fusco BM, Alessandri M. Analgesic Effect of Capsaicin in Idiopathic Trigeminal Neuralgia. Anesth Analg. 1992; 74:375–377

[13] Kanai A, Suzuki A, Kobayashi M, et al. Intranasal lidocaine 8% spray for second-division trigeminal neuralgia. Br J Anaesth. 2006; 97:559–563

[14] Poppen JL. An Atlas of Neurosurgical Techniques. Philadelphia: W. B. Saunders; 1960

[15] Sweet WH, Wepsic JG. Controlled Thermocoagulation of Trigeminal Ganglion and Rootlets for Differential Destruction of Pain Fibers. Part I. Trigeminal Neuralgia. J Neurosurg. 1974; 40:143–156

[16] Hakanson S. Trigeminal Neuralgia Treated by the Injection of Glycerol into the Trigeminal Cistern. Neurosurgery. 1981; 9:638–646

[17] Sweet WH, Poletti CE, Macon JB. Treatment of Trigeminal Neuralgia and Other Facial Pains by the Retrogasserian Injection of Glycerol. Neurosurgery 1981; 9:647–653

[18] Lunsford LD, Apfelbaum RI. Choice of Surgical Therapeutic Modalities for Treatment of Trigemina Neuralgia. Clin Neurosurg. 1985; 32:319–333

[19] Young RF. Glycerol Rhizolysis for Treatment of Trigeminal Neuralgia. J Neurosurg. 1988; 69:39–45

[20] Mullan S, Lichtor T. Percutaneous Microcompression of the Trigeminal Ganglion for Trigeminal Neuralgia. J Neurosurg. 1983; 59:1007–1012

[21] Belber CJ, Rak RA. Balloon Compression Rhizolysis in the Surgical Management of Trigeminal Neuralgia. Neurosurgery. 1987; 20:908–913

[22] Lichtor T, Mullan JF. A 10-Year Follow-Up Review of Percutaneous Microcompression of the Trigeminal Ganglion. Journal of Neurosurgery. 1990; 72:49–54

[23] Taarnhoj P. Decompression of the Posterior Trigeminal Root in Trigeminal Neuralgia. J Neurosurg. 1982 57:14–17

[24] Henderson JM, Lad SP. Motor cortex stimulation and neuropathic facial pain. Neurosurgical Focus 2006; 21

[25] van Loveren H, Greenberg MS. Tampa 2009

[26] Murali R, Rovit RL. Are peripheral neurectomies of value in the treatment of trigeminal neuralgia? An

analysis of new cases and cases involving previous radiofrequency Gasserian thermocoagulation. Journal of Neurosurgery. 1996; 85:435–437

[27] Wilkins RH, Burchiel KJ. Trigeminal neuralgia: Historical overview, with emphasis on surgical treatment. In: Surgical Management of Pain. New York: Thieme Medical Publishers, Inc.; 2002:288–301

[28] Tew JM, van Loveren H, Schmidek HH, et al. Percutaneous Rhizotomy in the Treatment of Intractable Facial Pain (Trigeminal, Glossopharyngeal, and Vagal Nerves). In: Operative Neurosurgical Techniques. 2nd ed. Philadelphia: W B Saunders; 1988:1111–1123

[29] Brown JA, Preul MC. Percutaneous Trigeminal Ganglion Compression for Trigeminal Neuralgia. Experience in 22 Cases and Review of the Literature. Journal of Neurosurgery. 1989; 70:900–904

[30] Menzel J, Piotrowski W, Penzholz H. Long-Term Results of Gasserian Ganglion Electrocoagulation. J Neurosurg. 1975; 42:140–143

[31] Wepsic JG. Complications of Percutaneous Surgery for Pain. Clinical Neurosurgery. 1976; 23:454–464

[32] Tew JM, Keller JT. The Treatment of Trigeminal Neuralgia by Percutaneous Radiofrequency Technique. Clinical Neurosurgery. 1977; 24:557–578

[33] Luksic I, Sestan-Crnek S, Virag M, et al. Trigeminal trophic syndrome of all three nerve branches: an underrecognized complication after brain surgery. Journal of Neurosurgery. 2008; 108:170–173

[34] Setyadi HG, Cohen PR, Schulze KE, et al. Trigeminal trophic syndrome. Southern Medical Journal. 2007; 100:43–48

[35] Kaplan M, Erol FS, Ozveren MF, et al. Review of complications due to foramen ovale puncture. J Clin Neurosci. 2007; 14:563–568

[36] Sekhar L, Heros RC, Kerber CW. Carotid-Cavernous Fistula Following Percutaneous Retrogasserian Procedures. Journal of Neurosurgery. 1979; 51:700–706

[37] Kuether TA, O'Neill OR, Nesbit GM, et al. Direct Carotid Cavernous Fistula After Trigeminal Balloon Microcompression Gangliolysis: Case Report. Neurosurgery. 1996; 39:853–856

[38] Agazzi S, Chang S, Drucker MD, et al. Sudden blindness as a complication of percutaneous trigeminal procedures: mechanism analysis and prevention. Journal of Neurosurgery. 2009; 110:638–641

[39] Kanpolat Y, Savas A, Bekar A, et al. Percutaneous controlled radiofrequency trigeminal rhizotomy for the treatment of idiopathic trigeminal neuralgia: 25-year experience with 1,600 patients. Neurosurgery. 2001; 48:524–32; discussion 532-4

[40] Tobler WD, Tew JM, Cosman E, et al. Improved outcome in the treatment of trigeminal neuralgia by percutaneous stereotactic rhizotomy with a new, curved tip electrode. Neurosurgery. 1983; 12:313–317

[41] Lunsford LD. Comment on Taha J M and Tew J M: Comparison of Surgical Treatments for Trigeminal Neuralgia: Reevaluation of Radiofrequency Rhizotomy. Neurosurgery. 1996; 38

[42] Brisman R. Gamma knife surgery with a dose of 75 to 76.8 Gray for trigeminal neuralgia. Journal of Neurosurgery. 2004; 100:848–854

[43] Pollock BE, Phuong LK, Foote RL, et al. High-dose trigeminal neuralgia radiosurgery associated with increased risk of trigeminal nerve dysfunction. Neurosurgery. 2001; 49:58–62; discussion 62-4

[44] Kondziolka D, Lunsford LD, Flickinger JC. Stereotactic radiosurgery for the treatment of trigeminal neuralgia. Clin J Pain. 2002; 18:42–47

[45] Massager N, Lorenzoni J, Devriendt D, et al. Gamma knife surgery for idiopathic trigeminal neuralgia performed using a far-anterior cisternal target and a high dose of radiation. J Neurosurg. 2004; 100:597–605

[46] Urgosik D, Liscak R, Novotny J,Jr, et al. Treatment of essential trigeminal neuralgia with gamma knife surgery. J Neurosurg. 2005; 102 Suppl:29–33

[47] Maesawa S, Salame C, Flickinger JC, et al. Clinical outcomes after stereotactic radiosurgery for idiopathic trigeminal neuralgia. J Neurosurg. 2001; 94:14–20

[48] Barba D, Alksne JF. Success of Microvascular Decompression with and without Prior Surgical Therapy

for Trigeminal Neuralgia. J Neurosurg. 1984; 60:104–107

[49] Schmidek HH, Sweet WH. Operative Neurosurgical Techniques. New York 1982

[50] Onofrio BM. Radiofrequency Percutaneous Gasserian Ganglion Lesions: Results in 140 Patients with Trigeminal Pain. J Neurosurg. 1975; 42:132–139

[51] Kondziolka D, Lunsford LD, Bissonette DJ. Long-Term Results After Glycerol Rhizotomy for Multiple Sclerosis-Related Trigeminal Neuralgia. Can J Neurol Sci. 1994; 21:137–140

[52] Burchiel KJ, Favre J. Current Techniques for Pain Control. Contemporary Neurosurgery. 1997; 19:1–6

[53] McLaughlin MR, Jannetta PJ, Clyde BL, et al. Microvascular decompression of cranial nerves: Lessons learned after 4400 operations. J Neurosurg. 1999; 90:1–8

[54] Tew JM, van Loveren HR. Atlas of Operative Microneurosurgery. Philadelphia: W. B. Saunders; 1994; 1: Aneurysms and Arteriovenous Malformations

[55] Day JD, Tschabitscher M. Anatomic position of the asterion. Neurosurgery. 1998; 42:198–199

[56] Pathmanaban ON, O'Brien F, Al-Tamimi YZ, et al. Safety of Superior Petrosal Vein Sacrifice During Microvascular Decompression of the Trigeminal Nerve. World Neurosurg. 2017; 103:84–87

[57] Liebelt BD, Barber SM, Desai VR, et al. Superior Petrosal Vein Sacrifice During Microvascular Decompression: Perioperative Complication Rates and Comparison with Venous Preservation. World Neurosurg. 2017; 104:788–794

[58] Anichini Giulio, Iqbal Mazhar, Rafiq Nasir Muhammad, et al. Sacrificing the superior petrosal vein during microvascular decompression. Is it safe? Learning the hard way. Case report and review of literature. Surgical Neurology International. 2016; 7:S415–S420

[59] Bederson JB, Wilson CB. Evaluation of Microvascular Decompression and Partial Sensory Rhizotomty in 252 Cases of Trigeminal Neuralgia. J Neurosurg. 1989; 71:359–367

[60] Avildsen JG. The Karate Kid. 1984

[61] Jannetta PJ. Microsurgical Management of Trigeminal Neuralgia. Arch Neurol. 1985; 42

[62] Burchiel KJ, Clarke H, Haglund M, et al. Long-Term Efficacy of Microvascular Decompression in Trigeminal Neuralgia. J Neurosurg. 1988; 69:35–38

[63] Schmidek HH, Sweet WH. Operative Neurosurgical Techniques. Philadelphia 1988

[64] Hanakita J, Kondo A. Serious Complications of Microvascular Decompression Operations for Trigeminal Neuralgia and Hemifacial Spasm. Neurosurgery. 1988; 22:348–352

[65] Moller MB, Moller AR. Loss of Auditory Function in Microvascular Decompression for Hemifacial Spasm: Results in 143 Consecutive Cases. J Neurosurg. 1985; 63:17–20

[66] Tew JM, Yeh HS. Hemifacial Spasm. Neurosurgery (Japan). 1983; 2:267–278

[67] Yeh HS, Tew JM, Ramirez RM. Microsurgical Treatment of Intractable Hemifacial Spasm. Neurosurgery. 1981; 9:383–386

[68] Martin RG, Grant JL, Peace D, et al. Microsurgical Relationships of the Anterior Inferior Cerebellar Artery and the Facial-vestibulocochlear Nerve Complex. Neurosurgery. 1980; 6:483–507

[69] Wilkins RH, Rengachary SS. Neurosurgery. New York 1985

[70] Moller AR, Jannetta PJ. Microvascular Decompression in Hemifacial Spasm: Intraoperative Electrophysiological Observations. Neurosurgery. 1985; 16:612–618

[71] Moller AR, Jannetta PJ. Hemifacial Spasm: Results of Electrophysiologic Recording During Microvascular Decompression Operations. Neurology. 1985; 35:969–974

[72] Dutton JJ, Buckley EG. Botulinum toxin in the management of blepharospasm. Arch Neurol. 1986; 43:380–382

[73] Kennedy RH, Bartley GB, Flanagan JC, et al. Treatment of Blepharospasm With Botulinum Toxin. Mayo Clin Proc. 1989; 64:1085–1090

112

[74] Rhoton AL. Comment on Payner T D and Tew J M: Recurrence of Hemifacial Spasm After Microvascular Decompression. Neurosurgery. 1996; 38

[75] Auger RG, Peipgras DG, Laws ER. Hemifacial Spasm: Results of Microvascular Decompression of the Facial Nerve in 54 Patients. Mayo Clinic Proceedings. 1986; 61:640–644

[76] Friedman WA, Kaplan BJ, Gravenstein D, et al. Intraoperative Brain-Stem Auditory Evoked Potentials During Posterior Fossa Microvascular Decompression. J Neurosurg. 1985; 62:552–557

[77] Moller AR, Jannetta PJ. Monitoring Auditory Functions During Cranial Nerve Microvascular Decompression Operations by Direct Recording from the Eighth Nerve. J Neurosurg. 1983; 59:493–499

[78] Fukushima T, Carter LP, Spetzler RF, et al. Microvascular Decompression for Hemifacial Spasm: Results in 2890 Cases. In: Neurovascular Surgery. New York: McGraw-Hill; 1995:1133–1145

[79] Rhoton AL. Microsurgical Anatomy of the Brainstem Surface Facing an Acoustic Neuroma. Surg Neurol. 1986; 25:326–339

[80] Jannetta PJ. Neurovascular Compression in Cranial Nerve and Systemic Disease. Ann Surg. 1980; 192:518–525

[81] Loeser JD, Chen J. Hemifacial Spasm: Treatment by Microsurgical Facial Nerve Decompression. Neurosurgery. 1983; 13:141–146

[82] Huang CI, Chen IH, Lee LS. Microvascular Decompression for Hemifacial Spasm: Analyses of Operative Findings and Results in 310 Patients. Neurosurgery. 1992; 30:53–57

[83] Payner TD, Tew JM. Recurrence of Hemifacial Spasm After Microvascular Decompression. Neurosurgery. 1996; 38:686–691

[84] Yeh HS, Tew JM. Tic Convulsif, the Combination of Geniculate Neuralgia and Hemifacial Spasm Relieved by Vascular Decompression. Neurology. 1984; 34:682–683

[85] Lovely TJ, Jannetta PJ. Surgical management of geniculate neuralgia. Am J Otol. 1997; 18:512–517

[86] Pulec JL. Geniculate neuralgia: diagnosis and surgical management. Laryngoscope. 1976; 86:955–964

[87] Jannetta PJ, Moller MB, Moller AR. Disabling Positional Vertigo. N Engl J Med. 1984; 310:1700–1705

[88] Youmans JR. Neurological Surgery. Philadelphia 1982

[89] Weinstein RE, Herec D, Friedman JH. Hypotension due to Glossopharyngeal Neuralgia. Arch Neurol. 1986; 43:90–92

[90] Ferrante L, Artico M, Nardacci B, et al. Glossopharyngeal Neuralgia with Cardiac Syncope. Neurosurgery. 1995; 36:58–63

[91] O'Neill BP, Aronson AE, Pearson BW, et al. Superior laryngeal neuralgia: carotidynia or just another pain in the neck? Headache. 1982; 22:6–9

113 Pain Procedures

113.1 Prerequisites for pain procedures

Medical therapy must be maximized before a patient is a candidate for a pain procedure. Usually this requires escalating the dose of oral narcotic pain medications until the point that the pain is relieved or the side effects (usually somnolence or hallucinations) are intolerable (e.g., up to 300–400 mg/day of MS Contin may sometimes be necessary).

113.2 Choice of pain procedure

▶ Table 113.1 shows some pain procedures that may be used for various indications (the list is not intended to be all-inclusive, but is rather to serve as a starting point for organizing pain procedures). In general, nonablative procedures are exhausted before resorting to ablative procedures.

Table 113.1 Choice of pain procedures[a]

Unilateral pain		Bilateral or midline pain	
Head, face, neck, UE	Pain at or below C5 dermatome	Below diaphragm	Above diaphragm
DBS stereotactic mesencephal- otomy	cordotomy[b]	spinal IT narcotics ↓ commissural myelotomy	intraventricular narcotics

[a]abbreviations: IT = intrathecal; UE or LE = upper or lower extremity
[b]cordotomy (open or percutaneous) if pain is unresponsive to or too high for spinal IT narcotics

113.3 Types of pain procedures

See pain procedures particular to trigeminal neuralgia (p. 1861).
Techniques for other conditions include:
1. electrical stimulation
   a) deep brain stimulation (p. 1839)[1]: targets include thalamus and periaqueductal or periventricular gray matter
   b) spinal cord stimulation (p. 1883)
2. direct drug administration into the CNS:
   a) different routes: spinal (p. 1881), epidural or intrathecal, intraventricular (p. 1882)
   b) different agents: local anesthetics, narcotics (without motor, sensory, or sympathetic impairment seen with local anesthetics) (p. 1881)
3. intracranial ablative procedures:
   a) cingulotomy: theoretically reduces the unpleasant effect of pain without eliminating the pain. Must be done bilaterally, recently with MRI. Intolerable pain usually recurs after ≈ 3 mos. 10–30% develop flattened affect
   b) medial thalamotomy: no longer used (presented for historical reasons). Controversial. Was used for some for nociceptive cancer pain. Performed stereotactically
   c) **stereotactic mesencephalotomy**[2]: for unilateral head, neck, face, and/or UE pain. Use MRI to create lesion 5 mm lateral to Sylvian aqueduct at the level of the inferior colliculus. Unlike spinal cordotomy, the lesion is not near any motor tracts. Main complication is diplopia due to interference with vertical eye movement, often transient
4. spinal ablative surgical procedures
   a) cordotomy: see below
      • open
      • percutaneous
   b) cordectomy
   c) commissural myelotomy: for bilateral pain (p. 1880)
   d) punctate midline myelotomy: for relief of visceral cancer pain
   e) dorsal root entry zone lesion (p. 1886)
   f) dorsal rhizotomy: not useful for large areas of involvement
   g) dorsal root ganglionectomy (an extraspinal procedure)

113

h) sacral cordotomy: for patients with pelvic pain who have colostomy and ileostomy. A ligature is tied around the dural sac below S1 nerve roots

5. sympathectomy: possibly for causalgia major; see Sympathectomy (p. 1853) and Complex regional pain syndrome (CRPS) (p. 525)

6. peripheral nerve procedures
   a) nerve block[3]:
      - neurolytic: injection of neurodestructive agents (e.g., phenol or absolute alcohol) on or near the target nerve
      - nonneurolytic: using local anesthetics, sometimes in combination with corticosteroids
   b) neurectomy: (e.g., intercostal neurectomy for pain due to infiltration of chest wall by malignancy). Performed open or percutaneously with radiofrequency lesion. May sacrifice motor function with mixed nerves
   c) peripheral nerve stimulators: rarely discussed

113.4 Cordotomy

113.4.1 General information

Interruption of the lateral spinothalamic tract fibers in the spinal cord. Cordotomy is the procedure of choice for *unilateral* pain below the C5 dermatomal level (≈ nipple; occasionally pain as high up as the mandible may be treated), in a terminally ill patient. Better for aching pain, poor for central pain, dysesthesias, causalgia (deafferentation pain), midline visceral pain. May be performed as an open procedure, but is more easily performed percutaneously at the C1–2 interspace (which limits the procedure to the cervical region). If there is any contralateral pain, it will tend to be magnified following the procedure and often leads to dissatisfaction with cordotomy. If there is any bladder dysfunction, it will usually be worse following cordotomy. Bilateral cervical cordotomies carry a risk of the loss of automaticity of breathing[4] (one form of sleep apnea, so-called Ondine's curse[5]). Therefore if bilateral cordotomies are desired, the second should be staged after normal respiratory function and CO_2 responsiveness are verified following the first procedure, or the second stage may be done as an open procedure in the thoracic region.

Review the cross-sectional spinal cord anatomy for relationships of the critical tracts (spinothalamic and corticospinal) to the dentate ligament, the anterior spinal artery, respiratory (▶ Fig. 1.15) and bladder areas (▶ Fig. 3.2).

113.4.2 Pre-op evaluation

Spirometric measurement of minute volume before and after breathing a mixture of 5% CO_2 and 95% O_2 for 5 minutes. If the MV decreases, these patients are at increased risk of having sleep apnea (usually transient), no increased risk if MV increases or stays the same. Also, patients with < 50% of predicted values on PFTs are not candidates.

In patients with pulmonary cancer contralateral to the planned side of cordotomy, check that the contralateral diaphragm is functioning with fluoroscopy; otherwise, if the ipsilateral diaphragm is lost due to cordotomy, the patient may be hypopneic.

113.4.3 Percutaneous cordotomy

General information

Indicated for unilateral pain below ≈ C4–5 in a terminally ill patient. Radiofrequency current is used to lesion the lateral spinothalamic tract.

Technique

Patient does not need to be NPO. Usual pain medications should be given. The patient must be awake and cooperative (any movement with the needle in the cord may lacerate the cord); however, one may give e.g., hydroxyzine (Vistaril®) 50 mg IM on call to procedure for relaxation.

The procedure is performed in the X-ray department with either fluoroscopic or CT guidance. For fluoroscopy, the head is placed in a Rosomoff head-holder with the height adjusted to keep the mastoid process in the same horizontal plane as the acromioclavicular joint. Working on the side contralateral to the pain, local anesthetic without epinephrine is infiltrated 1 cm caudal to the mastoid tip. An 18 gauge lumbar puncture needle is inserted perfectly horizontal aiming halfway between

he posterior margin of the body of C2 and the anterior portion of the C2 spinous process. Stay ros-
ral to the C2 lamina to avoid the nerve (which is painful).

The dura will be penetrated at about the time that the tip of the needle is approximately even with
he midline of the odontoid process on AP fluoro. A few ml of CSF are aspirated and shaken in a syringe
ogether with a few ml of Pantopaque®, and several ml of the mixture are injected into the subarachnoid space under lateral fluoro guidance (**note**: Pantopaque is no longer available, and water-soluble
agents are less effective). A needle endoscopic technique may be able to localize the spinal cord ante-
ior to the dentate ligaments. Some dye will layer on the anterior cord, some on the dentate ligament,
and most in the posterior thecal space. The dye will only stay momentarily on the dentate ligament,
thus be ready to immediately advance the needle just barely anterior to this while monitoring the tip
mpedance, which will jump from ≈ 300–500 Ω (ohms) in the CSF to ≈ 1200–1500 Ω as the spinal cord
s penetrated.

Stimulation at 100 Hz should produce contralateral tingling at a threshold of ≤ 1 volt. No motor
response should be elicited with 100 Hz in the spinothalamic tract, and if muscle tetany occurs,
esioning must *not* be performed. If tingling is in the arm, lesioning will usually render from the arm
and below analgesic. If tingling is in the lower extremity it will render only that limb analgesic. Stimulation at 2 Hz should produce ipsilateral twitching of the arm or neck at ≈ 1–3 volts.

Radiofrequency lesioning is performed for 30 seconds while the patient sustains contraction of
the *ipsilateral* hand and the voltage is gradually increased from zero. Any twitching of the hand is an
ndication to back down on the voltage. A second lesion is performed in the same region and is usully less painful. The appropriate body area is then checked for analgesia to pinprick.

If the procedure is performed satisfactorily, an ipsilateral Horner syndrome usually occurs.

Complications

or complications, see ▶ Table 113.2.

Table 113.2 Post-cordotomy complications

Complication	Frequency
ataxia	20%
ipsilateral paresis	5% total 3% permanent
bladder dysfunction	10% total 2% permanent
postcordotomy dysesthesia	8%
sleep-induced apnea	0.3% unilateral cordotomy 3% bilateral cordotomy
death (respiratory failure)	0.3% unilateral cordotomy 1.6% bilateral cordotomy

113

Outcome

n experienced hands, 94% will achieve at least significant pain relief at the time of hospital dis-
harge. The level of analgesia falls with time. At 1 year 60% will be pain-free, and at 2 years this will
e only 40%.

Post-procedure management

SF leakage will cease spontaneously. Patient is kept supine for 24 hrs to prevent "spinal" (post-LP)
eadache. Pain medication appropriate to postoperative management is prescribed. If successful,
ne can rapidly stop the narcotics for the primary pain; withdrawal syndromes occur only rarely.

13.4.4 Open cervical cordotomy (Schwartz technique)

General information

relatively quick method for open cervical cordotomy.[6] Can theoretically be done under local for
atients who cannot tolerate general anesthesia.

Technique

Position: prone; face carefully placed on padded horseshoe headrest, neck slightly flexed to open the interlaminar spaces and to lower the head to prevent accumulation of intracranial air.

Skin incision: midline from occiput to C3. Working only on the side *contralateral* to the pain muscles are stripped off the posterior lip of the foramen magnum, and from the lamina of C1 and C2 A Schwartz or Gelpi retractor is engaged between the occiput and C2. To increase exposure, the inferior half of C1 and superior half of C2 lamina are removed with a punch.

Dural incision: the ligamentum flavum is thin between C1–2, and can usually be opened with the dura in a linear incision from the lamina of C1 to C2 placed in the lateral third of the exposure, taking care to avoid bleeding from epidural veins. An angle is cut in the incision at either end to allow increased dural retraction. Tack-up sutures are placed in the dura, the arachnoid is opened, the dentate ligament is located and is gripped with a hemostat and divided between the hemostat and the dura.

Cordotomy: the dentate ligament is used to slightly rotate the spinal cord. A cordotomy knife (o 11 blade) with bone wax placed at 5 mm, is inserted into the cord in an avascular area just anterio to the dentate ligament, sharp side down. The anterolateral quadrant of the cord is cut with the following caveats:

- do not go posterior to the dentate ligament (to avoid corticospinal tract)
- do not cross the midline of the spinal cord
- do not injure the anterior spinal artery
- for patients with lower extremity pain, be sure to start exactly at the dentate ligament (to avoid missing lumbar and sacral fibers).

113.5 Commissural myelotomy

113.5.1 General information

AKA mediolongitudinal myelotomy. Interrupts pain fibers crossing in the anterior commissure o their way to the lateral spinothalamic tract.

113.5.2 Indications

Bilateral or midline pain, primarily below the thoracic levels (including abdomen, pelvis, perineum and lower extremities).

113.5.3 Technique

Laminectomy must extend at least 3 levels above the highest dermatome involved in pain. The dur is opened longitudinally and the operating microscope is then used to identify the midline sulcu (this is usually very difficult to see, and is then estimated as being halfway between where the dors roots enter the cord). Veins in the midline are sacrificed for the length of the proposed incision. number 11 scalpel blade is then placed in a hemostat with 6–7 mm of the tip exposed. The blade inserted in the midline at the upper end of the desired incision and is then passed caudally for th length of the planned incision (usually 3–4 cm).

113.5.4 Outcome

60% of patients have complete pain relief, 28% have partial, and 8% have none.

113.5.5 Complications

Weakness in the lower extremities occurs in ≈ 8% (usually lower motor neuron, presumably due injury to anterior horn motor neurons). Dysesthesias occur in almost all patients, but persist > a fe days in ≈ 16% (these patients also have impaired joint position sense, all of which are presumab due to posterior column injury). Bladder dysfunction is seen in ≈ 12%. Sexual dysfunction may al occur. There is a risk of injury to the anterior spinal artery (rare).

113.6 CNS narcotic administration

113.6.1 Intraspinal narcotics

General information

Spinal narcotics may be administered epidurally or intrathecally for pain relief. Satisfactory pain control can usually be achieved for pain below the neck, although for pain above the diaphragm/umbilicus some recommend intraventricular morphine (p. 1882).[7] May also be performed on a "one-time" basis e.g., injection into epidural space following a lumbar laminectomy. Or, it may be given on a short-term continuous basis, via an external epidural or intrathecal catheter. It may also be performed on an intermediate-term basis (< 60 days) with the use of a subcutaneous reservoir[8] or on a long-term basis with an implantable drug infusion pump[9] (e.g., Infusaid® or Medtronic® pump). Advantages over systemic narcotics include less sedation and/or confusion, less interference with GI motility (constipation), and possibly less N/V. The effectiveness is usually limited to ≈ 1 year and is thus not indicated for chronic benign pain. With time, increased doses are required because of the development of tolerance and/or progression of disease[10] with the concomitant development of the usual narcotic side effects.

Agents to use

Must be preservative-free (for either intrathecal or epidural use). This may be prepared by a pharmacist (e.g., add enough preservative-free 0.9% saline to 1 or 3 gm morphine sulfate powder to yield a total of 100 ml produces 10 or 30 mg/ml solution respectively, and then filter this through a 0.22 mcm filter[11]). Alternatively, commercially available preparations include Duramorph® (available as 0.5 or 1 mg/ml) and Infumorph® (available in 20 ml ampules of 10 or 25 mg/ml), any of which may be diluted to a lower strength with preservative-free diluent (normal saline). Cross-tolerance to systemic narcotics does occur, and spinal narcotics are more effective in patients who have not been on continuous high-dose IV opiates (patients on high-dose IV narcotics need higher initial intraspinal narcotic doses).

▶ **Side effects.** Include pruritus (often diffuse, and may be experienced most intensely in the nose), respiratory depression (the respiratory depression with spinal narcotics is usually very gradual, and is often easily detected by monitoring respiratory rate q 1 hr and taking action if the rate decreases), urinary retention, and N/V.

Trial injection

Before implanting a permanent delivery system, a test injection should be performed to verify pain relief and tolerance for medication. Administered via a percutaneously inserted epidural or intrathecal catheter connected to an external pump. Doses required for intrathecal catheters are usually ≈ 5–10 times lower than those for epidural catheters.

Sample post-injection orders after a one-time injection:
1. use no other narcotics for ≈ 24 hrs (with a continuous infusion additional narcotics should be withheld until the effect of the spinal narcotics has been determined)
2. 2 ampules (0.4 mg each) of naloxone (Narcan®) and syringe taped to patient's bed (for the first 24 hrs after a single injection; at all times with continuous infusion)
3. head of bed elevated ≥ 10° for 24 hrs
4. record respiratory rate q 1 hr for 24 hrs; if asleep and respiratory rate < 10 breaths/min, awaken patient. If unable to awaken, administer naloxone 0.4 mg IV and notify physician. Repeat naloxone 0.4 mg IV q 2 min PRN
5. **optional**: pulse oximeter for 24 hrs
6. diphenhydramine (Benadryl®) 25 mg IV q 1 hr PRN itching
7. droperidol (Inapsine®) 0.625 mg (which is 0.25 ml of the 2.5 mg/ml standard concentration available) IV q 30–60 mins PRN nausea
8. PRN supplemental pain medication:
    a) narcotic agonist/antagonist: e.g., nalbuphine (Nubain®) 1–4 mg IV q 3 hrs, OR
    b) ketorolac tromethamine (Toradol®) 15 mg IV or IM or 30 mg IM q 6 hrs (use lower dose for weight < 50 kg, age > 65 yrs, or reduced renal function)

113

Implantable drug delivery pumps

Although satisfactory pain control can be achieved with either epidural or intrathecal narcotics (morphine diffuses easily through the dura to the CSF where it gains access to pain receptors), epidural catheters commonly develop problems with scarring and may become less effective sooner than intrathecal catheters. Pumps should only be implanted if patients have successful pain control with test injection of spinal epidural (5–10 mg) or intrathecal (0.5–2 mg) morphine. A life expectancy of > 3 months is recommended for implantable pumps (if shorter longevity is anticipated, an external pump may be used).

One such series of commonly used implantable drug delivery pumps is manufactured by Infusaid Inc. The only needle that should be used with their devices are special 22 gauge Huber (non-coring) needles. Delivery rates increase with body temperature 10–13% per °C above 37 °C, they decrease by the same amount for every °C below 37 °C, and they also become inaccurate at ≤ 4 ml of reservoir fluid. These pumps should never be allowed to run until empty, as this may permanently affect accuracy and reliability of drug delivery. In addition to the pump reservoir port, most models have one or more side "bolus" ports that deliver injected fluid directly to the outlet tubing. One should not aspirate when accessing either port.

Medtronic produces a programmable pump.

Surgical insertion

Similar to the insertion of a lumbar-peritoneal shunt (p. 1829). The patient is placed in the lateral position, such as on a bean-bag device. The pump is inserted into a subcutaneous pocket, created with a slightly curved 8–10 cm skin incision. The pump may be sutured to the fascia of the abdomen (in obese patients, it may be sutured to the subcutaneous tissue). Excess tubing should be coiled underneath the pump to prevent inadvertent puncture when accessing either reservoir.

The spinal catheter is inserted through a Tuohy needle inserted between lumbar spinous processes either percutaneously or via a small incision 2–3 mm lateral to the spinous processes. Alternatively, it may be inserted directly via a hemilaminectomy. Fluoroscopy may be used intraoperatively to verify rostral placement of the catheter; radiographic visualization of the catheter may be aided by filling it with iodinated contrast, e.g., Omnipaque-300 (p. 230). All bends in the tubing should be very gradual to avoid kinking.

Post-op pain management

Although the pump will be infusing when the patient leaves the operating room, unless they have been on intraspinal narcotics up until the time of surgery, it will usually take several days for the drug to reach equilibrium in the CSF before the level of pain control will be adequate. This can be mitigated by a bolus infusion (3–4 mg morphine for epidural catheters, or 0.2–0.4 mg for intrathecal catheters).

Complications

Meningitis and respiratory failure are rare complications. CSF fistula and spinal H/A may occur. Disconnection or dislodgment of catheter tip may result in failure to control pain, but can usually be surgically corrected.

Outcome

Cancer pain is significantly improved in up to 90%. Success rate for neuropathic pain (e.g., postherpetic neuralgia, painful diabetic sensory neuropathy): 25–50%.

113.6.2 Intraventricular narcotics

Indications

May be used for cancer pain (especially head and neck)[12] unresponsive to other methods in patients with a life expectancy < 6 mos.

Technique

An intraventricular catheter is connected to a ventricular access device (p. 1831). 0.5–1 mg of intrathecal morphine is injected via the VAD and usually provides ≈ 24 hrs of analgesia.

Complications

▶ **Side effects.** Common ones include dizziness, N/V. The risk of respiratory depression is minimized by using correct dosing. Complications in a series of 52 patients[12]: bacterial colonization of reservoir (4%), dislodged catheter (2%), blocked catheter (6%), postoperative meningitis (2%).

Outcome

Pain is successfully controlled in 70% at 2 mos, but thereafter the effectiveness diminishes as a result of tolerance to the narcotics.

113.7 Spinal cord stimulation (SCS)

113.7.1 General information

Spinal cord stimulation (SCS) is an invasive pain management technique that is useful in treatment of selected cases of chronic limb or axial pain. Has superseded the technique known as dorsal column stimulation (DCS). Pain relief with SCS can be achieved with ventral stimulation and is not reliant on stimulation-induced paresthesias as with DCS. Pain relief can persist even after the cessation of stimulations, and is not reversed by naloxone. The exact mechanism of action is undetermined.

Consultation

If seeing a consultation for a new SCS, for best results:
1. failure of multidisciplinary approach to adequately control pain
2. screen for appropriate indications (e.g., neuropathic pain, FBSS etc.)
3. chronic neuropathic limb pain without high-yield structural pathology that can be remedied with definitive surgery
4. permanent implant only if patient undergoes a successful trial

If a patient already has an SCS system and they have experienced a change in stimulation:
1. obtain radiographs to see if the lead has changed position or fractured
2. interrogate the generator and/or leads for functionality
3. if system functionality confirmed, re-program
4. if re-programming unsuccessful, consider revision

113

113.7.2 Indications/contraindications

The most common SCS application is for relief of neuropathic leg pain.
FDA-approved indications include:
1. failed back surgery syndrome (p. 1884) (FBSS)[13]: especially if LE pain > back pain
2. complex regional pain syndrome (p. 1885) (CRPS), formerly "reflex sympathetic dystrophy"

Possible indications include:
1. diabetic neuropathy (p. 1886)
2. refractory angina pectoris (p. 1886)
3. postthoracotomy pain (intercostal neuralgia)
4. postherpetic neuralgia
5. painful limb ischemia from inoperable peripheral vascular disease (p. 1885)
6. functional: spastic hemiparesis, dystonia, bladder dysfunction

Relative contraindications include:
1. cancer pain
2. patients with limited life expectancy
3. patients with untreated depression
4. primarily nociceptive pain (p. 518)
5. patients with polysubstance abuse
6. patients with psychosis

113.7.3 Technique

The implant trial procedure is performed with the patient awake, under local anesthetic, to confirm appropriate stimulation coverage.[14]

Two techniques are used to place electrodes in the *epidural* space:
1. wire-like electrodes placed percutaneously with a Tuohy needle.
2. "paddle electrodes" placed via laminotomy

SCS leads have been placed anywhere from C1–5:
- leads at C1–2 usually provide coverage for neck, shoulder, or arm pain
- midline truncal stimulation between the neck and low back for pain is often difficult to achieve
- posterior column stimulation evokes tingling paresthesias targeted to overlay the area of pain and electrodes are always positioned in the dorsal epidural space
- leads are usually inserted under fluoroscopic guidance in the midline; however, if the symptoms are lateralized, leads can be placed eccentrically toward the affected side
- thoracic percutaneous leads are introduced into the epidural space via a Tuohy needle puncture at some level below the conus. They are threaded rostrally until the desired coverage is achieved. Wide distribution can be attained
- thoracic paddle leads are placed by performing a laminotomy at T9–10 with the lead passed rostrally to the T8–9 vertebral body level[14]

Following electrode placement, a trial with an external generator over several days is used to determine if there is a response. A trial is considered successful if there is greater than 50% pain reduction on visual analog scale (VAS). Responders undergo subsequent conversion to a permanent system with internalization of an implanted pulse generator (IPG). IPGs may be primary cell devices or rechargeable and are placed in a subcutaneous pocket in the flank, buttock, or lower abdominal quadrant. The IPG can be externally reprogrammed to "fine-tune" stimulation.

113.7.4 Complications

Overall risk of device-related complications is 32%.[14,15,16] Potential complications include:
1. lead migration: 13%. More common in percutaneous and cervical stimulators
2. lead breakage: 9.1%
3. infection: 3.5% incidence. Treated with electrode and/or IPG removal and antibiotics
4. hardware malfunction: 2.9%
5. unwanted stimulation: 2.4%
6. less common complications: CSF leak, radicular pain, intermittent interference with cardiac pacemakers, and neurologic deficit.

113.7.5 Outcome

The primary measure of success is a sustained reduction in pain > 50%.

Secondary goals may include: improved health-related quality of life, reduction in pain medication requirement, increased functional capacity, and return to work.

In a retrospective report on 410 patients with SCS implantation for a variety of indications followed for a mean of 96 months, successful therapy thus defined was achieved in 74%.[17]

113.7.6 Specific syndromes treated

Failed back surgery syndrome (FBSS)

Σ: Effectiveness of spinal cord stimulators for failed back surgery syndrome

The addition of SCS improves pain control over either PT or medical management alone for FBSS. At 24 months, SCS is as effective as reoperation in treating radicular pain, with no difference in ADLs or work status.

PROCESS trial[18] (Prospective Randomized Controlled Multicenter Trial of the Effectiveness of Spinal Cord Stimulation): 100 FBSS patients were randomized to SCS placement plus conventional medical management (CMM) (52 patients) vs. CMM alone (48 patients). The health-related quality of life, measured using EuroQol-5D questionnaire, was greater in the SCS group despite a higher total health care cost at 6 months.[15] In 24-month follow-up, the primary outcome was achieved in 37% of patients that were randomized to SCS plus CMM and 2% of patients that were randomized to CMM only. Patients were allowed to cross over. After crossover, the primary outcome was achieved in 47% of patients (34 of 72) who had SCS plus medical management as final treatment versus 7% of patients (1 of 15) in the other group (P=0.02).[19]

In another randomized prospective study, patients with persistent or recurrent radicular pain after lumbosacral surgery were randomized to reoperation vs. SCS. On an average of 3-year follow-up, the SCS group required fewer opiate analgesics. 9 of 19 patients in the SCS group compared to only 3 of 26 patients reoperated had self-reported pain relief and satisfaction (P<0.01), and there was no difference in ADLs and work status. Patients in the SCS group were less likely to crossover to undergo reoperation (5 of 24 patients from the SCS group versus 14 of 26 patients in the reoperation group, P=0.02).[20]

In a study evaluating the cost-effectiveness of SCS, the initial cost of SCS is offset by future reductions in healthcare resource utilization. The medium- to long-term costs of SCS seem to be economically favorable compared to other therapies for FBSS.[21]

Complex regional pain syndrome (CRPS)

Σ: Effectiveness of SCS for CRPS

SCS may be effective for treating CRPS during the first couple of years, but no significant benefit was evident at 5-year follow-up.

CRPS is a chronic pain condition marked by continuous disabling intense aching or burning pain. Type I is nonspecific soft-tissue pain with no known nerve injury. Type II (p.525) follows a nerve injury. Spontaneous pain, hyperpathia, and allodynia disproportionate to the inciting stimulus are hallmarks of CRPS. The pathophysiology leading to disproportional pain response is unknown and treatment options are limited. In a randomized clinical trial,[22] patients with CRPS Type I were randomized to receive SCS plus physical therapy (PT) (36 patients) or PT alone (18 patients). 24 of 36 patients had successful SCS trial and underwent implantation. At 6 months, in the group that received SCS plus PT, pain intensity reduced by 2.4 cm on the visual-analogue scale as opposed to an increase of 0.2 cm in the PT-only group (P<0.001). In addition, 39% of patients in the SCS group had "much improved" globally perceived effect vs. 6% (P=0.01). The health-related quality of life only improved in the SCS group. At 2-year follow-up, pain intensity in the SCS group reduced by 2.1 vs. 1.0 cm in the PT group compared to baseline (P<0.001) and global perceived effect was "much improved" in 43% vs. 6% (P=0.001).[23] However, these benefits were no longer significant in 5 years.[24]

Peripheral vascular disease

Σ: SCS for peripheral vascular disease

SCS does help with pain due to inoperable limb ischemia. It may or may not improve healing of pressure ulcers.

Peripheral vascular disease may result in clinical limb pain or ischemic ulcers.

A review of six controlled studies of nearly 450 patients, SCS+medical treatment was compared to medical treatment alone. Although there was no significant difference in ulcer healing, the use of analgesics was less and limb salvage after 12 months was significantly higher in the SCS group (relative risk = 0.71).[25]

113

Angina pectoris

Σ: SCS for angina pectoris

SCS was as effective as CABG in controlling refractory angina and protecting against MIs. SCS improves exercise capacity by an unknown mechanism.

In select patients SCS can reduce anginal pain and improve exercise capacity.

In a prospective study of 104 patients who underwent SCS placement for refractory angina pectoris (average follow-up ≈ 13 months), 73% had > 50% reduction of weekly anginal episodes compared to baseline.[26]

Diabetic neuropathy

Σ: SCS for diabetic neuropathy

Available data is limited, but SCS may be a viable modality for refractory pain from diabetic neuropathy. Further study is needed.

No good clinical data are available. A few studies with small numbers of patients suggest SCS can provide significant pain relief in most patients with diabetic neuropathy who have failed conservative management.[27,28,29]

A small prospective, open-label study reported 9 of 11 patients with diabetic neuropathy that failed conservative treatment had significant pain relief after SCS implantation at 6 months. Pain score on visual analogue scale decreased from 77 to 34. Microcirculatory perfusion did not change significantly from baseline.[29]

113.8 Deep brain stimulation (DBS)

Deafferentation pain syndromes (anesthesia dolorosa, pain from spinal cord injury, or thalamic pain syndromes) may benefit from stimulation of sensory thalamus (ventral posteromedial (VPM) or ventral posterolateral (VPL)). DBS for chronic neuropathic pain produces a 40–50% reduction in pain in about 25–60% of patients.[30]

Nociceptive pain syndromes are more likely to benefit from stimulation of periventricular gray matter (PVG) or periaqueductal gray matter (PAG), although PAG stimulation is rarely used because it often produces unpleasant side effects. Still, response rate has been only ≈ 20%,[31] resulting in failure of the FDA to approve these devices for pain.

Cluster headaches: may respond to hypothalamic stimulation, but larger trials with longer follow-up are needed.[30]

113.9 Dorsal root entry zone (DREZ) lesions

113.9.1 General information

Although use has been reported for a variety of indications, DREZ lesions appear to be most effective in treating the following:

1. deafferentation pain resulting from nerve root avulsion.[32,33,34] This most commonly occurs in motorcycle accidents
2. spinal cord injuries (SCI) with pain around the lowest spared dermatome with caudal extension of pain restricted to a few dermatomes (SCI with diffuse pain involving the entire body and limb below the injury is less responsive)
3. postherpetic neuralgia (p.522): usually good initial response, but early recurrence in ≤ few months is common, and only 25% have long-term relief of pain
4. postamputation phantom limb pain: there is some support for this in the literature, but others feel this is not a good indication[35]
5. ✖ generally not used for cancer pain

113

13.9.2 Technique

A laminectomy is performed over the involved segment(s) using radiographic localization. The dura is opened, and the DREZ is identified under microscope magnification using intact posterior rootlets above or below for orientation (contralateral rootlets may also be used to estimate the mirror-image location). Lesions are created ipsilateral to the avulsed nerve roots by radiofrequency current (approximately 50–60 lesions are required for several segments, each lesion is done at 75° for ≈ 15 seconds) or selective incisions extending from the last completely normal rootlet at the rostral end to the first normal rootlet caudally. The lesioning needle or knife blade is angled 30–45° medially and inserted to a depth of 2–3 mm. DREZ lesions may be combined with a cordectomy at the level of anatomic cord disruption in paraplegic patients.[35]

13.9.3 Post-op management

Bed rest for 3 days may reduce the risk of CSF leakage. Analgesics appropriate for a multilevel laminectomy are administered.

13.9.4 Complications

Ipsilateral weakness (related to corticospinal tract) or loss of proprioception (dorsal columns) occurs in 10% of patients, and is permanent in ≈ half (i.e., 5%).

13.9.5 Outcome

In pain related to brachial plexus avulsion, 80–90% long-term significant improvement can be expected. Paraplegics with pain limited to the region of injury have an 80% rate of improvement, compared to 30% for those with pain involving the entire body below the lesion.

References

[1] Young RF, Kroening R, Fulton W, et al. Electrical Stimulation of the Brain in Treatment of Chronic Pain: Experience Over 5 Years. Journal of Neurosurgery. 1985; 62:389–396

[2] Shieff C, Nashold BS. Stereotactic Mesencephalotomy. Neurosurgery Clinics of North America. 1990; 1:825–839

[3] Marshall KA. Managing Cancer Pain: Basic Principles and Invasive Treatment. Mayo Clinic Proceedings. 1996; 71:472–477

[4] Krieger AJ, Rosomoff HL. Sleep-Induced Apnea. Part 1: A Respiratory and Autonomic Dysfunction Syndrome Following Bilateral Percutaneous Cervical Cordotomy. J Neurosurg. 1974; 39:168–180

[5] Sugar O. In Search of Ondine's Curse. Journal of the American Medical Association. 1978; 240:236–237

[6] Schwartz HG. High Cervical Cordotomy. J Neurosurg. 1967; 26:452–455

[7] Lobato RD, Madrid JL, Fatela LV, et al. Intraventricular Morphine for Intractable Cancer Pain: Rationale, Methods, Clinical Results. Acta Anaesthesiologica Scandinavica. Supplementum. 1987; 85:68–74

[8] Brazenor GA. Long Term Intrathecal Administration of Morphine: A Comparison of Bolus Injection via Reservoir with Continuous Infusion by Implantable Pump. Neurosurgery. 1987; 21:484–491

[9] Penn RD, Paice JA. Chronic Intrathecal Morphine for Intractable Pain. J Neurosurg. 1987; 67:182–186

[10] Shetter AG, Hadley MN, Wilkinson E. Administration of Intraspinal Morphine Sulfate for the Treatment of Intractable Cancer Pain. Neurosurgery. 1986; 18:740–747

[11] Rippe ES, Kresel JJ. Preparation of Morphine Sulfate Solutions for Intraspinal Administration. Am J Hosp Pharm. 1986; 43:1420–1421

[12] Cramond T, Stuart G. Intraventricular Morphine for Intractable Pain of Advanced Cancer. Journal of Pain & Symptom Management. 1993; 8:465–473

[13] Kumar K, Nath R, Wyant GM. Treatment of Chronic Pain by Epidural Spinal Cord Stimulation. Journal of Neurosurgery. 1991; 75:402–407

[14] North RB, Ewend MG, Lawton MT, et al. Spinal cord stimulation for chronic, intractable pain: superiority of "multi-channel" devices. Pain. 1991; 44:119–130

[15] Kumar K, Taylor RS, Jacques L, et al. Spinal cord stimulation versus conventional medical management for neuropathic pain: a multicentre randomised controlled trial in patients with failed back surgery syndrome. Pain. 2007; 132:179–188

[16] Cameron T. Safety and efficacy of spinal cord stimulation for the treatment of chronic pain: a 20-year literature review. J Neurosurg. 2004; 100:254–267

[17] North RB, Kidd DH, Zahurak M, et al. Spinal Cord Stimulation for Chronic, Intractable Pain: Experience Over Two Decades. Neurosurgery. 1993; 32:384–395

[18] Manca A, Kumar K, Taylor RS, et al. Quality of life, resource consumption and costs of spinal cord stimulation versus conventional medical management in neuropathic pain patients with failed back surgery syndrome (PROCESS trial). Eur J Pain. 2008; 12:1047–1058

[19] Kumar K, Taylor RS, Jacques L, et al. The effects of spinal cord stimulation in neuropathic pain are sustained: a 24-month follow-up of the prospective randomized controlled multicenter trial of the effectiveness of spinal cord stimulation. Neurosurgery. 2008; 63:762–70; discussion 770

[20] North RB, Kidd DH, Farrokhi F, et al. Spinal cord stimulation versus repeated lumbosacral spine surgery for chronic pain: a randomized, controlled trial. Neurosurgery. 2005; 56:98–106; discussion 106-7

[21] Taylor RS, Taylor RJ, Van Buyten JP, et al. The cost effectiveness of spinal cord stimulation in the treatment of pain: a systematic review of the literature. J Pain Symptom Manage. 2004; 27:370–378

[22] Kemler MA, Barendse GA, van Kleef M, et al. Spinal cord stimulation in patients with chronic reflex sympathetic dystrophy. New England Journal of Medicine. 2000; 343:618–624

113

[23] Kemler MA, De Vet HC, Barendse GA, et al. The effect of spinal cord stimulation in patients with chronic reflex sympathetic dystrophy: two years' follow-up of the randomized controlled trial. Annals of Neurology. 2004; 55:13–18

[24] Kemler MA, de Vet HC, Barendse GA, et al. Effect of spinal cord stimulation for chronic complex regional pain syndrome Type I: five-year final follow-up of patients in a randomized controlled trial. Journal of Neurosurgery. 2008; 108:292–298

[25] Ubbink DT, Vermeulen H. Spinal cord stimulation for non-reconstructable chronic critical leg ischaemia. Cochrane Database Syst Rev. 2005. DOI: 10.1002/14651858.CD004001.pub2

[26] Di Pede F, Lanza GA, Zuin G, et al. Immediate and long-term clinical outcome after spinal cord stimulation for refractory stable angina pectoris. American Journal of Cardiology. 2003; 91:951–955

[27] Tesfaye S, Watt J, Benbow SJ, et al. Electrical spinal-cord stimulation for painful diabetic peripheral neuropathy. Lancet. 1996; 348:1698–1701

[28] Daousi C, Benbow SJ, MacFarlane IA. Electrical spinal cord stimulation in the long-term treatment of chronic painful diabetic neuropathy. Diabetic Medicine. 2005; 22:393–398

[29] de Vos CC, Rajan V, Steenbergen W, et al. Effect and safety of spinal cord stimulation for treatment of chronic pain caused by diabetic neuropathy. Journal of Diabetes and Its Complications. 2009; 23:40–45

[30] Awan NR, Lozano A, Hamani C. Deep brain stimulation: current and future perspectives. Neurosurgical Focus. 2009; 27. DOI: 10.3171/2009.4.FOCUS0982

[31] Coffey RJ. Deep brain stimulation for chronic pain: results of two multicenter trials and a structured review. Pain Med. 2001; 2:183–192

[32] Thomas DGT, Jones SJ. Dorsal Root Entry Zone Lesions (Nashold's Procedure) in Brachial Plexus Avulsion. Neurosurgery. 1986; 15:966–968

[33] Nashold BS. Current Status of the DREZ Operation 1984. Neurosurgery. 1984; 15:942–944

[34] Friedman AH, Nashold BS. Dorsal Root Entry Zone Lesions for the Treatment of Brachial Plexus Avulsion Injuries: A Follow-up Study. Neurosurgery 1988; 22:369–373

[35] Burchiel KJ, Favre J. Current Techniques for Pain Control. Contemporary Neurosurgery. 1997; 19:1–

114 Seizure Surgery

114.1 Indications for seizure surgery

114.1.1 General information

20-36% of patients continue to have seizures despite rigorous attempt at medical management with ASMs. Many of these patients may be candidates for surgical procedures to control their seizures.[1,2]

Epilepsy treatment should be aggressive to reduce: brain damage, development of secondary seizure foci, psychosocial distress and mortality (p. 480). Seizure surgery is associated with a reduction in mortality rate in medically refractory epilepsy, and while the reduction was highest when seizures are abolished, mortality is also reduced with significant reduction of tonic-clonic seizure frequency.[3] Unfortunately, many patients who would benefit from surgical treatment are not referred or are referred late for surgery due to the misconception surgery should be a last resort.[4]

The seizure disorder must be severe, debilitating, or socally disruptive to the patient.

114.1.2 Types of seizures amenable to surgery

The three general categories of seizure types suitable for seizure surgery[5]:
1. focal onset seizures (see below for criteria)
   a) temporal origin: the largest group of surgical candidates (especially mesial temporal lobe epilepsy (MTLE), ▶ Table 26.1, which is often medically refractory)
   b) extratemporal origin
2. symptomatic generalized seizures: e.g., for Lennox-Gastaut (p. 484) syndrome, corpus callosotmy may reduce the incidence of drop attacks
3. unilateral, multifocal epilepsy associated with infantile hemiplegia syndrome

114.1.3 Surgical candidates for focal onset seizures

There is no standard, widely accepted criteria for resective/ablative seizure surgery. Therefore patient selection differs between centers.[6]

A literature review found that most epilepsy centers define surgical candidacy by seizure frequency and medically refratory seizures, but that the definition of these terms varies.[6] The most common criteria found were: seizure frequency ≥ 1 seizure per month, and failure of ≥ 2 ASMs. They also point out that even "infrequent seizures may still pose significant risks and impair quality-of-life".[6]

Medically refractory epilepsy: most centers rely upon failure of at least 2 adequate trials of 2 simultaneous tolerable ASMs (the probability of control after 2 failures is 9.6%[2]). The ILAE recommends seizure freedom (Category 1 outcome) for whichever of the following is *longer*[7]:
- 12 months or
- 3 times the longest pre-intervention time between seizures during the past 12 months

114

114.2 Definitions

In addition to the classification of seizure (p. 480), the following terms & concepts are particularly relevant to seizure surgery.[8]

Epileptogenic lesion: a structural lesion believed to be producing the seizure, e.g., area of abnormal cortical development, or cavernous malformation.

Ictal onset zone (AKA seizure onset zone): the area that actually generates the seizure. Typically identified depth electrode recording (scalp electrodes can often give an approximation).

Symptomatogenic zone: region of cortex that produces the observed symptoms when activated by a seizure.

Irritative zone: region of cortex that produces interictal spikes detected on scalp or invasive EEG, magnetoencephalography (MEG), or triggered fMRI. Isolated spikes generally do not produce clinical symptoms.

Epileptogenic zone: region of cortex essential for the generation of a clinical seizure. Unlike the irritative zone, it can also be detected by single photon emission CT (SPECT).

Functional deficit zone: area of cortex that is impaired in the interictal period, either by destruction by a lesion or by functional inhibition.

114.3 Pre-surgical evaluation for seizure surgery

114.3.1 General information

All patients should undergo high-resolution MRI study to rule out e.g., neoplasm, AVM, cavernous malformations, mesial temporal sclerosis, or hippocampal lesion. Noninvasive techniques allow localization in the majority of cases.

25% of patients referred to specialized epilepsy clinics do not have epilepsy.[9,10] See ▶ Table 28.2 for some etiologies.

114.3.2 Noninvasive evaluation techniques

▶ **Video-EEG monitoring.** Preoperative long-term inpatient video-EEG monitoring (surface electrodes) to correlate the clinically disabling seizure with appropriate electrical abnormalities and possibly to identify the seizure focus is required.

▶ **High-resolution MRI.** The imaging modality of choice. Extremely good for detecting hippocampal asymmetry of mesial temporal sclerosis (MTS), and neuronal developmental abnormalities (e.g., cortical dysplasia) that may produce complex partial seizures (CPS).[11]

▶ **CAT scan.** A seizure focus may enhance with IV contrast shortly following a seizure. Subtle enhancement may be present on the side of the focus on interictal CT scan.[12]

▶ **PET scan (positron emission tomography).** Interictal PET scan using 18-fluorodeoxyglucose (18FDG) shows *hypo*metabolism lateralized to the side of temporal lobe focus in 70% of patients with medically refractory CPS (does not show actual *site* of origin). Useful when MRI and EEG cannot localize.

▶ **SPECT scan (single-photon emission computed tomography).** Used to demonstrate increased blood flow during a seizure to help localize site of onset. [99m]Technetium (Tc) hexamethyl-propylene-amine-oxime (HMPAO) is usually administered immediately after onset of seizure, and the scan may be obtained within several hours.[13]

▶ **MEG (magnetoencephalography).** Functional imaging technique for mapping brain activity by recording magnetic fields created by neuronal activity (electrical current).[14] Synchronized neuronal currents induce a weak magnetic field. Clinical uses include detecting and localizing pathological activity in patients with epilepsy and in localizing eloquent cortex for preoperative surgical planning. Requires a magnetically shielded room.

114.3.3 Mildly invasive techniques

▶ **Wada test.**[15] AKA intracarotid amytal test. Localizes dominant hemisphere (side of language function) and assesses ability of hemisphere without lesion to maintain memory when isolated. Usually reserved for candidates for large resections.[16] Each cerebral hemisphere is individually anesthetized via selective carotid catheterization (usually by a neurointerventionalist) and injection of short acting barbiturate.

Start with angiogram to assess cross-flow and to R/O persistent trigeminal artery (p. 83). Significant cross-flow is a relative contraindication to anesthetizing the side of dominant supply (patient goes to sleep).

Wada test may be grossly inaccurate with high-flow AVM. Also, portions of hippocampus may be supplied by posterior circulation (not anesthetized by ICA injection).

EEG monitoring is usually performed during the test when it is being done for seizure surgery. Patient will show delta waves during deepest level of anesthesia.

Technique:
- instruct patient as to what is expected
- catheterize ICA: usually start on side of lesion
- have patient hold contralateral arm in air, and instruct them to hold it there
- inject 100–125 mg sodium *amobarbital* (Amytal®) rapidly into internal carotid artery (effect starts almost instantaneously, begins to subside after ≈ 8 minutes; may subside in ≈ 2 minutes with AVM where flow rates are high)
- determine adequacy of injection by assessing motor function in elevated arm (should be ≈ flaccid)
- assess language skills by showing patient pictures of objects and asking them to name each one out loud and remember each one

- assess memory function by asking patient to name as many of the pictures as they can ≈ 15 minutes after test: if they have difficulty, ask them to pick out pictures from a group that contains additional ones not shown to patient
- repeat procedure on other side (use lower Amytal doses with each subsequent injection)

114.3.4 Evaluation techniques requiring surgery

▶ **EEG obtained with invasive electrodes.** Indications: Lack of lateralizing or localizing electrophysiology in preoperative evaluation requires invasive electrodes for better definition of seizure focus. Surgical options:
- depth electrodes
  - electrodes are placed stereotactically
  - stereoencephalography (sEEG): popularized in Europe by J. Talairach and J. Bancaud during the 1950s for invasive mapping of refractory focal epilepsy. The technique requires the placement of multiple depth electrodes in an orthogonal orientation to localize seizure onset.[17,18,19]
  - 2–3% risk of intracerebral hemorrhage.[16] Risk of infection with depth electrodes[16]: 2–10%.
- subdural grids or strips
  - grids are frequently used for extraoperative functional mapping (helpful in children or in the mentally retarded). Subdural grid electrodes are placed with a craniotomy.
  - surface strip electrodes may be placed through a burr hole
  - useful technique for intraoperative functional mapping

114.4 Surgical techniques

114.4.1 Basic procedures

Three basic types of procedure: resections, disconnections, and stimulation.[1] The chances of being seizure free after surgery are two to three times higher when a lesion is identified on histopathology or MRI.[20]

- **resections**
  a) resection of epileptic focus: higher chance of completely controlling seizures. Performed in noneloquent brain. Seizures must have focal onset (resection is discouraged if multifocal onset). Includes:
     - anterior temporal lobectomy or selective amygdalo-hippocampectomy for MTLE (p. 1893)
     - neocortical resections: especially with neuronal migration abnormalities
  b) resection of lesion in secondary epilepsy (lesional epilepsy e.g., tumor, AVM, cavernous malformation[21]…). In most cases the seizure focus is in or near the lesion, but some structural lesions are not responsible for the seizures. For seizure foci within the mesial temporal lobe, seizure control is better when lesionectomy is accompanied by amygdalo-hippocampectomy[22]
- **disconnections**: used when eloquent brain is involved, or to separate the electrical activity of the two cerebral hemispheres
  a) section of corpus callosum (callosotomy): when drop attacks are the most disabling seizure type or for multiple bilateral foci (see below)
  b) hemispherectomy: for unilateral seizures with widespread hemispheric lesions and profound contralateral neurologic deficit. If any cortex is left, must make sure it is functionally deafferented (disconnected)
     - anatomic hemispherectomy
     - functional hemispherectomy: preservation of the basal ganglia isolates the abnormal side with ≈ 80% seizure control rate (similar to anatomic hemispherectomy, but with lower complication rate)
  c) multiple subpial transections[23,24]: for partial seizure originating in eloquent cortical areas (e.g., sensorimotor cortex). The cortex is transected at 5 mm intervals leaving the pia and surface vessels intact, thus interrupting the horizontal spread of the seizure while sparing the vertically oriented functional fibers. Produced seizure freedom in 55% when combined with resection and in 24% when used alone
- **stimulation**: a reversible and modifiable (via programming changes) mode of therapy which may be particularly advantageous for poorly localized seizure foci or for seizure foci in areas of eloquent brain. 30–40% seizure reduction for most patients. Risks include hardware failure, hemorrhage (not typically seen with VNS), infection, and stimulation-induced side effects
  a) open-loop stimulation: blind stimulation continuously or intermittently
     1. vagus nerve stimulation (p. 1895) (VNS): side effects include voice changes
     2. deep brain stimulation (DBS). Targets:

114

centromedian nucleus of the thalamus[25]: better for generalized tonic-clonic seizures
bilateral anterior nucleus of the thalamus: for partial seizures (SANTE trial).[26] At 5 years 68% had ≥ 60% fewer seizures, 16% of 110 patients were seizure free for 6 months
hippocampus[25]: for partial seizures

b) closed-loop stimulation: stimulation in response to detection of a seizure, e.g., responsive neurostimulation (RNS®)[27,28] (NeuroPace). Shortcoming: detection of sezure can be difficult and imprecise, and may require extra (detection) leads. In 111 patients with MTLE, median seizure reduction was 70%, and 29% of patients had at least 6months seizure free, and 15% had no seizures for ≥ 1 year.[28] This modality may be best for patient with unilateral or bilatera MTE who are not eligible for resection or have failed previous resection. Risks include soft-tissue infections with a rate of 0.03 per implant year
c) chronic subthreshold cortical stimulation (CSCS or CS²)[29]: continuous (or intermittent) cortical stimulation at low levels to suppress a seizure focus

114.4.2 Anesthetic considerations

If intraoperative electrocorticography is to be performed:
- under local anesthesia: the only anesthetic agents that may be used are narcotics (usually fentanyl) and droperidol
- under general anesthesia: *avoid* benzodiazepines and barbiturates

114.4.3 Intraoperative electrocorticography (ECoG)

Subdural strips and/or grids are useful for ECoG and motor/speech mapping.
Methohexital (Brevitol®) may be given to try to provoke a seizure: observe for ↓ fast activity in suspected focus.

114.4.4 Intraoperative cortical mapping

See techniques of cortical mapping (p.1732).

114.5 Surgical procedures

114.5.1 Corpus callosotomy

Indications and contraindications

Partial (typically anterior 2/3) or total section may be most effective for generalized major moto seizures. Of little benefit for simple or complex seizures. Benefit has been supported for:
1. frequent episodes of *atonic seizures* ("drop attacks") where loss of postural tone → falls and injuries[30] (70% reduction with callosotomy), typically seen in Lennox-Gastaut syndrome
2. possibly for generalized seizure disorder with unilateral hemisphere damage (e.g., infantile hemiplegia syndrome); hemicortical resection may be better for this type, whereas callosotomy may promote partial seizures.
   Note: a "functional hemispherectomy" is recommended over "anatomically complete" hemispherectomy to reduce morbidity and mortality[5]
3. some patients with generalized seizures without identifiable, resectable focus
4. ✖ contraindication: major behavioral and/or language deficits may occur even with partial division in patients with speech and dominant handedness located in *opposite* hemispheres ("crosse dominance"). Thus, Wada test is recommended in all left-handed patients

Technical details

Division of the anterior two-thirds of the corpus callosum (CC) (minimizes the risk of disconnectio syndrome, see below) may be advantageous over complete callosotomy (controversial). Some advo cate sectioning the CC with intraoperative EEG until the typical bisynchronous discharges that ar usually seen become asynchronous.[31] No need to section anterior commissure. Can usually be pe formed via a bifrontal craniotomy utilizing a bicoronal skin incision.
May produce post-op ↓ verbalization or akinetic mutism that usually resolves in weeks.
Callosotomy has been reported in a small number of patients using laser interstitial thermal the apy (LITT) alone, or as a technique to extend a previous surgical callosotomy.[32,33]

114

MRI sagittal cuts are ideal for assessing extent of division of the CC.[34]

Disconnection syndrome

In a patient with a dominant left hemisphere, consists of left tactile anomia, left-sided dyspraxia (may resemble hemiparesis), pseudohemianopsia, right-sided anomia for smell, impaired spatial synthesis of right hand resulting in difficulty copying complex figures, decreased spontaneity of speech, incontinence.

More common with larger surgical sections of the CC. Risk is less if the anterior commissure is spared. Patients usually adapt after 2–3 months, with final function normal for most daily activities (deficits may show up on neuropsychological testing).

114.5.2 Mesial temporal lobe epilepsy (MTLE)

General information

80% of patients with medically intractable temporal seizures have a demonstrable focus in the anterior-mesial temporal lobe. Most patients have neuronal loss and gliosis of mesial temporal structures (mesial temporal sclerosis (p. 482) (MTS)). For this, a standard resection of temporal tip (with amygdalo-hippocampectomy) may be performed. In a randomized trial, anterior temporal lobectomy (ATL) was shown to be superior to medical management for treatment of medically resistant epilepsy. Results at one year show seizure reduction and improved quality of life in those patients who underwent ATL versus medical management alone for intractable epilepsy.[35]

Limits of resection (without significant neurologic deficit) with ATL

Note that these values are generally considered safe; however, variations occur from patient to patient and only intraoperative mapping can reliably determine the location of language centers.[36] Most centers spare the superior temporal gyrus.[37] The following measurements are made along the *middle* temporal gyrus:

* *dominant* temporal lobe: up to 4–5 cm may be removed. Over-resection may injure speech centers, which cannot be reliably localized visually
* *non-dominant* temporal lobe: 6–7 cm may be resected. Slight over-resection may → partial contralateral upper quadrant homonymous hemianopsia; resection of 8–9 cm → complete quadrantanopsia

Alternatively, intraoperative electrocorticography may be used to guide resection of electrically abnormal areas.

Resection should be performed in subpial plane to prevent injury to vascular branches.

114

114.5.3 Selective amygdalo-hippocampectomy (SAH)

Anterior temporal lobectomy was the initial surgery for temporal lobe epilepsy described by Penfield and Baldwin. In 1958, Niemeyer described a more selective approach to the hippocampus and amygdala through the middle temporal gyrus.[38] It would be almost thirty years until selective amygdalo-hippocampectomy (SAH) was later modified. The goal of SAH is to remove the epileptogenic focus while minimizing disruption of nearby neurovascular structures and white matter tracts. Image guidance is very helpful for these techniques. More recent studies have compared standard ATL to SAH and found that both techniques have similar outcome with regard to seizure freedom but suggest an improved neuropsychological outcome with SAH versus ATL.[39,40]

Three basic approaches:

1. transcortical: inferior temporal gyrus (ITG) approach. This technique uses a minimal-access approach via a trephine craniotomy for SAH[41]
2. transsylvian: approach requires a pterional craniotomy. More restrictive and greater risk of injury to M1 portion of MCA within Sylvian fissure[42]
3. subtemporal: uses a temporal fossa approach to access mesial structures[43,44]

114.6 Risks of seizure surgery

Major risks are related to[45]:

1. removal of essential areas of cortex

2. injury to medullary core underlying cortical resection (projection fibers, association fibers, and/or commissural fibers): the most common deficit after temporal lobectomy is a contralateral (homonymous) superior quadrantanopsia (so-called "pie-in-the-sky" defect, due to an injury to Meyer's loop wherein the fibers for the superior visual field of the optic radiation take a slight rostral "detour" towards the temporal tip; see ▶ Fig. 33.2)
3. injury to vessels in area of resection → ischemic damage to areas supplied: especially Sylvian branches during temporal lobectomy, anterior choroidal artery resulting in hemiparesis during mesial temporal lobe resection, or ACA branches with corpus callosotomy
4. injury to nearby cranial nerves: especially third nerve during hippocampectomy where it lies medial to tentorium

114.7 Other ablation techniques

114.7.1 Radiofrequency ablation (RF ablation)

Electric current is passed through depth electrodes to create small localized lesions approximately 4 mm diameter with the patient awake. Can be performed at the patient's bedside.

114.7.2 MRI-guided laser interstitial thermal therapy (MRGLITT)

Laser-induced thermal therapy uses thermal energy transmitted through a fiberoptic probe to induce cell death by damaging DNA and causing protein denaturation. The current therapy is performed with simultaneous MRI stereotactic guidance and real-time feedback from the ablated lesion.[46,47] It is considered less invasive than microsurgery. Main advantage is a shorter postoperative recovery period. Technique has been used for lesional (e.g., cavernous malformation) and nonlesional epilepsy. 82% of 17 patients > 1 year follow-up (mean 30 months) were seizure-free at 1 year (59% Engel class 1A, ▶ Table 114.1, 31% off all ASMs),[48] and ablations targeting more anterior, medial and inferior temporal lobe structures were more likely to be associated with Engel I outcomes.[49] Longer-term data is pending. LITT has been used to perform corpus callosotomy (see above).

114.7.3 Stereotactic radiosurgery (SRS) of mesial temporal lobe

The Radiosurgery or Open Surgery for Epilepsy (ROSE) trial found better seizure control with open anterior temporal lobectomy (78%) than with 24 Gy SRS (52%).[50] SRS had about a year latency before benefits were realized. The safety profile was similar. The conclusion was that SRS could be an option for patient who are not operative candidates or who choose not to have surgery.[50]

114.8 Postoperative management for seizure surgery (epilepsy surgery)

1. ICU for observation (24 hrs)
2. for seizures in the immediate post-op period ("honeymoon seizures"), not necessary to treat only one brief generalized seizure, otherwise load appropriately with IV Keppra or phenytoin
3. 10 mg dexamethasone (Decadron®) IV before surgery followed by q 8 hrs as necessary (longer taper for laser ablation and radiosurgery)
4. antiseizure medications are continued × 1–2 years even if no post-op seizures occur
5. after discharge: neuropsychiatric evaluation 6–12 months after surgery

114.9 Outcome

The modified Engel classification and the International Leage Against Epilepsy (ILAE) of outcome following seizure surgery are shown in ▶ Table 114.1.[51,52]

114.9.1 Outcome with resection of seizure focus

The greatest effect of seizure surgery is *reduction of seizure frequency*[37]; however, any surgical procedure may fail to have a beneficial effect.

Seizure control is usually assessed at 1, 3, & 6 mos post-op, and then annually. A post-op MRI is usually obtained at 3 mos post-op to assess extent of surgical resection. Most patients take anti-epileptic drugs (ASMs) for 2 years post-op, and then may be discontinued in those free of seizures.

Table 114.1 Modified Engel & ILAE classification of seizure surgery outcome[52]

Engel Class	General Description	Detailed Engel Description	ILAE Classification
I	seizure-free or residual auras	I-A: completely seizure free since surgery	Class 1. Completely seizure free; no auras.
		I-B: nondisabling simple partial seizures only since surgery	Class 1a. Completely seizure free since surgery; no auras.
		I-C: some disabling seizures after seizures surgery, but free from disabling seizures for 2 yrs	Class 2. only auras; no other seizures
		I-D: generalized convulsions with ASM discontinuation only	
II	rare disabling seizures (< 3 complex partial seizures per year)	II-A: initially free from disabling seizures, but still has rare seizures	Class 3. 1-3 seizure days/yr; ± auras
		II-B: rare disabling seizures since surgery	
		II-C: occasional disabling seizures since surgery, but rare seizures for the last 2 yrs	
		II-D: nocturnal seizures only	
III	worthwhile improvement	III-A: worthwhile seizure reduction	Class 4. 4 seizure days/yr - 50% reduction in baseline nuber of seizure days; ± auras
		III-B: prolonged seizure-free intervals of seizure days; auras amounting to 50% of follow-up period, but not 2 yrs	
IV	no worthwhile seizure improvement	IV-A: significant seizure reduction	Class 5. < 50% reduction in baseline number of seizure days - 100% of baseline number of seizure days; ± auras
		IV-B: no appreciable change	
		IV-C: seizures worse	Class 6. > 100% increase in baseline number of seizure days; ± auras

Recurrent seizures: although late seizures may occur, 90% of seizures that recur do so within 2 years.

2 years post-op in patients maintained on ASMs: 50% are seizure-free, and 80% have over 50% reduction of seizure frequency.

For temporal lobectomies in the dominant hemisphere without intraoperative monitoring, there is a 6% risk of mild dysphasia. Significant memory deficits occur in ≈ 2%.

14.9.2 Radiosurgery for epilepsy

Stereotactic radiosurgery has been suggested to be an effective treatment for pharmacoresistant epilepsy with the potential for less morbidity than resection.[53,54] Seizure-free outcomes ≈ 65% for MTLE (delayed response to therapy ≈ 6–12 months). Potential for long-term complications remains a concern (radionecrosis).[55]

14.9.3 Vagus nerve stimulation (VNS)

Electrodes wrapped around the *left* vagus nerve in the neck are connected to an implanted programmable generator to stimulate the nerve to reduce seizure frequency. As is also true with many ASMs, the mechanism of action is not well understood.

Indications: Although it has been used (off-label) for treatment-resistant depression and other psychiatric conditions, the FDA-approved indication is for adjunctive therapy for patients > 12 years old with partial-onset seizures refractory to medical treatment.

Complications: Main risk of surgery is transient or permanent vocal cord paralysis. Infection necessitating removal of the device occurred in 0.6%.[56]

Outcome: In an 11-year retrospective review of VNS in 400 patients, seizure control ≥ 90% occurred in 22% of patients, control ≥ 75% in 40%, control ≥ 50% in 64%.[56]

References

[1] Engel JJ. Surgery for Seizures. New England Journal of Medicine. 1996; 334:647–652

[2] Kwan P, Brodie MJ. Early identification of refractory epilepsy. N Engl J Med. 2000; 342:314–319

[3] Sperling MR, Barshow S, Nei M, et al. A reappraisal of mortality after epilepsy surgery. Neurology. 2016; 86:1938–1944

[4] Burneo JG, Shariff SZ, Liu K, et al. Disparities in surgery among patients with intractable epilepsy in a universal health system. Neurology. 2016; 86:72–78

[5] National Institutes of Health Consensus Development Conference. Surgery for Epilepsy. JAMA. 1990; 264:729–733

[6] Kwon CS, Neal J, Tellez-Zenteno J, et al. Resective focal epilepsy surgery - Has selection of candidates changed? A systematic review. Epilepsy Res. 2016; 122:37–43

[7] Kwan P, Arzimanoglou A, Berg AT, et al. Definition of drug resistant epilepsy: consensus proposal by the ad hoc Task Force of the ILAE Commission on Therapeutic Strategies. Epilepsia. 2010; 51:1069–1077

[8] Rosenow F, Luders H. Presurgical evaluation of epilepsy. Brain. 2001; 124:1683–1700

[9] Scheepers B, Clough P, Pickles C. The misdiagnosis of epilepsy: findings of a population study. Seizure. 1998; 7:403–406

[10] Smith D, Defalla BA, Chadwick DW. The misdiagnosis of epilepsy and the management of refractory epilepsy in a specialist clinic. QJM. 1999; 92:15–23

[11] Barkovich AJ, Rowley HA, Anderman F. MR in Partial Epilepsy: Value of High-Resolution Volumetric Techniques. American Journal of Neuroradiology. 1995; 16:339–343

[12] Oakley J, Ojemann GA, Ojemann LM, et al. Identifying Epileptic Foci on Contrast-Enhanced CAT Scans. Arch Neurol. 1979; 36:669–671

[13] Harvey AS, Hopkins IJ, Bowe JM, et al. Frontal Lobe Epilepsy: Clinical Seizure Characteristics and Localization with Ictal [99mTc-HMPAO SPECT. Neurology. 1993; 43:1966–1980

[14] Tovar-Spinoza ZS, Ochi A, Rutka JT, et al. The role of magnetoencephalography in epilepsy surgery. Neurosurg Focus. 2008; 25. DOI: 10.3171/FOC/2008/25/9/E16

[15] Wada J, Rasmussen T. Intracranial Injection of Amytal for the Lateralization of Cerebral Speech Dominance. J Neurosurg. 1960; 17:266–282

[16] Queenan JV, Germano IM. Advances in the Neurosurgical Management of Adult Epilepsy. Contemporary Neurosurgery. 1997; 19:1–6

[17] Bancaud J, Angelergues R, Bernouilli C, et al. Functional stereotaxic exploration (SEEG) of epilepsy. Electroencephalogr Clin Neurophysiol. 1970; 28:85–86

[18] Talairach J, Bancaud J, Bonis A, et al. Surgical therapy for frontal epilepsies. Adv Neurol. 1992; 57:707–732

[19] Gonzalez-Martinez J, Mullin J, Vadera S, et al. Stereotactic placement of depth electrodes in medically intractable epilepsy. J Neurosurg. 2014; 120:639–644

[20] Tellez-Zenteno J F, Hernandez Ronquillo L, Moien-Afshari F, et al. Surgical outcomes in lesional and non-lesional epilepsy: a systematic review and meta-analysis. Epilepsy Res. 2010; 89:310–318

[21] Cohen DS, Zubay GP, Goodman RR. Seizure outcome after lesionectomy for cavernous malformations. Journal of Neurosurgery. 1995; 83:237–242

[22] Jooma R, Yeh H-S, Privitera MD, et al. Lesionectomy versus Electrophysiologically Guided Resection for Temporal Lobe Tumors Manifesting with Complex Partial Seizures. Journal of Neurosurgery. 1995; 83:231–236

[23] Morrell F, Whisler WW, Bleck TP. Multiple subpial transection: A new approach to the surgical treatment of focal epilepsy. Journal of Neurosurgery. 1989; 70:231–239

[24] Rolston JD, Deng H, Wang DD, et al. Multiple Subpial Transections for Medically Refractory Epilepsy:

A Disaggregated Review of Patient-Level Data. Neurosurgery. 2018; 82:613–620

[25] Velasco M, Velasco F, Velasco AL. Centromedian-thalamic and hippocampal electrical stimulation for the control of intractable epileptic seizures. Journal of Clinical Neurophysiology. 2001; 18:495–513

[26] Salanova V, Witt T, Worth R, et al. Long-term efficacy and safety of thalamic stimulation for drug-resistant partial epilepsy. Neurology. 2015; 84:1017–1025

[27] Morrell MJ. Responsive cortical stimulation for the treatment of medically intractable partial epilepsy. Neurology. 2011; 77:1295–1304

[28] Geller EB, Skarpaas TL, Gross RE, et al. Brain-responsive neurostimulation in patients with medically intractable mesial temporal lobe epilepsy. Epilepsia. 2017; 58:994–1004

[29] Kerezoudis P, Grewal SS, Stead M, et al. Chronic subthreshold cortical stimulation for adult drug-resistant focal epilepsy: safety, feasibility, and technique. J Neurosurg. 2018; 129:533–543

[30] Gates JR, Leppik IE, Yap J, et al. Corpus Callosotomy Clinical and Electroencephalographic Effects. Epilepsia. 1984; 25:308–316

[31] Marino R, Ragazzo PC, Reeves AG. Epilepsy and the Corpus Callosum. New York: Plenum Press 1985:281–302

[32] Tao JX, Issa NP, Wu S, et al. Interstitial Stereotactic Laser Anterior Corpus Callosotomy: A Report of 2 Cases with Operative Technique and Effectiveness. Neurosurgery. 2019; 85:E569–E574

[33] Lehner KR, Yeagle EM, Argyelan M, et al. Validation of corpus callosotomy after laser interstitial thermal therapy: a multimodal approach. J Neurosurg 2018:1–11

[34] Bogen JE, Schultz DH, Vogel PJ. Completeness of Callosotomy Shown by MRI in the Long Term. Arch Neurol. 1988; 45:1203–1205

[35] Wiebe S, Blume WT, Girvin JP, et al. A randomized controlled trial of surgery for temporal-lobe epilepsy. N Engl J Med. 2001; 345:311–318

[36] Ojemann GA, Engel J. Surgical Treatment of the Epilepsies. New York: Raven Press; 1987:635–639

[37] Ojemann GA. Surgical Therapy for Medically Intractable Epilepsy. J Neurosurg. 1987; 66:489–499

[38] Niemeyer P, Baldwin M, Bailey P. The transventricular amygdala-hippocampectomy in temporal lobe epilepsy. In: Temporal Lobe Epilepsy. Springfield Charles C Thomas; 1958:461–482

[39] Paglioli E, Palmini A, Portuguez M, et al. Seizure and memory outcome following temporal lobe surgery: selective compared with nonselective approaches for hippocampal sclerosis. J Neurosurg. 2006 104:70–78

[40] Wendling AS, Hirsch E, Wisniewski I, et al. Selective amygdalohippocampectomy versus standard temporal lobectomy in patients with mesial temporal lobe epilepsy and unilateral hippocampal sclerosis. Epilepsy Res. 2013; 104:94–104

[41] Duckworth EA, Vale FL. Trephine epilepsy surgery: the inferior temporal gyrus approach. Neurosurgery. 2008; 63:ONS156–60; discussion ONS160-1

[42] Yasargil MG, Krayenbuhl N, Roth P, et al. The selective amygdalohippocampectomy for intractable temporal limbic seizures. J Neurosurg. 2010 112:168–185

[43] Hori T, Tabuchi S, Kurosaki M, et al. Subtemporal amygdalohippocampectomy for treating medically intractable temporal lobe epilepsy. Neurosurger 1993; 33:50–6; discussion 56-7

[44] Park TS, Bourgeois BF, Silbergeld DL, et al. Subtemporal transparahippocampal amygdalohippocampectomy for surgical treatment of mesial temporal lobe epilepsy. Technical note. J Neurosurg. 199 85:1172–1176

[45] Crandall PH, Engel J. Cortical Resections. In: Surgical Treatment of the Epilepsies. New York: Raven Press 1987:377–404

[46] Willie JT, Laxpati NG, Drane DL, et al. Real-time magnetic resonance-guided stereotactic lase

amygdalohippocampotomy for mesial temporal lobe epilepsy. Neurosurgery. 2014; 74:569–84; discussion 584-5

[47] Curry DJ, Gowda A, McNichols RJ, et al. MR-guided stereotactic laser ablation of epileptogenic foci in children. Epilepsy Behav. 2012; 24:408–414

[48] Willie JT, Malcolm JG, Stern MA, et al. Safety and effectiveness of stereotactic laser ablation for epileptogenic cerebral cavernous malformations. Epilepsia. 2019; 60:220–232

[49] Wu C, Jermakowicz WJ, Chakravorti S, et al. Effects of surgical targeting in laser interstitial thermal therapy for mesial temporal lobe epilepsy: A multicenter study of 234 patients. Epilepsia. 2019; 60:1171–1183

[50] Barbaro NM, Quigg M, Ward MM, et al. Radiosurgery versus open surgery for mesial temporal lobe epilepsy: The randomized, controlled ROSE trial. Epilepsia. 2018; 59:1198–1207

[51] Engel J, Van Ness PC, Rasmussen TB, et al. Outcome with respect to epileptic seizures. In: Surgical Treatment of the Epilepsies. 2nd ed. New York: Raven Press; 1993:609–621

[52] Wieser HG, Ortega M, Friedman A, et al. Long-term seizure outcomes following amygdalohippocampectomy. J Neurosurg. 2003; 98:751–763

[53] Barbaro NM, Quigg M, Broshek DK, et al. A multicenter, prospective pilot study of gamma knife radiosurgery for mesial temporal lobe epilepsy: seizure response, adverse events, and verbal memory. Ann Neurol. 2009; 65:167–175

[54] Regis J, Rey M, Bartolomei F, et al. Gamma knife surgery in mesial temporal lobe epilepsy: a prospective multicenter study. Epilepsia. 2004; 45:504–515

[55] Vale FL, Bozorg AM, Schoenberg MR, et al. Long-term radiosurgery effects in the treatment of temporal lobe epilepsy. J Neurosurg. 2012; 117:962–969

[56] Elliott RE, Morsi A, Kalhorn SP, et al. Vagus nerve stimulation in 436 consecutive patients with treatment-resistant epilepsy: long-term outcomes and predictors of response. Epilepsy Behav. 2011; 20:57–63

114

115 Radiation Therapy (XRT)

115.1 Introduction

Ionizing radiation comprises a portion of the electromagnetic spectrum and includes X-rays and gamma rays (both of which are electromagnetic radiation and transmit their energy via photons) and particulate radiation (e.g., protons). The goal of radiation therapy (XRT) in treating tumors is to cause cell death or to stop cell replication. Photons impart critical energy to achieve this result by the photoelectric effect (at lower energies, < 0.05 MeV), by Compton scattering (at higher energies of 0.1–10 MeV, e.g., in linear accelerators and Gamma knives), or by pair-production (at the highest energies).[1] In the Compton effect, the initial collision of the photon with an atom creates a free electron which then ionizes other atoms and breaks chemical bonds. The absorption of radiation by indirect ionization in the presence of water produces free radicals (containing an unpaired electron), which causes cellular injury (usually by damaging DNA) within the tumor.

See discussion of radiation dosage and units (p. 234).

115.2 Conventional external beam radiation

115.2.1 Fractionation

The practice in which the total radiation dose is delivered in a series of smaller brief applications. This is one means of increasing the therapeutic ratio (the ratio of the effectiveness of XRT on tumor cells to that of normal cells). Radiation injury is a function of the dose, the exposure time, and the area exposed. Radiation oncologists refer to the four "R's" of radiobiology[2]:
1. Repair of sublethal damage
2. Reoxygenation of tumor cells that were hypoxic before XRT: oxygenated cells are more sensitive than hypoxic cells because oxygen combines with unpaired electrons to form peroxides, which are more stable and lethal than free radicals
3. Repopulation of tumor cells following treatment
4. Redistribution (or reassortment) of cells within the cell cycle: cells in the mitotic phase are the most sensitive

115.2.2 Dosing

The biologically effective dose of fractionated radiation is often modeled by the linear-quadratic equation (LQ-model) shown in Eq (115.1), where n = the number of doses, d = dose per fraction, and the factors α & β are used to describe the cell response to radiation. A high α/β ratio ≥ 10 is designated as early-responding tissue such as tumor cells, and a ratio ≤ 3 is considered late-responding tissue (mitotically quiescent), such as normal brain and also AVMs.

Linear quadratic equation:

$$\text{biologically effective dose (BED) (Gy)} = n \times d \times \left[1 + \frac{d}{\alpha/\beta}\right] \tag{115.1}$$

115.3 Cranial radiation

Following surgery for tumor (craniotomy or spinal surgery), most surgeons wait $\approx$ 7–10 days before instituting XRT to the surgical site (allows initiation of healing from surgery).

CNS tumors that are very radiosensitive include:
1. lymphoma – they "melt away" with XRT but tend to recur later
2. germ cell tumors
3. metastatic small cell lung cancer

For specific indications and doses, see the appropriate section (e.g., GBM, metastasis…).

For side effects, see Radiation injury and necrosis (p. 1899).

115.4 Spinal radiation

115.4.1 General information

Most spine tumors are metastatic cancer. There is no proof that any treatment for spinal metastases will prolong survival. Treatment goals, regardless of the treatment modality, are pain relief and preservation of function.

Radiation therapy (XRT) is the main treatment modality for radiosensitive spinal metastases. Even tumors that are considered "radioresistant" can respond to XRT.

115.4.2 Typical spinal radiation

For most metastatic spine tumors treated with conventional radiation therapy (i.e., not stereotactic radiosurgery), the usual fractionation is 30 Gy administered over 10 fractions.

115.4.3 Emergency spinal radiation

For acute spinal cord paralysis from tumor, if emergency surgery is not a consideration, 8 Gy can be administered in the 1st fraction for lymphoma, multiple myeloma, and (although this is not standard) it could be considered for small-cell (neuroendocrine) carcinoma since it is so radiosensitive.

115.4.4 Side effects

1. radiation myelopathy (p. 1901)
2. due to overlap, radiation injury to GI tract: N/V, diarrhea
3. bone marrow suppression
4. growth retardation in children[3]
5. risk of developing cavernous malformations of the spinal cord (p. 1525)

115.5 Radiation injury and necrosis

115.5.1 General information

Radiation necrosis (RN) may mimic recurrent (or denovo) tumor both clinically and radiographically. Differences in prognosis and treatment make it important to distinguish between tumor and RN.

115.5.2 Pathophysiology

As radiation is selectively toxic to more rapidly dividing cells, the two normal cell types within the CNS most vulnerable to RN are vascular endothelium (which has a turnover time of ≈ 6–10 mos) and oligodendroglial cells. Vascular injury may be the primary limiting factor to the tolerance of cranial XRT.[4] Injury from XRT occurs at lower doses when given concurrently with chemotherapy (especially methotrexate).

115.5.3 Etiology of side effects

The mechanism(s) by which XRT causes side effects is not known with certainty, but may be due to:
1. damage to vascular endothelium: effects on cerebral vasculature may differ substantially from effects on systemic vessels[4]
2. glial injury
3. immune system effect

Radiation effects are divided into 3 phases[5]:
1. *acute*: occur during treatment. Rare. Usually an exacerbation of symptoms already present. Probably secondary to edema. Treat with ↑ steroids
2. *early delayed*: few weeks to 2–3 mos following completion of XRT. In spinal cord → Lhermitte's sign. In brain → post-irradiation lethargy & memory difficulties
3. *late delayed*: 3 mos–12 yrs (most within 3 years). Due to small artery injury → thrombotic occlusion → white matter atrophy or frank coagulative necrosis

115

Manifestations of radiation effects:

1. decreased cognition
    a) dementia may develop following XRT[6] in as little as 1 year post-XRT. Incidence was higher when doses of 25–39 Gy were given in fractions > 300 cGy[7]
    b) children: may attain lower IQ by ≈ 25 points, especially with > 40 Gy whole-brain XRT. Measurable IQ differences occur in children radiated before age 7, but more subtle deficits occur even in older children[8]
2. radiation necrosis
3. injury to anterior optic pathways
4. injury to hypothalamic-pituitary axis → hypopituitarism → growth retardation in children; see radiation injury to pituitary (p.893)
5. primary hypothyroidism (especially in children)
6. may induce formation of new tumor: tumors most commonly identified as having increased incidence following radiation treatment are gliomas (including glioblastoma[9]), meningiomas,[10] and nerve sheath tumors.[11] Skull base tumors have been reported following EBRT[12]
7. malignant transformation: e.g., after SRS for vestibular schwannomas (p.799)
8. leukoencephalopathy: profound demyelinating/necrotizing reaction 4–12 mos after combined RTX and methotrexate, especially in children with acute lymphoblastic leukemia (ALL) and adults with primary CNS tumors

115.5.4 Evaluation (differentiating RN from recurrent tumor)

Greenberg IMHO

Over the years many methods have been championed to differentiate radiation necrosis from recurrent high-grade glioma. Some are listed below. None have proven adequately reliable, and this may not even be a useful exercise. Tumor cells are frequently found on biopsy. The decision whether to reoperate is usually based on whether there is progressive mass effect (regardless of whether it is necrosis or tumor), taking into consideration the patient's neurologic condition, projected longevity, patient desires…

CT and MRI

Cannot reliably differentiate some cases of RN from tumor (especially astrocytoma; RN occasionally resembles glioblastoma).

MR spectroscopy (p.244) was reliable in distinguishing pure tumor (elevated choline) from pure RN (low choline), but was less definitive with mixed tumor/necrosis.[13]

DWI: mean ADCs were lower with recurrence ($1.18 \pm 0.13 \times 10^{-3}$ mm/s) vs. necrosis ($1.4 \pm 0.17 \times 10^{-3}$ mm/s)[14] (not all cases biopsy proven).

Nuclear brain scan

Some reports of success with thallium-201 and technetium-99 m brain scans.

Computerized radionuclide studies

PET (positron emission tomography) scan: because positron-emitting isotopes have short half-lives, PET scanning requires a nearby cyclotron to generate the radiopharmaceuticals at great expense. Utilizing 18-fluorodeoxyglucose (18FDG), regional glucose metabolism is imaged and is generally increased with recurrent tumor, and is decreased with RN. Specificity for distinguishing RN from tumor recurrence is > 90%, but sensitivity may be too low to make it reliable.[15] Amino acid tracers such as [11C]methionine and [18F]tyrosine are taken up by most brain tumors,[16] especially gliomas and may also be used to help differentiate tumor from necrosis. Accuracy may be increased by fusing PET scan with MRI.[17]

SPECT (single-photon emission computed tomography): "poor man's PET scan." Uses radio-labeled amphetamine. Uptake depends on presence of intact neurons and the condition of cerebral blood vessels (including blood-brain barrier). Decreased radionuclide uptake indicates necrosis, whereas tumor recurrence has no decreased uptake.

115

115.5.5 Treatment

1. steroids: symptoms from any form of radiation toxicity often respond initially to steroids (gluco-corticoids) or to an increased dose of steroids. Some patients may be "steroid-dependent" in that they manifest symptoms when attempts are made to wean steroids. Most symptoms can be mitigated with dexamethasone 2 mg PO TID to QID
2. bevacizumab (Avastin®): may be considered for refractory cases. May work by decreasing capillary leakage.
   The "MD Anderson protocol"[18]: bevacizumab 7.5 mg/kg IV q 3 weeks
3. reoperation and excision: appropriate if there is deterioration from mass effect, regardless of whether the mass effect is from recurrent tumor or RN. The decision to reoperate should be based on the patient's Karnofsky rating (p. 1640). Although some benefit has been shown, most reoperation studies are biased because they often select the patients who are doing better
4. other contentious therapies include: hyperbaric oxygen and anticoagulation
5. patients with documented tumor recurrence (as opposed to RN) may also be considered for additional radiation (external beam, interstitial brachytherapy, or stereotactic radiosurgery (SRS)) or chemotherapy

115.5.6 Prevention

Injury is dependent on total radiation dose, number of treatments or fractions (less damage occurs with more frequent small treatments), and volume treated.

Various studies to determine the tolerance of *normal* brain to XRT have estimated that 65–75 Gy given over 6.5–8 wks in 5 fractions/week is usually tolerated (radiation necrosis will occur in ≈ 5% after 60 Gy fractionated in 30 treatments over 6 weeks). Other studies have shown tolerance to 45 Gy for 10 fractions, 60 Gy for 35 fractions, and 70 Gy for 60 fractions.[5]

115.5.7 Radiation myelopathy

Radiation myelopathy (RM) typically occurs in patients with spinal cord included in radiation therapy (XRT) ports used to treat cancer outside the spinal cord. This includes breast, lung, thyroid, and epidural mets. Radiation (brachial) plexopathy (p. 571) may occur with irradiation in the region of the axilla for carcinoma of the breast. In the lower extremities, XRT for pelvic or bone tumors (e.g., of the femur) may produce lumbar plexopathy. In addition to permanent changes, radiation therapy may also produce spinal cord edema, which may resolve after completion of radiation therapy.

Epidemiology

Incidence difficult to estimate due to the fact that the onset is typically delayed, together with the poor survival of patients with malignant disease requiring XRT.

Most cases reported involve the cervical cord in spite of the higher frequency with which the thoracic cord is exposed to XRT (perhaps due to higher XRT doses to the head and neck and longer survival than with lung Ca).[19] Delay between completion of XRT and onset of symptoms is usually ≈ 1 yr (reported range: 1 mo–5 yrs).

Important factors relating to the occurrence of RM include[19]:
1. rate of application (probably the most important factor)
2. total radiation dose
3. extent of cord shielding
4. individual susceptibility and variability
5. amount of tissue radiated
6. vascular supply to the region radiated
7. source of radiation

Pathophysiology

Effects of XRT on the spinal cord that lead to RM are:
1. direct injury to cells (including neurons)
2. vascular changes, including endothelial cell proliferation → thrombosis
3. hyalinization of collagen fibers

Clinical

Clinical types of radiation myelopathy

Four clinical types have been described and are shown in ▶ Table 115.1.

Onset is usually insidious, but abruptness has also been described; the presentation often mimics epidural mets. First symptoms: usually paresthesias and hypesthesia of LEs, and Lhermitte's sign. Then spastic weakness of LEs with hyperreflexia develops. A Brown-Séquard syndrome is not uncommon.

Approximately 50% of patients developing RM also have dysphagia from esophageal strictures requiring dilatations (the dysphagia often predates the myelopathy).

Table 115.1 Types of radiation myelopathy

Type	Description
1	benign form; commonly several mos following XRT (reported as late as 1 yr). Usually resolves completely within several mos. Mild sensory symptoms (frequently limited to a Lhermitte's sign) without objective neurological findings
2	injury to anterior horn cells → lower motor neuron signs in arms or legs
3	described only in experimental animals after doses larger than normal XRT. Complete cord lesion within hours due to injury to blood vessels
4	the type commonly reported. Chronic, progressive myelopathy (see text)

Evaluation

Essentially a diagnosis of exclusion. Radiographic imaging (CT, myelography) will be normal. MRI may show spinal cord infarction. The history of previous radiation is key. The differential diagnosis is included in Acute paraplegia or quadriplegia (p. 1702).

Prognosis

Prognosis for Type 4 RM is poor. Usually progresses to complete (or near-complete) cord lesion. Paraplegia and/or sphincter involvement are poor signs.

Prevention

Maximum recommended cord radiation dose depends on size of port, and varies with investigator. With large-field techniques (> 10 cm of cord), the risk of RM is negligible with ≤ 3.3 Gy in 42 days (0.55 Gy/wk), and with small-field techniques ≤ 4.3 Gy in 42 days (0.717 Gy/wk). Larger doses may possibly be given safely if fractionated over longer periods. Recommended upper limit: 0.2 Gy/fraction.

115.6 Stereotactic radiosurgery and radiotherapy

115.6.1 General information

Key concepts

- stereotactic radiosurgery (SRS): the application of a single large dose of radiation to a stereotactically localized target usually ≤ 3 cm diameter with minimal radiation delivered to surrounding tissue. May be a single treatment or up to 5 treatment fractions
- stereotactic radiotherapy (SRT) is similar but employs hypofractionated dosing (2–5 treatment fractions) e.g., with a positioning mask, which can allow for larger targets
- both SRS and SRT may be performed with properly equipped linear accelerators (LINAC Scalpel, CyberKnife®...), collimated beams from multiple radioactive sources (Gamma Knife®), or less commonly, protons and heavy charged particle beams

115

Stereotactic radiosurgery (SRS)

Lars Leksell coined the term "radiosurgery" in 1951.[20] His concept was to replace the use of electrodes or "knives" (scalpels) with multiple intersecting beams of radiation to converge on an intracranial target through an intact skull. The dose of radiation at the point of intersection (the "isocenter") is higher than outside of the isocenter where the dose falls off sharply such that adjacent tissues receive only minimal radiation from each individual incident beam. When combined with a reliable method for aiming the beams at an intracranial target (e.g., using a stereotactic frame system and three-dimensional imaging) the technique came to be known as stereotactic radiosurgery.

Initially developed to create a necrotic lesion in specific nuclei or pathways for functional disorders, it has subsequently been proven that subnecrotic doses could trigger cellular reactions in tumors and vasculature that would lead to tumor shrinkage or control and obliteration of vascular malformations.

With conventional radiation treatments, the "R's" of radiobiology (p. 1898) are exploited. In contrast, with SRS, precision and accuracy are used to affect the target (e.g., damage tumor or thrombose AVM) and spare normal tissue.

Stereotactic radiotherapy (SRT)

Methods of immobilization and point-of-delivery imaging technologies have since made it practical to deliver stereotactic radiation spread out over several individual treatment sessions (known as fractions) when desirable. Many authors refer to this as stereotactic radiation therapy (SRT). The precise definition of SRT has evolved over time, with some publications describing it as using a conventional fractionation scheme (1.8–2 Gy/fraction). However the majority of authors refer to SRT in terms of a hypofractionated approach, generally limited to five treatment fractions (see below).

Fractionation capitalizes on the differential response of normal tissue from tumors to radiation insult; see the Four "R's" of radiobiology (p. 1898). The value of fractionation is more apparent for tissues with high rates of proliferation and less capability to repair sublethal DNA damage (high α/β ratio in Eq (115.1)).[21] However these models apply more directly in conventional fractionation schemes; their use in single- or hypo-fractionated schemes is a subject of current research.

Treatment over multiple fractions renders impractical the traditional stereotactic frame. SRT therefore employs various techniques for patient immobilization, including thermoplastic masks, dental-impression–based bite-blocks, and other relocatable frame systems. Displacement errors can be as high as 2–8 mm with mask systems; however, these uncertainties can be reduced with in-room imaging systems such as cone-beam CT (CBCT) which can assist in patient localization, as well as intra-fraction motion monitoring techniques such as orthogonal kilovoltage X-rays, surface tracking systems, and infrared marker tracking systems.

Blurred lines between SRS and SRT

Although some purists insist that SRS is performed in a single session, the current definition was expanded by AANS/CNS/ASTRO in 2007 to include radiosurgical procedures "using a rigidly attached stereotactic guiding device, other immobilization device, and/or a stereotactic image-guidance system ... performed in a limited number of sessions, up to a maximum of five."[22]

To further muddy the waters, for billing purposes in the U.S., the cpt codes used by Medicare for SRS (for brain and spine)[23,24] describe treatment in one session, whereas SBRT (stereotactic body radiation therapy) allows treatment delivery not to exceed 5 fractions within the body. For 5 or more fractions, Medicare considers it to be intensity-modulated radiation therapy (IMRT).

Comparison of SRS technologies

Various methods for delivering SRS/SRT are clinically available. Three main categories (based on sources of radiation) are Gamma Knife, linear accelerator-based, and heavy charged particle radiosurgery. Fundamentally, there is no difference between a photon created by radioactive decay (gamma ray) and a photon created using electrical energy in a linear accelerator (X-ray).

Gamma knife radiosurgery. In the original Gamma Knife (GK), the source of radiation is gamma decay of 201 cobalt-60 sources that align with an inner collimator to direct the resulting photon beams. A treatment couch includes a mount for an external collimation "helmet," each of which has either a 4-, 8-, 14-, or 18-mm diameter beam aperture for each source. The stereotactic frame affixed to the patient's head is positioned within the collimator helmet so the area to be treated is at the focus point of treatment unit. Several dwell positions (also called "shots" or "isocenters") may be defined to match dose distributions to irregularly shaped targets.

115

In the newer GK model Perfexion®, 192 cobalt-60 sources are distributed on 8 sectors attached to sector drive motors to move the sources along a fully internalized tungsten collimator. This allows each sector to move from "home," 4-, 8-, 16-mm collimators or shielded positions. The design makes possible composite use of different beam diameters to help optimize dose distribution. The Gamma Knife is specifically designed for cranial and upper cervical lesions, and is best suited for smaller lesions (< 3 cm diameter).

As the gamma sources age, output declines, and treatment times necessarily become longer. Eventually, the sources must be replaced, which is a time-consuming and expensive process.

▶ **Linear accelerator-based radiosurgery.** Linear accelerators (linacs) generate X-rays by accelerating electrons and directing them to strike a target of a substance with a high atomic number. The X-ray source and beam collimation is mounted on a rotating gantry, creating a fixed isocenter in space. Beam convergence is achieved via rotating arcs with the isocenter fixated on the target. The target is aligned to the isocenter using a treatment table that is adjustable in up to 6 degrees of freedom (6 dof, 3 translations, 3 rotations). Beams are collimated using either narrow-aperture cones (SRS cones) or multileaf collimators (MLCs), the latter of which use banks of computerized leaves to shape the treatment field and may be modulated to achieve specific dose distributions. Linacs are more versatile than GK in that they can treat cranial and extracranial targets, they often have built-in CBCT imaging to assist with patient setup and target localization, and they can have a higher dose rate (and thus potentially faster treatment). However, they are generally technically more complicated than GK and require substantially more quality assurance to maintain technical confidence. The Cyberknife is an SRS-specific linac that uses a robotic arm rather than an isocentrically-mounted linac to achieve 6 dof targeting.

▶ **Heavy charged particle radiosurgery.** Heavy charged particles (protons or helium ions) from a cyclotron can be used for radiosurgery.[25] Unlike high-energy photons (gamma and X-rays), which deposit the majority of their energy upon entrance into tissue and continue to deposit decreasing amounts of energy as they travel through the body, heavy charged particle beams have a shorter, bounded range of penetration wherein particles sharply increase energy deposition near the terminal depth of penetration (Bragg peak effect). Particle radiosurgery achieves a well-localized volume of high-dose radiation by taking advantage of cross-firing of a number of beams as well as the Bragg peak. Due to the expense and increased complexity of heavy charged particle SRS, this therapy is only available in a few centers in the world.

115.6.2 Indications

In general, SRS is useful for well-circumscribed lesions less than approximately 3 cm diameter. For larger lesions, the radiation dose must be reduced because of anatomic and radiobiological constraints.

Published uses of SRS include:
1. vascular lesions
   a) AVMs (including dural arteriovenous fistulas)
   b) cavernous malformations
2. tumors
   a) metastases
      1. as primary treatment (p. 1907)
      2. to treat resection cavity after surgery (p. 1908)
   b) vestibular schwannomas
   c) meningiomas
   d) PitNET/adenomas
   e) gliomas
   f) others: craniopharyngioma, pineal tumors, etc.
3. functional disorders
   a) trigeminal neuralgia[26,27]
   b) intractable chronic pain: thalamotomy[28]
   c) movement disorders: pallidotomy for Parkinson's disease or thalamotomy for tremor (usually not a technique of choice because of inability to perform physiologic stimulation prior to lesioning. May be a consideration for the rare patients who cannot undergo placement of a stimulator/lesioning needle)
   d) psychiatric diseases (e.g., obsessive-compulsive disorder)
   e) epilepsy[29]

115.6.3 Contraindications

Compressive tumors of the spinal cord, brainstem or optic structures: even with the sharp falloff of radiation dose, there remains radiation delivered within a few millimeters of the margins of the isocenter. This, together with post-radiation swelling, might create significant risk of neurologic injury. Surgical removal should be considered in these situations, especially for benign lesions in young individuals.

115.6.4 Treatment procedure

The treatment procedure includes placement of stereotactic frame (in framed-based SRS), obtaining stereotactic images, target definition, treatment planning and execution of treatment.

Target localization

MRI is the predominant imaging modality for SRS procedures given its superior soft tissue and tumor contrast. Typical MRI protocols include T1-weighted pre- and post-contrast images using 3D pulse sequences. If visualization of structures in surrounding CSF (trigeminal nerves, CPA tumors) is required, special sequences such as constructive interference in steady state (CISS) is useful. Fat-saturation sequences are used in cases with previously resected skull base tumors. NB: there is a 1–2 mm shift due to spatial distortion artifact from the MRI magnet. This effect is more prominent in high field strength MRI.

CT accuracy is never better than 0.6 mm, which is the pixel size. Usually is used when MRI is contraindicated or in cases where distortion in MRI may be a concern (dental brace, shunt). CT does not suffer susceptibility distortion as MRI and one can use a stereotactic CT to merge with nonstereotactic MRI for treatment planning.

Stereotactic angiography remains the best method to define the AVM nidi and their arterial supply and venous drainage. Given that angiograms provide only two sets of orthogonal images (usually AP and lateral images), CTA and/or MRI/MRA can be used as an adjunct to provide vascular anatomy on axial plane.

Treatment planning

Treatment planning is the process by which a dose distribution is created with the goal of adequately treating the target areas while largely sparing normal surrounding structures. In GK treatment, a dose distribution is created by defining one or more isocenters (shots). Each isocenter can make use of full complement beams of various diameters; however, in certain cases one or more of the beams can be blocked to shape the dose distribution for irregular targets and protect adjacent critical structures. For linac-based SRS, treatment planning is accomplished using computer simulation programs to help select the number of arcs or beams with certain orientation. Also, static and dynamic collimators have been developed. Intensity modulation is also a means of delivering the desired dose to a target while decreasing the dose given to surrounding structures.

Lesions that are not round or ellipsoid in shape are not a problem when using linac, but with older GKs, multiple isocenters must be used to conform to an irregular surface. This results in multiple "hotspots." This problem is eliminated with the GK Perfexion, which can create a single isocenter using different beam diameters. In the case of multiple metastases, it can generate individually shaped isocenters for each tumor and thus avoid having to change the helmet or add isocenters during a treatment.[30]

▶ **Normal tissue tolerance.** Cranial nerves: Damage to small nutrient vessels and Schwann cells or oligodendroglia are the possible mechanisms of radiation injury to cranial nerves. Special sensory nerves (optic, vestibulocochlear) are the most radiosensitive. The precise dose tolerance of cranial nerve is unclear; the optic nerve can probably tolerate doses lower than 8–10 Gy. Nerves in the parasellar region, the facial nerve and lower cranial nerves tend to tolerate higher doses.

SRS treatment may also have a deleterious effect in structures sensitive to swelling, such as brainstem. However, the structures at highest risk are those within the higher isodose lines immediately adjacent to the lesion.

▶ Table 115.2 shows maximum recommended doses of various organs for a single fraction. In the brain, critical radiation-sensitive structures include: optic vitreous, nerve, and chiasm, brainstem, pituitary gland, and cochlea.

▶ **Dose.** Dose is usually prescribed as a particular dose (in units of Gray) to the periphery of target. The periphery of the target is usually defined as the isodose curve, which covers the substantial (usually 95–100%) of the target. The isodose curve is the curve of equal dose usually defined as a

Table 115.2 Maximum recommended radiation dose of critical organs (delivered in a single fraction)

Structure	Maximum dose (cGy)	% of maximum (at a prescribed dose of 50 Gy)
eye lens (cataract induction begins at 500 cGy)	100	2%
optic nerve[31]	100	2%
skin in beam	50	1%
thyroid	10	0.2%

percentage of the maximum dose point. Traditionally, treatment planning for GK uses the 50% iso-dose line because for a single isocenter this is the location of steepest dose gradient. Linac-based SRS used higher isodose line (70–90%) to increase homogeneity of dose distribution.

Dose-volume relation: The dose of radiation that can be tolerated is highly dependent on the volume being treated (larger treatment volumes require lower doses to avoid radiation injury). Dose selection is made based on known information or is estimated from dose-volume relationship. If uncertain, err on the side of a lower dose or slightly underdose the margin of tumor. Previous radiotherapy must also be taken into account by the treatment team, as local structures are more sensitive.

115.6.5 Lesion-specific issues

Arteriovenous malformations

SRS is best accepted for the treatment of small to moderate-sized (<3 cm) AVMs that are deep or border on eloquent brain and have a "compact" (i.e., sharply demarcated) nidus, or for patients who are too high-risk for surgery due to medical comorbidities. The radiation induces endothelial cell damage, smooth muscle cell proliferation, thickening of the vascular wall, and ultimately obliteration of the lumen over a period of 1–3 years (latency period).[32] During the latency period, the annual risk of hemorrhage is ≈ 1–3% which is the same as the natural history.[33]

▶ **Dose.** Early study from Karlsson et al demonstrated increased obliteration rate with increased margin dose.[34] The effect reached the plateau at 25 Gy and a higher dose produced more complications without extra benefits. The optimal dose for AVMs generally ranges between 23–25 Gy. The dose might be reduced for nidi at critical locations or with a large volume. At McGill with linac SRS they use 25–50 Gy delivered to the 90% isodose curve at the edge of the nidus. With Bragg-peak complications occurred less frequently with doses < 19.2 Gy compared to doses above that (this may reduce the obliteration rate or increase the latency period).[35]

▶ **Results.** SRS has an overall obliteration rate of 70–80% across all cases of AVMs treated.[36] At 1 year, 46–61% of AVMs were completely obliterated on angiography, and at 2 years 86% were obliterated. There was no reduction in size in < 2% of cases. Smaller lesions have higher obliteration rates (with Bragg-peak in AVMs < 2 cm diameter, 94% thrombosed at 2 years, and 100% at 3 years).[35] AVMs > 25 mm in diameter have only ≈ 50% chance of obliteration with 1 SRS treatment. Angiographic features associated with high-flow AVMs predict a lower obliteration rate with SRS.[37]

▶ **Grading system.** SRS-based grading systems have been developed to predict patient outcomes since scales developed for surgical resection (e.g., the Spetzler-Martin scale) have not proven applicable for AVM radiosurgery. Long-term outcomes of 1012 patients treated with GK at UVA were analyzed to create the Virginia Radiosurgery AVM Scale (VRAS)(▶ Table 115.3 and ▶ Table 115.4).[38]

Table 115.3 Virginia Radiosurgery AVM Scale (VRAS)[36]: variables and points

Variable		Points	Score
AVM volume (cm³)	<2	0	(0 - 2)
	2–4	1	
	>4	2	
Eloquent location	no	0	(0 - 1)
	yes	1	
History of hemorrhage	no	0	(0 - 1)
	yes	1	
VRAS → TOTAL			(0 – 4)

115

Table 115.4 Virginia Radiosurgery AVM Scale (VRAS)[36]: total points and % favorable outcome

Total points	Favorable outcome (%)
0	83
1	79
2	70
3	48
4	39

Multivariate analysis showed that AVM volume, non-eloquent location, and no history of hemorrhage were independent predictors of AVM obliteration without post-treatment hemorrhage or permanent neurologic deficits.

► **Embolization.** Controversy exists as to whether embolization is helpful or harmful prior to SRS. Some experts find that target definition after embolization is extraordinarily difficult because of multiple small residual nidi. Experimental studies have shown attenuation of radiation effect by embolic material.[38] However, for large AVMs, embolization remains an effective adjunct to reduce the size of nidi to make AVMs amenable to SRS. Additionally, pre-SRS embolization should be considered for high-flow fistulas, which are more radioresistant, and intranidal/perinidal aneurysms, which are at risk for rupture.

► **Large AVMs.** Large AVMs ($> 10\,cm^3$) remain a significant challenge to treat with any modality. Single-stage SRS has resulted in low obliteration and high complication rates. To maximize the dose/volume response, SRS can be performed in a volume-staged fashion. The Pittsburgh group reported overall rates of total obliteration of 18%, 45%, and 56% at 5, 7, and 10 years, respectively, in a group of 47 patients with large AVMs. Ten patients had hemorrhage after SRS, and 5 of these patients died.[39]

► **Residual lesions after SRS.** Factors associated with treatment failures include: incomplete angiographic definition of the nidus (the most frequent factor, responsible for 57% of cases), recanalization of the nidus (7%), masking of nidus by hematoma, and a theorized "radiobiological resistance."[40] In some, no discernible reason for failure could be identified. In this series, the complete obliteration rate was ≈ 64%. If AVMs persist, retreatment with SRS 2–3 years later is an option.[40]

The ultimate goal of radiosurgery for AVMs is elimination of risk of hemorrhage. An imperfect surrogate marker for this goal has been total obliteration of the nidus on imaging. Reduced, unchanged, or increased hemorrhagic rates during the latency period have been reported. Proton beam treatment of AVMs affords no protection against hemorrhage in the first 12–14 months following treatment[25]; this is similar to the 12–24 month latency for photon radiation.[41] Hemorrhages may occur during the latency period even in AVMs that had never bled before,[35] and the question has been raised whether a partially thrombosed AVM is more likely to bleed because of increased outflow resistance. Yen et al reviewed a large group of AVM patients undergoing radiosurgery and reported that the hemorrhagic rates reduced from 6.6% before SRS to 2.5% after SRS. The protective effect is more significant in those AVMs that had a prior hemorrhage (10.4% to 2.8%).[42]

Vascular lesions other than AVMs

Dural arteriovenous fistulas (AVFs) have also shown promising response to SRS.[43] However, dural AVFs with cortical drainage should not be treated with SRS because these AVFs pose a high risk of hemorrhage. SRS is of no benefit for venous angiomas.[44] SRS for cavernous malformations remains controversial, as the lesions could not be precisely evaluated with MRI or angiography. However, published retrospective studies have demonstrated reduction of hemorrhage rates following SRS.[45,46]

Metastases, primary treatment

The gold standard and level 1 recommendation for a single brain metastasis amenable to surgical resection is surgery followed by WBRT.[47,48] This does not apply to extremely radiosensitive tumors such as lymphoma, small cell lung cancer, germ cell tumors, and multiple myeloma. There has not been a randomized study to compare surgery alone to SRS alone. A prospective randomized study by Muacevic et al showed comparable survival and local tumor control between SRS and surgery plus WBRT in patients with a single brain metastasis but a higher incidence of distant recurrence in the SRS arm.[49] When tissue is required for diagnosis, surgery should be considered. Tumors with

115

significant mass effect should also be resected if the patients are fit for surgery. In patients with ≤ 3 mets, single-dose SRS provides superior survival advantage as compared to WBRT (level III recommendation). Radiographic local control rate of ≈ 88% (reported range: 82–100%) has been cited.[50]

No significant difference has been found with SRS between tumors considered "radiosensitive" and those that are "radioresistant" as defined by standards developed for EBRT (see ▶ Table 55.7; however, histology may affect the rate of response). The lack of significance of "radioresistance" may be due in part to the fact that the sharp dose drop-off with SRS allows higher doses to be delivered to tumors than would be used with EBRT.

General guidelines for when to consider SRS for brain metastases are:

- total tumor number ≤ 10
- total tumor volume ≤ 15 cm³
- single tumor volume < 10 cm³, and
- no leptomeningeal disease present.

Recent studies on SRS for brain metastases have shown that total tumor volume is a better predictor of overall survival, local control, and even distant failure than tumor number.[51,52,53]

▶ **Dose.** RTOG 90–05 study recommended 24 Gy as the maximum tolerated doses of single-fraction SRS for tumors ≤ 20 mm in maximum diameter; 18 Gy for 21–30 mm; and 15 Gy for 31–40 mm.[54]

Metastases, post-resection treatment

SRS may be used for cavity treatment following removal of a metastasis. In analyzing treatment failures of post-op SRS, 25% of local failures occurred at the margin, and per-op dural involvment was very common.[55] For treatment planning, the following contouring guidelines are suggested:

1. the circumference of the contour should extend 2 mm beyond the cavity walls[56]
2. the surgical tract should be included in the treatment plan (even for deep lesions)[55]
3. for tumors that were in contact with the dura pre-operatively, the contour should extend a few mm along the dura[55]
4. for tumors that were in contact a dural venous sinus per-op, the contour should extend a few mm beyond the initial sinus contact[55]

Vestibular schwannomas (VS)

Possible indications of SRS for VS are: poor surgical candidates (due to poor medical condition and/or advanced age, some use > 65 or 70 years as a cutoff), patient refusing surgery, bilateral VS, postoperative treatment of incompletely removed VS that continue to grow on serial imaging, or recurrences following surgical removal. See the Management algorithm (p. 787) under Vestibular schwannomas for strategies that take into account the natural history.

▶ **Dose.** As there is little difference in radiographic control at different doses, single-dose SRS < 13 Gy is recommended for hearing preservation and to minimize new onset or worsening of cranial nerve deficits (Level III[57])

Meningiomas

In a large series of meningiomas treated with SRS by the Pittsburgh group,[58] among 942 patients with 1045 tumors treated, the control rate for patients with surgically verified WHO grade 1 meningiomas was 93%. Control rate for presumed meningiomas based on imaging (no prior histological confirmation) was 97%. The control rates for WHO grades II and III tumors were 50% and 17% respectively.

▶ **Dose.** The authors used a mean dose of 14 Gy to the tumor margin.[58]

PitNET/adenomas

Surgery is the mainstay of management for the majority of pituitary tumors (major exception: prolactinomas (p. 888)), especially for symptomatic nonsecretory (nonfunctioning) tumors (p. 887) and secretory tumors that fail medical treatment. For residual/recurrent secretory or nonsecretory tumors, SRS is an appropriate tool to arrest tumor growth and/or normalize hormonal function. In a large series of 418 patients with residual/recurrence PitNET/adenomas treated with GK at UVA,[59] th overall tumor control rate was 90% in patients with imaging follow-up available. The endocrine remission rates are 53% for acromegaly, 54% for Cushing's disease, and 26% for prolactinomas.

▶ **Dose.** The usual dose for nonsecretory tumors is ≈ 16–18 Gy, and a higher dose is required for secretory tumor ≈ 25 Gy.

▶ **Results.** Early studies of SRS showed limited numbers of hypopituitarism and cranial nerve injuries. Available long-term follow-up studies now demonstrate a 20–30% rate of new endocrinopathy after SRS and a low but not negligible risk of cranial nerve damage.[59]

Infiltrating tumors

SRS is generally not indicated as a primary treatment for infiltrating tumors, e.g., gliomas, due to the lack of a definable capsule and very close relationship between target volume and tolerated radiation dose. SRS has been used for recurrent lesions following standard treatment (surgical excision and adjuvant EBRT 60 Gy and temozolomide). One of the arguments for SRS in these tumors is the fact that 90% of recurrences are within the original radiographic solid tumor volume.[60] However, support for SRS boost declined after a 2004 RTOG trial 9305 showing no survival benefit in newly diagnosed GBM patients with upfront use of SRS followed by EBRT and BCNU chemotherapy. SRS can be used as a salvage treatment for small (< 10 cm^3), recurrent GBM after standard treatment. Kong et al showed SRS salvage treatment in these cases prolonged OS to 23 from 12 months.[61]

115.6.6 Treatment morbidity and mortality

Immediate morbidity and mortality

Immediate mortality from the actual treatments themselves is probably zero. Morbidity: all but ≈ 2.5% of patients were discharged home within 24 hours. Many centers do not admit patients overnight. Some immediate adverse reactions include[62]:
- 16% of patients require analgesics for post-procedural headaches and antiemetics for nausea/vomiting
- at least 10% of patients with subcortical AVMs had focal or generalized seizures within 24 hrs of treatment (only one was on subtherapeutic ASMs. All were controllable with additional ASMs.)

Premedication

The Pittsburgh Gamma Knife group gives methylprednisolone 40 mg IV and phenobarbital 90 mg IV immediately after the radiation dose to patients with tumors or AVMs to reduce these adverse effects.[62] For small lesions and patients without prior history of seizures, premedication with steroids or antiepileptics are probably not necessary.

Delayed morbidity

Long-term morbidity directly related to the radiation may occur, and just as with conventional XRT, is more frequent with larger doses and treatment volumes. Radiation complications include:
- radiation-induced changes, high intensity on MRI T2WI, or low density on CT: usually occur ≈ 13 months after SRS for AVMs. The incidence is 34% with 8.6% having imaging changes associated with neurological symptoms (focal deficits, seizures, or headache) and 1.8% developing radiation necrosis and permanent deficits.[63] The possible mechanisms of this side effect include glial cell damage, breakdown of blood-brain barrier, or early venous thrombosis. Premature venous thrombosis or occlusion before obliteration of AVM nidus can produce venous hyperemia or intracranial hemorrhage[64]
- vasculopathy: diagnosed by narrowing seen on angiography or by ischemic changes on imaging in ≈ 5% of cases
- cranial nerve deficits: occur in ≈ 1% of all cases. Incidence is higher with tumors of CPA or skull base
- radiation-induced tumors: only a few case reports of newly formed malignant tumors (glioblastomas) or malignant transformation of a benign tumor (vestibular schwannoma). Loeffler reported 6 cases over 80,000 radiosurgical procedures for benign diseases.[65] Radiation-induced meningioma is a well-known complication of radiation therapy.[66] In a large series of AVM patients treated with SRS, the incidence of radiation-induced meningioma was estimated to be 0.7%[67]

115.7 Interstitial brachytherapy

115.7.1 General information

Technique whereby radioactive implants are used to deliver locally high doses of radiation directly to tumors while exposing nearby normal brain to less toxic doses. At present, the numbers are too small and the follow-up too short to determine the efficacy of interstitial brachytherapy.[68]

Interstitial brachytherapy (IB) may reduce the rate of tumor growth, but it rarely produces clinical improvement. Patients are generally not considered for IB unless their Karnofsky score is ≥ 70.

115.7.2 Techniques

Techniques include:
1. insertion of high-activity iodine-125 pellets which remain in place (either by conventional open surgery or by stereotactic technique)
2. insertion of catheters (so-called afterloading catheters) containing radioactive source (such as gold or I-125) by stereotactic technique, which are then removed at a predetermined time (usually 1–7 days)
3. instillation of radioactive liquids (e.g., phosphorous isotope) into a cyst cavity

I-125 has several characteristics that favor its use: it emits low-energy gamma rays, which are absorbed by surrounding tissues minimizing radiation exposure of the normal brain, medical personnel, and visitors. It is available as low-activity (< 5 mCi) or high-activity (5–40 mCi) seeds.

Treatment planning is devised to deliver 60 Gy to the edge of a volume that extends 1 cm beyond the contrast-enhancing tumor, with variations included to spare radiosensitive structures (e.g., optic chiasm). Usual delivery rates are 40–50 cGy/hr to the tumor margin (30 cGy/hr is the critical dose for cessation of human tumor growth) requiring that the seeds stay in the afterloading catheter ≈ 6 days.

115.7.3 Radiation necrosis

Symptomatic radiation necrosis (RN) occurs in ≈ 40% of cases, and may occur as early as several months after IB. It may be impossible to differentiate from recurrent tumor in many cases. Symptomatic treatment is often achieved with increased corticosteroid dosages. Continued neurologic deterioration may require craniotomy.

115.7.4 Outcome

IB is often used as a "last-ditch" effort in a patient with a recurrent malignant tumor who has received maximal external beam irradiation and who is not a candidate for reoperation (as expected, the results in patients with such poor prognoses are not good). However, patients eligible for IB are usually better than those who are not candidates, and this may bias the results towards a better outcome.[69] Some studies with early (primary treatment) use have shown possible benefit.[70]

References

[1] Thompson TP, Maitz AH, Kondziolka D, et al. Radiation, Radiobiology, and Neurosurgery. Contemporary Neurosurgery. 1999; 21:1–5

[2] Hall EJ, Cox JD, Cox JD. Physical and Biologic Basis of Radiation Therapy. In: Moss' Radiation Oncology. 7th ed. St. Louis, Missouri: Mosby-Year Book, Inc.; 1994:3–66

[3] Tomita T, McLone DG. Medulloblastoma in Childhood: Results of Radical Resection and Low-Dose Radiation Therapy. J Neurosurg. 1986; 64:238–242

[4] O'Connor MM, Mayberg MR. Effects of Radiation on Cerebral Vasculature: A Review. Neurosurgery. 2000; 46:138–151

[5] Leibel SA, Sheline GE. Radiation Therapy for Neoplasms of the Brain. J Neurosurg. 1987; 66:1–22

[6] Duffner PK, Cohen ME, Thomas P. Late Effects of Treatment on the Intelligence of Children with Posterior Fossa Tumors. Cancer. 1983; 51:233–237

[7] DeAngelis LM, Delattre JY, Posner JB. Radiation-induced dementia in patients cured of brain metastases. Neurology. 1989; 39:789–796

[8] Radcliffe J, Packer RJ, Atkins TE, et al. Three- and Four-Year Cognitive Outcome in Children with Noncortical Brain Tumors Treated with Whole-Brain Radiotherapy. Annals of Neurology. 1992; 32:551–554

[9] Zuccarello M, Sawaya R, deCourten-Myers. Glioblastoma Occurring After Radiation Therapy for Meningioma: Case Report and Review of Literature. Neurosurgery. 1986; 19:114–119

[10] Mack EE, Wilson CB. Meningiomas Induced by High-Dose Cranial Irradiation. Journal of Neurosurgery. 1993; 79:28–31

[11] Ron E, Modan B, Boice JD, et al. Tumors of the Brain and Nervous System After Radiotherapy in Childhood. New England Journal of Medicine. 1988; 319:1033–1039

[12] Lustig LR, Jackler RK, Lanser MJ. Radiation-Induced Tumors of the Temporal Bone. Am J Otol. 1997; 18:230–235

[13] Rock JP, Hearshen D, Scarpace L, et al. Correlation between magnetic resonance spectroscopy and

[14] Hein PA, Eskey CJ, Dunn JF, et al. Diffusion-weighted imaging in the follow-up of treated high-grade gliomas: tumor recurrence versus radiation injury. AJNR Am J Neuroradiol. 2004; 25:201–209

[15] Thompson TP, Lunsford LD, Kondziolka D. Distinguishing recurrent tumor and radiation necrosis with positron emission tomography versus stereotactic biopsy. Stereotact Funct Neurosurg. 1999; 73:9–14

[16] Ericson K, Lilja A, Bergstrom M, et al. Positron emission tomography with ([11C]methyl)-L-methionine, [11C]D-glucose, and [68Ga]EDTA in supratentorial tumors. Journal of Computer Assisted Tomography. 1985; 9:683–689

[17] Thiel A, Pietrzyk U, Sturm V, et al. Enhanced Accuracy in Differential Diagnosis of Radiation Necrosis by Positron Emission Tomography-Magnetic Resonance Imaging Coregistration: Technical Case Report. Neurosurgery. 2000; 46:232–234

[18] Gonzalez J, Kumar AJ, Conrad CA, et al. Effect of bevacizumab on radiation necrosis of the brain. Int J Radiat Oncol Biol Phys. 2007; 67:323–326

[19] Eyster EF, Wilson CB. Radiation Myelopathy. J Neurosurg. 1970; 32:414–420

[20] Leksell L. The Stereotaxic Method and Radiosurgery of the Brain. Acta Chir Scand. 1951; 102:316–319

[21] Dale RG, Jones B. The assessment of RBE effects using the concept of biologically effective dose. Int J Radiat Oncol Biol Phys. 1999; 43:639–645

[22] Barnett GH, Linskey ME, Adler JR, et al. Stereotactic radiosurgery–an organized neurosurgery-sanctioned definition. J Neurosurg. 2007; 106:1–5

[23] Tipton KN, Sullivan N, Bruening W, et al. Stereotactic Body Radiation Therapy. Technical Brief No. 6. (Prepared by ECRI Institute Evidence-based Practice Center under Contract No. HHSA-290-02-0019.) AHRQ Publication No. 10 (11)-EHC058-EF. Rockville, MD 2011. https://effectivehealthcare.ahrq.gov/topics/stereotactic-body-radiation/technical-brief

[24] Stereotactic radiotherapy (SRS)/stereotactic radiation therapy (SBRT) for Medicare plans Policy # SURGERY 0581 T3. Trumbull CT 2009. https://www.oxhp.com/

[25] Kjellberg RN, Hanamura T, Davis KR, et al. Bragg-Peak Proton-Beam Therapy for Arteriovenous Malformations of the Brain. N Engl J Med. 1983; 309:269–274

[26] Leksell L. Stereotactic Radiosurgery in Trigeminal Neuralgia. Acta Chir Scand. 1971; 137:311–314

[27] Regis J, Metellus P, Hayashi M, et al. Prospective controlled trial of gamma knife surgery for essential trigeminal neuralgia. J Neurosurg. 2006; 104:913–924

[28] Steiner L, Forster D, Leksell L, et al. Gammathalamotomy in Intractable Pain. Acta Neurochirurgica. 1980; 52:173–184

[29] Barbaro NM, Quigg M, Broshek DK, et al. A multicenter, prospective pilot study of gamma knife radiosurgery for mesial temporal lobe epilepsy: seizure response, adverse events, and verbal memory. Ann Neurol. 2009; 65:167–175

[30] Lindquist C, Paddick I. The Leksell Gamma Knife Perfexion and comparisons with its predecessors. Neurosurgery. 2007; 61:130–40; discussion 140-1

[31] Leber KA, Berglöff J, Pendi G. Dose-Response Tolerance of the Visual Pathways and Cranial Nerves of the Cavernous Sinus to Stereotactic Radiosurgery. Journal of Neurosurgery. 1998; 88:43–50

[32] Schneider BF, Eberhard DA, Steiner LE. Histopathology of arteriovenous malformations after gamma knife radiosurgery. J Neurosurg. 1997; 87:352–357

[33] Derdeyn CP, Zipfel GJ, Albuquerque FC, et al. Management of Brain Arteriovenous Malformations: A Scientific Statement for Healthcare Professionals From the American Heart Association/American Stroke Association. Stroke. 2017; 48:e200–e224

[34] Karlsson B, Lindquist C, Steiner L. Prediction of obliteration after gamma knife surgery for cerebral arteriovenous malformations. Neurosurgery. 1997; 40:425–30; discussion 430-1

[35] Steinberg GK, Fabrikant JI, Marks MP, et al. Stereotactic Heavy-Charged-Particle Bragg-Peak Radiation for Intracranial Arteriovenous Malformations. N Engl J Med. 1990; 323:96–101

[36] Starke RM, Yen CP, Ding D, et al. A practical grading scale for predicting outcome after radiosurgery for arteriovenous malformations: analysis of 1012 treated patients. J Neurosurg. 2013; 119:981–987

[37] Taeshineetanakul P, Krings T, Geibprasert S, et al. Angioarchitecture determines obliteration rate after radiosurgery in brain arteriovenous malformations. Neurosurgery. 2012; 71:1071–8; discussion 1079

[38] Andrade-Souza YM, Ramani M, Beachey DJ, et al. Liquid embolisation material reduces the delivered radiation dose: a physical experiment. Acta Neurochir (Wien). 2008; 150:161–4; discussion 164

[39] Kano H, Kondziolka D, Flickinger JC, et al. Stereotactic radiosurgery for arteriovenous malformations, Part 6: multistaged volumetric management of large arteriovenous malformations. J Neurosurg. 2012; 116:54–65

[40] Pollock BE, Kondziolka D, Lunsford LD, et al. Repeat Stereotactic Radiosurgery of Arteriovenous Malformations: Factors Associated with Incomplete Outcomes. Neurosurgery. 1996; 38:318–324

[41] Saunders WM, Winston KR, Siddon RL, et al. Radiosurgery for Arteriovenous Malformations of the Brain Using a Standard Linear Accelerator: Rationale and Technique. International Journal of Radiation Oncology and Biological Physics. 1988; 13:441–447

[42] Yen CP, Sheehan JP, Schwyzer L, et al. Hemorrhage risk of cerebral arteriovenous malformations before and during the latency period after GAMMA knife radiosurgery. Stroke. 2011; 42:1691–1696

[43] Pan DH, Lee CC, Wu HM, et al. Gamma Knife radiosurgery for the management of intracranial dural arteriovenous fistulas. Acta Neurochir Suppl. 2013; 116:113–119

[44] Lindquist C, Guo W-Y, Kerlsson B, et al. Radiosurgery for Venous Angiomas. Journal of Neurosurgery. 1993; 78:531–536

[45] Lunsford LD, Khan AA, Niranjan A, et al. Stereotactic radiosurgery for symptomatic solitary cerebral cavernous malformations considered high risk for resection. J Neurosurg. 2010; 113:23–29

[46] Liscak R, Vladyka V, Simonova G, et al. Gamma knife surgery of brain cavernous hemangiomas. J Neurosurg. 2005; 102 Suppl:207–213

[47] Patchell RA, Tibbs PA, Walsh JW, et al. A Randomized Trial of Surgery in the Treatment of Single Metastases to the Brain. New England Journal of Medicine. 1990; 322:494–500

[48] Patchell RA, Tibbs PA, Regine WF, et al. Postoperative radiotherapy in the treatment of single metastases to the brain: a randomized trial. JAMA. 1998; 280:1485–1489

[49] Muacevic A, Wowra B, Siefert A, et al. Microsurgery plus whole brain irradiation versus Gamma Knife surgery alone for treatment of single metastases to the brain: a randomized controlled multicentre phase III trial. J Neurooncol. 2008; 87:299–307

[50] Fuller BG, Kaplan ID, Adler J, et al. Stereotactic Radiosurgery for Brain Metastases: The Importance of Adjuvant Whole Brain Irradiation. International Journal of Radiation Oncology and Biological Physics. 1992; 23:413–418

[51] Baschnagel AM, Meyer KD, Chen PY, et al. Tumor volume as a predictor of survival and local control in patients with brain metastases treated with Gamma Knife surgery. J Neurosurg. 2013; 119:1139–1144

[52] Bhatnagar AK, Flickinger JC, Kondziolka D, et al. Stereotactic radiosurgery for four or more intracranial metastases. Int J Radiat Oncol Biol Phys. 2006; 64:898–903

[53] Likhacheva A, Pinnix CC, Parikh NR, et al. Predictors of survival in contemporary practice after initial radiosurgery for brain metastases. Int J Radiat Oncol Biol Phys. 2013; 85:656–661

[54] Shaw E, Scott C, Souhami L, et al. Single dose radiosurgical treatment of recurrent previously irradiated primary brain tumors and brain metastases:

final report of RTOG protocol 90-05. Int J Radiat Oncol Biol Phys. 2000; 47:291–298

[55] Soliman H, Ruschin M, Angelov L, et al. Consensus Contouring Guidelines for Postoperative Completely Resected Cavity Stereotactic Radiosurgery for Brain Metastases. Int J Radiat Oncol Biol Phys. 2018; 100:436–442

[56] Brown PD, Ballman KV, Cerhan JH, et al. Postoperative stereotactic radiosurgery compared with whole brain radiotherapy for resected metastatic brain disease (NCCTG N107C/CEC.3): a multicentre, randomised, controlled, phase 3 trial. Lancet Oncol. 2017; 18:1049–1060

[57] Germano IM, Sheehan J, Parish J, et al. Congress of Neurological Surgeons Systematic Review and Evidence-Based Guidelines on the Role of Radiosurgery and Radiation Therapy in the Management of Patients With Vestibular Schwannomas. Neurosurgery. 2018; 82:E49–E51

[58] Kondziolka D, Mathieu D, Lunsford LD, et al. Radiosurgery as definitive management of intracranial meningiomas. Neurosurgery. 2008; 62:53–8; discussion 58-60

[59] Sheehan JP, Pouratian N, Steiner L, et al. Gamma Knife surgery for pituitary adenomas: factors related to radiological and endocrine outcomes. J Neurosurg. 2011; 114:303–309

[60] Choucair AK, Levin VA, Gutin PH, et al. Development of Multiple Lesions During Radiation Therapy and Chemotherapy. J Neurosurg. 1986; 65:654–658

[61] Kong DS, Lee JI, Park K, et al. Efficacy of stereotactic radiosurgery as a salvage treatment for recurrent malignant gliomas. Cancer. 2008; 112:2046–2051

[62] Lunsford LD, Flickinger J, Coffey RJ. Stereotactic Gamma Knife Radiosurgery. Initial North American Experience in 207 Patients. Arch Neurol. 1990; 47:169–175

[63] Yen CP, Matsumoto JA, Wintermark M, et al. Radiation-induced imaging changes following Gamma Knife surgery for cerebral arteriovenous malformations. J Neurosurg. 2013; 118:63–73

[64] Yen CP, Khaled MA, Schwyzer L, et al. Early draining vein occlusion after gamma knife surgery for arteriovenous malformations. Neurosurgery. 2010; 67:1293–302; discussion 1302

[65] Loeffler JS, Niemierko A, Chapman PH. Second tumors after radiosurgery: tip of the iceberg or a bump in the road? Neurosurgery. 2003; 52:1436–40; discussion 1440-2

[66] Brada M, Ford D, Ashley S, et al. Risk of second brain tumour after conservative surgery and radiotherapy for pituitary adenoma. BMJ. 1992; 304:1343–1346

[67] Sheehan J, Yen CP, Steiner L. Gamma Knife surgery-induced meningioma: Report of two cases and review of the literature. Journal of Neurosurgery 2006; 105:325–329

[68] Bernstein M, Laperriere N, Leung P, et al. Interstitial Brachytherapy for Malignant Brain Tumors: Preliminary Results. Neurosurgery. 1990; 26:371–380

[69] Florell RC, Macdonald DR, Irish WD, et al. Selection Bias, Survival, and Brachytherapy for Glioma. Journal of Neurosurgery. 1992; 76:179–183

[70] Gutin PH, Prados MD, Phillips TL, et al. External Irradiation Followed by an Interstitial High Activity Iodine-125 Implant "Boost" in the Initial Treatment of Malignant Gliomas: NCOG Study 6G-82-2. International Journal of Radiation Oncology and Biological Physics. 1991; 21:601–606

116 Endovascular Intervention

116.1 Introduction

AKA endovascular neurosurgery, neuroendovascular surgery, endovascular and surgical neuroradiology (ESNR), interventional neuroradiology (INR) or interventional neurology (IN), combines catheter-based techniques and imaging for the diagnosis and treatment of specific cerebral and spine conditions. Training is certified by the Committee on Advanced Subspecialty Training (CAST).

116.2 Indications/conditions treated

Endovascular intervention includes diagnosis as well as treatment of the following:
* aneurysms: coiling (± stent or balloon assistance), flow-diverting stents e.g., Pipeline, parent vessel sacrifice
* arteriovenous malformations (**AVM**s): embolization (preoperative or curative)
* dural arteriovenous fistula (**DAVF**): curative or palliative embolization
* spinal AVMs: embolization
* arteriovenous fistulas: e.g., carotid-cavernous fistulas (CCF)
* acute embolic stroke: intra-arterial thrombectomy, angioplasty, stenting, chemical thrombolysis
* cerebral venous thrombosis (**CVT**): thrombolysis or mechanical thrombectomy
* cerebrovascular arterial dissections: stenting or parent artery sacrifice
* common and internal carotid artery stenosis: angioplasty/stenting
* tumors: embolization. Primarily used before surgery as an adjunct to decrease vascularity e.g., with some meningiomas and hemangioblastomas
* intracranial atherosclerosis
* vasospasm
* chronic subdural hematoma: embolization of middle meningeal artery
* transverse sinus stenosis: stenting as may be indicated in pseudotumor cerebri (p. 955)
* inferior petrosal sinus sampling for localizing pituitary macroadenomas
* iatrogenic vascular injuries: stenting or embolization to achieve hemostasis
* refractory epistaxis: embolization to achieve hemostasis
* Wada testing: evaluation for language and memory localization (e.g., epilepsy patients being considered for surgery)
* intra-arterial chemotherapy: e.g., retinoblastoma
* intraoperative angiography (p. 1466): typically used in aneurysm surgery to confirm exclusion of the aneurysm and patency of parent vessels, and during AVM surgery to confirm elimination of nidus

116.3 Contraindications

* uncorrected (life-threatening) bleeding disorders
* relative contraindications:
  ○ poor renal function (due to iodine dye load): hemodialysis can be arranged in emergent situations; alternatively, patient may be hydrated and monitored for return to baseline creatinine
  ○ connective tissue disorder that predisposes to vessel dissection
  ○ severe allergy to iodine contrast: requires prior administration of "dye allergy prep" (p. 232)
  ○ major atheroma of aortic arch or plaque/atherosclerosis of great vessels (innominate, subclavian, common carotid artery) due to high risk for thromboembolic complications
  ○ for spinal angiography: thoracic aortic aneurysm (relative contraindication)

116.4 Risks of cerebral angiography

Risk varies with the nature of the pathology being investigated and with the experience of the angiography team. Overall risk of a complication resulting in a permanent neurologic deficit[1,2]: 0.1%. In ACAS, there was a 1.2% complication rate (p. 1549).

Risks include:
1. arterial dissection
2. perforation of artery or aneurysm
3. embolic thrombus

116

4. air embolism (p. 1738) : extremely rare (incidence of 0.08% in one series[3]). This incidence is likely higher with endovascular procedures (which may use pressurized arterial lines) than with diagnostic angio.[3] Treatment recommendations: elevate BP, ventilate with 100% O_2, consider hyperbaric oxygen[3]
5. puncture site complications
   a) hematoma at the puncture site
   b) embolism distal to the puncture site, e.g., that may compromise blood supply to the lower extremity

116.5 Miscellaneous angiography

▶ **Tumors.** While angiography is no longer used diagnostically for tumors, there are a few general principles that may be useful. Typically, non-vascular deep lesions cause changes in venous structures, whereas superficial lesions affect arterial structures. Malignant neoplasm (e.g., glioblastoma): the classic feature on angiography is an early draining vein. Meningiomas: the stain (contrast) "arrives early, stays late" (appears early in arterial phase, blush persists beyond venous phase); see also other angiographic findings with meningiomas (p. 812).

▶ **Allcock test.** Evaluates flow through the posterior communicating arteries by vertebral injection with simultaneous common carotid artery compression in the neck.

116.6 Pharmacologic agents

116.6.1 General information

This section presents drugs as they are used in neuroendovascular procedures.[4] The indications cited are specific to endovascular intervention.

116.6.2 Abciximab (ReoPro)

General information

The Fab fragment of an antibody. Prevents binding of fibrinogen to platelet GP IIb/IIIa receptors. Platelet inhibition lasts up to 48 hours.

Indications and case selection

- acute endoarterial thrombus during endovascular intervention
- dissection with thrombus adherent to intimal flap
- prophylaxis for intracranial or extracranial stent implantation

Contraindications

Do not administer concurrently with tPA (p. 1564).

Dosing

℞: bolus with 0.25 mg/kg IV over 10–60 minutes (shorter duration for the acute complications during intervention), followed by infusion of 0.125 mcg/kg/min (max. 10 mcg/min) for 12 hours.

Reversal

Discontinue abciximab infusion. Allow 10–30 minutes for clearance of the drug from plasma, followed by platelet transfusion. Surgical intervention should be delayed for 12–24 hours after discontinuation.

116.6.3 Aspirin

General information

Irreversibly inactivates cyclooxygenase (COX), resulting in platelet inhibition by preventing formation of prostaglandins from arachidonic acid that persists through the lifespan of the exposed platelets.

Indications and case selection

- Intra- (short-term) and postprocedural (short- + long-term) prophylaxis of thromboembolic events, e.g., during
  - diagnostic cerebral angiography
  - coil embolization of aneurysms
  - stent implantation (typically with a second antiplatelet agent)
  - balloon test occlusions
  - therapeutic occlusion of large arteries
- Subacute management of procedural complications, e.g.
  - parent artery coil herniations
  - thrombus or clot on coil phenomena
  - in-stent thrombus (alone or in combination with a second agent)

Dosing

R: typical dose does not exceed 325 mg PO daily

Uncoated Aspirin (ASA) achieves peak plasma concentrations within 30–40 minutes.[5,6] Enteric-coated ASA achieves peak plasma concentrations in up to 6 hours.[7]

Data on the prevalence of ASA resistance in neurointerventional procedures is scarce and the assessment is highly assay-dependent. A dose-related effect (i.e., improved response to increasing the dose) indicates that ASA also exerts antiplatelet effects through non-cyclooxygenase pathways.[8]

24–28% of patients are classified as aspirin-resistant.[9,10] However, results are conflicting on whether aspirin (or clopidogrel) resistance results in higher rates of thrombotic complications in patients undergoing neuroendovascular procedures.[11,12,13]

Reversal

ASA inhibition of COX is irreversible. Therefore, reversal is achieved by platelet transfusion.

116.6.4 Clopidogrel (Plavix™)

General information

A platelet ADP receptor antagonist.

Indications and case selection

- prevention of intraprocedural and short-term postprocedural (4–12 weeks) thromboembolic events related to endovascular procedures including
  - coil embolization of wide-neck cerebral aneurysms where stent will be used
  - stent implantation (with a second antiplatelet agent)
  - therapeutic occlusion of large arteries (often with a second antiplatelet agent)
- subacute management of procedural complications (alone or in combination with a second agent)
  - parent artery coil prolapse/herniation
  - thrombus or clot on coil phenomena
  - in-stent thrombus (may be more effective than other agents)

116

Dosing

R: 75 mg PO daily. Start 7–10 days prior to the actual procedure because there is a 3–7-day latency period to full therapeutic effect

LD: 300–600 mg PO, if there was no time to achieve therapeutic effect over a course of days. A therapeutic effect can usually be achieved within 2 to 3 hours of LD.

Reversal

Platelet transfusion.

116.6.5 Eptifibatide (Integrilin®)

General information

A reversible inhibitor of platelet aggregation by preventing the binding of fibrinogen, von Willebrand factor, and other adhesive ligands to GP IIb/IIIa. Platelet aggregation inhibition appears dose- and concentration-dependent and is reversible following discontinuation of eptifibatide. It causes a 5-fold increase in bleeding time and has no measurable effect on PT or aPTT.

Indications and case selection

These are the same as for abciximab (p. 1914).

Dosing

R: bolus 180 mcg/kg IV (max 22.6 mg) over 1–2 minutes followed by infusion of 2 mcg/kg/min.

Reversal

- discontinue drug. Significant reduction of anti-platelet effects occurs in 2–4 hours[14]
- for clinical signs or imaging evidence of hemorrhage:
  - for ICH, hemodynamic compromise, or decrease in Hb > 5 g/dl or decrease in HCT > 15%, give platelet transfusion
  - for a decrease in Hb < 5 g/dl or decrease in HCT < 15%, give desmopressin R: 0.3 mcg/kg × 1.

116.6.6 Heparin

General information

A glycosaminoglycan that indirectly inhibits thrombin by modulating antithrombin III (AT III) activity. It also indirectly inactivates factors IXa, Xa, XIa, and XIIa and restores electronegativity to endothelial surfaces. It prevents thrombin-platelet aggregation and inhibits von Willebrand factor. The anticoagulant effects are immediate. The half-life of IV heparin is approximately 1.5 hours.[15,16]

Indications and case selection

- prophylaxis during diagnostic angiography (used in flush solutions only)[4,17]
- almost all neuroendovascular procedures (except for diagnostic angiograms) including:
  - embolization of intracranial aneurysms (coil or Pipeline stent)
  - therapeutic occlusion of carotid, vertebral, or other large cerebral artery
  - embolization of brain AVM or dural AVF
  - cervical and intracranial angioplasty
  - intra- or extracranial stent implantation
  - balloon test occlusion of carotid, vertebral, or other large cerebral artery

Dosing

R: **Flush systems**: 4000–6000 i.u. per liter of 0.9% normal saline (typically 5000, yielding 5 i.u. per cc) for flush systems used in neuroendovascular procedures. For intraoperative angiography: 2500 i.u. per 1 liter of 0.9% normal saline (2.5 i.u. per cc) (lower dosage during surgery is a precaution against excessive bleeding from operative sites, e.g., during craniotomy, but intra-op angios generally use very little flush).

Endovascular interventions:

Aneurysm (coil, stent-assisted coil, flow diversion) embolization for unruptured aneurysm: bolus 60–70 units per kg of patient weight. Check the activated clotting time (ACT) 3–5 minutes after bolus and then hourly. Administer heparin 0–5000 units hourly PRN to maintain ACT between 250 and 300.

Coil embolization for ruptured aneurysm: several protocols exist.

- place the first (framing coil) prior to heparin bolus
- if balloon-assisted coiling is anticipated, IV heparin may be given sooner
- some interventionalists give 2000–3000 units as a bolus, followed by additional heparin bolus after placement of 1st coil

Stroke thrombectomy: because most thrombectomy procedures with modern devices can be performed rather quickly, many interventionalists no longer administer heparin bolus prior to thrombectomy.

Carotid artery stenting: similar to unruptured aneurysm embolization.

Balloon-test occlusion or prolonged stent-assisted coiling: for procedures with significant stasis of blood flow and thus increased risk of thrombus formation, higher ACT range of 300–350 may be utilized.

▶ **Post-procedure heparinization.** Generally not done unless acute clot formed. For aneurysm embolization, one of the following regimens are recommended:
   Heparin dosing for post coiling neurosurgery patients
- University of Cincinnati Protocol[18]: devised to administer a safe dose of heparin that does not require repeat blood draws and titration to ACT or aPTT
  - weight-based dosing
    - weight ≤ 75 kg: 900 units/hour, no bolus doses, for 12 hrs
    - weight > 75 kg: 1300 units/hour, no bolus doses, for 12 hrs
  - labs: no ACT or other laboratory draws required.
- *alternative:* the most commonly used heparin weight-based protocol (NB: this differs from dosing, e.g., for coronary indications or treatment of DVT or PE[19]): bolus dose of 60–70 units/kg followed by a maintenance IV infusion rate of 18 units/kg/hour

Reversal

IV protamine sulfate at 1 mg per 100 units of circulating heparin (not to exceed 50 mg total).
   A preloaded syringe of 50 mg should be available at all times. Normally protamine is administered as an IV infusion over 10–30 minutes, to prevent idiosyncratic hypotension and anaphylactoid symptoms. In an emergency, e.g., vessel or intracranial aneurysm perforation, anticoagulation must be immediately reversed by rapid IV bolus of 10 mg protamine over 1–3 minutes.

116.6.7 Nitroglycerine

General information

Produces strong and immediate vasodilatation by stimulation of cGMP, which results in vascular smooth muscle relaxation.

Indications and case selection

Vessel spasm during catheterization.

Dosing

℞: 100–300 mcg through the catheter.

116.6.8 Papaverine

General information

A benzylisoquinolone alkaloid that vasodilates by inhibition of cAMP and cGMP phosphodiesterases in smooth muscle, leading to increased intracellular levels of cAMP and cGMP. It may also inhibit the release of calcium from the intracellular space by blocking calcium ion channels in the cell membrane. Papaverine is short-acting, with half-life of less than 1 hour.

Indications and case selection

Pre-treatment for angioplasty. The resulting vasodilatation will assist with balloon catheter placement. Due to its short duration of action necessitating repeated administration, other agents e.g., verapamil, are generally preferred.

Dosing

℞: 300 mg of 3% papaverine (30 mg/ml) at pH 3.3, is diluted in 100 ml of normal saline to obtain a 0.3% concentration. It is administered intra-arterially through the microcatheter, which is positioned just proximal to the affected vascular segment at a rate of 3 ml/minute.
   ✱ Do not mix Papaverine with contrast agents or heparin, which may result in precipitation of crystals.

116

116.6.9 Sodium amytal

General information

A barbiturate derivative that activates GABA$_A$ receptors. When it is administered into cerebral vasculature during Wada test, it temporarily anesthetizes the perfused region, resulting in isolation of the contralateral hemisphere, permitting assessment of cortical functions including language and memory. It blocks neuronal activity, and in conjunction with lidocaine, which blocks axonal activity, it is administered as a test injection in procedures such as spinal AVM embolization, or embolization of spinal tumors, prior to the injection of the embolic agent.[20]

Indications and case selection

Wada test
Test injection prior to embolization of feeder vessel of AVM. In order to suppress both neuronal and axonal activity, amytal injection is followed by xylocaine injection.

Dosing

℞: 50–100 mg per test injection via catheter.
For administration, dilute 500 mg sodium amytal in 20 cc 0.9% NS to yield a concentration of 25 mg/cc of sodium amytal.
For Wada test, after catheterization of vessel of interest, 100 mg of sodium amytal (4 cc of the preparation described above) are injected through the catheter. Additional boluses of 25 mg (1 cc) or modification of the original bolus may be required, per the neurologist's request.

116.6.10 Tissue plasminogen activator (tPA, alteplase)

General information

A fibrin-specific thrombolytic protease that converts plasminogen to plasmin.

Indications for intravenous (IV) thrombolysis with tPA

The use of IV tPA has decreased due to superior results of mechanical clot removal (p. 1932) in situations when it is available. When IV tPA is employed, the following information is provided.[21]
Inclusion criteria:
- diagnosis of ischemic stroke causing measurable neurological deficit
- onset of symptoms ≤ 3 hrs before treatment begins (up to 4.5 hrs is supported by data with slightly lower level of evidence)
- age ≥ 18 years

✖ **Exclusion criteria:**
- arterial puncture at noncompressible site in previous 7 days
- history of previous intracranial hemorrhage
- intracranial neoplasm, AVM, or aneurysm
- recent intracranial or intraspinal surgery
- active internal bleeding
- elevated blood pressure (systolic > 185 mm Hg or diastolic > 110 mm Hg)
- acute bleeding diathesis including but not limited to:
  ○ platelet count < 100 X10^3/mm^3
  ○ heparin received within 48 hours resulting in an APTT above normal
  ○ current use of anticoagulant with an elevated PT (> 15 sec) or INR (> 1.7)
  ○ current use of direct thrombin inhibitors (desirudin, bivalirudin, argatroban)[22] or direct factor Xa inhibitors (rivaroxaban, edoxaban, betrixaban)[23] with elevated sensitive laboratory tests (e.g., aPTT, INR, platelet count, Ecarin Clotting Time (ECT), TT, or appropriate factor Xa activity assays)
- blood glucose concentration < 50 mg/dL (2.7 mmol/L)
- CT demonstrates multilobar infarction (hypodensity > 1/3 cerebral hemisphere)

Relative exclusion criteria:
- only minor or rapidly improving symptoms of stroke
- pregnancy

- seizure at onset with postictal residual neurological impairments
- major surgery or serious trauma within 14 days
- history of GI or urinary tract hemorrhage within 21 days
- recent acute myocardial infarction (within previous 3 months)

Dosing

℞: Intravenous: 0.9 mg/kg (max. 90 mg). The first 10% of the calculated dose is administered as an IV bolus over 1 minute and the remainder is infused starting *immediately* afterwards over an hour as long as the initial bolus is given within the 4.5-hour window.

℞: Intra-arterial thrombolysis with tPA: The dose is independent of any previously administered intravenous dose if IV tPA was given first. Rarely used as primary endovascular treatment nowadays given its low efficacy and high adverse event risk in comparison to other methods of thrombectomy. IA tPA is mainly used as adjunct treatment after thrombectomy if more distal emboli are noted angiographically.

First, 1–2 mg tPA is administered manually proximal to or within the clot, then an infusion of 0.5 mg/ml at 20 ml/hr (10 mg/hr). If not effective in lysing the clot, the infusion is prepared by mixing 10 mg of tPA in 20 ml in normal saline, resulting in a concentration of 1 mg tPA per 2 ml saline (or 0.5 mg/ml). An infusion pump may be used for more precise administration.

Frequent angiography is performed to determine angiographic response.
Discontinue tPA if
- adequate recanalization is achieved
- extravasation of contrast material is noted on angiography
- the maximum dose has been administered, or the administered dose approaches the maximum dose without clinical or angiographic improvement

℞ Cerebral venous thrombosis (CVT)

Similar to arterial stroke thrombectomy, chemical thrombolysis is rarely used as a sole treatment but rather as an adjunct to mechanical clot extraction. The bolus is usually 2–5 mg administered locally via a microcatheter into the thrombus. If unsuccessful, the microcatheter is left inside the affected sinus and then an infusion is started at a rate of 1 mg/hr, usually for 12–24 hours with repeat daily angiograms to determine the degree of response to thrombolysis. If a clot burden is still present on angiography, a longer duration of administration until the clot resolves is a consideration; however, after 24 hours bleeding complications become more frequent.

Reversal

If symptomatic intracranial bleeding is suspected[21]:
- immediately stop tPA infusion
- diagnostics:
  - bloodwork: CBC, PT (INR), aPTT, fibrinogen level, and type- and cross-match
  - STAT non-contrast head CT
- cryoprecipitate (includes factor VIII): 10 U infused over 10–30 min (onset: 1 hr, peak: 12 hrs), additional dose for fibrinogen level of < 200 mg/dL
- tranexamic acid (TXA) 1000 mg IV infused over 10 min OR ε-aminocaproic acid 4–5 g over 1 hour, followed by 1 g IV until bleeding is controlled. There is a risk of seizures with TXA, especially in renal failure
- hematology and neurosurgery consult as appropriate

116

16.6.11 Verapamil

General information

A nondihydropyridine calcium channel blocker that reduces the influx of calcium through L-type calcium channels in smooth-muscle cells, enabling vasodilation. Half-life is about 3–7 hours.

Indications and case selection

before balloon angioplasty: chemical vasodilatation prior to mechanical vasodilatation may enable a smoother and safer angioplasty
mild vasospasm, that does not warrant angioplasty
moderate vasospasm, that cannot be safely treated with angioplasty

Dosing

R: 5–10 mg IA. It is slowly infiltrated (over 2–10 minutes) into the vasospastic vessel via a microcatheter into the intracranial vessel, and/or via diagnostic or guide catheter into larger vessels, e.g., ICA or VA.

Reversal

For clinically significant hypotension or high degree AV block: treat with vasopressors and cardiac pacing, e.g., epinephrine, norepinephrine, and vasopressin infusions. Calcium chloride infusion is given in large doses, e.g., 1 gm/hr for more than 24 hours. 20% intralipid infusion (100 ml bolus followed by continuous infusion at 0.5 ml/kg/hr) may also be useful.[24] Atropine may be administered for bradycardia. Hemodialysis is ineffective.

116.6.12 Xylocaine

General information

Blocks the fast voltage-gated Na^+ channels in neuronal cell membranes. There may be inhibition of postsynaptic neurons and, consequently, action potentials.

Indications and case selection

As a local anesthetic prior to arteriotomy. Preparations with or without epinephrine may be used.
Cardiac xylocaine is used to test axonal function. It may be used alone or in conjunction with amobarbital.
Used for functional testing in case of spinal vascular disorders.
Provocative functional testing in cerebral AVMs.

Dosing

R: for local anesthesia: Approximately 5 ml of 2% lidocaine (max. 4 mg/ml to 280 mg; 14 ml)
R: for neurophysiological testing (Wada test): 10–40 mg i.a. of cardiac lidocaine.

Reversal

Lidocaine overdose[25]: intravenous bolus of 20% lipid emulsion 1.5 ml/kg over 1 min and start IV infusion at 15 ml/kg/hr. The bolus may be repeated twice at 5 min intervals, if cardiovascular stability is not restored. Additionally, the infusion may be doubled to 30 ml/kg/hr if instability persists after 5 minutes. Lipid emulsion is continued until cardiovascular stability is restored or maximum dose administered.[25] Do not exceed the maximum cumulative dose of 12 ml/kg.
Concurrent supportive care includes following ACLS protocols, e.g., securing airway, hemodynamic support, etc.
✗ Propofol is not a substitute for lipid emulsion in such cases. It has only 10% lipids, which is too low to be of benefit, and the cardio-depressant properties of propofol may be counterproductive in such situations.

116.7 Neuroendovascular procedure basics

116.7.1 Vascular access

General information

Most commonly, vascular access is obtained through femoral artery. If femoral access is not possible then the radial artery, brachial artery, or carotid artery (least common) may be used.

Femoral artery access

After prepping and draping the groin, place the left little finger on anterior superior iliac spine and span with thumb to the pubic symphysis. This approximately demarcates the ilioinguinal ligament. Bisect this line with the other hand and palpate the femoral pulse. The site of access is 3 fingerbreadth below the point of bisection, to ensure the vessel puncture site is *below* the ilioinguinal ligament and therefore compressible. A marker (e.g., hemostat) can be placed over the pulse and a fluoro shot taken to confirm that the planned access site is situated over the middle of the femoral head.

A small, superficial stab incision in the skin is made at the selected point, after infiltration of local anesthesia. In an elective case, a micropuncture set with a 7-cm 21- or 23-gauge needle may be used for vessel puncture. In an emergency (e.g., stroke) a larger 18 G single wall needle may be used to minimize the amount of time required to obtain femoral access. The artery is palpated and immobilized between the index and middle finger of one hand, while the needle is introduced through the stab at 45°. Once the artery is accessed, blood will emanate through the needle hub. An exchange over wires is made using modified Seldinger technique to place the sheath of desired size. Angiography is performed to confirm successful positioning of the sheath and ensure no local vasospasm, dissection, or active contrast extravasation is seen. The sheath is connected to a continuously running flush of heparinized saline and secured with adhesive or suture to prevent dislodgement.

Radial artery access

First perform Allen's test with pulse oximetry to ensure the hand has satisfactory vascular supply, in case the procedure results in radial artery occlusion.

Allen's test: Palpate the radial and ulnar arteries and place a pulse oximeter on the thumb or index finger. Make the patient flex and extend their fingers repeatedly. With digital pressure, compress both the radial and ulnar arteries during finger extension and maintain the compression until the oximetry pulse is lost. The wrist is maintained in approximately 20° flexion in order to avoid false positive test when the wrist is in hyperextension. Release the pressure on the ulnar artery. Measure the time taken to achieve visual capillary refill in finger pads and at least 92% oxygen saturation. Normal capillary refill time is < 5 sec, refill times of 5–15 secs are considered equivocal. A refill time longer than 15 sec is abnormal. Allen's test can also be performed using ultrasonography.

Reverse Allen's test: It should be performed when the radial artery is being subjected to a repeat procedure. Compress both the radial and ulnar arteries with digital pressure during finger extension and maintain the compression. Release the pressure on the *radial* artery. Measure the time taken to achieve visual capillary refill in finger pads and at least 92% oxygen saturation, as indicated above.

During access, the following modifications are made from the technique described above. A shorter 21 G needle (e.g., 3 cm instead of 7 cm) is used. Avoid entering the artery at a steep angle, as this may cause difficulties in threading the wire through the artery.

Advance a 0.018" wire through the needle hub into the radial artery and remove the needle. Make a nick in the skin over the wire, to aid in smoother insertion of larger sheaths. A 4 or 5 Fr (5 Fr because most diagnostic catheters for neuro procedures are still 5 Fr) micropuncture sheath (with dilator) is advanced over the wire and then the wire and dilator are removed. A cocktail of heparin (5000 IU/ml), verapamil (2.5 mg), 2% lidocaine (1.0 ml), and nitroglycerin (0.1 mg) are administered through the introducer sheath to relieve and/or prevent vasospasm. The patient should be forewarned about a transient but uncomfortable sensation of severe burning, as the cocktail is injected into the artery. The standard 0.035" wire is advanced through the sheath. The desired sheath size is then placed.

Note: After completion of the procedure, a closure device *is not* used for radial artery. Only manual compression for 15–20 minutes is applied. Alternatively, compression devices such as TR Band (Terumo) can be used instead of manual compression to achieve hemostasis.

16.7.2 Sheath management

Once placed, the sheath is connected to a continuously running heparinized saline solution at a rate of 30 ml/hr. The flush consists of 5000 units of heparin in 1000 ml of 0.9% saline bag (5 units/ml). The saline bag is placed in a pressure infuser which is inflated to 300 mm Hg. It is important that the sheath be continuously irrigated and the saline bag be under a pressure greater than the patient's own arterial pressure. The patient's leg on the side of the sheath is kept straight to prevent kinking of the sheath. If the intention is to maintain the sheath for several hours or a few days, it should be secured by suturing to the patient's skin.

16.7.3 Arteriotomy closure

After completion of the procedure, if vascular access will not be required within next few days, the sheath is removed. To do this, the following options are available:

pressure
  o *manual pressure:* palpate the artery proximal to site of arteriotomy, remove sheath and apply manual pressure for 15–30 minutes and gradually decreasing pressure every 5 minutes
  o Femostop™: prior to application, ensure ACT is < 150 and BP is under control. The inner circle of the Femostop dome should be positioned 1 cm superior and 1 cm medial to the actual puncture

site and over the femoral artery. Inflate the Femostop to 20–30 mm Hg above the patient's systolic pressure. If this does not result in hemostasis, inflate to higher pressures until distal pulses
are occluded. Maintain distal pulse occlusion for 5–7 minutes, then readjust the manometer
pressure until good pedal pulse and good color of extremities is achieved.
Continue to progressively decrease the applied pressure over the course of several hours, until
the device can be discontinued entirely. Usually, a Femostop is maintained for 6–12 hours.
- percutaneous closure devices
  - ✖ neither of the following should be used below the common femoral artery bifurcation if the
    vessel diameter is too small (typically < 4–5 mm) or if significant atherosclerosis is present
  - Angioseal™: effects closure by deposition of fibrin plug in the vessel which is then pulled back
    into the arteriotomy defect of the vessel wall. Angioseal is available in 6 and 8 Fr sizes. Deployed
    by exchanging it with the sheath over a wire. After deployment, the patient remains supine for
    2 hours (with pillow under the head) with the leg on the side of Angioseal kept straight. Patient
    is mobilized thereafter
  - Mynx™: a bio-absorbable intravascular sealant that is deposited in the arteriotomy defect.
    Available in 5, 6, 7 Fr sizes. Tends to be the least painful
  - Starclose™: Also exchanged with the sheath over a wire. Deployment results in stitch closure of
    the arteriotomy defect. Tends to be more painful

116.8 Diagnostic angiography for cerebral subarachnoid hemorrhage

116.8.1 General information

Objective: diagnose source of hemorrhage, assess supplying blood vessels and collateral vessels (may
require additional provocative maneuvers), assess vessels for possible bypass, assess for vasospasm.
  The most common cause of nontraumatic SAH is ruptured cerebral aneurysms. Other causes
include AVM (cerebral or spinal), vasculitis, pre-truncal nonaneurysmal subarachnoid hemorrhage,
arterial dissection, dural sinus thrombosis, pituitary apoplexy, bleeding dyscrasias, sickle cell disease,
and cocaine abuse. In 14–22%, a cause for SAH is not found on angiography.[26]

116.8.2 Setup

A sheath is placed in the femoral artery, connected to a continuously running flush of heparinized
saline. A diagnostic catheter is attached to a continuously running flush of heparinized saline. A
introduced into the vasculature via the sheath and advanced over the guidewire through the aorta to
the target vessel. The catheter is advanced with the guidewire leading and pulled back with the
guide wire completely retracted into the catheter. Once the catheter is in the desired position,
the guidewire is withdrawn completely and angiography performed, by using manual injections o
the auto-injector.

116.8.3 Planning

Pre-planning the procedure will save time, amount of contrast administered, and radiation exposure
Standard views (half Towne's and lateral for anterior circulation; Towne's and lateral for posterio
circulation) are obtained. Additionally, the images in appropriate projections are obtained, keeping
in mind the patient's pathology. Typically, a six-vessel angiogram, including bilateral internal, external carotid, and vertebral arteries, is performed to determine the source of the SAH. In certain case:
a spinal angiogram may also be needed. As needed, rotational angiography is performed and the 3I
reconstruction manipulated for further examination, as well as selection of further projections fo
angiography.

116.9 Disease-specific intervention

116.9.1 Aneurysms

General information

Endovascular therapy (coiling, and more recently, flow diversion) vs. clip debate is a moving targe
especially given the fact that as long-term data about endovascular treatment is becoming availabl
the technology continues to evolve, which renders the data obsolete. While there will always be

ole for surgical clipping, endovascular therapy has emerged as a first line therapy for most aneur-
sms (particularly ruptured aneurysms or in poor surgical candidates). Surgery still remains a strong
ption for MCA aneurysms and PICA aneurysms.

ndications

he selection of aneurysm for treatment depends upon the following considerations:

Ruptured vs. unruptured. A ruptured aneurysm needs to be treated urgently, as the risk or re-
upture is 2–3%/day in the first few days and 20% in 2 weeks. The risk of morbidity and mortality of
n untreated ruptured aneurysm is 45–50%.[27,28]

Symptoms other than rupture. Aneurysms that present with symptoms, e.g., cranial nerve palsy,
oss of vision or ischemia, may be at a higher risk of rupture than asymptomatic aneurysms (some
ymptoms may be due to acute expansion).[29,30,31,32,33,34]

Size. Large aneurysms (> 7–10 mm) are more likely to rupture than small (< 7 mm) aneurysms.[34,35]

Shape. An irregularly shaped aneurysm may be at a greater risk of rupture than a spherical saccu-
ar aneurysm. Irregular shape includes morphological characteristics such as daughter blebs, or
regular borders.[36]

Aspect ratio. In addition to size, the aspect ratio (aneurysm depth/neck width) may predict the
neurysms at risk of rupture. An aspect ratio greater than 1.6 may create low flow conditions in the
ome of the aneurysm that lead to stasis, thrombosis, and a fibrinolytic cascade that results in
reakdown of the intima.[37] A retrospective evaluation of 75 ruptured and 107 unruptured aneur-
sms demonstrated the mean aspect ratio to be 2.7 for ruptured and 1.8 for unruptured aneurysms
) < 0.001). The mean depth of aneurysm was also greater in ruptured aneurysms (7.7 ± 4.9 mm vs.
.1 ± 4.5 mm). 75% of the ruptured aneurysms were < 10 mm, and 62% of these had aspect
atio > 1.6.[38]

Location. The ISUIA studies demonstrated posterior circulation aneurysms had a higher risk of
upture compared to anterior circulation.[29,39] Conversely, cavernous segment aneurysms had a 0%
sk of rupture until they reached a size of 13–24 mm, when the 5-year cumulative risk became 3%.

Choice of treatment. The choice of treatment should take all of the above in addition to individ-
al patient considerations, e.g., age and overall health.
Wide necked aneurysms were previously thought better suited for clipping, but the availability of
ents that may act as scaffolding for coils, e.g., Enterprise™ stent, or act as vascular reconstruction
evices, e.g., Pipeline, has greatly increased the spectrum of aneurysms amenable to endovascular
eatment. Additionally, small aneurysms (< 4 mm in size) may be less favorable for coiling.

ndovascular options

Coiling. This is the treatment of first choice for most narrow-necked aneurysms. The first one or
vo coils (framing coils) used are equal to the average size of aneurysm (calculated as height +
vidth/2). The coils are progressively downsized and changed in softness as embolization progresses.
he goal is to maximally pack the aneurysm such that no contrast is seen entering it and without
using any loop to herniate into the vessel lumen. Even after maximal packing as seen angiographi-
lly, the actual packing is about 20–30%.[40]

Coiling with stenting. For wide-necked aneurysms, a stent may be used to prevent the coils from
erniating out of the aneurysm into the blood vessel. When a stent is used, the patient is required to
e on ASA (most commonly indefinitely, although certain centers stop all antiplatelet drugs after 1
ear) and clopidogrel or alternative agents such as ticagrelor or prasugrel (typically for 3–6 months).
herefore, stent assisted coiling is generally avoided in ruptured aneurysms, in part due to the fact
at if an EVD, ventricular shunt, or craniotomy is needed it may require temporary reversal of anti-
atelet medication, which increases the risk of acute in-stent thrombosis. However, it has also been
ndertaken successfully in ruptured cases, with 93% technical success, clinically significant ICH in 8%
ncluding 10% known to have EVDs), and significant thromboembolic events in 6%.[41]

Balloon-assisted coiling. This technique may be used for wide necked aneurysms where stenting
deemed less desirable, e.g., ruptured aneurysm, since it bypasses the need for dual anti-platelet

116

therapy. A balloon catheter is selected based on the diameter of the parent artery and the width of the aneurysm neck. The balloon segment of the catheter (indicated by radiopaque markers) is positioned across the neck and kept inflated during coil deposition into the aneurysm. It is deflated prior to coil detachment and the stability of the deposited coil assessed. If the coil appears stable, it is detached. This inflation-deflation technique is continued as required, until the aneurysm has been completely coiled. Close attention should be paid to ACT as prolonged balloon inflation times and local blood stasis may trigger local thrombus formation. It is typically not recommended to keep the balloon inflated for more than 3–5 minutes.

▶ **Dual catheter technique.** In this case two microcatheters are placed in the aneurysm. Coil loops are deposited alternatively from each. The technique is proposed to decrease the risk of coil loop prolapse/herniation in wide-neck aneurysms.

▶ **Coil types. Bare platinum coils**: detachable coils that come in various diameters (mm), length (cm), shapes (3D, box coils, helical), and degrees of softness. Framing coils are typically more "stiff" and will provide a solid frame, whereas finishing coils are very "soft" and will find vacant compartments within the coil mass.
Hydrocoils: platinum coils coated with hydrogel, which expands upon contact with blood filling the residual space between loops. These are typically used as "finishing" coils and are believed to reduce the risk of aneurysm recurrence/residual.

▶ **Pipeline Embolization Device (PED).** The woven design of this particular stent makes it low porosity, which attenuates blood entry into the aneurysm and therefore encourages stasis. If needed, two or more of these may be deployed within each other across the neck of the aneurysm to cause adequate flow stasis in the aneurysm. Angiography immediately post-deployment demonstrates contrast stasis in the aneurysm. Six-month follow-up angiography usually demonstrates complete obliteration of the aneurysm, such that it is no longer visualized. Once an aneurysm is successfully treated with PED, there is a 0% recurrence rate. The most recent iteration of the device known as Pipeline Flex™ is a 48-braid device that is somewhat easier to deploy than the earlier version. It is available in diameters from 2.5–5 mm. Sometimes, coil deployment in the aneurysm may also be required to encourage aneurysm thrombosis.

A strategy used in case of ruptured aneurysms is to "undercoil" the aneurysm to address the risk of re-rupture and then complete treatment with PED when it becomes safe to use dual antiplatelet therapy

In case of ruptured blister aneurysms, Pipeline device has been used with success by administering an abciximab bolus (0.125 mcg/kg) IV, approx. 10 minutes prior to device deployment.[42,43]

Indications:
- Large or giant wide-necked ICA aneurysms, from petrous to the superior hypophyseal segments
- Presently, patients must be 22 years of age or older
- PED has been used in cases outside the established indications, e.g., in MCA, and vertebral and basilar arteries[44,45,46]

Contraindications:
- Ruptured aneurysm (due to requirement of pre-embolization dual anti-platelet therapy). However, it has been used in ruptured blister aneurysms[42,43]
- Patients in whom dual anti-platelet therapy is contraindicated
- Patients who have not received dual anti-platelet therapy (ASA and clopidogrel) prior to procedure
- Active bacterial infection
- Metal allergy to cobalt, chromium, platinum or tungsten
- Patients with pre-existing stent in the parent artery at the target aneurysm location (relative contraindication)

Treatment of aneurysmal rupture during coiling

- notify anesthesia: for assistance with critical care management and in case you need to go to the O.R.
- immediately lower the blood pressure
- inflate balloon if balloon-assisted coiling
- immediately reverse anticoagulation. Give 50 mg of protamine (protamine should always be available during the procedure)

- do not remove the coil that caused the perforation; continue deploying it and follow with additional coils in rapid succession
- insert an extraventricular drain (EVD)

116.9.2 Endovascular management of vasospasm

General information

A ruptured aneurysm needs to be secured by coiling or clipping prior to hyperdynamic therapy or endovascular intervention for vasospasm.

Indications

Failure of resolution, or worsening of symptoms of vasospasm with hyperdynamic therapy for 12–24 hours.

Patients with conditions such as congestive heart failure, cardiac ischemia, or pulmonary edema that limit the institution of hyperdynamic therapy.[47]

Treatment options

In addition to pharmacological (hyperdynamic or triple-H) therapy, endovascular options for management of vasospasm include intra-arterial chemical spasmolysis, utilizing selective catheterization of the involved segment, and mechanical spasmolysis using angioplasty.

▶ **Chemical spasmolysis.** Verapamil: Drug of first choice for spasmolysis in many centers. Its advantage is a relatively long half–life (6–12 hours).

Indications:
- Mild to moderate vasospasm that does not warrant angioplasty. Or, when angioplasty cannot be used safely
- Vasospasm consequent to manipulation during endovascular intervention
- Prior to performing angioplasty, so that the dilatation is performed on the relaxed dilated artery rather than a relatively rigid vasoconstricted one

Dose: 5–10 mg injected gradually (over 2–10 minutes) via microcatheter, as the microcatheter is withdrawn through the spasmodic segment. Up to 20 mg may be given into each arterial tree. It is injected gradually to prevent a significant drop in BP or bradycardia.

Other drugs used for chemical spasmolysis include nicardipine, papaverine and nitroglycerine. Similar to verapamil, nicardipine has a relatively long half–life (9 hours). Papaverine (< 1 hour) and nitroglycerine (minutes) are comparatively short acting.

▶ **Angioplasty.** A balloon mounted catheter is positioned across the arterial segment in spasm. The balloon is gradually inflated under fluoroscopic visualization to the desired width (equal to or less than the caliber of the adjacent non-spastic segment). The rate of balloon inflation is at a rate ≤ 1 atm/15 sec (to "stretch," not "crack" the vessel).

A combination of chemical and mechanical spasmolysis may also be used such that initially the spastic segment is dilated using verapamil infiltration, followed by balloon angioplasty.

Balloon dilatation produces durable results. However, even verapamil induced spasmolysis has been noted to persist on angiographies performed 48–72 hours post treatment.

Angioplasty is performed under direct fluoroscopic visualization. To this effect, contrast media is admixed with normal saline (50:50 to 2/3–1/3 ratio) that is used to inflate the balloon.

Precautions during angioplasty:
- Avoid inflating the balloon beyond the normal caliber of the vessel
- Inflate gradually at a rate ≤ 1 atm/15 sec (to "stretch," not "crack" the vessel)
- Do not inflate the balloon beyond its indicated "burst pressure." This can also be avoided by selecting a balloon catheter with the appropriate width of the particular vessel and length of the segment in spasm

Complications and management. Vessel rupture. This can be avoided by not inflating the balloon beyond the normal caliber of the vessel. Following rupture, reverse therapeutic heparinization by administration of protamine 1 mg per 100 units of heparin (max. 50 mg). In such an emergency, rapid IV bolus of protamine (10 mg over 1–3 minutes) is delivered rather than over 10–30 minutes, which is usually done to prevent idiosyncratic hypotension and anaphylactoid symptoms.

116

Maintain wire (0.014") access across the injured vessel. Exchange for a balloon catheter 1 mm smaller in size and inflate it for about 20 minutes. Then deflate and perform angiography to see if bleeding has been controlled. If necessary, sacrifice the involved vessel using coils. With this approach, e.g., in the M2 segment of MCA, the complication of stroke is accepted with the aim of saving the patient's life. Additionally, decompressive craniotomy and evacuation of the clot may be required.

▶ **Dissection.** If it is minor, non-flow limiting and without a raised intimal flap, no intervention may be necessary. The dissection may be re-examined after an interval to verify resolution. If managed conservatively, place the patient on aspirin, with or without Plavix.

In case of a significant dissection, place a stent across the affected segment and start patient on ASA and plavix. Plavix 75 mg PO daily is usually administered for a month while ASA is continued indefinitely.

▶ **Thromboembolic complications.** A thrombus consequent to hardware, vessel injury blood stagnation or inadequate heparinization is apparent as a filling defect on control angiography. This can usually be readily addressed by administration of abciximab bolus of 0.25 mg/kg IV over 10–15 minutes, followed by infusion of 0.125 mcg/kg/min (max. 10 mcg/min) for 12 hours. Repeat angiography 15 minutes following the initiation of abciximab. If the thrombus persists, an angioplasty may be performed to flatten the thrombus against the wall of the vessel. Once blood flow is restored, its lytic properties, as well as the abciximab, may resolve the thrombus. Another consideration is to deploy a stent to restore lumen and blood flow.

▶ **ICH.** This may happen due to causes including vessel injury, bleeding into a previous area of infarct, hyperperfusion in a previously compromised area, or hypertension. When detected, discontinue and reverse the heparinization using protamine. Monitor patient closely. A decompressive craniotomy or craniectomy may be required if the hemorrhage is significant.

▶ **Surveillance and follow-up.** In addition to diligent monitoring in NICU, the progress or resolution of vasospasm can also be assessed by performing serial TCDs. Depending upon extent of availability, these can be daily, every other day or at least bi-weekly (e.g., q Monday and Thursday). The TCDs may be discontinued when resolution of vasospasm is apparent clinically and radiologically.

Angiography may be repeated approximately 3 days following initial intervention, or when there is significant change indicating worsening vasospasm. It need not be repeated, if the patient is obviously improving. Alternatively, CTA may be used for surveillance. At the time of surveillance angiography, additional treatments with chemical spasmolysis and/or balloon angioplasty may be considered. Therefore, start off with a larger sheath (usu. 6 Fr) to enable intervention.

Usually, the patient will remain in the NSICU for approximately 10–14 days, considering that vasospasm is maximal by 7–8 days and usually resolves by 14 days.[48,49,50,51]

116.9.3 Arteriovenous malformation

Indications for endovascular intervention

- the most common form of endovascular intervention for AVM is preoperative embolization to facilitate surgical AVM resection
- presence of associated lesions, e.g., aneurysm or pseudoaneurysm on the feeding pedicle or nidus, venous thrombosis, venous outflow restriction, venous pouches, or dilatations
- a small surgically inaccessible AVM, or where surgery carries a high risk of morbidity and mortality. Curative AVM embolization is rare and limited to small lesions with simple angioarchitecture. The small surgically inaccessible AVM can also be treated with radiosurgery, which has a better track record than curative AVM embolization attempts
- as a palliative treatment in an AVM that is not completely treatable by any approach or their combination, due to location and/or diffuse morphology, but is symptomatic. Use with caution: data suggests that partial embolization of complex AVMs may increase rupture rate and worsen outcome

AVM embolization

This can be performed using numerous agents (or their combination).

The agents include coils, onyx, NBCA, and PVA.

▶ **Coils.** These may be used to close down a vessel supplying the AVM, an AVM pouch, or aneurysm on the arteries associated with AVM. However, it cannot be relied upon to completely obliterate the AVM nidus or effect a cure.

▶ **Onyx™.** A "lava-like" liquid embolic agent—Ethylene vinyl alcohol (EVOH) copolymer; ethylene and vinyl alcohol dissolved in dimethyl sulfoxide (DMSO) with micronize tantalum (for radiopacity)—that solidifies through the process of precipitation, which is initiated when it comes into contact with an aqueous solution (e.g., blood, body fluids, normal saline, water) to form a cast. Not an adhesive. Amongst all agents currently available, it has the best and most controlled penetration of the AVM nidus. Therefore, Onyx has the greatest likelihood of achieving complete cure. Complete cure rates with onyx alone are possible in 20–51% of highly selected patients.[52,53,54] Supplied in premixed ready-to-use vials of Onyx-18, Onyx-34 and Onyx-500 in which the number (e.g., 18 for Onyx-18) corresponds to the nominal viscosity (as measured in centistokes), which the manufacturer controls by altering the EVOH concentration. Prior to use, the product must be shaken on a mixer for at least 20 minutes. Higher numbers indicate greater viscosity. Onyx 18 is most commonly used, Onyx 34 is used for very high flow AVMs.

Onyx is used with DMSO compatible microcatheters (marathon, echelon, XT-17, Duo) or balloon microcatheter (Scepter C) that have been primed with approximately 0.3 to 0.8 ml of DMSO injected slowly through the microcatheter (depending on the deadspace of the microcatheter) prior to injecting Onyx itself. This is done to eliminate any contrast, saline, or blood within the microcatheter that will cause the onyx to solidify in the catheter. The microcatheter tip is wedged in an arterial branch supplying the AVM, as close to the nidus as possible. It is ensured that the branch is exclusively supplying the AVM, by performing angiography through the microcatheter. The microcatheter is then primed with DMSO and Onyx embolization commenced under fluoroscopy. The onyx is visible due to admixed tantalum powder. It is injected slowly and continuously, avoiding too much force, as this could cause the Onyx to reflux instead of flowing forward, and prematurely close off access to the nidus. No more than 1 cm of Onyx reflux on the microcatheter should usually be allowed, as it may make the removal of catheter difficult later and may well cause disastrous complications (this is obviated with detachable 1-cm and 3-cm tip Apollo microcatheters which tolerate greater Onyx reflux). If reflux is noted, wait for 1–2 minutes and then continue with the injection. The already deposited Onyx will form a plug around the microcatheter causing the new deposit of Onyx to flow forward. The injection is stopped once Onyx is noted only to reflux and not flow into the nidus. Care is taken not to allow the Onyx to flow into the major draining vein or sinus, especially before the entire arterial supply is interrupted. The concept is the same as in surgical removal of AVMs, where major draining veins are occluded only after eliminating the arterial supply of AVM. Otherwise, the result is the same with ensuing venous hypertension resulting in AVM rupture and catastrophic ICH. In case of a large AVM, it is sometimes best to stage the procedure, addressing one major arterial tree at a time.

Intravenous or combined IV, and IA embolization of AVMs has been performed in a select group of small, deep seated AVMs, with single deep drainage.[55]

▶ **NBCA.** N-butyl cyanoacrylate is an embolic agent that is a glue which rapidly solidifies when it comes in contact with blood. Since the introduction of Onyx, its use has declined considerably due to the drawbacks of very short working time, greater risk of embolization into venous sinuses, and adhesion to catheters, rendering their extraction following embolization difficult. Such adhesion may cause intracranial bleeds or inadvertent catheter fractures with retained foreign body.

▶ **PVA.** Polyvinyl alcohol (PVA) particles are available in sizes ranging from 50 to 1000 mcm. While it may be useful in temporarily devascularizing the AVM, e.g., in preparation of craniotomy and surgical resection of AVM, the endovascular treatment with PVA alone is not durable.

116

Postoperative management

Post-op orders:
- admit the patient to NSICU
- keep leg on side used for procedure straight X 2 hrs (in case of Angioseal closure) or 6–8 hours (in case manual compression was applied), with HOB elevated 15°
- postprocedure heparinization is not required with AVMs because most ischemic events occur during the procedure and are related to the passage of embolic materials into normal blood vessels[15]
- check groins, DPs, vitals and neuro checks q 15 min X 4 hr, q 30 min X 4 hr, then q hr
- maintain mild hypotension for 12–72 hours, especially in case of larger AVMs, and monitor the patient for perfusion pressure break through bleeding, seizures, and other possible complications
- review/resume preprocedure medications (hold metformin for 48 hours after intervention; hold all oral hypoglycemics until good PO intake is established)[56]

Follow-up:
- outpatient appointment in 4 weeks

- follow-up angiography at 3 months. In case of staged AVM embolization, the interval between sessions is at the discretion of the interventionist, e.g., 1–4 weeks apart

116.9.4 Dural arteriovenous fistulae (DAVF)

General information

These are abnormal direct arteriovenous shunts within the leaflets of the dura.

Classification

There are numerous DAVF classifications. Borden (p.1517) and Cognard (p.1517) are amongst the more widely used.

Indications for endovascular intervention

- DAVF with "aggressive" features (▶ Table 116.1) are always considered for treatment. Due to the high annual mortality rate (10.4%) and annual hemorrhage rate (8.1%), the treatment should be expeditious.[57]
- DAVF with angiographic findings including:
  - selective contrast injection into ICA or VA demonstrating delayed cerebral circulation time. This is indicative of venous congestive encephalopathy.
  - pseudophlebitic pattern: Brain surface demonstrating tortuous, dilated collateral veins in the venous phase of the angiogram. This finding is associated with a greater risk of hemorrhage or non-hemorrhagic neurological deficit.
  - cortical venous reflux (CVR): To ensure that this is not missed, always perform selective (rather than global, non-selective) angiography when assessing for DAVF. Venous stenosis or obstruction is commonly found in patients with CVR.

If a DAVF is detected, look for additional fistulae, as they are multiple in up to 8%.

Those with "benign" features (see ▶ Table 116.1), may be considered for treatment if the symptoms are causing considerable discomfort to the patient, or are angiographically progressive. In many cases the treatment is palliative, i.e., the symptoms are reduced but the fistula is not completely obliterated. The benign type of DAVF should continue to be followed, even when treatment is not indicated because of the risk of conversion to a more aggressive form with CVR. The follow-up may be clinical, with radiological assessment for any change in symptoms. A suggested protocol is to perform MRA with gadolinium annually, with follow-up conventional catheter angiography at 3 years. If there is any change in the patient's clinical condition, whether it is worsening, improvement, or resolution of the symptoms, perform standard angiography to assess for CVR.

Asymptomatic DAVF can usually be followed.

Table 116.1 Differentiating aggressive from benign DAVF

"Aggressive" symptoms	"Benign" symptoms
• Cortical venous reflux (CVR): the hallmark of an aggressive DAVF • Intracerebral hemorrhage • Focal neurological deficit • Dementia • Papilledema • Increased intraocular pressure	• Pulsatile bruit • Orbital congestion (without increased intraocular pressure) • Cranial nerve palsy • Chronic headaches

Contraindications to endovascular intervention

Most contraindications are relative, and a risk-benefit assessment is performed on a case-by-case basis:
- *NBCA* should not be used in those with allergy to cyanoacrylates, ethiodol, or iodine. Premedication in those with iodine allergies is a consideration.
- *PVA* should not be used as a therapeutic option (other than in cases of epistaxis). It is usually indicated for pre-surgical devascularization of the lesion.

DAVF embolization

The approach can be transarterial, transvenous, or a combination. When feasible, a transvenous approach is preferred, as the probability of fistula obliteration is greater via the venous route. Ver infrequently, it is possible to access the venous side from the arterial route because of a large connection between the dural artery and adjacent vein, e.g., in traumatic DAVF.

For transvenous route, consider the potential outcome of venous occlusion, e.g., venous infarct, if the sinus being occluded is also the main source of drainage for normal veins. In such a situation, consider highly selective occlusion that will spare the normal drainage. Alternatively, instead of performing a complete occlusion, consider partial treatment only such that CVR is eliminated, converting the fistula into the benign Borden type I.

When using the venous route, ascertain that the venous channel is not tenuous (e.g., acute DAVF), rendering it prone to rupture during manipulation. The venous walls become sturdier when the fistula has been present for a while.

▶ **Coils.** Measure the maximum width of the fistulous site to be occluded and select the appropriate sized coils. Deposit as many coils as necessary to occlude the fistula.

Sometimes a "combined" strategy may be used, in which coils are initially deposited to slow the rapid blood flow through the fistula, followed by occlusion using a liquid embolic agent. If this strategy is used, start off with or exchange for a microcatheter compatible with the liquid embolic agent.

▶ **Onyx.** During transarterial embolization with liquid embolic agents, wedge the catheter as close as possible to the fistula. The technique of deposition is the same as for AVM (see AVM section (p. 1927)). It is important to disrupt the fistulous connection to achieve cure. Therefore, Onyx must penetrate into the venous aspect of the DAVF.

▶ **NBCA.** It is used less frequently since the availability of Onyx, for reasons described above.

▶ **PVA.** It really has no significant role in the treatment of DAVF.

116.9.5 Carotid-cavernous fistulae (CCF)

General information

CCF are categorized as direct and indirect. The direct CCF are usually posttraumatic and are a high-flow single shunt between the ICA and the cavernous sinus. Indirect CCF are low-flow from meningeal branches. The section below describes management of the direct type.

Indications for endovascular intervention

Direct fistulae usually require treatment as they frequently do not resolve spontaneously. Other indications: corneal exposure, diplopia, proptosis, intolerable bruits, or headaches.

Timing of treatment

If the patient is stable, treatment may usually be performed within a couple of days of the diagnosis (i.e., treatment does not have to be emergent).

Indications for urgent treatment: ICH, epistaxis, increased IOP, decreased visual acuity, rapidly progressive proptosis, cerebral ischemia, and enlargement of traumatic aneurysm beyond the cavernous sinus.

CCF embolization

The treatment goal is to eliminate the fistula.

Angiography is performed to identify the exact location and size of the fistula and its venous drainage. To address the high flow, consider angiography at 7.5 fps, instead of the usual 2–4 fps. In addition to the CCF, also look for other vascular injuries/anomalies.

Selective catheterization of both ECAs and ICAs is performed to assess their contribution to the CCF. Angiography is also performed after manual compression of the CCA on the side of fistula, to better assess cross-flow from the contralateral side. The digital compression will attenuate the high blood flow to the fistula, enabling its visualization. Do not compress both carotids simultaneously.

Rotational angiography with 3D reformatting may be performed to study the fistula and select appropriate working views for intervention. It is important to be cognizant of the venous involvement, including cavernous sinuses, superior and inferior ophthalmic veins, sphenoparietal sinus, superior and inferior petrosal sinuses, and the pterygoid plexi.

The following routes may be utilized for treating CCF: transarterial, transvenous, and via the superior ophthalmic vein (if conventional routes are not available). Other indications: corneal exposure, diplopia, proptosis, intolerable bruits, or headaches.[58]

▶ **Coils.** Currently, the method of choice is transarterial coil embolization of the CCF.

Using roadmapping images, the microcatheter is advanced over microwire into the cavernous sinus via the fistula. This may take some effort. Coils are then deployed and detached, as previously described for aneurysms. Periodic angiography is performed and further coils are placed until the cavernous sinus (CS) is completely occluded. Complete occlusion is indicated by no further contrast entering the CS.

▶ **Onyx.** Refer to AVM section (p.1927) for details regarding usage. In case of a high-flow fistula, prior to Onyx deposition, it may be advisable to initially deposit coils into the CS to slow the blood flow. This will prevent the inadvertent embolization of Onyx into the draining veins and sinuses. A balloon can be inflated within the parent ICA in order to protect it as Onyx is being injected into the cavernous sinus.

▶ **NBCA.** NBCA should be used with great caution, preferably after having slowed the flow through the CCF in order to prevent untoward deposition in the venous sinuses.

There is also potential for reflux into the carotid artery, which could cause a stroke. This may particularly occur when the CCF closure is near completion and the pressure gradient between the carotid artery and the CS is lowered. As with Onyx, a balloon can be inflated in the parent artery to protect it.

▶ **Coil occlusion of the ICA.** The desirable treatment for CCF is the occlusion of the fistula itself, essentially resulting in ICA reconstruction. This is frequently not possible. If the CCF is not amenable to treatment by any other route, sacrifice of the involved ICA is an option, especially if satisfactory supply has been confirmed from the contralateral ICA via anterior communicating and/or supply via the posterior communicating arteries.

Postoperative management and follow-up

Post-op orders:
- admit the patient to NSICU for overnight observation. Further ICU stay will depend upon the patient's clinical condition
- consult or arrange follow-up with ophthalmic surgery
- 0.9% NS + 20 meq KCl @ 150 cc/hr X 2 hrs, then decrease to 100 cc/hr if patient is NPO overnight, then advance diet as tolerated
- keep the leg that was used for procedure straight for 2 hrs in case of Angioseal closure, or 6–8 hours when manual compression was applied. May elevate 15° HOB, e.g., a pillow under the head
- check groin, DPs, vitals, and neuro checks q 15 min X 4 hrs, q 30 min X 4 hrs, then q hr
- review/resume preprocedure medications (hold metformin for 48 hours after intervention; hold all oral hypoglycemics until good PO intake is established)

Follow-up:
- D/C home the next morning after mobilizing, if there are no complications/other ongoing medical concerns requiring hospitalization
- follow-up on outpatient basis in 4 weeks
- follow-up angiography at 3 months

116.9.6 Vertebrojugular fistulae (VJF)

Etiologies

- Iatrogenic, e.g., during spine surgery or angiography, chiropractic manipulation, nerve block injection, or radiation therapy[59,60]
- Trauma, e.g., penetrating injury or GSW
- Vasculitis

Endovascular management of VJF

▶ **Stenting.** A polytetrafluoroethylene (PTFE) covered stent, e.g., Jostent, may be used to cover th ostia of the fistula.[59]

▶ **Coil occlusion.** In the presence of adequate blood flow through contralateral healthy vertebra artery, the fistulous artery may be occluded with coils.[61] Verify that the arterial wall with the fistu lous connection is part of the occluded segment.

► **NBCA occlusion.** Rarely, NBCA occlusion has been performed when stenting or coil occlusion were not possible.[62] Onyx may also be used similarly.

116.9.7 Carotid dissection

General information

See General information on arterial dissections (p. 1576).

Angiographic features

Luminal stenosis (65%), occlusion (28%), pseudoaneurysm (28%), luminal irregularity (13%), embolic distal branch occlusion (13%), intimal flap (12%), and slow ICA-MCA flow (11%).[63]

Management

The CADISS randomized trial showed no difference in efficacy of antiplatelet agents versus anticoagulation at preventing stroke and death in patients with symptomatic carotid and vertebral artery dissection.[64] Because the management with heparin and Coumadin is more complex, most physicians now favor the use of antiplatelets such as Aspirin. If anticoagulation is indicated, for example based on comorbid conditions such as atrial fibrillation or the presence of flow limiting thrombus, the following protocol may be considered.

The initial management in the absence of ICH is intravenous heparin for 12 hrs–7 days followed by warfarin.[65] The goal aPTT with heparin is 1.5–2.0 times the control value (50–80 sec). Warfarin is continued for 3–6 months with target INR range of 2.0–3.0.

Indications for endovascular intervention

persistent, worsening, or recurrent ischemic symptoms despite anticoagulation therapy
flow-limiting lesion with hemodynamic compromise

Stenting with/without coiling

The endovascular treatment for carotid dissection is stenting, including the use of flow diversion stents if needed. In case of intimal flap, the stent will appose the flap back to the arterial wall. Pseudoaneurysms have also been successfully occluded with stenting. Both uncovered and covered stents have been used successfully.[66] JoStent is a PTFE covered stent that is available in US. A vein covered stent has also been used.[67]

In case of a pseudoaneurysm that continues to show significant residual filling after stenting, coiling of the pseudoaneurysm will cause occlusion.[66]

After stenting, the patient remains on dual antiplatelet therapy (ASA + Plavix) for at least a month and ASA alone indefinitely.

Follow-up

Follow-up should be arranged for patients on warfarin (e.g., "Coumadin clinic").

Follow-up study in 3–6 months, which could be CTA, Doppler ultrasonography, or catheter angiogram.

116.9.8 Subclavian artery stenosis

General information

Radiologically demonstrable stenosis of the subclavian or innominate artery is present in approximately 17%. Of these, 2.5% have angiographic flow reversal in vertebral artery. Only 5.3% of those with angiographic steal have neurologic symptoms.[68]

Symptoms. The 5 D's of VBI (i.e., diplopia, dysarthria, defective vision, dizziness, and drop attacks). Other symptoms include headache, nystagmus, hearing loss, and focal seizures.[69,70]

The arterial stenosis is proximal to the origin of VA. Symptoms are induced by exercise or exertion using the arm ipsilateral to the stenosis. The increased flow demand due to the exertion results in retrograde blood flow through the VA. The neurological symptoms may be because of continuous brainstem ischemia or more commonly, ischemia due to ipsilateral arm exercise or exertion.[71]

116

Indications for endovascular intervention

Symptomatic subclavian artery stenosis (i.e., stenosis resulting in subclavian steal syndrome).

Endovascular intervention

This includes angioplasty and stenting. A balloon-mounted stent may be used, as the stent is deployed concurrently with angioplasty.[72] However, if the stenosis is particularly severe (e.g. <2 mm), pre-dilatation may be performed by a smaller balloon to achieve a caliber of 4 mm at site o stenosis. Normal antegrade blood flow is restored following successful angioplasty and stenting Radial or brachial access is frequently used for such cases.

Postoperative management

The patient is monitored at least overnight in NSICU.

After stenting, the patient remains on dual antiplatelet therapy (ASA + Plavix) for at least 1 month and ASA alone indefinitely.

Follow-up study in 3–6 months, which could be CTA, Doppler ultrasonography, or catheter angiogram.

Complications of angioplasty and stenting

The frequency of complications is 17.8% (of 73 procedures) for innominate and VA angioplasty and stenting. These include access-site bleeding and distal embolization.[73]

116.9.9 Ischemic stroke

IV tPA

The target for IV tPA administration ("door-to-needle time") is to administer within 60 minutes from time of arrival to hospital in ≥ 50% of patients.[21] However, IV tPA can be administered up to 4.5 hour after the onset of symptoms if the patient does not have any contraindications.[74] Candidates for IV tPA should receive it even if endovascular therapy is being considered (Level I[21]).

Dose: 0.9 mg/kg (max 90 mg) with 10% of the dose administered as a bolus over 1 minute and the rest infused over 60 minutes.

Do not wait for a patient with suspected stroke from large vessel occlusion to "improve" after IV tPA initiation (possible harm[21]). Once the IV tPA drip is started, the patient should be immediately taken to the angiography suite or transported to a center with neuroendovascular capabilities, prefer ably a comprehensive stroke center. An ongoing debate is whether IV tPA is "futile" in cases with large vessel occlusion given the low chance of large clot lysis, increased risk profile with the use of systemic tPA, and time delay to the initiation of thrombectomy. Trials to address this issue are cur rently underway in Europe.

Endovascular intervention

116

General information

Endovascular intervention is extremely safe and effective when performed up to 24 hours from strok symptom onset, including "wake-up" strokes. The number needed to treat (NNT) (the number o patients to which a treatment must be administered before either a single patient achieves a benefit o one adverse event is prevented) with thrombectomy is 2–4, compared to 3–19 for IV tPA in acu ischemic stroke (AIS). Trials favor rapid endovascular intervention in AIS with anterior circulatio proximal vessel occlusion, small infarct core, and moderate-to-good collateral circulation.[75,76,77,78,79,8] Meta-analysis of these randomized trials shows that even large core infarcts or more distal occlusion still benefit from thrombectomy.[81]

For AHA guidelines for mechanical thrombectomy, see Practice guideline: Mechanical thrombec tomy for acute ischemic stroke (AIS) (p. 1562).

Indications and case selection for intra-arterial tPA (IA-tPA)

- not recommended as primary therapy given widespread use of mechanical thrombectomy and data supporting its high safety and efficacy. A clinically beneficial dose has not been established (Level I[21])
- as adjunct treatment after mechanical thrombectomy for more distal clots

- primary endovascular treatment for very distal clots or for use within the first 6 hours of major ischemic stroke due to MCA occlusion (Level I[21]), although it is frequently used up to 24 hours as long as imaging did not show a large core infarct

Contraindications to intervention

Most contraindications are relative and have to be weighed against the risk of not intervening. These contraindications include:

- hemorrhagic infarct or ICH
- CT demonstrating hypodensity or mass effect consistent with evolving infarct of more than one-third of middle cerebral artery territory
- recent major surgery
- pregnancy
- when considering stenting, contraindication to anticoagulants and/or thrombolytics

Preprocedural management

This may be under the supervision of a stroke neurologist, or the neurosurgeon. Ensure the following:

- rapid transfer of patient to a facility with endovascular capabilities such as a comprehensive stroke center (CSC). Thrombectomy-capable stroke centers (TSC) have been recently introduced by the AHA/Joint Commission and are the subject of heated debate regarding its validity
- ABC's take precedence
- ensure patient has two intravenous lines, preferably 18G or larger. Start monitoring BP, pulse oximetry, ECG, O_2 saturation, cardiac rate and rhythm, respiratory rate
- insert a Foley catheter
- verify laboratory values including: platelet count, BUN, CR, APTT, PT/INR. β-HCG for females of reproductive age group
- maintain MAP ≥ 90 mm Hg
- non-contrast head CT scan: To rule out ICH and to determine the Alberta Stroke Program Early CT Score (ASPECTS) (p. 1559).[82] The score ranges from 0 to 10. A higher number corresponds to smaller stroke core burden. Score 6–10 is considered a "favorable" profile for endovascular therapy
- CTA: to assess location of the clot (hyperdense artery sign (p. 1560)), collaterals & vascular tortuosity
- MRI of the head is rarely indicated (may be obtained in select cases)
- if available and can be done without delay, then perfusion studies, e.g., CTP or MRP, especially in cases of wake-up strokes or when symptom onset is over 6 hours prior. These perfusion studies will demonstrate viable brain (penumbra) vs. completed stroke to help in selecting patients for thrombectomy
- in centers where available, CT, CTA, and CTP all are performed during the same session on CT scanner
- be cognizant of renal insufficiency, diabetes, congestive heart failure, etc., in which case consider diluted non-ionic contrast agent and carefully pre-plan to minimize contrast load
- the goal of intervention is to re-establish successful recanalization, defined as mTICI score[83] 2b/3 (▶ Table 116.2), as soon as possible

116

Table 116.2 Modified Treatment in Cerebral Ischemia (mTICI) scale[83]

Grade	Description
0	no perfusion
1	antegrade perfusion past the initial occlusion, but limited distal branch filling with little or slow distal reperfusion
2a	antegrade perfusion of < 50% of the ischemic territory of the occluded target artery (e.g., in 1 major division of the MCA & its territory)
2b	antegrade perfusion of > 50% of the ischemic territory of the occluded target artery (e.g., in 2 major divisions of the MCA & their territories)
3	complete antegrade reperfusion of the ischemic territory of the occluded target artery, with absence of visualized occlusion in all distal branches

Abbreviations: MCA = middle cerebral artery.

Techniques

▶ **Stent retrievers.** Due to a high success rate, stent retrievers became the method of first choice for clot removal in embolic stroke. The successful recanalization rate is 70–85%.[84,85,86,87] The two devices most commonly employed currently in the U.S. are Solitaire and Trevo. Also available in the U.S.: Penumbra System® 3D™ Revascularization Device and EmboTrap®.

A 7 or 8 Fr sheath is placed in the femoral artery, through which a guide sheath or a balloon-guide catheter is positioned in the cervical ICA (for anterior circulation strokes). The balloon-guide catheter increases the rate of successful recanalization, decreases the number of thrombectomy passes, and reduces the risk of distal embolic formation with thrombectomy. Angiography is performed to identify the site of occlusion. Using fluoroscopy and road mapping, a microcatheter is advanced over a microwire, across the site of occlusion. The microwire is removed and the stent retriever is advanced through the microcatheter such that it extends proximal and distal to the clot. The stent retriever is unsheathed by retracting the microcatheter as the retriever is maintained stationary. The stent retriever expands to its actual size and this results in restoration of flow in the occluded artery. After five minutes, if a balloon catheter is used, the balloon on the guide catheter is inflated to arrest blood flow. Maintaining gentle aspiration on the guide catheter, the stent retriever and microcatheter are retracted simultaneously. Once both the microcatheter and retriever are within the guide catheter, vigorous aspiration is applied as the two devices are concurrently retracted and removed from the patient. Angiography is performed to confirm reconstitution of circulation. Some operators utilize a distal aspiration catheter to capture the clot proximally and apply aspiration while removing the stent retriever. This approach is called "Solumbra" or "Trenumbra".[88]

Vessel perforation during stent retriever withdrawal has been reported.[89] The risk of perforation is believed to increase with treatment of more distal small occlusions.[90] Distal aspiration alone (discussed in the next paragraph) may be a preferable approach in such cases.

▶ **Primary aspiration.** Primary aspiration has emerged as a faster and cheaper alternative to primary stent retriever thrombectomy. This approach was first introduced as the ADAPT technique (A Direct Aspiration first Pass Technique). A large-bore catheter is placed in direct contact with the thrombus and aspiration is applied using a pump or manually with a syringe to extract the clot.[91] If unsuccessful alone, a stent retriever is introduced through the aspiration catheter as a rescue treatment to remove the clot. This approach is now also called "direct aspiration," "contact aspiration," and "primary aspiration" with a variety of catheters of different length and diameter available on the market to accommodate vessels of various sizes and locations ranging from the ICA terminus to the middle cerebral artery M2 and 3 segments. 3 recent randomized trials (ASTER, 3D, and COMPASS) showed equal safety and efficacy of both approaches in achieving successful recanalization.[92,93,94] The COMPASS trial also demonstrated significant cost-effectiveness and shorter time to recanalization with primary aspiration vs. stent retriever use.

▶ **Intra-arterial tPA.** This may be the simplest endovascular technique; however, on its own, recanalization rates are inferior compared to the above-mentioned mechanical techniques[95,96] (although it may be better than IV tPA). Currently, IA tPA is used primarily in conjunction with other techniques in ischemic stroke.

▶ **Other techniques.** Other techniques to extract thrombus have also been employed with mixed results including: aspiration with a simple syringe attached to a microcatheter, snares, angioplasty at the site of thrombus, stenting, etc.

Stent retrievers are preferred to the MERCI device (Level I[21]), as well as to other devices which may be reasonable in some circumstances (Level II[21]).

116.9.10 Cerebral venous thrombosis (CVT)

General information

Also see Cerebral venous thrombosis (p. 1594).

Hydration with IV fluids and IV anticoagulation with heparin or low-molecular-weight heparin (LMWH) are part of the initial treatment for cerebral venous thrombosis (CVT), even in the face of parenchymal venous hemorrhagic infarcts. Prior to initiation of treatment, blood for hypercoagulopathy tests is drawn.

Indications for endovascular intervention

1. clinical deterioration despite anticoagulation

2. contraindications to anticoagulation: bleeding diathesis, thrombocytopenia (< 100 K), or recent GI hemorrhage
3. coma
4. deep CVT
5. intracerebral hemorrhage (ICH)

Endovascular treatment

Chemical thrombolysis (tPA): A catheter may be advanced to the involved sinus or close to it, through the femoral vein. The advantage of local administration is that a larger amount of tPA actually reaches the clot vs. systemic administration through a peripheral vein. Usually, 2–5 mg are administered through the thrombus and then an infusion started at a rate of 1–2 mg/hr, usually for 12–24 hours. Bleeding complications increase after ≈ 24 hours. Repeat angio in 24 hours. If clot burden is still present on angiography, the infusion may be continued for longer, until the clot resolves.

For CVT, the infusion may be prepared in a concentration of 1 mg/10 ml (0.1 mg/ml), for a rate of 10 ml/hr.

Mechanical thrombectomy: Similar to arterial embolic stroke, devices such as Stentriever or Penumbra may be used for clot extraction. Additionally, devices intended for other sites, e.g., clot extraction from dialysis fistula, have also been used in cranial sinuses.[97] The challenge during endovascular intervention is negotiating the sigmoid-transverse sinus junction, especially when using bulkier catheters, e.g., AngioJet (very stiff).

116.9.11 Chronic subdural hematoma

Middle meningeal artery (MMA) embolization is a minimally invasive potential option for treating chronic SDH (CSDH). Membranes of the CSDH contain friable neovasculature[98] that may be responsible for repeated rebleeding into the subdural space and may contribute to recurrence after surgical evacuation. It has been shown to be safe and effective in small series as treatment for recurrent CSDH[99,100] as well as for primary treatment,[101] and larger trials are anticipated.

Technique (summary): angiography of the common and external carotid arteries is performed on the affected side. The distal MMA vasculature may exhibit irregular wispiness.[102] The MMA is selectively catheterized using a microcatheter, and 150–250-micron diameter polyvinyl alcohol particles[101] or 15–20% n-butyl-2-cyanoacrylate[99] is injected under fluoro roadmap until there is flow stasis. Post-injection angio confirms effective MMA embolization.

Branches to avoid: potential ophthalmic artery collaterals and branches supplying cranial nerves.

116.9.12 Tumor embolization

Indications

Preoperative devascularization of vascular tumors, including
• meningiomas: embolization for meningiomas is location-specific, size-dependent, institution-dependent, and potentially controversial. May be best reserved for large hypervascular convexity meningiomas. Usually performed 24 hours to 1 week preoperatively. The devascularization causes attenuation in intraoperative blood loss and the resultant necrosis frequently renders the tumor softer and easier to remove. However, tumor swelling may occur and occasionally an emergency craniotomy may be required
• hemangiopericytomas
• juvenile nasopharyngeal angiofibromas
• glomus jugulare tumors
• hemangioblastomas
• vascular metastases

Technique

A sheath is placed in the femoral artery and a guide catheter is positioned as close as possible to the vessels of interest, e.g., in case of a meningioma, the guide catheter tip is positioned in the proximal ECA. Angiography and roadmapping are performed through the guide catheter. Using fluoroscopy and road mapping, a microcatheter is advanced over wire into the branches supplying the tumor. Angiography is performed through the microcatheter to ascertain which branch supplies the tumor and that no concerning collaterals with intracranial circulation exist. A blank road map is obtained and embolization commenced. PVA particles or Onyx may be used for embolization. In case of Onyx, a DMSO-compatible catheter must be used. PVA may be cheaper and quicker to use for tumor

116

embolization. However, the devascularization is not durable and the occluded vessels may recanalize; therefore, with PVA the surgery should be performed within a few days of the embolization.

116.9.13 Refractory epistaxis

Indications

Epistaxis that has not responded to treatment including manual compression, nasal packing, local vasoconstrictors, endoscopic cauterization, or surgical ligation of sphenopalatine arteries.

Preoperative management

Verify lab values, including platelet count, BUN, CR, APTT, PT/INR, and β-HCG for females of reproductive age group. In renal insufficiency, diabetes, CHF, etc., use diluted non-ionic contrast agent and pre-plan carefully to maintain contrast load to minimum.

Liquids only on morning of procedure. NPO (for ≈ 6 hours) when procedure performed under general anesthesia.

Obtain informed consent for angiography and embolization of ECA branches.

Ensure two IV lines inserted. Insert Foley. The patient will be more comfortable and cooperative with an empty bladder, if the procedure becomes prolonged.

▶ **Technique.** Position patient on the neuroangiography table. Attach pulse oximetry and ECG leads for monitoring O_2 saturation, HR, cardiac rhythm respiratory rate, and BP.

A sheath is placed in the femoral artery. A guide catheter is positioned in the proximal ECA on the side of bleeding or pathology. Angiography and roadmapping are performed through the guide catheter. Using fluoroscopy and road mapping, a microcatheter is advanced over the wire into the sphenopalatine branches. Angiography is performed through the microcatheter to ascertain appropriate positioning and to ensure no concerning collaterals with intracranial circulation exist. Contrast extravasation, tumor blush, or pseudoaneurysms may be detected. A blank road map is obtained and embolization of the offending vessel commenced. PVA particles (250–300 mcg) or Onyx (18 or 34) may be used. In case of Onyx, a DMSO-compatible catheter is used. PVA may be cheaper and quicker to use. Monitor for dangerous anastomosis with the ICA, and especially the ophthalmic artery as Onyx may cause blindness via penetrating even the smallest collaterals.

Postoperative management

Post-op orders:

- admit to ICU for overnight observation. If nasal packing is used, typically removed for inspection for bleeding the next day, or managed by ENT if they are involved
- IV: 0.9% NS + 20 meq KCl @ 150 cc/hr X 2 hrs, then decrease to 100 cc/hr, if patient is NPO
- activity: keep right/left leg (whichever side was used for procedure) straight for 2 hrs (in case of Angioseal closure), or 6–8 hours (in case manual compression was applied), with HOB elevated 15°. This is achieved by placing a pillow under the patient's head. There should be no flexion in the femoral region. If more head elevation is required, place bed in reverse-Trendelenburg position
- check groin, DPs, vitals, and neuro checks q 15 min X 4 hrs, q 30 min X 4 hrs, then q hr
- advance diet as tolerated. Review/resume preprocedure medications (except oral hypoglycemics, until good PO intake is established)

References

[1] Dion JE, Gates PC, Fox AJ, et al. Clinical Events Following Neuroangiography: A Prospective Study. Stroke. 1987; 18:997–1004

[2] Earnest F, Forbes G, Sandok BA, et al. Complications of Cerebral Angiography: Prospective Assessment of Risk. American Journal of Radiology. 1984; 142:247–253

[3] Gupta R, Vora N, Thomas A, et al. Symptomatic cerebral air embolism during neuro-angiographic procedures: incidence and problem avoidance. Neurocrit Care. 2007; 7:241–246

[4] Khan SH, Abruzzo TA, Sangha KS, et al. Use of Antiplatelet, Anticoagulant and Thrombolytic Agents in Endovascular Procedures. Contemporary Neurosurgery. 2008; 29:1–7

[5] Kershaw RA, Mays DC, Bianchine JR, et al. Disposition of aspirin and its metabolites in the semen of man. J Clin Pharmacol. 1987; 27:304–309

[6] Patrignani P, Filabozzi P, Patrono C. Selective cumulative inhibition of platelet thromboxane production by low-dose aspirin in healthy subjects. J Clin Invest. 1982; 69:1366–1372

[7] Ross-Lee LM, Elms MJ, Cham BE, et al. Plasma levels of aspirin following effervescent and enteric coated tablets, and their effect on platelet function. Eur J Clin Pharmacol. 1982; 23:545–551

[8] Gurbel PA, Bliden KP, DiChiara J, et al. Evaluation of dose-related effects of aspirin on platelet function: results from the Aspirin-Induced Platelet Effect (ASPECT) study. Circulation. 2007; 115:3156–316

[9] Krasopoulos G, Brister SJ, Beattie WS, et al. Aspirin "resistance" and risk of cardiovascular morbidity: systematic review and meta-analysis. BMJ. 2008; 336:195–198

[10] Hovens MM, Snoep JD, Eikenboom JC, et al. Prevalence of persistent platelet reactivity despite use of aspirin: a systematic review. Am Heart J. 2007; 153:175–181

[11] Song J, Shin YS. Antiplatelet drug resistance did not increase the thromboembolic events after stent-assisted coiling of unruptured intracranial aneurysm: a single center experience of 99 cases. Neurol Sci. 2017; 38:879–885

[12] Kim BJ, Kwon JY, Jung JM, et al. Association between silent embolic cerebral infarction and continuous increase of P2Y12 reaction units after neurovascular stenting. J Neurosurg. 2014; 121:891–898

[13] Kim MS, Jo KI, Yeon JY, et al. Association between Postprocedural Infarction and Antiplatelet Drug Resistance after Coiling for Unruptured Intracranial Aneurysms. AJNR Am J Neuroradiol. 2016; 37:1099–1105

[14] Tcheng JE. Clinical challenges of platelet glycoprotein IIb/IIIa receptor inhibitor therapy: bleeding, reversal, thrombocytopenia, and retreatment. Am Heart J. 2000; 139:S38–S45

[15] Qureshi AI, Luft AR, Sharma M, et al. Prevention and treatment of thromboembolic and ischemic complications associated with endovascular procedures: Part II–Clinical aspects and recommendations. Neurosurgery. 2000; 46:1360–75; discussion 1375-6

[16] Hirsh J. Heparin. N Engl J Med. 1991; 324:1565–1574

[17] Khan SH, Ringer AJ. Handbook of neuroendovascular techniques. U.K.: Taylor and Francis;

[18] University of Cincinnati post-endovascular heparin dosing protocol. 2008

[19] Garcia DA, Baglin TP, Weitz JI, et al. Parenteral anticoagulants: Antithrombotic Therapy and Prevention of Thrombosis, 9th ed: American College of Chest Physicians Evidence-Based Clinical Practice Guidelines. Chest. 2012; 141:e24S–e43S

[20] Berenstein A, Lasjaunias P, Ter Brugge KG. Surgical neuroangiography. 2nd ed. Berlin: Springer; 2004; 1

[21] Powers WJ, Rabinstein AA, Ackerson T, et al. 2018 Guidelines for the Early Management of Patients With Acute Ischemic Stroke: A Guideline for Healthcare Professionals From the American Heart Association/American Stroke Association. Stroke. 2018; 49:e46–e110

[22] Lee CJ, Ansell JE. Direct thrombin inhibitors. Br J Clin Pharmacol. 2011; 72:581–592

[23] Davis EM, Packard KA, Knezevich JT, et al. New and emerging anticoagulant therapy for atrial fibrillation and acute coronary syndrome. Pharmacotherapy. 2011; 31:975–1016

[24] Liang CW, Diamond SJ, Hagg DS. Lipid rescue of massive verapamil overdose: a case report. J Med Case Rep. 2011; 5. DOI: 10.1186/1752-1947-5-399

[25] Ciechanowicz S, Patil V. Lipid emulsion for local anesthetic systemic toxicity. Anesthesiol Res Pract. 2012; 2012. DOI: 10.1155/2012/131784

[26] Yu DW, Jung YJ, Choi BY, et al. Subarachnoid hemorrhage with negative baseline digital subtraction angiography: is repeat digital subtraction angiography necessary? J Cerebrovasc Endovasc Neurosurg. 2012; 14:210–215

[27] Keedy A. An overview of intracranial aneurysms. Mcgill J Med. 2006; 9:141–146

[28] Wardlaw JM, White PM. The detection and management of unruptured intracranial aneurysms. Brain. 2000; 123 (Pt 2):205–221

[29] Wiebers DO, Whisnant JP, Huston J,3rd, et al. Unruptured intracranial aneurysms: natural history, clinical outcome, and risks of surgical and endovascular treatment. Lancet. 2003; 362:103–110

[30] Friedman JA, Piepgras DG, Pichelmann MA, et al. Small cerebral aneurysms presenting with symptoms other than rupture. Neurology. 2001; 57:1212–1216

[31] Juvela S, Porras M, Heiskanen O. Natural history of unruptured intracranial aneurysms: a long-term follow-up study. J Neurosurg. 1993; 79:174–182

[32] Hashimoto N, Handa H. The fate of untreated symptomatic cerebral aneurysms: analysis of 26 patients with clinical course of more than five years. Surg Neurol. 1982; 18:21–26

[33] Asari S, Ohmoto T. Natural history and risk factors of unruptured cerebral aneurysms. Clin Neurol Neurosurg. 1993; 95:205–214

[34] Locksley HB, Sahs AL, Sandler R. Report on the cooperative study of intracranial aneurysms and subarachnoid hemorrhage. 3. Subarachnoid hemorrhage unrelated to intracranial aneurysm and A-V malformation. A study of associated diseases and prognosis. J Neurosurg. 1966; 24:1034–1056

[35] Ferguson GG, Peerless SJ, Drake CG. Natural history of intracranial aneurysms. N Engl J Med. 1981; 305. DOI: 10.1056/NEJM198107093050211

[36] Ecker RD, Hopkins LN. Natural history of unruptured intracranial aneurysms. Neurosurg Focus. 2004; 17

[37] Ujiie H, Tamano Y, Sasaki K, et al. Is the aspect ratio a reliable index for predicting the rupture of a saccular aneurysm? Neurosurgery. 2001; 48:495–502; discussion 502-3

[38] Nader-Sepahi A, Casimiro M, Sen J, et al. Is aspect ratio a reliable predictor of intracranial aneurysm rupture? Neurosurgery. 2004; 54:1343–7; discussion 1347-8

[39] The International Study Group of Unruptured Intracranial Aneurysms Investigators (ISUIA). Unruptured Intracranial Aneurysms - Risk of Rupture and Risks of Surgical Intervention. New England Journal of Medicine. 1998; 339:1725–1733

[40] van Rooij WJ, Sluzewski M. Packing density in coiling of small intracranial aneurysms. AJNR Am J Neuroradiol. 2006; 27:725–6; author reply 726

[41] Bodily KD, Cloft HJ, Lanzino G, et al. Stent-assisted coiling in acutely ruptured intracranial aneurysms: a qualitative, systematic review of the literature. AJNR Am J Neuroradiol. 2011; 32:1232–1236

[42] Hu YC, Chugh C, Mehta H, et al. Early angiographic occlusion of ruptured blister aneurysms of the internal carotid artery using the Pipeline Embolization Device as a primary treatment option. J Neurointerv Surg. 2014; 6:740–743

[43] Yoon JW, Siddiqui AH, Dumont TM, et al. Feasibility and safety of pipeline embolization device in patients with ruptured carotid blister aneurysms. Neurosurgery. 2014; 75:419–29; discussion 429

[44] Fischer S, Vajda Z, Aguilar Perez M, et al. Pipeline embolization device (PED) for neurovascular reconstruction: initial experience in the treatment of 101 intracranial aneurysms and dissections. Neuroradiology. 2012; 54:369–382

[45] Saatci I, Yavuz K, Ozer C, et al. Treatment of intracranial aneurysms using the pipeline flow-diverter embolization device: a single-center experience with long-term follow-up results. AJNR Am J Neuroradiol. 2012; 33:1436–1446

[46] Yavuz K, Geyik S, Saatci I, et al. Endovascular treatment of middle cerebral artery aneurysms with flow modification with the use of the pipeline embolization device. AJNR Am J Neuroradiol. 2014; 35:529–535

[47] Jun P, Ko NU, English JD, et al. Endovascular treatment of medically refractory cerebral vasospasm following aneurysmal subarachnoid hemorrhage. AJNR Am J Neuroradiol. 2010; 31:1911–1916

[48] Kwak R, Niizuma H, Ohi T, et al. Angiographic study of cerebral vasospasm following rupture of intracranial aneurysms: Part I. Time of the appearance. Surg Neurol. 1979; 11:257–262

[49] Bergvall U, Galera R. Time relationship between subarachnoid haemorrhage, arterial spasm, changes in cerebral circulation and posthaemorrhagic hydrocephalus. Acta Radiol Diagn (Stockh). 1969; 9:229–237

[50] Graf CJ, Nibbelink DW. Cooperative study of intracranial aneurysms and subarachnoid hemorrhage. Report on a randomized treatment study. 3. Intracranial surgery. Stroke. 1974; 5:557–601

116

[51] Weir B, Grace M, Hansen J, et al. Time Course of Vasospasm in Man. J Neurosurg. 1978; 48:173–178

[52] Weber W, Kis B, Siekmann R, et al. Endovascular treatment of intracranial arteriovenous malformations with onyx: technical aspects. AJNR Am J Neuroradiol. 2007; 28:371–377

[53] Strauss I, Frolov V, Buchbut D, et al. Critical appraisal of endovascular treatment of brain arteriovenous malformation using Onyx in a series of 92 consecutive patients. Acta Neurochir (Wien). 2013; 155:611–617

[54] Saatci I, Geyik S, Yavuz K, et al. Endovascular treatment of brain arteriovenous malformations with prolonged intranidal Onyx injection technique: long-term results in 350 consecutive patients with completed endovascular treatment course. J Neurosurg. 2011; 115:78–88

[55] Consoli A, Renieri L, Nappini S, et al. Endovascular treatment of deep hemorrhagic brain arteriovenous malformations with transvenous onyx embolization. AJNR Am J Neuroradiol. 2013; 34:1805–1811

[56] Rasuli P, Hammond DI. Metformin and contrast media: where is the conflict? Can Assoc Radiol J. 1998; 49:161–166

[57] van Dijk JM, terBrugge KG, Willinsky RA, et al. Clinical course of cranial dural arteriovenous fistulas with long-term persistent cortical venous reflux. Stroke. 2002; 33:1233–1236

[58] Chalouhi N, Dumont AS, Tjoumakaris S, et al. The superior ophthalmic vein approach for the treatment of carotid-cavernous fistulas: a novel technique using Onyx. Neurosurg Focus. 2012; 32. DOI: 10.3171/2012.1.FOCUS123

[59] Sancak T, Bilgic S, Ustuner E. Endovascular stent-graft treatment of a traumatic vertebral artery pseudoaneurysm and vertebrojugular fistula. Korean J Radiol. 2008; 9 Suppl:S68–S72

[60] Nagashima C, Iwasaki T, Kawanuma S, et al. Traumatic arteriovenous fistula of the vertebral artery with spinal cord symptoms. Case report. J Neurosurg. 1977; 46:681–687

[61] O'Shaughnessy B A, Bendok BR, Parkinson RJ, et al. Transarterial coil embolization of a high-flow vertebrojugular fistula due to penetrating craniocervical trauma: case report. Surg Neurol. 2005; 64:335–40; discussion 340

[62] Jayaraman MV, Do HM, Marks MP. Treatment of traumatic cervical arteriovenous fistulas with N-butyl-2-cyanoacrylate. AJNR Am J Neuroradiol. 2007; 28:352–354

[63] Anson J, Crowell RM. Cervicocranial Arterial Dissection. Neurosurgery. 1991; 29:89–96

[64] Markus HS, Hayter E, Levi C, et al. Antiplatelet treatment compared with anticoagulation treatment for cervical artery dissection (CADISS): a randomised trial. Lancet Neurol. 2015; 14:361–367

[65] Hart RG, Easton JD. Dissections of Cervical and Cerebral Arteries. Neurol Clin North Am. 1983; 1:255–282

[66] Liu AY, Paulsen RD, Marcellus ML, et al. Long-term outcomes after carotid stent placement treatment of carotid artery dissection. Neurosurgery. 1999; 45:1368–73; discussion 1373-4

[67] Marotta TR, Buller C, Taylor D, et al. Autologous vein-covered stent repair of a cervical internal carotid artery pseudoaneurysm: technical case report. Neurosurgery. 1998; 42:408–12; discussion 412-3

[68] Fields WS, Lemak NA. Joint Study of extracranial arterial occlusion. VII. Subclavian steal—a review of 168 cases. JAMA. 1972; 222:1139–1143

[69] Fields WS. Reflections on "the subclavian steal". Stroke. 1970; 1:320–324

[70] Smith JM, Koury HI, Hafner CD, et al. Subclavian steal syndrome. A review of 59 consecutive cases. J Cardiovasc Surg (Torino). 1994; 35:11–14

[71] Brook I. Bacteriology of Intracranial Abscess in Children. J Neurosurg. 1981; 54:484–488

[72] Khan SH, Young PH, Ringer AJ. Endovascular treatment of subclavian artery stenosis associated with

vertebral artery pseudoaneurysm. Clin Neurol Neurosurg. 2012; 114:754–757

[73] Sullivan TM, Gray BH, Bacharach JM, et al. Angioplasty and primary stenting of the subclavian, innominate, and common carotid arteries in 83 patients. J Vasc Surg. 1998; 28:1059–1065

[74] Del Zoppo GJ, Saver JL, Jauch EC, et al. Expansion of the time window for treatment of acute ischemic stroke with intravenous tissue plasminogen activator: a science advisory from the American Heart Association/American Stroke Association. Stroke. 2009; 40:2945–2948

[75] Campbell BC, Mitchell PJ, Kleinig TJ, et al. Endovascular therapy for ischemic stroke with perfusion-imaging selection. N Engl J Med. 2015; 372:1009–1018

[76] Goyal M, Demchuk AM, Menon BK, et al. Randomized assessment of rapid endovascular treatment of ischemic stroke. N Engl J Med. 2015; 372:1019–1030

[77] Berkhemer OA, Fransen PS, Beumer D, et al. A randomized trial of intraarterial treatment for acute ischemic stroke. N Engl J Med. 2015; 372:11–20

[78] Fransen PS, Beumer D, Berkhemer OA, et al. MR CLEAN, a multicenter randomized clinical trial of endovascular treatment for acute ischemic stroke in the Netherlands: study protocol for a randomized controlled trial. Trials. 2014; 15. DOI: 10.1186/1745-6215-15-343

[79] Nogueira RG, Jadhav AP, Haussen DC, et al. Thrombectomy 6 to 24 Hours after Stroke with a Mismatch between Deficit and Infarct. N Engl J Med. 2018; 378:11–21

[80] Albers GW, Marks MP, Kemp S, et al. Thrombectomy for Stroke at 6 to 16 Hours with Selection by Perfusion Imaging. N Engl J Med. 2018; 378:708–718

[81] Goyal M, Menon BK, van Zwam WH, et al. Endovascular thrombectomy after large-vessel ischaemic stroke: a meta-analysis of individual patient data from five randomised trials. Lancet. 2016; 387:1723–1731

[82] Pexman JH, Barber PA, Hill MD, et al. Use of the Alberta Stroke Program Early CT Score (ASPECTS) for assessing CT scans in patients with acute stroke. AJNR Am J Neuroradiol. 2001; 22:1534–1542

[83] Zaidat OO, Yoo AJ, Khatri P, et al. Recommendations on angiographic revascularization grading standards for acute ischemic stroke: a consensus statement. Stroke. 2013; 44:2650–2663

[84] Stampfl S, Hartmann M, Ringleb PA, et al. Stent placement for flow restoration in acute ischemic stroke: a single-center experience with the Solitaire stent system. AJNR Am J Neuroradiol. 2011 32:1245–1248

[85] Mordasini P, Brekenfeld C, Byrne JV, et al. Experimental evaluation of immediate recanalization effect and recanalization efficacy of a new thrombus retriever for acute stroke treatment in vivo. AJNR Am J Neuroradiol. 2013; 34:153–158

[86] Wehrschuetz M, Wehrschuetz E, Augustin M, et al. Early single center experience with the solitaire thrombectomy device for the treatment of acute ischemic stroke. Interv Neuroradiol. 2011 17:235–240

[87] Hausegger KA, Hauser M, Kau T. Mechanical thrombectomy with stent retrievers in acute ischemic stroke. Cardiovasc Intervent Radiol. 2014; 37:863–874

[88] Dumont TM, Mokin M, Sorkin GC, et al. Aspiration thrombectomy in concert with stent thrombectomy. J Neurointerv Surg. 2014; 6. DOI: 10.1136/eurintsurg-2012-010624.rep

[89] Leishangthem L, Satti SR. Vessel perforation during withdrawal of Trevo ProVue stent retriever during mechanical thrombectomy for acute ischemic stroke. J Neurosurg. 2014; 121:995–998

[90] Mokin M, Fargen KM, Primiani CT, et al. Vessel perforation during stent retriever thrombectomy for acute ischemic stroke: technical details an

clinical outcomes. J Neurointerv Surg. 2017; 9:922–928

[91] Turk AS, Spiotta A, Frei D, et al. Initial clinical experience with the ADAPT technique: a direct aspiration first pass technique for stroke thrombectomy. J Neurointerv Surg. 2014; 6:231–237

[92] Lapergue B, Blanc R, Gory B, et al. Effect of Endovascular Contact Aspiration vs Stent Retriever on Revascularization in Patients With Acute Ischemic Stroke and Large Vessel Occlusion: The ASTER Randomized Clinical Trial. JAMA. 2017; 318:443–452

[93] Nogueira RG, Frei D, Kirmani JF, et al. Safety and Efficacy of a 3-Dimensional Stent Retriever With Aspiration-Based Thrombectomy vs Aspiration-Based Thrombectomy Alone in Acute Ischemic Stroke Intervention: A Randomized Clinical Trial. JAMA Neurol. 2018; 75:304–311

[94] Turk AS, Siddiqui AH, Mocco J. A comparison of direct aspiration versus stent retriever as a first approach ('COMPASS'): protocol. J Neurointerv Surg. 2018. DOI: 10.1136/neurintsurg-2017-013722

[95] Ernst R, Pancioli A, Tomsick T, et al. Combined intravenous and intra-arterial recombinant tissue plasminogen activator in acute ischemic stroke. Stroke. 2000; 31:2552–2557

[96] Intra-arterial thrombolysis. AJNR Am J Neuroradiol. 2001; 22:S18–S21

[97] Khan SH, Adeoye O, Abruzzo TA, et al. Intracranial dural sinus thrombosis: novel use of a mechanical thrombectomy catheter and review of management strategies. Clin Med Res. 2009; 7:157–165

[98] Tanaka T, Kaimori M. [Histological study of vascular structure between the dura mater and the outer membrane in chronic subdural hematoma in an adult]. No Shinkei Geka. 1999; 27:431–436

[99] Hashimoto T, Ohashi T, Watanabe D, et al. Usefulness of embolization of the middle meningeal artery for refractory chronic subdural hematomas. Surg Neurol Int. 2013; 4. DOI: 10.4103/2152-7806.116679

[100] Link TW, Schwarz JT, Paine SM, et al. Middle Meningeal Artery Embolization for Recurrent Chronic Subdural Hematoma: A Case Series. World Neurosurg. 2018; 118:e570–e574

[101] Link TW, Boddu S, Marcus J, et al. Middle Meningeal Artery Embolization as Treatment for Chronic Subdural Hematoma: A Case Series. Oper Neurosurg (Hagerstown). 2018; 14:556–562

[102] Link TW, Rapoport BI, Paine SM, et al. Middle meningeal artery embolization for chronic subdural hematoma: Endovascular technique and radiographic findings. Interv Neuroradiol. 2018; 24:455–462

Index